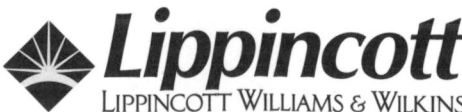

Maternal & Child Health Nursing

Care of the Childbearing & Childrearing Family

Maternal & Child Health Nursing

Care of the Childbearing & Childrearing Family

FOURTH EDITION

Adele Pillitteri, PhD, RN, PNP

Associate Professor
Department of Nursing
University of Southern California
Los Angeles, California
Former Director, Neonatal Nurse Practitioner Program
State University of New York at Buffalo
Buffalo, New York

Lippincott Williams & Wilkins
A Wolters Kluwer Company
Philadelphia • Baltimore • New York • London
Buenos Aires • Hong Kong • Sydney • Tokyo

Acquisitions Editor: Elizabeth Nieginski
Managing Editor: Barclay Cunningham
Editorial Assistant: Jean Otsuki
Senior Project Editor: Tom Gibbons
Senior Production Manager: Helen Ewan
Art Director: Carolyn O'Brien
Interior Design: Holly Reid McLaughlin
Manufacturing Manager: William Alberti
Indexer: Maria Coughlin
Compositor: Circle Graphics
Printer: Quebecor-Versailles

4th Edition

9 8 7 6 5 4 3 2 1

Library of Congress Cataloging-in Publication Data

Pillitteri, Adele.
Maternal & child health nursing : care of the childbearing & childrearing family / Adele Pillitteri.—4th ed.
p. cm.
Includes bibliographical references and index.
ISBN 0-7817-3628-5 (cloth : alk. paper)
1. Maternity nursing. 2. Pediatric nursing. I. Title: Maternal and child health nursing. II. Title.

RG951 .P637 2002
610′.73′678—dc21

2002066121

To my family:

Joseph, Rusty, Dawn, Bill, Heather, J.J., Lauren, and Lynn

with love

Reviewers

Civita Allard, MSN
Associate Professor
Department of Health Services—Nursing
Mohawk Valley Community College
Utica, New York

Denza Bruss, MSN
Assistant Professor
Department of Nursing
Utah Valley State University
Orem, Utah

Laurie Caton-Lemos, MS, RN
Lecturer/Clinical Instructor of Nursing
College of Nursing and Health Professions
University of Southern Maine
Portland, Maine

D'ann Dennis, MS, RN
Instructor of Nursing
Crowder College
Neosho, Missouri

Cathleen Dowe, RN
Lecturer
Department of Nursing
Jefferson Community College
Watertown, New York

Marcia Gasper, RNC, MSN, EdD(c)
Assistant Professor
Department of Nursing
Cedar Crest College
Allentown, Pennsylvania

Rebecca Gesler, MSN, RN
Instructor
Department of Nursing
St. Catharine College
St. Catharine, Kentucky

Sandra Grinnell, RN, MSN, CIMI
Assistant Professor, Maternal Child Health
Medcenter One College of Nursing
Bismarck, North Dakota

Elizabeth Jackson, MSN, RNC
Assistant Professor
Louisiana State University—Alexandria
Alexandria, Louisiana

Nancy Johnston, RN, MSN, CNRP, PhD(c)
Department of Nursing
Cedar Crest College
Allentown, Pennsylvania

Emma MacKay, MEd
Instructor, Faculty of Nursing
University of New Brunswick, Fredericton Campus
Fredericton, New Brunswick

Tami McCune-Pageler, MSN, RN
Associate Professor
Department of Nursing
Huron University
Huron, South Dakota

Edna McKim, MN
Associate Professor
School of Nursing
Memorial University of Newfoundland
St. Johns, Newfoundland

Donna Miracle, MS
Assistant Professor
Department of Nursing
Anderson University
Anderson, Indiana

Gloria Pearson, MA, RN
Assistant Professor
College of St. Scholastica
Duluth, Minnesota

Karen Reach, MS, RN
Instructor
Ellis Hospital School of Nursing
Schenectady, New York

Nancy A. Ryan-Winger, PhD, RN, CPNP
Professor
College of Nursing
Ohio State University
Columbus, Ohio

Dana Sandifer, MSN, RN
Department of Nursing
Hopkinsville Community College
Hopkinsville, Kentucky

Preface

Maternal-newborn and child health nursing are expanding areas as a result of the broadening scope of practice within the nursing profession and the recognized need for better preventive and restorative care in these areas. The importance of this need is reflected in the fact that many of the year 2010 health goals for the nation focus on these areas of nursing.

At the same time that the information in these areas of nursing is increasing, less time is available in nursing programs to cover it. Students experience difficulty reading all of the material contained in two separate textbooks.

Maternal and Child Health Nursing: Care of the Childbearing and Childrearing Family, Fourth Edition, is written with this challenge in mind. It views maternal-newborn and child health care not as two separate disciplines but as a continuum of knowledge. It is designed to present the content of the two disciplines comprehensively but not redundantly. It is based on a philosophy of nursing care that respects clients as individuals yet views them as part of families and society.

The book is designed for undergraduate student use for a combined course in maternal-newborn and child health, or for a curriculum in which these courses are taught separately but integrated. It provides a comprehensive, in-depth discussion of the many facets of maternal and child health nursing, while promoting a sensitive, holistic outlook on nursing practice. As such, the book will also be useful for graduate students who are interested in reviewing or expanding their knowledge in these areas.

Basic themes that are integrated into this text include the experience of wellness and illness as family-centered events, the perception of pregnancy and childbirth as periods of wellness in the life of a woman, and the importance of knowledge in the area of child development in the planning of nursing care. Also included are themes reflective of changes in health care delivery and the importance of meeting the needs of a culturally diverse population.

The Changing Health Care Scene

Managed care has drastically changed the health care delivery system, increasing the role of the nurse from a minor to a major player. Educational changes have to keep pace with health care reform so that nurses are prepared for this new level of responsibility. An increasingly multicultural population will continue to be reflected among both nurses and their clients, necessitating fine-tuning of culturally sensitive care.

New nursing curricula that are in keeping with this spirit of change emphasize outcomes, a greater focus on communication, therapeutic interventions, critical thinking, and nursing process.

Nursing issues that grow out of the current climate of change include the following:

- **The importance of health teaching with families as a cornerstone of nursing responsibility:** The teaching role of the nurse has greater significance in the new health care milieu as the emphasis on preventive care and short stays in the acute care setting creates the need for families to be better educated in their own care. Focus on Family Empowerment displays throughout the text address this issue.
- **An emphasis on National Health Goals:** As a way to focus care and research, National Health Goals have gained wider attention at a time when there is a greater need than ever to be wise in the choice of how dollars are spent. Students can familiarize themselves with these goals by referring to the Focus on National Health Goals display that appears at the beginning of each chapter.
- **The importance of individualizing care according to sociocultural uniqueness:** This is a reflection of both greater cultural sensitivity and an increasingly diverse population of caregivers and care recipients. Greater emphasis is being placed on the implications of multiple sociocultural factors in terms of how they affect the patient's response. Focus on Cultural Competence displays throughout the text show how cultural factors can be given greater consideration in the planning of care.
- **Changing areas of practice:** The variety of new care settings, as well as the diversity of roles in which nurses can practice, is reflected both in the proliferation of community-based nursing facilities and in the increase in the numbers of nurse-midwives and pediatric and neonatal nurse practitioners. This new edition places emphasis on the specific needs of clients related to the various health care settings in which they find themselves today. Focus on Multidisciplinary Care and Focus on Evidence-Based Practice boxes expand this area.

Organization of the Text

Maternal and Child Health Nursing follows the family from the pregnancy period, through labor, delivery, and the postpartal period; it then follows the child in the family from birth through adolescence. Coverage includes ambulatory and in-patient care and focuses on primary as well as secondary and tertiary care.

The book is organized in nine units:

Unit I provides an introduction to maternal and child health nursing. A framework for practice is presented, as well as current trends and the importance of considering childbearing and childrearing within a family context.

Unit II examines the nursing role in preparing families for childbearing and childrearing. Reproductive and sexual health, reproductive life planning, and the concerns of the infertile family are discussed.

Unit III presents the nursing role in caring for the pregnant family. Care of the woman during pregnancy and of the growing fetus is discussed. Separate chapters address the role of the nurse when the woman has a preexisting illness, develops a complication of pregnancy, has a special need, or will be cared for at home during pregnancy. Additional chapters detail the role of the nurse as a genetic counselor and an advocate for fetal health.

Unit IV addresses the nursing role in caring for the family during labor and birth. Separate chapters detail the labor process, the role of the nurse in providing comfort during labor, the nursing role when a woman develops a complication of labor and birth, and cesarean birth.

Unit V describes the nursing role in caring for the family during the postpartal period. Separate chapters discuss the care of the woman and her family, the newborn, and the changing role when a complication for either the woman or the newborn develops.

Unit VI discusses the nursing role in health promotion during childhood. The chapters in this unit cover principles of growth and development and care of the child from infancy through adolescence, including child health assessment and communication and health teaching with children and families.

Unit VII presents the nursing role in supporting the health of children and their families. The effects of illness on children and their families, diagnostic and therapeutic procedures, medication administration, and pain management are addressed, with respect to care of the child and family in hospital, home, and ambulatory settings.

Unit VIII examines the nursing role in restoring and maintaining the health of children and families when illness occurs. Disorders are presented according to body systems so that students have a ready orientation for locating content.

Unit IX discusses the nursing role in restoring and maintaining the mental health of children and families. Separate chapters discuss the role of the nurse when intimate partner or child abuse or mental, long-term, or fatal illness is present.

Pedagogic Features

Each chapter in the text is organized to provide a complete learning experience for the student. Numerous pedagogic features help the student understand and increase retention. Important elements include the following:

- **Chapter Objectives:** Learning objectives are included at the beginning of each chapter to identify the outcomes expected after the material in the chapter has been mastered.
- **Key Terms:** Terms that would be new to the student are listed at the beginning of each chapter in a ready reference list. The terms first appear in boldface type to draw the student's attention to them, are defined as they are used, and appear again in the Glossary.
- **Clinical Vignettes:** Short scenarios appear at the beginning of each chapter. These vignettes provide a taste of what is to come in the chapter, preparing the learner for the material to be presented and applying information that was covered previously. At the end of the chapter, Critical Thinking questions related to the scenario connect and bring the chapter full circle.
- **Tables and Displays:** Numerous tables and displays summarize important information and provide detail on some topics so that the student has a ready reference.
- **Checkpoint Questions:** Throughout the text, Checkpoint Questions appear to help readers check their progress and remain focused on the topic at hand. They ask readers to use the knowledge just gained in the last few pages, thus helping them remember this information. Answers are supplied at the end of the book.
- **"What If" Questions:** "What If" or critical-thinking questions also appear periodically throughout the text. These ask readers to apply the information just acquired in an "actual" situation. The readers must process the information and apply it to the new situation, thus maximizing learning and emphasizing critical thinking.
- **Key Points:** A review of important points is highlighted at the end of each chapter, to help students monitor their own comprehension.
- **Critical Thinking Exercises:** To involve the student in the decision-making realities of the clinical setting, several questions are posed at the end of each chapter. They can also serve as a basis for conference or class discussion.
- **References and Suggested Readings:** These provide the student with the information needed to do more in-depth reading of the sources noted in the text, as well as other relevant articles on the topics included in the chapter.
- **Appendices:** Appendices provide a quick reference to care pathways, laboratory values, growth charts, vital sign parameters, nutrition pyramids, drugs safe for use during lactation, and more.

Nursing Process

The nursing process format found throughout this text provides a strong theoretical underpinning for this important concept and helps the student understand how to use the nursing process in clinical practice.

- **Nursing Process Overview:** Each chapter begins with a review of nursing process in which specific suggestions, such as examples of nursing diagnoses and outcome criteria helpful to modifying care in the area under discussion, are given. These reviews improve students' preparation in clinical areas so that they can focus their care planning and apply principles to practice.
- **Nursing Diagnoses and Related Interventions:** A consistent format highlights the nursing diagnoses and related interventions throughout the text. A special heading draws the students' attention to these sections where individual nursing diagnoses, outcome

identification, and outcome evaluation are detailed for the major conditions and disorders discussed.

- **Nursing Care Plans:** Nursing care plans are written for specific clients to stress the importance of individualized care planning. The care plans are written with an emphasis on aiding students to apply theory to practice and to make use of critical thinking skills. Appendix L supplies examples of care pathways to further aid application.

Recurring Displays

Boxed displays throughout the text help the student focus on important information or provide additional insights.

- **Focus on National Health Goals:** To emphasize the nursing role in accomplishing the health care goals of our nation, these displays state specific ways in which maternal and child health nursing can provide better outcomes for both mother and child. They help the student to appreciate the importance of national health planning and the influence that nurses can have in creating a healthier nation.
- **Focus on Evidence-Based Practice:** These displays summarize research on topics related to maternal and child health nursing. They appear throughout the text to accentuate the use of evidence-based practice as the basis for nursing care.
- **Focus on Communication:** This feature presents case examples of less effective communication and more effective communication, illustrating for the student how an awareness of communication can improve the patient's understanding and positively impact outcomes.
- **Focus on Cultural Competence:** These displays serve to broaden the student's perspective on the many specific cultural influences that can affect the goals and interventions that nurses provide in the maternal and child health setting. They stress the need for nursing care to be modified to meet individualized needs.
- **Focus on Family Empowerment:** These boxes present detailed health teaching information for the family, emphasizing the importance of a partnership between nurses and clients in the management of health and illness.
- **Focus on Multidisciplinary Care:** In response to a changing health care environment, these boxes present practical information to help the nurse work with the numerous health care personnel who constitute the health care team or delegate appropriate responsibilities to unlicensed assistive personnel.
- **Focus on Pharmacology:** These boxes provide quick reference for medications that are commonly used for the health problems described in the text. They give the drug name (brand and generic, if applicable), dosage, pregnancy category, side effects, and nursing implications.
- **Nursing Procedures:** Techniques of procedures specific to maternal and child health care are boxed in an easy-to-follow two-column format, often enhanced with color figures.
- **Assessing the Client:** These visual guides provide head-to-toe assessment information for overall health status or specific disorders or conditions.

New to the Fourth Edition

This edition of *Maternal and Child Health Nursing* includes several new features:

- Focus on Evidence-Based Practice boxes highlighting research related to evidence-based practice
- A new chapter—Nursing Care of the Child Undergoing Medication Administration and Intravenous Therapy (Chapter 37)
- An expanded chapter—Communication and Teaching With Children and Families (Chapter 34)—to help students learn effective health teaching
- Photographic features depicting the labor process and a day in the life of a family with preschool- and school-age children

Ancillary Package

A complete learning and teaching package includes the following:

- **Connections Website:** Features a major care study with related student questions for student review and learning.
- **Free Interactive Self-Study CD-Rom:** Stored on the inside back cover of each book, 300 multiple-choice NCLEX-style questions challenge the student's comprehension and application of important material. Feedback is provided for each answer.
- **Instructor's Manual:** The perfect complement to classroom teaching strategies, this resource contains useful discussion topics, case studies, and critical thinking exercises.
- **Computerized Test Bank:** One thousand multiple-choice NCLEX-style questions.
- **Overhead Transparencies:** Full-color acetate transparencies illustrating important material enhance student understanding and facilitate classroom discussion.
- **Study Guide:** This companion to the text challenges the student's retention of key concepts and encourages critical thinking and application of information to actual nursing situations.

Adele Pillitteri, PhD, RN, PNP

Acknowledgments

I would like to express my sincere appreciation to Developmental Editor Maryann Foley; Elizabeth Nieginski, Acquisitions Editor; Barclay Cunningham, Managing Editor; Helen Ewan, Senior Production Manager; Tom Gibbons, Senior Project Editor; Carolyn O'Brien, Art Director; all the members of the Production Services Group involved with this text for their assistance and guidance throughout the project; and the countless nursing reviewers who generously added their expertise to this new edition.

A.P.

Contents

UNIT VI The Nursing Role in Health Promotion for the Childrearing Family

UNIT VII The Nursing Role in Supporting the Health of Ill Children and Their Families

Maternal & Child Health Nursing

Care of the Childbearing & Childrearing Family

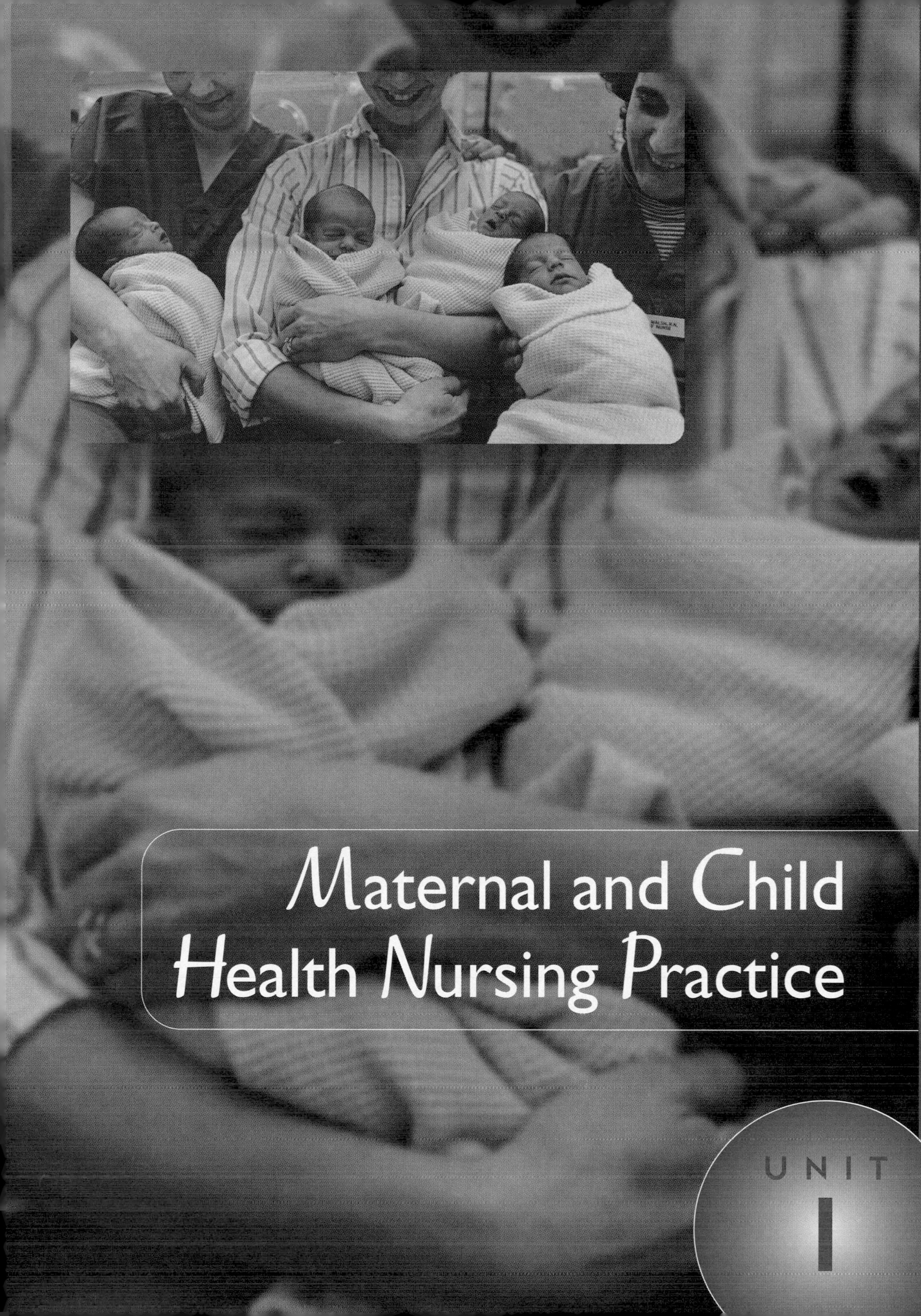

Maternal and Child Health Nursing Practice

UNIT

I

1

CHAPTER

A Framework for Maternal and Child Health Nursing

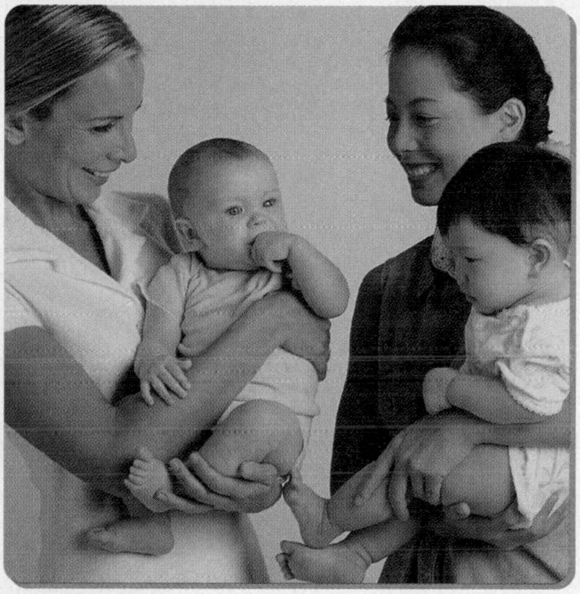

Key Terms

- clinical nurse specialist
- evidence-based practice
- family nurse practitioner
- fertility rate
- maternal and child health nursing
- mortality rate
- neonatal nurse practitioner
- neonate
- nurse-midwife
- nursing research
- pediatric nurse practitioner
- puerperium
- scope of practice
- women's health nurse practitioner

Objectives

After mastering the contents of this chapter, you should be able to:

1. Identify the goals and philosophy of maternal and child health nursing.
2. Describe the evolution, scope, and professional roles for nurses in maternal and child health nursing.
3. Define common statistical terms used in the field, such as infant and maternal mortality.
4. Discuss the implications of the common standards of maternal and child health nursing and the health goals for the nation for maternal and child health nursing.
5. Discuss the interplay of nursing process, evidence-based practice, and nursing theory as they relate to the future of maternal and child health nursing practice.
6. Use critical thinking to identify areas of care that could benefit from additional research or application of evidence-based practice.
7. Integrate knowledge of trends in maternal and child health care with the nursing process to achieve quality maternal and child health nursing care.

Anna Melendez is a premature neonate who must be transported to the regional center for care about 30 miles from the local hospital. Her parents, Melissa and Roberto, have many concerns. They don't want to be so far from their daughter, and they don't know how they will pay for her special care. Also, Melissa doesn't believe she is ready to leave the hospital so soon after having a cesarean birth. She recalls staying in the hospital much longer after having her first child, Miguel. Miguel, now 6 years old, is scared he will never see Anna again. What are some health care issues evident in this scenario? How has modern cost containment and managed care changed this scenario?

This chapter discusses standards and philosophies of maternal-child health care and how these standards and philosophies affect care.

After you've studied the chapter, answer the Critical Thinking Exercises at the end of the chapter and then access the on-line study activities (http://connection.lww.com) *to further sharpen your skills and test your knowledge.*

The care of childbearing and childrearing families is a major focus of nursing practice. To have healthy children, it is important to promote the health of the childbearing woman and her family from the time before children are born until they reach adulthood. Prenatal care and guidance are essential to the health of the woman and fetus and to the family's emotional preparation for childrearing. As children grow, the family needs continued health supervision and support. As children reach maturity, a new cycle begins and new support becomes necessary. The nurse's role in all these phases focuses on promoting healthy growth and development of the child and family in health and in illness.

Although the field of nursing typically divides its concerns for families during childbearing and childrearing into two separate entities, maternity and child health, the full scope of nursing practice in this area is not two separate entities, but one: maternal and child health nursing (Fig. 1-1).

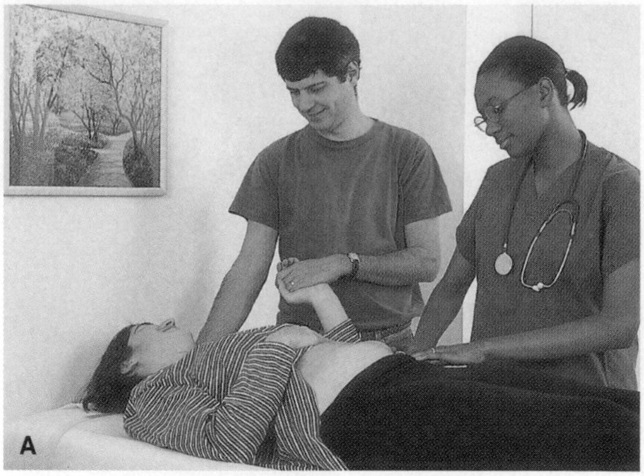

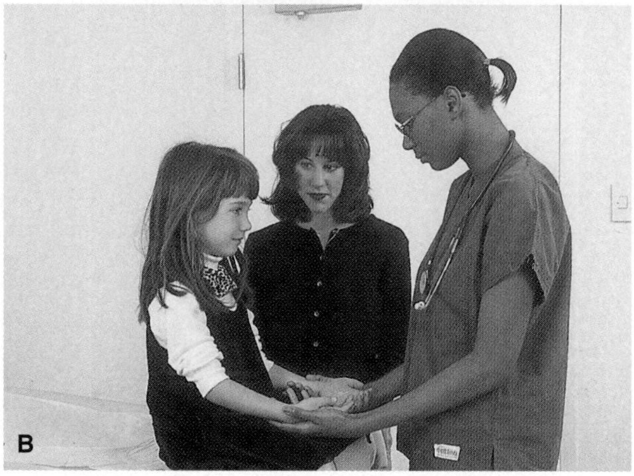

FIGURE 1.1 Maternal and child health nursing includes care of the pregnant woman, child, and family. (*A*) During a routine prenatal visit, a maternal child health nurse palpates a pregnant woman's fundus. (*B*) During a health maintenance visit, a maternal child health nurse assesses a pediatric client.

GOALS AND PHILOSOPHIES OF MATERNAL AND CHILD HEALTH NURSING

The primary goal of **maternal and child health nursing** care can be stated simply as the promotion and maintenance of optimal family health to ensure cycles of optimal childbearing and childrearing. Major philosophical assumptions about maternal and child health nursing are listed in Box 1-1. The goals of maternal and child health nursing care are necessarily broad because the scope of practice is so broad. The range of practice includes:

- Preconceptual health care
- Care of women during three trimesters of pregnancy and the **puerperium** (the 6 weeks after childbirth, sometimes termed the fourth trimester of pregnancy)
- Care of children during the perinatal period (6 weeks before conception to 6 weeks after birth)
- Care of children from infancy through adolescence
- Care in settings as varied as the birthing room, pediatric intensive care unit, and the home

In all settings and types of care, keeping the family at the center of care delivery is an essential goal. Maternal and child health nursing is always family-centered, which means the family is considered the primary unit of care. The level of family functioning affects the health status of individuals. If the family's level of functioning is low, the emotional, physical, and social health and potential of individuals in that family can be adversely affected. A healthy family, on the other hand, establishes an environment conducive to growth and health-promoting behaviors that sustain family members during crises. Similarly, the health of individuals and the ability to function strongly influences the health of family members and overall family functioning. Thus, a family-centered approach enables the nurse to better understand an individual and, in turn, provide holistic care. Box 1-2 provides a summary of key measures for the delivery of family-centered child health care.

BOX 1.1

PHILOSOPHY OF MATERNAL AND CHILD HEALTH NURSING

- Maternal and child health nursing is family-centered; assessment data must include a family and individual assessment.
- Maternal and child health nursing is community-centered; the health of families depends on and influences the health of communities.
- Maternal and child health nursing is research-oriented because research is the means whereby critical knowledge increases.
- Nursing theory and evidence-based practice provide a foundation for nursing care.
- A maternal and child health nurse serves as an advocate to protect the rights of all family members, including the fetus.
- Maternal and child health nursing uses a high degree of independent nursing functions because teaching and counseling are so frequently required.
- Promoting health is an important nursing role because this protects the health of the next generation.
- Pregnancy or childhood illness can be stressful and can alter family life in both subtle and extensive ways.
- Personal, cultural, and religious attitudes and beliefs influence the meaning of illness and its impact on the family. Circumstances such as illness or pregnancy are meaningful only in the context of a total life.
- Maternal and child health nursing is a challenging role for the nurse and is a major factor in promoting high-level wellness in families.

BOX 1.2

COMMON MEASURES TO ENSURE FAMILY-CENTERED MATERNAL AND CHILD HEALTH CARE

Principle

- The family is the basic unit of society.
- Families represent racial, ethnic, cultural, and socioeconomic diversity.
- Children grow both individually and as part of a family.

Nursing Interventions

- Encourage families to use community services so that family members are not separated by care needs.
- Encourage rooming-in in both maternal and child health hospital settings.
- Participate in early discharge programs to reunite families as soon as possible.
- Encourage family and sibling visits to promote family contacts.
- Assess families for strengths and specific needs.
- Respect diversity in families as a unique quality of that family.
- Include developmental stimulation in care.
- Encourage families to give care to a newborn or ill child.
- Share or initiate information on health planning with family members so care is family-oriented.

STANDARDS OF MATERNAL AND CHILD HEALTH NURSING PRACTICE

The importance a society places on caring can best be measured by the concern it places on its most vulnerable members or its elderly, disadvantaged, and young citizens. Specialty organizations develop standards of care to promote consistency and ensure quality nursing care in their areas of nursing practice. In maternal-child health, standards were developed in the 1980s by the Division of Maternal-Child Health Nursing Practice of the American Nurses Association to provide important guidelines for planning care and devising outcome criteria for the evaluation of nursing care. Updated in connection with the Society of Pediatric Nurses, these standards are shown in Box 1-3.

Several other specialty groups have developed guidelines for practice and education in this area. The Association of Women's Health, Obstetric, and Neonatal Nurses (AWHONN) has developed standards for the nursing care of women and newborns, summarized in Box 1-4.

A FRAMEWORK FOR MATERNAL AND CHILD HEALTH NURSING CARE

Maternal and child health nursing can be visualized within a framework in which nurses, using nursing process, nursing theory, and nursing research, care for families during childbearing and childrearing years through four phases of health care:

- Health promotion
- Health maintenance
- Health restoration
- Health rehabilitation

Examples of these phases of health care as they relate to maternal and child health are shown in Table 1-1.

The Nursing Process

Nursing care, at its best, is designed and implemented in a thorough manner, using an organized series of steps, to ensure quality and consistency of care. The nursing process, a proven form of problem solving based on the scientific method, serves as the basis for assessing, planning, and organizing care. That the nursing process is applicable to all health care settings, from the prenatal clinic to the pediatric intensive care unit, is proof that the method is broad enough to serve as the basis for all of nursing care (Carpenito, 2001).

BOX 1.3

AMERICAN NURSES ASSOCIATION/SOCIETY OF PEDIATRIC NURSES STANDARDS OF CARE AND PROFESSIONAL PERFORMANCE

Standards of Care

Comprehensive pediatric nursing care focuses on helping children and their families and communities achieve their optimum health potentials. This is best achieved within the framework of family-centered care and the nursing process, including primary, secondary, and tertiary care coordinated across health care and community settings.

Standard I: Assessment
The pediatric nurse collects health data.

Standard II: Diagnosis
The pediatric nurse analyzes the assessment data in determining diagnoses.

Standard III: Outcome Identification
The pediatric nurse identifies expected outcomes individualized to the client.

Standard IV: Planning
The pediatric nurse develops a plan of care that prescribes interventions to obtain expected outcomes.

Standard V: Implementation
The pediatric nurse implements the interventions identified in the plan of care.

Standard VI: Evaluation
The pediatric nurse evaluates the child's and family's progress toward attainment of outcomes.

Standards of Professional Performance

Standard I: Quality of Care
The pediatric nurse systematically evaluates the quality and effectiveness of pediatric nursing practice.

Standard II: Performance Appraisal
The pediatric nurse evaluates his or her own nursing practice in relation to professional practice standards and relevant statutes and regulations.

Standard III: Education
The pediatric nurse acquires and maintains current knowledge in pediatric nursing practice.

Standard IV: Collegiality
The pediatric nurse contributes to the professional development of peers, colleagues, and others.

Standard V: Ethics
The pediatric nurse's decisions and actions on behalf of children and their families are determined in an ethical manner.

Standard VI: Collaboration
The pediatric nurse collaborates with the child, family, and health care provider in providing client care.

Standard VII: Research
The pediatric nurse uses research findings in practice.

Standard VIII: Resource Utilization
The pediatric nurse considers factors related to safety, effectiveness, and cost in planning and delivering care.

American Nurses Association and the Society of Pediatric Nurses. (1996). *Statement on the scope and standards of pediatric clinical practice.* Washington, DC: American Nurses Publishing House.

The nursing process consists of five steps:

1. Assessment
2. Nursing diagnosis
3. Outcome identification and planning
4. Implementation
5. Outcome evaluation

All subsequent chapters in this book begin with a Nursing Process Overview that summarizes the major nursing concerns in each step of the process for the content of that particular chapter. Nursing care plans or care pathways throughout demonstrate the use of the nursing process for a selected client, provide examples of critical thinking in nursing, and clarify nursing care for specific client needs. In addition, selected chapters also identify specific nursing outcomes using the terminology presented in the Nursing Outcomes Classification (NOC) and nursing interventions and related activities using the terminology presented in the Nursing Intervention Classification (NIC) developed by the Iowa Intervention Project (Johnson, Maas, and Moorhead, 2000; McCloskey and Bulechek, 2000). These outcomes and interventions, specific to maternal and child health nursing, are highlighted in a box.

Evidence-Based Practice

Evidence-based practice involves the use of research or controlled investigation of a problem using a scientific method in conjunction with clinical expertise as acquired through experience and practice as a foundation for action. Bodies of professional knowledge grow and expand to the extent that people in that profession plan and carry out research. **Nursing research,** the controlled investigation of problems that have implications for nursing practice, is the method by which the foundation of nursing grows, expands, and improves, thus providing evidence for practice. In addition, evidence-based practice provides the justification for implementing activities for outcome achievement, ultimately resulting in improved, cost-effective patient care.

A classic example of how the results of nursing research can influence nursing practice is the application of the research carried out by Rubin (1963) on a mother's approach to her newborn. Before this published study, nurses

BOX 1.4

ASSOCIATION OF WOMEN'S HEALTH, OBSTETRIC, AND NEONATAL NURSES STANDARDS AND GUIDELINES

STANDARDS OF PROFESSIONAL PERFORMANCE

Standard I: Quality of Care
The nurse systematically evaluates the quality and effectiveness of nursing practice.

Standard II: Performance Appraisal
The nurse evaluates his/her own nursing practice in relation to professional practice standards and relevant statutes and regulations.

Standard III: Education
The nurse acquires and maintains current knowledge in nursing practice.

Standard IV: Collegiality
The nurse contributes to the professional development of peers, colleagues, and others.

Standard V: Ethics
The nurse's decisions and actions on behalf of patients are determined in an ethical manner.

Standard VI: Collaboration
The nurse collaborates with the patient, significant others, and health care providers in providing patient care.

Standard VII: Research
The nurse uses research findings in practice.

Standard VIII: Resource Utilization
The nurse considers factors related to safety, effectiveness, and cost in planning and delivering patient care.

Standard IX: Practice Environment
The nurse contributes to the environment of care delivery within the practice settings.

Standard X: Accountability
The nurse is professionally and legally accountable for his/her practice. The professional registered nurse may delegate to and supervise qualified personnel who provide patient care.

Association of Women's Health, Obstetric, and Neonatal Nurses. (1998). *Standards for the nursing care of women and newborns* (5th ed.). Washington, DC: Author.

assumed that a woman who did not immediately hold and cuddle her infant at birth was a "cold" or unfeeling mother. Rubin concluded that attachment is not a spontaneous procedure; rather, it more commonly begins with only fingertip touching. Armed with Rubin's finding and integrating these findings into practice, nurses became better able to differentiate healthy from unhealthy bonding behavior in postpartum women and their newborns. Thus, women following this step-by-step pattern of attachment were no longer recognized as unfeeling, but normal. By documenting these normal parameters, women who do not follow such a pattern can be identified and interventions can be planned and instituted to help these mothers gain a stronger attachment to their new infant. Additional nursing research in this area (discussed in Chap. 22) has provided further substantiation about the importance of this original investigation.

Evidence-based practice requires ongoing research to substantiate current actions as well as to provide guidelines for future actions. Some examples of current questions that warrant nursing investigation in the area of maternal and child health nursing include:

- What is the best stimulus to encourage women to come for prenatal care or parents to bring children for health maintenance care?
- How can nurses be instrumental in fostering multidisciplinary care?
- What are the special needs of women discharged from a hospital or birthing center within a short time after childbirth?
- How much self-care should young children be expected (or encouraged) to provide during illness?
- What is the effect of market-driven care on the quality of nursing care?
- What active measures can nurses take to reduce the incidence of child or intimate partner abuse?
- What are the effects of long-term home care on parents' or children's mental health?
- How is high self-esteem maintained in couples who are infertile, or in health-challenged children?
- How can nurses be active in helping prevent violence in schools?
- What do maternal-child health nurses need to know about alternative therapies such as herbal remedies?

The answers to these and other questions provided by research help to bolster the foundation from which to develop specific actions and activities for the improvement of maternal and child health. In selected chapters throughout this text, Focus on Evidence-Based Practice boxes contain summaries of current maternal and child health research pertinent to nursing care. The content of these boxes is designed to assist you in developing a questioning attitude regarding current nursing practice and in thinking of ways to incorporate research findings into care.

Nursing Theory

One of the requirements of a profession (together with other critical determinants, such as member self-set standards, monitoring of practice quality, and participation in research) is that the concentration of a discipline's knowledge flows from a base of established theory.

TABLE 1.1 Definitions and Examples of Phases of Health Care

TERM	DEFINITION	EXAMPLES
Health promotion	Educating clients to be aware of good health through teaching and role modeling	Teaching women the importance of rubella immunization before pregnancy; teaching children the importance of actions such as safer sex practices
Health maintenance	Intervening to maintain health when risk of illness is present	Encouraging women to come for prenatal care; teaching parents the importance of safeguarding their home by childproofing it against poisoning
Health restoration	Promptly diagnosing and treating illness using interventions that will return client to wellness most rapidly	Caring for a woman during a complication of pregnancy or a child during a respiratory illness
Health rehabilitation	Preventing further complications from an illness; bringing ill client back to optimal state of wellness or helping client to accept inevitable death	Helping a woman with trophoblastic disease to continue therapy or a child with chronic renal disease to continue to attend school

Nursing theorists offer helpful ways to view clients and nurses so nursing activities can best meet client needs (e.g., by seeing the client not simply as a physical form but as a dynamic force with important psychosocial needs). In maternal and child health nursing, viewing clients as extensions or active members of a family as well as holistic beings is vital. Only with this broad focus can nurses appreciate the significant effect on a family of a child's illness or of the introduction of a new member.

Another issue most nursing theorists address is how nurses should be viewed or what the goals of nursing care should be. At one time, the goal of nursing care could have been stated as providing care and comfort to injured and ill people. Most nurses today would perceive this view as a limited one, because they are equipped to do much more. Extensive changes in the scope of maternal and child health nursing have occurred as health promotion, or keeping parents and children well, becomes more important.

A third issue addressed by nurse theorists concerns the activities of nursing care; as goals become broader, so do activities. For example, when the primary goal of nursing was considered to be caring for ill people, nursing actions were limited to bathing, feeding, and providing comfort. Currently, with health promotion as a major nursing goal, teaching, counseling, supporting, and advocacy are also common roles. With new technologies available, nurses are caring for clients who are sicker than ever before. Because care of women during pregnancy and children during their developing years helps protect not only current health but also the health of the next generation, maternal-child health nurses fill these expanded roles to a unique and special degree.

Table 1-2 summarizes the tenets of a number of common nursing theorists and suggests ways these could be applied to maternal-child health care through the situation of one child. The third column of the table ("Emphasis of Care") demonstrates that although the theoretical bases of these theories differ, the result of any one of them is to provide a higher level of care. These different theories, therefore, do not contradict but rather complement each other in the planning and implementation of holistic nursing care.

✔ **CHECKPOINT QUESTIONS**

1. What is the primary goal of maternal and child health nursing?
2. What is the advantage of maternal and child health nursing being family-centered?
3. What features besides conducting research are the mark of a profession?

MATERNAL AND CHILD HEALTH NURSING TODAY

At the beginning of the 20th century, the infant mortality rate (the number of infants per 1,000 births who die during the first year of life) was over 100 per 1,000. In response to efforts to lower this rate, health care shifted from a treatment focus to a preventive one, dramatically changing the scope of maternal and child health nursing. Research on the benefits of early prenatal care led to the first major national effort to provide prenatal care to all pregnant women through prenatal nursing services (home visits) and clinics. Today, thanks to these and other community health measures (such as efforts to encourage breast-feeding, increased immunization, and injury prevention) as well as many technological advances, the infant mortality rate has fallen from 100 per 1,000 to 6.9 per 1,000 (National Center for Health Statistics [NCHS], 2000a).

Medical technology has contributed to a number of important advances in maternal and child health: childhood diseases such as measles and poliomyelitis are almost eradicated; specific genetic markers and genes responsible for many inherited diseases have been identified, possibly revolutionizing medical therapy in the coming years; new fertility drugs and techniques are allowing more couples than ever before to conceive; and the ability to delay preterm birth and improve life for premature infants has grown substantially. In addition, a growing trend toward health care consumerism, or self-care, has made many childbearing and childrearing families active participants

TABLE 1.2 Summary of Nursing Theories

Terry is a 7-year-old girl who is hospitalized because her right arm was severely injured in an automobile accident. There is a high probability she will never have full use of the arm again. Terry's mother is concerned because Terry showed promise in art. Previously happy and active in Girl Scouts, Terry has spent most of every day since the accident sitting in her hospital bed silently watching television.

THEORIST	MAJOR CONCEPTS OF THEORY	EMPHASIS OF CARE
Faye Abdellah	The role of the nurse is to identify and to correct needs according to 21 identified areas; needs may be overt (apparent) or covert (hidden or unknown to the client).	Assess Terry's health care needs according to the 21 areas of concern; care is incomplete until all needs are met.
Patricia Benner	Nursing is a caring relationship. Nurses grow from novice to expert as they practice in clinical settings.	Assess Terry as a whole. An expert nurse is able to do this intuitively from knowledge gained from practice.
Dorothy Johnson	A person comprises subsystems that must remain in balance for optimal functioning. Any actual or potential threat to this system balance is a nursing concern.	Assess the effect of lack of arm function on Terry as a whole; modify care to maintain function to all systems, not just musculoskeletal.
Imogene King	Nursing is a process of action, reaction, interaction, and transaction; needs are identified based on client's social system perceptions, and health; the role of the nurse is to help the client achieve goal attainment.	Discuss with Terry the way she views herself and illness. She views herself as a well child, active in Girl Scouts and school; structure care to help her meet these perceptions.
Madeleine Leininger	The essence of nursing is care. To provide transcultural care, the nurse focuses on the study and analysis of different cultures with respect to caring behavior.	Assess Terry's family for beliefs about healing. Incorporate these into care.
Florence Nightingale	The role of the nurse is viewed as changing or structuring elements of the environment such as ventilation, temperature, odors, noise, and light to put the client into the best opportunity for recovery.	Turn Terry's bed into the sunlight; provide adequate covers for warmth; leave her comfortable with electronic game to occupy her time.
Betty Neuman	A person is an open system that interacts with the environment; nursing is aimed at reducing stressors through primary, secondary, and tertiary prevention.	Assess for stressors such as loss of self-esteem and derive ways to prevent further loss such as praising her for combing her own hair.
Dorothea Orem	The focus of nursing is on the individual; clients are assessed in terms of ability to complete self-care. Care given may be wholly compensatory (client has no role); partly compensatory (client participates in care); or supportive-educational (client performs own care).	Arrange overbed table so Terry can feed herself; urge her to participate in care by doing as much for herself as she can.
Ida Jean Orlando	The focus of the nurse is interaction with the client; effectiveness of care depends on client's behavior, nurse's reaction to that behavior. The client should define own needs.	Ask Terry what she feels is her main need. Terry says that returning to school is what she wants most. Stress activities that allow her to maintain contact with school such as doing homework or telephoning friends.
Rosemarie Rizzo Parse	Nursing is a human science. Health is a lived experience. Man-living-health as a single unit guides practice.	Ask Terry what being sick means to her. Allow her to participate in care decisions based on this.
Hildegard Peplau	The promotion of health is viewed as the forward movement of the personality; this is accomplished through an interpersonal process including orientation, identification, exploitation, and resolution.	Plan care together with Terry. Encourage her to speak of school and accomplishments in Girl Scouts to retain self-esteem.
Martha Rogers	The purpose of nursing is to move the client toward optimal health; the nurse should view the client as whole and constantly changing and help people to interact in the best way possible with the environment.	Help Terry to make use of her left side as much as possible so she returns to school and previous level of functioning as soon as possible.
Sister Callistra Roy	The role of the nurse is to aid clients to adapt to the change caused by illness; levels of adaptation depend on the degree of environmental change and state of coping ability; full adaptation includes physiologic interdependence.	Assess Terry's ability to use her left hand to replace her right-hand functions, which are now lost; direct nursing care toward replacing deficit with other factors, self-concept, role function, and skills.

in their own health monitoring and care. Health care consumerism has also moved care from hospital to community sites and from long-term hospital stays to overnight surgical and ambulatory settings.

Even in light of these changes, much more still needs to be done. National health care goals established in 1999 for the year 2010 continue to stress the importance of maternal and child health to overall community health (Department of Health and Human Services [DHHS], 2000a). Although health care may be more advanced, it is still not accessible to everyone. These and other social changes and trends have expanded the roles of nurses in maternal and child health care and, at the same time, have made the delivery of quality maternal and child health nursing care a continuing challenge.

National Health Goals

In 1979, the U.S. Public Health Service initiated the formulation of health care objectives to be achieved by 1990. Many of these objectives directly involved maternal and child health care, because improving the health of this young age group has long-term effects. Many of these goals were not met by 1995 due to the limited time period available for problem solving. Health care goals have been reestablished, therefore, for the year 2010 (DHHS, 2000a). Goals specific for each content area are highlighted in subsequent chapters. The nation's priority goals (leading health indicators) are shown in the Focus on National Health Goals Box. Leading health indicators are intended to help everyone more easily understand the importance of health promotion and disease prevention and to encourage wide participation in improving health in the next decade. Maternal and child health nurses need to be familiar with these goals because they serve as the basis for grant funding and financing evidence-based practice. Nurses play a vital role in helping the nation achieve these objectives through both practice and research.

Trends in the Maternal and Child Health Nursing Population

The maternal and child population is constantly changing, along with changes in social structure, variations in family lifestyle, increased health care costs, improvements in medical technology, and changing patterns of illness. Table 1-3 summarizes some of the social changes that have occurred over the past 20 to 30 years that have altered health care priorities for maternal and child health nurses. Today, client advocacy, a philosophy of managed care, an increased focus on health education, and case management have made pronounced changes in nursing care for the maternal and child population.

Measuring Maternal and Child Health

Measuring maternal and child health is not as simple as defining a client as ill or well. Individual clients and health care practitioners may all have different perspectives on illness and wellness. For example, some children with chronic but controllable asthma think of themselves as well; others with the same degree of involvement consider themselves ill. Although pregnancy is generally considered a well state, some women think of themselves as ill during this period. A more objective view of health is provided by national health statistics.

A number of statistical terms are used to express the outcome of pregnancies and births and to describe child health (Box 1-5). The statistics that these terms encompass require accurate collection and analysis to provide a descriptive picture of the nation's health. Such a description is useful for comparison and planning of future health care needs.

Birth Rate

The birth rate in the United States has remained fairly constant for the past 10 years. As of 2000, the birth rate was 14.8 per 1,000 population (Hoyert et al., 2001; Fig. 1-2). Currently, the average family in the United States has 1.2 children. Boys are born more often than girls, at a rate of 1,053 boys to every 1,000 girls (NCHS, 2000b).

Fertility Rate

The term **fertility rate** reflects what proportion of women who could have babies are having them. The fertility rate for 2000 was 67%, a healthy reproductive rate for a country (NCHS, 2000b).

Fetal Death Rate

Fetal death is defined as the death in utero of a child (fetus) weighing 500 g or more, roughly the weight of a fetus of 20 weeks' or more gestation. Fetal deaths may occur because of maternal factors (e.g., maternal disease, premature cervical dilation, or maternal malnutrition) or fetal factors (e.g., fetal disease, chromosome abnormality, or poor placental attachment). Many fetal deaths occur for reasons yet unknown. The fetal death rate of a nation is important in evaluating health care because it reflects the overall quality of maternal health and prenatal care. The emphasis on both preconceptual and prenatal care has helped to reduce this rate from a number as high as 18% in 1950 to below 7% in 2000 (NCHS, 2000a).

Neonatal Death Rate

The first 28 days of life are known as the neonatal period, and the child during this time is known as a **neonate.** The neonatal death rate reflects not only the quality of care available to women during pregnancy and childbirth but also the quality of care available to infants during the first month of life.

The leading causes of infant mortality during the first 4 weeks of life are prematurity (early gestational age), low birthweight (a weight less than 2,500 g), and congenital anomalies. Approximately 80% of infants who die within 48 hours of birth weigh less than 2,500 g (5.5 lb). The proportion of infants born with low birthweight is about 7% of all births. This number rises slightly each year as better prenatal care allows infants who would have died in utero (fetal death) to be born and survive (Guyer, 2000).

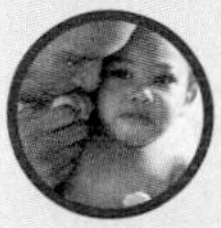

FOCUS ON NATIONAL HEALTH GOALS

LEADING HEALTH INDICATORS

Physical Activity

Regular physical activity throughout life is important for maintaining a healthy body, enhancing psychologic well-being, and preventing premature death. The objectives selected to measure progress in this area are:

- Increase the proportion of adolescents who engage in vigorous physical activity that promotes cardiorespiratory fitness 3 or more days per week for 20 or more minutes per occasion.
- Increase the proportion of adults who engage regularly, preferably daily, in moderate physical activity for at least 30 minutes per day.

Overweight and Obesity

Overweight and obesity are major contributors to many preventable causes of death. The objectives selected to measure progress in this area are:

- Reduce the proportion of children and adolescents who are overweight or obese.
- Reduce the proportion of adults who are obese.

Tobacco Use

Cigarette smoking is the single most preventable cause of disease and death in the United States. Smoking results in more deaths each year in the United States than AIDS, alcohol, cocaine, heroin, homicide, suicide, motor vehicle crashes, and fires—combined. The objectives selected to measure progress in this area are:

- Reduce cigarette smoking by adolescents.
- Reduce cigarette smoking by adults.

Substance Abuse

Alcohol and illicit drug use are associated with many of this country's most serious problems, including violence, injury, and HIV infection. The objectives selected to measure progress in this area are:

- Increase the proportion of adolescents not using alcohol or any illicit drugs during the past 30 days.
- Reduce the proportion of adults using any illicit drug during the past 30 days.
- Reduce the proportion of adults engaging in binge drinking of alcoholic beverages during the past month.

Responsible Sexual Behavior

Unintended pregnancies and sexually transmitted diseases (STDs), including infection with the human immunodeficiency virus that causes AIDS, can result from unprotected sexual behavior. The objectives selected to measure progress in this area are:

- Increase the proportion of adolescents who abstain from sexual intercourse or use condoms if currently sexually active.
- Increase the proportion of sexually active persons who use condoms.

Mental Health

Approximately 20% of the U.S. population is affected by mental illness during a given year; no one is immune. Of all mental illnesses, depression is the most common disorder. More than 19 million adults in the United States suffer from depression. Major depression is the leading cause of disability and is the cause of more than two thirds of suicides each year. The objective selected to measure progress in this area is:

- Increase the proportion of adults with recognized depression who receive treatment.

Injury and Violence

More than 400 Americans die each day from injuries, due primarily to motor vehicle crashes, firearms, poisonings, suffocation, falls, fires, and drowning. The risk of injury is so great that most persons sustain a significant injury at some time during their lives. The objectives selected to measure progress in this area are:

- Reduce deaths caused by motor vehicle crashes.
- Reduce homicides.

Environmental Quality

An estimated 25% of preventable illnesses worldwide can be attributed to poor environmental quality. In the United States, air pollution alone is estimated to be associated with 50,000 premature deaths and an estimated $40 billion to $50 billion in health-related costs annually. The objectives selected to measure progress in this area are:

- Reduce the proportion of persons exposed to air that does not meet the U.S. Environmental Protection Agency's health-based standards for ozone.
- Reduce the proportion of nonsmokers exposed to environmental tobacco smoke.

Immunization

Vaccines are among the greatest public health achievements of the 20th century. Immunizations can prevent disability and death from infectious diseases for individuals and can help control the spread of infections within communities. The objectives selected to measure progress in this area are:

- Increase the proportion of young children who receive all vaccines that have been recommended for universal administration for at least 5 years.
- Increase the proportion of noninstitutionalized adults who are vaccinated annually against influenza and ever vaccinated against pneumococcal disease.

Access to Health Care

Strong predictors of access to quality health care include having health insurance, a higher income level, and a regular primary care provider or other source of ongoing health care. Use of clinical preventive services, such as early prenatal care, can serve as indicators of access to quality health care services. The objectives selected to measure progress in this area are:

- Increase the proportion of persons with health insurance.
- Increase the proportion of persons who have a specific source of ongoing care.
- Increase the proportion of pregnant women who begin prenatal care in the first trimester of pregnancy.

Department of Health and Human Services. (2000). Leading health indicators. *Healthy people 2010.* Washington, D.C.: DHHS.

TABLE 1.3 Trends in Maternal and Child Health Care and Implications for Nurses

TREND	IMPLICATIONS FOR NURSING
Families are smaller than in previous decades.	Fewer family members are present as support in a time of crisis. Nurses must fulfill this role more than ever before.
Single parents are increasing in number.	A single parent may have fewer financial resources; this is more likely if the parent is a woman. Nurses need to inform parents of care options and to serve as a backup opinion when needed.
An increasing number of mothers work outside the home.	Health care must be scheduled at times a working parent can bring a child for care. Problems of latch-key children and the selection of child care centers need to be discussed.
Families are more mobile than previously; there is an increase in the number of homeless women and children.	Good interviewing is necessary with mobile families so a health database can be established; education for health monitoring is important.
Abuse is more common than ever before.	Screening for child or intimate partner abuse should be included in family contacts. Be aware of the legal responsibilities for reporting abuse.
Families are more health-conscious than previously.	Families are ripe for health education; providing this can be a major nursing role.
Health care must respect cost containment.	Comprehensive care is necessary in primary care settings because referral to specialists may no longer be an option.

Perinatal Death Rate

The perinatal period is defined in a number of different ways. Statistically, the period is defined as the time beginning when the fetus reaches 500 g (about week 20 of pregnancy) and ending about 4 weeks after birth. The perinatal death rate is the sum of the fetal and neonatal rates.

BOX 1.5

STATISTICAL TERMS USED TO REPORT MATERNAL AND CHILD HEALTH

Birth rate: The number of births per 1,000 population.

Fertility rate: The number of pregnancies per 1,000 women of child-bearing age.

Fetal death rate: The number of fetal deaths (over 500 g) per 1,000 live births.

Neonatal death rate: The number of deaths per 1,000 live births occurring at birth or in the first 28 days of life.

Perinatal death rate: The number of deaths of fetuses more than 500 g and in the first 28 days of life per 1,000 live births.

Maternal mortality rate: The number of maternal deaths per 100,000 live births that occur as a direct result of the reproductive process.

Infant mortality rate: The number of deaths per 1,000 live births occurring at birth or in the first 12 months of life.

Childhood mortality rate: The number of deaths per 1,000 population in children, 1 to 14 years of age.

Maternal Mortality Rate

Mortality rate is the rate of deaths from a specific cause. Early in the 20th century, the maternal mortality rate (death from childbirth) reached levels as high as 600 per 100,000 live births. Currently, the maternal mortality rate has declined to a low of 6.5 per 100,000 live births (NCHS, 2000a; Fig. 1-3). This dramatic decrease can be attributed to improved preconceptual, prenatal, labor and delivery, and postpartum care, such as:

- Greater detection of disorders such as ectopic pregnancy or placenta previa and prevention of related complications through the use of ultrasound
- Increased control of complications associated with hypertension of pregnancy
- Decreased use of anesthesia with childbirth

For most of the 20th century, uterine hemorrhage and infection were the leading causes of death during pregnancy and childbirth. This has changed owing to the increased ability to prevent or control hemorrhage and infection, so that hypertensive disorders currently are the leading causes of death in childbirth. Pregnancy-induced hypertension adds to preexisting hypertensive disorders, especially in older women. Nurses who are alert to the signs and symptoms of hypertension are invaluable guardians of the health of pregnant and postpartum women.

Infant Mortality Rate

The infant mortality rate of a country is an index of its general health. This rate is the traditional standard used to compare national health care to that of previous years and to that of other countries.

Thanks to medical advances and improvements in child care, the infant mortality rate in the United States has been steadily declining in recent years; it reached a record low in 2000 of 6.9 per 1,000 population (NCHS, 2000a). Unfortunately, infant mortality is not equal for all people.

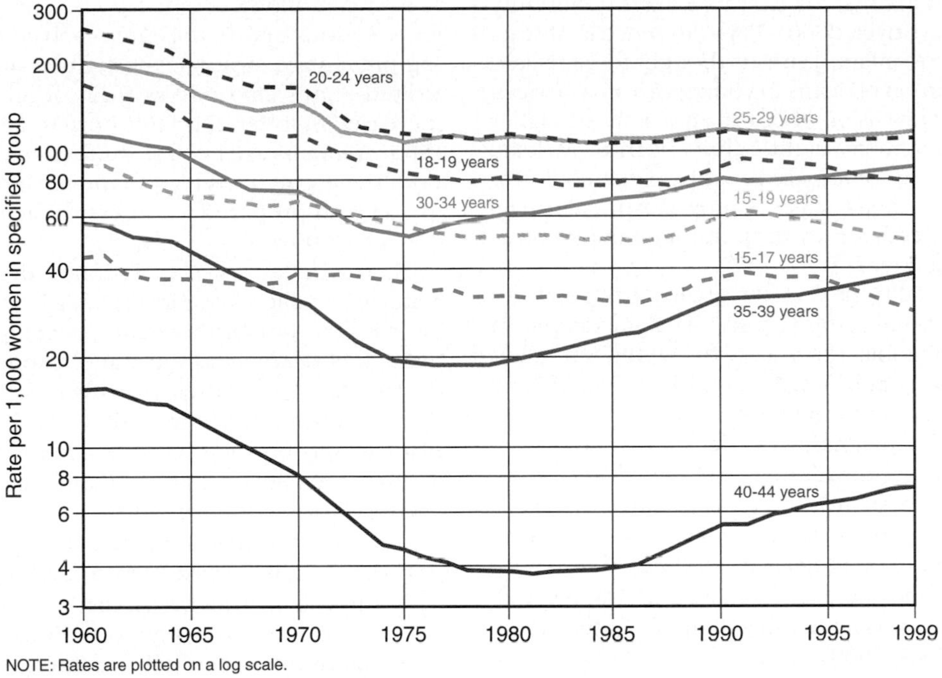

FIGURE 1.2 Birth rates by age of mother: United States, 1960–1999. (National Center for Health Statistics. [2001]. Births, marriages, divorces and deaths. *National Vital Statistics Report, 49*(1), 6. Hyattsville, MD: U.S. Public Health Service.)

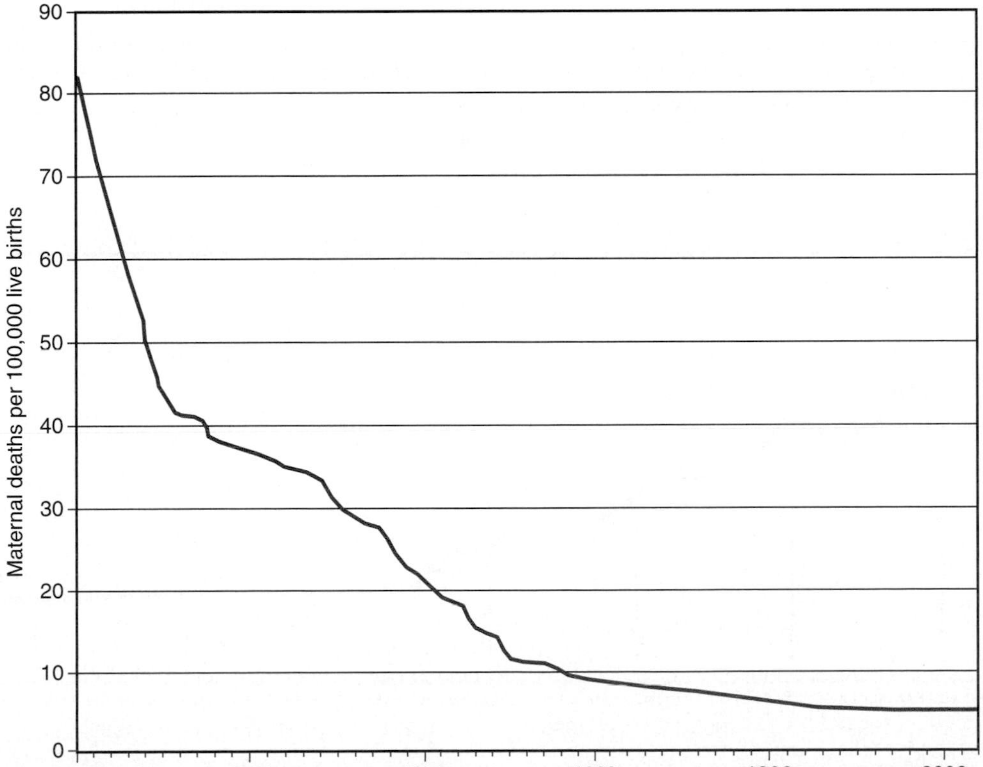

FIGURE 1.3 Maternal mortality rates, 2002. (National Center for Health Statistics [2002]. *National Vital Statistics Report, 50*(1), 3. Hyattsville, MD: U.S. Public Health Service.)

African-American infants, for example, have a mortality rate of almost 15% (Guyer, 2000). This difference in African-American and white infant deaths is thought to be related to the high proportion of births to young African-American mothers, unequal provision of health care, and the higher percentage of low-birthweight babies born to African-American women: 12% compared to approximately 5% for white and Asian women (Guyer, 2000). Despite this negative trend, the overall steady drop in total infant mortality is encouraging (Fig. 1-4).

The infant mortality rate varies greatly from state to state within the United States (Table 1-4). For example, in the District of Columbia, the area with the highest infant mortality, the rate is more than three times that in New Hampshire, the state with the lowest rate.

Table 1-5 shows the ranking of the United States compared to that of other developed countries. One would expect that a country such as the United States, which has one of the highest gross national products in the world and is known for its technological capabilities, would have the lowest infant mortality. However, in 2000, the U.S. infant mortality rate was higher than that of 27 other countries (United Nations, 2000).

One factor that may contribute to national differences in infant mortality is the type of health care available. In Sweden, for example, a comprehensive health care program provides free maternal and child health care to all residents. Women who attend prenatal clinics early in pregnancy receive a monetary award for early attendance; this almost guarantees that all women will come for prenatal care. Many people believe that a guaranteed health care system would lead to lower infant mortality in the United States.

Fortunately, the number of women who receive prenatal care in the United States is increasing. About 80% of women begin care in the first trimester (Guyer, 2000). Lack of early care allows complications of pregnancy to become more serious before they are resolved rather than allowing preventive strategies to reduce their intensity. The United States also differs from other countries in the increased number of infants born to adolescent mothers (30% of infants are born to mothers under 20 years old). Both these concerns lead to the birth of infants who are not as well prepared as others to face extrauterine life (Guyer, 2000).

The main causes of early infant death in the United States are problems occurring at birth or shortly thereafter. Prematurity, low birthweight, congenital anomalies, sudden infant death syndrome, and respiratory distress syndrome are major causes. However, the recommendation that the American Academy of Pediatrics made in 1992 to place infants on their back or side to sleep has led to an almost 50% decrease in the incidence of sudden infant death syndrome (Guyer, 2000).

Before antibiotics and formula sterilization practices, gastrointestinal disease was a leading cause of infant death. By advocating breast-feeding and teaching mothers strict adherence to good sanitary practices, health care practitioners can help ensure that gastrointestinal infection does not again become a major factor in infant mortality.

✔ CHECKPOINT QUESTIONS

4. What are social changes that have most greatly influenced maternal and child health care?
5. How has sudden infant death syndrome affected the infant mortality rate?
6. What health statistic is used for international comparisons of the health of countries?

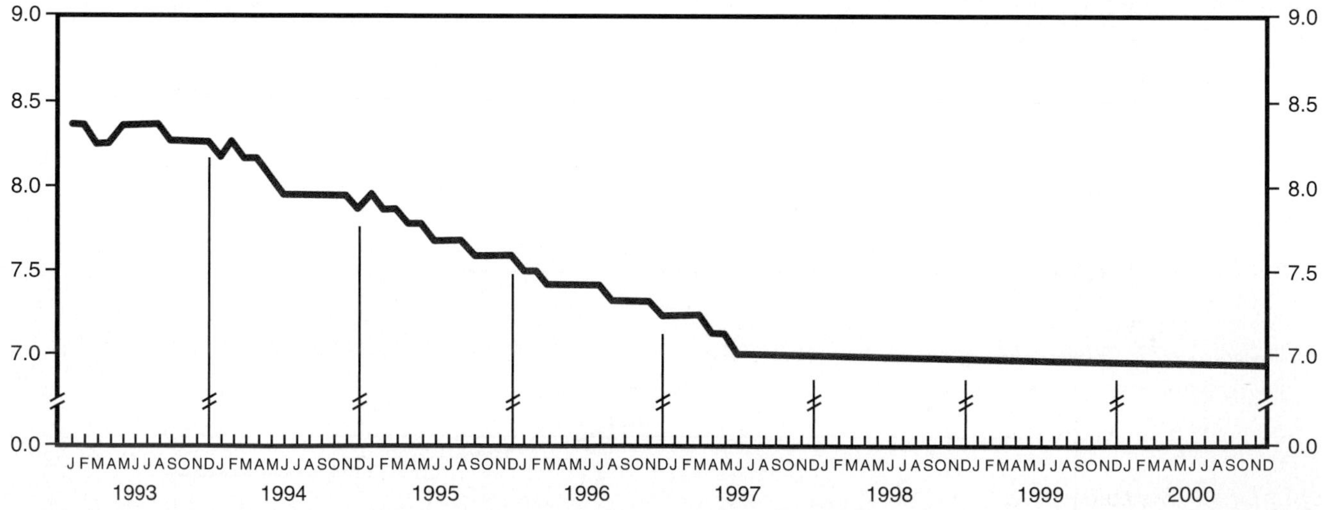

FIGURE 1.4 Infant mortality rates per 1,000 live births for successive 12-month periods ending with month indicated: United States, 2000. (National Center for Health Statistics. [2002]. Births, marriages, divorce and deaths. *National Vital Statistics Report, 50*(1), 2. Hyattsville, MD: U.S. Public Health Service.)

TABLE 1.4 Infant Mortality Rates per 1,000 by State

STATE	RATE
New Hampshire	4.8
Massachusetts	5.2
Washington	5.4
Utah	5.4
Maine	5.5
Oregon	5.6
California	5.7
Minnesota	6.0
Iowa	6.1
Vermont	6.2
Texas	6.3
New York	6.4
New Jersey	6.5
Alaska	6.5
Connecticut	6.7
New Mexico	6.7
Rhode Island	6.7
Wyoming	6.7
Colorado	6.8
Idaho	6.8
Nevada	6.8
Wisconsin	6.8
Hawaii	6.9
Montana	7.0
Arizona	7.1
Florida	7.2
Nebraska	7.2
Kansas	7.3
North Dakota	7.3
Kentucky	7.4
Pennsylvania	7.4
Virginia	7.5
Missouri	7.6
Indiana	7.9
Ohio	8.0
Michigan	8.1
Oklahoma	8.2
Tennessee	8.2
Delaware	8.3
West Virginia	8.3
Georgia	8.4
Arkansas	8.5
Illinois	8.5
South Dakota	8.5
Maryland	8.6
North Carolina	9.2
Louisiana	9.3
Alabama	9.8
South Carolina	9.8
Mississippi	10.3
District of Columbia	14.1

National Institute of Health Statistics (2002). *National Vital Statistics Report, 50*(4), 1.

Childhood Mortality Rate

Overall, the childhood mortality rate in the United States has decreased. In 1980, the childhood mortality rate was about 6.4% for children aged 1 to 4 years and 3.1% for children aged 4 to 14 years. In 2000, it was 3.2% and 1.8%, respec-

TABLE 1.5 Infant Mortality per 1,000 Live Births for Selected Countries, 2002

COUNTRY	INFANT MORTALITY: GIRLS	INFANT MORTALITY: BOYS
1. Japan	3	4
2. Sweden	3	4
3. Finland	4	4
4. Hong Kong SAR	4	4
5. Austria	4	5
6. Belgium	4	5
7. Germany	4	5
8. Iceland	4	5
9. Netherlands	4	5
10. Norway	4	5
11. Singapore	4	5
12. Switzerland	4	5
13. Czech Republic	5	5
14. Denmark	5	5
15. France	5	5
16. Australia	5	6
17. Canada	5	6
18. Italy	5	6
19. Slovenia	5	6
20. Spain	5	6
21. United Kingdom	5	6
22. Ireland	6	6
23. Israel	6	6
24. Luxembourg	6	6
25. New Zealand	6	6
26. Greece	6	7
27. Portugal	6	7
28. United States	7	7

United Nations Statistics Division. (2000). Infant mortality. *The world's women 2000: Trends and statistics.* New York: Author.

TABLE 1.6 Major Causes of Death in Childhood (by Percent)

CAUSE	AGE GROUP: *1 to 4 years*	*5 to 14 years*	*15 to 24 years*
Accidents (other than motor vehicle)	9.3	3.9	9.0
Motor vehicle accidents	5.2	5.2	29.5
Congenital anomalies	4.4	1.2	1.2
Malignant neoplasms	3.1	2.6	5.0
Homicide	2.6	1.5	20.3
Diseases of the heart	1.6	0.8	2.9
Human immuno-deficiency virus	1.3	0.5	1.7
Pneumonia and influenza	1.0	0.3	0.6
Suicide	0.0	0.9	13.3

National Center for Health Statistics (2000). Deaths and death rates for the 10 leading causes of death in specific age groups. *National Vital Statistics Report, 49*(12), 20.

tively (Guyer, 2000). The risk of death in the first year of life is higher than that in any other year under age 55. Children in the prepubescent period (age 5 to 14 years) have the lowest mortality of any child age group (Guyer, 2000).

The most frequent causes of childhood death are shown in Table 1-6. Motor vehicle accidents are a leading cause of death in children, but many accidents are largely preventable through education on the value of car seats and seat belt use, the dangers of drinking/drug abuse and driving, and the importance of pedestrian safety (Edgerton et al., 2002).

In addition, there is a high incidence of suicide in the 15-to-24-year-old age group (more girls than boys attempt suicide, but boys are more successful). Sadly, the incidence of suicide is increasing in the 5-to-14-year-old age group. Although school-age children and adolescents may not voice feelings of depression or anger during a health care visit, such underlying feelings may actually be a primary concern. Nurses need to be alert to cues of depression or anger because these feelings can lead to suicide. The high incidence of homicide (1.5% in school-age children and 20% in adolescents) and an increase in the number of adolescents infected with human immunodeficiency virus (HIV) are also growing concerns.

Childhood Morbidity Rate

Health problems occurring in large proportions of children today include respiratory disorders (including asthma and tuberculosis), gastrointestinal disturbances, and consequences of injuries. As more immunizations become available, fewer children in the United States are affected by common childhood communicable diseases. For instance, the incidence of poliomyelitis (once a major killer of children) is now extremely low (almost extinct), because nearly all children in the United States are immunized against it (NCHS, 2000a). Measles flared in incidence in the early 1990s but now is scheduled as a disease to be completely eradicated by 2005. Measles encephalitis can be as destructive and lethal as poliomyelitis, which underscores the importance of continued health education about measles immunization. Continued education about the benefits of immunization against rubella (German measles) is also needed. If women contract this form of measles during pregnancy, their infants can be born with severe congenital anomalies.

Although the decline in the overall incidence of preventable childhood diseases is encouraging, as many as 50% of children under 4 years of age in some communities are still not fully immunized (NCHS, 2000a). Childhood infectious diseases will increase again if immunization is not maintained as a high national priority.

The advent of HIV has changed care considerations in all areas of nursing, but it has particular implications for maternal and child health nursing: childbearing women and sexually active teenagers are at risk for becoming infected with HIV through sexual contact or exposure to blood and blood products; infected women may transmit the virus to a fetus during pregnancy through placental exchange. To help prevent the spread of HIV, adolescents and young adults must be educated about safe sexual practices. Standard precautions must be strictly followed in maternal and child health nursing as in other areas of nursing practice to safeguard health care providers and other clients.

Other infectious diseases growing in incidence include syphilis, genital herpes, hepatitis A and B, and tuberculosis. The rise in syphilis and genital herpes probably stems from an increase in nonmonogamous sexual relationships and lack of safe sex practices. The increase in hepatitis B is due largely to drug abuse and the use of infected injection equipment. One reason for the increase in hepatitis A is shared diaper-changing facilities in day care centers. Tuberculosis, once considered close to eradication, has experienced a resurgence, occurring today at approximately the same rate as measles in young adults. One form, occurring as an opportunistic disease in HIV-positive persons, is particularly resistant to the usual therapy (Guyer, 2000).

Trends in Health Care Environment

The settings for maternal and child health care are changing to better meet the needs of increasingly well-informed and vocal consumers.

Managed Care

Managed care refers to a system of health care delivery that focuses on reducing the cost of health care by closely monitoring the cost of personnel, use and brands of supplies, length of hospital stays, number of procedures carried out, and number of referrals requested. Before managed care, health care insurance paid separately for each procedure or piece of equipment the client received. Under managed care, the agency receives a certain sum of money for the client's care, no matter how many supplies, procedures, or personnel are used in care. In a managed care environment, helping to curtail cost is an important nursing function. Suggestions such as using generic-brand supplies, never breaking into kits of supplies to remove a single item, and urging the use of disposable supplies so personnel time will not be spent cleaning and sterilizing are welcome, cost-effective suggestions.

Managed care has had dramatic effects on health care, most noticeably limiting the number of hospital days and distribution of personnel. Before managed care, women stayed 3 or 4 days after childbirth; today, they rarely stay over 48 hours. Before managed care, nurses completed all care procedures for patients, no matter how small or unskilled the task. With managed care, ancillary personnel, such as unlicensed assistive personnel, perform many tasks under the supervision of the nurse. This system is designed to move the registered nurse (RN) to a higher level of function because it makes the RN accountable for a fuller range of services to patients. It also increases the accountability and responsibility of RNs to delegate tasks appropriately. As a result of managed care, the new advanced-practice role of case manager has been created.

It is important to know the legal aspects of delegation as identified in individual state nursing practice acts because some address specific tasks and activities that RNs may or may not delegate in that state. Accountability for completion and quality of the task remains with the nurse, so the nurse is responsible for knowing that the condition of the patient and the skill level of the assistive person are conducive to safe delegation. Four rules to follow when delegating are:

- Right task for the situation
- Right person to complete the task
- Right communication concerning what is to be done
- Right feedback or evaluation that the task was completed

Examples of delegation responsibility that can occur in maternal and child health are highlighted in the Focus on Multidisciplinary Care boxes located throughout the text.

When managed care was introduced, it was viewed as a system that could lead to poor-quality nursing care because it limits the number of supplies and time available for care. In settings where it works well, however, it has increased opportunities for nurses because it rewards creativity.

Alternative Settings and Styles for Health Care

This century has seen several major shifts in settings for maternity care. At the turn of the century, most births took place in the home, with only the very poor or ill giving birth in "lying-in" hospitals. By 1940 about 40% of live births occurred in hospitals and by 2000 the figure had risen to 98% (DHHS, 2000b). Today, a less dramatic but no less important trend is occurring as an increasing number of families are once more choosing childbirth at home or in alternative birth settings rather than hospitals. These alternative settings provide families with increased control in the birth experience and options for birth surroundings unavailable in hospitals. One strength of this movement is its encouragement of family involvement in birth. It also increases nursing responsibility for assessment and professional judgment and provides expanded roles for nurse practitioners, such as the nurse-midwife. Of all births in the United States, 5% currently are attended by midwives rather than physicians (Guyer, 2000).

Hospitals have responded to consumers' demand for a more natural childbirth environment by refitting labor and delivery suites as birthing rooms, often called LDR (labor-delivery-recovery) or LDRP (labor-delivery-recovery-postpartum) rooms. Partners, family, and other support people may remain in the room, which is designed to be a homelike environment, and participate in the childbirth experience (Fig. 1-5). Couplet care, care for both the mother and newborn by the primary nurse, is also encouraged. LDRP rooms promote a holistic, family-centered approach to maternal and child health care and are appealing to many families who might otherwise have opted against a hospital birth. However, LDRPs are not without fault. It has been argued that they are less private for laboring families, tend to be less relaxing for postpartum families, and make it difficult for nurses to manage the needs of both. Many hospitals are continuing to search for the best labor, delivery, and postpartum options. Whether at home, in a birthing center, or in a hospital, the goal is to keep childbirth as natural as a family desires in a setting where experienced nurse-midwives or physicians can provide professional care.

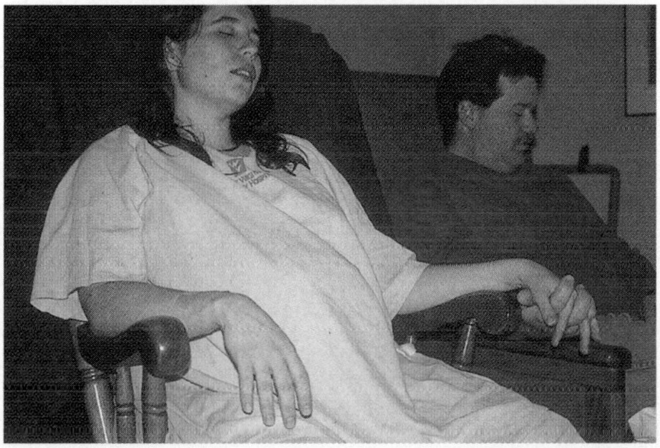

FIGURE 1.5 Mother and father share a close moment in a birthing room.

Health care settings for children are also changing. The home, community centers, outpatient clinics, well-baby clinics, schools, and group homes are some settings where comprehensive health care may be administered. In these settings, the nurse may provide immunizations, screenings, health and safety education, counseling, crisis intervention for teens, parenting classes, and care of the ill child and family. Community-based care can provide cost-effective health promotion, disease prevention, and patient care to a large number of children and families in an environment that is familiar to them.

Strengthening the Ambulatory Care System

The ambulatory care system has broadened its base so more and more people who might have been admitted to a hospital are now being cared for in ambulatory clinics or at home. This option has proved especially important in the care of sick children and women who are experiencing a pregnancy complication or who want early discharge after childbirth. Separating a child from his or her family during an illness has been shown to be potentially harmful to the child's development, so any effort to reduce the incidence of separation should have a positive effect (see Chap. 35). Avoiding long hospital stays for women during pregnancy is also a preferable method of care because it helps to maintain family contact.

WHAT IF? What if a woman must remain in the hospital after the birth of a new baby but the newborn has been discharged? Would it be better for the newborn to stay in the hospital or go home to be cared for by others?

Shortening Hospital Stays

Many hospitals perform children's surgery such as tonsillectomy or umbilical or inguinal hernia repair without requiring an overnight stay. Early on the morning of surgery, the parent and child arrive at the hospital, and the child receives a preoperative physical examination and medication. After surgery, the child is sent to a recovery room and then to a short-term observation unit. If the child is doing well and shows no complications by about 4 hours after surgery, he or she can be discharged. Similarly, women who have begun preterm labor stay in the hospital while labor is halted, and then are allowed to return home on medication with continued monitoring. The routine hospital stay for mothers and newborns after an uncomplicated delivery is now 2 days or less.

Short-term hospital stays require intensive health teaching by the nursing staff and follow-up by home care nurses. Parents must be taught to watch for danger signs in the child without being frightened. A woman with a complication of pregnancy must be taught to watch for signs that warrant immediate attention. New parents must be taught about their newborn's nutritional needs, umbilical cord care, bathing, and safety considerations, all before the euphoria and fatigue of birth have begun to wear off. This type of teaching is difficult because it includes not only imparting the facts of self-care but also providing support and reassurance that the client or parents are capable of this level of care.

Including the Family in the Health Care Setting

Many hospitals have developed policies that minimize the effects of separation from parents when children must be admitted for extended stays. Open visiting hours allow parents to visit as much as possible and sleep overnight in a bed next to their child. Parents also are allowed and encouraged to do as much for the child as they wish during a hospital stay, such as feeding and bathing the child or administering oral medicine. Most of a parent's time, however, is usually spent simply being close by to provide a comfortable, secure influence on the child to maintain normal growth and development. For the same reasons, parents on a maternity unit are encouraged to room-in and give total care to their well newborn.

Because parents are so important to their child's hospital experience and overall well-being, family-centered nursing is vital. Thus, the nurse's client load will not be just four children, for example, but four children plus four sets of parents; not just a single newborn, but his or her two parents as well.

Increase in the Number of Intensive Care Units

Over the past 20 years, care of infants and children has become more intensive. It is generally assumed that newborns with a term birthweight (more than 2,500 g or 5.5 lb) will thrive at birth. However, many infants are born each year with birthweights lower than 2,500 g or who are ill at birth and do not thrive. Such infants are regularly transferred to a neonatal intensive care unit (NICU) or intensive care nursery (ICN). Children undergoing cardiac surgery or recovering from near-drownings or multi-injury accidents are cared for in a pediatric intensive care unit (PICU). Intensive care at this early point in life is one of the most costly types of hospitalization. Expenses of $1,000 a day or $20,000 to $100,000 for a total hospital stay are not rare for care during a high-risk pregnancy and care for a high-risk infant. As the number of these settings increases, the opportunities for advanced-practice nursing also increase.

Regionalization of Intensive Care

To avoid duplication of care sites, it is an accepted practice for a community to establish centralized maternal or pediatric health services. Ill newborns may be transported to a central high-risk nursery when necessary. Likewise, high-risk women and children may be cared for in a regional setting with specialized resources for the diagnosis and treatment of their specific health problem. Through such planning, there is always one site that is properly staffed and equipped for every potential problem. However, when a newborn, older child, or parent is hospitalized in a regional center, the family members who have been left behind need a great deal of support. They may feel they have "lost" their infant, child, or parent unless health care personnel keep them abreast of the ill family member's progress by means of phone calls and snapshots and encourage the family to visit as soon as possible.

When regionalization concepts of newborn care first became accepted, transporting the ill or premature newborn to the regional care facility was the method of choice (Fig. 1-6). Today, however, when it is known in advance that a child may be born with a life-threatening condition, it may be safer to transport the mother to the regional center during pregnancy, because the uterus has advantages as a transport incubator that far exceed any commercial incubator yet designed.

An important argument against regionalization for pediatric care is that children will feel homesick in strange settings, overwhelmed by the number of sick children they see, and frightened because they are miles from home. An important argument against regionalization of maternal care is that being away from her community and support network places a great deal of stress on the pregnant woman and her family and limits her own doctor's participation in her care. These are important considerations. Because nurses more than any other health care group set the tone for hospitals, they are responsible for ensuring

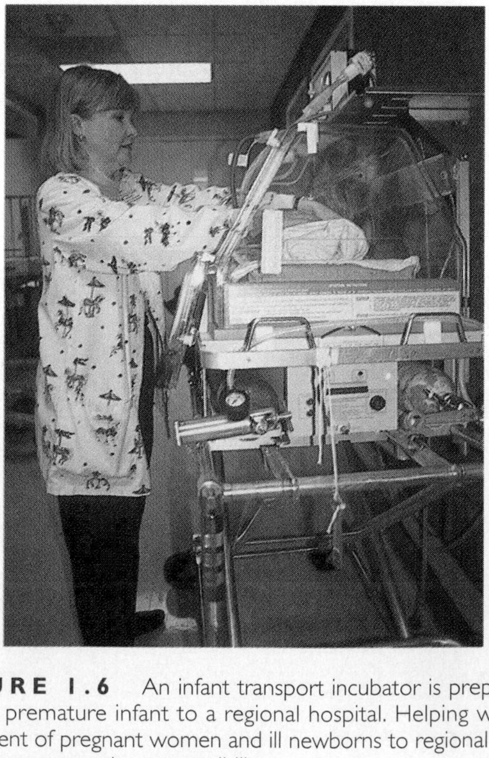

FIGURE 1.6 An infant transport incubator is prepared to move a premature infant to a regional hospital. Helping with safe movement of pregnant women and ill newborns to regional centers is an important nursing responsibility.

that clients and families feel as welcome in the regional centers as they would have been in a small hospital. Staffing should be adequate to allow sufficient time for nurses to comfort frightened children and prepare them for new experiences or support the pregnant woman and her family. Documenting the importance of such actions allows them to be incorporated in critical pathways and preserves the importance of the nurse's role.

Increased Reliance on Comprehensive Care Settings

Comprehensive health care is designed to meet all of a child's needs in one setting. In the past, care of children tended to be specialized. For example, a child with a congenital anomaly such as myelomeningocele or cerebral palsy might have been followed by a team of specialists for each facet of the problem. Such a team might include a neurologist, a physical therapist, an occupational therapist, a psychologist for intelligence quotient testing, a speech therapist, an orthopedic surgeon, and finally a special education teacher. The parents might need to find a special dentist who would accept clients with multiple disabilities. Each specialist would look at only one area of the child's needs rather than the whole child's development. Without extra guidance, parents would find themselves lost in a maze of visits to different health care personnel. If they were not receiving financial support for their child's care, they might not have been able to afford all the necessary services at one time. It might have been difficult to decide which of the child's problems needed to be treated immediately and which could be left untreated without worsening and developing into a permanent disability. Although specialists are still important to a child's care, a trusted primary care provider to help parents coordinate these specialized services is essential in today's managed care environment. In many settings, this primary care provider who follows the child through all phases of care is an advanced-practice nurse such as a family nurse practitioner, pediatric nurse practitioner, or a women's health nurse practitioner. Nurses can be helpful in seeing that both parents and children have all their needs met by a primary health care provider in this way. The family must become empowered to seek out a family-centered setting that will be best for their health (see Focus on Family Empowerment).

Increased Use of Alternative Treatment Modalities

There is a growing tendency for families to consult providers of alternative forms of therapy such as acupuncture or therapeutic touch in addition to, or instead of, traditional health care providers. Nurses have an increasing obligation to be aware of alternative therapies, which have the potential to either enhance or detract from the effectiveness of traditional therapy (see Focus on Cultural Competence).

In addition, health care providers who are unaware of the existence of some alternative forms of therapy may lose an important opportunity to capitalize on the positive features of that particular therapy. For instance, it would be important to know that an adolescent who is about to undergo a painful procedure is experienced at meditation. Asking the adolescent if she wanted to meditate before the procedure could help her relax. Not only could this decrease the child's discomfort, but it could also offer the child a feeling of control over a difficult situation. People are using an increasing number of herbal remedies, so asking about these at health assessment becomes more and more important (Waddell et al., 2001). For example, many women are taking ginger during pregnancy to alleviate morning sickness.

Increased Reliance on Home Care

Early hospital discharge has resulted in many women and children returning home before they are fully ready to care for themselves. Ill children and women with complications of pregnancy may choose to remain at home for care rather than be hospitalized. This has created a "second system" of

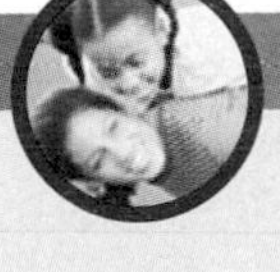

FOCUS ON FAMILY EMPOWERMENT
Tips for Selecting a Health Care Setting

Q. There are so many health care choices and settings available; which one should we choose?

A. When selecting a health care setting, use the following as a guide to help you decide what is best for your family:

- Can it be reached easily (going for preventive care when well or for care when ill should not be chores)?
- Will the staff provide continuity of care so you'll always see the same primary care provider if possible?
- Does the physical set-up of the facility provide for a sense of privacy yet a sense that health care providers share pertinent information so you do not have to repeat your history at each visit?
- Is the cost of care and the number of referrals to specialists explained clearly?
- Are preventive care and health education stressed (keeping well is as important as recovering from illness)?
- Do health care providers respect your opinion and ask for your input on health care decisions?
- Do health care providers show a personal interest in you?
- Is health education done at your learning level?
- Is the facility handicapped accessible?

FOCUS ON CULTURAL COMPETENCE

Cultural Variations and Alternative Therapies Affecting Health Care

The term *alternative health care practices* refers to therapies such as acupuncture, homeopathy, therapeutic touch, herbalism, and chiropractic care or nontraditional sources of health care such as tribal medicine or *yerberos* or *curanderos.* Some people seek these types of therapy or alternative providers before consulting a traditional health care provider; others consult them after what they perceive to be inadequate care by a traditional provider.

Respecting these forms of care can be instrumental in showing families that their sociocultural traditions and needs are important. Assessing what nontraditional measures are being used is important because the action can interfere with prescribed medications. For instance, the consumption of traditional ethnic remedies such as *jin bu huan,* a Chinese herbal medicine used to relieve pain, can cause adverse effects such as life-threatening bradycardia and respiratory depression. Lead poisoning has resulted from ingestion of *greta,* a traditional Mexican remedy used as a laxative.

care requiring many additional care providers. Nurses are instrumental in assessing women and children on hospital discharge to help plan the best type of continuing care, devising and modifying procedures for home care, and sustaining clients' morale and interest in health care during such situations as home monitoring to prevent premature labor. Because home care is a unique and expanding area in maternal and child health nursing, it is discussed in relation to maternal care in Chapter 16 and in relation to children in Chapter 35.

Increased Use of Technology

The use of technology is increasing in all health care settings. Charting by computer, seeking information on the Internet, and monitoring fetal heart rates by Doppler are a few examples. In addition to learning these technologies, maternal and child health nurses must be able to explain technology use and its advantages to clients. Otherwise, clients can find new technology more frightening than helpful to them.

Health Care Concerns and Attitudes

The 1980s brought about considerable change in the health care system and particularly in maternal and child health. As we enter the 21st century, there are likely to be even more changes as the United States actively works toward effective health goals and guaranteed health care for all citizens.

Increasing Concern Regarding Health Care Costs

The advent of managed care has concentrated efforts on reducing the cost of health care. This has direct implications for maternal and child health nursing because nurses must become more cost-conscious about supplies and services. Lack of financial ability to pay and insensitivity to cultural values are major reasons that women do not obtain prenatal care. For example, the woman may fear that changing jobs or not working during pregnancy may lead to loss of insurance coverage, thereby reducing her ability to pay for services. As a result, she may continue to work long hours or in unfit conditions during pregnancy to ensure insurance coverage. Early prenatal care, for example, is the single most important determinant of neonatal health. Thus, nurses are challenged to help to reduce costs while maintaining quality care.

Increasing Emphasis on Preventive Care

A generally accepted theory is that it is better to keep individuals well than to restore health after they have become ill. Counseling parents on ways to keep their homes safe for children is an important form of illness prevention in maternal and child health nursing. Research supporting the facts that accidents are still a major cause of death in children and that women still do not receive preconceptual or prenatal care are testaments to the need for much more anticipatory guidance in this area.

Increasing Emphasis on Family-Centered Care

Health promotion with families during pregnancy or childrearing is a family-centered event because teaching health awareness and good health habits is accomplished chiefly by role modeling. Illness in a child is automatically a family-centered event: parents may need to adjust work schedules to allow one of them to stay with the ill child, siblings may have to sacrifice an activity such as a birthday party or having a parent watch their school play, and family finances may have to be readjusted to pay for hospital and medical bills. When a mother is pregnant, family roles or activities may have to change to safeguard her health. A family may feel drawn together by the fright and concern of an acute illness; unfortunately, when an illness becomes chronic, it may pull a family apart or destroy it.

In recent years, the U.S. government has recognized that the care of individual family members is a family-centered event. The Family Medical Leave Act of 1993 is a federal law that requires employers with 50 or more employees to provide a minimum of 12 weeks of unpaid, job-protected leave to employees under four circumstances crucial to family life:

- Birth of the employee's child
- Adoption or foster placement of a child with the employee
- Need for the employee to care for a parent, spouse, or child with a serious health condition
- Inability of the employee to perform his or her functions because of a serious health condition

A serious health condition is defined as "an illness, injury, impairment, or physical or mental condition involving such circumstances as inpatient care or incapacity requiring 3 workdays' absence." Specifically mentioned in the law is any period of incapacity due to pregnancy or for prenatal care with or without treatment. Illness must be documented by a health care provider. Nurse practitioners and nurse-midwives are specifically listed as those who can document a health condition.

By adopting a view of pregnancy, childbirth, or illness as a family event, nurses are well equipped to provide family-centered care. Nurses can be instrumental in including family members in events from which they were once totally excluded, such as an unplanned cesarean birth. They can help child health care to be family-centered by consulting with family members about a plan of care and providing clear health teaching so family members can monitor their own care (Fig. 1-7). Nurses play an active role in both health promotion teaching and sustaining families through a child's illness. Nurses can educate families about the Family Medical Leave Act; many people are still not aware that they can take time off from work during pregnancy or to spend with a new baby, to care for a loved one with a serious health condition, or to tend to a personal health crisis (U.S. Department of Labor, 1995). Nurse practitioners or nurse-midwives can help ensure that the criteria of the Family Medical Leave Act are met by appropriately documenting a client's health condition.

Increasing Concern for the Quality of Life

In the past, health care of women and children was focused on maintaining physical health. More recently, however, a growing awareness that the quality of life is as important as physical health has expanded the scope of health care to include the assessment of psychosocial facets of life in such areas as self-esteem and independence. Good interviewing skills are necessary to elicit this information at health care visits. Nurses can be instrumental in assessing for such information and also in planning ways to improve the quality of life in the areas the client considers most important.

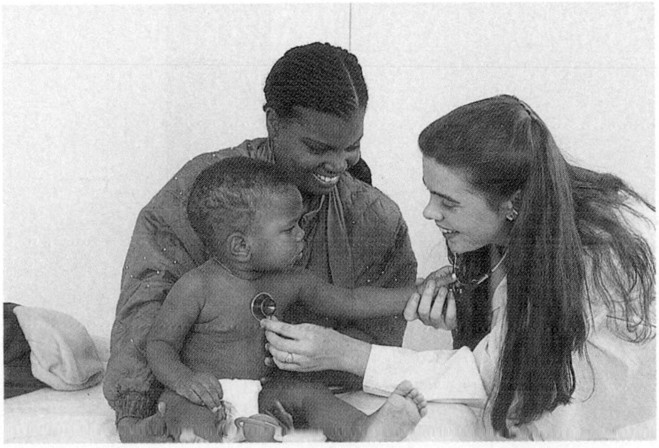

FIGURE 1.7 Family-centered care: The nurse involves the family in the care of the child.

One way in which the quality of life is being improved for children with chronic illness is the national mandate to allow them to attend regular schools, guaranteeing entrance despite severe illness or use of medical equipment such as a ventilator (Public Law 99-452). Nurses, serving as school nurses or consultants to schools, play important roles in making these efforts possible.

Increasing Awareness of the Individuality of Clients

Maternal and child clients today do not fit readily into any set category. Varying family structures, cultural backgrounds, socioeconomic levels, and individual circumstances lead to unique and diverse clients. Some women having children are younger than ever before, and an increasing number of women are experiencing their first pregnancies after the age of 35. Many women are having children outside of marriage. Homosexual couples are also beginning to raise families together, conceiving children through artificial insemination or adoption. As a result of advances in research and treatments, women who were once unable to have children, such as those with cystic fibrosis, are now able to manage a full-term pregnancy. Individuals with mental and physical challenges are also establishing families and rearing children.

Many families who have come from foreign countries enter the U.S. health care system for the first time during a pregnancy or with a sick child. This requires a greater sensitivity on the part of the health care provider to the sociocultural aspects of care. As the level of violence in the world increases, more and more families are exposed to living in violent communities. The incidence of abused children and pregnant women is also increasing. All of these concerns require increased nursing concern.

Empowerment of Health Care Consumers

Due in part to the influence of market-driven care and a strengthened focus on health promotion and disease prevention, individuals and families have recently begun to take increased responsibility for their own health. This begins with learning preventive measures to stay well. For some families, it means following a more nutritious diet and planning regular exercise; for others, it can mean an entire change in lifestyle. When a family member is ill, empowerment means learning more about the illness, participating in the treatment plan, and preventing the illness from returning. Families are very interested in participating in decision making regarding their childbearing options. Parents want to accompany their ill children into the hospital for overnight stays. They are eager for information about their child's health and want to contribute to the decision-making process. They may question treatments or care plans that they believe are not in their child's best interest. When health care providers do not provide answers to a client's questions or are insensitive to needs, many health care consumers are willing to take their business to another health care setting.

Nurses can be instrumental in promoting empowerment of parents and children by respecting their views and concerns, addressing clients by name, and regarding parents as important participants in their child's health, keeping them informed and helping them to make decisions about their child's care. Although the nurse may have seen 25 clients already in a particular day, he or she can make each client feel as important as the first by showing a warm manner and keen interest. Family empowerment displays are presented throughout the text to provide insight into ways in which the nurse may help empower the family.

WHAT IF? In the past, children with pneumonia were always hospitalized. What if a parent demands that her child, recently diagnosed with pneumonia, be hospitalized, even though it is your clinic's policy to have such children cared for at home by their parents? Would you advocate for hospitalization or not?

ADVANCED PRACTICE ROLES FOR NURSES IN MATERNAL AND CHILD HEALTH

As trends in maternal and child health care change, so do the roles of maternal and child health nurses. All maternal and child health nurses function in a variety of settings as caregivers, client advocates, researchers, case managers, and educators.

Maternal and child health nurses function in a variety of advanced-practice roles. In addition, staff nurses with a specified number of years of direct patient contact and validation supporting completion of pertinent continuing education programs can become certified in a specialty. This certification recognizes clinical expertise. The field of maternal and child health nursing has numerous opportunities for certification.

Women's Health Nurse Practitioner

A **women's health nurse practitioner** is a nurse with advanced study in the promotion of health and prevention of illness in women. Such a nurse plays a vital role in educating women about their bodies and sharing with them methods to prevent illness; they care for women with illnesses such as sexually transmitted diseases and counsel them about and offer information regarding reproductive life planning. They play a large role in helping women remain well so they can enter a pregnancy in good health and maintain their health throughout life.

Family Nurse Practitioner

A **family nurse practitioner** (FNP) is an advanced-practice role that provides health care not only to women but also to all persons throughout the age span. In conjunction with a physician, an FNP can provide prenatal care for the woman with an uncomplicated pregnancy. The FNP takes the health and pregnancy history, performs physical and obstetric examinations, orders appropriate diagnostic and laboratory tests, and plans continued care through pregnancy and for the family afterward. FNPs then follow the family indefinitely to promote health and optimal family functioning.

Neonatal Nurse Practitioner

The **neonatal nurse practitioner** (NNP) is skilled in the care of newborns, both well and ill. NNPs may work in level 1, 2, or 3 newborn nurseries, neonatal intensive care units, neonatal follow-up clinics, or physician groups, or in transporting the ill infant. The NNP's responsibilities include managing patient care in an intensive care unit, conducting normal newborn assessments and physical examinations, and providing high-risk follow-up discharge planning.

Pediatric Nurse Practitioner

A **pediatric nurse practitioner** (PNP) is a nurse prepared with extensive skills in physical assessment, interviewing, and well-child counseling and care. In this role, a nurse interviews parents as part of an extensive health history and performs a physical assessment of the child. If the nurse's diagnosis is that the child is well, he or she discusses with the parents any childrearing problems mentioned in the interview, gives any immunizations needed, offers necessary anticipatory guidance (based on the plan of care), and arranges a return appointment for the next well-child checkup. The nurse serves as a primary health caregiver or as the sole health care person the parents and child see at all visits.

If the PNP determines that a child has a common illness (e.g., iron deficiency anemia), he or she orders the necessary laboratory tests and prescribes appropriate drugs for therapy (Fig. 1-8). If the PNP determines that the child has a major illness (e.g., congenital subluxated hip, kidney disease, or heart disease), he or she consults with an associated pediatrician; together, they decide what further care is necessary. Nurse practitioners may also work in inpatient or specialty settings providing continuity of care to hospitalized children. As school nurse practitioners, they provide care to all children in a given community or school setting.

Nurse-Midwife

Throughout history, the **nurse-midwife,** an individual educated in the discipline of nursing and midwifery and licensed according to the requirements of the American

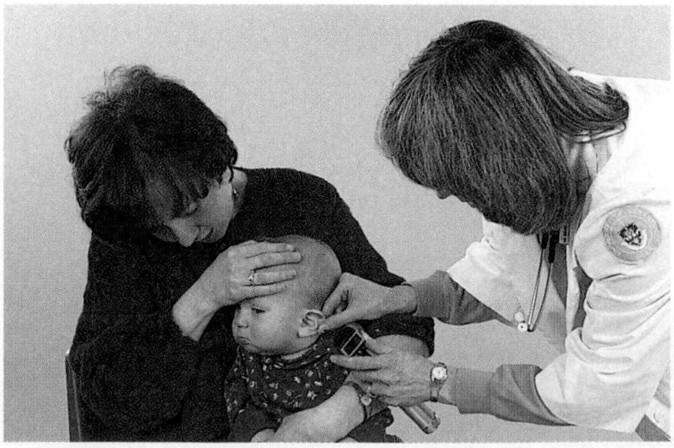

FIGURE 1.8 Pediatric nurse practitioner is an extended role for nurses.

College of Nurse-Midwives (ACNM), has played an important role in assisting women with pregnancy and childbearing. Either independently or in association with an obstetrician, the nurse-midwife can assume full responsibility for the care and management of women with uncomplicated pregnancies. Nurse-midwives play a large role in making birth an unforgettable family event as well as helping to ensure a healthy outcome for both mother and child (Fig. 1-9).

Clinical Nurse Specialists

Clinical nurse specialists are nurses prepared at the master's-degree level who are capable of acting as consultants in their area of expertise, as well as serving as role models, researchers, and teachers of quality nursing care. Examples of areas of specialization are neonatal, maternal, child and adolescent health care; childbirth education; and lactation consultation.

Consider, for example, how a child health clinician might intervene to help in the care of a 4-year-old child with diabetes mellitus who has been admitted to the hospital. The child is difficult to care for because he is so fearful of hospitalization and perplexed because his parents are having difficulty accepting his diagnosis. A child health clinician could be instrumental in helping a primary nurse organize care and meet with the parents to help them accept what is happening. Neonatal clinicians manage infants' care at birth and in intensive care settings; they provide home follow-up care to ensure the newborn remains well. Childbirth educators teach families about normal birth and how to prepare for labor and delivery. Lactation consultants educate women about breast-feeding and support them while they learn how to breast-feed.

Case Manager

A case manager is a graduate-level nurse who supervises a group of patients from the time they enter a health care setting until they are discharged from the setting, monitoring the effectiveness and cost and satisfaction of their health care. Case management can be a vastly satisfying nursing role because if the health care setting is one with "seamless walls," or follows people both during an illness and on their return to the community, it involves long-term contacts and lasting relationships.

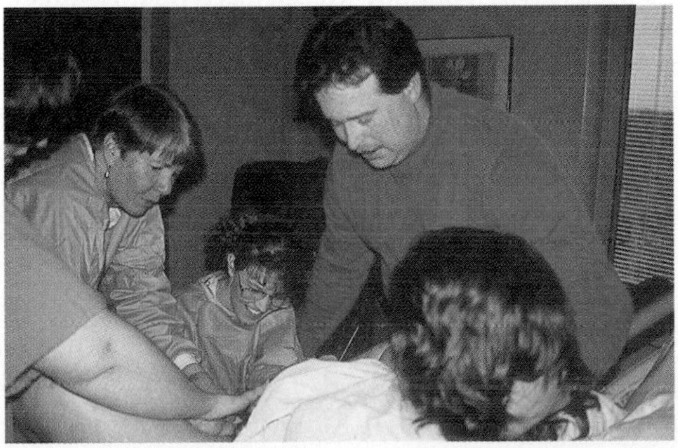

FIGURE 1.9 A nurse-midwife plays an important role in ensuring a safe birth.

LEGAL CONSIDERATIONS OF PRACTICE

Legal concerns arise in all areas of health care. Maternal and child health nursing carries some legal concerns that extend above and beyond other areas of nursing, because care is often given to an "unseen client"—the fetus—or to clients who are not of legal age for giving consent for medical procedures. In addition, labor, delivery, and birth of a neonate are considered "normal" events, so the risks for a lawsuit are greater when things go wrong. Nurses are legally responsible for protecting the rights of their clients, including confidentiality, and are accountable for the quality of their individual nursing care and that of other health care team members. Understanding the **scope of practice** (the range of services and care that may be provided by the nurse based on state requirements) and standards of care can help nurses practice within appropriate legal parameters.

Informing clients about their rights and responsibilities is helpful in protecting them. In a society in which child abuse is of national concern, nurses are becoming increasingly responsible for identifying and reporting incidents of suspected abuse in children.

Documentation is essential in protecting the nurse and justifying his or her actions. This concern is long-lasting, because children who feel they were wronged by health care personnel can bring a lawsuit at the time they reach legal age. This means that a nursing note written today may need to be defended as many as 21 years in the future. Nurses need to be conscientious about obtaining informed consent for invasive procedures and in determining that pregnant women are aware of any risk to the fetus involved with a procedure or test. In divorced or blended families (those in which two adults with children from previous relationships now live together), it is important to establish who has the right to give consent for health care. Personal liability insurance is strongly recommended for all nurses so they do not incur great financial losses during a malpractice or professional negligence suit.

If a nurse knows that the care provided by another practitioner was inappropriate or insufficient, he or she is legally responsible for reporting the incident. Failure to do so can lead to a charge of negligence or breach of duty.

The specific legal ramifications of procedures or care are discussed in later chapters with procedures or treatment modalities.

ETHICAL CONSIDERATIONS OF PRACTICE

Ethical issues are increasing in frequency in health care today. Some of the most difficult decisions in health care settings are those that involve children and their families. Just a few of the major potential conflicts include:

- Conception issues, especially those related to in vitro fertilization, embryo transfer, ownership of frozen oocytes or sperm, cloning, stem cell research, and surrogate mothers
- Abortion, particularly partial-birth abortions
- Fetal rights versus rights of the mother
- Use of fetal tissue for research
- Resuscitation (how long should it be continued?)
- The number of procedures or degree of pain that a child should be asked to endure to achieve a degree of better health
- The balance between modern technology and quality of life

Legal and ethical aspects of issues are often intertwined, which makes the decision-making process complex. Because maternal and child health nursing is so strongly family-centered, it is common to encounter some situations in which the interests of one family member are in conflict with those of another. It is not unusual for the values of a client not to match those of a health care provider. For example, when a pregnancy causes a woman to develop a serious illness, the family must make a decision either to terminate the pregnancy and lose the child or keep the pregnancy and work to support the mother through the crisis. If the fetus is also at risk from the illness, the decision may be easier to make; however, the circumstances are usually not clear-cut and the decisions that need to be made are difficult. These and other issues are bound to emerge during the course of practice. Nurses can help clients facing such difficult decisions by providing factual information and supportive listening and by helping the family in clarification of values.

The Pregnant Woman's Bill of Rights and the United Nations Declaration of Rights of the Child (see Appendix A) provide guidelines for determining the rights of clients in regard to health care.

✔ CHECKPOINT QUESTIONS

7. How does the Family Medical Leave Act support family-centered care?
8. Why has empowerment of the health care consumer become increasingly important?
9. Why has the family nurse practitioner become a popular advanced-practice role?

KEY POINTS

Standards of maternal and child health nursing practice have been formulated by the American Nurses Association and the Association of Women's Health, Obstetric and Neonatal Nurses (AWHONN) to serve as guidelines for practice.

Nursing theory and use of evidence-based practice are methods by which maternal and child health nursing expands and improves.

The most significant measure of maternal and child health is the infant mortality rate. It is the number of deaths in infants from birth to 1 year of age per 1,000 live births. This rate is declining steadily, but in the United States it is still higher than that of 20 other nations.

Trends in maternal and child health nursing include changes in the settings of care, increased concern about health care costs, improved preventive care, and family-centered care.

Advanced-practice roles in maternal and child health nursing include women's health, family, neonatal, and pediatric nurse practitioners; nurse-midwives; clinical nurse specialists; and case managers. All of these expanded roles contribute to making maternal and child health care an important area of nursing and health care.

Maternal and child health care has both legal and ethical considerations and responsibilities over and above those in other areas of practice because of the role of the fetus and child.

CRITICAL THINKING EXERCISES

1. How might family-centered care help the Melendez family, described in the beginning of the chapter? How can you explain the changes in health care so Melissa might understand why her hospital stay is so much shorter this time? How can you empower the family so they feel more in control of what is happening to them?
2. Other countries throughout the world have a health care delivery system based not on profit but on provision of care for all citizens through a tax-supported program. The infant mortality rate in many of these countries is lower than that in the United States. What are some reasons that might contribute to this?
3. The age of women having their first baby is increasing. For many women this is now 35 years and above.
   a. How do you anticipate this will change health care in the future?
   b. Are there special services that should be provided for such women?
   c. How will this trend influence childrearing in the future?

REFERENCES

American Nurses Association and Society of Pediatric Nurses. (1996). *Statement on the scope and standards of pediatric clinical practice.* Washington, D.C.: Authors.

Carpenito, L. J. (2001). *Handbook of nursing diagnosis* (9th ed.). Philadelphia: Lippincott Williams & Wilkins.

Department of Health and Human Services (2000a). *Healthy people 2010.* Washington, D.C.: DHHS.
Department of Health and Human Services (2000b). Births, marriages, divorces, and deaths for 2000. *Monthly Vital Statistics Report, 49*(12), 1.
Guyer, B. (2000). Annual summary of vital statistics. *Pediatrics, 106*(6), 1307–1317.
Hoyert, D. L., et al. (2001). Annual summary of vital statistics. *Pediatrics, 108*(6), 1241–1255.
Johnson, M., Maas, M., & Moorhead, S. (2000). *Nursing outcomes classification* (2d ed.). St. Louis: Mosby.
McCloskey, J., & Bulechek, G. (2000). *Nursing interventions classification* (3d ed.). St. Louis: Mosby.
National Center for Health Statistics (2000a). Trends and current status in childhood mortality. *Vital and Health Statistics, 49*(3), 21.
National Center for Health Statistics (2000b). Births, marriages, divorces and deaths. *Monthly Vital Statistics Report, 49*(7), 4.
Rubin, R. (1963). Maternal touch. *Nursing Outlook, 11,* 828.
United Nations Statistics Division. (2000). Infant mortality. *The world's women 2000: Trends and statistics.* New York: Author.
U.S. Department of Labor. (1995). Family Medical Leave Act. *Federal Register, 60*(4), 2179.
Waddell, D. L., Hummel, M. E., & Sumners, A. D. (2001). Three herbs you should get to know. *American Journal of Nursing, 101*(4), 48–53.

SUGGESTED READINGS

Carlisle, J. B., & Cull, V. V. (2001). Developmental care of children: Are nurses avoiding the issue? *American Journal of Nursing, 101*(3), 11–13.
Covington, C. Y., et al. (2001). Preventing obesity among urban children. *American Journal of Nursing, 101*(3), 73–82.
Evans, B. C. (2000). Clinical teaching strategies for a caring curriculum. *Nursing & Health Care Perspectives, 21*(3), 133–138.
Gellin, B. G., Maibach, E. W., & Marcuse, E. K. (2000). Do parents understand immunizations? A national telephone survey. *Pediatrics, 106*(5), 1097–1102.
Llahana, S. V., Poulton, B. C., & Coates, V. E. (2001). The pediatric diabetes specialist nurse and diabetes education in childhood. *Journal of Advanced Nursing, 33*(3), 296–306.
Mohr, W. K., et al. (2001). A reflection on values in turbulent times. *Nursing Outlook, 49*(1), 30–36.
Nehring, W. M. (2000). Violence in our schools: sources of prevention for pediatric nurses. *Journal of Child & Family Nursing, 3*(2), 159–162.
Purnell, M. J., et al. (2001). The nursing shortage: Revisioning the future. *Journal of Nursing Administration, 31*(4), 179–186.
Twycross, A. (2000). Education about pain: A neglected area? *Nurse Education Today, 20*(3), 244–253.
Ward, J. D. (2000). Pediatric cancer survivors: Assessment of late effects. *Nurse Practitioner, 25*(12), 18–39.
Yancey, A. K., et al. (2002). Role models, ethnic identity, and health-risk behaviors in urban adolescents. *Archives of Pediatrics and Adolescent Medicine, 156*(1), 55–61.

2

CHAPTER

The Childbearing and Childrearing Family and Community

Key Terms

- **community**
- **ecomap**
- **family**
- **family nursing**
- **family of orientation**
- **family of procreation**
- **family theory**
- **genogram**

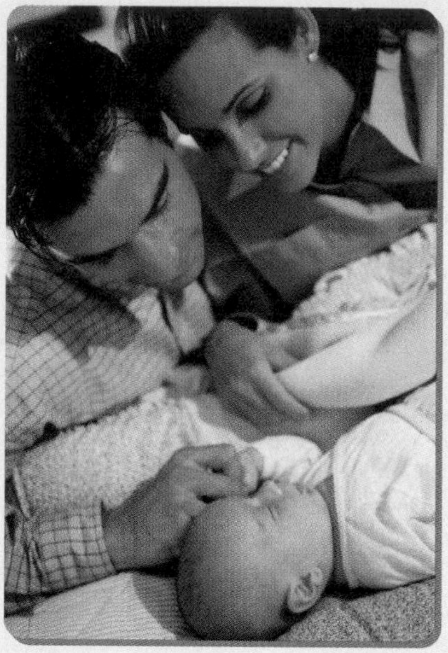

Objectives

After mastering the contents of this chapter, you should be able to:

1. Describe family structure, function, and family roles.
2. Assess a family for structure and health.
3. Formulate nursing diagnoses related to family health.
4. Develop expected outcomes to help a family achieve optimal health.
5. Plan health teaching strategies, such as helping a family modify its lifestyle to accommodate an ill child.
6. Implement nursing care, such as teaching a family more effective wellness behaviors.
7. Evaluate outcome criteria for achievement and effectiveness of nursing care to be certain that goals have been achieved.
8. Identify National Health Goals related to the family and specific ways that nurses can help the nation achieve these goals.
9. Identify areas of care related to family nursing that could benefit from additional nursing research or the application of evidence-based practice.
10. Use critical thinking to analyze additional ways that nursing care can be more family-centered or that client care can better include family members.
11. Integrate knowledge of family nursing with nursing process to promote quality maternal and child health nursing care.

Marlo Hanavan is a 32-year-old bookkeeper who is pregnant with her second child. Her first child, Carey, age 2 years, has just been diagnosed by the family health practitioner as having cerebral palsy. Carey needs long-term physical therapy and is bused daily to a special preschool. Mr. Hanavan is unemployed because of an accident at work 2 years ago. He has some income from selling woodworking products at craft shows. Mrs. Hanavan states that on many weeks she is forced to choose between health care and groceries. Is the Hanavan family a well family?

The previous chapter discussed the philosophy of maternal and child health nursing and the many roles that nurses fulfill in this area. This chapter adds information about families and communities that helps to ensure a healthy outcome for families. This is important information because inadequate parenting due to a dysfunctional family structure or a lack of community resources can contribute to poor pregnancy outcomes and poor child-rearing practices.

After you've studied the chapter, answer the Critical Thinking Exercises at the end of the chapter and then access the on-line study activities (http://connection.lww.com) *to further sharpen your skills and test your knowledge.*

FOCUS ON NATIONAL HEALTH GOALS

A number of National Health Goals speak directly to achieving healthy family and community life. The following goals are representative of these:

- Lower the current baseline of 25.2 children per 1,000 younger than age 18 who are maltreated.
- Reduce physical abuse directed at women by male partners to no more than 27 per 1,000 couples from a current baseline of 30 per 1,000 couples.
- Eliminate the prevalence of blood lead levels exceeding 10 ug/dL in children aged 1 month to 6 years from a baseline of 4.4% (DHHS, 2000).

Nurses can be instrumental in helping to see that goals such as these for healthier family living are met by assessing families and their environment to identify families at risk, assisting with counseling or further testing, and maintaining contact with families to ensure that long-term measures for care can be instituted. Intimate partner violence is further discussed in Chapter 14 and child abuse in Chapter 55; lead poisoning from excessive lead in the environment is discussed in Chapter 52.

No social group has the potential to provide the same level of support and long-lasting emotional ties as one's own family. Maintaining healthy family life is so important to the health and welfare of the nation that several National Health Goals speak directly to maintaining healthy family and community life (see Focus on National Health Goals box). Because the family has such an influence on the individual, nursing care that considers the family, not the individual (**family nursing**), has become a focus of modern nursing practice (Martin-Arafeh et al., 1999). **Family theory** details a set of perspectives from the family's point of view that can help nurses address the important health issues of the child-bearing and child-rearing family.

For instance, for a family to adjust to a new family member, the family's structure and roles must be flexible enough to adjust to the changes that pregnancy and a newborn will bring. An ill family member or one who is going through a difficult developmental period, such as adolescence, can put a tremendous strain on a family. The roles individuals assume in the family and their ability to adjust to new roles can influence a family's perception of a child's illness, as well as the family's ability to adjust to these situations and have a positive influence on their outcome. Because families do not live in isolation, the family's ability to thrive in a community and gain strength from the community is equally important. Thus, the modern concept of maternal and child health nursing is not limited to assessing individuals or individual circumstances, but rather examining them from a family/community standpoint.

For all these reasons, family/community-centered maternal and child health nursing considers the strengths, vulnerabilities, and patterns of family and community function to support families during childbirth and childrearing and to encourage healthy coping mechanisms in families facing a crisis. Health assessment and intervention planning should include consideration of the family's social, emotional, spiritual, and financial resources, as well as the physical and emotional condition of the home and the community environment.

NURSING PROCESS OVERVIEW

For Promotion of Family Health

Assessment

Family/community assessment provides information on the meaning of a current health situation or the ability to remain well to a family and the emotional support that the individual can expect from the family or community. This is vital to understanding what a pregnancy or childhood illness means to different members of the family, especially if not all members are in agreement. Family structure and function both need to be considered (see Focus on Multidisciplinary Care).

Nursing Diagnosis

Nursing diagnoses used in connection with families and communities generally relate to the family's ability to handle stress and to provide a positive environment for individual growth and development. Examples include:

- Parental role conflict related to prolonged separation from child during long hospital stay
- Interrupted family processes related to emergency hospital admission of oldest child
- Impaired parenting related to unplanned pregnancy

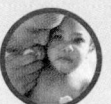

FOCUS ON MULTIDISCIPLINARY CARE

Unlicensed assistive personnel have many opportunities to interact with families in waiting rooms at ambulatory health care visits, in emergency rooms, or when families are waiting for a member to return from surgery. Teach such personnel to use these occasions not for simple chatting but to observe family interactions and report this information to you. Families often relate easily to such people and share information with them that they may not share as readily with professional health care providers (perceiving wrongly that health care providers are too busy to listen). When families develop health problems, many different health care professionals team together to give care. Help everyone to assess both the strengths of these families and the challenges facing them.

- Ineffective family coping related to inability to adjust to child's illness
- Readiness for enhanced family coping related to improved perceptions of child's capabilities
- Health-seeking behaviors related to birth of first child

"Impaired parenting" and "parental role conflict" are diagnoses that suggest that parents need additional help with parenting. The first family coping diagnosis ("ineffective family coping") indicates that a family is not functioning at an optimal level; the second ("readiness for enhanced family coping") is used for a well family or one that is exhibiting enhanced growth because of a specific event, such as the sudden diagnosis of illness in a child or an unplanned pregnancy. "Readiness for enhanced parenting" and "health-seeking behaviors" are diagnoses that apply to families who are investigating more effective ways to manage stress and improve family/community functioning.

Outcome Identification and Planning

Planning for nursing care must include a design that is family-centered and appropriate and desired by the majority of family members; otherwise, family members may have difficulty following the plan. The plan must also consider the community. For example, it is not helpful to suggest that a family take regular walks together to encourage shared decision-making and improve family communication if walking in their neighborhood is unsafe; participation in a family gym class at a local YMCA might be more practical in this instance.

Implementation

A plan for improving family/community health should flow smoothly if family members have agreed on it out of support for one another. It may be necessary in some instances to encourage family members to agree on a plan or to abide by a chosen plan. Otherwise, they may expend needless energy carrying out an activity that is counterproductive or in direct opposition to their major goal.

Outcome Evaluation

Evaluation should reveal not only that a goal was achieved but also that the family feels more cohesive after working together toward the goal. If evaluation does not reveal these two factors, reassessment is necessary to determine whether further interventions are required. Examples of expected outcomes that might be established are:

- Family members state they are adapting well to the presence of a newborn.
- Mother states she feels prepared to manage home care of her ill child.
- Father states he has arranged the family finances to accommodate new health care expenses for the family.

THE FAMILY

How well a family works together and how well it can organize itself against potential threats depend on its structure (who its members consist of) and its function (the activities or roles family members carry out).

Defining the Concept of Family

A **family** is defined by the U.S. Census Bureau (2000) as "a group of people related by blood, marriage, or adoption living together." This definition is workable for gathering comparative statistics but is limited when assessing a family for its health concerns or the support people available because some families are made up of unrelated couples, and at certain points in life not all family members may live together. Spradley and Allender (2000) define the family in a much broader context as "two or more people who live in the same household (usually), share a common emotional bond, and perform certain interrelated social tasks." This is a better definition for health care providers because it addresses the broad range of types of families that health care providers encounter.

Family Types

Many types of families exist, and a family type may change over time as it is affected by birth, work, death, divorce, and the growth of family members (see Focus on Cultural Competence). For the purposes of describing families in maternal and child health nursing, two basic family structures can be described:

- **Family of orientation** (the family one is born into; or oneself, mother, father, and siblings, if any)
- **Family of procreation** (a family one establishes; or oneself, spouse or significant other, and children)

More specific descriptions of family types vary greatly depending on family roles, generational issues, means of family support, and sociocultural influences. Almost all families, no matter what type, share common activities.

FOCUS ON CULTURAL COMPETENCE

How Do Cultural Traditions Affect Families? Families tend to display characteristics of their culture and community. Knowing some of the basic norms and taboos of different cultural groups is an important part of a nurse's knowledge base. This basic knowledge of a family's cultural background helps you to understand the family's value system and the degree of support family members have available.

The types of families that live in communities tend to be culturally determined: some cultures have extended families; others consist of single-parent families. Some cultures respect elderly family members and depend on them for advice; others are more oriented to the present and so treat older family members with less respect. Whether families are headed by men or women is also culturally determined.

Poverty is a major problem for many nondominant ethnic groups. Characteristic responses that are sometimes described as cultural limitations are actually the consequences of poverty—for example, a mother seeking medical care for her child late in the course of an illness or late in pregnancy for herself. Solving some problems may be a question of locating financial resources rather than overcoming cultural influences.

The Dyad Family

A dyad family refers to two people living together, usually a woman and man, without children. Many single young adults live together as a dyad in shared apartments, dormitories, or homes for companionship and financial security while completing school or beginning their careers. Dyad families are generally viewed as temporary arrangements, but if the couple chooses child-free living this can also refer to a lifetime arrangement.

The Nuclear Family

The traditional nuclear family structure is composed of a husband, wife, and children. After World War II, the nuclear family became the most common family structure. Today, however, the number of nuclear families in the United States has declined to about 50% of families due to the increase in divorce, single parenthood, and remarriage and the greater acceptance of alternative lifestyles. Increasing in incidence is the single-headed family (an increase from 10% of all families in 1960 to nearly 26% in 2001) (NCHS, 2000). An advantage of a nuclear family is its ability to provide support to family members because with its small size, people feel genuine affection for each other. In a time of crisis, this same characteristic may become a family weakness (there are few family members to share the burden and offer support). This makes helping nuclear families locate and reach out to support people during a crisis an important nursing responsibility.

A woman might choose to keep her birth name when marrying or to hyphenate her name with her spouse's. This can create challenges for interviewing, especially if the family is a blended one and children in a family and parents all have different last names.

The Cohabitation Family

Cohabitation families are composed of heterosexual couples who live together like a nuclear family but remain unmarried. Although such a relationship may be temporary, it may also be as long-lasting and as meaningful as a more traditional alliance and therefore offer as much psychological comfort and financial security as a marriage. Long-term cohabitation unions are growing in number because of the pressure to adhere to a monogamous relationship to avoid contracting the human immunodeficiency virus (HIV) or other sexually transmitted diseases, and a more widespread acceptance of cohabitation by society. Because cohabitation unions simulate nuclear families, the strengths and weaknesses of these families are the same as those of nuclear unions.

The Extended (Multigenerational) Family

The extended family includes not only the nuclear family but also other family members such as grandmothers, grandfathers, aunts, uncles, cousins, and grandchildren. An advantage of such a family is that it contains more people to serve as resources during crises and provides more role models for behavior or values. A possible disadvantage of an extended family is that family resources, both financial and psychological, must be stretched to accommodate all members. When assessing such families, remember that because of the many members present, a parent's strongest support person may not be a spouse or intimate partner, and a child's primary caregiver may not be his or her mother or father The grandmother or an aunt or another sibling, for example, may provide the largest amount of support or childcare, even though spouses and the child's parents are also present every day.

The Single-Parent Family

In as many as 50% to 60% of families with school-age children today, only one parent lives in the home. Of those families, 15% (increased from 4% in the last census) have a man as the single parent (NCHS, 2000). This increase in single-parent families is due both to the high rate of divorce and to the increasingly common practice of women raising children outside marriage. A health problem in a single-parent family is almost always compounded because if the parent is ill, there is no back-up person for childcare. If a child is ill, there is no close support person to give reassurance or a second opinion on whether the child's health is worsening or improving.

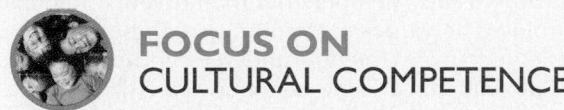

Low income is often an additional problem encountered by single-parent families, because the parent is most often a woman and women's incomes are lower than men's by about 30%. Single parents also may have difficulty with role modeling or identifying their own role in the family (they must provide duplicate roles, or financial support as well as childcare). Trying to fulfill several central roles this way is not only time-consuming but also mentally and physically exhausting and, in many instances, not rewarded. Such a parent may develop low self-esteem (if a spouse left or if the other parent refuses to help with child support). Single-parent fathers may have difficulty in addition with home management or childcare if they had little experience with these roles before the separation. Such feelings can interfere with decision-making and can impede daily functioning.

A single-parent family has the advantage of offering a child a special parent–child relationship and increased opportunities for self-reliance and independence. If there has been a divorce, one parent may have been given legal custody of the children, or both parents may have joint custody. Either way, both parents often participate in decision-making. At a time of illness, both may visit the ill child and may be eager to receive reports of the child's progress. Identifying who is the custodial parent is especially important when consent forms for care are signed.

The Blended Family

In a blended family, or remarriage or reconstituted family, a divorced or widowed person with children marries someone who also has children. Advantages of blended families are increased security and resources for the new family. Another benefit is that the children of blended families are exposed to different ways of life and may become more adaptable to new situations.

Childrearing problems may arise in this type of family from rivalry among the children for the attention of a parent or competition with the stepparent for the love of the biologic parent. In addition, each spouse may encounter difficulties helping rear the other's children. Often stepparents believe they are thrust into a limited or challenged role of authority. Children may not welcome a stepparent because they have not yet resolved their feelings about the separation of their biologic parents (either through divorce or death); the stepparent may differ from their biologic parents, particularly in terms of discipline and caregiving; or they may believe that the stepparent threatens their relationship with their biologic parent. They may have heard so many stories about evil stepparents that they come to the new family prejudiced against their new parent. They may also become distressed at seeing their other biologic parent move into another home and become a stepparent to other children.

Moreover, although financial difficulties may lessen in this type of family, finances also can be severely limited. One parent may be obligated to pay child support for children from a previous marriage while supporting the children of the current marriage. If there is economic disparity between the biologic parents, conflicts and distorted expectations can occur. Nurses can be instrumental in offering emotional support to members of a remarriage family until the adjustments for mutual living have been made.

The Communal Family

Communes comprise groups of people who have chosen to live together as an extended family. Their relationship to each other is motivated by social or religious values rather than kinship. Members often fulfill few traditional family roles. The values of commune members may be more oriented toward freedom and free choice than those of a traditional family. Some communes are described as cults or comprise a group of people who follow a charismatic leader. Adolescents, because they are in the process of determining what values to adopt for their future life, may find this type of commune particularly appealing (Aronoff et al., 2000).

People living in a commune may not wish to follow traditional health care regimens, preferring instead alternative therapies (health care may be seen as an established system that they are rejecting). On the other hand, people who reject traditional values may be the most creative people in a community, the most interested in participating in their own care and ripe for health teaching and learning.

The Gay or Lesbian Family

In homosexual unions, individuals of the same sex live together as partners for companionship, financial security, and sexual fulfillment. Such a relationship offers support in times of crisis comparable to that offered by a nuclear or cohabitation family. Some lesbian and gay families include children from previous heterosexual marriages or through the use of artificial insemination, adoption, or surrogate motherhood. Laws governing homosexual partners can affect health care if they limit health insurance coverage. Lack of understanding by health care providers of the strength and richness of these unions can further impede health care (Blackwell & Blackwell, 2000).

The Foster Family

Children whose parents can no longer care for them may be placed in a foster or substitute home by a child protection agency (Gottesman, 2001). Foster parents may or may not have children of their own. They receive remuneration for their care and concern of the foster child. Foster home placement is theoretically temporary until children can be returned to their own parents. If return is impossible or is not imminent, children may be raised to adulthood in foster care. Such children may experience almost constant insecurity, concerned that soon they will have to move again. They may have some emotional difficulties related to the reason they were removed from their original home (Horwitz et al., 2000).

When caring for children from foster homes, it is important to determine who has legal responsibility to sign for health care for the child (a foster parent may or may not have this responsibility). Most foster parents are as concerned with health care as biologic parents and can be depended on to follow health care instructions conscientiously.

The Adoptive Family

Families of a great many types (nuclear, extended, single-parent, gay and lesbian) adopt children today. No matter what the family structure, adopting brings a number of challenges to the adopting parents and the child, as well as to any other children in the family.

Methods of Adoption

Agency Adoption. In traditional agency adoption, a couple usually contacts an agency by first attending an informational meeting. If the couple decides to apply to the agency, they are then put on a waiting list for processing. A process that includes extensive interviewing and a home visit by an agency social worker determines whether the couple can be relied on to provide a safe and nurturing environment for an adopted child. Once approved by the agency, the couple is placed on a second waiting list. When a child has been located for them, the agency notifies the couple. Depending on the area of the country and the couple's particular requests, this may take anywhere from less than a year to 5 or 6 years. There are children in every state who are waiting for adoption and can be placed almost immediately into adopting homes, but most of these children are older and have lived with many foster families or have gone back and forth between the homes of their birth parents and foster care. Many others have special health care needs or are learning challenged. Although this is not an option that is appealing for every couple, adoption of such children can be a very rewarding experience for the right couple and will achieve a family for them.

Historically, there was little or no communication between the woman placing her baby for adoption and the adopting couple. In the past, this was seen as an advantage because the birth mother could then not interfere in the new couple's lives. Today, the disadvantage of this for the child is being realized: should a child want to learn his or her birth family's name or medical history or location, this information is not available. This had led to "open adoption" procedures in which the identity of neither the birth mother nor the adoptive parents is kept secret, allowing as much interaction as desired between the two sets of parents.

International Adoption. International adoption can often provide a baby in less time than a traditional agency adoption, but there may be unanswered questions about prenatal health care or the birth parent's background with this method. In addition, countries willing to permit abandoned or orphaned children to be adopted internationally are often economically disadvantaged or war-torn, meaning the child's health or development may have suffered. War conditions may allow children to be released from the country one day but not the next. This means couples who are waiting for an international adoption must be ready at a moment's notice either to travel to the foreign country or a neutral location to pick up their child or to give up the adoption because political reforms have stopped the release of children.

A home visit from a local agency and a significant amount of paperwork and communication with the international agency are usually required before a family can be approved for this type of adoption. Typically, the adoption is final before the child enters the country, or shortly after entering. The parents must examine their feelings ahead of time about how they will feel about having a child from a different culture. They should be encouraged to explore ways to respect the child's natural heritage and deal with possible prejudice toward the child by their neighbors and family who are not as culturally competent as they are. Local support groups consisting of other families who have gone through international adoption can be helpful to couples considering this option. In addition, many of the international adoption agencies provide follow-up support. It may be difficult for internationally adopted children to learn about or locate their natural parents in years to come because records of their birth may have been destroyed or changed in their native countries. In some countries, the birth certificate is deliberately changed to reflect the adoptive couple as the birth parents.

Private Adoption. For families who have exhausted other options or who cannot wait for the traditional agency adoption process, private adoption is another alternative. With private adoption, the adopting parents usually agree to pay a certain amount of money, part of which presumably goes toward the birth mother's prenatal and medical expenses. Sometimes, strict anonymity is maintained between the two parties; in other instances, the adopting couple and birth mother come to know each other well. Some pregnant women prefer to place their child for adoption directly with a couple this way rather than through an agency, so they can approve of the couple and maintain contact with the child afterward. The adopting parents might even attend the child's birth if the birth mother wishes.

The Internet has become a source where women wanting to place a baby for adoption can contact couples who want to adopt. Usually, a lawyer serves as the go-between to make certain all the legal ramifications of adoption have been considered by each party.

In some instances, close familiarity between the two parties creates difficulties later on: some couples may want to have the birth mother or father play a continued role in their lives, but others do not. If not, the birth mother may find it difficult to lose contact not only with the baby she has carried for 9 months but also with her new friends, who may have been extremely supportive of her during her pregnancy. These issues must be worked out legally well in advance of the birth because it is possible for a birth mother to change her mind about giving the baby up before the adoption is settled. There is little that an adopting couple can do in this circumstance, because court decisions tend to favor the rights of the birth mother. Parents who adopt by this route may live in fear for years that the birth mother will change her mind. Although many states have laws that place a time limit on the period during which the birth mother can change her mind, many courts have ruled in favor of returning an adopted child to the birth mother no matter what period has elapsed.

Caring for Adoptive Families

Regardless of the type of adoption, the new parents should visit a health care facility shortly after the child is placed in their home so that a base of health information on the child can be obtained, potential problems can be discussed, and solutions explored. If the birth mother of an adopted child ate an inadequate diet and received little prenatal care, for example, the adopted child may be at a higher risk for abnormal neurologic development. Children from countries that are war-torn or poverty-stricken have a greater risk of having illnesses such as hepatitis B, intestinal parasites, and growth retardation. They may lack immunizations (Johnson, 2000).

When assessing a family with a newly adopted child, determine the stage of parenting the parents have reached. The average parents have 9 months to prepare physically and emotionally for a coming baby. Although adoptive parents may have been planning on a baby for much longer than 9 months, the actual appearance of a child can occur suddenly. In a few days' time, the adoptive parents are asked to make the mental steps toward parenthood that biologic parents make over 9 months. There may be a great need at health care visits to explore their feelings about this change in their lives and their feelings about being parents so suddenly. If they have low self-esteem because they were unable to conceive or married a partner who was unable to conceive, they may need reassurance at health care visits that they are functioning well as parents. With the increase in foreign adoptions, parents often express a conflict between trying to preserve the child's native culture while socializing him or her to the community.

Also assess siblings' responses to the adopted child. Biologic children (whether born before or after the adoption) may feel inferior to the adopted child because they were "just born," not "chosen." On the other hand, they may feel superior because they are the "real" children of the parents. These feelings can interfere with their relationship with the adopted child as well as their parents.

It is generally accepted that adopted children should be told as early as they can understand that they are adopted. Knowing this from early childhood is not nearly as stressful as accidentally stumbling onto the information when they are school-aged or adolescents. By age 3 years, children are old enough to understand the story of their adoption: they grew inside the tummy of another woman who, because she could not care for them after they were born, gave them to the adopting parent to raise and love. It is important for parents not to criticize the birth mother as part of the explanation. Children need to know for their own self-esteem that their birth parents were good people and they were capable of being loved by them, but things just didn't work out that way.

When children are first told they are adopted, they may exhibit "honeymoon behavior" or may try to behave perfectly for fear of being given away again. Following this honeymoon period, children may deliberately test their parents to see whether, despite bad behavior such as disobeying or even shoplifting, the parents will still keep them. It helps parents to put this behavior in perspective if they are aware that it may happen and that nonadoptive children use the same testing strategies on some occasions.

As adopted children enter puberty and begin to think about having children of their own, they may need to express their feelings about being adopted. Some adopted children of this age have difficulty establishing a sense of identity because they do not know who their birth parents were. It is common for them to spend time tracing records and trying to locate their birth parents. Counsel adopting parents that this is not a rejection of them, but a normal consequence of being adopted. Children seek their birth parents not because they do not love their adoptive parents, but because they need that information to know where they fit into the eternal scheme of civilization.

Counseling an adopted child or forming a relationship with one as a health care provider carries an additional responsibility: making certain that the relationship is not ended abruptly or thoughtlessly. The person who will continue health supervision should be introduced to the child so he or she does not feel abandoned. When hospitalized, all preschoolers worry about being abandoned and left in the hospital. However, preschoolers who have just been told that they are adopted, that they were chosen by their adoptive parents "from all the babies in the hospital nursery," may be terribly afraid that they are now being returned to the hospital to be given back. Parents of an adopted child may need additional help in preparing the child for the hospital experience and also encouragement to stay with the child in the hospital as much as possible to reduce fear.

✔ **CHECKPOINT QUESTIONS**

1. What is an important strength of a single-parent family?
2. Suppose two gay men adopt a child. Would their family most resemble a nuclear or a single-parent family?
3. How soon should adopted children be told that they're adopted?

FAMILY FUNCTIONS AND ROLES

A family is a small community group, and, as a group, it works best if it designates certain people to complete certain tasks. Otherwise, work can be duplicated or never completed. Usually, the family roles that people view as appropriate are the ones they saw their own parents fulfilling. As each new generation takes on the values of the previous generation, traditions and culture pass from generation to generation.

An important part of family assessment is to identify the roles that family members assume, because family roles are changing and often not as well defined as in the past. Most families, for example, can identify an individual who serves as the wage earner or who supplies the bulk of the income for the family. This may be the mother, not the father. Also identified can be a financial manager (the person who pays the bills), a problem-solver, a decision-maker, a nurturer, a health manager, and a gatekeeper (the person who allows information into and out of the family). Knowing who fulfills these roles in a family helps you to work most effectively with the family.

If a hospitalized child will need continued care after he or she returns home, for example, it would be important to identify and contact the nurturing member of the family, because it will probably be this person who will supervise or give the needed care at home. Do not make assumptions about role fulfillment based on gender or stereotyping, because every family operates differently. For example, although nurturing has typically been thought of as a female characteristic, in some families men fulfill this role.

If a pregnancy will cause a major change in lifestyle for the family, it might be good to identify and contact the person in the family who is the decision-maker and the person who is the problem-solver (not necessarily the same person). If a child's illness will involve increased family expense, then identifying and contacting the wage earner or financial manager of the family would be important. Before introducing a change such as a new pattern of nutrition, it is important to identify the family's safety and health officer.

Box 2-1 highlights an appropriate outcome and intervention using the terminology identified by the Nursing Outcomes Classification and Nursing Interventions Classification (NOC and NIC).

Family Tasks

Duvall and Miller (1990) have identified eight tasks that are essential for a family to perform to survive as a healthy unit. These tasks differ in degree from family to family and depend on the growth stage of the family, but they are usually present to some extent in all families. Wellness behaviors such as these may decrease during periods of heightened stress. Assessing families for these characteristics, therefore, is helpful in establishing the extent of stress on a family and empowering the family to move toward healthier behaviors.

- Physical maintenance: A healthy family provides food, shelter, clothing, and health care for its members. Being certain that a family has enough resources to provide for a new or ill member is important in maternal and child health nursing.
- Socialization of family members: This task involves preparing children to live in the community and to interact with people outside the family. A family that lives in a community with a culture or values different from its own may find this a difficult task.
- Allocation of resources: Determining which family needs will be met and their order of priority is called allocation of resources. In healthy families, there is justification, consistency, and fairness in the distribution. Resources include not only financial wealth but also material goods, affection, and space. In some families, resources are limited, so no one has new shoes. A danger sign would be a family in which one child is barefoot while the others wear $100 sneakers.
- Maintenance of order: This task includes opening an effective means of communication between family members, establishing family values, and enforcing common regulations for all family members (see Focus on Family Empowerment). Determining the place of a new infant and what rules he or she will need to follow may be an important task for a developing family. In healthy families, members know the family rules and respect and follow them.
- Division of labor: The issue here is who will fulfill certain roles, such as family provider, caregiver, and home manager. Pregnancy or an illness of a

BOX 2.1

NURSING OUTCOMES CLASSIFICATION AND NURSING INTERVENTIONS CLASSIFICATION: FAMILY FUNCTION

NOC: Family Functioning

Family functioning is defined as the ability of the family to meet the needs of its members through developmental transitions (Johnson, Maas, & Moorhead, 2000). Some specific indicators suggesting achievement of this outcome include demonstration of the following:

- Socialization of new family members
- Regulation of members' behavior with performance of expected roles
- Adaptation to developmental transitions and unexpected crises
- Creation of environment for free expression by members
- Support of and assistance for one another
- Expression of loyalty to family
- Participation in community activities
- Involvement in problem-solving and conflict resolution
- Acceptance of diversity among members

NIC: Family Integrity Promotion, Childbearing Family

Family integrity promotion, childbearing family, is defined as facilitating the growth of individuals or families who are adding an infant to the family unit (McCloskey & Bulechek, 2000). Some important activities involved when implementing this intervention include:

- Creating an atmosphere to facilitate trust and promote acceptance
- Offering to be a listener
- Spending time with parents to convey acceptance and contribute to feelings of self-worth
- Monitoring the family's current situation, including psychosocial status and effects of newborn on family structure and couple's relationship after birth of the infant
- Identifying each member's and family's coping mechanisms
- Preparing parents for expected role changes and responsibilities of parenthood
- Reinforcing positive parenting behaviors

FOCUS ON FAMILY EMPOWERMENT
Tips to Improve Family Communication

Q. My family doesn't communicate well. How can I improve this?

A. Traditionally, families gathered for an evening meal, and this allowed a set period each day for interaction and problem-solving while problems were still small. If this isn't possible because of busy work or school schedules, suggestions for better communication might be:

- Set up a bulletin board or a chalk board that family members check each day for messages.
- Use a telephone answering tape or video camera to leave messages.
- Plan an earlier wake-up time one morning a week so all family members can have breakfast together.
- Reserve one night a week as "family night," when the family plans a special activity to do together.
- Join in each other's activities (if one is playing in a ball game, all come and watch).

child may change this arrangement and cause the family to rethink this task.

- Reproduction, recruitment, and release of family members: Often not a great deal of thought is given to this task: who lives in a family often happens more by changing circumstances than by true choice. Having to accept a new infant into an already crowded household may make a pregnancy a less-than-welcome event or cause reworking of this task.
- Placement of members into the larger society: This task consists of selecting community activities, such as school, religious affiliation, or a political group, that correlate with the family's beliefs and values. Selecting a birth setting, instituting health promotion, or choosing a hospital or hospice setting is part of this task.
- Maintenance of motivation and morale: A sense of pride in the family group, when created, helps members defend the family against threats and serve as support people to each other during crises. Assessing to see whether this feeling is present helps in planning care.

Family Life Cycles

Families, like individuals, pass through predictable developmental stages (Duvall & Miller, 1990). To predict the likelihood that a family is using health promotion activities, therefore, it is helpful to assess its developmental stage. The age of the oldest child marks the stage. Because families are delaying the age at which they have a first child and parents are living longer, the length of stages 1, 7, and 8 is growing. Box 2-2 highlights an appropriate outcome and intervention for families using the nursing outcomes and interventions classifications.

Stage 1: Marriage and the Family

Although Duvall refers to this stage as marriage, what occurs during it is also applicable to couples forming cohabitation, lesbian, gay or single alliances when formal marriage does not occur. During this first stage of family development, members work to achieve three tasks:

- Establish a mutually satisfying relationship
- Learn to relate well to their families of orientation
- If applicable, engage in reproductive life planning

Establishing a mutually satisfying relationship includes merging the values that a couple bring into the relationship from their families of orientation. This means not only adjusting to each other in terms of routines (e.g., sleeping, eating, or housecleaning) but also sexual and economic aspects. This first stage of family development is a tenuous one, as evidenced by the high rate of divorce or separation of partners at this stage. The illness of a family member or an unplanned pregnancy at this stage may be enough to destroy the still lightly formed bonds if the partners do not receive support from their former family members or alert health care providers to a problem.

Stage 2: The Early Child-Bearing Family

The birth or adoption of a first baby is usually an exciting yet stressful event that requires economic and social role changes. An important nursing role during this period is health education about well-child care and how to integrate a new member into a family. It is a further developmental step to change from being able to care for a well baby to caring for an ill one. One way of determining whether a parent has made this change is to ask what the new parent has tried to do to solve a childrearing or health problem. Even if what the person answers is not therapeutic or the best solution to the problem, as long as it is sensible (not "I don't do anything when the baby's sick; just take her right to my mother" but instead "I've been trying to give her a little water and keep her temperature down"), it probably means the parent has mastered this developmental step. Parents who have difficulty with this step need a great deal of support and counseling from health care providers to be able to care for an ill child at home or to manage a difficult pregnancy.

Stage 3: The Family With Preschool Children

A family with preschool children is a busy family because children at this age demand a great deal of time related to their growth and developmental needs and safety

BOX 2.2

NURSING OUTCOMES CLASSIFICATION AND NURSING INTERVENTIONS CLASSIFICATION: CHILDBEARING FAMILY

NOC: Parenting

Parenting is defined as the provision of an environment that promotes optimum growth and development of dependent children (Johnson, Maas, and Moorhead, 2000). Some specific indicators suggesting achievement of this outcome include the parent's ability to do the following:

- Provide for the child's physical needs, including regular preventive and episodic health care
- Eliminate controllable environmental hazards
- Stimulate social, cognitive, and emotional growth and development
- Use appropriate behavior management and discipline
- Demonstrate empathy toward, a loving relationship with, and positive attributes of the child
- Express realistic expectations of and satisfaction with the parental role

NIC: Risk Identification, Childbearing Family

Risk identification, childbearing family, is defined as the identification of an individual or family likely to experience difficulties in parenting and prioritization of strategies to prevent parenting problems (McCloskey & Bulechek, 2000). Some important activities involved when implementing this intervention include:

- Determining the age of the mother, developmental stage of the parent, parity of the mother, family's economic and educational status, mother's marital status, and literacy level
- Reviewing prenatal and intrapartal records for signs of prenatal attachment and complications
- Reviewing history, both maternal and prenatal, for abnormalities, stressors, and possible chemical dependency
- Ascertaining if pregnancy is planned or unplanned and degree of family approval and support
- Noting any medications, anesthesia, or analgesics administered during the intrapartal period, along with any signs of fetal distress or infant hypoxia
- Monitoring parent–infant interactions, with referral to community agency for follow-up as necessary
- Prioritizing areas for risk reduction and planning for risk-reduction activities

considerations as unintentional injuries (accidents) become a major health concern. If a child is hospitalized because of an accident, parents may have difficulty giving care because they feel they should have done more to prevent the child's injury. It may be difficult for parents to visit the hospital because they must care for other young children at home. If the child returns home for further care, a family in this stage may need continued support and help from a community health nurse to provide necessary health care for the ill member.

Stage 4: The Family With School-Age Children

Parents of school-age children have the important responsibility of preparing their children to be able to function in a complex world while at the same time maintaining their own satisfying marriage relationship. For many families, this is a trying time. Illness imposed at this stage adds to the burdens already present and may be enough to dissolve the marriage. Support systems within a family may be deceptive: family members may be physically present but provide little or no emotional support if internal tension exists. Many families during this period need to turn to a tertiary level of support such as friends, a religious affiliation, or counseling for adequate support.

Important nursing concerns during this family stage are monitoring children's health in terms of immunization, dental care, and health care assessments, monitoring child safety related to home or automobile accidents, and encouraging a meaningful school experience that will make learning a lifetime concern, not to be abandoned after a mere 12 years.

Stage 5: The Family With Adolescent Children

The primary goal for a family with teenagers differs considerably from the goal of the family in previous stages, which was to strengthen family ties and maintain family unity. Now the family must loosen family ties to allow adolescents more freedom and prepare them for life on their own. As technology advances at a rapid rate, the gap between generations increases; life when the parents were young was very different from what it is for their teenagers. This makes stage 5 a trying stage for both children and adults.

Violence—accidents, homicide, and suicide—is the major cause of death in adolescents. As adolescents become sexually active, they risk contracting sexually transmitted diseases such as HIV infection and gonorrhea. The nurse working with families at this stage, therefore, needs to spend time counseling members on safety (driving defensively and not under the influence of alcohol; safer sex practices; proper care and respect for firearms) and the dangers of drug abuse. If there is a "generation gap" between the parents and the children, the children may not be able to talk to their parents about these problems, particularly those of a controversial nature such as sexual responsibility. A nurse is a neutral person who can assist families at this stage when communication is difficult.

Stage 6: The Launching Center Family

For many families, the stage at which children leave to establish their own households is the most difficult stage because it appears to represent the breaking up of the family. Parental roles change from those of mother or father to once-removed support people or guideposts. The stage may represent a loss of self-esteem for parents, who feel themselves being replaced by other people in their children's lives. They may feel old for the first time and less able to cope with responsibilities. Illness imposed on a family at this stage may be detrimental to the family structure, breaking up an already disorganized and noncohesive group.

A nurse, again, can serve as a counselor to such a family. He or she can help the parents to see that what their children are doing is what they have spent a long time preparing them to do, and that leaving home is a positive, not a negative, step.

State 7: The Family of Middle Years

When a family returns to a two-partner nuclear unit, as it was before child-bearing, the partners may view this stage either as the prime time of their lives (an opportunity to travel, economic independence, and time to spend on hobbies) or as a period of gradual decline (lacking the constant activity and stimulation of children in the home, finding life boring without them, or experiencing "empty nest" syndrome). Because the family has returned to a two-partner union, support people may not be as plentiful as they were. Having a baby at this point in life may be viewed as exciting or worrisome, depending on individual circumstances.

Stage 8: The Family in Retirement or Older Age

The number of families of retirement age is approximately 15% to 20% of the population. These individuals are more apt to suffer from chronic and disabling conditions than younger persons. Although families at this stage are not having children, they remain important because they can offer a great deal of support and advice to young adults who are just beginning their families. Many grandparents care for their grandchildren while the parents are at work. This can be a strain on older adults: an analysis showed that women solely raising grandchildren have worse health than women of a similar age living in other family structures and considerably worse health than women with spouses raising grandchildren (Solomon & Marx, 1999).

WHAT IF? What if a family has a school-aged child and a newborn baby? What would be their family stage? What type of stressors might jeopardize this family's well-being?

Changing Patterns of Family Life

Family life has changed significantly in the United States during the past 50 years due to many complex and interrelated factors, such as the increased mobility of families, an increase in the number of families where both parents work outside the house, an increase in the number of one-parent families, and an increase in shared child-rearing responsibilities. Some women (the "sandwich generation") play dual roles by caring for children and aging parents at the same time. Many couples delay marriage and childrearing until they are finished with school and established in their careers. This delay has implications for fertility and the need for assisted reproduction strategies. Some parents, believing they were finished with childrearing, find their grown children returning home after college to live with them. Understanding the impact these changes have on family structure and family life can help you create care plans that are realistic and meet the needs of today's families (see Focus on Communication).

FOCUS ON COMMUNICATION

The Bennett family is composed of Ms. Bennett and her three children: Mark, 4; Bryan, 2; and Deanne, 2 months. You are concerned because the family has missed so many health maintenance visits that the children are underimmunized.

Less Effective Communication

Nurse: It's good to see you in clinic today, Ms. Bennett. I know money is a problem, but you've got to start coming more often until your children get caught up with their immunizations.

Ms. Bennett: It's hard with three children—

Nurse: I can't tell you enough how important immunizations are. Mark, you know, can't start school if he isn't immunized.

Ms. Bennett: It's hard—

Nurse: Babies, you know, have almost no natural immunity. That's why they need immunizations.

Ms. Bennett: It's hard—

Nurse: There's no reason important enough not to get them immunized.

Ms. Bennett: I'll do better. I promise.

More Effective Communication

Nurse: It's good to see you in clinic today, Ms. Bennett. I know money is a problem, but you've got to start coming more often until your children get caught up with their immunizations.

Ms. Bennett: It's hard with three children—

Nurse: I am sure it's hard to bring three children. What could I do to make coming to the clinic easier for you?

Ms. Bennett: I only have two car seats, so I can only bring two kids at one time.

Nurse: Let me give you the number of an agency to call to borrow an extra seat, not only so you can come to the clinic but so you can take them out safely other times.

In our zeal to educate people about good health practices, it is easy to rush in and teach without first assessing a family's most important needs. Unless these needs are met, people may agree to comply with a better health regimen but then be unable to do so because their original need was not met.

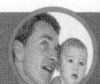

Mobility Patterns

Population movement has an important influence on the quality of family life. During the 20th century, vast numbers of rural families moved to urban communities; many urban families moved to the suburbs. This pattern of mobility is expected to continue into the future. This means that an area with many maternal and child health care facilities may find itself with few women or children to use them in the future; conversely, areas with many women or children may have few facilities for their care. Parents will travel a great distance to obtain health care for an ill child or during a pregnancy with complications, but they are less likely to do so for health maintenance or health promotion; thus, prenatal care or routine immunizations can be neglected. Families need to be asked if convenient health care is available.

Families of migrant farm workers have difficulty finding consistent health care because of their constant movement (Wilson et al., 2000). Children from these families have been identified as being at high risk for intestinal parasites, low socioeconomic status, and lack of immunizations. New immigrants must adjust not only to a new country but also to a different health care system. If laws limit their access to health care, their ability to find health care can be further compromised. Ensuring their access to health care may require both increased health education and community outreach. Nurses can be instrumental in seeing that health care organizations consider these issues and institute innovative measures, such as providing transportation to facilities, changing locales or services so facilities and needs remain balanced, or setting up outreach and translator programs so residents who do not speak English can receive adequate health care.

Poverty

Although the United States is a large and wealthy country, extreme poverty still exists, and in some areas it seems to be growing. As many as 20% of families with children have incomes that fall below the poverty line. Poverty places children and families at risk for a variety of health problems. The pregnant woman living in poverty, for example, is less likely to receive prenatal care or to take important prenatal vitamins if finances are a problem.

A family who must choose between buying groceries and paying for a child's immunizations will obviously buy groceries; the child's immunizations must wait until another time. If the family is forced to make this same choice week after week, the child could reach adulthood without protection against a number of potentially lethal diseases such as measles. Poverty allows acute illness to become chronic, forces families to live in dangerous neighborhoods, and, because of the high stress level always present, may increase the incidence of intimate partner abuse.

Reduced Government Aid Programs

The current trend toward reducing the length of government assistance to families and encouraging people receiving such assistance to begin or return to work stimulates parental productivity but also can create childcare problems (see Focus on Evidence-Based Practice).

FOCUS ON EVIDENCE-BASED PRACTICE

What Factors Are Most Apt to Impede Single Mothers on Welfare Support From Obtaining Gainful Employment?

For this study, focus group interviews were held with nine single mothers to explore what it was like to be a single mother and what barriers they perceived to obtaining full-time employment. Results of the interviews showed that women felt a sense of obligation to care for their children to optimize their growth and development. Problems they anticipated in obtaining employment included lack of adequate childcare and lack of support from the child's father, relatives, and friends for their efforts toward securing employment. Although this sample was small, the study suggests that moving single mothers from welfare to employment has inherent problems that must be addressed before such programs can be successful.

Youngblut, J. M., Brady, N. R., Brooten, D., & Thomas, D. J. (2000). Factors influencing single mothers' employment status. *Health Care for Women International, 21*(2), 125–136.

The new laws restricting the number of families eligible for federal assistance can add to poverty, although some families who ordinarily would not qualify for Medicaid funding will qualify if the mother is pregnant.

Health care providers can be instrumental in helping families secure benefits such as food stamps or funding from the Women, Infants and Children Special Supplemental Food Program (WIC). Families can be referred to free or scaled-payment health care programs so they can obtain health care despite their limited financial resources (Fig. 2-1) (Oken & Lightdale, 2000).

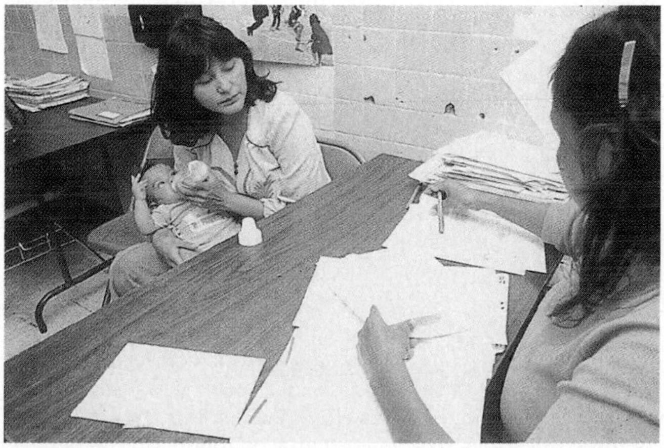

FIGURE 2.1 Community health nurses can be instrumental in helping a new parent gain access to area programs to improve child care.

The Homeless Family

It is estimated that more than 3 million people in the United States today are homeless. Although there is diversity in homeless families as in all others, they have a number of common characteristics. Many homeless families are headed by a woman, and an increasing number are headed by pregnant and parenting adolescents. Such families may not use health care providers or community agencies as effectively as other families. The frequency of drug and alcohol abuse and severe psychiatric problems is greater in homeless families (Ryan et al., 2000). Many mothers in homeless families were physically abused as children and have been battered by an intimate partner.

At least half of homeless children are under 5 years of age. Because of decreased environmental stimulation and lack of exposure to normal play activities, such children tend to perform worse than others on standard screening tests such as the Denver II. They have more physical illnesses, such as anemia, pneumonia, and dental problems. They may have inadequate growth.

When caring for homeless families, it is important to remember that every day represents a struggle for them (Kissman, 1999). They often lack support people, so they may need a health care provider to serve in this capacity to promote a healthier lifestyle or during times of stress such as illness.

Increasing Number of One-Parent Families

One-parent families are increasing in number because of the high divorce rate and the number of women having children outside of marriage. An increasing number of children are being raised by male or gay or lesbian single parents. Nurses can be instrumental in helping single parents strengthen their parenting skills and can provide a second opinion on a course of action or care to prevent parenting responsibilities from becoming overwhelming.

Increasing Divorce

Divorce is rarely easy for the people involved. Because they are so emotionally involved and their perceptions of their roles are changing so drastically, parents may be unable to give their children the support they need during a divorce. This can leave marked long-term, negative effects on children or make the loss of a parent through divorce little different than the loss of a parent through death. Severing ties with grandparents can be also difficult.

Children react in different ways to divorce depending on their age and understanding of what is happening and the explanations that parents give. Divorce, as a rule, has three separate phases, and children's responses follow a course similar to grief. The first phase of divorce is an antagonistic phase when parents realize they are no longer compatible; this is a time of quarreling, hurt feelings, and often whispered conversations. This can be an upsetting period for children because they don't understand what is happening. They may react with denial or anger and can believe that the impending divorce is their fault (Bryner, 2001).

The second phase of divorce is the actual separation stage. Everyone in the family is asked to take on an unfamiliar role and perhaps a new home and a marked difference in financial arrangements. It is a time for grieving for the missing parent. Although it is comforting to be free from a house filled with tension and arguing, children may also wish they had their old life back (similar to the bargaining stage of grieving).

The third phase of divorce involves reshaping. Parents may remarry; financial arrangements stabilize. Children realize that their lives are permanently changed and they cannot go back to the time before the divorce (similar to the acceptance stage of grieving).

Children may manifest their grief with physical symptoms such as nausea or fatigue. Their school performance may suffer. Boys generally have more emotional trauma from divorce than girls, probably because they lose their gender role model if the mother becomes the parent with custody.

Although divorce is a stressful time for children, a redeeming feature may be that the period following a divorce may be less stressful to children than living in a home where there was a high level of conflict between parents (Clarke-Stewart et al., 2000). Children need an explanation of why the divorce has occurred and assurance that it was not their fault. Children may have difficulty thinking of themselves as good people if they believe that one of their parents is bad or that they are responsible for the divorce. The parent who will now be raising them may need help in avoiding playing the role of the injured party and portraying the former partner as dishonorable, selfish, and unreliable. The parent may need time to discuss this issue. You can help by showing the parent that although the former spouse was not a good marriage partner, he or she may have been a good parent and may be well loved by the children.

Decreasing Family Size

The birth rate in the United States has declined steadily from 1900 to the present. The United States is now at a point below zero population growth, which means there are fewer births each year than deaths. Although small families mean there are fewer childcare requirements for parents, they also limit the parents' experience in childrearing, so the amount of childrearing counseling time per parent may increase.

Dual-Parent Employment

As many as 60% of women of childbearing age work at a full-time job outside the home today, and as many as 90% work at least part-time. The implication of this trend for health care providers is that health care facilities must schedule appointments at times when parents are free to come (parents are willing to miss work if their child is sick and needs to see a health care provider, but not necessarily for a health maintenance or a routine prenatal visit). Instructions about how to take medications must take into account a parent's work schedule. For instance, the directions should not state just "three times a day" but should be tailored to the times when a parent will be home to supervise the administration (e.g., before breakfast, after the parent returns from work, and at bedtime).

Dual-parent employment has increased the number of children attending day care centers or after-school programs. This may have an impact on health care because children attending day care centers have an increased incidence of infections such as acute diarrhea. You can help parents to choose a quality day care center that takes the necessary precautions against infection. School-age children often return home from school before the parents return from work. Helping parents prevent loneliness in these "latchkey" children and helping children make good use of their time alone is a nursing responsibility.

Increased Family Responsibility for Health Monitoring

In the past, parents relied on health care providers to monitor their children's health, and they accepted advice about health care without asking questions or expressing opinions. Today, most parents take (and should be encouraged to take) an active role in monitoring their children's health and participating in planning and goal setting. Changes in health care such as shortened hospital stays and an increased focus on health promotion and maintenance have added to the increased responsibilities for families to monitor their own health.

Because of consumer awareness, nurses have an increased responsibility to include parents and children in health care decisions. Using the nursing process for planning helps to accomplish this because the goal-setting step encourages patient participation. Health teaching, such as reducing smoking in the home or increasing the fiber content in meals, becomes more effective if the learners are interested in improving their health.

Increased Abuse in Families

An alarming statistic is that the incidence of domestic abuse (both child and intimate partner) is increasing yearly. This is apparently related to both an increased stress level in the population as a whole and better reporting of abuse. Detecting abuse begins with the awareness that it does occur. Careful screening at family contacts is essential (Kramer, 2002).

✔ CHECKPOINT QUESTIONS

4. How does smaller family size affect parenting?
5. What are common health problems of children adopted from foreign countries?
6. How does dual-parent employment change the way you might instruct parents to give a q.i.d. medicine to a child?

ASSESSMENT OF FAMILY STRUCTURE AND FUNCTION

Family health can be assessed on a variety of levels and in varying degrees of detail. The type of family data collected and the method of collection should match the way in which the assessment data will be used.

General characteristics of family type and functioning can be assessed using observation and general history questions (Table 2-1). When more detailed information about family environment and roles is required, using an assessment tool specifically developed for that purpose is most effective.

TABLE 2.1 Family Assessment

AREA OF ASSESSMENT	QUESTIONS TO ASK
Type of family	Who lives in the home? Is the family nuclear, extended, or other?
Family finances	Are finances adequate? Is money divided evenly among family members?
Safety	Is the home safe from fire or unintentional injuries (has smoke alarms, police and fire numbers posted?)
Health	Does the family eat a nutritious diet? Do they receive adequate sleep? Are immunizations current? Is there a balance between work and recreation? Can they cope with problems adequately?
Emotional support	
Within family	Do members eat together or spend an equal amount of time with each other daily? Do they band together to defend each other from outsiders?
Outside family	Is the family active in community organizations or activities? Do they visit (or are they visited by) friends and relatives? Can the family name one outside person they can always rely on for help in a time of crisis?
Family roles	
Nurturing figure	Who is the primary caregiver to children or any physically or cognitively challenged member?
Provider	Who brings in the bulk of the family's income?
Decision-maker	Who makes decisions, particularly in the area of lifestyle and leisure time?
Financial manager	Who supervises the family finances (pays the bills, provides for future savings?)
Problem-solver	Who does the family depend on to provide the solution for problems?
Health manager	Who ensures that family members keep health appointments, immunizations are kept current, and preventive care such as a mammogram for the mother is scheduled?
Gatekeeper	Who determines what information will be released from the family or what new information can be introduced?

The Well Family

Assessment of psychosocial family wellness requires measurement of how the family relates and interacts as a unit, including communication patterns, bonding, roles and role relationships, division of tasks and activities, governance of the family structure, decision-making and problem-solving, and leadership within the family unit. Assessment also looks at how the family relates to the outside community.

The **genogram,** a diagram that details family structure, provides information about the family's history and the roles of various family members over time, usually through several generations (Fig. 2-2). The genogram provides a basis for discussion and analysis of family interaction.

The Family APGAR (Smilkstein, 1978) is a screening tool of the family environment (Fig. 2-3). A family APGAR form is administered to each family member, and their scores are compared. The tool is easy to use and can complement the history.

The Family in Crisis

Nursing assessment of the family often occurs when the family is in crisis. The way families react to a crisis depends largely on the particular crisis, their past experiences with problem-solving, their perception of the event (whether they can clearly see what is the problem), and the resources available to them to help solve the problem. McCubbin et al. (2000) have suggested that assessing these factors is vital to predicting the probable extent of the crisis for the family. A crisis can change the family's perceptions and the resources available to them, so renewed assessment is therefore necessary to see how the family is weathering the impact (a double ABCX model of assessment; Fig. 2-4).

To use this model, first assess what is the stressor (an event or transition that has the potential to influence the family's dynamics) that is affecting the family. A house fire would be an example. Next, assess the family's perception of the stressor. If the family states that they had adequate insurance so everything can be replaced, for example, the stressor may have little effect, but if they feel overwhelmed by the loss of their home and possessions, it is having a major effect. The third step is to evaluate the resources available to the family, both internal and external. What is the family type? What are their vulnerabilities? Do they have friends who can help replace their possessions? Do they belong to a church or synagogue that will help? Every family will make some kind of adjustment to a problem. This adjustment and then the family's changed perception of the event lead to a need for further assessment.

This model is a useful one for family assessment because it does not assume that just because a stressor happens, an automatic outcome will occur. It respects the individuality of families, an important factor to remember in family assessment.

Listing a family's strengths and coping abilities as well as its areas of vulnerability helps to plan care; in addition, this process actually strengthens the family. Family assessment carried out with the family together in this way will bring out insights and better prepare family members to cope with the current level of stress and the difficult decisions that may be ahead. The Focus on Family Empowerment display provides practical suggestions to help families enduring a crisis.

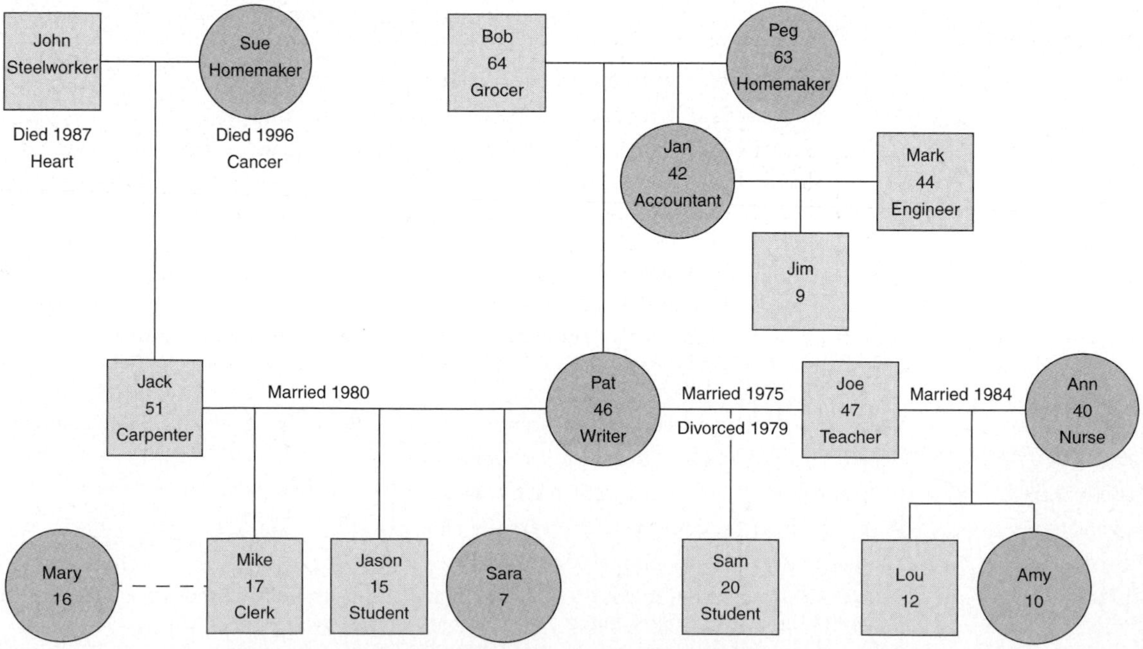

FIGURE 2.2 A family genogram showing three generations. Males are shown by squares, females by circles. Each family member's name, age, and occupation are supplied.

The Family APGAR Questionnaire

	Almost always	Some of the time	Hardly ever
I am satisfied with the help that I receive from my family* when something is troubling me.	______	______	______
I am satisfied with the way my family discusses items of common interest and shares problem solving with me.	______	______	______
I find that my family accepts my wishes to take on new activities or make changes in my lifestyle.	______	______	______
I am satisfied with the way my family expresses affection and responds to my feelings such as anger, sorrow and love.	______	______	______
I am satisfied with the way my family and I spend time together.	______	______	______

SCORING

Scoring: The patient checks one of three choices, which are scored as follows: 2 points for "Almost always," 1 point for "Some of the time" and 0 for "Hardly ever." The scores for each of the five questions are then totaled. A score of 7 to 10 suggests a highly functional family. A score of 4 to 6 suggests a moderately dysfunctional family. A score of 0 to 3 suggests a severely dysfunctional family.

WHAT IS MEASURED

Adaptation	How resources are shared, or the member's satisfaction with the assistance received when family resources are needed.
Partnership	How decisions are shared, or the member's satisfaction with mutuality in family communication and problem solving.
Growth	How nurturing is shared, or the member's satisfaction with the freedom available within the family to change roles and attain physical and emotional growth or maturation.
Affection	How emotional experiences are shared, or the member's satisfaction with the intimacy and emotional interaction within the family.
Resolve	How time* is shared, or the member's satisfaction with the time commitment that has been made to the family by its members.

*Besides sharing time, family members usually have a commitment to share space and money. Because of its primacy, time was the only item included in the Family APGAR; however, the nurse who is concerned with family function will enlarge understanding of the family's resolve by inquiring about family member's satisfaction with shared space and money.

FIGURE 2.3 The Family Apgar Questionnaire. (Smilkstein, G. [1978]. The Family APGAR, *Journal of Family Practice, 6,* 1231.)

THE FAMILY AS PART OF A COMMUNITY

Community can be defined in many ways, but it is generally accepted to refer to a limited geographic area in which the residents relate to and interact among themselves. When asked what community they are from, people may mention an entire city, a school district, a geographic district ("the East Side"), a street name ("Pine Street area"), or a natural marking ("the Lower Creek area").

Because the health of individuals is influenced by the health of their community, it is important to become acquainted with the community in which you practice. If you are caring for a client or family from a community unknown to you, then assess that community to see if there are aspects about it that contributed to an illness (and therefore need to be corrected) and to determine whether the person will be able to return to such a community without extra help and counseling after recovering from an illness (Fig. 2-5).

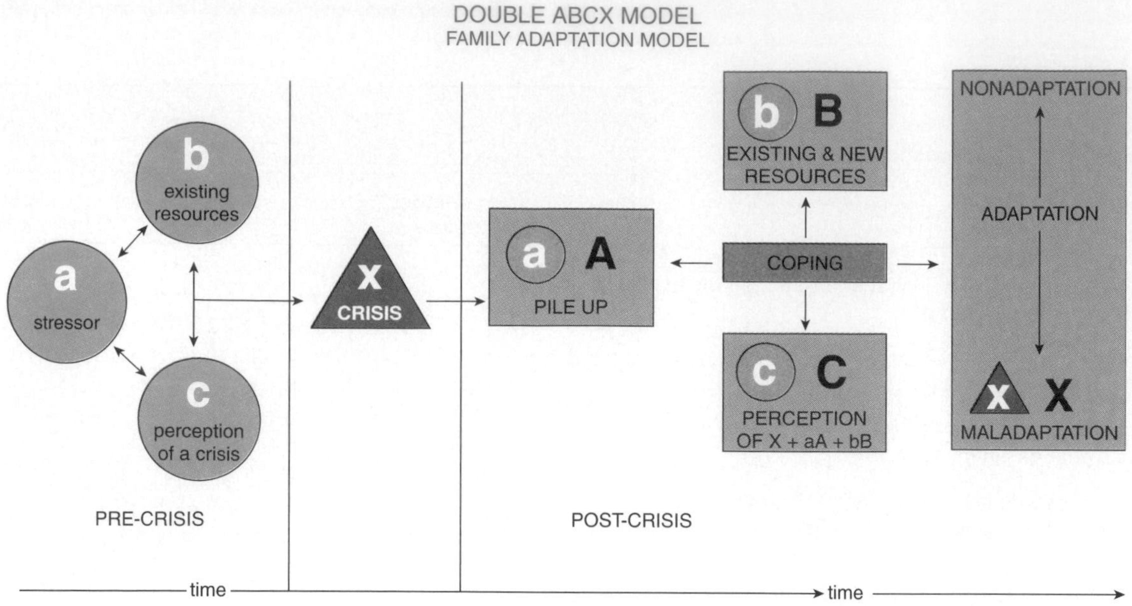

FIGURE 2.4 The ABCX System for Family Assessment. (McCubbin, H. I., Thompson, E. A., Thompson, A. L. & Futrell, J. A. [2000]. *The dynamics of resilient families.* Thousand Oaks, CA: Sage Publications.)

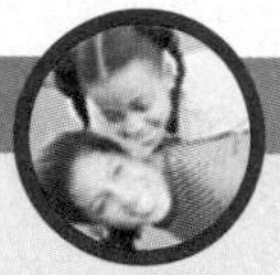

FOCUS ON FAMILY EMPOWERMENT

Tips for Reducing Family Stress

Q. How can my family better manage stress?

A. Managing stress calls for interventions specific to each family, but these are some suggestions:

1. Recognize that stress levels differ from person to person. Because one person is not upset by some condition does not mean that another person will not be annoyed or upset. On the other hand, if a situation does not annoy a person, that person should not feel that he or she has to react to it just because someone else does.
2. Learn to change those things you cannot accept and accept those things you cannot change. Trial and error is often required to determine the difference.
3. Often a total change is unnecessary; a simple modification will be ample to make the difference.
4. State your personal reactions to stress. Almost nothing limits the extent of a threat more than being able to describe it accurately.
5. Reach out for support. People under stress are often so involved in their problems that they do not realize that people around them want to help. Sometimes the people closest to the person feeling stress are under a similar threat and so are no longer able to offer support. When this happens, the person must call on second- or third-level support people (family or community) for help.
6. Reach out to give support when others are being threatened. Survival is a collaborative function of social groups; a favor offered now can be called in when you are in need at a later date.
7. Face a situation as honestly as possible. As a rule, knowing the exact nature of a threat is less stressful than a "something-is-out-there" feeling. On the other hand, do not feel compelled to face intense threats, such as a serious complication of pregnancy or a fatal illness in a child, until you have had time to mobilize your defenses, or you may be overwhelmed.
8. Do not rush decisions or make final adaptive outcomes to a stressful situation. As a rule, major decisions should be delayed at least 6 weeks after an event; 6 months is even better.
9. Anticipate life events and plan for them to the extent possible. Anticipatory guidance will not totally prepare you for a coming event but will at least serve notice that distress over the situation is normal.
10. Remember that unintentional injuries increase when people are under stress. A person worrying about a complication of pregnancy, for example, is more apt to have an automobile accident than a person who is stress-free. Children are more apt to poison themselves when the family is under stress.
11. Action feels good during stress because doing something brings a sense of control over feelings of helplessness and disorganization. Action often is so satisfying that people do things such as write threatening letters or shout harmful remarks that they later regret. Channel your energy into therapeutic action (such as going for a long walk) instead.

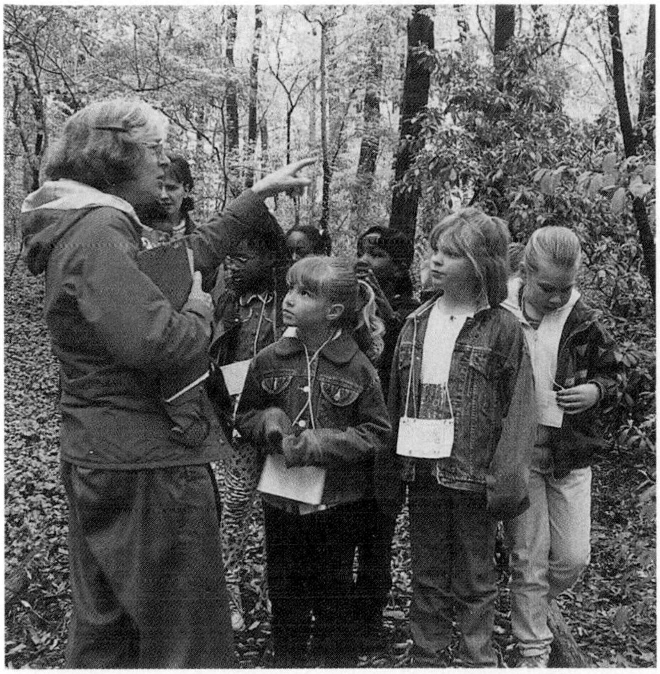

FIGURE 2.5 Community experiences can be a rich source of learning for children. Here a naturalist guides children on a walk through a community park.

Community assessment consists of examining the various systems that are present in almost all communities to see if they are functioning adequately. Knowing the individual aspects of families or community can help you understand why some children reach the illness level they do before parents bring them in for health care. In addition, such knowledge can set the stage for care (e.g., a woman living alone in a city has no transportation available to her until her husband comes home from work so she cannot come for prenatal care; a 5-year-old child develops measles because there are no free immunization services in the community).

It is easier for you to prepare a woman or child for return to a community after childbirth or a hospital stay if, for example, you know the specific features of the community where the family lives. (Does the Pine Street area have well or city water? How many flights of stairs does someone from the Stevens Plaza area have to walk to reach an apartment? Is there public transportation so the mother can return for her 2-week and 6-week visits with the baby?) Table 2-2 summarizes areas of community assessment to use in discharge planning.

WHAT IF? What if the assessment of one patient ready for hospital discharge shows that his family has multiple connections with the community, and the assessment of another shows only the hospital as a connection? Which family might need more discharge planning?

A second aspect of community assessment is to determine the health problems in particular communities and the relationship of the family to the community. This is done by means of an **ecomap,** a diagram of family and community relationships (Fig. 2-6). Such a map helps to assess the emotional support available to a family from the community. A family whom you assess as having few

TABLE 2.2 Community Assessment

AREA OF ASSESSMENT	QUESTIONS TO ASK
Age span	Is the family within the usual age span of the community and thereby assured of support people?
Education	If the family has school-age children, are there schools nearby? Is there a public library for self-education? Is there easy access to such places if the person is physically challenged? If a special program such as diet counseling is needed, does it exist?
Environment	Are environmental risks present, such as air pollution? Busy highways? Train yards? Pools of water where drowning could occur? Will hypothermia be a problem?
Financial status	Is there a high rate of unemployment in the community? What is the average occupation? Will this family have adequate finances to manage comfortably in this neighborhood? Are supplemental aid programs available?
Health care	Is there a health care agency the family can use for comprehensive care? Is it convenient, in terms of finances and time?
Housing	Are houses mainly privately owned or apartments? Are homes close enough together to afford easy contact? Are they in good repair? Will new construction or deteriorated housing be a safety problem?
Political	Is the community active politically? Can adults reach a local polling place to vote, or do they know how to apply for absentee ballots?
Recreational	Are recreational activities of interest available? Are they economically feasible?
Religion	Is there a facility where the family can worship as they choose? Is there easy transportation to it?
Safety	Is there adequate protection so family members can feel safe to leave home or remain home alone? Do they know about available hotlines and local police and fire department numbers? Are there smoke alarms in the bedrooms and near the kitchen?
Sociocultural	What is the dominant culture in the community? Does the family fit into this environment? Are foods that are culturally significant available?
Transportation	Is there public transportation? Will family members have access to it if they are physically challenged?

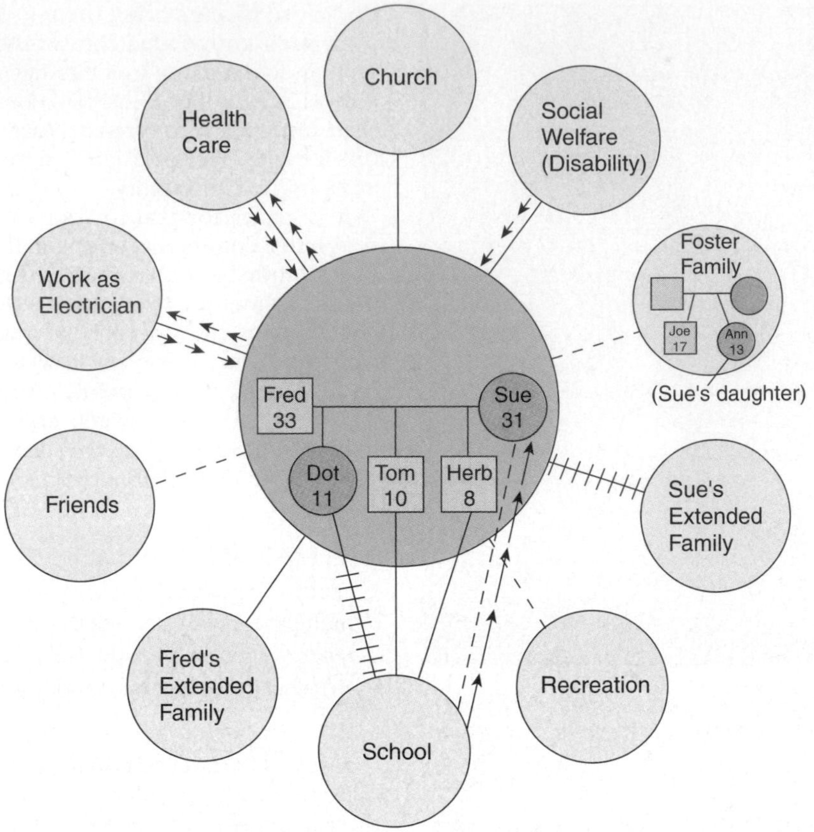

FIGURE 2.6 An ecomap of a family's relationship to its environment. The family members and their ages are shown in the center circle: the outer circles show community contacts. Lines indicate types of connections: *solid lines,* strong; *dotted lines,* tenuous; *lines with cross bars,* stressful. *Arrows* signify energy or resource flow, and absence of lines indicates no connection. (Spradley, B. W. & Allender, J. A. [2000]. *Community health nursing: Concepts and practice* [5th ed.]. Philadelphia: Lippincott Williams & Wilkins, with permission.)

connecting lines between its members and the community may need increased nursing contact and support to remain a well family. Focus on Nursing Care Planning demonstrates both family and community assessment.

✔ CHECKPOINT QUESTIONS

7. How does a genogram differ from an ecomap?
8. What is a family APGAR?
9. Why is assessing transportation in a community important in regard to health care?

KEY POINTS

A family is a group of people who share a common emotional bond and perform certain interrelated social tasks.

Common types of families include nuclear, extended, single-parent, blended, cohabitation, single alliance, gay and lesbian, foster, and adopted families.

Common family tasks are physical maintenance, socialization of family members, allocation of resources, maintenance of order, division of labor, reproduction, recruitment and release of members, placement of members into the larger society, and maintenance of motivation and morale.

Common life stages of families are marriage, early childbearing, families with preschool, school-age, and adolescent children, launching stage, middle-years families, and the family in retirement.

Changes in patterns of family life that are occurring are increased mobility, one-parent families, dual-parent employment, divorce, social problems such as abuse and poverty, and reduced family size. Considering a family as a unit (a single client) helps to plan nursing care that meets the family's total needs.

Families exist within communities; assessment of the community and the family's place in the community yields further information on family functioning and abilities.

FOCUS ON *Nursing Care Planning*

A FAMILY WITH AN ILL CHILD

A 12-year-old boy with cystic fibrosis is brought to the child development clinic for evaluation. His parents state, "He's been acting out in school quite a bit and he doesn't always take his medicines or do his treatments like he's supposed to." Client states, "Everybody's so busy, nobody has time for me. I'm not like the other kids. I'm always sick. Things will get even worse when the new baby comes."

Assessment: Blended family. Client oldest child with one stepsister, age 8 years; middle-class family living in modest three-bedroom home in the suburbs. Father works two jobs and does not participate in community activities: "Who has time?" Mother attending college full time with financial aid; 5 months pregnant and active in local government. Family takes weekly trips to the local high school pool for swimming; client refuses to go. Daily household chores done primarily by client with some help from sister. Client home alone after school until dinner time. Client and family have few close friends. Two neighbors available in case of emergency. Numerous community activities available for children and parents.

Client's respiratory rate 26; thin and pale. Productive cough with tenacious sputum. Last medications taken yesterday morning. Lungs with fine bilateral crackles.

Nursing Diagnosis: Interrupted family processes related to impact of child's illness and situational stressors

Outcome Identification: Family will verbalize improved family functioning and interaction by 3 months' time.

Outcome Evaluation: Family states participation in at least one group activity per week; family reports sitting down to a family meal at least twice a week; family demonstrates positive methods of communication.

Interventions	Rationale
1. Meet with family to identify areas of needed support. Encourage family members to verbalize needs and feelings.	1. Expression of feelings provides a safe outlet for emotions and helps to increase other family members' awareness of the needs.
2. Complete a family APGAR and genogram. Prioritize needs for each family member.	2. Family APGAR provides information about how families relate and interact. A genogram details family structure and roles. Priority setting promotes more focused, directed care for outcome achievement.
3. Develop strategies to assist each family member in meeting priority needs. Instruct in measures such as communication, relaxation, time management, and contracting.	3. Use of therapeutic measures assists in clarifying the needs and expectations and helps reduce stress.
4. Ascertain a common activity enjoyed by all members. Encourage participation in this activity, initially once a month, then twice a month, then weekly.	4. Participation in a group activity fosters bonding. Gradually increasing the frequency of the activity promotes integration into the family routine.
5. Encourage joint cooperation in meal planning and cleanup at least once per week.	5. Working together on a common task fosters interaction, communication, and trust.
6. Investigate outside community resources available. Encourage the family to use the services.	6. Community resources provide additional support in areas of need.

Nursing Diagnosis: Social isolation related to illness and family stressors

Outcome Identification: Client will participate in outside activities.

Outcome Evaluation: Client reports joining a local youth organization; states a friend visits after school at least once a week.

(continued)

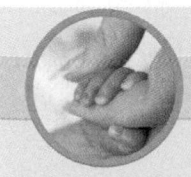

Interventions	Rationale
1. Explore with client outside activities that he might like or dislike. Develop a list of activities in which he would be willing to participate.	1. Exploration of likes and dislikes provides a baseline from which to build suggestions.
2. Evaluate family's ecomap. Contact local community organizations with client and set up a visit. Enlist the aid of the school nurse and guidance counselor in providing contacts.	2. Ecomapping helps to assess the emotional support available to the family. Contacting the organization with the client offers support and helps reduce his possible anxiety with new situations. School personnel provide additional support and reassurance.
3. Encourage client to participate in outside activities chosen.	3. Participation diminishes feelings of loneliness and isolation.

Nursing Diagnosis: Ineffective therapeutic regimen management related to family stressors and feelings of being different

Outcome Identification: The client will adhere to prescribed treatment program.

Outcome Evaluation: The client takes medications as prescribed; performs respiratory treatments as scheduled; demonstrates behaviors to reduce the risk of complications and exacerbations of cystic fibrosis. Respiratory rate within age-acceptable parameters; absence of cough; lungs clear or with minimal rales; sputum clear.

Interventions	Rationale
1. Listen to client's concerns about being sick and different from others.	1. Listening provides clues to understanding client's motivation for behavior.
2. Provide explanations of illness and rationale for treatment based on client's knowledge base.	2. Building on a client's knowledge base facilitates teaching and learning and minimizes repetition.
3. Review medication regimen and procedures for respiratory treatments. Demonstrate procedures, if necessary, and have client return demonstrate. Look for ways to incorporate treatment regimen into client's usual routine.	3. Review and redemonstration helps to reinforce measures and ensure client is doing them correctly. Incorporation of regimen into client's routine helps to promote positive adjustment and decrease feelings of being different.
4. Enlist the aid of parents and sister in regimen. Encourage each to assist with one aspect of the treatment program.	4. Family participation helps to increase client cooperation and promote positive adjustment to the experience. Family involvement in one aspect divides the responsibility so as not to overwhelm them, thus minimizing the risk of added stress on the family system.
5. Assess respiratory status for changes.	5. Follow-up assessment provides clues about the effectiveness of and client's adherence to treatment.
6. Encourage client and family participation in cystic fibrosis support groups.	6. Support groups help to minimize the feeling of being alone and different.

Because families work as a unit, the unmet needs of any member can spread to become the unmet needs of all family members.

Families do not always function at their highest level during periods of crisis; reassessing them during a period of stability may reveal a stronger family than it appeared on first assessment.

CRITICAL THINKING EXERCISES

1. The Hanavans are the family you met at the beginning of the chapter. Why is this a particularly unfortunate time for the Hanavans to have to choose between health care and groceries?

How would their needs change if they were an extended family? A single-parent family? A cohabitation family?

2. What family stage, according to Duvall, has the Hanavan family reached? What would a genogram of this family look like? An ecomap? What other health care providers would it be helpful to include in a team approach for problem-solving with this family?
3. As communities change, a family may find that it is the only family with children on a street or the only family who doesn't work at the local factory. What if you discovered a family "out of sync" with a community this way? How could health care providers help such a family?
4. Examine the National Health Goals related to the family. Most government-sponsored money for nursing research is allotted based on these goals. What would be a possible research topic to explore pertinent to these goals that would be fundable and would advance evidence-based practice?

REFERENCES

Aronoff, J., Lynn, S. J., & Malinoski, P. (2000). Are cultic environments psychologically harmful? *Clinical Psychology Review, 20*(1), 91–111.

Blackwell, D. A., & Blackwell, J. T. (2000). Building alternative families: Helping lesbian couples find the path to parenthood. *AWHONN Lifelines, 3*(5), 45–48.

Bryner, C. L. (2001). Children of divorce. *Journal of the American Board of Family Practice, 14*(3), 201–210.

Clarke-Stewart, K. A., et al. (2000). Effects of parental separation and divorce on very young children. *Journal of Family Psychology, 14*(2), 304–326.

Department of Health and Human Services. (2000). *Healthy people, 2010.* Washington, D.C.: DHHS.

Duvall, E. M., & Miller, B. (1990). *Marriage and family development.* Philadelphia: J.B. Lippincott.

Gottesman, M. M. (2001). Children in foster care: A nursing perspective on research, policy, and child health issues. *Journal of the Society of Pediatric Nurses, 6*(2), 55–64.

Horwitz, S. M., et al. (2000). Specialized assessments for children in foster care. *Pediatrics, 106*(1.1), 59–66.

Johnson, D. E. (2000). Long-term medical issues in international adoptees. *Pediatric Annals, 29*(4), 234–241.

Johnson, M., Maas, M., & Moorhead, S. (2000). *Nursing outcomes classification* (2d ed.). St. Louis: Mosby, Inc.

Kissman, K. (1999). Respite from stress and other service needs of homeless families. *Community Mental Health Journal, 35*(3), 241–249.

Kramer, A. (2002). Domestic violence: How to ask and how to listen. *Nursing Clinics of North America, 37*(1), 189–210.

Martin-Arafeh, J. M., Watson, C. L., & Baird, S. M. (1999). Promoting family-centered care in high-risk pregnancy. *Journal of Perinatal & Neonatal Nursing, 13*(1), 27–42.

McCloskey, J., & Bulechek, G. (2000). *Nursing interventions classification* (3d ed.), St. Louis: Mosby Inc.

McCubbin, H. I., Thompson, E. A., Thompson, A. L., & Futrell, J. A. (2000). *The dynamics of resilient families.* Thousand Oaks, CA: Sage Publications.

National Center for Health Statistics. (2000). Prevalence of intimate partner violence and injuries. *Morbidity & Mortality Weekly Report, 49*(26), 589–592.

Oken, E., & Lightdale, J. R. (2000). Updates in pediatric nutrition. *Current Opinion in Pediatrics, 12*(3), 282–290.

Ryan, K. D., et al. (2000). Psychological consequences of child maltreatment in homeless adolescents: Untangling the unique effects of maltreatment and family environment. *Child Abuse & Neglect, 24*(3), 333–352.

Smilkstein, G. (1978). The family APGAR. *Journal of Family Practice, 6,* 1231.

Solomon, J. C., & Marx, J. (1999). Who cares: Grandparent/grandchild households. *Journal of Women & Aging, 11*(1), 3–25.

Spradley, B. W., & Allender, J. A. (2000). *Community health nursing: Concepts and practice* (5th ed.). Philadelphia: J.B. Lippincott.

United States Census Bureau. (2000). *Statistical abstract of the U.S.* Washington, D.C.: U.S. Department of Commerce.

Wilson, A. H., Pittman, K., & Wold, J. L. (2000). Listening to the quiet voices of Hispanic migrant children about health. *Journal of Pediatric Nursing, 15*(3), 137–147.

Youngblut, J. M, et al. (2000). Factors influencing single mother's employment status. *Health Care for Women International, 21*(2), 125–136.

SUGGESTED READINGS

Altemeier, W. A. (2000). Growth charts, low birth weight, and international adoption. *Pediatric Annals, 29*(4), 204–205.

Anda, R. F., et al. (2000). Adverse childhood experiences and smoking during adolescence and adulthood. *Journal of the American Medical Association, 283*(15), 1958–1959.

Ayerst, S. L. (1999). Depression and stress in street youth. *Adolescence, 34*(135), 567–575.

Brien, M. J., Lillard, L. A., & Waite, L. J. (1999). Interrelated family-building behaviors: Cohabitation, marriage, and nonmarital conception. *Demography, 36*(4), 535–551.

Case, A., & Paxson, C. (2002). Parental behavior and child health. *Health Affairs, 21*(2), 164–178.

Miller, L. C., & Hendrie, N. W. (2000). Health of children adopted from China. *Pediatrics, 105*(6), E76–E79.

Rodriquez, R. (2000). The power of the collective battered migrant: Farmworker women creating safe spaces. *Health Care for Women International, 20*(4), 417–426.

Silverstein, D. N., & Roszia, S. K. (1999). Openness: A critical component of special needs adoption. *Child Welfare, 78*(5), 637–651.

Smit, E. M. (2000). Maternal stress during hospitalization of the adopted child. *MCN: American Journal of Maternal Child Nursing, 25*(1), 37–42.

Solomon, M. (2000). The fruits of their labors: A longitudinal exploration of parent personality and adjustment in their adult children. *Journal of Personality, 68*(2), 1308.

CHAPTER 3

Sociocultural Aspects of Maternal and Child Health Nursing

Key Terms

- **acculturation**
- **assimilation**
- **cultural values**
- **culture**
- **ethnicity**
- **ethnocentrism**
- **mores**
- **norms**
- **pain threshold**
- **pain tolerance**
- **stereotyping**
- **taboos**
- **threshold sensation**
- **transcultural nursing**

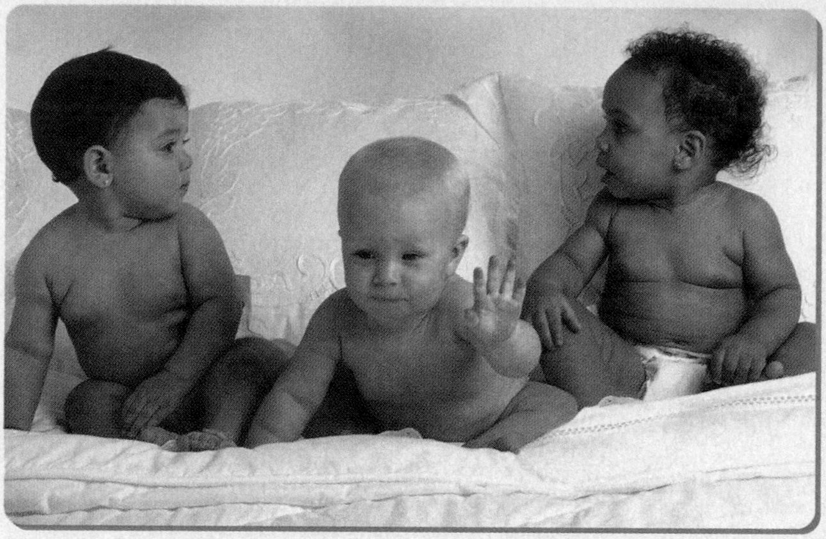

Objectives

After mastering the contents of this chapter, you should be able to:

1. Describe ways that sociocultural influences affect maternal and child health nursing care.
2. Assess a family for sociocultural influences that might influence the way it responds to childbearing and childrearing.
3. Formulate nursing diagnoses related to culturally appropriate aspects of nursing care.
4. Develop outcomes to assist families who have specific cultural needs to thrive in their community.
5. Plan and implement nursing care that respects the sociocultural needs and wishes of families.
6. Evaluate outcome criteria to be certain that goals of care related to sociocultural aspects have been achieved.
7. Identify National Health Goals related to sociocultural considerations that nurses could be instrumental in helping the nation achieve.
8. Identify areas of care related to sociocultural considerations that could benefit from additional nursing research or application of evidence-based practice.
9. Use critical thinking to analyze how the sociocultural aspects of care affect family functioning and develop ways to make nursing care more family-centered.
10. Integrate sociocultural aspects of care with nursing process to achieve quality maternal and child health nursing care.

Anna Rodriques is a 12-year-old child who is hospitalized for surgical repair of a broken tibia. She has a cast on her right leg and will be on bedrest for 3 days, then gradually will be allowed to learn crutch walking.

In planning care for her, you assume that because her culture is Hispanic, her family orientation will be male-dominant, her time focus will be on the present rather than the future, and nutrition preferences will be Mexican American. Based on this, you consult with Anna's father regarding the major aspects of her care. You concentrate on talking mainly about her current problem (bedrest) rather than future care at home. You speak to the dietitian about avoiding milk because lactase deficiency is present in many Mexican Americans.

You are surprised to hear Anna tell you on the second day of her hospital stay that she feels like a second-class person because her father has been asked for more input about her care than she has. She says she is particularly concerned that bone healing will not take place because she has had little milk to drink. She doesn't feel bedrest is a problem but is more concerned about being able to play soccer by next month.

What went wrong with Anna's care? If you had actually planned care in this way, of what would you have been guilty? What would have been a better approach for determining this family's cultural preferences?

Previous chapters described the standards and philosophy of maternal and child health nursing and family structure and function. This chapter adds information on how to care for people from diverse cultures. This is important information because it can enrich care and helps protect the health of both women and children.

After you've studied the chapter, answer the Critical Thinking Exercises at the end of the chapter and then access the on-line study activities (http://connection.lww.com) *to further sharpen your skills and test your knowledge.*

Nurses need to assess sociocultural status, ethnicity, and cultural beliefs to understand why people take preventive health measures or seek care for illness: these factors can strongly influence their responses (Josten et al., 2002).

Ethnicity refers to the cultural group into which a person was born, although the term is sometimes used in a narrower context to mean only race. **Culture** is a view of the world and a set of traditions that a specific social group uses and transmits to the next generation. **Cultural values** are preferred ways of acting based on those traditions. The way people react to health care is a cultural value.

Cultural values differ from nation to nation because they often arise from environmental conditions (for instance, in a country where water is scarce, daily bathing is not valued; in a country where meat is scarce, ethnic recipes use little meat). The usual values of a group are termed **mores** or **norms.** Expecting women to come for prenatal care and for parents to bring children for immunizations are examples of norms in the United States, but these are not beliefs worldwide. Actions that are not acceptable to a culture are called **taboos.** Three taboos that are universal are murder, incest, and cannibalism. Issues such as abortion and robbery are controversial because these are taboos only to some people, not all people.

Cultural values influence the manner in which people plan for childbearing and childrearing and respond to health and illness. In a culture in which men are the authority figures, for example, it might be expected that the father rather than the mother answers questions about an ill child. If you are from a culture in which women are expected to provide all childcare, you might find it annoying to hear a man taking over the responses at a health interview. A nurse who has been culturally influenced to believe that stoic behavior is the "proper" response to pain may be impatient with a woman who has been influenced to believe that expressing discomfort during childbirth is "proper." Nurses need to include all cultural groups in nursing research samples so more can be learned about cultural preferences in relation to nursing interventions and care.

Cultural differences occur across not only different ethnic backgrounds but also different lifestyles. Adolescents, urban youth, the hearing-challenged, and gays or lesbians have separate cultures from the mainstream, for instance. A parent who has been deaf since birth, for example, expects her deaf culture to be respected by having health care professionals attempt to communicate with her in her language. A lesbian mother could become irritated if she is asked, "Where is your husband?"

The United States is a country of such varied cultural groups and socioeconomic conditions that you are likely to see a wide range of behaviors exhibited (Fig. 3-1). Given the cultural mix, almost any behavior can be considered appropriate for some individuals at some time and place. Nursing care that is guided by cultural aspects and respects individual differences is termed **transcultural nursing** (Leininger, 2001).

Stereotyping means expecting a person to act in a characteristic way without regard to his or her individual characteristics. It is generally derogatory in nature. Statements such as, "Men never diaper babies well" or "Japanese women are never assertive" are examples of stereotyping. Stereotyping occurs largely because of lack of exposure to enough people in a particular group and, consequently, a lack of understanding of the wide range of differences among people. In the above examples, the first speaker, having seen one man change diapers poorly, assumes that this represents the entire male population. The second example demonstrates lack of knowledge of a changing culture. If this person were exposed to more Japanese women, she or he certainly would find that the statement is not true. Using such stereotypes, you could plan health care that would be inappropriate and would be resisted.

On the other hand, it is important not to ignore cultural characteristics, because most people are proud of their cultural heritage. It is possible to acknowledge and celebrate a client's culture without stereotyping by assessing the way in which he or she expresses cultural characteristics. Culture influences health so much that several National Health Goals have been established in reference to sociocultural aspects of care (see the Focus on National Health Goals).

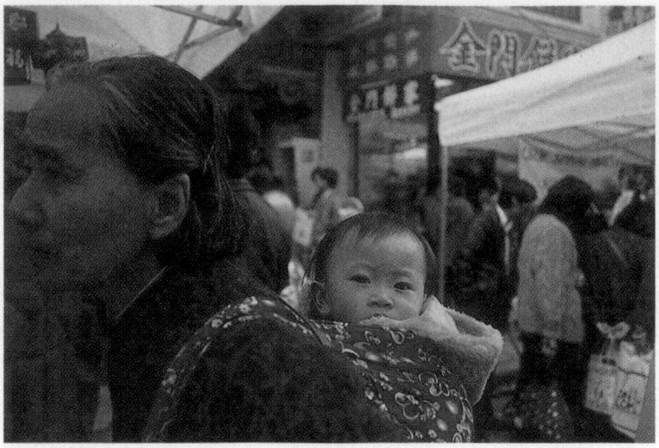

FIGURE 3.1 Various cultural preferences are evident in childrearing. In some cultures, extended family members such as grandparents take an active role in caring for the child. Learning about different ways is important in care planning.

FOCUS ON NATIONAL HEALTH GOALS

A number of National Health Goals are concerned with health practices that may be influenced by cultural factors. These are:

- Increase the proportion of pregnant women who receive early and adequate prenatal care from a baseline of 74% to a target of 90%.
- Increase the proportion of mothers who breastfeed their babies in the early postpartum period from a baseline of 64% to a target of 75%, and increase the number who continue to breastfeed until their babies are 6 months of age from a baseline of 29% to a target of 50%.
- Increase the proportion of healthy full-term infants who are put down to sleep on their backs from a baseline of 35% to a target of 70%.
- Increase the proportion of young children who receive all vaccines that have been recommended for universal administration from a baseline of 73% to a target of 80% (DHHS, 2000).

Nurses can be instrumental in helping the nation achieve these goals by designing prenatal and childcare services that take into account the cultural diversity in our country and by promoting the nutritional and immunologic advantages of breastfeeding in a culturally sensitive manner. Additional nursing research is needed on ways to make prenatal care and child health services more appealing to culturally diverse populations and on the education methods to best reach people who do not speak English.

NURSING PROCESS OVERVIEW

That Respects Sociocultural Aspects of Care

Assessment

Assessment of sociocultural factors is important to be certain that care is planned based not on predetermined assumptions but on the actual preferences of the family. To do this, assess each client as an individual, not merely as one of a group. Note the cultural characteristics of the client that differ from the cultural expectations in which care is being provided so that potential conflicts may be acknowledged and culturally competent care can be planned. Learn as much as you can about different cultures by reading about or talking to members of as many different ethnic groups as possible. Specific areas to assess, along with important findings in these areas, are shown in the Cultural Assessment Tool in Table 3-1.

Assessing the culture of a community is as important as assessing individual families because families are intrinsically joined to their community. An important area to assess is whether the family matches the dominant culture in the community. This is important because the type of foods stocked in supermarkets, the type of entertainment events that are planned, and the values and history that are stressed in schools and work settings are all influenced by the dominant culture.

Communities age the same as families. When homes are first built, many families tend to be young adults with children. Over the years, these families "settle in" to middle age and then are filled with families at retirement.

Older adults may find it difficult to relate if they move into a "young" community. A family who moves into a retirement-age community with young children may feel equally out of place. In all instances, a family that is of a culture other than the dominant one may have strong ties within the family but may have difficulty making strong, effective relationships in the community; they may be more isolated than they would like to be. Community assessment is further discussed in Chapter 2.

Nursing Diagnosis

Several nursing diagnoses speak to the consequences of ignoring cultural preferences in care. Examples are:

- Powerlessness related to expectations of care not being respected
- Powerlessness related to sociocultural isolation
- Impaired verbal communication related to English not being primary language
- Nutrition, less than body requirements, related to cultural preferences
- Anxiety related to a cultural preference for not bathing while ill
- Fear related to inability to buy food due to poor economic status

Outcome Identification and Planning

Planning needs to be very specific for the family and circumstances involved because sociocultural preferences tend to be very personal. Care may begin

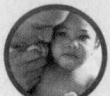

TABLE 3.1 Assessing for Cultural Values

AREA OF ASSESSMENT	QUESTIONS TO ASK OR OBSERVATIONS TO MAKE
Ethnicity	What country or race is the family from?
Communication	What's the main language used in the home?
Touch	Does the family typically touch each other? Do they use intimate or conversational space?
Time	Is being on time important? Is the family planning for the future?
Occupation	Is work important to the family? Do they plan leisure time or leave it unstructured?
Pain	Does the family express pain or remain stoic in the face of it? What do they believe relieves pain best?
Family structure	Is the family nuclear? Extended? Single-parent? Are family roles clear? Can an individual name a family member he/she would call on for support in a crisis?
Male and female roles	Is the family male or female dominant?
Religion	What is the family's religion? Do they actively practice their religion?
Health beliefs	What does the family believe about health? What do they believe causes illness? Makes illness better? Do they use alternative therapies or established practices?
Nutrition	Does the family eat an ethnic diet? Are the foods they enjoy available in their community?
Community	Is the predominant culture in the community the same as the family's? Can they name a neighbor they could call on in a crisis? Is the community a "young," a "settled-in," or a "retired" one? Is the culture one of immigration or stability?

with in-service education for health care providers who are unfamiliar with a particular cultural practice and its importance to the specific family involved. It may include arranging for variations in policy, such as the length of family visiting hours, types of food served, or kind of childcare. Such planning is beneficial because it can make health care more acceptable to a child or family and can also motivate providers to examine policies and question the rationale behind them (see Focus on Multidisciplinary Care).

Implementation

Appreciate that cultural values are ingrained and usually very difficult to change (in yourself and in others). An example of implementing care might be making arrangements for a new Native American mother to take home the placenta if that is important to her, or planning home care for a Chinese-American child whose family believes in herbal medicine. It might be establishing a network of health care agency personnel or personnel from a nearby university or importing firm to serve as interpreters. It might be educating a child, family, or community about the reason for a hospital practice. Do not feel that you and the health care agency are always the ones who must adapt; a particular situation may call for both sides to adjust (cultural negotiation).

Outcome Evaluation

Evaluation by assessing whether outcomes have been met should reveal that a family's sociocultural preferences were considered and respected during care. If this was not achieved, procedures may need to be modified until this can be realized. Examples of expected outcomes that might be established are:

- Parents list three ways they are attempting to preserve cultural traditions in their children.
- Child states she no longer feels socially isolated because of cultural differences.
- Family members state they have learned to substitute easily purchased foods for traditional foods unavailable in local stores in order to obtain adequate nutrition.
- Child with severe hearing impairment writes that he feels communication with ambulatory care staff has been adequate.

FOCUS ON MULTIDISCIPLINARY CARE

Many different health care professionals participate in the care of families. An advantage of having people from various cultures is that they can supply multiple solutions to problems, each drawing on a different background. They also can serve as multilingual interpreters.

You may need to conduct in-service meetings to educate other health care providers about a particular client's cultural preferences if they do not seem to recognize the importance of respecting different cultural values. Unlicensed assistive personnel may be from a variety of different cultural backgrounds. This means you have to help them respect cultural differences of clients and also those of fellow personnel. Unlicensed assistive personnel often serve food trays to clients. Be certain they respect cultural preferences while doing this and do not urge people to eat foods they believe will not be good for them or will harm them in some way.

SOCIOCULTURAL DIFFERENCES AND THEIR IMPLICATIONS FOR MATERNAL AND CHILD HEALTH NURSING

Respecting sociocultural values is important in maternal and child health because childbearing and childrearing are both times in life surrounded by many cultural traditions. Nurses can better provide multicultural care by understanding cultural concepts and sociocultural influences on families (Munoz, 2001).

Changing Cultural Concepts

Until recently, the United States was viewed as a giant cultural "melting pot" where all new arrivals gave up their native country's traditions and values and became "Americans." **Assimilation** or **acculturation** refers to this trade of ethnic traditions for those of the dominant culture. The process of assimilation means that cultural expression is lost by taking on the customs of the dominant culture.

In the past, any behavior that was not like that of middle-class Americans was viewed as strange and inferior. Many Americans were intolerant of these behaviors because they believed that the American way (which actually was the northern European way) was the "best" way. The belief that one's own culture is superior to all others is referred to as **ethnocentrism.** Ethnocentrism can lead to prejudice because the feelings and ways of other cultures cannot be understood or appreciated without the philosophy that the world is large enough to accommodate a diversity of ideas and behaviors and that there is probably no "best" way (see Focus on Evidence-Based Practice).

Historically, people whose cultures differed most drastically from the American ideal suffered the greatest amount of rejection because they were least able to assimilate. On the other hand, mutual cultural assimilation occurs in many communities. For example, when many Italians moved into American communities in the early 1900s, the average Italian family learned to speak English and the average American family learned to cook spaghetti with Italian sauce.

Today, many people question the idea that America ever was a melting pot; instead, the preferred concept is that of a "salad bowl" in which cultural traditions and values are tossed together, with all their crispness and flavor retained, to make a perfect mix. Retaining ethnic traditions strengthens and enriches family life. It provides security to younger family members to realize that they are one of a continuing line of people who have a past and will have a future (Fig. 3-2) (see Focus on Cultural Competence).

Cultural competence, the integration of cultural elements to enhance communication and work effectively with people, is a goal to strive for (Mayberry et al., 1999). However, numerous levels of cultural intolerance or acceptance persist because many people continue to hold different beliefs along the cultural competence continuum (Fig. 3-3).

When planning nursing care, it is important not only to respect people's cultural differences but also to help people share their cultural beliefs with health care providers

> **FOCUS ON EVIDENCE-BASED PRACTICE**
>
> ***Does Exposure to a Diverse Population Foster Acceptance of Diversity?***
>
> For this study, 349 students from four medical schools returned questionnaires describing the diversity proportions and diversity issues at their schools. Results showed that women students placed more value on the inclusion of diversity issues in the curriculum than did men students. African-American students were the least likely to think that the curriculum contained adequate information about diversity. The researchers concluded that students' perceptions of diversity were influenced by their own demographic characteristics and those of their school. The more diverse the school, the more comfortable students appeared to be with diversity and the more they valued its contribution to their education.
>
> Elam, C. L., Johnson, M. M., Wiggs, J. S., Messmer, J. M., Brown, P. I., & Hinkley, R. (2001). Diversity in medical school: Perceptions of first-year students at four southeastern U.S. medical schools. *Academic Medicine, 76* (1), 60–65.

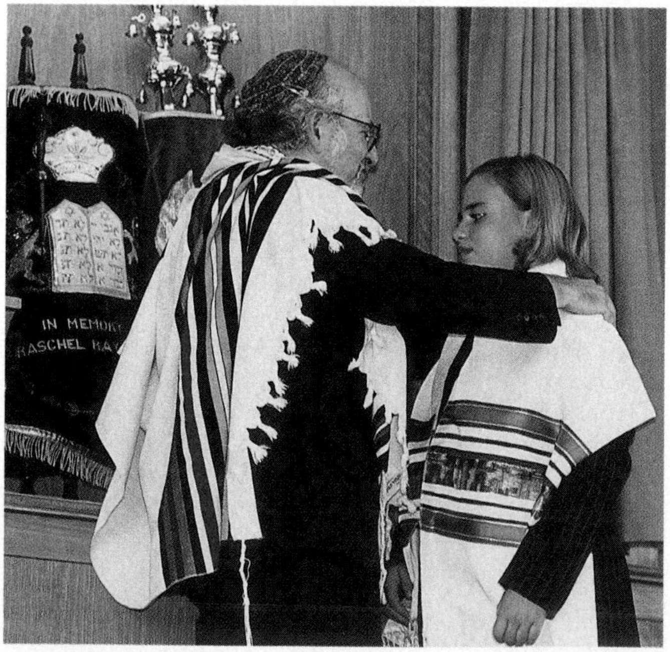

FIGURE 3.2 Cultural traditions offer a sense of security to children.

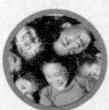

FOCUS ON CULTURAL COMPETENCE

How Can I Help My Family Preserve Our Cultural Heritage?

Preserving your cultural heritage when living in another culture calls for creative planning. Some suggestions for doing this are:

- Plan an "ethnic night" once a week when only ethnic food is served. Encourage children to invite friends for the meal and discuss the traditions behind the various foods.
- If a foreign language is part of your traditions, reserve one night a week when family members speak only the native language.
- Choose books for children that are written by authors from your culture or that advantageously describe the culture. Read them together.
- Monitor television for programs that focus on your culture. Watch them with your children.
- Talk to your children about your childhood and traditions and values that differ from those of other families as bedtime stories or "talk time."
- Celebrate holidays in the traditional manner. Including cultural influences in holiday celebrations adds a rich ingredient to these occasions.

so their beliefs can be considered and respected. As a nurse, you will have the opportunity to meet many people who hold cultural values different from your own. Throughout this text, Focus on Cultural Competence boxes feature specific cultural preferences as they relate to health care or nursing. Important sociocultural differences to assess or consider include various aspects of lifestyle.

✔ CHECKPOINT QUESTIONS

1. What is a cultural more?
2. What is stereotyping?
3. What is cultural competence?
4. What is transcultural nursing?
5. What is ethnocentrism?

Sociocultural Assessment

When assessing families as to whether socioeconomic or cultural influences are present that will make special considerations of care necessary, several categories of information related to the structure (composition) and function (roles and actions) of the family need to be examined.

Communication Patterns

Communication patterns (not only what people say, but also how they say it) are determined by culture and are increasingly important during times of stress (Copeland & Douglas, 1999). People who ordinarily associate only with members of their own culture, speaking their native language, may have great difficulty detailing a health history in English to a health care provider. Language barriers can be particularly significant for people who must give health histories when they or their child is ill, because their ability to cope and to express themselves in English may be at a low point. Even if people are able to converse well in English at work or in stores, they may not be able to recall the English words for symptoms such as nausea or dizziness, because these are not words that are commonly used. This person might omit mentioning a symptom rather than try to pantomime it or describe it in a different way.

Children who are embarrassed or bashful about speaking may simply not talk, and thus their needs may go unmet. As a general rule, it is unfair to ask children to inter-

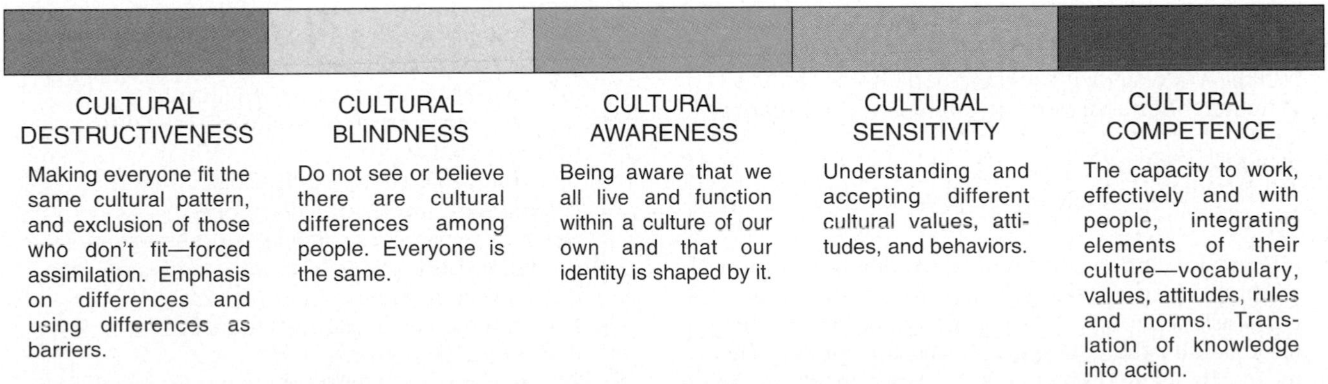

CULTURAL DESTRUCTIVENESS
Making everyone fit the same cultural pattern, and exclusion of those who don't fit—forced assimilation. Emphasis on differences and using differences as barriers.
CULTURAL BLINDNESS
Do not see or believe there are cultural differences among people. Everyone is the same.
CULTURAL AWARENESS
Being aware that we all live and function within a culture of our own and that our identity is shaped by it.
CULTURAL SENSITIVITY
Understanding and accepting different cultural values, attitudes, and behaviors.
CULTURAL COMPETENCE
The capacity to work, effectively and with people, integrating elements of their culture—vocabulary, values, attitudes, rules and norms. Translation of knowledge into action.

FIGURE 3.3 Cultural competence continuum. (Courtesy of the National Council of La Raza.)

pret for their parents. If a child is frequently asked to interpret for his or her parents, he or she may be forced to miss days of school. Translating also can place a child in situations that require adult judgment. In some cultures, it might be unacceptable for a younger person to serve as an interpreter for an older person, because this shifts authority (see Focus on Communication).

The terms "Hispanic" and "Latina" or "Latino" refer to people who identify with a Spanish culture. There are about 16 million documented persons of Mexican, Puerto Rican, Cuban, or other Spanish-speaking origin in the United States. When added to the number of Spanish-speaking people who are undocumented or living illegally in the country, this group numbers close to 25 million, or about 12% of the total U.S. population (U.S. Census Bureau, 2000). Health care providers and Hispanic communities are encouraged to work together to bridge communication gaps.

Communication problems arise not only from foreign languages but also from dialects within a country. Something as simple as a New Englander adding an "r" sound to the end of words ("idear" instead of "idea") may make an explanation difficult to follow. The slow cadence of a person from the South may seem strange to someone used to the rapid speech pattern of residents of New York City. Inner-city residents often speak a dialect unique to them. To care for such clients, it is important to learn their dialect's cadence and common words without attempting to use them yourself, unless that is your dialect. Trying to speak in a dialect not your own could be misinterpreted as mockery.

Touch is a form of communication. Whether people greet one another with hugs and kisses or do not touch each other at all is culturally determined. Not all people like to be touched or even to shake hands. For instance, some Vietnamese Americans feel that rumpling the hair or palpating fontanelles is an intrusive gesture because they believe the head is the seat of the body's spirit and should not be touched.

Whether people look at one another when talking is also culturally determined. Chinese Americans, for example, may not make eye contact during a conversation. This social custom shows respect for the position of the health care professional and is a compliment, not an avoidance issue (Box 3-1).

Be certain that cultural variations are respected in written as well as oral communications. In many instances, written communication can be even more problematic than oral communication: many people can speak a second language but cannot write or read it. Using short, easy sentences and being certain not to use words with double meanings are effective techniques.

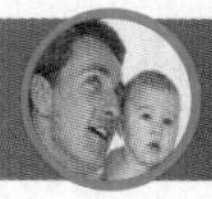

FOCUS ON COMMUNICATION

Anna Polinski is a Russian immigrant who brings her 6-year-old daughter, Lisinka, to a pediatric clinic because she thinks the child has an ear infection. Anna does not speak English. She has brought a neighbor as an interpreter.

Less Effective Communication

Nurse: What's the reason you're here today?
Neighbor: She thinks her daughter has an ear infection.
Nurse: Is Lisinka pulling or tugging at it?
Neighbor: Not that I've seen.
Nurse: Does she have any pain?
Neighbor: She hasn't said anything about that.
Nurse: Well, I'll take her temperature, but I doubt it's an infection.

More Effective Communication

Nurse: What's the reason you're here today?
Neighbor: She thinks her daughter has an ear infection.
Nurse: Ask the mother if Lisinka has been pulling or tugging at it.
Neighbor: I haven't seen her doing that.
Nurse: Ask her mother.
[The neighbor addresses the mother and then reports back.]
Neighbor: She says Lisinka was pulling at it all morning.
Nurse: Ask Lisinka if she has any pain.
[The neighbor addresses the child and then reports back.]
Neighbor: She says yes.
Nurse: Those are symptoms of an ear infection, all right.

Effectively using an interpreter adds additional responsibility to history taking. The nurse in the first scenario asked her first question of the mother but then directed all other questions to the interpreter. This means she secured a secondary history. When using an interpreter, be certain the interpreter is "interpreting," not giving the history.

BOX 3.1

METHODS TO IMPROVE HEALTH CARE WHEN CLIENTS DO NOT SPEAK ENGLISH AS THEIR PRIMARY LANGUAGE

1. Reading printed material may be difficult for the client. Assess the reading level and rewrite information at an easier reading level.
2. Ask an interpreter to translate material into other languages.
3. Be certain that rooms such as bathrooms are labeled with international symbols.
4. Learn a few phrases, such as "Good morning" or "This won't hurt," from other languages, and use them in interactions with clients.
5. Use hand gestures or draw a figure to communicate better.
6. When using an interpreter, do not ignore the person seeking health care in preference to the interpreter.

Use of Conversational Space

People of different cultures use the space around them differently. In the Western world, physical examinations are conducted in a very tight (intimate) space because palpation is a part of the examination. Conversation, on the other hand, is usually held at a distance of between 18 inches and 4 feet. Business is most often conducted at a 4-foot distance. People from Eastern cultures may not be comfortable in this same space. Being aware that use of space is culturally determined helps you to respect the use of space for clients.

Respect for modesty is a way to respect close space. Be aware that women from some Middle Eastern cultures adhere to a level of modesty exceeding what one may be used to.

Time Orientation

The cultural pattern in the United States is geared toward punctuality regarding appointments. "Time is money" is an often-quoted axiom. Other cultures may not have this concern for time. They may have, instead, a concept that time is to be enjoyed. For such a person, there is no such thing as wasted time. In some South Asian cultures, being late for appointments is a sign of respect (giving the person you are meeting time to organize and be prepared for your arrival). Women who do not have a strict time orientation may view as strange the hospital's practice of feeding infants at designated times (e.g., 10 AM, 2 PM). People who are not accustomed to adhering to schedules this way may have difficulty following a strict medical regimen. If they are told, for example, to give a child a medication at 8 AM, noon, and 6 PM daily and to return for another appointment at 2 PM in a week's time, you may have to stress that the medication should be taken three times a day, not necessarily at the specific times, but that returning for a checkup at a set time is important because the physician is in the health care facility only at that time.

Another way that time orientation differs is in whether a culture concentrates on the past, the present, or the future. The dominant U.S. culture is oriented to the present and future. People are expected not only to take care of themselves at the present moment but also to make plans for the future. Other cultures are oriented toward the past: they carefully preserve traditions, allowing only the slightest change or variations in practices. Others are oriented toward the present; saving money for college (a future-oriented action) may not be a high priority in these cultures. If a family's orientation is for the present or the past, members may have difficulty accepting a long-term rehabilitation plan (e.g., by 6 months a brain-injured boy will be walking with crutches, and it will be a full year before he will be fully ambulatory again). They may need to be motivated by present indications of progress (e.g., this afternoon the child will be allowed to sit up for the first time; this evening he can begin to have periods of time without oxygen).

The Amish are an example of a past-oriented culture: they adhere to time-honored traditions and do not accept modern technological advances such as immunizations. Some Native Americans also hold a past orientation. People from lower socioeconomic groups tend to be more present-oriented than those in middle or higher socioeconomic groups because of the struggle just to get through each day. People with strong religious convictions may be future-oriented (looking forward to a future existence better than their present one). Knowledge of these time orientations helps to plan effective care.

Work Orientation

The predominant culture in the United States stresses that everyone should be employed productively (called the Protestant work ethic) and that work should be a pleasure and valued in itself (as important as the product of the work). Other cultures do not value work in itself but see it as a means to an end (you work to get money or food, not satisfaction). A woman with this latter orientation might be more distressed to learn that bedrest during pregnancy will interfere with her ability to continue a hobby (going to baseball games) than with her occupation (teaching). Do not interpret this behavior as lazy or unproductive; it is merely a cultural or individual variation.

Family Orientation

Family structure and the roles of family members may be culturally determined. In most cultures, the nuclear family (mother, father, and children) is most common. In other cultures, extended families (nuclear family plus grandparents, aunts, uncles, and cousins) and single-parent families (single parent and child) may be more common. When caring for children, be certain to identify a child's primary caregiver before giving health care instructions if the family is not typical. Spouses serve as important support people during labor, so knowing whether someone fulfills this role is important (Sagrestano et al., 1999). Identifying the family decision-maker is also important because it may differ from the family member who provides support. Information about a family may be carefully guarded and not given freely at health care visits as a way of keeping the family intact and unique (and as a reflection of mistrust for health care providers).

Male and Female Roles

In most cultures, the man is the dominant figure. In such a culture, if approval for hospital admission or therapy is needed, it would be the man who would give this approval. In a culture where men are very dominant and women are extremely passive, a woman may be unable to offer an opinion of her own health or might be embarrassed to submit to a physical examination, especially from a male physician or nurse practitioner, unless a female nurse is also present. The incidence of intimate partner violence may be higher in male-dominant cultures (Alkon et al., 2001). In an extremely male-dominated family, a woman's pregnancy may have resulted not from a mutual decision but from sexual relations she felt she could not refuse.

In contrast, in some cultures, the woman may be the dominant person in the family. The oldest woman in the home would be the person who would give consent for treatment or hospital admission.

It is important to evaluate male and female roles because knowing the identity of the dominant person in the household also helps you to understand the impact of the illness on the family. If a woman is the family's dominant person and can no longer make her usual decisions because she is ill during pregnancy, for example, the entire family may be thrown into confusion. If the woman is a nondominant member, you may have to act as an advocate for her rights with a more dominant person.

In most hospitals today, the nursing staff expects the father to play an active role during labor and during a child's hospital stay. However, a man who does not maintain this role expectation or custom may be uncomfortable participating in labor or playing with a child. Awareness that male roles differ from country to country can help you find a middle ground for male participation in labor and childcare.

WHAT IF? What if a father says he wants to take no role in labor? Would you encourage him to time contractions (a typical role for fathers) or allow him to sit quietly in a corner of the room, as he prefers?

Religion

Religion is culturally determined, although there are wide variations in what religions people practice. Because religion guides a person's overall life philosophy, it influences how he or she feels about health and illness. Knowing what religion a family practices helps you locate a support person when needed, because this differs according to religion. It helps you in planning care because many nutrition practices, such as whether the family eats meat, can be dictated by religious beliefs. It can have important implications for decision-making during a difficult pregnancy or for childhood terminal care (Callister et al., 1999).

Health Beliefs

Health beliefs are not universal. Most people are familiar with the current controversy about whether male circumcision is necessary, for example. More surprising to most people is a belief that female circumcision (amputation of the clitoris and perhaps a portion of the vulva) is thought to be necessary in some cultures (Fourcroy, 1999).

It is generally assumed in the United States that illness is caused by documented factors such as bacteria, viruses, or trauma. In other cultures, however, illness may be viewed primarily as a punishment from God, an evil spirit, or the work of a person who wishes harm to the sick person. An example of this is a belief among some Hispanics that an evil eye (*mal ojo*) can cause illness. People who believe that their own sins caused an illness may not be highly motivated to take medication or other measures to get well again (such a woman when ill during a pregnancy does not believe that a spoonful of penicillin will cure her). People from some cultures may receive more comfort from a spiritualist or "witch doctor" than from their physician or nurse practitioner. They may believe it is necessary to suffer pain to be rid of the illness. People with this belief might be reluctant to ask for pain medication. Understanding different beliefs this way allows you to understand cultural differences and to work out mutual goals, even when the patient's views are not those you would choose for yourself or a member of your family (see Focus on Nursing Care Planning).

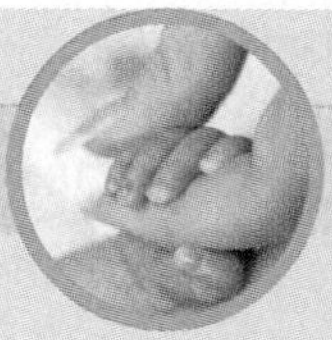

FOCUS ON *Nursing Care Planning*

A CHILD REQUIRING SOCIOCULTURAL CARE

An 8-year-old Chinese-American boy undergoes surgery for a ruptured appendix. Now, 36 hours after surgery, the child is started on a clear liquid diet with orders to advance as tolerated. He has not asked for any pain medication since returning from surgery.

Assessment: Temperature, 99.4°F; pulse, 96; respirations, 24. Seen lying on side with knees and hips flexed toward abdomen. Hands clenched and eyes tearing. When asked about pain, quietly stated, "I'm okay." Incisional dressing clean, dry, and intact. Bowel sounds active in all four quadrants. Intravenous fluids infusing without difficulty at keep vein open rate; intravenous antibiotics given every 6 hours. Diet progressed to soft. Oral intake primarily tea and soup. Client's mother states, "I want him to eat 'hot' foods." Family members and visitors present.

Nursing Diagnosis: Pain related to tissue trauma of surgery and cultural belief of not voicing concerns

Outcome Identification: Client will demonstrate pain level is within tolerable limits nonverbally.

Outcome Evaluation: Client accepts pain medication when offered; nonverbal expressions of pain are minimal to absent.

(continued)

Interventions	Rationale
1. Assess for nonverbal indicators of pain.	1. Verbalizing pain is culturally determined.
2. Offer pain medication as ordered.	2. Offering medications alleviates the need for the client to ask for relief when his belief is that he should not complain. It also allows the child to have some choice and control in his care.
3. Explain the concept of pain and why the client is experiencing it.	3. Explanations help a child of this age understand what is happening to him, thus minimizing any fears.
4. Assess the child's response to medications given.	4. Follow-up assessment is necessary to determine the degree of relief obtained.
5. Assist the child in using nonpharmacologic measures, such as guided imagery and deep breathing.	5. Nonpharmacologic methods are an effective means of pain control.

Nursing Diagnosis: Imbalanced nutrition, less than body requirements, related to limited caloric intake postoperatively and cultural beliefs about food and illness

Outcome Identification: Client will ingest culturally appropriate, nutritionally adequate foods.

Outcome Evaluation: Client verbalizes food likes and dislikes; ingests at least ¾ of food supplied on his meal trays. Family identifies culturally appropriate food selections.

Interventions	Rationale
1. Explain to the child and family the need for adequate consumption of nutrients and calories.	1. Adequate nutrition postoperatively is essential for optimal wound healing.
2. Question the child about likes and dislikes. Investigate the meaning of "hot" foods with the child's mother.	2. Ascertaining the child's likes and dislikes and information about "hot" foods provides a baseline for food suggestions.
3. Obtain a dietary consult to assist with menu planning. Encourage the family to bring foods from home.	3. Assistance from the dietitian ensures a nutritionally sound diet with culturally acceptable foods. Allowing the family to bring in foods demonstrates respect for the culture and increases the possibility that the child will increase his intake.

Women's concept of whether pregnancy is a time of wellness or illness differs in various cultures. Many American women visit health care facilities early in pregnancy, follow prenatal directives, and, at birth, allow a health care provider to supervise the birth. In other cultures, pregnancy and childbearing are considered such natural processes that a health care provider is unnecessary. The woman knows the special rules and taboos she must follow to ensure a safe birth and healthy child, and she is an active participant in labor and birth. She may plan to breastfeed until the next child is born, or as long as 1 to 5 years. Unless differences such as these are respected, it is difficult to plan prenatal care that meets the woman's needs.

The type of health care provider chosen is yet another trait that is not uniform across cultures. The health care delivery system in Mexico, for example, is less structured than the one in the United States. There are few physicians for the total population. Many drugs are available without prescription; therefore, a local pharmacist rather than a physician may serve as the main health care resource for many families. Families may first seek help for illness from a trusted family member. Such a member is termed *el que sabe* (the one who knows). During an illness, this person's approval of therapy is crucial; if it is not given, the ill person cannot comply with therapy. Outside the family structure are *yerberos* (herbalists) who grow and instruct people in the use of herbs or cures. Another advice source is a *curandero,* or one who heals by the use of herbs or diet. Others healers are *experitualistos,* who can treat supernaturally caused illnesses, and *brujos,* who not only revoke evil spells but also turn them around onto others. *Parteras* are midwives who care for women during pregnancy and birth. For many people, turning to a *yerbero* or *curandero* is preferable to professional health care because these people do not charge a fee but only accept donations or an exchange of goods or services. Also, relating health problems to them is not difficult because there is no language problem.

✔ CHECKPOINT QUESTIONS

6. Is touching someone a comforting gesture in all cultures?
7. How can differing time orientations interfere with health care?

Nutrition Practices

Foods and their methods of preparation are strongly culturally related (O'Dea, 1999). In many instances, hospitalized children cannot find on the menu any foods that appeal to them because of cultural preferences. A Japanese diet, for example, includes many vegetables such as bean sprouts, broccoli, mushrooms, water chestnuts, and alfalfa. Children with this preference could tire very quickly of the corn and peas common to a middle-class American diet. Fortunately, in most instances, a child's family can provide food that is appealing culturally and is still within prescribed dietary limitations (Fig. 3-4).

When counseling a woman about good nutrition during pregnancy, remember that respect for culturally preferred foods is important. Mexican-American women, for example, tend not to eat a large amount of meat compared with other cultures. Adequate protein can be ingested, however, by mixing sources of incomplete protein such as beans and rice. Some women may omit various foods during pregnancy because they believe a particular food will mark a baby (strawberries cause birthmarks, raisins cause brown spots) or they believe that it is necessary to eat "hot" or "cold" foods to ensure fetal growth. Pregnancy is considered a "hot" condition and pork is considered a "hot" food. It may be difficult for a woman who is trying to eat only "cold" foods to agree to increase her intake of meat, including pork, during pregnancy. Asian women may believe in a similar pattern of required balances (yin and yang).

Be aware of what is available in local food stores. Women who cannot buy the foods you recommend in their own neighborhood may not eat well because of the inconvenience involved in shopping elsewhere.

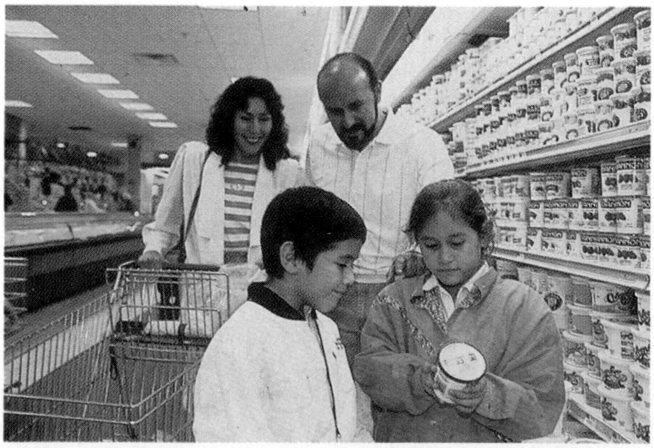

FIGURE 3.4 Families differ as to what food selections they prefer because of sociocultural preferences.

Another trait that is ethnically determined is lactose intolerance. This is the absence of lactase, the enzyme that breaks down the sugar (lactose) in milk so it can be used by the body. People with lactose intolerance (many Asians and blacks) cannot drink milk because of lactase deficiency.

Pain Responses

A person's response to pain is both individually and culturally determined. Although people may all have the same **threshold sensation** (the amount of stimulus that results in pain), their **pain threshold** (the point at which the individual reports that a stimulus is painful) and **pain tolerance** (the point at which an individual withdraws from a stimulus) vary greatly.

A person's culture dictates attitudes toward pain and the proper response to pain. One woman in labor, therefore, might report labor contractions as "agonizing" and scream each time she feels one, whereas the woman in the bed next to her might report her pain as tolerable and barely change her facial expression with contractions.

Caring for a person having pain can be problematic when the caregiver's concept of "proper" responses to pain differs from the patient's. Because there are so many possible responses to pain, it is important to assess each person individually. Further assessment of pain and its meaning to people is discussed in Chapters 19 and 38.

WHAT IF? What if a child shows no expression on his face after a bad burn (which you know must be painful)? How would you determine if he is really not feeling pain or if he is just not expressing it?

KEY POINTS

Culture is an organized structure that guides behavior into acceptable ways for that group. Usual customs are termed mores or norms. Actions that are not acceptable to a culture are taboos.

Each culture differs to some degree from every other. Most people are proud of these differences or cultural traits.

Culture is transmitted by both formal and informal ways from generation to generation.

Although cultural concepts adapt from time to time, they tend to remain constant.

Cultural practices arise from environmental conditions.

There is wide variation within a culture concerning values and actions because individuals make up the group and individually express their cultural heritage.

People bring cultural values and beliefs to nursing interactions, and these affect nursing and health care.

Cultural aspects that are important to assess are communication patterns; use of conversational space; response to pain; time, work, and family orientation; and social organization, including nutrition, family roles, and health beliefs.

CRITICAL THINKING EXERCISES

1. Anna Rodriques is the 12-year-old child you met at the beginning of the chapter. What went wrong with her care? If you had actually planned care in this way, of what would you have been guilty? What would have been a better approach for determining this family's cultural preferences? Supposing Anna is present-oriented: how would you approach discussions of a long-term rehabilitation program for her?
2. During a home visit with a woman who is 30 weeks' pregnant, you inquire why she has not gone yet for prenatal care. She states that before coming to the clinic she wants to visit a herbalist who will both predict her child's sex and guarantee a safe birth. Would recommending that she have a sonogram (which also could predict the fetal sex) be likely to be as satisfying for her?
3. Describe a situation when you had a conflict with a person of another culture. List your behaviors. List the behaviors of the other person. Identify the cultural values that prompted you to have these feelings and expectations, and consider the cultural values that may have prompted the other person to behave as he or she did.
4. Examine the National Health Goals related to sociocultural aspects of health care. Most government-sponsored money for nursing research is allotted based on these goals. What would be a possible research topic to explore pertinent to these goals that would be fundable and would advance evidence-based practice?

REFERENCES

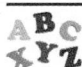

Alkon, A., et al. (2001). A violence-prevention and evaluation project with ethnically diverse populations. *American Journal of Preventive Medicine, 20*(1), 48–55.

Callister, L. C., Semenic, S., & Foster, J. C. (1999). Cultural and spiritual meanings of childbirth: Orthodox Jewish and Mormon women. *Journal of Holistic Nursing, 17*(3), 280–295.

Copeland, D. B., & Douglas, D. (1999). Communication strategies for the intrapartum nurse. *Journal of Obstetric, Gynecologic & Neonatal Nursing, 28*(6), 579–586.

Department of Health and Human Services. (2000). *Healthy people 2010.* Washington, D.C.: DHHS.

Elam, C. L. et al. (2001). Diversity in medical school. *Academic Medicine, 76*(1), 60–65.

Fourcroy, J. L. (1999). Female circumcision. *American Family Physician, 60*(2), 657–658.

Josten, L. E. et al. (2002). Dropping out of maternal and child home visits. *Public Health Nursing, 19*(1), 3–10.

Leininger, M. M. (Ed.). (2001). *Culture, care, diversity, and universality: A theory of nursing.* Sudbury, MA: Jones & Bartlett.

Mayberry, L. J., Affonso, D. D., Shibuya, J., & Clemmens, D. (1999). Integrating cultural values, beliefs, and customs into pregnancy and postpartum care. *Journal of Perinatal & Neonatal Nursing, 13*(1), 15–26.

Munoz, R. A. (2001). Rethinking ethnicity and health care: A sociocultural perspective. *American Journal of Psychiatry, 158*(1), 156–162.

O'Dea, J. A. (1999). Children and adolescents identify food concerns, forbidden foods, and food-related beliefs. *Journal of the American Dietetic Association, 99*(8), 970–973.

Sagrestano, L. M. et al. (1999). Ethnicity and social support during pregnancy. *American Journal of Community Psychology, 27*(6), 869–898.

U.S. Census Bureau. (2000). *Population projection program.* Washington, D.C.: Population Division.

SUGGESTED READINGS

Berry, A. B. (1999). Mexican American women's expressions of the meaning of culturally congruent perinatal care. *Journal of Transcultural Nursing, 10*(3), 203–212.

Gichia, J. E. (2000). Mothers and others: African American women's preparation for motherhood. *MCN, American Journal of Maternal Child Nursing, 25*(2), 86–91.

Greenfield, P. M., Quiroz, B., & Raeff, C. (2000). Cross-cultural conflict and harmony in the social construction of the child. *New Directions for Child & Adolescent Development, 1*(87), 93–108.

Hickey, C. A. (2000). Sociocultural and behavioral influences on weight gain during pregnancy. *American Journal of Clinical Nutrition, 71*(5 Suppl), 1364S–1370S.

Lipman, E. L. et al. (2002). Child well-being in single-mother families. *Journal of the American Academy of Child & Adolescent Psychiatry, 41*(1), 75–82.

Mann, R. J., Abercrombie, P. D., DeJoseph, J., Norbeck, J. S., & Smith, R. T. (1999). The personal experience of pregnancy for African-American women. *Journal of Transcultural Nursing, 10*(4), 297–305.

Willis, W. O. (1999). Culturally competent nursing care during the prenatal period. *Journal of Perinatal & Neonatal Nursing, 13*(3), 45–59.

Wilson, A. H., & Robledo, L. (1999). Listening to Hispanic mothers: Guidelines for teaching. *Journal of the Society of Pediatric Nurses, 4*(3), 125–127.

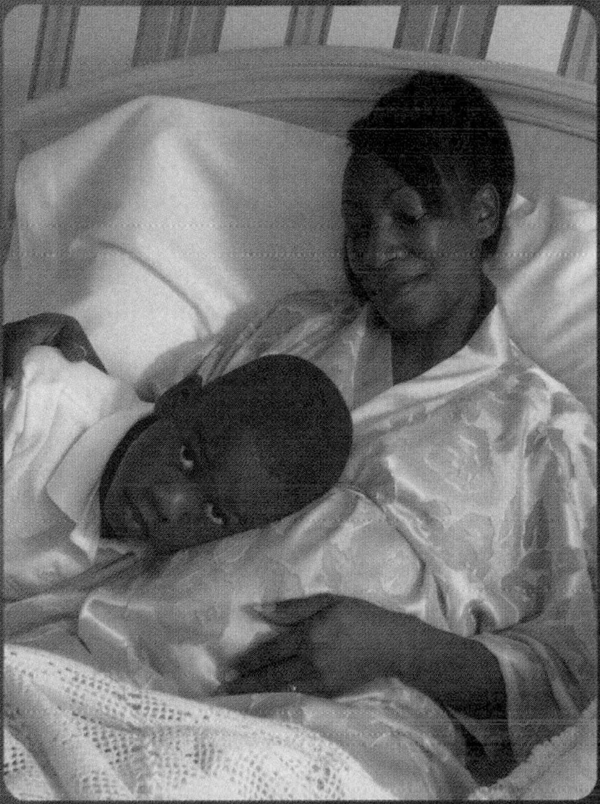

The Nursing Role in Preparing Families for Childbearing and Childrearing

UNIT

II

4

CHAPTER

Reproductive and Sexual Health

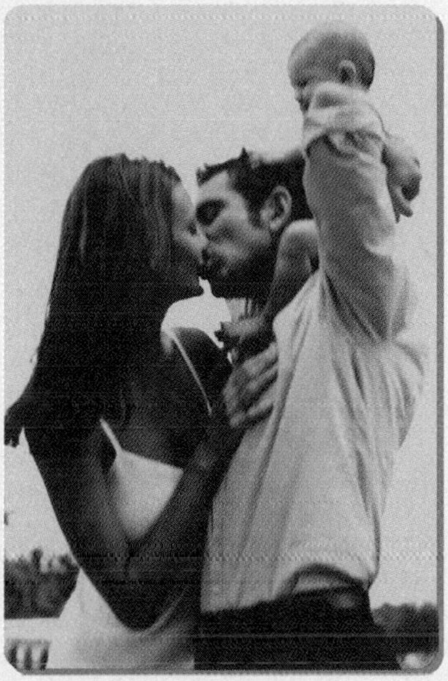

Key Terms

- adrenarche
- andrology
- anteflexion
- anteversion
- aspermia
- bicornuate uterus
- biologic gender
- culdoscopy
- cystocele
- dyspareunia
- endocervix
- endometrium
- erectile dysfunction
- gender identity
- gender role
- gonad
- gynecology
- gynecomastia
- heterosexual
- homosexual
- laparoscopy
- lesbian
- menarche
- menorrhagia
- metrorrhagia
- myometrium
- menopause
- oocyte
- perimetrium
- premature ejaculation
- rectocele
- retroflexion
- retroversion
- thelarche
- transsexual
- transvestite
- vaginismus
- voyeurism

Objectives

After mastering the contents of this chapter, you should be able to:

1. Describe anatomy and physiology necessary for reproductive and sexual health.
2. Assess a couple for anatomic and physiologic readiness for child-bearing, biologic gender, gender role, and gender identity.
3. Formulate nursing diagnoses related to reproductive or sexual health.
4. Identify appropriate outcomes for reproductive and sexual health education.
5. Plan nursing care related to anatomic and physiologic readiness for child-bearing or sexual health, such as helping adolescents discuss concerns in these areas.
6. Implement nursing care related to reproductive health, such as educating about menstruation.
7. Evaluate outcome criteria for achievement and effectiveness of care.
8. Identify National Health Goals related to reproductive health and sexuality and specific ways that nurses can help the nation achieve these goals.
9. Identify areas of care in relation to reproductive and sexual health that could benefit from additional nursing research or application of evidence-based practice.
10. Use critical thinking to analyze ways that clients' reproductive and sexual health can be improved for healthier childbearing and adult health.
11. Integrate knowledge of reproductive health and sexuality with nursing process to achieve quality maternal and child health nursing care.

You have been asked to teach a class on sexual and reproductive health to eighth-grade students. A boy in the first row asks why he has to learn about female reproduction. A girl who hasn't begun menstruation as yet asks you to predict when she will have her first period. The boy behind her says he doesn't believe sex education should be taught in school. How would you respond to these questions?

Previous chapters presented the scope of maternal and child health and how the structure and function of families can have an impact on health. This chapter adds information about how to educate children, women, and their partners about anatomy, physiology, and sexuality to your knowledge base.

After you've studied the chapter, answer the Critical Thinking Exercises at the end of the chapter and then access the on-line study activities (http://connection.lww.com) *to further sharpen your skills and test your knowledge.*

Whether people are planning on childbearing or not, everyone is wiser by being familiar with reproductive anatomy and physiology and his or her own body's reproductive and sexual health. Women and their partners who are planning for childbearing may be especially curious about reproductive physiology and the changes the pregnant woman will undergo, so this is an opportune time to educate both partners about reproductive and gynecologic health.

Sexuality, in particular, is a major area of concern for adolescents and individuals or families of childbearing age. The nurse who cares for childbearing or childrearing families can be asked a variety of detailed questions about sexuality.

Although the general public is becoming increasingly sophisticated about their bodies, misunderstandings about sexuality, conception (preventing or promoting), and childbearing still abound. For instance, many young adults want to know what is considered a "normal" sexual response or the "normal" expected frequency for sexual relations. A general rule of thumb in answering this question is that normal sexual behavior includes any act mutually satisfying to both sexual partners. Actual frequency and type of sexual activity vary widely.

One of the biggest contributions nurses can make is to encourage clients to ask questions about sexual and reproductive functioning. With this attitude, problems of sexuality and reproduction are brought out into the open and made as resolvable as other health concerns or problems (see Focus on Multidisciplinary Care).

Nurses who can clearly explain the physical and emotional changes of puberty to the adolescent, the physiologic changes of pregnancy to a young adult couple, or the expected changes of menopause to a middle-aged woman provide much-needed health teaching information. A number of National Health Goals that speak directly to improving reproductive or sexual health are shown in the Focus on National Health Goals.

NURSING PROCESS OVERVIEW

For Promotion of Reproductive and Sexual Health

Assessment

Problems of sexuality or reproductive health may not be evident on first meeting a client because it may be difficult for that person to bring up the topic until he or she feels more secure. Good follow-through and planning are important because a person may find the courage to discuss a problem once but then be unable to do so again. If the problem is ignored or forgotten through a change in caregivers, it may never be addressed again.

Any change in physical appearance (such as happens with puberty or with pregnancy) can intensify or create a sexual or reproductive concern. The person with a sexually transmitted disease (STD), excessive weight loss or gain, a disfiguring scar from surgery or an accident, hair loss such as occurs with chemotherapy, surgery or inflammation or infection of reproductive organs, chronic fatigue or pain, spinal cord injury, or the presence of a retention catheter needs to be assessed for problems regarding his or her sexual role as well as other important areas of reproductive functioning.

This may not be a routine part of every health assessment. However, it should be included when appropriate, such as when discussing adolescent development or before providing reproductive life planning information, during pregnancy, or after childbirth. At other times, it is wise to listen for verbal or nonverbal clues that suggest a person wants to discuss a sexual or reproductive concern. These clues are often subtle: "I guess marriage isn't for

FOCUS ON MULTIDISCIPLINARY CARE

Unlicensed assistive personnel are often assigned to help with patient care, so are often the people who are asked questions about value-laden topics such as sexuality or sexual preference. Educate unlicensed assistive personnel that people need to know about their body's anatomy and physiology and to have their questions about sexuality answered without bias. Teach them to reply to a question they do not know the answer to with, "I don't know the answer to that, but I'll ask your nurse and find out."

Questions about sexual functioning may also be asked of health care partners such as physical or occupational therapists. Help them alert you to the type of questions your patients are asking to keep you informed and possibly identify a topic where you need to initiate a discussion.

FOCUS ON NATIONAL HEALTH GOALS

A number of National Health Goals speak directly to reproductive and sexual health. Here are some of them:

- Reduce the proportion of adolescents who have engaged in sexual intercourse to no more than 15% by age 15 from a baseline of 27% of girls and 33% of boys.
- Increase to at least 50% the proportion of sexually active, unmarried people who used a condom at last sexual intercourse from a baseline of 19%.
- Reduce deaths from cancer of the uterine cervix to no more than 1.3 per 100,000 women from a baseline of 2.8 per 100,000.
- Reduce breast cancer deaths to no more than 20.6 per 100,000 women from a baseline of 23 per 100,000 (DHHS, 2000).

Nurses can be instrumental in helping the nation achieve these goals by educating adolescents about abstinence and refusal skills, safer sex practices, and the need to participate in screening activities such as breast or testicular self-examination as they grow into adulthood, as well as conduct research to investigate better ways to teach self-examination.

everyone"; "I'm not the woman I used to be"; "Are there ever funny effects from this medicine I'm taking?" Telling a seemingly inappropriate sexual joke may be yet another clue. Nonverbal clues may include extreme modesty or obvious embarrassment in response to a question about voiding or perineal pain or stitches.

Assessment in the area of reproductive health begins with interviewing clients to determine what they know about the reproductive process and STDs. Any concerns they might have about their own reproductive functioning or safe sex practices should be explored. This area of health interviewing takes practice and the conviction that exploring sexual health is as important as exploring less emotionally involved areas of health, such as dietary intake or activity level. The 14-year-old girl who is not yet menstruating, for instance, may be anxious about that fact but may be reluctant to say so unless asked directly. A statement such as the following invites discussion: "Although many of your friends at school may be menstruating already, it's not at all uncommon for some girls not to begin their periods until age 15 or 16. How do you feel about not yet having your period?" This combination of providing information and questioning may encourage the girl to discuss not only her possible concern about delayed menarche, but other areas that will show her knowledge or lack of knowledge about reproductive health. Specific questions to include in a sexual history are shown in Box 4-1.

Important steps to include in physical examination are to observe for normal distribution of body hair (i.e., hair on arms, axilla, and triangle-shaped pubic hair in women; diamond-shaped pubic hair in men) and normal genital and breast development. Also, observe for signs and symptoms of STDs. Many STDs are asymptomatic, so it is important to assess whether the client is at risk for contracting a STD (see Chap. 32 for documentation of stages of sexual development and signs of STDs).

Nursing Diagnosis

Common nursing diagnoses used in regard to reproductive health are:

- Health-seeking behaviors related to reproductive functioning
- Anxiety related to inability to conceive after 6 months without birth control
- Pain related to uterine cramping from menstruation
- Disturbance in body image related to early development of secondary sex characteristics

Diagnoses relevant to sexuality include:

- Sexual dysfunction related to as yet unknown cause
- Altered sexuality patterns related to chronic illness
- Self-esteem disturbance related to recent reproductive tract surgery
- Altered sexuality patterns related to fear of harming the fetus
- Anxiety related to fear of contracting an STD
- Health-seeking behavior related to learning responsible sexual practices

BOX 4.1

SPECIFIC QUESTIONS TO INCLUDE IN A SEXUAL HISTORY

Are you sexually active?
Is your sexual partner of the same or different gender?
How many sexual partners have you had in the past 6 months?
Are you satisfied with your sex life? If not, why not?
Do you have any concerns about your sex life? If so, what are they?
Do you practice "safer sex"?
Have you ever contracted a sexually transmitted disease or been worried that you have one?
Have you ever experienced a problem such as erectile dysfunction, failure to achieve orgasm, or pain during intercourse?
Are you using a method to prevent pregnancy or sexually transmitted diseases?
Are you satisfied with your current family planning method, or do you have any questions about it?

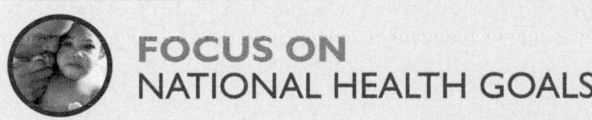

Outcome Identification and Planning

A major part of nursing care in this area is to empower clients to feel control over their bodies. Thus, health teaching should be planned to provide clients with knowledge about the reproductive system and specific information about ways to alleviate discomfort or prevent reproductive disease. It may also be important to plan interventions to strengthen the person's gender identity or role behavior. It is essential to design care that demonstrates acceptance of all lifestyles equally.

Implementation

The primary role of the nurse concerning reproductive anatomy and physiology is education. This is a major role because both female and male clients may feel more comfortable asking questions of nurses than other health care providers. To help clients understand reproductive functioning and sexual health throughout their life, specific teaching might include:

- Explaining to a school-age boy that nocturnal emissions are normal
- Teaching an early adolescent what is normal and abnormal in relation to menstrual function
- Teaching an adolescent safer sex practices
- Explaining reproductive physiology to the couple who wishes to become pregnant

Teaching is often enhanced by the use of illustrations from books or journals, clips from videos or compact disks, or models of internal and external reproductive systems. Nursing interventions in this area, however, include much more than just distributing educational materials. For example, empathy for a woman's concern of increased tension before menstruation may help validate her concern that she has premenstrual dysphoric syndrome. Serving as a role model for gender roles can also be a valuable intervention, particularly for young clients. Discussing the subject of reproduction in a matter-of-fact way, or treating menstruation as a positive sign of growth as a woman rather than as a burden, may help clients assume a positive attitude about these subjects from the start.

Interventions that strengthen an individual's sense of maleness or femaleness may improve a client's gender identity or role behavior. A woman who believes that part of a female role is to be assertive needs opportunities in her care plan for making decisions and self-care; a hospitalized adolescent who views a man's role as being a person who watches Monday night football needs time structured for this activity at the same priority level as other activities. Unless such activities are structured, they can be easily omitted by busy health care providers.

Homosexual clients, or others with alternative lifestyles, usually reveal their sexual orientation to health care providers because they want help dealing with friends or family who are having difficulty accepting their gender identity. A helpful referral organization is the Children of Lesbians and Gays Everywhere group (*www.colage.org*). In addition to support, provide health education that addresses potential concerns of gay or lesbian clients. For example, include a discussion about anal or oral-genital sex practices when presenting information on safer sex.

Evaluation

Evaluation in the area of reproductive health must be ongoing because health education needs change with circumstances and increased maturity. For example, the needs of a woman at the beginning of a pregnancy may be totally different than her needs at the end.

How people feel about themselves sexually has a great deal to do with how quickly they recover from an illness, how quickly they are ready to begin self-care after childbirth, or even how well motivated they are as adolescents to accomplish activities in other life phases that depend on being sure of sexuality or gender role.

Examples of expected outcomes are:

- Client states he is no longer fearful of contracting an STD.
- Client states she is better able to control symptoms of premenstrual dysphoric syndrome.
- Couple states they have achieved a mutually satisfying sexual relationship.
- Client states he is ready to tell family about gay gender identity.

REPRODUCTIVE DEVELOPMENT

Physiologic readiness for childbearing begins during intrauterine life; full function is initiated at puberty when the hypothalamus synthesizes and releases gonadotropin-releasing factor stimulator (GnRf), which in turn triggers the anterior pituitary to begin to release follicle-stimulating hormone (FSH) and luteinizing hormone (LH). FSH and LH initiate the production of androgen and estrogen, which in turn initiate visible signs of maturity or secondary sex characteristics.

Intrauterine Development

The sex of an individual is determined at the moment of conception by the chromosome information of the particular ovum and sperm that joined to create the new life. A **gonad** is a body organ that produces sex cells (the ovary in females and the testis in males). At approximately week 5 of intrauterine life, primitive gonadal tissue is already formed. In both sexes, two undifferentiated ducts, the mesonephric (wolffian) and paramesonephric (müllerian) ducts, are present. By week 7 or 8, in chromosomal males, this early gonadal tissue differentiates into primitive testes and begins formation of testosterone. Under the influence of testosterone, the mesonephric duct begins to develop into the male reproductive organs and the paramesonephric duct regresses. If testosterone is not present by week 10, the gonadal tissue differentiates into ovaries and the paramesonephric duct develops into female reproductive organs. All the **oocytes** (cells that will develop into eggs throughout the woman's mature years) are already formed in ovaries at this stage.

At around week 12, under the influence of testosterone, the external genitals become visible as penile tissue elongates and the urogenital fold on the ventral surface of the penis closes to form the urethra; in females, with no testosterone present, the urogenital fold remains open to form the labia minora; what would be formed as scrotal tissue in the male becomes the labia majora in the female. If for some reason testosterone secretion is halted in utero, a chromosomal male could be born with female-appearing genitalia. If a woman should be prescribed a form of testosterone during pregnancy or if the woman, because of a metabolic abnormality, produces a high level of testosterone, a chromosomal female could be born with male-appearing genitalia.

Pubertal Development

Puberty is the stage of life at which secondary sex changes begin. Girls are beginning dramatic development and maturation of reproductive organs at earlier ages than ever before (9 to 12 years; for boys, 12 to 14 years). Although the mechanism that initiates this dramatic change in appearance is not well understood, the hypothalamus, under the direction of the central nervous system, may serve as a gonadostat or regulation mechanism set to "turn on" gonad functioning at this age. Although not proven, the theory is that a girl must reach a critical weight of approximately 95 lb (43 kg) or develop a critical mass of fat before the hypothalamus is triggered to send initial stimulation to the anterior pituitary gland to begin gonadotropic hormone formation. Studies of female athletes and dancers reveal that a lack of fat can delay or halt menstruation (Berkey et al., 2000; Chang et al., 2000). The phenomenon of why puberty occurs is even less understood in boys.

Role of Androgen

Androgenic hormones are the hormones responsible for muscular development, physical growth, and the increase in sebaceous gland secretions that causes typical acne in both boys and girls. In males, androgenic hormones are produced by the adrenal cortex and the testes; in females, by the adrenal cortex and the ovaries.

Levels of the primary androgenic hormone, testosterone, are low in males until puberty (approximately age 12 to 14 years). At that time, testosterone levels rise to influence the development of the testes, scrotum, penis, prostate, and seminal vesicles; the appearance of male pubic, axillary, and facial hair; laryngeal enlargement and its accompanying voice change; maturation of spermatozoa; and closure of growth in long bones.

In girls, testosterone influences enlargement of the labia majora and clitoris and formation of axillary and pubic hair. This development of pubic and axillary hair due to androgen stimulation is termed **adrenarche.**

Role of Estrogen

When triggered at puberty, ovarian follicles in females begin to excrete a high level of the hormone estrogen. This hormone is actually not one substance but three compounds (estrone [E1], estradiol [E2], and estriol [E3]). It can be considered a single substance, however, in terms of action.

The increase in estrogen levels in the female at puberty influences the development of the uterus, fallopian tubes, and vagina; typical female fat distribution and hair patterns; breast development; and an end to growth because it closes the epiphyses of long bones. The beginning of breast development is termed **thelarche.**

Secondary Sex Characteristics

Adolescent sexual development has been categorized into stages (Tanner, 1990). There is wide variation in the times that adolescents move through these developmental stages; however, the sequential order is fairly constant. In girls, pubertal changes typically occur as follows:

1. Growth spurt
2. Increase in the transverse diameter of the pelvis
3. Breast development
4. Growth of pubic hair
5. Onset of menstruation
6. Growth of axillary hair
7. Vaginal secretions

The average age at which **menarche** (the first menstrual period) occurs is 12.5 years. It may occur as early as age 9 or as late as age 17, however, and still be within a normal age range. Irregular menstrual periods are the rule rather than the exception for the first year. Menstrual periods do not become regular until ovulation consistently occurs with them (menstruation is not dependent on ovulation), and this does not tend to happen until 1 to 2 years after menarche. This is one reason why estrogen-based oral contraceptives are not commonly recommended until a girl's menstrual periods have become stabilized or are ovulatory (to prevent administration of a compound to halt ovulation before it is firmly established).

Production of spermatozoa does not begin in intrauterine life as does the production of ova, nor are spermatozoa produced in a cyclic pattern as are ova; rather, they are produced in a continuous process. Sperm production continues from puberty throughout the male's life span; in contrast, the production of mature ova stops at menopause.

Secondary sex characteristics of boys usually occur in the following order:

1. Increase in weight
2. Growth of testes
3. Growth of face, axillary, and pubic hair
4. Voice changes
5. Penile growth
6. Increase in height
7. Spermatogenesis

ANATOMY AND PHYSIOLOGY OF THE REPRODUCTIVE SYSTEM

Although the structures of the female and male reproductive systems differ greatly in both appearance and function, they are homologues (that is, they arise from the same embryonic origin; Fig. 4-1). The study of the female reproductive organs is called **gynecology. Andrology** is the study of the male reproductive organs.

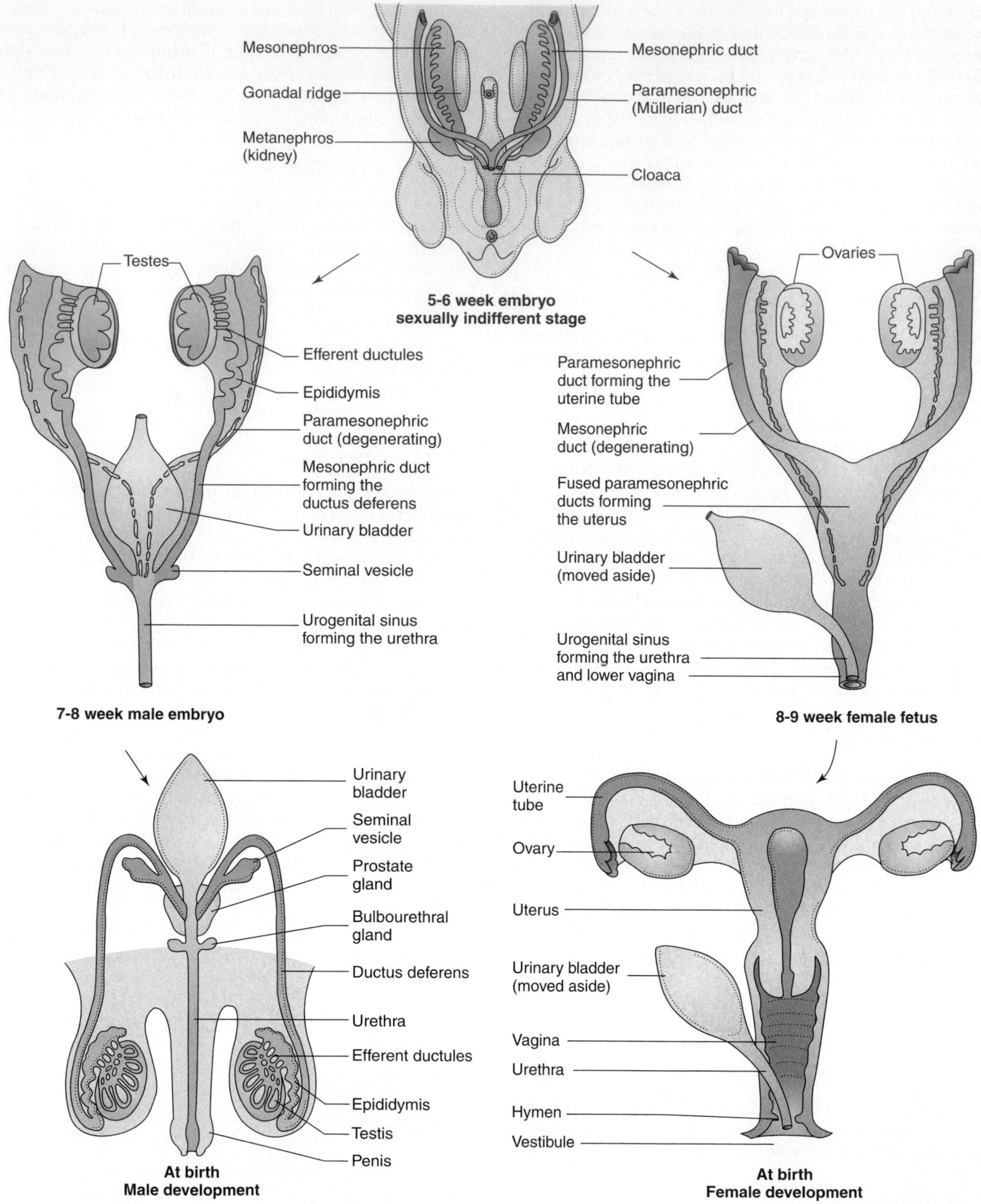

FIGURE 4.1 Development of the internal reproductive organs. *(continued)*

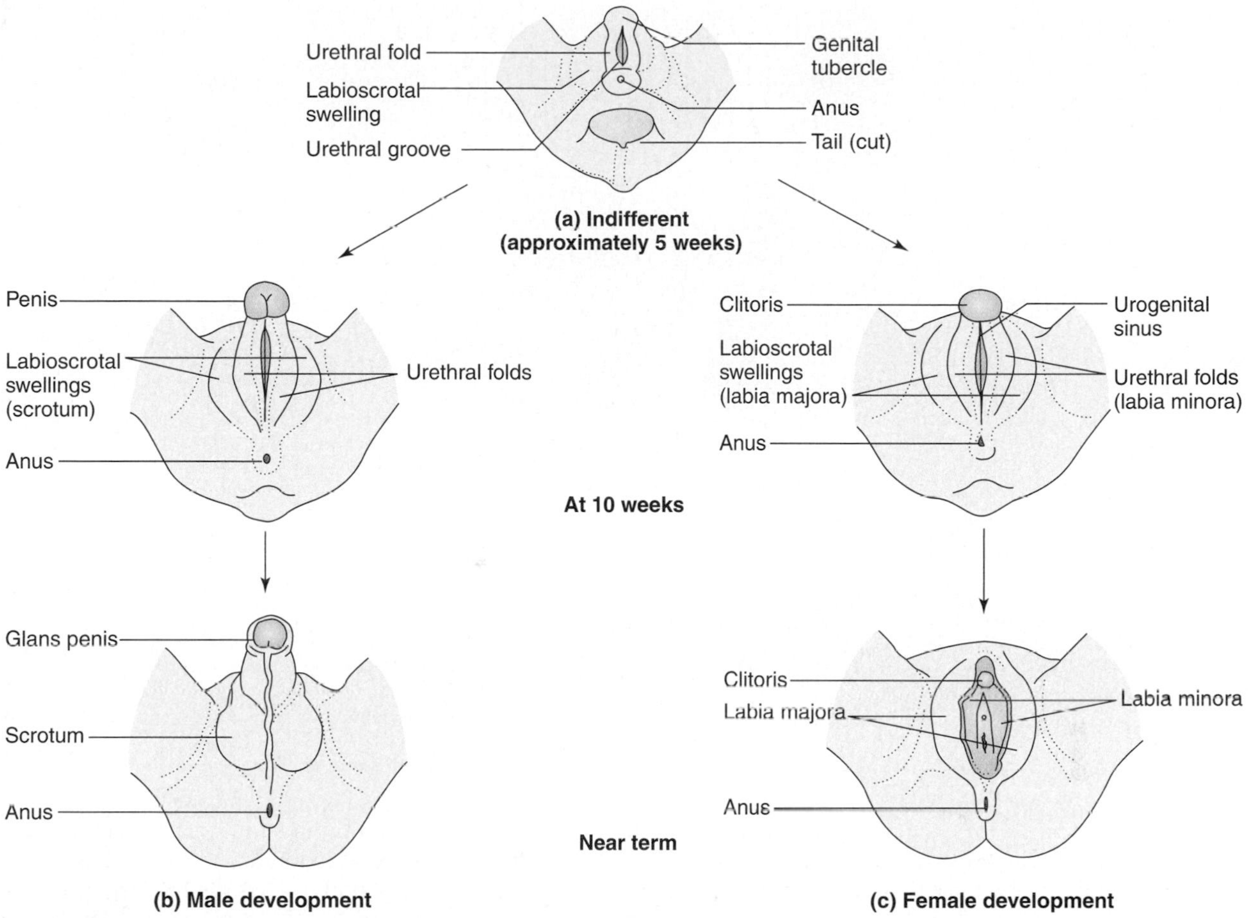

FIGURE 4.1 *(continued)* Development of the internal reproductive organs.

Male Reproductive System

Understanding the male reproductive system is necessary to appreciate the process of conception and human sexuality.

Male External Structures

External genital organs of the male include the penis, the scrotum, and the testes (which are encased in the scrotal sac). Spermatozoa are produced in the testes and reach maturity, surrounded by semen, in the external structures. Semen is derived from the prostate gland (60%), the seminal vesicles (30%), the epididymis (5%), and the bulbourethral glands (5%). It is alkaline and contains a basic sugar and mucin (protein). Figure 4-2 illustrates external and internal male reproductive anatomy.

Penis. The penis is composed of three cylindrical masses of erectile tissue: two termed the corpus cavernosa, and a third, termed corpus spongiosum, contained in the shaft. The urethra passes through these layers of erectile tissue to make the penis serve as the outlet for both the urinary and the reproductive tracts in men. With sexual excitement, nitric acid is released from the endothelium of blood vessels. This results in engorgement, or an increase in the blood flow to the arteries of the penis. The ischiocavernosus muscle at the penis base then contracts, trapping both venous and arterial blood in the three sections of erectile tissue and leading to distention and erection of the penis. At the distal end of the organ is a bulging sensitive ridge of tissue, the glans. A retractable casing of skin or prepuce protects the nerve-sensitive glans at birth. Many infants in the United States undergo circumcision, or surgical removal of the prepuce, shortly after birth (Fig. 4-3). The penile artery, a branch of the pudendal artery, provides the blood supply for the penis. Penile erection is stimulated by parasympathetic nerve innervation (Pentyala et al., 2001).

Scrotum. The scrotum is a rugated, skin-covered muscular pouch suspended from the perineum. It contains the testes, epididymis, and the lower portion of the spermatic cord. Its function is to support the testes and help regulate the temperature of sperm through contraction or relaxation and moving testes closer to or further away from the perineum (Weber et al., 2002).

Testes. The testes are two ovoid glands 2 to 3 cm wide that lie in the scrotum. Each testis is encased by a protective white fibrous capsule and is composed of a number of lobules, each lobule containing interstitial cells (Leydig's cells) and a seminiferous tubule. Seminiferous tubules produce spermatozoa. Leydig's cells are responsible for production of the male hormone testosterone.

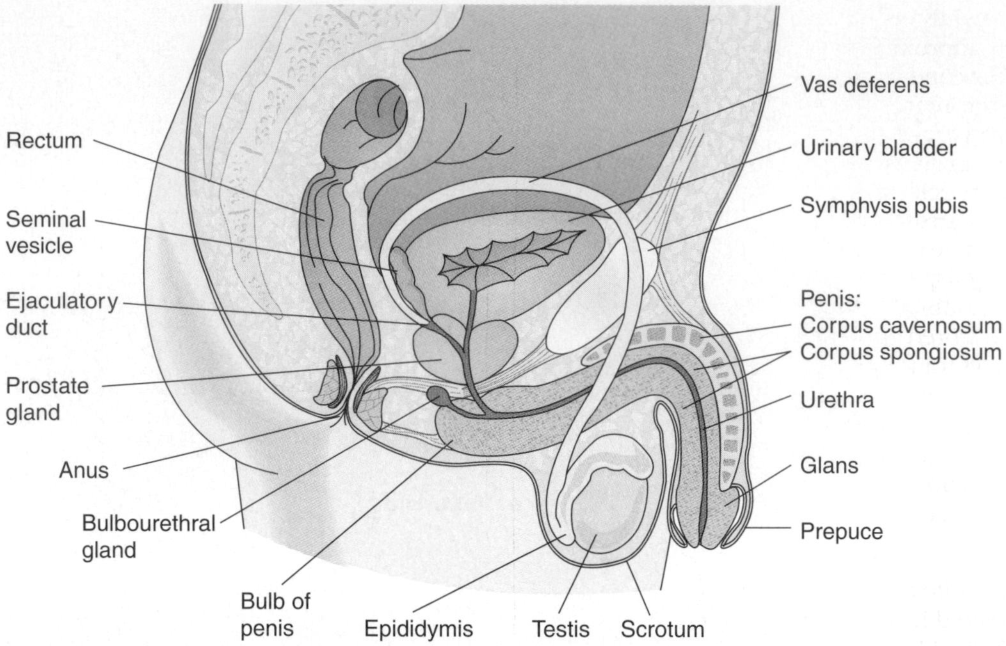

FIGURE 4.2 Male internal and external reproductive organs.

Testes first form in utero in the pelvic cavity. They descend, late in pregnancy (about the 34th to 38th week) into the scrotal sac. Because this descent occurs so late in pregnancy, many male preterm infants are born with undescended testes. These children need to be followed closely to see that the testes descend when the infant reaches what would have been the 34th to 38th week of gestational age, because testicular descent does not occur as readily in extrauterine life as it would in utero.

Spermatozoa are produced through a complex sequence of regulatory events. First, the hypothalamus releases gonadotropin-releasing hormone (GnRH), which in turn influences the anterior pituitary gland to release FSH and LH. FSH is then responsible for the release of androgen-binding protein (ABP), whereas LH is responsible for the release of testosterone. Finally, ABP binding of testosterone promotes spermatogenesis. Once in the bloodstream, increased amounts of testosterone have a feedback effect on the hypothalamus and anterior pituitary gland, thereby decreasing the production of the FSH and LH.

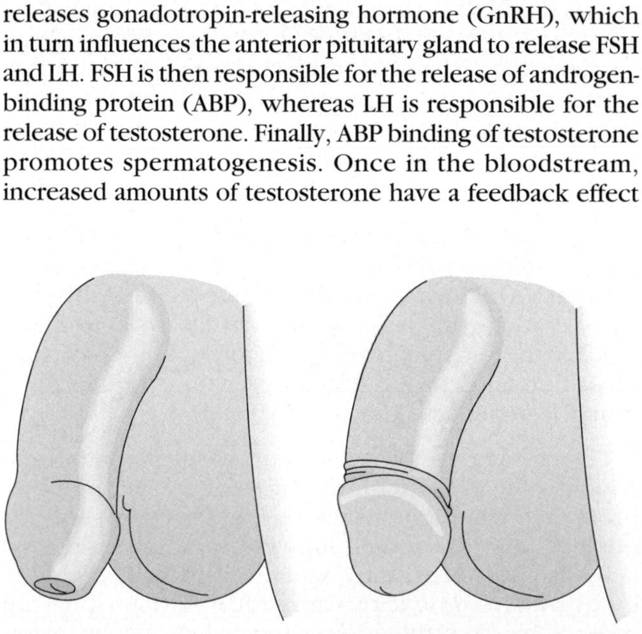

FIGURE 4.3 Uncircumcised and circumcised penis.

In most males, one testis is slightly larger than the other and is suspended slightly lower in the scrotum than the other (usually the left one). Because of this, the testes tend to slide past each other more readily on sitting or muscular activity, and there is less possibility of trauma to them. Most body structures of importance are more protected than are the testes (the heart, kidneys, and lungs are surrounded by ribs of hard bone, for example). Because spermatozoa do not survive at body temperature, however, the testes are suspended outside the body, where the temperature is approximately 1°F lower than body temperature and sperm survival can be ensured.

Beginning in early adolescence, boys need to learn testicular self-examination (see Chap. 33). Testes should feel firm, smooth, and egg-shaped. The epididymis can be palpated as a firm swelling on the superior aspect of the testes. Caution boys not to mistake this for an abnormal growth.

In very cold weather, the scrotal muscle contracts to bring the testes closer to the body; in very hot weather, or in the presence of fever, the muscle relaxes, allowing the testes to fall away from the body. In this way, the temperature of the testes can remain as even as possible to promote the production and viability of sperm.

Male Internal Structures

The male internal reproductive organs are the epididymis, the vas deferens, the seminal vesicles, the ejaculatory ducts, the prostate gland, the urethra, and the bulbourethral glands (see Fig. 4-2).

Epididymis. The seminiferous tubule of each testis leads to a tightly coiled tube, the epididymis. Because each epididymis is so tightly coiled, its length is extremely deceptive: it's actually approximately 20 ft long. The epididymis is responsible for conducting sperm from the testis to the vas deferens, the next step in the passage to the outside. Some sperm are stored in the epididymis, and a part of the fluid that surrounds sperm (semen, or seminal fluid) is produced by the cells lining the epididymis. Because the epididymis is so narrow along its entire length, infection (epididymitis) can lead to easy scarring of the lumen and prohibit passage of sperm beyond the scarred point.

Sperm are immobile and incapable of fertilization as they pass or are stored at the epididymis level. It takes at least 12 to 20 days for them to travel the length of the epididymis, and a total of 64 days for them to reach maturity. This is one reason that **aspermia** (absence of sperm) and oligospermia (fewer than 20 million sperm per milliliter) are problems that do not appear to respond immediately to therapy but rather only after 2 months.

Vas Deferens (Ductus Deferens). The vas deferens is an additional hollow tube surrounded by arteries and veins and protected by a thick fibrous coating. It carries sperm from the epididymis through the inguinal canal into the abdominal cavity, where it ends at the seminal vesicles and the ejaculatory ducts. Sperm mature as they pass through the vas deferens. They are not mobile at this point, however, probably due to the fairly acidic medium of the semen produced at this level. The blood vessels and vas deferens together are referred to as the spermatic cord. A varicocele, or a varicosity of the internal spermatic vein, can contribute to male infertility by causing congestion with increased warmth in the testes. Vasectomy (severing of the vas deferens) is a popular means of male birth control.

Seminal Vesicles. The seminal vesicles are two convoluted pouches that lie along the lower portion of the posterior surface of the bladder and empty into the urethra by way of the ejaculatory ducts. These glands secrete a viscous portion of the semen, which has a high content of a basic sugar, protein, and prostaglandins and is alkaline. Sperm become increasingly motile with this added fluid because it surrounds them with nutrients and a more favorable pH.

Ejaculatory Ducts. The two ejaculatory ducts pass through the prostate gland and join the seminal vesicles with the urethra.

Prostate Gland. The prostate is a chestnut-sized gland that lies just below the bladder. The urethra passes through the center of it, like the hole in a doughnut. The prostate gland secretes a thin alkaline fluid. When added to the secretion from the seminal vesicles and the accompanying sperm from the epididymis, this alkaline fluid further protects sperm from being immobilized by the naturally low pH level of the urethra. In middle life, many men develop hypertrophy of the prostate. This swelling interferes with both fertility and urination. It can be relieved by medical therapy or surgery.

Bulbourethral Glands. Two bulbourethral or Cowper's glands lie beside the prostate gland and by short ducts empty into the urethra. Like the prostate gland and seminal vesicles, they secrete an alkaline fluid that helps counteract the acid secretion of the urethra and ensure the safe passage of spermatozoa.

Urethra. The urethra is a hollow tube leading from the base of the bladder, which, after passing through the prostate gland, continues to the outside through the shaft and glans of the penis. It is approximately 8 in (18 to 20 cm) long. As with other urinary tract structures, it is lined with mucous membrane.

✔ CHECKPOINT QUESTIONS

1. What hormone influences male facial hair development at puberty?
2. What is the first menstrual period termed? The beginning of breast development?
3. Vasectomy is the cutting of what structure?

Female Reproductive System

The female reproductive system, like the male system, has both external and internal components.

Female External Structures

The structures that form the female external genitalia are termed the vulva (from the Latin word for covering) and are illustrated in Figure 4-4.

Mons Veneris. The mons veneris is a pad of adipose tissue located over the symphysis pubis, the pubic bone joint. It is covered by a triangle of coarse, curly hairs. The purpose of the mons veneris is to protect the junction of the public bone from trauma.

Labia Minora. Just posterior to the mons veneris spreads two hairless folds of connective tissue, the labia minora. Before menarche, these folds are fairly small; by childbearing age, they are firm and full; after menopause, they atrophy and again become much smaller. Normally the folds of the labia minora are pink; the internal surface is covered with mucous membrane, the external surface with skin. The area is abundant with sebaceous glands, so localized sebaceous cysts may occur here.

Labia Majora. The labia majora are two folds of adipose tissue covered by loose connective tissue and epithelium; they are positioned lateral to the labia minora. Covered by pubic hair, the labia majora serve as protection for the external genitalia and the distal urethra and vagina. They are fused anteriorly but separated posteriorly. Trauma to the area, such as occurs from childbirth or rape, can lead to extensive edema formation in the area because of the looseness of the connective tissue base.

Other External Organs. The vestibule is the flattened, smooth surface inside the labia. The openings to the bladder (the urethra) and the uterus (the vagina) both arise from the vestibule. The clitoris is a small (approximately 1 to 2 cm) rounded organ of erectile tissue at the forward junction of the labia minora. It is covered by a

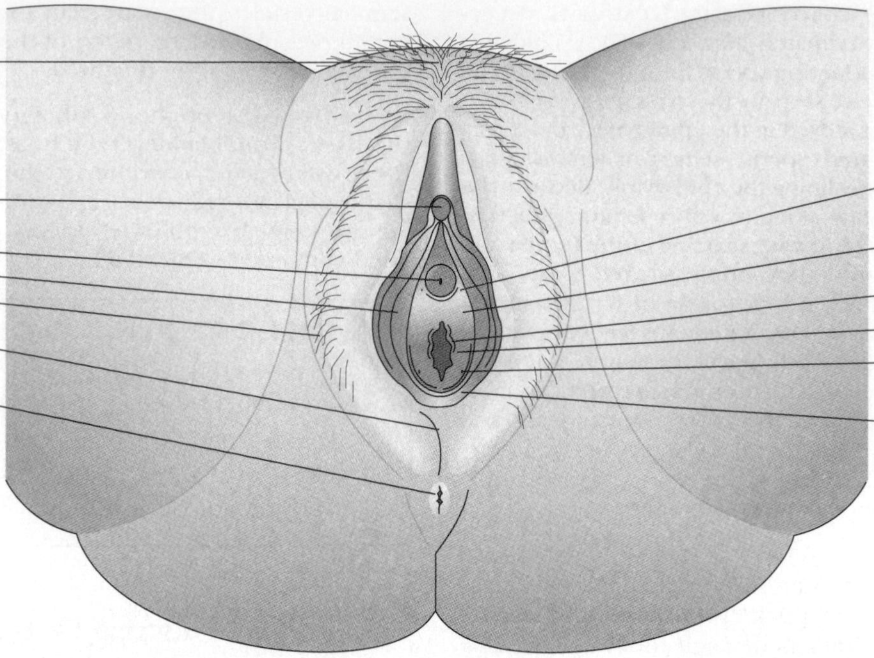

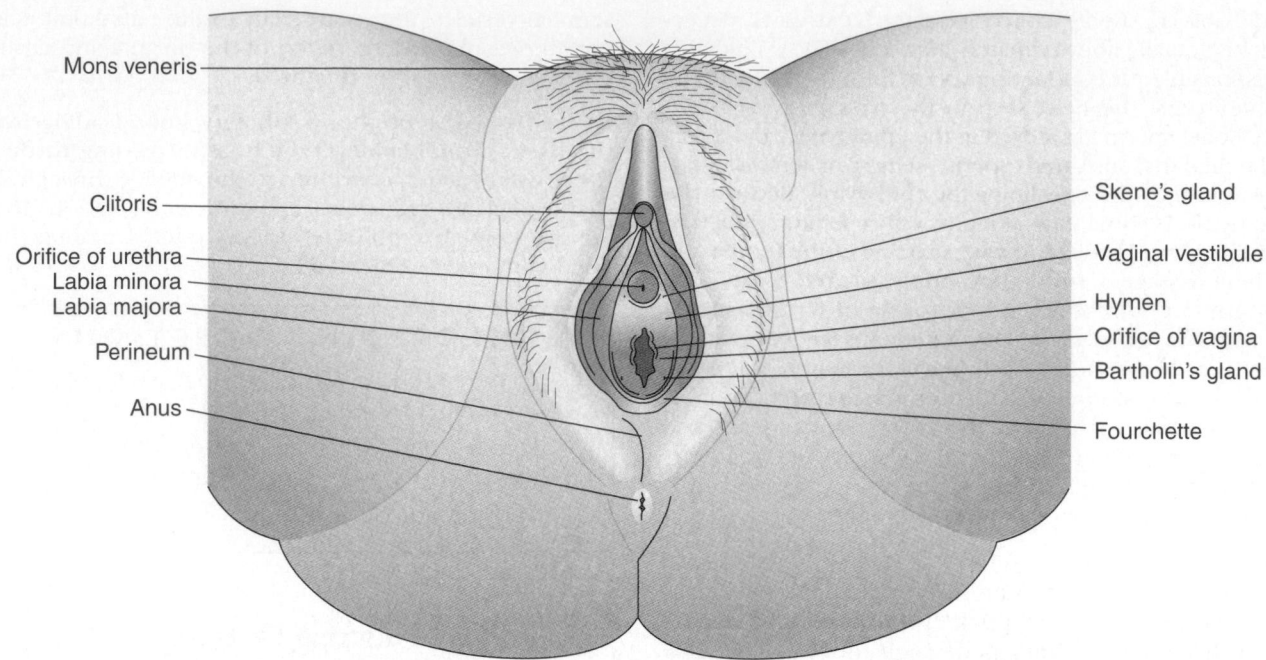

FIGURE 4.4 Female external genitalia.

fold of skin, the prepuce. The clitoris is sensitive to touch and temperature and is the center of sexual arousal and orgasm in the female. Arterial blood supply for the clitoris is plentiful. When the ischiocavernosus muscle surrounding it contracts with sexual arousal, the venous outflow for the clitoris is blocked, leading to clitoral erection.

Two Skene's glands (paraurethral glands) are located just lateral to the urinary meatus, one on each side. The ducts open into the urethra. Bartholin's glands (vulvovaginal glands) are located just lateral to the vaginal opening on both sides. Their ducts open into the distal vagina. Secretions from both these glands help to lubricate the external genitalia during coitus. The alkaline pH of their secretion helps to improve sperm survival in the vagina. Both Skene's glands and Bartholin's glands may become infected and produce a discharge and local pain.

The fourchette is the ridge of tissue formed by the posterior joining of the two labia minora and the labia majora. This is the structure that is sometimes cut (episiotomy) during childbirth to enlarge the vaginal opening.

Posterior to the fourchette is the perineal muscle or the perineal body. Because this is a muscular area, it is easily stretched during childbirth to allow enlargement of the vagina and passage of the fetal head. Many exercises (such as Kegel's, squatting, and tailor-sitting) are aimed at making the perineal muscle more relaxed and more expandable to allow easy expansion during birth without the tearing of this tissue.

The hymen is a tough but elastic semicircle of tissue that covers the opening to the vagina in childhood. It is often torn during the time of first sexual intercourse. However, due to the use of tampons and active sports participation, many girls who have not had sexual relations do not have intact hymens at the time of their first pelvic examination. Occasionally, a girl will have an imperforate hymen, or a hymen so complete it does not allow passage of menstrual blood from the vagina or allow for sexual relations until it is surgically incised.

Vulvar Blood Supply. The blood supply of the external genitalia is mainly from the pudendal artery and a portion of the inferior rectus artery. Venous return is through the pudendal vein. Pressure on this vein by the fetal head may cause extensive back-pressure and development of varicosities (distended veins) in the labia majora. Because of the rich blood supply, trauma to the area, such as occurs from pressure during childbirth, can cause large hematomas. This ready blood supply also, fortunately, contributes to the rapid healing of any tears in the area following childbirth.

Vulvar Nerve Supply. The anterior portion of the vulva derives its nerve supply from the ilioinguinal and genitofemoral nerves (L1 level). The posterior portions of the vulva and vagina are supplied by the pudendal nerve (S3 level). Such a rich nerve supply makes the area extremely sensitive to touch, pressure, pain, and temperature. Anesthesia for childbirth may be administered locally to block the pudendal nerve; this eliminates pain sensation at the perineum during birth. Normal stretching of the perineum with childbirth causes temporary loss of sensation in the area.

Female Internal Structures

Female internal reproductive organs (Fig. 4-5) are the ovaries, the fallopian tubes, the uterus, and the vagina.

Ovaries. The ovaries are approximately 4 cm long by 2 cm in diameter and approximately 1.5 cm thick, or the size and shape of almonds. They are grayish-white and

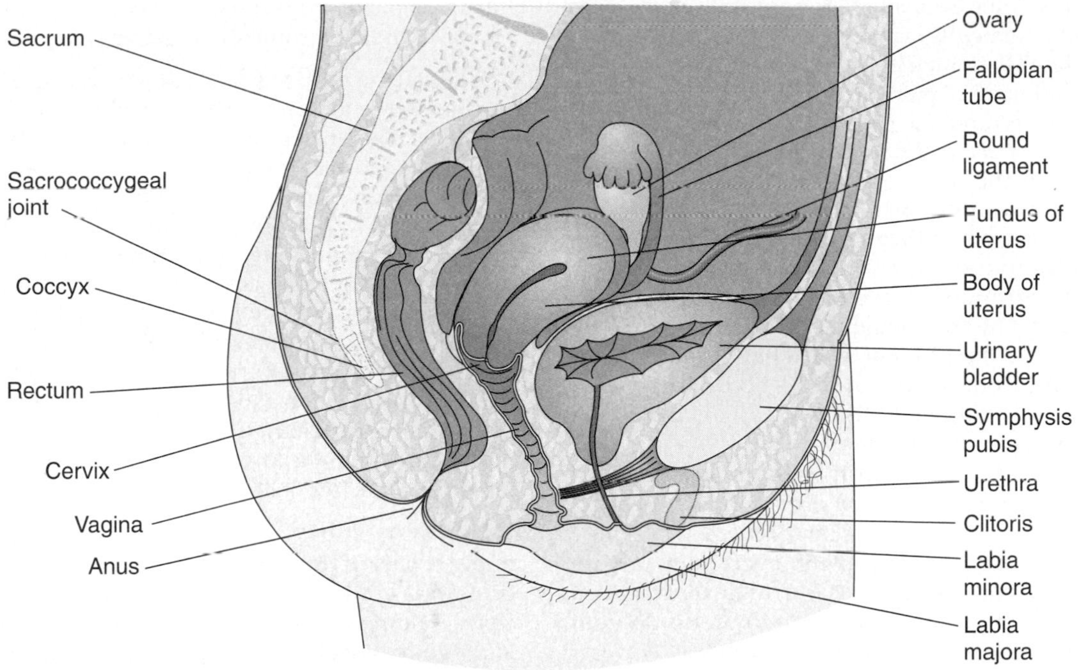

FIGURE 4.5 Female internal reproductive organs.

appear pitted, or with minute indentations on the surface. An unruptured, glistening, clear, fluid-filled graafian follicle (an ovum about to be discharged) or a miniature yellow corpus luteum (the structure left after the ovum has been discharged) often can be observed on the surface of the ovary.

Ovaries are located close to and on both sides of the uterus in the lower abdomen. It is difficult to locate them by abdominal palpation because they are located so low. If an abnormality is present, such as an enlarging ovarian cyst, however, the tenderness this causes may be evident on lower-left or lower-right abdominal palpation.

The function of the two ovaries (the female gonads) is to produce, mature, and discharge ova (the egg cells). In the process, the ovaries produce estrogen and progesterone and initiate and regulate menstrual cycles. If the ovaries are removed before puberty (or are nonfunctional), the resulting absence of estrogen will prevent breasts from maturing at puberty; in addition, pubic hair distribution will assume a more male pattern than normal. After menopause, or cessation of ovarian function, the uterus, breasts, and ovaries themselves undergo atrophy or a reduction in size because of a lack of estrogen. Ovarian function, therefore, is necessary for maturation and maintenance of secondary sex characteristics in females. The estrogen secreted by ovaries is also important to prevent osteoporosis, or weakness of bones, because of withdrawal of calcium from bones. This frequently occurs in women after menopause, making them prone to serious spinal, hip, and wrist fractures. Because cholesterol is incorporated into estrogen, the production of estrogen is thought to keep cholesterol levels reduced and so limit the effects of atherosclerosis (artery disease) in women. Estrogen may be prescribed for women at menopause to help prevent osteoporosis and cardiovascular disease. However, the benefits of estrogen must be carefully weighed against potential risks of endometrial cancer (Ling & Duff, 2001).

Ovaries are held in suspended positions and kept in close contact with the ends of the fallopian tubes by three strong supporting ligaments attached to the uterus or the pelvic wall. They are unique among pelvic structures in that they are not covered by a layer of peritoneum. Because they are not encased this way, ova can escape from them and enter the uterus by way of the fallopian tubes. Because they are suspended in position rather than being firmly fixed in place, an abnormal tumor or cyst growing on them can enlarge to a size easily twice that of the organ before pressure on surrounding organs or the ovarian blood supply leads to symptoms of compression. This is the reason that ovarian cancer continues to be one of the leading causes of death from cancer in women (the tumor grows without symptoms for such an extended period).

Ovaries are formed with three principal divisions:

1. A protective layer of surface epithelium
2. The cortex, filled with the ovarian and graafian follicles. Here the immature (primordial) follicles mature into ova and produce large amounts of estrogen and progesterone.
3. The central medulla, containing the nerves, blood vessels, lymphatic tissue, and some smooth muscle tissue

Division of Reproductive Cells (Gametes). At birth, each ovary contains approximately 2 million immature ova (oocytes), which were formed during the first 5 months of intrauterine life. Although these cells have the unique ability to produce a new individual, they basically contain the usual cell components: a cell membrane, an area of clear cytoplasm, and a nucleus containing chromosomes.

The oocytes differ from all other body cells in the number of chromosomes they contain in the nucleus. The nucleus of all other human body cells contains 46 chromosomes, consisting of 22 pairs of autosomes (paired matching chromosomes) and one pair of sex chromosomes (two X sex chromosomes in the female and an X and a Y sex chromosome in the male). Reproductive cells (ova and spermatozoa) have only half the usual number of chromosomes so that, when they combine (fertilization), the new individual formed from them will have the normal number of 46 chromosomes. If both the ova and spermatozoa carried the full complement of chromosomes, a new individual formed out of them would have twice the normal amount of chromosome material. There is a difference in the way reproductive cells divide that causes this change in chromosome number.

Cells in the body, such as skin cells, undergo cell division by mitosis, or daughter cell division. In this type of division, all the chromosomes are duplicated in each new cell just before cell division, giving every new cell the same number of chromosomes as the original parent cell. Oocytes divide in intrauterine life by mitotic division. Division activity then appears to halt until at least puberty, when a second type of cell division, meiosis (cell reduction division), occurs. In the male, this reduction division occurs just before the spermatozoa mature. In the female, it occurs just before ovulation. Following this division, an ovum has 22 autosomes and an X sex chromosome; a spermatozoon has 22 autosomes and either an X or a Y sex chromosome. A new individual formed from the union of an ovum and an X-carrying spermatozoon will be female (an XX chromosome pattern); an individual formed from the union of an ovum and a Y-carrying spermatozoon will be male (an XY chromosome pattern).

Maturation of Oocytes. Each oocyte lies in the ovary surrounded by a protective sac, or thin layer of cells, called a follicle. The structure in this underdeveloped state is called a primordial follicle. Five to 7 million of these are first formed in utero. The maturation of these primitive follicles appears to stop approximately at month 5 of intrauterine life. The majority never develop beyond the primitive state and actually atrophy, so that by birth there are only 2 million present; by age 7 years, only approximately 500,000 are present in each ovary; by 22 years, there are approximately 300,000; by menopause, or the end of the fertile period in females, none are left (all have either matured or atrophied). "The point at which no functioning oocytes remain in the ovaries" is one definition of menopause (Seifer et al., 2001).

Fallopian Tubes. The fallopian tubes arise from each upper corner of the uterine body and extend outward and backward until each opens at the distal end next to an ovary. Fallopian tubes are approximately 10 cm in length in a mature woman. Their function is to convey the ovum from the ovaries to the uterus and to provide a place for fertilization of the ovum by sperm.

Although a fallopian tube is a smooth, hollow tunnel, it is anatomically divided into four separate parts (Fig. 4-6). The most proximal division, the interstitial portion, is that part of the tube that lies within the uterine wall. This portion is only approximately 1 cm in length; the lumen of the tube is only 1 mm in diameter at this point. The isthmus is the next distal portion. It is, like the interstitial

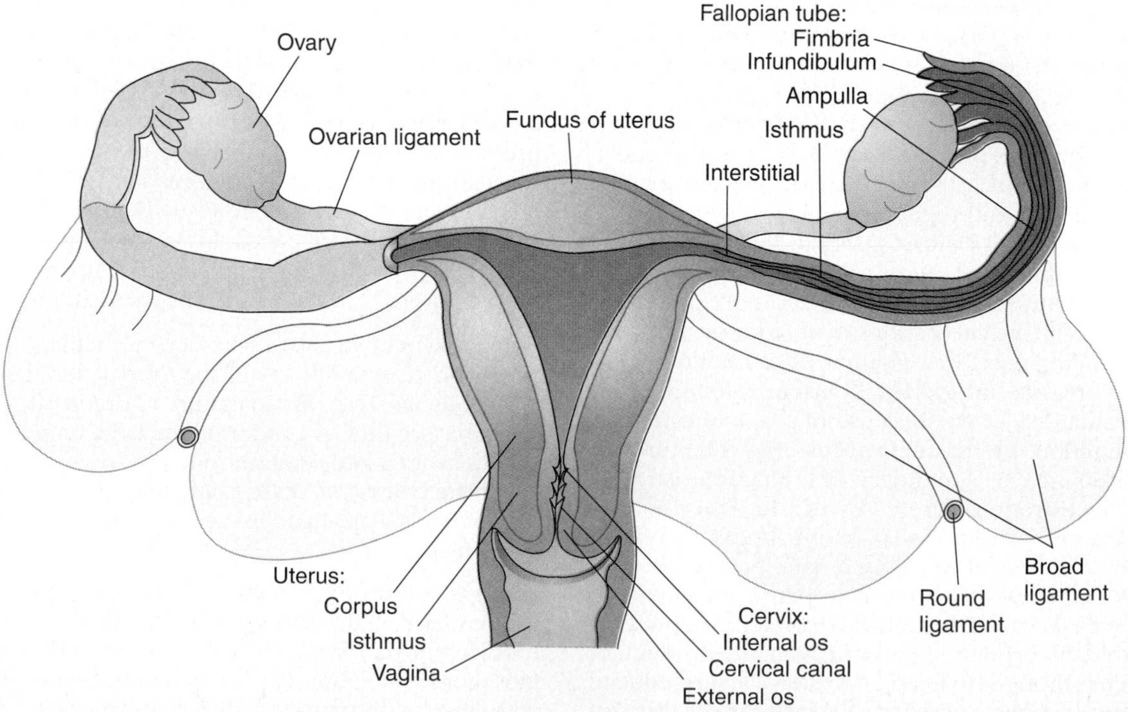

FIGURE 4.6 Anterior view of female reproductive organs showing relationship of fallopian tubes and body of the uterus.

tube, extremely narrow. This segment is approximately 2 cm in length. This is the portion of the tube that is cut or sealed in a tubal ligation, or tubal sterilization procedure. The ampulla is the third and also the longest portion of the tube. It is approximately 5 cm in length. It is in this ampullar portion that fertilization of an ovum usually occurs. The infundibular portion is the most distal segment of the tube. It is approximately 2 cm long and is funnel-shaped. The rim of the funnel is covered by fimbria (small hairs) that help to guide the ovum into the fallopian tube.

The lining of the entire fallopian tube is composed of mucous membrane, which contains both mucus-secreting and ciliated (hair-covered) cells. Beneath the mucous lining are connective tissue and a circular muscle layer. The muscle layer of the tube produces peristaltic motions that conduct the ovum the length of the tube. This migration of the ovum is aided by the action of the ciliated lining and the mucus, which acts as a lubricant. The mucus produced may also act as a source of nourishment for the fertilized egg because it contains protein, water, and salts.

Because the fallopian tubes are open at the distal end, a direct pathway from the external organs through the vagina to the uterus and tubes exists. This pathway makes conception possible. Unfortunately, it can also lead to infection of the peritoneum (peritonitis) if disease spreads from the tubes to the peritoneum. For this reason, careful, clean technique must be used during pelvic examination or treatment. Vaginal examinations during labor and birth are done with sterile technique to ensure that no organisms can enter.

Uterus. The uterus is a hollow, muscular, pear-shaped organ located in the lower pelvis, posterior to the bladder and anterior to the rectum. During childhood, it is approximately the size of an olive, and its proportions are reversed from what they are later on, the cervix being the largest portion of the organ. At approximately age 8 years, an increase in the size of the uterus begins. The maximum increase in size occurs by approximately age 17 years, which may be a factor contributing to the low-birthweight babies typically born to adolescents younger than this age.

With maturity, a uterus is approximately 5 to 7 cm long, 5 cm wide, and in its widest upper part 2.5 cm deep. In a nonpregnant state, it weighs approximately 60 g. The function of the uterus is to receive the ovum from the fallopian tube; provide a place for implantation and nourishment during fetal growth; furnish protection to a growing fetus; and at maturity of the fetus, expel it from the woman's body.

After a pregnancy, the uterus never returns to its nonpregnant size. Therefore, in the woman who has borne a child, uterine dimensions are closer to 9 cm long, 6 cm wide, 3 cm thick, and 80 g in weight. Anatomically, the uterus consists of three divisions: the body or corpus, the isthmus, and the cervix.

The body of the uterus is the uppermost part and forms the bulk of the uterus. The lining of the cavity is continuous with that of the fallopian tubes, which fuse at its upper aspects (the cornua). The portion of the uterus between the points of attachment of the fallopian tubes is the fundus. During pregnancy, the body of the uterus is the portion of the structure that expands to contain the growing fetus. The fundus is the portion that can be palpated abdominally to determine the amount of uterine growth occurring during pregnancy, to measure the force of uterine contractions during labor, and to assess that the uterus is returning to its nonpregnant state after childbirth.

The isthmus of the uterus is a short segment between the body and the cervix. In the nonpregnant uterus, it is only 1 to 2 mm in length. During pregnancy, this portion also enlarges greatly to aid in accommodating the growing fetus. It is the portion of the uterus that is most commonly cut when a fetus is born by a cesarean birth.

The cervix is the lowest portion of the uterus. It represents approximately one third of the total uterus size, or approximately 2 to 5 cm long. Approximately half of it lies above the vagina and half extends into the vagina. The cavity is termed the cervical canal. The junction of the canal at the isthmus is the internal cervical os; the distal opening to the vagina is the external cervical os. The level of the external os is at the level of the ischial spines (an important relationship in estimating the level of the fetus in the birth canal).

Uterine and Cervical Coats. The uterine wall consists of three separate coats or layers of tissue: an inner one of mucous membrane (the endometrium), a middle one of muscle fibers (the myometrium), and an outer one of connective tissue (the perimetrium).

The **endometrium** layer of the uterus is important in terms of menstrual function and childbearing. It is not a single structure but is rather formed by two layers of cells. The layer closest to the uterine wall, or the basal layer, is not much influenced by hormones. The inner second glandular layer is greatly influenced by both estrogen and progesterone. This is the layer that grows and becomes so thick and responsive each month under the influence of estrogen and progesterone that it is capable of supporting a pregnancy. If pregnancy does not occur, this is the layer that is shed as the menstrual flow.

The mucous membrane lining of the cervix is termed the **endocervix.** The endocervix, continuous with the endometrium, is also affected by hormones, but changes are manifested in a more subtle way. The cells of the cervical lining secrete mucus to provide a lubricated surface so spermatozoa can readily pass through the cervix; the efficiency of this lubrication increases or wanes depending on hormone stimulation. At the point in the menstrual cycle when estrogen production is at its peak, as much as 700 mL of mucus per day is produced; at the point that estrogen is very low, only a few milliliters are produced. Because mucus is alkaline, it helps to decrease the acidity of the upper vagina, aiding in sperm survival. During pregnancy, the endocervix becomes plugged with mucus, forming a seal to keep out ascending infections.

The lower surface of the cervix and the lower third of the cervical canal are lined not with mucous membrane but with stratified squamous epithelium similar to that lining the vagina. Locating the point at which this tissue changes from epithelium to mucous membrane is important when obtaining a Papanicolaou smear (a test for cervical cancer) because this tissue interface is most often the origin of cervical cancer.

The **myometrium,** or muscle layer of the uterus, is composed of three interwoven layers of smooth muscle, the fibers of which are arranged in longitudinal, transverse, and oblique directions. This network offers extreme strength to the organ. The myometrium serves the important function of constricting the tubal junctions and preventing regurgitation of menstrual blood into the tubes. It also holds the internal cervical os closed during pregnancy to prevent a preterm birth. When the uterus contracts at the end of pregnancy to expel the fetus, equal pressure is exerted at all points throughout the cavity because of this unique arrangement of muscle fibers. After childbirth, this interlacing network of fibers is able to constrict the blood vessels coursing through the layers, thus limiting loss of blood in the woman. Myomas, or benign uterine tumors, arise from the myometrium. The **perimetrium,** or the outermost layer of the uterus, offers added strength and support to the structure.

Uterine Blood Supply. The large descending abdominal aorta divides to form two iliac arteries; main divisions of the iliac arteries are the hypogastric arteries. These further divide to form the uterine arteries and supply the uterus. Because the uterine blood supply is not far removed from the aorta, it is copious and adequate to supply the growing needs of a fetus. As an additional safeguard, after supplying the ovary with blood, the ovarian artery (a direct subdivision of the aorta) joins the uterine artery as a fail-safe system to ensure that the uterus will have an adequate blood supply. The blood vessels that supply the cells and lining of the uterus are tortuous against the sides of the uterine body in nonpregnant women. As a uterus enlarges with pregnancy, the vessels "unwind" and so can stretch to maintain an adequate blood supply as the organ enlarges. The uterine veins follow the same twisting course as the arteries; they empty into the internal iliac veins.

An important organ relationship to be aware of is the association of uterine vessels and the ureters. The ureters from the kidneys pass directly in back of the ovarian vessels near the fallopian tubes; as shown in Figure 4-7, they cross just beneath the uterine vessels before they enter the bladder. This close anatomic relationship has implications in procedures such as tubal ligation, cesarean birth, and hysterectomy (removal of the uterus), because a ureter may be injured by a clamp if bleeding is controlled by clamping the uterine or ovarian vessels.

WHAT IF? What if a woman returns from a tubal ligation procedure (clamping of the fallopian tubes) and has had no urine output for 6 hours? Why is observing women for urine output after uterine or fallopian tube surgery always a critical assessment?

Uterine Nerve Supply. The uterus is supplied by both afferent (sensory) and efferent (motor) nerves. The efferent nerves arise from T5 through T10 spinal ganglia. The afferent nerves join the hypogastric plexus and enter the spinal column at T11 and T12. The fact that sensory innervation from the uterus registers lower in the spinal column than does motor control has implications in controlling pain in labor. An anesthetic solution can be injected near

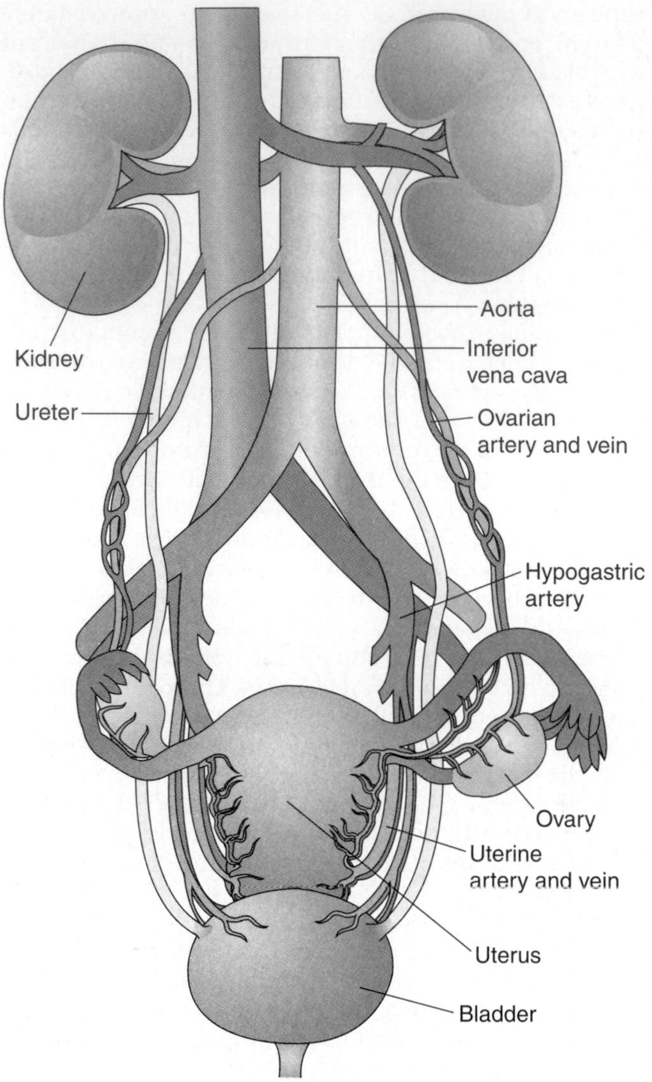

FIGURE 4.7 Blood supply to the uterus.

the spinal column and stop the pain of uterine contractions at the T11 and T12 levels without stopping motor control or contractions (registered above this at the T5 to T10 level). This is the principle of epidural anesthesia (see Chap. 19).

Uterine Supports. The uterus is suspended in the pelvic cavity by a number of ligaments and is supported by a combination of fascia and muscle. Because it is not fixed in one location, it is free to enlarge without discomfort during pregnancy. If these supports become overstretched during pregnancy, they may not support the bladder well afterward, and the bladder can then herniate into the anterior vagina (a **cystocele**). A **rectocele** may develop in the same way if the rectum pouches toward the vaginal wall (Fig. 4-8).

A fold of peritoneum behind the uterus is the posterior ligament. This forms a pouch (Douglas' cul-de-sac) between the rectum and uterus. Because this is the lowest point of the pelvis, any fluid such as blood in the pelvis tends to collect in this space. The space can be examined for the presence of fluid by inserting a culdoscope

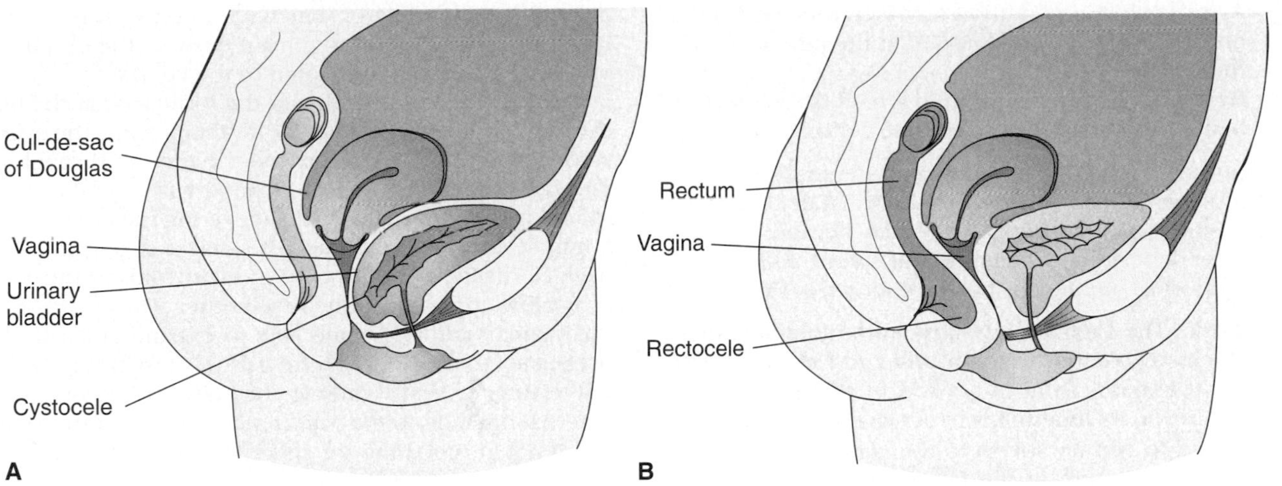

FIGURE 4.8 (*A*) Cystocele. The bladder has herniated into the anterior wall of the vagina. (*B*) Rectocele. The posterior of the vagina is herniated.

through the posterior vaginal wall (**culdoscopy**) or a laparoscope through the abdominal wall (**laparoscopy**).

The broad ligaments are two folds of peritoneum that cover the uterus front and back and extend to the pelvic sides. The round ligaments are two fibrous muscular cords that pass from the body of the uterus near the attachments of the fallopian tubes through the broad ligaments into the inguinal canal and insert into the fascia of the vulva. The round ligaments act as "stays" to steady the uterus. If a pregnant woman moves quickly, she may pull one of these ligaments and feel a quick, sharp pain of frightening intensity in one of her lower abdominal quadrants.

Uterine Deviations. A number of uterine deviations relating to shape and position may interfere with fertility or pregnancy. In the fetus, the uterus first forms with a septum or a fibrous division, longitudinally separating it into two portions. As the fetus matures, this septum dissolves, so that typically at birth no remnant of the division remains. In some women, the septum never atrophies, and so the uterus remains as two separate compartments. In others, half of the septum is still present. Still other women have oddly shaped "horns" at the junction of the fallopian tubes, termed a **bicornuate uterus.** All these malformations may decrease the ability to conceive or to carry a pregnancy to term. Some variations of uterine formation are shown in Figure 4-9. The specific effects of these deviations on fertility and pregnancy are discussed in later chapters.

Ordinarily, the body of the uterus is tipped slightly forward. However, a deviation in the positioning of the uterus may exist. Positional deviations of the uterus include:

- **Anteversion,** a condition in which the fundus is tipped forward
- **Retroversion,** a condition in which the fundus is tipped back

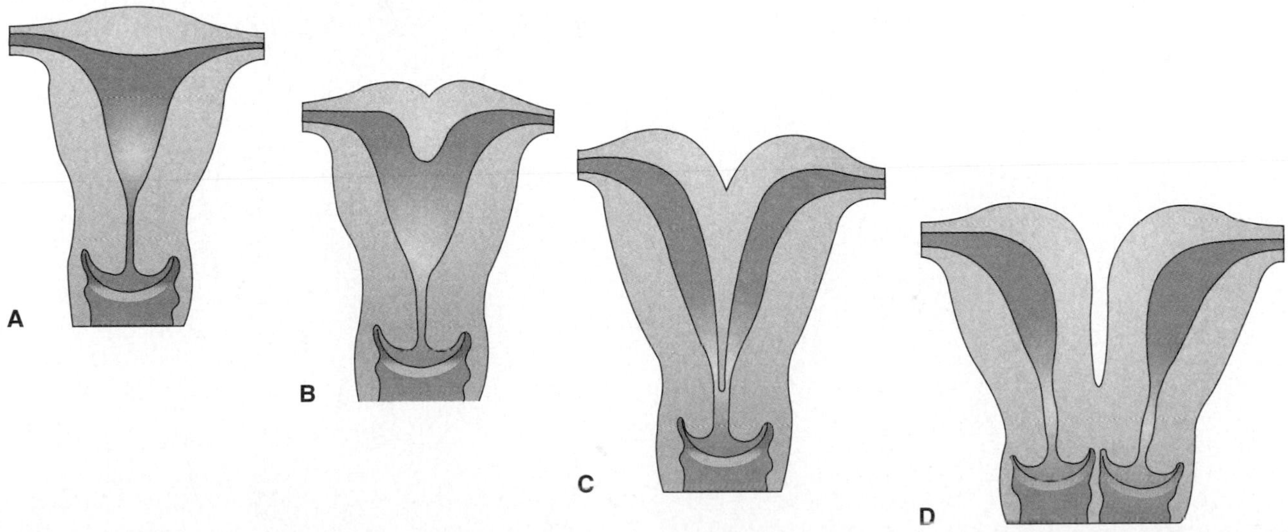

FIGURE 4.9 (*A*) Normal uterus. (*B*) Bicornuate uterus. (*C*) Septum dividing uterus. (*D*) Double uterus. Abnormal shapes of uterus allow less placenta implantation space.

- **Anteflexion,** a condition in which the body of the uterus is bent sharply forward at the junction with the cervix
- **Retroflexion,** a condition in which the body is bent sharply back just above the cervix

Minor variations of these positions generally cause no reproductive problems. Extreme abnormal flexion or version positions may interfere with fertility because they may block the deposition or migration of sperm. Examples of these abnormal uterine positions are shown in Figure 4-10.

Vagina. The vagina is a hollow musculomembranous canal located posterior to the bladder and anterior to the rectum. It extends from the cervix of the uterus to the external vulva. Its function is to act as the organ of intercourse and to convey sperm to the cervix so sperm can meet with the ovum in the fallopian tube. With childbirth, it expands to serve as the birth canal.

When a woman is lying on her back as she does for a pelvic examination, the course of the vagina is inward and downward. Because of this downward slant and the insertion of the uterine cervix into the distal portion, the length of the anterior wall of the vagina is approximately 6 to 7 cm long; the posterior wall is 8 to 9 cm. At the uterine end of the structure, there are recesses on all sides of the cervix termed fornices. Behind the cervix is the posterior fornix; at the front, the anterior fornix; and at the sides, the lateral fornices. The posterior fornix serves as a place for the pooling of semen after coitus; this allows a large number of sperm to remain close to the cervix and encourages sperm migration into the cervix.

The vaginal wall is so thin at the fornices that the bladder can be palpated through the anterior fornix, the ovaries through the lateral fornices, and the rectum through the posterior fornix. The vagina is lined with stratified squamous epithelium similar to that covering the cervix. It has a middle connective tissue layer and a strong muscular wall. Normally, the walls contain many folds or rugae and lie in close approximation to each other. These folds make the vagina very elastic and able to expand at the end of pregnancy to allow a full-term baby to pass through without tearing. A circular muscle, the bulbocavernosus, at the external opening to the vagina acts as a voluntary sphincter. Women preparing for childbirth are advised to relax and tense this external vaginal sphincter muscle a set number of times each day to make it more supple for birth and to help maintain tone after birth (Kegel's exercises).

The blood supply to the vagina is furnished by the vaginal artery, a branch of the internal iliac artery. Vaginal tears at childbirth tend to bleed profusely because of this rich blood supply. This rich blood supply, however, is also the reason that healing of any vaginal trauma at birth occurs rapidly.

The vagina has both sympathetic and parasympathetic nerve innervations originating at the S1 to S3 levels. It is not an extremely sensitive organ, however. Sexual excite-

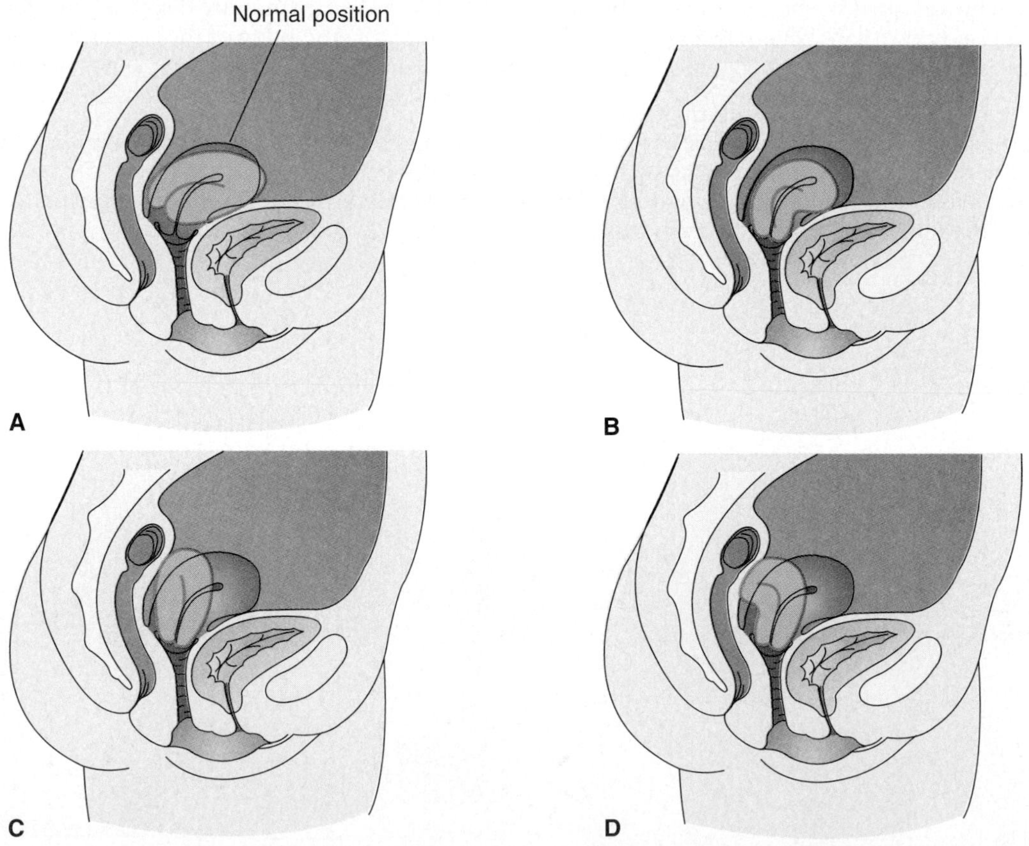

FIGURE 4.10 Uterine flexion and version. (*A*) Anteversion. (*B*) Anteflexion. (*C*) Retroversion. (*D*) Retroflexion.

ment, often attributed to vaginal stimulation, is influenced mainly by clitoral stimulation.

The mucus produced by the vaginal lining has a rich glycogen content. When this glycogen is broken down by the lactose-fermenting bacteria (Döderlein's bacillus) that frequent the vagina, lactic acid is formed. This makes the usual pH of the vagina acid, a condition detrimental to the growth of pathologic bacteria, so that even though the vagina connects directly to the external surface, infection is not usually present. Under normal circumstances, women should be instructed not to use vaginal douches or sprays as a daily hygiene measure, because this may clean away the natural acid medium of the vagina and, in turn, invite vaginal infections. Following menopause, the pH of the vagina becomes closer to 7.5 or slightly alkaline, a reason that vulvovaginitis infections occur more frequently in women in this age group.

✔ CHECKPOINT QUESTIONS

4. Do all women who have never had sexual relations have intact hymens?
5. What is the point in the cervix at which cervical cancer is most apt to occur?
6. How does uterine retroversion differ from uterine retroflexion?

Breasts

The mammary glands, or breasts, arise from ectodermic tissue early in utero. They remain, however, in a halted stage of development until a rise in estrogen at puberty produces a marked increase in size from increased connective tissue and deposition of fat in girls and a transient increase in boys. The glandular tissue of the breasts, necessary for successful breast-feeding, remains undeveloped until a first pregnancy begins. Increase in male breast size is termed **gynecomastia.** If boys are not prepared that this is a normal change of puberty, they can be concerned that they are developing abnormally. Gynecomastia is most evident in obese boys.

Breasts are located anterior to the pectoral muscle (Fig. 4-11). In many women, breast tissue extends well into the axilla. Women should be taught to always include this region in breast self-examination or some breast tissue will be missed. Milk glands of breasts are divided by connective tissue partitions into approximately 20 lobes. All the glands in each lobe produce milk by acinar cells and deliver it to the nipple by a lactiferous duct. The nipple has approximately 20 small openings through which milk is secreted. An ampulla portion of the duct just posterior to the nipple serves as a reservoir for milk before breast-feeding.

A nipple is composed of smooth muscle that is capable of erection on manual or sucking stimulation. On stimulation, it transmits sensations to the posterior pituitary gland to release oxytocin. Oxytocin acts to constrict milk gland cells and push milk forward into the ducts that lead to the nipple. The nipple is surrounded by a darkly pigmented area of epithelium approximately 4 cm in diameter termed the areola; the areola appears rough on the surface owing to many sebaceous glands, called Montgomery's tubercles.

The blood supply to the breasts is profuse because it is formed by thoracic branches of the axillary, internal mammary, and intercostal arteries. This effective blood supply is important in bringing nutrients to the milk glands and makes possible a plentiful supply of milk for breast-feeding. It also, unfortunately, aids in the metastasis of breast cancer if this is not discovered early by breast self-examination or mammography.

Pelvis

The pelvis serves both to support and protect the reproductive and other pelvic organs. It is a bony ring formed by four united bones: the two innominate (flaring hip) bones that form the anterior and lateral portion of the ring,

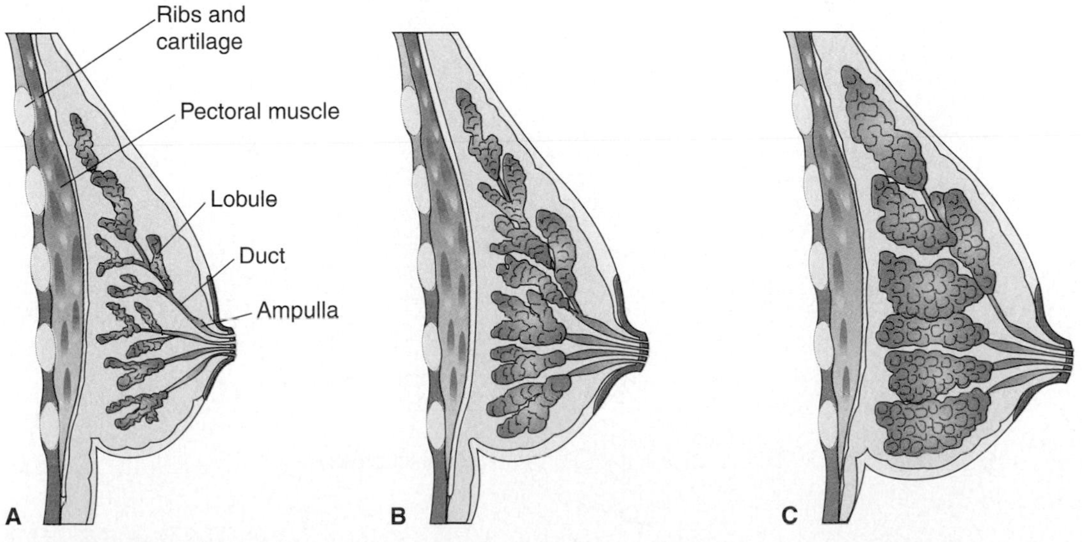

FIGURE 4.11 Anatomy of the breast. (*A*) Nonpregnant. (*B*) Pregnant. (*C*) During lactation.

and the coccyx and sacrum, which form the posterior aspect (Fig. 4-12).

Each innominate bone is divided into three parts: ilium, ischium, and pubis. The ilium forms the upper and lateral portion. The flaring superior border of this bone is what forms the prominence of the hip (the crest of the ilium). The ischium is the inferior portion. At the lowest portion of the ischium are two projections: the ischial tuberosities. This is the portion of bone on which a person sits. These projections are important markers used to determine lower pelvic width. The ischial spines are small projections that extend from the lateral aspects into the pelvic cavity. They mark the midpoint of the pelvis. The pubis is the anterior portion of the innominate bone. The symphysis pubis is the junction of the innominate bones at the front of the pelvis.

The sacrum forms the upper posterior portion of the pelvic ring. There is a marked anterior projection (the sacral prominence) of this bone at the point where it touches the lower lumbar vertebrae. This is a landmark to identify when securing pelvic measurements.

The coccyx, just below the sacrum, is composed of five very small bones fused together. Although it is stiff, there is a degree of movement possible in the joint between the sacrum and the coccyx (the sacrococcygeal joint). This is important movement because it permits the coccyx to be pressed backward, allowing more room for the fetal head as it passes through the bony pelvic ring at birth.

For obstetric purposes, the pelvis is further divided into the false pelvis (the superior half) and the true pelvis (the inferior half; Fig. 4-13). The false pelvis supports the uterus during the late months of pregnancy and aids in directing the fetus into the true pelvis for birth. The false pelvis is divided from the true pelvis only by an imaginary line: the linea terminalis. This imaginary line is drawn from the sacral prominence at the back to the superior aspect of the symphysis pubis at the front of the pelvis. Above the line is the false pelvis; below it, the true pelvis.

Other important terms in relation to the pelvis are the inlet, the pelvic cavity, and the outlet. The inlet is the entrance to the true pelvis, or the upper ring of bone through which the fetus must first pass to be born vaginally. It is at the level of the linea terminalis or is marked by the sacral prominence in the back, the ilium on the sides, and the superior aspect of the symphysis pubis in the front. If one looks down at the pelvic inlet, the passageway at this point appears heart-shaped because of the jutting sacral prominence. It is wider transversely (sideways) than in the anteroposterior dimension.

The outlet is the inferior portion of the pelvis, or that portion bounded in the back by the coccyx, on the sides by the ischial tuberosities, and in the front by the inferior aspect of the symphysis pubis. In contrast to the inlet of the pelvis, the greatest diameter of the outlet is its anteroposterior diameter.

The pelvic cavity is the space between the inlet and the outlet. This space is not a straight but a curved passage. There are physiologic reasons for this design. The curve slows and controls the speed of birth and therefore reduces sudden pressure changes in the fetal head, which might rupture cerebral arteries. The snugness of the cavity compresses the chest of the fetus as he or she passes through, helping to expel lung fluid and mucus and thereby better prepare the lungs for good aeration at birth.

The level of the ischial spines marks the midplane or midpoint of the pelvis. This marker is used to assess the level to which the fetus has descended into the birth canal during labor. For a baby to be delivered vaginally, he or she must be able to pass through the ring of pelvic bone. Therefore, the pelvic opening must be sufficient, or the infant will be too large to be born except by cesarean birth. This is not a problem for the average woman; it may

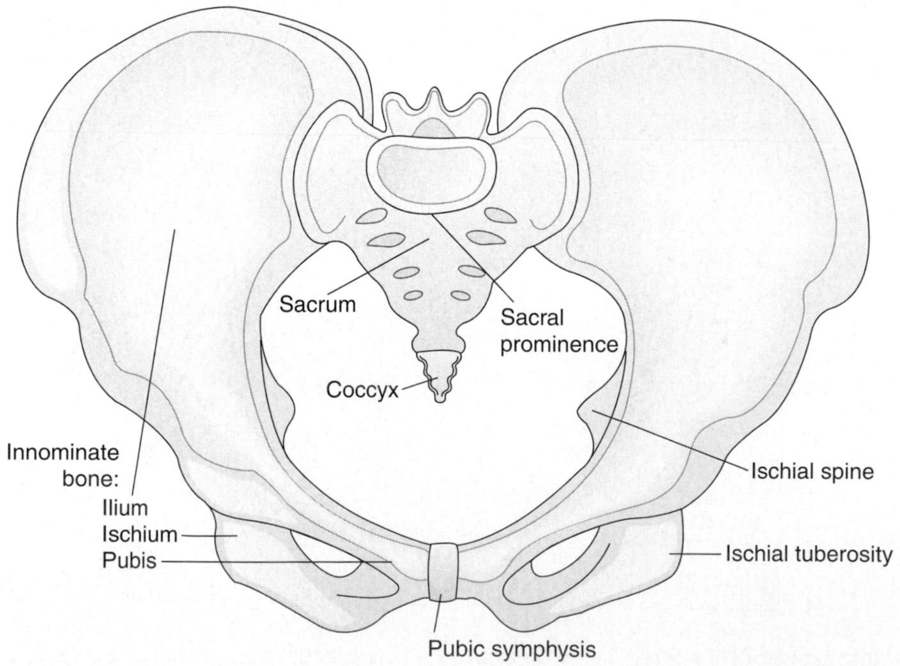

FIGURE 4.12 Structure of the pelvis.

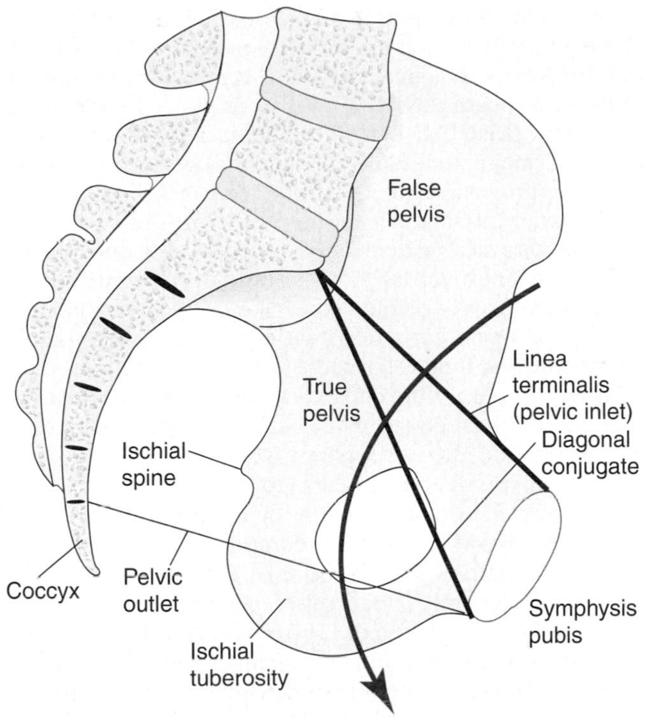

FIGURE 4.13 True and false pelvis. Portion above linea terminalis is false pelvis; portion below is true pelvis. *Arrow* shows "stovepipe" curve that the fetus must follow to be born.

be a problem for the young adolescent girl who has not yet achieved full pelvic growth (girls younger than age 14 years are most prone to this difficulty) or a woman who has had a pelvic injury such as from an automobile accident. Different pelvic types and an assessment of pelvic size are discussed in detail in Chapter 10.

MENSTRUATION

A menstrual cycle (also termed a female reproductive cycle) can be defined as episodic uterine bleeding in response to cyclic hormonal changes. It is the process that allows for conception and implantation of a new life. The purpose of a menstrual cycle is to bring an ovum to maturity and renew a uterine tissue bed that will be responsible for its growth should it be fertilized. Menarche, the first menstrual period in girls, may occur as early as age 8 or 9 or as late as age 17 and still be within normal limits. Because menarche may occur as early as age 9 years, it is good to include health teaching information on menstruation to both girls and their parents as early as fourth grade as part of routine care. It is a poor introduction to sexuality and womanhood for a girl to begin menstruation unwarned and unprepared for the important internal function it represents (Frank & Williams, 1999).

The length of menstrual cycles differs from woman to woman, but the accepted average length is 28 days (from the beginning of one menstrual flow to the beginning of the next). However, it is not unusual for cycles to be as short as 23 days or as long as 35 days. The length of the average menstrual flow (termed menses) is 2 to 7 days, although women may have periods as short as 1 day or as long as 9 days.

Because there is such variation in length, frequency, and amount of menstrual flow and such variation in the onset of menarche, many women have questions about what is considered normal. Contact with health care personnel during a yearly health examination or prenatal visit is often the first opportunity some women have to ask questions they have had for some time. Table 4-1 summarizes the normal characteristics of menstruation for quick reference.

Physiology of Menstruation

Four body structures are involved in the physiology of the menstrual cycle: the hypothalamus, the pituitary gland, the ovaries, and the uterus. For a menstrual cycle to be complete, all four structures must contribute their part; inactivity from any part will result in an incomplete or ineffective cycle (Fig. 4-14).

Hypothalamus

The release of luteinizing hormone-releasing hormone (LHRH, sometimes abbreviated GnRH for gonadotropin-releasing hormone) by the hypothalamus initiates the menstrual cycle; the presence of estrogen represses the hormone. During childhood, the hypothalamus is apparently so sensitive to the small amount of estrogen produced by the adrenal glands that release of the hormone is suppressed. Beginning with puberty it becomes less sensitive to estrogen feedback; this causes the initiation every month in females of the hormone LHRH. This is transmitted from

TABLE 4.1 Characteristics of Normal Menstrual Cycles

CHARACTERISTIC	DESCRIPTION
Beginning (menarche)	Average age of onset, 12 or 13 years; average range of age, 9–17 years
Interval between cycles	Average 28 days; cycles of 23 to 35 days not unusual
Duration of menstrual flow	Average flow, 2–7 days; ranges of 1–9 days not abnormal
Amount of menstrual flow	Difficult to estimate; average 30 to 80 mL per menstrual period; saturating pad or tampon in less than an hour is heavy bleeding
Color of menstrual flow	Dark red; a combination of blood, mucus, and endometrial cells
Odor	Similar to that of marigolds

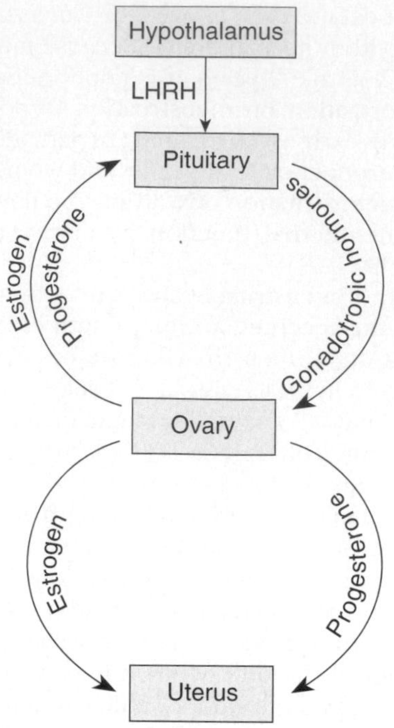

FIGURE 4.14 The interaction of pituitary-uterine-ovarian functions in a menstrual cycle.

the hypothalamus to the anterior pituitary gland and signals the anterior pituitary gland to begin producing the gonadotropic hormones follicle-stimulating hormone and luteinizing hormone (FSH and LH). Because production of LHRH is cyclical, menstrual periods also cycle.

Diseases of the hypothalamus causing deficiency of this releasing factor result in delayed puberty. Diseases causing early activation of the releasing factor lead to abnormally early sexual development or precocious puberty (see Chap. 47). When hormones secreted by the ovary such as estrogen and progesterone rise in amount each month, they create an inhibitory feedback mechanism that halts production of the releasing factor for the remainder of the month. This also occurs when high levels of pituitary-based hormones such as prolactin, FSH, or LH are present.

Pituitary Gland

Under the influence of LHRH, the anterior lobe of the pituitary gland (the adenohypophysis) produces two hormones that act on the ovaries to further influence the menstrual cycle: (1) FSH, a hormone that is active early in the cycle and is responsible for maturation of the ovum, and (2) LH, a hormone that becomes most active at the midpoint of the cycle and is responsible for ovulation, or release of the mature egg cell from the ovary, and growth of the uterine lining during the second half of the menstrual cycle.

Ovary

Under the influence of FSH and LH, called gonadotropic hormones because they cause growth (trophy) in the gonads (ovaries), one ovum matures in one or the other ovary and is discharged from it each month.

During the fertile period of a woman's life (from menarche to menopause) every month, one of the ovary's primordial follicles is activated by FSH secreted by the anterior pituitary to begin to grow and mature. Its cells produce a clear fluid (follicular fluid) containing a high content of estrogen (mainly estradiol) and some progesterone. As the structure grows in size, it is propelled toward the surface of the ovary. At maturity, it is visible on the surface of the ovary as a clear water blister approximately one-quarter or one-half inch across. At this stage of maturation, the small ovum (barely visible to the naked eye, approximately the size of a printed period) with its surrounding follicle membrane and fluid is termed a graafian follicle.

By day 14 before the end of a menstrual cycle (the midpoint of a typical 28-day cycle), the ovum has divided by mitotic division into two separate bodies: a primary oocyte, which contains the bulk of the cytoplasm, and a secondary oocyte, which contains so little cytoplasm it is not functional. The structure also has accomplished its meiotic division or has reduced its number of chromosomes to its haploid (having only one member of a pair) number of 23.

Following an upsurge of LH from the pituitary, prostaglandins are released and the graafian follicle ruptures. The ovum is set free from the surface of the ovary, a process termed ovulation. It is swept into the open end of a fallopian tube. It is important to teach women that ovulation occurs on approximately the 14th day before the onset of the next cycle. Because ovulation happens at the midpoint of a 28-day cycle, many women think incorrectly that the midpoint of their cycle will be the time of ovulation. If the cycle is only 20 days long, however, their day of ovulation would be day 6, not the 10th or middle day. If a cycle is 44 days long, ovulation would occur on day 30, not day 22.

After the ovum and the follicular fluid have been discharged from the ovary, the cells of the follicle remain in the form of a hollow, empty pit. The FSH has done its work at this point and now decreases in amount. The second pituitary hormone, LH, continues to rise in amount and acts on the follicle cells of the ovary. The LH causes the ovary to produce lutein, a bright-yellow fluid, instead of follicular fluid. The lutein is high in progesterone with some estrogen, whereas the follicular fluid was high in estrogen with some progesterone. This yellow fluid fills the empty follicle, which is then termed a corpus luteum (yellow body).

The basal body temperature of a woman drops slightly (0.5° to 1°F) just before the day of ovulation because of the extremely low level of progesterone present at that time. It rises 1°F the day after ovulation because of the concentration of progesterone (which is thermogenic) that is present at that time. The woman's temperature remains at this level until approximately day 24 of the menstrual cycle, when the progesterone level again decreases.

If conception (fertilization by a spermatozoon) occurs as the ovum proceeds down a fallopian tube, and the fertilized ovum implants on the endometrium of the uterus, the corpus luteum will remain throughout the major portion of the pregnancy (approximately 16 to 20 weeks). If conception does not occur, the unfertilized ovum atrophies after 4 or 5 days, and the corpus luteum (called a "false" corpus luteum) will then remain for only approximately

8 to 10 days. As the corpus luteum regresses, it is gradually replaced by white fibrous tissue, and the resulting structure is termed a corpus albicans (white body). Figure 4-15 shows the times when ovarian hormones are secreted at peak levels during a typical 28-day menstrual cycle.

Uterus

Stimulation from the hormones produced by the ovaries causes specific monthly effects on the uterus. Figure 4-15 illustrates the uterine changes during the menstrual cycle. These changes are also detailed below.

First Phase of Menstrual Cycle (Proliferative). Immediately after a menstrual flow (occurring the first 4 or 5 days of a cycle), the endometrium, or lining of the uterus, is very thin, only approximately one cell layer in depth. As the ovary begins to produce estrogen (in the follicular fluid, under the direction of the pituitary FSH), the endometrium begins to proliferate. This growth is very rapid and increases the thickness of the endometrium approximately eightfold. This increase continues for the first half of the menstrual cycle (from approximately day 5 to day 14). This half of a menstrual cycle is termed interchangeably the proliferative, estrogenic, follicular, or postmenstrual phase.

Second Phase of Menstrual Cycle (Secretory). After ovulation, the formation of progesterone in the corpus luteum (under the direction of LH) causes the glands of the uterine endometrium to become corkscrew or twisted in appearance and dilated with quantities of glycogen and mucin, an elementary sugar and protein. The capillaries of

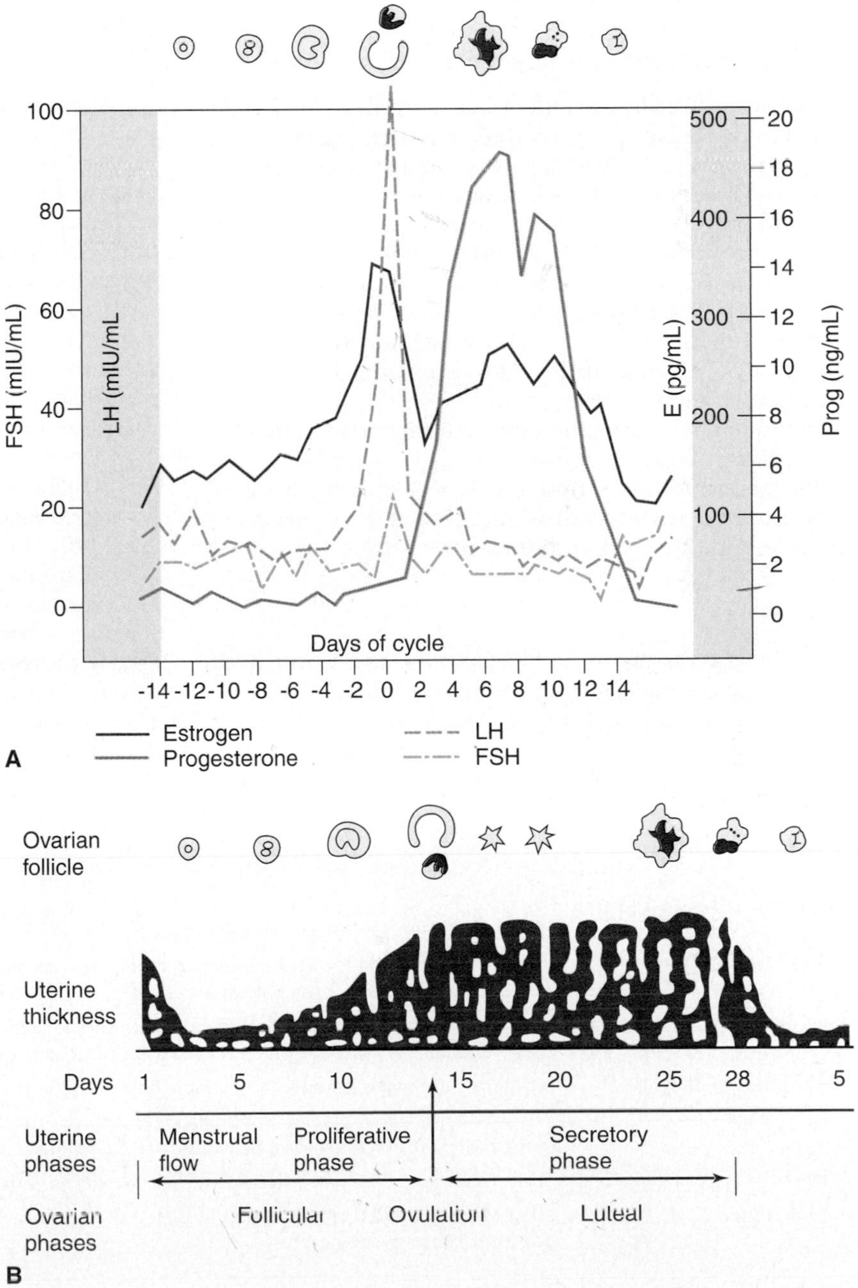

FIGURE 4.15 (*A*) Plasma hormone concentrations in the normal female reproductive cycle. (*B*) Ovarian events and uterine changes during the menstrual cycle.

the endometrium increase in amount until the lining takes on the appearance of rich, spongy velvet. This second phase of the menstrual cycle is termed the progestational, luteal, premenstrual, or secretory phase.

Third Phase of Menstrual Cycle (Ischemic). If fertilization does not occur, the corpus luteum in the ovary begins to regress after 8 to 10 days. As it regresses, the production of progesterone and estrogen decreases. With the withdrawal of progesterone stimulation, the endometrium of the uterus begins to degenerate (at approximately day 24 or day 25 of the cycle). The capillaries rupture, with minute hemorrhages, and the endometrium sloughs off.

Menses: Final Phase of a Menstrual Cycle. The following products are discharged from the uterus as the menstrual flow or menses:

- Blood from the ruptured capillaries
- Mucin from the glands
- Fragments of endometrial tissue
- The microscopic, atrophied, and unfertilized ovum

Menses is actually the end of an arbitrarily defined menstrual cycle. Because it is the only external marker of the cycle, however, the first day of menstrual flow is used to mark the beginning day of a new menstrual cycle.

Contrary to common belief, menstrual flow contains only approximately 30 to 80 mL of blood; it may seem more because of the accompanying mucus and endometrial shreds. The iron loss in a menstrual flow is approximately 11 mg. This is enough loss that many women need to take a daily iron supplement to prevent iron depletion during their menstruating years.

In women who are going through menopause, menses may typically be a few days of spotting before a heavy flow or heavy flow followed by a few days of spotting, because progesterone withdrawal is more sluggish or tends to "staircase" rather than withdraw smoothly.

Cervix

The mucus of the uterine cervix as well as the uterine body lining changes each month during the menstrual cycle. During the first half of the cycle, when hormone secretion from the ovary is low, cervical mucus is thick and scant. Sperm survival in this type of mucus is poor. At the time of ovulation, when the estrogen level is high, cervical mucus becomes thin and copious. Sperm penetration and survival at the time of ovulation in this thin mucus are excellent. As progesterone becomes the major influencing hormone during the second half of the cycle, cervical mucus again becomes thick and sperm survival is again poor.

Additional changes in cervical mucus are described in Chapter 6, because changes in cervical mucus are helpful in establishing fertility. Nursing education regarding cervical mucus changes can help women plan coitus to coincide with ovulation so they can increase their chances of pregnancy, or to avoid coitus at the time of ovulation to prevent pregnancy (see Chap. 5).

Education Regarding Menstruation

Education regarding menstruation is an important aspect of comprehensive sexuality education. Many myths about menstruation still exist, such as during menses women should not get a permanent; they should not plant vegetables because the vegetables will die; or they should not eat sour foods because this can cause cramping. Early preparation for menstruation to dispel these myths is vital to girls' future child-bearing and their concept of themselves as women because it teaches them to trust their body or think of menstruation as a mark of pride or growing up. Education regarding menstruation is equally important for boys so they can appreciate the cyclic process that a woman's reproductive system activates and can be active participants in helping plan or prevent the conception of children.

Girls who are well prepared for menstruation and view it as a positive happening are more likely to cope with menstrual discomforts and pain effectively, thus missing fewer school days than those who view menstruation as an ill time. Important teaching points for girls at menarche regarding menstruation are summarized in Table 4-2. Menstrual disorders including dysmenorrhea (painful menstruation), **menorrhagia** (abnormally heavy menstrual flows), **metrorrhagia** (bleeding between menstrual periods), and premenstrual dysphoric syndrome (Long, 2000) are discussed in Chapter 47 with other reproductive tract disorders.

TABLE 4.2 Teaching About Menstrual Health

AREA OF CONCERN	TEACHING POINTS
Exercise	It's good to continue moderate exercise during menses because it increases abdominal tone. Sustained excessive exercise, such as professional athletes maintain, can cause amenorrhea.
Sexual relations	Not contraindicated during menses (the male should wear a condom to prevent exposure to body fluid). Heightened or decreased sexual arousal may be noticed during menses. Orgasm may increase menstrual flow.
Activities of daily life	Nothing is contraindicated (many people believe incorrectly that things like washing hair are harmful).
Pain relief	Any mild analgesic is helpful. Prostaglandin inhibitors such as ibuprofen (Motrin) are specific for menstrual pain. Applying local heat may also be helpful.
Rest	More rest may be helpful if dysmenorrhea interferes with sleep at night.
Nutrition	Many women need iron supplementation to replace iron lost in menses. Eating pickles or cold food does not cause dysmenorrhea.

✔ **CHECKPOINT QUESTIONS**

7. Is the pelvic inlet wider in the anteroposterior or transverse diameter? Is the pelvic outlet the same?
8. What two hormones, important for a complete menstrual cycle, are secreted by the pituitary?
9. On what day of a menstrual cycle does ovulation typically occur?

Menopause

Menopause is the cessation of menstrual cycles. The postmenopausal period is the time of life following menopause. Perimenopausal is a term used to denote the period during which menopausal changes are occurring. The age range at which menopause occurs is wide, between 40 and 55 years. Both the age of menarche and the age of menopause tend to be familial (if menarche occurred early in a mother, it will probably occur early in her daughter; if menopause began early in a mother, it may begin early in her daughter). The earlier the age of menarche, the earlier menopause tends to occur. Women need health teaching to learn the normal parameters of menopause so they may continue to monitor their own health during this time (Dell & Stewart, 2000).

Women often refer to this period as a "change of life" because it marks the end of their ability to bear children and the beginning of a new phase of life. It can be a time of stress because of this role change, especially when this is coupled with other psychologically threatening happenings or vulnerability (Becker et al., 2001). Through health teaching, nurses can help women appreciate that loss of uterine function may make almost no change in their life and, for the woman with dysmenorrhea (painful menstruation) or with no desire for more children, may be a welcome change. Many women today begin hormone replacement therapy with menopause to help reduce symptoms such as hot flashes and decrease the possibility of osteoporosis developing with a decrease in estrogen. Hormone replacement is controversial, however, because there is some association between estrogen replacement and uterine cancer; see the Focus on Pharmacology: Estrogen (Premarin and Prempro). To reduce the risk of endometrial cancer, drug compounds of estrogen with progesterone added for the last 10 days of a month (Prempro) have been devised.

FOCUS ON PHARMACOLOGY

Conjugated Estrogen (Premarin and Prempro)

Classification: Female hormone; estrogen

Action: Conjugated estrogen is used for relief of vasomotor symptoms associated with menopause.

Pregnancy category: X

Dosage: 0.625–1.25 mg/d PO taken either on a cycle of 3 weeks on/1 week off or continuously. Therapy is initiated on the fifth day of menstruation or any time after 2 months of amenorrhea.

Possible adverse reactions: Headaches, dizziness, mental depression, nausea, vomiting, abdominal cramps, bloating, breakthrough bleeding, changes in menstrual patterns, dysmenorrhea, symptoms like premenstrual dysphoric syndrome, photosensitivity, peripheral edema, chloasma, cancers, blood clots, and liver disease

Nursing Implications

- Encourage the client to schedule frequent follow-up visits throughout therapy.
- Instruct the patient to take the drug cyclically or for a short term.
- Explain the possible side effects.
- Caution patient to use contraception during treatment to prevent pregnancy.
- Warn the client to report pain in the groin or calves; weakness or numbness in the extremities; chest pain or sudden shortness of breath; severe sudden headaches, dizziness, fainting, or mental depression; changes in speech or vision; yellowing of the skin and eyes; abnormal vaginal bleeding; or severe abdominal pain.
- Prempro is 0.625 mg of estrogen and 5 mg medroxyprogesterone; it has an advantage over Premarin of lowering the risk of endometrial cancer because it more accurately simulates normal endometrial growth.

SEXUALITY AND SEXUAL IDENTITY

Sexuality is a multidimensional phenomenon that includes feelings, attitudes, and actions. It has both biologic and cultural components. It encompasses and gives direction to a person's physical, emotional, social, and intellectual responses throughout life. Each person is born a sexual being, and his or her gender identity and gender role behavior evolve from and usually conform to the societal expectations within that person's culture. Nurses can play a major role in promoting sexual health through education and discussion. Box 4-2 highlights appropriate outcomes and interventions using the terminology identified by the Nursing Outcome Classification and Nursing Intervention Classification.

Biologic gender is the term used to denote chromosomal sexual development: male (XY) or female (XX). **Gender identity** or sexual identity is the inner sense a person has of being male or female, which may be the same as or different from biologic gender. **Gender role** is the behavior a person conveys about being male or female, which, again, may or may not be the same as biologic gender or gender identity.

Development of Gender Identity

Whether gender identity arises from primarily a biologic or psychosocial focus is controversial. The amount of testosterone secreted in utero (a process termed sex typing) may affect this characteristic. How appealing parents or other adult role models portray their gender roles may

BOX 4.2

NURSING OUTCOMES AND NURSING INTERVENTIONS CLASSIFICATION: SEX AND SEXUALITY

NOC: Knowledge, Sexual Functioning

Knowledge, sexual functioning is defined as the extent of understanding conveyed about sexual development and responsible sexual practices (Johnson et al., 2000). Some specific indicators suggesting achievement of this outcome include the client's ability to describe the following:

- Function of specific reproductive body parts
- Physical and emotional changes associated with puberty
- Reproduction
- Societal influences on sexual behavior
- Safe sex practices
- Effective contraception
- Measures to prevent sexually transmitted diseases

NIC: Teaching, Safe Sex

Teaching, safe sex is defined as providing instruction about sexual protection during sexual activity (McCloskey & Bulechek, 2000). Some important activities involved when implementing this intervention include:

- Discussing client's attitudes about birth control methods and instructing on the use of effective methods as appropriate
- Encouraging client to be selective in choosing sexual partners
- Instructing on low-risk sexual practices, importance of good hygiene, lubrication, and voiding after intercourse
- Endorsing the use of condoms, including ways for client to convince partners to use them
- Providing client with condoms and spermicidal products as appropriate
- Encouraging clients at high risk for STDs to seek regular examinations
- Planning sex education classes for groups of clients as appropriate

NIC: Teaching, Sexuality

Teaching, sexuality is defined as assisting individuals to understand physical and psychosocial dimensions of sexual growth and development (McCloskey & Bulechek, 2000). Some important activities involved when implementing this intervention include:

- Creating a nonjudgmental, accepting atmosphere
- Explaining human anatomy and physiology of the male and female body and human reproduction
- Discussing signs of fertility, such as ovulation and menstruation
- Supporting parents' role as primary sexuality educators for their children
- Educating parents on sexual growth and development
- Using appropriate questions for client's self-reflection
- Exploring the meaning of sexual roles
- Discussing sexual behavior and appropriate ways to express one's feelings and needs
- Informing children and adolescents of the benefits to postponing sexual activity and on the negative consequences of early child-bearing
- Teaching about STDs, including AIDS
- Educating children and adolescents about effective contraception, including assisting adolescents in choosing a method as appropriate
- Facilitating role-playing to aid in resisting peer and social pressures of sexual activity
- Enhancing self-esteem through peer role-modeling and role-playing

also influence how a child envisions himself or herself. For example, both sons and daughters often relate better to whichever parent is kinder and more caring. This may result in a son assuming characteristics often regarded as feminine or daughters developing interests typically regarded as masculine.

Gender role is also culturally influenced. In Western society, women have in the past been viewed as kind and nurturing, with sole responsibility for childrearing and homemaking. Men were viewed as financial providers for the family. Fortunately, gender roles today are more interchangeable than they once were: women pursue all kinds of jobs and careers without loss of femininity; men participate (some as primary homemakers) with childrearing and household duties without loss of masculinity.

An individual's sense of gender identity develops throughout an entire life span, but the stage is set by expectations even before a child is born. Although parents usually respond to the question, "Do you want a boy or a girl?" with the answer, "It doesn't matter as long as it's healthy," many parents actually do have strong preferences for a male or female child. Although some parents may be disappointed if the child is not the gender they hoped for, most adapt quickly and will say later that they always wanted that sex child. Children who suspect that their parents wanted a child of the opposite sex are more likely to adopt roles of the opposite sex than if they are confident their parents are pleased with them as they are.

Infancy

From the day of birth, female and male babies are treated differently by their parents. People generally bring girls dainty rattles and dresses with ruffles; on the whole, they are treated more gently by parents and held and rocked more than male babies. People tend to buy boys bigger rattles and sports-related jogging suits. Admonitions given babies can be different. A girl might be told, "Don't cry. You don't look pretty when you cry." A boy might be told, "You've got to learn to be tougher than that if you're ever going to make it in this world." By the end of the first year, differences in play are usually strongly evident. Boys appear to demonstrate more innate aggression at this stage than girls.

Preschool Period

Children can distinguish between males and females as early as age 2 years. By age 3 or 4 years, they know what sex they are, and they have absorbed cultural expectations of that sex role. Often, boys will play rough-and-tumble games with other boys, and girls will play more quietly with each other, although the two frequently mix at this age.

Sex role modeling is reinforced through behavior toward and expectations of the child as well as from watching television, the color and décor of the child's room, and the child's clothing. Social contacts between the child and significant adults contribute to sexual identification and should be encouraged in this developmental period. A positive self-concept grows from parental love, effective relationships with others, success in play activities, and gaining skills and self-control.

Most American parents are not too rigid about what clothing or colors are appropriate for boys and girls. They strive to teach both sons and daughters about expressing feelings, performing household tasks, and engaging in the same play activities. However, some parents have fixed role identifications. They tend to foster quiet, domestic behavior in their daughters and tough, aggressive behaviors in their sons and have more definite ideas regarding gender-related play and apparel. Comments such as, "What kind of mommy are you going to be, treating a doll that way?" or "Is that the way a lady sits?" from parents and well-meaning friends help to govern their choice of actions. Common sayings such as "all boy" or "boys will be boys" represent the differences expected between the two sexes. The suggestions in the Focus on Family Empowerment can help parents promote a positive gender identity in their child.

Although the development of an Oedipus complex (the strong emotional attachment of a preschool boy for his mother or a preschool girl for her father) may have been overstated by Freud as a result of sexual bias, many children manifest indications that such a phenomenon is occurring. The preschool boy begins to show signs of competing with his father for his mother's love and attention; the preschool girl begins to compete with the mother for the father's attention and love. Parents may need reassurance that this phenomenon of competition and romance in preschoolers is normal and is one step in the development of their child's gender role identity.

School-Age Child

Early school-age children typically spend play time imitating adult roles as a way of learning gender roles (Fig. 4-16). They start to form strong impressions of what a female or male role should be. Where once schools promoted differences in boys and girls by separating activities and through such beliefs as expecting boys to be poorer readers, to write less neatly, and to act rougher in the school hallways, grade schools have become more attuned to unisex activities.

Girls may participate in activities that were once male-dominated such as Little League or shop and auto repair courses; boys can take cooking courses or ballet lessons, formerly the province of girls.

Adolescent

At puberty, as the adolescent begins the process of establishing a sense of identity, the problem of final gender role identification surfaces again. Most early adolescents maintain strong ties to their gender group; boys with boys,

FOCUS ON FAMILY EMPOWERMENT

Gender Identity

Sexuality and reproductive function can be areas of care that families have many questions about yet are hesitant to ask. Helping parents to feel comfortable asking this type of question is a major point in health teaching. Here are two commonly asked questions:

Q. Is it all right to call body parts by nicknames such as "peter," or should we use the anatomic name?

A. Although this is strictly up to parents, using anatomic names is usually advised. This prevents children from thinking of one part of the body as so different from others (and perhaps dirty or suspect) that it can't be called by its real name.

Q. Is it important to give our children unisex toys? Can't girls play with dolls and boys with trucks anymore?

A. Developing a sense of gender is more involved than what toys children use for play. If parents are concerned with instituting unisex roles in children, they need to begin by monitoring their own perspective on what they believe are female and male roles. Once they project a feeling that roles are interchangeable, no one action but rather the general home milieu will teach this to children in their family.

The way people manifest maleness and femaleness is culturally influenced. For example, in certain cultures, a man may be expected to maintain an air of "machismo" or a distance while his partner is in labor rather than move closer to her and be more comforting. Being aware of cultural differences in this way helps you to view people as individuals and better understand their actions in situations.

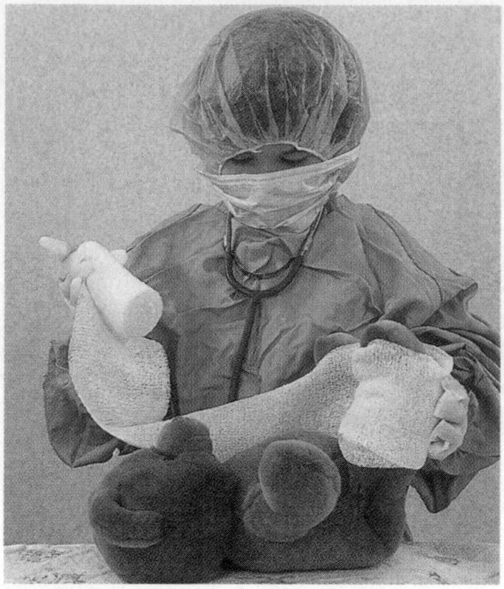

FIGURE 4.16 Early school-age children imitate adult roles to learn more about them. Here a girl "tries on" what being a doctor will feel like.

girls with girls. The advent of menstruation may provide a common bond for girls at this stage. Some adolescents choose a child of their own gender a few years older than themselves to use as their model of gender role behavior. This is a way that adolescents can be certain that they understand and feel comfortable with their own sex before they are ready to reach out and interact with members of the opposite sex (Lammers et al., 2000).

Interviewing adolescents for a sexual history needs to be done tactfully and with confidentiality, because this is a new and sensitive area for them. As many as 50% of ninth-grade boys and 30% of ninth-grade girls are already sexually active. As many as 75% of college sophomores are sexually active. This means they need guidelines for safer sex (Box 4-3). Including such instructions in sexual counseling should help to reduce the incidence of STDs as well as empower adolescents with better self-care skills. It is important when discussing safer sex practices to be certain that adolescents not only understand when but how they will incorporate them into their lifestyle. One of the reasons that preventive measures for human immunodeficiency virus (HIV) and other STDs have not been as successful as first predicted may be that adolescents' total lifestyle and interpretation of sexuality were not at first considered (see the Focus on Communication).

Adolescence can be a very stressful time for the boy who first realizes that he is gay or the girl who first realizes that she is lesbian. Part of the reason for the high suicide rate in adolescence may be because homosexual teenagers feel so lost in a heterosexual-dominant culture (La Sala, 2000).

Young Adult

When young adults move away from home to attend college or establish their own home, they choose the way they will express their sexuality along with other life patterns. Many young adults marry with a commitment to one sexual partner. Others establish relationships (cohabitation) less binding by legal definitions but perhaps equally binding in concern and support. Young adults may view cohabitation as a means of learning more about a possible marriage partner on a day-to-day basis in the hope that a future marriage will then be stronger and more lasting. Homosexuality or bisexuality may be overtly expressed for the first time during this period (Beeler & DiProva, 1999).

Gender identity can affect parenting roles. Individuals may have firmly fixed notions by the age of parenthood regarding their gender roles in the care of children. These individuals may strongly embrace or reject male or female roles in parenting. Other individuals may have difficulty in assuming parenting roles or may be flexible about them. Generally, gender roles in parenting are influenced by the way an individual was raised.

Conflicts in parenting can occur if an individual's gender roles do not meet the needs of his or her child and family situation or an individual's partner has different expectations regarding gender roles. Parents-to-be need to take time to discuss some of the views they have on parenting and see whether they agree on male and female roles and their relationship with their children. A single parent may be concerned about how both roles can be fulfilled and can benefit from talking with a health care provider about how to discuss this area of concern with a child. Conflicts in the role parents have chosen often come to light for the first time during pregnancy as they worry about what type of parent they are going to be or if they are adequately prepared to be a parent. Being able to talk to health care personnel about the gender role they have adopted in life can be a major step in resolving feelings of inadequacy and preparing themselves to raise a child.

Middle-Age Adult

For many women and men in midlife, sexuality has achieved a degree of stability. A sense of masculinity or femininity and comfortable patterns of behavior have been established. This increased security in identity can promote greater intimacy in sexual and social relationships. This may also be a time when adults allow themselves more freedom in exploring and satisfying sexual needs.

Although menopause alters reproductive functioning, it does not physically inhibit sexual functioning. Generally, a woman with a strong self-image, positive sexual and social relationships, and knowledge regarding her body and menopause is likely to progress through this natural biologic stage without problems and remain sexually active and satisfied. Nurses can be instrumental in teaching women about what to expect at menopause so it is not a surprise and helping them maintain self-esteem through this natural process.

During mid-life, men may begin to experience changes in sperm production, erectile power, achievement of orgasm, and sex drive, although these changes generally do not significantly alter reproductive or sexual functioning. Some men feel that these changes threaten their sexuality and "maleness" and may respond negatively. Other men feel these changes make sex more pleasurable and

BOX 4.3

GUIDELINES FOR SAFER SEX PRACTICES

1. Be selective in choosing sexual partners. When you have sex, you are exposing yourself to the infections of everyone with whom your partner has ever had sex. The more partners you have relations with, the greater your danger of contracting a sexually transmitted disease.
2. Don't be reluctant to ask a sexual partner about his or her sexual lifestyle before engaging in sexual relations. If a partner has a history of casual contacts or bisexual or unprotected sex, there is a greater hazard of infection for you than if your partner is also choosy about partners.
3. Avoid sexual relations with IV drug users or prostitutes (male or female) or sexual partners who have had sexual relations with such people, because such people have a greater than usual chance of carrying HIV and hepatitis B infections.
4. Inspect your sexual partner for any lesions or abnormal drainage in the genital area. Do not engage in sexual relations with anyone who exhibits these signs.
5. The use of a condom is the best protection against infection. Condoms should be latex; the chance of the condom tearing is less if it is a prelubricated brand. Those coated with the spermicide nonoxynol-9 appear to be effective in destroying HIV, herpes, gonorrhea, and chlamydia. Use water-based lubricants such as KY Jelly on condoms, because oil-based lubricants can weaken the rubber. Spermicidal cream or jelly with nonoxynol-9 provide not only lubrication but also some additional protection against infectious agents.
6. Condoms should be protected from excessive heat to avoid rubber deterioration and should be inspected to be certain they are intact before use. Do not inflate condoms before use to test for intactness because this weakens the rubber.
7. Condoms should be fitted over the erect penis with a small space left at the end to accept semen. The condom should be held against the sides of the penis while the penis is withdrawn to prevent spillage of semen.
8. Voiding immediately after sexual relations may aid in washing away contaminants on the vulva or in the urinary tract.
9. Anal intercourse carries a high risk for HIV and hepatitis B infection as well as infection from intestinal organisms. Use lubricants for anal penetration to keep bleeding and condom resistance to a minimum.
10. Do not engage in oral-penile sex unless the male wears a condom, because even preejaculatory fluid may contain viruses and bacteria. For safer oral-vaginal sex, a condom split in two or a plastic dental dam like that used for pediatric dentistry and covering the mouth should be used to protect against the exchange of body fluids.
11. Hand-to-genital contact may be hazardous if open cuts are present on hands. Use a latex glove or finger cot for protection.
12. To decrease the possibility of transferring germs, do not share sexual aids such as vibrators.
13. If you think you have contracted a sexually transmitted disease, do not engage in sexual relations until you have contacted a health care provider and are again disease-free. Alert any recent sexual partners that you might have an infection so they also can receive treatment.

intimate and often respond positively. Actual sexual dysfunctions, as a result of physical or psychosocial changes, may arise at this time. Teaching men about normal biophysical changes, providing them with methods to improve sexual functioning, and offering them support are important nursing roles.

Mid-life is often a time when both men and women reexamine life goals, careers, accomplishments, value systems, and familial and social relationships. As a result, some people adapt, whereas others experience stress or a crisis. This reexamination can positively or negatively affect an individual's gender identity and sexuality. For example, a woman may realize that she is not able to be both a homemaker and career person. She may either modify her belief that it is important for a woman to assume both roles or try harder to achieve this goal, believing that she has personally failed. The increased incidence of sexual encounters that men have with younger women at this age is seen by many as the man's way of reassuring himself of his attractiveness and virility and denying the fear of aging.

Certain medications such as antihypertensives, antianxiety agents, and narcotics may diminish sexual response in both men and women. Being aware of this is important not only for clients, so they can understand that it is an expected response, but also for their partners.

A woman who undergoes surgery on her reproductive organs, such as hysterectomy (removal of the uterus), needs sensitive nurses to listen to her concerns about the meaning of the experience to her. For some women, the loss of a uterus can be synonymous with the loss of femininity. If both ovaries are also removed (oophorectomy), an immediate surgical menopause occurs. The hormonal changes occurring with the removal of both ovaries must be dealt with openly. Limited hormonal replacement is often a means of simulating the naturally decreasing hormone levels of natural menopause. Education about the risks and benefits of hormone replacement therapy is important.

FOCUS ON COMMUNICATION

Mark is a 16-year-old boy visiting the health care clinic. He states he has had painful urination all day. He is sexually active. A culture is taken to determine if he has an STD.

Less Effective Communication

Nurse: Mark, you may have a sexually transmitted disease, so I'll need to ask you a few questions.
Mark: Uh-huh.
Nurse: Do you practice safe sex?
Mark: Uh, yeah.
Nurse: I assume that means you always use a condom.
Mark: Right.
Nurse: It would be hard to contract an STD if you always do.
Mark: Guess I'm just unlucky.

More Effective Communication

Nurse: Mark, you may have a sexually transmitted disease, so I'll need to ask you a few questions.
Mark: Uh-huh.
Nurse: What do you consider to be safe sex?
Mark: Using birth control, like the pill or a condom.
Nurse: What method do you use?
Mark: My girlfriend's on the pill, so we don't need to use anything else.
Nurse: The pill will help prevent pregnancy, but it won't protect you from contracting an STD.
Mark: No kidding.
Nurse: Let's talk about the different protection needed to prevent pregnancy and STDs.

Adolescents are often concerned about adults respecting their privacy. Usually, they offer as little information as possible, especially in regards to sexual issues. Asking them specific, open-ended questions is important to ensure a positive exchange of information and effective health teaching. As they offer details, it is important to remain nonjudgmental and to encourage them so they continue to elaborate.

The individual who comments about the need to maintain a reduced activity level at work or a reduced social schedule may also be seeking information and direction in other important areas of life such as sexual relations.

Older Adult

Both male and female older adults can enjoy active sexual relationships. Some men experience lesser erectile firmness or ejaculatory force than when they were younger, but others discover that they are able to maintain an erection longer. Both sexes need to follow safer sex practices throughout life. Because males remain fertile throughout life, they must continue to be responsible sex partners in terms of reproductive planning. Older women may have less vaginal secretions because they have less estrogen after menopause. Using a water-soluble lubricant before sexual intercourse may enhance their comfort and enjoyment. An estrogen supplement also often corrects this.

The Individual Who is Physically Challenged

Individuals who are physically challenged have sexual desires and needs the same as others. They may have difficulty, though, with sexual identity or sexual enjoyment due to the effects of their condition. Males with upper spinal cord injury may have difficulty with erection and ejaculation, because these actions are governed at the spinal level. Manual stimulation of the penis or psychological stimulation achieves erection in most men with spinal cord lesions, allowing the man a satisfying sexual relationship with his partner. Women with most spinal cord injuries cannot experience orgasm but are able to conceive and have children.

Those who interpret a procedure such as a colostomy as disfiguring may be reluctant to participate in sexual activities, fearing that the sight of an apparatus will diminish their partner's satisfaction or enjoyment. People with chronic pain such as arthritis may be too uncomfortable to enjoy sex. Individuals with urinary catheters may be concerned about their ability to enjoy coitus with the catheter in place. For women, a retention catheter should not interfere with coitus. Males can be taught how to replace their own catheter so they can remove it for sexual relations. In all instances in which one sexual partner is disabled in some way, the response of a loving partner does much to enhance the body image and feelings and adequacy of a mate. Encouraging them to ask questions and work on specific difficulties is a nursing role.

Sexuality is a facet of rehabilitation that has not always received attention. In the past, if a person could accomplish activities of daily living such as eating, elimination, and mobility, then that person was considered to be leading a normal or near-normal life. Today, establishment of a satisfying sexual relationship is considered an activity of daily living and should be included as such in assessment of clients in rehabilitation programs.

HUMAN SEXUAL RESPONSE

Sexuality has always been a part of human life, but it is only in the past few decades that it has been studied scientifically by experts in the field of sex research. One common finding of researchers has been that feelings and attitudes about sex vary widely: the sexual experience is unique to each individual, but sexual physiology (that is, how the body responds to sexual arousal) has common features.

Sexual Response Cycle

Two of the earliest researchers of sexual response were Masters and Johnson. In 1966, they published the results of a major study of sexual physiology based on more than 10,000 episodes of sexual activity among more than 600 men and women (Masters,1998). In this study, they described the human sexual response as a cycle with four discrete stages: excitement, plateau, orgasm, and resolution.

Excitement

Excitement occurs with physical and psychological (i.e., sight, sound, emotion, or thought) stimulation that causes parasympathetic nerve stimulation. This leads to arterial dilation and venous constriction in the genital area; the blood supply to this area increases, with resulting vasocongestion and increasing muscular tension. In women, this vasocongestion causes the clitoris to increase in size and mucoid fluid to appear on vaginal walls as lubrication. The vagina widens in diameter and increases in length. The nipples become erect. In men, erection occurs; there is scrotal thickening and elevation of the testes. In both sexes, there is an increase in heart and respiratory rates and blood pressure.

Plateau

The plateau stage is reached just before orgasm. In the woman, the clitoris is drawn forward and retracts under the clitoral prepuce; the lower part of the vagina becomes extremely congested (formation of the orgasmic platform), and there is increased nipple engorgement.

In men, the vasocongestion leads to full distention of the penis. Heart rate increases to 100 to 175 beats per minute and respiratory rate to approximately 40 respirations per minute.

Orgasm

Orgasm occurs when stimulation proceeds through the plateau stage to a point at which the body suddenly discharges accumulated sexual tension. A vigorous contraction of muscles in the pelvic area expels or dissipates blood and fluid from the area of congestion. The average number of contractions for the woman is 8 to 15 contractions at intervals of one every 0.8 seconds. In men, muscle contractions surrounding the seminal vessels and prostate project semen into the proximal urethra. These contractions are followed immediately by three to seven propulsive ejaculatory contractions, occurring at the same time interval as in the woman, which force semen from the penis.

As the shortest stage in the sexual response cycle, orgasm is usually experienced as intense pleasure affecting the whole body, not just the pelvic area. It is also a highly personal experience; descriptions of orgasms vary greatly from person to person.

Resolution

Resolution is the period during which the external and internal genital organs return to an unaroused state. For the male, a refractory period occurs during which further orgasm is impossible. Women do not go through this refractory period, so it is possible for women who are interested and properly stimulated to have additional orgasms immediately after the first. The resolution period generally takes 30 minutes for both men and women.

Controversies About Female Orgasm

The female orgasm has been a topic of much controversy over the years, beginning with Freud who posited that there were two types of female orgasms, clitoral and vaginal. He believed that clitoral orgasms (originating from masturbation or other noncoital acts) represented sexual immaturity and that only vaginal orgasms were the authentic, mature form of sexual behavior in women. Accordingly, he considered women to be neurotic if they did not achieve orgasm through intercourse.

Masters (1998) showed that there is no physiologic difference between an orgasm achieved through intercourse and one achieved by stimulating the clitoris directly. Women have reported a difference in the intensity and character between orgasms achieved through coitus and through other means, and some prefer one to the other, but there is no physiologic difference between them. For most women, adequate time for foreplay is essential for them to be orgasmic.

In recent years, a subject of controversy regarding female sexuality has arisen: the existence or not of "the G spot." First described in 1950 by the German physician Grafenberg, the G spot, presumably located on the inner portion of the vaginal wall, halfway between the pubic bone and the cervix, has been recently promoted as an area of heightened erotic sensitivity. Several studies carried out in the past 10 years have not been able to verify the existence of this particular anatomic site, although some women do claim to possess such an erotic trigger (Masters, 1998).

Influence of the Menstrual Cycle on Sexual Response

During the second half of the menstrual cycle—the luteal phase—there is increased fluid retention and vasocongestion in the woman's lower pelvis. Because some vasocongestion is already present at the beginning of the excitement stage of the sexual response, women appear to reach the plateau stage more quickly and achieve orgasm more readily during this time. Women also seem to be more interested in initiating sexual relations at this time.

Influence of Pregnancy on Sexual Response

Pregnancy is another time in life when, because of the rapidly growing fetus in the lower pelvic area, vasocongestion of the area occurs. Some women experience their first orgasm during their first pregnancy due to this phenomenon. After a pregnancy, many women experience increased sexual interest because the new growth of blood vessels during pregnancy lasts for some time and continues to facilitate pelvic vasocongestion (see the Focus on Evidence-Based Practice). This is why discussing sexual relationships is an important part of health teaching during pregnancy. At a time when a woman may want sexual contact very much, she needs to be free of myths and misconceptions such as orgasm will cause a spontaneous miscarriage (see Focus on Nursing Care Planning). Although the level of oxytocin does appear to rise in women following orgasm, it is not enough to cause concern in the average woman.

For some women, the increased breast engorgement that accompanies pregnancy may result in extreme breast sensitivity during coitus. Foreplay that includes sucking

FOCUS ON EVIDENCE-BASED PRACTICE

Does Women's Sexual Activity Increase or Decrease During Pregnancy?

For this study, to explore women's sexual experiences during pregnancy, 141 pregnant women from the offices of obstetricians at a tertiary care university hospital in Canada were asked to complete questionnaires. Results showed that vaginal intercourse and sexual activity overall decreased throughout pregnancy. Most women reported a decrease in sexual desire (58%). Forty-nine percent of women worried that sexual intercourse could harm the pregnancy. Although women had sexual concerns, only 29% discussed sexual activity in pregnancy with their doctor, and 49% raised the issue first. Of those women who did not discuss the topic with their doctors, 76% wished it had been discussed.

This is an important study for nurses because it reveals that most women have concerns over sexual activity during pregnancy, showing how much this topic needs to be discussed at prenatal visits.

Bartellas, E., Crane, J. M., Daley, M., Bennett, K. A., & Hutchens, D. (2000). Sexuality and sexual activity in pregnancy. *BJOG: International Journal of Obstetrics & Gynecology, 107*(8), 964–968.

or massaging breasts is not contraindicated unless the woman has a history of premature labor.

Types of Sexual Orientation

Sexual gratification is experienced in a number of ways. One's culture determines acceptable forms of sexual expression. What is considered normal varies greatly among cultures, although general components of accepted sexual activity are that privacy, consent, and lack of force are included. Most individual value systems are closely aligned to the cultural norm.

Heterosexuality

A **heterosexual** is one who finds sexual fulfillment with a member of the opposite gender. Because interest in the opposite sex and sexual relationships may begin as early as the beginning of puberty (age 10 to 12 years), health care providers need to provide information on safer sex practices and ways an individual plans to use these as early as this for the knowledge to be most helpful.

Homosexuality

A **homosexual** is a person who finds sexual fulfillment with a member of his or her own sex. Many homosexual men prefer to use the term "gay." **Lesbian** refers to a homosexual woman.

Why homosexual gender identity develops is unknown, although evidence that this is genetically determined or develops because of the effect of an abnormal level of estrogen or testosterone in utero is increasing. Even before puberty, most individuals who are homosexual report a realization that they are "different" in that they are not interested in opposite-sex classmates. It is probably during adolescence, in seeking a sense of identity, that they realize the reason they feel "different" is because they are homosexual. This can be a frightening time because a homosexual identity is not usually easily revealed to family or friends. Some people refuse to associate with homosexuals to such an extent that a fear termed homophobia exits.

Although gay and lesbian children have often demonstrated behavior that is inconsistent with expected gender roles from early childhood, young adulthood is the time most persons begin to assume a homosexual lifestyle. Many young adults are worried about the stigma of being labeled a homosexual and so keep their identity secret from heterosexual acquaintances. Others "commit" or "come out" or are able to reveal to friends and family that they are homosexual (Santelli et al., 2000).

Because the period of identity confusion during adolescence can be so traumatic to a homosexual youth, it is important for health care providers to be sensitive to their needs in the area of identity formation. The adolescent suicide rate is high in gay and lesbian adolescents because it is such a time of turmoil. Gay youths may need additional counseling to help them avoid acquiring HIV and other STDs because issues such as avoiding contact through anal intercourse may not be routinely covered in such education. Lesbians may be at less risk for STDs than males because of the low incidence of these diseases in the lesbian population. Securing a sexual history and providing information on the prevention of STDs and their signs and symptoms are important responsibilities for health care providers caring for gay and lesbian, as well as heterosexual, youths.

With children being raised by gay and lesbian couples today, an important part of health guidance is allowing couples to discuss their sexual concerns and wishes for their children.

Bisexuality

People are bisexual if they achieve sexual satisfaction from both homosexual and heterosexual relationships. Gay and bisexual men may be at greater risk for HIV and STDs than others. Female partners of bisexual men need to be aware of this increased risk.

Transsexuality

A **transsexual** is an individual who, although of one biologic gender, feels as if he or she should be of the opposite gender. Such people may have sex change operations so they appear cosmetically as the sex they envision themselves to be. However, such operations do not change the person's chromosomal structure. Although capable of sexual relations in this new role (a synthetic vagina or penis is created), the person is incapable of reproduction. The incidence of sex change operations has decreased in recent years because of potential disappointment follow-

FOCUS ON *Nursing Care Planning*

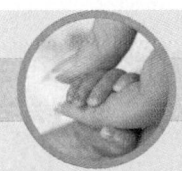

A PREGNANT COUPLE WITH CONCERNS ABOUT SEXUAL ACTIVITY

A couple, 12 weeks pregnant, comes to the antepartal clinic for a routine visit. The wife, in tears, states, "My husband doesn't seem interested in me anymore. We haven't had sex since I became pregnant." Husband states, "I'm afraid I'll hurt the baby."

Assessment: Client 12 weeks pregnant with history of spontaneous miscarriage 2 years ago. Prior to conception, couple engaged in coitus approximately two or three times per week. Prenatal exam within acceptable limits.

Nursing Diagnosis: Altered sexuality patterns related to prenatal changes and fear of harming fetus

Outcome Identification: Couple will state resumption of mutually satisfying sexual relationship by next visit.

Outcome Criteria: Couple verbalizes positive sexual contact; reports engaging in sexual intercourse and pleasurable noncoital activities.

Interventions	Rationale
1. Assess the couple's lifestyle and concerns since becoming pregnant. Encourage the couple to verbalize their needs and feelings.	1. Assessment of lifestyle and concerns provides a baseline from which to build. Verbalization of feelings provides a safe outlet for emotions and helps to increase the other partner's awareness.
2. Explore misinformation and misconceptions. Use anatomic charts, illustrations, and other materials as appropriate.	2. Exploration of these areas provides opportunities to correct them and also helps to open the lines of communication between the partners.
3. Explain that sexual intercourse is allowed during pregnancy until labor begins. Use charts and illustrations to show how the fetus is protected in utero.	3. Barring complications, couples can engage in sexual intercourse to the extent that it is comfortable and desired. Visual aids enhance learning.
4. Inform the couple that contractions may occur after orgasm but these are not harmful to the fetus and will subside.	4. Alerting the couple to this possibility prepares them and eliminates the fear that may occur, thinking that their actions caused labor to begin.
5. Continue to encourage the couple to talk openly about their feelings, concerns, desires, and changes in interest to each other throughout the pregnancy.	5. Physical and psychological changes occur in both the pregnant woman and her partner throughout pregnancy. Open communication enhances the relationship.
6. Review alternative sexual positions and other pleasurable activities such as cuddling, stroking, and massaging. Reinforce on next visit.	6. As pregnancy progresses, the discomforts, fatigue, and increasing abdominal size and pressure may interfere with a satisfying sexual relationship. Advance planning prepares the couple for adaptations that may be necessary.

ing the surgery: despite a new outward appearance, the person realizes that he or she is still not totally the person he or she wished to become.

Types of Sexual Expression

Because people are individuals, types of sexual expression are individualized.

Celibacy

Celibacy is abstinence from sexual activity. Celibacy is the avowed state of certain religious orders. It is also a way of life for many adults and one becoming fashionable among a growing number of young adults. The theoretical advantage of celibacy is the ability to concentrate on means of giving and receiving love other than through sexual expression.

Masturbation

Masturbation is self-stimulation for erotic pleasure; it can also be a mutually enjoyable activity for sexual partners. It offers sexual release, which may be interpreted by the person as overall tension or anxiety relief. Masters (1998) reported that women may find masturbation to orgasm the most satisfying sexual expression and use it more commonly than men. Children between ages 2 and 6 years discover masturbation as an enjoyable activity as they explore their bodies. Children under a high level of tension may become accustomed to using masturbation as a means of falling asleep at night or at naptime. They do this without any attempt at concealment because they have not yet been affected by society's view that such activity is private.

School-age children continue to use masturbation for enjoyment or to relieve tension but perform such activities in private. Counseling parents about what is normal or to be expected is discussed in Chapters 30 to 32. In a hospital setting, a school-age child may assume that he or she has more privacy than actually exists, and thus may be discovered masturbating if someone walks unannounced into the room.

Following reproductive tract surgery or childbirth, many adult men and women are concerned with how soon they will be able to have sexual relations again without feeling pain. They may masturbate to orgasm to test whether everything in their body is still functional, much as the preschooler does.

Erotic Stimulation

Erotic stimulation is the use of visual materials such as magazines or photographs for sexual arousal. Although this is thought of as mostly a male phenomenon, there is increasing interest in centerfold photographs in magazines marketed primarily to women. Some parents of adolescents may need to be assured that an interest in this type of material is developmental and normal. Respect this type of reading material when straightening patient rooms in a health care facility.

Fetishism

Fetishism is sexual arousal by the use of certain objects or situations. Leather, rubber, shoes, and feet are frequently perceived to have erotic qualities. The object of stimulation does not just enhance the experience; rather, it becomes a focus of arousal. A person may come to require the object or situation for stimulation.

> **WHAT IF?** What if, on unpacking a patient's suitcase on hospital admission, you discover that your new patient has brought a wardrobe of unusual rubber articles of clothing or photographs of people wearing rubber? What would you do?

Transvestism

A **transvestite** is an individual who dresses to take on the role of the opposite sex. Transvestites can be heterosexual, homosexual, or bisexual. Some transvestites, particularly married heterosexuals, may be under a great deal of strain to keep their lifestyle a secret from friends and neighbors.

Voyeurism

Voyeurism is sexual arousal by looking at another's body. Almost all children and adolescents pass through a stage when voyeurism is appealing; this passes with more active sexual expressions. That some voyeurism exists in almost everyone is illustrated by the large number of R-rated movies shown on television and in movie theaters and by the erotic descriptions in modern novels. Voyeurism may be practiced to the exclusion of other sexual experiences, but such an extreme probably reflects great insecurity or the inability to feel confident enough to relate to others on more personal levels.

Sadomasochism

Sadomasochism involves inflicting pain (sadism) or receiving pain (masochism) to achieve sexual satisfaction. It is a practice generally considered to be within the limits of normal sexual expression as long as the pain involved is minimal and the experience is satisfying to both sexual partners.

Autoerotic asphyxia is a practice of producing oxygen deficiency (usually by hanging) during masturbation to produce a feeling of extreme sexual excitement. Not aware that the act can be fatal (from hanging), a number of adolescents are killed by this practice each year.

Other Types of Sexual Expression

A multitude of other types of sexual expression exist (e.g., exhibitionism, obscene phone calling, pedophilia, and bestiality). Exhibitionism is revealing one's genitals in public. Pedophiles are individuals interested in sexual encounters with children. Known pedophiles are registered sex offenders. When they move into a new community, families are notified of the move according to Megan's Law, a national law designed to alert citizens to the presence of a sex offender in a community. Ways to keep children safe from sex offenders are discussed in Chapter 30 with other aspects of community safety.

DISORDERS OF SEXUAL FUNCTIONING

Disorders involving sexual functioning can have a psychogenic origin (produced by psychic factors rather than organic factors), a biogenic origin (produced by biologic processes), or both. They are also categorized as primary (a lifelong condition) or secondary (occurring after the person has experienced a period of normal functioning).

Primary Sexual Dysfunction

There are several types of primary sexual dysfunction. Careful assessment can help to clarify whether the cause is related to physical factors, psychological factors, or a combination of both.

Erectile Dysfunction

Erectile dysfunction (ED), formerly referred to as impotence, is the inability to produce or maintain an erection long enough for vaginal penetration or partner satisfaction. The majority of reasons why this occurs are physical, such as aging and atherosclerosis. A debilitating disease such as diabetes can also play a role. The problem is compounded by doubt about the ability to perform and reluctance to discuss the problem with health care providers. The drug of choice today for erectile dysfunction is sildenafil (Viagra) taken up to once a day to stimulate penile erection (Karch, 2001; see the Focus on Pharmacology: Sildenafil [Viagra]). If this is not successful (it is contradicted in men with a risk of cardiovascular illness or who are taking medications that contain nitrates), surgical implants to aid erection and the use of vacuum pressure are possible alternatives. Testosterone injections may be helpful in some men. In all instances, frank discussion about the cause of the problem and current therapy available is helpful.

Premature Ejaculation

Premature ejaculation is ejaculation before penile-vaginal contact. The term is often used to mean ejaculation before the sexual partner's satisfaction as well. Premature ejaculation can be unsatisfactory and frustrating for both partners.

The cause of premature ejaculation, like that of erectile dysfunction, can be psychological. Masturbating to orgasm (in which orgasm is achieved quickly owing to lack of time) may play a role. Other reasons suggested are doubt about masculinity and fear of impregnating the woman, which prevents the man from sustaining an erection. Serotonergic antidepressants may be helpful. Sexual counseling for both partners to reduce stress may be helpful in alleviating the problem.

Failure to Achieve Orgasm or Decreased Sexual Desire

The failure of a woman to achieve orgasm can be due to poor sexual technique, concentrating too hard on achievement, or possible negative attitudes toward sexual relationships. Treatment is aimed at relieving the underlying cause. It may include instruction and counseling for the couple about sexual feelings and needs. Some women experience a decrease in sexual desire during perimenopause. Administration of estrogen and androgen may be effective in enhancing libido in these women (Barbieri, 2000). Sildenafil (Viagra) is not FDA-approved for women, but administration of this or dopamine is a future possibility.

Vaginismus

Vaginismus is involuntary contraction of the muscles at the outlet of the vagina when coitus is attempted. This muscle contraction prohibits penile penetration. Vaginismus may occur in women who have been raped. It can also be the result of early learning patterns in which sexual relations were viewed as bad or sinful. As with other sexual problems, sexual or psychological counseling to reduce this response may be necessary (Phillips, 2000).

Dyspareunia

Dyspareunia is pain during coitus. It can occur due to endometriosis (abnormal placement of endometrial tissue), vaginal infection, or hormonal changes such as those that occur with menopause. It can be psychological. Treatment is aimed at the underlying cause (Canavan & Heckman, 2000).

Inhibited Sexual Desire

Lack of a desire for sexual relations may be a concern of young or middle-aged adults. Health teaching can reassure such clients that this is normal in circumstances such as following the death of a family member, divorce, or a stressful job change. It can be a side effect of medicines. Support of a caring sexual partner or relief of the tension causing the stress allows a return to sexual interest.

Secondary Sexual Dysfunction

Chronic diseases, such as peptic ulcers, or chronic pulmonary disorders that cause frequent pain or discomfort may interfere with a man or woman's overall well-being and interest in sexual activity. Obese men and women may have difficulty achieving deep penetration because of the bulk of their abdomen. An individual with an STD such as genital herpes may forgo sexual relations rather than inform a partner of the disease. Encouraging open communication between sexual partners is a nursing intervention that proves useful in all these situations.

FOCUS ON PHARMACOLOGY

Sildenafil Citrate (Viagra)

Classification: Therapy for erectile dysfunction

Action: Causes smooth muscle relaxation and inflow of blood to the corpus cavernosum of the penis, achieving erection

Dosage: 50 mg P.O. prn 1 hour before sexual activity, up to one dose per day

Possible Adverse Reactions: Headache, dizziness, ventricular arrhythmia, impairment of blue/green discrimination

Nursing Implications

- Assess patient for preexisting cardiovascular risk.
- Caution patient that dose should be limited to one time per day; use is contradicted if the patient is taking nitrates.
- Erection lasting more than 4 hours and priapism can occur. This can lead to penile tissue damage.
- Caution patient that this drug does not protect against sexually transmitted diseases or pregnancy, so he must use safe sex practices.

✔ CHECKPOINT QUESTIONS

10. You discover a preschooler masturbating when you go to wake her from a nap. Is this unusual?
11. What percentage of adolescents are sexually active?
12. Should sexual partners of bisexual males insist their partner use a condom?

KEY POINTS

The reproductive and sexual organs form early in intrauterine life; full functioning becomes possible at puberty.

The female internal organs of reproduction include the ovaries, fallopian tubes, uterus, and vagina.

The female external organs of reproduction include the mons veneris, labia minora and majora, vestibule, clitoris, fourchette, perineal body, hymen, and Skene's and Bartholin's glands.

The male external reproductive structures are the penis, scrotum, and testes. Internal organs are the epididymis, vas deferens, seminal vesicles, ejaculatory ducts, prostate gland, urethra, and bulbourethral glands.

A menstrual cycle is periodic uterine bleeding in response to cyclic hormones. Menarche is the first menstrual period. Menstrual cycles are possible because of the interplay between the hypothalamus, pituitary, ovaries, and uterus.

Biologic gender is determined by chromosomal content (XX or XY) and is set at conception. Gender identity is a person's concept of being male or female. This develops over a lifetime. Gender role is yet a third aspect and is the behavior a person assumes based on his or her gender identity as male or female.

Masters and Johnson have identified a sexual response cycle consisting of excitement, plateau, orgasm, and resolution stages. Disorders of sexual dysfunction include failure to achieve orgasm, vaginismus, dyspareunia, inhibited sexual desire, premature ejaculation and erectile dysfunction.

People present with varying sexual orientations, such as heterosexual, homosexual or bisexual. Common sexual expressions are voyeurism, fetishism, and celibacy.

Educating people about reproductive function is an important primary prevention measure because it teaches them to better monitor their own health through breast and vulvar or testicular self-examination.

Adolescents should be taught that with sexual maturity comes sexual responsibility. The best protection against either an STD or an unintentional pregnancy is the practice of abstinence or safer sex.

CRITICAL THINKING EXERCISES

1. At the beginning of the chapter, you were asked to teach an eighth-grade class on sexual and reproductive health. A boy in the first row asks why he has to learn about female reproduction. A girl who hasn't begun menstruation yet asks you to predict when she will have her first period. The boy behind her says he doesn't believe sex education should be taught in school. How would you respond to these questions?
2. A 15-year-old boy whom you see in your role as a school nurse is concerned because a number of his friends have sexually transmitted diseases. What would you advise him regarding safer sex practices?
3. A mother is concerned because her daughter, age 7, seems to be a "tomboy." She asks you how she can convince her daughter to be more of a "lady." What advice would you give her? Suppose her daughter was 17? Would your advice be different? Suppose she was concerned because a son was not "boy" enough? Would your answer be any different?
4. Examine the National Health Goals related to reproductive tract or sexual functioning. Most government-sponsored money for nursing research is allotted based on these goals. What would be a possible research topic to explore pertinent to these goals?

REFERENCES

Barbieri, R. L. (2000). Approach to sexual dysfunction in the female. In H. D. Humes (Ed.). *Kelly's textbook of internal medicine.* Philadelphia: Lippincott Williams & Wilkins.

Bartellas, E. et al. (2000). Sexuality and sexual activity in pregnancy. *BJOG: International Journal of Obstetrics & Gynecology, 107*(8), 964–968.

Becker, D., et al. (2001). Psychological distress around menopause. *Psychosomatics, 42*(3), 252–257.

Beeler, J., & DiProva, V. (1999). Family adjustment following disclosure of homosexuality by a member: Themes discerned in narrative accounts. *Journal of Marital & Family Therapy, 25*(4), 443–459.

Berkey, C. S., et al. (2000). Relation of childhood diet and body size to menarche and adolescent growth in girls. *American Journal of Epidemiology, 152*(5), 446–452.

Canavan, T. P., & Heckman, C. D. (2000). Dyspareunia in women: Breaking the silence is the first step toward treatment. *Postgraduate Medicine, 108*(2), 149–152.

Chang, S. H., et al. (2000). Height and weight change across menarche of schoolgirls with early menarche. *Archives of Pediatrics & Adolescent Medicine, 154*(9), 880–884.

Dell, D. L., & Stewart, D. E. (2000). Menopause and mood: Is depression linked with hormone changes? *Postgraduate Medicine, 108*(3), 34–36.

Department of Health and Human Services. (2000). *Healthy people 2010.* Washington, D.C.: DHHS.

Frank, D., & Williams, T. (1999). Attitudes about menstruation among fifth-, sixth-, and seventh-grade pre- and post-menarcheal girls. *Journal of School Nursing, 15*(4), 25–31.

Johnson, M., Maas, M., & Moorhead, S. (2000). *Nursing outcomes classification* (2d ed.). St. Louis: Mosby, Inc.

Karch, A. M. (2001). *Lippincott's nursing drug guide.* Philadelphia: Lippincott Williams & Wilkins.

Lammers, C. et al. (2000). Influences on adolescents' decision to postpone onset of sexual intercourse: A survey analysis of virginity among youths aged 13 to 18 years. *Journal of Adolescent Health, 26*(1), 42–48.

La Sala, M. C. (2000). Lesbians, gay men, and their parents: Family therapy for the coming-out crisis. *Family Process, 39*(1), 67–81.

Ling, F. W., & Duff, P. (2001). *Obstetrics and gynecology: Principles for practice.* New York: McGraw-Hill.

Long, F. W. (2000). Recognizing and treating premenstrual dysphoric disorder in the obstetric, gynecologic and primary care practices. *Journal of Clinical Psychiatry, 61*(12 suppl), 9–16.

Masters, W. H. (1998). *Heterosexuality.* New York: Smithmark.

McCloskey, J., & Bulechek, G. (2000). *Nursing interventions classification* (3d ed.). St. Louis: Mosby, Inc.

Pentyala, S., et al. (2001). Be prepared for patients who need help for erectile dysfunction. *Patient Care for the Nurse Practitioner, 4*(3), 13–27.

Phillips, N. A. (2000). Female sexual dysfunction: Evaluation and treatment. *American Family Physician, 62*(1), 127–136.

Santelli, J. S., et al. (2000). The association of sexual behaviors with socioeconomic status, family structure, and race/ethnicity among U.S. adolescents. *American Journal of Public Health, 90*(10), 1582–1588.

Seifer, D. B., Samuels, P., & Kniss, D. A. (2001). *The physiologic basis of gynecology and obstetrics.* Philadelphia: Lippincott Williams & Wilkins.

Tanner, J. M. (1990). Fetus into man. In *Physical growth from conception to maturity* (2nd ed.). Cambridge, MA: Harvard University Press.

Weber, R. F. A. et al. (2002). Environmental influences on male reproduction. *BJU International, 89*(2), 143–148.

SUGGESTED READINGS

Avery, M. D., Duckett, L., & Frantzich, C. R. (2000). The experience of sexuality during breastfeeding among primiparous women. *Journal of Midwifery & Women's Health, 45*(3), 227–237.

Barber, M. D. et al. (2002). Sexual function in women with urinary incontinence and pelvic organ prolapse. *Obstetrics & Gynecology, 99*(2), 281–289.

Benazzi, F. (2000). Female depression before and after menopause. *Psychotherapy & Psychosomatics, 69*(5), 280–283.

Blythe, M. J., & Rosenthal, S. L. (2000). Female adolescent sexuality: promoting healthy sexual development. *Obstetrics & Gynecology Clinics of North America, 27*(1), 125–141.

Brown, J. D. (2000). Adolescents' sexual media diets. *Journal of Adolescent Health, 27*(2 suppl), 35–40.

Carvajal, S. C. (1999). Psychosocial predictors of delay of first sexual intercourse by adolescents. *Health Psychology, 18*(5), 443–452.

Fergusson, D. M., Horwood, L. J., & Beautrasis, A. L. (1999). Is sexual orientation related to mental health problems and suicidality in young people? *Archives of General Psychiatry, 56*(10), 876–880.

Geller, S. E., Harlow, S. D., & Bernstein, S. J. (1999). Differences in menstrual bleeding characteristics, functional status, and attitudes toward menstruation in three groups of women. *Journal of Women's Health & Gender-Based Medicine, 8*(4), 533–540.

Griffin, C. M. (1999). Reframing menarche education: A developmental perspective. *Advance for Nurse Practitioners, 7*(11), 53–57.

Hogan, D. P., Sun, R., & Cornwell, G. T. (2000). Sexual and fertility behaviors of American females aged 15–19 years. *American Journal of Public Health, 90*(9), 1421–1425.

Obermeyer, C. M. (2000). Menopause across cultures: A review of the evidence. *Menopause, 7*(3), 184–192.

Zillmann, D. (2000). Influence of unrestrained access to erotica on adolescents' and young adults' dispositions toward sexuality. *Journal of Adolescent Health, 27*(2 suppl), 41–44.

5

CHAPTER

Reproductive Life Planning

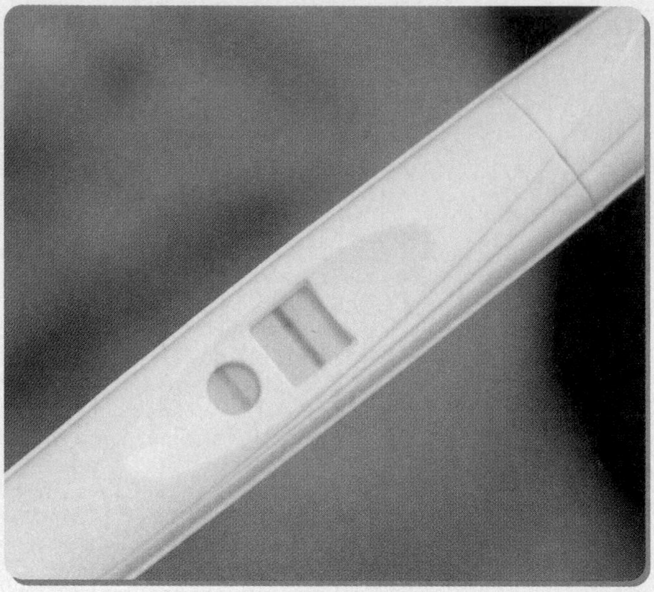

Key Terms

- abstinence
- barrier method
- basal body temperature method
- calendar method
- cervical cap
- coitus interruptus
- condom
- contraceptive
- diaphragm
- elective termination of pregnancy
- fertility awareness
- intrauterine device
- laparoscopy
- monophasic
- natural family planning
- reproductive life planning
- triphasic
- tubal ligation
- vasectomy

Objectives

After mastering the contents of this chapter, you should be able to:

1. Describe common methods of reproductive life planning and the advantages, disadvantages, and risk factors associated with each.
2. Assess clients for reproductive life planning needs.
3. Formulate nursing diagnoses related to reproductive life planning concerns.
4. Identify expected outcomes for couples desiring reproductive life planning.
5. Plan nursing care related to reproductive life planning, such as helping a client select a suitable family planning measure.
6. Implement nursing care related to reproductive life planning, such as educating adolescents about the use of condoms as a safer sex practice as well as to prevent unwanted pregnancy.
7. Evaluate outcome criteria for achievement and effectiveness of care.
8. Identify National Health Goals related to reproductive life planning that nurses can be instrumental in helping the nation achieve.
9. Identify areas related to reproductive life planning that could benefit from additional nursing research or application of evidence-based practice.
10. Use critical thinking to analyze methods that could be used to promote reproductive health within a family-centered framework.
11. Integrate reproductive life planning with nursing process to achieve quality maternal and child health nursing care.

Seventeen-year-old Dana Crews has come to a community health clinic for a pelvic examination and Pap smear. During the assessment interview, Dana states that she is sexually active. She and her boyfriend sometimes use a condom. She trusts her boyfriend will "stop in time" when they aren't using one. She doesn't want to take the pill because she can't afford it and she's afraid her parents will find out that she's having sex. Does Dana need any additional health teaching to be well informed about reproductive life planning?

Previous chapters described the anatomy and physiology of the male and female reproductive systems. This chapter adds information about ways to prevent pregnancy or plan and space children. This is important information because it builds a base for care and health teaching about safer sex practices.

After you've studied the chapter, answer the Critical Thinking Exercises at the end of the chapter and then access the on-line study activities (http://connection.lww.com) *to further sharpen your skills and test your knowledge.*

Reproductive life planning includes all the decisions an individual or couple make about having children. These decisions usually include if and when to have children, how many children to have, and how they are spaced. Couples often need counseling about how to avoid conception. Others need information on increasing fertility. Some couples need counseling because contraception has failed.

It's important for the health of children that as many pregnancies as possible are intended. When a pregnancy is unintended, the mother is less likely to seek prenatal care, less likely to breast-feed, and more likely to expose the fetus to harmful substances. The child of such a pregnancy is at greater risk of low birthweight, dying in the first year, being abused, and not receiving sufficient resources for healthy development. A disproportionate share of the women who bear children whose conception was unintended are unmarried, less apt to complete high school or college, and more likely to require public assistance and to live in poverty than their peers who are not mothers (DHHS, 2000; Felton & Bartoces, 2002).

Not so long ago, **contraceptive** products (products to prevent pregnancy) were not all that reliable or could not be easily purchased. Today, people have numerous contraceptive choices, which range in reliability and accessibility from fair to good. Reproductive health has become so important that a number of National Health Goals speak directly to this area of care (see the Focus on National Health Goals).

An individual's or a couple's choice of contraceptive method should be made carefully, with complete knowledge about the advantages, disadvantages, and side effects of the various options (see Focus on Communication). Important things to consider are:

- Personal values
- Ability to use a method correctly
- How the method will affect sexual enjoyment
- Financial factors
- Status of a couple's relationship
- Prior experiences
- Future plans

FOCUS ON NATIONAL HEALTH GOALS

A number of National Health Goals speak directly to reproductive life planning. These are:

- Reduce the proportion of females experiencing pregnancy despite use of a reversible contraceptive method from a baseline of 13% to a target of 7%.
- Increase the proportion of pregnancies that are intended from a baseline of 51% to a target of 70%.
- Decrease the proportion of births occurring within 24 months of a previous birth from a baseline of 11% to a target of 6%.
- Increase the proportion of females at risk for unintended pregnancy (and their partners) who use contraception from a baseline of 93% to a target of 100%.
- Increase the number of health care providers who provide emergency contraception.
- Increase male involvement in pregnancy prevention and family planning efforts (new goal; baseline to be determined) (DHHS, 2000).

Nurses can be instrumental in helping the nation achieve these objectives by teaching people, especially adolescents, about contraceptive options. This must be done carefully to avoid indirectly encouraging sexual activity among teens. Investigation as to what contraceptives adolescents prefer or why they make the choices they do could be an important area of nursing research.

The widespread use of contraceptives in recent years points to both an increased awareness of the responsibility for contraception and the options available. Understanding how various methods of contraception work and how they compare in terms of benefits and disadvantages is necessary for successful nursing counseling. It is also important to be able to answer questions about elective termination of pregnancy with accurate, up-to-date knowledge and objectivity for couples whose contraceptive has failed. Legal and ethical issues (e.g., enforced use of contraception for the physically or mentally challenged) must also be considered when counseling clients on the use of contraceptives. With information and the ability to discuss specific concerns, clients are better prepared to make the decisions that are right for them (Shaban et al., 2001).

NURSING PROCESS OVERVIEW

For Reproductive Health

Assessment

As a result of changing social values and lifestyles, many people are able to talk easily about reproductive life planning. Remember, however, that others are

FOCUS ON COMMUNICATION

Mrs. Irving is a 30-year-old woman who gave birth to her first child, an 8-lb boy, yesterday. You notice her sitting by her hospital bed, dressed ready to go home, reading a brochure on birth control.

Less Effective Communication

Nurse: Is that pamphlet helpful? Tell you everything you need to know?

Mrs. Irving: I'm kind of in the dark here. I had such endometriosis I had trouble getting pregnant, so I've never used anything.

Nurse: You'll need to start. You don't want to get pregnant again for at least 2 years.

More Effective Communication

Nurse: Is that pamphlet helpful? Tell you everything you need to know?

Mrs. Irving: I'm kind of in the dark here. I had such endometriosis I had trouble getting pregnant, so I've never used anything.

Nurse: But you want to start using something now?

Mrs. Irving: Not really. My doctor told me to only wait 6 months after this baby to try and have another because the endometriosis could grow back.

Nurse: That's good planning. And good to see you considering your individual lifestyle before making a choice.

Reproductive life planning measures must be individualized to fit a person's lifestyle; otherwise, they will be quickly discontinued. Using time with a woman to help her assess her lifestyle is better than just giving advice with a "one size fits all" philosophy.

ASSESSING the Client for Possible Contraindications to Contraceptive Use

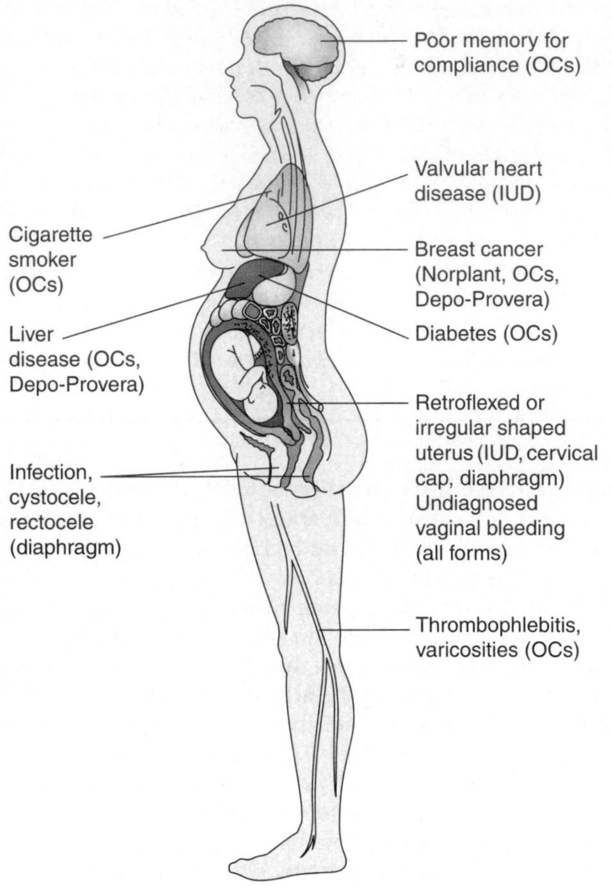

uncomfortable with this topic and may not voice their interest in the subject independently. For this reason, at health assessments, clients need to be asked if they want more information or need any help with reproductive life planning. Important assessments before the initiation of a contraceptive method include:

- A Pap smear, pregnancy test, gonococcal and chlamydial screening, and perhaps hemoglobin for detection of anemia
- Obstetric history such as sexually transmitted diseases (STDs), past pregnancies, previous elective abortions, failure of previously used methods, and compliance record
- Subjective assessment of the client's desires, needs, feelings, and understanding of conception (e.g., teens may believe that nothing can happen to them; many women in the immediate postpartal period may believe that they cannot conceive immediately, especially if they are breast-feeding)
- Sexual practices such as frequency, number of partners, feelings about sex and body image (see Assessing the Client for Possible Contraindications to Contraceptive Use)

Nursing Diagnosis

Nursing diagnoses applicable to reproductive life planning may include:

- Health-seeking behaviors regarding contraception options related to desire to prevent pregnancy
- Deficient knowledge related to use of diaphragm
- Decisional conflict regarding choice of birth control because of health concern
- Decisional conflict related to unwanted pregnancy
- Powerlessness related to failure of chosen contraceptive
- Ineffective sexuality patterns related to fear of pregnancy

Planning and Implementation

When establishing goals for care in this area, be certain that they are realistic for the individual. If a woman has a history of poor compliance with medication, for instance, it might not be realistic for her to plan to take an oral contraceptive every day. It is important, too, to be sensitive to and explore a couple's religious, cultural, and moral beliefs before suggesting possible methods. It is equally important to explore your own beliefs and values. This not only helps develop a self-awareness of how these beliefs affect nursing care but in turn allows you to become more sensitive to the beliefs of others.

Education is an important nursing role in this area. Some couples cannot make realistic plans about contraception because they are uninformed or misinformed about the options. An organization helpful for referral for reproductive life planning is Planned Parenthood (*www.plannedparenthood.org*). When counseling, be certain to emphasize safer sex measures as well as contraceptive ones (see Guidelines for Safer Sex Practices, Box 4-3). For example, although many contraceptive options offer reliable pregnancy prevention, only condoms provide protection against STDs, an important concern if the relationship is not a monogamous one (see Focus on Multidisciplinary Care).

It is important for clients to provide informed consent for surgical contraceptive methods or procedures. The risks, benefits, alternatives, and proper use of the method and the client's understanding of his or her rights and responsibilities are recorded on the consent form. Always obtain the client's signature in the presence of a witness. Informed consent helps ensure that clients have weighed their options and chosen a method that best meets their needs.

Outcome Evaluation

Evaluation is important in reproductive life planning because anything that causes clients to discontinue or misuse a particular method will leave them at risk of pregnancy. It is important to reassess early (within 1 to 3 weeks) after a couple begins a new method of contraception to prevent such an occurrence. Evaluation is much broader than simply ensuring that no unwanted conception occurs, however. The satisfaction of a woman and her sexual partner with the method chosen is also important. Examples of expected outcomes include:

- Client voices confidence in chosen method by next visit.
- Client expresses satisfaction with chosen method at follow-up visit.
- Client consistently uses chosen method without pregnancy for next year.

FOCUS ON MULTIDISCIPLINARY CARE

Many health care facilities print information on contraception, which they distribute to women to read before discharge. Women are then invited to ask questions as necessary about the material. Read them to see that they're accurate, and if suggestions are needed, make them to the correct health care committee. Be certain that unlicensed assistive personnel understand that if a woman has a question about the written material, their job is not to answer it but to refer the woman to someone such as a nurse who is more knowledgeable about the subject. Otherwise, they may suggest what method works for them rather than offering unbiased advice. This can result in a woman choosing a contraceptive method that is not appropriate for her lifestyle and that may then be ineffective for her.

CONTRACEPTIVES

As many as 40 million women in the United States use some form of contraception; this represents three fourths of women of childbearing age (Speroff & Darney, 2001). An ideal contraceptive should be:

- Safe
- 100% effective
- Free of side effects
- Easily obtainable
- Affordable
- Acceptable to the user and sexual partner
- Free of effects on future pregnancies

The effectiveness of various contraceptive measures is shown in Table 5-1. This table gives the failure rates for each method in the first year of use. The failure rate represents the number of pregnancies that occur among couples who use the method consistently and correctly.

Focus on Nursing Care Planning provides details on how to implement a plan of care for an adolescent seeking contraceptive information. Box 5-1 highlights appropriate outcomes and interventions using the terminology identified by the Nursing Outcomes Classification and Nursing Interventions Classification. Focus on Evidence-Based Practice addresses the question of whether women are as well informed about birth control options as they want to be.

Abstinence

Obviously, the most effective way to protect against conception is to abstain from sexual intercourse (**abstinence**). This has a 0% failure rate. Abstinence is also the most effective way to prevent STDs. However, clients, particularly adolescents, may find it difficult to comply with abstinence or may completely overlook it as an option (Thomas, 2000). In a moment of passion, many otherwise responsible people may fail to consider this as an option. It is important to present abstinence as a contraceptive option, however, and provide information on ways to comply with this method (see Focus on Family Empowerment).

Natural Family Planning

Natural family planning methods are those, as the name implies, that involve no chemical or foreign material being introduced into the body (Tommaselli et al., 2000).

Many people hold religious beliefs that rule out the use of birth control pills or devices; others simply prefer these methods because no expense or foreign substance is involved; still others simply believe that a "natural" way

TABLE 5.1 Contraceptive Failure Rates

TYPE OF CONTRACEPTIVE	FAILURE RATE (%)*	ADVANTAGES	DISADVANTAGES
None	85	No motivation necessary	Highly unreliable
Spermicides	21	No major health risk; no prescription necessary	Unaesthetic to some; must be properly inserted
Periodic abstinence	20	No cost; acceptable to Roman Catholic church	Requires high motivation and periods of abstinence
Withdrawal	18	No cost	Requires motivation
Cervical cap	18	Can use for several days if desired	May be difficult to insert; can irritate cervix
Diaphragm	18	No major health risks; easy to use	Insertion may be difficult
Female condom	15	Protection against STDs	Insertion may be difficult
Male condom	12	Protects against STDs; male responsibility; no prescription necessary	Requires interruption of sexual activity
IUD	3	No memory or motivation needed	Cramping, bleeding; expulsion possible; possible risk of PID
Pill	3	Coitus independent	Continual cost; possible side effects
Injectable progesterone	0.3	Coitus independent; dependable for 4 to 12 weeks	Continual cost; continual injections
Implanted progesterone	0.04	Coitus independent; dependable for 5 years	Initial cost; appearance on arm
Female sterilization	0.4	Permanent and highly reliable	Initial cost; irreversible
Male sterilization	0.1	Permanent and highly reliable	Initial cost; irreversible

*Among couples who use the method consistently and correctly during a year's time.
Modified from Speroff, L., & Darney, P. D. (2001). *A clinical guide for contraception.* Philadelphia: Lippincott Williams & Wilkins.

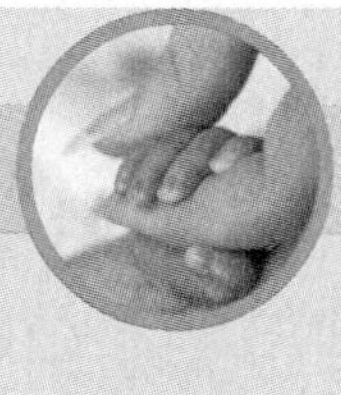

FOCUS ON *Nursing Care Planning*

AN ADOLESCENT SEEKING CONTRACEPTIVE INFORMATION

A 16-year-old girl comes to the clinic asking about contraception. She states, "I have to do something so I don't get pregnant, but I don't know what."

Assessment: Past medical history negative for major health problems. Menarche at age 12. Menstrual cycle ranging from 28 to 35 days with moderately heavy flow lasting 5 to 7 days with cramping. "I usually have to stay home from school for a day." Last menstrual flow 1 week ago. Sexually active for past 3 months without use of any form of contraception. Denies history of sexually transmitted diseases or other reproductive problems. Weight appropriate for height. All secondary sex characteristics present.

Nursing Diagnosis: Health-seeking behaviors related to knowledge deficit about contraception

Outcome Identification: Client will choose and use a method of contraception within 1 month's time.

Outcome Evaluation: Client identifies options available; states valid reasons for method chosen; demonstrates correct use of and appropriate follow-up care for method chosen; voices satisfaction with method chosen.

(continued)

Interventions	Rationale
1. Assess client's lifestyle; review possible options for contraception.	1. Assessing lifestyle provides clues to possible reasons for excluding some methods. Poor compliance by adolescents may leave some methods in doubt.
2. Instruct the client about the method selected, including any specific measures such as insertion, removal, cleaning, or how and when to take or use the method. Have client repeat information or return demonstrate technique.	2. Instruction provides an opportunity for learning to improve compliance.
3. Review and discuss the need for safer sex practices.	3. Safer sex practices promote health, empower the client, and minimize the risk of sexually transmitted diseases. Discussion provides additional feedback and support and permits a safe outlet for expression of concerns and feelings.
4. Explain the need for routine follow-up, including yearly pelvic examinations and routine screening.	4. Follow-up is essential for evaluating compliance and satisfaction and reducing the risk of possible complications.

of planning pregnancies is best for them. These people, therefore, become the candidates for natural family planning methods. The effectiveness of these methods varies greatly, depending mainly on the couple's ability to refrain from having sex on fertile days. Failure rates usually range from 10% to 20% (Speroff & Darney, 2001), although the theoretical failure rate is as low as 1% or 2%. If pregnancy should occur, the continued use of these methods poses no risk to the fetus.

Fertility Awareness Methods

Fertility awareness methods rely on detecting when the woman will be capable of impregnation (fertile) and using periods of abstinence or contraceptive use during that time. Couples are then free to go without contraception during the rest of the month (Speroff & Darney, 2001). As described below, there are a variety of ways to determine a fertile period. Couples may do this by calculating the

BOX 5.1

NURSING OUTCOMES AND NURSING INTERVENTIONS CLASSIFICATION: CONTRACEPTION

NOC: Knowledge, Conception Prevention
Knowledge, conception prevention, is defined as the extent of understanding conveyed about pregnancy prevention (Johnson et al., 2000). Some specific indicators suggesting achievement of this outcome include the client's ability to describe the following:

- Various methods such as periodic abstinence, chemical and mechanical barriers, hormonal therapy, and surgical intervention
- Method for how chosen contraceptive works
- Correct use of chosen method (including a demonstration of its use)
- Effectiveness on STD transmission
- How conception occurs
- Advantages and disadvantages of having a child
- Influence of personal and religious values on contraception

NIC: Family Planning, Contraception
Family planning, contraception, is defined as the facilitation of pregnancy prevention by providing information about the physiology of reproduction and methods to control conception (McCloskey & Bulechek, 2000). Some important activities involved when implementing this intervention include:

- Determining the need for family planning
- Explaining reasons for most unplanned pregnancies
- Determining ability and motivation of client and partner to use contraception correctly and regularly
- Appraising client's knowledge of contraception and plans for selecting a method
- Explaining female reproductive cycle and advantages and disadvantages of methods
- Assisting female client to determine ovulation through basal body temperature, changes in vaginal secretions, and other physiologic indicators
- Instructing client in use of chemical, hormonal, or mechanical contraceptives
- Referring client to community resources for family planning

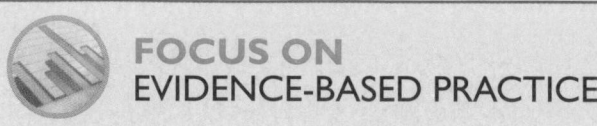

FOCUS ON EVIDENCE-BASED PRACTICE

Are Women as Well Informed About Birth Control Options as They Want to Be?

To answer this question, researchers interviewed 330 randomly selected women who were currently using a birth control measure. Most of the study participants were African-American or Hispanic. The most commonly used methods of birth control were condoms (28%), oral contraceptives (19%), and Depo-Provera implants (13%). The main problems that women voiced about the contraceptives they were using were weight gain, breakthrough bleeding, nausea, and vomiting. Young women expressed a greater desire to learn more about birth control than did older women. The abortion rate was significantly higher in younger women. To reduce this higher abortion rate and the risk of unplanned or unwanted pregnancies in the younger age group, the researchers suggest increased counseling is needed.

This is an important study for nurses because nurses are the people who perform a high percentage of reproductive life planning counseling. Knowing that younger women are interested in learning more about methods and how to use them effectively can open up teaching opportunities.

Shaban, D. W., et al. (2001). The knowledge and use of birth control in the year 2000: The future needs of minority women. *Obstetrics & Gynecology, 97*(4), S17–S22.

period based on a set formula, the woman's body temperature, the consistency of cervical mucus, use of an over-the-counter ovulation test kit, or a combination of these methods.

Calendar (Rhythm) Method. The **calendar method** requires a couple to abstain from coitus on the days of a menstrual cycle when the woman is most likely to conceive (3 or 4 days before until 3 or 4 days after ovulation). To plan for this, a woman should keep a diary of six menstrual cycles. To calculate "safe" days, she subtracts 18 from the shortest cycle documented. This number represents her first fertile day. She subtracts 11 from her longest cycle. This is her last fertile day. If she had six menstrual cycles ranging from 25 to 29 days, her fertile period would be from the 7th day (25 minus 18) to the 18th day (29 minus 11). To avoid pregnancy, she would avoid coitus or use a contraceptive such as vaginal foam during these days (Fig. 5-1*A*).

Basal Body Temperature Method. The basis of the **basal body temperature (BBT) method** is that just before the day of ovulation, a woman's BBT falls about half a degree. At the time of ovulation, her BBT rises a full degree because of the influence of progesterone. This higher level is then maintained for the rest of her menstrual cycle.

To use this method, the woman takes her temperature each morning immediately after waking, before she undertakes any activity. This is her BBT. As soon as she notices a slight dip in temperature followed by an increase, she knows that she has ovulated. She refrains from having sex for the next 3 days (the life of the discharged ovum). Sperm can survive for at least 4 days in the female reproductive tract; thus, combining this method with a calendar method is usually recommended so the couple abstains for a few days before ovulation as well. For more information on BBT and its use in aiding fertility, see Chapter 6 and Figure 6-2.

A problem with this method is that many factors can affect BBT. For example, a temperature rise from illness could be mistaken as the signal of ovulation. If this happens, a woman could mistake a fertile day for a safe one. Changes in the woman's daily schedule, such as starting an aerobic program, can also influence the BBT.

Cervical Mucus (Billings) Method. Another method to predict ovulation is to use the changes in cervical mucus that occur naturally with ovulation. Before ovulation each month, the cervical mucus is thick and does not stretch when pulled between the thumb and finger (known as spinnbarkeit). Just before ovulation, mucus secretion increases. With ovulation (the peak day), cervical mucus becomes copious, thin, watery, and transparent. It feels slippery and stretches at least 1 inch before the strand breaks. In addition, breast tenderness and an anterior tilt

FOCUS ON FAMILY EMPOWERMENT

Suggestions for Promoting Abstinence

Q. I'm only 16. How can I avoid being intimidated into unwanted sex?

A. A few suggestions are:

- Discuss with your partner in advance what sexual activities you will permit and what you will not.
- Try to avoid high-pressure situations (e.g., a party with known drug use, excessive alcohol consumption, and no adult supervision).
- If pressured, say "no" as if you mean it.
- Be certain your partner understands that you consider being forced into relations against your wishes the same as rape, not simply irresponsible conduct.
- Don't accept any drugs to "help you relax" or "be cool," as such a drug would impair your judgment. The drug could also be the "date rape" drug, flunitrazepam (Rohypnol).

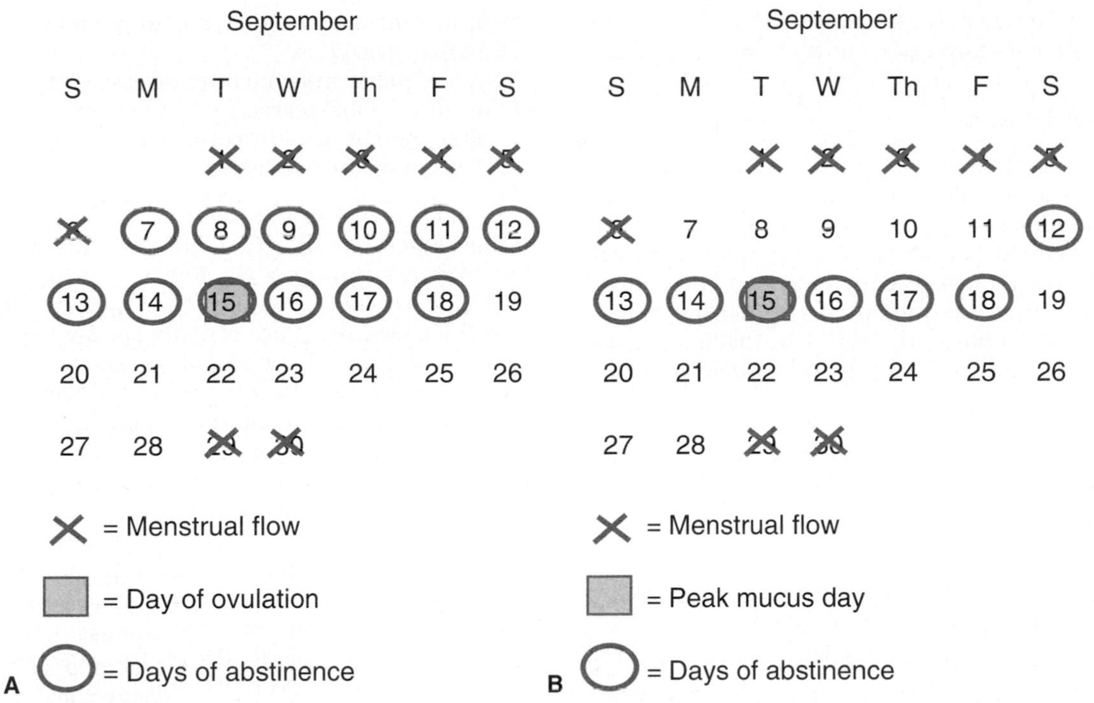

FIGURE 5.1 (A) A typical month using the calendar method as a natural family planning method. (B) A typical month using the cervical mucus method of natural family planning. Unmarked days are those safe for sexual relations.

to the cervix occur. All the days the mucus is copious and the 3 days after the peak day are considered to be fertile days, or days the woman should abstain from sex to avoid conception.

The woman using this method must be conscientious about assessing her vaginal secretions daily, or she will miss the changing cervical secretions. The feel of vaginal secretions after sexual relations is unreliable because seminal fluid (the fluid containing sperm from the male) has a watery, postovulatory consistency and can be confused with ovulatory mucus. Figure 5-1*B* shows a hypothetical month using this method.

Symptothermal Method. The symptothermal method of birth control combines the cervical mucus and BBT methods. The woman takes her temperature daily, watching for the rise in temperature that marks ovulation. She also analyzes her cervical mucus daily. The couple must abstain from intercourse until 3 days after the rise in temperature or the fourth day after the peak of mucus change because these are the woman's fertile days. The symptothermal method is more effective than either the BBT or cervical mucus method alone.

Ovulation Awareness. Yet another method to predict ovulation is the use of an over-the-counter ovulation detection kit. These kits detect the midcycle surge of luteinizing hormone that can be detected in urine 12 to 24 hours before ovulation. Such kits are about 98% to 100% accurate in predicting ovulation. Although fairly expensive, using such a kit in place of cervical mucus testing makes this form of natural family planning more attractive to many women.

Lactation Amenorrhea Method. As long as a woman is breast-feeding an infant, there is some natural suppression of ovulation. However, the use of lactation as a birth control method is not dependable. Because women may ovulate but not menstruate while breast-feeding, the woman may still be fertile even if she has not had a period since childbirth. After 6 months of breast-feeding, the woman should be advised to choose another method of contraception.

Coitus Interruptus. **Coitus interruptus** is one of the oldest known methods of contraception. The couple proceeds with coitus until the moment of ejaculation. Then the man withdraws and spermatozoa are emitted outside the vagina. Unfortunately, ejaculation may occur before withdrawal is complete and, despite the care used, some spermatozoa may be deposited in the vagina. Because there may be a few spermatozoa in pre-ejaculation fluid, even though withdrawal seems controlled, fertilization may occur. For these reasons, coitus interruptus offers little protection against conception. Adolescent boys often lack the control or experience to use the method (Everett et al., 2000).

Effect on Sexual Enjoyment

Once a couple is certain of the woman's nonfertile days using one of the natural planning methods, more spontaneity in sexual relations is possible than with methods that involve vaginal insertion products. On the other hand, the required days of abstinence may make a natural planning method unsatisfactory and unenjoyable for a couple.

Coitus interruptus may be unenjoyable because of the need to withdraw before ejaculation.

Use by the Adolescent

Natural methods of family planning (with the exception of abstinence) are usually not the contraceptive method of choice for adolescents. Girls tend to have occasional anovulatory menstrual cycles for several years after menarche, and they do not always experience definite cervical changes or an elevated body temperature. Also, these methods require adolescents to say "no" to sexual intercourse on fertile days, a difficult task to do under peer pressure.

> ✔ **CHECKPOINT QUESTIONS**
>
> 1. Why are fertility awareness methods so attractive to many women?
> 2. What is the best way to maximize the effectiveness of a fertility awareness method?
> 3. Why is coitus interruptus usually ineffective?

Oral Contraception

Oral contraceptives, commonly known as the pill or OCs, are composed of varying amounts of synthetic estrogen combined with a small amount of synthetic progesterone (Blackburn et al., 2000). The estrogen acts to suppress follicle-stimulating hormone and luteinizing hormone, thereby suppressing ovulation. The progesterone action complements that of estrogen by causing a decrease in the permeability of cervical mucus, thereby limiting sperm motility and access to ova. Progesterone also interferes with endometrial proliferation to such a degree that the possibility of implantation is significantly decreased (Ling & Duff, 2001).

Popular OCs prescribed in the United States are **monophasic** (provide fixed doses of both estrogen and progestin throughout the 21-day cycle). Biphasic preparations deliver a constant amount of estrogen throughout the cycle but an increased amount of progestin during the last 11 days. **Triphasic** preparations vary both estrogen and progestin content throughout the cycle. Triphasic types more closely mimic a natural cycle, thereby reducing breakthrough bleeding (bleeding outside the normal menstrual flow).

OCs must be prescribed by a physician, nurse practitioner, or nurse-midwife following a pelvic examination and a Papanicolaou (Pap) smear. When used correctly, they are 99.5% effective in preventing conception. Because women occasionally forget to take them and there are individual differences in women's physiology, the typical failure rate is around 3%.

Noncontraceptive benefits to women who take OCs include decreased incidences of:

- Dysmenorrhea, due to lack of ovulation
- Premenstrual dysphoric syndrome, because of the increased progesterone levels
- Iron deficiency anemia, due to the reduced amount of menstrual flow
- Acute pelvic inflammatory disease (PID) with resulting tubal scarring
- Endometrial and ovarian cancer and ovarian cysts
- Fibrocystic breast disease

Although there has been a fair amount of publicity about the increased risk of breast cancer in pill users, this is unproven (Blackburn et al., 2000).

OCs are packaged in convenient dispensers. The instructions for taking them are roughly similar for all brands. They are packaged 21 or 28 pills to a container. It is generally recommended that the first pill be taken on a Sunday (the first Sunday following the beginning of a menstrual flow). However, the woman may choose to take her first pill on any day she chooses. After childbirth, a woman should start the contraceptive on the Sunday closest to 2 weeks after delivery; if after an abortion, then on the first Sunday following the procedure. Because pills are not effective for the first 7 days, she is advised to use a second form of contraception during the initial 7 days she takes pills. The woman prescribed a 21-day cycle brand takes a pill at the same time every day for 21 days. Pill taking by this regimen will end on a Saturday. The woman would then not take any pills for 1 week. She would restart a new month's supply of pills on the Sunday 1 week after she stopped. A menstrual flow begins about 4 days after the woman finishes a cycle of pills (Fig. 5-2).

To eliminate having to count days between pill cycles, certain brands of oral contraceptives are packaged with 28 pills—21 active pills and 7 placebo pills for a total of 28 pills. With these brands, a woman starts a second dispenser of pills the day after finishing the first dispenser. There is no need to skip days because of the placebo tablets. Menstrual flow begins during the days of the 7 placebo tablets.

Women who do not want to have menstrual flows can eliminate them by beginning a new 21-day cycle of pills immediately after finishing a first one rather than waiting

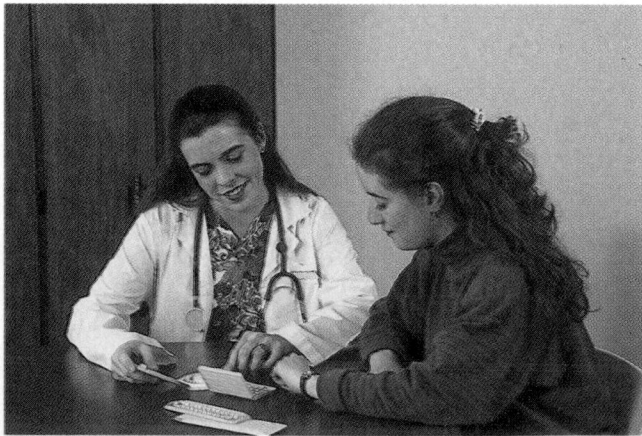

FIGURE 5.2 Counseling women on how to follow an oral contraceptive schedule and what to do if they miss a day or more is an important nursing responsibility.

FOCUS ON FAMILY EMPOWERMENT
Suggestions on Oral Contraceptive Management

Q. What should I do if I forget to take an oral contraceptive pill?

A. Your actions may differ:

1. If you forget to take one pill, take it as soon as you remember. Continue the following day with your usual schedule. This might mean taking two pills on one day, if you don't remember until the second day. *Missing one pill this way should not initiate ovulation.*
2. If you miss two consecutive pills, take two pills as soon as you remember and two pills again the following day. Then continue the following day with your usual schedule. You may experience some breakthrough bleeding (vaginal spotting) with two forgotten pills. Do not mistake this bleeding for your menstrual flow. *Missing two pills may allow for ovulation, so an added contraceptive should be used for the remainder of the month.*
3. If you miss three or more pills in a row, throw out the rest of the pack and start a new pack of pills the following Sunday. *You might not have a period because of this routine and should use extra protection until 7 days after starting a new pack of pills.*

the usual 7 days to begin a new cycle (with the 28-day cycle regimens, omitting taking the placebo pills and immediately beginning a new dispenser). It is not advised that women do this on a continual basis, but the advice can be helpful to cover certain special occasions.

For ovulation suppressants to be effective, they must be taken consistently and conscientiously. Some women leave them in plain sight on the bathroom counter or kitchen counter so they are easily reminded to take them. Women with young children in the house need to be cautioned that this is a dangerous practice. Poisoning with increased blood clotting from the high estrogen content could result if a small child ingested the pills accidentally. Women who have difficulty remembering to take a contraceptive in the morning may find it easier to take a daily pill at bedtime or with a meal (the time of day makes no difference; it is the consistency that is important). Also, some women find that taking pills at bedtime rather than in the morning eliminates any nausea they otherwise experience (see Focus on Family Empowerment).

Side Effects and Contraindications

For a listing of risk factors and contraindications associated with OCs, see Box 5-2. The main side effects that women may experience are:

- Nausea
- Weight gain
- Headache
- Breast tenderness
- Breakthrough bleeding (spotting outside the menstrual period)
- Monilial vaginal infections
- Mild hypertension
- Depression

These side effects usually subside after a few months of use or may be managed by using a different routine or brand of contraceptive.

Although it is no longer believed that the use of OCs leads to an increased risk of myocardial infarction, the pill is not routinely prescribed for women with a history of thromboembolic disease or a family history of cerebral or cardiovascular accident because of the increased tendency toward clotting as an effect of increased estrogen.

All women taking OCs are advised to notify their health care provider if the following symptoms, which are indicative of myocardial or thromboembolic complications, occur:

- Chest pain (pulmonary embolus or myocardial infarction)
- Shortness of breath (pulmonary embolus)
- Severe headaches (cerebrovascular accident)

BOX 5.2

ABSOLUTE AND POSSIBLE CONTRAINDICATIONS TO ORAL CONTRACEPTIVE USE

Absolute

Breast-feeding
Family history of cerebrovascular accident or coronary artery disease
History of thromboembolic disease
History of liver disease
Undiagnosed vaginal bleeding

Possible

Age 40+
Breast or reproductive tract malignancy
Diabetes mellitus
Elevated cholesterol or triglycerides
High blood pressure
Mental depression
Migraine or other vascular-type headaches
Obesity
Pregnancy
Seizure disorders
Sickle cell or other hemoglobinopathies
Smoking
Use of medication or drug with interaction effect

- Severe leg pain (thrombophlebitis)
- Eye problems such as blurred vision (hypertension, cerebrovascular accident)

Early studies found that breast-fed infants had lower weight gains when the mother was taking an oral contraceptive containing a high level of estrogen during breast-feeding, because the estrogen content decreased the woman's milk supply. Although there is less estrogen in today's preparations, it is still not recommended that breast-feeding women take estrogen-based OCs until their milk supply is well established. Women may take progesterone-only pills (mini-pills) during breast-feeding (see below).

OCs have been known to interfere with glucose metabolism. For this reason, women with diabetes mellitus or a history of liver disease, including hepatitis, should be evaluated individually before OCs are prescribed.

A number of drugs such as barbiturates, griseofulvin, isoniazid, penicillin, and tetracycline decrease the effectiveness of OCs, so women might want to change their contraceptive temporarily while taking these drugs (Burroughs & Chambliss, 2000). OCs may interact with a number of drugs such as acetaminophen, anticoagulants, and some anticonvulsants, reducing their therapeutic effect. Typically, OCs increase or strengthen the action of caffeine and corticosteroids.

The cost of oral contraceptives and the woman's ability to follow instructions faithfully must both be considered before prescribing OCs. The woman using OCs should return for a follow-up visit yearly for a pelvic examination, Pap smear, and breast examination as long as she continues to use this form of birth control. Women without risk factors may continue to take low-dose oral contraceptives until they reach menopause.

Effect on Sexual Enjoyment

For the most part, not having to worry about pregnancy because the contraceptive being used is so reliable makes sexual relations more enjoyable for couples. Some women appear to lose interest in coitus after taking the pill for about 18 months, possibly because of the long-term effect of altered hormones in their body. Sexual interest increases again after they change to another form of contraception. Some women experience nausea with the pill and find this interferes with sexual enjoyment as well as with other activities. If they are having side effects with one brand, they might be able to take another brand that has a different strength of estrogen without problems.

Effect on Pregnancy

If the woman taking an OC suspects that she has become pregnant, she should discontinue taking the pill if she intends to continue the pregnancy. High levels of estrogen or progesterone might be teratogenic to a growing fetus (Speroff & Darney, 2001).

Use by the Adolescent

It is usually recommended that adolescent girls have well-established menstrual cycles for at least 2 years before beginning OCs. This reduces the chance that the OC will cause permanent suppression of pituitary-regulating activity. Estrogen has the side effect of causing the epiphyses of long bones to close and growth to halt; therefore, waiting at least 2 years will also ensure that the preadolescent growth spurt will not be halted. Because adolescents' compliance with most medications is low, adolescent girls may not take pills reliably enough to make them effective. In addition, the cost of a continuing supply of pills may be prohibitive for teens. OCs have side benefits of improving facial acne in some girls because of the increased estrogen/androgen ratio created, and of decreasing dysmenorrhea, a problem for many adolescents. The pill may be prescribed to some adolescents specifically to decrease dysmenorrhea, especially if endometriosis is present (see Chap. 7).

Discontinuing Use

After a woman stops taking an OC, she may not be able to become pregnant for 1 or 2 months, and possibly 6 to 8 months, because the pituitary gland requires a recovery period to begin cyclic gonadotropin stimulation again. If ovulation does not return spontaneously after this time, it can be stimulated by clomiphene citrate (Clomid) therapy.

Mini-Pills

OCs containing only progesterone are popularly called mini-pills. Without estrogen content, ovulation may occur, but because the progestins have not allowed the endometrium to develop fully, implantation will not take place. Such a pill has advantages for the woman who cannot take an estrogen-based pill because of the danger of thrombophlebitis but who wants high-level contraception assurance. This type of pill is taken every day even through the menstrual flow. Because it doesn't interfere with milk production, it may be taken during breast-feeding.

Emergency Postcoital Contraception

A number of regimens are available for emergency postcoital contraception. The Yuzpe regimen consists of the administration of two fixed-dose combination pills (usually Ovral), taken within 72 hours of unprotected intercourse (Wellbery, 2000). This is followed by two additional pills in 12 hours. This high dose of estrogen (200 mcg) will almost always cause nausea and vomiting, If a pill is vomited within 2 hours of administration, it should be repeated. Pretreatment with an antiemetic such as 50 mg meclizine (Bonine) is usually recommended to decrease the possibility of vomiting.

A specially designed emergency contraceptive kit (Preven) is available for use (over the counter in some states) after unprotected sexual intercourse, particularly after a sexual assault has occurred. These are often referred to as "morning-after pills." The kit consists of a urine pregnancy test to determine whether pregnancy has occurred and four pills that contain concentrations of estrogen/progestin (the first two taken within 72 hours of intercourse and the next two 12 hours later). The high level of estrogen interferes with the production of progesterone and therefore prohibits good implantation (Ho, 2000).

A progestin-only method termed "Plan B" is also available. With this plan, two pills containing high doses of levonorgestrel are taken (one pill immediately and one 12 hours later). This plan results in less nausea and may actually prevent more pregnancies than the estrogen-based regimen (Grimes et al., 2001).

Overall, the rate of effectiveness for emergency postcoital methods of contraception is about 98%. The method should always be used cautiously because high levels of estrogen are associated with congenital anomalies if the pregnancy is not prevented. Mifepristone, discussed below as an abortifacient, may also be prescribed for emergency postcoital contraception.

✔ CHECKPOINT QUESTIONS

4. What is the method by which OCs act?
5. What are the common side effects associated with OCs?
6. What are the danger signs that women taking OCs should be instructed to report?

Subcutaneous Implants

Norplant consists of six nonbiodegradable Silastic implants, about the width of a pencil lead, that are filled with levonorgestrel (a synthetic progesterone) and embedded just under the skin on the inside of the upper arm (Fig. 5-3). Once embedded, the implants appear only as irregular lines on the skin, simulating small veins. Over the next 5 years, the implants slowly release the hormone, suppressing ovulation, stimulating thick cervical mucus, and changing the endometrium so implantation is difficult.

The implants are inserted using a local anesthetic during the menses or no later than day 7 of the menstrual cycle to be certain that the woman is not pregnant at the time of insertion. They can be inserted immediately after an abortion or 6 weeks after birth of a baby. The failure rate is 1% for the first year and about 3% by the fifth year of use. The implants are removed under local anesthesia (Speroff & Darney, 2001).

A disadvantage of the implants is cost ($500 on average). The following are possible side effects:

- Weight gain
- Irregular menstrual cycle, which includes spotting, breakthrough bleeding, amenorrhea, or prolonged periods
- Hair loss

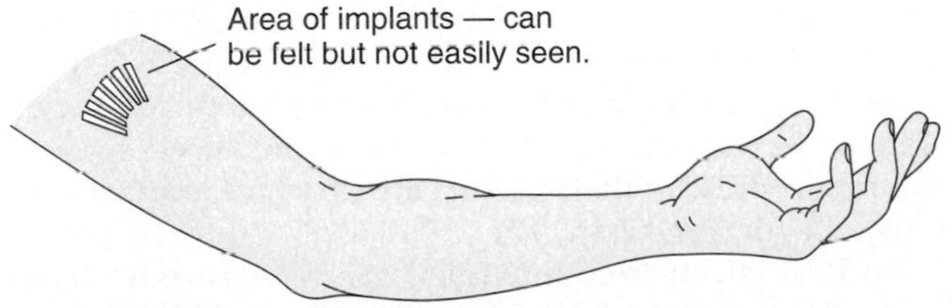
Area of implants — can
be felt but not easily seen.

FIGURE 5.3 The appearance of Norplant implants placed under the skin.

- Depression
- Scarring at the insertion site
- Need for removal

A major advantage of this long-term reversible contraceptive is that it offers an effective and reliable alternative to OCs and their estrogen-related side effects. Compliance issues associated with OCs are eliminated. Sexual enjoyment is not inhibited, as may be the case with condoms, spermicides, diaphragms, and natural family planning. Implants can be used during breast-feeding without an effect on milk production. Also, implants can be used safely in adolescents. The rapid return to fertility (about 3 months after removal) is an advantage for women who wish to have children.

Contraindications to Norplant are pregnancy, desire to be pregnant within 1 to 2 years, and undiagnosed uterine bleeding. A complication (rare) that can occur is an infection at the insertion site. If pregnancy does occur with the rods in place, they should be removed to reduce the possibility of birth defects in the fetus.

Intramuscular Injections

A single injection of medroxyprogesterone acetate (DMPA or Depo-Provera) given every 12 weeks or Lunelle injections (a synthetic estrogen and progesterone given every 30 days) inhibit ovulation, alter the endometrium, and change the cervical mucus. The effectiveness rate of these methods is nearly 100%, making them an increasingly popular contraceptive method. Potential side effects are similar to those of subcutaneous implants: irregular menstrual cycle, headache, weight gain, and depression. Depo-Provera may impair glucose tolerance in women at risk for diabetes. Because there also may be a slight increase in the risk for osteoporosis, women should be advised to include an adequate amount of calcium in their diet (up to 1,200 mg/day) and engage in weight-bearing exercise daily to minimize this risk.

Like subcutaneous implants, intramuscular injections have the same advantage of longer-term reliability without many of the side effects and contraindications associated with OCs. An advantage of intramuscular injections over implants is that there is no visible sign that a birth control measure is being used. Depo-Provera can be used during breast-feeding. Two disadvantages are that the woman must return to a health care provider for a new injection every 4 to 12 weeks for the method to remain reliable, and the return to fertility is often delayed by about 6 to 12 months. A reminder system such as a postcard mailed by the prescribing agency may be necessary to be certain that women return on time for their next injection; see the Focus on Pharmacology: Medroxyprogesterone Acetate (Depo-Provera). Alternative methods of administration, such as allowing pharmacists to give the injections or selling them over the counter so women can inject themselves, are being studied.

Intrauterine Devices

The **intrauterine device** (IUD) is a small plastic object inserted into the uterus through the vagina. IUDs became popular as a method of birth control in the 1980s but are

FOCUS ON PHARMACOLOGY

Medroxyprogesterone Acetate (Depo-Provera)

Classification: Contraceptive

Action: Medroxyprogesterone acetate (Depo-Provera) is a progesterone derivative, which inhibits the secretion of pituitary gonadotropins, thereby altering the endometrium and preventing follicular maturation and ovulation.

Pregnancy Category: X

Dosage: 150 mg intramuscular injection every 3 months

Possible Side Effects: Spotting, breakthrough bleeding, amenorrhea, irregular menstrual flow, headaches, weight fluctuations, fluid retention, edema, rash or acne, abdominal discomfort, glucose intolerance, pain at injection site

Nursing Implications

- Advise client to have an annual physical examination that includes breast examination, pelvic examination, and Pap smear.
- Caution the client about potential side effects.
- Advise the client to report pain or swelling of the legs, acute chest pain or shortness of breath, tingling or numbness in the extremities, loss of vision, sudden severe headaches, dizziness, or fainting; these are signs of cardiovascular complications.

used by only 1% of U.S. women today because few manufacturers continue to provide them following a number of lawsuits in association with the increased incidence of PID (infection of the pelvic organs) in women using one particular brand (Vanos, 1999).

Although the insertion of foreign objects into the uterus for contraceptive purposes dates back several thousand years, the mechanism of action for this method is still not fully understood. Originally, it was thought that the presence of a foreign substance in the uterus interfered with the ability of an ovum to develop as it traversed the fallopian tube. Another possibility was that a local sterile inflammatory action resulted and prevented implantation. Newer information suggests that IUDs interfere with fertilization. When copper is added to the device, sperm mobility appears to be effected. This decreases the possibility of sperm successfully traversing the uterine space and reaching the ovum.

An IUD must be fitted by a physician, nurse practitioner, or nurse-midwife, who first performs a pelvic examination following a Pap test. The device is inserted before the client has had coitus after a menstrual flow so the health care provider can be assured that the woman is not pregnant at the time of insertion. Insertion may be done immediately after childbirth: an IUD inserted this soon after childbirth does not affect uterine involution or return to a prepregnant uterine size.

The insertion procedure is performed in an ambulatory setting such as a physician's office or a reproductive planning clinic. It is inserted in a collapsed position, then enlarged to its final shape in the uterus when the inserter is withdrawn. The woman may feel a sharp cramp as the device is passed through the internal cervical os, but she will not feel the IUD after it is in place. Properly fitted, such devices are contained wholly within the uterus, although the string attached protrudes through the cervix into the vagina.

Three common types of IUDs used in the United States are the Copper T380 (ParaGard), a T-shaped plastic device wound with copper, and Progestasert and Mirena, which hold a drug reservoir of progesterone in the stem (Fig. 5-4). The progesterone in the drug reservoir gradually diffuses into the uterus through the plastic and prevents endometrium proliferation and thickens cervical mucus. The Progestasert must be changed yearly or the progesterone supply will become depleted. The newer Mirena type is effective for 5 years (possibly 7). Both have a failure rate as low as 1% to 2%. The Copper T380, because of the added copper, has a failure rate less than 1%. It is effective for 8 years, after which time it should be removed and replaced with a new IUD.

IUDs have several advantages over other contraceptives. Only one insertion is necessary, so there is no continuing expense. They are also more convenient because they do not need daily attention or interfere with sexual enjoyment. There is some indication they may decrease the incidence of endometrial cancer. They are appropriate for women who are at risk for developing complications associated with OCs or who wish to avoid some of the systemic hormonal side effects. The woman should regularly check after each menstrual flow to make sure the IUD string is in place, and obtain a yearly pelvic examination.

Side Effects and Contraindications

A woman may notice some spotting or uterine cramping the first 2 or 3 weeks after insertion; as long as this is present, she should use an additional form of contraception such as vaginal foam. A woman with an IUD in place has a higher than usual risk for PID, although the copper-wound devices may actually have a lower risk. There is also a higher risk of ectopic (tubal) pregnancy. Some women have a heavier than usual menstrual flow for 2 or 3 months and experience more dysmenorrhea than other women. Ibuprofen, a prostaglandin inhibitor, is helpful in relieving the pain. Occasionally, a woman continues to have cramping and spotting following insertion; in these instances, she is likely to expel the device spontaneously. Women with IUDs in place should take active steps to avoid toxic shock syndrome (staphylococcal infection from the use of tampons), because infection might travel by the IUD string into the uterus to cause uterine infection. They also need to know the most common symptoms of PID (fever, lower abdominal tenderness, and pain on intercourse) so they can report these to their health care provider immediately if they occur (see Chap. 47).

An IUD is not recommended for women who have never been pregnant (their small uterus could be punctured with insertion), who have multiple sexual partners, or who have a history of PID. If PID is suspected, the

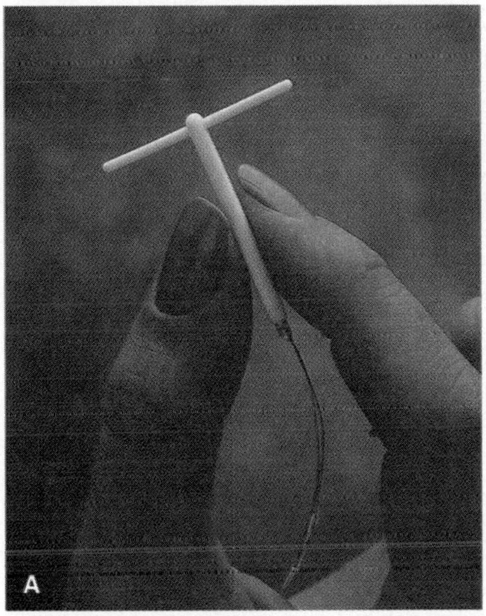

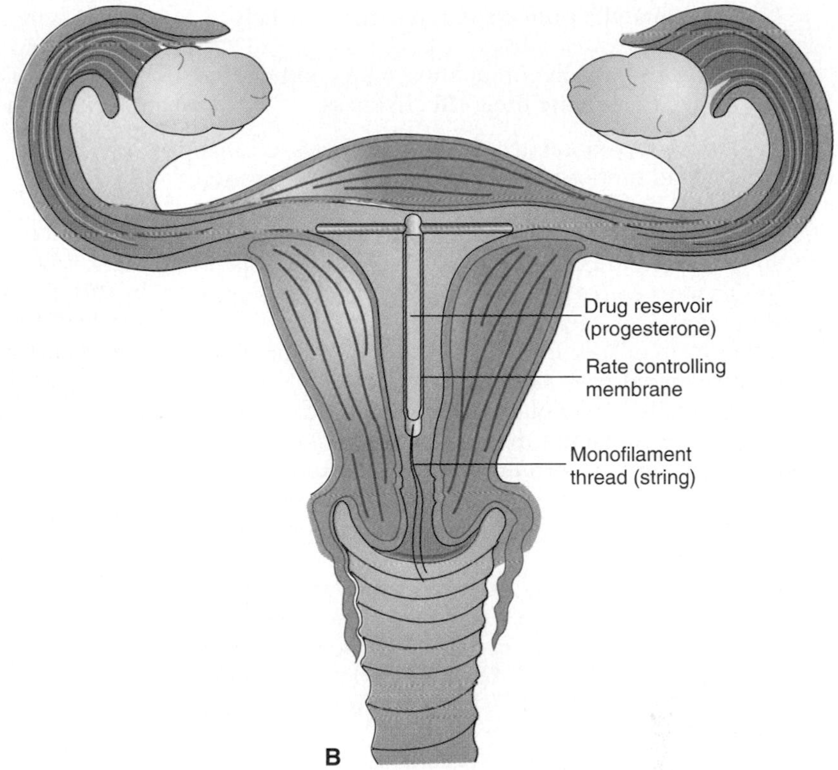

FIGURE 5.4 (*A*) Intrauterine device; (*B*) an IUD in place in the uterus.

device should be removed and the woman should receive antibiotic therapy to treat the infection.

IUDs are also contraindicated in the woman whose uterus is distorted in shape (the device might perforate an abnormally shaped uterus). They are not advised for women with severe dysmenorrhea (painful menstruation), menorrhagia (bleeding between menstrual periods), or a history of ectopic (tubal) pregnancy, because their use may increase the symptoms or incidence of these conditions. Women with valvular heart disease may be advised against the use of an IUD because the increased risk of PID may lead to accompanying valvular involvement from bacterial endocarditis. Because IUDs cause a heavier than usual menstrual flow, a woman with anemia is also generally not considered to be a good candidate for IUD use.

Effect on Pregnancy

If a woman with an IUD in place suspects that she is pregnant, she should alert her primary health care provider. Although the IUD may be left in place during the pregnancy, it is usually removed vaginally to prevent the possibility of infection or spontaneous abortion during the pregnancy. The woman should receive an early sonogram to rule out ectopic pregnancy, as there is an increased incidence of this in IUD users.

Use by the Adolescent

IUDs are rarely prescribed for adolescents because teens tend to have variable sexual partners and no prior pregnancies, contraindications to IUD use.

✔ CHECKPOINT QUESTIONS

7. What are two advantages of subcutaneous implants and intramuscular injections over OCs?
8. For how long are subcutaneous implants effective? Intramuscular injections?
9. How does an IUD prevent conception?

Barrier Methods

Barrier methods are forms of birth control that work by the placement of a chemical or other barrier between the cervix and advancing sperm so sperm cannot enter the uterus or fallopian tubes and fertilize the ovum. A major advantage of barrier methods is that they lack the hormonal side effects associated with OCs. However, compared to OCs, failure rates are higher and sexual enjoyment may be lessened.

Vaginally Inserted Spermicidal Products

Spermicidal agents cause the death of spermatozoa before they can enter the cervix. These agents are not only actively spermicidal but also change the vaginal pH to a strong acid level, a condition not conducive to sperm survival. In addition to the general benefits for barrier contraceptives, some advantages of spermicides are:

- They may be purchased without a prescription or healthcare provider appointment, so they allow for greater independence and lower costs.

- Nonoxynol-9, the preferred ingredient, may help prevent STDs.
- They may be used in conjunction with another contraceptive to increase their effectiveness.

The various preparations available include gels, creams, films, foams, and suppositories. Gels or creams are inserted into the vagina before coitus with an applicator (Fig. 5-5). The woman should do this no more than 1 hour before coitus for the most effective results. She should not douche for 6 hours after coitus to ensure that the agent has completed its spermicidal action.

Another form of spermicidal protection is a film of glycerin impregnated with nonoxynol-9 that is folded and inserted vaginally. On contact with vaginal secretions or precoital penile emissions, the film dissolves and a carbon dioxide foam forms to protect the cervix against invading spermatozoa. The use of these is not recommended in women near menopause, a time in life when vaginal secretions are lessening.

Still other vaginal products are cocoa butter- and glycerin-based vaginal suppositories filled with nonoxynol-9. Inserted vaginally, these dissolve and release the spermicidal ingredients. Because it may take about 15 minutes for a suppository to dissolve, it must be inserted 15 minutes before coitus.

Side Effects and Contraindications. Vaginally inserted spermicidal products are contraindicated in women with acute cervicitis because they might further irritate the cervix. They are generally inappropriate for couples who must prevent conception (perhaps the woman is taking a drug that is teratogenic, or the couple absolutely does not want the responsibility of children) because the overall failure rate of all forms of these products is about 20%. Some women find the vaginal leakage after use of these products bothersome. Vaginal suppositories, because of the cocoa butter or glycerin base, are the most bothersome in this regard.

Effect on Sexual Enjoyment. Although spermicidal products must be inserted fairly close to the time of coitus, they also are so easily purchased over the counter that many couples find the inconvenience of insertion only a minor problem. If a couple is concerned that the method does not offer enough protection, worry about becoming pregnant may interfere with sexual enjoyment. Some couples find the foam or moisture irritating to vaginal and penile tissue during coitus and so are unable to use them.

Effect on Pregnancy. If conception should occur, there is no reason to think that the fetus will be affected by the spermicide. Some women worry that a sperm that survived the spermicide must have been weakened by migrating through it and will, therefore, produce a defective child. They can be assured that conception occurred most likely because the product did not completely cover the cervical os, so the sperm that reached the uterus is free of the product and unharmed.

Use by the Adolescent. Many adolescents use vaginal products as their chief method of birth control because no parental permission or extensive expense is involved. Adolescents should be cautioned that this method has a high failure rate (20%). All women need to be cautioned that preparations labeled "feminine hygiene" products are for vaginal cleanliness and are not spermicidal; thus, they are not effective contraceptives.

Because of the nontraditional settings in which adolescents may engage in coitus (e.g., in cars or on couches), some young women find inserting the product awkward and consequently do not use it, even though they have purchased it and intended to be more cautious.

Diaphragms

A **diaphragm** is a circular rubber disk that is placed over the cervix prior to intercourse; it forms a barricade against the entrance of spermatozoa (Fig. 5-6). Although

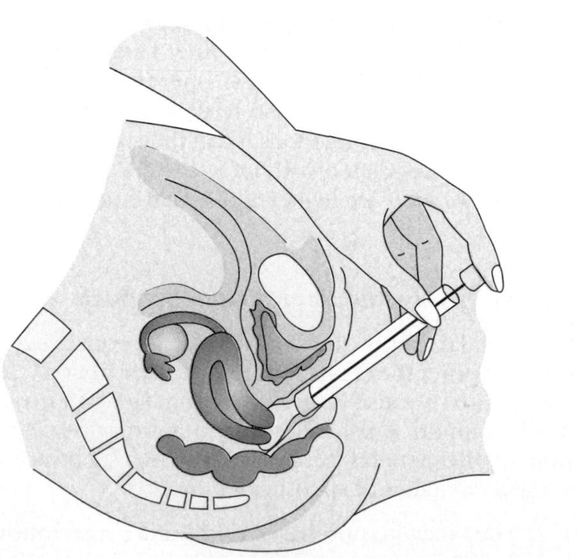

FIGURE 5.5 Vaginal insertion of a spermicidal agent.

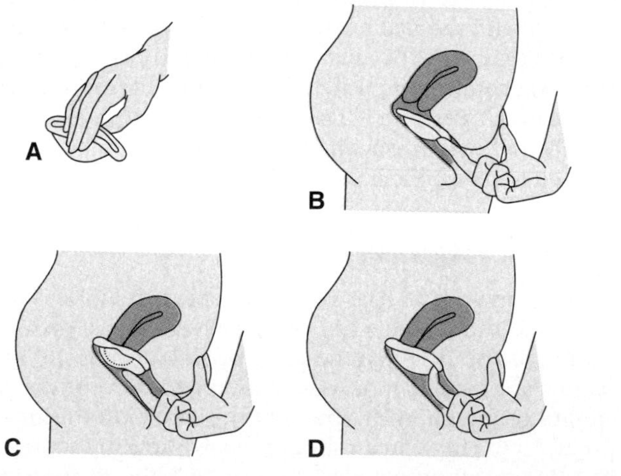

FIGURE 5.6 Proper insertion of a diaphragm. (*A*) After spermicidal jelly or cream is applied to the rim, the diaphragm is pinched between the fingers and thumb. (*B*) The folded diaphragm is then gently inserted into the vagina and pushed backward as far as it will go. (*C*) To check for proper positioning, the woman should feel the cervix to be certain it is completely covered by the soft rubber dome of the diaphragm. (*D*) To remove the diaphragm, a finger is hooked under the forward rim and the diaphragm is pulled down and out.

newer studies demonstrate that a spermicide may not be required, using a spermicidal gel with a diaphragm combines a barrier and a chemical method of contraception. A diaphragm is prescribed and fitted initially by a physician, nurse practitioner, or nurse-midwife to ensure a correct fit. Because the shape of the cervix changes with pregnancy, miscarriage, cervical surgery (dilatation and curettage [D&C]), or therapeutic abortion, a woman must return for a second fitting if any of these occur. The woman should also have the fit checked after gaining or losing more than 15 lb, which may change the pelvic and vaginal contours.

The failure rate of the diaphragm may be as low as 5% to 6% if the woman uses it with spermicidal jelly, checks it with a finger after insertion to be certain it is fitted well up over the cervix, and cares for it properly and inspects it periodically to see that the rubber is not deteriorating. See Focus on Family Empowerment for more information on the proper use and care of diaphragms.

Side Effects and Contraindications. Users of diaphragms may experience a higher number of urinary tract infections (UTIs) than nonusers, probably because of pressure on the urethra. Diaphragms may not be effective if the uterus is prolapsed, retroflexed, or anteflexed to such a degree that the cervix is also displaced in relation to the vagina. Intrusion on the vagina by a cystocele or rectocele (walls of the vagina are displaced by bladder or bowel) may make inserting a diaphragm difficult. Diaphragms should not be used in the presence of acute cervicitis, because the close contact of the rubber and the use of a spermicide may cause additional irritation. Other contraindications include:

- History of toxic shock syndrome
- Allergy to rubber or spermicides
- History of recurrent UTIs

Effect on Sexual Enjoyment. Some women dislike using diaphragms because they must be inserted before coitus (although they may be inserted up to 2 hours beforehand, minimizing this problem) and they should be left in place for 6 hours afterward. Use of a vibrator as a part of foreplay, frequent penile insertion, or the woman-superior position during coitus may dislodge the diaphragm, so it may not be the contraceptive of choice for some couples. If coitus is repeated before 6 hours, the diaphragm should not be removed and replaced, but more spermicidal gel should be added. Some couples may find this precaution restricting. An advantage of the diaphragm is that it allows sexual relations during menses (although see the precaution on toxic shock syndrome below). It may offer some protection against STDs. If a woman should become pregnant while using a diaphragm, there is no risk of harm to the fetus.

Use by the Adolescent. Adolescents may be fitted for diaphragms. However, because an adolescent girl's vagina will vary in size as she matures and starts sexual relations, the device may not remain as effective as it does with older women. Adolescents may need to be reminded that continuing pelvic examinations are necessary to ensure that it continues to fit properly. Some adolescents may not know

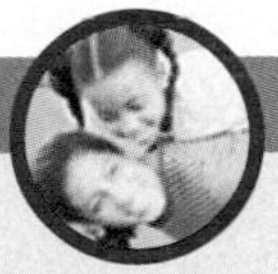

FOCUS ON FAMILY EMPOWERMENT

Guidelines for Diaphragm Insertion

Q. What are the best guidelines for inserting and caring for a diaphragm?

A. To insert and care for a diaphragm, follow these steps:

1. Before coitus, coat the rim of the diaphragm with a contraceptive jelly.
2. Squat, elevate one leg, or lie in a supine position.
3. Insert the diaphragm into the vagina, sliding it along the posterior wall and pressing it up against the cervix so it is held in place by the vaginal fornices.
4. Check that it is secure against the cervix by palpating the cervical os through the diaphragm (see Fig. 5-6).
5. Keep the diaphragm in place for at least 6 hours after coitus because spermatozoa remain viable in the vagina for that duration. The diaphragm may be left in place for as long as 24 hours. If it is left in the vagina longer than this, the stasis of fluid may cause cervical inflammation (erosion) or urethral irritation.
6. Remove the diaphragm by inserting a finger into the vagina and loosening the diaphragm by pressing against the anterior rim, and withdrawing it vaginally.
7. Wash the diaphragm in mild soap and water. Dry it gently and store it in its protective case. If this step is followed, the diaphragm will last for 2 to 3 years.

To prevent toxic shock syndrome (a staphylococcal infection introduced through the vagina) while using a diaphragm, it is important to follow these steps:

1. Wash your hands thoroughly with soap and water before insertion and removal of a diaphragm or cervical cap.
2. Don't use either a diaphragm or cervical cap during a menstrual period.
3. Don't leave the diaphragm or cervical cap in place longer than 24 hours.
4. Be aware of the symptoms of toxic shock syndrome, such as elevated temperature, diarrhea, vomiting, muscle aches, and a sunburn-like rash.
5. If the above symptoms should occur, immediately remove the diaphragm or cervical cap and telephone your health care provider.

where their cervix is or how to feel for it when checking the placement of the diaphragm; an anatomic diagram can be used for education, or they can be shown the cervix during a pelvic examination by use of a mirror.

WHAT IF? What if two teenage girls tell you they plan on sharing a diaphragm because they don't have enough money for each to buy one? What would you recommend? Why?

Cervical Caps

A **cervical cap** is yet another barrier method of contraception. Caps are made of soft rubber, are shaped like a thimble, and fit snugly over the uterine cervix (Fig. 5-7). The lowest reported failure rate of the cervical cap is 8%, although the typical rate of failure is estimated to be as high as 18% (Speroff & Darney, 2001).

Many women cannot use cervical caps because their cervix is too short for the cap to fit properly. Also, caps tend to dislodge more readily than diaphragms during coitus. An advantage is that cervical caps can remain in place longer than diaphragms because they do not put pressure on the vaginal walls or urethra; however, this length of time should not exceed 24 hours to prevent cervical irritation. Cervical caps, like diaphragms, must be fitted individually by a health care provider. They are contraindicated in clients with:

- An abnormally short or long cervix
- A previous abnormal Pap smear
- A history of toxic shock syndrome
- An allergy to latex or spermicide
- A history of PID, cervicitis, or papillomavirus infection
- A history of cervical cancer
- Undiagnosed vaginal bleeding

Vaginal Rings

Vaginal rings (NuvaRings) are a new type of protection that consists of a thin, flexible plastic ring about 2 inches across that contains a combination of estrogen and progestin. It is inserted into the vagina and left in place for 21 days, then removed for 7 days. Following menses, a new ring is inserted. The ring releases lower doses of estrogen than the lowest dose of oral contraceptive on the market, so it supplies an estrogen-based method with very few side effects. Women may need to make out a calendar that they post conspicuously to remind themselves to remove and replace the ring.

Male Condoms

A **condom** is a latex rubber or synthetic sheath that is placed over the erect penis before coitus (Fig. 5-8). It prevents pregnancy because spermatozoa are deposited not in the vagina but in the tip of the condom. The use of condoms has an ideal failure rate of 2% and a typical failure rate of about 12%, as breakage or spillage occurs in up to 12% of uses. A big advantage of condoms is that they are one of the few "male-responsibility" birth control measures available, and no health care visit or prescription is needed. Latex condoms have the additional potential of preventing the spread of STDs, and their use has become a major part of the fight against human immunodeficiency virus (HIV) infection. It is recommended that they always be worn during coitus between partners who do not maintain a monogamous relationship.

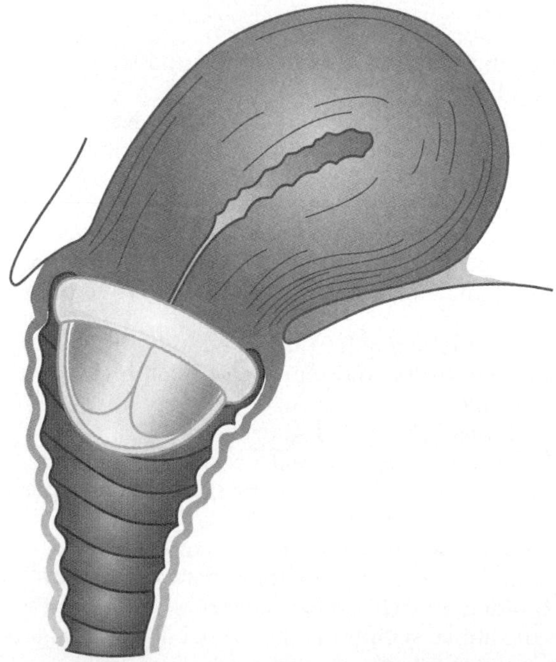

FIGURE 5.7 A cervical cap is placed over the cervix and used with a spermicidal jelly the same as a diaphragm.

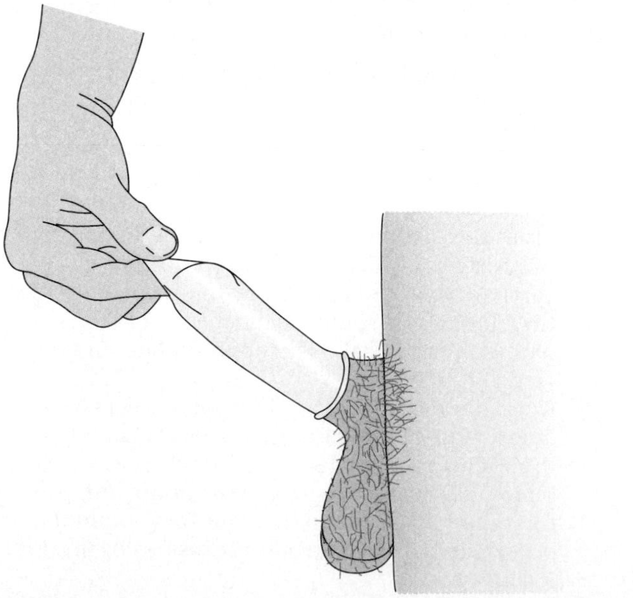

FIGURE 5.8 Male condom. Being certain that space is left at the tip helps to ensure the condom will not break with ejaculation.

Side Effects and Contraindications. There are no contraindications to the use of condoms except for a sensitivity to latex.

Effect on Sexual Enjoyment. To be effective, condoms must be applied before any penile-vulvar contact, because even pre-ejaculation fluid may contain some sperm. The condom should be positioned so it is loose enough at the penis tip to collect the ejaculate without placing undue pressure on the condom. The penis (with the condom held carefully in place) must be withdrawn before it begins to become flaccid after ejaculation. If it is not withdrawn at this time, sperm may leak from the now loosely fitting sheath into the vagina. Some men find that condoms dull their enjoyment of coitus; some couples do not like that the male must withdraw promptly after ejaculation. Concern that the condom may break or slip may also inhibit sexual pleasure.

Use by the Adolescent. Male adolescents are showing an increase in their ability to use condoms responsibly. Adolescent boys who have infrequent coitus may use condoms that they have owned and stored for a long time. The effectiveness of these old condoms, especially if they are carried in a warm pocket, is questionable. Adolescents may need to be cautioned that condoms should never be reused, because even a pinpoint hole can allow thousands of sperm to escape. For many adolescent couples, use of a vaginally inserted spermicide by the girl and a condom by her partner is the preferred method of birth control. The effectiveness of these two methods used in conjunction becomes about 95%.

Female Condoms

Condoms for females are latex sheaths made of polyurethane and lubricated with nonoxynol-9. The inner ring (closed end) covers the cervix, and the outer ring (open end) rests against the vaginal opening. The sheath may be inserted any time before sexual activity and then removed after ejaculation occurs. Like male condoms, they are intended for one-time use and offer protection against both conception and STDs (Fig. 5-9). Female condoms can be purchased over the counter but are more expensive than male condoms. Male and female condoms should not be used together. Although female condoms are still being tested, the failure rate in preliminary studies was somewhat greater than the failure rate for male condoms, about 15%. Most of these pregnancies occurred because of incorrect or inconsistent use. They have not gained great popularity because women have found them difficult to use.

✔ CHECKPOINT QUESTIONS

10. What are the major advantages and disadvantages of diaphragms?
11. What is the ingredient in spermicides that protects against STDs?
12. Why is the female condom less popular than other contraceptive methods?

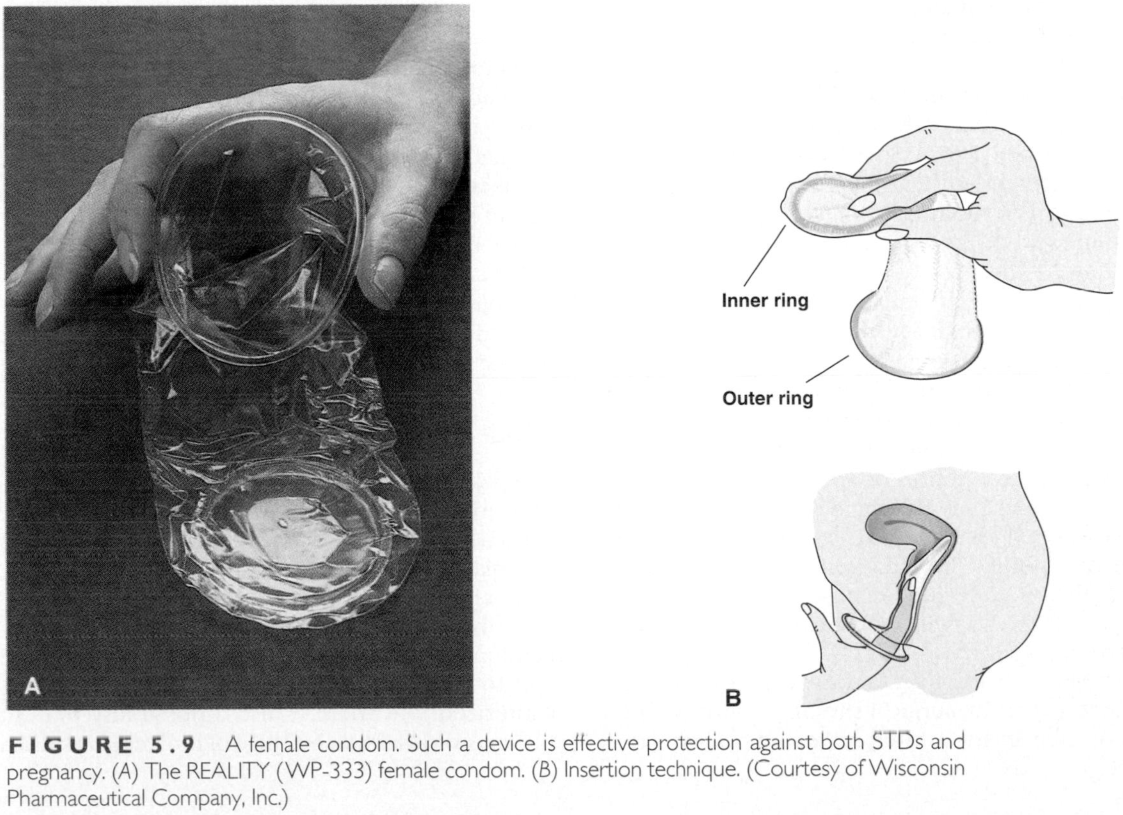

FIGURE 5.9 A female condom. Such a device is effective protection against both STDs and pregnancy. (*A*) The REALITY (WP-333) female condom. (*B*) Insertion technique. (Courtesy of Wisconsin Pharmaceutical Company, Inc.)

Surgical Methods of Reproductive Life Planning

Surgical methods of reproductive life planning include sterilization (**tubal ligation** for women and **vasectomy** for men). About 14% of all women in the United States of childbearing age choose a sterilization procedure to prevent unwanted pregnancy. Vasectomy is the contraceptive method of choice for about 10% of men, making these two procedures the most frequently used methods of contraception in the United States for couples over 30 years of age. So many people choose these surgical methods because they are the most effective methods of contraception besides abstinence and they have no effect on sexuality.

Although procedures for the reversal of both male and female sterilization do exist, such techniques are much more complicated and expensive than the sterilization itself, and success rates vary greatly. For this reason, surgical methods should be chosen with great thought and care and should be considered a permanent method. Counseling should be especially intensive for men and women under age 25 as the possibility of divorce, death of a sexual partner, loss of a child, or remarriage could change their philosophy toward child-bearing in the future. In addition, sterilization is not recommended for individuals whose fertility is important to their self-esteem.

Vasectomy

In a vasectomy, a small incision is made in each side of the scrotum. The vas deferens at that point is then cut and tied, cauterized, or plugged, blocking the passage of spermatozoa (Greek, 2000; Fig. 5-10). Vasectomy can be done under local anesthesia in an ambulatory setting such as a physician's office or a reproductive life planning clinic. The man experiences a small amount of local pain afterward, which can be managed by taking a mild analgesic and applying ice to the site. The procedure is 99.9% effective (Speroff & Darney, 2001). Spermatozoa that were present in the vas deferens at the time of surgery may remain viable for as long as 6 months, however, so although the man can resume sexual intercourse within 1 week, an additional birth control method should be used until two negative sperm reports have been examined (proof that all sperm in the vas deferens have been eliminated, usually requiring 10 to 20 ejaculations).

Some men resist the concept of vasectomy because they are not sufficiently aware of their anatomy to know exactly what the procedure involves. Vasectomy does not interfere with the production of sperm; the testes continue to produce sperm as always, but the sperm simply do not pass beyond the severed vas deferens and are absorbed at that point. The man will still have full erection and ejaculation capacity. Because he also continues to form seminal fluid, he will ejaculate seminal fluid, only it will not contain sperm.

There are very few complications associated with vasectomy. A hematoma at the surgical site may occur. Six percent to 7% of men in the United States who have had a

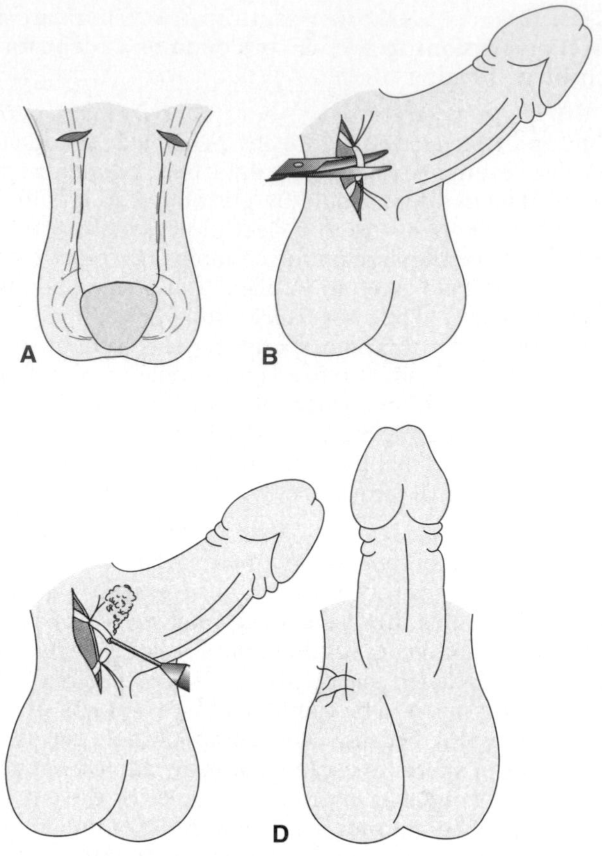

FIGURE 5.10 Vasectomy. (*A*) Site of vasectomy incisions. (*B*) The vas deferens being cut with surgical scissors. (*C*) Cut ends of the vas deferens are cauterized to completely ensure blockage of the passage of sperm. (*D*) Final skin suture.

vasectomy seek a reversal of the procedure. Unfortunately, the success rate for reanastomosis is only 45% to 60%. Some men develop autoimmunity or form antibodies against sperm, so that even if reconstruction of the vas deferens is successful at a later date, the sperm they produce do not have good mobility and are incapable of fertilization (Speroff & Darney, 2001).

Vasectomy may be associated with the development of urolithiasis (kidney stones). A few men develop chronic pain after vasectomy (postvasectomy pain syndrome); having the procedure reversed will relieve this.

Tubal Ligation

Sterilization of women could include removal of the uterus or ovaries (hysterectomy), but it generally refers to a minor surgical procedure, such as tubal ligation, whereby the fallopian tubes are occluded by cautery, crushing, clamping, or blocking the tubes and thereby preventing passage of both sperm and ova (Westhoff & Davis, 2000). Tubal ligation has a 99.9% effectiveness rate. Not only is it difficult to reconstruct fallopian tubes after they have been cauterized, but there is also a possibility that afterward the anastomosis site, because of its irregular surface, could cause an ectopic (tubal) pregnancy. If a silicone gel is instilled into the tubes as a blocking agent, this can be removed at a later date to reverse the procedure. Even this technique, however, as with vasectomy, should not be undertaken unless the woman does view it as a permanent, irreversible procedure.

Although the reason why it occurs is not clear, tubal ligation is associated with a decreased incidence of ovarian cancer. The most common operation to achieve tubal ligation is **laparoscopy.** After a menstrual flow and before ovulation, an incision as small as 1 cm is made just under the woman's umbilicus with the woman under general or local anesthesia. A lighted laparoscope is inserted through the incision. Carbon dioxide is then pumped into the incision to lift the abdominal wall upward out of the line of vision. The surgeon locates the fallopian tubes by viewing the field through the laparoscope. An electrical current to coagulate tissue is then passed through the instrument for about 3 to 5 seconds, or the tubes are clamped and cut or filled with a silicone gel to seal them (Fig. 5-11). The procedure can also be done by culdoscopy (a tube inserted through the posterior fornix of the vagina) and colpotomy (incision through the vagina), but the incidence of pelvic infection is higher with these procedures and visualization is less.

The woman is discharged in a few hours following the procedure. She may notice abdominal bloating after the procedure for the first 24 hours until the carbon dioxide infused at the beginning of the procedure is absorbed. Until this is absorbed, she may notice sharp diaphragmatic or shoulder pain if some of the carbon dioxide escapes under the diaphragm and presses on ascending nerves.

Women need to be certain that they have no unprotected coitus before the procedure (sperm trapped in the tube could fertilize an ovum there and cause an ectopic pregnancy). A woman may return to having coitus as soon as 2 to 3 days after the procedure; thus, this procedure provides immediate contraception. Women need to be informed before the procedure that laparoscopy, unlike a hysterectomy, will not affect the menstrual cycle, so they will still have a monthly menstrual flow. Complications include the risk of bowel perforation, hemorrhage, and the risks of general anesthesia with the procedure.

Contraindications to laparoscopy are an umbilical hernia, because bowel perforation might result, and extensive obesity, which would probably require a full laparotomy to allow adequate visualization. A number of women develop vaginal spotting, intermittent vaginal bleeding, and even severe lower abdominal cramping after tubal ligation, symptoms labeled posttubal ligation syndrome. Removing the fallopian tubes appears to relieve the symptoms.

Tubal ligation can be done as soon as 4 to 6 hours following the birth of a baby or an abortion, although it is more often done at 12 to 24 hours after birth. The abdominal distention at this time may make locating the tubes difficult, so a minilaparotomy may be used. Such procedures can be done in an ambulatory surgery department under local anesthesia. An incision is made 2 to 3 cm transversely just above the pubic hair. The fallopian tubes are pulled to the surface and lifted out of the incision to be visualized. Metal or plastic clips or rubber rings are then used to seal the tubes. Clips cause necrosis at that point in the tubes. The woman may notice a day or two of abdominal discomfort caused by the local necrosis at the clip site. A fimbriectomy, or removal of the fimbria at the distal end of the tubes, is yet another technique.

Effect on Sexual Enjoyment

Both tubal ligation and vasectomy may lead to increased sexual enjoyment because they largely eliminate the possibility of pregnancy. If either partner changes his or her mind about having children, however, the surgery may become an issue between them that interferes not only with sexual enjoyment but also with other aspects of their relationship as well.

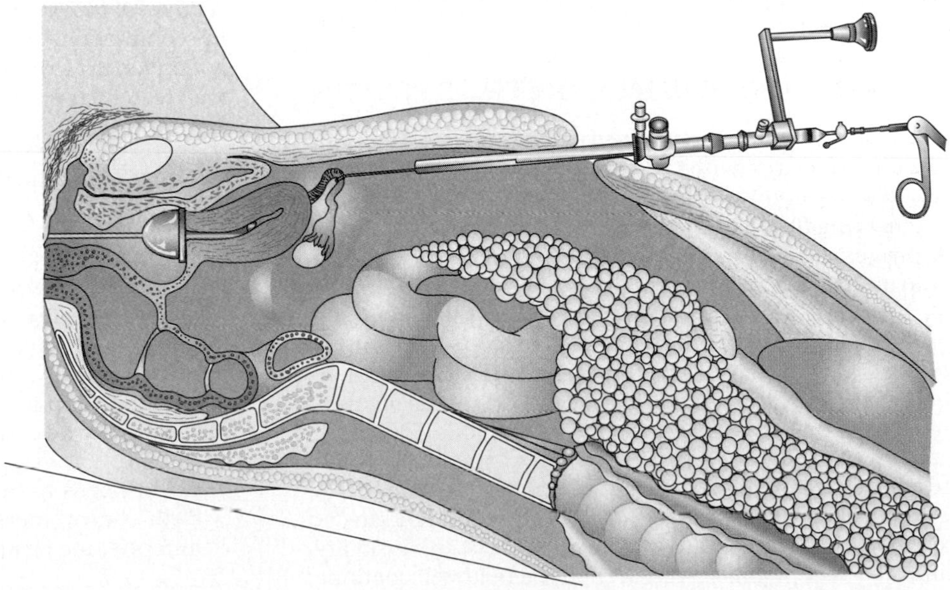

FIGURE 5.11 Laparoscopy for tubal sterilization. (From Richard Wolf Medical Instruments Corporation, with permission).

Use by the Adolescent

Sterilization is not advised for adolescents because their future goals may change so drastically that what they wanted at age 16 or 18 may not be what they want at all at age 30. Adolescents should be counseled to use more temporary forms of birth control. Later, if they still feel vasectomy or tubal ligation is the method of reproductive life planning for them, the option is still available.

> **✔ CHECKPOINT QUESTIONS**
>
> 13. What is a vasectomy?
> 14. Why do some women experience sharp shoulder pain after a tubal ligation done by laparoscopy?
> 15. Why is it important that a couple view surgical methods of reproductive life planning as permanent?

THE COUPLE WITH A PHYSICAL CHALLENGE

A couple with a physical challenge should be asked at health care visits if reproductive life planning is a concern. A man, for example, who has unsteady coordination might not have adequate hand coordination to place a condom effectively. A woman with a similar handicap might have difficulty inserting a diaphragm or cervical cap; a woman who is cognitively challenged might not understand the need to take OCs daily. For these reasons, subcutaneous implants or Depo-Provera may be the ideal contraceptives for many couples with a disability.

> **WHAT IF?** What if Dana Crews, the 17-year-old girl described at the beginning of the chapter, tells you the reason she wants a birth control method prescribed is to stop menstrual cramps? What advice would you give her?

FUTURE TRENDS IN CONTRACEPTION

Because estrogen is responsible for most of the side effects associated with OCs, studies are being conducted of even lower-dose estrogen pills. A progesterone-filled vaginal ring that is permanently implanted is a possibility. A progesterone-impregnated diaphragm and biodegradable implants that do not have to be removed may be used in the future. Transdermal progestin patches will soon be approved by the FDA and will be on the market. A birth control vaccine consisting of antibodies against human chorionic gonadotropin hormone and injections of testosterone for males (which halt sperm production, the same as estrogen halts ova production in women) are being tested at major centers. Until some method satisfies all the criteria for an ideal contraceptive (i.e., completely safe, no side effects, low cost, easy availability, easy reversibility, and user acceptability), research in the field will continue.

ELECTIVE TERMINATION OF PREGNANCY

An **elective termination of pregnancy** is a procedure performed to deliberately end a pregnancy before fetal viability. Such procedures are also referred to as therapeutic, medical, or induced abortions. Nurses employed in a health care agency where induced abortions are performed or who work for physicians or clinics who perform them are asked to assist with the procedures as a part of their duties. In the past, elective abortion was exclusively a surgical procedure. In 2000, the FDA approved the use of mifepristone (Mifegyne), a drug taken orally to induce abortion; see Focus on Pharmacology: Mifepristone (Mifegyne).

Induced abortions are done for a number of reasons:

- To end a pregnancy that threatens a woman's life (e.g., pregnancy in a woman with class IV heart disease)
- To end a pregnancy that involves a fetus found on amniocentesis to have a chromosomal defect
- To end a pregnancy that is unwanted because it is the result of rape or incest
- To terminate the pregnancy of a woman who chooses not to have a child at this time in her life. The majority of induced abortions are done for this reason.

Women having induced abortions have laboratory studies performed before the procedure, including a pregnancy test, complete blood count, blood typing (including Rh factor), a gonococcal smear, a serologic test for syphilis, a urinalysis, and a Pap smear. Pregnancies are dated by sonogram (Lichtenberg et al., 2001).

> **FOCUS ON PHARMACOLOGY**
>
> **Mifepristone (Mifegyne)**
>
> *Classification:* Abortifacient
>
> *Action:* A progesterone antagonist that stimulates uterine contractions and sloughing of endometrium, causing an implanted trophoblast to loosen from the placental wall (can be used up to 49 days' gestational age)
>
> *Pregnancy Category:* X
>
> *Dosage:* One-time dose of 600 mg P.O.
>
> *Possible Adverse Effects:* Headache, vomiting, diarrhea, heavy uterine bleeding
>
> *Nursing Interventions*
> - Drug may cause such nausea that client may appreciate being premedicated with an antiemetic.
> - Drug is usually followed within 48 hours with a prostaglandin for greater effect.
> - Client may need a D&C if heavy bleeding does not resolve.
> - Client needs to be counseled regarding effective birth control measures to avoid having to take mifepristone again in the future.

In 1973, the U.S. Supreme Court ruled that induced abortions must be legal in all states as long as the pregnancy is under 12 weeks. Individual states can regulate abortion in a second-trimester pregnancy and prohibit abortion in a third-trimester pregnancy that is not life-threatening. They can also mandate additional regulations regarding the procedure, such as requiring a 24-hour waiting period for counseling or requiring parental approval for minors. Whether a particular institution or health care provider provides abortion services depends on the policy and choice of that institution or individual. The federal government continues to debate the legal status of near-birth or partial-birth abortions.

About 28 in every 1,000 U.S. women will elect to terminate a pregnancy in their lifetime (one abortion occurs for every three live births in the U.S. yearly) (DHHS, 2000). The majority of these are done when the pregnancy is less than 12 weeks in length. The maternal mortality of surgical abortion is 0.6 per 100,000 abortions performed (statistics are not yet compiled for U.S. medical abortions). This makes abortion about 11 times safer for women than childbirth, for which the mortality rate is closer to 6 per 100,000 births. Box 5-3 highlights appropriate outcomes and interventions using the terminology identified by the Nursing Outcomes Classification and Nursing Interventions Classification.

Medically Induced Abortion

Mifepristone (a progesterone antagonist) is a compound that blocks the effect of progesterone, preventing implantation of the fertilized ovum and therefore causing abortion. The compound is taken as a single oral dose of 600 mg any time within 49 days of gestational age. Rh_oD-negative women should receive (D) immune globulin at this same time. If pregnancy expulsion does not occur from this drug alone, 3 days later, misoprostol 400 µg (a prostaglandin E1 analog) is administered in a single oral or vaginal dose. This causes uterine contraction with mild cramping and pregnancy expulsion. Mifepristone

BOX 5.3

NURSING OUTCOMES AND NURSING INTERVENTIONS CLASSIFICATION: PREGNANCY TERMINATION

NOC: Knowledge, Conception Prevention

Knowledge, conception prevention, is defined as the extent of understanding conveyed about pregnancy prevention (Johnson et al., 2000). Some specific indicators suggesting achievement of this outcome include the client's ability to describe the following:

- Various methods of contraception, such as periodic abstinence, chemical and mechanical barriers, hormonal therapy, and surgical intervention
- How conception occurs
- Advantages and disadvantages of having a child

NIC: Unplanned Pregnancy

Unplanned pregnancy is defined as the facilitation of decision making regarding pregnancy outcome (Johnson et al., 2000). Some important activities involved when implementing this intervention include:

- Determining if client has made a choice about the outcome of pregnancy
- Encouraging client and significant other to explore options regarding outcomes
- Discussing alternatives to abortion
- Discussing factors related to unplanned pregnancy
- Assisting client in identifying support system, encouraging client to involve support system during decision making
- Supporting client and significant other in decision about pregnancy outcome
- Clarifying misinformation about contraceptive use
- Referring to community agencies with services that will support client on decision making about pregnancy outcome

NIC: Pregnancy Termination Care

Pregnancy termination care is defined as managing the physical and psychological needs of the woman undergoing a spontaneous or elective abortion (McCloskey & Bulechek, 2000). Some important activities involved when implementing this intervention include:

- Preparing client physically and psychologically for abortion procedure, including explaining any sensations that client may feel, and signs to report
- Providing analgesics and antiemetics as needed
- Administering medication to terminate pregnancy as appropriate
- Encouraging significant other to support client before, during, or after the abortion
- Monitoring for bleeding and cramps
- Initiating intravenous access as necessary
- Observing for signs of spontaneous abortion
- Performing vaginal examination as appropriate
- Monitoring physiologic parameters, such as vital signs and observing for signs of shock, and completing delivery record and death report, sending any specimens for genetic studies as appropriate
- Saving all tissue passed
- Administering oxytocics after delivery, if appropriate
- Administering Rh_o(D) immune globulin if client is Rh negative
- Providing anticipatory guidance about grief reaction

has a 90% effectiveness rate when it is administered alone within 49 days of the last menstrual period and 95% when it is followed by a prostaglandin (i.e., misoprostol). See the Focus on Pharmacology: Mifepristone (Mifegyne).

It is important that women be taught to watch for signs of complications and know how to contact a health care practitioner if any are apparent (Table 5-2). Most women notice continued bleeding indistinguishable from a spontaneous miscarriage for up to 2 weeks.

Medical abortion is contraindicated under the following circumstances:

- Confirmed or suspected ectopic pregnancy
- An intrauterine device is in place
- Chronic adrenal failure
- Current long-term systemic corticosteroid therapy
- History of allergy to mifepristone, misoprostol, or other prostaglandins
- Hemorrhagic disorders or concurrent anticoagulant therapy (Newhall & Winikoff, 2000)

Advantages of medical abortion are the decreased risk of damage to the uterus through instrument insertion and decreased use of anesthesia necessary for surgically performed abortions. Most practitioners require the woman to return for postprocedure ultrasonography or a pregnancy test to ensure that the pregnancy is ended. The complications of medical abortion are incomplete abortion and the possibility of prolonged bleeding. To reduce patient risk, women should have access to emergency care facilities during the procedure. Research is being conducted on whether the dose of either mifepristone or misoprostol can be reduced while still producing satisfactory results. Whether women can independently take these medicines at home is also being investigated (Christin-Maitre et al., 2000).

Mifepristone has additional applications, such as regression of uterine leiomyomas, labor induction, and detoxification in cocaine overdose. As a group, women who undergo medical abortion prefer it to surgical abortion (Jensen et al., 2000). It is important that women receive contraceptive counseling following the procedure so they can avoid having to undergo such a procedure again in the future.

Surgically Induced Abortion Procedures

Elective abortions involve a number of techniques, depending on the gestation age at the time the abortion is performed.

Menstrual Extraction

Menstrual extraction or suction evacuation is the simplest type of surgical abortion procedure. It is performed on an ambulatory basis 5 to 7 weeks after the last menstrual period. The woman voids, and her perineum is washed with an antiseptic (shaving is unnecessary). A speculum is then introduced vaginally, the cervix is stabilized by a tenaculum, and a narrow polyethylene catheter is introduced through the vagina into the cervix and uterus (Fig. 5-12*A*). The lining of the uterus that would be shed with a normal menstrual flow is then suctioned and removed by means of the vacuum pressure of a syringe. Menstrual extraction is completed quickly and with a minimum of discomfort (some abdominal cramping may occur as the tenaculum grasps the cervix or as the last of the endometrium is suctioned away). The woman should remain supine for about 15 minutes after the procedure until uterine cramping quiets to prevent hypotension on standing. She may be given oral oxytocin to ensure full uterine contraction after the procedure. It is important she be taught to watch for signs and symptoms of complications and know how to contact a health care practitioner if any are apparent (see Table 5-2). Because a pliable catheter is used, uterine puncture is unlikely. However, the possibility of hemorrhage and infection is the same as in other surgical abortion procedures.

Women can expect some vaginal bleeding, similar to a normal menstrual flow, for a week after the procedure; they may have occasional spotting for up to 2 weeks. Women should be advised not to douche, use tampons, or resume coitus until 1 week after the procedure to avoid introducing infection. Plans should be made for a return visit in 2 weeks. This visit should include a pelvic examination and pregnancy test to be certain that the procedure was successful and the pregnancy was terminated. It is important that women receive contraceptive counseling following the procedure so they can avoid having to undergo such a procedure again in the future.

Dilatation and Curettage

If the gestational age of the pregnancy is under 13 weeks, a dilatation and curettage (D&C) procedure may be used. This procedure is usually done in an ambulatory setting using a paracervical block. A paracervical block does not eliminate pain but limits what the woman experiences to cramping and a feeling of pressure at her cervix.

TABLE 5.2 Signs and Symptoms of Complications After Elective Termination of Pregnancy

SIGN/SYMPTOM	POSSIBLE MEANING
Heavy vaginal bleeding (more than two pads saturated in 1 hour)	Hemorrhage
Passing of clots	Hemorrhage
Abdominal pain or tenderness (endometritis)	Infection
Fever over 100.4°F	Infection (endometritis)
Severe depression	Inadequate coping ability

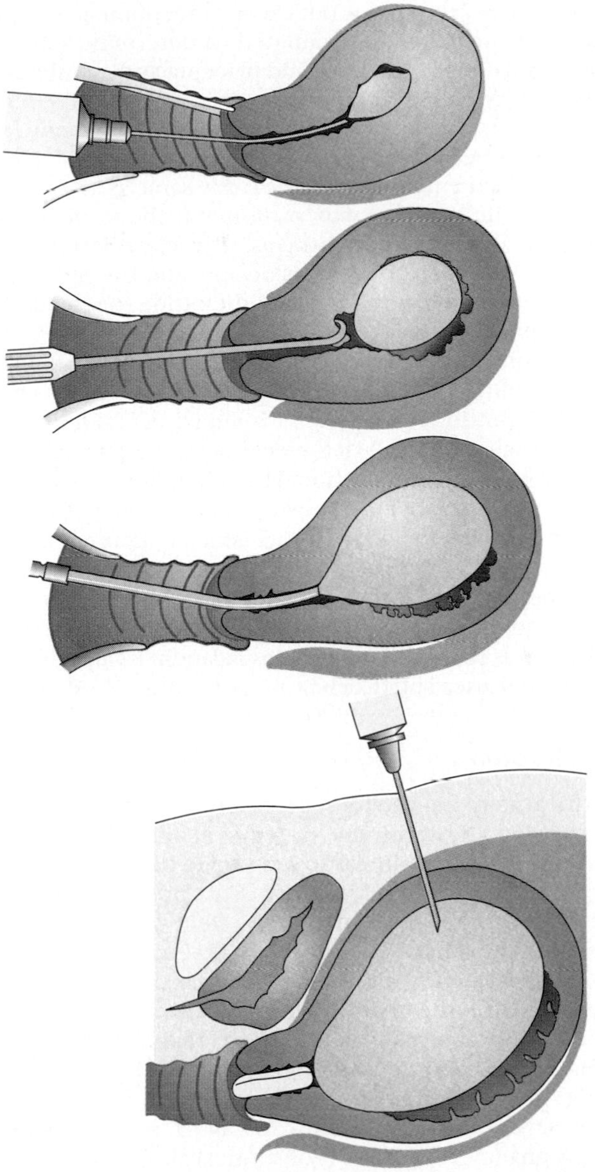

A B C D

FIGURE 5.12 Techniques of surgical elective termination of pregnancy. (*A*) Vacuum extraction. (*B*) Dilatation and curettage (D&C). (*C*) Dilatation and vacuum extraction (D&E). (*D*) Saline induction.

In preparation for the procedure the woman voids, the perineum is washed, the anesthetic block is administered, and the cervix is dilated. The uterus is then scraped clean with the curette, removing the zygote and trophoblast cells with the uterine lining (see Fig. 5-12*B*). After the procedure, the woman remains in the hospital or clinic for 1 to 4 hours with careful assessment of vital signs and perineal care. She may be given oxytocin to ensure firm uterine contraction and minimize bleeding. If there are no complications, she can return home after approximately 4 hours. She needs to be instructed on the signs and symptoms of complications (see Table 5-2) and offered contraceptive counseling so she can avoid a repeat procedure.

A D&C has the potential risk of uterine puncture from the instruments used and carries an increased risk of uterine infection compared to menstrual extraction because of greater cervical dilatation used. A woman may be given prophylactic antibiotics to prevent infection.

Dilatation and Vacuum Extraction

Most second-trimester abortions (those between 12 and 16 weeks) are done by dilatation and vacuum extraction (D&E), which can be either an inpatient or an ambulatory procedure. In some centers, dilatation of the cervix is begun the day before the procedure by insertion of a laminaria tent (seaweed that has been dried and sterilized) into the cervix under sterile conditions. In a moist body part such as the cervix, the seaweed begins to absorb fluid and swell in size. Over a 24-hour period, gradually, painlessly, and without trauma, it dilates the cervix enough for a vacuum extraction tip to be inserted. There is some concern that frequent dilatation of the cervix can lead to an incompetent cervix, or one that dilates so easily that it will not remain contracted during a subsequent pregnancy. Therefore, laminaria dilatation is often chosen for young women who may have more than one abortion in their lifetime, as the gradual dilation of the cervix by this method helps to safeguard their childbearing potential. Antibiotic prophylaxis may be initiated at the time of the laminaria insertion to protect against infection. The woman is cautioned not to have sexual relations until the abortion is complete to further reduce the possibility of infection.

After either laminaria dilatation or dilatation by traditional dilators, a narrow suction tip specially designed for the incompletely dilated cervix is introduced into the cervix (see Fig. 5-12*C*). The negative pressure of a suction pump or vacuum container then gently evacuates the uterine contents over a 15-minute period. The woman will feel pain as the cervical dilatation is performed and some pressure and cramps similar to menstrual cramps during suction, but it is not a markedly painful procedure.

After the procedure, the woman lies flat for at least 15 minutes. She remains in the hospital or clinic for about 4 hours for careful assessment of vital signs and perineal care. She usually receives oxytocin to ensure firm uterine contraction and minimize bleeding. She should also receive appropriate contraceptive counseling. She can expect to have bleeding comparable to a menstrual flow for the first week afterward, and spotting up to 2 or 3 weeks afterward. Cramping may continue for up to 24 to 48 hours; she can take a mild analgesic such as acetaminophen (Tylenol) or Ibuprofen (Advil or Motrin) for discomfort. She should be taught the danger signals shown in Table 5-2. If none of these signals is present, she can resume normal activities within 24 hours after the procedure. She should be advised not to douche, use tampons, or resume coitus until she returns in 2 weeks for a follow-up examination.

D&E has the potential for uterine puncture, although this is rare, because a rigid cannula is used for the procedure. Because the cervix was dilated, there is a potential, as in all surgical abortion procedures, for postprocedure infection.

Saline Induction

Saline induction is a method used if a pregnancy is between 16 and 24 weeks (see Fig. 5-12*D*). It is based on the principle that hypertonic (20%) saline causes fluid shifts and sloughing of the placenta and endometrium. It is an inpatient or ambulatory procedure.

The woman is admitted to a same-day surgery unit and has laminaria inserted to help prepare the cervix for dilatation. Four hours later, she voids to reduce the size of her bladder so it will not be accidentally punctured by the saline injection. Her abdominal wall is then prepared with an antiseptic solution and a local anesthetic is administered. A sterile spinal needle is inserted into the uterus through the anesthetized abdominal wall, and 100 to 200 mL of amniotic fluid is removed by a sterile syringe with amniocentesis technique (see Chap. 8). A 20% hypertonic saline solution of up to 200 mL is then injected through the same needle through the abdominal wall into the amniotic fluid. The needle is then withdrawn. Within 12 to 36 hours after the injection, labor contractions begin. The labor (which takes an additional 12 to 36 hours) may be shortened by administration of a dilute intravenous solution of oxytocin. Because the products of conception are small, the actual delivery causes only a momentary stinging pain as the perineum is stretched.

The woman needs the same care as any woman in labor:

- Frequent explanations of what is happening
- Medication for discomfort; breathing exercises may be helpful to minimize this
- Presence of people important to her and health care personnel for support

A serious potential complication of saline abortion is hypernatremia from accidental injection of the hypertonic saline solution into a blood vessel within the uterine cavity. The presence of such a concentrated salt solution in the bloodstream could cause body fluid to shift into the blood vessels in an attempt to equalize osmotic pressure. Serious dehydration of tissue could result. If an intravascular puncture should occur, the woman immediately experiences an increased pulse rate, a flushed face, and a severe headache. If such symptoms should occur, the injection must be stopped immediately and an intravenous solution such as 5% dextrose begun to dilute the saline solution and restore fluid balance.

If large amounts of oxytocin are necessary to induce labor with a saline abortion, the woman must be observed closely for signs of water intoxication, or body fluid accumulating in body tissue, the same side effect of oxytocin administration that can occur when it is used with term birth. Signs of water intoxication are severe headache, confusion, drowsiness, edema, and decreased urinary output. These symptoms occur subtly at first, then grow in severity. If such symptoms occur, the oxytocin drip should be stopped immediately. The symptoms will then decrease as body fluid shifts back to normal compartments. Always infuse oxytocin using a piggyback method during an abortion procedure, the same as with a woman in term labor, so it is possible to stop the infusion of oxytocin quickly yet maintain a fluid line for emergency drugs or fluid.

After delivery of the products of conception, it is important that the tissue be examined to determine whether the entire conceptus (fetus and placenta and membranes) has been delivered. If the woman wishes to see the fetus, wrap it as if it were a full-term infant and allow her to see it. Women need to be carefully observed for vaginal hemorrhage following the procedure, the same as after a term birth. If the delivery was prolonged, the woman may develop disseminated intravascular coagulation from trauma (see Chap. 15); if this occurs, she is very susceptible to hemorrhage as her blood clotting mechanism is compromised.

All women should receive contraception counseling following saline inductions. The woman can expect to have vaginal spotting for as long as 2 weeks. A first menstrual flow usually occurs 2 to 8 weeks after the procedure. A follow-up examination should be scheduled 2 to 4 weeks after the procedure for assessment of reproductive organs. Sexual relations and douching are generally contraindicated until the time of this postabortion checkup, or for 2 weeks.

A method similar to saline induction is the injection of intra-amniotic urea or prostaglandin F2-alpha. Urea is not as effective as saline induction; prostaglandin F2-alpha causes extreme nausea and diarrhea as unpleasant side effects.

Hysterotomy

If the gestational age for a pregnancy is more than 16 to 18 weeks, a hysterotomy, or removal of the fetus by surgical intervention similar to a cesarean birth, may be performed. Surgery is necessary at this point because the uterus becomes resistant to the effect of oxytocin as it reaches this phase of pregnancy and may not respond to saline induction, even with the assistance of oxytocin. Furthermore, the chance is great at this gestational age, because the uterus is so enlarged, that the uterus will not respond and contract afterward, leading to hemorrhage. The technique for hysterotomy is identical to that of cesarean birth (see Chap. 20). Because this is so late in pregnancy, less than 1% of surgical abortions are done using this technique.

"Partial Birth Abortion"

"Partial birth abortion" is a surgical technique used during the last 3 months of pregnancy when the fetus has been discovered to have a congenital anomaly that will be incompatible with life or will result in a severely compromised child, such as one with an encephalocele or high meningocele. Labor is induced by a combination of oxytocin and cervical ripening. The fetus is turned so that the breech presents to the birth canal. A clamp is then inserted into the base of the fetal skull, the head contents are destroyed, and the head is collapsed and then delivered. "Partial birth abortion" remains legal in the United States because it is believed that the procedure is sometimes necessary to protect the health of the mother. In reality, it is rarely used for that purpose, because a cesarean birth at that point in pregnancy or delivery of a preterm infant would accomplish the same thing. It is a type of procedure that raises ethical and political questions, particularly in relation to abortion rights.

Isoimmunization

Whenever a placenta is dislodged, either by spontaneous delivery or surgical or medical intervention at any point in pregnancy, blood from the placental villi (the fetal blood) may enter the maternal circulation. This has implications for the Rh-negative woman. Enough Rh-positive blood may enter her circulation to cause isoimmunization, the production by her immunologic system of antibodies against Rh-positive blood. If her next child should have Rh-positive blood, these antibodies would attempt to destroy the red blood cells of the infant during the months in utero.

After either a medically or surgically induced abortion, because the blood type of the conceptus is unknown, all women with Rh-negative blood should receive $Rh_0(D)$ immune globulin (RhoGAM or RHIG) within 72 hours of the procedure to prevent the buildup of antibodies in the event the conceptus was Rh positive (see Chap. 26 for a full discussion of Rh disease).

Psychological Aspects of Elective Termination of Pregnancy

Women of all ages, married or unmarried, with or without children, request induced abortions. The usual profile of a woman who is having such a procedure is young, unmarried, with no previous live births and undergoing the procedure for the first time to end an unwanted pregnancy.

Women having induced abortion need the same kind of explanations and support that women in labor receive (often more so, because women do not share abortion experiences with each other as they share labor experiences, so they usually have received little advance preparation).

Most women feel anxious when they appear at the hospital or clinic for an abortion. Some of the anxiety comes from having made a difficult decision to reach this step; some comes from having to face the unknown; some may come from feelings of loss or shame and sadness that they had to make a decision with which they are not totally comfortable. Remembering that this is not a decision taken lightly helps to plan nursing care aimed at making an abortion as nontraumatic as possible (Major et al., 2000).

A few women express sadness and guilt after abortion. These women may need to be referred for professional counseling so they can integrate and accept this event in their lives.

✔ CHECKPOINT QUESTIONS

16. Why is abortion safer early in pregnancy than later?
17. What threat does frequent dilatation of the cervix pose? What method of dilatation can be used to reduce this risk?
18. What signs and symptoms indicate a complication after an abortion?

KEY POINTS

Reproductive life planning involves personal decisions based on each individual's background, experiences, and sociocultural beliefs. It involves thorough planning to be certain that the method chosen is acceptable and can be used effectively.

Natural family planning (periodic abstinence) methods are varied but involve determining the fertile period each month and then avoiding sexual relations during that time.

Oral contraceptives are combinations of estrogen and progesterone. They provide one of the most reliable forms of contraception outside of abstinence. Women older than 40 years who smoke are not candidates for oral contraceptive use because of the danger of cardiovascular complications. Counsel them to find a form of contraception that is reliable and allows them to remain sexually active.

Subcutaneous implants (renewed every 5 years) and subcutaneous injections (renewed every 3 months) are new methods of contraception. They are almost 100% effective.

Intrauterine devices are placed in the uterus to prevent fertilization and implantation. Women with IUDs are at greater risk for pelvic inflammatory disease than others. Counsel them to limit the number of sexual partners and be aware of the signs and symptoms of PID.

Barrier methods include the diaphragm, cervical cap, vaginal spermicides, diaphragm, and condom (male and female). Such methods are low in cost but are not as effective as ovulation suppressant methods. Use of diaphragms has been associated with UTIs.

"Morning after" protection involves administration of a high dose of estrogen that prevents FSH release, preventing ovulation.

Surgical methods of contraception are tubal ligation in women and vasectomy in men. Counsel individuals who wish to undergo these procedures that they are largely irreversible.

Elective termination of pregnancy can be accomplished by menstrual extraction, dilatation and curettage, dilatation and evacuation, saline induction, administration of mifepristone (Mifegyne), or hysterotomy. Counsel women not to think of elective termination of pregnancy as a contraceptive method; it is a recourse to be used only when preventive measures fail. Women who are Rh negative need to receive $Rh_0(D)$ immune globulin following these procedures.

When counseling clients about reproductive life planning, nurses have a responsibility to counsel them regarding safer sex practices as well, such as using a condom during sexual intercourse to avoid sexually transmitted diseases or HIV infection.

CRITICAL THINKING EXERCISES

1. What patient education information would you provide for Dana Crews, the 17-year-old described at the beginning of this chapter? What method of reproductive life planning would you recommend for her? Would your teaching and recommendations differ if Dana were 39 years old and afraid to use OCs because of possible side effects?
2. A young adult male is interested in taking an active role in reproductive life planning and does not want to contract a sexually transmitted disease. He has no regular sexual partners at present. What recommendations would you make? Would this be different if he had a monogamous relationship?
3. A 16-year-old girl has been admitted to the hospital for a saline induction for an elective termination of pregnancy. Her mother asks you to give her only a minimum of analgesia so she remembers the experience as painful and therefore won't get pregnant again. Do you agree with this philosophy? Are there other measures you could take to help her avoid future pregnancy?
4. Examine the National Health Goals related to reproductive life planning. Most government-sponsored money for nursing research is allotted based on these goals. What would be a possible research topic to explore pertinent to these goals that would be fundable and would advance evidence-based practice?

REFERENCES

Blackburn, R. D., Cunkelman, A., & Zlidar, V. M. (2000). Oral contraceptives: An update. *Population Reports, Series A; Oral Contraceptives, 28*(1),1-16.

Burroughs, K. E., & Chambliss, M. L. (2000). Antibiotics and oral contraceptive failure. *Archives of Family Medicine, 9*(1), 81-82.

Christin-Maitre, S., Bouchard, P., & Spitz, I. M. (2000). Medical termination of pregnancy. *New England Journal of Medicine, 342*(13), 946-956.

Department of Health and Human Services. (2000). *Healthy people 2010.* Washington, D.C.: DHHS.

Everett, S. A., et al. (2000). Use of birth control pills, condoms, and withdrawal among U.S. high school students. *Journal of Adolescent Health, 27*(2), 112-118.

Felton, G. M., & Bartoces, M. (2002). Predictions of initiation of early sex in black and white adolescent females. *Public Health Nursing, 19*(1), 59-67.

Greek, G. (2000). Vasectomy: A safe, effective, economical means of sterilization. *Postgraduate Medicine, 108*(2), 173-179.

Grimes, D. A., Hanson, V., & Sondheimer, S. (2001). New approaches to emergency contraception. *Patient Care for the Nurse Practitioner, 4*(3), 44-54.

Ho, P. C. (2000). Emergency contraception: Methods and efficacy. *Current Opinion in Obstetrics & Gynecology, 12*(3), 175-179.

Jensen, J. T., Harvey, S. M., & Beckman, L. J. (2000). Acceptability of suction curettage and mifepristone abortion in the United States: A prospective comparison study. *American Journal of Obstetrics & Gynecology, 182*(6), 1292-1299.

Johnson, M., Maas, M., & Moorhead, S. (2000). *Nursing outcomes classification* (2d ed.). St. Louis: Mosby, Inc.

Lichtenberg, E. S. et al. (2001). First trimester surgical abortion practices. *Contraception, 64*(6), 345-352.

Ling, F. W., & Duff, P. (Eds.). (2001). *Obstetrics and gynecology: Principles for practice.* New York: McGraw-Hill.

Major, B., et al. (2000). Psychological responses of women after first-trimester abortion. *Archives of General Psychiatry, 57*(8), 777-784.

McCloskey, J., & Bulechek, G. (2000). *Nursing interventions classification* (3d ed.). St. Louis: Mosby Inc.

Newhall, E. P., & Winikoff, B. (2000). Abortion with mifepristone and misoprostol: Regimens, efficacy, acceptability and future directions. *American Journal of Obstetrics & Gynecology, 183*(2 suppl), S44-53.

Shaban, D. W., et al. (2001). The knowledge and use of birth control in the year 2000: The future needs of minority women. *Obstetrics & Gynecology, 97*(4), S17-S22.

Speroff, L., & Darney, P. D. (2001). *A clinical guide for contraception.* Philadelphia: Lippincott Williams & Wilkins.

Thomas, M. H. (2000). Abstinence-based programs for prevention of adolescent pregnancies: A review. *Journal of Adolescent Health, 26*(1), 5-17.

Tommaselli, G. A., et al. (2000). The importance of user compliance on the effectiveness of natural family planning programs. *Gynecologic Endocrinology, 14*(2), 81-89.

Vanos, W. A. (1999). The intrauterine device and its dynamics. *Advances in Contraception, 15*(2), 119-132.

Wellbery, C. (2000). Emergency contraception. *Archives of Family Medicine, 9*(7), 642-646.

Westhoff, C., & Davis, A. (2000). Tubal sterilization: Focus on the U.S. experience. *Fertility & Sterility, 73*(5), 913-922.

SUGGESTED READINGS

Alderman, P. M., & Morrison, G. E. (2000). Standard incision or no-scalpel vasectomy? *Journal of Family Practice, 48*(9), 719-721.

Arevalo, M., Sinai, I., & Jennings, V. (1999). A fixed formula to define the fertile window of the menstrual cycle as the

basis of a simple method of natural family planning. *Contraception, 60*(6), 357-360.
Breitbart, V. (2000). Counseling for medical abortion. *American Journal of Obstetrics & Gynecology, 183* (2 suppl), S26-33.
Bumpass, L. L., Thomson, E., & Godecker, A. L. (2000). Women, men, and contraceptive sterilization. *Fertility & Sterility, 73*(5), 937-946.
Clark, S., Ellertson, C., & Winikoff, B. (2000). Is medical abortion acceptable to all American women: The impact of sociodemographic characteristics on the acceptability of mifepristone-misoprostol abortion. *Journal of the American Medical Women's Association, 55*(3 suppl), 177-182.
Darroch, J. E. et al. (2002). Differences in teenage pregnancy rates among five developed countries: The roles of sexual activity and contraceptive use. *Family Planning Perspectives, 33*(6), 244-250.
Hacker, K. A., et al. (2000). Listening to youth: Teen perspectives on pregnancy prevention. *Journal of Adolescent Health, 26*(4), 279-288.
Jaccard, J., & Dittus, P. J. (2000). Adolescent perceptions of maternal approval of birth control and sexual risk behavior. *American Journal of Public Health, 90*(9), 1426-1430.
Kruse, B., et al. (2000). Management of side effects and complications in medical abortion. *American Journal of Obstetrics and Gynecology, 183*(2 suppl), S65-75.
Parsons, J. T., et al. (2000). Perceptions of the benefits and costs associated with condom use and unprotected sex among late adolescent college students. *Journal of Adolescence, 23*(4), 377-391.
Pymar, H. C., & Creinin, M. D. (2000). Alternatives to mifepristone regimens for medical abortion. *American Journal of Obstetrics & Gynecology, 183*(2), S54-S64.
Templeman, C. L., et al. (2000). Postpartum contraceptive use among adolescent mothers. *Obstetrics & Gynecology, 95*(5), 770-776.

6

The Infertile Couple

CHAPTER

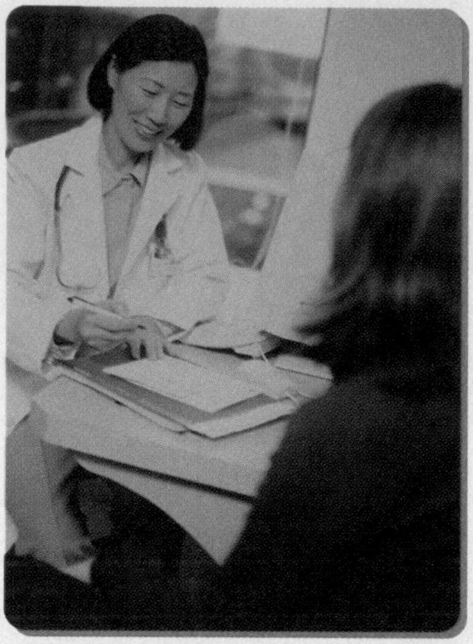

Key Terms

- **anovulation**
- **cryptorchidism**
- **endometriosis**
- **erectile dysfunction**
- **infertility**
- **mumps orchitis**
- **primary infertility**
- **secondary infertility**
- **sperm count**
- **sperm motility**
- **spermatogenesis**
- **varicocele**

Objectives

After mastering the contents of this chapter, you should be able to:

1. Describe common causes of infertility in men and women.
2. Describe common assessments necessary to detect infertility.
3. Formulate nursing diagnoses related to infertility.
4. Identify appropriate expected outcomes for the infertile couple.
5. Plan interventions to meet the needs of the couple with a diagnosis of infertility.
6. Assist with interventions associated with the diagnosis of infertility or measures to promote fertility, such as health teaching.
7. Evaluate outcomes for achievement and effectiveness of care.
8. Identify National Health Goals related to infertility that nurses can participate in helping the nation achieve.
9. Identify areas of nursing care related to fertility that could benefit from additional nursing research or application of evidence-based practice.
10. Use critical thinking to analyze nursing strategies that can be used to support a couple through a fertility assessment.
11. Integrate knowledge about infertility with the nursing process to achieve quality maternal and child health nursing care.

Mr. and Mrs. Carl, married when they were both 25, planned to wait 5 years before beginning their family so they would have time to save money for a house. At the end of 5 years, they bought the house. On the day they moved in, Mrs. Carl stopped taking her birth control pills. At the end of a year, however, she still was not pregnant. Three years later, the Carls began fertility testing. They are now undergoing their second cycle of in vitro fertilization and embryo transfer. The Carls have applied for a second mortgage on their house to finance the fertility testing and fertilization procedures. At her last visit, Mrs. Carl stated, "This is my fault because I'm so rigid. I can't relax enough to get pregnant. Look at the way I had to buy the house before I could even consider getting pregnant, and now we'll probably lose it. Besides that, it feels like our whole life revolves around trying to get pregnant."

Previous chapters described the process of normal ovulation and conception. This chapter adds information to expand your knowledge base about care of the couple who is unable to conceive.

After you've studied the chapter, answer the Critical Thinking Exercises at the end of the chapter and then access the on-line study activities (http://connection.lww.com) *to further sharpen your skills and test your knowledge.*

FOCUS ON NATIONAL HEALTH GOALS

One of the National Health Goals identified by the *Healthy People 2010* directly addresses the problem of infertility:

- Reduce the proportion of married couples whose ability to conceive or maintain a pregnancy is impaired from a baseline of 13% to a target of 10% (DHHS, 2000).

To meet this health goal, nurses need to be active in health promotion and early identification of problems that could lead to infertility. In addition, nurses need to play an active role in teaching clients about safer sex practices (see Chap. 4) to help reduce the incidence of sexually transmitted diseases and pelvic inflammatory disease, which can contribute to infertility. Nursing research to investigate areas such as how to help women better recognize the symptoms of pelvic inflammatory disease is also necessary.

Infertility, or the inability to conceive a child or sustain a pregnancy to childbirth, affects as many as 10% to 15% of couples who desire children (Hammond & Stillman, 2000). Couples exploring fertility testing come in all different patterns: many are married couples; some have plans to marry; some desire to remain single but bear a child; some are gay or lesbian. When a couple pursues fertility counseling, they usually have fears and anxieties not only about their inability to conceive but what this condition means to their future and their family. Without information about the cause of their infertility, each may blame himself or herself or carry unexpressed anger toward the partner. In addition, the couple may strongly desire a child but also feel the normal anxieties associated with impending parenthood, such as loss of independence and an established lifestyle that a child will bring. For all these reasons, infertility screening and counseling can be an emotionally difficult and physically demanding process, often creating a high level of strain on a couple's relationship (Adamson et al., 2001).

Many marriage customs, such as throwing rice, originate from old rituals to promote fertility. The existence of such common rituals provides evidence about the importance of having children for the average couple and society as a whole.

One National Health Goal aimed at reducing infertility is shown in the Focus on National Health Goals box. Because most fertility tests are conducted in ambulatory settings, nurses play key roles in educating the couple about the variety of tests and procedures that may be performed. They are important members of fertility health care teams, often assuming responsibility for health assessment, client education and counseling, helping clients identify and express their feelings about the desire to have a child, how far they are willing to go in terms of testing and procedures to achieve this desire, and how they might feel if they can't have a child. In addition, educating clients about the available procedures, many of which are complex and demand knowledgeable, ongoing participation, and participating in the complex planning and implementation of treatment strategies are also important roles. When pregnancy cannot be achieved, nurses can counsel clients about available alternatives, such as adoption or child-free living.

NURSING PROCESS OVERVIEW

For the Couple With Infertility

Assessment

Infertility assessment requires a series of laboratory and physical examinations, which may affect the core of a couple's self-image and self-esteem. Nursing assessment often reveals that one or both partners feel inadequate or angry and frustrated. It may be possible to detect such feelings while gathering information for the history. Questions such as, "How do you feel about what has happened?" or "How do you think your partner feels about not being able to conceive?" may be enough to encourage partners to express their concerns. Talking with both partners together may be advantageous because they may feel more comfortable speaking about their problem together. On the other hand, it is important to spend some time alone with each client in case there is anything a partner wishes to discuss privately. This might be the only opportunity one of them has to ask that one "silly" question or voice a fear that they believe is too foolish to ask or bring up in front of their partner.

Nursing Diagnosis

Nursing diagnoses related to problems of infertility are likely to focus on psychosocial issues associated with the inability to conceive and the long, arduous process of fertility testing and management. Possible diagnoses include:

- Fear related to outcome of infertility studies
- Situational low self-esteem related to the inability to conceive
- Anxiety related to the heavy schedule and timing of planned testing
- Deficient knowledge related to measures to promote fertility
- Anticipatory grieving related to failure to conceive or sustain a pregnancy

If a specific problem is revealed in this area or if testing and therapy become so overwhelming for a couple that their relationship (including sexual patterns) begins to unravel, "Sexual dysfunction related to command performance of infertility therapy" might be applicable. "Powerlessness related to repeated unsuccessful attempts at achieving conception" and "Hopelessness related to perception of no viable alternatives to usual conception" may also be relevant.

Outcome Identification and Planning

In establishing expected outcomes with a couple undergoing fertility testing and counseling, attempt to ensure that the couple realizes that because testing takes a long time, results will not be instantaneous. A couple may need to change or modify their goals if tests begin to show that what they first wanted, to have a child without medical intervention, is impossible. Box 6-1 highlights appropriate outcomes and interventions using the terminology identified by the Nursing Outcomes Classification (NOC) and Nursing Interventions Classification (NIC).

Implementation

Fertility testing can be costly, and some health insurance programs do not provide reimbursement for fertility testing. However, surgery such as that to relieve endometriosis would be covered because this is a health concern. Because of this, couples need to know beforehand about the specific estimates for the cost of

BOX 6.1

NURSING OUTCOMES AND NURSING INTERVENTIONS CLASSIFICATION: INFERTILITY

NOC: Knowledge, Fertility Promotion

Knowledge, fertility promotion is defined as the extent of understanding conveyed about fertility testing and conditions affecting conception (Johnson, Maas, & Moorhead, 2000). Some specific indicators suggesting achievement of this outcome include the client's ability to describe the following:

- Effects of age, coital frequency, nutrition, physical anomalies, environmental conditions, pelvic surgeries or infections, and hormone levels on fertility
- Methods used to test fertility, including ultrasonography, sperm count, and postcoital test
- Methods used to detect ovulation, such as basal body temperature

NIC: Fertility Preservation

Fertility preservation is defined as providing the information, counseling, and treatment that facilitate reproductive health and the ability to conceive (McCloskey & Bulechek, 2000). Some important activities involved when implementing this intervention include:

- Discussing factors related to infertility
- Assessing reproductive status, including pelvic examination and cervical cultures, as appropriate
- Teaching about prevention of sexually transmitted diseases including signs and symptoms and need for early, aggressive treatment
- Discussing the effects of various contraceptive methods on fertility
- Referring client for thorough physical examination for health problems affecting fertility, such as endometriosis
- Reviewing lifestyle habits that may affect fertility such as smoking, substance use, alcohol consumption, nutritional patterns, exercise, and sexual behavior
- Instituting a referral for client with history indicative of possible fertility problems for early diagnosis and treatment

NIC: Family Planning, Infertility

Family planning, infertility is defined as the management, education, and support of the client and significant other undergoing evaluation and treatment for infertility (McCloskey & Bulechek, 2000). Some important activities involved when implementing this intervention include:

- Explaining about the reproductive cycle
- Assisting the female client in measures to detect ovulation
- Determining the client's understanding of test results and recommended therapy
- Supporting the client through the infertility history and evaluation
- Assisting with expressions of grief, disappointment, and expressions of failure
- Referring the client to support groups as appropriate
- Determining the effect of infertility on the couple's relationship

testing or therapy. They also may need help budgeting and planning their resources accordingly.

Suggesting that a couple combine involvement with fertility testing with ongoing activities or begin a new activity together such as taking a night school course, planting a garden, or learning a new sport or hobby at the same time they begin fertility testing is a way of helping them reduce the feeling that their entire existence revolves around the testing procedures. This also may help provide them with time for sharing experiences and increasing intimacy, helping to compensate for any decreased enjoyment that comes from "scheduled" sexual relations.

Throughout testing, couples need thorough education about the various procedures. Make sure to review any specific instructions about pre- and post-procedural care. Depending on their motivations, a couple's reaction to study results may vary from relief to stoic acceptance to grief for children never to be born. Each partner may wonder whether the other will be able to continue the relationship if he or she turns out to be the "infertile" one. Couples need the support of health care personnel throughout the course of infertility studies, from the first day they braced themselves to ask, "Exactly why are we childless?" until the end, regardless of the results.

Participation in a support group may allow a couple to work through the stress that fertility testing places on their lives. Resolve (*www.resolve.org*), a national support group for couples with infertility, can be helpful in offering referral sources and support that a couple can use in planning. Another organization is the American Society of Reproductive Medicine (*www.asrm.org*).

Outcome Evaluation

Examples of expected outcomes in this area might be:

- Client rearranges work plans to manage heavy schedule of testing by 1 month's time.
- Couple verbalizes appropriate information in preparation for testing.
- Couple demonstrates a high level of self-esteem after fertility studies, even in the face of disappointing study outcomes.

For the couple with problems involving infertility, evaluation must be ongoing because, as circumstances around them change, so may their goals and desires. Until they can accept an alternative method of having children, such as adoption or artificial insemination, former plans have been crushed. It is not unusual to see a couple move through steps of denial, anger, bargaining, and depression before they reach a level of acceptance that they are different in this one area of life from others, but not limited in their ability to achieve in other areas. With acceptance, they are able to make adjustments in their wants or plans to feel fulfilled again.

Future evaluation is also important, because a couple who decides at age 20 to choose child-free living may change their minds at a later date. A couple who chooses artificial insemination may decide after a number of unsuccessful attempts that they are no longer interested in this method of conception. Keeping evaluation an ongoing process allows such a plan to be modified as necessary. Couples seen for fertility testing can be encouraged to telephone or visit every 6 months to 1 year to inquire about new discoveries in the field of fertility and how these apply to their situation.

INFERTILITY

Infertility is said to exist when a pregnancy has not occurred after at least 1 year of engaging in unprotected coitus. In **primary infertility,** there have been no previous conceptions; in **secondary infertility,** there has been a previous viable pregnancy but the couple is unable to conceive at present. Sterility refers to the inability to conceive because of a known condition, such as the absence of a uterus.

Between 13% and 20% of couples in the United States are infertile. In about 40% of couples with an infertility problem, the cause of infertility is multifactorial; in about 30% of couples, it is the man who is infertile; 20% to 30% of couples experience ovulatory failure; and 20% to 40% experience tubal, vaginal, or uterine problems as the cause of their infertility. In as many as 15% of couples, no known cause for the infertility can be discovered despite all the diagnostic tests currently available (Hammond & Stillman, 2000).

Some couples, because they are unaware of the average length of time it takes to achieve a pregnancy, may worry that they are infertile when they are not. When engaging in coitus an average of four times per week, 50% of couples take 6 months to conceive; after 12 months, 85% of couples will conceive. These periods are longer if sexual relations are less frequent (Adamson et al., 2001).

Couples who engage in coitus daily, hoping to cause early impregnation, may actually have more difficulty conceiving than those who space coitus to every other day. This is because too-frequent coitus can lower a man's spermatozoa count to a level below optimal fertility. Couples who focus their sexual relations on trying to increase sperm/ovum exposure may find their lives governed by temperature charts and "good days" and "bad days" to such an extent that their relationship suffers.

The chance of infertility increases with age. Because of this gradual decline in fertility, women who defer pregnancy to their late thirties are apt to have more difficulty getting pregnant than their younger counterparts. Women using medroxyprogesterone (Depo-Provera) or levonorgestrel (Norplant) for contraception should know that they may have difficulty becoming pregnant for several months after discontinuing the medication, often anywhere between 2 to 7 months on average to possibly 1 year, because it takes this long to restore normal body functioning. This recovery period is shorter for women taking an oral contraceptive. Once normal menses resume, usually by the next month, pregnancy is possible.

Male Infertility Factors

A number of factors typically lead to male infertility:

- Disturbance in **spermatogenesis** (production of sperm cells)
- Obstruction in the seminiferous tubules, ducts, or vessels preventing movement of spermatozoa

- Qualitative or quantitative changes in the seminal fluid preventing **sperm motility** (movement of sperm)
- Development of autoimmunity that immobilizes sperm
- Problems in ejaculation or deposition preventing spermatozoa from being placed close enough to the woman's cervix to allow ready penetration and fertilization

Inadequate Sperm Count

The **sperm count** is the number of sperm in a single ejaculation or milliliter of semen. The minimum sperm count considered normal is 20 million per milliliter of seminal fluid, or 50 million per ejaculation. At least 60% of sperm should be motile, and 60% should be normal in shape and form. Spermatozoa must be produced and maintained at a temperature slightly lower than body temperature to become normal and fully motile (Sandlow, 2000). Therefore, any condition that significantly increases body temperature can affect sperm count. This is why the testes, in which sperm are produced and stored, are suspended in the scrotal sac away from body heat. Actions that increase scrotal heat, such as working at desk jobs or driving a great deal every day (e.g., salesmen or motorcyclists) may lower sperm counts in men compared to those whose occupations allow them to be ambulatory at least part of each day. Frequent use of hot tubs or saunas may also lower sperm counts appreciably. Another reason for an inadequate sperm count is a chronic infection, such as tuberculosis or recurrent sinusitis, due to the elevated temperature that may accompany such infections.

Congenital abnormalities such as **cryptorchidism** (undescended testes) may lead to lowered sperm production if surgical repair of this problem was not completed until after puberty, or if the spermatic cord became twisted after the surgery (Weidner et al., 1999). Sons of women who took diethylstilbestrol (DES), an estrogen prescribed in the past to sustain pregnancies, have an increased chance of producing abnormal sperm.

Yet another cause of male infertility is **varicocele** (varicosity of the spermatic vein). This varicosity increases the temperature within the testes, so spermatogenesis can be slowed or disrupted. Surgery to repair the varicocele increases the chances for conception.

Other conditions that may inhibit sperm production include trauma to the testes; surgery on or near the testicles that results in impaired testicular circulation; and endocrine imbalances, particularly with the thyroid, pancreas, and pituitary glands. Drug or excessive alcohol use and environmental factors such as excessive exposure to x-rays or radioactive substances have also been found to negatively affect spermatogenesis (Sinclair, 2000). Men exposed to radioactive substances on the job should have adequate protection of the testes. When undergoing pelvic x-rays, men should always be furnished with a protective lead shield.

Obstruction or Impaired Sperm Motility

Obstruction may occur at any point along the pathway that spermatozoa must travel to reach the outside: the seminiferous tubules, the epididymis, the vas deferens, the ejaculatory duct, or the urethra (see Fig. 4-2). Diseases such as **mumps orchitis** (testicular inflammation and scarring due to the mumps virus), epididymitis (inflammation of the epididymis), and tubal infections such as gonorrhea or ascending urethral infection may cause adhesions and occlusions, interfering with sperm transport. Congenital stricture of a spermatic duct is sometimes seen. Hypertrophy of the prostate gland occurs in many men beginning at about age 50 years. Pressure from this on the vas deferens can interfere with sperm transport. Infection of the prostate gland, through which the seminal fluid must pass, or infection of the seminal vesicles (spread from urinary tract infections) can change the composition of the seminal fluid enough to reduce sperm motility.

It has been shown that men who have vasectomies may develop an autoimmune reaction or may form antibodies that immobilize their own sperm. It is conceivable that men with obstruction in the vas deferens from other causes, such as scarring following an infection, could also develop an autoimmune reaction that immobilizes sperm the same way.

Anomalies of the penis, such as *hypospadias* (urethral opening on the ventral surface of the penis) or *epispadias* (urethral opening on the dorsal surface), may cause deposition of spermatozoa too far from the sexual partner's cervix to allow optimal cervical penetration. Extreme obesity in a male may also interfere with penetration.

Ejaculation Problems

Psychological problems, debilitating diseases such as a cerebrovascular accident or Parkinson's disease, and some medications, such as certain antihypertensive agents, may result in **erectile dysfunction** (formerly called impotence). This is primary if the man has never been able to achieve erection and ejaculation and secondary if the man has been able to achieve ejaculation in the past but now has difficulty. Erectile dysfunction may be a difficult problem to solve if it is associated with stress, as this is usually not easily relieved. If the erectile dysfunction is caused by a psychological issue (psychogenic infertility), a solution to the problem can include psychological or sexual counseling and may involve long-term care.

Premature ejaculation (ejaculation before penetration) may interfere with the proper deposition of sperm. It is another problem often attributed to psychological causes. Adolescents may experience it until they become more experienced in sexual techniques.

✔ CHECKPOINT QUESTIONS

1. When is infertility said to exist?
2. What congenital condition may impair spermatogenesis if not repaired before puberty?

Female Infertility Factors

The factors that cause infertility in women are analogous to those causing infertility in men: **anovulation** (faulty or inadequate production of ova), problems of ova transport through the fallopian tubes to the uterus, uterine factors such as tumors or poor endometrial development, and cervical and vaginal factors that immobilize spermatozoa (Rosene-Montella et al., 2000).

Anovulation

Anovulation (absence of ovulation), the most common cause of infertility in women, may occur from a genetic abnormality such as Turner's syndrome (hypogonadism) in which there are no ovaries to produce ova. It may also occur as a result of a hormonal imbalance caused by a condition such as hypothyroidism interfering with hypothalamus-pituitary-ovarian interaction. Ovarian tumors may produce anovulation due to feedback stimulation on the pituitary. Chronic or excessive exposure to x-rays or radioactive substances, general ill health, poor diet, or stress may all contribute to poor ovarian function. Stress affects the ovaries by reducing hypothalamic secretion of gonadotropin-releasing hormone (GnRH), which then lowers luteinizing hormone (LH) and follicle-stimulating hormone (FSH) production. Decreased body weight, or a body/fat ratio of less than 10%, as in female athletes (for example, competitive runners) or in women who are excessively lean or anorexic, can reduce pituitary hormones such as FSH and LH and halt ovulation.

In addition, natural ovulatory patterns vary greatly among women, thus affecting fertility. Some women may ovulate only a few times a year. Sometimes this can be detected by examining the menstrual history, but even if a woman experiences regular monthly menstruation, it does not necessarily indicate that she is also ovulating on a regular basis. A recent study has shown that ova discharged from the right ovary may favor fertilization more than left-sided ones (Fukuda et al., 2000).

Tubal Transport Problems

Difficulty with tubal transport usually occurs because scarring has developed in the fallopian tubes. This usually occurs from chronic salpingitis (chronic pelvic inflammatory disease [PID]) or else results from a ruptured appendix or abdominal surgery involving infection and subsequent adhesion formation in the fallopian tubes.

Pelvic Inflammatory Disease. PID is infection of the pelvic organs: the uterus, fallopian tubes, ovaries, and their supporting structures. The infection can be extensive, causing pelvic peritonitis. Many organisms can be the cause of PID, but chlamydia and gonorrhea are the most frequent causative organisms. PID occurs at a rate of 25 per 100; in other words, one fourth of all women will experience this type of infection in a lifetime (Eschenbach, 2000). The rate of infection is highest in teenagers. The increase in the younger age group is due to the overall high prevalence of sexually transmitted infections. More than 100,000 women become infertile each year as a result of PID (National Institute of Allergy and Infectious Disease, 1998).

Although sexual transmittal accounts for the majority of all PID, infections with organisms such as *Escherichia coli* and *Streptococcus* are also recognized as possible causes. There is also a higher incidence of PID in women using intrauterine devices (IUDs), perhaps because the presence of the IUD causes a mild inflammation.

PID usually begins with a cervical infection that spreads by surface invasion along the endometrium and then out to the fallopian tubes and ovaries. Bacterial invasion is most apt to occur at the end of a menstrual period because menstrual blood provides an excellent growth medium. There also is loss of the normal cervical mucous barrier at this time, thus increasing the risk for initial invasion. When left unrecognized and untreated, PID enters a chronic phase, which then results in the scarring that can lead to stricture of the fallopian tubes and resulting fertility problems. After a single incidence of PID, about 20% of women are left with significant tube blockage to reduce fertility. The more episodes of PID a woman has, the greater her risk of infertility (Zondervan & Barlow, 2000).

Uterine Problems

Tumors such as fibromas (leiomyomas) may be a rare cause of infertility if they block the entrance of the fallopian tubes into the uterus or limit the space available on the uterine wall for effective implantation. A congenitally deformed uterine cavity may limit implantation sites, but this also is rare. Use of DES has been linked to malformations of the uterus, such as a T-shaped uterus. Because this drug is no longer prescribed during pregnancy, women of childbearing age with this anomaly are now rarely seen.

Poor secretion of estrogen or progesterone from the ovary can result in inadequate endometrium formation (over- or underproduction), which interferes with implantation and embryo growth. Endometriosis also can interfere with uterine fertility.

Endometriosis. **Endometriosis** refers to the implantation of uterine endometrium, or nodules, that have spread from the interior of the uterus to locations outside the uterus. The most common sites of endometrium spread include Douglas's cul-de-sac, the ovaries, the uterine ligaments, and the outer surface of the uterus and bowel (Wellbery, 1999; Fig. 6-1).

Endometriosis occurs in as many as 25% of women, occurring most probably from regurgitation through the fallopian tubes at the time of menstruation. Viable particles of endometrium that have regurgitated this way begin to proliferate and grow at the new sites, impeding fertility in a variety of ways. When growths occur in the fallopian tube, tubal obstruction may result or adhesions forming from these growths may displace fallopian tubes away from the ovaries, preventing the entrance of ova into the tubes. The presence of peritoneal macrophages drawn to the distant sites when the abnormal tissue is recognized can destroy sperm. The occurrence of endometriosis may indicate this endometrial tissue has different or more friable qualities than normal endometrium (perhaps due to a luteal phase defect) and so is a type of endometrium that doesn't support embryo implantation as well as usual. Endometriosis can be treated both medically and surgically (Vercellini et al., 2000; see Chap. 47 for the treatment of endometriosis).

Cervical Problems

At the time of ovulation, the cervical mucus is thin and watery and can be easily penetrated by spermatozoa for a period of 12 to 72 hours. If coitus is not synchronized

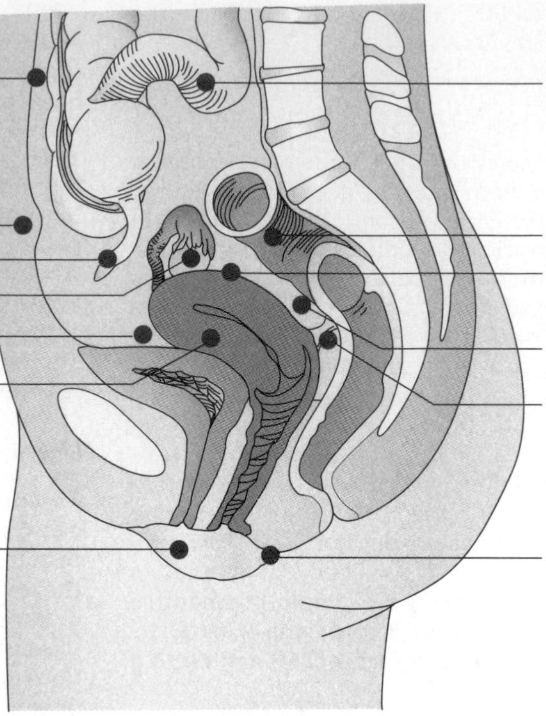

FIGURE 6.1 Common sites of endometriosis formation.

with this time period, the cervical mucus may be too thick to allow spermatozoa to penetrate the cervix. Infection or inflammation of the cervix (erosion) may cause so much thickening in cervical mucus that spermatozoa cannot penetrate it easily or survive in it. A stenotic cervical os or obstruction of the os by a polyp may compromise penetration. However, this is rarely enough of a problem to be the sole cause of infertility. A woman who has undergone dilatation and curettage (D&C) procedures several times or cervical conization (cervical surgery) should be evaluated in light of the possibility that scar tissue and tightening of the cervical os may have occurred.

Vaginal Problems

Infection of the vagina may cause the pH of the vaginal secretions to become acidotic, limiting or destroying the motility of spermatozoa. Some women appear to have sperm-immobilizing or sperm-agglutinating antibodies in their blood plasma that act to destroy sperm cells in the vagina or cervix. Both or either of these problems can limit the ability of sperm to enter the uterus.

Unexplained Infertility

In a small proportion of couples, no known cause for infertility can be discovered. Possibly the problems of either partner alone are not significant, but when combined they become sufficient to create infertility. It is obviously discouraging for couples to complete a fertility evaluation and be told that their inability to conceive cannot be explained. Such couples need support from health care providers to find alternative solutions, such as continuing to try to conceive, choosing to adopt, or agreeing to a child-free life.

✔ CHECKPOINT QUESTIONS

3. What two organisms are most commonly associated with PID?
4. How does endometriosis affect fertility?

FERTILITY ASSESSMENT

Not all couples who desire fertility testing want to have children immediately. Some just want to know for their own peace of mind that they are fertile. Others want to know that they are indeed infertile so they can discontinue contraceptive measures (although they need to be cautioned that they still need to maintain safer sex practices).

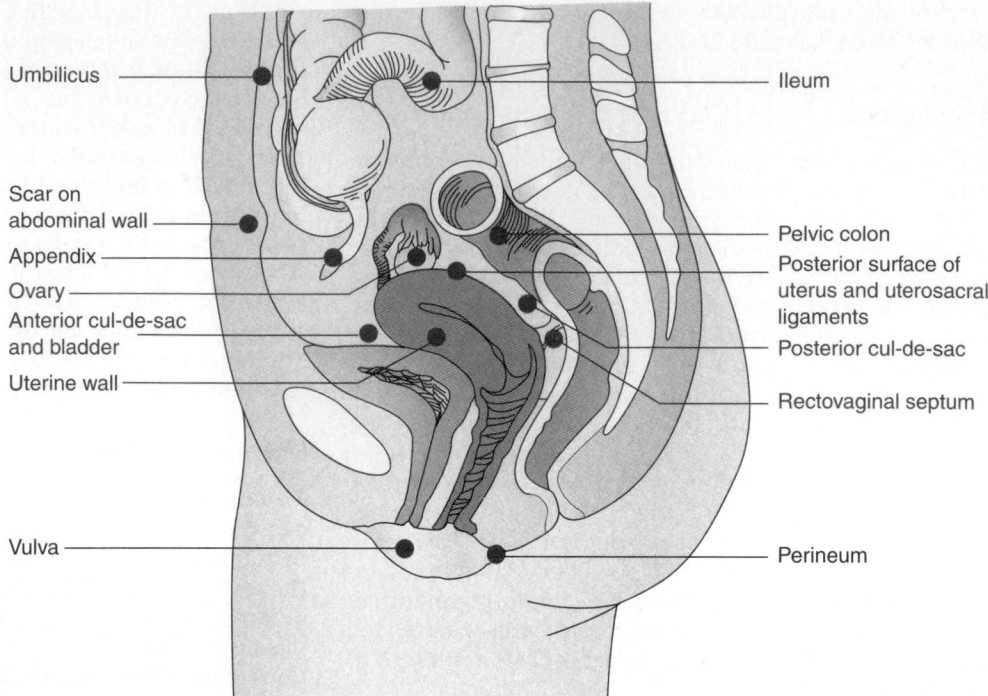

The age of the couple and the degree of apprehension they feel about possible infertility make a difference in determining when they should be referred for fertility evaluation. Although some health care plans or specific settings set limits on the age that fertility testing can be scheduled (e.g., not under age 18 years, not over age 45 years), other settings do not establish such limits, allowing couples of any age to benefit from assessment. As a rule of thumb, if the woman is younger than age 35 years, she should be referred for evaluation after 1 year of infertility and if older than age 35 years, after 6 months of infertility. Referral is recommended sooner for woman over 35 because of possible age limitations associated with adoption, artificial insemination, and embryo transfer, the alternatives to natural child-bearing (besides child-free living, which must not be discounted). It would be doubly unfortunate if a couple delayed fertility testing past the point of not only being able to conceive, but also to a point at which an adoption agency would consider them "too old" to be prospective parents. If the couple is extremely apprehensive over their apparent infertility, studies should never be delayed, regardless of the couple's age.

Because infertility may be a problem of either partner, fertility studies involve both partners. Nurses play key roles in preparing couples for these tests, helping them schedule the studies appropriately and supporting them while they wait for results. It is important that all personnel involved work cooperatively so couples do not receive conflicting reports to add to their stress level.

History

Nurses often assume the responsibility for initial history taking with the infertile couple. Because of the wide variety of factors that may be responsible for infertility, it is important that the history be thorough. A minimum history for the man should include:

- General health
- Nutrition
- Alcohol, drug, or tobacco use
- Congenital health problems such as hypospadias or cryptorchidism
- Illnesses such as mumps orchitis, urinary tract infection, or sexually transmitted diseases
- Operations such as surgical repair of a hernia, which could have resulted in a blood compromise to the testes
- Current illnesses, particularly endocrine illnesses or low-grade infections
- Past and current occupation and work habits (e.g., does his job involve sitting at a desk all day or exposure to x-rays or other forms of radiation?)

It is important to document sexual practices such as the frequency of coitus and masturbation, failure to achieve ejaculation, premature ejaculation, coital positions used, use of lubricants and past contraceptive measures, and existence of any children produced from a previous relationship. The man's cultural or religious values that may affect sexual practices should also be obtained (see Focus on Cultural Competence). It may be difficult for men to discuss this area of their life, especially if the interviewer is a woman. Thus, skillful interviewing is crucial.

Most people believe that infertility is a woman's problem. Many women, even after careful explanation that the problem is their male partner's and not theirs, continue to show low self-esteem, as if the fault rests with them. A woman should be asked about current or past reproductive tract problems, such as infections; her overall health, emphasizing endocrine problems such as galactorrhea (breast nipple secretions) or symptoms of thyroid dysfunction; and any abdominal or pelvic operations she has had that could have compromised blood flow to pelvic organs. Additional questions focus on the frequency of using douches or intravaginal medication or sprays (these may interfere with vaginal pH); exposure to occupational hazards such as x-rays or toxic substances; and nutrition, especially folic acid intake (de Weerd, 2002).

Also obtain information from the woman about whether she can detect ovulation. Pay particular attention to the typical symptoms, such as breast tenderness and midcycle "wetness," that indicate ovulation.

In addition to the above, a menstrual history should be obtained, including:

- Age of menarche
- Length, regularity, and frequency of menstrual periods
- Amount of flow
- Any difficulties experienced, such as dysmenorrhea or premenstrual dysphoric disorder
- History of contraceptive use
- History of any previous pregnancies or abortions

While obtaining the history, take time with each partner individually and as a couple to encourage questions and to discuss overall attitudes toward sexual relations, pregnancy, and parenting. A frank discussion centered on resolving the couple's fears and clearing up any longstanding confusion or misinformation will help to set a positive tone for future interactions, establish a feeling of trust with health care personnel, and increase self-esteem. Talking with both partners can also help them clarify their feelings about infertility and why they are seeking help in this area (see Focus on Nursing Care Planning).

FOCUS ON CULTURAL COMPETENCE

Do Cultural Traditions Ever Interfere With Fertility?

Obtaining a sexual history, which is necessary for a fertility evaluation, is often difficult to obtain because couples may not be comfortable discussing this part of their life due to cultural taboos. Factors as simple as how often couples engage in sexual relations, however, are influenced by culture and religion. According to Orthodox Jewish law, for example, a couple may not engage in sexual relations for 7 days following menstruation (the *nida* period). This can result in fertility problems if the woman ovulates within the 7-day period. Being aware that cultural differences can influence how a couple reacts to a diagnosis of infertility can help you appreciate the meaning of this diagnosis to an individual couple.

Physical Assessment

After a thorough history, both men and women need a complete physical examination. Inspect, in particular, for secondary sexual characteristics and genital abnormalities, such as the absence of a vas deferens or the presence of undescended testes or a varicocele (enlargement of a testicular vein). The presence of a hydrocele (collection of fluid in the tunica vaginalis of the scrotum) is rarely associated with infertility but should be documented if present.

For the woman, a thorough physical assessment including breast and thyroid examination is necessary to rule out current illness. Of particular importance are secondary sex characteristics, which indicate maturity and good pituitary

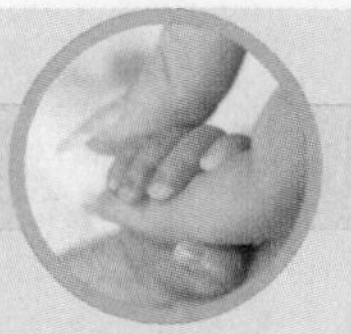

FOCUS ON *Nursing Care Planning*

THE FAMILY SEEKING A FERTILITY EVALUATION

A 28-year-old married woman comes to the health care facility for a fertility evaluation. She states, "We've been trying to have a baby now for over a year, but no luck. All of our other friends have had babies without any problems. Why can't I? What's wrong with me?"

Assessment: Past medical history negative for any major health problems; reports a menstrual cycle of 5 days' duration with moderate flow every 30 to 32 days; moderate dysmenorrhea for the first 2 days of her menses. Oral contraceptive use for 6 years; discontinued 1.5 years ago. Baseline laboratory studies and vital signs within normal limits.

Nursing Diagnosis: Situational low self-esteem disturbance related to inability to conceive

Outcome Identification: Client will express positive feelings about herself.

Outcome Evaluation: Client verbalizes feelings about possible infertility and effect on self-esteem; participates actively in care and treatment decisions; states she has some control over situation and required treatment.

Interventions	Rationale
1. Attempt to identify the meaning of fertility to the client.	1. Identifying the meaning of fertility assists in determining the impact that a diagnosis of infertility may have on the client.
2. Encourage client to express feelings and thoughts about self, fertility, and infertility.	2. Sharing of feelings and concerns permits a safe outlet for emotions and also aids in highlighting the client's awareness of possible impact on self-esteem.
3. Review and reinforce with client positive attributes about self.	3. Positive attributes provide a foundation for rebuilding self-esteem.
4. Clarify any misconceptions client may have about fertility and infertility.	4. Misconceptions can reduce self-esteem.
5. Assist with measures to increase independent role functioning and encourage active participation in decision making.	5. Independence and ability to perform one's role promotes self-esteem; active participation enhances the feeling of control over situations.
6. Discuss possible support persons and groups; include spouse as appropriate.	6. Additional support can assist in reinforcing positive attributes, thus enhancing self-esteem.

Nursing Diagnosis: Deficient knowledge related to reproductive functions and infertility

Outcome Evaluation: Client will express accurate information about reproductive functioning and infertility.

Outcome Evaluation: Client verbalizes information about reproductive structures and normal function, fertilization, and conception; discusses possible factors associated with infertility; exhibits understanding of measures involved with evaluation of and treatment for infertility.

Interventions	Rationale
1. Assess client's current knowledge level about reproductive functioning and infertility.	1. Obtaining a baseline knowledge assessment provides a foundation on which to build future teaching strategies.
2. Review structure and function of male and female reproductive systems, including fertile periods, fertilization, and conception; clarify any misconceptions.	2. Reviewing helps to enhance learning and strengthen understanding.

(continued)

Interventions	Rationale
3. Discuss possible factors associated with fertility and infertility; include spouse in discussion as appropriate.	3. Discussing factors assists in providing a baseline for understanding possible diagnostic tests and treatments. Including the client's spouse helps promote family-centered care.
4. Instruct the client and spouse about recommended tests and possible long-term treatment.	4. Teaching helps to increase the client's awareness and lessen anxiety and fears, preparing the client and spouse for what is to come.
5. Provide ample time for questions and concerns.	5. Providing time for questions and concerns helps clarify information, individualize information, and promote a feeling of control and trust.

function (see Chap. 32 for a discussion of Tanner stages). A complete pelvic examination (see Chap. 10) is needed to rule out anatomic defects and infection.

Fertility Testing

Typically, laboratory testing for men includes a semen analysis, urinalysis, and some blood tests. Often, one of the first tests performed for the man is semen analysis. If this is abnormal, then further testing such as a complete blood count; blood typing, including Rh factor; a serologic test for syphilis; sedimentation rate (an increased rate indicates inflammation); protein-bound iodine (a test for thyroid function); cholesterol level (arterial plaques could interfere with pelvic blood flow); and gonadotropin, prolactin, and testosterone levels may be obtained. Testing for the presence of human immunodeficiency virus (HIV) infection is also crucial (Crosignani & Rubin, 2000).

To determine the woman's general state of health, laboratory tests similar to those done on the man will be ordered. Typically, these include a Pap smear, rubella titer, and HIV evaluation. Serum or urine hormone levels and a serologic test for syphilis may be necessary. If the client has symptoms of thyroid dysfunction, a thyroid uptake determination and thyroid-stimulating hormone levels may be ordered. If the woman has a history of menstrual irregularities, blood will be assayed for FSH, estrogen, LH, and progesterone levels. If the client has galactorrhea, a serum prolactin level will be obtained. A pelvic sonogram may be performed to rule out ovarian, tubal, or uterine structural disorders.

Semen Analysis

For a semen analysis, after 2 to 4 days of sexual abstinence, the man ejaculates by masturbation into a clean, dry specimen jar, and the spermatozoa are examined under a microscope within 1 hour (see Focus on Family Empowerment). The number of spermatozoa in the specimen are counted, and their appearance and motility are noted. An average ejaculation should produce 2.5 to 5.0 mL of semen and should contain a minimum of 20 million spermatozoa per milliliter of fluid (the average normal sperm count is 50 to 200 million per milliliter). The analysis may need to be repeated in 2 or 3 more months because spermatogenesis is an ongoing process, requiring 30 to 90 days for new sperm to reach maturity.

Sperm Penetration Assay and Antisperm Antibody Testing

For impregnation to take place, sperm must be mobile enough and have the capacity to reach and enter the ova. One reason for poor sperm mobility may be the presence

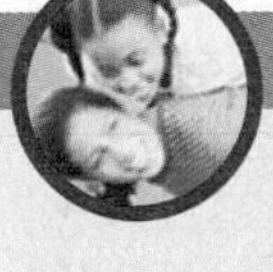

FOCUS ON FAMILY EMPOWERMENT

Tips for Ensuring an Accurate Semen Analysis

Q. What can I do to make sure that the analysis of my semen sample is as accurate as possible?

A. To ensure accuracy of the results, use the following guidelines when obtaining a semen sample for analysis:

- Use a clean, dry plastic or glass container with a secure lid to collect the sample.
- Collect the specimen as close as possible to your usual schedule of sexual activity.
- Avoid using any lubricants when you collect the specimen.
- After you've collected the specimen in the container, close it securely and write down the time you collected it.
- Keep the specimen at body temperature while transporting it. Carrying it next to your chest is one way to do this.
- Take the specimen to the laboratory or health care provider's office immediately so it can be analyzed within 1 hour of collection.

of antisperm antibodies, which tend to cause agglutination of sperm. These can exist in the woman so that sperm, when deposited, are agglutinated in her vagina and cannot travel to the fallopian tubes for fertilization of the ovum. They also can develop in men who have had reversed vasectomies or experienced an obstruction in the epididymis so that sperm are never fully mobile. It is possible to test for these by laboratory analysis to determine whether such antibodies are present.

Sperm penetration studies are laboratory tests to determine whether sperm, once they reach the ova, can penetrate the ova. Using an artificial reproductive technique such as in vitro fertilization, poorly mobile sperm or those with poor penetration can be injected into the woman's ovum under laboratory conditions (intracytoplasmic sperm injection), bypassing the need for sperm to be fully mobile (Check et al., 2000).

Ovulation Determination by Basal Body Temperature

One of the first tests ordered for women is the recording of basal body temperature (BBT), a simple test for ovulation. It documents the slight temperature increase (from 0.4° to 1.0°F) that normally occurs with the release of progesterone following ovulation. To determine this, the woman takes her temperature before getting out of bed each morning or engaging in any activity, eating, or drinking, using a special BBT or ear thermometer. She plots this daily temperature on a monthly graph, noticing conditions that might affect her temperature (e.g., colds, other infections, or sleeplessness). At the time of ovulation, the basal temperature can be seen to dip slightly (about 0.5°F), then rise to a level no higher than normal body temperature and stay at that level until 3 or 4 days before the next menstrual flow. This increase in BBT marks the time of ovulation because it occurs immediately after ovulation (actually the beginning of the luteal phase of the menstrual cycle, which can occur only if ovulation occurred). A temperature rise should last approximately 10 days. If not, a luteal phase defect is suggested (progesterone production begins but is not sustained). Typical graphs of basal body temperature are shown in Figure 6-2.

WHAT IF? A woman has been asked to record a daily basal body temperature. What if she tells you she works nights as a cocktail waitress, going to bed at 4 AM? She wakes at 6 AM to drive her husband to work. At noon, she sleeps for 4 or 5 hours until getting up to go to work. When during the day should she record her basal body temperature?

Ovulation Determination by Test Strip

Various brands of commercial kits are available for assessing the upsurge of LH that occurs just before ovulation. These can be used in place of obtaining BBT. The woman dips a test strip into a midmorning urine specimen and then compares it with the kit instructions for a color change. Such kits are purchased over the counter, are easy to use, and have the advantage of marking the point just before

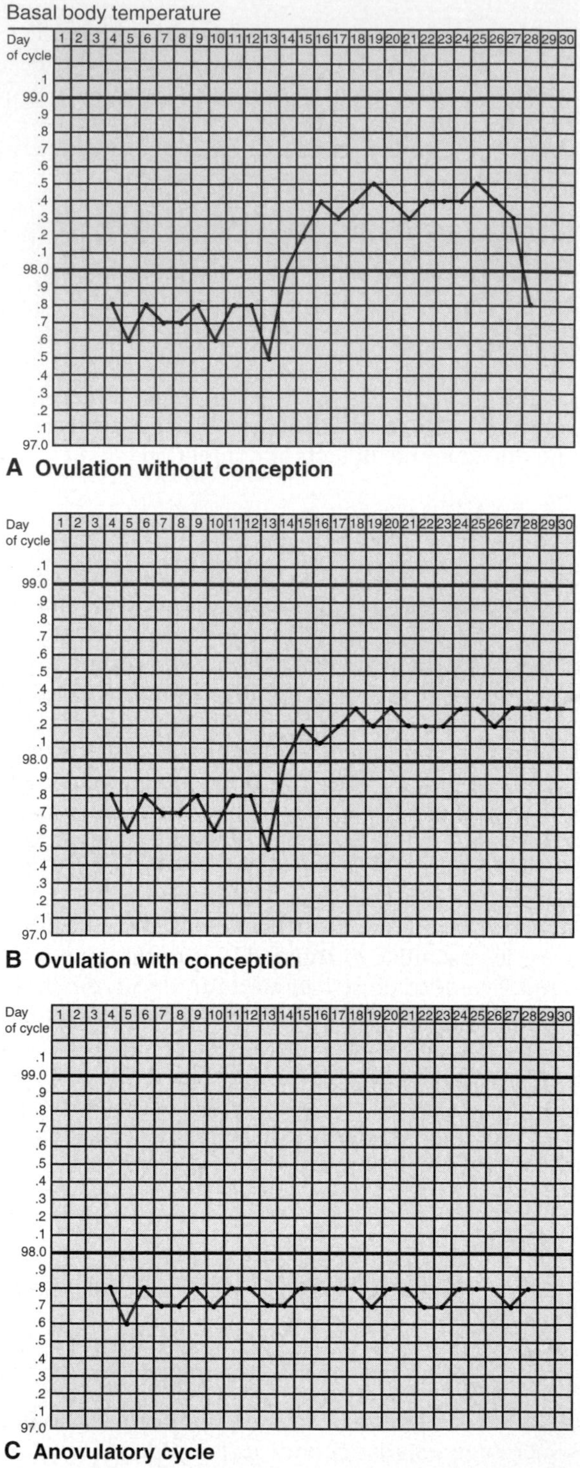

FIGURE 6.2 Basal body temperature graph. (*A*) The woman's temperature dips slightly at midpoint in the menstrual cycle, then rises sharply, an indication of ovulation. Toward the end of the cycle (the 24th day), her temperature begins to decline, indicating that progesterone levels are falling and that she did not conceive. (*B*) The woman's temperature rises at the midpoint in the cycle and remains at that elevated level past the time of her normal menstrual flow, suggesting that pregnancy has occurred. (*C*) There is no preovulatory dip, and no rise of temperature anywhere during the cycle. This is the typical pattern of a woman who does not ovulate.

ovulation occurs rather than after ovulation, as is the case with BBT. They are not as economical as simple temperature recording but are advantageous for women with irregular work or daily activity schedules (e.g., working the night shift or arising at different times in the morning).

Ovulation Determination by Cervical Mucus Assessment

At the height of estrogen stimulation, cervical mucus is copious and thin and has a low viscosity and cellularity. It "ferns" or forms a distinct pattern when allowed to dry. This is an easy test of hormonal influences.

Fern Test. When high levels of estrogen are present in the body, as they are just before ovulation, the cervical mucus forms fernlike patterns when it is placed on a glass slide and allowed to dry. The patterns are due to the crystallization of sodium chloride on mucus fibers. This is known as arborization or ferning (Fig. 6-3). When progesterone is the dominant hormone, as it is just after ovulation, when the luteal phase of the menstrual cycle is beginning, a fern pattern is no longer discernible. Cervical mucus is examined at midcycle to detect that ferning or a high estrogen surge is present. Women who do not ovulate continue to show the fern pattern throughout the menstrual cycle (progesterone levels never become dominant), or they never demonstrate it because their estrogen levels never rise.

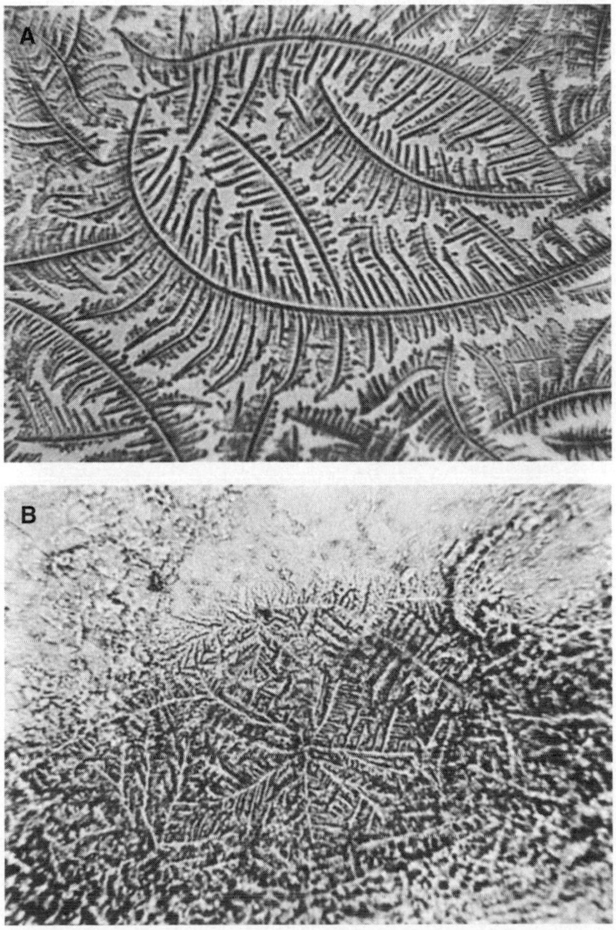

FIGURE 6.3 (*A*) A ferning pattern of cervical mucus occurs with high estrogen levels. (*B*) Incomplete ferning during secretory phase of cycle.

Spinnbarkeit Test. At the height of estrogen secretion, the cervical mucus not only becomes thin and watery, but it also can be stretched into long strands. This stretchability is in contrast to its thick, viscous state when progesterone is the dominant hormone. Performing this test, known as spinnbarkeit, at the midpoint of a menstrual cycle is another way to demonstrate that high levels of estrogen are being produced and, by implication, that ovulation is about to occur. A woman can do this herself by stretching the sample between thumb and finger, or it can be tested in an examining room by smearing a cervical mucus specimen on a slide and stretching the mucus between the slide and cover slip (Fig. 6-4).

Postcoital Test

A postcoital test combines both ovulation detection and semen analysis. For such a test, the time of ovulation is predicted from the woman's BBT chart or a commercial ovulation predictor kit. The couple has coitus at this time, and then the woman reports to the health care facility within 2 to 8 hours. With the woman in a lithotomy position, a specimen of cervical mucus is removed and examined microscopically for ferning, spinnbarkeit, cell count, and viable spermatozoa. The postcoital test shows the presence of sperm and how they interact with the woman's vaginal and cervical environment.

A good result shows abundant, elastic mucus with a high number of motile sperm. If sperm are found to be clumped and immobile or if the mucus is very thick, this may indicate a problem with timing or possibly point to a sperm antibody problem. A finding of no sperm could indicate azoospermia. If white blood cells are present in the cervical mucus, an endocervical or endometrial infection is suggested, requiring treatment with an appropriate antibiotic. Once a mainstay of infertility testing, postcoital tests are

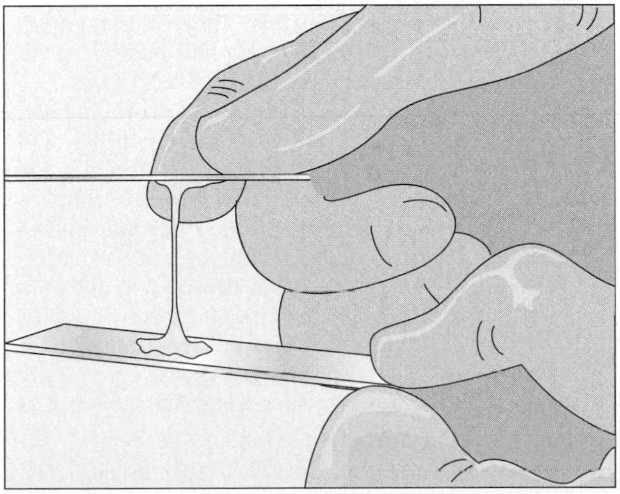

FIGURE 6.4 Spinnbarkeit is the property of cervical mucus to stretch a distance before breaking.

not used as much now as formerly because their scheduling is difficult and they may yield little more information than a single sperm or cervical mucus analysis would reveal (see Focus on Evidence-Based Practice).

Ultrasonography and X-Ray Imaging

Ultrasound and x-ray imaging can be used to determine the patency of fallopian tubes and assess the depth and consistency of the endometrial lining.

Sonohysterography. Sonohysterography is an ultrasound technique designed for inspecting the uterus. The uterus is filled with sterile saline introduced through a narrow catheter inserted into the uterine cervix. A transvaginal ultrasound transducer is then inserted into the vagina to inspect the uterus for abnormalities such as septal deviation or the presence of a myoma. Because this is a minimally invasive technique, it can be done at any time during the menstrual cycle.

Hysterosalpingography. Hysterosalpingography (uterosalpingography) is a radiologic examination of the fallopian tubes using a radiopaque medium. It is done immediately after the menstrual flow to avoid reflux of menstrual debris up the tubes and unintentional irradiation of a growing zygote. It is contraindicated if infection of the vagina, cervix, or uterus is present (infectious organisms might be forced into the pelvic cavity). For the procedure, radiopaque material (iodine-based) is introduced into the cervix under pressure (Fig. 6-5). The radiopaque material outlines the uterus and both tubes, provided the tubes are patent. Because the medium is thick, it distends the uterus and tubes slightly, causing momentary painful uterine cramping. After the study, the contrast medium drains out through the vagina. The instillation of radiopaque material may be therapeutic as well as diagnostic: the pressure of the solution may actually break up adhesions as it passes through the fallopian tubes, thereby increasing their patency. The procedure carries a small risk of infection, allergic reaction to the contrast medium, and embolism from dye entering a uterine blood vessel.

Surgical Evaluation

If the above assessments do not reveal the cause of infertility, a number of surgical procedures may be scheduled.

Uterine Endometrial Biopsy

Uterine endometrial biopsy may be used as a test for ovulation or to reveal an endometrial problem such as a luteal phase defect. If the endometrium resembles a corkscrew (a typical progesterone-dominated endometrium), this suggests that ovulation has occurred. Endometrial biopsies are being performed less commonly, being replaced with serum progesterone level evaluations.

The biopsy is usually done 2 or 3 days before the expected menstrual flow (day 25 or 26 of a typical 28-day menstrual cycle). After a paracervical block, a thin probe and biopsy forceps are introduced through the cervix. The woman may experience mild to moderate discomfort from the maneuvering of the instruments. There may be

FOCUS ON EVIDENCE-BASED PRACTICE

Are Postcoital Tests Good Predictors of Fertility?
To answer this question, researchers studied the results of postcoital tests in 207 couples who had been infertile for at least 12 months. Results of this analysis showed that 68% of couples who had been infertile for less than 3 years and who had a positive postcoital test (healthy sperm and good survival times) conceived within 2 years following the test. This was in comparison to only 14% in couples who had positive postcoital tests but had been infertile for over 3 years.

The researchers concluded that the postcoital test can be used to help predict whether couples will conceive. Couples who experience infertility for over 3 years may have true unexplained infertility.

This study is significant for nurses because nurses are the health care providers that many couples undergoing fertility testing turn to for information and support. As the postcoital test is difficult for busy couples to schedule, it is a test that couples frequently ask if they should have done. Knowing that it can supply important information provides additional evidence as a basis for your response.

Glazener, C. M., Ford, W. C., & Hull, M. G. (2000). The prognostic power of the post-coital test for natural conception depends on duration of infertility. *Human Reproduction, 15*(9), 1953–1957.

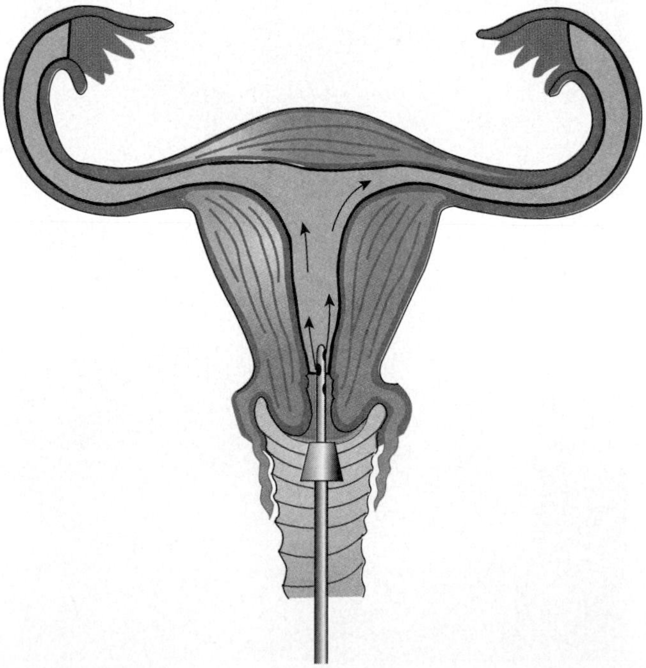

FIGURE 6.5 Insertion of a dye for a hysterosalpingogram. The contrast dye outlines the uterus and fallopian tubes on x-ray to demonstrate patency.

a moment of sharp pain as the biopsy specimen is taken from the anterior or posterior uterine wall. Possible complications include pain, excessive bleeding, infection, or uterine perforation. This procedure is contraindicated if pregnancy is suspected (although the chance it would interfere with a pregnancy is probably under 10%) and also if an infection such as acute PID or cervicitis is present. The woman should be cautioned to expect a small amount of vaginal spotting after the procedure. She should be instructed to call her primary care provider if she develops a temperature of more than 101°F, has a large amount of bleeding, or passes clots. It is important to advise the woman to telephone the health care agency when she has her next menstrual flow. This helps "date" the endometrium and the accuracy of the analysis.

Hysteroscopy

Hysteroscopy is visual inspection of the uterus through the insertion of a hysteroscope, a thin hollow tube, through the cervix. This is helpful if uterine adhesions or other abnormalities were discovered on the hysterosalpingogram.

Laparoscopy

Laparoscopy is the introduction of a thin, hollow, lighted tube (a fiberoptic telescope or laparoscope) through a small incision in the abdomen just under the umbilicus to examine the position and state of the fallopian tubes and ovaries. Typically, it is rarely done except when uterosalpingography is abnormal. It is scheduled during the follicular phase of a menstrual period and done under general anesthesia because the extensive maneuvering causes pain. This also allows for good relaxation and a steep Trendelenburg position (which brings the reproductive organs down out of the pelvis). Carbon dioxide is introduced into the abdomen to cause the abdominal wall to move outward and offer better visualization. Women may feel a bloating of their abdomen after such a procedure. If some carbon dioxide escapes under the diaphragm, they may feel extremely sharp shoulder pain from pressure.

The laparoscopy technique (see Fig. 5-11) may be used to view the proximity of the ovaries to the fallopian tubes. If the distance is too great, the discharged ovum cannot enter the tube. During the procedure, dye can be injected into the uterus through a polyethylene cannula placed in the cervix to assess tubal patency. Tubes are patent if the dye appears in the abdominal cavity. A scope may be passed directly into the fallopian tubes to reveal information about the presence and condition of the fimbria and endometrium lining the tubes. If fimbria have been destroyed from PID, the chance for normal conception is in doubt, because ova seem unable to enter the tube when fimbrial currents are absent.

> **✔ CHECKPOINT QUESTIONS**
>
> 5. Which test includes an x-ray of the fallopian tubes using a contrast medium?
> 6. Following a laparoscopy, what two discomforts voiced by the client are common?

INFERTILITY MANAGEMENT

Management of infertility focuses on correction of the underlying problems that were discovered on assessment. In the meantime, all couples can benefit from some practical information on how to increase the chances of achieving conception on their own. Some suggestions to discuss with a couple are included in the accompanying Focus on Family Empowerment display.

Correction of the Underlying Problem

The overall management of infertility involves treating such underlying causes as chronic disease, inadequate hormone production, endometriosis, or infection. If correcting these problems does not yield success, infertility management focuses on achieving conception through assisted reproductive techniques such as in vitro fertilization or sperm donation.

Increasing Sperm Count and Motility

If sperm cannot be motile because the vas deferens is obstructed, the obstruction is, unfortunately, usually extensive and difficult or impossible to relieve by surgery. If spermatozoa are present but the total count is low, a man might be advised to abstain from coitus for 7 to 10 days to increase the count. Ligation of a varicocele (if present) and advising changes in lifestyle, such as wearing looser clothing, avoiding long periods of sitting, and avoiding prolonged hot baths, may be helpful to reduce scrotal heat and increase the sperm count.

Administration of clomiphene citrate (Clomid), an estrogen antagonist, may successfully increase an inadequate sperm count. Aromatase inhibitors to increase testosterone-to-estrogen ratio (Ramon & Schlegel, 2002) or testosterone and human chorionic gonadotropin also may be used.

If spermatozoa appear to be immobilized by vaginal secretions due to an immunologic factor, the response can be reduced by abstinence or condom use for about 6 months. However, to avoid this prolonged time interval, washing of the spermatozoa and intrauterine insemination may be preferred. The administration of corticosteroids to the woman may have some effect in decreasing sperm immobilization because it reduces her immune response and antibody production.

Reducing the Presence of Infection

If a vaginal infection is present, the infection will be treated according to the causative organism based on culture reports (see Chap. 14). Vaginal infections such as trichomoniasis and moniliasis tend to recur, requiring close supervision and follow-up. The possibility that the sexual partner is reinfecting the woman needs to be considered. Women who are prescribed metronidazole (Flagyl) for a trichomonal infection should be cautioned that it may be teratogenic early in pregnancy and so should not be continued if a pregnancy is suspected.

Hormone Therapy

If the problem appears to be a disturbance of ovulation, hormone therapy with clomiphene citrate (Clomid, Sero-

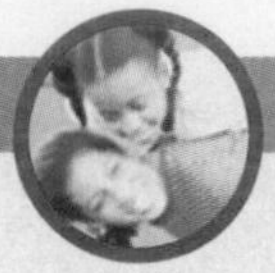

FOCUS ON FAMILY EMPOWERMENT
Suggestions to Aid Conception

Q. Is there anything that we can do to help increase our chances for conception?

A. Use the following suggestions to help aid conception:

- Couples can determine the woman's time of ovulation through the use of basal body temperature, analysis of cervical secretions, or a commercial ovulation determination kit. Planning sexual relations for every other day around the time of ovulation is ideal.
- Although frequent intercourse may stimulate sperm production, men need sperm recovery time after ejaculation to maintain an adequate sperm count. This is why coitus every other day, rather than every day, during the fertile period will probably yield faster results.
- The male-superior position is the best position for intercourse to achieve conception because it places sperm closest to the cervical opening.
- The male should try for deep penetration so ejaculation places sperm as close as possible to the cervix. Elevating the woman's hips on a small pillow is another way to facilitate sperm collection near the opening to the cervix.
- The woman should remain on her back with knees drawn up for at least 20 minutes after ejaculation to help sperm remain near the cervix.
- No artificial lubricants should be used because they may interfere with sperm motility.
- No douching or lubricants should be used before or after intercourse so vaginal pH is unaltered.

phene) is the treatment of choice to stimulate ovulation (see Focus on Pharmacology: Clomiphene). In other women, ovarian follicular growth can be stimulated by the administration of human menopausal gonadotropins (Pergonal) in conjunction with administration of human chorionic gonadotropin (HCG) to produce ovulation (see Focus on Pharmacology: Menotropins). Human menopausal gonadotropins (derived from postmenopausal urine) are combinations of FSH and LH. If increased prolactin levels are identified, bromocriptine (Parlodel) is added to the medication regimen to reduce prolactin levels and allow for the rise of gonadotropins (Leibowitz & Hoffman, 2000).

Administration of either clomiphene citrate or human menopausal gonadotropins may overstimulate an ovary, causing multiple ova to come to maturity and possibly resulting in multiple births. Women who receive these agents should be counseled that this is a possibility, although this is less of a problem when follicular growth is monitored by ultrasound. If spermatozoa do not appear to survive in the vaginal secretions because secretions are too scant or tenacious, the woman may be placed on low-dose estrogen therapy to increase mucus production during days 5 to 10 of her cycle. Conjugated estrogen (Premarin) is a type of estrogen used for this purpose.

If the problem appears to be a luteal phase defect, this may be corrected by progesterone vaginal suppositories begun on the third day of the temperature rise and continued for the next 6 weeks if pregnancy occurs or until the menstrual flow resumes. Oral progesterone is not prescribed because it may cause fetal reproductive tract abnormalities should pregnancy occur.

Surgery

If a myoma (fibroid tumor) is interfering with fertility, a myomectomy, or removal of the tumor by surgery, may be necessary. Myomectomy may be done by a hysteroscopic ambulatory procedure if the growth is small. Uterine adhesions may also be lysed by hysteroscopy. After this procedure, an IUD may be inserted for 3 months to prevent the uterine sides from touching and estrogen is administered to prevent adhesions from reforming. This treatment may be difficult for the woman to accept because preventing pregnancy (using an IUD) is exactly what she does not want to do.

For problems of abnormal uterine formation, such as a septate uterus, surgery is also available. These defects, however, are generally related to early pregnancy loss, not infertility.

If the problem is tubal insufficiency from inflammation, diathermy or steroid administration may be helpful in reducing adhesions. Hysterosalpingography may be repeated to see whether it can produce a therapeutic effect. Canalization of the fallopian tubes and plastic surgical repair (microsurgery) are possible treatments. If peritoneal adhesions or nodules of endometriosis are holding the tubes fixed and away from the ovaries, these can be removed by laparoscopy or laser surgery. Additional therapy for endometriosis, including severing the uterine nerve to reduce pain, is discussed in Chapter 47.

Assisted Reproductive Techniques

If ovulation, sperm production, or sperm mobility problems cannot be corrected, assisted reproductive strategies are available (Cramer et al., 2000). Box 6-2 highlights an appropriate outcomes and interventions using the terminology identified by the Nursing Outcome Classification and Nursing Intervention Classification.

Artificial Insemination

Artificial insemination is the instillation of sperm into the female reproductive tract to aid conception. The sperm can be instilled into the cervix (intracervical insemination) or into the uterus (intrauterine insemination). Either the husband's sperm (artificial insemination by husband) or donor sperm (artificial insemination by donor or therapeutic donor insemination) can be used. These techniques

FOCUS ON PHARMACOLOGY

Clomiphene Citrate (Clomid)

Action: Clomiphene citrate (Clomid) is an estrogen agonist used to stimulate the ovary. The drug binds to estrogen receptors, decreasing the number of available estrogen receptors and falsely signaling the hypothalamus to increase FSH and LH secretion.

Pregnancy category: X

Dosage: Initially, 50 mg/day orally for 5 days (started anytime if no recent uterine bleeding or about the fifth day of the cycle if uterine bleeding occurs) followed by 100 mg/day for 5 days, started as early as 30 days after the initial course of therapy. This second course may be repeated one more time.

Possible adverse reactions: Abdominal discomfort, distention, bloating, nausea, vomiting, breast tenderness, vasomotor flushing, ovarian enlargement, ovarian overstimulation, multiple births, visual disturbances.

Nursing Implications:
- Ensure that the woman has had a pelvic examination and baseline hormonal studies before therapy.
- Instruct the client in medication scheduling. Use a calendar to mark treatment schedule and plot ovulation. Remind client that timing intercourse with ovulation is important for achieving pregnancy.
- Explain about the signs of estrogen and progesterone activity.
- Advise the client that 24-hour urine samples may be necessary periodically.
- Caution client to report any bloating, stomach pain, blurred vision, unusual bleeding, bruising, or visual changes.
- Inform the client that therapy may be repeated for a total of three courses; if no results are obtained, therapy will be discontinued at that point.

FOCUS ON PHARMACOLOGY

Menotropins (Pergonal, Humegon)

Action: Menotropins are a purified preparation of human gonadotropins that produces ovarian follicular development and growth. When followed by administration of human chorionic gonadotropin (HCG), they produce ovulation.

Pregnancy category: C

Dosage: To achieve ovulation, 5 IU FSH/7.5 IU LH intramuscularly daily for 9 to 12 days, followed by administration of 10,000 IU HCG 1 day later.

Possible adverse reactions: Ovarian enlargement, hyperstimulation syndrome, febrile reactions, multiple pregnancies.

Nursing Implications:
- Explain the drug's action so that the client understands the importance of coordinating sexual relations with ovulation.
- Instruct the client and partner in the procedure for intramuscular injection, if appropriate.
- Monitor the client at least every other day during treatment and for 2 weeks afterward for signs of possible ovarian enlargement. If it occurs, discontinue the drug and notify the primary health care provider. Prepare the client for possible admission to the health care facility.
- Assist client in preparing a calendar to show treatment schedule to assist with compliance.
- Provide explanations about the signs of estrogen and progesterone activity to watch for.
- Advise the client to have intercourse daily beginning on the day before HCG therapy to achieve the desired effects.
- Counsel the client and partner about possible breast enlargement and also about the possibility of multiple births.

may be used when the man has an inadequate sperm count or the woman has a vaginal or cervical factor interfering with sperm motility. They are also used when the man has a known genetic disorder he does not want transmitted to offspring or the woman has no male partner. It is useful for men who, feeling their family was complete, underwent a vasectomy that cannot be reversed, but who now wish to have children. In the past, men who underwent chemotherapy or radiation for testicular cancer had to accept being child-free afterward when they were no longer able to produce sperm. Today, sperm can be cryopreserved (frozen) in a sperm bank before radiation or chemotherapy, and then used for insemination afterward.

One disadvantage of using frozen sperm is that it tends to have slower motility than unfrozen specimens. However, although the rate of conception may be lower from this source, there appears to be no increase in the incidence of congenital anomalies in children conceived by this method. An advantage of cryopreserved sperm is that it can be used even after years of storage. However, this has resulted in ethical, legal, and religious dilemmas.

WHAT IF? What would happen if a couple divorces or dies before cryopreserved sperm is used? To whom would the cryopreserved sperm belong at that point?

To prepare for artificial insemination, the woman must record her BBT, assess her cervical mucus, or use an ovulation predictor kit to be able to predict her likely day of ovulation. On the day after ovulation, the seminal fluid is delivered to the cervix using a device similar to a cervical cap or diaphragm or injected directly into the uterus using a flexible catheter (Fig. 6-6).

If therapeutic donor insemination is selected, the donors are usually volunteers who have no history of disease and

BOX 6.2

NURSING OUTCOMES AND NURSING INTERVENTIONS CLASSIFICATION: REPRODUCTIVE TECHNOLOGIES

NOC: Knowledge, Treatment Procedures

Knowledge, treatment procedures is defined as the extent of understanding conveyed about procedures required as part of a treatment regimen (Johnson, Maas, & Moorhead, 2000). Some specific indicators suggesting achievement of this outcome include the client's ability to describe the following:

- Treatment procedure and purpose
- Steps of the procedure, including how the procedure works
- Any restrictions or precautions for or care associated with the procedure
- Possible complications, including any actions to take should complications arise

NIC: Reproductive Technology Management

Reproductive technology management is defined as assisting a client through the steps of complex infertility treatment (McCloskey & Bulechek, 2000). Some important activities involved when implementing this intervention include:

- Providing education about the various treatment modalities
- Discussing ethical dilemmas before initiating a particular modality
- Teaching ovulation prediction and detection techniques and administration of ovulatory stimulants
- Assisting with fertilization procedures
- Providing anticipatory guidance for client about typical emotional reactions associated with fertilization procedures
- Discussing the risks associated with a planned procedure
- Performing pregnancy tests, including providing support when implantation fails
- Scheduling follow-up medications, tests, and examinations
- Referring to an infertility support group as needed

no family history of possible inheritable disorders. The blood type, or at least the Rh factor, can be matched with the woman's to prevent Rh incompatibility. If a woman desires, frozen sperm from sperm banks can be selected according to desired physical or mental characteristics.

With artificial insemination, especially therapeutic donor insemination, legal issues must be considered. Some states have specific laws regarding inheritance, child support, and responsibility concerning children conceived by this method. Some couples have religious or ethical beliefs that prohibit them from using artificial insemination. In addition, because artificial insemination takes an average of 6 months to achieve conception, it may be a discouraging process for couples.

✔ **CHECKPOINT QUESTIONS**

7. When would AIH (artificial insemination by the husband) be used?
8. What is an advantage of using frozen sperm for artificial insemination?

In Vitro Fertilization and Embryo Transfer

In vitro fertilization (IVF) refers to removing one or more mature oocytes from a woman's ovary by laparoscopy and then fertilizing them by exposing them to sperm under laboratory conditions outside the woman's body. Embryo transfer (ET, also called ova transfer) refers to the insertion of the laboratory-grown fertilized ovum into the woman's uterus approximately 40 hours after fertilization, where ideally one or more of them will implant and grow.

IVF-ET is most often used for couples who have not been able to conceive because the woman has blocked or damaged fallopian tubes. It is also used when the man has oligospermia or a low sperm count, because the controlled concentrated conditions in the laboratory require fewer sperm for fertilization (perhaps as few as 50,000, whereas nearly 50 million are normally required). IVF-ET may be helpful to couples when an absence of cervical mucus prevents sperm from traveling to or entering the cervix, or antisperm antibodies cause immobilization of sperm. In addition, couples with unexplained infertility of long duration may be helped by IVF-ET.

A donor ovum, rather than the woman's own ovum, also can be used for the woman who does not ovulate or who carries a sex-linked disease that she does not want to pass on to her children.

Before the procedure, the woman is given an ovulation agent such as clomiphene citrate (Clomid) or human menopausal gonadotropin (Pergonal). Beginning about the 10th day of the menstrual cycle, the ovaries are examined daily by sonography to assess the number and size of developing ovarian follicles. When a follicle appears to be mature, the woman is given an injection of HCG hormone, causing ovulation in 38 to 42 hours.

A needle is then introduced intravaginally, guided by ultrasound, and the oocyte is aspirated through a sterile tube from its follicle. Often, many oocytes ripen at once, and perhaps as many as 3 to 12 can be removed. The oocytes are incubated for at least 8 hours to ensure viability. In the meantime, the husband or donor supplies a fresh semen specimen. The sperm cells and oocytes are mixed and allowed to incubate in a growth medium.

Even fewer sperm would be necessary if there were some way to help sperm make their way through the resistant zona pellucida surrounding the ovum. A number of techniques, such as creating passages through the resistant cells (zona drilling), have been discovered to help sperm cross the zona. In some instances, it has been possible to inject sperm directly under the zona pellucida (intracytoplasmic sperm injection). This technique is so effective that theoretically only one sperm is necessary to achieve fertilization.

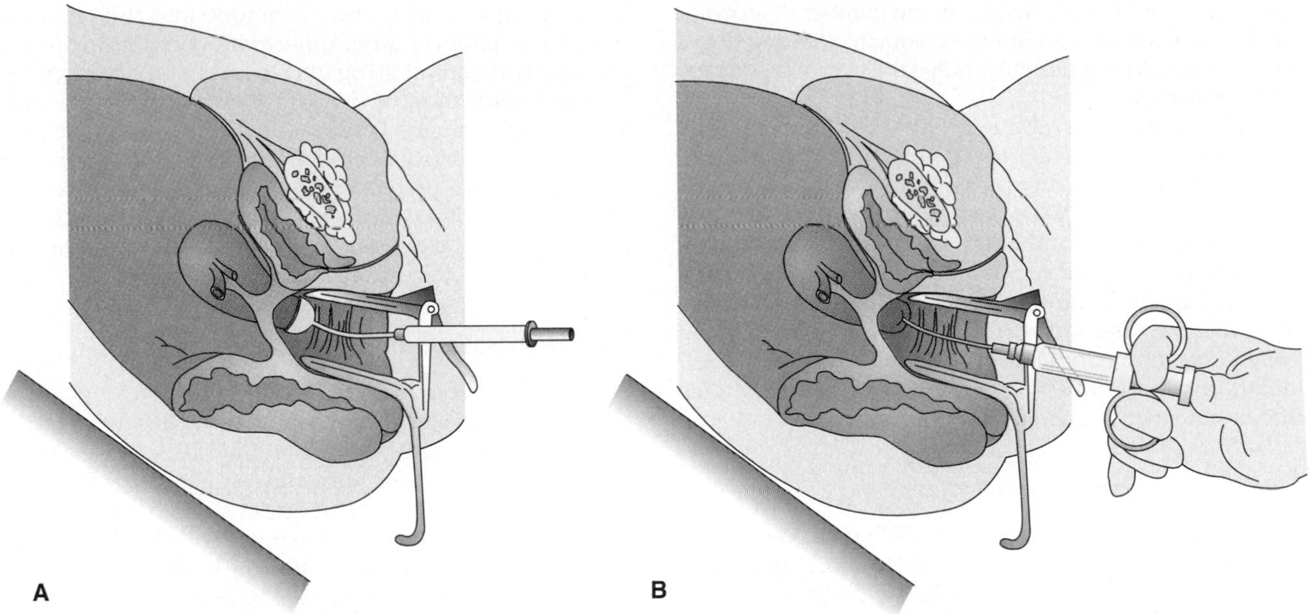

FIGURE 6.6 Artificial insemination. Sperm are deposited next to the cervix (*A*) or injected directly into the uterine cavity (*B*).

When fertilization of the chosen oocytes occurs, the zygotes formed almost immediately begin to divide and grow. By 40 hours after fertilization, they will have undergone their first cell division. The fertilized eggs are examined and, if normal, a chosen number are transferred back to the uterine cavity through the cervix using a thin catheter (Fig. 6-7). If the couple desires, any eggs not used can be frozen for use at a later time. However, like sperm cryopreservation, egg cryopreservation presents a range of ethical and religious dilemmas.

A lack of progesterone can occur if the corpus luteum was injured by the aspiration of the follicle. Progesterone may be given to the woman if it is believed she will not produce enough to support implantation. Proof that the zygote has implanted can be demonstrated by a routine serum pregnancy test as early as 11 days after transfer.

In some centers, nurse practitioners are the health care providers who complete oocyte removal and transfer. In all centers, nurses need to supply support and counseling to sustain the couple through the process. The recovery rate for harvesting ripened eggs is high (about 90%), as is the ability to fertilize eggs by sperm in vitro. However, the overall pregnancy rate by IVF-ET is as low as 20% to 30% per treatment cycle. Although IVF-ET programs do not result in an increase in birth defects, about 25% of pregnancies end in spontaneous abortion (the same rate as for natural pregnancies). Once a pregnancy has been successfully implanted, the woman's prenatal care is the same as that for any pregnancy. Research has shown that because the couple was so committed to the procedure, they adjust to pregnancy and parenthood well.

If a sonogram reveals that a multiple pregnancy of more than two or three zygotes has been achieved, selective termination of gestational sacs until only two are remaining may be recommended. This is done by the intra-abdominal injection of potassium chloride into the gestational sacs

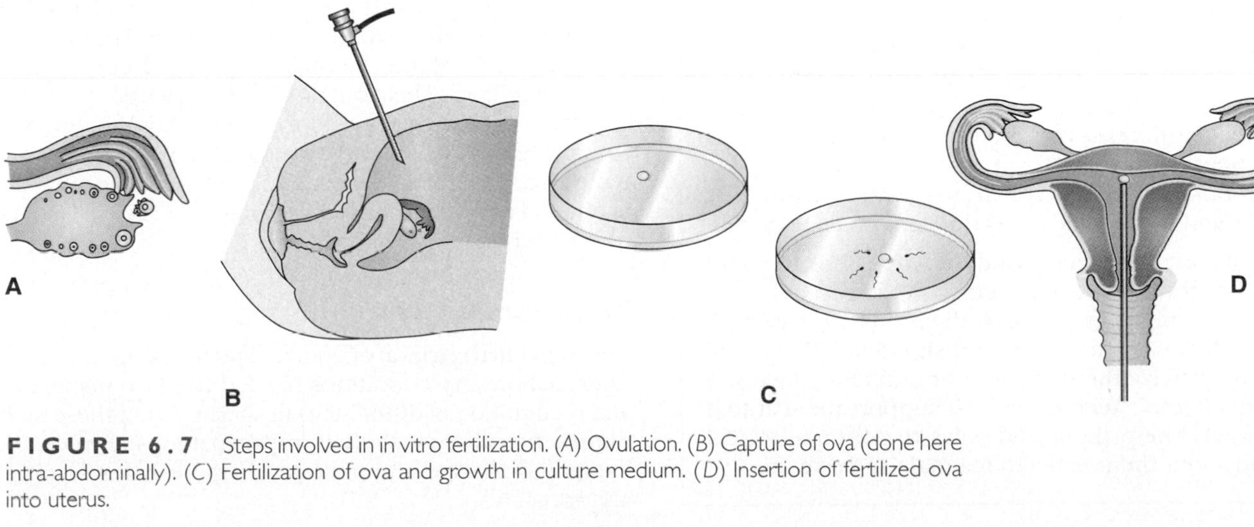

FIGURE 6.7 Steps involved in in vitro fertilization. (*A*) Ovulation. (*B*) Capture of ova (done here intra-abdominally). (*C*) Fertilization of ova and growth in culture medium. (*D*) Insertion of fertilized ova into uterus.

chosen to be eliminated. Reducing the number of growing embryos in this way to a number a woman could expect to carry to term without difficulty helps to ensure the success of the pregnancy.

IVF-ET is expensive (about $10,000 a cycle) and available only at specialized centers. There is a risk that if bacteria are introduced at any point in the transfer, maternal infection could occur. Waiting to be accepted by a center's program and waiting for the steps of obtaining the oocyte, laboratory growth, and pregnancy success is a major psychological strain. Couples report a feeling of social isolation during this time and weariness answering friends' and family's questions about the procedure. Couples need empathic support from health care providers through this difficult time (see Focus on Communication).

Gamete Intrafallopian Transfer

In gamete intrafallopian transfer (GIFT) procedures, ova are obtained from ovaries exactly as in IVF-ET. Instead of waiting for fertilization to occur in the laboratory, however, both ova and sperm are instilled within a matter of hours using a laparoscopic technique into the open end of a patent fallopian tube. Some centers are opting to perform this procedure using ultrasound to guide the collection and instillation of ova and sperm rather than using laparoscopic surgery. Fertilization then occurs in the tube, and the zygote moves to the uterus for implantation. This procedure has a pregnancy rate slightly higher than that of IVF-ET. The procedure is contraindicated if the woman's fallopian tubes are blocked, because this could lead to ectopic (tubal) pregnancy (Farhi et al., 2000).

Zygote Intrafallopian Transfer

Zygote intrafallopian transfer (ZIFT) involves oocyte retrieval by transvaginal, ultrasound-guided aspiration, followed by culture and insemination of the oocytes in the laboratory. Within 24 hours, the fertilized eggs are transferred by laparoscopic technique into the end of a waiting fallopian tube. ZIFT differs from GIFT in that fertilization takes place outside the body, allowing health care providers to be certain that impregnation has occurred before the growing structure is reintroduced. As in GIFT, a woman must have one functioning fallopian tube for the technique to be successful because the zygotes are implanted into the fimbriated end of a tube rather than into the uterus.

Surrogate Embryo Transfer

Surrogate embryo transfer is an assisted reproductive technique for the woman who does not ovulate. The process involves an oocyte donated by a friend or provided by an anonymous oocyte donor. The menstrual cycles of the donor and recipient are synchronized by administration of gonadotropic hormones. At the time of ovulation, the donor's ovum is removed by a transvaginal, ultrasound-guided procedure. The oocyte is then fertilized by the recipient woman's male partner's sperm (or donor sperm) and placed in the recipient woman's uterus by ET or GIFT. Once pregnancy occurs, it will progress the same as an unassisted pregnancy.

Intravaginal Culture

Intravaginal culture is another reproductive technique that uses the woman's own body as an incubator-like device. Ova are obtained from the woman and placed with the sperm in a sterile, hermetically sealed container of culture medium. This container is then placed inside the woman's vagina, being held there by a diaphragm. As a result, the ova and sperm are maintained at normal body temperatures. After approximately 48 hours, the container is opened and any fertilized dividing eggs are transferred to the uterus.

Blastomere Analysis

The individual retrieval of oocytes and fertilization of them under laboratory conditions has led to close inspection and recognition of differences in sperm. Using these techniques, before the oocyte is impregnated, sperm can be examined for specific genetic characteristics or other abnormalities.

FOCUS ON COMMUNICATION

Mrs. Baker is a 33-year-old woman who has been trying to get pregnant for 6 years. She and her husband have agreed to in vitro fertilization at a cost of approximately $10,000 per month even though her religion does not approve of this technique. Every time you see her at the fertility clinic, she seems sadder than the previous time.

Less Effective Communication

Nurse: How is everything going, Mrs. Baker?

Mrs. Baker: Fine, except it's been six years.

Nurse: That's your fault, Mrs. Baker. Instead of moving quickly through infertility management, you've stalled at every step. You didn't want to take Clomid, then you didn't want to pay for in vitro. . . .

Mrs. Baker: Making wise choices is difficult for me. I'll probably make a lousy parent if I ever do get pregnant.

More Effective Communication

Nurse: How is everything going, Mrs. Baker?

Mrs. Baker: Fine, except it's been six years.

Nurse: Six years? In the face of such a long time period, I think you've done very well. Infertility management is always difficult.

Mrs. Baker: I've learned to be patient. I figure that will stand me in good stead the day I do have a child.

Clients often may not make the same choices about fertility testing or management that a health care provider might make; such decisions are based on individual circumstances and situations. Be careful not to criticize them for poor or different choices. A more effective technique is to support them at that point and help them find ways to continue to feel good about themselves to maintain self-esteem.

Approximately 200 genetic diseases such as hemophilia are known to be sex-linked or transmitted to male offspring by the woman on the X chromosome. These illnesses could be prevented if a woman who carried the X-linked gene had only girls as offspring. The thought that people can preselect the sex of their children (have only boys or only girls) has been appealing to people not only for this reason but also for simple preference.

A number of methods to differentiate X-carrying from Y-carrying sperm have been identified. Couples participating in intrauterine transfer and artificial insemination can have sex predetermined using these methods. Such techniques can be useful because popular methods to influence the sex of a child (such as douching with a baking soda mixture before coitus to have a boy or with a vinegar solution to have a girl) have proved to be more folklore than scientific fact.

ALTERNATIVES TO CHILDBIRTH

For some couples, even treatment for infertility with procedures such as IVF-ET will not be successful. These couples need to consider still other options.

Surrogate Mothers

A surrogate mother is a woman who agrees to carry a pregnancy to term for an infertile couple. The surrogate may provide the ova and be impregnated by the man's sperm. In other instances, the ova and sperm both may be donated by the infertile couple, or donor ova and sperm may be used. Surrogate mothers are often friends or family members who assume the role out of friendship or compassion, or they can be referred to the couple through an agency or attorney and receive monetary reimbursement for their service. The infertile couple can enjoy the pregnancy as they watch it progress in the surrogate.

A number of ethical and legal problems can arise with surrogate motherhood if the surrogate mother decides at the end of pregnancy that she has formed an attachment to the fetus and wants to keep the baby despite the prepregnancy agreement she signed. Court decisions have been split on whether the surrogate or infertile couple has the right to the child. Another potential problem occurs if the child is born imperfect and the infertile couple then no longer wants the child. Who should have responsibility in this instance? For these reasons, couples and the surrogate mother must be certain they have given adequate thought to the process and what will be the outcome should these problems occur before attempting it.

Adoption

Adoption, once a ready alternative for infertile couples, is still a viable alternative, although there are fewer children available for adoption today from official agencies than formerly. Often it takes longer to find a child for adoption than it once did unless the couple considers foreign-born or physically or cognitively challenged children. Also, like other alternatives, adoption may not be right for every couple. Issues of adoptive families are discussed in Chapter 2.

Child-Free Living

Child-free living is an alternative lifestyle available to both fertile and infertile couples. For many infertile couples who have been through the rigors and frustrations of infertility testing and unsuccessful treatment regimens, child-free living may emerge as the option they finally wish to pursue. A couple in the midst of fertility testing may begin to reexamine their motives for pursuing pregnancy and decide that pregnancy and parenting are not worth the emotional or financial cost of future treatments. They may decide that the additional stress of going through an adoption is not for them, or a couple may simply decide that children are not necessary for them to fulfill their family unit. For these couples, child-free living is a positive choice (Fernandes, 1999).

Child-free living has advantages for a couple in that it allows time for both to pursue careers. They can travel more or have more time to pursue hobbies or continue their education. If a couple still wishes to include children in their lives in some way, many opportunities are available to do this: through family connections (most parents welcome offers from siblings or other family members to share in childrearing), through volunteer organizations (such as Big Brother or Big Sister programs), or through local schools and town recreational programs.

Child-free living can be as fulfilling as having children because it allows a couple more time to help other people and to contribute to society through personal accomplishments. Many couples today who feel that overpopulation is a major concern are choosing child-free living, even when infertility is not present.

✔ CHECKPOINT QUESTIONS

9. What must be present in the woman for GIFT to be effective?
10. How does GIFT differ from ZIFT?

KEY POINTS

- Infertility is said to exist when a pregnancy has not occurred after 1 year of unprotected coitus. Sterility refers to the inability to conceive because of a known condition.
- About 10% to 15% of couples today experience infertility. The incidence increases with the age of the couple.
- Infertility testing is an intense psychological stress for couples. Support from health care personnel is necessary during this time not only to help couples through the experience on an individual basis but also to help them maintain their relationship as a couple.
- Couples who are told that an infertility problem has been discovered are apt to suffer a great loss of self-esteem. The nursing role includes offering

support to help them look at other aspects of their lives where they do achieve to help them feel that they are productive, healthy people in many ways.

Male factors that contribute to infertility are inadequate sperm count, obstruction or impaired sperm motility, and problems with ejaculation. Female factors that cause infertility are problems with ovulation, tubal transport, impaired implantation, or interference with sperm motility.

Infertility assessment procedures consist of a health history, physical examination, laboratory tests to document general health, and specific tests for semen, ovulation, tubal patency, and hormone analysis.

Measures to induce fertility are aimed at improving sperm number and transport, decreasing infections, stimulating ovulation, and regulating hormones.

Artificial insemination, donor egg transfer, in vitro fertilization, adoption, surrogate motherhood, and child-free living are all possible solutions for infertility.

CRITICAL THINKING EXERCISES

1. Mrs. Carl, whom you met at the beginning of the chapter, stated that she believed her infertility problem was her fault because she was too rigid. She says, "It feels like our whole life revolves around trying to get pregnant." What measures could you suggest to make the process easier for them?
2. A 30-year-old woman who has just been married states that she wants to have a child as soon as possible. What advice would you give her to help increase her chances of conceiving quickly?
3. A woman is scheduled for a hysterosalpingogram. How would you prepare her for this procedure? What should she expect when the procedure is over?
4. Examine the national health goals related to infertility. Most government-sponsored money for nursing research is allotted based on these goals. Propose a possible research topic to explore pertinent to these goals that would be both fundable and advance evidence-based practice.

REFERENCES

Adamson, D., et al. (2001). A model for initial care of the infertile couple. *Journal of Reproductive Medicine, 46*(4 Suppl), 409–426.

Check, M. L., et al. (2000). ICSI as an effective therapy for male factor with antisperm antibodies. *Archives of Andrology, 45*(3), 125–130.

Cramer, D. W., et al. (2000). Recent trends in assisted reproductive techniques and associated outcomes. *Obstetrics & Gynecology, 95*(1), 61–66.

Crosignani, P. G., & Rubin, B. L. (2000). Optimal use of infertility diagnostic tests and treatment. *Human Reproduction, 15*(3), 723–732.

Department of Health and Human Services. (2000). *Healthy people 2010.* Washington, DC: DHHS.

de Weerd, S., et al. (2002). Preconception counseling improves folate status of women planning pregnancy. *Obstetrics & Gynecology, 99*(1), 45–50.

Eschenbach, D. A. (2000). Pelvic infections and sexually transmitted diseases. In Scott, J. R., et al. *Danforth's obstetrics & gynecology* (pp. 579–600). Philadelphia: Lippincott Williams & Wilkins.

Farhi, J., et al. (2000). Zygote intrafallopian transfer in patients with tubal factor infertility after repeated failure of implantation with in vitro fertilization-embryo transfer. *Fertility & Sterility, 74*(2), 390–393.

Fernandes, L. (1999). Fertility treatment: How do you tell couples it's time to stop? *Nursing Standard, 13*(49), 14–15.

Fukuda, M., et al. (2000). Right-sided ovulation favors pregnancy more than left-sided ovulation. *Human Reproduction, 15*(9), 1921–1926.

Glazener, C. M., Ford, W. C., & Hull, M. G. (2000). The prognostic power of the post-coital test for natural conception depends on duration of infertility. *Human Reproduction, 15*(9), 1953–1957.

Hammond, C. B. & Stillman, R. J. (2000). Infertility and assisted reproduction. In Scott, J. R., et al. *Danforth's obstetrics & gynecology.* Philadelphia: Lippincott Williams & Wilkins.

Johnson, M., Maas, M., & Moorhead, S. (2000). *Nursing outcomes classification* (2d ed.). St. Louis: Mosby.

Leibowitz, D., & Hoffman, J. (2000). Fertility drug therapies: Past, present, and future. *Journal of Obstetric, Gynecologic & Neonatal Nursing, 29*(2), 201–210.

McCloskey, J., & Bulechek, G. (2000). *Nursing interventions classification* (3rd ed.). St. Louis: Mosby.

National Institute of Allergy and Infectious Disease, National Institutes of Health. (1998). *Fact sheet, pelvic inflammatory disease.* Washington, DC: Public Health Service, U.S. Department of Health and Human Services.

Raman, J. D., & Schlegel, P. N. (2002). Aromatase inhibitors for male infertility. *Journal of Urology, 167*(2.1) 624–629.

Rosene-Montella, K., et al. (2000). Evaluation and management of infertility in women. *Annals of Internal Medicine, 132*(12), 973–981.

Sandlow, J. I. (2000). Shattering the myths about male infertility. *Postgraduate Medicine, 107*(2), 235–239.

Sinclair, S. (2000). Male infertility: Nutritional and environmental considerations. *Alternative Medicine Review, 5*(1), 28–38.

Vercellini, P., et al. (2000). Surgical management of endometriosis. *Best Practice & Research in Clinical Obstetrics & Gynecology, 14*(3), 501–523.

Weidner, I. S., et al. (1999). Risk factors for cryptorchidism and hypospadias. *Journal of Urology, 161*(5), 1606–1609.

Wellbery, C. (1999). Diagnosis and treatment of endometriosis. *American Family Physician, 60*(6), 1753–1762.

Zondervan, K., & Barlow, D. H. (2000). Epidemiology of chronic pelvic pain. *Best Practice & Research in Clinical Obstetrics & Gynaecology, 14*(3), 403–414.

SUGGESTED READINGS

Daya, S. (2000). Cost-effective, evidence-based infertility care. *Current Opinion in Obstetrics & Gynecology, 12*(3), 199–200.

Dokras, A., & Olive, D. L. (1999). Endometriosis and assisted reproductive technologies. *Clinical Obstetrics & Gynecology, 42*(3), 687–698.

Ferrara, I., et al. (2000). Intrauterine donor insemination in single women and lesbian couples: A comparative study of pregnancy rates. *Human Reproduction, 15*(3), 621–625.

Goldfarb, J. M., et al. (2000). Fifteen years experience with an in-vitro fertilization surrogate gestational pregnancy programme. *Human Reproduction, 15*(5), 1075–1078.

Golombok, S., et al. (1999). Social versus biological parenting: family functioning and the socioemotional development of children conceived by egg or sperm donation. *Journal of Child Psychology & Psychiatry & Allied Disciplines, 40*(4), 519–527.

Lapp, T. (2000). ACOG issues: Recommendations for the management of endometriosis. *American Family Physician, 62*(6), 1431–1434.

Nagler, H. M., et al. (2002). The natural history of partial ejaculatory duct obstruction. *Journal of Urology, 167*(1), 253–254.

Reame, N. (1999). Informed consent issues in assisted reproduction. *Journal of Obstetric, Gynecologic & Neonatal Nursing, 28*(3), 331–338.

Sanders, K. A., & Bruce, N. W. (1999). Psychosocial stress and treatment outcome following assisted reproductive technology. *Human Reproduction, 14*(6), 1656–1662.

Simpson, J. L., & Carson, S. A. (1999). The reproductive option of sex selection. *Human Reproduction, 14*(4), 870–872.

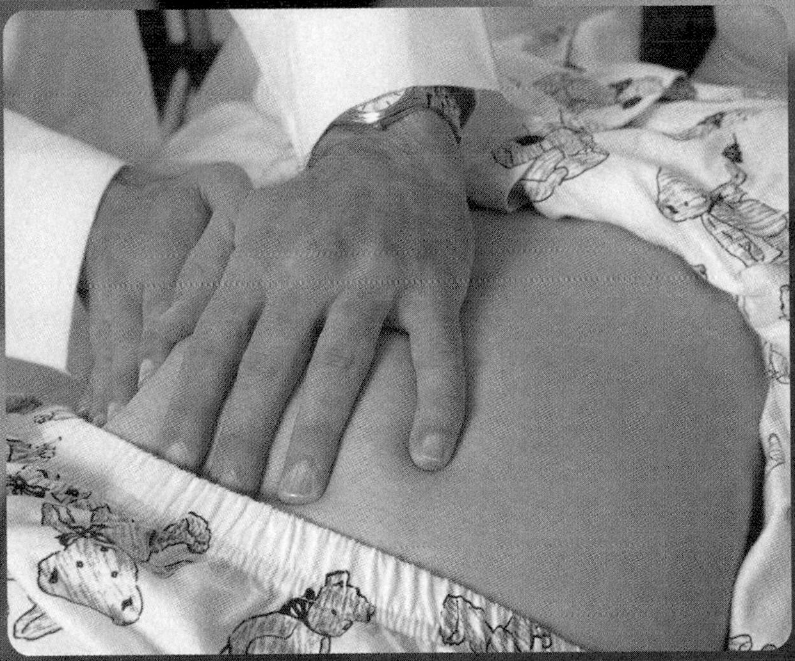

The Nursing Role in Caring for the Pregnant Family

UNIT III

Genetic Assessment and Counseling

CHAPTER 7

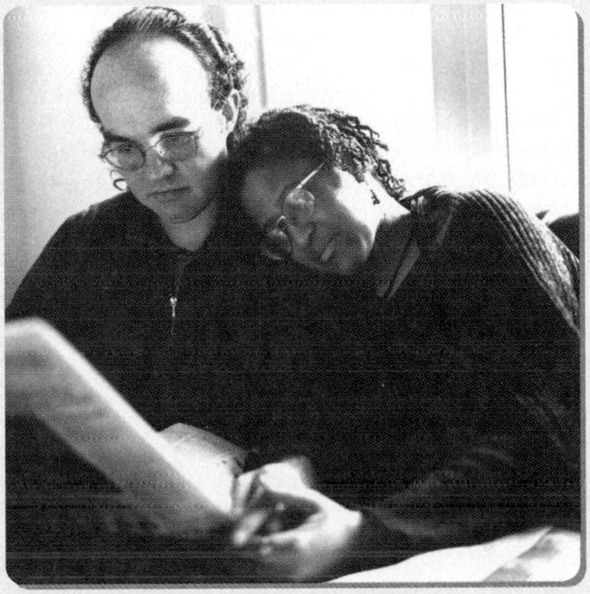

Key Terms

- alleles
- chromosomes
- dermatoglyphics
- dominant gene
- genes
- genetics
- genome
- genotype
- heterozygous trait
- homozygous trait
- imprinting
- karyotyping
- meiosis
- nondisjunction
- phenotype
- recessive gene

Objectives

After mastering the contents of this chapter, you should be able to:

1. Describe the nature of inheritance, patterns of recessive and dominant mendelian inheritance, and common chromosomal aberrations such as nondisjunction syndromes.
2. Assess a family for the probability of inheriting a genetic disorder.
3. Formulate nursing diagnoses related to genetic disorders.
4. Establish expected outcomes that meet the needs of the pregnant family undergoing genetic assessment and counseling.
5. Plan nursing care related to an alteration in genetic health, such as assisting with an amniocentesis.
6. Implement nursing care related to identification of or counseling for a genetic disorder.
7. Evaluate outcomes for achievement and effectiveness of nursing care.
8. Identify National Health Goals and specific measures related to genetic disorders that nurses can take to help the nation achieve these goals.
9. Identify areas related to genetic assessment that could benefit from additional nursing research or application of evidence-based practice.
10. Use critical thinking to analyze ways that nurses can contribute to health education and counseling for genetic issues.
11. Integrate knowledge of genetic inheritance with nursing process to achieve quality maternal and child health nursing care.

Mrs. Alvarez is a woman you meet at a genetic counseling center. She was adopted as a newborn and never felt a need to locate her birth parents because her adoptive parents provided a "close to perfect" childhood for her. After college, she married the most eligible bachelor in her hometown. She is now pregnant with her first child. At 15 weeks into the pregnancy, she has been advised her child may have translocation Down syndrome. She asks you, "Why is this happening? There's no disease in either of our families." How would you answer her?

Previous chapters described techniques for caring for women and their families preparing for childbearing and childrearing. This chapter discusses the basic principles by which disorders are inherited and information about the necessary assessments, care, and guidelines for counseling for the woman and her family when it is discovered there is a possibility of a genetic disorder in a child. This is important information because it can influence the health of a family for generations to come.

After you have studied this chapter, answer the Critical Thinking Exercises at the end of this chapter, then access the on-line study activities (http://connection.lww.com) *to further sharpen your skills and test your knowledge.*

The possibility that a child could have a genetic disorder crosses the minds of most pregnant women and their partners at some point in a pregnancy, whether or not there is any family history of genetic disorders. Many pregnant couples ask health care providers about their chances of having a child with a genetic disorder and about genetic testing as advances in screening techniques have made genetic testing a common feature of prenatal care. The importance of the national genome program and the necessity to improve techniques for screening for genetic disorders have become a national priority (see Focus on National Health Goals). Nurses can be instrumental in fostering the achievement of these goals through stressing the importance of the national genome program and supporting families during genetic testing.

Most women are offered routine screening of alphafetoprotein (AFP) levels at the 15th week of a pregnancy to evaluate for neural tube or chromosome defects in the fetus. Chorionic villi sampling (CVS) and amniocentesis are follow-up techniques that may be offered to women over the age of 35 years or if the AFP level is abnormal to further screen for genetic disorders. Couples who already know of the existence of a genetic disorder in their family or those who have had a previous child born with a congenital anomaly often require still additional, more extensive testing. After a positive test for a genetic disorder, they will almost certainly undergo an emotional period of decision making. Informative and sensitive genetic counseling by health care providers educated in the specialty of genetics is essential for these couples. Because most screening takes place in an ambulatory setting, the nurse plays a vital role as educator, supporter, and communicator for the family (Lam & MacKenzie, 2002).

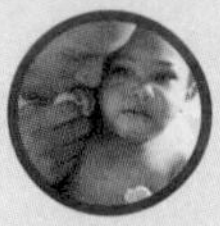

FOCUS ON NATIONAL HEALTH GOALS

Two National Health Goals speak directly to genetic disease and screening:

- Increase to at least 90% the proportion of women enrolled in prenatal care who are offered screening and counseling for prenatal detection of fetal abnormalities.
- Increase to at least 95% the proportion of newborns screened by state-sponsored programs for genetic disorders and other disabling conditions and to 90% the proportion of newborns testing positive for disease who receive appropriate treatment (DHHS, 2000).

Nurses can be instrumental in helping achieve these goals by being sensitive to the need for genetic screening and counseling in prenatal and birth settings. Answers to questions provided by nursing research, such as when are people most responsive to genetic counseling or what effect on bonding occurs, if any, when the parents learn about an alpha-fetoprotein level during pregnancy, can also help meet these goals.

NURSING PROCESS OVERVIEW

For Genetic Assessment and Counseling

Assessment

Assessment is a crucial step in any nursing intervention, but it plays an especially vital role in genetic screening and counseling. Assessment measures include a detailed family history, physical examination of both the parents and the affected child, and an ever-growing series of laboratory assays of blood, amniotic fluid, and maternal and fetal cells. Nurses serve as members of genetic assessment and counseling teams in many roles, especially when helping to obtain the initial family history, assist with the preliminary physical examination, obtain blood serum for analysis, or assist with procedures, such as amniocentesis.

Nursing Diagnosis

Typical nursing diagnoses related to the area of genetic disorders are:

- Decisional conflict related to testing for an untreatable genetic disorder
- Fear related to outcome of genetic screening tests
- Situational low self-esteem related to identified chromosomal abnormality
- Deficient knowledge related to inheritance pattern of the family's inherited disorder
- Health-seeking behaviors related to potential for genetic transmission of disease

- Ineffective sexuality pattern related to fear of conceiving a child with a genetic disorder

Outcome Identification and Planning

Outcome identification and planning for families involved with genetic assessment differ according to the type of assessments performed and the results obtained. They may include determining what information the couple needs to know before testing can proceed or helping couples to arrange for further assessment measures during a pregnancy. Goals must be realistic and consistent with the individual's or couple's lifestyle (not all people want to be totally informed about family illnesses).

Implementation

Parental reaction to the knowledge that their child has a possible genetic disorder or to the birth of a child with a genetically inherited disorder usually involves a grief reaction, similar to that experienced by parents whose child dies at birth. Both must work through the stages of shock and denial ("This cannot be true"), anger ("It's not fair this happened to us"), and bargaining ("If only this would go away") to reorganization and acceptance ("It has happened to us and it is all right"). For some couples, a genetic disorder may not be diagnosed during the pregnancy. In fact, it may not be discovered until birth, or possibly not even until school age. For these parents, the reaction will occur at that later point of diagnosis.

As a rule, when parents are under stress, the focus is on helping the parents concentrate on short-term goals and actions. Look first at the immediate needs of the family, fetus, and newborn and later on at what type of continued follow-up will be necessary; for instance, after the birth, will the baby need to be hospitalized for immediate surgical correction of accompanying congenital anomalies? Will the parents take the baby home or will he or she be placed temporarily in foster care? What kind of decisions about the child's education need to be made?

Identifying support people who can be helpful to the parents during their time of disorganization and shock is also important. These people may be the usual family resources, such as grandparents or other family members. In some families, these people may be as disturbed by the diagnosis as the parents and so cannot offer their usual support. Secondary support sources may be necessary, including organizations such as the March of Dimes Birth Defects Foundation (*www. modimes.org*), the American Association of Klinefelter Syndrome Information & Support (*www. AAKSIS.org*), the National Fragile X Foundation (*www.NFXF.org*), the National Down Syndrome Society (*www. ndss.org*), and the Turner's Syndrome Society (*www. Turner-syndrome-us.org*). Not all parents are ready to talk to members of such organizations at the time of diagnosis. To join the organization makes the diagnosis "real" or moves them out of denial before they may be ready.

Identifying health care personnel with whom the parents will need to maintain contact during the next few months can offer additional support. Consistent, clear communication among all health care team members is essential. At some point, decisions will need to be made about the future, such as schooling, surgical procedures, behavior problems, or future development. Ensuring that the parents have health care providers whom they know they can turn to, especially when they are moving out of denial, helps to keep the family safe.

Outcome Evaluation

Examples of expected outcomes for the family with a known genetic disorder may include the following:

- Couple states they feel capable of coping no matter what the outcome of genetic testing.
- Client accurately states the chances of a genetic disorder occurring in her next child.
- Couple states they have resolved their feelings of low self-esteem related to birth of a child with a genetic disorder.

A couple's decisions about genetic testing and childbearing may change over time. For example, at age 25, a decision made not to have children because of a potential genetic disorder may be difficult to maintain as the couple, now age 30, sees many of their friends with growing families. Individuals and couples who have asked for genetic counseling should be given the phone number of a genetic counselor and should be urged to call periodically for news of recent advances in genetic screening techniques or disease treatments so they can remain current.

GENETIC DISORDERS

Inherited or genetic disorders are disorders that can be passed from one generation to the next. They result from some disorder in gene or chromosome structure. **Genetics** is the study of the way such disorders occur.

Genetic abnormalities can occur at the moment of ovum and sperm fusion or even earlier, in the meiotic division phase of the gametes (ovum and sperm). Some genetic abnormalities are so severe that normal fetal growth cannot continue. This results in early spontaneous abortion. Genetic disorders are so common that as many as 50% of first-trimester spontaneous miscarriages may be the result of chromosomal abnormalities. Other genetic disorders do not affect life in utero, and the result of the disorder becomes apparent only at the time of fetal testing or after birth. In the near future, it may be possible not only to identify aberrant genes for disorders but also to insert healthy genes in their place. Gene replacement therapy has already been used with some success in the treatment of blood and immunodeficiency syndromes.

Nature of Inheritance

Genes are the basic units of heredity that determine both the physical and mental characteristics of people. Composed of segments of DNA (deoxyribonucleic acid), they direct protein synthesis. Genes are woven into strands in the nucleus of all body cells to form **chromosomes.**

In humans, each cell, with the exception of the sperm and ovum, contains 46 chromosomes (44 autosomes and 2 sex chromosomes). The spermatozoa and ova each carry only half of the chromosome number, or 23 chromosomes. For each chromosome in the sperm cell, there is a like chromosome of similar size and shape and function (autosomes, or homologous chromosomes) in the ovum. Because genes are always located at fixed positions on chromosomes, two like genes (**alleles**) for every trait are represented in the ovum and sperm on autosomes. The one chromosome in which this does not occur is the chromosome for determining sex. If the sex chromosomes are both type X (large symmetric) in the zygote formed from the union of a sperm and ovum, the individual is female (Fig. 7-1*A*). If one sex chromosome is an X and one a Y (a smaller type), the individual is a male (Fig. 7-1*B*).

A person's **phenotype** refers to his or her outward appearance or the expression of the genes. A person's **genotype** refers to his or her actual gene composition. A person's **genome** is the complete set of genes present (about 50,000 to 100,000). A normal genome is abbreviated as 46XX or 46XY (designation of the total number of chromosomes plus a graphic description of the sex chromosomes present). If a chromosomal aberration exists, it is listed after the sex chromosome pattern. In such abbreviations, the letter *p* stands for short arm defects and *q* stands for the long arm of chromosomes. The abbreviation 46XX5p–, for example, is the abbreviation for a female with 46 total chromosomes but with the short arm of chromosome 5 missing (cri-du-chat syndrome). In Down syndrome, the person has an extra chromosome 21, which is abbreviated as 47XX21+ or 47XY21+.

Mendelian Inheritance: Dominant and Recessive Patterns

The principles of genetic inheritance of disease are the same as those that govern genetic inheritance of other physical characteristics, such as eye or hair color. These principles were discovered and described by Gregor Mendel, an Austrian naturalist, and are known as *mendelian laws.*

A person who has two like genes for a trait—for blue eyes, for example (one from the mother and one from the father)—on two like chromosomes is said to be **homozygous** for that trait. If the genes differ (a gene for blue eyes from the mother and a gene for brown eyes from the father, or vice versa), the person is said to be **heterozygous** for that trait. Many genes are dominant in their action over others; that is, when paired with other genes, **dominant genes** are always expressed in preference to the other genes. A gene that is not dominant is **recessive.** For example, brown eye color is dominant over blue, so a person with a heterozygous pattern would appear to have brown eyes. An individual with two homozygous genes for a dominant trait is said to be *homozygous dominant;* the individual with two genes for a recessive trait is *homozygous recessive.*

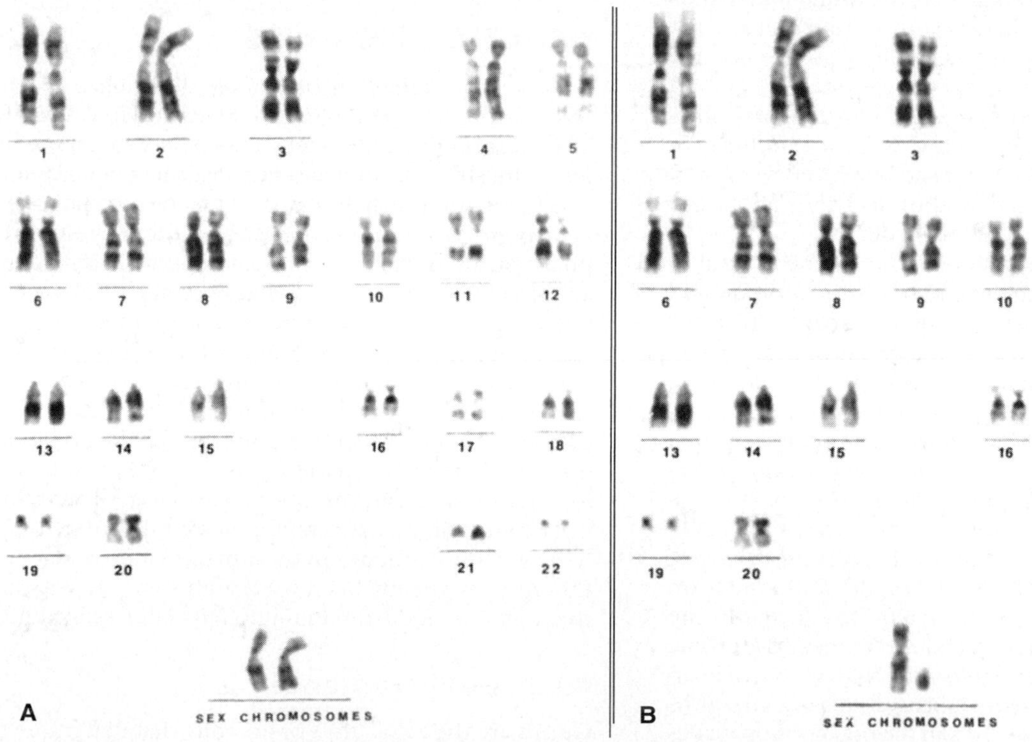

FIGURE 7.1 Photomicrographs of human chromosomes (karyotypes [photograph of chromosomes arranged in a standard classification]). If a blood sample is taken from a child or adult and the white blood cells are examined at the mitotic division phase of reproduction, transferred to slides, and photographed under high-power magnification, the individual chromosomes can be cut from the photograph and arranged according to size and shape. (*A*) Normal female karyotype. (*B*) Normal male karyotype.

Mendelian laws permit the prediction of inheritance of traits, such as eye color, or the chance that a child born to parents with a certain genotype will be born with a disorder. Inheritance patterns for eye color or hair color provide a useful example of these principles. If the father is homozygous dominant (has two dominant genes for brown eye color) and the mother is homozygous recessive (has two genes for blue eye color), it can be predicted that their children have a 100% chance of being heterozygous for the trait (Fig. 7-2*A*); they will appear brown-eyed (the phenotype) but will carry a recessive gene for blue eyes (the genotype). If the father, however, is heterozygous (has one dominant gene and one recessive gene), a child born to this couple will now have an equal chance of being brown-eyed or blue-eyed (Fig. 7-2*B*).

Suppose the mother is heterozygous instead of homozygous recessive and the father is homozygous dominant. When this pairing occurs, the chances are equal that their child will be homozygous dominant like the father or heterozygous like the mother. All the children's phenotypes will be brown eyes (Fig. 7-2*C*).

Suppose both parents are heterozygous. There is a 25% chance of their children being homozygous recessive (appear blue-eyed), a 50% chance of their being heterozygous (appear brown-eyed), and a 25% chance of their being homozygous dominant (appear brown-eyed). This is how two brown-eyed parents can produce a blue-eyed child (Fig. 7-2*D*).

This is also true for hair color, with brown hair the dominant gene and blonde hair the recessive gene. Using mendelian laws, for example, two brunette parents can produce a blonde child. However, it is impossible to predict a person's genotype from the phenotype, or outward appearance.

Inheritance of Disease

The same principles governing inheritance are applicable to predicting inherited disorders. Disorders may be transmitted as either dominant or recessive traits.

Autosomal Dominant Disorders

Although there are over 1,000 autosomal disorders known, only a few are commonly seen. A person with a dominant gene for a disease is usually heterozygous (has a corresponding healthy recessive gene for the trait). For example, Huntington disease, a progressive neurologic disorder that usually begins between ages 35 and 45 years and is characterized by loss of motor control and intellectual deterioration, is an example of a dominantly inherited disorder. It is now possible to detect people who will develop this disorder by analyzing for a specific gene on chromosome 4. Unfortunately, there is no cure for the disorder, which means potentially affected individuals must make a difficult choice in deciding to undergo the analysis when they can do nothing if the result is positive.

Other examples of dominantly inherited disorders include facioscapulohumeral muscular dystrophy, a form of *osteogenesis imperfecta* (a disorder in which bones are exceedingly brittle), and Marfan syndrome (a disorder of connective tissue in which the child is thinner and taller than normal and has associated heart defects). If a person with a dominant disorder trait such as facioscapulohumeral muscular dystrophy mates with a person who does not have the trait, as shown in Figure 7-3*A*, the chances are even (50%) that a child would be born with the disorder or be disease- and carrier-free.

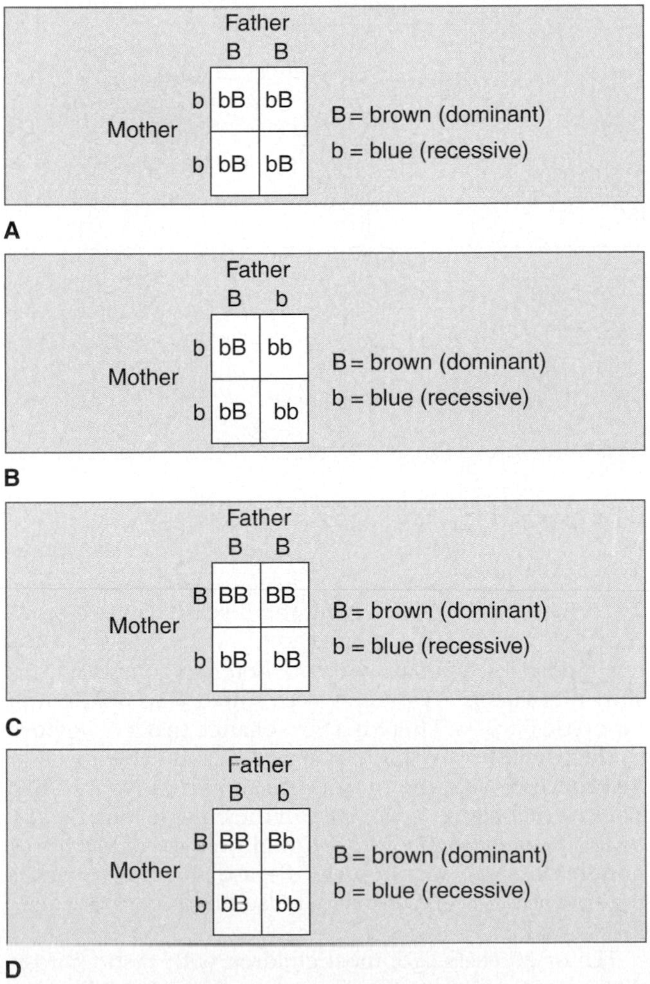

FIGURE 7.2 Possible inheritance of eye color.

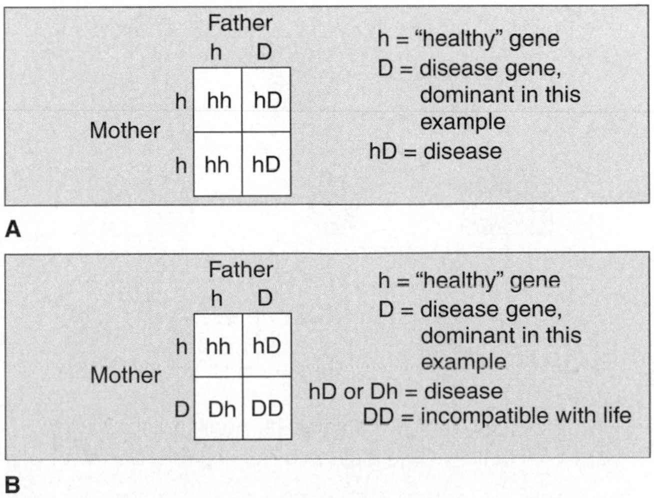

FIGURE 7.3 Autosomal dominant inheritance.

Two people with a dominantly inherited disorder are unlikely to choose each other as reproductive partners. If they do, however, their chances of having children free from the disorder decline (Fig. 7-3*B*): there would be only a 25% chance of a child being disease- and carrier-free, a 50% chance the child would have the disorder like they do, and a 25% chance that a child would be homozygous dominant (have two dominant disorder genes), a condition that is probably incompatible with life.

In assessing family pedigrees (maps of family relationships) for the incidence of inherited disorders, a number of common findings are usually discovered when a dominantly inherited pattern is present in the family:

1. One of the parents of a child with the disorder also will have the disorder.
2. The sex of the affected individual is unimportant in terms of inheritance.
3. There is usually a history of the disorder in other family members.

Figure 7-4 shows a typical pedigree of a family with a dominantly inherited autosomal disorder.

Autosomal Recessive Inheritance

Most genetic disorders are inherited as recessive, not dominant, traits. Such diseases do not occur unless two genes for the disease are present (that is, a homozygous recessive pattern). Many inborn errors of metabolism are recessively inherited this way. Examples include cystic fibrosis, adrenogenital syndrome, albinism, Tay-Sachs disease, galactosemia, phenylketonuria, limb-girdle muscular dystrophy, and Rh-factor incompatibility problems that arise with pregnancy.

An example of autosomal recessive inheritance is shown in Figure 7-5*A*, in which both parents are disease-free. Both are heterozygous in genotype, however, and thus carry a recessive gene for cystic fibrosis. There is a 25% chance of a child born to them being disease- and carrier-free (homozygous dominant for healthy genes), a 50% chance of a child being, like themselves, free of disease but carrying the unexpressed disease gene (heterozygous), and a 25% chance of a child having the disease (homozygous recessive).

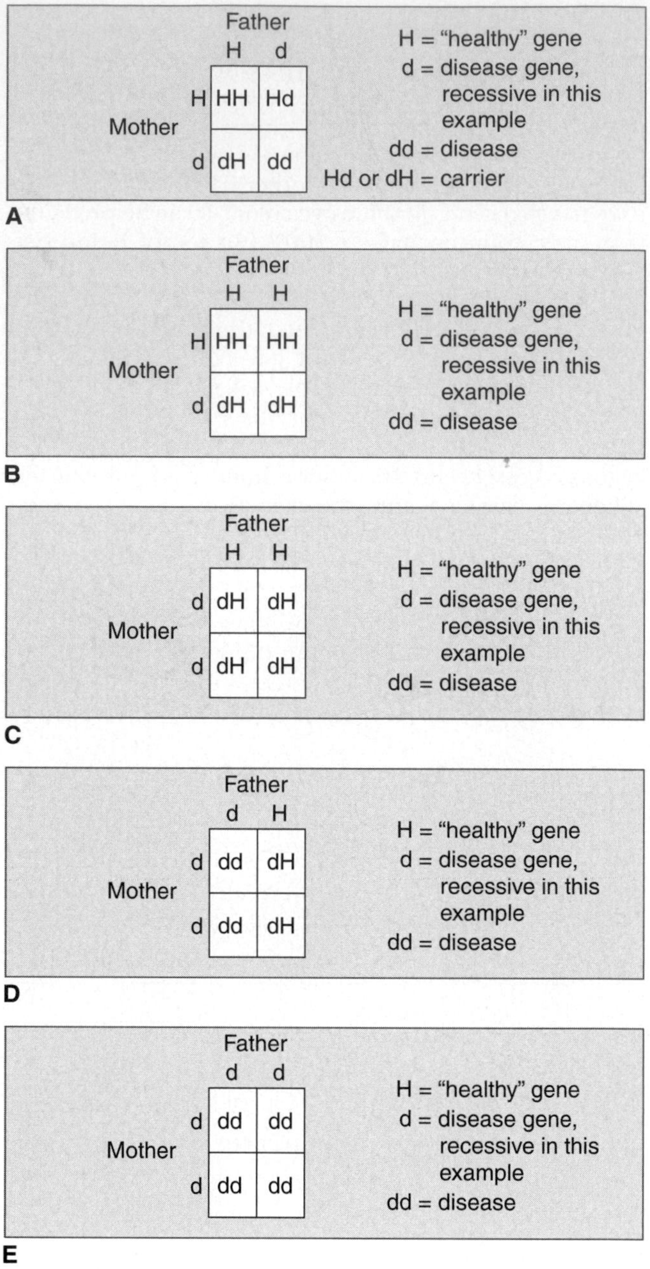

FIGURE 7.5 Autosomal recessive inheritance.

Suppose the woman with the heterozygous genotype shown in Figure 7-5*A* mates with a man who has no trait for cystic fibrosis. There is a 50% chance that a child born to them will be completely disorder- and carrier-free or heterozygous like the mother, as shown in Figure 7-5*B*. There is no chance in this case of the child having the disorder. However, the child should be aware that his or her children may manifest the disease if he or she carries the trait and if a sexual partner also has a recessive gene for the trait.

Ten or 20 years ago, most children with cystic fibrosis died in early childhood and so never reached childbearing age. Today, with good management, some live to have chil-

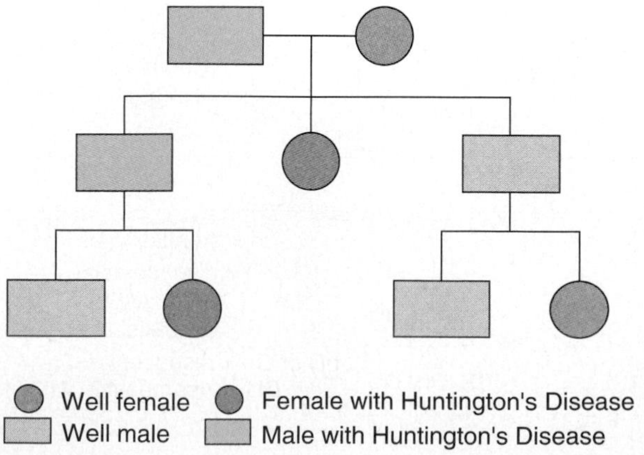

FIGURE 7.4 Family pedigree: autosomal dominant inheritance.

dren of their own. If a person with cystic fibrosis should choose a sexual partner without the trait, all their children would be free of the disorder. However, they all would carry a recessive gene for the disorder (see Fig. 7-5*C*).

If the person with cystic fibrosis mated with a person with an unexpressed gene for the disease, there would be a 50% chance that a child would have the disorder or would carry a recessive gene for the disorder (see Fig. 7-5*D*). If a person with the disorder mated with a person who also had the disorder, as shown in Figure 7-5*E,* there is a 100% chance that a child would have the disorder.

When family pedigrees are assessed for the incidence of inherited disease, situations commonly discovered when a recessively inherited disease is present in the family include the following:

1. Both parents of a child with the disorder are clinically free of the disorder.
2. The sex of the affected individual is unimportant in terms of inheritance.
3. The family history for the disorder is negative (no one can identify anyone else who had it).
4. A known common ancestor between the parents sometimes exists. This is how both male and female have come to possess a like gene for the disorder.

Figure 7-6 shows a typical pedigree of a family with an autosomal recessive inherited disorder.

> ✔ **CHECKPOINT QUESTIONS**
>
> 1. How does a person's phenotype differ from his or her genotype?
> 2. How many chromosomes are found in a sperm cell?
> 3. What type of genetic disorder is cystic fibrosis?

X-Linked Dominant Inheritance

Some genes for disorders are located on, and therefore transmitted only by, the female sex chromosome (the X chromosome). This is called X-linked inheritance. When the gene is dominant, it need be present on only one of the X chromosomes for symptoms of the disorder to be manifested (Fig. 7-7*A*). Family characteristics seen with this type of inheritance include:

1. All individuals with the gene are affected.
2. Female children of affected men are all affected; male children of affected men are unaffected.
3. It appears in every generation.
4. All children of homozygous affected women are affected. Fifty percent of heterozygous affected women are affected (Fig. 7-8). An example of a disease in this group is hypophosphatemia.

X-Linked Recessive Inheritance

The majority of X-linked inherited disorders are recessive. With this, the mother will be the carrier for the disorder. Any time a normal gene also is present, as in her female children, the expression of the disease will be blocked. However, if the gene is not paired, as in her male children, the disease will be manifested.

Hemophilia A, Christmas disease (a blood-factor deficiency), color blindness, Duchenne (pseudohypertrophic) muscular dystrophy, and fragile X syndrome are examples of this type of inheritance. Such a pattern is shown in Figure 7-7*B,* in which the mother has the affected gene on one of her X chromosomes and the father is disease-free. The chances are 50% that a male child will manifest the disease and 50% that a female child will carry the disease gene. If the father has the disease and chooses a sexual partner who is free of the disease gene, the chances are 100% that

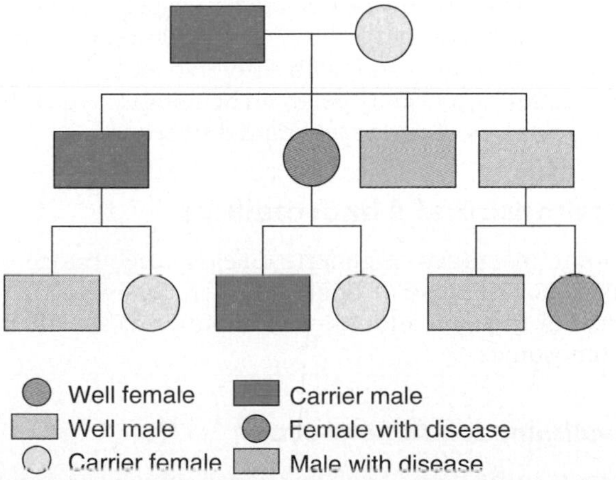

FIGURE 7.6 Family pedigree: autosomal recessive inheritance.

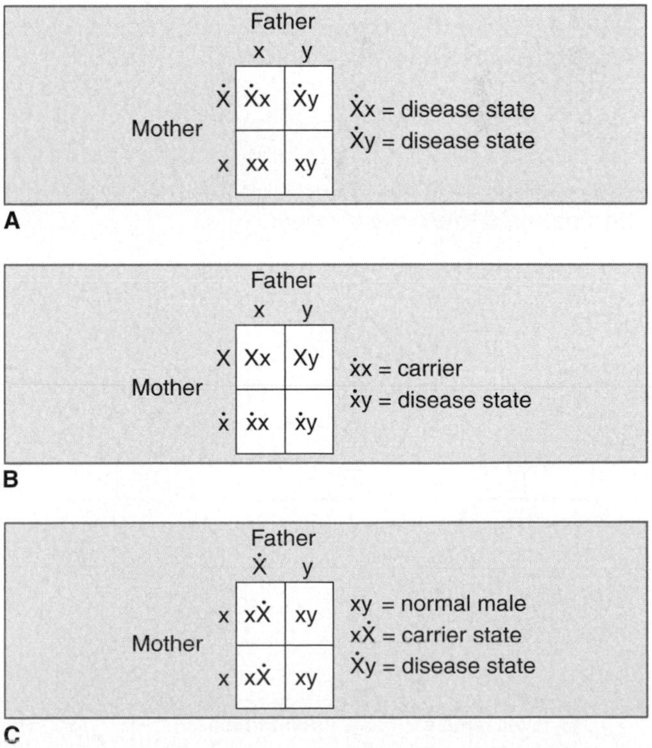

FIGURE 7.7 Sex-linked inheritance: (*A*) sex-linked dominant; (*B, C*) sex-linked recessive.

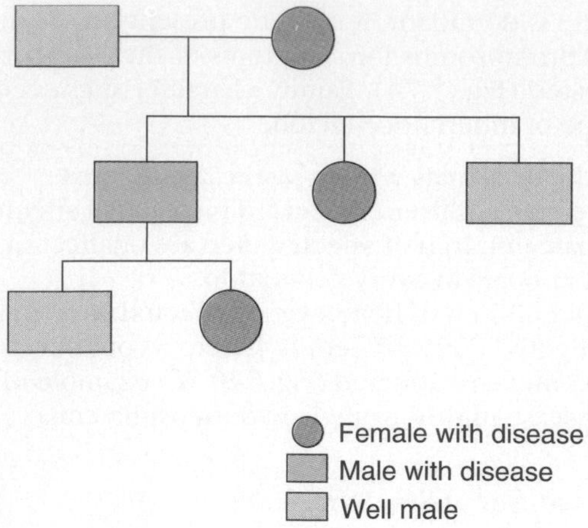

FIGURE 7.8 Family pedigree: X-linked dominant inheritance.

a daughter will have the sex-linked recessive gene. There is no chance a son will have the disease (see Fig. 7-7*C*).

When family pedigrees are assessed for inherited disorders, the following findings usually are apparent if an X-linked recessive inheritance disorder is present in the family:

1. Only males in the family will have the disorder.
2. A history of girls dying at birth for unknown reasons often exists (females who had the affected gene on both X chromosomes, a condition incompatible with life).
3. Sons of an affected man are unaffected.
4. The parents of affected children do not have the disorder.

Figure 7-9 shows a typical family pedigree in which there is an X-linked recessive inheritance pattern.

WHAT IF? What if a woman, knowing that she carries a recessive X-linked chromosome disorder, says she wants to have all boys because they will not show symptoms? Is she well informed?

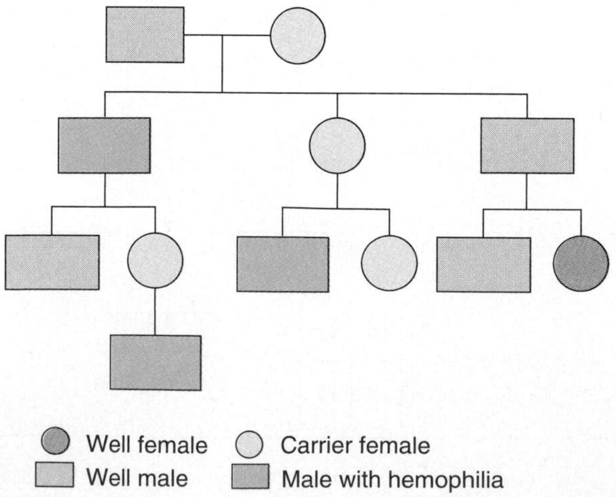

FIGURE 7.9 Family pedigree: X-linked recessive inheritance.

Multifactorial (Polygenic) Inheritance

Many congenital disorders (disorders present at birth) such as heart disease, diabetes, pyloric stenosis, cleft lip and palate, neural tube disorders, hypertension, and mental illness tend to have a higher-than-usual incidence in some families. Diabetes is one example that has been studied closely. Certain human lymphocyte antigens (HLAs) inherited from both parents appear to play a role in genetic susceptibility to diabetes mellitus. Children who will develop diabetes mellitus can be shown to have an increased frequency of HLA B8, B15, DR3, and DR4 on chromosome 6. They lack DR2, an HLA that appears to be protective against diabetes mellitus.

Diseases caused by multifactorial reasons do not follow the mendelian laws of inheritance, probably because more than a single gene or HLA is involved. Environmental influences may be instrumental in determining whether the disorder is expressed. It is difficult to counsel parents regarding these disorders because their occurrence is so unpredictable. A family history, for instance, reveals no set pattern. Some of these conditions have a predisposition to occur more frequently in one sex (e.g., cleft palate occurs more often in girls), but they can occur in either sex.

Imprinting

Imprinting refers to the differential expression of genetic material and allows researchers to identify whether the chromosomal material has come from the male or female parent. In some instances, such as hydatidiform molc (see Chap. 15), it can be shown that no maternal contribution is made to a fertilized ovum. In Prader-Willis syndrome, a chromosome 15 abnormality in which children are severely cognitively challenged, no paternal contribution is present.

Genetic Markers

A *genetic marker* is a specific point on a chromosome that, if present, marks the location of a missing or abnormal gene. Chromosomal markers can be identified in varying types of pediatric illnesses, such as leukemias and lymphomas, suggesting that a genetic basis exists for some of these illnesses. Cystic fibrosis can now be detected prenatally because of a gene marker on chromosome 7. In the future, more markers will be identified and, with recombinant DNA processing techniques, a healthy gene can be reimplanted at these sites as a means of curing inherited diseases.

Chromosomal Abnormalities

In some instances of genetic disease, the abnormality occurs not because of dominant or recessive gene patterns but through a fault in the number or structure of chromosomes.

Nondisjunction Abnormalities

Meiosis is the type of cell division in which the number of chromosomes in the cell is reduced to the haploid (half) number for reproduction (23 rather than 46 chromosomes). All sperm and ova initially undergo a meiosis cell division early in formation. During this division, half of the chromosomes are attracted to one pole of the cell and half to the other pole. The cell then divides cleanly, with 23 chromosomes in the first new cell and 23 chromosomes in the second new cell. Chromosomal abnormalities occur when the division is uneven (**nondisjunction**). The result may be that one new sperm cell or ovum has 24 chromosomes and the second only 22 (Fig. 7-10). If a defective spermatozoon or ovum fuses with a normal spermatozoon or ovum, the zygote (sperm and ovum combined) will have 47 or 45 chromosomes, not the normal 46. The presence of 45 chromosomes does not appear to be compatible with life, and the embryo or fetus probably will be aborted. Down syndrome (trisomy 21) (47XX21+ or 47XY21+) is an example of a disease in which the individual has 47 chromosomes. There are three rather than two of chromosome 21 (Fig. 7-11).

The incidence of Down syndrome increases with increasing age and is highest if the mother is over age 35 and the father is over age 55. Thus, aging seems to present an obstacle to clean cell division. The incidence is 1:100 in women over age 40 compared to 1:1,500 in women under age 20 (Chung, 2000). Other examples of cell nondisjunction include trisomy 13 (Fig. 7-12) and trisomy 18 (cognitive challenge syndromes).

When nondisjunction occurs in the sex chromosomes, other types of abnormalities occur. Turner and Klinefelter syndromes are the most common types. In Turner syndrome (45XO), marked by webbed neck, short stature, sterility, and possible cognitive challenge, the individual, although female, has only one X chromosome or has two X chromosomes but one is defective. She appears to be female (female phenotype) because of the one X chromosome. In Klinefelter syndrome (marked by sterility and possibly cognitive challenge), the individual has male genitals but the sex chromosomal pattern is 47XXY.

Deletion Abnormalities

Deletion abnormalities are a form of chromosome disorder in which part of a chromosome breaks during cell division, causing the affected person to have the normal number of chromosomes plus or minus an extra portion of a chromosome, such as 45.75 chromosomes or 47.5. For example, in cri-du-chat syndrome (46XY5q–), one portion of chromosome 5 is missing (see discussion later in this chapter).

Translocation Abnormalities

Translocation abnormalities are perplexing situations in which a child gains an additional chromosome through another route. A form of Down syndrome occurs as a translocation abnormality. In this instance, one parent of the child has the correct number of chromosomes (46), but chromosome 21 is misplaced and abnormally attached to chromosome 14. The parent's appearance and functioning are normal because the total chromosome count is a normal 46. He or she is termed a *balanced translocation carrier.*

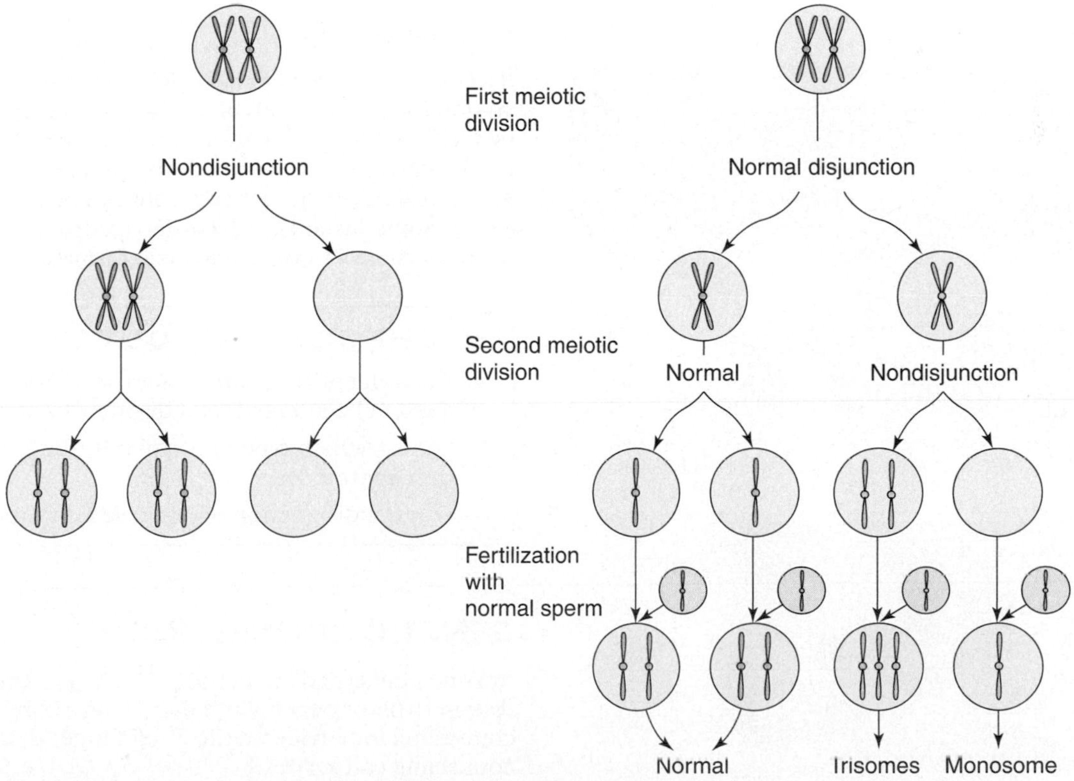

FIGURE 7.10 Process of nondisjunction at the first and second meiotic divisions of the ovum and fertilization with normal sperm.

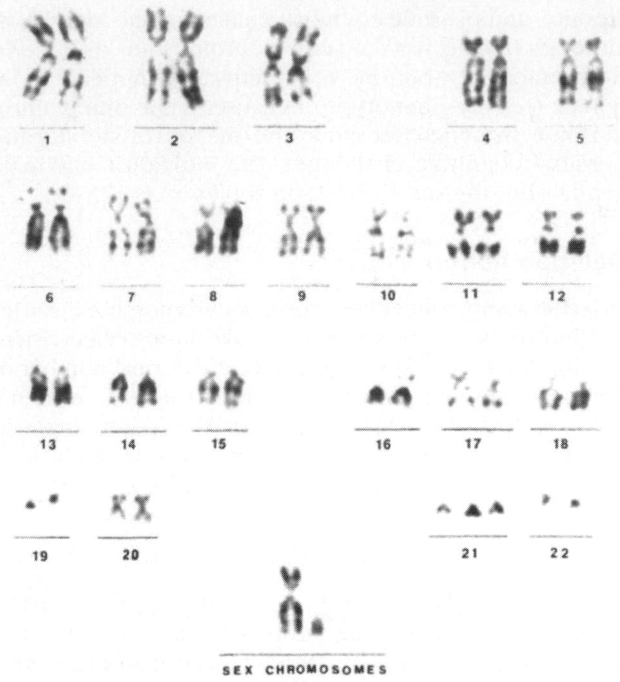

FIGURE 7.11 Karyotype of trisomy 21.

However, if during meiosis, this abnormal chromosome 14 (carrying the extra 21 chromosome) and the normal chromosome 21 are both included in one sperm or ovum, the resulting child will have a total of 47 chromosomes, including the extra number 21. The child is said to have an *unbalanced translocation syndrome.* The phenotype (appearance) of the child will be indistinguishable from the form of Down syndrome that occurs from nondisjunction.

About 2% to 5% of children with Down syndrome have this type of chromosome pattern. It is important to identify parents who are translocation carriers because their chance of having a child born with Down syndrome is higher than normal. If the father is the carrier, this risk is about 5%; if the mother is the carrier, the risk is about 15%. As many as 15% of couples who have frequent early spontaneous miscarriages may have this type of chromosomal aberration (Qumsiyeh et al., 2001).

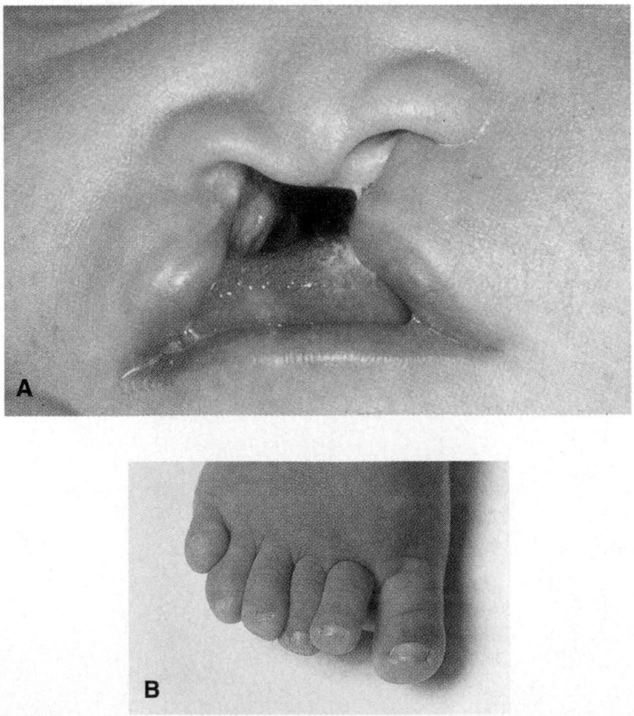

FIGURE 7.12 An infant with trisomy 13 has (*A*) a cleft palate and (*B*) supernumerary digits (polydactyly).

Mosaicism

Normally, a nondisjunction abnormality occurs during the meiosis stage of cell division, when sperm and ova halve their number of chromosomes. Mosaicism is an abnormal condition that is present when the nondisjunction disorder occurs after fertilization of the ovum as the structure begins mitotic (daughter-cell) division. When this occurs, different cells in the body will have different chromosome counts. The extent of the disorder depends on the proportion of tissue with normal chromosome structure to tissue with abnormal chromosome constitution. Children with Down syndrome who have near-normal intelligence may have this type of pattern. The occurrence of such a phenomenon at this stage of development suggests that a teratogenic (harmful to the fetus) condition, such as x-ray or drug exposure, existed at that point to disturb normal cell division. This genetic pattern in a female would be abbreviated as 46XX/47XX21+.

Isochromosomes

If a chromosome accidentally divides not by a vertical separation but by a horizontal one, a new chromosome with mismatched long and short arms can result. This is an isochromosome. It has much the same effect as a translocation abnormality when an entire extra chromosome exists. Some instances of Turner syndrome (45XO) may occur because of isochromosome formation.

✔ CHECKPOINT QUESTIONS

4. Does an entire chromosome, or only a part, need to be affected for a disorder to occur?
5. During which type of division is nondisjunction thought to occur?
6. Can nondisjunction occur in sex chromosomes?

GENETIC COUNSELING

Anyone concerned about the possibility of transmitting a disease to his or her children should have access to genetic counseling for advice on the inheritance of disease. Such counseling can serve to:

- Reassure people who are concerned about their children inheriting a particular disorder and

provide concrete, accurate information (if what they are concerned about is not an inherited disorder, for example)
- Allow people who are affected by inherited disorders to make informed choices about future reproduction
- Educate people about inherited disorders and the process of inheritance
- Offer support by skilled health care professionals to people who are affected by genetic disorders

Confidentiality of information revealed in genetic screening is essential and must be maintained. Such information could be used to damage a person's reputation or harm a future career or relationship. The necessity to maintain confidentiality prevents the health care provider from alerting other family members unless the member requesting genetic assessment has given consent. In some instances, a history reveals new information, such as that a child has been adopted or is the result of artificial insemination, or that the child's father is not the current husband. The member of the family seeking counseling has the right to decide whether this information may be shared with other family members (Johnson & Brensinger, 2000).

The timing of genetic counseling is important. The ideal time is before the first pregnancy. Some couples take this step before committing themselves to marriage, offering out of compassion for the partner not to involve him or her in a marriage commitment if children of the marriage would be subject to an inherited disorder. Other couples first become aware of a need for genetic counseling after the birth of a child with a disorder. Couples who seek counseling after a first affected child is born need counseling before a second pregnancy occurs. They are not ready for this, however, until the initial shock of their first child's condition and the grief reaction that may accompany it have run their course. Only then are they ready for information and decision making (see Focus on Family Empowerment).

Even if a couple decides not to have any more children, it is important they know that genetic counseling is available should their decision change. They also should be aware that as their children reach reproductive age, they too may benefit from genetic counseling. Couples who might benefit from a referral for genetic counseling may include the following:

- *A couple who has a child with a congenital abnormality or an inborn error of metabolism.* Many congenital abnormalities occur because of teratogenic invasion during pregnancy that is often unrecognized. Learning that the abnormality occurred by chance rather than inheritance is important so the couple does not have to spend the remainder of their child-bearing years in fear that another of their children may be born this way (although a chance circumstance could occur again). If a definite teratogenic agent, such as a

FOCUS ON FAMILY EMPOWERMENT
Genetic Screening

Q. Why do I have to wait so late in pregnancy for genetic studies by amniocentesis?

A. Genetic analysis is done on skin cells obtained from amniotic fluid. The test cannot be scheduled until enough amniotic fluid is present for analysis. Fortunately, this now can be done as early as the 12th week of pregnancy.

Q. Why do laboratories take so long to return karyotyping results?

A. Karyotyping has traditionally (and by necessity) been done on cells at the metaphase (center phase) of division. This means the laboratory has to delay testing until the cells grow to reach this phase. New techniques now allow analysis to be done immediately so that results are available much sooner.

Q. There are no inherited diseases that we know of in our family, but should my husband and I have a karyotype done "just to be sure" before we have our first baby?

A. A genetic analysis is not routinely recommended unless there is evidence or suspicion of disease in the family. Remember that karyotyping only reveals diseases that are present on chromosomes. A "perfect" karyotype doesn't guarantee that a newborn will not be ill in a noninherited way.

Q. If chorionic villi are part of the placenta, how does testing them reveal the chromosome picture of the fetus?

A. Because the fetus and all accessory structures arise from the same single ovum and sperm, the placenta contains the same cells as the fetus.

Q. Do some genetic disorders occur more frequently in some ethnic groups than others?

A. Yes, certain genetic disorders are more commonly found in some ethnic groups because people often marry within their same racial or ethnic group. β-Thalassemia, for example, occurs most frequently in families of Greek or Italian background. α-Thalassemia occurs most often in persons from the Philippines or Southeast Asia. Sickle cell anemia occurs more often in African Americans. Tay-Sachs disease occurs most often in people of Jewish ancestry. It is important that a family at high risk for a particular genetic disorder in this way be informed of the incidence of these disorders and offered genetic screening as appropriate.

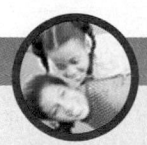

drug the woman took during pregnancy, can be identified, the couple can be advised about preventing this in a future pregnancy.

- *A couple whose close relatives have a child with a genetic disorder, including those with a child who has a congenital abnormality or inborn error of metabolism* (see Focus on Nursing Care Planning).

Many conditions are caused by multifactorial inheritance. It is difficult to predict the expected occurrence of these "familial" or multifactorial disorders. Therefore, counseling should be aimed at educating the couple about the disorder, available treatment,

FOCUS ON *Nursing Care Planning*

A COUPLE CONCERNED ABOUT GENETIC DISORDERS IN FUTURE OFFSPRING

A woman, 29 years of age, comes to the clinic with her spouse. She states, "We want to have a child, but we're concerned that there might be a problem. My brother has hemophilia."

Assessment: Client's past medical history is without evidence of major health problems. One sibling, a brother with hemophilia A. Client's parents without history of disorder or other major health problems. Spouse's past medical history without evidence of problems. States, "My parents, two brothers and sister are all healthy."

Nursing Diagnosis: Health-seeking behaviors related to knowledge of possible genetic disorder inheritance.

Outcome Identification: Couple will verbalize the possible risk for hemophilia in offspring based on results of testing.

Outcome Evaluation: Couple identifies factors associated with risk for hemophilia; voices understanding of genetic testing necessary; states the chances for offspring to have hemophilia.

Interventions	Rationale
1. Obtain a detailed history and physical examination of the client and spouse, including information about family and other relatives. Develop a family pedigree for client and spouse.	1. A thorough history and physical examination provide baseline information to direct the need for follow-up testing. A family pedigree provides additional information about the client's and spouse's family history.
2. Review with the couple the mode of transmission and chances for manifesting hemophilia.	2. Hemophilia is an X-linked recessive disorder with the mother as the carrier of the affected gene on one of her X chromosomes.
3. Prepare the client for genetic counseling and testing. Instruct the couple in the need to evaluate their parents also.	3. Although the parents deny a history of problems, there is the possibility that the client's mother is a carrier for the gene. Genetic counseling and testing will reveal if the client is also a carrier for the disorder.
4. Provide emotional support and guidance to the couple throughout testing. Encourage the use of community resources for additional help.	4. Emotional support from a variety of sources helps to alleviate some of the stress and anxiety associated with genetic testing.

Nursing Diagnosis: Fear related to the outcome of genetic testing.

Outcome Identification: Couple will state that they are able to cope with the results of genetic testing.

Outcome Evaluation: Couple accurately states the chances of offspring having hemophilia; demonstrates positive coping mechanisms throughout testing; actively questions to make informed decisions about child-bearing.

(continued)

Interventions	Rationale
1. Explore the meaning of genetic testing with the couple. Encourage them to verbalize their feelings and concerns. Allow time for questions and answers.	1. Exploration, verbalization, and active questioning provide a safe outlet for feelings, help to increase the other partner's awareness of needs, and open lines of communication.
2. Instruct the couple in positive coping mechanisms. Include activities such as sharing of information, relaxation and breathing exercises, and physical activity.	2. Positive coping mechanisms assist in controlling fear and minimizing its intensity, thus promoting effective problem solving.
3. Review results of testing as available and provide explanations.	3. Explanation enhances the couple's understanding of the implications of the results.
4. Refer couple for additional counseling and to appropriate community resources.	4. Additional counseling and support is necessary for informed decision making. Use of community resources provides additional support and helps reduce feelings of isolation and loneliness.

and the prognosis or outcome. Based on this information, the couple can make an informed reproductive choice.

- *Any individual who is a known balanced translocation carrier.* Understanding of his or her own chromosome structure and the process by which future children could be affected can help the individual make an informed choice about reproduction or can alert him or her to the likely importance of fetal karyotyping during any future pregnancy.
- *Any individual who has an inborn error of metabolism or chromosomal disorder.* Any person with a disease should know the inheritance pattern of the disease and, like those who are balanced translocation carriers, should be aware of prenatal diagnosis, if possible, for his or her particular disorder.
- *A consanguineous (closely related) couple.* The more closely related two people are, the more genes they have in common, so the more likely it is that a recessively inherited disease will be expressed. A brother and sister, for example, have about 50% of their genes in common; first cousins have about 12% of their genes in common.
- *Any woman over 35 years of age and any man over 45 years of age.* This is directly related to the association between advanced parental age and the occurrence of Down syndrome.
- *Couples of ethnic backgrounds in which specific illnesses are known to occur.*

Genetic counseling may result in making individuals feel "well" or free of guilt for the first time in their lives. They may discover that the disorder they were worried about was not an inherited one but was rather a chance occurrence.

In other instances, counseling results in informing individuals that they are carriers of a trait that is responsible for a child's condition. Even when people understand that they have no control over this, knowledge about passing along a genetic abnormality can cause guilt and self-blame. Marriages and relationships can suffer unless both partners are given adequate support.

Nursing Responsibilities

Nurses play important roles in assessing for genetic disorders, in offering support to individuals who seek genetic counseling, and in helping with reproductive genetic testing procedures. Nurses can be instrumental in the following:

- Alerting a couple to what procedures they can expect to undergo
- Explaining how different genetic screening tests are done and when they are usually offered
- Supporting a couple during the wait for test results
- Assisting couples in values clarification, planning, and decision making based on test results

A great deal of time may need to be spent offering support for a grieving couple confronted with the reality of how tragically the laws of inheritance have affected their lives.

Genetic counseling is a role for nurses only if they are adequately prepared in the study of genetics, a curriculum at the graduate level. Without this background, genetic counseling can be dangerous and destructive (see Focus on Multidisciplinary Care).

Whether one is acting as a nursing member of a genetic counseling team or as a genetics counselor, some common principles apply. First, the individual or couple being counseled needs a clear understanding of the information provided. People may listen to the statistics of their situation ("Your child has a 25% chance of having this disease") and misinterpret what they hear. They can construe a "25% chance" to mean that if they have one child with the disease, they can then have three normal children without any worry. A 25% chance, however, means that with each pregnancy, there is a 25% chance the child will have the disease (chance has no "memory" of what has already happened). It is as if the couple has four cards, all aces, with the ace of spades representing the disease. When a card is drawn from the set of four, the chance of its being the ace of spades is 1 in 4 (25%). This principle applies to the first pregnancy and any future pregnancies. When the couple is ready to have a second child, it is as

FOCUS ON MULTIDISCIPLINARY CARE

There are many myths about genetic inheritance. Be certain that other health care personnel, such as unlicensed assistive personnel or laboratory technicians, do not try to interpret the incidence of disorders to couples who are at a health care facility for genetic counseling. A counselor must know the entire circumstances of the disorder for information to be accurate. All health care personnel can help by ensuring that all of a couple's questions have been answered before they leave by alerting and informing the counselor that the couple needs more information, thus facilitating further communication. You can act to ensure that the couple knows the correct number to call and the appropriate person to contact should they have additional questions after they return home or in the future.

FOCUS ON COMMUNICATION

Jill Meier is a 20-year-old woman who is planning on getting married in another month. She is worried because the only two children of her sister were born with cystic fibrosis. Her sister has advised Jill not to have children rather than risk having a child with the disorder.

Less Effective Communication

Nurse: Hello, Miss Meier. What's the reason you've come to the clinic today?

Miss Meier: I'm in kind of a hurry, but I'd like to know what is the chance that my children will have cystic fibrosis, like my sister's children do?

Nurse: If you carry the trait, cystic fibrosis will occur in 25% of your children. That's a rule.

Miss Meier: But if it's already happened twice in my family, doesn't that mean it won't happen as often with my children?

Nurse: Actually, I'd guess there would be a greater chance than normal that your children could get it because it's happened twice to your sister.

Miss Meier: Thanks. It's good to get good information.

More Effective Communication

Nurse: Hello, Miss Meier. What's the reason you've come to the clinic today?

Miss Meier: I'm in kind of a hurry, but I'd like to know what is the chance that my children will have cystic fibrosis, like my sister's children do?

Nurse: Unfortunately, that isn't the kind of question that can be answered off the top of my head in a hurry. Let me ask the nurse practitioner if she can take a family history to get you started toward an answer.

Because we live in an age in which information flows freely, people may believe that predictions about the inheritance of disorders can also be supplied quickly. More important than getting information to people quickly is being certain they are getting it accurately, because people make life-long decisions based on this information.

if the card drawn during the first round is returned to the set, so the chance of drawing the ace of spades in the second draw is exactly the same as in the first draw. Similarly, the couple's chances of having a child with the disease remain 1 in 4 in the second pregnancy.

Second, it is never appropriate for any health care provider to impose his or her own values or opinions on others. Individuals with known inherited diseases in their family must face difficult decisions, such as how much genetic testing to undergo or whether to terminate a pregnancy that will result in a child with a specific genetic disease. Couples need to be made aware of all the options available to them. Then they need to think about the options and make their own decisions. Couples always should understand that nobody is judging their decision, because it must be one with which they can live (see Focus on Communication).

Assessment for the Presence of Genetic Disorders

Genetic counseling begins with careful assessment of the pattern of inheritance in the family. History, physical examination of family members, and laboratory analysis, such as **karyotyping** (a visual presentation of chromosomes), are performed to define the extent of the problem and the chance of inheritance.

History

A detailed family history is obtained to see if any disorders are present in family members. The mother's age is important because some disorders increase in incidence with age. Ethnic background also is important because certain disorders occur more commonly in some ethnic groups than others. If the couple seeking counseling is unfamiliar with the family history, ask them to talk to senior family members about grandparents, aunts, uncles, and so forth before they come for an interview. Ask specifically for instances of spontaneous miscarriage or children in the family who died at birth. In many instances, these children died of unknown chromosomal disorders or were miscarried because of one of the 70 or more known chromosomal abnormalities inconsistent with life.

An extensive prenatal history of any affected person should be obtained to determine if environmental conditions could account for the condition. A family pedigree is done (see Fig. 7-6) to attempt to diagnose the trend of inheritance. Such a diagram not only identifies the possibility of a chromosomal disorder occurring in a particular couple's children but also helps to identify other family members who might benefit from genetic counseling.

Taking a health history for a genetic pedigree determination is often difficult because the facts detailed may evoke uncomfortable emotions such as sorrow, guilt, or inadequacy. Many people may have only sketchy information about their families, such as, "The baby had some kind of nervous disease" or "Her heart didn't work right." Attempt to obtain more information by asking the couple to describe the appearance or activities of the affected individual or asking for permission to obtain health records.

When a child is born dead, parents are advised to have a chromosomal analysis and autopsy performed on the infant. If at some future date they wish genetic counseling, this would allow their genetic counselor to have accurate medical information available.

Physical Assessment

Because genetic disorders often occur in various degrees of expression, a careful physical assessment of any family member with a disorder, that child's siblings, and the couple seeking counseling is needed. It is possible for an individual to have a minimal expression of a disorder and to have gone undiagnosed up to that point. During inspection, pay particular attention to certain body areas, such as the space between the eyes; the height, contour, and shape of ears; and the number of fingers and toes and the presence of webbing. **Dermatoglyphics** (the study of surface markings of the skin) should also be done, noting any abnormal fingerprints or palmar creases, which appear with some disorders. Abnormal hair whorls or coloring can also be present.

Careful inspection of newborns is often sufficient to identify a child with a potential chromosomal disorder. Infants with multiple congenital anomalies, those born at less than 35 weeks' gestation, and those whose parents have had previous children with chromosomal disorders need extremely close assessment. Table 7-1 lists the physical characteristics suggestive of some common inherited syndromes in children.

TABLE 7.1 Common Physical Characteristics of Children With Chromosomal Syndromes

CHARACTERISTIC	PROBABLE SYNDROME
Late closure of fontanelles	Down syndrome
Bossing (prominent forehead)	Fragile X syndrome
Microcephaly	Trisomy 18, trisomy 13
Low-set ears	Trisomy 18, trisomy 13
Slant of eyes	Down syndrome
Epicanthal fold	Down syndrome
Abnormal iris color	Down syndrome
Large tongue	Down syndrome
Prominent jaw	Fragile X syndrome
Low-set hairline	Turner syndrome
Multiple hair whorls	Trisomy 18, trisomy 13
Webbed neck	Turner syndrome
Wide-set nipples	Trisomy 13
Heart abnormalities	Many syndromes
Large hands	Fragile X syndrome
Clinodactyly	Down syndrome
Overriding of fingers	Trisomy 18
Rocker-bottom feet	Trisomy 13
Abnormal dermatoglyphics	Down syndrome
Simian crease on palm	Down syndrome
Absence of secondary sex characteristics	Klinefelter and Turner syndromes

Diagnostic Testing

For genetic counseling to be effective, the exact type of genetic disorder must be identified accurately. Many diagnostic tests are available to provide important clues about possible disorders. Before pregnancy, karyotyping of both parents and an already affected child provides a picture of the chromosome pattern that can be used to predict future children. Once a woman is pregnant, several other tests may be performed to help in the prenatal diagnosis of a genetic disorder. These include AFP analysis, CVS, amniocentesis, percutaneous umbilical blood sampling, sonography, and fetoscopy.

Karyotyping. A karyotype is a visual presentation of the chromosome pattern of an individual. For karyotyping, a sample of peripheral venous blood or a scraping of cells from the buccal membrane is taken. Cells are allowed to grow until they reach a stage of metaphase or are at their most easily observed phase. Then they are stained, placed under a microscope, and photographed. Chromosomes are identified according to size and shape and stain, cut from the photograph, and arranged as in Figure 7-1. Any additional, lacking, or abnormal chromosomes can be visualized by this method.

A new method allows karyotyping to be done immediately, rather than waiting for the cells to reach metaphase. *Fluorescence in situ hybridization (FISH)* staining can be done in interphase as well. This makes it possible for a report to be obtained in only 1 day. New techniques also are available for identifying what cells to use for analysis. A few fetal cells circulate in the maternal bloodstream, most noticeably trophoblasts, lymphocytes, and granulocytes. They are present but few in number during the first and second trimesters but plentiful during the third trimester. There is increasing evidence that such cells can be cultured and used for genetic testing for such disorders as the trisomies.

Barr Body Determination. If a child is born with ambiguous genitalia (it is difficult to determine whether the child is male or female from outward appearance), a Barr body determination, a quick test to evaluate whether the child has two X chromosomes (female), can be done. Only one X chromosome is functional in females; the nondominant one appears to be uninvolved in cell metabolism. Cells are scraped from the buccal membrane of the inner surface of the child's cheek, stained, and then magnified. After staining, the presence of this nondominant X chromosome will appear as a black dot on the edge of the nucleus. It is called a *Barr body*. The presence of a Barr body confirms that the child is chromosomally female. After this quick procedure, the child will need further chromosomal investigation, including a complete karyotype, to reveal his or her complete chromosomal pattern. To be certain the cell stain was adequately absorbed, a known female's buccal membrane scraping is examined as well. Often, this is the mother.

Alpha-fetoprotein Analysis. AFP is a glycoprotein produced by the fetal liver. The level of AFP present in amniotic fluid or maternal serum will differentiate from normal if a chromosomal or a spinal cord disorder is present. Most pregnant women have a serum test done at the 15th week of pregnancy. If the result is abnormal, the amniotic fluid will be assessed. The level is elevated in spinal cord disease (twice the value of the mean for that gestational age) and is decreased in a chromosomal disorder such as trisomy 21. Unfortunately, AFP measured in maternal serum has a false-positive rate of about 30% if the date of conception is not well documented. Use of a "triple study" (AFP, estriol, and hCG) reduces this false-positive rate (Fischbach, 2002). Analysis of a pregnancy-associated plasma protein A that is also increased with a Down syndrome pregnancy and measurement of the fetal neck thickness by sonogram are still other measures used for analysis if a maternal serum AFP test is positive (see Focus on Evidence-Based Practice). Women with an elevated serum result need confirmation by sonogram or amniocentesis and psychological support to face what may be a very grave finding in their infant. Receiving a false-positive report can be devastating to a family during the pregnancy, potentially interfering with bonding with the infant (Hall, Bobrow, & Marteau, 2000; Tercyak et al., 2001).

Chorionic Villi Sampling. CVS involves the retrieval and analysis of chorionic villi for chromosome analysis. Although this procedure may be done as early as week 5 of pregnancy, it is more commonly done at 8 to 10 weeks. With this technique, the chorion cells are located by ultrasound. A thin catheter is then inserted vaginally or a biopsy needle is inserted abdominally or intravaginally, and a number of chorionic cells are removed for analysis (Wilson, 2000; Fig. 7-13). CVS carries a small risk (about 2% to 4%) of causing excessive bleeding, leading to pregnancy loss, and parents should be informed about this risk before the procedure. There also have been some instances of children being born with missing limbs after the procedure (limb reduction syndrome). This has occurred with a high enough frequency that use of the procedure is now limited.

After CVS, the woman should be instructed to report chills or fever suggestive of infection or symptoms of threatened miscarriage (uterine contractions or vaginal bleeding). Women with an Rh-negative blood type need Rh immune globulin administration after the procedure to guard against isoimmunization in the fetus. Amazingly accurate, one test yields no more false-positive results than amniocentesis.

The cells removed in CVS are karyotyped or submitted for DNA analysis to reveal whether the fetus has a genetic disorder. Because chorionic villi cells are rapidly dividing, results are available quickly, perhaps as soon as the fol-

FOCUS ON EVIDENCE-BASED PRACTICE

Should Additional Components Be Added to Triple-Screen Analysis to Reduce False-Positive Findings for Down Syndrome?

The usual screening procedure for Down syndrome during pregnancy consists of analyzing serum levels of alpha-fetoprotein (AFP), unconjugated estriol (E3), and human chorionic gonadotropin (hCG). Unfortunately, AFP testing is associated with false-positive results. To see if additional studies would improve the accuracy of identifying the presence of a Down syndrome baby in utero, researchers added a sonogram scan for humerus length and nuchal thickness (humerus length is shortened in Down syndrome; nuchal thickness is increased). The women used as subjects in this study were all 35 years of age or older. Results of the study showed that 46 cases of Down syndrome were identified in the 2,437 pregnancies (1.9%) examined. Triple-screen analysis alone detected the abnormal pregnancy only 45% of the time. This detection rate rose to 80% for the four-marker method. The researchers suggest that humerus length and nuchal thickness measurement be added to traditional triple-screen measurement as an additional component of pregnancy screening.

Because all women are offered screening for AFP level during pregnancy to attempt to identify open spinal defects or chromosomal abnormalities, nurses working with these women need to be cognizant of the problem involving false-positive results, particularly showing lower-than-normal AFP levels. With this scenario, the woman is told that her fetus may have Down syndrome. To rule this out, she then is asked to have an amniocentesis with karyotyping. In a number of instances, the fetus is shown to be normal; for an unidentified reason, the AFP level was lower than the statistical average. Even though the woman is assured at that point in pregnancy that her fetus is normal, she cannot help but worry throughout the pregnancy that something might still be wrong. Even after the baby is born, women continue to "study" the baby to be certain that the first test was not the accurate one. Thus, any tests that would help rule out these false-positives could have a dramatic effect on the woman's acceptance of her pregnancy.

Since nurses often are the individuals who interact with the parents frequently and who may be asked to convey test results to parents, knowledge of the possibility of false-positive test results for AFP provides a sound evidence base for providing support to the family and helping them understand what is happening as they go through the additional testing that will follow.

Bahado-Singh, R. O., Oz, A. U., Gomez, K., Hunter, D., Copel, J., Baumgarten, A., & Mahoney, M. J. (2000). Combined ultrasound biometry, serum markers and age for Down syndrome risk estimation. *Ultrasound in Obstetrics & Gynecology, 15*(3), 199–204.

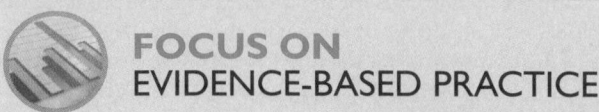

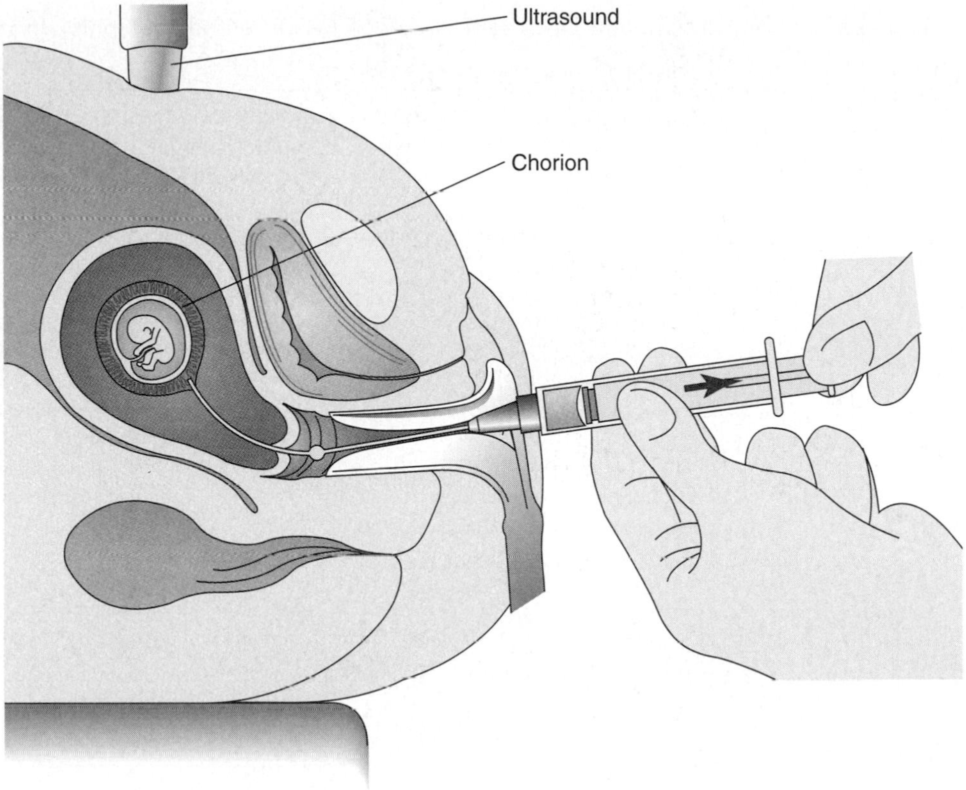

FIGURE 7.13 Chorionic villi sampling. Since the villi arise from trophoblast cells, their chromosome structure is the same as the fetus's.

lowing day. If a twin or multiple pregnancy is present, with two or more separate placentas, cells should be removed separately from each placenta. Because fraternal twins are derived from separate ova, one twin could have a chromosomal abnormality while the other is normal (Jenkins & Wapner, 2000).

Not all inherited diseases can be detected by CVS. Parents need to know that only those disorders involving abnormal chromosomes, nondisjunction, or those whose gene location or specific DNA disorder is known can be identified by CVS. The test does not reveal the extent of spinal cord abnormalities.

Table 7-2 shows common chromosomal nondisjunction disorders that can be diagnosed prenatally through karyotyping. Other conditions, such as cystic fibrosis, muscular dystrophy, and Huntington chorea, are identified by gene markers on individual chromosomes.

The decision to undergo CVS is a major one for a couple. As a rule, they are not making a decision simply for CVS. If the CVS reveals that their child is abnormal, they will be asked to make a decision about the future of the pregnancy.

Deciding to terminate a pregnancy is rarely easy. The couple may need a great deal of support with their decision, both to carry it through and afterward. Also, if they decide not to terminate the pregnancy, they will need support during the remainder of the pregnancy and in the days after birth. It may be difficult for a couple to believe that what the test showed is true. Only when they inspect the baby and see that the test was accurate—that the child does have Down syndrome, for example—do they see the reality. The result may be a long-lasting depression.

Amniocentesis. Amniocentesis is the withdrawal of amniotic fluid through the abdominal wall for analysis at the 14th to 16th week of pregnancy. Analysis may include the karyotyping of skin cells obtained or analysis of AFP or acetylcholinesterase. Assessing for acetylcholinesterase, a breakdown product of blood, helps to reduce false-positive results. If the acetylcholinesterase result is negative, it confirms that an elevated AFP level is not a false-positive reading from blood in the fluid. Some disorders, such as Tay-Sachs disease, can be identified by the lack of a specific enzyme, such as hexosaminidase A, in amniotic fluid. Because amniocentesis is also a common assessment for fetal maturity, it is discussed further in Chapter 8 (see also Fig. 8-14).

New techniques of amniocentesis allow it to be done as early as the 12th week of pregnancy. Although less amniotic fluid can be removed at this time (only about 2 mL compared to the 5-mL sample obtained later), it is enough fluid for genetic testing. For the procedure, a pocket of amniotic fluid is located by sonography. Then a needle is inserted transabdominally and fluid is aspirated. Skin cells in the fluid are karyotyped for chromosomal number and structure. The level of AFP is analyzed. Amniocentesis has the advantage over CVS of carrying only a 0.5% risk of spontaneous miscarriage. Unfortunately, it is usually not done until the 14th to 16th week of pregnancy. This may prove to be a difficult time because by this date, the

TABLE 7.2 Chromosomal Nondisjunction Disorders That Can Be Detected by Amniocentesis or CVS

SYNDROME	CHROMOSOMAL CHARACTERISTICS	CLINICAL SIGNS
Down syndrome	Extra chromosome 21	Cognitively challenged Protruding tongue Epicanthal folds Hypotonia
Translocation Down syndrome	Translocation of a chromosome, perhaps 14/21	Same clinical signs as trisomy 21
Trisomy 18	Extra chromosome 18	Cognitively challenged Congenital malformations
Trisomy 13	Extra chromosome 13	Cognitively challenged Multiple congenital malformations Eye agenesis
Cri-du-chat syndrome	Deletion of short arm of chromosome 5	Cognitively challenged Facial structure anomalies Peculiar cat-like cry
Fragile X syndrome	Distortion of the X chromosome	Cognitively challenged
Philadelphia chromosome	Deletion of one arm of chromosome 21	Chronic granulocytic leukemia
Turner syndrome	Only one X chromosome present	Short stature Streak gonads Infertility Webbed neck
Klinefelter syndrome	An extra X chromosome present (XXY)	Small testes Gynecomastia Infertility

woman is beginning to accept her pregnancy and bond with the fetus. In addition, termination of pregnancy during the second trimester can be difficult. Women need support to wait for the procedure, to wait for test results, and to make a decision about the pregnancy. Women with an Rh-negative blood type need Rh immune globulin administration after the procedure to protect against isoimmunization in the fetus. All women need to be observed for about 30 minutes after the procedure to be certain that labor contractions are not beginning and that the fetal heart rate remains within normal limits.

Percutaneous Umbilical Blood Sampling. Percutaneous umbilical blood sampling (PUBS) is the removal of blood from the umbilical cord using an amniocentesis technique (Fig. 7-14). This allows more rapid karyotyping than is possible when only skin cells are removed (Tongsong et al., 2000). PUBS is discussed further in Chapter 8.

Sonography. Sonography is a diagnostic tool that is helpful in assessing a fetus for general size and structural disorders of the internal organs, spine, and limbs. Because some genetic disorders are associated with congenital defects, sonography may be helpful. Sonography may be used concurrently with amniocentesis because it causes no apparent risk to the fetus.

Fetoscopy. Fetoscopy is the insertion of a fiberoptic fetoscope through a small incision in the mother's abdomen into the uterus and membranes to inspect the fetus for gross abnormalities. It can be used to confirm a sonography finding, remove skin cells for DNA analysis, or perform surgery for a congenital defect such as a stenosed urethra.

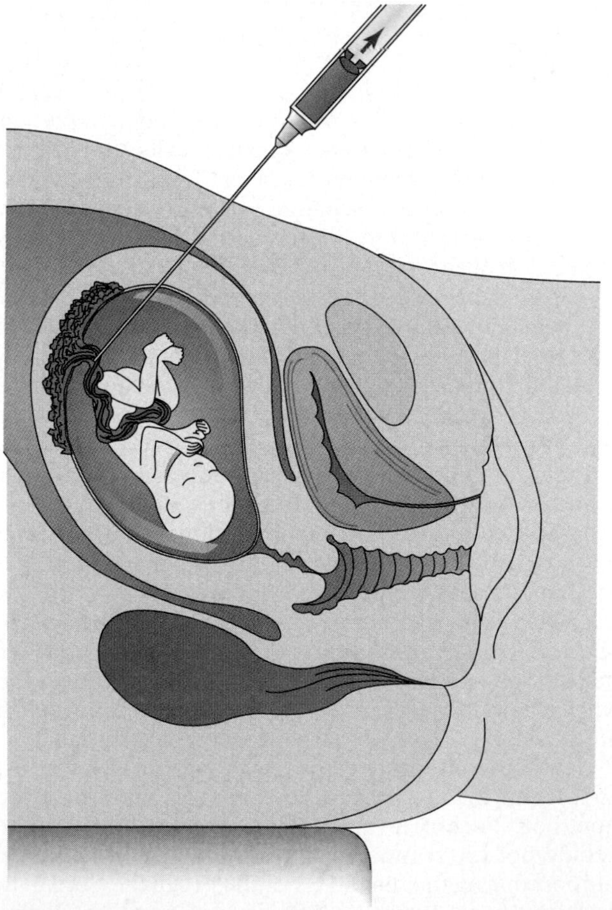

FIGURE 7.14 Percutaneous umbilical blood sampling. Blood is withdrawn from the cord using amniocentesis technique.

Preimplantation Diagnosis. Although currently not recommended, in the future it may be possible for a fertilized embryo to be removed from the uterus by lavage before implantation, with cells from the zona pellucida removed and biopsied for DNA or cell analysis. The ovum would then be reinserted or not, depending on the findings and the parents' wishes. This would provide genetic information extremely early in a pregnancy. The technique is currently possible with the embryo transfer procedures used in fertility treatment. This technique may also allow healthy genes to be inserted to correct underlying disorders very early in pregnancy.

✔ CHECKPOINT QUESTIONS

7. When is the ideal time for genetic counseling?
8. What two principles apply to all genetic counseling?
9. Which diagnostic test provides a visual presentation of an individual's chromosomal pattern?
10. Why is CVS used less today than formerly?

Reproductive Alternatives

Some couples are reluctant to seek genetic counseling because they are afraid they will be told it would be unwise to have children. Helping them to realize that viable alternatives for having a family exist for them allows them to seek the help they need.

Artificial insemination by donor (AID) is an option for couples in whom the genetic disorder is one inherited by the male partner or is a recessively inherited disorder carried by both partners. AID is available in all major communities and may permit the couple to experience the satisfaction and enjoyment of a normal pregnancy.

If the inherited problem is one arising from the female partner, use of a surrogate mother (a woman who agrees to be artificially inseminated by the male partner's sperm and bear a child for the couple) is a possibility. Donor egg transfer (an ovum is taken from a donor, fertilized in the laboratory by the husband's sperm, and then implanted in the wife's uterus) is another possibility. Like AID, donor embryo transfer offers the couple a chance to experience a normal pregnancy. All these procedures are expensive and, depending on individual circumstances, may have disappointing success rates. They are discussed in more detail in Chapter 6.

Termination of a pregnancy that reveals a chromosomal or metabolic abnormality is another option. Diagnosis of a disorder during pregnancy and prompt treatment at birth to minimize the prognosis and outcome of the disorder is another possibility.

Adoption is an alternative many couples find rewarding (see Chaps. 2 and 6). Also, choosing to remain child-free should not be discounted as a viable option. Many couples who have every reason to think they would have normal children choose this alternative because they believe their existence is full and rewarding without the presence of children.

Couples need support from health care personnel to decide on the alternative that is correct for them. It is most important for a couple to select the option that is right for them, not one that they sense a counselor feels would be best. They may need to consider the ethical philosophy or beliefs of other family members when making their decision, although ultimately they must do what they believe is best.

Legal and Ethical Aspects of Genetic Screening and Counseling

Nurses can be instrumental in seeing that couples who seek genetic counseling receive results in a timely manner and with compassion about what the results may mean to future child-bearing. Nurses who participate in genetic screening or counseling must keep in mind several legal responsibilities (Carson, 2000), including the following:

- Participation in genetic screening must be elective.
- People desiring genetic screening must sign an informed consent for the procedures.
- Results must be interpreted correctly and provided to the individuals as quickly as possible.
- The results must not be withheld from the individuals and must be given only to those persons directly involved.
- After genetic counseling, persons must not be coerced to undergo procedures such as abortion or sterilization. Any procedure must be a free and individual decision.

Failure to heed these guidelines could result in charges of invasion of privacy, breach of confidentiality, or psychological injury caused by "labeling" someone or imparting unwarranted fear and worry about the significance of a disease or carrier state. All couples who seek counseling and are identified as being at risk for having a child with a genetic disorder must be informed of the risk and offered appropriate diagnostic procedures such as amniocentesis. "Wrongful birth" lawsuits have been initiated against health care providers for not making this information available to couples.

Genetic screening and counseling can raise serious ethical questions for a couple, particularly when they choose to terminate a pregnancy based on CVS or amniocentesis findings. Some people argue that a decision to abort a child based just on the strong possibility that the child would be mentally or physically challenged is unethical. The problem becomes even more difficult when a disorder that affects only male or only female offspring is present. For instance, a woman who carries the gene for an X-linked disorder for which there is no prenatal screening test might choose to abort all male fetuses, although each will have a 50% chance of not inheriting the disease. Another dilemma can occur if it is discovered that a twin pregnancy includes one normal and one affected child.

It is important to remember that the choice to be made is the couple's, not the counselor's. A useful place to start counseling might be with values clarification, to be certain the couple understands what is most important to them.

WHAT IF? A woman is pregnant with twins. One twin fetus is diagnosed as having Down syndrome and the other is not. Would it be ethical for her to attempt to abort the affected child when the procedure also might endanger the child without the disorder?

COMMON CHROMOSOMAL DISORDERS RESULTING IN PHYSICAL OR COGNITIVE DEVELOPMENTAL DISORDERS

A number of chromosomal disorders may be detected at birth on physical examination. The most common chromosomal disorders revealed this way are nondisjunction syndromes. Many of these disorders leave children cognitively challenged. Care of the child who is cognitively challenged is discussed in Chapter 54.

Trisomy 13 Syndrome

In *trisomy 13 syndrome* (Patau syndrome), children have an extra chromosome 13 and are severely cognitively challenged. The incidence is low, approximately 0.45 per 1,000 live births. Midline body disorders are present, and common findings include microcephaly with abnormalities of the forebrain and forehead; eyes that are smaller than normal (microphthalmos) or absent; cleft lip and palate; low-set ears; heart defects, particularly ventricular septal defects; and abnormal genitalia. Most of these children do not survive beyond early childhood (see Fig. 7-12).

Trisomy 18 Syndrome

Children with *trisomy 18 syndrome* have three number-18 chromosomes. They are severely cognitively challenged. The incidence is approximately 0.23 per 1,000 live births. These children tend to be small for gestational age at birth and have markedly low-set ears, a small jaw, congenital heart defects, and misshapen fingers and toes (the index finger tends to deviate or cross over other fingers). Also, the soles of their feet are often rounded instead of flat (rocker-bottom feet). Most of these children do not survive beyond early infancy.

Cri-du-Chat Syndrome

Cri-du-chat syndrome is the result of a missing portion of chromosome 5. In addition to an abnormal cry, which is much more like the sound of a cat's than a human infant's, children with cri-du-chat syndrome tend to have a small head, wide-set eyes, and a downward slant to the palpebral fissure of the eye. They are severely cognitively challenged.

Turner Syndrome

The child with *Turner syndrome* (gonadal dysgenesis; 45XO) has only one functional X chromosome. The child is short in stature. The hairline at the nape of the neck is low-set, and the neck may appear to be webbed and short (Muscari, 2001). The newborn may have appreciable edema of the hands and feet and a number of congenital anomalies, most frequently coarctation (stricture) of the aorta and kidney disorders. The child has only streak (small and nonfunctional) gonads, so that with the exception of pubic hair secondary sex characteristics do not develop at puberty. Lack of ovarian function results in sterility. The incidence is approximately 1 per 10,000 live births. With Barr body determination on karyotyping, the child is shown to have only one X chromosome (no Barr body present).

Although children with Turner syndrome may be severely cognitively challenged, difficulties in this area are more commonly limited to learning disabilities. Socioemotional adjustment problems often accompany the syndrome as well because of the lack of fertility and if the nuchal folds are prominent.

Growth hormone may help children with Turner syndrome to achieve additional height. If treatment with estrogen is begun at approximately age 13 years, secondary sex characteristics will appear. If females continue taking estrogen for 3 out of every 4 weeks, they will have withdrawal bleeding that results in a menstrual flow. This flow, however, does not correct the problem of sterility. Gonadal tissue is scant and inadequate for ovulation because of the basic chromosomal aberration.

Klinefelter Syndrome

Infants with *Klinefelter syndrome* are males with an XXY chromosome pattern (47XXY). Characteristics of the syndrome may not be noticeable at birth. At puberty, the child has poorly developed secondary sex characteristics and small testes that produce ineffective sperm. Affected individuals tend to develop gynecomastia (increased breast size). The incidence is about 1 per 1,000 live births. Karyotyping can be used to reveal the additional X chromosome present (Rogers, 2000).

Fragile X Syndrome

Fragile X syndrome is an X-linked pattern of inheritance in which one long arm of an X chromosome is defective (Welch & Williams, 1999). The incidence is about 1 in 1,000 live births. It is the most common cause of cognitive challenge in boys.

Before puberty, boys with fragile X syndrome typically have maladaptive behaviors such as hyperactivity and autism. They have reduced intellectual functioning, with marked deficits in speech and arithmetic. They may be identified by the presence of a large head, a long face with a high forehead, a prominent lower jaw, and large protruding ears. Hyperextensive joints and cardiac disorders may also be present. After puberty, enlarged testicles may become evident. Affected individuals are fertile and can reproduce.

Carrier females may show some evidence of the physical and cognitive characteristics. Although intellectual function from the syndrome cannot be improved, both folic acid and phenothiazine administration may improve symptoms of poor concentration and impulsivity.

Down Syndrome (Trisomy 21)

Trisomy 21, the most frequent chromosomal abnormality, occurs in about 1 in 800 live births. It occurs most frequently in the pregnancies of women who are over 35 years of age (the incidence is as high as 1 in 100 live births for these women). Paternal age (over 55) may also contribute to the increased incidence in this age group (Chung, 2000).

The physical features of children with Down syndrome are so marked that fetal diagnosis is possible by sonography in utero. The nose is broad and flat. The eyelids have an extra fold of tissue at the inner canthus (an epicanthal fold), and the palpebral fissure (opening between the eyelids) tends to slant laterally upward. The iris of the eye may have white specks in it, called Brushfield spots. Even in the newborn, the tongue may protrude from the mouth because the oral cavity is smaller than normal. The back of the head is flat, the neck is short, and an extra pad of fat at the base of the head causes the skin to be so loose it can be lifted up (like a puppy's neck). The ears may be low-set. Muscle tone is poor, giving the baby a rag-doll appearance. This can be so lax that the child's toe can be touched against the nose (not possible in the average mature newborn). The fingers of many children with Down syndrome are short and thick, and the little finger is often curved inward. There may be a wide space between the first and second toes and first and second fingers. The palm of the hand shows a peculiar crease (a simian line) or a horizontal palm crease rather than the normal three creases in the palm (Fig. 7-15).

Children with Down syndrome usually are cognitively challenged to some degree. The challenge can range from that of an educable child (intelligence quotient [IQ] of 50 to 70) to one who is profoundly affected (IQ less than 20). The extent of the cognitive challenge is not evident at birth. Educable children may represent mosaic chromosomal patterns. The fact that the brain is not developing well is evidenced by a head size that is generally under the 10th or 20th percentile at well-child visits.

These children appear to have altered immune function and thus are prone to upper respiratory infections. Congenital heart disease, especially atrioventricular defects, is common. Stenosis or atresia of the duodenum, strabismus, and cataract disorders are also common. For unknown reasons, acute lymphocytic leukemia occurs approximately 20 times more frequently in children with Down syndrome than in the general population. Even if children are born without an accompanying disorder such as heart disease, their lifespan generally is only 40 to 50 years because aging seems to occur faster than normal.

Children with Down syndrome need to be exposed to early educational and play opportunities (Freeman & Kasari, 2002; see Chap. 54). Because they are prone to infections, sensible precautions such as using good handwashing technique are important when caring for them. The enlarged tongue may interfere with swallowing and cause choking unless the child is fed slowly. As with all newborns, these infants need physical examination at birth to enable detection of the genetic disorder and initiation of parental counseling and support.

✔ CHECKPOINT QUESTIONS

11. What is the genetic abnormality seen with Turner syndrome?
12. Are all children with Down syndrome severely cognitively challenged?

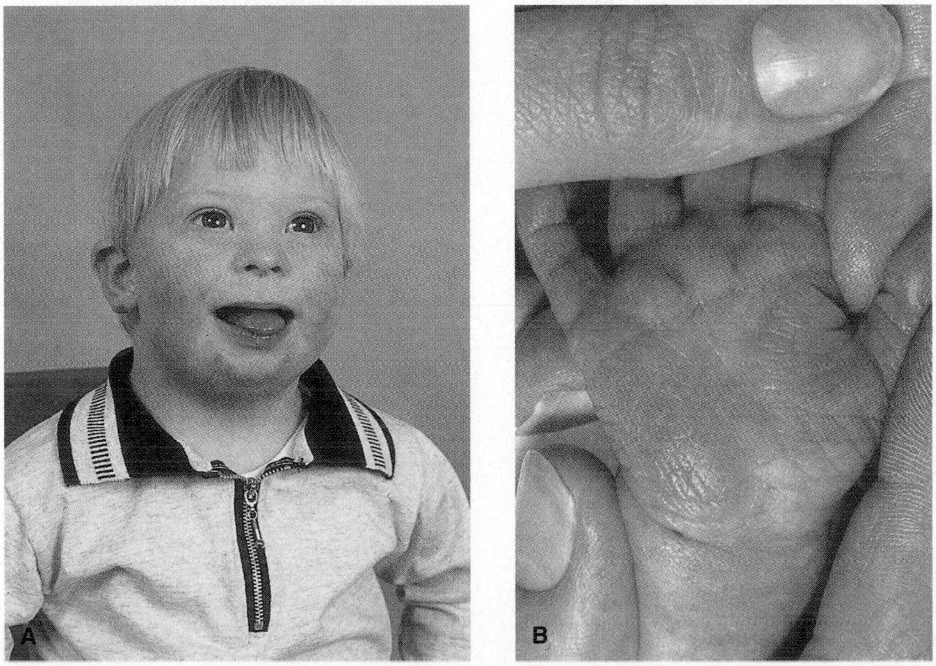

FIGURE 7.15 (*A*) Typical facial features of the child with Down syndrome. (*B*) A simian line, a horizontal crease seen in children with Down syndrome.

KEY POINTS

Genetic disorders are disorders resulting from a defect in structure or number of genes or chromosomes. Genetics is the study of how and why such disorders occur.

A phenotype is a person's outward appearance. Genotype refers to the actual gene composition. A person's genome is the complete set of genes present. A karyotype is a graphic representation of chromosomes present.

A person is homozygous if he or she has two like genes for a trait and heterozygous if he or she has two unlike genes for a trait.

Mendelian laws can predict the likely incidence of recessive or dominant diseases in offspring. Division disorders including nondisjunction abnormalities, deletion, translocation, and mosaicism also create genetic disorders.

Genetic counseling can be a role for nurses if they receive proper preparation and education. Assessment of genetic disorders consists of a health history, physical examination, and diagnostic studies such as chorionic villi sampling, amniocentesis, alpha-fetoprotein analysis, and Barr body determinations.

Some karyotyping tests, such as chorionic villi sampling and amniocentesis, introduce a risk of spontaneous or threatened miscarriage. Be certain that women undergoing these tests remain in the health care facility for at least 30 minutes after a procedure to be certain that a complication such as vaginal bleeding, uterine cramping, or abnormal fetal heart rates is not present. Women with an Rh-negative blood type need Rh immune globulin administration after these procedures.

An important aspect of genetic counseling is respecting a couple's right to privacy. Be certain that information remains confidential and is not given indiscriminately to others, including other family members.

People who are told that a genetic abnormality does exist in their family may suffer a loss of self-esteem. Offering support to help them deal with the feelings they experience is an important nursing intervention.

Common nondisjunction genetic disorders include Down syndrome (trisomy 21), trisomy 13, trisomy 18, Turner syndrome, and Klinefelter syndrome. Most of these syndromes include some degree of cognitive challenge.

CRITICAL THINKING EXERCISES

1. Mrs. Alvarez, whom you met at the beginning of the chapter, didn't know her family history. What questions would you want to ask about her husband's family? Suppose Mr. Alvarez tells you that he had two brothers who died at birth. Would that finding be important?
2. Suppose a couple knows that they both carry a gene for a recessively inherited disorder, yet they have had five children and none of the children shows symptoms of the disorder. Is it possible for them to have had five children without any symptoms of the disease? What are the chances their sixth child will also be disease-free?
3. A 26-year-old woman seen in a prenatal clinic has a twin sister with Down syndrome. The client has been afraid until now to have a child because of the chance her child will also have the syndrome. She states, "My family has always been so ashamed that a genetic defect could happen in our family."
   a. Why would a genetic syndrome appear in one twin and not the other this way?
   b. What does the client's statement about her family feeling ashamed reveal about her knowledge of genetic disorders?
   c. Would it be realistic to assure the client that her child will not have Down syndrome?
   d. What genetic tests would you anticipate that the client will have ordered during pregnancy to detect the possibility of Down syndrome in her child?
   e. Suppose the client is so worried that her child has the syndrome that she decides to abort her fetus and remain childless rather than undergo genetic testing. Is this her right? What would be her fetus' rights?
4. Examine the National Health Goals related to genetics or genetic counseling. Most government-sponsored money for nursing research is allotted based on these goals. What would be a possible research topic to explore pertinent to these goals that would be fundable and would advance evidence-based practice?

REFERENCES

Bahado-Singh, R.O., et al. (2000). Combined ultrasound biometry, serum markers and age for Down syndrome risk estimation. *Ultrasound in Obstetrics & Gynecology, 15*(3), 199–204.

Carson, W. Y. (2000). Legal issues associated with genetics. *Nursing Clinics of North America, 35*(3), 719–729.

Chung, E. K. (2000). Down (Trisomy 21) syndrome. In M. W. Schwartz. *The 5-minute pediatric consult* (pp. 336–337). Philadelphia: Lippincott Williams & Wilkins.

Department of Health and Human Services. (2000). *Healthy people 2010.* Washington, DC: DHHS.
Fischbach, F. (2002). *A manual of laboratory and diagnostic tests* (3rd ed.). Philadelphia: Lippincott Williams & Wilkins.
Freeman, S. F. & Kasari, C. (2002). Characteristics and qualities of the play dates of children with Down syndrome. *American Journal of Mental Retardation, 107*(1), 16-31.
Hall, S., Bobrow, M., & Marteau, T. M. (2000). Psychological consequences for parents of false negative results on prenatal screening for Down's syndrome: Retrospective interview study. *British Medical Journal, 320*(7232), 407-412.
Jenkins, T. M., & Wapner, R. J. (2000). The challenge of prenatal diagnosis in twin pregnancies. *Current Opinion in Obstetrics & Gynecology, 12*(2), 87-92.
Johnson, K. A., & Brensinger, J. D. (2000). Genetic counseling and testing: Implications for clinical practice. *Nursing Clinics of North America, 35*(3), 615-626.
Lam, L. W. & MacKenzie, A. E. (2002). Coping with a child with Down syndrome. *Qualitative Health Research, 12*(2), 223-237.
Muscari, M. E. (2001). *Advanced pediatric clinical assessment.* Philadelphia: Lippincott Williams & Wilkins.
Qumsiyeh, M. B., et al. (2001). Cytogenetics. In Elzouki, A. Y., Harfi, H. A. & Nazer, H. M. *Textbook of clinical pediatrics* (pp. 20-32). Philadelphia: Lippincott Williams & Wilkins.
Rogers, M. A. (2000). Understanding Klinefelter's syndrome. *Nurse Practitioner, 25*(5), 116-119.
Tercyak, K. P., et al. (2001). Psychological response to prenatal genetic counseling and amniocentesis. *Patient Education & Counseling, 43*(1), 73-84.
Tongsong, T. et al. (2000). Cordocentesis at 16-24 weeks of gestation: Experience of 1,320 cases. *Prenatal Diagnosis, 20*(3), 224-228.
Welch, J. L., & Williams, J. K. (1999). Fragile X syndrome. *Neonatal Network, 18*(6), 15-22.
Wilson, R. D. (2000). Amniocentesis and chorionic villus sampling. *Current Opinion in Obstetrics & Gynecology, 12*(2), 81-86.

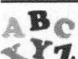

ABC XYZ SUGGESTED READINGS

Antsaklis, A., et al. (2000). Genetic amniocentesis in women 20-34 years old: Associated risks. *Prenatal Diagnosis, 20*(23), 247-250.
Bourguignon, A., Briscoe, B., & Nemzer, L. (1999). Genetic abortion: Considerations for patient care. *Journal of Perinatal & Neonatal Nursing, 13*(2), 47-58.
Cate, S. & Ball, S. (2000). Multiple marker screening for Down syndrome: Whom should we screen? *Journal of the American Board of Family Practice, 12*(5), 367-374.
Davis, J., Krasnewich, D., & Puck, J. M. (2000). Genetic testing and screening in pediatric populations. *Nursing Clinics of North America, 35*(3), 643-651.
Grimes, D. A., & Snively, G. R. (1999). Patients' understanding of the medical risks: Implications for genetic counseling. *Obstetrics & Gynecology, 93*(6), 910-914.
Kenner, C., & Dreyer, L. A. (2000). Prenatal and neonatal testing and screening: A double-edged sword. *Nursing Clinics of North America, 35*(3), 627-642.
Kocun, C. C., et al. (2000). Changing trends in patient decisions concerning genetic amniocentesis. *American Journal of Obstetrics & Gynecology, 182*(5), 1018-1020.
Lewin, M. B. (2000). The genetic basis of congenital heart disease. *Pediatric Annals, 29*(8), 469-481.
Matthews, A. L. (1999). Chromosomal abnormalities: Trisomy 18, trisomy 13, deletions, and microdeletions. *Journal of Perinatal & Neonatal Nursing, 13*(2), 59-75.
Newberger, D. S. (2000). Down syndrome: Perinatal risk assessment and diagnosis. *American Family Physician, 62*(4), 825-832.
Ross, J., Zinn, A., & McCauley, E. (2000). Neurodevelopmental and psychosocial aspects of Turner syndrome. *Mental Retardation & Developmental Disabilities Research Reviews, 6*(2), 135-141.
Wertz, D. C. & Knoppers, B. M. (2002). Serious genetic disorders: Can or should they be defined? *American Journal of Medical Genetics, 108*(1), 29-35.

The Growing Fetus

CHAPTER 8

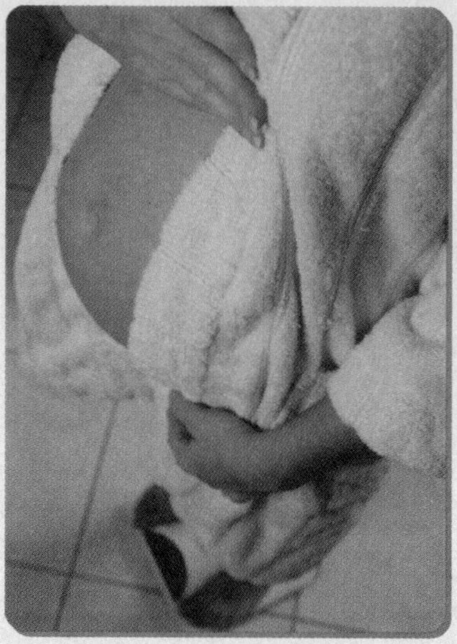

Key Terms

- amniocentesis
- amniotic cavity
- amniotic membrane
- blastocyst
- cephalocaudal
- chorionic membrane
- chorionic villi
- coelocentesis
- corona radiata
- cotyledons
- decidua basalis
- decidua capsularis
- decidua vera
- ductus arteriosus
- ductus venosus
- ectoderm
- embryo
- entoderm
- estimated date of birth
- fertilization
- fetoscopy
- fetus
- foramen ovale
- hydramnios
- implantation
- lightening
- McDonald's Rule
- mesoderm
- morula
- neural plate
- nonstress test
- oligohydramnios
- organogenesis
- quickening
- surfactant
- trophoblast
- umbilical cord
- Wharton's jelly
- yolk sac
- zona pellucida
- zygote

Objectives

After mastering the contents of this chapter, you should be able to:

1. Describe the growth and development of the fetus by gestation week.
2. Assess fetal growth and development through maternal and pregnancy landmarks.
3. Formulate nursing diagnoses related to the needs of the pregnant woman and the fetus.
4. Establish outcome criteria that meet the needs of the growing fetus.
5. Plan nursing care that promotes healthy fetal growth.
6. Implement nursing care to help ensure a safe pregnancy outcome and a safe fetal environment.
7. Evaluate expected outcomes for achievement and effectiveness of care.
8. Identify National Health Goals related to fetal growth that nurses can help the nation to achieve.
9. Identify areas of fetal health that could benefit from additional nursing research or application of evidence-based practice.
10. Use critical thinking to analyze ways to promote fetal growth and development.
11. Integrate knowledge of fetal growth and development with nursing process to achieve quality maternal and child health nursing care.

Liz Calhorn, an 18-year-old, is 20 weeks pregnant. Although she says she knows she should stop smoking during pregnancy, she has not been able to do this. Twice during the pregnancy (at the 4th and 10th week), she drank beer at summer picnics. Today, at a clinic visit, she tells you that she has felt her fetus move. She states, "Feeling the baby move made me realize there's someone inside me, you know what I mean? I didn't think of this as having a baby before, just being pregnant. It made me know it's time I started being more careful with what I do."

Feeling a fetus move this way is often the trigger that makes having a baby "real" for many women. The more women know about fetal development, the easier it is for them to begin to think of the pregnancy not as something interesting happening to them, but as something that is producing a separate life.

Previous chapters described preparation for childbearing, including health promotion, infertility, and genetics. This chapter adds information about fetal growth and development and assessment of fetal health.

After you've studied the chapter, answer the Critical Thinking Exercises at the end of the chapter and then access the on-line study activities (http://connection.lww.com) *to further sharpen your skills and test your knowledge.*

FOCUS ON NATIONAL HEALTH GOALS

A number of National Health Goals address fetal growth. These are:

- Reduce the fetal death rate (death below 20 or more weeks of gestation) to no more than 5 per 1,000 live births from a baseline of 7.6/1,000.
- Reduce low birthweight to an incidence of no more than 5% of live births and very low birthweight to no more than 1% of live births from baselines of 6.8% and 1.2% (DHHS, 2000).

Nurses can be instrumental in helping the nation achieve these goals by urging women to plan their pregnancies so they can enter a pregnancy in good health. Educating women about the importance of attending prenatal care is another vital role. Nursing research in such areas as why women avoid prenatal care or how soon women make lifestyle changes during pregnancy could help lead to achievement of these National Health Goals.

Throughout history, different societies have held a variety of beliefs and superstitions about the way the **fetus** (the infant during intrauterine life) grows. Medieval artists depicted the child in utero completely formed as a miniature man. Leonardo da Vinci, in his notebooks of 1510 to 1512, made several sketches of unborn infants that indicated he believed the fetus was immobile and essentially a part of the mother, sharing her blood and internal organs. During the 17th and 18th centuries, a baby was thought to form to a miniature size in the mother's ovaries; when male cells were introduced, the baby expanded to birth size. A second theory was that the child existed in the head of the sperm cell as a fully formed being, the uterus serving only as an incubator in which it grew. It was not until 1758 that Kaspar Wolff proposed that both parents contribute equally to the structure of the baby. Thanks to the work of modern medical researchers and photographers who have been able to capture the process of fertilization and fetal development using enhanced, high-tech photography, there is now a clear idea of what the fetus looks like from the moment of conception until birth. Surveillance of the fetus by ultrasound documents this growth process.

The fetus grows and develops steadily during this time. To increase the health of fetuses during pregnancy, several National Health Goals have been devised (see Focus on National Health Goals).

NURSING PROCESS OVERVIEW

For Helping Ensure Fetal Health

Assessment

The predictable stages of fetal development provide a guide for determining the well-being of an individual fetus. Health care providers can also use these stages as guidelines to predict more accurately the expected date of birth. For the expectant family, knowledge about fetal growth and development can provide an important frame of reference, helping the mother to understand some of the changes going on in her body and allowing all family members to begin thinking about and accepting the newest member of their family before the baby actually arrives. Conveying the findings gained from fetal assessment in as much detail as parents request is an important nursing role.

Nursing Diagnosis

Common nursing diagnoses related to growth and development of the fetus focus on the mother and family as well as the fetus. Examples include:

- Health-seeking behaviors related to knowledge of normal fetal development
- Anxiety related to lack of fetal movement
- Deficient knowledge related to need for good prenatal care for healthy fetal development

Outcome Identification and Planning

Goals and outcome criteria established for teaching about fetal growth should be realistic and based on the parents' knowledge and desire for information. When additional assessment measures are necessary, such as an amniocentesis or an ultrasound examination, it is important to include this material in the teaching plan, explaining why further assessment is necessary and what the parents can expect.

Implementation

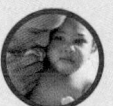

Teaching parents about fetal growth and development helps them to visualize the fetus at each stage of development. This, in turn, helps them to understand the importance of implementing healthy behaviors, such as eating well and avoiding substances that may be dangerous to the fetus. Viewing a sonogram may help initiate bonding between the parents and the infant. Chapters 11 and 12 discuss specific health maintenance teaching measures that are vital to fetal health and well-being.

Outcome Evaluation

Outcome evaluation related to fetal growth and development usually focuses on determining whether the mother or family has made any changes in lifestyle to ensure fetal growth and whether the mother voices confidence that her baby is healthy and growing normally. Examples of expected outcomes are:

- Parents describe smoke-free living at next prenatal visit.
- Client records number of movements of fetus for 1 hour daily.
- Couple attends prenatal care regularly.

STAGES OF FETAL DEVELOPMENT

In just 38 weeks, a fertilized egg matures from a single cell carrying all the necessary genetic material to a fully developed fetus ready to be born. Table 8-1 lists common terms used to describe the fetus at various stages in this growth.

Fetal growth and development is typically divided into three periods: pre-embryonic (first 2 weeks, beginning with fertilization), embryonic (weeks 3 through 8), and fetal (from week 8 through birth).

Fertilization: The Beginning of Pregnancy

Fertilization is the union of the ovum and a spermatozoon. Other terms used to describe this phenomenon are conception, impregnation, or fecundation. Fertilization usually occurs in the outer third of a fallopian tube, the ampullar portion. Because the functional life of a spermatozoon is about 48 hours, possibly as long as 72 hours, the total critical time span during which fertilization may occur is about 72 hours (48 hours before ovulation plus 24 hours afterward).

After ovulation, as the ovum is extruded from the graafian follicle, it is surrounded by a ring of mucopolysaccharide fluid (the **zona pellucida**) and a circle of cells (the **corona radiata**). These structures increase the bulk of the ovum, facilitating its migration to the uterus. They probably also serve as protection from injury. The ovum and surrounding cells are propelled into the near fallopian tube by currents initiated by the fimbriae, the fine, hairlike structures that line the openings of the fallopian tubes. Peristaltic action of the tube and movement of the tube cilia help propel the ovum along the length of the tube. Usually only one ovum reaches maturity each month. Once released, fertilization must occur fairly quickly because an ovum is capable of fertilization for only 24 hours (48 hours at the most). After that time, it atrophies and becomes nonfunctional.

Normally, an ejaculation of semen averages 2.5 mL of fluid containing 50 to 200 million spermatozoa per milliliter, or an average of 400 million per ejaculation. At the time of ovulation, there is a reduction in the viscosity (thickness) of the cervical mucus, making it easier for spermatozoa to penetrate it. Sperm transport is so efficient close to ovulation that spermatozoa deposited in the vagina during intercourse generally reach the cervix within 80 seconds and the outer end of a fallopian tube within 5 minutes after deposition. This is one reason why douching is not an effective contraceptive measure.

Spermatozoa move by means of their flagella (tails) and uterine contractions through the cervix and the body of the uterus and into the fallopian tubes toward the waiting ovum. The mechanism whereby spermatozoa are drawn toward an ovum is probably a species-specific reaction, similar to an antibody–antigen reaction. Capacitation is a final process that sperm must undergo to be ready for fertilization. This process, which happens as the sperm move toward the ovum, consists of changes in the plasma membrane of the sperm head, which reveals the sperm-binding receptor sites.

All the spermatozoa that achieve capacitation reach the ovum and cluster around the protective layer of corona cells. Hyaluronidase (a proteolytic enzyme) is apparently released by the spermatozoa and acts to dissolve the layer of cells protecting the ovum. It is believed that the large numbers of sperm contained in an ejaculation provide enough enzymes to dissolve the corona cells. Under ordinary circumstances, only one spermatozoon is able to penetrate the cell membrane of the ovum. Once it penetrates the zona pellucida, the cell membrane becomes impervious to other spermatozoa. An exception to this is the formation of hydatidiform mole, in which multiple sperm enter; this leads to abnormal growth (see Chap. 15).

Immediately after penetration of the ovum, the chromosomal material of the ovum and spermatozoon fuse. The resulting structure is called a **zygote.** Because the spermatozoon and ovum each carried 23 chromosomes (22 autosomes and 1 sex chromosome), a fertilized ovum has 46 chromosomes. If an X-carrying spermatozoon enters the ovum, the resulting child will have two X chromosomes and will be female (XX). If a Y-carrying spermatozoon fertilizes the ovum, the resulting child will have an X and a Y chromosome and will be male (XY).

Fertilization is never a certain occurrence because it depends on at least three separate factors: maturation of both sperm and ovum, the ability of sperm to reach the ovum, and the ability of the sperm to penetrate the zona pellucida and cell membrane and achieve fertilization.

TABLE 8.1 Terms Used to Denote Fetal Growth

NAME	TIME PERIOD
Ovum	From ovulation to fertilization
Zygote	From fertilization to implantation
Embryo	From implantation to 5–8 weeks
Fetus	From 5–8 weeks until term
Conceptus	Developing embryo or fetus and placental structures throughout pregnancy

From the fertilized ovum (the zygote), the future child and also the accessory structures needed for support during intrauterine life, such as the placenta, fetal membranes, amniotic fluid, and umbilical cord, are formed.

> ✔ **CHECKPOINT QUESTIONS**
>
> 1. What helps to propel the ovum from the ovary to the fallopian tube?
> 2. What term is used to refer to the implanted fertilized ovum?

Implantation

Once fertilization is complete, the zygote migrates toward the body of the uterus, aided by the currents initiated by the muscular contractions of the fallopian tubes. It takes 3 or 4 days for the zygote to reach the body of the uterus. During this time, mitotic cell division, or cleavage, begins. The first cleavage occurs at about 24 hours; cleavage divisions continue to occur at a rate of one about every 22 hours. By the time the zygote reaches the body of the uterus, it consists of 16 to 50 cells. At this stage, because of its bumpy outward appearance, it is termed a **morula** (from the Latin word *morus,* meaning mulberry).

The morula continues to multiply as it floats free in the uterine cavity for 3 or 4 more days. Large cells tend to collect at the periphery of the ball, leaving a fluid space surrounding an inner cell mass. At this stage, the structure is termed a **blastocyst.** It is this structure that attaches to the uterine endometrium. The cells in the outer ring are known as **trophoblast** cells. They are the part of the structure that will later form the placenta and membranes. The inner cell mass (embryoblast cells) is the portion of the structure that will later form the embryo.

Implantation, or contact between the growing structure and the uterine endometrium, occurs approximately 8 to 10 days after fertilization. After the 3rd or 4th day of free floating (about 8 days from ovulation), the last residues of the corona and zona pellucida are shed by the growing structure. The blastocyst brushes against the rich uterine endometrium (in the second [secretory] phase of the menstrual cycle), a process termed apposition. It attaches to the surface of the endometrium (adhesion) and settles down into its soft folds (invasion). Stages to this point are depicted in Figure 8-1.

The blastocyst is able to invade the endometrium because as the trophoblast cells on the outside of the structure touch the endometrium, they produce proteolytic enzymes that dissolve the tissue they touch. This action allows the blastocyst to burrow deeply into the endometrium and receive some basic nourishment of glycogen and mucoprotein from the endometrial glands. As invasion continues, the structure establishes an effective communication network with the blood system of the endometrium. The touching or implantation point is usually high in the uterus, on the posterior surface. If the point of implantation is low in the uterus, the growing placenta may occlude the cervix and make birth of the child difficult (placenta previa).

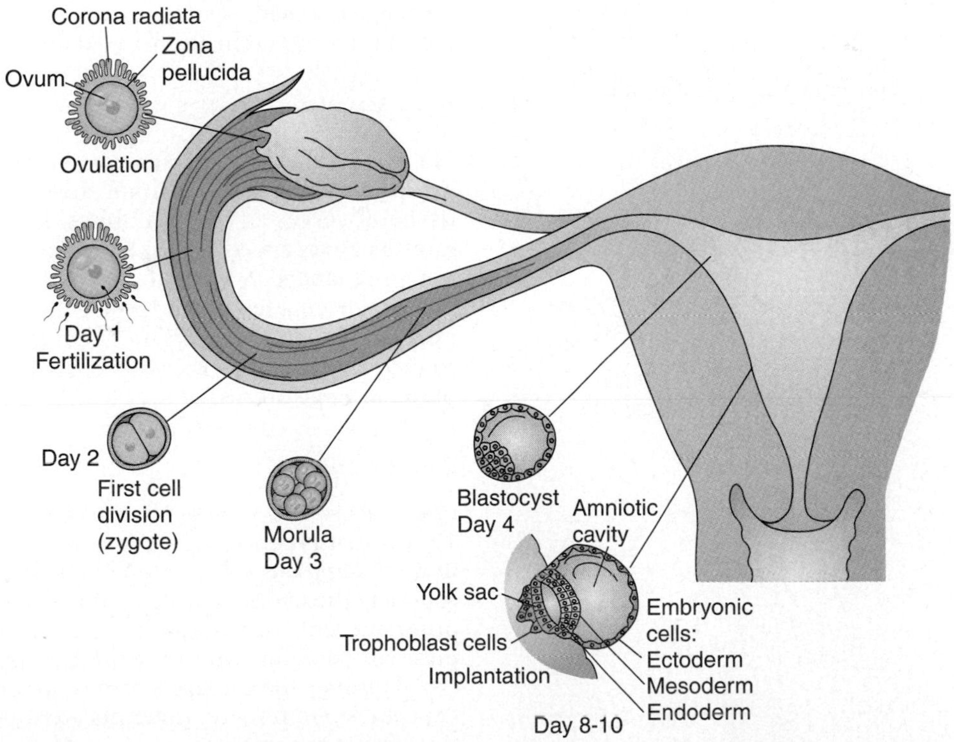

FIGURE 8.1 Schema of ovulation, fertilization, and implantation. At the time of implantation, the blastocyst is already differentiated into germ layers (ectoderm, mesoderm, and endoderm). Cells at the periphery of the structure are trophoblast cells that mature into the placenta.

Implantation is an important step in pregnancy because as many as 50% of zygotes never achieve it. In these instances, a pregnancy ends as early as 8 to 10 days after conception, often before the woman is even aware it had begun. Occasionally, a small amount of vaginal spotting appears with implantation because capillaries are ruptured by the implanting trophoblast cells. A woman who normally has a particularly scant menstrual flow may mistake implantation bleeding for her menstrual period. If this happens, the predicted date of birth of her baby (based on the time of her last menstrual period) will then be calculated 4 weeks late. Once implanted, the zygote is called an **embryo.**

EMBRYONIC AND FETAL STRUCTURES

The Decidua

After fertilization, the corpus luteum in the ovary continues to function rather than to atrophy because of the influence of human chorionic gonadotropin (hCG) hormone secreted by the trophoblast cells. Thus, the uterine endometrium, instead of sloughing off as in a normal menstrual cycle, continues to grow in thickness and vascularity. The endometrium is now termed decidua (the Latin word for falling off) because it will be discarded after the birth of the child. The decidua has three separate areas:

1. **Decidua basalis,** the part of the endometrium lying directly under the embryo (or the portion where the trophoblast cells are establishing communication with maternal blood vessels)
2. **Decidua capsularis,** the portion of the endometrium that stretches or encapsulates the surface of the trophoblast
3. **Decidua vera,** the remaining portion of the uterine lining (Fig. 8-2)

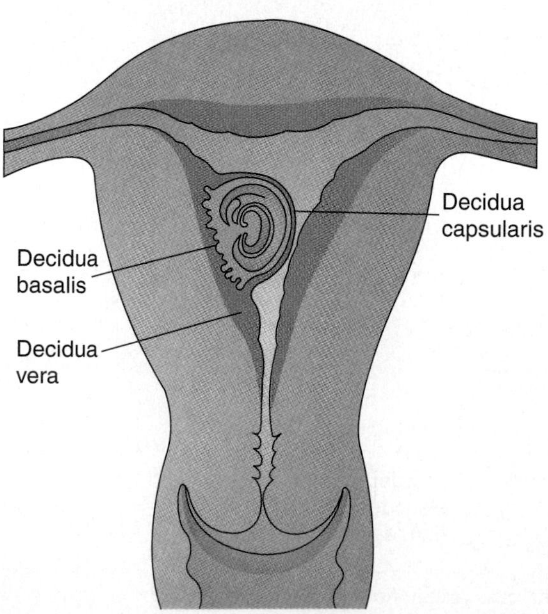

FIGURE 8.2 Division of uterine decidua into three areas.

As the embryo continues to grow, it pushes the decidua capsularis before it like a blanket. Eventually, enlargement brings the structure into contact with the opposite uterine wall. Here, the decidua capsularis fuses with the endometrium of the opposite wall. This is why at birth, the entire inner surface of the uterus is stripped away, leaving the organ highly susceptible to hemorrhage and infection (Seifer et al., 2001).

Chorionic Villi

Once implantation is achieved, the trophoblastic layer of cells of the blastocyst begins to mature rapidly. As early as the 11th or 12th day, miniature villi, or probing "fingers," termed **chorionic villi,** reach out from the single layer of cells into the uterine endometrium. At term, nearly 200 such villi will have formed.

Chorionic villi have a central core of loose connective tissue surrounded by a double layer of trophoblast cells. The central core of connective tissue contains fetal capillaries. The outer of the two covering layers is termed the syncytiotrophoblast, or the syncytial layer. This layer of cells is instrumental in the production of various placental hormones, such as hCG, somatomammotropin (human placental lactogen [HPL]), estrogen, and progesterone. The inner layer, known as the cytotrophoblast or Langhans' layer, is present as early as 12 days' gestation. It appears to function early in pregnancy to protect the growing embryo and fetus from certain infectious organisms such as the spirochete of syphilis. However, this layer of cells disappears between the 20th and 24th week. This is why syphilis is considered to have a high potential for fetal damage late in pregnancy, when cytotrophoblast cells are no longer present. Unfortunately, the layer appears to offer little protection against viral invasion at any point.

The Placenta

The placenta, Latin for pancake, which is descriptive of its size and appearance at term, arises out of trophoblast tissue. It serves as the fetal lungs, kidneys, and gastrointestinal tract and as a separate endocrine organ throughout pregnancy. Its growth parallels that of the fetus, growing from a few identifiable cells at the beginning of pregnancy to an organ 15 to 20 cm in diameter and 2 to 3 cm in depth at term. It covers about half the surface area of the internal uterus.

Circulation

Placental circulation is depicted in Figure 8-3. As early as the 12th day of pregnancy, maternal blood begins to collect in the intervillous spaces of the uterine endometrium surrounding the chorionic villi. By the 3rd week, oxygen and other nutrients, such as glucose, amino acids, fatty acids, minerals, vitamins, and water, diffuse from the maternal blood through the cell layers of the chorionic villi to the villi capillaries. From there, nutrients are transported back to the developing embryo.

For practical purposes, there is no direct exchange of blood between the embryo and the mother during pregnancy. The exchange is carried out only by selective

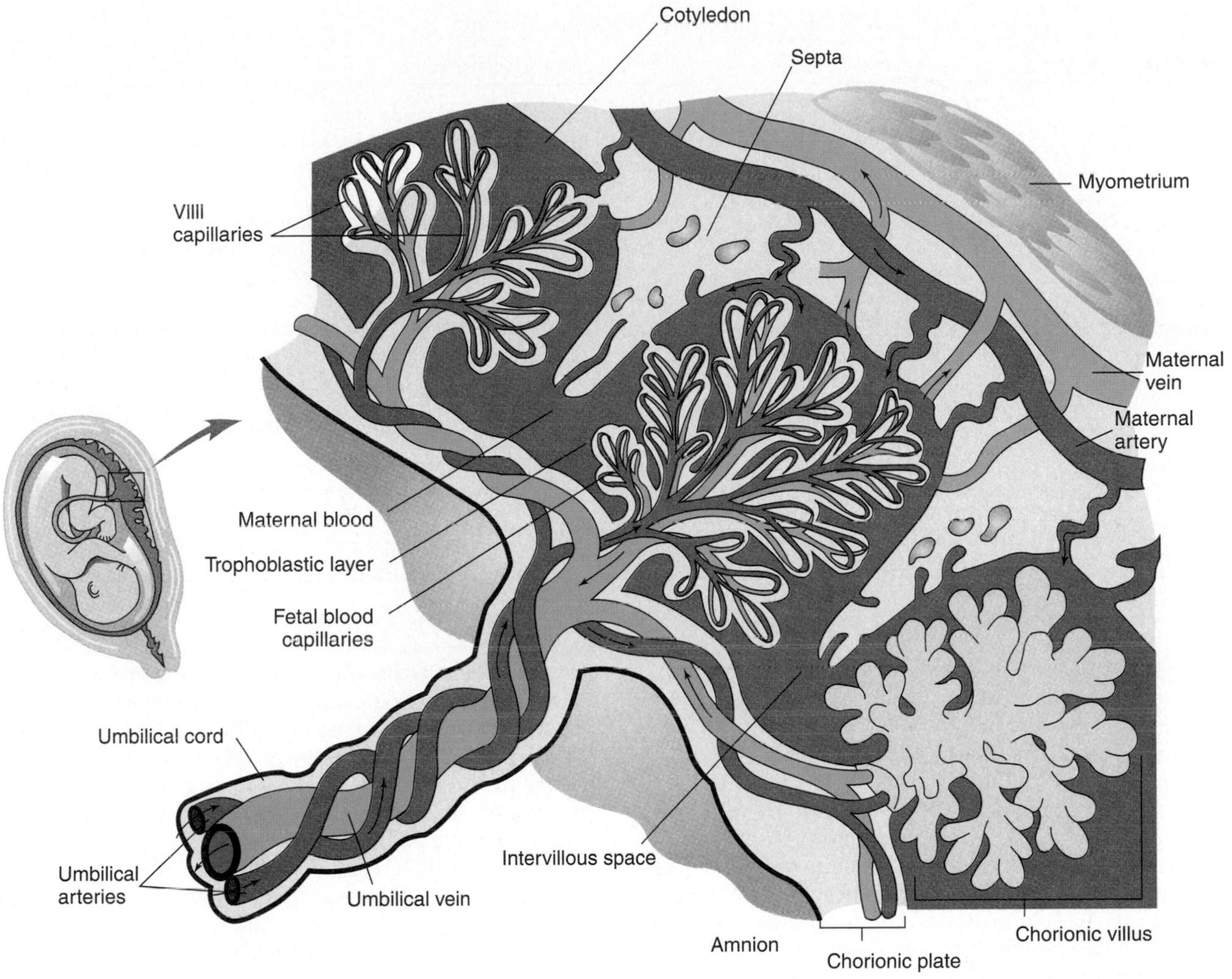

FIGURE 8.3 Placental circulation.

osmosis through the chorionic villi. However, because the chorionic villi layer is only one cell thick, minute breaks do allow occasional cells to cross. Placenta osmosis is so effective that all but a few substances are able to cross the placenta into the fetal circulation. Because almost all drugs are able to cross into the fetal circulation, it is important that a woman take no drugs (including alcohol and nicotine) other than those prescribed for her during pregnancy. Specific mechanisms allow nutrients to cross the placenta (Table 8-2). All these processes are affected by maternal blood pressure and the pH of the fetal and maternal plasma. Specific transport of nutrients is discussed in Chapter 11.

As the number of chorionic villi increases with pregnancy, the villi form an increasingly complex communication network with the maternal blood. Intervillous spaces grow larger and larger, becoming separated by a series of partitions or septa. In a mature placenta, there are as many as 30 separate segments, called **cotyledons.** These compartments are what make the maternal side of the placenta at term look rough and uneven.

About 100 maternal uterine arteries supply the mature placenta. To provide enough blood for exchange, the rate of uteroplacental blood flow in pregnancy increases from about 50 mL/min at 10 weeks to 500 to 600 mL/min at term. No additional maternal arteries appear after the first 3 months of pregnancy. However, to accommodate the increased blood flow, the arteries increase in size. Systemically, the mother's heart rate, total cardiac output, and blood volume increase to supply the placenta (Uckan & Townsend, 1999).

In the intervillous spaces, maternal blood jets from the coiled or spiral arteries in streams or spurts and then is propelled from compartment to compartment by the currents initiated. As the blood circulates around the villi and nutrients osmose from maternal blood into the villi, the maternal blood gradually loses its momentum and settles to the floor of the cotyledons. From there, it enters the orifices of maternal veins located in the cotyledons and is returned to the maternal circulation. Braxton Hicks contractions, the barely noticeable uterine contractions that are present from about the 12th week of pregnancy, aid in maintaining pressure in the intervillous spaces by closing off the uterine veins momentarily with each contraction.

Uterine perfusion, and thus placental circulation, is most efficient when the mother lies on her left side. This position lifts the uterus away from the inferior vena cava, pre-

TABLE 8.2 Mechanisms by Which Nutrients Cross the Placenta

MECHANISM	DESCRIPTION
Diffusion	When there is a greater concentration of a substance on one side of a semipermeable membrane than on the other, substances of correct molecular weight cross the membrane from the area of higher concentration to the area of lower concentration. Oxygen, carbon dioxide, sodium, and chloride cross the placenta by simple diffusion.
Facilitated diffusion	To ensure that the fetus receives enough concentrations of necessary growth substances, some substances cross the placenta more rapidly or more easily without the expenditure of energy than would occur if only simple diffusion were operating. A carrier moves the substance into and through the membrane. Glucose is an example of a substance that crosses by this process.
Active transport	This process requires energy and action of an enzyme to facilitate transport. Essential amino acids and water-soluble vitamins cross the placenta against the pressure gradient or from an area of lower molecular concentration to an area of greater molecular concentration. Amino acid concentrations in the fetal plasma are twice what they are in the mother, a situation that must occur to provide building substances for active fetal growth.
Pinocytosis	Absorption by the cellular membrane of microdroplets of plasma and dissolved substances. Gamma globulin, lipoproteins, phospholipids, and other molecular structures that are too large for diffusion and that cannot participate in active transport cross in this manner. Unfortunately, viruses that then infect the fetus may also cross in this manner.

venting blood from being trapped in the lower extremities. If the mother lies on her back and the weight of the uterus compresses the vena cava, placental circulation can be so sharply reduced that supine hypotension occurs.

At term, the placental circulatory network is so extensive that a placenta weighs 400 to 600 g (1 lb) and is one-sixth the weight of the baby. If a placenta is smaller than this, it suggests that circulation to the fetus may have been inadequate. Interestingly, a placenta heavier than this also may indicate that circulation to the fetus was threatened because the placenta was forced to spread out in an unusual manner to maintain a sufficient blood supply. The fetus of a woman with diabetes may develop a larger-than-usual placenta, probably from excess fluid collected between cells.

Endocrine Function

Aside from serving as the source of oxygen and nutrients for the fetus, the syncytial (outer) layer of the chorionic villi develops into a separate, important hormone-producing system.

Human Chorionic Gonadotropin. The first hormone to be produced is hCG. This hormone can be found in maternal blood and urine as early as the first missed menstrual period (shortly after implantation has occurred) through about the 100th day of pregnancy. Because this is the hormone analyzed by pregnancy tests, a false-negative result from a pregnancy test may be reported before or after this period. The mother's serum will be completely negative for hCG within 1 to 2 weeks after delivery. Testing for hCG after delivery can be used as proof that all the placental tissue has been delivered.

hCG acts as a fail-safe measure to ensure that the corpus luteum of the ovary continues to produce progesterone and estrogen. If the corpus luteum should fail and the level of progesterone should fall, this would cause endometrial sloughing, with loss of the pregnancy followed by a rise of pituitary gonadotropins to induce a new menstrual cycle. hCG also may play a role in suppressing the maternal immunologic response so placental tissue is not rejected. Because the structure of hCG is similar to luteinizing hormone of the pituitary gland, if the fetus is male, it exerts an effect on the fetal testes to begin testosterone production. The presence of testosterone causes the maturation of the male reproductive tract.

At about the 8th week of pregnancy, the outer layer of cells of the developing placenta begins to produce progesterone. At this point, the corpus luteum is no longer needed so the production of hCG, which sustained it, begins to decrease.

Estrogen. Estrogen (primarily estriol) is produced as a second product of the syncytial cells of the placenta. Estrogen contributes to the mother's mammary gland development in preparation for lactation and stimulates uterine growth to accommodate the developing fetus. Assessing the amount of estriol in maternal serum was used in the past to test fetal well-being.

Progesterone. Estrogen is often referred to as the "hormone of women," progesterone as the "hormone of mothers." Progesterone is necessary to maintain the endometrial lining of the uterus during pregnancy. It is present in serum as early as the 4th week of pregnancy as a result of the continuation of the corpus luteum. When placental synthesis begins (at around the 12th week), the level rises progressively during the remainder of the pregnancy. This hormone also appears to reduce the contractility of the uterine musculature during pregnancy, which prevents premature labor. Such reduced contractility is probably produced by a change in electrolytes (notably potassium and calcium), which decreases the action potential of the uterus.

Human Placental Lactogen (Human Chorionic Somatomammotropin). Human placental lactogen (HPL) is a hormone with both growth-promoting and lactogenic (milk-producing) properties. It is produced by the placenta beginning as early as the 6th week of pregnancy, increasing to a peak level at term. It can be assayed in both maternal serum and urine. It promotes mammary gland (breast) growth in preparation for lactation in the mother. It also serves the important role of regulating maternal glucose, protein, and fat levels so adequate amounts of these are always available to the fetus.

The Umbilical Cord

The **umbilical cord** is formed from the amnion and chorion and provides a circulatory pathway connecting the embryo to the chorionic villi. The function of the cord is to transport oxygen and nutrients to the fetus from the placenta and to return waste products from the fetus to the placenta. The umbilical cord is about 53 cm (21 in) in length at term. It is about 2 cm (¾ in) thick. It contains one vein (carrying blood from the placental villi to the fetus) and two arteries (carrying blood from the fetus back to the placental villi). The remnant of the yolk sac may be found in the fetal end of the cord as a white fibrous streak at term. The bulk of the cord is a gelatinous mucopolysaccharide called **Wharton's jelly,** which gives the cord body and prevents pressure on the vein and arteries. The outer surface is covered with amniotic membrane.

The number of veins and arteries in the cord is always assessed at birth. Normally, there are two umbilical arteries and one umbilical vein. About 1% of all infants are born with a cord that contains only a single vein and artery. About 15% of these infants are found to have accompanying congenital anomalies, particularly of the kidney and heart.

Blood can be withdrawn from the umbilical vein or transfused into the vein during intrauterine life for fetal assessment or treatment (termed percutaneous umbilical blood sampling). The rate of blood flow through an umbilical cord is rapid (350 mL/min at term). Whether an adequate blood flow (blood velocity) is present in the cord can be determined by ultrasound. Both systolic and diastolic pressure can be determined by this method.

The rapid rate of blood flow through the cord makes it unlikely that a cord will twist or knot enough to interfere with the fetal oxygen supply. In about 20% of all births, a loose loop of cord is found around the fetal neck (a nuchal cord). If this loop of cord is removed before the newborn's shoulders are extruded, so there is no traction on it, the oxygen supply to the fetus remains unimpaired.

Smooth muscle is abundant in the arteries of the cord. Constriction of these muscles after birth contributes to hemostasis and helps prevent hemorrhage of the newborn through the cord. Because the umbilical cord contains no nerve supply, it can be cut at birth without discomfort to the child or mother.

✔ CHECKPOINT QUESTIONS

3. What structure in the blastocyst goes on to develop into the placenta?
4. How many arteries and veins are usually found in the umbilical cord?
5. Why is it important to stress avoiding alcohol and tobacco early in pregnancy?

The Membranes and Amniotic Fluid

The chorionic villi on the medial surface of the trophoblast (those that are not involved in implantation because they do not touch the endometrium) gradually thin and leave the medial surface of the structure smooth (the chorion laeve, or smooth chorion). The smooth chorion eventually becomes the **chorionic membrane,** the outermost fetal membrane. Once it becomes smooth, it offers support to the sac that contains the amniotic fluid. A second membrane lining the chorionic membrane, the **amniotic membrane** or amnion, forms beneath the chorion (Fig. 8-4). Early in pregnancy, these membranes become so adherent that they seem as one at term. These membranes cover the fetal surface of the placenta and give that surface its typically shiny appearance. Like the umbilical cord, they have no nerve supply. Thus, when they rupture at term, neither mother nor child experiences any pain.

Unlike the chorionic membrane, the amniotic membrane not only offers support to amniotic fluid but also actually produces the fluid. In addition, it produces a phospholipid that initiates the formation of prostaglandins, which cause uterine contractions and may be the trigger that initiates labor.

Amniotic fluid is constantly being newly formed and reabsorbed, so it is never stagnant within the membranes. Because the fetus continually swallows the fluid, it is absorbed across the fetal intestine into the fetal bloodstream. From there, the umbilical arteries exchange it across the placenta. Some fluid is probably absorbed by direct contact with the fetal surface of the placenta. At term, the amount of amniotic fluid ranges from 800 to 1,200 mL. If for any reason the fetus is unable to swallow

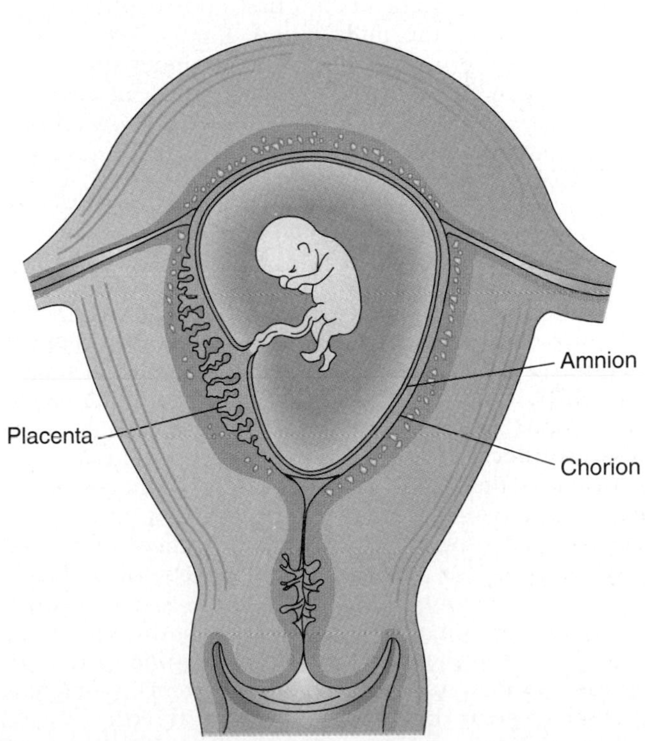

FIGURE 8.4 Membranes, with embryo lying within amniotic sac.

(esophageal atresia or anencephaly are the two most common reasons), excessive amniotic fluid or **hydramnios** (more than 2,000 mL total or pockets of fluid larger than 8 cm on ultrasound) will result. Hydramnios also tends to occur in women with diabetes because hyperglycemia causes excessive fluid shift into the amniotic space. Early in fetal life, as soon as the fetal kidneys become active, fetal urine adds to the quantity of the amniotic fluid. A disturbance of kidney function may cause **oligohydramnios,** or a reduction in the amount of amniotic fluid (less than 300 mL total or no pocket on ultrasound larger than 1 cm).

Amniotic fluid is an important protective mechanism for the fetus. It shields against pressure or a blow to the mother's abdomen. It protects the fetus from changes in temperature, because liquid changes temperature more slowly than air. It probably aids in muscular development, because it allows the fetus freedom to move. Finally, it protects the umbilical cord from pressure, protecting fetal oxygenation.

Even if the membranes rupture before birth and the bulk of the amniotic fluid is lost, some will always surround the fetus in utero because new fluid is constantly being formed. Amniotic fluid is slightly alkaline, with a pH of about 7.2. Checking the pH of the fluid at the time of rupture helps to differentiate it from urine, which is acidic (pH 5.0 to 5.5).

ORIGIN AND DEVELOPMENT OF ORGAN SYSTEMS

From the beginning of fetal growth, development proceeds in a **cephalocaudal** (head-to-tail) direction; that is, head development occurs first and is followed by development of the middle and, finally, lower body parts. This pattern of development continues after birth, evidenced by newborns lifting up their head approximately a year before walking. As a fetus grows, body organ systems develop from specific tissue layers called germ layers.

Primary Germ Layers

At the time of implantation, the blastocyst already has differentiated to a point at which two separate cavities appear in the inner structure: (1) a large one, the **amniotic cavity,** which is lined with a distinctive layer of cells, the **ectoderm,** and (2) a smaller cavity, the **yolk sac,** which is lined with **entoderm** cells (see Fig. 8-1).

In chicks, the yolk sac serves as a supply of nourishment for the embryo throughout its development. In humans, the yolk sac appears to supply nourishment only until implantation. After that, it provides a source of red blood cells until the embryo's hematopoietic system is mature enough to perform this function (at about the 12th week of intrauterine life). The yolk sac atrophies after the hematopoietic function is complete and remains only as a thin white streak discernible in the cord at birth.

Between the amniotic cavity and the yolk sac, a third layer of primary cells, the **mesoderm,** forms. The embryo will begin to develop (from an embryonic shield) at the point where the three cell layers (ectoderm, entoderm, mesoderm) meet. Each germ layer of primary tissue develops into specific body systems (Table 8-3). Knowing which structures arise from each germ layer is important because coexisting congenital defects found in newborns usually arise from the same layer. For example, a fistula between the trachea and the esophagus (both organs arising from the entoderm) is a common birth anomaly. Heart and kidney defects (both organs arising from the mesoderm) are also commonly seen together. It is rare, however, to see a newborn with a heart malformation (arises from the mesoderm) and a lower urinary malformation (bladder and urethra arise from the entoderm). One reason rubella infection is always serious in pregnancy is because this virus is capable of affecting all the germ layers, thereby causing congenital anomalies in a myriad of body systems, regardless of the primary germ layer of origin.

Knowing the origins of body structures also helps to explain why certain screening procedures are ordered for newborns with congenital malformations. A kidney x-ray examination, for example, may be ordered for a child born with a heart defect. A child with a malformation of the urinary tract is often investigated for reproductive abnormalities as well (Freedman et al., 2000).

All organ systems are complete, at least in a rudimentary form, at 8 weeks' gestation (the end of the embryonic

TABLE 8.3 Origin of Body Tissue

GERM LAYER	BODY PORTIONS FORMED
Ectoderm	Central nervous system (brain and spinal cord)
	Peripheral nervous system
	Skin, hair, and nails
	Sebaceous glands
	Sense organs
	Mucous membranes of the anus, mouth, and nose
	Tooth enamel
	Mammary glands
Mesoderm	Supporting structures of the body (connective tissue, bones, cartilage, muscle, ligaments, and tendons)
	Dentin of teeth
	Upper portion of the urinary system (kidneys and ureters)
	Reproductive system
	Heart
	Circulatory system
	Blood cells
	Lymph vessels
Entoderm	Lining of pericardial, pleura, and peritoneal cavities
	Lining of the gastrointestinal tract, respiratory tract, tonsils, parathyroid, thyroid, thymus glands
	Lower urinary system (bladder and urethra)

period). During this early time of **organogenesis** (organ formation), the growing structure is most vulnerable to invasion by teratogens (any factor that affects the fertilized ovum, embryo, or fetus adversely, such as alcohol or a chemotherapy drug). Women need to know how to minimize their exposure to these teratogens (see Focus on Family Empowerment). Figure 8-5 illustrates critical periods of fetal growth. Teratogens are discussed in Chapter 11.

Cardiovascular System

The cardiovascular system is one of the first systems to become functional in intrauterine life. Simple blood cells joined to the walls of the yolk sac progress to a network of blood vessels and to a single heart tube forming as early as the 16th day of life, beating as early as the 24th day. The septum that divides the heart into chambers develops during the 6th or 7th week. Heart valves begin to develop in the 7th week. The heartbeat may be heard with a Doppler as early as the 10th to 12th week of pregnancy. An electrocardiogram (ECG) may be recorded on a fetus as early as the 11th week, although the accuracy of such ECGs is in doubt until about the 20th week of pregnancy, when conduction is more regulated.

The heart rate of a fetus is affected by fetal oxygen level, body activity, and circulating blood volume, just as in adult life. After the 28th week of pregnancy, when the sympathetic nervous system has matured, the heart rate begins to show a baseline variability of about 5 beats per minute on a fetal heart rate rhythm strip.

Fetal Circulation

As early as the 3rd week of intrauterine life, fetal blood has begun to exchange nutrients with the maternal circulation across the chorionic villi. Fetal circulation (Fig. 8-6) differs from extrauterine circulation in several respects. During intrauterine life, the fetus derives oxygen and excretes carbon dioxide not from oxygen exchange in the lungs but from the placenta. Blood does enter the lungs while the child is in utero, but this blood flow is to supply the cells of the lungs themselves, not for oxygen exchange. Specialized structures present in the fetus shunt blood flow to supply the most important organs: the brain, liver, heart, and kidneys.

Blood arriving at the fetus from the placenta is highly oxygenated. This blood enters the fetus through the umbilical vein (called a vein even though it carries oxygenated blood, because the direction of the blood is toward the fetal heart). The umbilical vein carries the blood to the inferior vena cava through an accessory structure, the **ductus venosus.** The ductus venosus receives most of the oxygenated blood from the umbilical vein to supply the fetal liver. It then empties into the inferior vena cava. From the inferior vena cava, blood is carried to the right side of the heart. As the blood enters the right atrium, the bulk of it is shunted into the left atrium through an opening in the atrial septum, the **foramen ovale.** From the left atrium, it follows the course of normal circulation into the left ventricle and into the aorta.

Deoxygenated blood from the body is returned to the heart by the vena cava. The blood enters the right atrium and leaves it by the normal circulatory route; that is, through the tricuspid valve into the right ventricle, then into the pulmonary artery in the normal manner. A small portion of this blood flow services the lung tissue. However, the larger portion is shunted away from the lungs through an additional structure, the **ductus arteriosus,** directly into the aorta and then into the descending aorta.

Most of the blood flow from the descending aorta is transported by the umbilical arteries (called arteries, even though they are now transporting deoxygenated blood, because they are carrying blood away from the fetal heart) back through the umbilical cord to the placental villi, where new oxygen exchange takes place.

The blood oxygen saturation level of the fetus is about 80% of the newborn's saturation level. The rapid fetal heart rate during pregnancy (120 to 160 beats per minute) is necessary to supply oxygen to cells when red blood cells are never fully saturated. Despite a low blood oxygen saturation level, carbon dioxide does not accumulate in the fetal system because of its rapid diffusion into maternal blood across a favorable placental pressure gradient.

Fetal Hemoglobin

Fetal hemoglobin differs from adult hemoglobin in several ways. It has a different composition (two alpha and two gamma chains, compared with two alpha and two beta chains of adult hemoglobin). Fetal hemoglobin has greater oxygen affinity, which increases its efficiency, and is more concentrated. At birth, a newborn's hemoglobin level is about 17.1 g/100 mL, compared with an adult's normal level of 11 g/100 mL; a newborn's hematocrit is about 53%, compared with an adult's normal level of 45%.

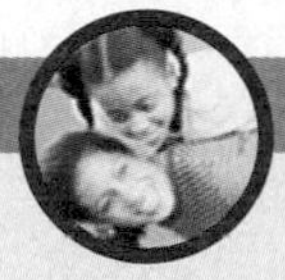

FOCUS ON FAMILY EMPOWERMENT
Avoiding Fetal Teratogens

Q. How can I guard against fetal teratogens at work?

A. Here are a number of helpful tips:

- Avoid rooms where smokers gather, such as coffee rooms.
- Refrain from drinking alcohol, a frequent accompaniment to work lunches or social functions; make sure that nonalcoholic drinks are available.
- Ask your employer for a statement on hazardous substances at your work site; discuss your need to avoid these during pregnancy.

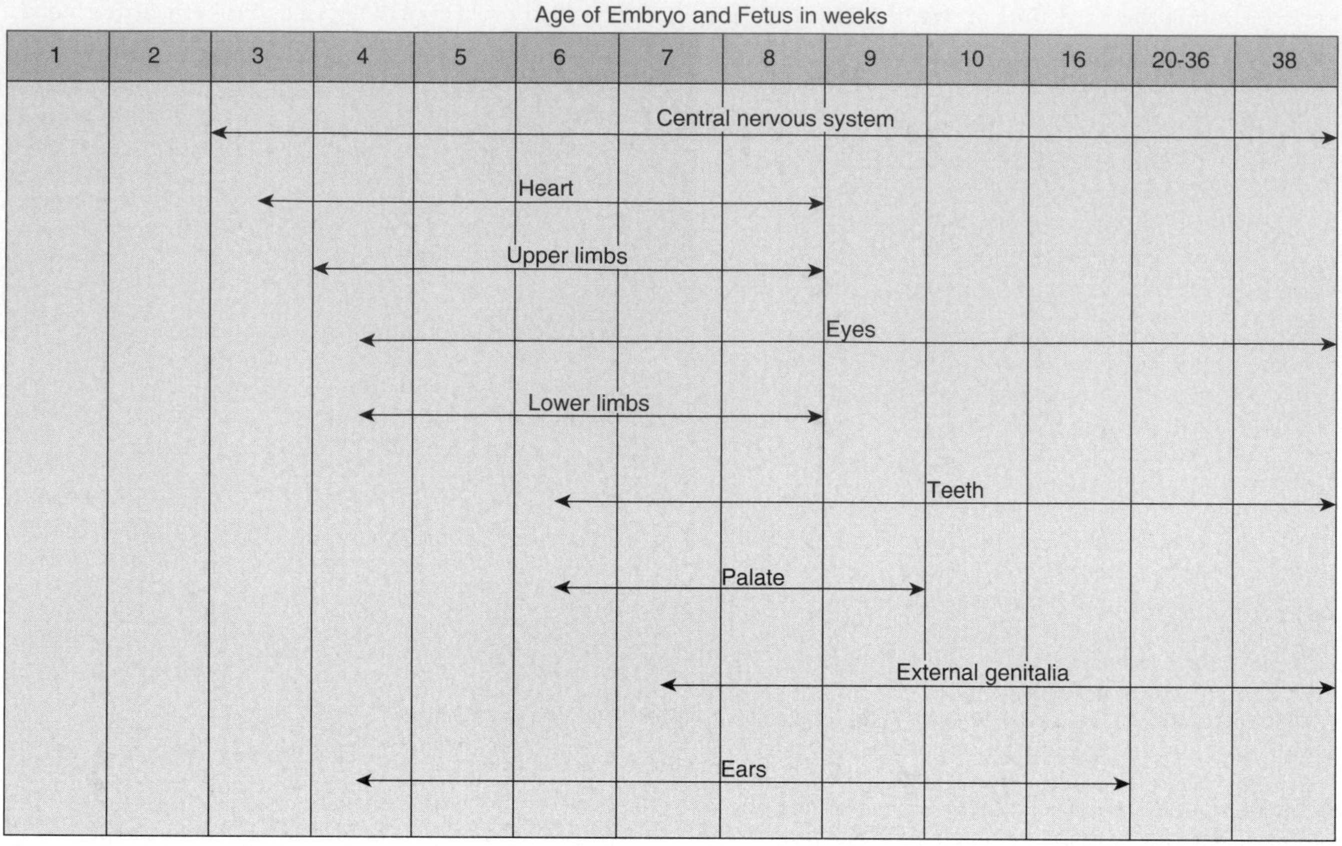

FIGURE 8.5 Critical periods of fetal growth.

The change from fetal to adult hemoglobin levels begins before birth and accelerates after birth. The major blood dyscrasias, such as sickle cell anemia, are defects of the beta hemoglobin chain. Therefore, clinical symptoms do not become apparent until the bulk of fetal hemoglobin has matured to adult hemoglobin composition at about 6 months of age.

Respiratory System

At the 3rd week of intrauterine life, the respiratory and digestive tracts exist as a single tube. Like all body tubes, initially it is a solid structure, which then canalizes (hollows out). By the end of the 4th week, a septum begins to divide the esophagus from the trachea. At the same time, lung buds appear on the trachea.

Until the 7th week of life, the diaphragm does not completely divide the thoracic cavity from the abdomen. During the 6th week of life, lung buds may extend down into the abdomen, re-entering the chest only as the chest's longitudinal dimension increases and the diaphragm becomes complete (at the end of the 7th week). If the diaphragm fails to close completely, the stomach, spleen, liver, or intestines may enter the thoracic cavity. The child may be born with a diaphragmatic hernia, compromising the lungs and perhaps displacing the heart.

Important respiratory development milestones include:

- Alveoli and capillaries begin to form between the 24th and 28th weeks. Both capillary and alveoli development must be complete before gas exchange can occur in the fetal lungs.
- Spontaneous respiratory movements begin as early as 3 months of pregnancy, continuing throughout pregnancy.
- Specific lung fluid with a low surface tension and low viscosity forms in alveoli to aid in expansion of alveoli at birth; it is rapidly absorbed after birth.
- **Surfactant,** a phospholipid substance, is formed and excreted by the alveolar cells at about the 24th week of pregnancy. This decreases alveolar surface tension on expiration, preventing alveolar collapse and improving the infant's ability to maintain respirations in the outside environment.

Surfactant has two components: lecithin and sphingomyelin. Early in the formation of surfactant, sphingomyelin is the chief component. At about 35 weeks, there is a surge in the production of lecithin. This then becomes the chief component by a ratio of 2:1. With fetal lung movements, surfactant mixes with amniotic fluid. Analysis of the lecithin/sphingomyelin (L/S) ratio by an amniocentesis technique is one of the primary tests of fetal maturity. Lack of surfactant is a factor associated with the development of respiratory distress syndrome (see Chap. 26). Any interference with the blood supply to the fetus, such as occurs with placental insufficiency from hypertension, appears to enhance surfactant development. This type of stress probably increases steroid levels in the

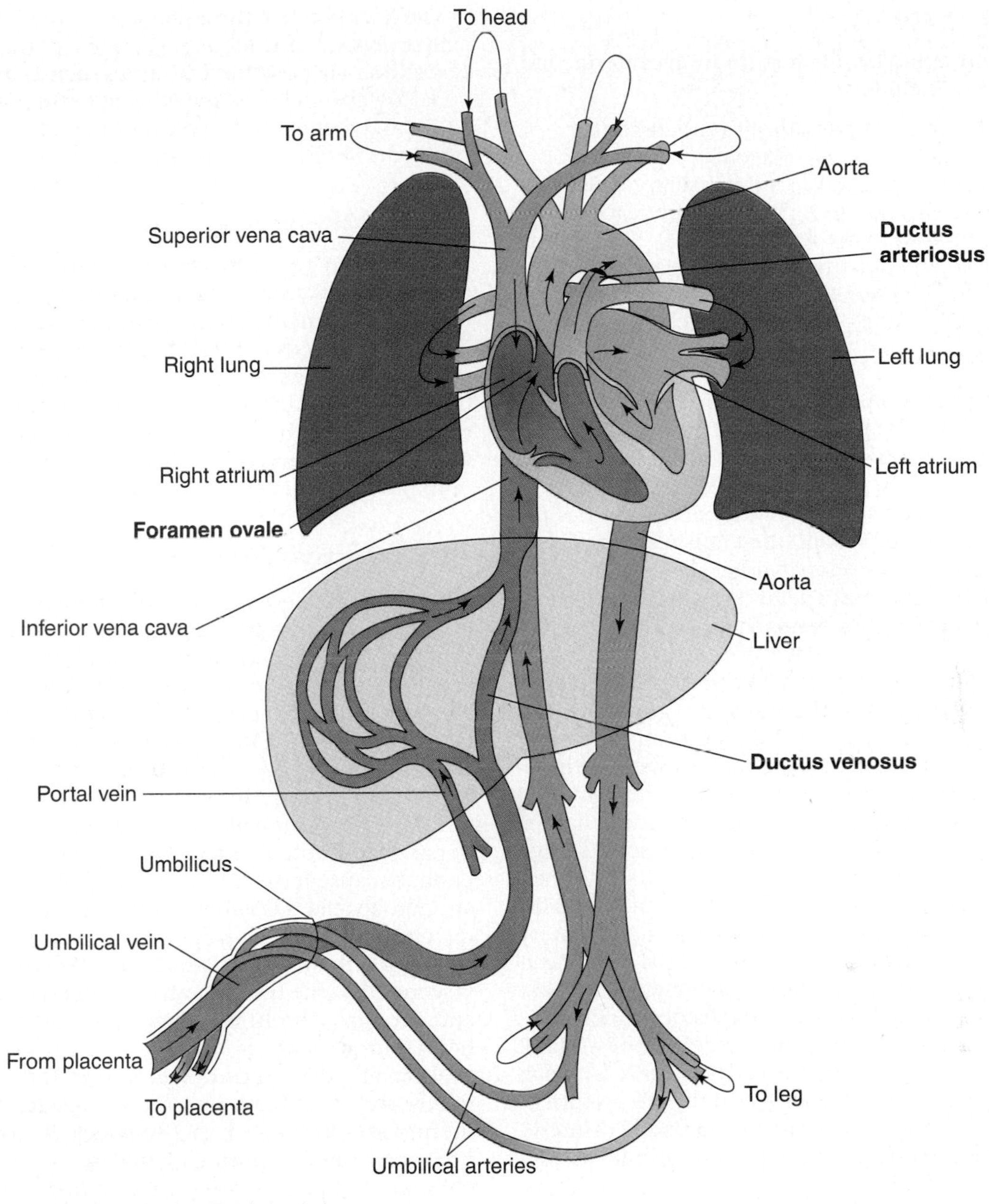

FIGURE 8.6 Fetal circulation.

fetus. Increased steroid levels are associated with alveolar maturation (Ling & Duff, 2001).

Nervous System

Like the circulatory system, the nervous system begins to develop extremely early in pregnancy. During the 3rd and 4th weeks of life, possibly before the woman even realizes that she is pregnant, active formation of the nervous system and sense organs has already begun.

- A **neural plate** (a thickened portion of the ectoderm) is apparent by the 3rd week of gestation. Its top portion differentiates into the neural tube, which will form the central nervous system (brain and spinal cord), and the neural crest, which will develop into the peripheral nervous system.
- Brain waves can be detected on an electroencephalogram (EEG) by the 8th week.
- All parts of the brain (cerebrum, cerebellum, pons, and medulla oblongata) form in utero, although they are not completely mature at birth. Growth continues to occur rapidly during the 1st year and continues at high levels until 5 or 6 years of age.
- Eye and inner ear develop as projections of the original neural tube.
- By 24 weeks, the ear is capable of responding to sound; the eyes exhibit a pupillary reaction, indicating sight is present.

The neurologic system seems particularly prone to insult during the early weeks of the embryonic period. All during pregnancy and at birth, the system is vulnerable to damage from anoxia.

Endocrine System

As soon as endocrine organs mature in intrauterine life, function begins, including:

- The fetal adrenal glands supply a precursor for estrogen synthesis by the placenta.
- The fetal pancreas produces the insulin needed by the fetus (insulin does not cross the placenta from the mother to the fetus).
- The thyroid and parathyroid glands play vital roles in metabolic function and calcium balance.

Digestive System

The digestive tract is separated from the respiratory tract at about the 4th week. After this time, the intestinal tract grows extremely rapidly. Initially solid, the tubes canalize (hollow out) to become patent. Later, the endothelial cells of the gastrointestinal tract proliferate extensively, occluding the lumens once more, and they must canalize again. Atresia or stenosis can develop if either the first or second canalization does not occur. The proliferation of cells shed in the second recanalization forms the basis for meconium (see below).

Because the abdomen becomes too small to contain the intestine, a portion of the intestine, guided by the vitelline membrane (a part of the yolk sac), enters the base of the umbilical cord during the 6th week of intrauterine life. Intestine remains in the base of the cord until about the 10th week. At this time, the fetal trunk has extended and enlarged the abdominal cavity so it is large enough to accommodate all the intestinal mass. As the intestine returns to the abdominal cavity, it must rotate 180 degrees. Failure to do so can result in inadequate mesentery attachments, possibly leading to volvulus of the intestine. If any intestinal coils remain outside the abdomen, in the base of the cord, a congenital anomaly, omphalocele, develops. A similar defect, gastroschisis, occurs when the original midline fusion that occurred at the early cell stage is incomplete. If the vitelline duct does not atrophy after return of the intestines, a Meckel's diverticulum (a pouch of intestinal tissue) or an opening between the intestine and the umbilicus can result.

Meconium forms in the intestines as early as the 16th week. It consists of cellular wastes, bile, fats, mucoproteins, mucopolysaccharides, and portions of the vernix caseosa, the lubricating substance that forms on the fetal skin. Meconium is black or dark green (obtaining its color from bile pigment) and sticky.

The gastrointestinal tract is sterile before birth. Because vitamin K is synthesized by the action of bacteria in the intestines, this can cause vitamin K levels to be low in the newborn. Sucking and swallowing reflexes are not mature until the fetus is about 32 weeks or the fetus weighs 1,500 g.

The ability of the gastrointestinal tract to secrete enzymes essential to carbohydrate and protein digestion is mature at 36 weeks. However, amylase, an enzyme found in saliva and necessary for digestion of complex starches, is not mature until 3 months after birth. Many newborns have not yet developed lipase, an enzyme needed for fat digestion.

The liver is active throughout gestation, functioning as a filter between the incoming blood and the fetal circulation and as a deposit for fetal stores such as iron and glycogen. However, it is still immature at birth, possibly leading to hypoglycemia and hyperbilirubinemia, two serious problems in the first 24 hours after birth.

Musculoskeletal System

The fetus can be seen to move on ultrasound as early as the 11th week, although the mother usually does not feel this movement (**quickening**) until nearly 20 weeks. In the first 2 weeks of fetal life, cartilage prototypes provide position and support. Ossification of bone tissue begins about the 12th week. The ossification process continues all through fetal life and actually until adulthood. Carpals, tarsals, and sternal bones generally do not ossify until birth is imminent.

Reproductive System

A child's sex is determined at the moment of conception by a spermatozoon carrying an X or a Y chromosome and can be determined as early as 8 weeks by chromosomal analysis. At about the 6th week of life, the gonads (ovaries or testes) form. If testes form, testosterone is secreted, apparently influencing the sexually neutral genital duct to form other male organs (maturity of the wolffian, or mesonephric, duct). In the absence of testosterone secretion, female organs will form (maturation of the müllerian, or paramesonephric, duct). This is an important phenomenon, because if the mother should take an androgen or an androgen-like substance during this stage of pregnancy, the child, although chromosomally female, would appear more male than female at birth. If deficient testosterone is secreted by the testes, both the müllerian (female) duct and the male (wolffian) duct could develop (pseudohermaphroditism).

Normally, the testes descend from the pelvic cavity, where they first form into the scrotal sac late in intrauterine life, at the 34th to 38th week. Thus, many male preterm infants are born with undescended testes. These children should be followed closely to see that the testes descend when the child reaches what would have been the 34th to 38th week of gestational age, because testicular descent does not occur as readily in extrauterine life as it would in utero.

Urinary System

Although rudimentary kidneys are present as early as the end of the 4th week, they do not appear to be essential for life before birth. Urine is formed by the 12th week and is excreted into the amniotic fluid by the 16th week of gestation. At term, fetal urine is being excreted at the rate of 500 mL/day. An amount of amniotic fluid that is less than normal (oligohydramnios) suggests that fetal kidneys are not secreting adequate urine.

The complex structure of the kidneys is gradually developed during pregnancy and for months afterward. The loop of Henle, for example, is not fully differentiated until the child is born. Glomerular filtration and concentration of urine in the newborn are not efficient because the kidneys are not fully mature even by birth.

Early in the embryonic stage of urinary system development, the bladder extends to the umbilical region. On rare occasions, an open lumen between the urinary bladder and the umbilicus fails to close. Termed a patent urachus, this is discovered at birth by the persistent drainage of a clear, acid-pH fluid (urine) from the umbilicus.

Integumentary System

The skin of a fetus appears thin and almost translucent until subcutaneous fat begins to be deposited at about 36 weeks. Skin is covered by soft downy hairs (lanugo) and a cream cheese–like substance, vernix caseosa, which is important for lubrication and keeping the skin from macerating.

Immune System

IgG maternal antibodies cross the placenta into the fetus primarily during the third trimester of pregnancy, giving a fetus temporary passive immunity against diseases for which the mother has antibodies. These often include poliomyelitis, rubella (German measles), rubeola (regular measles), diphtheria, tetanus, infectious parotitis (mumps), and pertussis (whooping cough). Little or no immunity to the herpes virus (the virus of cold sores and genital herpes) is transferred to the fetus; thus, the average newborn is potentially susceptible to these diseases.

The level of passive IgG immunoglobulins peaks at birth and then decreases over the next 8 months while infants begin to build up their own stores of IgG as well as IgA and IgM. Because the passive immunity received by the newborn has already declined substantially by about 2 months, immunization against diphtheria, tetanus, pertussis, poliomyelitis, and *H. influenzae* is typically started. Passive antibodies to measles have been demonstrated to last over a year. Consequently, the immunization for measles is not given until an extrauterine age of 15 months.

It has been shown that a fetus is capable of active antibody production late in a pregnancy. Generally, this is not necessary, however, because antibodies are manufactured only when stimulated by an invading antigen, and antigens rarely invade the intrauterine space. However, infants whose mothers have had an infection such as rubella during pregnancy typically have IgM antibodies to rubella in their blood serum at birth. Because IgA and IgM antibodies cannot cross the placenta, their presence in a newborn is proof that the fetus has been exposed to the disease.

✔ CHECKPOINT QUESTIONS

6. When does surfactant excretion by alveolar cells begin?
7. What two conditions may occur within the first 24 hours after birth because of the infant's immature liver?
8. Which immunoglobulin crosses the placenta?

Milestones of Fetal Growth and Development

During pregnancy, couples ask many questions about their baby's appearance and age. To answer these questions effectively and to plan care that safeguards fetal growth, it is helpful to be able to describe the developmental milestones by weeks of intrauterine life.

This can be confusing because the life of the fetus is generally measured from the time of ovulation or fertilization (ovulation age), but the length of the pregnancy is generally measured from the first day of the last menstrual period (gestational age). Because ovulation and fertilization take place about 2 weeks after the last menstrual period, the ovulation age of the fetus is always 2 weeks less than the length of the pregnancy or the gestational age.

Both ovulation and gestational age are also sometimes measured in lunar months (4-week periods) or in trimesters (3-month periods) rather than in weeks. In lunar months, a pregnancy is 10 months (40 weeks or 280 days) long; a fetus grows in utero 9.5 lunar months or three full trimesters (38 weeks or 266 days).

The following discussion of fetal developmental milestones is based on gestation weeks because it is helpful when talking to expectant parents to be able to correlate fetal development to the way they measure pregnancy: from the first day of the last menstrual period. Figure 8-7 illustrates the comparative size and appearance of human embryos and fetuses at different stages.

End of 4 Gestation Weeks

At the end of the 4th week of gestation, the human embryo is a rapidly growing formation of cells but does not resemble a human being yet.

- Length: 0.75 to 1 cm.
- Weight: 400 mg.
- The spinal cord is formed and fused at the midpoint.
- Lateral wings that will form the body are folded forward to fuse at the midline.
- Head folds forward, becoming prominent, representing about one third of the entire structure.
- The back is bent so the head almost touches the tip of the tail.
- The rudimentary heart appears as a prominent bulge on the anterior surface.
- Arms and legs are budlike structures.
- Rudimentary eyes, ears, and nose are discernible.

End of 8 Gestation Weeks

- Length: 2.5 cm (1 in).
- Weight: 20 g.
- Organogenesis is complete.
- The heart, with a septum and valves, is beating rhythmically.
- Facial features are definitely discernible.
- Extremities have developed.
- External genitalia are present, but sex is not distinguishable by simple observation.
- The primitive tail is regressing.

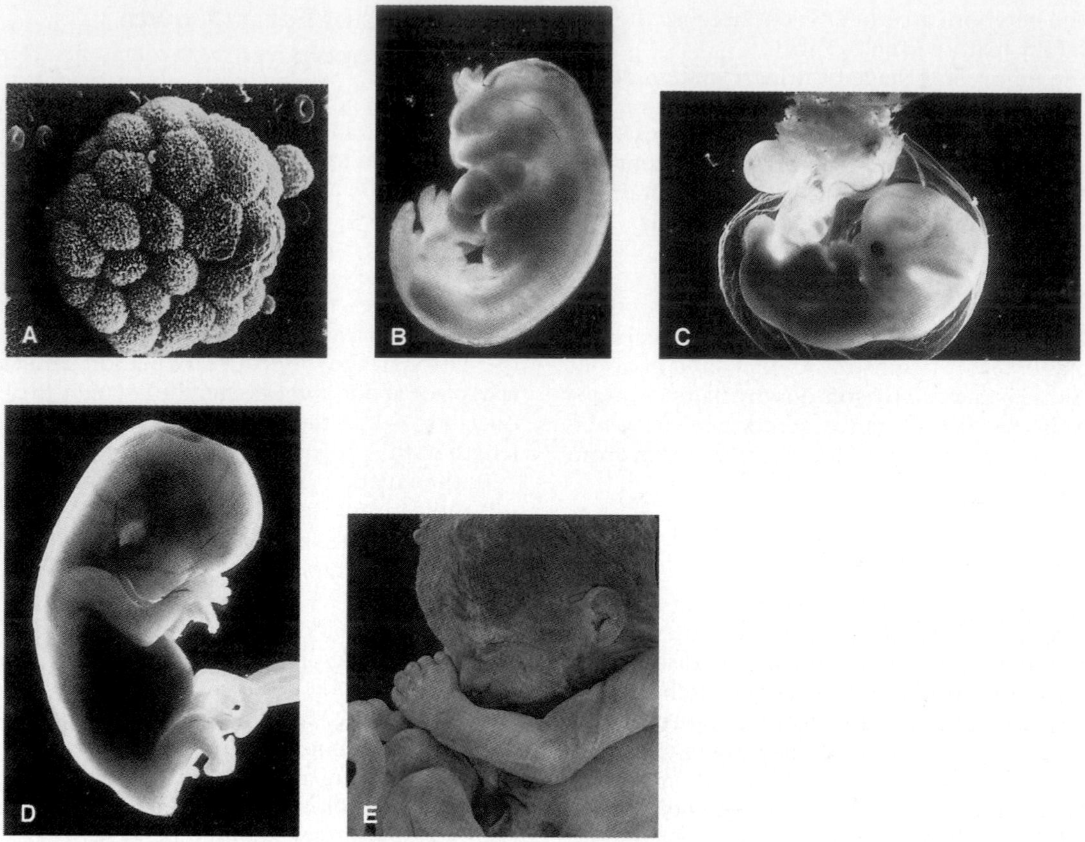

FIGURE 8.7 Human embryos at different stages of life: (*A*) Implantation in uterus 7 to 8 days after conception. (*B*) Embryo at 32 days. (*C*) At 37 days. (*D*) At 41 days. (*E*) Between 12–15 weeks.

- Abdomen appears large as the fetal intestine is growing rapidly.
- Sonogram shows a gestational sac, diagnostic of pregnancy (Fig. 8-8).

End of 12 Gestation Weeks (First Trimester)

- Length: 7 to 8 cm.
- Weight: 45 g.
- Nail beds are forming on fingers and toes.
- Spontaneous movements are possible, although usually too faint to be felt by the mother.
- Some reflexes, such as Babinski reflex, are present.
- Bone ossification centers are forming.
- Tooth buds are present.
- Sex is distinguishable by outward appearance.
- Kidney secretion has begun, although urine may not yet be evident in amniotic fluid.
- Heartbeat is audible by a Doppler.

End of 16 Gestation Weeks

- Length: 10 to 17 cm.
- Weight: 55 to 120 g.
- Fetal heart sounds are audible with an ordinary stethoscope.
- Lanugo (the fine, downy hair on the back and arms of newborns, apparently serving as a source of insulation for body heat) is well formed.
- Liver and pancreas are functioning.
- Fetus actively swallows amniotic fluid, demonstrating an intact but uncoordinated swallowing reflex; urine is present in amniotic fluid.
- Sex can be determined by ultrasound.

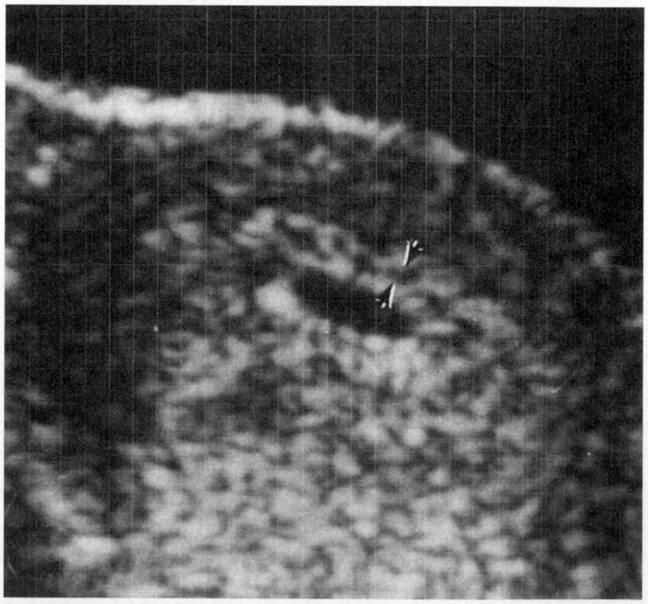

FIGURE 8.8 Sonogram showing the characteristic circle diagnostic of pregnancy (the gestational sac).

End of 20 Gestation Weeks

- Length: 25 cm.
- Weight: 223 g.
- Spontaneous fetal movements can be sensed by the mother.
- Antibody production is possible.
- Hair forms, extending to include eyebrows and hair on the head.
- Meconium is present in the upper intestine.
- Brown fat, a special fat that will aid in temperature regulation at birth, begins to be formed behind the kidneys, sternum, and posterior neck.
- Fetal heartbeat is strong enough to be audible through the abdomen with an ordinary stethoscope.
- Vernix caseosa, a cream cheese-like substance produced by the sebaceous glands that serves as a protective skin covering during intrauterine life, begins to form.
- Definite sleeping and activity patterns are distinguishable (the fetus has developed biorhythms that will guide sleep/wake patterns throughout life).

End of 24 Gestation Weeks (Second Trimester)

- Length: 28 to 36 cm.
- Weight: 550 g.
- Passive antibody transfer from mother to fetus probably begins as early as the 20th week of gestation, certainly by the 24th week of gestation. Infants born before antibody transfer has taken place have no natural immunity and need more than the usual protection against infectious disease in the newborn period until the infant's own store of immunoglobulins can build up.
- Meconium is present as far as the rectum.
- Active production of lung surfactant begins.
- Eyebrows and eyelashes are well defined.
- Eyelids, previously fused since the 12th week, are now open.
- Pupils are capable of reacting to light.
- When fetuses reach 24 weeks, or 601 g, they have achieved a practical low-end age of viability if they are cared for after birth in a modern intensive care facility.
- Hearing can be demonstrated by response to sudden sound.

End of 28 Gestation Weeks

- Length: 35 to 38 cm.
- Weight: 1,200 g.
- Lung alveoli begin to mature, and surfactant can be demonstrated in amniotic fluid.
- Testes begin to descend into the scrotal sac from the lower abdominal cavity.
- The blood vessels of the retina are extremely susceptible to damage from high oxygen concentrations (an important consideration when caring for preterm infants who need oxygen).
- The eyes open.

End of 32 Gestation Weeks

- Length: 38 to 43 cm.
- Weight: 1,600 g.
- Subcutaneous fat begins to be deposited (the former stringy, "little old man" appearance is lost).
- Fetus is aware of sounds outside the mother's body.
- Active Moro reflex is present.
- Birth position (vertex or breech) may be assumed.
- Iron stores that provide iron for the time during which the neonate will ingest only milk after birth are beginning to be developed.
- Fingernails grow to reach the end of fingertips.

End of 36 Gestation Weeks

- Length: 42 to 48 cm.
- Weight: 1,800 to 2,700 g (5 to 6 lb).
- Body stores of glycogen, iron, carbohydrate, and calcium are augmented.
- Additional amounts of subcutaneous fat are deposited.
- Sole of the foot has only one or two crisscross creases compared with the full crisscross pattern that will be evident at term.
- Amount of lanugo begins to diminish.
- Most babies turn into a vertex or head-down presentation during this month.

End of 40 Gestation Weeks (Third Trimester)

- Length: 48 to 52 cm (crown to rump, 35 to 37 cm).
- Weight: 3,000 g (7 to 7.5 lb).
- Fetus kicks actively, hard enough to cause the mother considerable discomfort.
- Fetal hemoglobin begins its conversion to adult hemoglobin. The conversion is so rapid that, at birth, about 20% of hemoglobin will be adult in character.
- Vernix caseosa is fully formed.
- Fingernails extend over the fingertips.
- Creases on the soles of the feet cover at least two thirds of the surface.

In primiparas (women having their first baby), the fetus often sinks into the birth canal during the last 2 weeks, giving the mother a feeling that her load is being lightened. This event is termed **lightening.** It is a fetal announcement that the third trimester of pregnancy has ended and birth is at hand.

Determination of Estimated Birth Date

It is impossible to predict the day of birth with a high degree of accuracy. Traditionally, this date has been referred to as the EDC, for estimated date of confinement. Because women are no longer "confined" after childbirth, EDB (**estimated date of birth**) or EDD (estimated date of delivery) is more commonly used today.

Fewer than 5% of pregnancies end exactly 280 days from the last menstrual period; fewer than half end within 1 week of the 280th day. Nagele's rule is the standard method used to predict the length of a pregnancy

(Box 8-1). Gestation age wheels or birth date calculators, which can be used to predict a birth date, are also available.

If fertilization occurs early in a menstrual cycle, the pregnancy will probably end "early"; if ovulation and fertilization occur later in the cycle, the pregnancy will end "late." Because of these normal variations, a pregnancy ending 2 weeks before or 2 weeks after the estimated calculated date of birth is considered well within the normal limit (a pregnancy of 38 to 42 weeks in length).

WHAT IF? Liz Calhorn, the young woman you met at the beginning of the chapter, first came to your prenatal clinic on August 5. What if she tells you she had her last menstrual period March 13 to 18? What would be her estimated date of birth?

ASSESSMENT OF FETAL GROWTH AND DEVELOPMENT

Much information about the size and health of the unborn child can be gathered through a variety of assessment techniques. Nursing responsibility for these assessment procedures includes seeing that a signed consent form has been obtained as needed, scheduling the procedure, explaining the procedure to the woman and her support person, preparing the woman physically and psychologically, providing support during the procedure, assessing both fetal and maternal responses to the procedure, providing follow-up care to the woman, and managing equipment and specimens (see Focus on Multidisciplinary Care).

Additional consent to perform a procedure is necessary if the procedure poses any risk to the mother or fetus that would not otherwise be present. Information must be provided about what the procedure entails and what the possible risks are.

FOCUS ON MULTIDISCIPLINARY CARE

During pregnancy, women may interact with a host of health care personnel. Unlicensed assistive personnel may assist with such assessments as taking a woman's blood pressure or doing urine testing. While they are doing these procedures, a pregnant woman may ask them questions about her pregnancy or voice a concern that her fetus does not seem to be moving as much as previously.

Be certain that unlicensed assistive personnel recognize that conversing with a pregnant woman while they perform simple assessments is helpful, but answering some questions, such as what is normal fetal growth or fetal movement, requires professional judgment. Otherwise, a woman's concerns about fetal growth can be missed and necessary further assessment not carried out.

Estimating Fetal Growth

McDonald's rule is a method of determining, during midpregnancy, that the fetus is growing in utero by measuring fundal (uterine) height. Typically, the distance from the fundus to the symphysis in centimeters is equal to the week of gestation between the 20th and 31st weeks of pregnancy. The measurement is made from the notch of the symphysis pubis to over the top of the uterine fundus as the woman lies supine (Fig. 8-9). McDonald's rule becomes inaccurate during the third trimester of pregnancy because the fetus is growing more in weight than height during this time. Until then, a fundal height much greater than this standard suggests multiple pregnancy, a miscalculated due date, a large-for-gestational-age infant, hydramnios (increased amniotic fluid volume), or hydatidiform mole (see Chap. 15). A fundal measurement much less than this suggests that either the fetus is failing to thrive (small for gestational age), the pregnancy length is miscalculated, or an anomaly, such as anencephaly, is developing.

Recording that the fundus reaches typical milestone measurements, such as over the symphysis pubis at 12 weeks, at the umbilicus at 20 weeks, and at the xiphoid process at 36 weeks, is also a helpful determination.

Assessing Fetal Well-Being

A number of actions or procedures are helpful in detecting and documenting fetal well-being.

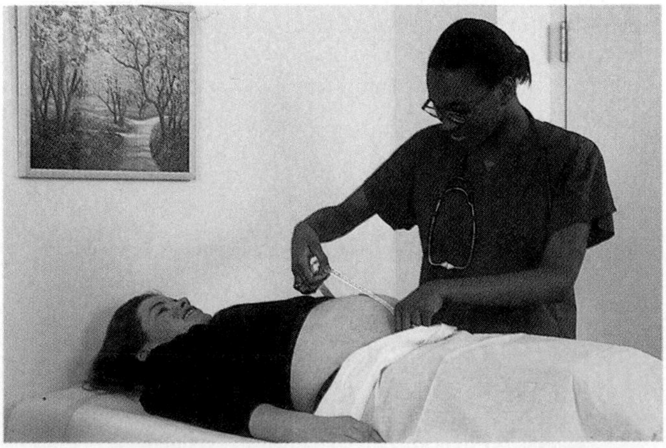

FIGURE 8.9 Measuring fundal height from the superior aspect of the pubis to the fundal crest. The nurse places the tape flat against the abdomen for the measurement.

BOX 8.1

NAGELE'S RULE

To calculate the date of birth by this rule, count backward 3 calendar months from the first day of the last menstrual period and add 7 days. For example, if the last menstrual period began May 15, you would count back 3 months (April 15, March 15, February 15) and add 7 days, to arrive at a date of birth of February 22.

Fetal Movement

Fetal movement that can be felt by the mother (quickening) begins at approximately 18 to 20 weeks of pregnancy and peaks at 28 to 38 weeks. A healthy fetus moves with a degree of consistency, but a fetus affected by placental insufficiency will show greatly decreased movements. Asking the mother to observe and record the number of movements the fetus makes daily offers a gross assessment of fetal well-being. A healthy fetus moves at least 10 times a day.

Because of variations in movements among normal, healthy fetuses as well as variations in different health care providers' level of confidence in the technique, a variety of protocols have been developed by different institutions. There also is great variety in what is accepted as normal in different areas of the country. One popular way to approach this assessment is to ask the mother to lie in a left recumbent position after a meal and record how many fetal movements she feels over the next hour (the Sandovsky method). A fetus normally moves a minimum of twice every 10 minutes or an average of 10 to 12 times an hour. The mother is instructed to telephone her health care provider if she has felt fewer than five (half the normal number) during the chosen hour. Another protocol is "Count-to-Ten" (the Cardiff method). For this, the mother records the time interval it takes for her to feel ten fetal movements. Usually, this occurs within 60 minutes. Make sure to instruct the client that fetal movements do vary, especially in relation to sleep cycles of the fetus and the mother's activity during the observation time. Otherwise, she can become unduly anxious that the fetus may be in jeopardy.

WHAT IF? You give instructions to Liz Calhorn, the mother described at the beginning of the chapter, to count fetal movements for 1 hour three times a day after meals. What if she tells you that she snacks all day long rather than eats at regular times? How would you modify your instructions? Which is more important, that she count movements after meals or that she does it three times a day?

Fetal Heart Rate

The fetal heart rate should be 120 to 160 beats per minute throughout pregnancy. Fetal heart sounds can be heard and counted as early as the 10th to 11th week of pregnancy by the use of an ultrasonic Doppler technique (Fig. 8-10). Box 8-2 highlights an appropriate outcome and intervention using terminology identified by the Nursing Outcomes Classification (NOC) and Nursing Interventions Classification (NIC).

Rhythm Strip Testing. The term "rhythm strip testing" has come to mean assessment of the fetal heart rate in terms of baseline and long- and short-term variability. For the test, the woman is placed in a semi-Fowler's position (either in a comfortable lounge chair or on an examining table or bed with an elevated backrest) to prevent supine hypotension syndrome during the test. External fetal heart rate and uterine contraction monitors are attached abdominally (Fig. 8-11*A*) and record the fetal heart rate for 20 minutes.

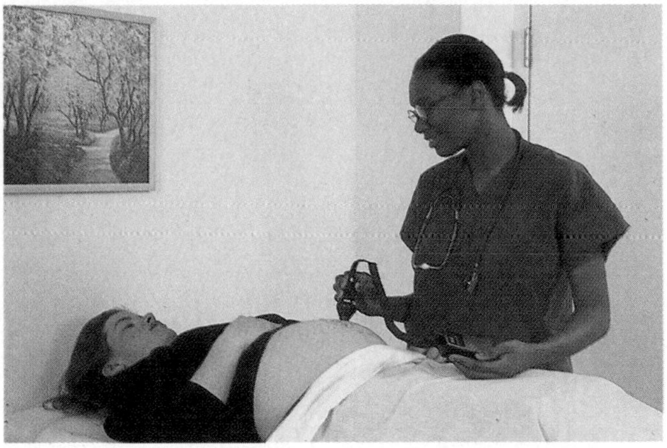

FIGURE 8.10 Measuring fetal heart rate with a Doppler transducer, which detects and broadcasts the fetal heart rate so the parents-to-be as well as you can hear it.

The baseline reading refers to the average rate of the fetal heartbeat per minute. Short-term variability (also called beat-to-beat variability) denotes the small changes in rate that occur from second to second if the fetal parasympathetic nervous system is receiving adequate oxygen and nutrients. In the rhythm strip in Figure 8-11*B*, for example, the baseline (average) of the fetal heartbeat would be 130 beats per minute. Beat-to-beat variability is present.

Long-term variability denotes the differences in heart rate that occur over the 20-minute time period. Note in Figure 8-11*B* how the heart rate varies from 150 to 120. Because the average fetus moves about twice every 10 minutes, and movement causes the heart rate to increase, there will typically be two or more instances of fetal heart rate acceleration in a 20-minute rhythm strip. Long-term variability this way reflects the state of the fetal sympathetic nervous system.

Rhythm strip testing requires the mother to remain in a fairly fixed position for 20 minutes. Keep her well informed of the purpose of the test, how it is interpreted, and the meaning of results. The more she understands about the process, the better she can cooperate to make it successful.

Nonstress Testing. A **nonstress test** measures the response of the fetal heart rate to fetal movement. The woman is positioned and the fetal heart rate and uterine contraction monitors are attached as for obtaining a rhythm strip. The woman pushes a button attached to the monitor (similar to a call bell) whenever she feels the fetus move. The paper tracing is marked by a dark line at these points.

When the fetus moves, the fetal heart rate should increase about 15 beats per minute and remain elevated for 15 seconds. It should decrease to its average rate again as the fetus quiets (see Fig. 8-11*C*). If no increase in beats per minute is noticeable on fetal movement, poor oxygen perfusion of the fetus is suggested.

A nonstress test usually is done for 10 to 20 minutes. The test is reactive if two accelerations of fetal heart rate (15 beats or more) lasting for 15 seconds occur after movement within the chosen time period. The test is non-

BOX 8.2

NURSING OUTCOMES AND NURSING INTERVENTIONS CLASSIFICATION

NOC: Fetal Status, Antepartum

Fetal status, antepartum, is defined as the conditions indicative of fetal physical well-being from conception to the onset of labor (Johnson, Maas, & Moorhead, 2000). Some specific indicators suggesting achievement of this outcome include the following parameters demonstrated within the expected range:

- Fetal heart rate
- Deceleration patterns
- Variability
- Fetal ultrasound growth measurements
- Fetal movement frequency and pattern
- Nonstress test
- Contraction stress test
- Biophysical profile score
- Amniotic fluid sample findings
- Umbilical artery blood flow velocity

NIC: Electronic Fetal Monitoring, Antepartum

Electronic fetal monitoring, antepartum, is defined as the electronic evaluation of fetal heart rate response to movement, external stimuli, or uterine contractions during antepartal testing (McCloskey & Bulechek, 2000). Some important activities involved when implementing this intervention include:

- Reviewing obstetric history for risk factors requiring antepartal testing
- Determining client's knowledge about reasons for testing
- Assessing maternal vital signs and inquiring about oral intake
- Verifying maternal and fetal heart rates before initiating electronic fetal monitoring
- Instructing client about reasons for monitoring
- Performing Leopold maneuver to determine fetal position
- Applying transducer as appropriate
- Distinguishing and differentiating among multiple fetuses
- Reassuring mother about normal fetal heart rate signs; adjusting monitors to achieve and maintain tracing clarity
- Obtaining baseline fetal heart rate tracing per protocol
- Interpreting electronic monitor strip for baseline heart rate, long-term variability, and presence of spontaneous accelerations, decelerations, or contractions
- Initiating intravenous infusion, ultrasound, or vibroacoustic stimulation as per protocol
- Interpreting tracing based on test
- Providing anticipatory guidance for abnormal test results
- Providing written discharge instructions for future testing and return for follow-up as indicated

reactive if no accelerations occur with the fetal movements. The results also can be interpreted as nonreactive if no fetal movement occurs or there is low short-term fetal heart rate variability (less than 6 beats per minute) throughout the testing period (Devoe, 1999).

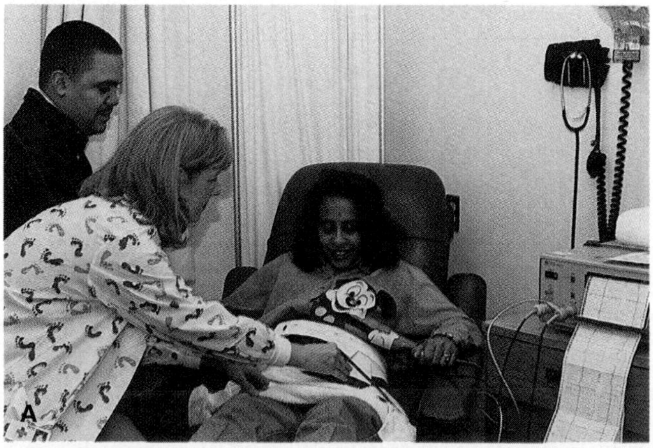

FIGURE 8.11 Rhythm strip and nonstress testing of fetal heart rate. (A) The woman sits in a comfortable chair to avoid supine hypotension. Both a uterine contraction monitor and fetal heart rate monitor are in place on her abdomen. (*continued on next page*)

If a 20-minute period passes without any fetal movement, it may mean only that the fetus is sleeping. If the mother is given an oral carbohydrate snack, such as orange juice, her blood glucose level may increase enough to cause fetal movement. The fetus may be stimulated by a loud sound (see Vibroacoustic Stimulation below).

Because both rhythm strip and nonstress testing are noninvasive procedures and cause no risk to either mother or fetus, they can be used as screening procedures in all pregnancies. They can be done at home daily as part of a home monitoring program for the mother who is having a complication of pregnancy (see Chap. 16).

If a nonstress test is nonreactive, additional fetal assessment, such as a contraction stress test or biophysical profile test, will be scheduled.

Vibroacoustic Stimulation. In acoustic (sound) stimulation, an instrument such as an artificial larynx or a specially designed acoustic stimulator is applied to the mother's abdomen to produce a sharp sound, startling and waking the fetus. The instrument emits a sound level of approximately 80 dB at a frequency of 80 Hz.

During a standard nonstress test, if a spontaneous acceleration has not occurred within 5 minutes, a single 1- to 2-second sound stimulation is applied to the lower abdomen. This could be repeated again at the end of

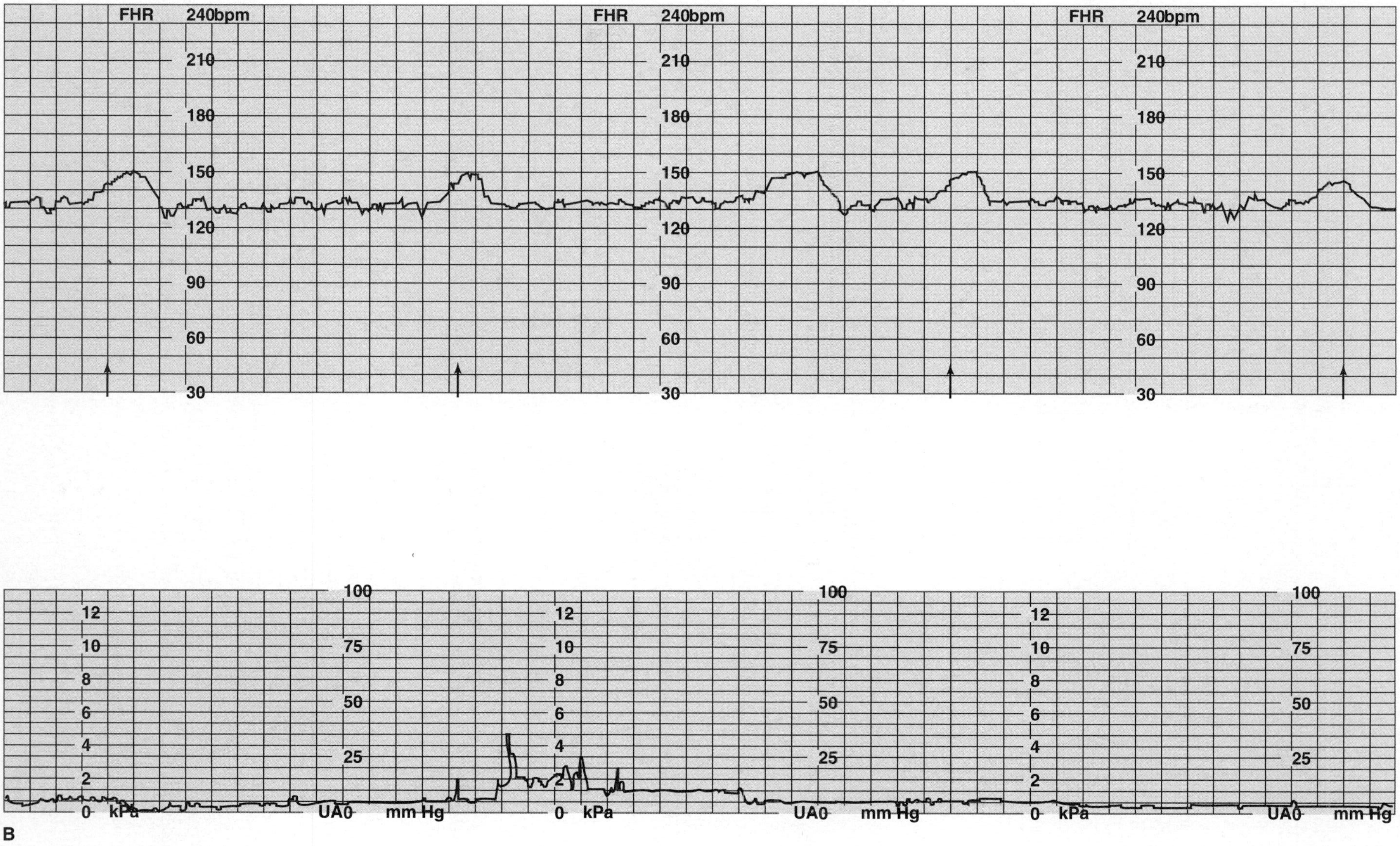

FIGURE 8.11 (*continued*) (*B*) A rhythm strip. The upper strip signifies heart rate; the lower strip indicates uterine activity. *Arrows* signal fetal movement. (*Continued on next page*)

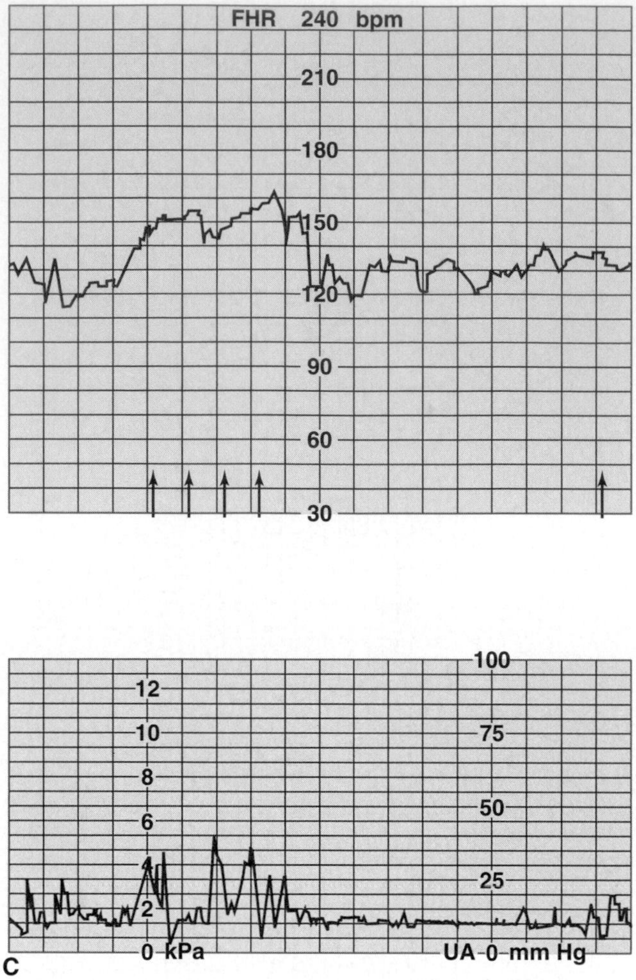

C

FIGURE 8.11 *(continued)* (C) Baseline fetal heart rate is 130–132. This strip shows fetal heart rate acceleration in response to fetal movement.

10 minutes if no further spontaneous movement occurs, so two movements within the 10-minute window can be evaluated (Mandeville & Troiano, 1999).

Contraction Stress Testing. With contraction stress testing, the fetal heart rate is analyzed in conjunction with contractions. When this test was first developed, contractions were initiated by the intravenous infusion of oxytocin. However, once started, contractions begun this way were sometimes difficult to stop and led to preterm labor. For this reason, a source of oxytocin for current contraction stress testing is achieved by nipple stimulation. Gentle stimulation of the nipples releases oxytocin in the same way as happens with breast-feeding.

With external uterine contraction and fetal heart rate monitors in place, the baseline fetal heart rate is obtained. Next, the mother rolls a nipple between her finger and thumb until uterine contractions begin, which are recorded by a uterine monitor. Three contractions with a duration of 40 seconds or more must be present in a 10-minute window before the test can be interpreted. The test is negative (normal) when no fetal heart rate decelerations are present with contractions. It is positive (abnormal) when 50% or more of contractions cause a late deceleration (a dip in fetal heart rate that occurs toward the end of a contraction and continues after the contraction). See Chapter 18 for further discussion of fetal heart rate monitoring with labor contractions.

Nonstress tests and contraction stress tests are compared in Table 8-4. After a contraction stress test, encourage the woman to remain in the health care facility for about 30 minutes to be certain that contractions have quieted and preterm labor is not a risk.

Ultrasound

Ultrasound, or the response of sound waves against objects, is a much-used tool in modern obstetrics, although the recommendations for its use are changing because of unproven benefits in the face of added expense. It can be used to:

- Diagnose pregnancy as early as 6 weeks' gestation
- Confirm the presence, size, and location of the placenta and amniotic fluid
- Establish that the fetus is growing and has no gross defects, such as hydrocephalus, anencephaly, or spinal cord, heart, kidney, and bladder defects
- Establish the presentation and position of the fetus (sex can be diagnosed if a penis is revealed)
- Predict maturity by measurement of the biparietal diameter

TABLE 8.4 Comparison of Nonstress and Contraction Tests

ASSESSMENT	NONSTRESS	CONTRACTION
What is measured	Response of fetal heart rate in relation to fetal movements	Response of fetal heart rate in relation to uterine contractions produced by nipple stimulation
Normal findings	Two or more accelerations of fetal heart rate of 15 beats/min lasting 15 sec or more following fetal movements in a 20-min period	No late decelerations with contractions
Safety considerations	Woman should not lie supine to prevent supine hypotension syndrome	In addition to supine hypotension syndrome, observe woman for 30 min afterward to see that contractions are quiet and preterm labor does not begin

Ultrasound is also used to discover complications of pregnancy, such as the presence of an intrauterine device, hydramnios or oligohydramnios, ectopic pregnancy, missed miscarriage, abdominal pregnancy, placenta previa, premature separation of the placenta, coexisting uterine tumors, multiple pregnancy, or genetic abnormalities such as Down syndrome. Fetal anomalies such as neural tube defects, diaphragmatic hernia, or urethral stenosis also can be diagnosed. Fetal death can be revealed by a lack of heartbeat and respiratory movement. After birth, a sonogram may be used to detect a retained placenta or poor uterine involution.

With ultrasound, intermittent sound waves of high frequency (above the audible range) are projected toward the uterus by a transducer placed on the abdomen or in the vagina. The sound frequencies that bounce back can be displayed on an oscilloscope screen as a visual image. The frequencies returning from tissues of various thicknesses and properties present distinct appearances. A permanent record can be made of the scan.

The intricacy of the image obtained depends on the type or mode of process used. B-mode scanning is the process most frequently used and generally what people refer to as a sonogram. This mode allows patterns to merge and form a picture similar to a black-and-white television picture (called gray-scale imaging). Real-time mode involves the use of multiple waves that allow the screen picture to move. On this type of sonogram, the fetal heart can be seen to move, and even movement of extremities, such as the fetus bringing a hand to the mouth to suck a thumb, can be seen. A parent who is in doubt that her fetus is well or whole can be reassured by viewing a real-time sonogram image.

Before an ultrasound, the woman needs a good explanation of what will happen and assurance that the process does not involve x-rays (see Focus on Communication). This means it is also safe for the father of the child to remain in the room during the test.

For the sound waves to reflect best and the uterus to be held stable, it is helpful if the mother has a full bladder at the time of the procedure. To ensure this, she should drink a full glass of water every 15 minutes beginning an hour and a half before the procedure and then not void before the procedure.

For the actual procedure, the mother lies on an examining table and is draped for privacy, but with her abdomen exposed. (To prevent supine hypotension syndrome, place a towel under her right buttock to tip her body slightly so the uterus will roll away from the vena cava.) A gel is applied to her abdomen to improve the contact of the transducer. (Be certain the gel is room temperature or even slightly warmer, or it can cause uncomfortable uterine cramping.) The transducer is then applied to her abdomen and moved both horizontally and vertically until the uterus and its contents are fully scanned (Fig. 8-12). Ultrasound also may be done using an intravaginal technique.

Although the long-term effects of ultrasound are not yet known, the technique appears to be safe for both mother and fetus. It appears to involve no discomfort for the fetus. Usually, the only discomfort for the mother is that the contact lubricant may be messy and she may experience a strong desire to void before the scan is completed. Taking home a photograph of the sonogram image can enhance bonding because it is proof that the pregnancy exists and the fetus appears well (see Focus on Evidence-Based Practice).

FOCUS ON COMMUNICATION

Mrs. Hunda is a young woman in her 7th month of pregnancy who is about to have an ultrasound.

Less Effective Communication

Nurse: Do you have any questions, Mrs. Hunda?

Mrs. Hunda: I'm wondering if I want to know the baby's sex or not.

Nurse: Most people do these days. It helps them plan for an individual person, not just any baby.

Mrs. Hunda: I think I'd like to be surprised. I know I don't want another boy.

Nurse: If it were me, I'd want to know. I think it would be helpful.

Mrs. Hunda: Okay, tell me what the ultrasound shows.

More Effective Communication

Nurse: Do you have any questions, Mrs. Hunda?

Mrs. Hunda: I'm wondering if I want to know the baby's sex or not.

Nurse: That's an individual decision. What things are you thinking about?

Mrs. Hunda: I think I'd like to be surprised. I know I don't want another boy.

Nurse: Tell me about that. Why is that?

Mrs. Hunda: My son has cerebral palsy. I don't want that to happen again.

Becoming so engrossed in giving advice, the nurse in the first example forgot to assess the exact information that the client wanted. Taking the time to assess this, such as was done in the second example, revealed that the sex of the child was only a small part of what the mother was afraid to learn.

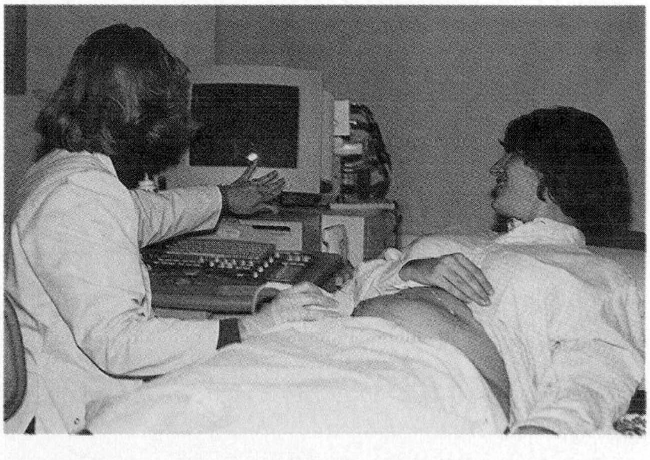

FIGURE 8.12 A sonogram being recorded. Notice the mother's interest in being able to see her baby's first picture.

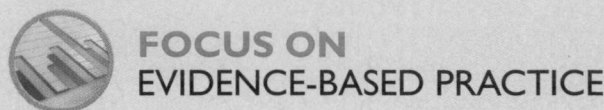

FOCUS ON EVIDENCE-BASED PRACTICE

Does the Average Woman Want a Sonogram During Pregnancy?

Most women in the United States have a routine sonogram done during pregnancy. To determine women's beliefs about this test, 150 prenatal patients coming for maternity care at a large military medical center were asked if they wanted a sonogram, and why, and their willingness to pay for the examination. Of the 150 subjects, 135 (88%) said they wanted to have a sonogram. Only 37%, however, said they would be willing to pay for the procedure. The most common reasons women gave for wanting sonograms were to ensure that the fetus was healthy and growing well and to determine the fetal sex. The researchers concluded that most women want a sonogram during pregnancy, but their reasons for wanting the exam may differ from the medical reason that dictates such a procedure.

This is an important study for nurses because nurses are frequently intimately involved in care and counseling of the pregnant woman. Nurses should be aware that these women are very concerned about the health of the fetus and can be curious about the sex of their baby.

Stephens, M. B., Montefalcon, R., & Lane, D. A. (2000). The maternal perspective on prenatal ultrasound. *Journal of Family Practice, 48* (7), 601—604.

✔ CHECKPOINT QUESTIONS

9. At 26 weeks' gestation, what would you expect a fundal height measurement to be?
10. When is a nonstress test considered nonreactive (abnormal)?
11. When an ultrasound is being done for fetal assessment, what must the woman do to ensure the best sound wave transmission?

Biparietal Diameter. Ultrasound may be used to predict fetal maturity by measuring the biparietal diameter (side-to-side measurement) of the fetal head. In 80% of pregnancies, when the biparietal diameter of the fetal head is 8.5 cm or more, the infant will weigh more than 2,500 g (5.5 lb). A biparietal diameter of 8.5 cm indicates a fetal age of 40 weeks. Figure 8-13 is a sonogram showing the biparietal diameter of a fetus at 24 weeks.

Two other measurements commonly made by sonography are head circumference (34.5 cm is a 40-week fetus) and femoral length.

Doppler Umbilical Velocimetry. Doppler ultrasonography measures the velocity at which red blood cells in the uterine and fetal vessels are traveling. Assessment of the blood flow through uterine blood vessels in this way is helpful in determining the vascular resistance present in women with diabetes or hypertension of pregnancy and the resultant placental insufficiency that may occur. Decreased velocity is an important predictor of poor neonatal outcome.

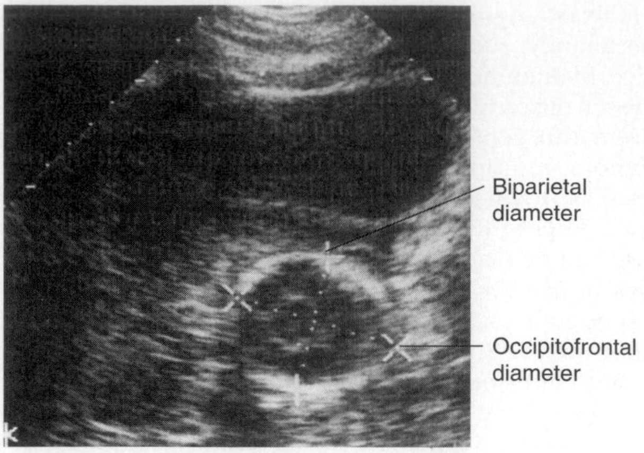

FIGURE 8.13 A sonogram at 24 weeks' gestation showing measurement of the biparietal diameter. (Courtesy of the Department of Medical Photography, Children's Hospital, Buffalo, NY.)

Placental Grading. Based particularly on the amount of calcium deposits in the base of the placenta, placentas can be graded by ultrasound as 0 (a placenta 12 to 24 weeks), 1 (30 to 32 weeks), 2 (36 weeks), and 3 (38 weeks). Because fetal lungs are apt to be mature at 38 weeks, a grade 3 placenta suggests that the fetus is mature.

Amniotic Fluid Volume Assessment. The amount of amniotic fluid present is an important fetal assessment measure because a portion of the fluid is formed by fetal kidney output. If a fetus is becoming stressed in utero so that circulatory and kidney functions are failing, urine output and, consequently, the volume of amniotic fluid also will decrease. A decrease in amniotic fluid volume puts the fetus at risk for compression of the umbilical cord and interference with nutrition (Magann et al., 2000).

For gestations of less than 20 weeks, the uterus is hypothetically divided along the linea nigra into two vertical halves. The vertical diameter of the largest pocket of amniotic fluid present is measured in centimeters on each side. The amniotic volume index (total) is the sum of the two measurements.

For gestations of 20 weeks or more, the uterus is divided into four quadrants, using the linea nigra again as the vertical dividing line and the level of the umbilicus as the horizontal dividing line. The vertical diameter of the largest pocket of fluid in each quadrant is obtained, and the four values are then added to produce the amniotic fluid index. The average index is approximately 15 cm between 28 and 40 weeks. An index greater than 20 to 24 cm indicates hydramnios (excessive fluid, perhaps caused by inability of the fetus to swallow); an index less than 5 to 6 cm indicates oligohydramnios (decreased amniotic fluid, perhaps caused by poor perfusion and kidney failure).

Electrocardiography

Fetal ECGs may be recorded as early as the 11th week of pregnancy. The ECG is inaccurate before the 20th week, however, because until this time fetal electrical conduction is so weak that it is easily masked by the mother's ECG tracing. It is rarely used unless a specific heart anomaly is suspected.

Magnetic Resonance Imaging

Magnetic resonance imaging (MRI) also may be used to assess the fetus. Because the technique apparently causes no harmful effects to the fetus or mother (although extensive long-term testing is not yet available), MRI has the potential to replace or complement ultrasound as a fetal assessment technique. It may be most helpful in diagnosing complications such as ectopic pregnancy or trophoblastic disease (see Chap. 15).

Maternal Serum Alpha-Fetoprotein

Alpha-fetoprotein is a substance produced by the fetal liver that is present in amniotic fluid and maternal serum. The level is abnormally high in the maternal serum if the fetus has an open spinal or abdominal defect, because the open defect allows more alpha-fetoprotein to appear. The level is low if the fetus has a chromosomal defect, such as Down syndrome; the reason is unknown. Alpha-fetoprotein levels begin to rise at 11 weeks' gestation and then steadily increase until term. Traditionally assessed at the 15th week of pregnancy, due to new analysis techniques it is now feasible to analyze this as early as the 11th week of pregnancy. Between 85% and 90% of neural tube defects and 20% of Down syndrome babies can be detected by this method.

Triple Screening

Triple screening, or analysis of three indicators (maternal serum for alpha-fetoprotein, unconjugated estriol, and hCG), may be performed in place of alpha-fetoprotein testing alone to yield more reliable results (60% to 70% of Down syndrome babies). Like measuring maternal serum for alpha-fetoprotein, it requires only a simple venipuncture.

Chorionic Villi Sampling

Chorionic villi sampling (CVS) is a biopsy and analysis of chorionic villi for chromosomal analysis done at 10 to 12 weeks of pregnancy. Because this is used almost exclusively for chromosomal analysis, it is discussed in Chapter 7. **Coelocentesis** (transvaginal aspiration of fluid from the extraembryonic cavity) is an alternative method to remove cells for fetal analysis.

Amniocentesis

Amniocentesis (from the Greek *amnion* for sac and *kentesis* for puncture) is the aspiration of amniotic fluid from the pregnant uterus for examination. The procedure can be done in a physician's office or an ambulatory clinic as early as the 12th to 13th week of pregnancy. Formerly, the procedure was delayed until the 14th to 16th week to allow for a generous amount of amniotic fluid to form. Refined analysis requires only 1 mL of fluid for analysis, so earlier intervention is possible. Amniocentesis also is used late in pregnancy to test for fetal maturity.

Amniocentesis is a technically easy procedure, but it can be frightening to a woman. Because it involves penetrating the integrity of the amniotic sac, there also is a risk to the fetus, although this is low. It can lead to complications such as hemorrhage from penetration of the placenta, infection of the amniotic fluid, and puncture of the fetus. There is some suggestion the procedure is associated with decreased lung function in the newborn. It can lead to irritation of the uterus, causing premature labor.

In preparation for amniocentesis, ask the woman to void (to reduce the size of the bladder, thus preventing inadvertent puncture). Place her in a supine position on the examining table and drape her appropriately, exposing only her abdomen. Place a folded towel under her right buttock to tip her body slightly to the left and move the uterus off the vena cava to prevent supine hypotension syndrome. Attach fetal heart rate and uterine contraction monitors. Take the maternal blood pressure and the fetal heart rate for baseline levels.

Explain that a sonogram will be done to determine the position of the fetus, a pocket of amniotic fluid, and the placenta. Then her abdomen will be washed with an antiseptic solution, and a local anesthetic will be given. Warn the client that she may feel a sensation of pressure as the needle used for aspiration, a 3- or 4-in, 20- to 22-gauge spinal needle, is introduced. Do not suggest that she take a deep breath and hold it as a distraction against discomfort: this lowers the diaphragm against the uterus and shifts intrauterine contents.

The needle is inserted into the amniotic cavity over a pool of amniotic fluid, carefully avoiding the fetus and placenta (Fig. 8-14). A syringe is attached, and a chosen amount of amniotic fluid is withdrawn. The needle is then removed, and the woman rests quietly for about 30 minutes. During the procedure and for the 30 minutes afterward, assess the fetal heart rate monitor and uterine contraction monitor to be certain the fetal heart rate remains normal and no uterine contractions are occurring.

If the woman has Rh-negative blood, Rho(D) immune globulin (RhIG; RhoGAM) may be administered after the procedure to prevent fetal isoimmunization. This is to ensure that maternal antibodies will not form against any placental red blood cells that accidentally were released during the procedure.

Amniocentesis can provide information in a number of areas, described below.

Color. Normal amniotic fluid is the color of water; late in pregnancy, it may have a slightly yellow tinge. A strong yellow color suggests a blood incompatibility (the yellow results from the presence of bilirubin released with the hemolysis of red blood cells). A green color suggests meconium staining, a phenomenon associated with fetal distress.

Lecithin/Sphingomyelin Ratio. Lecithin and sphingomyelin are the protein components of the lung enzyme

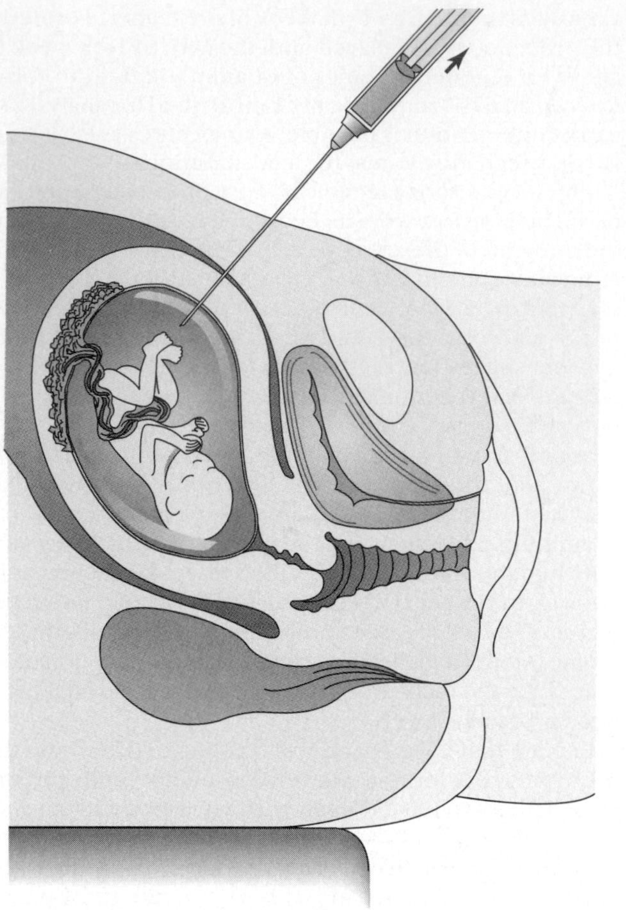

FIGURE 8.14 Amniocentesis. A pocket of amniotic fluid is located by sonogram. A small amount of fluid is removed by aspiration.

surfactant that the alveoli begin to form about the 22nd to 24th weeks of pregnancy. After amniocentesis, the lecithin/sphingomyelin ratio may be determined quickly by a shake test or sent for laboratory analysis. A ratio of 2 to 1 is traditionally accepted as lung maturity.

Infants of mothers with severe diabetes may have false-mature readings of lecithin because the stress to the infant in utero tends to mature lecithin pathways early. Fetal values must be considered in light of the presence of maternal diabetes, or the infant may be born with mature lung function but be immature overall (fragile giants) and thus may not do well in postnatal life. Some laboratories interpret a ratio of 2.5:1 or 3:1 as a mature indicator in these infants.

Phosphatidyl Glycerol and Desaturated Phosphatidylcholine. These are other compounds, in addition to lecithin and sphingomyelin, that are found in surfactant. Pathways for these compounds mature at 35 to 36 weeks. Because they are present only with mature lung function, when they are present in the sample of amniotic fluid obtained by amniocentesis, it can be predicted that respiratory distress syndrome will not occur.

Bilirubin Determination. The presence of bilirubin may be analyzed if a blood incompatibility is suspected. If bilirubin is going to be analyzed, the specimen must be blood-free or a false-positive reading will occur.

Chromosome Analysis. A few fetal skin cells are always present in amniotic fluid. These cells may be cultured and stained for karyotyping. The chromosomal diseases that can be detected by prenatal amniocentesis and their significance to health are discussed in Chapter 7.

Fetal Fibronectin. Fibronectin is a glycoprotein that plays a part in helping the placenta attach to the uterine decidua. It can be found in abundant amounts in the amniotic fluid. Early in pregnancy, it can be assessed in the woman's cervical mucus, but the amount then fades until after 20 weeks of pregnancy, it is no longer present. As labor approaches and cervical dilatation begins, it can be assessed again in cervical or vaginal fluid. Damage to fetal membranes releases a great deal of the substance, so detection of fibronectin in the woman's vagina can serve as an announcement that preterm labor may be beginning (Miller & Paul, 2000).

Inborn Errors of Metabolism. Some inherited diseases caused by inborn errors of metabolism can be detected by amniocentesis. For a condition to be identified this way, the enzyme defect must be present in the amniotic fluid as early as the time of the procedure. Examples of illnesses that can be detected this way are cystinosis and maple syrup urine disease (amino acid disorders).

Alpha-Fetoprotein. If the fetus has an open body defect, such as anencephaly, myelomeningocele, or omphalocele, increased levels of alpha-fetoprotein will be present in the amniotic fluid because of leakage of alpha-fetoprotein into the amniotic fluid. The level will be decreased in the fluid of fetuses with chromosomal defects such as Down syndrome. Acetylcholinesterase is a similar compound obtained from amniotic fluid in high levels if a neural tube defect is present.

Percutaneous Umbilical Blood Sampling

Percutaneous umbilical blood sampling (also called cordocentesis or funicentesis) is the aspiration of blood from the umbilical vein for analysis. After locating the umbilical cord by sonography, a thin needle is inserted by amniocentesis technique into the uterus and is guided by ultrasound until it pierces the umbilical vein. A sample of blood is then removed for blood studies, such as a complete blood count, direct Coombs' test, blood gases, and karyotyping. To ensure that the blood obtained is fetal blood, it is submitted to a Kleihauer-Betke test. If a fetus is found to be anemic, blood may be transfused using this same technique. Because the umbilical vein continues to ooze for a moment after the procedure, fetal blood could enter the maternal circulation, so RhIG is given to Rh-negative women to prevent sensitization. The fetus is monitored by a nonstress test before and after the procedure to be certain uterine contractions are not present and by ultrasound to see that no bleeding is evident. This procedure carries little additional risk to the fetus or mother over amniocentesis and can yield information not available by any other means, especially about blood dyscrasias.

Amnioscopy

Amnioscopy is the visual inspection of the amniotic fluid through the cervix and membranes with an amnioscope (a small fetoscope). The main use of the technique is to detect meconium staining. It carries some risk of membrane rupture.

Fetoscopy

Fetoscopy, visualizing the fetus by inspection through a fetoscope (an extremely narrow, hollow tube inserted by amniocentesis technique), is sometimes helpful in assessing fetal well-being. A photograph can be taken through the fetoscope to assure the parents that their infant is well and perfectly formed. The procedure may be used to:

- Confirm the intactness of the spinal column
- Obtain biopsy samples of fetal tissue and fetal blood samples
- Perform elemental surgery, such as inserting a polyethylene shunt into the fetal ventricles to relieve hydrocephalus or anteriorly into the fetal bladder to relieve a stenosed urethra

The 16th or 17th week of pregnancy is about the earliest time in pregnancy that fetoscopy can be performed. For the procedure, the mother is prepared and draped as for amniocentesis. A local anesthetic is injected into the abdominal skin. The fetoscope is then inserted after a minor abdominal incision. If the fetus is very active, meperidine (Demerol) may be administered to the mother to avoid fetal injury by the scope and to allow better observation. This drug crosses the placenta and sedates the fetus.

Fetoscopy carries a small risk of premature labor. Amnionitis (infection of the amniotic fluid) may occur. To avoid this, the mother may be prescribed 10 days of antibiotic therapy after the procedure. The number of procedures performed by fetoscopy is limited because of the manipulation involved and the ethical quandary of the mother's autonomy being compromised by the fetal needs if further procedures are necessary (e.g., asking the mother to undergo general anesthesia so the fetus can have surgery).

Biophysical Profile

A biophysical profile combines four to six parameters (fetal breathing movements, fetal movement, fetal tone, amniotic fluid volume, placental grading, fetal heart reactivity) into one assessment. The scoring for a complete profile is shown in Table 8-5. By this system, each item has the potential for scoring a 2, so 12 would be the highest score possible. If only four parameters are used, 8 is a perfect score. A biophysical profile is more accurate in predicting fetal well-being than any single assessment. Because the scoring system is similar to that of the Apgar score determined at birth on infants, it is popularly called a fetal Apgar.

Biophysical profiles may be done as often as daily during a high-risk pregnancy. If the fetus score on a complete profile is 8 to 10, the fetus is considered to be doing well. A score of 4 to 6 denotes a fetus in jeopardy. More recently, some centers use only two assessments (the amniotic fluid index and nonstress test) for assessment. Referred to as a modified biophysical profile, it predicts short-term viability by the nonstress test and long-term viability by the amniotic fluid index. Nurses play a large role in obtaining the information for both the modified and full biophysical profile by obtaining either the nonstress test or the sonogram reading (Manning, 1999; Tongsong et al., 1999).

✔ CHECKPOINT QUESTIONS

12. What does an elevated maternal serum alpha-fetoprotein level suggest?
13. Why do women need to void just before an amniocentesis?

KEY POINTS

The union of a single sperm and egg (fertilization) signals the beginning of pregnancy. The fertilized ovum (a zygote) travels by way of a fallopian tube to the uterus, where implantation takes place in about 8 days. From implantation to 5 to 8 weeks,

TABLE 8.5 Biophysical Profile Scoring

ASSESSMENT	INSTRUMENT	CRITERIA FOR A SCORE OF 2
Fetal breathing	Sonogram	At least one episode of 30 sec of sustained fetal breathing movements within 30 min of observation
Fetal movement	Sonogram	At least three separate episodes of fetal limb or trunk movement within a 30-min observation
Fetal tone	Sonogram	The fetus must extend and then flex the extremities or spine at least once in 30 min
Amniotic fluid volume	Sonogram	A pocket of amniotic fluid measuring more than 1 cm in vertical diameter must be present
Placental grade	Sonogram	Placenta is grade 3; grading is based on structure and amount of calcium present
Fetal heart reactivity	Nonstress test	Two or more fetal heart rate accelerations of at least 15 beats/min above baseline and of 15 sec duration occur with fetal movement over a 20-min time period

the growing structure is called an embryo. The period following this until birth is the fetal period.

Growth of the umbilical cord, amniotic fluid, and amniotic membranes proceeds in concert with fetal growth. The placenta produces a number of important hormones: estrogen, progesterone, chorionic somatomammotropin, and human chorionic gonadotropin.

Various methods to assess fetal growth and development include fundal height, fetal movement, fetal heart tones, ultrasound, magnetic resonance imaging, alpha-fetoprotein analysis, amniocentesis, percutaneous umbilical blood sampling, amnioscopy, and fetoscopy.

A biophysical profile is a combination of fetal assessments that better predicts fetal well-being than single parameters.

CRITICAL THINKING EXERCISES

1. Liz Calhorn, whom you met at the beginning of the chapter, has stated that her feelings have changed since she felt her baby move inside her. How would you modify your health teaching with her because of this?
2. A client is scheduled for an ultrasound at 20 weeks' gestation to assess fetal growth. She states that she does not want to know the sex of her fetus. Why do some women want to know the sex of a fetus and some do not? Is there an advantage to knowing or not knowing?
3. Late in pregnancy, a client is scheduled for weekly nonstress tests. She states that she hates to have these done because they are time-consuming and boring. How could you make such tests more appealing and so increase compliance?
4. Examine the National Health Goals related to fetal health. Most government-sponsored money for nursing research is allotted based on these goals. What would be a research topic to explore pertinent to these goals that would be fundable and would advance evidence-based practice?

REFERENCES

Department of Health and Human Services. (2000). *Healthy people 2010.* Washington, D.C.: DHHS.

Devoe, L. D. (1999). Nonstress testing and contraction stress testing. *Obstetrics & Gynecology Clinics of North America, 26*(4), 535–556.

Freedman, A. L., Johnson, M. P., & Gonzalez, R. (2000). Fetal therapy for obstructive uropathy: Past, present, future. *Pediatric Nephrology, 14*(2), 167–176.

Johnson, M., Mass, M. & Moorhead, S. (2000). *Nursing outcomes classification* (2nd ed.). St. Louis: Mosby.

Ling, F. W., & Duff, P. (2001). *Obstetrics and gynecology: Principles for practice.* New York: McGraw-Hill.

Magann, E. F., et al. (2000). Amniotic fluid volume estimation and the biophysical profile: A confusion of criteria. *Obstetrics & Gynecology, 86*(4), 640–642.

Mandeville, L. K., & Troiano, N. H. (1999). Guidelines for fetal acoustic stimulation. In *High-risk and critical care intrapartum nursing* (p. 418). Philadelphia: Lippincott-Raven.

Manning, F. A. (1999). Fetal biophysical profile. *Obstetrics & Gynecology Clinics of North America, 26*(4), 557–577.

McCloskey, J. & Bulechek, G. (2000). *Nursing interventions classification* (3rd ed.). St. Louis Mosby.

Miller, D. A. & Paul, R. (2000). Antepartum-intrapartum fetal monitoring. In Scott, J. R., et al. *Danforth's obstetrics and gynecology* (8th ed., pp. 243–256). Philadelphia: Lippincott Williams & Wilkins.

Seifer, D. B., Samuels, P., & Kniss, D. A. (2001). *The physiologic basis of gynecology and obstetrics.* Philadelphia: Lippincott Williams & Wilkins.

Sheridan, E., et al. (2002). Congenital rubella syndrome: A risk in immigrant populations. *Lancet, 359*(9307), 674–4675.

Stephens, M. B., Montefalcon, R. & Lane, D. A. (2000). The maternal perspective on prenatal ultrasound. *Journal of Family Practice, 48*(7), 601–604.

Tongsong, T., et al. (1999). The rapid biophysical profile for assessment of fetal well-being. *Journal of Obstetrics & Gynaecology Research, 25*(6), 431–436.

Uckan, E. M., & Townsend, N. S. (1999). Fetal adaptation. In L. K. Mandeville & N. H. Troiano. *High-risk and critical care intrapartum nursing* (pp. 32–50). Philadelphia: Lippincott-Raven.

SUGGESTED READINGS

Christensen, F. C., & Rayburn, W. F. (1999). Fetal movement counts. *Obstetrics & Gynecology Clinics of North America, 26*(4), 607–621.

Cuneo, B. F., & Strasburger, J. F. (2000). Management strategy for fetal tachycardia. *Obstetrics & Gynecology, 86*(4), 575–581.

Flaxman, S. M., & Sherman, P. W. (2000). Morning sickness: A mechanism for protecting mother and embryo. *Quarterly Review of Biology, 75*(2), 113–148.

Hepner, D. L., et al. (2002). Herbal medicine use in parturients. *Anesthesia & Analgesia, 94*(3), 690–693.

Kamel, H. S., Makhlouf, A. M., & Youssef, A. A. (1999). Simplified biophysical profile: An antepartum fetal screening test. *Gynecologic & Obstetric Investigation, 47*(4), 223–228.

Kamel, H. S., et al. (1999). Psychological and obstetrical responses of mothers following antenatal fetal sex identification. *Journal of Obstetrics & Gynaecology Research, 25*(1), 43–50.

Kelly, M. K., et al. (2000). Effect of antenatal steroid administration on the fetal biophysical profile. *Journal of Clinical Ultrasound, 28*(5), 224–226.

Mori, A., Iwabuchi, M., & Makino, T. (2000). Fetal haemodynamic changes in fetuses during fetal development evaluated by arterial pressure pulse and blood flow velocity waveforms. *BJOG: International Journal of Obstetrics & Gynaecology, 107*(5), 668–677.

9

CHAPTER

Psychological and Physiologic Changes of Pregnancy

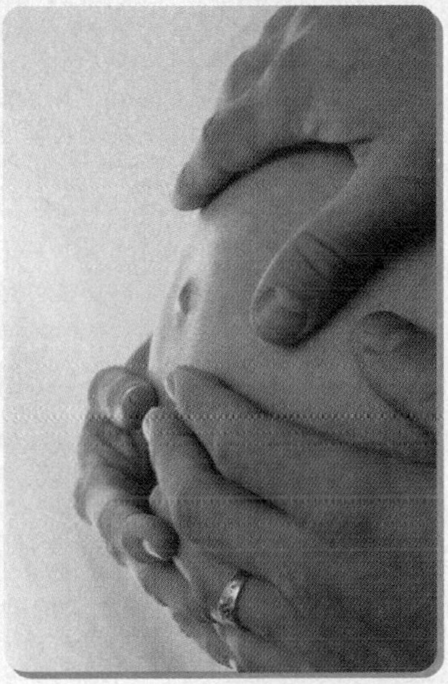

Key Terms

* ballottement
* Braxton Hicks contractions
* Chadwick's sign
* couvade syndrome
* diastasis
* Goodell's sign
* Hegar's sign
* hyperptyalism
* lightening
* melasma
* Montgomery's tubercles
* multipara
* operculum
* polyuria
* positive signs of pregnancy
* presumptive signs of pregnancy
* primigravida
* probable signs of pregnancy
* pseudoanemia
* striae gravidarum

Objectives

After mastering the contents of this chapter, you should be able to:

1. Describe common psychological and physiologic changes that occur with pregnancy, the underlying principles for these changes, and the relationship of the changes to the pregnancy diagnosis.
2. Assess a woman for the psychological and physical changes that occur with pregnancy through health history and physical examination.
3. Formulate nursing diagnoses related to the psychological and physical changes of pregnancy.
4. Identify outcome criteria for the family's psychological and physical adaptation to pregnancy.
5. Plan nursing care related to the changes and diagnosis of pregnancy, such as helping the woman plan to get adequate rest.
6. Implement nursing care, such as health teaching related to the expected changes of pregnancy.
7. Evaluate outcome criteria for the achievement and effectiveness of care.
8. Identify National Health Goals that nurses could be instrumental in helping the nation achieve.
9. Identify areas of nursing care related to the psychological and physiologic changes of pregnancy that could benefit from additional nursing research or application of evidence-based practice.
10. Use critical thinking to analyze how the physical and psychological changes of pregnancy affect family functioning, and develop ways to make nursing care more family-centered.
11. Integrate knowledge of the psychological and physiologic changes of pregnancy with nursing process to achieve quality maternal and child health nursing care.

Lauren Maxwell is a part-time model who has come to your clinic for her first prenatal visit. She tells you that she missed her period 4 weeks ago and immediately took a home pregnancy test. It was positive! She's excited because she and her husband have been trying for several months to get pregnant. She is also anxious: "I know there's no turning back now, but I wonder what this will do to my career," she tells you. She says that her husband doesn't seem a bit scared: "I don't know if that's a good thing or not," she confides. She's also worried about being a good parent: "I'd die," she says, "if I turned into the same kind of parent my parents were."

In addition to the positive home pregnancy test, Lauren presents with amenorrhea, breast tenderness, fatigue, and morning sickness. A pregnancy test has been ordered. Lauren is interested in knowing when she will begin to look pregnant and what she can do for the morning sickness.

Previous chapters discussed normal anatomy and physiology before pregnancy. This chapter adds information to your knowledge base about the physical and psychological changes that occur in both a woman and her partner during pregnancy. This is important information because it can help protect the health of both the woman and the newborn.

After you've studied the chapter, answer the Critical Thinking Exercises at the end of the chapter and then access the on-line study activities (http://connection.lww.com) *to further sharpen your skills and test your knowledge.*

Pregnancy brings both psychological and physical changes to the woman and her partner. Clients are often interested in the changes pregnancy brings, because these changes verify the reality and mark the progress of a pregnancy.

The physiologic changes of pregnancy occur gradually but eventually affect all organ systems of the woman's body. Psychological changes occur in response not only to the physiologic alterations that are occurring but also to the increased responsibility associated with welcoming a new and completely dependent person to the family. The changes occur in order for the woman to provide oxygen and nutrients for the growing fetus, as well as extra nutrients for her own increased metabolism during the pregnancy. They ready her body for labor and birth and for lactation once the baby is born. Although the physiologic changes that occur with pregnancy are extensive, they are also temporary; when pregnancy ends, the woman's body returns virtually to its prepregnant state.

Despite the magnitude of some of these changes, it cannot be stressed enough that they are extensions of normal physiology. This means that pregnancy represents wellness, not illness. Because of this, the major responsibility of the nurse caring for the pregnant woman and family is to help the family maintain a state of wellness throughout the pregnancy and into early parenthood. A National Health Goal relevant to this issue is shown in the Focus on National Health Goals box.

FOCUS ON NATIONAL HEALTH GOALS

At least one National Health Goal speaks directly to the physiologic and psychological changes of pregnancy:

- Increase to at least 60% the proportion of primary care providers who provide age-appropriate preconception care and counseling (DHHS, 2000).

Nurses can be instrumental in helping the nation achieve this objective by being certain that adolescents receive counseling in nutrition and safer sex practices so they can enter intended pregnancies in good health. Nursing research to identify the best way to reach mature women with preconception counseling is also important.

NURSING PROCESS OVERVIEW

For Healthy Adaptation to Pregnancy

Assessment

Ideally, assessment for pregnancy begins before the pregnancy. During a preconception assessment, it is important to evaluate the woman's health status, nutritional intake (e.g., sufficient intake of folic acid), and lifestyle (e.g., drinking and smoking habits); identify any potential problems (e.g., potential for ectopic pregnancy resulting from tubal scarring); and identify the woman's understanding and expectations of conception, pregnancy, and parenthood.

In early pregnancy, be certain that you establish a trusting relationship with a woman so she will see you as a person who is capable of counseling her and helping her solve problems and in whom she is willing to confide. It is important to assess the woman's health and nutritional status, as well as the well-being of the fetus, throughout pregnancy. Document the woman's physiologic adaptation and the family's psychological adaptation to pregnancy, noting any abnormal findings. Physical findings are gained through the health history, physical assessment, and laboratory tests. Assessment in psychological areas is obtained primarily through interviewing and should include societal, cultural, family, and personal influences on the client's physiologic and psychological adaptation to pregnancy.

Nursing Diagnosis

Nursing diagnoses involving the changes that occur with pregnancy may include:

- Anxiety related to unexpected pregnancy
- Ineffective breathing pattern related to respiratory system changes of pregnancy
- Disturbed body image related to weight gain with pregnancy
- Deficient knowledge related to normal changes of pregnancy
- Imbalanced nutrition, less than body requirements, related to morning sickness

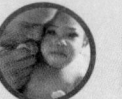

Outcome Identification and Planning
Although a woman may have read pamphlets or talked to her friends about the physiologic changes of pregnancy, she is often surprised to see these changes occurring in herself. She may say, "I knew I'd be tired, but I never guessed it would be this bad," or "I've read about a brown line forming on my abdomen, but is it normal for it to be this dark? Will this go away?"

Planning nursing care in connection with the physiologic and psychological changes of pregnancy should involve a plan to review this type of concern with the woman as well as a plan to ask about the individual responses she is experiencing.

Implementation
The changes of pregnancy may appear insignificant if taken one by one, but together they add up to major changes.

Most women of childbearing age have a mental picture of themselves. A woman has a good idea how she will look in a dress before she tries it on in a store. She participates in sports or other activities that conform to her self-image. Then, in 9 months, she gains 25 to 30 lb and her figure changes so drastically that none of her prepregnancy clothes fit. At the beginning of pregnancy, she may feel constantly nauseated. Toward the end of pregnancy, the extra weight and the strain of waiting may make her feel tired and short of breath. Endocrine changes make her moody and perhaps quick to cry. She may never have been concerned with her health before; now, every month (and toward the end of pregnancy, every week), she must report for a prenatal checkup. She may worry that she will never lose all the weight she has gained, that the stretch marks on her abdomen will remain forever, and that she will always be as tired or as nauseated as she feels during various stages of her pregnancy.

At prenatal visits, women need help in voicing their concerns about these physiologic changes of pregnancy. The worry brought on by these changes may compound an already stressful situation if the woman is not aware that the changes are a normal but transitory part of pregnancy. She needs suggestions on exercise and nutrition to prepare for pregnancy and to follow during pregnancy. For many women, pregnancy is the first time they have seen a health care provider since childhood. Nursing interventions can be instrumental in not only guiding a woman safely through pregnancy but also connecting her with ongoing health care.

Outcome Evaluation
Evaluation should determine if the woman has really "heard" your teaching. Pregnancy may be a time of stress for the woman and her partner. People under stress do not always comprehend well, so it is not unusual for a woman to pocket away information, thinking, "I'll concentrate on what that means when it happens to me, not now." Then, when a particular change has happened, she realizes that she has forgotten what you said. Evaluation that reveals learning did not take place confirms that pregnancy is a period of stress more often than it reflects the quality of teaching. Examples of outcome criteria you might strive for are:

- Client states that she is able to continue her usual lifestyle through pregnancy.
- Family members describe ways they have adjusted their lifestyles to accommodate the mother's fatigue.
- Couple states they accept the physiologic changes of pregnancy as normal.

THE DIAGNOSIS OF PREGNANCY

The diagnosis of pregnancy marks a major life milestone. If a pregnancy was planned, the diagnosis produces a feeling of intense fulfillment and achievement; if it was not planned or not desired, it can result in an equally extreme crisis state. The medical diagnosis of pregnancy serves to date the expected birth and help predict the existence of a high-risk status.

From the day the pregnancy is confirmed, most women try to eat a proper diet, give up cigarette smoking and alcohol ingestion, and stop taking over-the-counter medication. Because a woman may not take these measures before confirmation of her pregnancy, early diagnosis is important. If the woman does not wish to continue the pregnancy, early diagnosis is imperative; elective termination of pregnancy always should be carried out at the earliest stage possible for the safest outcome.

When a sexually active woman is scheduled for diagnostic testing that includes a pelvic x-ray such as an intravenous pyelogram, you might suggest that she first have a rapid serum pregnancy test to rule out pregnancy as a possibility, to avoid exposing a fetus to radiation.

Most women who come to a health care facility for a diagnosis of pregnancy have already guessed that they are pregnant based on a multitude of presumptive signs. Often, they have already done a home pregnancy test to see if they are pregnant (Shew et al., 2000).

Pregnancy is officially diagnosed on the basis of the symptoms reported by the woman and the signs elicited by a health care provider. These signs and symptoms are traditionally divided into three classifications: presumptive, probable, and positive (Table 9-1).

Presumptive Signs of Pregnancy

Presumptive signs of pregnancy are those that are least indicative of pregnancy; taken as single entities, they could easily indicate other conditions. These findings, discussed in connection with the body system in which they occur, are largely subjective in that they are experienced by the woman but cannot be documented by the examiner (see Assessing the Client for Presumptive Signs of Pregnancy).

Probable Signs of Pregnancy

In contrast to presumptive signs, **probable signs of pregnancy** can be documented by the examiner. Although they are more reliable than the presumptive signs, they still

TABLE 9.1 Presumptive, Probable, and Positive Signs of Pregnancy

TIME FROM IMPLANTATION (WEEKS)	PRESUMPTIVE FINDING	PROBABLE FINDING	POSITIVE FINDING	DESCRIPTION
1		Serum laboratory tests		Tests of blood serum reveal the presence of human chorionic gonadotropin hormone.
2	Breast changes			Feeling of tenderness, fullness, or tingling; enlargement and darkening of areola
2	Nausea, vomiting			Nausea or vomiting on arising
2	Amenorrhea			Absence of menstruation
3	Frequent urination			Sense of having to void frequently
6		Chadwick's sign		Color change of the vagina from pink to violet
6		Goodell's sign		Softening of the cervix
6		Hegar's sign		Softening of the lower uterine segment
6		Sonographic evidence of gestational sac		Characteristic ring is evident.
8			Sonographic evidence of fetal outline	Fetal outline can be seen and measured by sonogram.
10–12			Fetal heart audible	Doppler ultrasound reveals heart beat.
12	Fatigue			General feeling of tiredness
12	Uterine enlargement			Uterus can be palpated over symphysis pubis.
16		Ballottement		When lower uterine segment is tapped on a bimanual examination, the fetus can be felt to rise against abdominal wall.
18	Quickening			Fetal movement felt by woman
20			Fetal movement felt by examiner	Fetal movement can be palpated through abdomen.
20		Braxton Hicks sign		Periodic uterine tightening occurs.
20		Fetal outline felt by examiner		Fetal outline can be palpated through abdomen.
24	Linea nigra			Line of dark pigment on the abdomen
24	Melasma			Dark pigment on face
24	Striae gravidarum			Red streaks on abdomen

are not positive or true diagnostic findings (see Assessing the Client for Probable Signs of Pregnancy). They are also discussed in connection with the body system in which they occur.

Laboratory Tests

The commonly used laboratory tests for pregnancy are based on detecting the presence of human chorionic gonadotropin (hCG), a hormone created by the chorionic villi of the placenta, in the urine or blood serum of the pregnant woman. Because all laboratory tests for pregnancy are accurate in diagnosing pregnancy only 95% to 98% of the time, positive results from these tests are considered probable rather than positive signs.

These tests are performed by radioimmunoassay (RIA), enzyme-linked immunosorbent assay (ELISA), or radioreceptor assay (RRA) techniques. For these tests, hCG is measured in international units. In the nonpregnant woman, no units will be detectable because there are no trophoblast cells producing hCG. In the pregnant woman, trace amounts of hCG appear in the serum as early as 24 to 48 hours after implantation. They reach a measurable level (about 50 mIU/mL) 7 to 9 days after conception. Levels peak at about 100 mIU/mL between the 60th and 80th day of gestation. After this point, the level declines

ASSESSING the Client for Presumptive Signs of Pregnancy

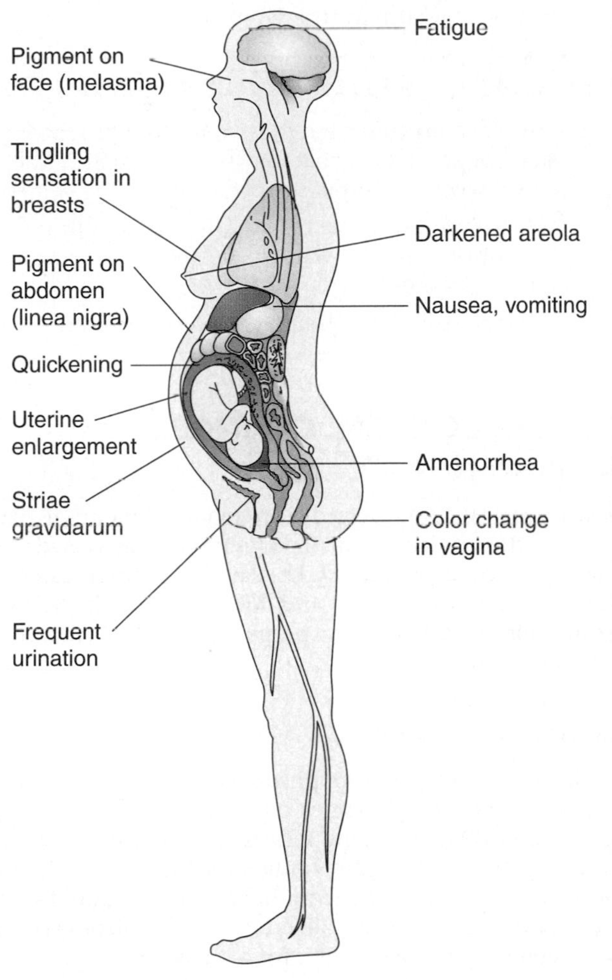

ASSESSING the Client for Probable Signs of Pregnancy

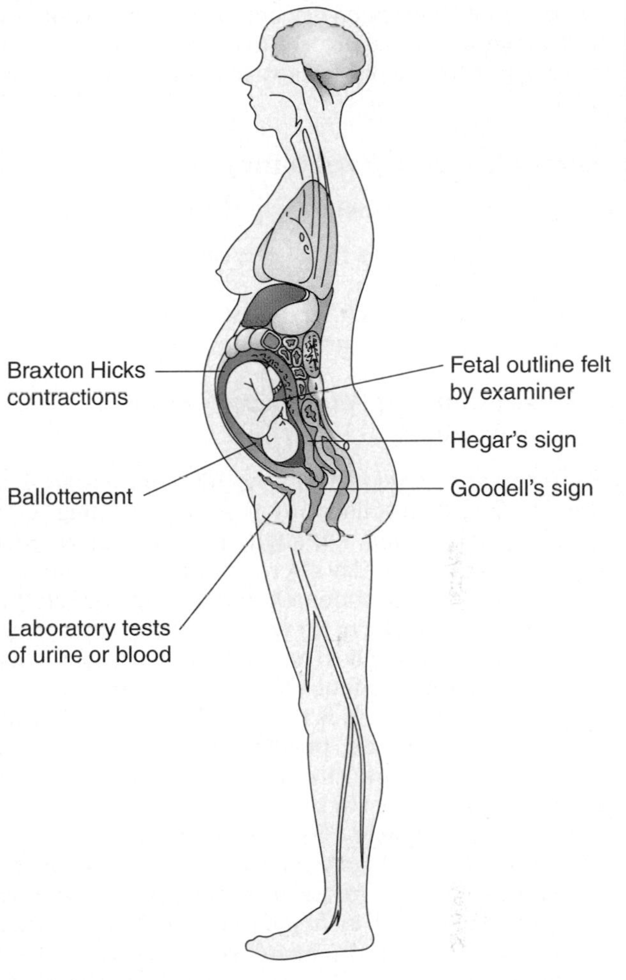

again so that, at term, it is barely detectable in serum or urine.

Urine, formerly used extensively for pregnancy testing, is now used only rarely in health care settings because blood serum tests give earlier results. Urine tests still form the basis of home pregnancy tests. Any woman who thinks she might be pregnant but gets a negative result from a pregnancy test should be advised to have a repeat test 1 week later if she is still experiencing amenorrhea. If she is not pregnant, she might have a condition such as an ovarian tumor causing the amenorrhea and would need appropriate therapy.

Home Pregnancy Tests

Several brand-name kits for pregnancy testing based on immunologic reactions are available over the counter. These tests have a high degree of accuracy (about 97%) if the instructions are followed exactly. They are convenient because waiting for a health care appointment to have a pregnancy test is an anxious, stressful time for many women. For this type of test, the woman dips a reagent strip into her stream of urine. A color change on the strip denotes pregnancy. Home tests can detect as little as 50 to 150 mIU/mL of hCG. They take 3 to 5 minutes to perform. Most manufacturers suggest the woman wait until the day of the missed menstrual period to test.

In the past, one of the chief reasons women sought early prenatal care was to obtain an official diagnosis of pregnancy rather than for reasons of health. Now that women can diagnose their pregnancies at home by means of a test kit, they may not seek prenatal care until something seems to be wrong with the pregnancy or until they are far along and feel they should do something about arranging medical coverage for the birth. Caution women that early and regular prenatal care is important to safeguard the pregnancy outcome. After a positive pregnancy test, the next step should be to arrange for prenatal care (Wheeler, 1999).

Women taking psychotropic drugs (e.g., antianxiety agents) may have false-positive results on pregnancy tests. Women taking oral contraceptives also may have false-positive results; for such a test to be accurate, oral contraceptives should have been discontinued 5 days before the test. Women who have proteinuria, are postmenopausal, or have hyperthyroid disease also may show false-positive results.

Positive Signs of Pregnancy

There are only three **positive signs of pregnancy:**

- Demonstration of a fetal heart separate from the mother's
- Fetal movements felt by the examiner
- Visualization of the fetus by ultrasound

Demonstration of a Fetal Heart Separate From the Mother's

The presence of a fetal heart can be demonstrated by hearing its sound (auscultation) or seeing it beating on an ultrasound examination. Although the fetal heart has been beating since the 24th day after conception, it is audible by auscultation of the abdomen with an ordinary stethoscope only at about 18 to 20 weeks of pregnancy. Fetal heart sounds are difficult to hear when the abdomen has a great deal of subcutaneous fat or a larger than normal amount of amniotic fluid is present (hydramnios). They are heard best when the position of the fetus is determined by palpation and the stethoscope is placed over the area of the fetus's back. The fetal heart rate usually ranges between 120 and 160 beats per minute.

Ultrasonic monitoring systems that convert ultrasonic frequencies to audible frequencies (Doppler technique) are extremely helpful in detecting fetal heart sounds. Fetal heart sounds may be heard as early as the 10th to 12th week of gestation by this method. Echocardiography can demonstrate a heartbeat as early as 5 weeks.

Fetal Movements Felt by the Examiner

Fetal movements may be felt by the woman as early as 16 to 20 weeks of pregnancy. Those felt by an objective examiner are considered much more reliable and constitute a positive sign of pregnancy. Such movements may be felt by the 20th to 24th week of pregnancy unless the woman is extremely obese.

Visualization of Fetus by Ultrasound

High-frequency sound waves projected toward a woman's abdomen are useful in diagnosing pregnancy. If the woman is pregnant, a characteristic ring, indicating the gestational sac, will be revealed on the oscilloscope as early as the 4th to 6th week of pregnancy. This method also gives information about the site of implantation and whether a multiple pregnancy exists. By the 8th week, a fetal outline can be seen so clearly within the sac that the crown-to-rump length can be measured to establish the gestational age of the pregnancy. By using a real-time technique of ultrasound, fetal heart movement may be demonstrated as early as the 6th week with transvaginal sonography and the 7th week with transabdominal sonography. Seeing or hearing a fetal heartbeat is proof of a pregnancy for the health care provider and also for the woman.

> ✔ **CHECKPOINT QUESTIONS**
>
> 1. List three presumptive signs and three probable signs of pregnancy that may be noted within the first 6 weeks of implantation.
> 2. What is the hormone tested for by a laboratory test for pregnancy? What may cause false-positive results?
> 3. What are the three positive signs of pregnancy?

PSYCHOLOGICAL CHANGES OF PREGNANCY

A woman's attitude toward a pregnancy depends a great deal on the environment in which she was raised, the messages about pregnancy her family communicated to her as a child, the society and culture in which she lives as an adult, and whether the pregnancy has come at a good time in her life.

Social Influences

Until recently, the heavy emphasis on medical management for women during pregnancy conveyed the idea that pregnancy was a 9-month-long illness. The pregnant woman went alone to a physician's office for care; at the time of birth, she was separated from her family and admitted to a hospital. She was hospitalized in seclusion from visitors and even from the new baby for a week afterward.

Today, our society has come to view pregnancy more in terms of health. Nurses have played an important role in helping to convince other health care providers that certain long-standing protocols are no longer appropriate. As a result, women are being encouraged to participate in all aspects of the experience. Instead of coming alone for prenatal care, they now bring their families. Instead of being given general anesthetics so they can "sleep through" labor and birth, women are urged to participate actively in childbirth. Many alternatives to the traditional in-hospital labor and birth experience now exist, both inside and outside of hospitals. The addition of birthing rooms and an emphasis on family-centered care have helped involve families, not just the woman, in childbirth.

The way the pregnant woman and her partner feel about pregnancy and childbirth may be affected by their cultural background, their personal experiences, and the experiences of friends and relatives, as well as by the current public philosophy of childbirth. People's opinions about adolescent pregnancies, "late in life" pregnancies, or pregnancies in lesbians have changed markedly. Encouraging women to be active, rather than to rest, during pregnancy has dramatically changed how women accept pregnancy and may influence birth outcomes (see Focus on Evidence-Based Practice). By informing women about their options and continuing to work with other health care providers to "demedicalize" childbirth, nurses can help make pregnancy and childbirth more enjoyable for their clients and families.

Cultural Influences

A woman's cultural background may strongly influence how active a role she wants to take in her pregnancy. Certain beliefs and taboos may place restrictions on her behavior and activities (Andrews & Boyle, 2002). The Focus on Family Empowerment box lists some common cultural beliefs about activities considered appropriate during pregnancy. However, these beliefs may not be held by all members of a particular group. To learn about the beliefs of a woman and her partner, ask at prenatal visits if there is anything they believe should or should not be done to keep the baby healthy. Supporting these beliefs is important and shows respect for the individuality of the woman (Hartmann & Bung, 1999).

FOCUS ON EVIDENCE-BASED PRACTICE

Can Exercise During Pregnancy Influence the Type of Birth?

To answer this question, 137 women in their first pregnancy were followed throughout their pregnancy as to their type and amount of exercise. At birth, the type of delivery was documented. The results of the study showed that sedentary women were four times more likely to need a cesarean birth than active women.

This study has important implications for nurses because nurses are often the people who counsel women during pregnancy on exercise or who conduct exercise programs for pregnant women.

Bungum, T. J., Peaslee, D. L., Jackson, A. W., & Perez, M. A. (2000). Exercise during pregnancy and type of delivery in nulliparae. *Journal of Obstetric, Gynecologic & Neonatal Nursing, 29*(3), 258–264.

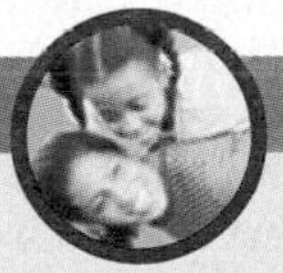

FOCUS ON FAMILY EMPOWERMENT

Beliefs About Pregnancy

Q. Where do people get their beliefs about pregnancy?

A. They come from a variety of sources:

Prescriptive Beliefs

- Remain active during pregnancy to aid the baby's circulation (Crow Indian).
- Remain happy to bring the baby joy and good fortune (Pueblo and Navajo Indians, Mexican, Japanese).
- Sleep flat on your back to protect the baby (Mexican).
- Keep active during pregnancy to ensure a small baby and an easy birth (Mexican).
- Continue sexual intercourse to lubricate the birth canal and prevent dry labor (Haitian, Mexican).
- Continue daily baths and frequent shampoos during pregnancy to produce a clean baby (Filipino).

Restrictive Beliefs

- Avoid cold air during pregnancy (Mexican, Haitian, Asian).
- Do not reach over your head or the cord will wrap around the baby's neck (Black, Hispanic, White, Asian).
- Avoid weddings and funerals or you will bring bad fortune to the baby (Vietnamese).
- Do not continue sexual intercourse or harm will come to you and the baby (Vietnamese, Filipino, Samoan).
- Do not tie knots or braid or allow the baby's father to do so, as it will cause difficult labor (Navajo Indian).
- Do not sew (Pueblo Indian, Asian).

Taboos

- Avoid lunar eclipses and moonlight or the baby may be born with a deformity (Mexican).
- Don't walk on the streets at noon or five o'clock, as this may make the spirits angry (Vietnamese).
- Don't join in traditional ceremonies like Yei or Squaw dances or spirits will harm the baby (Navajo Indian).
- Don't get involved with persons who cast spells or the baby will be eaten in the womb (Haitian).
- Don't say the baby's name before the naming ceremony or harm might come to the baby (Orthodox Jewish).
- Don't have your picture taken because it might cause stillbirth (Black).

Andrews, M., & Boyle, J. (2002). *Transcultural concepts in nursing care* (4th ed.). Philadelphia: Lippincott Williams & Wilkins.

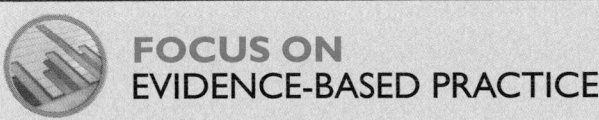

Family Influences

The family in which a woman was raised can be as influential to her beliefs about pregnancy as her cultural environment. If she and her siblings were loved and were seen as the pleasant outcome of a happy marriage, she is more likely to have a positive attitude toward her pregnancy than if she and her siblings were seen as intruders or were blamed for the breakup of a marriage. No matter how often a woman is told that pregnancy is natural and simple, she will not be overjoyed to find herself pregnant if all she has heard are stories about excruciating pain and endless suffering in labor. If her mother constantly reminded her, "If you hadn't come along, I could have gone to college" or "I could have had a career," the daughter may view pregnancy as disastrous.

"People love as they have been loved" is said so often it has become a cliché. It is highly relevant, however, to whether pregnancy and childbirth will be viewed in a positive or a negative light. If a woman has had difficulty loving others because she has not received love, she may have difficulty loving and accepting the fetus growing within her. To mother her baby well, she should be able to feel a pleasurable anticipation at the prospect of rearing a child; becoming a mother is a second adjustment above and beyond being pregnant. The woman who views mothering as a positive activity is more likely to be pleased when she becomes pregnant than one who devalues mothering.

Individual Influences

A woman's ability to cope with or adapt to stress plays a major role in how she will resolve conflict and adapt to new life contingencies. This ability to adapt—to being a mother without needing mothering, to loving a child as well as a husband, to becoming a mother of each new child—depends, in part, on her basic temperament, on whether she adapts to new situations quickly or slowly, whether she faces them with intensity or maintains a low-key approach, and whether she has had experiences coping with change and stress.

The extent to which a woman feels secure in her relationship with the people around her, especially the father of her child, is usually important to her acceptance of a pregnancy. Acceptance will be easier if she has confidence in the stability of her relationship with the child's father and knows that he will be there to give her emotional support. On the other hand, she may be uneasy about being pregnant if her partner may disappear shortly, leaving her alone to raise the child.

A woman who thinks of brides as young but mothers as old may believe that pregnancy will rob her of her youth. If she thinks children are sticky-fingered and time-consuming, she may view the pregnancy as taking away her freedom. If she has heard that pregnancy will permanently stretch her abdomen and breasts, her concern may be that she will lose her looks. She may feel that pregnancy will rob her financially and ruin her chances of job promotion. These are real feelings and must be taken seriously when counseling pregnant women. Such concerns cannot be shrugged off with simple clichés ("One door closes, another one opens") or with repression ("You shouldn't think that way; you'll love having a baby in the house"). The woman needs an opportunity to express these feelings and become aware of their intensity to resolve them. Women who do not have a supportive partner need to locate a support person during pregnancy. Often this is another woman who relates to the wonder and excitement of pregnancy and birth.

Whether a father of a child is able to accept the pregnancy and the coming child depends on the same factors that affect the woman: cultural background, past experience, and relationship with family members. If he was raised to believe that men should not show their emotions, he may not be able to say easily, "I want this baby" or "I'm glad" when his partner tells him of the positive diagnosis. He may not be able to say such things as, "It's great to feel it kick."

Although he might be inarticulate in these ways, he may be able to convey such emotions by a touch or a caress, one reason his presence is always desirable at a prenatal visit and certainly in a birthing room. His partner will know that his hand on hers is as meaningful an expression of emotion as a spoken word.

THE PSYCHOLOGICAL TASKS OF PREGNANCY

During the 9 months of pregnancy, a woman and her partner run a gamut of emotions ranging from surprise at finding out the woman is pregnant (or wishing she were not) to pleasure and acceptance of the fact as they begin to identify with the child, to fear for themselves and the child, to impatience with the process near the end of pregnancy (Table 9-2). Once the child is born, the woman and her partner may feel surprised again that it really happened and that the mother has really given birth.

TABLE 9.2 Common Psychosocial Changes That Occur With Pregnancy

PSYCHOSOCIAL CHANGE	DESCRIPTION
First Trimester	
Task: Accepting the pregnancy	Woman and partner both spend time recovering from shock of learning they are pregnant and concentrate on what it feels like to be pregnant. A common reaction is ambivalence, or feeling both pleased and not pleased at the pregnancy.
Second Trimester	
Task: Accepting the baby	Woman and partner move through emotions such as narcissism and introversion as they concentrate on what it will feel like to be a parent. Role-playing and increased dreaming are common.
Third Trimester	
Task: Preparing for the baby and end of pregnancy	Woman and partner grow impatient with pregnancy as they ready themselves for birth.

From a physiologic standpoint, it is fortunate that a pregnancy is 9 months long, because this gives the fetus time to mature and be prepared for life outside the protective uterine environment. From a psychological standpoint, the 9-month period is fortunate for the family, giving it time to prepare emotionally as well. How well a woman adjusts to the potential stress of pregnancy can affect her relationship with the child and may even influence whether she is able to carry the pregnancy to term.

First Trimester: Accepting the Pregnancy

The Woman

Most cultures structure their celebrations around important life events. Coming of age, marriages, birthdays, and deaths all have rituals to help individuals take a step forward or accept the coming change in their lives. A diagnosis of pregnancy is a similar rite of passage. This aura of initiation into one of the large mysteries of life gives special meaning to the health care visit in which the diagnosis of pregnancy is confirmed, making it more than an ordinary visit to a health care facility.

The availability of family planning measures today, in theory, would seem to prevent the diagnosis of pregnancy from being a surprise. In reality, as many as 50% of pregnancies are unintended, unwanted, or mistimed. Every pregnancy is a surprise to some extent, either because the woman had not planned on becoming pregnant or had been looking forward to being pregnant but cannot believe it has happened so quickly. No woman is absolutely confident in advance that she will be able to conceive until it happens. If pregnancy announced itself with more reliable signs than a missed period, slight breast tenderness, or vague nausea and tiredness, women could become more certain how they feel about being pregnant sooner. Home pregnancy test kits have helped women in this regard by confirming pregnancy early on. Until it is verified by a home test or a health care visit, however, the uncertainty of the symptoms makes pregnancy a vague theoretical possibility and leaves room for denial (Wessel & Buscher, 2002).

Often women immediately experience something less than pleasure and closer to disappointment or anxiety at the news. This emotional response of ambivalence is further discussed below. Fortunately, most women are able to change their attitude toward the pregnancy by the time they feel the child move inside them. Some health care plans provide for a routine sonogram at 4 months of pregnancy. Seeing a fetal outline on the monitor screen during a sonogram can promote acceptance.

The Partner

Once partners were forgotten in the childbearing process. Unwed fathers, in particular, were often dismissed as not interested in the pregnancy or the woman's health. However, today it is recognized that all partners have an important role and should be encouraged to have an emotional interest in the pregnancy. This means that as the woman adapts to pregnancy, her partner may go through some of the same psychological changes.

For partners, accepting the pregnancy means not only accepting the certainty of the pregnancy and the reality of the child to come but also accepting the woman in her changed state. A partner should try to give the woman emotional support while she is learning to accept the reality of pregnancy, and she should reciprocate when the partner begins to go through the process.

Like women, partners' feelings regarding the pregnancy vary. Often partners are proud and happy about the pregnancy, facilitating acceptance of the pregnancy. However, partners may experience some feelings that make this task more difficult. It is not unusual for a partner to feel somewhat jealous of the growing baby, who, although not yet physically apparent, seems to be taking up a great deal of his partner's time and thought.

An unwed father may have a great deal of difficulty accepting a pregnancy unless he is actively involved in prenatal care. He tries to picture himself as a father but then realizes that if he does not marry his partner, he may never play a full father role to this child; the image disappears again. Because the unwed father can relate to the fact that he fathered the child, however, he may feel a deep sense of loss if the woman decides to have an abortion or if the baby is born less than perfect. In addition, he may not have anyone to turn to for support because no one recognizes his loss, and so he must suffer alone.

Second Trimester: Accepting the Baby

The Woman

A second turning point in pregnancy is often quickening, or the first moment the woman feels fetal movement. Until a woman experiences for herself this proof of the child's existence, she may think of the life inside her as an integral part of herself rather than as a separate entity. She knows it is there; she eats to meet its needs and takes special vitamins to help it grow, but it seems just another part of her body. With quickening, however, she is able to give the child an identity. She begins to imagine how she will feel at the birth when the physician or midwife announces, "It's a boy!" or "It's a girl!" She begins to imagine herself as a mother, perhaps teaching her child the alphabet or how to ride a bicycle. This anticipatory role-playing is an important task for the pregnant woman. It leads her to a larger concept of her condition. It helps her realize that not only is she pregnant but also there is a child inside her.

The woman may continue to use the term "fetus." This does not necessarily mean that she has not yet accepted the pregnancy or still considers the baby an inanimate object. Some women believe that referring to the child as "she" or "he" will bring bad luck or disappointment if the child is of the opposite sex. Although a sonogram can reveal the sex of the child, some women choose not to know because they fear being misled by an inaccurate sonogram reading or they simply wish to be surprised about the sex of their child at birth. If the woman chooses not to know, it makes sense for her to keep an open mind regarding the sex of the child, especially if one sex is desired more than the other.

Most women can pinpoint a moment during each pregnancy when they knew definitely that they wanted the child. For a woman who carefully planned the pregnancy, this moment of awareness may occur as soon as she recovers from the surprise of learning she has actually conceived. For others, it may come when she announces the news to her parents and hears them express their joy or when she sees a look of pride on her partner's face. It might be the moment of quickening, when she realizes that the fetus inside her is not passive but is an active being. Shopping for baby clothes for the first time, setting up the crib, seeing a blurry outline on a sonogram screen: any of these small actions may suddenly make the coming baby seem real and desired (Fig. 9-1).

On the other hand, accepting the baby as a welcome family addition might not come until labor has begun or after several hours of labor. It might even be the moment she first hears the baby's cry or first touches or feeds the newborn. It could take several weeks after the baby is born for the woman to accept her new reality. Unfortunately, some women have great difficulty coming to terms with motherhood, especially if they have a complication of pregnancy, are having financial difficulty, or lack emotional support. The tremendous emotional and physical upheaval brought about by the hormonal changes of pregnancy and impending childbirth can lead to postpartum depression or, in rare instances, even psychosis.

A good way to measure the level of a woman's acceptance of the coming baby is to measure how well she follows prenatal instructions. Until a woman views the growing structure inside her as something desired, it may be difficult for her to discipline herself to follow a proper diet. If she wants very much to be pregnant but is not yet convinced that she is, she may have difficulty eliminating her favorite high-carbohydrate, low-protein food from her diet. After all, gaining weight may be the most certain proof she has of being pregnant (see Focus on Communication).

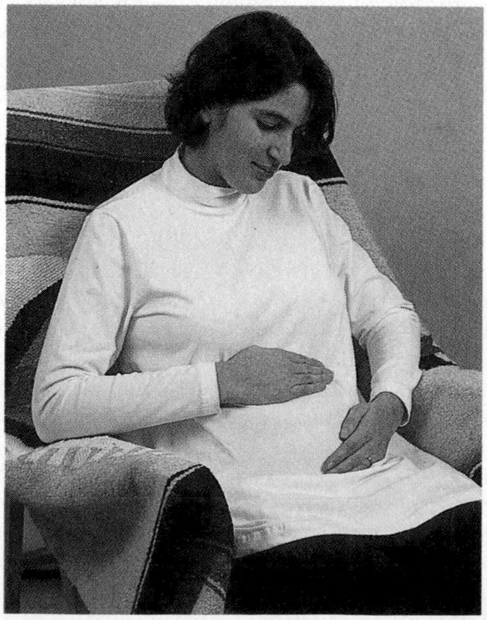

FIGURE 9.1 A growing abdomen and fluttering fetal movements help to make the pregnancy a reality.

FOCUS ON COMMUNICATION

Mrs. Peters is a 30-year-old woman you have seen in a prenatal clinic every month for the last 3 months. She answers questions at visits when asked but never volunteers any information. You'd like her to talk more about how she feels about being pregnant and her plans for the new baby.

Less Effective Communication

Nurse: Good morning, Mrs. Peters. How are you today?

Mrs. Peters: Tired.

Nurse: So am I. Working full time isn't fun, is it? Do you have any problems?

Mrs. Peters: No.

Nurse: That's good. Saves me writing. Have you felt the baby move yet?

Mrs. Peters: Yes.

Nurse: That must be so exciting. I can't wait until I have my first child and can feel that. Have you started plans for the baby? A crib? Clothing?

Mrs. Peters: No.

Nurse: There's a big sale at the mall starting Saturday. Better not miss it.

More Effective Communication

Nurse: Good morning. Mrs. Peters. How are you today?

Mrs. Peters: Tired.

Nurse: Tell me about that.

Mrs. Peters: I am so tired by noon every day that I can barely get my work done. I should never have gotten pregnant.

Nurse: You're so tired you can barely get your work done?

Mrs. Peters: No one in our financial situation should be having a baby.

Some people are naturally shy and are not interested in casual conversations at health care visits. Others are not talkative because they are not aware that health care providers are interested in them as individuals. In the first example, the nurse actually cuts off conversation because she is so busy talking about her own needs and expectations that the client does not want to compete. Focusing on the client's concerns, as happens in the second example, allows the woman to feel the health care provider's concern and interest in helping her solve her problem.

The Partner

As the woman begins to actively prepare for the coming baby, the partner may feel as if he is left standing in the wings, waiting to be asked to take part in the event. To compensate for this feeling, the partner may become overly absorbed in his work, striving to produce something concrete on the job or to earn enough money to demonstrate that he, too, is capable of creating something. This preoccupation with work may limit the amount of time the partner spends with the family, just when the pregnant woman most needs emotional support.

Some men may have difficulty enjoying the pregnancy if they have been misinformed about sexuality, pregnancy, and women's health. A man might believe, for example, that breastfeeding will make his wife's breasts no longer attractive and will advise against it. He may believe that childbirth will stretch his wife's vagina so much that sexual relations will no longer be enjoyable and will advocate for a cesarean birth. Such a man needs education to correct misinformation. Many men comment that the information they receive about childbirth and pregnancy is too concerned with their partner or the child and not enough with how they feel or what they know.

Third Trimester: Preparing for Parenthood

During the third trimester, couples usually begin "nest-building" activities, such as planning the infant's sleeping arrangements, buying clothes, choosing names for the infant, and "ensuring safe passage" by learning about birth.

Couples at this point are interested in attending prenatal classes or preparation for childbirth classes. It is helpful to ask the couple what specifically they are doing to get ready for birth in order to document how prepared they will be for the baby's arrival.

Certain external life contingencies may slow the mental work of pregnancy on the part of the woman or her partner (Box 9-1). During prenatal visits, such difficulties might be revealed by asking, "How does your partner feel about your being pregnant?" or "Has anything changed in your home life since you last came to the clinic?" It is unrealistic to believe that one health care professional has all the solutions to the problems that couples can develop during pregnancy. A multidisciplinary approach (e.g., referral to the nutritionist, nurse practitioner, or social services) is often necessary to help solve some of these multifaceted problems.

It is helpful for couples to attend childbirth education classes or classes on preparing for parenthood. Attending these classes can help a couple accept the pregnancy, expose them to other parents as role models, and provide practical information about pregnancy and childcare. The education in these classes, however, must be individualized to be meaningful to couples.

To be ready to be parents, a couple must complete a number of specific tasks. These steps, discussed in the following sections, are important with each pregnancy, not just the first one. (For more information on childbirth education classes and planning for parenthood, see Chap. 13.)

Reworking Developmental Tasks

One of the tasks of pregnancy is working through previous life experiences. Needs and wishes that have been repressed for years may surface to be studied and reworked, often to an extreme extent.

Primary among these life experiences is the woman's relationship with her parents, particularly with her mother. For the first time in her life, she finds she can empathize with her mother and the way she used to worry when she came home later than expected. The pregnant woman has already begun to worry about her child, to the point that she wonders if something is wrong when she feels no movement for a few hours, even though she is only 5 months into the pregnancy.

Fear of dying is a common childhood fear that can be revived during pregnancy. Although the likelihood of this happening is remote, it is not entirely unrealistic.

For the woman to work through past fears and conflicts of this kind, she needs to think about them when she is alone as well as to discuss them with others. She may throw out comments to her partner, friends, or health care personnel to test their reactions to these thoughts. A typical opening statement is, "I really hated my mother when I was a kid." If the response to this remark is a therapeutic, open-ended one (e.g., "You hated her?"), the woman may feel able to reveal the intensity of her conflict with her mother and how she cannot bear to think of the child inside her feeling that way about her. Teenagers who are pregnant need to resolve the conflict of being both a child and a mother. Unless these feelings are resolved, they may continue to have a negative impact on the woman's view of becoming a mother.

Other cues that signal a woman's distress about pregnancy and childbirth may be more subtle, such as, "Am I ever going to make it through this?" This expression might mean simply that she is tired of her backache, but it also might be a plea for reassurance that she will survive this event in her life.

BOX 9.1

EVENTS THAT COULD CONTRIBUTE TO DIFFICULTY ACCEPTING PREGNANCY

- Learning that the pregnancy is a multiple pregnancy
- Learning that the fetus has a developmental abnormality
- Pregnancy less than a year after a previous one
- Relocation during pregnancy (involves a need to find new support people)
- Moving away from the family or back to the family for economic reasons
- Role reversal (a previously supporting person who becomes dependent, or vice versa)
- Job loss
- Marital infidelity
- Illness in self, husband, or a relative
- Loss of a significant other
- Complications of pregnancy
- Having friends or relatives who have had children born with health disorders
- A series of devaluing experiences (e.g., failure in school or work)
- History of previous miscarriages, fertility problems, traumatic births
- Previous fetal or neonatal loss

A woman needs to have confidence in those who provide health care for her during pregnancy so she can express some of these disturbing thoughts and work through them. As a rule, a woman who is comfortable seeking information experiences less anxiety than those unable to do this.

The pregnant woman's partner needs to do the same reworking of old values and forgotten developmental tasks. A man may rethink his relationship with his father to understand better what kind of father he will be. Some men may have had emotionally distant fathers and wish to be more emotionally available to their own children. These men may have to reconcile feelings toward their fathers and learn a new pattern of behavior.

Role-Playing and Fantasizing

The second step in preparing for parenthood is role-playing, or fantasizing about what it will be like to be a parent. Just as a preschooler learns what to do by following her mother as she sets a table or balances her checkbook, the pregnant woman begins to spend time with other pregnant women or mothers of young children to learn how to be a mother. She is drawn into a world of talk about babies and pregnancy with these women. She may find that her own mother becomes more important to her, and a new, more equal relationship often develops. A pregnant woman may offer to babysit for a neighbor or relative so she can "practice" caring for a new baby. As a part of the role-playing process, women's dreams tend to focus on the pregnancy and concerns about keeping themselves and their coming child safe.

Although role-playing may be difficult for a pregnant teen who has not yet made the transition to adulthood, it is an important one in helping her become a mother. If the only role models she has are other girls her age, who typically are not interested in the commitment to mothering, or if the role model is her own mother, who might be unable to cope with problems such as poverty, too many children, or an ineffectual husband, then the young girl will probably assume the same role. She needs exposure to good role models (in classes for mothers, at the health care agency, in a social agency) to be able to find a maternal role that will be worth copying and integrating into her own behavior.

The father-to-be also has role-playing to do during pregnancy. He has to imagine himself as the father of a boy and as the father of a girl. A first-time father may have to change his view of himself as a carefree individual to a significant member of a family unit. If he already is a father, he has to cast aside a father-of-one identity to accept a father-of-two image, and so forth. Many fathers want or need to take on the role of nurturer but have had little or no experience caring for newborns or infants. Newborn care classes provided before or after the birth can help fathers assume this role.

Other support persons who will have an active role in raising the child (e.g., grandparents, lesbian partners) also have to work out their roles in regard to the pregnancy and parenthood. This may be particularly difficult because the roles for these support persons may not be clearly defined, and no role model may be apparent.

> ✔ **CHECKPOINT QUESTIONS**
>
> 4. How has the view of pregnancy as a time of wellness influenced the pregnancy and birth experience?
> 5. What individual influences play a major role in a woman's ability to adapt to pregnancy and parenting?
> 6. What are three psychological tasks of pregnancy?

Emotional Responses to Pregnancy

Emotional responses to pregnancy can vary greatly, but common reactions include ambivalence, grief, narcissism, introversion or extroversion, body image and boundary concerns, couvade syndrome, stress, mood swings, and changes in sexual desire. It is helpful to caution the pregnant woman and her partner about the changes they can expect. Otherwise, they might misinterpret the woman's mood swings, decreased sexual interest, introversion, or narcissism not as changes of pregnancy but as loss of interest in their relationship.

Ambivalence

Pregnancy is an intrusive process that cannot be ignored. A separate individual is growing inside the woman's body, and she is undergoing many psychological and physiologic changes. She may want to be pregnant, and yet she may not be enjoying it. This leads to some degree of ambivalence. Ambivalence toward pregnancy does not mean that positive feelings counteract negative feelings so that the woman is left feeling almost nothing toward her pregnancy. It does, however, refer to the interwoven feelings of wanting and not wanting that always exist at high levels. It is important to emphasize that this ambivalence is normal. Otherwise, if a poor outcome should result, the woman may recall her ambivalence and feel guilty.

Partners also experience ambivalence, sometimes more so than pregnant women. Partners may experience ambivalence because they are afraid to voice their concerns, thinking they ought to already know about certain things and not wanting to compound the pregnant woman's anxieties by appearing anxious themselves. Partners may also feel ambivalent if they are not well prepared for parenthood or have had little experience with children. Often it is harder for partners to resolve their feelings of ambivalence because they do not experience the physical and physiologic changes of pregnancy and often do not have a strong support network. To help partners resolve some ambivalence, provide an outlet for them to discuss concerns and offer parenting information.

Grief

The thought that grief could be associated with such a positive process as childbirth seems at first out of place. But before a woman can take on a mothering role, she has to give up or alter her present roles. She will never be a daughter in exactly the same way again. She must incorporate her new role as a mother into her other roles as a daughter, wife, or friend. Her partner must incorporate a new role as a father into his other roles of son, husband, or friend.

Narcissism

A woman's reaction to the intrusion of pregnancy can be manifested in many ways. Self-centeredness is generally an early reaction to pregnancy. A woman who previously was barely conscious of her body, who dressed in the morning with little thought about what to wear, who was unconcerned about her posture or her weight, suddenly begins to concentrate on these aspects of her life. She dresses so her pregnancy will or will not show, and dressing becomes a time-consuming, mirror-studying procedure. She makes a ceremony out of fixing her meals. She may lose interest in her job or community events because the work seems alien to the events taking place in her body, which constantly remind her that a new round of life is beginning.

A woman sometimes manifests narcissism by a change in her activities. She may stop playing tennis, even though her physician tells her it will do no harm in moderation. She may also criticize her husband's driving when it never bothered her before. She does these things to unconsciously protect her body and thus her baby. Men may demonstrate the same behavior by reducing risky activities such as mountain biking, trying to ensure they will be present to raise the child.

When caring for the pregnant woman, it is important to remember that she may feel a need to protect her body in this way, that her own self is important. This means she may regard unnecessary nudity as a threat to her body (as her nurse, be sure to drape her properly for pelvic and abdominal examinations). She may resent casual remarks such as, "Oh my, you've gained weight" (a threat to her appearance) or, "You don't like milk?" (a threat to her judgment).

There is a tendency to organize health instruction during pregnancy around the baby: "Be sure and keep this appointment. You want to have a healthy baby." "You really ought to drink more milk for the baby's sake." This approach may be particularly inappropriate early in pregnancy, before the fetus stirs and before the woman is convinced not only that she is pregnant but also that there is a baby inside her who is going to be born. At this stage, a woman may be much more interested in doing things for herself because it is her body, her tiredness, and her well-being that will be directly affected.

An increased interest in health on the pregnant woman's part allows you an opportunity to assess the woman's overall health status and health care beliefs and to provide general health teaching. This may influence the pregnant woman's long-term health as well as the health of the entire family unit. It may be particularly important to take advantage of this opportunity when caring for a woman who does not frequently visit the health care facility for checkups.

Introversion Versus Extroversion

Introversion, or turning inward to concentrate on oneself and one's body, is a common finding during pregnancy. Some women, however, react in an entirely opposite fashion and become more extroverted. They become more active, appear healthier than ever before, and are more outgoing. This tends to occur in women who are finding unexpected fulfillment in pregnancy, perhaps who had seriously doubted they would be lucky enough or fertile enough to conceive. Such a woman regards her expanding abdomen as proof that she is equal to her sisters. Although such a woman may become more varied in her interests during pregnancy, she may surprise those around her who previously regarded her as quiet and self-contained.

Body Image and Boundary

Body image (the way your body appears to yourself) and body boundary (a zone of separation you perceive between yourself and objects or other people) change during pregnancy as the woman begins to envision herself as a mother in addition to being a daughter or wife. This change in body image is part of the basis for narcissism and introversion. How the woman feels about her body as pregnancy progresses may influence decisions such as whether to breastfeed. Changes in the body boundary concept lead to a firmer distinction between objects, yet at the same time the boundary is perceived as extremely vulnerable, as if the body were delicate and easily harmed. This change in boundary perception is so startling that pregnant women may walk far away from an object such as a table in order to avoid it.

Stress

Pregnancy is a time of stress for many women. This stress of pregnancy, like any stress, can make it difficult for the woman to meet her daily responsibilities. People who were dependent on her before pregnancy may feel hurt, because now that she is pregnant she seems to have strength only for herself. If signs of preterm birth occur, the stress level can become intolerable (May & Salyer, 1999).

To help families keep their perspective, remind them that a decrease in the responsibilities that a pregnant woman takes on is a reaction to the stress of pregnancy, not the pregnancy itself. Many nonpregnant women and men function at work under just as much stress due to marital discord or a loved one's illness or death and have just as much difficulty with making decisions in these circumstances. Pregnancy may actually be less stressful than these situations because of its predictable 9-month outcome.

A woman with few support people around her almost automatically has more difficulty adjusting to and accepting a pregnancy and a new child than if she had more support. During pregnancy, she may feel especially stressed, leading to acute loneliness, depression, and a further inability to function. A woman who begins a pregnancy with a strong support person and then loses that person through trauma, illness, separation, or divorce needs special attention in regard to loneliness. She should be evaluated carefully and given extra support because her loneliness is likely to be extremely acute. A loss of this kind has the potential to interfere not only with her own health but also with parent–child bonding.

A common effect of stress is decreased decision-making ability. Determining whether the twinges she feels in her back are beginning labor contractions or just backache, and whether she should telephone her primary care provider, are difficult decisions to make for someone who is stressed. Knowing that she has supportive health care providers she can call on when needed is important.

Couvade Syndrome

Many men experience physical symptoms such as nausea, vomiting, and backache to the same degree or even more intensely than their partners do. These symptoms are often the result of stress, anxiety, and empathy for the pregnant woman. This is common enough that it has been given a name: **couvade syndrome.** The more the partner is involved in or attuned to the changes of the pregnancy, the more symptoms he may experience. As the woman's abdomen begins to grow, the father may perceive himself as growing larger, too, as if he were the one who was pregnant. For the most part, these are healthy happenings and require psychological attention only if the man becomes emotionally disturbed or delusional.

WHAT IF? What if you find yourself doing twice your normal work because a male coworker whose wife is 5 months pregnant calls in sick at least 3 days a week because of "flu symptoms"? Could you assume this is couvade syndrome?

Emotional Lability

Mood changes occur frequently in a pregnant woman, partly as a manifestation of narcissism (her feelings are easily hurt by remarks that would have been laughed off before) and partly because of hormonal changes, particularly the sustained increase in estrogen and progesterone. Mood swings are so common they may make a woman's reaction to her family and to health care routines unpredictable. What she finds acceptable one week she may find intolerable the next. She may cry over her children's bad table manners at one meal and find the situation amusing and even charming the next. Women and their partners and families need to be cautioned that such mood swings occur, beginning with early pregnancy, so that they can accept them as part of pregnancy (see Focus on Family Empowerment).

Changes in Sexual Desire

Most women report that their sexual desire changes, at least to some degree, during pregnancy. For women who were worried about becoming pregnant, they might truly enjoy sex for the first time during pregnancy. Others may feel a loss of desire due to the estrogen increase or may unconsciously view sexual relations as a threat to the fetus they must protect. Some may worry that having sex may bring on early labor.

During the first trimester, most women report a decrease in libido because of the nausea, fatigue, and breast tenderness that accompany early pregnancy. During the second trimester, as blood flow to the pelvic area increases to supply the placenta, libido and sexual enjoyment rise markedly. During the third trimester, it may remain high or decrease because of difficulty finding a comfortable position and increasing abdominal size. When a couple knows early in pregnancy that such changes may occur, they can be interpreted in the correct light (i.e., as a difference, not as loss of interest in the sexual partner). Suggestions for helping women and their partners adjust to these circumstances are discussed in Chapter 11.

Changes in the Expectant Family

Most parents are aware that their older children need preparation when a new baby is on the way; however, knowing that such preparation is called for and being able to give it are two different things. For this reason, some couples appreciate suggestions from health care personnel as to how this task can be accomplished.

Preparing a child for the birth of a sibling is discussed in Chapters 13 and 30. Both preschool and school-age children need to be reassured periodically during preg-

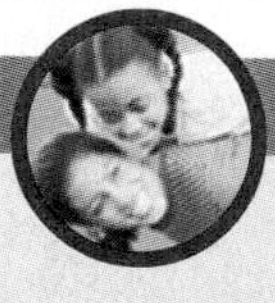

FOCUS ON FAMILY EMPOWERMENT
Mood Swings During Pregnancy

Q. I have so many mood swings. How can I reduce these?

A. The following suggestions should help reduce the occurrence of mood swings:

- Try to avoid fatigue, because this is when your normal defenses are most likely to be down (ask yourself if everything you're doing really needs to be done).
- Try to reduce your level of stress by setting priorities.
- Don't let little problems grow into big ones; attack them when they first occur.
- Try to see situations from other persons' perspective (they're not as involved in your pregnancy as you). Things that don't seem important to you may be important to them.
- Let others know you're aware you're having trouble with emotions since you became pregnant. Your family and friends will be more than willing to help you through this time if they realize it is of concern to you.

nancy that a new baby is adding to the family and will not replace them in their parents' affection.

> **✔ CHECKPOINT QUESTIONS**
>
> 7. When does the woman usually begin to think of the fetus as a separate entity? Why might the partner have a harder time accepting the pregnancy than the woman?
> 8. What tasks are involved in preparing for parenthood?
> 9. How do a woman and her partner manifest narcissism?

PHYSIOLOGIC CHANGES OF PREGNANCY

Physiologic changes that occur during pregnancy can be categorized as local (confined to the reproductive organs) or systemic (affecting the entire body). Both the symptoms (subjective findings) and signs (objective findings) of the physiologic changes of pregnancy are used to diagnose and mark the progress of pregnancy. Table 9-3 summarizes the physiologic changes that occur during a typical 40-week pregnancy.

Reproductive System Changes

Reproductive tract changes are those involving the uterus, ovaries, vagina, and breasts.

Uterine Changes

The most obvious alteration in the woman's body during pregnancy is the increase in the size of the uterus to accommodate the growing fetus. Over the 10 lunar months of pregnancy, the uterus increases in length, depth, width, weight, wall thickness, and volume.

- Length grows from approximately 6.5 to 32 cm.
- Depth increases from 2.5 to 22 cm.
- Width expands from 4 to 24 cm.
- Weight increases from 50 to 1,000 g.
- The uterine wall thickens from about 1 cm to about 2 cm; by the end of pregnancy, the wall thins so it is supple and only about 0.5 cm thick.
- The volume of the uterus increases from about 2 mL to more than 1,000 mL. The uterus can hold a 7-lb (3,175 g) fetus plus 1,000 mL of amniotic fluid for a total of about 4,000 g.

This great uterine growth is due partly to formation of a few new muscle fibers in the uterine myometrium, but principally to the stretching of existing muscle fibers: by the end of pregnancy, muscle fibers in the uterus are two to seven times longer than they were before pregnancy. The uterus is able to withstand this stretching of its muscle fibers because of the formation of extra fibroelastic tissue between fibers, which binds them closely together. Because uterine fibers only stretch during pregnancy and are not newly built, the uterus is able to return to its prepregnant state at the end of the pregnancy with little difficulty and almost no destruction of tissue (Ling & Duff, 2001).

TABLE 9.3 Timetable for Physiologic Changes of Pregnancy

LOCATION OF CHANGE	BODY OCCURRENCE		
	1st Trimester	*2nd Trimester*	*3rd Trimester*
Cardiovascular	Blood volume increasing →		→
	Pseudoanemia	Blood pressure slightly decreased	Blood pressure returns to prepregnancy levels
	Clotting factors increasing →		→
Ovarian	Corpus luteum active —	Corpus luteum fading	
Uterine	Increased growth →		→
		Placenta forming estrogen and progesterone →	→
Cervix	Softening progressive →		→ "Ripe"
Vaginal	White discharge present →		Increasing →
Musculoskeletal		Progressive cartilage softening →	→
		Lordosis increasing →	→
Pigmentation		Progressively increasing →	→
Kidney	Glomerular filtration rate increasing →		→
		Glycosuria →	→
	Aldosterone increased, increasing sodium and fluid →		→
Gastrointestinal		Slowed peristalsis →	→
Thyroid	Increased metabolic rate →		→

The woman becomes aware of the growing uterus early in pregnancy; by the end of the 12th week of pregnancy, it is large enough to be palpated as a firm spheroid under the abdominal wall, just above the symphysis pubis. An important factor to assess regarding uterine growth is its constant, steady, predictable increase in size. By the 20th or 22nd week of pregnancy, for example, it should reach the level of the umbilicus. By the 36th week, it should touch the xiphoid process and can make breathing difficult. About 2 weeks before term (the 38th week) for a **primigravida,** a woman in her first pregnancy, the fetal head settles into the pelvis to prepare for birth, and the uterus returns to the height it was at 36 weeks. This is termed **lightening** because of the better lung expansion and easier breathing patterns that seem to lighten the woman's load. When lightening will occur is not predictable in the **multipara** (a woman who has had one or more children). In these women, it may not be experienced until labor begins.

Changes in fundal height during pregnancy are shown in Figure 9-2. Uterine height is measured from the top of the symphysis pubis over the top of the fundus. Because a uterine tumor could mimic this steady growth, uterine growth is only a presumptive sign of pregnancy.

The exact shape of the expanding uterus is influenced by the position of the fetus inside. The fundus of the uterus usually remains in the midline during pregnancy, although it may be pushed slightly to the right side because of the larger bulk of the sigmoid colon on the left. As the uterus increases in size, it pushes the intestines to the sides of the abdomen, elevates the diaphragm and liver, compresses the stomach, and puts pressure on the bladder. The woman may worry that there will not be enough room inside her abdomen for the increase in size. She can be assured that the abdominal contents shift readily to accommodate uterine enlargement (Fig. 9-3).

Uterine blood flow increases during pregnancy as the placenta grows and requires more and more blood for perfusion. Before pregnancy, uterine blood flow is 15 to 20 mL/min. By the end of pregnancy, it is as much as 500 to 750 mL/min, with 75% of that volume going to the placenta. One method for measuring and monitoring uterine blood velocity during pregnancy is Doppler ultrasound. One sixth of the total body blood supply is circulating through the uterus at any given time; thus, uterine bleeding in pregnancy is always potentially serious because it could result in a major blood loss. Women should be warned that blood loss poses a major health risk and should be instructed to contact the health care practitioner if this should occur (Seifer et al., 2001).

A bimanual examination (one finger of the examiner is placed in the vagina, the other hand on the abdomen) demonstrates that, with pregnancy, the uterus is more anteflexed, larger, and softer to the touch than usual. At about the 6th week of pregnancy (at the time of the second missed menstrual period), the lower uterine segment just above the cervix becomes so soft that when it is compressed between the examining fingers on bimanual examination, the wall cannot be felt or it feels as thin as tissue paper. This extreme softening of the lower uterine segment is known as **Hegar's sign** (Fig. 9-4).

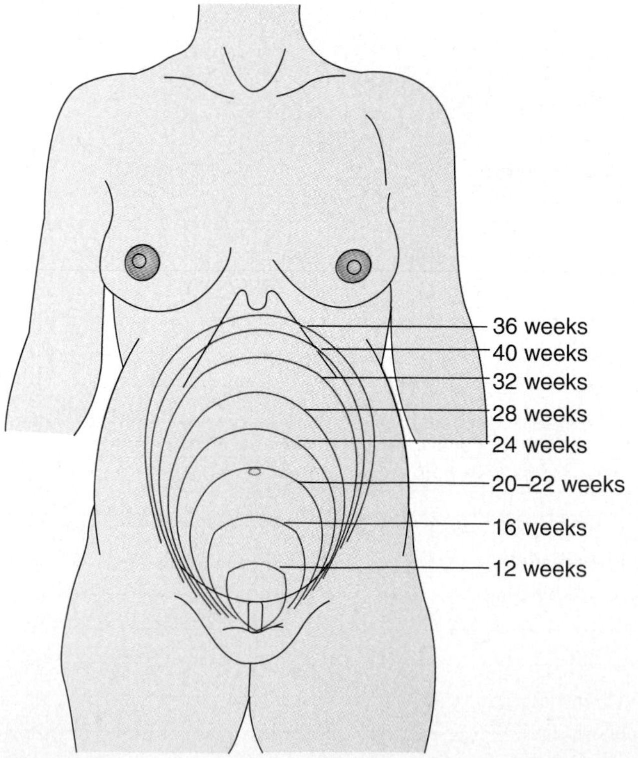

FIGURE 9.2 Fundus height at various weeks of pregnancy.

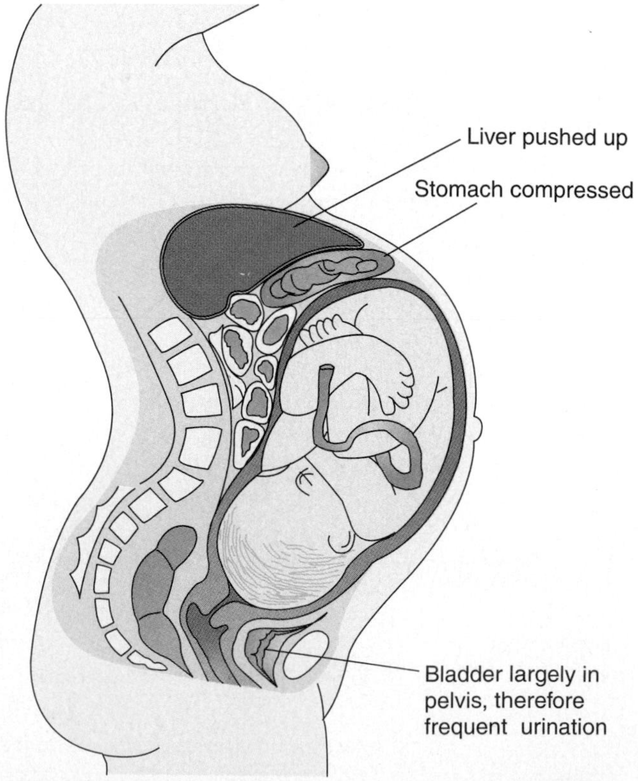

FIGURE 9.3 Crowding of abdominal contents late in pregnancy.

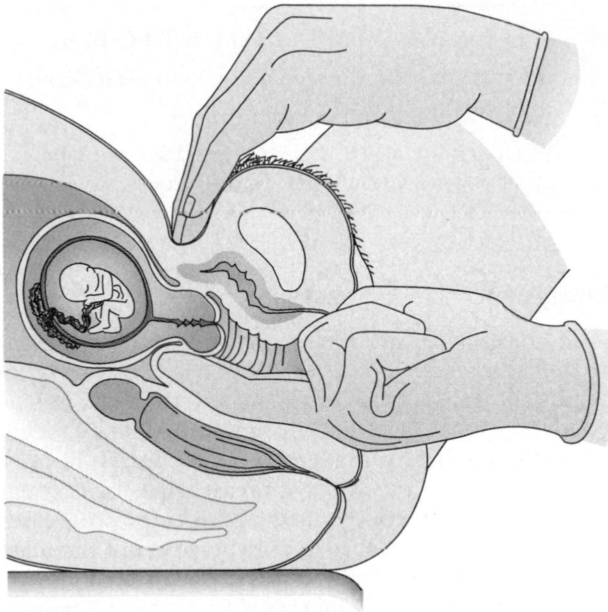

FIGURE 9.4 Examining for Hegar's sign. If the sign is present, the wall of the uterus is softer than normal.

During the 16th to 20th week of pregnancy, when the fetus is still small in relation to the amount of amniotic fluid present, **ballottement** (from the French word *balloter,* meaning to toss about) may be demonstrated. On bimanual examination, if the lower uterine segment is tapped sharply by the lower hand, the fetus can be felt to bounce or rise in the amniotic fluid up against the top examining hand. This phenomenon is interesting; again, however, it may be simulated by a uterine tumor, so it is no more than a probable sign of pregnancy. Between the 20th and 24th week of pregnancy, the uterine wall has become thinned to such a degree that a fetal outline within the uterus may be palpated by a skilled examiner. Because a tumor with calcium deposits could simulate a fetal outline, palpation of a uterine mass does not constitute a confirmation of pregnancy.

Uterine contractions begin early in pregnancy, at least by the 12th week, and are present throughout the rest of pregnancy, becoming stronger and harder as the pregnancy advances. They may be felt by a woman as waves of hardness or tightening across her abdomen. An examining hand may be able to feel a contraction as well, and an electronic monitor will be able to measure the frequency and length of such contractions. These "practice" contractions, termed **Braxton Hicks contractions,** serve as warm-up exercises for labor and increase placental perfusion. They may become so strong and noticeable in the last month of pregnancy that they are mistaken for labor contractions (false labor). They can be differentiated from true labor contractions on internal examination because they do not cause cervical dilation. Although these contractions are always present with pregnancy, they also could accompany any growing uterine mass; so, like ballottement, they are no more than a probable sign of pregnancy.

Amenorrhea

Amenorrhea (absence of menstruation) occurs with pregnancy because of the suppression of follicle-stimulating hormone (FSH). In a healthy woman who has menstruated previously, the absence of menstruation strongly suggests that impregnation has occurred. Amenorrhea, however, also heralds the onset of menopause or could result from delayed menstruation due to unrelated reasons, such as uterine infection, climate change, worry (perhaps over becoming pregnant), a chronic illness such as severe anemia, or stress. It occurs in athletes who train strenuously, especially in long-distance runners whose percentage of body fat drops below a critical point. Amenorrhea is therefore only a presumptive sign of pregnancy.

Cervical Changes

In response to the increased level of circulating estrogen from the placenta during pregnancy, the cervix of the uterus becomes more vascular and edematous. Increased fluid between cells causes the cervix to soften in consistency, and increased vascularity causes it to darken from a pale pink to a violet hue. The glands of the endocervix undergo both hypertrophy and hyperplasia as they increase in number and distend with mucus. A tenacious coating of mucus fills the cervical canal. This mucous plug, called the **operculum,** will act to seal out bacteria during pregnancy and so help prevent infection in the fetus and membranes.

Softening of the cervix in pregnancy (**Goodell's sign**) is marked. The consistency of a nonpregnant cervix may be compared with that of the nose, whereas the consistency of a pregnant cervix more closely resembles that of an earlobe. This softening is so marked it is rated as a probable diagnostic sign of pregnancy. Just before labor, the cervix becomes so soft that it takes on the consistency of butter and is said to be "ripe" for birth.

Vaginal Changes

Under the influence of estrogen, the vaginal epithelium and underlying tissue become hypertrophic and enriched with glycogen; they loosen from their connective tissue attachment in preparation for great distention at birth. This increase in the activity of the epithelial cells results in a white vaginal discharge throughout pregnancy.

An increase in the vascularity of the vagina, beginning early in pregnancy, parallels the vascular changes in the uterus. The resulting increase in circulation to the vagina changes the color of the vaginal walls from the normal light pink to a deep violet (**Chadwick's sign**).

Vaginal secretions during pregnancy fall from a pH of over 7 (an alkaline pH) to 4 or 5 (an acid pH). This occurs because of the action of *Lactobacillus acidophilus,* bacteria that grow freely in the increased glycogen environment and by so doing increase the lactic acid content of secretions. This changing acid content makes the vagina resistant to bacterial invasion for the length of the pregnancy. This change in pH also, unfortunately, favors the growth of *Candida albicans,* a species of yeastlike fungi.

A candidal infection is manifested by an itching, burning sensation in addition to a cream cheese-like discharge. A nonpregnant woman needs medication for such an infection to relieve discomfort. A pregnant woman needs medication not only to relieve discomfort but also to prevent transmission of the infection to the infant as it passes through the birth canal at term. Candidal infection in the newborn is termed thrush or oral monilia. Therapy for this is discussed in Chapter 43.

Ovarian Changes

Ovulation stops with pregnancy because of the active feedback mechanism of estrogen and progesterone produced by the corpus luteum early in pregnancy and the placenta later in pregnancy. This feedback causes the pituitary gland to halt production of FSH and luteinizing hormone (LH). Without stimulation from these, ovulation will not occur.

The corpus luteum that was created following the ovulation that led to the pregnancy continues to increase in size on the surface of the ovary until about the 16th week of pregnancy, by which time the placenta has taken over as the chief provider of progesterone and estrogen. The corpus luteum, no longer essential for the continuation of the pregnancy at this time, regresses in size to become indistinct.

✔ CHECKPOINT QUESTIONS

10. What is Chadwick's sign and why does it occur?
11. What are Braxton Hicks contractions?
12. What are the advantage and the disadvantage of a lowered vaginal pH during pregnancy?

Changes in the Breasts

Subtle changes in the breasts that occur as a result of estrogen and progesterone production may be one of the first physiologic changes of pregnancy a woman notices (at about 6 weeks; Fig. 9-5). She may experience a feeling of fullness, tingling, or tenderness in her breasts because of the increased stimulation of breast tissue by the high estrogen level in the body. As the pregnancy progresses, breast size increases because of hyperplasia of the mammary alveoli and fat deposits. The areola of the nipple darkens and its diameter increases from about 3.5 cm to 5 or 7.5 cm (1.5 in to 2 to 3 in). There is additional darkening of the skin surrounding the areola in some women, forming a secondary areola. As vascularity of the breasts increases, blue veins may become prominent over the surface of the breasts. The sebaceous glands of the areola (**Montgomery's tubercles**) enlarge and become pro-

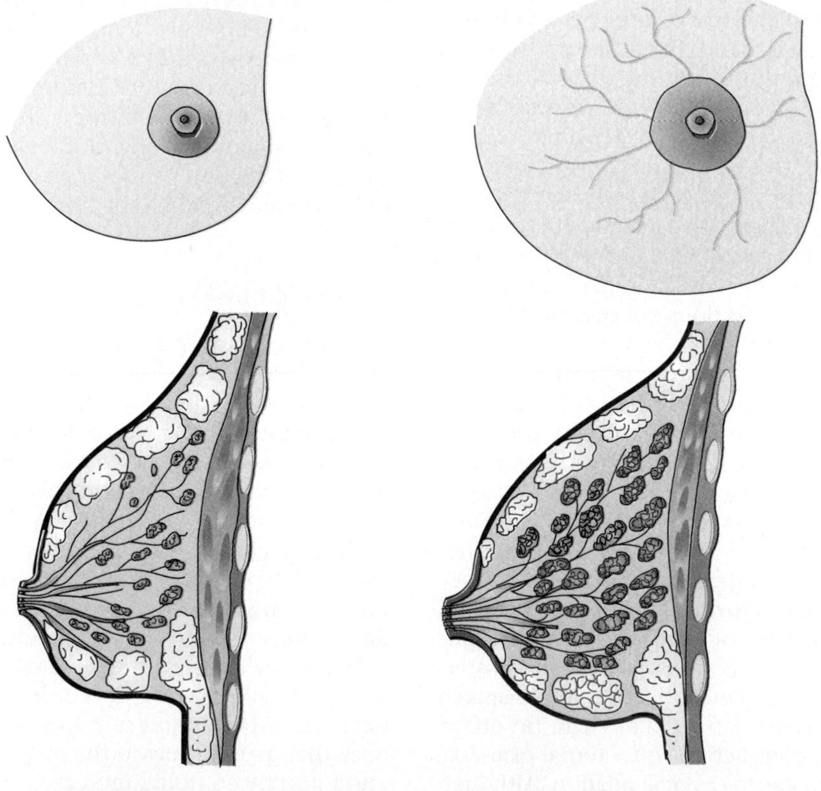

FIGURE 9.5 Comparison of non-pregnant and pregnant breasts.

tuberant. The secretions from these glands keep the nipple supple and help to prevent the nipples from cracking and drying during lactation.

Early in pregnancy, the breasts begin readying themselves for the secretion of milk. By the 16th week, colostrum, the thin, watery, high-protein fluid that is the precursor of breast milk, can be expelled from the nipples.

Systemic Changes

Although the physiologic changes first noticed by a woman are apt to be those of the reproductive system and breasts, changes are occurring in almost all body systems.

Integumentary System

As the uterus increases in size, the abdominal wall must stretch to accommodate it. This stretching (plus possibly increased adrenal cortex activity) can cause rupture and atrophy of small segments of the connective layer of the skin. This leads to pink or reddish streaks (**striae gravidarum**) appearing on the sides of the abdominal wall and sometimes on the thighs (Fig. 9-6). In the weeks after birth, striae gravidarum lighten to a silvery-white color

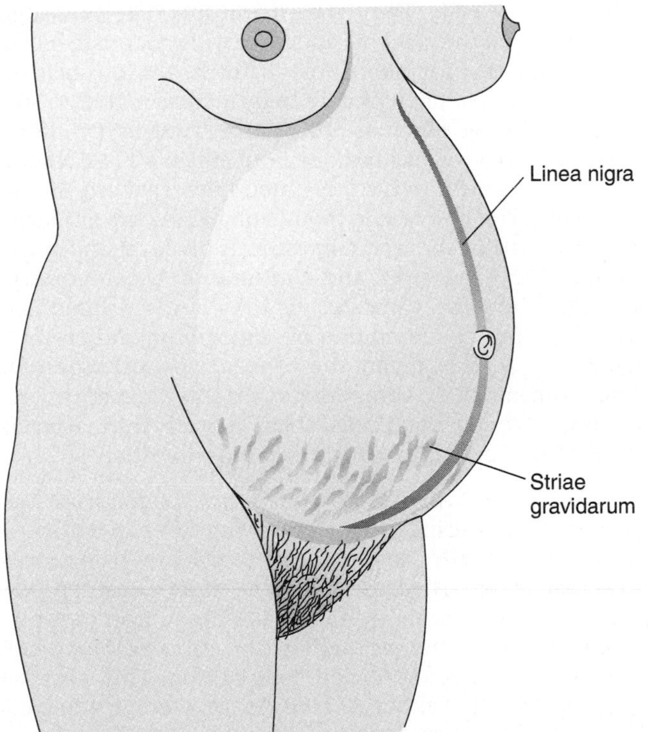

FIGURE 9.6 Skin changes in pregnancy. In the later months of pregnancy, reddish, slightly depressed streaks called striae gravidarum often develop in the skin of the abdomen and, sometimes, the breasts and thighs. Following pregnancy, these fade to glistening, silvery lines. In many pregnancies, the abdominal skin at the midline becomes markedly pigmented, assuming a brownish-black color, referred to as a linea nigra.

(striae albicantes or atrophicae) and, although permanent, become barely noticeable.

Occasionally, the abdominal wall has difficulty stretching enough to accommodate the growing fetus, causing the rectus muscles to actually separate, a condition known as **diastasis.** If this happens, it will appear after pregnancy as a bluish groove at the site of separation.

The umbilicus is stretched by pregnancy to such an extent that by the 28th week, its depression becomes obliterated and smooth because it has been pushed so far outward. In most women, it may appear as if it has turned inside out, protruding as a round bump at the center of the abdominal wall.

Extra pigmentation generally appears on the abdominal wall. A brown line (linea nigra) may be present, running from the umbilicus to the symphysis pubis and separating the abdomen into a right and left hemisphere (see Fig. 9-6). Darkened areas may appear on the face, particularly on the cheeks and across the nose. This is known as **melasma** (chloasma) or the "mask of pregnancy." These increases in pigmentation are due to melanocyte-stimulating hormone secreted by the pituitary. With the decrease in the level of the hormone after pregnancy, these areas lighten and again disappear. Vascular spiders (small, fiery-red branching spots) are sometimes seen on the skin of pregnant women, particularly on the thighs. These probably result from the increased level of estrogen in the body. These may fade but not completely disappear after pregnancy. The activity of sweat glands increases throughout the body during pregnancy. This is manifested as an increase in perspiration. Palmar erythema (redness and itching) may occur on the hands from the increased estrogen level. Fewer hairs on the head enter a resting phase due to overall increased metabolism, so scalp hair growth is increased.

Respiratory System

Most women notice some shortness of breath as pregnancy progresses. The total respiratory changes and the compensating mechanisms that occur in the respiratory system can be described as a chronic respiratory alkalosis fully compensated by a chronic metabolic acidosis.

As the uterus enlarges during pregnancy, a great deal of pressure is put on the diaphragm and, ultimately, on the lungs. The diaphragm may be displaced by as much as 4 cm upward. This crowding of the chest cavity causes an acute sensation of shortness of breath late in pregnancy, until lightening relieves the pressure.

Even with all this crowding, vital capacity (the maximum volume exhaled following a maximum inspiration) of the woman does not decrease during pregnancy because, although they are crowded in the vertical dimension, the lungs can expand horizontally. Residual volume (the amount of air remaining in the lungs following expiration) is decreased up to 20% by the pressure of the diaphragm. Tidal volume (the volume of air inspired) is increased up to 40% as the woman draws in extra volume to increase the effectiveness of air exchange. Total oxygen consumption increases by as much as 20%.

The increased level of progesterone during pregnancy appears to set a new level in the hypothalamus for acceptable blood carbon dioxide levels (PCO_2) because during pregnancy a woman's body tends to maintain a PCO_2 at closer to 32 mm Hg than the normal 40 mm Hg.

This low PCO_2 level causes a favorable CO_2 gradient at the placenta (the fetal CO_2 level is higher than that in the mother, allowing CO_2 to cross readily from the fetus to the mother).

To keep the mother's pH level from becoming acid from the load of CO_2 being shifted to her by the fetus, increased ventilation (mild hyperventilation) to blow off excess CO_2 begins early in pregnancy. At full term, a woman's total ventilation capacity may have risen by as much as 40%. This increased ventilation may become so extreme that the woman develops a respiratory alkalosis. To compensate for this, plasma bicarbonate is excreted by the kidneys. This results in increased urination or **polyuria,** an early sign of pregnancy. With greater urine output, both additional sodium and additional water are lost.

The slight increase in pH in serum due to the changed expiratory effort is advantageous because it slightly increases the binding capacity of maternal hemoglobin and thereby raises the oxygen content of maternal blood (the level of PO_2) from a normal level of about 92 mm Hg to a level of 106 mm Hg early in pregnancy. This is advantageous to fetal growth by allowing good placental exchange.

The cumulative effect of these respiratory changes is often experienced by the woman as chronic shortness of breath. She will need a clear explanation that although her breathing rate is more rapid than normal (18 to 20 breaths per minute), this is normal for pregnancy.

A local change that often occurs in the respiratory system is marked congestion, or "stuffiness," of the nasopharynx, a response to increased estrogen levels (Ellegard et al., 2000). Women may worry that this stuffiness indicates an allergy or a cold. Not realizing that it is happening because they are pregnant, some women, unfortunately, may take over-the-counter cold medications or antihistamines in an effort to relieve the congestion. Some continue to take the medication after pregnancy is confirmed, not mentioning it to their physician because they think the stuffiness is a separate problem and not related to the pregnancy. Asking a woman at prenatal visits if she is taking any kind of medicine or if she has noticed nasal stuffiness is an important nursing responsibility.

Changes in respiratory function during pregnancy are summarized in Table 9-4.

Temperature

Early in pregnancy, body temperature increases slightly because of the secretion of progesterone from the corpus luteum (the temperature, which increased at ovulation, remains elevated). As the placenta takes over the function of the corpus luteum at about 16 weeks, the temperature generally decreases to normal.

Some women may mistakenly assume this slight rise in temperature (99.6°F orally), associated with pregnancy-related nasal congestion, is a sure sign of a cold, and may think they need medication. It is important to explain the reason for these changes to allow a woman to accept them without worrying.

TABLE 9.4 Respiratory Changes During Pregnancy

VARIABLE	CHANGE
Vital capacity	No change
Tidal volume	Increased by 30%–40%
Respiratory rate	Increased, 1 or 2/minute
Residual volume	Decreased by 20%
Plasma PCO_2	Decreased to about 27–32 mm Hg
Plasma pH	Increased to 7.40–7.45
Plasma PO_2	Increased to 104–108 mm Hg
Respiratory minute volume	Increased by 40%
Expiratory reserve	Decreased by 20%

Cardiovascular System

Changes in the circulatory system are extremely significant to the health of the fetus because they are important for adequate placental and fetal circulation. Table 9-5 summarizes the changes that are described in the following sections.

Blood Volume. To provide for an adequate exchange of nutrients in the placenta and to provide adequate blood to compensate for blood loss at birth, the circulatory blood volume of the woman's body increases at least 30% (and possibly as much as 50%) during pregnancy. Blood loss at a normal vaginal birth is about 300 to 400 mL; blood loss from a cesarean birth is much higher, about 800 to 1,000 mL. The increase in blood volume occurs gradually near the end of the first trimester. It peaks at about the 28th to the 32nd week and continues at this high level through the third trimester. As the plasma volume first increases, the concentration of hemoglobin and erythrocytes may decline, giving the woman a **pseudoanemia.** The woman's body compensates for this change by producing more red blood cells, creating nearly normal levels of red blood cells again by the second trimester.

Iron Needs. Almost all women need some iron supplementation during pregnancy owing to a variety of factors. They usually have comparatively low iron stores (less than 500 mg) because of their monthly menstrual loss. The fetus requires about 350 to 400 mg of iron to grow. The increases in the mother's circulatory red blood cell mass require an additional 400 mg of iron. This is a total increased need of about 800 mg. As the average woman's store of iron is less than this (about 500 mg), and iron absorption may be impaired during pregnancy as a result of decreased gastric acidity (iron is absorbed best from an acid medium), additional iron is often prescribed during pregnancy to prevent a true anemia.

Either a hemoglobin concentration of less than 11.5 g/100 mL or a hematocrit value below 30% is generally considered true anemia, for which iron therapy above normal supplementation is advocated. (See Chap. 14 for additional information on anemia in pregnancy.) The need for folic acid increases even more during pregnancy, or else mega-

TABLE 9.5 Changes in the Cardiovascular System During Pregnancy

ASSESSMENT FACTOR	PREPREGNANCY	PREGNANCY
Cardiac output		25%–50% increase
Heart rate	70–80	80–90
Plasma volume (mL)	2,600	3,600
Blood volume (mL)	4,000	5,250
Red blood cell mass (mm^3)	4,200,000	4,650,000
Leukocytes (mm^3)	7,000	20,500
Total protein (g/dL)	7.0	5.5–6.0
Fibrinogen (mg/dL)	300	450
Blood pressure		Decreases in 2nd trimester, at prepregnancy level in 3rd trimester

lohemoglobinemia (large, nonfunctioning red blood cells) will result. Folic acid has also been linked to a reduced risk for neural tube defects in fetuses. Prenatal vitamins include folic acid. Women should be certain to eat foods high in folic acid such as spinach, asparagus, and legumes during both the prepregnancy period and pregnancy.

Heart. To handle the increase in blood volume in the circulatory system, a woman's cardiac output increases significantly by 25% to 50%; the heart rate increases by 10 beats per minute. Like the circulating volume increase, the bulk of the cardiac work increase occurs during the second trimester, with a small increase in the third trimester. This rise in circulating load has implications for the woman with cardiac disease. Although the average woman's heart is able to adjust to these changes readily, a woman whose heart has difficulty handling her normal circulating load may be overwhelmed by the requirements placed on it when she is pregnant. The average woman may be unaware of the significant circulatory system changes that are occurring inside her to supply adequate blood to the placenta.

Because the diaphragm is elevated by the growing uterus late in pregnancy, the heart is shifted to a more transverse position in the chest cavity and may appear enlarged on x-ray examination. Some women have audible functional (innocent) heart murmurs during pregnancy, probably because of the altered heart position.

Palpitations of the heart are not uncommon during pregnancy, particularly on quick motion. The woman should be cautioned that if palpitations do occur, she should not be frightened. Palpitations in the early months of pregnancy are probably caused by sympathetic nervous system stimulation; in later months, they may result from increased thoracic pressure caused by the pressure of the uterus against the diaphragm.

Regional Blood Flow. During the third trimester, blood flow to the lower extremities is impaired by the pressure of the expanding uterus on veins and arteries, which slows circulation. This decrease in blood flow in the venous system leads to edema and varicosities of the vulva, rectum, and legs.

Blood Pressure. Despite the hypervolemia of pregnancy, the blood pressure does not normally rise because the increased heart action takes care of the greater amount of circulating blood. Average blood pressures for adult women are shown in Appendix G.

In most women, blood pressure actually decreases slightly during the second trimester because of the lowered peripheral resistance to circulation as the placenta expands rapidly. If this occurs, during the third trimester, the blood pressure rises again to first-trimester levels (Fig. 9-7).

Supine Hypotension Syndrome. When a pregnant woman lies supine, the weight of the growing uterus presses the vena cava against the vertebrae, obstructing blood flow from the lower extremities. This causes a decrease in blood return to the heart and, consequently, immediately decreased cardiac output and hypotension (Fig. 9-8). The woman experiences this as lightheadedness, faintness, and palpitations. Maternal hypotension is potentially dangerous because it can cause fetal hypoxia.

Supine hypotension syndrome can be corrected easily by having the woman turn onto her side (preferably the left side) to enhance blood flow through the vena cava. To lessen the possibility of this phenomenon, women have an increase in collateral blood circulation during pregnancy.

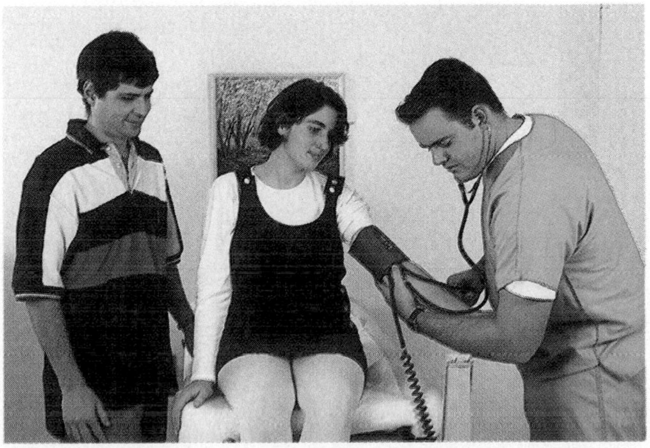

FIGURE 9.7 Blood pressure determination is an important assessment during pregnancy; normally, this does not elevate during pregnancy.

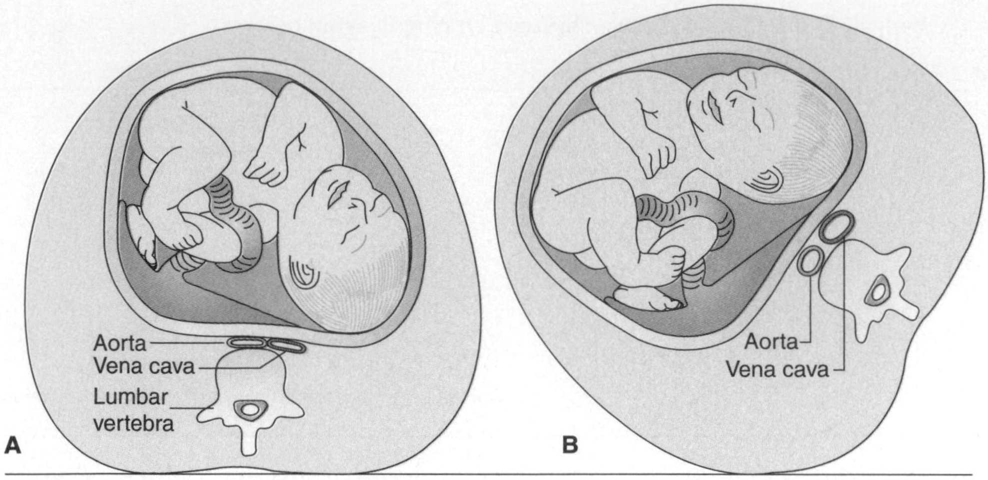

FIGURE 9.8 Supine hypotension can occur if a pregnant woman lies on her back. (*A*) The weight of the uterus compresses the vena cava, trapping blood in the lower extremities. (*B*) If a woman turns on her side, pressure is lifted off of the vena cava.

Teach women always to rest on their left side rather than their back, because even with additional collateral circulation, a supine position tends to lead to hypotension.

Blood Constitution. The level of circulating fibrinogen, a constituent of the blood necessary for clotting, increases as much as 50% during pregnancy, probably because of the increased level of estrogen. Other clotting factors, such as factors VII, VIII, IX, and X, and the platelet count also increase. These increases are a safeguard against major bleeding should the placenta be dislodged and the uterine arteries or veins be opened. Total white blood cell count rises slightly as both a protective mechanism and a reflection of the woman's total blood volume (up to about 20,000/mm^3). The total protein level of blood decreases, perhaps indicating the amount of protein being taken by the fetus. Because the circulating system has a lowered total protein load and hypervolemia, fluid readily leaves the intravascular spaces to equalize osmotic and hydrostatic pressure. This causes the common ankle and foot edema of pregnancy (not to be confused with nondependent or generalized edema, which is a symptom of pregnancy-induced hypertension).

Overall, blood lipids increase by one third; cholesterol serum level increases 90% to 100%. These increases provide a ready supply of available energy for the fetus.

WHAT IF? Lauren Maxwell, the woman you met at the beginning of this chapter, stated that some of her concerns were morning sickness and fatigue. What if you discovered she was homeless? Would your advice for her be any different?

Gastrointestinal System

As the uterus increases in size, it tends to displace the stomach and intestines toward the back and sides of the abdomen. At about the midpoint of pregnancy, the pressure may be sufficient to slow intestinal peristalsis and the emptying time of the stomach, leading to heartburn, constipation, and flatulence. Relaxin, a hormone produced by the ovary, may contribute to decreased gastric motility; this natural slowing is helpful as blood supply may be reduced to the gastrointestinal tract (blood is drawn to the uterus). Progesterone also has an effect on smooth muscle, such as that in the intestine, making it less active.

At least 50% of women experience some nausea and vomiting early in pregnancy. This is one of the first sensations the woman may experience with pregnancy (sometimes noticed even before the first missed menstrual period). It is most apparent early in the morning on rising or if she becomes fatigued during the day. It is more frequent in women who smoke cigarettes. Known as morning sickness, nausea and vomiting begin to be noticed at the time that levels of hCG and progesterone begin to rise. It may occur as a systemic reaction to increased estrogen levels or decreased glucose levels, because glucose is being utilized in great quantities by the growing fetus. Common interventions to decrease nausea and vomiting are discussed in Chapter 12.

This common feeling of nausea usually subsides after the first 3 months, after which the woman may have a voracious appetite. Although the acidity of stomach secretions decreases during pregnancy, heartburn may result from the reflux of stomach contents into the esophagus as a result of upward displacement of the stomach by the uterus and a relaxed cardioesophageal sphincter due to the action of relaxin. Interventions for heartburn are also discussed in Chapter 12.

Due to the gradual slowing of the gastrointestinal tract, decreased emptying of bile from the gallbladder may result. This can lead to reabsorption of bilirubin into the maternal bloodstream, giving rise to the symptom of generalized itching (subclinical jaundice). A woman who has had gallstones may have an increased tendency to stone formation during pregnancy as a result of the increased plasma cholesterol level and additional cholesterol incorporated in bile. Women with peptic ulcers generally find their condition improved during pregnancy because the acidity of the stomach is decreased.

Some women notice hypertrophy at their gumlines and bleeding of gingival tissue when they brush their teeth. There may be increased saliva formation (**hyperptyalism**), probably as a local response to increased levels of estrogen. This is an annoying but not serious problem. A lower than normal pH of saliva may lead to increased tooth decay if tooth brushing is not done conscientiously. This can be a problem in homeless women who do not have frequent access to a place to brush their teeth.

Urinary System

The urinary system undergoes many physiologic changes during pregnancy. These include alterations in fluid retention and renal, ureter, and bladder function. Changes in the urinary system are summarized in Table 9-6. Changes of the urinary system result from:

- Effects of estrogen and progesterone activity
- Compression of the bladder and ureters by the growing uterus
- Increased blood volume
- Postural influences

Fluid Retention. To provide sufficient fluid volume for effective placental exchange, total body water increases to 7.5 L; this requires the body to increase its sodium reabsorption in the tubules to maintain osmolarity. Under the influence of progesterone, there is an increased response of the angiotensin-renin system in the kidney, which leads to an increase in aldosterone production. Aldosterone aids sodium reabsorption. Progesterone appears to be potassium-sparing, so that even with an increased urine output, potassium levels remain adequate.

Water is retained during pregnancy to aid the increase in blood volume and to serve as a ready source of nutrients to the fetus. Because nutrients can pass to the fetus only when dissolved in or carried by fluid, this ready fluid supply is a fetal safeguard.

TABLE 9.6 Urinary Tract Changes During Pregnancy

VARIABLE	CHANGE
Glomerular filtration rate	Increased by 50%
Renal plasma flow	Increased by 25%–80%
Blood urea nitrogen	Decreased by 25%
Plasma creatinine level	Decreased by 25%
Renal threshold for sugar	Decreased to allow slight spillage
Bladder capacity	Increased by 1,000 mL
Diameter of ureters	Increased by 25%
Frequency of urination	Increased 1st trimester, last 2 weeks of pregnancy to 10–12 times/day

At one time, pregnant women were administered diuretics to help clear this excess fluid from their system. A sodium-restricted diet was also recommended. Today, it is recognized that these practices are potentially harmful because the fluid has physiologic benefits for the fetus. In addition, the excess fluid can serve to replenish the mother's own blood volume should hemorrhage occur.

Renal Function. During pregnancy, the woman's kidneys must excrete not only the waste products of her body but also those of the growing fetus. Also, the kidneys must be able to excrete additional fluid and manage the demands of increased renal blood flow. The kidneys may increase in size, changing their structure and ultimately affecting their function.

During pregnancy, urinary output gradually increases (about 60% to 80%). The specific gravity decreases. Glomerular filtration rate (GFR) and renal plasma flow begin to increase in early pregnancy to meet the increased needs of the circulatory system. By the second trimester, both the GFR and the renal plasma flow have increased by 30% to 50% and remain at this level for the duration of the pregnancy. This rise is consistent with that of the circulatory system increase, peaking at about 24 weeks. This efficient GFR level leads to a lowered blood urea nitrogen (BUN) and low creatinine levels in maternal plasma. A BUN of 15 mg/100 mL or higher and a serum creatinine over 1 mg/100 mL are considered abnormal and reflect the kidney's difficulty in handling the increased blood load. The higher GFR leads to increased filtration of glucose into the renal tubules. Because reabsorption of glucose by the tubule cells occurs at a fixed rate, this means there will be some accidental spilling of glucose into the urine during pregnancy. Lactose, which is being produced by the mammary glands but is not used during pregnancy, will also be spilled into the urine. Although minimal spilling of glucose into the urine may occur, the finding of more than a trace of glucose in a routine sample of urine from a pregnant woman is considered abnormal until proven otherwise, because this can occur with gestational diabetes (see Chap. 14).

Creatinine clearance has become the standard test for renal function during pregnancy, because creatinine is cleared from the body at a steady rate in relation to GFR. A normal pregnancy value is 90 to 180 mL/min. This is analyzed from a 24-hour urine sample.

Ureter and Bladder Function. Due to the increased level of progesterone during pregnancy, the ureters increase in diameter and the bladder capacity increases to about 1,500 mL. The uterus tends to rise on the right side of the abdomen because it is pushed slightly in that direction by the greater bulk of the sigmoid colon. As a result, pressure on the right ureter may lead to urinary stasis and pyelonephritis if not relieved. Pressure on the urethra may lead to poor bladder emptying and bladder infection. Such infections are potentially dangerous to the pregnant woman because they can ascend to become kidney infections. They are potentially dangerous to the fetus because urinary tract infections are associated with preterm labor (Delzell & Lefevre, 2000).

The pregnant woman may notice an increase in urinary frequency during the first 3 months of pregnancy until the uterus rises out of the pelvis and relieves pressure on the bladder. Frequency of urination may return at the end of pregnancy as lightening occurs and the fetal head exerts renewed pressure on the bladder.

Skeletal System

Calcium and phosphorus needs are increased during pregnancy because the fetal skeleton must be built. As pregnancy advances, there is a gradual softening of the pelvic ligaments and joints to create pliability and to facilitate passage of the baby through the pelvis at birth. This softening is probably due to the influence of the ovarian hormone relaxin and placental progesterone. Excessive mobility of the joints may cause discomfort. A wide separation of the symphysis pubis, as much as 3 to 4 mm by 32 weeks of pregnancy, may occur. This makes women walk with difficulty.

To change her center of gravity and make ambulation easier, the pregnant woman tends to stand straighter and taller than usual. This stance is sometimes referred to as the "pride of pregnancy." Standing this way, unfortunately, with the shoulders back and the abdomen forward, creates a lordosis (forward curve of the lumbar spine), which may lead to backache (see Focus on Family Empowerment).

Endocrine System

Almost all aspects of the endocrine system increase during pregnancy (Table 9-7).

Placenta. The most striking change in the endocrine system during pregnancy is the addition of the placenta as an endocrine organ that produces large amounts of estrogen, progesterone, hCG, human placental lactogen (hPL), relaxin, and prostaglandins. Estrogen causes breast and uterine enlargement. Palmar erythema during early pregnancy may also be a response to the high circulating estrogen levels. Progesterone has a major role in maintaining the endometrium, inhibiting uterine contractility, and aiding in the development of the breasts for lactation. Relaxin, secreted primarily by the corpus luteum, is responsible for helping inhibit uterine activity and soften the cervix and the collagen in joints. Softening of the cervix allows for dilatation at delivery; softening of collagen allows for laxness in the lower spine and helps enlarge the birth canal. hCG is secreted by the trophoblast cells of the placenta in early pregnancy. It stimulates progesterone and estrogen synthesis until the placenta can assume this role. hPL, also known as human chorionic somatomammotropin, is also produced by the placenta. It serves as an antagonist to insulin, freeing fatty acids for energy so glucose becomes available for the fetal growth.

In addition to the above, prostaglandins are found in high concentrations in the female reproductive tract and the decidua during pregnancy. Prostaglandins affect smooth muscle contractility to such an extent they may be the trigger that initiates labor at term.

Pituitary Gland. The pituitary gland is affected by pregnancy because there is a halt in the production of FSH and LH brought on by the high estrogen and progesterone levels of the placenta. There is increased production of growth hormone and melanocyte-stimulating hormone (causing skin pigment changes). Late in pregnancy, the posterior pituitary begins to produce oxytocin, which will be needed to aid labor. Prolactin production is also begun late in pregnancy as the breasts prepare for lactation.

Thyroid and Parathyroid Glands. The thyroid gland is altered significantly. The gland enlarges in early pregnancy to such an extent that the basal body metabolic rate increases by about 20%. Levels of protein-bound iodine, butanol-extractable iodine, and thyroxine are all elevated in blood serum. If a sufficient supply of iodine is not present during pregnancy, goiter (thyroid hypertrophy) can occur as the gland intensifies its productive effort.

These thyroid changes, along with emotional lability, tachycardia, palpitations, and increased perspiration, may lead to a mistaken diagnosis of hyperthyroidism if pregnancy has not been determined.

The parathyroid glands, which are necessary for the metabolism of calcium, also increase in size during pregnancy. Because calcium is important for fetal growth, the hypertrophy is probably necessary to satisfy the increased requirement of calcium.

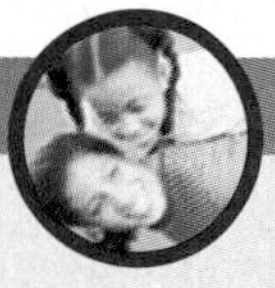

FOCUS ON FAMILY EMPOWERMENT
Backache During Pregnancy

Q. I had terrible backache with my last pregnancy. How can I avoid it with this one?

A. Backache is a common symptom of pregnancy owing to the strain on lower vertebrae from carrying extra weight. It may be serious if:

- It is experienced as waves of pain (could be preterm labor).
- There are accompanying urinary symptoms such as frequency and pain on urination (could be a urinary tract infection).
- The back is tender at the point of backache (could be pyelonephritis or a kidney infection).
- Rest doesn't relieve it (could be a muscle strain).

Measures to relieve backache in pregnancy are:

- Limit the use of high heels because they add to the natural lordosis of pregnancy.
- Try to rest daily with feet elevated.
- Walk with head high, pelvis straight.
- Pelvic rocking at the end of the day may relieve pain for the night.

TABLE 9.7 Endocrine Gland Changes and Effects During Pregnancy

GLAND	CHANGE	EFFECT
Thyroid gland	Slight enlargement	Increased basal metabolism rate
	Increased thyroid hormone production	Increased oxygen consumption
Parathyroid gland	Slight enlargement	Better utilization of calcium and vitamin D
	Increased parathyroid hormone production	
Pancreas	Early in pregnancy, decreased insulin production because of heavy fetal demand for glucose	Additional glucose is available for fetal growth
	After first trimester, increased insulin production because of insulin antagonist properties of estrogen, progesterone, and human placental lactogen	
Pituitary gland	FSH and LH decreased	Anovulation
	Prolactin increased	Breasts prepared for lactation
	Melanocyte-stimulating hormone increased	Increased skin pigment
	Human growth hormone increased	
Placenta	Estrogen and progesterone produced	Uterine and breast enlargement, fat deposits
		Increased blood coagulation, sodium and water retention
	Relaxin increased	Softening of cervix and collagen of joints
	Human placental lactogen	Increases glucose available for fetus
		Decreases utilization of protein for energy, increasing protein available for fetal growth

Adrenal Glands. Adrenal gland activity increases in pregnancy as elevated levels of corticosteroids and aldosterone are produced. It is assumed that this increased level aids in suppressing an inflammatory reaction or helps to reduce the possibility of the woman's body rejecting the foreign protein of the fetus, the same as it would automatically do for a foreign-tissue transplant. It also helps to regulate glucose metabolism in the woman. The increased level of aldosterone aids in promoting sodium reabsorption and maintaining osmolarity in the amount of fluid retained. This indirectly helps to safeguard the blood volume and provide adequate perfusion pressure across the placenta.

Pancreas. The pancreas increases production of insulin in response to the higher levels of glucocorticoid produced by the adrenal glands. Insulin is less effective than normal, however, because estrogen, progesterone, and hPL are all antagonists to insulin. Thus, a woman who is diabetic and taking insulin before pregnancy will need more insulin during pregnancy. A woman who is prediabetic may develop overt diabetes for the first time during pregnancy. Overall, the effect of diminishing the action of insulin is beneficial because it ensures a ready supply of glucose for fetal growth.

The glucose level of a fetus is about 30 mg/100 mL below the maternal glucose level. To prevent fetal hypoglycemia, with resultant cell destruction or lack of fetal growth, a maternal glucose level is usually at a higher than normal level during pregnancy. A number of fail-safe physiologic measures are effected to achieve this.

As mentioned, although the pancreas secretes an increased level of insulin throughout pregnancy, it appears to be not as effective. With insulin that is less effective, fat stores of the woman are utilized as well as available glucose. This maintains maternal glucose levels at a fairly steady level despite long intervals between meals or days of increased activity. To ensure against hypoglycemia, a pregnant woman should keep her diet high in calories and should never go longer than 12 hours between meals. Because the rapidly developing fetus uses so much glucose in early pregnancy, a fasting blood glucose level at this time is generally low (80 to 85 mg/100 mL).

Immune System

Immunologic competency during pregnancy apparently decreases, probably to prevent the woman's body from rejecting the fetus as if it were a transplanted organ. IgG production is particularly decreased; this may make the woman more prone to infection during pregnancy. A simultaneous increase in the white blood cell count may help to counteract the decrease in IgG response.

✔ CHECKPOINT QUESTIONS

13. Insulin is less effective than usual during pregnancy. How does this safeguard the fetus?
14. What is the most effective test of renal function during pregnancy?
15. What is the effect of melanocyte-stimulating hormone during pregnancy?

KEY POINTS

The diagnosis of pregnancy is based on three types of findings: presumptive, probable, and positive.

The positive signs of pregnancy are demonstration of a fetal heart separate from the mother's, fetal movement felt by an examiner, and visualization of the fetus by ultrasound.

Women may have read about the expected psychological and physiologic changes of pregnancy, but once these changes are actually being experienced, they may find them more intense than anticipated.

Although a woman may be in a physician's office or prenatal clinic for only an hour, if her pregnancy was confirmed at that visit, she invariably feels "more pregnant" when she leaves. Early diagnosis is important so the woman can begin to change unhealthy habits or, if she desires, have adequate time to carry out an elective termination.

The ability of a woman to accept a pregnancy depends on social, cultural, family, and individual influences.

The psychological tasks of pregnancy are centered on ensuring safe passage for the fetus. These consist of: in the first trimester; accepting the pregnancy; in the second trimester, accepting the baby; and in the third trimester, preparing for parenthood.

Common emotional responses that occur with pregnancy can be grief, narcissism, introversion or extroversion, stress, couvade syndrome, body image and boundary confusion, emotional lability, and changes in sexual desire.

Common emotional responses that occur with pregnancy can be grief, narcissism, introversion or extroversion, stress, couvade syndrome, body image and boundary confusion, emotional lability, and changes in sexual desire.

Physiologic changes that occur with pregnancy are both local (uterine, ovarian, and vaginal) and systemic changes (respiratory, cardiovascular, urinary, and skin changes).

CRITICAL THINKING EXERCISES

1. Lauren Maxwell, the woman described at the beginning of this chapter, said she felt scared of being pregnant because she "would die" if she thought she might be the same type of parent her parents were. Is being scared a common reaction to learning about a pregnancy? She says her partner is not scared. Would it be better or worse if he felt the same way? Has she completed the psychological development tasks of pregnancy? What suggestions could you make to help her be a better parent?
2. Your neighbor used a home test kit to determine that she is pregnant. She has not been to a health care setting because she says the most important reason for going would be to learn whether she is pregnant, and she already knows that. What argument could you use to convince her that prenatal care is important for more than pregnancy diagnosis?
3. You notice that a 60-year-old father-to-be rarely accompanies his new 24-year-old wife to the prenatal clinic for care. He says this is because doing that is only for "young guys." How would you advise him?
4. Examine the National Health Goals related to health during pregnancy. Most government-sponsored money for nursing research is allotted based on these goals. What would be a possible research topic to explore pertinent to these goals that would be fundable and would advance evidence-based practice?

REFERENCES

Andrews, M., & Boyle, J. (2002). *Transcultural concepts in nursing care* (4th ed.). Philadelphia: Lippincott Williams & Wilkins.

Bungum, T. J., et al. (2000). Exercise during pregnancy and type of delivery in nulliparae. *Journal of Obstetric, Gynecologic & Neonatal Nursing, 29*(3), 258–264.

Delzell, J. E. Jr., & Lefevre, M. L. (2000). Urinary tract infections during pregnancy. *American Family Physician, 61*(3), 713–721.

Department of Health and Human Services (2000). *Healthy people 2010.* Washington, D.C.: DHHS.

Ellegard, E., et al. (2000). The incidence of pregnancy rhinitis. *Gynecologic & Obstetric Investigation, 49*(2), 98–101.

Hartmann, S., & Bung, P. (1999). Physical exercise during pregnancy: Physiological considerations and recommendations. *Journal of Perinatal Medicine, 27*(3), 204–215.

Ling, F. W., & Duff, P. (2001). *Obstetrics and gynecology: Principles for practice.* New York: McGraw-Hill.

May, K. A., & Salyer, S. J. (1999). Psychosocial implications of high-risk intrapartum care. In L. K. Mandeville & N. H. Troiano. *High-risk and critical care intrapartum nursing* (pp. 51–64). Philadelphia: Lippincott-Raven.

Seifer, D. B., Samuels, P., & Kniss, D. A. (2001). *The physiologic basis of gynecology and obstetrics.* Philadelphia: Lippincott Williams & Wilkins.

Shew, M. L., et al. (2000). Prevalence of home pregnancy testing among adolescents. *American Journal of Public Health, 90*(6), 974–976.

Wessel, J., & Buscher, U. (2002). Denial of pregnancy. *BMJ: British Medical Journal, 324*(7335), 458.
Wheeler, M. (1999). Home and laboratory pregnancy-testing kits. *Professional Nurse, 14*(8), 571-576.

SUGGESTED READINGS

Devine, C. M., Bove, C. F., & Olson, C. M. (2000). Continuity and change in women's weight orientations and lifestyle practices through pregnancy and the postpartum period: The influence of life course trajectories and transitional events. *Social Science & Medicine, 50*(4), 567-582.
Hepner, D. L., et al. (2002). Herbal medicine use in parturients. *Anesthesia & Analgesia, 94*(3), 690-693.
Klerman, L. V., & Rooks, J. P. (1999). A simple, effective method that midwives can use to help pregnant women stop smoking. *Journal of Nurse-Midwifery, 4*(2), 118-123.
McDermott, S., et al. (2000). Urinary tract infections during pregnancy and mental retardation and developmental delay. *Obstetrics & Gynecology, 96*(1), 113-119.
Pastore, L. M., et al. (1999). Predictors of symptomatic urinary tract infection after 20 weeks gestation. *Journal of Perinatology, 19*(7), 488-493.
Schieve, L. A., et al. (2000). Prepregnancy body mass index and pregnancy weight gain: Associations with preterm delivery. *Obstetrics & Gynecology, 96*(2), 194-200.
Soltani, H., & Fraser, R. B. (2000). A longitudinal study of maternal anthropometric changes in normal weight, overweight, and obese women during pregnancy and postpartum. *British Journal of Nutrition, 84*(1), 95-101.
Varga, I., et al. (2000). Analysis of maternal circulation and renal function in physiologic pregnancies: Parallel examinations of the changes in the cardiac output and the glomerular filtration rate. *Journal of Maternal-Fetal Medicine, 9*(2), 97-104.
Walker, L. O., Cooney, A. T., & Riggs, M. W. (1999). Psychosocial and demographic factors related to health behaviors in the 1st trimester. *Journal of Obstetric, Gynecologic & Neonatal Nursing, 28*(6), 606-614.
Willis, F. R., et al. (2000). Children of renal transplant recipient mothers. *Journal of Paediatrics & Child Health, 36*(3), 230-235.

CHAPTER 10

Assessing Fetal and Maternal Health: The First Prenatal Visit

Key Terms

- abortion
- age of viability
- chloasma
- conjugate vera
- diagonal conjugate
- erosion
- gravida
- ischial tuberosity
- lithotomy position
- multigravida
- multipara
- nulligravida
- para
- primigravida
- primipara
- speculum
- true conjugate

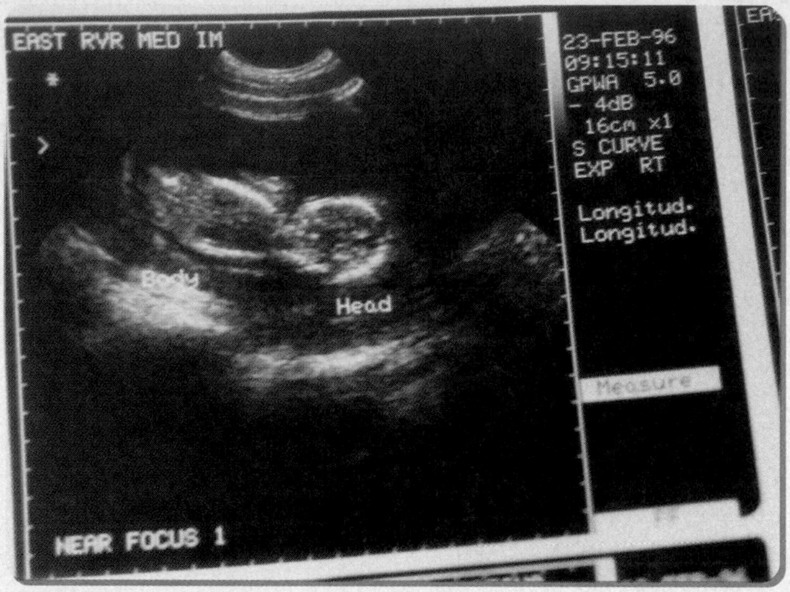

Objectives

After mastering the contents of this chapter, you should be able to:

1. Describe the areas of health assessment commonly included in a first prenatal visit.
2. Assess a pregnant woman's health status.
3. Formulate nursing diagnoses related to health status of pregnancy.
4. Identify expected outcomes for achieving a healthy pregnancy.
5. Plan nursing care such as preparing a woman for a pelvic examination or fundal measurement.
6. Implement nursing care such as establishing a risk score for pregnancy.
7. Evaluate outcomes related to fetal or maternal health for achievement and effectiveness of care.
8. Identify National Health Goals nurses can be instrumental in helping the nation to achieve.
9. Identify areas of prenatal care that could benefit from additional nursing research or application of evidence-based practice.
10. Use critical thinking to analyze ways to ensure family-centered prenatal care.
11. Integrate knowledge of pregnancy health assessment with nursing process to achieve quality maternal and child health care.

Sandra Czerinski is a 29-year-old woman, 16 weeks pregnant, who comes for a first prenatal visit. She is concerned because she didn't realize she was pregnant until a week ago. Because of this, she has been actively dieting (two diet drinks plus one meal of mainly vegetables daily) plus lifting weights at a health club. She says she won't need her urine tested because she knows she doesn't have a urinary tract infection. "Trust me," she says, "I know what one of those feels like." She does not want any blood work done because she doesn't have health insurance. She hasn't had a pelvic examination since she was in high school, when she had a vaginal infection. She remembers that as being very painful. What type of support or counseling does Sandra need?

Previous chapters described normal anatomy and physiology of the reproductive tract and the changes of pregnancy. This chapter adds information about prenatal care that helps to ensure a healthy outcome for both a woman and her child. This is important information because prenatal care is directly responsible for protecting the health of both women and newborns.

After reading this chapter, answer the Critical Thinking Exercises at the end of the chapter and then access the on-line study activities (http://connection.lww.com) *to further sharpen your skills and test your knowledge.*

Prenatal care, essential for ensuring the overall health of newborns and their mothers, is a major strategy for helping to reduce the number of low-birthweight babies born yearly. It is seen as so important that a number of National Health Goals speak directly to it (see Focus on National Health Goals). Ideally, prenatal care begins during the mother's childhood. It includes balanced nutrition with adequate intake of calcium and vitamin D during infancy and childhood to prevent rickets (which can distort pelvic size); adequate immunizations against contagious diseases for protection against viral diseases such as rubella during pregnancy; and a healthy daily diet to ensure the best state of health possible for a woman and her partner when entering pregnancy (Reifsnider & Gill, 2000).

Promoting prenatal health also includes developing positive attitudes about sexuality, womanhood, and childbearing. Once a woman becomes sexually active, preparation for a successful pregnancy includes practicing safer sex, regular pelvic examinations, and prompt treatment of any sexually transmitted disease to prevent complications that could lead to infertility. Acquisition and use of reproductive life planning information may help to ensure that each pregnancy is planned. These are steps involved with preconceptual care.

Women who maintain a healthy lifestyle come to a first prenatal visit prepared to follow health-promotion strategies. For many women, this visit may be the first time they have been to a health care facility since the routine health maintenance visits of childhood. It also may be the first time they have had an appointment that focuses more on health promotion than on the diagnosis of disease. A woman may have a specific reason (her agenda) for coming to the first prenatal visit (e.g., to confirm the diagnosis of pregnancy). This makes the visit an ideal time to impress on her the necessity for additional health promotion visits during pregnancy (your agenda). Ideally, her motivation will allow you to provide the information, counseling, and care necessary during pregnancy and also promote development of a positive pattern of healthy behaviors for the family to use in the future. Because the majority of prenatal care occurs in ambulatory settings, education is crucial. What and how much is needed varies depending on the age and parity of the woman and her degree of family support. Box 10-1 highlights appropriate outcomes and interventions for preconception care using the terminology identified by the Nursing Outcomes Classification (NOC) and Nursing Interventions Classification (NIC).

FOCUS ON NATIONAL HEALTH GOALS

A number of National Health Goals speak directly to the importance of prenatal care:

- Increase to at least 80% the proportion of primary care providers who provide age-appropriate preconception care and counseling.
- Increase to at least 90% the proportion of all pregnant women who receive prenatal care in the first trimester of pregnancy from a baseline of 76% (DHHS, 2000).

Nurses can be instrumental in helping the nation to achieve these goals by educating women and their families about the importance of prenatal care and by making sites of prenatal care receptive to women and families. Additional nursing research to investigate ways to promote prenatal care or to enlarge the scope of nursing involvement in prenatal care would be important to help the nation meet these goals.

NURSING PROCESS OVERVIEW

For the First Prenatal Visit

Assessment

The first prenatal visit is a time to establish baseline data relevant to planning health-promotion strategies now and with every subsequent visit. Explaining why specific assessment data are relevant to the pregnancy may be the first step in this process. For instance, when weighing the woman, discussing what routine weight gain is to be expected in the next couple of months supplies important information while showing that weight measurement is an important routine procedure. Relating assessment information and health-promotion activities throughout the pregnancy helps keep the woman and her family well informed and eager to comply with further health care recommendations. Obtaining a health history, including screening for the presence of teratogens (any factor that may adversely affect the fetus) and any problems the woman may be experiencing, is important initially and at subsequent visits.

BOX 10.1

NURSING OUTCOMES AND NURSING INTERVENTIONS CLASSIFICATION: PRECONCEPTION

NOC: Knowledge, Preconception
Knowledge, preconception is defined as the extent of understanding conveyed about maternal health prior to conception to ensure a healthy pregnancy (Johnson, Maas, & Moorhead, 2000). Some specific indicators suggesting achievement of this outcome include the client's ability to:

- Describe factors to consider when deciding about pregnancy
- Describe components of a healthy pregnancy, including healthy diet, appropriate rest and exercise, and potential adverse effects of alcohol, tobacco, and drug use
- Identify maternal risk factors associated with pregnancy and fetal development, environmental hazards, and risk for hereditary diseases
- Describe potential personal and family adjustments to pregnancy and addition of new family member

NIC: Preconception Counseling
Preconception counseling is defined as screening and providing information and support to individuals of child-bearing age before pregnancy to promote health and reduce risks (McCloskey & Bulechek, 2000). Some important activities involved when implementing this intervention include:

- Obtaining client history, including thorough sexual history, and determining readiness for pregnancy with both partners
- Providing information about risk factors
- Referring for genetic counseling or prenatal diagnostic testing as needed
- Encouraging dental examination to minimize exposure to x-ray examinations and anesthetics
- Instructing about the relationships among early fetal development and personal habits, medication use, teratogens, and self-care needs
- Recommending self-care measures needed during the preconception period
- Educating about ways to avoid teratogens
- Discussing ways to prepare for pregnancy socially, financially, and psychologically
- Identifying real and perceived barriers to family planning services
- Encouraging contraception until prepared for pregnancy
- Discussing methods of identifying fertility, signs of pregnancy and ways to confirm pregnancy
- Encouraging the need for early and continued prenatal care once pregnant

Chapter 11 discusses important assessments later in pregnancy.

Nursing Diagnosis

Nursing diagnoses appropriate to early pregnancy include:

- Health-seeking behaviors related to guidelines for nutrition and activity during pregnancy
- Deficient knowledge regarding exposure to teratogens during pregnancy
- Risk for injury to fetus related to current lifestyle behaviors

In addition, although most women probably have used a home pregnancy detection kit to find out if they are pregnant, the first prenatal visit officially serves to confirm this, so nursing diagnoses may focus on the response of the woman and her family to that information. For example:

- Decisional conflict related to desire to be pregnant
- Risk for ineffective coping related to confirmation of unplanned pregnancy

Outcome Identification and Planning

Sufficient time should be reserved for a first prenatal visit so it can be thorough, allowing enough time to set realistic goals and expected outcomes with both the woman and her partner, if desired. Make sure that a woman leaving an initial prenatal visit schedules an appointment for a following visit, as this may not occur to a woman who may be excited or overwhelmed by all the new things that are happening to her and her family. Establishing a pattern of regular appointments is crucial to providing adequate prenatal care. During a normal pregnancy, return appointments are usually scheduled every 4 weeks through the 32nd week of pregnancy, every 2 weeks through the 36th week, and then every week until birth. Women categorized as high risk are followed more closely.

Implementation

The purposes of prenatal care are to:

- Establish a baseline of present health
- Determine the gestational age of the fetus
- Monitor fetal development
- Identify the woman at risk for complications
- Minimize the risk of possible complications by anticipating and preventing problems before they occur
- Provide time for education about pregnancy and possible dangers

During the first visit, much time is spent on client teaching about prenatal care. In addition, it may be helpful to give the woman and her partner pamphlets or books that cover the same topics. Be sure you have read all the printed material you give families. This helps ensure that their advice is consistent with what you have already said and with the views of their primary care physician or nurse-midwife. A beautiful picture on the cover of a pamphlet does not ensure the quality of the advice inside. In addition, reinforce instructions that the woman may call the health care setting if she has any problems or questions during the coming months. Some women may feel reluctant to "bother" a health care provider outside of scheduled visits unless you give them permission to do this.

Outcome Evaluation

Evaluation during the first prenatal visit should concentrate on the woman's initial progress toward understanding goals of care for pregnancy and assessing outcomes established for specific diagnoses. Examples of expected outcomes might include:

- Client states she feels well informed about the common discomforts of pregnancy.
- Client lists the dangers of exposure to teratogens during pregnancy.
- Couple verbalizes they have reached a decision about maintaining or discontinuing the pregnancy.

HEALTH PROMOTION DURING PREGNANCY

The Preconceptual Visit

Ideally, women schedule appointments with a physician or nurse-midwife before becoming pregnant to obtain accurate reproductive life planning information, receive reassurance about fertility (as much as can be given based on a health history and a routine physical examination), and detect any problems that may need correction through a health history, pelvic examination, and Papanicolaou (Pap) test. At this visit, hemoglobin level and blood type (including Rh factor) can be determined; minor vaginal infections such as those arising from *Candida* can be corrected to help ensure fertility; and the woman can be counseled on the importance of a good protein diet, adequate intake of folic acid, and early prenatal care in the event she does become pregnant (de Weerd et al., 2002). More often, however, women arriving for their first prenatal visit will not have had a recent health care appointment oriented toward reproduction. Thus, the first prenatal visit usually covers a wide range of assessment criteria.

Choosing a Health Care Provider for Pregnancy and Childbirth

Once a woman is or suspects that she may be pregnant, she chooses a primary health care provider to care for her throughout the pregnancy and birth. Various options are available, including a prenatal clinic, her HMO health care provider, a nurse-midwife, an obstetrician, or a family practitioner. Regardless of the type of health care provider chosen, prenatal care needs to be initiated early and continued throughout pregnancy.

Nurses can contribute to the success of prenatal care by listening, counseling, and teaching, three areas of nursing expertise. Many clinics and group practices provide an initial educational seminar for women in the early stages of their pregnancy, often led by a nurse or nurse practitioner. Box 10-2 summarizes ways that prenatal care can be improved and individualized so that all women are interested in obtaining it.

HEALTH ASSESSMENT DURING THE FIRST PRENATAL VISIT

Prenatal care is important because lack of it is associated with the birth of preterm infants and various complications for the woman. The major causes of death during pregnancy today for women are ectopic pregnancy, hypertension, hemorrhage, embolism, infection, and anesthesia-related complications such as intrapartum cardiac arrest (DHHS, 2000). An important focus of all prenatal visits, therefore, is to screen for danger signs that might reveal any of these conditions are occurring (see Chap. 11).

Box 10-3 highlights appropriate outcomes and interventions for prenatal care using the terminology identified by the Nursing Outcomes Classification and Nursing Interventions Classification.

The first visit includes an extensive health history, a complete physical examination, including a pelvic examination, and blood and urine specimens for laboratory work. Manual pelvic measurements can be taken to determine pelvic adequacy. Following this, time should be set aside to begin health education about pregnancy (see Focus on Nursing Care Planning).

> ✔ **CHECKPOINT QUESTIONS**
>
> 1. What three areas of nursing expertise contribute to the success of prenatal care?
> 2. What information is obtained at the first prenatal visit?

The Initial Interview

Interviewing expectant women often elicits contradictory information. Women are likely to want to talk about their past health and current pregnancy, so interviewing them should go smoothly and be productive. On the other hand, pregnancy symptoms are subtle, so a woman may not regard certain information as important, providing vague answers to questions about these areas. Perhaps she is unaware that she is the only person who knows the answers to a number of vital questions ("How do you feel about being pregnant?" or "What have you been taking for your morning nausea?"). Outside pressures, such as having to report for work or older children coming home from school, may interfere with the effectiveness of the interview. Late in pregnancy, a woman may feel uncomfortable sitting for a long time.

Interviewing is best accomplished in a private, quiet setting. Trying to talk to a woman in a crowded hallway or a full waiting room is rarely effective. Pregnancy is too private an affair to be discussed under these circumstances.

(text continues on page 234)

BOX 10.2

SUGGESTIONS FOR IMPROVING PRENATAL CARE SERVICES

- Schedule appointments for women within a week after they first call the health care setting. This initial contact can be done through a group orientation session, individually by a health team member, or, if risk status warrants, by a physician. Try to schedule further appointments at times convenient for the client and her support people to encourage attendance.
- Make waiting time educational by providing materials such as pamphlets or videotapes in the waiting room.
- Provide privacy for assessments such as blood pressure, weight, and urine checks.
- Encourage women to feel responsible for their health record. If a woman's first language is not English, make sure to record pregnancy information so she can read it.
- Be certain that pregnant women meet health care providers while fully clothed and upright, not naked and in a lithotomy position on an examining table.
- Encourage family members and friends to accompany the woman for prenatal care. Allow them to enter the examination room and participate in all aspects of care to the extent they and the client desire.
- Schedule appointments to provide continuity of care. Be certain that women have a specific person's name as a phone contact for pregnancy-related questions. Without this, they tend not to call.
- Educate pregnant women about care options and encourage them to participate in making decisions about their care.

BOX 10.3

NURSING INTERVENTIONS AND NURSING OUTCOMES CLASSIFICATION: PRENATAL CARE

NOC: Knowledge, Pregnancy

Knowledge, pregnancy is defined as the extent of understanding conveyed about maintenance of a healthy pregnancy and prevention of complications (Johnson, Maas, & Moorhead, 2000). Some specific indicators suggesting achievement of this outcome include evidence of the following:

- Acknowledgment of the importance of prenatal care and prenatal education along with discussion of options for providing prenatal health care and childbirth
- Identification of the danger signs of pregnancy and possible complications
- Description of the following: major fetal developmental milestones; physical and psychological changes of pregnancy; appropriate health-promotion behaviors such as proper body mechanics, adequate rest and sleep, and exercise; measures to promote self-care for discomforts of pregnancy; healthy weight gain patterns and correct use of dietary supplements; importance of dental care; safe sex practices; and proper use of safety devices in an automobile
- Description of the signs of labor and techniques to facilitate effective labor
- Identification of possible fetal teratogens and environmental hazards
- Discussion of ways to prepare family members

NIC: Prenatal Care

Prenatal care is defined as the monitoring and managing of a patient during pregnancy to prevent complications and promote a healthy outcome for both the mother and infant (McCloskey & Bulechek, 2000). Some important activities involved when implementing this intervention include:

- Instructing client on importance of regular prenatal care throughout pregnancy, necessary nutrition, exercise, rest, desired weight gain, danger signs, fetal growth and development, self-care strategies for common discomforts, and harmful effects of teratogens
- Encouraging client's partner to participate in prenatal care, including attending prenatal classes
- Monitoring physiologic parameters including nutritional status, blood pressure, laboratory studies such as urine glucose and protein and hemoglobin, edema of ankles, hands and face, deep tendon reflexes
- Measuring fundal height with comparison to gestational age
- Assessing fetal heart rate and fetal growth and development
- Providing anticipatory guidance about physical and psychological changes during pregnancy
- Monitoring psychological adjustment of client and family, along with counseling client about changes in sexuality and body image during pregnancy
- Assessing social support system and assisting client to develop and use social support
- Instructing client on how to monitor fetal activity
- Guiding client in imaging her unborn child as appropriate
- Providing parents with opportunity to hear fetal heart tones and see ultrasound image of the fetus
- Referring client to childbirth preparation and child care and parenting classes as appropriate

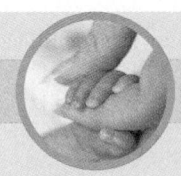

FOCUS ON *Nursing Care Planning*

THE FIRST PRENATAL VISIT FOR A CLIENT

A 31-year-old African-American woman comes to the obstetrician's office for evaluation. She states, "I think I'm pregnant. I did one of those home pregnancy tests and it was positive. Plus I'm late with my period and I feel like I did when I was pregnant with my first child. Oh, I hope it's not as bad as my last pregnancy."

Assessment: Gravida 2, Para 1. Last menstrual period 6 weeks ago. Reports fatigue and nausea for the last 2 weeks. Previous pregnancy required bed rest during the last trimester for preterm labor. "Those last weeks were so scary. I had to stop working and I felt so alone. My husband is away from home a lot because of his job." Delivered healthy female infant, 6 lbs 8 oz, at 37 weeks' gestation vaginally.

Menarche at age 11; menstrual cycle every 29 days, 6 days' duration with moderate flow and mild cramps. Past history positive for sinusitis and appendectomy at age 12 years. Smokes about half pack per day, "more when I'm stressed at work"; employed full time as executive director at local advertising agency. Denies alcohol use. "I drink club soda with lime or mineral water."

ROS: Height 5 feet 6 inches; weight 160 lb. Slight gingival hyperplasia; breasts full and slightly tender.

Pelvic examination by nurse-midwife: cervical os slitlike, clean, and slightly soft; uterus enlarged and soft; + Chadwick's sign, + Hegar's sign, and + Goodell's sign. Uterine height palpable at symphysis. Fetal heart rate via Doppler at 152 beats per minute.

Remainder of physical examination within normal limits. Serum hCG and ultrasound positive for pregnancy.

Nursing Diagnosis: Health-seeking behaviors related to guidelines for second pregnancy

Outcome Identification: Client will demonstrate positive behaviors to ensure successful outcome at each visit.

Outcome Evaluation: Client states the need to stop smoking; identifies measures to promote optimal fetal growth and development; makes appointments for follow-up visits and testing.

Interventions	Rationale
1. Assist with and perform initial assessment, including vital signs, height and weight measurement, and history and physical examination.	1. Initial assessment provides a baseline for future comparison and identification of factors that may place the client at risk for problems.
2. Assess the client's knowledge about guidelines for healthy pregnancy and antepartal care.	2. Although the guidelines for each pregnancy are usually similar, each pregnancy experience is different. Assessment of client's knowledge provides a baseline to identify teaching needs.
3. Review the plans for antepartal care visits, examinations, and laboratory testing. Include information about physiologic and psychological changes of pregnancy. Assist client with setting up appointments for visits and tests to evaluate fetal well-being as necessary.	3. Reviewing information provides reinforcement of what is to come and helps to alleviate fears and anxieties related to pregnancy. Assisting with appointment setting helps to ensure compliance.
4. Instruct the client about the effects of smoking on the fetus. Assist client with methods to reduce and stop, if possible.	4. Nicotine in cigarettes has been shown to be teratogenic to the fetus.
5. Discuss with the client the increased nutritional needs during pregnancy. Provide information about a well-balanced diet, including food selections, such as fresh fruits and vegetables, calcium sources, and high-protein foods, fluid intake, and prenatal vitamin supplementation.	5. A well-balanced diet with adequate fluid intake and use of prenatal vitamins helps to ensure an optimal environment for fetal growth and development.

(continued)

Interventions	Rationale
6. Compare prepregnancy and baseline weights. Monitor weight at every visit.	6. A baseline weight is necessary for future comparison. Adequate weight gain during pregnancy (typically 25 to 30 lb) is necessary for optimal fetal growth and development.
7. Discuss with the client her expectations about this pregnancy, including the impact on the family, her partner's attitude, and any religious or cultural beliefs.	7. Psychosocial assessment is important to assist the client in identifying areas of need and adapting psychologically to the pregnancy to ensure the optimal outcome for the mother, fetus, and family.

Nursing Diagnosis: Anxiety related to pregnancy course based on experience with first pregnancy

Outcome Identification: Client will state that feelings of anxiety have diminished by next visit.

Outcome Evaluation: Client accurately identifies signs and symptoms of her own anxiety; verbalizes confidence in ability to cope with pregnancy; demonstrates use of positive coping mechanisms.

Interventions	Rationale
1. Review the client's past pregnancy history.	1. Evaluation of previous pregnancy may reveal clues to possible factors placing the client at risk for problems.
2. Allow client to verbalize concerns about her past and current pregnancies. Acknowledge her anxieties and provide feedback.	2. Verbalization provides a safe outlet for concerns and helps to increase the client's awareness of them and their possible impact on this pregnancy. Acknowledging the client's anxieties validates her feelings; feedback helps to correct any misinformation.
3. Reinforce guidelines related to prenatal care and follow-up and measures to ensure a healthy pregnancy.	3. Reinforcement enhances learning and clarifies misconceptions to provide the client with a sense of control and promote optimal fetal growth and development.
4. Assist client in identifying how she feels when she is anxious.	4. The ability to identify signs and symptoms of anxiety is the first step in controlling it.
5. Instruct the client in measures to decrease anxiety, such as relaxation techniques, breathing exercises, and activity. Praise the client for use of effective coping mechanisms.	5. Measures to decrease anxiety help to enhance the client's control over the situation. Praising helps to reinforce use of positive coping mechanisms in the future.
6. Encourage the client to have her partner accompany her on some future visits.	6. Partner participation in the pregnancy offers the client additional support and promotes a sharing partnership, thus enhancing family-centered care.
7. Instruct the client about possible danger signs to report immediately. Emphasize that although these signs are important, they do not necessarily mean that something is wrong.	7. Knowledge of possible danger signs allows for early detection and prompt interventions should they be necessary.
8. Ensure that the client has a name and number to call should any problems arise.	8. Having a contact person readily available helps to reassure the client that she is not alone and help is always available.

It is helpful if the person scheduling the appointment cautions the woman that the first visit may be long. This prevents her from trying to fit the visit in between other errands or from having to terminate the interview because of another appointment.

Be certain to ask what name a woman wants you to use when addressing her in a prenatal setting, and make certain that she knows your name and understands your role correctly. If she views you as a secretary, she will be willing to discuss superficial facts (name, address, phone number, and the like) but will resist discussing more intimate things (her feelings toward this pregnancy, the difficulty she has reworking old fears, how scared she is about birth).

Because initial health history taking is often time-consuming, the woman may be asked to complete some of the forms. However, many women feel this is callous and depersonalizing. Thus, good interviewing techniques are important to obtain thorough and meaningful health histories within time constraints. The rapport established by face-to-face interviewing gives a woman the feeling that she is more than just a client number or chart. It may be as much a reason she returns for follow-up care as her desire to be assured that her pregnancy is progressing normally.

Components of the Health History

An initial interview serves several purposes:

- Establishing rapport
- Gaining information about the woman's physical and psychosocial health
- Obtaining a basis for anticipatory guidance for the pregnancy

Establishing a baseline health picture at the initial pregnancy visit is important. If on subsequent visits a symptom is mentioned, you can then check your records to verify that it is truly a new symptom. It may be that the woman is just becoming more aware of it. General interviewing techniques are discussed in Chapter 33. Included in the following section are the elements pertinent to a pregnancy history.

Demographic Data

Demographic data usually obtained include name, age, address, telephone number, religion, and health insurance information.

Chief Concern

The chief concern is the reason the woman has come to the health care setting—in this instance, the fact that she is or thinks she is pregnant.

Inquire about the date of her last menstrual period and whether she has had a pregnancy test or used a home test kit. Elicit information about the signs of early pregnancy, such as nausea, vomiting, breast changes, or fatigue. Question her about any discomforts of pregnancy, such as constipation, backache, or frequent urination. Has she been exposed to any contagious diseases? Has she taken any medicine that might be harmful to fetal growth? Also, ask about any danger signs of pregnancy, such as bleeding, continuous headache, visual disturbances, or swelling of the hands and face.

Ask if the pregnancy was planned. If you feel uncomfortable asking directly, using a statement such as, "All pregnancies are a bit of a surprise. Is that how it was with this one?" may help provide you with this information. Another way to word such a question would be, "Some couples plan on having children right away; some plan on waiting. How was it with you?" If the woman says the pregnancy was not planned, explore to learn if she has reached a decision about whether to continue with the pregnancy. A question such as, "Some women change their mind about wanting a baby once they realize they are pregnant; some don't. How has it been for you?" may be effective for obtaining this type of information because it says either option is possible. You just want her to tell you which is happening.

Family Profile

In the past, the social history or family setting history (family profile) was left until the end of a health interview. More often, it is now obtained at the beginning of the interview, following the chief concern. Doing so may help you get to know the woman earlier, identify support persons, and shape the nature and kind of questions asked and evaluate the possible impact of the client's culture on care (see Focus on Cultural Competence). Inquiring about marital status may be awkward. One way to do this is to ask, "Who else lives at home with you?" The married woman may answer, "My husband and my 4-year-old son." The single woman may answer, "No one," "My parents and my brothers and sisters," or "My boyfriend." As a rule, most unmarried women want you to know they are unmarried to alert you that they may not have support people readily available.

It is important to know the size of the apartment or house in which a woman lives because you will be talking with her in the coming months about a bedroom or space for a baby's bed. It also is important to know whether the essential rooms are on the ground floor or upstairs in case she is restricted from climbing stairs more than once or twice a day during the last part of pregnancy or after birth.

Before you can begin to offer a woman any more than stereotyped health care instruction, get to know her and her sexual partner's age (additional testing such as genetic screening may be necessary if her age is over 35), their educational levels (offers an estimation of how well they will be able to understand teaching), and occupation (does the woman's involve heavy lifting, long hours of standing in one position, handling of a toxic substance?).

Adaptation to pregnancy is highly individualized. A change in status from independence to dependence be-

FOCUS ON CULTURAL COMPETENCE

How Do Cultural Variations Affect Attendance at Prenatal Care?

Hispanic women constitute one of the fastest-growing and most diverse groups in the United States, representing many countries of origin and cultural practices. Low birthweight is frequently associated with Hispanic women. They may have difficulty coming in for prenatal care because of inability to use public transportation and difficulty communicating with agency personnel. They may need interdisciplinary and culturally sensitive prenatal care to ensure well-being and optimal birth outcome.

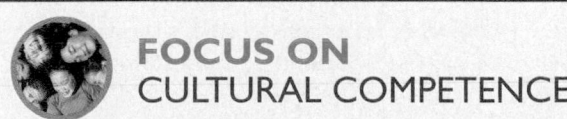

cause of stopping work, chronic illness at home, the death or loss of a significant person during pregnancy, geographic moves, financial hardship, and lack of support people are examples of situations that can hinder a woman's ability to accept her pregnancy and child. No one in the health care setting will be aware of these potentially harmful situations unless questions about family profile are asked.

History of Past Illnesses

Questions about the past medical history are an important part of an interview because a past condition may become active during or immediately following pregnancy. Representative diseases that can pose a potential difficulty during pregnancy include kidney disease, heart disease (coarctation of the aorta and rheumatic fever cause problems most often), hypertension, sexually transmitted diseases (including hepatitis B and human immunodeficiency virus [HIV]), diabetes, thyroid disease, recurrent seizures, gallbladder disease, urinary tract infections, varicosities, phenylketonuria, tuberculosis, and asthma. It is important to find out whether a woman had childhood diseases such as chickenpox (varicella), mumps (epidemic parotitis), measles (rubeola), German measles (rubella), or poliomyelitis. From this information, you can estimate the degree of antibody protection the client has against these diseases if she is exposed to them during her pregnancy. While pregnant, she can be immunized against poliomyelitis by the Salk (killed virus) vaccine. However, she cannot be immunized against the other diseases because the vaccines against these contain live viruses, as does the oral Sabin poliomyelitis vaccine. Live virus vaccines could be harmful to the fetus if the virus crosses the placenta.

Also ask about any allergies, including any drug sensitivities. As a rule, women with allergies of any magnitude should breast-feed rather than bottle-feed their infants to avoid possible milk allergy in the infant (Cunningham et al., 2001). Any past surgical procedures are also important because adhesions resulting from past abdominal surgery may interfere with uterine growth.

WHAT IF? What if a woman states she has no idea what childhood diseases or immunizations she had? How would you suggest she obtain this information?

History of Family Illnesses

A family history documents illnesses that occur frequently in the family and helps to identify potential problems in the mother during pregnancy or in the infant at birth. Ask specifically about cardiovascular and renal disease, cognitive impairment, blood disorders, or any known inherited disease or congenital anomalies.

Day History/Social Profile

Information about a woman's current nutrition, elimination, sleep, recreation, and interpersonal interactions can be elicited best by asking the woman to describe a typical day of her life. If any of this information is not reported spontaneously as she describes her day, ask for additional details.

Nutrition is an important part of a day history to obtain, particularly in light of the number of young adults with eating disorders today (Little & Lowkes, 2000). A "24-hour recall" is helpful in obtaining accurate nutrition information because the woman tells you what she actually ate, not what she should have eaten (see Focus on Communication).

Ask about the type, amount, and frequency of exercise to determine her routine pattern and whether it will be consistent with a recommended level for pregnancy (ACOG, 2002). If she hikes or camps, she is at risk for exposure to Lyme disease. Ask about hobbies. Certain hobbies, such as working with lead-based glazes and ceramics, might not be wise to continue during pregnancy because lead is teratogenic.

FOCUS ON COMMUNICATION

Ms. Scott is a young woman who has come to her obstetrician's office for a first prenatal visit.

Less Effective Communication

Nurse: The next thing I need, Ms. Scott, is for you to tell me what a typical day is like for you.

Ms. Scott: I don't usually have typical ones. Or very interesting ones.

Nurse: What about yesterday? Could you describe that to me?

Ms. Scott: Okay. I was up at 7:00, was at work by 9:00. A friend picked me up after work and we celebrated his birthday. I was back home and in bed by 10:00. That's pretty much the day.

Nurse: You're right. It doesn't sound very interesting. Next, let me ask you about your family medical history.

More Effective Communication

Nurse: The next thing I need, Ms. Scott, is for you to tell me what a typical day is like for you.

Ms. Scott: I don't usually have typical ones. Or very interesting ones.

Nurse: What about yesterday? Could you describe that to me?

Ms. Scott: Okay. I was up at 7:00, was at work by 9:00. A friend picked me up after work and we celebrated his birthday. I was back home and in bed by 10:00. That's pretty much the day.

Nurse: What did you have for breakfast?

Ms. Scott: Nothing. I was too rushed to eat.

Nurse: Dinner?

Ms. Scott: We were celebrating at a bar. Cheese blintzes, I think. And beer. A lot of beer.

Most people are not aware how much information can be revealed by a day history, so they give only a scant description of their day. Asking additional questions to make them elaborate on various parts often reveals poor nutrition, poor exercise, or risky behavior patterns.

A social profile provides information on the woman's overall lifestyle. Because smoking cigarettes can lead to reduced fetal weight gain (Klerman & Rooks, 1999; Valanis et al., 2001), obtain information about the client's smoking and drinking habits. Smoke, whether first-hand or second-hand, has been shown to be harmful to fetal growth. Identifying family smoking habits can lead to interventions to reduce or discontinue smoking. Excessive alcohol intake may lead to poor nutrition or be directly responsible for fetal alcohol syndrome. If a woman answers vaguely, "I drink socially" or "I only smoke occasionally," attempt to determine exactly what she means so you can accurately evaluate the frequency of these events (Autti-Ramo, 2000).

Pregnant women, especially adolescents, are at an increased risk for intimate partner abuse (see Focus on Evidence-Based Practice). Ask enough questions to be certain this is not happening.

A medication history is also important. Ask whether the woman takes any medications, prescribed or over-the-counter, because their effect on a growing fetus will have to be evaluated. This also includes any herbal preparations that the woman might be using. Even seemingly innocent medications for simple conditions can be detrimental during pregnancy. For example, isotretinoin (Accutane), a vitamin A preparation taken for acne, is associated with spontaneous miscarriage and congenital anomalies. Fenugreek, an herbal supplement used to treat constipation and indigestion, is associated with stimulating uterine contractions and thus should not be used during pregnancy.

Be sure to include the use of any recreational drugs, such as marijuana or cocaine. These also can be deleterious to fetal growth. Also include intravenous drug use because of the increased risk for exposure to HIV or hepatitis B. Although this type of information is not readily revealed by people, most women will answer these questions honestly during pregnancy because they are concerned about protecting the health of the fetus.

FOCUS ON EVIDENCE-BASED PRACTICE

Is Prenatal Violence a Risk Factor for Preterm Birth in Pregnant Teenage Girls?

To examine this problem, the amount of violence documented by pregnant teens who attended a county health department prenatal care program was compared to that reported by adult women. Among the teenagers, 16% reported prenatal violence, including 9% who reported severe violence such as hitting, kicking, or stabbing. Among adult women, only 11% reported prenatal violence, with only 4.8% reported as severe. Teenagers were more apt to report abdominal trauma (56% vs. 22% in older women) and violence perpetrated by a relative (23% vs. 5%). At the end of pregnancies, teens who reported severe prenatal violence were significantly more likely to deliver preterm infants than those who reported less or no prenatal violence.

This study is significant for nurses because it reinforces the importance of asking about intimate partner abuse at prenatal visits. Based on this study, this type of questioning is important for all pregnant women, but especially pregnant teenagers. Therefore, nurses need to ensure that adequate time is provided for interviewing women alone, without their intimate partner, so that they can feel free to discuss the subject. Many women do not report abuse or do so only when asked directly about it. Only when such abuse is detected can it be stopped and the health of the woman and fetus protected.

Covington, D. L., Justason, B. J., & Wright L. N. (2001). Severity, manifestations, and consequences of violence among pregnant adolescents. *Journal of Adolescent Health, 28*(1), 55-61.

Gynecologic History

In the past, most women had children early in their childbearing years, and the number of reproductive tract or women's health problems, such as breast disease, that they had experienced before pregnancy were few. Today, however, women often delay conception of their first child past 30 years of age. Therefore, it is not unusual to discover a woman who has had a reproductive tract or breast problem. Table 10-1 lists common gynecologic illnesses and their possible significance in pregnancy.

A woman's past experience with her reproductive system may have some influence on how well she accepts a pregnancy. Obtain information about her age of menarche (first menstrual period) and how well she was prepared for it as a normal part of life. Ask about her usual cycle, including the interval, duration, amount of menstrual flow, and any discomfort she feels. Ascertain her degree of discomfort, including when it occurs, how long it lasts, and what she does to relieve it. If she describes menstrual cramps as "horrible" and wonders "how I live through them some months," anticipate the need for additional counseling to help her prepare for labor. Some women with severe dysmenorrhea look forward to pregnancy as 9 months without discomfort. Anticipate their need for counseling in the postpartal period about active ways to relieve their menstrual discomfort (see Chap. 47). Also ask if a woman does a monthly breast and/or perineum self-examination (see Chap. 33 for these techniques) to evaluate her interest in self-care.

Be certain to ask about past surgery on the reproductive tract. For example, if a woman has had tubal surgery, such as for an ectopic pregnancy, the statistical risk of another tubal pregnancy increases. If she has had uterine surgery, a cesarean birth may be necessary because her uterus may not be able to expand and contract as efficiently as usual. If she has undergone frequent dilatation and curettage of the uterus, her cervix may be incompetent or unable to remain closed for 9 months. This could lead to premature birth unless she has a surgical procedure (cerclage) for this (see Chap. 15).

Question the client about what reproductive planning methods, if any, have been used. Occasionally, a woman may become pregnant with an intrauterine device (IUD) in place. If this occurs, it will have to be removed to prevent infection during pregnancy. Another woman, not

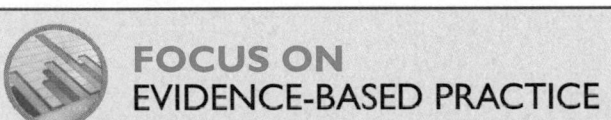

TABLE 10.1 Gynecologic Disorders

DISORDER	POSSIBLE SYMPTOMS	SIGNIFICANCE AND SUGGESTED THERAPY
Vulva		
Cysts of Skene's or Bartholin's glands	Asymptomatic swelling at the sides of the urinary meatus or vestibule	Such cysts are surgically incised to prevent blockage of gland duct.
Condylomata acuminata	Cauliflower-like lesion on vulva	This lesion tends to occur in women with chronic vaginitis. Caused by the epidermatrophic virus that causes common warts. Removed by cryocautery or knife excision.
Lichen sclerosus	Whitish papules on the vulva; asymptomatic	There is no need for removal; the area is biopsied because leukoplakia, a potentially cancerous condition, has an almost identical appearance.
Leukoplakia	Thick, gray, patchy epithelium that cracks; possibly a premalignant state and infects easily, accompanied by itching and pain	Therapy involves hydrocortisone and frequent return visits to health care personnel (every 6 months) for observation to detect any changes suggestive of carcinoma.
Carcinoma of the vulva	A shallow vulvar ulcer that does not heal	Vulvar cancer occurs most often in postmenopausal women; represents only 3% to 4% of all reproductive tract cancers in women. Therapy is vulvectomy—vagina is left intact, and sexual relations and pregnancy with cesarean birth to prevent tearing of fibrotic vulvar tissue may be possible.
Vagina and Cervix		
Adenosis	Asymptomatic vaginal cysts with columnar rather than squamous epithelium present on vaginal walls	This condition is caused by diethylstilbestrol (DES) administration while in utero. Has the potential for becoming malignant (clear cell adenocarcinoma). If adenosis is present, an examination two or three times a year with a Pap test and Lugol's staining is necessary, and the woman should not use estrogen sources such as oral contraceptives. If adenocarcinoma occurs, local destruction of atypical cells can be achieved by excision, cautery, or cryosurgery. This condition is rarely seen today because DES is no longer prescribed during pregnancy.
Cervical polyp	Red, vascular, protruding pedunculated tissue that bleeds readily with trauma	A polyp may be discovered because of vaginal spotting on coitus, tampon insertion, or vaginal examination. Removed vaginally by excision. Often associated with chronic cervical inflammation.
Cervicitis (erosion)	Reddened cervical tissue with a whitish exudate	Douching with a vinegar solution aids healing. May be treated with cryosurgery if extensive.
Nabothian cyst	Clear shining circles on cervix from blocked gland ducts	No therapy is necessary.
Cervical carcinoma	Postcoital spotting, unexplained vaginal discharge or spotting between menstrual periods	Cervical cancer is the most frequent type of reproductive tract malignancy; risk factors include coitus with multiple partners or uncircumcised males, herpes type II infections, or DES use during pregnancy. Diagnosed by Pap test or colposcopy. Therapy is conization, radiation, or surgical excision. Pregnancy is possible following cervical carcinoma; cesarean birth may be necessary because of fibrotic cervical tissue.
Ovaries		
Endometrial cyst	Chocolate-brown cyst on tender enlarged ovary; may cause acute pain if rupture occurs	Endometriosis is the cause; occurs in women aged 20 to 40 years. Therapy is surgical excision; ovary may or may not be removed depending on extent of cyst.
Follicular cyst	Amenorrhea and possibly dyspareunia; ovary tender and enlarged	Cysts typically regress after 1 or 2 months; low-dose oral contraceptive may be prescribed for 6 to 12 weeks to suppress ovarian activity; estrogen may be continued for 6 months.
Polycystic disease	Multiple follicular cysts of both ovaries	Excess adrenal supply of estrogen leads to inhibition of follicle-stimulating hormone and anovulation. Clomiphene citrate therapy to induce ovulation or wedge resection of the ovaries is used as therapy.
Corpus luteum cyst	Delayed menstrual flow followed by prolonged bleeding; ovary enlarged and tender	A corpus luteum has persisted rather than atrophied. Most regress in about 2 months; a low-dose oral contraceptive may be prescribed for 6 weeks to suppress ovarian activity.

(continued)

TABLE 10.1 Gynecologic Disorders *(Continued)*

DISORDER	POSSIBLE SYMPTOMS	SIGNIFICANCE AND SUGGESTED THERAPY
Dermoid cyst	Asymptomatic; ovary enlarged on examination	Cyst originates from embryonic tissue; may contain hair, cartilage, and fat. Most common ovarian tumor of childhood; also occurs at 30 to 50 years. Therapy is surgical resection.
Serous cystadenoma	Bilateral; asymptomatic except for signs of pelvic pressure	This is the most common type of benign ovarian cyst; high malignancy rate of 20% to 30%. Therapy is surgical resection.
Carcinoma	Asymptomatic; intermenstrual bleeding	Ovarian cancer originates in epithelial tissue most often in women over 50 years of age. Tendency may be inherited; environmental contamination may play a role in development. Therapy is hysterectomy and salpingo-oophorectomy.
Uterus		
Endometrial polyp	Intermenstrual bleeding	Polyp is removed by dilatation and curettage.
Leiomyomas (fibroids)	Asymptomatic or with increased menstrual flow	Muscle and fibrous connective tissue form in response to estrogen stimulation. May increase in size during pregnancy; may cause interference with cervical dilatation and result in postpartal hemorrhage. Stress to the myometrium by uterine contractions may be the original cause of formation. Therapy is surgical resection (myomectomy) or hysterectomy if childbearing is complete.
Endometrial carcinoma	Vaginal bleeding between menstrual periods	Diagnosis is by endometrial washing, not Pap test. Therapy is hysterectomy.
Uterine prolapse	Vaginal pressure and low back pain	The uterus has descended in the vagina due to overstretching of uterine supports and trauma to the levator ani muscle. Occurs most often in women who had insufficient prenatal care, birth of a large infant, a prolonged second stage of labor, bearing-down efforts or extraction of a baby before full dilatation, instrument birth, and poor healing of perineal tissue postpartally. Therapy is surgery to repair uterine supports or placement of a pessary, a plastic uterine support. Women with pessaries in place need to return for a pelvic examination every 3 months to have the pessary removed, cleaned, and replaced and the vagina inspected; otherwise, vaginal infection or erosion of the vaginal walls can result.

realizing that she is pregnant, may continue to take an oral contraceptive for some time into the pregnancy. Document if this occurred because there is some evidence that estrogen can harm fetal growth. Be certain to include a sexual history, including the number of sexual partners and use of safer sex practices.

As part of any woman's gynecologic history, assess for the possibility of stress incontinence (incontinence of urine on laughing, coughing, deep inspiration, jogging, or running). With these actions, the diaphragm descends, increasing abdominal pressure, which increases bladder tension and causes emptying. Stress incontinence occurs from lack of strength in the perineal muscles and bladder supports. Commonly, weakness occurs from difficult births, the birth of large infants, grand multiparity, and instrument births. Some women accept stress incontinence as a normal consequence of childbearing and may not report it unless asked. During pregnancy, stress incontinence can be intensified from the increasing abdominal pressure.

Stress incontinence may be prevented and relieved to some degree by strengthening the perineal muscles with the use of Kegel exercises (periodic tightening of the perineal muscles; see Chap. 11). Surgical correction to increase support to the bladder neck also may be performed.

Obstetric History

Do not assume that the current pregnancy is a woman's first pregnancy simply because she is very young or says she has only recently been married. For each previous pregnancy, document the child's sex and the place and date of birth. Review the pregnancy briefly:

- Was it planned?
- Did she have any complications, such as spotting, swelling of her hands or feet, falls, or surgery?
- Did she take any medication? If so, what and why?
- Did she receive prenatal care? If so, when did she start?
- What was the duration of the pregnancy?
- What was the duration of labor?
- Was labor what she expected? Worse? Better?
- What was the type of birth?
- What type of anesthesia, if any, was used?
- Did she have stitches following birth?
- Did she have any complications, such as excessive bleeding or infection?
- What was the infant's birthweight?
- What was the condition of the infant at birth? Did the infant cry right away?

- What was the infant's Apgar score? (Some mothers know the infant's Apgar score and can tell you this.)
- Was any special care needed for the baby, such as suctioning, oxygen, or an incubator?
- Was the baby discharged from the health care setting with her?
- What is the child's present state of health?
- How was the pregnancy overall for her?

Ask about any previous miscarriages or abortions and whether she had any complications during or following them. **Abortion** is the medical term for any pregnancy terminated before the age of viability. The **age of viability** is the earliest age at which fetuses could survive if they were born at that time, generally accepted as 24 weeks, or fetuses weighing more than 400 g. If the woman's blood type is Rh negative, ask if she received Rh immune globulin (RhIG [RhoGAM]) after miscarriages or abortions or previous births so you will know whether Rh sensitization could have occurred. Ask if she had a blood transfusion to establish possible risk of hepatitis B or HIV exposure or Rh sensitization.

After a history of previous pregnancies is obtained, determine the woman's status with respect to the number of times she has been pregnant, including the present pregnancy (**gravida**), and the number of children above the age of viability she has previously birthed (**para**). Table 10-2 provides an explanation of these terms. For example, a woman who has had two previous pregnancies, has given birth to two term children, and is again pregnant is gravida 3, para 2. A woman who has had two miscarriages at 12 weeks (under the age of viability) and is again pregnant is a gravida 3, para 0.

A more comprehensive system for classifying pregnancy status (GTPAL or GTPALM) provides greater detail on the pregnancy history. By this system, the gravida classification remains the same, but para is broken down into:

T: The number of full-term infants born (infants born at 37 weeks or after)
P: The number of preterm infants born (infants born before 37 weeks)
A: The number of spontaneous or induced abortions
L: The number of living children
M: Multiple pregnancies

Using this system, the woman in the first example above would be gravida 3, para 2002 (GTPAL) or 320020 (GTPALM). A multigestation pregnancy is considered as one para. For example, a woman who had twins, then one preterm infant, and is now pregnant again would be a gravida 3, para 21031 (GTPALM).

A pregnant woman who had the following past history—a boy born at 39 weeks' gestation, now alive and well; a girl born at 40 weeks' gestation, now alive and well; a girl born at 33 weeks' gestation, now alive and well—would have her pregnancy information summarized as follows: gravida 4; para 21030 (GTPALM).

TABLE 10.2 Terms Related to Pregnancy Status

TERM	DEFINITION
Para	The number of pregnancies that reached viability, regardless of whether the infants were born alive or not
Gravida	A woman who is or has been pregnant
Primigravida	A woman who is pregnant for the first time
Primipara	A woman who has given birth to one child past age of viability
Multigravida	A woman who has been pregnant previously
Multipara	A woman who has carried two or more pregnancies to viability
Nulligravida	A woman who has never been and is not currently pregnant

Review of Systems

A review of systems completes the subjective information. Use a systematic approach, such as head to toe, and explain what you'll be doing. For example, "I'm going to start at the top of your head and go through to your toes, asking about body parts or systems and any diseases that you may have had." A review of systems helps women recall diseases they forgot to mention earlier, such as a urinary tract infection, a disease that can influence the outcome of pregnancy and so would be important to your history taking (McDermott et al., 2000).

The following body systems and questions about conditions constitute the minimum information to be addressed in a review of systems for a first prenatal visit:

- *Head:* Headache? Head injury? Seizures? Dizziness? Syncope?
- *Eyes:* Vision? Glasses needed? Diplopia? Infection? Glaucoma? Cataract? Pain? Recent changes?
- *Ears:* Infection? Discharge? Earache? Hearing loss? Tinnitus? Vertigo?
- *Nose:* Epistaxis (nose bleeds)? Discharge? How many colds a year? Allergy? Postnasal drainage? Sinus pain?
- *Mouth and pharynx:* Dentures? Condition of teeth? Toothaches? Any bleeding of gums? Hoarseness? Difficulty in swallowing? Tonsillectomy?
- *Neck:* Stiffness? Masses?
- *Breasts:* Lumps? Secretion? Pain? Tenderness? Does she know how to do a breast self-examination? Does she do this monthly?
- *Respiratory system:* Cough? Wheezing? Asthma? Shortness of breath? Pain? Serious chest illness, such as tuberculosis or pneumonia?
- *Cardiovascular system:* History of heart murmur? History of heart disease such as rheumatic fever or Kawasaki disease? Hypertension? Any pain? Palpitations? Anemia? Does she know her blood pressure? Has she ever had a blood transfusion?
- *Gastrointestinal system:* What was her prepregnancy weight? Vomiting? Diarrhea? Constipation? Change in bowel habits? Rectal pruritus? Hemorrhoids? Pain? Ulcer? Gallbladder disease? Hepatitis? Appendicitis?

- *Genitourinary system:* Urinary tract infection? Hematuria? Frequent urination? Sexually transmitted disease? Pelvic inflammatory disease? Hepatitis B? HIV?
- *Extremities:* Varicose veins? Pain or stiffness of joints? Any fractures or dislocations?
- *Skin:* Any rashes? Acne? Psoriasis?

Conclusion

End an interview by asking if there is something you have not covered that the woman wants to discuss. This gives her one more chance to ask any questions she has about this new life experience.

Support Person's Role

More and more partners accompany women for prenatal care today. Young children may accompany their mothers on these visits. Some women bring a female friend as their best support person. If family members are present, should they be included in an initial interview? As a whole, interviewing is most effective if it is a one-to-one interaction. A woman may be unwilling to mention certain concerns when her family is present for fear of worrying them. A husband may not be the father of her child, and she may be unable to voice her concern over this fact or alert you to the possibility she is worried about blood incompatibility because another man is the father.

If childbearing is to be a family affair, however, it is important to determine the partner's degree of acceptance of the pregnancy and of assuming a new role. Including siblings in a prenatal visit provides them with an opportunity to involve them with the pregnancy planning and coming baby. Interviewing the woman alone and then inviting the support person and family to join her while you talk about pregnancy symptoms with them as a family is an effective solution (Fig. 10-1). Providing some private interview time with a partner allows the partner to express any concerns or worries. The main areas you should investigate with the partner include his current health, his feelings and concerns about the pregnancy, and his knowledge of pregnancy and childbirth. If the woman wishes, the partner can accompany her during the physical examination. After the confirmation of pregnancy, the partner should be included when health care information is given (see Focus on Family Empowerment).

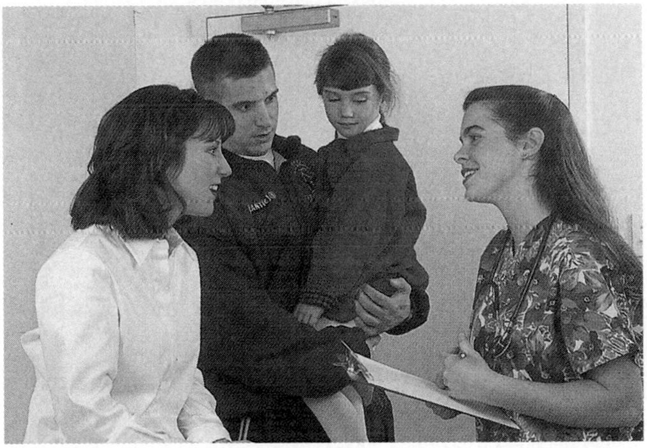

FIGURE 10.1 Include support people in a prenatal visit when appropriate or desired so that visits are family centered. Here a husband, wife, and child are included in the initial prenatal interview, making all feel a part of the pregnancy.

> **✔ CHECKPOINT QUESTIONS**
>
> 3. Why is information about past illnesses important?
> 4. What medical term is used to denote any pregnancy terminated before the age of viability?

Physical Examination

After the health history, a physical examination is performed. The woman should undress, put on a gown, and empty her bladder. Emptying the bladder will make the pelvic examination more comfortable for her, allow easier identification of pelvic organs, and provide a urine specimen for laboratory testing. This urine specimen should be

FOCUS ON FAMILY EMPOWERMENT
Suggestions for Encouraging Partner Participation in Prenatal Visits

Q. What can I do to make sure that my partner can be involved with this pregnancy?

A. Here are some suggestions for encouraging your partner's participation:

- Ask for appointments to be scheduled at a time that is convenient for both of you.
- Be certain that your partner reserves enough time so the visit doesn't become more of an inconvenience than an enjoyable event. A prenatal visit can be lengthy.
- Ask your partner to accompany you into the examining room at visits so you both can share progress or decisions.
- Be certain that the partner listens to the fetal heart at visits as soon as it can be heard.
- If a sonogram is scheduled, ask your partner to view this with you (it's an exciting moment to see your fetus moving).

obtained by a clean-catch technique so it can be examined for bacteriuria in addition to protein, glucose, and ketones. Nursing Procedure 10-1 reviews instructions for women on how to obtain a clean-catch urine sample.

A physical examination at a first prenatal visit typically includes inspection of body systems, with emphasis on the changes that occur with pregnancy or that could signal a developing problem. General techniques of physical examination are discussed in Chapter 33.

Baseline Height/Weight and Vital Sign Measurement

The woman's weight and height are obtained at a first prenatal visit to establish a baseline for future comparison. Record this assessment with her prepregnancy weight, if available, to determine how much weight she has already gained or lost (Fig. 10-2). When weighing, be certain to convey an air of "accuracy is what counts" instead of "minimal weight gain is important," so the woman feels free to gain 30 to 35 lb during pregnancy (many adolescents need to gain 40 lb).

Vital signs, including blood pressure, respiratory rate, and pulse rate, also are measured for baseline information. A sudden increase in blood pressure, like a sudden weight gain, is a danger sign of hypertension of pregnancy. A sudden increase in pulse or respirations may suggest bleeding. If close monitoring will be necessary during pregnancy, a support person or the woman herself can be taught the technique of blood pressure recording.

Assessment of Systems

General Appearance and Mental Status. Physical examination always begins with an inspection of general appearance to form an overall impression of the woman's health and well-being. General appearance is important because it reveals how people feel about themselves by the manner in which they dress, the way they speak, and the body posture they assume. Closely inspect for signs such as careless hygiene, unwashed hair, inappropriate or soiled clothing, and sad facial expression that may suggest fatigue or depression.

If the woman has any bandages and other dressings in place, be sure to remove and replace them because they could hide important findings. A growing problem, or perhaps one receiving increased recognition, is intimate partner abuse. Ask when and how any skin abnormality, such as an ecchymotic area, occurred. Most marks from battering occur on the face, the ulnar surfaces of the forearms (from a woman raising her arms to defend herself), the abdomen or buttocks (from being kicked), or the upper arms (from being grabbed and held forcefully). Noting the color of ecchymotic spots helps to date when they occurred. Such marks typically progress through purple to yellow changes.

Head and Scalp. Examine the head for symmetry, normal contour, and tenderness and the hair for presence, distribution, thickness, excessive dryness or oiliness, cleanliness, or the use of hair dye (hair dye may be carcinogenic over an extended period of time). Look for **chloasma** (extra pigment on the face), which may accompany pregnancy. Hair growth speeds up during pregnancy as a result of the overall increased metabolic rate, and women may comment they have noticed this. Dryness or sparseness of hair suggests poor nutrition. Lack of cleanliness may suggest fatigue, reflecting that the woman has not felt well enough to wash it recently. Urge women during pregnancy to let some other task go and save energy for self-care so they can continue to feel good about themselves. Dandruff shampoos may be used during pregnancy because they are not absorbed.

Eyes. Edema in the eyelids, spots before the eyes, or diplopia (double vision) may indicate pregnancy-induced hypertension (PIH). If an ophthalmoscopic examination is done, the optic disk may appear swollen from edema associated with PIH. Help pregnant women recognize symptoms of poor vision as danger signs of pregnancy that should be reported as soon as possible. If they do close desk work, caution them to take a break every hour so sensations of eyestrain are not confused with actual danger signs.

Nose. The increased level of estrogen associated with pregnancy may cause nasal congestion or the appearance of swollen nasal membranes. Even topical medicines such as nose drops or nasal sprays are absorbed to some degree. Advise a woman to avoid these during pregnancy without her physician's or nurse-midwife's knowledge and consent.

Ears. The nasal stuffiness that accompanies pregnancy may lead to blocked eustachian tubes and therefore a feeling of "fullness" or dampening of sound during early pregnancy. Usually this disappears as the body adjusts to the new estrogen level. Normal hearing level and normal tympanic landmarks should be present.

Sinuses. Sinuses should feel nontender. Establishing that tenderness over sinuses does not exist helps to evaluate a client's reports of headache during pregnancy (a danger sign until ruled otherwise).

Mouth, Teeth, and Throat. The pregnant woman is prone to vitamin deficiency because of the rapid growth of the fetus. Assess carefully for cracked corners of the mouth that would reveal vitamin A deficiency. Assess carefully for pinpoint lesions with an erythematous base on the lips; these suggest a herpes infection (a herpes lesion on the gumline is more often a shallow ulcer). Because newborns are susceptible to herpes infection, lesions present at birth may necessitate limiting the woman's contact with her newborn. Gingival (gum) hypertrophy may result from estrogen stimulation during pregnancy. The gums may be slightly swollen and tender to the touch, but not reddened.

Teach all women not to neglect good dental hygiene or yearly dental supervision visits while pregnant. They should maintain thorough toothbrushing (some stop thorough brushing because they notice slightly blood-tinged saliva due to gingival hypertrophy).

If many dental caries are obvious, the woman should be referred to a dentist or dental clinic. Carious teeth are a source of infection and should be treated before abscesses develop and cause more serious problems. Contrary to what many women believe, dental x-rays can be taken

NURSING PROCEDURE 10.1: OBTAINING A CLEAN-CATCH URINE SPECIMEN

Purpose
Helping a woman obtain a clean-catch urine specimen

Procedure	Principle
1. Ask the client to wash her hands.	1. Handwashing helps prevent the spread of microorganisms.
2. Have the client open the commercial clean-catch urine specimen kit and moisten the cotton balls with the antiseptic solution or open the prepared antiseptic wipes.	2. Preparation enhances efficiency and decreases the possibility of contamination during the procedure.

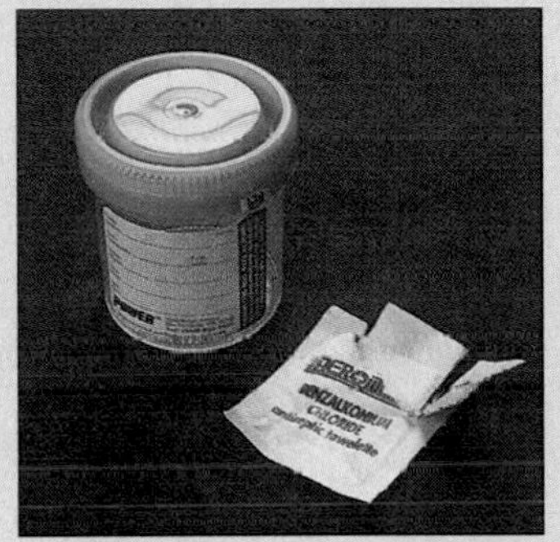

Procedure	Principle
3. a. Have the client sit on the commode and separate her labia with her nondominant hand.	3. Cleansing helps prevent microorganisms from entering the urine specimen. Cleansing from front to back prevents bringing rectal contamination forward and prevents transmission of microorganisms.

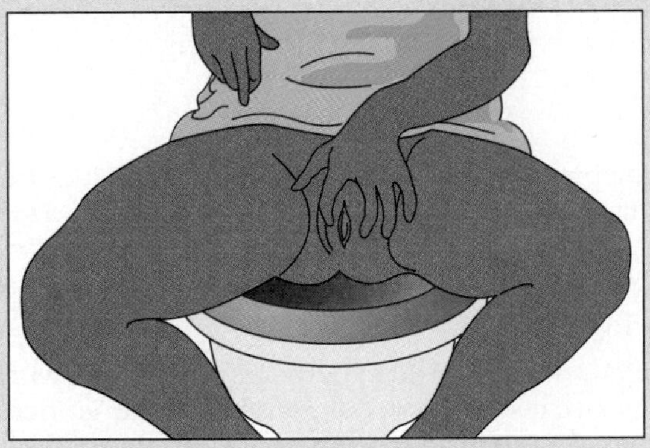

b. Tell her to cleanse her perineum, washing from front to back, using a cotton ball or wipe for only one stroke, then discarding it.

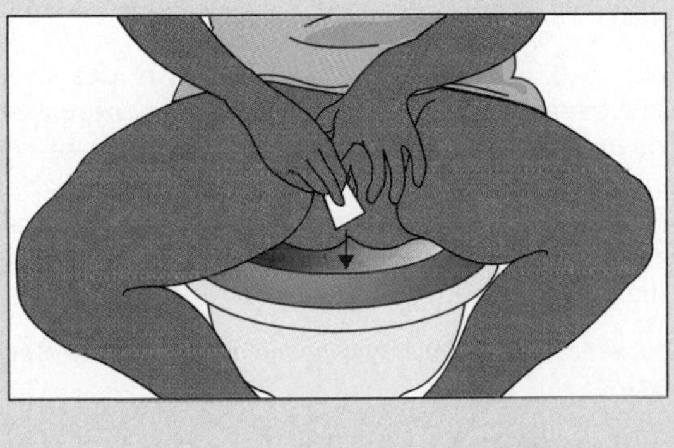

(continued)

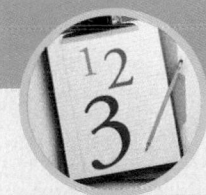

Procedure	Principle
4. Advise the client to avoid touching the inside of the container or cap.	4. Careful handling of equipment prevents contamination.
5. Ask her to begin urinating, allowing the first urine to flow into the toilet. Then tell her to hold the container under the urine stream to obtain the specimen, removing the container after approximately 10 to 20 mL has been obtained. Once obtained, advise the client to remove the container, release her hand from her labia, and finish voiding in the toilet. 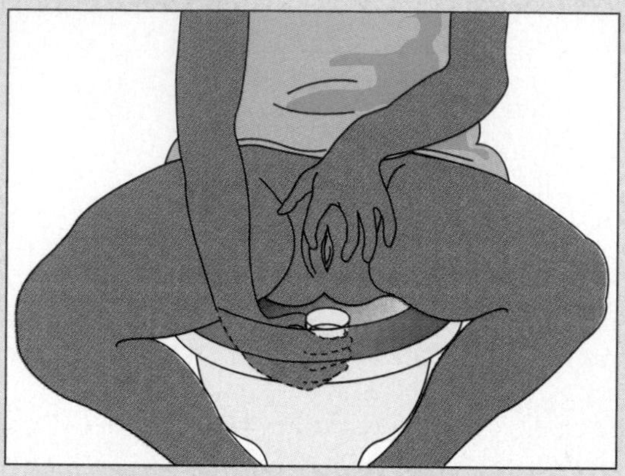	5. The first flow of urine washes microorganisms and debris from the urinary meatus. Collecting the specimen midstream ensures a sterile specimen is obtained.
6. Tell the woman to cap the specimen container, wash her hands, and bring it to you. Encourage her to report any pain on urination.	6. Capping the container prevents inadvertent spilling and possible contamination of the specimen. Pain on urination is a symptom of urinary tract infection.

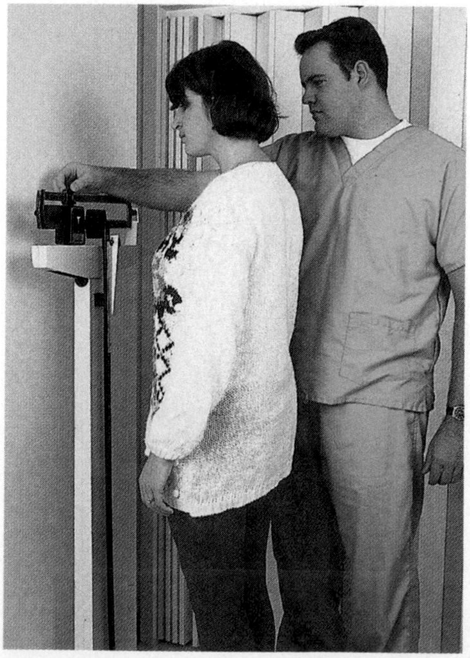

FIGURE 10.2 A woman weighs in at a prenatal visit. The pregnant woman may need reassurance that she is gaining an appropriate amount of weight.

during pregnancy as long as the woman reminds her dentist that she is pregnant and wears a lead apron. Extensive dental work requiring anesthesia should not be done during pregnancy without approval from the woman's primary care provider.

Neck. Slight thyroid hypertrophy may occur with pregnancy because the overall metabolic rate is increased. Encourage a woman to continue to use iodized salt during pregnancy and to eat seafood at least once weekly to supply enough iodine for thyroxine production with this increased rate. Without this precaution, some women will view iodine as an unnecessary additive and discontinue using it during pregnancy.

Lymph Nodes. No palpable lymph nodes should be present. Pregnant women may develop an increased number of upper respiratory infections because of reduced immunologic resistance. This could result in enlarged cervical lymph nodes. If they develop a tooth abscess from bacterial growth under hypertrophied gingival tissue, submaxillary lymph nodes may be palpable.

Breasts. As pregnancy begins, the breasts undergo the following:

- Breast areola darkens.
- Montgomery tubercles become prominent.

- Breast size increases.
- Breast tone firms.
- Secondary areola may develop surrounding the natural one.
- Blue streaking of veins becomes prominent.
- Colostrum may be expelled as early as the 16th week of pregnancy.
- Any supernumerary nipple also may become darker (assure the woman that this is a normal pregnancy change).

All women should be instructed on monthly breast self-examination. The day after the end of each monthly menstrual flow is a good marking point for the nonpregnant woman to use. This is also a time when hormonal influences on breast tissue are low, so breast tissue is normally not swollen or tender and examination is not uncomfortable. When pregnant, the woman should specify a certain day each month (the first day, the last day) for breast self-examination (see Focus on Family Empowerment in Chap. 33 for more information on breast self-examination). If she discovers a lesion on self-examination, she should report it promptly. Remind women that 90% of breast lesions are not cancer. Otherwise, they can become so afraid that they are "frozen" into immobility. Benign breast lesions that might be discovered on physical examination are discussed in Chapter 47.

Heart. Heart rate should range from 70 to 80 beats per minute. No accessory sounds or murmurs should be present. Because of the increase in breast size, it may be difficult to hear the woman's heart beat during pregnancy. Occasionally, a woman may develop an innocent (functional) heart murmur because of the increased vascular volume. If this occurs, she needs further evaluation to ensure that it is only a physiologic change of pregnancy and not a previously undetected heart condition. Many women notice occasional palpitations (heart skipping a beat) during pregnancy, especially when lying supine. Teach pregnant women always to rest or sleep on their side (left side is best) to avoid this problem (Lee, Zaffke, & McEnany, 2000).

Lungs. Assess respiratory rate and rhythm. Although lung tissue assumes a more horizontal position during pregnancy, vital capacity is not reduced. Late in pregnancy, diaphragmatic excursion (diaphragm movement) is lessened because the diaphragm cannot descend as fully as usual because of the distended uterus.

Back. Assess the spine for any abnormal curve that would suggest scoliosis. Young women with scoliosis may need a referral to their orthopedist during pregnancy to be certain that their condition is not worsening. The lumbar curve in many pregnant women is accentuated on standing so that they can maintain body posture in the face of increasing abdominal size. This response may cause considerable back pain during pregnancy.

Rectum. Assess the rectum closely for hemorrhoidal tissue, which commonly occurs from pelvic pressure preventing venous return. This can be very uncomfortable for women and worrisome if they are not assured that it is a normal discomfort of pregnancy.

Extremities and Skin. Assess the upper extremities. Many women develop palmar erythema and itching early in pregnancy from a high estrogen level and perhaps subclinical jaundice (jaundice that is not yet apparent by a color change). Assess the lower extremities carefully for varicosities, filling time of the toenails (should be under 5 seconds), and the presence of edema. Pelvic pressure interferes with venous return from the lower extremities. Any edema more than ankle swelling may be a danger sign of pregnancy.

Assess the gait of pregnant women to see that they are keeping their pelvis tucked under the weight of their abdomen. This position prevents them from developing muscle strains from abnormal abdominal muscle tension. Many pregnant women develop a "waddling" gait later in pregnancy from relaxation of the symphysis pubis. This may cause pain if the cartilage is actually so unstable that it moves on walking.

Measurement of Fundal Height and Fetal Heart Sounds

At about 12 to 14 weeks of pregnancy, the uterus is palpable over the symphysis pubis as a firm globular sphere. It reaches the umbilicus at 20 to 22 weeks and the xiphoid process at 36 weeks, and then often returns to about 4 cm below the xiphoid due to "lightening" at 40 weeks. If the woman is past 12 weeks of a pregnancy, palpate the fundus location, measure the fundal height (from the notch above the symphysis pubis to the superior aspect of the uterine fundus), and plot the height on a graph such as the one shown in Figure 10-3. Plotting uterine growth at each visit can help to detect any variations in fetal growth. If an abnormality is detected, further investigation with ultrasound can be made to determine the cause of the increase or decrease in growth.

Auscultate for fetal heart sounds (120 to 160 beats per minute). These can be heard at 10 to 12 weeks if a Doppler technique is used but not until 18 to 20 weeks if a regular stethoscope is used. Palpate for fetal outline and position after the 28th week.

> **✔ CHECKPOINT QUESTIONS**
>
> 5. What is the typical cause of nasal congestion during pregnancy?
> 6. Why might it be difficult to hear the client's heart beat during pregnancy?

Pelvic Examination

A pelvic examination reveals information on the health of both internal and external reproductive organs. It requires the following equipment: a **speculum** (a metal or plastic instrument with movable flat blades; Fig. 10-4), a spatula for cervical scraping, a clean examining glove, lubricant, a glass slide for plating the Pap smear, a culture tube, and two or three sterile cotton-tipped applicators for obtaining cervical cultures. A good examining light and a stool at correct sitting height are also necessary.

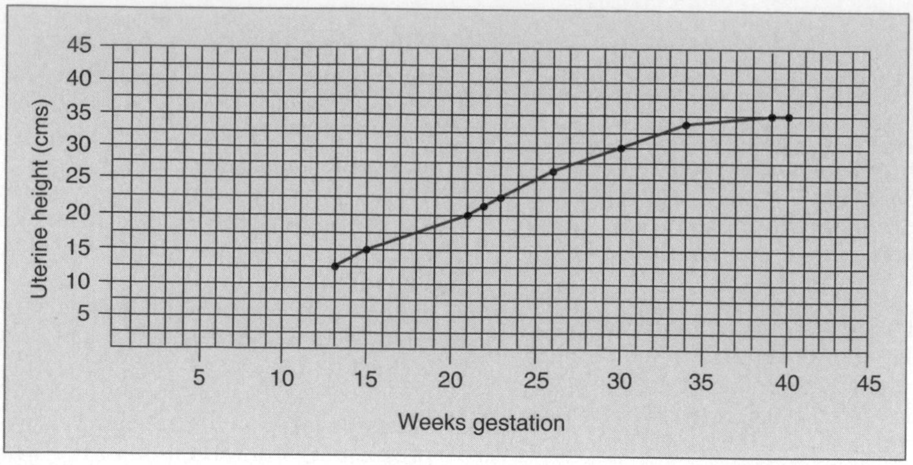

FIGURE 10.3 Plotting uterine height on such a graph at prenatal visits (typically after 12 weeks gestation) helps to monitor whether fundal height is adequate.

For a pelvic examination, the woman should void and then lie in a **lithotomy position** (on her back with her thighs flexed and her feet resting in the examining table stirrups (Fig. 10-5). Her buttocks should extend slightly beyond the end of the examining table. Her abdominal muscles will be more relaxed if she has a pillow under her head. Allow the woman the opportunity to talk with the person performing the examination while sitting up, before being placed in a lithotomy position. This may ease her discomfort and enhance her sense of self-esteem and control.

Properly drape the client with a draw sheet over the abdomen that extends over the legs. Pregnant women should remain in a lithotomy position for as short a time as possible to help prevent thromboembolism and supine hypotension.

Many women want their support person to remain with them at the head of the table during the examination. In addition, it is customary, especially on an initial visit, for a nurse or an unlicensed assistive person to be in the room with the woman for the pelvic examination to offer additional support. This is true whether the examiner is male or female (see Focus on Multidisciplinary Care).

Support is essential. If this is a first pregnancy, it may be the first time the woman has had a pelvic examination. In addition, hearing stories about how painful these examinations are may cause the woman to become tense just thinking about it. When the pelvic muscles are tight and tense, not only does the examination become painful, but also the examiner has difficulty assessing the status of the pelvic organs.

If desired, the woman may watch the pelvic examination with an overhead mirror or a mirror held by herself or the examiner. Seeing vaginal cervical pathology may help her to understand any kind of problem present and the interventions necessary to improve it. If not already doing so, women should be told how to do a monthly perineal examination (holding a mirror) just as they do a monthly breast self-examination.

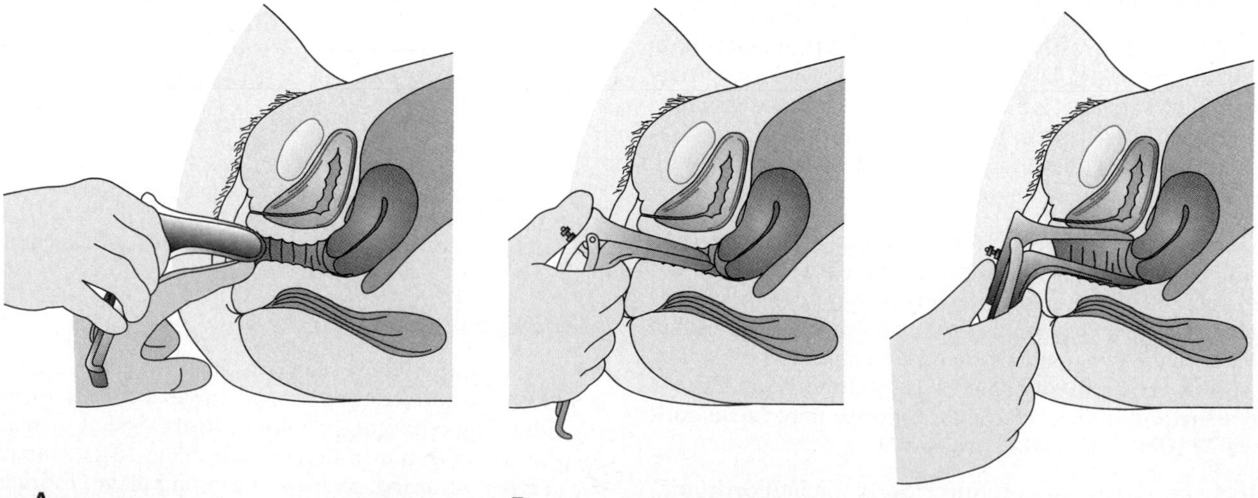

FIGURE 10.4 Insertion of a vaginal speculum. (*A*) Blades held obliquely on entering the vagina. (*B*) Blades rotated to horizontal position as they pass the introitus. (*C*) Blades separated by depressing thumbpiece and elevating handle. The position of the blades is maintained by adjusting a thumbscrew.

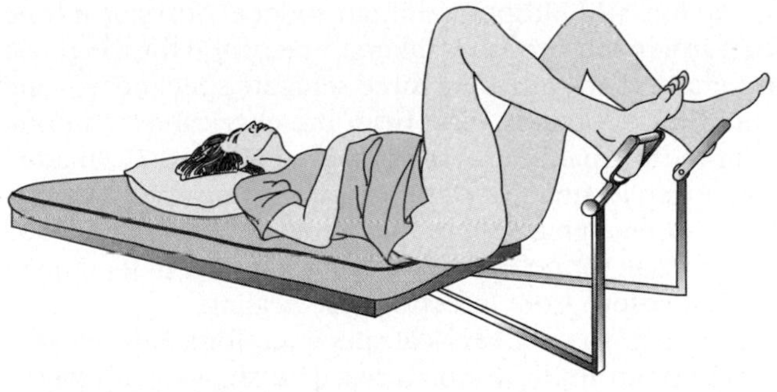

FIGURE 10.5 A lithotomy position used for a pelvic examination. Help position the woman with her buttocks just over the edge of the table for the actual examination. Drape appropriately for modesty.

WHAT IF? What if the foot of an examining table in a clinic faces the room door, leaving women to feel exposed should someone walk in unexpectedly? Is this the best position for the table? What could you do about this?

External Genitalia. A pelvic examination begins with inspection of the external genitalia. Any signs of inflammation, irritation, or infection, such as redness, ulcerations, or vaginal discharge, are noted.

A herpes simplex 2 virus infection appears as clustered, pinpoint vesicles on an erythematous (reddened) base on the vulva. These are painful when touched or irritated by underclothes. The presence of herpes lesions on the vulva or vagina at the time of birth may necessitate cesarean birth to prevent exposing the fetus to the virus during passage through the birth canal. There may be an association between cervical cancer and herpes simplex 2 infections.

FOCUS ON MULTIDISCIPLINARY CARE

Unlicensed assistive personnel may be asked to stay in the examining room with women undergoing a pelvic examination, both for comfort and support and to help them relax. Be certain they understand their role in the room is to remain at the head of the table as a support person, not to stand at the foot of the table as an observer. Being at the head of the table enables them to hold the woman's hand if she needs the support of physical contact. Explanations of what is happening or what the examiner is doing are also helpful. Meaningful conversation with the woman may be helpful, but conversation with the examiner over her head is not. Suggesting that a woman breathe in and out (not holding her breath as she is likely to do) is another technique to help her relax (holding her breath pushes the diaphragm down and makes the pelvic organs tense and unyielding).

Note in the record the presence of a herpes infection for future follow-up with cytologic (Pap) smears for cervical cancer.

The Skene glands are checked for infection. To do this, a sterile gloved finger is inserted into the vagina and pressed against the anterior vaginal wall to see if any pus can be extruded from the openings to the glands at the urethral opening. The woman is also evaluated for possible infection of the Bartholin glands. The sites of the Bartholin glands (5 and 7 o'clock positions) are palpated between the vaginal finger and the thumb of the same hand. If a discharge is produced from any of these gland ducts (Skene or Bartholin), a culture is obtained. Infection here could be caused by something as simple as streptococci. Often it is gonorrhea.

Problems with vascular muscle wall support, such as a rectocele (a forward pouching of the rectum and posterior vaginal wall due to loss of posterior vaginal muscular support) or a cystocele (an inward pouching of the bladder and anterior vaginal wall due to loss of vaginal muscular support), are also evaluated. To reveal these, while the labia are gently separated to allow a view of the vaginal walls, the woman is asked to bear down as if she were moving her bowels.

Internal Genitalia. To view the cervix, the vagina must be opened with a speculum. No lubricant other than warm water should be used over the speculum blades because even a water-soluble lubricant might interfere with the interpretation of the Pap smear that will be taken. Warm water rather than cold water should be used so the woman does not contract her vaginal muscles when she feels the cold instrument.

A speculum is introduced with the blades in a closed position and directed toward the posterior rather than the anterior vaginal wall because the posterior wall is less sensitive (see Fig. 10-4*A*). A speculum enters most readily if it is inserted at an oblique angle (the crease of the blades directed to 4 or 8 o'clock), then rotated to a horizontal position when fully inserted (the crease of the blades pointing to a 3 or 9 o'clock position) (see Fig. 10-4*B*). When fully inserted and rotated to a horizontal position, the blades are opened so the cervix is visible and are secured in the open position by tightening the thumb screw at the side (see Fig. 10-4*C*).

With the speculum in place, the cervix can be inspected for its position. Normally it is centered on the vagina; a retroverted uterus has a cervix positioned anteriorly, and an anteverted uterus has its cervix positioned posteriorly. Its color (a nonpregnant cervix is light pink; in pregnancy it changes to almost purple) and any lesions, ulcerations, discharge, or otherwise abnormal appearance are noted.

In a **nulligravida** (a woman who is not or never has been pregnant), the cervical os is round and small. In a woman who has had a previous pregnancy with a vaginal birth, the cervical os has much more of a slitlike appearance (Fig. 10-6*A*). If the woman had a cervical tear during a previous birth, the cervical os may appear as a transverse crease the width of the cervix or a typical starlike (stellate) formation. If a cervical infection is present, a mucus discharge may be present. With infection, the epithelium of

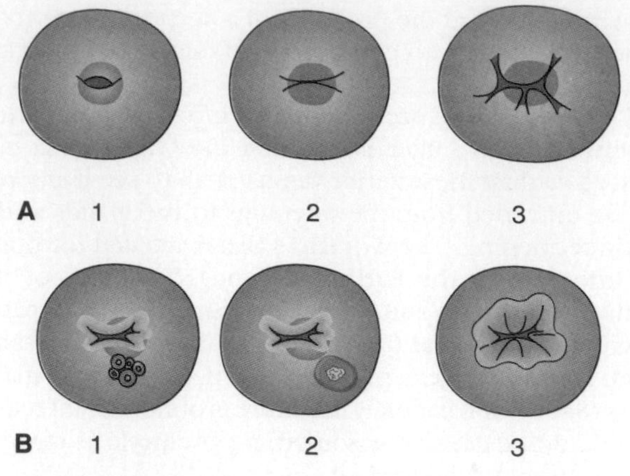

FIGURE 10.6 (*A*) Appearances of the cervix. (1) Nulligravida cervix. (2) Cervix after childbirth. (3) "Stellate" cervix seen after mild cervical tearing. (*B*) Possible cervical lesions. (1) Herpes II. (2) Chancre of syphilis. (3) Erosion or infection.

the cervical canal often enlarges and spreads onto the area surrounding the os, giving the cervix a reddened appearance (**erosion;** see Fig. 10-6*B*). This area bleeds readily if it is touched.

Trichomoniasis, a protozoal infection, generally gives signs of redness; a profuse, whitish, bubbly discharge; and petechial spots on the vaginal walls. Candidal (*Monilia*) infection typically presents with thick, white vaginal patches that may bleed if scraped away. A gonorrhea infection typically presents with a thick, greenish-yellow discharge and extreme inflammation. Chlamydia infection, in contrast, shows few symptoms.

Carcinoma of the cervix appears as an irregular, granular growth at the os. Cervical polyps (red, soft, pedunculated protrusions) also are occasionally seen at the os.

Pap Smear. Although only an endocervical smear (one from inside the cervix) is taken to be plated for a Pap test in some centers, in others three separate specimens—one from the endocervix, one from the cervical os, and one from the vaginal pool—are obtained (Fig. 10-7). In addition, a cervicogram (a photograph of the cervix) may be taken. Cervicograms serve as complements to Pap smears as a weapon for detecting cervical cancer and documenting that lesions from infections are healing.

To obtain an endocervical specimen for a Pap smear, a sterile cotton applicator or cervical brush, wet with saline, is inserted through the speculum into the os of the cervix and gently rotated, first clockwise, then counterclockwise (see Fig. 10-7*A*). It is then removed without touching the sides of the vagina. The specimen is then gently painted on a glass slide. The slide is sprayed with a fixative to preserve the cells.

To take a cervical os specimen, the uneven end of the spatula is inserted through the speculum and is pressed on the os of the cervix and rotated to scrape cells in a circle around the os (see Fig. 10-7*B*). After removal, the spatula is then smeared onto a slide and sprayed with fixative.

For the specimen from the vaginal pool, a cotton-tipped applicator or the opposite end of the spatula blade is placed at the posterior fornix just below the cervix (the vaginal pool; see Fig. 10-7*C*). The applicator or spatula is rolled gently to pick up secretions collected there. After careful removal, the specimen is placed on a third slide and sprayed with fixative.

The classification of Pap smears is constantly being revised as the meaning of abnormal cells is further defined. Two methods of classification are shown in Table 10-3. Be certain when discussing these reports with women that they do not overinterpret the classifications. Class I means only normal cells were found. Class II means that cells are inflamed because infection is present (the woman needs to be treated and reexamined in about

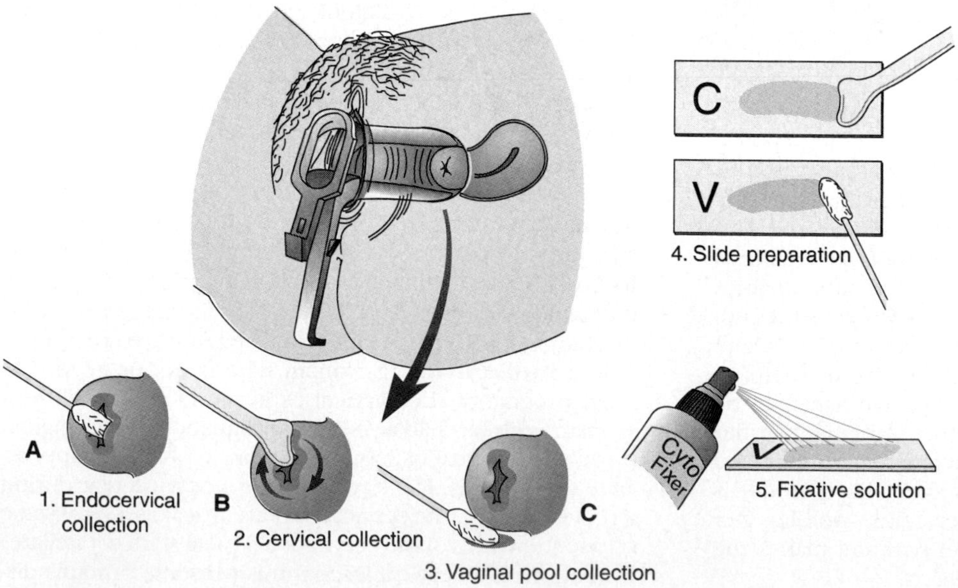

FIGURE 10.7 Obtaining a Pap smear. (*A*) Specimen taken from endocervix. (*B*) Specimen taken from cervix. (*C*) Specimen taken from vaginal pool.

TABLE 10.3 Classification of Pap Smears

ORIGINAL CLASS SYSTEM	BETHESDA SYSTEM (1988, 1991)
Class I—Normal	Normal
Class II—Slightly suspicious for malignancy	Atypical squamous cells of undetermined significance
Class III—Moderately suspicious for malignancy	Low-grade squamous intraepithelial lesion; equivalent to changes associated with human papilloma virus and CIN I
Class IV—Highly suspicious	High-grade squamous intraepithelial lesion; equivalent to CIN II or III
Class V—Diagnostic for malignancy	Invasive cancer

CIN, cervical intraepithelial neoplasia.

3 months). Cervical intraepithelial neoplasia (CIN) levels (class III) are moderately suspicious for malignancy. This level requires a colposcopy examination for further evaluation. Class IV identifies carcinoma in situ or precancerous cells that are present. Class V is indicative of squamous cell carcinoma.

Many women ask how often repeat Pap smears are necessary because the recommendations have changed and are confusing. The American Cancer Society recommends a Pap smear as infrequently as every 3 years in women who have had two consecutive negative tests a year apart. Women who should have them more frequently are those who were exposed to diethylstilbestrol (DES) in utero, who have multiple sexual partners, who have a history of human papillomavirus (HPV), who smoke cigarettes, or who were active sexually before age 21. Screening as infrequently as every 3 years could miss pathology in these women.

Vaginal Inspection. Before the speculum is removed, a culture for gonorrhea, chlamydia, or group B streptococcus may be taken. After gently swabbing the cervix using cotton-tipped applicators, the specimens obtained are then plated onto a medium to allow for their growth. All these organisms can cause disease in the newborn, so it is best if they can be eradicated during pregnancy.

A speculum must be unlocked and partially closed before removal; otherwise, pain from excessive stretching could occur. If the speculum is kept partially open as it is removed, it should not cause any pain, and the sides of the vagina can be inspected as it is withdrawn. In a nonpregnant woman, vaginal walls are light pink; pregnancy turns them dark blue to purple. Any areas of inflammation, ulceration, lesions, or discharge should be noted. A vaginal inspection is especially critical for a woman whose mother took DES during her pregnancy. Daughters of women who took DES are prone to develop adenosis, or overgrowth of cervical endothelium (which is possibly associated with vaginal cancer).

Examination of Pelvic Organs. Following the speculum examination, a bimanual (two-handed) examination is performed to assess the position, contour, consistency, and tenderness of pelvic organs (Fig. 10-8). The index and middle fingers of one gloved hand are lubricated and inserted into the vagina so the walls of the vagina can be palpated for abnormalities. The other hand is then placed on the woman's abdomen and pressed downward toward the hand still in the vagina until the uterus can be felt between them. If a uterus is extremely retroverted, it may not be palpable abdominally. Next, the right and left ovaries are identified by the same method. Ovaries are normally slightly tender, so the pressure caused by palpation may cause the woman some discomfort.

Abnormalities that can be noted by bimanual examination include ovarian cysts, enlarged fallopian tubes (perhaps from pelvic inflammatory disease), and an enlarged uterus (see Table 10-1). An early sign of pregnancy (Hegar's sign) is elicited on bimanual examination (see Fig. 9-5).

Rectovaginal Examination. After a bimanual pelvic examination, the hand is withdrawn from the vagina. The index finger is reinserted into the vagina and the middle finger into the rectum. By palpating the tissue between the examining fingers in this way, it is possible to assess the strength and irregularity of the posterior vaginal wall. This maneuver may be slightly uncomfortable for the woman because of the rectal pressure involved. Some examiners use a clean pair of gloves before they perform

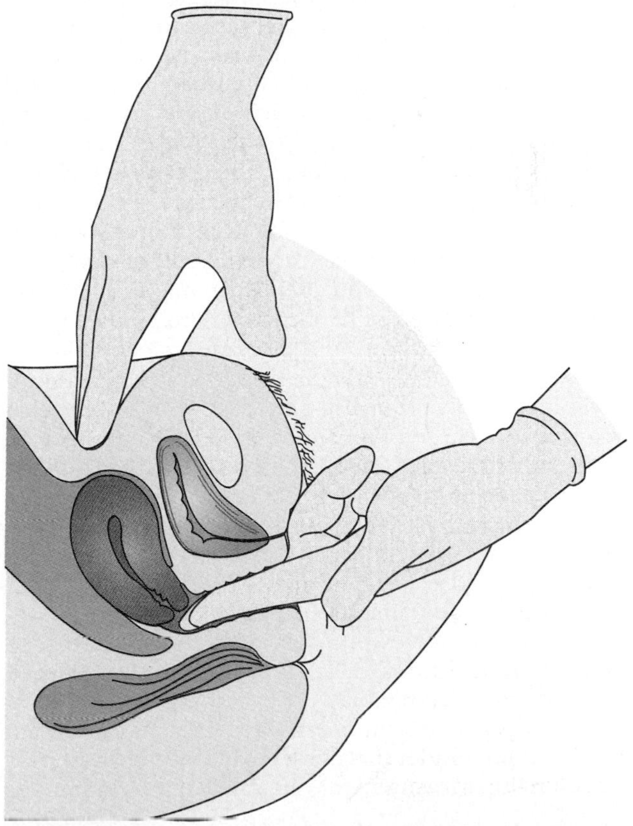

FIGURE 10.8 A bimanual examination to determine uterine size.

a vaginal-rectal examination so they will not spread an infection from the vagina to the rectum. After the rectal examination, if it is necessary to reexamine the vagina for any reason, the glove must be changed to avoid contaminating the vagina with fecal material.

After completing the examination, any excess lubricant is wiped away from the vaginal and rectal openings. It is important to wipe front to back to prevent bringing rectal contamination forward to the vaginal introitus.

✔ CHECKPOINT QUESTIONS

7. What two glands are evaluated during an examination of the external genitalia?
8. How does the nulligravida client's cervical os typically appear?
9. What three specimens typically are obtained for a Pap smear?

Estimating Pelvic Size

It is impossible to predict from the outward appearance of a woman whether her pelvis is adequate for the fetus to pass through its center. Some women look as if they have a wide pelvis but, in reality, have only wide iliac crests and a normal or even smaller-than-normal internal ring. Other women appear as if their pelvis will be small because the iliac crests are nonflaring, but the internal pelvis, the part that must be sufficiently large for childbirth, is of average size, allowing them to give birth vaginally without difficulty. Differences in pelvic contour and development occur mainly because of hereditary factors, but disease (e.g., rickets, now rarely seen in the United States, which may cause contraction of the pelvis) or injury (inadequate repair following an accident) also may play a role.

If on this initial visit the primary care provider establishes that the woman is pregnant, and if she has never given birth vaginally before, pelvic measurements may be taken. Some care providers prefer to take these measurements later in pregnancy, when the woman's pelvic muscles are more relaxed, making measurement easier. If a routine sonogram is scheduled, estimations may be made by a combination of pelvic pelvimetry and fetal sonography. Estimation of pelvic adequacy must be done at least by the 24th week of pregnancy, because by this time there is danger that the fetal head will reach a size that will interfere with safe passage and birth if the pelvic measurements are small.

Once a woman has given birth vaginally, her pelvis has been proved adequate. Thus, it is not necessary to take her pelvic measurements again unless she has had an intervening history of trauma to the pelvis.

The types of pelves found in women can be categorized into four groups (Fig. 10-9): android, anthropoid, gynecoid, and platypelloid.

Internal pelvic measurements give the actual diameters of the inlet and outlet through which the fetus must pass. The following measurements are made most commonly:

1. The **diagonal conjugate.** This is the distance between the anterior surface of the sacral prominence and the anterior surface of the inferior margin of the symphysis pubis (Fig. 10-10). The most useful measurement for estimation of pelvic size, it suggests the anteroposterior diameter of the pelvic inlet (the narrower diameter at that level, or the one that is most apt to cause a misfit with the fetal head). The diagonal conjugate is measured while the woman is in a lithotomy position. To measure it, two fingers are introduced vaginally and pressed inward and upward until the middle finger touches the sacral prominence. With the other hand, the part of the examining hand where it touches the symphysis pubis is marked (see Fig. 10-10*A*). After withdrawing the examining hand, the distance between the tip of the middle finger and the marked point on the glove on that hand is measured by comparing it with a ruler or, for greater accuracy, a pelvimeter. Warn the client that the measurement may be slightly painful. The woman may feel the pressure of the examining finger as it stretches to touch the sacral prominence. If the examiner's hand is small with short fingers, manual pelvic measurements may not be possible, because the fingers may not reach the sacral prominence. If the measurement obtained is more than 12.5 cm, the pelvic inlet is rated as adequate for childbirth (the diameter of the fetal head that must pass that point averages 9 cm in diameter).
2. The **true conjugate** or **conjugate vera** is the measurement between the anterior surface of the sacral prominence and the posterior surface of the inferior margin of the symphysis pubis. This measurement cannot be made directly, but it can be estimated from the measurement made of the diagonal conjugate. To do this, the usual depth of the symphysis pubis (assumed to be 1.2 to 2 cm) is subtracted from the diagonal conjugate measurement. The distance remaining will be the true conjugate, or the actual diameter of the pelvic inlet through which the fetal head must pass. The average true conjugate diameter is, therefore, 12.5 cm minus 1.5 or 2 cm, or 10.5 to 11 cm.
3. The **ischial tuberosity** diameter. This measurement is the distance between the ischial tuberosities, or the transverse diameter of the outlet (the narrowest diameter at that level, or the one most apt to cause a misfit). It is made at the medial and lowermost aspect of the ischial tuberosities at the level of the anus (see Fig. 10-10*B*). A pelvimeter is generally used, although the diameter can be measured by a ruler or by comparing it with a known hand span or clenched fist measurement. A diameter of 11 cm is considered adequate because it will allow the widest diameter of the fetal head, or 9 cm, to pass freely through the outlet.

Laboratory Assessment

A number of laboratory studies are included in assessment measures at a first prenatal visit to confirm general health and rule out sexually transmitted diseases that could injure the growing fetus. Normal levels for these studies are shown in Appendix F.

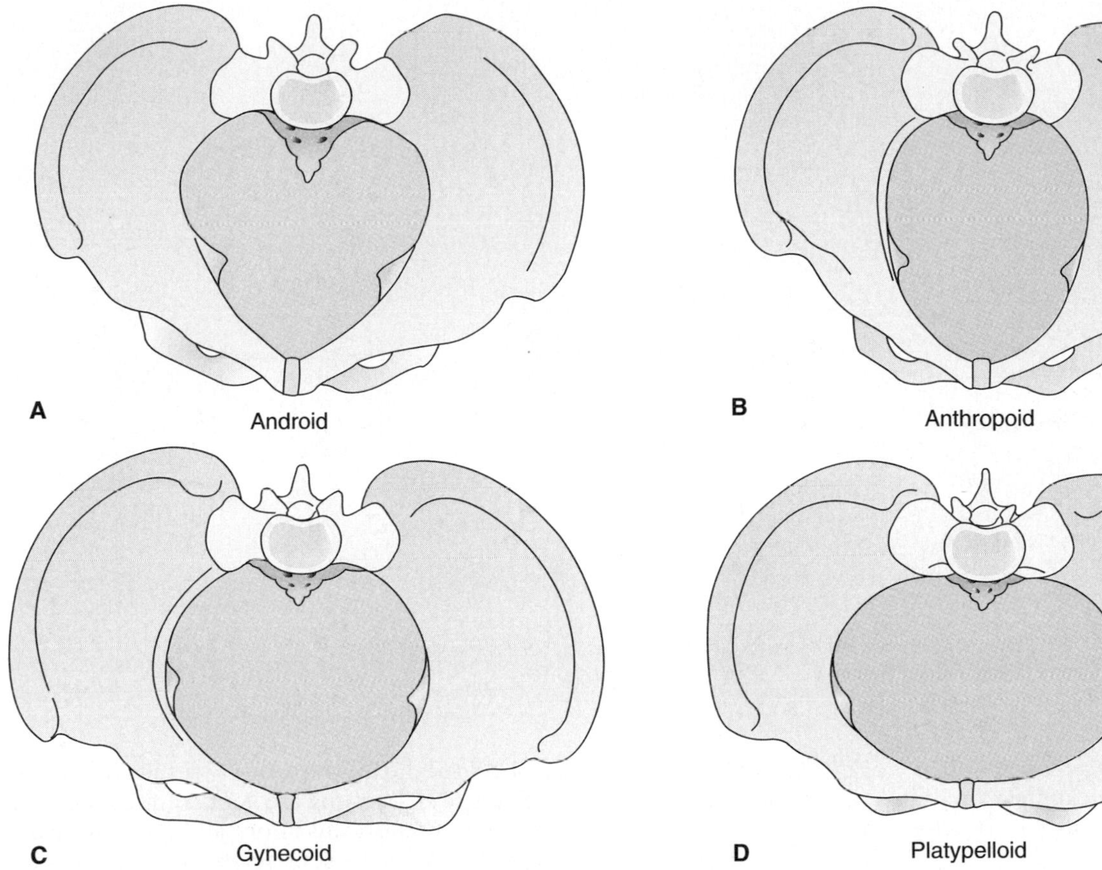

FIGURE 10.9 Types of pelves. (A) *Android* pelvis—"male" pelvis. The pubic arch in this pelvis type forms an acute angle, making the lower dimensions of the pelvis extremely narrow. A fetus may have difficulty exiting from this type of pelvis. (B) *Anthropoid* pelvis—"ape-like" pelvis. The transverse diameter is narrow, and the anteroposterior diameter of the inlet is larger than normal. This does not accommodate a fetal head as well as a gynecoid pelvis. (C) *Gynecoid* pelvis—"normal" female pelvis. The inlet is well rounded forward and backward; the pubic arch is wide. This pelvic type is ideal for childbirth. (D) *Platypelloid* pelvis—"flattened" pelvis. The inlet is an oval, smoothly curved, but the anteroposterior diameter is shallow. A fetal head might not be able to rotate to match the curves of the pelvic cavity in this type of pelvis.

Blood Studies

The following blood studies are usually done at the first prenatal visit:

1. A complete blood count, including hemoglobin or hematocrit and red cell index to determine the presence of anemia, a white blood cell count to determine infection, and a platelet count to estimate clotting ability. African-American women also may have a blood sample taken to test for sickle cell trait or disease and possibly glucose-6-phosphate dehydrogenase if they have not had this done before.
2. A serologic test for syphilis (VDRL or rapid plasma reagin test). Syphilis must be treated early in pregnancy before fetal damage occurs. A blood sample for a serologic test for gonorrhea may be drawn on women suspected of having the disease.
3. Blood typing (including Rh factor). Blood may have to be made available if the woman has bleeding early in her pregnancy.
4. Maternal serum for AFP. The level will be elevated if a neural tube or abdominal defect is present in the fetus; it may be decreased if a chromosomal anomaly is present in the fetus. This test is done at 16 to 18 weeks of pregnancy. The level in serum is expressed as "multiples of the mean" (MOM). A normal value is 2.5 MOM. If this is elevated, a sonogram will be ordered to assess for a fetal disorder.
5. An indirect Coombs' test (determination if Rh antibodies are present). This test is generally repeated at 28 weeks of pregnancy. If the titers are not elevated, an Rh-negative woman will receive RhIG (RhoGAM) at 28 weeks of pregnancy and after any procedure that might cause placental bleeding, such as amniocentesis or external version.
6. Antibody titers for rubella and hepatitis B (HBsAg). These tests determine whether the woman is protected against rubella if exposure should occur during pregnancy and whether a newborn will have the chance of developing hepatitis B. HBsAg

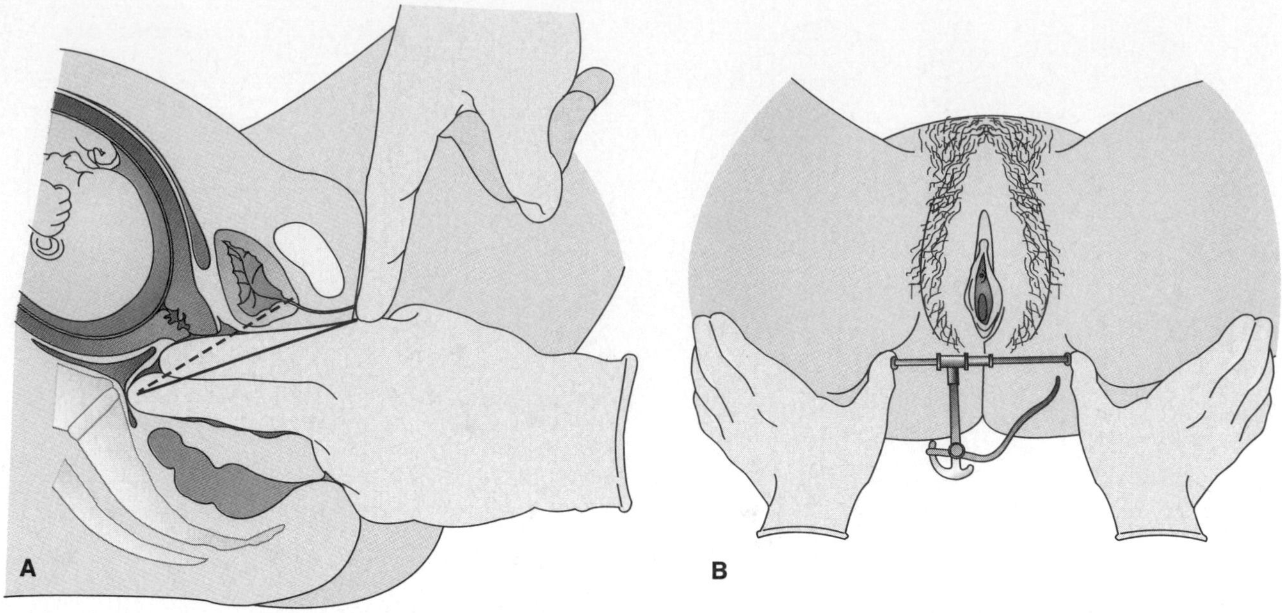

FIGURE 10.10 (A) Measurement of diagonal conjugate diameter. *Solid line* = diagonal conjugate; *dotted line* = true conjugate. (B) Measurement of ischial tuberosity diameter.

may be repeated at about 36 weeks. Antibodies for varicella (chickenpox) may also be assessed. Vaccine against this, like rubella, can be offered in the postpartal period.

7. HIV screening. All woman can be asked, and those at high risk for contracting HIV/AIDS should be asked, whether they want to be screened for this disease early in pregnancy. High-risk criteria include women who have used or are using intravenous drugs; have engaged in sex with multiple partners; have had sexual partners who are infected or are at risk because they are bisexual, intravenous drug abusers, or hemophiliacs; or received a blood transfusion between 1977 and 1985 (Minkoff, 2000).

   Screening is done by an enzyme-linked immunosorbent assay (ELISA) on a blood sample. If this is positive, the finding is confirmed by a second test (a Western blot). Testing for HIV early in pregnancy allows a woman found to be antibody positive the opportunity to begin therapy with zidovudine (AZT), which may decrease the risk of the infant developing the disease. It also allows the option of choosing to terminate a pregnancy to avoid giving birth to an infant who has a high risk of developing the disease.

   Because HIV is a fatal disease, some women may choose not to have a blood titer taken because they would rather not know that they have the illness. This is their option. Screening cannot be mandatory in prenatal settings. Health care providers need to be certain that test results given to clients are accurate (a high blood antibody titer means the person has been exposed to the disease, not that he or she necessarily has the disease) and are presented with tact and compassion with respect for the meaning of the results to the client. Results of HIV testing are kept confidential; be certain not to report this information to anyone other than the client. A client needs support when being told about an HIV-positive report because there is no cure as yet for the infection.

8. If the woman has a history of previously unexplained fetal loss, has a family history of diabetes, has had babies who were large for gestational age (9 lb or more at term), is obese, or has glycosuria, she will need to be scheduled for a 50-g oral 1-hour glucose loading or tolerance test toward the end of the first trimester to rule out gestational diabetes. If not, she will have this done routinely at the 24th to 28th week to evaluate insulin-antagonistic effects of placental hormones, which can register a noticeable effect at this time. The plasma glucose should not be above 140 mg/dL at 1 hour (see Chap. 14 for a discussion of diabetes in pregnancy).

Urinalysis

As mentioned, a urinalysis is performed to test for albuminuria, glycosuria, and pyuria. All three of these can be done by means of test strips and microscopic examination of the urine.

Tuberculosis Screening

The incidence of tuberculosis is on the rise, an increase related to the HIV epidemic. More people with lowered immune system resistance (i.e., those with HIV infection) are contracting tuberculosis and then spreading it to others in the population. In light of this, the physician or nurse-midwife may order a purified protein derivative

(PPD) tuberculin test to screen for tuberculosis. Any woman who has a positive reaction would then require a chest x-ray for further diagnosis.

If the woman has a history of tuberculosis, a tuberculin skin test should not be given because the reaction would be extreme. To assess her current disease status, a chest x-ray may be ordered. A woman is often reluctant to have this done because she knows radiation is harmful to a growing fetus. She needs to be assured that she will be given a lead apron to cover her abdomen to protect the fetus, exposing only her chest to radiation.

Screening for tuberculosis early in pregnancy is important because it is a chronic and debilitating disease that increases the risk of miscarriage. Further, the change in the shape of the lung tissue as the growing uterus presses on the lung may reactivate old lesions.

Ultrasonography

If the date of the last menstrual period is unknown, the woman will be scheduled for a sonogram to confirm the pregnancy length or document healthy fetal growth.

Risk Assessment

Table 10-4 summarizes necessary data assessment for a first prenatal visit. After this assessment, findings are analyzed to determine whether this pregnancy is apt to continue with a good outcome or there is some risk that it will end before term or with an unfavorable fetal or maternal outcome (a high-risk pregnancy).

Many factors enter into the categorization of high risk. Most health care agencies use some tool to determine high risk, but no tool is perfect because the concept of high risk is a very individualized one. Table 10-5 lists factors that would identify a pregnancy as being at high risk. The woman identified this way needs close observation during pregnancy to see that the pregnancy is progressing well; the infant born of a woman identified this way needs close observation in the neonatal period until it is confirmed that no anomalies exist.

The failure to identify risk potential in pregnancy leads to increased perinatal mortality. Risk assessment should be updated at each pregnancy visit. See Chapters 14 through 17 for a more detailed discussion of high-risk pregnancy and its management.

✔ CHECKPOINT QUESTIONS

10. What type of pelvis is considered best for vaginal birth?
11. Which measurement of pelvic diameter, if too small, is most apt to cause a problem with the fit of the fetal head?
12. An ischial tuberosity measurement of what size is considered adequate?

KEY POINTS

Prenatal care has the potential to reduce congenital anomalies and the infant mortality rate. Its purposes

TABLE 10.4 Assessments for a First Pregnancy Visit

Health History	
Demographic data	Name, address, age, telephone number, health insurance
Chief concern	Was pregnancy planned? When was last menstrual period? Any exposure to infectious diseases or ingestion of drugs since she thinks she has been pregnant?
Family and social profile	What is family composition? Who is her chief support person? What is her occupation? Source of income? Level of exercise? Hobbies? Recreational drug use? Living conditions? Nutrition? Sleep pattern?
Past medical history	Any abdominal surgery, kidney, heart, hypertension, sexually transmitted diseases, diabetes, allergies?
Gynecologic history	When was menarche? What is length and duration of menstrual cycle?
Obstetric history	Any previous pregnancies? When? Type and outcome of birth? Any history of previous miscarriages?
Review of systems	Brief review of all body systems
Physical Examination	
Baseline data	Height, weight, vital signs, fundal height measurements (after 12 weeks), fetal heart sounds
System assessment	Full physical examination to confirm general health
Pelvic examination	General assessment, Pap smear, cultures for chlamydia, gonorrhea, group B streptococcus, pelvic measurements
Laboratory Assessment	
Blood assessment	Complete blood count, serologic test for syphilis, blood type and Rh, alpha-fetoprotein, antibody titer against Rh, hepatitis B, HIV, rubella and possibly varicella
Urinalysis	Clean catch for glucose, protein, ketones and culture
Tuberculosis	PPD
Ultrasound	To date pregnancy or confirm fetal health (if date of last menstrual period is unknown)

TABLE 10.5 Assessments That Might Categorize a Pregnancy as At Risk

Obstetric History	History of infertility or grand multiparity Premature cervical dilatation Uterine or cervical anomaly Previous preterm labor or preterm birth or cesarean birth Previous macrosomic infant Two or more spontaneous or elective abortions Previous hydatidiform mole/choriocarcinoma Previous ectopic pregnancy or stillborn/neonatal death Previous multiple gestation Previous prolonged labor Previous low-birthweight infant Previous midforceps delivery DES exposure in utero Last pregnancy under 1 year Previous infant with neurologic deficit, birth injury, or congenital anomaly
Medical History	Cardiac or pulmonary disease, chronic hypertension Metabolic disease Renal disease, recent urinary tract infection, or bacteriuria Gastrointestinal disorders Seizure disorders Family history of severe inherited disorders Surgery during pregnancy Emotional disorders or cognitive challenge Previous surgeries, particularly involving reproductive organs Endocrine disorders Hemoglobinopathies Sexually transmitted diseases Reproductive tract anomalies, history of abnormal Pap smear, malignancy
Current Obstetric Status	Inadequate prenatal care Intrauterine growth-restricted fetus Large-for-gestational-age fetus Pregnancy-induced hypertension or preeclampsia Abnormal fetal surveillance tests Polyhydramnios Placenta previa Abnormal presentation Maternal anemia Weight gain under 10 lb or weight loss over 5 lb Over/underweight Fetal or placental malformation Rh sensitization Preterm labor Multiple gestation Premature rupture of membranes Abruptio placentae Postdate pregnancy Fibroid tumors Fetal manipulation Cervical cerclage Sexually transmitted disease Maternal infection Poor immunization status
Psychosocial Factors	Inadequate finances Social problems Adolescent Poor nutrition More than two children at home; no help Lack of acceptance of pregnancy Attempt or ideation of suicide Inadequate or poor housing Father of baby uninvolved Minority status

(continued)

TABLE 10.5 Assessments That Might Categorize a Pregnancy as At Risk *(Continued)*

	Dangerous occupation Inadequate support systems Dysfunctional grieving Psychiatric history
Demographic Factors	Maternal age under 16 or over 35 Education under 11 years
Lifestyle	Cigarette smoking greater than 10 cigarettes a day Substance abuse Long amounts of time spent commuting Nonuse of seatbelts Alcohol intake Heavy lifting or long periods of standing Unusual stress No in-home smoke detectors

include the following: establishing a baseline of present health, determining the gestational age of the fetus, monitoring fetal development, identifying the woman at risk for complications, minimizing the risk of possible complications by anticipating and preventing problems before they occur, and providing time for education about pregnancy and possible dangers.

A first prenatal visit not only confirms a pregnancy but also provides a time to assess the client's needs and to educate her about pregnancy. Assessments consist of a health history, physical examination, and laboratory tests. The physical examination could include measurement of fundal height and assessment of fetal heart sounds if the pregnancy is beyond 12 weeks, a pelvic examination (including a Pap test), and possibly an estimation of pelvic size.

A first prenatal visit sets the tone for visits to follow. Maintaining a supportive manner is helpful in establishing rapport and allowing the woman to feel comfortable to return for future care. Remember that a family, not a woman alone, is having a baby, and include family members in procedures and health teaching as desired.

Pregnant women should remain in a lithotomy position for as short a time as possible to help prevent thromboembolism and supine hypotension syndrome.

Common pelvic types include gynecoid (well rounded with wide pubic arch), anthropoid (narrow), platypelloid (flattened), and android (male or with a sharp pubic arch). A gynecoid pelvis is ideal for childbearing.

The true conjugate (conjugate vera) is the measurement between the anterior surface of the sacral prominence and the posterior surface of the inferior margin of the symphysis pubis (the anterior-posterior diameter of the pelvic inlet). The average is 10.5 to 11 cm. The ischial tuberosity diameter is the distance between the ischial tuberosities or the transverse diameter of the outlet. The average is 11 cm.

CRITICAL THINKING EXERCISES

1. Ms. Czerinski, whom you met at the beginning of the chapter, was worried about having a pelvic examination. How could you help relieve her concern?
2. Asking enough questions during a health history is important to be able to estimate health risks. Consider this situation: a client works as an elementary school teacher, teaching students in the third grade. Are there any special risks you can think of associated with this situation? Is there a greater opportunity than normal for her to develop upper respiratory infections, for example? Is this a job that probably keeps her on her feet for long periods? Is she apt to be exposed to toxic substances at work?
3. A woman you are caring for has no one with her at a prenatal visit. Another has a supportive husband. Would your role be different in these two situations?
4. Examine the national health goals related to prenatal care. Most government-sponsored money for nursing research is allotted based on these goals. What would be a possible research topic to explore pertinent to these goals that would be fundable and would advance evidence-based practice?

REFERENCES

ACOG Committee on Obstetric Practice. (2002). Exercise during pregnancy and the postpartum period. *Obstetrics & Gynecology, 99*(1), 171–173.

Autti-Ramo, I. (2000). Twelve-year follow-up of children exposed to alcohol in utero. *Developmental Medicine & Child Neurology, 42*(6), 406–411.

Covington, D. L., Justason, B. J. & Wright, N. (2001). Severity, manifestations, and consequences of violence among pregnant adolescents. *Journal of Adolescent Health, 28*(1), 55–61.

Cunningham, F. G. et al. (2001). *Williams obstetrics* (21st ed.). Stamford, CT: Appleton and Lange.

Department of Health and Human Services. (2000). *Healthy people 2010.* Washington, DC: DHHS.
de Weerd, S. et al. (2002). Preconception counseling improves folate status of women planning pregnancy. *Obstetrics & Gynecology, 99*(1), 45–50.
Johnson, M., Maas, M., & Moorhead, S. (2000). *Nursing outcomes classification* (2nd ed.). St. Louis: Mosby.
Klerman, L. V., & Rooks, J. P. (1999). A simple, effective method that midwives can use to help pregnant women stop smoking. *Journal of Nurse-Midwifery, 4*(2), 118–123.
Lee, K. A., Zaffke, M. E., & McEnany, G. (2000). Parity and sleep patterns during and after pregnancy. *Obstetrics & Gynecology, 95*(1), 14–18.
Little, L., & Lowkes, E. (2000). Critical issues in the care of pregnant women with eating disorders and the impact on their children. *Journal of Midwifery & Women's Health, 45*(4), 301–307.
McCloskey, J., & Bulechek, G. (2000). *Nursing interventions classification* (3rd ed.). St. Louis: Mosby.
McDermott, S. et al. (2000). Urinary tract infections during pregnancy and mental retardation and developmental delay. *Obstetrics & Gynecology, 96*(1), 113–119.
Minkoff, H. L. (2000). Human immunodeficiency virus and other perinatal infections. In Scott, J. R., et al. *Danforth's obstetrics and gynecology* (8th ed., pp. 393–406). Philadelphia: Lippincott Williams & Wilkins.
Reifsnider, E., & Gill, S. L. (2000). Nutrition for the childbearing years. *Journal of Obstetric, Gynecologic & Neonatal Nursing, 29*(1), 43–55.
Valanis, B., et al. (2001). Maternal smoking cessation and relapse prevention during health care visits. *American Journal of Preventive Medicine, 20*(1), 1–8.

SUGGESTED READINGS

Ances, B. M. (2002). New concerns about thalidomide. *Obstetrics & Gynecology, 99*(1), 125–128.
Bungum, T. J., Peaslee, D. L., Jackson, A. W., & Perez, M. A. (2000). Exercise during pregnancy and type of delivery in nulliparae. *Journal of Obstetric, Gynecologic & Neonatal Nursing, 29*(3), 258–264.
Carter, A. S., Baker, C. W., & Brownell, K. D. (2000). Body mass index, eating attitudes, and symptoms of depression and anxiety in pregnancy and the postpartum period. *Psychosomatic Medicine, 62*(2), 264–270.
Chez, R. A. (2000). Nutrition in pregnancy. *Journal of Obstetric, Gynecologic & Neonatal Nursing, 29*(3), 226.
Delzell, J. E. Jr., & Lefevre, M. L. (2000). Urinary tract infections during pregnancy. *American Family Physician, 61*(3), 713–721.
Devine, C. M., Bove, C. F., & Olson, C. M. (2000). Continuity and change in women's weight orientations and lifestyle practices through pregnancy and the postpartum period: The influence of life course trajectories and transitional events. *Social Science & Medicine, 50*(4), 567–582.
Ershoff, D. H., et al. (1999). The Kaiser Permanente prenatal smoking-cessation trial: When more isn't better, what is enough? *American Journal of Preventive Medicine, 17*(3), 161–168.
Foti, T., Davids, J. R., & Bagley, A. (2000). A biomechanical analysis of gait during pregnancy. *Journal of Bone & Joint Surgery, 82*(5), 625–632.
Schieve, L. A., et al. (2000). Prepregnancy body mass index and pregnancy weight gain: Associations with preterm delivery. *Obstetrics & Gynecology, 96*(2), 194–200.
Soltani, H., & Fraser, R. B. (2000). A longitudinal study of maternal anthropometric changes in normal weight, overweight, and obese women during pregnancy and postpartum. *British Journal of Nutrition, 84*(1), 95–101.
Walker, L. O., Cooney, A. T., & Riggs, M. W. (1999). Psychosocial and demographic factors related to health behaviors in the first trimester. *Journal of Obstetric, Gynecologic & Neonatal Nursing, 28*(6), 606–614.

Promoting Fetal and Maternal Health

CHAPTER 11

Key Terms

- Braxton Hicks contractions
- cytomegalovirus
- fetal alcohol syndrome
- leukorrhea
- Sims' position
- teratogen
- teratogenicity
- toxoplasmosis

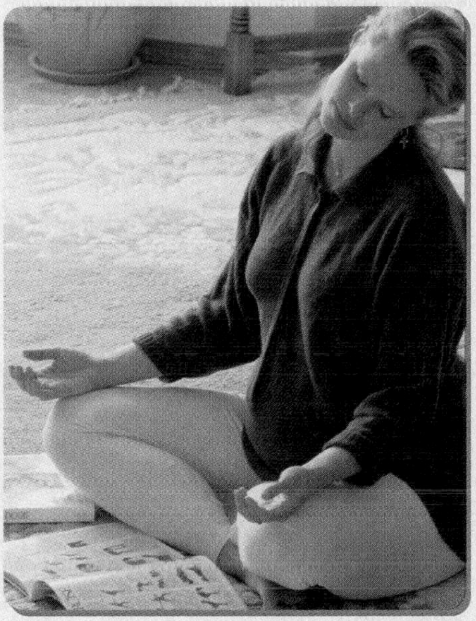

Objectives

After mastering the contents of this chapter, you should be able to:

1. Describe health practices important for a positive pregnancy outcome.
2. Assess a woman's health practices and concerns during pregnancy.
3. Formulate nursing diagnoses to promote a healthy pregnancy.
4. Identify expected outcomes to promote a healthy pregnancy.
5. Plan health-promotion strategies to limit exposure to teratogens or reduce the minor discomforts of pregnancy.
6. Implement care to promote positive health practices during pregnancy.
7. Evaluate outcomes for achievement and effectiveness of health promotion.
8. Identify National Health Goals related to pregnancy care that nurses can help the nation to achieve.
9. Identify areas of prenatal care that could benefit from additional nursing research or the application of evidence-based practice.
10. Use critical thinking to analyze ways to promote individualized and family-centered prenatal care.
11. Integrate knowledge of health-promotion strategies with the nursing process to achieve quality maternal and child health nursing care.

Julberry Adams, a single woman, is 4 months' pregnant when you see her in a prenatal clinic. She works as a curator for an art gallery. She is worried that she will not be able to work past 6 months of her pregnancy because her job involves a great deal of walking. She has already stopped volunteer work teaching children's swimming at the YMCA. She wonders how she will be able to afford her apartment if she has to quit work. She wants to travel to see her sister in St. Louis because her sister is very ill but has heard that pregnant women shouldn't drive over 100 miles. What additional health teaching does Ms. Adams need?

Previous chapters discussed normal anatomy and physiology and the changes of pregnancy. This chapter adds information about the health teaching that women need during pregnancy to ensure a healthy outcome for themselves and their child. This is important information because it can help protect the health of both women and newborns.

After you've studied the chapter, answer the Critical Thinking Exercises at the end of the chapter and then access the on-line study activities (http://connection.lww.com) *to further sharpen your skills and test your knowledge.*

FOCUS ON NATIONAL HEALTH GOALS

A number of National Health goals speak to the importance of prenatal care. These are:

- Increase to 94% the proportion of pregnant women who abstain from alcohol, cigarettes, and illicit drugs.
- Increase the proportion of pregnant females screened for sexually transmitted diseases during prenatal health care visits.
- Increase to at least 90% the proportion of all pregnant women who receive early and adequate prenatal care from a baseline of 74% (DHHS, 2000).

Because nurses are important members of prenatal health care teams, they play a significant role in seeing that services include preconceptual care and that women are aware that early pregnancy care is important. Evidence-based practice and nursing research to answer such questions as what aspects of preconceptual care are most important in reducing pregnancy complications, and what are effective incentives to make women come early for prenatal care, are important to help the nation meet these goals.

The health of the fetus and mother are inextricably linked. Generally, a woman who eats well and takes care of her own health provides a healthy environment for fetal growth and development. However, she may need instructions on exactly what constitutes a healthy lifestyle for herself and her baby. Most likely, she will have questions regarding how much extra rest she needs, what type of exercise she can continue, and whether all the changes going on in her body, some of which bring her daily discomfort, are normal. Therefore, a major role in promoting maternal and fetal health is education. Providing empathetic advice about ways to alleviate the minor discomforts of pregnancy, alerting the woman to the danger signs of pregnancy, and keeping abreast of the latest scientific studies done on maternal exposure to teratogens are all part of this role. National Health Goals have been established to increase the number of women receiving prenatal care (see Focus on National Health Goals).

NURSING PROCESS OVERVIEW

For Health Promotion of the Fetus and Mother

Assessment

A thorough health history, physical evaluation, and initial laboratory data are obtained at a first prenatal visit. Continuing assessment concentrates on screening for any abnormalities in physical or emotional health that might be occurring and for the presence of teratogens in the pregnant woman's environment. Encourage the pregnant woman to discuss whatever concerns she has during the visits. Although some of these concerns may represent minor common discomforts associated with normal pregnancy, others may be early indicators of potential problems (see Assessing the Client for Discomforts of Pregnancy). You need to know what is going on as soon as possible—first, so you can provide information and guidance on ways to alleviate the discomforts of pregnancy and, second, so you can alert the woman's physician or nurse-midwife of your findings early in the pregnancy. Early detection and continued monitoring of conditions such as pregnancy-induced hypertension (PIH) and diabetes reduce the risks of their danger.

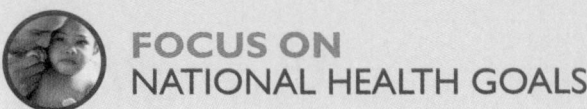

Unless women bring problems to the health care provider's attention early in pregnancy, they may not learn to take the necessary measures to prevent further discomfort during or after the pregnancy. Many women do not mention any concerns or discomforts unless specifically asked because they may not be aware of their significance or are reluctant to take up a busy health care provider's time for these things. For example, women experiencing constipation may not take care of the problem early or well enough to prevent the occurrence of hemorrhoids, which may become a long-term problem not only throughout the pregnancy but afterward as well.

Nursing Diagnosis

Examples of nursing diagnoses related to health promotion of the pregnant woman and fetus may include:

- Health-seeking behaviors related to interest in maintaining optimal health during pregnancy
- Anxiety related to minor symptoms of pregnancy
- Risk for deficient fluid volume related to nausea and vomiting of pregnancy

ASSESSING the Client for Discomforts of Pregnancy

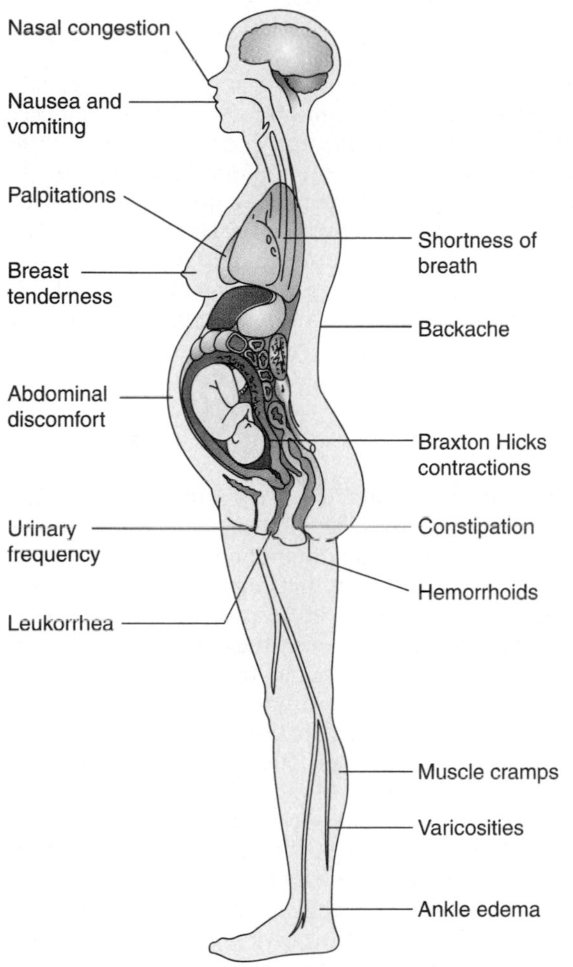

- Constipation related to reduced peristalsis during pregnancy
- Disturbed body image related to change of appearance with pregnancy
- Risk for ineffective sexuality patterns related to fear of harming fetus during pregnancy
- Disturbed sleep pattern related to frequent need to empty bladder during night
- Fatigue related to metabolic changes of pregnancy
- Risk for fetal injury related to maternal cigarette smoking

Outcome Identification and Planning

When establishing goals and outcomes, be certain that the plans are realistic for the woman's situation and family lifestyle (see Focus on Cultural Competence). Try to turn long-term goals into more manageable, short-term ones if possible. For example, a goal of reducing smoking during the pregnancy or giving up cigarettes just for the duration of the pregnancy may be more realistic than a goal of stopping smoking altogether. Eliminating the pressure of making a major permanent lifestyle change may help the woman concentrate her efforts on herself and the fetus over the next several months. Continued reinforcement of her progress may help her to continue reducing the number of cigarettes smoked or to quit smoking altogether after the baby is born, providing a smoke-free environment for her child. Similarly, you cannot set a goal for a woman to be free of the nausea of early pregnancy. The best you can expect to accomplish is to maintain good nutrition and adequate weight gain. Nor can you do much about the frequency of urination, backache, or fatigue that occur with pregnancy except to help the woman adapt her lifestyle to these symptoms (e.g., encourage her to drink more liquids during the day and less in the early evening; schedule regular rest periods if possible).

Often, helping a woman plan to avoid teratogens is difficult because a total change in lifestyle, such as not smoking, not drinking alcohol, or changing a work environment, may be involved. Fortunately, most women are highly motivated to complete a pregnancy satisfactorily. With this level of motivation, planning becomes the task of determining the best route to achieve a goal rather than educating about the need for goal achievement. The web site *www.orpheus.ucsd.edu/ctis* is a helpful site to answer questions about whether certain drugs are teratogenic.

When planning teaching strategies, the woman's receptiveness to instruction is key. Regardless of how

FOCUS ON CULTURAL COMPETENCE

Providing culturally competent care is vital to ensuring that as many families as possible participate in preconception and prenatal care (Leininger, 2001). Recent immigrants may not speak English, so providing meaningful prenatal education can be challenging. Women from cultures that view pregnancy as a wellness state do not seek care because they do not view pregnancy as a time when medical intervention is necessary. They may be extremely modest and may find pelvic examinations difficult, intrusive, and embarrassing. They may rely on herbs and folk remedies to manage the common discomforts of pregnancy. A belief that blood is not replaceable may prevent them from easily agreeing to laboratory blood studies. This variety of cultural backgrounds makes individualized assessment mandatory.

Planning prenatal care to meet the needs of all of the different cultures represented in the United States may include furnishing interpreters to aid in communication, providing classes in prenatal health, explaining how health-promotion regimens fit with women's cultural belief systems, and maintaining an attitude of advocacy to help women adjust to a formal health care system.

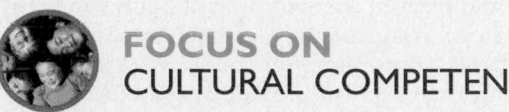

excited and pleased the woman is about being pregnant, she can assimilate only so much information at one particular time. Therefore, be selective about the health information you provide and include those points most relevant to the individual woman. For example, the need to discuss varicosity prevention would be greater for a woman with a history of varicosities in a former pregnancy than for one who is pregnant for the first time and is very athletic. Keep in mind that the health measures being taught must be maintained for an extended time—40 weeks. Choose priorities and give meaningful, individualized health advice to ensure that the woman follows these measures throughout this period. The chances for success with this kind of advice are much greater.

Remember that a basic tenet of teaching and learning is that learning is enhanced when the information has direct application to that person. Devise a plan to space the provision of health-promotion and health-maintenance information based on the changes associated with early and late pregnancy. Those measures that are immediately applicable are taught first; those that have relevance only toward the end of pregnancy are taught then.

Implementation

The major interventions associated with health promotion during pregnancy involve teaching. Although the average woman is aware that some discomforts may occur, these discomforts may seem different when they are happening to her. Often, adolescent girls are uninformed about the common discomforts of pregnancy because they lack a set of peers with pregnancy experience. One who knows that it is normal for breast tenderness to occur during pregnancy may not be sure that the amount of breast tenderness she is having is normal. A woman who had a mental image of herself as someone who would not gain much weight during pregnancy may be very concerned that she is, in fact, gaining a great deal of weight. It is crucial to any teaching to be certain all women understand that they should double-check with their primary care provider before taking any medication during pregnancy.

Other important interventions include good role modeling, such as not smoking in prenatal settings, and exhibiting a healthy lifestyle through nutrition and exercise.

Outcome Evaluation

Evaluation is an ongoing process aided by regular prenatal health care visits. Desired outcomes developed with the woman at one prenatal visit need to be assessed at the next. Examples of appropriate outcomes may include:

- The client verbalizes measures to manage the common discomforts of pregnancy.
- The client reports resting for a half-hour twice a day.
- The client verbalizes positive statements about her appearance.
- The client states that she has stopped smoking.
- The client documents that she walks the length of a city block daily.

HEALTH PROMOTION DURING PREGNANCY

Self-Care Needs

Because pregnancy is not an illness, few special care measures other than common sense about self-care are required. Many women, however, have heard different warnings about what they should or should not do during pregnancy. Thus, the average woman needs some help separating fact from fiction so that she can enjoy her pregnancy unhampered by unnecessary restrictions. Be alert to the common misunderstandings of pregnancy. In no other area of nursing, except for possibly infant feeding, do there seem to be as many misconceptions or inappropriate information available to women.

Bathing

At one time, tub baths were restricted during pregnancy because it was feared that bath water would enter the vagina and cervix and contaminate the uterine contents. Further, it was believed that hot water touching the abdomen might initiate labor. Because the vagina normally is in a closed position, however, the danger of tub bath water entering the cervix is minimal. In addition, the water temperature has no documented effect on initiating labor. During pregnancy, sweating tends to increase because the woman excretes waste products for herself and the fetus. She also has an increase in vaginal discharge. For these reasons, daily tub baths or showers are now recommended.

As pregnancy advances, the woman may have difficulty maintaining her balance when getting in and out of a bathtub. If so, she should change to showering or sponge bathing. If membranes rupture or vaginal bleeding is present, tub baths are contraindicated because then there would be a danger of contamination of uterine contents. During the last month of pregnancy, when the cervix may begin to dilate, some health care providers restrict tub bathing for the same reason.

Breast Care

A few precautions during pregnancy are helpful to prevent breast discomfort. A general rule is to wear a firm, supportive bra with wide straps to spread weight across the shoulders. The woman may need to buy a larger bra halfway through pregnancy to accommodate increased breast size.

At about the 16th week of pregnancy, colostrum secretion begins in the breasts. The sensation of a fluid discharge from the breasts can be frightening unless the woman is forewarned that this is a possibility. Instruct her to wash her breasts with clear tap water (no soap) daily to remove the colostrum, thus minimizing the risk of infection. Afterward, she should dry the nipples well by patting them.

If colostrum secretion is profuse, she may need to place gauze squares or breast pads inside her bra, changing them frequently to maintain dryness. Otherwise, constant moisture next to the breast nipple may cause nipple excoriation, pain, and fissuring.

Dental Care

Good toothbrushing habits should continue throughout pregnancy. Gingival tissue tends to hypertrophy during pregnancy. Unless the pregnant woman brushes well, pockets of plaque form readily between the enlarged gumline and teeth. In addition, encourage the pregnant woman to see her dentist regularly for routine examination and cleaning. Nine months is a fairly long time to be without preventive dental care. Although the pregnant woman should question the need for x-rays during pregnancy, if these are necessary for dental health, they can be done safely as long as the woman's abdomen is shielded with a lead apron.

Tooth decay occurs from the action of bacteria on sugar. This action lowers the pH of the mouth, creating an acid medium that leads to etching or destruction of the enamel of teeth. Encourage snacking on nutritious foods, such as fresh fruits and vegetables like apples and carrots to avoid sugar coming in contact with the teeth. If the client has trouble avoiding sweet snacks such as candy, suggest eating sweet snacks that dissolve easily (like a chocolate bar) rather than those (like chewy candy) that remain in the mouth a long time. This helps to minimize the levels of sugar in the mouth.

Perineal Hygiene

Although women have increased vaginal discharge during pregnancy, douching is contraindicated because the force of the irrigating fluid could cause it to enter the cervix and lead to infection. In addition, douching alters the pH of the vagina, leading to an increased risk of bacterial growth.

Dressing

The days when a woman had to purchase a completely new maternity wardrobe have disappeared. Although economically advantageous, this may be disappointing to a woman who wants to announce her pregnancy early by wearing maternity clothing.

The woman should avoid garters, extremely firm girdles with panty legs, and knee-high stockings because these may impede lower-extremity circulation. If she plans on breast-feeding her newborn, she might choose to buy bras suitable for breast-feeding so she can continue to use them after the baby's birth. Suggest wearing shoes with a moderate to low heel to minimize pelvic tilt and possible backache. Otherwise, the rules are common sense and comfort.

Sexual Activity

Some women are reluctant to ask questions about sexual relations during pregnancy. However, most women are concerned about whether sexual intercourse should be restricted. Many need information to refute some of the myths about sexual relations in pregnancy that still exist. Common myths include the following:

- "Coitus on the expected date of her period will initiate labor."
- "Orgasm will initiate labor, but participating in sexual relations without orgasm will not."
- "Coitus during the fertile days of a cycle will cause a second pregnancy or twins."
- "Coitus might cause rupture of the membranes."

None of these is true. Asking a woman at a prenatal visit if she has any questions about sexual activity allows her to voice such concerns (see Focus on Communication). Then you can help dispel these myths, allowing the woman to feel more comfortable and secure that coitus is not harming her child.

Women with a history of spontaneous miscarriage may be advised to avoid coitus during the time of the pregnancy when a previous miscarriage occurred. Women whose membranes have ruptured or who have vaginal spotting should be advised against coitus until examined to prevent possible infection. Advise caution about male oral–female genital contact, because accidental air embolism has been

FOCUS ON COMMUNICATION

Constance Murphy is a woman who is 6 months pregnant and has recently separated from her husband.

Less Effective Communication

Nurse: Has anything changed since your last visit, Mrs. Murphy?
Ms. Murphy: I'm not Mrs. Murphy anymore.
Nurse: What does that mean?
Ms. Murphy: I'm getting a divorce.
Nurse: I'm sorry. Is there anything I can do?
Ms. Murphy: Tell me how long into pregnancy I can have sex.
Nurse: Well, since you're separated, you won't need that kind of advice any longer. Let's talk instead about exercise and pregnancy.

More Effective Communication

Nurse: Has anything changed since your last visit, Mrs. Murphy?
Ms. Murphy: I'm not Mrs. Murphy anymore.
Nurse: What does that mean?
Ms. Murphy: I'm getting a divorce.
Nurse: I'm sorry. Is there anything I can do?
Ms. Murphy: Tell me how long into pregnancy I can have sex.
Nurse: Basically as long as you're comfortable and you don't have any complications.
Ms. Murphy: Good. My boyfriend made me promise to ask today.

Health teaching is an art separate from teaching morality. In the first scenario, the nurse cuts off communication by making a judgment and thus supplying the information that the nurse thinks the client needs. In the second scenario, the nurse actively listens to the client, focuses in on her needs and concerns, and supplies the information the client has requested.

reported from this act during pregnancy (Dickerson & Chez, 2000). Otherwise, there are no sexual restrictions during pregnancy.

Early in pregnancy, a woman may experience a decreased desire for coitus resulting from the increased estrogen level in her body. Breast tenderness may limit a usual pattern of sexual arousal. As pelvic congestion increases from the additional uterine blood supply, most women may notice increased clitoral sensation. Some women may experience orgasm for the first time during pregnancy because of the increased pelvic congestion. As pregnancy advances and the woman's abdomen increases in size, she and her sexual partner may need to use new positions for intercourse. A side-by-side position or the woman in a superior position may be more comfortable. As vaginal secretions change, the woman may find a water-soluble lubricant helpful. If she begins to experience discomfort from penile penetration, mutual masturbation or female oral–male genital relations might be satisfying to both partners. Caution women with a nonmonogamous sexual partner about the partner's need to use a condom to prevent transmission of a sexually transmitted disease during pregnancy (Genc & Ledger, 2000). Women also may use female condoms throughout pregnancy.

✔ CHECKPOINT QUESTIONS

1. When is tub bathing contraindicated during pregnancy?
2. What should the pregnant woman use to clean her breasts of colostrum?
3. Do women need to continue to use safer sex practices during pregnancy?

Exercise

Exercise during pregnancy is important to prevent circulatory stasis in the lower extremities. It also can offer a general feeling of well-being. For some women, teaching about exercise focuses on helping them realize the need for exercise and urging them to get enough. Others may need to be cautioned to restrict exercise or participation in contact sports.

Extreme exercise has been associated with a lower birth rate (Campbell & Mottola, 2001). The American College of Obstetricians and Gynecologists (ACOG) recommends that the average, well-nourished women should exercise during pregnancy every day for 30 consecutive minutes (ACOG, 2002). An exercise program should consist of 5 minutes of warm-up exercises, an active "stimulus" phase of 20 minutes, and then 5 minutes of cool-down exercises. The type of activity chosen depends on the woman's interests. Exercises that exercise large muscle groups rhythmically, such as walking, are best. The intensity of the exercise program depends on the woman's cardiopulmonary fitness. Before she begins any exercise program, make sure the woman has consulted her physician or nurse-midwife. If any complication of pregnancy should occur, such as bleeding or PIH, the woman should discontinue her exercise program until she rechecks with her primary health care provider about continuing the program.

Both pregnant and nonpregnant women should exercise at 70% to 85% of their maximum heart rate. The easiest way to calculate this is to subtract the woman's age from 220, then multiply this by 70% or 85%. For example, after exercise a 23-year-old woman should have a pulse range of 137 to 167 (220 minus 23 times 70% and 85%). For a woman of 35, this target range would be 129 to 157.

Teach the client how to assess quickly if she is exercising too strenuously by evaluating her ability to continue talking while exercising. If she is too short of breath to do this, she is exercising beyond her target heart rate.

A planned exercise program may have long-term benefits, such as weight control and a decrease in the incidence of ovarian cancer (Cottreau et al., 2000). Other benefits may include:

- Lowered cholesterol level
- Reduced risk of osteoporosis
- Increased energy level
- Maintenance of healthy body weight
- Decreased risk of heart disease
- Increased self-esteem and well-being
- Possible reduction in the rate of cesarean birth (see Focus on Evidence-Based Practice)

As a rule, a woman can continue any sport she participated in before pregnancy unless it was one that involved body contact, such as soccer. If a woman is a competent

FOCUS ON EVIDENCE-BASED PRACTICE

Can Exercise During Pregnancy Affect the Type of Birth?

To answer this question, nurse researchers interviewed 137 nulliparous women about the amount of aerobic exercise they had participated in during their pregnancy. Results showed that the 93 sedentary women who participated in the study were two to four times more likely to deliver by cesarean birth than the 44 women who participated in aerobic exercise. The researchers concluded that regular participation in physical activity during the first two trimesters of pregnancy may be associated with reduced risk for cesarean birth in nulliparous women.

This is an important study because women are participating in so many more active sports and exercise clubs than ever before, so knowing whether exercise during pregnancy is safe has become more important. Nurses can incorporate this information in their teaching plan for pregnant women when discussing activities and recommending appropriate exercises during the antepartal period.

Bungum, T.J., Peaslee, D.L., Jackson, A.W., & Perez, M.A. (2000). Exercise during pregnancy and type of delivery in nulliparae. *Journal of Obstetric, Gynecologic & Neonatal Nursing, 29*(3), 258–264.

horsewoman, for example, there is little reason for her to discontinue riding until it becomes uncomfortable (as long as she does not have a history of early miscarriage). Pregnancy is not the time to learn to ride, however, because a beginning rider is at greater risk for being thrown than an experienced one. The same principles apply to skiing and bicycling. An accomplished skier or bicyclist may continue the activity in moderation until balance becomes a problem. Pregnancy is not the time to learn to ski or ride a bicycle, however, because the lack of skill may result in many falls.

Swimming is a good activity for pregnant women and, like bathing, is not contraindicated as long as the membranes are intact. Long-distance swimming or any other activity carried out to a point of extreme fatigue should be avoided. A high-impact aerobics program is contraindicated because this is strenuous to both pelvic and knee joints. In addition, it may lead to hyperthermia for the mother and the fetus. Use of hot tubs and saunas after workouts longer than 15 minutes is contraindicated because these also could raise the internal fetal temperature. Fetal hyperthermia may be dangerous because it is associated with congenital anomalies (Niebyl, 2000).

Walking is the best exercise during pregnancy, and women should be encouraged to take a walk daily unless inclement weather, many levels of stairs, or an unsafe neighborhood are contraindications. Jogging, in contrast, is questioned because of the strain that the extra weight of pregnancy places on the knees. Late in pregnancy, jogging can cause pelvic pain from relaxed symphysis pubis movement. Guidelines for exercise during pregnancy are highlighted in the Focus on Family Empowerment box.

Sleep

The optimal condition for body growth occurs when growth hormone secretion is at its highest level—that is, during sleep. This, plus the overall increased metabolic demand, appears to be the physiologic reason pregnant women need an increased amount of sleep or at least rest to build new body cells during pregnancy.

Pregnant women rarely have difficulty falling asleep at night because of this increased physiologic need for sleep. If the woman has trouble falling asleep, drinking a glass of warm milk may help. Relaxation exercises (lying quietly, systematically relaxing neck muscles, shoulder muscles, arm muscles, and so on) also may be effective.

Late in pregnancy, a woman often finds herself awakened from sleep at short, frequent intervals by the activity of the fetus. Frequent waking this way leads to loss of REM

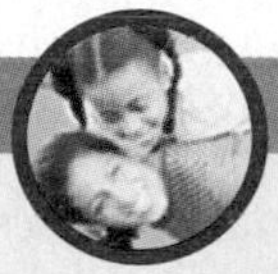

FOCUS ON FAMILY EMPOWERMENT
Guidelines for Exercise in Pregnancy

Q. Now that I'm pregnant, how can I exercise and what kinds of exercise should I do?

A. Use the following as guidelines for exercising while you are pregnant:

1. Perform regular exercise (about three times per week) rather than engage in intermittent activity.
2. Do not perform vigorous exercise in hot, humid weather or if you have a fever to avoid overexerting yourself or developing hyperthermia.
3. Avoid activities that require jumping, jarring motions, or rapid changes in direction, because your joints may be unstable.
4. Exercise on a wooden floor or a tightly carpeted surface to reduce shock to the abdomen or knees and provide a sure footing.
5. Avoid exercises and motions that involve deep flexion or joint extension, such as stretching with the toes extended, to avoid muscle cramping.
6. Always start your exercise program by warming up for approximately 5 minutes with activities such as slow walking or stationary cycling with low resistance.
7. End your exercise program with a period of gradually declining activity that includes gentle, stationary stretching. Because of the increased risk of joint injury, do not stretch to the point of maximum resistance.
8. Measure your heart rate at times of peak activity. Talk with your primary care provider about target heart rate and limits, and don't exceed them.
9. When getting up from lying on the floor, do so gradually to prevent dramatic blood pressure changes or stretching of the round ligament.
10. Drink liquids liberally before and after exercise to prevent dehydration. If necessary, interrupt your activity to replenish fluids.
11. If you were sedentary before pregnancy, begin your exercise program with physical activity of very low intensity and advance your activity level gradually.
12. Stop any activity and contact your primary care provider if any unusual symptoms appear.
13. Perform strenuous activities for no longer than 20 minutes.
14. Do not exercise in the supine position (lying down flat) after the 4th month of gestation to prevent supine hypotension.
15. Avoid exercises that employ the Valsalva maneuver (holding your breath, bearing down) because this decreases blood supply to the fetus.
16. Make sure your caloric intake is adequate to meet not only the extra energy needs of pregnancy but also those of the exercise performed.

(rapid eye movement) sleep. On arising, a woman may feel anxious or not well rested, although she has slept her usual number of hours. She also may awaken with dyspnea if she is lying flat. In this instance, sleeping on two pillows or on a couch with an armrest may be helpful.

To obtain enough sleep and rest during pregnancy, most pregnant women need a rest period during the afternoon as well as a full night of sleep. A good resting or sleeping position is a modified **Sims' position,** with the top leg forward (Fig. 11-1). This puts the weight of the fetus on the bed, not on the woman, and allows good circulation in the lower extremities.

Be certain women know to avoid resting in a supine position. Otherwise, they can develop supine hypotension syndrome (faintness, diaphoresis, and hypotension from the pressure of the expanding uterus on the inferior vena cava). Also be certain they know not to rest with their knees sharply bent either when sitting or lying down, because of the increased risk of venous stasis below the knee.

Employment

Unless jobs involve exposure to toxic substances, lifting heavy objects, other kinds of excessive physical strain, long periods of standing, or having to maintain body balance, there are few reasons women cannot continue to work throughout pregnancy (Frazier et al., 2001). Changes in public assistance laws have led to more women working during pregnancy than ever before (Youngblut et al., 2000). To protect women from loss of employment benefits during pregnancy, Congress passed an employment rights law in 1978 (Public Law 95-555). However, this law does not cover women who work for companies with fewer than 15 employees.

According to this law, an employer cannot:

- Deprive women of seniority rights, in pay or promotion, because they take a maternity leave
- Treat women returning from maternity leave as new hires, starting over on the eligibility period for pension and other benefits
- Force pregnant women to leave if they are able to and want to continue working
- Refuse to hire women just because they are pregnant or fire them for the same reason
- Refuse to cover employees' normal pregnancy and delivery expenses in the company health plan or pay less for pregnancy than for other medical conditions
- Refuse to pay sick leave or disability benefits to women whose difficult pregnancies keep them off the job

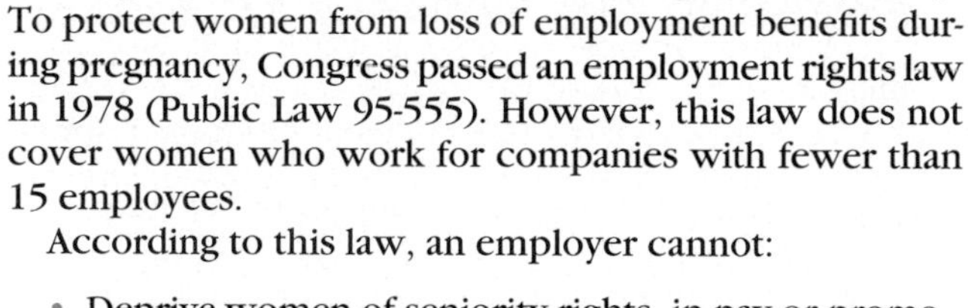

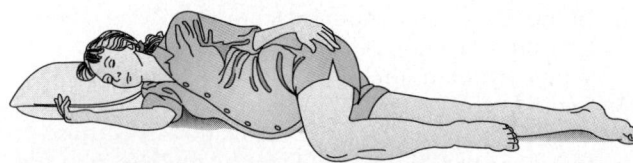

FIGURE 11.1 Modified Sims' position as a rest position during pregnancy. The knees and elbows should be slightly bent, the muscles limp, and the breathing slow and regular. Notice that the weight of the fetus is resting on the bed.

Passed in 1993, the Family Leave Act, a federal law, guarantees women the right to 12 weeks of unpaid, job-protected leave on the birth of a child, the adoption or foster placement of a child, when the woman is needed to care for a parent, spouse, or child with a serious health condition, or because of a serious health condition in herself (29 CFR 825.11). Specifically mentioned in the law is any period of incapacity due to pregnancy or for prenatal care (American Public Health Association, 2001). Families need to be educated about this important law because many women are still not aware that they can take time off from work during pregnancy or to spend with a new baby. In addition, some women may be able to qualify for provisions under the Americans with Disabilities Act (Pardeck, 2001).

Some occupations are hazardous because they bring women into contact with harmful substances. For example, nurses working with anesthetic gases in operating room suites or dental offices are reported to have a higher incidence of spontaneous miscarriage and, possibly, congenital anomalies in children than nurses working in other locales, probably due to exposure to nitrous oxide (National Institute of Occupational Safety and Health, 2000). This finding suggests that breathing even a low dose of anesthetic gases such as nitrous oxide can be a serious occupational hazard for these nurses. Nurses working with chemotherapy agents should wear gloves to protect themselves from exposure to these drugs, which are possibly teratogenic. Ribavirin (Virazole), an antibiotic used to treat respiratory syncytial infections, is also apparently teratogenic if inhaled by health care providers.

A number of studies suggest that spontaneous miscarriage may occur more frequently in women who work at strenuous jobs or those that require long periods of standing (Frazier et al., 2001). Other problems that can occur with employment include interference in adequate rest and nutrition. Urge the woman who works outside her home to put her feet up to rest when performing tasks that can be done in that position. Review what she eats at fast-food restaurants or packs for herself to be certain she understands that this type of lunch can be as nutritious as if she were eating at home if she takes the time to plan ahead.

Remember, most women work to augment or supply the family income. Even those who could afford to leave their jobs may not be willing to sacrifice the collegial relationships and sense of fulfillment derived from work, nor the lifestyle their income has allowed them to enjoy. Counseling them to reserve periods during the day for rest and to eat a proper diet is more effective than suggesting they resign from their jobs during pregnancy to get more rest (see Focus on Family Empowerment).

✔ CHECKPOINT QUESTIONS

4. What is considered one of the best exercises for a woman during pregnancy?
5. What condition can occur if a pregnant woman rests in a supine position?
6. What are two areas that women working outside the home often need good planning to accomplish?

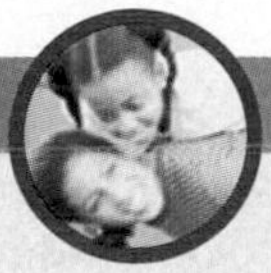

FOCUS ON FAMILY EMPOWERMENT
Guidelines for Pregnant Working Women

Q. Now that I'm pregnant, can I continue my normal job outside of the home?

A. Use the following as guidelines for safe pregnancy practices:

- Allow yourself to rest during your break periods rather than running errands, etc.
- Try to use at least part of your lunch hour to rest. Lie on your left side in a break room if possible. If this is not possible, then rest sitting with your legs elevated.
- If your job involves long periods of standing, think of times you could stop and elevate your legs (working in a low file drawer, reading time in a classroom, etc.).
- Walk around periodically to avoid prolonged standing in one position if possible; stretch your back periodically to avoid backache.
- Wear support hose to improve venous return to your lower extremities.
- Avoid excessive overtime or working longer than 8-hour shifts.
- Empty your bladder every 2 hours to help prevent bladder infection.
- Get extra rest on weekends or days off.
- Take great caution when working around equipment that requires good balance. Avoid ladders or climbing late in pregnancy, when balance may be a problem.
- Learn your target heart rate for exercise. If your job involves strenuous exercise, stop and rest at the point your target heart rate is exceeded.
- Be sure you are not relying on fast foods for meals. Take time to pack or purchase nutritious foods.

Travel

Most women have questions about travel during pregnancy (Thomas, 2000). Early in a normal pregnancy, there are no restrictions. If the woman is susceptible to motion sickness, she should not take any medication unless specifically prescribed or approved by her physician or nurse-midwife for this. Late in pregnancy, travel plans should take into consideration the possibility of early labor, requiring birth at a strange setting where the woman's obstetric history is unknown. In addition, at any time during the pregnancy when traveling, the woman should be encouraged to avoid eating uncooked fruits, vegetables, and meat or drinking unpurified water (Dickerson & Chez, 2000).

Regardless of the month of her pregnancy, if the woman plans to spend time at a remote location, such as a campsite, be certain she knows the location of a nearby health care facility should an unexpected complication occur. If she is going to be away from home for an extended time, she needs to make arrangements to visit a health care provider in that area so she can keep the schedule of her regular prenatal visits. Encourage her to make these plans far enough in advance to allow her records to be copied and taken with her or be forwarded to the interim health care provider. Be aware that you need her written permission to send records. Also, make sure she has enough of her prescribed vitamin supplement plus adequate prescriptions for refills as necessary.

Advise a woman who is taking a long trip by automobile to plan for frequent rest or stretch periods. Preferably every hour, but at least every 2 hours, she should get out of the car and walk a short distance. This will relieve stiffness and muscle ache and improve lower extremity circulation, helping to prevent varicosities and hemorrhoids.

Women may drive as long as they fit comfortably behind the steering wheel. While pregnant, they should use seat belts like everyone else. Occasionally, uterine rupture has been reported from seat belt use, but overall the evidence suggests that seat belts reduce maternal mortality in car accidents. Both shoulder harnesses and lap belts should be used. The lap belt should be worn as snugly as comfortable so that it fits under the abdominal bulge and across the pelvic bones. The shoulder harness should be snug but comfortable, worn across the shoulder, chest, and upper abdomen. A pad may be placed under the shoulder harness at the neck to avoid chafing (Fig. 11-2).

Pregnancy is also a time for a family to think about transportation safety for the newborn. Purchasing a car

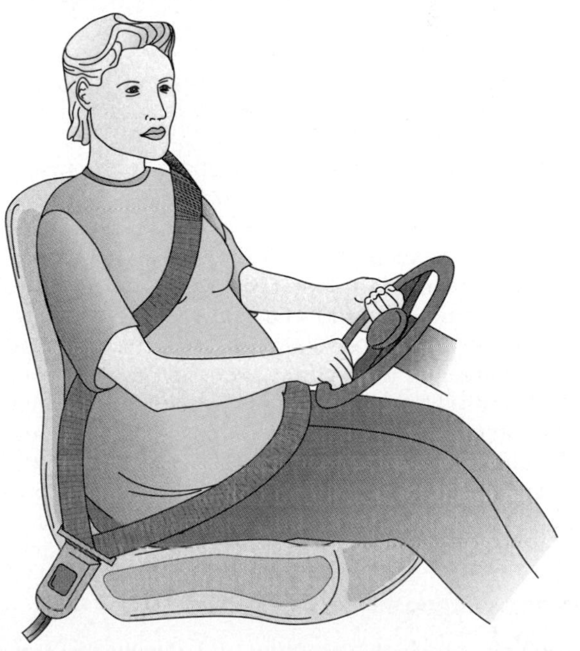

FIGURE 11.2 Proper seat belt position for a pregnant woman.

seat is an investment that is not only legally required for transporting infants but also helps guarantee their safety. Families who cannot afford to purchase an infant car seat may want to inquire among friends or relatives about the possibility of borrowing one no longer needed. Many hospitals and local Red Cross chapters also provide infant seats on a rental or loan basis for families who may find it difficult to obtain one in other ways.

Traveling by plane is not contraindicated as long as the plane has a well-pressurized cabin (true of commercial airlines but not of all small private planes). Some airlines do not permit women who are more than 7 months pregnant on board; others require written permission from the woman's primary caregiver. Advise the woman to investigate these restrictions by calling the airline or a travel agency before making travel plans.

With businesses becoming global, more women than ever before are asked to travel internationally. Women who are traveling abroad may need additional immunizations, such as an immunization for cholera, for entry into certain countries to safeguard their health. All live virus vaccines (measles, mumps, rubella, and yellow fever) are contraindicated during pregnancy and must not be administered unless the risk of the disease outweighs the risk to the pregnancy. Before any immunization, women should ask their primary care provider to verify it will be safe during pregnancy. Pregnancy does not alter indications for rabies vaccine because without the vaccine, a fatal disease could occur (Dickerson & Chez, 2000).

WHAT IF? A pregnant client tells you that as a sales representative for a toy company, she is required to travel all across the country, at least once a month, sometimes two or three times a month. Sometimes she drives or takes a train; other times she flies. She asks your advice about whether she should ask her employer for a change in her position. How would you respond?

Discomforts of Early Pregnancy: The First Trimester

Although most women are pleased to be pregnant, the symptoms of early pregnancy tend to cause discomfort to the woman rather than provide evidence that she is carrying a child. As such, the woman may become frustrated, expecting pregnancy to be a time of glowing good health. Providing empathetic and sound advice about measures to relieve these discomforts helps promote the overall health and well-being of a pregnant client. Although the symptoms discussed below are classified as minor, they may not seem minor to the woman who wakes up each morning feeling nauseated, wondering if she will ever feel like herself again. Also, each of these symptoms has the potential to lead to problems that are more serious.

Nursing Diagnoses

Listening, observing carefully, and developing nursing diagnoses based on assessment data are important steps in prenatal care. Examples of nursing diagnoses that might be developed for women experiencing the discomforts of early pregnancy are listed below. Keep in mind that although many women will experience one or several of these symptoms, each woman's experience is unique and nursing diagnoses must be developed according to each woman's individual needs. Possible examples may include:

- Health-seeking behaviors related to interest in using herbal remedies to relieve discomforts of pregnancy
- Disturbed body image related to breast and abdominal enlargement in pregnancy
- Constipation related to reduced peristalsis in pregnancy
- Fatigue related to increased physiologic need for sleep and rest during pregnancy
- Acute pain related to frequent muscle cramps secondary to physiologic changes of pregnancy
- Disturbed sleep pattern related to frequent need to empty bladder during night

Breast Tenderness

Breast tenderness is often one of the first symptoms noticed in early pregnancy; it may be most noticeable on exposure to cold air. For most women, the tenderness is minimal and transient, something they are aware of but not something that overly concerns them. If the tenderness is enough to cause discomfort, encourage the woman to wear a bra with a wide shoulder strap for support and to dress warmly to avoid cold drafts if cold increases symptoms. If actual pain exists, the presence of conditions such as nipple fissure or other explanations for the pain, such as breast abscess, should be ruled out.

Palmar Erythema

Palmar erythema, or palmar pruritus, occurs in early pregnancy and is probably caused by increased estrogen levels. Constant redness or itching of the palms may make the woman think she has an allergy. Explain that this is normal before she spends time and effort trying different soaps or detergents or attempting to implicate certain foods she has eaten. For some women, calamine lotion may be soothing. As soon as her body adjusts to the increased level of estrogen, the erythema and pruritus disappear.

Constipation

As the weight of the growing uterus presses against the bowel and peristalsis slows, constipation may occur. Discuss preventive measures with the woman early in pregnancy to help her avoid this problem. Encourage her to evacuate her bowels regularly (many women neglect this first simple rule); to increase the amount of roughage in her diet by eating raw fruits, bran, and vegetables; and to drink at least eight 8-oz glasses of water daily.

Some women find that their prescribed oral iron supplement contributes to constipation. Reinforce the need for this supplement to build fetal iron stores. Help the woman find a method to relieve or prevent constipation other than not taking the supplement.

Advise the woman not to use over-the-counter or herbal remedies to prevent constipation, especially mineral oil. Mineral oil interferes with the absorption of fat-soluble vitamins (A, D, K, and E), which are necessary for good fetal growth and maternal health.

Enemas also should be avoided because their action might initiate labor. Over-the-counter laxatives are contraindicated, as are all drugs during pregnancy unless specifically prescribed or sanctioned by the woman's physician or nurse-midwife (Dickerson & Chez, 2000). If dietary measures and attempts at regular bowel evacuation fail, a stool softener, such as docusate sodium (Colace), and evacuation suppositories, such as glycerin, may be prescribed. Some women have extensive flatulence accompanying constipation. Recommend avoiding gas-forming foods, such as cabbage or beans, to help control this problem.

Nausea, Vomiting, and Pyrosis

At least half of pregnant women experience enough gastrointestinal symptoms to cause discomfort in pregnancy. Because these symptoms also interfere with nutrition, they are discussed in Chapter 12.

Fatigue

Fatigue is extremely common in early pregnancy. It is probably due to increased metabolic requirements. Much of it can be relieved by increasing the amount of rest and sleep. Some women are reluctant to take time out of their day for rest. They know that pregnancy is not an illness, and so they proceed as if nothing is happening to them. Rarely is there justification during a normal pregnancy for women to take extra days off from work because of their condition, but it is also unrealistic to proceed as if nothing is happening. Fatigue can increase the amount of morning sickness a woman experiences. If she becomes too tired, she may not eat properly. If she remains on her feet without at least one break during the day, the risk for varicosities and the danger of thromboembolic complications increase.

For all these reasons, ask women at prenatal visits whether they manage to have at least one short rest period every day. A good resting position is a modified Sims' position, with the top leg forward (see Fig. 11-1). This puts the weight of the fetus on the bed, not on the woman, and allows good circulation in the lower extremities.

A woman who works outside her home at a job that requires her to be on her feet most of the day might use part of her lunch hour to sit with her feet elevated, such as on an adjoining chair (Fig. 11-3). After she returns home from work in the evening, she may need to modify her customary routine from typical activities such as cooking dinner or watching a child's soccer game to resting, then cooking dinner or going to the soccer game, or resting while her partner cooks dinner (part of "we are having a baby at our house" for a partner who does not usually share in household chores). Women who work at sedentary jobs, inside or outside their home, may, in contrast, need to use this time to increase their activity, such as taking a walk or using a treadmill.

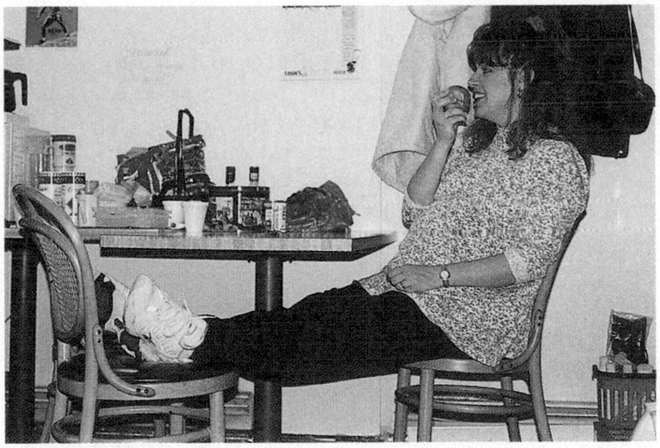

FIGURE 11.3 If at all possible, women need to arrange a "feet-up" period during their workday.

Muscle Cramps

Decreased serum calcium levels, increased serum phosphorus levels, and, possibly, interference with circulation commonly cause muscle cramps of the lower extremities during pregnancy. These problems are best relieved by the woman lying on her back momentarily and extending the involved leg while keeping her knee straight and dorsiflexing the foot until the pain is gone (Fig. 11-4).

If the woman is having frequent leg cramps, she may need a prescription for aluminum hydroxide gel (Amphojel), which binds phosphorus in the intestinal tract and thereby lowers its circulating level. Lowering milk intake to only a pint daily and supplementing this with calcium lactate may also help to reduce the phosphorus level. Elevating the lower extremities frequently during the day to improve circulation and avoiding full leg extension, such as stretching with the toes pointed, may be beneficial. Typically, muscle cramps are a minor symptom of pregnancy. However, the pain may be extreme and the intensity of the contraction can be frightening. Always ask at prenatal visits if this is a problem. Otherwise, women may not realize that cramping is pregnancy-related and so fail to report it unless asked.

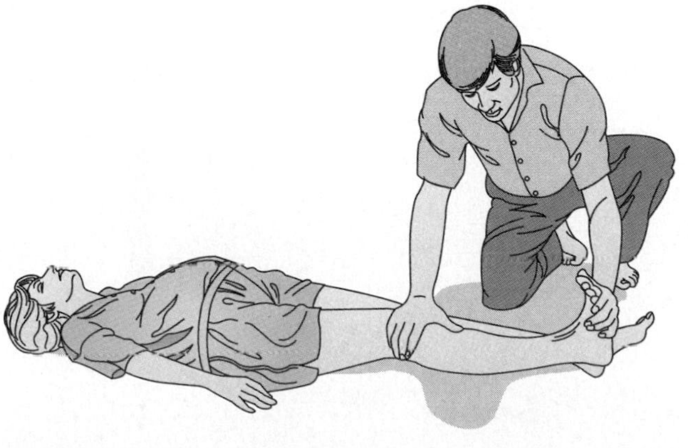

FIGURE 11.4 Relieving a leg cramp in pregnancy. Pressing down on the knee and pressing the toes backward (dorsiflexion) relieves most cramps. Here, the client's partner helps.

Hypotension

Supine hypotension is a symptom that occurs when a woman lies on her back and the uterus presses on the vena cava, impairing blood return to the heart. The woman experiences an irregular heart rate and a feeling of apprehension. Relieving the problem is simple: if the woman turns or is turned on her side, pressure is removed from the vena cava, blood flow is restored, and the symptoms quickly fade.

If a woman rises suddenly from a lying or sitting position or stands for an extended time in a warm or crowded area, she may faint from the same phenomenon (blood pooling in the pelvic area or lower extremities). Rising slowly and avoiding extended periods of standing prevent this problem. If the woman should feel faint, sitting with her head lowered—the same action as for any person who feels faint—will alleviate the problem.

Varicosities

Varicosities, or the development of tortuous leg veins, are common in pregnancy because the weight of the distended uterus puts pressure on the veins returning blood from the lower extremities. This causes pooling of blood in the vessels. The veins become engorged, inflamed, and painful. Although usually confined to the lower extremities, varicosities can extend to the vulva. They occur most frequently in women with a family history of varicose veins and those who have a large fetus or a multiple pregnancy. Urge such women to prevent varicosities early in pregnancy; if left until the second trimester, the best you can accomplish is relief of pain from already formed varicosities.

Resting in a Sims' position or on the back with the legs raised against the wall or elevated on a footstool for 15 to 20 minutes twice a day is a good precaution (Fig. 11-5). Caution women not to sit with their legs crossed or their knees bent. Constrictive knee-high hose or garters should be avoided.

Some women, especially those who developed varicosities during a previous pregnancy, may need elastic support stockings such as TEDS for relief of varicosities. When applied properly, the stockings should reach an area above the point of distention. The woman also should don the support stockings before she arises in the morning. Once she is on her feet, the pooling of blood has already begun, and the stockings will be less effective. Before a woman buys stockings, be certain she understands that the stockings should be labeled "medical support hose." Many pantyhose manufacturers advertise their stockings as giving "firm support," and the woman may assume erroneously that this is sufficient for her.

Because it stimulates venous return, exercise is as effective as rest periods at alleviating varicosities. Most women assume they do not need set exercise periods during pregnancy because they work hard at other activities. If they analyze the type of work they do, however, they will realize that a great deal of this work leads to venous stasis of the lower extremities. Women stand in one position to wash dishes, cook dinner, run a copying machine, defend a client in court, process a part on an assembly line, or teach a class. In addition, sitting at a desk for prolonged periods of time with the legs dependent also promotes venous stasis. Women need to break up these long periods of sitting or standing with a "walk break" at least twice a day. As a rule, their families benefit by accompanying them. Partners may discover that they, too, walk very little during their workday.

Vitamin C may be helpful in reducing the size of varicosities because it is involved in the formation of blood vessel collagen and endothelium. Ask at prenatal visits whether the woman includes fresh fruit in her diet.

Hemorrhoids

Hemorrhoids (varicosities of the rectal veins) occur commonly in pregnancy because of pressure on these veins from the bulk of the growing uterus. Preventive measures early in pregnancy may be effective in reducing their severity. Daily bowel evacuation helps to relieve constipation and also helps to prevent the formation of hemorrhoids. Resting in a modified Sims' position daily also is helpful. At day's end, assuming a knee-chest position (Fig. 11-6) for 10 to 15 minutes is an excellent way to reduce the pressure on rectal veins. Keep in mind that a knee-chest position may make a woman feel lightheaded initially. Therefore,

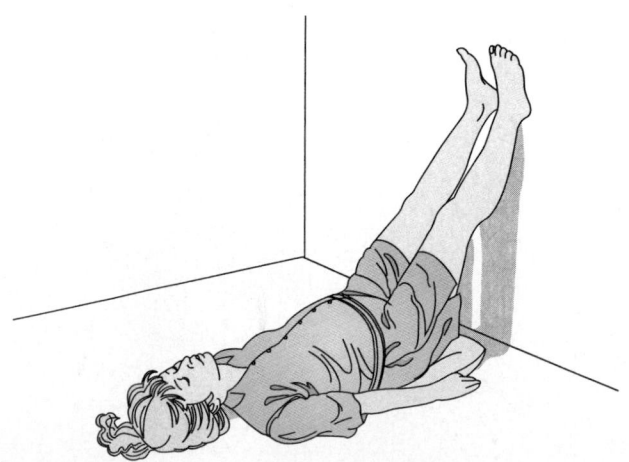

FIGURE 11.5 Position to relieve varicosities. The mother keeps a pad under her right hip to prevent supine hypotensive syndrome.

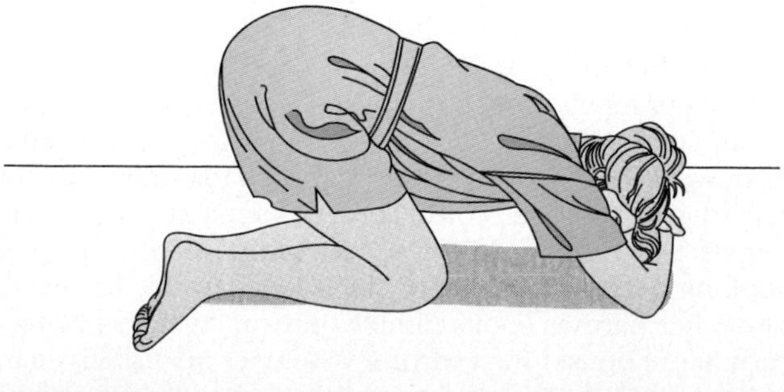

FIGURE 11.6 Knee–chest position. Because the weight of the uterus is shifted forward, this position allows for free flow of urine from the kidneys (preventing urinary tract stasis and infection) and better circulation in the rectal area (preventing hemorrhoids).

instruct her to remain in this position for only a few minutes at first, and then gradually increase the time until she can maintain the position comfortably for about 15 minutes. Stool softeners may be recommended for the woman who already has hemorrhoids. Applying witch hazel or cold compresses may help to relieve pain. Replacing hemorrhoids with gentle finger pressure can be helpful. As with varicosities, think prevention, not just providing help for already established hemorrhoids.

✔ CHECKPOINT QUESTIONS

7. Why is mineral oil contraindicated to relieve constipation of pregnancy?
8. What is the main cause of muscle cramps in pregnancy?
9. Why do hemorrhoids occur during pregnancy?

Heart Palpitations

On sudden movement, such as turning over in bed, a pregnant woman may experience a bounding palpitation of the heart. This is probably due to the circulatory adjustments necessary to accommodate her increased blood supply during pregnancy. Although only momentary, the sensation may be frightening because the heart seems to have skipped a beat. Gradual, slow movements will help prevent it from happening so frequently. It is reassuring for women to know that palpitations are normal and to be expected on occasion. Only if they occur very frequently or continuously or are accompanied by pain are they a concern.

Frequency of Urination

Frequency of urination occurs in early pregnancy due to the pressure of the growing uterus on the anterior bladder. The sensation may last for about 3 months, sometimes beginning as early as the first or second missed menstrual period, disappear in midpregnancy when the uterus rises above the bladder, and return again in late pregnancy as the fetal head presses against the bladder (Fig. 11-7).

When a woman describes frequency of urination, be certain this is the only urinary symptom that she has. Question her about any burning or pain on urination or whether she has noticed any blood in her urine. These are signs of urinary tract infection.

There are no solutions for decreasing the frequency of urination. Suggesting a woman reduce the amount of caffeine she is drinking may be helpful. Most importantly, the woman needs to understand that voiding more frequently is a normal phenomenon. Unless a woman is cautioned that the sensation of frequency returns after lightening (the settling of the fetal head into the inlet of the pelvis at pregnancy's end), she may think she has a urinary tract infection. This is less noticeable in women who have practiced Kegel exercises (alternately contracting and relaxing perineal muscles; Box 11-1) in preparation for birth.

Occasionally, a woman notices stress incontinence (involuntary loss of urine on coughing or sneezing) during pregnancy. Although this is largely unpreventable, doing Kegel exercises helps to strengthen urinary control, directly strengthens perineal muscles for birth, and decreases the possibility of stress incontinence.

Abdominal Discomfort

Some women experience uncomfortable feelings of abdominal pressure early in pregnancy. Women with a multiple pregnancy may notice this throughout pregnancy. Women learn to relieve the feeling by putting gentle pressure on the uterine fundus. Typically, pregnant women stand with their arms crossed in front because the weight of their arms resting on their abdomen relieves this discomfort.

When women stand up quickly, they may experience a pulling pain in the right or left lower abdomen from ten-

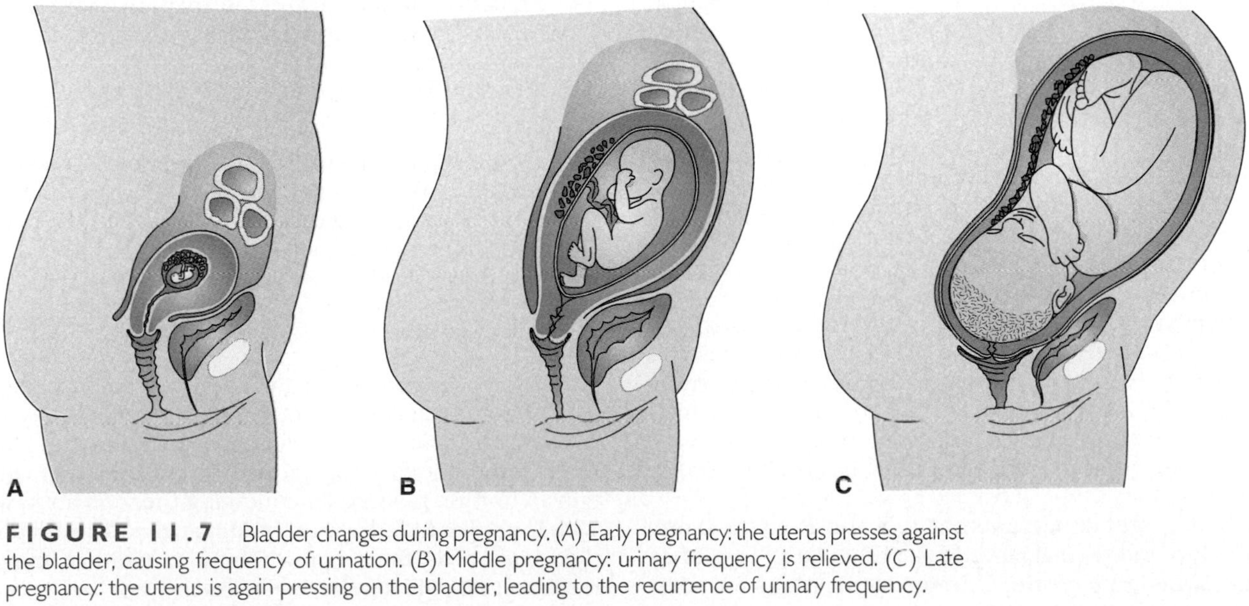

FIGURE 11.7 Bladder changes during pregnancy. (*A*) Early pregnancy: the uterus presses against the bladder, causing frequency of urination. (*B*) Middle pregnancy: urinary frequency is relieved. (*C*) Late pregnancy: the uterus is again pressing on the bladder, leading to the recurrence of urinary frequency.

BOX 11.1

KEGEL EXERCISES

Kegel exercises are exercises designed to strengthen the pubococcygeal muscles. Each is a separate exercise and should be done about three times a day. Exercises are as follows:

1. Squeeze the muscles surrounding the vagina as if stopping the flow of urine. Hold for 3 seconds. Relax. Repeat this sequence 10 times.
2. Contract and relax the muscles surrounding the vagina as rapidly as possible 10 to 25 times.
3. Imagine that you are sitting in a bathtub of water and squeeze muscles as if sucking water into the vagina. Hold for 3 seconds. Relax. Repeat this action 10 times.

It may take as long as 6 weeks of exercise before pubococcygeal muscles are strengthened. In addition to strengthening urinary control and preventing stress incontinence, Kegel exercises can lead to increased sexual enjoyment because of the tightened vaginal muscles.

sion on the round ligaments. The pain is sharp and frightening. They can prevent this by always rising slowly from a lying to a sitting, or from a sitting to a standing position. Because round ligament pain may simulate the abrupt pain that occurs with ruptured ectopic pregnancy, the client's description of the pain must be evaluated carefully.

Leukorrhea

Leukorrhea, a whitish, viscous vaginal discharge or an increase in the amount of normal vaginal secretions, occurs in response to the high estrogen levels and the increased blood supply to the vaginal epithelium and cervix in pregnancy. A daily bath or shower to wash away accumulated secretions and prevent vulvar excoriation usually controls this problem. Caution the woman not to douche; douching is contraindicated throughout pregnancy. Some women may wear perineal pads to control the discharge. Caution women not to use tampons, however, because this could lead to stasis of secretions and subsequent infection. Wearing cotton underpants and sleeping at night without underwear also are helpful in reducing moisture and possible vulvar excoriation. Advise women to contact their physician or nurse-midwife if there is a change in the color, odor, or character of this discharge, which might suggest infection.

A woman with vulvar pruritus needs evaluation because this strongly indicates infection. Be certain she is describing pruritus-like symptoms and is not describing burning on urination, a sign of an early bladder infection (which also needs therapy, but of a different type). Common vaginal infections that present with pruritus are discussed in Chapter 47.

Avoiding tight underpants and pantyhose may help prevent vulvar and vaginal infections, particularly yeast infections. Although over-the-counter medications for yeast infections are available, caution women to contact their health care provider rather than self-treat vaginal infections during pregnancy. Some medications (metronidazole [Flagyl], in particular) prescribed for trichomonas are not recommended during early pregnancy due to possible **teratogenicity** (fetal harm).

A woman who is uncomfortable about discussing this part of her body or who associates vaginal infections with poor hygiene or sexually transmitted disease may be reluctant to mention an irritating vaginal discharge. Therefore, at each prenatal visit, be sure to ask each woman specifically whether she is experiencing this problem.

WHAT IF? A pregnant woman nearing the end of her first trimester comes to the clinic concerned because she has urinary frequency. She also reports a white vaginal discharge. How would you go about evaluating this woman to determine whether she is experiencing a normal discomfort of pregnancy or a urinary tract infection?

Discomforts of Middle to Late Pregnancy

At approximately the 20th to 24th weeks, the midpoint of pregnancy, a woman is usually ready for further health teaching that relates to the new developments that will occur in the latter half of pregnancy. She should be informed of the signs and symptoms of beginning labor. As she starts to view the child within her as a separate person, she becomes interested in discussing and making plans for labor, birth, and the infant's care. The midpoint of a pregnancy also is a good time to review the precautionary measures to prevent constipation, varicosities, and hemorrhoids and to describe the new minor symptoms that may occur.

Nursing Diagnoses

Possible nursing diagnoses associated with the discomforts of middle to late pregnancy include the following:

- Health-seeking behaviors related to discomforts of middle to late pregnancy
- Acute pain related to postural changes in pregnancy
- Anxiety related to lack of information about shortness of breath resulting from expanding uterine pressure on diaphragm
- Deficient knowledge related to occurrence of Braxton Hicks contractions in late pregnancy

Box 11-2 highlights appropriate outcomes and interventions related to monitoring the mother in the later part of pregnancy, using the terminology identified by the Nursing Outcomes Classification (NOC) and Nursing Interventions Classification (NIC).

Backache

As pregnancy advances, a lumbar lordosis occurs and postural changes necessary to maintain balance may lead to backache. Wearing shoes with low to moderate heels reduces the amount of spinal curvature necessary to maintain an upright posture. Encouraging the woman to walk with her pelvis tilted forward (putting pelvic support under the weight of the fetus) is also helpful. In addition, applying local heat may aid in relieving backache.

BOX 11.2

NURSING OUTCOMES AND NURSING INTERVENTIONS CLASSIFICATION: MONITORING IN LATE PREGNANCY

NOC: Maternal Status, Antepartum

Maternal status, antepartum is defined as the conditions and behaviors indicating maternal well-being from conception to the onset of labor (Johnson, Maas, & Moorhead, 2000). Some specific indicators suggesting achievement of this outcome may include:

- Evidence of emotional attachment to the fetus
- Ability to cope with discomforts of pregnancy
- Weight change within expected range
- Vital signs within expected parameters
- Laboratory test results such as urine protein and glucose, blood glucose, hemoglobin, and liver enzymes within expected range

NOC: Fetal Status, Antepartum

Fetal status, antepartum is defined as the conditions indicating fetal physical well-being from conception to the onset of labor (Johnson, Maas, & Moorhead, 2000). Some specific indicators suggesting achievement of this outcome may include:

- Fetal heart rate between 120 and 160 beats per minute
- Fetal ultrasound growth and movement frequency and pattern within expected range

NIC: Surveillance, Late Pregnancy

Surveillance, late pregnancy is defined as the purposeful and ongoing acquisition, interpretation, and synthesis of maternal-fetal data for treatment, observation, or admission (McCloskey & Bulechek, 2000). Some important activities to include when implementing this intervention include:

- Determining maternal-fetal health risk(s) through client interview
- Monitoring maternal vital signs
- Inquiring about presence and quality of fetal movements
- Monitoring for signs of PIH, urinary tract infection, and preterm labor
- Assessing elimination patterns
- Interpreting results of diagnostic tests
- Monitoring comfort level, nutritional status, changes in sleep patterns, and uterine activity
- Obtaining history of sexually transmitted diseases and frequency of intercourse as appropriate
- Instituting appropriate treatment according to standard protocols

To avoid back strain, advise women to squat rather than bend over to pick up objects. Also encourage them always to lift objects by holding them close to the body. For some women, a firmer mattress during this time may be required. Sliding a board under the mattress is a cost-effective alternative for achieving a firmer sleeping surface. Pelvic rocking or tilting, an exercise described in Chapter 13, also helps to prevent and relieve backache.

Backache can be an initial sign of a bladder or kidney infection. Thus, obtaining a detailed account of the woman's symptoms is crucial to ensure that she is describing only backache. Too often, women are observed at a prenatal visit only lying in a lithotomy position on an examining table. Always assess the manner in which the woman walks and what type of shoes she is wearing as she moves from the waiting room to the examining room to evaluate whether her posture or shoes could be a cause.

Caution women not to take herbal remedies, muscle relaxants, or analgesics (or any other medication) for back pain without first consulting their physician or nurse-midwife. Generally, acetaminophen (Tylenol) is considered to be safe and effective for relieving this type of pain during pregnancy.

Headache

Many women experience headache during pregnancy, apparently from their expanding blood volume, which puts pressure on cerebral arteries. Trying to reduce any possible causative situations, such as eye strain or tension, may lessen the number of headaches they experience. Resting with cold towels on their forehead and taking usual adult doses of acetaminophen usually furnish adequate relief. Although a few women who have migraine headaches find these worsen during pregnancy, most women notice considerable improvement with this type of headache (see Chapter 49). Caution women that if a headache is unusually intense or continuous, they should report it to their primary care provider. This type of headache may be a danger sign of pregnancy.

Dyspnea

As the expanding uterus puts pressure on the diaphragm, causing some lung compression, shortness of breath may occur. A woman will notice this primarily at night when her body is flat. She also will definitely notice it on exertion. Sitting upright, allowing the weight of the uterus to fall away from the diaphragm, helps to relieve the problem. As pregnancy progresses, the woman may require two or more pillows to sleep on at night to avoid dyspnea. Caution her to limit her activities during the day before she becomes short of breath. Always question women about this important symptom at prenatal visits to be certain the sensation is not continuous, which describes more than usual involvement.

Ankle Edema

Most women experience some swelling of the ankles and feet during late pregnancy, most noticeably at the end of the day. Women are often conscious of this first when they kick off their shoes and then cannot put them on again comfortably.

As long as proteinuria and hypertension are absent, ankle edema of this nature is a normal occurrence of pregnancy. It is probably caused by reduced blood circulation in the lower extremities due to uterine pressure and general fluid retention. This simple edema can be relieved best by resting in a left side-lying position because this increases the kidney's glomerular filtration rate and allows good venous return. Sitting for half an hour in the afternoon and again in the evening with the legs elevated is also helpful. Women should avoid wearing constricting clothing such as panty girdles or knee-high stockings because these impede lower extremity circulation and venous return.

Some women need reassurance that ankle edema is normal during pregnancy. Otherwise, they worry that it is a beginning sign of PIH. On the other hand, do not dismiss a report of lower extremity edema lightly until you are certain the woman does not exhibit any signs of proteinuria or edema of other, nondependent parts, or has had a sudden increase in weight indicative of pregnancy-induced hypertension.

Braxton Hicks Contractions

Beginning as early as the 8th to 12th week of pregnancy, the uterus periodically contracts and then relaxes again. Early in pregnancy, these contractions, termed **Braxton Hicks contractions,** are not noticeable. In middle and late pregnancy, the contractions become stronger, and the woman who tenses at the sensation may even experience some minimal pain, similar to a hard menstrual cramp. Although these contractions are not a sign of beginning labor, women should telephone or e-mail their primary care provider to report them so that they can be evaluated. A rhythmic pattern of contractions can be a beginning sign of labor.

> ✔ **CHECKPOINT QUESTIONS**
>
> 10. Why might a pregnant woman experience shortness of breath?
> 11. What position is best for relieving ankle edema during pregnancy?

Danger Signs of Pregnancy

Assure the pregnant woman that you have no reason to think she is going to experience any serious problems, that you have every reason to believe she is going to have a normal, uncomplicated pregnancy (assuming that is true), but that if any of the things described below should occur she should inform her health care provider by telephone or e-mail immediately. Be certain you give her an alternate contact number to call if the health care facility is closed. Emphasize that if one of these danger signs should occur, it serves merely as a signal of the possibility that something may happen. It is important for her to report it immediately so it can be dealt with before something harmful does occur.

Vaginal Bleeding

A woman should report vaginal bleeding, no matter how slight, because some of the serious bleeding complications of pregnancy begin with slight spotting. When talking with the woman, ask her how she discovered the spotting. If she discovered it on toilet paper following a bowel movement, she may be reporting spotting from hemorrhoids. Until the bleeding is found to be innocent, all women with spotting need further evaluation.

Persistent Vomiting

Once- or twice-daily vomiting is not uncommon during the first trimester of pregnancy. However, persistent, frequent vomiting is not normal. Vomiting that continues past the 12th week of pregnancy is also extended vomiting. Persistent or extended vomiting depletes the nutritional supply available to the fetus and is a danger to the pregnancy. (See Chap. 12 for a discussion of persistent vomiting [hyperemesis gravidarum].)

Chills and Fever

Chills and fever may indicate an intrauterine infection, a serious complication for both the woman and the fetus. They also may be symptoms of a relatively benign gastroenteritis. However, because the woman cannot make a definite determination about the cause, further evaluation by a health care provider is necessary.

Sudden Escape of Clear Fluid From the Vagina

When clear fluid is discharged suddenly from the vagina, the membranes may have ruptured. Although this may be one of the first signs of labor, mother and fetus are now both threatened because the uterine cavity is no longer sealed against infection. If the fetus is small and the head does not fit snugly into the cervix, the umbilical cord may prolapse. If the cord is then compressed by the fetal head, the fetus is in immediate and grave danger. Alerting the health care provider to any sudden escape of fluid is crucial so a safe and controlled birth can be planned. Occasionally, a woman confuses stress incontinence (involuntary loss of urine on coughing or sneezing or lifting a heavy object) for this. In this situation, vaginal examination typically reveals that the membranes are still intact.

Abdominal or Chest Pain

Abdominal pain at any time is a signal that something is abnormal, so women should report it immediately. Some women may think that it is normal because the growing uterus is deflecting their other organs from the usual alignment, but they are wrong: the uterus expands painlessly. Abdominal pain is a sign of some other problem, such as a tubal (ectopic) pregnancy, separation of the placenta, preterm labor, or something unrelated to the pregnancy but perhaps equally as serious, such as appendicitis, ulcer, or pancreatitis. Chest pain may indicate a pulmonary embolus, a complication that may follow thrombophlebitis.

Pregnancy-Induced Hypertension (PIH)

PIH refers to a potentially severe and even fatal elevation of blood pressure during pregnancy. A number of symptoms signal that PIH is developing:

1. Rapid weight gain (over 2 lb per week in the second trimester, 1 lb per week in the third trimester)
2. Swelling of the face or fingers
3. Flashes of light or dots before the eyes
4. Dimness or blurring of vision
5. Severe, continuous headache
6. Decreased urine output

Some edema of the ankles during pregnancy is normal, particularly if it occurs after the woman has been on her feet for a long period of time. Swelling of the hands (ask if she has noticed that her rings are tight) or face (difficulty opening eyes in the morning due to edema of the eyelids) indicates edema too extensive to be normal. Visual disturbances or a continuous headache may signal cerebral edema or acute hypertension. Be certain the woman is not reporting symptoms she had before she became pregnant. If she had the same visual difficulties and headaches before pregnancy as she is reporting now, she may need to see an ophthalmologist rather than her obstetrician for help with the problem. (See Chap. 15 for more on PIH.)

Increase or Decrease in Fetal Movement

Because a fetus normally moves more or less the same amount every day, an unusual increase or decrease in movement suggests that the fetus is responding to the need for oxygen. Be sure to question the client about typical fetal movement and whether she has noticed any increase or decrease recently. Also emphasize the need for the client to report any changes so that further testing and follow-up can be done. Tests of fetal movement are discussed in Chapter 8.

PREVENTION OF FETAL EXPOSURE TO TERATOGENS

A **teratogen** is any factor, chemical or physical, that adversely affects the fertilized ovum, embryo, or fetus. To reach maturity in optimal health, a fetus needs sound genes (see Chap. 7) and a healthy intrauterine environment that protects it from the influence of teratogens.

At one time, it was assumed that a fetus in utero was protected from chemical or physical injury by the presence of the amniotic fluid and by the absence of any direct placental exchange between mother and fetus. When infants were born with disorders, it was often attributed to the influence of fate, bad luck, or, in some cultures, evil spirits. Today, it is acknowledged that a fetus is extremely vulnerable to environmental injury. Although many anomalies occurring in utero are still unknown, many teratogenic factors have been isolated (Ances, 2002).

Effects of Teratogens on the Fetus

Several factors influence the amount of damage a teratogen can cause. The strength of the teratogen is one factor. For example, radiation is a known teratogen. In small amounts (everyone is exposed to some radiation every day, such as from sun rays), it causes no damage. However, in large doses (e.g., the amount of radiation necessary to treat cancer of the cervix), serious fetal defects or death can occur.

The timing of the teratogenic insult is another factor that makes a significant difference. If a teratogen is introduced before implantation, either the zygote is destroyed or appears unaffected. If the insult occurs when the main body systems are being formed (in the 2nd to 8th weeks of embryonic life), the fetus is very vulnerable to injury. During the last trimester, the potential for harm again decreases because all the organs of the fetus are formed and are merely maturing. The times when different anatomic areas of the fetus are most likely to be affected by teratogens are shown in Figure 8-5.

Two known exceptions to the rule that deformities usually occur in early embryonic life are the effects caused by the organisms of syphilis and toxoplasmosis. These two infections can cause abnormalities in organs that were originally formed normally.

A third factor determining the effects of a teratogen is the teratogen's affinity for specific tissue. Lead, for instance, attacks and disables nervous tissue. Thalidomide causes limb defects. Tetracycline causes tooth enamel deficiencies and, possibly, long bone deformities. The rubella virus, on the other hand, can affect many organs: the eyes, ears, heart, and brain are the four most commonly attacked.

Nursing Diagnoses

It is important for nurses who care for women during pregnancy to be familiar with the various categories of teratogens. Much of the health history information obtained at prenatal visits helps to determine whether the woman has been exposed to a teratogen since the last visit.

Possible nursing diagnoses associated with maternal exposure to teratogens may include:

- Health-seeking behavior related to mother's interest in avoiding exposure to substances harmful to the fetus during pregnancy
- Risk for fetal injury related to lack of knowledge about teratogenicity of alcohol, drugs, and cigarettes
- Risk for infection related to fetal transmission from possible maternal exposure to genital herpes

Teratogenic Maternal Infections

Teratogenic maternal infections can involve either sexually transmitted or systemic infections. This group of diseases has been described collectively under the umbrella term TORCH, an abbreviation for toxoplasmosis, rubella, cytomegalovirus, and herpes simplex virus. (Some sources identify the O with "other infections," which could include syphilis, hepatitis B virus [HBV], and human immunodeficiency virus [HIV].) All these infections are known to cross the placenta and affect the fetus during pregnancy. The TORCH screen was developed as an immunologic survey to determine whether these infections exist in either the pregnant woman (to identify fetal risk factors) or the newborn (to detect if antibodies against the common infectious teratogens are present). Although it is now known that many more than the original four or five maternal infections can harm the fetus or newborn (a chlamydia or streptococcal B infection, for example, can cause pneumonia in the newborn [see Chap. 26]), the TORCH screen still provides a quick way to assess the potential risk of teratogenic infection in pregnant women and newborns.

Infections that cross the placenta can be viral, bacterial, or protozoan. Most cause relatively mild, flulike symptoms in a woman but can have much more serious effects on the fetus or newborn. Preventing and predicting fetal injury from infection is complicated because a disease may be subclinical (without symptoms in the mother) and yet may injure the fetus. The most common teratogenic infections are described in more detail below.

Toxoplasmosis

Toxoplasmosis, a protozoan infection, is spread most commonly through contact with uncooked meat, although it may also be contracted through handling cat stool in soil or cat litter (Cook et al., 2000). The woman experiences almost no symptoms of the disease except a few days of malaise and posterior cervical lymphadenopathy. If the infection crosses the placenta, the infant may be born with central nervous system damage, hydrocephalus, microcephaly, intracerebral calcification, and retinal deformities. If the diagnosis is established by serum analysis during pregnancy, therapy with sulfonamides may be prescribed. However, the prevention of fetal deformities is uncertain, and sulfa may lead to increased bilirubin levels in the newborn. Pyrimethamine, an antiprotozoal agent, may also be used. This drug is an antifolic acid drug, so it is not administered early in pregnancy to prevent reducing folic acid levels.

Prepregnancy serum analysis can be done to identify women who have never had the disease and so are susceptible (about 50% of women). Removing a cat from the home during pregnancy as a means of prevention is not necessary as long as the cat is healthy. On the other hand, taking in a new cat is unwise. Instruct pregnant women to avoid undercooked meat and also not to change a cat litter box or work in soil in an area where cats may defecate.

Rubella

The rubella virus usually causes only a mild rash and mild systemic illness in the mother, but the teratogenic effects on the fetus can be devastating. Fetal damage from maternal infection with rubella (German measles) includes deafness, mental and motor challenges, cataracts, cardiac defects (most commonly patent ductus arteriosus and pulmonary stenosis), retarded intrauterine growth (small for gestational age), thrombocytopenic purpura, and dental and facial clefts, such as cleft lip and palate (Lee & Bowden, 2000).

Typically, a rubella titer is obtained on the first prenatal visit. A titer greater than 1:8 suggests immunity to rubella. A titer of less than 1:8 suggests that the woman is susceptible to viral invasion. A titer that is greatly increased over a previous reading or is initially extremely high suggests that a recent infection has occurred.

A woman who is not immunized before pregnancy cannot be immunized during pregnancy because the vaccine uses a live virus that would have effects similar to those occurring with a subclinical case of rubella. After a rubella immunization, a woman is advised not to become pregnant for 3 months until the rubella virus is no longer active. Immediately after a pregnancy, all women with low rubella titers should be immunized to provide protection against rubella in future pregnancies.

An increasing concern is women who demonstrate antibodies against rubella yet become reinfected during pregnancy. Because of this, pregnant women should avoid contact with children with rashes. Infants who are born to mothers who had rubella during pregnancy may be capable of transmitting the disease for up to 8 months after birth. The infant needs to be isolated from other newborns during the newborn period. The mother should be made aware of the possibility that her infant might infect others, including pregnant women. Nurses should receive immunization against rubella to ensure that they neither spread nor contract the disease.

Cytomegalovirus

Cytomegalovirus (CMV), a member of the herpes virus family, is another teratogen that can cause extensive damage to a fetus while causing few symptoms in the woman. It is transmitted by droplet infection from person to person. Forty percent to 100% of women are estimated to have been infected with CMV before pregnancy (Minkoff, 2000). If a woman acquires a primary CMV infection during pregnancy and the virus crosses the placenta, congenital CMV infection can occur. Because the woman has almost no symptoms, she may not be aware that she has contracted an infection. However, the infant may be born severely neurologically challenged (hydrocephalus, microcephaly, spasticity), with eye damage (optic atrophy, chorioretinitis), deafness, or chronic liver disease. The child's skin may be covered with large petechiae ("blueberry-muffin" lesions). Diagnosis in the mother or infant can be established by the isolation of CMV antibodies in serum. Unfortunately, no treatment for the infection exists even if it presents in the mother with enough symptoms to allow detection. Because there is no treatment or vaccine for the disease, routine screening for CMV during pregnancy is not recommended. Women can help prevent exposure by thorough handwashing before eating and avoiding crowds of young children at daycare or nursery settings.

Like herpes simplex, a primary CMV infection may become latent and then reactivate periodically. These recurrences are not thought to have a teratogenic effect on the fetus, but they can cause infection of the newborn during birth from genital secretions, or postpartum from exposure to CMV-infected breast milk. CMV infection contracted at or shortly after birth is not associated with serious adverse effects except in babies of very low birthweight (1,200 g).

Herpes Simplex Virus (Genital Herpes Infection)

A primary, first-episode genital herpes infection in a pregnant woman poses a substantial risk to the fetus. The first time a woman contracts a genital herpes infection, systemic involvement occurs. The virus spreads into the bloodstream (viremia) and crosses the placenta to the fetus.

If the infection takes place in the first trimester, severe congenital anomalies or spontaneous miscarriage may occur. If the infection occurs during the second or third trimester, there is a high incidence of premature birth, intrauterine growth retardation, and continuing infection of the newborn at birth. Unless recognized and treated, the fetal mortality and morbidity rates are as high as 60% (Minkoff, 2000).

If the woman has had herpes simplex virus type 1 infections before the genital herpes invasion or if the genital herpes (type 2) infection is a recurrence, antibodies to the virus in her system prevent spread of the virus to the fetus across the placenta. If genital lesions are present at the time of birth, however, the fetus may contract the virus during birth. For women with a history of genital herpes and existing genital lesions, cesarean birth is often advised to reduce the risk of neonatal infection. This awareness of the placental spread of herpes simplex virus has increased the importance of obtaining information about exposure to genital herpes or any painful perineal or vaginal lesions that might indicate this infection at prenatal visits (Minkoff, 2000).

Intravenous or oral acyclovir (Zovirax) can be administered to women during pregnancy (Karch, 2001). The primary mechanism for protecting the fetus, however, focuses on disease prevention. Urging women to practice safer sex is important to lessen their exposure to this and other sexually transmitted diseases.

Other Viral Diseases

It has been difficult to demonstrate other viral teratogens, but rubeola (measles), coxsackievirus, mumps, varicella (chickenpox), poliomyelitis, influenza, and viral hepatitis all may be teratogenic. Parvovirus B19, the causative agent of erythema infectiosum (also called fifth disease), if contracted during pregnancy, can cross the placenta and attack the red blood cells of the fetus. Infection during early pregnancy is associated with fetal death. If the infection occurs late in pregnancy, the infant may be born with severe anemia and congenital heart disease (Ely et al., 2000).

Syphilis. Syphilis, a sexually transmitted infection, is of great concern for the maternal–fetal population despite the availability of accurate screening tests and proven medical treatment (Genc & Ledger, 2000). A syphilis infection during pregnancy can place the fetus at risk for congenital syphilis. The causative spirochete, *Treponema pallidum,* can extensively damage the fetus after the 16th to 18th week of intrauterine life, when the cytotrophoblastic layer of the placental villi has atrophied and no longer protects against it. If detected and treated before this time, the fetus is rarely affected. However, if left untreated beyond the 18th week of gestation, deafness, cognitive challenge, osteochondritis, and fetal death are possible.

Safer sex practices, early detection, and immediate treatment with antibiotics are the best ways to limit congenital syphilis. Serologic screening (either a VDRL or a rapid plasma reagin) should be done at the first prenatal visit; the test may then be repeated again close to term (the 8th month). Even when a woman has been treated with appropriate antibiotics, the serum titer remains high for more than 200 days; an increasing titer, however, suggests that reinfection has occurred. In an infant born to a woman with syphilis, the serologic test for syphilis may remain positive for up to 3 months even though the disease was treated during pregnancy. Benzathine penicillin is often used as therapy because it is long-acting and may be given safely during pregnancy.

The newborn with congenital syphilis may have congenital anomalies, extreme rhinitis (sniffles), and a characteristic syphilitic rash, all of which identify the baby as high-risk at birth. Medical and nursing care of the newborn with congenital syphilis is discussed in Chapter 26.

Lyme Disease. Lyme disease, a multisystem disease caused by the spirochete *Borrelia burgdorferi,* is spread by the bite of a deer tick. The highest incidence occurs in the summer and early fall. The largest outbreaks of the disease are found on the east coast of the United States (Hu & Klempner, 2001). After the tick bite, a typical skin rash, *erythema chronicum migrans* (large, macular lesions with a clear center), develops. Pain in large body joints such as the knee may be present. Infection in pregnancy can result in spontaneous miscarriage or severe congenital anomalies.

Women anticipating becoming pregnant or who are pregnant should avoid areas such as wooded or tall grassy areas where they are apt to be bitten by ticks. If hiking in these areas, a woman should avoid the use of tick repellents containing diethyltoluamide because this ingredient is teratogenic. Instead, she should wear long, light-colored slacks tucked into her socks to prevent her legs from being exposed. To spread the spirochete, the tick must be present on the body possibly as long as 24 hours. After returning home from an outing, the woman should inspect her body carefully and immediately remove any ticks found. If she has any symptoms that suggest Lyme disease or knows she has been bitten, she should contact her primary health care provider immediately. Treatment of Lyme disease for pregnant women differs from that for nonpregnant women. The drugs used for nonpregnant adults, tetracycline and doxycycline, cannot be used during pregnancy because they cause tooth discoloration and, possibly, long-bone malformation in the fetus. A course of penicillin will be prescribed to reduce symptoms in the pregnant woman.

Because the symptoms of Lyme disease are chronic but not dramatic (a migratory rash and joint pain), women may not report them at a prenatal visit unless they are educated about their importance and are asked at prenatal visits if such symptoms are present.

Infections That Cause Illness at Birth. A number of infections are not teratogenic to the fetus during pregnancy but are harmful if they are present at the time of birth. Gonorrhea, candidiasis, chlamydia, streptococcus B, and hepatitis B infections are examples of these. Chapters 26 and 47 discuss the effects of these infections on maternal, fetal, and neonatal health.

Potential Teratogenicity of Vaccines

Live virus vaccines, such as measles, mumps, rubella, and poliomyelitis (Sabin type), are contraindicated during pregnancy because they may transmit the viral infection to the fetus. Care must be taken in routine immunization programs to make sure that adolescents about to be vaccinated are not pregnant or do not become pregnant until about 3 months afterward. Women who work in biologic laboratories where vaccines are manufactured are well advised not to work with live virus products during pregnancy.

Teratogenicity of Drugs

Many women, assuming that the rule of being cautious with drugs during pregnancy applies only to prescription drugs, take over-the-counter drugs or herbal supplements freely. Although not all drugs cross the placenta (e.g., heparin does not because of its large molecular size), most do. Also, even though most herbs are safe, ginseng, for example, used to improve general well-being, or senna, used to relieve constipation, may not be safe (Allaire et al., 2000).

To identify drugs that are unsafe for ingestion during pregnancy, the U.S. Food and Drug Administration (FDA) has established five categories of safety (Table 11-1). It is important to recognize two principles related to drug intake during pregnancy:

- Any drug or herbal supplement, under certain circumstances, may be detrimental to fetal welfare. Therefore, during pregnancy, women should not take any drug or supplement not specifically prescribed or approved by their physician or nurse-midwife.
- A woman of childbearing age and ability should take no drugs other than those prescribed by a physician or nurse-midwife to avoid exposure to a drug should she become pregnant.

The classic teratogenic drug is thalidomide, once liberally prescribed for morning sickness in Europe. Never approved for use in the United States, thalidomide caused amelia or phocomelia (total or partial absence of extremities) in 100% of instances when taken between the 34th and 45th day of pregnancy. Isotretinoin (Accutane), a drug commonly prescribed for adolescent acne, is an example of a teratogenic drug still in use today. Other examples of drugs capable of being teratogenic are shown in Table 11-2.

The use of recreational drugs during pregnancy puts a fetus at risk in two ways: the drug may have a direct teratogenic effect, and intravenous drug use also risks exposure to diseases such as HIV and hepatitis B.

Narcotics such as meperidine (Demerol) and heroin have long been implicated as causing intrauterine growth retardation. The use of marijuana alone apparently does not, although the long-term effects of marijuana during pregnancy are still unstudied (Kozer & Koren, 2001). Cocaine, particularly its crack form, is harmful to the fetus because it causes vasoconstriction in the mother, compromising placental blood supply and so interfering with the fetal nutrient supply. Its use is associated with spontaneous miscarriage, preterm labor, meconium staining, and intrauterine growth retardation. Children of cocaine users may suffer long-term effects, such as learning disorders or poor attention span (Delaney-Black et al., 2000). However, studies are contradictory as to the extent of long-term effects (Frank et al., 2001). See Chapter 17 for more information on the hazards of cocaine or heroin use during pregnancy.

An area of recreational drug use that needs to be examined is that of inhalant abuse ("huffing"). Substances frequently used as inhalants include gasoline, butane lighter fluid, Freon, glue, and nitrous oxide. Although the teratogenic properties of inhalants are not well studied, they all carry the possibility of respiratory distress, which could limit the oxygen supply to the fetus (Kurtzman et al., 2001).

Teratogenicity of Alcohol

Evidence over the years has shown that when women consumed a large quantity of alcohol during pregnancy, their babies showed a high incidence of congenital deformities and cognitive impairment. It was assumed that these defects were the result of the mother's poor nutritional sta-

TABLE 11.1 Pregnancy Risk Categories of Drugs

CATEGORY	DESCRIPTION	EXAMPLE
A	Adequate studies in pregnant women have failed to show a risk to the fetus in the first trimester of pregnancy; there is no evidence of risk in later trimesters.	Thyroid hormone
B	Animal studies have not shown an adverse effect on the fetus, but there are no adequate clinical studies in pregnant women.	Insulin
C	Animal studies have shown an adverse effect on the fetus, but there are no adequate studies on humans, or there are no adequate studies in animals or humans. Pregnancy risk is unknown.	Docusate sodium (Colace)
D	There is evidence of risk to the human fetus, but the potential benefits of use in pregnant women may be acceptable despite potential risks.	Lithium citrate
X	Studies in animals or humans show fetal abnormalities, or adverse reaction reports indicate evidence of fetal risk. The risks involved clearly outweigh potential benefits.	Isotretinoin (Accutane)

Karch, A.M. (2001). *Lippincott's nursing drug guide.* Philadelphia: Lippincott Williams & Wilkins.

TABLE 11.2 Some Potentially or Positively Teratogenic Drugs

CATEGORY	DRUG	DRUG USE	TERATOGENIC EFFECT
Vitamin A derivatives	Isotretinoin (Accutane) Etretinate (Tegison)	Acne Psoriasis	Craniofacial, cardiac, CNS anomalies Craniofacial, cardiac, CNS anomalies
Alcohol	Wine, whiskey	Social use	Fetal alcohol syndrome
Analgesics	Acetylsalicylic acid (aspirin) NSAIDs	Minor pain relief	Prolonged pregnancy; maternal bleeding Patent ductus arteriosus
Antineoplastics	Methotrexate Cyclophosphamide (Cytoxan)	Chemotherapy Chemotherapy	Multiple anomalies Multiple anomalies
Androgens	Danazol	Endometriosis	Masculinization of female fetus
Anticonvulsants	Phenytoin (Dilantin) Valproic acid Carbamazepine Lamotrigine	Seizures	Fetal hydantoin syndrome Neural tube defects Neural tube defects Possibly fetal anomalies
Anticoagulants	Warfarin (Coumarin)	Anticoagulation	Fetal bleeding or anomalies
Antidepressants	Imipramine (Tofranil)	Elevate mood	Cardiovascular anomalies
Antischizophrenic	Lithium	Schizophrenia	Hydramnios
Antithyroid	Methimazole	Hypothyroidism	Hypothyroidism in fetus
Antibiotics	Ribavirin Sulfonamides Tetracycline	Respiratory infection Infection Infection	Multiple anomalies Hyperbilirubinemia in newborn Teeth and bone deformities
Antihelmintics	Lindane	Eradication of lice	Manufacturer recommendation of limiting exposure to 2 doses
Angiotensin-converting enzyme inhibitors	Enalapril (Vasotec) Captopril (Capoten)	Reduce hypertension	Oligohydramnios
Caffeine	Caffeine	Coffee, soft drinks, chocolate	Low birth weight
Hypoglycemics	Tolbutamide (Orinase)	Type II diabetes	Profound hypoglycemia in newborn
Nicotine		Cigarette smoke	Growth retardation
Radiopharmaceuticals	Iodide-131	Diagnostic studies	May destroy thyroid of fetus
Narcotics	Cocaine Heroin	Social pleasure	Dysmorphic and CNS anomalies Growth retardation; narcotic withdrawal in newborn
Tranquilizers	Benzodiazepine (diazepam)	Reduce anxiety	Growth retardation; CNS dysfunction Hypotonia, respiratory depression
Vaccines (live)	Rubella	Provide immunity	Possible infection in fetus

Niebyl, J.R. (2000). Teratology and drugs in pregnancy. In Scott, J.R., et al. *Danforth's obstetrics and gynecology* (8th ed., pp. 197–211). Philadelphia: Lippincott Williams & Wilkins.

tus (drinking alcohol rather than eating food), not necessarily the direct result of the alcohol. However, alcohol has now been firmly isolated as a teratogen. Fetuses cannot remove the breakdown products of alcohol from their body. The large buildup of these leads to vitamin B deficiency and accompanying neurologic damage.

It is important to screen women during pregnancy for alcohol use because an infant born with **fetal alcohol syndrome** is small for gestational age and cognitively challenged and has a characteristic craniofacial deformity including short palpebral fissures, a thin upper lip, and an upturned nose (Chasnoff et al., 2001). Because of individual variations in metabolism, it is impossible to define a safe level of alcohol consumption. Women are best advised, therefore, to abstain from alcohol completely. An important area for research is how to help women stop drinking alcohol (Hankin et al., 2000). Women with alcohol addiction should be referred to an alcohol treatment program as early in pregnancy as possible to help them reduce their alcohol intake (see Focus on Nursing Care Planning).

Teratogenicity of Cigarettes

Cigarette smoking is associated with infertility in women (Hruska et al., 2000). Cigarette smoking by a pregnant woman has been shown to have teratogenic effects on the fetus, especially growth retardation. In addition, these children are at greater risk than others for sudden infant death syndrome (Pollack, 2001). Low birthweight in infants of smoking mothers results from vasoconstriction of the uter-

FOCUS ON *Nursing Care Planning*

A PREGNANT WOMAN WITH THREATS TO FETAL HEALTH

A 20-year-old pregnant woman comes to the prenatal clinic reporting mild nausea and occasional vomiting in the morning. "Sometimes I just can't eat. My friend said that I should try smoking marijuana to help."

Assessment: Gravida 1, para 0. Unsure of date of last menstrual period—approximately 16 weeks ago. Uterine height at 2 cm above symphysis. Fetal heart rate at 148 beats per minute via Doppler. History of frequent sinus headaches. "I use Sudafed (pseudoephedrine) at least 3 to 4 times a week and Neo-synephrine nasal spray at least once every day." Smokes 2 packs of cigarettes per day. Started smoking at age 15 years. Drinks 2 to 3 beers/week "just to unwind." Denies history of marijuana or other recreational drug use.

Nursing Diagnosis: Risk for fetal injury related to knowledge deficit concerning possible fetal exposure to teratogens.

Outcome Identification: Client will demonstrate positive behaviors to reduce risk of injury to the fetus. Fetal growth and development will be within appropriate parameters.

Outcome Evaluation: Client reports a decrease in smoking to 10 cigarettes/day or less and no alcohol consumption; verbalizes no use of recreational drugs, including marijuana; demonstrates absence of behaviors indicative of alcohol or drug use; states contact with health care providers about use of sinus medications.

Interventions	Rationales
1. Review history of sinus headache for onset, type, duration, and relief obtained.	1. History review provides a baseline to determine future interventions and provides information of the severity of the client's condition.
2. Consult with client's primary and maternal health care providers about safety of over-the-counter (OTC) medications.	2. OTC medication use must be addressed to determine the degree of possible teratogenicity to the fetus.
3. Discuss with client possible nonpharmacologic measures to assist with sinus headache relief, including saline nasal sprays, humidification, and warm compresses to nasal area.	3. Nonpharmacologic comfort measures may provide symptomatic relief without danger to the fetus.
4. Discuss possible dangers of drug and alcohol use during pregnancy and instruct client about possible dangers.	4. Alcohol and drug use, including OTC medications, can be teratogenic to the fetus. Education provides valuable information to foster client's motivation for changing behaviors.
5. Encourage the client to decrease smoking and quit if possible. Offer suggestions to accomplish this, including use of sugar-free gums or candies, distraction, and activity. Refer to a smoking cessation group if appropriate.	5. Cigarette use during pregnancy can lead to fetal growth retardation. Support and suggestions provide concrete measures to assist client with cutting down and cessation.
6. Suggest client replace alcohol consumption with caffeine-free beverage intake.	6. Alcohol consumption during pregnancy is associated with fetal alcohol syndrome. Caffeine may be an associated fetal teratogen.
7. Review measures to combat nausea and vomiting, such as dry crackers, small frequent meals, and fluid intake. Encourage client to participate in discussion and offer suggestions appropriate for her lifestyle.	7. Adequate nutrition and hydration are important for fetal growth and development. Client participation helps to individualize care, increase feelings of control, and promote compliance.
8. Anticipate the need for follow-up ultrasound examination for fetal growth evaluation.	8. Follow-up ultrasound examination provides evidence for evaluation of fetal growth and development according to age-appropriate parameters.

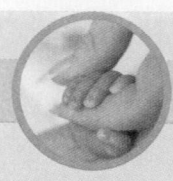

ine vessels, an effect of nicotine that limits the blood supply to the fetus. Another contributory effect may be related to inhaled carbon monoxide. Thus, inhaling the smoke of another person's cigarettes may be as harmful as actually smoking the cigarettes. All prenatal health care settings should be smoke-free environments for this reason.

If the woman cannot stop smoking during pregnancy (and, realistically, many women cannot), reducing the number of cigarettes smoked per day should help diminish adverse effects on the fetus. This should also serve to protect the woman's own health.

It is very difficult for the average woman to stop smoking. The best way to urge women to discontinue smoking is to educate them about the risks to themselves and their fetus at the first prenatal visit. When doing this teaching, keep in mind that varying cultures use cigarettes more than others. It may be effective to encourage women to sign a contract with a health care provider to try to stop or to join a smoking-cessation program. Be certain pregnant women know that they should not enter a stop-smoking program that uses drug therapy such as nicotine patches, because the substitute drug may be as harmful to the fetus as smoking.

Environmental Teratogens

Teratogens from environmental sources can be as lethal to the fetus as those that are directly or deliberately ingested. Women can be exposed to many of these through contact at outside jobs or care of their family. For example, washing children's hair with a shampoo such as lindane (Kwell) to remove lice should be limited to two exposures (Karch, 2001).

Metal and Chemical Hazards

Pesticides and carbon monoxide such as from automobile exhaust are examples of chemical teratogens that are harmful and should be avoided. Chemicals in a variety of work environments also can be quite dangerous, such as arsenic, a byproduct of copper and lead smelting, used in pesticides, paints, and leather processing; formaldehyde, used in paper manufacturing; and mercury, used in the manufacture of electrical apparatus. Additional information on specific chemicals can be obtained from the National Institute for Occupational Safety and Health (NIOSH) at their web site (*www.cdc.gov/NIOSH*).

Lead poisoning generally is considered a problem of early childhood, but it is also a fetal hazard because lead is teratogenic. Women may ingest lead by drinking water that travels through old pipes that are leaching lead or by "sniffing" gasoline. Lead ingestion during pregnancy may lead to a newborn who is cognitively or neurologically challenged.

Radiation

Rapidly growing cells are extremely vulnerable to destruction by radiation. Radiation has been proven to be a potent teratogen to unborn children because of the high proportion of rapidly growing cells present. It produces a range of malformations depending on the stage of development of the embryo or fetus and the strength and length of exposure. If the exposure occurs before implantation, the growing zygote apparently is killed. If the zygote is not killed, it survives apparently unharmed. The most damaging time for exposure and subsequent damage is from implantation to 6 weeks after conception (when many women are not yet aware that they are pregnant). The nervous system, brain, and the retinal innervation are most affected.

As a rule, therefore, all women of childbearing age should be exposed to pelvic x-rays only in the first 10 days of a menstrual cycle (when pregnancy is unlikely because ovulation has not yet occurred), except in emergency situations. A serum pregnancy test can be done on all women who have reason to believe they might be pregnant before diagnostic tests involving x-rays are performed.

Radiation of the pelvis should be avoided during pregnancy if at all possible. It should be undertaken only at term if the data are important for birth and cannot be obtained by any other means. Sonography and magnetic resonance imaging have replaced x-ray examination for confirmation of situations such as multiple pregnancy because these do not appear to be teratogenic.

In addition to immediate fetal damage, evidence exists that radiation can have long-lasting effects on the health of the child. There appears to be an increased risk of cancer in children exposed to radiation in utero. Exposure of the fetal gonads could lead to a genetic mutation that will not be evident until the next generation (Schwartz, 2000).

If the woman needs nonpelvic radiation during pregnancy (e.g., dental x-rays, limb x-ray after a fall), a lead apron is required to shield her pelvis during the procedure. Even fluoroscopy, which uses lower radiation doses than regular x-ray photography, can cause fetal deformities and should be avoided during pregnancy—again, except in an emergency. Although still being investigated, long-term use of slight radiation sources, such as a word processor, computer, or cellular phone, does not appear to be teratogenic.

Hyperthermia and Hypothermia

Hyperthermia to the fetus may be detrimental to growth because it interferes with cell metabolism. Hyperthermia can occur from the use of saunas, hot tubs, or tanning beds, or from a work environment next to a furnace, such as in welding or steel making. For this reason, pregnant women who use a hot tub at 40°C should not stay in it for longer than 10 minutes at one time (Niebyl, 2000). Maternal fever early in pregnancy (4 to 6 weeks) may cause abnormal fetal brain development and possibly seizure disorders, hypotonia, and skeletal deformities.

The effect of hypothermia on pregnancy is not well known. Because the uterus is an internal organ, the woman's body temperature would have to be lowered significantly before a great deal of fetal change would result.

Teratogenicity of Maternal Stress

Many myths exist about the effect of being frightened or surprised while pregnancy. For example:

- "If a woman sees a mouse during pregnancy, her child will be born with a furry or molelike birthmark."

- "Eating strawberries causes strawberry birthmarks."
- "Looking at a handicapped child while pregnant will cause a child in utero to be handicapped the same way."

Common sense and awareness of fetal–maternal physiology have dispelled these superstitions. There is some evidence, however, that an emotionally disturbed pregnancy, one filled with anxiety and worry beyond the usual amount associated with pregnancy, could produce physiologic changes through its effect on the sympathetic division of the autonomic nervous system. The primary changes include an increase in heart rate, constriction of the peripheral blood vessels, a decrease in gastrointestinal motility, and dilation of coronary vessels (the fight-or-flight syndrome). If the anxiety is prolonged, the constriction of uterine vessels could interfere with the blood and nutrient supply to the fetus.

These phenomena are characteristic only of long-term, extreme stress, not of the normal anxiety of pregnancy. Illness or death of one's partner, difficulty with relatives, marital discord, and illness or death of another child are examples of stressful situations that might provoke excessive anxiety.

Helping a woman resolve these complex problems during pregnancy is not easy. If maternal stress is severe, however, securing counseling is as important as ensuring good physical care.

PREPARATION FOR LABOR

At about the midpoint of pregnancy, it is time to review the events that signal the beginning of labor so that women will not be surprised by these happenings or dismiss them as something other than what they are.

Lightening

Lightening is the settling of the fetal head into the inlet of the true pelvis. It occurs approximately 2 weeks before labor in primiparas but at unpredictable times in multiparas. The woman notices that she is not as short of breath as she was. Her abdominal contour is definitely changed, and on standing she may experience frequency of urination or sciatic pain (pain across her buttock radiating down her leg) from the lowered fetal position.

Show

Show is the common term used to denote the release of the cervical plug (operculum) that formed during pregnancy. It consists of a mucous, often blood-streaked vaginal discharge and indicates the beginning of cervical dilatation.

Rupture of the Membranes

A sudden gush of clear fluid (amniotic fluid) from the vagina indicates rupture of the membranes. The woman should telephone her primary care provider immediately when this occurs. After rupture of the membranes, there is a danger of cord prolapse and uterine infection.

Excess Energy

Feeling extremely energetic is a sign of labor important for women to recognize. It occurs as part of the body's physiologic preparation for labor. If the woman does not recognize the sensation for what it is, she may use this burst of energy to clean her house or finish paperwork at the office and exhaust herself before labor begins. If she can recognize this symptom as an initial sign of labor, she can conserve her energy in preparation for labor.

Uterine Contractions

For most women, labor begins with contractions. True labor contractions usually start in the back and sweep forward across the abdomen like the tightening of a band. They gradually increase in frequency and intensity. Advise a woman to telephone her primary care provider when contractions begin to alert health care personnel that she is in labor. Inform her at what point in labor her physician or nurse-midwife wants her to come to the health care facility (such as when contractions are 5 minutes apart). Be certain she knows this is not a hard-and-fast rule. If she should become exceptionally anxious, be home alone, or have a long drive, she should be given the option of using common sense to determine when to leave home.

✔ CHECKPOINT QUESTIONS

12. How might a pregnant client contract toxoplasmosis?
13. What types of vaccine are contraindicated during pregnancy?
14. Which FDA pregnancy risk category is associated with fetal abnormalities and drugs whose risks clearly outweigh the benefits?

KEY POINTS

Prenatal education is an important part of prenatal care. The more women know about measures they should take during pregnancy to safeguard their health, the more likely they will avoid substances or activities harmful to fetal growth.

Urge women to find the best way for them to modify their lifestyle for pregnancy. Pregnancy is 9 months long, so modifications must be agreeable to a woman or she will not maintain them over such a long time span.

Discussion and health-teaching periods during pregnancy should cover self-care topics such as bathing, sexual activity, sleep, and exercise.

Women need to make provisions for rest periods during their day and to be aware of any potential teratogens at a work site, such as exposure to radiation or heavy metals.

Women who travel should plan for break periods to avoid congestion in the lower extremities. Seatbelts should be used when traveling by car.

Common discomforts of early pregnancy include breast tenderness, constipation, palmar erythema, nausea and vomiting, fatigue, muscle cramps, pain from varicosities or hemorrhoids, heart palpitations, frequency of urination, vulvar pruritus, and leukorrhea. If women know that these symptoms may occur, they will not interpret them as complications.

Minor discomforts of middle or late pregnancy include backache, dyspnea, ankle edema, and Braxton Hicks contractions. Women need to be cautioned that contractions could be a sign of labor.

Danger signs for women to report during pregnancy are vaginal bleeding, persistent vomiting, chills and fever, escape of fluid from the vagina, abdominal or chest pain, swelling of the face and fingers, vision changes or continuous headache, rhythmic cramping, burning with urination, or a pronounced decrease in fetal movement.

Women should be aware of the danger to the fetus from infectious diseases such as rubella, HIV, cytomegalovirus, herpes simplex virus, syphilis, Lyme disease, and toxoplasmosis during pregnancy and should be taught how to avoid these illnesses.

All women should also be counseled about the necessity to avoid the use of any drugs or herbal supplements not specifically approved by their physician or nurse-midwife during pregnancy, as well as alcohol and cigarettes.

It is almost impossible for a woman to modify a behavior, such as smoking, if her support person does not agree to change. Including the family in care is an important way of helping support persons understand the necessity for the modification and increase cooperation.

Beginning signs of labor for the pregnant woman to be alert for include lightening, show, excess energy, rupture of membranes, and uterine contractions.

CRITICAL THINKING EXERCISES

1. Julberry Adams, the woman you met at the beginning of the chapter, voiced a number of concerns, including whether she should stop work and whether it would be safe to take a long trip. What advice would you give her regarding this?
2. A 19-year-old college student comes to see you in a prenatal clinic. She is unmarried and lives in a college dormitory. She admits she has not been taking her prenatal vitamins and describes a day to you that involves long periods of sitting with almost no exercise.
   a. What would be some recommendations specifically related to college life you could make to help this client increase her exercise level?
   b. What suggestions could you make to improve her medication compliance?
   c. The client mentioned no support person on whom she could rely for advice during pregnancy. Would you make any recommendations about whom she might consult on a college campus for this?
3. Examine the National Health Goals related to health promotion during pregnancy. Most government-sponsored money for nursing research is allotted based on these goals. What would be a possible research topic to explore pertinent to these goals that would be fundable and would advance evidence-based practice?

REFERENCES

ACOG Committee on Obstetrics Practice. (2002). Exercise during pregnancy and the postpartum period. *Obstetrics & Gynecology, 99*(1), 171–173.

Allaire, A. D., Moos, M. K., & Wells, S. R. (2000). Complementary and alternative medicine in pregnancy: A survey of North Carolina certified nurse-midwives. *Obstetrics & Gynecology, 95*(1), 19–23.

American College of Obstetricians & Gynecologists. (2000). *Recommendations for exercise in pregnancy.* Washington, DC: ACOG.

American Public Health Association. (2001). Expanded family and medical leave. *American Journal of Public Health, 91*(3), 477–478.

Ances, B. M. (2002). New concerns about thalidomide. *Obstetrics & Gynecology, 99*(1), 125–128.

Bungum, T. J. et al. (2000). Exercise during pregnancy and type of delivery in nulliparae. *Journal of Obstetric, Gynecologic & Neonatal Nursing, 29*(3), 258–264.

Campbell, M. K., & Mottola, M. F. (2001). Recreational exercise and occupational activity during pregnancy and birth weight: A case-control study. *American Journal of Obstetrics & Gynecology, 184*(3), 403–408.

Chasnoff, I. J., et al. (2001). Screening for substance use in pregnancy: A practical approach for the primary care physician. *American Journal of Obstetrics & Gynecology, 184*(4), 752–758.

Cook, A. J., et al. (2000). Sources of toxoplasma infection in pregnant women. *British Medical Journal, 321*(7254), 142–147.

Cottreau, C. M., Ness, R. B., & Kriska, A. M. (2000). Physical activity and reduced risk of ovarian cancer. *Obstetrics & Gynecology, 96*(4), 609–614.

Delaney-Black, V., et al. (2000). Teacher-assessed behavior of children prenatally exposed to cocaine. *Pediatrics, 106*(4), 782–791.

Department of Health and Human Services. (2000). *Healthy people 2010.* Washington, DC: DHHS.

Dickerson, V. M., & Chez, R. A. (2000). Normal pregnancy and prenatal care. In Scott, J. R., et al. *Danforth's obstetrics and gynecology* (8th ed., pp 65–90). Philadelphia: Lippincott Williams & Wilkins.

Ely, J. W., Yankowitz, J., & Bowdler, N. C. (2000). Evaluation of pregnant women exposed to respiratory viruses. *American Family Physician, 61*(10), 3065–3074.

Frank, D. A., et al. (2001). Growth, development, and behavior in early childhood following prenatal cocaine exposure: A systematic review. *JAMA, 285*(12), 1613–1625.

Frazier, L. M., Golbeck, A. L., & Lipscomb, L. (2001). Medically recommended cessation of employment among pregnant women. *Obstetrics & Gynecology, 97*(6), 971–975.

Genc, M., & Ledger, W. J. (2000). Syphilis in pregnancy. *Sexually Transmitted Infections, 76*(2), 73–79.

Hankin, J., McCaul, M. E. & Heussner, J. (2000). Pregnant, alcohol-abusing women. *Alcoholism: Clinical & Experimental Research, 24*(8), 1276–1286.

Hruska, K. S., et al. (2000). Environmental factors in infertility. *Clinical Obstetrics & Gynecology, 43*(4), 821–829.

Hu, L. T., & Klempner, M. S. (2001). Update on the prevention, diagnosis, and treatment of Lyme disease. *Advances in Internal Medicine, 46*(2), 247–275.

Johnson, M., Maas, M., & Moorhead, S. (2000). *Nursing outcomes classification* (2nd ed.). St. Louis: Mosby.

Karch, A. M. (2001). *Lippincott's nursing drug guide.* Philadelphia: Lippincott Williams & Wilkins.

Kozer, E., & Koren, G. (2001). Effects of prenatal exposure to marijuana. *Canadian Family Physician, 47*(2), 263–264.

Kurtzman, T. L., Otsuka, K. N., & Wahl, R. A. (2001). Inhalant abuse by adolescents. *Journal of Adolescent Health, 28*(3), 170–180.

Lee, J. Y., & Bowden, D. S. (2000). Rubella virus replication and links to teratogenicity. *Clinical Microbiology Reviews, 13*(4), 571–587.

Leininger, M. M. (Ed.). (2001). *Culture, care, diversity, and universality: A theory of nursing.* Sudbury, MA: Jones & Bartlett.

McCloskey, J., & Bulechek, G. (2000). *Nursing interventions classification* (3rd ed.). St. Louis: Mosby.

Minkoff, H. L. (2000). Human immunodeficiency virus and other perinatal infections. In Scott, J. R., et al. *Danforth's obstetrics and gynecology* (8th ed., pp 393–406). Philadelphia: Lippincott Williams & Wilkins.

Niebyl, J. R. (2000). Teratology and drugs in pregnancy. In Scott, J. R., et al. *Danforth's obstetrics and gynecology* (8th ed., pp 197–211). Philadelphia: Lippincott Williams & Wilkins.

National Institute of Occupational Safety & Health. (2000). *Nitrous oxide.* DHHS Publication #99-105. Washington, DC: DHHS.

Pardeck, J. T. (2001). Update on the Americans with Disabilities Act: Implication for health and human services delivery. *Journal of Health & Social Policy, 13*(4), 1–15.

Pollack, H. A. (2001). Sudden infant death syndrome, maternal smoking during pregnancy, and the cost-effectiveness of smoking cessation intervention. *American Journal of Public Health, 91*(3), 432–436.

Schwartz, M. W. (2000). *The 5-minute pediatric consult* (2nd ed.). Philadelphia: Lippincott Wilkins & Wilkins.

Thomas, R. E. (2000). Preparing patients to travel abroad safely. *Canadian Family Physician, 46*(1), 132–138.

Youngblut, J. M., et al. (2000). Employment patterns and timing of birth in women with high-risk pregnancies. *Journal of Obstetric, Gynecologic & Neonatal Nursing, 29*(2), 137–144.

SUGGESTED READINGS

Albrecht, S. A., Higgins, L. W., & Lebow, H. (2000). Knowledge about the deleterious effects of smoking and its relationship to smoking cessation among pregnant adolescents. *Adolescence, 35*(140), 709–716.

Carpenter, M. W. (2000). The role of exercise in pregnant women with diabetes mellitus. *Clinical Obstetrics & Gynecology, 43*(1), 56–64.

Clapp, J. F., et al. (2000). Portal vein blood flow-effects of pregnancy, gravity and exercise. *American Journal of Obstetrics & Gynecology, 183*(1), 167–172.

de Weerd, S. et al (2002). Preconceptual counseling improves folate status of women planning pregnancy. *Obstetrics & Gynecology, 99*(1), 45–50.

Ebrahim, S. H., et al. (2000). Trends in pregnancy-related smoking rates in the United States. *JAMA, 283*(3), 361–366.

Flaxman, S. M., & Sherman, P. W. (2000). Morning sickness: A mechanism for protecting mother and embryo. *Quarterly Review of Biology, 75*(2), 113–148.

Heenan, A. P., Wolfe, L. A., & Davies, G. A. (2001). Maximal exercise testing in late gestation: Maternal responses. *Obstetrics & Gynecology, 97*(1), 127–134.

Marquez-Sterling, S., et al. (2000). Physical and psychological changes with vigorous exercise in sedentary primigravidae. *Medicine & Science in Sports & Exercise, 32*(1), 58–62.

Morrison, E. H. (2000). Periconception care. *Primary Care: Clinics in Office Practice, 27*(1), 1–12.

Reilly, K. (2000). Nutrition, exercise, work, and sex in pregnancy. *Primary Care: Clinics in Office Practice, 27*(1), 105–115.

Rolater, S., Winslow, E., & Jacobson, A. F. (2000). One drink too many. *American Journal of Nursing, 100*(5), 64–66.

Stephansson, O., et al. (2001). Maternal weight, pregnancy weight gain, and the risk of antepartum stillbirth. *American Journal of Obstetrics & Gynecology, 184*(3), 463–469.

Promoting Nutritional Health During Pregnancy

12

CHAPTER

Key Terms

- **body mass index**
- **complete protein**
- **Hawthorne effect**
- **hypercholesterolemia**
- **hyperplasia**
- **hypertrophy**
- **incomplete protein**
- **lactase**
- **obese**
- **overweight**
- **pica**
- **pyrosis**
- **underweight**

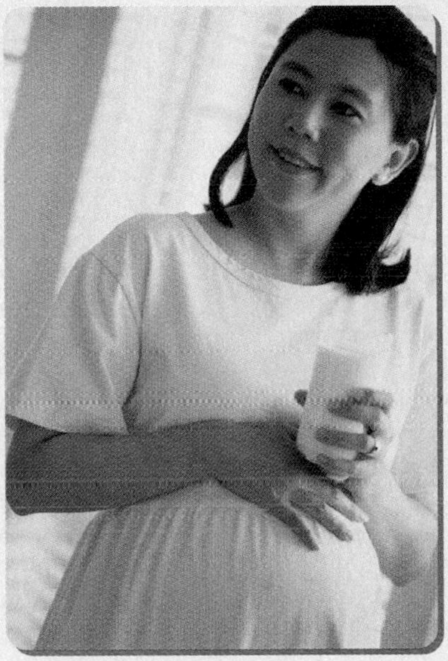

Objectives

After mastering the contents of this chapter, you should be able to:

1. Describe the requirements for healthy nutrition during pregnancy.
2. Assess a woman's nutrition during pregnancy.
3. Formulate nursing diagnoses related to nutritional concerns during pregnancy.
4. Develop expected outcomes to assist the pregnant woman to achieve optimal nutrition during pregnancy.
5. Plan health teaching strategies such as ways to increase iron and calcium intake to promote optimal nutritional intake during pregnancy.
6. Implement nursing care that encourages healthy nutritional practices during pregnancy.
7. Evaluate expected outcomes for achievement and effectiveness of nutritional care.
8. Identify National Health Goals related to nutrition and pregnancy that nurses can be instrumental in helping the nation achieve.
9. Identify areas related to nutrition and pregnancy that could benefit from additional nursing research or application of evidence-based practice.
10. Use critical thinking to analyze the effects of different life situations on nutrition patterns to create ways nutritional health can be improved and family-centered.
11. Integrate nutrition knowledge with nursing process to achieve quality maternal and child health nursing care.

Tori Alarino is 4 months pregnant and works at a fast-food restaurant during the day. She eats her breakfast and lunch at work. Her husband works four evenings a week, so she cooks for herself on those evenings. She dislikes milk, so she drinks milkshakes as a source of calcium. She is concerned because she has already gained 23 lb. She craves oranges, eating six to eight of them a day. She tells you, "I thought pregnant women always craved pickles and ice cream. What's wrong with me?" What nutrition counseling does Ms. Alarino need?

Previous chapters described normal anatomy and physiology, the changes associated with pregnancy, and common discomforts and danger signs of pregnancy. This chapter adds information about prenatal nutrition that can help to ensure a healthy outcome for both a woman and her child. This is important information because inadequate nutrition during pregnancy can be responsible for poor pregnancy outcome.

After you've studied the chapter, answer the Critical Thinking Exercises at the end of the chapter and then access the on-line study activities (http://connection.lww.com) *to further sharpen your skills and test your knowledge.*

Although a good diet cannot guarantee a good pregnancy outcome, it certainly makes an important contribution. A poor diet, such as one deficient in folic acid, can cause birth anomalies in the fetus. Both the nutritional state that a woman brings into pregnancy and her nutrition during pregnancy have a direct bearing on her health and on fetal growth and development.

Early in pregnancy, fetal growth occurs largely by an increase in the number of cells formed (**hyperplasia**); late in pregnancy it occurs mainly by enlargement of existing cells (**hypertrophy**). A fetus deprived of adequate nutrition early in pregnancy may be small for gestational age because of an inadequate number of cells in the body. Later on, although the number of cells may be normal, retarded growth may occur because these cells are smaller than the usual size. To ensure that early pregnancy deficiencies do not occur, encourage women of childbearing age to follow a balanced diet before pregnancy (preconceptual care) that specifically supplies adequate folic acid (400 μg/day). Otherwise, in the time before they recognize that they are pregnant (about 6 weeks), their poor diet and lack of important nutrient stores could seriously impair fetal growth (Reifsnider & Gill, 2000). Good nutrition during pregnancy is so important that the subject is addressed in National Health Goals (see the Focus on National Health Goals).

FOCUS ON NATIONAL HEALTH GOALS

A number of National Health Goals speak to nutrition in pregnancy. These are:

- Reduce anemia among low-income pregnant females in their third trimester from a baseline of 29% to a target of 20%.
- Increase the proportion of pregnancies begun with an optimum folic acid level from a baseline of 21% to a target of 80%.
- Increase the proportion of mothers who achieve a recommended weight gain during their pregnancies (DHHS, 2000).

Nurses can be instrumental in helping the nation achieve these goals by stressing the importance of a balanced diet for all people so women enter pregnancy with adequate nutritional stores. They can help pregnant women plan ways to ingest adequate iron daily and to remember to take their prenatal vitamin (which contains an iron and folic acid supplement) daily. Nursing research on such problems as what are effective methods to help people remember to take daily medications, how women who cannot drink milk can obtain adequate calcium, and in what ways women can be helped to gain weight in pregnancy by eating high-protein, not empty-carbohydrate foods, could add important information in this area of care.

NURSING PROCESS OVERVIEW

For Promoting Nutritional Health in the Pregnant Woman

Assessment

Assessment begins with a woman's preconceptual as well as postconceptual nutrition patterns before any nutritional planning can begin. From this assessment, determine whether the client is eating a balanced diet as represented by the food pyramid. Also evaluate any cultural, environmental, and social lifestyle factors that may affect eating habits. A 24-hour recall history is the best way to secure necessary information, confirm a well-balanced diet, and identify areas for teaching and learning.

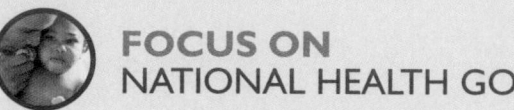

Nursing Diagnosis

Nursing diagnoses related to nutritional status of the pregnant woman must consider the desired health and growth of both the fetus and the mother. Both inadequate intake of nutrients to sustain fetal growth and inappropriate intake of nutrients, such as overuse of vitamins, can lead to poor fetal growth. The woman who is eating large amounts of nutritionally inferior food and the woman who has a problem eating because of nausea and vomiting or fatigue may be at risk for the same problems. Being sensitive to a client's concern about maintaining her own appearance in light of her need to gain sufficient weight helps her keep a healthy perspective on "eating for two." Common nursing diagnoses include:

- Imbalanced nutrition, less than body requirements, related to increased physiologic needs
- Imbalanced nutrition, less than body requirements, related to nausea every morning
- Health-seeking behaviors related to determining best food choices in pregnancy

- Imbalanced nutrition, more than body requirements, related to chronic poor eating habits
- Deficient knowledge related to need for increased intake of nutrients and calories during pregnancy

Outcome Identification and Planning

In large health centers, nutritionists are available to meet with women prenatally and help them plan nutrition during pregnancy. In other settings, a nutritionist may be available only for women with special needs, so the responsibility falls directly on nurses. When helping a woman set expected outcomes for improving nutritional patterns, be certain to consider all the cultural and lifestyle factors that give different meanings to food. Because food is an expensive commodity, financial resources must also be considered. Teaching about long-term outcomes such as rebuilding iron stores or muscle mass is important. Eating an improved diet for a week will probably not make a radical change. However, continuing a healthy eating pattern throughout the pregnancy (and maintaining it throughout life) will bring about important changes.

Implementation

As everyone who has tried to lose weight or change nutritional patterns knows, this can be a lonely and seemingly unrewarding endeavor. Begin by emphasizing the physiologic basis for nutritional needs. Based on this, explain what nutritional deficits you have found, and then show the pregnant woman how to change her nutritional patterns to improve this situation. Pregnant women are usually highly motivated to adopt healthy behaviors for the sake of their baby's health, although they still need support and encouragement because this can involve a major life change. For example, you could use a telephone conversation or person-to-person contact to encourage the client to eat a different lunch than others around her are eating; to get up 15 minutes earlier in the morning to prepare breakfast rather than just dashing to work with only coffee; or to resist having a soft drink with dinner and drink orange juice or milk instead. Asking women to list what foods they eat daily and to bring in the chart to show you at a health maintenance visit is an effective motivating technique for many people. In research studies, this is called a **Hawthorne effect,** in which people who are being watched do better than those who are not. With this system, the average woman will eat better than she usually does so her list looks better when she presents it. As soon as she realizes that better eating patterns are making her feel better, it is hoped that she will continue them indefinitely.

Be careful with issuing general statements such as, "Eat high-protein foods." Food in the supermarket is not labeled "high-protein," so provide advice in more specific terms: for example, "Eat three servings of some type of meat or fish every day."

The word "diet" has come to mean a form of unpleasant food denial. Rather than a "pregnancy diet," therefore, it is better to talk about the "foods that are best for you during pregnancy" or "pregnancy nutrition." These statements are more positive and refer more closely to foods you are encouraging the woman to eat. Giving the woman a clearly written list of suggested foods may help. Be sure the list is short, clear, and specific. Complicated lists of foods or a list of don'ts can be overwhelming and confusing and therefore may be ignored.

Outcome Evaluation

When evaluating whether the client's nutritional pattern has been improved, rely on the most important assessments: weight, energy level, general appearance, bowel function, and, when available, hemoglobin and urinalysis findings. Urge women to be honest about whether they are actually following the nutrition plan. If they are not, it probably means that the plan did not fit their lifestyle or degree of motivation. Examples of outcomes that would demonstrate improved nutrition are:

- Client plans weekly menus that include three main meals and two snacks per day.
- By next prenatal visit, client demonstrates knowledge of meat and nonmeat sources of protein by providing menus of meals eaten in the last week that include fish, eggs, beans, or peanut butter.
- Client verbalizes correct information about calcium needs during pregnancy.
- Client states she is able to make up later in each day meals missed because of nausea.
- Client's food lists for 1 week include three sources of calcium per day.
- Client describes pattern she is using to increase fluid intake to six glasses daily.

Remember that people have some degree of "backsliding," especially at holidays and special events. To prevent this, help the woman make definite, concrete plans for an upcoming holiday or event. Also, be certain to comment on the things the woman is doing correctly. Positive reinforcement, a basic rule of teaching, enhances learning, self-esteem, and compliance.

RELATIONSHIP OF MATERNAL DIET TO INFANT HEALTH

During pregnancy, the woman must eat adequately to supply enough nutrients to the fetus so it can grow as well as to support her own nutrition. Adequate protein intake is important, as it may help prevent complications of pregnancy such as pregnancy-induced hypertension or preterm birth. Deficiencies or overuse of vitamins may contribute to birth defects. Folic acid deficiency is associated with neural tube abnormalities (Bailey, 2000).

Recommended Weight Gain During Pregnancy

A weight gain of 11.2 to 16 kg (25 to 40 lb) is currently recommended as an average weight gain in pregnancy. If a woman is at high risk for nutritional deficits, a more precise estimation of adequate weight gain can be calculated. This is done by computing **body mass index** (BMI), the ratio of weight to height (Box 12-1; see also Appendix E). Women who are high or low in weight for their height (BMI below 19.8 or above 26.1) need to have expected outcomes for weight gain adjusted.

Weight gain in pregnancy occurs from both fetal growth and accumulation of maternal stores (see Assessing Maternal Weight Gain) and occurs at approximately 0.4 kg (1 lb) per month during the first trimester and then 0.4 kg (1 lb) per week during the last two trimesters (a trimester pattern of 3-12-12). In the average woman, weight gain is considered excessive if it is more than 3 kg (6.6 lb) a month during the second and third trimesters; it is less than usual if it is under 1 kg (2.2 lb) per month during the second and third trimesters. Women can be assured that most of the weight gained with pregnancy will be lost afterward.

Women who are underweight coming into pregnancy should gain slightly more weight than the average woman during pregnancy (0.5 kg per month or week rather than 0.4, or 30 to 40 lb). An obese woman might be advised to gain less than average (0.3 kg or 15 lb). However, to ensure adequate fetal nutrition, women should be advised not to diet to lose weight during pregnancy. Weight gain should be higher for a multiple pregnancy than for a single pregnancy. Women pregnant with twins should be encouraged to gain at least 1 lb per week for a total of 40 to 45 lb (Dudek, 2001). Sudden increases in weight that suggest fluid retention or polyhydramnios or a loss of weight that suggests illness should be carefully evaluated at prenatal visits.

BOX 12.1

CALCULATING BODY MASS INDEX

To calculate body mass index (BMI):

1. Convert weight into kilograms (divide weight in lb by 2.2).
2. Convert height into centimeters (multiply height in inches by 2.5).
3. Convert centimeters into meters (divide result by 100).
4. Square height in meters.
5. Divide weight in kilograms by height in meters squared.

For example: Mrs. Adams is 5′6″ tall and weighs 150 lbs. To determine her BMI:

1. Convert weight into kilograms: 150 lb ÷ 2.2 = 68 kg.
2. Convert height into centimeters: 5′6″ = 66″ (5 × 12 = 60 + 6 = 66 inches)
   66 × 2.5 = 165 cm
   165 ÷ 100 = 1.65 m
3. Square height in meters (1.65 × 1.65 = 2.72).
4. Divide weight (kg) by m² (68 ÷ 2.72 = 25 BMI).

Normal Prepregnancy BMI

Underweight	Under 19.8
Normal weight	19.8–26.0
Overweight	26.1–29.0
Obese	Above 29.0

ASSESSING Maternal Weight Gain

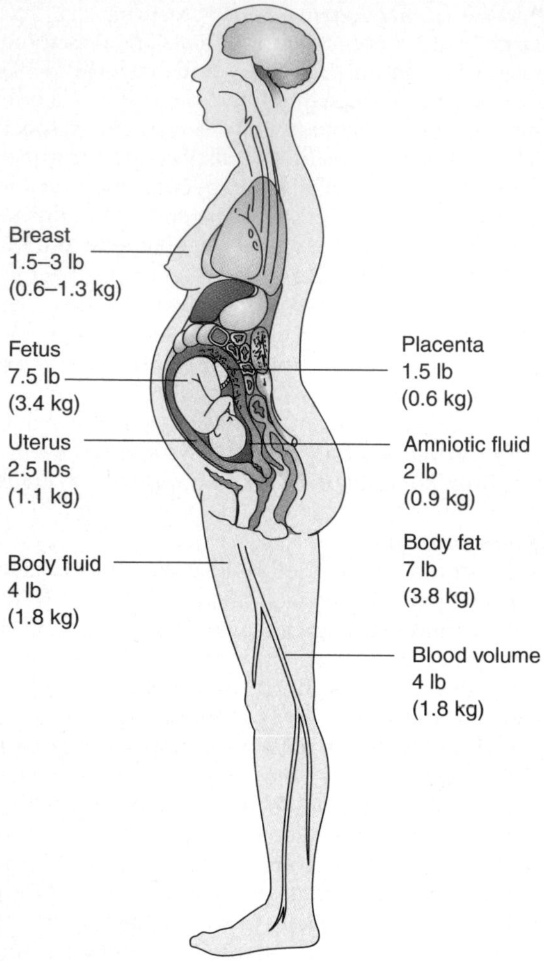

Components of Healthy Nutrition for the Pregnant Woman

The old saying that a pregnant woman must "eat for two" is not a myth; it is a scientific fact. However, this does not mean that the woman needs to eat enough for two adults, just enough to provide nutrients for the growing fetus. To do this, many women will not have to increase by much the quantity of food eaten, but they will have to increase the quality of their intake.

The recommended daily dietary allowances (RDA) for girls and women and the requirements for pregnancy were revised in 1989 (Table 12-1). Foods eaten should represent the food groups in a food pyramid (Fig. 12-1). When discussing nutrition, refer to servings of food rather than milligrams or percentages, because this is how women measure amounts.

TABLE 12.1 Recommended Daily Dietary Allowances for Pregnant and Nonpregnant Women

	NONPREGNANT WOMEN			PREGNANT WOMEN
	Age 11–14	***Age 15–18***	***Age 19–30***	
Calories (kcal)	2,200	2,200	2,200	2,500
Protein (g)	46	44	46	60
Fat-Soluble Vitamins				
Vitamin A (μg)	800	800	800	800
Vitamin D (μg)	10	10	5	5
Vitamin E (mg)	8	8	15	15
Water-Soluble Vitamins				
Ascorbic acid (mg) Vitamin C	50	60	75	85
Folic acid (μg)	150	180	400	600
Niacin (mg)	15	15	14	17
Riboflavin (mg)	1.3	1.3	1.3	1.6
Thiamine (mg) (B_1)	1.1	1.1	1.1	1.4
Vitamin B_{12} (μg)	2.0	2.0	2.4	2.6
Vitamin B_6 (mg)	1.4	1.5	1.3	2.0
Minerals				
Calcium (mg)	1,200	1,200	1,200	1,200
Phosphorus (mg)	1,200	1,200	700	700
Iodine (μg)	150	150	150	175
Iron (mg)	15	15	15	30
Magnesium (mg)	280	300	310	350
Zinc (mg)	12	12	12	15

National Research Council, National Academy of Sciences, Food and Nutrition Board (1989). *Recommended dietary allowances* (10th ed.). Washington, DC: National Academy Press.

Calorie Needs

The RDA of calories for women of childbearing age is 2,200. An additional 300 calories, or a total caloric intake of 2,500 calories, is recommended to meet the increased needs of pregnancy. In addition to supplying energy for the fetus and placenta, this increase provides calories to sustain an elevated metabolic rate from increased thyroid function and an increased workload from the extra weight the woman must carry. An inadequate intake of carbohydrates may lead to protein breakdown for energy, depriving the fetus of essential protein, and possibly resulting in ketoacidosis and neurologic defects. The use of sugar substitutes is not recommended because the woman needs sugar to maintain carbohydrate levels. Even obese women should never consume fewer than 1,500 calories per day.

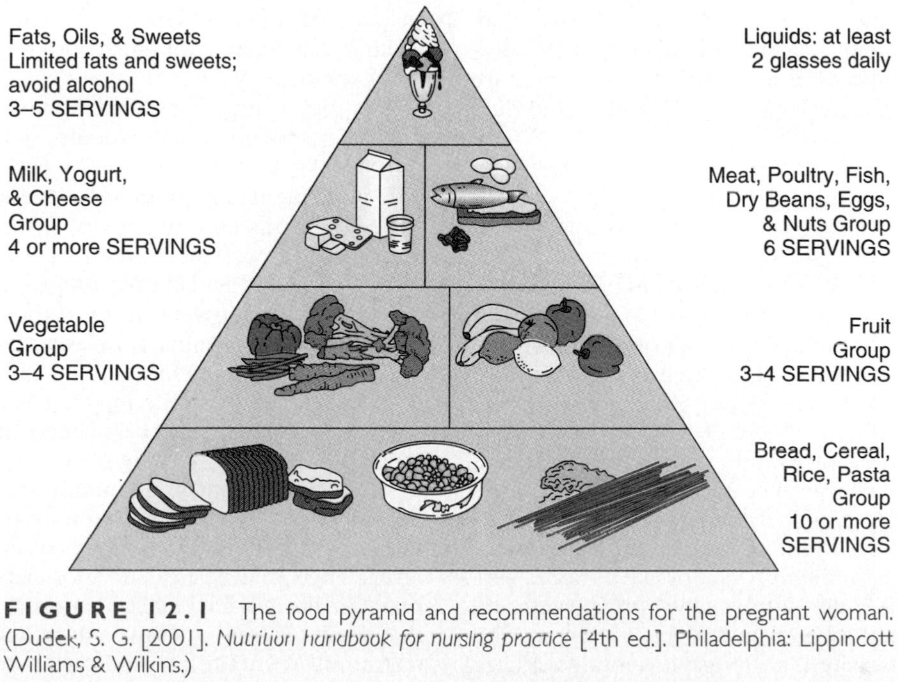

FIGURE 12.1 The food pyramid and recommendations for the pregnant woman. (Dudek, S. G. [2001]. *Nutrition handbook for nursing practice* [4th ed.]. Philadelphia: Lippincott Williams & Wilkins.)

When helping a woman plan an increased caloric intake, consider her lifestyle. For example, many women commonly skip meals, have erratic eating patterns, or rely on fast and convenience foods. Be certain that they plan to add calories by eating foods rich in protein, iron, and other essential nutrients rather than eating more fast-food, empty-calorie foods such as pretzels and doughnuts. Suggest preparing snacks such as carrot sticks or cheese and crackers early in the day when fatigue is usually less, keeping them readily available in the refrigerator. Otherwise, later in the day when they are tired, they may snack on empty-calorie food simply because it takes no preparation.

The easiest method for determining if the woman's caloric intake is adequate is assessing the weight that she is gaining. Keep in mind that the weight gain pattern is as important as the total weight gain. Even if the woman has surpassed her target weight before the end of the third trimester, encourage her not to restrict her caloric intake. She should continue to gain weight because the fetus is growing rapidly during this time.

Protein Needs

The RDA for protein in women is 44 to 46 g. During pregnancy, the intake of protein increases to 60 g daily. If protein needs are met, overall nutritional needs are likely to be met as well (with the possible exceptions of ascorbic acid, vitamin A, and vitamin D) because of the high incorporation of other nutrients with protein foods. If protein intake is inadequate, iron, B vitamins, calcium, and phosphorus also will probably be inadequate. Vitamin B_{12} is found almost exclusively in animal protein. If animal protein is totally excluded from the diet, a vitamin B_{12} deficiency is likely unless this is supplemented.

Extra protein is best supplied by meat, poultry, fish, yogurt, eggs, and milk, because the protein in these forms contains all nine essential amino acids, or is **complete protein.** The protein in nonanimal sources does not contain all essential amino acids (and thus is **incomplete protein**). It is possible to provide all amino acids by combining nonanimal proteins. Proteins that when cooked together provide all essential amino acids are termed complementary proteins. Examples are beans and rice, legumes and rice, or beans and wheat.

A woman with a family history of high cholesterol levels (**hypercholesterolemia**) probably should not eat more than two or three eggs per week because of the high cholesterol content of eggs. Encourage such women to eat lean meat, to cook with olive oil instead of lard or butter, and to remove the skin from poultry to reduce its fat content. Lunch meats such as bologna or salami should not be included as staples because their protein content may not be high and their fat content is invariably exceptionally high.

Milk is a rich source of protein. Unfortunately, some women resist drinking it because it can be high in calories as well as fat. Others cannot drink it because of lactose intolerance. Some women find it difficult to drink a quart of milk a day because they simply do not like its taste. Nonfat milk, either liquid or dry, supplies the same protein and half the calories as regular milk and is very low in fat. Buttermilk can be substituted, although it contains a large amount of sodium, or chocolate or another flavoring can be added to make milk palatable. Yogurt or cheese may also be substituted for milk, or milk may be incorporated into custards, eggnogs, or cream soups. Women who are lactose intolerant can add a lactase supplement purchased over the counter, which predigests milk and makes it palatable.

✔ **CHECKPOINT QUESTIONS**

1. What is the current recommendation for weight gain during pregnancy?
2. During the third trimester, approximately how much weight should the woman gain per week?
3. What is a complete protein?

Fat Needs

Only linoleic acid, an essential fatty acid necessary for new cell growth, cannot be manufactured in the body from other sources. Thus, women must be concerned about consuming a source of this during pregnancy. Vegetable oils are a good source. In addition, using vegetable oils (e.g., safflower, corn, olive, peanut, and cottonseed) that have a low cholesterol content rather than animal oils (lard) is recommended for all adults as a means of preventing hypercholesterolemia and coronary heart disease.

Vitamin Needs

The intake of vitamins as a daily dietary supplement has become so common that their importance may be underestimated by some women. Requirements for both fat-soluble and water-soluble vitamins increase during pregnancy to support the growth of new fetal cells (see Table 12-1). Vitamin deficiency can result in several problems. Severe folate deficiency can lead to megaloblastic anemia in the woman as well as fetal neural tube defects (see below). Vitamin D, essential for calcium absorption, when lacking, can begin to diminish both fetal and maternal mineral bone density.

Although vitamin needs do increase during pregnancy, most of the vitamin intake requirements (with the exception of folic acid) can be met by eating a healthy, varied diet with plenty of fruits and vegetables. Women who were taking oral contraceptives before they became pregnant should be certain to include good sources of vitamins A and B and folic acid in early pregnancy because oral contraceptives may deplete stores of these vitamins. Counsel women not to use mineral oil as a laxative because it can prevent absorption of fat-soluble vitamins from the gastrointestinal tract, thus hindering their availability to the body.

Commonly, a specially designed multivitamin supplement is prescribed; see the Focus on Pharmacology: Prenatal Vitamins (Natalins). Caution women to avoid taking megadoses of vitamins. The fat-soluble vitamins are stored in the body rather than excreted and thus can reach toxic levels. There may be an association between excessive vitamin A intake and fetal malformation. It is well documented that the intake of excessive vitamin A in the form of isotretinoin (Accutane), a medication prescribed for acne,

FOCUS ON PHARMACOLOGY

Prenatal Vitamins (Natalins)

Action: Supplements nutrition to ensure adequate intake of vitamins and minerals during pregnancy. The folic acid content helps prevent megaloblastic anemia in the mother and neural tube defects in the fetus.

Ingredients: Vitamin A (4,000 U), vitamin D (400 U), vitamin E (15 U), vitamin C (80 mg), vitamin B_1 (1.5 mg), vitamin B_2 (2.0 mg), vitamin B_6 (4 mg), vitamin B_{12} (2.5 μg), niacin (17 mg), folic acid (1.0 mg), pantothenic acid (7 mg), calcium (200 mg), iron (54 mg), copper (3 mg), zinc (25 mg), and magnesium (100 mg)

Dosage: One tablet daily

Possible Adverse Reactions: None known. Folic acid may mask the signs of pernicious anemia.

Nursing Implications

- Encourage women to take the medication exactly as prescribed; caution women not to exceed the recommended dosage.
- Assist with ways to remind women to take the medication, such as a note on the refrigerator.
- Advise women to keep vitamins, like all medications, out of the reach of small children to prevent accidental poisoning.

causes congenital anomalies (Karch, 2001). The mechanism of placental transfer of water-soluble vitamins makes fetal blood levels regularly higher than maternal blood levels, so a maternal overdosage can potentially cause fetal toxicity. Megadoses of vitamin C may cause withdrawal scurvy in the infant at birth.

When cautioning women about vitamin use, advise them not to leave prenatal vitamins within reach of small children. Excessive folic acid and iron can cause poisoning in small children.

Although folic acid (folacin) belongs to the B vitamin group, its importance during pregnancy warrants a separate discussion. Found predominately in fresh fruits and vegetables, folic acid is necessary for red blood cell formation. As the woman's blood volume doubles during pregnancy, her folic acid needs increase substantially. Without adequate folic acid, a megaloblastic anemia (large but ineffective red blood cells) may develop. If the woman manifests such symptoms at the time of birth, the infant may be affected as well.

For these reasons, as well as its importance in preventing neural tube defects, women should eat foods high in folic acid such as vegetables and fruit and should take a prenatal vitamin that contains a folic acid supplement of 0.4 to 1.0 mg (Dudek, 2001).

Mineral Needs

Minerals are necessary for new cell building in the fetus. Because they are found in so many foods and because mineral absorption improves during pregnancy, mineral deficiency, with the exceptions of calcium, iodine, and iron, is rare (Ladipo, 2000).

Calcium and Phosphorus. The skeleton and teeth constitute a major portion of the fetus. Tooth formation begins as early as 8 weeks in utero. Bones begin to calcify at 12 weeks. To supply adequate calcium and phosphorus for bone formation, pregnant women need to eat foods high in calcium and vitamin D (necessary for calcium to be absorbed from the gastrointestinal tract and to enter bones). The recommended amount of calcium during pregnancy is 1,200 to 1,500 mg. If a woman cannot drink milk or eat milk products such as cheese, she can be prescribed a daily calcium supplement. Most foods high in protein are also high in phosphorus, so by eating high-protein foods, women receive enough phosphorus.

Before nutrition counseling in pregnancy became common, women expected to lose "a tooth a child." That is, they believed the fetus, as he or she grew, would drain calcium from their teeth. Although it is unlikely that a woman will lose a tooth with pregnancy today, the concern reflected in this myth about the fetus taking calcium from the mother is well founded. However, the calcium in teeth is not as readily absorbed as that of bone. It is more likely that inadequate calcium intake will result in diminished maternal bone density rather than weakened teeth. With an adequate calcium intake during pregnancy, the fetus will receive the needed calcium for growth and mineralization of the fetal skeleton without taking any away from the maternal bones or teeth.

Iodine. Iodine is essential for the formation of thyroxine and, therefore, for the proper functioning of the thyroid gland. It is important that the woman ingests enough during pregnancy to supply the needs of her increased thyroid gland function during this time. If iodine deficiency occurs, it may cause thyroid enlargement (goiter) in the woman or fetus. In extreme instances, it may cause hypothyroidism in the fetus. Thyroid enlargement in the fetus at birth is serious because the increased pressure of the enlarged gland on the airway could lead to early respiratory distress. If not discovered at birth, hypothyroidism may lead to the infant's being cognitively challenged. The RDA for iodine is 175 μg daily during pregnancy. Seafood is the best source.

In areas where the water and soil are known to be deficient in iodine, it is suggested that women use iodized salt and include a serving of seafood in their diet at least once a week.

Iron. A fetus at term has a hemoglobin level of 17 to 21 g per 100 mL of blood, a level that is necessary to oxygenate the blood during intrauterine life. Iron is needed to build this high level of hemoglobin. In addition, after week 20 of pregnancy, the fetus begins to store iron in the liver to last through the first 3 months of life, when intake will consist mainly of milk, typically low in iron. In addition to supplying fetal needs, the woman needs iron to build an increased red cell volume for herself and to protect against iron lost in blood at delivery.

The RDA for iron for pregnant women is 30 mg. An average diet supplies about 6 mg iron per 1,000 calories. If the woman eats a 2,500-calorie diet daily, her daily intake is about 15 mg of iron. Because only 10% to 20% of dietary iron is absorbed, however, she is actually taking in less than this amount (closer to 1.5 mg to 3 mg). Therefore, dietary supplementation with 15 mg iron per day helps ensure that adequate iron is ingested and absorbed. Stress to women that iron supplementation is intended as a supplement to, not a replacement for, iron-rich foods.

Women with low incomes may find it difficult to eat adequate iron-rich foods, because the foods richest in iron (e.g., organ meats; eggs; green, leafy vegetables; whole grain; enriched breads; dried fruits) are also expensive. Iron absorption increases in an acid environment. Thus, eating iron-rich foods with orange juice may increase absorption. Oral iron compounds turn stools black and cause constipation in some women. Urge women not to stop taking the iron compound because of constipation; increasing fluid intake or fiber is a better way to relieve the constipation. Some women may need a prescribed stool softener such as docusate sodium (Colace); this stool softener is not associated with teratogenic action, so it can be taken safely during pregnancy.

Fluoride. Because fluoride aids in the formation of sound teeth, a pregnant woman should drink fluoridated water. In an area where the water is not fluoridated either naturally or artificially, supplemental fluoride may be recommended. Fluoride in large amounts causes brown-stained teeth, so the woman should not take the supplement more often than prescribed or if tap water in her area is already fluoridated.

Sodium. Sodium is the major electrolyte that acts to maintain fluid balance in the body. When sodium is retained rather than excreted by the kidneys, an equal or balancing amount of fluid is also retained. Retaining enough fluid during pregnancy in the maternal circulation is important to ensure a pressure gradient to allow optimal exchange of nutrients across the placenta.

Unless the woman is hypertensive or has heart disease with required sodium restriction when she enters pregnancy, she should continue to salt foods as usual during pregnancy. However, she should use moderation with foods that are extremely salty, such as lunch meats or potato chips, and with the additive monosodium glutamate. Too much salt could result in retention of excessive amounts of fluid, putting a strain on her heart as blood volume doubles.

Zinc. Zinc is necessary for the synthesis of DNA and RNA. Although not well proved, zinc deficiency may be associated with preterm birth. The RDA for zinc during pregnancy is 15 mg, or an increase of 3 mg over prepregnancy needs. Most people who take in adequate protein also take in adequate zinc because zinc is contained in foods such as meat, liver, eggs, and seafood. It is a component of prenatal vitamins to help ensure an adequate intake.

Fluid Needs

Extra amounts of water are needed during pregnancy to promote kidney function because the woman must excrete waste products for two. Two glasses of fluid daily over and above a daily quart of milk is a common recommendation.

Fiber Needs

Constipation can occur during pregnancy from slowed peristalsis due to the pressure of the uterus on the intestine. Eating fiber-rich foods, foods consisting of parts of the plant cell wall resistant to normal digestive enzymes of the small intestine, such as broccoli and asparagus, are a natural way of preventing constipation, because the bulk of the fiber left in the intestine aids evacuation. Fiber also has the advantage of lowering cholesterol levels and may remove carcinogenic contaminants from the intestine. Encourage women to eat plenty of fresh fruits and vegetables, especially green, leafy vegetables, to provide fiber. Eating fiber-rich foods this way is a better choice for preventing constipation than taking a fiber laxative. Doing so allows the woman to receive nutrients from the food as well as preventing constipation.

Foods to Avoid in Pregnancy

As discussed in Chapter 11, alcoholic beverages should not be ingested by the pregnant woman because of their potentially teratogenic effects on the fetus. Other foods to be avoided are those that contain food additives, because the effect of many of these is unknown.

Foods With Caffeine

Caffeine is thought of by many women as just an incidental ingredient in beverages. Actually, it is a central nervous system stimulant capable of increasing heart rate, urine production in the kidney, and secretion of acid in the stomach (Dudek, 2001).

A daily intake of caffeine of two or three cups of coffee has not been associated with low birthweight, but excessive intake of caffeine should be limited. To limit their caffeine intake, women may not only have to limit the amount of coffee they drink but also other sources of caffeine as well, such as chocolate, soft drinks, and tea. If a woman has difficulty omitting these common foods from her diet, she can still reduce the amount of caffeine she ingests by modifying their preparation. For example, instant coffee has less caffeine than brewed coffee; percolated coffee has less caffeine than dripped coffee. Decaffeinated coffee, as the name implies, contains almost no caffeine.

Tea, like coffee, varies in caffeine content depending on the type and time of brewing. The longer tea brews, the greater the caffeine content. Green tea has less caffeine than black tea. Both herbal teas and decaffeinated tea are available.

The cocoa bean that is used to make chocolate and cocoa is yet another natural source of caffeine. Chocolate sources tend to be low in caffeine, however, when compared with coffee. A cup of coffee contains approximately 120 mg of caffeine, whereas a cup of hot chocolate contains only 10 mg. Baking chocolate, used for cake frostings and glazes, is proportionately higher, containing about 35 mg of caffeine per ounce.

Soft drinks do not naturally contain caffeine. It is added to improve their appeal. To limit the amount of caffeine consumed, encourage pregnant women to choose caffeine-free types.

Artificial Sweeteners

Artificial sweeteners are used to improve the taste and limit the caloric content of foods. Federal controls regulate the use of these ingredients, but it is probably safest for pregnant women to reduce their intake of these substances. For instance, although the sweetener aspartame has been approved by the FDA for consumption and is apparently safe during pregnancy, large amounts of the compound should be avoided by pregnant women until its safety is confirmed. The use of saccharine is not recommended during pregnancy because it is eliminated slowly from the fetal bloodstream. In any event, pregnant women need carbohydrates furnished by sugar rather than artificial substances (Dudek, 2001).

WHAT IF? What if your pregnant client states, "Boy, am I in trouble. I love coffee. There's always a pot brewing at my office. And I have a cup of cappuccino for lunch." What suggestions could you make to help her reduce her caffeine intake?

Weight Loss Diets

As a rule, reducing diets and calorie restrictions are contraindicated during pregnancy because they may lead to fetal ketoacidosis and possibly neurologic defects. If women have been following such diets before becoming pregnant, they may have few nutritional stores, and additional vitamin supplementation may be necessary.

✔ CHECKPOINT QUESTIONS

4. Which essential fatty acid cannot be manufactured by the body?
5. What is the primary function of folic acid?
6. What can women do to enhance absorption of iron?

ASSESSMENT OF NUTRITIONAL HEALTH

The best method for assessing nutritional intake is to ask for a "typical day" history or a 24-hour nutrition recall to isolate usual patterns and possible nutritional risk factors (Table 12-2). First, ask if yesterday was a typical day. If it was, then ask the woman to list all the food she ate within the past 24 hours, starting with when she awakened until she went to sleep. Be certain she includes all the snack foods she ate, as well as sit-down meals. This method of history taking yields much more accurate information about actual intake than if the woman is asked how often during the week she eats citrus fruit, or how much milk she drinks every day. A woman who knows how much milk she ought to drink a day will probably say she drinks a quart a day during pregnancy. However, if asked to list the foods she ate the day before, she may report that she drank only one glass of milk all day.

After obtaining the day's list of food, compare the types and amounts on the list with those shown in Figure 12-1 to see if all food groups and adequate amounts are included. Comparing foods from the person's 24-hour recall with a guide is a helpful way to show clients that what they thought was a "perfect" intake is imperfect, or what they thought was a "little" problem actually involves the loss of an entire food group. Once a woman sees that an actual deficit exists, she may be more motivated to improve her nutrition. Such a picture also offers an instant reward for the woman who is ingesting adequate foods.

In addition to actual food intake, ask the woman if she thinks she has any problem with nutrition (such as cravings). Also, assess the circumstances of eating, such as cultural preferences, who prepares food in the family, and how many meals are eaten outside the home weekly. Table 12-3 summarizes this additional information.

To strengthen history findings, assess the woman's prepregnancy weight and calculate her BMI. People with poor nutrition are over- or underweight and show typical physical signs. Table 12-4 lists important physical exami-

TABLE 12.2 Nutritional Risk Factors During Pregnancy

RISK	RATIONALE
Adolescent (less than 18 years old at LMP)	An adolescent has increased nutritional needs.
Short intervals between pregnancies	The woman's body has not had time to replace nutritional stores depleted during previous pregnancy(ies).
Low income	Family may not have resources to purchase adequate foods to meet pregnancy nutritional needs.
Follows food fads	Foods eaten may not be those adequate for pregnancy. (Some diets may be lacking in essential nutrients.)
Drug use (including cigarettes and alcohol)	Drugs may be ingested in preference to healthy foods.
Existence of a chronic illness requiring a special diet	Intake may be low in an essential substance such as carbohydrate or protein.
Underweight or overweight	Underweight and overweight status may indicate chronic inadequate dietary patterns.
Multiple pregnancy	The woman must supply enough nutrition for multiple fetal development.
Anemic at conception	The woman has no iron stores for fetal growth.
Lactose intolerance	The woman may not be ingesting adequate calcium for fetal skeletal growth.

TABLE 12.3 Areas to Be Assessed for a Total Nutrition History

AREA OF ASSESSMENT	PERTINENT QUESTIONS
Food preparation	Who does the cooking?
	How many people does the woman cook for?
	How are foods usually prepared (fried or baked)?
	What spices or condiments are commonly used?
	What type oil is used for frying (saturated or unsaturated)?
Food pattern	How many meals are eaten a day?
	Which is the biggest meal?
	What types of food are eaten?
	How many snacks are eaten a day? What are they?
	How many meals are eaten outside the home?
	Where are they eaten? Cafeteria? Fast-food store? Restaurant? Bagged lunch?
	Any foods that she cannot or will not eat? Why?
Financial concerns	Is there enough money for food?
	Who does the shopping?
	Would the woman eat differently if more money were available?
	Is any supplementary financial program used?
Activity level	Is she normally active or sedentary? (Could increase calorie need.)
Health	Does she know of any allergies to food?
	Does she have any trouble with chewing or digestion?
	What is bowel movement frequency?
	Was she taking oral contraceptives before pregnancy?
	Does she take supplemental vitamins? What type? How many?
	Does she drink alcohol? What type? How much?
	Does she smoke cigarettes?
	What is her stress level? Does this affect her appetite?
Personal food preferences	Are there any foods she particularly enjoys or dislikes?
	Are there any foods she feels are harmful or particularly beneficial to her?
	Are there any cultural or religious preferences?
Family dietary patterns	Does anyone in the family eat a special diet?
	Is anyone obviously overweight or underweight?
	Does the family eat meals together?
	Is mealtime a social time?

nation assessments that suggest a good nutritional intake or evidence of poor nutrition.

Hemoglobin or hematocrit determinations (see Appendix F) are also important assessments of good nutrition. These may reveal smoking habits, as cigarette smokers have higher HgB levels than nonsmokers. These values are measured early in pregnancy and then usually repeated close to term and again at birth. A urinalysis can also be important because a finding such as elevated urine specific gravity could suggest a disturbed fluid balance, and elevated urine glucose suggests gestational diabetes (see Chap. 14).

PROMOTING NUTRITIONAL HEALTH DURING PREGNANCY

Setting Nutritional Outcomes

Plans for improving nutritional patterns must take into account the woman's lifestyle, family preferences, financial resources, customs, and cultural desires, because she and her family must follow them for 9 months (Fig. 12-2; see also Focus on Nursing Care Planning).

Family Considerations

Meal planning must involve the entire family. Even if a woman is receptive to changing her eating habits, she may have difficulty carrying out recommendations if her family resists such changes. With an adolescent, it is important to speak with the person who prepares the meals at home to effect a change. In families in which a member has a special nutritional need, such as restricted sodium, the change may be even more difficult.

Financial Considerations

Food is costly. To provide the extra servings required during pregnancy, a woman must spend more on food for herself per week than she is used to spending. Women generally view this increased expense as an investment in their child's health and do not regard it as a burden. However, the family with a marginal income, although they may be willing to shoulder the additional cost, may have trouble actually doing so. If this occurs, review what foods the woman is eating to be certain she is not buying only starchy foods because they are more filling and less expensive than protein foods. Help her secure available financial assistance such as food stamps, or inform her about nutritional aid programs such as the Women, Infants and Children Special Supplemental Food Program (WIC).

Under the food stamp program, a family with a low income can buy stamps that can be redeemed at grocery stores for any food items except alcohol or pet food. The cost of stamps varies but can increase a family's buying power as much as $150 a month.

The advantage of this type of program is that it helps to supplement the cost of food but places almost no restrictions on what foods can be selected and purchased. It can make the difference for a low-income family between being able to eat meat or living on a starchy diet. Rules concerning eligibility for these programs are changing because

TABLE 12.4 Physical Signs and Symptoms of Adequate Pregnancy Nutrition

ASSESSMENT AREA	SIGNS OF GOOD NUTRITION	SIGNS OF POOR NUTRITION
Hair	Shiny; strong with good body	Hair dull and lifeless
Eyes	Good eyesight, particularly at night; conjunctiva moist and pink	Pale and dry conjunctiva; difficulty with night vision
Mouth	No cavities in teeth; no swollen or inflamed gingiva; no cracks or fissures at corners of mouth; mucous membrane moist and pink; tongue smooth and nontender	Fissures at corners of mouth; tongue rough and tender; mucous membrane pale
Neck	Normal contour of thyroid gland	Thyroid gland enlarged
Skin	Smooth, with normal color and turgor; no ecchymotic or petechial areas present	Rough texture; poor turgor
Extremities	Normal muscle mass and circumference; normal strength and mobility; edema limited to slight ankle involvement; normal reflexes	Poor muscle tone; diminished reflexes
Finger- and toenails	Smooth; pink; normal contour	Pale; break easily; little growth
Weight	Within normal limits of ideal weight before pregnancy; following normal pattern of pregnancy weight gain	Over- or underweight; unusually slow or rapid weight gain
Blood pressure	Within normal limits for length of pregnancy	Decreased from anemia; increased from hypertension

of new government restrictions that allow persons to remain on this type of assistance for a limited time only.

The WIC program is a federal program that provides nutritional support for low-income women and children. Established in 1972 as a pilot program, WIC is funded by the Food and Nutrition Service of the U.S. Department of Agriculture (Swensen et al., 2001). The program supplies supplemental foods and nutrition education for:

- Pregnant women
- Postpartal women up to 6 months
- Nursing mothers up to 1 year
- Children from birth to age 5

Eligibility for the program is based on income level, geographic area, and nutritional risk. Each state defines the income eligibility level. To receive food, clients must live in an area that has been designated as a funding area. The nurse or nutritionist in the health care facility determines possible risk and nutritional need. Factors considered that put pregnant women at nutritional risk include age (adolescent or woman over 40); poor obstetric history such as previous spontaneous miscarriage, a short period between pregnancies, previous low-birthweight infant, or gestational diabetes; anemia; poor weight gain; or inadequate consumption of food by nutrition history.

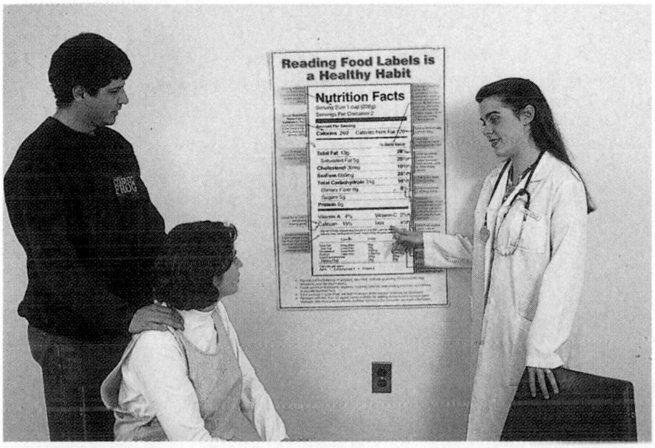

FIGURE 12.2 Encourage pregnant women and their partners to eat a varied diet with a high iron and protein content. This may be difficult for the woman early in pregnancy because of nausea, late in pregnancy because of fatigue.

For the pregnant woman, foods typically offered by the program include those with high-quality protein, iron, calcium, and vitamins A and C, such as fruit juice, eggs, milk, and cheese. At predetermined intervals, WIC clients are reevaluated to see if the program supplements are still necessary. WIC has been successful in improving nutrition during pregnancy because it supplies additional food to recipients and because the periodic evaluations provide time for nutritional counseling. The WIC program not only reduces the risk of low birthweight but also reduces medical costs by preventing costly newborn care.

School lunch programs are yet another way that some pregnant adolescents can receive help with nutrition. Millions of school children qualify for free or reduced-price school lunches. A school lunch (type A) is designed to provide one third of a child's RDA. For many adolescents, these school lunches may be the most nutritious meal they eat in a day.

Cultural Considerations

Women during pregnancy may have difficulty changing from familiar patterns of food preparation because asking them to change their intake also involves changing the food patterns of other family members. Culture also may affect what foods are prepared. This may positively or negatively impact the woman's nutritional patterns during

FOCUS ON *Nursing Care Planning*

A PREGNANT CLIENT WITH INADEQUATE NUTRITIONAL PATTERN

A 26-year-old pregnant Asian-American woman comes to the antepartal health care facility for a visit. She states, "I don't want to gain too much weight."

Assessment: Primigravida; LMP 9 weeks ago. Height 5′6″. Prepregnancy weight: 110 lb (10 lb under desirable weight for height); BMI 14. Weight today: 111 lb. History of weight problem during adolescence; currently controlling weight by eating one main meal per day. 24-hour dietary recall: Breakfast—1 cup decaffeinated tea with 1 slice of toast with jelly; lunch—none; dinner—one serving of broccoli with 1 ounce of meat stir-fried, ½ cup of steamed rice, 1 cup of tea; snacks—8 ounces of iced tea, saltine crackers. States she has felt fatigued and constipated for last 3 weeks.

Nursing Diagnosis: Imbalanced nutrition, less than body requirements, related to inadequate intake of calories and desire to control weight

Outcome Identification: Client will verbalize daily dietary intake of appropriate number of calories and minerals.

Outcome Evaluation: Client's dietary recall demonstrates increased caloric consumption with high-quality nutritious foods. Client reports intake of foods high in calories, iron, calcium, and protein; demonstrates weight gain appropriate for stage of pregnancy and prepregnancy weight.

Interventions	Rationale
1. Explain the need for adequate consumption of nutrients and calories while listening to client's concern about weight gain.	1. Adequate nutrition is essential for optimal fetal growth and development. Listening to client's concerns aids in validating the client's feelings and establishing trust.
2. Question client about food likes and dislikes. Investigate any cultural influences on food choices.	2. Ascertaining food preferences and cultural influences on food provides a baseline for future food selections and suggestions.
3. Consult with the dietitian and maternal health care provider about recommended caloric and mineral requirements.	3. Caloric recommendations may need to be increased in light of client's BMI and prepregnancy and current weight.
4. Assist client with food suggestions. Enlist the aid of a dietitian to assist with meal planning and culturally acceptable food choices. Provide written information as needed.	4. Assistance from a dietitian ensures a nutritionally sound diet with culturally acceptable food choices. Printed information enhances learning.
5. Instruct client to keep a diet journal recording all food and fluid intake for 1 week, and review with client on next visit.	5. Keeping a journal provides concrete evidence of client's compliance with nutritional plan.
6. Arrange for a follow-up appointment in 1 week.	6. Scheduling close follow-up provides an opportunity for evaluation and reinstruction. Changing nutritional habits and behaviors can be difficult.

Nursing Diagnosis: Fatigue related to increased physiologic demands of pregnancy and inadequate nutritional intake

Outcome Identification: Client will report improved energy level within 1 month.

Outcome Evaluation: Client states causes of fatigue; demonstrates improved nutritional intake; reports measures to balance activity and rest periods; exhibits hemoglobin level above 11 g/100 mL.

(continued)

Interventions	Rationale
1. Assess client's pattern of daily activity.	1. Assessment of client's daily activity patterns provides possible clues to underlying contributory factors for fatigue and a baseline for future suggestions.
2. Review the physiologic changes associated with pregnancy and their impact on client's fatigue. Also review nutritional impact on fatigue level.	2. Increased metabolic requirements of pregnancy and inadequate nutrition may result in fatigue.
3. Consult with maternal health care provider about necessary laboratory tests, such as hemoglobin and serum iron levels.	3. Inadequate nutrition and being underweight may deplete nutritional stores, predisposing the client to iron-deficiency anemia.
4. Institute measures to improve nutrition, such as eating lunch and a bigger breakfast.	4. Adequate nutrition is essential for a healthy outcome for the mother and fetus.
5. Instruct the client in the need for increased rest periods and pacing activities. Teach energy conservation measures.	5. A balance of activity and rest minimizes metabolic demands and helps allow sufficient energy for activities, including meal preparation.

Nursing Diagnosis: Constipation related to physiologic changes of pregnancy and inadequate fiber intake

Outcome Identification: Client will report that constipation has been relieved.

Outcome Evaluation: Client describes food high in fiber that she eats daily; reports bowel movement at least every other day.

Interventions	Rationale
1. Counsel client regarding causes of constipation with pregnancy, such as pressure on bowel and slowed motility.	1. Information about contributory causes can provide a basis for action.
2. Remind client of the need for a regular time for bowel evacuation.	2. Bowel evacuation is stimulated by habit.
3. Assist client to continue to include fiber foods in diet.	3. Fiber mechanically stimulates peristalsis and aids in bowel evacuation.
4. Help the client find ways to increase fluid in diet.	4. Fluids aid in distending the bowel, thus promoting bowel evacuation.
5. Encourage client to increase activity level within limits of available energy	5. Activity promotes peristalsis. Increasing activity within the client's limits minimizes the risk of additional fatigue.

pregnancy. Common cultural differences that are important to be aware of in nutritional counseling are shown in the Focus on Cultural Competence (see also Appendix K).

✔ CHECKPOINT QUESTIONS

7. What is the best way to obtain a nutrition history?
8. If a woman qualifies for WIC, for approximately how long is she eligible for services if she is breast-feeding?

Managing Common Problems Affecting Nutritional Health

Specific nutrition problems in pregnancy may result from a number of factors or circumstances. Discomforts such as constipation and flatulence have already been discussed (see Chap. 11).

Nausea and Vomiting

As many as 50% of pregnant women report nausea and vomiting. No definite cause has been established for this symptom of early pregnancy, but it may be related to:

- Sensitivity to the high levels of chorionic gonadotropin hormone produced by the trophoblast
- High estrogen or progesterone levels
- Lowered maternal blood sugar caused by the needs of the developing embryo
- Lack of pyridoxine (vitamin B_6)
- Diminished gastric motility

Nausea is aggravated by fatigue and may be aggravated by emotional disturbance (Flaxman and Sherman, 2000).

Most women notice the sensation as early as the first missed menstrual period, and it lasts the first 3 months of

FOCUS ON CULTURAL COMPETENCE

CHARACTERISTICS OF CERTAIN ETHNIC DIETS

Group and Place of Origin	*Staple Foods*	*Comments*
Hispanic Americans from Puerto Rico	Steamed white rice; many varieties of beans; wheat breads; starchy vegetables such as cassavas, yams, breadfruit, plantains, and green bananas; green peppers; tomatoes; garlic; dried, salted fish; salt pork, bacon; lard; olive oil; sugar; jams and jellies, sweet pastries; sugared fruit juices; cafe con leche (coffee and hot milk)	Milk is rarely consumed as a beverage. Most food is cooked for long periods of time or fried. Malt beer is believed to be nutritious and may be given to children and breast-feeding mothers.
Hispanic Americans from Mexico, Central America	Many varieties of beans; steamed rice; corn products such as tortillas made from lime-soaked cornmeal; chili peppers, tomatoes; mangoes; prickly pear fruit; potatoes; meat and sausages; fish; poultry; eggs; milk cheeses; milk custards and bread puddings; lard; sweet chocolate and coffee drinks; cakes, pastries	Most vegetables are cooked so long that they lose most of their nutritional value. Diet is high in fiber and starch. Animal fat is frequently added during food preparation. Because milk, green leafy vegetables, and fruit intakes are low, diet may be inadequate in calcium, iron, vitamin A, and vitamin C. Obesity is common.
Hispanic Americans from Cuba	Stews and casseroles flavored with sage, parsley, bay leaf, thyme, cinnamon, curry, capers, onion, cloves, garlic, saffron. Soup is served daily. Fried foods, especially fish, poultry, eggs; rice; many varieties of beans	Fruits and vegetables are not eaten on a regular basis. Main meal is usually served at lunch.
Southern African-Americans from West Africa (many generations in United States)	Hominy grits; biscuits; cornmeal and corn bread; rice; legumes; potatoes; onions; tomatoes; hot peppers; green leafy vegetables cooked in fatback or salt pork; okra; sweet potatoes; squashes; corn; cabbage; melons; peaches; pecans; all parts of a pig; fresh meats and poultry; fish; thick stews; butter, shortening, and lard; sugar; bread puddings; pies and sweets	African-American food patterns are similar to whites in same region. Northern African-Americans may be unfamiliar with "soul food." Frying is common; diet tends to be high in fat and salt, low in calcium. High rate of obesity.
Chinese Americans (diets vary sometimes with region)	Rice and rice gruel; wheat noodles; corn; green vegetables, especially from the cabbage family; squashes; cucumbers; eggplant; leafy vegetables; various shoots, including bamboo, mung, and soy; sweet potatoes; radishes; onions; peas and pods; mushrooms; roots; many local, seasonal vegetables; pickled vegetables; sea vegetables; plums; peaches; tangerines; kumquats and other citrus fruits; litchis; longans; mangoes; papayas; pomegranates; soybean products such as tofu (soybean curd), soy sauces, bean noodles, and soy milk; tiny portions of meat, fish with bones, or poultry; seafood; soup or tea as beverage; sugar as seasoning	Yin (feminine)–yang (masculine) concept of balancing intake; moderation is valued. Obesity is rare. Regional differences in food choices exist. Rice symbolizes life and fertility. Raw vegetables are rarely served. Diet is high in fiber and many nutrients, is low in fat, and may be low in protein.
Japanese Americans	Rice; vegetables; pickled vegetables; soy as miso (soup), tofu, bean paste, and soy sauce; fruits; salads; fish with bones; sugar as seasoning; sea vegetables; seafood; ginseng; green tea	Common preparation methods include broiling, steaming, boiling, and stir-frying. Meat portions are small. Milk is rarely used by adults. Diet is low in fat, rich in nutrients, high in sodium.

Vietnamese Americans	Rice, rice noodles; French bread and croissants with butter; hot peppers; curries of asparagus and potatoes; salads; tropical fruits and vegetables; lemons and limes; small portions of poultry; eggs; fish pats; nuoc nam (a strong, fermented fish sauce added to almost every cooked dish); sweets, candies, sweetened drinks; coffee; tea	Rice may be eaten at every meal. Fresh milk is not readily available; lactose intolerance is common. Little fat is used in preparation. Diet may be low in iron and calcium.
Native Americans	Southeast: corn; cornmeal; coontie (flour from a palmlike plant); fried breads; swamp cabbage (now illegal to harvest); pumpkins; squashes; papayas; alligator, snake, wild hog, duck, fish, and shellfish. Northeast: blueberries; cranberries; beans; corn; pumpkins; fish; lobster; wild game; maple syrup. Midwest: bison; beans; corn; melons; squashes; tomatoes. Southwest: corn (many colors and varieties); beans; squash; pumpkins; chili peppers; melons; pinenuts; cactus. Northwest: salmon; caviar; other fish; otter; seal; whale; bear; elk; other game; wild fruits; acorns (and other wild nuts); wild greens	Food has great religious and social significance. Corn is a status food for most tribes. Milk is seldom used; calcium intake is usually low. Diets on some reservations are considered poor. High rate of obesity.

Dudek, S. (2001). *Nutrition handbook for nursing practice* (4th ed.). Philadelphia: Lippincott Williams & Wilkins.

pregnancy. The sensation is usually most intense on arising but may occur while the woman is preparing meals or smelling food. Vomiting at least once a day is common. Women who work nights and sleep days often experience "evening sickness," because that is when they arise.

Methods such as acupressure, antimotion sickness wrist bands, or avoiding fluid with meals are effective for some women. Increasing carbohydrate intake seems to relieve nausea better than any other nutrition remedy. The traditional solution is for women to keep dry crackers, such as saltines, by the bedside and eat a few before rising; sourball candies may serve the same purpose. The woman can then eat a light breakfast or delay breakfast until 10 or 11 AM, past the time her nausea seems to persist. She must maintain a good food intake during pregnancy even in light of nausea, so she must compensate for any missed meals later in the day. If preparing food for others makes her feel queasy, she should try to give these responsibilities to another family member, at least through the worst phase of this symptom. Preparing and freezing meals ahead of time, perhaps at night when the nausea is less bothersome, may also help.

It is a good rule for women not to go longer than 12 hours between meals during pregnancy to prevent hypoglycemia. Thus, a woman may need to include a late-evening snack in her meals to compensate for a late breakfast. She may be able to tolerate fruit and raw vegetables during the morning before other food. Urge her to experiment with soups or vegetable drinks that she may not usually think of as breakfast foods but that will give her early-morning calories.

Caution women against self-medicating for nausea by taking antacids. Excessive use of antacids containing sodium bicarbonate may cause fluid retention because of the sodium content. Remember that a woman should not take any medication during pregnancy unless prescribed by her physician or nurse-midwife (see the Focus on Family Empowerment).

Fortunately, nausea usually disappears spontaneously as the woman enters her fourth month of pregnancy. If it persists beyond this month or is so extreme in early pregnancy that it interferes with nutrition, it may indicate the development of hyperemesis gravidarum, a complication of pregnancy (see discussion later in this chapter)

Cravings

Cravings for food or aversions to certain foods during pregnancy are so common that they are considered a normal part of adaptation to pregnancy. It was formerly considered that these strange desires for food reflected a woman's need to call attention to the pregnancy or were a reaction to her imposed dependent state. However, cravings are actually more likely the result of a physiologic need for more carbohydrates or particular vitamins and minerals.

Now that recommended pregnancy nutrition allows for more calories and a greater pregnancy weight gain is encouraged, cravings are seen less often than before. When taking a nutritional history, ask if the woman notices any particular cravings. As long as this is a healthy type of food, help her plan a nutrition intake that includes the food, at least in moderation. This is a positive approach to nutrition counseling. It allows her to enjoy her pregnancy without feeling guilty because she is eating foods she craves.

During pregnancy, some women report an abnormal craving for nonfood substances (termed **pica** from the Latin for magpie, a bird that is an indiscriminate eater). The most common form of pica in the past was a craving

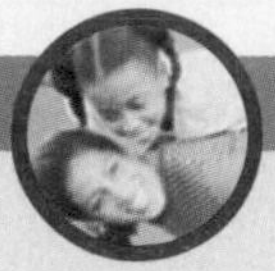

FOCUS ON FAMILY EMPOWERMENT
Measures to Reduce and Evaluate Nausea During Pregnancy

Q. I've been nauseated ever since I became pregnant. How can I reduce this?

A. Medications are rarely prescribed to relieve nausea with pregnancy because they can have an effect on fetal growth. Common nonpharmacologic measures you can take to reduce nausea are:

- Be aware that at least 50% of women experience nausea during pregnancy, so what you are experiencing is normal.
- Eat a few dry crackers, toast, or a sourball before you get out of bed in the morning to increase your carbohydrate intake.
- Eat small but frequent meals rather than large infrequent ones.
- Avoid greasy or highly seasoned food.
- Delay breakfast until nausea passes (dinner if it is evening nausea).
- Make up missed meals at some other time of the day to maintain nutrition.
- Avoid sudden movements and fatigue because these may increase or cause nausea.
- Eat a snack before bedtime so delaying breakfast won't cause you to go a long time between meals.
- Purchase a wrist acupressure band (purchased in travel stores for motion sickness).

If nausea is present:

- Try sipping a carbonated beverage, water, or an herbal noncaffeinated tea.
- Try a walk outside in the fresh air or take deep breaths through an open window.

Notify your health care provider if:

- You are losing weight rather than gaining it.
- You have not gained the projected amount of weight for your week of pregnancy.
- You are unable to make up for lost meals some other time of the day.
- You have signs of dehydration such as little urine output.
- Nausea has lasted past 12 weeks of pregnancy.
- You vomit more than once daily.

for laundry starch. Currently, pica may be a craving for clay, dirt, cornstarch, or ice cubes (Simpson et al., 2000). Although some of these items can do no harm in themselves, the ingestion of large quantities can leave the woman deficient in protein, iron, and calcium, nutrients essential for a healthy pregnancy outcome.

Always question women at prenatal visits if they crave any nonfood items. Most women do not supply this information unless asked directly. They worry that you will find their behavior odd, or they may not realize their habit is pregnancy-related as much as being a nervous habit.

Encouraging a woman to stop eating the nonfood substance may not be effective because the habit may be deeply ingrained. Because pica is a symptom that often accompanies iron-deficiency anemia, correcting the underlying problem with an iron supplement may correct the pica. At subsequent visits, however, be certain to assess the woman for this and ask her if she notices any difference in her cravings.

Pyrosis

Pyrosis (heartburn) is a burning sensation along the esophagus caused by regurgitation of gastric contents into the lower esophagus. In pregnancy, it may accompany nausea, but it may persist beyond the resolution of nausea and even increase in severity as pregnancy advances.

Pyrosis is probably caused by decreased gastric motility that slows gastric emptying. It may be relieved by eating small meals frequently and by not lying down immediately after eating, to help prevent reflux. Aluminum hydroxide (Amphojel) or a combination of aluminum and magnesium hydroxide (Maalox) may be prescribed for relief. Be certain a woman understands that this "chest" pain is from her gastrointestinal tract and that, although it is called heartburn, it has nothing to do with her heart.

Hypercholesterolemia

Women with a family history of hypercholesterolemia may enter pregnancy with an elevated cholesterol level. During pregnancy, increasing progesterone levels cause a further elevation of cholesterol. This can lead to an increased risk for gallstone formation (cholelithiasis) and cardiovascular disease. Preventing cholelithiasis during pregnancy is important because this causes extremely sharp pain. Surgery to remove gallstones during pregnancy can threaten the fetus because of the necessary anesthesia, even with new ambulatory laparotomy techniques.

A woman who has had difficulty with hypercholesterolemia before pregnancy may need to continue to eat only moderate amounts of fat during pregnancy to prevent any increase in cholesterol. Helpful ways to reduce cholesterol may include:

- Exercising daily
- Eating oat bran
- Broiling meat rather than frying it
- Eating fish high in omega-3 oil, such as salmon or tuna
- Using a minimum of salad oils
- Substituting new omega-3 products for butter

Urge women to check with their health care provider about the wisdom of continuing to take cholesterol-lowering drugs during pregnancy, because these may be teratogenic. A low-cholesterol diet will automatically be lower in calories than the average diet, because oils and fats add many calories. Therefore, assess these women carefully for adequate weight gain during pregnancy. Make sure that a woman does include some oil daily (perhaps as olive oil on a salad) so she has included a source of linoleic acid in her daily intake.

> **✔ CHECKPOINT QUESTIONS**
>
> 9. When does nausea usually disappear during pregnancy?
> 10. What is pica?
> 11. If a pregnant woman has hypercholesterolemia, for what conditions is she at risk?

Promoting Nutritional Health in Women With Special Needs

The Adolescent

The pregnant adolescent needs a high caloric intake (2,500 calories per day) to supply energy for her high level of activity and growth. The nutrients most often lacking from a typical adolescent diet tend to be calcium, iron, folic acid, and total calories. Look for sources of these when analyzing a teenager's pregnancy intake.

Good nutrition can be a problem with pregnant teenagers because of the dual demands of consuming enough food to provide for fetal growth and their own continuing growth. Often adolescents, in their search for identity, avoid foods that their parents see as important for them (e.g., milk, warm cereal, vegetables, or fruit), indulging instead in foods such as soft drinks, potato chips, and French fries. To help the adolescent plan nutritional intake for pregnancy, respect her right to reject traditional foods as long as her diet includes sufficient nutrients. A cheese and sausage pizza, a glass of milk, and an apple is a lunch that provides all basic food groups (meat: sausage; bread: pizza crust; vegetable: tomato sauce; dairy: cheese and milk; fruit: apple). A hamburger "with everything" plus a tangerine and milk provides the same (see Focus on Communication). Focus on Evidence-Based Practice discusses self-efficacy and the pregnant adolescent.

Most adolescents snack frequently during the day. Toward the end of pregnancy, when fatigue may be a problem, they may begin to eat more and more "junk food" because preparing nutritious snacks takes more effort. Advise them to prepare some nutritious snacks such as carrot sticks or cheese bites early each day when they have more energy so that later in the day, when they are tired, eating a nutritious snack will not involve much effort.

Counseling adolescents may be difficult because they often are not responsible for cooking the food they eat. You may need to speak to their parents or support persons (with permission) about certain foods to prepare before you can alter their nutrition pattern. If possible, suggest a number of foods that would fill a deficit and let the adolescent choose from them to provide a sense of control (Lenders et al., 2000).

> **FOCUS ON COMMUNICATION**
>
> Geraldine is a 16-year-old girl who comes to the prenatal clinic for her first visit. You want to obtain a nutrition history from her.
>
> ***Less Effective Communication***
>
> *Nurse:* Are you eating a nutritious diet?
> *Geraldine:* Sure. My mom's a good cook.
> *Nurse:* Did you learn about the food pyramid in school? Are you eating all the different kinds of food it shows?
> *Geraldine:* Sure. Grain is at the bottom; fat is on the top.
> *Nurse:* You need to drink at least a quart of milk a day. Are you doing that?
> *Geraldine:* Sure. Easy. I like milk.
> *Nurse:* That's great. Good nutrition is so important during pregnancy. I'm glad you're so aware of it.
>
> ***More Effective Communication***
>
> *Nurse:* Are you eating a nutritious diet?
> *Geraldine:* Sure. My mom's a good cook.
> *Nurse:* Tell me what you ate yesterday.
> *Geraldine:* A muffin for breakfast, pizza for lunch, ravioli for supper. Ice cream before bed.
> *Nurse:* What did you drink with meals?
> *Geraldine:* Root beer for breakfast and lunch. Kool-aid for supper.
> *Nurse:* Would you mind if I talked to your mother about ways you could eat more fruit? And more milk?
> *Geraldine:* I rarely listen to her. If I did, I wouldn't be pregnant, would I?
>
> Most people believe they eat well, so if just asked general questions about nutrition, they respond that their nutrition is adequate. Only when asked to actually describe what they ate during one day is the truth revealed. Here, questioning also reveals that this adolescent needs direct nutrition counseling because she may not listen to advice given by a parent.

The Woman Over Age 40

Today, many women are older than 40 by the time they have their first child, and many more are older than 40 when they have their second or third child. The nutritional needs of women in this age group are poorly studied, but these women should maintain the same careful pregnancy nutrition as younger women. Because women in this age group may have slightly decreased kidney function, they should maintain a high fluid intake to remove waste products for themselves and for the fetus. Many women at this point in life are caring for elderly parents, and many have delayed child-bearing to establish a career; they may eat whatever they are preparing for elderly parents or depend on packed or fast-food lunches for at least part of their nutrition each week. Focus your nutrition counseling on maintaining adequate nutrition during pregnancy, based on the woman's lifestyle.

The Woman With Decreased Nutritional Stores

A woman with high parity or a short interval between pregnancies or one who has been dieting rigorously to lose weight before pregnancy may enter pregnancy with such depleted nutritional reserves that she has little to

FOCUS ON EVIDENCE-BASED PRACTICE

If Adolescents Gain Self-Efficacy, Could It Improve Their Nutrition?

Self-efficacy is the power to be personally effective. It is a concept closely aligned with self-concept or feeling able to accomplish. One of the concerns with adolescents who are pregnant is that they will "follow the crowd" rather than be independent enough to change to healthier eating habits.

To see if specific interactions by health care professionals could improve self-efficacy for adolescents during pregnancy, researchers divided a sample of 28 urban pregnant adolescents (94% African-American, 4% white, 2% other) between a control and an experimental group. The control group of teenagers received routine prenatal care. The second group had increased interventions with health care personnel aimed at strengthening their feelings about themselves. Self-efficacy was measured when the adolescents entered prenatal care and again in the postpartal period. Results of the study showed that all adolescents improved in self-efficacy during pregnancy whether they received special interventions or not (as if the total experience of pregnancy is so great, it caused a change in everyone). Among those adolescents who received special interventions, interventions such as peer support and small group sessions showed the most positive effects.

This is an important study for nurses because nurses are the health care professionals who may spend the most time with adolescents while they are pregnant. Knowing that peer support and group interactions are effective techniques to use with adolescents can guide how information is presented.

Ford, K., et al. (2001). Effects of a prenatal care intervention on the self-concept and self-efficacy of adolescent mothers. *Journal of Perinatal Education, 10*(2), 15–22.

draw on during the first part of pregnancy. This is critical during the time she may not be able to eat well because of the normal nausea and vomiting of pregnancy. In addition, nutritional stores may be affected by other variables. Be alert to the following:

- Women from low-income families may enter pregnancy with anemia.
- Women who used diuretics for a dieting program may be deficient in potassium.
- Women who have been taking oral contraceptives may have decreased folate stores.
- Women who were using intrauterine devices or who have menorrhagia may be deficient in iron from excessive blood loss with menstrual flows.
- Women who drink alcohol excessively may be deficient in thiamine.

Women with these decreased nutritional stores need to be identified early in pregnancy through history taking so you can provide specific nutritional counseling early in the pregnancy. They may need additional supplements during pregnancy to restore a particular nutrient.

The Woman Who Is Underweight

Today's emphasis on slim, model-like female figures makes it easy to overlook the health problem of a woman who is underweight. A woman who enters a pregnancy underweight, however, needs nutritional counseling just as much as any pregnant client.

In pregnancy, **underweight** can be defined as a state in which a woman's weight is 10% to 15% less than the ideal weight for her height, or a BMI of less than 19.8. Being underweight usually occurs because of a long-standing poor nutritional pattern, or it may signify underlying disease. Most women who are underweight tire easily and have an accompanying iron-deficiency anemia and reduced resistance to disease. As a consequence, they have a higher than usual incidence of low-birthweight infants.

Being underweight may occur for a variety of reasons in addition to dieting for weight loss:

- Poverty and the inability to buy adequate food (however, many poor women are obese, not underweight, because starchy foods are less expensive than those that have a higher protein content, such as meat and eggs)
- Excessive worry or stress, emotions that can lead to a loss of appetite
- Depression, which causes a chronic loss of appetite
- An eating disorder, such as anorexia nervosa or bulimia, conditions in which the woman has developed a revulsion to food (see Chap. 54)

However, the major reason for being underweight is insufficient intake of food due to chronic poor nutritional habits.

Nutritional counseling with underweight women may be difficult because the woman is being asked to change lifelong eating habits. Counseling also can be challenging because during the first trimester of pregnancy, when fetal need is greatest and at a time when she has nausea and vomiting, possibly losing all desire to eat, you are asking her to take in additional food.

Begin counseling by asking the woman for a 24-hour nutrition recall. If she is asked if she eats well, she will usually say that she does (it seems adequate to her because it is her usual pattern).

Total daily caloric intake for the underweight woman may need to be 3,500 calories (500 to 1,000 calories more than the usual specified daily amount). Work with women to develop menus based on well-planned meals rather than on quick take-out foods. Suggest additional calories in the form of a concentrated formula such as an instant liquid breakfast drink. Be certain the woman understands this should not be a high-protein drink used for high-protein dieting regimens. Such diet drinks deliver a concentrated solute load (breakdown products of protein) to the kidney (already working to capacity because of the pregnancy) and provide so little carbohydrate in proportion to protein that they encourage the breakdown of protein for body energy, a process that results in acidosis. High-protein diets of this nature are not recommended for long-term use by anyone, but they should be totally avoided by women during pregnancy.

A 500-calorie increase over normal requirements should result in a weight gain of an additional pound per week. Be certain to plan for this additional gain when the total weight gain during pregnancy is calculated at each office visit. Otherwise, the total weight gain of the woman may seem excessive when it is actually healthy.

If a lack of nutritional stores makes the woman feel tired, urge her to schedule adequate rest periods daily so she can feel sufficiently energetic to prepare nutritious meals. Be certain she is taking her prescribed vitamin and iron supplements. Additional nutritional counseling in the postpartal period may be necessary so she can maintain better nutrition throughout her life and can enter a subsequent pregnancy (if there is one) in a state of nutritional health.

Even when underweight women gain excessive weight during pregnancy, they still tend to have a higher than usual incidence of low-birthweight infants, probably because of depleted nutrient stores at the pregnancy's beginning. This is one reason that preconceptual health care visits and assessment are so important (Stephenson & Symonds, 2002).

The Woman Who Is Overweight

During pregnancy, a woman is considered **overweight** if she is 20% above ideal weight or has a BMI over 26.1. She is considered **obese** if she weighs more than 200 pounds, she is 50% above ideal body weight for height, or her BMI is above 29. Although obesity may occur from hypothyroidism, it most often occurs as a result of excessive caloric intake and decreased energy expenditure.

As many as 10% of pregnant women in the United States are overweight. Less-educated women and those living in poverty tend to be more overweight than others.

Obesity becomes a problem during pregnancy for a variety of reasons:

- Pregnancy causes circulatory volume to increase 20% to 50% and metabolism to increase to meet the demands of the pregnancy, placing additional stress on a possibly already overworked body.
- Obesity is associated with an increased incidence of gestational diabetes and increased risk for pregnancy-induced hypertension.
- It is often difficult to hear fetal heart tones in an obese woman; palpating for position and size of the fetus at birth is also difficult.
- Obese women are at an increased risk for giving birth to infants with macrosomia (excessive fetal growth); this increases the incidence of cesarean births in this population.
- The pregnancies of obese women are more apt to be prolonged, leading to postmature infants.
- Performing a cesarean birth, if necessary, may be difficult because of the excessive adipose tissue that must be incised to reach the uterus.
- Ambulating during pregnancy and immediately afterward is more difficult because of the increased energy expenditure necessary, increasing the risk for complications such as thrombophlebitis and pneumonia.

Nutritional counseling with obese women during pregnancy may be difficult because overeating has many causes. For some women, overeating is a coping mechanism for stress; whenever they feel tense or worried, they have something "comforting" to eat. Therefore, because pregnancy is stressful, it may be difficult for a woman to change her food intake patterns at this time. Other women overeat because their parents did, and they were raised to consume a high-calorie diet. Changing this pattern means changing a lifelong habit. If the woman's family also enjoys an excessive intake of calories, then the entire family may have to change their eating patterns to effect a change in the woman's intake.

Dieting to reduce weight is not recommended during pregnancy because if carbohydrates are reduced too much, the body will use protein and fat for energy. This can deprive the fetus of protein and lead to ketoacidosis. Although the long-term effects of mild ketoacidosis on the fetus are not well studied, it can be avoided if the daily caloric intake, even in the most obese woman, does not go below 1,500 to 1,800 per day.

Overweight women tend to exercise less than women of normal weight. Exercising is more awkward and more tiring, and they may feel self-conscious. Try to encourage them to engage in at least a minimum activity program, such as walking around the block once a day, in conjunction with lessened carbohydrate intake.

Helping a woman look at her nutrition in terms of empty-calorie versus nutritious foods may help her to eat more sensibly. Early in pregnancy, when she is eager to appear pregnant, she may resist limiting her intake. Stress that a fetus grows best on nutritious foods, not necessarily those with the most calories. Provide additional nutritional counseling in the postpartal period so she can prepare more nutritious meals in the future for herself and her growing family. If successful, she will not enter another pregnancy severely overweight.

The Woman Who Is a Vegetarian

There are over 10 million vegetarians in the United States. Since 1995, the U.S. government has endorsed vegetarianism as consistent with the Dietary Guidelines for Americans. Most women vegetarians are closer to their ideal weight and have lower serum cholesterol levels and lower blood pressure levels than women who eat a more typical American diet. Nurses may find that many pregnant women, therefore, will want to exclude meat from their diets. There are many different types of vegetarians: lacto-ovo-vegetarians (no animal flesh or fish is eaten, but dairy products and eggs are), lactovegetarians (no meat, fish, or eggs are eaten, but dairy products are), and vegans (nothing derived from an animal is eaten). Most vegetarians are knowledgeable about their diets and can discuss what foods are high in various nutrients and how they incorporate such foods in their daily intake.

A vegetarian food pyramid is identical to a usual one, except it contains no meat (see Appendix K). Women should try to eat three or more servings a day of both fruits and vegetables, six or more servings per day of grains, and two or more servings per day of legumes such as kidney, black, or lima beans.

Special concerns for pregnant vegetarians include lack of vitamin B_{12} (meat is the chief source of this) and an inadequate intake of calcium (recommend dark-green vegetables as sources) and vitamin D (fortified milk and sunlight are the main sources of this). Urge women who are vegetarians to take a daily prenatal supplement, like all women, to ensure adequate iron and folic acid.

The Woman With Phenylketonuria

Phenylketonuria (PKU), named because the breakdown product of phenylalanine is excreted in the urine in this form, is an inherited disorder in which a person cannot convert the essential amino acid phenylalanine into tyrosine, the form used for cell growth. Without conversion, phenylalanine accumulates in the person's serum, eventually leaving the bloodstream to invade body cells. When brain cells are invaded, severe cognitive challenge and accompanying neurologic damage, such as recurrent seizures, may develop (see Chap. 48). The fetus of a woman with uncontrolled PKU can develop microcephaly, intrauterine growth restriction, and neurologic damage as well.

Children with PKU follow a diet with restricted phenylalanine intake until at least past adolescence. A woman with PKU should consult her internist when she is planning to become pregnant and should plan to return to a low-phenylalanine diet for at least 3 months before she becomes pregnant. Foods high in phenylalanine are high in protein; examples of foods low in phenylalanine are fruits and vegetables such as orange juice, bananas, squash, spinach, and peas. The woman typically follows this low-phenylalanine diet during the pregnancy and afterward as long as she is breast-feeding.

The woman with PKU needs support during pregnancy to adhere to these nutritional restrictions. It is particularly disappointing for a woman if she does not become pregnant immediately after starting the restricted diet, because each month that she is "prepregnant" extends the period she must follow the restrictions. A woman with PKU is usually well informed about her particular nutritional needs. She is aware that phenylalanine is destructive to developing brain cells and that not following her restricted plan could leave her future child severely cognitively challenged (Waisbren et al., 2000).

The Woman With a Multiple Pregnancy

The woman with a multiple pregnancy gains more weight overall and with greater speed than the woman carrying a single child because of the increased fetal weight. To sustain her own nutrition stores, she must ingest high levels of protein and carbohydrate. In particular, there is an increased burden on maternal iron and folic acid stores. It is important that multiple pregnancy be recognized early and nutrition supplements be added as needed.

WHAT IF? What if a woman with a multiple pregnancy tells you she is "eating for four," so takes four desserts every day for lunch? Will this hurt her or just add on a few extra pounds?

The Woman Who Smokes or Uses Drugs or Alcohol

The specific effects of alcohol, cigarette smoking, and drug use on fetal growth are discussed in Chapter 11. In addition to specific teratogenic fetal effects, these substances can lead to general nutrition problems because the woman is ingesting these substances rather than eating nutritious foods.

The Woman With Concurrent Health Problems

Any health concern that requires rigid salt, protein, or carbohydrate restriction poses a potential threat to fetal nutrition during pregnancy. Women who have medical problems such as kidney disease, diabetes, tuberculosis, bulimia, or anorexia nervosa need special dietary considerations during pregnancy because of the specific metabolic disorders that occur with these diseases. A malabsorption syndrome such as inflammatory bowel disease or celiac disease can also pose a threat (Mighty & Atkins, 2000). Nursing interventions and nutrition concerns for women with health problems such as these are discussed in Chapters 14 and 17.

The Woman Who Eats Many Fast-Food Meals

As many as 90% of women of child-bearing age work at least part-time outside their homes. This means that nutritional counseling must involve helping women who rely on packed lunches or fast-food meals to maintain adequate pregnancy nutrition. The difficulty with fast-food restaurants is the limited choice of food available. This can cause a woman to grow tired of the same thing and thus eat little. Unless there is a salad bar, there is likely to be a limited menu of fruits and vegetables. Fast-food restaurants have also been associated with outbreaks of infection due to undercooked hamburger or contaminated salad bars. This could lead to severe gastrointestinal symptoms such as vomiting and diarrhea and possible electrolyte imbalance.

A packed lunch poses few problems in pregnancy as long as the woman uses some creativity in preparation so she does not grow so tired of packed lunches that she reduces her noontime intake. Packing a lunch at bedtime rather than in the morning, when she may feel nauseous (and therefore packs little because nothing looks good), is a good recommendation early in pregnancy. Late in pregnancy, a woman may feel too tired at bedtime to do this and should change to preparing it in the morning, when she has more energy. Including a thermos with a cream soup is a good way to add milk and calcium to the diet. Packing carrot sticks or sliced cucumbers, tomatoes, or apples helps make the lunch nutritious and also provides a midmorning or midafternoon snack. Having snacks available this way prevents her from going long stretches of time without eating.

✔ CHECKPOINT QUESTIONS

12. Why might counseling an underweight client be difficult in early pregnancy?
13. A pregnant vegetarian is at risk for what nutritional deficiencies?

The Woman With Lactose Intolerance

The sugar in milk is lactose. In the intestine, lactose is broken down into glucose and galactose by the enzyme **lactase.** In most of the world's population, lactase is present in infants but disappears by school age. After this point, many people have difficulty digesting lactose or are lactose intolerant. African-Americans, Native Americans, and Asians tend to have the highest percentage of lactose intolerance (approximately 70% of African-American adults cannot drink milk). Those most able to tolerate milk are Northern Europeans and their descendants.

When people who are lactose intolerant drink milk, they report nausea, diarrhea, cramps, gas, and a general feeling of bloatedness. Some express these symptoms as simply, "I don't like milk." The intestinal slowing that accompanies pregnancy may allow women to handle lactose better during pregnancy than they usually do.

Women who cannot drink milk because of lactose intolerance may be able to eat cheese because the processing of cheese changes the lactose content; yogurt may also be tolerated. Fortified soy milk is another possible substitute. Lactase tablets can be prescribed to supplement absent lactase. Typically, the woman chews these before ingesting milk products. Even with this, however, a calcium supplement (1,200 mg daily) and a vitamin D supplement (400 IU) may be necessary. This is because the amount of cheese or yogurt needed to replace the calcium of milk is too large to be practical. Because milk is a good source of protein, be sure to assess whether, without milk, the woman's intake of protein is adequate.

Many baby magazines, television advertisements, and government pamphlets on pregnancy mention repeatedly that it is important to drink milk during pregnancy. It may be necessary to explain that as long as a woman ingests the same nutrients from other foods, the actual drinking of milk is not important.

The Woman With Hyperemesis Gravidarum

Hyperemesis gravidarum (sometimes called pernicious vomiting) is nausea and vomiting of pregnancy that is prolonged past week 12 of pregnancy or is so severe that dehydration, ketonuria, and significant weight loss occur within the first 12 weeks. The cause is unknown, but women with the disorder may have increased thyroid function due to the thyroid-stimulating properties of human chorionic gonadotropin. It occurs at an incidence of 1 in 200 to 300 women.

Assessment. With hyperemesis gravidarum, the woman's nausea and vomiting are so severe that she cannot maintain her usual nutrition. She may show an elevated hematocrit concentration at her monthly prenatal visit because her inability to retain fluid has resulted in hemoconcentration. Concentrations of sodium, potassium, and chloride may be reduced from low intake, and hypokalemic alkalosis may result if vomiting is severe during the day or persists for an extended period. In some women, polyneuritis, due to a deficiency of B vitamins, develops. Weight loss can be severe. Urine may test positive for ketones, evidence that the woman's body is breaking down stored fat and protein for cell growth. If left untreated, the condition is associated with intrauterine growth restriction or preterm birth if the woman becomes dehydrated and can no longer provide the fetus with essential nutrients for growth. Prolonged hospitalization or home care with this disorder may result in social isolation.

Determine how much nausea and vomiting women are having during pregnancy. Ask a woman to describe the events of the day before if she says it was a typical day. How late into the day did the nausea last? How many times did she vomit, and how much? What was the total amount of food she was able to eat?

Therapeutic Management. Women with hyperemesis gravidarum usually need to be hospitalized for approximately 24 hours to monitor intake, output, and blood chemistries and to prevent dehydration.

All oral food and fluids are usually withheld. Intravenous fluid (3,000 mL Ringer's lactate with added vitamin B, for example) may be administered to increase hydration. An antiemetic, such as metoclopramide (Reglan), may be prescribed to control vomiting. Throughout this period, carefully measure intake and output, including the amount of vomitus.

If there is no vomiting after the first 24 hours of oral restriction, small amounts of clear fluid may be begun and the woman is discharged home, usually with a referral for home care. If clear fluid is tolerated, small quantities of dry toast, crackers, or cereal may be taken every 2 or 3 hours, then the woman can be gradually advanced to a soft diet, then to a normal diet. If vomiting returns at any point, enteral or total parenteral nutrition may be attempted. Home care follow-up provides further information about the client's status after hospital discharge (see Chap. 16).

NURSING DIAGNOSES AND RELATED INTERVENTIONS

A woman with hyperemesis gravidarum needs the opportunity to express how she feels about the strange thing that is happening to her, how it feels to be pregnant and live with the ever-present nausea. Some women are under such psychosocial stress that counseling is necessary to help them decide whether to terminate the pregnancy or allow it to go to completion. An appropriate nursing diagnosis may be Ineffective coping related to stress of pregnancy or concurrent life events. Be certain that the outcomes established are realistic. It may not be possible to stop vomiting completely, but enough supplemental fluid to counteract the loss of fluid with vomiting can be supplied.

Nursing Diagnosis: Risk for deficient fluid volume related to vomiting secondary to hyperemesis gravidarum

Outcome Identification: Client will maintain adequate hydration for her own and fetal needs.

Outcome Evaluation: Client remains free of signs and symptoms of dehydration (i.e., poor skin turgor or dry skin or mucous membranes); urine output is greater than 30 mL/h; urine specific gravity ranges between 1.003 and 1.030; no further episodes of vomiting occur.

Like the typical nausea and vomiting of pregnancy, the vomiting of hyperemesis gravidarum may be precipitated by fatigue and the smell of cooking. Encourage the woman to serve herself small portions so the amount on her plate does not appear overwhelming. It is best if foods are presented attractively. Hot foods should be hot, and cold foods should be cold.

An emesis basin is an important piece of equipment for the woman who is vomiting. While she is hospitalized, put it out of sight and not on the bedside table, however, so she is not constantly reminded of vomiting. Try to limit her exposure to food odors. Be sure that food carts smelling of food such as fish, bacon, or coffee are not parked outside her door at mealtimes. Be sure to reinforce these instructions with other health care providers (see the Focus on Multidisciplinary Care).

Nursing Diagnosis: Imbalanced nutrition, less than body requirements, related to prolonged vomiting

Outcome Identification: Client will ingest enough nutrients orally or intravenously to sustain herself and growing fetus for remainder of pregnancy.

Outcome Evaluation: Client eats at least 2,500 calories daily.

Some women have such extreme symptoms that vomiting recurs with the introduction of food. To maintain adequate nutrition to support fetal growth, the woman may need to be maintained on total parenteral nutrition or enteral feedings. While she is receiving total parenteral nutrition at home, instruct her to check her urine for glucose and ketones twice daily. If there is glucose in the urine, this suggests that the infusion solution contains more glucose than the body's metabolism can use. Ketones in the urine mean that the body is not receiving enough nutrients and it is breaking down protein. If either of these findings is positive, she should telephone her health care provider because she needs a nutrition reassessment.

Fortunately, despite its extreme symptoms, excessive vomiting during pregnancy rarely leads to pregnancy loss or low-birthweight newborns when it is treated (Wenstrom & Malee, 2000).

✔ CHECKPOINT QUESTIONS

14. What is the greatest danger associated with hyperemesis?
15. If vomiting continues even with cessation of oral intake or resumes with oral intake, what treatment may be prescribed?

FOCUS ON MULTIDISCIPLINARY CARE

Many different health care providers contact women during pregnancy—physicians, nurse-midwives, sonogram technicians, pediatricians, nurse practitioners, and nutritionists, for example—and all have opportunities to talk to women about pregnancy nutrition.

Unlicensed assistive personnel may be assigned to help care for a woman with hyperemesis gravidarum while in the hospital or at home. Be certain that they understand that the woman is not experiencing the usual nausea and vomiting of pregnancy, but a serious illness that can be life-threatening. Caution them not to talk about food while they work (e.g., "What's the soup of the day in the cafeteria?") or to urge the woman to "Eat just a little more. You're starving your baby." Urging women with hyperemesis gravidarum to eat this way can cause them to feel guilty on top of feeling so nauseated that they cannot eat.

KEY POINTS

Assessment of nutritional health involves a health history (24-hour recall) and physical examination.

Pregnant women should increase their intake of calories, protein, and certain vitamins and minerals during pregnancy to help ensure fetal growth.

Nutrition during pregnancy should include about 300 additional daily calories to provide energy, spare protein, and provide for fetal growth requirements.

Important minerals necessary for pregnancy include iron, iodine, calcium, fluoride, sodium, and zinc. Most women need to take an iron supplement to prevent iron-deficiency anemia.

Women should consider their intake of caffeine and artificial sweeteners during pregnancy.

Prenatal vitamins contain additional folic acid supplements and iron, so these should be used instead of over-the-counter vitamins during pregnancy. Be certain that women regard pregnancy vitamins as medication and follow the medication rule: take nothing other than medications specifically recommended by the primary care provider, or else toxicity could result.

Advise pregnant women not to go longer than 12 hours between meals, to avoid hypoglycemia.

Women who are at high risk for inadequate nutrition include those who are adolescent or over age 40; those who have decreased nutrition stores; those with a multiple pregnancy; those who are lactose intolerant; those who are underweight or overweight; those on a special diet; those using drugs, including alcohol or cigarettes; and those with hyperemesis gravidarum (extreme nausea and vomiting).

Common nutrition concerns associated with pregnancy include nausea and vomiting, constipation, cravings (including pica), and pyrosis.

Hyperemesis gravidarum is nausea and vomiting of pregnancy that extends past 12 weeks of pregnancy or is too extreme to allow for adequate nutrition. Women with this condition may need their nutrition supplemented by total parenteral nutrition or enteral feedings.

CRITICAL THINKING EXERCISES

1. Ms. Alarino, whom you met at the beginning of the chapter, was drinking milkshakes as a source of calcium. Was this a wise choice? Why do you think she craved oranges?
2. A 30-year-old woman who is 2 months pregnant comes for her routine prenatal visit. She works as a supermarket cashier. She states she is too

nauseated in the morning to eat before she leaves for work, and she is too tired of seeing food go by her to prepare a good meal after work. What suggestions could you give to help her increase her food intake?

3. A 21-year-old pregnant client reports that she rarely eats vegetables; when she does, she fries them in butter. How would you use a food pyramid to explain better pregnancy nutrition to her?
4. A 19-year-old pregnant college student adheres to a food plan that provides for only lunch and dinner. Both of these must be obtained from the college cafeteria. What suggestions could you make to ensure that she obtains adequate nutrition during pregnancy?
5. Examine the National Health Goals related to nutrition and pregnancy. Most government-sponsored money for nursing research is allotted based on these goals. What would be a possible research topic to explore pertinent to these goals that would be fundable and would advance evidence-based practice?

REFERENCES

Bailey, L. B. (2000). New standard for dietary folate intake in pregnant women. *American Journal of Clinical Nutrition, 71*(5), 1304S–1307S.

Department of Health and Human Services. (2000). *Healthy people 2010.* Washington, D.C.: DHHS.

Dudek, S. G. (2001). *Nutrition handbook for nursing practice* (4th ed.). Philadelphia: Lippincott Williams & Wilkins.

Flaxman, S. M., & Sherman, P. W. (2000). Morning sickness. *Quarterly Review of Biology, 75*(2), 113–148.

Ford, K, et al. (2001). Effects of a prenatal care intervention on the self-concept and self-efficacy of adolescent mothers. *Journal of Perinatal Education, 10*(2), 15–22.

Karch, A. M. (2001). *Lippincott's nursing drug guide.* Philadelphia: Lippincott Williams & Wilkins.

Ladipo, O. A. (2000). Nutrition in pregnancy: Mineral and vitamin supplements. *American Journal of Clinical Nutrition, 72*(1), 280S–290S.

Lenders, C. M., McElrath, T. F., & Scholl, T. O. (2000). Nutrition in adolescent pregnancy. *Current Opinion in Pediatrics, 12*(3), 291–296.

Mighty, H. E., & Atkins, D. (2000). Pregnancy and inflammatory bowel disease: Current management. *Journal of the Association for Academic Minority Physicians, 11*(2-3), 38–43.

Reifsnider, E., & Gill, S. L. (2000). Nutrition for the childbearing years. *Journal of Obstetric, Gynecologic & Neonatal Nursing, 29*(1), 43–55.

Simpson, E., et al. (2000). Pica during pregnancy in low-income women born in Mexico. *Western Journal of Medicine, 173*(1), 20–24.

Stephenson, T. & Symonds, M.E. (2002). Maternal nutrition as a determinant of birth weight. *Archives of Disease in Childhood, 86*(1), 4–6.

Swensen, A. R., et al. (2001). Nutritional assessment of pregnant women enrolled in the Special Supplemental Program for Women, Infants and Children (WIC). *Journal of the American Dietetic Association, 101*(8), 903–908.

Waisbren, S. E., et al. (2000). Outcome at age 4 years in offspring of women with maternal phenylketonuria: The Maternal PKU Collaborative Study. *Journal of the American Medical Association, 283*(6), 756–762.

Wenstrum, K. D., & Malee, M. P. (2000). Medical and surgical complications of pregnancy. In J. R. Scott, et al. *Danforth's obstetrics and gynecology* (8th ed., pp. 327–391). Philadelphia: Lippincott Williams & Wilkins.

SUGGESTED READINGS

Carter, A. S., Baker, C. W., & Brownell, K. D. (2000). Body mass index, eating attitudes, and symptoms of depression and anxiety in pregnancy and the postpartum period. *Psychosomatic Medicine, 62*(2), 264–270.

Centers for Disease Control (2001). Knowledge and use of folic acid among women of reproductive age. *MMWR, 50*(10), 185–189.

Godfrey, K. M., & Barker, D. J. (2000). Fetal nutrition and adult disease. *American Journal of Clinical Nutrition, 71*(5), 1344S–1352S.

Hun, D. J. et al. (2002). Effects of nutrition education programs on anthropometric measurements and pregnancy outcomes of adolescents. *Journal of the American Dietetic Association, 102*(3), S100–S102.

Huxley, R. R. (2000). Nausea and vomiting in early pregnancy: Its role in placental development. *Obstetrics & Gynecology, 95*(5), 779–782.

King, J. C. (2000). Physiology of pregnancy and nutrition metabolism. *American Journal of Clinical Nutrition, 71*(5), 1218S–1225S.

Lacroix, R., Eason, E., & Malzack, R. (2000). Nausea and vomiting during pregnancy: A prospective study of its frequency, intensity, and patterns of change. *American Journal of Obstetrics & Gynecology, 182*(4), 931–937.

Little, L., & Lowkes, E. (2000). Critical issues in the care of pregnant women with eating disorders and the impact on their children. *Journal of Midwifery & Women's Health, 45*(4), 301–307.

Maine, D. (2000). Role of nutrition in the prevention of toxemia. *American Journal of Clinical Nutrition, 72*(1), 298S–300S.

Mazzotta, P., & Magee, L. A. (2000). A risk-benefit assessment of pharmacological and nonpharmacological treatments for nausea and vomiting or pregnancy. *Drugs, 59*(4), 781–800.

Roseboom, T. J., et al. (2001). Maternal nutrition during gestation and blood pressure in later life. *Journal of Hypertension, 19*(1), 29S–34S.

Rouse, B., et al. (2000). Maternal phenylketonuria syndrome: Congenital heart defects, microcephaly, and developmental outcomes. *Journal of Pediatrics, 136*(1), 57–61.

Schieve, L. A., et al. (2000). Prepregnancy body mass index and pregnancy weight gain: Associations with preterm delivery. *Obstetrics & Gynecology, 96*(2), 194–200.

13

CHAPTER

Preparation for Childbirth and Parenting

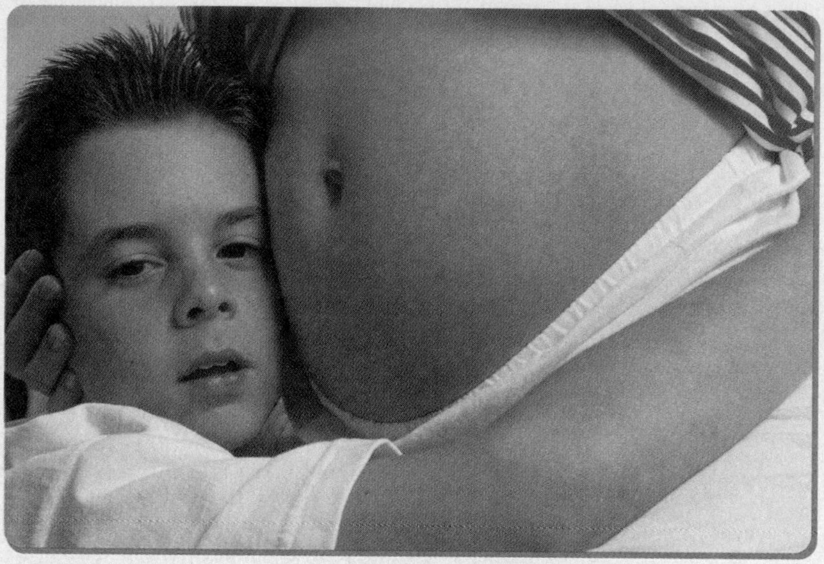

Key Terms

- alternative birthing centers (ABC)
- birthing bed
- birthing chairs
- birthing room
- cleansing breath
- conditioned reflexes
- consciously controlled breathing
- conscious relaxation
- distraction
- effleurage
- gate control theory of pain perception
- labor-delivery-recovery-postpartum rooms (LDRP)
- labor-delivery-recovery rooms (LDR)
- Leboyer method
- psychoprophylactic
- vaginal birth after cesarean birth (VBAC)

Objectives

After mastering the contents of this chapter, you should be able to:

1. Describe common alternative settings for birth and preparation necessary for childbirth and parenting.
2. Assess a couple for readiness for childbirth in regard to choice of birth attendant, preparation for labor, and setting.
3. Formulate nursing diagnoses related to preparation for childbirth and parenting.
4. Identify expected outcomes for the couple preparing for childbirth and parenting.
5. Plan nursing care such as teaching exercises that are effective for strengthening abdominal and perineal muscles for childbirth.
6. Implement nursing care such as supporting a woman during labor by the Lamaze method of prepared childbirth or helping a couple select and prepare for an alternative birth setting such as the home.
7. Evaluate outcome criteria for achievement and effectiveness of care.
8. Identify National Health Goals related to preparation for parenthood that nurses could be instrumental in helping the nation to achieve.
9. Identify areas related to preparation for childbirth that could benefit from additional nursing research or application of evidence-based practice.
10. Use critical thinking to analyze ways that birth can be made more family-centered through the use of prepared childbirth classes and alternative birth settings.
11. Integrate the principles of prepared childbirth with nursing process to achieve quality maternal and child health nursing care.

Julia Marco is pregnant with her second child. During her first pregnancy, she did not attend childbirth classes. She received an epidural for the birth. During a prenatal visit, Julia tells you that she would now like to have a natural birth in a birthing center. She asks you for information on childbirth education courses. Her husband, Joe, wants Julia to go to the hospital and have an epidural like the last time. He insists, "The doctors know what they are doing. We should just let them do their job." After further speaking with Joe, you discover that he doesn't want Julia to go through the pain of natural childbirth and fears that he will not be able to help her during labor. How can you help alleviate some of Joe's concerns and best advise the Marcos on preparations for childbirth?

Previous chapters discussed normal anatomy, physiology, and nursing care necessary during pregnancy. This chapter adds information about the education couples need to make labor and birth a satisfying experience. This is important information because it can help protect the health of both women and children throughout the continuum of pregnancy, birth, and childrearing.

After you've studied the chapter, answer the Critical Thinking Exercises at the end of the chapter and then access the on-line study activities (http://connection.lww.com) *to further sharpen your skills and test your knowledge.*

As active consumers of health care, expectant families are faced with a wide array of choices about a childbirth experience and preparation for parenting. Two of the most important decisions they need to make involve the choice of birth attendant and setting. For example, the woman may elect to have her family doctor, obstetrician, or nurse-midwife attend the birth and to be supported by her husband, partner, family member, friend, or doula (a woman who is experienced in childbirth and provides continuous emotional and physical support). A woman may also choose to give birth at a birthing center or in the hospital. Birthing centers and birthing rooms within hospitals provide environments for families who desire a childbirth experience that is relaxed, "homey," and "family-centered" yet close to medical sources should any complication arise during the birth or early postpartal period. Low-risk families may plan to have a nurse-midwife attend a home birth.

No matter what setting a woman or couple chooses, expectant parents need to be prepared for childbirth. Childbirth preparation courses help prepare expectant couples for the physical and emotional aspects of childbirth and teach nonpharmacologic methods of pain relief during labor. Courses are individualized to meet parents' needs and may be divided into classes for women with special needs such as adolescents, career women, women who are physically challenged, or those experiencing a high-risk pregnancy. Also available are classes to help prepare siblings and classes for grandparents to learn more about their role. Women having a **vaginal birth after cesarean birth** (VBAC) or women who know they will need a cesarean birth also can attend specially designed classes. In some communities, classes are offered at work or school sites. Classes offered at work sites benefit the employer as much as the employee because prenatal care and guidance are correlated with healthier pregnancy outcome and fewer lost workdays.

Although parenting is unarguably the most important of occupations, it is one of the few that requires no formal education, no examination to test a person's ability to take on such a role, and no refresher course to ensure that a parent is following healthy standards of child-rearing. Encouraging preparation is a nursing role because educating families about both childbirth and parenting is important in making childbirth a satisfying experience, helping a family bond with its new member, and promoting wellness behaviors that could last throughout the family's life cycle. National Health Goals related to preparation for parenting are shown in the Focus on National Health Goals box.

NURSING PROCESS OVERVIEW

For Childbirth and Parenting Education

Assessment

Some couples have a clear idea of where and how they wish their child's birth to occur. Others cannot even consider the actual birth until they have adjusted to the idea of pregnancy. Assessing each woman's or couple's readiness for decision making, as well as providing information early in the process, helps the woman or couple make this kind of decision. For couples who have chosen what may be considered an alternative birthing option such as home birth, it is important that they understand both the physical and emotional requirements of such a choice. Whether she is a primipara or multipara, it is also important to

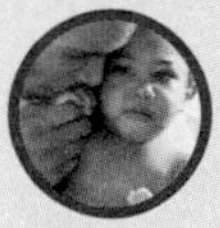

FOCUS ON NATIONAL HEALTH GOALS

Preparation for childbirth classes supply information not only on how to prepare for childbirth but also on how to parent. A number of National Health Goals speak directly to such classes:

- Increase the proportion of pregnant women who attend a series of prepared childbirth classes.
- Increase the proportion of pregnant women who receive early and adequate prenatal care from a baseline of 74% to a target level of 90% (DHHS, 2000).

Nurses actively participate as instructors in preparation for childbirth and parenting classes and help supervise prenatal care, so they have direct roles in helping the nation achieve these objectives. Nursing research that addresses such issues as what is the best timing during pregnancy for education about birth, what teaching techniques help parents retain information best, and what support parents want most from nurses during labor would be helpful to better identify the needs for preparation for labor.

ascertain whether a woman and her support person need childbirth or parenting courses and to provide appropriate information so they can participate in such a course. (See Assessing the Client's Preparation for Labor.)

Nursing Diagnosis

A typical nursing diagnosis for this area of nursing care is:

- Health-seeking behaviors related to a lack of information about childbirth and newborn care

If there is a lack of support people, diagnoses that might apply are:

- Ineffective coping related to lack of support people
- Anxiety related to absence of significant other

For the couple unable to make a decision about a childbirth setting, an appropriate diagnosis might be:

ASSESSING the Client's Preparation for Labor

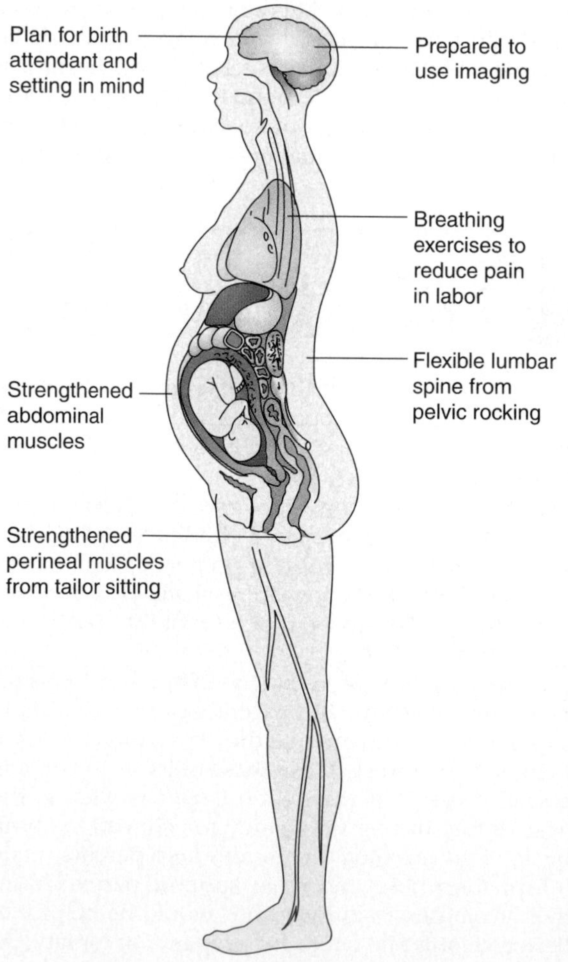

- Decisional conflict related to lack of information regarding advantages and disadvantages of childbirth settings

If there are older children in the family, a nursing diagnosis might be:

- Anxiety related to role in pending birth event and ability to welcome a sibling

Outcome Identification and Planning

Be certain when planning with couples for labor and birth that the goals they set are realistic and flexible. Not all women want to go through labor without any analgesia, but most would like to participate as fully as possible. Some women may be reluctant to attend a childbirth preparation course because they fear that would mean committing themselves to a medication-free birth. They can be assured that learning about "natural childbirth" methods does not preclude learning about what medications are available for pain relief and using those medications if desired. At the same time a couple is planning goals for childbirth, it is best to encourage them to be flexible in expectations for themselves. A woman who has decided ahead of time that she absolutely will not take any medication during labor and birth may find the intensity or duration of labor to be so severe that she will need an analgesic or epidural block to make the experience tolerable. If she and her support person have made the goal of medication-free labor too strict, they may believe they have failed when medication becomes necessary. A birth plan (discussed below) that includes information regarding the woman's or couple's preferences for labor, birth, immediate care of the newborn, and actions to be taken if complications should arise can help the woman and her support person set realistic outcomes.

Finally, it is important to establish with the woman or couple that the ultimate goal of childbirth is a healthy baby and healthy parents. This will prevent them from concentrating on limited goals such as not having fetal monitoring or a particular birthing position and concentrate instead on doing whatever is required to make the birth safest for both them and the baby.

The following organizations are helpful referral sources for couples:

Maternity Center Association (*www.maternity.org*)
Lamaze International (*www.lamaze-childbirth.com*)
International Childbirth Education Association (*www.icea.org*)
La Leche League International (*www.lalecheleague.org*)

Implementation

Nurses play vital roles in preparing parents for childbirth. Box 13-1 highlights appropriate outcomes and interventions using the terminology identified by the Nursing Outcomes Classification and Nursing Interventions Classification. It is important to provide a woman and her partner with information on the benefits and drawbacks of birthing options, without

BOX 13.1

NURSING OUTCOMES AND NURSING INTERVENTIONS CLASSIFICATION: PARENTAL PREPARATION

NOC: Knowledge, Labor and Delivery

Knowledge, labor and delivery, is defined as the extent of understanding about labor and delivery (Johnson et al., 2000). Some specific indicators suggesting achievement of this outcome include the ability to describe the following:

- Birthing options
- Role of support person/coach
- Signs and symptoms of labor, stages and phases of labor
- Pain-control methods and effective breathing and relaxation techniques
- Potential medication and procedures needed during labor and complications
- Effective pushing techniques

NIC: Childbirth Preparation

Childbirth preparation is defined as the provision of information and support to facilitate childbirth and enhance an individual's ability to develop and perform the parental role (McCloskey & Bulechek, 2000). Some important activities involved when implementing this intervention include:

- Exploring options for prenatal care and labor and delivery
- Informing client about option for delivery over intact perineum and circumstances requiring an episiotomy
- Preparing client for delivery options if complications arise
- Teaching client and partner breathing and relaxation techniques and comfort measures
- Instructing partner in coaching
- Promoting client's self-esteem in assuming parental role
- Providing anticipatory guidance for parenthood
- Assisting parents in preparing siblings for birth, with referral for sibling preparation classes as necessary

FOCUS ON MULTIDISCIPLINARY CARE

Many different health care providers are involved in providing prenatal care, including physicians, nurse practitioners, sonogram technicians, nurse-midwives, nutritionists, and health educators. Be certain that everyone discusses childbirth as a positive, growth-enhancing experience, not merely an experience to be endured.

Unlicensed assistive personnel may have roles in prenatal clinics such as showing women into examining rooms and arranging for return appointments. While doing these things, clients may ask them about what preparation for labor or parenting classes the clinic or hospital sponsors. Not realizing that something that was good for them may not be right for everybody, some unlicensed assistive personnel may give women advice such as, "Ask for an epidural so you can ease through the whole thing. It's the only way to go." To make childbirth an individual experience, women need more individualized advice than this. They need to know all their options so they can make informed choices.

influencing them in a particular direction. To remain objective, it is important to examine your own attitudes, cultural influences, and values related to childbirth and explore how these beliefs might differ from those of your clients. With referral to a childbirth preparation course, many questions can be answered in a sympathetic group setting, where feelings and anxieties can be shared as well. Be familiar with the content of courses in your community so you can be certain that the courses you suggest present adequate and accurate information and are appropriate for individual couples (see the Focus on Multidisciplinary Care).

Be certain to review the arrangements the woman needs to make for labor and birth at a midpoint in pregnancy. No matter how calm a woman seems when discussing these details, many women have some fear that at the last minute they will forget what they need to do when labor begins. In addition, the woman should be encouraged to work out arrangements for transportation to the hospital or birthing center and to arrange for childcare if she has other children at home. The woman who anticipates a home birth must organize her home and purchase supplies well in advance of her expected due date.

Outcome Evaluation

Evaluation of whether expected outcomes for childbirth education have been achieved should be carried out during the last few prenatal visits. By the last trimester, the woman or couple should know where the baby will be born and should have worked out transportation and childcare details. Women who will be coached through childbirth by their husbands or another support person should be encouraged to continue practicing breathing and relaxation techniques together up to the time of birth so they do not lose these skills.

Examples of expected outcomes that would demonstrate the success of interventions are:

- Couple states they feel prepared for childbirth.
- Client states she feels confident she can use breathing exercises to get through contractions as long as 70 seconds.
- Client has made preparations for a doula to support her during labor.

- Sibling states she is ready to welcome a new brother or sister into the family.

CHILDBIRTH EDUCATION

Childbirth education courses began initially to encourage women to attend to prenatal care. They continue because they fulfill an important second need for education about labor and childbirth. The overall goals of childbirth education are to prepare expectant parents emotionally and physically for childbirth while promoting wellness behaviors that can be used by parents and families for life. Specific goals of preparation for childbirth classes are to:

- Prepare the expectant mother and her support person for the childbirth experience
- Create clients who are knowledgeable consumers of obstetric care
- Help clients reduce and manage pain with both pharmacologic and nonpharmacologic methods
- Help increase couples' overall enjoyment of and satisfaction with the childbirth experience

Childbirth Educators and Methods of Teaching

Childbirth educators are health care providers who usually have a professional degree in the helping professions as well as a certificate from a course specifically on childbirth education. They teach expectant parents about the physical and emotional aspects of pregnancy, childbirth, and early parenthood and present coping skills and labor support techniques. Although childbirth education is an interdisciplinary field, it has historically been associated with nursing, as nurses play a major role in designing and teaching childbirth education courses. Most classes are taught in a group format; most incorporate a variety of teaching techniques such as videotapes and slides, lecture, and demonstration (especially for content on relaxation and breathing techniques). One of the most important aspects of these courses, however, is group interaction. Women and their partners enjoy the opportunity to share their fears and hopes about their pregnancy and upcoming birth with others as they learn together.

Efficacy of Childbirth Education Courses

Many studies have been done to determine just how effective childbirth courses are in reducing the pain of childbirth, shortening the length of labor, decreasing the amount of medication used, and increasing overall enjoyment of the experience. Because of the variability in courses offered, however, it is often difficult to compare results of attending childbirth classes versus not attending classes. This is partly because participants already have a high degree of positive motivation, which may skew the results. Despite these difficulties with measurement, it is generally accepted that preparation courses can increase satisfaction, reduce the amount of reported pain, and increase feelings of control (Lowe, 2000).

Cultural and Socioeconomic Factors

Whether women want or are able to take a childbirth and parenting preparation course depends a great deal on cultural and socioeconomic factors and individual choices (see the Focus on Communication). A course may not be helpful if suggestions made regarding infant clothing and supplies, formula or breast-feeding, or maternal nutrition and health are not culturally appropriate. In some cultures, the advice of a friend or family member carries more weight than the advice of a professional health care practitioner. Asking each woman separately whether she is interested in a course and being certain that women are fully informed of the options are two ways to avoid cultural stereotyping and to be certain that all women receive the advice and knowledge they need for a positive birth experience. Providing childbirth and parenting information that takes into account the cultural practices and financial needs of individual clients is the best approach to ensure that the information is understood and accepted.

FOCUS ON COMMUNICATION

Mrs. Briggs is a primigravida you meet at a prenatal clinic. She is in the 16th week of an uncomplicated pregnancy.

Less Effective Communication

Nurse: Have you signed up for childbirth preparation class yet, Mrs. Briggs?
Mrs. Briggs: No.
Nurse: Don't wait too much longer. You're already in your fourth month.
Mrs. Briggs: I'm not sure I'm going to sign up.
Nurse: Everyone can benefit from childbirth preparation. I'll write the telephone number down for you so you remember to call.

More Effective Communication

Nurse: Have you signed up for childbirth preparation class yet, Mrs. Briggs?
Mrs. Briggs: No.
Nurse: Don't wait too much longer. You're already in your fourth month.
Mrs. Briggs: I'm not sure I'm going to sign up.
Nurse: Why is that?
Mrs. Briggs: I read the brochure and the classes are all at the wrong time. And cost too much.
Nurse: Let's work together to find a course that's right for you. We can use the Internet to find out what other options might be available.

It is so important for couples to attend preparation for labor classes that it is easy to ignore the reasons they present for not wanting to attend them. Careful listening often reveals that time or money concerns are reasons why couples choose not to attend a course. Helping to investigate the many options is the beginning of problem solving.

Perineal and Abdominal Exercises

Women are encouraged to maintain an overall active exercise program during pregnancy, as this may help prevent the need for cesarean birth (Bungum et al., 2000). In childbirth preparation classes, women learn exercises to strengthen their pelvic and abdominal muscles and make these more supple. Supple perineal muscles allow for ready stretching during birth, reducing discomfort; strengthened muscles more quickly revert to their normal condition and function quickly and efficiently after childbirth (Magann et al., 2002).

A woman may begin exercises as early in pregnancy as she likes; however, women enrolled in Lamaze preparation programs generally do not begin until the last 8 to 10 weeks of pregnancy. This time frame allows for learning the conditioned responses necessary for prepared labor closer to the time they will be used, but it limits the total amount of time directed to perineal exercises. If labor begins early, the woman may have had little or no practice with the perineal exercises.

Women should not participate in a formal exercise program without their physician's or nurse-midwife's approval. They should not attempt to exercise if any of the danger signs of pregnancy appear, and they should never exercise to a point of fatigue. Common safety precautions for preparation for childbirth exercises in pregnancy are summarized in the Focus on Family Empowerment.

Many exercises can be incorporated into daily activities so they take little time from a woman's day. It is best, however, for the woman to set aside a specific time each day for the task; otherwise, participation is apt to be sporadic. Initially, women should do each exercise only a few times, gradually increasing the number at each session.

Tailor Sitting

Although many woman may be familiar with tailor sitting, they may have to be retaught the position so it is done in a way that stretches the perineal muscles without occluding blood supply to the lower legs. The woman should not put one ankle on top of the other but should place one leg in front of the other (Fig. 13-1). As she sits in this position, she should gently push on her knees (pushing them toward the floor) until she feels her perineum stretch. This is a good position to use to watch television, read, or talk to friends. It is good to plan on sitting in this position for at least 15 minutes every day. By the end of pregnancy, the woman's perineum should be so supple that when she tailor-sits, her knees will almost touch the floor if pushed.

Squatting

Squatting (Fig. 13-2) also stretches the perineal muscles and can be a useful position for second-stage labor, so a woman should also practice this position for about 15 minutes a day. Most women need a demonstration of effective squatting; otherwise, they tend to squat on their tiptoes. For the pelvic muscles to stretch, the woman must keep her feet flat on the floor. Incorporating squatting into daily activities such as picking up toys from the floor reduces the amount of time a woman must devote to daily exercises.

Pelvic Floor Contractions (Kegel Exercises)

Pelvic floor contractions are another activity that can be done during daily activities. While sitting at her desk or working around the house, the woman can tighten the muscles of the perineum by doing Kegel exercises (see Box 11-1). Such perineal muscle-strengthening exercises will be helpful in the postpartum period; they also promote perineal healing, increase sexual responsiveness, and help prevent stress incontinence in later life.

Abdominal Muscle Contractions

Abdominal muscle contractions help strengthen the abdominal muscles during pregnancy and therefore help prevent constipation as well as help restore abdominal tone after pregnancy. Strong abdominal muscles can also

FOCUS ON FAMILY EMPOWERMENT
Exercise Guidelines for Labor Preparation

Q. How can I be sure the exercises I'm doing in pregnancy won't hurt me or my baby?

A. Try following these guidelines:

- Never exercise to a point of fatigue.
- Always rise from the floor slowly to prevent orthostatic hypotension.
- To rise from the floor, roll over to the side first and then push up to avoid strain on the abdominal muscles.
- For leg exercises, to prevent leg cramps, never point the toes (extend the heel).
- To prevent muscle strain, do not attempt exercises that hyperextend the lower back.
- Do not hold your breath while exercising because this increases intra-abdominal and intrauterine pressure.
- Do not continue with exercises if any danger signal of pregnancy occurs.
- Do not practice second-stage pushing. Pushing increases intrauterine pressure and could rupture membranes.

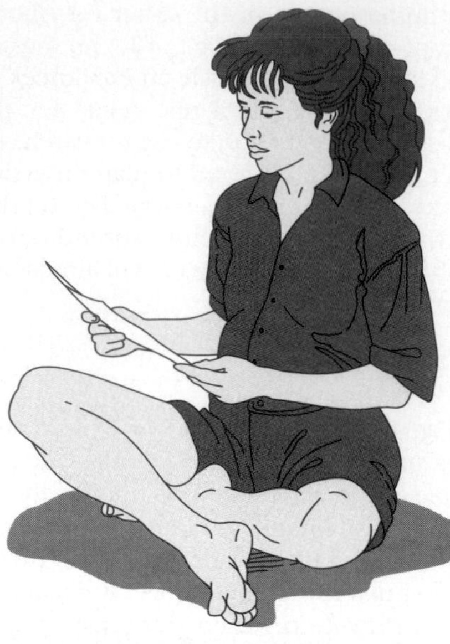

FIGURE 13.1 Tailor sitting strengthens the thighs and stretches perineal muscles to make them more supple. Notice that the legs are parallel so that one does not compress the other. A woman could use this position for television watching, telephone conversations, or playing with an older child.

contribute to effective second-stage pushing during labor. Abdominal contractions can be done in a standing or lying position along with pelvic floor contractions. The woman merely tightens her abdominal muscles, then relaxes them. She can repeat the exercise as often as she wishes during the day.

Another way to do the same thing is to practice "blowing out a candle." The woman takes a fairly deep inspiration, then exhales normally. Holding her finger about 6 inches in front of herself, as if it were a candle, she then exhales forcibly, pushing out residual air from her lungs. She can feel her abdominal muscles contract as she reaches the end of her forcible exhalation.

Pelvic Rocking

Pelvic rocking (Fig. 13-3) helps relieve backache during pregnancy and early labor by making the lumbar spine more flexible. It can be done in a variety of positions: on hands and knees, lying down, sitting, or standing. The woman arches her back, trying to lengthen or stretch her spine. She holds the position for 1 minute, then hollows her back. A woman can do this at the end of the day about five times to relieve back pain and make herself more comfortable for the night.

✔ CHECKPOINT QUESTIONS

1. Why is it important to strengthen the perineal muscles? Which exercises help do this best?
2. Why is it important to strengthen the abdominal muscles? Which exercise helps strengthen these muscles?
3. At what point in any one session should a pregnant woman stop exercising?

Methods for Pain Management

Beginning in the late 1950s, many specific methods for nonpharmacologic pain reduction during labor were developed. These included the Lamaze, Dick-Read, and Bradley methods, all named after the professionals who developed them. More recently, however, childbirth education has been moving away from the strict method approach to a more eclectic one. Much research is being done to verify the effectiveness of each of these many techniques, and in practice many educators are using a variety of approaches in their courses (see the Focus on Cultural Competence).

Most of the methods advocated are based on three premises:

1. Discomfort during labor can be minimized if the woman comes into labor informed about what is happening and prepared with breathing exercises

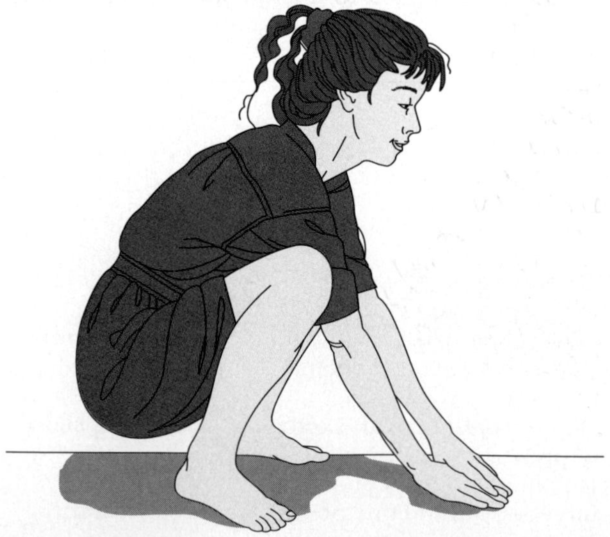

FIGURE 13.2 Squatting helps to stretch the muscles of the pelvic floor. Notice that the feet are flat on the floor for optimum stretching.

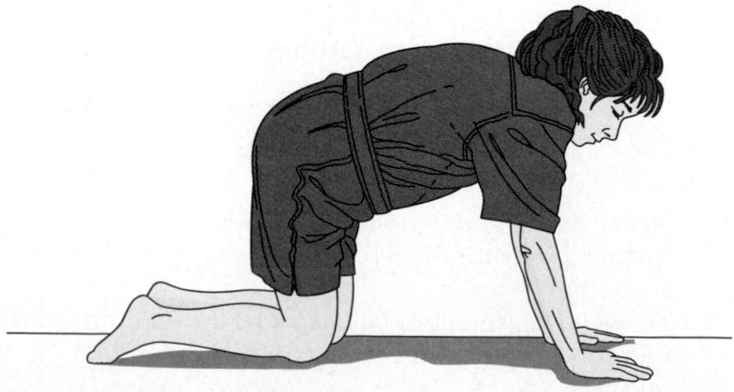

FIGURE 13.3 Pelvic rocking is helpful in relieving backache during pregnancy and labor. The woman hollows her back and then arches it.

FOCUS ON CULTURAL COMPETENCE

The plans that women make for childbirth can be culturally influenced. A woman from a culture in which modesty is stressed, for example, may not want to have a mirror positioned over a birthing bed. Some women want to use aromatherapy to help them relax. A very old Native American belief is that a knife placed under the mattress will "cut the pain" better than a Lamaze program. Whom women choose as a support person or coach in labor can also differ, depending on their cultural background. Mexican Americans, for example, may choose a female relative or friend rather than a male partner. Asian women may prefer a family member experienced in childbirth rather than an inexperienced male partner. Assess each couple individually to be certain that cultural preferences such as these are respected.

to use during contractions. In classes, therefore, the woman learns about her body's response in labor, the mechanisms involved in childbirth, and breathing exercises she can use during labor.

2. Discomfort during labor can be minimized if the woman's abdomen is relaxed and the uterus is allowed to rise freely against the abdominal wall with contractions. Childbirth methods differ only in the manner by which they achieve this relaxation.
3. Pain perception can be altered by **distraction** techniques or by the **gate control theory of pain perception** (Box 13-2).

The Bradley (Partner-Coached) Method

The Bradley method of childbirth, originated by Robert Bradley (1981), is based on the premise that childbirth is a joyful natural process and stresses the important role of the husband during pregnancy, labor, and the early newborn period. During pregnancy, the woman performs muscle-toning exercises and limits or omits foods that contain preservatives, animal fat, or a high salt content. Pain is reduced in labor by abdominal breathing. In addition, the woman is encouraged to walk during labor and to use an internal focus point as a disassociation technique. The Bradley method is used widely in some areas of the United States and at specific centers.

The Psychosexual Method

The psychosexual method of childbirth was developed by Sheila Kitzinger (1990) in England during the 1950s. The method stresses that pregnancy, labor and birth, and the early newborn period are important points in the woman's life cycle. It includes a program of conscientious relaxation and levels of progressive breathing that encour-

BOX 13.2

GATE CONTROL MECHANISMS

Pain Pathway

- The endings of small peripheral nerve fibers detect a stimulus.
- They transmit it to cells in the dorsal horn of the spinal cord.
- Impulses pass through a dense, interfacing network of cells in the spinal cord (the substantia gelatinosa).
- Immediately, a synapse occurs that returns the transmission to the peripheral site through a motor nerve. For example, a person touches a candle flame; the impulse travels to the spinal cord and back, and the person jerks his or her hand away from the flame.
- After this short-circuit synapse, the impulse then continues in the spinal cord to reach the hypothalamus and cortex of the brain.
- The impulse is interpreted (the candle is hot) and perceived as pain.

Gating Theory of Pain Control

The gating theory of pain refers to the gate control mechanisms in the substantia gelatinosa that are capable of halting an impulse at the level of the spinal cord so the impulse is never perceived at the brain level as pain, or a process similar to closing a gate.

Techniques to Assist Gating Mechanisms

- **Cutaneous Stimulation.** If large peripheral nerves next to an injury site are stimulated, the ability of the small nerve fibers at the injury site to transmit pain impulses appears to decrease. Therefore, rubbing an injured part or applying transcutaneous electrical nerve stimulation (TENS) or heat or cold to the site (cutaneous stimulation) is an effective maneuver to suppress pain. Effleurage, or light massage used in the Lamaze method, accomplishes this.
- **Distraction.** If the cells of the brain stem that register an impulse as pain are preoccupied with other stimuli, a pain impulse cannot register. Distraction or imagery accomplishes this. Different childbirth classes use different breathing, vocalization, or focusing techniques to accomplish this. (Breathing techniques are most often employed in childbirth classes because they increase oxygenation to the mother and fetus as well as decrease pain.)
- **Reduction of Anxiety.** Pain impulses are perceived more quickly if anxiety is also present. Thus, the third technique of gating is to reduce patient anxiety as much as possible. Teaching a woman what to expect during labor is a means of achieving this.

ages the woman to "flow with" rather than struggle against contractions.

The Dick-Read Method

The Dick-Read (1987) method is based on the approach proposed by Grantly Dick-Read, an English physician. The premise is that fear leads to tension, which leads to pain. If one can prevent this chain of events from occurring, or break the chain between fear and tension or tension and pain, then one can reduce the pain of contractions. The woman achieves relaxation and reduced pain by using abdominal breathing during contractions.

The Lamaze Method

The Lamaze method of prepared childbirth is the method most often taught in the United States today. It is based on the theory that through stimulus-response conditioning women can learn to use controlled breathing and therefore reduce pain during labor. The Lamaze method was previously termed the **psychoprophylactic** method, which means preventing pain in labor (prophylaxis) by use of the mind (psyche), because the method concentrates on helping women relax to make labor a manageable experience.

The method was developed in Russia based on Pavlov's conditioning studies but was popularized by a French physician, Ferdinand Lamaze. Formal classes are organized by Lamaze International or the International Childbirth Education Association. Many other classes teach variations on the Lamaze method.

Three main premises are taught in the prenatal period related to the gate control method of pain relief:

1. Pain occurs to a lesser extent if the woman is relaxed. Much time in class is spent reviewing or teaching reproductive anatomy and physiology and the process of labor and birth. If they are familiar with what will happen to the woman in labor and the nature of contractions, the couple may enter labor with decreased tension.
2. Sensations such as uterine contractions can be inhibited from reaching the brain cortex and registering as pain. The woman is taught to concentrate on breathing patterns and to use imagery or focusing (concentrating) on a specified object to block incoming pain sensations. The effectiveness of focusing can be observed in athletes who hurt themselves in basketball or football games but do not feel the pain until after the game because they are so focused on winning.
3. Conditioned reflexes are a positive action to use to displace pain during labor. Time in class is spent on learning **conditioned reflexes,** or reflexes that automatically occur in response to a stimulus. Conditioned responses were first noted by Pavlov while conducting studies on salivation in dogs. The same training technique is applied to the birth process in the Lamaze method. The woman is conditioned to relax automatically on hearing a command ("contraction beginning") or on the feel of a contraction beginning. The responses to contractions must be recently conditioned to be effective (because conditioned responses fade if not reinforced). It is generally recommended, therefore, that women attend class in the last trimester of pregnancy.

Classes are kept small so that there is time for individual instruction and attention to each couple (Fig. 13-4). A woman is advised to bring to class a support person who will act as her coach in labor. Classes focus on learning and practicing breathing exercises and relaxation techniques. Exercises vary from teacher to teacher, especially in terms of complexity, but have common features shown below. In addition, information to guide the woman and her coach through pregnancy (e.g., prenatal nutrition, exercises, and common discomforts of pregnancy) and prepare them for unexpected circumstances (e.g., malpresentation, cesarean birth, or the need for analgesia or anesthesia) is provided. Supplies that the woman or couple might pack in advance to bring to the hospital may also be discussed (Table 13-1).

Conscious Relaxation. **Conscious relaxation** is learning to relax body portions deliberately so that, unknowingly, the woman does not remain tense and cause unnecessary muscle strain and fatigue during labor. She practices relaxation during pregnancy by deliberately relaxing one set of muscles, then another and another until her body is completely relaxed. The support person concentrates on noticing symptoms of tension such as a wrinkled brow, clenched fists, or a stiffly held arm. By either placing a comforting hand on the tense body area or telling the woman to relax that area, the support person helps her to achieve complete relaxation.

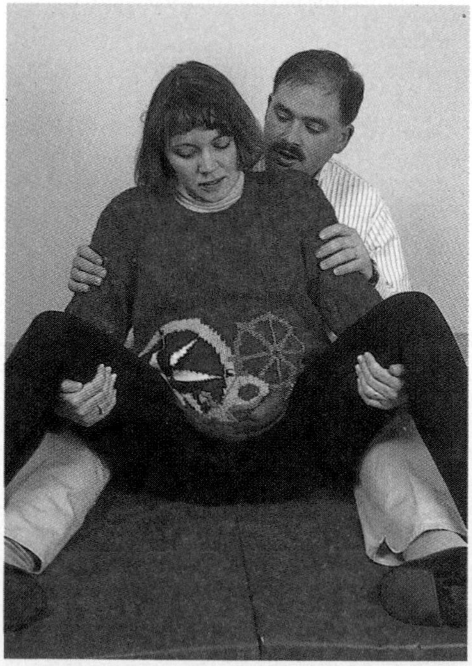

FIGURE 13.4 Every woman needs to be well prepared for birth. Here a couple practices positions for pushing in a childbirth preparation class.

TABLE 13.1 Supplies to Prepare for Labor

ITEM	PURPOSE
Lip balm	To prevent dry lips
Mouthwash	For rinsing dry mouth
Toothbrush and toothpaste	To prevent dry mouth
Warm socks	Comfort
Small rolling pin covered with soft cloth	Back massage
Focal point	To increase concentration
Busy work (e.g., knitting or magazines)	To pass time
Paper bag	To correct hyperventilation
Extra pillow	For semi-Fowler's position in labor
Watch	For timing contractions
Baby powder	For reducing friction of effleurage
Lollipops	For energy and dry mouth
Snacks (e.g., apples or potato chips)	For coach's comfort
Tapes or compact discs and player	To increase relaxation

The Cleansing Breath. To begin all breathing exercises, the woman breathes in deeply and then exhales deeply (a **cleansing breath**). To end each exercise, she repeats this step. It is an important step to take because it limits the possibility of hyperventilation with rapid breathing patterns; it helps ensure an adequate fetal oxygen supply. It is also part of the conditioned response.

Consciously Controlled Breathing. Using **consciously controlled breathing,** or set breathing patterns at specific rates, prevents the diaphragm from descending fully and therefore prevents it from putting pressure on the expanding uterus. To practice, the woman inhales comfortably but fully, then exhales, with her exhalation a little stronger than her inhalation. She practices breathing in this manner at a controlled pace, depending on the intensity of contractions. Various levels of breathing are:

Level 1. Slow chest breathing at this level consists of comfortable but full respirations at a rate of 6 to 12 breaths per minute. The level is used for early contractions.

Level 2. For this level, breathing is lighter than level 1. The rib cage should expand but be so light the diaphragm barely moves. The rate of respirations is up to 40 per minute. This is a good level of breathing for contractions when cervical dilation is between 4 and 6 cm.

Level 3. Breathing at this level is even more shallow, mostly at the sternum. The rate is 50 to 70 breaths per minute. As the respirations become faster, the exhalation must be a little stronger than the inhalation to allow good air exchange and to prevent hyperventilation. If the woman practices saying "out" with each exhalation, she almost inevitably will make exhalation stronger than inhalation. The woman uses this level for transition contractions. Keeping the tip of her tongue against the roof of her mouth helps prevent the oral mucosa from drying out during such rapid breathing.

Level 4. At this level, the woman uses a "pant-blow" pattern, such as taking three or four quick breaths (in and out), then a forceful exhalation. Because this type of breathing sounds like a train (breath-breath-breath-huff), it is sometimes referred to as "choo-choo" breathing or "hee-hee-hee-hoo" breathing.

Level 5. The woman pants at this level. Chest panting is continuous, very shallow panting at about 60 breaths per minute. It can be used during strong contractions or during the second stage of labor to prevent the woman from pushing before full dilatation.

Some courses stop teaching at the point a woman has mastered the levels of breathing; others have her learn to shift from one level to the other on command or at the point she feels a need for more pain relief. To do this, at the sound of "contraction beginning," she breathes at 12 breaths a minute; at the sound of "contraction getting harder," 40 breaths a minute; "harder still," 70 breaths a minute; and so on, imitating basic shifts she will use in labor.

A woman who can successfully perform the various levels of breathing and maintain relaxation is prepared to handle all labor contractions up to the second stage of labor.

Figure 13-5 illustrates the use of levels of breathing. An early labor contraction is mild. When the contraction begins, the coach says, "contraction beginning." The woman takes a cleansing breath, then breathes at level 1; she feels no bite from the contraction and so does not need to change to a more involved breathing pattern. Later in labor, the contraction is stronger and longer. Now, at the sound of "contraction beginning," the woman takes a cleansing breath, then begins level 1 breathing (3 breaths); shifts to level 2 (4 to 6 breaths); then shifts to level 3 (10 breaths). The contraction is lessening. She shifts down to level 2 (4 to 6 breaths), then to level 1 (3 or 4 breaths). The contraction is gone. She takes a final cleansing breath. During actual labor, her coach can tell the strength of contractions by resting a hand on her abdomen or observing a uterine contraction monitor. The coach can tell the woman when to shift breathing levels depending on the coach's estimation of the strength of the contraction with words such as, "contraction beginning, getting stronger, now getting weaker, gone." In the time before transition to the second stage of labor, when contractions are longest and strongest, the woman may need to use her level 4 breathing or continuous light panting as well.

Effleurage. One additional technique to encourage relaxation and displace pain in the Lamaze method is **effleurage,** which is light abdominal massage, done with just enough pressure to avoid tickling. To do this, the woman traces a pattern on her abdomen with her fingertips (Fig. 13-6). The rate of effleurage should remain constant even though breathing rates change. Effleurage serves

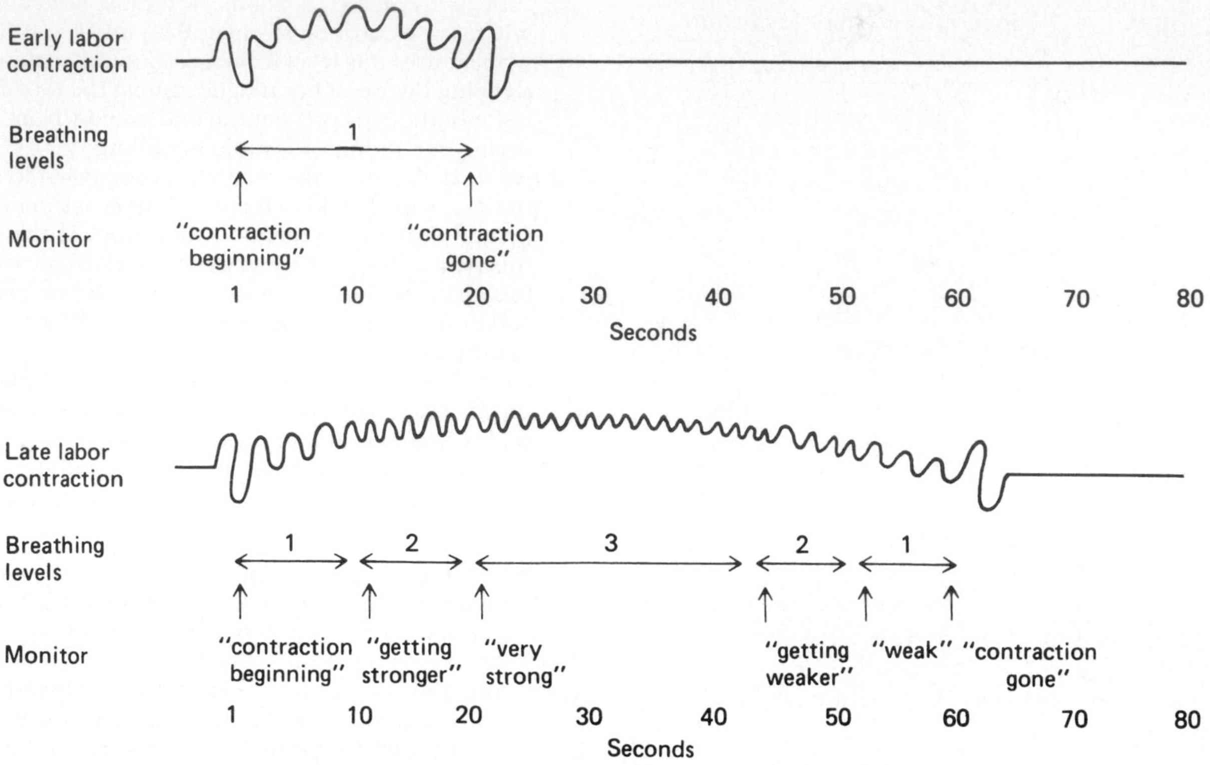

FIGURE 13.5 Example of differing breathing patterns during a single contraction. 1, 2, and 3 are levels of breathing. A cleansing breath is taken at the beginning and end of the contraction.

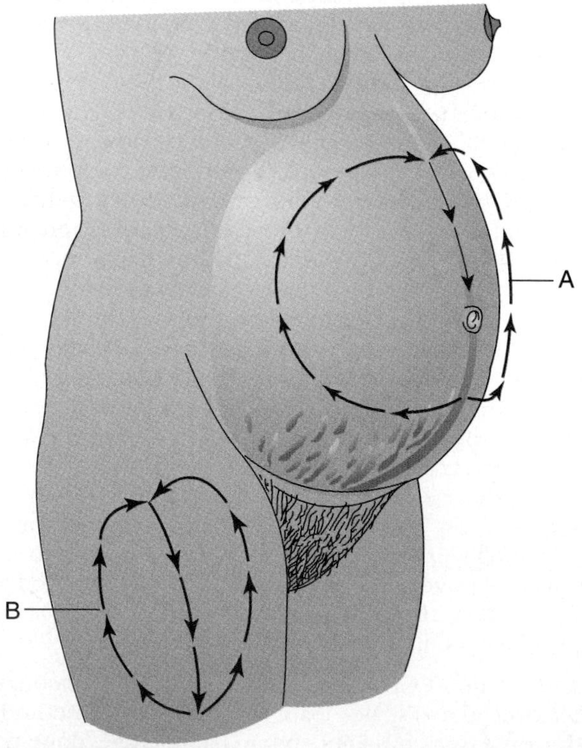

FIGURE 13.6 Effleurage patterns. (*A*) During uterine contractions, a woman traces the pattern on her bare abdomen with her fingers. (*B*) If electronic fetal monitoring is being used, effleurage may be performed on the thigh.

as a distraction technique and decreases sensory stimuli transmission from the abdominal wall, helping limit local discomfort. If an external electronic monitor is in place on the abdomen, effleurage can be done superior or inferior to it or even on the thighs. Effleurage can also be done by the support person.

Focusing or Imagery. Focusing intently on an object (sometimes called "sensate focus") is another method of keeping sensory input from reaching the cortex of the brain. The woman brings into labor a photograph of her partner or children, a graphic design, or just something that appeals to her (Fig. 13-7). She concentrates on it during contractions. Be careful not to step into the woman's line of vision during a contraction and break her concentration. Other women use imagery by concentrating on an image such as watching waves rolling onto a beach or relaxing on a porch swing. Do not ask questions or talk to women using this technique because you will break their concentration.

Second-Stage Breathing. During the second stage of labor, when the baby is actually pushed down the birth canal, the type of breathing that is best to use is controversial. In the past, women were told to hold their breath while they pushed. Now it is believed that holding the breath for a prolonged time impairs blood return from the vena cava (a Valsalva maneuver), so this is now discouraged. Teaching women to breathe out while pushing may be helpful. This is called physiologic pushing. Other instructors suggest women breathe any way that is natural for them, except holding their breath.

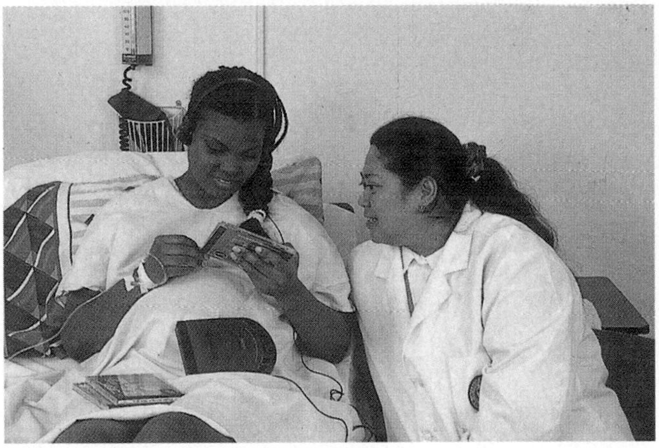

FIGURE 13.7 A woman chooses what object she wishes to focus on during labor. Here, a woman and nurse listen to the taped music the woman will focus on during contractions.

Women should not practice pushing. The possibility that they would rupture membranes by doing this is too great. They can practice assuming a good position for pushing (squatting, sitting upright, leaning on partner) but should always be cautioned not to actually push.

✔ CHECKPOINT QUESTIONS

4. What are the three basic premises of the Lamaze method?
5. What are the principles of the gate control theory of pain relief?
6. How do effleurage and focusing/imagery help reduce pain?

Preparation for Cesarean Birth

The fact that cesarean birth may be necessary to ensure a safe birth is covered in most childbirth classes. In some communities, cesarean birth is offered to women as an alternative to vaginal birth to help prevent uterine prolapse or urinary incontinence in later years (Bost, 2000). The woman who knows that she is to have a cesarean birth due to a pelvic abnormality or because she is a candidate for a repeat cesarean birth needs specific preparation; see Chapter 20.

EXPECTANT PARENTING CLASSES

A number of other types of courses are offered to expectant parents that focus on concepts other than preparing for the actual labor and birth. Hospitals, health maintenance organizations, and community health services may provide classes for women and their families that focus on family health. These include sibling preparation classes, refresher classes for repeat parents or grandparents, classes for expectant adoptive parents, preparation for parenting specially geared toward adolescents, breast-feeding classes, and many others. The most common of these courses is the expectant parenting class, which generally covers the normal stages of pregnancy and newborn care.

Most preparation for parenthood programs are planned to cover 4 to 8 hours of content spaced over a 4- to 8-week period. Both women and their support people are invited, and the curriculum is individualized for the group and its needs. If all the women in the group already have children, for example, they may not need a tour of a maternity unit as part of the program; instead, they may want to learn what is new in baby food or childcare. If all the women in the class work at least part-time, discussion of "brown bag nutrition" and how to include rest periods during work might be useful. If all the women are teenagers, they may be most interested in what is going to happen to their bodies during pregnancy, or what sports are safe to continue during pregnancy. They may also need more information on what to expect when their baby is born. They probably will want a tour of the maternity unit (Fig. 13-8). A typical course plan for 8 weeks is shown in Box 13-3.

Sibling Education Classes

Sibling classes are organized to acquaint older brothers and sisters with what happens during birth and how they can expect a newborn to look and act. The classes review how babies grow and things children can do to help their mother during a pregnancy, such as not leaving toys on the floor that need to be picked up and helping her eat healthy foods.

If the classes are held at a hospital, a tour of a newborn nursery is included so children can see how small their new sibling will be. A hospital room like the one their mother will occupy may be visited.

For sibling classes to be successful, age-appropriate information and activities must be provided. See Chapters 28 to 32 for growth and development expectations by age group. Younger children may need reassurance that their parents will continue to love them after the new baby arrives. Older children may be interested in learning about newborn care and being a part of planning for the newborn.

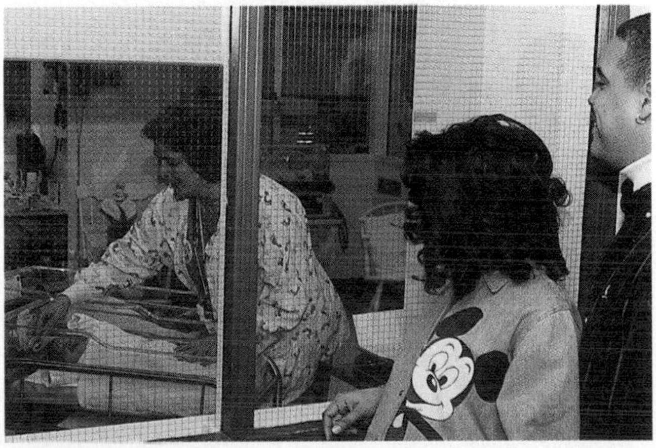

FIGURE 13.8 An enjoyable part of a preparation-for-parenthood class is touring a maternity service. Here, parents-to-be view a newborn nursery.

BOX 13.3

SAMPLE CONTENT FOR EXPECTANT PARENTS CLASS

Lesson 1 Review of Physiologic Changes of Pregnancy and Fetal Growth
Lesson 2 Personal Care During Pregnancy
- Nutrition
- Hygiene
- Exercise
- Rest

Lesson 3 Emotional Changes During Pregnancy
Lesson 4 Labor and Delivery
- The Process of Birth
- Exercises and Breathing Techniques
- Medication in Labor

Lesson 5 The Postpartum Period
Lesson 6 Infant Care
- Nutrition
- Hygiene

Lesson 7 Plans for Birth
- Birth Settings Available
- Supplies to Take to Birth Settings
- Tour or Film of a Typical Setting

Lesson 8 Reproductive Life Planning

THE CHILDBIRTH PLAN

Key among the decisions a couple must make during pregnancy is the choice of setting and birth attendant. The expectant woman and her partner should also think about other issues, such as the extent of family participation they wish during labor, specific labor procedures, birthing positions, medication options, plans for the immediate postbirth period and baby care, and the postpartum stay and family visitation. Some suggestions for a woman and her partner to consider in planning these specific childbirth details are shown in the Focus on Family Empowerment.

Birth planning is usually part of the curriculum for childbirth education classes because a group setting may be the best way for couples to sort out their questions and feelings about how to plan for a healthy and enjoyable birth. Urge couples to make decisions about these issues before the day of birth, or else decisions could be determined by agency policy or the circumstances of the moment without the couple's input. If the expectant family has a strong desire in a certain area, planning ahead will allow them to communicate this so their wish can be accommodated if possible. Be certain all couples understand, however, that the birth plan should be flexible because a complication or change of plans may arise. For example, in the event of a complication of labor or birth that requires an emergency cesarean birth, a preference to have the baby without anesthesia will need to be modified. Box 13-4 illustrates a sample birth plan.

WHAT IF? What if a woman tells you that the father of her baby will not be with her during labor? She asks you if it is really important to have someone with her. How would you advise her?

THE BIRTH SETTING

The setting for birth that a couple chooses depends on the woman's health and that of the fetus as well as the couple's preferences on how much supervision they desire at the birth. Although hospitals are the usual site for birth

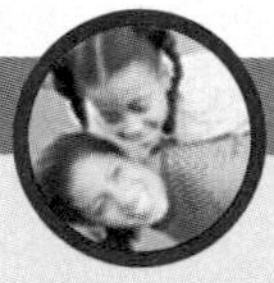

FOCUS ON FAMILY EMPOWERMENT
Choosing a Birth Setting

Q. There are so many options available for a birth setting. How do I decide which to choose?

A. Choosing a birth setting is a personal decision. Some questions you might want to ask are:

- What type of caregiver will supervise my prenatal care and labor and birth? Nurse-midwife? Family doctor? Obstetrician?
- Will the same person be present at prenatal visits as for birth? Does the setting offer preparation for childbirth or child-rearing classes?
- What setting can I choose from? A birthing room? An alternative birthing center? My home?
- Will I be allowed to choose a birth position? Will I have input into the amount of anesthesia used? Will administration of ophthalmic ointment for the baby be delayed? Can I begin breast-feeding immediately? Will nurses who are supportive and informed about breast-feeding be available? Can I use a doula?
- Will the setting allow my partner to participate? Will he or she be allowed to be with me through labor and birth? Could he or she cut the cord or help deliver the baby? Can older children participate? Can I record the birth on videotape or by photograph?
- Is early discharge available? Will a follow-up home visit be included in care?
- If I should have a complication during labor or birth, are there adequate supplies and personnel available for emergency care? If the baby should have a complication, is there provision for immediate emergency care or transport to a high-risk facility?

BOX 13.4

BIRTH PLAN: NORMA ANDERSON

Birth Attendant
Alexander Coppin, MD, or nurse-midwife Kaitlin Brandywine, whoever is on call for the big day.

Birth Setting
Birthing Room Number 1 at Huntington General

Support Person
Husband Donald (if out of town, my sister Adrienne)

Activities During Labor
I want to walk or rock in the rocking chair or play Monopoly.
I want to wear my own nightgown, and listen to Simon and Garfunkel Central Park Concert tape.
Husband wants to videotape birth.

Birth
Position for birth: squatting
No episiotomy
Husband wants to cut cord.

Postpartum
I want to breastfeed immediately.
I want to use kangaroo care to keep baby warm.
I want to room in.
Husband wants to sleep over on bedside cot.

today, that has not always been the case. Up until the late 1800s, childbirth was conducted in the home. Analgesia or anesthesia for childbirth was unpopular until Queen Victoria delivered Prince Leopold under chloroform in 1853. Unfortunately, this extensive level of anesthesia for childbirth led to additional interventions, because under anesthesia women were no longer able to push effectively during the second stage of labor. It became necessary to use a lithotomy position and an episiotomy and forceps for birth as well.

Part of the reason for so much anesthesia during birth can be attributed to physicians misinterpreting the types of pain in childbirth. It was assumed that the moment of birth was the major time of discomfort. As a result, women were allowed to labor without any pain medication and then were given anesthesia or analgesia right before the baby was born. In reality, women may not be as uncomfortable during that time as they are early in labor. Although the pain felt during the second stage of labor is intense, it is also the most fulfilling and even most exhilarating time, and it is directly followed by the birth of the baby.

Fortunately, birthing practices have changed to incorporate women's needs based on their descriptions of the pain of childbirth. There is also an economic incentive for change. If women choose physicians or hospitals who subscribe to more progressive birth practices over the services of more traditional facilities, the overall standard of care in communities leans toward the more progressive settings. The addition of birthing rooms to hospitals in the past 20 years is an example of this change. Nurses are in a strong position to advocate for making childbirth a "natural" process in the least restrictive setting possible. At the same time, nurses have a strong responsibility to encourage parents to maintain enough restrictions that birth remains safe.

Choosing the Appropriate Setting

Women may choose hospitals, birthing centers, or their homes as settings for birth. Women with high-risk pregnancies have less choice; most nurse-midwives and physicians insist that women with potential complications give birth at hospitals, where immediate emergency care is available.

Choosing a Birth Attendant and Support Person

In the United States, most births are supervised by an obstetrician, a physician specializing in labor and birth. As the tendency for specialized physician practice declines, it is becoming more common, however, for family medicine practitioners to serve as birth attendants. It is also becoming more common for nurse-midwives to attend births, especially at alternative birth centers (see the Focus on Evidence-Based Practice) (Galotti et al., 2000).

In addition to selecting who will medically supervise the baby's birth, a woman needs to choose who will support her in labor. In years past, this support was offered by experienced women in the community. In the 1960s, the role was given to the father of the baby. Today, both men and women offer this type of support. In addition to having the father of their baby present, many women are

FOCUS ON EVIDENCE-BASED PRACTICE

Which Women are Most Apt to Choose a Midwife Rather Than a Physician as Their Birth Attendant?
To answer this question, 88 women from differing education backgrounds were interviewed about what criteria they used to choose a birth attendant. Women who selected a midwife reported feeling more in agreement with alternative birth philosophies, more knowledgeable about birth attendants, and more in control over the birth attendant decision than others. Following the birth, they were more satisfied about their delivery decisions and more satisfied with their pain medication decisions.

These are not surprising results (women who are more knowledgeable of choices make more choices), but they have important implications for nurses because nurses are the people most apt to be talking to women about birth decisions. It is important to supply women with up-to-date information so they can make informed decisions.

Galotti, K. M., et al. (2000). Midwife or doctor: A study of pregnant women making delivery decisions. *Journal of Midwifery & Women's Health, 45*(4), 320–329.

choosing a doula, or a person specially prepared to assist with birth. Fathers may find it hard to provide doula-type support during labor because of their own emotional involvement in the birth. Having such a person present frees the father to enjoy the birth rather than feeling occupied with coaching instructions. Although research in the subject is not extensive, there are suggestions that rates of oxytocin augmentation, epidural anesthesia, and cesarean birth can be reduced by doula support.

Hospital Birth

Advantages and disadvantages of hospital birth are summarized in Box 13-5. A hospital has the advantage of having ready supplies and expert personnel if the mother or fetus or newborn should have a complication of birth.

In evaluating studies that compare the complications of birthing centers or home births to hospitals, be sure to consider that high-risk mothers give birth at hospitals; thus, the number of complications in hospital settings is bound to be higher than in other settings.

A woman usually comes to the hospital when her contractions are approximately 5 minutes apart and regular in pattern. If she has preregistered at the hospital, she is admitted to a **birthing room** without any separation time from her support person. Birthing rooms are also called **labor-delivery-recovery rooms** (LDRs) or **labor-delivery-recovery-postpartum rooms** (LDRPs). Such rooms are decorated in a homelike atmosphere; couples can bring favorite music or reading materials with them to use during labor; and the bed can be used as a labor bed until birth, when it converts into a birthing bed or a lithotomy position bed (Fig. 13-9). Women are expected to use a prepared method of childbirth with a minimum of analgesia and anesthesia (although an advantage of a hospital birth is that anesthesia such as an epidural is readily available if needed). An important aspect of birthing rooms is that the support person and often other family members can stay with the woman for the entire length of labor and birth, allowing the laboring couple and family to have more control over their birth experience.

Most hospitals screen women in early labor with an external monitor for both fetal heart rate and uterine contractions. If the fetal heart rate is good, such a monitor can usually be removed and used again only for periodic screening as labor progresses. The woman may have intravenous access started as a prophylactic measure. If this is done, the needle can be inserted in a dorsal hand vein so it causes little discomfort and inconvenience for her.

At the time of birth, additional cabinets in the room are opened and converted into a space for baby care. A support person remains with the woman during birth and in some settings can cut the umbilical cord if desired. Women can choose a birthing position: lithotomy, squatting, supine recumbent, or side-lying.

Birthing chairs (Fig. 13-10) are comfortable reclining chairs with a slide-away seat that allow a woman to assume a comfortable position during labor and also furnish perineal exposure so a birth attendant can assist with the birth. They have the advantage of maintaining the woman in a semi-Fowler's position, a position that acts with gravity and thus may speed the second stage of labor.

If a woman chooses to use a supine recumbent position (on her back with knees flexed) rather than a lithotomy position (legs elevated into stirrups) for birth, she uses a

BOX 13.5

ADVANTAGES AND DISADVANTAGES OF HOSPITAL BIRTH

Advantages

- The woman is encouraged to be prepared to control the discomfort of labor through nonmedication measures such as controlled breathing.
- The woman is encouraged to be knowledgeable about the labor process and make decisions about procedures performed.
- The woman is encouraged to consider breastfeeding to aid uterine contraction and infant bonding.
- Labor, birth, and immediate postpartal care can all be scheduled in a single room.
- The woman is attended by skilled professionals during labor and birth and the postpartal period.
- Emergency care and extended high-risk care are immediately available.

Disadvantages

- Separation of the family for at least one night.
- Mother may not feel as much in control of the childbirth experience as she may wish.
- Care may be fragmented, particularly if the woman's physician is not present during the entire labor and birth, or if labor nurses change shifts in the middle of labor. (Many nurse-midwives and physicians make it a point, however, to remain with their client throughout the entire childbirth experience.)

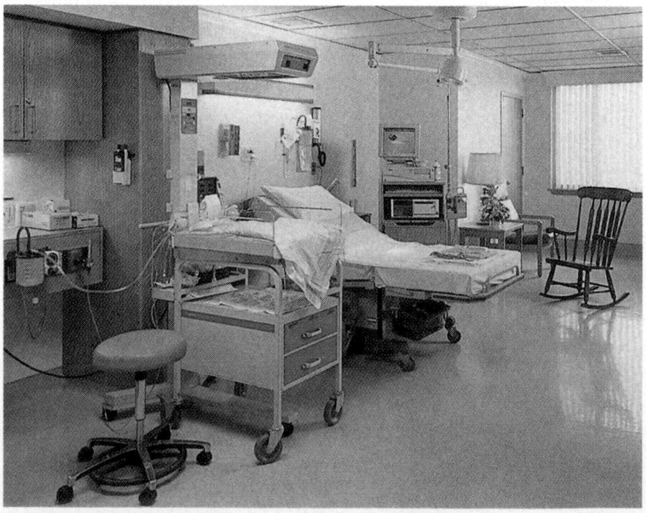

FIGURE 13.9 A birthing (labor-birth-recovery) room designed to maintain a home-like atmosphere in a hospital setting.

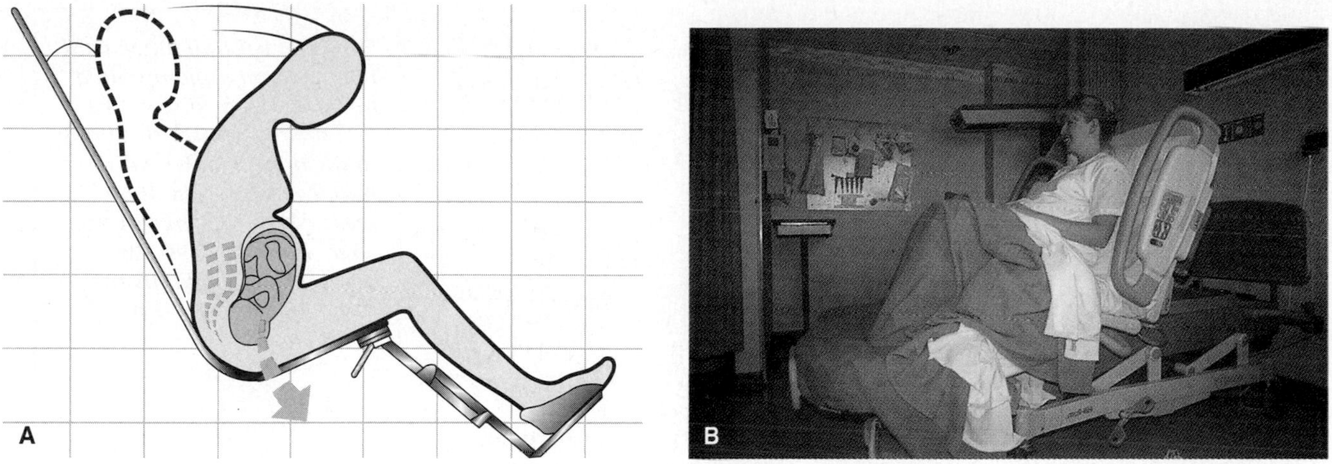

FIGURE 13.10 (*A*) A birthing chair allows the woman to maintain a semi-Fowler's position. (*B*) A birthing chair used during labor.

birthing bed. Such a position reduces tension on the perineum and may result in fewer perineal tears than with a lithotomy position.

Postpartal Care

After birth, mothers may breast-feed immediately. The infant remains with the parents so they have a chance to become acquainted. Women giving birth in LDRPs remain there with their families for the rest of the hospital stay. Women giving birth in birthing rooms may be transferred to the postpartal unit after birth; they remain there for the length of their hospital stay. Because hospital stays are so short today, the more women and their babies are together, the better, so both LDRPs and postpartal units serve as "rooming-in" units in which the infant remains in the mother's room for most of the day. Breast-feeding on demand for infants should be the rule. There should be no restrictions on visiting for the primary support person; in many institutions, a rollaway bed is provided so this person can remain constantly. Siblings of the newborn should be allowed to visit at least once and touch and become acquainted with the newborn.

Alternative Birthing Centers

Alternative birthing centers (ABCs) are wellness-oriented childbirth facilities designed to remove childbirth from the acute care hospital setting while providing enough medical resources for emergency care should a complication of labor and birth arise (see Focus on Nursing Care Planning). Such a setting is established within or near a hospital, or at least within an easy distance of one. Because it is located outside an acute care setting, where infections abound, the risk of nosocomial infection to the mother is thought to be reduced. The birth attendants tend to be nurse-midwives. Women who deliver in ABCs are screened for complications before being admitted. Because women are carefully screened, the mortality rate of mothers and infants is no higher and may be lower in these out-of-hospital settings than in hospital settings.

Like hospitals, ABCs have LDRP rooms where a woman and her support person can invite friends and siblings to participate in the birth. In some centers, a central play area for siblings and cooking facilities are also available. ABCs encourage the woman to express her own needs and wishes during the labor process. A minimum of analgesia and anesthesia is provided, and she can choose a birth position. She can bring her own music or distraction objects, and the partner can perform such tasks as cutting the umbilical cord if he or she chooses. Advantages and disadvantages of ABCs are summarized in Box 13-6.

Women remain in an ABC from 4 to 24 hours after birth. Because a minimum of analgesia or anesthesia is used, a woman recovers quickly after birth and is prepared to be discharged this early.

> **WHAT IF?** What if a woman and her partner are having a serious disagreement about whether to plan for a home or hospital birth? What issues would you suggest they explore? If they cannot agree, how could they compromise?

Home Birth

Home birth is the usual mode of birth in developing countries. Under the supervision of nurse-midwives, it is a popular choice for birth in Europe, but only about 1% of women in the United States choose this method (Hoyert et al., 2001). The Frontier Nursing Service of Kentucky is an example of an organization in the United States that maintains an active and well-accepted program of home birth. Home birth may be supervised by a physician, but nurse-midwives are the more likely choice as birth attendants in this setting.

Most women who choose home birth in the United States are well educated and from middle-income families.

During a routine antepartal visit, a client, accompanied by her partner, states, "We don't want to have this baby in the hospital. There are too many germs. What about these alternative birth centers?" Partner states, "We don't have medical insurance. A hospital is just too expensive."

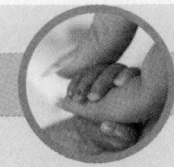

FOCUS ON *Nursing Care Planning*

A FAMILY WHO DESIRES BIRTH AT AN ALTERNATIVE BIRTH CENTER

Assessment: Client verbalizing use of alternative birth center (ABC) to avoid hospitalization; reports concern over previous hospital birth of son. "I had a urinary tract infection afterward." Son now 4 years old. "We want him to be part of this." Limited financial resources with no medical insurance. Partner states, "An alternative birth center would be less expensive." Birth attendant to be a nurse-midwife, with neighbor acting as client's doula. No childbirth education classes attended with previous pregnancy; not enrolled in any with this pregnancy at present. Pregnancy progressing normally without evidence of problems or complications. Gravida 2, para 1, 24 weeks' gestation.

Nursing Diagnosis: Decisional conflict related to choice of birth setting and birth process

Outcome Identification: Client and partner will verbalize an agreed-upon birth setting choice by 3 weeks.

Outcome Evaluation: Client and partner state advantages and disadvantages of birth setting options; verbalize goal of healthy mother and baby as motivation for choice of birth setting; discuss plans for birth based on birth setting chosen.

Interventions	Rationale
1. Explore with client and partner past experiences with childbirth and current expectations and beliefs. Encourage couple to verbalize feelings, concerns, and needs.	1. Exploration provides a baseline from which to provide future instructions. Verbalization of feelings permits a safe outlet for emotions and assists in increasing the other person's awareness.
2. Urge the couple to discuss plans and goals with each other.	2. Discussion promotes sharing and working toward common goals.
3. Review the requirements, advantages, and disadvantages for birth setting choices.	3. Review of options allows the couple to make an informed decision appropriate for their needs.
4. Obtain information about local childbirth education classes and assist couple with selecting class that fits their resources.	4. Education and preparation enhance the chances of a positive childbirth experience. Assistance with choosing a program that fits the couple's resources helps to promote compliance.
5. Request the couple find a caretaker for son during the birth.	5. A caretaker is important to enhance the experience for the older child, thus promoting a positive, family-centered event.
6. Instruct the couple and caretaker to attend classes on sibling preparation for birth.	6. Adequate preparation for all involved improves the chances of a positive experience.
7. Encourage the couple to discuss the role of doula with the neighbor. Have each person identify his or her roles and responsibilities.	7. Advance discussion of roles and responsibilities reduces the possibility of conflicts during labor.
8. Provide the couple with information about contracts for finances and emergency care with the birth setting.	8. Contracting for services safeguards the well-being of all involved should unexpected circumstances arise.

BOX 13.6

ADVANTAGES AND DISADVANTAGES OF ABCs

Advantages

- The woman is encouraged to be prepared to control the discomfort of labor through non-medication measures such as controlled breathing.
- The woman is encouraged to be knowledgeable about the labor process and to help care providers with decision making.
- The woman is encouraged to breast-feed to aid uterine contraction and infant bonding.
- Family integrity can be maintained because family members may accompany her to the birthing center.
- The woman is attended by skilled professionals during labor and delivery.
- Emergency care is immediately available. Extended high-risk care is easily arranged.

Disadvantages

- Extended high-risk care is not immediately available.
- The woman may be fatigued after birth because of early discharge.
- She must independently monitor her postpartal status because of early discharge.

BOX 13.7

ADVANTAGES AND DISADVANTAGES OF HOME BIRTH

Advantages

- The woman is encouraged to become knowledgeable about the birth process and be an active participant in independently reducing the discomfort of labor.
- The woman has the greatest freedom for expressing her individuality.
- There is no separation of the family at birth.

Disadvantages

- Adequate equipment other than first-line emergency equipment is unavailable.
- An abrupt change of goals is necessary if hospitalization is required.
- Exhaustion of the woman and support person may occur because of the responsibility placed on them.
- Interference with the "taking-in phase" may occur postpartally because the woman must "take hold."
- The woman must independently monitor her postpartal status.

They choose home birth so they can have the baby close by after birth, can have more control over the childbirth experience, and can give birth in familiar, low-cost surroundings (Anderson & Anderson, 1999).

The main advantage of a home birth is that it allows for family integrity: the woman and her family are not separated. On the other hand, it puts the responsibility on the woman to prepare her home for the birth (difficult if she is exhausted toward the end of pregnancy) and to take care of the infant after birth. Some people, however willing, may be unable to take on these roles in a crisis situation such as childbirth. Many women passing through their first postpartal phase, or a "taking-in" phase, may be happier maintaining a dependent passive role than taking responsibility for the infant's care. Advantages and disadvantages of home birth are summarized in Box 13-7.

To be a candidate for a home birth, a woman must be in good health, must be able to adjust to changing circumstances, and must have an adequate system of support people who will sustain her during labor and assist her for the first few days after birth. Women with any complication of pregnancy are not candidates for home birth.

Children Attending the Birth

Most birthing centers and some hospitals allow children to view the birth of a sibling. If older children will be present, a person separate from the main support person needs to be designated to provide entertainment, explanations, food, and sleep for them. The mother must not be expected to provide such supervision during labor, when she becomes introverted and has concern only for herself. A child who is without supervision during this time can remember the experience as a time of rejection rather than an exciting, happy experience.

Help couples consider if the birth experience will be a positive and enjoyable one for the child. This decision is often based on the developmental level of the child. Allowing a child to witness the birth of kittens or puppies in some instances might be a more appropriate way to expose a child to birth. In addition, attendance at sibling classes designed to prepare children to witness the birth is often required.

ALTERNATIVE METHODS OF BIRTH

In addition to setting, a number of different methods of childbirth have become popular in the past 15 to 20 years. These include alternative birth methods such as the Leboyer method and birth under water.

Leboyer Method

Frederick Leboyer (1975) is a French obstetrician who postulated that moving from a warm, fluid-filled intrauterine environment to a noisy, air-filled, brightly lighted birth room is a major shock to a newborn. With the **Leboyer method**, the birthing room is darkened so there is no sudden contrast in light; it is kept pleasantly warm, not chilled. There should be soft music playing, or at least no harsh noises in the room. The infant should be handled gently; the cord is cut late; and the infant is placed immediately after birth into a warm-water bath.

These principles are not drastically different from the usual practice, as infants are always handled gently at birth. Some neonatologists question the wisdom of a warm bath because it may reduce spontaneous respirations and allow a high level of acidosis to occur. Late cutting of a cord may lead to excess blood viscosity in the newborn. Certainly, soft music, gentle handling, and a welcome atmosphere are important ingredients for all birth attendants to try to incorporate into birth. Providing dim lights (or at least not bright, glaring ones) could be given more consideration in most institutions.

Hydrotherapy and Water Birth

Reclining or sitting in warm water during labor can be soothing; the feeling of weightlessness that occurs under water as well as the relaxation from the warm water both can contribute to reduce discomfort in labor. Using this principle, a number of birthing centers allow women to labor and give birth in spa tubs of warm water. The baby is born under water and then immediately brought to the surface for a first breath. Some potential difficulties with underwater birth are contamination of the bath water with feces expelled with pushing efforts during the second stage of labor (this could lead to uterine infection), aspiration of bath water by the fetus, and maternal chilling when she leaves the water. Women choosing this method should be advised that research on the safety and wisdom of the method is ongoing (Nikodem, 2000).

✔ CHECKPOINT QUESTIONS

7. If a mother has a complication of pregnancy, which birth setting should she choose?
8. What should be the basic goal of all birth settings?
9. What is a doula?

KEY POINTS

Couples should be encouraged to make a childbirth plan early in pregnancy that includes birth attendant and setting.

Common exercises taught in pregnancy to strengthen perineal muscles are tailor sitting, squatting, and Kegel exercises. Abdominal muscle-contraction and pelvic rocking exercises strengthen the abdominal muscles and help relieve backache.

Types of childbirth preparation include the Bradley (partner-coached), psychosexual (Kitzinger), Dick-Read, and Lamaze methods. Lamaze is the most common method practiced in the United States.

Commonly used nonpharmacologic techniques for pain relief in labor are conscious relaxation, consciously controlled breathing, effleurage, focusing, imagery, and hydrotherapy.

Expectant parents' classes provide information on pregnancy, birth, and childcare.

Common sites for childbirth include hospitals, alternative birthing centers, and home.

CRITICAL THINKING EXERCISES

1. Recall Joe Marco in the beginning of this chapter. How would you convey to him that natural childbirth can be a positive experience for him and his wife Julia? How would you assure him that he and Julia can have a safe and active part in the birth of their child?
2. A 19-year-old woman who is expecting her first baby tells you she does not intend to attend a preparation for labor class because she wants to have epidural anesthesia as soon as she is admitted to the hospital in labor. Would you advise her to attend a class or not?
3. A couple having their third child ask you if they should allow their oldest child to view the birth. How would you advise them? What further information would you need before you could give informed advice?
4. A couple wants to have a Leboyer birth. How would you prepare the birthing room?
5. Examine the National Health Goals related to childbirth. Most government-sponsored money for nursing research is allotted based on these goals. What would be a possible research topic to explore pertinent to these goals that would be fundable and would advance evidence-based practice?

REFERENCES

Anderson, R. E., & Anderson, D. A. (1999). The cost-effectiveness of homebirth. *Journal of Nurse-Midwifery, 4*(1), 30–35.

Bost, B. W. (2000). Should elective cesarean birth be offered at term as an alternative to labor and delivery for prevention of complications, including symptomatic pelvic prolapse, as well as stress urinary and fecal incontinence? *Obstetrics & Gynecology, 95*(4), S46.

Bradley, R. (1981). *Husband-coached childbirth* (3rd ed.). New York: Harper Collins.

Bungum, T. J., et al. (2000). Exercise during pregnancy and type of delivery in nulliparae. *Journal of Obstetric, Gynecologic & Neonatal Nursing, 29*(3), 258–264.

Department of Health and Human Services. (2000). *Healthy people 2010.* Washington, D.C.: DHHS.

Dick-Read, G. (1987). *Childbirth without fear: The original approach to natural childbirth* (5th ed.). New York: Harper Collins.

Galotti, K. M., et al. (2000). Midwife or doctor: A study of pregnant women making delivery decisions. *Journal of Midwifery & Women's Health, 45*(4), 320–329.

Hoyert, D. L. et al. (2001). Annual summary of vital statistics. *Pediatrics, 108*(6), 1241–1255.

Johnson, M., Maas, M., & Moorhead, S. (2000). *Nursing outcomes classification* (2d ed.). St. Louis: Mosby.

Kitzinger, S. (1990). *The experience of childbirth.* New York: Viking Penguin.

Leboyer, F. (1975). *Birth without violence.* New York: Alfred A. Knopf.

Lowe, N. K. (2000). Self-efficacy for labor and childbirth fears in nulliparous pregnant women. *Journal of Psychosomatic Obstetrics & Gynecology, 21*(4), 219–224.

Magann, E. F. et al. (2002). Antepartum, intrapartum, and neonatal significance of exercise on healthy low-risk pregnant working women. *Obstetrics & Gynecology, 99*(3), 466–472.

McCloskey, J., & Bulechek, G. (2000). *Nursing interventions classification* (3rd ed.). St. Louis: Mosby.

Nikodem, V. C. (2000). Immersion in water in pregnancy, labour and birth. *Cochrane Database of Systematic Reviews, 2*, CD000111.

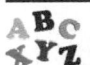

SUGGESTED READINGS

Chen, C. H., et al. (2001). Women's perceptions of helpful and unhelpful nursing behaviors during labor: A study in Taiwan. *Birth, 28*(3), 180–185.

Clapp, J. F. et al. (2002). Continuing regular exercise during pregnancy. *American Journal of Obstetrics & Gynecology, 186*(1), 142–147.

Gagnon, A. J. (2000). Individual or group antenatal education for childbirth/parenthood. Cochrane Database of Systematic Reviews, 4:CD002869.

Johnson, T. R., et al. (2000). A competency-based approach to comprehensive pregnancy care. *Women's Health Issues, 10*(5), 240–247.

Logan, K. (2001). Audit of advice provided on pelvic floor exercises. *Professional Nurse, 16*(9), 1369–1372.

Morison, S., et al. (1999). Birthing at home: The resolution of expectations. *Midwifery, 15*(1), 32–39.

Stone, P. W., et al. (2000). Economic analysis of two models of low-risk maternity care: A freestanding birth center compared to traditional care. *Research in Nursing & Health, 23*(4), 279–289.

Van Hoover, C. (2000). Pain and suffering in childbirth. *Midwifery Today, 55*(1), 39–42.

Wickham, S. (2000). Homebirth: What are the issues? *Midwifery Today, 6*(50), 16–18.

High-Risk Pregnancy: The Woman With a Preexisting or Newly Acquired Illness

14

CHAPTER

Key Terms

- deep vein thrombosis
- glucose tolerance test
- glycosuria
- glycosylated hemoglobin
- high-risk pregnancy
- hyperglycemia
- hypoglycemia
- insulin pump
- megaloblastic anemia
- orthopnea
- paroxysmal nocturnal dyspnea
- peripartal cardiomyopathy
- proteinuria
- sexually transmitted disease

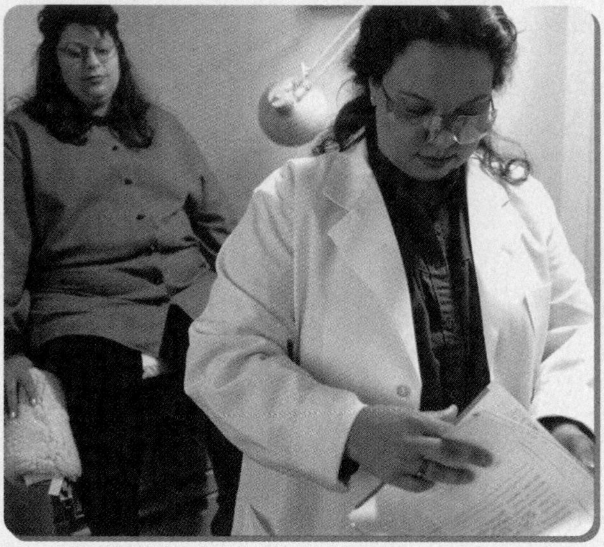

Objectives

After mastering the contents of this chapter, you should be able to:

1. Define *high-risk pregnancy*, including factors that contribute to its development.
2. Describe common illnesses such as cardiovascular disease, diabetes mellitus, or renal and blood disorders that can result in complications when they exist with pregnancy.
3. Assess the woman with an illness during pregnancy for changes occurring because of the pregnancy.
4. Formulate nursing diagnoses related to the effect of a preexisting or newly acquired illness on pregnancy.
5. Identify expected outcomes that will contribute to a safe pregnancy outcome when illness occurs with pregnancy (e.g., planning ways a woman can secure more rest).
6. Plan nursing care for the woman with an illness during pregnancy (e.g., teaching insulin administration to a woman newly diagnosed with gestational diabetes).
7. Implement nursing care for the woman when illness complicates pregnancy.
8. Evaluate outcomes to determine achievement and effectiveness of care.
9. Identify National Health Goals related to complications of pregnancy that nurses can be instrumental in helping the nation achieve.
10. Identify areas related to illness and pregnancy that could benefit from additional nursing research or application of evidence-based practice.
11. Use critical thinking to analyze ways that nursing care can remain family-centered when a preexisting or newly acquired illness develops.
12. Integrate knowledge of high-risk pregnancy and nursing process to achieve quality maternal and child health nursing care.

Angelina Pellegoso is a 42-year-old woman pregnant with her first child. She developed gestational diabetes early in pregnancy, but because she eats out frequently as part of her job (a fundraiser for a movie producer), by the 30th week of pregnancy she has already been hospitalized twice for hyperglycemia. This morning while driving to work on the freeway, her compact car was struck by an 18-wheel truck. Both of Angelina's legs were broken, and she suffered head and abdominal trauma. In the emergency room, her serum glucose was found to be 207 mg/dL. Her blood pressure was 90/40; her pulse was 130/min; the fetal heart rate was 180/min. An abdominal monitor showed moderate-strength uterine contractions 2 minutes apart.

She tells you, "I know everything is going to be all right. I was wearing my seat belt." Does Angelina have a realistic outlook on her condition? Do you think she realizes that pregnancy often becomes high risk, not for any one factor, but an accumulation of them?

Previous chapters discussed normal pregnancy. This chapter adds information about illnesses that can complicate pregnancy when they occur in women of childbearing age.

After you've studied the chapter, answer the Critical Thinking Exercises at the end of the chapter and then access the on-line study activities (http://connection.lww.com) *to further sharpen your skills and test your knowledge.*

When a woman enters pregnancy with a chronic condition such as cardiovascular or kidney disease, both she and the fetus are at risk for complications. The course of a normal pregnancy can complicate the disease; plus, the disease can cause complications that can affect the baby or leave the woman less equipped to function in the future or undergo a future pregnancy. Nursing care for the woman with a preexisting illness focuses on close observation of maternal health and fetal well-being, education of the woman and her family about danger signs to watch for during pregnancy, and actions to minimize complications whenever possible.

In addition to preexisting illnesses, the pregnant woman, like any other person, may develop non-pregnancy-related illnesses or suffer from trauma during a pregnancy. When this occurs, the illness or injury can adversely affect not only the woman but the unborn child as well. Nursing care for the well, pregnant woman focuses on preventing illness and trauma by promoting an especially healthy lifestyle. When accidents and illness occur despite these safeguards, nursing care must focus on:

- Preventing such disorders from affecting the health of the fetus
- Helping the mother regain her health as quickly as possible so she can continue a healthy pregnancy and prepare herself psychologically and physically for labor and birth and the arrival of her newborn

Conditions that cause severe symptoms such as a marked change in fluid and electrolyte balance, altered cardiovascular or respiratory function, or severe blood loss are especially dangerous to a fetus. Some infections, notably toxoplasmosis (see Chap. 11) and some of the sexually transmitted infections, can be devastating to the unborn child and need to be addressed as soon as they are discovered. National Health Goals related to complications of pregnancy are shown in the Focus on National Health Goals box.

Although pregnancy can be a stressful time, generally women experience overall good health during their pregnancies, perhaps in part because of the extra care and concern in keeping healthy for two. This extra motivation also encourages the woman with a high-risk pregnancy to carefully follow the therapeutic regimen established to keep her and her fetus safe.

NURSING PROCESS OVERVIEW

For Care of the Woman With a Preexisting or Newly Acquired Illness

Assessment

Accurate prenatal assessment of the woman with a preexisting or newly acquired illness requires a thor-

---

FOCUS ON NATIONAL HEALTH GOALS

A number of National Health Goals are aimed at reducing complications of pregnancy from existing or newly acquired disorders. These are:

- Reduce HIV infections in adolescent and young adult females (13 to 24 years of age) to one new case per 100,000 live births from a baseline of 17 per 100,000.
- Reduce gonorrhea to an incidence of no more than 19 new cases per 100,000 people from a baseline of 123 per 100,000.
- Eliminate primary and secondary syphilis to an incidence of no more than 0.2 per 100,000 from a baseline of 3.2 per 100,000.
- Reduce genital herpes and genital warts to 14% from a baseline of 17%.
- Reduce fetal deaths to 4.1 per 1000 live births from a baseline of 6.8 per 1,000.
- Reduce maternal deaths to 3.3 per 100,000 live births from a baseline of 7.1 per 100,000.
- Reduce maternal illness during pregnancy to 24 per 100 births from a baseline of 31.2 per 100 (DHHS, 2000).

Nurses can be instrumental in helping the nation reach these goals by educating women about the dangers of and ways to prevent STDs such as syphilis, gonorrhea, and HIV infection. In addition, nurses can help women who have diabetes mellitus understand the importance of prepregnancy care so they enter pregnancy without hyperglycemia, an important effort in reducing congenital anomalies in newborns.

Evidence-based practice and nursing research in areas such as the best way to prevent STDs, how to educate HIV-positive women of the danger to a newborn, and specific effects of illnesses on pregnancy or the fetus are needed.

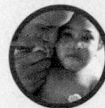

ough understanding of the signs and symptoms of illnesses, such as cardiovascular disease or diabetes mellitus, in addition to an understanding of the course of a normal pregnancy. Assessment techniques include objective measures such as establishing baseline vital signs as well as subjective factors such as the extent of edema or exhaustion (Fig. 14-1). Such assessment is best made by health care personnel who care for the woman consistently throughout the pregnancy so subtle changes in data can be best recognized. In the absence of a consistent care provider, teach the woman to assess her health in relation to objective parameters. Teach her to report exhaustion, for example, in relation to daily activity (e.g., "Two weeks ago I could walk a block without being short of breath. Today I could walk only half a block"; "The last time I was in for a checkup, edema didn't occur until bedtime. Now I notice it every afternoon by the time my son comes home from school").

Nursing Diagnosis

Nursing diagnoses developed for the woman with a high-risk pregnancy address the specific, disease-related conditions as well as any therapeutic restrictions such conditions might require. Possible nursing diagnoses may include:

- Risk for infection transmission related to lack of knowledge of safer sex practices
- Ineffective tissue perfusion (cardiopulmonary) related to mitral valve prolapse during pregnancy
- Pain related to pyelonephritis
- Social isolation related to prescribed bed rest during pregnancy secondary to concurrent illness
- Ineffective role performance related to increasing level of daily restrictions secondary to chronic illness and pregnancy
- Knowledge deficit related to normal changes of pregnancy versus illness complications
- Fear regarding pregnancy outcome related to chronic illness

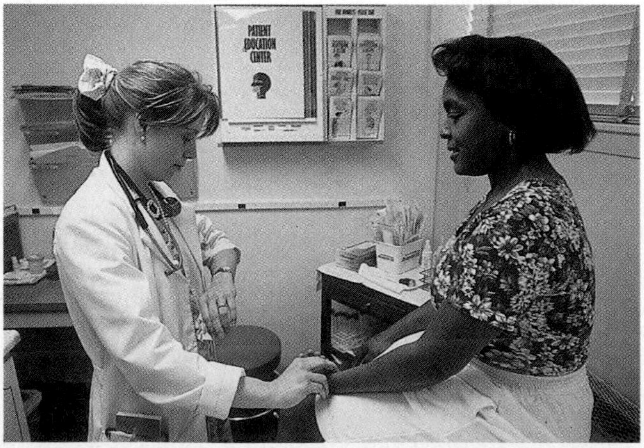

FIGURE 14.1 It is important to establish baseline vital signs in order to later identify a complication related to a preexisting condition.

- Health-seeking behaviors related to the increasing knowledge of the effects of illness on pregnancy
- Situational low self-esteem related to diagnosis of HIV infection

Outcome Identification and Planning

Be certain that the outcomes and goals established are realistic in light of the mother's health and the restrictions placed on her by her health. One family member with illness affects all family members; therefore, outcomes should relate to the entire family's health.

Planning with the woman with a preexisting medical condition should be done based on the pattern of her life before the pregnancy. For example, to ensure that the pregnant woman receives adequate rest during pregnancy, planning for two rest periods a day would be appropriate. However, for a woman with cardiac disease who took two rest periods a day before pregnancy, this would be ineffective because she needs more rest than others. Remember that the additional health supervision needed during pregnancy may involve increased expenses for the family; the family may need to develop new ways to meet these expenses. Thus, a major goal for a woman with a severe chronic condition might be to maintain her health during pregnancy so she can remain at home as long as possible, thereby minimizing hospitalization and family disruptions.

Planning after trauma may be difficult for a woman because of the shock of the accident. Be careful, however, not to make plans completely for her (e.g., "Your best plan would be to allow the doctor to put a cast in place"). Instead, give the woman the available alternatives (e.g., "As the doctor explained, there are two separate therapies for a dislocated knee; let me review with you the advantages and disadvantages of each therapy"). Allowing the woman to choose among alternatives helps her to participate in planning care and maintain self-esteem, thus helping her to move a step toward parenthood and assuming care for her family.

Implementation

Nursing interventions for the pregnant woman with an illness unrelated to her pregnancy may focus on teaching her new or additional measures to maintain health. Imaginative solutions to problems must be created or, after a time, the woman may be unable to adjust to the changes she must make.

Provide the pregnant woman who sustained trauma with an opportunity to talk about the event after the emergency care is complete. She may feel guilty that she was not more careful. In some instances, her support person may have been responsible for causing the injury (e.g., by driving carelessly). She may feel both anger at that person's carelessness and yet relief that he or she was not injured and is there to offer support.

A woman and her partner can usually work through these emotions satisfactorily if the pregnancy progresses normally after this point and the fetus was uninjured. If the fetus was injured or the pregnancy disrupted, the event may cause a great deal of stress, and counseling may be needed to help the woman and her partner overcome feelings of guilt and anger regarding the event.

Outcome Evaluation

If evaluation of outcomes at health care visits reveals that an outcome is not being met, new assessment, analysis, and planning need to be done. In some instances, an outcome is not met because the woman did not understand the need for the additional pregnancy measure. Evaluation may reveal that the woman needs more psychological support to continue to follow a pregnancy routine consistently. Nine months is a long time to adhere to restrictions. Make evaluation ongoing to ensure that you know throughout the pregnancy whether interventions are successful. Some examples of outcomes that might be established are:

- Client states she rests for 2 hours morning and afternoon; dependent edema remains at 1+ or less at next prenatal visit.
- Family members state they are all participating in exercise program since mother developed gestational diabetes.
- Client reports no increase in burning on urination or flank pain at next prenatal visit.

IDENTIFYING THE HIGH-RISK PREGNANCY

A **high-risk pregnancy** is one in which a concurrent disorder, pregnancy-related complication, or external factor jeopardizes the health of the mother, the fetus, or both.

Some women enter pregnancy with a chronic illness that, when superimposed on the pregnancy, makes it high risk. Other women enter pregnancy in good health but then develop a complication of pregnancy that causes it to become high risk. In some instances, a combination of particular circumstances—poverty, lack of support people, poor coping mechanisms, genetic inheritance, or past history of pregnancy complications—can cause a pregnancy to be categorized as high risk (see Focus on Cultural Competence).

In most instances, more than one factor contributes to the classification of a pregnancy as high risk. The pregnancy of a woman who is diabetic, for example, is automatically termed one with greater than normal risk because the fetus is growing in an environment in which **hyperglycemia** (increased serum glucose) is the rule. During the pregnancy, the woman, worrying that something will happen to her baby, may fail to begin the "pregnancy work" that she must do so bonding can take place. At birth, the child is in double jeopardy: not only is the baby born with an illness, but he or she also is at high risk for poor maternal–child attachment.

The preterm infant born to a teenage girl, likewise, has a double problem. Not only is the infant immature (and at risk for all the complications that accompany immaturity), but also he or she has a mother who often is immature as well (see Chap. 17 for discussion of the special needs of the pregnant adolescent).

FOCUS ON CULTURAL COMPETENCE

An illness during pregnancy can complicate not only a pregnancy but also a woman's entire lifestyle and that of her family. Women who think of pregnancy as a time of wellness may have a great deal of difficulty accepting a medical regimen such as daily blood glucose monitoring because this is contradictory to their primary belief. Women in extended families may have an easier time accepting hospitalization during pregnancy than those living in nuclear families because more people are available to take over their role at home. Conversely, women in extended families may have more difficulty with hospitalization because more people are depending on them to be at home.

Assessing all families individually and asking about the effect of an illness during pregnancy on the entire family helps to identify problems and leads to timely problem solving.

Table 14-1 lists common psychological, social, and physical factors that can cause a pregnancy to be categorized as high risk. Categorizing the risks as minimal, moderate, or extensive differs with each woman because of her individual coping mechanisms and level of support. For example, a woman living in extreme poverty who does not have access to community support would be at high risk for poor nutritional intake during pregnancy, whereas a woman with a similar income who could depend on a nutritional assistance program such as WIC and counseling from a community health nurse might be only at minimal risk.

Remembering that the term "high risk" rarely refers to just one causative factor helps in the planning of holistic and ultimately effective nursing care. Box 14-1 highlights appropriate outcomes and interventions related to high-risk pregnancy care using the terminology identified by the Nursing Outcomes Classification (NOC) and Nursing Interventions Classification (NIC).

Preexisting or newly acquired maternal illnesses that can make a pregnancy high risk are covered in this chapter. Chapter 15 discusses pregnancy-related conditions and illnesses that can make a pregnancy high risk. Chapter 17 covers populations that are at high risk due to age (younger than 18 years or older than 40 years), the presence of a disability, or drug abuse.

SEXUALLY TRANSMITTED DISEASES AND PREGNANCY

Sexually transmitted diseases (STDs) are those spread through sexual contact with an infected partner. This chapter provides a brief overview of those STDs most important to identify during pregnancy because of their

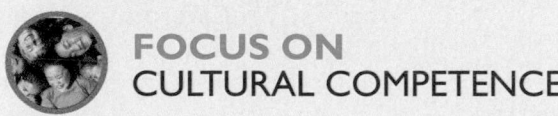

TABLE 14.1 Factors That Categorize a Pregnancy as High Risk

PSYCHOLOGICAL	SOCIAL	PHYSICAL
Prepregnancy		
History of drug dependence (including alcohol) History of intimate partner abuse History of mental illness History of poor coping mechanisms Cognitively challenged Survivor of childhood sexual abuse	Occupation involving handling of toxic substances (including radiation and anesthesia gases) Environmental contaminants at home Isolated Lower economic level Poor access to transportation for care High altitude Highly mobile lifestyle Poor housing Lack of support people	Visual or hearing challenges Pelvic inadequacy or misshape Uterine incompetency, position, or structure Secondary major illness (heart disease, diabetes mellitus, kidney disease, hypertension, chronic infection such as tuberculosis, hemopoietic or blood disorder, malignancy) Poor gynecologic or obstetric history History of previous poor pregnancy outcome (miscarriage, stillbirth, intrauterine fetal death) History of child with congenital anomalies Obesity Pelvic inflammatory disease History of inherited disorder Small stature Potential of blood incompatibility Younger than age 18 years or older than 35 years Cigarette smoker Substance abuser
Pregnancy		
Loss of support person Illness of a family member Decrease in self-esteem Drug abuse (including alcohol and cigarette smoking) Poor acceptance of pregnancy	Refusal of or neglected prenatal care Exposure to environmental teratogens Disruptive family incident Decreased economic support Conception under 1 year from last pregnancy or pregnancy within 12 months of the first pregnancy	Subject to trauma Fluid or electrolyte imbalance Intake of teratogen such as a drug Multiple gestation A bleeding disruption Poor placental formation or position Gestational diabetes Nutritional deficiency of iron, folic acid, or protein Poor weight gain Pregnancy-induced hypertension Infection Amniotic fluid abnormality Postmaturity
Labor and Delivery		
Severely frightened by labor and delivery experience Inability to participate due to anesthesia Separation of infant at birth Lack of preparation for labor Birth of infant who is disappointing in some way (e.g., sex, appearance, or congenital anomalies) Illness in newborn	Lack of support person Inadequate home for infant care Unplanned cesarean birth Lack of access to continued health care Lack of access to emergency personnel or equipment	Hemorrhage Infection Fluid and electrolyte imbalance Dystocia Precipitous birth Lacerations of cervix or vagina Cephalopelvic disproportion Internal fetal monitoring Retained placenta

potential effect on the pregnancy, fetus, or newborn. Chapter 26 discusses additional specific effects on the fetus or newborn.

All STDs can be prevented to some extent by the use of safer sex practices (see Chap. 4), including use of a condom and a spermicide containing nonoxynol-9 for sexual relations. Little disease immunity is developed against a STD once it has been contracted, so it is possible to become reinfected if prevention measures are not followed. In most instances, an infected partner should also be treated

BOX 14.1

NURSING OUTCOMES AND NURSING INTERVENTIONS CLASSIFICATION: HIGH-RISK PREGNANCY

NOC: Fetal status, Antepartum
Fetal status, antepartum is defined as the conditions indicating fetal physical well-being from conception to the onset of labor (Johnson, Maas, & Moorhead, 2000). Some specific indicators suggesting achievement of this outcome include the following:

- Fetal heart rate within range of 120 to 160 beats per minute
- Fetal ultrasound growth measurements, movement frequency, and movement pattern within expected range
- Variability and deceleration patterns in electronic fetal monitor findings within expected parameters

NOC: Maternal status, Antepartum
Maternal status, antepartum is defined as the conditions and behaviors indicating maternal well-being from conception to the onset of labor (Johnson, Maas, & Moorhead, 2000). Some specific indicators suggesting achievement of this outcome include the woman's ability to:

- Demonstrate emotional attachment to the fetus
- Cope with discomforts of pregnancy
- Exhibit neurologic reflexes, vital signs, urine protein and glucose, blood glucose, hemoglobin levels, and other laboratory test results as indicated within expected parameters

NIC: High-risk pregnancy care
High-risk pregnancy care is defined as the identification and management of a high-risk pregnancy to promote healthy outcomes for the mother and baby (McCloskey & Bulechek, 2000). Some important activities involved when implementing this intervention include:

- Determining factors related to poor pregnancy outcomes, including medical risk factors, past pregnancy risk factors, and social and demographic risk factors
- Identifying the woman's knowledge base about potential risk factors
- Providing education to minimize risk factors in conjunction with usual prenatal teaching and self-care activities
- Referring to appropriate support programs as needed
- Instructing on the use of self-monitoring techniques and procedures, including medication therapy
- Providing written guidelines for signs and symptoms that require immediate attention

or the disease can recur from cross-infection (Weisbord et al., 2001).

Treatment of most STDs begins with determining the causative organism so that the appropriate antimicrobial or antifungal agent can be prescribed. Women need to be educated about the mode of transmission for these diseases and about measures to reduce the vulvar or vaginal irritation they frequently cause (see Chap. 47).

NURSING DIAGNOSES AND RELATED INTERVENTIONS

Nursing Diagnosis: Pain related to vulvar irritation secondary to existence of STD.

Outcome Identification: Client will be free of symptoms of infection, instituting measures to prevent contracting this or other STDs in the future.

Outcome Evaluation: No vaginal discharge or pruritus is present by history or examination. Client reports she is using safer sex practices.

The Woman With Candidiasis

Candidiasis causes a vaginal infection spread by the fungus *Candida*. The woman notices a thick vaginal discharge that resembles cream cheese and extreme pruritus. The vagina appears red and irritated. Candidiasis occurs more frequently during pregnancy than normally because of the increased estrogen level present during pregnancy, which causes the vaginal pH to be less acidic. It occurs most frequently in women being treated with an antibiotic for another infection, in women with gestational diabetes, and in women with HIV infection. Women with repeated infections should have their urine tested for glucose to detect gestational diabetes.

The disease is diagnosed by microscopic analysis of the vaginal discharge mounted on a wet slide. It is treated by the vaginal application of an over-the-counter antifungal cream such as miconazole (Monistat) for 7 days or a single dose of oral fluconazole (Diflucan). Treating the infection during pregnancy is important because the profuse vaginal discharge and pruritus can be very uncomfortable for the woman. In addition, if infection is present in the vagina at the time of childbirth, it may cause a candidal infection, or thrush, in the newborn (see Chap. 43). Caution pregnant women to telephone their primary health care provider before using an over-the-counter product to be certain the product is safe to use during pregnancy and also so that her primary care provider can know that vaginal infections are occurring (Cunningham et al., 2001).

The Woman With Trichomoniasis

Trichomoniasis is an infection caused by a single-cell protozoan that is spread by coitus. The woman notices a yellow-gray, frothy, odorous vaginal discharge. The infection is diagnosed by examination of vaginal secretions on a wet slide that has been treated with potassium hydroxide

(KOH). It is important that trichomoniasis infections are identified because they may be associated with preterm labor, premature rupture of membranes, and postcesarean infection (Eschenbach, 2000).

The drug of choice for the disorder, metronidazole (Flagyl), may be teratogenic if used during the first trimester of pregnancy. Thus, the disorder is usually treated with topical clotrimazole, a drug with a lesser effect.

The Woman With Bacterial Vaginosis

Bacterial vaginosis is local infection of the vagina by the invasion, most commonly, of *Gardnerella vaginalis* organisms. The associated discharge is gray and has a fishy odor. Pruritus may be intense. The treatment for nonpregnant women is metronidazole, either orally as Flagyl or topically as a vaginal cream. Because metronidazole is not usually recommended for use during the first trimester of pregnancy, women are usually treated with a topical cream late in pregnancy. Assure women that a topical cream will be safe to use at this later time so that they will finish the full prescription. Untreated *G. vaginalis* infections are associated with amniotic fluid infections and, perhaps, preterm labor and premature ruptured membranes (Eschenbach, 2000).

The Woman With Chlamydia

Chlamydia is one of the most common types of vaginal infections seen during pregnancy. Usually, screening for this infection via a vaginal culture occurs during the woman's first prenatal visit. If the woman has multiple sexual partners, screening occurs again in the third trimester. The infection, caused by a gram-negative intracellular parasite, causes a heavy, gray-white vaginal discharge. Diagnosis is made by culture of the organism from vaginal secretions using a specific chlamydia culture kit. Therapy for nonpregnant women is usually with doxycycline (Vibramycin), a tetracycline. This is contraindicated during pregnancy because of possible fetal long-bone deformities; azithromycin (Zithromax) or amoxicillin (Amoxil) is used instead. There is a high association between gonorrhea and chlamydia; therefore, if a chlamydia infection is documented, women are usually tested for gonorrhea as well. The woman's partner also should be treated to prevent the woman from becoming reinfected.

Chlamydia infections must be treated because they are associated with premature rupture of the membranes, preterm labor, and endometritis in the postpartal period. An infant who is born while a chlamydia infection is present in the vagina can suffer conjunctivitis or pneumonia after birth (see Chaps. 40 and 50).

The Woman With Syphilis

Syphilis is a systemic disease caused by the spirochete *Treponema pallidum.* Unlike most diseases, it is currently increasing in frequency in the United States. The first stage of syphilis results in a painless ulcer (chancre) on the vulva or vagina. Early in pregnancy (before week 18), the placenta appears to provide some protection against the disease. After this time, however, the spirochete crosses the placenta freely and may be responsible for spontaneous miscarriage, preterm labor, stillbirth, or congenital anomalies in the newborn (see Chap. 26). All pregnant women are screened for syphilis at the first prenatal visit by a VDRL, ART, or FTA-ABS antibody reaction test. Those who have multiple sexual partners are tested again at about week 36 of pregnancy. In some institutions, women are screened again at the beginning of labor and newborns are screened for congenital syphilis by a cord blood sample.

One injection of benzathine penicillin G is the drug of choice for the treatment of syphilis during pregnancy. After therapy, the woman may experience a sudden episode of hypotension, fever, tachycardia, and muscle aches. This is called a Jarisch-Herxheimer reaction and is caused by the sudden destruction of spirochetes. The reaction lasts about 24 hours and then fades (Genc and Ledger, 2000).

The Woman With a Herpes Simplex Virus Type 2 Infection

Genital herpes infection is a sexually transmitted disease caused by the herpes simplex virus (HSV) type 2. The first time that a woman contracts the infection, painful, small, pinpoint vesicles surrounded by erythema develop on the vulva or in the vagina, accompanied by a low-grade fever 3 to 7 days after exposure. There may be a genetic susceptibility to the herpes virus; some women appear to be more prone to infection than others. Although the symptoms fade in a few days, the virus remains in local nerve ganglions, becoming activated by a break in the skin or possibly stress.

If the woman has a primary infection, herpes can be transmitted across the placenta to cause congenital infection in the newborn. If the woman has primary or secondary active lesions in the vagina or on the vulva at the time of birth, herpes infection can be transmitted to the newborn at birth. When infection in the newborn occurs, congenital herpes, a severe systemic infection that is often fatal, can result (see Chap. 26). To help avoid transmission, women with active lesions are usually scheduled for a cesarean birth. If no lesions are present, a vaginal birth is preferable.

Diagnosis is made by the appearance of the lesions, Pap smear, and enzyme-linked immunosorbent assay (ELISA). The drug of choice for the treatment of herpes infection is acyclovir (Zovirax) in an ointment or oral form (Karch, 2001). Acyclovir is classified as a pregnancy category C drug. Women can reduce the pain of the lesions by taking sitz baths or applying warm, moist tea bags to the area. Condom use by the woman's partner or by the woman (female condom) is strongly urged to prevent transmission of the virus to the woman's partner.

The Woman With Gonorrhea

Gonorrhea is an STD caused by the gram-negative coccus *Neisseria gonorrhoeae.* A yellow-green vaginal discharge may be present, or the woman may be asymptomatic. The male partner usually has severe symptoms of pain on urination and a purulent yellow penile discharge. Despite safer sex practices and effective therapy, this disease is being spread at an epidemic rate among young adults.

Gonorrhea is associated with spontaneous miscarriage, preterm birth, and endometritis in the postpartal period. It is also a major cause of pelvic infectious disease (PID) and infertility. Diagnosis is made by culture of the organism from the vagina, rectum, or urethra. Although gonorrhea has traditionally been treated with amoxicillin and probenecid, the incidence of penicillinase-producing strains has made this traditional therapy ineffective. Therefore, cefixime (Suprax) as a one-time intramuscular injection is the current recommended therapy. This drug can be safely administered during pregnancy (pregnancy risk category B). Sexual partners also should be treated to prevent reinfection. Because most people who contract gonorrhea also are found to have a chlamydial infection, nonpregnant women should receive doxycycline therapy at the same time. If the woman is pregnant, she should receive amoxicillin.

It is important that gonorrhea be identified and treated during pregnancy because if the infection is present at the time of birth, it can cause a severe eye infection that can lead to blindness in the newborn (ophthalmia neonatorum; see Chap. 26).

The Woman With Human Papillomavirus Infection

The human papillomavirus (HPV) causes fibrous tissue overgrowth on the external vulva (condyloma acuminatum). The infection may be present in as many as 10% to 30% of women and most often in women who have multiple sexual partners. At first, lesions appear as discrete papillary structures; they then spread, enlarge, and coalesce to form large, cauliflower-like lesions. These tend to increase in size during pregnancy because of the high vascular flow in the pelvic area. They may become secondarily ulcerated and infected; when this occurs, a foul vulvar odor may develop.

Therapy for such lesions is aimed at dissolving the lesions and also ending any secondary infection present. Podophyllum (Podofin) applied directly to lesions is the drug of choice for nonpregnant women but is contraindicated during pregnancy because of possible toxic effects on the fetus. Trichloroacetic acid (TCA) or bichloracetic acid (BCA) applied to the lesions weekly may be effective and can be used during pregnancy. Large lesions may be removed by laser therapy, cryocautery, or knife excision. With cryocautery, edema at the site is evident immediately; lesions become gangrenous and sloughing occurs in 7 days. Healing will be complete in 4 to 6 weeks with only slight depigmentation at the site. Sitz baths and a lidocaine cream may be soothing during the healing period. Unless they are bothersome, lesions may be left in place during pregnancy and removed during the postpartal period.

The presence of vulvar lesions appears to have no effect on the fetus during pregnancy, but if they are present at the time of birth and obstruct the birth canal, a cesarean birth may be necessary. HPV infections are serious because they are associated with the development of cervical cancer later in life. Women who have had one episode of infection should be conscientious about having yearly Pap tests for the rest of their lives.

The Woman With a Group B Streptococcal Infection

Although a less publicized disease than STDs such as herpes type 2 or gonorrhea, streptococcus B infection may occur at a higher incidence during pregnancy than those diseases or in as many as 15% to 35% of pregnant women (Gilson et al., 2000). Although infection develops within the cervix or vagina, the mother usually experiences no symptoms. Consequences can be urinary tract infection (UTI), intra-amniotic infection leading to preterm birth, and postpartal endometritis.

The Centers for Disease Control and Prevention (CDC) recommends that all pregnant women be screened for streptococcus B at 35 to 38 weeks of pregnancy This is important because approximately 40% to 70% of neonates whose mothers have an active infection will become infected from placental transfer or from direct contact with the organisms at birth. Infected neonates may develop severe pneumonia, sepsis, respiratory distress syndrome, or meningitis (see Chap. 26).

A broad-spectrum penicillin such as ampicillin is the treatment of choice (McDuffie, 2000). Women who experience rupture of membranes at less than 37 weeks of pregnancy may be treated with intravenous ampicillin to reduce the risk of spreading the infection to the newborn.

The Woman with Hepatitis B or C

Hepatitis B and C are both STDs that are increasing in incidence. These are discussed further in Chapter 45.

The Woman With HIV Infection

The human immunodeficiency virus (HIV), the organism responsible for acquired immunodeficiency syndrome (AIDS), is the most serious of the STDs because it may be fatal to both mother and child. Women are contracting this at much faster rates than formerly; in many areas, they are the fastest-growing category of HIV-infected persons. It has become the leading cause of death in women 25 to 44 years of age. One percent to 2% of every 1,000 women giving birth are HIV positive. Pregnancy does not appear to accelerate the progression of the disease (Minkoff, 2000).

The disorder is caused by a retrovirus that infects and disables T lymphocytes. Without T lymphocytes, the body cannot fight infection through T-cell and B-cell activity (see Chap. 42). The virus may be contracted through sexual intercourse, by exposure to infected blood, by vertical transmission across the placenta to the fetus at birth, or by breast milk to the newborn. Risk factors include:

- Multiple sexual partners of the individual or sexual partner
- Bisexual partners

- Intravenous drug use by the individual or sexual partner
- Blood transfusions (rare)

Assessment

When the HIV virus invades T lymphocytes (T4 cells), it substitutes its own RNA and DNA for the cell's DNA. T4 cells die, reducing the woman's immune system functioning. A CD4 cell count in the laboratory determines how many T4 cells are present and functioning. When this count falls below 500 cells/mm^3 or the viral load rises above 5,000 copies/mL, it is difficult to resist opportunistic infections.

Unlike other STDs, HIV rarely begins with reproductive tract irritation. Instead, early symptoms are more subtle and often difficult to differentiate from those of other diseases or even from the symptoms of early pregnancy (e.g., fatigue, anemia, diarrhea, and weight loss).

Without therapy, HIV infection may progress through the following stages:

- The initial invasion of the virus, which may be accompanied by mild, flulike symptoms
- Seroconversion, in which the woman converts from having no HIV antibodies in blood serum (HIV serum negative) to having antibodies positive for HIV (HIV serum positive). This happens 6 weeks to 1 year after exposure.
- An asymptomatic period during which the woman appears to be disease-free except for symptoms such as weight loss and fatigue (a wasting syndrome), although the virus can be replicating during this time. The length of the period varies but averages 2 to 6 years.
- A symptomatic period during which the woman develops opportunistic infections and possible malignancies (e.g., toxoplasmosis, oral and vaginal candidiasis, gastrointestinal illness, herpes simplex, *Pneumocystis carinii* pneumonia [PCP], *Candida* esophagitis, Kaposi sarcoma, and HIV-associated dementia). At this point, the CD4 count is usually below 200 cells/mm^3.

Although women are not as yet routinely screened for this infection during pregnancy (as a rule, no screening program is initiated for any disease until there is a cure for the disease [Lo et al., 2000]), women who practice high-risk behaviors should be asked if they want to be screened. The woman with HIV may also have contracted other STDs such as syphilis, gonorrhea, chlamydia, and hepatitis B, and so should be screened for these as well. Because HIV-positive women are at higher risk for developing toxoplasmosis and cytomegalovirus infections, the history should include questions about cat ownership and ingestion of raw meat, and mild, flulike symptoms (see Chap. 8). Ordinarily, toxoplasmosis presents with few symptoms. However, in the HIV-positive woman, it may invade the cerebrospinal fluid and cause extreme neurologic involvement. Tuberculosis occurs at a higher rate in people with HIV than others and may worsen during pregnancy; thus, a test for this should also be included.

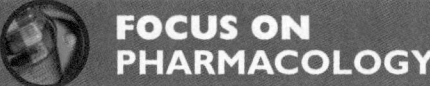

Testing for HIV is done by an ELISA antibody reaction; for confirmation, a Western blot analysis is required. If a woman is found to be HIV positive (has developed antibodies from having been exposed to the virus), the issues of safer sex practices, testing of sexual contacts, continuation or termination of the pregnancy, and treatment during pregnancy need to be addressed. HIV is associated with low birthweight and preterm birth. If the woman is untreated, 20% to 50% of infants born to HIV-positive women will develop AIDS in the first year of life. If zidovudine (ZVD) is administered beginning with the 14th week of pregnancy and the newborn receives the drug for 6 weeks, the risk of perinatal transmission can be reduced to only 8% to 10% (Minkoff, 2000; see Focus On Pharmacology: Zidovudine).

Therapeutic Management

Women who are identified as HIV positive are usually advised not to become pregnant until more is learned about how to prevent transmission to a fetus. Often, however, the existence of HIV is discovered only after pregnancy is

FOCUS ON PHARMACOLOGY

Zidovudine (ZVD)

Action: A thymidine analog effective in inhibiting replication of some retroviruses, notably HIV. Used to help block transmission of HIV from pregnant woman to fetus.

Pregnancy Category: C

Dosage: 100 mg five times a day from the 14th week of gestation to the beginning of labor

Possible Adverse Reactions: Fatigue, headache, nausea, vomiting, skin rash, agranulocytopenia, loss of feeling or sensation, paresthesias

Nursing Implications

- Monitor hematologic indices every 2 weeks. Help woman arrange her schedule so that she can adhere to plan for follow-up laboratory testing.
- Advise women they must be certain to take the drug around the clock; otherwise they tend to omit the fifth dose of the day.
- Tell the woman that opportunistic infections such as vaginal candidiasis may continue to occur. Advise her to inform her primary care provider of such infections.
- Offer advice on ways to continue adequate intake, such as small frequent meals, despite nausea that may occur.
- Help the woman to analyze her lifestyle if loss of feeling or sensation occurs to minimize the risk for injury, such as being burned while cooking.
- Caution the woman that taking zidovudine does not reduce the risk of transmission of HIV to others by sexual contact or blood contamination. Instruct in continued need for safer sex practices.

already present. Progression of the disease is determined by frequent CD4 cell counts and viral load levels.

A goal of therapy is to maintain the CD4 cell count at greater than 500 cells/mm^3 and the viral load at less than 5,000 copies/mL by administering a protease inhibitor such as ritonavir (Norvir). Zidovudine should be administered to help reduce mother-to-fetal transmission. Typically, zidovudine is prescribed as 100 mg orally five times per day during pregnancy. During labor it is given intravenously. The newborn then receives the drug in syrup form (2 mg/kg every 6 hours) for 6 weeks.

If PCP develops, the woman is treated with trimethoprim with sulfamethoxazole (Bactrim). Trimethoprim may be teratogenic in early pregnancy; sulfamethoxazole (Gantanol) may lead to increased bilirubin levels in the newborn if administered late in pregnancy. Pentamidine (Pentam), the drug of choice for PCP in nonpregnant women, may be administered by aerosol (NebuPent).

Kaposi sarcoma, a rare malignancy that tends to occur with AIDS, is normally treated with chemotherapy. Chemotherapy is contraindicated during early pregnancy because of the potential for fetal injury but can be used later in pregnancy to halt these malignant growths.

Thrombocytopenia (lowered platelet count) may be present as a part of the disease pathology or as a response to zidovudine therapy. This may make the woman a poor candidate for an epidural injection for anesthesia during labor or for episiotomy. She may need a platelet transfusion to restore coagulation ability. To reduce the risk of mother-to-newborn transmission, women are offered the option of cesarean birth.

Follow-up testing of newborns being treated with zidovudine for the first 6 weeks is important. If the child has two negative HIV cultures at 4 months of age, HIV can be reasonably excluded (Samuel and Suh, 2000).

NURSING DIAGNOSES AND RELATED INTERVENTIONS

In addition to the risk for infection transmission, which is a consideration for all STDs, an important nursing diagnosis and related intervention for the pregnant woman who is HIV positive is:

Nursing Diagnosis: Risk for infection (opportunistic) related to dysfunction of the immune system secondary to invasion of HIV.

Outcome Identification: Client will exhibit no signs and symptoms of a severe opportunistic infection during the remainder of pregnancy.

Outcome Evaluation: CD4 counts remain above 500/mm^3; viral load less than 5,000 copies/mL; no symptoms of lung, vaginal, esophageal, or central nervous system infections are present.

Women who have CD4 counts below 200/mm^3 may be prescribed drugs to help prevent opportunistic infections. Such drugs include acyclovir (Zovirax) for herpes simplex, clotrimazole troches (Mycelex) for oral thrush, pyrimethamine (Daraprim) and sulfadiazine for toxoplasmosis, and trimethoprim with sulfamethoxazole (Bactrim) for PCP. They may be immunized against pneumonia, influenza, and hepatitis B.

During pregnancy and at birth, active interventions are necessary to reduce the possibility of fetal exposure to maternal blood, often the mode of transmission to the fetus. Amniocentesis, for example, presents a risk for exposure to maternal blood and therefore should be avoided for diagnosing fetal maturity. During labor, internal fetal monitors, scalp blood sampling, forceps, and vacuum extraction are avoided to prevent the creation of a source of bleeding (that is, an open lesion on the fetal scalp). Episiotomy also is avoided to limit this as a possible blood source. Breast milk may transmit HIV and also increases the incidence of mastitis, so generally the woman is advised not to breast-feed her infant (Semba, 2000). Breastfeeding could also be exhausting for a debilitated woman.

Women who are HIV positive need to be aware that they can still spread this illness to others through unprotected sexual relations or unintentional contamination by blood, even though they are being treated with antibiotics or zidovudine. Nurses can help reduce this risk by providing patient education information about the mode of HIV transmission and safer sex practices.

Health care providers must take care to use standard precautions (see Chap. 43) to protect against the spread of HIV. This includes the use of gloves when there is a possibility of contact with body secretions; cover gowns if clothing will be exposed to secretions; and goggles at birth, when there may be splashing of amniotic fluid. Gloves should be worn when handling the newborn until all maternal blood has been removed by a first bath. No blood sampling or injections should be completed on the neonate until after a first bath and the removal of maternal blood.

Caring for the woman who is HIV positive during pregnancy and childbirth calls for great sensitivity to respect the woman as a patient with a possibly fatal disease while at the same time encouraging her to continue with prenatal care. Because research into the cause and treatment of this disease is ongoing and constantly changing, nurses need to remain current on recommendations for therapy or prevention.

✔ CHECKPOINT QUESTIONS

1. What two groups of pregnant women are most likely to develop *Candida* infections?
2. The usual drug of choice for trichomoniasis is metronidazole (Flagyl). Why may this drug not be the drug of choice for treating these infections early in pregnancy?
3. What is the advantage to the fetus when zidovudine is administered to a woman who is HIV positive?

HEMATOLOGIC DISORDERS AND PREGNANCY

Hematologic disorders during pregnancy involve either blood formation or coagulation disorders.

Anemia and Pregnancy

Because the blood volume expands during pregnancy slightly ahead of the red cell count, most women have a pseudoanemia of early pregnancy. This is normal and should not be confused with the true anemia that can occur as a complication of pregnancy.

NURSING DIAGNOSES AND RELATED INTERVENTIONS

Nursing Diagnosis: Risk for ineffective tissue perfusion related to maternal anemia during pregnancy.

Outcome Identification: Client will demonstrate adequate measures to guard against anemia during pregnancy and exhibit signs of adequate tissue perfusion during pregnancy.

Outcome Evaluation: Client takes prenatal supplement daily; hemoglobin is above 11 mg/dL; fetal heart rate is 120 to 160 bpm.

The Woman With Iron-Deficiency Anemia

Iron-deficiency anemia is the most common anemia of pregnancy, complicating as many as 15% to 25% of all pregnancies. Many women enter pregnancy with a deficit of iron stores resulting from a diet low in iron, heavy menstrual periods, or unwise weight-reducing programs. Iron stores are apt to be low in women experiencing a short period (less than 2 years) between pregnancies or those from low socioeconomic communities. When the hemoglobin level is below 10 mg/dL (hematocrit under 33%), iron deficiency is suspected (Xiong et al., 2000).

Iron is made available to the body by absorption from the duodenum into the bloodstream, where it is bound to transferrin for transport to the liver, spleen, and bone marrow. At these sites, it is incorporated into hemoglobin or stored as ferritin.

Iron-deficiency anemia is characteristically a microcytic (small red blood cell), hypochromic (less hemoglobin than the average red cell) anemia because when an inadequate supply of iron is ingested, iron is unavailable for incorporation into red blood cells. As a result, cells are not as large or as rich in hemoglobin as they normally are. Both hematocrit and hemoglobin will be reduced (under 33% and 10 mg/dL, respectively). Serum transferrin will be under 100 mg/dL, the transferrin saturation level will be under 5%, serum iron will be under 30 μg/dL, and mean corpuscular hemoglobin concentration will be under 30; iron-binding capacity, in contrast, will be increased (over 400 μg/dL). Iron-deficiency anemia is associated with low birthweight and preterm birth. Because the body recognizes that it needs increased nutrients, some women develop pica, or the eating of substances such as ice or starch. The woman experiences extreme fatigue and poor exercise tolerance.

All women should take prenatal vitamins containing an iron supplement of 60 mg elemental iron as prophylactic therapy against iron-deficiency anemia during pregnancy. Women with iron-deficiency anemia will be prescribed therapeutic levels of medication (120 to 180 mg elemental iron/day), usually prescribed as ferrous sulfate or ferrous gluconate. Iron is best absorbed in an acid medium. Therefore, advise women to take iron supplements with orange juice or a vitamin C supplement. In addition, they need to eat a diet high in iron and vitamins (green leafy vegetables, meat, legumes, fruit). If they are not already enrolled in a WIC program but are eligible, a referral should be made to help ensure a better diet. When women begin to take a prescribed iron supplement, new red blood cells should begin to increase or the reticulocyte count should rise from a normal range of 0.5% to 1.5% to 3% to 4% by 2 weeks' time. Some women report constipation or gastric irritation when taking oral iron supplements. Increasing roughage in the diet and always taking the pills with food help reduce these symptoms.

If iron-deficiency anemia is severe and a woman is noncompliant with oral iron therapy, intramuscular or intravenous iron dextran can be administered.

The Woman With Folic Acid-Deficiency Anemia

Folic acid, or folacin, one of the B vitamins, is necessary for the normal formation of red blood cells in the mother and has been associated with preventing neural tube defects in the fetus. Folic acid-deficiency anemia is seen in 1% to 5% of pregnancies (Wenstrom & Malee, 2000). It occurs most often in multiple pregnancies because of the increased fetal demand; in women with a secondary hemolytic illness in which there is rapid destruction and production of red blood cells; in women who are taking hydantoin, an anticonvulsant agent that interferes with folate absorption; and in women who have been taking oral contraceptives. The anemia that develops is a **megaloblastic anemia** (enlarged red blood cells). The mean corpuscular volume will be elevated, in contrast to the lowered level seen with iron-deficiency anemia. The deficiency may take a number of weeks to develop, so it often becomes most apparent during the second trimester of pregnancy. It may be a contributory factor in early miscarriage or premature separation of the placenta.

Because the fetal effects of deficiency occur in the first few weeks of fetal development, women expecting to become pregnant should be advised to begin a vitamin supplement (over-the-counter) or be conscious about eating folacin-rich foods during this time (green leafy vegetables, oranges, dried beans). All women of childbearing age should take a supplement of 400 μg folic acid daily (DHHS, 2000). Over-the-counter multivitamin preparations generally do not contain adequate folic acid for pregnancy, when the requirement increases to 600 μg/day, whereas vitamins specifically designed for pregnancy do. Women who develop folic acid-deficiency anemia are prescribed therapeutic levels of folic acid. At prenatal visits, ask whether the woman is taking her prescribed vitamin. To save money, women may not have a prescription filled and may be using over-the-counter, less expensive types, not aware of the difference.

The Woman With Sickle Cell Anemia

Sickle cell anemia is a recessively inherited hemolytic anemia caused by an abnormal amino acid in the beta chain of hemoglobin. If the abnormal amino acid replaces the amino acid valine, sickle hemoglobin (HbS) results; if it is substituted for the amino acid lysine, nonsickling hemoglobin (HbC) results. An individual who is heterozygous (has only one gene in which the abnormal substitution has occurred) has the sickle cell trait (HbAS). If the person is homozygous (has two genes in which the substitution has occurred), sickle cell disease (HbSS) results.

With the disease, the majority of red blood cells are irregular or sickle-shaped. They cannot carry as much hemoglobin as normally shaped red blood cells. When oxygen tension becomes reduced, as happens at high altitudes, or blood becomes more viscid than usual (dehydration), the cells tend to clump because of the irregular shape. This clumping can result in vessel blockage and organ infarcts. The cells then will hemolyze, reducing the number available or causing a severe anemia.

Approximately 1 in every 10 African Americans has the sickle cell trait (i.e., carries a recessive gene for S hemoglobin but is asymptomatic); 1 in every 400 African Americans theoretically has the disease. Although the sickle cell trait does not appear to influence the course of pregnancy in terms of pregnancy-induced hypertension, prematurity, miscarriage, or perinatal mortality, women with the trait do seem to have an increased incidence of asymptomatic bacteriuria, resulting in an increased incidence of pyelonephritis.

At any time in life, sickle cell anemia is a threat to life if vital blood vessels such as those to the liver, kidneys, heart, lungs, or brain become blocked. In pregnancy, blockage to the placental circulation can directly compromise the fetus, causing low birthweight and possibly death.

Assessment. All African-American woman who have not been previously tested should be screened for sickle cell anemia at the first prenatal visit. Hemoglobin levels for all women with sickle cell disease should be obtained frequently. A woman with sickle cell disease may normally have a hemoglobin level of 6 to 8 mg/100 mL. Unless she receives active interventions to raise this level, she will maintain it during pregnancy, possibly with harm to the fetus. Hemolysis in a sickle cell crisis may occur so rapidly that a woman's hemoglobin level can fall to 5 or 6 mg/100 mL in a few hours. There is an accompanying rise in her indirect bilirubin level because she cannot conjugate the bilirubin released from red blood cells so quickly destroyed.

Because the pregnant woman with sickle cell anemia is more susceptible to bacteriuria than other women, a clean-catch urine sample should be collected periodically during pregnancy to detect developing bacteriuria while the woman is still asymptomatic.

Throughout pregnancy, monitor the woman's diet to be certain she is consuming sufficient amounts of folic acid and possibly an additional folic acid supplement, which may be necessary to build new red blood cells. Her fluid intake should also be carefully monitored. She should consume at least eight glasses of fluids daily. Early in pregnancy, when she may be nauseated, her fluid intake can easily decrease, and dehydration and a subsequent sickle cell crisis may occur.

Assess the woman's lower extremities at prenatal visits for pooling of blood. This is apt to occur from uterine pressure as pregnancy advances. Such pooling and pressure can lead to red cell destruction. Standing for long periods during the day increases this pressure, whereas sitting on a chair with the legs elevated or lying on the side in a modified Sims' position encourages venous return from the lower extremities. Help a woman plan her day so she has limited long periods of standing.

Fetal health is usually monitored during pregnancy by an ultrasound examination at 16 to 24 weeks to assess for intrauterine growth restriction and by weekly nonstress or ultrasound examinations beginning at about 30 weeks. Blood flow through the uterus and placenta may be measured by blood flow velocity. If blood flow velocity is reduced, the chance of intrauterine growth restriction is increased.

Therapeutic Management. Interventions to prevent sickle cell crisis can include periodic exchange transfusions throughout pregnancy to replace the sickle cells with normal cells. An exchange transfusion serves a secondary purpose of removing a quantity of the increased bilirubin resulting from the breakdown of red blood cells as well as restoring the hemoglobin level (Mahomed, 2000). If a crisis occurs, controlling pain, administering oxygen as needed, and increasing the fluid volume of the circulatory system to lower viscosity are important interventions (see Chap. 44 for further discussion of therapy of sickle cell anemia). The fluid administered is often hypotonic (0.45 saline) to keep plasma tension low because of the difficulty the woman has concentrating urine to remove large amounts of fluid. As a rule, women with sickle cell disease are not given an iron supplement during pregnancy. The cells cannot incorporate iron in the usual manner that normal cells can, so excessive iron buildup may result. Women do need a folic acid supplement to keep the new cells produced from being megaloblastic (Cunningham et al., 2001).

If the woman develops an infection that raises her temperature and causes her to perspire more than normally (creates dehydration) or contracts a respiratory infection that compromises air exchange so that her PO_2 is lowered, hospitalization for observation may be necessary to rule out the development of a sickle cell crisis and subsequent hemolysis of crowded cells.

When the fetus is mature, the time and method of birth are individualized. Keep the woman well hydrated in labor. If an operative birth is necessary, she generally receives nerve block anesthesia rather than a general anesthetic to avoid hypoxia.

Women generally are interested in determining at birth whether their child has inherited the disease. Because the disorder is recessively inherited, if one of the parents has the disease and the other is free of the disease and trait, the chances that the child will inherit the disease are zero. If the woman has the disease and her partner has the trait, the chances that the child will be born with the disease are 50% (see Chap. 7). If both parents have the disease, all their children will also have the disease.

Symptoms of sickle cell disease do not become clinically apparent until the child's fetal hemoglobin has converted to a largely adult pattern (in 3 to 6 months). Fetal hemoglobin comprises two alpha and two gamma chains; adult hemoglobin comprises two alpha and two beta chains. Because the sickle cell trait is carried on the beta chain, it will not be manifested clinically until this chain appears. Electrophoresis of red blood cells obtained during fetal life by percutaneous umbilical blood sampling or amniocentesis, however, can reveal the presence of the disease on the few beta chains present early in pregnancy. Newborns have approximately 15% adult hemoglobin at birth, so electrophoresis testing at birth can also reveal if the disease is present. Nursing care of the child with sickle cell disease is discussed in Chapter 44.

Coagulation Disorders and Pregnancy

Most coagulation disorders are sex-linked or occur only in males, so have little effect on pregnancies. However, Von Willebrand disease is a coagulation disorder inherited as an autosomal dominant trait that does occur in women. The woman notices symptoms of menorrhagia and frequent episodes of epistaxis. If the symptoms are not severe, the condition may go undiagnosed until pregnancy, when the woman experiences a spontaneous miscarriage or postpartal hemorrhage.

Women with the disorder have normal platelet counts, but bleeding time is prolonged. Factor VIII-related antigen (VIII-R) and factor VIII coagulation activity (VIII-C) are both reduced. Replacement of these factors by infusion of cryoprecipitate or fresh-frozen plasma may be necessary before labor to prevent excessive bleeding.

Hemophilia B (Christmas disease, factor IX deficiency) is a sex-linked disorder, so the actual disease occurs only in males. However, female carriers may have such a reduced level of factor IX (only 33% of normal) that hemorrhage with labor or a spontaneous miscarriage can be a serious complication. Carriers of the disorder need to be identified before pregnancy. Restoration of factor IX levels can be done by infusion of factor IX concentrate or fresh-frozen plasma.

Percutaneous umbilical blood sampling can be used to detect whether a male fetus has hemophilia. Before an internal fetal heart rate monitor is attached or fetal scalp blood sampling is done during labor, the fetal status needs to be determined. If the fetus has a coagulation disorder, these procedures would be contraindicated because they could result in extensive fetal blood loss.

Idiopathic thrombocytopenic purpura (ITP), a decreased number of platelets, can occur in women. The cause is unknown, but it is assumed to be an autoimmune illness (an antiplatelet antibody that destroys platelets is apparently released). Symptoms of the illness usually occur shortly after a viral invasion such as an upper respiratory infection.

Without an adequate level of platelets, minute petechiae or large ecchymoses appear on the woman's body. Frequent nosebleeds may occur. Laboratory studies reveal a marked thrombocytopenia (platelet count may be as low as 20,000/mm^3).

The illness typically runs a 1- to 3-month limited course. A platelet transfusion may be administered to temporarily increase the platelet count. Oral prednisone is also effective. Women with the phenomenon need to be identified during pregnancy because the decreased platelet count can lead to increased bleeding at birth. In addition, the antiplatelet factor can cross the placenta and cause accompanying platelet destruction in the newborn, or allow the newborn to be born with the illness (see Chap. 44 for care of the child with ITP).

✔ CHECKPOINT QUESTIONS

4. Why are prescription vitamin supplements better than over-the-counter ones for pregnant women?
5. Why is it important for women to have a sufficient amount of folic acid intake early in pregnancy or before conception?
6. Should women with sickle cell disease routinely take an iron supplement during pregnancy?

RENAL AND URINARY DISORDERS AND PREGNANCY

Adequate kidney function is important to successful pregnancy outcome because the woman is excreting waste products for herself and also the fetus. Therefore, any condition that interferes with kidney or urinary function is potentially serious.

The Woman With a Urinary Tract Infection

As many as 4% to 10% of nonpregnant women have asymptomatic bacteriuria (organisms are present without symptoms of infection). In the pregnant woman, because the ureters dilate from the effect of progesterone, stasis of urine occurs. The minimal glucosuria that occurs with pregnancy allows more than the usual number of organisms to grow. This causes asymptomatic urinary tract infections (UTIs) in as many as 10% to 15% of pregnant women (Cunningham et al., 2001). Women with known vesicoureteral reflux (backflow of urine up the ureters) tend to develop UTIs or pyelonephritis more often than others do. A danger of asymptomatic infections is that they can progress to pyelonephritis (infection of the pelvis of the kidney). An increased incidence of preterm labor, premature rupture of membranes, and fetal loss may be associated with pyelonephritis. The organism most commonly responsible for UTI is *Escherichia coli* from an ascending infection. A UTI can also occur as a descending infection, or begin in the kidneys from the filtration of organisms present from other body infections. If the infectious organism is determined to be streptococcus B, it indicates the woman has an extensive infection. Vaginal cultures should be obtained because streptococcal B infection of the genital tract is associated with pneumonia in newborns.

Assessment

A UTI typically is manifested by frequency and pain on urination. With pyelonephritis, the woman develops pain in the lumbar region (usually on the right side) that radiates downward. The area feels tender to palpation. She may have accompanying nausea and vomiting, malaise, pain, and frequency of urination. Her temperature may be elevated only slightly or may be as high as 103° to 104°F (39° to 40°C). The infection usually occurs on the right side because there is greater compression and urinary stasis on the right ureter from the uterus being pushed that way by the large bulk of the intestine on the left side. A urine culture will reveal over 100,000 organisms per milliliter of urine, a level diagnostic of infection.

Therapeutic Management

Obtain a clean-catch urine sample for culture and sensitivity on women with possible symptoms (see Nursing Procedure 10-1). Many health care agencies ask women for clean-catch urine specimens at intervals during pregnancy (tested by a rapid dipstick method) to detect infection before it becomes symptomatic. A sensitivity test after a culture will determine which antibiotic needs to be prescribed to combat the infection. Amoxicillin, ampicillin, and cephalosporins are effective against most organisms causing UTIs and are considered safe antibiotics during pregnancy. The sulfonamides can be used early in pregnancy but not near term because they interfere with protein binding of bilirubin, which can lead to hyperbilirubinemia in the newborn. Tetracyclines are contraindicated in pregnancy; they cause retardation of bone growth and staining of the fetal teeth (Karch, 2001).

NURSING DIAGNOSES AND RELATED INTERVENTIONS

Nursing Diagnosis: Risk for infection related to stasis of urine with pregnancy.

Outcome Identification: Client will demonstrate no signs of infection during pregnancy.

Outcome Evaluation: Oral temperature is below 100.4°F (38°C), and a clean-catch urine specimen has a bacteria count below 100,000 colonies per milliliter.

All women during pregnancy can be reminded of common measures to prevent UTIs, such as:

- Voiding frequently (at least every 2 hours)
- Wiping front to back after bowel movements
- Wearing cotton, not synthetic fiber, underwear
- Voiding immediately after sexual intercourse

The pregnant woman with a UTI needs to take some additional measures, such as drinking an increased amount of fluid to flush out the infection from the urinary tract. Do not merely tell her to "push fluids" or "drink lots of water." Give her a specific amount to drink every day (up to 3 to 4 L per 24 hours) to make certain that her fluid intake will be sufficiently increased.

A woman can promote urine drainage by assuming a knee–chest position for 15 minutes morning and evening. In this position, the weight of the uterus is shifted forward, releasing the pressure on the ureters and allowing urine to drain more freely.

If the woman has one UTI during pregnancy, the chances are high that she will develop another late in pregnancy, when urinary stasis tends to be greater. She may therefore be kept on prophylactic antibiotics throughout the remainder of the pregnancy. Ask at prenatal visits whether she is continuing to take this type of prophylactic medicine. When women have pain and symptoms of urinary frequency, they take medication well. When they no longer have any clinical evidence that they are sick, their compliance rate, like any other adult's, begins to fall dramatically. The woman may need to post a chart on her refrigerator door or in her bathroom to remind herself to take the medication. Leaving the medicine on a counter to remind herself to take it is not a good habit to develop because soon she will have a new baby in the house; encourage her to keep medicine out of sight and reach to get into the habit of "childproofing" at this early stage.

The woman who develops pyelonephritis may be hospitalized for 24 to 48 hours, then placed on home care and treated with intravenous antibiotics. After this acute episode, she may be maintained on a drug such as oral nitrofurantoin (Macrodantin) for the remainder of the pregnancy. Acidifying urine by the use of ascorbic acid (vitamin C), which is often recommended in nonpregnant women, is not recommended during pregnancy because the newborn can develop scurvy in the immediate neonatal period from withdrawal.

After birth, the woman who developed more than one UTI may have an intravenous pyelogram scheduled to help detect any urinary tract abnormality that might be present, such as vesicoureteral reflux, to help prevent future infections.

The Woman With Chronic Renal Disease

In the past, children with chronic renal disease did not reach childbearing age or were advised not to have children because of their high risk during pregnancy. Today, women with chronic renal disease are having children because pregnancy does not appear to cause progressive deterioration of kidney lesions. With conscientious prenatal care, women who have had renal transplants can expect to have healthy pregnancies and healthy children (Willis et al., 2000).

Pregnancy increases the workload of the kidneys because they must excrete waste products not only for the woman but also for the fetus for 40 weeks. Many women with renal disease take a corticosteroid (prednisone) at a maintenance level. This drug therapy typically is continued throughout the pregnancy. Although reports of animal studies have shown an increased incidence of cleft palate from corticosteroid use during pregnancy, this does not appear to happen in humans. However, the infant may be hyperglycemic at birth because of the suppression of insulin activity by corticosteroids. Women may develop severe anemia because their diseased kidneys do not produce erythropoietin. Fortunately, synthetic erythropoietin is now available and is safe to take during pregnancy (Karch, 2001).

Because the glomerular filtration rate normally increases during pregnancy, the woman is able to clear waste products from her body for both herself and the fetus with such efficiency that her serum creatinine level is actually slightly below normal during pregnancy. The normal serum creatinine level is 0.7 mg per 100 mL; during pregnancy, it falls to about 0.5 mg per 100 mL. Women with kidney disease who normally have a serum creatinine level of more than 2.0 mg/dL may be advised not to undertake a pregnancy lest the increased strain on already damaged kidneys lead to kidney failure.

However, it is difficult to interpret kidney function during pregnancy based on nonpregnant values (see Assessing the Pregnant Woman With Renal Disease). Trace amounts of glucose and protein in the urine are common during pregnancy because of increased glomerular permeability. If the woman is told about this possibility, she will understand that it is an expected change of pregnancy, not a forecast of changing kidney function. **Proteinuria** must be compared to her individualized prepregnancy level to be meaningful. Many women with renal disease have elevated blood pressure. To be meaningful, their blood pressure levels during pregnancy must therefore also be compared with prepregnancy levels as well as to a normal level.

ASSESSING the Pregnant Woman With Renal Disease

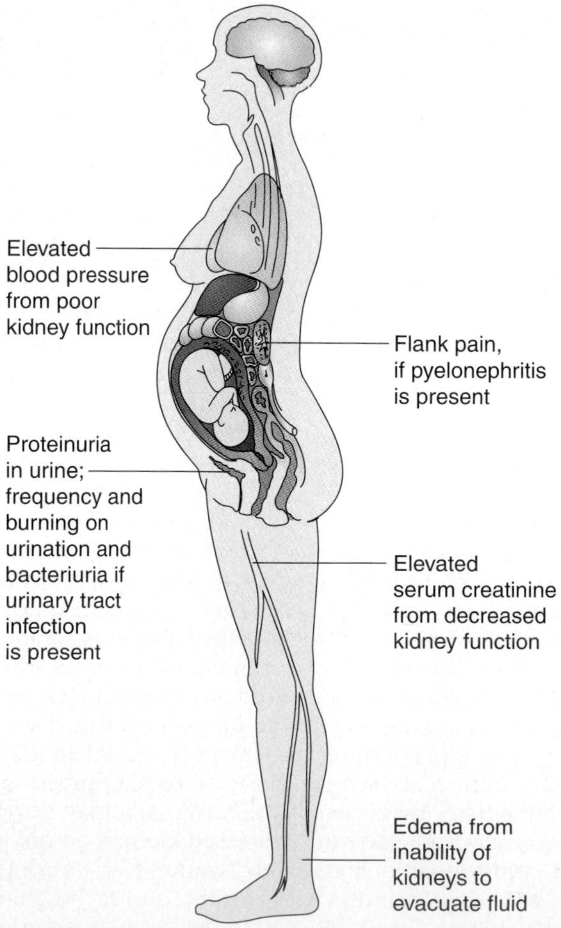

Although successful pregnancy in women with kidney transplants is to be expected, women should be considered individually to determine whether they will be able to carry a pregnancy to term before a pregnancy is initiated. Criteria to be evaluated include:

- The woman's general health and the time since the transplant (preferably more than 2 years)
- The woman's serum creatinine level
- The presence of proteinuria or hypertension or signs of graft rejection
- Medication taken to reduce graft rejection

It is helpful if the drugs the woman is taking are limited to prednisone and azathioprine (an antimetabolite [Imuran], but with no reports of fetal compromise from its use). Women with severe renal disease may require dialysis to aid kidney function during pregnancy. This is associated with a risk of preterm labor, perhaps because progesterone is removed with the dialysis. To prevent this complication, progesterone may be administered intramuscularly before dialysis. If hemodialysis is used, it should be scheduled frequently and for short durations to avoid acute fluid shifts. The heparin administered in connection with hemodialysis is safe during pregnancy because it does not cross the placenta. Even in light of the expanding uterine size, peritoneal dialysis is actually preferred because it normally causes less drastic fluid shifts. This can be accomplished on an ambulatory basis (continuous ambulatory peritoneal dialysis) throughout pregnancy.

Women with renal disease need a great deal of support during pregnancy. They are aware that kidneys are vital for life and that the stress of pregnancy on damaged kidneys may cause them to fail. They are aware that they are risking not only the life of the child growing inside them but also their own lives. They may need extra support and information to know how the fetus is doing. They may need extra time with their infant at birth for bonding because they may have been too concerned during pregnancy to begin this process.

RESPIRATORY DISORDERS AND PREGNANCY

Respiratory diseases range from the mild, such as the common cold, to the severe, such as active tuberculosis. Chronic respiratory conditions may worsen in pregnancy because the rising uterus compresses the diaphragm, reducing the size of the thoracic cavity and available lung space just when increased lung function is needed to provide adequate oxygen exchange for the fetus and mother. Any respiratory disorder can pose serious hazards to the fetus if allowed to progress to the point where the mother's oxygen–carbon dioxide exchange is altered.

NURSING DIAGNOSES AND RELATED INTERVENTIONS

Nursing Diagnosis: Risk for ineffective breathing pattern related to respiratory disorder during pregnancy.

Outcome Identification: Client will maintain an adequate, if altered, breathing pattern during pregnancy.

Outcome Evaluation: Respiratory rate is 16 to 20 per minute, PO_2 is above 80 mm Hg, PCO_2 is below 40 mm Hg, and fetal heart rate is 120 to 160 bpm with good variability.

The Woman With Acute Nasopharyngitis

Acute nasopharyngitis (common cold) tends to be more severe during pregnancy than at other times because during pregnancy, estrogen stimulation normally causes some degree of nasal congestion. With even a minor cold, therefore, the woman finds it difficult to breathe. Women should be cautioned that unless they have a fever with the cold, taking acetaminophen (Tylenol) is unnecessary. Aspirin should be avoided during pregnancy because of possible interference with blood clotting in both mother and fetus and the possibility of prolonged pregnancy at term. Because common colds are invariably caused by a virus, antibiotic therapy is unnecessary except to prevent a secondary infection. Although most simple cough syrups contain no ingredients that would make them unsafe for use during pregnancy, women should check with their health care provider before taking any over-the-counter medication for a cold (see Focus on Family Empowerment).

The Woman With Influenza

Influenza is caused by a virus, identified as type A, B, or C. The disease spreads in epidemic form and is accompanied by high fever, extreme prostration, aching pains in the back and extremities, and generally a sore, raw throat. Influenza infection has not been clearly correlated with congenital anomalies in children, although it has been correlated with preterm labor and spontaneous miscarriage. Treatment includes an antipyretic such as acetaminophen (Tylenol) to control fever and oseltamivir (TamiFlu), an antiviral drug. Because the influenza vaccines are made from killed virus, women may be immunized safely against influenza during pregnancy (Ie et al., 2002).

The Woman With Pneumonia

Pneumonia is the bacterial or viral invasion of lung tissue. After the invasion, an acute inflammatory response occurs with exudate of red blood cells, fibrin, and polymorphonuclear leukocytes into the alveoli. This process confines the bacteria or virus within segments of the lobes of the lungs. Pneumonia is a serious complication of pregnancy because the fluid that collects in the alveolar spaces limits oxygen–carbon dioxide exchange in the lungs. If the collection of fluid is extreme, it can limit the oxygen available to the fetus. Therapy usually involves the use of an appropriate antibiotic and perhaps oxygen administration. With severe disease, ventilation support may be necessary. There is a tendency for women with pneumonia late in pregnancy to begin preterm labor (Cunningham et al., 2001). During labor, oxygen should be administered so the fetus has adequate oxygen resources during contractions.

The Woman With Asthma

Asthma is a disorder marked by reversible airflow obstruction, airway hyperreactivity, and airway inflammation. An attack is often triggered by an irritant such as an inhaled allergen. It complicates about 1% of pregnancies. With inhalation of the allergen, there is an immediate release of bioactive mediators such as histamine and leukotrienes from an IgE immunoglobulin interaction. This results in constriction of the bronchial smooth muscle, marked mucosal inflammation and swelling, and the production of thick bronchial secretions. These three processes cause a marked reduction in the size of the lumen of air passages. The woman has difficulty with air exchange; on exhalation, she makes a high-pitched whistling sound (bronchial wheezing) from air being pushed past the bronchial narrowing. Asthma has the potential of reducing the oxygen supply to the fetus if a major attack should occur during pregnancy. Although many women find that their asthma

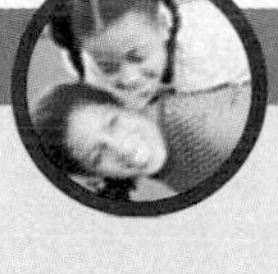

FOCUS ON FAMILY EMPOWERMENT
Relieving Cold Symptoms During Pregnancy

Q. I'm 3 months pregnant and I feel as if I'm beginning to get a cold. What should I do?

A. Use the following guidelines to help combat cold symptoms during pregnancy:

- Be sure to get extra rest and sleep and eat a light diet high in vitamin C (orange juice and fruit) to help boost the immune system.
- If you experience any aches and pains, take acetaminophen (Tylenol) every 4 hours.
- Use a room humidifier, especially at night, to moisten nasal secretions and help mucus drain.
- Use only over-the-counter cough drops or syrups that contain natural ingredients such as honey and lemon to help reduce coughing. Check with your health care provider regarding other types of over-the-counter cough drops or syrups.
- Apply a medicated vapor rub to your chest if you prefer to help relieve nasal congestion.
- Use cool or warm compresses to relieve sinus headaches. Check with your health care provider regarding the use of over-the-counter decongestants.

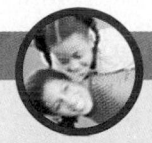

is improved during pregnancy due to the high circulating levels of corticosteroids that are present during pregnancy, women with asthma have a higher rate of preterm birth and intrauterine growth restriction than other women do. A woman should check with her physician or nurse-midwife about the safety of the medications she routinely takes for this disorder before pregnancy to be certain it will be safe to continue use during pregnancy and breast-feeding.

Beta-adrenergic agonists such as terbutaline and albuterol are the drugs of choice and the ones taken by most women prenatally for asthma. Beta-adrenergic agonists have the potential to reduce labor contractions and thus are tapered close to term if possible (Karch, 2001).

If beta-adrenergic agonists become ineffective, an inhaled glucocorticoid such as beclomethasone (Beclovent, Vancenase) or fluticasone (Flovent), an oral corticosteroid such as prednisone, or a mast cell stabilizer such as cromolyn sodium (Intal) may be added to the regimen (Wenstrom and Malee, 2000). Many adolescents with asthma are prescribed antileukotriene receptor antagonists such as montelukast sodium (Singulair) or zafirlukast (Accolate). These are oral medications (pregnancy category B) and may be continued during pregnancy (Nelson-Piercy, 2001). Women who have been taking a corticosteroid during pregnancy may need parenteral administration of hydrocortisone during labor because of the added stress during this time.

WHAT IF? Corticosteroids should never be discontinued abruptly because they are necessary to help the body manage stress, and after use the adrenal glands may need time to readjust to cortisone production. What if a woman with asthma told you she suddenly discontinued the daily prednisone she has been taking for 5 years? What would you recommend she do?

The Woman With Tuberculosis

Tuberculosis is a disease that should have been eradicated in view of the effective treatment available. However, in highly populated areas, the incidence has actually increased and in some areas is at epidemic proportions. Worldwide, it is still one of the leading causes of death (Llewelyn et al., 2000).

With tuberculosis, lung tissue is invaded by *Mycobacterium tuberculosis,* an acid-fast bacillus. Macrophages and T lymphocytes surround the bacillus, but rather than actually killing it, they merely surround and confine it. Fibrosis, calcification, and a final ring of collagenous scar tissue develop, effectively sealing off the organisms from the body and any further invasion or spread. Antibodies developed will thereafter cause a positive response when tested such as with the Mantoux (purified protein derivative [PPD]) test.

Assessment

In high-risk areas, women should undergo skin testing (a PPD test) at their first prenatal visit. A follow-up chest x-ray can be done for women who show positive reactions. Women need to be cautioned that a positive reaction does not necessarily mean that they have the disease; it can mean that they have at some time been exposed to tuberculosis and so have antibodies in their system. A chest x-ray to confirm the diagnosis can be done safely in pregnancy if the abdomen is shielded. Symptoms of tuberculosis include:

- Chronic cough
- Weight loss
- Hemoptysis
- Night sweats
- Low-grade fever
- Chronic fatigue

Therapeutic Management

Women with active tuberculosis need treatment during pregnancy. Isoniazid (INH) and ethambutol hydrochloride (Myambutol), the drugs of choice for tuberculosis, may be given without apparent teratogenic effects. INH may result in a peripheral neuritis if the woman does not take supplemental pyridoxine (vitamin B) as well. Ethambutol may cause optic nerve involvement (optic atrophy and loss of green color recognition) in the mother. To detect this, test the woman monthly using a Snellen (eye test) chart. If symptoms develop, expect to discontinue the drug.

The woman who has active tuberculosis must be especially careful to maintain an adequate level of calcium during pregnancy to ensure that tuberculosis pockets form or are not broken down. With tuberculosis, a woman is usually advised to wait 1 to 2 years after the infection becomes inactive before attempting to conceive. This is because recent inactive tuberculosis can become active during pregnancy. Pressure on the diaphragm from below changes the shape of the lung, and an incompletely sealed pocket may be broken in this process. Pushing during labor may increase intrapulmonary pressure and cause the same phenomenon. Recent inactive tuberculosis may also become active during the postpartal period as the lung suddenly returns to its more vertical prepregnant position, allowing calcium deposits to break open.

Although tuberculosis can be spread by the placenta to the fetus, it usually is spread to the infant after birth. A woman with a recent history of tuberculosis should have at least three negative sputum cultures before she holds or cares for her infant. If these are negative, there is no need to isolate the infant from the mother; she can even breast-feed. If active tuberculosis is in the home, the infant is generally discharged on prophylactic INH to prevent infection, with follow-up skin testing at 3-month intervals. If the infant is to be placed on INH, a mother also taking INH should not breast-feed. Otherwise, the combined dosage the infant receives (INH is found in breast milk) might be toxic to the infant.

The Woman With Cystic Fibrosis

Cystic fibrosis is a recessively inherited disease in which there is generalized dysfunction of the exocrine glands. This dysfunction leads to mucous secretions, particularly in the pancreas and lungs, becoming so viscid or thick that normal lung and pancreatic function is compromised.

DNA markers have been used to localize a gene mutation for this disease to chromosome 7. The presence of cystic fibrosis may be identified by chorionic villi sampling or amniocentesis and identification of the gene marker (a technique called restriction fragment length polymorphism) during pregnancy. Many men with cystic fibrosis are sterile because the semen is so thick that sperm cannot be mobile. Fertility may be lessened in women with the disorder because sperm cannot migrate through the viscid cervical mucus. Thus, conception may be a concern. Reproductive technologies such as artificial insemination or in vitro fertilization may be necessary for conception so sperm are not obstructed by cervical mucus or fallopian tubal transport is not impaired.

Persons with the disease typically develop symptoms of chronic respiratory infection and overinflation of their lungs from the thickened mucus as well as an inability to digest fat and protein because the pancreas cannot release amylase. Because of poor pulmonary function that results in inadequate oxygen supply to the fetus, there is an increased risk for preterm labor and perinatal death during pregnancy (Cunningham et al., 2001).

Therapy for the illness consists of pancrelipase (Pancrease) to supplement pancreatic enzymes and a bronchodilator or antibiotic to reduce pulmonary symptoms. Although pancrelipase is a pregnancy risk category C drug (teratogenic effects are unknown), it does not appear to affect the fetus. In addition to pharmacologic measures, women with cystic fibrosis must perform chest physiotherapy daily to reduce a buildup of lung secretions.

Modifications for Pregnancy

Because pancrelipase may interfere with iron absorption, the woman is at greater risk for iron-deficiency anemia during pregnancy than other women are. Therefore, an iron supplement usually is prescribed. Persons with cystic fibrosis have a higher-than-usual incidence of developing diabetes mellitus due to pancreas involvement; therefore, women need close monitoring of serum glucose levels at prenatal visits to detect the development of gestational diabetes.

Chest physiotherapy becomes difficult late in pregnancy because the process is exhausting. Moving to new positions is difficult, and lying prone, a position used frequently in postural drainage, is contraindicated in late pregnancy. The woman may need to plan more frequent and shorter sessions in modified positions (other than prone) to prevent exhaustion (Fig. 14-2). Fetal health will be monitored by ultrasound and nonstress tests to identify intrauterine growth restriction.

Modifications for the Postpartal Period

Help the woman plan how to conserve her energy for infant care in the immediate postpartal period so she does not become exhausted and can enjoy her newborn. Breastfeeding is usually not recommended because the breast milk of women with cystic fibrosis may contain more fatty acid than usual, and it is tiring for the mother.

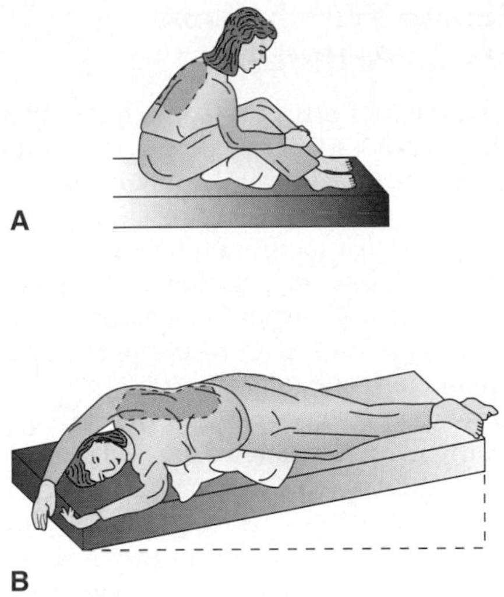

FIGURE 14.2 Modified positions for chest physiotherapy during pregnancy: (A) chest physiotherapy for the upper lobes; (B) chest physiotherapy for the lower lobes.

✔ CHECKPOINT QUESTIONS

7. Why are women prone to develop urinary tract infections during pregnancy?
8. Should women who have had tuberculosis in the past ingest more or less milk or other sources of calcium during pregnancy?
9. Should women with cystic fibrosis continue to take a pancreatic enzyme during pregnancy?

RHEUMATIC DISORDERS AND PREGNANCY

A number of rheumatic disorders occur in young adult women and thus are seen during pregnancy. Because most of these illnesses result in discomfort, potential or actual pain related to disease pathology is the primary nursing diagnosis used. Women may not achieve a pain-free outcome because of the nature of these illnesses, but outcomes should center on the woman stating that her pain level is tolerable.

NURSING DIAGNOSES AND RELATED INTERVENTIONS

Nursing Diagnosis: Pain related to rheumatic disorder during pregnancy

Outcome Identification: Client will report a decrease in pain to a tolerable level during pregnancy.

Outcome Evaluation: Client states that she is moderately comfortable and is able to maintain her usual level of daily activity.

The Woman With Juvenile Rheumatoid Arthritis

Juvenile rheumatoid arthritis (sometimes referred to as chronic rheumatoid arthritis), a disease of connective tissue with joint inflammation and contracture, is most likely the result of an autoimmune response. The disease pathology involves synovial membrane destruction. Inflammation with effusion, swelling, erythema, and painful motion of the joints occurs. Over time, formation of granulation tissue can fill the joint space, resulting in permanent disfigurement and loss of joint motion.

Symptoms of the disease may improve during pregnancy because of the naturally increased circulating level of corticosteroids in the maternal bloodstream during pregnancy (Cunningham et al., 2001). During the postpartal period, when the woman's corticosteroid levels fall to prepregnancy levels again, arthritis symptoms will probably recur.

Women with juvenile rheumatoid arthritis frequently take corticosteroids and nonsteroidal antiinflammatory drugs (NSAIDs) to prevent joint pain and loss of mobility. Some women may be taking oral aspirin therapy. Although they should continue to take these medications during pregnancy to prevent joint damage, large amounts of salicylates may lead to prolonged pregnancy (salicylate interferes with prostaglandin synthesis, so labor contractions are not initiated). The infant may have a bleeding defect due to the high salicylate level and may also experience premature closure of the ductus arteriosus due to the drug's effects. For this reason, the woman is asked to decrease her intake of salicylates approximately 2 weeks before term. A few women may be taking low-dose methotrexate, a carcinogen (pregnancy risk category X). They should consult their health care practitioner before becoming pregnant about the advisability of discontinuing this drug during pregnancy.

In the postpartal period, the determination as to the safety of breast-feeding must be individualized based on the medication that each woman is taking. Those taking an NSAID such as ibuprofen can breast-feed. Those taking large doses of aspirin may be advised not to breastfeed because of the danger of increased bleeding in the infant.

The Woman With Systemic Lupus Erythematosus

Systemic lupus erythematosus (SLE) is a multisystem chronic disease of connective tissue that can occur in women of childbearing age: its highest incidence is in women ages 20 to 40 years (Kuper & Failla, 2000). Widespread degeneration of connective tissue (especially of the heart, kidneys, blood vessels, spleen, skin, and retroperitoneal tissue) occurs with onset of the illness. The most marked skin change is a characteristic erythematous butterfly-shaped rash on the face. In the kidneys, fibrin deposits develop, plugging and blocking the glomeruli and leading to necrosis and scarring. The thickening of collagen tissue in the blood vessels causes vessel obstruction. This could be life-threatening to the woman if blood flow to vital organs becomes compromised and life-threatening to the fetus if blood flow to the placenta is obstructed. Many women with SLE have antiphospholipid antibodies, which increase the tendency for thrombi to form. The woman may be taking a corticosteroid, NSAIDs, heparin and salicylates to reduce disease symptoms (Empson et al., 2002).

The naturally increased circulation of corticosteroids during pregnancy may lessen symptoms in some women. In others, the chief complication of the disorder—acute nephritis with glomerular destruction—may occur for the first time during pregnancy.

With associated nephritis, the woman's blood pressure will rise. She will develop hematuria and decreased urine output. Proteinuria and edema may begin. It is difficult to differentiate these symptoms from the symptoms of pregnancy-induced hypertension, except that with pregnancy-induced hypertension there is no hematuria. Frequent monitoring of serum creatinine levels is necessary to assess kidney function. If this value is over 1.5 mg/dL and proteinuria and a decreased creatinine clearance value are also present, the fetus is seriously threatened. Dialysis or plasmapheresis may be necessary.

Women are asked to decrease salicylate use close to birth to reduce the possibility of bleeding in the newborn. Intravenous hydrocortisone may be administered during labor to help the woman adjust to the stress at this time. During the postpartal period, there may be an acute exacerbation of symptoms in the woman as corticosteroid levels again fall to normal. Infants of women with SLE tend to be small for gestational age due to the decreased blood flow to the placenta. There is a greater than usual incidence of spontaneous miscarriage and preterm birth. Infants may be born with a lupus-like rash, anemia, and thrombocytopenia (low platelet count). Newborn symptoms last about 6 months and then fade. Congenital heart block, for which a pacemaker may be necessary, can occur in the newborn. Screening for the exact type of autoantibodies present may be helpful in predicting which newborns are susceptible to this.

GASTROINTESTINAL DISORDERS AND PREGNANCY

Although minor gastrointestinal discomfort (e.g., nausea, heartburn, constipation) is common during pregnancy, acute abdominal pain and protracted vomiting are causes for concern. Pregnancy complications such as abruptio placentae or ectopic pregnancy often manifest with acute abdominal pain, so differentiating the cause of abdominal pain is important. In some instances, abdominal pain is associated with a condition completely unrelated to the pregnancy such as ulcerative colitis, hepatitis, hiatal hernia, or cholecystitis. These conditions may be known to the woman before she becomes pregnant, or they may develop or be discovered during her pregnancy. Women who have colostomies complete pregnancy without difficulty. Even a previous liver transplant is not a contraindication to pregnancy.

NURSING DIAGNOSES AND RELATED INTERVENTIONS

Nursing Diagnosis: Imbalanced nutrition, less than body requirements related to a gastrointestinal disorder during pregnancy

Outcome Identification: Client will ingest adequate nutrition during pregnancy.

Outcome Evaluation: Client's weight gain is 25 to 30 lb for pregnancy; hemoglobin is above 11 mg/dL; specific gravity of urine is below 1.030.

The Woman With Appendicitis

Appendicitis is inflammation of the appendix. Its incidence is high in young adults, occurring as frequently as approximately 1 in 1,500 to 2,000 pregnancies (Cunningham et al., 2001).

Assessment

History taking is important. Appendicitis usually begins with a few hours of nausea, and then an hour or two of generalized abdominal discomfort follows. The woman may have vomiting during this time. Then comes the typical sharp, peristaltic, lower right quadrant pain of acute appendicitis.

The pain associated with appendicitis is different from the pain that occurs suddenly from an overstretched round ligament during pregnancy. Pain from an overstretched ligament may cause sharp lower quadrant pain if the woman stands up suddenly, but the pain is only transient. Appendicitis pain is also different from that of ectopic pregnancy. With ectopic pregnancy, the woman may have morning sickness but not the same extended nausea and vomiting. The pain of ectopic pregnancy may be either diffuse or sharp. In the nonpregnant woman, the sharp localized pain of appendicitis appears at McBurney's point (a point halfway between the umbilicus and the iliac crest on the lower right abdomen). In the pregnant woman, the appendix is often displaced so far up in the abdomen that the localized pain may resemble the pain of gallbladder disease (Fig. 14-3). A complete blood count will reveal leukocytosis. However, because pregnant women have an elevated white blood cell count, this increased finding is not as helpful in pregnancy as it might be otherwise. Her temperature may be elevated. There are typically ketones in the urine. A sonogram may reveal the inflamed appendix.

Advise the woman not to take food, liquid, or laxatives while she is waiting to be evaluated for possible appendicitis, because increasing peristalsis tends to cause an inflamed appendix to rupture.

Therapeutic Management

If the woman is near term (past 36 weeks) and the fetus is believed to be mature, a cesarean birth may be performed to deliver the baby and then remove the inflamed appendix. If appendicitis occurs early in pregnancy, the inflamed appendix is removed by laparoscopy. As long as the anesthesiologist is aware that the woman is pregnant and carefully controls oxygen levels during anesthesia administration, the outcome of the pregnancy will be good.

If the appendix ruptures before surgery, the risk to both mother and fetus increases dramatically. This is because with rupture, infected material is free in the peritoneum and can spread by the fallopian tubes to the fetus. Generalized peritonitis is such an overwhelming infection that it

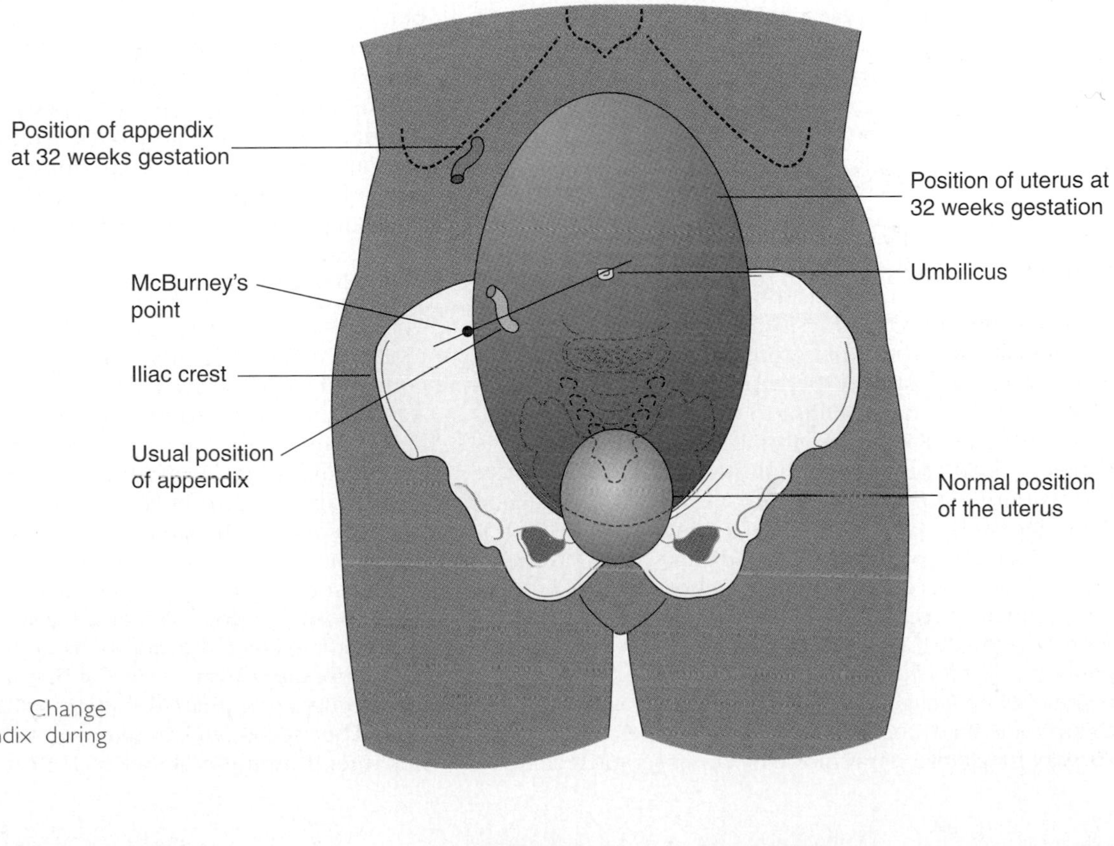

FIGURE 14.3 Change in position of appendix during pregnancy.

is difficult for the woman's body to combat it effectively and also maintain the pregnancy. In addition, peritoneal adhesions may develop after an appendix ruptures, resulting in infertility due to changes in the placement of fallopian tubes.

The Woman With Gastroesophageal Reflux Disease or Hiatal Hernia

Gastroesophageal reflux disease (GERD) refers to the reflux of acid stomach secretions into the esophagus. Hiatal hernia is a condition in which a portion of the stomach extends and protrudes up through the diaphragm into the chest cavity, trapping stomach acid and causing it to reflux into the esophagus. Although these conditions can be present constantly, symptoms most often occur only sporadically after increased peristaltic action. Both conditions may generate symptoms for the first time during pregnancy as the uterus pushes the stomach up against the esophagus and increases the reflux of acid or the hernia. Symptoms include:

- Heartburn, which is particularly extreme when lying supine after a full meal
- Gastric regurgitation
- Dysphagia (difficulty swallowing)
- Possible weight loss due to the inability to eat
- Hematemesis (vomiting of blood) if esophageal irritation occurs from the reflux of hydrochloric acid

During pregnancy, these conditions are usually diagnosed by direct endoscopy or ultrasound to avoid exposing the woman to barium x-rays. Antacids may be prescribed to help relieve pain. A histamine receptor antagonist, such as ranitidine, may be prescribed to inhibit gastric acid production and thus help minimize pain. Advise the woman to sleep with her head elevated to help confine stomach secretions. After pregnancy, as the uterine pressure is decreased, the symptoms generally become less noticeable or disappear.

The Woman With Cholecystitis and Cholelithiasis

Cholecystitis (gallbladder inflammation) and cholelithiasis (gallstone formation) are most frequently associated with age older than 40 years, obesity, multiparity, and ingestion of a high-fat diet. Symptoms (constant aching and pressure in the right epigastrium, perhaps accompanied by jaundice), therefore, are more apt to occur in the older pregnant woman. Gallstones are formed from cholesterol. It is debated whether the hypercholesterolemia that naturally occurs during pregnancy leads to an increased incidence of cholecystitis or cholelithiasis (Cunningham et al., 2001).

Medical therapy for both conditions is to lower fat intake. A woman can eat a low-fat but not a fat-free diet during pregnancy because of the importance of linoleic acid for fetal growth. Cholecystitis can be diagnosed by sonogram. If an acute episode occurs during pregnancy, it can generally be managed by administering intravenous fluids to provide fluid and nutrients and analgesics for pain. Surgery for gallbladder removal by laparoscopic technique may be done during pregnancy if the woman's symptoms cannot be controlled by conservative management.

The Woman With Hepatitis

Hepatitis is a liver disease that may occur from invasion of the A, B, C, D, or E virus. Hepatitis A is spread mainly by fecal–oral contact (children in day-care settings have a high incidence) or by ingestion of fecally contaminated water or shellfish after an incubation period of 2 to 6 weeks. Pregnant women exposed to hepatitis A may be given prophylactic gamma globulin to try to prevent the disease after exposure. This form follows a rather benign course and is not known to be transmitted to the fetus.

Hepatitis B and C are spread by exposure to contaminated blood or blood products. These two types also can be spread by contact with contaminated semen or vaginal secretions and thus are considered STDs. Hepatitis D and E are apparently spread by the same methods as hepatitis B but are rarely seen in pregnant women.

Hepatitis B has an incubation period of 6 weeks to 6 months. It occurs in both an acute and chronic form, leading to liver cell necrosis with scarring and inability to convert indirect to direct bilirubin or excrete direct bilirubin. Women exposed to the virus receive immune globulin for prophylaxis; hepatitis B vaccine may be administered to those who are at high risk, such as women who handle blood products. Hepatitis C may not demonstrate symptoms for 12 months.

Assessment

With all forms of hepatitis, the woman may notice symptoms of nausea and vomiting. Her liver area may feel tender to palpation. Urine will be dark yellow from excretion of bilirubin; stools will be light-colored from lack of bilirubin. Jaundice occurs as a late symptom. On physical examination, hepatomegaly (enlargement of the liver) is noted. The bilirubin level is elevated. Levels of liver enzymes such as transaminase are increased. Specific antibodies against the virus can be detected in the blood serum, so women are routinely screened for this during pregnancy. If a liver biopsy is necessary for diagnosis, this can be performed safely during pregnancy (Graham, 2001).

Therapeutic Management

The woman is usually prescribed bed rest and encouraged to eat a high-calorie diet because her liver has difficulty converting stored glycogen into glucose in its diseased state. Follow standard precautions to avoid contact with body fluids.

Hepatitis during pregnancy may lead to spontaneous miscarriage or preterm labor. The later in pregnancy the mother contracts hepatitis B infection, the greater the risk the infant will be affected or develop hepatitis B. This is a serious consequence in newborns because a proportion of HB Ag-positive infants will develop liver cirrhosis or carcinoma later in life. If the mother has anti-HB antibodies present (antibodies toward a virus subgroup), the incidence of this occurring appears to be less. After birth, the infant should be washed well to remove any maternal blood, and hepatitis B immune globulin (HBIG) and immunization against hepatitis B should be administered (see Chap. 23 for additional newborn care). The infant needs to be observed carefully for symptoms of infection during the first few months of life. The mother is advised not to breastfeed because HB Ag antigens can be recovered from breast milk.

The Woman With Inflammatory Bowel Disease

Crohn's disease (inflammation of the terminal ileus) and ulcerative colitis (inflammation of the distal colon) occur most often in young adults between ages 12 and 30 years (childbearing years). The cause of these diseases is unknown, but an autoimmune process is thought to be responsible. In both diseases, the bowel develops shallow ulcers. The woman experiences chronic diarrhea, weight loss, occult blood in stool, and nausea and vomiting. If extreme, obstruction and fistula formation with peritonitis can occur. With Crohn's disease, malabsorption, particularly of vitamin B (a substance whose absorption occurs almost entirely in the ileum), occurs.

These diseases obviously have the potential for interfering with fetal growth if extreme malabsorption occurs. Therapy for the disorders is total rest for the gastrointestinal tract by administration of total parenteral nutrition. Although it is possible to sustain a pregnancy by this route, it is obviously not a desirable nutrition pattern. Sulfasalazine (Azulfidine), an anti-inflammatory and a mainstay of therapy, may be continued during pregnancy without fetal injury (Karch, 2001). Close to birth, the dosage of sulfasalazine is reduced because it may interfere with bilirubin binding sites and cause neonatal jaundice.

NEUROLOGIC DISORDERS AND PREGNANCY

Neurologic illness is not a common problem affecting women of childbearing age. However, any neurologic disease with symptoms of seizures must be carefully managed during pregnancy because the anoxia caused by severe seizures could deprive the fetus of oxygen, with serious outcomes.

NURSING DIAGNOSES AND RELATED INTERVENTIONS

Nursing Diagnosis: Risk for injury (maternal) related to recurrent seizures

Outcome Identification: Client will remain free of any injury related to occurrence of a seizure.

Outcome Evaluation: Client states she is injury-free, with no signs and symptoms of injury; no automobile or other accidents are documented.

The Woman With a Seizure Disorder

Recurrent seizures have a number of causes, such as head trauma or meningitis. The causes of most instances of recurrent seizures, however, are unknown (idiopathic).

Recurrent seizures were at one time so incapacitating that women who experienced them were generally advised not to have children. Today, however, no contraindication to pregnancy exists for women with seizures (Wenstrom and Malee, 2000).

Therapeutic Management

In the early months of pregnancy, women with recurrent seizures need to be cautioned to continue taking their seizure control medications despite the nausea or vomiting of pregnancy. Be certain they understand that the rule "Do not take medication during pregnancy" does not apply to their seizure control medications. Since some anticonvulsant medications are mildly teratogenic, the woman is in the difficult position of having to take drugs to safeguard her own health, but by taking them she may not be safeguarding the health of the fetus. The risk of adverse maternal or fetal outcome from seizures during pregnancy, however, is greater than the risk of teratogenicity from taking anticonvulsant drugs (Karch, 2001).

All women should have evaluations of serum drug levels before pregnancy or early in pregnancy. As the blood volume increases with pregnancy, some women may need their dosage increased. Common drugs prescribed for the control of seizures and their potential effects on the fetus include the following:

- Phenytoin sodium (Dilantin), a pregnancy risk category D drug, can result in a Dilantin syndrome (cognitive impairment and a peculiar facial proportion not unlike that of the fetal alcohol syndrome). This may occur because of competition for folic acid binding sites. Some infants may have an increased danger of neural tube disorders as a result of this folic acid displacement. A sonogram can confirm that a neural tube defect has not occurred.
- Trimethadione (Tridione) is associated with cognitive challenges and physical deformities; it is pregnancy risk category D.
- Valproic acid (sodium valproate and divalproex sodium) is pregnancy risk category D or of proven risk.
- Carbamazepine (Tegretol) is a pregnancy risk category C drug.
- Ethosuximide (Zarontin), a drug often used to control absence seizures, is a pregnancy risk category C drug.

Women who have been taking phenytoin (Dilantin) may have chronic hypertension. For these women, a baseline blood pressure should be established early in pregnancy so that later changes can be interpreted in terms of this already elevated pressure.

Infants are also prone to hemorrhagic disease of the newborn because of decreased vitamin K coagulation factors at birth. To counteract this, women may be prescribed vitamin K during labor or the last 4 weeks of gestation.

NURSING DIAGNOSES AND RELATED INTERVENTIONS

Nursing Diagnosis: Risk for ineffective tissue (placental) perfusion related to hypoxia resulting from maternal seizure

Outcome Identification: Client will take prescribed anticonvulsant therapy during pregnancy and will be prepared for emergency management of seizures. Adequate fetal oxygenation will be maintained throughout pregnancy.

Outcome Evaluation: Client informs health care personnel about history of seizures; states importance of immediate care and oxygen therapy should she begin a seizure. Apgar score at birth is 7 to 10, with no apparent birth anomalies.

Absence seizures (often just a rapid fluttering of the eyelids or a moment's staring into space) will have no effect on the woman or fetus. Tonic-clonic seizures (sustained, full-body involvement) could conceivably affect the fetus because spasm of the chest muscles may lead to hypoxia. If a seizure should occur, the woman must be evaluated to ascertain that the cause of the seizure was from the underlying disease, not from beginning hypertension of pregnancy. Nonpregnant women experiencing tonic-clonic seizures do not need oxygen administered to them during a seizure. In pregnancy, administering oxygen by mask is good prophylaxis to ensure adequate fetal oxygenation.

Urge the woman to alert hospital personnel at the time of labor that she has recurrent seizures and to report the type of medication she is taking. She should continue to take the medication during labor. If a general anesthetic should be necessary, the anesthesiologist needs to know about her condition before administering anesthesia; otherwise, during the excitement phase of anesthesia induction, a seizure may occur.

Nursing Diagnosis: Risk for impaired parenting related to maternal feelings of low self-esteem and fear that her child will inherit seizure disorder

Outcome Identification: Client will voice the low statistical probability that her child will inherit her disorder and will demonstrate confidence in her ability to care for the infant by discharge.

Outcome Evaluation: Client accurately states the nature of her disorder (acquired or idiopathic) and the statistical chances of her child inheriting the disorder. After child is born, client identifies sudden jerking movements in her newborn (such as Moro reflex) as healthy newborn characteristics.

A woman who has recurrent seizures may worry that her child will have seizures as the child grows older. If the woman's seizures are the result of an acquired disorder (i.e., infection, such as meningitis or head trauma), the woman can be assured that her child's risk for seizures is no greater than that for any other child. If the etiology of her seizures is unknown, the chance that her child also will have them is slightly higher than in the normal population. This prediction is only theoretical, however, and cannot be made without a thorough review of the onset and nature of the woman's disorder (Cunningham et al., 2001). Be certain the woman has her newborn with her for long periods so she can become acquainted with the sudden jerking motions that occur such as when a newborn is startled (Moro reflex) or quivering of the jaw with prolonged crying. Otherwise she may interpret these normal movements as seizure activity.

The Woman With Myasthenia Gravis

Myasthenia gravis is an autoimmune disorder characterized by the presence of an IgG antibody against acetylcholine receptors in striated muscle. This causes failure of the striated muscles to contract, particularly those of the oropharyngeal, facial, and extraocular groups (Cunningham et al., 2001).

Myasthenia gravis is treated by the administration of anticholinesterase drugs such as pyridostigmine (Mestinon) or neostigmine (Prostigmin) and possibly the corticosteroid prednisone. These medications may be continued during pregnancy. Plasmapheresis to remove immune complexes from the bloodstream may be prescribed to reduce symptoms further. Plasmapheresis must be carried out gradually during pregnancy to reduce the risk of fluid overload or hypotension. Because smooth muscle is not affected by the disease, labor should occur normally. Magnesium sulfate should be avoided because it can diminish the acetylcholine effect and therefore increase disease symptoms. The fetus will experience no effects from maternal drugs.

An infant born to a woman with myasthenia gravis may demonstrate disease symptoms at birth due to the transfer of antibodies. This is further discussed in Chapter 51.

The Woman With Multiple Sclerosis

Multiple sclerosis (MS) occurs predominantly in women of child-bearing age, usually between 20 and 40 years of age (Wenstrom & Malee, 2000). With MS, nerve fibers become demyelinated and therefore lose function. Women develop symptoms of fatigue, numbness, blurred vision, and loss of coordination. Women are commonly administered ACTH or a corticosteroid to strengthen nerve conduction. These can be administered safely during pregnancy. Cyclosporine (Sandimmune), azathioprine (Imuran), and cyclophosphamide (Cytoxan), drugs also frequently administered, are not safe for use during pregnancy. Interferon is untested as to pregnancy safety and as such is classified as a pregnancy category C drug. Women may continue with plasmapheresis (withdrawal and replacement of plasma), another treatment regimen during pregnancy, as long as the volume is well controlled. Although pregnancy does not affect the course of MS, women with the disorder grow increasingly fatigued as pregnancy progresses. UTIs tend to occur as a poorly defined consequence of the illness.

A painless precipitous birth may occur at term if the woman has quadriplegia. Also during labor, women may be prone to autonomic dysreflexia from the pain of labor. This leads to severe hypertension, headache, diaphoresis, and bradycardia. Administration of an epidural anesthetic may decrease the risk of this occurring.

MUSCULOSKELETAL DISORDERS AND PREGNANCY

Women of childbearing age have few common musculoskeletal disorders. One that may be seen is scoliosis.

The Woman With Scoliosis

Scoliosis (lateral curvature of the spine) occurs most often in girls between 12 and 14 years of age. If it is uncorrected at this time, the curvature progresses until it causes deformity, interfering with respiration and heart action because of chest compression. Pelvic distortion can interfere with childbirth, especially at the pelvic inlet. If the woman's spine is extremely curved, spinal or epidural anesthesia may be more difficult to administer.

Girls with scoliosis may wear a brace such as a Milwaukee brace during their adolescent years to maintain an erect posture. Although these braces are not as bulky as they once were, unless they are modified, they cannot be continued during the last half of pregnancy. Other girls have stainless-steel rods (Harrington rods) implanted on both sides of their vertebrae to strengthen and straighten the spine. Such rod implantations do not interfere with pregnancy; the woman will notice some back pain from tension on the back muscles similar to that experienced by the average pregnant woman. If the woman's pelvis is distorted, a cesarean birth may be necessary to ensure a safe birth. Vaginal birth, if permitted, requires the same management as for any woman; the woman must be closely observed for progression of labor. Plot the course of labor on a labor graph so an unusually long first stage, suggesting cephalopelvic disproportion, can be recognized. Chapter 51 discusses in detail the nursing care of adolescents with scoliosis.

✔ CHECKPOINT QUESTIONS

10. If a woman with a rheumatic disease is taking salicylates during pregnancy, why will she be asked to decrease her salicylate intake late in pregnancy?
11. What is the usual way a woman contracts hepatitis B during pregnancy?
12. Phenytoin sodium (Dilantin) is a drug commonly prescribed for seizures. What pregnancy risk category is this drug?

CARDIOVASCULAR DISORDERS AND PREGNANCY

The number of women of childbearing age who have heart disease is diminishing as more and more congenital heart anomalies (discussed in Chap. 41) are corrected in early infancy. Also, rheumatic fever is being more actively prevented and treated so that cardiac damage from this disorder is reduced. Therefore, cardiovascular disease complicates only approximately 1% of all pregnancies (Cunningham et al., 2001). Cardiovascular disease is still a problem in pregnancy, however, because improved management of women with these diseases has enabled women who might never have risked pregnancy in the past to do so now. Even women who have had heart transplants can be expected to have successful pregnancies (Meller & Goldman, 2000).

The majority of cardiovascular problems that cause difficulty with pregnancy are valvular damage caused by rheumatic fever or Kawasaki disease and congenital anomalies such as atrial septal defect or uncorrected coarctation of the aorta (Franklin et al., 2002). The age at which women are becoming pregnant is increasing, so there is a corresponding increase in the incidence of coronary artery disease and varicosities during pregnancy. In contrast, heart disease that occurs specifically with pregnancy (peripartal heart disease) rarely occurs.

A woman with cardiovascular disease needs a team approach to care during pregnancy, combining the talents of an internist, obstetrician, and nurse. Ideally, the woman should visit her obstetrician or family physician before conception so the health care team can become familiar with her state of health when she is not pregnant and establish baseline evaluations of her heart function, such as with echocardiograms. The woman should begin prenatal care as soon as she suspects she is pregnant (1 week after the first missed menstrual period) so close assessment of her general condition and circulatory system can be maintained.

Pregnancy taxes the circulatory system of every woman, even without cardiac disease, because both the blood volume and cardiac output increase approximately 30% (perhaps as much as 50%). Most of this increase occurs in the first 28 weeks of pregnancy, and then this greater blood volume continues to be maintained for the remainder of pregnancy.

Because of the increased blood flow past valves, heart murmurs are identified in many women during pregnancy. These functional (innocent) and transient murmurs disappear after the pregnancy. Heart palpitations on sudden exertion are also normal in pregnancy. Neither of these symptoms is a sign of cardiovascular disease, but merely an indication of the normal physiologic adjustment to pregnancy.

The danger of pregnancy in a woman with cardiac disease occurs mainly due to the increase in circulatory volume. The most dangerous time for the woman is in weeks 28 to 32, just after the blood volume reaches its peak. However, if heart disease is severe, symptoms can occur almost immediately. The woman's heart may become so overwhelmed by the increase in blood volume that her cardiac output falls to the point that vital organs (including the placenta) are no longer perfused adequately. When this happens, neither the oxygen nor nutritional requirements of her cells and those of the fetus are met.

The determination of whether a woman with cardiovascular disease can complete a pregnancy depends on the type and extent of her disease. As a rule, a woman with artificial but well-functioning heart valves can be expected to complete a pregnancy without difficulty as long as she has consistent prenatal and postpartal care. The occasional woman with a pacemaker implant can also expect to complete pregnancy. To predict pregnancy outcome, heart disease is divided into four categories based on the criteria established by the New York State Heart Association (Table 14-2). The woman with class I or II heart disease can expect to experience a normal pregnancy and birth. Women with class III can complete a

TABLE 14.2 Classification of Heart Disease

CLASS	DESCRIPTION
I	Uncompromised. Women have no limitation of physical activity. Ordinary physical activity causes no discomfort. They have no symptoms of cardiac insufficiency and no anginal pain.
II	Slightly compromised. Women have slight limitation of physical activity. Ordinary physical activity causes excessive fatigue, palpitation, and dyspnea or anginal pain.
III	Markedly compromised. Women have a moderate to marked limitation of physical activity. During less than ordinary activity, they experience excessive fatigue, palpitations, dyspnea, or anginal pain.
IV	Severely compromised. Women are unable to carry out any physical activity without experiencing discomfort. Even at rest they experience symptoms of cardiac insufficiency or anginal pain.

Criteria Committee of the New York State Heart Association. (1979). *Nomenclature and criteria for diagnosis of disease of the heart and blood vessels* (8th ed.). Boston: Little, Brown; with permission.

pregnancy by maintaining almost complete bed rest. Women with class IV heart disease are poor candidates for pregnancy because they are in cardiac failure even at rest and when they are not pregnant; they are usually advised to avoid pregnancy.

The Woman With Cardiac Disease

The Woman With Left-Sided Heart Failure

Left-sided heart failure occurs in conditions such as mitral stenosis, mitral insufficiency, and aortic coarctation. The left ventricle cannot move the volume of blood forward that is received by the left atrium from the pulmonary circulation. The reason for the failure is often at the level of the mitral valve. The normal physiologic tachycardia of pregnancy shortens diastole (atrial contraction) and decreases the time available for blood to flow across this valve. The inability of the mitral valve to push blood forward causes back-pressure on the pulmonary circulation, causing it to become distended; systemic blood pressure decreases in the face of lowered cardiac output, and pulmonary hypertension occurs. When pressure in the pulmonary vein reaches a point of about 25 mm Hg, fluid begins to pass from the pulmonary capillary membranes into the interstitial spaces surrounding the alveoli and then into the alveoli themselves (pulmonary edema). The normal decrease in serum albumin that occurs with pregnancy can cause pulmonary edema to form at an even lower capillary pressure than usual. Pulmonary edema interferes with oxygen–carbon dioxide exchange because the fluid coats the alveolar exchange space. If pulmonary capillaries rupture under the pressure, small amounts of blood leak into the alveoli. This is manifested by a productive cough of blood-speckled sputum. Women with pulmonary hypertension are at an extremely high risk for spontaneous miscarriage, preterm labor, and maternal death during pregnancy.

As the oxygen saturation of the blood decreases from dysfunction of the alveoli, chemoreceptors stimulate the respiratory center to increase the respiratory rate. At first this is noticeable only on exertion, then finally with rest also. Body cells receive little oxygen, and the woman experiences increased fatigue, weakness, and dizziness (specifically from lack of oxygen in the brain cells). As the systemic decrease in blood pressure registers on the pressoreceptors in the aorta, the heart rate increases and peripheral vasoconstriction occurs in an attempt to increase the systemic blood pressure. As the fall in blood pressure is registered with the renal angiotensin system, both sodium and water retention occur.

As pulmonary edema becomes severe, the woman cannot sleep in any position except with her chest and head elevated (**orthopnea**). Elevating her chest allows edema to settle to the bottom of her lungs, thus freeing space for gas exchange. She may also notice **paroxysmal nocturnal dyspnea**—suddenly waking at night short of breath. This occurs because heart action is more effective when she is at rest. With the more effective heart action, interstitial fluid is returned to the circulation. This overburdens the circulation, causing increased left-side failure and increased pulmonary edema. The end result of severe heart failure is poor placental perfusion with intrauterine growth restriction.

If mitral stenosis is present, it is so difficult for blood to leave the left atrium that a secondary problem of thrombus formation can occur. If coarctation of the aorta is causing the difficulty, both dissection of the aorta and thrombus formation can be secondary problems. The woman may be prescribed antihypertensives to control blood pressure, diuretics to reduce blood volume, and beta blockers to improve ventricular filling. A low-sodium diet also may be indicated. If blood flow to the uterus is impaired by the aortic constriction, fetal mortality will be high. The woman needs serial ultrasound and nonstress tests done after weeks 30 to 32 of pregnancy to monitor fetal health. Balloon valve angioplasty to loosen mitral valve adhesions can be performed safely during pregnancy (Meller & Goldman, 2000). If an anticoagulant is required, heparin is the drug of choice.

The Woman With Right-Sided Heart Failure

Congenital heart defects such as pulmonary valve stenosis and atrial and ventricular septal defects may result in right-sided heart failure. Right-sided failure occurs when the output of the right ventricle is less than the blood volume received by the right atrium from the vena cava or venous circulation. Back-pressure from this results in congestion of the systemic venous circulation and decreases cardiac output to the lungs. Blood pressure decreases in the aorta because less blood is reaching it; pressure is high in the vena cava; both jugular venous distention and increased portal circulation occur. The liver and spleen become distended. Distention of abdominal vessels can lead to exudate of fluid from the vessels into the peritoneal cavity (ascites). Fluid moves from the systemic circulation into the interstitial spaces (peripheral edema). Liver enlargement can cause extreme dyspnea and pain in a pregnant woman because the enlarged liver, as it is pressed upward by the enlarged uterus, puts extreme pressure on the diaphragm.

The congenital anomaly most apt to cause right-sided failure in women of reproductive age is Eisenmenger syndrome (a right-to-left atrial or ventricular septal defect with an accompanying pulmonary stenosis). Women who have an uncorrected anomaly of this type can be expected to be hospitalized during pregnancy. They need oxygen administration and frequent arterial blood gas assessments to ensure fetal growth. During labor, they may need a pulmonary artery catheter inserted to monitor pulmonary pressure. They need extremely close monitoring after epidural anesthesia to minimize the risk of hypotension.

The Woman With Peripartal Heart Disease

An extremely rare condition, **peripartal cardiomyopathy** can originate late in pregnancy in women with no previous history of heart disease. Although the cause is unknown, it is apparently due to the effect of the pregnancy on the circulatory system. In many instances it may occur from previously undetected heart disease; it occurs most often in African-American multiparas in conjunction with hypertension of pregnancy (Cunningham et al., 2001). Late in pregnancy, the woman develops signs of myocardial failure (i.e., shortness of breath, chest pain, and edema). Her heart begins to increase in size (cardiomegaly). If this occurs, her activity must be sharply reduced. Many women need diuretic and digitalis therapy. Low-dose heparin may be administered to decrease the risk of thromboembolism. Immunosuppressive therapy may improve the symptoms.

If the cardiomegaly persists past the postpartal period, it is generally suggested that the woman not attempt any further pregnancies because the condition tends to recur in future pregnancies. Oral contraceptives are contraindicated because of the danger of thromboembolism with this method. The disease may progress to the point that following pregnancy, the woman may need a heart transplant.

Assessment of the Woman With Cardiac Disease

Nurses play a major role in the care of the pregnant woman with cardiovascular disease. Continuous assessment of the woman's health status, health education, and health-promotion activities are essential. Assessment of the woman with cardiac disease begins with a thorough health history to document her prepregnancy cardiac status (see Assessing the Pregnant Woman With Heart Disease). Ask about her level of exercise performance (what level can she do before growing short of breath and what physical symptoms does she experience, such as cyanosis of the lips or nail beds). Ask if she normally has a cough and edema. Every woman with cardiac disease should be instructed to report coughing during pregnancy and should be seen even if she assumes it is just a simple upper respiratory infection, because pulmonary edema from heart failure may first manifest as a cough.

Edema in women with heart disease must never be taken lightly. A decision is necessary to determine if edema is the normal edema of pregnancy (innocent), the beginning of pregnancy-induced hypertension (serious), or the edema of heart failure (serious). The normal edema of pregnancy involves only the feet and ankles. Edema of either pregnancy-induced hypertension or heart failure may begin as ankle edema. Edema of pregnancy-induced hypertension usually begins after week 20. If the edema is a sign of heart failure, it can begin at any time and other symptoms will probably also be present: irregular pulse, rapid or difficult respirations, and perhaps chest pain on exertion. Be certain to record a baseline blood pressure, pulse rate, and respiratory rate in either a sitting or lying position; then, at future health visits, always take these in the same position for a most accurate comparison. Making comparison assessments for nail bed filling (should be

ASSESSING the Pregnant Woman With Heart Disease

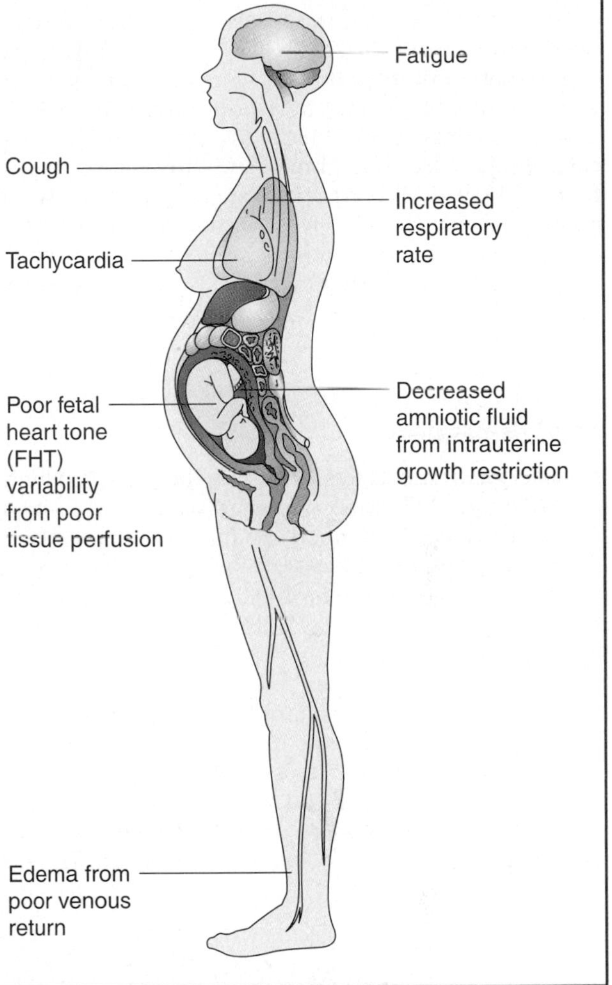

under 5 seconds) and jugular venous distention is helpful throughout pregnancy. If a woman's heart disease involves right-sided heart failure, assessment of liver size at visits is helpful. Keep in mind that liver assessment becomes difficult and probably inaccurate late in pregnancy because the enlarged uterus presses the liver upward.

For additional cardiac status assessment, the woman may need an electrocardiogram (ECG), chest x-ray, or echocardiogram done at periodic points in pregnancy. Assure her that an ECG merely measures cardiac electrical discharge and thus does not harm the fetus in any way. Echocardiography uses sonography and thus will not harm the fetus. Chest x-ray is considered safe as long as the woman's abdomen is covered by a lead apron during the exposure. An ECG may become less accurate late in pregnancy (demonstrates left axis deviation) because the enlarged uterus presses upward on the diaphragm and displaces the heart laterally.

Fetal Assessment

Cardiac failure affects fetal growth at the point at which the maternal blood pressure becomes insufficient to provide an adequate supply of blood and nutrients to the placenta. For this reason, the infants of women with severe heart disease tend to have low birthweights because not enough nutrients are available. This poor perfusion level may lead to severe fetal distress if the blood flow is inadequate for carbon dioxide exchange, ultimately resulting in an acidotic environment for the fetus (Cunningham et al., 2001). Preterm labor also may occur. This exposes the infant to the hazards of immaturity as well as low birthweight. The infant may not respond well to labor (evidenced by late deceleration patterns on a fetal heart monitor) if cardiac decompensation has reached a point of placental incompetency.

NURSING DIAGNOSES AND RELATED INTERVENTIONS

Nursing Diagnosis: Deficient knowledge regarding the effects of maternal cardiovascular disease on the pregnancy and fetus

Outcome Identification: Client will demonstrate understanding of danger signs and need to contact physician.

Outcome Evaluation: Client identifies danger signs and steps to take when they occur; maternal blood pressure is maintained above 100/60 mm Hg and fetal heart rate at 120 to 160 bpm.

Be certain that the goals and outcomes established are realistic. Not all women with heart disease will be able to complete a pregnancy; some infants of women with severe involvement will be born with the effects of placental insufficiency, such as neurologic involvement or cognitive challenge. However, there are positive actions the woman with heart disease can take to reduce or eliminate complications during pregnancy. These include measures to rest and strengthen heart action. Nursing interventions are concerned with helping her to achieve these measures (see Focus on Nursing Care Planning).

Promote Rest. A woman with cardiac disease needs more rest during pregnancy than the average woman to lessen the strain of the increased burden of the pregnancy on her heart. Remember that when cardiac output is not enough to meet systemic body demands, peripheral vasoconstriction occurs. Because the uterus is a peripheral organ, this causes uterine/placental constriction. Therefore, a rest program must be carefully designed so the woman stops exercising before this point is reached. Exactly how much rest she is to have should be carefully detailed for her. She may need to discontinue work early in pregnancy rather than work until the end of pregnancy, as the average woman usually plans to do. Exactly how much she will be allowed to do should be detailed as well. Allowing "normally heavy" housework may mean nothing more strenuous than dusting to some women. To others, it may mean washing windows, turning mattresses, and shoveling snow. Make certain the woman's definition of "heavy work" is the same as yours and her physician's or nurse-midwife's.

Many women need two rest periods a day (fully resting, not getting up frequently to answer the door or telephone) and a full night's sleep (not tossing and turning because of excess noise or heat in the room) to obtain adequate rest. Rest should be in the left lateral recumbent position to prevent supine hypotension syndrome and increased heart effort.

Promote Healthy Nutrition. The woman with cardiac disease may need closer supervision of nutrition during pregnancy than does the average woman. She must gain enough weight to ensure a healthy pregnancy and a healthy baby. However, she must not gain so much excess weight that she has to supply additional cells with nutrients, because this could overburden her heart and circulatory system.

Be certain that she is taking her prenatal vitamins, because these contain an iron supplement to help prevent anemia. Anemia requires the body to circulate blood more vigorously to distribute oxygen to all body cells; if her heart is already taxed, she cannot do this. If the woman was following a sodium-restricted diet before pregnancy, this may be continued during pregnancy. Sodium is necessary for maintaining fluid volume and balance. Allowing the woman's body to retain enough blood volume to supply blood to the placenta is important. Typically, the woman's sodium intake is limited but not severely restricted during pregnancy.

WHAT IF? What if a woman with cardiac disease tells you she tries to eat absolutely no salt in an attempt to control her tendency toward edema? What would you do?

Educate Regarding Medication. Women taking cardiac medication before pregnancy may need to increase

FOCUS ON *Nursing Care Planning*

THE PREGNANT WOMAN WITH HEART DISEASE

A 30-year-old client with a history of heart disease comes to the clinic for evaluation. She states, "I think I'm pregnant. I just want to make sure everything goes okay with the pregnancy."

Assessment: Well-nourished female with history of class I heart disease. Weight appropriate for height. Vital signs within acceptable parameters. Last menstrual period 6 weeks ago. Reports slight nausea and breast fullness. Serum hCG level positive for pregnancy.

Nursing Diagnosis: Health-seeking behaviors related to effect of heart disease on pregnancy.

Outcome Identification: Client will demonstrate measures to promote the health and well-being of herself and her fetus during pregnancy.

Outcome Evaluation: Client describes physiologic changes of pregnancy and effects on heart disease; verbalizes factors that increase cardiac demands; identifies danger signs and symptoms.

Interventions	Rationale
1. Assist with and perform initial assessment, including vital signs and height and weight, comparing to prepregnancy levels.	1. Initial assessment provides a baseline for future comparison and identifies factors placing the client at risk.
2. Assess client's knowledge of heart disease and changes of pregnancy. Evaluate lifestyle and activity level.	2. Assessment of client's knowledge provides a baseline from which to build future teaching strategies. Lifestyle and activity levels can be affected, depending on the degree of cardiac compromise.
3. Review plans for laboratory testing and scheduling of antepartal care visits.	3. Reviewing information reinforces what is to come and helps to alleviate fears and anxiety. More frequent antepartal visits may be necessary to ensure optimal fetal and maternal well-being.
4. Coordinate care with maternal and cardiac health care provider.	4. Collaboration with maternal and cardiac health care providers is essential to ensure a healthy outcome for the mother and fetus.
5. Educate the client about need for adequate rest and pacing of activities with energy-conservation measures. Check with cardiac health care provider about any possible activity restrictions.	5. Increased metabolic demands of pregnancy increase cardiac workload, placing the client at risk for possible cardiac decompensation. Activity restrictions may be necessary to prevent uteroplacental insufficiency.
6. Encourage the client to rest in the lateral recumbent position.	6. Lateral recumbent position prevents supine hypotension syndrome.
7. Counsel the client about nutritional requirements and adequate weight gain. Monitor weight gain at each visit.	7. Adequate nutrition is essential for optimal fetal growth and development. However, too much weight gain places an added strain on the heart.
8. Advise client to remind cardiac health care providers that she is pregnant. Warn client to check with health care providers before taking any over-the-counter medications.	8. Maintenance medications for cardiac function may need to be increased because of the expanded blood volume in pregnancy. Any drug may be teratogenic to the fetus.
9. Instruct client in measures to prevent infection and to notify health care provider at the first sign of any infection.	9. Infection increases energy expenditure, metabolic rate, and cardiac output, placing additional workload on the heart.
10. Assist client with measures to relax and reduce stress.	10. Anxiety and stressors can increase the workload of the heart.
11. Instruct client in danger signs and symptoms of cardiac decompensation.	11. Knowledge of danger signs allows for early recognition and prompt intervention, minimizing the risk to the mother and fetus.
12. Arrange for referrals to appropriate community resources to assist with pregnancy and household management.	12. Community resources provide additional support and help reduce possible stressors.

their maintenance dose because of the expanded blood volume during pregnancy. A woman who needed digoxin before pregnancy will continue to require it (and can take it safely) during pregnancy. A woman who was not digoxin-dependent before pregnancy may need such therapy prescribed as pregnancy advances and her cardiac output has to be increased or strengthened. To aid the woman in continuing to think of herself as a fully functioning person, help her to understand that this does not mean her heart function is weakening, but rather that it is being stressed further by the increased circulatory load of pregnancy. Digoxin is sometimes administered to a woman during pregnancy to slow the fetal heart if fetal tachycardia is present. Propranolol (Inderal), a beta-adrenergic blocker frequently used for cardiac arrhythmias, is a pregnancy category C drug (unstudied in pregnancy) but apparently does not cause fetal abnormalities. Nitroglycerin, a compound often prescribed for angina, is also a category C drug but is apparently safe.

A woman who was taking penicillin prophylactically after rheumatic fever to prevent a recurrence (often taken for 10 years after the occurrence of rheumatic fever, or at least until age 18 years) should continue to take this drug during pregnancy because penicillin is not known to be a fetal teratogen (a category B drug). Close to the anticipated day of birth, some physicians begin a course of an antibiotic such as penicillin for women with heart disease. This is because the postpartal period always involves some mild invasion of bacteria from the denuded placental site on the uterus into the bloodstream. Since this invading bacteria may be streptococci, the bacteria often responsible for subacute bacterial endocarditis, a course of ampicillin, gentamicin (Garamycin), amoxicillin (Amoxil), or clindamycin (Cleocin) at this time offers women needed protection.

It is often difficult to keep healthy women from taking over-the-counter medicines during pregnancy; conversely, it can be just as difficult to encourage them to take the medicine they need during pregnancy. Help them understand that there are valid exceptions to the rule of "no medicine during pregnancy."

Educate Regarding Avoidance of Infection. A systemic infection almost automatically increases body temperature, causing a woman to have to expend more energy and increase her cardiac output. This insult may be too much for the woman with heart disease to withstand. Caution the client to avoid visiting or being visited by people with infections. She should alert health care personnel at the first indication of an upper respiratory tract infection or UTI so that, if warranted, antibiotic therapy can be begun early in the course of the infection. Monthly screening for bacteriuria with a clean-catch urine test may be recommended.

Nursing Interventions During Labor and Birth

The anesthetic of choice during labor for women with heart disease is often an epidural, because this can make both labor and birth less taxing. Many women with heart disease should not push with contractions; pushing requires more effort than they should expend. If an epidural anesthetic is used, low forceps or a vacuum extractor can be used for birth. A woman may be disappointed that her birth is not more "natural." Stress that these measures can help her achieve her ultimate goals, which are a healthy newborn and a mother able to care for her new baby.

Fetal heart rate and uterine contractions should be closely monitored during labor on all women with heart disease. The mother's blood pressure, pulse, and respirations are assessed frequently. A rapidly increasing pulse rate (more than 100 bpm) is an indication that her heart is pumping ineffectively and has increased its rate in an effort to compensate. Advise the woman to assume a side-lying position to reduce the possibility of supine hypotension syndrome. If she has some pulmonary edema, it may be necessary for her to have her chest and head elevated (semi-Fowler's position) to ease the work of breathing. Remember that fatigue is a symptom of heart decompensation. If this occurs in labor, evaluate the client carefully to determine whether the fatigue is heart- or labor-related.

Postpartal Nursing Interventions

The period immediately after birth may be the most critical time for the woman with heart disease (Cunningham et al., 2001). With delivery of the placenta, the blood that supplied the placenta is now released into the general circulation, subsequently increasing the blood volume 20% to 40%. During pregnancy, the increase in blood volume occurred over a 6-month period, so the heart had time to adjust to this change gradually. After birth, the increase in pressure takes place within 5 minutes, so the heart must make a rapid and major adjustment.

If the woman is in severe congestive failure after birth, she needs a program of decreased activity and possibly anticoagulant and digoxin therapy until her circulation stabilizes. As soon as possible, have her ambulate to avoid the formation of emboli. Antiembolic stockings may be needed to increase venous return from the legs. If prophylactic antibiotics had not been started prior to birth, they will be started immediately after birth to discourage subacute bacterial endocarditis caused by introduction of microorganisms through the placental site.

A woman with heart disease is often interested in close inspection of her baby immediately after birth because she wants to know that her infant does not have a heart defect or was not harmed by any medication she took. Be sure to point out that acrocyanosis is normal in newborns, so she does not interpret her baby's severe peripheral cyanosis as cardiac inadequacy.

In the postpartal period, agents to encourage uterine involution such as oxytocin (Pitocin) must be used with caution because they tend to increase blood pressure, and this necessitates increased heart action. As a rule, the woman with heart disease can breast-feed without difficulty. However, the woman needs an individualized assessment to ensure that this is the best decision for her. Postpartal exercises to improve abdominal tone should not be undertaken until her physician or nurse-midwife approves them. Kegel exercises are acceptable for perineal strengthening. Suggest a stool softener if it has not been prescribed to prevent straining with bowel movements.

Before discharge, be certain the woman has thought through what help she will need at home so she can continue getting periods of adequate rest. Also ensure that she schedules a return appointment for a postpartal checkup for both her gynecologic health and cardiac status.

The Woman With an Artificial Valve Prosthesis

Once women with a heart valve prostheses were advised not to become pregnant. Today, caring for a woman with a valve prosthesis during pregnancy would not be unusual. One potential problem involves the use of oral anticoagulants such as Coumarin derivatives to prevent the formation of clots at the valve site. Unfortunately, these medications may increase the risk of congenital anomalies in infants (pregnancy risk category D). Women, therefore, are usually placed on heparin therapy before becoming pregnant to reduce this risk. Heparin does not cross the placenta and thus does not interfere with fetal development or fetal coagulation (category C). Subclinical bleeding from the anticoagulant in the mother may cause placental dislodgement. Be sure to observe the woman closely for signs of premature separation of the placenta during pregnancy and labor.

The Woman With Chronic Hypertensive Vascular Disease

Women with chronic hypertensive disease come into pregnancy with an elevated blood pressure (140/90 mm Hg or above). Hypertension of this kind is usually associated with arteriosclerosis or renal disease, making it a problem of the older pregnant woman. Chronic hypertension places the mother and fetus at high risk because fetal well-being may be compromised by poor placental perfusion during the pregnancy. Management is similar to that of the woman with pregnancy-induced hypertension (Lockwood & Paidas, 2000; see Chap. 15).

The Woman With Venous Thromboembolic Disease

The incidence of venous thromboembolic disease increases during pregnancy due to a combination of stasis of blood in the lower extremities from uterine pressure and hypercoagulability (the effect of increased estrogen; see Assessing the Pregnant Woman With Venous Thromboembolic Disease). When the pressure of the fetal head at birth puts additional pressure on lower extremity veins, damage can occur to the walls of vessels. When this triad of effects is in place (stasis, vessel damage, and hypercoagulation), the stage is set for thrombus formation in the lower extremities. The likelihood of **deep vein thrombosis** (DVT) leading to pulmonary emboli increases for women 30 years of age or older because increased age is yet another risk factor for thrombosis formation (Cunningham et al., 2001).

Symptoms of pulmonary embolism include:

ASSESSING the Pregnant Woman With Venous Thromboembolic Disease

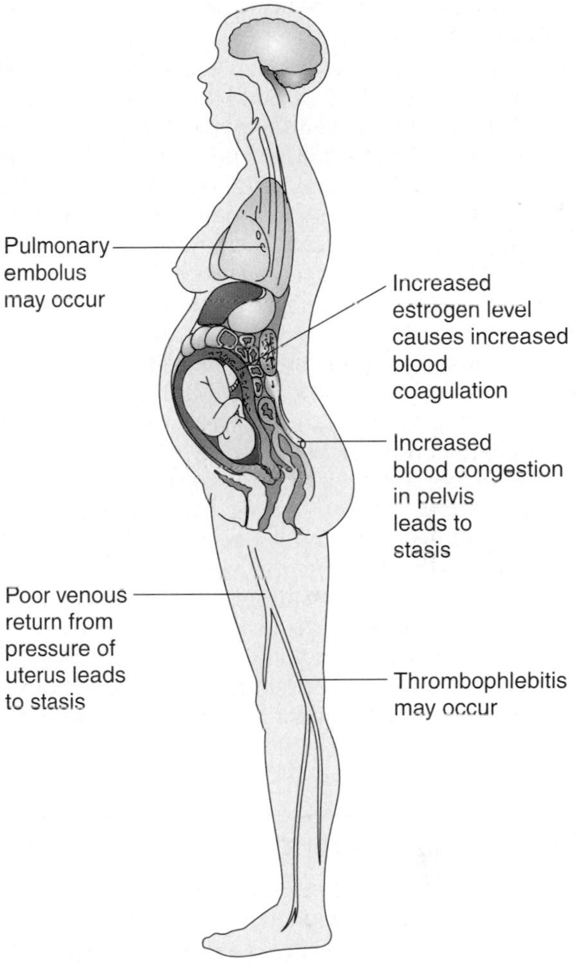
Pulmonary embolus may occur
Increased estrogen level causes increased blood coagulation
Increased blood congestion in pelvis leads to stasis
Poor venous return from pressure of uterus leads to stasis
Thrombophlebitis may occur

- Chest pain
- Sudden onset of dyspnea
- Cough with hemoptysis
- Tachycardia or missed beats
- Severe dizziness or fainting from lowered blood pressure.

Pulmonary embolism is an emergency. Care measures are discussed in Chapter 15.

The risk of thrombus formation can be reduced through common-sense measures such as avoiding the use of constrictive knee-high stockings, not sitting with legs crossed at the knee, and avoiding standing in one position for a long period. If a thrombus does occur during pregnancy, it is diagnosed by the woman's history and Doppler ultrasonography. The woman will be treated with bed rest and intravenous heparin for 24 to 48 hours. After this, she may be prescribed subcutaneous heparin every 12 or 24 hours for the duration of the pregnancy. It is generally recommended that the lower abdomen be used for rotating sites for subcutaneous heparin administration. With pregnancy, however, this site is usually avoided and the injection sites are limited to the arms and thighs. Heparin dosage is regulated by frequent partial thromboplastin time (PTT) determinations (Toglia, 2000). Additional measures of care for the woman with DVT, such as heat, elevation, and bed rest, are discussed in Chapter 25 because 50% of cases occur in the postpartal period.

A particular group of women has been identified as being more susceptible to thrombi formation, spontaneous miscarriage, fetal death, and hypertension of pregnancy: women with antiphospholipid antibodies (aPLA) (Esplin, 2001). It is not known why aPLA occurs in some clients and not in others, but these antibodies probably represent an autoimmune process. Women who are identified as aPLA positive may be started on a prophylactic program of aspirin or subcutaneous heparin during pregnancy and continued postpartally to reduce the possibility of DVT. Administration of a corticosteroid helps to reduce the formation of additional antibodies and thus may also be prescribed. After pregnancy, such women should not begin an oral contraceptive, which can increase blood coagulation and the possibility of thrombi formation.

Women taking heparin during pregnancy should not take any additional injections once labor begins to help reduce the possibility of hemorrhage at birth; they are not candidates for routine episiotomy or epidural anesthesia for this same reason unless at least 4 hours has passed since the last heparin dose was given. PTT determinations should be continued during labor. Heparin or sodium warfarin (Coumadin) administration is resumed after birth (Esplin, 2001).

✔ CHECKPOINT QUESTIONS

13. Can women with cardiac disease safely take digoxin during pregnancy?
14. Should women who are taking prophylactic penicillin after rheumatic fever continue to take this during pregnancy?
15. When a woman with deep vein thrombosis takes heparin during pregnancy, will the infant be born with a bleeding disorder?

ENDOCRINE DISORDERS AND PREGNANCY

Endocrine disorders can be serious in pregnancy because enzymes or hormones control so many specific body functions.

The Woman With a Thyroid Dysfunction

As a normal effect of pregnancy, the thyroid gland enlarges (hypertrophies) slightly due to increased vascularity. The woman with preexisting thyroid problems may have difficulty making this pregnancy transition.

NURSING DIAGNOSES AND RELATED INTERVENTIONS

Nursing Diagnosis: Risk for maternal and fetal injury related to preexisting thyroid disorder and drug therapy during pregnancy

Outcome Identification: Mother and fetus will suffer no adverse effects from maternal hormonal imbalance and drug therapy.

Outcome Evaluation: No congenital anomalies are present in infant at birth; Apgar score is 7 to 10. Mother is able to continue prepregnancy activities.

The Woman With Hypothyroidism

Hypothyroidism is a rare condition in young adults and especially in pregnancy because women with symptoms of untreated hypothyroidism may be anovulatory and unable to conceive. The woman with hypothyroidism has difficulty increasing thyroid functioning to a pregnancy level. Thus, the pregnant woman with hypothyroidism often has a history of early spontaneous miscarriage. She fatigues easily and tends to be obese; her skin is dry (myxedema) and she has little tolerance for cold. Hypothyroidism is associated with extreme nausea and vomiting during pregnancy (hyperemesis gravidarum).

Most women with hypothyroidism take levothyroxine (Synthroid) to supplement their lack of thyroid hormone. A woman who is taking levothyroxine needs to consult with her obstetrician and internist when she is planning on becoming pregnant. She needs to come for early diagnosis and close follow-up as soon as she suspects she is pregnant (1 week past her missed menstrual period). As a rule, her dose of levothyroxine will be increased for the duration of the pregnancy to simulate the effect that would normally occur in pregnancy (Vettraino & Welch, 2000). Be certain that the woman realizes the importance of taking this increased dose.

After the pregnancy, the dose of levothyroxine prescribed for pregnancy must be gradually tapered back to the prepregnancy level. Be certain the woman does not continue to take her pregnancy dose (trying to be economical and use up her higher-dose pills), or she will pass beyond normal thyroid function and develop hyperthyroidism.

The Woman With Hyperthyroidism

Hyperthyroidism causes the following symptoms:

- Rapid heart rate
- Exophthalmos (protruding eyeballs)
- Heat intolerance
- Nervousness
- Heart palpitations
- Weight loss

Hyperthyroidism is more apt to be seen in pregnancy than hypothyroidism. If undiagnosed, the woman may develop heart failure during pregnancy because her rapid heart rate cannot adjust to the increasing blood volume occurring with pregnancy. She is more prone to symptoms of hypertension of pregnancy, fetal growth restriction, and preterm labor than the average woman is (Davies & Cobin, 2000).

Hyperthyroidism is normally diagnosed by a nuclear medicine imaging study involving the radioactive uptake of ^{131}I subtype. This diagnostic procedure should not be used during pregnancy because the fetal thyroid will also incorporate this drug, possibly resulting in destruction of the fetal thyroid.

Treatment for hyperthyroidism is with thioamides (methimazole [Tapazole] or propylthiouracil [PTU]) to reduce thyroid activity. These drugs are, unfortunately, teratogens. They cross the placenta and can lead to congenital hypothyroidism and consequently an enlarged thyroid gland (a goiter) in the fetus. If this abnormal neck growth enlarges enough, it can obstruct the airway and make resuscitation difficult for the infant at birth. The woman should be regulated on the lowest dose possible and cautioned to keep a careful record of doses taken so she does not forget or accidentally duplicate a dose. Surgical treatment to reduce the functioning of the maternal thyroid gland can be accomplished, but this is generally not the treatment of choice during pregnancy due to the need for general anesthesia. After a pregnancy, if the woman desires other children, the procedure might be possible as an interpregnancy procedure.

If the woman's thyroid function was not regulated during pregnancy, the infant may be born with symptoms of hyperthyroidism because of the excess stimulation he or she received in utero. An assay of fetal cord blood will reveal the level of T4 and thyroid-stimulating hormone and the need for therapy. If the infant appears jittery, tachypnea and tachycardia may be present. Women receiving smaller or minimal doses of antithyroid drugs may breast-feed successfully, although women receiving large doses of antithyroid drugs may be advised not to breast-feed because these drugs are excreted in breast milk (Karch, 2001).

The Woman With Diabetes Mellitus

Diabetes mellitus is an endocrine disorder in which the pancreas cannot produce adequate insulin to regulate body glucose levels. The disorder affects 20 to 50 per 1,000 pregnancies (Langer, 2000). Before insulin was produced synthetically in 1921, women with diabetes failed to survive to reach childbearing age, were infertile, or had spontaneous miscarriages early in pregnancy. Now that diabetes can be controlled, three new problems have developed:

1. How to bring a woman with diabetes through a pregnancy with good glucose and insulin control
2. How to protect her infant in utero from the adverse effects of the disease
3. How to care for the infant in the first 24-hour period after birth until the infant's insulin-glucose regulatory mechanism stabilizes

Reproductive planning may be a fourth concern for a woman with diabetes. She may not be a candidate for oral contraceptives because progesterone interferes with insulin activity and therefore increases blood glucose levels. The estrogen in contraceptives has the potential for increasing lipid and cholesterol levels and the risk for increased blood coagulation. Intrauterine devices have been implicated in higher-than-usual rates of pelvic inflammatory disease (Cunningham et al., 2001); because women with diabetes have difficulty fighting infections, these are not usually advised either. Norplant (subcutaneous implanted progestin) or Depo-Provera may be good choices (see Chap. 5).

Pathophysiology and Clinical Manifestations

The possible etiology and pathology of diabetes mellitus are discussed in detail in Chapter 48. The primary problem of any woman with this disorder is controlling the balance between insulin and blood glucose levels to prevent hyperglycemia or hypoglycemia. Both of these conditions are dangerous during pregnancy because they are threats to normal fetal growth.

If a woman's insulin amount is insufficient, glucose cannot be used by body cells. The cells register their glucose want, and the liver quickly converts stored glycogen to glucose to increase the serum glucose level. Because of the insulin insufficiency, however, the body cells still cannot use the glucose, and the serum glucose levels continue to rise (hyperglycemia). When the level of blood sugar rises to 150 mg/100 mL (normal is 80 to 120 mg/dL), the kidneys begin to excrete quantities of glucose in the urine (**glycosuria**) in an attempt to lower the level. During pregnancy, the point at which this happens may be even lower than 150 mg/100 mL. Because of osmotic action, the increased amount of glucose in the urine reduces fluid absorption in the kidney, and large quantities of fluid are lost in urine (polyuria).

Dehydration begins to occur; the blood serum becomes concentrated and the blood volume may fall. With the reduced blood flow, cells do not receive adequate oxygen, and anaerobic metabolic reactions cause large stores of lactic acid to pour out of muscle into the bloodstream. Fat is mobilized from fat stores and metabolized for energy, and large amounts of ketone bodies are poured into the bloodstream. Ketone bodies are acidic (the best example is acetone). These two acid sources lower the pH of the blood, and a metabolic acidosis develops.

Next, protein stores are tapped by the body as it attempts to find a source of energy for body cells. Protein catabolism reduces the supply of protein to body cells. Cell catabolism also results in the loss of potassium and sodium from the body. Long-term effects of diabetes mellitus are vascular narrowing, leading to kidney and retinal dysfunction and increasing blood pressure (Spellacy, 2000).

Diabetes During Pregnancy

Even a woman who has successful regulation of glucose and insulin metabolism before pregnancy is apt to develop less-than-optimal control during pregnancy because all women experience a number of changes in the glucose-insulin regulatory system as pregnancy progresses. Glomerular filtration of glucose is increased (the glomerular excretion threshold is lowered), causing slight glycosuria. The rate of insulin secretion is increased, and the fasting blood sugar is lowered. All women appear to develop an insulin resistance as pregnancy progresses (i.e., insulin does not seem normally effective during pregnancy), a phenomenon that is probably caused by the presence of the hormone human placental lactogen (chorionic somatomammotropin) and high levels of cortisol, estrogen, progesterone, and catecholamines. Placental insulinase may cause increased breakdown or degradation of insulin. This resistance to or destruction of insulin is helpful in a normal pregnancy because it prevents the blood glucose from falling to dangerous limits, despite the increased insulin secretion that occurs. It causes difficulty for a diabetic pregnant woman in that she must increase her insulin dosage beginning at about week 24 of pregnancy to prevent hyperglycemia.

At the same time, the continued use of glucose by the fetus may lead to **hypoglycemia** (lowered serum glucose levels) for the mother between meals; this is most apt to occur overnight. A low maternal level of glucogenic amino acids (used by the liver to produce glucose) compounds this. She may become ketoacidotic from the breakdown of stored fat between meals, most likely occurring during the second and third trimesters. An increase in the amount of amniotic fluid occurs in at least 25% of diabetic women, probably due to hyperglycemia in the fetus that causes increased urine production. Amniocentesis may be done to decrease the level of amniotic fluid. Unfortunately, this exposes the woman to infection and possible preterm labor and is only a temporary measure because amniotic fluid is continually produced. If the woman has preexisting kidney disease (revealed by proteinuria, decreased creatinine clearance, and hypertension), the risk of fetal growth restriction, asphyxia, stillbirth, and maternal pregnancy-induced hypertension rises markedly (Cunningham et al., 2001).

When glucose regulation is poor, the woman is at greater risk for pregnancy-induced hypertension and infection (particularly monilial infection) than other women are. Infants of women with poorly controlled diabetes tend to be large (more than 10 lb) because the increased insulin the fetus must produce to counteract the overload of glucose he or she receives acts as a growth stimulant. The increased glucose adds subcutaneous fat deposits. A macrosomic infant may create birth problems at the end of the pregnancy due to cephalopelvic disproportion. This, combined with an increased risk for shoulder dystocia, may make it necessary for infants of women with diabetes to be born by cesarean birth.

There is a high incidence of congenital anomaly, especially caudal regression syndrome, spontaneous miscarriage, and stillbirth in infants of women with uncontrolled diabetes. At birth, the neonates are more prone to hypoglycemia, respiratory distress syndrome, hypocalcemia, and hyperbilirubinemia. The first trimester of pregnancy is the most critical time for fetal development; if the woman can be kept from becoming hyperglycemic during this time, the chances of a congenital anomaly are greatly lessened (Cunningham et al., 2001).

The Woman With Gestational Diabetes

Approximately 2% to 3% of all women who do not begin a pregnancy with diabetes become diabetic during pregnancy, usually at the midpoint of pregnancy when insulin resistance becomes most noticeable. This is termed gestational diabetes mellitus. The symptoms fade again at the completion of pregnancy, but the risk of developing type 2 diabetes may be as high as 50% to 60% later in life (Cunningham et al., 2001). It is unknown whether gestational diabetes results from inadequate insulin response to carbohydrate or from excessive resistance to insulin; a combination of both may occur. Risk factors for gestational diabetes include:

- Obesity
- Age over 25 years
- History of large babies (10 lb or more)
- History of unexplained fetal or perinatal loss
- History of congenital anomalies in previous pregnancies
- Family history of diabetes (one close relative or two distant ones)
- Member of a population with a high risk for diabetes (Native American, Hispanic, Asian; American Diabetes Association, 2001)

Classification of Diabetes Mellitus

Diabetes is divided into various categories that can be used to predict pregnancy outcome (Table 14-3).

Assessment

All women should be screened during pregnancy for gestational diabetes. This is usually done using a 50-g oral glucose challenge test at weeks 24 to 28 of pregnancy. It may be repeated at 32 weeks if the woman is obese or over age 40 years. Women who are considered at high risk for developing gestational diabetes should be screened at their first prenatal visit and again at 24 to 28 weeks (see Assessing the Pregnant Woman With Diabetes Mellitus).

The new recommendations by the American Diabetes Association have set the values for diagnosis at levels lower than ever before. After the oral 50-g glucose load is ingested, a venous blood sample is taken for glucose determination 60 minutes later. If the serum glucose at 1 hour is more than 140 mg/dL, women are scheduled for a 100-g, 3-hour fasting **glucose tolerance test.** If two of the four blood samples collected are abnormal or the fasting value is above 95 mg/dL, a diagnosis of diabetes can be made. The values that confirm diabetes are shown in Table 14-4.

Monitoring the Woman With Diabetes

The woman with pregestational diabetes (type 1 or type 2) should come to her obstetrician for care before she becomes pregnant; during this waiting period, her condition can be well regulated so that hyperglycemia does not develop during the early weeks of pregnancy, when the tendency for congenital anomalies in the fetus is highest (Holing, 2000). The woman should use a home test kit to determine she is pregnant at the earliest possible time. The best insulin control program for her during pregnancy can then be determined. The measurement of **glycosylated hemoglobin** is used to detect the degree of hyperglycemia present. This is a measure of the amount of

TABLE 14.3 Classification of Diabetes Mellitus

CLASS	DESCRIPTION
Type 1	Formerly known as insulin-dependent diabetes mellitus. A state characterized by the destruction of the beta cells in the pancreas that usually leads to absolute insulin deficiency. a. Immune-mediated diabetes mellitus results from autoimmune destruction of the beta cells. b. Idiopathic type 1 refers to forms that have no known cause.
Type 2	Formerly known as non-insulin-dependent diabetes mellitus. A state that usually arises because of insulin resistance combined with a relative deficiency in the production of insulin.
Gestational diabetes	A condition of abnormal glucose metabolism that arises during pregnancy. Possible signal of an increased risk for type 2 diabetes later in life.
Impaired glucose homeostasis	A state between "normal" and "diabetes" in which the body is no longer using and/or secreting insulin properly. a. Impaired fasting glucose: A state when fasting plasma glucose is 110 but under 126 mg/dL. b. Impaired glucose tolerance: A state when results of the oral glucose tolerance test are 140 but under 200 mg/dL in the 2-hour sample.

American Diabetes Association. (2001). *New classifications and recommendations for diabetes mellitus.* New York: ADA.

ASSESSING the Pregnant Woman With Diabetes Mellitus

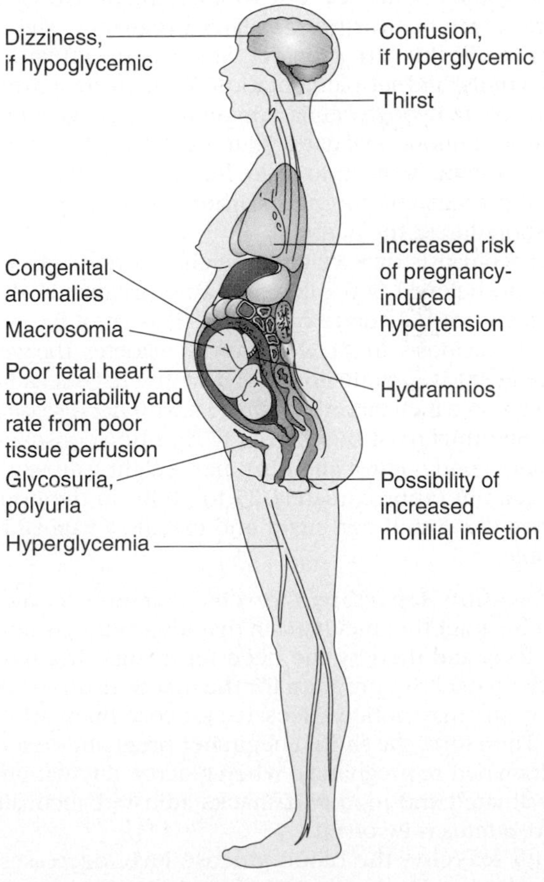

glucose attached to hemoglobin. As glucose circulates in the bloodstream, it binds to a portion of the total hemoglobin in the blood. The amount of glucose that attaches to hemoglobin in this way will be high if the hemoglobin has been exposed to a greater level of glucose than normally present. Measuring glycosylated hemoglobin reflects the average blood glucose level over the past 4 to 6 weeks (the time the red blood cells were picking up the glucose). The upper normal level of HbA is 6% of total hemoglobin.

A urine culture may be done each trimester to detect asymptomatic UTI.

Ophthalmic examination should be done once during pregnancy for the woman with gestational diabetes and at each trimester for women with known diabetes. Background retinal changes, such as increased exudate (Fig. 14-4), dot hemorrhage, and macular edema, progress or originate during pregnancy. If proliferation retinopathy was present before pregnancy, this also progresses and can lead to blindness. Laser therapy to halt these changes can be done during pregnancy without risk to the fetus.

TABLE 14.4 Oral Glucose Challenge Test Values (Fasting Plasma Glucose Values) for Pregnancy

TEST TYPE	PREGNANT GLUCOSE LEVEL (mg/dL)*
Fasting	95
1 hour	180
2 hours	155
3 hours	140

*Following a 100-g glucose load. Rate is abnormal if two values are exceeded.
Fischbach, F. (2001). *A manual of laboratory and diagnostic tests* (6th ed.). Philadelphia: Lippincott Williams & Wilkins.

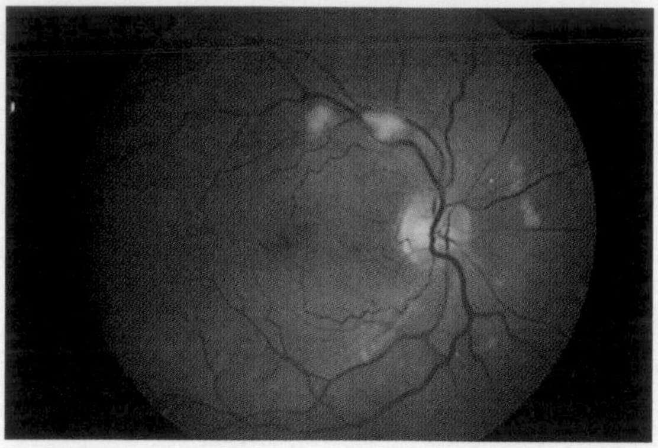

FIGURE 14.4 Increased exudate in the retina can occur with progressing diabetes during pregnancy. It appears as a "cloud-like" finding obscuring a retinal vessel.

NURSING DIAGNOSES AND RELATED INTERVENTIONS

Because diabetes is such a complex disorder, associated nursing diagnoses are many and varied. They include but are not limited to:

- Risk for ineffective tissue perfusion related to reduced vascular flow
- Imbalanced nutrition, less than body requirements, related to inability to use glucose
- Risk for ineffective coping related to required change in lifestyle
- Risk for infection related to impaired healing accompanying condition
- Deficient fluid volume related to polyuria accompanying disorder
- Deficient knowledge related to difficult and complex health problem
- Health-seeking behaviors related to voiced need to learn home glucose monitoring
- Noncompliance related to discouragement or misunderstanding or fear of therapeutic measures

The following nursing diagnoses and related interventions illustrate one of the most important facets of the nurse's role in caring for the pregnant client with diabetes: health teaching.

Nursing Diagnosis: Deficient knowledge related to therapeutic regimen necessary during pregnancy

Outcome Identification: Client will demonstrate knowledge about effects of pregnancy on diabetic condition and vice versa by 1 month.

Outcome Evaluation: Woman states importance of careful attention to nutrition, exercise, and home monitoring of glucose levels during pregnancy; describes nutrition and exercise program; states intention to keep nutrition and exercise constant.

Nurses can be instrumental in teaching women with diabetes how to change their therapeutic regimen during pregnancy (or begin one if newly diagnosed). Important topics include nutrition, exercise, insulin administration, blood glucose monitoring, and explanations of the various fetal assessment tests that will be done.

Education Regarding Nutrition During Pregnancy. Many women of childbearing age who have had diabetes since early childhood do not follow a strict diabetic diet but eat sensibly, covering any excess food eaten with the administration of additional insulin. This type of regimen is apt to require excessive insulin administration during pregnancy as a woman begins to "eat for two." Therefore, the woman is well advised to alert her health care providers about the prospects of beginning a pregnancy. In this way, she can begin a stricter diabetic diet before she becomes pregnant. Women who develop gestational diabetes should begin a diabetic diet as soon as they are diagnosed (see Focus on Communication).

Dietary control, or maintaining an adequate glucose intake so hypoglycemia does not occur, may be extremely difficult early in pregnancy because of nausea and vomiting. An 1,800- to 2,200-calorie diet (or one calculated at 35 Kcal per kg of ideal weight), divided into three meals and three snacks, is a usual regimen for a woman with diabetes during pregnancy. Keeping calories evenly distributed this way during the day helps to keep the serum glucose constant.

In addition, her diet should include a reduced amount of saturated fats and cholesterol and an increased amount of dietary fiber. Increased fiber decreases postprandial hyperglycemia and thus lowers insulin requirements. Of dietary calories, 20% to 30% should be from protein, 40% to 60% from carbohydrate, and 25% to 40% from fat.

If a woman cannot eat due to vomiting or nausea early in pregnancy or heartburn in later pregnancy, she must notify her health care provider. She may need temporary intravenous fluid supplementation. Women are extremely vulnerable to hypoglycemia at night during pregnancy due to the continuous fetal use of glucose during the time they sleep. Urge the woman to make her final snack of the day one of protein and complex carbohydrate to allow slow digestion during the night.

If a woman is overweight, she should not reduce her intake to below 1,800 calories during pregnancy. A diet this low in carbohydrate causes breakdown of fat, which produces acidosis. In the woman with diabetes, the weight of the infant is directly correlated with what she gains in pregnancy (which directly correlates with her disease control). She thus must be extremely nutrition-conscious to maintain good control and keep her weight gain to a suitable amount (approximately 25 to 30 lb) in the hope of limiting the size of her infant and making a vaginal birth possible.

Education Regarding Exercise During Pregnancy. Exercise is another mechanism that lowers the serum glucose level and thereby the need for insulin. If a woman begins an exercise program for the first time during pregnancy, she may notice excessive glucose fluctuations at first. Therefore, she should begin her pregnancy exercise program before pregnancy, when glucose fluctuation can be evaluated and food and snacks adjusted accordingly before a fetus is involved.

With exercise, the blood glucose level decreases because the muscles increase their uptake of glucose. This

FOCUS ON COMMUNICATION

Ms. Gomez is a 25-year-old woman, 24 weeks pregnant, who has pregestational diabetes. Her history shows she moved from Guadalajara, Mexico, only a year ago.

Less Effective Communication

Nurse: *Buenos dias,* Ms. Gomez. *Coma esta' usted?*
Ms. Gomez: *Bien. Gracias.*
Nurse: Oh, that was fun. I love practicing Spanish with patients. I don't understand much, though. If you'd said anything other than a one-word answer, I wouldn't have known what you meant. How's your diet going? Are you having any trouble following the diet the nutritionist gave you?
Ms. Gomez: No.
Nurse: Do you get out for a walk every day?
Ms. Gomez: *Si.*
Nurse: Any trouble doing your blood sugar? Your *azucar de sangre?*
Ms. Gomez: No.
Nurse: Good. Glad you're doing well. It was fun talking to you.

More Effective Communication

Nurse: *Buenos dias,* Ms. Gomez. *Coma esta' usted?*
Ms. Gomez: *Bien. Gracias.*
Nurse: Oh, that was fun. I love practicing Spanish with patients. I've noticed that sometimes when people answer that question with "bien, gracias," though, they're only being polite. Do you really feel well?
Ms. Gomez: I feel tired all the time.
Nurse: Tell me more about that.
Ms. Gomez: I'm so tired by nightfall, I can't cook. So I haven't been eating much.

Women who develop a complication of pregnancy have an added stress to their life. In the example above, the nurse made an admirable attempt to communicate with a patient in the patient's primary language. She forgot, however, that people under stress don't necessarily process new information well, and if she was having trouble interpreting Spanish, a patient might have equal trouble interpreting her English. This patient interpreted the instruction that she couldn't understand more than a one-word answer to mean she shouldn't answer with more than one word. Learning a second language can be important in inner-city communities. This nurse would have communicated better, however, if she had remembered that the purpose of a nurse–patient exchange was not for her to have fun but for effective assessment.

effect lasts for at least 12 hours after exercise. If the arm in which she injected insulin is actively exercised, the insulin is released quickly and hypoglycemia can be marked. To avoid this phenomenon, the woman should eat a snack consisting of protein or complex carbohydrate before exercise and should maintain a consistent exercise program (she should not do aerobic exercises one day and then none the next, but rather 30 minutes of walking every day). In the woman with poor blood glucose control, extreme exercise will cause hyperglycemia and ketoacidosis as the liver both releases glucose and breaks down fatty acids in an attempt to supply enough energy for the exercise (yet the body cannot use them because of inadequate insulin).

Therapeutic Management

Both women with gestational diabetes and those with overt diabetes need more frequent prenatal visits than usual to ensure close monitoring of their conditions and that of the fetus. Keeping blood glucose levels near normal helps minimize the risk of maternal and fetal complications (Kuzuga, 2000).

Insulin. Early in pregnancy, a woman with diabetes may need less insulin because the fetus is using so much glucose for rapid cell growth. Later in pregnancy, she will need an increased amount because her metabolic rate and need increase. If she has been taking one particular kind of insulin and a specified dosage for a long time before the pregnancy, changing the type and dosage may be unnerving for her. Be certain she understands that reregulation is a necessity because of the changes in her metabolism. Women with gestational diabetes will be started on insulin therapy if diet alone is unsuccessful in regulating glucose values.

The dosage and type of insulin are specific for each woman. The insulin chosen is usually a short-acting insulin (regular) combined with an intermediate type. Two thirds of the total amount of the day's insulin is given in the morning; the other third is given in the evening. This is self-administered 30 minutes before breakfast in a ratio of 2 : 1 (intermediate to regular) and again just before dinner in a ratio of 1 : 1. Human insulin is recommended because it has the potential for provoking a lesser antibody response than beef or pork insulins. Use of a very-short-acting insulin such as Lispro, which has a 1-hour peak time, can lead to more fluctuations in blood glucose levels. Oral hypoglycemia agents are not used for regulation because, unlike insulin, they cross the placenta and are potentially teratogenic.

Help the woman plan her day based on the time interval their insulin takes to reach its peak. For example, an intermediate insulin given before breakfast reaches its peak after lunch or late in the afternoon just before dinner. Regular insulin given before breakfast reaches its peak just after breakfast. An intermediate insulin given in the evening reaches its peak into the next day before breakfast; the evening regular insulin injection peaks after dinner or at bedtime. Knowing when insulin reaches its peak level makes serum glucose monitoring meaningful and alerts women to the time of the day when they are most apt to be hypoglycemic (see Chap. 48).

Be certain the woman is using an injection technique of stretching the skin taut and injecting at a 90-degree angle. Although this is normally intramuscular injection technique, insulin syringes have such short needles ($\frac{5}{8}$ in) that this places the insulin in the subcutaneous tissue. Most women prefer not to use abdominal sites during pregnancy. Because insulin is absorbed more slowly from the thigh than the upper arm, the woman should maintain a consistent rotating injection routine (such as using all sites in one limb before using another or rotating limbs) to maintain as consistent a level of absorption as possible. Insulin is adjusted to keep a fasting blood glucose level below 95 to 100 mg/dL and a 2-hour postprandial level below 120 mg/dL (Langer, 2000).

Insulin Pump Therapy (Continuous Subcutaneous Insulin Infusion). Because a woman will have some periods of relative hyperglycemia and hypoglycemia no matter how carefully she maintains her diet and balances her exercise level, an effective method to keep serum glucose constant is to administer insulin by a continuous pump during pregnancy (Gabbe et al., 2000). An **insulin pump** is an automatic pump about the size of a transistor radio. A syringe of regular insulin is placed in the pump chamber and a small-gauge needle is attached to thin polyethylene tubing implanted into the subcutaneous tissue of the woman's abdomen or thigh (Fig. 14-5). Day and night, at a continuous rate of about 1 U per hour, the pump edges the syringe barrel forward, infusing insulin continually into the subcutaneous tissue. Depending on the individual prescription, before a snack and before a meal, the woman can dial or press a button on the pump; the pump then pushes the syringe barrel forward to administer the bolus. The site of the pump insertion is cleaned daily and covered with sterile gauze; the site is changed every 24 to 48 hours to ensure absorption remains optimal.

Several restrictions are necessary when using an insulin pump. The pump must not be allowed to become wet; therefore, the woman should remove the pump (not the syringe and tubing) when showering and remove the complete apparatus (pump, syringe, and tubing) to bathe or swim (caution her not to leave it disconnected for more than 1 hour). The woman might prefer to wear clothing that hides the pump's outline (it can either be held against her abdomen by an over-the-shoulder sling or hung from a belt around her waist). To assess that the pump is delivering insulin at the designated rate, the woman must do blood glucose determinations about four times throughout the day (fasting and 1 hour after each meal). When pump therapy first begins, she must wake at night and do a 2 AM blood glucose determination because this is a time when she is vulnerable for hypoglycemia.

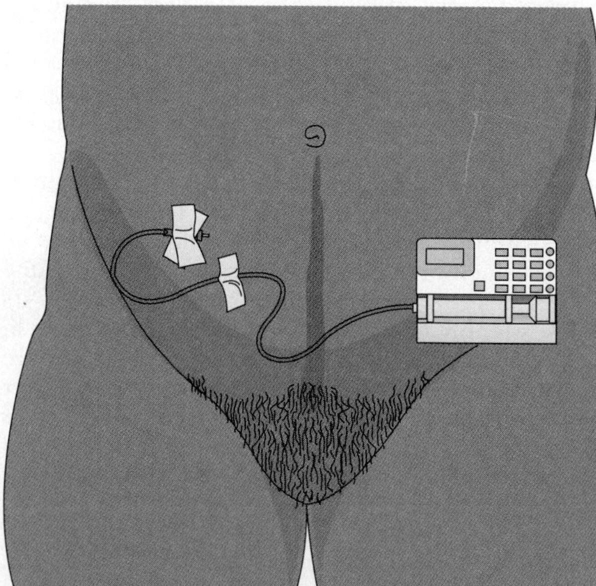

FIGURE 14.5 Using an insulin pump during pregnancy is the best assurance that insulin levels will remain constant.

Blood Glucose Monitoring. All women with diabetes can be taught to do blood glucose monitoring to determine if hyperglycemia or hypoglycemia exists. Women with preexisting diabetes use this technique every day; women with gestational diabetes may assess blood glucose levels only once a week. For this, the woman uses a fingerstick technique, using one of her fingertips as the site of lancet puncture. The strip is then inserted into a glucose meter that determines the glucose level. A fasting blood glucose level below 95 to 100 mg/dL and a 2-hour postprandial level below 120 mg/dL are well-adjusted values.

When a woman discovers hypoglycemia is present, she should ingest some form of sustained carbohydrate such as a glass of milk and some crackers. Taking a less-concentrated fluid such as milk rather than orange juice and including a complex carbohydrate helps prevent a rebound phenomenon in which a high glucose level is created that produces even more pronounced hypoglycemia.

If the woman discovers an elevated blood glucose level, she should assess her urine for ketones. The finding of ketones in two separate specimens should be reported to a health care provider. Acidosis during pregnancy must be prevented because maternal acidosis leads to fetal anoxia due to fetal inability to use oxygen when body cells are acidotic. The most common time during pregnancy for hypoglycemia is the 2nd and 3rd month, before insulin resistance peaks; for hyperglycemia, it is the 6th month, or the time insulin resistance is becoming most pronounced.

Tests for Placental Function and Fetal Well-Being. Monitoring of fetal well-being is individualized depending on the health care team and the woman's level of involvement (Jovanovic, 2000). Because women with diabetes tend to have infants with a higher-than-normal incidence of birth anomalies, the woman may have a serum alphafetoprotein level obtained at 15 to 17 weeks to assess for a neural tube defect and an ultrasound examination performed at approximately 18 to 20 weeks' gestation to detect gross abnormalities. A creatinine clearance test may be ordered each trimester. A normal creatinine clearance rate suggests that the woman's vascular system is intact and uterine perfusion is adequate. Placental functioning may also be assessed by a weekly nonstress test or biophysical profile (see Chap. 8) if the woman is in good control or a daily nonstress test if her regulation is poor.

A woman may be asked to self-monitor fetal well-being by recording how many movements occur an hour. Be certain she knows that fetal activity varies depending on her activity and meal patterns to prevent her from becoming frightened by normal variations. The healthy fetus makes approximately 10 movements per hour (see Chap. 8). Sonography to determine fetal growth, amniotic fluid volume, placental location, and biparietal diameter may be taken at week 28 and then again at weeks 36 to 38. Oligohydramnios (small amount of amniotic fluid) may indicate fetal growth restriction or fetal renal abnormality, whereas hydramnios (excessive amount of amniotic fluid) may indicate gastrointestinal malformation or poorly controlled disease. The lecithin–sphingomyelin ratio by amniocentesis is performed by week 36 of pregnancy to assess fetal maturity. In pregnancies complicated by diabetes, this ratio tends not to show maturity as early as in other pregnancies because the synthesis of phosphatidyl glycerol, the compound that stabilizes surfactant, is delayed in a diabetes-complicated pregnancy.

Because lung surfactant does not appear to form as early in these fetuses as others (due to the decreased level of cortisone present because of high serum glucose levels), the presence of phosphatidyl glycerol is used to indicate lung maturity. Although it is known that administering corticosteroids to the mother during the last week of pregnancy can hasten lung maturity, corticosteroids may also impair fetal insulin release and perhaps fetal islet development. Therefore, with a fetus who already has a risk at birth from poor glucose control, corticosteroid use to improve lung maturity is not usually attempted.

Fetal surveillance is difficult for the woman. Having to wait during each weekly test to hear how the fetus is doing is emotionally draining. The woman may believe it is somehow her fault (it is, after all, her diabetes) if the monitoring equipment shows fetal distress.

The woman's partner may be unable to accompany her once or twice a week while she is having these tests (it may be difficult enough for her to schedule this time). She needs health care personnel with her who can help her to minimize the feeling that she is alone.

Timing for Birth. Before women with diabetes were managed with maximum control during pregnancy, the timing of the birth was a chief concern. Among the most hazardous times for the fetus are weeks 36 to 40 of pregnancy (when the fetus is drawing large stores of maternal nutrients because of its large size). In the past, many pregnancies were terminated early enough to prevent fetal loss from placental insufficiency due to poor perfusion during these weeks; it was hoped that this was not so early that immaturity posed further complications.

To accomplish early birth, for many years cesarean birth was almost routinely performed in pregnant diabetic women at approximately 37 weeks' gestation. Cesarean birth was chosen because it is difficult to induce labor this early in pregnancy because the cervix is not yet ripe or responsive to labor contractions. Further, babies of diabetic women may be large, making vaginal delivery difficult. Moreover, a fetus suffering placental dysfunction or insufficiency, which may occur with maternal diabetes, will not do well in labor and may die. Early cesarean births, however, often resulted in immature infants who died in the neonatal period because of respiratory distress syndrome (infants of diabetic women may be more prone to this than usual even without a cesarean birth).

Today, when accurate assessment of fetal age is available and the pregnancy can be maintained within safe limits by the use of nonstress testing for a longer period, the last weeks of pregnancy are not as hazardous as before, and the timing of birth is much more individualized.

Vaginal birth is preferred if at all possible. Cesarean birth always presents a higher risk than vaginal birth for the fetus, and because of the difficulty of glucose regulation, the fetus of a diabetic mother is already under enough stress. Labor is induced by rupture of the membranes or an oxytocin infusion after measures to induce cervical ripening (see Chap. 21). Both labor contractions and fetal heart sounds should be monitored continuously during labor to ensure early detection of placental dysfunction. An internal fetal monitor may be used with scalp pH recordings. The woman's glucose level is regulated during labor by an intravenous infusion of regular insulin, with a blood glucose assay every hour. Regulating the glucose level carefully during labor reduces the possibility of rebound hypoglycemia in the newborn (see Chap. 26 for care of the infant of a diabetic woman at birth).

If the woman will be given an epidural anesthetic, use of an intravenous glucose solution as a plasma volume expander is avoided or additional insulin is added to the intravenous solution to counteract the effects of the glucose infused.

Postpartal Adjustment. During the postpartal period, a woman with pregestational diabetes must undergo another readjustment to insulin regulation. With insulin resistance gone, often she needs no insulin during the immediate postpartal period; in another few days, she will then return to her prepregnant insulin requirements. Blood glucose will be regulated in conjunction with 1- or 2-hour postprandial blood glucose determinations. The woman with gestational diabetes usually demonstrates normal glucose values by 24 hours after birth and needs no further diet or insulin therapy. She requires careful observation, however, during the immediate postpartal period because if hydramnios was present during pregnancy, she is at risk of hemorrhage from poor uterine contraction. Women with diabetes may breast-feed because insulin is one of the few substances that does not pass into breast milk from the bloodstream (Karch, 2001).

Because the woman who has had gestational diabetes is at risk for developing type 2 diabetes later in life, glucose testing should be done during health maintenance visits throughout life. Be certain that women have contraceptive information as appropriate. Remind women with pregestational diabetes that before they plan a second pregnancy, they will need to be certain that their disease is stabilized and in good control (the first trimester of pregnancy is a crucial fetal developmental time).

✔ CHECKPOINT QUESTIONS

16. What is the effect of hyperglycemia on early fetal growth?
17. Would you advise women with diabetes to exercise during pregnancy?
18. Why is nighttime a particularly hazardous time for the fetus of a woman with diabetes receiving continuous insulin pump therapy?

CANCER AND PREGNANCY

Malignancies most commonly seen with pregnancy are those that occur frequently during childbearing years (Blackwell et al., 2000):

- Cervical
- Breast
- Ovarian
- Thyroid
- Leukemia
- Melanoma
- Lymphomas

As women delay having their first child, the incidence of malignancy during pregnancy is expected to rise.

Although immunologic mechanisms are altered during pregnancy, there is no proof that pregnant women are more prone to cancer than other women are, that pregnancy changes the course of an existing disease, or that maternal cancer spreads to the fetus (Scott & Branch, 2000). If a woman is in the first trimester when the malignancy is diagnosed, she and her partner are asked to make a difficult decision: to delay treatment to avoid teratogenic risks to a fetus (possibly increasing the woman's risk); to abort the pregnancy to allow chemotherapy or radiation treatment; or to choose chemotherapy or radiation treatment with the almost certain knowledge that they will cause birth anomalies in the fetus.

As a rule, women can receive chemotherapy in the second and third trimesters without adverse fetal effects. Radiation therapy, in contrast, another modality that is a mainstay of cancer therapy, puts the fetus at risk throughout pregnancy if the fetus is directly exposed.

Surgery to remove a tumor can be completed during pregnancy with the understanding that the fetus is at possible risk for anoxia during anesthesia. The woman is at more than the usual risk of thrombus formation postoperatively due to the increased coagulation process accompanying pregnancy. Cervical conization has a particularly high fetal risk because the surgery may directly disrupt the pregnancy.

Cancer in the woman does not appear to metastasize to the fetus. This is because the placenta serves as an effective barrier against this spread and also because the fetus may be capable of resisting the invasion of the foreign cells.

MENTAL ILLNESS AND PREGNANCY

Mental illness may precede or occur with pregnancy. Schizophrenia tends to occur in adolescence and thus may occur in pregnant women. Depression occurs almost four times more commonly in women than in men, so it is the most common mental illness seen in pregnant women (Nolan, 2000).

Stress makes it more difficult to use coping mechanisms, and pregnancy or childbirth may be the stress that reveals mental illness for the first time. It is important that any psychotropic medication being taken by a pregnant woman be evaluated for possible fetal harm. For example, lithium, a mainstay of therapy for mood disorders such as bipolar disorder (manic depression), is a teratogen. The woman with a psychiatric disorder should be cared for by both a psychiatric care team and a prenatal care group to ensure that the stress of pregnancy is not exacerbating the mental illness, and that distorted perceptions or depression are not complicating the pregnancy.

Mental illness may also occur in the postpartal period (postpartal depression or psychosis; see Chap. 25).

TRAUMA AND PREGNANCY

Trauma (injury by force) is a phenomenon that seems remote from pregnancy because pregnant women usually take extra safety precautions to protect their body from harm. However, trauma in women occurs at a high incidence during the childbearing years because, for this age group, automobile accidents, homicide, and suicide are among the leading causes of death. During pregnancy, the incidence of trauma is 6% to 7% (as many as 250,000 pregnant women experience trauma per year). A high incidence occurs during the last trimester due to clumsiness, fainting, and hyperventilation. Orthopedic injuries such as broken wrists or sprained ankles occur because the pregnant woman's sense of balance is altered. In an automobile accident, a pregnant woman is often the front-seat passenger, and this is the passenger who often receives the most severe injury in an accident. Other women seen in emergency rooms have suffered intimate partner abuse.

Preventing Accidents

Accidents occur more frequently in people under stress than in those with little stress in their lives. Because pregnancy is a life event that may cause stress in a family's life, a woman and her family should take sensible precautions for safety. Pregnancy counseling should include education about ways to avoid accidents and trauma (see Focus on Family Empowerment).

Physiologic Changes in Pregnancy That Affect Trauma Care

In an emergency situation, the physiologic changes that normally occur with pregnancy must be considered for physical assessment to be meaningful. A primary rule to remember is that after a traumatic injury, a woman's body will maintain her own homeostasis at the expense of the fetus. To maintain blood pressure in the face of hemorrhage, for example, the woman's body will use peripheral vasoconstriction. The uterus is a peripheral organ in a shock response, so the blood supply to the uterus will be greatly diminished and the nutrient supply to the fetus greatly compromised (see Assessing the Effects of Trauma in the Pregnant Woman).

The woman's total plasma volume increases during pregnancy from approximately 2,600 mL to 4,000 mL at term. This increase serves as a safeguard to the woman if trauma with bleeding should occur because the woman can lose more blood than normal (up to 30% of her blood volume) before hypovolemia is clinically evident. This also means, however, that fluid replacement volume will undoubtedly have to be high because the woman needs more fluid than the nonpregnant woman to restore her circulatory volume. The central venous pressure (normal is 0 to 5 cm H_2O in a

FOCUS ON FAMILY EMPOWERMENT

Preventive Measures to Reduce Accidents During Pregnancy

Q. I feel so clumsy since I'm pregnant. What can I do to make sure that I don't have an accident?

A. To help reduce your risk for accidental injury during pregnancy, follow these guidelines:

- Don't stand on stepstools or stepladders (it is difficult to maintain balance on a narrow base).
- Keep small items such as toys out of pathways (a pregnant woman has difficulty seeing her feet).
- Avoid throw rugs without a nonskid backing.
- Use caution stepping in and out of a bathtub.
- Do not overload electrical circuits (it is difficult for a pregnant woman to escape a fire because of poor mobility).
- Do not smoke so falling asleep with a cigarette will not be a problem.
- Do not take medicine in the dark so an error is not apt to occur.
- Avoid handling any toxic substances at work.
- Avoid working to a point of fatigue, because this lowers judgment.
- Avoid long periods of standing, because this can lead to a drop in your blood pressure, causing you to feel dizzy and faint.
- Always use a seatbelt while driving or as a passenger in an automobile.
- Refuse to ride with anyone who has been drinking alcohol or whose judgment might be impaired.

ASSESSING the Effects of Trauma in the Pregnant Woman

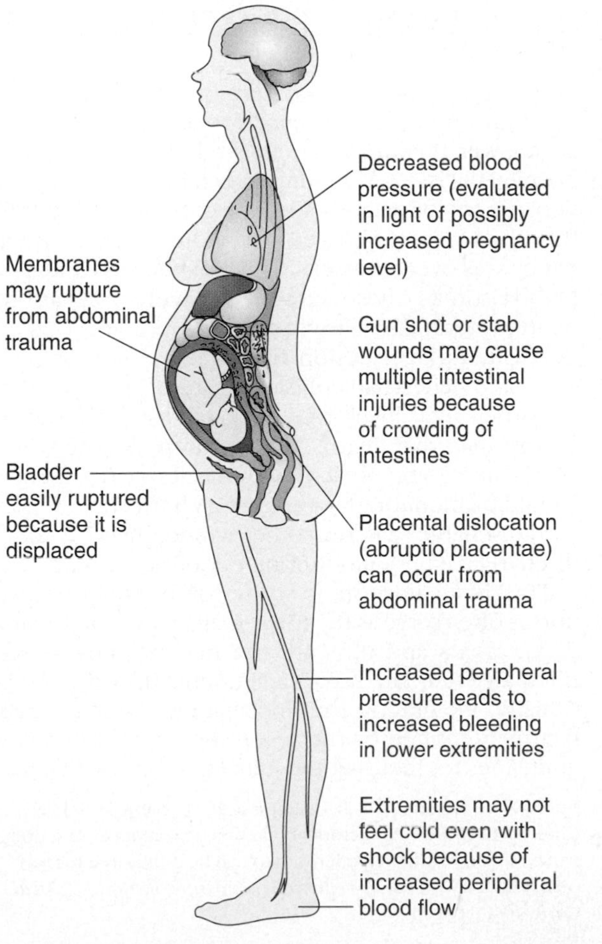
Decreased blood pressure (evaluated in light of possibly increased pregnancy level)
Membranes may rupture from abdominal trauma
Gun shot or stab wounds may cause multiple intestinal injuries because of crowding of intestines
Bladder easily ruptured because it is displaced
Placental dislocation (abruptio placentae) can occur from abdominal trauma
Increased peripheral pressure leads to increased bleeding in lower extremities
Extremities may not feel cold even with shock because of increased peripheral blood flow

nonpregnant state) is increased to 2 to 7 cm H_2O. Although the woman needs a large amount of replacement fluid, this means her circulation can also be overwhelmed more easily than normal by intravenous fluid infusion.

To accommodate the increased vascular load of pregnancy, cardiac output increases from 1 L/min early in pregnancy to 6 to 7 L/min in the second trimester. This volume circulates through the placenta at a rapid rate: approximately one sixth of the total blood volume is present in the placenta at all times. Thus, a uterine laceration is always serious because up to one sixth of blood volume can be quickly lost.

To move this increased blood volume adequately through the circulation, the heart rate increases 15 to 20 beats above normal, so a pulse rate of 80 to 95 is normal. Thus, do not automatically assume that a rapid pulse rate indicates hemorrhage. In addition, since the heart is displaced by the elevated diaphragm, an ECG will show a left axis deviation.

Peripheral venous pressure in the pregnant woman is unchanged. However, it tends to be higher in the lower extremities because of compression of the vena cava and back pressure. As a result, lacerations of the legs or perineum bleed much more profusely than usual. Peripheral blood flow in general is increased due to decreased peripheral vascular resistance (the effect of estrogen and decreased sympathetic activity all through pregnancy). As a result, the pregnant woman can be in severe shock, yet her extremities will still not feel cold and clammy.

During pregnancy, the leukocyte count rises (to 20,000 mm^3 at term). Thus, it is difficult to use this determination as a sign of infection after an open wound. The serum albumin level decreases during pregnancy, making the large loss that normally occurs with burns a more serious response than usual. Serum liver enzyme levels (i.e., serum glutamic-oxaloacetic transaminase, serum glutamate pyruvate transaminase, and lactate dehydrogenase) remain the same during pregnancy. If these are elevated after trauma, liver trauma can be detected. Since levels of alkaline phosphatase, a substance also usually helpful in detecting liver trauma, are three to four times greater in the pregnant woman at term than normally (from placental origin), this marker loses its importance. Because pancreatic amylase levels remain unchanged during pregnancy, the pancreas can be evaluated as usual.

Abdominal pain is difficult to localize during pregnancy because organs are pushed aside by the growing uterus. The abdomen often feels tense during pregnancy, so guarding and rigidity of the abdominal wall may be lost as important findings. Bleeding into the abdominal cavity with an abdominal injury is apt to be forceful and extreme because of the increased pressure in the pelvic vessels. A procedure such as a needle paracentesis to assess for bleeding into the abdominal cavity is dangerous because the bowel, dislocated from its usual position, can be easily punctured. Culdocentesis, or needle aspiration through the posterior vaginal fornix into the peritoneal cavity, may be done. Peritoneal lavage (the process of inserting a peritoneal dialysis catheter into the abdominal cavity, adding a liter of an isotonic solution, aspirating it again, and analyzing it for blood or urine) may reveal bleeding or bladder rupture best.

The bladder of a pregnant woman is susceptible to rupture because it is the most anterior organ and is elevated abnormally. After abdominal trauma, an indwelling bladder catheter is often inserted to assess for blood in the urine.

Psychosocial Considerations

When a pregnant woman is seen at a health care facility after an accident, she is apprehensive and frightened, both for herself and for the health of the fetus. She is worried not only about what has happened but also about what could have happened (if the knife had slipped an inch farther, if the automobile accident had been worse, if she had fallen from farther up the stepladder) and about what medical care will be required (does she need an x-ray?; if she does, will this be safe for the fetus?). She may feel guilty about her carelessness (if she were really a good mother she would have had her seatbelt fastened or not tried to stand on a stepladder to hang drapes alone). A feeling of guilt lowers her self-esteem and increases her level of stress. Remember that people under stress do not process information well and so may not perceive correctly the information given to them. Always try to review information with a woman at a later date to be certain that she does have the facts of her injury and has an accurate understanding of the follow-up care needed.

Assessment

Assessment of the injured pregnant woman must be done quickly yet thoroughly and must include both her psychological and physical status. A pregnant woman may be so concerned with her fetus' health that she does not realize she is injured. Another woman might not even consider the possibility that her fetus could be injured until someone asks if she has felt the fetus move since the accident (not realizing that a loss of blood from her leg would affect uterine blood flow). Assessment should be done concurrently with supportive reassurance ("Your blood pressure is low but the fetal heart beat sounds good") to try to relieve her fear of fetal damage. Use a Doppler method of assessing fetal heart tones if possible to demonstrate to the woman and yourself that the fetus still appears to be well. External monitoring of fetal heart rate and uterine contractions best rules out fetal distress and preterm labor (see Focus on Evidence-Based Practice).

In an emergency situation, a woman needs her support people around her. Locate them as necessary and also assess their reaction to the trauma.

Health History

In an emergency situation, a few minutes spent attempting to calm the woman and move her past her initial fright is time well spent unless symptoms of major body system disturbances require that immediate efforts need to be directed elsewhere. Reducing the woman's level of anxiety will enhance her ability to cooperate with the history and physical assessment.

Take a brief pregnancy history as well as a trauma history (i.e., length of pregnancy or any complications). Ask specifically if fetal heart tones have been heard by an examiner during the pregnancy, if she has felt the fetus move since the accident, if she has any sensation of tightening or pain in her abdomen that could be uterine contractions, and if she knows what her prepregnancy and

FOCUS ON EVIDENCE-BASED PRACTICE

Following Trauma, Which Pregnant Women Are Most Apt to Begin Preterm Labor?

To answer this question, researchers reviewed the hospital charts of 271 women seen in the emergency department following some type of trauma. Results of this chart review showed that women whose pregnancy was over 35 weeks who had been assaulted or involved in a pedestrian collision were most apt to be in preterm labor. Factors most predictive of fetal death included ejection from the vehicle, motorcycle and pedestrian collision, maternal tachycardia, abnormal fetal heart rate, lack of restraint, and of course maternal death. The researchers concluded that women who present with the above risk factors should be monitored for at least 24 hours before hospital discharge, whereas other women may be safely discharged after a monitoring period of 6 hours.

This is an important study for nurses because nurses often serve as the triage manager in emergency departments and thus are the first persons to see trauma victims and take initial trauma histories. Additionally, integrating the information about the risk factors identified by the researchers provides some guidelines for focusing the initial trauma assessment.

Curet, M. J., Schermer, C. R., Demarest, B. G., Bieneik, E. J., & Curet, L. B. (2000). Predictors of outcome in trauma during pregnancy: Identification of patients who can be monitored for less than 6 hours. *Journal of Trauma-Injury Infection and Critical Care, 49*(1), 18–25.

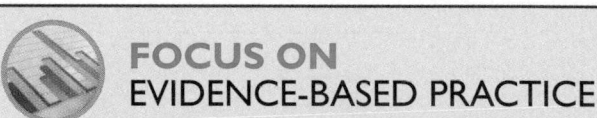

pregnancy blood pressures have been to help evaluate the extent of blood loss from the trauma.

Document the circumstances of the trauma: what happened, the time that has passed since the injury, signs and symptoms of injury the woman is experiencing, and actions she has taken to counteract these.

If the woman fell, for example, how far did she fall? (A fall from the top of a stepladder is more likely to be serious than a fall from a low rung.) What body part did she land on? (Landing on her abdomen may be very serious, although she may be in less pain than if she injured a wrist in the fall.) For an automobile accident, ask how fast the car was traveling, if she was thrown from the car, or if the windshield broke (generally in automobile accidents, windshields are broken from the impact of a head striking the windshield; thus, the woman needs to be assessed for a head injury).

As a final measure, assess whether the woman's degree of injury is in proportion to the history. Injuries out of proportion to the history (a woman states that she tripped on her front steps, but you notice that all her extremities are ecchymotic and her jaw is broken) suggest intimate partner abuse rather than a simple accident. Analyze also whether the woman seemed to be using a sensible degree of caution for the circumstances. If not, assess her awareness of safety precautions. In rare situations, a woman may self-inflict injury in an attempt to end an unwanted pregnancy; this too must be determined. A naive adolescent, for example, may attempt to end a pregnancy by a deliberate fall or poisoning, which she then reports as an accident.

Physical Examination

Accidents become fatal when lung, heart, kidney, or brain function becomes inadequate; fetal health is in jeopardy when uteroplacental function is impaired. Therefore, it is important to evaluate these body systems first (Table 14-5).

With multiple trauma, a nasogastric tube is usually passed to empty the stomach. A Foley catheter is inserted to assess urine output and to rule out a ruptured bladder (blood would return or urine would be blood-tinged if bleeding were occurring).

To prevent supine hypotension syndrome, be certain the woman does not lie supine for an examination. If it is necessary for her to lie on her back, manually displace the uterus from the vena cava by placing rolled towels or a blanket under her right side to tip her body approximately 15 degrees to the side. If surgery is necessary, the operating room table can be tipped to achieve this same effect.

TABLE 14.5 Initial Assessments After Trauma During Pregnancy

BODY SYSTEM	ASSESSMENT
Respiratory system	Quality of respirations (labored or even?)
	Rate of respirations
	Sounds of obstruction (wheezing, retractions, coughing?)
	Color (cyanotic?)
	Oxygen hunger (inability to lie flat, nasal flaring?)
Cardiovascular system	Color (pallor from hemorrhage?)
	Gross bleeding
	Pulse rate (increases with hemorrhage)
	Blood pressure (decreases with hemorrhage)
	Feeling of apprehension from altered vascular pressure?
Nervous system	Level of consciousness (woman answers questions coherently?)
	Pupils (equal and reacting to light?)
	Bruises or bump on head or spinal column
	Loss of motion or sensory function in a body part
Renal system	Bruising on anterior abdominal wall over bladder or on back over kidneys
	Blood in urine
Uterine-fetal system	Bradycardia, tachycardia, or absence of fetal heart tones or loss of variability on fetal monitor
	Vaginal bleeding
	Clear (amniotic) fluid leaking from vagina
	Bruising on abdomen over uterus

NURSING DIAGNOSES AND RELATED INTERVENTIONS

Nursing care during the initial phase of an emergency focuses on stabilizing the woman and protecting the fetus. Examples of nursing diagnoses that would be appropriate are:

- Fear related to threat of injury to the fetus
- Risk for fetal injury related to apparent suicide attempt
- Ineffective tissue perfusion related to severed artery
- Ineffective breathing pattern related to lung lacerated by gunshot wound

Once the immediate emergency phase has passed, nursing diagnoses will focus on prevention of more severe injury and alleviation of emotional distress and will depend on the type of injury received. Examples are:

- Risk for infection related to loss of skin integrity or wound contamination
- Situational low self-esteem related to occurrence of accident
- Powerlessness related to seriousness of the injury sustained or inability to prevent accident from occurring

Therapeutic Management

Planning in an emergency always involves two phases: planning for immediate care to stabilize the client and planning for continuing care once the emergency has passed.

Implementations in emergency situations must be done quickly yet always remembering that the woman's primary health condition is that she is pregnant.

If respirations are not present or are ineffective, cardiopulmonary resuscitation (CPR) should begin the same as with any person after trauma (see Nursing Procedure 14-1). To be certain the woman has not just fainted, try to rouse her by calling her name or shaking her shoulders. If this is unsuccessful, assess whether her airway is obstructed by holding your cheek next to her nostrils and assessing for air exchange, and look in her mouth for a foreign object. If she is not breathing, pull her chin forward and, using a resuscitation bag, administer two breaths. Although an enlarged uterus puts considerable pressure on the diaphragm and consequently the lungs, only normal pressure is necessary to inflate the lungs fully in a resuscitation attempt. Assess cardiovascular function by palpating the carotid pulse. If this is not palpable or the pupils are fixed, heart function must also be supplemented. Begin external heart massage at a rate of two breaths to every 15 heart compressions (one rescuer) or one breath to 5 cardiac compressions for two rescuers (the same as for all adults). Cardiac massage may be awkward late in pregnancy because of the size of the uterus, but undue pressure should not be necessary to create heart action. Cardioversion is done according to the usual agency protocol.

After assessment of the level of consciousness and cardiovascular and respiratory status, if there has been blood loss, a central venous pressure line may be inserted and lactated Ringer's or another isotonic solution infused to restore fluid volume or provide an open line for emergency medication.

If hypotension is present, it must be corrected quickly to maintain a pressure gradient across the placenta. However, any antihypotensive agent that achieves increased blood pressure by causing peripheral vasoconstriction is contraindicated (vessels in the uterus would constrict). Ephedrine is the drug of choice with a pregnant woman to restore blood pressure because it has a minimal peripheral vasoconstrictive effect. Dopamine in low doses is a second drug that can be used. After emergency interventions, care depends on the specific injury or trauma present.

NURSING DIAGNOSES AND RELATED INTERVENTIONS

Nursing Diagnosis: Risk for ineffective tissue perfusion related to blood loss from trauma

Outcome Identification: Client will demonstrate signs of adequate tissue perfusion for the next 24 hours.

Outcome Evaluation: Client's blood pressure is above 100/60 mm Hg; pulse below 100 bpm; no signs of labor are present; fetal heart rate is 120 to 160 bpm; nonstress test shows good variability.

NURSING PROCEDURE 14.1: CPR DURING PREGNANCY

Purpose
To restore respiratory and cardiac function.

Plan	Principle
1. Shake the woman's shoulders and shout.	1. Shaking the shoulders and shouting are an attempt to determine unconsciousness and to rouse the woman to ensure that she has not fainted.
2. Lift the chin to position the airway.	2. Lifting the chin aids in straightening the airway to ensure that it is patent.
3. Establish lack of respirations by listening and feeling for air movement.	3. Listening and feeling for air movement provides evidence of breathing.
4. Begin rescue breathing with administration of 2 quick breathing-bag breaths.	4. Rescue breathing introduces oxygen for gas exchange.
5. Assess carotid pulse.	5. Presence of carotid pulse indicates cardiac function.
6. Begin chest compressions if there is no carotid pulse. Continue until resuscitation is complete. a. With one rescuer, place both hands on the lower sternum just above xiphoid process and deliver 15 chest compressions followed by 2 rescue breaths until cardiopulmonary function returns. b. With two rescuers, deliver 5 chest compressions followed by 1 breath.	6. External chest compressions simulate the action of the heart to maintain tissue perfusion.
7. Place a rolled or folded towel under the woman's hips.	7. A towel placed under one hip helps to prevent uterine compression of the vena cava.

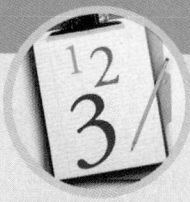

Open Wounds

A number of types of wounds occur with trauma.

Lacerations. A laceration (a jagged cut) may involve only the skin layer or may penetrate to deeper subcutaneous tissue or tendons. Lacerations generally bleed profusely. Bleeding should be halted by pressure on the edge of the laceration (this is difficult to achieve in lower extremities because venous pressure is greatly increased in pregnancy). After cleaning, the area is sutured through each layer of tissue involved to approximate the edges. For sutures to be used, a local anesthetic such as Xylocaine is necessary. Because this has only a local effect, it is safe to use during pregnancy. If the laceration is superficial and the woman is nervous about the use of an anesthetic, the edges can be approximated with a butterfly strip made from a commercial adhesive strip. This will allow it to heal, although with a slightly more noticeable scar. Antishock trousers should be used with caution to halt lower extremity bleeding because the top of these trousers may exert pressure on the uterus, pressing it against the vena cava and causing a supine hypotension syndrome.

Because the white blood cell count is normally elevated during pregnancy, a single count is a poor indicator of the presence or extent of infection in wounds. However, serial measurements can be valuable.

Puncture Wounds. A puncture wound results from penetration of a sharp object such as a nail, splinter, nail file, or knife. Puncture wounds bleed little—an advantage in terms of minimizing blood loss but not in terms of wound cleaning. A puncture wound is usually not sutured because suturing would create a sealed, unoxygenated cavity below the sutures with a space where tetanus bacilli can grow. If the woman has had a tetanus immunization within the past 10 years, tetanus toxoid is administered. If the woman did not have a tetanus immunization within 10 years (the usual condition), tetanus toxoid plus immune tetanus globulin is administered. These are both considered safe to administer during pregnancy.

Puncture wounds are frightening because the average woman knows they can have severe consequences from tetanus. This type of wound also usually occurs in association with a degree of violence.

Knife wounds cause deep penetration and are often directed into the abdomen. They may easily reach the depth of the uterus, possibly directly injuring the fetus. Most stab wounds of the abdomen, however, occur in the upper quadrants of the abdomen, above the height of the uterus. To determine the depth and extent of the wound, a fistulogram may be done. This involves insertion of a thin catheter into the wound; the wound is then filled with radiopaque solution. An x-ray of the area filled by the solution will reveal the extent of the puncture. If the peritoneal cavity was perforated, dye will outline the intestines. If there is a suspicion of bleeding into the abdominal cavity, a celiotomy or an exploratory surgical procedure into the abdominal cavity may be performed. Surgery this close to the uterus usually does not result in disruption of the pregnancy. If the diaphragm was cut, the intestines may herniate into the chest cavity (diaphragmatic hernia) due to the increased abdominal pressure from the enlarged uterus. After surgical repair of an injured diaphragm, cesarean birth may be planned to avoid strain on a newly repaired diaphragm during labor. The uterus appears to have a natural resistance to infection, so even if it is punctured, infection in the uterus rarely occurs.

Animal Bites. Pregnant women are rarely bitten by any animal but a dog. Animal bites are a form of puncture wound, so if the rabies immunization status of the dog is known, the wound is washed and treated as a puncture wound. If the dog cannot be located or is proved to be rabid after 48 hours of observation, the woman must be administered rabies immune globulin and vaccine. Pregnancy is not a contraindication to rabies immunization because contracting the disease would be much more serious.

Pregnant women should be advised to use caution and avoid contact with unfamiliar dogs. Also, if the woman is camping in a remote location, for example, she should be cautioned to avoid feeding any wild animals such as squirrels and raccoons.

Blunt Abdominal Trauma

Blunt trauma occurs generally from automobile accidents, when the woman's abdomen strikes the steering wheel or dashboard, or from someone deliberately kicking or punching her abdomen. No visible break is present in the skin. After the injury, the underlying tissue becomes edematous; broken underlying blood vessels may ooze and form ecchymosis or a hematoma at the site. To assess if there is abdominal bleeding, a diagnostic peritoneal lavage may be done by introducing a small amount of normal saline by a syringe and then withdrawing it to see if blood is evident. Ultrasound may also be used.

Careful assessment that the pregnancy has not been harmed must be made because a traumatic blow to the abdomen could cause dislodgement of the placenta (abruptio placentae) or preterm labor. Palpate the uterus for any abnormal contours that would suggest edema or internal bleeding, and count fetal heart tones. Using a Doppler instrument is helpful to assure the woman that her fetus is unharmed. Real-time sonography may also be helpful in showing that the uterus and placenta are intact. A pelvic examination is usually performed to assess for vaginal bleeding or seepage of clear fluid that would suggest rupture of the amniotic membranes. If the woman reports uterine contractions, uterine and fetal monitoring is necessary to estimate the strength and effect of contractions on the fetal heart rate and also determine if preterm labor has begun. Magnesium sulfate is usually selected to halt preterm labor after trauma because it has fewer hemodynamic effects than beta-mimetic drugs (see Chap. 15 for a full discussion of these drugs).

The possibility that placental blood will enter the maternal circulation with uterine trauma is a threat to the Rh-negative woman. Rh-negative women are therefore typically administered Rh immune globulin after trauma. The presence of fetal blood cells in the maternal bloodstream can be documented by a Kleihauer-Betke test (on staining, maternal cells remain colorless; fetal cells turn purple-pink).

Gunshot Wounds

A woman may receive a gunshot wound as an intended victim or an innocent bystander; occasionally, a woman attempts suicide by a gunshot wound. Assessment of the wound includes inspection for the point where the bullet entered the body and also the point where the bullet exited (the entry wound is small but the exit wound is large because as a bullet slows, it begins to tumble, enlarging the space it occupies). The uterine wall is so thick during pregnancy that it may trap a bullet; thus, there may be no exit point from her body if the uterus was punctured. If the bullet entered high in the abdomen, the intestines will surely be injured; because so much is compressed above the uterus, the intestines may sustain many tears from one bullet.

Gunshot wounds are surgically cleaned and debrided, and the woman is treated with a high-dose antibiotic. Ampicillin, a drug safe during pregnancy, is frequently prescribed. If a bullet enters the uterus, the incidence of fetal mortality is high, especially if the placenta is torn by the bullet. After providing emergency care to the woman for the injury, it is important to investigate carefully the circumstances of the injury. Gunshot wounds must be reported to the police. Stay with the woman as necessary while she recounts her history of the accident again for law enforcement officers.

Poisoning

Pregnant women are not apt to swallow a poison, although this can occur accidentally, especially if a woman wakes at night and attempts to take medicine in the dark. Food poisoning from inadequately refrigerated or undercooked foods can occur. Poisoning can reflect a suicide attempt.

Poisoning in the pregnant woman is managed the same as in any individual. The woman should telephone the local poison control center, state that she is pregnant and what she accidentally swallowed, and follow the specific recommendation of personnel at the poison control center. Syrup of ipecac (15 mL followed by a glass of water) is the best emetic to cause vomiting and discharge of the poison from her body and is safe for use during pregnancy. However, no ipecac should be taken until the woman has checked with the poison control center because some poisons can be more harmful if vomited than if allowed to remain in the body. Activated charcoal may also be used.

After the woman has been treated and the emergency of the poisoning is over, investigate carefully the circumstances of the poisoning to help the woman learn about safety with medications or to discover possible suicidal intent.

Choking

If a pregnant woman chokes on a piece of meat or any foreign object blocks the airway, attempting to dislodge the object with a sudden upward thrust to the upper abdomen (a Heimlich maneuver) is difficult. This is because of a lack of space between the uterus and the end of the sternum and because a person cannot reach from the rear around the woman's enlarged abdomen. Late in pregnancy, therefore, a rescuer might use successive chest thrusts instead. Nursing Procedure 14-2 describes how to perform chest thrusts for a pregnant woman.

Orthopedic Injuries

Because a woman has poor balance late in pregnancy, she may trip more readily than usual; when she falls, she automatically reaches out a hand to cushion the fall and to prevent landing on her abdomen. Due to her extra weight, this may result in a serious wrist injury. Apply ice to the area to decrease swelling as an immediate first-aid measure. An x-ray may be necessary to determine whether a fracture is present. Assure the woman that an x-ray of an extremity is safe during pregnancy as long as her abdomen is shielded during the radiation exposure. Delegate someone to accompany her to the x-ray department and remain with her (outside the actual x-ray room) to ensure that lead protection is offered to her. Also caution this person to be alert if signs of preterm labor should suddenly develop as a result of an undetected injury.

Because women of childbearing age are usually healthy, healing of fractures or torn ligaments generally occurs quickly and without complications. Be certain a woman can identify good calcium food sources if she has a fracture so both she and the fetus can have adequate calcium for new bone growth.

Because many more adolescent girls and young adult women participate in sports today than ever before, an increasing number of women of childbearing age have weakened knee cartilage from having dislocated a knee joint during active sports play (formerly thought of only as a football injury). During pregnancy, when all body cartilage softens, combined with the excessive abdominal weight the woman carries, the woman may dislocate her knee again.

Any woman who has had a previous knee injury should have it reevaluated early in pregnancy. A support device such as a knee immobilizer may be required for the last 3 months of pregnancy to keep the joint from dislocating again. Discuss with her the advantage of prevention because if the knee cartilage cannot sustain her added weight and dislocates again, she may fall. In addition, she may then need to wear an immobilizer for approximately 6 weeks for therapy. Preventing the dislocation minimizes the risk for possible injury due to a fall and will allow her to be fully mobile at the time she has a new child to care for. She can be assured that a knee immobilizer in place at the time of birth will not interfere with birth; if a lithotomy position and stirrups for birth are necessary, a modified stirrups position can be devised for her.

The laxness of body cartilage may also cause separation of the symphysis pubis if a woman falls with her legs outspread. Many women experience some nagging suprapubic joint pain during pregnancy. A suture separation this way, however, is very painful, especially on walking or turning. To avoid pain and allow the cartilage to heal, the woman needs to remain on bed rest at home for 4 to

NURSING PROCEDURE 14.2: CHEST THRUSTS FOR THE PREGNANT WOMAN

Purpose
To relieve tracheal aspiration.

Plan	Principle
For Conscious Victim in Standing Position	***For Conscious Victim in Standing Position***
1. Stand behind the woman and encircle her chest with your arms.	1. Proper positioning ensures proper placement of chest pressure and prevents inadvertent injury to underlying body structures.

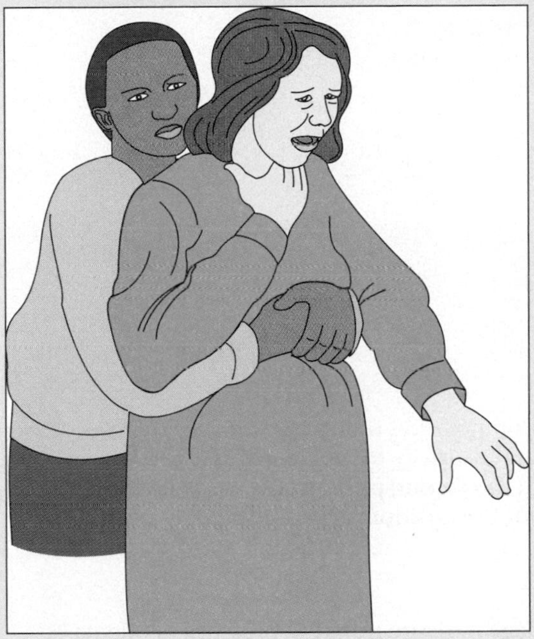

Plan	Principle
2. Place the thumb side of your fist on the middle of the woman's sternum.	2. Placement of fist against the chest ensures a solid structure for compression.

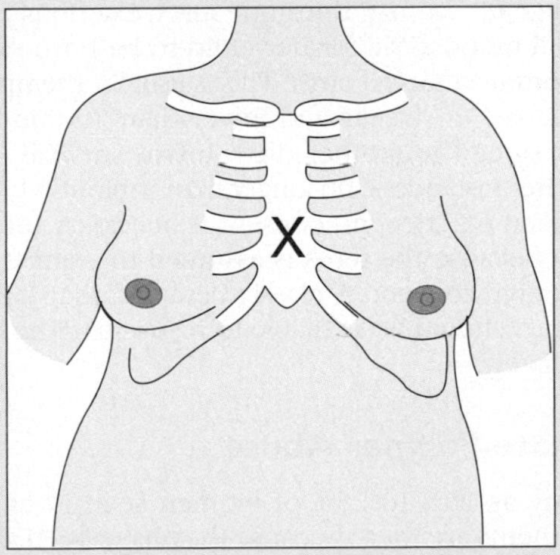

Plan	Principle
3. Grab the fist with the other hand and perform backward thrusts until the foreign body is expelled.	3. Pressure on the chest compresses the ribs, increasing chest and lung pressure. This increased pressure forces an object lodged in the airway to move upward.

(continued)

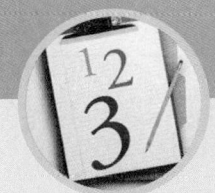

Plan	Principle
For Unconscious Victim in Supine Position	***For Unconscious Victim in Supine Position***
1. Place the woman in the same position as for external heart compressions (heel of the hand on the lower sternum). 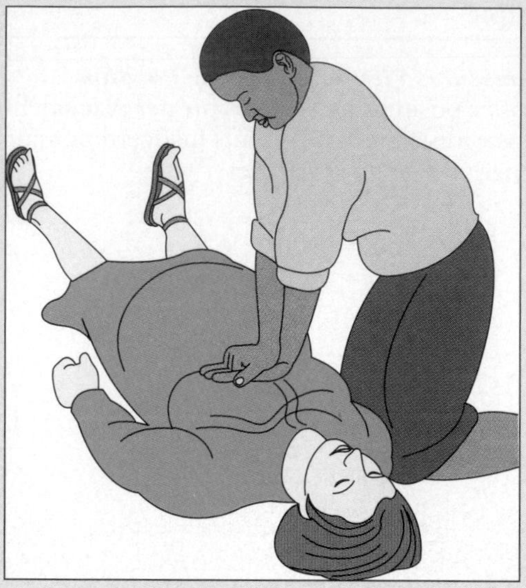	1. Loss of consciousness interferes with the woman's ability to maintain an upright position.
2. Follow Steps 2 and 3 as with standing victim.	2. Compression of the chest forces the object lodged in the airway to move upward. Chest compression in the supine position can be as effective in the supine position as in the standing position.

6 weeks. If separation of the symphysis pubis is present at the time of birth, this may make labor more painful, especially the pelvic division of labor as the fetus is pushed through the pelvic ring.

Burns

Burns are dangerous to the pregnant woman because of both the thermal injury that occurs and the inhalation of carbon monoxide gases from the fire, which can lead to extreme fetal hypoxia as carbon monoxide crosses the placenta in place of oxygen (Taggart & Parry, 1999). Smoke is irritating to lung tissue and can result in extensive lung edema; this can cause additional fetal hypoxia due to the lack of oxygen–carbon dioxide exchange space. Because the fluid and electrolyte loss can be great with burns, hypotension from hypovolemia or an electrolyte imbalance can occur. In response to a severe trauma such as a burn, prostaglandins are produced, possibly causing preterm labor. Both maternal and fetal prognoses are poor if burns cover more than 50% of body surface area. Fortunately, few women of childbearing age experience this degree of burn in the United States.

Interestingly, burn tissue heals more quickly than normal during pregnancy. This is probably related to the overall increased metabolism and possibly to the increased corticosteroid serum level that prevents inflammation and damage to tissue from the pressure of edema.

Postmortem Cesarean Birth

If a pregnant woman does not survive serious trauma, it may still be possible for her child to be born safely by a postmortem cesarean birth. This is usually attempted if the fetus is past 24 weeks and fewer than 20 minutes have passed since the mother died. Infant survival is best in these circumstances if no longer than 5 minutes has passed. By general practice, no consent is necessary for this procedure because the fetus is assumed to want to live but cannot give consent. A classic cesarean incision is used. Personnel should be available to resuscitate the newborn immediately.

Intimate Partner Abuse

As many as 20% to 25% of women seen in emergency departments are there because they have been abused by their intimate partner (Campbell et al., 2000). Abused women may be pregnant because they were unable to resist sexual advances from an abusive partner. The woman may desire the pregnancy very much because she thinks that having a child will change the partner and make him a better person. She may be grateful, thinking that by having an infant she will have someone to love her. Intimate partner abuse may increase during pregnancy because stress is often a trigger to beatings, and pregnancy, with all that an expected new child entails (another mouth to feed, body to clothe, or dependent to protect), can increase stress.

Although it is impossible to predict how any individual woman will respond to pregnancy, abused women may demonstrate behaviors that reveal abuse. An abused woman may come for care late in pregnancy or not at all because her partner may control her transportation or money; she may fear that a health care provider will identify and report the abuse; or she may have been pretending that the pregnancy did not exist to reduce stress in her home. She may be noticeable in a prenatal setting because she has purchased no maternity clothing (she has no funds for herself and asking for money may incite violence). She may decline laboratory tests if they involve transportation or money.

The abused woman may have difficulty following a recommended pregnancy diet (she must cook what her partner wants or she will be beaten). She may leave before the nurse-midwife or physician sees her at a prenatal setting, or she may grow anxious if her appointment is running late (she must be home to cook dinner or risk a beating).

She may call and cancel appointments frequently (or simply not keep appointments) because she has an obvious black eye or a bleeding facial laceration she does not want to reveal. She may dress inappropriately for warm weather, wearing long-sleeved, tight-necked blouses to cover up bruises on her neck or arms. When undressed for a physical examination, there may be bruises or lacerations on her breasts, abdomen, or back that she cannot explain. Her neck may reveal linear bruises from strangulation. Ask any woman with bruises to account for them. Listen to see whether the explanation seems to correlate with the extent and placement of a bruise or laceration (see Assessing the Abused Pregnant Woman).

The woman who has experienced abuse may be anxious to listen to the baby's heartbeat at prenatal visits because her partner recently punched or kicked her abdomen and she is worried that the fetus has been hurt. Minimal placental infarcts from blunt abdominal trauma may lead to poor placental perfusion and low birthweight. If abdominal trauma is suspected, a sonogram may be done because this is the most accurate method of assessing fetal health after trauma. Fetal heart tones and fundal height should also be recorded.

ASSESSING the Abused Pregnant Woman

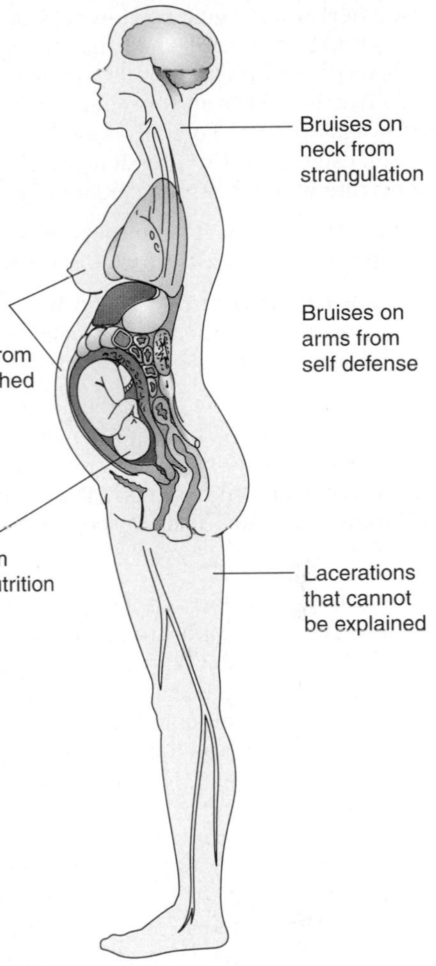

NURSING DIAGNOSES AND RELATED INTERVENTIONS

Nursing diagnoses for the abused woman may pertain to physical injuries sustained, but they should also address the emotional manifestations of abuse and suggest her need to seek help. Some examples include:

- Powerlessness related to perception that it is impossible to break away from abusing partner
- Fear related to constant threat of violence
- Social isolation related to client's need to hide evidence of her abuse
- Ineffective denial related to inability to face the fact that partner is abusive
- Compromised family coping related to dysfunctional relationship between client and abusive partner

Goals of care should address ways to keep the woman safe from further abuse. Expected outcomes should be specific tasks the woman could accomplish to meet the goals, such as:

- Client carries phone number of home for abused women with her.
- Client and abusive partner continue to attend counseling sessions.
- Client states she has filed restraining order against abusive partner.
- Client states she feels secure living at safe house.

It may be difficult to work with an abused woman who will not leave an abusive situation because it is hard to understand why she stays in the situation. A common finding is that the woman is immobilized and unable to leave from fear of the abusive person (he has threatened that if she leaves, he will find her and kill her) and the guilt and low self-esteem she feels (he has told her so many times that this is her fault and she deserves to be treated this way that she believes it). To free herself from this emotional paralysis, she needs outside help. To compound the problem, her low self-esteem and depression lead her to believe that no one would be interested in helping her.

Nursing Diagnosis: Chronic low self-esteem related to continuing physical and mental abuse

Outcome Identification: Client will express positive aspects about herself, realistically describing the situation she is in by 3 months' time.

Outcome Evaluation: Client identifies positive traits about self; begins to discuss possible reasons why she has remained in an abusive situation; makes concrete, realistic plans for future; states that she feels able, with continuing help and outside resources, to protect herself in future.

Until she can develop better self-esteem, the abused woman may need support to make even simple decisions. Support any ability to make constructive decisions that she has left. Be familiar with safe shelters for abused women in the community; discuss with her how she can call the police at any time and they will take her to the shelter. Help her obtain a restraining order to keep the abusive person from coming near her again if this is necessary.

After the birth of the child, assuming the woman moved away from the abuser, she may begin to feel depressed because she is lonely. This may lead to her having unreal expectations of the child, trying to make the infant smile at her and interact with her more than a newborn is capable of in order to have someone to love her. Caution her that her newborn does love her but she has to give the child time to grow. Demonstrate all the things the child can do, such as attend to the sound of her voice or cuddle against her. Without this awareness, her unreal expectations can lead to disappointment and can interfere with mothering. Do not leave an abused woman without a support system after the birth of the child. If she was depending on prenatal personnel during her pregnancy, the gap must be filled with another support system. This could be a social agency that deals specifically with abused women in the community; it could be a community health nurse who will be visiting her after she returns home. If she is left without a support person, her low self-esteem may not allow her to reach out and seek help. She may decide that suicide or returning to the abuser is her best recourse. If a woman does return to live with an abusive partner, both the woman and the infant need frequent health care visits scheduled so their health and welfare can be monitored. A child raised in a home where the mother is abused will learn that this is acceptable conduct, and the abuse may extend to yet another generation (see Chap. 55).

✔ CHECKPOINT QUESTIONS

19. Why are lacerations of lower extremities potentially more serious in pregnant women than others?
20. Syrup of ipecac or activated charcoal is the usual therapy for poisoning. Are these safe to administer during pregnancy?
21. What are two common reasons abused women stay with their abusers?

KEY POINTS

A high-risk pregnancy is one in which a concurrent disorder, pregnancy-related complication, or external factor jeopardizes the health of the mother, the fetus, or both.

Pregnancy is a stress to any family because it involves financial expenses plus changes in family roles. If a complication of pregnancy develops, this stress is almost automatically intensified. Families need support during this time to be able to cope with the increased burden.

When women with a preexisting disease become pregnant, a thorough history and physical examination are crucial to obtain at the first prenatal visit to establish a baseline of information on the condition. Documentation of any medication being taken for a secondary condition is also necessary to protect against adverse drug interactions and the possibility of teratogenic action on the fetus.

Teaching is an important nursing intervention because the woman with a preexisting illness must make modifications in her usual therapy to adjust to pregnancy. Pregnancy often stimulates women to learn more about their primary disease as well.

Women who have a complication early in pregnancy may continue to worry about the health of their fetus all during pregnancy. They need to be assured (appropriately) that the episode was temporary and that, with continued monitoring, the fetus should not suffer harm. After giving birth, they may need additional time to spend with their newborns to convince themselves that the infants are healthy so bonding can begin.

Sexually transmitted diseases such as candidiasis, trichomoniasis, chlamydia, syphilis, herpes type 2, gonorrhea, papilloma, and HIV may occur during pregnancy. These illnesses need prompt treatment. Women need to follow safer sex practices to help prevent these diseases.

Because blood volume increases by as much as 50% during pregnancy, cardiac function may become inadequate if cardiovascular disease is present. Illnesses that cause difficulty can be either acquired disorders such as Kawasaki disease and rheumatic fever or congenital disorders such as mitral valve stenosis and coarctation of the aorta.

Various forms of anemia can cause complications of pregnancy; iron-deficiency anemia, sickle cell anemia, and folic acid deficiency-anemia are examples. All these anemias can result in fetal distress because of inadequate oxygen transport.

Urinary tract disorders can lead to pregnancy complications because pregnancy increases the workload of the kidneys. UTIs and chronic renal disease are two disorders that may lead to early pregnancy loss.

Acute nasopharyngitis, asthma, pneumonia, influenza, and tuberculosis are respiratory disorders seen in pregnancy. The incidence of tuberculosis is on the increase, and these patients need special assessment and care.

Juvenile rheumatoid arthritis and systemic lupus erythematosus are examples of rheumatic disorders seen in pregnancy. These disorders generally require large doses of NSAIDs for therapy. Women taking salicylates are advised to decrease use 2 weeks before birth to avoid bleeding disorders in the newborn.

Some gastrointestinal illnesses that occur with pregnancy are hiatal hernia, cholecystitis, viral hepatitis, inflammatory bowel disease, and appendicitis. If surgery is necessary for conditions such as cholecystitis or appendicitis, it can be scheduled during pregnancy but may result in preterm labor.

Recurrent seizure is the most frequently seen neurologic condition during pregnancy. Many drugs used to control seizures are teratogenic; women need to have their medical regimen evaluated before pregnancy to be certain that they are regulated on the fewest medications possible.

The major endocrine disorder seen during pregnancy is diabetes mellitus. Gestational diabetes is diabetes that occurs during pregnancy and fades after it.

Trauma in pregnancy includes automobile accidents and falls. Women with traumatic injuries need to be carefully assessed to determine if intimate partner abuse was the cause of the trauma.

CRITICAL THINKING EXERCISES

1. Angelina Pellegoso, the woman you met at the beginning of the chapter, was seen in an emergency room after an automobile accident. She has multiple injuries. Following a severe injury of this kind, what body systems would you assess first?
2. A 23-year-old woman you care for has gestational diabetes. She is resistant to learning about her condition because she knows that the condition is only temporary and will fade at the end of pregnancy. What type of teaching plan would you devise to help her learn in the face of this attitude?
3. One of the most devastating medical diagnoses today is that of HIV (AIDS). How is this illness a threat to the newborn as well as the mother? Summarize measures nurses can use to help prevent the spread of this disorder. Are there changes a prenatal clinic would have to make to care for an HIV-positive woman?
4. Examine the national health goals related to the family with a complication of pregnancy. Most government-sponsored money for nursing research is allotted based on these goals. What would be a possible research topic to explore pertinent to these goals that would be fundable and would advance evidence-based practice?

REFERENCES

American Diabetes Association. (2001). *New classifications and recommendations for diabetes mellitus.* New York: ADA.

Blackwell, D. A., Elam, S., & Blackwell, J. T. (2000). Cancer and pregnancy; a health care dilemma. *Journal of Obstetric, Gynecologic, & Neonatal Nursing, 29*(4), 405–412.

Campbell, J. C., et al. (2000). Reproductive health consequences of intimate partner violence. *Clinical Nursing Research, 9*(3), 217–237.

Cunningham, F. G., et al. (2001). *Williams obstetrics* (21st ed.). Stamford, CT: Appleton & Lange.

Curet, M. J. et al. (2000). Predictors of outcomes in trauma during pregnancy. *Journal of Trauma-Injury Infection and Critical Care, 49*(1), 18–25.

Davies, T. F., & Cobin, R. H. (2000). Thyroid diseases in pregnancy and the postpartum period. In Ransom, S. B., et al. *Practical strategies in obstetrics and gynecology* (pp. 393–411). Philadelphia: Saunders.

Department of Health and Human Services. (2000). *Healthy people 2010.* Washington, DC: DHHS.

Empson, M. et al. (2002). Recurrent pregnancy loss with antiphospholipid antibody. *Obstetrics & Gynecology, 99*(1), 135–144.

Eschenbach, D. A. (2000). Pelvic infections and sexually transmitted diseases. In Scott, J. R., et al. *Danforth's obstetrics and gynecology* (8th ed., pp. 579–600). Philadelphia: Lippincott Williams & Wilkins.

Esplin, M. S. (2001). Management of antiphospholipid syndrome during pregnancy. *Clinical Obstetrics & Gynecology, 44*(1), 20–28.

Gabbe, S. G., et al. (2000). Benefits, risks, costs, and patient satisfaction associated with insulin pump therapy for the pregnancy complicated by type I diabetes mellitus. *American Journal of Obstetrics & Gynecology, 182*(6), 1283–1291.

Genc, M., & Ledger, W. J. (2000). Syphilis in pregnancy. *Sexually Transmitted Infections, 76*(2), 73–79.

Gilson, G. J., et al. (2000). Prevention of group B streptococcus early-onset neonatal sepsis. *Journal of Perinatology, 20*(8), 491–495.

Graham, E. M. (2001). Infectious complications of pregnancy: maternal and fetal. In Seifer, D. B., Samuels, P., & Kniss, D. A. (Eds.). *The physiologic basis of gynecology and obstetrics.* Philadelphia: Lippincott Williams & Wilkins.

Holing, E. V. (2000). Preconception care of women with diabetes: the unrevealed obstacles. *Journal of Maternal-Fetal Medicine, 9*(1), 10–13.

Ie, S., et al. (2002). Respiratory complications of pregnancy. *Obstetrical & Gynecological Survey, 57*(1), 39–46.

Johnson, M., Maas, M., & Moorhead, S. (2000). *Nursing outcomes classification* (2nd ed.). St. Louis: Mosby.

Jovanovic, L. (2000). Medical emergencies in the patient with diabetes during pregnancy. *Endocrinology & Metabolism Clinics of North America, 29*(4), 771–787.

Karch, A. M. (2001). *Lippincott's nursing drug guide.* Philadelphia: Lippincott Williams & Wilkins.

Kuper, B. C., & Failla, S. (2000). Systemic lupus erythematosus: A multisystem autoimmune disorder. *Nursing Clinics of North America, 35*(1), 253–265.

Kuzuga, T. (2000). Early diagnosis, early treatment and the new diagnostic criteria of diabetes mellitus. *British Journal of Nutrition, 84*(2 supp), S177–181.

Langer, O. (2000). Diabetes. In Ransom, S. B., et al. *Practical strategies in obstetrics and gynecology* (pp. 413–427). Philadelphia: Saunders.

Llewelyn, M., et al. (2000). Tuberculosis diagnosed during pregnancy. *Thorax, 55*(2), 129–132.

Lo, B., et al. (2000). Ethical issues in early detection of HIV infection to reduce vertical transmission. *Journal of Acquired Immune Deficiency Syndromes, 25*(2S), S136–S143.

Lockwood, C. J., & Paidas, M. J. (2000). Preeclampsia and hypertensive disorders. In Cohen, W. R. (Ed.) *Complications of pregnancy* (5th ed., pp. 207–219). Philadelphia: Lippincott Williams & Wilkins.

Mahomed, K. (2000). Prophylactic versus selective blood transfusion for sickle cell anaemia during pregnancy. *Cochrane Database of Systematic Reviews* (2): CD000040.

McCloskey, J., & Bulechek, G. (2000). *Nursing interventions classification* (3rd ed.). St. Louis: Mosby.

McDuffie, R. S. (2000). Screening techniques for group B streptococcal infection. *Contemporary OB/GYN, 45*(12), 95–100.

Meller, J., & Goldman, M. E. (2000). Cardiopulmonary disorders. In Cohen, W. R. (ed.). *Complications of pregnancy* (5th ed., pp. 189–205). Philadelphia: Lippincott Williams & Wilkins.

Minkoff, H. L. (2000). Human immunodeficiency virus and other perinatal infections. In Scott, J. R., et al. *Danforth's obstetrics and gynecology* (8th ed., pp. 393–406). Philadelphia: Lippincott Williams & Wilkins.

Nelson-Piercy, C. (2001). Asthma in pregnancy. *Thorax, 56*(4), 325–328.

Nolan, T. E. (2000). Primary care in gynecology. In Scott, J. R., et al. *Danforth's obstetrics and gynecology* (8th ed., pp. 485–515). Philadelphia: Lippincott Williams & Wilkins.

Samuel, R. & Suh, B. (2000). Antiretroviral therapy 2000. *Archives of Pharmaceutical Research, 23*(5), 425–437.

Scott, J. R., & Branch, D. W. (2000). Immunologic disorders in pregnancy. In Scott, J. R., et al. *Danforth's obstetrics and gynecology* (8th ed., pp. 363–392). Philadelphia: Lippincott Williams & Wilkins.

Semba, R. D. (2000). Mastitis and transmission of human immunodeficiency virus through breast milk. *Annals of the New York Academy of Sciences, 918*(11), 156–162.

Spellacy, W. N. (2000). Diabetes mellitus and pregnancy. In Scott, J. R., et al. *Danforth's obstetrics and gynecology* (8th ed., pp. 301–308). Philadelphia: Lippincott Williams & Wilkins.

Taggart, S., & Parry, D. (1999). When one is two. *Journal of Burn Care & Rehabilitation, 20*(1), 71–76.

Toglia, M. R. (2000). Venous disease and thromboembolism. In Cohen, W. R. (ed.). *Complications of pregnancy* (5th ed., pp. 267–276). Philadelphia: Lippincott Williams & Wilkins.

Vettraino, I. M., & Welch, R. A. (2000). Drug therapy in pregnancy. In Ransom, S. B., et al. *Practical strategies in obstetrics and gynecology* (pp. 424–435). Philadelphia: Saunders.

Weisbord, J. S., et al. (2001). Sexually transmitted diseases during pregnancy: Screening, diagnostic, and treatment practices among prenatal care providers. *Georgia. Southern Medical Journal, 94*(1), 47–53.

Wenstrom, K. D., & Malee, M. (2000). Medical and surgical complications of pregnancy. In Scott, J. R., et al. *Danforth's obstetrics and gynecology* (8th ed., pp. 327–362). Philadelphia: Lippincott Williams & Wilkins.

Willis, F. R. et al. (2000). Children of renal transplant recipient mothers. *Journal of Paediatrics & Child Health, 36*(3), 230–235.

Xiong, X., et al. (2000). Anemia during pregnancy and birth outcome: A meta-analysis. *American Journal of Perinatology, 17*(3), 137–146.

ABC XYZ SUGGESTED READINGS

Angelini, D. J. (1999). Obstetric triage: Management of acute nonobstetric abdominal pain in pregnancy. *Journal of Nurse-Midwifery, 44*(6), 572–584.

Borg, W. P., & Sherwin, R. S. (2000). Classification of diabetes mellitus. *Advances in Internal Medicine, 45,* 279–295.

Cousins, L. (1999). Fetal oxygenation, assessment of fetal well-being, and obstetric management of the pregnant patient with asthma. *Journal of Allergy & Clinical Immunology, 103*(2), S343–349.

Delzell, J. E., & Lefevre, M. L. (2000). Urinary tract infections during pregnancy. *American Family Physician, 61*(3), 713–721.

deWeerd, S, et al. (2002). Preconception counseling improves folate status of women planning pregnancy. *Obstetrics & Gynecology, 99*(1), 45–50.

Drapkin Lyerly, A., & Anderson, J. (2001). Human immunodeficiency virus and assisted reproduction: reconsidering evidence, reframing ethics. *Fertility & Sterility, 75*(5), 843–858.

Franklin, O., et al. (2002). Prenatal diagnosis of coarctation of the aorta improves survival and reduces morbidity. *Heart, 87*(1), 67–69.

Fullerton, J. T. (1999). Surgery during pregnancy. *Seminars in Perioperative Nursing, 8*(3), 101–108.

Lin, F. Y., et al. (2001). The effectiveness of risk-based intrapartum chemoprophylaxis for the prevention of early-onset neonatal group B streptococcal disease. *American Journal of Obstetrics & Gynecology, 184*(6), 1204–1210.

Litmanovitz, I. et al. (2000). Fetal intrathoracic injuries following mild maternal motor vehicle accident. *Journal of Perinatal Medicine, 28*(2), 158–160.

Luppi, C. J. (1999). Cardiopulmonary resuscitation in pregnancy. *AWHONN Lifelines, 3*(3), 41–45.

Moodley, P., & Sturm, A. W. (2000). Sexually transmitted infections, adverse pregnancy and neonatal infection. *Seminars in Neonatology, 5*(3), 255–269.

Mourad, J., et al. (2000). Appendicitis in pregnancy. New information that contradicts long-held clinical beliefs. *American Journal of Obstetrics & Gynecology, 182*(5), 1027–1029.

Murakami, S., et al. (2000). Renal disease in women with severe preeclampsia or gestational proteinuria. *Obstetrics & Gynecology, 96*(6), 945–949.

Ovalle, A., & Levancini, M. (2001). Urinary tract infections in pregnancy. *Current Opinion in Urology, 11*(1), 55–59.

Scanlon, K. S. et al. (2000). High and low hemoglobin levels during pregnancy: Differential risks for preterm birth and small for gestational age. *Obstetrics & Gynecology, 96*(5), 741–748.

Schatz, M. (1999). Interrelationships between asthma and pregnancy: A literature review. *Journal of Allergy & Clinical Immunology, 103*(2), S330–S336.

Sellman, J. S., & Holman, L. (2000). Thromboembolism during pregnancy. *Postgraduate Medicine, 108*(4), 71–77.

Sheffield, J. S., & Cunningham, F. G. (2001). Detecting and treating septic pelvic thrombophlebitis. *Contemporary OB/GYN, 46*(3), 15–23.

Sifakis, S., & Pharmakides, G. (2000). Anemia in pregnancy. *Annals of the New York Academy of Sciences, 900,* 125–136.

Sivanesaratnam, V. (2000). The acute abdomen and the obstetrician. *Best Practice & Research in Clinical Obstetrics & Gynaecology, 14* (1), 89–102.

Taha, T. E., & Gray, R. H. (2000). Genital tract infections and perinatal transmission of HIV. *Annals of the New York Academy of Sciences, 918*(2), 84–98.

Torres, S., et al. (2000). Abuse during and before pregnancy: prevalence and cultural correlates. *Violence & Victims, 15*(3), 303–321.

Walker, I. D. (2000). Thrombophilia in pregnancy. *Journal of Clinical Pathology, 53*(8), 573–580.

15

CHAPTER

High-Risk Pregnancy: The Woman Who Develops a Complication of Pregnancy

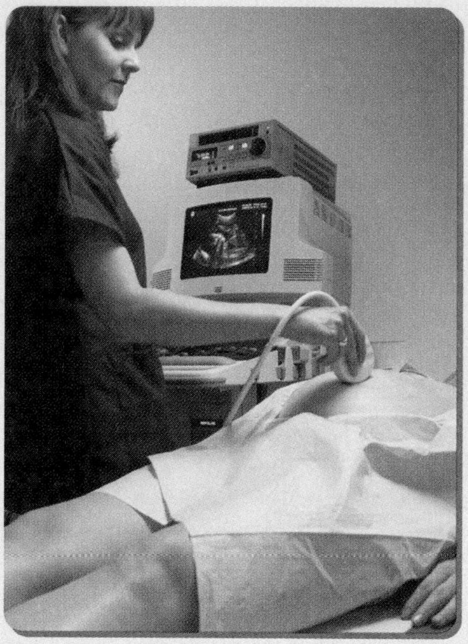

Key Terms

- abortion
- ankle clonus
- cervical cerclage
- chorioamnionitis
- complete miscarriage
- couvelaire uterus
- eclampsia
- ectopic pregnancy
- erythroblastosis fetalis
- gestational trophoblastic disease
- HELLP syndrome
- hemolytic disease of the newborn
- hydramnios
- imminent miscarriage
- incompetent cervix
- incomplete miscarriage
- isoimmunization
- miscarriage
- missed miscarriage
- placenta previa
- postterm pregnancy
- preeclampsia
- premature cervical dilatation
- premature separation of the placenta
- preterm labor
- preterm rupture of membranes
- pseudocyesis
- recurrent pregnancy loss
- Rh incompatibility
- spontaneous miscarriage
- threatened miscarriage
- tocolytic agent

Objectives

After mastering the contents of this chapter, you should be able to:

1. Describe complications of pregnancy that place the pregnant woman and her fetus at high risk.
2. Assess the woman who is experiencing a complication of pregnancy.
3. Formulate nursing diagnoses that address the needs of the woman and her family experiencing a complication of pregnancy.
4. Identify expected outcomes to minimize the risks to the pregnant woman and her fetus.
5. Plan nursing interventions to meet the needs and promote optimal outcome for the woman and her family.
6. Implement nursing actions specific to the woman who has developed a complication of pregnancy.
7. Evaluate outcomes for effectiveness and achievement.
8. Identify National Health Goals related to complications of pregnancy and specific measures nurses can take to help the nation achieve these goals.
9. Identify areas of nursing care related to high-risk pregnancy that could benefit from additional nursing research or the application of evidence-based practice.
10. Use critical thinking to analyze ways that nurses can help prevent complications of pregnancy.
11. Integrate knowledge of complications of pregnancy with nursing process to achieve quality maternal and child health nursing care.

Beverly Muzuki is a 20-year-old primipara, 34 weeks pregnant, whom you see in a prenatal clinic. She has had symptoms of a urinary tract infection for the past few days but didn't call the clinic because she knew she had an appointment today and thought getting some help for it could wait until she came in. Yesterday she noticed some mild abdominal pain but thought it was irritation from the bladder infection. During the night, she woke twice because of a nagging backache. This morning, her membranes ruptured and now she has intermittent sharp uterine contractions. "Why did this happen?" she asks you. "I didn't do anything wrong." Were Beverly's actions as informed as they could have been? What additional health teaching might have prevented her from starting labor so early?

Previous chapters described normal pregnancy and preexisting and newly acquired conditions that can complicate pregnancy. This chapter adds to your knowledge base information about complications directly related to the pregnancy that can occur.

After you've studied the chapter, answer the Critical Thinking Exercises at the end of the chapter and then access the on-line study activities (http://connection.lww.com) *to further sharpen your skills and test your knowledge.*

Most women enter pregnancy in apparent good health and achieve a normal pregnancy and birth without complications. In a few women, however, for reasons that usually are unclear, unexpected deviations or complications from the course of normal pregnancy occur. When this happens, it can place a severe burden on the woman and her family. All families benefit from the support and skill of a professional nurse who helps them work through the tasks of pregnancy, accept it, and prepare to become new parents. The support and skill of a professional nurse are essential to a family who, in addition to the usual tasks of pregnancy, must take special care to ensure the continuation of the pregnancy and who may be very concerned that the baby cannot be carried to term. Initially, if a pregnant woman develops a complication, hospitalization may be necessary. Once stabilized, the woman may be a candidate for continued follow-up with home care (see Chap. 16).

The leading causes of maternal death during pregnancy are thromboembolism, hemorrhage, infection, hypertension of pregnancy, anesthesia complications, ectopic pregnancy, and heart disease (Cunningham et al., 2001). When any of these complications occurs, it has the potential to threaten the life of the mother and the fetus directly and, indirectly, the health of the family. National Health Goals to reduce complications of pregnancy are shown in the Focus on National Health Goals box.

FOCUS ON NATIONAL HEALTH GOALS

Preventing complications of pregnancy is viewed as so important by the majority of people that this is included in National Health Goals. Four of these goals are:

- Reduce maternal deaths from pregnancy-related causes to 3.3 per 100,000 live births from a baseline of 7.1 per 100,000.
- Reduce maternal illness and complications due to pregnancy to 24 per 100 births from a baseline of 31 per 100 births.
- Reduce preterm births to 7.6% from a baseline of 11.6%.
- Reduce low birthweight to an incidence of no more than 5% of live births from a baseline of 7.6% and very low birthweight to no more than 0.9% of live births from a baseline of 1.4% (DHHS, 2000).

Nurses working in prenatal settings can be helpful in seeing that women are well informed about the normal course of pregnancy so they can recognize and alert health care providers when a complication is occurring. They can actively participate in risk assessment at prenatal visits. Nursing research is needed in areas such as what is the best way to determine each woman's individual needs so prenatal instructions can be specifically planned, or whether increasing the number of prenatal visits for high-risk women reduces complications during pregnancy.

NURSING PROCESS OVERVIEW

For Care of the Woman Who Develops a Complication of Pregnancy

Assessment

Nurses often are the first ones to discover a complication of pregnancy because they talk to clients first at prenatal visits. At prenatal visits, ask women about any symptoms that might indicate potential complications. Provide enough time for a thorough health history so problems such as headache, blurred vision, or vaginal spotting can be uncovered and investigated thoroughly.

In addition, at the close of the visit, review these symptoms with the woman so she can recognize potential problems and contact the health care center if problems occur. Assure women when giving this information that they are free to call whenever they are concerned. Otherwise, they may wait until their symptoms are acute rather than call when they first notice them.

Nursing Diagnosis

Many nursing diagnoses pertain to the woman with a pregnancy complication. Some examples may include:

- Anxiety related to guarded pregnancy outcome
- Deficient fluid volume related to third-trimester bleeding
- Risk for infection related to incomplete miscarriage
- Ineffective tissue perfusion related to hypertension of pregnancy
- Deficient knowledge related to signs and symptoms of possible complications

Outcome Identification and Planning

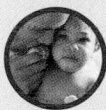

When a complication of pregnancy is an emergency situation, outcomes focus on a short time frame. These outcomes must address fetal and maternal welfare, often reflecting family welfare. Treatment protocols, such as those related to bleeding, preterm labor, and hypertension of pregnancy, once established should be regularly updated and maintained so they remain current. Be certain that they reflect a current nursing management level so nurses can act swiftly and independently. Once the woman's condition stabilizes, outcome identification can then focus on long-term objectives.

Many women who develop a pregnancy complication may spend a few days in the hospital for therapy and monitoring followed by discharge to the home, where they may be required to maintain bed rest for a long time. Waiting for a pregnancy to come to term this way can be a difficult and anxious time. Readmission to the health care facility, especially when some new complication has occurred that might threaten the pregnancy outcome, only serves to compound these feelings. Planning must consider the many feelings this experience may cause.

Implementation

Interventions for the woman experiencing a complication of pregnancy include measures to maintain the following:

- Physiologic functioning of the pregnancy
- The woman's and family's psychological acceptance
- The duration of pregnancy as long as possible for the mother and fetus

Maintaining an optimistic attitude of fetal progress is important so thc woman does not begin anticipatory grieving for the fetus and halt the growth of bonding. If the complication can be contained and the pregnancy continues uninterrupted, this will help protect the mental health of the family. If the pregnancy cannot be continued, be available to offer support to the family who grieves for the loss of the unborn child and, in rare instances, loss of future childbearing potential or the woman herself.

After a pregnancy with complications, the mother has reason to be especially worried about the infant's health at the time of birth. Be certain she spends enough time with the child to see that although perhaps born before term, the infant is well and healthy. It is helpful to assess the infant for such things as ability to follow a light and respond to a voice while the woman is present. This helps to demonstrate that the infant is well. If an infant is ill at birth, the mother needs to spend time with the child as well, visiting in an intensive care nursery. This may be difficult because she still may be ill herself.

Outcome Evaluation

Although the success or failure of some nursing interventions cannot be fully evaluated until the child is born or even into the postnatal period, outcomes should be evaluated throughout the pregnancy. Be aware that after a complication of early pregnancy, a woman cannot help but worry during the remainder of the pregnancy that the complication will recur or that the original insult to the fetus was severe enough to cause long-term effects. Evaluate the woman's psychological attitude and physical status at each continuing health care visit to be certain she is coping with the situation and the fear and strain she lives under until the child is born.

Not all fetal outcomes will be optimal. Evaluation will then include the ability of the family to adjust to care of an ill infant. Examples suggesting achievement of outcomes might include:

- Client's blood pressure is maintained within acceptable parameters.
- Couple state they feel able to cope with anxiety associated with the pregnancy complication.
- Client remains free of signs and symptoms of pregnancy-induced hypertension.
- Client accurately verbalizes crucial signs and symptoms to report to the health care provider immediately.

BLEEDING DURING PREGNANCY

Vaginal bleeding is a deviation from the normal that may occur at any time during pregnancy. It is never normal, and it is always frightening. It may or may not be serious, but it must always be carefully investigated because if it occurs in sufficient amount or for sufficient cause it can impair both the outcome of the pregnancy and the woman's life or health. The primary causes of bleeding during pregnancy are summarized in Table 15-1.

Bleeding and the Development of Shock

Any degree of vaginal bleeding during pregnancy is potentially serious because the amount visualized may be only a fraction of the blood actually lost. This happens because an undilated cervix and intact membranes can be effective in containing blood within the uterus. A woman with any degree of bleeding, therefore, needs to be evaluated for the possibility that she is experiencing a significant blood loss and for hypovolemic shock.

The process of shock due to blood loss is shown in Figure 15-1. Note that because the uterus is a nonessential body organ, danger to the fetal blood supply occurs when the woman's body begins to decrease blood flow to peripheral organs (although the increased blood volume of pregnancy allows more than normal blood loss before hypovolemic shock occurs). Signs of hypovolemic shock (Table 15-2) occur when 10% of blood volume, or approximately two units of blood, have been lost; fetal distress occurs when 25% of blood volume is lost (see Assessing the Pregnant Woman With Hypovolemic Shock). Because "normal" blood pressure varies from woman to woman, it is important to know the baseline blood pressure for a pregnant woman to evaluate shock. Women should be informed of their blood pressure at prenatal visits; for example, "Your blood pressure is 110 over 70—that's normal," not just "Your pressure is normal." Then if blood loss should occur, the woman can be helpful in offering her baseline pressure.

TABLE 15.1 Summary of Causes of Bleeding During Pregnancy

TIME	TYPE	CAUSE	ASSESSMENT	CAUTIONS
First trimester	Threatened miscarriage (early—under 16 weeks; late—16 to 24 weeks)	Unknown; possibly chromosomal, uterine abnormalities	Vaginal spotting, perhaps slight cramping	
	Imminent (inevitable) miscarriage		Vaginal spotting, cramping, cervical dilatation	
	Missed miscarriage		Vaginal spotting, perhaps slight cramping; no apparent loss of pregnancy	Disseminated intravascular coagulation associated with missed miscarriage
	Incomplete miscarriage		Vaginal spotting, cramping, cervical dilatation, but incomplete expulsion of uterine contents	
	Complete miscarriage		Vaginal spotting, cramping, cervical dilatation, and complete expulsion of uterine contents	
	Ectopic (tubal) pregnancy	Implantation of zygote at site other than in uterus; tubal constricture, adhesions associated	Sudden unilateral lower abdominal quadrant pain; minimal vaginal bleeding, possible signs of shock or hemorrhage	May have repeat ectopic pregnancy in future if tubal scarring is bilateral
Second trimester	Hydatidiform mole (gestational trophoblastic disease)	Abnormal proliferation of trophoblast tissue; fertilization or division defect	Overgrowth of uterus; highly positive human chorionic gonadotropin (hCG) test; no fetus present on sonogram; bleeding from vagina of old or fresh blood accompanied by cyst formation	Retained trophoblast tissue may become malignant (choriocarcinoma); follow for 6 months to 1 year with hCG testing
	Premature cervical dilation	Cervix begins to dilate and pregnancy is lost at about 20 weeks; unknown cause, but cervical trauma from dilatation and curettage (D&C) may be associated	Painless bleeding leading to expulsion of fetus	Can have cervical sutures placed to ensure a second pregnancy
Third trimester	Placenta previa	Low implantation of placenta possibly due to uterine abnormality	Painless bleeding at beginning of cervical dilatation	No vaginal examinations to minimize placental trauma
	Premature separation of the placenta (abruptio placentae)	Unknown cause; associated with hypertension; placenta separates from uterus	Sharp abdominal pain followed by uterine tenderness; vaginal bleeding; signs of maternal shock, fetal distress	Disseminated intravascular coagulation associated with condition
	Preterm labor	Many possible etiologic factors such as trauma, substance abuse, pregnancy-induced hypertension or cervicitis; increased chance in multiple gestation, maternal illness	Show (pink-stained vaginal discharge) accompanied by uterine contractions becoming regular and effective	Preterm labor may be halted if the cervix is less than 4 cm dilated and the membranes are intact

NURSING DIAGNOSES AND RELATED INTERVENTIONS

Nursing Diagnosis: Risk for deficient fluid volume related to bleeding during pregnancy

Outcome Identification: Client will exhibit signs of adequate fluid balance during pregnancy.

Outcome Evaluation: Client's blood pressure is maintained at at least 100/60 mm Hg, pulse rate is below 100 beats per minute; only minimal bleeding is apparent; fetal heart rate is maintained at 120 to 160 bpm, with adequate short-term and long-term variability; urine output is greater than 30 mL/hour.

Therapy for hypovolemic shock is aimed at restoring blood volume and halting the source of hemorrhage (Table 15-3). A woman suspected of serious bleeding needs intravenous fluid replacement. Use a large-gauge angiocath (16 or 18) for rapid fluid

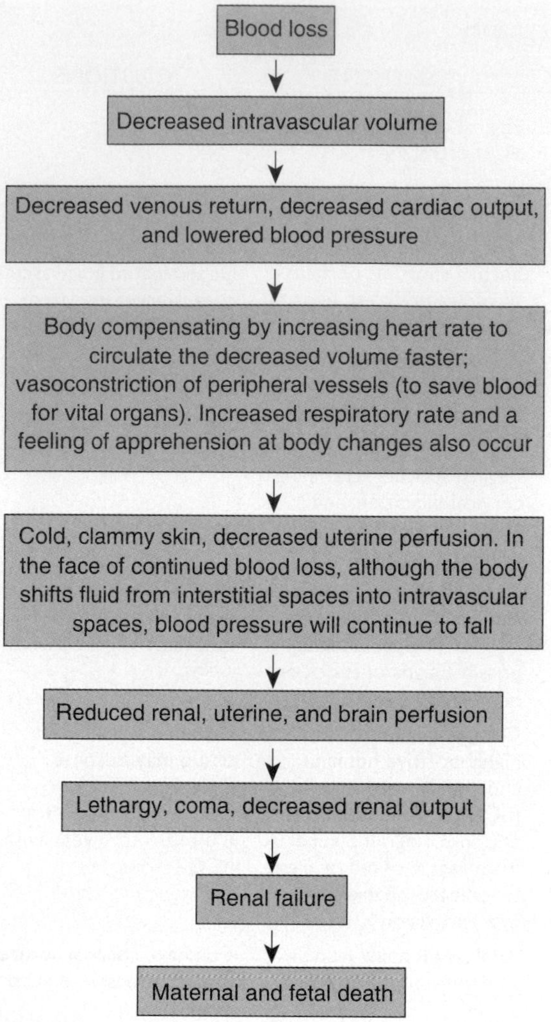

FIGURE 15.1 The process of shock due to blood loss (*hypovolemia*).

TABLE 15.2 Signs and Symptoms of Hypovolemic Shock

ASSESSMENT	SIGNIFICANCE
Increased pulse rate	Heart attempting to circulate decreased blood volume
Decreased blood pressure	Less peripheral resistance because of decreased blood volume
Increased respiratory rate	Increases gas exchange to better oxygenate decreased red blood cell volume
Cold, clammy skin	Vasoconstriction occurs to maintain blood volume in central body core
Decreased urine output	Inadequate blood is entering kidney due to decreased blood volume
Dizziness or decreased level of consciousness	Inadequate blood is reaching cerebrum due to decreased blood volume
Decreased central venous pressure	Decreased blood is returning to heart due to reduced blood volume

ASSESSING the Pregnant Woman With Hypovolemic Shock

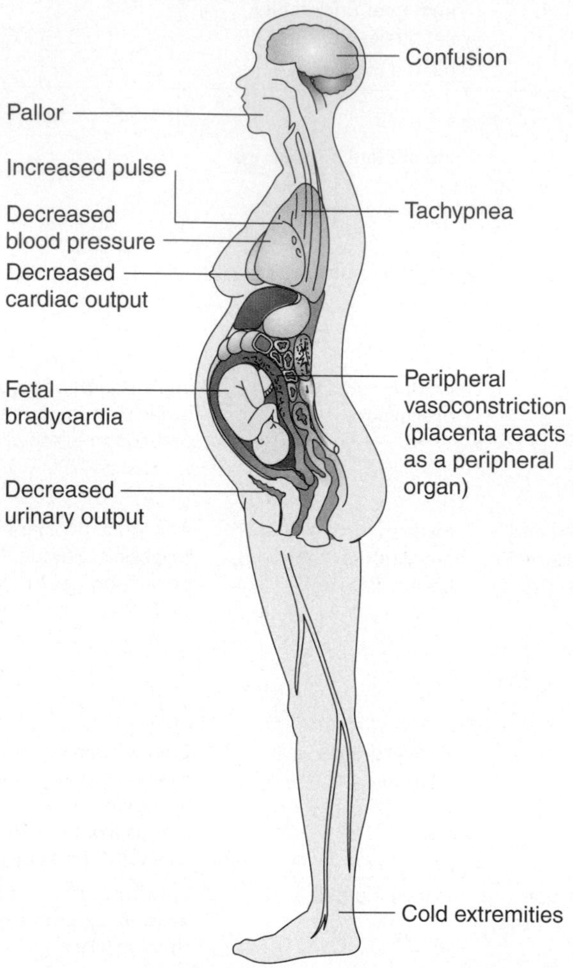

expansion with a solution such as Ringer's lactate. This allows a blood transfusion to be administered through the same site as soon as blood is available. Obtaining hemoglobin and hematocrit levels and securing a sample for typing or cross-matching of blood are essential. The woman may have a central venous pressure or a pulmonary artery catheter (to measure pulmonary capillary wedge pressure) inserted (see Chap. 41). During pregnancy, these values differ from the average, so they should be evaluated in light of the pregnancy. A central venous pressure during pregnancy is 2 to 7 mm Hg; pulmonary capillary wedge pressure is 6 to 10 mm Hg. If respirations are rapid, administer oxygen by mask and monitor oxygen saturation levels by pulse oximetry. Obtain arterial blood gases as ordered. Frequent assessments of vital signs and continuous fetal monitoring by an external monitoring device should be started. Urge the woman to lie in a lateral position.

TABLE 15.3 Emergency Interventions for Bleeding in Pregnancy

INTERVENTION	RATIONALE
Alert health care team of emergency situation.	Provides maximum coordination of care
Place woman flat in bed on her side.	Maintains optimal placental and renal function
Begin intravenous fluid such as lactated Ringer's with a 16 or 18 angiocath.	Replaces intravascular fluid volume; intravenous line is established if blood replacement will be needed
Administer oxygen as necessary at 6–10 L/min by face mask.	Provides adequate fetal oxygenation despite lowered maternal circulating blood volume
Monitor uterine contractions and fetal heart rate by external monitor.	Assesses whether labor is present and fetal status; external system avoids cervical trauma
Omit vaginal examination.	Prevents tearing of placenta if placenta previa is cause of bleeding
Withhold oral fluid.	Anticipates need for emergency surgery
Order type and cross-match of two units whole blood.	Allows for restoring circulating maternal blood volume if needed
Measure intake and output.	Enables assessment of renal function (will decrease to under 30 mL/hour with massive circulating volume loss)
Assess vital signs (pulse, respirations, and blood pressure every 15 min; apply pulse oximeter and automatic blood pressure cuff as necessary).	Provides baseline data on maternal response to blood loss
Assist with placement of central venous pressure or pulmonary artery catheter and blood determinations.	Provides more accurate data on maternal hemodynamic state
Measure maternal blood loss by weighing perineal pads; save any tissue passed.	Provides objective evidence of amount of bleeding. Saturating a sanitary pad in less than 1 hour is heavy blood loss; tissue may be abnormal trophoblast tissue.
Set aside 5 mL of blood drawn intravenously in a clean test tube; observe in 5 min for clot formation.	Tests for possible blood coagulation problem (disseminated intravascular coagulation; suspect this if no clot forms within time limit)
Assist with ultrasound examination.	Supplies information on placental and fetal well-being
Maintain a positive attitude about fetal outcome.	Supports mother–child bonding
Support woman's self-esteem; provide emotional support to woman and her support person.	Assists problem solving because this is lessened by poor self-esteem.

If this is not possible, position her on her back, with a wedge under one hip. Doing so minimizes uterine pressure on the vena cava and blood being trapped in the lower extremities (supine hypotension syndrome).

CONDITIONS ASSOCIATED WITH FIRST-TRIMESTER BLEEDING

The time during pregnancy at which bleeding occurs helps to identify its cause. The two most common causes of bleeding during the first trimester are spontaneous miscarriage and ectopic pregnancy.

Spontaneous Miscarriage

An **abortion** is defined as any interruption of a pregnancy before the fetus is viable (a stage of development that will enable the fetus to survive outside the uterus if born at that time). When a pregnancy is medically or surgically interrupted, this is typically termed abortion. When the interruption occurs spontaneously, it is clearer to refer to it as a **miscarriage**.

A nonviable fetus is usually defined as a fetus of 20 to 24 weeks of gestation or weighing 500 g or less. A fetus born at this point is considered a premature or immature birth (Cunningham et al., 2001).

Spontaneous miscarriage occurs in 15% to 30% of all pregnancies and occurs from natural causes (Scott, 2000a). Elective abortion, discussed in Chapter 5, is the planned medical termination of a pregnancy.

A spontaneous miscarriage is an early miscarriage if it occurs before week 16 of pregnancy and a late miscarriage if it occurs between weeks 16 and 24. For the first 6 weeks of pregnancy, the developing placenta is tentatively attached to the decidua of the uterus; during weeks 6 to 12, a moderate degree of attachment to the myometrium is accomplished. After week 12, the attachment is penetrating and deep. Because of the degrees of attachment achieved at different weeks of pregnancy, it is important to attempt to establish the week of the pregnancy at which bleeding has become apparent. Bleeding before week 6 is rarely severe; bleeding after week 12 can be profuse because the placenta is implanted deeply. Fortunately, at this time, with such deep placental implantation, the fetus is expelled as in natural childbirth before the placenta separates. Uterine contraction then helps to control placental bleeding as it does postpartally. For some women, then, the stage of attachment between weeks 6 and 12 can lead to the most severe bleeding and threat to their lives.

Causes of Spontaneous Miscarriage

The most frequent cause of miscarriage in the first trimester of pregnancy is abnormal fetal formation, due either to a teratogenic factor or to a chromosomal aberration. Approximately 60% of fetuses aborted early have structural abnormalities (Scott, 2000a). In other miscarriages, immunologic factors may be present or "rejection" of the embryo through an immune response may occur.

Another common cause of early miscarriage involves implantation abnormalities. Approximately 50% of zygotes are never implanted (Cunningham et al., 2001). With inadequate implantation, the placental circulation cannot function adequately and fetal nutrition will be inadequate. Poor implantation may result from inadequate endometrial formation or from an inappropriate site of implantation.

Miscarriage may also occur if the corpus luteum fails to produce enough progesterone to maintain the decidua basalis. Progesterone therapy may be attempted to prevent this if this cause is documented.

Infection in the woman may be yet another cause of miscarriage. Rubella, syphilis, poliomyelitis, cytomegalovirus, and toxoplasmosis infections readily cross the placenta, possibly causing fetal death. Urinary tract infection also increases the incidence of a miscarriage. With an infection, if the fetus fails to grow, estrogen and progesterone production by the placenta falls. This leads to endometrial sloughing. With the sloughing, prostaglandins are released, leading to uterine contraction and cervical dilatation along with expulsion of the products of conception.

Ingestion of a teratogenic drug is another cause. For example, isotretinoin (Accutane), if taken early in pregnancy, can lead to miscarriage or fetal abnormality (Karch, 2001). Because miscarriage can occur from so many causes and because the cause is unlikely to be determined with an early miscarriage, couples may have difficulty understanding why it happened to them (see Focus on Family Empowerment).

Assessment

The presenting symptom of spontaneous miscarriage is almost always vaginal spotting. At the first indication of vaginal spotting, a woman should telephone her health care provider and describe what is happening. Because a nurse often takes this initial call, nurses need to be aware of guidelines for assessing vaginal bleeding quickly during pregnancy (Table 15-4).

The history of the episode is important in helping the physician or nurse-midwife diagnose the cause. Knowledge of the woman's actions is important to ensure she did not attempt to self-abort. She may prefer not to mention such an attempt, but usually will if asked directly. Ask what she has done about the bleeding to be certain she has not inserted a tampon to stop bleeding. If she has, although reporting only slight spotting, she actually has an unknown amount of blood loss.

Therapeutic Management

Depending on the symptoms and the description of the bleeding or spotting the woman gives, the physician or nurse-midwife will decide whether the woman needs to be seen and, if so, in an ambulatory setting or the hospital.

Threatened Miscarriage

Threatened miscarriage is manifested by vaginal bleeding, initially beginning as scant bleeding, and usually bright red. There may be slight cramping, but no cervical dilatation is present on vaginal examination. The woman may be asked to come to the clinic or office to have a sonogram done to evaluate the viability of the fetus. Blood for human chorionic gonadotropin hormone (hCG) may be drawn at the start of bleeding and again in 48 hours (if the placenta is still intact, the level of this in the bloodstream should double in this time). Limiting activity to no strenuous activity for 24 to 48 hours is the key intervention, assuming the threatened abortion involves a live fetus and presumed placental bleeding. Complete bed rest is usually not indicated. Bed rest may stop the vaginal bleeding, but only because blood is pooling vaginally. When the woman does ambulate again, bleeding will recur.

Women are apt to be extremely worried at the sight of bleeding and perhaps watching a pregnancy end. They need some time to talk with a sympathetic support person about how distressed they feel. It is important to convey concerned reassurance that miscarriages happen

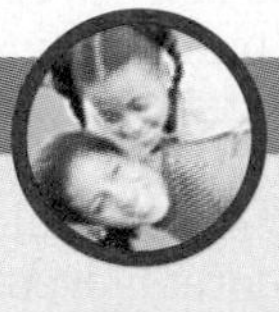

FOCUS ON FAMILY EMPOWERMENT
Coping With a Spontaneous Miscarriage

Q. My doctor has told me that I had an abortion, but I thought I had a miscarriage. What's the difference?

A. Abortion is the medical term for any pregnancy loss before the fetus could have lived outside the uterus. Think of the word as interchangeable with miscarriage.

Q. Did I do something wrong to cause this miscarriage?

A. Early miscarriage is largely unpreventable because it is caused by such things as abnormal chromosome formation or poor uterine implantation—things over which you have no control. Following sensible guidelines such as eating a nutritious diet so you enter a pregnancy in good health and avoiding cigarette smoking or drinking alcohol are sensible recommendations to reduce your risk of complications. If you had extensive blood loss with your miscarriage, you might want to be certain to eat iron-rich foods (meat, green vegetables) to help restore red blood cells for a second pregnancy.

TABLE 15.4 Immediate Assessment of Vaginal Bleeding During Pregnancy

ASSESSMENT FACTOR	SPECIFIC QUESTIONS TO ASK
Confirmation of pregnancy	Does the woman know for certain that she is pregnant (positive pregnancy test or physician/nurse-midwife confirmation)? A woman who has been pregnant before and states that she is sure she is pregnant is probably right, even if she has not yet had this confirmed.
Pregnancy length	What is the length of the pregnancy in weeks?
Duration	How long did the bleeding episode last? Is it continuing?
Intensity	How much bleeding occurred? (Ask the woman to compare it to a common measure [e.g., a tablespoon, a cup].)
Description	Was it mixed with amniotic fluid or mucus? Was it bright red (fresh blood) or dark (old blood)? Was it accompanied by tissue fragments? Was it odorous?
Frequency	Steady spotting? A single episode?
Associated symptoms	Cramping? Sharp pain? Dull pain? Has she ever had cervical surgery?
Action	What was happening when the bleeding started? What has she done (if anything) to control bleeding?
Blood type	Does she know this? (Rh-negative women will need Rh immune globulin to prevent Rh isoimmunization.)

spontaneously, not because of anything the woman did. Women with threatened miscarriages look for reasons why this could have happened, such as running up a flight of stairs, forgetting to take an iron pill, or getting angry with an older child. Being told that none of these events causes miscarriages may help to minimize the guilt that many women feel.

Most women are disappointed to learn that there is no cure to "hold the pregnancy." In the past, estrogen in the form of diethylstilbestrol (DES) was prescribed for this purpose, but there is no conclusive evidence that this helps. Daughters born of DES-aided pregnancies had a high incidence of vaginal cancer (Cunningham et al., 2001), and sons were more susceptible to cystic testicular development and possible infertility.

If the spotting with threatened miscarriage is going to stop, it usually does so within 24 to 48 hours after the woman reduces her activity. When bleeding stops, she can gradually resume normal activities. Coitus is usually restricted for 2 weeks after the bleeding episode to prevent infection and to avoid inducing further bleeding.

As many as 50% of women with threatened miscarriage continue the pregnancy; for the other 50%, unfortunately, the threatened miscarriage changes to imminent or inevitable miscarriage (Cunningham et al., 2001).

Imminent (Inevitable) Miscarriage

A threatened miscarriage becomes an **imminent (inevitable) miscarriage** if uterine contractions and cervical dilation occur. With cervical dilation, the loss of the products of conception cannot be halted. A woman who reports cramping or uterine contractions is usually asked to come to the hospital or office, where she is examined. She should save any tissue fragments she has passed and bring them with her so they can be examined. If no fetal heart sounds are detected and a sonogram reveals an empty uterus or nonviable fetus, the physician may perform a dilation and curettage (D&C) to ensure that all the products of conception are removed. Be certain the woman has been told that the pregnancy was already lost and that all procedures, such as a suction curettage, are to clean the uterus and prevent further complications, such as infection. Any tissue fragments passed in the labor room, along with any the woman passed at home, should be saved so they can be examined for an abnormality such as gestational trophoblastic disease (hydatidiform mole; see below) or for assurance that all the products of conception have been removed from the uterus. After the D&C, the woman will assess vaginal bleeding by recording the number of pads used. Saturating more than one pad per hour is abnormally heavy bleeding.

Complete Miscarriage

In a **complete miscarriage,** the entire products of conception (fetus, membranes, and placenta) are expelled spontaneously without any assistance. The bleeding usually slows within 2 hours and then ceases within a few days after passage of the products of conception.

Incomplete Miscarriage

In an **incomplete miscarriage,** part of the conceptus (usually the fetus) is expelled, but the membranes or placenta is retained in the uterus. The term incomplete can be confusing for women. They may interpret it as indicating that because the miscarriage is only partial, the pregnancy can continue. Be careful not to encourage false hopes by also misinterpreting this term.

In an incomplete miscarriage, there is a danger of maternal hemorrhage as long as part of the conceptus is retained in the uterus because the uterus cannot contract effectively in this condition. The physician will usually perform a D&C or suction curettage to evacuate the remainder of the pregnancy from the uterus. Be certain the woman knows that the pregnancy is already lost and that the procedure is being done only to protect her from hemorrhage and infection, not to end the pregnancy.

Missed Miscarriage

In a **missed miscarriage,** now more commonly referred to as early pregnancy failure, the fetus dies in utero but is not expelled. Women may find this term misleading because it seems that if a miscarriage is "missed," then the pregnancy can continue. A missed miscarriage is usually discovered at a prenatal examination when the fundal height is measured and no increase in size can be demonstrated, or when previously heard fetal heart sounds cannot be heard. The woman may have had symptoms of a threatened miscarriage (painless vaginal bleeding), or she may have had no prior clinical symptoms.

A sonogram can establish that the fetus is dead. Often the embryo actually died 4 to 6 weeks before the onset of miscarriage symptoms or failure of growth was noted. After the sonogram, a D&C most commonly will be done. If the pregnancy is over 14 weeks, labor may be induced by a prostaglandin suppository or misoprostol (Cytotec) to dilate the cervix, followed by oxytocin stimulation or administration of mifepristone (Demetroulis et al., 2001). If the pregnancy is not actively terminated, miscarriage usually occurs spontaneously within 2 weeks. There is a danger of allowing this normal course to happen, however, because disseminated intravascular coagulation (DIC), a coagulation defect, may develop if the dead (and possibly toxic) fetus remains too long in utero.

Most women hope, until the moment the sonogram shows that their fetus is dead, that their baby is alive. They may need support in accepting the reality of the situation (see Focus on Communication) and need counseling to accept a future pregnancy because of fears that whatever force struck silently and strangely in one pregnancy might strike again.

Recurrent Pregnancy Loss

In the past, women who had three spontaneous miscarriages that occurred at the same gestational age were called "habitual aborters." They were often advised that they were apparently too "nervous" or that something was so wrong with their hormones that childbearing was not for them. Today, the term **recurrent pregnancy loss** is used to describe this miscarriage pattern. A thorough investigation is done to discover the cause of the loss and help ensure the outcome of a future pregnancy (Cunningham et al., 2001). Recurrent pregnancy loss occurs in about 1% of women who want to be pregnant (Scott, 2000a). Although many occur for unknown reasons, possible causes may include:

- Defective spermatozoa or ova
- Endocrine factors such as lowered levels of protein-bound iodine (PBI), butanol-extractable iodine (BEI), and globulin-bound iodine (GBI), poor thyroid function, or luteal phase defect
- Deviations of the uterus, such as septate or bicornate uterus
- Infection
- Autoimmune disorders such as those involving lupus anticoagulant and antiphospholipid antibodies (Vaquero et al., 2001; Empson et al., 2002)

Complications of Miscarriage

As with full-term childbirth, hemorrhage and infection are two of the most likely complications after miscarriage. The risk for isoimmunization and the woman's psychological state also need to be considered.

FOCUS ON COMMUNICATION

Amy Bueller is 16 weeks pregnant. She had some vaginal spotting a week ago that stopped spontaneously. Her private doctor saw her today for a prenatal visit. The doctor was unable to hear fetal heart tones. A sonogram revealed a missed miscarriage. Amy is now admitted for a D&C. You approach her to take admission vital signs.

Less Effective Communication

Nurse: Hello, Amy. All right if I take your temperature and pulse?
Amy: I'm sure they're fine. I feel fine.
Nurse: I'm sorry for you that this happened. It must be upsetting.
Amy: The bleeding was scary. Made me really nervous that something was wrong with the baby.
Nurse: Bleeding is always scary. I hate to see it.
Amy: All I want to do now is get this surgery over with so I can get on with having a baby.
Nurse: That's the advantage of being young. There's lots of time for babies. Both temperature and pulse are good. You were right—they are fine.

More Effective Communication

Nurse: Hello, Amy. All right if I take your temperature and pulse?
Amy: I'm sure they're fine. I feel fine.
Nurse: I'm sorry for you that this happened. It must be upsetting.
Amy: The bleeding was scary. Made me really nervous that something was wrong with the baby.
Nurse: Did the doctor talk to you about what she thought the bleeding meant? Or what the sonogram showed?
Amy: She said I missed having a miscarriage. I feel really lucky for that.
Nurse: I'll ask your doctor to re-explain what she meant by a missed miscarriage. That can be very confusing.

Because many women want so badly to be pregnant, it can be easy for them to "miss" bad information about a pregnancy. In the above scenario, the nurse was so intent on chatting that she failed to realize that the client was misinformed. Better listening skills in the second example revealed a serious misunderstanding of what missed abortion means.

Hemorrhage. With a complete spontaneous miscarriage, serious or fatal hemorrhage is rare. With an incomplete miscarriage or in the woman who develops an accompanying coagulation defect (usually DIC), major hemorrhage is a possibility. If excessive vaginal bleeding is occurring, immediately position the woman flat and massage the uterine fundus to aid contraction (see Chap. 22). This may be impossible with an early pregnancy because of the small uterine size. The woman may need a D&C to empty the uterus of the material that is preventing it from contracting and achieving hemostasis. Monitor vital signs for changes to detect possible hypovolemic shock. A transfusion may be necessary to replace blood loss. Direct replacement of fibrinogen may be used to aid coagulation.

After a self-limiting complete miscarriage, the woman needs clear instructions on how much bleeding is abnormal (a rule of thumb is that more than one sanitary pad per hour is excessive); what color changes she should expect in bleeding (gradually changing to a dark color and then to the color of serous fluid as it does with the postpartal woman); and that any unusual odor or passing of large clots is also abnormal. If the physician has prescribed an oral medication such as methylergonovine maleate (Methergine) to aid with contraction, be sure the woman understands why it is being prescribed and the importance of taking it. Some women repress their feelings, anxious to forget the experience as quickly as possible. Repression helps them to handle their anger or grief at the loss of the pregnancy. Be careful that in repressing the experience, the woman does not also repress the memory of her medication and leave herself open to hemorrhage.

Infection. The possibility of infection is minimal when pregnancy loss occurs over a short period, bleeding is self-limiting, and instrumentation is limited. However, it may occur.

After a miscarriage, be certain the woman knows the danger signs of infection, such as fever, abdominal pain or tenderness, and a foul vaginal discharge. Fever can be a transient reaction to a period of decreased fluid intake that preceded the miscarriage. In other instances, the fever may be a systemic reaction to the miscarriage process. All fevers of more than 100.4°F (38.0°C) require careful evaluation to avoid overlooking the possibility of infection.

Infection tends to occur in women who have lost appreciable amounts of blood, most likely from the debilitating effect of blood loss. Such women need especially close observation to rule out this second and possibly fatal complication.

The organism responsible for infection after miscarriage is usually *Escherichia coli* (spread from the rectum forward into the vagina). Caution the woman to wipe the perineal area from front to back after voiding and particularly after defecation to prevent the spread of bacteria from the rectal area. Caution her not to use tampons to control vaginal discharge, because stasis of any body fluid increases the risk of infection. Be careful about using statements such as, "You'll have some vaginal flow now, almost exactly like a menstrual flow." Otherwise, the woman might treat it as a menstrual flow and use tampons.

If infection occurs, endometritis (infection of the uterine lining) is the type that usually occurs. It may be more extensive, however, and parametritis, peritonitis, thrombophlebitis, and septicemia can occur. The management of these infections is the same as if they were occurring after the safe delivery of a child (see Chap. 25).

Septic Abortion. A septic abortion is an abortion that is complicated by infection. Infection can happen after a spontaneous miscarriage, but more frequently it occurs in women who have tried to self-abort or were aborted illegally using a nonsterile instrument such as a knitting needle. Because the uterus is a warm, moist, dark cavity, infectious organisms, once introduced, grow rapidly in this environment, particularly if products of conception such as necrotic membranes are still present.

The woman has symptoms of fever and crampy abdominal pain, and her uterus feels tender to palpation. Left untreated, such an infection can lead to toxic shock syndrome, septicemia, kidney failure, and death.

Women with septic abortion need immediate, intensive assessment and treatment. Typically, complete blood count, serum electrolytes, serum creatinine, blood type and cross-match, and cervical, vaginal, and urine cultures are obtained. An indwelling urinary (Foley) catheter may be inserted to monitor urine output hourly. Intravenous fluid to restore fluid volume and provide a route for high-dose, broad-spectrum antibiotic therapy is started. A combination of penicillin (gram-positive coverage), gentamicin (gram-negative aerobic coverage), and clindamycin (gram-negative anaerobic coverage) is commonly used.

A central venous pressure or pulmonary artery catheter may be inserted to monitor left atrial filling pressure and hemodynamic status. The removal of all infected or necrotic tissue from the uterus is important, so a D&C will be performed. Tetanus toxoid given subcutaneously or tetanus immune globulin given intramuscularly will be administered for prophylaxis against tetanus.

Infection can be so severe that the woman is admitted to an intensive care setting for continuing care. Dopamine and digitalis may be necessary to maintain sufficient cardiac output. Oxygen and perhaps ventilatory support may be necessary to maintain respiratory function.

Assuming the woman recovers from the intense episode, septic abortion may lead to future infertility due to uterine scarring or fibrotic scarring of the fallopian tubes. If the woman caused the infection by trying to self-abort, she needs follow-up counseling to assist her to learn better problem solving.

Isoimmunization. Whenever a placenta is dislodged, either by spontaneous birth or by a D&C at any point in pregnancy, some blood from the placental villi (the fetal blood) may enter the maternal circulation. If the woman is Rh negative, enough Rh-positive fetal blood may enter her circulation to cause **isoimmunization**—the production of antibodies against Rh-positive blood by her immunologic system. If her next child should have Rh-positive blood, these antibodies would attempt to destroy the red blood cells of the next infant during the months the infant is in utero.

After a miscarriage, because the blood type of the conceptus is unknown, all women with Rh-negative blood should receive Rh (D antigen) immune globulin (RhIG) to prevent the buildup of antibodies in the event the conceptus was Rh positive.

Powerlessness. As with pregnancy loss for any reason, the woman's adjustment to a spontaneous miscarriage must be assessed. Sadness and grief over the loss or a feeling that she has lost control of her life is to be expected. Spontaneous miscarriage can be particularly heartbreaking for the older woman because she realizes that her window of childbearing is limited.

✔ CHECKPOINT QUESTIONS

1. What is usually the first presenting sign of a spontaneous miscarriage?
2. The woman with a missed miscarriage who does not abort spontaneously is at risk for what two conditions?

Ectopic Pregnancy

An **ectopic pregnancy** is one in which implantation occurs outside the uterine cavity. The implantation may occur on the surface of the ovary or in the cervix. The most common site (in approximately 95% of such pregnancies) is in a fallopian tube (Fig. 15-2). Of these fallopian tube sites, approximately 80% occur in the ampullar portion, 12% occur in the isthmus, and 8% are interstitial or fimbrial.

With ectopic pregnancy, fertilization occurs as usual in the distal third of the fallopian tube. Immediately after the union of ovum and spermatozoon, the zygote begins to divide and grow normally. Unfortunately, because an obstruction is present, such as an adhesion of the fallopian tube from a previous infection (chronic salpingitis or pelvic inflammatory disease), congenital malformations, scars from tubal surgery, or a uterine tumor pressing on the proximal end of the tube, the zygote cannot travel the length of the tube. It lodges at the strictured site along the tube and implants there instead of in the uterus.

Approximately 2% of pregnancies are ectopic; ectopic pregnancy is the second most frequent cause of bleeding early in pregnancy (Pisarska & Carson, 2000). The incidence is increasing because of the increasing rate of pelvic inflammatory disease, which leads to tubal scarring (Cunningham et al., 2001). Ectopic pregnancy occurs more frequently in women who smoke compared to those who do not. It also occurs more frequently in women who douche, possibly due to the risk of introducing an infection (Pisarska & Carson, 2000). There is some evidence that intrauterine devices (IUDs) used for contraception may slow the transport of the zygote and lead to tubal or ovarian implantation. The incidence also increases following in vitro fertilization. Women who have one ectopic pregnancy have a 10% to 20% chance that a subsequent pregnancy will also be ectopic (Cunningham et al., 2001). This is because salpingitis that leaves scarring is usually bilateral. Congenital anomalies such as webbing (fibrous bands) may also be bilateral. Oral contraceptives may reduce the possibility of ectopic pregnancy (Burkman, 2001).

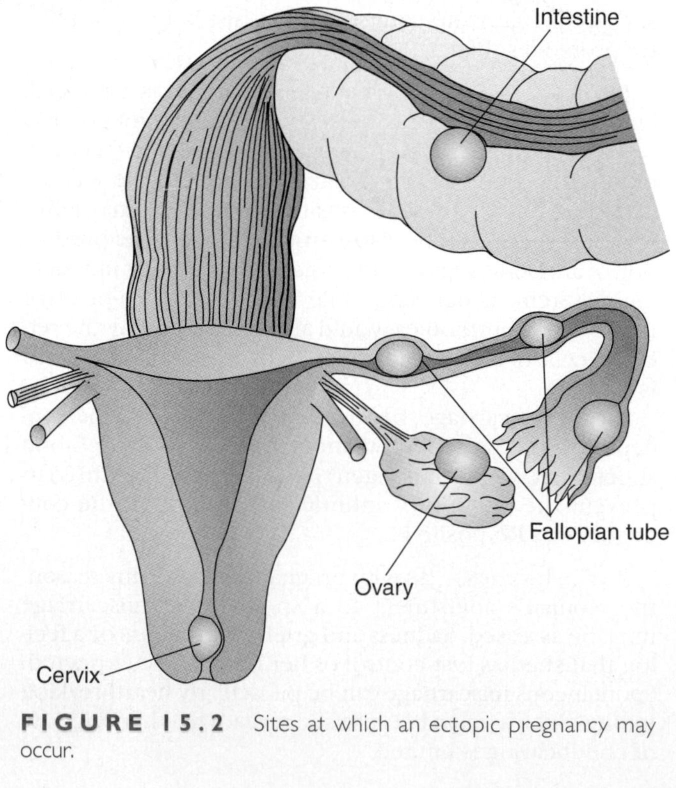

FIGURE 15.2 Sites at which an ectopic pregnancy may occur.

Assessment

With ectopic pregnancy, there are no unusual symptoms at the time of implantation. The corpus luteum of the ovary continues to function as if the implantation were in the uterus. No menstrual flow occurs. The woman may experience the nausea and vomiting of early pregnancy, and a pregnancy test for hCG will be positive.

At weeks 6 to 12 of pregnancy (2 to 8 weeks after a missed menstrual period), the zygote grows large enough to rupture the slender fallopian tube or the trophoblast cells break through the narrow base. Tearing and destruction of the blood vessels in the tube result. The extent of the bleeding that occurs depends on the number and size of the ruptured vessels. If implantation is in the interstitial portion of the tube (where the tube joins the uterus), rupture can cause severe intraperitoneal bleeding. Fortunately, the incidence of tubal pregnancies is highest in the ampullar area (the distal third), where the blood vessels are smaller and profuse hemorrhage is less likely. However, continued bleeding from this area may in time result in a large amount of blood loss. Therefore, a ruptured ectopic pregnancy is serious regardless of the site of implantation.

The woman usually experiences a sharp, stabbing pain in one of the lower abdominal quadrants at the time of rupture, followed by scant vaginal spotting. With placental dislodgment, progesterone secretion stops and the uterine decidua begins to slough, causing bleeding. The amount of bleeding evident with a ruptured ectopic pregnancy often does not reveal the actual amount present. This is because the products of conception from the ruptured tube and the accompanying blood may be expelled into the pelvic cavity rather than into the uterus. Therefore, blood does not reach the vagina to become evident. If internal bleeding progresses to acute hemorrhage, the woman may experience lightheadedness and rapid pulse, signs of shock.

When helping determine the possibility of an ectopic pregnancy, ask the woman whether she has pain or vaginal bleeding. Any woman with sharp abdominal pain and vaginal spotting must be evaluated to rule out the possibility of ectopic pregnancy. Occasionally, a woman will move suddenly and pull one of the round ligaments, the anterior uterine supports. This can cause a sharp, momentary, innocent lower quadrant pain. However, it would be rare for this phenomenon to be reported in connection with vaginal spotting.

By the time the woman with a ruptured ectopic pregnancy arrives at the hospital or physician's office, she may be experiencing severe shock as evidenced by a rapid, thready pulse, rapid respirations, and falling blood pressure. Leukocytosis may be present, not from infection but from the trauma. Temperature is usually normal. A transvaginal sonogram will demonstrate the ruptured tube and collecting pelvic fluid. Either a falling hCG or serum progesterone level suggests that the pregnancy has ended. If the diagnosis of ectopic pregnancy is in doubt, the physician may insert a needle through the postvaginal fornix into the cul-de-sac under sterile conditions to see whether blood that has collected there from internal bleeding can be aspirated. A laparoscopy or culdoscopy can be used to visualize the fallopian tube if the symptoms alone do not reveal a clear picture of what has happened. However, sonography alone usually reveals a clear-cut diagnostic picture (Gracia & Barnhart, 2001).

If the woman waits before seeking help, gradually her abdomen becomes rigid from peritoneal irritation. If blood is slowly seeping into the peritoneal cavity, the umbilicus may develop a bluish tinge (Cullen's sign). The woman may have continuing extensive or dull vaginal and abdominal pain; movement of the cervix on pelvic examination may cause excruciating pain. There may be pain in her shoulders from blood in the peritoneal cavity causing irritation to the phrenic nerve. A tender mass is usually palpable in Douglas' cul-de-sac on vaginal examination.

Therapeutic Management

Although some ectopic pregnancies spontaneously resolve, requiring no treatment, it is difficult to predict when this will happen (Atri et al., 2001). Once an ectopic pregnancy ruptures, it is an emergency situation and the woman's condition must be evaluated quickly. Keep in mind that the amount of blood evident is a poor estimate of the actual blood loss. Blood needs to be drawn immediately for hemoglobin level, typing and cross-matching, and possibly hCG level for immediate pregnancy testing, if pregnancy has not been confirmed. Intravenous fluid using a large-gauge catheter to restore intravascular volume is begun. Blood also can be administered through this same line if necessary.

The therapy for a ruptured ectopic pregnancy is laparoscopy to ligate the bleeding vessels and to remove or repair the damaged fallopian tube. A rough suture line on a fallopian tube may lead to another tubal pregnancy, so either the tube will be removed or suturing on the tube is done with microsurgical technique.

If a tube is removed, the woman is theoretically only 50% fertile, because every other month, when she ovulates from the ovary next to the removed tube, sperm cannot reach the ovum on that side. However, this is not a reliable contraceptive measure. Research in rabbits has shown that translocation of ova can occur—that is, an ovum released from the right ovary can pass through the pelvic cavity to the opposite (left) fallopian tube and become fertilized, and vice versa (Cunningham et al., 2001).

As with miscarriage, women with Rh-negative blood should receive Rh (D) immune globulin (RhIG) after an ectopic pregnancy for isoimmunization protection in future childbearing.

If an ectopic pregnancy can be diagnosed by a routine sonogram before the tube has ruptured, it can be treated medically by the oral administration of methotrexate followed by leucovorin. Methotrexate, a folic acid antagonist chemotherapeutic agent, attacks and destroys fast-growing cells. Because trophoblast and zygote growth is rapid, the drug is drawn to the site of the ectopic pregnancy (see Chap. 53 for a general discussion of chemotherapy agents). Women are treated until a negative hCG titer is achieved. A hysterosalpingogram or sonogram is usually performed after the chemotherapy to assess whether the tube is fully patent. Mifepristone, an abortifacient, is also effective at causing sloughing of the tubal implantation site. The advantage of these therapies is that the tube is left intact, with no surgical scarring (Tulandi & Sammour, 2000).

NURSING DIAGNOSES AND RELATED INTERVENTIONS

Nursing Diagnosis: Powerlessness related to early loss of pregnancy secondary to ectopic pregnancy

Outcome Identification: Client will regain sense of self-worth by 6 months.

Outcome Evaluation: Client states she feels sad at pregnancy loss but is able to deal with situation; has returned to work and has forward-thinking plans.

A woman who has had an ectopic pregnancy not only has grief stages to work through (she has lost a child) but also may have problems of diminished self-image and a sense of powerlessness to resolve if surgery included removal of a fallopian tube. She may believe that she is now half a woman if she equated reproductive structures and childbearing with being a woman. She needs to verbalize concerns about this and future childbearing. The process of working through grief and role images takes weeks to months. It should begin in the hospital, however, where the woman has professional people to help her through the first days and estimate whether she will need counseling.

Abdominal Pregnancy

Very rarely after ectopic pregnancy rupture—so rarely that the instances are difficult to document—the product of conception is expelled into the pelvic cavity with a minimum of bleeding. The placenta continues to grow in the fallopian tube, spreading perhaps into the uterus for a better blood supply; or it may escape into the pelvic cavity and implant on an organ such as an intestine. The fetus will grow in the pelvic cavity (an abdominal pregnancy).

In an abdominal pregnancy, the fetal outline is easily palpable because it is directly below the abdominal wall, not inside the uterus. The woman may not be as aware of movements as she would be normally, or she may experience painful fetal movements and abdominal cramping with fetal movements.

The woman's past history may include uterine surgery or the sudden pain of ectopic pregnancy earlier in the pregnancy. A sonogram or magnetic resonance imaging is used to reveal the fetus outside the uterus.

The danger of abdominal pregnancy is that the placenta will infiltrate and erode a major blood vessel in the abdomen, leading to hemorrhage. If implanted on the intestine, it may erode so deeply that it causes bowel perforation and peritonitis. The fetus is also at high risk because without a good uterine blood supply, nutrients may not reach the fetus in adequate amounts. The survival rate in an abdominal pregnancy is only approximately 60% because of poor nutrient supply. In infants who do survive, there is an increased incidence of fetal deformity from inadequate nutrient supply (Pisarska & Carson, 2000).

At term, the infant must be born by laparotomy. The placenta is often difficult to remove after birth if it is implanted on an abdominal organ such as the intestine. It may be left in place and allowed to be absorbed spontaneously in 2 or 3 months. A follow-up sonogram can be used to detect whether this has occurred, or the woman can be treated with methotrexate. However, this therapy may not be effective because the remaining trophoblasts are no longer fast-growing.

✔ CHECKPOINT QUESTIONS

3. Where are the majority of ectopic pregnancies located?
4. What is the usual treatment for a ruptured ectopic pregnancy?

CONDITIONS ASSOCIATED WITH SECOND-TRIMESTER BLEEDING

There are two main causes of bleeding during the second trimester: gestational trophoblastic disease and premature cervical dilation.

Gestational Trophoblastic Disease (Hydatidiform Mole)

Gestational trophoblastic disease is proliferation and degeneration of the trophoblastic villi (Cunningham et al., 2001). As the cells degenerate, they become filled with fluid and appear as fluid-filled, grape-sized vesicles. With this condition, the embryo fails to develop beyond a primitive start. Such structures must be identified because they are associated with choriocarcinoma, a rapidly metastasizing malignancy (Fig. 15-3).

The incidence of gestational trophoblastic disease is approximately 1 in every 2,000 pregnancies. The condition tends to occur most often in women who have a low protein intake, in young women (under age 18 years), in women older than age 35 years, and in women of Asian heritage (Hammond, 2000).

Two types of molar growth can be identified by chromosome analysis. With a complete mole, all trophoblastic villi swell and become cystic. If an embryo forms, it dies early at only 1 to 2 mm in size with no fetal blood present

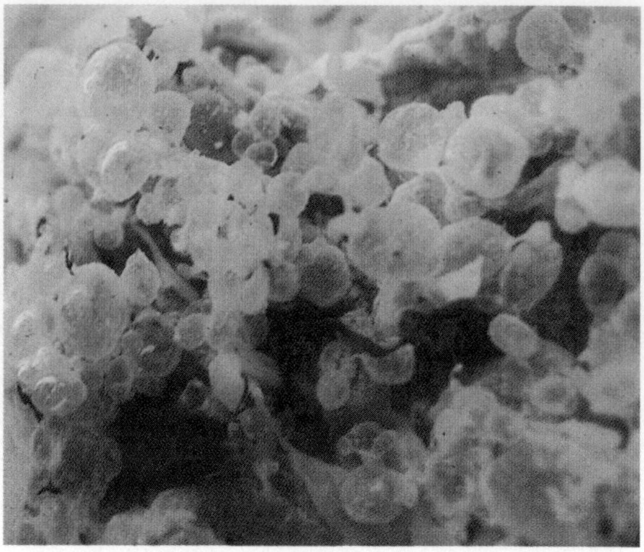

FIGURE 15.3 Gestational trophoblastic disease.

in the villi. On chromosomal analysis, although the karyotype is a normal 46XX or 46XY, this chromosome component was contributed only by the father or an "empty ovum" was fertilized and the chromosome material was duplicated (Fig. 15-4A).

With a partial mole, some of the villi form normally. The syncytiotrophoblastic layer of villi, however, is swollen and misshapen. Although no embryo is present, fetal blood may be present in the villi. A macerated embryo of approximately 9 weeks' gestation may be present. A partial mole has 69 chromosomes (a triploid formation in which there are three chromosomes instead of two for every pair,

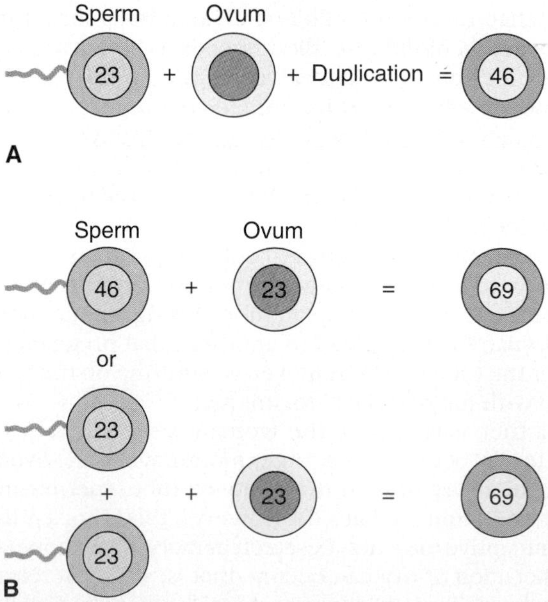

FIGURE 15.4 Formation of gestational trophoblastic disease. (A) Complete mole. (B) Partial mole.

one set supplied by an ovum that apparently was fertilized by two sperm or an ovum fertilized by one sperm in which meiosis or reduction division did not occur). This could also occur if one set of 23 chromosomes was supplied by one sperm and an ovum that did not undergo reduction division supplied 46 (see Fig. 15-4*B*).

In contrast to complete moles, partial moles rarely lead to choriocarcinoma. Although still above average, hCG titers are lower in partial than in complete moles; they also return to normal faster after mole evacuation.

Assessment

Because proliferation of the trophoblast cells occurs so rapidly with this condition, the uterus tends to expand faster than normally. This causes the uterus to reach its landmarks (just over the symphysis brim at 12 weeks, at the umbilicus at 20 to 24 weeks) before the usual time. This rapid development is also diagnostic of multiple pregnancy or a miscalculated due date, however, so this finding must be evaluated carefully. No fetal heart sounds are heard because there is no viable fetus. Because hCG is produced by the trophoblast cells that are overgrowing, a serum or urine test of hCG for pregnancy will be strongly positive (1 to 2 million IU compared with a normal pregnancy level of 400,000 IU).

Results continue to be strongly positive after day 100 of pregnancy, when the level of hCG normally would begin to decline. This fact must be evaluated carefully also, because highly positive test results can be characteristic of multiple pregnancies with more than one placenta. The nausea and vomiting of early pregnancy is usually marked, probably due to the high hCG level present. Symptoms of hypertension of pregnancy (i.e., hypertension, edema, and proteinuria) are ordinarily not present before week 20 of pregnancy. With gestational trophoblastic disease, they may appear before this time. A sonogram will show dense growth (typically a snowflake pattern) but no fetal growth in the uterus.

At approximately week 16 of pregnancy, if the structure was not identified earlier by sonogram, it will identify itself with vaginal bleeding. This may begin as vaginal spotting of dark-brown blood or as a profuse fresh flow. As the bleeding progresses, it is accompanied by discharge of the clear-fluid-filled vesicles. This is why it is important for any woman who begins to miscarry at home to bring any clots or tissue passed to the hospital with her. The presence of clear-fluid-filled cysts changes the diagnosis to gestational trophoblastic disease.

Therapeutic Management

Therapy for gestational trophoblastic disease is suction curettage to evacuate the mole. After surgery, hCG levels remain high. Half of women still have a positive reading at 3 weeks; one fourth still have a positive test result at 40 days.

Following mole extraction women should have a baseline pelvic examination, a chest x-ray, and a serum test for the beta subunit of hCG. The hCG is analyzed every 1 to 2 weeks until levels are again normal. Thereafter, serum hCG levels are assessed every 2 to 4 weeks for 6 months. Gradually declining hCG titers suggest no complication. Levels that plateau for three times or increase in amount suggest malignant transformation. The woman should be instructed to use a reliable contraceptive method such as an oral contraceptive agent for 6 months so that a positive pregnancy test (the presence of hCG) resulting from a new pregnancy will not be confused with increasing levels and a developing malignancy. Some physicians give women who have had gestational trophoblastic disease a prophylactic course of methotrexate, the drug of choice for choriocarcinoma. However, because the drug interferes with white blood cell formation (leukopenia), prophylactic use must be weighed carefully. If malignancy should occur, it can be treated effectively in most instances with methotrexate at that time.

After 6 months, if hCG levels are still negative, the woman is theoretically free of the risk of a malignancy developing. Thus, she could plan a second pregnancy. Although the development of gestational trophoblastic disease means that a pregnancy never materialized and that a fetus never formed, the woman may experience the same feeling of loss after its evacuation that she would have experienced after the loss of a true pregnancy. She did, after all, believe that she was pregnant. In addition, she is faced with the possibility that a malignancy may develop. She also must delay her childbearing plans for half a year. If she has already put off having a child for some time, this may seem unbearably long.

Women need the opportunity to express their anger and sense of unfairness at this type of event. They may feel inadequate because something went wrong with the pregnancy. They may wonder whether it will happen again, whether they will ever be able to have children. Unfortunately, women who have one incidence of gestational trophoblastic disease have a four- to fivefold increased risk of a second molar pregnancy (Hammond, 2000). They need early screening with ultrasound during a second pregnancy to be certain this is not happening again.

WHAT IF? What if a woman diagnosed as having had a hydatidiform mole tells you she doesn't believe in birth control and does not intend to take the oral contraceptives prescribed following her mole evacuation? How would you advise her?

Premature Cervical Dilatation

Premature cervical dilatation, previously termed an **incompetent cervix,** refers to a cervix that dilates prematurely and therefore cannot hold a fetus until term (Tulandi & Sammour, 2000). The dilation is usually painless. Often the first symptom is show (a pink-stained vaginal discharge) or increased pelvic pressure, which may be followed by rupture of the membranes and discharge of the amniotic fluid. Uterine contractions begin, and after a short labor the fetus is born. Unfortunately, this commonly occurs at approximately week 20 of pregnancy, and the fetus is too immature to survive. Early dilatation is relatively rare, occurring in about 1% of women (Scott, 2000a).

It is often difficult to explain in a particular instance what caused premature dilatation. It is associated with increased maternal age, congenital structural defects, and trauma to the cervix such as might have occurred with a cone biopsy or repeated D&Cs. Although it may be diagnosed by an early sonogram before symptoms occur, it is usually diagnosed only after the pregnancy is lost.

After the loss of one child due to premature cervical dilatation, a surgical operation termed **cervical cerclage** can be performed to prevent this from happening again. As soon as a sonogram confirms that the fetus of a second pregnancy is healthy, at approximately weeks 12 to 14, purse-string sutures are placed in the cervix by the vaginal route under regional anesthesia. This procedure is called a McDonald or a Shirodkar procedure after the surgeons who perfected the technique. The sutures serve to strengthen the cervix and prevent it from dilating (Fig. 15-5).

In a McDonald procedure, nylon sutures are placed horizontally and vertically across the cervix and pulled tight to reduce the cervical canal to a few millimeters in diameter. With a Shirodkar technique, sterile tape is threaded in a purse-string manner under the submucous layer of the cervix and sutured in place to achieve a closed cervix. Although routinely accomplished by a vaginal route, sutures may be placed by a transabdominal route.

With these procedures, the sutures may be removed at weeks 37 to 38 of pregnancy so the fetus may be delivered vaginally. When a transabdominal approach is used, the sutures may be left in place and a cesarean birth is performed (Ecker, 2001).

Be certain to ask women who are reporting painless bleeding (the symptoms of spontaneous miscarriage also) whether they have had past cervical operations.

Still newer techniques allow purse-string sutures to be set before the woman becomes pregnant, providing added assurance that she will not begin miscarrying before week 14 of pregnancy. Women who are discovered to have cervical dilatation but with membranes still intact at a prenatal visit may have emergent cerclage sutures placed in the cervix even at that point as prophylaxis against preterm birth. The success of this procedure is limited (Matijevic et al., 2001).

Currently, the prognosis for a successful pregnancy after surgical correction for premature cervical dilatation is very

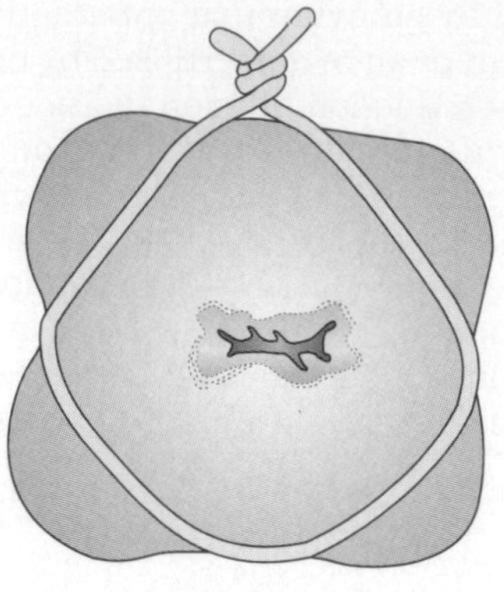

FIGURE 15.5 Shirodkar suture for cervical cerclage.

favorable. The success rate with both types of cerclage techniques is 80% to 90% (Cunningham et al., 2001). After cerclage surgery, women remain on bed rest (perhaps in a slight or modified Trendelenburg position) for a few days to decrease pressure on the new sutures. Sexual relations can be resumed in most instances after this rest period.

CONDITIONS ASSOCIATED WITH THIRD-TRIMESTER BLEEDING

Slight spotting late in pregnancy can be caused by trauma from a pelvic examination or coitus, so this could be an innocent finding. Bleeding during late pregnancy usually occurs, however, from placenta previa, premature separation of the placenta (abruptio placentae), or preterm labor, all of which are serious conditions.

Placenta Previa

Placenta previa (Fig. 15-6) is low implantation of the placenta. It occurs in four degrees: implantation in the lower rather than in the upper portion of the uterus (low-lying placenta); marginal implantation (the placenta edge approaches that of the cervical os); implantation that occludes

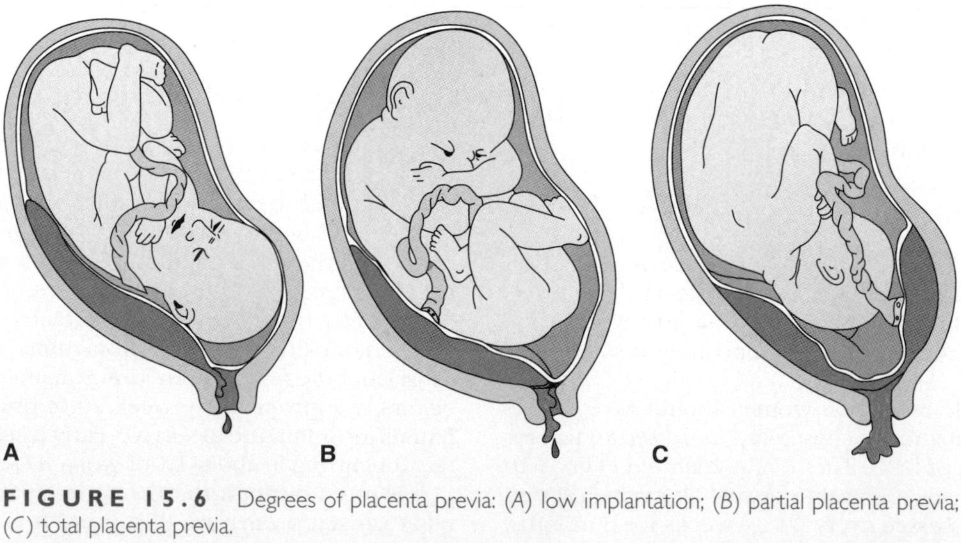

FIGURE 15.6 Degrees of placenta previa: (*A*) low implantation; (*B*) partial placenta previa; (*C*) total placenta previa.

a portion of the cervical os (partial placenta previa); and implantation that totally obstructs the cervical os (total placenta previa). The degree to which the placenta covers the internal cervical os is generally estimated in percentages: 100%, 75%, 30%, and so forth.

Increased parity, advanced maternal age, past cesarean births, past uterine curettage, and multiple gestation are all associated with placenta previa. The incidence is approximately 5 per 1,000 pregnancies (Scott, 2000b). It is thought to occur whenever the placenta is forced to spread to find an adequate exchange surface. An increase in congenital fetal anomalies may occur if the low implantation does not allow optimal fetal nutrition or oxygenation.

Assessment

Because routine sonograms are performed so frequently during pregnancy, most instances of placenta previa are diagnosed today before any symptoms occur. In these instances, the condition is explained to the woman and she is cautioned to avoid coitus, get adequate rest, and telephone her health care provider at any sign of vaginal bleeding. Bleeding with placenta previa occurs when the lower uterine segment begins to differentiate from the upper segment late in pregnancy (approximately week 30) and the cervix begins to dilate. The bleeding results from the placenta's inability to stretch to accommodate the differing shape of the lower uterine segment or the cervix. The bleeding that occurs is usually abrupt, painless, and bright red and sudden enough to frighten the woman. It is not associated with increased activity or participation in sports. It may stop as abruptly as it began, so that by the time the woman is seen at the health care site she is no longer bleeding, or it may slow after the initial hemorrhage but continue as continuous spotting.

Therapeutic Management

The bleeding of placenta previa, like that of ectopic pregnancy, is an emergency situation. The site of bleeding, the uterine decidua (maternal blood), places the mother at risk for hemorrhage. Because the placenta is loosened, the fetal oxygen supply may be compromised, placing the fetus at risk also. With the placenta loosening, preterm labor may begin, posing an additional threat to the fetus.

Immediate Care Measures. To ensure an adequate blood supply to the woman and fetus, place the woman immediately on bed rest in a side-lying position. Be sure to assess the following:

- Duration of the pregnancy
- Time the bleeding began
- Woman's estimation of the amount of blood—ask her to estimate in terms of cups or tablespoons (a cup is 240 mL; a tablespoon is 15 mL)
- Whether there was accompanying pain
- Color of the blood (redder blood indicates that the bleeding is fresher or is continuing)
- What she has done for the bleeding (if she inserted a tampon to halt the bleeding, there may be hidden bleeding)
- Whether there were prior episodes of bleeding during the pregnancy
- Whether she had prior cervical surgery for premature cervical dilatation

Inspect the perineum for bleeding. Estimate the present rate of blood loss. Weighing perineal pads before and after use and calculating the difference by subtraction is a good method to determine vaginal blood loss. An Apt or Kleihauer-Betke test (test strip procedures) is used to detect whether the blood is of fetal or maternal origin. Never attempt a pelvic or rectal examination with painless bleeding late in pregnancy because any agitation of the cervix when there is a placenta previa may initiate massive hemorrhage, fatal to both mother and child. Obtain baseline vital signs to determine whether symptoms of shock are present. Continue to assess blood pressure every 5 to 15 minutes or continuously with an electronic cuff. Begin intravenous fluid therapy using a large-gauge catheter and monitor urine output frequently, as often as every hour, as an indicator of blood volume adequacy. Attach an external fetal monitor and begin recording fetal heart sounds and uterine contractions. Obviously, an internal monitor that requires invasion of the cervix is contraindicated. Hemoglobin, hematocrit, prothrombin time, partial thromboplastin time, fibrinogen, platelet count, and type and cross-match and antibody screen should be assessed to establish baselines, detect a possible clotting disorder, and ready blood for replacement if necessary. Vaginal birth is always safest for an infant. Therefore, it is essential to determine the placenta's location as accurately as possible in the hope that its position will make vaginal birth feasible. If the previa is under 30%, it may be possible for the fetus to be born past it. If over 30%, and the fetus is mature, the safest birth method for both mother and baby is often a cesarean birth.

The abdominal examination may reveal that the fetal head is not engaged because of the interfering placenta. However, this finding gives little indication of how much of the placenta is obscuring the os and thus preventing the head from engaging. Anticipate the order for a transvaginal sonogram to detect this. If no previa is detected, the physician may attempt a careful speculum examination of the vagina and cervix to rule out a source of bleeding such as ruptured varices or cervical trauma.

Vaginal examinations (actual investigation of dilation) to determine whether placenta previa exists are done in an operating room or a fully equipped birthing room so that if hemorrhage does occur with the manipulation, an immediate cesarean birth can be carried out to remove the child and the bleeding placenta and contract the uterus.

Have oxygen equipment available in case the fetal heart sounds indicate fetal distress, such as bradycardia or tachycardia, late deceleration, or variable decelerations.

Continuing Care Measures. The point at which a diagnosis of placenta previa is made and the age of the gestation dictate the final management. If labor has begun, bleeding is continuing, or the fetus is being compromised (measured by the response of the fetal heart rate to contractions), birth must be accomplished regardless of gestational age. If the bleeding has stopped, the fetal heart sounds are of good quality, maternal vital signs are good, and the fetus is not yet 36 weeks of age, the woman is usually managed by expectant watching. As many as half of all women with bleeding from placenta previa are managed this way.

Typically, the woman remains in the hospital on bed rest for close observation for 48 hours. If the bleeding stops, she will be sent home with a referral for bed rest and home care. Careful assessment of fetal heart sounds is made and laboratory tests, such as hemoglobin or hematocrit, are frequently obtained. Betamethasone, a steroid that hastens fetal lung maturity, may be prescribed for the mother to encourage the maturity of fetal lungs if the fetus is less than 34 weeks' gestation (see Focus on Pharmacology).

NURSING DIAGNOSES AND RELATED INTERVENTIONS

Because the diagnosis of placenta previa with bleeding is an emergency situation, all goals should reflect the emergency condition and a short time frame for resolution.

Nursing Diagnosis: Fear related to outcome of pregnancy after episode of placenta previa bleeding

Outcome Identification: Client expresses her fears about the baby openly and continues making positive statements about the baby.

Outcome Evaluation: Client discusses concerns with nurse and other health care providers; states that hearing fetal heart beat helps to reassure her about baby's health.

Often it is difficult for the woman who has experienced bleeding late in a pregnancy to wait for the baby to come to term, wondering whether her infant is all right. Regardless of her outward appearance, most likely she is experiencing severe emotional stress. She cannot help but wonder if the next bleeding she experiences may kill her, the infant, or both. She may become so worried about the safety of her child that she begins to think of the baby as already dead. She might begin to neglect her diet or her supplementary vitamins because "it doesn't matter any more." Listening to fetal heart sounds and being reassured that they are in a healthy range are helpful. She also needs to be able to talk to someone about her fears so she doesn't feel alone with her concerns.

FOCUS ON PHARMACOLOGY

Betamethasone (Celestone)

Action: Betamethasone is a corticosteroid that acts as an anti-inflammatory and immunosuppressive agent. It is given to pregnant women 12 to 24 hours before delivery to hasten fetal lung maturity and thus help prevent respiratory distress syndrome in the newborn.

Pregnancy Risk Category: C

Dosage: 12.5 mg IM initially; may be repeated in 24 hours and again in 1 to 2 weeks

Possible Adverse Effects: Burning, itching, and irritation at the injection site. Swelling, tachycardia, headache, dizziness, weight gain, sodium and fluid retention. Increased risk of infection if used long term

Nursing Implications

- Explain the purpose of the drug to the woman.
- Administer the initial dose IM. Anticipate the need for repeat dosing within 24 hours and again in 1 to 2 weeks.
- Assist with measures to halt preterm labor if indicated.
- Continue to monitor client's vital signs and fetal heart rate for changes.
- If the woman is also receiving a tocolytic agent, be alert for possible cardiac decompensation as a result of a drug–drug interaction. Observe for signs such as increased pulse, decreased blood pressure, and presence of edema.
- Assess for signs and symptoms of possible infection with long-term use.
- Instruct the woman about the possibility of repeat doses.

Birth

As soon as the fetus reaches 37 weeks of age (2,500 g), an amniocentesis analysis for lung maturity shows a positive result (a favorable lecithin–sphingomyelin ratio), bleeding occurs again, labor begins, or the fetus shows symptoms of distress, the fetus will be delivered. Be sure to advise the woman during her weeks or days of waiting that a cesarean birth will probably be necessary because of the low implantation of the placenta. If the pregnancy is not yet at term, inform her that her baby probably will have a low birth weight.

On the day of birth, a woman needs a great deal of support. It is one thing to talk about being ready for surgery; it is another to be truly ready. She may be as frightened as she was the evening her bleeding began. If at the time of the initial bleeding the pregnancy is past 36 weeks, a birth decision will generally be made immediately. If the placenta previa is found to be total, delivery through the placenta is impossible and the baby must be delivered by cesarean birth. If the placenta previa is partial, the amount of the blood loss, the condition of the fetus, and the woman's parity will influence the birth decision. With a cesarean birth for placenta previa, although the skin incision is still a transverse (bikini) one, the uterine cut must be made high, possibly vertically above the low implantation site of the placenta. If a sonogram clearly reveals the placental location, a transverse uterine incision may be possible.

After birth, the mother inspects her child carefully. She may think that because of the problems with placental implantation, there might be something wrong with her child. During the postpartal period, she needs frequent visits with her child to be certain he or she is all right.

Any woman who has had a placenta previa is more prone than normal to postpartal hemorrhage because the placental site is in the lower uterine segment, which does not contract as efficiently as the upper segment. Also, because the uterine blood supply is less in the lower segment, the placenta tends to grow larger than it would normally, leaving a larger denuded surface area when it is removed. As a second complication, the woman is more likely to develop endometritis because the placental site is close to the cervix, the portal of cntry for pathogens.

Premature Separation of the Placenta (Abruptio Placentae)

Unlike placenta previa, in **premature separation of the placenta** (also called abruptio placentae; Fig. 15-7), the placenta appears to have been implanted correctly. Suddenly, however, it begins to separate and bleeding results. This generally occurs late in pregnancy; it may occur as late as during the first or second stage of labor. Because premature separation of the placenta may occur during an otherwise normal labor, it is important to always be alert to the amount and kind of vaginal discharge a woman is having in labor. Listen to her description of the kind of pain she is having to detect this grave complication. Premature separation of the placenta occurs in about 10% of pregnancies and is the most frequent cause of perinatal death (Scott, 2000b).

The primary cause of premature separation is unknown, but certain predisposing factors have been identified, including high parity, a short umbilical cord, chronic hypertensive disease, hypertension of pregnancy, direct trauma (as from an automobile accident), and vasoconstriction from cocaine use. Cigarette smoking is also an associated factor (Scott, 2000b).

Premature separation of the placenta may follow a rapid decrease in uterine volume, such as occurs with sudden release of amniotic fluid. Usually the fetal head is low enough in the pelvis that it prevents loss of the total volume of the amniotic fluid at one time. Thus, normally a rapid reduction in amniotic fluid this way does not occur.

Assessment

The woman experiences a sharp, stabbing pain high in the uterine fundus as the initial separation occurs. If labor begins with the separation, each contraction will be accompanied by pain over and above the pain of the contraction. In some women, the pain is not evident with contractions but tenderness is felt on uterine palpation.

Heavy bleeding usually accompanies premature separation of the placenta, although it may not be readily apparent. There will be external bleeding if the placenta separates first at the edges and blood escapes freely from the cervix. If the center of the placenta separates first, however, blood will pool under the placenta and be hidden from view. Blood may infiltrate the uterine musculature (**couvelaire uterus** or uteroplacental apoplexy), forming a hard, boardlike uterus with no apparent, or minimally apparent, bleeding present. Signs of shock usually follow quickly because of the blood loss. The uterus becomes tense and rigid to the touch. If bleeding is extensive, the woman's reserve of blood fibrinogen may be used up in her body's attempt to accomplish effective clot formation, and DIC syndrome occurs (see below).

If the woman is being admitted to the hospital after experiencing symptoms at home, assess the time the bleeding began, whether pain accompanied it, the amount and kind of bleeding, and the woman's actions. Initial blood work should include hemoglobin level, typing and cross-matching, and a fibrinogen level and fibrin breakdown products to detect the occurrence of DIC. For a quick assessment of blood clotting ability, draw 5 mL and place it in a clean, dry test tube. Stand it aside untouched for 5 minutes. At the end of this time, if a clot has not formed, suspect an interference with blood coagulation.

Therapeutic Management

On admission, the woman needs a large-gauge intravenous catheter inserted for fluid replacement and oxygen by mask to limit fetal anoxia. Monitor fetal heart sounds externally and record maternal vital signs every 5 to 15 minutes to establish baselines and observe progress. The baseline fibrinogen determination is followed by additional determinations up to the time of delivery. Keep the woman in a lateral, not supine, position to prevent pressure on the vena cava and additional interference with fetal circulation. It is important not to disturb the injured placenta any further. Therefore, do not perform any vaginal or pelvic examination or give an enema to the woman with a diagnosed or suspected placental separation.

For better prediction of fetal and maternal outcome, the degrees of placental separation are graded (Table 15-5) (Sorokin, 2000). Unless the separation is minimal (grades 0 and 1), the pregnancy must be terminated because the fetus cannot obtain adequate oxygen and nutrients. If the pre-

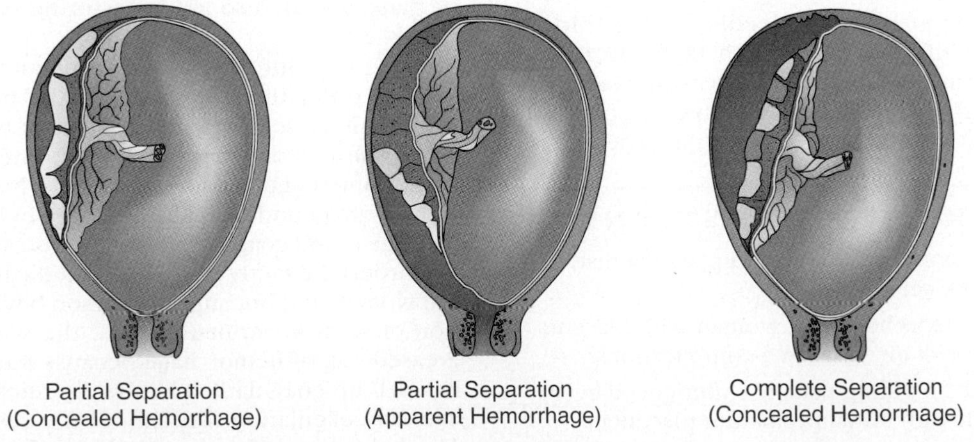

FIGURE 15.7 Premature separation of the placenta.

TABLE 15.5 Premature Separation of the Placenta: Degrees of Separation

GRADE	CRITERIA
0	No symptoms of separation were apparent from maternal or fetal signs; the diagnosis that a slight separation did occur is made after birth, when the placenta is examined and a segment of the placenta shows a recent adherent clot on the maternal surface.
1	This is minimal separation, but enough to cause vaginal bleeding and changes in the maternal vital signs; no fetal distress or hemorrhagic shock occurs, however.
2	This is moderate separation; there is evidence of fetal distress; the uterus is tense and painful on palpation.
3	This is extreme separation; without immediate interventions, maternal shock and fetal death will result.

mature separation occurs during active labor, rupturing the membranes or augmenting labor with intravenous oxytocin may be the method of choice to hasten birth. Rupturing the membranes prevents large amounts of blood from being trapped in the myometrium, which, if allowed to accumulate, could prevent uterine contraction. Because artificially rupturing the membranes allows a slow, steady escape of amniotic fluid, a sudden change in uterine pressure does not encourage more separation. If birth does not seem imminent, cesarean birth is the delivery method of choice.

If DIC has developed, surgery may pose a grave risk because of the possibility of hemorrhage during the surgery and later from the surgical incision. Intravenous administration of fibrinogen or cryoprecipitate (which contains fibrinogen) may be used to elevate her fibrinogen level.

Fetal prognosis depends on the extent of the placental separation and the degree of fetal hypoxia. Maternal prognosis depends on how promptly treatment is instituted. Death can occur from massive hemorrhage leading to shock and circulatory collapse or renal failure from the circulatory collapse.

Any woman who has had bleeding before birth is more prone to infection after birth than the average woman. A woman with a history of premature separation of the placenta, therefore, needs to be observed closely for the development of infection in the postpartal period.

✔ CHECKPOINT QUESTIONS

5. What term is used to describe a placenta that occludes the cervical os?
6. After her baby is born, the woman with placenta previa is at risk for what two complications?
7. What is the first thing usually experienced by the woman with initial premature placental separation?

Disseminated Intravascular Coagulation

DIC is an acquired disorder of blood clotting. Symptoms include easy bruising or bleeding from an intravenous site (Cunningham et al., 2001). Conditions such as premature separation of the placenta, hypertension of pregnancy, amniotic fluid embolism, placental retention, septic abortion, and retention of a dead fetus are associated with its development. Normally, platelets quickly form a seal over a point of bleeding to prevent further loss of blood. Intrinsic and extrinsic clotting pathways are activated, and this plug is strengthened by fibrin threads into a firm, fixed structure. To prevent too much clotting from occurring, at the same time the clot is being formed, thrombin activates fibrinolysin, a proteolytic enzyme, to begin to digest excess fibrin threads (anticoagulation). This lysis results in the release of fibrin degradation products.

DIC occurs when there is extreme bleeding and so many platelets and fibrin from the general circulation rush to the site that there are not enough left for further clotting. The high thrombin level continues to encourage anticoagulation. This results in a paradox: at one point, the person has increased coagulation, but throughout the rest of the system, a bleeding defect exists. DIC is an emergency situation because it can result in extreme blood loss. Goals must reflect the presence of the emergency.

To stop the process of DIC, the underlying insult that began the phenomenon must be halted. When the insult was a complication of pregnancy such as premature separation of the placenta, ending the pregnancy by delivering the fetus and placenta is part of the answer. Next, the marked coagulation must be stopped so that coagulation factors can be freed and restore normal clotting function. This is accomplished by the intravenous administration of heparin to halt the clotting cascade. Heparin must be given cautiously close to birth or postpartal hemorrhage can occur after delivery of the placenta. If bleeding during pregnancy was the stimulus for DIC, a blood or platelet transfusion may be necessary to replace blood or platelet loss. This administration may be delayed, however, until after heparin therapy so the new blood factors are also not consumed by the coagulation process. Antithrombin III factor, fibrinogen, or cryoprecipitate (which contains fibrinogen) can also be used to restore blood clotting. If these are not available, fresh-frozen plasma or platelets can also aid in restoring clotting function (Clark, 2000).

It can be confusing for the woman with a disorder such as premature separation of the placenta to have her physician tell her one minute that bleeding is what he or she is worried about and the next minute hear that an anticoagulant such as heparin has been ordered. If the woman understands the action of heparin—to discourage blood coagulation—it seems as if the physician has ordered exactly the wrong medication. Be certain the woman and her support person have a full explanation of what is happening (i.e., the woman has an increased risk of hemorrhage because part of her system has tied up coagulation factors; by releasing them, you can aid coagulation throughout the rest of her body). This helps to instill and maintain confidence in her caregivers.

Evaluation focuses on determining whether the woman's blood coagulation studies are returning to normal and if any anoxia has occurred, particularly in renal or brain cells from occluded coagulated capillaries. Fetal and newborn assessment is important to evaluate the sufficiency of the placental circulation.

WHAT IF? What if a pregnant client who you are caring for is receiving subcutaneous heparin and asks why can't she take this drug orally? How would you answer her? Does she need to be sure that the infant receives assessment for blood coagulation ability at birth?

PRETERM LABOR

Preterm labor is labor that occurs before the end of week 37 of gestation. It occurs in approximately 9% to 10% of all pregnancies. Any woman having persistent uterine contractions (four every 20 minutes) should be considered to be in labor (Colombo & Iams, 2000). A woman is documented as being in actual labor if she is having uterine contractions that cause cervical effacement over 80% and dilation over 1 cm. Preterm labor is always serious because if it results in the infant's birth, the infant may be premature. Preterm births are responsible for almost two thirds of all infant deaths in the neonatal period (Colombo & Iams, 2000).

Some women wait to seek help for preterm labor, unwilling to face the fact that labor contractions have started. Some diagnose their contractions as nothing more than extremely hard Braxton Hicks contractions and so do not seek help early. Currently, when there is treatment available to delay labor until the fetus reaches a level of maturity that will allow him or her to survive in the outside environment, evaluation and the institution of therapy before membranes rupture are vital.

Why labor begins before the fetus is mature is unclear in most instances. Preterm labor often occurs for unknown reasons but it is associated with dehydration, urinary tract infection, and **chorioamnionitis** (infection of the fetal membranes and fluid). African-American women, adolescents, and those who receive inadequate prenatal care are most susceptible (Parsons & Spellacy, 2000). Women who continue to work at strenuous jobs during pregnancy or perform shift work that leads to extreme fatigue may have a higher incidence than others.

Common symptoms of early preterm labor include a persistent, dull, low backache; vaginal spotting; a feeling of pelvic pressure or abdominal tightening; menstrual-like cramping; increased vaginal discharge; uterine contractions; and intestinal cramping. Any woman who has these symptoms or believes she is in preterm labor for any reason needs to be carefully evaluated because symptoms of labor are subtle and best recognized by the woman herself. Be certain all women receive information on the signs and symptoms of preterm labor so they do not overlook the more subtle signs.

Therapeutic Management

Although a number of diagnostic tests are being evaluated, it is not possible to predict which pregnancies will end early with preterm labor. It is possible to analyze changes in vaginal mucus, such as the presence of fetal fibronectin, a protein produced by trophoblast cells. If this is present in vaginal mucus, it may predict that preterm contractions are occurring (Rinehart et al., 2001). A shortened cervix, revealed by sonography, may be predictive. Medical attempts can be made to stop labor if the fetal membranes intact, fetal distress is absent, there is no evidence that bleeding is occurring, the cervix is not dilated more than 4 to 5 cm, and effacement is not more than 50%. Box 15-1 highlights appropriate outcomes and interventions using the terminology identified by the Nursing Outcomes Classification and Nursing Interventions Classification.

A woman who is in preterm labor is usually first admitted to the hospital and placed on bed rest to relieve the pressure of the fetus on the cervix. Intravenous fluid therapy to keep the woman well hydrated is initiated because hydration may have an influence on stopping contractions, although this has not been scientifically documented (Parsons & Spellacy, 2000). If the woman is dehydrated, the pituitary gland is activated to secrete antidiuretic hormone, and it may also release oxytocin. Oxytocin strengthens uterine contractions. By keeping her well hydrated, the release of oxytocin may be minimized.

Vaginal and cervical cultures and a clean-catch urine sample are obtained to rule out infection. Assuring the woman that everything that can be done is being done is important. Following initial therapy, women in preterm labor can be safely cared for at home as long as they can dependably remain on almost complete bed rest, drink enough fluid to remain well hydrated, and take an oral **tocolytic agent** (a drug to halt labor) such as oral terbutaline (see Focus on Family Empowerment, and see Chap. 16 for a discussion of home care). It is important that women also maintain adequate nutrition and do not smoke cigarettes (poor nutrition and smoking put them at high risk for preterm birth).

Drug Administration

Women in preterm labor may receive an antibiotic for group B streptococcus prophylaxis. For reasons not clearly understood, the administration of a corticosteroid to the fetus appears to accelerate the formation of lung surfactant. During the time labor is being chemically halted, therefore, if the pregnancy is under 34 weeks, the woman may be given a steroid (betamethasone) to attempt to hasten fetal lung maturity (two doses of 12 mg betamethasone given intramuscularly 24 hours apart, or four doses of 6 mg dexamethasone given intramuscularly 12 hours apart; Colombo & Iams, 2000). It takes about 24 hours for betamethasone to have an effect, so it is important that labor be halted for at least this long. The effect lasts approximately 7 days. If the fetus is not born within that time span, the dose of betamethasone will be repeated.

Although calcium channel blockers such as nifedipine (Procardia) or a prostaglandin antagonist such as indo-

BOX 15.1

NURSING OUTCOMES AND NURSING INTERVENTIONS CLASSIFICATION: HALTING PRETERM LABOR

NOC: Maternal Status, Intrapartum

Maternal status, intrapartum is defined as the conditions and behaviors indicating maternal well-being from the onset of labor to delivery (Johnson, Maas, & Moorhead, 2000). Some specific indicators suggesting achievement of this outcome include the following:

- Adequate coping mechanisms
- Uterine contraction frequency, duration, and intensity within expected range
- Progression of cervical dilation within accepted parameters
- Vital signs and laboratory test results within expected range

NIC: Labor Suppression

Labor suppression is defined as the control of uterine contractions prior to 37 weeks' gestation to prevent preterm birth (McCloskey & Bulechek, 2000). Some important activities involved when implementing this intervention include:

- Determining fetal age based on last menstrual period, sonogram, fundal height measurements, and date of quickening and audible fetal heart tones
- Ascertaining information about onset and duration of preterm labor symptoms, including any activities that preceded the onset
- Evaluating the status of amniotic membranes
- Assessing uterine activity
- Palpating for fetal position, presentation, and station
- Performing cervical exam for dilation, effacement, softening, and position
- Initiating hydration measures and monitoring intake and output
- Initiating tocolytic therapy
- Monitoring vital signs, fetal heart rate, and uterine activity as a baseline and every 15 minutes during tocolytic therapy
- Assessing for possible side effects of tocolytic therapy
- Preparing client and family for discharge to home care, including medication regimen, activity restrictions, diet, hydration, sexual activity, contraction palpation techniques, and signs and symptoms to notify physician
- Providing referrals for assistance with activities at home such as child care and home maintenance

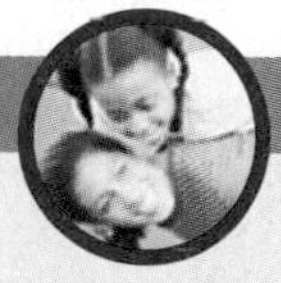

FOCUS ON FAMILY EMPOWERMENT

Measures to Help Prevent a Recurrence of Preterm Labor for Women on Bed Rest

Q. My doctor has put me on bed rest to help stop my labor. What else can I do?

A. To help prevent a recurrence of preterm labor, follow these helpful guidelines:

- Remain on bed rest except to use the bathroom (use a bed or feet up on a couch or lounge).
- Drink eight to ten glasses of fluids daily (keep a pitcher by your bed so you don't have to get up to get some).
- Be certain to take your prescribed tocolytic medication on time to maintain a constant blood level. Set an alarm clock as necessary, especially at night.
- Monitor fetal heart rate and uterine contractions daily.
- Keep mentally active by reading or working on a project to prevent boredom.
- Avoid activities that could stimulate labor, such as nipple stimulation.
- Consult your primary care provider as to whether sexual relations should be restricted.
- Immediately report signs of ruptured membranes (sudden gush of vaginal fluid) or vaginal bleeding.
- Report signs of urinary tract or vaginal infection (burning or frequency of urination; vaginal itching or pain).
- Report symptoms of pulmonary congestion (cough and difficulty breathing unless upright), which can be effects of tocolytic drugs.
- Keep appointments for prenatal care.

If uterine contractions recur:

- Empty your bladder to relieve pressure on the uterus.
- Lie down on your left or right side to encourage blood return to the uterus.
- Attach the fetal and uterine contraction monitor.
- Drink two to three glasses of fluid to increase hydration.
- Telephone your health care provider to report incident and ask for further care measures.

methacin (Indocin) can be used as tocolytic agents, these are not the drugs of choice due to their side effects. For example, there is a danger of decreased fetal urine output, resulting in oligohydramnios and premature closure of the fetal ductus arteriosus with resultant fetal pulmonary hypertension, after indomethacin administration.

Magnesium sulfate is often the first drug used to halt contractions. Classified as a cathartic, it also has a central nervous system depressant action that slows and halts uterine contractions (see Focus on Pharmacology).

In addition to magnesium sulfate, beta-sympathomimetic drugs may also be used. Beta-1 receptor sites are found in adipose tissue, heart, liver, pancreatic islet cells, and gastrointestinal smooth muscle. Beta-2 receptor sites are found in uterine smooth muscle, bronchial smooth muscle, and blood vessels. Beta-adrenergic drugs act to halt contractions by coupling with adrenergic receptors on the outer surface of the membrane of myometrial cells. This releases adenylcyclase, which triggers the conversion of adenosine triphosphate into cyclic adenosine monophosphate. This substance is responsible for reducing the intracellular concentration of calcium through protein binding. With a lowered intracellular calcium concentration, muscle contraction is ineffective and uterine contractions halt. An ideal tocolytic drug is one that acts entirely on beta-2 receptor sites and does not cause any heart or gastrointestinal symptoms.

Ritodrine hydrochloride (Yutopar) and terbutaline (Brethine) are two drugs that act almost entirely on beta-2 receptor sites and so exert only mild hypotensive and tachycardiac effects. Of these two drugs, terbutaline is more frequently used. As a beta-2 receptor, it causes blood vessels and bronchi to relax along with the uterine muscle. As a result, hypotension can occur. This causes the heart rate to increase to move blood more effectively. Hypokalemia may occur from a shift of potassium into cells, and blood glucose and accompanying plasma insulin levels may increase. Pulmonary edema may occur (Karch, 2001). Headache, due to the dilatation of cerebral blood vessels, is a common side effect; nausea and emesis also may occur. Headache, nausea, and vomiting are side effects to be observed for but are not reasons to discontinue therapy. Terbutaline should be used cautiously with clients with diabetes mellitus and thyroid dysfunction. In a woman who is predisposed to develop gestational diabetes, terbutaline can raise her blood sugar level so much that she becomes overtly diabetic. This further complicates her pregnancy.

Before a tocolytic drug is administered, obtain baseline blood data (hematocrit, serum glucose, potassium, sodium chloride, carbon dioxide) and possibly an electrocardiogram. An external uterine and fetal monitor should be in place (see Focus on Nursing Care Planning).

When administering terbutaline, mix the drug with Ringer's lactate rather than a dextrose solution to prevent any unnecessary hyperglycemia. Administer it as a piggyback connected to a main intravenous solution so that it can be stopped immediately if effects such as tachycardia or arrhythmias occur. Use microdrip tubing and an infusion pump to ensure a consistent, accurate flow rate.

After an initial flow rate is calculated and started, this rate may be increased every 10 minutes until uterine activity halts or side effects become extreme. Assess pulse and blood pressure approximately every 15 minutes while the flow rate is being increased and thereafter every 30 minutes until contractions halt. Assess also for chest pain and dyspnea. Auscultate the lungs for crackles (rales) to detect signs of pulmonary edema. Promptly report a pulse rate

FOCUS ON PHARMACOLOGY

Magnesium Sulfate

Action: Magnesium sulfate is a central nervous system depressant that acts to block neuromuscular transmission to halt convulsions. It can also be used to halt premature labor (unlabeled use).

Pregnancy Risk Category: B

Dosage: Initially, 4–6 g administered IV as a bolus followed by individually calculated IV infusion at a rate to maintain designated serum levels.

- Therapeutic range: 5.0–8.0 mg/100 mL
- Patellar reflex disappears: 8–10 mg/100 mL
- Respiratory depression occurs: 15–20 mg/100 mL
- Cardiac conduction defects occur: More than 20 mg/100 mL

Possible Adverse Effects: Flushing, thirst. With toxicity, absence of deep tendon reflexes, respiratory depression, cardiac arrhythmias, cardiac arrest, and decreased urine output.

Nursing Implications

- Administer continuous infusion piggybacked into a main IV line so it can be discontinued immediately without interfering with fluid administration.
- Always use an infusion control device to maintain a regular flow rate.
- Assess maternal blood pressure and fetal heart rate continuously with bolus IV administration.
- Assess deep tendon reflexes every 1–4 hours during continuous infusion. Use patellar reflex. If patient has received epidural anesthesia, use biceps reflex.
- Monitor intake and output every hour during continuous infusion. Urine output should be 30 mL/hour or greater.
- Assess client's level of consciousness, including ability to respond to questions, every hour.
- Obtain serum magnesium levels as indicated, usually every 6 to 8 hours.
- Keep calcium gluconate, the antidote for toxicity, readily available at the bedside.
- Maintain serum blood levels (for anticonvulsant use) at 5–8 mg/100 mL. If blood serum levels rise above this, respiratory depression, cardiac arrhythmias, and cardiac arrest can occur.
- Do not administer additional doses and stop infusion if deep tendon reflexes are absent or if respiratory rate is less than 14 or urine output is less than 30 mL/hour.
- This drug may cause respiratory depression in the newborn if administered close to birth. Alert the neonatal care personnel about this possibility.

FOCUS ON *Nursing Care Planning*

THE WOMAN IN PRETERM LABOR

A 22-year-old single woman at 28 weeks' gestation with twins is admitted in preterm labor. Tears in her eyes, she states, "I'm so scared. I don't want to lose my babies."

Assessment: G1P0 female; twin gestation at 28 weeks; fetal heart rates 136 and 142 beats per minute; reports positive fetal movements. Uterine contractions every 7 minutes lasting 40 seconds. L/S ratio less than 2:1. Heart rate 88 beats per minute; respirations 22; blood pressure 130/78. Intravenous tocolytic therapy with terbutaline ordered.

Nursing Diagnosis: Risk for injury (maternal and fetal) related to effects of preterm labor and tocolytic therapy.

Outcome Identification: Client will exhibit cessation of uterine contractions, carrying fetuses to as close to term as possible.

Outcome Evaluation: Contractions cease after treatment with tocolytic; fetal heart rates remain within acceptable parameters; fetal lung maturity improves as evidenced by rising L/S ratio; client remains free of signs and symptoms of adverse effects of tocolytic therapy.

Interventions	Rationale
1. Assess status of client and fetus. Obtain laboratory studies, including complete blood count, hemoglobin and hematocrit, serum electrolytes; anticipate need for ECG. Obtain urine, vaginal, and cervical cultures as ordered.	1. Assessment provides a baseline for future comparisons. Urine, vaginal, and cervical cultures help to rule out infection as a causative factor for preterm labor.
2. Institute bed rest with client in side-lying position. Apply external uterine and fetal monitoring.	2. Bed rest relieves pressure of the fetus on the cervix. Side-lying position enhances uterine perfusion. Uterine and fetal monitoring provides evidence of maternal and fetal well-being.
3. Begin intravenous fluid therapy as ordered. Assist with or insert an intravenous line.	3. Intravenous fluid improves hydration, which may help to minimize contractions.
4. Administer terbutaline intravenously as ordered, initially 10 μg/minute, increasing every 10 minutes to a maximum dosage of 80 μg/min, until desired effect.	4. Terbutaline is a beta-2 selective agonist that acts as a uterine relaxant, helping to halt preterm contractions.
5. Administer terbutaline as an intravenous piggyback solution with a main intravenous infusion. Use microdrip tubing and an infusion pump.	5. Piggyback administration allows for stoppage of tocolytic should adverse effects occur. Using microdrip tubing and an infusion pump allows for a consistent, accurate flow rate.
6. Monitor client's vital signs closely, every 15 minutes during adjustment of flow rate and then every 30 minutes until contractions cease. Auscultate lungs for changes in breath sounds. Assess for chest pain and dyspnea. Monitor fetal heart rates and patterns every 15 to 30 minutes.	6. Maternal pulse over 120 beats per minute or persistent tachycardia or tachypnea, chest pain, dyspnea, or adventitious breath sounds may indicate impending pulmonary edema. Fetal tachycardia or late or variable decelerations indicate possible uterine bleeding or fetal distress, which requires emergency birth.
7. Obtain hematocrit and serum electrolyte levels every 4 hours or as ordered. Monitor intake and output every hour during infusion, keeping intake to 100 mL/hour or less.	7. Hematocrit, electrolyte levels, and hourly measurements of intake and output provide evidence of the client's fluid volume status. If intake is greater than 100 mL/hour, fluid overload may occur. placing the client at risk for pulmonary edema.
8. Anticipate administration of betamethasone as ordered.	8. Betamethasone may be administered to hasten fetal lung maturity, helping to decrease the risk of respiratory distress syndrome should birth of the fetuses become necessary.

(continued)

Interventions	Rationale
9. Instruct client to report any feelings of chest pain, dizziness, nervousness, or irregular heartbeats.	9. Early recognition of possible adverse effects allows for prompt intervention.
10. Have propranolol (Inderal) readily available.	10. Propranolol (Inderal) is a beta-adrenergic blocking agent that may be used to counteract possible episodes of hypotension caused by infusion.
11. Monitor uterine contractions, including frequency and duration. Continue infusion for 12–24 hours after cessation of contractions. Anticipate switch to oral tocolytic therapy, administering first oral dose 30 minutes before discontinuing intravenous infusion.	11. Monitoring of uterine contractions provides evidence of effectiveness of therapy. Administering oral dose prior to discontinuation of intravenous infusion maintains consistent serum drug concentrations for effective control.
12. Continue to monitor client's and fetuses' status. Instruct client in measures to control preterm labor, including drug therapy.	12. Continued assessment is necessary to evaluate effectiveness of therapy. Education enhances understanding of the situation and promotes compliance with therapy, improving the chances for a successful outcome.

Nursing Diagnosis: Fear related to uncertainty of outcome.

Outcome Identification: Client will demonstrate positive coping behaviors to deal with situation.

Outcome Evaluation: Client verbalizes concerns and fears; works with caregivers in measures to control preterm labor; participates in decision making and relaxation measures.

Interventions	Rationale
1. Allow client to verbalize feelings and concerns. Assess for possible feelings related to cause of preterm labor.	1. Verbalization and assessment of feelings provide a safe outlet for emotions and help to dispel any misconceptions about the cause of preterm labor.
2. Approach the client in a calm, consistent, unhurried manner. Explain all actions and procedures. Attempt to minimize environmental stimuli.	2. Using a calm, consistent, unhurried approach with explanations helps to minimize the threat of the situation. Minimizing environmental stimuli can help reduce fear and anxiety.
3. Include client in treatment process and inform her about things ahead of time if possible.	3. Client participation enhances client's control over the situation and may help to instill hope and promote decision making.
4. Question client about the possibility of notifying a close friend or family member to be with her.	4. The presence of a friend or family member can offer additional support to the client.
5. Assist client with using relaxation techniques, such as muscle relaxation, breathing, and music.	5. Relaxation techniques help to decrease feelings of anxiety and fear, enhancing feelings of control.
6. Provide frequent updates about the client's and fetuses' progress.	6. Frequent updates about progress help to minimize feelings of fear about the unknown.

of more than 120 bpm, blood pressure below 90/60, chest pain, dyspnea, rales, or cardiac arrhythmias. Obtain hematocrit and serum electrolyte levels every 4 hours or as ordered during administration. Be certain to assess the total parenteral intake. If this exceeds 100 to 125 mL/hour, the woman may develop a fluid overload, which also can lead to pulmonary edema. Measure intake and output every hour during the active infusion, then every 4 hours after the infusion. Also obtain daily weights. Daily weights are important because an increasing daily weight suggests retention of fluid or accumulation of edema. Observe the fetal heart rate closely for tachycardia (heart rate over 160 bpm), late decelerations, or variable decelerations that suggest possible uterine bleeding or the need for emergency birth of the fetus rather than continuation of the pregnancy.

After the halt of contractions, the infusion usually is continued for 12 to 24 hours, then oral administration of terbutaline is begun. The first oral dose is given 30 minutes before the intravenous infusion is discontinued to prevent any drop in serum concentration. After this initial stabilization, the woman continues to take an oral tocolytic until 37 weeks' gestation or fetal lung maturity is established by amniocentesis. Before hospital discharge, teach the woman how to take her pulse before each dose of medication and to call if the pulse rate is more than 120 bpm or if she experiences palpitations or extreme nervousness.

Women must set their alarm clocks so they awaken at night to take the dose prescribed. Otherwise, their serum level of medication in the morning will be too low to be effective. Caution them that if they forget a dose, they must take a pill as soon as they remember and then space their doses accordingly from that time. They should not double the dose to make up for the missed pill because extreme tachycardia could result.

Terbutaline may also be administered subcutaneously by continuous pump. This allows for home drug administration using lower doses of medicine. Oral terbutaline therapy has the potential of prolonging labor an average of 2 weeks. With subcutaneous pump infusions, labor can be delayed an average of 8 to 9 weeks. Similar to an insulin pump, a terbutaline pump contains a syringe filled with the drug. A small polyethylene catheter leads from the pump to a subcutaneous needle. When the needle is inserted into the subcutaneous tissue of the abdomen or the thigh, the pump automatically injects a continuous low dose of medication subcutaneously. The pump can be set to "bolus" an injection of the drug at the time of day when contractions tend to occur the most. A woman could manually trigger the pump to inject extra medicine (within set limits) if she should begin to feel contractions. The pump can be carried in a sash around the waist or kept in a pocket of clothing. Pumps should never get wet, so the syringe should be removed from the pump while the woman showers. For tub bathing, she should remove both the pump and needle and replace it immediately afterward.

Fetal Assessment

In addition to supervising tocolytic therapy, it is important to assess overall fetal welfare daily in the woman trying to delay preterm labor. Women may be instructed to use a daily fetal movement count or "count to 10" test. The woman should be taught how to do this before discharge and then continue it when she is at home. The typical fetus moves 10 times in an hour. To evaluate fetal movement, the woman lies down on her left side and times the number of minutes it takes for her to feel 10 fetal movements (about an hour) or counts the number of fetal movements she feels in 1 hour (the average is 10 to 12). If the time it takes to feel 10 fetal movements is twice what it was the day before or if she feels fewer than 5 movements during an hour (half of what she should feel), she monitors again for a second hour. If at the end of this second hour fetal activity is still under 10 per hour, she should report it immediately. Because of the variation of movements among normal, healthy fetuses, different perinatal centers use different protocols for counting fetal movements. What standard is accepted as normal also varies.

Labor That Cannot Be Halted

In some women, preterm labor is too far advanced when they are first seen in a health care facility for it to be halted. Usually, if membranes have ruptured or the cervix is more than 50% effaced and 3 to 4 cm dilated, it is unlikely that labor can be halted. The rupturing of membranes, especially, can be thought of as a point of no return in stopping or delaying labor because of the increased risk of infection that begins from that point.

If the fetus is very immature at the time labor cannot be halted, a cesarean birth may be planned to reduce pressure on the fetal head and reduce the possibility of subdural or intraventricular hemorrhage.

Most women assume that if the fetus is preterm, labor will be shorter than normal because the infant is still so small. This is not necessarily true because the first stage of labor, the longest stage, proceeds exactly as it would with a term pregnancy. The second stage of labor may be shorter because a small infant can be pushed through the dilated cervix and the birth canal much more easily. Because the second stage takes at most 1 hour, however, this means the difference will not be more than 30 minutes to 1 hour. Unless a woman is given this explanation, she may worry not only that her labor is preterm but also that something is going wrong because it is lasting so long.

Because of the increased risk for prolapse of the cord around a small head, artificial rupture of the membranes is not done as a rule in preterm labor until the fetal head is firmly engaged. Delaying rupture of the membranes may prolong the first stage of labor.

Analgesic agents are administered with caution during preterm labor because of the immaturity of the fetus. The immature infant will have enough difficulty breathing at birth without the additional burden of being sedated from a drug such as meperidine (Demerol). If the woman wants pain relief, an epidural is preferable.

Uterine contractions and fetal heart sounds should be continuously monitored during labor. The woman can feel reassured by the evidence of the monitor screen or graph or the projected sound that, although her infant is likely to be small, heart tones seem to be of good quality and the infant is reacting well to labor.

Women may assume that because the infant's head is small, an episiotomy will be unnecessary for birth, and they will therefore escape the discomfort of postpartal stitches. Although the head of a preterm infant is smaller than that of a mature infant, it is also more fragile. Excessive pressure might result in a subdural or intraventricular hemorrhage that could be fatal. Therefore, the woman may actually need an episiotomy incision larger than usual. Forceps may also be used at delivery to reduce pressure on the fetal head.

The cord of the preterm infant is usually clamped immediately rather than waiting for pulsations to stop. This is because an immature infant has a difficult time excreting the large amount of bilirubin that will be formed if this extra blood is added to the circulation. The extra amount of blood may also overburden the circulatory system.

NURSING DIAGNOSES AND RELATED INTERVENTIONS

Examples of nursing diagnoses for the woman with preterm labor that cannot be halted include:

- Fear related to uncertain outcome of pregnancy
- Pain related to labor contractions

- Situational low self-esteem related to inability to carry pregnancy to term
- Risk for fetal injury related to preterm birth

Be certain that the outcomes established for care are realistic. Although many measures are available to help the preterm baby adjust to birth, the baby born preterm will be at risk for a variety of medical problems (see Chap. 26).

Nursing Diagnosis: Situational low self-esteem related to feelings of responsibility for preterm labor

Outcome Identification: Client demonstrates understanding of areas of pregnancy over which she does and does not have control (i.e., labor beginning); will express positive hopes for future.

Outcome Evaluation: Client expresses feelings and worries to nurse; states that it is unknown why labor begins but that she knows she is not responsible for her labor beginning prematurely.

A woman in preterm labor is undergoing an extreme crisis situation. She cannot help asking herself, "What did I do to cause this?" Time spent taking the initial history or timing contractions presents an opportunity to bring the concern out in the open: "Did Dr. Smith explain to you that labor sometimes begins early this way without any reason? Some women worry that they did something to bring on preterm labor, but this isn't true. Have you had any thoughts like that?"

A woman in preterm labor that cannot be halted needs a support person with her because she is apt to be more concerned than the average person about labor. She needs frequent assurance during labor that she is breathing well with contractions or just that she is "doing well." She may not be mentally prepared for labor because it has come unexpectedly. During the postpartal period, a woman may need continued reassurance. Helping rebuild self-esteem this way can better prepare her to be a mother to her preterm infant.

✔ CHECKPOINT QUESTIONS

8. What two interventions are important for the woman first diagnosed with preterm labor?
9. What is the beta-sympathomimetic agent most commonly used for tocolysis?

PRETERM RUPTURE OF MEMBRANES

Preterm rupture of membranes is rupture of fetal membranes with loss of amniotic fluid during pregnancy (Weitz, 2001). The cause of preterm rupture is unknown, but it is associated with infection of the membranes (chorioamnionitis). It occurs in 2% to 18% of pregnancies (Parsons & Spellacy, 2000). If rupture occurs early in pregnancy, it poses a major threat to the fetus. After rupture, the seal to the fetus is lost and uterine and fetal infection may occur. A second complication that can result from preterm membrane rupture is increased pressure on the umbilical cord from the loss of amniotic fluid, inhibiting the fetal nutrient supply, or cord prolapse (extension of the cord out of the uterine cavity into the vagina), a condition that could also interfere with fetal circulation. Cord prolapse is most apt to happen when the fetal head is still too small to fit the cervix firmly. Yet another risk to the fetus of remaining in a non-fluid-filled environment is the development of a Potter-like syndrome of distorted facial features and pulmonary hypoplasia from pressure. Preterm labor may follow rupture of the membranes. Inhibition of labor is rarely used after rupture of membranes because of the increased possibility of fetal infection after that point.

Assessment

Rupture of the membranes is suggested by the history. The woman usually describes a sudden gush of clear fluid from the vagina, with continued minimal leakage. Occasionally, a woman mistakes urinary incontinence caused by exertion for rupture of the membranes. Amniotic fluid cannot be differentiated from urine by appearance, so a sterile vaginal speculum examination is done to observe for vaginal pooling of fluid. If the fluid is tested with nitrazine paper, amniotic fluid causes an alkaline reaction on the paper (appears blue) and urine an acidic reaction (remains yellow). The fluid can also be tested for ferning, or the typical appearance of a high-estrogen fluid on microscopic examination. If there is still a question as to whether the membranes have ruptured, a sonogram may be ordered to assess the amniotic fluid index. Because preterm rupture of membranes is associated with vaginal infection, cultures for *Neisseria gonorrhoeae,* beta-streptococci, and *Chlamydia* are usually taken. Blood is drawn for white blood count and C-reactive protein. Avoid doing routine vaginal examinations because the risk of infection rises significantly when digital examinations are performed after preterm rupture of membranes.

If the fetus is estimated to be mature enough to survive in an extrauterine environment at the time of rupture and labor does not begin within 24 hours, labor contractions are usually induced by intravenous administration of oxytocin.

Therapeutic Management

If labor does not begin and the fetus is too young to survive outside the uterus, the woman will be placed on bed rest either in the hospital or at home (Parsons & Spellacy, 2000). The time between rupture and birth of the infant is called the latency period. Prophylactic administration of broad-spectrum antibiotics during this period may delay the onset of labor and reduce the risk of infection in the newborn. Women positive for streptococcus B need intravenous administration of penicillin or ampicillin to reduce the possibility of this infection in the newborn. It is usually not necessary to administer a corticosteroid to accelerate fetal lung maturity after preterm rupture of membranes because the lack of amniotic fluid causes early maturation of lung tissue by itself. Administration of a corticosteroid may also increase the possibility of maternal infection and is not proven to be effective with preterm rupture (Weitz, 2001).

It may be possible to apply a fibrin-based sealant to ruptured membranes so they are again intact. This is done by application of commercial fibrin sealant through the vagina into the cervix. To prevent infection from being introduced with the procedure, women may receive a course of antibiotics following resealing (Sciscione et al., 2001).

NURSING DIAGNOSES AND RELATED INTERVENTIONS

Nursing Diagnosis: Risk for infection related to preterm rupture of membranes without accompanying labor

Outcome Identification: Client will remain free of signs and symptoms of infection during the period between membrane rupture and birth of the baby.

Outcome Evaluation: Maternal white blood cell count remains within acceptable parameters; maternal temperature is less than 100.4°F (38.0°C).

An infection can be dangerous for both the mother and fetus. If at home, a woman is instructed to take her temperature twice a day and to report a fever (a temperature greater than 100.4°F [38.0°C]), uterine tenderness, or odorous vaginal discharge. She should refrain from tub bathing, douching, and coitus because of the danger of introducing infection. The white cell count will need to be assessed frequently, perhaps as often as daily. A count of more than 18,000 to 20,000/mm^3 suggests infection.

Before the woman is discharged to home care, be certain she knows how to read a thermometer, that she has specific instructions as to what degree of temperature she should report, and that she understands that bed rest should be strictly followed. Help her make arrangements for the daily white blood cell count through a laboratory service or home care nurse.

Many misconceptions about the difficulty of labor after preterm rupture of the membranes (dry labor) exist. Every day, the woman hopes the fetus is ready to be born, ending the long wait, yet she is also afraid to begin labor. She needs support for the remainder of the pregnancy and reassurance that because amniotic fluid is always being formed, there is no such thing as a dry labor. Intrauterine amnioinfusion may be used to supply additional uterine fluid and help protect the umbilical cord from compression and the fetus from compression deformities or pulmonary hypoplasia (see Chap. 18).

PREGNANCY-INDUCED HYPERTENSION

Pregnancy-induced hypertension (PIH) is a condition in which vasospasm occurs during pregnancy. Signs of hypertension, proteinuria, and edema develop. It is unique to pregnancy and occurs in 5% to 10% of pregnancies in the United States (Abramovici et al., 2000). Despite years of research, the cause of the disorder is still unknown. Originally it was called toxemia because researchers pictured a toxin of some kind being produced by the woman in response to the foreign protein of the growing fetus, the toxin leading to the typical symptoms. No such toxin has ever been identified.

PIH, a condition separate from chronic hypertension, tends to occur most frequently in primiparas younger than age 20 years or older than 40 years, women from a low socioeconomic background (perhaps because of poor nutrition), women who have had five or more pregnancies, women of color, women with a multiple pregnancy, women with hydramnios, and women with underlying disease such as heart disease, diabetes with vessel or renal involvement, and essential hypertension. The condition may be associated with poor calcium or magnesium intake (see Focus on Evidence-Based Practice).

Pathophysiologic Events

PIH occurs from systemic peripheral vascular spasm and affects almost all organs. The vascular spasm may be caused by increased cardiac output that injures the endothelial cells of the arteries and the action of prostaglandins (notably decreased prostacyclin and increased thromboxane). Normally, blood vessels during pregnancy are resistant to the effects of pressor substances such as angiotensin and norepinephrine, so blood pressure remains normal during pregnancy. With PIH, this reduced responsiveness to blood pressure changes appears to be lost. Vasoconstriction occurs and blood pressure increases dramatically (Branch & Porter, 2000).

With hypertension, the cardiac system can become overwhelmed because the heart is forced to pump against rising peripheral resistance. This reduces the blood supply to organs, most markedly the kidney, pancreas, liver, brain,

FOCUS ON EVIDENCE-BASED PRACTICE

Could Genetics Contribute to Preeclampsia?

To answer this question, researchers interviewed 298 men and 237 women whose mothers had experienced preeclampsia and compared them to twice as many men and women whose mothers did not experience preeclampsia. Results showed that men whose mothers had experienced preeclampsia were twice as likely to father a child whose birth was complicated by the disorder as were those whose mother had a pregnancy without the complication.

Women whose own births were complicated by preeclampsia were three times as likely to suffer the illness during their own pregnancies as others. These results suggest a genetic component to the disorder.

This is an important research study for nurses because nurses are often the people who obtain past medical and pregnancy histories and thus are the people who document preeclampsia in previous pregnancies. Knowing that some women are more susceptible to this condition than others sets the stage for effective health teaching and close monitoring for early detection and prompt intervention.

Esplin, M.S. et al. (2001). Paternal and maternal components of the predisposition to preeclampsia. *New England Journal of Medicine, 344*(12), 867–872.

and placenta. Tissue hypoxia may follow in the maternal vital organs; poor placental perfusion may reduce the fetal nutrient and oxygen supply. Ischemia in the pancreas may result in epigastric pain and an elevated amylase–creatinine ratio. Spasm of the arteries in the retina leads to vision changes. If retinal hemorrhages occur, blindness can result.

Vasospasm in the kidney increases blood flow resistance. Degenerative changes develop in kidney glomeruli because of the back-pressure. This leads to increased permeability of the glomerular membrane, allowing the serum proteins albumin and globulin to escape into the urine (proteinuria). The degenerative changes also result in decreased glomerular filtration, so there is lowered urine output and clearance of creatinine. Increased tubular reabsorption of sodium occurs. Because sodium retains fluid, edema results. Edema is further increased because as more protein is lost, the osmotic pressure of the circulating blood falls and fluid diffuses from the circulatory system into the denser interstitial spaces to equalize the pressure (edema; Fig. 15-8). Extreme edema can lead to cerebral and pulmonary edema and seizures (**eclampsia**).

The arterial spasm causes the bulk of the blood volume in the maternal circulation to be pooled in the venous circulation, so the woman has a deceptively low arterial intravascular volume. In addition, thrombocytopenia or a lowered platelet count occurs as platelets cluster at the sites of endothelial damage. Measuring hematocrit levels helps to assess the extent of plasma loss to the interstitial space or the extent of the edema (the higher the hematocrit, the more is being lost). A hematocrit level above 40% suggests significant fluid loss.

Assessment

Although women may have additional symptoms such as vision changes, typically hypertension, proteinuria, and edema are considered the classic signs of PIH. However, not all three need to be present for its diagnosis. Of the three, hypertension and proteinuria are the most significant. Edema is significant only if hypertension and proteinuria or signs of multiorgan system involvement are present. Symptoms rarely occur before 20 weeks of pregnancy (see Assessing the Woman With Pregnancy-Induced Hypertension).

PIH is classified as gestational hypertension, mild preeclampsia, severe preeclampsia, and eclampsia, depending on how far advanced it has become (Table 15-6). Any woman who falls into one of the high-risk categories for PIH should be observed carefully for symptoms at prenatal visits. She needs instructions about what symptoms to watch for so she can alert prenatal personnel if additional symptoms occur between visits.

Gestational Hypertension

A woman is said to have gestational hypertension when she develops an elevated blood pressure (140/90 mm Hg) but has no proteinuria or edema. Perinatal mortality is not increased with simple gestational hypertension, so no drug therapy is necessary. Some women are prescribed low-dose aspirin therapy because of its antiplatelet function. Although difficult to document, this therapy may help to prevent increased blood pressure (Heyborne, 2000). Chronic hypertension may develop in these women later in life, however.

Mild Preeclampsia

If a seizure from hypertension of pregnancy occurs, the woman has eclampsia, but any status before that point is **preeclampsia.** A woman is said to be mildly preeclamptic when her blood pressure rises to 140/90 mm Hg, taken on two occasions at least 6 hours apart. The diastolic value of blood pressure is extremely important to note because

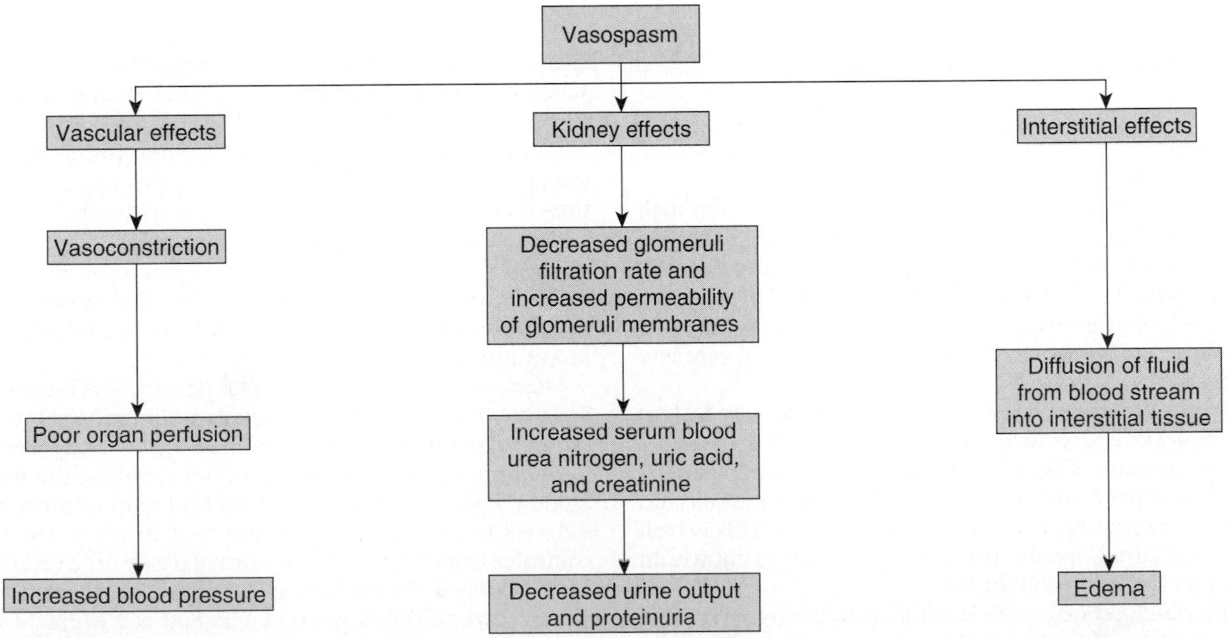

FIGURE 15.8 Physiologic changes with pregnancy-induced hypertension.

ASSESSING the Woman With Pregnancy-Induced Hypertension

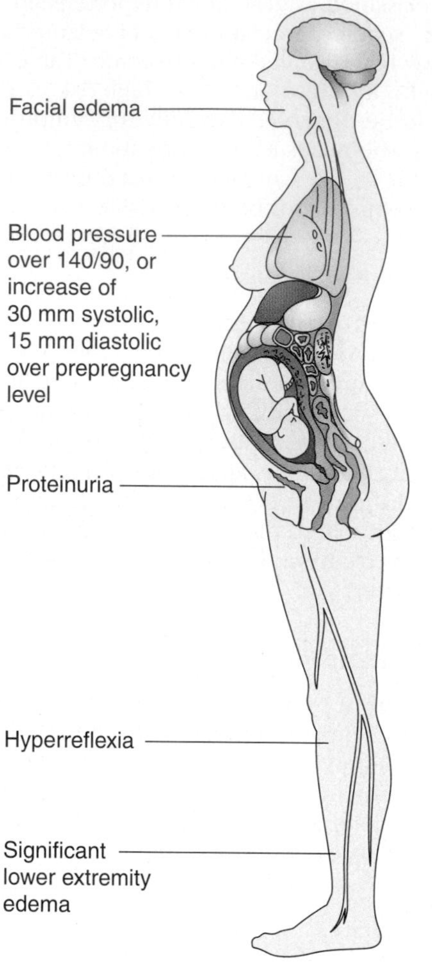

TABLE 15.6 Symptoms of Pregnancy-Induced Hypertension

HYPERTENSION TYPE	SYMPTOMS
Gestational hypertension	Blood pressure 140/90 or systolic pressure elevated 30 mm Hg or diastolic pressure elevated 15 mm Hg above prepregnancy level; no proteinuria or edema; blood pressure returns to normal after birth
Mild preeclampsia	Blood pressure 140/90 or systolic pressure elevated 30 mm Hg or diastolic pressure elevated 15 mm Hg above prepregnancy level; proteinuria of 1–2+ on a random sample; weight gain over 2 lb per wk in second trimester and 1 lb per wk in third trimester; mild edema in upper extremities or face
Severe preeclampsia	Blood pressure of 160/110; proteinuria 3–4+ on a random sample and 5 g on a 24-hour sample; oliguria (500 mL or under in 24 hours or altered renal function tests; elevated serum creatinine more than 1.2 mg/dL); cerebral or visual disturbances (headache, blurred vision); pulmonary or cardiac involvement; extensive peripheral edema; hepatic dysfunction; thrombocytopenia; epigastric pain
Eclampsia	Convulsion or coma accompanied by signs and symptoms of preeclampsia

it is this pressure that best indicates the degree of peripheral arterial spasm present.

A second criterion is systolic blood pressure greater than 30 mm Hg and diastolic pressure greater than 15 mm Hg above prepregnancy values. This rule is helpful, but the value of 140/90 mm Hg is a more useful cutoff point, however, and must be used when there are no baseline data available, such as when a woman seeks prenatal care late in pregnancy.

Average blood pressures in American women are shown in Appendix G. A woman younger than age 20 could have a blood pressure of 98/61 and still be within normal limits. If her blood pressure were elevated 30 mm Hg systolic and 15 mm Hg diastolic, it would be only 128/76. This is well beneath the traditional warning point of 140/90 but would represent hypertension for her.

With mild preeclampsia, in addition to the hypertension the woman has proteinuria (1+ or 2+ on a reagent test strip on a random sample). Many women show a trace of protein during pregnancy. Actual proteinuria is said to exist when it registers as at least 1+ or more (this represents a loss of 1 g/L).

Occasionally women have orthostatic proteinuria (on long periods of standing, they excrete protein; at bed rest, they do not). If proteinuria is present without other signs of PIH (no hypertension and no edema), check to see when the specimen was tested. Ask her to bring in a first morning urine sample. This may reveal that orthostatic proteinuria, not preeclampsia, may be the cause of protein in her urine.

Edema also may be present. This develops, as mentioned, because of the protein loss, sodium retention, and lowered glomerular filtration rate. Edema begins to accumulate in the upper part of the body, rather than just the typical ankle edema of pregnancy. A weight gain of more than 2 lb/wk in the second trimester or 1 lb/wk in the third trimester usually indicates abnormal tissue fluid retention. This is likely to be the first symptom to appear and is discovered when the woman is weighed at a prenatal visit. Noticeable edema may or may not be present when this sudden increase in weight first occurs.

Severe Preeclampsia

A woman has passed from mild to severe preeclampsia when her blood pressure has risen to 160 mm Hg systolic and 110 mm Hg diastolic or above on at least two occasions 6 hours apart at bed rest (the position in which blood pressure is lowest) or her diastolic pressure is 30 mm Hg above the prepregnancy level. Marked proteinuria, 3+ or 4+ on a random urine sample or more than 5 g in a 24-hour sample, and extensive edema are also present.

With severe preeclampsia, the extreme edema will be noticeable in the woman's face and hands as puffiness. It is most readily palpated over bony surfaces, such as over the tibia on the anterior leg, the ulnar surface of the forearm, and the cheekbones, where the sponginess of fluid-filled tissue can be palpated best. If there is swelling or puffiness at these points to a palpating finger but the swelling cannot be indented with finger pressure, the edema is nonpitting. If the tissue can be indented slightly, this is 1+ pitting edema; moderate indentation is 2+; deep indentation is 3+; and indentation so deep it remains after removal of the finger is 4+ pitting edema.

Further assess edema by asking the woman if she has noticed any edema. Most women at the end of pregnancy have edema of the feet at the end of the day. They report this as difficulty fitting into their bedroom slippers, or kicking off their shoes at dinnertime and then not being able to put them back on again. This is a normal discomfort of pregnancy. However, edema that has progressed to the upper extremities or the face is abnormal. Women report upper extremity edema as "my rings are so tight that I can't get them off" and facial edema as "when I wake in the morning, my eyes are swollen shut" or "I can't talk until I walk around awhile." This accumulating edema will reduce their urine output to approximately 400 to 600 mL per 24 hours.

Some women have severe epigastric pain and nausea and vomiting, possibly due to abdominal edema or ischemia to the pancreas and liver. If pulmonary edema develops, the woman may report feeling short of breath. If cerebral edema occurs, reports of visual disturbances such as blurred vision or seeing spots before their eyes may be voiced. Cerebral edema also produces symptoms of severe headache and marked hyperreflexia and perhaps muscle clonus.

Eclampsia

This is the most severe classification of hypertension of pregnancy. A woman has passed into this third stage when cerebral edema is so acute that a seizure or coma occurs. With eclampsia, maternal mortality is as high as 20% from causes such as cerebral hemorrhage, circulatory collapse, or renal failure (Cunningham et al., 2001).

The fetal prognosis in eclampsia is poor because of hypoxia and consequent fetal acidosis. If premature separation of the placenta from vasospasm occurs, the prognosis is even more grave. If the fetus must be delivered before term, all the risks of the immature infant will be faced. In preeclampsia, fetal mortality is approximately 10%. If eclampsia develops, the mortality increases to as high as 25% (Cunningham et al., 2001).

Nursing Diagnoses

The nursing diagnoses used with PIH are numerous because the disease has such wide-ranging effects. Some possible nursing diagnoses may include:

- Ineffective tissue perfusion related to vasoconstriction of blood vessels
- Deficient fluid volume related to fluid loss to subcutaneous tissue
- Risk for fetal injury related to reduced placental perfusion secondary to vasospasm
- Social isolation related to prescribed bed rest

Nursing Interventions for the Woman With Mild Hypertension of Pregnancy

Clients with mild preeclampsia can be managed at home with frequent follow-up care (see Chap. 16). Regardless of the setting, the care is similar.

Promote Bed Rest. When the body is in a recumbent position, sodium tends to be excreted at a faster rate than during activity. Bed rest, therefore, is the best method of aiding increased evacuation of sodium and encouraging diuresis. Rest should always be in a lateral recumbent position to avoid uterine pressure on the vena cava and prevent supine hypotension syndrome.

Promote Good Nutrition. The woman needs to continue her usual pregnancy diet. At one time, stringent restriction of salt was advised to reduce edema. This is no longer true because stringent sodium restriction may activate the renin-angiotensin-aldosterone system and result in increased blood pressure, compounding the problem.

Provide Emotional Support. It is difficult for a woman with preeclampsia to appreciate the potential seriousness of symptoms because they are still so vague. Neither high blood pressure nor protein in urine is something she can see or feel. She may be aware that edema is present, but it seems unrelated to the pregnancy: it is her hands that are swollen, not a body area near her growing child.

Women are also used to having severe disorders treated with some form of medication. With mild preeclampsia, no medication is prescribed. This can make her underestimate the severity of the situation. She may take instructions such as getting rest rather lightly. In addition, it is not always easy to comply with an instruction such as to get additional rest during the day. Ninety percent of women of childbearing age work outside the home. Approximately half the women with PIH, therefore, are being asked to take a leave of absence from work. Most working women contribute financially to the running of the household, such as providing a part of the mortgage or rent or car payments. If a woman is unmarried, her income is probably her sole support. Thus, it could be difficult to ask her to temporarily leave work on the basis of a few vague symptoms—a little swelling or a little headache—when she may receive reduced wages.

Health care providers cannot solve financial problems, but be certain to ask enough questions at health care visits so that financial need, if present, can be documented. Questions such as, "What will it mean to your family if you have to be on bed rest?" and "How long a maternity leave does your work allow?" bring concerns out into the open.

A woman with small children must usually make child care arrangements to get additional rest when receiving home care. The mother who spends considerable time chauffeuring school-age children to activities may have to investigate car pooling as an alternative. A mother may have to discontinue being a volunteer leader or ask her family for more help around the house, such as cleaning or cooking. Ask, "What will it mean to your other children or your husband if you have to rest?" to allow her to face this problem. Remember that having a wife or mother on bed rest is a stress on the total family, so other family members may need support as well.

Women with beginning signs of hypertension will be seen approximately weekly or more frequently for the remainder of pregnancy. Be certain the woman understands that if symptoms worsen before her next health care visit, she should call and report them immediately. Because there is no cure for preeclampsia, adherence to bed rest and attempts to reduce symptoms early are crucial.

Nursing Interventions for the Woman With Severe Hypertension of Pregnancy

If the preeclampsia is severe (i.e., systolic blood pressure of more than 160 mm Hg, diastolic blood pressure of more than 110 mm Hg, or both on two occasions 6 hours apart after the woman has been on bed rest; extensive edema; marked proteinuria [3+ to 4+]; cerebral or visual disturbances; marked hyperreflexia; or oliguria [500 mL per 24 hours or less]), the woman may be admitted to the health care facility. If the pregnancy is 36 weeks or more in length, or fetal lung maturity can be confirmed by amniocentesis, labor can be induced to end the pregnancy at this point. If the pregnancy is less than 36 weeks, or the amniocentesis reveals immature lung function, interventions will be instituted to attempt to alleviate the severe symptoms and allow the fetus to come to term.

Support Bed Rest. With hospitalization, bed rest can be enforced and the woman can be observed more closely than she was on home care. Because a loud noise such as a crying baby or a dropped tray of equipment may be sufficient to trigger a seizure initiating eclampsia, the woman with severe preeclampsia should be admitted to a private room so she can rest as undisturbed as possible. Raise side rails to help prevent injury if a seizure should occur.

The room should be darkened because a bright light can also trigger seizures. However, the room should not be so dark that caregivers need to use a flashlight to make assessments. Shining a flashlight beam into the woman's eyes is the kind of sudden stimulation to be avoided. Visitors are usually restricted to support people (e.g., husband, father of the child, mother, or older children).

Stress is another stimulus capable of increasing blood pressure and evoking seizures in the woman with severe preeclampsia. Be certain the woman receives clear explanations of what is happening and what is planned. Clear explanations help her to accept the need for visitor restrictions and not to "cheat" on bed rest. Allow her opportunities to express her feelings about what is happening or how bewildered she is because the few simple symptoms she noticed 2 weeks ago (increase in weight or increasing edema) have now developed into a syndrome that may be lethal to her baby and possibly to her.

Monitor Maternal Well-Being. The woman's blood pressure should be taken frequently (at least every 4 hours) or with a continuous monitoring device to detect any increase, which is a warning that her condition is worsening. Obtain blood studies as ordered (i.e., complete blood count, platelet count, liver function, blood urea nitrogen, and creatine and fibrin degradation products) to assess for renal and liver function and the development of DIC, which often accompanies severe vasospasm. Because she is at high risk for premature separation of the placenta and resulting hemorrhage, a type and cross-match for blood is usually drawn.

Obtain daily hematocrit levels as ordered to monitor blood concentration. This level will rise if increased fluid is leaving the bloodstream for interstitial tissue. Also, anticipate the need for frequent plasma estriol and electrolyte levels. The woman's optic fundus is assessed daily for signs of arterial spasm, edema, or hemorrhage.

An indwelling urinary catheter may be inserted to allow accurate recording of output and comparison with intake. Urinary output should be more than 600 mL per 24 hours (more than 30 mL/hour); an output lower than this suggests oliguria. Urinary proteins and specific gravity should be measured and recorded with voiding or hourly if an indwelling catheter is present. A 24-hour urine sample may be collected for protein and creatinine clearance determinations to evaluate kidney function. A woman with mild preeclampsia spills between 0.5 g and 1 g of protein every 24 hours (1+ on a random sample); a woman with severe preeclampsia spills approximately 5 g per 24 hours (3+ to 4+ on an individual specimen).

Obtain daily weights at the same time each day for evaluation of tissue fluid retention. Ensure that the woman is wearing approximately the same amount of clothing at each weighing so any change in weight is not influenced by a change in the weight of her clothing.

Monitor Fetal Well-Being. Generally, single Doppler auscultation at approximately 4-hour intervals is sufficient at this stage of management. However, the fetal heart rate may be assessed continuously with an external fetal monitor. The woman may have a nonstress test or biophysical profile done daily to assess uteroplacental sufficiency (see Chap. 8). Oxygen administration to the mother may be necessary to maintain adequate fetal oxygenation and prevent bradycardia.

Support a Nutritious Diet. The woman needs a moderate- to high-protein, moderate-sodium diet to compensate for the protein she is losing in urine. An intravenous fluid line should be initiated and maintained to serve as an emergency route for drug administration as well as to administer fluid to reduce hemoconcentration and hypovolemia.

Administer Medications to Prevent Eclampsia. A hypotensive drug such as hydralazine (Apresoline) or labetalol (Normodyne) may be prescribed to reduce hypertension. These drugs act to lower blood pressure by peripheral dilatation without interfering with placental circulation. They can cause tachycardia. Therefore, assess pulse and blood pressure after administration. Diastolic pressure should not be lowered below 80 to 90 mm Hg or inadequate placental perfusion may occur.

Despite these new drugs, magnesium sulfate remains the drug of choice to prevent eclampsia (Table 15-7). The drug, classified as a cathartic, reduces edema by causing a shift in fluid from the extracellular spaces into the intestine. It also has a central nervous system depressant action (it blocks peripheral neuromuscular transmissions), which lessens the possibility of seizures (Karch, 2001).

To achieve immediate reduction of the blood pressure, magnesium sulfate is first given intravenously in a loading or bolus dose. Given intravenously over 15 minutes, the drug begins to act almost immediately; unfortunately, the effect lasts only 30 to 60 minutes, so administration must continue.

For magnesium sulfate to act as an anticonvulsant, blood serum levels are maintained at 5 to 8 mg/100 mL. If the blood serum level rises above this, respiratory depression, cardiac arrhythmias, and cardiac arrest can occur. The importance of different serum levels is shown in the Focus on Pharmacology box for this drug earlier in the chapter.

The most evident symptoms of overdose from magnesium sulfate administration include decreased urine output, depressed respirations, reduced consciousness, and decreased deep tendon reflexes. Because magnesium is excreted from the body almost entirely through the urine, urine output must be monitored closely to ensure adequate elimination. If severe oliguria should occur (less than 100 mL in 4 hours), excessively high serum levels of magnesium can result. Before further magnesium sulfate is administered, therefore, urine output should be above 25 to 30 mL/hour with a specific gravity of 1.010 or lower. Respirations should be above 12 per minute, the woman should be able to answer questions asked of her, **ankle clonus** (a continued motion of the foot) should be minimal, and deep tendon reflexes should be present. These assessments should be made every hour if a continuous intravenous infusion is being used.

The easiest deep tendon reflex to assess is the patellar reflex (knee jerk). Instructions for initiating this reflex and ankle clonus are shown in Box 15-2. If an epidural block has been given for labor anesthesia, assess the biceps or triceps reflex (see Chap. 33).

In addition to making the above assessments when magnesium sulfate is being given, a solution of 10 mL of a 10% calcium gluconate solution (1 g) should be kept ready nearby for immediate intravenous administration should the woman develop signs and symptoms of magnesium toxicity. Calcium is the specific antidote for magnesium toxicity. Severe oliguria may be treated by the intravenous infusion of salt-poor albumin. This high-colloid solution will call fluid into the intravascular space by osmotic pressure; the kidneys will then excrete the extra fluid along with magnesium sulfate levels.

TABLE 15.7 Drugs Used in Pregnancy-Induced Hypertension

DRUG	INDICATION	DOSAGE	COMMENTS
Magnesium sulfate Pregnancy risk category B	Muscle relaxant; prevents seizures	Loading dose 4–6 g Maintenance dose 1–2 g/h IV	Infuse loading dose slowly over 15–30 min. Always administer as a piggyback infusion Assess respiratory rate, urine output, deep tendon reflexes, and clonus every hour. Keep in mind that urine output should be over 30 mL/hour and respiratory rate over 12/min. Serum magnesium level should remain below 7.5 mEq/L. Observe for CNS depression and hypotonia in infant at birth.
Hydralazine (Apresoline) Pregnancy risk category C	Antihypertensive (peripheral vasodilator); used to decrease hypertension	5–10 mg/IV	Administer slowly to avoid sudden fall in blood pressure. Maintain diastolic pressure over 90 mm Hg to ensure adequate placental filling.
Diazepam (Valium) Pregnancy risk category D	Halt seizures	5–10 mg/IV	Administer slowly. Dose may be repeated q 5–10 min (up to 30 mg/hour). Observe for respiratory depression or hypotension in mother and respiratory depression and hypotonia in infant at birth.
Calcium gluconate Pregnancy risk category C	Antidote for magnesium intoxication	1 g/IV (10 mL of a 10% solution)	Have prepared at bedside when administering magnesium sulfate. Administer at 5 mL/min.

Karch, A. M. (2001). *Lippincott's nursing drug guide.* Philadelphia: Lippincott Williams & Wilkins.

BOX 15.2

ELICITING A PATELLAR REFLEX AND ANKLE CLONUS

Patellar Reflex

With the woman in a supine position, ask her to bend her knee slightly. Place your hand under her knee to support the leg. Locate the patellar tendon in the midline just below the knee cap. Strike it firmly and quickly with a reflex hammer or the side of your hand. If the leg and foot move, a patellar reflex is present. The reflex is scored as:

0 = No response; hypoactive; abnormal
1+ = Somewhat diminished response but not abnormal
2+ = Average response
3+ = Brisker than average but not abnormal
4+ = Hyperactive; very brisk; abnormal

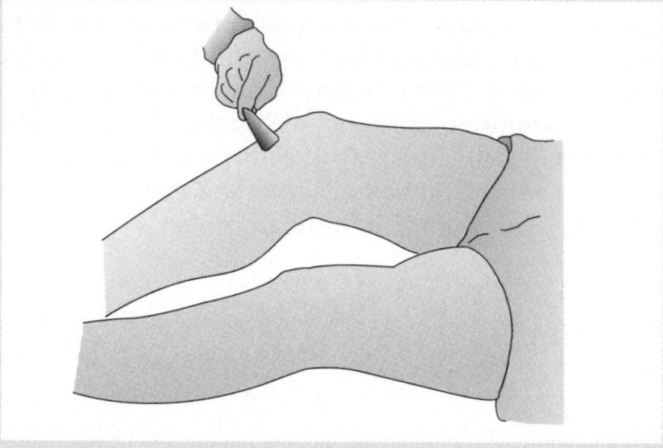

Ankle Clonus

To elicit ankle clonus, dorsiflex the woman's foot three times in rapid succession. As you take your hand away, observe the foot. If no further motion is present, no ankle clonus is present. If the foot continues to move involuntarily, clonus is present. Although usually just rated as present or absent, it can be rated as:

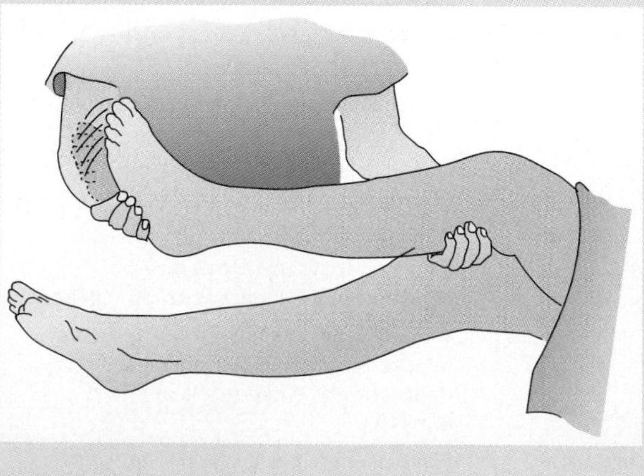

Mild (2 movements)
Moderate (3–5 movements)
Severe (over 6 movements)

On the day of birth, the anesthesiologist must be alerted to the fact that the woman has been receiving magnesium sulfate. If magnesium sulfate is given intravenously within 2 hours of the baby's birth, the baby may be born with respiratory depression because the drug crosses the placenta. A fetal heart rate monitor may show loss of variability of heartbeat immediately after magnesium therapy; the sonogram may reveal reduced fetal breathing movements. Observe carefully for other signs of fetal effects, such as late deceleration with labor contractions. Magnesium sulfate is continued for 12 to 24 hours after birth to prevent eclampsia from occurring during this period. The dose is then tapered and discontinued. Breast-feeding usually is delayed until the medication is discontinued.

Nursing Interventions for the Woman With Eclampsia

Degeneration of the woman's condition from severe preeclampsia to eclampsia occurs when cerebral irritation from increasing cerebral edema becomes so acute that a seizure results. This usually occurs late in pregnancy but can happen up to 48 hours after childbirth. Immediately before a seizure, the woman's blood pressure rises suddenly from additional vasospasm. Her temperature rises sharply to 103° to 104°F (39.4° to 40°C) from increased cerebral pressure. She notices blurring of vision or severe headache (from the increased cerebral edema) and her reflexes become hyperactive. She may experience a premonition that "something is happening." Vascular congestion of the liver or pancreas can lead to epigastric pain and nausea. Urinary output may decrease abruptly to less than 30 mL/hour. Eclampsia has actually occurred, however, only when the woman experiences a seizure.

Tonic-Clonic Seizures. An eclamptic seizure is a tonic-clonic type that occurs in stages. After the preliminary signal or aura, all the muscles of the body contract. Her back arches, her arms and legs stiffen, and her jaw closes abruptly. She may bite her tongue from the rapid closing of her jaw. Respirations halt because her thoracic muscles are held in contraction. This phase of the seizure, called the tonic phase, lasts approximately 20 seconds. It may seem longer because the woman may grow slightly cyanotic from the cessation of respirations.

The priority care for the woman with a seizure is to maintain a patent airway. Administer oxygen by face mask to protect the fetus during this interval. Assess oxygen saturation via a pulse oximeter. Apply an external fetal heart monitor if one is not already in place to assess the condition of the fetus. To prevent aspiration, turn the woman on her side to allow secretions to drain from her mouth.

After the tonic phase of the seizure, all the muscles of the body contract and relax repeatedly, causing her extremities to flail wildly (clonic phase). She inhales and exhales irregularly as her thoracic muscles contract and relax. She may aspirate the saliva that collected in her mouth during the tonic phase if she was not placed on her side.

Her bladder and bowel muscles contract and relax; incontinence of urine and feces may occur. Although she begins to breathe during this stage, the breathing is not entirely effective. She may remain cyanotic and may need continued oxygen therapy, not for herself but for the fetus. The clonic stage of a seizure lasts up to 1 minute. Magnesium sulfate or diazepam (Valium) may be administered intravenously as an emergency measure at this time.

The third stage of the seizure is the postictal state. During this stage, the woman is semicomatose and cannot be roused except by painful stimuli for 1 to 4 hours. Extremely close observation is as necessary during the postictal stage, as it was during the first two stages, because if the seizure caused premature separation of the placenta, labor may begin during this period and the woman will be unable to report the sensation of contractions. Also, the painful stimulus of contractions may initiate another seizure. Keep the woman on her side so secretions can drain from her mouth. Give her nothing to eat or drink by mouth. In coma, hearing is the last sense lost and the first one regained, so remember when talking at her bedside that she may be able to hear even though she does not respond. Continuously assess fetal heart sounds and uterine contractions. Check for vaginal bleeding every 15 minutes. Evidence that placental separation may have occurred will appear first on the fetal heart record; vaginal bleeding will strengthen the presumption.

Birth. If the gestational age of the pregnancy is more than 24 weeks, a decision about delivery will be made as soon as the woman's condition stabilizes, usually 12 to 24 hours after the seizure. There is some evidence that the fetus does not continue to grow after eclampsia occurs. Thus, terminating the pregnancy at this point is appropriate for both mother and child. For an unexplained reason, fetal lung maturity appears to advance rapidly with PIH (possibly from the intrauterine stress), so even though the fetus is younger than 36 weeks, the lecithin-sphingomyelin ratio may indicate fetal lung maturity.

Cesarean birth is always more hazardous for the fetus because of the association of retained lung fluid (see Chap. 26). Further, the woman with eclampsia is not a good candidate for surgery. Because the vascular system is low in volume, she may become hypotensive with regional anesthesia, such as an epidural block. The preferred method for birth, therefore, is vaginal. If labor does not begin spontaneously, rupture of the membranes or induction of labor with intravenous oxytocin may be instituted. If this is ineffective and the fetus appears to be in imminent danger, cesarean birth is indicated.

Postpartal Hypertension. Postpartal hypertension may occur up to 10 to 14 days after birth, although most cases occur in the first 48 hours after birth. Monitoring blood pressure in the postpartal period is essential to detect residual hypertensive or renal disease. Women who had an elevation of blood pressure during pregnancy should be instructed to return for a postpartal checkup to have their postpregnancy blood pressure evaluated to be certain it has returned to normal.

> **✔ CHECKPOINT QUESTIONS**
>
> 10. What are the three major symptoms of pregnancy-induced hypertension?
> 11. What is the drug of choice for the treatment of severe preeclampsia?

HELLP Syndrome

HELLP syndrome is a variation of PIH named for the common symptoms that occur: *h*emolysis, *e*levated *l*iver enzymes, and *l*ow *p*latelets. The syndrome occurs in 4% to 12% of patients with PIH, or approximately 1 in every 150 births. It is a serious syndrome because it results in a maternal mortality as high as 24% and an infant mortality as high as 35% (Cunningham et al, 2001).

Why some women with severe preeclampsia also develop the HELLP syndrome is unknown. It occurs in both primigravidas and multigravidas. The first symptoms are usually nausea, epigastric pain, general malaise, and right upper quadrant tenderness. Laboratory studies reveal hemolysis of red blood cells (they appear fragmented on a peripheral blood smear), thrombocytopenia (a platelet count below 100,000/mm^3), and elevated liver enzymes (alanine aminotransferase [ALT] and serum aspartate aminotransferase [AST]). The liver enzyme levels are elevated from hemorrhage and necrosis of the liver. Women with the HELLP syndrome need close observation for bleeding, in addition to the observations necessary for preeclampsia.

Therapy for the condition is to improve the platelet count by transfusion of fresh-frozen plasma or platelets. Complications associated with the syndrome are subcapsular liver hematoma, hyponatremia, renal failure, and hypoglycemia. If hypoglycemia is present, this is corrected by an intravenous dextrose infusion. The infant is delivered as soon as feasible by either vaginal or cesarean birth. Maternal hemorrhage may occur at birth because of poor clotting ability. Epidural anesthesia may not be possible because of the low platelet count and the high possibility of bleeding at the epidural site (Abramovici et al., 2000). Laboratory results return to normal after birth, the same as preeclamptic symptoms generally fade.

MULTIPLE PREGNANCY

Multiple gestation is considered a complication of pregnancy because the woman's body must adjust to the effects of more than one fetus. The incidence of multiple births has increased dramatically because of the use of fertility drugs (Gorrill et al., 2001). Where once it was as low as 0.5% to 1% of pregnancies, multiple births now account for almost 2%. The rate of twinning in the United States is 1 in 84 births; triplets, 1 in 6,400 (Spellacy, 2000a).

Identical (monozygotic) twins begin with a single ovum and spermatozoon. In the process of fusion, or in one of the first cell divisions, the zygote divides into two identical individuals. Single-ovum twins usually have one placenta, one chorion, two amnions, and two umbilical cords. The twins are always of the same sex. Fraternal (dizygotic, nonidentical) twins are the result of the fertilization of two separate ova by two separate spermatozoa (possibly not from the same sexual partner). Double-ova twins have two placentas, two chorions, two amnions, and two umbilical cords. The twins may be of the same or different sex (Fig. 15-9). Two thirds of twins are dizygotic. It is sometimes difficult to determine by sonogram or at delivery whether twins are identical or fraternal because the two fraternal placentas may fuse and appear as one large placenta.

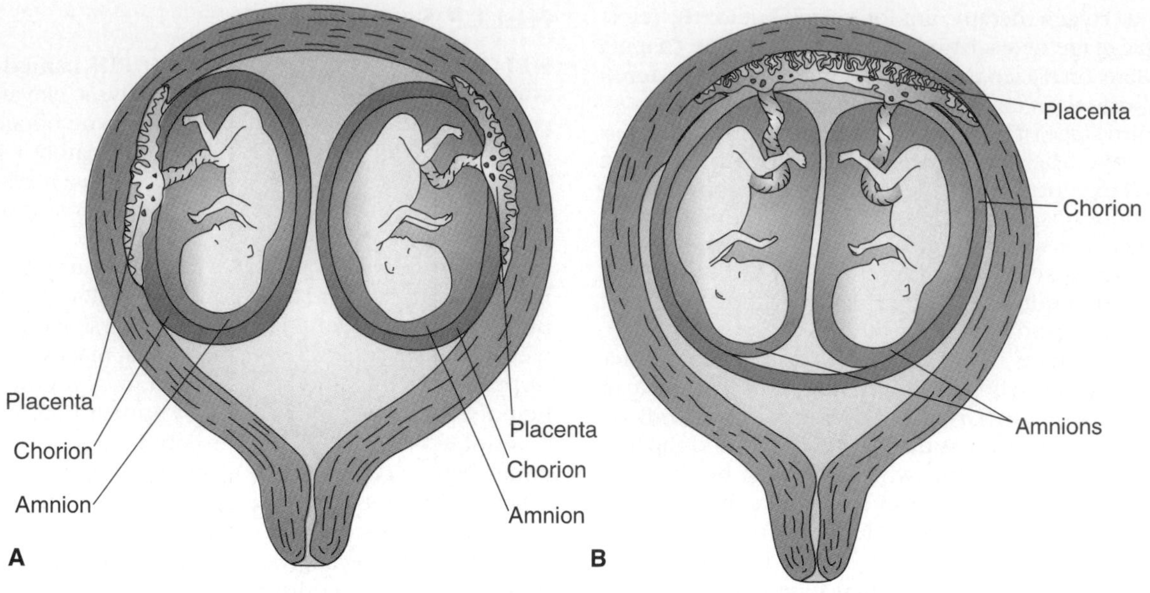

FIGURE 15.9 Multiple gestations. (*A*) Dizygotic twins showing two placentas, two chorions, and two amnions. (*B*) Monozygotic twins with one placenta, one chorion, and two amnions.

Multiple pregnancies of three, four, five, six, or seven children may be single-ovum conceptions, multiple-ova conceptions, or a combination of the two types. Naturally occurring multiple pregnancies are more frequent in nonwhites than in whites. The higher a woman's parity and age, the more likely she is to have a multiple gestation. Inheritance appears to play a role in natural dizygotic twinning; this has a familial maternal pattern of occurrence (Rodis, 2001).

Assessment

Multiple gestation is suspected early in pregnancy, when the uterus begins to increase in size at a rate faster than usual. Alpha-fetoprotein levels are elevated. A sonogram reveals multiple gestation sacs. In some instances, early ultrasound examinations reveal multiple amniotic sacs but then later in pregnancy, only one remains (vanishing twin syndrome). At the time of quickening, the woman may report flurries of action at different portions of her abdomen rather than at one consistent spot (where the feet are located) or more than the expected amount of fetal activity. On auscultation of the abdomen, multiple sets of fetal heart sounds may be heard, but if one or more fetuses has his or her back positioned toward the woman's back, only one fetal heart sound may be heard.

Therapeutic Management

Women with a multiple gestation are more susceptible to complications of pregnancy such as PIH, hydramnios, placenta previa, preterm labor, and anemia than are women carrying one fetus. They also are more prone to postpartal bleeding because of the additional uterine stretching (Rodis, 2001). Because a multiple pregnancy usually ends before the normal term, immaturity of the newborns is a crisis superimposed at birth. There is a higher risk of congenital anomalies in twins, such as spinal cord defect, than with single births. There is a higher incidence of velamentous cord insertion (the cord inserted into the fetal membranes) with twins than with single births, so bleeding at the time of delivery from a torn cord is increased. With monozygotic twins, the fetuses can share vascular communication, possibly leading to overgrowth of one fetus and undergrowth of the second (a twin-to-twin transfusion), resulting in discordant infants (Spellacy, 2000a). If a single amnion is present, there can be knotting and twisting of umbilical cords, causing fetal distress or difficulty with birth. The woman needs closer prenatal supervision than the woman with a single gestation to detect these problems as early as possible.

NURSING DIAGNOSES AND RELATED INTERVENTIONS

Nursing Diagnosis: Fatigue related to increased stress on body functioning secondary to multiple gestation

Outcome Identification: Client states the correct cause of fatigue and establishes regular rest periods to counteract exhaustion for remainder of pregnancy.

Outcome Evaluation: Client states that she is tired but identifies steps she has taken to minimize fatigue.

Spend time at health care visits reviewing with the woman her need for extra rest, especially in the side-lying position during the day, to increase tissue perfusion.

Because the woman is carrying a double weight during pregnancy, she may notice extreme fatigue and backache. She may have more difficulty resting or sleeping than the average woman because of greater discomfort and increased fetal activity. As the growing uterus compresses her stomach, she may find her appetite decreasing and her intake falling. To compensate and maintain nutrition, she may need to eat six small meals a day rather than three large ones. She must take her iron, folic acid, and vitamin supplement.

Toward the end of pregnancy, the woman may have extreme difficulty ambulating because of fatigue and backache. Her abdomen may become so stretched that she feels as if she is going to burst.

Many women with a multiple pregnancy are prescribed bed rest at home during the last 2 or 3 months of pregnancy to decrease the risk of preterm labor and increase the possibility that the pregnancy will come to term, or at least pass week 34, when the chances for survival of the fetuses rise markedly. She may be asked to come to a health care facility for monthly ultrasound examinations or weekly nonstress tests to document normal fetal growth beginning with the 28th week of pregnancy. However, this may not be necessary if the pregnancy is going well and the fetuses are growing consistently. If these tests are necessary, be certain that these appointments are scheduled to conserve her energy as much as possible.

Nursing Diagnosis: Parental role conflict related to recent discovery of multiple (as opposed to single) pregnancy

Outcome Identification: Client demonstrates positive attitude about event of multiple birth and demonstrates behaviors indicative of the formation of close bonds with multiple infants.

Outcome Evaluation: Client states that she is looking forward to multiple infants (may express concern about her ability to manage their arrival); client identifies changes she is making in preparation now that more than one baby is expected.

The woman with a multiple pregnancy has to work through two role changes during pregnancy rather than one. First, she must work to accept the fact that she is pregnant. Suddenly, at a routine office visit, two or more gestational sacs are seen on ultrasound or two or more sets of heart sounds are heard. She is told that she has a multiple pregnancy. Now she has to work through a second role change—for example, becoming a mother of two, not of one, or a mother of four or five. This role change may be difficult to complete, especially if the pregnancy ends early. The woman may need extra help postpartally to form a close mother–child relationship with her newborns.

Nursing Diagnosis: Fear concerning her own and the babies' health related to risks of multiple pregnancy

Outcome Identification: Client expresses her fears and is able to manage them well enough to keep a positive outlook on pregnancy.

Outcome Evaluation: Client accurately states risks of multiple pregnancy; expresses confidence in health care team's ability to care for her and her babies through pregnancy and birth.

In addition to having to work through a role change, the woman with a multiple pregnancy has more reason to fear for her life and the life of her babies than does the average woman. Every woman has heard stories about twins being born so prematurely that they did not survive, and about the special danger for the last infant born. If she has not already heard these stories, she will most probably hear them before her due date. Unfortunately, all these risks cannot simply be filed away under the heading of untrue stories. Both prematurity and high risk to the last born infant are real hazards in multiple gestation. Help the woman deal with her fears as positively as possible. It is helpful to tell her that there is no indication so far that her babies are in any danger; that right now it is best to continue doing the things that have to be done; that if any problems should arise, the health care team and the woman's family will be there to support her.

Sometimes a woman is so fearful that her infants will be born too small to survive that she makes no preparations for the infants. This is an indication that she lacks confidence in herself. She cannot imagine that she will be lucky enough or "good" enough to be able to carry a multiple pregnancy to completion. She needs assurance during pregnancy that she is managing well so her self-esteem is maintained at as high a level as possible. When her babies are born and all are healthy, the proof she needs that she "deserved" this or was capable of it will be present in her arms.

Nursing care at the birth of multiple infants is discussed in Chapter 21.

✔ CHECKPOINT QUESTIONS

12. What does HELLP stand for?
13. Typically, single-ovum twins have how many placentas and how many umbilical cords?

HYDRAMNIOS

Hydramnios is excessive amniotic fluid formation. Usually the amniotic fluid volume is 500 to 1,000 mL at term. More than 2,000 mL or an amniotic fluid index above 24 cm is considered hydramnios. Hydramnios can cause fetal malpresentation because of the extra uterine space for the fetus to turn that it provides. It also can lead to premature rupture of the membranes followed by preterm labor from the increased pressure and possible prostaglandin release. Preterm rupture of the membranes adds the additional risks of both infection and prolapsed cord.

Assessment

Amniotic fluid is formed by the cells of the amniotic membrane and from fetal urine. It is swallowed by the fetus, absorbed across the intestinal membrane into the fetal bloodstream, and transferred across the placenta. Although hydramnios can occur separate from fetal involvement, accumulation of amniotic fluid suggests difficulty with the fetus' ability to swallow or absorb or excessive urine production. Inability to swallow occurs in infants who are anencephalic or who have tracheoesophageal fistula with stenosis or intestinal obstruction. Excessive urine output occurs in the fetuses of diabetic women (hyperglycemia in the fetus causes increased urine production).

The first sign of hydramnios may be an unusually rapid enlargement of the uterus. The small parts of the fetus are difficult to palpate because the uterus is unusually tense. Auscultating the fetal heart rate is difficult because of the increased amount of fluid surrounding the fetus.

The woman may begin to notice extreme shortness of breath as the overly distended uterus pushes up against her diaphragm. She may develop lower extremity varicosities and hemorrhoids because of poor venous return from the extensive uterine pressure. She will have increased weight gain. Generally, a sonogram will be ordered to attempt to document the presence of hydramnios and to discover a reason for the excessive amount of fluid (Cunningham et al., 2001).

Therapeutic Management

Women with severe hydramnios may be admitted to the hospital for bed rest and further evaluation or may be cared for at home. Regardless of the setting, maintaining bed rest helps to increase uteroplacental circulation and reduces pressure on the cervix, which may help prevent preterm labor. Educate the woman to report any sign of ruptured membranes or uterine contractions. Although not common, there is a possibility that straining to defecate could increase uterine pressure and cause rupture of membranes. Help her avoid constipation by encouraging her to eat a high-fiber diet. Suggest that a stool softener be prescribed if diet alone is ineffective.

Assess vital signs and lower extremity edema frequently, because the extremely tense uterus puts unusual pressure on the diaphragm and vessels of the pelvis.

It is possible for amniocentesis to be performed to remove some of the extra amniotic fluid. Because amniotic fluid is replaced rapidly, however, this is only a temporary measure unless it is repeated daily. Indomethacin may be prescribed to reduce total volume. If contractions begin, tocolysis with magnesium sulfate may be begun to prevent or halt preterm labor.

In most instances of hydramnios, there is preterm rupture of the membranes due to excessive pressure, followed by preterm labor. To prevent the sudden loss of fluid and an accompanying prolapsed cord, membranes can be "needled" (a thin needle is inserted vaginally to pierce them) to allow a slow, controlled release of fluid. After birth, the infant must be assessed carefully for factors that may have interfered with the ability to swallow in utero.

POST-TERM PREGNANCY

A term pregnancy is 38 to 42 weeks long. A pregnancy that exceeds these limits is prolonged (**post-term pregnancy,** *postmature,* or *postdate*). The infant of such a pregnancy is considered postmature, or dysmature, if there is evidence that placental insufficiency has interfered with fetal growth (Spellacy, 2000b).

Post-term pregnancy occurs in 3% to 12% of all pregnancies (Cunningham et al., 2001). Included in this group are some pregnancies that appear to extend beyond the due date set for them because of a faulty due date. Women who have long menstrual cycles (40 to 45 days) do not ovulate on day 14 as in a typical menstrual cycle. They ovulate 14 days from the end of their cycle, or on day 26 or 31. Thus, their child will be "late" by 12 to 17 days.

In other instances, the pregnancy is truly overdue. For some reason, the trigger that initiates labor did not turn on. Prolonged pregnancy can occur in a woman receiving a high dose of salicylates (for severe sinus headaches or rheumatoid arthritis) because salicylate interferes with the synthesis of prostaglandins, which may be responsible for the initiation of labor. It is also associated with myometrial quiescence, or a uterus that does not respond to normal labor stimulation.

It is dangerous for a fetus to remain in utero more than 2 weeks beyond term for a number of reasons. Meconium aspiration is more apt to occur as fetal intestinal contents are more likely to reach the rectum. If the fetus continues to grow, macrosomia will create a birth problem. However, the usual effect of being post-term is lack of growth. A placenta seems to have a growth potential for only 40 to 42 weeks. After that time, it acquires calcium deposits (becomes grade 3) and cannot function adequately. A fetus still in utero will be exposed to decreased blood perfusion. Oligohydramnios (a decreased amount of amniotic fluid) leading to variable decelerations from cord compression may occur. The fetus may suffer from a lack of oxygen, fluid, and nutrients.

If labor has not begun by 41 weeks, a maternal vaginal fibronectin level, a nonstress test, and/or a biophysical profile may be done to document the state of placental perfusion and the amount of amniotic fluid. If normal, then the due date has probably been miscalculated. If the test results are abnormal or the physical examination or biparietal diameter measured on sonography suggests that the fetus is term size, the infant will be delivered by inducing labor. Prostaglandin gel or misoprostol (Cytotec) applied to the cervix to initiate ripening, or stripping of membranes followed by an oxytocin infusion is a common method used to induce labor. If oxytocin is ineffective, cesarean birth will be necessary. The fetal heart rate must be monitored closely during labor to be certain that placental insufficiency is not occurring from aging of the placenta. Nursing care for the post-term infant at birth is discussed in Chapter 26.

PSEUDOCYESIS

In **pseudocyesis** (false pregnancy), nausea and vomiting, amenorrhea, and enlargement of the abdomen occur in a nonpregnant woman. It can also be seen in men (Cunningham et al., 2001). There are a number of theories as to why the phenomenon occurs: wish-fulfillment theory suggests that the woman's desire to be pregnant actually causes physiologic changes to occur; conflict theory suggests that a desire for and fear of pregnancy create an internal conflict leading to changes; and depression theory attributes the cause to major depression. In any event, the woman's body responds with physiologic symptoms. In some women, the abdomen becomes so enlarged that they appear to be 7 or 8 months pregnant. On physical examination, it is obvious, however, that the uterus is not pregnant. Sonographic imaging will rule out pregnancy. Both men and women with the disorder need psychological counseling to learn how to better handle their needs.

ISOIMMUNIZATION (RH INCOMPATIBILITY)

Approximately 15% of whites and 10% of African Americans in the United States are missing the Rh (D) factor in their blood or have an Rh-negative blood type (Cunningham et al., 2001). If a woman who is Rh negative carries an Rh-positive fetus, a blood incompatibility between mother and fetus may result. Although this is basically a problem that affects the fetus, it causes such concern and apprehension in the woman during pregnancy that it becomes a maternal problem as well (Crowther & Middleton, 2000).

Rh incompatibility occurs only when an Rh-negative mother (one negative for a D antigen or one with a dd genotype) is carrying a fetus with an Rh-positive blood type (DD or Dd genotype). For such a situation to occur, the father of the child must either be homozygous (DD) or heterozygous (Dd) Rh positive. If the father of the child is homozygous (DD) for the factor, 100% of the couple's children will be Rh positive (Dd). If the father is heterozygous for the trait, 50% of their children can be expected to be Rh positive (Dd).

It is easiest to understand how the Rh factor can endanger the fetus if one thinks of it as an antigen (which it is). People who have Rh-positive blood have a protein factor (the D antigen) that Rh-negative people do not. When an Rh-positive fetus begins to grow inside an Rh-negative mother who is sensitized, it is as though her body is being invaded by a foreign agent, or antigen. Her body reacts in the same manner it would if the invading factor were a foreign substance such as measles or mumps virus. As a result, she forms antibodies against the invading substance. The Rh factor exists as a portion of the red blood cell. In the case of Rh invasion, therefore, to destroy the antigen, the entire red cell must be destroyed. The maternal antibodies formed cross the placenta and cause red blood cell destruction (hemolysis) of fetal red blood cells (Fig. 15-10). The fetus becomes so deficient in red blood cells that sufficient oxygen transport to body cells cannot be maintained. This condition is termed **hemolytic disease of the newborn** or **erythroblastosis fetalis.** Management of the infant born with this condition is discussed in Chapter 26.

Theoretically, there is no connection between fetal blood and maternal blood during pregnancy, so the mother should not be exposed to fetal blood. However, an occasional villus ruptures, allowing a drop or two of fetal blood to enter the maternal circulation. Procedures such as amniocentesis or percutaneous umbilical blood sampling can also cause this. As the placenta separates after birth of the child, there is an active exchange of fetal and maternal blood from damaged villi. Therefore, most of the maternal antibodies formed against the Rh-positive blood are formed by the Rh-negative woman in the first 72 hours after birth.

Assessment

All women with Rh-negative blood should have an anti-D antibody titer done at a first pregnancy visit. If the results are normal or the titer is minimal (normal is 0; a ratio below 1:8 is minimal), the test will be repeated at week 28 of pregnancy. No therapy is needed.

If the woman's anti-D antibody titer is elevated at a first assessment (1:16 or greater), showing Rh sensitization, the titer will be monitored approximately every 2 weeks during the remainder of the pregnancy. The well-being of the fetus in this potentially toxic environment will be monitored every 2 weeks (or more often) by amniocentesis (see Chap. 8). Spectrophotometer readings are made of

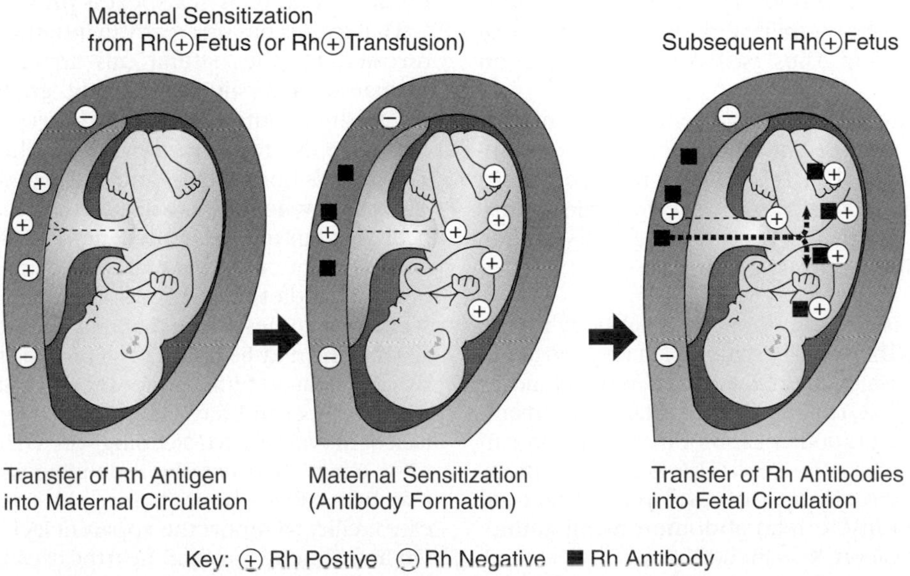

FIGURE 15.10 Maternal antibody formation preceding sensitization of the fetus to Rh antigen.

the amniotic fluid obtained by this technique to reveal the fluid density. If the readings (at 450-fm optical density) are plotted on a graph and correlated with gestational age, the extent of involvement and the amount of bilirubin present can be judged.

If the fluid density remains low (zone 1), the fetus either is in no distress or, more likely, is an Rh-negative fetus. If the spectrophotometer reading is moderate (zone 2), preterm birth by induction of labor at fetal maturity is indicated. If the reading is high (zone 3), the fetus is in imminent danger, and immediate birth will be carried out or intrauterine transfusion begun (Scott & Branch, 2000).

Therapeutic Management

Today, with the discovery of Rh (D) immune globulin (RhIG), the problem of maternal isoimmunization to an Rh-positive fetus should be eliminated. RhIG, a commercial preparation of passive antibodies against the Rh factor, is administered to women at 28 weeks of pregnancy. It does not cross the placenta late in pregnancy and destroy fetal red blood cells because the antibodies are not the IgG class, the only type that crosses the placenta. If this is given again by injection to the mother in the first 72 hours after delivery of an Rh-positive child, the mother forms no natural antibodies. Because RhIG is passive antibody protection, it is transient, and in 2 weeks to 2 months, the passive antibodies are destroyed. Only those few antibodies that were formed during pregnancy are left. Thus, every pregnancy is like a first pregnancy in terms of the number of antibodies present, ensuring a safe intrauterine environment for any future pregnancies.

If there was no change in the woman's antibody-D titer at week 28 of pregnancy, no special therapy during pregnancy needs to be undertaken. After birth, the infant's blood type will be determined from a sample of the cord blood. If it is Rh positive—Coombs' negative, indicating that a large number of antibodies are not present in the mother—the mother will receive an RhIG injection. If the newborn's blood type is Rh negative, no antibodies have been formed in the mother's circulation during pregnancy and none will form. Thus, passive antibody injection is unnecessary.

Although in future years the problem of Rh sensitization will be greatly reduced, it currently remains a complication of pregnancy. This is because a few women do not receive RhIG injections after induced abortions, miscarriages, ectopic pregnancy, or amniocentesis as they should, and so antibody formation begins.

Intrauterine Transfusion. A high Rh-antibody titer in the woman suggests that rapid destruction of fetal red blood cells is occurring. Women may be administered high doses of gamma globulin (IVIG) to help reduce fetal involvement.

To restore fetal red blood cells, blood transfusion can be performed on the fetus in utero. This is done by injecting red blood cells directly into a vessel in the fetal cord or depositing them in the fetal abdomen using amniocentesis technique (Scott & Branch, 2000).

Blood used for transfusion in utero is either the fetus' own type (determined by percutaneous blood sampling) or group O negative if the fetal blood type is unknown. From 75 to 150 mL of washed red cells will be used, depending on the age of the fetus. After deposition of the blood in the cord, the cannula is withdrawn and the woman is urged to rest for approximately 30 minutes while fetal heart sounds and uterine activity are monitored.

Obviously, intrauterine transfusion is not without risk. A cord blood vessel may be lacerated by the needle, or the uterus may be so irritated by the invasive procedure that labor contractions begin. For the fetus who is severely affected by isoimmunization, however, such a risk is no greater than that of leaving the fetus untreated in the intrauterine environment. The mother receives an RhIG injection after the transfusion to help reduce increased sensitization from the amniocentesis. Transfusion is sometimes done only once during pregnancy, or it may be repeated five or six times every 2 weeks. As soon as fetal maturity is reached, as shown by a mature lecithin–sphingomyelin ratio, delivery will be induced.

After birth, the infant may require an exchange transfusion to remove hemolyzed red blood cells and replace them with healthy blood cells (see Chap. 26). The woman needs to discuss her plans for further childbearing and to be provided with contraceptive information if she believes that the strain of this pregnancy, the constant feeling of wishing that everything was all right but never being certain that it was, is more than she wants to endure again.

FETAL DEATH

Obviously, one of the most severe complications of pregnancy that can occur is fetal death. The most likely causes include chromosomal abnormalities, congenital malformations, infections such as hepatitis B, immunologic causes, and complications of maternal disease. If fetal death happens before the time of quickening, the woman will not be aware that the fetus has died because she was not able to feel fetal movements. This type of fetal death may be discovered at a routine prenatal visit when no fetal heartbeat can be heard. A real-time sonogram will reveal that no fetal heartbeat is present.

That a fetus has died early in intrauterine life may first be revealed by the natural miscarriage that occurs. The woman begins painless spotting, gradually accompanied by uterine contractions with cervical effacement and dilatation. No fetal heartbeat can be heard on assessment. The fetus is born lifeless and emaciated. Carefully observe all women who deliver a dead fetus because if the fetus has been dead in utero for any length of time, the risk for the development of DIC increases.

If a fetus dies in utero past the point of quickening, the woman becomes aware that fetal movements are suddenly absent. She may lie down or sit in a position that she knows usually causes fetal movement. Unable to believe that something could have happened, she may attribute the lack of movement to "sleeping" or "saving enough strength to be born." Because she is denying what is happening, it may be a full 24 hours before she telephones the health care facility to report the apparent lack of fetal movement. On assessment, no fetal heartbeat can be heard. A sonogram also will confirm the absence of a fetal heartbeat.

If labor does not begin spontaneously, it will be induced through a combination of prostaglandin gel such as misoprostol (Cytotec) applied to the cervix to effect cervical ripening and oxytocin administration to begin uterine contractions. Blood for coagulation studies to detect DIC should be obtained.

NURSING DIAGNOSES AND RELATED INTERVENTIONS

Nursing Diagnosis: Powerlessness related to fetal death

Outcome Identification: Client and family will express and share feelings among themselves and with significant others.

Outcome Evaluation: Client and support person express meaning of pregnancy loss to them; identify other support people/family with whom they can share grief.

Going through labor knowing that the fetus is dead is difficult. The woman grieves for both her dead child and her inability to carry a pregnancy to completion. She may wonder what she did to cause this (e.g., forgot an iron supplement or painted a crib) or may believe that she is not as good a woman as others. Give her opportunities to express how she feels about this loss. "This must be a very difficult day for you" is the kind of statement that opens up the topic for discussion. If there are older children, it might be a help to explore how the woman plans to explain the fetal death to them.

Remember that the support person is grieving too (Armstrong, 2001). Encourage a support person to remain with the woman during labor. Although this is a difficult time, it makes the birth real, ends the pregnancy, and allows the couple to begin active grieving. Ask if the couple want the support of clergy.

Labor involving a dead fetus is the same as for a live fetus because every fetus is basically a passive participant during labor. It may be difficult for the woman to use controlled breathing exercises, although encouraging her to use them is helpful in making the experience one of controllable pain. If the woman wishes a high level of analgesia, she may have it because there is no fetus to protect from narcotic effects, although too much may lead to poor uterine involution in the postpartal period.

Ask if the parents wish to see the child. If they do, wash away obvious blood, swaddle the baby as if he or she were a well newborn, and bring the baby to them. Point out particularly endearing features of the child that may provide a focus for memories. Some parents want to keep a lock of the child's hair. Others want to keep the hospital identification bracelet or to take a photograph. Encourage the parents to name the child to make him or her more real. All of these measures are helpful in making the death real to parents and letting them begin the healthy process of grieving.

If the child has a congenital anomaly that led to the death, prepare them for this before bringing the child to them, and explain how the anomaly affected the child. Explain hospital procedures such as when the body will be released or what additional permission for autopsy is needed. Ask them about their desire for clergy or religious rites, such as baptism. Different communities have different laws concerning whether burial for an immature fetus is necessary. Consult local health department regulations so you can serve as a resource person for parents concerning this.

The woman need only remain for a short stay in the hospital, assuming no complications with labor developed. Many couples ask if it will be safe for them to have another child. They need to consult with their obstetrician or nurse-midwife about why this fetal death occurred to learn that answer. Some ask if it would be best if they have another baby right away. For some couples, this is a good recommendation, providing no physical health problem intervenes. For others, waiting for an interval of time (perhaps 6 months) may be necessary so they can work through their grief before starting a new pregnancy. This helps prevent the new baby from becoming a "replacement baby" or someone to take the place of the dead infant rather than a unique individual in his or her own right. This is important because replacement children are rarely able to live up to the image of what the dead baby would have been if only she or he had lived.

Prepare the couple for the possibility that they may feel sad on the day the infant would have been born if the pregnancy had been carried to term, or if they visit a friend's child of the age their child would have been. Be certain before the woman is discharged from the hospital that she has a support person she can rely on during the following week or month, when the full impact of the fetal loss registers. Be certain she has a return appointment for a gynecologic checkup so her physiologic and psychological health can be evaluated at that time.

✔ CHECKPOINT QUESTIONS

14. What amount of amniotic fluid characterizes hydramnios?
15. What is the chief effect of an Rh incompatibility on the fetus?

KEY POINTS

Bleeding is a major complication that can occur during pregnancy. The bleeding evident during pregnancy may not be indicative of the actual amount of bleeding occurring because so much internal bleeding may also be happening. As a rule, women with bleeding of pregnancy should be positioned on their side to improve placental circulation.

Vaginal bleeding during pregnancy is always serious until ruled otherwise because it has the potential to diminish the blood supply of both the mother and fetus.

Spontaneous miscarriage is the loss of a pregnancy before viability of the fetus (20 to 24 weeks). The majority of these early pregnancy losses are attributed to chromosomal abnormality. Miscarriages are classified as threatened, imminent, complete, incomplete, missed, or recurrent pregnancy loss. Women who have a spontaneous miscarriage at home should bring any tissue passed to the hospital for an analysis for gestational trophoblastic disease.

Ectopic pregnancy is pregnancy implantation outside the uterus, usually in a fallopian tube. If discovered before the tube ruptures, this can be treated with methotrexate or mifepristone. If not discovered early, it produces sharp lower quadrant pain at about 6 to 12 weeks as the tube ruptures. Surgery is done to remove or repair the tube to halt bleeding.

Gestational trophoblastic disease is abnormal growth of the trophoblast tissue. If not discovered by sonogram before this, bleeding usually occurs at about the 16th week of pregnancy. Women need close follow-up after this because it can lead to choriocarcinoma, a malignancy.

Premature cervical dilatation occurs when the cervix dilates early in pregnancy, before viability of the fetus. Sutures (cervical cerclage) can be placed to prevent the cervix from dilating prematurely in a second pregnancy.

Placenta previa is low implantation of the placenta so that it crosses the cervical os. If it is not discovered before labor, cervical dilatation may cause the placenta to tear, causing severe blood loss. Women who have symptoms of placenta previa (painless vaginal bleeding in the third trimester) should not have vaginal examinations done to prevent disruption of the low-implanted placenta.

Premature separation of the placenta (abruptio placentae), placental separation from the uterus before the fetus is born, usually occurs late in pregnancy. This separation immediately cuts off blood supply to the fetus. Women with increased parity, those with previous uterine surgery, and those who use cocaine are at highest risk for this. Often it is manifested by sudden, sharp fundal pain, then a continuing dull pain and vaginal bleeding.

Disseminated intravascular coagulation is a blood disorder that may occur with any trauma. It can accompany such conditions as premature separation of the placenta and pregnancy-induced hypertension. Blood coagulation is so extreme at one point in the circulatory system that clotting factors are used up, resulting in their absence in the remainder of the system. Beginning symptoms of this include easy bruising, petechiae, and oozing from intravenous sites. Heparin is used to stop the coagulation and free up clotting factors for systemic use.

Preterm labor is labor that occurs after 20 weeks and before the end of the 37th week of pregnancy. A woman is said to be in preterm labor when she has had uterine contractions every 10 minutes for 1 hour and cervical dilatation begins.

Tocolytics, drugs that can halt labor, include magnesium sulfate and beta-sympathomimetic agents such as terbutaline (Brethine).

Preterm rupture of the membranes, tearing of the fetal membranes with loss of amniotic fluid before the pregnancy is at term, is a serious complication. After rupture, there is a high risk of fetal and uterine infection (chorioamnionitis).

Pregnancy-induced hypertension is a unique disorder that occurs with pregnancy with three classic symptoms: hypertension, edema, and proteinuria. It is categorized as preeclampsia or eclampsia. If mild (blood pressure not over 140/90), treatment is bed rest. If severe (blood pressure over 160/110), bed rest plus administration of magnesium sulfate is necessary. If a seizure occurs, the condition is termed eclampsia. The mortality of the fetus is high after eclampsia. Helping prevent the disease from progressing to this stage is an important nursing responsibility.

The HELLP syndrome is a unique form of pregnancy-induced hypertension marked by hemolysis of red blood cells, elevated liver enzymes, and a low platelet count.

Multiple gestation puts an additional strain on a woman's physical resources and may lead to birth complications or immaturity of the infants. Helping a woman obtain adequate nutrition and rest during pregnancy are nursing responsibilities.

Post-term pregnancy is pregnancy that extends beyond 42 weeks. As the placenta deteriorates at this time, the fetus may receive decreased nutrients.

Hydramnios is overproduction of amniotic fluid (above 2,000 mL). This can lead to premature labor from ruptured membranes because of increased intrauterine pressure.

Isoimmunization (Rh incompatibility) is a possibility when the woman who is Rh negative becomes sensitized, and the fetus is Rh positive. Maternal antibodies have formed that can destroy fetal red blood cells, leading to anemia, edema, and jaundice in the newborn. Being certain that women are screened for blood type early in pregnancy is a nursing responsibility.

CRITICAL THINKING EXERCISES

1. Beverly Muzuki is the woman you met at the beginning of the chapter who was in preterm labor at 34 weeks of pregnancy. Beverly discounted the symptoms she was having as not being early labor. What are the signs of early labor

that you would have liked her to have been more aware of?

2. A 30-year-old woman (G1P0) is admitted to the labor service with a probable diagnosis of placenta previa. Everyone else on the unit is at lunch, so you are alone. You know you should not do a pelvic examination with a placenta previa. How would you estimate her amount of blood loss? How would you determine that blood loss was not affecting the fetus?
3. An 18-year-old woman is on bed rest at home after preterm rupture of membranes at 32 weeks of pregnancy. What assessments would you want to do to ensure that she is not developing chorioamnionitis? What signs and symptoms of preterm labor would you want her to be aware of? Suppose she tells you that she is too busy to stay on bed rest. What suggestions would you give her so she could best achieve bed rest? Does she have an ethical obligation to her fetus to rest? What about a legal obligation?
4. Examine the National Health Goals related to complications of pregnancy. Most government-sponsored money for nursing research is allotted based on these goals. What would be a possible research topic to explore pertinent to these goals that would be fundable and would advance evidence-based practice?

REFERENCES

Abramovici, D., Mattar, F., & Sibai, B. M. (2000). Hypertensive disorders in pregnancy. In Dombrowski, M. P., et al. *Practical strategies in obstetrics and gynecology* (pp. 380–389). Philadelphia: W. B. Saunders.

Armstrong, D. (2001). Exploring fathers' experiences of pregnancy after a prior perinatal loss. *MCN: American Journal of Maternal Child Nursing, 26*(3), 147–153.

Atri, M., et al. (2001). Expectant treatment of ectopic pregnancies: Clinical and sonographic predictors. *AJR American Journal of Roentgenology, 176*(1), 123–127.

Branch, D. W., & Porter, T. F. (2000). Hypertensive disorders of pregnancy. In Scott, J. R., et al. *Danforth's obstetrics and gynecology* (8th ed., pp. 309–326). Philadelphia: Lippincott Williams & Wilkins.

Burkman, R. T. (2001). Oral contraceptives: Current status. *Clinical Obstetrics & Gynecology, 44*(1), 62–72.

Clark, S. L. (2000). Critical care obstetrics. In Scott, J. R., et al. *Danforth's obstetrics and gynecology* (8th ed., pp. 471–484). Philadelphia: Lippincott Williams & Wilkins.

Colombo, D. R., & Iams, J. D. (2000). Preterm birth. In Ransom, S. B., et al. *Practical strategies in obstetrics and gynecology* (pp. 344–352). Philadelphia: Saunders.

Crowther, C., & Middleton, P. (2000). Anti-D administration after childbirth for preventing Rhesus alloimmunisation. *Cochrane Database of Systematic Reviews, 2*, CD000021.

Cunningham, F. G., et al. (2001). Obstetrical hemorrhage. In Cunningham, F. G., et al. *William's obstetrics* (21st ed., pp. 619–669). New York: McGraw-Hill.

Demetroulis, C., et al. (2001). A prospective randomized control trial comparing medical and surgical treatment for early pregnancy failure. *Human Reproduction, 16*(2), 365–369.

Department of Health and Human Services (2000). *Healthy people, 2010.* Washington, DC: DHHS.

Ecker, J. L. (2001). The incompetent cervix and cervical cerclage. In Gershenson, D. M., et al. *Operative gynecology* (2d ed., pp. 837–850). Philadelphia: W.B. Saunders.

Empson, M., et al. (2002). Recurrent pregnancy loss with antiphospholipid antibody: A systematic review of therapeutic trials. *Obstetrics & Gynecology, 99*(1), 135–14.

Esplin, M. S., et al. (2001). Paternal and maternal components of preeclampsia. *New England Journal of Medicine, 344*(12), 867–872.

Gorrill, M. J., et al. (2001). Multiple gestations in assisted reproductive technology. *American Journal of Obstetrics & Gynecology, 184*(7), 1471–1475.

Gracia, C. R., & Barnhart, K. T. (2001). Diagnosing ectopic pregnancy: Decision analysis comparing six strategies. *Obstetrics & Gynecology, 97*(3), 464–470.

Hammond, C. B. (2000). Gestational trophoblastic neoplasms. In Scott, J. R., et al. *Danforth's obstetrics and gynecology* (8th ed., pp. 927–937). Philadelphia: Lippincott Williams & Wilkins.

Heyborne, K. (2000). Preeclampsia prevention: Lessons from the low-dose aspirin therapy trials. *American Journal of Obstetrics & Gynecology, 183*(3), 523–528.

Johnson, M., Maas, M., & Moorhead, S. (2000). *Nursing outcomes classification* (2nd ed.). St. Louis: Mosby.

Karch, A. M. (2001). *Lippincott's nursing drug guide.* Philadelphia: Lippincott Williams & Wilkins.

Matijevic, R., et al. (2001). Cervical incompetence: The use of selective and emergency cerclage. *Journal of Perinatal Medicine, 29*(1), 31–35.

McCloskey, J., & Bulechek, G. (2000). *Nursing interventions classification* (3rd ed.). St. Louis: Mosby.

Parsons, M. T., & Spellacy, W. N. (2000). Preterm labor. n Scott, J. R., et al. *Danforth's obstetrics and gynecology* (8th ed., pp. 257–267). Philadelphia: Lippincott Williams & Wilkins.

Pisarska, M. E., & Carson, S. A. (2000). Ectopic pregnancy. In Scott, J. R., et al. *Danforth's obstetrics and gynecology* (8th ed., pp. 155–172). Philadelphia: Lippincott Williams & Wilkins.

Rinehart, B. K., et al. (2001). Pregnancy outcome in women with preterm labor symptoms without cervical change. *American Journal of Obstetrics & Gynecology, 184*(5), 1004–1007.

Rodis, J. (2001). Multiple gestation. In Seifer, D. B., et al. (Eds). *The physiologic basis of gynecology and obstetrics.* Philadelphia: Lippincott Wilkins & Williams.

Sciscione, A. C., et al. (2001). Intracervical fibrin sealants: A potential treatment for early preterm premature rupture of the membranes. *American Journal of Obstetrics & Gynecology, 184*(3), 368–373.

Scott, J. R. (2000a). Early pregnancy loss. In Scott, J. R., et al. *Danforth's obstetrics and gynecology* (8th ed., pp. 143–153). Philadelphia: Lippincott Williams & Wilkins.

Scott, J. R. (2000b). Placenta previa and abruption. In Scott, J. R., et al. *Danforth's obstetrics and gynecology* (8th ed., pp. 407–418). Philadelphia: Lippincott Williams & Wilkins.

Scott, J. R., & Branch, D. W. (2000). Immunologic disorders in pregnancy. In Scott, J. R., et al. *Danforth's obstetrics and gynecology* (8th ed., pp. 363–392). Philadelphia: Lippincott Williams & Wilkins.

Sorokin, Y. (2000). Obstetric hemorrhage. In Ransom, S. B., et al. *Practical strategies in obstetrics and gynecology* (pp. 311–320). Philadelphia: W.B. Saunders.

Spellacy, W. N. (2000a). Multiple pregnancies. In Scott, J. R., et al. *Danforth's obstetrics and gynecology* (8th ed., pp. 293–300). Philadelphia: Lippincott Williams & Wilkins.

Spellacy, W. N. (2000b). Postdate pregnancy. In Scott, J. R., et al. *Danforth's obstetrics and gynecology* (8th ed., pp. 287-292). Philadelphia: Lippincott Williams & Wilkins.

Tulandi, T., & Sammour, A. (2000). Evidence-based management of ectopic pregnancy. *Current Opinion in Obstetrics & Gynecology, 12*(4), 289-292.

Vaquero, E. et al. (2001). Pregnancy outcome in recurrent spontaneous abortion associated with antiphospholipid antibodies. *American Journal of Reproductive Immunology, 45*(3), 174-179.

Weitz, B. W. (2001). Premature rupture of the fetal membranes. *MCN: American Journal of Maternal Child Nursing, 26*(2), 86-92.

SUGGESTED READINGS

Angelini, D. J. (1999). Obstetric triage: Management of acute nonobstetric abdominal pain in pregnancy. *Journal of Nurse-Midwifery, 44*(6), 572-584.

Bar, J., et al. (2000). Low-molecular-weight heparin for thrombophilia in pregnant women. *International Journal of Gynaecology & Obstetrics, 69*(3), 209-213.

Bick, R. L. (2000). Syndromes of disseminated intravascular coagulation in obstetrics, pregnancy, and gynecology. *Hematology-Oncology Clinics of North America, 14*(5), 999-1044.

Creinin, M. D., et al. (2001). Early pregnancy failure: Current management concepts. *Obstetrics & Gynecologic Survey, 56*(2), 105-113.

Carp, H., et al. (2001). Karyotype of the abortus in recurrent miscarriage. *Fertility & Sterility, 75*(4), 678-682.

Dasari, P., & Devi, S. (2000). Primary peritoneal pregnancy: A case report. *Journal of Obstetrics & Gynaecology Research, 26*(1), 45-47.

de Weerd, S., et al. (2002). Preconception counseling improves folate status of women planning pregnancy. *Obstetrics & Gynecology, 99*(1), 45-50.

Haddad, B., et al. (2000). Risk factors for adverse maternal outcomes among women with HELLP (hemolysis, elevated liver enzymes, and low platelet count) syndrome. *American Journal of Obstetrics & Gynecology, 183*(2), 444-448.

Kauffman, D. E., & Caritis, S. Post-term pregnancy. In Ransom, S. B., et al. *Practical strategies in obstetrics and gynecology* (pp. 353-359). Philadelphia: Saunders.

Krause, S. A., & Graves, B. W. (1999). Midwifery triage of first trimester bleeding. *Journal of Nurse-Midwifery, 44*(6), 537-548.

Lipscomb, G. H., et al. (2000). Nonsurgical treatment of ectopic pregnancy. *New England Journal of Medicine, 343*(18), 1325-1329.

Lurie, S., Feinstein, M., & Mamet, Y. (2000). Disseminated intravascular coagulopathy in pregnancy. *Archives of Gynecology & Obstetrics, 263*(3), 126-130.

Lydon-Rochelle, M., et al. (2001). First-birth cesarean and placental abruption or previa at second birth. *Obstetrics & Gynecology, 97*(5), 765-769.

Lynch, A. et al. (2001). Assisted reproductive interventions and multiple birth. *Obstetrics & Gynecology, 97*(2), 195-200.

Newton, R., & Rutherford, A. J. (2001). Early pregnancy loss. *Practitioner, 245* (1621), 266-268.

Palinski, W., & Napoli, C. (1999). Pathophysiological events during pregnancy influence the development of atherosclerosis in humans. *Trends in Cardiovascular Medicine, 9*(7), 205-214.

Park, J. S., et al. (2001) The relationship between oligohydramnios and the onset of preterm labor in preterm premature rupture of membranes. *American Journal of Obstetrics & Gynecology, 184*(3), 459-462.

Rath, W., Faridi, A., & Dudenhausen, J. W. (2000). HELLP syndrome. *Journal of Perinatal Medicine, 28*(4), 249-260.

Wilson, W. (2000). An A&E nurse's fast-track for potential miscarriage patients. *Accident & Emergency Nursing, 8*(1), 9-12.

CHAPTER 16

Home Care of the Pregnant Client

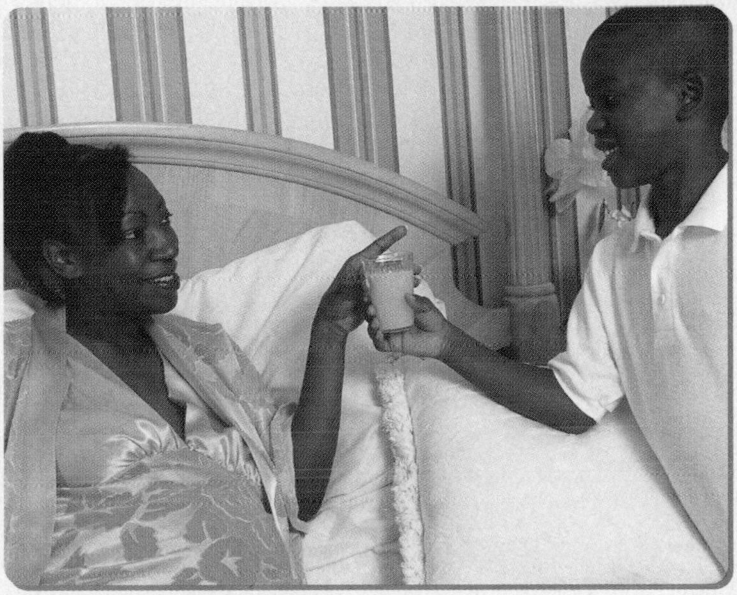

Key Terms

- **home care**
- **perinatal home care**
- **skilled home nursing care**

Objectives

After mastering the contents of this chapter, you should be able to:

1. Describe common health concerns requiring home care during pregnancy.
2. Assess the pregnant woman receiving home care.
3. Formulate nursing diagnoses related to care of the pregnant client at home.
4. Identify expected outcomes for the woman and family requiring home care.
5. Plan nursing care appropriate to meet the needs of the pregnant home care client.
6. Implement nursing care to meet the needs of the pregnant home care client.
7. Evaluate outcomes for effectiveness and achievement of a satisfying home care experience for the woman and her family.
8. Identify National Health Goals related to home care during pregnancy that nurses can be instrumental in helping the nation to achieve.
9. Identify areas of home care nursing that could benefit from additional nursing research or application of evidence-based practice.
10. Use critical thinking to analyze how home care influences family functioning, and develop ways to make nursing care more family-centered.
11. Integrate knowledge of home care with nursing process to achieve quality maternal and child health nursing care.

Lee Puente, a 20-year-old woman who is 20 weeks pregnant, began preterm labor. After this was successfully halted, she was placed on a program of fetal surveillance and uterine monitoring including bedrest at home. She tells you it's impossible for her to rest at home. She has two preschool children who constantly need her care and interrupt her rest. She has missed three doses of her tocolytic agent because she forgot to take them. She wants to be hospitalized instead for care.

Was Ms. Puente a good candidate for home care? What additional interventions does she need to help her make home care more successful?

Previous chapters described both normal pregnancy and complications of pregnancy that require a level of care usually available only in an acute care facility. This chapter adds information about illnesses that complicate pregnancy but can be managed with a combination of home and ambulatory care.

After you've studied the chapter, answer the Critical Thinking Exercises at the end of the chapter and then access the on-line study activities (http://connection.lww.com) *to further sharpen your skills and test your knowledge.*

In the past, when complications occurred during pregnancy, women were required to spend weeks or even months in the hospital on bedrest so their condition could be closely monitored. Today, many women can remain at home on **home care.**

Perinatal home care is care of pregnant women in their homes, provided by or supervised through a home health care or community health care agency (Koniak-Griffin et al., 2002). Home care agencies can be either freestanding or allied with a health care facility. Specialized services such as providing supplies for total parenteral nutrition, fetal monitoring, or laboratory analysis may be furnished by special service companies. Voluntary agencies often provide services such as transportation to and from health care agency assessments.

Nursing care is considered **skilled home nursing care** if it includes physician-prescribed procedures such as dressing changes, administration of medication, health teaching, or observation of the woman's progress or status through such activities as monitoring vital signs or fetal heart rate (FHR). Whether nursing care is categorized as skilled or not is important because it can determine whether it will be paid for by third-party reimbursement.

Many health departments have maternal-newborn projects that provide home care during pregnancy, allowing women to maintain contact with their families. Perinatal home care works best when a woman is strongly committed to home care and well prepared to work in conjunction with health care providers. Women with complications such as preterm labor that has been halted, hyperemesis gravidarum (excessive nausea and vomiting of pregnancy), hypertension of pregnancy, and multiple gestation are examples of women usually able to remain at home with supervision and periodic visits by a community or home care nurse. Women with diagnosed placenta previa may also be good candidates for home monitoring. There may be an advantage of placing women with premature ruptured membranes on home care rather than hospital care because of the decreased exposure to infection their own home offers. It is possible that having a caring person such as a visiting nurse take an interest in a woman during pregnancy to the extent involved in home care may have long-term effects, such as lowering the incidence of child abuse and child injury (Kitzman et al., 2000).

Home care visits vary in frequency depending on the client's condition, ability to comply with home care, and ability to contact the nurse to ask questions. In some settings, telephone contacts and e-mail and chat room contacts are used to link health care providers with women during home care.

Home care of the pregnant women has numerous advantages. It prevents extensive disruption of the family unit because the woman can remain at home with her family. It can increase a woman's self-confidence because it allows her more participation in and often more control of her circumstances. Often, a woman can be better assessed in her own setting than in a strange agency environment. Family interactions, values, and priorities are more obvious than in a health care setting. Home visiting provides a private, one-on-one opportunity for health teaching. In addition, home care has been shown to reduce the cost of monitoring women during high-risk pregnancies, with no differences in pregnancy outcomes. In today's health care climate of cost containment and shortened hospital stays, home care for the pregnant client will increase in frequency. This calls for nurses to be certain that nursing standards and protocols for home care are created and followed to ensure client safety.

Home carc is not without its disadvantages, however. It can actually increase the cost for an individual family if the family's insurance does not cover the cost of nursing visits or necessary supplies. It also can cause increased anxiety and concern because women are asked to assume a much greater responsibility for monitoring their own condition. Orienting families to home care, making home visits, supervising and coordinating home health personnel, providing health teaching in relation to pregnancy and childrearing, and evaluating whether home care remains appropriate during the remainder of a pregnancy are all important nursing responsibilities.

Low birthweight occurs in newborns when preterm labor cannot be halted. Nurses can be instrumental in seeing that women who are candidates for home care receive enough orientation and support that they are able to remain on home care as a means of preventing low birthweight. They can be instrumental in seeing that time spent during home care is not wasted time for a woman, but a time of preparation for birth and child-rearing.

It is well documented that women who receive prenatal care have better pregnancy outcomes than those who don't. Because home care can be a means of increasing prenatal care, especially in the areas of additional health teaching and monitoring, National Health Goals that speak to prenatal care also apply to home care (see the Focus on National Health Goals).

FOCUS ON NATIONAL HEALTH GOALS

National Health Goals are concerned with reducing complications of pregnancy by better monitoring during pregnancy. Such monitoring can be done by prenatal care visits or home care visits. National Health Goals speak directly to the necessity of preventing preterm birth, a condition frequently managed by home care. These goals are:

- Increase to at least 90% the proportion of all pregnant women who receive early and adequate prenatal care from a baseline of 74%.
- Reduce low birthweight (infants born weighing less than 2,500 g) to an incidence of no more than 5% of live births from a baseline of 7.6%, and very low birthweight (infants weighing less than 1,500 g) to no more than 0.9% of live births from a baseline of 1.4%.
- Reduce preterm births from a baseline of 11% to a target of 7.6% (DHHS, 2000).

Nurses can be instrumental in helping the nation achieve these goals by helping women better accept and adhere to home care during pregnancy. Nursing research topics to address in this area are: What are the most effective ways to relieve a woman's anxiety about home care? What is the ideal frequency for home visits? When nursing care time is included in costs, is home care cost-effective?

NURSING PROCESS OVERVIEW

For the Pregnant Woman on Home Care

Assessment

Most women who will be scheduled for home care are first seen in an ambulatory health care setting or an acute care facility for initial diagnosis and then discharged from that facility with a referral to a home care program.

Home care is not a level of care adequate for everyone or every situation, so evaluating whether the woman is a good candidate for home care is the first assessment needed. Figure 16-1 shows a typical assessment tool used to qualify women for home care. Using this tool, women can be divided into three levels of care based on the identification of factors, both physical and psychosocial, that may affect the pregnancy and its outcome. Those categorized as low risk (level I) probably need only weekly visits during pregnancy; those at intermediate risk (level II), one to three visits per week; and those at high risk (level III), as many as four to seven visits per week. All women need to be re-evaluated about every 30 days to see if their risk level has changed and therefore the number of home visits needed has changed.

Important assessments to be made at visits include the woman's current status, whether she will be able to continue to effectively monitor her own health at home, and what other services or resources she needs to ensure that her care is optimal.

The term "resources" refers not only to material objects (e.g., hospital bed, glucometer to test for serum glucose, fetal home monitor) but also whether the woman and her family are able to deal with the chronic stress of home care. Women often have to quit work to become home care patients. This can reduce the family's income dramatically. Environmental considerations also can add to the stress of the situation. Assess if the woman's physical surroundings are adequate for home care. Is there enough floor space for a hospital bed if required? Is there space for a uterine or fetal monitor? Is there a telephone that can be brought close to where the woman will rest? Is there adequate heat or air conditioning so she can be comfortable?

Typically, women are taught how to self-assess various parameters such as blood pressure, temperature, pulse, perhaps urine for protein or glucose, fundal height, fetal movement and heart rate, and uterine contractions in preparation for home care. When teaching these assessments, be certain to spend enough time with the woman so that she thoroughly understands both the reason for the assessment and the procedure for doing it. The nurse who visits in the home, then, not only continues this health teaching but may also carry out many of the assessments.

A first home visit usually includes a thorough health history and physical examination; environmental, community, and social assessment; assessment of compliance with medical, preventive, or medication regimens; and evaluation of the need for the services of a home health care aide or further nursing visits. Future visits focus on continuing assessment and evaluation of patient progress, compliance, and readiness to move to another level of health care.

Nursing Diagnosis

Nursing diagnoses for home care may address the physiologic reason for supervised home care or the effect of the experience on the family, such as:

- Deficient knowledge related to complication of pregnancy and necessary procedures and treatments
- Interrupted family processes related to need for home care
- Ineffective role performance related to bedrest at home
- Social isolation related to need for home care
- Anxiety related to complication of pregnancy requiring home care

Outcome Identification and Planning

Outcome identification and planning for home care require close collaboration between the health care

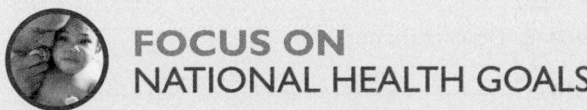

Client Data

Client's name ____________________

Nickname ____________________

Client's DOB __/__/__ Client's Age ____

Client's ins. type & no. ____________________

Client's SS no. ____________________

Client's race __ White __ Black

__ Hispanic __ Other

EDC ____ Weeks gestation ____________

Primary language ____________________

__ Home __ Shelter __ Homeless

__ Staying with relatives

Current residence address:

____
Street

____
City Zip

Phone ____________________

Best time to contact ____________________

Diagnoses

1. ____________________
2. ____________________
3. ____________________

Exacerbating potentials:

Emergency Contact Person/s

Name ____________________
Age

Relationship ____________________

Phone ____________________

Address ____________________
Street

____
City Zip

Doctor (must use PCP if applicable)

Name ____________________

Hospital ____________________

Phone ____________________

Address ____________________
Street

____
City Zip

Consulting Doctors on Care

Phone ____________________

1. ____________________
2. ____________________
3. ____________________

Other consultants:

1. SW ____________________
2. other ____________________

____

1. Planned hospital for delivery ____________________
2. History of prenatal care this pregnancy ____________________
3. Planned delivery:

Vaginal C-section

____

I. Prior OB history: G ________ P ________

FIGURE 16.1 Perinatal home needs assessment tool. *(continued)*

PIH ________ GDM ________ IDDM ________ Eclampsia ________

No. of children living with her, and their ages: ________________________________

____

Any children in foster care, or living elsewhere: ________________________________

____

____

II. Current State of Health:
1. Physical
2. Mental
3. Emotional
4. Social
5. Hospitalizations/Surgeries
6. Diet/Nutrition/weight prior to pregnancy; weight gain so far
7. Activity
8. Physical limitations
9. Support systems
10. Limitations
11. Medications—Time, Frequency, Amount, Purpose, Side effects
12. Teaching Needed

__ Transportation __ Self-treatment

__ Changes during pregnancy

__ Nutrition __ Home Safety __ Community Resources

- __ utilities
- __ phone
- __ housing
- __ cooking
- __ water
- __ respite
- __ ref.
- __ others

__ Growth/Dev.

__ Parenting Education

__ Budgeting of financial resources

__ Parenting skills __ Parenting education

__ Gestational diabetes __ Premature labor

__ Rupture of membranes __ Signs/Symptoms of Labor

13. Referrals already made: ________________________________
14. Referrals needed: ________________________________

__ WIC __ Wheels

____

FIGURE 16.1 (*continued*) Perinatal home needs assessment tool.

IV. Family Data/Support Network:
1. Other household members (name, age, medical issues)
2. Other significant others/extended family members
   Are they available to assist with care of child—when delivered?
3. Summary of household function—Do people work together?
   Do they get along? Who is in charge?
4. Evidence of drug/ETOH use
5. Smoker

Housing Information
1. Current residence ___ Permanent ___ Temporary
2. Type of residence ___ House ___ Apt. ___ Shelter ___ Other explain ____________
3. Length of time in current residence ____________
4. Are there Plans to Move? ___ Yes ___ No ___ When? ____________
   New Address: ____________
5. Layout of House:
   no. of bedrooms _____ no. of bathrooms _____
   ___ Kitchen ___ Dining area ___ Living area ___ Furniture
   Condition of House: ____________
   Safety Issues at House:
   Outlets: ___ 2 Prong ___ 3 Prong ___ Adeq. nos.
   ___ Inadeq. nos.
   Smoke alarms: ___ Yes ___ No no. of alarms: ____________
   Stable railings: ___ Yes ___ No
   Adequate lighting: ___ Yes ___ No (specify)
   Emergency nos. Posted: ___ Yes ___ No
   Sanitation: no. of Bathrooms: ___
   A. Is kitchen sanitary? ___ Yes ___ No (specify)
   B. Pest Control: Are the following present:
      ___ Roaches ___ Rats/Mice ___ Flies
   C. Plumbing problems ____________
      Medication storage: Specify plan for storage, if refrigeration needed
      Infection control needs surrounding care:
      Summary of client home needs assessment
      ____
      Problem list—Preliminary
      ____
      Plan

FIGURE 16.1 *(continued)* Perinatal home needs assessment tool.

providers at a health care agency and those providing care through the home care or community agency. Typically, the initial referral from the health care agency provides the foundation from which the home care nurse develops a plan of care. A major portion of this planning involves reviewing with the woman and her family exactly what their needs are, what will be expected of them, and what they can expect of the nurse, and developing outcomes that address these needs and expectations. If this is not carefully done, some women, for example, will assume that staying at home is all that is required of them, when what is actually required is complete bedrest. "Walking through a day" with them helps them to determine at what points during the day they will need additional assistance to be able to remain in bed at home. For example, the woman on bedrest may need assistance with meal preparation or hygiene while her partner is at work. In this situation, a referral for a home health aide would probably be appropriate. She may need help with transporting her children to school or activities. Discussing these issues with her helps her call on resources such as other family members, neighbors, or community volunteer groups.

Determining family roles (see Chap. 2), such as who is the wage earner, the decision maker, the nurturer, or the problem solver, is also important. Home care is most successful when these family roles are not disrupted but strengthened to support whatever new activities or concerns need to be addressed.

Implementation

Women receiving home care have the advantage over hospitalized women of being in their own environment with their families. Because home care provides only intermittent visits, however, there is the possible disadvantage of not being constantly supervised by health care personnel. Be certain to reassure the woman and her family after assessment that her condition has not changed and it is safe for her to remain at home on the present program. If changes have occurred, introduce new interventions and evaluate their effectiveness. Interventions performed for the pregnant client at home are little different from those performed in an acute care facility. They can range from teaching and counseling to hands-on care. The only difference is that they are done in the client's home. This means home care nurses need to have the same background and level of expertise as acute care nurses. In addition, they may need to be more flexible and adaptable because each home visit may be very different from the one just before or after.

Outcome Evaluation

Outcome evaluation for the pregnant woman receiving home care includes determining whether the woman and fetus are remaining well at home and whether the woman feels comfortable and secure with the arrangement. For many women, successful home care can mean the difference between too early a birth and a successful term pregnancy.

Examples of outcome criteria include:

- Client demonstrates adequate skill in performing home monitoring procedures.
- Client verbalizes changes in condition she will need to report to her health care provider.
- Client participates as a member of the family within limitations imposed by pregnancy complication.
- Family members state they have adjusted to home care of mother.
- Client states she is able to maintain contact with friends and family despite complete bedrest at home.

HOME CARE

Discharge planners in acute care settings can be instrumental in setting the stage for home care by discussing the need for continued health supervision with women and helping them to begin establishing personal goals for home care. A number of steps are then necessary for the actual home visit to be successful (see the Focus on Cultural Competence). These steps can be divided into previsit, visit, and postvisit phases.

Preparing for a Home Visit

Typically, a first home visit is made within 24 hours of discharge from an acute care facility or after notice from the ambulatory care facility. Be certain to obtain a copy of the client's referral form to familiarize yourself with her treat-

FOCUS ON CULTURAL COMPETENCE

Because the structure of families is culturally determined, home care of a woman during pregnancy will be easier for some than for others. If the family is extended, for example, the woman may be so involved in the care of other family members, such as an older adult, that she is unable to rest adequately at home. On the other hand, in such a family, there may be many people to offer care and support, so rest at home is ideal.

In some cultures males are very dominant, so the thought of the man giving care to his wife is exactly the opposite of a usual pattern. If a woman is the dominant member of the household, becoming a passive, cared-for partner may be extremely difficult for her.

Some cultures stress that women must be active during pregnancy to help ensure a small baby and therefore an easier birth. The culture of a particular community might oppose the use of technology, so a woman living there might not like having to use home monitoring equipment. Assess each family individually to determine how home care may affect that particular family.

ment course and her plan of care. Obtain any supplies that may be needed for the visit. Keep in mind that you are going to be a guest in the client's home. Respect for the client's and family's privacy, beliefs, lifestyles, routines, culture, and requests is crucial. As a part of this, it is best to telephone the client in advance to arrange a time for the visit so it will be convenient for her and her family. Obtain necessary instructions to reach the home. To avoid disrupting family routines, try not to visit at mealtime unless observing what the woman is eating for a typical meal is necessary for assessment. Be alert to possible environmental, social, and cultural factors identified on the referral that may require nursing creativity. Keep in mind that the ethical and legal aspects of nursing care, such as confidentiality, informed consent, decision making, and client rights, commonly associated with acute care nursing are also applicable to home care. Remember this when transporting a chart or notes on a client or when discussing the visit with others.

Ensuring Personal Safety

Because home care nurses work alone, they should take measures to ensure their personal safety on the way to the client's home, during the visit, and afterward. Safety tips for traveling in an unfamiliar community are shown in Box 16-1.

BOX 16.1

SAFETY TIPS FOR HOME HEALTH CARE TRAVEL

- Plan your trip in advance using a reliable map of the area.
- Let someone know where you are going and the expected time of your return.
- Keep your automobile in good repair and filled with gasoline so you can avoid having to make stops at unfamiliar service stations.
- Lock any valuables in the trunk of your car *before* you leave the health care agency, not after you park in front of a home to visit.
- Learn the location of public phones in the area, or keep a cellular phone with you.
- If you suspect that someone is following you in your car, drive to the nearest police or fire station.
- If you suspect that someone is following you while you are walking, walk into a business establishment.
- Carry only minimal supplies so your hands are free and your appearance does not suggest that you carry drugs or valuables.
- Drive or walk on main or busy streets; avoid shortcuts through alleys or unoccupied areas.
- Walk determinedly, as if you have a purpose and are in charge of your environment and situation.

✔ CHECKPOINT QUESTIONS

1. Is home care more or less cost-effective than hospital care for women with complications of pregnancy?
2. Why is it important to assess family roles before providing home care?
3. When is a first home care visit typically made?

Making the Visit

Depending on the location of the client's home, the facilities and resources available may vary. The setting may be a house, apartment, mobile home, or shelter. On arrival at the client's home, knock or ring the bell and wait for someone to let you in. Greet the client and any other family members present. Greet family pets if they come to greet you (but don't pet strange dogs). Dogs typically serve a guard function and you want them to view you as a friendly, not a threatening, visitor. Sometimes special advance arrangements, such as having a neighbor let you in, may be necessary if the client is alone and cannot walk down a stairway or a long hallway to answer the door.

As in any health care setting, wash your hands before touching the client for assessment, and follow standard precautions while caring for the client. Ask permission to use the kitchen or bathroom sink to wash. Many home care nurses carry liquid soap and paper towels or disposable wipes with them for handwashing if the client's facilities are inconvenient or unavailable.

WHAT IF? What if the client you are visiting lives in a shelter for homeless women or a shelter for abused women? How would you anticipate that your visit would differ from visiting a client's home?

Assessing the Client

Typically on a first visit, a thorough health assessment, including a review of systems and evaluation of the social environment, medications, nutrition, safety, and compliance with treatment thus far, is necessary. In addition, a consent for treatment and release of information form may need to be signed by the client (Fig. 16-2).

Provide privacy and confidentiality when obtaining the health history and performing a physical examination in the home. Some homes may be too cool early in the morning for physical assessment because the heat has been turned down during the night. Arranging for a visit later in the day may alleviate this problem. If a home has few rooms, finding a private location can be difficult. Include assessment not only of physical aspects but of mental or psychosocial ones as well. Women receiving home care are usually anxious to have a nurse confirm that they are well and that the self-assessments they have been making have been accurate (Fig. 16-3).

If the woman is on bedrest, ask how she occupies her time. A woman is not really resting if she is concerned

Client Name: ____________________

Address: ____________________

City: __________ State: __________ Zip: __________ Phone: ( ) __________

Insurance Company: ____________________ Insurance I.D.#

I, the __________ (of the patient), intending to be legally bound, hereby:

1. Consent to such care and treatment by , and its employees and agents (collectively, the "Agency"), as prescribed by the client's physician or dictated by the client's condition.
2. Authorize the Agency to release any medical records in its possession concerning the client as may be required by law or to pay benefits on the client's behalf. I authorize the client's physicians, insurors, and hospitals to release such medical records to the Agency at the Agency's request.
3. Authorize my insuror to disclose to the Agency the terms and extent of my coverage, and the amount of payments made to me for services provided by the Agency.
4. Assign, transfer and set over to the Agency all of my or the client's rights to insurance proceeds or other funds to which I am or the patient is or will become entitled as a result of the services rendered by the Agency.
5. Consent to and authorize payment, which would otherwise be payable to me or the client, to be made directly to the Agency. The Agency may issue a receipt for such payment which shall discharge the insurance company of its obligations under the policy to the extent of such payment.
6. Agree that I remain individually responsible to pay the Agency for all charges not paid for any reason by the insurer or other third-party payor. I understand that payment in full is due upon receipt of my bill. If payment for the Agency's service is made directly to me by my insuror, I agree to endorse the check to and forward it to the Agency within three days of receipt.

A photocopy of this document, if executed, shall be considered as effective and valid as the original.

The effect of this form and the Client's Rights and Responsibilities on the back of this form have been explained to me by the Agency and I understand its content and significance.

Date: __________ Signature: __________

Name: __________

(Please Print)

FIGURE 16.2 Form for consent for treatment, release of information, assignment of benefits, and notice of client rights.

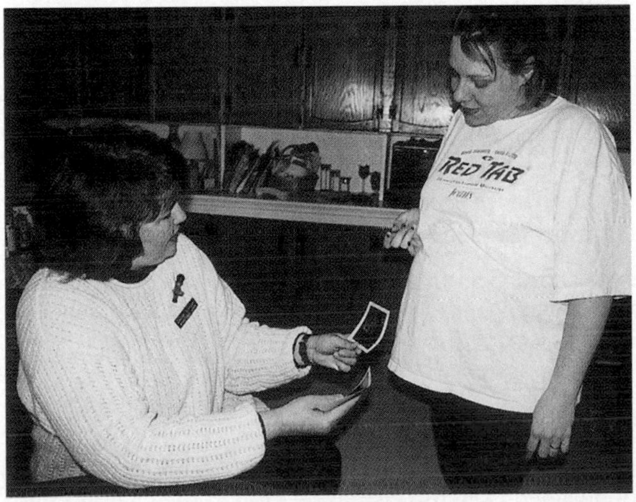

FIGURE 16.3 The home health nurse assesses the pregnant woman and provides reassurance.

about her family or finances, is caring for older children, or is bored. Evaluate her understanding of her condition and make sure she knows the danger signs to report immediately. Be certain that the woman has a means of obtaining refills on prescriptions and knows what measures to take if her condition should worsen, such as telephoning 911, a hospital, or her primary care provider. Be certain that she knows the importance of keeping health care appointments and has transportation to them. At all times, despite the informality of the setting, good interviewing and physical assessment skills are important (see the Focus on Communication). Throughout the assessment, evaluate the client's needs and provide instructions and reinforcement about any specific areas that are necessary.

Assessing the Environment

During a visit, observe whether the house is safe for home care. This means adequate water, electricity, heat, and refrigeration. Are there smoke detectors in the home?

FOCUS ON COMMUNICATION

Francine Gregory is receiving home care because of hyperemesis of pregnancy. She lost 15 pounds at the beginning of pregnancy but now, at 25 weeks, has gained back the lost pounds plus 2 extra after beginning supplemental enteral feedings every day. A home health aide visits her three times a week to supervise her nutrition. She always seems pleased to be visited by a home care nurse.

Less Effective Communication

Nurse: Hello, Francine. Is everything going all right?
Francine: Good.
Nurse: Are you eating everything you're supposed to?
Francine: Sure.
Nurse: Not throwing up any more, are you?
Francine: No.
Nurse: Good. I'm glad you're doing so well.

More Effective Communication

Nurse: Hello, Francine. How is everything?
Francine: All right.
Nurse: What did you eat for breakfast?
Francine: A slice of toast.
Nurse: What happened afterward?
Francine: I threw it up. I do that about once—maybe twice—a day.
Nurse: I need to do a more thorough assessment.

Because home settings are more informal than those of health care agencies, it is easy to forget that a home is a health care setting and let a relationship become more relaxed than therapeutic. In the first scenario, the nurse lapsed into using leading questions rather than structured ones for a health interview. Francine responded to the leading questions by supplying answers she thought the nurse wanted to hear, not necessarily the true answers.

FOCUS ON MULTIDISCIPLINARY CARE

Effective home care requires a team of health care providers, including the supervising physician, home care nurses, health equipment suppliers, home care aides, and participating, informed clients. Home health aides are an invaluable help in providing home health care because they can supply the bulk of personal care services, such as assisting with or providing hygiene, assisting with ambulation, and providing adequate nutrition. Home health aides have varied levels of education depending on the home health care or community health care agency policies and the level of care they are being asked to provide. Keep in mind the following guidelines:

- When working with unlicensed assistive personnel, be sure you are familiar with their level of ability and education so you do not assign a task to them that is above their ability or one that prevents them from using their full potential.
- When making assignments, be certain they understand that making an assessment (e.g., recording a blood pressure) is not the same as evaluating the meaning of the assessment. That requires professional expertise.
- When they are in a client's house, remind them that they are a guest in the house and need to respect the values and patterns of that household.
- When a client no longer needs home care and the time comes to terminate the relationship, know that they may need your help with ending the relationship and saying good-bye because, often, their services have been of such a personal nature.

Are they in working order? Are there drafts or broken windows? Are there rodents or insects in the house? Is the room that will be the new baby's free of lead-based paint?

If the woman is on bedrest, do the arrangements seem adequate or is it likely that she will be getting up every few minutes to care for small children or answer the telephone? Evaluate how far the bathroom is from the woman's bed. A bedside commode may be necessary to avoid a long walk. Check that there is a telephone nearby the client so she has a means of calling someone, both to prevent loneliness and to secure emergency help. If the woman needs assistance with personal hygiene, evaluate the need for a referral for a home health aide to help her (see the Focus on Multidisciplinary Care).

Before leaving the home, set the date and time of the next visit and review any signs and symptoms that she should report immediately to the agency or health care provider rather than waiting for the next visit. Be sure she has the home care agency's and health care provider's phone numbers. Many clients feel more comfortable calling the home care agency rather than the primary care provider's office if the agency has nurses on call around the clock. The nurse on call can then help the client determine what action would be best to take.

WHAT IF? What if you discover large mouse holes in the room that will be used by your pregnant client's new baby? What would you do?

Maintaining Personal Safety

Evaluation as to whether a home is a safe place to visit needs to be ongoing during a visit. Safety tips to keep in mind during home care visits are shown in Box 16-2.

Postvisit Planning

Postvisit planning consists of documenting all information gained from the visit in relation to the client's condition, completing agency forms so billing for supplies and nursing time can be accurate, and evaluating the client's current status and future needs. It may include commu-

BOX 16.2

SAFETY TIPS DURING HOME CARE VISITS

- Do not carry a purse or backpack that suggests you are carrying a large sum of money or other valuables.
- Park your car in a well-lighted, busy area. Lock the car door.
- Do not leave valuable objects such as an expensive CD player in your car, so it is not a target for car thieves.
- Avoid approaching homes by a dark back alley; use the front door or a busy hallway.
- Use special caution in stairwells and elevators. Leave a stairwell or elevator if a potentially threatening person enters, with an excuse such as, "I've forgotten my red pen."
- When you first enter the home, assess it for personal safety. Ask who is at home. If there are animals in the house, ask if they are friendly.
- If there are animals, take precautions to avoid getting flea bites (sit on a kitchen chair, not an upholstered chair).
- Be cautious about accepting food or drink if you are not certain about the hygiene of the dishes or food. Decline it gracefully with an excuse such as, "I'm trying to cut down on the amount of coffee I drink," or "It's against my agency's rules."
- Leave a home immediately if you feel threatened or unsafe.
- Have your car keys in your hand when you leave the house so you can unlock and enter your car rapidly.
- Look under your car when approaching it and in the back seat of your car before entering it to be certain no one is there. Relock your car door immediately once inside.
- If both you and the client are in personal danger, call the community emergency number, such as 911, for help.

nicating a change in status to the primary health care provider, asking for a renewal of orders, or updating and revising the plan of care. Accurate documentation is essential. Although the forms may vary, the rules for documentation in home care are the same as for any health care facility.

Follow-Up Visits

Subsequent home visits are planned depending on the woman's circumstances and the amount of health education and supervision needed. A second visit could be scheduled as often as the next day or as infrequently as once a month. Frequent assessments accomplished at subsequent visits include vital signs, FHR, nutrition assessment, assessment of the possibility of beginning labor, and nursing care actions such as health education or medication compliance.

✔ CHECKPOINT QUESTIONS

4. When interviewing a home care client who has a dog, where should you sit?
5. What should you do if, in the middle of a home visit, a woman's former partner arrives and threatens you?
6. What is a tactful way to refuse a cup of coffee offered during a home visit?

NURSING RESPONSIBILITIES FOR HOME CARE

Nursing responsibilities for women receiving home care during pregnancy vary because the reason for home care during pregnancy also varies. Typical actions or interventions carried out in homes are discussed below.

Promoting a Therapeutic Environment

Home care is most successful if there are effective support people to help the client. Otherwise, the woman can experience a sense of loneliness and low self-esteem that may interfere with her compliance with the treatment program, such as maintaining bedrest long enough to sustain a pregnancy.

Women on bedrest during pregnancy can react in a number of ways, but many report feeling "tied down," "like a prisoner," and "like I'm missing out." One way women can cope with the stress of the experience is by keeping busy or using their time to learn a new skill. Most women can identify activities for stimulation by themselves. A few may need a stimulation program to prevent them from passing the time simply by watching television or napping. For example, if the woman likes to read but doesn't always have the time to do so, bedrest at home may provide an ideal time for her to catch up on her reading. If she has other children, she can spend part of her time reading to them. She could also use the time to take a home-study course, learn a new hobby, write a short story, or study for a certifying examination related to her work. In any event, helping her plan meaningful activities such as these can help her view home care not as wasted time, but as time invested in her family or career (see the Focus on Family Empowerment).

Promoting Healthy Family Functioning

Many women fulfill multiple roles in their family, such as financial manager, peacemaker, problem solver, nurturer, and decision maker. Even when a woman is on bedrest, help her to continue in these roles to ensure the family's usual functioning, because support people often have great difficulty assuming these roles in her place. As a rule, support people can be supportive only if they understand the need for the home care program and the importance of their role. Arranging for a homemaker service to care for children or an aging parent or to help with light housework may be necessary to prevent support people from feeling stretched so thin they cannot function. Often support people are not present at the time of a home visit because they work during the day. Ask the woman at home visits how

FOCUS ON FAMILY EMPOWERMENT

Suggestions for Best Use of Time While on Bedrest

Q. I feel like I'm wasting my time just being home this way. What can I do to keep busy?

A. Try these suggestions:

- Renew an old hobby or begin a new one.
- Ask someone to bring you books on newborn care from the library so you can pass the time reading.
- Telephone friends. Rest next to a telephone so friends know they won't be disturbing you when they return calls.
- Catch up on your correspondence. Friends and family will be surprised and delighted to hear from you.
- Investigate if there is a local community project you could work on while on bedrest (e.g., telephoning for a political campaign, urging neighbors to write letters of support for a new playground).
- If you worked outside your home prior to this, ask your employer if there is a project you could work on from bedrest.
- If you have Internet access, spend time online looking for information about pregnancy, childbirth, childrearing, or just chatting with friends or others (be conscious of the telephone bill that might result).
- Learn a second language; there are many books available on this.
- Take a mail-order course on something you want to learn more about (e.g., creative writing; learning to be a paralegal).
- Ask your home care nurse about preparation for childbirth information. By conscientiously practicing breathing exercises while on bedrest, you can become well prepared for labor and birth.

her support people are coping and if there are ways this experience could be made easier for them as well as for her (see the Focus on Evidence-Based Practice).

Health Teaching

A home care visit can provide many more opportunities for one-on-one health teaching than a health care agency setting. An important aspect of teaching may be providing childbirth education, because the woman on bedrest will not be able to attend formal classes (Josten et al., 2002).

Medicine Administration

Many pregnant women receiving home care need to take some type of medicine, such as a tocolytic to halt preterm labor or an antibiotic to prevent a uterine infection, in addition to the usual prenatal vitamin supplementation. They may be taking an antihypertensive for hypertension of pregnancy (Branch & Porter, 2000). Review the rules of safe medication administration to minimize mistakes such as taking the medicine more frequently than prescribed or forgetting to take it. (Common safeguards for home administration of medicine are shown in Chap. 36.) If the woman does not have a support person who will remind her to take medicine, help her make out a written schedule or calendar for administration so she can remind herself. Encourage the woman to use this as a practical tool, crossing off each time she has taken the medication. This helps to eliminate confusion and allows the home care nurse to evaluate the client's compliance with therapy.

Providing for Adequate Nutrition and Hydration

A woman who is receiving home care often needs help maintaining adequate nutrition. She may be the person who plans menus, shops for food, and cooks for the fam-

FOCUS ON EVIDENCE-BASED PRACTICE

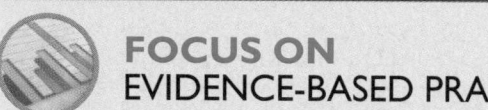

Can Preterm Labor Be Halted if Pregnant Women Receive Home Care?

For this study, 250 women experiencing preterm labor were randomly assigned to home care or hospital care management. A perinatal information form was used to collect data on demographic and pregnancy variables. Three separate stress inventories were used to measure the woman's perception of care and family functioning. These were administered at the time women were assigned to a study group and at 1 week and 2 weeks of the study. Results revealed that women in both groups felt reduced anxiety by the third week of the study over the time of randomization. Women in the home care group were more satisfied with support from their male partner. There was no significant difference between the two groups in family functioning. At the time of birth, gestational age and birthweight of newborns from the two groups were similar. The researchers concluded that home care management is a safe and efficacious method of health care for women experiencing preterm labor.

Nurses frequently provide care for women in home care situations. This study shows the importance of this form of management of preterm labor for the woman, her family, and the infant. Nurses in a home care environment are in a position to care for the family as well as the woman and to help the woman's family and partner provide support.

Goulet, C., et al. (2001). A controlled clinical trial of home care management versus hospital care management for preterm labour. *International Journal of Nursing Studies, 38*(3), 259–269.

ily. With her on bedrest, other family members must assume these roles. Otherwise, the entire family, including the pregnant woman, can find themselves not maintaining good nutrition. Instruct family members about healthy nutrition practices, emphasizing the client's specific nutritional needs. Assist with meal planning and suggestions for healthy snacks.

All women during pregnancy should drink six to eight full glasses of fluid a day to obtain adequate fluid for effective kidney function and placental exchange (Parsons & Spellacy, 2000). Be certain women on bedrest have a supply of fluid close to their bed.

Intravenous Administration

Pregnant women may be receiving intravenous therapy as a means of medication administration or, especially for women with hyperemesis gravidarum, as a means of hydration. Women with sickle cell anemia may receive blood transfusions in the home.

Intravenous medication and fluid administration is accomplished using either a peripheral or central insertion site. Because peripheral intravenous lines frequently become dislodged, in the home setting intravenous fluid is often administered by a central line or a peripherally inserted catheter threaded to a central blood vessel (a PICC line). Specially pressurized fluid containers allow for fast and easy administration of special solutions. To help women infuse large amounts of fluid slowly and accurately, an intravenous infusion pump is strongly recommended. Women can receive antibiotics through "piggyback" infusions they keep frozen until the time of administration. Be certain the woman knows how to monitor intravenous insertion sites for inflammation and infiltration, how to protect the site from becoming infected (e.g., cover it with plastic rather than letting it get wet), and how to monitor the amount and kind of fluid or medication infused.

Home Enteral Nutrition

Women who have hyperemesis gravidarum may also receive nutrition by a nasogastric tube. The supplies necessary for enteral feedings such as feeding tubes and enteral pumps are available for rent or purchase through pharmacies or medical supply houses or the home care agency. Such tubes are usually changed every 2 to 4 weeks. The home care nurse will most likely be the person responsible for changing the tube, but this depends on the home care agency's policies. In addition to assessing the client, be sure the woman is familiar with all aspects of care for the tube, equipment, and administration of the feeding. Encourage the woman to monitor the supply of formula for the feedings so it doesn't run out, especially over weekends. She probably will need to weigh herself daily and record the weight. Be certain she knows when to call for advice if she is having difficulty or is unsure if her weight is remaining adequate.

Total Parenteral Nutrition

Total parenteral nutrition (TPN) may be used to supply complete nutrition and fluid to women with hyperemesis gravidarum on home care. Usually the home care agency or a separate private vendor will furnish and deliver the formula, tubing, clean dressings, and an infusion pump. The formula, which consists of amino acids, hypertonic glucose, vitamins, and minerals in solution, should be stored in the client's refrigerator until 1 to 2 hours before use; it is then removed from the refrigerator and allowed to warm to room temperature. Women requiring this type of intravenous nutritional therapy usually have a central venous access device such as a central venous catheter or PICC inserted. The catheter may be inserted before the woman is discharged from the acute care facility or as an outpatient procedure if the woman is already at home. The home care nurse plays a key role in teaching the woman about the therapy and also in assessing her response to therapy.

Throughout the therapy, the client needs instruction about monitoring the infusion of the solution and the patency of the tube. She needs to know the correct frequency of feedings (whether continuous or intermittent) and the interval at which she should have blood work scheduled. She also needs to be taught to change dressings, observe the insertion site, and assess her temperature for signs of possible infection. She must be aware of any restrictions she should adhere to (e.g., no baths if the water level will rise above the catheter insertion site). Because TPN solutions are hypertonic, instruct the woman how to obtain fingerstick blood glucose levels as necessary, usually every 6 hours. Encourage her to record these finding so they can be evaluated on the next visit. Be sure she knows what findings should be reported immediately.

Promoting Elimination

Promoting elimination in the woman receiving home care can call for advance planning. The site where the woman is going to rest is often determined by the location of a bathroom. If strict bedrest is required, a bedside commode may be necessary.

Constipation occurs at a high rate during pregnancy and may occur even more frequently in women on bedrest from lack of exercise. Encourage women to eat a diet high in fiber and to drink at least eight glasses of fluid daily in an attempt to minimize this problem.

Teaching Self-Monitoring of Vital Signs

Monitoring vital signs in the home does not differ from monitoring them in a health care agency. Mercury thermometers may be used in place of electronic thermometers. If a woman will be using a mercury/glass thermometer, caution her that mercury is a toxic contaminant if the thermometer breaks. Remind women that this type of thermometer takes a full 3 minutes to register rather than the more convenient few seconds needed by electronic thermometers. For consistency, the woman should take her blood pressure in the same position (lying down or sitting up) and on the same arm. Encourage the client to keep a record of the readings so you can evaluate them on your next visit. Using an automated cuff simplifies taking blood pressure. Results obtained by self-monitoring are as predictive of hypertension of pregnancy as those taken by health care providers in a clinic setting (see Focus on Nursing Care Planning)

FOCUS ON *Nursing Care Planning*

A PREGNANT WOMAN AT HOME ON BEDREST

A 32-year-old female client, 30 weeks pregnant, is placed on home bedrest after her last prenatal visit to prevent further hypertension of pregnancy. On your home visit, she states, "I don't know how I can stay in bed for the next 10 weeks. I have to work and keep an eye on two small children."

Assessment: Client primary wage earner in the family; works full time as a travel agent. Lives with husband and 2 children, 2 years and 4 years of age, in a two-story home. Client's bedroom on second floor with bathroom located next to bedroom, approximately 20 feet from client's bed. "We just bought this house over a year ago. How are we going to make the mortgage payments?" Husband is full-time doctoral student receiving only a student stipend. "He leaves about 9:30 A.M. and gets home around 4 P.M. every day but Thursday. Then he gets home around 6:30 P.M." Four-year-old child goes to half-day nursery school 3 days a week. Two-year-old home with mom, currently being potty trained.

Vital signs: Temperature 98.4°F; pulse 76; respirations 22; blood pressure 144/94; FHR 148. Mild facial edema; +1 protein in urine; 2-pound weight gain in 1 week.

Nursing Diagnosis: Anxiety related to bedrest and interference with family and financial responsibilities

Outcome Identification: Client will demonstrate positive behaviors to maintain bedrest and role responsibilities until minimum fetal maturity is reached.

Outcome Evaluation: Client identifies methods to participate in work and child care while maintaining bedrest; verbalizes increased comfort with imposed bedrest; maintains bedrest for at least 6 weeks.

Interventions	Rationale
1. Discuss with client areas of concern about finances, roles, home management, and childcare.	1. Discussion provides baseline information to identify client's needs, beliefs, and responsibilities.
2. Check with maternal health care provider regarding the degree of activity limitation and extent of bedrest required.	2. Varying degrees of bedrest may be ordered to control hypertension of pregnancy.
3. Review with client specific activity restrictions, such as complete bedrest, bedrest with bathroom privileges, stairs, and the reasons for them. Arrange for a bedside commode if necessary.	3. Review provides reinforcement and enhances understanding of the rationale for bedrest, thus promoting compliance.
4. Assist client with planning effective childcare; discuss possible help from friends and family. Arrange for a home health care aide to assist with household management and childcare.	4. Planning effective methods for childcare and home management helps to alleviate two of the stressors associated with the client's anxiety about bedrest.
5. Have client check with employer about personnel policies regarding pregnancy problems. Review with client possible work activities she could continue at home.	5. Personnel policies should allow for financial compensation for pregnancy problems. Continuing some work from home may also help to relieve some of the financial stress, which is important in relieving the client's overall anxiety level.
6. Urge couple to arrange for telephone connection next to client's bed, both for communication and for possible computer/modem connection to continue work activities.	6. Helping establish a means of communication provides both stimulation and contact with others and also a possibility for continuing work.

(continued)

Interventions	Rationale
7. Encourage client to plan frequent periods of quiet time. Suggest activities such as reading and listening to music. Advise client to lie on her side.	7. Planning quiet activities helps prevent the client from overdoing work-related activities and enhances the effectiveness of bedrest. Side lying enhances placental perfusion.
8. Suggest client arrange for time each day to spend with children in quiet activities, such as reading to them or playing a game.	8. Quiet activities with the children enhance family bonding and decrease feelings of isolation in the children while still allowing the client to maintain bedrest.

Nursing Diagnosis: Risk for injury (maternal and fetal) related to effects of hypertension of pregnancy

Outcome Identification: Client's systolic and diastolic blood pressure will remain within prescribed pregnancy parameters for the duration of her pregnancy.

Outcome Evaluation: Blood pressure remains 140/90 or less; FHR within acceptable parameters; urine for protein remains +1 or less; weight gain limited to 1 lb/week; edema limited and without increase.

Interventions	Rationale
1. Assess vital signs, including heart rate, blood pressure, and FHR, at every visit.	1. Assessment of vital signs, especially blood pressure and FHR, provides a baseline for future comparison and evidence of the client's and fetus' status.
2. Check random urine specimen for protein at each visit. Instruct client to check urine specimen daily and report any values > +1.	2. Proteinuria > +3 indicates severe preeclampsia.
3. Monitor daily weights and intake and output. Instruct client to weigh herself every day at the same time with approximately the same amount of clothing. Also teach her how to measure and record intake and output.	3. Weight and intake and output provide evidence of tissue fluid retention. Consistency with measurements ensures accuracy.
4. Teach client to assess for edema, including location, amount, and degree of pitting.	4. Increasing edema, especially of the face and upper extremities, indicates severe preeclampsia.
5. Question client about fetal movements. Instruct client in methods to count fetal movements and estimate uterine weight.	5. Fetal movements and uterine self-assessment provide information about fetal well-being and growth.
6. Instruct client and husband how to take client's blood pressure daily and record.	6. Daily blood pressure checks provide objective data about the client's status for evaluation by the nurse on follow-up visits.
7. Encourage a diet high in protein and adequate fluid intake.	7. Protein, which is being lost in the urine, needs to be replaced to ensure optimal fetal growth and development.
8. Instruct client and family members in signs and symptoms of increased hypertension, such as increased edema, increased protein in urine, headache, dizziness, blurred vision, increased weight gain, or decreased urine output. Advise client to call the home care agency or health care provider if any occur.	8. Knowledge of the danger signs and symptoms allows for early identification and prompt intervention to prevent threats to the mother and fetus.

Teaching Self-Monitoring of Uterine Height, Contractions, and Fetal Heart Rate

Fundal height is measured by using a paper tape measure according to McDonald's rule (see Chap. 8). If the woman is asked to record serial fundal height measurements, demonstrate the correct technique and have her give a return demonstration, as this measurement varies greatly depending on where the tape measure is placed. Be sure the client is measuring the height in the same location each time. It may be necessary to mark the points with an indelible pen to ensure consistent and accurate measurements.

Many women conduct count-to-10 assessments daily (count the number of fetal movements they feel in a designated time period; see Chap. 8) to help assess fetal well-being (Miller & Paul, 2000). FHR is usually checked at each home visit. In addition, the client may be taught how to obtain this herself. FHR can be recorded by listening with a Doppler, a fetoscope, a regular stethoscope (although FHR may be very difficult to hear), or an electronic monitoring device supplied as part of her home care program.

The client can self-monitor uterine contractions using a uterine monitor, the same as in a health care facility, or by palpation. Instruct her to measure the time from the beginning to the end of each contraction and determine the interval between contractions (from the beginning of one contraction to the beginning of the next). Advise her to count and time contractions for 30 to 60 minutes. As a general rule, tell her to call the home care agency or health care provider if contractions are 10 minutes apart or less, or if they last 30 seconds or more.

A rhythm strip or nonstress test can be conducted using a portable monitor approximately the size of a transistor radio. The woman straps this device to her abdomen, positioning the sensor approximately 2 to 3 fingerbreadths below the umbilicus or at the top of the fundus, for 20 to 30 minutes at a set time every day, or at any time she feels contractions or is concerned about the lack of fetal movement (Fig. 16-4). The monitor records both uterine contractions and FHR. At the conclusion of the monitoring period, the monitor is held next to a telephone and the tracing is transmitted to a central facility for evaluation. Home monitoring thus can provide ready evaluation of contractions, possibly resulting in improved pregnancy outcomes, therefore decreasing the need for neonatal intensive care.

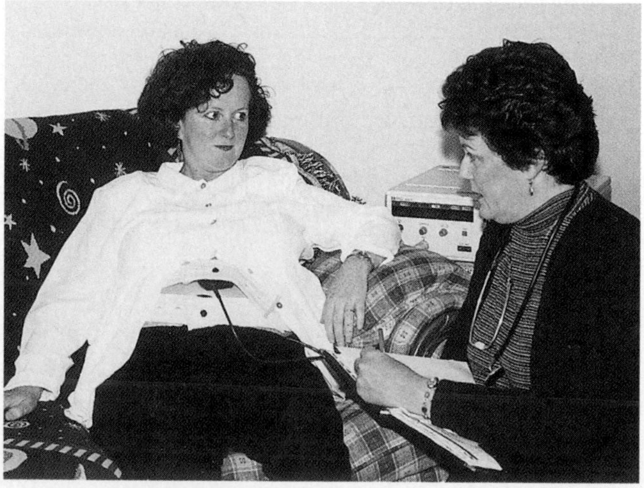

FIGURE 16.4 Fetal heart rate and uterine contractions can be recorded successfully by women at home.

Teaching Self-Monitoring by Serum or Urine Testing

Women who develop diabetes mellitus during pregnancy may be required to monitor serum glucose levels using a test strip and glucometer at least once daily (typically, four times a day) (Spellacy, 2000). Many women are reluctant to learn this procedure because they don't like the thought of having to pierce the skin of a finger to draw blood. Automated lancet devices and even skin sensors are available to help with this. Pregnant women can be taught to perform this procedure effectively and successfully in the home.

✔ CHECKPOINT QUESTIONS

7. Why is constipation apt to be a problem for a woman on bedrest at home?
8. How much fluid should a pregnant woman receiving home care drink daily?

KEY POINTS

Home care can be more cost-effective than hospital care for women with a pregnancy complication or women considered at high risk for complications.

Home care, like hospital care, can be costly for people without health insurance. However, it has the advantage of preventing extensive disruption of a family.

Home care requires careful planning and a combined effort between the home care agency and the health care provider to ensure collaboration and continuity.

Frequent conditions for which women may require home care are preterm labor, hyperemesis gravidarum, diabetes mellitus, and hypertension of pregnancy.

CRITICAL THINKING EXERCISES

1. Lee Puente is the woman you met at the beginning of the chapter. Was she a good candidate for home care? What additional interventions would she need to make home care more successful for her?
2. When you are visiting a home care client, do standard precautions to prevent the spread of infection apply? Explain your answer.

3. A home care client you visit is 18 years old. She is home alone most of the day because both of her parents work. Her boyfriend visits between 9 and 10 AM daily, and school friends visit in the afternoon. What would be the best time of the day to schedule a home visit?
4. Examine the National Health Goals related to pregnancy and home care. Most government-sponsored money for nursing research is allotted based on these goals. What would be a possible research topic to explore pertinent to these goals that would be fundable and would advance evidence-based practice?

REFERENCES

Branch, D. W., & Porter, T. F. (2000). Hypertensive disorders of pregnancy. In J. R. Scott, et al. *Danforth's obstetrics and gynecology* (8th ed., pp. 309-329). Philadelphia: Lippincott Williams & Wilkins.

Department of Health and Human Services. (2000). *Healthy people 2010.* Washington, DC: DHHS.

Goulet, C. et al. (2001). A controlled clinical trial of home care management versus hospital care management for preterm labour. *International Journal of Nursing Studies, 38*(3), 259-269.

Josten, L. E., et al. (2002). Dropping out of maternal and child home visits. *Public Health Nursing, 19*(1), 3-10.

Kitzman, H., et al. (2000). Enduring effects of nurse home visitation on maternal life course. *JAMA, 283*(4), 1983-1989.

Koniak-Griffin, D. et al. (2002). Public health nursing care for adolescent mothers: Impact on infant health and selected maternal outcomes at 1 year postbirth. *Journal of Adolescent Health, 30*(1), 44-54.

Miller, D. A., & Paul, R. (2000). Antepartum-intrapartum fetal monitoring. In J. R. Scott, et al. *Danforth's obstetrics and gynecology* (8th ed., pp. 243-256). Philadelphia: Lippincott Williams & Wilkins.

Parsons, M. T., & Spellacy, W. N. (2000). Preterm labor. In J. R. Scott, et al. *Danforth's obstetrics and gynecology* (8th ed., pp. 257-267). Philadelphia: Lippincott Williams & Wilkins.

Spellacy, W. N. (2000). Diabetes mellitus and pregnancy. In J. R. Scott, et al. *Danforth's obstetrics and gynecology* (8th ed., pp. 301-307). Philadelphia: Lippincott Williams & Wilkins.

SUGGESTED READINGS

Eaton, M. K. (2002). Home health access dilemma. *Journal of Nursing Administration, 32*(1), 9-11.

Hannah, M. E., et al. (2000). Prelabor rupture of the membranes at term: Expectant management at home or hospital? *Obstetrics & Gynecology, 96*(4), 533-538.

Hayward, S. (2000). Nurse home visits during pregnancy and early childhood had positive effects on aspects of maternal life course 3 years later. *Evidence-Based Nursing, 3*(4), 115.

Krause, S. A., & Graves, B. W. (1999). Midwifery triage of first trimester bleeding. *Journal of Nurse-Midwifery, 44*(6), 537-548.

Manfredi, C., et al. (2000). Minimal smoking cessation interventions in prenatal, family planning and well-child public health clinics. *American Journal of Public Health, 90*(3), 423 427.

Meyers, K., Johnson, M., & Langdon, R. (2001). Coping styles of pregnant adolescents. *Public Heath Nursing, 18*(1), 24-32.

Wheat, S. (2001). Breastfeeding initiative. *Community Practitioner, 4*(3), 90-99.

CHAPTER 17

High-Risk Pregnancy: The Woman With Special Needs

Key Terms

- **autonomic dysreflexia**
- **emancipated minor**
- **substance dependent**

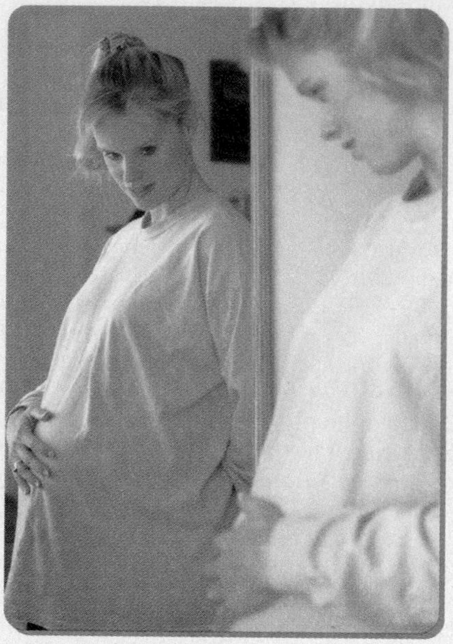

Objectives

After mastering the contents of this chapter, you should be able to:

1. Identify the characteristics of the pregnant woman who has special needs.
2. Describe the risks of pregnancy for the woman with special needs.
3. Assess the woman with special needs during pregnancy.
4. Formulate nursing diagnoses related to pregnancy for the woman with special needs.
5. Identify expected outcomes for the pregnant woman with special needs.
6. Plan nursing care to address the special growth and development needs of the adolescent and the woman over age 40, and the specific strengths and weaknesses of the woman who is physically or cognitively challenged or drug dependent during pregnancy.
7. Implement nursing care for a woman with special needs.
8. Evaluate outcomes to ensure that goals for care have been achieved.
9. Identify National Health Goals related to the woman with a special need that nurses can be instrumental in helping the nation to achieve.
10. Identify areas related to care of the woman with special needs during pregnancy that would benefit from additional nursing research or application of evidence-based practice.
11. Use critical thinking to analyze ways that nursing care of the pregnant woman with a special need can be optimally family centered.
12. Integrate knowledge of the risks of pregnancy with age extremes, drug use, and physical or cognitive challenges with the nursing process to achieve quality maternal and child health nursing care.

Mindy Carson, a 14-year-old girl, is 20 weeks pregnant. The father of Mindy's baby is a college student. He doesn't want Mindy to keep her baby after the birth because he doesn't want to get married until he finishes graduate school, which is 4 years away. Mindy insists she is old enough to be a parent and wants to keep the baby very much. You find Mindy's mother arguing with the baby's father in the middle of a prenatal clinic's waiting room. Mindy's mother says Mindy won't be able to support a child. The father says the state's generous welfare laws will support her. They both turn to you and ask you what you would recommend. Is Mindy old enough to be a parent? What qualities would you look for in her to discover if she is ready to parent? What are the implications of new child welfare laws for teenage mothers? What type of referral does Mindy need?

Typically, many women seen in a prenatal care setting do not fit the description of the average pregnant woman—a well young adult who maintains healthy patterns of living. Previous chapters discussed high-risk pregnancies for women who are ill when they become pregnant, for those who develop an illness while pregnant, and for those who develop a complication related to the pregnancy. This chapter presents information to add to your knowledge base about high-risk pregnancy in women with other special needs—those who are at the two age extremes (very young adolescents and women who have waited until midlife to have their first child); those who are physically or cognitively challenged (such as with a spinal cord injury or hearing challenge); and those who are drug dependent.

After you've studied the chapter, answer the Critical Thinking Exercises at the end of the chapter and then access the on-line study activities (http://connection.lww.com) *to sharpen your skills and test your knowledge.*

Among adolescents, the pregnancy rate, although still high, is decreasing slightly. It is increasing in women over age 40 (DHHS, 2000). Adolescents require special consideration during pregnancy because they are physically and psychosocially immature. Women over age 40 may need special consideration because, at this time in life, they may have difficulty adjusting psychosocially to a first pregnancy and the family changes that requires.

The pregnancy rate also is increasing among women who are physically or cognitively challenged, including those with conditions such as cerebral palsy that might have precluded pregnancy a few years ago. Physical and cognitive conditions present a challenge to childbearing and childrearing, but do not necessarily prevent women from establishing their own families. Supportive nursing care that considers the limitations imposed by a particular disability, while focusing on the normal aspects of childbearing and childrearing, is vital to these women.

The pregnancies of women who are drug dependent also require a great deal of nursing support and care. Ideally, a woman would give up substance abuse for the health of the fetus, but that may not be possible. When this happens, every effort must be made to provide enough prenatal care and attention to protect the fetus in other ways.

These women with special needs have become a focus of attention as evidenced by the National Health Goals (see Focus on National Health Goals). The Department of Health and Human Services (DHHS) also has initiated a special program to help reduce teenage pregnancy (*www.girlpower.gov*).

NURSING PROCESS OVERVIEW

For Care of the Pregnant Woman With Special Needs

Assessment

Assessing the strengths and weaknesses of individual clients is always crucial to establishing accurate nursing diagnoses and realistic outcomes and planning effective nursing interventions. When a client has a special need, this part of the assessment becomes even more essential. Establishing as thorough a database as possible early in pregnancy helps to predict the possible risks a woman may be exposed to when pregnancy is affected by age extremes, physical or cognitive challenges, or unhealthy lifestyle.

When caring for the woman who is physically challenged, keep in mind that physical disabilities occur in degrees; therefore, first establish the impact of the disability on the woman's life before offering any care or guidance for care measures during pregnancy. Be cer-

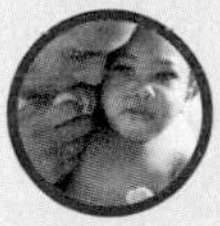

FOCUS ON NATIONAL HEALTH GOALS

A number of National Health Goals have been formulated to improve the health of women with special needs during pregnancy. These are:

- Reduce pregnancy among adolescent females to no more than 43/1000 adolescents from a baseline of 68/1000.
- Increase abstinence from alcohol, cigarettes, and illicit drugs among pregnant women to 100% from a baseline of 86% (alcohol), 99% (binge drinking), and 98% (illicit drugs) (DHHS, 2000).

Nurses can be instrumental in helping the nation achieve these goals by teaching adolescents about the dangers of substance abuse and the complications, both psychological and physical, of teenage pregnancy.

Nurses can add to this knowledge base by being active research investigators. Special topics for possible investigation and areas of evidence-based practice may include the most effective way to impress adolescents about the dangers of substance abuse, and the ideal birth control measure for adolescents (ie, one that would actually be used). As more and more women over age 40 are becoming pregnant, the effects of pregnancy on this age group and their adjustment to it also need to be investigated.

tain to assess physical limitations and abilities and psychosocial or emotional strengths. The capacity of the woman with special needs to adapt to pregnancy depends both on her physical capabilities and on the ability to persevere against odds and overcome what the average woman might think of as insurmountable obstacles. For example, the woman with a spinal cord injury is likely to have developed ways of coping in daily life that may never occur to someone who has not experienced that disability.

For some drug-dependent women, pregnancy may be the impetus for breaking a drug habit. Other women cannot accomplish this. Your main goal should be to encourage the woman to keep coming for prenatal care. As long as she feels comfortable with you during regular visits, you may be able to establish a trusting relationship that could eventually provide her with the confidence to try a more healthful pattern of living.

Nursing Diagnosis

Nursing diagnoses established for pregnant women with special needs differ in degree, but not substance, from the nursing diagnoses established for all pregnant women. For example, if a pregnant adolescent is still growing, nutrition is an important issue for her and for the fetus. Examples of appropriate nursing diagnoses may include:

- Risk for imbalanced nutrition related to combined needs of adolescence and pregnancy
- Risk for fetal injury related to drug and alcohol use
- Impaired physical mobility related to physical disability
- Risk for injury related to unstable balance
- Impaired verbal communication related to spastic muscle functioning
- Impaired home maintenance related to a sensory challenge
- Readiness of enhanced family coping, related to commitment to have a child in the face of a disabling condition

Outcome Identification and Planning

As with any client, be especially careful to establish realistic outcomes, given a woman's particular condition or situation. The adolescent, for instance, cannot achieve independent decision making if her family is still making decisions for her. A woman who is visually challenged may not be able to read a digital display on a glucometer or use a wall clock to time contractions.

Often, the pregnant woman with a special need already has significant stressors to deal with in her life. Adolescence is a period of growth and change that can be stressful for the teenager and her family. The physically challenged woman constantly copes with a condition that must be considered in all activities, even if she has adjusted completely to the limitations such a disability imposes. The drug-dependent woman is confined by a life-threatening habit.

Pregnancy brings with it a whole new set of stressors that can be overwhelming if the woman has no outside support. Planning for the pregnant woman with a special need, therefore, often involves identifying support people to help with this added stress. This support can consist of family, friends, and health care providers. If the woman is not totally independent in her care, some planning may be required with her support person, who may be the person who actually carries out the proposed action. At the same time, be sure not to ignore the woman and plan around her. Only if she approves of the plan can pregnancy be the enjoyable experience it should be. This principle applies to any woman, but especially one with special needs.

A major problem encountered when planning with the pregnant adolescent is that she may have difficulty accepting the reality of the pregnancy, and so may not be interested in pursuing prenatal care.

Some primiparas older than 40 years may have delayed pregnancy to pursue further education or a career, or to solidify a loving, stable relationship. Remember that the woman who has been submerged in a career instead of the world of babies and homemaking may, like the adolescent, be less informed about normal pregnancy findings or healthful pregnancy practices than the younger woman. Be certain that you do not equate a woman's knowledge in one field, such as chemistry or law, with her knowledge of prenatal care.

Plans should include ways to strengthen confidence and self-esteem, crucial attributes for a mother. These also are areas in which the woman with a special need, especially one who perceives herself as too young or too old or who has experienced physical dysfunction, may not have developed fully. Drug dependence may be related to feelings of lowered self-worth, which may have been strengthened if the drug-dependent woman has tried unsuccessfully to limit her drug intake in the past.

Being certain that plans are established in a wide range of areas helps to ensure that planning is comprehensive. Remember to include safe care of the newborn in plans for all women with special needs. Once the infant is born, it may be too late to make these plans in a comprehensive manner.

Implementation

For the high-risk pregnant woman, promoting a healthy pregnancy and preventing pregnancy complications are crucial. Care focuses on teaching and encouraging the woman with any special need to determine how best to manage her pregnancy according to her particular situation.

Unfortunately, a high proportion of adolescents do not seek prenatal care early in pregnancy because they deny that they are, in fact, pregnant. Others may not feel comfortable in a health care facility. The same may be true of the woman with a drug dependency who fears reprisals from health care providers regarding her drug use. A nonjudgmental, welcoming attitude that focuses on the pregnancy and the baby, while avoiding recriminations about the woman's youth or circumstances, is essential to attracting such women to prenatal care and keeping them coming for regular visits. (They may hear from a friend that the staff members at the clinic are helpful, not judgmental, and then take the first step into the facility.)

For women who are physically challenged, modifications may be necessary for some interventions associated with typical pregnancy-related procedures. For example, it may be necessary to modify a pelvic examination when a woman is not able to place her legs in table stirrups. Modifying procedures promotes individualized care for all women, improving overall nursing care.

Outcome Evaluation

Evaluation of nursing interventions in the care of the pregnant woman with a special need often focus on the woman's physical and emotional readiness for childbearing, maintenance of fetal health, and ability of the woman to provide a safe and healthy environment for her newborn. The following are examples that can be used to evaluate the success of a specific outcome:

- Client states she will use walker to maintain balance during pregnancy.
- Adolescent lists intake of adequate nutrition, even with frequent meals at fast-food restaurants.
- Family members state they have been able to adjust to changing demands of pregnancy in mother who is physically challenged.

THE PREGNANT ADOLESCENT

Adolescent pregnancy is not a new phenomenon. Historically, it was common for women to marry at an early age and have a first baby during adolescence. In today's society, however, marriage during the teenage years is not encouraged. Thus, teenage pregnancy is not encouraged. New educational programs on the importance of delaying pregnancy have decreased the number of births in the United States to girls under age 18 years by 3% to 6%, resulting in a rate of 55/100. Although decreased, this number is still higher than that of other developed countries (DHHS, 2000). A combination of factors contributes to the inability to eradicate teenage pregnancy. These include:

- Earlier age of menarche in girls (many girls begin menstruating at age 10, so are ovulating and able to conceive by age 11)
- Increase in the rate of sexual activity among teenagers
- Lack of knowledge about (or failure to use) contraceptives
- Desire by young girls to have a child

In addition, some adolescents become pregnant as the result of rape or incest (Wiemann et al., 2000).

The failure of adolescents to obtain adequate knowledge of contraceptive measures is an issue that can be addressed by the health care profession. Unfortunately, providing information does not always resolve the problem entirely because adolescents often lack money to purchase protection such as birth control pills or a diaphragm. In addition, the egocentric phenomenon of adolescence makes the sexually active teenager believe that she just will not become pregnant. In other words, "It won't happen to me." On the other hand, some adolescent girls actually plan pregnancy. They believe that being pregnant will free them from an intolerable school or home situation and will give them someone to love. This phenomenon must be recognized because it puts a tremendous responsibility on a newborn baby to furnish love and change a girl's life. Child abuse can occur when the newborn cannot meet such expectations.

At one time, pregnant unmarried girls were sent to a "secret" home or shelter where they would stay through the pregnancy, give birth, place the child for adoption, and return home as if nothing had happened to them. But something did happen, as much as the girl and her family wanted to pretend it did not. Often, the girl was impacted psychologically, because she developed a relationship with the stranger inside her and then had to give the newborn away and never mention him or her again. Today, pregnant girls attend prenatal clinics or come to physician's offices just as older women do. They deliver in birthing rooms at hospitals, and as many as 90% keep their babies (DHHS, 2000). Few give birth in alternative birth centers because adolescent pregnancies are considered high risk. Home birth is not recommended for the same reason. Offering increased guidance during pregnancy and for the following year can be an important nursing role (Koniak-Griffin et al., 2002).

Developmental Crises of Adolescence

Adolescence is a vulnerable time for pregnancy because the developmental tasks of pregnancy are superimposed on those of adolescence. The developmental tasks of the average adolescent are fourfold: to establish a sense of self-worth and a value system; to establish lasting relationships; to emancipate from parents; and to choose a vocation (Erikson, 1963). A girl in the process of separating from her parents may be devastated by the knowledge that in less than a year someone will be dependent on her. When she realizes she is pregnant, she may have decreased ability to separate from her parents because she needs their financial help more than ever to obtain prenatal care and buy prenatal vitamins. If she must depend on her parent's health insurance, she may feel virtually trapped into dependence. Helping adolescents to make their own health care decisions at health care visits helps to foster a sense of independence in the middle of this forced dependency. Consider, for example, the decision that the adolescent must make about where to place a medication reminder chart: if it hangs in the kitchen, her mother may monitor it; in her bedroom or in her school locker, she alone will monitor it. An adolescent may not be able to choose when she comes for care (her mother has the car to drive her only on Tuesday afternoons), but during a visit she can do many things to feel independent, such as weigh herself, hold a mirror to view her pelvic examination, or be interviewed apart from her parent.

Parents may have difficulty allowing a daughter to participate in making her own health care decisions this way. You may need to remind them that a pregnant adolescent is regarded as an **emancipated minor**—or a person capable of health care decisions—and so may sign permission for her own care. Soon she will be caring for an infant, so she needs this practice in independence.

Pregnancy may interfere with the development of a healthy sexual relationship and cause difficulty in establishing future intimate relationships if the girl realizes that her current relationship has led to a situation detrimental to her. To prevent this, it is useful to help her view the pregnancy as a growth-producing experience. Most people can point to a day in their life when they "grew up" (perhaps a day a parent became ill or the day they left home for college). This pregnancy can be a "growing-up" revelation or a growth-producing experience for her.

Establishing a value system or sense of identity can be difficult if health care personnel treat a pregnant adolescent as though she were irresponsible. Encouraging her to continue school is crucial to her self-esteem and to her future, as well as to the future of her unborn child. High school personnel today encourage adolescents to stay in school. Many schools have special programs that include aspects of prenatal care (see Focus on Nursing Care Planning).

Prenatal Assessment

Adolescents are considered high-risk clients because they have a high incidence of pregnancy-induced hypertension and iron-deficiency anemia. They also have a higher incidence of preterm birth, with low-birth-weight infants. In

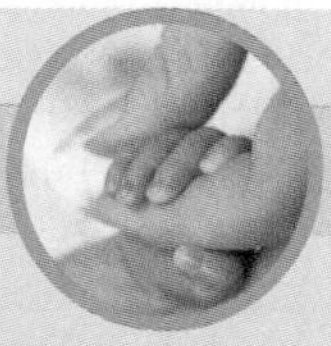

FOCUS ON *Nursing Care Planning*

THE PREGNANT ADOLESCENT

An adolescent female, 15 years old, comes to the clinic. She has noticed weight gain and has been feeling nauseated in the early morning for the past 3 months.

Assessment: Pale, tired-appearing female; LMP approximately 3 months ago. Sexually active for past 8 months with use of contraception. HCG level positive for pregnancy. On learning results, client states, "What are my parents going to say? I don't know how my boyfriend's going to react." Verbalizing her desire to continue with pregnancy, she continues, "Now I can eat anything I want since I'm eating for two. But I guess I'll have to quit school."

Lives with family in second-floor apartment above snack shop, which parents own and run. Client currently caring for 5-year-old sister after school while parents work downstairs.

Dietary recall reveals: no intake for breakfast; tuna sandwich, cola, and banana for lunch; one serving each of roast beef, potatoes, and corn, 8 ounces iced tea for dinner; candy bar for snack after school; chips for after-dinner snack.

Nursing Diagnosis: Imbalanced nutrition related to increased nutritional demands of pregnancy superimposed on adolescent nutritional needs.

Outcome Identification: Client will demonstrate intake of adequate nutrients to support adolescent and pregnancy needs.

Outcome Evaluation: Client identifies appropriate food choices; reports intake of foods high in calories, iron, calcium, and protein as evidenced by written dietary record; demonstrates weight gain appropriate for stage of pregnancy. Dietary recall demonstrates intake of nutritionally adequate foods.

Interventions	Rationale
1. Assess client's nutritional habits; discuss with client ideas and beliefs about "eating for two."	1. Assessment provides a baseline from which to develop future suggestions and teaching strategies. Discussion about eating for two provides information about client's knowledge base.
2. Explain the need for consumption of adequate nutrients.	2. Adequate nutrient intake is essential for both the client's and fetus' optimal growth and development.
3. Question the client about food likes and dislikes.	3. Ascertaining food preferences helps to determine suggestions that the client would be more apt to comply with.

(continued)

Interventions	Rationale
4. Consult with the dietitian and maternal health care provider about recommendations for calorie requirements. Contact possible community resources such as Women, Infant, Children (WIC) program for assistance.	4. Calorie requirements may need to be increased from normal pregnancy requirements in light of client's dietary habits. WIC program can provide additional nutritional support and education.
5. Assist client with food suggestions and selections. Enlist the aid of the dietitian to assist with meal planning. Offer choices for food selections based on the adolescent's school and activity lifestyle. Provide written information as appropriate.	5. Assistance from the dietitian ensures a nutritionally sound diet. Offering choices individualizes care and allows the adolescent some control with decision making, thus increasing the possibility for compliance. Written materials enhance learning and provide a means for review and reinforcement.
6. Instruct client to keep a daily dietary journal, recording all food and fluid intake until next visit. Schedule return visit for 1 week.	6. Journal recordings provide the adolescent with a concrete activity for participating in care and also aid in evaluating the client's understanding of and compliance with nutritional plan. Scheduling a return visit within a short time provides additional opportunities for evaluation, review, and education.

Nursing Diagnosis: Interrupted family processes related to the stress of adolescent pregnancy and parenting.

Outcome Identification: Client and family demonstrate positive coping mechanisms to handle stress effectively.

Outcome Evaluation: Client and family members communicate expectations openly; client identifies plans for self, infant, and family; clarifies relationship desired with father of child. Baby's father participates in pregnancy activities as desired.

Interventions	Rationale
1. Assess client's relationship with parents. Encourage client to tell parents about pregnancy. Use role playing and simulation to aid adolescent in talking with parents.	1. Assessment of parental relationship provides clues about the client's home life, aiding in identifying appropriate methods for informing the parents.
2. Urge the client to inform the baby's father about the pregnancy. Encourage the client to include him at prenatal visits if both parties agree.	2. Involvement of the father, if desired, provides an additional source of support for the client and allows the father to define his role, promoting adaptation.
3. Schedule a return visit with the client, boyfriend, and family to discuss all parties' needs and concerns.	3. A follow-up visit is essential to encourage communication among all parties involved.
4. Encourage open discussion of parental concerns with the client. Enlist the aid of a social worker as appropriate.	4. Open communication provides a safe outlet for expression of feelings and assists with family adaptation. Social service provides additional support and assistance with decision making.
5. Assist client and those involved with ways to adapt to changes of pregnancy. Reinforce understanding of those involved about the client's need for support. Instruct in ways to offer support.	5. Adolescence is a highly stressful time; additional help may be required to cope with the added demands of pregnancy.
6. Discuss with the client and those involved future plans for the client, infant, and family. Encourage continued participation in school.	6. Discussion promotes active problem solving and positive adaptation. Continuing school aids in enhancing the client's self-esteem, maintaining peer relationships and promoting positive coping.
7. Set up follow-up visits with client and support persons; plan teaching strategies as appropriate.	7. Close, continued supervision and education are essential because the adolescent pregnant client is at risk for complications of pregnancy.

addition, they may have a high rate of intimate partner abuse (Wiemann et al., 2000). Early and consistent prenatal care is essential to their health and the health of their baby.

Unfortunately, many adolescents do not seek prenatal care until late in their pregnancies. In part, this may be due to the girl's denial of the pregnancy. Not seeking prenatal care is also a way of protecting the pregnancy—if she doesn't tell anyone, no one can suggest that she terminate it. After the 6th month, abortion is no longer a possibility so she can feel free to come for care without being subjected to this pressure.

Other factors contributing to the lack of prenatal care include lack of knowledge of the importance of prenatal care and dependence on others for transportation. The girl may feel awkward in a prenatal setting (as an adult setting) and frightened about her first pelvic examination. In addition, adolescents have a difficult time relating to authority figures. A primary nursing or case management approach that minimizes the number of health care providers the girl is exposed to may be the most effective method for providing care during the prenatal period for adolescents. Ideally, every community should have a facility that is designed especially for adolescents. If this is not possible, all settings should accommodate adolescents' needs so this last reason for poor prenatal care can be eliminated.

Health History

A detailed health history should be taken at the first prenatal health care visit. It is best to take this history without the girl's parents present. The girl needs practice in being responsible for her own health, and having to account for her health practices helps her do this. It also helps prevent her from fabricating an answer to please a parent.

Some adolescents come to the facility with concerns such as "weight gain" or "feeling tired all the time," hoping that health care providers think of pregnancy as a possible reason for their symptoms. This is part of denial or pregnancy protection. Always be alert to the possibility of pregnancy when an adolescent describes symptoms that are vague and hard to define. If the importance of what she is saying when she mentions feeling "tired" or "nauseated" is missed, she may ask if someone will feel her stomach. If told that this is not necessary for any of the symptoms she has mentioned, she may describe bigger symptoms, such as "terrible stomach pain." Think of possible pregnancy when you hear such a "growing" history.

Many adolescents believe their world is totally separate from the adult world and, to keep it separate, they do not voluntarily share information. When interviewing adolescents, be certain to press for the responses needed to assess safely. Do not accept statements such as "I eat okay" as a nutrition history or "I'm a very active person" as a history of rest and activity.

If the adolescent delayed seeking health care, ask for the reason at her first prenatal visit. Acknowledge that "protecting" the pregnancy is a desirable motive, but that continuing with prenatal care is much more beneficial.

If a parent does accompany the girl, ask the parent separately what, if any, concerns he or she wishes to discuss. A young adolescent is still a daughter, and a parent may be as concerned about her health during this pregnancy as he or she was at health visits when the girl was being seen for a cold or injury.

The baby's father may accompany the girl into the clinic or office to have the diagnosis established. Because he is not married to the adolescent, he does not have a legal right to participate in the girl's decision concerning pregnancy, abortion, or whether the child will be adopted at the pregnancy's end. But he may not be devoid of feelings for either the girl or the conceived child. If he is an adolescent, he may feel sorrow that because of his age he cannot provide adequately for the girl and baby. If a complication occurs, he may feel genuine grief. The concept of the boy as irresponsible reveals a lack of understanding of human behavior, especially that of adolescents. Allowing him to offer support in the current pregnancy helps him to better define his role. Be sure he receives compassionate education on preventing further pregnancies.

Often, adolescent girls have not been exposed to many pregnant women, so they may need extra teaching to help them become aware of common pregnancy symptoms such as urinary frequency, fatigue, and vaginal discharge. Asking what symptoms an adolescent is having, and reassuring her that they are part of a normal pregnancy, will help prevent her from attempting to treat them with potentially teratogenic over-the-counter medications.

As pregnancy progresses, listen for signs of "nest-building" behavior during a pregnancy history. An adolescent girl may not have the financial resources to buy clothing or a baby bed. She may reveal nest-building feelings by asking an increasing number of questions about newborns. Offer suggestions, such as making one article of clothing for the baby or saving her own money for one article—activities that promote active involvement in the pregnancy and provide a measure of nest-building potential (the girl who, week after week, spends her money on something else is probably not as involved in the pregnancy as the girl who puts away even one dollar each week toward a pair of baby shoes).

Some adolescents have difficulty telling their parents about the pregnancy. They need help in knowing how to tell someone what is happening. Role-playing or simulation may be an effective technique for this. Some girls report on a second visit that their parents were not nearly as angry as they had anticipated. Instead, they reacted as if they had been waiting to hear this news, having accepted it as inevitable months before.

Family Profile. Adolescents may leave home if their family disapproves of the pregnancy, joining the ranks of homeless or adolescent runaways. Others do not leave home, but separate themselves emotionally from their family. Trying to manage by themselves leaves young girls with tremendous financial strain and a devastating sense of loneliness. Ask the girl at prenatal visits where she is living, what is the source of her income, and whom she would call if she suddenly became ill.

Asking about home life may reveal a dysfunctional family or an incest relationship as the cause of the pregnancy. If the girl is under legal age, incest is considered child abuse. Know your local and state laws on this topic and make the necessary report.

Because of family relationship problems, a girl may need help in making arrangements for the next few months. Will her parents allow her to live at home during the pregnancy? If not, is there a relative that she may go to? What kind of financial support does she need? Family and social supports for pregnant adolescents have been shown to be important influences on the maintenance of a healthy pregnancy lifestyle and, thus, prevention of low birth weight in their children.

Ask if the girl is planning to continue with school. Pregnancy is an egocentric time when outside interests do not always seem important. Help her to see that the months of pregnancy will go faster if she is busy. Remaining in and doing well in school is a way of keeping busy. It also is important in preparing the adolescent for the future, because a high school education is necessary to obtain marketable skills to support herself and her baby. Once she has given birth, returning to school may be difficult because she may have child care problems and because she may feel she is more mature than the other girls (or the other girls may make her feel this way). Any school that obtains federal money cannot discriminate against students because they are physically challenged. Many states interpret pregnancy as physically challenging, so in those states a girl cannot be forced to leave school (or even asked to go to an alternate school) because of pregnancy. You may need to advocate for the girl with the school committee for a proper school placement.

Day History. Few adolescents are willing to provide detailed day histories unless the purpose of a day history is well explained. Tell her the purpose of the history is to learn more about her as a whole person, not to discover if she is doing things during the day she should not do. Adolescents are private people; to allow you to walk through their adolescent world for a day is a breach of adolescent philosophy.

Ask in particular about nutritional practices, sleep, daily activity, use of drugs, and whether they have friends who can support them through this experience.

Be certain to include questions about her medication history. Ask if she is taking anything over the counter. Some adolescents take acne medication that is potentially teratogenic, such as tetracycline or isotretinoin (Accutane). Some take frequent doses of over-the-counter cold remedies. Impress upon adolescents the importance of not taking any medication—even nonprescription—without prior approval from her physician or nurse-midwife.

Physical Examination

Physical examination procedures with pertinent adolescent findings are discussed in Chapter 33. A statement such as "Oh, you're starting to have colostrum," a positive finding of pregnancy, may be frightening to an adolescent who does not know what colostrum is.

A better way to phrase such a finding might be "Your breasts are healthy. You are already beginning to produce early breast milk. Later on we'll talk about the importance of breast milk for newborns." This kind of feedback makes the health examination a learning experience, relieves anxiety for adolescents who tend to be very concerned about body appearance, and provides a way of encouraging healthy behavior patterns.

Adolescents are at an increased risk for pregnancy-induced hypertension, probably due to immature blood vessels (Branch & Porter, 2000). Obtain a baseline blood pressure determination at the first prenatal visit. Few adolescents are told the results of blood pressure determinations at health maintenance visits, so they will not know what their typical finding is. Make a point of informing them of their blood pressure reading to encourage active health care participation in the future. Adolescents are often active in a waiting room—walking to get a magazine, returning it, looking out the window; be certain that the girl has 15 minutes of rest before you take a blood pressure or the recording will be falsely high.

Use a Doppler technique to obtain fetal heart tones, if possible, because hearing the fetal heart helps the adolescent acknowledge the reality of her pregnancy. For the same reason, make a point of assessing fundal height growth from visit to visit to show that the baby is growing.

Adolescents who use drugs may be reluctant to supply a urine specimen for testing because they are afraid you are secretly looking for evidence of drug use. In this instance, you may receive a cupful of water in place of a urine specimen. If in doubt as to the substance you are testing, check the specific gravity. The specific gravity of water is 1.000, whereas urine specific gravity ranges from 1.003 to 1.030.

Many adolescents like to weigh themselves at prenatal visits. Weight gain in early pregnancy is proof that they are pregnant. It is good practice to make a note of the clothing the girl is wearing the first time she is weighed (eg, jeans, T-shirt) so later weight determinations can be compared accurately.

> **✔ CHECKPOINT QUESTIONS**
>
> 1. What are three factors that contribute to the rising rate of teenage pregnancy?
> 2. What are the four developmental tasks associated with adolescence that a pregnant adolescent needs to complete?

NURSING DIAGNOSES AND RELATED INTERVENTIONS

Nursing Diagnosis: Health-seeking behaviors related to special care necessary for healthy adolescent pregnancy

Outcome Identification: Client will obtain necessary information on self-care during pregnancy.

Outcome Evaluation: Client states she feels confident in her ability to take care of herself and avoid pregnancy complications, and actively asks questions about her pregnancy.

Prenatal Health Teaching. Adolescents need a great deal of health teaching during pregnancy because they do not know many common measures of care that the older woman may have learned from experience. They are often unwilling to follow health care advice, however, that makes them different in any way from their peers. On the other hand, adolescents often do not have well-established health practices, so they are adaptable to a well-health approach.

Adolescent girls may respond to health teaching that is directed to their own health more than to that of the fetus inside them: "Eat a high-protein diet because protein makes your hair shiny (or prevents split fingernails)" often leads to better compliance than a statement that protein is good for the baby. "Taking the iron supplement should make you feel less tired" is better than "It will help build the baby's blood supply," for the same reason. These are truthful statements and they appeal to an adolescent's preoccupation with self. In addition, this type of health teaching is the only form to which the adolescent who is denying her pregnancy can respond.

Be certain to include information on the effects of all drugs on fetal welfare, including over-the-counter medications, herbal preparations, and recreational drugs. Pregnancy can become an important growth experience if it provides the motivation some adolescents need to withdraw from recreational drug use.

Adolescents also need instructions about possible discomforts and changes associated with pregnancy, and measures to relieve them. (See Chapter 11 for a complete discussion.) Many adolescents develop hemorrhoids during pregnancy because the disproportion of their body size to the fetus puts extra pressure on pelvic vessels, causing blood to pool in rectal veins. Reassure them that this is a pregnancy-related phenomenon that will resolve when the pregnancy is over.

Adolescents may also develop many striae across the sides of the abdomen because so much stretching of the abdominal skin occurs. Assure them that, because of skin elasticity, these marks will probably fade after pregnancy. Chloasma, excess pigment deposition on the face and neck, appears at the same rate in adolescents as in older women. Adolescents, however, may be more conscious of this pigment because, overall, they are more conscious and concerned about their facial appearance. Suggesting a cover makeup and offering reassurance that the pigmentation will fade after pregnancy may help.

Nutrition. Good nutrition is a major problem during adolescent pregnancy because many enter pregnancy with poor nutritional stores from years of eating a less-than-optimal diet. Lack of good nutrition can result in low-birth-weight newborns and preterm births (Lenders, McElrath, & Scholl, 2000). The younger the girl is, the more likely she is to have a low-birth-weight infant. To prevent these complications, the girl's diet must be sufficient to maintain her own health, allow for growth of the fetus, and also to provide for the needs of her own growing body. This means that she may need to gain more weight than the mature women does during pregnancy (Buschman et al., 2001). Protein, iron, folic acid, and vitamin A and C deficiencies may become acute. Besides eating larger amounts of food, the pregnant adolescent must eat the proper foods, possibly abandoning the food fads she has been following. Some girls are so peer oriented that they balk at substituting a glass of orange juice for a cola beverage because no one else they know drinks orange juice. The best you may be able to accomplish is to secure her agreement to switch to noncaffeinated soft drinks.

Many adolescent girls eat poorly during pregnancy because they simply do not know what constitutes a good diet. Some girls have little choice in what foods are prepared at home. To change a dietary pattern, you may have to talk to the person who does the cooking in the family.

Many adolescents eat at least one meal a week at a fast-food restaurant. Remember that if the girl is attending school, she eats at least one meal away from home each day. If she travels by school bus, she may have to leave by 6:00 or 7:00 in the morning, so she needs suggestions on how to construct a quick but healthy breakfast. If she leaves home this early, she will have a long wait until lunchtime. Suggest midmorning snacks, such as fruit, that are not just empty calories. Be certain that nutrition education includes how to "brown-bag" or buy a nutritious cafeteria lunch (type A school lunches are discussed in Chapter 31).

WHAT IF? What if an adolescent tells you that her daily nutrition consists of a liquid diet beverage for breakfast and lunch and pizza for dinner? Will this typical teenage diet be adequate for her during pregnancy?

Adolescents traditionally demonstrate poor compliance to medication. They may need frequent reminders that vitamin and iron supplements during pregnancy must not only be purchased but also must be taken. Be sure the girl posts a medication reminder chart at home or in her school locker to help increase compliance.

Activity and Rest. Adolescents vary greatly in their preferred level of activity. Assess the girl's participation in sports activities and determine which ones (if any) should be discontinued during pregnancy (diving, gymnastics, touch football). Many girls practice sports not for the enjoyment of the sport but for the feeling of "team" or companionship. You may need to suggest alternative activities (joining the drama or language club, inviting friends over once a week to watch a movie) or they will suffer from the loss of companionship.

Adolescent girls may not plan enough rest time during pregnancy, especially if they are acting as if nothing is happening to them. It may help to explore their typical day and suggest ways to rest without compromising social relationships.

Pregnancy Information. A young girl may have distorted beliefs about her body. Despite all the health information given to children in school, it is not uncommon to find an adolescent who thinks that her baby is growing in her stomach. Such a girl is unwilling to eat large meals during pregnancy for fear of suffocating the fetus. All adolescent girls need substantial education on the physiologic changes that occur during pregnancy. In addition, specific information about labor and delivery is essential to counteract all the scare stories they may have heard from their peers. Gaining knowledge is another way that pregnancy can be a growth experience. At the end of the pregnancy, this adolescent will know a great deal more about her body and her ability to monitor her health than her average classmate.

Childbirth Preparation. Adolescents have a strong need for peer companionship. When they become pregnant, they often are cut off from fellow adolescents. This makes them "ripe," therefore, to join a class of adolescents in preparation for childbirth. They are excellent students because being a student is age appropriate for them. They have enough childish magical belief operating that they are not skeptical about whether prepared childbirth will work for them. In fact, believing that prepared childbirth will work is an important component in a successful prepared childbirth experience, so this becomes a self-fulfilling prophecy.

Birth Decisions. Pelvic measurements should be taken early and carefully in adolescent girls. Cephalopelvic disproportion is a real possibility because of the girl's incomplete pelvic growth (Dudley, 2000). Most girls who are told that their baby will have to be born by cesarean birth respond well to the news, and many are relieved, because surgery seems controlled and simple compared with the agonies of labor that they imagine. The decision on the method of birth should be shared with the girl and her parents when the health care team reaches it. This is part of being honest with the girl. Adolescents, for the most part, want to know the truth. They tend to regard the withholding of information not as protection, but as an indication that they are being treated like children.

Plans for the Baby. Adolescents may need additional time at prenatal visits to talk to a good listener concerning their feelings about being pregnant and becoming a mother. Scared? Bewildered? Numb? Happy? Be certain they know all the options available to them: keeping the baby, or placing the baby in a temporary foster home or for adoption. Adolescents should be encouraged to breastfeed. Breast tissue matures with pregnancy, so even the very young adolescent is physically capable of breastfeeding (Volpe & Bear, 2000).

ASSESSING the Pregnant Adolescent for Complication Risk

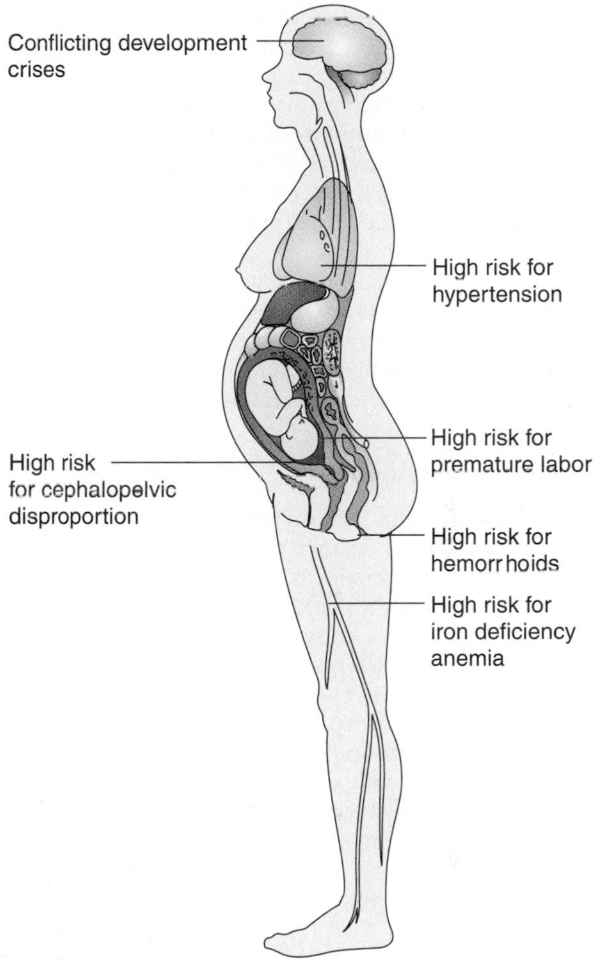

Complications of Adolescent Pregnancy

Adolescent pregnancy carries an increased incidence of pregnancy-induced hypertension, iron-deficiency anemia, preterm labor, and cephalopelvic disproportion (see Assessing the Pregnant Adolescent for Complication Risk). Cephalopelvic disproportion leads to an increased incidence of cesarean birth. With conscientious prenatal care, complications can be minimized (Jolly et al., 2000).

Pregnancy-Induced Hypertension

Because adolescents are more prone to pregnancy-induced hypertension than the average woman (see Chapter 15), establishing a baseline blood pressure is important because some adolescents may not have had their blood pressure measured since a preschool or school-age checkup as long as 10 years earlier.

The best intervention for reducing an increasing blood pressure during pregnancy is bedrest, preferably in a side-lying position. Bedrest may be difficult for a teenager because she easily grows bored on bedrest, and being confined to bed limits her interactions with peers and school activities. Many girls on bedrest at home may rest better if they are lying on the living room couch, where they can be aware of household activity, rather than in an upstairs bedroom where they have to get up time and again to see what is happening. Also, it is easier for a parent to encourage bedrest if the girl is within eyesight. If called too many times to the distant bedroom for small tasks, a parent tends to say, "Get up and get it yourself this time."

Help to establish a specific routine of bedrest—does it mean being strictly confined to bed or sitting up part of the day in a lounge chair with legs elevated? Can she take a shower once a day? Use the bathroom? Knowing the exact rules from the beginning helps prevent misunderstandings and hurt feelings.

Girls on bedrest need activities to keep them busy. These can include homework or listening to music. If the end of the pregnancy is near, she may be able to have a friend bring her homework assignments. If the bedrest period will be longer than 2 weeks, however, she may need to make arrangements for home tutoring. You may need to advocate for her with the school system for this service (remembering that only rarely can it be denied on the basis of pregnancy). "Assignments" from the health care agency, such as reading about appropriate toys and games for infants, may provide a way to occupy time. Frequent telephone calls from the health care facility show concern and offer an opportunity to enforce health teaching points. Be certain the girl does not interpret being placed on bedrest as being ill. This may cause her to reduce her nutritional intake or to curtail body hygiene.

Low-dose aspirin therapy also may be prescribed. Keep in mind that adolescents often are not reliable at taking daily medicine, particularly if it seems as unimportant as aspirin. Help the girl make a medicine reminder chart to promote adherence and compliance with this aspect of care.

If the hypertension continues after a period of bedrest at home (or if the symptoms of pregnancy-induced hypertension are acute when they are first discovered), the girl may be admitted to the hospital so bedrest can be better enforced. As soon as the fetus is mature, labor is induced.

Iron-Deficiency Anemia

Many adolescent girls are iron deficient because their low protein intake cannot balance the amount of iron lost with menstrual flows. Deficiency is revealed by chronic fatigue, pale mucous membranes, and a hemoglobin level less than 11 g/dL. As if the girl's body has identified a mineral lack, iron-deficiency anemia is associated with pica, or the ingestion of inedible substances. Cravings for ice cubes or candy bars may develop because of this.

A pregnancy compounds iron-deficiency anemia because the girl must now supply enough iron for fetal growth and her increasing blood volume. All women should take an iron and folic acid supplement (folic acid is important for red blood cell growth and prevention of neural tube defects) during pregnancy. This is especially important for the adolescent.

Help the girl plan a daily time for taking the nutrition supplement. Review with her how many iron-rich foods she needs to eat daily. An iron supplement is not a supplement until her dietary intake is already strong in iron-rich foods.

As soon as the body has iron, it will begin forming immature red blood cells (reticulocytes) rapidly. A reticulocyte count may be obtained in 2 weeks to evaluate these levels and provide evidence that the iron supplement is being taken. If the reticulocyte count is not elevated by 2 weeks, it implies the girl did not take the supplement. Taking a stool swab and assessing it for the black tinge of an iron supplement is another method of assessment for medicine compliance.

Preterm Labor

Adolescents are at high risk for preterm labor (Jolly, 2000). Review the signs of labor with them by the 3rd month of pregnancy. Stress that labor contractions begin as only a sweeping contraction no more intense than menstrual cramps. Stress that any vaginal bleeding is suspicious until ruled otherwise. Adolescent girls have gained much of their knowledge of labor from television (where a woman suddenly announces she is in labor and within 15 minutes gives birth). Therefore, they may dismiss light contractions as simple discomfort, not realizing they might be the start of labor. Adolescents who recognize labor contractions early on can seek care to have premature labor halted.

Complications and Concerns of Labor, Birth, and the Postpartal Period

Cephalopelvic Disproportion

Because their own development is still immature, adolescents are prone to cephalopelvic disproportion (Phipps & Sowers, 2002). Cephalopelvic disproportion is suggested by lack of engagement at the beginning of labor, a prolonged first stage of labor, and, finally, poor fetal descent. Adolescent labor does not differ from labor in the older woman if cephalopelvic disproportion is absent. Graphing labor progress is a good way to detect labor that is becoming abnormal at these points. Be certain that the adolescent has a support person with her in labor so she can relax and breathe effectively with contractions. If this person is also an adolescent, you may need to serve as the true support person during labor, or at least spend considerable time coaching so he or she can effectively support the girl in labor.

Postpartal Hemorrhage

Young adolescents are more prone to postpartal hemorrhage than the average woman because if the girl's uterus is not yet fully developed, it becomes overdistended by pregnancy. An overdistended uterus does not contract as readily as a normally distended uterus in the postpartal period. Adolescents also may have more frequent or deeper perineal and cervical lacerations because of the size of the infant in relation to their body. On the other hand, young adolescents are generally healthy and have supple body tissue that allows for adequate perineal stretching. If a laceration does occur, it usually heals readily without complication.

Inability to Adapt Postpartally

The immediate postpartal period may be an almost unreal time for an adolescent. Giving birth is such a stress and a major crisis that all women have difficulty integrating it into their life. It may be particularly difficult for the adolescent. The girl may "block out" the hours of labor as if they didn't happen. If she was particularly frightened by labor, she may have received a narcotic, so her memory of the labor hours is not clear. Urge her to talk about labor and birth to make the happening real to her. Otherwise, a high proportion of postpartum depression can occur.

Lack of Knowledge About Infant Care

Adolescents show the same positive bonding behavior with their infants as their more mature counterparts (Fig. 17-1). They may, however, lack knowledge of infant care. Although they may consider themselves to be knowledgeable in child care because they baby-sat for a neighbor's child or a younger sibling, they may be overwhelmed in the

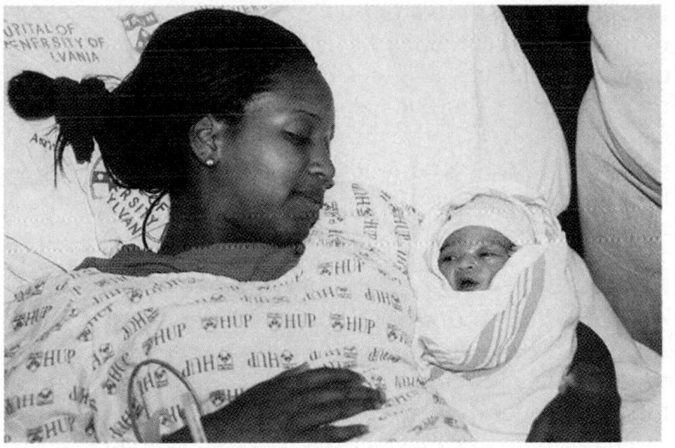

FIGURE 17.1 A new adolescent mother begins to bond with her infant.

postpartal period to realize that when the baby is their own, child care is not as simple as it once seemed. For example, when the child cries, they cannot hand it to someone else; at the end of 4 hours, when they are tired of caring for the baby, they cannot leave and walk away. Although these things were most likely discussed with her during her pregnancy, these feelings may not arise until the child is actually born. Spend time with the girl observing how she handles the infant. Demonstrate bathing and changing the baby as appropriate. Model good parenting behaviors whenever possible by being aware of how you hold and care for the child.

Unfortunately, most adolescent mothers do not breastfeed (Volpe & Bear, 2000). This is related to their perception of breastfeeding as something that will "tie them down" and the reality (in many instances) that they will be returning to a full-time school program soon after birth. Better education about the importance of breastfeeding and tips for how to incorporate it into a busy lifestyle can increase the numbers of adolescents who breastfeed their newborns (see Chapter 24). Help young mothers who do not choose to breastfeed to find a feeding method that is satisfying to them and safe for the infant.

✔ CHECKPOINT QUESTIONS

3. What are common complications associated with adolescent pregnancy?
4. What blood test can be used to demonstrate compliance with the use of iron supplements?

THE PREGNANT WOMAN OVER AGE 40

The incidence of women delaying their first pregnancy until their late 30s or early 40s is increasing (see Focus on Cultural Competence). Seven percent of births in the United States today are to women over age 35; 2 to 3% are to women over age 40 (DHHS, 2000). In the past, it was assumed that a woman of this age was past the optimum age for childbearing and was at risk for many complica-

FOCUS ON CULTURAL COMPETENCE

What is perceived as the best time in life to have children is culturally influenced. In developing countries, many people believe that having children young allows parents to grow with children. In other cultures, such as the United States, many believe that delaying childbirth until a family is financially secure is best. What you believe, therefore, may not be the belief of a family for whom you are caring. What may be a catastrophe to you may seem like a blessing to someone else (and vice versa). Assess couples by history and observation to determine if childbearing appears to be timed correctly for them. If not, they may need extra time to accept a pregnancy and adapt to becoming parents.

tions. With the exception of greater chromosomal abnormality, there is little evidence of increasing complications in women older than age 35 as long as prenatal care is begun early in the pregnancy (Abu-Heija et al., 2000).

The woman over age 40 is more likely than a younger woman to have a previously diagnosed condition, such as hypertension, varicosities, or hemorrhoids. In addition, by age 40 a woman usually has a major role change to undertake during pregnancy, because she often is well established in a career or has an accustomed routine at home or in her community. She needs to think through how this pregnancy and childrearing are going to fit into and change her life. Although she may feel rich in the number of support people she perceives around her, she may discover she has few "pregnancy support" people because she does not have many friends her age who are also having babies—some may be close to becoming grandmothers. The only things these friends remember of pregnancy and labor are their particular highs and lows, and they don't reflect current practice. This may leave her without access to the daily "shop talk" of other pregnant women, or someone to turn to with questions such as whether the backache she is experiencing or frequent need to urinate is normal. On the other hand, because many women delay childbearing today, she may be one of a sizable group of women in the community experiencing pregnancy at this stage of life.

Childbirth education classes oriented toward the older woman provide important information on pregnancy and can bring these women and their support people together. The woman over age 40, like any other pregnant woman, needs access to health care personnel who can supply her with factual information during pregnancy. She also needs additional support while she works through this role change in her life.

Developmental Tasks and Pregnancy

The developmental challenge of the over-40 age group is to expand their awareness or develop generativity—that is, a sense of moving away from themselves and becoming involved with the world or community (Erikson, 1963). Some people assume that, once they reach adulthood, the way they are is the way they always will be. They are surprised to see that changes still occur. They are amazed to find that their bodies change (e.g., men may lose their hair; women and men both gain weight) and so do their interests. They find themselves joining committees and clubs, coaching Little League teams, or organizing fundraising or community events.

A woman in this age group who is pregnant may begin to feel ambivalent during pregnancy, because she may want to continue with community activities, yet also wants to concentrate on the fetus inside her. You may need to help her balance her life so she can manage crossing two life phases this way.

Many adults over the age of 40 years are caring for aging parents. This additional responsibility may make it difficult for women to complete the psychological work of pregnancy. It also may create extra strain on the woman's finances and time.

Prenatal Assessment

The woman over age 40, like all women, should begin prenatal care early in pregnancy. Fortunately, most women of this age group are well informed about the advisability of early prenatal care and have adequate health insurance, so they do seek an early appointment. A few mistakenly believe that their lack of menstruation is the result of early menopause, so they do not seek an early health care consultation.

Health History

Ask women in this age group about their present symptoms of pregnancy, and how they feel about the pregnancy and how it fits into their lifestyle. If the woman did not realize that she was pregnant, she may have self-medicated. Ask if she has been taking any medication or herbal remedies to relieve reported symptoms, such as nausea or fatigue. Because a woman is functioning well in a business world does not mean she has a healthy pregnancy lifestyle. Don't accept answers such as "I drink socially" or "I take the usual drugs" without exploring what the phrases mean specifically.

Family Profile. Some women over age 40 who are pregnant for the first time have recently changed their life pattern (married or became involved in a long-term sexual relationship), or have decided to have a child without a marriage partner before they are no longer able to conceive. Whereas the younger woman often waits a while after marrying to become pregnant, the woman over age 40 often plans to become pregnant immediately after marriage because she senses her reproductive years are running out. Because of this, she may find herself making many adjustments at once (not only to a new life partner, house or apartment, and perhaps community, but also to a pregnancy).

Identify her source of income. For example, if she has a well-paying job, stopping work because of a pregnancy complication may reduce the family's income greatly. Also evaluate how many people are financially or emotionally dependent on her (such as children from a former marriage, elderly parents, an elderly neighbor, or fellow workers who count on her). During pregnancy, when a woman often needs extra emotional support, feeling responsible for so many people can be difficult (see Focus on Communication).

Day History. Ask specifically about a woman's job and estimate the amount of walking or back strain it entails. Ask about recent diet or exercise programs. If she belongs to a health club, remind her that the use of saunas and hot tubs for longer than 10 minutes at a time are contraindicated during pregnancy because of possible hyperthermia and teratogenic effects of extreme heat on the developing fetus. Identify personal habits, such as cigarette smoking and alcohol consumption, that may be detrimental to the fetus to determine if counseling to halt or decrease these habits could be effective.

FOCUS ON COMMUNICATION

Becky Kramer is a 42-year-old woman who is pregnant with her first baby.

Less Effective Communication

Nurse: Hello, Mrs. Kramer. How are you feeling?
Ms. Kramer: Good, but always tired. You know.
Nurse: You should try and rest more.
Ms. Kramer: Right.
Nurse: Ask your husband to help you more.
Ms. Kramer: I'll do that.
Nurse: Or stop work. That'll leave you time to rest more.
Ms. Kramer: Right. Great solution.
Nurse: Glad I could be of help.

More Effective Communication

Nurse: Hello, Mrs. Kramer. How are you feeling?
Ms. Kramer: Good, but always tired. You know.
Nurse: Are you getting enough rest and sleep?
Ms. Kramer: How can I? I have to work.
Nurse: Is there anyone who could help you out more? A husband? A friend?
Ms. Kramer: I'm pretty much alone since I got pregnant. And I don't have a husband.
Nurse: As long as you're coming to this clinic, you're not alone. Tell me about a typical day and let's investigate together what could be done.

It is easy to think of a single woman's pregnancy as something that happens only to adolescents or at least to young adults. In truth, it can happen at any age. In the first scenario, the nurse was so intent on problem solving that she forgot the first step of effective problem solving—identify the exact problem that needs solving. In the second scenario, when the nurse continues to assess rather than offer advice, she is able to identify the problem.

Physical Examination

The woman over age 40 needs a thorough physical examination at her first prenatal visit to establish her general health and to identify any problems, particularly circulatory disturbances. Inspect lower extremities thoroughly for varicosities, because these are more common in women over age 40. Be certain to obtain a urine specimen, and test for specific gravity, glucose, and protein to evaluate overall renal function.

Assess the woman's breasts for any abnormalities. Urge her to continue breast self-examination during pregnancy since women over age 40 are in a higher-risk group for breast cancer than younger women are. Pregnant women may have a tendency to neglect this because they lack a menstrual period marker as a reminder. In addition, be certain to assess for fetal heart sounds and fetal movement at prenatal visits because hydatidiform mole has a higher than usual incidence in the woman over age 40 (see Chapter 15).

Chromosomal Assessment

Women over age 40 may be offered the opportunity for chorionic villi sampling at 8 to 10 weeks of pregnancy or an amniocentesis at the 14th to 16th week of pregnancy to detect chromosomal abnormalities. A triple-screen (alpha-fetoprotein [AFP], human chorionic gonadotropin, and unconjugated estriol levels) drawn on blood serum at the 15th week of pregnancy also is recommended to detect an open spinal cord or chromosomal defect. Be certain the woman is prepared for these studies and receives support during them. Alert her about the possibility of false-positive results with AFP testing, which will require additional follow-up. Many women of this age group do not begin nest building until these tests confirm that the child will be healthy.

NURSING DIAGNOSES AND RELATED INTERVENTIONS

Nursing Diagnosis: Health-seeking behaviors related to special care necessary for healthy pregnancy

Outcome Identification: Client actively inquires about information necessary for health care practices.

Outcome Evaluation: Client states she feels confident in self-care and her ability to decrease complications of pregnancy.

Be certain to adapt prenatal teaching to fit the woman's lifestyle. If she has not planned on ever being pregnant, she may have isolated herself through the years from "mothering" activities and so, despite her years, knows little about pregnancy and newborn care. In terms of knowledge, this puts her at the same level as the adolescent. Others have read so extensively that they may know more theoretical information than the woman who has already given birth. Also, review information about possible discomforts. (For a complete discussion, see Chapter 11.) The woman over age 40 is prone to hemorrhoids because she may have some rectal varicosities present at the beginning of pregnancy. Pain from rectal distention may, in fact, be one of the primary symptoms that she reports at a first visit. Review measures to reduce these and increase comfort.

Varicosities, like hemorrhoids, develop readily in the woman over age 40 because she may have had some tendency toward them even before the pregnancy. As with hemorrhoids, her best approach during pregnancy is to prevent varicosities rather than to allow them to develop (see Focus on Family Empowerment).

Be certain to record on the woman's chart any degree of varicosity formation during pregnancy so nurses caring for her during the postpartal period can take special precautions to prevent thrombophlebitis. With venous stasis present after birth, the woman is even more prone to develop this complication.

Nutrition. Assess the number of meals the woman eats outside her home each week, including those she packs as a lunch or eats in restaurants. She may need tips on how to adjust pregnancy nutrition so she can obtain the same nutrition whether she prepares meals at home or eats them at

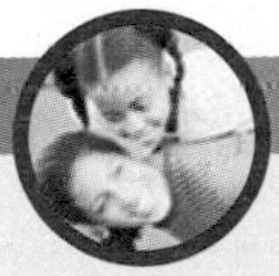

FOCUS ON FAMILY EMPOWERMENT
Tips on Preventing Varicose Veins

Q. My friend developed terrible varicose veins when she was pregnant. Is there anything that I can do so this won't happen to me?

A. Although not foolproof, incorporate the following activities in your day to help prevent the development of varicose veins:

- Find opportunities at work to elevate your legs, such as a coffee or lunch break.
- Be certain your diet includes vitamin C because this is important to strengthen vein walls.
- Rest in a side-lying position with your body tipped slightly forward (Sims' position). This allows leg veins to drain and empty.
- Avoid long periods of standing in one place by taking "walk breaks"; active muscle contraction helps venous return.
- Avoid sitting with your legs crossed.
- Don't wear anything constricting on your lower legs, such as knee-high stockings.
- Wear support hose. Be certain to put them on before you get out of bed in the morning, before veins become swollen, for best results.

an office or community function. Urge her to substitute a caffeine-free soft drink in place of alcoholic beverages. In some offices, large amounts of coffee are consumed. Urge her to substitute milk or juice. Many women this age normally drink little milk. Rather than getting used to milk again, she may appreciate suggestions on other ways to ingest calcium, such as puddings or yogurt.

Prenatal Classes. Because a pregnant woman over age 40 may be unique in her circle of friends, she may feel shut out of her usual group because of the pregnancy. She may be ready, therefore, to join a childbirth preparation or prenatal exercise class where she is "one of the group" (Fig. 17-2).

Be certain the woman plans (or the couple plans together) to set aside a specific time every day to do breathing exercises in preparation for labor. Otherwise, she may never find time to get to them in a busy day and will be unprepared in labor.

Complications of Pregnancy for the Woman Over Age 40

The complications of pregnancy most likely to occur in a woman over age 40 are those related to the phenomenon that her circulatory system may not be as competent as when she was younger or her body tissues may not be as elastic as they once were (see Assessing the Pregnant Woman Over 40 for Complications). These complications may include hypertension of pregnancy, preterm or post-term birth, and cesarean birth (Parsons & Spellacy, 2000; Branch & Porter, 2000).

ASSESSING the Pregnant Woman Over 40 for Complications

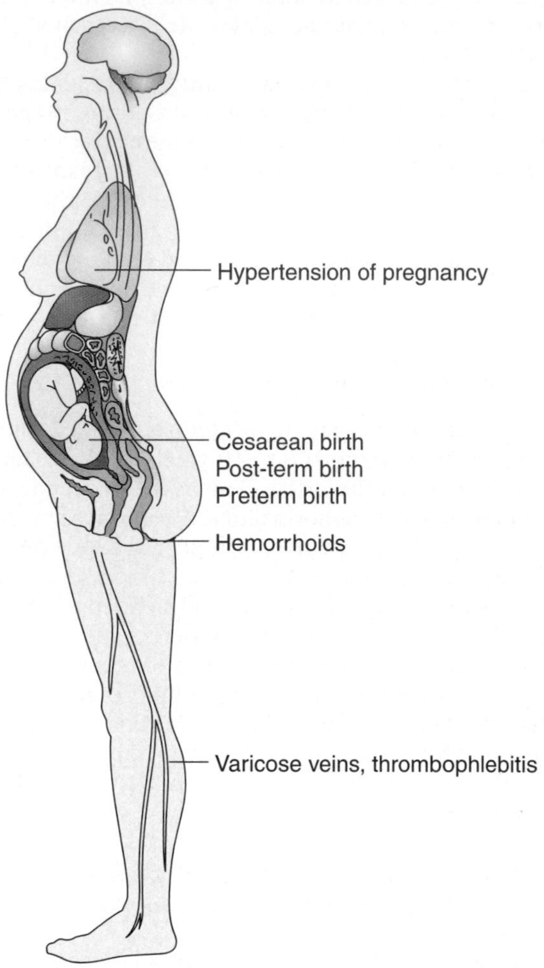

Pregnancy-Induced Hypertension

A woman over age 40 may have a higher incidence of pregnancy-induced hypertension than a younger woman, possibly related to blood vessel inelasticity or because hypertension tends to occur more frequently in nulliparas than multiparas or those with already elevated blood pressure (Branch & Porter, 2000). As with any woman, the best way to reduce the symptoms of pregnancy-induced hypertension is for her to rest for a good portion of each day. If the woman works full-time, stopping work may be difficult for her, not only because she believes she may miss out on a promotion or risk losing her job, but also because she is used to being productive, not merely resting all day. To allow her to rest effectively, you may need to help her plan activities she can accomplish on bedrest, such as reworking a school course outline, restructuring her office filing system, or working at a hobby that she has wanted to pursue but never had time for before.

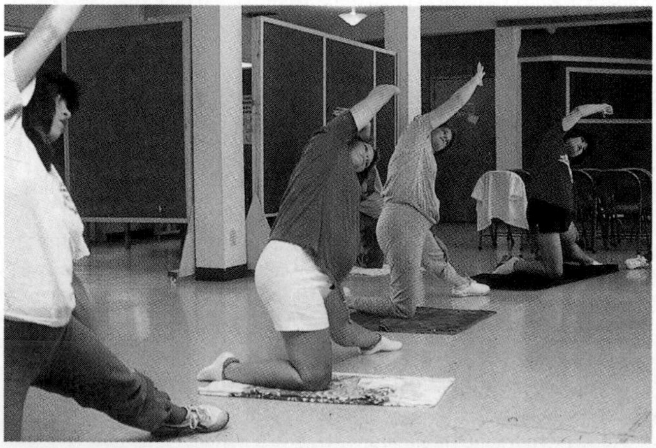

FIGURE 17.2 Exercise classes during pregnancy provide women with an opportunity to interact with other pregnant women while benefitting from a carefully monitored work-out.

Complications and Concerns of Labor, Birth, and the Postpartal Period

Complications that occur with the woman over age 40 related to birth or the immediate period after delivery also are the results of a body that may not be as elastic as it was when the woman was younger.

Failure to Progress in Labor

Labor in the older primipara may be prolonged because cervical dilatation may not occur as spontaneously as in the younger woman, probably because of decreased elasticity in cells. Graphing labor progress is a good method of determining when labor is becoming prolonged. Many women this age may need a cesarean birth if labor is overly prolonged and places the fetus at risk. Encourage the woman to verbalize how she is feeling about her progress throughout labor to allow for reassurance and prompt intervention should problems arise. Urge the support person to be present for the birth to offer needed support. Keep in mind that some older men may not be as comfortable with this as their younger counterparts would be.

Difficulty Accepting the Event

Women over age 40 may begin to have second thoughts about planning a pregnancy this late in life as the reality of a new baby registers with them during the intrapartal and postpartal period. Although they may have read a great deal about babies during pregnancy, they may wish they had read more or were as confident with this phase of their life as they are about other areas such as their home, office, or classroom. Review plans for child care and postpartal rest, with an emphasis on helping women learn to balance their lives. They most likely will need this help, especially if they are planning on returning to work soon after the birth.

Postpartal Hemorrhage

Just as the cervix may not dilate as readily during the older woman's labor, the uterus may not contract as readily in the postpartal period due to inelasticity. Therefore, the older woman is at higher risk for postpartal hemorrhage. Close observation is essential. Because the woman over age 40 may be an independent woman who is interested in self-care, she may ask for little help. Be sure to assess the amount of lochial flow to detect this complication.

✔ CHECKPOINT QUESTIONS

5. Why might the woman over age 40 be at higher risk for pregnancy-induced hypertension than others?
6. For what reason is the woman over age 40 at greater risk for postpartal hemorrhage?

THE PREGNANT WOMAN WHO IS PHYSICALLY OR COGNITIVELY CHALLENGED

In the past, women with conditions such as vision, hearing, cognitive, spinal cord, or orthopedic challenges were sheltered by their families to such an extent that women with even moderate physically challenging conditions did not meet potential sexual or marriage partners and so did not become pregnant. In addition, most people believed that these individuals should not become pregnant. Although care of women who are challenged in other ways has always been important to nursing, there has been little application of that care to the maternal–child health area. Today, women with varying degrees of disability attend public schools, work in offices, join community organizations, establish sexual relationships, marry, and plan pregnancies. Because these women (and in some instances, their support persons also) face special problems related to their conditions, nursing care during pregnancy must be designed with these special concerns in mind so the woman's and family's problems and needs are addressed (Lipson & Rogers, 2000).

Table 17-1 lists general areas of care that are important in planning for the physically or cognitively challenged woman who is pregnant.

TABLE 17.1 Areas of Planning With Physically or Cognitively Challenged Women During Pregnancy

AREA	ASSESSMENT AND PLANNING GUIDELINES
Transportation	Ask if the woman has transportation for prenatal care and for emergencies.
Pregnancy counseling	Assess the special modifications of care that will need to be made depending on the woman's special challenge. Use additional visual or auditory aids to make your teaching points clear.
Support person	Assess who is the woman's support person. In some instances, the woman's condition requires so much assistance during pregnancy that one support person will not be enough. If necessary, contact community agencies to lend additional support with her consent.
Health	Don't lose track of the woman's primary health problem. For example, the woman with cerebral palsy needs to continue an active muscle exercise program during pregnancy for her primary illness.
Work	Assess whether the woman works outside her home and, if this is discontinued during pregnancy, what she could substitute for a social contact activity. Women with physical or cognitive challenges may be lonely because they do not have a wide range of friends or social contacts.
Recreation	Assess whether her level of activity is adequate, and make concrete suggestions within her limitations for increasing it. Many women with a physically challenging condition lead a rather sedentary life (partly because they do not have many social contacts).
Self-esteem	Assess the woman's level of self-esteem: it may be low because of repeated failures in her life. Give praise at prenatal visits and help her make pregnancy a growth experience.

Rights of the Physically or Cognitively Challenged Person

By federal law, physically disabled persons must have freedom of access to public buildings by means of ramps or handrails. All public health care facilities should be in compliance with these laws both in terms of physical facilities and in the true spirit of the law. That is, people are made to feel psychologically welcome as well as physically able to reach the inside of the building. By the same law, a hospital cannot deny care to a person with a disability even though the disabling condition complicates treatment considerably, possibly requiring extra personnel and time. A woman with a disability has full rights to her child, so the baby cannot be taken from her at birth without her full consent. Likewise, she cannot be forced to terminate the pregnancy or undergo sterilization unless that is her informed decision.

Modifications for Pregnancy

Most women with some degree of challenge need modifications of their care during pregnancy. Explore with them at a first prenatal visit the exact nature of their disability and their general self-image. Some women who are physically or cognitively challenged maintain high self-esteem despite severe limitations, and are able to modify, grow, and learn with a pregnancy, whereas others have a poor sense of self-esteem that will make this particularly difficult for them. For many of them, pregnancy will become a special event, a 9-month announcement to everyone that, despite their seeming limitations, they are equal to other women and capable of participating in one of life's miracles.

Safety Measures to Explore

Safety is a key area of concern when caring for the pregnant woman who is physically or cognitively challenged. Be sure to assess areas such as emergency contact persons, suppliers of transportation, and individual considerations, such as mobility, elimination, and possible autonomic responses.

Emergency Contacts. Evaluate the client's ability to contact someone in case of an emergency. Does the woman have a telephone she can reach readily, and know how to activate the emergency medical system (911) in her community? Some women with limited mobility, such as those with spinal cord injury or cerebral palsy, have a specially designed telephone contact system in their home that connects them to a paramedic or hospital emergency service through a beeper system. Check that they intend to maintain this throughout pregnancy. Women who are hearing challenged use a specially equipped telephone (a TDD device) that prints out messages for them. If a woman's speech is not clear, evaluate whether she will be understood while using the telephone to call for help in an emergency.

Transportation. Assess the client's ability to access medical care if an emergency occurs. If a woman depends on a support person for transportation to a health care facility, appointments may have to be arranged according to that person's schedule to prevent missed appointments. If a woman does not drive, who would transport her if a pregnancy emergency should occur? Women with cognitive or vision challenges, for example, do not qualify for a driver's license and may need someone, such as a family member or friend, to drive. Women with spinal cord injury may have difficulty transferring into the specially equipped, hand-controlled car they usually drive as the pregnancy progresses.

Mobility. All women who use wheelchairs are taught to press with their arms against the armrests and lift their buttocks up off the wheelchair seat for 5 seconds every hour. This prevents the formation of pressure ulcers on the buttocks and posterior thighs. Encourage women to continue to perform this maneuver during pregnancy. The increased weight of the fetus increases their risk for pressure ulcer formation from compression. In addition, severe hip flexion from sitting in a wheelchair limits venous return from the lower extremities. For at least 1 hour every morning and afternoon, encourage women who ambulate by wheelchair to decrease the sharp bend at the knees that results from sitting in the chair, to promote venous return and help prevent varicosities and thrombi formation. Adjusting the footrests of the wheelchair so a woman's legs are not sharply bent at the knees is helpful.

If balance is a problem, a woman may need reevaluation at the midpoint of pregnancy as the weight of her abdomen increases. This may necessitate the use of crutches if she did not use them before, or use of a wheelchair if she was ambulatory with crutches or a walker before pregnancy. Keep in mind that the woman who is physically challenged achieved the degree of ambulation that she first presents usually only after years of physical therapy and strengthening of leg and arm muscles. Help her see that reducing her degree of independence during pregnancy is not a step backward for her but a step forward, allowing her to have a safe pregnancy without the danger of falling (Fig. 17-3).

Elimination. When mobility is an effort, a woman may not drink as much as usual or use a bathroom as frequently

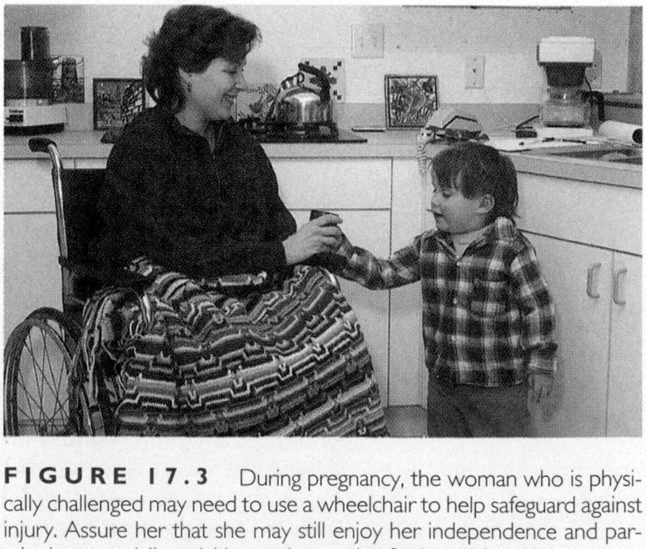

FIGURE 17.3 During pregnancy, the woman who is physically challenged may need to use a wheelchair to help safeguard against injury. Assure her that she may still enjoy her independence and partake in many daily activities, such as caring for her older child.

as she would if those actions were effortless. Encourage a high fluid intake and frequent voiding to prevent urinary tract infections. Women with spinal cord injury who use an indwelling catheter are at especially high risk for contracting urinary tract infections during pregnancy. Women who perform self-catheterization or change their own indwelling catheter may be unable to continue to do this late in pregnancy because the increasing size of their abdomen interferes with ability to see or reach the perineum comfortably. It may be necessary for her to arrange for a support person, a home care nurse, or a home health aide to do this.

Autonomic Responses. In a woman who has a high spinal cord injury (cervical or high thoracic), observe for **autonomic dysreflexia** during pregnancy, labor, and the immediate postpartal period. This is an exaggerated autonomic response to stimuli. Any irritating condition, such as a distended bladder, increasing uterine size, or breastfeeding, may initiate the response. Without upper motor neuron control to reverse the phenomenon, extreme symptoms can occur. Manifestations may include severe hypertension (300/160 mm Hg); throbbing headache; flushing of the skin and profuse diaphoresis above the level of the spinal lesion; nausea; and bradycardia. Immediate action is necessary to protect against cerebral vascular accident or intraocular damage. Elevate the woman's head to reduce cerebral pressure and locate the irritating stimulus (usually a distended bladder or bowel). If bladder distention is the cause, remove the bladder pressure by catheterization if an indwelling catheter is not in place. If a catheter is in place, check to see why it is not draining, then encourage it to drain by unkinking or flushing to allow urine to flow freely again. Anticipate the need for an antihypertensive agent to alleviate the extreme hypertension, although as soon as the source of irritation is removed, symptoms typically fade quickly (Wenstrom & Malee, 2000).

Prenatal Care Modifications to Meet Specific Needs

Physical examination may need to be modified depending on individual circumstances (Welner, 2000). Although women with disabilities have been followed by health care providers most of their life, they may never have had a pelvic examination before and so need clear instructions about why it is needed and what it will consist of. Many obstetric examining tables, for example, are built for the comfort of the examiner and are too high for a woman to transfer to from a wheelchair by simply sliding onto the table. To help a woman move to the table, a ramp from the physical therapy department may be necessary so the wheelchair can be elevated to the level of the table. Woman with spinal cord injury or cerebral palsy may be unable to maintain their legs in a lithotomy position because of either hip flexion contracture or laxness of leg support. A dorsal recumbent, rather than a lithotomy, position may be required for a pelvic examination.

Women who are cognitively challenged may not be aware how they became pregnant. If the woman became pregnant because she was taken advantage of sexually, she may need some time to talk and work through this experience before she can allow a pelvic examination.

If a visually challenged woman brings a guide dog with her to the health care visit, remember that, although the dog's chief function is to offer direction, its natural instinct causes it to become the woman's protector. In this role, the dog may feel threatened by people who try to pet it. Petting a guide dog also distracts it from safeguarding its owner. When interviewing or teaching visually challenged women, do not use your hands to illustrate points ("I'll need a urine sample of at least this much urine [measured with your fingers]"). Do not use colors as descriptions of objects ("put on the blue gown"). Use demonstration aids that allow the woman to feel or touch. When helping with or performing physical assessment, make a point that you are closing the door or drawing a curtain to ensure privacy. Always alert the woman that you are going to touch her, so as not to startle her. Otherwise, you may find yourself facing a growling guide dog that rises to protect her.

If the woman is hearing impaired, remember that she may not be able to see the examiner's face during a pelvic examination. This means any question asked of her during this time will not be understood because she cannot see the examiner's lips to lip read.

Pregnancy Education

Modify health teaching to meet the woman's specific needs. As stated previously, avoid references to colors or using your hands when explaining something to a visually challenged woman. Enlist the aid of her other senses, such as touch. For a woman who is cognitively challenged, instructions about pregnancy may need to be limited to those few items crucial for safety, such as "do not drink alcohol or take any medicine."

If a woman and her support person are both visually challenged, use of pamphlets about pregnancy care is limited. If the woman's support person has vision, offer the pamphlets to the support person, suggesting the partner read them to her as a shared activity. This will be helpful for her and also makes the partner a more informed support person. Many visually challenged women have tape recorders supplied by Recording for the Blind and Dyslexic (*www.rfbd.org*), a national, nonprofit, voluntary organization. Telephone the local association and ask if they have any material already recorded on pregnancy or breastfeeding that they could supply. If not, make a tape recording of any information you particularly want the woman to remember or she seems concerned about. Supply the health care facility telephone number at the beginning of the tape for an easy reminder in an emergency, and perhaps the date of her next visit as well.

Plan nutritional education based on the client's specific challenge and usual routine. Explore what the woman normally eats. A visually challenged woman or one who ambulates by wheelchair, for example, may prepare her own breakfast and lunch, meals that do not necessarily require a stove. The only hot meal the woman may eat is one a support person cooks in the evening. Nutrition counseling for two meals daily, therefore, needs to center on foods that can be prepared without cooking.

Activity and exercise, important for any pregnant woman, are crucial for the woman who is physically challenged. Evaluate the amount of exercise the woman gets daily. If mobility is a concern, exercise can be very reduced in bad weather. In this case, be sure the woman understands that walking around her home or apartment can provide the same level of exercise as if she were walking around the block or exercising in a health club.

Although labor and the child's birth may be modified somewhat because of a woman's physical condition, gaining general knowledge about labor and birth and participating in a shared experience with her life partner are still valuable. Urge women who are challenged in some way to attend childbirth preparation classes. If the woman is not working outside her home, she may have more time than others to practice breathing exercises and enter labor more adept at using such a method to control pain in labor than other women.

If the woman is severely hearing challenged, remember that she may not have heard the many spot television announcements on not smoking or drinking alcohol during pregnancy; she may need more time at prenatal visits so these can be discussed. In addition, lip reading is a difficult skill to learn, so many hearing-challenged persons are unable to do this with ease. Even if a woman is skilled at this, new words such as amniotic, gestation, or edema cannot be easily deciphered. Show the woman the printed words so she can see what your lip motion represents when presenting new pregnancy terms. If a woman uses sign language, she may bring an interpreter with her to translate. Be certain to talk to her, not the interpreter, when interviewing.

Modifications for Labor and Birth Preparation

Women who are physically or cognitively challenged will need adaptations in preparation for labor and birth. Keep in mind the following:

- A woman with a spinal cord injury may not be able to feel uterine contractions. Late in pregnancy, she will need to palpate her abdomen periodically for tightening or the presence of contractions so she is aware of beginning labor.
- Women with muscle spasticity or spinal cord injury may not be able to push effectively for the second stage of labor and so may need a higher percentage of cesarean birth or forceps birth than others.
- If a woman cannot assume a lithotomy position because of hip contracture, vaginal delivery from a Sims or dorsal recumbent position can be used.
- Braille watches used by visually challenged persons may not have second hands. They may need to time the length of contractions by counting rather than timing them by a watch.
- During labor, the hearing-challenged woman cannot hear information on how she is progressing if you are not directly facing her. If she needs to communicate with her support person in sign language, act as an advocate to keep her hands unencumbered by equipment such as intravenous lines. Remember that she cannot hear the infant cry at birth. Hand the infant to her as soon as possible after birth so she can see that the baby is crying and breathing well.
- Be certain to identify the usual sounds of birthing rooms (the beeping of a monitor, the swish of a central supply routing system, and so forth) for visually challenged woman. Hearing sounds and not being able to identify them is frightening.

Modifications for Postpartum Care

After birth, be sure to include the following:

- Ask whether the woman desires contraceptive information.
- Be certain the woman has a return appointment for both herself and the infant for follow-up care and that the arrangements seem to be within the limitations of her capabilities, transportation, and understanding.

Modifications for Planning Child Care

Allow for extra time during the first days postpartum for mother–child interaction. For example, after birth, a woman who is cognitively challenged may need extra time to understand the transition from "being pregnant" to "having a baby." She may have difficulty learning to judge when the infant is hungry. She may need extra supervision to be certain she doesn't leave the baby unprotected on a bed. A woman with a spinal cord disability may be particularly interested in inspecting her baby's back. A visually challenged woman will probably want to reassure herself that the baby can see. Be sure to give the baby to her as soon as possible so she can touch the baby and feel for intact body parts. If the birthing room is cold, explain to her that you want to rewrap the baby to prevent chilling, not because her touching is wrong or because you are trying to hide an imperfection in the baby.

Breastfeeding has special advantages for women who are physically or cognitively challenged because it is the method of feeding that is not only best for the baby, but also requires the least preparation effort on the mother's part. For the woman who is visually challenged and unable to read printed instructions, for example, breastfeeding eliminates formula errors. For the woman who is ambulatory by wheelchair, it eliminates trips to the refrigerator. However, breastfeeding may not be possible for a woman with muscle spasticity because the let-down reflex, which depends on muscle relaxation, may not occur. Be certain that women who are cognitively challenged understand that they need to feed until the infant is satisfied, not until they are tired of feeding.

Review with the woman any modifications in equipment that may be necessary. Many women need a referral for home care follow-up and possibly the use of a home health aide.

Encourage women to think through what baby care equipment will be best for them. Some infant crib rails lower by pressure on a foot pedal. Others use a waist-high lever. The woman who ambulates by wheelchair usually finds the waist-high lever most convenient because she can reach this most easily.

If the woman has difficulty with mobility, ask how she anticipates carrying the infant. Using an anterior baby sling is usually effective with a wheelchair. Women who are mobile by crutches or a walker can place the baby in a small wagon and pull it. Some women lie on their back on the floor, place the baby on their chest, and scoot across the floor. The important point is not how she carries the baby, but that she has thought through a safe and comfortable way to do this.

Urge a visually challenged woman to make eye contact with her infant when talking to him. Many visually challenged people do not turn on lights in their home because they do not perceive the difference between light and dark. Encourage the woman to develop a habit of turning on lights after dinner because her infant will need light to develop vision. If her support person also is visually challenged, suggest she check with a close friend or neighbor monthly to see that light bulbs have not burned out.

One of the biggest worries for the hearing-impaired woman is that she will not be able to hear her baby crying. Help her plan to bring the infant's crib or bassinet close to her bed so she can feel the vibration of the baby's stirring and waking. Urge her to talk to the infant as she gives care so the infant is introduced to sounds and words. Some women whose speech is severely affected by their hearing disorder are reluctant to speak to strangers. Assure her that her infant is not a stranger and will quiet readily to the sound of her voice. The child may develop her speech pattern because of this. Being spoken to and sung to during the first year is important for overall development, however, so this is still preferable to living in a world of silence.

Some women who are cognitively challenged may have been raised in a group home and only recently discharged to their own apartment. Unlike those raised at home, these women may have unusual difficulty making plans for child care because they have never seen the care of young children. You have a legal obligation to investigate whether a newborn will receive safe care before hospital discharge. Be certain to ask enough questions so that you are sure that a woman who is severely cognitively challenged, for example, has a responsible friend or partner to help her with child care.

✔ CHECKPOINT QUESTIONS

7. For what reason is the pregnant woman with a spinal cord injury at increased risk for pressure ulcers?
8. A pregnant woman with a high thoracic spinal cord injury is at risk for what problem related to an irritating stimulus?
9. What is apt to be one of the biggest child care concerns of a hearing-challenged woman?
10. Why is it important for visually challenged women to turn on house lights when providing infant care?

THE WOMAN WHO IS SUBSTANCE DEPENDENT

Substance dependence is a growing health problem in women of childbearing age; thus, its incidence during pregnancy is increasing. As many as 10 to 20% of pregnant women use illegal drugs during pregnancy (DHHS, 2000). Cocaine, amphetamine, and multiple drug use have increased dramatically in recent years. Adolescents have an increased rate of inhalant abuse.

Substance abuse is the inability to meet major role obligations, legal problems and an increase in risk-taking behavior or exposure to hazardous situations. A person is **substance dependent** when they have withdrawal symptoms following discontinuation of the substance, combined with abandonment of important activities, spending increased time in activities related to substance use, using substances for a longer time than planned, and continued use despite worsening problems due to substance use (Bukstein, 2000).

Typically, substance-dependent women are thought to be in the younger age group as the overall incidence of drug use is highest in this group and they have less traditional lifestyles than others. However, any woman could be substance dependent. Therefore, all pregnant women need to be assessed for the possibility of substance abuse.

A woman with a substance abuse problem may come late in the pregnancy for prenatal care because she is afraid her drug use will be discovered and she will be reported to authorities. She may have difficulty following prenatal instructions for proper nutrition because although she may desire to eat well, she may lack sufficient money for both drugs and nutritious food. If she chooses drugs, her nutrition is apt to be inadequate. She may not have money for supplemental vitamins or iron preparations for the same reason. If she is using a drug that sustains her for only a few hours, she cannot wait long at a health care facility to be seen for an appointment.

Illicit drugs tend to be of small molecular weight, so they cross the placenta readily. As a result, the fetus of an addicted mother has a drug concentration of about 50% that of the mother. Because this can lead to fetal effects, drug abuse can account for fetal abnormalities or preterm birth. If a woman uses injected drugs, the risk for hepatitis B or human immunodeficiency virus (HIV) infection increases. Additionally, prostitution is a major means for securing money to buy drugs. Thus the risk for sexually transmitted diseases is increased, posing an additional threat to the fetus.

NURSING DIAGNOSES AND RELATED INTERVENTIONS

Nursing Diagnosis: Risk for injury to self and fetus related to chronic substance abuse

Outcome Identification: Client will decrease substance abuse during pregnancy.

Outcome Evaluation: Client states that she has enrolled in a substance abuse treatment program and consequently is no longer abusing drugs.

Women who are substance dependent need anticipatory guidance and nursing support during pregnancy. Often, women who abuse substances have few effective support people with whom they feel free to discuss their problems or concerns or who can answer their questions about pregnancy. Because of their numerous needs, they require the multidisciplinary team approach offered by formal substance abuse treatment programs. Fortunately, with good support and active participation in a treatment program, pregnancy can become a stimulus for drug withdrawal and a maturing and growth experience for a woman.

If the woman is still abusing a drug by the time she begins labor, the infant may experience drug withdrawal symptoms after birth (usually nervousness, irritability or lethargy, and possibly seizures; see Chapter 26). Breastfeeding is usually not encouraged because, just as all drugs cross the placenta to some extent, they also are all excreted into breast milk. The woman who is still abusing a drug at this time needs additional referral so she can secure help. In some states, women who test positive for drug abuse, either during pregnancy or at the time of birth, are reported to state child protective agencies; they may be accused of child abuse and jailed, and their infant may be placed in foster care. Be certain you are familiar with agency and state policy concerning these directives.

WHAT IF? What if a pregnant woman tells you she is not using drugs during pregnancy, but as you are helping her undress for a physical examination, you notice several packets of white powder fall out of her pocket? What would you do?

ASSESSING the Pregnant Cocaine-Abusing Woman

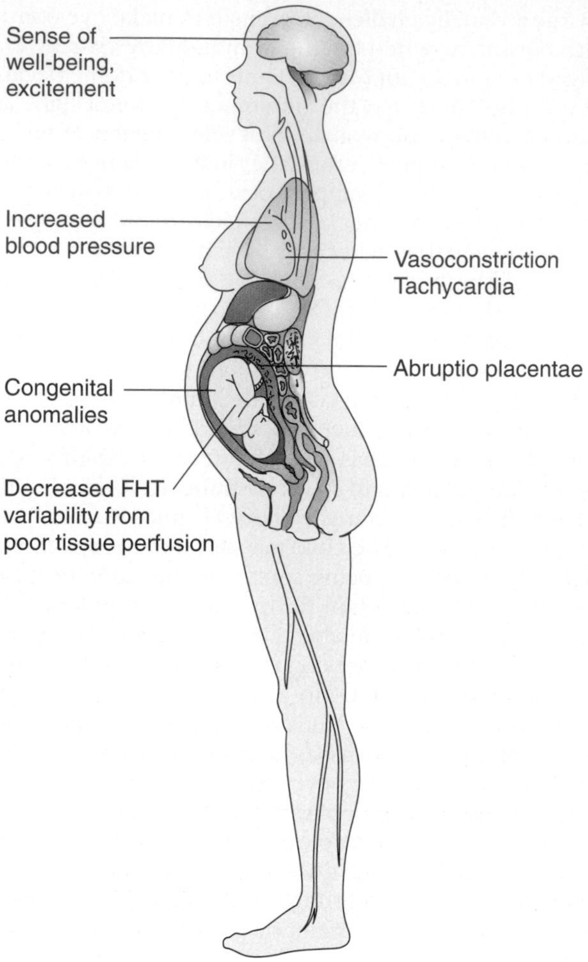

Drugs Commonly Used During Pregnancy

Recreational drugs commonly used in pregnancy are those commonly used by women in their childbearing years. These may include cocaine, amphetamines, marijuana, phencyclidine, inhalants, and opiates.

Cocaine

Cocaine is derived from *Erythroxylon coca,* a plant grown almost exclusively in South America. When sniffed into the nose or smoked in a pipe, cocaine is absorbed across the mucous membranes, affecting the central nervous system. As a result, sudden vasoconstriction occurs. Respiratory and cardiac rates and blood pressure increase rapidly in response to the vasoconstriction. Immediate death may result from cardiac failure. Alkaloidal cocaine (crack), a concentrated mixture, produces an even more rapid and intense "high" when inhaled.

Cocaine has become one of the most frequently abused drugs during pregnancy. Its use is exceptionally harmful during pregnancy because the extreme vasoconstriction that occurs can severely compromise placental circulation, leading to abruptio placentae, or a tearing loose of the placenta, which can result in preterm labor or fetal death (see Assessing the Pregnant Cocaine-Abusing Woman). Infants born of cocaine-dependent women may suffer the immediate effects of intracranial hemorrhage and a withdrawal syndrome of tremulousness, irritability, and muscle rigidity. Long-term effects are not well documented but learning defects are suspected (Delaney-Black et al., 2000; Smith et al., 2001).

Counseling women to discontinue cocaine use during pregnancy is often disappointing. The effects of the drug are so intense that it is difficult for addicted women to withdraw. Cocaine use can be detected by urinalysis because the metabolites of cocaine can be detected in urine up to 1 week after use.

Amphetamines

Methamphetamine (speed) has a pharmacologic effect similar to cocaine. Its use is increasing in incidence because it is easily and cheaply manufactured. Ice, a rock type of methamphetamine that is smoked, has the potential for causing high concentrations of drug in the maternal circulation. Newborns whose mothers used the drug show signs of jitteriness and poor feeding at birth (Anglin et al., 2000).

Marijuana and Hashish

Both marijuana and hashish are obtained from the hemp plant, cannabis. When smoked, they produce tachycardia and a sense of well-being. These drugs are frequently part of polydrug abuse, and thus their singular effects are not well documented. They are associated with loss of short-term memory and increased respiratory infection in adults (Chasnoff, 2001). A frequent user may not be able to breastfeed because of reduced milk production and the risk to the newborn from excretion of the drug in the milk.

Phencyclidine

Phencyclidine (PCP) is an animal tranquilizer that is a frequently used street drug in polydrug abuse. It causes increased cardiac output and a sense of euphoria. It has the potential for causing long-term hallucinations (flashback episodes) in the user. PCP tends to leave the maternal circulation and concentrate in fetal cells, so it has the potential to be particularly injurious to the fetus.

Narcotic Agonists

Narcotic agonists, used for the treatment of pain (e.g., morphine or meperidine [Demerol]) and cough suppression (codeine), are also widely abused because of their potent analgesic and euphoric effect. Heroin, a raw opiate, is the main opiate used recreationally to the point of dependence. Its use is increasing in incidence in young adults. A short-acting narcotic, heroin is inactive until it crosses the blood-brain barrier (which it does more quickly than morphine). It may be administered intradermally ("skin popping"), through inhalation ("snorting"), or intravenously ("shooting"). It produces an immediate and short-lived feeling of euphoria (high) followed by sedation. Pregnancy complications related to its use include pregnancy-induced hypertension, phlebitis, subacute bacterial endocarditis, and, because narcotics are often injected with shared needles, hepatitis B and HIV infection.

Withdrawal symptoms include nausea, vomiting, diarrhea, abdominal pain, hypertension, restlessness, shivering, insomnia, body aches, and muscle jerks. Withdrawal symptoms may begin as soon as 6 hours after the last drug dose and can continue for several days. Their severity and duration depend on the amount of drug used daily and length of the dependence period (Kelly et al., 2000).

Heroin abuse in the pregnant woman can result in fetal opiate dependence and severe withdrawal symptoms at birth. Infants of opiate-abusing women tend to be small for gestational age and have an increased incidence of fetal distress and meconium aspiration. They will have the same withdrawal symptoms after birth as the mother would if she abruptly stopped taking the drug.

Because the fetus is exposed to drugs that must be processed by the liver during pregnancy, the fetal liver is forced to mature faster than normal. For this reason, newborns of substance-abusing women seem better able to cope with bilirubin at birth than other babies; hyperbilirubinemia is, therefore, rarely a problem. Fetal lung tissue also appears to mature more rapidly than normal, apparently from the stress of intrauterine drug exposure. Thus, although the infant is born preterm, the chance that he will develop a condition such as respiratory distress syndrome is less than average (Cunningham et al., 2001).

If at all possible, the opiate-dependent woman should be enrolled in a methadone maintenance program during pregnancy. Infants of women on methadone do not escape withdrawal symptoms, and some infants appear to have more severe reactions to methadone withdrawal than to heroin withdrawal. Because the woman is being provided an oral drug legally, however, the fetus is at least ensured better nutrition, better prenatal care, and less exposure to pathogens such as hepatitis B and HIV. Drug withdrawal symptoms of the newborn and accompanying nursing care are discussed in Chapter 26.

Inhalants

Inhalant abuse refers to the "sniffing" or "huffing" of aerosol drugs. Frequently abused substances include airplane glue, cooking sprays, or computer keyboard cleaners. Most of these substances contain Freon as the propellant, and can lead to severe respiratory and cardiac irregularities. The effect of these drugs during pregnancy is not well documented, but the respiratory depression they can cause could be enough to limit the fetal oxygen supply to a serious level (Kurtzman et al., 2001) (see Focus on Evidence-Based Practice).

✔ CHECKPOINT QUESTIONS

11. Why is cocaine so destructive to fetal growth?
12. The fetus of a drug-addicted mother has approximately what percentage of the mother's drug concentration?

FOCUS ON EVIDENCE-BASED PRACTICE

What Substances Do Adolescents Abuse as Inhalants That Could Affect Pregnancy Outcomes?

For this study, adolescents were asked what substances they frequently abused. Results showed that white youths were more apt to use inhalants than black youths. The most likely age for first-time abuse of inhalants was 13 years. As many youths reported only experimenting with inhalants as those who were heavy users. The majority of youths reported using inhalants with friends present. Sites where they reported abuse was a friend's home (68%); their own home (54%); on the street (40%); at parties (28%); on school grounds (26%); and at school (18%). Substances frequently used as inhalants included gasoline (57%), Freon (40%), butane lighter fluid (38%), glue (29%), and nitrous oxide (23%).

This is an important study for nurses because it identifies how many adolescents may be abusing inhalants and how young they are when they start. Teenagers at

(continued)

the age of 13 are in middle schools. This means that school nurses must be aware of the potential for this type of drug abuse well before high school. Information from this study can be used to develop specific school education programs about the use of inhalants. In addition, this study provides an impetus for further research to directly study the effects of these substances on pregnancy and the fetus.

Kurtzman, T. L., Otsuka, K. N., & Wahl, R. A. (2001). Inhalant abuse by adolescents. *Journal of Adolescent Health, 28*(3), 170–180.

KEY POINTS

Adolescent pregnancy is a major problem because it occurs at such a high rate and can interfere with the development of both the adolescent and fetus. Nursing care needs to be individualized to meet the prepartal, intrapartal, and postpartal needs of this age group. Helping adolescents to view a pregnancy as a growth experience can help them mature in their ability to parent.

Women who delay childbearing until age 40 may need additional discussion time at prenatal visits to help them incorporate a pregnancy into their lifestyle. They may need reminders to save time during the day for rest, particularly if at risk for pregnancy-induced hypertension.

Women who are physically, cognitively, visually, or hearing challenged or who have a spinal cord injury are apt to have special needs during pregnancy, which must be addressed by health care providers. Providing time for discussion early in pregnancy so these needs can be identified and anticipated is an important role for nurses.

Women who are physically or cognitively challenged may need help in adjusting their usual regimen to pregnancy. Be certain they are aware of how to contact help in an emergency. Assess that all medications they are taking for their primary disorder are safe for use during pregnancy.

The woman who is substance dependent presents a unique challenge during pregnancy. Encouraging the woman to decrease or halt her drug intake to safeguard the health of the fetus is a short-term goal. Addressing the need for the woman to decrease drug intake for the remainder of her life so she can be a quality parent for her child is a long-term goal.

The fetus of a woman who is substance dependent is at high risk because of the direct effects of the drug and the indirect effects of an unhealthy lifestyle. Women addicted to opiates should be encouraged to join methadone maintenance programs if possible to reduce fetal risk.

CRITICAL THINKING EXERCISES

1. Mindy, the 14-year-old girl you met at the beginning of the chapter who is 20 weeks pregnant, tells you that she is old enough to be a responsible parent and plans on keeping her baby. What clues would you look for in her to see if her evaluation of herself is correct?
2. A 44-year-old woman who was recently married is pregnant after in vitro fertilization. She works out at a health spa daily and flies 3 days every week to out-of-state locations for work. Outline a plan of care for this client to help her avoid complications of pregnancy. Suppose she had a very sedentary life. Would your advice be different?
3. A 22-year-old woman who is substance dependent on methamphetamine comes to the clinic for a prenatal visit. You suspect she supports her drug habit by prostitution. She refuses to wait for care if she has to wait over 15 minutes. Describe modifications to this client's plan of care that are necessary to ensure consistent prenatal care. What specific advice would you want to stress with her to avoid complications of pregnancy?
4. Examine the National Health Goals related to women with special needs. Most government-sponsored money for nursing research is allotted based on these goals. What would be a possible research topic to explore pertinent to these goals that would be both fundable and helpful in advancing evidence-based practice?

REFERENCES

Abu-Heija, A. T., Jallad, M. F., & Abukteish, F. (2000). Maternal and perinatal outcome of pregnancies after the age of 45. *Journal of Obstetrics & Gynaecology Research, 26*(1), 27–30.

Anglin, M. D. et al. (2000). History of the methamphetamine problem. *Journal of Psychoactive Drugs, 32*(2), 137–141.

Branch, D. W. & Porter, T. F. (2000). Hypertensive disorders of pregnancy. In J. R. Scott et al. (Eds.). *Danforth's obstetrics and gynecology* (8th ed., pp. 309–326). Philadelphia: Lippincott Williams & Wilkins.

Bukstein, O. G. (2000). Adolescent substance abuse. In H. I. Kaplan et al. (Eds.). *Comprehensive textbook of psychiatry.* Philadelphia: Lippincott Williams & Wilkins.

Buschman, N. A., Foster, G., & Vickers, P. (2001). Adolescent girls and their babies: Achieving optimal birthweight. *Child: Care, Health & Development, 27*(2), 163–171.

Chasnoff, I. J. et al. (2001). Screening for substance use in pregnancy: A practical approach for the primary care physician. *American Journal of Obstetrics & Gynecology, 184*(4), 752–758.

Cunningham, F. G., et al. (2001). *Williams obstetrics* (21st ed.). Stamford, CT: Appleton and Lange.

Delaney-Black, V. et al. (2000). Teacher-assessed behavior of children prenatally exposed to cocaine. *Pediatrics, 106*(4), 782–791.

Department of Health and Human Services. (2000). *Healthy people 2010.* Washington, DC: Author.

Dudley, D. J. (2000). Complications of labor. In J. R. Scott et al. (Eds.). *Danforth's obstetrics and gynecology* (8th ed., pp. 437–455). Philadelphia: Lippincott, Williams & Wilkins.

Erikson, E. (1963). *Childhood and society.* New York: Norton.

Jolly, M. C. et al. (2000). Obstetric risks of pregnancy in women less than 18 years old. *Obstetrics & Gynecology, 96*(6), 962–966.

Kelly, J. J. et al. (2000). The drug epidemic: Effects on newborn infants and health resource consumption at a tertiary perinatal centre. *Journal of Paediatrics & Child Health, 36*(3), 262–264.

Kurtzman, T. L., Otsuka, K. N., & Wahl, R. A. (2001). Inhalant abuse by adolescents. *Journal of Adolescent Health, 28*(3), 170–180.

Lenders, C. M., McElrath, T. F., & Scholl, T. O. (2000). Nutrition in adolescent pregnancy. *Current Opinion in Pediatrics, 12*(3), 291–296.

Lipson, J. G. & Rogers, J. G. (2000). Pregnancy, birth, and disability: Women's health care experiences. *Health Care for Women International, 21*(1), 11–26.

Parsons, M. T., & Spellacy, W. N. (2000). Preterm labor. In J. R. Scott et al. (Eds.). *Danforth's obstetrics and gynecology* (8th ed., pp. 257–268). Philadelphia: Lippincott Williams & Wilkins.

Phipps, M. G., & Sowers, M. (2002). Defining early adolescent childbearing. *American Journal of Public Health, 92*(1), 125–128.

Smith, L. M. et al. (2001). Brain proton magnetic resonance spectroscopy and imaging in children exposed to cocaine in utero. *Pediatrics 107*(2), 227–231.

Volpe, E. M. & Bear, M. (2000). Enhancing breastfeeding initiation in adolescent mothers through the Breastfeeding Educated and Supported Teen (BEST) Club. *Journal of Human Lactation, 16*(3), 196–200.

Welner, S. (2000). Pregnancy in women with disabilities. In W. R. Cohen (Ed.). *Complications of pregnancy* (5th ed.). Philadelphia: Lippincott Williams & Wilkins.

Wenstrom, K. D. & Malee, M. P. (2000). Medical and surgical complications of pregnancy. In J. R. Scott et al. (Eds.). *Danforth's obstetrics and gynecology* (8th ed., pp. 327–362). Philadelphia: Lippincott Williams & Wilkins.

Wiemann C. M., et al. (2001). Pregnant adolescents: Experiences and behavior associated with physical assault by an intimate partner. *Maternal & Child Health Journal, 4*(2), 93–101.

SUGGESTED READINGS

Albrecht, S. A., Higgins, L. W., & Lebow, H. (2000). Knowledge about the deleterious effects of smoking and its relationship to smoking cessation among pregnant adolescents. *Adolescence, 35*(140), 709–716.

Anda, R. F. et al. (2001). Abused boys, battered mothers, and male involvement in teen pregnancy. *Pediatrics, 107*(2), E19–26.

Blythe, M. J. & Rosenthal, S. L. (2000). Female adolescent sexuality: Promoting healthy sexual development. *Obstetrics & Gynecology Clinics of North America, 27*(1), 125–141.

Gilmore, H. T. (2001). Peyote use during pregnancy. *South Dakota Journal of Medicine, 54*(1), 27–29.

Greydanus, D. E., Patel, D. R., & Rimsza, M. E. (2001). Contraception in the adolescent: An update. *Pediatrics, 107*(3), 562–573.

Harner, H. M. Burgess, A. W., & Asher, J. B. (2001). Caring for pregnant teenagers: Medicolegal issues for nurses. *Journal of Obstetric, Gynecologic & Neonatal Nursing, 30*(2), 139–147.

Key, J. D., Barbosa, A., & Owens, V. J. (2001). The Second Chance Club: Repeat adolescent pregnancy prevention with a school-based intervention. *Journal of Adolescent Health, 28*(3), 167–169.

Kozer, E. & Koren, G. (2001). Effects of prenatal exposure to marijuana. *Canadian Family Physician, 47*(2), 263–264.

Kralewski, J. & Stevens-Simon, C. (2000). Does mothering a doll change teens' thoughts about pregnancy? *Pediatrics, 105*(3), E30–35.

Margolin, A. et al. (2002). Acupuncture for the treatment of cocaine addiction. *JAMA, 287*(1), 55–63.

Michels, T. M. (2000). "Patients like us": Pregnant and parenting teens view the health care system. *Public Health Reports, 115*(6), 557–575.

Myors, K., Johnson, M., & Langdon, R. (2001). Coping styles of pregnant adolescents. *Public Health Nursing, 18*(1), 24–32.

Ostrea, E. M. et al. (2001). Estimates of illicit drug use during pregnancy by maternal interview, hair analysis, and meconium analysis. *Journal of Pediatrics, 138*(3), 344–348.

Ricciardi, R. (2000). First pelvic examination in the adolescent. *Nurse Practitioner Forum, 11*(3), 161–169.

Templeman, C. L., et al. (2000). Postpartum contraceptive use among adolescent mothers. *Obstetrics & Gynecology, 95*(5), 770–776.

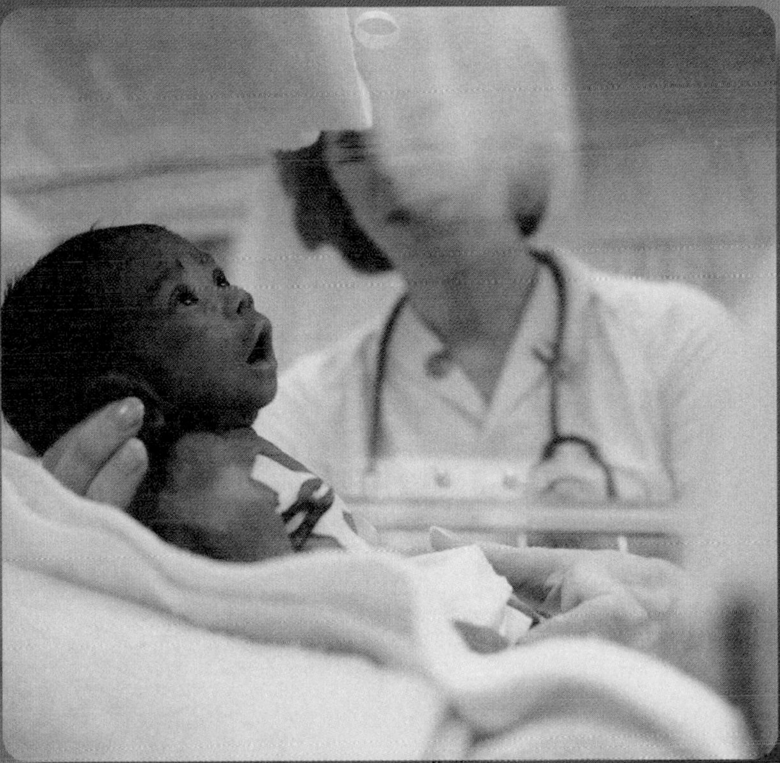

The Nursing Role in Caring for the Family During Labor and Birth

UNIT IV

The Labor Process

18

CHAPTER

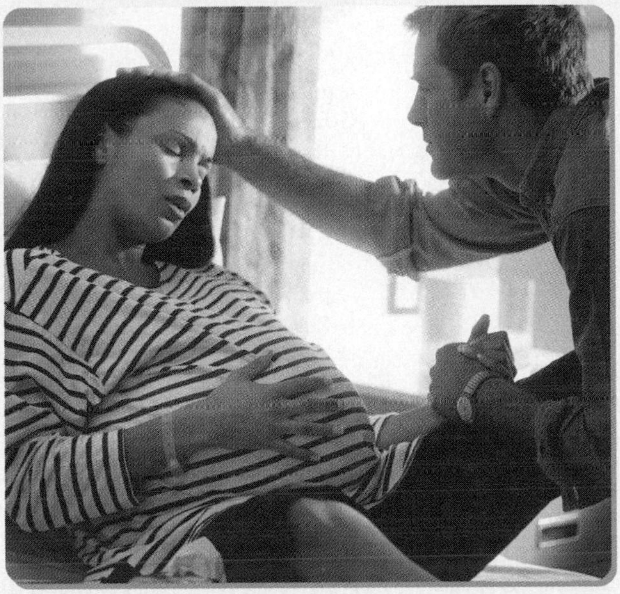

Key Terms

- amnioinfusion
- attitude
- breech presentation
- cardinal movements of labor
- cephalic presentation
- crowning
- dilatation
- effacement
- engagement
- episiotomy
- fetal descent
- Leopold's maneuvers
- lie
- lightening
- molding
- passage
- passenger
- pathologic retraction ring
- physiologic retraction ring
- position
- powers
- ripening
- station
- transition

Objectives

After mastering the contents of this chapter, you should be able to:

1. Describe the common theories explaining the onset of labor.
2. Discuss the role of the components of labor: passenger, the passage, and powers.
3. Assess a woman in labor, identifying the stage and progression.
4. Formulate nursing diagnoses related to the physiologic and psychological aspects.
5. Establish outcomes to meet the needs of the woman throughout the labor process.
6. Implement nursing care for the family during labor.
7. Evaluate outcomes for achievement and effectiveness of nursing care.
8. Identify National Health Goals related to a safe labor and birth that nurses can be instrumental in helping the nation to achieve.
9. Identify areas related to labor and birth that could benefit from additional nursing research or application of evidence-based practice.
10. Use critical thinking to analyze the effectiveness of nursing care measures in meeting the needs of women and their families in labor.
11. Integrate knowledge of nursing care in labor with nursing process to achieve quality maternal and child health nursing care.

Linda Bailey is a 26-year-old you admit to a birthing room. She is having labor contractions of 45 seconds' duration, 3 minutes apart. Her husband is not with her because he is out of town at an Army Reserve camp. Linda has a sister who lives two blocks from the hospital, but Linda doesn't want her called. She asks if she can call her mother on the telephone. As you finish assessing contractions, she screams with pain and shouts, "This can't be right! I've had pain cutting through me like this for 6 hours!" What type of support does Linda need most?

Previous chapters described the anatomic and physiologic changes that occur in pregnancy as well as effective steps women can take to prepare for labor. This chapter adds information about the labor process and how to explain this to women and their support person. This is important information because labor can be a frightening process if support people are not present.

After you've studied the chapter, answer the Critical Thinking Exercises at the end of the chapter and then access the on-line study activities (http://connection.lww.com) *to further sharpen your skills and test your knowledge.*

Labor is the series of events by which uterine contractions and abdominal pressure expel the fetus and placenta from the woman's body. Regular contractions cause progressive dilatation of the cervix and sufficient muscular force to allow the baby to be pushed to the outside. It is a time of change, both an ending and a beginning, for the woman, the fetus, and the family.

Labor and birth require the woman to use all the psychological and physical coping methods she has available. Regardless of the amount of childbirth preparation and the number of times she has been through the experience previously, she needs family-focused nursing care, because childbirth marks the beginning of a new family structure. This is further emphasized by the National Health Goals (see the Focus on National Health Goals).

FOCUS ON NATIONAL HEALTH GOALS

As labor and birth are both high-risk times for the fetus and the mother, a number of National Health Goals speak directly to them. These goals are:

- Reduce maternal deaths to no more than 3.3/100,000 live births from a baseline of 7.1/100,000.
- Reduce fetal deaths at 20 or more weeks' gestation to no more than 4.1/1000 live births from a baseline of 6.8/1000.
- Reduce fetal and infant deaths during the perinatal period (28 weeks' gestation to 7 days after birth) to no more than 4.5/1,000 live births from a baseline of 7.5/1,000 live births (DHHS, 2000).

Nurses can be instrumental in helping the nation achieve these goals by closely monitoring women during labor and birth and by teaching women as much as possible about labor so they are able to use as little analgesia and anesthesia as possible. The less anesthesia and analgesia used, the fewer the complications that can result in fetal or maternal death.

Topics that could benefit from additional nursing research in this area are advantages and disadvantages of different birthing settings; the best way to teach unprepared women to learn breathing patterns for labor; how support people can best be prepared for their role; and advantages and disadvantages of different birthing or labor positions.

NURSING PROCESS OVERVIEW

For the Woman in Labor

Labor and birth are enormous emotional and physiologic accomplishments not only for a woman but for her support person as well. For this reason, support persons should be treated with respect and should be included in all phases of the process whenever possible. Interventions that make the experience more positive and memorable for them help to contribute to future family interactions.

Assessment

Assessment of a woman in labor must be done quickly yet thoroughly and gently. The woman is keenly aware of words spoken around her and the manner with which procedures are carried out. Because of this sensitivity, she may perceive a venipuncture as a very painful experience. She may have difficulty relaxing for a vaginal examination if she fears pressure on the fetal head will cause her pain. Remember that pain is a subjective symptom. Only the woman can evaluate how much she is experiencing or how much she will be able to endure.

Assess how much discomfort a woman in labor is having not only by what she voices, but also by subtle signs of pain such as facial tenseness, flushing or paleness of the face, hands clenched in a fist, rapid breathing, or rapid pulse rate. Knowing the extent of the woman's discomfort helps guide the choice of comfort interventions she may need.

Nursing Diagnosis

Common nursing diagnoses used during labor include:

- Pain related to labor contractions
- Anxiety related to process of labor and birth
- Health-seeking behaviors related to management of discomfort of labor
- Situational low self-esteem related to inability to use prepared childbirth method

Although the discomfort of labor is commonly referred to as "contractions" rather than "pain," do not omit the word "pain" from a nursing diagnosis because the term strengthens an understanding of the problem.

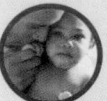

Outcome Identification and Planning
When establishing outcomes with the woman in labor and her partner, be certain they are realistic. Usually, labor takes place over a relatively short time (an average of 12 hours). Therefore, outcomes must be met within this period. On the other hand, it is important not to project a definite time limit for labor to be completed. The length of labor can vary greatly from person to person and still be within normal limits. It is necessary also to appreciate the magnitude of labor. It is unlikely that all the fear or anxiety during the woman's labor can be alleviated. Often, because it is such an unusual and significant experience, the average couple may need assistance with using additional coping measures.

Be certain to incorporate both the woman and her support person in planning so the experience is a shared one. Planning may include review and education of the normal labor process. Although a couple may have learned this during pregnancy, the reality of labor may seem much different from what they imagined. Planning also must be flexible, changing with the progress of labor, and individualized, allowing the woman to experience the significance of the event for herself.

Comfort promotion is vital. A plan addressing the discomforts of labor includes planning for education, validation, and response to the woman's pain to help her maintain realistic perceptions about it. Be certain to include planning for comfort measures such as changing a wet sheet or offering a moisturizing cream for dry lips.

Implementation
Interventions in labor must always be carried out between contractions if possible so the woman is free to use a prepared childbirth technique to limit the discomfort of contractions. This calls for good coordination of care among health care providers and planning with the woman and her support person.

Outcome Evaluation
During labor, evaluation must be ongoing to preserve the safety of the woman and her child. After birth, evaluation helps to determine the woman's opinion of her experience with labor and birth. Ideally, the experience should be one that she was not only able to endure but one that allowed her self-esteem to grow and the family to grow through a shared experience. It is advantageous to talk to women in the early postpartal period about their labor experience. Doing so serves as a means of evaluating nursing care during labor. It also provides the woman the chance to "work through" this experience and incorporate it into her self-image. Examples of possible outcome criteria may include:

- Client states pain during labor was tolerable because of her advance preparation.
- Client verbalizes that her need for additional comfort measures was met.
- Client and family members voice that the labor and birth experience was a positive growth experience for them, both individually and as a family.

THEORIES OF LABOR ONSET

Labor normally begins when a fetus is sufficiently mature to cope with extrauterine life, yet not too large to cause mechanical difficulties with birth. The trigger that converts the random, painless Braxton Hicks contractions into strong, coordinated, productive labor contractions, however, is unknown. In some instances, labor begins before the fetus is mature (preterm birth). In others, labor is delayed until the fetus and the placenta have both passed beyond the optimal point for birth (postterm birth).

Although a number of theories have been proposed to explain why labor begins, it is believed that labor is influenced by a combination of factors from the mother and fetus. These factors include:

- Uterine muscle stretching, which results in prostaglandin release
- Pressure on the cervix, which stimulates the release of oxytocin from the posterior pituitary
- Oxytocin stimulation, which works together with prostaglandin to initiate contractions
- Change in the ratio of estrogen to progesterone (increasing estrogen in relation to progesterone stimulates uterine contractions)
- Placental age, which triggers contractions at a set point
- Rising fetal cortisol levels, which reduce progesterone formation and increase prostaglandin formation
- Fetal membrane production of prostaglandin, which stimulates contractions
- Seasonal and time influences (Farrington & Ward, 2000)

SIGNS OF LABOR

Preliminary Signs of Labor

Before labor, the woman often experiences subtle signs that can signal the onset of labor. All pregnant women should be taught how to recognize these.

Lightening

In primiparas, **lightening,** or descent of the fetal presenting part into the pelvis, occurs approximately 10 to 14 days before labor begins. This changes the woman's abdominal contour as the uterus becomes lower and more anterior. Lightening gives the woman relief from the diaphragmatic pressure and shortness of breath she has been experiencing and thus "lightens" her load. Lightening probably occurs early in primiparas because of tight abdominal muscles. In multiparas, it is not as dramatic and usually occurs on the day of labor or even after labor has begun. With lightening, however, abdominal pressure increases, and this may result in reports of shooting leg pains from the pressure on the sciatic nerve, increased amounts of vaginal discharge, and urinary frequency from pressure on the bladder.

Increase in Level of Activity

A woman may wake on the morning of labor full of energy, in contrast to her feelings during the previous month. This increase in activity is due to an increase in epinephrine release that is initiated by a decrease in progesterone produced by the placenta. Additional epinephrine prepares the woman's body for the work of labor ahead.

Braxton Hicks Contractions

In the last week or days before labor begins, the woman usually notices extremely strong Braxton Hicks contractions, which she may interpret as true labor contractions. Table 18-1 summarizes the ways these contractions can be differentiated from true labor.

Primiparas may have great difficulty in distinguishing between the two forms of contractions. A woman may be admitted to the labor unit of a hospital or birthing center because false contractions so closely simulate true labor. It is discouraging for a woman who is having what seem like contractions (and strong Braxton Hicks cause real discomfort) to be told that she is not in true labor and should return home. When this happens, women need sympathetic support. They can be reassured that misinterpreting labor signals is common. Remind them that if false contractions have become strong enough to be mistaken for true labor, then true labor must not be far away.

Ripening of the Cervix

Ripening of the cervix is an internal sign seen only on pelvic examination. Throughout pregnancy, the cervix feels softer than normal, like the consistency of an earlobe (Goodell's sign). At term, the cervix becomes still softer and can be described as "butter-soft," and it tips forward. Ripening is an internal announcement that labor is close at hand.

Signs of True Labor

Signs of true labor involve uterine and cervical changes. The more women know about true labor signs, the better, because then they will be better able to recognize them. This is helpful both in preventing preterm birth and being able to feel secure during labor.

TABLE 18.1 Differentiation Between True and False Labor Contractions

FALSE CONTRACTIONS	TRUE CONTRACTIONS
Begin and remain irregular.	Begin irregularly but become regular and predictable.
Felt first abdominally and remain confined to the abdomen and groin.	Felt first in lower back and sweep around to the abdomen in a wave.
Often disappear with ambulation and sleep.	Continue no matter what the woman's level of activity.
Do not increase in duration, frequency, or intensity.	Increase in duration, frequency, and intensity.
Do not achieve cervical dilatation.	Achieve cervical dilatation.

Uterine Contractions

The surest sign that labor has begun is the initiation of effective, productive, involuntary uterine contractions. Because contractions are involuntary and come without warning, they can be frightening in early labor. Helping women appreciate that they can predict their pattern and can control the degree of discomfort they feel by using breathing exercises offers them a sense of control.

Show

As the cervix softens and ripens, the mucus plug that filled the cervical canal during pregnancy is expelled. The exposed cervical capillaries seep blood as a result of pressure exerted by the fetus. The blood, mixed with mucus, takes on a pink tinge and is referred to as "show" or "bloody show." Women need to be aware of this event so they don't think that they are bleeding abnormally.

Rupture of the Membranes

Labor may begin with rupture of the membranes, experienced as either a sudden gush or scanty, slow seeping of clear fluid from the vagina. Some women may worry when labor begins with rupture of the membranes because they believe labor will then be "dry" and thus will be difficult and long. Actually, amniotic fluid continues to be produced until delivery of the membranes after the birth of the fetus; thus, no labor is ever "dry." Early rupture of the membranes can be advantageous if it causes the fetal head to settle snugly into the pelvis, because this can actually shorten labor.

Two risks associated with ruptured membranes are intrauterine infection and prolapse of the umbilical cord, which can cut off the oxygen supply to the fetus. In most instances, if labor has not spontaneously occurred by 24 hours after membrane rupture and the pregnancy is at term, labor will be induced to help reduce these risks.

✔ **CHECKPOINT QUESTIONS**

1. Where are false labor contractions usually felt initially?
2. What are the three major signs of true labor?

COMPONENTS OF LABOR

A successful labor depends on four integrated concepts: (1) the woman's pelvis (the **passage**) is of adequate size and contour; (2) the **passenger** (the fetus) is of appropriate size and in an advantageous position and presentation; (3) the **powers** of labor (uterine factors) are adequate; and (4) the woman's psyche is preserved so afterward labor can be viewed as a positive experience.

Passage

The passage refers to the route the fetus must travel from the uterus through the cervix and vagina to the external perineum. Because these organs are contained inside the pelvis, the fetus must also pass through the pelvic ring. (Pelvic anatomy is discussed in Chap. 4; see Figs. 4-12 and 4-13). For the fetus to pass through the pelvis, the pelvis must be of adequate size. Two pelvic measurements are important to determine the adequacy of the pelvic size: the diagonal conjugate (the anterior-posterior diameter of the inlet) and the transverse diameter of the outlet (see Figs. 10-10 and 10-11). At the pelvic inlet, the anteroposterior diameter is the narrowest diameter; at the outlet, the transverse diameter is the narrowest (Fig. 18-1).

In most instances, if a disproportion between the fetus and pelvis occurs, the pelvis is the structure at fault. When the fetus is causing the problem, it is often because the fetal head is presented to the birth canal at less than its narrowest diameter, not because the head is actually too large. Keep this in mind when discussing with parents why an infant cannot be born vaginally. In this situation, emphasize that the pelvis is too small, not that the head is too big. For parents to learn that a child cannot be born vaginally because the mother's pelvis is too small can be upsetting. However, to learn that the infant's head is too large implies that something is seriously wrong with the baby (which is generally not the case). Avoiding this type of negative thought helps promote good parent-child bonding.

Passenger

The passenger is the fetus. The body part of a fetus that has the widest diameter is the head, so this is the part least likely to be able to pass through the pelvic ring. Whether a fetal skull can pass depends on both its structure (bones, fontanelles, and suture lines) and its alignment with the pelvis.

Structure of the Fetal Skull

The cranium, the uppermost portion of the skull, comprises eight bones. The four superior bones—the frontal (actually two fused bones), the two parietal, and the occipital—are the important bones in childbirth. The area over the frontal bone is referred to as the sinciput. The area over the occipital bone is referred to as the occiput. The other four bones of the skull (sphenoid bone, ethmoid bone, and two temporal bones) lie at the base of the cranium. These bones are of little significance in childbirth because they are never presenting parts. The chin, referred to by its Latin name *mentum,* can be a presenting part.

The bones of the skull meet at suture lines. The sagittal suture, a membranous interspace, joins the two parietal bones of the skull. The coronal suture is the line of junction of the frontal bones and the two parietal bones. The lambdoid suture is the line of junction of the occipital bone and the two parietal bones. The suture lines are important in birth because they allow the cranial bones to move and overlap, thus molding or diminishing the size of the skull so it can pass through the birth canal more readily.

Significant membrane-covered spaces called the fontanelles are found at the junction of the main suture lines. The anterior fontanelle (sometimes referred to as the bregma) lies at the junction of the coronal and sagittal sutures. Because the frontal bone consists of two fused bones, four bones (counting the two parietal bones) are actually involved at this junction, making the anterior fontanelle diamond-shaped. Its anteroposterior diameter measures approximately 3 to 4 cm; its transverse diameter, 2 to 3 cm.

The posterior fontanelle lies at the junction of the lambdoidal and sagittal sutures. Because the two parietal bones and the occipital bone are involved at this junction, the posterior fontanelle is triangular. It is smaller than the anterior fontanelle, measuring approximately 2 cm across its widest part. Fontanelle spaces compress during birth to aid in molding of the fetal head. Their presence can be assessed on manual examination of the cervix after it has dilated during labor. This helps to establish the position of the fetal head and whether it is in a favorable position for birth. The space between the two fontanelles is referred to as the vertex (Fig. 18-2).

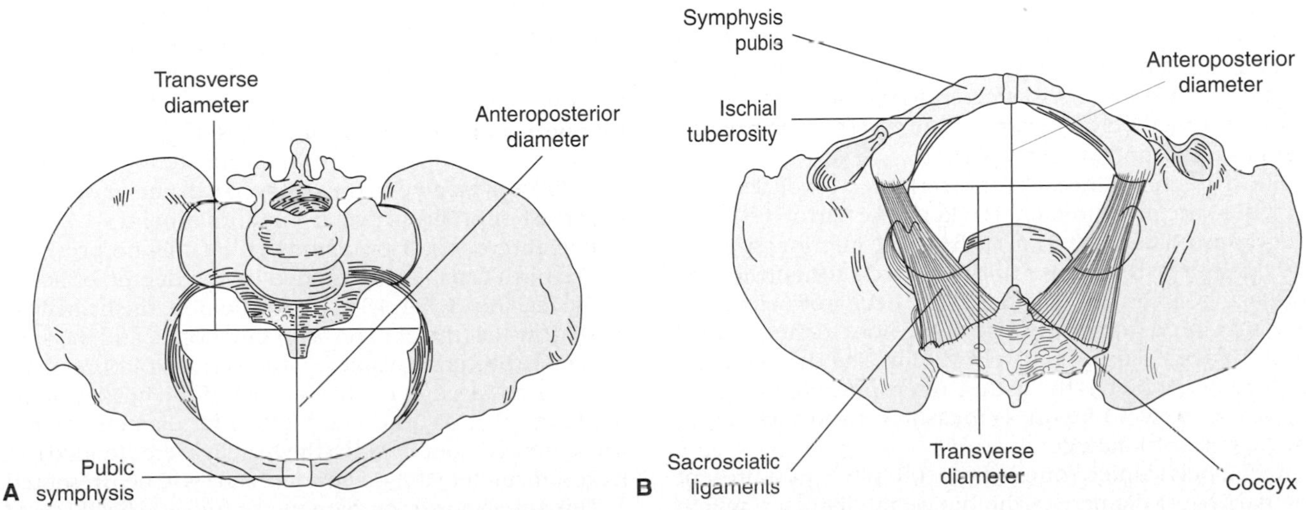

FIGURE 18.1 Views of the pelvic inlet and outlet: (*A*) pelvic inlet; (*B*) pelvic outlet.

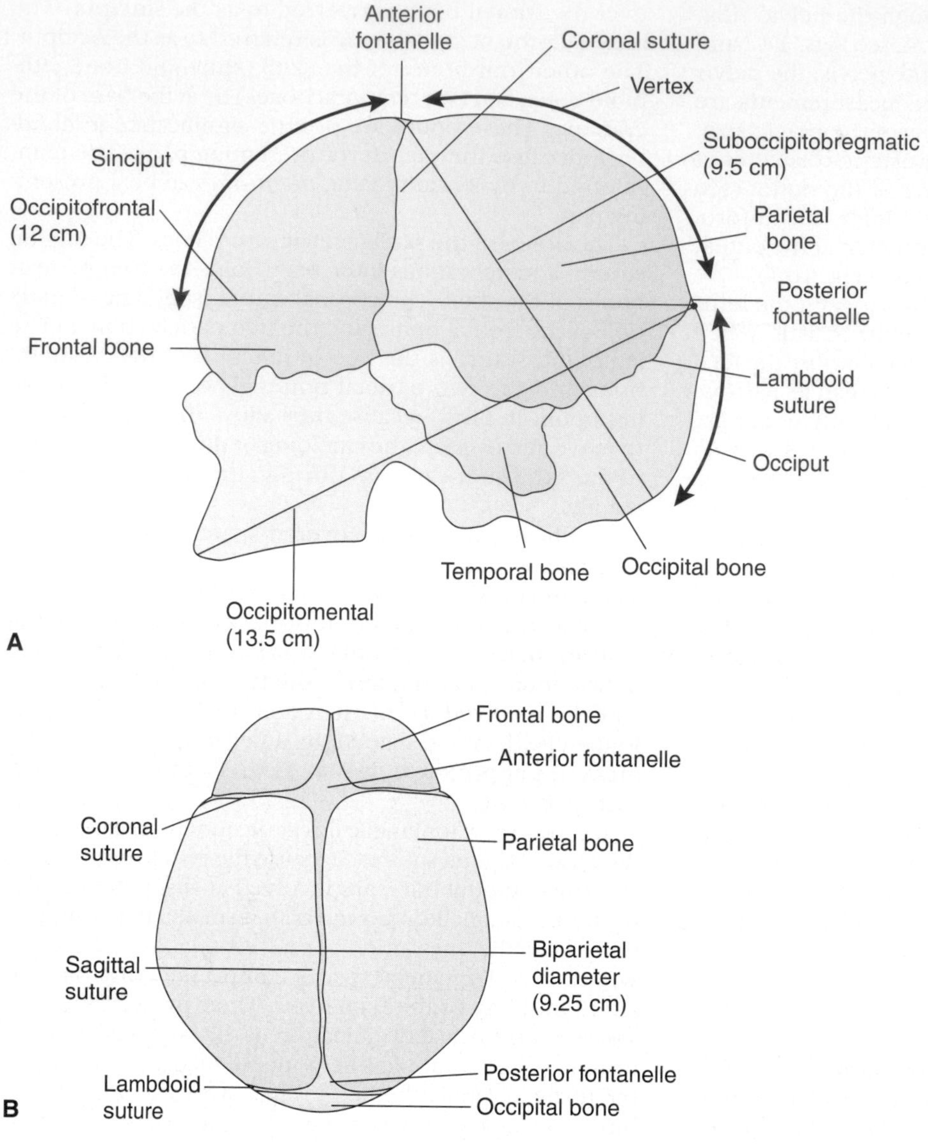

FIGURE 18.2 The fetal skull: (*A*) lateral view; (*B*) vertex view.

Diameters of the Fetal Skull

The shape of a fetal skull causes it to be wider in its anteroposterior diameter than in its transverse diameter. To fit through the birth canal, the fetus must present the smaller diameter (the transverse diameter) to the smaller diameter of the maternal pelvis; otherwise, progress may be halted and birth may not be accomplished.

The diameter of the anteroposterior fetal skull depends on where the measurement is taken. The narrowest diameter (approximately 9.5 cm) is from the inferior aspect of the occiput to the center of the anterior fontanelle (the suboccipitobregmatic diameter). The occipitofrontal diameter, measured from the bridge of the nose to the occipital prominence, is approximately 12 cm. The occipitomental diameter, which is the widest anteroposterior diameter (approximately 13.5 cm), is measured from the chin to the posterior fontanelle.

At the pelvic inlet, for example, the fetus must present the narrowest diameter—the biparietal diameter, which is approximately 9.25 cm (see Fig. 18-2*B*)—to the anteroposterior diameter of the pelvis, a space approximately 11 cm wide. At the outlet, this narrow diameter must be presented to the transverse diameter, a space approximately 11 cm wide. If the anteroposterior diameter of the skull (a measurement wider than the biparietal diameter) is presented to the anteroposterior diameter of the inlet, **engagement,** or the settling of the fetal head into the pelvis, may not occur. If the anteroposterior diameter of the skull is presented to the transverse diameter of the outlet, arrest of progress may occur at that point.

The anteroposterior diameter that will be presented to the birth canal is determined by the degree of flexion of the fetal head (Fig. 18-3). In full flexion, the head flexes so sharply that the chin rests on the thorax, and the smallest anteroposterior diameter, the suboccipitobregmatic, will be presented to the birth canal. If the head is held in moderate flexion, the occipitofrontal diameter will be presented. In poor flexion (the head hyperextended), the largest diameter (the occipitomental) will be presented.

This anteroposterior diameter of the fetal head must fit through the transverse diameter of the pelvic inlet, a

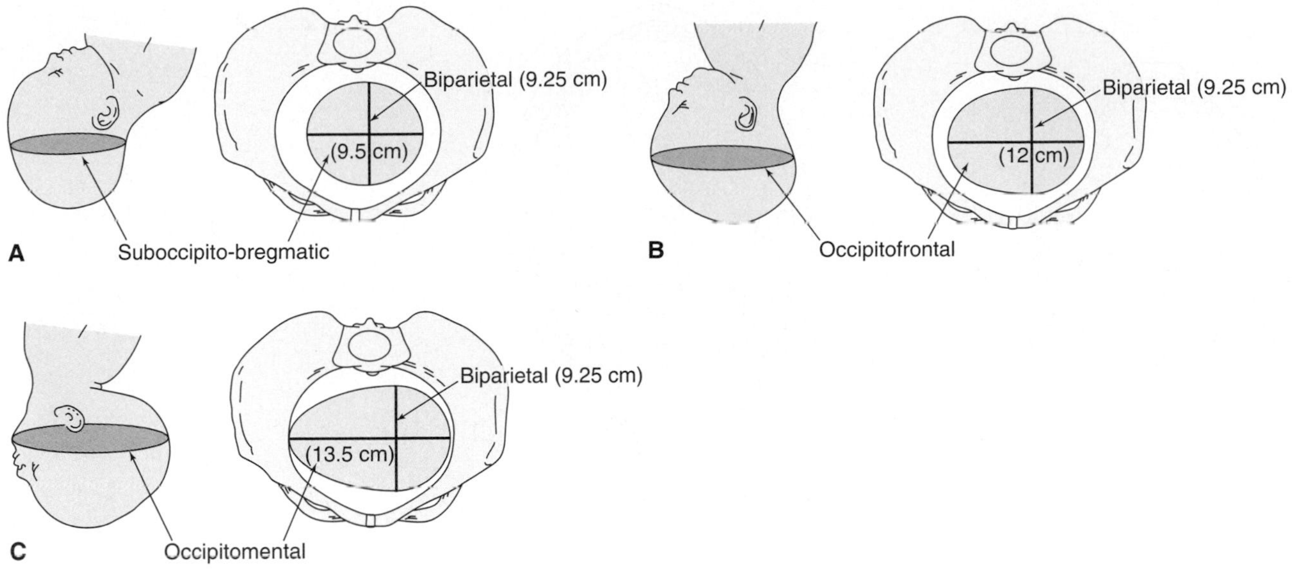

FIGURE 18.3 (*A*) Complete flexion allows the smallest diameter of the head to enter the pelvis. (*B*) Moderate flexion causes a larger diameter to enter the pelvis. (*C*) Poor flexion forces the largest diameter against the pelvic brim, but the head is too large to enter the pelvis.

space of approximately 12.4 to 13.5 cm; and at the outlet, through the anteroposterior diameter of the pelvis, a space of 9.5 to 11.5 cm. It follows that a fetal head presenting a diameter of 9.5 cm will fit through a pelvis much more readily than if the diameter is 12.0 or 13.5 cm.

Molding

Molding is the change in shape of the fetal skull produced by the force of uterine contractions pressing the vertex against the not-yet-dilated cervix. Because the bones of the fetal skull are not yet completely ossified and therefore do not form a rigid structure, they overlap and cause the head to become narrower but longer, facilitating its passage during birth. Molding is commonly seen in newborns. The overlapping of the sagittal suture line and generally the coronal suture line can be easily palpated in the newborn skull. Parents can be reassured that it only lasts a day or two and is not a permanent condition. There is little molding when the brow is the presenting part (described in the following section) because frontal bones are fused. No skull molding occurs when the fetus is breech because the buttocks, not the head, are presented first.

Fetal Presentation and Position

In addition to being familiar with the parts and diameters of the fetal head, it is important to understand the terms that describe fetal presentation and position.

Attitude. **Attitude** describes the degree of flexion the fetus assumes during labor or the relation of the fetal parts to each other (Fig. 18-4). A fetus in good attitude is in complete flexion: the spinal column is bowed forward, the head is flexed forward so much that the chin touches the sternum, the arms are flexed and folded on the chest, the thighs are flexed onto the abdomen, and the calves are pressed against the posterior aspect of the thighs (see Fig. 18-4*A*). This normal "fetal position" is advantageous for birth because it helps the fetus present the smallest anteroposterior diameter of the skull to the pelvis and also because it puts the whole body into an ovoid shape, occupying the smallest space possible.

A fetus is in moderate flexion if the chin is not touching the chest but is in an alert or "military position" (see Fig. 18-4*B*). This position causes the next-widest anteroposterior diameter, the occipital frontal diameter, to present to the birth canal. A fair number of fetuses assume a military position during the early part of labor. This does not usually interfere with labor because part of the mechanisms of labor (descent and flexion) causes the fetus to flex the head fully at that point.

The fetus in partial extension presents the "brow" of the head to the birth canal (see Fig. 18-4*C*). If a fetus is in poor flexion, the back is arched, the neck is extended, and the fetus is in complete extension, presenting the occipitomental diameter of the head to the birth canal (face presentation; see Fig. 18-4*D*). This is an unusual position. It presents too wide a skull diameter to the birth canal for normal birth. Such a position may occur if there is less than the normal amount of amniotic fluid present (oligohydramnios), which does not allow the fetus adequate movement. It also may reflect a neurologic abnormality that is causing spasticity.

Engagement. Engagement refers to the settling of the presenting part of the fetus far enough into the pelvis to be at the level of the ischial spines, a midpoint of the pelvis. Descent to this point means that the widest part of the fetus (the biparietal diameter in a cephalic presentation; the intertrochanteric diameter in a breech presentation) has passed through the pelvis or the pelvic inlet has been proven adequate for birth. In a primipara, nonengagement of the head at the beginning of labor indicates a possible complication, such as an abnormal presentation or

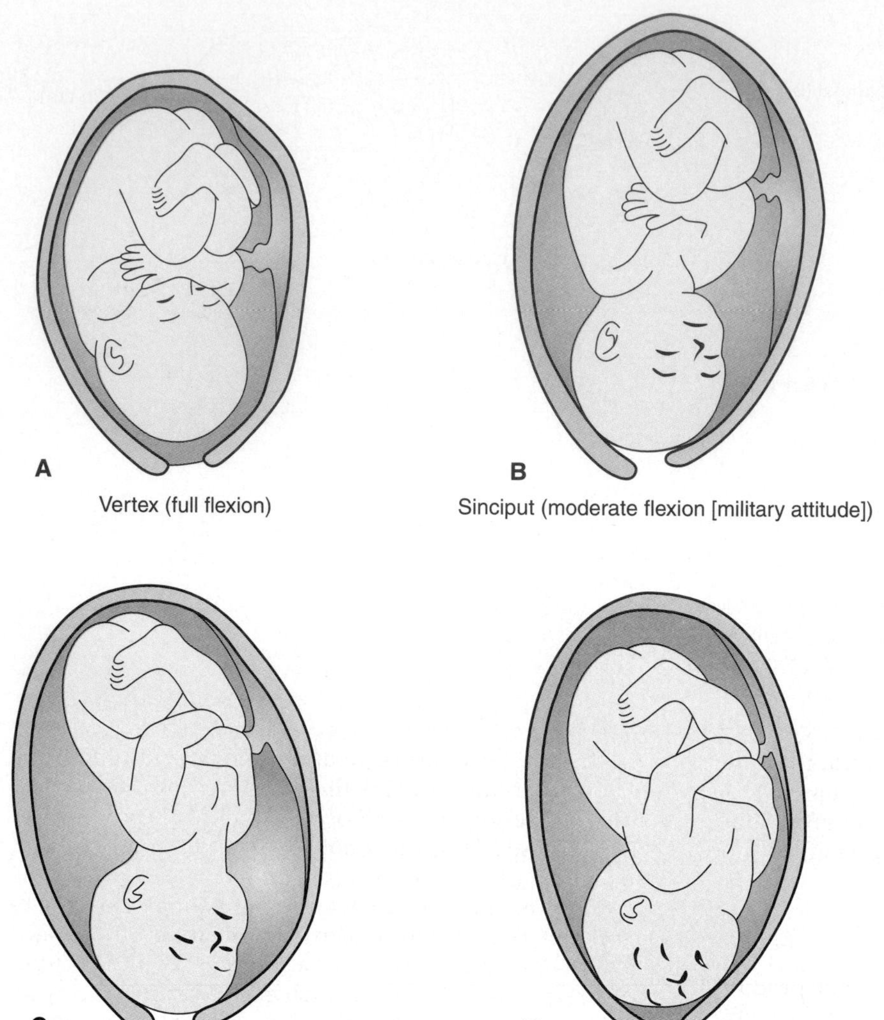

FIGURE 18.4 Fetal attitude. (*A*) Fetus in full flexion presents smallest (suboccipitobregmatic) anteroposterior diameter of skull to inlet in this good attitude (vertex presentation). (*B*) Fetus is not as well flexed (military attitude) as in *A* and presents occipitofrontal diameter to inlet (sinciput presentation). (*C*) Fetus in partial extension (brow presentation). (*D*) Fetus in complete extension presents wide (occipitomental) diameter (face presentation).

position, abnormality of the fetal head, or cephalopelvic disproportion. In multiparas, engagement may or may not be present at the beginning of labor. A presenting part that is not engaged is said to be "floating." One that is descending but has not yet reached the iliac spines can be said to be "dipping." The degree of engagement is assessed by vaginal and cervical examination.

Station. **Station** refers to the relationship of the presenting part of the fetus to the level of the ischial spines (Fig. 18-5). When the presenting part is at the level of the ischial spines, it is at a 0 station (synonymous with engagement). If the presenting part is above the spines, the distance is measured and described as minus stations, which range from −1 cm to −4 cm. If the presenting part is below the ischial spines, the distance is stated as plus stations (+1 cm to +4 cm). At a +3 or +4 station, the presenting part is at the perineum and can be seen if the vulva is separated (synonymous with **crowning**).

Fetal Lie. **Lie** is the relationship between the long (cephalocaudal) axis of the fetal body and the long (cephalocaudal) axis of the woman's body; in other words, whether the fetus is lying in a horizontal (transverse) or a vertical (longitudinal) position. Approximately 99% of fetuses assume a longitudinal lie (with their long axis parallel with the long axis of the woman). Longitudinal lies are further classified as cephalic, with the head as the first part to contact the cervix, or breech, with the breech, or buttocks, as the first portion to contact the cervix.

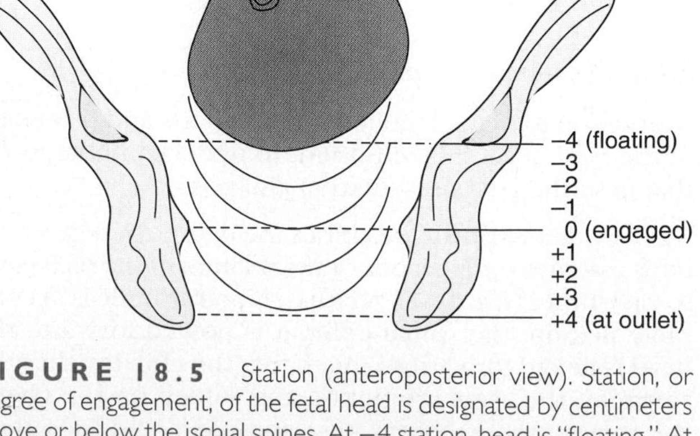

FIGURE 18.5 Station (anteroposterior view). Station, or degree of engagement, of the fetal head is designated by centimeters above or below the ischial spines. At −4 station, head is "floating." At 0 station, head is "engaged." At +4 station, head is "at outlet."

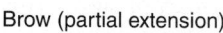

Types of Fetal Presentation

Fetal presentation denotes the body part that will first contact the cervix or deliver first. This is determined by fetal lie and the degree of flexion (attitude).

Cephalic Presentation. A **cephalic presentation** means that the head is the body part that first contacts the cervix. It is the most frequent type of presentation, occurring as often as 95% of the time. The four types of cephalic presentation (vertex, brow, face, and mentum) are described in Table 18-2. During labor, the area of the fetal skull that contacts the cervix often becomes edematous from the continued pressure against it. This edema is called a caput succedaneum. In the newborn, the point of presentation can be analyzed from the location of the caput.

Breech Presentation. A **breech presentation** means that either the buttocks or feet are the first body parts to contact the cervix. Breech presentations occur in approximately 3% of births and are affected by fetal attitude. A good attitude brings the fetal knees up against the umbilicus; a poor attitude does not. Breech presentations usually are difficult births, with the presenting point influencing the degree of difficulty. Three types of breech presentation (complete, frank, and footling) are possible (Table 18-3).

Shoulder Presentation. In a transverse lie, the fetus is lying horizontally in the pelvis so that its long axis is perpendicular to that of the mother. The presenting part usually becomes one of the shoulders (acromion process), an iliac crest, a hand, or an elbow (Fig. 18-6).

Fewer than 1% of fetuses lie transversely. This may be caused by relaxed abdominal walls from grand multiparity, allowing the uterus to be unsupported and fall forward. Another cause is pelvic contraction, in which the horizontal space is greater than the vertical space. Placenta previa (the placenta is located low in the uterus, obscuring some of the vertical space) may also limit the fetus' ability to turn, resulting in a transverse lie. When this occurs, the usual contour of the abdomen at term is distorted or is fuller side to side rather than top to bottom.

If an infant is preterm and smaller than usual, an attempt to turn the fetus may be made. Most infants in a transverse lie must be born by cesarean birth, however, because they are unable to deliver normally from this "wedged" position. Discovering a shoulder presentation is an important assessment because it almost automatically identifies a birth position that puts both mother and child in jeopardy unless skilled health care personnel are available to complete a cesarean birth.

Types of Fetal Position

Position is the relationship of the presenting part to a specific quadrant of the woman's pelvis. For convenience, the maternal pelvis is divided into four quadrants according to the mother's right and left: (1) right anterior, (2) left anterior, (3) right posterior, and (4) left posterior.

Four parts of the fetus have been chosen as landmarks to describe the relationship of the presenting part to one of the pelvic quadrants. In a vertex presentation, the occiput is the chosen point; in a face presentation, it is the chin (mentum); in a breech presentation, it is the sacrum; in a shoulder presentation, it is the scapula or the acromion process.

Position is marked by an abbreviation of three letters. The middle letter denotes the fetal landmark (O for occiput, M for mentum or chin, Sa for sacrum, and A for acromion process). The first letter defines whether the landmark is pointing to the mother's right (R) or left (L). The last letter defines whether the landmark points anteriorly (A), posteriorly (P), or transversely (T).

When the occiput of the fetus points to the left anterior quadrant in a vertex position, for example, this is termed left occipitoanterior (LOA). The fetus is in good attitude in a vertical cephalic lie. When the occiput points to the right posterior quadrant, the position is right occipitoposterior (ROP). LOA is the most common fetal position and right occipitoanterior (ROA) the second most frequent position. Box 18-1 summarizes possible positions. Six common positions in cephalic presentations are depicted in Figure 18-7.

Position is important because it influences the process and efficiency of labor. Typically, a fetus delivers fastest from an ROA or LOA position. Labor is considerably extended if the position is posterior (ROP or LOP). Posterior positions may also be more painful for the mother because the rotation of the fetal head puts pressure on the sacral nerves, causing sharp back pains.

TABLE 18.2 Types of Cephalic Presentations

TYPE	LIE	ATTITUDE	DESCRIPTION
Vertex	Longitudinal	Good (full flexion)	The head is sharply flexed, making the parietal bones or the space between the fontanelles (the vertex) the presenting part. This is the most common presentation and allows the suboccipitobregmatic diameter to present to the cervix.
Brow	Longitudinal	Moderate (military)	Because the head is only moderately flexed, the brow or sinciput becomes the presenting part.
Face	Longitudinal	Poor	The fetus has extended the head to make the face the presenting part. From this position, extreme edema and distortion of the face may occur. The presenting diameter (the occipitomental) is so wide birth may be impossible.
Mentum	Longitudinal	Very poor	The fetus has completely hyperextended the head to present the chin. The widest diameter (occipitomental) is presenting. As a rule, the fetus cannot enter the pelvis in this presentation.

TABLE 18.3 Types of Breech Presentations

TYPE	LIE	ATTITUDE	DESCRIPTION
Complete 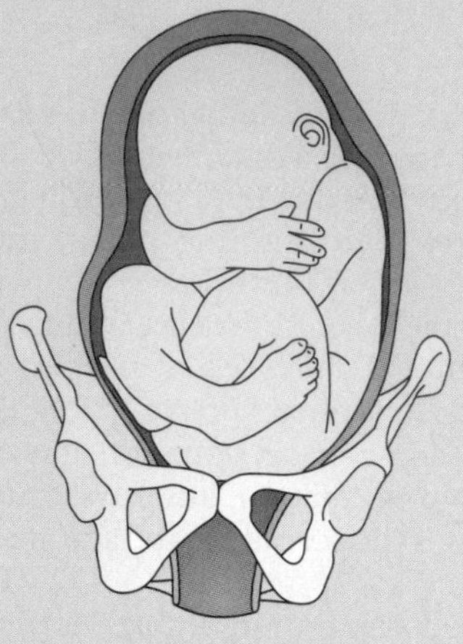	Longitudinal	Good (full flexion)	The fetus has thighs tightly flexed on the abdomen; both the buttocks and the tightly flexed feet present to the cervix.
Frank 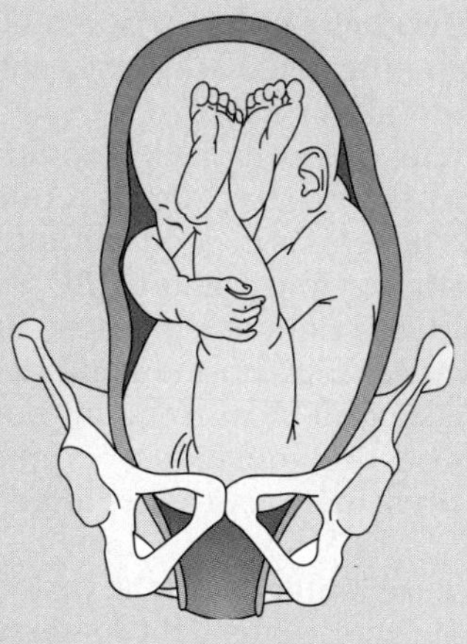	Longitudinal	Moderate	Attitude is moderate because the hips are flexed but the knees are extended to rest on the chest. The buttocks alone present to the cervix.
Footling 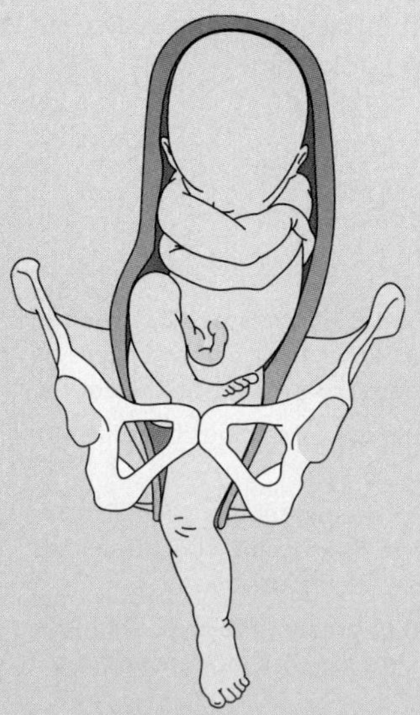	Longitudinal	Poor	Neither the thighs nor lower legs are flexed. If one foot presents, it is a single-footling breech; if both present, it is a double-footling breech.

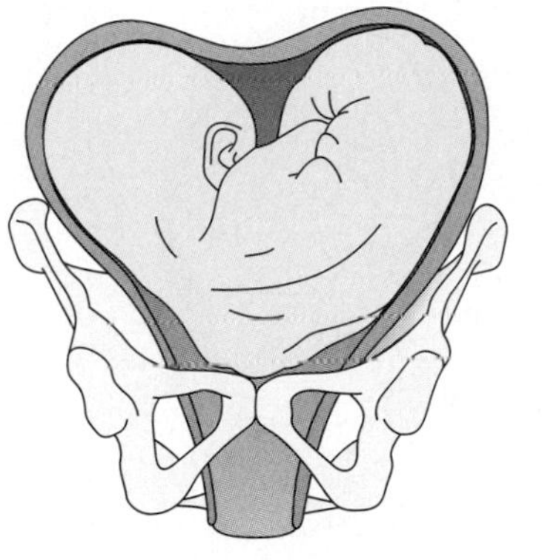

FIGURE 18.6 Transverse or shoulder presentation.

Never

Importance of Determining Fetal Presentation and Position

It is important to document presentation and position because the presentation of a body part other than the vertex puts the fetus at risk. It implies a proportional difference between the fetus and pelvis (the pelvis is too narrow to allow the fetus to pass through), making a cesarean birth necessary. The membranes also are more apt to rupture early, increasing the possibility of infection. The risk for fetal anoxia and meconium staining, complications that lead to respiratory distress at birth, are also increased.

Four methods are used to determine fetal position, presentation, and lie: (1) combined abdominal inspection and palpation, (2) vaginal examination, (3) auscultation of fetal heart tones, and (4) sonography.

The vertex is the ideal presenting part because the skull bones are capable of molding so effectively to accommodate the cervix. It also may actually aid in cervical dilatation and prevents complications such as a prolapsed cord (cord passing between the presenting part and the cervix and entering the vagina before the fetus). When a body part other than the vertex presents, labor is invariably longer due to ineffective descent of the fetus, ineffective dilatation of the cervix, and irregular and weak uterine contractions.

The less effective labor is, the longer it is, tiring the mother and reducing the excitement of the experience. If an operative birth is necessary and postoperative complications occur, the mother may require a longer hospital stay and have more pain and disability after the birth. If the fetus delivers vaginally after a complicated labor, there is an increased risk for perineal tears or cervical lacerations, which may also increase her disability and possibly interfere with her future child-bearing. When labor is threatening and unsatisfactory, it can interfere with maternal–child bonding.

BOX 18.1

POSSIBLE FETAL POSITIONS

Vertex Presentation (occiput)
LOA, left occipitoanterior
LOP, left occipitoposterior
LOT, left occipitotransverse
ROA, right occipitoanterior
ROP, right occipitoposterior
ROT, right occipitotransverse

Breech Presentation (sacrum)
LSaA, left sacroanterior
LSaP, left sacroposterior
LSaT, left sacrotransverse
RSaA, right sacroanterior
RSaP, right sacroposterior
RSaT, right sacrotransverse

Face Presentation (mentum)
LMA, left mentoanterior
LMP, left mentoposterior
LMT, left mentotransverse
RMA, right mentoanterior
RMP, right mentoposterior
RMT, right mentotransverse

Shoulder Presentation (acromion process)
LAA, left scapuloanterior
LAP, left scapuloposterior
RAA, right scapuloanterior
RAP, right scapuloposterior

✔ CHECKPOINT QUESTIONS

3. What are the four integrated components of labor?
4. Which pelvic diameter is narrowest at the pelvic outlet?
5. What structure lies at the junction of the coronal and sagittal sutures?
6. Which fetal skull diameter is the widest anteroposterior diameter?
7. What term is used to describe the relationship of the fetal presenting part to the level of the ischial spines?
8. Which presentation is considered ideal?

Mechanisms (Cardinal Movements) of Labor

Passage of the fetus through the birth canal involves a number of different position changes to keep the smallest diameter of the fetal head (in cephalic presentations) always presenting to the smallest diameter of the birth canal. These position changes are termed the **cardinal movements of labor:** descent, flexion, internal rotation, extension, external rotation, and expulsion (Fig. 18-8).

Descent. Descent is the downward movement of the biparietal diameter of the fetal head to within the pelvic inlet. Full descent occurs when the fetal head extrudes beyond the dilated cervix and touches the posterior vaginal floor. The pressure of the fetus on the sacral nerves causes the mother to experience a pushing sensation. Descent occurs because of pressure on the fetus by the uterine fundus. Full descent may be aided by abdominal muscle contraction.

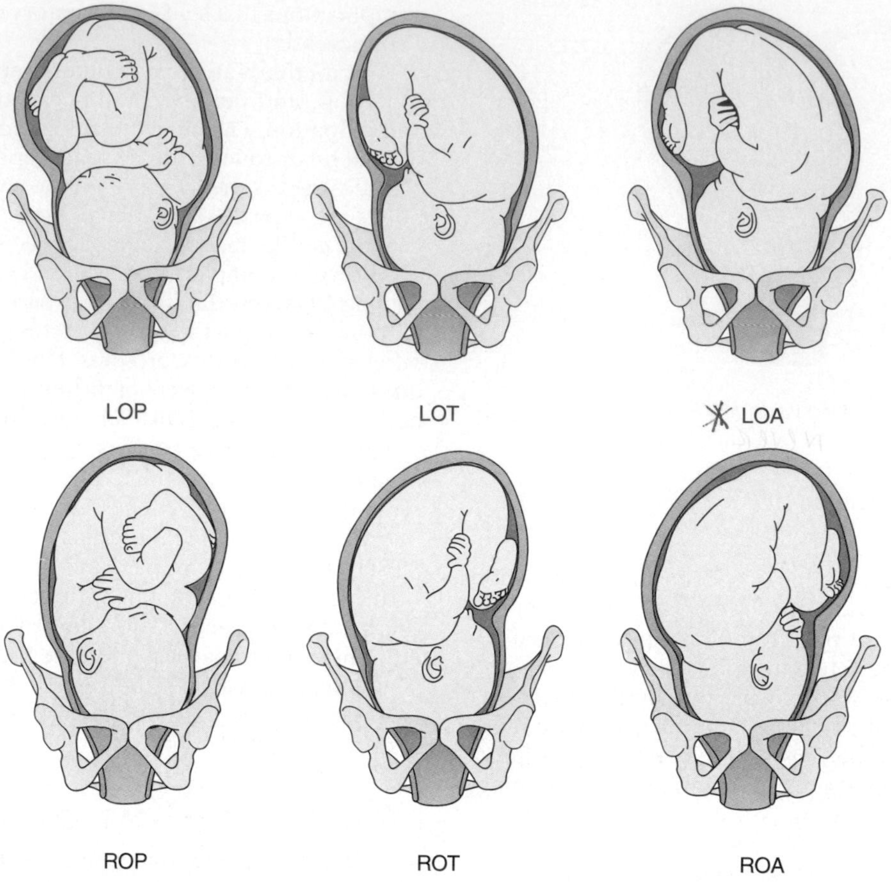

FIGURE 18.7 Fetal position. All are vertex presentations. A = anterior; L = left; O = occiput; P = posterior; R = right; T = transverse.

Flexion. As descent occurs, pressure from the pelvic floor causes the fetal head to bend forward onto the chest. The smallest anteroposterior diameter (the suboccipitobregmatic diameter) is the one presented to the birth canal in this flexed position. Flexion is aided by abdominal muscle contraction during pushing.

Internal Rotation. During descent, the head enters the pelvis with the fetal anteroposterior head diameter (suboccipitobregmatic, occipitomental, or occipitofrontal, depending on the amount of flexion) in a diagonal or transverse position. The head flexes as it touches the pelvic floor, and the occiput rotates until it is superior, or just below the symphysis pubis, bringing the head into the best diameter for the outlet of the pelvis (the anteroposterior diameter is now in the anteroposterior plane of the pelvis). This movement brings the shoulders, coming next, into the optimal position to enter the inlet or puts the widest diameter of the shoulders (a transverse one) in line with the wide transverse diameter of the inlet.

Extension. As the occiput is born, the back of the neck stops beneath the pubic arch and acts as a pivot for the rest of the head. The head thus extends, and the foremost parts of the head, the face and chin, are born.

External Rotation. In external rotation, almost immediately after the head of the infant is born, the head rotates (from the anteroposterior position it assumed to enter the outlet) back to the diagonal or transverse position of the early part of labor. The aftercoming shoulders are thus brought into an anteroposterior position, which is best for entering the outlet. The anterior shoulder is born first, assisted perhaps by downward flexion of the infant's head.

Expulsion. Once the shoulders are born, the rest of the baby is born easily and smoothly because of its smaller size. This is expulsion and is the end of the pelvic division of labor.

For a view of the complete birth sequence, see Figure 18-9.

Powers of Labor

The powers of labor, supplied by the fundus of the uterus, are implemented by uterine contractions, a process that causes cervical dilatation and then expulsion of the fetus from the uterus. After full dilatation of the cervix, the primary power is supplemented by the use of the abdominal muscles. It is important for women to understand they should not bear down with their abdominal muscles until the cervix is fully dilated. Doing so will impede the primary force or could cause fetal and cervical damage.

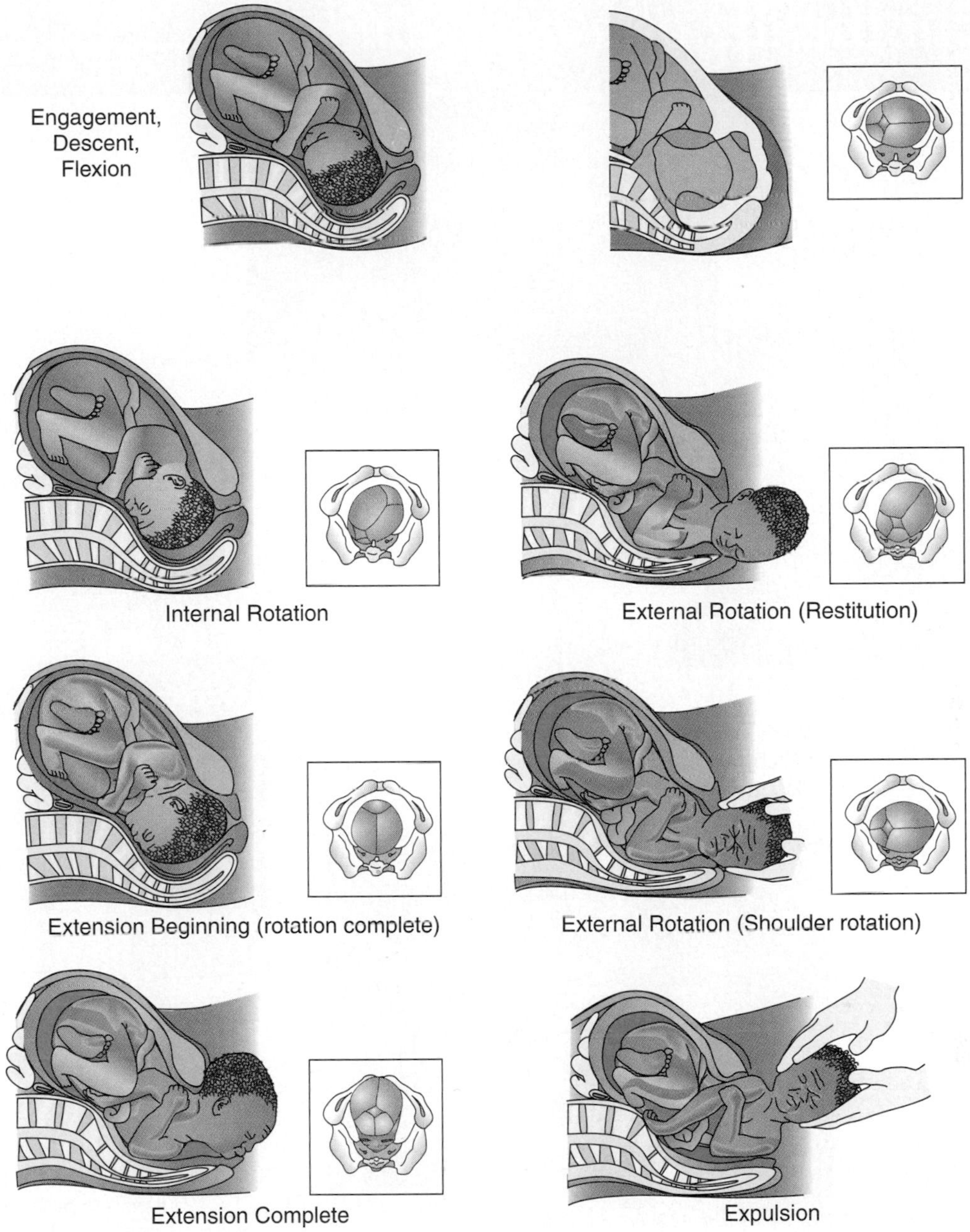

FIGURE 18.8 Mechanism of normal labor and cardinal positions of the fetus from a left occipitoanterior position.

Uterine Contractions

Origins. Like cardiac contractions, labor contractions begin at a "pacemaker" point located in the myometrium near one of the uterotubal junctions. Each contraction begins at that point and then sweeps down over the uterus as a wave. After a short rest period, another contraction is initiated and the downward sweep begins again.

In early labor, the uterotubal pacemaker may not be working in a synchronous manner. This makes contractions sometimes strong, sometimes weak, and irregular. This mild incoordination of early labor improves after a few hours as the pacemaker becomes more attuned to calcium concentrations in the myometrium and begins to function smoothly.

In some women, contractions appear to originate in the lower uterine segment rather than in the fundus. These are reverse, ineffective contractions, and actually cause tightening rather than dilatation of the cervix. That contractions are being initiated in a reverse pattern is difficult to tell from palpation. It can be suspected if a woman tells you that she feels pain in her lower abdomen before the contraction is readily palpated at the fundus. It is truly revealed only when cervical dilation does not occur.

Some women seem to have additional pacemaker sites in other portions of the uterus. If present, contractions will be uncoordinated. These may slow labor and may lead

FIGURE 18-9.

A day in the life of a new family.

6:00 AM: Early in labor, Linda is supported and comforted by her husband and her sister.

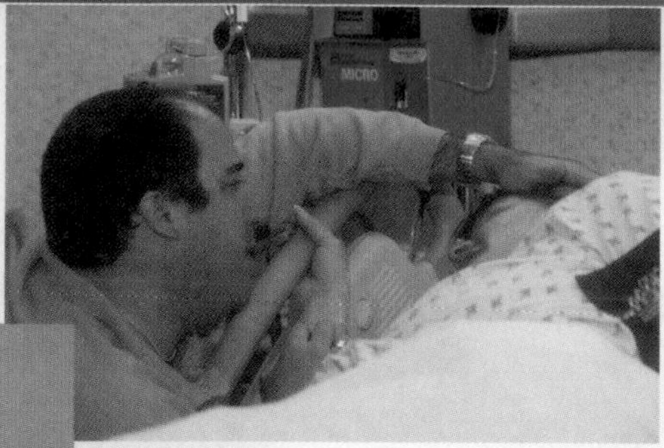

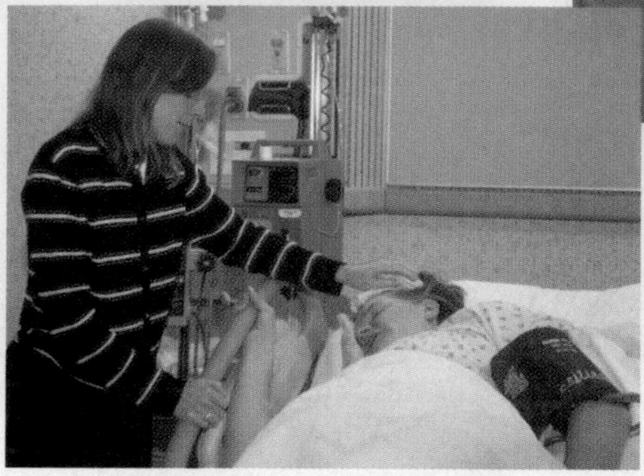

9:00 AM: The nurse checks the fetal monitor and documents Linda's status.

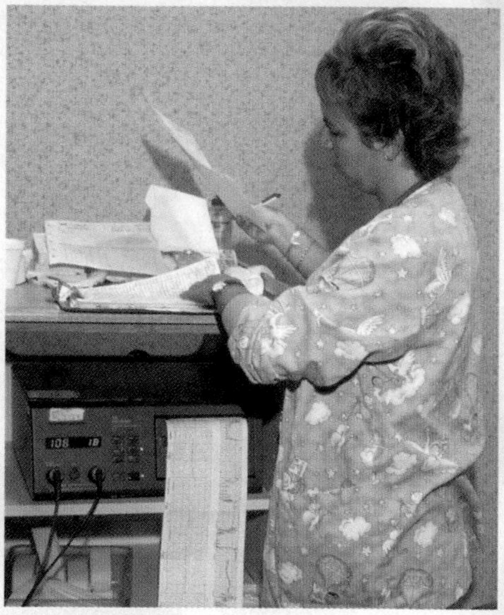

10:00 AM: The doctor makes a final check of cervical dilation and tells Linda it's time to push.

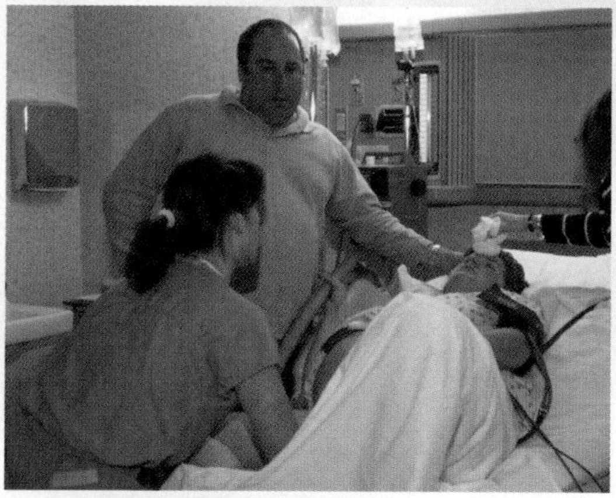

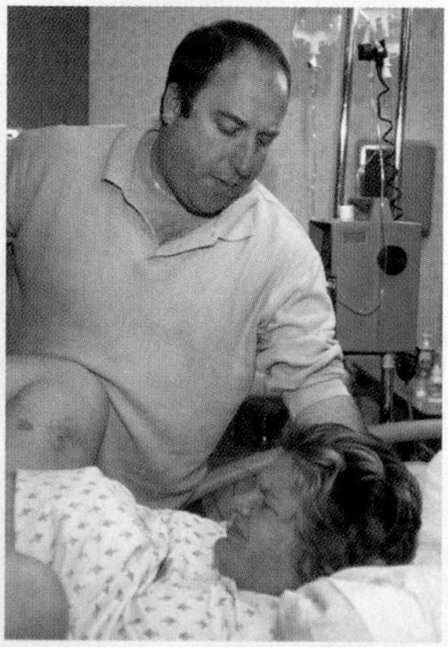

10:30 AM: Linda pushes in the lithotomy position, with Aaron as coach.

11:15 AM: Linda moves to an alternative position using the support bar to promote delivery.

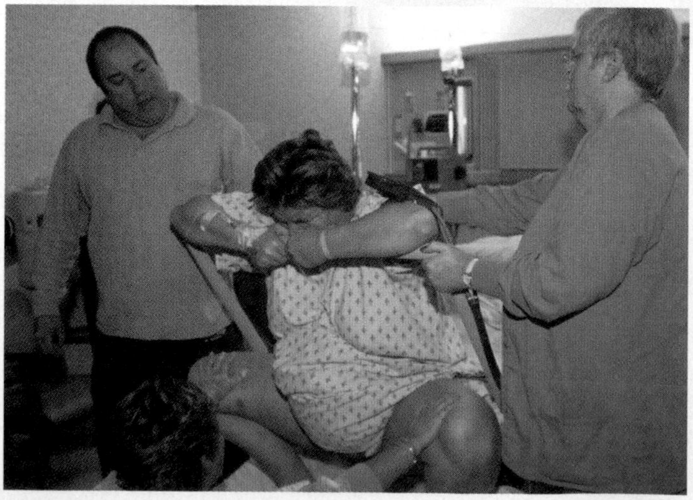

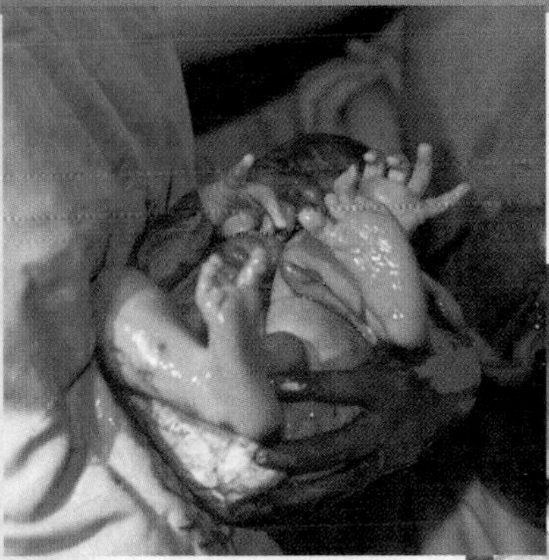

12:12 PM: Welcome Stephen! Dad cuts the cord.

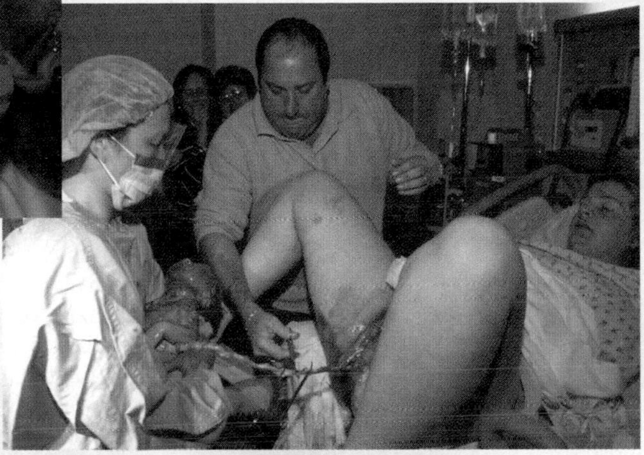

12:15 PM: Mom holds her son for the first time. Her mother and sister (now a grandmother and aunt!) look on.

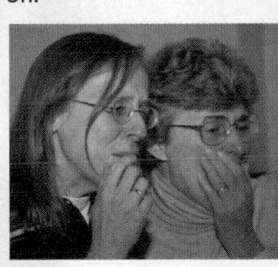

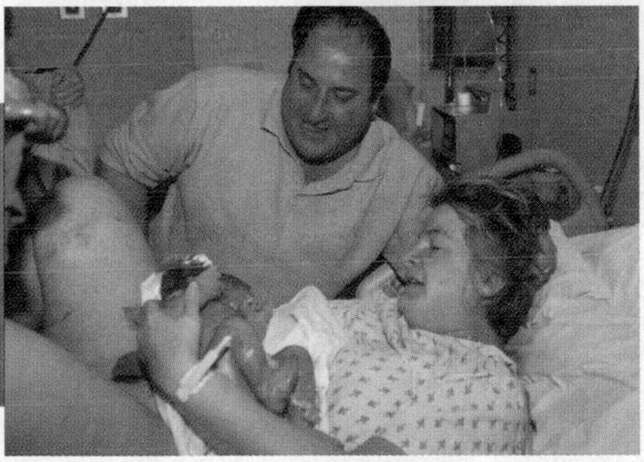

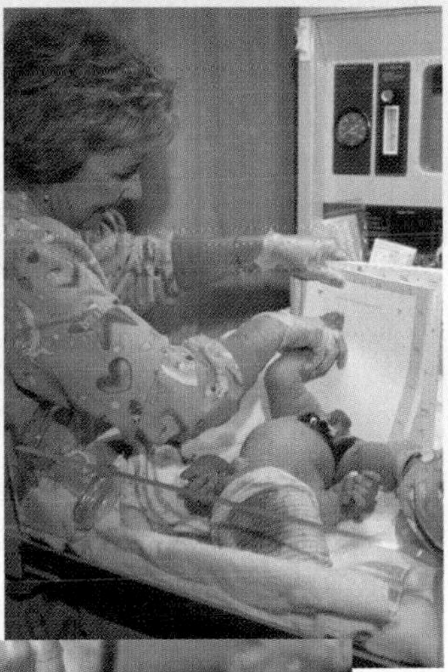

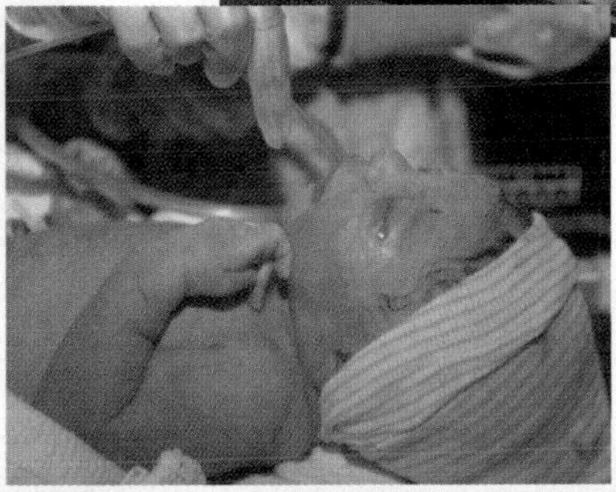

12:30 PM: The nurse performs suctioning to clear the airways and takes the baby's footprints.

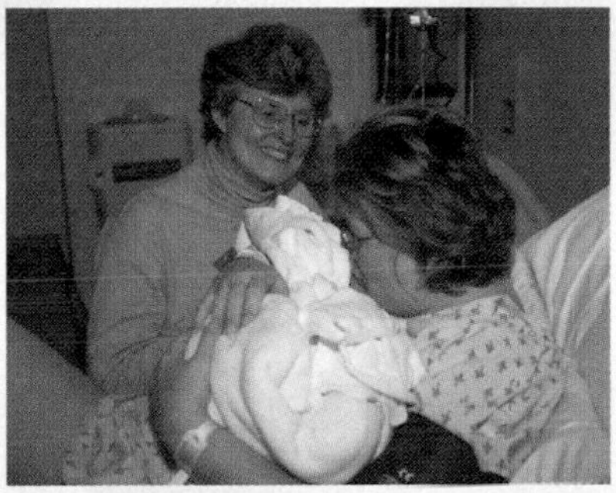

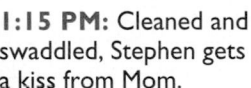

1:15 PM: Cleaned and swaddled, Stephen gets a kiss from Mom.

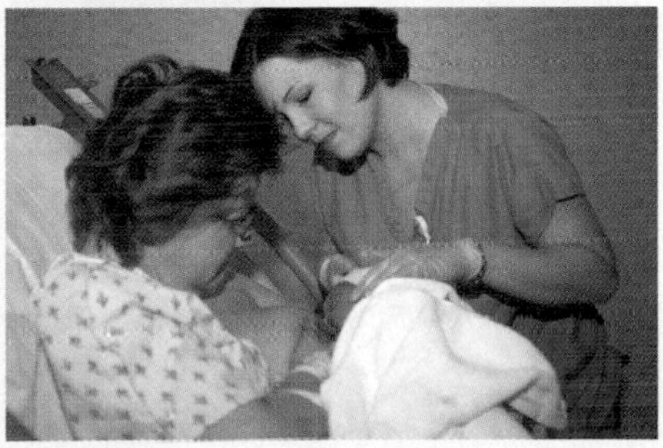

3:00 PM: Linda gives Stephen his first feeding, with a little help from the nurse.

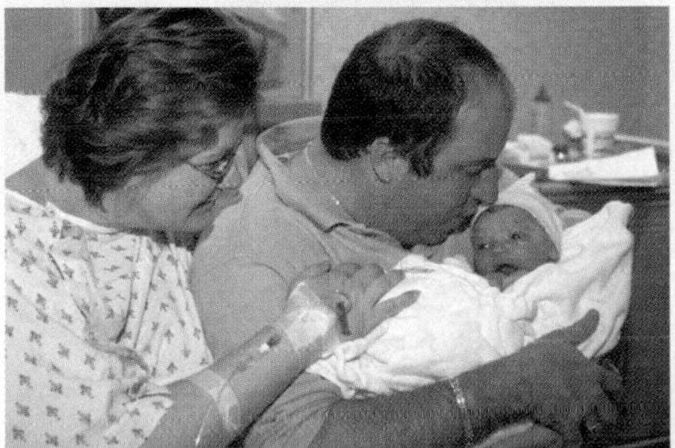

5:00 PM: Aaron and Linda bond with the new member of their family.

to failure to progress and fetal distress because they do not allow for adequate placental filling. All these possibilities make evaluating the rate, intensity, and pattern of uterine contractions an important nursing responsibility.

Phases. A contraction consists of three phases: the increment, when the intensity of the contraction increases; the acme, when the contraction is at its strongest; and the decrement, when the intensity decreases (Fig. 18-10). Between contractions the uterus relaxes. As labor progresses, the relaxation intervals decrease from 10 minutes early in labor to 2 to 3 minutes. The duration of contractions also changes, increasing from 20 to 30 seconds to a range of 60 to 90 seconds.

Contour Changes. As labor contractions progress and become regular and strong, the uterus gradually differentiates itself into two distinct functioning areas. The upper portion becomes thicker and active, preparing it to exert the strength necessary to expel the fetus when the expulsion phase of labor is reached. The lower segment becomes thin-walled, supple, and passive, so the fetus can be pushed out of the uterus easily. As these events occur, the boundary between the two portions becomes marked by a ridge on the inner uterine surface, the **physiologic retraction ring.**

The contour of the overall uterus also changes from a round, ovoid structure to an elongated one whose vertical diameter is markedly greater than its horizontal diameter. This lengthening serves to straighten the body of the fetus, placing it in better alignment to the cervix and pelvis. As the uterus contracts, the round ligaments move, keeping the fundus forward, again to assist with placing the fetus in good alignment with the cervix. The elongation of the uterus exerts pressure against the diaphragm and causes the often-expressed sensation that a uterus is "taking control" of the woman's body.

In a difficult labor, particularly when the fetus is larger than the birth canal, the round ligaments of the uterus become tense during dilatation and expulsion and may be palpable on the abdomen. The normal physiologic retraction ring may become prominent and observable as an abdominal indentation. Termed a **pathologic retraction ring** or Bandl's ring, it is a danger sign that signifies impending rupture of the lower uterine segment if the obstruction to labor is not relieved (Cunningham et al., 2001).

Cervical Changes

Even more marked than the changes in the body of the uterus are two changes that occur in the cervix: effacement (thinning) and dilatation (enlargement).

Effacement. **Effacement** is shortening and thinning of the cervical canal. Normally, the canal is approximately 1 to 2 cm long. With effacement, this canal virtually disappears (Fig. 18-11). This occurs because of longitudinal traction from the contracting uterine fundus.

In primiparas, effacement is accomplished before dilatation begins. Be sure to inform the woman of this. Otherwise, she may become discouraged if, for example, at noon after a cervical examination she is 2 cm dilated and then at 4 PM she is still 2 cm dilated. This type of report makes it seem to her that absolutely nothing has happened in 4 hours. However, effacement will have been occurring, and when complete, dilatation will then progress rapidly.

In multiparas, dilatation may proceed before effacement is complete. Effacement must occur at the end of dilatation, however, before the fetus can be safely pushed through the cervical canal or cervical tearing may result.

Dilatation. **Dilatation** refers to the enlargement of the cervical canal from an opening a few millimeters wide to one large enough (approximately 10 cm) to permit passage of the fetus (see Fig. 18-11).

Dilatation occurs for two reasons. First, uterine contractions gradually increase the diameter of the cervical canal lumen by pulling the cervix up over the presenting part of the fetus. Second, the fluid-filled membranes press against the cervix. If the membranes are intact, they push ahead of

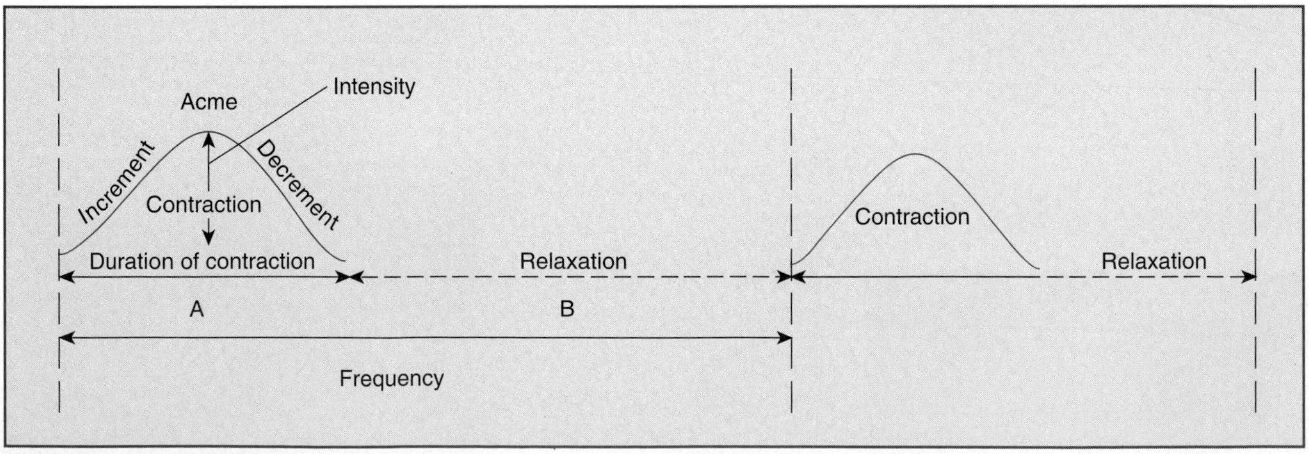

FIGURE 18.10 The interval and duration of uterine contractions. The frequency of contractions is the time from the beginning of one contraction to the beginning of the next contraction. It consists of two parts: (*A*) the duration of the contraction and (*B*) the period of relaxation. The *broken line* indicates an indeterminate period because the relaxation time (*B*) is usually of longer duration than the actual contraction (*A*).

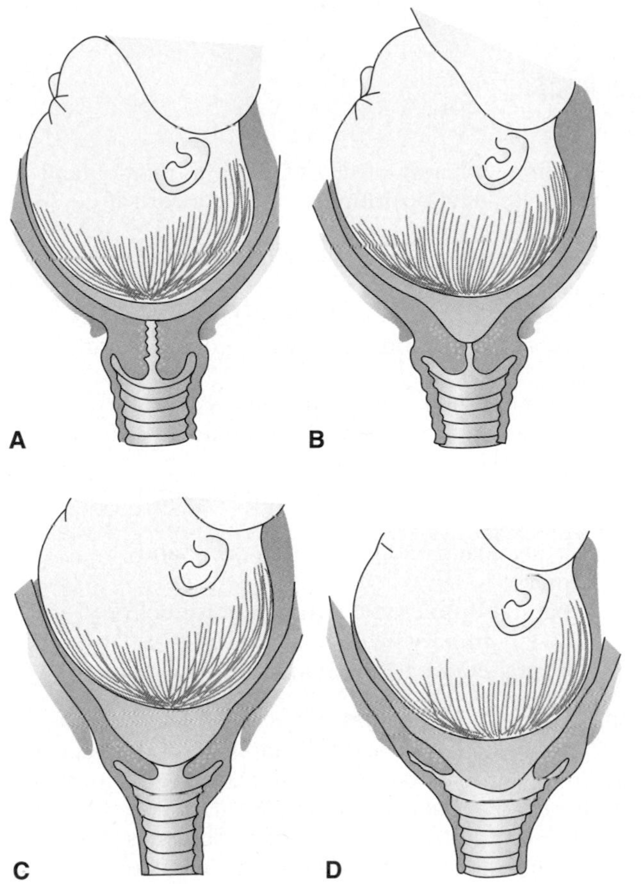

FIGURE 18.11 Effacement and dilatation of cervix. (*A*) Beginning labor. (*B*) Effacement is beginning; dilation is not apparent yet. (*C*) Effacement is almost complete. (*D*) After complete effacement, dilatation proceeds rapidly.

the fetus and serve as an opening wedge. If they are ruptured, the presenting part serves this same function.

As dilatation begins, there is an increase in the amount of vaginal secretions (termed show), because the last of the operculum or the mucus plug in the cervix is dislodged, and minute capillaries in the cervix rupture.

Psyche

The fourth "P," or "psyche," refers to the psychological state or feelings that women bring into labor with them. For many women, this is a feeling of apprehension or fright. For almost everyone, it includes a sense of excitement or awe.

Women who manage best in labor typically are those who have a strong sense of self-esteem and a meaningful support person. These allow women to feel in control of sensations and circumstances they have not experienced previously and are not at all what they pictured as happening (Moore, 2001).

Encouraging women to ask questions at prenatal visits and attend preparation for childbirth classes helps prepare them for labor. Encouraging them to share their experience after labor serves as "debriefing time" and helps them integrate the experience into their total life

✔ **CHECKPOINT QUESTIONS**

9. What are the six cardinal mechanisms of labor?
10. What term is used to describe the intensity of the contraction at its strongest point?
11. What two cervical changes occur during labor?

STAGES OF LABOR

In nursing literature, labor is traditionally divided into three stages: a first stage of dilatation, beginning with true labor contractions and ending when the cervix is fully dilated; a second stage, from the time of full dilatation until the infant is born; and a third or placental stage, from the time the infant is born until after the delivery of the placenta. The first 1 to 4 hours after birth of the placenta are sometimes termed the "fourth stage" to emphasize the importance of the close observation needed at this time. This designation can be helpful in planning nursing interventions to ensure the safety of both the mother and the fetus. Box 18-2 highlights appropriate outcomes and interventions using the terminology identified by the Nursing Outcomes Classification (NOC) and Nursing Interventions Classification (NIC).

Friedman (1978), a physician who studied the process of labor extensively, used data to identify two phases of labor: latent and active phases. He further divided the active phase into three parts. His data, when plotted in graph form, are useful in monitoring an individual woman's labor progress (Fig. 18-12). Friedman's terms—preparatory division, dilatational division, and pelvic division—correspond to the first and second stages of labor described here. Table 18-4 lists clinical features of the divisions of labor as described by Friedman. Because his "norms" refer to averages, an individual woman's labor can vary greatly from the ideal projected course of labor and still be normal for that woman.

Typically, a labor progress graph is labeled as follows:

- Left side numbered from 1 to 10 (representing the centimeters of cervical dilatation)
- Bottom line numbered to represent the number of hours of labor
- Right side numbered from –4 to +4 (representing the station of the presenting part)

After each cervical examination, cervical dilatation and **fetal descent** are plotted on the graph. The pattern of cervical dilatation usually plots as an S-shaped curve. The fetal descent pattern forms a downward curve. Both lines cross at the point of maximum cervical dilatation. A typical labor graph is shown in Figure 18-13.

First Stage

The first stage of labor is divided into three phases: the latent, the active, and the transition phases.

Latent Phase

The latent or preparatory phase begins at the onset of regularly perceived uterine contractions and ends when rapid cervical dilatation begins. Contractions during this

BOX 18.2

NURSING OUTCOMES CLASSIFICATION AND NURSING INTERVENTIONS CLASSIFICATION: INTRAPARTAL PERIOD

NOC: Maternal Status, Intrapartum

Maternal status, intrapartum, is defined as the conditions and behaviors indicating maternal well-being from the onset of labor to delivery (Johnson, Maas, & Moorhead, 2000). Some specific indicators suggesting achievement of this outcome include demonstration of the following:

- Coping mechanisms
- Techniques to facilitate labor
- Uterine contraction frequency, duration, and intensity within expected range
- Physiologic parameters such as vital signs, neurologic reflexes, urine output, and blood glucose levels within expected range
- Progressive cervical dilation

NOC: Fetal Status, Intrapartum

Fetal status, intrapartum, is defined as the conditions and behaviors indicating fetal well-being from the onset of labor to delivery (Johnson, Maas, & Moorhead, 2000). Some specific indicators suggesting achievement of this outcome include demonstration of the following:

- Fetal heart rate between 120 and 160 beats per minute
- Fetal position, presenting part, heart rate, and scalp blood pH within expected range
- Amniotic fluid color and amount within expected range
- Deceleration patterns and variability findings without deviation from expected

NIC: Intrapartal Care

Intrapartal care is defined as the monitoring and management of stages one and two of the birth process (McCloskey & Bulechek, 2000). Some important activities involved when implementing this intervention include:

- Admitting client to birthing area after determining that client is in labor
- Determining if client's membranes have ruptured
- Encouraging family participation as appropriate with the labor process
- Performing Leopold maneuver and vaginal exams as appropriate
- Monitoring maternal vital signs and fetal heart rate and patterns, reporting any deviations or abnormalities
- Applying electronic fetal monitor as appropriate (see next NIC)
- Assessing pain level, instituting positioning, breathing, relaxation, and other methods for pain control; administering analgesics as ordered
- Providing ice chips, wet washcloth, or hard candy
- Encouraging voiding at least every 2 hours
- Assisting with anesthetic administration
- Assisting with amniotomy with assessment of fetal heart rate, fetal positioning, and fetal cord after amniotomy
- Cleansing perineum and assisting with pad changes regularly
- Monitoring progress including vaginal discharge, cervical dilation and effacement, position, and fetal descent
- Performing vaginal examinations as necessary
- Encouraging spontaneous bearing-down efforts for second stage
- Evaluating pushing efforts and length of time in second stage
- Assisting coach and supporting client and partner
- Preparing supplies and equipment for delivery
- Notifying primary health care provider at appropriate time to scrub for attending delivery

NIC: Electronic Fetal Monitoring, Intrapartum

Electronic fetal monitoring, intrapartum, is defined as electronic evaluation of the fetal heart rate response to uterine contractions during intrapartal care (McCloskey & Bulechek, 2000). Some important activities involved when implementing this intervention include:

- Verifying maternal and fetal heart rate response to uterine contractions during intrapartal care
- Instructing client and partner about reasons for electronic monitoring
- Applying tocotransducer snugly after determining fetal position via Leopold maneuver
- Palpating to determine contraction intensity with tocotransducer use
- Differentiating among multiple fetuses by documenting on tracing and comparing data when simultaneous tracings are being used
- Discussing appearance of rhythm strip with client and support person
- Reassuring client about normal fetal heart rates
- Adjusting monitor to achieve and maintain clear tracing
- Interpreting rhythm strips when at least a 10-minute tracing has been obtained
- Documenting elements of external tracing and relevant intrapartal care
- Initiating fetal resuscitation interventions (see below) to treat abnormalities
- Documenting changes in fetal heart patterns after resuscitation
- Applying internal fetal electrode and internal uterine pressure catheter after rupture of membranes, when necessary
- Documenting maternal and fetal response to internal monitoring placement

continued on page 483

Continued

NURSING OUTCOMES CLASSIFICATION AND NURSING INTERVENTIONS CLASSIFICATION: INTRAPARTAL PERIOD

- Keeping primary health care provider informed of changes
- Continuing electronic monitoring through second-stage labor or up to time of cesarean delivery, with removal if cesarean delivery is necessary
- Documenting monitor interpretation, including providing safekeeping of intrapartal strip as part of the permanent record

NIC: Resuscitation, Fetus

Resuscitation, fetus, is defined as administering emergency measures to improve placental perfusion or correct fetal acid–base status (McCloskey & Bulechek, 2000). Some important activities involved when implementing this intervention include:

- Assessing fetal vital signs, including observation of abnormalities
- Repositioning client to lateral or hands-knees position
- Applying oxygen at 6 to 8 L/minute if positioning is ineffective
- Initiating intravenous therapy, including administration of fluid bolus, as ordered
- Performing vaginal examination with fetal scalp stimulation
- Documenting strip interpretation, including activities performed, and fetal and maternal response
- Reassuring client and support person
- Decreasing uterine activity by stopping oxytocin infusion or administering tocolytic medication as appropriate
- Performing amniotransfusion for abnormal variable decelerations or meconium-stained amniotic fluid
- Turning client to left lateral position for pushing during second stage
- Anticipating requirements for mode of delivery and neonatal support based on fetal responses to resuscitation techniques

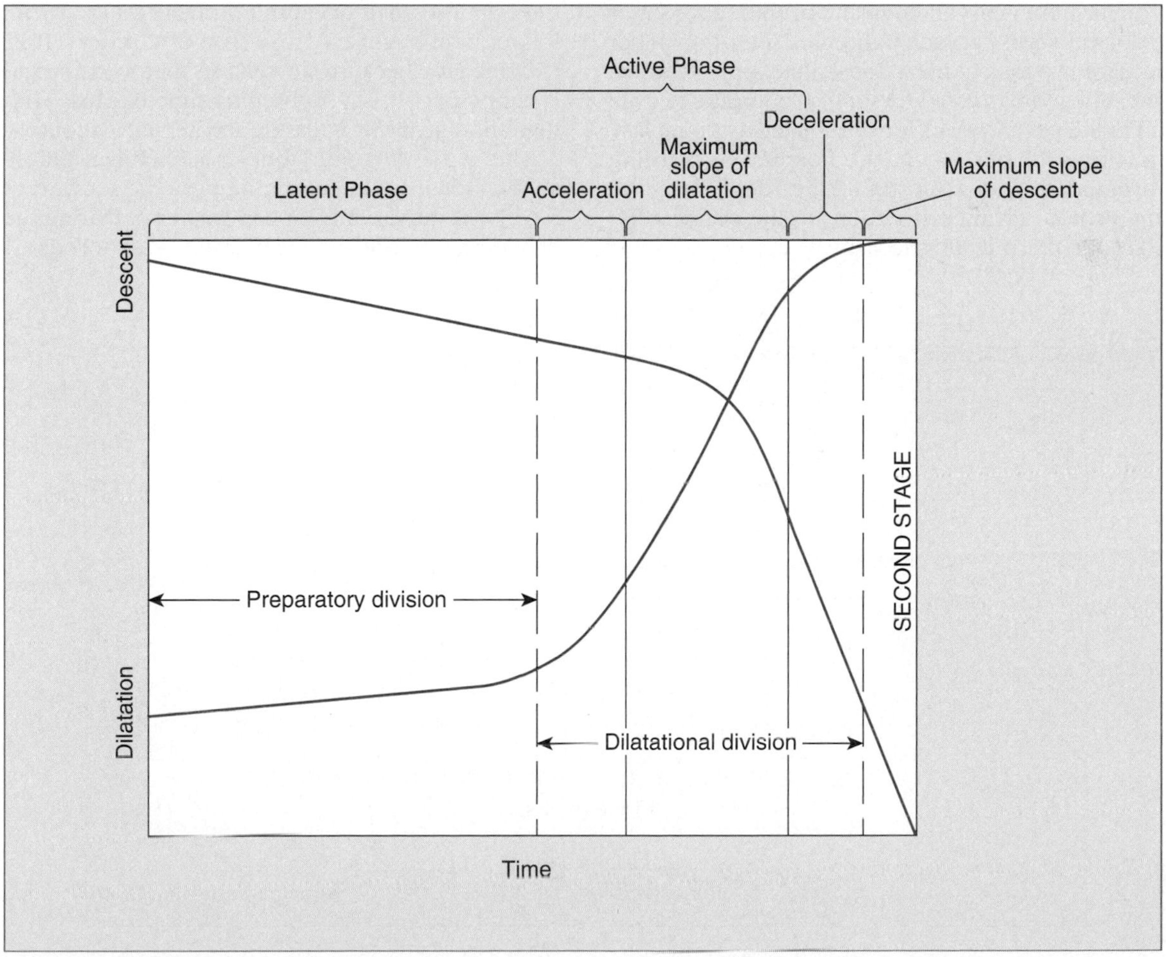

FIGURE 18.12 Divisions of labor.

TABLE 18.4 Principal Clinical Features of the Divisions of Labor

	FIRST STAGE		SECOND STAGE
FEATURE	*Preparatory Division*	*Dilatational Division*	*Pelvic Division*
Functions	Contractions coordinated, cervix prepared	Cervix actively dilating	Pelvis negotiated; mechanisms of labor; fetal descent; birth
Interval	Latent phase	Acceleration and phase of maximum slope	Deceleration phase and maximum descent
Measurement	Elapsed duration	Linear rate of dilatation	Linear rate of descent
Diagnosable disorders	Prolonged latent phase	Protracted dilatation; protracted descent	Prolonged deceleration; secondary arrest of dilatation; arrest of descent; failure of descent

From Friedman, E. (1978). *Labor, clinical evaluation and management* (2nd ed.). New York: Appleton-Century-Crofts, p. 54, with permission.

phase are mild and short, lasting 20 to 40 seconds. Cervical effacement occurs, and the cervix dilates from 0 to 3 cm. The phase lasts approximately 6 hours in a nullipara and 4.5 hours in a multipara. A woman who enters labor with a "nonripe" cervix will have a longer than usual latent phase. Analgesia given too early in labor will also prolong this phase. The latent phase may be prolonged if a cephalopelvic disproportion (a disproportion between the fetal head and pelvis) exists.

In a woman who is psychologically prepared for labor and who does not tense at each tightening sensation in her abdomen, latent phase contractions cause only minimal discomfort. The woman can (and should) continue to walk about and make preparations for birth, such as doing last-minute packing for her stay at the hospital or birthing center, preparing older children for her departure and upcoming birth, or giving instructions to the person who will take care of them while she is away.

Active Phase

During the active phase of labor, cervical dilatation occurs more rapidly, going from 4 cm to 7 cm. Contractions are stronger, lasting 40 to 60 seconds and occurring approximately every 3 to 5 minutes. This phase lasts approximately 3 hours in a nullipara and 2 hours in a multipara. Show (increased vaginal secretions) and perhaps spontaneous rupture of the membranes may occur. This can be a difficult time for a woman because contractions are stronger, last longer, and begin to cause true discomfort. It is also an exciting time because she realizes that something dramatic is happening. It is a frightening time because she realizes that labor is truly progressing and her life is about to change.

The active stage of labor in a Friedman graph can be subdivided into the following periods: acceleration (4 to 5 cm) and maximum slope (5 to 9 cm). During the period of maximum slope, cervical dilatation proceeds at its most

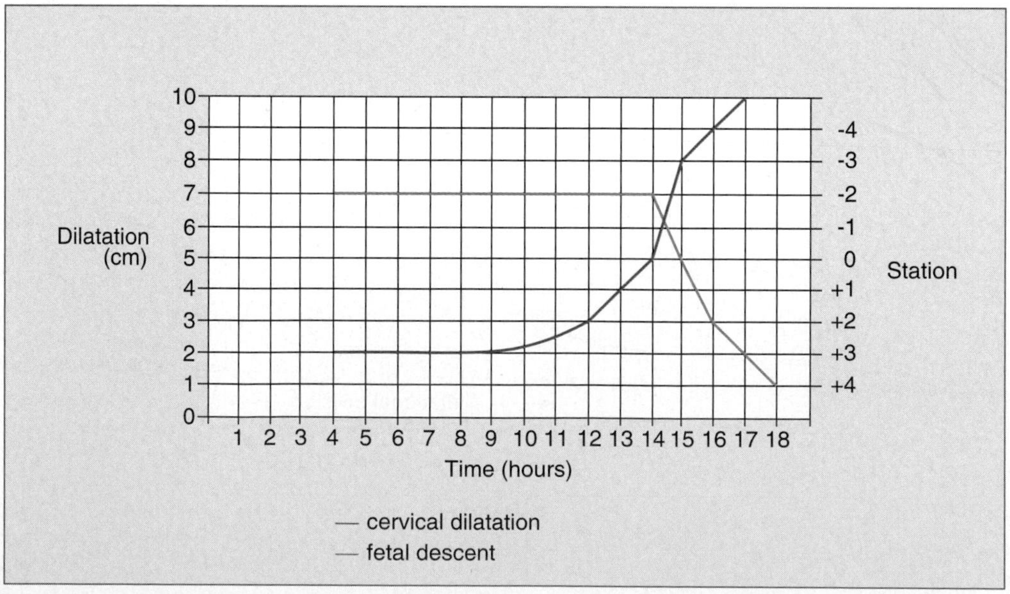

FIGURE 18.13 Normal labor graph. Fetal descent and cervical dilatation are occurring at the same time.

rapid pace, averaging 3.5 cm per hour in nulliparas and 5 to 9 cm per hour in multiparas. Administration of an analgesic at this point has little effect on the progress of labor.

Transition Phase

During the **transition** phase, maximum dilatation of 8 to 10 cm occurs, and contractions reach their peak of intensity, occurring every 2 to 3 minutes with a duration of 60 to 90 seconds. Dilatation continues at a rapid rate. If the membranes have not previously ruptured or been ruptured by amniotomy, they will rupture as a rule at full dilatation (10 cm). If it has not previously occurred, show will be present as the last of the mucus plug from the cervix is released. By the end of this phase, full dilatation (10 cm) and complete cervical effacement (obliteration of the cervix) have occurred.

During this phase, the woman may experience intense discomfort, so strong it is accompanied by nausea and vomiting. Because of the intensity and duration of the contractions, she may experience a feeling of loss of control, anxiety, panic, and irritability. The sensation in her abdomen may be so intense that it may seem as though labor has taken charge of her. A few minutes before, she enjoyed having her forehead wiped with a cool cloth. Now she may knock the wiper's hand away. A moment before, she enjoyed having her partner rub her back. Now she may resist being touched and push that person away. Her focus is entirely inward on the task of birthing her baby.

The peak of the transition phase can be identified by a slight slowing in the rate of cervical dilatation when 9 cm is reached (termed deceleration on a labor graph). As the woman reaches the end of this stage at 10 cm of dilatation, a new sensation (i.e., an irresistible urge to push) begins to occur.

Second Stage

The second stage of labor is the period from full dilatation and cervical effacement to birth of the infant. Contractions change from the characteristic crescendo–decrescendo pattern to an overwhelming, uncontrollable urge to push or bear down with contractions as if she had to move her bowels. The woman may experience momentary nausea or vomiting because pressure is no longer exerted on her stomach as the fetus descends in the pelvis. She pushes with such force that she perspires and the blood vessels in her neck may become distended.

As the fetal head touches the internal side of the perineum, the perineum begins to bulge and appear tense. The anus of the woman may appear everted. Stool may be expelled from the pressure exerted on it. As the fetal head is pushed still tighter against the perineum, the vaginal introitus opens and the fetal scalp becomes visible at the opening to the vagina. At first, this is a slitlike opening, which then becomes oval, then circular. The circle enlarges from the size of a dime to that of a quarter to that of a half-dollar. This is called crowning.

It takes a few contractions of this new type for the woman to realize that everything is still all right, just different, and to appreciate that it feels good, not frightening, to push with contractions. In fact, the need to push becomes so intense that she cannot stop herself. She barely hears the conversation in the room around her. All of her energy, her thoughts, her being are directed toward giving birth. As she pushes, using her abdominal muscles and the involuntary uterine contractions, the fetus is pushed out of the birth canal.

Third Stage

The third stage of labor, or the placental stage, begins with the birth of the infant and ends with the delivery of the placenta. Two separate phases are involved: placental separation and placental expulsion.

After the birth of the infant, the uterus can be palpated as a firm, round mass just inferior to the level of the umbilicus. After a few minutes of rest, uterine contractions begin again, and the organ assumes a discoid shape. It retains this new shape until the placenta has separated, approximately 5 minutes after the birth of the infant.

Placental Separation

Placental separation occurs automatically as the uterus resumes contractions. As the uterus contracts down on an almost empty interior, there is such a disproportion between the placenta and the contracting wall of the uterus that folding and separation of the placenta occur. Active bleeding on the maternal surface of the placenta begins with separation; the bleeding helps to separate the placenta still further by pushing it away from its attachment site. As separation is completed, the placenta sinks to the lower uterine segment or the upper vagina.

The following signs indicate that the placenta has loosened and is ready to deliver:

- Lengthening of the umbilical cord
- Sudden gush of vaginal blood
- Change in the shape of the uterus

If the placenta separates first at its center and last at its edges, it tends to fold on itself like an umbrella and will present at the vaginal opening with the fetal surface evident. Appearing shiny and glistening from the fetal membranes, it is called a Schultze's placenta. Approximately 80% of placentas separate and present in this way. If, however, the placenta separates first at its edges, it slides along the uterine surface and presents at the vagina with the maternal surface evident. It looks raw, red, and irregular with the ridges or cotyledons that separate blood collection spaces showing, and is called a Duncan placenta. A simple trick of remembering the presentations is associating "shiny" with Schultze (the fetal membrane surface) and "dirty" with Duncan (the irregular maternal surface) (Fig. 18-14).

Bleeding occurs as part of the normal consequence of placental separation, before the uterus contracts sufficiently to seal maternal sinuses. The normal blood loss is 300 to 500 mL.

Placental Expulsion

After separation, the placenta is delivered either by the natural bearing-down effort of the mother or by gentle pressure on the contracted uterine fundus by the physician or

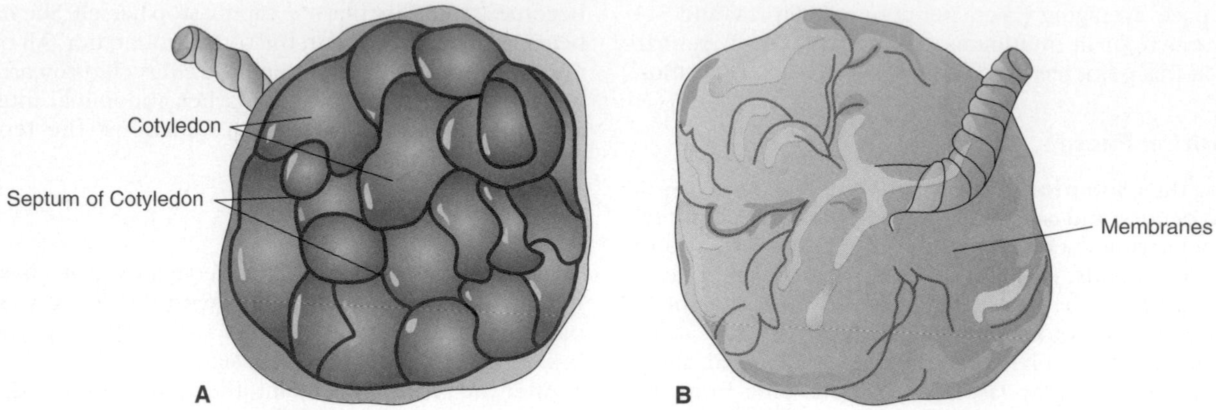

FIGURE 18.14 Maternal (*A*) and fetal (*B*) surface of the placenta.

nurse-midwife (Credé's maneuver). Pressure must never be applied to a uterus in a noncontracted state or the uterus may evert and hemorrhage. This is a grave complication of birth, because the maternal blood sinuses are open and gross hemorrhage occurs.

If the placenta does not deliver spontaneously, it can be removed manually. With delivery of the placenta, the third stage of labor is over. In some institutions, placentas are saved to have blood removed for stem cell research or the membranes may be used as temporary coverings for burns. In some cultures, parents want the placenta saved (see the Focus on Cultural Competence). Ask the parents if this is important to them before the placenta is destroyed.

✔ CHECKPOINT QUESTIONS

12. What are the three phases of the first stage of labor?
13. When does the second stage of labor begin?
14. What two phases are involved in the third stage of labor?

FOCUS ON CULTURAL COMPETENCE

For most health care providers in the United States, a placenta has little importance or meaning after its work of oxygenation is done and it is delivered. For many women, however, the placenta has continuing importance. For this reason, women may ask if they can take it home with them. In a number of Asian and Native American cultures, women bury the placenta to ensure that the child will continue to be healthy. In some parts of China, the placenta is cooked and eaten to ensure the continued health of the mother (Schneiderman, 1997). Be certain when supplying placentas to women that you respect standard precautions and hospital policy.

MATERNAL AND FETAL RESPONSES TO LABOR

Physiologic Effects of Labor on the Mother

Although labor is a local process that involves the abdomen and reproductive organs, its intensity is so great that almost all body systems are affected (Farrington & Ward, 2000).

Cardiovascular System

Labor involves strenuous work and effort, causing an increase in cardiac output, blood pressure, and pulse rate.

Cardiac Output. A contraction greatly decreases the blood flow to the uterus because it puts pressure against uterine arteries. This increases the amount of blood that remains in the general circulation, leading to an increase in peripheral resistance, which results in an increase in systolic and diastolic blood pressure. In addition, during pushing, the cardiac output may be increased as much as 40% to 50% above the prelabor level.

The average blood loss with birth (300 to 500 mL) is not detrimental to most women because of the blood volume increase that occurs during pregnancy. It actually plays a role in reducing blood volume to prepregnancy levels. Immediately after birth, with the weight and pressure removed from the pelvis, blood from the peripheral circulation may flood into the pelvic vasculature, momentarily dropping the pressure in the vena cava. The body quickly compensates for this, and a heavy load of blood is delivered to the heart, causing cardiac output to peak at 80% above prelabor levels. As pressure of the uterus against the vena cava is no longer present, within the first hour after delivery cardiac output will decrease from these high levels by about 50%. The average woman's heart adjusts well to even these changes. If she has a cardiac problem, however, these sudden hemodynamic changes can have implications for her (see Chap. 14).

Blood Pressure. With the increased cardiac output during contractions, systolic blood pressure rises an average of 15 mm Hg with each contraction. Higher increases could be a sign of pathology. When the woman lies in a supine position and pushes, her blood pressure can drop precipitously, leading to hypotension. An upright or side-lying position during the second stage of labor can help avoid such a problem.

Hemopoietic System

The major change in the blood-forming system that occurs during birth is the development of leukocytosis or a sharp increase in the number of circulating white blood cells, possibly as a result of stress and heavy exertion. At the end of labor, the average woman has a white blood cell count of 25,000/mm^3 to 30,000/mm^3 cells, compared with a normal of 5,000/mm^3 to 10,000/mm^3.

Respiratory System

Whenever there is an increase in cardiovascular parameters, the body responds by increasing respiratory rate to supply additional oxygen. This can result in hyperventilation. Using appropriate breathing patterns helps to avoid severe hyperventilation. Total oxygen consumption increases about 100% during the second stage of labor. This is comparable to that of a person performing a strenuous exercise such as running.

Temperature Regulation

The increased muscular activity associated with labor may result in a slight elevation (1°) in temperature. Diaphoresis occurs with accompanying evaporation to cool and limit excessive warming.

Fluid Balance

Because of the increase in rate and depth of respirations (which causes moisture to be lost with each breath) and diaphoresis, insensible water loss increases during labor. Fluid balance is further affected by the withholding of oral intake to only sips of fluid or ice cubes or hard candy. The combination of increased losses and decreased intake may make intravenous fluid replacement necessary if labor is prolonged.

Urinary System

With the decrease in fluid intake during labor and the increased insensible water loss, kidneys begin to concentrate urine to preserve both fluid and electrolytes. Specific gravity may rise to a high normal level of 1.020 to 1.030. It is not unusual for protein (trace to 1+) to be evident in urine from the breakdown of protein due to increased muscle activity. Pressure of the fetal head as it descends in the birth canal against the anterior bladder reduces bladder tone or the ability of the bladder to sense filling. Overfilling, unless the woman is asked to void approximately every 2 hours during labor, may occur, possibly decreasing bladder tone in the postpartal period.

Musculoskeletal System

All during pregnancy, relaxin, an ovarian-released hormone, has acted to soften the cartilage between bones. In the week before labor, considerable additional softening causes the symphysis pubis and sacral/coccyx joints to be even more relaxed and movable, allowing them to stretch apart to increase the size of the pelvic ring by as much as 2 cm. This increased pubic flexibility may be noted as increased back pain or irritating nagging pain at the pubis as the woman walks or turns in labor.

Gastrointestinal System

The gastrointestinal system becomes fairly inactive during labor. This is probably due to the shunting of blood to more life-sustaining organs and also to pressure on the stomach and intestine from the contracting uterus. Digestive and emptying time of the stomach is prolonged, explaining why eating during labor is usually restricted. Some women experience a loose bowel movement as contractions grow strong, similar to what they may experience with menstrual cramps.

Neurologic and Sensory Responses

The neurologic responses that occur during labor are those responses related to pain (increased pulse and respiratory rate). Early in labor, the contraction of the uterus and dilatation of the cervix cause the discomfort. This pain is registered at uterine and cervical nerve plexuses (at the level of the 11th and 12th thoracic nerves). At the moment of birth, the pain is centered on the perineum as it stretches to allow the fetus to move past it. Perineal pain is registered at S2 to S4 nerves.

Psychological Responses of the Woman to Labor

Labor can lead to emotional distress because it represents the beginning of a major life change for the woman and her partner. Even for the most organized woman, pain reduces the ability to cope and may make her short-tempered or quick to criticize things around her. Admitting her quickly to a birthing room in an environment free from outside interference will help her begin to control her breathing patterns and reduce the pain of early contractions, as well as begin to organize coping strategies.

Fatigue

By the time the date of birth approaches, a woman is generally tired from the burden of carrying so much extra weight with her. In addition, most women do not sleep well during the last month of pregnancy. Because they have backache in a side-lying position, they turn on their back and the fetus kicks and wakens them; they turn to their side and their back aches again, and so on. Sleep hunger from this discomfort can make it difficult for them to perceive situations clearly or to adjust rapidly to new situations. A little deficiency such as a wrinkled sheet can appear as a threatening discrepancy in their care. The process of labor can loom as an overwhelming, unendurable experience.

Fear

Women appreciate a review of the labor process early in labor because it serves as a reminder that childbirth is not a strange, bewildering experience but a predictable and well-documented one. Explain that contractions last a certain length and reach a certain firmness but always have a rest period in between.

Being taken by surprise—labor moving faster or slower than a woman thought it would—can be frightening. It brings to mind any horror stories of labor that a woman has heard. Compounding this, the woman may begin to worry that her infant may die or be born with an abnormality; she may be afraid she will not meet her own behavior expectations. Explain that labor is predictable, but also variable, to limit this kind of fear.

Cultural Influences

Cultural factors influence a woman's experience of labor. In the past, American women were accustomed to following hospital procedures and the medical model of care and so followed instructions with few questions. Today, women are educated to question modes of care. In addition, every woman in labor responds to cultural cues in some way. This makes her response to pain, her choice of nourishment, her preferred birthing position, the proximity and involvement of a support person, and customs related to the immediate postpartum period individualized (Moore, 2001).

To make labor a positive experience, be prepared to adapt your care to the woman's specific circumstances. A woman may have traditions that run counter to American hospital protocols. Address these differences and make arrangements to accommodate her beliefs or customs if possible (e.g., providing warm food or fluids during labor or saving the placenta for the mother to take home). If you do not speak the woman's language, arranging for an interpreter or working closely with a family member who can interpret may be necessary.

Fetal Responses to Labor

Although the fetus is basically a passive participant in labor, the effect of pressure and circulatory changes that occur with contractions cause detectable physiologic differences.

Neurologic System

Uterine contractions exert pressure on the fetal head, so the same response involved with that of any instance of increased intracranial pressure occurs. The fetal heart rate (FHR) decreases by as much as 5 bpm during a contraction as soon as contraction strength reaches 40 mm Hg. This decrease appears on a fetal heart monitor as an early deceleration pattern.

Cardiovascular System

The ability to respond to cardiovascular changes is usually mature enough that the average fetus is unaffected by the continual variations of heart rate that occur with labor—a slight slowing and then a return to normal (baseline) levels. During a contraction, the arteries of the uterus are sharply constricted and, therefore, the filling of cotyledons almost completely halts. The amount of nutrients, including oxygen, exchanged during this time is reduced, causing a slight but inconsequential fetal hypoxia. Increased intracranial pressure from uterine pressure on the fetal head serves to keep circulation from falling below normal during the duration of a contraction.

Integumentary System

The pressure involved in the birth process is often reflected in minimal petechiae or ecchymotic areas on the fetus (particularly the presenting part). There may also be edema of the presenting part (caput succedaneum).

Musculoskeletal System

The force of uterine contractions tends to push the fetus into a position of full flexion. A fully flexed position is the most advantageous for birth because it can speed labor.

Respiratory System

The process of labor appears to aid in the maturation of surfactant production by alveoli in the fetal lung. The pressure applied to the chest from contractions and passage through the birth canal clears it of lung fluid. Thus, the infant born vaginally tends to be able to establish respirations easier than the fetus born by cesarean birth (Cunningham et al., 2001).

Danger Signs of Labor

A wide variation exists among individual patterns of labor contractions and maternal responses to labor and birth. Certain signs, however, indicate that the course of events is deviating too far from normal. These signs, both fetal and maternal, are described below (see Assessing for Danger Signs of Labor). Nursing care of the woman experiencing a complication during labor or birth is addressed in Chapter 21.

Fetal Danger Signs

High or Low Fetal Heart Rate. As a rule, an FHR of more than 160 bpm (fetal tachycardia) or less than 110 bpm (fetal bradycardia) is a sign of possible fetal distress. An equally important sign is a late or variable deceleration pattern (described below) on the fetal monitor. The fetal heart rate may return to a normal range in between these irregular patterns and give a false sense of security if FHR is assessed only between contractions.

Meconium Staining. Meconium staining, a green color in the amniotic fluid, is not always a sign of fetal distress but is highly correlated with its occurrence. It reveals that the fetus has had an episode of loss of sphincter control, allowing meconium to pass into the amniotic fluid. It may indicate that the fetus has or is experiencing hypoxia, which stimulates the vagal reflex and leads to increased bowel motility. Although meconium staining may be normal in a breech presentation, as pressure on the buttocks causes meconium loss, it should always be reported immediately so its cause can be investigated.

Hyperactivity. Ordinarily, a fetus is quiet and barely moves during labor. Fetal hyperactivity may be a sign that

ASSESSING for Danger Signs of Labor

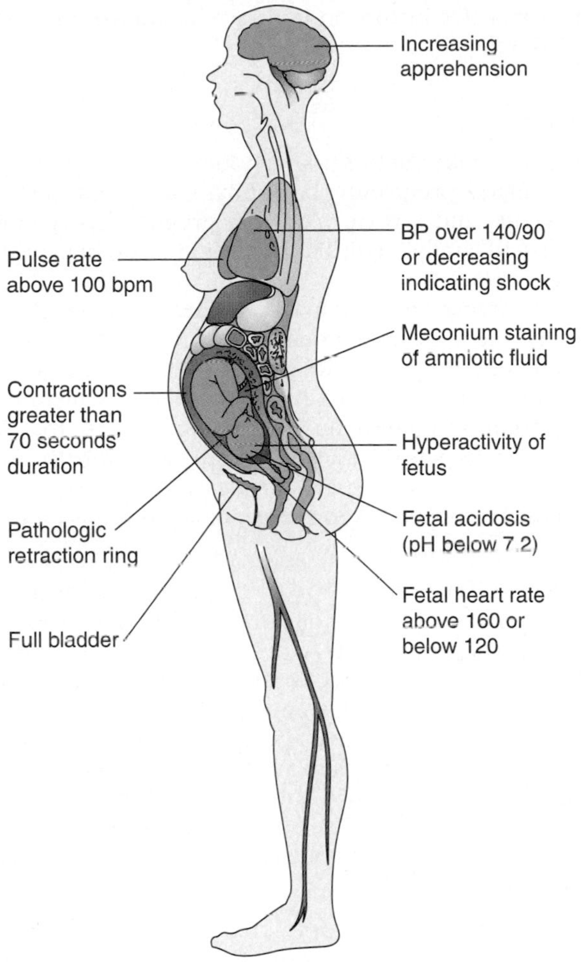

hypoxia is occurring because exertion is a common reaction to the need for oxygen.

Fetal Acidosis. When blood analyses are made on the fetus during labor by use of a scalp capillary technique, the finding of acidosis (blood pH below 7.2) is a certain sign that fetal well-being is becoming compromised.

Maternal Danger Signs

Rising or Falling Blood Pressure. Normally, maternal blood pressure rises slightly in the second (pelvic) stage of labor due to her pushing effort. A systolic pressure greater than 140 mm Hg and a diastolic pressure greater than 90 mm Hg, or an increase in the systolic pressure of more than 30 mm Hg and a diastolic pressure of more than 15 mm Hg (the basic criteria for pregnancy-induced hypertension), should be reported. Just as important to report is a falling blood pressure, because it may be the first sign of intrauterine hemorrhage. A falling blood pressure is often associated with other clinical signs of shock such as apprehension, increased pulse rate, and pallor.

Abnormal Pulse. Most pregnant women have an average pulse rate of 70 to 80 bpm. Pulse normally increases slightly during the second stage of labor due to the exertion involved. A maternal pulse greater than 100 bpm during the normal course of labor is unusual and should be reported. It may be another indication of hemorrhage.

Inadequate or Prolonged Contractions. Uterine contractions normally become more frequent, intense, and longer as labor progresses. If they become less frequent, less intense, or shorter in duration, this may indicate uterine exhaustion (inertia). If this problem cannot be corrected, a cesarean birth may be necessary.

A period of relaxation must be present between contractions so the intervillous spaces of the uterus can fill and maintain an adequate supply of oxygen and nutrients for the fetus. As a rule, uterine contractions lasting longer than 70 seconds should be reported because contractions of this length may begin to compromise fetal well-being by interfering with adequate uterine artery filling.

Pathologic Retraction Ring. An indentation across the woman's abdomen where the upper and lower segments of the uterus join may be a sign of extreme uterine stress and possible impending uterine rupture. For this reason, it is important to observe the contours of the abdomen periodically during labor. Fetal heartbeat auscultation automatically provides a regular opportunity to assess the woman's abdomen. If an electronic monitor is in place, it is necessary to make this observation deliberately.

Abnormal Lower Abdominal Contour. A full bladder during labor may be manifested as a round bulge on the lower anterior abdomen. This is a danger signal for two reasons: first, the bladder may be injured by the pressure of the fetal head; second, the pressure of the full bladder may not allow the fetal head to descend.

Increasing Apprehension. Warnings of psychological danger during labor are as important to consider in assessing maternal well-being as physical signs. A woman who is becoming increasingly apprehensive despite clear explanations of unfolding events may only be approaching the second stage of labor. She may, however, not be "hearing" because she has a concern that has not been met. Using an approach such as, "You seem more and more concerned. Could you tell me what is worrying you?" may be helpful. Increasing apprehension also needs to be investigated for physical reasons because it can be a sign of oxygen deprivation or internal hemorrhage.

✔ CHECKPOINT QUESTIONS

15. What is the average increase in systolic blood pressure during a contraction?
16. How rapid a pulse during labor is considered a danger sign?
17. What length of uterine contractions is long enough to compromise fetal well-being?

MATERNAL AND FETAL ASSESSMENT DURING LABOR

Immediate Assessment of the Woman in Stage One

A number of immediate assessment measures are necessary to safeguard maternal and fetal health once a woman arrives at a birthing facility. After the woman and her support person are oriented to the area, procedures focus on obtaining these vital assessment data (see the Focus on Family Empowerment). The same data need to be obtained for a home birth.

Initial Interview and Physical Examination

Important data that need to be obtained include the extent of the woman's labor, her general physical condition, and her preparedness for labor and birth.

For an initial interview, obtain information about the following areas:

- Expected date of birth
- Frequency, duration, and intensity of contractions
- Amount and character of show
- Rupture of membranes
- Vital signs (temperature, pulse, respirations, and blood pressure [assessed between contractions])
- Time the woman last ate
- Any known drug allergies
- Past pregnancy history and previous pregnancy outcomes
- Her birth plan or what individualized measures she has planned, such as no analgesia or who will cut the umbilical cord

This amount of information is scant but helps to establish whether the woman is in active labor and needs intense care or whether she has arrived at the hospital or birthing center in an earlier stage of labor and will benefit from paced interventions.

After initial assessment procedures, a woman is categorized by her risk for having difficulty in labor or risk to the newborn needing special care at birth.

Detailed Assessment During the First Stage

If the woman is in active labor, the history taken on arrival may be the only history obtained until after the baby is born. If the woman is not facing imminent delivery, a more extensive history and physical examination can be carried out.

History

The history taken at this point should include a review of the woman's pregnancy, both physical and psychological events, and a review of past pregnancies, general health, and family medical information to aid in planning nursing care.

Interviewing a woman in labor in detail can be difficult because the woman is constantly interrupted by labor contractions. Be patient. Remember that the longest contraction is rarely more than 60 seconds. A woman may concentrate so intently on a breathing exercise that she completely forgets the question asked just before the contraction. As the contraction subsides, repeat the question as if it had not been asked before, or act as if it is no trouble to ask it again.

Current Pregnancy History. Important information needed for a complete history is documentation of gravida and para; a description of the pregnancy (if it was planned or not, pattern and place of prenatal care, whether nutrition was adequate, if any complications such as spotting, falls, hypertension of pregnancy, infection, or alcohol or drug ingestion occurred); plans for labor (does she want medication for pain, will she use breathing exercises, will she have a support person with her); and childcare (will she breast-feed or bottle-feed? Has she chosen a pediatrician?).

Past Pregnancy History. Document prior pregnancies (numbers, dates, types of birth, any complications, and outcomes, including sex and birthweight of children). What is the current health status of the children?

Past Health History. Document any previous surgery (surgical adhesions might interfere with free fetal passage); heart disease or diabetes (she will need special pre-

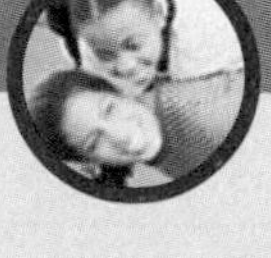

FOCUS ON FAMILY EMPOWERMENT

Admission Procedures for the Laboring Client

Q. What will happen when I arrive at a birthing center?

A. Every setting differs, but actions you can expect are:

- Orientation to a birthing room
- Baseline assessment of your temperature, pulse, respirations, and blood pressure
- Recording of your pregnancy history and physical examination
- Assessment of fetal heart rate
- A vaginal examination
- Urine and necessary blood samples obtained
- Explanation of fetal or uterine monitoring equipment to be used; connection of this equipment

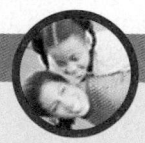

cautions during labor and birth); anemia (blood loss at birth may be more important than it is normally); tuberculosis (lung lesions may be reactivated at birth by changes in lung contour); kidney disease or hypertension (blood pressure will need to be watched even more carefully than it is normally); or a sexually transmitted disease such as herpes (the infant may be exposed to the disease by vaginal contact if the disease is still active). Determine if her lifestyle places her at high risk for human immunodeficiency virus (HIV) exposure.

Family Medical History. Ask if any family member has a heart disease, a blood dyscrasia, diabetes, kidney disease, cancer, allergies, seizures, congenital defects, or is cognitively challenged. Adequate preparation can then be made for a child who might have special needs.

Physical Examination

After history taking, the woman needs a thorough physical examination, including a pelvic examination, to confirm the presentation and position of the fetus and determine the stage of dilatation.

Physical assessment during labor begins, as does all physical assessment, with the woman's overall appearance and is similar to that for any woman. However, be prepared to adapt the techniques to the client's stage of labor and its progression. Does she appear tired? Pale? Ill? Frightened? Is there obvious edema or dehydration? Are there open lesions anywhere?

Palpate for enlargement of lymph nodes to detect the possibility of infection. Inspect the mucous membrane of the mouth and the conjunctiva of the eyes for color. Does the color (paleness) suggest anemia? What is the condition of her teeth? Are there any caries? Do any teeth appear abscessed (such a condition needs to be documented because it might account for a postpartum fever)? Examine the outer and inner surfaces of her lips carefully. Does she have herpes lesions (pinpoint vesicles on an erythematous base)? Type II (genital) virus can be lethal to newborns. If herpetic lesions are present anywhere, the woman will probably be isolated from her child until the lesions crust.

Assess lungs to be certain they are clear to auscultation. Listen for normal heart sounds and rhythms. Many pregnant women at term have a grade II to III systolic ejection murmur from the extra volume of blood that must cross the heart valves. Inspect and palpate her breasts. Are they free of cysts and lumps? Ask if she inspects her own breasts monthly. Do not try to teach breast self-examination while a woman is in labor. Most likely, she will be unable to concentrate on the instructions. If she needs education in this area, indicate it on her chart so the postpartum nursing staff can provide it before she is discharged.

Mark the chart also of a woman who has a palpable mass in her breasts for re-examination after labor and birth. This is probably an enlarged milk gland but needs further evaluation.

Abdominal Assessment. Assessing the abdomen is important for the woman in labor. Estimate fetal size by fundal height (should be at the level of the xiphoid process at term); assess presentation and position by Leopold's maneuvers (see below). Palpate and percuss the bladder area (over the symphysis pubis) to detect a full bladder. Assess for abdominal scars because abdominal or pelvic surgery can leave adhesions.

Finally, inspect the lower extremities for skin turgor for dehydration, edema, and varicose veins. Women with large varicosities are prone to thrombophlebitis after birth. Some physicians prefer not to use birth room stirrups if varicosities are prominent during labor, because the stirrups may press against them. Severe edema suggests hypertension of pregnancy, so the extent and intensity of edema must be assessed and correlated with the woman's blood pressure.

Leopold's Maneuvers

Leopold's maneuvers are a systematic method of observation and palpation to determine fetal presentation and position. They are described in Nursing Procedure 18-1.

Assessing Rupture of Membranes

One of every four labors begins with spontaneous rupture of the fetal membranes. When this occurs, there may be a sudden gush of amniotic fluid from the vagina. The woman may be startled by this sensation because it feels as if she has lost bladder control. She may be embarrassed before she realizes that the warm fluid on her perineum and legs is not urine but a sudden announcement that labor is beginning. In other women, rupture of membranes is more subtle, occurring as a slow loss of fluid. There may be a question whether the membranes have ruptured when this occurs.

A sterile vaginal examination using a sterile speculum usually reveals if amniotic fluid is present in the vagina. After vaginal secretions are obtained (usually by a sterile, cotton-tipped applicator), test them with a strip of Nitrazine paper. Vaginal secretions are acid; amniotic fluid is alkaline. If amniotic fluid has passed through the vagina recently, the pH of vaginal fluid will probably be alkaline (with a pH greater than 6.5) when tested by Nitrazine paper (appears blue-green or gray to deep blue). A false reading may occur in women with intact membranes who have a heavy bloody show, because blood is also alkaline. An additional test is a fern test (examination of vaginal secretions under a microscope). Because of its high estrogen content, amniotic fluid will show a fern pattern when dried and examined this way; urine will not.

For the woman whose membranes ruptured at home, ask her to describe the color of the amniotic fluid. It should be as clear as water. Yellow-stained fluid may indicate a blood incompatibility between mother and fetus (the amniotic fluid is bilirubin-stained from the breakdown of red blood cells). Green fluid indicates meconium staining. Although normal in breech deliveries because of buttocks compression, in a vertex presentation meconium staining may indicate fetal anoxia. A fetus with meconium staining needs immediate assessment to safeguard well-being. The infant will need continuing close assessment after birth because of possible meconium aspiration.

NURSING PROCEDURE 18.1: LEOPOLD'S MANEUVERS

Purpose

Systematically observing and palpating the abdomen to determine fetal presentation and position.

Procedure	Principle
1. Prepare the client.	
a. Explain the procedure.	a. Explanation reduces anxiety and enhances cooperation.
b. Instruct the client to empty her bladder.	b. Doing so promotes comfort and allows for more productive palpation because fetal contour will not be obscured by a distended bladder.
c. Position the woman supine with knees slightly flexed. Place a small pillow or rolled towel under one side.	c. Flexing the knees relaxes the abdominal muscles. Using a pillow or towel tilts the uterus off the vena cava, thus preventing supine hypotension syndrome.
d. Wash your hands using warm water.	d. Handwashing prevents the spread of possible infection. Using warm water aids in client comfort and prevents tightening of abdominal muscles.
e. Observe the woman's abdomen for longest diameter and where fetal movement is apparent.	e. The longest diameter (axis) is the length of the fetus. The location of activity most likely reflects the position of the feet.
2. Perform the first maneuver.	2. This maneuver determines whether fetal head or breech is in the fundus.
a. Stand at the foot of the client, facing her, and place both hands flat on her abdomen.	a. Proper positioning of hands ensures accurate findings.
b. Palpate the superior surface of the fundus. Determine consistency, shape, and mobility.	b. When palpating, a head feels more firm than a breech. A head is round and hard; the breech is less well defined. A head moves independently of the body; the breech moves only in conjunction with the body.

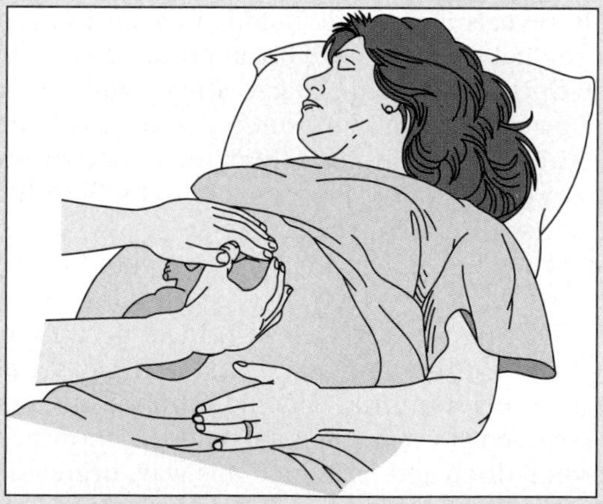

Procedure	Principle
3. Perform the second maneuver.	3. This maneuver locates the back of the fetus.
a. Face the client and place the palms of each hand on either side of the abdomen.	a. Proper positioning of hands ensures accurate findings.
b. Palpate the sides of the uterus. Hold the left hand stationary on the left side of the uterus while the right hand palpates the opposite side of the uterus from top to bottom. Then hold the right hand steady, and repeat palpation using the left hand on the left side.	b. This method is most successful to determine the direction the fetal back is facing. One hand will feel a smooth, hard, resistant surface (the back), while on the opposite side, a number of angular nodulations (the knees and elbows of the fetus) will be felt.

(continued)

Procedure	Principle
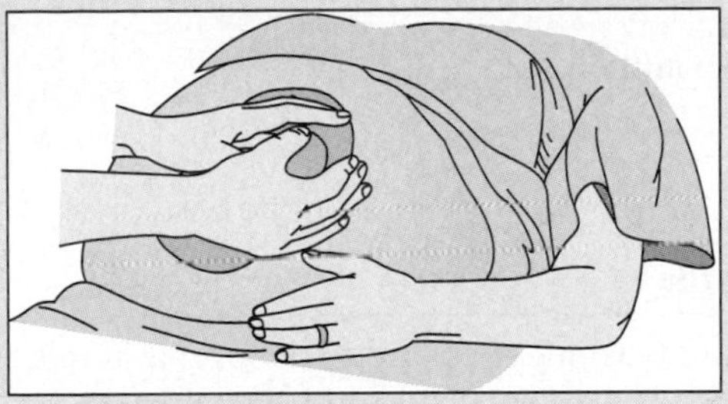	
4. Perform the third maneuver.	4. This maneuver determines the part of the fetus at the inlet and its mobility.
a. Gently grasp the lower portion of the abdomen just above the symphysis pubis between the thumb and index finger and try to press the thumb and finger together. Determine any movement and whether the part is firm or soft.	a. If the presenting part moves upward so an examiner's hands can be pressed together, the presenting part is not engaged (not firmly settled into the pelvis). If the part is firm, it is the head; if soft, then it is the breech.
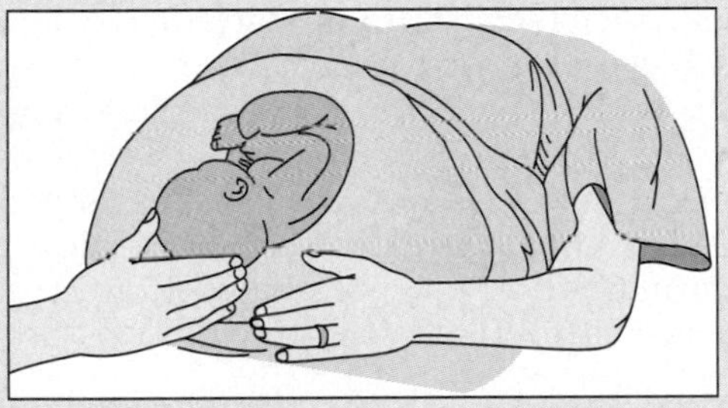	
5. Perform the fourth maneuver.	5. This maneuver determines fetal attitude and degree of fetal extension into the pelvis; should only be done if fetus is in cephalic presentation. Information about the infant's anteroposterior position may also be gained from this final maneuver.
a. Place fingers on both sides of the uterus approximately 2 inches above the inguinal ligaments, pressing downward and inward in the direction of the birth canal. Allow fingers to be carried downward. 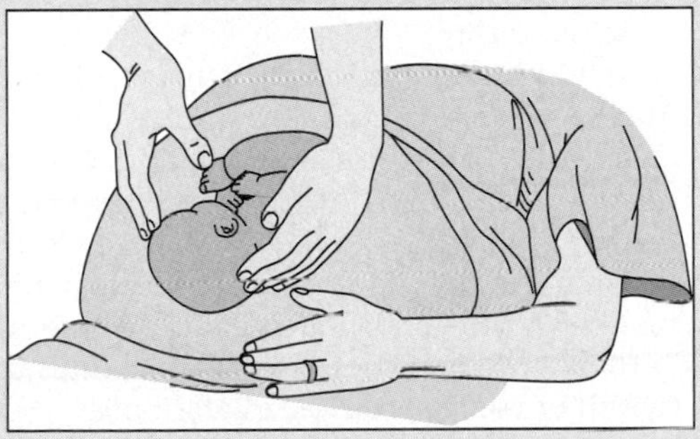	a. The fingers of one hand will slide along the uterine contour and meet no obstruction, indicating the back of the fetal neck. The other hand will meet an obstruction an inch or so above the ligament—this is the fetal brow. The position of the fetal brow should correspond to the side of the uterus that contained the elbows and knees of the fetus. If the fetus is in a poor attitude, the examining fingers will meet an obstruction on the same side as the fetal back. That is, the fingers will touch the hyperextended head. If the brow is very easily palpated (as if it lies just under the skin), the fetus is probably in a posterior position (the occiput is pointing toward the woman's back).

Vaginal Examination

A vaginal examination is necessary to determine the extent of cervical effacement and dilatation and to confirm the fetal presentation, position, and degree of descent. The technique for a vaginal examination in labor is shown in Nursing Procedure 18-2.

Vaginal examinations may be done either between contractions or during contractions. More fetal skull may be palpated during a contraction because the cervix retracts

NURSING PROCEDURE 18.2: VAGINAL EXAMINATION

Purpose

Determine cervical readiness and fetal position and presentation.

Procedure	Principle
1. Wash your hands; explain procedure to client. Provide privacy.	1. Handwashing helps prevent spread of microorganisms; explanations ensure client cooperation and compliance. Privacy enhances self-esteem.
2. Assess client status and adjust plan to individual client need.	2. Care is always individualized according to a client's needs.
3. Assemble equipment: sterile examining gloves, sterile lubricant, antiseptic solution. Ask the woman to turn onto back with knees flexed (a dorsal recumbent position). Put on sterile examining gloves.	3. Organization and planning improve efficiency. Positioning in this manner allows for good visualization of perineum. Using a sterile glove prevents contamination of birth canal.
4. Discard one drop of clean lubricating solution and drop an ample supply on tips of gloved fingers.	4. Discarding the first drop ensures that quantity used will not be contaminated.
5. Pour antiseptic solution over vulva using nondominant hand.	5. This prevents the spread of organisms from perineum to birth canal.
6. Place nondominant hand on the outer edges of the woman's vulva and spread her labia while inspecting the external genitalia for lesions. Look for red, irritated mucous membranes; open, ulcerated sores; clustered, pinpoint vesicles.	6. Positioning hands in this way allows for good perineal visualization. Presence of any lesions may indicate an infection and possibly preclude vaginal birth.
7. Look for escaping amniotic fluid or the presence of umbilical cord or bleeding.	7. Amniotic fluid implies membranes have ruptured and umbilical cord may have prolapsed. Bleeding may be a sign of placenta previa. *Do not do a vaginal examination if a possible placenta previa is present.*
8. If there is no bleeding or cord visible, introduce your index and middle fingers of dominant hand gently into the vagina, directing them toward the posterior vaginal wall.	8. The posterior vaginal wall is less sensitive than the anterior wall. Stabilize the uterus by placing your nondominant hand on the woman's abdomen.
9. Touch the cervix with your gloved examining fingers. a. Palpate for cervical consistency and rate if *firm* or *soft.*	9. a. The cervix feels like a circular rim of tissue around a center depression. Firm is similar to the tip of a nose; soft is as pliable as an earlobe. The anterior rim is usually the last portion to thin.
b. Measure the extent of dilatation; palpate for an anterior rim or lip of cervix. 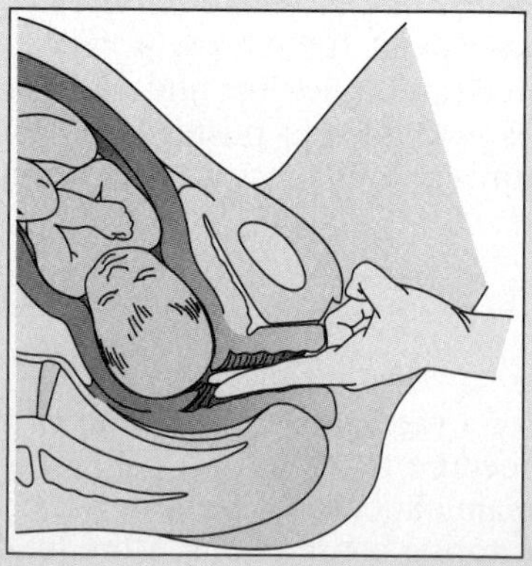	b. The width of the fingertip helps to estimate the degree of dilatation. An index finger averages about 1 cm; a middle finger about 1½ cm. If they can both enter the cervix, the cervix is dilated 2½ to 3 cm. If there would be room for double the width of your examining fingers in the cervix, the dilatation is about 5 to 6 cm. When the space is four times the width of your fingertips, dilatation is complete—10 cm. Measure the width of your fingertips on a centimeter scale if you are going to do vaginal examination so you know how wide your index and middle fingers are at the tip.

(continued)

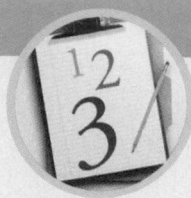

Procedure	Principle
10. Estimate the degree of effacement.	10. Effacement is estimated in percentage depending on thickness. A cervix before labor is 2 to 2½ cm thick. If it is only 1 cm thick now, it is 50% effaced. If it is tissue paper thin, it is 100% effaced. With a 100% effaced cervix, dilatation is difficult to feel for because the edges of the cervix are so thin.
11. Estimate whether membranes are intact.	11. The membranes (with a slight amount of amniotic fluid in front of the presenting part) are the shape of a watch crystal. With a contraction, they bulge forward and become prominent and can be felt much more readily.
12. Locate the ischial spines. Rate the station of the presenting part. Identify the presenting part.	12. Ischial spines are palpated as notches at the 4 and 8 o'clock positions at the pelvic outlet. Station is the number of centimeters above or below the spines where the presenting part is. Identifying the presenting part confirms findings obtained with Leopold's maneuvers. Differentiating a vertex from a breech may be more difficult than would first appear. A vertex has a hard, smooth surface. Fetal hair may be palpable but massed together and wet; it may be difficult to appreciate through gloves. Palpating the two fontanelles, one diamond-shaped and one triangular, helps the identification. Buttocks feel softer and give under fingertip pressure. Identifying the anus may be possible because the sphincter action will "trap" the index finger.
13. Establish the fetal position.	13. The fontanelle palpated is invariably the posterior one because the fetus maintains a flexed position, presenting the posterior not the anterior fontanelle. In an ROA position, the triangular fontanelle will point toward the right anterior pelvic quadrant. In an LOA position, the posterior fontanelle will point toward the left anterior pelvis. In a breech presentation, the anus can serve as a marker for position. When the anus is pointing toward the left anterior quadrant of the woman's pelvis, the position is LSA.
14. Withdraw your hand. Wipe the perineum front to back to remove secretions or examining solution. Leave client comfortable and turned to side.	14. Use as gentle a technique with withdrawal as insertion. Wiping front to back prevents moving rectal contamination forward to the vagina. Side-lying is the best position to prevent supine hypotension syndrome in labor.
15. Document procedure and assessment findings and how client tolerated procedure.	15. Documentation provides a means for communication and evaluation of care and client outcomes.

more at that time. However, examining during a contraction is more painful and rarely is justified by the additional amount of information gained. Palpating membranes during a contraction when they are under pressure may cause them to rupture.

Women are anxious to have frequent progress reports during labor to assure them that everything is progressing well. Tell the woman immediately after the examination about the progress of dilatation. Most women are aware of dilatation but not the word effacement. Just saying, "no further dilatation" is a depressing report. "You're not dilated a lot more, but a lot of thinning out is happening and that's just as important" is the same report given in a positive manner. After finishing a vaginal examination, plot the new degree of dilatation and descent of the presenting part on a labor progress graph as described earlier.

Do not do vaginal examinations in the presence of fresh bleeding, because this may indicate a placenta previa (implantation of the placenta so low in the uterus that it encroaches on the cervical os). Performing a vaginal examination in this instance might tear the placenta and cause hemorrhage, resulting in danger to both mother and fetus. If in doubt, err on the side of postponing a vaginal examination.

Assessment of Pelvic Adequacy

Evaluating pelvic adequacy using internal conjugate and ischial tuberosity diameters is generally done during pregnancy so that by weeks 32 to 36 of pregnancy, the nurse-midwife or physician is alerted that a cephalopelvic disproportion could occur. Women with this potential problem are cautioned not to attempt a home birth or use a birthing center without nearby hospital facilities.

Whether the pelvis is wide enough to allow the fetus to pass through the internal diameters can be reassessed during early labor. Because these procedures involve excessive vaginal manipulation and discomfort (and the diameters obtained during pregnancy have not changed), they are not retaken routinely. However, if the woman did not receive prenatal care, they need to be estimated at this time. (These procedures are described in Chapter 10.)

The suprapubic angle may be estimated early in labor to determine how readily the fetal head will deliver (if the angle is too steep, the fetal head can lock behind it). To estimate this angle, place the fingers vaginally and press up against the pubic arch. If the fingers cannot be separated in this position, the angle is unusually steep (less than 90 degrees). An unusually steep pubic arch may prevent the fetal head from delivering freely and increases the possibility that the perineal tissue may tear during birth as the fetal head is pushed posteriorly.

Sonography

Sonography may be used at term to determine the diameters of the fetal skull and to determine presentation, presenting part, position, flexion, and degree of descent of the fetus. If a woman is going to be transported to another department to have this done, someone should accompany her so if labor becomes more active, she can be returned quickly to the labor and birth service.

Vital Signs

Vital signs are taken at the beginning of labor and then repeated periodically as summarized in Table 18-5.

Temperature. Obtain the woman's temperature every 4 hours during labor. A temperature higher than 37.2°C (99°F) should be reported to the attending physician or nurse-midwife because it may indicate the development of infection. Unless there are accompanying symptoms, however, temperature elevation usually reflects dehydration in the woman who is taking no fluids by mouth. After rupture of membranes, temperature should be taken every 2 hours because the possibility for infection increases markedly after this time.

Pulse and Respiration. Pulse and respiration rate should be taken and recorded every 4 hours during labor. A woman's pulse may be rapid on admission because she is nervous and anxious. After she has become better acquainted with her surroundings and has been assured that everything is going well, her pulse usually ranges between 70 and 80 bpm. A persistent pulse rate of more than 100 bpm suggests tachycardia from dehydration or hemorrhage. Respiratory rate during labor is usually 18 to 20 breaths per minute. Do not count respirations during contractions, because women tend to breathe rapidly from pain. Conversely, if a woman is using controlled breathing to decrease pain in labor, her respirations will be abnormally slow.

Observe for hyperventilation (rapid, deep respirations). Prolonged hyperventilation leads to the "blowing off" of carbon dioxide and accompanying symptoms of dizziness and tingling of hands and feet. Rebreathing into a paper bag and reassurance help to reverse this process.

Blood Pressure. Blood pressure should be taken and recorded every 4 hours during labor. If the woman receives an analgesic agent (such as meperidine) that tends to be hypotensive, check her blood pressure approximately 15 minutes after administration. Take blood pressure between contractions, both for the woman's comfort and for accuracy, because blood pressure tends to rise 5 to 15 mm Hg during a contraction. An increase in blood pressure may indicate the development of pregnancy-induced hypertension. A decrease in blood pressure or a decrease in the pulse pressure (the difference between the systolic and diastolic pressures) may indicate hemorrhage.

Laboratory Analysis

Blood. Blood is drawn for hemoglobin and hematocrit, VDRL (serologic test for syphilis), hepatitis B antibodies, and blood typing to determine the woman's baseline level

TABLE 18.5 Time Intervals for Nursing Interventions During First Stage of Labor

INTERVENTION	ASSESSMENT ON ADMISSION	CONTINUED ASSESSMENTS
Assess and Record		
Temperature	X	q4h (unless membranes are ruptured, then q2h)
Pulse	X	q4h
Respirations	X	q4h
Blood pressure	X	q4h
Voiding	X	q2–4h
FHR	X	Continuously by monitor or q30min
Contractions	X	Continuously by monitor or q30min
Provide		
Ambulation	X	Until membranes rupture
Support	X	Continuously

of health. These findings can also alert the laboratory that a woman with a certain blood type is in labor and help predict whether a blood incompatibility is likely to exist in the newborn.

Urine. Obtain a urine specimen and test it immediately for protein and glucose, then send it to the laboratory for a complete urinalysis. If the woman reports any symptoms that suggest a urinary tract infection (e.g., burning on urination, blood in urine, extreme frequency, flank pain), obtain a clean-catch specimen for culture. A woman in labor is able to void most easily if she is allowed to use a bathroom. However, if the woman has reported ruptured membranes, do not allow her to ambulate to a bathroom until it is confirmed that the fetal head is engaged so gravity changes with walking do not cause a prolapsed cord. A bedpan or receptacle placed on the commode allows for collection of any material passed by the vagina.

Assessment of Uterine Contractions

Uterine contractions may be monitored intermittently by hand or continuously by an internal or external system. Most women are monitored continuously at least for a short period in early labor to screen for fetal well-being. Continuing to monitor the duration, strength, and interval between contractions can aid in tracking the progress of labor.

Length of Contractions. To determine the beginning of a contraction without a monitor, rest a hand on the woman's abdomen at the fundus of the uterus very gently to sense the gradual tensing and upward rising of the fundus that accompanies a contraction (Fig. 18-15). It is possible to palpate this tensing approximately 5 seconds before the woman is able to feel the contraction. (Contractions are palpable when the intrauterine pressure reaches approximately 20 mm Hg. The pain of a contraction is not usually felt until pressure reaches approximately 25 mm Hg.) The duration of a contraction is timed from the moment the uterus first tenses until it has relaxed again.

Intensity of Contractions. In addition to observing the duration of contractions, estimate the intensity or the strength of the contraction. Contractions are rated as mild (the uterus is contracting but does not become more than minimally tense); moderate (the uterus feels firm); or strong (the contraction is so intense the uterus feels as hard as a wooden board at the peak of the contraction). In a strong contraction, you will not be able to indent the uterus with your fingertips.

After estimating the intensity of contractions, check the fundus at the conclusion of the contraction to determine that it relaxes and becomes soft to the touch again. This demonstrates that the uterus is not in continuous contraction but is providing a relaxation time during which blood vessels can fill to supply the fetus with adequate oxygen.

Frequency of Contractions. Next, time the frequency of contractions. The frequency is timed from the beginning of one contraction to the beginning of the next (see Fig. 18-10).

Use as light a touch as possible on the woman's abdomen while timing contractions or estimating their strength.

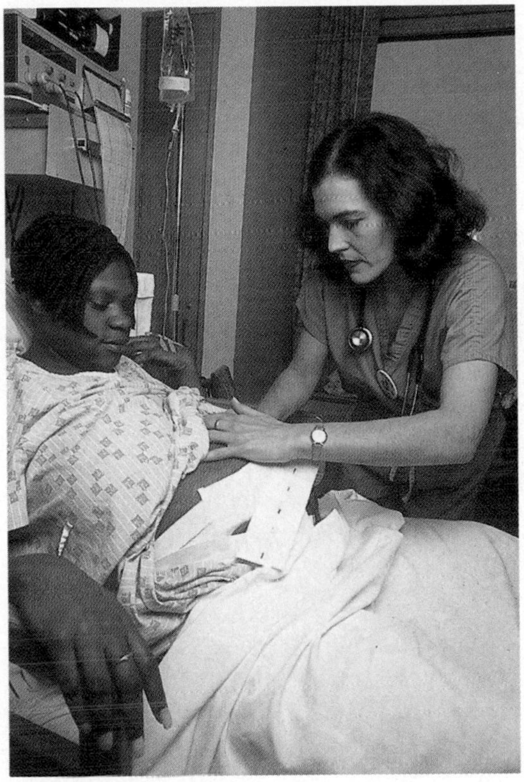

FIGURE 18.15 Contractions can be assessed by very gently placing the hand over the fundus of the uterus.

The fundus of the uterus becomes tender if it has to push against the extra weight of a hand with each contraction—unnecessary discomfort for a woman in labor.

Initial Fetal Assessment

Fetal assessment must be undertaken along with maternal assessment as soon as the woman is admitted to a labor unit. Although passive in labor, a fetus is subjected to extreme pressure by uterine contractions and passage through the birth canal. It is important to ascertain that FHR remains within normal limits despite these pressures.

Auscultation of Fetal Heart Sounds

Fetal heart sounds are transmitted through the convex portion of the fetus, because that is the part lying in close contact with the uterine wall. In a vertex or breech presentation, fetal heart sounds are best heard through the fetal back; in a face presentation, the back becomes concave and so the sounds are best heard through the more convex thorax. In breech presentations, fetal heart sounds are heard most clearly high in the uterus at the woman's umbilicus or above. In cephalic presentations, they are heard loudest low in the abdomen. In ROA position, the sounds are heard best in the right lower quadrant; in LOA position, in the left lower quadrant. In posterior positions (LOP or ROP), the heart sounds are loudest at the maternal side. Figure 18-16 shows how to locate heart sounds for different fetal positions.

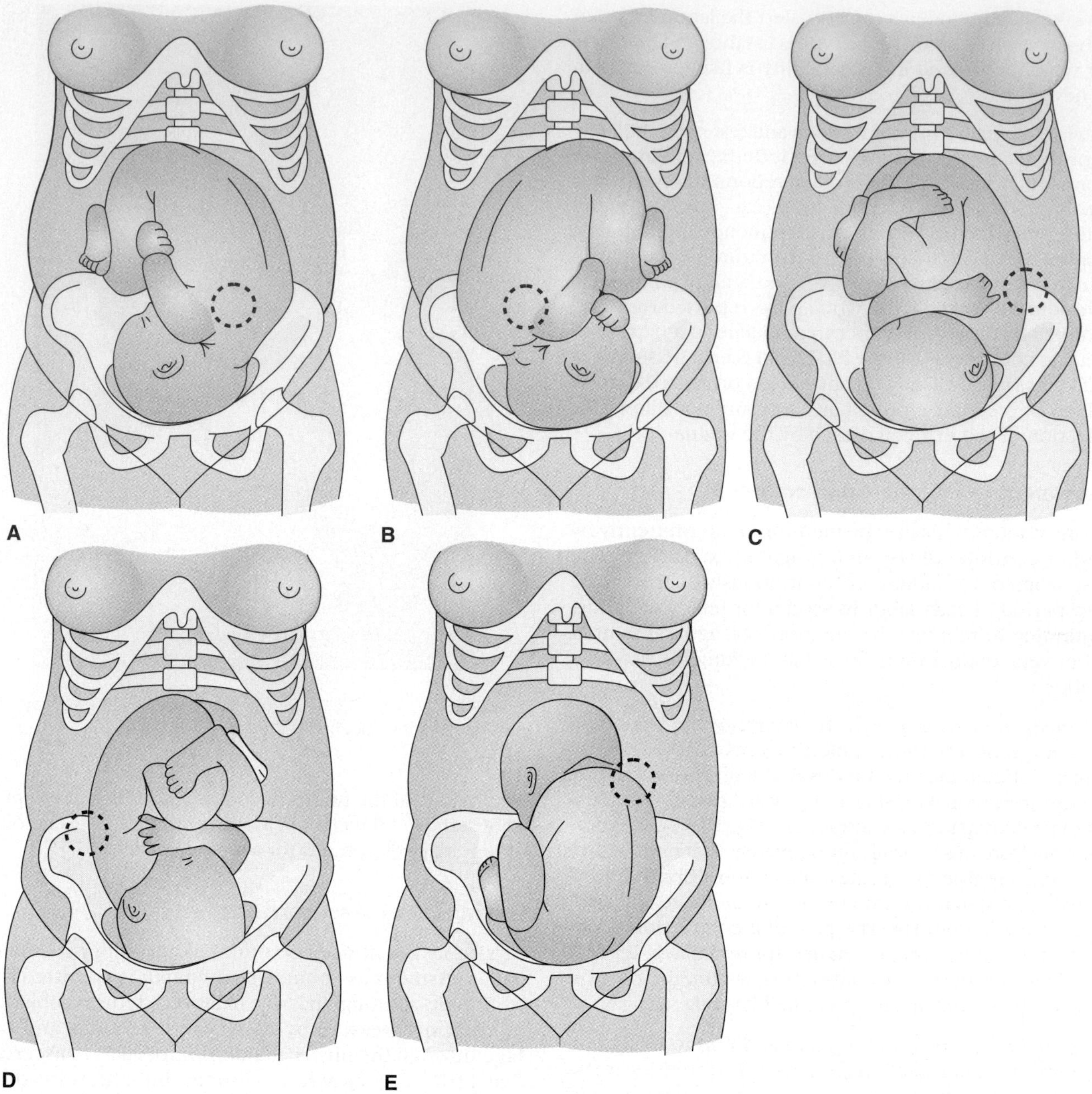

A B C D E

FIGURE 18.16 Locating fetal heart sounds by fetal position. (*A*) LOA, (*B*) ROA, (*C*) LOP, (*D*) ROP, (*E*) LSA.

Hearing the fetal heart sounds in these positions provides confirmatory information about fetal position. Conversely, recognizing the fetal position aids in locating fetal heart sounds.

Count FHR every 30 minutes during beginning labor, every 15 minutes during active labor, and every 5 minutes during the second stage of labor. This can be done by viewing the FHR monitoring strip or periodic auscultation.

To auscultate fetal heart sounds, use either a stethoscope or a fetoscope (a modified stethoscope attached to a headpiece) or obtain them with a Doppler unit, which uses ultrasound waves that bounce off the fetal heart to produce echoes or clicking noises (Fig. 18-17). These clicks reflect the rate of the fetal heart beat.

> **✔ CHECKPOINT QUESTIONS**
>
> 18. How often should the nurse assess vital signs for the woman in labor?
> 19. What are Leopold's maneuvers?
> 20. What is the usual pH of amniotic fluid?

ELECTRONIC MONITORING

In most settings, FHR is screened at least for a short time in early labor by an external electronic monitoring system. The monitor is left in place for continuous monitor-

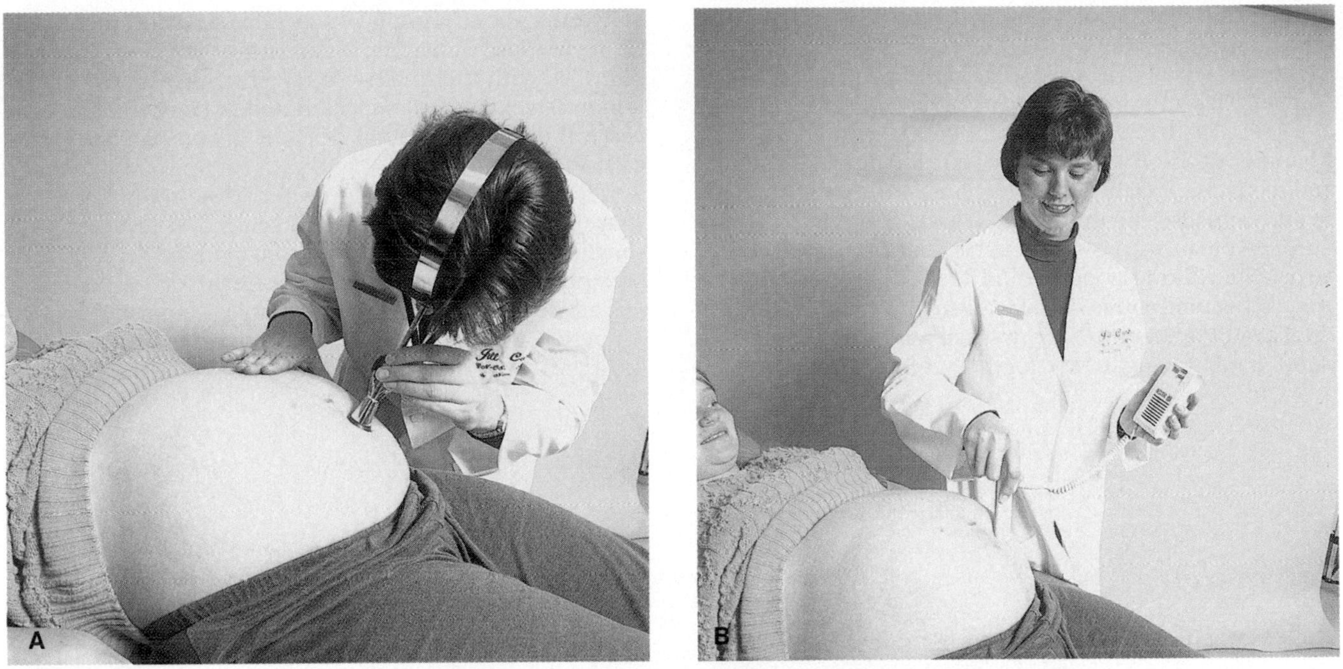

FIGURE 18.17 (*A*) Auscultation of the fetal heartbeat using the fetoscope. (*B*) A Doppler ultrasound device can be used to monitor fetal heart rate intermittently in low-risk labor.

ing on women who are categorized as high risk for any reason or who have oxytocin stimulation.

The use of fetal monitors has provoked one of the biggest controversies in modern obstetric health care. Monitors were widely adopted in the mid-1970s as a means of immediately detecting variations in FHR. However, prepared childbirth advocates have long criticized the overuse of monitoring devices, arguing that they intrude into the childbirth experience, causing needless discomfort and distraction to the mother. The medical profession readily admits that monitors have contributed to the growing number of cesarean births. Advocates of monitoring would say that the prevention of complications in even one baby is worth this increase. However, others believe that monitors often point to a problem where none exists, resulting in unnecessary cesarean births (which carries its own set of risks) and unnecessary frightening of parents (which could adversely affect early parent–infant bonding).

Monitoring does offer many advantages from a health care provider's standpoint. Observing FHR on a monitor is easier than listening with a stethoscope or fetoscope. In addition, most health care providers have grown accustomed to monitors and may feel insecure without them. Few people advocate the return to using stethoscopes for assessment; using monitors for periodic assessment rather than continuous monitoring is a compromise solution (Miller & Paul, 2000).

Tell the parents that FHR can vary greatly during labor, and the monitor is an aid only and should not be the focus of their attention. Parents can become so focused on what is happening on the monitor that they lose the ability to concentrate on previously learned relaxation and breathing techniques.

External Electronic Monitoring

External electronic monitoring can be used to monitor both uterine contractions and FHR continuously or intermittently. The information is obtained from sensors strapped to the woman's abdomen (Fig. 18-18).

Contractions are monitored by means of a pressure transducer or tocodynamometer (*toko* is Greek for contraction). The transducer must be placed over the uterine fundus or the area of greatest contractility. It is held in place by

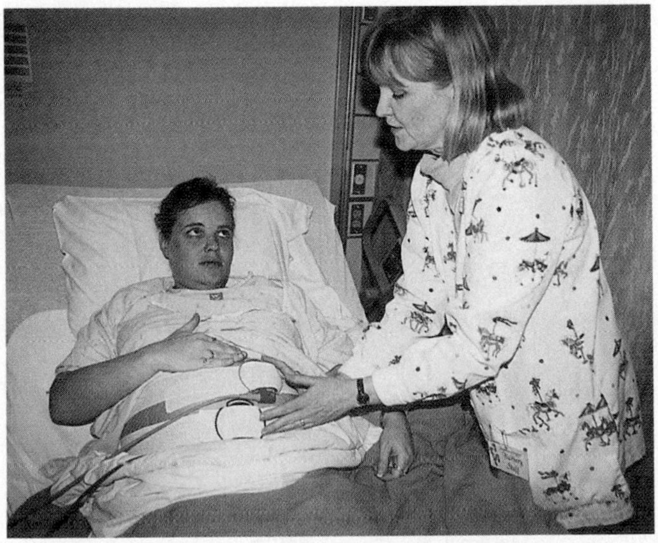

FIGURE 18.18 External electronic monitoring in place. Two devices (a transducer for the uterus and an ultrasound sensor for the fetus) are strapped to the woman's abdomen.

an adjustable strap or stockinette girdle (Fig. 18-19*A*). The transducer converts the pressure registered into an electronic signal that is recorded on graph paper.

The FHR is monitored using an ultrasonic sensor or monitor (see Fig. 18-19*A*) also strapped against the woman's abdomen at the level of the fetal chest. The small Doppler unit converts fetal heart movements into audible beeping sounds and also records them on graph paper.

The woman who is worried that something will happen to her child during labor will find it reassuring to listen to the regular beeping sound of the undistressed fetal heart from a fetal heart transducer. Many women ask for and can have a short graph tracing to save for their child's baby book.

External monitoring is not as reliable as internal monitoring because a change in maternal or fetal position may interfere with the quality of the tracing. However, it is noninvasive and easily applied and does not depend on cervical dilatation or fetal descent. It can be introduced early in labor.

Occasionally, a woman may feel discomfort from the strap holding an external monitoring unit in place. The snugness of the sensor head also may limit her ability to breathe deeply. Spreading talcum powder on the abdomen may make the strap more comfortable. Removing the sensor periodically and allowing for a position change is helpful. If the woman changes her position herself (and she will

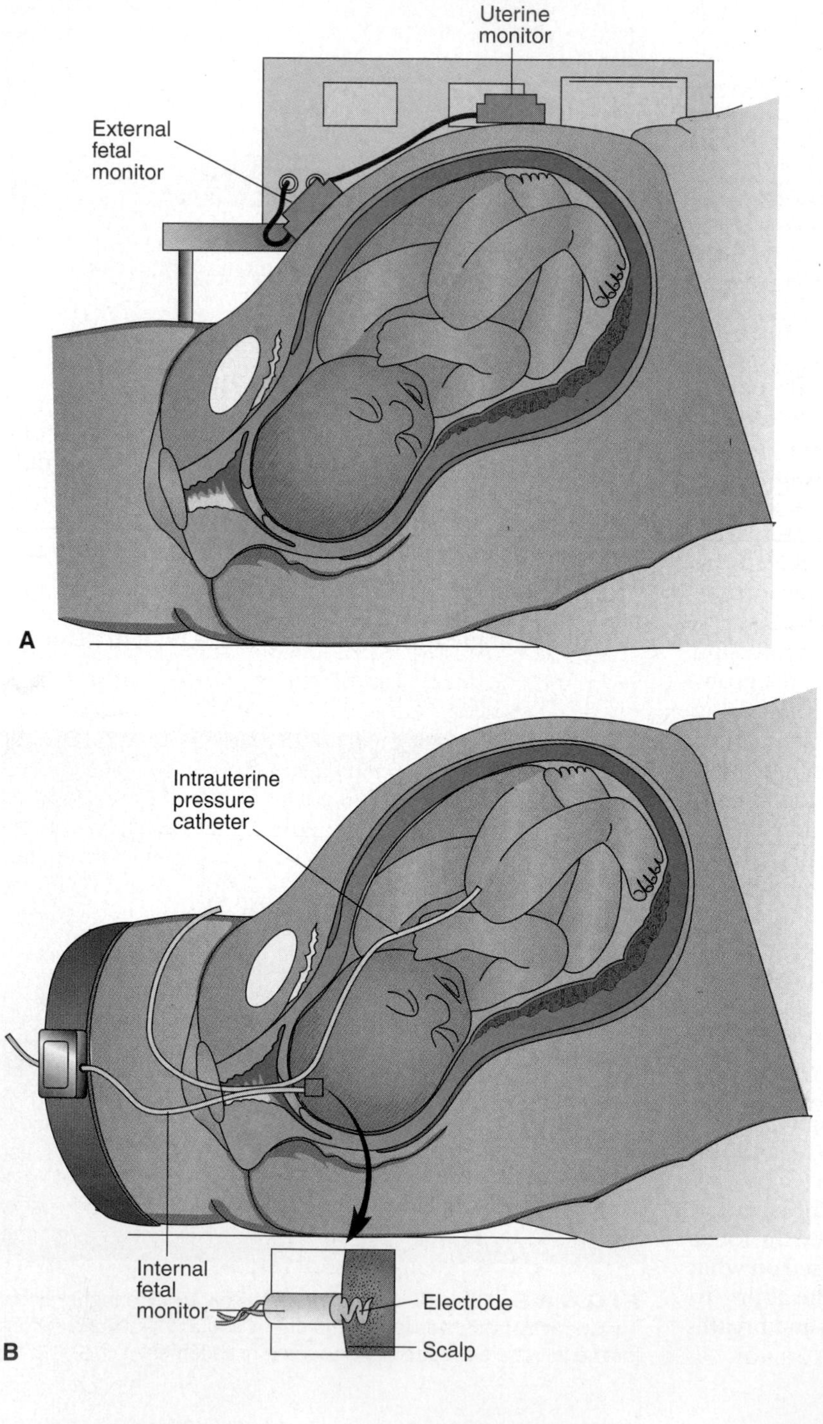

FIGURE 18.19 Placement of electronic monitoring leads. (*A*) External leads to monitor for FHR and uterine contractions. (*B*) An internal fetal heart rate lead in place on the fetal scalp. Uterine contractions are monitored by the intrauterine catheter.

change position often during labor), the sensor will need to be repositioned. Remind her that the accompanying fetal heart signal may stop when she changes position so she will not think her baby's heart has stopped.

Women do not need to lie on their backs for monitoring; thus, the likelihood of supine hypotension syndrome is not increased. With a monitor attached, be careful not to focus solely on the equipment. Be sure to communicate and offer support to the woman and her partner.

WHAT IF? What if you enter the client's room while she has an electronic monitor in place and discover that she is lying on her back, seemingly frozen in one position? Would you urge her to turn or, if comfortable, let her lie in a position of comfort for her?

Internal Electronic Monitoring

Internal electronic monitoring is the most precise method for assessing FHR and uterine contractions. A pressure-sensing catheter is passed through the vagina, alongside the fetus, into the uterine cavity after the membranes have ruptured and the cervix has dilated to at least 3 cm (see Fig. 18-19*B*). The end of the catheter extending from the vagina is attached to a pressure recorder. As each contraction puts pressure on the uterine contents, the pressure exerted on the catheter is recorded. When uterine contractions are monitored by an internal pressure gauge, the frequency, duration, baseline strength, and peak strength of contractions can all be evaluated. Strength of contractions is evaluated by the size of the peak of the contraction on the tracing. Equally important to evaluate is the return of the uterine tone to baseline strength between contractions. This ensures placental filling between contractions.

With contractions during the latent phase, the baseline level is under 5 mm Hg; with active contractions, it is approximately 12 mm Hg. During the second stage of labor, the baseline may be as high as 20 mm Hg. Baseline readings that do not return to 20 mm Hg or below indicate uterine hypertonia and a possible compromise of fetal well-being.

The FHR recording is obtained from a fetal scalp electrode. When the fetal head is engaged, the electrode is inserted vaginally and attached to the fetal scalp. A fetal electrocardiograph signal is obtained, amplified, and then fed into a cardiotachometer. The output from the cardiotachometer is recorded on permanent graph paper.

This level of information cannot be matched by external monitoring, which records only the frequency and duration of contractions. The detail on fetal heartbeats is also clearer with internal monitoring (described in the next section). On the other hand, internal monitoring is invasive, carries the risk of uterine infection, and limits the woman's movement. Thus, it is not used as routinely as external monitoring but is reserved for women who are categorized as high risk during labor.

Telemetry

Telemetry allows monitoring of both FHR and uterine contractions to be carried out free of connecting wires that could hamper a woman's movements in labor. An internal pressure uterine lead, as in internal monitoring, is inserted and a fetal scalp electrode is also attached. A miniature radio transmitter is then placed in the vagina to transmit the FHR and uterine contraction signals to a distant monitor. The major advantage of telemetry is that it allows the woman to ambulate while being internally monitored. Because it is more expensive than other equipment, not all birth settings use telemetry.

Fetal Heart Rate Tracing

Traditional FHR monitors trace both the FHR and the duration and interval of uterine contractions onto paper rolls (Fig. 18-20). Uterine contraction information is recorded on the bottom half of the paper, FHR on the top half. Time can be calculated by counting the number of bold vertical lines on the paper (the space between two bold lines represents 60 seconds).

Fetal Heart Rate Patterns

Assessing and interpreting FHR patterns involve evaluating three parameters: the baseline rate, variabilities in the baseline rate (long-term and short-term), and periodic changes in the rate (acceleration and deceleration).

Baseline FHR

A baseline FHR is determined by analyzing a range of fetal heartbeats recorded on a 10-minute tracing that is obtained between contractions. A normal rate is 120 to 160 bpm. The rate fluctuates slightly (5 to 15 bpm) when the fetus moves or sleeps. If an increase or decrease occurs and is sustained for a 10-minute period, then a new baseline or a baseline change is established. Abnormal patterns in the baseline rate include fetal bradycardia and fetal tachycardia.

Fetal bradycardia occurs when the FHR is below 120 bpm for 10 minutes. A moderate bradycardia of 100 to 119 is not considered serious and is probably due to a vagal response elicited by the fetal head being compressed during labor. Marked bradycardia (under 100 bpm) is a sign of hypoxia and is considered dangerous.

Fetal tachycardia occurs when the rate is 160 beats or more per minute (for a 10-minute period). Moderate tachycardia is 161 to 180 bpm. Marked tachycardia is more than 180 bpm. Marked fetal tachycardia may be due to fetal hypoxia, maternal fever, drugs, fetal arrhythmia, or maternal anemia or hyperthyroidism.

Variability

FHR variability is considered to be one of the most reliable indicators of fetal well-being. Baseline variability is variation or differing rhythmicity in the heart rate over time and is reflected on the FHR tracing as a slight irregularity or "jitter" to the wave. The degree of baseline variability increases when the fetus is stimulated and slows when the fetus sleeps. If no variability is present, it indicates that the natural pacemaker activity of the fetal heart (effects of sympathetic and parasympathetic nervous system) has been affected. The cause may be a response to narcotics or barbiturates administered to the woman in

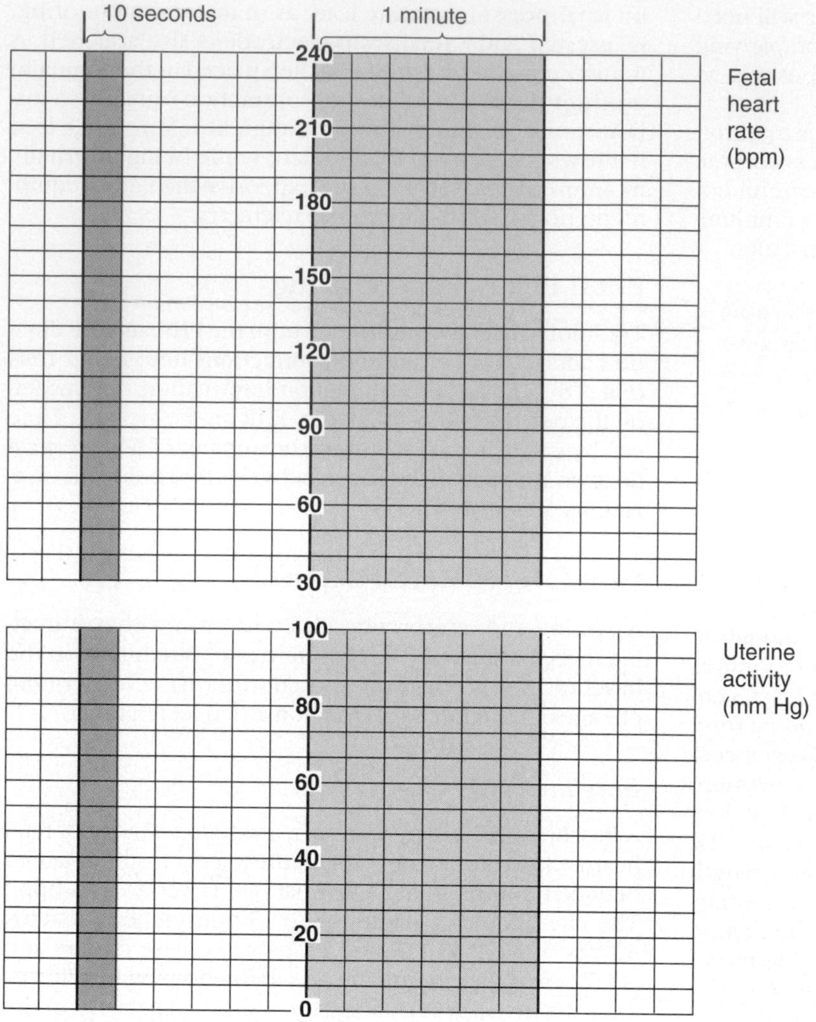

FIGURE 18.20 Paper strip for recording electronic fetal monitoring data.

labor, but the possibility of fetal hypoxia and acidosis must be investigated. Very immature fetuses will show diminished baseline variability because of a reduced nervous system response to stimulation and immature cardiac node function.

Baseline variability is defined as being long-term or short-term (beat-to-beat; Fig. 18-21). Long-term variability (LTV) is seen on a broad view of the recording and results from fluctuations in FHR of 6 to 10 beats occurring 3 to 10 times per minute. Short-term variability (STV) or beat-to-beat variability refers to the difference between successive heartbeats, usually about 3 to 5 bpm. These changes are very subtle and can be picked up only with internal electronic monitoring. Beat-to-beat variability can be rated

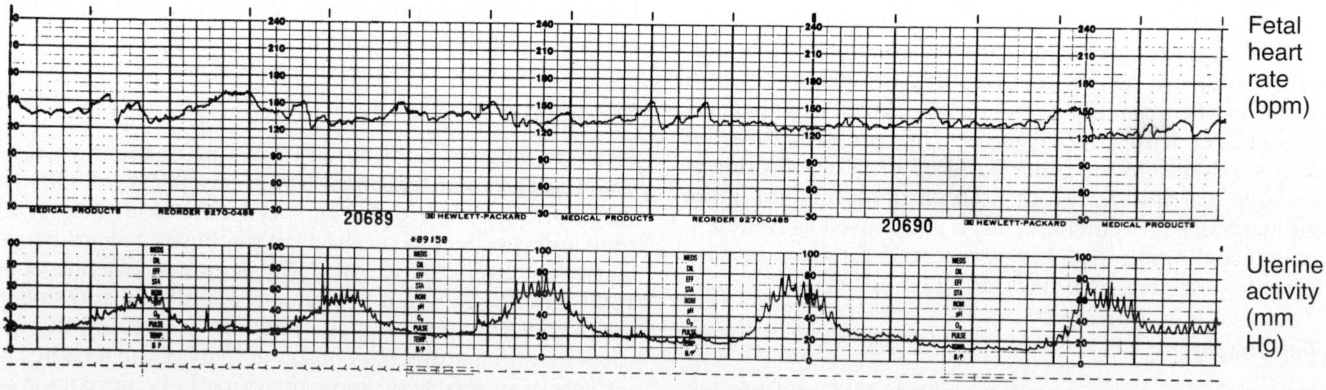

FIGURE 18.21 Fetal monitoring strip showing both long-term and short-term (beat-to-beat) variability.

as "present," "decreased," or "absent." Decreasing variability indicates the development of fetal distress. Absent variability is considered a severe sign, indicating that serious fetal compromise is present.

Periodic Changes

Periodic changes or fluctuations in FHR occur in response to contractions and fetal movement and are described in terms of accelerations or decelerations. Periodic changes are short-term changes in rate rather than baseline lasting a few seconds to 1 to 2 minutes. Four such responses are acceleration, early deceleration, late deceleration, and variable deceleration.

Accelerations. Accelerations are temporary normal increases in FHR due to fetal movement or compression of the umbilical vein during contraction.

Early Decelerations. Early decelerations are periodic decreases in FHR resulting from pressure on the fetal head during contractions. Parasympathetic stimulation in response to vagal nerve compression brings about a slowing of FHR. Early deceleration follows the pattern of the contraction, beginning when the contraction begins and ending when the contraction ends. However, the waveform of the FHR change is inverse to the contraction waveform, with the lowest point of the deceleration occurring with the peak of the contraction, thus serving as a mirror image of the contraction. The rate rarely falls below 100 bpm and returns quickly to between 120 and 160 beats at the end of the contraction (Fig. 18-22).

Early decelerations normally occur late in labor when the head has descended fairly low. As such, they are viewed as a normal pattern. However, if they occur early in labor before the head has fully descended, the head compression causing the waveform change could be the result of cephalopelvic disproportion and is a cause for concern.

Late Decelerations. Late decelerations are those that are delayed until 30 to 40 seconds after the onset of the contraction and continue beyond the end of the contraction (see Fig. 18-22). This is an ominous pattern in labor because it suggests uteroplacental insufficiency or decreased blood flow through the intervillous spaces of the uterus during uterine contractions. The lowest point of the deceleration (nadir) occurs near the end of the contraction instead of at the peak. This pattern may occur with marked hypertonia or with abnormal uterine tone caused by the administration of oxytocin. Immediate steps to correct the situation must be initiated. If oxytocin is being used, stop or slow the rate of administration. Change the woman's position from supine to lateral (to relieve pressure on the aorta and vena cava and to supply more blood to the uterus). Administer intravenous fluids or oxygen to the woman as prescribed. Prepare for possible prompt birth of the infant if the late decelerations persist and if FHR variability becomes abnormal (absent or decreased).

Prolonged decelerations are decelerations that last longer than 2 to 3 minutes but less than 10 minutes. They generally reflect an isolated occurrence, but they may signify a significant event such as cord compression or maternal hypotension. Thus, they need to be reported and documented.

Variable Decelerations. The pattern of variable decelerations refers to decelerations that occur at unpredictable times in relation to contractions; they indicate compression of the cord, which can be an ominous development in terms of fetal well-being (Fig. 18-23). Cord compression may occur because of a prolapsed cord but also may occur because the fetus is lying on the cord. It tends to occur more frequently after rupture of the membranes than when membranes are intact, or with oligohydramnios (less than a normal amount of amniotic fluid) such as occurs in postterm pregnancy or with intrauterine growth restriction. Because the pattern this produces is variable, often exhibited as U-, V-, or W-shaped waves, it can be completely missed if monitoring is not continuous. If this pattern is recognized on the monitor, change the woman's position from supine to lateral or to a Trendelenburg position to relieve pressure on the cord. Administer fluids and oxygen to the woman as prescribed. If variable decelerations are not relieved by these measures, amnioinfusion may be prescribed.

Amnioinfusion. **Amnioinfusion** is the addition of a sterile fluid into the uterus to supplement the amniotic fluid. The technique neither shortens nor prolongs labor; it just prevents additional cord compression. A sterile catheter is introduced through the cervix into the uterus after rupture of the membranes. It is attached to intravenous tubing and a solution of warmed normal saline or

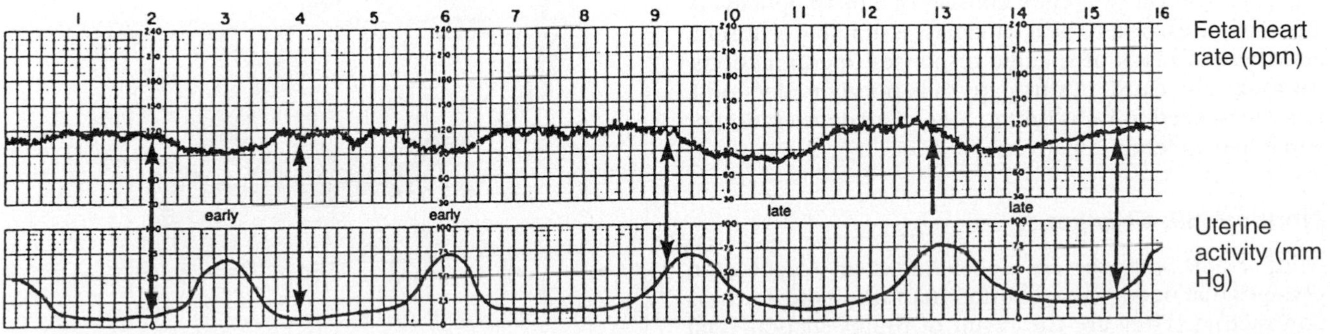

FIGURE 18.22 Schematic drawing of periodic FHR changes. Although the shape and depth of early and late decelerations are similar, note the differences in the onset of the decelerations and the recovery time to the baseline rate.

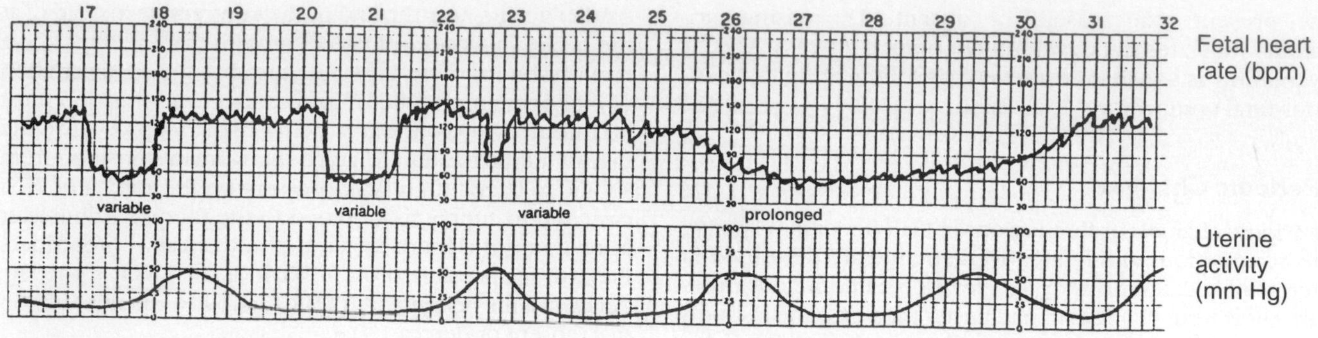

FIGURE 18.23 Schematic drawing of variable and prolonged decelerations. Note the abrupt drop in FHR in both types of decelerations. The variable decelerations return to baseline more quickly than the prolonged deceleration at 26–31 minutes, however.

lactated Ringer's solution is infused rapidly (Cunningham et al., 2001). Initially, approximately 500 mL is infused, and then the rate is adjusted to infuse the least amount necessary to maintain a monitor pattern without variable decelerations. Throughout the procedure, urge the woman to lie in a lateral recumbent position to prevent supine hypotension syndrome.

Help maintain strict aseptic technique during insertion and while caring for the catheter. Continuously monitor FHR and uterine contractions internally during the infusion. Record maternal temperature hourly to detect infection. Be sure the infusing solution is warmed to body temperature before the infusion to prevent chilling of the mother and fetus. This can be done by placing the bag of fluid on a radiant heat warmer or using a blood/fluid warmer before administration.

Because the mother will have a continuous flow of the infusing solution out of the vagina during the procedure, change her bed frequently. Also assess that there is constant drainage. If vaginal leakage should stop, it usually means the fetal head is firmly engaged and all fluid being infused is being held in the uterus. This is dangerous because it may lead to hydramnios (excessive amniotic fluid) and possibly uterine rupture.

Sinusoidal FHR Pattern

In a fetus who is severely anemic or hypoxic, central nervous system control of heart pacing may be so impaired that the FHR pattern resembles a frequently undulating wave. Long-term variability consists of 5 to 15 bpm every 3 to 5 minutes, beat-to-beat variability is minimal or absent, and there is a lack of specific responses to contractions. Although the cause of this pattern is poorly understood, it is recognized to be as ominous as a late deceleration or variable deceleration pattern.

Nonperiodic Changes

Nonperiodic changes are deceleration or acceleration changes that occur at times other than when the uterus is contracting. They are the result of things such as fetal movement, a change in maternal position, or administration of analgesia. Treatment may not be necessary; if it is, it depends on the causative factor.

OTHER ASSESSMENT TECHNIQUES

Scalp Stimulation

If FHR variability is depressed, the welfare of the fetus can be further assessed by scalp stimulation. This is done by applying pressure with fingers to the fetal scalp through the dilated cervix (Fig. 18-24). This causes a tactile response in the fetus that will momentarily increase FHR. If the fetus is in distress and becoming acidotic, however, FHR acceleration will not occur. Scalp stimulation, therefore, is an assessment of acid–base balance in the fetus.

Fetal Blood Sampling

By monitoring fetal blood composition, hypoxia in the fetus may be determined before it is apparent on an ECG or an external monitoring system. This is because changes in blood composition lead to alterations in FHR. It is unnecessary and impractical to monitor all fetuses by blood sampling during labor. The procedure is reserved for high-risk fetuses.

The oxygen saturation, Po_2, Pco_2, pH, bicarbonate excess, and hematocrit of fetal blood may all be determined during labor if a sample of capillary blood is taken from the fetal scalp as it presents at the dilated cervix. After

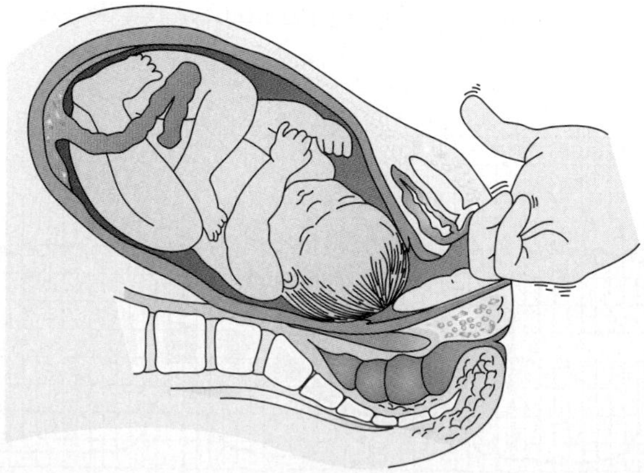

FIGURE 18.24 Technique for scalp stimulation. (Redrawn from *Journal of Perinatal and Neonatal Nursing, 1*, 16; with permission from Aspen Publishers, Inc.)

cervical dilatation of 3 to 4 cm and rupture of the membranes, the fetal head is visualized by the use of an amnioscope, a small, cone-shaped instrument with a light source at the far end. The scalp is cleaned with povidone-iodine and sprayed with silicon. A small scalpel is introduced vaginally into the cervix, and the fetal scalp is nicked. The silicon causes blood to form in beads, which are then caught by a capillary tube. The incision is then compressed until the bleeding has stopped. After the procedure, the mother must be observed after two contractions to be certain no new scalp bleeding occurs.

Although a blood sample obtained this way may be analyzed for many parameters, usually only the pH results are necessary. If a fetus is hypoxic, the pH will fall (become acidotic). A scalp blood pH greater than 7.25 is considered normal for a fetus during labor. A pH between 7.21 and 7.25 should be repeated in 30 minutes. A scalp blood pH below 7.20 is acidotic and recognized as a level of fetal distress. This technique may be used to verify a heart rate pattern on a monitor that is becoming ominous. It can also be used to verify that no acidosis is occurring, even when a monitor rate is showing decreased variability. Fetal scalp sampling is becoming less popular because it has been found that firm pressure against the fetal head by a finger inserted vaginally will increase monitor strip variability. If a variability increase occurs by this method, blood sampling is not necessary.

Fetal blood sampling involves no pain for the mother but may involve an uncomfortable sensation of pressure similar to an examining hand in the vagina. Infants who have had internal scalp blood samples taken should not be delivered by vacuum extraction because this can lead to renewed bleeding at the puncture site.

Acoustic Stimulation

Acoustic stimulation, or instrumentally producing a sharp sound next to the woman's abdomen, is used with nonstress tests during pregnancy to produce FHR acceleration. It can also be used during labor to demonstrate that the fetus is reactive.

> ✔ **CHECKPOINT QUESTIONS**
>
> 21. What two events must have taken place for internal electronic fetal monitoring to be used?
> 22. When do variable decelerations occur?
> 23. In relation to the contraction, when does a late deceleration begin?

CARE OF THE WOMAN DURING THE FIRST STAGE OF LABOR

The first stage of labor starts at the beginning of contractions and ends when the cervix has reached full dilation. Most women have had labor contractions for hours before they arrive at a birthing center because they deliberately stay at home until they are well into the first stage. Most likely, they have been experiencing pain and relying on their own judgment that everything is going well for a long time. One of their chief needs when they arrive at the birthing center, therefore, is to be assured that everything is going well. For the woman who has been unable to manage pain by breathing exercises, pain relief will be a priority need.

NURSING DIAGNOSES AND RELATED INTERVENTIONS

Care during the first stage of labor centers on helping the woman feel confident in her ability to control the pain and progress of labor and maintain physiologic stability. At first, it is exciting for the woman to feel labor contractions. They are little more than menstrual cramps and project a "this-is-really-happening" quality. Soon, however, if a woman is not concentrating on controlled breathing exercises, the contractions become biting in their intensity. Despite the fact that she is becoming more and more uncomfortable, however, nothing seems to be happening. A couple can begin to worry that something is going wrong and may think that because the 9 months are over victory is near, yet it is eluding them. Give couples frequent progress reports in labor so they do not become discouraged or fearful at this seeming lack of progress (see Focus on Nursing Care Planning).

Nursing Diagnosis: Powerlessness related to duration of labor

Outcome Identification: Client will demonstrate that she feels some control over the labor process after 30 minutes.

Outcome Evaluation: Client expresses preferences for position and techniques to control pain; asks questions about her progress and states feelings about what is happening.

A woman wants to feel that she has some control over her situation during labor. Most women accomplish this by stating their preferences, breathing with contractions, and changing their position to the one that makes them feel most comfortable. Some women handle the stress of labor by becoming extremely quiet. Others feel most comfortable when they can show their emotions by shouting or crying. Help the woman express her feelings in her own way, one that works the best for her.

Respect Contraction Time. Do not interrupt the woman in the middle of breathing exercises during labor. Once her concentration is disrupted, she feels the extent of the contraction. If she has been successfully using breathing exercises to reduce pain, suddenly feeling the full force of a contraction is frightening. She tenses, the pain becomes worse, and she may doubt her ability to breathe constructively in the face of such sharp pain with the next contraction. Allow the woman to finish breathing with her contraction, then ask questions or announce what procedure needs to be done next, or ask the question but wait patiently for the answer. (See Chap. 19 for a discussion of pain management techniques.)

Promote Change of Positions. In early labor, a woman may be out of bed walking or sitting up in bed or

FOCUS ON *Nursing Care Planning*

A WOMAN IN LABOR

A pregnant woman is now entering the active phase of the first stage of labor. Her husband states, "She's having stronger contractions now, more regular, and they're coming every 4 minutes. She was doing so well before with her breathing. Now I think she's losing it."

Assessment: Second pregnancy for client; first pregnancy ended in spontaneous miscarriage at 12 weeks. Spontaneous rupture of membranes 4 hours ago at home; reported clear fluid. Contractions now 50 seconds' duration, every 4 minutes with increasing intensity. Cervix dilated to 7 cm and 80% effaced. Vertex presentation in LOA position at +1 station. FHR 152 beats per minute with good variability. Client previously using breathing techniques and position changes learned in childbirth education classes with contractions. Now appears anxious and diaphoretic; pounding fists on the bed and pushing husband away. NPO except for ice chips and hard candy. Temperature 99.4°F (37.5°C); pulse 86; respirations 24; blood pressure 126/82.

Nursing Diagnosis: Powerlessness related to change in labor pattern and increase in contraction intensity and frequency

Outcome Identification: Couple will demonstrate ability to control situation by 20 minutes.

Outcome Evaluation: Couple identifies factors within their control; demonstrates positive behaviors to manage situation; participates in decisions when possible.

Interventions	Rationale
1. Assess couple for contributing factors related to feelings of loss of control.	1. Assessment of factors provides a baseline for developing future strategies.
2. Assist couple with using controlled breathing exercises and position changes. Reinforce information learned in childbirth education classes.	2. Use of controlled breathing and position changes helps to reduce pain of contractions and enhances feelings of control. Reinforcement of previous learning provides additional resources for the couple to use.
3. Slowly and clearly explain the events and changes occurring with the active stage of labor. Inform the couple of things that can and cannot be controlled.	3. Explanation provides the couple with an understanding of what is happening and why. Information about things that can be controlled provides a means for focused participation.
4. Reassure, as appropriate, that labor is proceeding without problems.	4. Reassurance helps to minimize anxiety and increase motivation and hope.
5. Allow opportunities for the couple to manipulate the environment. Offer couple options from which they can choose.	5. Opportunities and options allow for active participation in care and decision making.
6. Emphasize positive aspects of situation and what can be controlled.	6. Positive emphasis on controllable aspects helps to shift the focus of their fears, thus enhancing feelings of control.
7. Provide continued emotional support throughout labor and provide privacy as appropriate. Encourage the husband to continue to actively support his wife.	7. Emotional support assists in reinforcing positive behaviors, thus enhancing self-esteem. Privacy allows the couple to share their feelings and concerns openly with each other, helping to promote a shared experience.

(continued)

Nursing Diagnosis: Risk for infection related to early rupture of membranes

Outcome Identification: Client will remain free of signs and symptoms of infection.

Outcome Evaluation: Temperature remains below 100.4°F (38°C); pulse, respirations, and blood pressure remain within acceptable parameters of client's baseline values.

Interventions	Rationale
1. Obtain vital signs, including oral temperature, at least every 1 to 2 hours, and report any temperature above 100.4°F (38°C).	1. Changes in vital signs, especially an elevated temperature, may be an early indicator of infection.
2. Perform perineal care frequently, especially after each voiding and any bowel movements. Change bed linens and pads as soon as they become soiled or moist.	2. Perineal care and linen changes help to remove any possible drainage or secretions that may pose a risk for infection.
3. Use aseptic technique when performing or assisting with pelvic examination.	3. Aseptic technique reduces the risk of introducing organisms into the pelvic cavity.
4. Administer IV fluids as ordered to maintain fluid balance.	4. IV replacement fluids may be necessary to prevent dehydration, a possible causative factor for temperature elevation.

in a chair, kneeling, squatting, or in whatever position she prefers (Fig. 18-25). Because a bed is the main piece of furniture in a birthing room, most women assume they are expected to lie in bed and so must be assured otherwise (see the Focus on Communication).

A woman whose membranes have ruptured should lie on her side until a fetal monitor shows good baseline variability and no variable decelerations or she has been checked by a physician or nurse-midwife, because unless the head of the fetus is well engaged (firmly fitting into the pelvic inlet), the umbilical cord may prolapse into the vagina if she walks.

If medication such as a narcotic is given, a woman should remain in bed for approximately 15 minutes afterward to avoid a fall if she should become dizzy from the

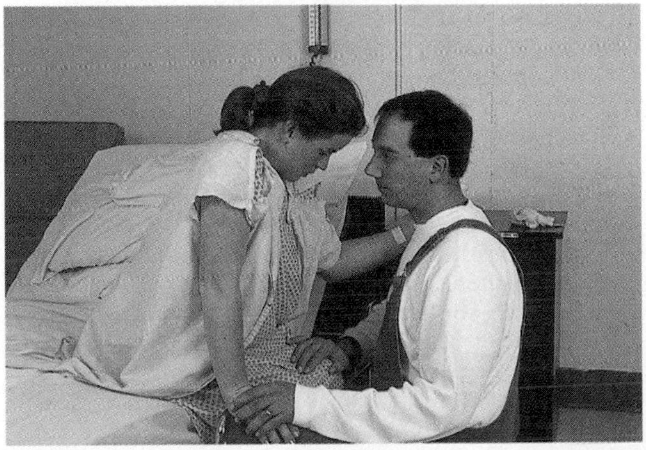

FIGURE 18.25 Finding a comfortable position during early labor is important. This woman prefers sitting on the edge of the bed, while leaning on her partner for support.

medication. As labor becomes advanced, remaining in bed and assuming a position of her choice are best so that if the birth is precipitous, the infant will not be born while she is walking, and suffer an injury. A squatting position is very effective for birth because it helps to align the fetal presenting part with the cervix and also uses the fetal weight to help bring about cervical dilation.

While the woman is in bed, encourage her to lie on her side, preferably the left side. This position causes the heavy uterus to tip forward away from the vena cava, allowing free blood return from the lower extremities and adequate placental filling and circulation. Most women are comfortable in this position and adjust to it readily. Position the chair for the support person facing the woman. Otherwise, she will keep turning to her back to talk.

Some women have learned to do breathing exercises in a supine position and may need additional coaching to do them in a side-lying position. If the woman must turn to her back during a contraction to make her breathing exercises effective, help her to remember to return to her side between contractions.

Promote Voiding and Provide Bladder Care. A full bladder or bowel can impede fetal descent. The relationship of a full bladder to descent of the fetus is shown in Figure 18-26. Encourage the woman to void, if possible, at least every 2 to 4 hours. Remind a woman to do this because she may misinterpret the discomfort of a full bladder as part of the sensations of labor. Assess for a full bladder by percussion (an empty bladder sounds dull; a full one sounds resonant). If she cannot void and the bladder is distended, she may need to be catheterized. Catheterizing a woman in labor is uncomfortable for her and difficult for the nurse: the vulva is edematous from the pressure of the fetal presenting part, making the urethra

FOCUS ON COMMUNICATION

Mrs. Gellan is a 19-year-old woman who is having her first baby. Her baby is in an occiput posterior position, so she has had extensive back pain since labor began.

Less Effective Communication
Nurse: You don't look very comfortable, Mrs. Gellan. Would you feel better if you sat in the rocking chair rather than stay in bed?
Mrs. Gellan: Can I do that?
Nurse: I told you on admission. You can do whatever is most comfortable for you.
Mrs. Gellan: Would it be all right if I walked over to the window?
Nurse: I told you on admission. Do whatever is most comfortable for you.
Mrs. Gellan: I guess I'm not being a very good patient.

More Effective Communication
Nurse: You don't look very comfortable, Mrs. Gellan. Would you feel better if you sat in the rocking chair rather than stay in bed?
Mrs. Gellan: Can I do that?
Nurse: You can use any position that is comfortable for you.
Mrs. Gellan: Would it be all right if I walked over to the window?
Nurse: Whatever is most comfortable for you.
Mrs. Gellan: Thank you. You're very understanding.

Most women in labor are enduring so much pain and are under so much stress that they don't "hear" or process instructions well. Reminding them that they have not processed information well is not therapeutic because it can lower their self-esteem and sense of self-control.

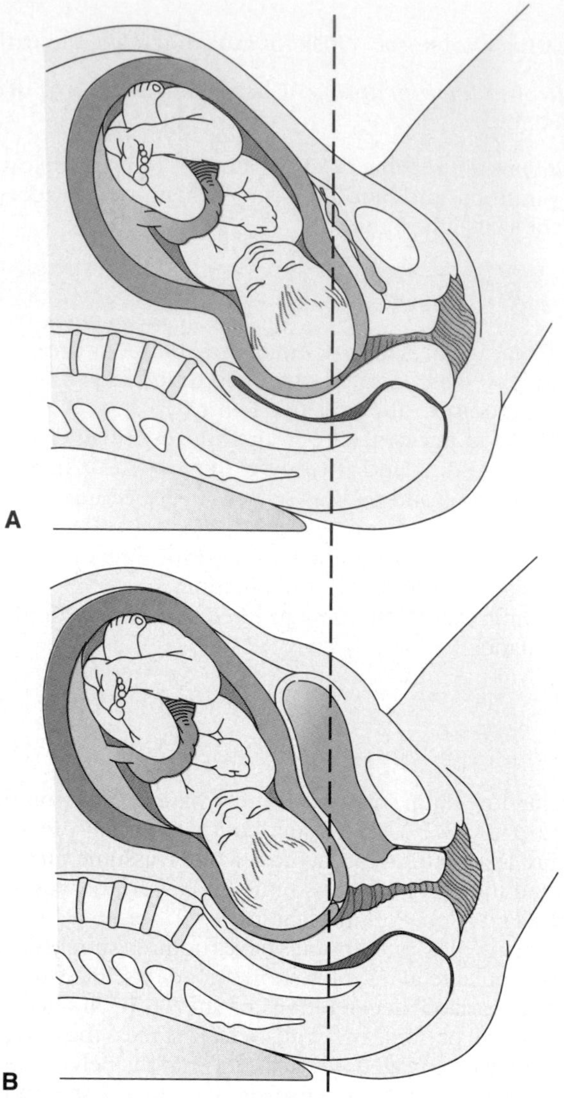

FIGURE 18.26 Effect of a full bladder on fetal descent. (*A*) Bladder is empty. (*B*) A full bladder impedes fetal progress.

difficult to locate and stretching the urethral canal downward. Use a small catheter (No. 12-14F), and insert it between contractions. Use extremely careful aseptic technique to avoid introducing any microorganisms that might result in a urinary tract infection.

Nursing Diagnosis: Risk for ineffective breathing pattern related to breathing exercises

Outcome Identification: Client will not experience hyperventilation when using breathing techniques during labor.

Outcome Evaluation: Client's respiratory rate is within normal limits; skin normal color, cool, and dry. No reports of lightheadedness or tingling/numbness in extremities.

Hyperventilation (an accelerated rate of respiration) occurs when a woman exhales more deeply than she inhales. As a result, extra carbon dioxide is blown off and respiratory alkalosis results. This can occur when a woman is practicing breathing exercises in preparation for labor but is more apt to occur during actual labor. She feels lightheaded and may have tingling or numbness in her toes and fingertips. If allowed to progress, this can lead to coma.

To halt hyperventilation, the woman should keep a paper bag nearby when doing breathing exercises. She can ward off symptoms of hyperventilation by breathing in and out into the paper bag. This causes her to rebreathe the carbon dioxide she exhales, thus replacing the carbon dioxide lost. If a paper bag is unavailable, she can use her cupped hands instead.

The best way to handle hyperventilation is to prevent it. Be certain that when the woman is breathing rapidly she is not hyperventilating, and that she ends all breathing sessions with a long cleansing breath to help restore carbon dioxide balance.

Nursing Diagnosis: Anxiety related to stress of labor

Outcome Identification: Client will manage the stress of situation with positive coping mechanisms.

Outcome Evaluation: Client states that she feels somewhat in control of her situation; she and her support person express confidence in themselves and health care personnel.

Labor is such an intense process that it creates a high level of emotional stress for both the woman and her support person. Ability to tolerate stress (to cope adequately) depends on a person's perception of the event, the support people available, and past experience in using coping mechanisms. Ways to reduce stress in labor, therefore, center around helping a woman to perceive labor clearly and providing the opportunity for her partner to provide support as well as being personally available to provide support to the woman and her partner throughout the labor process (see Focus on Evidence-Based Practice).

Offer Support. There is no substitute for personal touch and contact as a way to provide support during labor. Patting a woman's arm while telling her that she is progressing in labor, brushing a wisp of hair off her forehead, wiping her forehead with a cool cloth—these are indispensable methods of conveying concern. This caring attitude has several benefits. First, it may make the difference in helping the woman feel safe and able to continue in control. In addition, a woman who is touched, who experiences the warmth and friendliness of human contact during labor—a time when she is physically dependent—may handle her newborn (who is also physically dependent and undergoing an adjustment not unlike the one she has just gone through) more warmly and affectionately. On the other hand, not all women care for physical contact during labor. Enjoyment of touch can be culturally determined.

Respect and Promote the Support Person's Activities. Admit the support person to the birthing area with the woman and allow him or her to remain with the woman throughout birth (see Focus on Cultural Competence). Having someone with her during labor is important, because everything is new and she may not be used to the sensation of contractions. Acquaint the woman and the support person with the physical facilities and point out where supplies such as towels, washcloths, and ice chips are stored so the support person can get them when necessary. Review procedures so the support person can be assured early in labor that he or she is welcome there. Also be sure that all health care personnel are aware of who the support person is and make him or her feel welcome (see Focus on Multidisciplinary Care).

Often the support person will be acting as a labor coach. Ask both the woman and the support person if they have been to prepared childbirth classes and whether the support person plans to help the woman with her breathing. If so, support this person's role. When he or she is hesitant, it is better to review techniques than to take over. Offer praise not only for the woman but for the support person as well. Relieve the person as necessary so he or she can take a break and get something to eat or visit with older children (Fig. 18-27). If older children will view the birth, be certain they are oriented and have a childcare provider (Lynch, 2001).

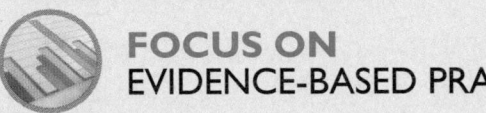

FOCUS ON EVIDENCE-BASED PRACTICE

What Actions of Nurses Do Women Value Most in Labor?

To answer this question, nurse researchers interviewed a convenience sample of 50 women following childbirth. The interviews were tape recorded and transcribed, then analyzed to identify themes. The women ranged in age from 21 to 40 years; all were married, all had more than 12 years of schooling, and 64% of them were employed.

Results of the study showed that 60% of the women reported having received only helpful nursing behavior during labor; 38%, however, reported having received both helpful and unhelpful nursing actions. Those nursing measures most valued by women were emotional support provider, comforter, information/advice provider, professional/technical skill provider, and advocate. Unhelpful nursing actions were failure to provide emotional support, comfort, or adequate or correct information or to perform needed technical duties.

This is an important study for nurses because it details nursing actions that are helpful and unhelpful to women during labor. Although this study was conducted in Taiwan, childbirth is such a universal phenomenon that the findings are relevant everywhere.

Chen, C. H. et al. (2001). Women's perceptions of helpful and unhelpful nursing behaviors during labor: A study in Taiwan. *Birth, 28*(3), 180–185.

FOCUS ON CULTURAL COMPETENCE

The person a woman chooses to stay with her during childbirth can be a husband, the father of the child, a sister or parent, or a close friend. Which of these persons a woman chooses is somewhat culturally determined. A Mexican-American woman, for example, might choose a female family member to accompany her instead of her male partner.

It is important for women to be able to understand what is happening to them during labor. If English is not the woman's primary language, make arrangements to locate an interpreter. If the woman is hearing impaired, it is the hospital's responsibility to provide an interpreter for her so she can receive adequate explanations of her progress. Remember that whether women enjoy being touched or not during labor is in part culturally determined. Assess early in a woman's labor whether she might benefit from such caring measures as having her hand held or her back rubbed.

FOCUS ON MULTIDISCIPLINARY CARE

Women on a busy obstetric service will receive care from a multitude of health care professionals. Unlicensed assistive personnel may be assigned to take routine vital signs such as blood pressure, pulse, and temperature of a woman in labor. They may be asked to help convert a labor room to a birthing room. They may be assigned to help with immediate postpartum care. Be certain that these providers are aware of the importance of the support person for a woman in labor. Otherwise, they may ask the person to leave the room unnecessarily or neglect thinking of ways that they could be helpful to this person as well as the woman in labor.

In addition to having the father of their baby present, many women choose a doula or another woman to be with them in labor (Jordan et al., 2001). Fathers may find it hard to provide doula-type support during labor because of their own emotional involvement in the birth. Having such a person present frees the father to enjoy the birth rather than feel occupied with coaching instructions. Although research in the subject is not extensive, there are suggestions that rates of oxytocin augmentation, epidural anesthesia, and cesarean birth can be reduced by doula support.

WHAT IF? What if a doula and the woman's partner disagree on whether a woman in labor needs additional medication for pain? Whose suggestion would you listen to most? How could you resolve the issue?

Support the Woman's Pain Management Efforts. Some women believe that using a prepared childbirth method will allow a pain-free labor. When they realize this is untrue, they may panic and lose the ability to use prepared breathing. Some support people are more nervous than they anticipated and have difficulty being supportive, leaving the woman to manage her anxiety on her own. In these instances, administering an analgesic might be effective in reducing anxiety or taking the edge off contractions. With this degree of relaxation, the woman is then able to return to effective breathing techniques. Sometimes simply the support of a person such as a nurse, who is confident that breathing can be effective in reducing the discomfort of labor, is all the woman needs to resume her breathing exercises with success.

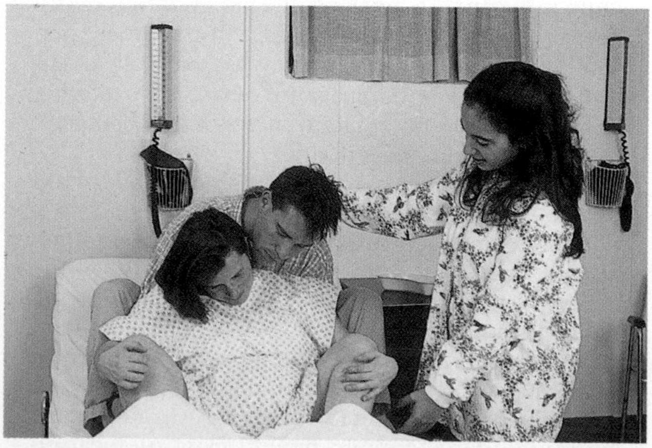

FIGURE 18.27 Encouraging the support person is an important nursing role, which enhances the childbirth experience.

Many women plan on using nonpharmacologic pain relief measures such as aromatherapy; ask what the woman has planned and what your role should be (see the Focus on Evidence-Based Practice).

Nursing Diagnosis: Risk for fluid volume deficit related to prolonged lack of oral intake and diaphoresis from the duration of labor

Outcome Identification: Client will not experience fluid volume deficit during labor.

Outcome Evaluation: Client states that she does not feel thirsty; voids at least 30 mL/h every 2 to 4 hours.

How much fluid or food a woman should ingest during labor is controversial. Most hospitals limit the amount of oral fluid or food intake during labor to ice chips or lollipops to prevent aspiration if, in an emergency, general anesthesia administration should be necessary. Because of this, the woman's mouth and

FOCUS ON EVIDENCE-BASED PRACTICE

What Complementary or Alternative Therapies Do Nurse-Midwives Suggest to Aid Labor Contractions?

To investigate the use of herbal preparations for cervical ripening and induction or augmentation of labor by nurse-midwives, researchers surveyed the 500 members of the American College of Nurse-Midwives.

The survey identified 90 CNMs who routinely prescribed or suggested alternative therapies in their practice. They tended to be younger and more likely to deliver women at home or in an out-of-hospital birthing center than in a hospital setting than those who did not use alternative therapies. Of the CNMs who used herbal preparations to stimulate labor, 64% used blue cohosh, 45% used black cohosh, 63% used red raspberry leaves, 93% used castor oil, and 60% used evening primrose oil.

This is an important study because it reveals how popular the use of alternative therapies is today. Be careful when recommending that women use such remedies during pregnancy because although they are all "natural," they are not all safe during pregnancy. Blue cohosh, for example, has been linked with cardiovascular emergencies in the woman and anoxia in the fetus.

McFarlin, B. L., Gibson, M. H., O'Rear, J., & Harman, P. (1999). A national survey of herbal preparations used by nurse-midwives for labor stimulation. *Journal of Nurse-Midwifery, 44*(3), 205–216.

lips may become dry from mouth breathing. Applying a cream to her lips or allowing her to suck on hard candy or ice chips is generally enough to relieve this discomfort. Women in prolonged labor may need isotonic sports drinks to prevent secondary uterine inertia (a cessation of labor contractions) as well as generalized dehydration and exhaustion (Kubli et al., 2002). If all oral fluids are contraindicated by the birth plan, intravenous glucose solutions may be administered to maintain caloric reserve.

Amniotomy

Amniotomy is the artificial rupturing of membranes. Rupturing membranes if they do not rupture spontaneously allows the fetal head to contact the cervix more directly and may increase the efficiency of contractions. For this, the woman's cervix must be dilated at least 3 cm. She is placed in a dorsal recumbent position; an amniohook (a long thin instrument) or a hemostat is passed vaginally. The membranes are torn, and amniotic fluid is allowed to escape. This puts the fetus momentarily at risk for cord prolapse because there is a possibility that a loop of cord will escape with the fluid. Always take FHR immediately after the rupture of membranes to determine that this did not happen (Cruikshank, 2000).

✔ CHECKPOINT QUESTIONS

24. How will a full bladder sound when percussed?
25. After an amniotomy, for what is the fetus at risk?

CARE OF THE WOMAN DURING THE SECOND STAGE OF LABOR

The second stage of labor is the time from full cervical dilation to birth of the newborn. Even women who have taken childbirth education classes are surprised at the intensity of the contractions in this phase of labor. Because the feeling to push is so strong, many women react by tensing their abdominal muscles and trying to resist, which makes the sensation more painful and frightening. Some women react to this change in contractions by growing increasingly argumentative and angry, or by crying and screaming.

The next hour will consist of sensations for the woman that are difficult to appreciate unless they have been experienced. The support person plays a vital role because all the preparations done up to this point may still not be enough to sustain a woman unless she has a support person with her. This sharing is also important later, after the birth, when the two can talk about it.

Women need to have an experienced health care person with them as well as they enter this stage of labor to reassure them that the change in contractions is normal and to give knowledgeable support that everything is all right.

Assess fetal heart sounds at the beginning of the second stage of labor to be certain that the start of the baby's passage in the birth canal is not occluding the cord and interfering with fetal circulation. A timetable for second-stage interventions is shown in Table 18-6.

Preparing the Place of Birth

Once women had little say as to the setting where their baby would be born, but today women are allowed a multitude of options. Some choose their own home. In the past, hospitals provided different rooms for labor (labor rooms), for delivery (delivery rooms), and rooms for recuperation (postpartum rooms). Today, these rooms are combined into labor-delivery-recovery-postpartum rooms (LDRP or LDR rooms). The setting is not as important as the provision of warm, supportive care.

Birthing Room

For a multipara, convert the birthing room into a birth room when the cervix is dilated to 7 to 9 cm. For a primipara, this can be delayed until the head has crowned to the size of a quarter or half-dollar (full dilatation and descent). Convert the room to a birth room by opening the sterile packs of supplies on waiting tables. The drapes and materials used for birth are sterile so no microorganisms are accidentally introduced into the uterus. A table set up with equipment, such as sponges, drapes, scissors, basins, clamps, bulb syringe, vaginal packing, and sterile gowns, gloves, and towels, and then covered can be left up to 8 hours. Open the

TABLE 18.6 Time Intervals for Nursing Interventions During Second Stage of Labor

INTERVENTION	BEGINNING OF SECOND STAGE	CONTINUED FREQUENCY	AFTER BIRTH OF INFANT	AFTER DELIVERY OF PLACENTA
Assess and Record				
Temperature	X	q2h		X
Pulse	X	q1h	X	X
Respirations	X	q1h	X	X
Blood pressure	Following anesthetic administration	q1h	X	X
FHR	X	Continuously by monitor or q5min		
Contractions	X	Continuously by monitor or q5min		
Provide				
Support	X	Continuously	Continuously	Continuously

partition at the end of the room to reveal the "baby island," or newborn care area. Such areas include a radiant heat warmer, equipment for suction and resuscitation, and supplies for eye care and identification of the newborn. Turn on the radiant heat warmer in advance so the bottom mattress is pleasantly warm to the touch at the time of birth. Place sterile towels and a blanket on the warmer so these will also be warm to use to dry and cover the infant.

Positioning for Birth

A variety of positions can be used for birth. At one time, the lithotomy position was the major position for birth, but it is no longer the position of choice in birthing rooms or alternative birth centers—although the labor beds in these locales usually have attached stirrups to allow birth in a lithotomy position. Alternative birth positions include the lateral or Sims' position, dorsal recumbent (on the back with knees flexed), semisitting, and squatting.

Nurse-midwives tend to favor these alternative birth positions for their clients because less tension seems to be placed on the perineum, resulting in fewer perineal tears. An episiotomy can be made in some alternative positions, although suturing is more difficult than in a lithotomy position.

If the physician prefers a lithotomy position for birth, position the woman into the stirrups while the physician is scrubbing and donning a sterile mask, gown, and gloves. Raise both legs at the same time to prevent strain on the woman's back and lower abdominal muscles. The strap holding the leg in the stirrups should be secured snugly but not so tightly that it causes constriction. Many women perceive stirrups as an unnatural position for birth, but they provide the best position for performing an episiotomy or a forceps-assisted birth or for viewing the perineum to detect lacerations or other problems at birth, and they are generally not uncomfortable. Pad the stirrups with abdominal pads if the woman has ankle edema; to prevent thrombophlebitis, be certain there is no pressure on her calves.

Because pushing becomes less effective in a lithotomy position, the top portion of the table can be raised to a 30- to 60-degree angle so the woman can continue to push effectively. Lying for longer than 1 hour in a lithotomy position leads to intense pelvic congestion because blood flow to the lower extremities is impeded. Pelvic congestion may lead to an increase in thrombophlebitis in the postpartal period. It may also contribute to excessive blood loss with birth and placental loosening. For these reasons, place the woman's legs in a lithotomy position only at the last moment.

Once the woman is in a lithotomy position, the table's lower half is folded downward ("broken") so the physician can be in close proximity to the birth outlet. Make sure there is always someone at the foot of a broken delivery room table so that if birth should occur precipitously, the infant will not fall and be injured.

Promoting Effective Second-Stage Pushing

For the most effective pushing during the second stage of labor, the woman must push with contractions and rest between them. The best approach is to allow her to push when she feels the urge and use the position and technique she feels are best for her. Pushing is usually best done from a semi-Fowler's, squatting, or "all-fours" position rather than lying flat, to allow gravity to aid the effort (Fig. 18-28). The woman can use short pushes or long, sustained ones, whichever are more comfortable. Holding her breath during a contraction could cause a Valsalva's maneuver or temporarily impede blood return to the heart because of increased intrathoracic pressure. This could also interfere with blood supply to the uterus. To prevent her from holding her breath during pushing, urge her to breathe out during a pushing effort.

In a multipara, to keep the second stage of labor from moving too fast, it may be necessary to prevent her from pushing. To accomplish this, ask her to pant with contractions. Because it is difficult to push effectively when she is using her diaphragm for panting, this limits pushing. Remember that pushing is involuntary. Regardless of how much a woman wants to cooperate, stopping this overwhelming urge to push is almost beyond her power. Demonstrating "panting like a puppy" and panting with her may be most effective. Be sure she is inhaling adequately. Otherwise, she might hyperventilate and become lightheaded while panting. Have her take deep cleansing breaths between contractions to prevent this.

Perineal Cleaning

Clean the perineum with a warmed antiseptic (cold causes cramping) and then rinse it with a designated solution before birth according to the policy of the physician, nurse-midwife, or agency. Clean from the vagina outward (so microorganisms are moved away from the vagina), using a clean compress for each stroke. Include a wide area (vulva, upper inner thighs, pubis, and anus). Figure 18-29 shows a typical pattern for cleaning. After cleaning, place sterile drapes around the perineum.

The pressure of the fetal head may cause fecal material to be expelled from the rectum. The physician or nurse-midwife will sponge this away as it occurs to prevent contamination of the birth canal.

Episiotomy

An **episiotomy** is a surgical incision of the perineum made to prevent tearing of the perineum with birth and to release pressure on the fetal head with birth. An episiotomy incision is made with blunt-tipped scissors in the midline of the perineum (a midline episiotomy) or begun in the midline but directed laterally away from the rectum (a mediolateral episiotomy; Fig. 18-30). Mediolateral episiotomies have the advantage over midline cuts in that if tearing occurs beyond the incision, it will be away from the rectum, with less danger of complication from rectal mucosal tears. However, midline episiotomies appear to heal more easily, cause less blood loss, and result in less postpartum discomfort.

Obstetric practice varies as to how often episiotomies are done. They were once done only when tearing seemed imminent, then were considered routine with a normal birth, and now are used less frequently. The advantage of an episiotomy is that it substitutes a clean cut for a ragged tear, minimizes pressure on the fetal head, and shortens

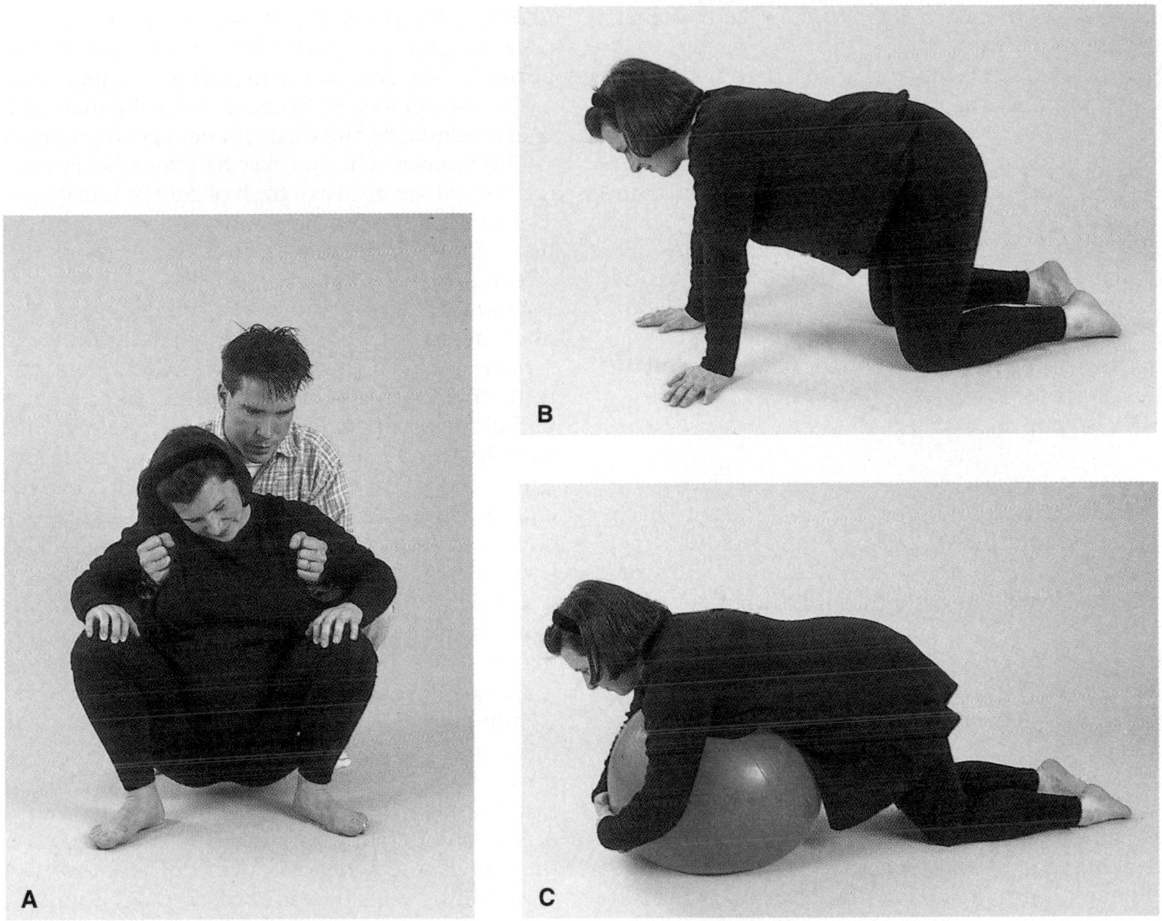

FIGURE 18.28 Positions for pushing during second stage labor: (*A*) squatting with support person; (*B*) all-fours; (*C*) all-fours with chest support.

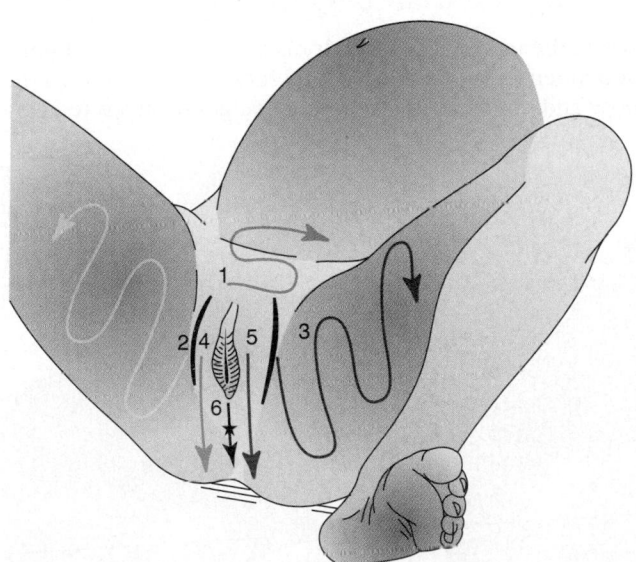

FIGURE 18.29 Pattern for cleaning perineum before birth. Cleaning from the birth canal outward moves bacteria away from, not into, the vagina. Numbers refer to steps of the procedure.

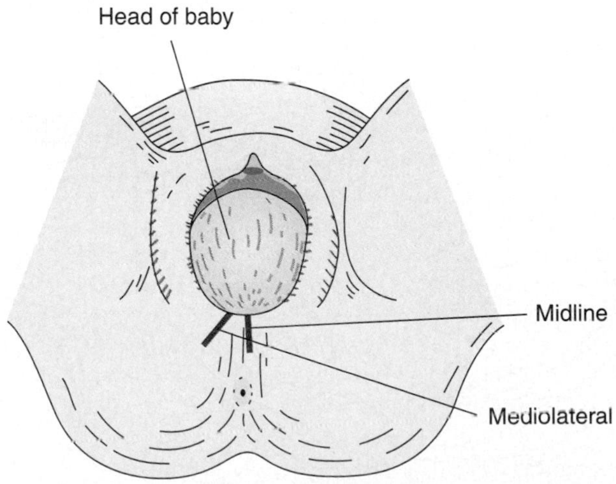

FIGURE 18.30 Position of episiotomy incision in a woman during second stage of labor. Baby's head is presenting to vagina outlet (crowning).

the last portion of the second stage of labor (Cunningham et al., 2001).

The pressure of the fetal presenting part against the perineum is so intense that the nerve endings in the perineum are momentarily deadened. Thus, an episiotomy may be done without anesthesia. However, in some cases a pudendal block is done; lidocaine is injected via a long needle through the vaginal wall near the ischial spine, numbing the lower vaginal area and the perineum.

At the time of the incision, there is a slight loss of blood, but the pressure of the presenting part serves to seal the cut edges and minimizes bleeding. The fetal head generally moves forward considerably once the tension on the perineum is relieved.

Birth

As soon as the head of the fetus is prominent (approximately 8 cm across), the physician or nurse-midwife may place a sterile towel over the rectum and press forward on the fetal chin while the other hand is pressed downward on the occiput (a Ritgen maneuver; Fig. 18-31). This helps the fetus achieve extension, so the head is born with the smallest diameter presenting. This also controls the rate at which the head is born. Pressure should never be applied to the fundus of the uterus to effect birth, because uterine rupture may occur.

The woman is asked to continue pushing until the occiput of the fetal head is firmly at the pubic arch. Then the head is born between contractions. This helps to prevent the head from being expelled too rapidly. It also helps to avoid perineal tears and a rapid change in pressure in the infant's head (which could rupture cerebral blood vessels). The woman may be asked to pant deliberately so she does not push during a contraction. She may be asked to push again without a contraction present to deliver the shoulders. Repeat instructions as necessary because often the mother is so involved with the coming birth that she does not hear. Offer guidance and support to the partner as well because he or she may be almost as overwhelmed by the birth process as the woman.

The woman who has not had anesthesia experiences the birth of the head as a flash of pain or burning sensation, as if someone had momentarily poured hot water on her perineum. It is a fleeting sensation but is not particularly uncomfortable.

Immediately after birth of the head, the physician or nurse-midwife suctions out the infant's mouth with a bulb syringe and then passes his or her fingers along the occiput to the newborn's neck to determine whether a loop of umbilical cord is encircling the neck. It is not uncommon for a single loop of cord to be positioned this way (termed a nuchal cord). If such a loop is felt, it is gently loosened and drawn down over the fetal head. If it is too tightly coiled to allow this, it must be clamped and cut before the shoulders are delivered. Otherwise, it could tear and interfere with the fetal oxygen supply.

After expulsion of the fetal head, external rotation occurs. The shoulders and the remainder of the newborn must now be delivered to free the chest for the first breath. Gentle pressure is exerted downward on the side of the infant's head, and the anterior shoulder is born. Slight upward pressure on the side of the head allows the anterior shoulder to nestle against the symphysis and the posterior shoulder to be born. The remainder of the body then slides free without any further difficulty.

A child is considered born when the whole body is delivered. This is the time that should be noted and recorded as the time of birth—a nursing responsibility. (Most physicians and nurse-midwives regard it as their responsibility or pleasure to announce the sex of the infant.) With the birth of the infant, the second stage of labor is complete (Fig. 18-32).

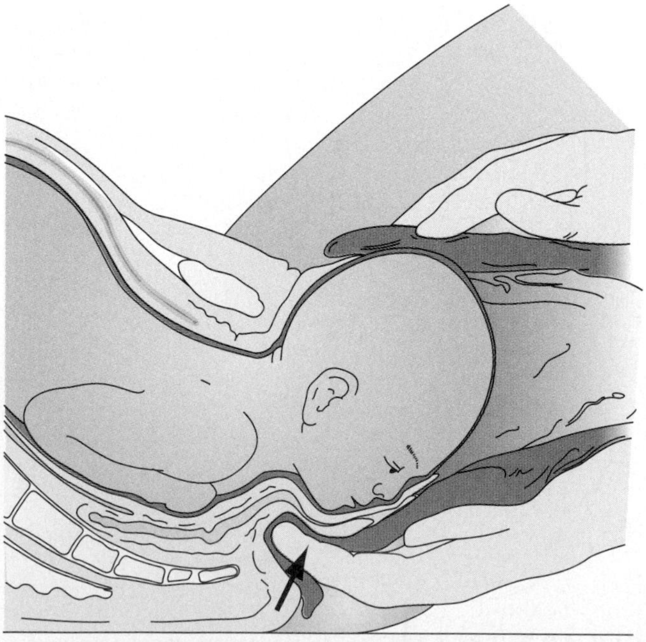

FIGURE 18.31 Ritgen's maneuver as it appears in median section. *Arrow* shows direction of pressure.

Cutting and Clamping the Cord

While the infant is held with his or her head in a slightly dependent position to allow secretions to drain from the nose and mouth, the mouth may be gently aspirated by a

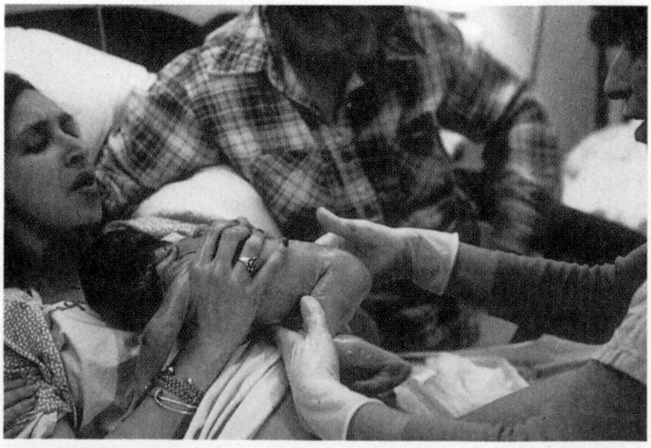

FIGURE 18.32 The nurse-midwife hands the baby to mom immediately after birth.

bulb syringe to remove additional secretions. The infant is then laid on the abdominal drape of the mother while the cord is cut. The cord will continue to pulsate for a few minutes after birth and then the pulsation ceases. There are a number of theories about the best time for cutting the cord and the best position of the infant. Delaying the cutting until pulsation ceases and maintaining the infant at a uterine level allows as much as 100 mL of blood to pass from the placenta into the fetus. On the other hand, late clamping of the cord may cause overinfusion with placental blood and the possibility of polycythemia and hyperbilirubinemia in the infant. This is a particular concern in preterm infants. Raising the infant on the abdomen may modify the amount of blood infused as well as allow the parents a free, unobstructed view of the new child. The timing of cord clamping therefore will vary depending on the physician or nurse-midwife's preference and the maturity of the infant.

The cord, clamped using two Kelly hemostats placed 8 to 10 in from the infant's umbilicus, is cut between them; an umbilical clamp is then applied (Fig. 18-33). A cord blood sample is obtained to provide a ready source of infant blood if blood typing or other emergency measures need to be done. The vessels in the cord are counted to see that three are present. In most births, the woman's partner may cut the cord.

Clamping the cord is part of the stimulus that initiates a first breath. With this, the infant's most important transition to the outside world, the establishment of independent respirations, is made.

Introducing the Infant

After the cord is cut, the infant is handed to a nurse who receives him or her in a sterile blanket. Be sure to hold the newborn firmly because he or she is covered with slippery amniotic fluid. Lay the infant on the radiant heat warmer and dry him or her well with a warmed towel. Cover the infant's head with a wrapped towel or cap. Wrap the infant snugly and, assuming that respirations are good, take the infant to the head of the table to visit with the mother and father.

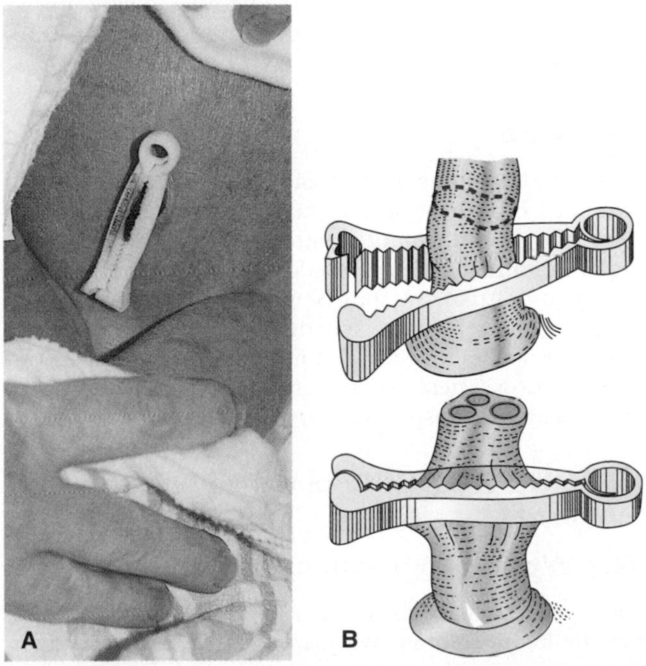

FIGURE 18.33 (*A*) Umbilical clamp applied to cord. (*B*) Placing clamp; locking clamp.

Both the mother and her partner usually want to see and touch their newborn immediately after birth. This assures them that the baby is well. It also is important in initiating a parent–child relationship. Prophylactic eye ointment should not be administered to the infant until after parents have had this chance to see their infant (and the infant has had a chance to see them). (See Chap. 23 for infant care after birth.) If the woman wishes to breastfeed, this is an optimal time for her to begin. An infant sucking at the breast stimulates the release of endogenous oxytocin. Although it is not well documented that this actually makes a difference, it theoretically aids in uterine contractions and involution, or the return of the uterus to its prepregnant stage.

CARE OF THE WOMAN DURING THE THIRD AND FOURTH STAGES

The third stage of labor is the time from the birth of the baby until the placenta is delivered. For most women, it is both a time of excitement and a time of feeling anticlimactic that the infant has been safely born. The fourth stage includes the first few hours after birth. It signals the beginning of dramatic changes because it marks the beginning of a new family.

Oxytocin

Once the placenta is delivered, oxytocin is generally ordered to be administered intramuscularly or intravenously. Such medication increases uterine contractions and therefore minimizes uterine bleeding.

Oxytocin (Pitocin) may be added to an existing intravenous line (4 U as a bolus and 20 to 30 U/L of intravenous fluid) to help contract the uterus. Methylergonovine maleate (Methergine), a semisynthetic derivative of ergonovine, may be administered intramuscularly (Karch, 2001). Methergine produces strong and effective contractions, and its effect lasts several hours; see Focus on Pharmacology: Methylergonovine Maleate (Methergine).

The administration of these drugs is a nursing responsibility in most health care facilities. Medication should not be given until the physician or nurse-midwife indicates that it is appropriate. Although it may be given as early as with the delivery of the fetal anterior shoulder, the physician or nurse-midwife may want to inspect the placenta first to ensure that it is intact and without gross abnormalities and that none of its cotyledons remains in the uterus. Because oxytocics cause hypertension by vasoconstriction, be sure to obtain a baseline blood pressure. They should not be used in women with elevated blood pressure. Document the administration of oxytocics given in the delivery or birthing room on the maternal record. Intravenous administration of oxytocin may be continued for up to 8 hours after birth to ensure uterine contraction. The next dose of medication to maintain

FOCUS ON PHARMACOLOGY

Methylergonovine Maleate (Methergine)

Action: Methylergonovine maleate is an ergot alkaloid that stimulates uterine contractions. It is primarily used to prevent and treat postpartum hemorrhage due to uterine atony.

Pregnancy category: C

Dosage: 0.2 mg IM after delivery of the placenta, then 0.2 mg orally every 6 to 12 h for 1 to 2 days after delivery.

Possible adverse reactions: Nausea, vomiting, hypertension; possible ergot toxicity

Nursing Implications

- Assess vital signs, especially blood pressure, before administering. Do not administer if blood pressure is 140/90 or greater.
- Continue to monitor vital signs as ordered after initial dose and throughout therapy.
- Assess the amount of vaginal bleeding and fundal consistency before administering to provide a baseline. Continue to assess these parameters frequently after administration. Monitor pad count.
- Assess for signs of ergot toxicity, including vomiting, diarrhea, headache, and dizziness. Be alert to marked vasoconstriction, which may be evidenced by coldness, paleness, and numbness of the feet and hands. Discontinue the drug and notify the physician immediately should any occur.

contraction cannot be given closer than 3 or 4 hours to this dose or severe hypertension can occur.

Placenta Delivery

If the placenta does not deliver spontaneously, the physician or nurse-midwife will need to remove it manually. After delivery, the placenta is inspected to be certain it is intact and normal in appearance and weight. Normally, a placenta is one-sixth the weight of the infant. If it is unusually large or small, you may be asked to weigh it.

Perineal Repair

After delivery of the placenta, any necessary perineal stitching is performed. This process can be a long, tedious one from the mother's perspective. She must lie on her back and wait for the procedure to be completed, while the attention of others is riveted on the newborn lying in the warmer off to one side. This can make the mother feel rejected. It is important to be sensitive to the mother's needs at this time. Be certain to include her in explanations and appreciate how anticlimactic she may feel.

If suturing of an episiotomy is done immediately after the birth of the placenta, a woman who delivered without anesthesia will theoretically still have so much natural-pressure anesthesia of the perineum that she will not require an anesthetic. In actuality, however, by the time the placenta is delivered (approximately 5 minutes), enough sensation has returned to the perineum that the woman will probably need some type of medication for comfort. Women who received a regional anesthetic during labor, such as a pudendal block, or those who have had epidural anesthesia will probably not need additional medication during episiotomy repair.

Immediate Postpartal Assessment and Nursing Care

Once the episiotomy repair is complete, the drapes are removed and the woman's legs are simultaneously and carefully lowered from the stirrups, if they were used, to prevent back injury.

Obtain vital signs (i.e., pulse, respirations, and blood pressure) every 15 minutes for 1 hour and then according to the agency's policy. Pulse and respirations may be fairly rapid (80 to 90 bpm and 20 to 24 respirations per minute) and blood pressure slightly elevated due to the excitement of the moment and recent oxytocin administration. Palpate the fundus for size, consistency, and position and observe the amount and characteristics of the lochia. Perform perineal care, and apply a perineal pad.

If the birth was in a birthing room, the birthing bed is returned to its original position. Offer a clean gown and a warmed blanket because a mother often experiences a chill and shaking sensation 10 to 15 minutes after birth. This may be due in part to the low temperature of a birthing room but may also be the result of the sudden release of pressure on pelvic nerves or excess epinephrine production during labor. It is a normal phenomenon but can be frightening to the mother. She may associate the shaking chill with fever or infection and worry that she will be ill at a time when she most wants to be well to care for her new child. Reassure her that this is a normal transitory sensation.

Aftercare

This is the beginning of the postpartal period or the fourth stage of labor. Because the uterus may be so exhausted from labor that it cannot maintain contraction, there is a high risk for hemorrhage. In addition, the woman often is so exhausted that she may be unable to assess her own condition or report any changes. Specific assessments done during this time are continued throughout the postpartal period. These assessments are discussed in Chapter 22 with other aspects of postpartal care.

UNIQUE CONCERNS OF THE WOMAN IN LABOR

The Woman Without a Support Person

Some women have chosen to reject or want to do without the infant's father, who is the usual support person during labor. Such women may appreciate having a family member or close friend act as their support person. A young girl who did not receive prenatal care may not be aware that she could have asked the father of her child to accompany her and may appreciate being told that she can telephone him and ask him to join her. If he chooses to be part of the labor experience, it will reflect his commitment to the mother of his child and his value to her as an important person in her life.

A woman whose acceptance of her pregnancy was slow to develop due to lack of adequate support people may not have completed the psychological tasks by the time she is in labor. This could make her more apprehensive about a new life role and calls for increased assessment of parent–child bonding in the immediate postpartal period. She needs a supportive nurse during labor.

The Woman Who Will Be Placing Her Baby for Adoption

Even if a woman has decided to place her baby for adoption, she needs to be an active participant in her labor and birth experience. She should watch the baby being born and be allowed to hold it as desired. Each state has a set number of days in which she must decide whether or not to keep the baby. Although the decision may have been easy to make during pregnancy, once she holds the baby in her arms, the prospect of giving up a child may be more painful than she realized. She needs support no matter what decision she eventually makes. Be certain to offer support, not influencing advice, because the woman is the only person who knows whether keeping this child is right for her.

Vaginal Birth After Cesarean Birth (VBAC)

Women who have had a previous cesarean birth that involved a low transverse uterine incision are often allowed a trial labor with their next pregnancy to see if vaginal birth will be possible. The length of labor in these women is usually comparable with that of primiparas, not multiparas, because it is their first vaginal birth. Most women are anxious for vaginal birth to be successful so they do not have to undergo surgery again. At the same time, they may be surprised and dismayed at the length and discomfort of normal labor and wish they could have another cesarean. Urge a woman to breathe with contractions, push effectively, and accept vaginal birth.

If during the previous labor a complication occurred that necessitated the cesarean birth, a woman cannot help but worry that this will happen again. The woman needs a support person with her and health care providers who are aware of her possible level of apprehension. Women having a VBAC usually have external electronic monitoring because of the risk for uterine rupture.

Fortunately, the outcome of VBAC is usually without complication. If necessary, oxytocin augmentation (see Chap. 21) can be used to strengthen uterine contractions as with any labor; vacuum extraction and forceps birth can be used as necessary.

Many women are reluctant to try a vaginal birth because they are concerned about the pain involved. Afterward, many are relieved to realize that although they did have more discomfort before birth, they had appreciably less pain afterward.

✔ CHECKPOINT QUESTIONS

26. How should you encourage the woman to breathe during pushing?
27. Which type of episiotomy appears to heal more easily, with less blood loss?
28. In the immediate postpartal period, how often should vital signs be assessed?

KEY POINTS

Labor is the series of events by which uterine contractions expel the fetus and placenta from the woman's body.

The exact reason why labor begins is unknown. It most likely occurs because of an interplay between fetal and uterine factors.

Effective labor depends on interactions between the passage, the passenger, the power of contractions, and the woman's psychological readiness ("psyche").

Labor is an almost overwhelming experience because it involves intense sensations and emotions. Women need support people with them to help them cope with this experience.

Fetal presentation (the fetal body part that will initially contact the cervix) and position (the relationship of the fetal presenting part to a specific quadrant of the woman's pelvis) are both important in determining the success of labor.

The first stage of labor lasts from the onset of cervical dilatation until completion (10 cm). The second stage is from the time of full dilatation until the infant is born. A third or placental stage is from the time the infant is born until after delivery of the placenta. A fourth stage is the first few hours after birth.

Danger signs of labor include abnormal FHR, meconium staining of amniotic fluid, abnormal maternal pulse or blood pressure, inadequate or prolonged contractions, formation of a pathologic retraction ring, development of an abnormal lower abdomen contour, and increasing apprehension.

Monitoring uterine contractions and FHR is an important nursing responsibility. Fetal bradycardia, tachycardia, and late and variable decelerations are important observations to make. Interventions such as keeping the woman on her left side and promoting voiding help prevent fetal distress. Offering psychological support is crucial to maternal well-being.

Pushing during the second stage of labor should be guided by the woman's need to push. Urge her to breathe out while pushing.

The placental stage follows birth and consists of placental separation and expulsion. Observe for excessive bleeding during this time. Do not pull on the cord to hasten separation because this can lead to uterine inversion.

A fetus is in potential danger when the membranes rupture because of the possibility of cord prolapse. Always assess FHR at this point to safeguard the fetus.

A woman is at potential risk for hemorrhage throughout labor because of the possibility that the placenta could be dislodged. Assess for vaginal bleeding and vital signs to be sure this is not occurring.

CRITICAL THINKING EXERCISES

1. Linda Bailey, the woman you met at the beginning of the chapter, was certain that her labor was not normal because it had lasted for 6 hours. Is this an unusually long time for a first stage of labor? Do you think she would have been comforted by learning the usual length?
2. A woman in active labor is admitted to a birthing room. She states that she has read nothing during her pregnancy about labor and has little idea of what to expect. Would it be better to educate her or let her follow her practice of not knowing? If you decide to teach her, what would you tell her early in labor? Midway in labor? Why might a woman enter labor without having read about it?
3. A fetus is in a vertex presentation and an occipito-posterior position and has a military attitude. Explain how this might affect the process of labor and what concerns you might anticipate in preparing the client for birth.
4. Most women today accept fetal monitoring equipment as an expected part of labor care. How would you care for a woman who states she does not want this type of fetal monitoring?
5. Examine the National Health Goals related to labor and childbirth. Most government-sponsored money for nursing research is allotted based on these goals. What would be a possible research topic to explore that would be fundable and would advance evidence-based practice?

REFERENCES

Cruikshank, D. P. (2000). Malpresentations and umbilical cord complications. In J. R. Scott, et al. *Danforth's obstetrics and gynecology* (8th ed., pp. 419–436). Philadelphia: Lippincott Williams & Wilkins.

Cunningham, F. G., et al. (2001). Mechanisms of normal labor. In F. G. Cunningham, et al. *William's obstetrics* (21st ed., pp. 291–308). New York: McGraw-Hill.

Department of Health and Human Services. (2000). *Healthy people 2010.* Washington, D.C.: DHHS.

Farrington, P. F., & Ward, K. (2000). Normal labor, delivery and puerperium. In J. R. Scott, et al. *Danforth's obstetrics and gynecology* (8th ed., pp. 91–110). Philadelphia: Lippincott Williams & Wilkins.

Friedman, E. (1978). *Labor, clinical evaluation and management* (2nd ed.). New York: Appleton-Century-Crofts.

Johnson, M., Maas, M., & Moorhead, S. (2000). *Nursing outcomes classification* (2d ed.). St. Louis: Mosby, Inc.

Jordan, E. T., et al. (2000). Educating undergraduate nursing students as birth companions. *Nursing & Health Care Perspectives, 22*(2), 89–91.

Karch, A. M. (2001). *Lippincott's nursing drug guide.* Philadelphia: Lippincott Williams & Wilkins.

Kubli, M., et al. (2002). An evaluation of isotonic "sports drinks" during labor. *Anesthesia & Analgesia, 94*(2), 404–408.

Lynch, M. (2001). Being there: Kids on hand at siblings' birth. *Nursing Spectrum 11*(6), 18–19.

McCloskey, J., & Bulechek, G. (2000). *Nursing interventions classification* (3d ed.). St. Louis: Mosby, Inc.

McFarlin, B. L., et al. (1999). A national survey of herbal preparations used by nurse-midwives for labor stimulation. *Journal of Nurse-Midwifery, 44*(3), 205–216.

Miller, D. A., & Paul, R. (2000). Antepartum-intrapartum fetal monitoring. In J. R. Scott, et al. *Danforth's obstetrics and gynecology* (8th ed., pp. 243–256). Philadelphia: Lippincott Williams & Wilkins.

Moore, M. L. (2001). Adopting birth philosophies to guide successful birth practices and outcomes. *Journal of Perinatal Education, 10*(2), 43–45.

Schneiderman, J. (1997). Cultural uses of placentas. *MCN: American Journal of Maternal Child Nursing, 23*(6), 256.

SUGGESTED READINGS

Browning, C. A. (2000). Using music during childbirth. *Birth, 27*(4), 272–276.

Cleeton, E. R. (2001). Attitudes and beliefs about childbirth among college students. *Birth, 28*(3), 192–201.

Corbett, C. A., & Callister L. C. (2000). Nursing support during labor. *Clinical Nursing Research, 9*(1), 70–83.

Gale, J., et al. (2001). Measuring nursing support during childbirth. *MCN: American Journal of Maternal Child Nursing, 26*(5), 264–271.

Hostetler, D. R., & Bosworth, M. F. (2000). Uterine inversion: A life-threatening obstetric emergency. *Journal of the American Board of Family Practice, 13*(2), 120–123.

Keenan, P. (2000). Benefits of massage therapy and use of a doula during labor and childbirth. *Alternative Therapies in Health & Medicine, 6*(1), 66–74.

Larimore, W. L., & Cline, M. K. (2000). Keeping normal labor normal. *Primary Care: Clinics in Office Practice, 27*(1), 221–236.

Manogin, T. W., et al. (2000). Caring behaviors by nurses: Women's perceptions during childbirth. *Journal of Obstetric, Gynecologic & Neonatal Nursing, 29*(2), 153–157.

Niven, C. A., & Murphy-Black, T. (2000). Memory for labor pain. *Birth, 27*(4), 244–253.

Perla, L. (2002). Patient compliance and satisfaction with nursing care during delivery and recovery. *Journal of Nursing Care Quality, 16*(2), 60–66.

19

CHAPTER

Providing Comfort During Labor and Birth

Key Terms

- analgesia
- anesthesia
- doula
- endorphins
- epidural anesthesia
- pain
- pressure anesthesia
- pudendal nerve block
- transcutaneous electrical nerve stimulation (TENS)

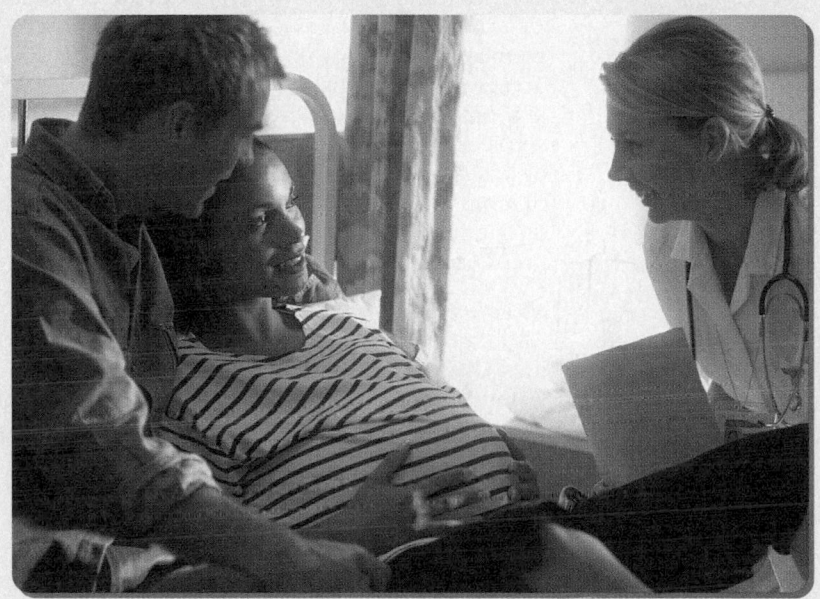

Objectives

After mastering the contents of this chapter, you should be able to:

1. Describe the physiologic basis of contractions during labor and birth and how they are related to theories of pain relief.
2. Identify complementary and alternative therapies that may be used to promote a woman's comfort during labor and birth.
3. Discuss the pharmacologic agents commonly used to provide analgesia and anesthesia.
4. Assess the degree and type of discomfort a woman is experiencing, including her ability to cope with it effectively during labor and birth.
5. Formulate nursing diagnoses related to the effect of pain during labor and birth.
6. Establish expected outcomes to meet the needs of the woman experiencing discomfort during labor and birth.
7. Plan nursing interventions to promote comfort during labor and birth.
8. Implement common complementary and pharmacologic measures for pain relief during labor and birth.
9. Evaluate outcomes for effectiveness of nursing care and achievement of a satisfying labor experience for the woman and her family.
10. Identify National Health Goals related to analgesia and anesthesia and childbirth that nurses can be instrumental in helping the nation to achieve.
11. Identify areas related to promoting comfort during labor that could benefit from additional nursing research or application of evidence-based practice.
12. Use critical thinking to analyze ways to maintain family-centered care when analgesia and anesthesia are used in childbirth.
13. Integrate knowledge of pain relief measures during labor and birth with the nursing process to achieve quality maternal and child health nursing care.

Jonny Baranca is a primipara you admit to a birthing unit in early labor. Her cervix is 4 cm dilated. She tells you her sister had epidural anesthesia for the birth of her baby 3 months ago. The sister told Jonny that preparation for labor really wasn't necessary because an epidural block completely obliterated her pain in labor. Based on her sister's experience, Jonny expected to be given an epidural block as soon as she arrived at the hospital. When you enter her room, you find her lying on her back in a birthing bed, crying. Her husband is standing outside in the hallway at the nursing desk, shouting that his wife deserves better care than this.

Was the advice that Jonny received from her sister realistic advice? What are some immediate interventions you could do to help her better manage her pain?

Previous chapters discussed the process of labor and care for the woman in labor. This chapter adds information to your knowledge base about how to promote comfort during labor. This is important information because it can help change labor from a possibly negative experience to a positive one.

After you've studied the chapter, answer the Critical Thinking Exercises at the end of the chapter and then access the on-line study activities (http://connection.lww.com) *to further sharpen your skills and test your knowledge.*

Concerns about the discomfort and pain involved in labor and birth can sometimes dominate a pregnant woman's or couple's thoughts about childbirth, particularly as the baby's due date approaches. Providing information during prenatal visits about the numerous methods for comfort promotion and pain control available to women can help allay some of these fears. As discussed in Chapter 13, prepared childbirth classes can provide couples with an opportunity to learn more about and to practice a variety of techniques, such as prepared childbirth breathing patterns. Often, however, the labor experience can be overwhelming, or greater than the couple expected. When this occurs, administration of an analgesic or a regional anesthetic can reduce discomfort sufficiently to allow the woman to regain control over the labor process and the childbirth experience. The result may be a satisfying, positive experience, which ultimately promotes the entire family's health. On the other hand, a woman may feel that she has failed because she required medication for pain relief. Therefore, careful explanation and support are essential to foster a positive outcome.

Much has been written in nursing literature about the benefits of using the neutral term *contractions* instead of labor pains. The theory is a sound one, not only because the woman is experiencing a *contracting* sensation but also because calling it *pain* could magnify her fear and tension. Tension, in turn, magnifies pain. Remember, however, that renaming it will not change its basic nature. By any name, discomfort accompanies labor. Fortunately, many nursing interventions can help reduce pain, so that labor is as fulfilling and rewarding an experience as the woman hoped it would be (Jimenez, 2000).

Making labor and birth a memorable experience for families is so important that National Health Goals have been established to address this topic. These are shown in the Focus on National Health Goals.

NURSING PROCESS OVERVIEW

For Pain Relief During Childbirth

Assessment

Pain, the sensation of discomfort, is a subjective, personal symptom; what the person says it is; and present when the person says it is (McCaffery & Pasero, 1999). It is unique to each individual so only the woman can describe or know the extent of her pain. To assess the amount of discomfort a woman is having in labor, listen to what she is saying. Also look for subtle signs of pain such as facial tenseness, flushing, or paleness, hands clenched in fists, rapid breathing, or rapid pulse rate. Knowing the extent of a woman's discomfort helps to guide nursing care (see Assessing the Woman in Pain Related to Labor).

Nursing Diagnosis

Although pain related to labor contractions is the most obvious nursing diagnosis applicable to labor, it is not the only relevant one during this time. Pain can create other problems for the laboring woman that can negatively affect the childbirth experience. If not resolved, these problems can intensify pain. Some women may become more concerned with their

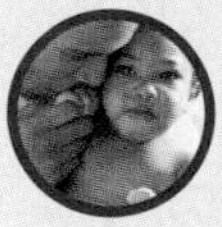

FOCUS ON NATIONAL HEALTH GOALS

As both analgesia and anesthesia administration during labor can increase both maternal and fetal mortality, several National Health Goals are related to the types of pain relief used in labor, for example:

- Reduce the maternal mortality rate to no more than 3.3 per 100,000 live births from a baseline of 7.1 per 100,000.
- Reduce the fetal death rate during the perinatal period (28 weeks of gestation to 7 days after birth) to no more than 4.5 per 1000 live births from a baseline of 7.5 per 1000 (DHHS, 2000).

Nurses can be instrumental in helping the nation achieve these goals by educating women about the advantages of prepared childbirth, helping them to use breathing patterns or other complementary and alternative therapies and techniques during labor so that they need a minimum of analgesia and anesthesia, and conscientiously monitoring women who receive analgesics and anesthesia during labor and birth.

Areas that could benefit from additional nursing research include satisfaction with complementary or alternative therapy comfort measures, women's satisfaction with regional anesthesia in labor, and their reasons why the prepared childbirth method they anticipated using was not adequate.

ASSESSING the Woman in Pain Related to Labor

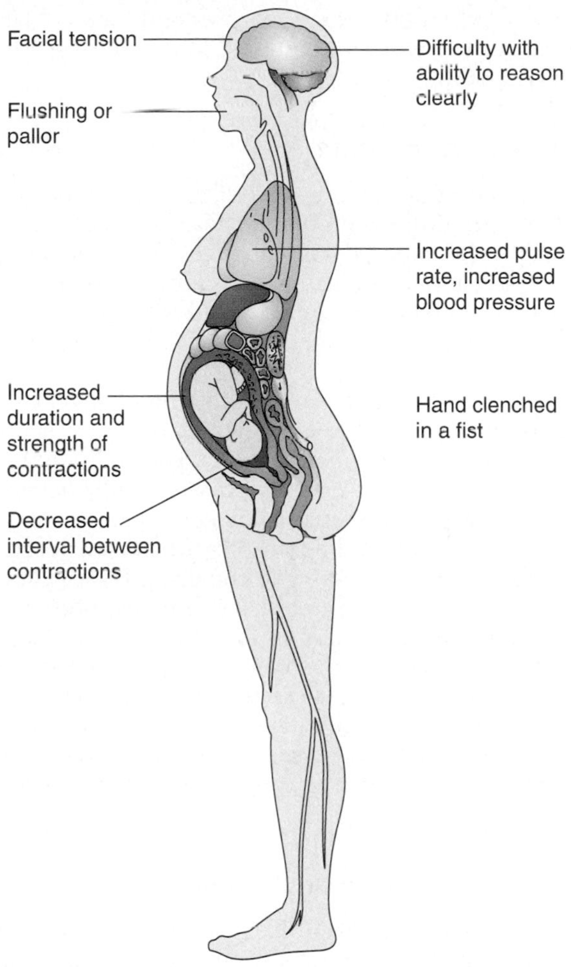

reaction to the pain than to the pain itself. Applicable nursing diagnoses may include:

- Pain related to labor contractions
- Powerlessness related to duration and intensity of labor
- Anxiety related to lack of knowledge about "normal" labor process
- Risk for situational low self-esteem related to ineffectiveness of prepared childbirth breathing exercises
- Decisional conflict related to use of analgesia or anesthesia during labor

Outcome Identification and Planning

When developing outcomes and planning interventions to manage discomfort, consider the woman's perceptions about childbirth, her past childbirth experiences, if any, and the amount and type of childbirth preparation she and her partner have had because the outcomes established must be realistic for the woman. An expectation for using no medication may be inappropriate.

Pharmacologic agents used during labor and birth may pose risks for both the mother (e.g., hypotension) and the fetus (e.g., bradycardia). Their use must always be weighed against the alternative risk to the mother (enduring a painful labor). The decision may also affect family functioning if the method chosen limits the partner's participation in the birth.

Implementation

Many interventions to promote comfort and relieve pain are available. Keeping the woman and her support person informed about the progress of labor is important. Simply knowing that birth is getting even a little closer can make the next few contractions easier to withstand. Supporting and encouraging the woman to use methods of complementary and alternative therapies for pain management, such as relaxation, also are helpful. Offering analgesia or assisting with anesthesia administration during labor or birth requires nursing judgment and a caring presence to help one woman accept analgesia when she needs it and to encourage another to experience childbirth without heavy sedation.

Outcome Evaluation

Evaluation is ongoing and generally must occur within a short time frame. The following are examples to indicate successful achievement of outcomes:

- Client states pain during labor was within a tolerable level for her.
- Couple report they felt in control throughout the labor process.
- Client states she does not feel intimidated by thoughts of pain during labor.

Long-term evaluation should reveal that a woman found labor and birth to be an experience that was not only endurable but allowed her to grow in self-esteem and the family to grow through a shared experience. Asking a woman to describe her labor experience in relation to pain aids evaluation and helps her work through this emotional period of life and integrate it into her previous experience.

EXPERIENCE OF PAIN DURING CHILDBIRTH

Etiology of Pain During Labor and Birth

Normally, contractions of the involuntary muscles, such as the heart, stomach, and intestine, do not cause pain. This concept makes uterine contractions unique because they do cause pain. Several explanations exist for why this happens. During contractions, blood vessels constrict, reducing the blood supply to uterine and cervical cells, resulting in anoxia to muscle fibers. This anoxia can cause pain in the same way that blockage of the cardiac arteries causes the pain of a heart attack. As labor progresses and contractions become longer and harder, the ischemia to cells increases, the anoxia increases, and the pain intensifies.

Pain also probably results from the stretching of the cervix and perineum. This phenomenon is the same as that causing intestinal pain when accumulating gas stretches the intestines. At the end of the transitional phase in labor, when stretching of the cervix is complete and the woman begins to feel she has to push, pain from the contractions often magically disappears as long as she is pushing, until the fetal presenting part causes the final stretching of the perineum (Cunningham et al., 2001).

Additional discomfort in labor may stem from the pressure of the fetal presenting part on tissues, including pressure on surrounding organs, such as the bladder, the urethra, and the lower colon. Pain at birth largely results from perineal tissue stretching.

Physiology of Pain

Pain is a basic protective mechanism that alerts a person to something harmful happening somewhere in the body. Pain sensation begins in nociceptors, the end points of afferent nerves, when they are activated by mechanical, chemical, or thermal stimuli. Nociceptors are located predominantly in the skin, bone periosteum, joint surfaces, and arterial walls. When end terminals are stimulated, chemical mediators such as prostaglandins, histamine, bradykinin, and serotonin are synthesized and sensitize the nociceptors. The pain impulse is transmitted along small unmyelinated (C-fibers) and large myelinated (A-delta fibers) to the spinal cord. The more numerous C-fibers conduct slowly and apparently carry dull, low-level pain; the fewer A-delta fibers apparently carry sharp, well-localized pain.

In the dorsal horn of the spinal cord, somatostatin, cholecystokinin, and substance P serve as neurotransmitters or assist the pain impulse across the synapse between the peripheral nerve and the spinal nerve. The pain impulse then ascends the spinal cord to the brain cortex where it is interpreted as pain.

The Melzack-Wall gate control theory of pain control (Melzack-Wall, 1965), the most widely accepted theory of pain response and control today, proposes that pain can be halted at three points: the peripheral end terminals, the synapse points in the dorsal horn, or the point the impulse is interpreted as pain in the brain cortex.

Pain in peripheral terminals is automatically reduced by the production of endorphins and enkephalins, naturally occurring opiates that act to limit transmission of pain from the end terminals. Pain can be reduced further by mechanically stimulating additional nerve fibers by actions such as rubbing the skin.

A major action of pain medications is to block spinal cord neurotransmitters, never allowing the pain impulse to cross to a spinal nerve. The brain cortex can be distracted from sensing impulses as pain by such techniques as imagery, thought stopping, aromatherapy, or yoga.

Sensory impulses from the uterus and cervix synapse at the spinal column at the level of T10 through T12 and L1. Pain relief measures for the first stage of labor, therefore, have to block these upper synapse sites. For the elimination of pain during cesarean birth, receptors at the level of T6 through T8 must be blocked so the upper and lower uterus is blocked.

Sensory impulses from the perineum are carried by the pudendal nerve to join the spinal column at S2, S3, and S4. Pain relief for birth, therefore, when the perineum is initiating the pain, must block these lower receptor sites. This is an important point to remember when talking to women in labor about pain relief. Some interventions relieve pain for both the first *and* second stages of labor, whereas others work for first *or* second stage but not for both (Fishburne, 2000).

Perception of Pain

The amount of discomfort a woman experiences during contractions differs according to her expectations of and preparation for labor, the length of the labor, the position of the fetus, and the availability of support people around her (Fig. 19-1). The discomfort a woman experiences can become compounded when fear and anxiety are also present (McCrea et al., 2000).

Pain is perceived differently by different individuals because of psychosocial, physiologic, and cultural responses (see Focus on Cultural Competence). The body's ability to produce and maintain **endorphins** (naturally occurring opiate-like substances) may influence a person's overall pain threshold and the amount of pain a person perceives at any given time. Women who come into labor believing the pain will be horrible are usually surprised afterward to realize that the agony they expected never materialized. On the other hand, expectations of pain may make a woman so tense during labor that her pain is worse than it would have been if she had been relaxed. A woman cannot relax simply because she is instructed to do so by another person, however. Some additional intervention must be used.

Factors Influencing Pain Perception

Fetal position is a physical variable that can influence pain. A woman with a fetus in an occiput posterior position, for example, often reports intense or nagging back pain during labor, even between contractions.

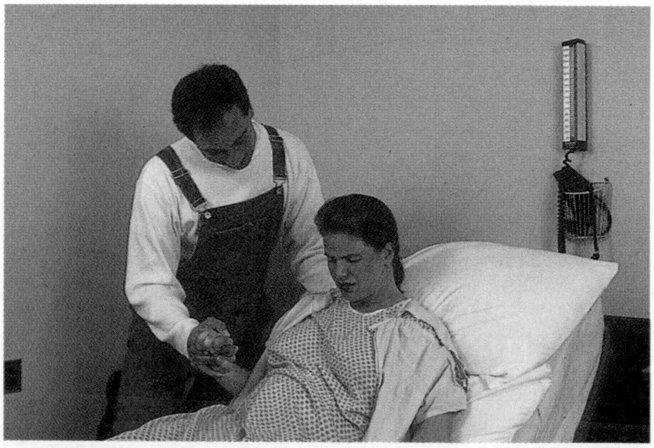

FIGURE 19.1 The discomfort a woman experiences during childbirth may be related to the amount of support she receives from her family or health care providers.

FOCUS ON CULTURAL COMPETENCE

Responses to pain are culturally determined. Based on this, some believe that being stoic and nonverbal is what is expected of them. Others believe that expressing their discomfort by screaming or actively verbalizing their feelings will best reduce pain. If English is not a woman's primary language, it may be particularly difficult for her to describe her level of distress. Assess each woman individually to determine not only what level of comfort she feels is right for her during labor but also the manner in which she feels most able to express discomfort. Depend on facial expression, body posture and tension, as well as voiced expressions to determine the comfort level of a client (McCaffery & Pasero, 1999).

The amount of analgesia that women desire or will accept is both situational and culturally determined. In a culture in which birth is seen as a "natural" process, less analgesia is generally desired. Women who have an effective support person with them may need less pharmacologic pain relief measures than those who do not. Therefore, providing nursing support can have a positive influence on pain relief in labor.

Psychological factors that influence pain include fear, anxiety, worry, expectation of pain, body image, and self-efficacy. Women who feel they can control their situation (have self-efficacy) are apt to report less pain than those who feel they have no control over their situation.

COMFORT AND PAIN RELIEF MEASURES

The pattern of interventions to promote comfort and manage pain in labor has swung from a philosophy of no intervention (none given), to a philosophy of drug intervention as an essential element (too much given), to a modern approach of empowering women and their partners with information so they can decide how to best relieve pain during labor, within the limits of medical safety. For centuries, in Western civilization, offering pain relief in labor was thought to be amoral because, according to the Biblical account, God commanded Eve, "I will greatly multiply thy sorrow and thy conception; in sorrow thou shalt bring forth children . . ." (Genesis 3:16). In the witch-burning period of American history, the concept that childbirth should be painful was so strongly ingrained that women were burned as witches for providing comfort to other women in labor.

With the discovery of ether and chloroform in the 1800s, it became apparent that childbirth could be managed completely pain free. Unfortunately, this goal was achieved by means of complete anesthesia or unconsciousness during labor and birth.

Current philosophy centers on informed decision making. Nurses play a key role in educating the woman and her support person about the numerous comfort and pain relief strategies available, making sure they understand the choices available to them along with the benefits and risks. Throughout their decision-making process, they need support for their choices. In addition, be sure that any other personnel involved in the client's care understand how their actions or statements can affect the woman's perception of pain during labor (see Focus on Multidisciplinary Care).

Support From a Doula or Coach

A woman's husband or the father of her child has traditionally served as the chief support person in labor. However, some husbands or fathers may find it difficult to provide effective coaching or support in labor because of their own emotional involvement in the birth. Women who are aware that they may not have effective one-to-one support in labor should be encouraged to identify another person who could come with them and provide this support. A **doula** is a woman without professional credentials who guides and assists a woman in labor in this way. Having a doula with a woman in labor can increase her self-esteem and decrease rates of oxytocin augmentation, epidural anesthesia, and cesarean birth the same as other support (Keenan, 2000).

✔ CHECKPOINT QUESTIONS

1. During the first stage of labor, what level of receptors must be blocked to achieve pain relief?
2. What substance naturally produced by the body helps to reduce pain?
3. What is a popular name for a non-medical person who helps support a woman in labor?

FOCUS ON MULTIDISCIPLINARY CARE

Although unlicensed assistive personnel and other members of the multidisciplinary health care team do not have direct responsibility for pain management for women in labor, they can be influential in setting the tone for how much pain management is offered to women in labor. Often, during labor, personnel may interact with the woman, describing their experiences with labor and birth. Be certain that if they recount their own experiences ("I had an epidural with my last baby; I'll never have anything else again"; "I've seen enough babies born to know the only sensible thing to do is to ask to be knocked out"), they are recounting a personal experience that applied to them and not offering informed advice. Be certain they do not discount complementary and alternative therapy measures for pain relief as unimportant. Women need to have confidence in measures to receive the most benefit from them.

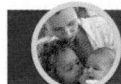

Complementary and Alternative Therapies for Pain Relief

Alternative and complementary therapies for pain relief involve nonpharmacologic measures that include interventions that may be used either as a woman's total pain management program or to complement pharmacologic interventions. Most of these interventions are based on the gate control theory concept that distraction can be effective in preventing the brain from processing pain sensations coming into the cortex.

Relaxation

The technique of relaxation, as discussed in Chapter 13, is taught in most preparation for childbirth classes. Relaxation keeps the abdominal wall from becoming tense, allowing the uterus to rise with contractions without pressing against the hard abdominal wall. It also serves as a distraction technique because, while concentrating on relaxing, the woman cannot concentrate on pain. In addition to conscious relaxation, having a woman shift position or find the position in labor that is most comfortable for her is helpful. Asking women to bring favorite music tapes or aromatherapy for them to enjoy in the birthing room are good ways to aid relaxation (Browning, 2000; Burns et al., 2000).

Focusing and Imagery

Concentrating intently on an object is another method of distraction, or keeping sensory input from reaching the cortex of the brain. For this technique, the woman uses a photograph of someone important to her or some image she finds appealing. She concentrates on it during contractions. Other women use imagery by concentrating on a mental image, such as watching waves rolling onto a beach. Do not ask questions or talk to women while they are using imagery or focusing because it breaks their concentration (Steffes, 2000).

Breathing Techniques

Breathing patterns are also taught in most preparation for childbirth classes (see Chapter 13). They are advantageous because they help to relax the abdomen. They are largely distraction techniques because a woman concentrating on slow-paced breathing cannot concentrate on her pain. Breathing strategies can be taught to a woman in labor if she is not familiar with their advantages before labor.

Herbal Preparations

Several herbal preparations have traditionally been used to reduce pain with dysmenorrhea or labor, although there is little factual support for their effectiveness. Examples that you may see people using include raspberry leaves, fennel, and life root. Blue cohosh (squaw root), used to induce uterine contractions, is not recommended because of the risk of acute toxic effects such as cerebral vascular accident to the mother or fetus (DerMarderosian, 2001).

Aromatherapy and Essential Oils

Aromatherapy is the use of aromatic essential oils to lead to emotional and physical well-being. Their use is based on the principle that the sense of smell plays a significant role in overall health. When an essential oil is inhaled, its molecules are transported via the olfactory system to the limbic system in the brain. The brain responds to particular aromas with emotional responses. When applied externally, they are absorbed by the skin and then carried throughout the body (Marks, 2000). When a drop of oil, such as lavender, is placed on the skin, you should be able to taste it within 15 seconds. The oils used may be able to penetrate cell walls and transport nutrients or oxygen to the inside of cells. Jasmine and lavender are oils thought to be responsible for an easier labor.

Heat or Cold Application

Heat and cold have always been used for pain relief after injuries such as minor burns or strained muscles. It is only lately that they have been considered an effective way to help relieve the pain of labor contractions. Women who are having back pain may find application of heat to their lower back by a heating pad or a moist compress very comforting.

Women who become warm from the exertion of labor find a cool washcloth to their forehead comforting. Ice chips to suck on to relieve mouth dryness are also refreshing.

Bathing or Hydrotherapy

Standing under a warm shower, or soaking in a tub of warm water, jet hydrotherapy tub, or whirlpool are other ways to apply heat to help reduce the pain of labor (Teschendorf & Evans, 2000). The temperature of water used should be between 95°F and 100°F (35.0°C and 37.8°C) to prevent hyperthermia (Benfield et al., 2001) (see Focus on Evidence-Based Practice). This type of pain relief measure usually is not recommended for women whose membranes have ruptured because of the risk of infection.

Therapeutic Touch and Massage

Therapeutic touch is the use of touch to comfort and relieve pain. It is based on the concept that the body contains energy fields that, when plentiful, lead to health and when in less supply, result in ill health. Krieger (1990), in a classic work, defines therapeutic touch as the laying on of hands to redirect the energy fields that lead to pain. Although the action is not well documented, touch and massage probably work to relieve pain by increasing the release of endorphins (Lothian, 2000). It also is a form of distraction. Effleurage, the technique of gentle abdominal massage often taught with Lamaze preparation for childbirth classes, is a form of therapeutic touch (Fig. 19-2).

Yoga

Yoga, a term derived from the Sanskrit word for union, denotes a series of exercises that were originally designed to bring people who practice it closer to their God. It

FOCUS ON EVIDENCE-BASED PRACTICE

Is Hydrotherapy Effective for Pain Relief in Labor?
To see if hydrotherapy can promote relaxation and decrease pain during labor, researchers assigned nine women in labor to an experimental group where they agreed to be immersed in a tub of water at a temperature of 37°C for 1 hour during early labor. Nine other women served as a control group and received no hydrotherapy during labor. By as little as 15 minutes' time, the bathing women reported their anxiety and pain scores were decreased compared to those of nonbathers. By the end of the hour, the amount of pain they were experiencing was still decreased. No significant differences were found in maternal or fetal complications.

This is an important study because, although the sample is small, it effectively shows the benefits of hydrotherapy for relieving short-term anxiety and pain during labor. As nurses are being asked more and more to participate in hospital design, knowing that alternative therapies such as this can be effective allows nurses to make suggestions for equipment such as hydrotherapy tubs or other alternative therapies. Additionally, this study can provide impetus for further research into this topic, for example, using a larger sample size.

Benfield, R. D., Herman, J., Katz, V. L., Wilson, S. P., & Davis, J. M. (2001). Hydrotherapy in labor. *Research in Nursing & Health, 24*(1), 57–67.

offers a significant variety of proven health benefits including increasing the efficiency of the heart, slowing the respiratory rate, improving fitness, lowering blood pressure, promoting relaxation, reducing stress, and allaying anxiety. Exercises consist of deep breathing exercises, body postures to stretch and strengthen muscles, and meditation to focus the mind and relax the body. It may be helpful in reducing the pain of labor through its ability to relax the body and possibly through the release of endorphins that may occur.

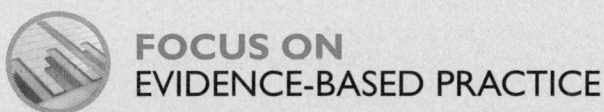

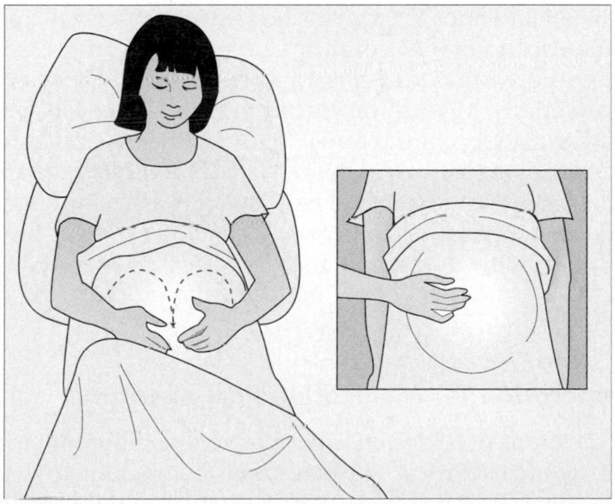

FIGURE 19.2 The laboring woman performs effleurage on her abdomen.

Reflexology

Reflexology is the practice of stimulating the hands, feet, and ears as a form of therapy. Professional reflexologists apply pressure to specific areas of the hands, feet, and ears to alleviate common ailments such as headaches, back pain, sinus colds, and stress. The theory behind reflexology is that each of the body's organs and glands are linked to corresponding areas of the hands and feet. The body is divided into 10 zones that run in longitudinal lines from the top of the head to the tips of the toes. Application of pressure to the specific area aims to restore energy to the body and improve the overall condition.

Crystal or Gemstone Therapy

Some gemstones or crystals are thought to have healing powers, and so women may bring these into a birthing room to use during labor. The woman who uses crystals or gemstones may believe that their healing power is magnified when they are positioned around her body. Be especially careful when changing bedding or rearranging equipment in a birthing room. Respect the position of these crystals because the woman may feel they do not work their healing powers in a different position (Marks, 2000).

Hypnosis

Hypnosis is yet another method of pain relief for labor. A woman who wants to use this modality needs to meet with her hypnotherapist during pregnancy. At these visits, she is evaluated for and further conditioned for susceptibility to hypnotic suggestion. At the last prenatal visit, she is given the posthypnotic suggestion that she will experience reduced pain or absence of pain during labor. For the woman who is susceptible to hypnotic suggestion, the method can provide a very satisfactory drug-free method of pain relief.

Biofeedback

Biofeedback is based on the belief that people have control and can regulate internal events such as heart rate and pain response. Women interested in using biofeedback for pain relief in labor must attend several sessions during pregnancy to condition themselves to regulate their pain response. During these sessions, a biofeedback apparatus is used to measure muscle tone or the ability of the woman to relax (DiFranco, 2000).

Transcutaneous Electrical Nerve Stimulation

Transcutaneous electrical nerve stimulation (TENS) relieves pain by counter irritation on nociceptors. With two pairs of electrodes attached to the woman's back to coincide with the T10–L1 nerve pathways, low-intensity electrical stimulation is given continuously or applied by the woman herself as a contraction begins. This stimulation blocks the afferent fibers, or prevents pain from traveling to the spinal cord synapses from the uterus. As labor progresses and the pelvic division begins, the electrodes are moved to stimulate the S2–4 level. High-intensity stimulation is generally needed to control the pain at this stage.

TENS can be as effective as epidural anesthesia for pain relief in labor (Van der Spank, 2000). Some women may object to being "tied down" to the equipment. Women with extreme back pain during labor may benefit the most from a TENS unit, because this type of pain is difficult to relieve with controlled breathing exercises. TENS is also discussed in Chapter 20 as it applies to the postoperative pain of a cesarean birth.

Acupressure and Acupuncture

Acupuncture is based on the concept that illness results from an imbalance of energy. To correct the imbalance, needles are inserted into the skin at designated susceptible body points (tsubos). The points are located along meridians that course throughout the body supplying organs of the body with energy. These points are not necessarily near the affected organ. Activation of these points apparently results in release of endorphins.

Acupressure, in contrast, is the application of pressure or massage at these points. A common point used for the woman in labor is Co4 (Hoku or Hegu point) located between the first and second metacarpal bones on the back of the hand. When a support person holds and squeezes a woman's hand in labor, he or she may be triggering this point.

Intracutaneous Nerve Stimulation

Intracutaneous nerve stimulation (INS) is a technique of counter-irritation involving the intradermal injection of sterile water or saline along the borders of the sacrum to relieve low back pain during labor (Fishburne, 2000). Some women find the technique helpful, while others prefer to bear back pain rather than submit to such an unnatural pain relief measure.

✔ CHECKPOINT QUESTIONS

4. For what type of pain are heat applications most effective during labor?
5. Which pregnant women should avoid the use of warm-water tub bathing for pain relief in labor?

Pharmacologic Pain Relief During Labor

Pharmacologic management of pain during labor and birth includes **analgesia,** which reduces or decreases awareness of pain, and **anesthesia,** which causes partial or compete loss of sensation. Many choices are available today. For the best results, women need to be included in the individual selection for them (Faucher & Brucker, 2000). Be certain to ask about allergies to any medications before administering them during labor.

Virtually all medication given during labor crosses the placenta and has some effect on the fetus. Thus, it is important that a woman receive as little systemic medication as possible during labor. On the other hand, labor should not test a woman to the limit of her endurance, especially since local anesthesia is available. Be sure to caution women not to take acetylsalicylic acid (aspirin) for pain in labor. Aspirin interferes with blood coagulation, increasing the risk for bleeding in the newborn or mother.

Goals of Pharmacologic Management of Pain During Labor

Medication effectively used during labor must relax the woman and relieve her discomfort, yet have minimal systemic effects on her uterine contractions, her pushing effort, or the fetus. Whether a drug affects the fetus depends on its ability to cross the placenta. Drugs with a molecular weight of more than 1000 cross poorly, whereas those with a molecular weight of less than 600 cross very readily. Drugs with highly charged molecules or molecules strongly bound to protein cross more slowly than others. Fat-soluble drugs cross most easily. A preterm fetus, which has an immature liver and is unable to metabolize or inactivate drugs, is generally more affected by drugs than a term fetus. If a drug causes a systemic response, such as hypotension, in the woman, it can result in a decreased PO_2 gradient across the placenta and fetal hypoxia. If it causes confusion or disorientation in the woman, she may be unable to work effectively with contractions, thus labor may be prolonged. If a medication causes changes in the fetus, such as a decreased heart rate or central nervous system (CNS) depression, it may be difficult for the newborn infant to initiate respirations at birth, severely compromising the infant in the important first minutes of life.

Because pain is a subjective sensation, women experience different levels during labor. Some women are most aware of pain early in labor, whereas some report the second stage of labor as the most difficult. The point at which pain medication is needed, therefore, also differs from one individual to another. Once labor is well underway, medication to relieve discomfort can speed its progress because the woman can relax and work with, not against, contractions. Medication given too early, however, tends to slow labor contractions. The American College of Obstetricians and Gynecologists (ACOG) currently recommends that women receive pain relief at the point they request it, regardless of cervical dilatation (ACOG, 2002). Unfortunately, no perfect analgesic agent exists for labor or birth that has no effect on labor, the mother, and the fetus.

Preparation for Medication Administration

Medications used during labor vary among different health care agencies. Research is constantly being done to determine the effectiveness and safety of new drugs for use during labor. To be safe, always remember the criteria that a drug must fulfill to be used in pregnancy, or expand the rule of basic medication administration from "Never give any drug unless you know it is safe for your individual client" to "Never give a drug in labor without knowing it is safe for both your clients: the mother and the fetus."

The preparations frequently used in labor and birth are shown in Table 19-1. Prepare the woman for the type of agent to be given: how it will be administered (e.g., "You'll need to lie on your side") and what she can expect to happen after administration (e.g., "I'll be taking your blood pressure frequently"). Women in labor are under stress. Experiencing surprising body sensations without preparation can be so frightening it defeats an individual's coping abilities. When a person struggles against medication administration because she does not understand what is going on, the risk of inadvertent problems increases.

WHAT IF? What if a woman in labor wants something for pain but has no idea what to ask for? How would you advise her? You notice her husband grips her hand very tightly during contractions. What possible pain relief measure is her husband's tight pressure providing for her?

Narcotic Analgesics

Narcotics are often given in labor because of their potent analgesic effect. Unfortunately, all the drugs in this category cause fetal CNS depression to some extent. Be sure

TABLE 19.1 Analgesics and Anesthetics Commonly Used in Labor and Birth

TYPE	DRUG	USUAL DOSAGE/ROUTE	EFFECT ON MOTHER	EFFECT ON LABOR PROGRESS	EFFECT ON FETUS OR NEWBORN
Narcotic analgesic	Meperidine (Demerol)	25 mg IV, 50–100 mg IM q3–4 h; also epidurally	Effective analgesic; feeling of well-being	Relaxation, possibly aiding progress during cervical relaxation. Slows labor contractions if given early.	Should be given 3 h before delivery to avoid respiratory depression in newborn. Decreases beat-to-beat variability in FHR.
	Nalbuphine (Nubain)	10–20 mg IM q3–6 h, 0.3–3 mg/kg over 10–15 min IV	Slowing of respiratory rate; effective analgesic	Mild maternal sedation	Results in some respiratory depression
	Butorphanol (Stadol)	1–2 mg IM or IV q3–4 h	Withdrawal symptoms if woman is opiate-dependent	Possible slowing of labor if given early	Results in some respiratory depression
	Morphine sulfate	Intrathecally 0.2–1 mg; 5 mg epidurally	Pruritus; effective analgesia	Possible slowing	Has minimal effect
	Fentanyl (Sublimaze)	50–100 µg IM or 25–50 µg IV; also epidurally	Hypotension; respiratory depression	Slowing of labor if given early	May result in respiratory depression
Lumbar epidural block	Local anesthetic Bupivacaine (Marcaine), Ropivacaine (Naropin)	Administered for first stage of labor; with continuous block, anesthesia will last through delivery; injected at L3–4; Fentanyl or morphine possibly added	Rapid onset, in minutes; lasting 60–90 min; loss of pain perception for labor contractions and delivery; possible maternal hypotension	Slowing of labor if given early; pushing feeling obliterated, resulting in possible prolonged second stage	May be some differences in response in first few days of life
Pudendal block	Local anesthetic Lidocaine (Xylocaine)	Administered just before delivery for perineal anesthesia; injected through vagina	Rapid anesthesia of perineum	None apparent	None apparent
Local infiltration of perineum	Local anesthetic Lidocaine (Xylocaine)	Injected just before for episiotomy incision	Anesthesia of perineum almost immediately	None apparent	None apparent
General intravenous anesthetic	Thiopental	Administered IV by anesthesiologist or nurse-anesthetist	Rapid anesthesia; also rapid recovery	Forceps required because abdominal pushing is no longer possible	Results in infant being born with CNS depression

Adapted from Karch, A. M. (2001). *Lippincott's nursing drug guide.* Philadelphia: Lippincott Williams & Wilkins.

to question an order for a narcotic if a woman is in preterm labor. Because of possible lung immaturity, a preterm infant may have extreme difficulty coping with the added insult of respiratory depression at birth.

Narcotic analgesics commonly used include meperidine hydrochloride (Demerol), morphine sulfate, nalbuphine (Nubain), fentanyl (Sublimaze), and butorphanol tartrate (Stadol). Meperidine is advantageous as an analgesic in labor because it has additional sedative and antispasmodic actions. Thus, it is effective in relieving pain, helping to relax the cervix, and giving a feeling of euphoria and well-being. Demerol may be given either intramuscularly or intravenously. The dose is 25 to 100 mg, depending on the woman's weight and route of administration. The drug begins to act about 30 minutes after intramuscular (IM) injection and about 5 minutes after intravenous (IV) administration. Its duration of action is 2 to 3 hours (Karch, 2001).

Demerol also may be self-administered by a patient-controlled analgesic (PCA) pump for low-dose but frequent administration during labor. Intrathecal administration (injected into the cerebral spinal fluid), although not successful with all women, is used less frequently.

Because Demerol crosses the placenta, it may cause respiratory depression in the fetus. The drug crosses the placenta minutes after being administered either IV or IM to the mother. Because the fetal liver takes 2 to 3 hours to activate the drug into the fetal system, however, the effect will not be registered in the fetus for 2 to 3 hours after administration. For this reason, Demerol is given when the mother is more than 3 hours away from birth. This allows the peak action of the drug in the fetus to have passed by the time of birth.

It may be puzzling to see a sleepy baby delivered to a woman who was given Demerol 2 hours before birth and an alert baby delivered to a woman who had Demerol within 1 hour of birth. In the second instance, however, the peak action or peak effect has not yet occurred in the infant. This newborn needs careful assessment for the next 4 hours until the drug reaches its peak.

Nalbuphine hydrochloride (Nubain) and butorphanol tartrate (Stadol) are synthetic narcotic analgesics also used in labor. The action of these agents is comparable to that of Demerol. Like Demerol, they may also leave a degree of respiratory depression in the newborn.

Whenever a narcotic is given during labor, a narcotic antagonist such as naloxone (Narcan) should be available for administration to the infant at birth (see Focus on Pharmacology). Carefully observe an infant who receives naloxone in the immediate birth period, because when the drug's effect wears off, the infant's respirations may become severely depressed again. If severe infant respiratory depression is anticipated, Narcan can be given to the mother just before birth. It readily crosses the placenta and, because it interferes with or competes for narcotic binding sites, it may increase the chance for spontaneous respiratory activity in the newborn.

WHAT IF? What if a woman in labor received no narcotics during labor, yet her newborn is very sleepy? Would you administer naloxone? Would asking the mother if she used recreational drugs be warranted?

FOCUS ON PHARMACOLOGY

Naloxone Hydrochloride (Narcan)

Action: Naloxone hydrochloride is a narcotic antagonist that counteracts the effect of narcotic analgesics

Pregnancy category: B

Dosage: 0.01 mg/kg IV via umbilical vein, SC, or IM; repeated at 2- to 3-minute intervals until response is obtained.

Possible adverse reactions: Hypotension, hypertension, tachycardia, diaphoresis, tremulousness

Nursing Implications

- Anticipate the need for resuscitative measures; have resuscitative equipment and emergency drugs readily available.
- If no IV access is available, prepare for possible administration via endotracheal tube.
- If no response is seen after two or three doses, question if respiratory depression is caused by narcotics.
- Continuously monitor all vital signs for changes.
- Remember that the pain-relieving effect of narcotics will be reversed; assess for pain in the neonate.

Intrathecal Narcotics. *Intrathecal* refers to injection into the spinal cord. With intrathecal narcotic injection, a catheter is introduced into the spinal canal (the subarachnoid space) and a narcotic such as morphine or fentanyl citrate is injected into the canal by way of the catheter. Both intrathecal morphine and fentanyl provide excellent pain relief for labor pain. The drug takes effect in 15 to 30 minutes. Pain relief lasts 4 to 7 hours. A woman is able to feel the urge to push at the second stage of labor, allowing her to actively participate in the birth. Because intrathecal injections are not as effective in reducing the pain of the actual birth, they may be supplemented with a pudendal block in late labor. Possible side effects of intrathecal morphine are intense pruritus, nausea, and vomiting. The pruritus can be treated with IV diphenhydramine (Benadryl) if it becomes too uncomfortable.

Additional Drugs

Additional drugs, such as tranquilizers, may be administered during labor to reduce anxiety or potentiate the action of a narcotic. Examples include hydroxyzine hydrochloride (Vistaril) and a phenothiazine derivative such as promethazine (Phenergan). Remember that these drugs do not relieve pain, so a woman in labor needs pain management measures in addition to these drugs.

Regional Anesthesia

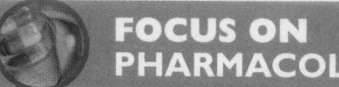

Regional anesthesia is the injection of a local anesthetic such as chloroprocaine (Nesacaine) or bupivacaine (Marcaine) to block specific nerve pathways. It achieves pain relief by blocking sodium and potassium transport in the nerve membrane, thereby stabilizing the nerve in a polarized resting state so it is unable to conduct sensations.

Depending on the region anesthetized, a woman may or may not continue to be aware of contractions. Various regional anesthetic injection sites are shown in Figure 19-3. Women with preeclampsia may have associated bleeding defects, and need to be assessed carefully before regional anesthesia is administered.

Because regional anesthetics are not introduced into the maternal circulation, it was once believed they had no effect on the fetus. Research has demonstrated that there is some uptake of these drugs by the fetus, however, possibly resulting in fetal heart rate decelerations and symptoms of flaccidity, bradycardia, and hypotension in the newborn (Karch, 2001). Effects are minimal when compared with those of systemic anesthetic agents, however. Most importantly, regional anesthesia allows the woman to be completely awake and aware of what is happening during birth. They do not depress uterine tone, leaving the uterus capable of optimal contraction after birth, thereby helping to prevent postpartal hemorrhage.

It is rare that an infant is born with symptoms of toxicity from a regional anesthetic. If it occurs, however, an exchange transfusion at birth will remove the anesthetic from the bloodstream. Gastric lavage also will remove a great deal of anesthetic, because anesthetics have a strong affinity for acid mediums such as stomach acid.

Epidural Anesthesia (Peridural Blocks). The nerves in the spinal cord are protected by several tissue layers. The pia mater is the membrane adhering to the nerve fibers. Surrounding this is the *cerebrospinal fluid* (CSF). Next comes the arachnoid membrane and outside that, the *dura mater.* Outside the dura mater is a vacant space (the *epidural space*). Beyond it is the *ligamentum flavum,* yet another protective shield to the vulnerable spinal cord.

An anesthetic agent introduced into the CSF in the subarachnoid space is called a spinal injection or spinal anesthesia. An anesthetic agent placed just inside the ligamentum flavum in the epidural space is **epidural anesthesia** (see Fig. 19-3). Anesthetic agents placed in the epidural space at the L4–5, L3–4, or L2–3 interspace block not only spinal nerve roots in the space but also the sympathetic nerve fibers that travel with them. Therefore, such a block provides pain relief for both labor and birth. Such a block may actually increase contraction strength and blood flow to the uterus. Because the woman no longer experiences pain, the release of catecholamines (epinephrine) with a beta-blocking effect from a pain response is decreased, making this a very effective pain relief measure for labor (Howell, 2000).

"Spinal headaches" occur rarely after epidural anesthesia. These headaches are caused by leakage of CSF or instillation of air into CSF. With epidural anesthesia, the CSF space is not entered. Because the injection technique is potentially frightening, women need continuous support during the process.

Epidural blocks, administered by an anesthesiologist or nurse anesthetist, are suitable for almost all women. They are advantageous for women with heart disease, pulmonary disease, diabetes, and sometimes severe pregnancy-induced hypertension, because they make labor virtually pain free and thus reduce stress from the discomfort of labor to a minimum. Because the woman does not feel contractions, her physical energy is preserved. Epidural blocks are acceptable for use in preterm labor because the drug has scant effect on the fetus. They allow for a controlled and gentle birth with less trauma to an immature fetal skull. Because the woman receives no systemic medication, the

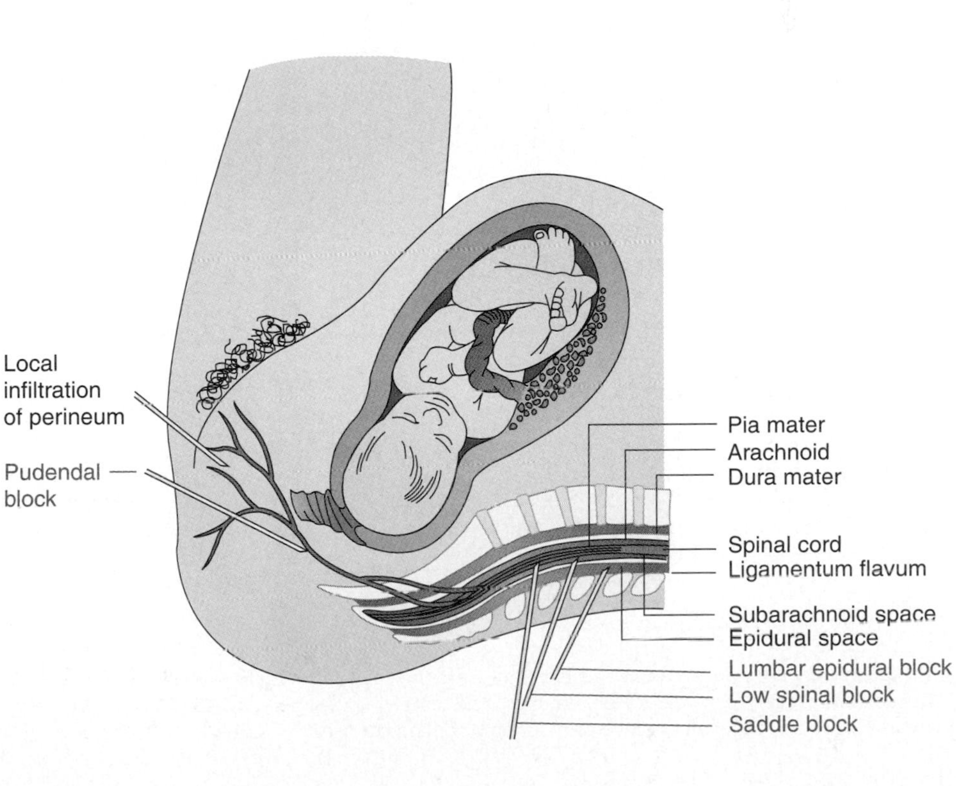

FIGURE 19.3 Anatomy of the spinal canal and sites of injection for regional anesthesia.

infant responds more quickly after birth than if systemic narcotic analgesics were used.

The chief concern with epidural anesthesia is its tendency to induce hypotension in the woman because of its blocking effect on the sympathetic fibers in the epidural space. This blocking leads to decreased peripheral resistance in the woman's circulatory system. Blood flows freely into peripheral vessels, and a pseudohypovolemia registering as hypotension occurs. However, the combined use of fentanyl and bupivacaine can lower the possibility of hypotension occurring. In addition, this possibility also can be reduced by ensuring that the woman is well hydrated with 500 to 1000 mL of IV fluid, such as Ringer's lactate, before the anesthetic is given. Ringer's lactate is preferable to a glucose solution, because too much maternal glucose can cause hyperglycemia with rebound hypoglycemia in the newborn. Be certain the woman does not lay supine, but remains on her side after an epidural to help prevent supine hypotension syndrome.

If hypotension does occur, raising the woman's legs and administering oxygen and additional IV fluid along with an agent such as ephedrine to elevate blood pressure may be necessary to stabilize cardiovascular status.

In rare instances, the anesthetic enters the blood circulation, as manifested by drowsiness, a metallic taste on the tongue, slurred speech, blurred vision, unconsciousness, and seizures leading to cardiac arrest. If such symptoms occur, it is an emergency situation. The woman needs oxygen, an anticonvulsant such as diazepam (Valium) or thiopental (Pentothal) IV followed by prompt delivery of the fetus.

The use of an epidural block tends to prolong the second stage of labor, but whether this leads to an increase in cesarean births is controversial (Fishburne, 2000). Descent can slow, for example, taking 3 hours rather than 2 hours, but if there is no indication that this is detrimental to the fetus, it should not lead to a greater need for vacuum extraction or cesarean birth. Relaxation of the levator ani muscle may impede internal rotation of the fetal head, further slowing labor or making the use of forceps necessary to effect rotation. This occurs primarily when the fetus is in an occiput-posterior position. Oxytocin may be given to shorten labor. Allowing an epidural to wear off by the second stage of labor so the woman can push with contractions is another option. However, experiencing contractions at this point can be overwhelming for the woman and counteracts the original reason for giving the anesthetic.

Technique for Administration. Lumbar epidural anesthesia is begun when the cervix is dilated 5 to 6 cm. An IV infusion and equipment for blood pressure monitoring should be in place. The woman is positioned on her side or sitting upright. Her back should not be flexed because this increases the possibility of puncturing the dura and accidentally giving the anesthetic as spinal, not epidural, anesthesia. The lumbar area of her back is cleaned with an antiseptic solution. A local anesthetic is injected into the skin to form a wheal over the L3–4 vertebra. A special 3- to 5-inch needle is then passed through the L3–4 interspace into the epidural space. After needle placement, a polyethylene catheter is passed through the needle into the space, and the needle is then withdrawn, leaving the catheter to be taped in place. A closed system (a syringe is attached) is established to prevent infection through the catheter (Fig. 19-4).

A small test dose of a local anesthetic solution is injected through the catheter. Five minutes later, the woman's legs are inspected for flushing and warmness, evidence that the anesthetic is in the epidural space (peripheral dilatation is

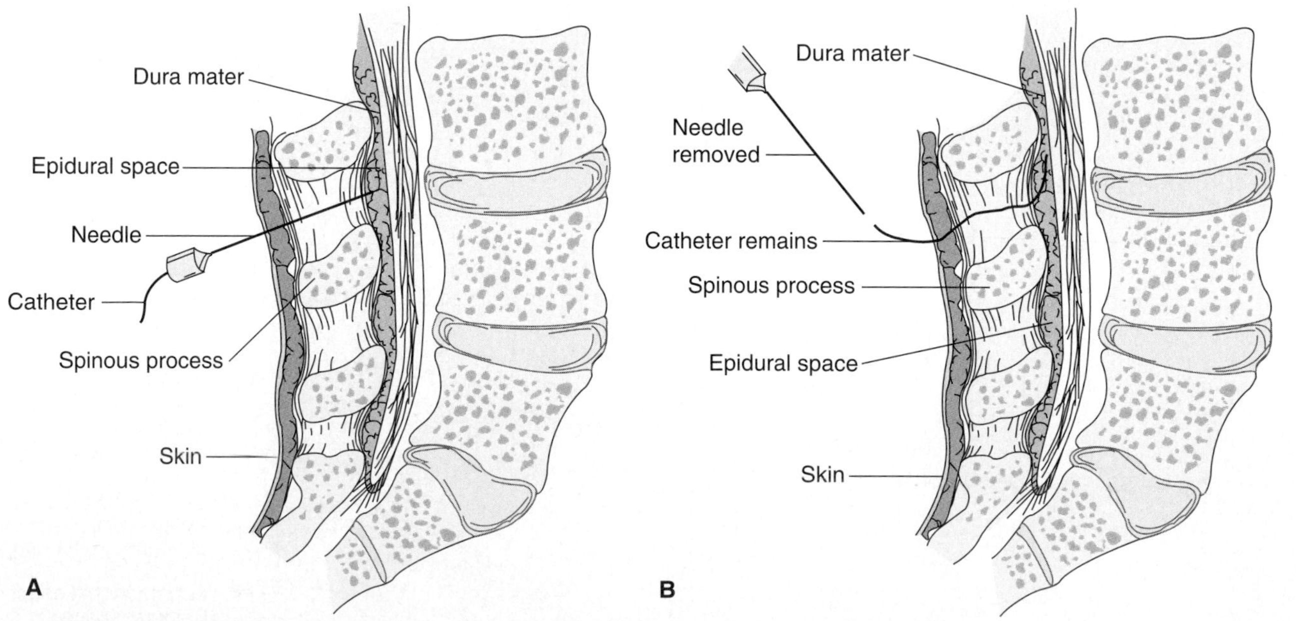

FIGURE 19.4 (*A*) A needle is inserted into the epidural space. (*B*) A catheter is threaded into the epidural space; the needle is then removed. The catheter allows medication to be administered intermittently or continuously to relieve pain during labor and childbirth.

beginning). Assess the woman's pulse and blood pressure. If the anesthetic was accidentally placed in a blood vessel, toxic symptoms of hypotension, slurred speech, and rapid pulse would be present. After assurance that the anesthetic is epidural, an initial dose of anesthetic is given through the catheter. This produces anesthesia up to the level of the umbilicus in 10 to 15 minutes. Unfortunately, the effect of the anesthetic is short lived (40 minutes to 2 hours). To keep the woman free from discomfort, periodically administer another dose of anesthetic, termed a top-up, or continually infuse additional anesthetic by an infusion pump.

Before an additional top-up dose is administered, the woman should be asked to both write and say out loud a phrase such as "I can do it" three times. If she is unable to do this (lack of fine motor coordination and slurred speech indicate a slowly occurring toxic reaction), the dose needs to be questioned.

Epidural anesthesia may also be given in a "segmented" fashion. With this technique, after the test dose, only a small dose (about 4 mL) is given. This provides anesthesia for uterine contractions but not perineal relaxation. Close to birth, if the woman sits up and an additional dose is given, perineal anesthesia will result. Leaving the lower anesthesia for late in labor in this way allows for better internal rotation of the fetal head, because the perineal muscle is not lax and there is less chance that forceps for rotation will be necessary.

A nurse should be in continuous attendance when an epidural anesthetic is given. Epidural anesthesia may cause a temporary elevation in temperature, so keep this in mind when evaluating the woman's temperature. To detect hypotension, continuously monitor the woman's blood pressure for the first 20 minutes after each new injection of anesthetic. Continue to monitor blood pressure throughout the time the anesthetic is in effect to be certain the systolic pressure does not fall below 100 mm Hg or decrease 20 mm Hg in a hypertensive woman. A drop greater than this may be life threatening to the fetus unless prompt, effective corrective measures are taken, such as repositioning and administering an antihypotensive agent. If such measures are instituted quickly, fetal outcome will not be compromised.

With an epidural block, the woman loses sensation of her bladder filling. Remind the woman to void every 2 hours, monitor intake and output, and observe and palpate for bladder distention. Be aware of the standards and policies of the health care agency related to adding additional anesthesia or removing the catheter.

Once initiated, epidural anesthesia also can be self-administered via patient-controlled epidural analgesia (PCEA). With this technique, an epidural catheter delivers an analgesic mixture when the client presses a button on a special pump. A lockout period follows each self-administration to avoid overdosage. This method of administration is advantageous because less anesthetic is required when compared to that associated with continuous epidural infusion (CEI).

Combined Spinal Epidural Technique. Some women feel a greater sense of control in labor if they can walk around in early labor. To make this possible, combined spinal epidural (CSE) technique was originated. To administer this, an anesthesiologist first inserts an epidural needle using usual epidural technique. He or she then inserts a very fine spinal needle through the epidural lumen into the subarachnoid space and the CSF, confirming that the second needle is into the CSF by allowing a drop of fluid to fall from the end of the needle. A narcotic agonist (e.g., fentanyl) is then added to the CSF, and the spinal needle is withdrawn. A catheter is inserted into the epidural needle, and the epidural needle is then removed and the catheter is taped in place.

The advantage of a CSE administration is immediate pain relief (where an epidural alone would take 20 to 30 minutes to accomplish that). In addition, it allows the woman to be ambulatory. Possible complications that can occur include hypotension, pruritus, urinary retention, nausea and vomiting, and a post-dura puncture headache (although all of these are rare).

Spinal (Subarachnoid) Anesthesia. Spinal anesthesia is used less frequently today in preference to lumbar epidural blocks. It may be used in an emergency, because the administration technique is simpler than that of an epidural and can be accomplished more rapidly.

For spinal anesthesia, a local anesthetic agent such as bupivacaine (Marcaine) or ropivacaine (Naropin) is injected using lumbar puncture technique into the subarachnoid space (into the CSF) at the third or fourth lumbar interspace. A narcotic agonist such as morphine or fentanyl may be added for additional pain relief. For administration, the woman is placed in a sitting position on the side of the birthing bed, with legs dangling and head bent. She is asked to bend her head forward so her back curves and the intravertebral spaces open. Be sure to support her in this position because she is "front-heavy" as a result of her pregnancy and could easily fall forward if not well supported.

After injection, the anesthetic normally rises to the level of T10. Anesthesia up to the umbilicus and including both legs will be achieved.

Spinal anesthetic agents may be "loaded" or "weighted" with glucose to make them heavier than CSF. This helps prevent them from rising too high in the spinal canal and interfering with the motor control of the uterus or with respiratory muscles.

After injection of the anesthetic, the anesthesiologist asks the woman to lie down again. It is important that she does lie down at this time, because if she sits up too long, the anesthetic will not rise high enough in the canal to achieve pain relief. On the other hand, she must not lie down before this time or the anesthetic will rise too high in the canal. Lying with a pillow under her head also helps ensure that the anesthesia will be confined to the lower spinal canal.

Hypotension from sympathetic blockage in the lower extremities can occur immediately after administration. This leads to vasodilation and a decrease in central blood pressure. If hypotension occurs, placental blood perfusion will be compromised. Turn the woman to her left side to reduce vena cava compression. Expect the anesthesiologist to quickly increase the rate of IV fluid to increase blood volume. A vasopressor, such as ephedrine, to increase blood pressure and oxygen also may be administered. Do not place a woman in a Trendelenburg position to help restore blood pressure after spinal anesthesia is given. This could make the anesthetic rise high in her spinal column, causing uterine contractions or respiratory function to cease.

To guard against hypotension, IV fluids such as lactated Ringer's solution are usually given before the injection to ensure hydration. Be certain the fluid is infusing well before the anesthesia is administered.

A late complication of spinal anesthesia is a postpartal dural puncture headache (PDPH) or "spinal headache." This occurs because of continuous leakage of spinal fluid from the needle insertion site and possibly from the irritation of a small amount of air that enters at the injection site. The shift in the pressure of CSF, causing strain on the cerebral meninges, initiates pain. The incidence of such headaches is reduced if a small-gauge needle is used for the injection and the woman drinks a quantity of fluid afterward, as a high fluid intake rapidly provides replacement of spinal fluid. Although usually encouraged, asking a woman to remain flat may no longer be necessary because of the routine use of small needles in most settings.

If a headache does occur, it can be relieved by having the woman lie flat and administering an analgesic. Some women find a cold cloth to their forehead helpful. If a headache is incapacitating, it can be treated with a blood patch technique. For this, 10 mL of blood is withdrawn from the woman's arm and then immediately injected into the epidural space over the spinal injection site. The blood injected then clots and seals off any further leakage of CSF (Fishburne, 2000).

✔ CHECKPOINT QUESTIONS

6. What are the goals of pharmacologic pain management during labor and birth?
7. What is a disadvantage of systemic meperidine during labor?
8. What are two concerns associated with epidural anesthesia?
9. Where is the anesthetic injected when spinal anesthesia is used?

Medication for Pain Relief During Birth

Stretching of the perineum causes pain during birth. The simplest form of pain relief for birth is the natural **pressure anesthesia** that results from the fetal head pressing against the stretched perineum. This natural anesthesia is often adequate to allow an episiotomy to be performed without concern that the woman will feel the cut. The pain she experiences as the fetal head is born, although intense and hot, occurs suddenly and is over quickly. Often, after the hours of hard contractions the woman has come through, this flash of pain seems minimal. For some women, however, additional medication may be needed to reduce the pain of birth.

Local Anesthetics

Local Infiltration. Local infiltration is the injection of an anesthetic such as lidocaine (Xylocaine) into the superficial nerves of the perineum. It is used when the fetal head is too low to allow for a pudendal block. The anesthetic is placed along the borders of the vulva. The effects last for approximately 1 hour, allowing for suturing of an episiotomy without additional anesthetic.

Pudendal Nerve Block. A **pudendal nerve block** (Fig. 19-5) is the injection of a local anesthetic such as chloroprocaine (Nesacaine) or bupivacaine (Marcaine) near the right and left pudendal nerves at the level of the ischial spine. The injection, made through the vagina with the woman in a lithotomy or dorsal recumbent position, provides relief of perineal pain in 2 to 10 minutes that lasts for approximately 1 hour. Anesthesia achieved with this method is sufficiently deep to allow the use of low forceps during birth and an episiotomy repair. Although the injection is only local, the fetal heart rate and the mother's blood pressure should be checked immediately after the injection in case maternal hypotension occurs.

General Anesthesia

General anesthesia administration is never preferred for childbirth, because it carries the dangers of hypoxia and possible inhalation of vomitus during administration (Fishburne, 2000). Pregnant women are particularly prone to gastric reflux because of increased stomach pressure from the weight of the full uterus beneath it. The gastroesophageal valve also may be displaced and possibly functioning improperly. Despite these risks, general anesthesia may be necessary in emergency situations such as abruptio placentae when an immediate cesarean birth is required.

For complete and rapid anesthesia during childbirth, thiopental sodium (Pentothal), a short-acting barbiturate, is usually the drug of choice. It causes rapid induction of anesthesia and minimal postpartal bleeding. After induction with thiopental sodium, the woman is intubated and anesthesia is then maintained by nitrous oxide and oxygen. Thiopental sodium crosses the placenta rapidly. Infants born of a woman anesthetized by this method, therefore, may be slow to respond at birth and may need resuscitation. However, in view of the degree of barbiturate intoxication demonstrable in the infant, his or her ability to respond and alertness at birth are always surprising.

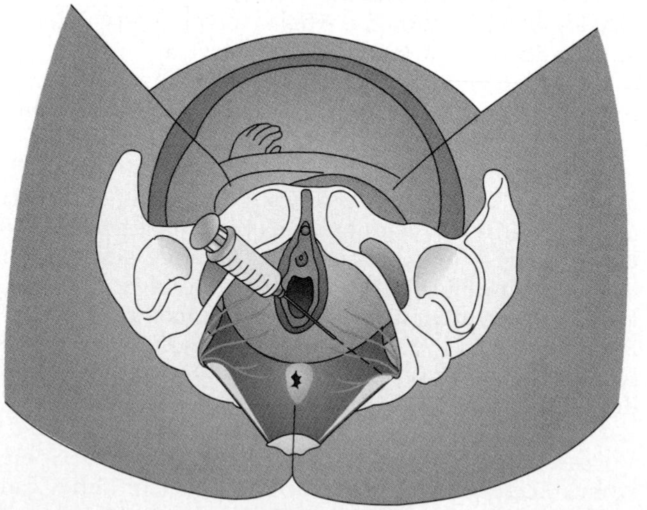

FIGURE 19.5 Pudendal nerve block.

All women who receive a general anesthesia must be observed closely in the postpartum period because of the possibility of uterine atony and hemorrhage. Most gases used for general anesthesia cause uterine relaxation, thereby reducing effective contractions and hemostasis postpartum. After having general anesthesia, some women may comment that their throat feels raw or sore. This is normal and is due to pain from insertion of the endotracheal tube. Using an anesthetic throat spray or gargle, sipping cold liquids, or sucking on ice chips (as soon as this is safe after general anesthesia) may help to relieve the discomfort.

Preparation for the Safe Administration of General Anesthesia. To ensure safe anesthesia administration, an anesthesiologist or nurse anesthetist needs a minimum of six drugs readily available: (1) ephedrine, to use in the event blood pressure falls; (2) atropine sulfate, to dry oral and respiratory secretions to prevent aspiration; (3) thiopental sodium (Pentothal), for rapid induction of a general anesthetic in an emergency; (4) succinylcholine (Anectine), to achieve laryngeal relaxation for intubation in an emergency; (5) diazepam (Valium), to control seizures, a possible reaction to anesthetics; and (6) isoproterenol (Isuprel), to reduce bronchospasm should aspiration occur. In addition to these medications, an adult laryngoscope, endotracheal tube, a breathing bag with a source of 100% oxygen, and a suction catheter and suction source should be at hand.

Aspiration of Vomitus. Inhalation of vomitus is a major problem associated with the use of general anesthesia in pregnant women due to pressure from the uterus on the stomach. It can be fatal if the woman's airway becomes occluded by foreign matter. Also, stomach contents have an acid pH that can cause chemical pneumonitis and secondary infection of the respiratory tract.

Some anesthesiologists may order ranitidine (Zantac) IV, or an oral antacid such as sodium citrate to be given to the woman before general anesthesia is administered, to reduce the level of acid in stomach contents should aspiration occur. Metoclopramide (Reglan) to increase gastric emptying may also be prescribed.

For general anesthesia administration, the woman should be placed on her back with a wedge under her right hip to displace the uterus from the vena cava. To prevent the occurrence of hypotension and to establish a line for emergency medications, IV fluid is begun. She is given a rapid-induction IV agent and is then intubated with a cuffed endotracheal tube. To prevent gastric reflux and aspiration before intubation is achieved, cricoid pressure (which seals off the esophagus by compressing it between the cricoid cartilage and the cervical vertebrae) must be applied as soon as the IV agent is begun until the cuff on the tube is in place.

The moments of induction of general anesthesia before the endotracheal tube is safely in place are critical ones for the anesthesiologist. Respect his or her need to concentrate until the task is achieved.

If aspiration of vomitus occurs in the delivery room, prompt attention is essential. The anesthesiologist suctions the trachea to remove as much foreign material as possible. The woman is intubated, if she was not previously, and given 100% oxygen. Intravenous isoproterenol to reduce bronchospasm and a corticosteroid to reduce an inflammatory reaction may be given. Positive-pressure ventilation may be started. Blood gases and a chest x-ray usually are done to determine the degree of aeration of which she is capable.

Usually, the woman will receive mechanical ventilation until her overall clinical condition improves, as shown by the chest x-ray films and blood gases. She is critically ill at the time of aspiration and often will be transferred to an intensive care unit for the special care she requires to survive this occurrence.

> ✔ **CHECKPOINT QUESTIONS**
>
> 10. What type of local anesthetic provides relief of perineal pain?
> 11. What two medications may be ordered to reduce gastric acidity and minimize the risks should aspiration of vomitus occur in the woman receiving general anesthesia?

NURSING CARE TO PROMOTE THE COMFORT OF THE WOMAN DURING LABOR

The best approach to pain management for women in labor combines both pharmacologic and complementary and alternative therapy measures.

NURSING DIAGNOSES AND RELATED INTERVENTIONS FOR PAIN RELIEF DURING LABOR

Nursing Diagnosis: Anxiety related to lack of knowledge about labor experience

Outcome Identification: Client will demonstrate good understanding of what is happening during her labor.

Outcome Evaluation: Client identifies beginning and ending of contractions; expresses confidence rather than confusion about ongoing process.

In addition to causing local discomfort, pain can evoke a general stress response (fight-or-flight syndrome). This releases epinephrine, which causes peripheral and uterine vasoconstriction. Therefore, the degree of pain experienced may increase because of the resulting increase in tissue anoxia. Reducing anxiety through relaxation techniques such as planned breathing exercises, or by administering medication to reduce anxiety, can reduce vasoconstriction, thus helping to reduce pain.

Reduce Anxiety With Explanations of Labor Process. Planning with women about their options for pain relief during labor should begin prenatally (see Focus on Family Empowerment). The pain in labor can be reduced by natural methods based on the gate control theory (see Chapter 13). Be sure to offer careful explanations of what

FOCUS ON FAMILY EMPOWERMENT
Learning More About Options for Pain Relief During Labor

Q. My friends have told me horror stories about pain during labor. What can I do so I won't hurt so much?

A. Here are some suggestions to help with pain relief:

- Ask your obstetrician or nurse-midwife about options early in pregnancy. The options your care provider suggests may actually influence your decision whether this is the optimal care provider for you.
- Attend childbirth preparation classes during pregnancy and conscientiously practice breathing or other relaxation exercises. These measures can be adequate all by themselves; if not, they complement pharmacologic methods of pain relief.
- Make a birth plan detailing what position for labor and other options you want to use. This helps give you a greater sense of control.
- Be certain a support person will be with you during labor. Name a second person or investigate a doula if you are uncertain your usual support person can fill this role.
- Late in pregnancy, if you are still concerned, let your primary care provider know. In addition to medication for pain relief during labor, medication to reduce anxiety is also available.
- On admission to the hospital, let the medical and nursing staff know you are concerned. The most commonly used options today are oral, intramuscular, or intravenous administration of narcotics and injection of regional anesthesia by epidural block. Ask questions about any method suggested that you do not understand.
- Be aware that the choice of receiving analgesia or anesthesia is yours. On the other hand, if a complication occurs, be ready to compromise in the interest of safety for yourself or your child.

is happening or what will happen once a woman begins labor. This can help alleviate anxiety and thereby reduce some discomfort.

Women in labor relax best if they have a clear understanding of what to expect. Be sure to explain the characteristics of contractions and reinstruct as necessary; for example, explain that labor contractions are rhythmic in nature and come and go repeatedly. Do not assume that the woman is aware of this because she is experiencing the contractions. Her pain experience may be such that she is unaware of any relief between contractions (see Focus on Communication). She may fear that things will worsen as labor progresses and that the pain will become continuous.

This on-off effect differentiates the pain of labor contractions from that of a toothache or headache, which is continuous. Sometimes, just knowing this can help the woman tolerate the pain even as it increases in intensity.

Do not assume everyone knows that the rupturing of membranes is painless, that a pink-stained show is normal, and that contractions change in character during the pelvic division of labor. A woman having her first child probably *does not know*. A woman having her second child *may not remember* or finds this time so different from the last time (even if it is well within normal limits) that she is frightened. Be certain to give explanations to the woman's husband or support person, too; otherwise, he or she may start to convey anxiety back to the woman.

Nursing Diagnosis: Ineffective coping related to combination of uterine contractions and anxiety

Outcome Identification: Client will actively participate in labor using positive coping strategies.

Outcome Evaluation: Client expresses confidence in her ability to maintain active participation during labor; demonstrates continued breathing techniques; expresses need to change position; and expresses confidence in labor nurse and other health care providers.

Provide Comfort Measures. Usually, anyone can tolerate a little discomfort from a backache, being thirsty, having dry lips, or a leg cramp. However, few people can tolerate having all of these discomforts simultaneously or feeling even one of them while experiencing labor contractions.

Assist the support person to provide to the woman in labor the usual comfort measures that are helpful for anyone with pain, such as reassurance or a change in position. For dry lips, ice chips to suck on, moistening the lips with a wet cloth, or moisturizing jelly may be helpful. A cool cloth to wipe perspiration from her forehead can avoid her feeling overheated.

Be aware of what is happening to the woman's bedclothes and clothing, which will wrinkle rapidly and stick to her skin because she is perspiring. If a waterproof pad is used under her buttocks, it will become soiled with vaginal secretions and feel hot and sticky. However, never apply sanitary pads in labor. Although they absorb vaginal secretions well, they tend to slip out of place, possibly carrying pathogens from the rectal area forward to the vaginal opening. Instead, change the waterproof pad frequently. At least halfway through the first stage of labor, or more frequently as indicated by the patient's condition, change the sheets and give the woman a clean gown. She could bathe or take a shower if that would be helpful. These measures help her to feel clean and refreshed and with a ready-to-go-again feeling.

Think of comfort measures for the woman's support person as well. Is the chair by the side of the bed com-

FOCUS ON COMMUNICATION

Mrs. Lorrie is a woman who stated in early labor that she didn't want to use any medication for pain relief. As soon as her contractions became 30 seconds in length, however, she requested some analgesia. Her physician prescribed meperidine, IM. Her contractions are now 40 seconds in duration and only moderately strong. She looks increasingly uncomfortable with each contraction.

Less Effective Communication

Nurse: How are you feeling, Mrs. Lorrie? Is there anything I can do for you?
Mrs. Lorrie: I need something else for pain. I can't stand this any longer.
Nurse: Didn't the medicine I gave you work at all?
Mrs. Lorrie: It's working for now, but it won't be enough by another half hour. I'll need something else by then.
Nurse: You won't be able to get anything for another 2 hours. I'm sorry.

More Effective Communication

Nurse: How are you feeling, Mrs. Lorrie? Is there anything I can do for you?
Mrs. Lorrie: I need something else for pain. I can't stand this any longer.
Nurse: On a scale of zero to 10, with zero being no pain and 10 being the worst pain ever, how would you rate your pain now?
Mrs. Lorrie: It's about a two now, but it'll be a 10 in another half-hour when my contractions will be constant and stronger. I won't be able to stand them when they don't let up at all.
Nurse: I'm sorry. I must not have explained that contractions always have a space in between them. Let's talk about that.

Because women in labor are under stress, they may not hear instructions as well as they normally would. First assess the pain. Asking the woman to rate her pain on a scale of zero to 10 is an effective method for pain assessment. Also be certain to assess that women have a clear understanding of the nature of labor contractions so they are well prepared to manage them.

fortable? Does he or she need to stretch or take a beverage or bathroom break? It is difficult for the support person to comfort the woman if he or she is uncomfortable from hours of sitting still in one position.

Nursing Diagnosis: Pain related to labor contractions

Outcome Identification: Client will be able to breathe through contractions or use other techniques (including pain medication) to reduce pain to tolerable level during labor and birth.

Outcome Evaluation: Client states pain is reduced to tolerable level with techniques used and is able to handle or "work with" contractions; demonstrates ability to listen and respond to questions and instructions.

Encourage Comfortable Positioning. An upright, sitting, or walking position may be most comfortable for the woman in early labor. Contractions also are most efficient in this position. Thus, before membranes have ruptured, a woman may be most comfortable either sitting in a chair or ambulating. After the membranes have ruptured, however, and if the fetal head is not engaged, there may be danger in walking about because the cord might prolapse and impede fetal circulation. If this is so, the woman should remain in bed. Urge her not to lie on her back to avoid supine hypotension syndrome.

Encouraging position changes from time to time is important. Assist her to find a satisfying position by moving bedclothes or monitor leads, if any are attached. If she wishes to walk and has no support person, walk with her. Pelvic rocking between contractions may relieve tense back muscles.

Position changes are also essential in the second stage of labor. Depending on medical protocols and barring any medical contraindications, the woman might prefer to sit, stand, kneel on hands and knees, lie in dorsal recumbent or lateral recumbent positions, or squat (see Chapter 18). Keep in mind that maintaining these positions often requires assistance from one or two support people.

Assist Woman With Prepared Childbirth Method. Depending on the type of childbirth preparation the woman and her support person have had, the method used may include breathing exercises, distraction by focusing on an external object, acupressure, therapeutic touch, music therapy, guided imagery, self-hypnosis, or a combination of these methods (see Chapter 13). Biofeedback is not well documented in labor but may be effective.

Often with the discomfort and stress of labor, it is easy to forget what was learned in the relaxed, fun setting of antepartal classes. As necessary, review previously learned breathing techniques with the woman. Urge her to begin these early in labor even before contractions become strong. It is not essential for women to use complex breathing patterns in labor; even the woman who has had no prior training in breathing exercises can use a simple breathing pattern to alleviate discomfort with just a little guidance from a nurse (see Focus on Nursing Care Planning).

Massage is another pain relief method that can be taught to a woman and her support person during labor. It may be especially useful if the woman is experiencing back pain from labor. Rubbing or massaging the sacral area often alleviates back pain. Firm counterpressure on the lower back, thighs, feet, hands, or shoulders can provide a relaxing distraction from the sensation of internal pressure and pain.

Provide Pharmacologic Pain Relief. Some women benefit from combined pain relief measures. Pharmacologic management of pain during labor and birth can be supplied by either analgesia or anesthesia, or a combination of the two. For example, a short-acting narcotic such as fentanyl (Sublimaze) may be administered epidurally in combination with a local anesthetic for additional pain relief. This increases the rate at which action from the anesthetic is achieved. With the addition of fentanyl, less local anesthetic may be necessary. This may increase the woman's ability to push effectively during the second stage of labor.

FOCUS ON *Nursing Care Planning*

A WOMAN WHO REQUIRES COMFORT MEASURES DURING LABOR AND BIRTH

A 32-year-old pregnant woman admitted in early labor states, "My contractions aren't too bad, but my back hurts. I want to try and do this as naturally as possible. I was asleep when my last baby was born 6 years ago."

Assessment: Gravida 2, para 1; accompanied by husband acting as support person and coach. Contractions of moderate intensity, every 6 to 7 minutes, 35 seconds' duration. Cervix dilated 3 cm, 60% effaced. Membranes intact. FHR 148; fetus in ROA position. Attended childbirth education classes; using breathing exercises and focusing on photograph of child at foot of the bed.

Nursing Diagnosis: Pain related to effects of uterine contractions and pressure on pelvic structures

Outcome Identification: Client will state that pain is within tolerable limits throughout duration of labor.

Outcome Evaluation: Client verbalizes discomfort is controlled with nonpharmacologic methods; responds to questions and instructions; identifies need for additional pain relief measures.

Interventions	Rationale
1. Assess level of client's pain from uterine contractions and pelvic pressure.	1. Assessment helps to identify areas of chief concern, providing a baseline for future interventions.
2. Provide a comfortable environment; change sheets frequently, adjust room temperature, offer cool washcloths to forehead, and close door.	2. A comfortable environment aids in relaxation and minimizes distractions, promoting effective coping to manage discomfort.
3. Encourage client to assume different positions and change them regularly. Allow client to walk or sit in chair, if not contraindicated.	3. Position changes promote comfort, reduce muscle tension, relieve pressure, and promote fetal descent.
4. Encourage husband to massage back area, using pressure as tolerated by client. Encourage the use of lotion when massaging the back.	4. Back massage aids in muscle relaxation. Pressure helps to counteract some of the pain. Lotion reduces friction and provides a soothing, relaxed feeling.
5. Respect the need for focusing during contractions. Refrain from intervening with client during a contraction.	5. Interrupting the client's focusing is distracting, making the technique ineffective as a pain relief measure.
6. Provide information, updating the couple on labor progress.	6. Frequent updates about the client's condition and progress help to alleviate any anxiety and fears that may exacerbate pain and help to increase willingness to continue to the desired end.
7. Inspect the client's suprapubic area and palpate for bladder distention. Encourage client to void every 2 hours.	7. A full bladder contributes to the client's discomfort and impedes fetal descent, possibly prolonging labor.
8. Allow client's husband to take occasional breaks. Stay with the client during this time, providing support.	8. Occasional relief breaks allow the client's husband to conserve energy and be refreshed, thus enhancing his ability to provide continued support throughout the duration of labor.
9. Assess for verbal and nonverbal indicators of pain and evaluate response to techniques used.	9. Follow-up assessment provides information about the effectiveness of comfort measures used and need for additional relief measures.
10. Inform the couple about possible pharmacologic relief methods available to them.	10. Providing the couple with information offers them choices, enhancing a sense of control.

Helping the woman decide if and when medication should be given requires an in-depth understanding of the available drugs, their effects on the mother and the fetus, and their mechanism and duration of action. It also requires sympathetic listening and counseling skills. Many women come into labor wishing to avoid drugs entirely. Once in labor, they may change their minds but hesitate to say so, especially if their partners also feel that a birth without the use of drugs is ideal. Other women may come into labor asking to receive something immediately to avoid experiencing any pain. In both instances, provide information about the use of drugs and their ultimate effects. Also maintain a supportive presence to help the woman make the best decision for herself and her baby. Some women require analgesia or anesthesia because of a complication. Helping these women and their support person understand why the medication is necessary calls for equal care and skill. As a rule, record a baseline fetal heart rate (FHR) and maternal blood pressure and pulse before administering medication; reassess 15 minutes later for fetal and maternal safety.

✔ CHECKPOINT QUESTIONS

12. What hormone is released with the general stress response associated with pain?
13. Which positions promote efficient uterine contractions in early labor?

KEY POINTS

Pain in labor occurs because of anoxia to uterine cells, stretching of the cervix and perineum, and pressure of the presenting part of the fetus on tissues.

Each person perceives pain differently. Only the woman herself can describe the extent of her pain.

The better prepared a woman is for childbirth, the less analgesia and anesthesia usually is necessary.

Complementary and alternative therapies, such as reducing anxiety, providing changes in position, increasing knowledge, and supporting prepared childbirth exercises should be encouraged in conjunction with prescribed analgesics.

Be certain to ask about allergy to medication before administering it in labor. Women under stress may omit mentioning this unless directly asked.

Women may lose their ability to use controlled breathing after systemic narcotic administration because of a "lightheaded" feeling. They may need additional support during this time to be able to continue with a breathing technique until the analgesic begins to have an effect.

Regional anesthesia such as epidural anesthesia can be extremely effective in relieving labor pain. Be certain the woman is well hydrated with IV fluid and that blood pressure is within normal limits before administration.

During regional or general anesthesia administration, if the woman must lie supine, she should have a wedge positioned under her right buttock to help prevent supine hypotension syndrome. If hypotension should occur after epidural anesthesia administration, elevating the woman's legs is an emergency measure to help relieve hypotension.

If a narcotic analgesic is used, naloxone (Narcan) must be available for possible newborn resuscitation.

General anesthesia is rarely administered for an uncomplicated labor because it has risks for both the mother and infant.

CRITICAL THINKING EXERCISES

1. Jonny, the patient you met at the beginning of the chapter, didn't attend any preparation for childbirth classes because she planned to rely totally on a regional block for pain relief. If you had met her during pregnancy, instead of when she was beginning labor, would you have supported this plan? Are there any complementary and alternative therapies that she could have planned for in addition to relying on a regional block?
2. A woman says she wants a general anesthetic for labor or she will leave the hospital. Her physician has said he cannot justify a general anesthetic for uncomplicated labor. You find the woman crying. She says her doctor won't give her anything for pain. How would you handle this situation?
3. A woman seemed well prepared for labor but, after an injection of meperidine early in labor, grows angry with her coach and refuses to use breathing exercises because she feels "lightheadedness and pain worse than before." How would you help her at this point?
4. Examine the National Health Goals related to comfort in labor. Most government-sponsored money for nursing research is allotted based on these goals. What would be a possible research topic to explore pertinent to these goals that would be both fundable and advance evidence-based practice?

REFERENCES

American College of Obstetricians & Gynecologists. (2002). Analgesia and cesarean delivery rates. *Obstetrics & Gynecology, 99*(2), 369–370.

Benfield, R. D., et al. (2001). Hydrotherapy in labor. *Research in Nursing & Health, 24*(1), 57–67.

Browning, C. A. (2000). Using music during childbirth. *Birth, 27*(4), 272–276.

Burns, E. E. et al. (2000). An investigation into the use of aromatherapy in intrapartum midwifery practice.

Journal of Alternative & Complementary Medicine, 6(2), 141–147.

Cunningham, F. G., et al. (2001). Analgesia and anesthesia. In F. G. Cunningham et al. (Eds.). *William's obstetrics* (21st ed., pp. 361–384). New York: McGraw-Hill.

Department of Health and Human Services. (2000). *Healthy people 2010.* Washington, DC: Author.

DerMarderosian, A. (2001). *The review of natural products.* Philadelphia: Lippincott Williams & Wilkins.

DiFranco, J. T. (2000). Biofeedback. In Nichols, F. H. & Humenick, S. S. (Eds.). *Childbirth education: Practice, research and theory* (2nd ed., pp. 200–212). Philadelphia: W. B. Saunders.

Faucher, M. A. & Brucker, M. C. (2000). Intrapartum pain: Pharmacologic management. *Journal of Obstetric, Gynecologic & Neonatal Nursing, 29*(2), 169–180.

Fishburne, J. I. (2000). Obstetric analgesia and anesthesia. In J. R. Scott et al. *Danforth's obstetrics and gynecology* (8th ed., pp. 65–90). Philadelphia: Lippincott Williams & Wilkins.

Howell, C. J. (2000). Epidural versus non-epidural analgesia for pain relief in labour. *Cochrane Database of Systematic Reviews, (2),* CD000331.

Jimenez, S. L. M. (2000). Comfort and pain management. In Nichols, F. H. & Humenick, S. S. (Eds.). *Childbirth education: Practice, research and theory* (2nd ed., pp. 137–177). Philadelphia: W.B. Saunders.

Karch, A. M. (2001). *Lippincott's nursing drug guide.* Philadelphia: Lippincott Williams & Wilkins.

Keenan, P. (2000). Benefits of massage therapy and use of a doula during labor and childbirth. *Alternative Therapies in Health & Medicine, 6*(1), 66–74.

Krieger, D. (1990). Therapeutic touch: Two decades of research, teaching, and clinical practice. *Imprint, 37*(3), 83–89.

Lothian, J. A. (2000). Touch. In Nichols, F. H. & Humenick, S. S. (Eds.). *Childbirth education: Practice, research and theory* (2nd ed., pp. 213–226). Philadelphia: W. B. Saunders.

Marks, G. K. (2000). Alternative therapies. In Nichols, F. H. & Humenick, S. S. (Eds.). *Childbirth education: Practice, research and theory* (2nd ed., pp. 376–398). Philadelphia: W. B. Saunders.

McCaffery, M. & Pasero, C. L. (1999). How can we improve the way we perform our pain assessments to meet the needs of patients from diverse cultures? *American Journal of Nursing, 99*(8), 18–22.

McCrea, H., Wright, M. E., & Stringer, M. (2000). Psychosocial factors influencing personal control in pain relief. *International Journal of Nursing Studies, 37*(6), 493–503.

Melzack, R. & Wall, P. (1965). Pain mechanisms: A new theory. *Science, 150*(2), 971–982.

Steffes, S. A. (2000). Relaxation: Imagery. In Nichols, F. H. & Humenick, S. S. (Eds.). *Childbirth education: Practice, research and theory* (2nd ed., pp. 227–252). Philadelphia: W. B. Saunders.

Teschendorf, M. E. & Evans, C. P. (2000). Hydrotherapy during labor: An example of developing a practice policy. *MCN: American Journal of Maternal Child Nursing, 25*(4), 198–203.

Van der Spank, J. T. et al. (2000). Pain relief in labor by transcutaneous electrical nerve stimulation (TENS). *Archives of Gynecology & Obstetrics, 264*(3), 131–136.

SUGGESTED READINGS

Corbett, C. A. & Callister, L. C. (2000). Nursing support during labor. *Clinical Nursing Research, 9*(1), 70–83.

Gomar, C. & Fernandez, C. (2000). Epidural analgesia-anaesthesia in obstetrics. *European Journal of Anaesthesiology, 17*(9), 542–558.

Janssen, P. A., Klein, M. C., & Soolsma, J. H. (2001). Differences in institutional cesarean delivery rates: The role of pain management. *Journal of Family Practice, 50*(3), 217–223.

Larimore, W. L. & Cline, M. K. (2000). Keeping normal labor normal. *Primary Care: Clinics in Office Practice 27*(1):221–236.

Lowe, N. K. (2000). Self-efficacy for labor and childbirth fears in nulliparous pregnant women. *Journal of Psychosomatic Obstetrics & Gynecology, 21*(4), 219–224.

Manogin, T. W., Bechtel, G. A., & Rami, J. S. (2000). Caring behaviors by nurses: Women's perceptions during childbirth. *Journal of Obstetric, Gynecologic & Neonatal Nursing, 29*(2), 153–157.

Nikodem, V. C. (2000). Immersion in water in pregnancy, labour and birth. *Cochrane Database of Systematic Reviews, 2,* CD000111.

Niven, C. A. & Murphy-Black, T. (2000). Memory for labor pain: A review of the literature. *Birth, 27*(4), 244–253.

Perla, L. (2002). Patient compliance and satisfaction with nursing care during delivery and recovery. *Journal of Nursing Care Quality, 16*(2), 60–66.

Van Hoover, C. (2000). Pain and suffering in childbirth. *Midwifery Today, 55*(1), 39–42.

20

CHAPTER

Cesarean Birth

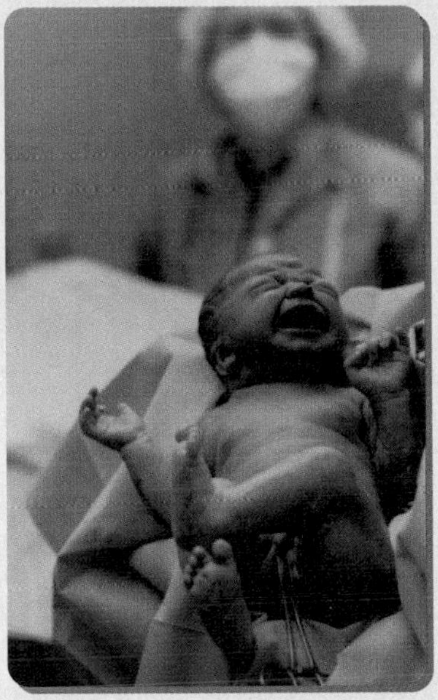

Key Terms

- **cesarean birth**
- **classic cesarean incision**
- **dehiscence**
- **low segment incision**
- **retractors**

Objectives

After mastering the contents of this chapter, you should be able to:

1. Describe the indications for cesarean birth.
2. Assess a woman scheduled for cesarean birth for effective preoperative, intraoperative, and postoperative needs.
3. Formulate nursing diagnoses related to cesarean birth.
4. Establish outcomes that meet the needs of a woman requiring a cesarean birth.
5. Plan appropriate nursing care to ensure family-centered care.
6. Implement common preoperative and postoperative care measures for cesarean birth.
7. Evaluate outcomes for achievement and effectiveness of nursing care.
8. Identify National Health Goals related to cesarean birth that nurses can be instrumental in helping the nation to achieve.
9. Identify areas related to cesarean birth that could benefit from additional nursing research or application of evidence-based practice.
10. Use critical thinking to analyze common complications of cesarean birth to develop preventive strategies.
11. Integrate knowledge of cesarean birth with the nursing process to achieve quality maternal and child health nursing care.

Moja is a 29-year-old woman who is pregnant with her first baby. Her labor began with ruptured membranes and dark green meconium-stained amniotic fluid. Moja telephoned her nurse-midwife, who asked her to come to the hospital immediately. Moja drove herself to the birthing center and arrived in 20 minutes. Fetal heart rate was 100 bpm. An obstetrician was consulted, and she scheduled Moja for an immediate cesarean birth. Moja reacted calmly to the news that she needed surgery until she realized her boyfriend would not be able to get to the hospital until her surgery was over. She refused to sign for permission, saying, "I can't. I just can't go through this alone."

Is Moja's response typical of a woman who is told she needs a surgical procedure for the birth of her baby? What action by a nurse would be best to help her accept this procedure without feeling so alone?

Previous chapters described the normal anatomy and physiology of labor and the sequence of usual birth. This chapter adds information about cesarean birth as a way to help a woman ensure a healthy outcome for both herself and her child.

After you've studied the chapter, answer the Critical Thinking Exercises at the end of the chapter, and then access the on-line study activities (http://connection.lww.com) *to further sharpen your skills and test your knowledge.*

Cesarean birth, birth accomplished through an abdominal incision into the uterus, is one of the oldest types of surgical procedures known. Unfortunately, it is a procedure always more hazardous than vaginal birth. Fortunately, when compared with other surgical procedures, it is one of the safest types of surgeries and one with few complications (Scott, 2000).

The word "cesarean" is derived from the Latin *caedore,* which means "to cut." At one time, there was a popular belief that Julius Caesar was delivered by a cesarean birth and that the procedure was named for him. However, because Caesar was born before antibiotics and sterile surgical technique, it seems unlikely that his mother (who is known to have been alive in his adult years) would have survived such a procedure. Currently, cesarean birth is used most often as a prophylactic measure, to alleviate problems of birth for conditions such as those listed in Box 20-1. It is generally contraindicated when there is a documented dead fetus (labor can be induced to avoid a surgical procedure).

The term *cesarean birth* rather than *cesarean delivery* is generally used to accentuate that this is a birth more than a surgical procedure. A major concern in maternal and child health nursing is the increasing number of cesarean births being performed annually (see Focus on National Health Goals). In 1970, only 5.5% of women in the United States had infants born by cesarean birth. Currently, the incidence is nearly 18% for first time mothers, over 70% for repeat procedures (DHHS, 2000). This rate results from the combination of the increased safety of cesarean birth and the use of fetal monitors, which provide for early detection of fetal problems (Gamble & Creedy, 2000). Its increase may also be related to the phenomenon that physicians skilled in doing cesareans have less experience with other methods

BOX 20.1

SELECTED INDICATIONS FOR CESAREAN BIRTH

Maternal Factors

Active genital herpes or papilloma
AIDS or HIV-positive status
Cephalopelvic disproportion
Cervical cerclage
Disabling conditions, such as severe hypertension of pregnancy, that prevent pushing to accomplish the pelvic division of labor
Failed induction or failure to progress in labor
Obstructive benign or malignant tumor
Previous cesarean birth by classic incision

Placenta Factors

Placenta previa
Premature separation of the placenta
Umbilical cord prolapse

Fetal Factors

Compound conditions such as macrosomic fetus in a breech lie
Extreme low birth weight
Fetal distress
Major fetal anomalies, such as hydrocephalus
Multigestation or conjoined twins
Transverse fetal lie

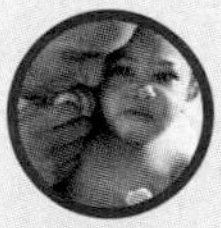

FOCUS ON NATIONAL HEALTH GOALS

Two National Health Goals speak directly to cesarean birth:

- Reduce cesarean births among low-risk (full-term, singleton, vertex presentation) women having their first child to 15% of live births from a baseline of 18%.
- Reduce cesarean births among women who have had a prior cesarean birth to 63% of live births from a baseline of 72% (DHHS, 2000).

Nurses can be instrumental in helping the nation achieve these goals by encouraging women who fulfill the criteria for vaginal birth after cesarean (VBAC) to attempt a vaginal birth with a second child.

Additional nursing research in this area could include studies and application of evidence-based practice on the effect of nursing practice and the cesarean birth rate, effective pain management for cesarean birth, and measures to help the family adjust smoothly from the hospital to home setting after a cesarean birth.

that might be used to solve a problem. It may also be related to physician fears of malpractice suits should a fetus be allowed to deliver vaginally and then be discovered to have suffered anoxia. A few women request cesarean birth with the thought of reducing birth stress, incontinence, or uterine prolapse (Bost, 2000). Although the present incidence of cesarean birth is a concern, this concern must be weighed against the potential for the procedure to reduce the incidence of infants being born cognitively or physically challenged or who die at birth. Few parents insist that giving birth vaginally is more important than ensuring the birth of a healthy baby by cesarean birth.

A number of legal and ethical issues have arisen in recent years when women have refused to undergo cesarean births in these instances. Because women do have a right to decide if they will undergo surgery, the right to refuse the procedure is respected. In some instances, however, a court order for the procedure has been obtained to save the fetus. Fortunately, most circumstances do not come to this point of conflict with health care providers. Maternal child care nurses should be aware of the opinion of their agency's ethics committee on this issue. As a rule, nurse-midwifery birthing services have a lower incidence of cesarean birth than hospital services do. Continuous support during labor also appears to decrease the incidence (Hodnett, 2001).

NURSING PROCESS OVERVIEW

For the Woman Having a Cesarean Birth

Assessment

Many women are informed during pregnancy that a cesarean birth may be necessary due to evidence of their smaller than usual pelvic diameters. Others learn during labor that a cesarean birth will be likely. Assessment as to whether the woman will be a good candidate for surgery can be done throughout the pregnancy or very quickly in an emergency. Assessment must include both physiologic and psychological status and preparedness.

Nursing Diagnosis

Nursing diagnoses specific to the woman having a cesarean birth are often related to common complications from surgery or patient/family concerns about surgical birth. Specific examples include:

- Risk for infection related to a surgical incision
- Fear related to impending surgery
- Pain related to a surgical incision
- Deficient fluid volume related to blood loss from surgery
- Powerlessness related to medical need for cesarean birth

Outcome Identification and Planning

The same outcome applies to the woman giving birth by cesarean as the woman giving birth vaginally: a healthy mother and child. Because cesarean birth decisions are sometimes made suddenly, planning may be limited to a few minutes. Whether or not the surgery is anticipated, however, certain presurgery steps such as preparation for anesthesia are necessary to prepare the woman and her support partner. Plans must include discharge instructions and home care because the woman will remain in the health care facility only 2 or 3 days.

Implementation

Every woman is aware that childbirth poses some risk to her health. When superimposing major surgery on top of this, it is imperative that the woman and her support person have confidence in the health care personnel caring for them. Otherwise, they could have difficulty coping with the insult of surgery. When giving care to any woman during labor, be certain to establish a helping relationship with both the woman and her support person. This relationship is especially advantageous should the birth method need to be altered. The nurse who cares for the woman during labor may or may not follow her to surgery, depending on hospital policy. For the woman who knows in advance that she will have a cesarean birth, the following organization can be helpful:

- International Cesarean Awareness Network (*www.ICAN-ONLINE.org*)

Many interventions focus on teaching and support. The more the woman understands about what is happening to her, the more she can accept and cooperate with the procedure. During surgery, sterile technique is essential. A postpartal infection can be devastating to the woman who already has made many other physical adaptations. After the procedure, provide adequate "talk time" to allow the woman time to review what happened and fit it in with what she and her partner expected.

Another important intervention includes coordination of health care team members (i.e., anesthesiologist, surgeon, pediatrician or neonatologist, and recovery room or nursery personnel). This is particularly important if the surgery will be performed in a hospital surgery department rather than in the labor and delivery suite, or if the infant will be transferred to an intensive care nursery or a distant site for intensive care after the birth.

Outcome Evaluation

Evaluation of outcomes is important in the care of a woman after cesarean birth to ensure the absence of complications. Such evaluations are sometimes difficult to do because of shortened hospital stays. It is especially important to consider the overall goals of a healthy baby and mother and the development of a positive mother–infant (or parent or family–infant) relationship. The following are examples that demonstrate successful achievement of the outcomes:

- Patient states that she understands the reason for a cesarean birth.
- Patient states that she felt well prepared for cesarean birth even in light of an emergency.
- Couple states that they feel able to cope with newborn care even with mother recovering from surgery.

- Patient remains free of any signs and symptoms of infection after cesarean birth.
- Patient states incisional pain is controlled and tolerable.

CESAREAN BIRTH

There are two types of cesarean birth: scheduled and emergency. In the first instance, there is time for thorough preparation for the experience throughout the antepartal period. Some women may have even taken a childbirth preparation class specifically for cesarean birth. With the second type, preparation must be done much more rapidly but with the same concern for fully informing the woman and her support person about what circumstances created the need for a cesarean birth and how the birth will proceed. Cesarean birth is mentioned in most childbirth classes, so any woman who has taken such classes may at least be familiar with the procedure should one become necessary for her. Box 20-2 highlights appropriate outcomes and interventions using the terminology identified by the Nursing Outcomes Classification (NOC) and Nursing Interventions Classification (NIC).

Scheduled Cesarean Birth

In the 1950s, cesarean birth became a status symbol when movie actresses asked to have cesarean births to save themselves the strain of labor and in some instances to schedule the birth conveniently between movie contracts. The average woman came to think of cesarean birth as an easy method of painless childbirth. Because the risk of injury from cesarean birth is higher than that from vaginal birth, this philosophy put both mothers and fetuses at greater risk than necessary. Scheduling cesarean births this freely also resulted in preterm births. A physical indication for a cesarean birth, such as a transverse presentation, genital herpes, cephalopelvic disproportion, or avoidance of post-procedure stress incontinence, must be documented before a cesarean procedure can be performed. Cesarean birth may reduce the transfer of HIV from mother to newborn (Read et al., 2001). With new surgical techniques, particularly the use of a low cervical incision, "once a cesarean, always a cesarean" no longer applies. Most women who have had a cesarean in the past 10 years are eligible to give birth vaginally in subsequent pregnancies if the circumstances otherwise are appropriate for vaginal birth. About 60% of women today have a vaginal birth after a cesarean birth (VBAC). VBACs are most successful if there is an interval greater than 19 months between the cesarean and the VBAC (Huong et al., 2002). For more information, see Chapter 18.

Emergency Cesarean Birth

Emergency cesarean births are done for reasons such as placenta previa, abruptio placentae, fetal distress, or failure to progress in labor. An emergency cesarean birth carries with it the risk of all emergency surgery: a woman who may not be a prime candidate for anesthesia and who is psychologically unprepared for the experience. In addition, the woman may have a fluid and electrolyte imbalance and be both physically and emotionally exhausted from a long labor.

BOX 20.2

NURSING OUTCOMES AND NURSING INTERVENTIONS CLASSIFICATION: CESAREAN BIRTH

NOC: Knowledge, Labor and Delivery

Knowledge, labor and delivery, is defined as the extent of understanding conveyed about labor and delivery (Johnson, Maas, & Moorhead, 2000). Some specific indicators suggesting achievement of this outcome may include the woman's ability to describe the following:

- Birthing options
- Role of support person
- Stages and phases of labor and delivery
- Methods of pain control
- Effective breathing techniques
- Potential complications

NIC: Cesarean Section Care

Cesarean section care is defined as the preparation and support of the client delivering a baby by cesarean section (McCloskey & Bulechek, 2000). Some important activities when implementing this intervention include:

- Determining client's perception and preparation
- Explaining reasons for unplanned cesarean birth
- Encouraging client to express feelings and urging support person to be present
- Setting up equipment for the procedure
- Providing information about the procedure and sensations afterward, progress during the procedure, and status of infant throughout the procedure
- Inspecting incisional site
- Encouraging early ambulation
- Administering pain medication as needed
- Discussing client's and support person's feelings about the procedure after birth

Effects of Surgery on the Woman

Cesarean birth, like any surgical procedure, has systemic effects.

Stress Response

Whenever the body is subjected to stress, either physical or psychosocial, it responds with measures to preserve the function of major body systems. A stress response results in release of epinephrine and norepinephrine from the adrenal medulla. Epinephrine causes an increased heart rate, bronchial dilatation, and elevation of the blood glucose level. Norepinephrine leads to peripheral vasoconstriction, which forces blood to the central circulation and increases blood pressure. These normally positive responses (the person is tensed or ready for action with good heart and lung function and glucose for energy) may antagonize anesthetic action, which is aimed at minimizing body activity. In the pregnant woman, such responses may minimize blood supply to her lower extremities. Already prone to thrombophlebitis from stasis of blood flow, these responses compound or greatly increase the risk of thrombophlebitis. Combined with interferences to major body systems, these effects can add to the risk of surgery.

Interference With Body Defenses

The skin serves as the primary line of defense against bacterial invasion. When skin is incised for a surgical procedure, this important line of defense is lost. Strict adherence to aseptic technique during surgery and in the days following the procedure are necessary to compensate for the impaired defense. If cesarean birth is performed after membranes have been ruptured for hours, the woman's risk for infection will be higher than if membranes were intact. Many women receive prophylactic antibiotics, such as ampicillin (Omnipen) to ensure protection against postsurgical endometritis (Spinnato et al., 2000).

Interference With Circulatory Function

Although incised vessels, required in even the simplest surgical procedures, are immediately clamped and ligated during surgery, some blood loss always occurs. Extensive blood loss leads to hypovolemia and lowered blood pressure. This could lead to ineffective perfusion of all body tissues if the problem is not quickly recognized and corrected. The amount of blood lost in cesarean birth is comparatively high. Pelvic vessels are congested with blood needed to supply the placenta, and with pressure on these vessels, blood loss occurs freely. During a vaginal birth, a woman loses 300 to 500 mL of blood. This loss increases to 500 to 1000 mL with a cesarean birth.

Interference With Body Organ Function

When any body organ is handled, cut, or repaired in surgery, it may respond with a temporary disruption in function. Pressure from edema or inflammation as fluid moves into the injured area will further impair function of the organ involved and that of surrounding organs. If blood vessels are compressed due to the edema, distant organs may be deprived of blood flow, leading to reduced function in those organs. Postoperatively, close assessment of the organ involved and total body function is necessary to determine the total degree of disruption.

During cesarean birth, the uterus is obviously handled and, thus, may not contract as well afterward. This may lead to postpartum hemorrhage. To reach the uterus, the bladder must be displaced anteriorly. As a result of this handling, the bladder may not sense filling as well following the procedure. Pressure is exerted on the intestine, which may lead to a paralytic ileus or halting of intestinal function. After a cesarean birth, therefore, uterine function, bladder, intestine, and lower circulatory function must be carefully assessed.

Interference With Self-Image or Self-Esteem

Surgery always leaves an incisional scar that will be noticeable to some extent afterward. If the resulting scar from cesarean birth (a horizontal one across the lower abdomen) is noticeable, its appearance may cause the woman to feel self-conscious later. Although most women accept cesarean birth well, a woman may feel a loss of self-esteem if she believes it marks her as a woman unable to give vaginal birth.

✔ CHECKPOINT QUESTIONS

1. What primary line of defense against infection is lost with cesarean birth?
2. What is the approximate amount of blood lost with cesarean birth?

NURSING CARE OF THE WOMAN ANTICIPATING A CESAREAN BIRTH

The woman admitted to the hospital for an anticipated cesarean birth may be more worried about the procedure, because she has had more time to worry than the woman who is told during labor that an emergency cesarean is necessary. After the woman is admitted to the health care facility, allow her time to talk about any fears she has. She needs encouragement to do as much as possible for herself preoperatively. Doing so helps a woman feel in control and may help to diminish her fear.

A woman undergoing surgery cannot begin to relax as long as her support person is nervous and worried. Make a point of including this person in all explanations and admission routines.

Preoperative Interview

Both the physician and anesthesiologist or nurse anesthetist will interview a woman preoperatively to obtain a health history and make an assessment and decision for safe anesthetic use. A nursing assessment is also essential. Be sure to ask about any past surgery, secondary illnesses, allergies to foods or drugs, and current medications to help establish surgical risk. Obtain additional information, including:

- Woman's knowledge about the procedure
- Length of the hospitalization anticipated
- Any postsurgical equipment to be used such as an indwelling catheter and intravenous fluid, and any necessary precautions for her infant

This information is important because it serves as a foundation for future teaching.

Operative Risk for the Woman

For any surgery to be performed safely, the person must be in the best possible physical and psychological state before surgery. People who are in less than optimal physical or psychological health are at risk for a complicated surgical outcome unless the risk factor is identified and special precautions are taken. Up to 25% of women experience some type of complication (Scott, 2000).

Poor Nutritional Status

A woman who is obese is at risk because such a condition interferes with wound healing. Tissue that contains an abundance of fatty cells is difficult to suture, so the incision may take longer to heal. A prolonged healing period increases the risk for infection and rupture of the incision (**dehiscence**). The person's heart may also have an increased workload. Therefore, the physiologic shock of surgery may place greater stress on an already overworked organ. In addition, an obese person often has more difficulty turning and ambulating postoperatively than a person of normal weight, and thus has an increased risk for developing respiratory or circulatory complications, such as pneumonia or thrombophlebitis (Baeten et al., 2001).

A woman with a protein or vitamin deficiency is also at risk for poorer healing. Protein and vitamins C and D are necessary for new cell formation at the incision site. Vitamin K is necessary for blood clotting to effect hemostasis after surgery. Although most pregnant women follow sound nutritional practices and take iron supplements, some may still be iron deficient (particularly women with a multiple gestation or women who have not taken supplements), placing them at high risk for extreme fatigue following surgery.

Age Variations

Age affects surgical risk because it can result in decreased circulatory and renal function. Most pregnant women fall within the young adult age group, making them excellent candidates for surgery. The young adolescent and the woman older than age 40 both fall into categories of slightly higher risk (Matsumoto & Resnik, 2001).

Altered General Health

A person who has a secondary illness (e.g., cardiac disease, diabetes mellitus, anemia, or kidney or liver disease) is at surgical risk, depending on the extent of disease. The pathology present from the secondary illness may interfere with the woman's ability to adjust physically to the demands of surgery. Women with a secondary illness may also have an accompanying nutritional or electrolyte imbalance related to their primary illness.

Therefore, asking about any secondary illnesses is an essential component of the preoperative nursing history. Before surgery, people are under stress, thus limiting their reasoning and decision-making abilities. It is not unusual for people admitted for any type of surgery to state that they are generally healthy and minutes later request insulin on the day of surgery because they are diabetic.

A medication history also is important because some drugs will increase surgical risk by interfering with the effect of the anesthetic or healing of tissue. Several drugs that pregnant women might be taking and their potential complications are shown in Table 20-1.

TABLE 20.1 Drugs That May Result in Complications of Surgery

TYPE OF DRUG	ACTION
Antibiotics	Specific antibiotics may predispose to renal insufficiency or increase neuromuscular blockage; can lead to opportunistic infections
Anticoagulants	May cause hemorrhage due to lack of hemostasis during surgery
Anticonvulsants	May increase liver action and metabolism of anesthetic agent
Antihypertensives	May result in hypotension after anesthesia
Corticosteroids	May block body's response to shock and lead to lack of adrenal function
Insulin	May lead to hypoglycemia during labor or hyperglycemia if a dextrose solution is administered
Antianxiety agents	May cause hypotension after anesthesia

Fluid and Electrolyte Imbalance

A woman who enters surgery with a lower than normal blood volume will feel the effect of surgical blood loss more than the woman with a normal blood volume. Hypovolemia may result from recent vomiting, diarrhea, or a poor fluid intake before surgery. The woman who began labor and now has been told she is to have a cesarean birth may easily fall into this category, because she may have had nothing to eat or drink for almost 24 hours. Intravenous fluid replacement therapy usually is initiated preoperatively and continued postoperatively to prevent fluid and electrolyte imbalances.

Fear

Women who are extremely worried need a very detailed explanation of the procedure before they can enter surgery without intense fear. Most cesarean births currently are performed under epidural anesthesia, so they are less frightening. If general anesthesia is used, however, the person who is frightened is at a greater risk for cardiac arrest than the person who is calm and relaxed.

In many instances, just helping a woman acknowledge that fear of surgery is normal may be helpful. The procedure does not become any less traumatic, but the woman can view her feelings as "normal" and expected, thus helping to enhance her self-esteem.

Operative Risk to the Newborn

Cesarean birth places the newborn at a greater risk than a vaginal birth does. When a fetus is pushed through the birth canal, pressure on the chest helps to rid the lungs of lung fluid. Thus respirations are more likely to be adequate at birth than if the fetus is not subjected to this pressure.

For this reason, more infants delivered by cesarean birth have some degree of respiratory difficulty for a day or two after birth than those that are born vaginally. See Chapter 26 for a discussion of this condition, often referred to as transient tachypnea of the newborn. In addition, some infants develop pulmonary hypertension, a serious cardiovascular complication (Levine et al., 2001).

Preoperative Diagnostic Procedures

For surgery to be performed safely, adequate circulatory and renal function must be documented immediately preoperatively. Preoperative diagnostic procedures for the woman who is to have a cesarean birth usually include:

- Vital sign determination
- Urinalysis
- Complete blood count
- Coagulation profile (PT, PTT)
- Serum electrolytes and pH
- Blood typing and cross matching
- Sonogram to determine fetal presentation and maturity

During pregnancy, a woman, and particularly one who was in prolonged labor, may have an elevated leukocyte count (up to 20,000/mm^3), so this finding is not as helpful an indicator for the presence of infection in the pregnant woman as it is with others.

Preoperative Teaching

Fear of the unknown is one of the hardest fears to conquer. Preoperative teaching is aimed at acquainting the woman with the procedure and any special equipment to be used, allowing her to be as informed as possible to reduce fear. Activities to help maintain respiratory and skeletal muscle function to prevent postsurgical complications should also be included in teaching.

Before beginning teaching, assess how much the woman already knows about the surgery. The woman who has had a cesarean birth for her first child and now is being admitted for a second procedure already knows many details. Even so, she will undoubtedly appreciate having her memory refreshed and recall confirmed. Answer all specific questions and fill in gaps in knowledge. Ensure that all information offered is accurate. It is confusing and potentially frightening for a woman to be told, for instance, that she will not have intravenous fluid after the surgery and then discover the intravenous line in place. Be certain not to use hospital jargon such as "NPO." People under stress do not process new information well. They cannot process information at all if they do not understand. Have the woman return demonstrate activities such as deep breathing to show that she understands the information and can do this well.

Explain preoperative measures that will be necessary, such as surgical skin preparation, eating nothing before the time of surgery, premedication (if this will be used), and method of transport. Review the necessity for an indwelling catheter, intravenous fluid, placement of an epidural catheter (if used for post procedural pain relief) and early ambulation afterward.

Throughout teaching, use visual aids as necessary. Draw pictures or show illustrations of anatomy, if necessary. Be careful not to leave textbooks about cesarean procedure techniques with the patient. Typically these books also describe complications. Knowledge of possible complications of the procedure is necessary for an informed consent, but reading about complications complete with color illustrations may be too overwhelming.

Teaching to Prevent Complications

Women who work to maintain good respiratory and circulatory function postoperatively will probably experience fewer postoperative respiratory and circulatory complications than those who do not. These preventive measures are best taught during the preoperative period, when the woman is free of pain and can concentrate on the teaching. Such teaching also gives the woman a positive outlook about surgery and a sense of control over the situation. By teaching about postoperative care, you are saying, "I'll see you and your new child safely back here in your room afterward," a message with a comforting subliminal message for the woman who has serious doubts that there will be an afterward or at least not one with a newborn.

Deep Breathing. Periodic deep breathing exercises fully aerate the lungs and help to prevent stasis of lung mucus, which tends to occur because of the prolonged time spent in the supine position during surgery. Because stasis always has the potential for causing infection, it must be prevented as much as possible.

Taking 5 to 10 deep breaths every hour postoperatively helps to increase lung function. A woman does this simply by inhaling as deeply as possible, holding her breath for a second or two, and then exhaling as deeply as possible. She must be certain that she inhales and exhales fully. Otherwise, she might experience lightheadedness from hyperventilation.

Incentive Spirometry. A common device used postoperatively to encourage deep breathing is the incentive spirometer. An incentive spirometer is fun to operate and gives a patient a sense of reward for the effort. Be sure to explain how to use the device. The initial impression is usually that the device works by blowing into the instrument. Because its purpose is to fully aerate lung spaces, most models are triggered by *inhalation,* not exhalation.

Turning. Women do not need to practice turning side to side before surgery because this activity is tiring for them to do while pregnant. However, they should understand that turning postoperatively is important to prevent both respiratory and circulatory stasis.

Ambulation. The most effective way to stimulate lower extremity circulation following a cesarean birth is with early ambulation. For this reason, most surgeons prefer the woman to be out of bed and walking by 4 hours after surgery (as soon as the effect of the epidural anesthesia has worn off). Helping women to do this can be difficult because the woman is both fatigued and in pain. She needs to understand just how important this action is. Ambulation is extremely important after cesarean birth, because the edema of the low pelvic surgery compresses circulation to the lower extremities, increasing the risk for lower extremity circulatory stasis. Women also may be prescribed antiembolic stockings (TEDS) to support venous return.

Immediate Preoperative Care Measures

A number of measures must be taken immediately before surgery to ensure a safe outcome.

Informed Consent

Obtaining operative consent is the surgeon's responsibility, but seeing that it is obtained is everyone's responsibility. Nurses may be asked to witness the woman's signature on such a form. Before signing as a witness, be certain it was *informed* consent, one in which the woman was explained the risks and benefits of the procedure in terms that she could understand.

The law differs from state to state regarding emancipated minors (girls under legal age but who are pregnant or the previous mother of a child). Emancipated minors can sign their own surgical permission although they are legally under age.

Overall Hygiene

Most women who are having planned cesarean births are admitted to the facility on the morning of surgery and usually have showered or bathed at home. On admission, provide a clean hospital gown. If the woman's hair is long, encourage her to braid it or put it into a ponytail so it will more easily fit under the surgical cap to be worn. Hair contained by a cap is less likely to spread microorganisms during surgery. Follow institutional procedure about removing nail polish, jewelry, contact lenses, or hair ornaments before surgery. A growing number of women wear acrylic fingernails and are reluctant to remove them for surgery. Therefore, ensure that the woman's toenails are free of polish and use the toenails to assess capillary refill.

> **WHAT IF?** What if a woman who is going to have epidural anesthesia refuses to remove her contact lenses even though it is hospital policy for anyone receiving anesthesia? She says, "Without them, I won't be able to see my baby being born." Would you ask the nurse anesthetist whether removing them is absolutely necessary or insist on the woman following procedure without question?

Gastrointestinal Tract Preparation

The physician may order an enema before surgery to empty the woman's bowel and allow the bowel to rest for a few days postsurgery. If an enema is ordered, be certain to administer it using gentle, gravity-only pressure. Provide a bedpan for her to expel the enema, or remain with her and accompany her to the bathroom so she does not injure herself by hurrying to reach a bathroom.

A gastric emptying agent such as metoclopramide (Reglan) to speed stomach emptying or a histamine blocker such as ranitidine (Zantac) to decrease stomach secretions may be ordered. An oral antacid such as sodium citrate (Bicitra) to neutralize the acid secretions of the stomach also may be prescribed. These precautions are necessary because the woman will be lying on her back during the procedure, and esophageal reflux and aspiration are highly possible.

Baseline Intake and Output Determinations

To reduce the anterior bladder size and keep it away from the surgical field, an indwelling urinary catheter may be inserted before transport for surgery or after arrival in the surgical suite. Catheterizing a pregnant woman is more difficult than catheterizing a nonpregnant woman, because the pressure of the fetal head puts pressure on the urethra. The vulva may be swollen and distorted in shape from vulval varicosities or edema. Use good lighting so the perineum is clearly revealed. After catheter insertion, be certain that urine is draining, because fetal pressure on the urethra may reduce the flow of urine considerably. During transport, keep the drainage bag below the level of the woman's bladder to prevent urine backflow and the introduction of microorganisms into the bladder.

If catheterization is difficult before surgery, do not traumatize the urethra by repeated attempts. Catheterization can be done in the birthing or delivery room after the anesthetic agent is given. If there is a delay between the catheter insertion time and surgery, mark the drainage bag just before surgery with the amount in the bag or empty it so presurgery urine output can be differentiated from postsurgery urine output. One of the gravest dangers of any surgical procedure is kidney failure from the physiologic stress of surgery or lack of blood flow to them due to decreased blood pressure. All reproductive tract surgery puts ureter flow at risk because of edema in the surgery area (Cunningham et al., 2001).

Hydration

Most women have an intravenous fluid line begun before surgery with a fluid such as lactated Ringer's solution. Doing so helps to ensure that they are fully hydrated and do not experience hypotension from epidural anesthesia administration, use of the supine position, or blood loss at birth. Be certain this line is started in the woman's nondominant hand to allow her to hold her newborn after surgery without interference. Use an appropriate size catheter (18 or 20 gauge) so blood replacement therapy can be administered if needed.

Preoperative Medication

A minimum of preoperative medication is used with a woman having a cesarean birth to prevent compromising the fetal blood supply and to ensure that the newborn is wide awake at birth and initiates respirations spontaneously.

Patient Chart and Presurgery Checklist

Documentation of nursing care up to the time the woman leaves the nursing care unit or labor room must be completed before the woman leaves for the surgical suite. Many hospitals use an additional preoperative checklist, such as that shown in Figure 20-1, as a reminder of all necessary measures to be taken. Checking and signing such a form indicate that the specific measures are complete.

Transport to Surgery

The woman may be transferred to surgery in her bed, or she may be helped to move to a stretcher. It is important to hold the stretcher tightly against the side of the bed for safe transfer, because the woman is awkward in her movements because of her pregnancy. Urge her to lie on her side to prevent supine hypotension syndrome during transport. Ensure safety by having the side rails up and the cart straps secure. Cover her with a blanket or sheet to prevent her from chilling. Make sure her chart with the surgical checklist accompanies her. Check that her identification is secure before she leaves the patient unit.

Role of the Support Person

In most instances, a woman's family can be as involved in the cesarean birth as they would be for a vaginal birth. A support person may need more encouragement to watch a cesarean birth than a vaginal one, because he or she may view the surgery as being much bloodier than it actually is. Helping family members realize that cesarean birth is little different from vaginal birth helps them progress to bonding with the infant and incorporating a new member into the family.

> ✔ **CHECKPOINT QUESTIONS**
>
> 3. What are five factors that place a pregnant woman at surgical risk?
> 4. What increases the risk of lower-extremity circulatory stasis during a cesarean birth?
> 5. What measure is used to reduce bladder size and keep it away from the surgical field?

NURSING CARE OF THE WOMAN HAVING AN EMERGENCY CESAREAN BIRTH

Many women who will have a cesarean birth have no warning during pregnancy that this will happen. During labor, when they develop a complication such as prolapsed cord or fetal distress, it becomes necessary.

The woman who is told during labor that an emergency procedure is necessary actually may be relieved that surgery has been suggested. If she was having severe pain with labor, this procedure will alleviate it. Another woman might feel great disappointment when told that her baby must be born by cesarean birth. In many women, both emotions are present.

Surgical risk in an emergency situation is determined from the baseline history and physical examination information previously obtained at the beginning of labor. Preoperative preparation measures such as vital signs, urinalysis, and blood work have also been obtained. Immediate preparation concerns such as informed consent, application of elastic stockings, if appropriate, gastrointestinal tract preparation, bladder catheterization, and

		Completed
Patient concerns		
Skin preparation		________
Identification in place		________
Temperature, pulse, respiration	________	________
Blood pressure	________	________
Height	________ Weight ________	________
Voided	________ Time ________ Amount ________	________
NPO after	________	
Hospital gown		________
Hairpins removed		________
Nail polish removed		________
Jewelry removed		________
Preoperative medication	________	________
Dentures removed	________ In place ________	________
Contact lenses removed	________	________
Prosthetic devices removed	________	________
Chart concerns		
Addressograph plate attached		________
Operative permit obtained		________
Urinalysis		________
Hematocrit or CBC		________
Blood order of	________	________
	Signature ________	R.N.

FIGURE 20.1 Preoperative checklist for cesarean birth. Checklists will vary from hospital to hospital.

establishing an intravenous line will be the same. Usually, there is little or no time for postoperative teaching, because the available time must be spent explaining the immediate procedures to the woman, such as transfer, abdominal preparation, and anesthesia. Document carefully what was taught so the nurse caring for the woman postoperatively will be aware of the need for additional teaching (see Focus on Communication).

INTRAOPERATIVE CARE MEASURES

Administration of Anesthesia

The surgical nurse will assist the woman to move from the transport stretcher or bed to the operating room table and remain with her while anesthesia is administered. If the woman has an epidural catheter in place, be careful not to dislodge it while she is being moved. If anesthesia administration will be delayed, encourage the woman to remain on her side or insert a pillow under her left hip to keep her body slightly tilted to the side to prevent supine hypotension syndrome. If she will have a spinal anesthetic (which may be used in an emergency), the anesthesiologist will generally administer this with the woman sitting up. The anesthesiologist may ask you to help the woman curve her back to separate the vertebrae and facilitate entry of the spinal needle. It is difficult for a woman having uterine contractions to remain in this position for long. Talking to her while gently restraining her and letting her lean against you is the most effective means of helping her maintain this position. Epidural anesthesia is generally administered with the woman lying on her side.

FOCUS ON COMMUNICATION

Mrs. Joles has been told she will need a cesarean birth because of cephalopelvic disproportion.

Less Effective Communication

Nurse: Mrs. Joles. Can I answer any questions for you?
Mrs. Joles: I want something to put me to sleep so I won't know anything.
Nurse: An epidural?
Mrs. Joles: That won't be good enough. I want to be asleep so I won't know what's happening.
Nurse: Most people . . .
Mrs. Joles: . . . don't have c-sections so what applies to them doesn't apply to me.
Nurse: I'll tell the anesthesiologist you want general anesthesia.

More Effective Communication

Nurse: Mrs. Joles. Can I answer any questions for you?
Mrs. Joles: I want something to put me to sleep so I won't know anything.
Nurse: An epidural?
Mrs. Joles: That won't be good enough. I want to be asleep so I won't know what's happening.
Nurse: Most people . . .
Mrs. Joles: . . . don't have c-sections so what applies to them doesn't apply to me.
Nurse: It sounds like you don't want to know what's happening.
Mrs. Joles: Asleep, I won't know if my baby is born dead.

Most women appreciate that cesarean births are done to prevent their infant from being harmed. Others interpret a cesarean birth as being done because the harm has already occurred. Some women interpret a cesarean birth as an announcement that they are somehow not as good as other women. Still others are relieved that labor is over. Be certain to ask enough questions so you can learn the importance or meaning of the event to the individual woman.

Skin Preparation

Reducing the number of bacteria on the skin before surgery automatically reduces the possibility of bacteria entering the incision at the time of surgery. Shaving away abdominal hair, if indicated, and washing the skin area over the incision site with soap and water accomplish this.

The skin preparation area for a cesarean birth varies among agencies. Some agencies require extensive skin preparation from above the umbilicus to below pubic hair, whereas others require only a limited preparation of the immediate incisional area.

Surgical Incision

After anesthetic administration, the woman is positioned with a towel under her left hip to move abdominal contents up and away from the surgical field and to lift her uterus off the vena cava. A screen may be placed at the patient's shoulder level and covered with a sterile drape to block the flow of bacteria from the woman's respiratory tract to the incision site. This also helps to block the patient's and support person's line of vision to prevent additional anxiety and fear from the sight of the incision. The support person is positioned at the patient's head to provide support. The incision area on the woman's abdomen is then scrubbed and appropriate drapes are placed around the area of incision so only a small area of skin is left exposed. Watching a cesarean birth is usually the first surgery the average father or support person has ever witnessed. Because of this, the person may be too overwhelmed by and interested in the procedure to be of optimum support. He or she may become concerned about the amount of manipulation and cutting that occurs before the uterus itself is cut (assuming fetal distress is not extreme). Prepare the patient and support person for the sights they might see or help talk them through it as they occur.

Types of Cesarean Incisions

There are two types of cesarean incisions. The type chosen depends on the presentation of the fetus and the speed with which the procedure will be performed (Figure 20-2). In a **classic cesarean incision**, the incision is made vertically through both the abdominal skin and the uterus. A classic incision is made high on the uterus so it can be used with a placenta previa to avoid cutting the placenta. However, it leaves a wide skin scar and runs through the active

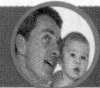

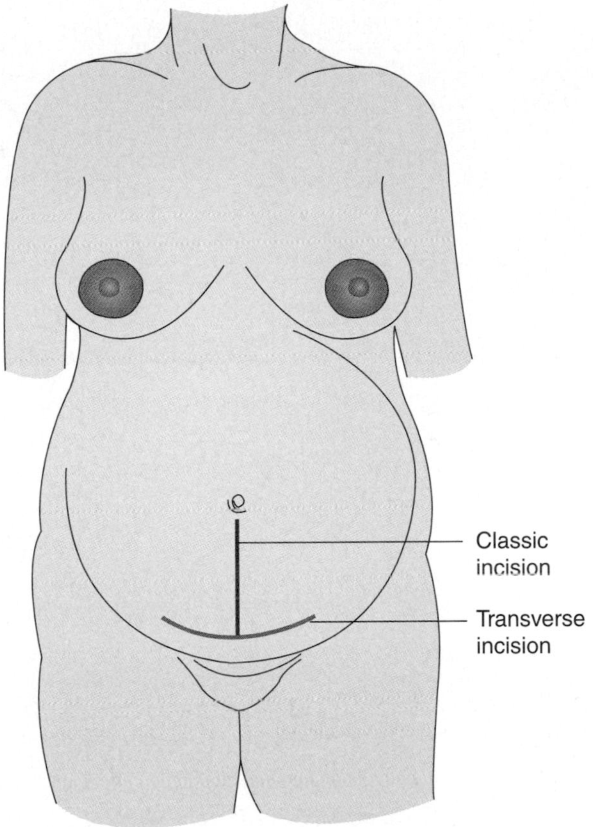

FIGURE 20.2 Types of cesarean incisions.

contractile portion of the uterus. Because this type of scar could rupture during labor, it is likely that the woman will not be able to have a subsequent vaginal birth.

A **low segment incision** is one made horizontally across the abdomen just over the symphysis pubis and also horizontally across the uterus just over the cervix. This is the most common type of cesarean incision currently done. It is also referred to as a Pfannenstiel incision or a "bikini" incision, because even a low-cut bathing suit would cover it. Because this type of incision is through the nonactive portion of the uterus (the part that contracts minimally), it is less likely to rupture in subsequent labors, making it possible for a woman to deliver vaginally with a future pregnancy. It also results in less blood loss, is easier to suture, decreases postpartal uterine infections, and is less likely to cause postpartal gastrointestinal complications. The major disadvantage of this incision is that it takes longer to perform, possibly making it impractical for an emergency cesarean birth. In a few instances, a skin incision is made horizontally and then the uterine incision is made vertically, or vice versa. For this reason, during a future pregnancy, do not assume that just because a woman has a small skin incision she will have a small uterine incision as well.

Birth of the Infant

Once the surgical incision is complete, **retractors** (long, curved, metal instruments) are slipped into the incision. Gentle traction on the handles by an assistant keeps the incision spread apart, allowing good visualization of the uterus and the internal incision. Sterile towels may be placed in the incision to separate the uterus from other organs. The uterus is then cut, and the child's head may be delivered manually or by the application of forceps (Fig. 20-3). The mouth and nose of the baby are suctioned by a bulb syringe, the same as in a vaginal birth, before the remainder of the child is delivered. Oxytocin is administered intravenously by the anesthesiologist as the child or placenta is delivered, to increase uterine contraction and reduce blood loss. In many instances, the woman's partner can be allowed to cut the umbilical cord. After full birth, the uterus is pulled forward onto the abdomen and covered with moist gauze. The internal cavity of the uterus is inspected, and the membranes and placenta are manually removed. If the woman wishes to have a tubal ligation, it can be done at this time. The uterus, subcutaneous tissue, and skin incisions are then closed. Be sure to remind the woman and her support person that closing the incision might be a long process and they should not become concerned that something is wrong. Metal staples are usually used on the exterior skin because they leave the least amount of scarring.

Observing the amount of abdominal manipulation that is accomplished during surgery increases understanding of how tender a woman's abdomen will be afterward. This also helps to explain why a post cesarean birth patient often has an overall "aching" feeling after surgery.

Introduction of the Newborn

Once it is determined that the newborn is breathing spontaneously, he or she is shown to the mother and support person, just as is done after a vaginal birth. The support person can hold the baby immediately. The mother may have difficulty doing this because she has intravenous fluid infusing into one hand and the surgical drapes are still in place. Assist her as necessary. Visiting with the newborn lays a foundation for bonding and also distracts the couple from the tedious process of incision closure. Breastfeeding is usually delayed until the woman has been moved to a recovery room, because it initiates uterine contraction and may interfere with suture placement. Breastfeeding also may be awkward with the anesthesia screen in place and because of the lack of privacy.

✔ **CHECKPOINT QUESTIONS**

6. Why are women given sodium citrate (Bicitra) or a drug such as metoclopramide (Reglan) before a cesarean birth?
7. Why are the two types of incisions used for cesarean birth?

POSTPARTAL CARE MEASURES

Women who deliver by cesarean birth have an additional care concern in the immediate postpartal period, because they are not only postpartal patients but postsurgical ones as well. Due to the strain of the unexpected procedure, they may have increased difficulty bonding with their new infant. There is little time for teaching because of shortened hospital stays. As with all postpartal women, the postpartal

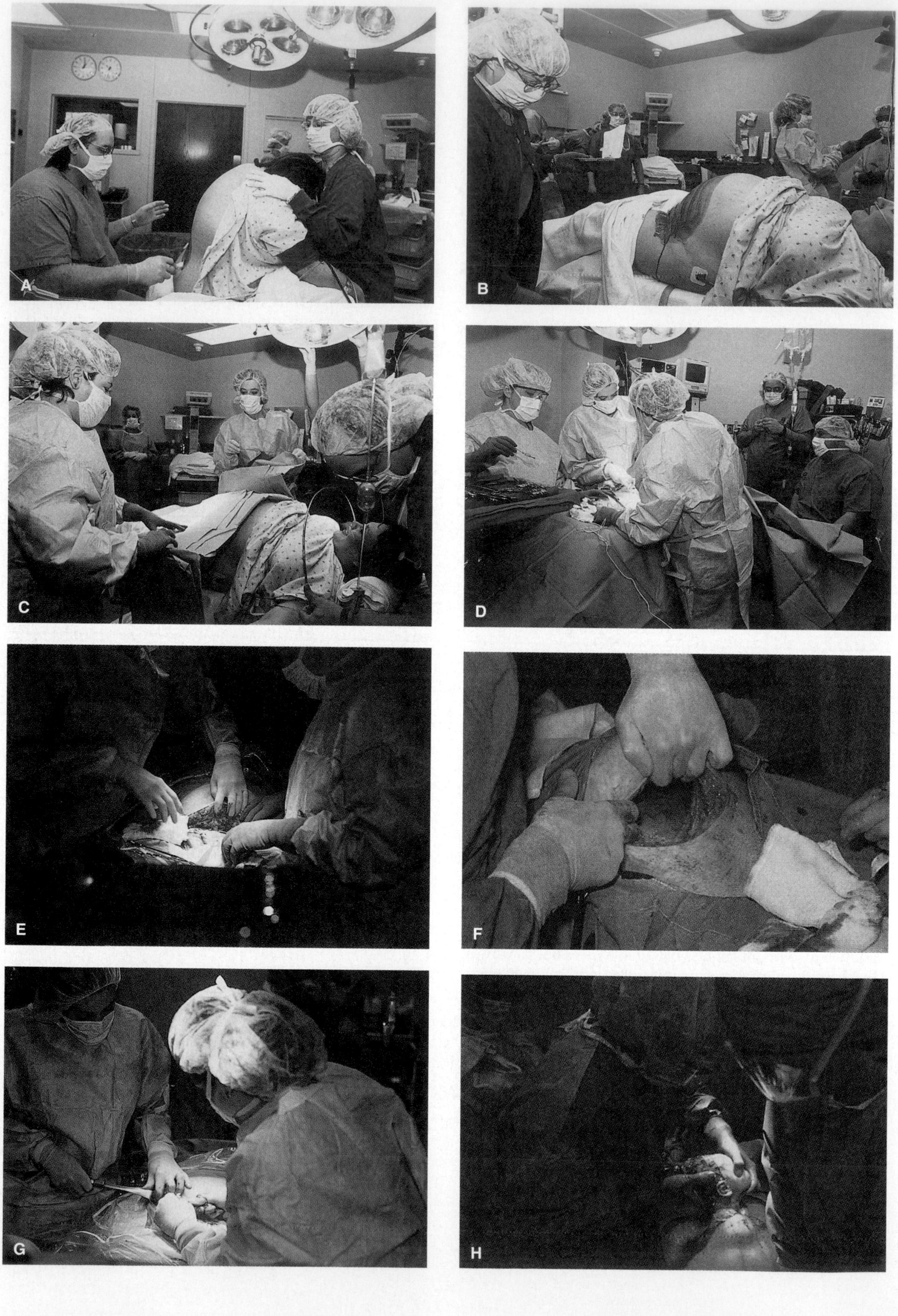
A
B
C
D
E
F
G
H

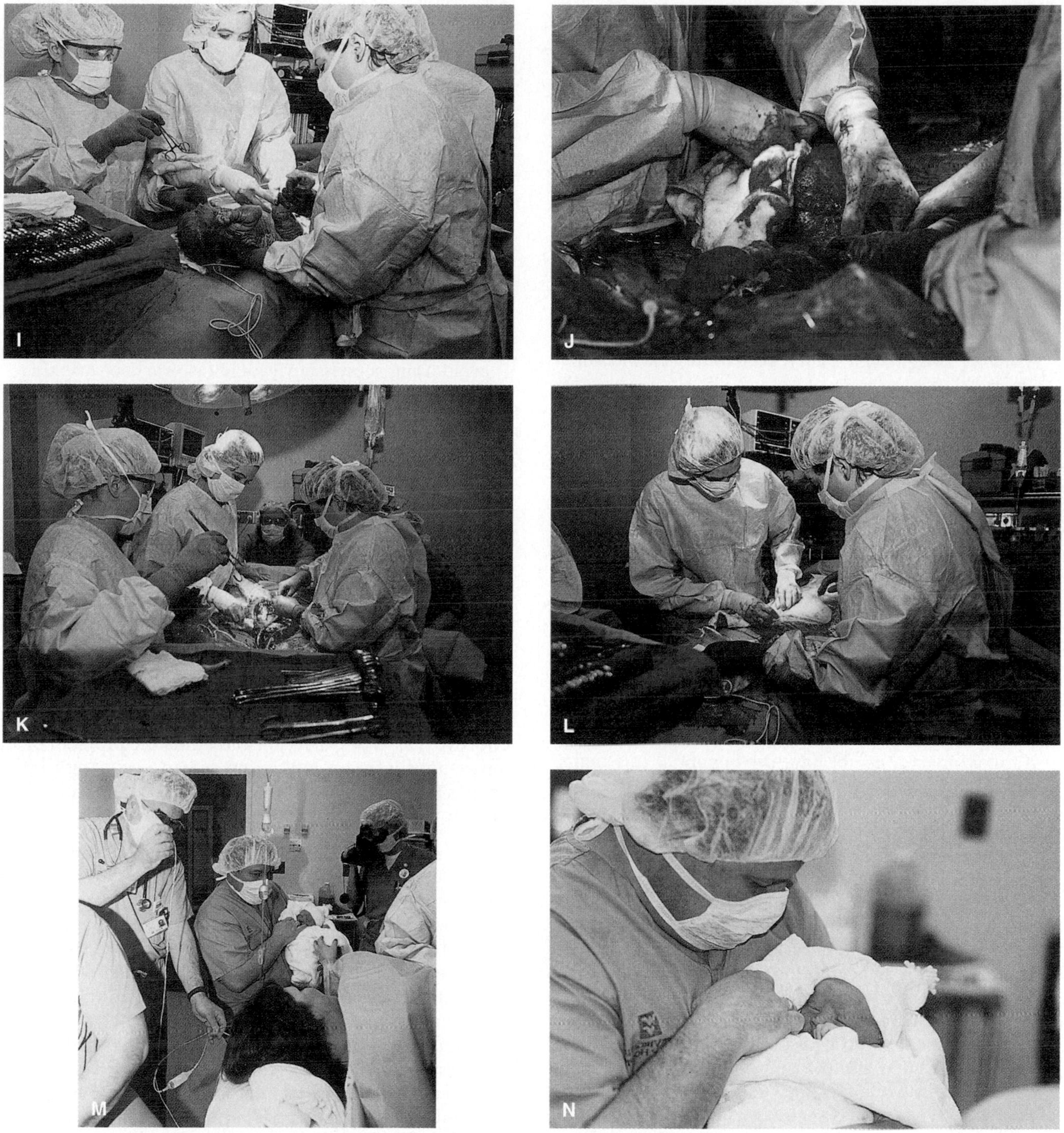

FIGURE 20.3 Cesarean birth. (*A*) Preparation for anesthesia. (*B*) Abdominal skin preparation. (*C*) Draping of operative site. (*D*) Preparation for initial incision. (*E*) Initial incision. (*F*) Opening of the peritoneum. (*G*) Retractors in place. (*H*) Delivery of head and posterior shoulder. (*I*) Infant born. (*J*) Suturing of uterus complete. (*K*) Suturing of abdominal layers. (*L*) Skin closure. (*M*) Family bonding with mother's first touch. (*N*) Father bonding with newborn.

phase for the woman who delivers by cesarean birth can be divided into an immediate recovery period (the so-called fourth stage of labor) and an extended postpartal period.

NURSING DIAGNOSES AND RELATED INTERVENTIONS DURING THE IMMEDIATE POSTPARTAL PERIOD

Immediately after surgery is completed, the woman is transferred by stretcher from the operating room table to the post anesthesia care unit (PACU) or postpartal room. If spinal anesthesia was used, remember that her legs are fully anesthetized so she will not be able to move them.

Nursing Diagnosis: Pain related to surgical incision

Outcome Identification: Patient will experience tolerable level of pain during postpartal period.

Outcome Evaluation: Patient verbalizes extent of pain and need for relief; states that level of pain is tolerable.

Pain control used to be a major problem after cesarean birth. Pain was so intense that it led to surgical complications, such as pneumonia or thrombophlebitis, because the pain interfered with the woman's ability to move and deep breathe. It impaired bonding with a newborn if holding him or her was painful. Today, women who have epidural anesthesia for cesarean birth have morphine (Duramorph) or fentanyl added to the epidural catheter after surgery. This keeps them pain free for the next 24 hours (see Chapter 19). If the woman does not have the benefit of this analgesia, pain assessment and pain management is very important. Use a pain rating scale. Nursing assessment without the use of a specific pain rating tool can be unreliable because the woman's overall excitement may interfere with the accuracy of the assessment. Generally, a narcotic analgesic is ordered to be given with a patient-controlled analgesia (PCA) pump for the first 24 to 48 hours after surgery, followed by a less strong analgesic such as acetaminophen (Tylenol) orally. Transcutaneous electrical nerve stimulation (TENS), intranasal butorphanol (Stadol), or intrathecal morphine or patient-controlled epidural anesthesia (PCEA) with fentanyl may also be used. A woman who is concerned about her infant may experience more pain than the woman who is assured that her infant is doing well, because anxiety and fear heighten the pain response and a tense body posture causes pressure on sutures.

Be certain when administering analgesics after surgery that you supplement them with other comfort measures, such as change of position or straightening of bed linen. Check for abdominal distention, which suggests intestinal gas pain rather than incision pain. Always ask the woman what type of pain she is experiencing to be certain she is describing incisional pain and not pain in a leg or some other body part that would suggest a complication. Pain from intestinal gas can be a major concern. Ambulation is effective in helping to relieve this pain.

Urge the woman to continue to take adequate analgesia to effectively manage her pain after she returns home. Many women who are breastfeeding are reluctant to accept an analgesic, especially just before breastfeeding, for fear of the analgesic being passed in breast milk to the infant. It is true that most analgesics do pass in breast milk, but the infant takes such a small amount of breast milk (mainly colostrum) during this time that the amount of analgesia received is negligible (Baka et al., 2002). Also, without the analgesic, the woman may be so uncomfortable that she is unable to hold the infant comfortably and enjoy having the infant with her. Placing a pillow over her lap will deflect the weight of the infant from the suture line and lessen pain. Be certain women understand to avoid using acetylsalicylic acid (aspirin) because this can interfere with blood clotting and healing.

Epidural Analgesia. Although epidural analgesia provides effective pain relief post-cesarean birth, side effects of epidural morphine administration, such as intense itching and nausea and vomiting can occur. An antihistamine such as diphenhydramine (Benadryl) may be given to reduce pruritus; an antiemetic such as metoclopramide (Reglan) may be administered to counteract nausea. The use of fentanyl reduces the risk for these side effects. Even with these annoying side effects, epidural analgesia can be a very effective means of pain control after cesarean birth.

On the postpartal unit, an infusion pump is connected to their epidural catheter and the woman can infuse a bolus of narcotic as she needs additional pain relief. This is an effective means of pain relief and omits the problem of an intravenous infusion infiltrating as can occur with intravenous PCA. Morphine and fentanyl are two narcotics frequently used in this way.

Patient-Controlled Analgesia. Patient-controlled analgesia (PCA) is a method of pain control in which patients administer doses of intravenous narcotic analgesia to themselves as needed (Reiff & Niziolek, 2001). Although it may be used during labor, it is most frequently used to control postsurgical pain. With a solution such as Ringer's lactate or 5% dextrose infusing, a PCA pump containing a locked syringe of narcotic (meperidine or morphine) is attached to the intravenous line at a port close to the patient. To receive a dose of analgesia, the patient pushes a button similar to a call bell. This alerts the automatic pump to deliver a set amount of narcotic into the intravenous line. The pump has a "lock-out" setting that prevents a patient from administering a larger dose than would be safe or doses more frequently than would be safe (e.g., every 8 minutes; Fig. 20-4).

With PCA, a fairly constant level of pain relief can be maintained. The pain and fear of injections are eliminated. Overall, women tend to use a much lower dosage with a PCA system than they would with intramuscular injections. PCA works well with postcesarean patients because they feel well enough to be interested in self-care and self-administration of analgesia.

Transcutaneous Electrical Nerve Stimulation. Transcutaneous electrical nerve stimulation (TENS) is, as the

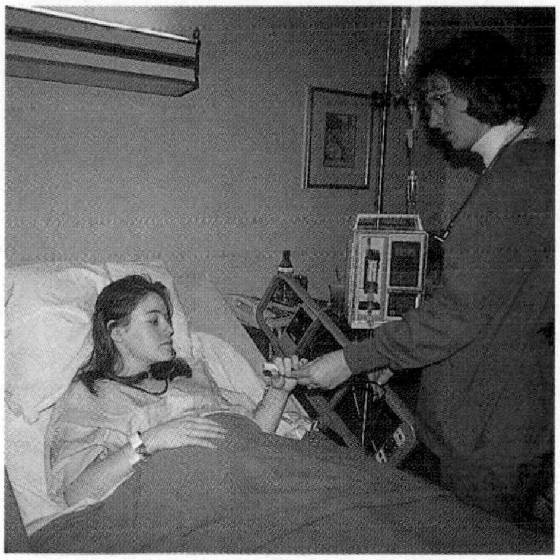

FIGURE 20.4 Patient-controlled analgesia (PCA) pump. By pushing the button, a client delivers a bolus of narcotic to herself.

name implies, the transmission of an electrical current across the skin. This is done by the application of electrodes to the skin surface. It is an effective method of controlling pain sensation because pain is carried by small affective (sensory) nerve fibers. Irritation or stimulation of the large afferent nerve fibers by the electrical stimulation blocks the ability of the cerebral cortex to interpret the incoming small afferent sensation (a gating control theory). This is the same phenomenon that rubbing or scratching skin at the point of pain achieves (see also Chapter 13). The use of TENS provides important pain relief following a cesarean birth in addition to giving the woman a sense of control over the situation.

WHAT IF? What if a woman refuses to allow you to assess her fundal height after a cesarean birth because she has so much pain? How would you approach this situation?

Nursing Diagnosis: Risk for deficient fluid volume related to blood loss during surgery

Outcome Identification: Patient will remain free of signs and symptoms of postsurgical hemorrhage.

Outcome Evaluation: Patient's blood pressure is 100/60 mm Hg or more; pulse is between 60 and 100 bpm; scant to no bleeding on surgical dressing is present.

The potential always exists for deficient fluid volume related to blood loss during surgery. The possibility of hemorrhage after surgery exists until all blood vessels cut and ligated during surgery have thrombosed, sclerosed, and permanently sealed closed. The risk doubles for the postpartum woman. She may hemorrhage vaginally from an uncontracted uterus as well as internally from "bleeders" or blood vessels that were not securely ligated. This danger is most acute in her first hour after surgery and remains an acute problem for the first 24 hours.

To detect the earliest signs of bleeding, monitor blood pressure, pulse, and respiratory rate every 15 minutes for the first hour after surgery, every 30 minutes for the next 2 hours, every hour for the next 4 hours, or as specifically ordered. Signs indicative of possible hemorrhage include:

- Falling blood pressure (more than 20 mm Hg) or a systolic blood pressure less than 80 mm Hg or a drop of 5 to 10 mm Hg over several readings
- Changes in pulse rate (over 110 bpm or below 60 bpm)
- Rapid respirations
- Restlessness and a sense of thirst

Inspect the dressing over the surgical incision for blood staining at the same time vital signs are assessed. Observe the perineal pad for lochia flow, and palpate the fundal height every time. Lochial discharge may be decreased in a woman after a cesarean birth because the uterus was cleaned during surgery, but some lochia will always be present. It follows a typical rubra, serosa, alba pattern. The woman who had either spinal or epidural anesthesia usually will not experience pain on uterine palpation until the anesthesia has worn off, approximately 4 to 24 hours. Therefore, uterine palpation should not increase her pain. Once the effect of the anesthesia or analgesia has decreased, always palpate gently but thoroughly enough to determine uterine consistency.

At the same time the uterus is assessed for firmness, assess the remainder of the abdomen for softness. A hard, "guarded" abdomen is one of the first signs of peritonitis (peritoneal infection), a complication that may occur with any abdominal surgical procedure. Be certain to turn the woman to look under her body for bleeding. Blood oozing from a surgical wound or vaginally can pool considerably under a patient before it is visible.

Oxytocin may be ordered to be added to the first 1 or 2 L of fluid after surgery to ensure firm uterine contraction. If the rate of fluid administration gets behind, be careful about "catch-up" administration. Oxytocin can elevate blood pressure by causing vasoconstriction. It may be safer to allow the fluid to remain behind for a time, rather than risk dangerously elevating blood pressure. Be aware that the woman is prone to hemorrhage at the point that the oxytocin is discontinued, because this is the first time the uterus is really asked to maintain contraction on its own after the surgery. Notify her surgeon of any changes in vital signs that might indicate hemorrhage, so prompt action can occur. Remember a minimal but continued change in vital signs (pulse steadily increasing, blood pressure steadily declining) is as ominous a sign of hemorrhage, as is a sudden alteration in these measurements.

NURSING DIAGNOSES AND RELATED INTERVENTIONS DURING THE EXTENDED POSTPARTAL PERIOD

The average woman who has delivered her child by cesarean birth will remain in the hospital from 48 hours to 4 days, depending on the woman's insurance carrier. During this period and until she returns to have her sutures or staples removed, several interventions are necessary to promote healing, prevent postoperative complications, and establish bonding with the new child. Common concerns of women include pain, fatigue, interference with gastrointestinal function, and reduced activity level.

Nursing Diagnosis: Risk for deficient fluid volume related to postsurgical fluid restriction

Outcome Identification: Patient will exhibit signs and symptoms of adequate fluid volume after surgery.

Outcome Evaluation: Patient's urine specific gravity is between 1.003 and 1.030; weight loss is not more than 5 to 10 lb; fluid intake equals 2 to 3 L/day.

Adequate fluid intake is important after surgery to replace blood loss from surgery and to maintain blood pressure and renal function. The handling of the intestine during surgery causes it to halt or slow in function. It takes approximately 24 to 48 hours before full function is restored and oral intake is possible. Administer intravenous fluids as ordered, and at a rate that is not too rapid (which could lead to cardiac overload) or too slow (which could lead to inadequate circulatory compensation). Keep an accurate intake and output record for at least the first 24 hours to ascertain an adequate fluid balance.

Help the woman learn to "guard" the intravenous fluid line, because she needs a high proportion of fluid during this time (all postpartal women undergo diuresis as a physiologic postpartal change). At the same time, do not urge such caution that the woman is afraid to turn or ambulate. Her risk for thrombophlebitis is high, so she must turn frequently when in bed and ambulate early in the postpartal period.

Assess the woman's abdomen at least once every 8 hours for bowel sounds, small "pinging" sounds heard on auscultation at a rate of 5 to 10 per minute, denoting air and fluid moving through the intestines. Passage of flatus is another indication that intestinal function is again active. As soon as these signs are present, intravenous fluid therapy is usually discontinued and the woman is allowed sips of fluid. After beginning oral intake, wait 1 hour before removing the intravenous line. Doing so ensures that the woman is not experiencing nausea and vomiting, which might require restarting intravenous therapy. Introduce oral fluid slowly, for example, ice chips for the first hour, then sips of clear fluid such as ginger ale, Jello, tea, or flavored frozen ice. Gradually advance the woman's diet to a soft and then regular diet as ordered. Some women assume that they will not be allowed to eat for a long time after surgery and are surprised (and suspicious) to learn that they can have ice chips only hours after surgery. Ice chips dissolve so slowly that the woman receives little fluid from them; they feel cool, however, and will quickly take away the dry "cottony" feeling in her mouth caused by lack of fluid.

Teach women to continue to drink a large quantity of fluid after they return home (at least six glasses daily), especially if they are breastfeeding.

Nursing Diagnosis: Constipation related to effects of abdominal surgery and anesthesia

Outcome Identification: Woman reports bowel movement without difficulty.

Outcome Evaluation: Woman voices that she has a bowel movement every 2 to 3 days.

Note carefully the time of a first bowel movement after surgery. If the woman has had no bowel movement by hospital discharge, the physician may order a stool softener, a suppository, or an enema to facilitate stool evacuation. Assure the woman who is not receiving much food yet that it is normal not to have bowel movements for 3 or 4 days postoperatively, especially if she had an enema administered before surgery.

Teach women to eat a diet high in roughage and fluid and to attempt to move their bowels at least every other day to avoid constipation after they return home. Some women will need a stool softener prescribed because incisional pain interferes with their ability to use their abdominal muscles effectively. Caution them not to strain to pass stools as this puts pressure on their incision.

Nursing Diagnosis: Risk for impaired urinary elimination related to surgical procedure

Outcome Identification: Patient will demonstrate adequate urinary output during postpartal period.

Outcome Evaluation: Urinary output is more than 30 mL/h; patient reports no pain, frequency, burning, or hesitancy on voiding.

Because the bladder was handled and displaced during surgery, its tone or ability to sense filling may be inadequate to initiate voiding after surgery. The indwelling catheter placed before surgery will usually be left in place for 4 to 24 hours to ensure good urine drainage. Assess that the catheter is draining (a postpartal woman has a urine output of 3000 to 5000 mL per 24 hours). Bladder distention will occur rapidly if the catheter becomes blocked.

Before catheter removal, a urine culture may be ordered to check for the possibility of a urinary tract infection. After removal of the catheter, the average woman voids in 4 to 8 hours. Assess for bladder filling by palpation, pressing lightly over the symphysis pubis to assess fullness (Fig. 20-5*A*) and by percussion. On percussion, an empty bladder sounds dull, a full bladder, resonant, and an extended bladder, hyperresonant (Fig. 20-5*B*). If a bladder has filled to capacity but cannot empty properly, the woman may have "retention with overflow" or void 30 to 60 mL of urine every 15 to 20 minutes. This voiding pattern is potentially dangerous because it means that the woman's bladder is held continuously under tension. This can result in permanent bladder damage if the condition goes undetected. In addition, the constantly full bladder may prevent the uterus from contracting, possibly increasing the risk of postpartal hemorrhage.

To help a woman void, administer her prescribed analgesic, which helps to relax abdominal musculature, or encourage her to keep her level under control by using her PCA or PCEA pump. In addition, provide

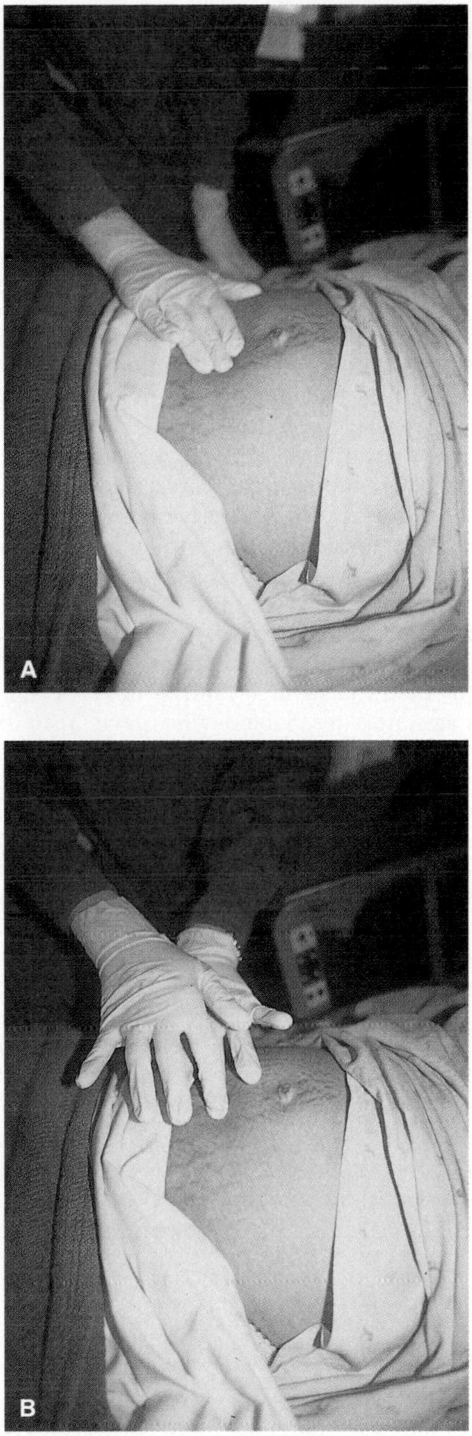

FIGURE 20.5 (A) Assessing bladder filling by palpation. (B) Assessing bladder filling by percussion.

privacy for voiding, and offer a bedpan or assist the woman to walk to the bathroom at least every 2 hours. Other measures that might be effective include pouring warm water over her vulva (measure the amount of water used so that it can be differentiated from urine) and running water from a tap within hearing distance of the woman.

Voiding after surgery provides evidence of adequate renal and circulatory function, because the kidneys must have adequate blood flow through them to function.

Teach women to continue to drink adequate fluid (at least five to six glasses daily) to ensure an adequate fluid output after they return home. Be certain they know to telephone their primary care provider if they should develop symptoms of a urinary tract infection, such as pain or frequency with voiding or blood in urine.

Nursing Diagnosis: Risk for ineffective peripheral tissue perfusion related to immobility during and after surgery

Outcome Identification: Patient will remain free of any signs and symptoms of significant cardiovascular effects from surgery.

Outcome Evaluation: Capillary refill less than 5 seconds; absence of calf pain, redness, edema, or areas of warmth on lower extremities.

Because a woman's abdominal muscles are lax from the stretching from pregnancy, abdominal contents tend to shift forward and put pressure on the suture line when sitting or standing, causing pain and an uncomfortable feeling often described as "everything falling out." She may feel more comfortable turning and sitting up if she supports her abdomen with one hand or splints the incision with a pillow.

Leg exercises, such as flexing and extending the knees, and early ambulation are the woman's best safeguards against lower extremity circulatory problems. Thromboembolitic stockings may be prescribed to help promote venous return and prevent venous stasis. Teach women to apply these before arising, while they are supine and venous distention is minimal. Always allow a woman to sit on the edge of the bed for a few minutes before helping her to a standing position, to prevent orthostatic hypotension. Assessing blood pressure before she gets out of bed for the first time is an additional safeguard. Before ambulation, also assess the lower extremities for pain in the calf on dorsiflexion of the foot (Homans' sign—which may or may not be reliable) or pain, edema, warmth, or redness in the calf to detect for the possibility of a thrombus. It is dangerous for a patient to ambulate if signs of a thrombus are present. A thrombus could shift, becoming an embolus, a potentially lethal situation.

Often, it is difficult for women to understand the importance of turning and ambulating as soon as possible after surgery (Fig. 20-6). Still experiencing the "taking in" postpartal phase, a woman may prefer to spend the first days after surgery just resting quietly in bed. Encourage her to use adequate analgesia during that time to enable her to move and ambulate with the least amount of pain. Also urge her to splint the incisional area. Reinforce the need for continued activity balanced with rest after discharge. Be certain she understands the signs and symptoms of complications, such as thrombophlebitis and pulmonary embolism.

Nursing Diagnosis: Risk for impaired parenting related to the emergency nature of birth or discomfort from surgery

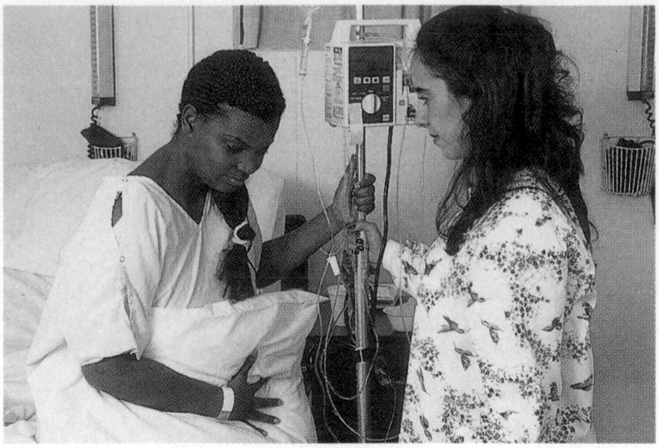

FIGURE 20.6 Encouraging women to be out of bed will help prevent complications from a cesarean birth. It is important to splint the incision area while getting up and ambulating.

Outcome Identification: Parents demonstrate adequate bonding behavior in the postpartal period.

Outcome Evaluation: Parents hold and feed child and voice positive comments about the infant.

When cesarean births are unscheduled, the woman does not have much time preoperatively to think about how she will feel after surgery. Most women are surprised to realize how well they feel overall but also how quickly they become fatigued and how painful a simple surgical incision can be. Being assured that they are recovering well and that surgery is a physiologic shock to their system helps them to accept temporary discomforts. It can help them bond with their newborn following a cesarean birth, just as women who give birth vaginally do (see Focus on Evidence-Based Practice).

If the woman's baby was born with a complication or has been placed in an intensive care nursery or transferred to a distant hospital for tertiary care, the postpartal course can be difficult because she experiences a sense of loss. Depression, which can slow all body functions and certainly her ability to "take hold" in the postpartal period, may occur.

Unless the baby was transferred to another site, be certain the woman has ample time to hold and feed her child. Most women can breastfeed satisfactorily. If equipment, such as intravenous lines or devices, is present, assist the woman with holding the newborn so the equipment doesn't interfere with the time spent with the infant. She may have some reason to think her baby is not quite perfect—after all, the baby was not born "perfectly"—so she may need additional time to inspect the baby and feel comfortable with him or her (Fig. 20-7) (see Focus on Nursing Care Planning).

Nursing Diagnosis: Fatigue related to effects of surgery

Outcome Identification: Patient gradually resumes self-care activities in the first 24 hours.

FOCUS ON EVIDENCE-BASED PRACTICE

Do Women Who Have Cesarean Births Bond as Well With Their Infants as Women Whose Infants Are Born Vaginally?

To answer this question, researchers assessed 74 mothers who gave birth vaginally and compared them to 37 women who gave birth by planned and 56 women who gave birth by unplanned cesarean birth as to psychosocial outcomes at 4 and 12 months postpartum.

Researchers had hypothesized that unplanned cesarean delivery would be related to less optimal outcomes and that this relationship would be influenced by the woman's opinion or feelings about the birth. Results of the study showed that there were no birth-related differences in mother–infant interactions between the groups with one exception: women who demonstrated few nervous habits (were low in neuroticism) who gave birth by unplanned cesarean showed less positive affect toward their infants at 4 months than did women high in neuroticism (who had many nervous habits) who gave birth by unplanned cesarean. Researchers concluded that there is little cause for concern about the quality of mother–infant interactions following cesarean births.

This is an important study for nurses because it provides some evidence about maternal–infant bonding. Because virtually no differences were found among the groups evaluated, nurses can continue to institute measures that promote bonding regardless of the method of birth. Additionally, this study could provide the foundation for further research into areas such as determining the most effective measures to promote bonding and key areas upon which to focus assessments for bonding at follow-up visits.

Durik, A. M., Hyde, J. S., & Clark, R. (2000). Sequelae of cesarean and vaginal deliveries: Psychosocial outcomes for mothers and infants. *Developmental Psychology, 36*(2), 251–260.

Outcome Evaluation: Patient voices that she is pleased with level of self-care; ambulates well by 24 hours, and sleeps restfully at night.

Although a woman needs activity and movement after surgery, she also needs adequate rest. Many women attempt to handle their own and their newborn's needs immediately after surgery, because their excitement over their baby and their new role makes them unaware of their underlying fatigue. Extreme fatigue interferes with healing, however, possibly increasing the risk for infection. It also can eventually interfere with bonding with the child. Help the woman plan a day that includes care of her new child and periods of rest for herself as well. Be certain at bedtime that she has adequate analgesic to allow her to be pain free for the night. Provide a time in the middle of the morning and again in the afternoon for un-

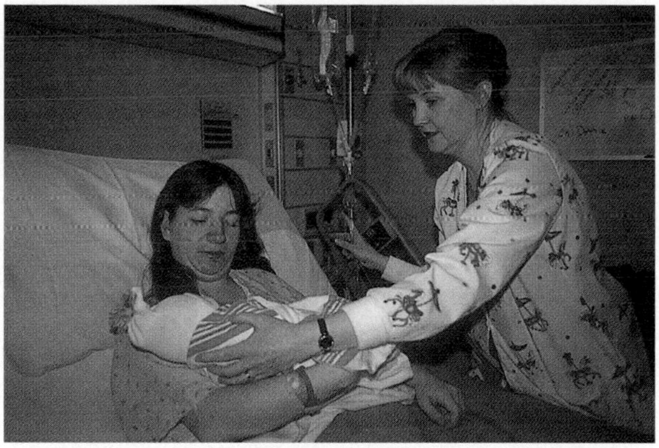

FIGURE 20.7 The nurse assists with holding the newborn and positioning the equipment so that the intravenous line does not interfere with mother–child interactions.

interrupted rest. Explore her plans for care at home to be certain her plans for rest seem realistic for a post-surgical-postpartal woman.

Rest is often best accomplished if women plan for it every time the newborn sleeps. Without adequate rest, they can notice increased uterine bleeding, which leads to excessive loss of fluid and iron stores.

Nursing Diagnosis: Impaired skin integrity related to surgical incision

Outcome Identification: Surgical incision exhibits signs and symptoms of healing without complication.

Outcome Evaluation: Incision line is clean, dry, intact without erythema; oral temperature is less than 38°C.

Surgical incisions heal by primary intention, or by the gradual removal and replacement of dead or damaged cells at the wound site with new cells produced by the surrounding tissue. Assess the surgical incision once during each nursing shift while a woman is hospitalized to ensure wound edges are approximated and no signs of infection, such as erythema, are present. As soon as she can walk steadily, she can take a shower after first removing the dressing. Warm, clean water on the incision is soothing. After this point, the woman usually makes the decision about continuing to wear a dressing. Lack of a dressing prevents moisture accumulation at the incision site and decreases the possibility of infection.

Teach women to continue to observe their incision daily at home. Instruct them in signs and symptoms of possible infection, including redness or the presence of a discharge, and to report any to their primary care provider. With a cesarean birth, healing will be adequate enough by day 4 or 5 that skin sutures or clamps

FOCUS ON *Nursing Care Planning*

THE WOMAN FOLLOWING AN EMERGENCY CESAREAN BIRTH

An 18-year-old primigravida underwent an emergency cesarean birth with epidural anesthesia for cephalopelvic disproportion after a failed trial labor. She gave birth to a healthy 8 lb, 2 oz baby girl. "It hurts so much all over. I can't move and I'm so tired. Take the baby away. I can't hold her right now."

Assessment: Post-cesarean birth 4 hours ago without problems. Estimated blood loss of 500 mL. Abdomen soft but tender with transverse incision. Bowel sounds sluggish but present. Incisional dressing clean, dry, and intact. Uterus firm, 1 fingerbreadth below umbilicus. Minimal lochia rubra vaginal drainage. Urine output 100 mL in last hour. Skin pink, warm, and dry. Skin turgor good. Intravenous solution infusing at 100 cc/h. IV site clean, dry, without signs of infiltration. Vital signs: temperature—98.4°F; pulse—78; respirations—23; blood pressure—130/76. Pulse, respirations, and blood pressure slightly elevated above baseline. Respirations shallow. Complaining of abdominal pain, especially at incisional area. "It hurts so much to even breathe." Holding hands over abdomen; barely moving in bed. Client's mother at bedside holding her hand and stroking her forehead. PCA pump in place but not being used by client.

Nursing Diagnosis: Pain related to tissue trauma from abdominal incision of cesarean birth

Outcome Identification: Client will report that pain level has decreased to tolerable levels.

Outcome Evaluation: Client identifies causes of pain; uses PCA appropriately; reports a decrease in pain with analgesic administration; pulse, respirations, and blood pressure return to baseline.

(continued)

Interventions	Rationale
1. Assess client's pain including type, location, and intensity. Use a 10-point rating scale.	1. Assessment provides clues to underlying cause of pain and provides a baseline for developing appropriate pain relief strategies.
2. Explain use of patient-controlled analgesia (PCA). Instruct client about method.	2. Analgesia provides effective pain relief. PCA provides continuous, consistent levels of pain relief without the need for repeated injections and promotes self care.
3. Inform client about pain relief measures, including how long it takes to achieve relief and how long to expect relief to last.	3. Pain is exacerbated by anxiety of the unknown. Providing information promotes relaxation, reduces fears, and enhances therapeutic effectiveness of the drug.
4. Institute additional comfort measures, such as changing position and bed linens frequently, splinting incision, applying cool compresses to the forehead, using pillows and blankets for support, and massaging and rubbing the back. Enlist the aid of the client's mother in providing comfort measures.	4. Comfort measures reduce stress and anxiety, elevate mood, and raise the pain threshold, thus enhancing the therapeutic effectiveness of the analgesia and the client's control over and ability to tolerate pain.
5. Assist client with slow, controlled deep breathing.	5. Deep breathing promotes relaxation and reduces muscle tension and also enhances lung expansion.
6. Assess client's response to pain relief measures and for possible adverse effects from narcotic analgesics.	6. Follow-up assessment is essential to determine the effectiveness of pain relief measures used and need for any change. Although rare, narcotic analgesics may cause sedation and respiratory depression.
7. Provide reinforcement for positive coping mechanisms.	7. Positive reinforcement enhances self-esteem and control.

Nursing Diagnosis: Risk for impaired parenting related to pain and fatigue

Outcome Identification: Client will demonstrate bonding behaviors with newborn prior to discharge.

Outcome Evaluation: Client holds infant warmly; maintains eye contact with infant; makes positive statements about the newborn.

Interventions	Rationale
1. Allow client some time for rest; encourage her to self-administer analgesics for pain relief.	1. Rest and pain relief help the client to regain control, thus improving the chance for positive interaction with the newborn.
2. Bring the child to the client and place a pillow over the client's lap to support the newborn. Assist the client with handling the newborn. Support breastfeeding efforts.	2. A pillow on the lap deflects the weight of the newborn off the suture line and lessens pain. Assistance provides physical and emotional support for a new experience, thus enhancing the client's confidence and self-esteem.
3. Review normal growth and development of a newborn and point out positive attributes. Encourage the client to look at, touch, and talk to the newborn.	3. Awareness of a newborn's appearance prepares the client for what she will see. Pointing out positive attributes and encouraging interaction promote bonding.
4. Praise the client for positive behaviors and interactions with the child in light of the client's pain and fatigue level.	4. Praise promotes self-esteem and confidence to manage new situations.
5. Encourage the client to keep the newborn in the room with her for extended periods as she is able.	5. Extended contact within the client's ability to tolerate the activity encourages bonding while minimizing the risk for additional fatigue.

Nursing Diagnosis: Ineffective breathing pattern related to postoperative pain

Outcome Identification: Client will achieve optimal respiratory function.

Outcome Evaluation: Client demonstrates coughing and deep breathing exercises and incentive spirometry every 2 hours. Lungs are clear to auscultation; respiratory rate is within acceptable parameters.

Interventions	Rationale
1. Assess client's respiratory status including rate, depth, and character of respirations. Auscultate lungs for adventitious sounds.	1. Respiratory assessment provides baseline information for evaluation of changes in the client's status.
2. Elevate the client's head of the bed 30 to 45 degrees and encourage the client to change positions frequently.	2. Elevation of the head of the bed causes abdominal organs to shift away from the diaphragm, thus promoting lung expansion. Frequent position changes promote lung expansion and mobilization of secretions.
3. Instruct the client in coughing and deep breathing exercises and use of incentive spirometry at least every 2 hours. As appropriate, suggest that client self-administer analgesic one half hour prior to activities and have client splint incision.	3. Coughing, deep breathing, and incentive spirometry promote lung expansion and prevent stasis of secretions, which could predispose the client to atelectasis or infection. Premedication prior to activities and splinting prevent pain from interfering with maximum lung expansion.
4. Ensure adequate fluid intake as tolerated.	4. Fluids help to liquefy secretions and aid in expectoration.
5. Assist the client to get out of bed to the chair and to ambulate.	5. Movement, including ambulation, facilitates movement of secretions, preventing respiratory compromise.
6. Continue to assess vital signs every 2 to 4 hours as indicated. Auscultate lungs for diminished or absent sounds or adventitious sounds.	6. A change in vital signs is an early indicator of possible infection. Decreased or absent breath sounds may indicate obstruction or atelectasis. Adventitious sounds may indicate a narrowing of the airways or fluid or air accumulation.

can be removed, although many are left in place until the woman returns for a follow-up appointment in 2 weeks.

Discharge Planning

The woman being discharged after cesarean birth takes home not only her new baby, but a fair amount of pain and discomfort as well. It is important to discuss home care arrangements, emphasizing the need for adequate help with the newborn and other responsibilities at home (see Focus on Family Empowerment). She should be aware of any restriction on exercise or activity (as a rule, she should not lift any object heavier than 10 lb for the first 2 weeks) as well as signs of possible complications directly related to the surgery, such as redness or drainage at the incision line, lochia heavier than a normal menstrual period, abdominal pain, temperature above 38°C (100.4°F), or frequency or burning on urination. She can resume coitus as soon as the act is comfortable for her, possibly as early as 1 week. Be sure that she has contraceptive information prior to discharge, if desired. Also ensure that she has an appointment for a return visit for health assessment with her health care provider, both for herself and her newborn (usually in 2 weeks).

Before discharge and again at the time of a second pregnancy, women need to be informed that they probably can have a second child by vaginal birth (see VBAC, Chapter 18). This not only makes them informed consumers of health care but also can influence whether they plan an additional pregnancy.

✔ CHECKPOINT QUESTIONS

8. What assessments are important to detect a possible lower extremity thrombus?
9. Other than bowel sounds, what else might you use to assess the return of intestinal function?
10. Typically, how much urine is eliminated by the postpartal woman in the first 24 hours?

FOCUS ON FAMILY EMPOWERMENT
Measures to Regain Energy After a Cesarean Birth

Q. I feel so tired after my cesarean. What can I do to feel stronger?

A. After a cesarean birth, women usually regain energy rapidly. This is because, unlike most people who have had surgery, you did not have it because you were ill, but because it was an alternative method to have a healthy baby. The following are measures that can help you regain your energy rapidly:

- Drink adequate fluid daily (at least six glasses). This helps prevent a urinary tract infection and also helps supply all the cells in your body with adequate nutrients.
- Rest twice a day for at least one half hour each time. This helps because your baby will probably wake you at least once during the night.
- Don't hesitate to accept help from family and friends for tasks such as house cleaning or grocery shopping.
- Limit the number of stairs that you climb daily to one flight once a day. Also limit the amount of weight you lift to the weight of your new baby.
- Don't attempt to be the "perfect" new mom. Relax and enjoy your new baby.

KEY POINTS

The term *cesarean "birth"* is preferred to *cesarean "section"* or delivery because this puts the focus on the childbirth rather than surgical elements of the procedure.

Cesarean birth may be either a scheduled or emergency procedure. It carries more risk for the mother and infant than vaginal birth does and is undertaken only when medically necessary.

Establishing surgical risk includes assessment of nutritional status, age, general health, fluid and electrolyte balance, and psychological condition.

Assessment measures before surgery usually include vital sign determination, urinalysis, blood studies such as complete blood count, electrolytes, blood typing and cross matching, and sonography.

The skin incision may be vertical (a classic incision), although it is usually a horizontal one just above the pubic hair. The internal incision into the uterus is also usually a horizontal incision into the lower uterine segment.

The old saying "Once a cesarean, always a cesarean" is no longer true, as long as cephalopelvic disproportion does not exist and the previous incision was a low transverse one.

Support people can lose a great deal of their ability to support if they feel intimidated and out of place in an operating room; offer them support as needed to make this a positive experience for them as well.

Cesarean birth is one of the safest types of surgery performed. To keep the woman safe after the procedure, remember that she is both a surgical and a postpartum patient. Make assessments to ensure neither postpartum nor postsurgical complications occur.

Adequate pain management is important to allow a woman a sense of control and comfort.

Women are physically exhausted after cesarean birth and may be psychologically exhausted because of the emergency nature of the experience. Provide rest time to relieve the physical strain and a chance to verbalize the experience to help relieve the psychological strain.

A major intervention after cesarean birth is early ambulation to prevent complications. Incisional pain may make this difficult, so strong nursing support and adequate pain management are necessary.

CRITICAL THINKING EXERCISES

1. Moja, the woman you met at the beginning of the chapter, was afraid to have a cesarean birth because she didn't want to be alone. What actions could you take to make her situation easier to accept?

2. A woman is receiving patient-controlled epidural anesthesia (PCEA) after a cesarean birth. She tells you she is not interested in this and would rather have injections for pain. Describe and explain the action you might take. Would you advocate for use of PCEA or advocate with her physician for a changed order?

3. A woman's husband tells you he cannot possibly stay with his wife in the operating room while she has a cesarean birth. He states he will feel nauseated and probably faint. His wife wants very badly to have him come with her. How would you intervene to promote family-centered care and meet the couple's needs?

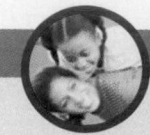

4. Examine the National Health Goals related to cesarean birth. Most government-sponsored money for nursing research is allotted based on these goals. What would be a possible research topic to explore pertinent to these goals that would be both fundable and advance evidence-based practice?

REFERENCES

Baeten, J. M., Bukusi, E. A., & Lambe, M. (2001). Pregnancy complications and outcomes among overweight and obese nulliparous women. *American Journal of Public Health, 91*(3), 436–440.

Baka, N. E., et al. (2002). Colostrum morphine concentrations during postcesarean intravenous patient-controlled analgesia. *Anesthesia & Analgesia, 94*(1), 184–187.

Bost, B. W. (2000). Should elective cesarean birth be offered at term as an alternative to labor and delivery for prevention of complications, including symptomatic pelvic prolapse, as well as stress urinary and fecal incontinence? *Obstetrics & Gynecology, 95*(4), S46.

Cunningham, F. G., et al. (2001). Cesarean section and postpartum hysterectomy. In F. G. Cunningham et al. (Eds.). *William's obstetrics* (21st ed., pp. 537–564). New York: McGraw-Hill.

Department of Health and Human Services. (2000). *Healthy people* 2010. Washington, DC: Author.

Durik, A. M., Hyde, J. S., & Clark, R. (2000). Sequelae of cesarean and vaginal deliveries: Psychosocial outcomes for mothers and infants. *Developmental Psychology, 36*(2), 251–260.

Gamble, J. A. & Creedy, D. K. (2000). Women's request for a cesarean section: A critique of the literature. *Birth, 27*(4), 256–263.

Hodnett, E. D. (2002). Caregiver support for women during childbirth. *Cochrane Database of Systematic Reviews, 1*(1).

Huang, W. H., et al. (2002). Interdelivery interval and the success of vaginal birth after cesarean delivery. *Obstetrics & Gynecology, 99*(1), 41–44.

Johnson, M., Maas, M., & Moorhead, S. (2000). Nursing outcomes classification (2nd ed.). St. Louis: Mosby.

Levine, E. M., et al. (2001). Mode of delivery and risk of respiratory diseases in newborns. Obstetrics & Gynecology, *97*(3), 439–442.

Matsumoto, L. C. & Resnik, R. (2001). Cesarean delivery and surgery in the pregnant patient. In Gershenson, D. M., DeCherney, A. H., Curry, S. L., & Brubaker, L. (Eds.). *Operative gynecology* (2nd ed., pp. 851–862). Philadelphia: W.B. Saunders.

McCloskey, J. & Bulechek, G. (2000). *Nursing interventions classification* (3rd ed.). St. Louis: Mosby.

Read, J. S., et al. (2001). Mode of delivery and postpartum morbidity among HIV-infected women: the women and infants transmission study. *Journal of Acquired Immune Deficiency Syndromes, 26*(3), 236–245.

Reiff, P. A. & Niziolek, M. M. (2001). Troubleshooting tips for PCA. *RN, 64*(4), 33–37.

Scott, J. R. (2000). Cesarean delivery. In Scott, J. R., et al. (Eds.). *Danforth's obstetrics and gynecology* (8th ed., pp. 65–90). Philadelphia: Lippincott Williams & Wilkins.

Spinnato, J. A., et al. (2000). Antibiotic prophylaxis at cesarean delivery. *Journal of Maternal-Fetal Medicine, 9*(6), 348–350.

SUGGESTED READINGS

Chauhan, S. P., et al. (2000). Cesarean delivery for suspected fetal distress among preterm parturients. *Journal of Reproductive Medicine, 45*(5), 395–402.

Chelmow, D., Ruehli, M. S., & Huang, E. (2001). Prophylactic use of antibiotics for nonlaboring patients undergoing cesarean delivery with intact membranes; a meta-analysis. *American Journal of Obstetrics & Gynecology, 184*(4), 656–661.

Garcia, F. A., et al. (2001). Effect of academic affiliation and obstetric volume on clinical outcome and cost of childbirth. *Obstetrics & Gynecology, 97*(4), 567–576.

Gregory, K. D. (2000). Monitoring, risk adjustment and strategies to decrease cesarean rate. *Current Opinion in Obstetrics & Gynecology, 12*(6), 481–486.

Hannah, M. E., et al. (2000). Planned caesarean section versus planned vaginal birth for breech presentation at term. *Lancet, 356*(9239), 1375–1383.

Hofmeyr, G. J. & Hannah, M. E. (2002). Planned caesarean section for term breech delivery. *Cochrane Database of Systematic Reviews, 1*(1).

Main, D. M., et al. (2000). The relationship between maternal age and uterine dysfunction: A continuous effect throughout reproductive life. *American Journal of Obstetrics & Gynecology, 182*(6), 1312–1320.

Perla, L. (2002). Patient compliance and satisfaction with nursing care during delivery and recovery. *Journal of Nursing Care Quality, 16*(2), 60–66.

Ramsey, P. S., Ramin, K. D., & Ramin, S. M. (2000). Labor induction. *Current Opinion in Obstetrics & Gynecology, 12*(6), 463–473.

Schulz-Lobmeyr, I. & Wenzl, R. (2000). Complications of elective cesarean delivery necessitating postpartum hysterectomy. *American Journal of Obstetrics & Gynecology, 182*(3), 729–730.

21 CHAPTER

The Woman Who Develops a Complication During Labor and Birth

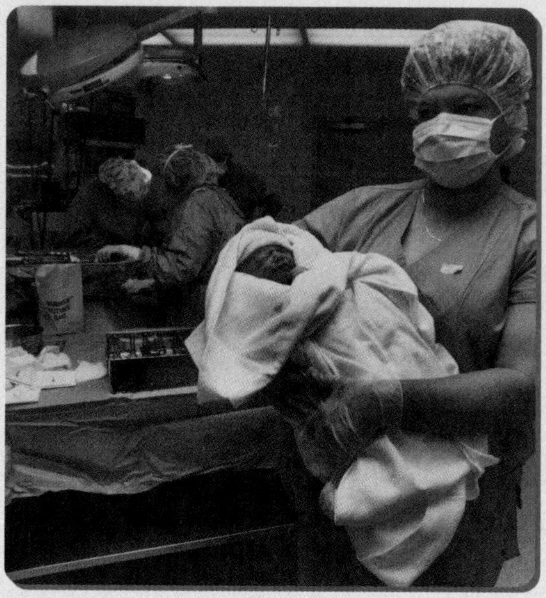

Key Terms

- amniotic fluid embolism
- augmentation of labor
- battledore placenta
- dysfunctional labor
- dystocia
- external cephalic version
- forceps birth
- hypertonic uterine contractions
- hypotonic uterine contractions
- induction of labor
- oxytocin
- pathologic retraction ring
- placenta accreta
- placenta circumvallata
- placenta marginata
- placenta succenturiata
- precipitate labor
- umbilical cord prolapse
- uterine inversion
- vacuum extraction

Objectives

After mastering the contents of this chapter, you should be able to:

1. Define the terms *dystocia* and *dysfunctional labor*.
2. Describe the common deviations in the power (force of labor), the passage, or the passenger that can cause dystocia or dysfunctional labor.
3. Assess the woman in labor and during birth for deviations from the normal labor process.
4. Formulate nursing diagnoses related to deviations from normal in labor and birth.
5. Identify expected outcomes associated with deviations in normal labor and birth and resultant complications.
6. Plan nursing interventions that will help the family meet established outcomes.
7. Implement care related to potential complications in labor or birth.
8. Evaluate outcomes for achievement and effectiveness of care.
9. Identify National Health Goals related to complications of labor that nurses could be instrumental in helping the nation achieve.
10. Identify areas related to complications of labor that could benefit from additional nursing research or application of evidence-based practice.
11. Use critical thinking to analyze ways to maintain family-centered nursing care when deviations from the normal in labor and birth occur.
12. Integrate the knowledge of deviations of normal in labor and birth with nursing process to achieve quality maternal and child health nursing care.

Roseann Bigalow, a 24-year-old woman about to give birth to her first baby, is admitted to a birthing room. Her contractions are 5 minutes apart. She states she feels more pain in her back than in her abdomen, "like my spine is tearing apart." A sonogram shows that her baby is above average in weight and in an occipitoposterior position. Her husband tells you he has heard that large babies deliver slower than average-size ones. He asks you if a posterior position could make his wife's labor even longer. What would you tell the Bigalows?

Previous chapters discussed normal labor and birth. This chapter adds information about what happens when complications of labor occur. This is important information to know because the sooner a complication in labor is recognized, the better the chance is that the situation can be corrected and that both fetal and maternal health can be protected.

After you've studied the chapter, answer the Critical Thinking Exercises at the end of the chapter, and then access the on-line study activities (http://connection.lww.com) *to further sharpen your skills and test your knowledge.*

Although labor usually proceeds without any deviations from the normal, many potential complications can occur. It is estimated that a potential complication occurs in as many as 31% of all births (DHHS, 2000). A difficult labor—**dystocia**—can arise from any of the three main components of the labor process: (1) the power (force that propels the fetus [uterine contractions]); (2) the passenger (the fetus); or (3) the passageway (the birth canal). In addition, medical interventions used to prevent or manage certain complications can cause difficulties of their own.

Because complications can occur at any point in the process, continuous monitoring of the laboring woman and fetus and providing emotional support for her and her partner are essential. The hours of labor are stressful even when everything proceeds normally. The laboring woman needs to be assured periodically that everything is going smoothly and that both she and the fetus appear to be doing well. When a complication arises and assurances cannot be given as freely, the stress for the woman and her support person can increase tremendously.

Nurses play a key role in providing skilled physical and emotional care during labor. The woman who is experiencing a complication in labor needs someone who is knowledgeable about the deviation and its treatment and understands the woman's fears and feelings of helplessness.

Complications of labor and birth can lead to infant mortality. National Health Goals related to attempts to decrease birth injury are shown in Focus on National Health Goals.

FOCUS ON NATIONAL HEALTH GOALS

A number of National Health Goals speak directly to complications of labor. These are:

- Reduce cesarean births among low-risk women to no more than 15 per 100 deliveries from a baseline of 18 per 100.
- Reduce the maternal mortality rate to no more than 3.3 per 100,000 live births from a baseline of 7.1 per 100,000.
- Reduce maternal complications during hospitalized labor and delivery to no more than 24 per 100 births from a baseline of 31.2 per 100 births (DHHS, 2000).

Nurses can be instrumental in helping the nation to achieve these goals by helping to identify women in labor who have a fetus presenting occipitoposteriorly and to initiate position changes that may speed the rotation of the fetus, thereby avoiding cesarean birth; and by being alert to the preliminary symptoms of uterine rupture, which accounts for a substantial number of maternal deaths during labor.

Further nursing research is needed as to whether breech and occipitoposterior positions can be prevented by position changes during pregnancy.

NURSING PROCESS OVERVIEW

For the Woman With a Labor or Birth Complication

Assessment

One of the major assessments used to detect deviations from normal in labor and birth is fetal and uterine monitoring. Working with such apparatus involves explaining its importance to parents, winning their cooperation, and using judgment in reading the various patterns. Typically, monitoring women in labor entails problems not found in other high-risk areas such as an intensive care unit (ICU). In an ICU, the person being monitored has been admitted to the unit because he or she is seriously ill. The person, recognizing the seriousness of the illness, accepts almost any monitoring or other procedure without protest. He or she lies still to prevent artifacts on the tracing. However, a woman in labor, who is otherwise well but develops a complication, may be less accepting of technologic or pharmacologic intervention. She moves because she is in pain. Her movement may cause artifacts on tracings, requiring frequent adjustment of equipment to achieve a clear tracing. Understanding that this is a normal consequence of labor is essential for effective assessment and continued care.

Nursing Diagnosis

Common nursing diagnoses specific to the woman experiencing a complication during labor or birth refer to specific problems. Some examples may include the following:

- Fear related to uncertainty of pregnancy outcome
- Anxiety related to medical procedures and apparatus necessary for ensuring health of mother and fetus
- Fatigue related to loss of glucose stores through work and duration of labor
- Risk for ineffective tissue perfusion related to excessive loss of blood

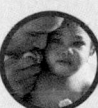

- Risk for injury (maternal or fetal) related to development of complication, effect on mother and fetus, and treatment required
- Risk for injury (maternal or fetal) related to labor involving a multiple gestation pregnancy
- Anticipatory grieving related to nonviable monitoring pattern of fetus

Outcome Identification and Planning

When a complication occurs, outcome identification may be difficult because the outcome may not be what the woman in labor desires. Encouraging a couple to clarify their priorities is helpful. For example, early in labor, a woman might say that her goals are to avoid monitoring equipment or an episiotomy. However, if fetal bradycardia occurs, monitoring and a cesarean birth may be necessary. If this happens, reminding the woman that the primary goal is to have a healthy baby may help her accept changes, including whatever interventions are necessary to achieve her ultimate objective.

Implementation

When a woman develops a complication of labor or birth, a priority, possibly an emergency, situation exists. Interventions must be planned and performed efficiently and effectively, based on the individual circumstances. All actions must safeguard both the woman and the fetus while providing psychological reassurance for the woman and her support person.

Evaluation

Evaluation of client outcomes may reveal unhappiness because not every woman who experiences a deviation from the normal in labor and birth will be able to give birth to a healthy child. Some deviations will be too great. Some interventions will not be maximally effective because of individual circumstances. Some infants will die; a few women may even be left unable to bear future children. Evaluation may lead to new analysis that the couple's chief need at that point is to grieve for the child or for a lifestyle that can no longer be theirs. When the outcome is more positive, the couple needs to be evaluated for signs that they are able to begin interaction with the child after a harrowing experience.

Examples of outcome achievement might be:

- Client voices confidence she can cope with fear.
- Client demonstrates adequate energy during course of labor to maintain effective breathing patterns.
- Client's blood pressure remains above 110/60 in spite of excessive blood loss with placenta delivery.
- Client begins positive grieving behaviors in response to loss of newborn.

PROBLEMS WITH THE POWER (THE FORCE OF LABOR)

Inertia is a time-honored term to denote that sluggishness of contractions, or the force of labor, has occurred. A more current term is **dysfunctional labor.** Dysfunction can occur at any point in labor but is generally classified as primary (occurring at the onset of labor) or *secondary* (occurring later in labor). The risk of maternal postpartal infection and hemorrhage and infant mortality is higher in women who have a prolonged labor than in those who do not. Therefore, it is vital to recognize and prevent dysfunctional labor (Dudley, 2000).

Prolonged labor appears to result from several factors. Hypotonic, hypertonic, and uncoordinated contractions all play roles (Box 21-1). It is likely to occur if the fetus is large (Hogberg & Lekas, 2000).

Ineffective Uterine Force

Uterine contractions are the basic force moving the fetus through the birth canal. As described in Chapter 18, uterine contractions occur because of the interplay of contractile hormones (adenosine triphosphate, estrogen, and progesterone) and the influence of major electrolytes such as calcium, sodium, and potassium, specific contractile proteins (actin and myosin), epinephrine and norepinephrine, oxytocin, and prostaglandins. About 95% of labors are completed with contractions that follow a predictable, normal course. However, abnormal contractions may occur, including (1) hypotonic contractions, (2) hypertonic contractions, and (3) uncoordinated contractions. These types of contractions can be ineffective, resulting in an ineffective labor.

Electronic uterine monitoring, external or internal, is used to monitor the duration, strength, and interval between contractions. Another method of evaluating the adequacy of uterine activity is to evaluate contractions based on Montevideo units. Montevideo units are calculated by adding the sum total, in mm Hg of height over the baseline, of all contractions that occur during a 10-minute window. For example, suppose that four contractions

BOX 21.1

COMMON CAUSES OF DYSFUNCTIONAL LABOR

Inappropriate use of analgesia (excessive or too early administration)
Pelvic bone contraction that has narrowed the pelvic diameter so that the fetus cannot pass, such as might have occurred in a client with rickets
Poor fetal position (posterior rather than anterior position)
Extension rather than flexion of the fetal head
Overdistention of the uterus, as with multiple pregnancy, hydramnios, or an excessively oversized fetus
Cervical rigidity
Presence of a full rectum or urinary bladder that impedes fetal descent
Mother becoming exhausted from labor
Primigravida status

occur in a 10-minute window, each 50 mm Hg above the baseline. This would total 200 Montevideo units. A total of 180 to 200 units suggests adequate uterine activity (Miller & Paul, 2000).

Hypotonic Contractions

Figure 21-1*A* illustrates the appearance of normal uterine contractions. With **hypotonic uterine contractions,** the number of contractions is usually low or infrequent (not increasing beyond two or three in a 10-minute period). The resting tone of the uterus remains below 10 mm Hg, and the strength of contractions does not rise above 25 mm Hg (Fig. 21-1*B*). Hypotonic contractions are most apt to occur during the active phase of labor. They may occur when analgesia has been administered too early (before cervical dilatation of 3 to 4 cm) or when bowel or bladder distention prevents descent or firm engagement. They may occur in a uterus overstretched by a multiple gestation, a larger-than-usual single fetus, or hydramnios, or in a uterus lax from grand multiparity. Such contractions are not exceedingly painful, because of the lack of intensity. Keep in mind, however, that the strength of a contraction is a subjective symptom. Some women may interpret these contractions as very painful.

Hypotonic contractions increase the length of labor, because more of them are necessary to achieve cervical dilatation. During the postpartal period, the uterus can be exhausted from a long labor and may not continue to contract as effectively, thus increasing the woman's chance for postpartal hemorrhage. With the cervix dilated for a long period, both the uterus and the fetus are at greater risk for infection.

For these reasons, after ultrasonic confirmation rules out cephalopelvic disproportion, an oxytocin infusion to augment labor usually is started to strengthen contractions and increase their effectiveness. Membranes may be artificially ruptured (amniotomy) to further speed labor. In the first hour postpartum, palpate the uterus and assess lochia every 15 minutes to ensure that postpartal contractions are not also hypotonic and therefore inadequate to halt bleeding.

Hypertonic Contractions

Hypertonic uterine contractions are marked by an increase in resting tone to more than 15 mm Hg (Fig. 21-1*C*). However, the intensity of the contraction may be no stronger than that associated with hypotonic contractions. Hypertonic contractions tend to occur frequently; they are most commonly seen in the latent phase of labor. Hypertonic contractions occur because the muscle fibers of the myometrium do not repolarize after a contraction, thereby "wiping it clean" to accept a new pacemaker stimulus. They are believed to occur because more than one pacemaker is stimulating the contractions. Hypertonic contractions tend to be painful, because the myometrium becomes tender from constant lack of relaxation and resultant anoxia to uterine cells. The woman may become frustrated or disappointed with her breathing exercises for childbirth, because they are ineffective in achieving pain relief.

The lack of relaxation between contractions does not allow optimal uterine artery filling, which may lead to fetal anoxia early in the latent phase of labor. Any woman whose pain seems out of proportion to the quality of her contractions should have both a uterine and fetal external monitor applied for at least a 15-minute interval to ensure the resting phase of the contractions is adequate and the fetal pattern is not showing late deceleration. Manage-

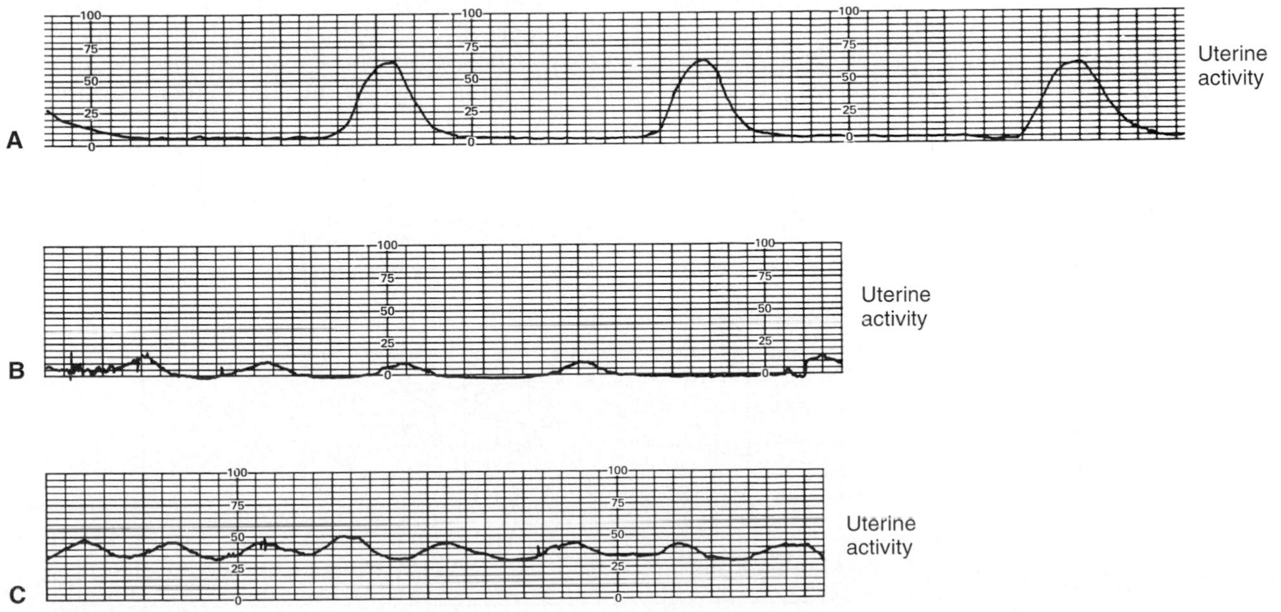

FIGURE 21.1 (*A*) Normal uterine contractions. (*B*) Hypotonic contractions; notice rise in pressure no more than 10 mm Hg. (*C*) Hypertonic contractions; notice the high resting pressure (40–50 mm Hg).

TABLE 21.1 Comparison of Hypotonic and Hypertonic Contractions

CRITERIA	HYPERTONIC	HYPOTONIC
Phase of labor	Latent	Active
Symptoms	Painful	Painless
Medication		
Oxytocin	Unfavorable reaction	Favorable reaction
Sedation	Helpful	Little value

ment of hypertonic contractions involves rest and pain relief with a drug such as morphine sulfate. Changing the linen and the client's gown, darkening room lights, and decreasing noise and stimulation are also helpful. If deceleration in the fetal heart rate (FHR), an abnormally long first stage of labor, or lack of progress with pushing ("second stage arrest") occurs, cesarean birth may be necessary. Both the woman and her support person need to understand that, although the contractions are strong, they are, in reality, ineffective and are not achieving cervical dilatation. Hypotonic and hypertonic contractions are compared in Table 21-1.

Uncoordinated Contractions

Normally, all contractions are initiated at one pacemaker point in the uterus. A contraction sweeps down over the uterus, encircling it; repolarization occurs, a low resting tone is achieved, and another pacemaker-activated contraction begins. With uncoordinated contractions, more than one pacemaker may be initiating contractions, or receptor points in the myometrium are acting independently of the pacemaker. Uncoordinated contractions may occur so closely together that they do not allow good cotyledon filling. Because they occur so erratically (one on top of another and then a long period without any), it may be difficult for the woman to rest or use breathing exercises between contractions.

Applying a fetal and uterine external monitor and assessing the rate, pattern, resting tone, and fetal response to contractions for at least a 15-minute interval (a longer time may be necessary to show the disorganized pattern in early labor) reveals the abnormal pattern. Oxytocin administration may be helpful in uncoordinated labor to stimulate a more effective and consistent pattern of contractions with a better, lower resting tone.

Dysfunctional Labor and Associated Stages of Labor

As stated previously, dysfunctional or ineffective labor can occur at any point in labor. For a graphic illustration of these times, see Figure 21-2. Regardless of when dysfunctional labor occurs, the effect on the woman and her support person will be the same: anxiety, fear, or discouragement. The woman needs a continuous explanation of what is happening: "We're going to take a sonogram to check the baby's position." "This is a drug to urge your uterus into stronger contractions." "I know resting is the last thing you feel like doing, but that is what I want you to try to do."

Dysfunction at the First Stage of Labor

Prolonged Latent Phase. The major dysfunction that can occur in the first stage of labor is a prolonged latent phase.

The normal parameters for the stages of labor are highlighted in Table 21-2. A *prolonged latent phase,* as defined by Friedman (1978), is a latent phase that is longer than 20 hours in a nullipara and 14 hours in a multipara. This may occur if the cervix is not "ripe" at the beginning of labor and time has to be spent getting truly ready for labor. It may occur if there is excessive use of an analgesic early in labor. With a prolonged latent phase, the uterus tends to be in a hypertonic state. Relaxation between

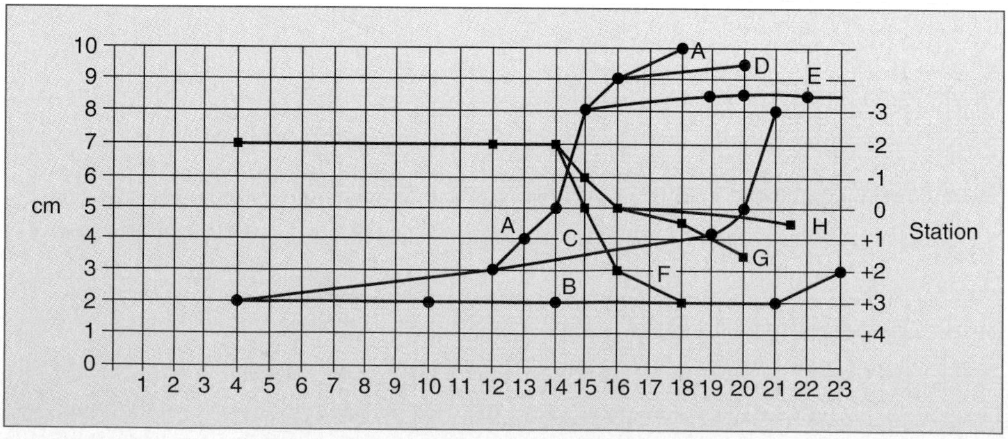

FIGURE 21.2 Graph showing types of abnormal labor. (*A*) Normal labor curve. (*B*) Prolonged latent phase. (*C*) Protracted active-phase dilatation. (*D*) Prolonged deceleration phase. (*E*) Secondary arrest of dilatation. (*F*) Normal descent. (*G*) Prolonged descent. (*H*) Arrest of descent.

TABLE 21.2 Lengths of Phases of Stages of Normal Labor in Hours

	NULLIPARA		MULTIPARA	
PHASE	*Average*	*Upper Normal*	*Average*	*Upper Normal*
Latent phase	8.6	20.0	5.3	14.0
Active phase	5.8	12.0	2.5	6.0
Second stage	1	1.5	0.25	1

contractions is inadequate, and the contractions are only mild (less than 15 mm Hg on a monitor printout) and therefore ineffective. One segment of the uterus may contract with more force than another segment.

Management of a prolonged latent phase in labor includes helping the uterus to rest and administering adequate fluid to the woman to prevent dehydration. Administration of morphine may relax hypertonicity. This usually allows labor to become effective and begin to progress. If it does not, a cesarean birth or amniotomy and oxytocin infusion to assist labor may be necessary.

Protracted Active Phase. A protracted active phase is usually associated with cephalopelvic disproportion (CPD) or fetal malposition, although it may reflect ineffective myometrial activity. This phase is prolonged if cervical dilatation does not occur at a rate of 1.2 cm/h or more in a nullipara or 1.5 cm/h or more in a multipara or if the active phase lasts over 12 hours in a primigravida, 6 hours in a multigravida (see Fig. 21-2). If the cause of the delay in dilatation is fetal malposition or CPD, cesarean birth may be necessary. Dysfunctional labor during the dilatational division tends to be hypotonic in contrast to the hypertonic action at the beginning of labor. After a sonogram to show that cephalopelvic disproportion is not present, oxytocin may be prescribed to augment labor.

Prolonged Deceleration Phase. A deceleration phase has become prolonged when it extends beyond 3 hours in a nullipara and 1 hour in a multipara. Prolonged deceleration phase most often results from abnormal fetal head position. A cesarean birth is frequently required.

Secondary Arrest of Dilatation. A secondary arrest of dilatation has occurred when there is no progress in cervical dilatation for more than 2 hours.

Prolonged Descent. *Prolonged descent* of the fetus occurs if the rate of descent is less than 1.0 cm/h in a nullipara or less than 2.0 cm/h in a multipara.

With both a prolonged active phase of dilatation and prolonged descent, contractions have been of good quality and proper duration, and effacement and beginning dilatation have occurred. But then, the contractions become infrequent and of poor quality, and dilatation stops. If everything except the suddenly faulty contractions is normal (CPD or poor fetal presentation has been ruled out by sonogram), then rest and fluid intake, as advocated for hypertonic contractions, also apply. If membranes have not ruptured, rupturing them at this point may be helpful. Intravenous oxytocin may be used to induce the uterus to contract effectively. A semi-Fowler's position, squatting, kneeling, or more effective pushing may speed descent.

Dysfunction at the Second Stage of Labor

Arrest of Descent. *Arrest of descent* results when no descent has occurred for 1 hour in a multipara, or 2 hours in a nullipara. Failure of descent has occurred when expected descent of the fetus does not begin (engagement or movement beyond 0 station has not occurred).

The most likely cause for arrest in labor during the second stage is CPD. Cesarean birth is generally the method of choice for delivery. If there is no contraindication to vaginal birth, oxytocin may be used to assist in labor.

NURSING DIAGNOSES AND RELATED INTERVENTIONS FOR DYSFUNCTIONAL LABOR

It is impossible to prevent all dysfunctional labor, just as it is impossible to predict the functioning of anyone's hormonal system or individual response to labor. However, a number of nursing interventions can contribute to the progression of normal labor and help change a dysfunctional labor to a functional one.

Nursing Diagnosis: Fatigue related to prolonged labor

Outcome Identification: Client will maintain adequate energy for continued labor.

Outcome Evaluation: Woman states she is able to continue active participation in labor; maintains effective breathing with contractions.

Because labor is work, it can cause a woman to deplete her glucose stores. On a client's admission to a birthing room, assess how likely this might be by asking the time of her last meal. If she ate breakfast at 8 am and then began labor by 2 PM, she is only 6 hours away from a full meal. If, however, she last ate at 5 PM the preceding evening and did not eat breakfast because she awoke with labor this morning, she is 11 hours away from a full meal. Alert the physician or nurse-midwife to this situation. If the client is still in early labor, she may be allowed to drink some high-carbohydrate fluid such as orange juice. Intravenous fluid therapy also may be initiated to provide glucose for energy (see Focus on Evidence-Based Practice).

Many women react negatively to the idea of intravenous fluid therapy during labor, possibly perceiving it as loss of control over their bodies or removal of the "naturalness" of labor and birth. Introduce the idea of intravenous fluid therapy, explaining its purpose *before* arriving with the bag of fluid and tubing. When inserting the intravenous catheter device, try

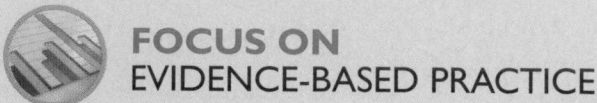

FOCUS ON EVIDENCE-BASED PRACTICE

Does Eating During Labor Reduce the Incidence of Instrument Delivery?

In the United States, most women are advised not to eat or drink during labor. In contrast, in Europe, most women are allowed to continue eating and drinking. For this study, 211 nulliparous women in the Netherlands, following the birth of their infants, were asked what they had been advised about eating and drinking during labor, what they consumed, and whether they had followed the advice given to them. Results showed that 66% of the women said that they had not been given advice. Seventy-five percent of them ate solid food during labor. The incidence of instrument delivery due to a nonprogressing second stage of labor was lower in these women with a caloric intake (13%) when compared to women who did not have a caloric intake (24%).

This is an important study for nurses because it supplies information about differences in labor practices and gives new information on the possible importance of caloric intake during labor. A third interesting finding was that the average woman followed the advice given to her by a health care professional, thus documenting evidence of the influence that nurses can have on health teaching.

Scheepers, H. C., Thans, M. C., deJong, P. A., Essed, G. G., Le Cessie, S., and Kanhaie, H. H. (2001). Eating and drinking in labor: The influence of caregiver advice on women's behavior. *Birth, 28*(2), 119–123.

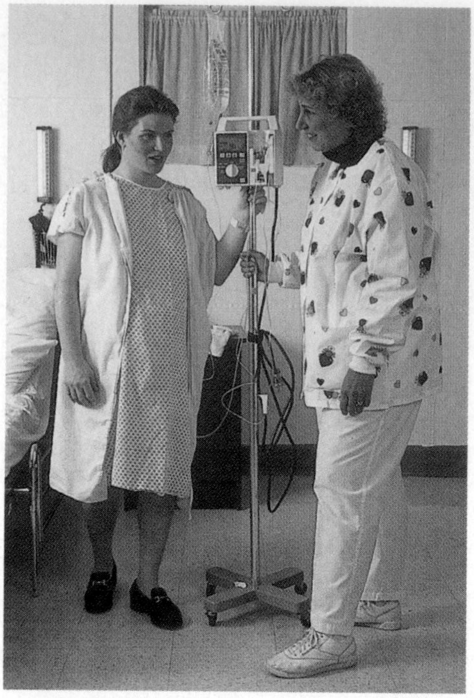

FIGURE 21.3 An intravenous line, a common piece of equipment for women in labor, does not need to limit mobility.

to use an insertion site in the woman's nondominant hand and, if necessary, only a small "reminder" handboard. Assure the woman that she can be out of bed and walking, can turn freely, squat, sit, or use whatever position she prefers during labor. None of these acts will interfere with the infusion (Fig. 21-3). Most physicians and nurse-midwives also allow women to have lollipops or hard candy to suck on during labor to supply additional glucose.

Although difficult to document, if the woman is neither tense nor frightened during labor, her cervix appears to dilate more rapidly and therefore shorten normal labor. Manage stress by making the transfer from home to health care facility as least traumatic as possible. Ask directly if the woman has any concerns. Offer explanations of all procedures. Make the support person just as welcome and comfortable as the woman herself. A question such as "Is labor what you thought it would be?" to both the woman and her support person often helps them to express different concerns.

Remember that pain is an exhausting phenomenon. Encourage the use of nonpharmacologic comfort measures. Breathe with the woman, give back rubs, change sheets, use cool washcloths, and so forth. If breathing exercises or complementary therapies such as aromatherapy or music can be effective, the need for analgesia (which can lead to hypotonic contractions) can be reduced (Burns, 2000).

To increase the blood supply to the uterus and prevent hypotension, urge the woman to lie on her side so the uterus is lifted off the vena cava. If a woman insists on lying supine, place a hip roll under one or the other buttock to cause her pelvis to "tip" and, at least to some extent, move the uterus to the side.

A full bladder prevents descent of the fetus and may impede uterine contractions. Urge the woman in labor to void every 2 hours to keep the bladder empty and to aid progress.

WHAT IF? What if a woman's doctor tells her not to eat in labor because she may need general anesthesia for a cesarean birth, but you find her eating potato chips because she doesn't want general anesthesia? What would you do?

Nursing Diagnosis: Risk for deficient fluid volume related to length and work of labor and accompanying vomiting and diarrhea

Outcome Identification: Client will exhibit signs and symptoms of adequate fluid and electrolyte balance during labor.

Outcome Evaluation: Urine is without evidence of ketones; specific gravity is between 1.003 and 1.030; skin turgor and serum electrolyte levels are within acceptable parameters.

Low levels of serum electrolytes or body fluid can occur in labor for the same reason as a decreased glucose level, that is, there has been a long interval between eating and the end of labor. Additionally, vomiting and diarrhea that occasionally accompany labor can increase fluid and electrolyte losses. Question the woman about any vomiting or diarrhea and determine the extent (eg, one episode of a small amount of diarrhea or vomiting that lasted on and off for 30 minutes). Profuse diaphoresis and hyperventilation that occur with labor can further increase fluid and electrolyte losses through insensible water loss. Test voidings frequently during labor for glucose, protein, ketones, and specific gravity (place a urine collector container on the bathroom toilet if the woman is going to use the toilet). Ketones in the urine suggest starvation ketosis. A concentrated specific gravity suggests a lack of fluid. Extreme dehydration may lead to increased blood viscosity, possibly increasing the risk for thrombophlebitis during the postpartal period.

✔ CHECKPOINT QUESTIONS

1. During which phase of labor do hypotonic contractions usually occur?
2. When is the deceleration phase considered to be prolonged?
3. What is the most common cause for arrest of descent during the second stage of labor?

Contraction Rings

Two types of contraction rings can occur in a dysfunctional labor. A simple type is a constriction ring, which can occur at any point in the myometrium and at any time during labor. The most common is a **pathologic retraction ring** (Bandl's ring) that occurs at the juncture of the upper and lower uterine segments. This is a warning sign that severe dysfunctional labor is occurring. The ring usually appears during the second stage of labor as a horizontal indentation across the abdomen (Fig. 21-4). It is formed by excessive retraction of the upper uterine segment; the uterine myometrium is much thicker above than below the ring.

When a pathologic retraction ring occurs in early labor, it is usually from uncoordinated contractions. In the pelvic division of labor, it is usually caused by obstetric manipulation or the result of the administration of oxytocin. The fetus is gripped by the retraction ring and cannot advance beyond that point. The undelivered placenta will also be held at that point.

Contraction rings often can be identified by sonogram. Such a finding is extremely serious and should be reported promptly. Administration of intravenous morphine sulfate or the inhalation of amyl nitrite may relieve the retraction ring. A tocolytic may be administered to halt contractions. If the situation is not relieved, uterine rupture and death of the fetus may occur. In the placental stage, massive maternal hemorrhage may result, because the placenta is loosened but then cannot deliver, preventing the uterus from contracting.

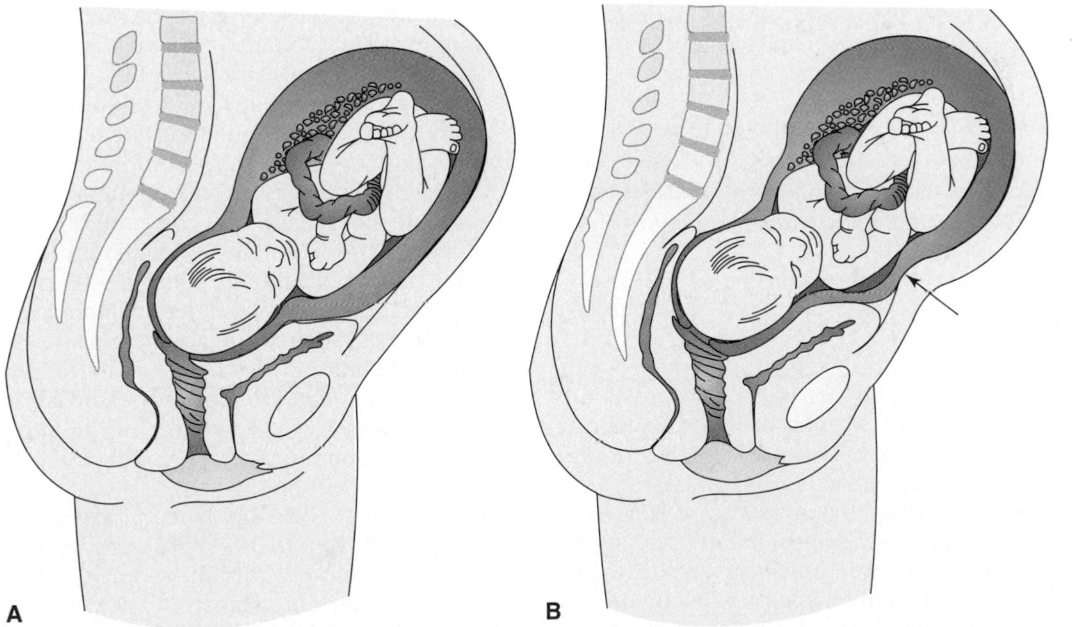

FIGURE 21.4 Pathologic retraction ring. (*A*) Uterus in the normal second stage of labor. Notice how the upper uterine segment is becoming thicker and the lower uterine segment is thinning. A physiologic retraction ring is normally formed at the division of the upper and lower uterine segments. (*B*) Uterus with a pathologic retraction ring (Bandl's ring). The wall below the ring is thin and the abdomen shows an indentation. This constriction is caused by obstructed labor and is a warning sign that if the obstruction is not relieved, the lower segment may rupture.

Most likely, a cesarean birth will be necessary to ensure safe birth of the fetus. Manual removal of the placenta under general anesthesia may be required if the retraction ring does not allow the placenta to be delivered.

Precipitate Labor

Precipitate labor and birth occur when uterine contractions are so strong that the woman gives birth with only a few rapidly occurring contractions. It is often defined as a labor that is completed in fewer than 3 hours (Cunningham et al., 2001). Such rapid labor is likely to occur with multiparity or may follow induction of labor by oxytocin or amniotomy. Contractions may be so forceful they lead to premature separation of the placenta, placing the mother and fetus at risk for hemorrhage. Rapid labor also poses a risk to the fetus because subdural hemorrhage may result from the sudden release of pressure on the head. The woman may sustain lacerations of the birth canal from the forceful birth. She also can feel overwhelmed by the speed of labor.

A precipitate labor can be predicted from a labor graph if, during the active phase of dilatation, the rate is greater than 5 cm/h (1 cm every 12 minutes) in a nullipara and more than 10 cm/h (1 cm every 6 minutes) in a multipara. If this is occurring, a tocolytic may be administered to reduce the force and frequency of contractions.

Inform the multiparous woman by week 28 of pregnancy that her labor might be shorter than a previous one. This allows her to plan for appropriately timed transportation to the hospital or alternative birthing center. When labor begins, alert women who had a prior precipitate labor and birth that they may well deliver this way again. Both grand multiparas and women with histories of precipitate labor should have the birthing room converted to birth readiness before full dilatation. Then, birth can be accomplished in a controlled surrounding.

WHAT IF? What if a woman told you she was in labor only 1 hour with her last baby but is planning to spend her last days of this pregnancy in a mountain cabin 60 miles from the hospital? What would you do?

Uterine Rupture

Rupture of the uterus during labor, although rare (occurring only in about 1 in 1500 births), is always a possibility (Cunningham et al., 2001). A uterus ruptures when it undergoes more strain than it is capable of sustaining. Rupture occurs most commonly when a vertical scar from a previous cesarean birth or hysterotomy repair tears. Contributing factors may include prolonged labor, faulty presentation, multiple gestation, unwise use of oxytocin, obstructed labor, and traumatic maneuvers using forceps or traction. Uterine rupture accounts for as many as 5% of all maternal deaths. When it occurs, fetal death will occur unless immediate cesarean birth can be accomplished. In these instances, fetal outcome can be optimal (Yap, Kim, & Laros, 2001).

Impending rupture is preceded by a pathologic retraction ring (an indentation is apparent across the abdomen over the uterus) and strong uterine contractions without any cervical dilatation. To prevent rupture when these symptoms are present, anticipate the need for an immediate cesarean birth. If a uterus should rupture, the woman experiences a sudden, severe pain during a strong labor contraction. She may report a "tearing" sensation. Rupture can be complete, going through endometrium, myometrium, and peritoneum, or incomplete, leaving the peritoneum intact. With a complete rupture, uterine contractions will stop. There is hemorrhage from the torn uterus into the abdominal cavity and possibly into the vagina. Signs of shock begin, including rapid, weak pulse, falling blood pressure, cold and clammy skin, and dilatation of the nostrils from air hunger. The woman's abdomen will change in contour. Two distinct swellings will be visible: the retracted uterus and the extrauterine fetus. Fetal heart sounds become absent. If the rupture is incomplete, the signs are less evident than in complete rupture. With an incomplete rupture, the woman may experience only a localized tenderness and a persistent aching pain over the area of the lower segment. Fetal heart sounds, a lack of contractions, and the woman's vital signs will gradually reveal fetal and maternal distress (see Assessing the Pregnant Woman With a Complete Uterine Rupture).

Because the uterus at the end of pregnancy is such a vascular organ, uterine rupture is an immediate emergency situation comparable to splenic or hepatic rupture. Administer emergency fluid replacement therapy as ordered. Anticipate use of intravenous oxytocin to attempt to contract the uterus and minimize bleeding. Prepare the woman for a possible laparotomy as an emergency measure to control bleeding and effect a repair. The viability of the fetus will depend on the extent of the rupture and the time that elapses between the rupture and abdominal extraction. The woman's prognosis will depend on the extent of the rupture and blood loss.

It is inadvisable for a woman to conceive again after a rupture of the uterus unless it occurred in the inactive lower segment. Therefore, the physician, with consent, may perform a hysterectomy (removal of the damaged uterus) or tubal ligation at the time of the laparotomy. Both procedures result in loss of childbearing ability. The woman may have difficulty giving her consent at this time because it is unknown whether the fetus will live. If blood loss was acute, she may be non-responsive because of decreased cerebral perfusion secondary to hypotension. If this has happened, her support person must be the one who gives this consent, relying on the information provided by the operating surgeon to decide whether a functioning uterus can be saved.

Be prepared to offer information to the support person and to inform him or her about the fetal outcome, the extent of the surgery, and the woman's safety as soon as possible. Initially, the woman and her support person will probably be thankful because her life was saved. However, they may become almost immediately angry that the rupture occurred, especially if the fetus died and the woman will no longer be able to have children. Allow them time to express these emotions without feeling threatened. They may grieve both for the loss of the child and their fertility as a couple.

ASSESSING the Pregnant Woman with Complete Uterine Rupture

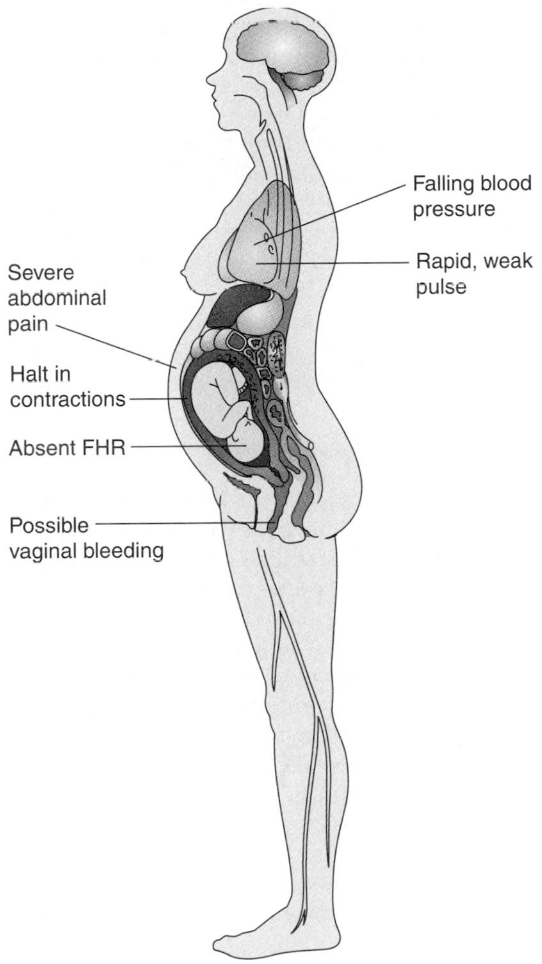

Inversion of the Uterus

Uterine inversion is a rare phenomenon, occurring in about 1 in 15,000 births, in which the uterus turns inside out (Calder, 2000). It may occur after the birth of the infant if traction is applied to the umbilical cord to remove the placenta or if pressure is applied to the uterine fundus when the uterus is not contracted. It may also occur when the placenta attaches at the fundus, so that during birth, the passage of the fetus pulls the fundus down.

Inversion occurs in various degrees. The inverted fundus may lie within the uterine cavity or the vagina or, as in total inversion, protrude from the vagina. When an inversion occurs, a large amount of blood suddenly gushes from the vagina. The fundus is not palpable in the abdomen. If the loss of blood continues unchecked for more than a few minutes, the woman will immediately show signs of blood loss: hypotension, dizziness, paleness, or diaphoresis. Since the uterus is not contracted in this position, bleeding continues. A woman could exsanguinate within a period as short as 10 minutes.

Never attempt to replace the inversion because handling may increase the bleeding. Never attempt to remove the placenta if it is still attached, because this will only create a larger surface area for bleeding. In addition, administering an oxytocic drug only compounds the inversion. An intravenous fluid line needs to be started, if one is not already present (if doing this, use a large-gauge needle because blood will need to be replaced); if a line is already in place, it should be opened to achieve optimal flow of fluid to try to restore fluid volume. Administer oxygen by mask, and assess vital signs. Be prepared to perform cardiopulmonary resuscitation (CPR) if the woman's heart should fail from the sudden blood loss. The woman will be given general anesthesia or possibly nitroglycerin or a tocolytic drug intravenously immediately to relax the uterus (Hostetler & Bosworth, 2000). The delivering physician or nurse-midwife then replaces the fundus manually. Administration of oxytocin after manual replacement helps the uterus to contract and remain in its natural place. Because the uterine endometrium was exposed, the woman will need antibiotic therapy postpartum to prevent infection.

Amniotic Fluid Embolism

Amniotic fluid embolism occurs when amniotic fluid is forced into an open maternal uterine blood sinus through some defect in the membranes or after membrane rupture or partial premature separation of the placenta. Previously, it was thought that particles such as meconium or shed fetal skin cells in the amniotic fluid entered the maternal circulation and reached the lungs as small emboli. Now, it is recognized that a humoral or anaphylactoid response is the more likely cause (Clark, 2000). This condition may occur during labor or in the postpartal period. The incidence is no more than 1 in 8000 births; it is not preventable because it cannot be predicted. Possible risk factors include oxytocin administration, abruptio placentae, and hydramnios.

The clinical picture is dramatic. The woman, in strong labor, sits up suddenly and grasps her chest because of sharp pain and inability to breathe (secondary to pulmonary artery constriction). She becomes pale and then turns the typical bluish gray associated with pulmonary embolism and lack of blood flow to the lungs. The immediate management is oxygen administration by facemask or cannula. Within minutes, the woman will need CPR. CPR may be ineffective, because these procedures (inflating the lungs and massaging the heart) do not relieve the pulmonary constriction. Therefore, blood still cannot circulate to the lungs. Death may occur in minutes.

The woman's prognosis depends on the size of the embolism and the skill and speed of emergency interventions. Even if she survives the initial insult, the risk for disseminated intravascular coagulation (DIC) developing is high, further compounding her condition (Bick, 2000). In this event, she will need continued management that includes endotracheal intubation to maintain pulmonary function and therapy with fibrinogen to counteract DIC. The woman most likely will be transferred to an ICU. The prognosis for the fetus is guarded, because reduced placental perfusion results from the severe drop in maternal blood pressure. Labor often begins or the fetus is delivered immediately by cesarean birth.

> **✔ CHECKPOINT QUESTIONS**
>
> 4. When a woman experiences a complete uterine rupture, what type of pain does she typically report?
> 5. With uterine inversion, why should the placenta never be removed if it is still attached?

PROBLEMS WITH THE PASSENGER

Birth complications may arise if the maternal pelvis is undersized, such as in early adolescence or in women with altered bone growth, for example, from rickets (Konje & Ladipo, 2000). It also can occur if the umbilical cord prolapses, if more than one fetus is present, or if the fetus is too large for or is malpositioned in the birth canal.

Prolapse of the Umbilical Cord

In **umbilical cord prolapse,** a loop of the umbilical cord slips down in front of the presenting fetal part (Fig. 21-5). Prolapse may occur at any time after the membranes rupture if the presenting part is not fitted firmly into the cervix. It tends to occur most often with the following conditions:

- Premature rupture of membranes
- Fetal presentation other than cephalic
- Placenta previa
- Intrauterine tumors preventing the presenting part from engaging
- A small fetus
- Cephalopelvic disproportion preventing firm engagement
- Hydramnios
- Multiple gestation

The incidence is 0.2 to 0.6% of births (Cruikshank, 2000).

Assessment

In rare instances, the cord may be felt as the presenting part on an initial vaginal examination during labor. It may be identified in this position on sonogram. In this event, cesarean birth will be necessary before rupture of the membranes occurs. Otherwise, with rupture, the cord will slide down into the vagina from the pressure exerted by the amniotic fluid. More often, however, cord prolapse is first discovered only after membranes have ruptured, when a variable deceleration FHR pattern suddenly becomes apparent. The cord may then be visible at the vulva.

To rule out cord prolapse, always assess fetal heart sounds immediately after rupture of the membranes occurring either spontaneously or by amniotomy.

Therapeutic Management

Cord prolapse automatically leads to cord compression, because the fetal presenting part presses against the cord at the pelvic brim. Management is aimed toward relieving pressure on the cord, thereby relieving the compression and the resulting fetal anoxia. This may be done by placing a gloved hand in the vagina and manually elevating the fetal head off the cord, or by placing the woman in a knee-chest or Trendelenburg position, which causes the fetal head to fall back from the cord. Administering oxygen at 10 L/min by facemask to the mother is also helpful to improve oxygenation to the fetus. A tocolytic agent may be used to reduce uterine activity and pressure on the fetus.

If the cord has prolapsed to the extent that it is exposed to room air, drying will begin, leading to atrophy of the

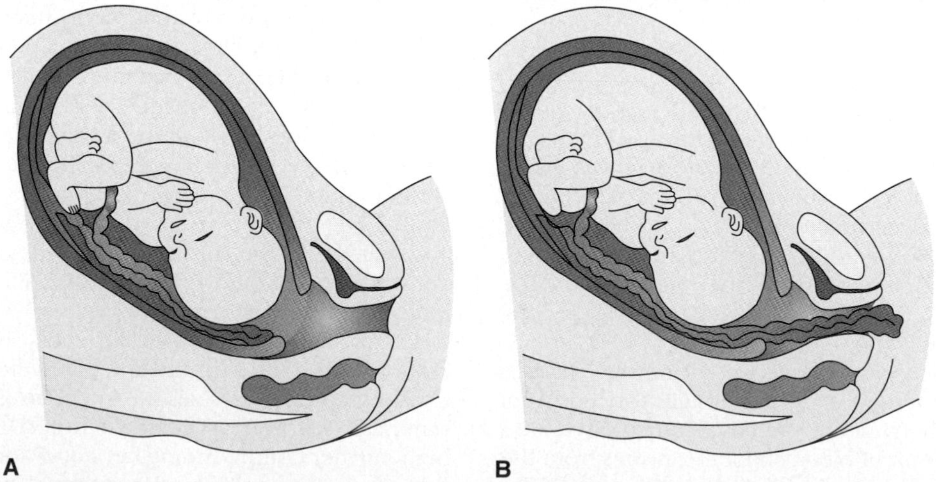

FIGURE 21.5 Prolapse of the umbilical cord. (*A*) The cord is prolapsed but still within the uterus. (*B*) The cord is visible at the vulva. In both instances the fetal nutrient supply is being compromised, although only a cord such as that shown in *B* would be visible. Both prolapses could be detected by fetal monitoring.

umbilical vessels. Do not attempt to push any exposed cord back into the vagina. This may add to the compression by causing knotting or kinking. Instead, cover any exposed portion with a sterile saline compress to prevent drying.

If the cervix is fully dilated at the time of the prolapse, the physician may choose to deliver the infant quickly, possibly with forceps, to prevent fetal anoxia. If dilatation is incomplete, the birth method of choice is upward pressure on the presenting part by a practitioner's hand in the woman's vagina to keep pressure off the cord until the baby can be delivered by cesarean birth.

Multiple Gestation

A woman with a multiple gestation usually causes a flurry of excitement in a birthing room. Additional personnel are needed for the birth (as many nurses to attend to possibly immature infants as there are infants, plus additional pediatricians or neonatal nurse practitioners). In the middle of all the preparatory activity, it is easy to forget that the woman may be more frightened than excited. Be sure to focus on her needs and those of the babies. Twins may be born by cesarean birth to decrease the risk that the second fetus will experience anoxia; this also is often the situation in multiple gestations of three or more because of the increased incidence of cord entanglement and premature separation of a placenta.

If a woman with a multiple gestation will be giving birth vaginally, she is usually instructed to come to the hospital early in labor. The first stage of labor will not differ greatly from that of a mother with a single-gestation pregnancy. Coming to a hospital this early in labor, however, will make labor seem long. Urge the woman to spend the early hours of labor engaged in an activity such as playing cards to make the time pass more quickly. Analgesia administration should be conservative so it will not compound any respiratory difficulties the infants may have at birth because of their immaturity. Support the woman's breathing exercises to minimize the need for analgesia or anesthesia. Multiple pregnancies often end before full term, so the woman may not yet have practiced breathing exercises. The early hours of labor can be used for this as well.

If possible, monitor each FHR by a separate fetal monitor during labor. Because the babies are usually small, firm head engagement may not occur, increasing the risk for cord prolapse after rupture of the membranes. Uterine dysfunction from a long labor, an overstretched uterus, and premature separation of the placenta after the birth of the first child may be more common. Because of the multiple fetuses, abnormal fetal presentation may occur. Anemia and hypertension of pregnancy occur at higher-than-usual incidences during multiple gestations. Be certain to assess the woman's hematocrit level and blood pressure closely during labor because of this. Box 21-2 highlights appropriate outcomes and interventions for a woman at risk for injury related to multiple gestation using the terminology of the Nursing Outcomes Classification (NOC) and Nursing Interventions Classification (NIC).

With a multiple gestation, the first fetus usually presents vertex. After the first infant is born, both ends of the baby's cord will be tied or clamped permanently rather than with cord clamps, which could slip. This will prevent hemorrhage through an open cord end if additional infants have shared the placenta. The first infant is identified as *A*, and newborn care is started for him or her. Oxytocin, usually given to immediately halt the uterus and minimize bleeding as an infant is born, will not be given to the woman to avoid compromising the circulation of the infants not yet born.

Most twin pregnancies present with both twins vertex. This is followed in frequency by vertex and breech,

BOX 21.2

NURSING OUTCOMES AND NURSING INTERVENTIONS CLASSIFICATION: MULTIPLE GESTATION

NOC: Maternal Status, Intrapartum

Maternal status, intrapartum is defined as the conditions and behaviors indicating maternal well-being from the initiation of labor through delivery (Johnson, Maas, & Moorhead, 2000). Some specific indicators suggesting achievement of this outcome include the following:

- Vital signs, neurologic status, and urine output are within expected range
- Frequency, duration, and intensity of uterine contractions are within expected range
- Cervical dilation is progressing as expected.
- Client demonstrates use of techniques to facilitate and cope with labor

NIC: Intrapartum Care, High-Risk Delivery

Intrapartum care, high-risk delivery is defined as assisting with the vaginal birth of multiple or malpositioned fetuses (McCloskey & Bulechek, 2000). Some important activities involved when implementing this intervention for the woman with multiple gestation include:

- Informing the client and her support person about the additional procedures and techniques that may be necessary during the delivery process.
- Preparing additional equipment and personnel for delivery
- Assisting with amniotomy, ultrasonography, forceps or vacuum extraction application as needed
- Recording the time of birth for the first neonate and any subsequent neonates delivered
- Assisting with neonatal resuscitation, if necessary.
- Explaining any newborn characteristics related to the high-risk birth, such as forcep marks or bruising
- Encouraging parental interaction with neonates immediately after delivery.

breech and vertex, and then breech and breech (Cunningham et al., 2001; Fig. 21-6). Multiple gestations of three or more have extremely varied presentations. After the birth of the first child, the lie of the second fetus is determined by external abdominal palpation and sonogram. If the presentation is not vertex, external version is attempted to make it so. If this is not successful, a decision for a breech delivery or cesarean birth will be made. If the infant will be born vaginally, an oxytocin infusion may be begun at this point to assist uterine contractions, thereby shortening the time span between births. Nitroglycerin may be administered to relax the uterus.

Occasionally, the placenta of the first infant separates before the second fetus is born, and there is sudden, profuse bleeding at the vagina. This creates a risk for the woman. The uterus cannot contract as it normally would, thereby halting the bleeding, because it is still filled with the additional fetus. If the separation of the first placenta caused loosening of the additional placentas, or if a common placenta is involved, the fetal heart sounds of the other fetuses will register distress immediately. They need to be born at once if they are to survive. This is why, with most multiple gestations today, if all of the fetuses are not vertex presentations, they will be delivered by cesarean birth (Spellacy, 2000).

Parents usually want to inspect multiple-gestation infants thoroughly after the birth. The time allowed for this inspection depends on the infants' weight and condition. Some parents worry that the hospital will confuse their infants through improper identification. Review with them the measures used to ensure correct identification.

Even though women have known for months that they are having multiple infants, many women have difficulty believing that this has really happened. They feel a need to recount over and over their surprise and to view all their infants together to prove to themselves that it is true. If parents are unable to inspect the infants thoroughly immediately after the birth because of the infants' low birth weight and the danger of chilling, they need the opportunity to do so as soon as possible to dispel any fears they had throughout pregnancy that the babies would be born less than perfect.

Assess the mother carefully in the immediate postpartal period because the overly distended uterus (due to the multiple gestation) may have more difficulty contracting than usual, placing her at risk for hemorrhage from uterine atony. In addition, the risk for uterine infection increases if labor or birth was prolonged. The infants need careful assessment to determine their true gestational age and

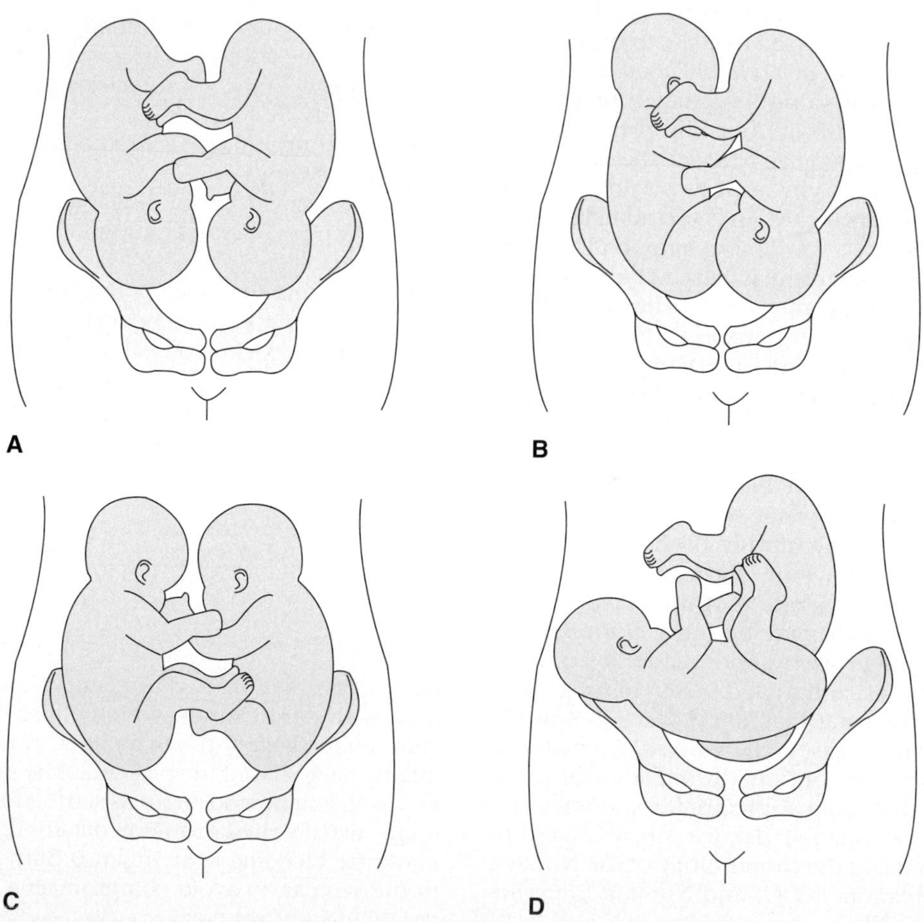

FIGURE 21.6 Four different twin presentations. (*A*) Both infants vertex. (*B*) One infant vertex and one breech. (*C*) Both infants breech. (*D*) One infant vertex and one in a transverse lie.

whether a phenomenon such as twin-to-twin transfusion has occurred (see Chapter 26).

✔ CHECKPOINT QUESTIONS

6. What is the best immediate action if a prolapsed cord is exposed to room air?
7. How do most twin fetuses usually present?

Problems With Position, Presentation, or Size

Occipitoposterior Position

In approximately one tenth of all labors, the fetal position is posterior rather than anterior. That is, the occiput (assuming the presentation is vertex) is directed diagonally and posteriorly, right occipitoposterior (ROP) or left occipitoposterior (LOP; Cunningham et al., 2001). In these positions, during internal rotation, the fetal head must rotate not through a 90-degree arc (Fig. 21-7) but through an arc of approximately 135 degrees (Fig. 21-8).

Posterior positions tend to occur in women with android, anthropoid, or contracted pelves. A posterior position is suggested by a dysfunctional labor pattern such as a prolonged active phase, arrested descent, or fetal heart sounds heard best at the lateral sides of the abdomen.

A posteriorly presenting head does not fit the cervix as snugly as one in an anterior position. Because this increases the risk of umbilical cord prolapse, the position of the fetus is confirmed on vaginal examination or by sonogram. The majority of fetuses presenting in posterior positions, if they are of average size and in good flexion and aided by forceful uterine contractions, will rotate through the large arc and arrive at a good birth position for the pelvic outlet, and will be born satisfactorily with only increased molding and caput formation. Because the arc of rotation is greater, it is usual for the labor to be somewhat prolonged. Because the fetal head rotates against the sacrum, the woman may experience pressure and pain in her lower back due to sacral nerve compression. These sensations may be so intense that she asks for medication for relief, not for her contractions but for the intense back pressure and pain. Pressure on the sacrum, such as with a back rub or a change of position, may be helpful in relieving a portion of the pain (Fig. 21-9). Applying heat or cold, whichever feels best, also may help. Lying on the side opposite the fetal back or maintaining a hands-and-knees position may help the fetus rotate. During a long labor, be certain that the woman voids approximately every 2 hours to keep the bladder empty, because a full bladder impedes descent of the fetus. Be aware how long it has been since she last ate. During a long labor, she may need intravenous glucose solutions to replace glucose stores used for energy.

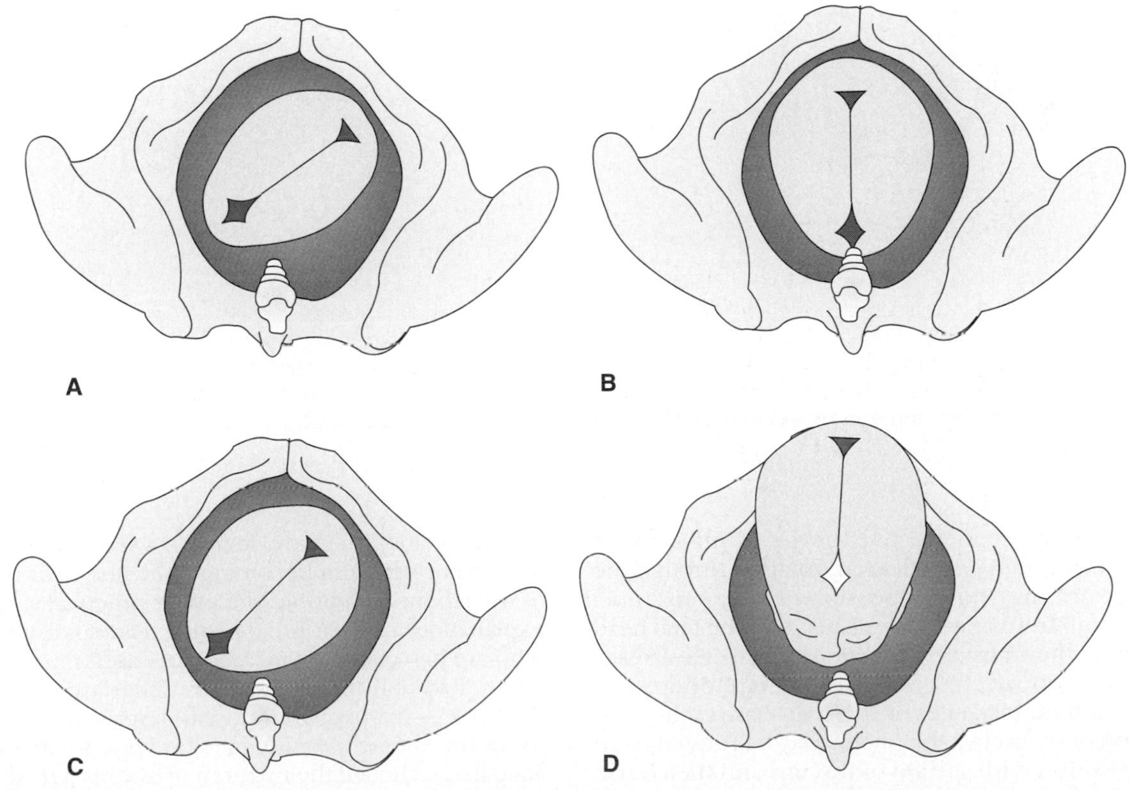

FIGURE 21.7 Left occipitoanterior (LOA) rotation. (*A*) A fetus in a cephalic presentation, LOA position. View is from the outlet. The fetus rotates 90 degrees from this position. (*B*) Descent and flexion. (*C*) Internal rotation complete. (*D*) Extension; the face and chin are born.

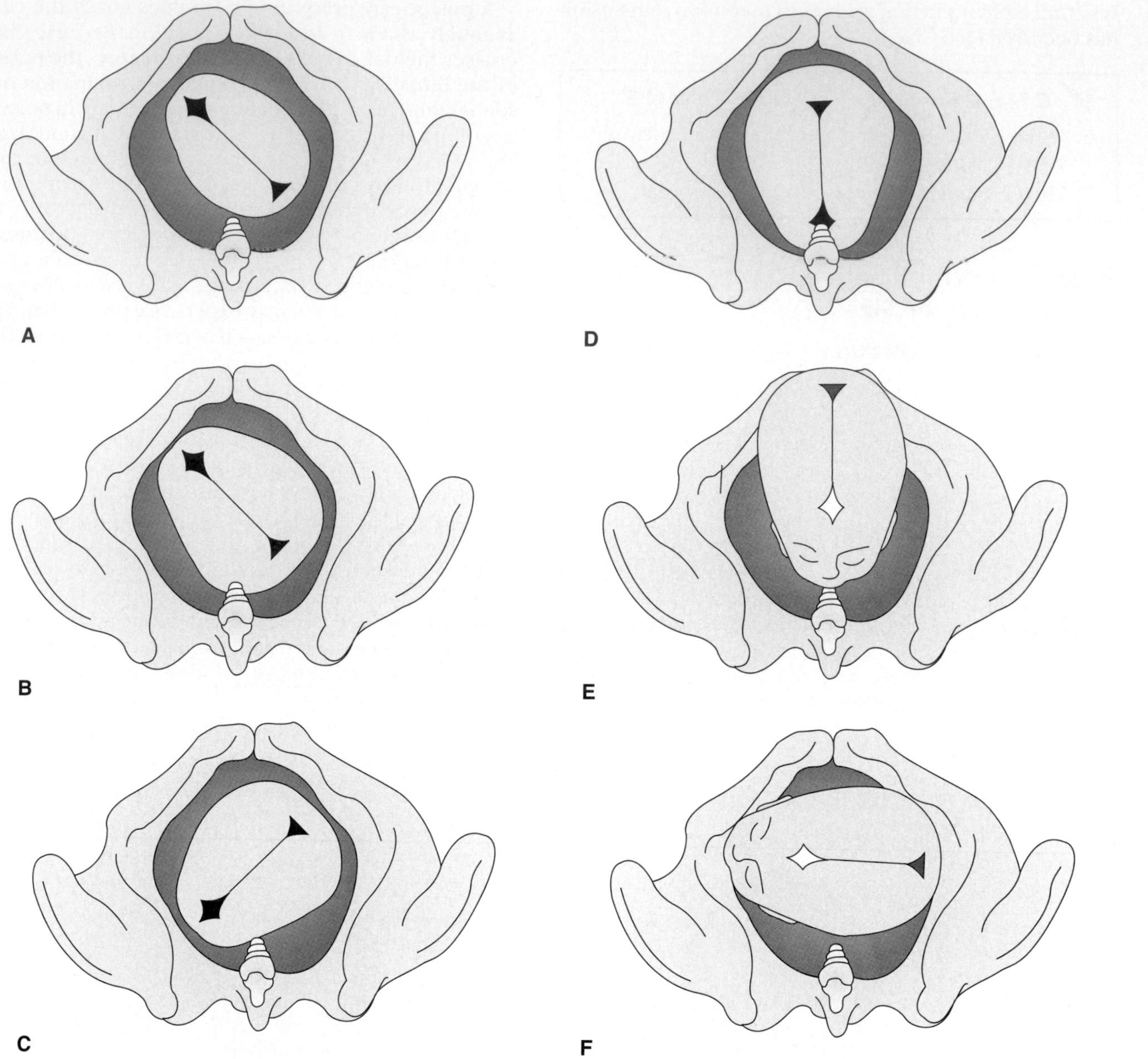

FIGURE 21.8 Left occipitoposterior (LOP) rotation. (*A*) Fetus in a cephalic presentation, LOP position. View is from outlet. The fetus rotates 135 degrees from this position. (*B*) Descent and flexion. (*C*) Internal rotation beginning. Because of the posterior position, the head will rotate in a longer arc than if it were in an anterior position. (*D*) Internal rotation complete. (*E*) Extension; the face and chin are born. (*F*) External rotation; the fetus rotates to place the shoulders in an anteroposterior position.

If contractions are ineffective, or the infant is above average size or not in good flexion, rotation through the 135-degree arc may not be possible. Uterine dysfunction may result from maternal exhaustion. The fetal head may arrest in the transverse position (transverse arrest). Rotation may not occur (persistent occipitoposterior position). In both instances, if the fetus has reached the midportion of the pelvis, he or she may be rotated to an anterior position with the aid of forceps and then born. Cesarean birth may be used instead, because the risk of a midforceps maneuver exceeds the risk of a cesarean birth.

During labor, the woman needs a great deal of support to prevent her from becoming panicked over the length of the labor. In addition, she needs practical step-by-step explanations of what is happening. Paradoxically, women who are best prepared for labor are often most frightened when deviations occur, because things are not going "by the book"—not happening just as described by the instructor of the course they attended. Provide frequent reassurance that, although their pattern of labor is not "textbook," it is within safe, controlled limits. If forceps are used for birth, the woman is at risk for reproductive tract lacerations, hemorrhage, and infection in the postpartum period.

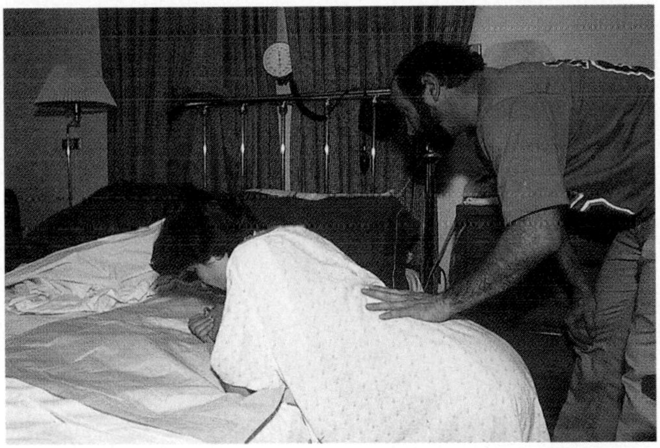

FIGURE 21.9 With a posterior fetal position, the woman may feel extensive back pressure. Pressure on her lower back by her support person may help relieve this problem.

Breech Presentation

Most fetuses are in a breech presentation early in pregnancy. However, by week 38 of gestation, the fetus normally turns to a cephalic presentation. Although the fetal head is the widest single diameter, the fetus's buttocks (breech), plus the lower extremities, actually take up more space. The fundus, being the largest part of the uterus, probably accounts for the fact that in approximately 97% of all pregnancies, the fetus turns so that the buttocks and lower extremities are in the fundus.

There are several types of breech presentations (see Chapter 18). Breech presentation may occur for any of the reasons shown in Box 21-3. Breech presentation is more hazardous than a cephalic presentation because there is a higher risk of the following:

- Anoxia from a prolapsed cord
- Traumatic injury to the aftercoming head (can result in intracranial hemorrhage or anoxia)
- Fracture of the spine or arm
- Dysfunctional labor

Early rupture of the membranes tends to occur because of the poor fit of the presenting part. The inevitable contraction of the fetal buttocks from cervical pressure often causes meconium to be extruded into the amniotic fluid before birth. This, unlike meconium staining that occurs from fetal anoxia, is not a sign of fetal distress but is expected from the buttock pressure. Such meconium excretion, however, can lead to meconium aspiration if the infant inhales amniotic fluid.

Assessment. With a breech presentation, the fetal heart sounds usually are heard high in the abdomen. Leopold's maneuvers, a vaginal examination, and ultrasound will reveal the presentation. If the breech is complete and firmly engaged, the tightly stretched gluteal muscles may be mistaken on vaginal examination for a head; the cleft between the buttocks may be mistaken for the sagittal suture line. Sonography confirms a breech presentation. Such a study also gives information on pelvic diameters, fetal skull diameters, and evidence of possible placenta previa.

In a breech birth, the same stages of flexion, descent, internal rotation, expulsion, and external rotation occur as in a vertex birth. Always monitor FHR and uterine contractions continuously if possible. This allows early detection of fetal distress from a complication, such as a prolapsed cord, and prompt intervention.

Birth Technique. If the infant will be born vaginally, when full dilatation is reached, the woman is allowed to push, and the breech, trunk, and shoulders are born (Fig. 21-10). As the breech spontaneously emerges from the birth canal, it is steadied and supported by a sterile towel held against the infant's inferior surface (Fig. 21-10*C*). The shoulders present to the outlet with their widest diameter anteroposterior. If they do not deliver readily, the arm of the posterior shoulder may be drawn down by passing two fingers over the infant's shoulder and down the arm to the elbow, then sweeping the flexed arm across the infant's face and chest and out. The other arm is delivered in the same way. External rotation is allowed to occur to bring the head into the best outlet diameter.

Birth of the head is the most hazardous part of a breech birth. Because the umbilicus precedes the head, a loop of cord passes down alongside the head. The pressure of the head against the pelvic brim will automatically compress this loop of cord.

A second danger of a breech birth is intracranial hemorrhage. With a cephalic presentation, molding to the confines of the birth canal occurs over hours. With a breech birth, pressure changes occur instantaneously. Tentorial tears, which can cause gross motor and mental incapacity

BOX 21.3

CAUSES OF BREECH PRESENTATION

- Gestational age under 40 weeks
- Abnormality in the fetus, such as anencephaly, hydrocephalus, or meningocele. (In a fetus with hydrocephalus, the widest fetal diameter is the head, and so it retains the most "comfortable" position.)
- Hydramnios that allows for free fetal movement, so that the fetus does not have to make a "most comfortable" choice
- Congenital anomaly of the uterus, such as midseptum, that traps the fetus in a breech position
- Any space-occupying mass in the pelvis, such as a fibroid tumor of the uterus or a placenta previa, that does not allow the head to present
- Pendulous abdomen. If the abdominal muscles are lax, the uterus may fall so far forward that the fetal head comes to lie outside the pelvic brim, causing a breech presentation.
- Multiple gestation. The presenting infant cannot turn to a vertex position.
- Unknown factors

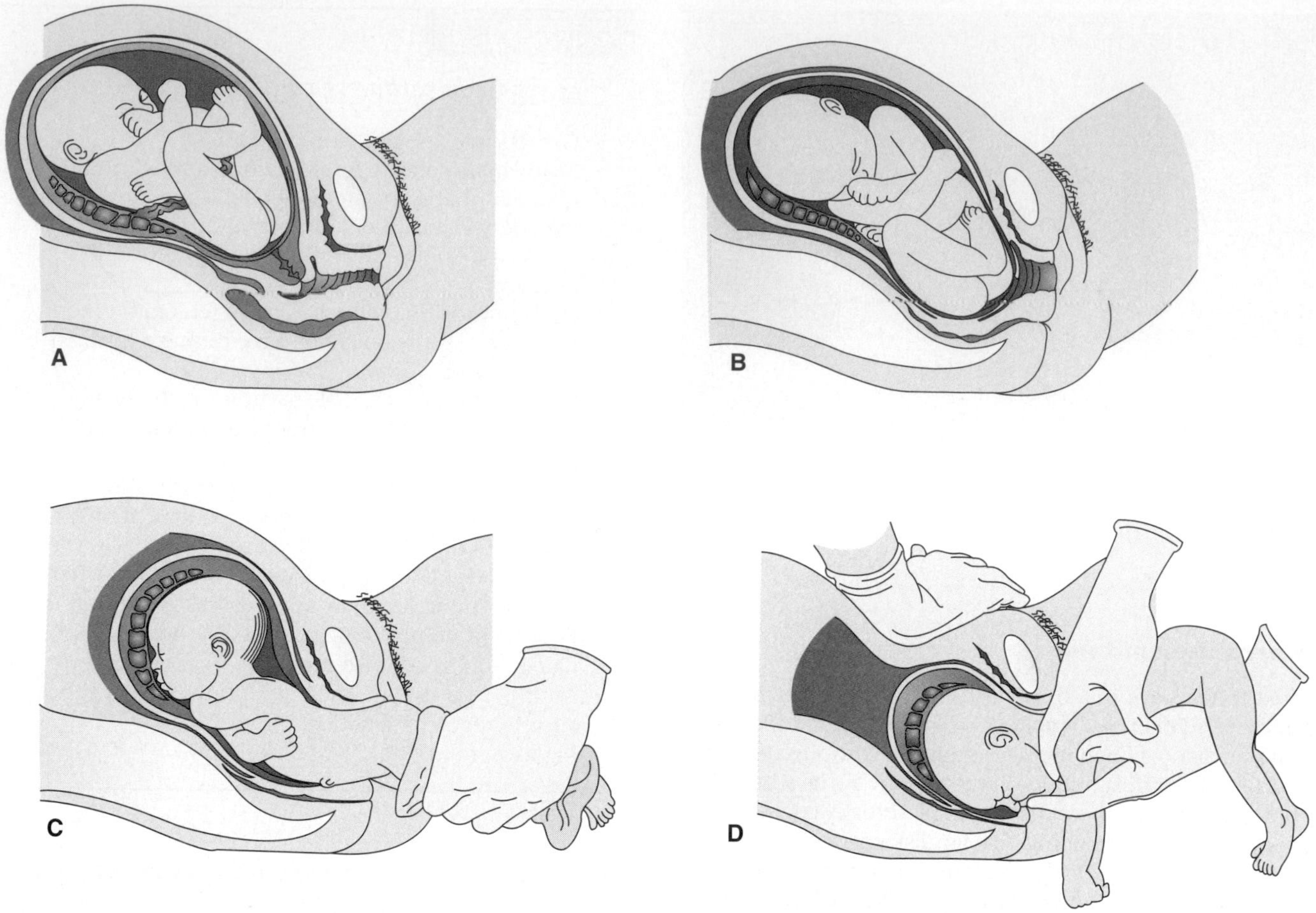

FIGURE 21.10 Breech birth. (*A*) Position before labor; left sacroposterior. (*B*) Descent and internal rotation. (*C*) Legs being born; the shoulders turn to present to the anteroposterior diameter. (*D*) The head is born. External rotation has put the anteroposterior diameter of the head in line with the anteroposterior diameter of the mother's pelvis. The head is delivered by gentle pressure to flex the head fully and by gentle traction to the shoulders upward and outward. Additional pressure might be applied by an assistant to the abdominal wall to ensure head flexion.

or lethal damage to the fetus, may result. The infant who is delivered suddenly to reduce the amount of time that the cord is compressed may therefore suffer an intracranial hemorrhage. In contrast, the infant who is delivered gradually to reduce the possibility of intracranial injury may suffer hypoxia. Thus, birth of an aftercoming head involves precise judgment and skill.

To aid in delivery of the head, the trunk of the infant is usually straddled over the physician's right forearm (Fig. 21-10*D*). Two fingers of the physician's right hand are placed in the infant's mouth. The left hand is slid into the mother's vagina, palm down, along the infant's back. Pressure is applied to the occiput to flex the head fully. Gentle traction applied to the shoulders (upward and outward) delivers the head. An aftercoming head may also be delivered by the aid of Piper forceps to control the flexion and rate of descent (Fig. 21-11).

Parents usually inspect a breech baby after the birth a little more closely than do the average parents. They, as well as the person who makes the initial physical assessment of the infant, are looking for the reason that made the presentation breech. An infant who was delivered in a frank breech position may tend to keep his or her legs extended and at the level of the face for the first 2 or 3 days of life. The infant who was a footling breech may tend to keep the legs extended in a footling position for the first few days. Be sure to point this out to the parents, so they do not misinterpret the strange posture of the infant.

Face Presentation

A fetal head presenting at a different angle than expected is termed *asynclitism.* Face and brow presentations are examples. Face (chin, or mentum) presentation is rare, but when it does occur, the diameter that the fetus presents to the pelvis is often too large for birth to proceed. A head that feels more prominent than normal with no engagement apparent on Leopold's maneuvers suggests a face presentation. It is also suggested when the head and back are both felt on the same side of the uterus with Leopold's maneuvers. The back is difficult to outline

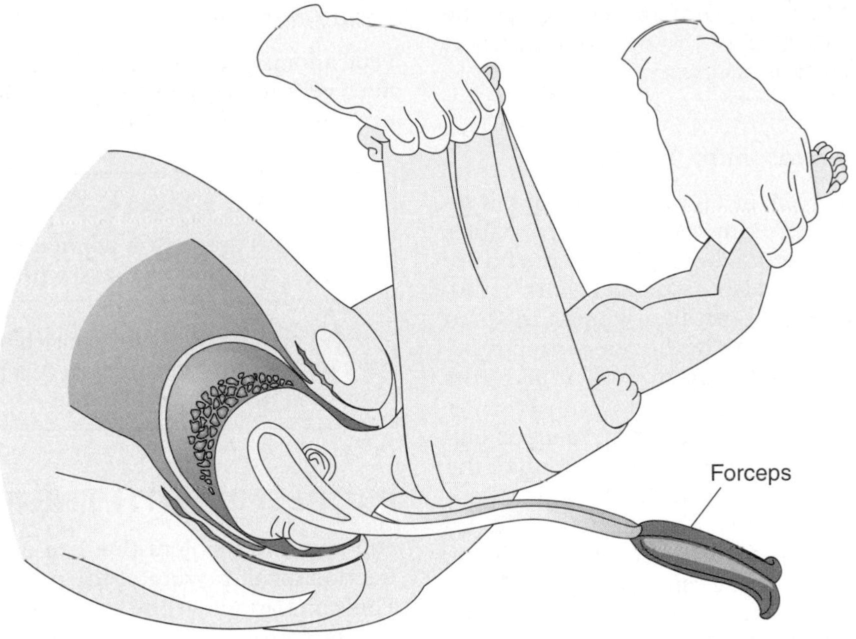

FIGURE 21.11 With Piper forceps used for a breech birth, traction is applied directly to the head, and damage to the infant's neck is avoided.

in this presentation because it is concave. If the back is extremely concave, fetal heart tones may be transmitted to the forward-thrust chest and heard on the side of the fetus where feet and arms can be palpated. A face presentation is confirmed by vaginal examination when the nose, mouth, or chin can be felt as the presenting part.

A fetus in a posterior position, instead of flexing the head as labor proceeds, may extend the head, resulting in a face (chin) presentation, usually occurring in a woman with a contracted pelvis or placenta previa. It also may occur in the relaxed uterus of a multipara, with prematurity, hydramnios, and fetal malformation. It is a warning signal. Something abnormal is causing the chin presentation.

When a face presentation is suspected, a sonogram is done to confirm it; if indicated, the pelvic diameters are measured. If the chin is anterior and the pelvic diameters are within normal limits, the infant may be delivered without difficulty (perhaps after a long first stage of labor, because the face does not mold well to make a snugly engaging part). If the chin is posterior, cesarean birth may be the choice of birth. Otherwise, it would be necessary to wait for a long posterior-to-anterior rotation to occur. Such rotation can result in uterine dysfunction or a transverse arrest.

Babies born after a chin presentation have a great deal of facial edema and may be purple from ecchymotic bruising. Lip edema may be so severe that the infant is unable to suck for a day or two. The infant may need gavage feedings to obtain enough fluid until he or she can suck effectively. The infant must be observed closely for a patent airway. Thus, for the first 24 hours, the infant usually is transferred to an intensive care nursery. The parents need to be assured that the edema is transient and will disappear in a few days, with no aftermath.

Brow Presentation

A brow presentation is the rarest of the presentations. It occurs with a multipara or a woman with relaxed abdominal muscles. It almost invariably results in obstructed labor, because the head becomes jammed in the brim of the pelvis as the occipitomental diameter presents. Unless the presentation spontaneously corrects, cesarean birth will be necessary to deliver the infant safely. Brow presentations also leave the infant with extreme ecchymotic bruising on the face. Upon seeing this bruising over the same area as the anterior fontanelle or "soft spot," parents may need additional reassurance that the child is well after birth.

Transverse Lie

Transverse lie occurs in women with pendulous abdomens, with uterine masses such as fibroid tumors that obstruct the lower uterine segment, with contraction of the pelvic brim, with congenital abnormalities of the uterus, or with hydramnios. It may occur in infants with hydrocephalus or other gross abnormalities that prevent the head from engaging. It may also occur in prematurity, when the infant has room for free movement, in multiple gestation (particularly in a second twin), or when there is a short umbilical cord.

A transverse lie is usually obvious on inspection, when the ovoid of the uterus is found to be more horizontal than vertical. The abnormal presentation can be detected by means of Leopold's maneuvers. A sonogram may be taken to confirm the abnormal lie and to give information such as pelvic size.

A mature fetus cannot be delivered vaginally from this presentation. Often, the membranes rupture at the beginning of labor. Because there is no firm presenting part, the cord or an arm may prolapse, or the shoulder obstructs the cervix. Cesarean birth is necessary.

Oversized Fetus (Macrosomia)

Size may become a problem in a fetus who weighs more than 4000 to 4500 g (approximately 9 to 10 lb). Babies of this size are most frequently born to women who are diabetic. Large babies are also associated with multiparity, because each infant born to a woman tends to be slightly heavier and larger than the one born just before. Macrosomia complicates up to 10% of all births (Zamorski & Biggs, 2001).

An oversized infant may cause uterine dysfunction during labor or at birth owing to the overstretching of the fibers of the myometrium. The wide shoulders may pose a problem at birth, because they cause fetal pelvic disproportion or even uterine rupture from obstruction. If the infant is so oversized that he or she cannot deliver vaginally, cesarean birth becomes the birth method of choice. The large size of the fetus may be missed in an obese woman because the fetal contours are difficult to palpate. Being obese does not mean that she has a larger-than-usual pelvis. Pelvimetry or sonography can be used to compare the fetal size with the woman's pelvic capacity.

The perinatal mortality of larger infants is substantially increased (15% versus the normal 4%). The large infant born vaginally has a higher-than-normal risk of cervical nerve palsy, diaphragmatic nerve injury, or fractured clavicle because of shoulder dystocia. Postpartally, the mother has an increased risk of hemorrhage because the overdistended uterus may not contract as readily (Cunningham et al., 2001).

Shoulder Dystocia

Shoulder dystocia is a delivery problem that is increasing in incidence along with the increasing average weight of infants. The problem occurs at the second stage of labor when the fetal head is born but the shoulders are too broad to enter and be delivered through the pelvic outlet. This is hazardous to the mother because it can result in vaginal or cervical tears. It is hazardous to the fetus because the cord is compressed between the fetal body and the bony pelvis, possibly resulting in a fractured clavicle or a brachial plexus injury.

Shoulder dystocia is most apt to occur in women with diabetes, in multiparas, and in post-date pregnancies. The problem is often not identified until the head has been born. Then the wide anterior shoulder locks beneath the symphysis pubis. The condition may be suspected earlier if the second stage of labor is prolonged, if there is arrest of descent, or if, when the head appears on the perineum (crowning), it retracts instead of protruding with each contraction (a turtle sign).

Asking the woman to flex her thighs sharply on her abdomen (McRobert's maneuver) widens the pelvic outlet and may let the anterior shoulder deliver (Gherman et al., 2000). Applying suprapubic pressure may help the shoulder escape from beneath the symphysis pubis.

Fetal Anomalies

Fetal anomalies of the head such as hydrocephalus (fluid-filled ventricles) or anencephaly (absence of the cranium) can also complicate birth (see Chapter 39).

> ✔ **CHECKPOINT QUESTIONS**
>
> 8. What is the reason women experience lower back pain and pressure with an occipito-posterior position?
> 9. Which fetus is most apt to have shoulder dystocia—a term female of a primipara or a post-term male of a multipara?

PROBLEMS WITH THE PASSAGE

Still another problem that can cause dystocia is a contraction or narrowing of the passageway or birth canal. This can happen at the inlet, the midpelvis, or the outlet. The narrowing causes CPD, or a disproportion between the size of the normal fetal head and the pelvic diameters. This results in failure to progress in labor.

Inlet Contraction

Inlet contraction, narrowing of the anteroposterior diameter to less than 11 cm, or a maximum transverse diameter of 12 cm or less, is ordinarily due to rickets in early life or an inherited small pelvis. In primigravidas, the fetal head normally engages at weeks 36 to 38 of pregnancy. When this event occurs before labor begins, it is proof that the pelvic inlet is adequate. Following the general rule that "what goes in, comes out," a head that engages or proves it fits into the pelvic brim will probably also be able to pass through the midpelvis and through the outlet.

When engagement does not occur in a primigravida, then either a fetal abnormality (larger-than-usual head) or a pelvic abnormality (smaller-than-usual pelvis) should be suspected. As a rule, engagement does not occur in multigravidas until labor begins. Previous birth of a full-term infant vaginally without problems is proof that the birth canal is adequate.

Every primigravida should have pelvic measurements taken and recorded before week 24 of pregnancy. Based on these measurements and the assumption that the fetus will be of average size, a birth decision can then be made.

With CPD, because the fetus does not engage but remains "floating," malposition may occur, further complicating an already difficult situation. Should membranes rupture, the possibility of cord prolapse increases greatly.

Outlet Contraction

Outlet contraction is defined as the narrowing of the transverse diameter at the outlet to less than 11 cm. This is the distance between the ischial tuberosities, a measurement that is easy to make during a prenatal visit and thus can be anticipated before labor begins. It is also easily done during labor (see Chapter 18).

Trial Labor

If a woman has a borderline (just adequate) inlet measurement, and the fetal lie and position are good, her physician or nurse-midwife may allow her a "trial" labor to determine whether labor can progress normally. A trial labor continues as long as descent of the presenting part and dilatation of the cervix are occurring. Monitor fetal heart sounds and uterine contractions continuously if possible. Be sure that the woman's urinary bladder is kept as empty as possible to allow the fetal head to use all the space available. Urge her to void every 2 hours. After rupture of the membranes, assess FHR carefully, because if the fetal head is still high, there is an increased danger of prolapsed cord and anoxia in the fetus. If after a definite period (6 to 12 hours) adequate progress in labor cannot be documented or at any time fetal distress occurs, the woman will be scheduled for a cesarean birth.

It may be difficult for women to undertake a labor they know they may be unable to complete because they believe they are being needlessly subjected to pain. Emphasize, but do not overstress, that it is best for the baby to be born vaginally. If the trial labor fails and cesarean birth is scheduled, provide an explanation about why a cesarean birth is necessary and now best for the baby (see Focus on Communication).

Some women having a trial labor feel as if they themselves are on trial. When dilatation does not occur, they feel discouraged and inadequate, as if they are somehow at fault. A woman may not be aware how much she wanted the trial labor to work until she is told that it is not working. The support person also may be as frightened and feel as helpless as the woman when a deviation occurs in labor. The couple needs assurance from health care personnel that a cesarean birth is an alternative, not inferior, method of birth. In this instance, it is the method of choice, allowing them to achieve their goal of a healthy mother and a healthy child.

External Cephalic Version

External cephalic version is the turning of a fetus from a breech to a cephalic position before birth (Cunningham et al., 2001). For the procedure, FHR and possibly ultrasound should be recorded continuously. A tocolytic agent may be administered to help relax the uterus. The breech and vertex of the fetus are located and grasped transabdominally by an examiner's hands on the woman's abdomen. Gentle pressure is then exerted to rotate the fetus in a forward direction to a cephalic lie (Fig. 21-12). The use of external version can decrease the number of cesarean births necessary from breech presentations. Contraindications to the procedure include multiple gestation, severe oligohydramnios, contraindications to vaginal birth, a cord that wraps around the neck, and unexplained third-trimester bleeding, which might be a placenta previa. External version may be uncomfortable because of the feeling of pressure. Therefore, the woman needs support to tolerate this. Women who are Rh negative should receive Rh immunoglobulin in case minimal bleeding occurs.

FOCUS ON COMMUNICATION

Marilee Olsen is a 30-year-old woman having her first baby. Her physician told her she has a small pelvis and so she may not be able to deliver vaginally.

Less Effective Communication

Nurse: Hello, Mrs. Olsen. Is it all right if I attach a fetal heart rate and uterine contraction monitor so we can observe you closely during labor?
Ms. Olsen: Sure. Although I don't intend to be in labor long. I'm going to do this quick.
Nurse: Has your doctor talked to you about the fact that you have a pelvis a little smaller than some women?
Ms. Olsen: Sure. But it hasn't interfered with anything during my pregnancy.
Nurse: I'm glad you have a positive outlook. That always makes labor seem to go faster.

More Effective Communication

Nurse: Hello, Mrs. Olsen. Is it all right if I attach a fetal heart rate and uterine contraction monitor so we can observe you closely during labor?
Ms. Olsen: Sure. Although I don't intend to be in labor long. I'm going to do this quick.
Nurse: Has your doctor talked to you about the fact that you have a pelvis a little smaller than some women?
Ms. Olsen: Sure. But it hasn't interfered with anything during my pregnancy.
Nurse: Did she explain that a small pelvis doesn't mean there is a problem during pregnancy? That the problem often occurs during labor?
Ms. Olsen: She said labor would be a trial.
Nurse: Let's talk about what that means.

When a woman develops a complication of pregnancy that is referred to by a strange name, it is almost expected that a couple will not understand the term and will need it thoroughly explained. When a condition has a common name such as protracted pelvis or trial labor, however, it is easy to assume that the condition doesn't need much explanation because the term will be clear to them. In reality, couples need explanations about all conditions because what is common to health care personnel is not common to everyone. In the first scenario, the nurse assumed she and the client were talking about the same thing. In the second scenario, the nurse explored a little further and discovered the client was assuming that the problem was resolved when it actually had just begun.

✔ CHECKPOINT QUESTIONS

10. What two conditions usually cause inlet contraction?
11. What external procedure can be used to turn a fetus from a breech to a cephalic position?

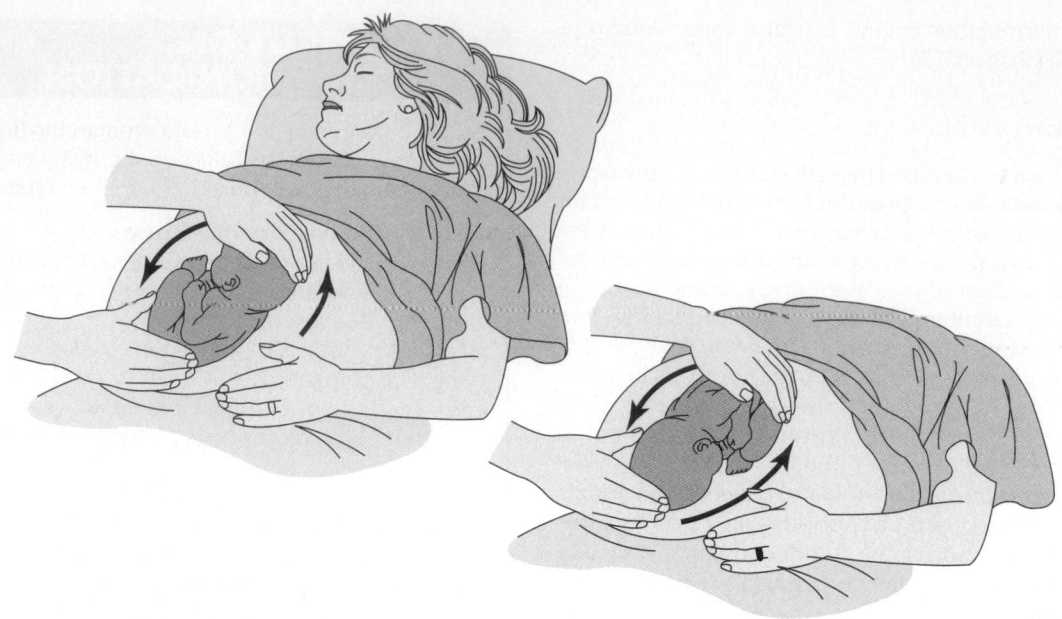

FIGURE 21.12 External cephalic version. The fetus is rotated by external pressure to a cephalic lie.

THERAPEUTIC MANAGEMENT OF PROBLEMS OR POTENTIAL PROBLEMS IN LABOR AND BIRTH

When labor contractions are ineffective, several interventions, such as induction and augmentation of labor with oxytocin or *amniotomy* (artificial rupture of the membranes), may be initiated to strengthen them. Because amniotomy is also used in uncomplicated labor, it is discussed in Chapter 18.

Induction and Augmentation of Labor

Induction of labor means that labor is artificially started. **Augmentation of labor** refers to assisting labor that has started spontaneously to be more effective. It may be necessary to initiate labor before the time when it would have occurred spontaneously because a fetus is in danger or because labor does not occur spontaneously and the fetus appears to be at term. The primary reasons for inducing labor include the presence of preeclampsia, eclampsia, severe hypertension or diabetes, Rh sensitization, prolonged rupture of the membranes, intrauterine growth restriction, and postmaturity (a pregnancy lasting beyond 42 weeks)—all situations that increase the risk for the fetus to remain in utero. Augmentation of labor or assistance to make uterine contractions stronger may be necessary when contractions are hypotonic or too weak or infrequent to be effective.

Because the procedure carries a risk of uterine rupture, a decrease in the fetal blood supply from poor cotyledon filling, and premature separation of the placenta, it is used cautiously with multiple gestation, hydramnios, grand parity, maternal age older than 40 years of age, and the presence of previous uterine scars.

Before induction of labor is begun, the following conditions must be present:

- The fetus is in a longitudinal lie.
- The cervix is ripe, or ready for birth.
- A presenting part is engaged.
- There is no cephalopelvic disproportion.
- The fetus is estimated to be mature by date, demonstrated by a lecithin–sphingomyelin ratio or sonogram biparietal diameter to rule out preterm birth.

Cervical Ripening

Cervical ripening, or a change in the cervical consistency from firm to soft, is the first step the uterus must complete in early labor. Such softness is necessary for dilatation and coordination of uterine contractions. To determine whether a cervix is "ripe," or ready for dilation, Bishop (1964) established criteria for scoring (Table 21-3). Using

TABLE 21.3 Scoring of Cervix for Readiness for Elective Induction

SCORING FACTOR	SCORE 0	1	2	3
Dilation (cm)	0	1–2	3–4	3–4
Effacement (%)	0–30	40–50	60–70	80
Station	−3	−2	−1–0	+1–+2
Consistency	Firm	Medium	Soft	
Position	Posterior	Mid position	Anterior	

Adapted with permission from Bishop, E. H. (1964). Pelvic scoring for elective induction. *Obstetrics and Gynecology, 24,* 266.

this scale, if a woman's total score is eight or more, the cervix is considered ready for birth and should respond to induction. To "ripen" a cervix, various methods can be instituted. One is "stripping the membranes" or separating the membranes from the lower uterine segment. This is an easy office visit procedure. Possible complications of this mechanical method include bleeding from an undetected low-lying placenta, inadvertent rupture of membranes, and the introduction of infection if membranes should rupture. Hygroscopic suppositories (suppositories of seaweed that swell on contact with cervical secretions) can be inserted to gradually and gently urge dilation (laminaria technique). These are held in place by gauze sponges saturated with povidone-iodine or an antifungal cream. Documenting how many dilators and sponges were placed is important so it can be documented afterward that none remain.

A commonly used method of speeding cervical ripening is the application of a prostaglandin gel to the interior surface of the cervix by a catheter or suppository, or the external surface by applying it to a diaphragm and then placing the diaphragm against the cervix (Sanchez-Ramos et al., 2002). Additional doses may be applied every 6 hours. Two or three doses are usually adequate to cause ripening. Women should remain flat to prevent leakage of the medication, and FHR should be monitored continuously for at least 30 minutes after each application, perhaps up to 2 hours after vaginal insertion. Side effects are vomiting, fever, diarrhea, and hypertension, so these should be observed. Oxytocin induction can be started 6 to 12 hours after the last prostaglandin dose (beginning it sooner might lead to hyperstimulation of the uterus [Karch, 2001]).

Prostaglandins should be used with caution in women with asthma, renal or cardiovascular disease, or glaucoma (Focus on Pharmacology: Misoprostol).

FOCUS ON PHARMACOLOGY

Misoprostol (Cytotec)

Action: Misoprostol is a synthetic prostaglandin (PGE1 analog) that produces cervical dilation.

Pregnancy Risk Category: X

Dosage: 50 to 100 μg orally or 25 to 50 μg placed intravaginally in the posterior fornix.

Possible Adverse Effects: Uterine hyperstimulation, nonreassuring fetal heart rate pattern, nausea, diarrhea, flatulence, headache.

Nursing Implications

- Keep in mind that this drug has not received approval from the federal Food and Drug Administration (FDA) for use as a cervical ripening agent and that cervical dilation is identified as an unlabeled use for this drug.
- Ensure that the woman is rated safe for cervical dilation and vaginal birth (such as absence of placenta previa, and cephalopelvic disproportion, mature fetus) before administration.
- Anticipate the need for a nonstress test to ensure fetal health before drug is used.
- Continuously monitor uterine activity and fetal heart rate.
- Have an intravenous fluid line and terbutaline readily available should uterine hyperstimulation occur (Wilson, 2000).

Induction of Labor by Oxytocin

Administration of **oxytocin,** a synthetic form of the naturally occurring pituitary hormone, initiates contractions in a uterus at pregnancy term. Oxytocin is administered intravenously so its effect can be quickly discontinued to avoid hyperstimulation. The half-life of oxytocin is approximately 3 minutes; thus, with intravenous administration, the serum level and effects will end hyperstimulation quickly.

Induction is begun by the dilute administration of an intravenous form of oxytocin, such as Pitocin or Syntocinon. The drug is traditionally mixed in the proportion of 10 IU in 1000 mL of Ringer's lactate. Ten IU of oxytocin is the same as 10,000 milliunits (mU), so each milliliter of this solution will contain 10 mU of oxytocin. An alternative dilution method is to add 15 IU of oxytocin to 250 mL of an intravenous solution. This yields a concentration of 60 mU/1 mL. Physician's orders for administration of oxytocin for induction generally designate the number of milliunits to be administered per minute. Be sure to know the dilution used and recognize the concentration in each milliliter (see Focus on Pharmacology: Oxytocin for Labor Induction).

When administering the infusion, "piggyback" the oxytocin solution with a maintenance intravenous solution such as 5% dextrose and water. Then, if the oxytocin needs to be discontinued quickly during the induction, the main intravenous line will be maintained. Always use the infusion port closest to the client. This way, if it is stopped, little remains in the tubing. Using an infusion pump helps control the infusion rate, ensuring a uniform rate even when the woman changes position. A physician should be immediately available during the entire procedure to ensure safety. Box 21-4 highlights an appropriate outcome and intervention for the woman at risk for injury related to induction with oxytocin using the terminology from the Nursing Outcomes Classification and Nursing Interventions Classification.

Infusions are usually begun at a rate of 0.5 mU/min to 1 mU/min. If there is no response from this, the infusion is gradually increased in amount every 15 minutes to 60 minutes by small increments of 1 to 2 mU until contractions begin (ACOG, 1995). Many women respond with as little as 4 mU/min; most women respond at 16 mU/min. An administration rate of more than this will likely cause tetanic contractions. The rate should not be increased to more than 20 mU/min without checking for further instructions. Aggressive induction (an increment of 6 mU/min instead of the usual 1 to 2 mU/min) has been suggested as a way to shorten labor, and may be used in some research facilities. When cervical dilatation reaches 4 cm, artificial rupture of the membranes may be performed to further induce labor, and the infusion may be discontinued at that point. For some women, the infusion will be continued through full dilatation (Rouse et al., 2000).

FOCUS ON PHARMACOLOGY

Oxytocin for Labor Induction

Action: Oxytocin is a synthetic form of the naturally occurring posterior pituitary hormone used to initiate uterine contractions in a term pregnancy.

Pregnancy Risk Category: C

Dosage: Initially 1 to 2 mU/min by IV infusion increased at a rate no more than 1 to 2 U/min at 15- to 30-minute intervals until a contraction pattern similar to normal labor is achieved.

Possible Adverse Effects: Nausea, vomiting, cardiac arrhythmias, uterine hypertonicity, tetanic contractions, uterine rupture (with excessive dosages), severe water intoxication, and fetal bradycardia

Nursing Implications

- Prepare IV solution by adding 1 mL (10 IU) to 1000 mL of 0.9% aqueous sodium chloride or other IV fluid (resulting solution contains 10 mU/mL).
- Use an infusion pump to ensure accurate control of rate.
- Regulate infusion rate to establish uterine contractions similar to a normal labor pattern.
- Monitor frequency, duration, and strength of contractions.
- Assess maternal pulse and blood pressure, and watch for possible hypertension. If hypertension occurs, discontinue the drug and notify the physician.
- Continuously monitor fetal heart rate for signs of fetal distress.
- Monitor intake and output and watch for signs of possible water intoxication, such as headache, vomiting. Limit IV fluids to 150 mL/h.
- Prepare client for birth (Karch, 2001)

BOX 21.4

NURSING OUTCOMES AND NURSING INTERVENTIONS CLASSIFICATION: INDUCTION WITH OXYTOCIN

NOC: Maternal Status, Intrapartum

Maternal status, intrapartum is defined as conditions and behaviors indicating maternal well being from the onset of labor to delivery (Johnson, Maas, & Moorhead, 2000). Some specific indicators suggesting achievement of this outcome include the following:

- Blood pressure, pulse rate, and urine output remain within expected ranges
- Intensity, frequency, and duration of uterine contractions do not deviate from expected findings
- Cervical dilation progresses as expected
- No complaints of headache are reported by the client

NIC: Labor induction

Labor induction is defined as the initiation or augmentation of labor by mechanical or pharmacological methods (McCloskey & Bulechek, 2000). Some important activities involved when implementing this intervention include:

- Monitoring maternal and fetal vital signs before induction
- Initiating IV medication to stimulate uterine activity after physician consultation
- Observing for onset or change in uterine activity
- Monitoring labor progress, closely observing for signs of abnormal labor progress
- Avoiding uterine hyperstimulation by infusing oxytocin to achieve adequate contraction, frequency, duration, and relaxation
- Monitoring for signs of uteroplacental insufficiency during the process of induction
- Reducing or increasing oxytocin as per protocol until birth is imminent.

Continuously monitor FHR and uterine contractions during the procedure (see Assessing the Pregnant Woman for Danger Signs of Oxytocin Administration). Peripheral vessel dilatation, a side effect of oxytocin, may cause extreme hypotension. Excessive stimulation of the uterus by oxytocin may lead to tonic uterine contractions with fetal death or, in extreme instances, rupture of the uterus. The woman's pulse and blood pressure should be taken every 15 minutes. Contractions should occur no more than every 2 minutes, should not be stronger than 50 mm Hg pressure, and should last no longer than 70 seconds. The resting pressure between contractions should not exceed 15 mm Hg by monitor (Fig. 21-13). If contractions become more frequent or longer in duration than these safe limits, or if signs of fetal distress occur, stop the intravenous infusion and seek help immediately. Anticipate the need for oxygen administration, if necessary. It is better for contractions to slow from a period of inadequate oxytocin administration because the infusion was stopped unnecessarily than for tonic contractions to continue. Because of the short half-life of oxytocin, stopping the flow rate almost immediately stops the oxytocin effect. If this is not effective, a beta-adrenergic receptor drug such as terbutaline sulfate (Brethine) may be ordered to decrease myometrial activity.

Oxytocin has an antidiuretic effect resulting in decreased urine flow, possibly leading to water intoxication. Water intoxication is first manifested by headache and vomiting. If these danger signs are observed in the woman during induction of labor, they should be reported immediately and the infusion should be discontinued. Water intoxication in its severest form can lead to seizures, coma, and death because it causes a shift in interstitial tissue fluid. Keep an accurate intake and output record, and test and record urine specific gravity to detect discrepancies in the pattern. Limit the amount of intravenous fluid being given to 150 mL/h by ensuring that the main intravenous fluid line is infusing at a rate not more than 2.5 mL/min.

Women may have heard that induced labor is more painful or "so different" from normal labor that breathing exercises are worthless, or that it goes so fast it will be harmful to the fetus (see Focus on Family Empowerment).

ASSESSING the Pregnant Woman for Danger Signs of Oxytocin Administration

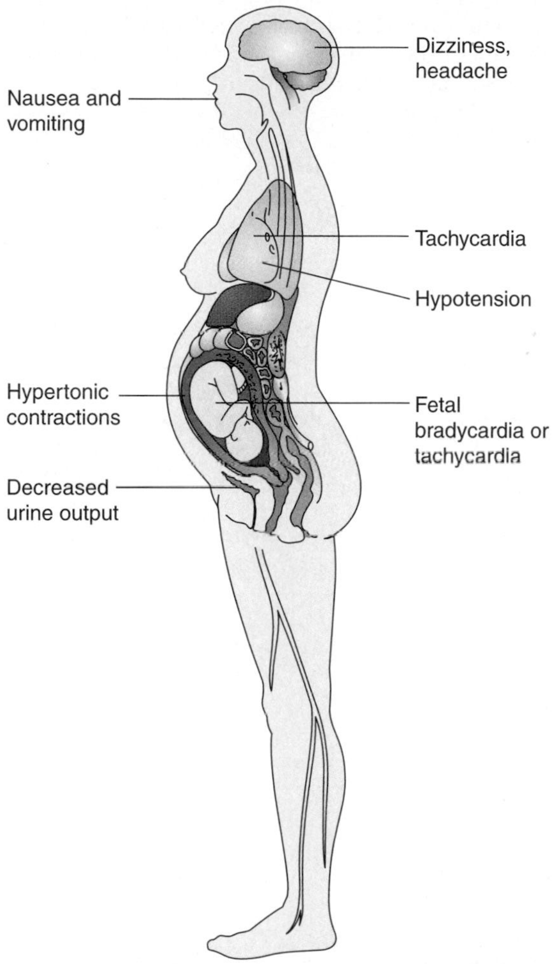

Induced labors do tend to have a slightly shorter first stage than the average unassisted labor. This is an advantage to the woman, however, not a disadvantage. Once contractions begin by this method, they are basically normal uterine contractions. The woman can be assured of this so that she does not fight the contractions or become unnecessarily tense, which would prevent her from using her breathing techniques effectively. Induction of labor with oxytocin may predispose the newborn to hyperbilirubinemia and jaundice. Observe the infant closely for this in the first few days of life.

Augmentation by Oxytocin

Augmentation of labor is required when labor contractions begin spontaneously but then become so weak, irregular, or ineffective (hypotonic) that assistance is needed to strengthen them (see Focus on Nursing Care Planning).

Precautions regarding oxytocin augmentation are the same as for its use for primary induction of labor. A uterus may be very responsive or respond very effectively to oxytocin when it is used as augmentation. Be certain that the drug is increased in small increments only, and that fetal heart sounds are well monitored during the procedure.

Active Management of Labor

A technique of active management of labor began in Europe and has spread to some centers in the United States. It includes the aggressive administration of oxytocin (increases of 6 mU/min rather than 1 or 2 mU to shorten labor to 12 hours and hopefully reduce the incidence of cesarean birth and postpartal infection (Dudley, 2000). The maximum dosage of oxytocin used may be as high as 36 to 40 mU/min. Active management is controversial because it violates the tradition of birth as a normal, procedure-free process. Because it can shorten labor, it has the potential to reduce the number of postpartal fevers that occur.

Forceps Birth

At one time, babies were routinely delivered with forceps. Today, forceps are rarely used because they may lead to increased urinary stress incontinence in women (Van

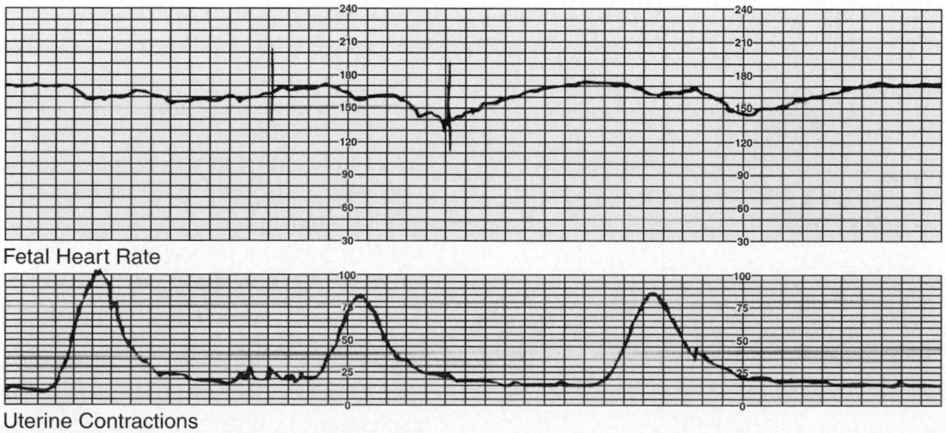

FIGURE 21.13 Hypertonic uterine contractions caused by an oxytocin infusion. Contractions are as high as 100 mm Hg in intensity. Late decelerations and an FHR of 170 bpm baseline are present.

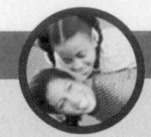

FOCUS ON FAMILY EMPOWERMENT
Understanding Augmentation of Labor

Q. My doctor mentioned something about helping my labor along. What does she mean?

A. Augmentation of labor is used when labor contractions are ineffective. It can shorten labor and avoid the necessity of cesarean birth. The drug used is oxytocin, a synthetic form of the hormone naturally released by your body during labor. It is administered intravenously. Once labor contractions begin by this method, they are the same as naturally occurring contractions. You will be able to use your prepared breathing exercises with them.

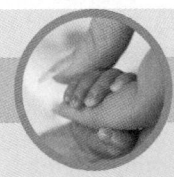

FOCUS ON *Nursing Care Planning*
A WOMAN EXPERIENCING DYSFUNCTIONAL LABOR

A 33-year-old multipara has been in labor for the past 13 hours. Her partner states, "Why is it taking so long?" The client asks, "Is the baby okay?" The primary health care provider orders an oxytocin infusion to assist with contractions.

Assessment: Client G5P3 in latent stage of labor. Membranes artificially ruptured approximately 1 hour ago. Cervix dilated 4 cm, 80% effaced. Internal electronic fetal monitoring in place. Contractions every 3 minutes, with peak strength at 20–25 mm Hg and a duration of 10 seconds. FHR at 130 to 140 beats per minute with beat-to-beat variability present. Client and partner visibly apprehensive, watching monitor intensely.

Client vital signs within acceptable parameters. Ringer's lactate intravenous solution infusing at 150 mL/hour via infusion pump. Client NPO, asking for something to eat "to keep up strength." Pelvic ultrasound reveals no difficulty with fetal presentation or position. Oxytocin ordered at 1 mU/min; increase 1 mU/min at 15-min intervals.

Nursing Diagnosis: Risk for injury (maternal and fetal) related to prolonged labor with ineffective contractions and use of oxytocin

Outcome Identification: Client will deliver healthy newborn vaginally without further problems or complications.

Outcome Evaluation: Client's vital signs within acceptable parameters; FHR and fetal heart patterns within acceptable limits; contractions increase after oxytocin administration without becoming hypertonic; labor progresses without signs and symptoms of maternal or fetal distress.

Interventions	Rationale
1. Assess vital signs, fetal heart rate and pattern, and contractions. Explain all procedures, equipment, and treatments to be used.	1. Assessment provides a baseline for future comparisons. Explanation helps to allay the couple's anxiety, helping them to view these items as an aid to a positive outcome.
2. Administer intravenous fluids as ordered. Use an infusion pump.	2. Intravenous fluid replacement helps to prevent possible dehydration secondary to prolonged labor. An infusion pump ensures an accurate flow rate and decreases the risk of possible fluid overload.
3. Maintain client's NPO status.	3. Withholding food and fluids minimizes the risk for aspiration should anesthesia be necessary.

(continued)

Interventions	Rationale
4. Encourage the client to lie on her side as much as possible.	4. A side-lying position enhances placental perfusion.
5. Begin intravenous oxytocin administration as ordered using an infusion control device. Administer it as a secondary infusion piggybacked into a port of the main intravenous solution that is closest to the client.	5. Oxytocin stimulates uterine contractions. Piggybacking the solution with an infusion control device allows for accurate dosing. Should an emergency arise, the infusion can be stopped immediately.
6. Assess FHR, maternal vital signs, and contractions every 15 minutes during infusion. Manually palpate the uterine fundus between contractions and evaluate peak strength of contractions via internal electronic monitoring.	6. Continued close monitoring provides evidence of maternal and fetal well being. Manual palpation and evaluation of peak strength provide information about uterine resting tone, which, if increased, can impair placental perfusion. Manual palpation also provides evidence of possible pathologic retraction ring, an obstetric emergency.
7. Gradually increase the oxytocin infusion at a rate of 1 mU/min every 15 minutes as ordered.	7. Gradual dosage increases continue to stimulate uterine contractions while minimizing the risk for possible oxytocin toxicity.
8. Notify the maternal health care provider if the client's blood pressure is more than 150/90; resting contraction pressure is more than 15 mm Hg or frequency is more than 2 every 2 minutes; FHR less than 120 or more than 160 beats per minute; or late deceleration occurs. Stop the oxytocin infusion immediately.	8. Oxytocin toxicity can lead to hypertonic uterine contractions with possible fetal death and uterine rupture. Oxytocin has a short half-life. Stopping the infusion halts the effect of oxytocin almost immediately.
9. Anticipate the need for administering oxygen and a beta 2 receptor agent, such as terbutaline.	9. Supplemental oxygen improves the maternal supply of oxygen to the fetus. Terbutaline decreases myometrial activity, reducing hypertonic uterine contractions.

Nursing Diagnosis: Risk for excess fluid volume related to oxytocin administration

Outcome Identification: Client will remain free of signs and symptoms of fluid overload throughout labor.

Outcome Evaluation: Client's vital signs and cardiopulmonary status within acceptable parameters; client remains alert and oriented to person, place, and time; urine output is at least 30 mL/hour; urine specific gravity 1.010–1.030.

Interventions	Rationale
1. Assess vital signs and auscultate heart and lung sounds for changes. Note any bounding pulse, tachypnea, shallow or labored breathing, shortness of breath, or dyspnea. Inspect sacral area and extremities for edema.	1. Oxytocin exerts antidiuretic effects, which may result in water intoxication possibly leading to hypertension, and peripheral and pulmonary edema.
2. Assess neurologic status for changes, such as headache, lethargy, confusion, or a change in the client's level of consciousness.	2. Water intoxication causes a shift in interstitial fluid affecting all major organs, including the brain, which would lead to cerebral edema.
3. Assess intake and output and test urine for specific gravity. Monitor the intravenous fluid infusion and adjust rate as ordered.	3. Intake and output and urine specific gravity provide reliable indicators about a client's fluid volume status. Inadvertent administration of too rapid a rate or too great an amount of intravenous fluid can increase the risk of fluid overload.
4. Anticipate the need for fluid restrictions.	4. Fluid restrictions may be necessary to minimize the risk for increasing fluid overload.

(continued)

Nursing Diagnosis: Anxiety related to pregnancy outcome resulting from prolonged labor and need for oxytocin

Outcome Identification: Client and partner will verbalize feelings about the progress of labor and outcome.

Outcome Evaluation: Couple state concerns; demonstrate positive coping mechanisms; actively question to make informed decisions.

Interventions	Rationale
1. Explore the meaning of prolonged labor with the couple. Encourage them to verbalize their feelings and concerns. Allow time for questions and answers. Assess for possible feelings related to "cause" of prolonged labor.	1. Exploration, verbalization, and active questioning provide a safe outlet for feelings, help to increase the other partner's awareness of needs, and open lines of communication.
2. Approach the client in a calm, consistent, unhurried manner. Explain all actions and procedures. Attempt to minimize environmental stimuli.	2. Using a calm, consistent, unhurried approach with explanations helps to minimize the threat of the situation. Minimizing environmental stimuli can help reduce fear and anxiety.
3. Include couple in the treatment process and inform them about things ahead of time, if possible.	3. Couple's participation enhances their control over the situation and may help to instill hope and promote decision making.
4. Instruct the couple in positive coping mechanisms. Include activities such as sharing of information, relaxation and breathing exercises, and physical activity.	4. Positive coping mechanisms assist in controlling fear and minimizing its intensity, thus promoting effective problem solving.
5. Provide frequent updates about the progress of the client and fetus.	5. Frequent updates about progress help to minimize the feelings of fear about the unknown.

Kessel et al., 2001). They may be necessary if the following conditions occur:

- A woman is unable to push with contractions in the pelvic division of labor, such as after regional anesthesia or a woman with a spinal cord injury.
- Cessation of progress in the second stage of labor occurs.
- The fetus is in an abnormal position or is immature.

Forceps are steel instruments constructed of two blades that slide together at their shaft to form a handle. They are applied first by one blade being slipped into a woman's vagina next to the fetal head, and then the other side being slipped into place. Next, the shafts of the instrument are brought together in the midline to form the handle.

Forceps are designed to prevent pressure from being exerted on the fetal head as well as aid birth. Reducing pressure can avoid subdural hemorrhage in the fetus as the fetal head reaches the perineum. A fetus in distress from a complication such as prolapsed cord can be delivered more quickly by the use of forceps.

A **forceps birth** is a forceps outlet procedure when the forceps are applied after the fetal head reaches the perineum. The term *low forceps birth* may be used to indicate the fetal head is at a +2 station or more. If the fetal head is engaged but at less than +2 station, this is a *midforceps birth.* This type has been associated with birth trauma. Because cesarean birth involves less risk to the fetus than the use of midforceps, such a procedure is rarely used today. Some anesthesia, at least a pudendal block, is necessary for forceps application to achieve pelvic relaxation and reduce pain. Usually, an episiotomy is used to prevent perineal tearing due to pressure on the perineum.

Before forceps are applied,

- Membranes must be ruptured.
- Cephalopelvic disproportion must not be present.
- Cervix must be fully dilated.
- Woman's bladder must be empty.

Record FHR before forceps application. Because there is a danger that the cord could be compressed between the blade and the fetal head, assess FHR again immediately after application. The woman's cervix needs to be carefully assessed after forceps birth to be certain that no laceration occurred. To rule out bladder injury, record the time and amount of the first voiding. In addition, assess the newborn to be certain that no facial palsy or subdural hematoma exists. Explain to the parents that a forceps birth may leave a transient erythematous mark on the newborn's cheek (see Chap. 33). This will fade in 1 to 2 days.

Vacuum Extraction

A fetus, if positioned far enough down the birth canal, may be born by **vacuum extraction** (Miksovsky & Watson, 2001). With the fetal head at the perineum, a disk-shaped cup is pressed against the fetal scalp over the posterior fontanelle. When vacuum pressure is applied, air beneath

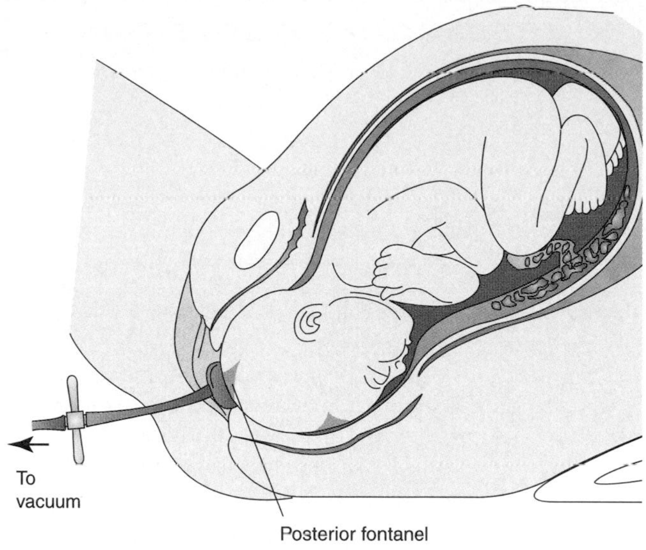

FIGURE 21.14 Vacuum extraction.

the cup is sucked out and the cup then adheres so tightly to the fetal scalp that traction on the cord leading to the cup will deliver the fetus (Fig. 21-14).

Vacuum extraction has advantages over forceps birth in that little anesthesia is necessary (making the fetus less depressed at birth) and fewer lacerations of the birth canal occur. Its major disadvantage is that it causes a marked caput that may be noticeable as long as 7 days after birth. Tentorial tears from extreme pressure also have occurred. A mother may need reassurance that the caput swelling is harmless to her infant and will decrease rapidly. Vacuum extraction should not be used as a method of birth if scalp blood sampling was done, because the suction pressure can cause severe bleeding at the sampling site. Moreover, vacuum extraction is not advantageous for preterm infants because of the softness of the preterm skull.

✔ CHECKPOINT QUESTIONS

12. What are the first symptoms of water intoxication to observe for during oxytocin induction of labor?
13. Is fetal blood sampling a contraindication to vacuum extraction?

ANOMALIES OF THE PLACENTA AND CORD

Anomalies of the Placenta

The placenta and cord are always examined for the presence of anomalies after birth. The normal placenta weighs approximately 500 g and is 15 to 20 cm in diameter and 1.5 to 3.0 cm thick. Its weight is approximately one sixth that of the fetus. A placenta may be unusually enlarged in women with diabetes. In certain diseases, such as syphilis or erythroblastosis, the placenta may be so large that it weighs half as much as the fetus. If the uterus has scars or a septum, the placenta may be wide in diameter, because it was forced to spread out to find implantation space.

Placenta Succenturiata

A **placenta succenturiata** (Fig. 21-15*A*) has one or more accessory lobes connected to the main placenta by blood vessels. No fetal abnormality is associated with it. However, it is important that it be recognized, because the small lobes may be retained in the uterus after birth, leading to severe maternal hemorrhage. On inspection, the placenta will appear torn at the edge, or torn blood vessels may extend beyond the edge of the placenta. The remaining lobes must be removed from the uterus manually to prevent maternal hemorrhage from poor uterine contraction.

Placenta Circumvallata

Ordinarily, the chorion membrane begins at the edge of the placenta and spreads to envelop the fetus; no chorion covers the fetal side of the placenta. In **placenta circumvallata,** the fetal side of the placenta is covered to some extent with chorion (Fig. 21-15*B*). The umbilical cord enters the placenta at the usual midpoint, and large vessels spread out from there. They end abruptly at the point where the chorion folds back onto the surface, however. (In **placenta marginata,** the fold of chorion reaches just to the edge of the placenta.) Although no abnormalities are associated with this type of placenta, its presence should be noted.

Battledore Placenta

In a **battledore placenta,** the cord is inserted marginally rather than centrally (Fig. 21-15*C*). This anomaly is rare and has no known clinical significance.

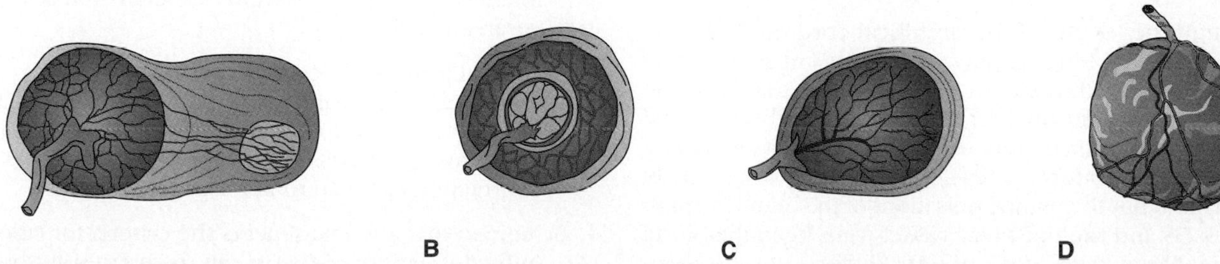

FIGURE 21.15 Abnormal placental formation. (*A*) Placenta succenturiata. (*B*) Placenta circumvallata. (*C*) Battledore placenta. (*D*) Velamentous cord insertion.

Velamentous Insertion of the Cord

Velamentous insertion of the cord is a situation in which the cord, instead of entering the placenta directly, separates into small vessels that reach the placenta by spreading across a fold of amnion (Fig. 21-15*D*). This form of cord insertion is most frequently found with multiple pregnancy. It may be associated with fetal anomalies.

Vasa Previa

In *vasa previa,* the umbilical vessels of a velamentous cord insertion cross the cervical os, so they would deliver before the fetus. The vessels may tear with cervical dilatation, the same as a placenta previa may tear. Before inserting any instrument such as an internal fetal monitor, structures should be identified to prevent accidental tearing of a vasa previa. Tearing would result in sudden fetal blood loss. If sudden painless bleeding occurs with the beginning of cervical dilation, vasa previa should be suspected. It can be confirmed by sonogram. If this is identified, the infant will need to be born by cesarean birth.

Placenta Accreta

Placenta accreta is an unusually deep attachment of the placenta to the uterine myometrium (ACOG, 2002). The placenta will not loosen and deliver. Attempts to remove it manually may lead to extreme hemorrhage because of the deep attachment. Hysterectomy or treatment with methotrexate to destroy the still-attached tissue may be necessary.

Anomalies of the Cord

Two-Vessel Cord

A normal cord contains one vein and two arteries. The absence of one of the umbilical arteries is associated with congenital heart and kidney anomalies, because the insult that caused the loss of the vessel probably led to other mesoderm germ layer structures as well (Cunningham et al., 2001). Inspection of a cord must be made immediately at birth before it begins to dry, because drying will distort the appearance. Document the number of vessels present. The child with only two vessels needs to be observed carefully for other anomalies during the newborn period.

Unusual Cord Length

Although the length of the umbilical cord rarely varies, some abnormal lengths may occur. An unusually short umbilical cord can result in premature separation of the placenta or an abnormal fetal lie. An unusually long cord can be compromised more easily because of its tendency to twist or knot more. Occasionally, a cord will actually form a knot, but the natural pulsations of the blood through the vessels and the muscular vessel walls keep the blood flow adequate. Also, it is not unusual for a cord to wrap once around the fetal neck but, again, with no interference to fetal circulation.

✔ CHECKPOINT QUESTIONS

14. Approximately how much does a placenta weigh?
15. In which type of placenta is the cord inserted marginally rather than centrally?

KEY POINTS

Complications of labor arise from problems with the force of labor, the passage, or the passenger. Hypotonic, hypertonic, and uncoordinated contractions all can occur, resulting in ineffective first or second stages of labor.

Precipitate labor is birth that is completed in less than 3 hours. It can be responsible for subdural hemorrhage in the fetus and cervical lacerations in the mother.

Uterine rupture, although rare, is suggested by a pathologic retraction ring (shown by an indentation across the abdomen over the uterus).

Uterine inversion is a grave complication. If the situation is not immediately corrected, emergency hysterectomy is necessary to save the woman's life. Almost all occurrences of uterine inversion can be avoided by two axioms of care: *Do not put pressure on an uncontracted fundus immediately postpartum* (massage first to cause it to contract); and *do not exert pressure on an umbilical cord to achieve placental delivery.*

Amniotic fluid embolism occurs when amniotic fluid is forced into an open maternal uterine blood sinus. The woman notices chest pain and dyspnea. Administer oxygen and notify the woman's primary care provider of this emergency.

Prolapse of the umbilical cord is an emergency situation that requires prompt action. Position the woman quickly into either a Trendelenburg or knee-chest position to relieve cord compression or apply manual pressure vaginally to lift the head away from the cord; notify the woman's primary caregiver of the emergency.

Multiple gestations can complicate birth. Many infants of multiple gestations are delivered by cesarean birth.

Abnormal position, presentation, or size of the fetus (e.g., occipitoposterior position, breech, face, or brow presentation, and transverse lie) as well as problems of the passage such as inlet and outlet contraction can lead to labor complications.

Be certain that a woman meets the criteria for labor induction before preparing an oxytocin solution. These criteria include engagement of the fetal head, a "ripe" cervix, and absence of cephalopelvic disproportion. Question an order if the above criteria are not present.

Always prepare oxytocin as a "piggyback" solution, being extremely careful of the dose used. Both a uterine and FHR monitor should be used continuously during labor induction. Observe that contractions occur no less than 2 minutes apart and are no longer than 70 seconds in duration.

Vacuum extraction and forceps are methods to assist birth. Both mother and infant need special observation after these procedures to detect cervical or vaginal tearing.

Anomalies of the placenta and cord, such as placenta succenturiata, placenta circumvallata, battledore placenta, or a two-vessel cord, can lead to birth complications.

CRITICAL THINKING EXERCISES

1. Roseann Bigalow is the woman you met at the beginning of the chapter. Her fetus is in a posterior position, and she has severe back pain. What actions could her husband take to help relieve his wife's pain from this posterior fetal position?
2. A young couple is having their first child. After rupture of membranes, you notice that the fetal monitor shows variable decelerations. On inspection, you are able to see the cord at the vaginal opening. You are aware that this is a fetal emergency. How would you proceed, in order of priority, to address this situation?
3. One woman under your care began labor spontaneously at 10 AM. Another woman had an oxytocin infusion for induction of labor at 10 AM because her pregnancy had extended 2 weeks beyond her expected due date. How would you develop a plan of care addressing the following factors: (1) whether both women will be able to use breathing exercises with contractions, and (2) what the priority observations are for each woman?
4. Examine the National Health Goals related to complications of childbirth. Most government-sponsored money for nursing research is allotted based on these goals. What would be a possible research topic to explore pertinent to these goals that would be both fundable and advance evidence-based practice?

REFERENCES

American College of Obstetricians & Gynecologists. (2002). ACOG committee opinion: Placenta accreta. *Obstetrics & Gynecology, 99*(1), 169–170.

Bick, R. L. (2000). Syndromes of disseminated intravascular coagulation in obstetrics, pregnancy, and gynecology. *Hematology-Oncology Clinics of North America, 14*(5), 999–1044.

Bishop, E. H. (1964). Pelvic scoring for elective induction. *Obstetrics & Gynecology, 24*(2), 266–269.

Burns, E., et al. (2000). The use of aromatherapy in intrapartum midwifery practice: An observational study. *Complementary Therapies in Nursing & Midwifery, 6*(1), 33–34.

Calder, A. A. (2000). Emergencies in operative obstetrics. *Best Practice & Research in Clinical Obstetrics & Gynaecology, 14*(1), 43–55.

Clark, S. L. (2000). Critical care obstetrics. In J. R. Scott, et al. (Eds.). *Danforth's obstetrics and gynecology* (8th ed., pp. 471–484). Philadelphia: Lippincott Williams & Wilkins.

Cruikshank, D. P. (2000). Malpresentations and umbilical cord complications. In J. R. Scott, et al. (Eds.). *Danforth's obstetrics and gynecology* (8th ed., pp. 419–436). Philadelphia: Lippincott Williams & Wilkins.

Cunningham, F. G. (Ed.) (2001). *William's obstetrics.* New York: McGraw-Hill.

Department of Health and Human Services. (2000). *Healthy people 2010.* Washington, DC: Author.

Dudley, D. J. (2000). Complications of labor. In J. R. Scott, et al. (Eds.). *Danforth's obstetrics and gynecology* (8th ed., pp. 437–455). Philadelphia: Lippincott Williams & Wilkins.

Friedman, E. A. (1978). *Labor: Clinical evaluation and management* (2nd ed.). New York: Appleton.

Gherman, R. B., et al. (2000). Analysis of McRoberts' maneuver by x-ray pelvimetry. *Obstetrics & Gynecology, 95*(1), 43–47.

Hogberg, U. & Lekas, B. M. (2000). Prolonged labour attributed to large fetus. *Gynecologic & Obstetric Investigation, 49*(3), 160–164.

Hostetler, D. R. & Bosworth, M. F. (2000). Uterine inversion: A life-threatening obstetric emergency. *Journal of the American Board of Family Practice, 13*(2), 20–123.

Johnson, M., Maas, M. & Moorhead, S. (2000). *Nursing outcomes classification* (2nd ed.). St. Louis: Mosby.

Karch, A. M. (2001). *Lippincott's nursing drug guide.* Philadelphia: Lippincott Williams & Wilkins.

Konje, J. C. & Ladipo, O. A. (2000). Nutrition and obstructed labor. *American Journal of Clinical Nutrition, 72*(1 Suppl), 291S–297S.

McCloskey, J. & Bulechek, G. (2000). *Nursing interventions classification* (3rd ed.). St. Louis: Mosby.

Miksovsky, P. & Watson, W. J. (2001). Obstetric vacuum extraction: State of the art in the new millennium. *Obstetrical & Gynecological Survey, 56*(11), 736–751.

Miller, D. A. & Paul, R. (2000). Antepartum-intrapartum fetal monitoring. In J. R. Scott, et al. (Eds.). *Danforth's obstetrics and gynecology* (8th ed., pp. 243–256). Philadelphia: Lippincott Williams & Wilkins.

Rouse, D. J. et al. (2000). Criteria for failed labor induction. *Obstetrics & Gynecology, 96*(5.1), 671–677.

Sanchez-Ramos, L., et al. (2002). Labor induction with 25 micrograms versus 50 micrograms intra vaginal misoprostol. *Obstetrics & Gynecology, 99*(1), 145–151.

Scheepers, H. C., et al. (2001). Eating and drinking in labor: The influence of caregiver advice on women's behavior. *Birth, 28*(2), 119–123.

Spellacy, W. N. (2000). Multiple pregnancies. In J. R. Scott, et al. (Eds.). *Danforth's obstetrics and gynecology* (8th ed., pp. 293–307). Philadelphia: Lippincott Williams & Wilkins.

Van Kessel, et al. (2001). The second stage of labor and stress urinary incontinence. *American Journal of Obstetrics & Gynecology, 184*(7), 1571–1575.

Wilson, C. (2000). The nurse's role in misoprostol induction: A proposed protocol. *Journal of Obstetric, Gynecologic & Neonatal Nursing, 29*(6), 574–583.

Yap, O. W., Kim, E. S., & Laros, R. K. (2001). Maternal and neonatal outcomes after uterine rupture in labor. *American Journal of Obstetrics & Gynecology, 184*(7), 1576–1581.

Zamorski, M. A. & Biggs, W. S. (2001). Management of suspected fetal macrosomia. *American Family Physician, 63*(2), 302–306.

SUGGESTED READINGS

Davies, S. (2001). Amniotic fluid embolus: A review of the literature. *Canadian Journal of Anaesthesia, 48*(1), 88–98.

Brauer-Rieke, G. (2000). Shoulder dystocia. *Midwifery Today, 55*(1), 28–29.

Green, B. T. & Umana, E. (2000). Amniotic fluid embolism. *Southern Medical Journal, 93*(7), 721–723.

Hogg, B. B. & Owen, J. (2001). Laminaria versus extra-amniotic saline solution infusion for cervical ripening in second-trimester labor inductions. *American Journal of Obstetrics & Gynecology, 184*(6), 1145–1148.

Kabiru, W. N., et al. (2001). Trends in operative vaginal delivery rates and associated maternal complication rates in an inner-city hospital. *American Journal of Obstetrics & Gynecology, 184*(6), 1112–1114.

Koniak-Griffin, D. (1999). Strategies for reducing the risk of malpractice litigation in perinatal nursing. *Journal of Obstetric, Gynecologic & Neonatal Nursing, 28*(3), 291–299.

Luckas, M. & Bricker, L. (2000). Intravenous prostaglandin for induction of labour. *Cochrane Database of Systematic Reviews* (4), CD002864.

Penn, Z. & Ghaem-Maghami, S. (2001). Indications for caesarean section. *Best Practice & Research in Clinical Obstetrics & Gynaecology, 15*(1), 1–15.

Perla, L. (2002). Patient compliance and satisfaction with nursing care during delivery and recovery. *Journal of Nursing Care Quality, 16*(2), 60–66.

Ramsey, P. S., Ramin, K. D., & Field, C. S. (2000). Shoulder dystocia: Rotational maneuvers revisited. *Journal of Reproductive Medicine, 45*(2), 85–88.

Stamp, G., Kruzins, G., & Crowther, C. (2001). Perineal massage in labour and prevention of perineal trauma: Randomized controlled trial. *BMJ, 322*(7297), 1277–1280.

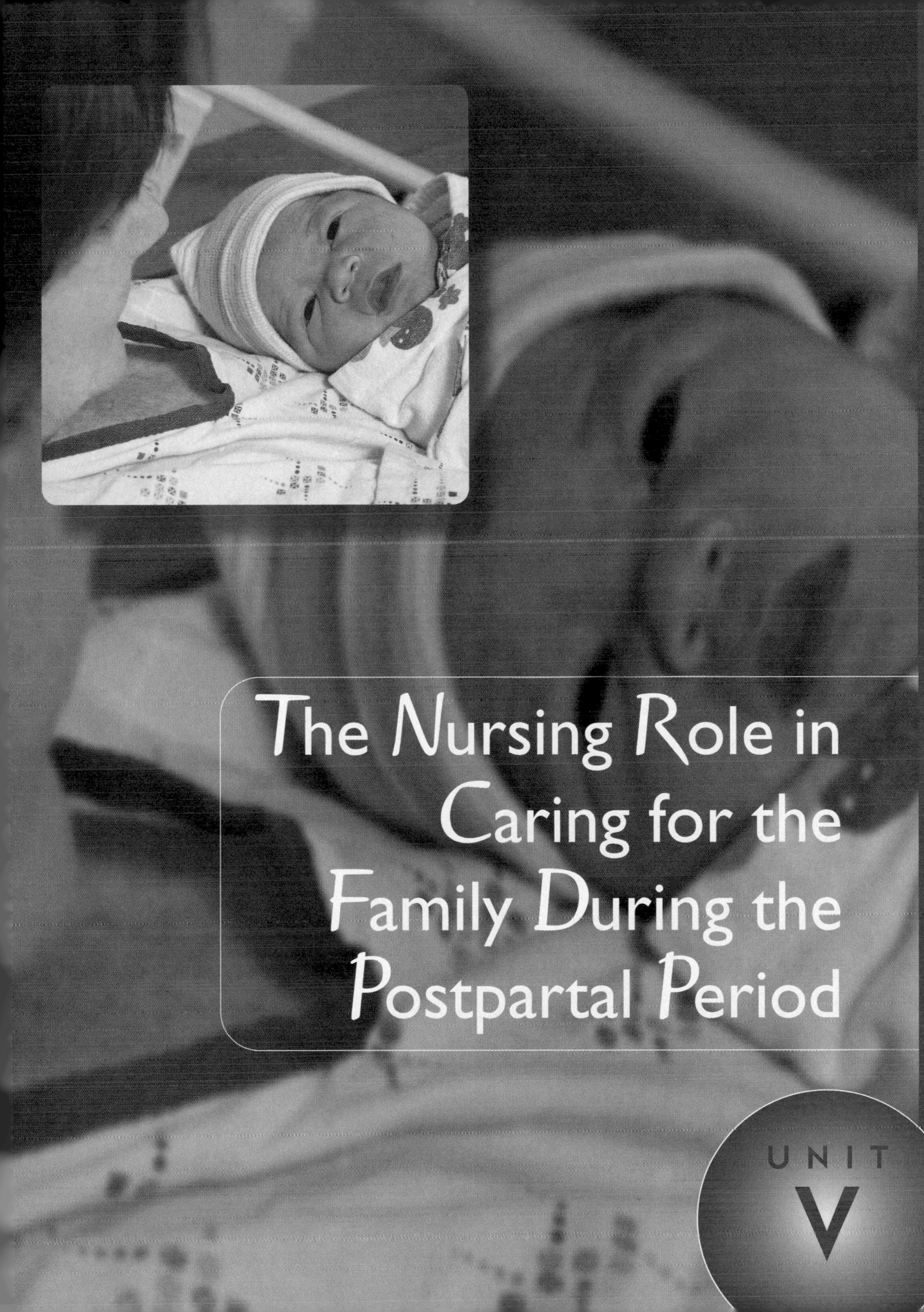

The Nursing Role in Caring for the Family During the Postpartal Period

UNIT

V

22

CHAPTER

Nursing Care of the Postpartal Woman and Family

Key Terms

- **afterpains**
- **diastasis recti**
- **en face position**
- **engrossment**
- **Homans' sign**
- **involution**
- **letting-go phase**
- **lochia**
- **lochia alba**
- **lochia rubra**
- **lochia serosa**
- **primary engorgement**
- **rooming-in**
- **sitz bath**
- **taking-hold phase**
- **taking-in phase**
- **uterine atony**

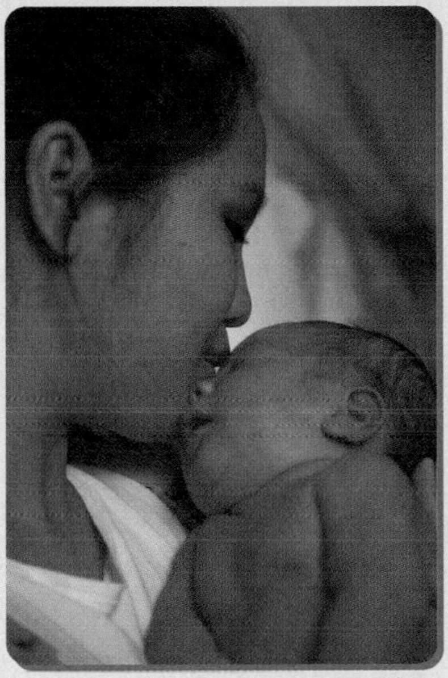

Objectives

After mastering the contents of this chapter, you should be able to:

1. Describe the psychological and physiologic changes that occur in the postpartal woman.
2. Assess a woman and her family for physiologic and psychological changes after childbirth.
3. Formulate nursing diagnoses related to physiologic and psychological transitions of the postpartal period.
4. Identify expected outcomes for the postpartal woman and family related to the changes during this period.
5. Plan nursing care such as measures to aid uterine involution or encourage bonding.
6. Implement nursing care to aid the progression of physiologic and psychological transitions occurring in the client and family.
7. Evaluate outcomes to determine effectiveness of nursing care and achievement of outcomes.
8. Identify National Health Goals related to the postpartal period that nurses can be instrumental in helping the nation to achieve.
9. Identify areas related to care of the postpartal family that could benefit from additional nursing research or application of evidence-based practice.
10. Use critical thinking to analyze ways that postpartum nursing care can be more family centered.
11. Integrate knowledge of the physiologic and psychological changes of the postpartal period with the nursing process to achieve quality maternal and child health nursing care.

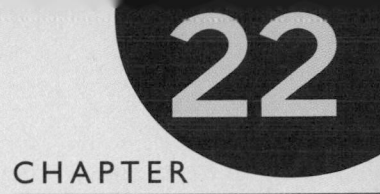

As the nurse working in a postpartum unit, you are caring for Mike and Joan Cooper who have just become parents of an 8 lb, 2 oz baby girl. Mike will be taking a week off from work to spend time with Joan and the new baby. Joan is on maternity leave from her job.

As you prepare them for discharge, you notice that they seem overwhelmed with much of the information they have been provided. Joan says, trying to get the baby to nurse, "Maybe my breasts are too small and the baby can't get enough milk. I'm hoping that if I breastfeed, I won't have to worry about birth control for a while, but I'm having so much trouble." Mike is concerned that if Joan breastfeeds the baby, he will feel left out. He pulls you aside and says, "Sometimes, I see my wife crying for no reason. Isn't she as happy as I am?"

Previous chapters discussed caring for the pregnant woman and family during the antepartal and intrapartal periods. This chapter adds information about caring for the postpartal woman and family to your knowledge base. Many physiologic and psychological changes occur during this period, enabling nurses to play major roles in assessment, comfort promotion, and education.

After you've studied this chapter, answer the Critical Thinking Exercises at the end of the chapter, and then access the on-line study activities (http://connection.lww.com) *to further sharpen your skills and test your knowledge.*

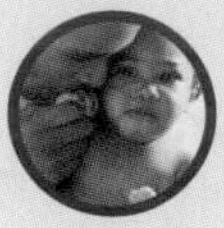

FOCUS ON NATIONAL HEALTH GOALS

The first hour postpartum is an extremely dangerous one for hemorrhage. It is also the optimum period when breastfeeding should begin. National Health Goals that involve this time period include the following:

- Reduce the maternal mortality rate to no more than 3.3/100,000 live births from a baseline of 7.1/100,000.
- Reduce the proportion of births occurring within 24 months of a previous birth to 6% from a baseline of 11%.
- Increase to at least 75% the proportion of mothers who breastfeed their babies in the early postpartum period from a baseline of 64% (DHHS, 2000).

Nurses can be instrumental in helping the nation to achieve these goals by maintaining close observation in the immediate postpartal period to detect maternal hemorrhage, encouraging and supporting women who breastfeed, and ensuring that women receive reproductive life planning information.

Areas that could benefit from additional nursing research include discovering effective means to encourage women to maintain breastfeeding and effective ways to teach women to monitor their own health in the postpartal period, particularly when, because of early discharge, they may be home when uterine hemorrhage occurs.

The postpartal period, or *puerperium* (from the Latin *puer,* "child," and *parere,* "to bring forth"), refers to the 6-week period after childbirth. This is a time of maternal changes that are retrogressive (involution of the uterus and vagina) and progressive (production of milk for lactation, restoration of the normal menstrual cycle, and beginning of a parenting role). Protecting a woman's health as these changes occur is important for preserving her future childbearing function and for ensuring that she is physically well enough to incorporate her new child into the family. This period is popularly termed the *fourth trimester of pregnancy.*

The physical care a woman receives during the postpartal period can influence her health for the rest of her life. The emotional support she receives can influence the emotional health of her child and family and so can be felt into the next generation. National Health Goals related to the postpartal period that nurses can be instrumental in helping the nation achieve are shown in the Focus on National Health Goals.

NURSING PROCESS OVERVIEW

For the Postpartal Woman and Family

Assessment

During the puerperium, assessment of a woman is accomplished with health interview, physical examination, and analysis of laboratory data. Assessment of a woman's psychological adjustment begins with her reaction at birth (is she disappointed with the sex of the baby? is she happy to be through with the pregnancy or still longing to be back in it?) and continues with every contact with the family during and after the hospital stay. Assess the extent and quality of the woman's interaction with the child (does she hold the infant and talk to him or her?), her overall mood (do you observe her crying? does she have long periods of staring into space or not talking?), and her ability to begin infant care. Observe also for self-care. If a woman feels good about herself, even though she is exhausted from childbirth, she will generally try to maintain her appearance. If she is depressed, she probably has little energy to do things such as comb her hair or worry about her appearance.

It is also important to ensure that physical changes, such as uterine involution, are occurring by evaluating uterine size and consistency and lochia flow amount (see Assessing the Postpartal Woman).

Nursing Diagnosis

Nursing diagnoses during the postpartal period usually are concerned with either the family's inability to accept and bond with the new child or physiologic considerations. Examples include:

- Risk for impaired parenting related to disappointment in the sex of the child

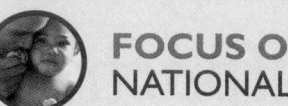

ASSESSING the Postpartal Woman

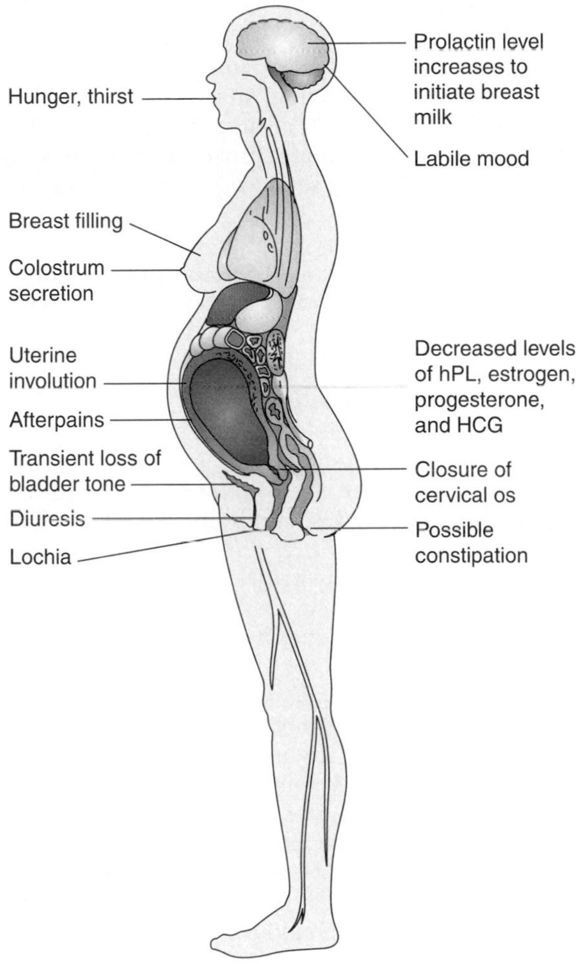

- Fear related to lack of preparation for child care
- Risk for deficient fluid volume related to postpartal hemorrhage

Outcome Identification and Planning

Be certain that outcomes established during this time are realistic in light of the woman's changed life pattern. Most postpartum families remain in the hospital for a relatively short time, ranging from 48 to 72 hours. The postpartum stay in an alternative birth center can be as short as 4 hours. Therefore, outcomes must be devised that can be accomplished and evaluated during this short period of client contact. Inability to accomplish certain outcomes may require follow-up home care.

When planning care in the postpartal period, try to arrange procedures to allow optimal time for family-infant interaction and yet allow adequate time for rest to relieve exhaustion. Relief of exhaustion allows for improved coping abilities and better planning for self-care. After adequate instruction, women should be able to monitor their own health.

Planning should include ample time for health teaching. An important part of teaching related to care of the newborn is preparation for the unexpected and the need for flexibility, because parents don't yet know what their new life will be like (whether their child will sleep deeply or fitfully at night, whether their child will become hungry at long or short intervals) or how tired they will become after being awakened during the night. Brainstorming—practicing to produce at least three different methods of reaching a particular goal—is excellent practice for parenting.

Implementation

All interventions in the postpartal period should be family centered to enhance family functioning and bonding.

Interventions also are geared toward increasing the woman's self-esteem and allowing her to view herself as a new mother and the infant as part of her family. Teaching new mothers is important, but it is also important to explore what they already know about child care and what they think would be a sensible solution to a problem. Giving advice only solves an immediate problem; helping the woman to learn good problem-solving techniques enhances her ability to handle the many challenges that may arise more effectively. Teaching takes on an even greater role when the woman is discharged soon after birth. Follow-up home care visits may be required to ascertain family–infant bonding and additional health care needs.

Outcome Evaluation

If the woman fails to make an adequate adjustment in the postpartal period, she may have difficulty integrating the infant into the family. The child's mental health, self-esteem, and ability to form a sense of trust will be affected. Follow-up evaluation must be done either by telephone or at home visits and at postpartal and well-child return visits.

Evaluation in the postpartal period involves being certain not only that the woman and her baby are safe but also that the woman knows how to maintain her health after returning home from a health care facility.

Examples of outcome achievement include:

- Parents spontaneously make at least one positive comment about child's characteristics before hospital discharge.
- Client states she believes she will be able to manage newborn care with support of significant other.
- Client's lochial flow is no more than one saturated perineal pad (50 mL) every 3 hours.

PSYCHOLOGICAL CHANGES OF THE POSTPARTAL PERIOD

A transition is a movement or passage from one position or concept to another. It is a pause between what was and what is to be or the internal process experienced by people when change occurs. In a classic presentation of what transition entails, Bridges (1994) states this as change is something that happens to people and transition is how they respond to change.

People move through several predictable stages during transition: the act of ending old ways of thinking or believing (letting go); a neutral zone during which the old way is gone but the new way is not yet comfortable; and a new beginning during which new ideas and concepts are put into action (Bridges, 1994). The postpartum period is a time of transition during which the couple gives up concepts such as "childless" or "parents of one" and moves to the new beginning of parenthood. The immediate postpartal period is a neutral time during which the couple tries out the new role and attempts to "fit" their expectations for that role. Nurses can be instrumental in helping couples acknowledge the extent of the change to help them gain closure on their previous lifestyle. Opening channels for communication, anticipating new needs, and highlighting potential gains that will occur because of the change are important actions.

Phases of the Puerperium

In her classic work on maternal behavior, Reva Rubin, a nurse, divided the puerperium into three separate phases (Rubin, 1977). She viewed the first of these, called the **taking-in phase,** as encompassing the first 2 or 3 days. The subsequent phases, called **taking-hold** and **letting-go,** are times of renewed action and forward movement. At the time that these phases of the puerperium were identified, women were hospitalized for 5 to 7 days after childbirth and moved in a paced manner from one step to the next. Today, with hospitalization as short as a few hours, women appear to move through these phases much more quickly and may be experiencing two different phases at once.

Taking-In Phase

The taking-in phase, the first phase experienced, is a time of reflection for a woman. During this period, the woman is largely passive. She prefers having a nurse minister to her, to get her a bath towel or a clean nightgown, and make decisions for her rather than doing these things herself. This dependence is due partly to her physical discomfort from possible perineal stitches, afterpains, or hemorrhoids; partly to her uncertainty in caring for a newborn; and partly from the extreme exhaustion that follows childbirth.

As a part of thinking and pondering about her new role, a woman usually wants to talk about her pregnancy, especially about her labor and birth. She holds the child with a sense of wonder. Can this child really be hers? Is birth really over? Could she be this lucky? She needs time to rest and regain her physical strength and to calm and contain her swirling thoughts. Encouraging her to talk about the birth helps her do this (see Focus on Communication).

FOCUS ON COMMUNICATION

Mrs. Cooper is 6 hours post childbirth. You want to assess her for postpartal pain, so you enter her hospital room. She is wearing a hospital gown and sitting in the chair by her bed.

Less Effective Communication

Nurse: How are you feeling, Mrs. Cooper?

Mrs. Cooper: Like I'm still rushing around. I called my husband as soon as my water broke. He hit a truck on the way home, though, so never got home. I tried to call—

Nurse: Do you have any pain?

Mrs. Cooper: It's not bad. I tried to call my mother, but she couldn't come over because she didn't have a car. Our neighbor—

Nurse: Okay, then let me check your stitches.

More Effective Communication

Nurse: How are you feeling, Mrs. Cooper?

Mrs. Cooper: Like I'm still rushing around. I called my husband as soon as my water broke. He hit a truck on the way home, though, so never got home. I tried to call—

Nurse: Do you have any pain?

Mrs. Cooper: It's not bad. I tried to call my mother, but she couldn't come over because she didn't have a car. Our neighbor—

Nurse: Go on. I didn't mean to interrupt.

Mrs. Cooper: Our neighbor said he'd drive me but then discovered his wife had his car keys. It was a three-ring circus of problems.

Nurse: "A three-ring circus"?

Mrs. Cooper: Yes. Finally, my husband made it home, but then there was such a bad accident on the freeway we had to drive all the way around the lake. I thought I'd have the baby in the middle of the bridge.

Nurse: That must have been terrifying for you.

Most women are interested in discussing their labor and birth experience in the days immediately after birth. Repeating a story of how worried they were when labor started, how much pain they had, or how scared they were when their membranes broke helps them put these sensations into perspective and integrate these experiences into their life. Communication that encourages women to elaborate on a story is therapeutic; communication that discourages storytelling is not. Allowing and even encouraging Mrs. Cooper to elaborate on her story helps to "debrief" her concern about not reaching the hospital on time. After talking about what concerned her most, then returning to a discussion and assessment of her pain would be appropriate.

Taking-Hold Phase

After the time of passive dependence, a woman begins to initiate action. She prefers to get her own washcloth and to make her own decisions. Women who give birth without any anesthesia may reach this second phase in a matter of hours after birth.

During the taking-in period, a woman may have expressed little interest in caring for her child. Now, she begins to take a strong interest. As a rule, therefore, it is always best to give the woman brief demonstrations of baby care and then allow her to care for the child herself—with watchful guidance.

Although a woman's actions suggest strong independence during this time, she often still feels insecure about her ability to care for her new child. She needs praise for the things she does well to give her confidence, for example, supporting the baby's head, beginning breastfeeding, and bubbling the baby correctly. This positive reinforcement begins in the care facility and continues after discharge, at home and at postpartum and well-baby visits.

Do not rush a woman through the phase of taking-in or prevent her from taking hold when she reaches that point. For many young mothers, learning to make decisions about their child's welfare is one of the most difficult phases of motherhood. It helps if the woman has practice in making such decisions in a sheltered setting rather than first taking on that level of responsibility when she is on her own.

Letting-Go Phase

In the third phase, called letting-go, the woman finally redefines her new role. She gives up the fantasized image of her child and accepts the real one; she gives up her old role of being childless or the mother of only one or two (or however many children she had before this birth). This process requires some grief work and readjustment of relationships similar to what occurred during pregnancy. It is extended, and continues during the child's growing years. A woman who has reached this phase is well into her new role.

> ✔ **CHECKPOINT QUESTIONS**
>
> 1. What are the three phases of the puerperium as described by Reva Rubin?
> 2. During which phase does the mother begin to demonstrate a strong interest in child care?

Development of Parental Love and Positive Family Relationships

During pregnancy, almost every woman worries about her ability to be a "good" mother. This concern doesn't evaporate as soon as the baby is born. Some women seem able to recognize a newborn's needs immediately and to give care with confident understanding right from the start. More often, however, a woman enters into a relationship with her newborn tentatively and with qualms and conflicts that must be addressed before the relationship can be meaningful. This is because parental love is only partly instinctive. A major portion develops gradually, in stages: planning the pregnancy, hearing the pregnancy confirmed, feeling the child move in utero, birthing, seeing the baby, touching the baby, and, finally, caring for the child. Factors such as a difficult labor or transport and separation from the newborn may slow the process or interfere with the woman's ability to bond with her baby.

Many women may not experience maternal feelings for their infants until days or even weeks after giving birth. Some fathers admit they have difficulty "claiming" or bonding with an infant (feeling fatherly toward the new child) until as late as 3 months after the birth, when the child can smile or coo and interact more directly with them. Both parents' ability to reach out can be strengthened by allowing them to touch and spend time with the new child in the first few hours of life.

Forming a strong bond with a child is not a problem only for first-time parents. Experienced parents can have just as much difficulty—they know they love 4-year-old Johnny and 2-year-old Sue at home, but worry that their hearts may not be big enough to love a new child, too.

Because of these mixed feelings, parents may not show genuine warmth the first time they hold their infant. Although a woman carried an infant inside her for 9 months, she now approaches her newborn as she would a stranger. The first time she holds the infant, she may touch only tentatively. She may hold him or her, but she touches only the blanket and never makes physical contact. If she unfolds the blanket to examine the baby or count the fingers or toes, she may use only her fingertips (Fig. 22-1).

Gradually, as a woman holds her child more, she begins to express more warmth, touching the child with the palm of her hand rather than with her fingertips. She holds her newborn tightly, in a more motherly way. She smooths the baby's hair, brushes a cheek, plays with toes, and lets the baby's fingers clasp hers. Soon, she feels comfortable enough to press her cheek against the baby's or kiss the infant's nose or mouth; she has become a mother tending to her child. This identification process is termed *claiming* or *bonding* (Lvoff, Lvoff, & Klaus, 2000). Looking directly at her newborn's face, with direct eye contact (termed an **en face position**), is a sign that the woman is beginning effective interaction. Many fathers can be observed staring at a newborn for long intervals in this same way. Often termed **engrossment,** this action alerts caregivers to how actively the father, as well as the mother, makes an active contribution to bonding (Fig. 22-2). The length of time parents take to bond with a child depends on the circumstances of the pregnancy and birth, the wellness and ability of the child to meet the parent's expectations, reciprocal

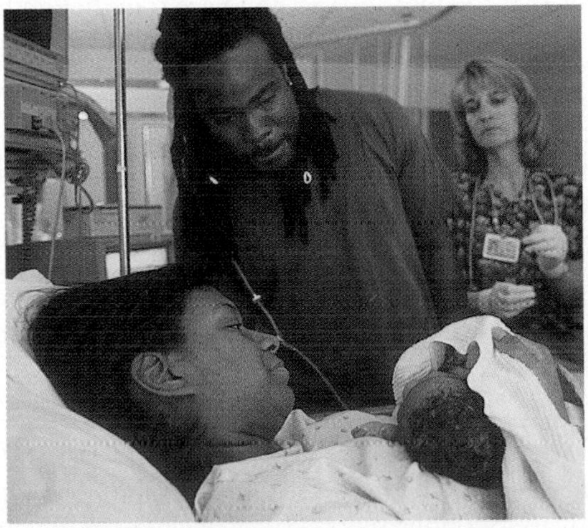

FIGURE 22.1 A mom and dad beginning interaction with their newborn immediately after birth. At first some parents are tentative, but gradually they will bond.

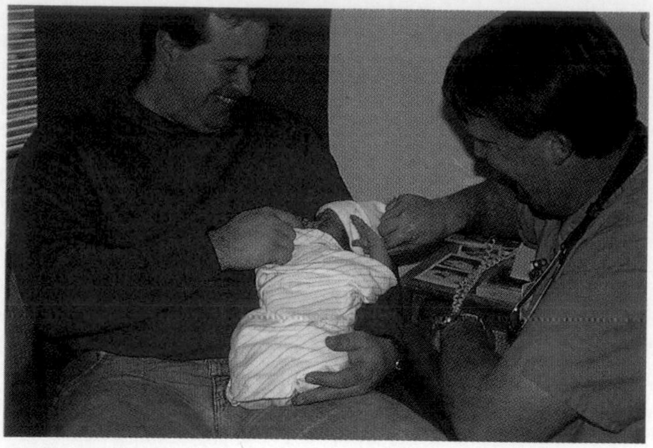

FIGURE 22.2 A nurse encourages a father as he interacts and bonds with his newborn.

actions by the newborn, and the opportunities the parents have to interact with the child. Freedom from stringent rules helps in developing good parent–child relationships. To help parents sort out their feelings about being a mother or father and about their new responsibility, provide a supportive presence and offer anticipatory guidance when necessary.

Rooming-In

The more time a woman has to spend with her baby, the sooner she may feel competent in child care, and therefore is most likely to form a sound mother–child relationship. Because the average postpartal hospital stay usually ranges from 1 to 2 days, a woman has very little time to become acquainted with her newborn before going home. If the infant stays in the room with her (called **rooming-in**) rather than in a central nursery, she can become better acquainted with her child and begin to feel more confident in her ability to care for him or her after discharge. In many settings, the father can stay overnight, or room-in, as well.

There are two types of rooming-in: *complete,* which implies that the mother and child are together 24 hours a day, and *partial,* in which the infant remains in the woman's room for part of the time, perhaps from 10:00 AM to 9:00 PM, after which he or she is taken to a small nursery near the woman's room or returned to a central nursery for the night. With both complete and partial rooming-in, the father and siblings can also hold and feed the infant.

Rooming-in also may allow a couple to retain anticipatory guidance and instructions in newborn care better because a nurse has demonstrated bathing, feeding, changing, and so forth on their child (see Focus on Evidence-Based Practice).

> **FOCUS ON EVIDENCE-BASED PRACTICE**
>
> ***Does Rooming-In Increase Maternal–Newborn Bonding?***
>
> It is difficult to evaluate this question in the United States because rooming-in to encourage bonding is routinely arranged in most hospitals. To answer the question, therefore, researchers went to a maternity hospital in Russia that had recently changed its newborn care practices to a Baby-Friendly Initiative that encouraged early contact, breastfeeding, and rooming-in of the mother and infant from birth until the time of discharge. Mothers included in the study were mostly from urban working-class communities with most of them having received prenatal care. Researchers discovered that the infant abandonment rate at the hospital decreased from 50/10,000 births before the new interventions to 27/10,000 after the baby-friendly initiatives. They concluded that early mother–infant contact with breastfeeding and rooming-in is a simple, low-cost method for increasing mother–child bonding.
>
> This is an important study for nurses because nurses are health care professionals who control or influence many of the procedures or philosophy of postpartal care. This study provides evidence for instituting a cost-effective method that benefits the clients, both mother and infant. Knowing that such measures are important can help nurses be stronger advocates for such measures at their work site.
>
> Lvoff, N. M., Lvoff, V., & Klaus, M. H. (2000). Effect of the baby-friendly initiative on infant abandonment in a Russian hospital. *Archives of Pediatrics & Adolescent Medicine, 154*(5), 474–477.

Sibling Visitation

Waiting at home, separated from their mother and listening only to telephone reports of what a new brother or sister looks like, is difficult for children. They may picture the new baby as much older than he or she actually is. "He is eating well" may produce an image of a child sitting at a table using a fork and spoon. "He weighs 8 pounds" can be meaningless information. A chance to visit the hospital and see the new baby and mother reduces feelings that a mother cares more about the new baby than about them. It also helps to integrate the baby into the family (Fig. 22-3).

Children should be free of contagious diseases (upper respiratory illnesses, recent exposure to chickenpox) when they visit. After this is ensured, the children should wash their hands and then be encouraged actually to hold or touch the newborn with parental assistance. Some hospitals may require siblings to wear a cover gown as well.

Separation from children is often as painful for a mother as it is for children. Allowing siblings to visit can help to relieve some of the impact of separation. Keep in mind that you may need to caution a woman that a sibling's opinions of a new brother or sister, for example, those of a preschooler, may not be complimentary. This baby with little hair is not their idea of a "pretty baby." If they thought the new baby would be big enough to play with, they may not feel he is a "big baby." Seeing the baby, however, even if his or her appearance is not what they expected, is helpful in establishing strong relationships and should be encouraged.

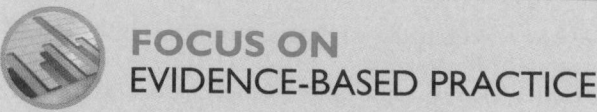

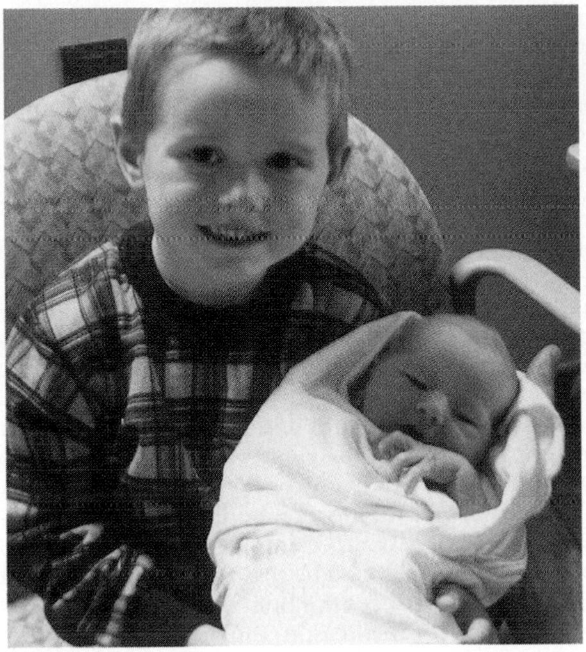

FIGURE 22.3 Sibling visiting is important to bring a family together.

Maternal Concerns and Feelings in the Postpartal Period

Traditionally, the assumption has been that most of a woman's concerns in the postpartal period center on the care of the infant. Classes in the postpartal period have focused on teaching how to breastfeed and bathe infants. Although these are concerns for many mothers, they are not necessarily their chief concerns. A woman has come through a tremendous psychological experience during pregnancy and birth of a child. She has made a complete role change. It is only to be expected, then, that some of her attention and interest during this time will be directed inward as she tries to view herself in this new role.

Major issues identified by postpartum women include breast soreness; regaining their figure; regulating the demands of housework, their partner, and their children; coping with emotional tension and sibling jealousy; and fatigue.

Abandonment

Many mothers, if given the opportunity, admit to feeling abandoned and less important after birth. Only hours before, they were the center of attention, with everyone asking about their health and well-being. Now, suddenly, the baby is the chief interest. Everyone asks about the baby; the gifts are all for the baby. Even her obstetrician, who has made her feel so important for the last 9 months, may ask during a visit, "How's that healthy 8-pound boy?" The woman may feel confused by a sensation very close to jealousy. How can a good mother be jealous of her own baby?

You can help the woman by verbalizing the problem: "How things have changed! Everyone's asking about the baby today and not about you, aren't they? How does that make you feel?" These are welcome words for a woman to hear. It is reassuring to know the sensation she is experiencing, while still uncomfortable, is normal.

When a newborn comes home, the father may have much the same feelings. He may become resentful of the time his wife spends with the infant. Perhaps the two used to sit at the table after dinner discussing the day or the future. Now she hurries away to feed the baby. She used to watch the late show with him at night. Now she goes to bed earlier because she knows she will be up again at 2:00 AM.

This is a good subject to discuss with new parents. Both motherhood and fatherhood involve some compromising in favor of the baby's interests. Examination of competitive feelings should start during pregnancy or early in the postpartal period. Making infant care a shared responsibility helps to make both partners feel equally involved in the baby's care and can help alleviate these feelings.

Disappointment

Another common feeling parents may experience is disappointment in the baby. All during pregnancy, they pictured a chubby-cheeked, curly-haired, smiling girl or boy. They have instead a skinny baby, without any hair, who is crying constantly.

It can be difficult for parents to feel positive immediately about a child who does not meet their expectations in this way. It can cause parents to remember their adolescence, when they felt gangly and unattractive, or experience feelings of inadequacy all over again.

You can never change the sex, size, or look of a child, but in the short time that you care for a postpartal family, you can help to change a mother's or father's feelings about the infant. Handle the child warmly to show that you find the infant satisfactory or even special. Comment on the child's good points, such as long fingers, lovely eyes, and good appetite. During periods of crisis like childbearing, it is possible for a key person such as a nurse to offer support that can tip the scale toward acceptance or at least help the person involved to take a clearer look at his or her situation and begin to cope with the new circumstances.

Postpartal Blues

During the puerperium, as many as 50% of women experience some feelings of overwhelming sadness for which they cannot account (Cunningham et al., 2001). They burst into tears easily or may feel let down or be irritable. This temporary feeling after birth has long been known as the *baby blues.*

This phenomenon may be due to hormonal changes, particularly the decrease in estrogen and progesterone that occurs with the delivery of the placenta. For some women, it may be a response to dependence and low self-esteem caused by exhaustion, being away from home, physical discomfort, and the tension engendered by assuming a new role, especially if the woman does not receive support from her partner (Leathers & Kelley, 2000). The syndrome is evidenced by tearfulness, feelings of inadequacy, mood lability, anorexia, and sleep disturbance.

A woman needs assurance that sudden crying episodes are normal; otherwise, she will not understand what is happening to her. Her support person also needs such assurance, or he may think that she is unhappy with him or with the baby or is keeping some terrible secret about the baby from him.

Anticipatory guidance and individualized support from health care personnel are important to help the parents understand what is happening and that this response is normal. It is also important to give a woman a chance to verbalize her feelings: "I know there's absolutely no reason for me to be crying, but I cannot stop." Allowing her to make as many decisions as possible can help give her a sense of control over her life.

Remember, however, that not all postpartal women cry because they have baby blues. A woman sometimes has other reasons to feel sad during this time. Perhaps problems at home have become overwhelming. Her husband may have been laid off from his job just when they most need the money. A parent may be ill, or their house may have been damaged in some way. Keeping the lines of communication open with postpartal women is important to help differentiate between problems that can be handled best with discussion and concerned understanding, and those that should be referred to the social service department or a community health agency.

Thirty percent of women experience postpartal depression. Serious depression requiring formal counseling or psychiatric care occurs in about 12% of women during the postpartal period (Beck & Gable, 2001). Postpartal depression and psychosis are discussed in Chapter 25.

✔ CHECKPOINT QUESTIONS

3. What typical position does a mother who is relating well with her new infant use when holding him or her?
4. Why do so many postpartal women demonstrate emotional lability?

PHYSIOLOGIC CHANGES OF THE POSTPARTAL PERIOD

Retrogressive physiologic changes occurring during the postpartal period include those related specifically to the reproductive system and other systemic changes (Harrison, 2000).

Reproductive System Changes

Involution is the process whereby the reproductive organs return to their nonpregnant state. The woman is in danger of hemorrhage from the uterus until involution is complete.

The Uterus

Involution of the uterus involves two main processes. First, the area where the placenta was implanted is sealed off, preventing bleeding. Second, the organ is reduced to its approximate pregestational size.

The sealing of the placenta site is accomplished by rapid contraction of the uterus immediately after the delivery of the placenta. This contraction pinches the blood vessels entering the 7-cm-wide area left denuded by the placenta and controls bleeding. With time, thrombi form within the uterine sinuses and permanently seal the area. Eventually, endometrial tissue undermines the site and obliterates the organized thrombi, completely covering and healing the area. This process leaves no scar tissue within the uterus, so it does not compromise future implantation sites.

The same contraction process reduces the bulk of the uterus. Devoid of the placenta and the membranes, the walls of the uterus thicken and contract, gradually reducing the uterus from being a container large enough to hold a full-term fetus to one the size of a grapefruit. Uterine contraction can be compared with a rubber band that has been stretched for many months and now is regaining its normal contour. None of the rubber band is destroyed; the shape is simply altered. A few cells of the uterine wall are broken down into their protein components by an autolytic process. These components are then absorbed by the bloodstream and excreted by the body in urine. The main mechanism that reduces the bulk of the uterus, however, is contraction. For this reason, the postpartal period, like pregnancy, is not a period of illness, of necrosing cells being evacuated, but primarily a period of healthy change.

With involution, the uterus will never completely return to its prepregnancy state. However, its reduction in size is dramatic. Immediately after birth the uterus weighs about 1000 g. At the end of the first week, it weighs 500 g. By the time involution is complete (6 weeks), it will weigh approximately 50 g, its prepregnant weight.

Uterine contraction begins immediately after placental delivery. The fundus of the uterus may be palpated through the abdominal wall halfway between the umbilicus and the symphysis pubis within a few minutes after birth. One hour later, it has risen to the level of the umbilicus, where it remains for approximately the next 24 hours. From then on, it will decrease one fingerbreadth (1 cm) a day in size. On the first postpartal day, the fundus of the uterus will be palpable one fingerbreadth below the umbilicus; on the second, two fingerbreadths below the umbilicus; and so on. Because a fingerbreadth is about 1 cm, this can be recorded as 1 cm below the umbilicus, 2 cm below it, and so forth. In the average woman, by the ninth or tenth day, the uterus will have contracted so much that it has withdrawn into the pelvis and can no longer be detected by abdominal palpation (Fig. 22-4). Because oxytocin, which stimulates uterine contractions, is released with breastfeeding, the uterus of the breastfeeding woman may contract even more quickly. However, breastfeeding does not protect against postpartum hemorrhage.

Typically, on palpation, the fundus should be midline in the abdomen. Occasionally, it is found slightly to the right, because the bulk of the sigmoid colon forced it to the right during pregnancy and it tends to remain in that position. Assessment of fundal height should be made shortly after the woman's bladder has been emptied, because a full bladder will keep the uterus from contracting, pushing it upward and possibly deviating it from the midline, due to the laxness of the uterine ligaments, giving an inaccurate reading.

Uterine involution may be delayed by a condition such as birth of multiple fetuses, hydramnios, exhaustion from

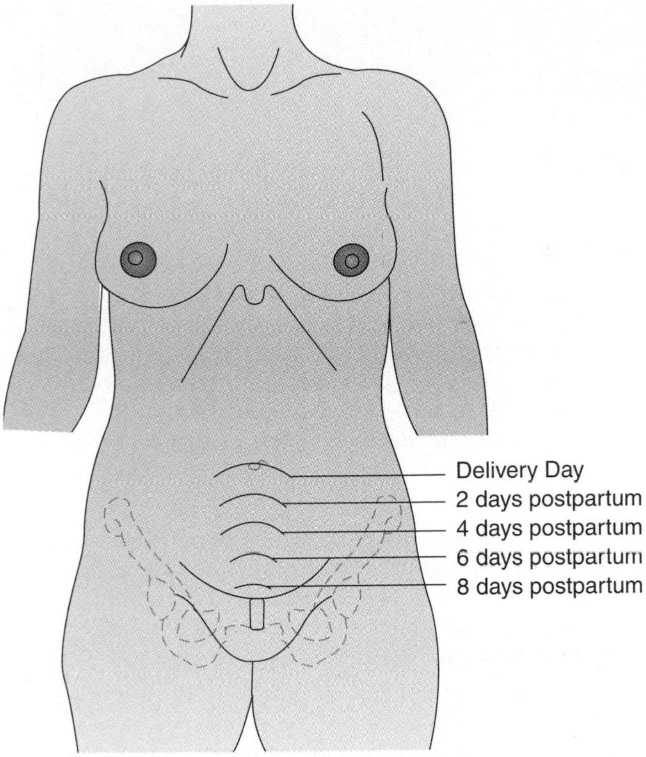

FIGURE 22.4 Uterine involution. The uterus decreases in size at a predictable rate during the postpartal period. After 10 days, it recedes under the pubic bone and is no longer palpable.

prolonged labor or a difficult birth, grand multiparity, or physiologic effects of excessive analgesia. Contraction may be difficult when there is retained placenta or membranes or a full bladder. Involution will occur most dependably in a woman who is well nourished and who ambulates early after birth (gravity may play a role).

An estimation of the consistency of the postpartal uterus is as important as measurement of its height. A well-contracted fundus feels firm. It can be compared with a grapefruit in size and tenseness, or consistency. Whenever the fundus feels boggy (soft or flabby), it is not as contracted as it should be, despite its position in the abdomen.

The first hour postpartum is potentially the most dangerous time for the woman. If the uterus should become relaxed during this time (**uterine atony**), the woman will lose blood very rapidly, because no permanent thrombi have yet formed at the placental site.

In some women, the contraction of the uterus after birth causes intermittent cramping similar to that accompanying a menstrual period. These are termed **afterpains.** They tend to be noticed most by multiparas rather than primiparas and in mothers who have given birth to large babies or had an overdistended uterus for any other reason. In these situations, the uterus must contract more forcefully to regain its prepregnancy size and has difficulty maintaining a steady contracted state. These sensations are noticed most intensely with breastfeeding, because the infant's sucking causes a release of oxytocin from the posterior pituitary, increasing the strength of the contractions.

Lochia

The separation of the placenta and membranes occurs in the spongy layer or outer portion of the decidua basalis. By the second day after birth, the layer of decidua remaining under the placental site (an area 7 cm wide) and throughout the uterus differentiates into two distinct layers. The inner layer attached to the muscular wall of the uterus remains, serving as the foundation from which a new layer of endometrium will be formed. The layer adjacent to the uterine cavity will become necrotic, being cast off as a uterine discharge similar to a menstrual flow. This uterine flow, consisting of blood, fragments of decidua, white blood cells, mucus, and some bacteria, is known as **lochia.**

The portion of the uterus where the placenta was not attached will be fully cleansed by this sloughing process and will be in a reproductive state in about 3 weeks. The placental implantation site will take approximately 6 weeks (the entire postpartal period) to be cleansed and healed.

For the first 3 days after birth, a lochia discharge consists almost entirely of blood, with only small particles of decidua and mucus. Because of its red color, it is termed **lochia rubra.** As the amount of blood involved in the cast-off tissue decreases (about the fourth day), and leukocytes begin to invade the area as they do any healing surface, the flow becomes pink or brownish in color (**lochia serosa**). On about the tenth day, the amount of the flow decreases and becomes colorless or white (**lochia alba**). Lochia alba is present in most women until the third week after birth, although it is not unusual for a lochia flow to last the entire 6 weeks of the puerperium. Characteristics of lochia are summarized in Table 22-1. Several rules for judging whether lochia flow is normal are summarized in the Focus on Family Empowerment.

The Cervix

Immediately after birth, the cervix is soft and malleable. Both the internal and external os are open. Like contraction of the fundus of the uterus, contraction of the cervix begins at once. By the end of 7 days, the external os is narrowed to the size of a pencil opening, and the cervix feels firm and nongravid again.

TABLE 22.1 Characteristics of Lochia

TYPE OF LOCHIA	COLOR	DURATION (DAY)	COMPOSITION
Lochia rubra	Red	1–3	Blood, fragments of decidua, and mucus
Lochia serosa	Pink	3–10	Blood, mucus, and invading leukocytes
Lochia alba	White	10–14 (may last 6 weeks)	Largely mucus; leukocyte count high

FOCUS ON FAMILY EMPOWERMENT
Evaluating a Lochia Flow

Q. How do I know if my lochia is normal?

A. A number of guidelines are helpful for evaluating a lochia flow. These are:

Amount: Lochia amount will vary from woman to woman. Mothers who breastfeed tend to have less lochial discharge than those who do not, because the natural release of the hormone oxytocin during breastfeeding strengthens uterine contractions. Conservation of fluid for lactation also may be a factor. Lochial flow increases on exertion, especially the first few times you are out of bed, but decreases again with rest. The increase in amount that occurs with ambulation, however, is the result of vaginal discharge of pooled lochia, not a true increase in amount. Lochia amount truly does increase on strenuous exercise, such as lifting a heavy weight or walking up stairs. Saturating a perineal pad in less than an hour is considered an abnormally heavy flow and should be reported.

Consistency: Lochia should contain no large clots. Clots may indicate that a portion of the placenta has been retained and is preventing closure of the maternal uterine blood sinuses. In any event, large clots denote poor uterine contraction, which needs to be corrected.

Pattern: Lochia is red for the first 1 to 3 days (lochia rubra), pinkish-brown from days 4 to 10 (lochia serosa), and then white (lochia alba) for as long as 6 weeks after birth. The pattern of lochia (rubra to serosa to alba) should not reverse. A red flow after it has turned pink or white may indicate that placental fragments have been retained or that uterine contraction is decreasing and new bleeding is beginning.

Odor: Lochia should not have an offensive odor. Lochia has the same odor as menstrual blood. An offensive odor usually indicates that the uterus has become infected. Immediate intervention is needed to halt postpartal infection.

Absence: Lochia should never be absent during the first 1 to 3 weeks. Absence of lochia, like presence of an offensive odor, may indicate postpartal infection. Lochia may be scant in amount after cesarean birth, but it is never altogether absent.

The process in the cervix does involve the formation of new muscle cells. This is in contrast to the process of uterine involution in which the changes consist primarily of old cells being returned to their former position by contraction. Like the fundus, however, the cervix does not return exactly to its prepregnant state. The internal os will close as before, but assuming that the birth was vaginal, the external os will usually remain slightly open and appear slitlike or stellate (star shaped), when previously it was round. Finding this pattern on pelvic examination suggests that childbearing has taken place.

The Vagina

After a vaginal birth, the vagina is soft with few rugae. Its diameter is considerably greater than normal. The hymen is permanently torn and heals with small separate tags of tissue. It takes the entire postpartal period for the vagina to involute (as in the uterus, by contraction) until it gradually returns to its approximate prepregnant state. Thickening of the walls also appears to depend on renewed estrogen stimulation from the ovaries; a woman who is breastfeeding and in whom ovulation is delayed may continue to have thin-walled or fragile vaginal cells that cause slight vaginal bleeding during sexual intercourse until about 6 weeks' time. Like the cervix, the vaginal outlet will remain slightly more distended than before; if the woman practices Kegel exercises, the strength and tone of the vagina will increase more rapidly (see Chapter 11). This may be important for both the woman and her partner's sexual enjoyment.

The Perineum

Due to the great deal of pressure experienced during birth, the perineum responds by developing edema and generalized tenderness. Portions of the perineum may show ecchymosis from the rupture of surface capillaries. The labia majora and labia minora typically remain atrophic and softened in a woman, never returning to their prepregnant state.

Systemic Changes

The same body systems involved in pregnancy are involved in postpartal changes as the body returns to its prepregnant state.

The Hormonal System

Pregnancy hormones begin to decrease as soon as the placenta is no longer present. Levels of human chorionic gonadotropin (HCG) and human placental lactogen (hPL) are almost negligible by 24 hours. By week 1, progestin, estrone, and estradiol are at pre-pregnancy levels. Estrol may be elevated for an additional week before it reaches prepregnancy levels. Follicle-stimulating hormone (FSH) remains low for about 12 days, and then begins to rise to initiate a new menstrual cycle (Cunningham et al, 2001).

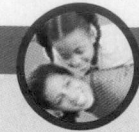

The Urinary System

During a vaginal birth, the fetal head exerts a great deal of pressure on the bladder and urethra as it passes on the bladder's underside. This pressure may leave the bladder with a transient loss of tone, and edema surrounding the urethra makes voiding difficult. Although a bladder fills rapidly and becomes distended, the woman may have no sensation of having to void. The woman who has had an epidural, a spinal, or a general anesthetic for birth can feel no sensation in the bladder area until the anesthetic has worn off.

To prevent permanent damage to the bladder from overdistention, assess the woman's abdomen frequently in the immediate postpartal period. On palpation, a full bladder is felt as a hard or firm area just above the symphysis pubis. On percussion (placing one finger flat on the woman's abdomen over the bladder and tapping it with the middle finger of the other hand), a full bladder sounds resonant in contrast to the dull, thudding sound of non-fluid-filled tissue. Pressure on this area may make the woman feel as if she has to void, but she is then unable to do so. As the bladder fills, it displaces the uterus; uterine position is thus a good gauge of whether the bladder is full or empty. If the uterus is becoming uncontracted, evidenced as softness on palpation, is boggy, and is being pushed to the side, the usual cause is an overfilled bladder.

The hydronephrosis or increased size of ureters that occurred during pregnancy remains present for about 4 weeks postpartum. The increased size of these structures in conjunction with reduced bladder sensitivity increases the possibility of urinary stasis and urinary tract infection in the postpartal period (Nel et al., 2001).

During pregnancy, as much as 2000 mL to 3000 mL excess fluid accumulates in the body. An extensive diuresis begins to take place almost immediately after birth to rid the body of this fluid, thus increasing the daily output of the postpartal woman greatly. Urinary volume may easily rise from a normal level of 1500 mL/day to as much as 3000 mL/day during the second to fifth day after birth. This marked increase in urine production causes the bladder to fill rapidly.

In the postpartal period, urine tends to contain more nitrogen than normal. This is probably due in part to the woman's increased muscle activity during labor and in part to the breakdown of protein in a portion of the uterine muscle that occurs during involution. Lactose levels in the urine are the same as during pregnancy, as the body prepares for breastfeeding. Diaphoresis (excessive sweating) is another way by which the body rids itself of excess fluid. This is noticeable in women soon after birth.

The Circulatory System

The diuresis evident between the second and fifth days postpartum plus the blood loss at birth act to reduce the added blood volume the woman accumulated during pregnancy. This reduction occurs so rapidly that by the first or second week postpartum, the blood volume has returned to its normal prepregnancy level.

Usual blood loss is 300 mL to 500 mL with a vaginal birth and 500 mL to 1000 mL with a cesarean birth. A four-point decrease in hematocrit (proportion of red blood cells to proportion of circulating plasma), and a 1-g decrease in hemoglobin value will occur with each 250 mL of blood lost. If the average woman enters labor with a hematocrit of 37%, therefore, it will be about 33% on the first postpartal day. Hemoglobin will fall from 11 g to 10 g/dL. If the woman was anemic during pregnancy, she can expect to continue to be anemic postpartum. As excess fluid is excreted, the hematocrit will gradually rise due to hemoconcentration, eventually reaching prepregnancy levels by 6 weeks.

Women generally continue to have the same high level of plasma fibrinogen during the first postpartal weeks as they did during pregnancy. This is a protective measure against hemorrhage. However, this high level also increases the risk of thrombus formation (Salonen et al., 2001). There is also an increase in the number of leukocytes in the blood. The white blood cell count may be as high as 30,000/mm^3 total (mainly granulocytes), particularly if the woman had a long or difficult labor. This, too, is part of the body's defense system, a defense against infection and an aid to healing.

Varicosities present will recede, but rarely will return to a completely prepregnant appearance. Although vascular blemishes, such as spider angiomas, fade slightly, they may not disappear completely either.

The Gastrointestinal System

Digestion and absorption begin to be active again soon after birth. Almost immediately, the woman feels hungry from the glucose used during labor and thirsty from the long period of restricted fluid plus the beginning diaphoresis. Unless she has the after effects of general anesthesia, she can eat without difficulty from nausea or vomiting during this time.

Hemorrhoids (distended rectal veins) that have been pushed out of the rectum due to the effort of pelvic-stage pushing often are present. Bowel sounds are active, but passage of stool through the bowel may be slow because of the still-present effect of relaxin on the bowel. Bowel evacuation also may be difficult due to pain of episiotomy sutures or hemorrhoids.

The Integumentary System

After birth, the stretch marks on the abdomen (striae gravidarum) still appear reddened and may be even more prominent than during pregnancy, when they were tightly stretched. Typically, in a Caucasian woman, these will fade to a pale white over the next 3 to 6 months; in an African-American woman, they will be revealed as only slightly darker pigment. Excessive pigment on the face and neck (chloasma) and on the abdomen (linea nigra) will be barely detectable in 6 weeks' time. If **diastasis recti** (overstretching and separation of the abdominal musculature) are present, the area will appear slightly indented. If the separation is large, it will appear as a bluish area in the abdominal midline. Modified sit-ups help to strengthen abdominal muscles and return abdominal support to its prepregnant level.

Both the abdominal wall and the ligaments that support the uterus that were obviously stretched during pregnancy usually require the full 6 weeks of the puerperium to return to their former state.

> ✔ **CHECKPOINT QUESTIONS**
>
> 5. By the fourth day postpartum, where on her abdomen would you expect to palpate a woman's fundus?
> 6. How much blood loss does a woman usually experience with a vaginal delivery? What effect does this have on her hemoglobin level?

Effects of Retrogressive Changes

The overall effects of the postpartal changes discussed above are exhaustion and weight loss.

Exhaustion

As soon as birth is completed, the woman experiences total exhaustion. For the last several months of pregnancy, she probably has experienced some difficulty sleeping. Near the end of pregnancy, she was unable to find a comfortable position in bed because of the fetus' activity or the presence of back or leg pain. All during labor, she has eaten very little, if anything, and has worked very hard with little or no sleep. Now she has sleep hunger, which may make it difficult for her to cope with new experiences and stressful situations (Perla, 2002).

Weight Loss

The rapid diuresis and diaphoresis during the second to fifth day postpartum will ordinarily result in a weight loss of an additional 5 lb (2 kg to 4 kg) over the approximately 12 lb (5.8 kg) that the woman lost at birth. Lochia flow will cause an additional 2- to 3-lb (1-kg) loss for a total weight loss of about 19 lb. Additional weight loss is most dependent on the amount of pregnancy weight gain and whether the woman takes active measures to lose weight. It is also influenced by nutrition, exercise, and breastfeeding. The weight a woman reaches at 6 weeks post birth will be her baseline postpartal weight. In many women, this is above their prepregnancy weight.

Vital Sign Changes

Vital sign changes in the postpartum period reflect the internal adjustments occurring as the woman's body begins its return to its prepregnant state.

Temperature

Temperature is always taken orally or tympanically during the puerperium because of the danger of vaginal contamination and the discomfort involved in rectal intrusion.

A woman may show a slight increase in temperature during the first 24 hours of the puerperium due to dehydration occurring during labor. If she receives adequate fluid during the first 24 hours, the temperature will return to normal. As stated, most women are thirsty immediately after birth and so are eager to drink. Drinking a large quantity of fluid is not a problem unless the woman is nauseated from a birth anesthetic.

Any woman whose oral temperature rises above 100.4°F (38°C), excluding the first 24-hour period, is considered by criteria of the Joint Commission on Maternal Welfare to be febrile, and a postpartal infection should be suspected.

Occasionally, on the third or fourth day postpartum, when the breasts fill with milk, the woman's temperature rises for a period of hours because of the increased vascular activity involved. If the elevation in temperature lasts more than a few hours, however, infection is a more likely reason for the fever. Infection is a major cause of postpartal mortality and morbidity, and nurses play a major role in early detection of postpartum infections.

Pulse

The pulse rate during the postpartal period is generally slightly slower than normal. During pregnancy, the distended uterus obstructed the amount of venous blood returning to the heart. After birth, stroke volume increases to accommodate the increased blood volume returning to the heart. The increased stroke volume reduces the pulse rate to between 60 and 70 bpm. As diuresis diminishes, the blood volume and blood pressure fall, and the pulse rate increases accordingly. By the end of the first week, the pulse rate has returned to normal.

Pulse rate should be evaluated carefully in the postpartal period because a rapid and thready pulse is a possible sign of hemorrhage. Be certain that you are comparing the woman's pulse rate with the normal range of the postpartal period, not with the normal pulse rate in the general population. Otherwise, you may misinterpret the finding.

Blood Pressure

Blood pressure should be monitored carefully during the postpartal period because it also can indicate bleeding. A woman's blood pressure reading should be compared with that of her prepregnancy level, rather than with standard blood pressure ranges, because blood pressure can vary in pregnant women.

A reading above 140 mm Hg systolic or 90 mm Hg diastolic may indicate the development of postpartal pregnancy-induced hypertension, an unusual but serious complication of the puerperium (see Chapter 15). Oxytocics, drugs frequently administered during the postpartal period to achieve uterine contraction, cause contraction of all smooth muscle, including blood vessels. Consequently, these drugs can increase blood pressure. Always take a blood pressure before administering one of these agents. If blood pressure is over 140/90, withhold the agent and notify the physician or nurse-midwife to prevent hypertension and possible cerebrovascular accident.

A major complication of acute blood loss is orthostatic hypotension, or dizziness that occurs on standing, which results from the lack of adequate blood volume to maintain nourishment of brain cells. To test if a woman will be susceptible to this, assess her blood pressure and pulse with her lying supine. Next, raise the head of the bed fully upright, wait 2 or 3 minutes, and then reassess these values. If pulse rate is increased more than 20 bpm and blood pressure is 15 to 20 mm Hg lower than formerly, the woman will be susceptible to dizziness and possibly falling when she ambulates. Advise her to sit up slowly and "dangle" on the side of her bed before attempting to walk. If she notices obvious dizziness on sitting upright, support her during ambulation to avoid the possibility of her falling. Inform the physician or nurse-midwife of these findings. Caution her not to attempt to walk carrying her newborn until her cardiovascular status adjusts better to her blood loss.

WHAT IF? Your client, Joan Cooper, is now 12 hours postpartum. She has an oral temperature of 99°F (40.2°C) and is uncomfortable from profuse diaphoresis and extreme fatigue. What actions would you take?

Progressive Changes

Two physiologic changes during the puerperium involve progressive changes or the building of new tissue. Because new tissue building requires good nutrition, strict dieting that limits cell-building ability is contraindicated in the first 6 weeks after childbirth.

Lactation

The formation of breast milk (lactation) is initiated in a woman whether or not she plans to breastfeed.

Early in pregnancy, the increased estrogen level produced by the placenta stimulated the growth of milk glands and growth in breast size from accumulated fluid and extra adipose tissue. For the first 2 days postpartum, the average woman notices little change in her breasts from the way they were during pregnancy. Since midway through pregnancy, she has been secreting colostrum, a thin, watery, pre-lactation secretion. She continues to excrete this fluid the first 2 days postpartum. On the third day, her breasts tend to become full and feel tense or tender as milk forms within breast ducts.

Breast milk forms in response to the fall in estrogen and progesterone levels that follows delivery of the placenta (which causes an increase in prolactin and stimulates milk production). When the production of milk begins, the milk ducts become distended. Nipple secretion changes to bluish white, the typical color of breast milk. The breasts become fuller, larger, and firmer. In many women, breast distention becomes marked, often accompanied by a feeling of heat or throbbing pain. Breast tissue may appear reddened, its appearance simulating that of an acute inflammatory or infectious process. The distention is not limited to the milk ducts but occurs in the surrounding tissue as well, because blood and lymph enter the area to contribute fluid to the formation of milk. This feeling of tension in the breasts on the third or fourth day postpartum is termed **primary engorgement.** It fades as the infant begins effective sucking and empties the breasts of milk. Whether milk production continues depends on nipple stimulation (which releases oxytocin), the infant sucking at the breasts, use of a breast pump, and the ability of milk to come forward in the breasts (a let-down reflex). Whether women continue to breastfeed after hospital discharge is influenced by such factors as employment, personal habits, and how important they view breastfeeding to be (Milligan et al., 2000). Postpartum care of breasts and breastfeeding are discussed in Chapter 24.

Return of Menstrual Flow

With the delivery of the placenta, the production of placental estrogen and progesterone is no longer available to the woman; this decrease in hormones causes a rise in the production of FSH by the pituitary and, therefore, with only a slight delay, the return of ovulation. This will initiate prepregnancy menstrual cycles.

If the woman is not breastfeeding, she can expect her menstrual flow to return in 6 to 10 weeks after birth. If she is breastfeeding, menstrual flow may not return for 3 or 4 months or, in some women, for the entire lactation period. The absence of a menstrual flow, however, does not guarantee that a woman will not conceive during this time. She may ovulate well before menstruation returns.

NURSING CARE OF THE WOMAN AND FAMILY IN THE FIRST 24 HOURS POSTPARTUM

Women usually remain in a birthing or recovery room for the first hour postpartum for careful assessment. After this initial hour, they are encouraged to shower, are taught perineal care, and then remain in the room as a postpartal patient or are transferred to a postpartal room. The most dangerous hour in childbearing has passed. Box 22-1 highlights an appropriate outcome and intervention for the postpartal woman using the terminology from the Nursing Outcomes Classification (NOC) and Nursing Interventions Classification (NIC).

A woman's care must be completed conscientiously because during the entire first 24 hours after birth, the uterus is prone to hemorrhaging until the myometrial vessels have healed. For a couple giving birth at home, one of the worries is that they will not appreciate how dangerous a time this is for the mother. With attention focused more on the newborn than the mother, postpartal hemorrhage could occur. In the hospital, various health care personnel may be involved in caring for the woman. Be sure that all members of the health care team are knowledgeable about this danger as well (see Focus on Multidisciplinary Care).

Assessment

Health History

As with all health assessment, postpartal assessment begins with history taking. Technical aspects of pregnancy, labor, and birth can be learned from the woman's pregnancy, labor, and birth chart. Most of this information is best obtained from the woman, however, because this supplies not only information on events of her pregnancy or labor but also her emotions and impressions about them. If you

BOX 22.1

NURSING OUTCOMES AND NURSING INTERVENTIONS CLASSIFICATION: THE POSTPARTAL WOMAN

NOC: Maternal Status, Postpartum

Maternal status, postpartum is defined as the condition and behaviors indicating maternal well-being from delivery of the placenta to completion of involution (Johnson, Maas, & Moorhead, 2000). Some specific indicators suggesting achievement of this outcome include the following:

- Temperature, heart rate, and blood pressure within expected range
- Uterine fundal height and lochia characteristics as expected
- Urinary and bowel elimination status within expected range
- Evidence of perineal healing
- Physical activity and endurance within expected range

NIC: Postpartal Care

Postpartal care is defined as the monitoring and management of the patient who has recently given birth (McCloskey & Bulechek, 2000). Some important activities involved when implementing this intervention include:

- Monitoring vital signs, lochia (character, amount, odor, and presence of clots), fundal height, and status of episiotomy
- Gently massaging fundus until firm, as needed
- Reinforcing appropriate perineal hygiene techniques
- Applying ice to perineum to minimize swelling
- Administering analgesics PRN
- Encouraging early ambulation and beginning postpartal exercises with resumption of normal activities as tolerated
- Monitoring for symptoms of postpartum depression
- Determining how patient feels about changes in body after delivery
- Providing anticipatory guidance about sexuality and family planning
- Scheduling follow-up examinations for newborn and mother
- Performing discharge teaching
- Arranging for follow-up home care if necessary

FOCUS ON MULTIDISCIPLINARY CARE

Unlicensed assistive personnel may be called upon to obtain vital signs and help with ambulating, bathing, and perineal care, and providing comfort measures. When delegating tasks to unlicensed assistive personnel, be certain that tasks are within their capability to perform. Advise caregivers to wear gloves to protect against contact with body fluids when assessing women's perineum and lochia; applying ice packs or topical anesthetic sprays to the perineum; changing perineal or breast pads; assessing the breasts if there is leakage of colostrum or milk; and handling clothing, perineal pads, and/or bedding contaminated with lochia.

For women's and infants' safety, remind caregivers to support women the first time they are out of bed because they grow lightheaded easily from blood loss at delivery; always take women's temperature by the oral or tympanic route to avoid perineal trauma; and remind women not to leave their newborn unattended. Even newborns can roll over far enough to fall off a bed or counter.

Other health care providers may also be involved in the woman's care. For example, if physical therapy is involved, help the therapists to schedule visits at times so that they don't interfere with breastfeeding or the woman's rest.

previously cared for the woman during labor and birth, it is unnecessary to obtain this information again.

Family Profile. Information needed includes age, support persons, other children, type of housing and community setting, occupation, education level, and socioeconomic level. This information is necessary to evaluate the impact that this new child will have on the woman and her family. It lays a foundation for teaching of self- and child care that is specific to her knowledge level and needs.

Pregnancy History. Information needed includes para and gravida (and the reason for any discrepancy), expected date of birth, whether the pregnancy was planned, and problems or complications such as spotting or hypertension of pregnancy. This information helps you to know the woman's potential for bonding, because an unplanned pregnancy or complications arising during pregnancy may interfere greatly with this.

Labor and Birth History. The length of labor, position of fetus, type of birth, any analgesia and anesthesia used, problems during labor such as fetal distress, supine hypotension syndrome, and perineal sutures are all important information to gather. This information helps plan for necessary procedures.

Infant Data. The sex and weight of the infant, any difficulty at birth, such as the need for resuscitation, plans to breastfeed or formula feed, and any congenital anomalies present are the major facts to obtain. This information helps you to plan care for the infant and promote bonding with the parents.

Postpartal Course. Ask about general health; activity level since birth; a description of lochia; presence of perineal, abdominal, or breast pain; difficulty with elimination; success with infant feeding; and response of her support person to parenting. This information helps in planning anticipatory guidance for home care.

Laboratory Data

Women routinely have a hemoglobin and hematocrit level done 12 to 24 hours after birth to determine whether blood loss at birth has left them anemic. If the hemoglobin is below 10 g/100 mL, supplementary iron is usually prescribed. Take note of the laboratory reports on postpartal women and make certain that any abnormal finding, such as low hemoglobin, is brought to the attention of the physician or nurse-midwife. The responsibilities of the new mother coupled with the additional burden of an undetected low hemoglobin level can severely tax her energy levels.

If the woman required catheterization during labor or had a urinary tract infection during pregnancy, a urinalysis or urine culture may be ordered in the postpartal period. A urine specimen should be obtained during this time with a clean-catch technique using a sterile cotton ball tucked in the vagina introitus to prevent lochia from contaminating the specimen. In some cases, it may be necessary to obtain a specimen by urinary catheterization.

FOCUS ON CULTURAL COMPETENCE

In the United States, the postpartal period is generally regarded as a time of wellness; early ambulation and eating a varied diet are encouraged. In other cultures, the period after childbirth may be regarded primarily as a time of rest. Cultural differences involving dietary restrictions, activity levels, and taboos and rituals are not uncommon. In traditional Japan, for example, a woman would remain inside for as long as 100 days; she might not bathe or wash her hair for a week after birth. In Korea, women avoid exposure to cold, including air conditioning, and try to eat warm foods only. Mexican women traditionally follow these same actions of keeping warm, avoiding baths, and eating only warm foods to "dry the womb."

Assessing women in the postpartal period for cultural variations is important because such variations explain why a woman might be reluctant to ambulate or why she leaves a lunch of cold salad and iced tea uneaten although she said she was hungry.

Physical Assessment

During early labor, a woman is given a fairly complete physical examination. During the immediate postpartal period, repetition of this complete examination is not necessary. However, crucial assessments examining particular aspects of health such as an estimation of nutrition and fluid state, energy level, presence or absence of pain, breast health, fundal height and consistency, lochia amount and character, perineal integrity, and circulatory adequacy are required.

General Appearance. A woman's general appearance in the postpartal period reveals a great deal about her energy level, her self-esteem, and whether she is moving into the taking-hold phase of recovery. Before assessing the client, ask her to void so she has an empty bladder. Observe how much energy she uses when reaching for her robe or walking to the bathroom—does she struggle or move listlessly, or does she accomplish this task quickly? Observe for a cringing expression or hand pressure against her abdomen that suggests pain on movement. Observe whether she has combed her hair, applied makeup, and put on her own clothing or an agency gown. Many women choose to sleep in an agency gown to prevent getting lochia stains on their own clothing, but a woman who is pleased with herself, her pregnancy, and her birth experience is usually anxious to wear her own clothing and "fuss" with her appearance within an hour after birth. A woman who is extremely exhausted or depressed probably will not bother with her appearance (Farrington & Ward, 2000). Keep in mind, however, that a woman whose labor progressed rapidly and who came to the health care agency as an emergency admission may not have had time to pack a comb and brush or her own clothing. Cultural variations will also affect appearances (see Focus on Cultural Competence).

Hair. Palpate the woman's hair to determine its firmness and strength. When a diet is deficient in nutrients, hair becomes listless and "stringy." A woman who had good nutritional intake during pregnancy has firm, crisp hair. Many women begin to lose a quantity of hair in the postpartal period. During pregnancy, metabolism was increased and hair growth was rapid, with many hairs reaching maturity at the same time. As a woman's body returns to a normal metabolism level, this hair is lost. You may need to assure her that this is not a sign of illness but just another aspect of returning to her prepregnant state.

Face. Assess the woman's face for evidence of edema, most apparent early in the morning because the woman has been lying supine with her head level during the night. Edema is manifested as puffy eyelids or a prominent fold of tissue inferior to the lower eyelid. Normally, this is negligible. However, in the woman who had hypertension of pregnancy, so accumulated excessive fluid, it may be evident. It also will become evident in the woman who is developing postpartal pregnancy-induced hypertension, although this condition is rare.

Eyes. Inspect the color of the inner conjunctiva, normally pink and moist. The conjunctiva of the woman who is anemic from poor pregnancy nutrition or excessive blood loss at birth will have a pale conjunctiva. If the woman is dehydrated, the area will appear dry. Check the hematocrit level of any woman with pale conjunctivae. Be alert to possible variations because of skin color. The conjunctiva always appears lightly shaded in fair-skinned women. Dark-skinned women may have a ruddy conjunctiva appearance even with anemia.

Breasts. Using a bra in the postpartal period supports breast tissue that has increased fluid accumulation in preparation for breastfeeding. It also aids in comfort. Check to make sure that the bra is adequate and comfortable. Properly fitted, the straps should not leave erythemic marks on the shoulders. In addition, it should fit firmly and snugly, but not so tightly as to leave red marks on the skin. Breast tissue increases in size as breast milk forms, so a bra that was adequate during pregnancy may no longer be adequate by the second or third postpartal day. Advise women to buy a nursing bra for the postpartal period that is one to two sizes larger than their pregnancy size to allow for this size increase.

Ask the woman to remove the bra and cover her breasts with a towel or folded sheet to protect modesty. Ask the woman to raise her hands over her head and tuck them under her head as this stretches and thins breast tissue. Inspect and then palpate for breast size, shape, and color.

Breast tissue feels soft on palpation the first and second day. On the third, it feels firm and warm (described as *filling*). On the third or fourth day, breasts appear large and reddened, with taut, shiny skin (engorgement). On palpation, they may feel hard, tense, and painful. Normally, engorgement causes the entire breast to feel warm or appear reddened. If only one portion of a breast is warm or reddened, mastitis or inflammation and, possibly, infection of glands or milk ducts are suggested (Fiorica, 2000).

Occasionally, a firm nodule is detected on palpation. Usually, this is only a temporarily blocked milk duct or milk contained in a gland that is not flowing forward to the nipple. However, the location of the nodule should be noted, reported to the physician or nurse-midwife, and reassessed before discharge. Such blocking of breast milk generally is relieved by the infant sucking. Any nodule needs reassessment, however, because a fibrocystic or malignant growth unrelated to the pregnancy could be present.

Note whether the nipple is normally erect and not inverted. Assess the nipple for a crack, fissure, or presence of caked milk. Avoid squeezing the nipple because this can be painful, especially to sensitive nipples. Unnecessary nipple manipulation also may increase the risk of mastitis by providing a portal for infection (Fiorica, 2000).

Uterus. For uterine assessment, position the client supine so the height of the uterus is not influenced by an elevated position. Observe the woman's abdomen for contour to detect distention and the appearance of striae or a diastasis. If a diastasis is present (appears as a slightly indented, possibly bluish-tinged groove in the midline of the abdomen), measure the width and length by fingerbreadths. Palpate the fundus of the uterus by placing a hand on the base of the uterus just above the symphysis pubis and the other at the umbilicus. Press in and downward with the hand on the umbilicus until you "bump" against a firm globular mass in the abdomen: the uterine fundus (Fig. 22-5). For the first hour after birth, the height of the fundus is at the umbilicus or even slightly above it. Assess the fundus for consistency (firm, soft, or boggy), location (midline), and height. Measure in fingerbreadths (eg, 2 F↓ umbilicus, or 2 cm beneath the umbilicus). Although this measurement seems less scientific than a measurement of the height of the uterus from the pubis, it is the most useful measurement because it shows the gradual decline in size or distance from the umbilicus.

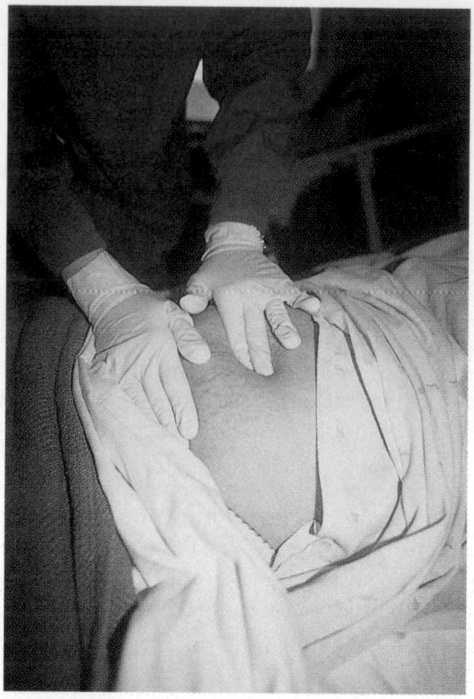

FIGURE 22.5 To palpate the uterus, be certain to place one hand at the base of the uterus. This fundus is about 2 fingerbreadths below the umbilicus.

Never palpate a uterus without supporting the lower segment, because the uterus potentially can invert (and in so doing cause a massive hemorrhage).

Palpating the fundus should not cause pain as long as the action is done gently. If the uterus is not firm on palpation, massage it gently with the examining hand. This generally causes it to contract and become firm immediately. Massage is a gentle rotating motion of the hand. It should never be hard or forceful, lest it be painful to the mother or cause the uterus to expend excess energy. If the fundus does not grow firm with massage, extreme atony, possibly retained placenta fragments, or an excess amount of blood loss may be occurring. Notify the woman's physician or nurse-midwife. Administer oxytocin as ordered PRN. In addition, placing the infant at breast will cause endogenous release of oxytocin and achieve the same effect as oxytocin administration.

If the woman received no oxytocin after birth to help her uterus contract, assess the fundus every 10 to 15 minutes to assist the fundus to contract should it become soft or relaxed during the first hour. If massage appears ineffective, a clot may be present in the cavity of the uterus. The clot may be expressed from the uterus using gentle pressure on the fundus, but only after the uterus has been massaged. If the uterus is totally relaxed, fundal pressure could cause inversion of the uterus, an extremely serious complication that leads to rapid hemorrhage, possibly necessitating an emergency hysterectomy to save the woman's life. Another reason the uterus may not be well contracted is because a rapidly filling bladder is preventing contraction. If contraction remains inadequate, a uterine sonogram may be ordered to help detect any abnormalities.

After the first hour after birth, the uterus may be evaluated for height and consistency less frequently, depending on the institution's policy. By the ninth or tenth day postpartum, the uterus will have become so small that it is no longer palpable above the symphysis pubis.

Lochia. A woman can expect to have lochia for 2 to 6 weeks. Characteristics of normal lochia and the change in pattern from red to pink to white are described in Table 22-1.

During the first hour postpartum, when the fundus is checked every 15 minutes, also remove the mother's perineal pad and evaluate lochia character, amount, color (rubra, serosa, or alba), odor, and presence of any clots. Be certain the pad is not adhering to perineal stitches before removing.

When you turn the woman to inspect her perineum, be sure to check under her buttocks to avoid missing any bleeding that may be pooling below her. If you observe a constant trickle of vaginal flow or the woman is soaking through a pad every 60 minutes, she is losing more than the average amount of blood. She needs to be checked by a physician or nurse-midwife to be certain there is no cervical or vaginal tear.

While the woman is at a health care facility, you need to inspect her lochia discharge once every 15 minutes for the first hour, and then according to the institution's policy. Make certain a woman understands that she must wash her hands after handling pads and must use only her own personal care equipment so she does not contract or spread infection. Demonstrate good role modeling for handwashing and equipment use. Women should be encouraged to change perineal pads frequently as they begin self-care. Lochia is an excellent medium for bacterial growth that could spread through the vagina to the uterus. The presence of constantly wet pads against an episiotomy suture line also slows healing. Often this is not a problem for the woman while she is at a health care facility, but the woman who is trying to save money may try to conserve on the number of pads she uses at home. Be certain she knows not to use tampons until she returns for her postpartal checkup to prevent the risk for infection and toxic shock syndrome. Ensure that women know the criteria for judging the amount and type of normal lochia (see Focus on Family Empowerment earlier in the chapter).

WHAT IF? Your client, Joan Cooper, at 18 hours postpartum states that she has had to change her perineal pad twice in the last 30 minutes because they were saturated. She noticed two large clots on the last pad. What assessment should you first perform on her and why?

Perineum. When lochia is evaluated, the perineum also should be inspected. Ask the woman to turn on her side into a Sims' position with her back toward you. If a midline episiotomy was performed, position the mother on either side. If a mediolateral incision is present, turning so the incision is on the bottom buttock often causes less pain and offers better visibility. Gently lift the upper buttock and inspect the perineum. Observe for ecchymosis, hematoma, erythema, edema, intactness, and presence of drainage or bleeding from any episiotomy stitches.

An episiotomy is usually 1 or 2 in long. However, if a laceration was involved, stitches may extend from the vagina back to the rectum. Rarely, they extend forward toward the urethra. An episiotomy incision is generally fused (edges sealed) by 24 hours after birth; if it is a midline incision, it may be almost invisible because the perineal fold obscures it. A hematoma (blood-filled, protruding sphere) could be present if surface capillaries were broken during the pressure of birth; note this as a potential complication. If there is clotted lochia along the incision, the woman probably needs a review of postpartal perineal care so this does not continue to occur. Before discharge, a woman who has perineal stitches can be taught to lie on her back and view her perineum with a hand-held mirror. Once a day while at home, she should inspect for redness, sloughing of sutures, pus formation, or drainage at the suture line.

After perineal assessment, assess the rectal area for the presence of hemorrhoids. Note the number, appearance, and size in centimeters.

✔ CHECKPOINT QUESTIONS

7. Which hormone is responsible for stimulating milk production?
8. How will normal lochia appear during the first hour postpartum?

NURSING DIAGNOSES AND RELATED INTERVENTIONS

Nursing Diagnosis: Pain related to uterine cramping (afterpains) or perineal sutures

Outcome Identification: Client will report pain at a tolerable level during postpartal period.

Outcome Evaluation: Client states that degree of pain is tolerable; demonstrates knowledge of measures for adequate pain relief.

Provide Pain Relief for Afterpains. Women can be assured that discomfort from afterpains is normal and rarely lasts more than 3 days. If necessary, either ibuprofen (e.g., Motrin), an NSAID effective for relief of afterpains because of its anti-inflammatory properties, or a common analgesic such as acetaminophen (e.g., Tylenol) can be taken for relief. As with any abdominal pain, heat to the abdomen should be avoided because it could cause relaxation of the uterus and subsequent uterine bleeding.

Relieve Muscular Aches. Many women feel sore and aching after labor and birth because of the excessive energy they used for pushing during the pelvic division of labor. They say they feel as if they have "run for miles." The woman may need a mild analgesic such as acetaminophen (Tylenol) for the pain. A backrub is effective for relieving aching shoulders or back. Carefully assess the woman who states she has pain on standing. Pain in the calf of the leg on standing (a position that dorsiflexes the foot) is a sign similar to a Homans' sign suggesting thrombophlebitis (see the section entitled Assess Peripheral Circulation).

Give Episiotomy Care. Although the frequency of performing an episiotomy is decreasing, 30% to 50% of women may still receive one. Sutures for this can be sore and painful. Although relatively small in size, an episiotomy can cause considerable discomfort because the perineum is an extremely tender area. The muscles of the perineum are involved in many activities (sitting, walking, stooping, squatting, bending, urinating, defecating). Thus, an incision in this area causes a great deal of discomfort.

Most women expect labor to be painful. However, they usually do not anticipate the pulling pain from perineal stitches in the postpartal period. This discomfort interferes with their rest and sleep, with eating, and with being able to sit and hold the baby comfortably.

Because the perineal area heals rapidly, women can be assured that this discomfort is normal and, fortunately, does not usually last more than 5 or 6 days. Many physicians and nurse-midwives order a soothing cream or anesthetic spray to be applied to a suture line to reduce discomfort. A cortisone-based cream or sitz bath helps to decrease inflammation and, thus, tension in the area. Because of their cooling effect, witch hazel preparations are a mainstay for relief of both perineal and hemorrhoidal discomfort. A woman may worry that she will experience additional discomfort when the episiotomy sutures are removed. Explain to her that these are made of an absorbable material that will not need to be removed, and usually dissolve within 10 days.

Promote Perineal Exercises. Some women find that carrying out perineal exercises three or four times a day greatly relieves episiotomy discomfort. The exercise consists of contracting and relaxing the muscles of the perineum five to ten times in succession as if trying to stop voiding (Kegel exercises). This improves circulation to the area and so helps decrease edema. When repeated frequently, Kegel exercises help the woman regain her prepregnant muscle tone and form (Meyer et al., 2001).

Administer Cold and Hot Therapy. Applying an ice bag or cold pack to the perineum during the first 24 hours reduces perineal edema and the possibility of hematoma formation, and therefore reduces pain and promotes healing and comfort. Be certain not to place ice or plastic directly on the perineum. Wrap the ice bag first in a towel or disposable pad to decrease the chance of a thermal injury (risk of injury increases because the perineum has decreased sensation from edema). Commercial cold packs combined with perineal pads also are available. Partially filling a rubber glove with ice chips is a low-cost alternative, if latex allergy is not a concern.

Ice to the perineum after the first 24 hours is no longer therapeutic. After this time, healing increases best if circulation to the area is encouraged by the use of heat. Dry heat in the form of a perineal hot pack or moist heat with a sitz bath is an effective way of increasing circulation to the perineum, providing comfort, reducing edema, and promoting healing.

Commercial hot packs that grow warm after they are "cracked" and the chemicals in them are combined are available. Caution women to use a washcloth or gauze square between the pack and their skin to prevent a possible burn when applied.

Administer Sitz Baths. A **sitz bath** is a portable basin that fits on a toilet seat. A reservoir filled with water provides a constant supply of swirling water to the basin. The movement of water soothes healing tissue, decreases inflammation by vasodilation to the area, and therefore effectively reduces discomfort and promotes healing.

Sitz baths usually use water that is maintained at 100°F to 105°F (38°C to 41°C). Be certain the water in the sitz bath is not too hot before you help a woman to use it. The woman will not be sensitive to the temperature because healing surfaces are not good indicators of temperature. This caution applies particularly to the woman who is using an analgesic cream or spray on the perineum or who has a great deal of generalized perineal edema. Both situations make her prone to burns from scalding water unless you act to protect her (see Nursing Procedure 22-1).

A sitz bath should be used three to four times per day for a maximum of 20 minutes each time. Because of the soothing effect of the warm water and the sitting position, the woman may feel extremely tired and unsteady on her feet after using a sitz bath and may need help in getting back to bed.

Provide Pain Management. Several topical medications with Xylocaine bases, such as gels or sprays, are available to relieve perineal pain. These are applied to the incision line with a clean gauze square or via a spray. Because of their anesthetic action, they instantly reduce incision line pain. Be certain the woman understands how to use any cream or suture-line spray ordered for her. Tucks, a commercial form of soft pads impregnated with witch hazel, which can be tucked between the perineum and a sanitary pad, also are effective in relieving perineal pain. Some women doubt the efficacy of suture-line medications or worry that applying the cream will hurt more than not applying it. They may need extra encouragement to try these helpful aids.

Many women who have had an episiotomy require an oral or parenteral analgesic to relieve their perineal discomfort. Most physicians and nurse-midwives order a moderate strength analgesic such as propoxyphene/acetaminophen (Darvocet) or codeine for the first 24 hours, then a milder one such as acetaminophen for the remainder of the first week. Ibuprofen also is widely used. Aspirin is not used routinely for pain during the postpartal period because it interferes with blood clotting and may increase the woman's risk for hemorrhage from the denuded placental site (Karch, 2001).

Nursing Diagnosis: Risk for infection (uterine) related to lochia and episiotomy

Outcome Identification: Client will remain free of any symptoms of infection during postpartal period.

Outcome Evaluation: Client's temperature remains below 100.4°F; no redness or abnormal discharge is present at an episiotomy line; lochia without foul odor.

Provide Perineal Care. Every woman needs attention to perineal cleanliness in the postpartal period to prevent infection (Cunningham et al., 2001). Women are particu-

NURSING PROCEDURE 22.1: SITZ BATHS

Purpose
To aid healing of the perineum through application of moist heat

Procedure	Principle
1. Wash your hands; identify client and explain procedure.	1. Handwashing prevents the spread of infection; identification ensures that procedure is performed on correct client, thus promoting safety; explanation assists in alleviating any anxiety.
2. Assess client's condition; ascertain whether client is able to ambulate to bathroom; assist and modify as necessary.	2. A sitz bath can make a woman feel lightheaded, increasing her risk of injury. Fatigue and exhaustion may interfere with client's ability to ambulate or tolerate procedure, also increasing her risk for injury.
3. Assemble equipment, including sitz bath, clean towel, perineal pad.	3. Organization of equipment increases efficiency of the procedure.
4. Place sitz bath on toilet seat. Fill collecting bag with warm water at a temperature of 100°F to 105°F (38°C to 41°C). Hang the bag overhead so a steady stream of water will flow from the bag, through the tubing, and into the basin.	4. Using correct temperature of water eliminates risk of thermal injury. Adequate flow of warm water increases circulation to the perineum, thereby reducing inflammation and aiding healing.

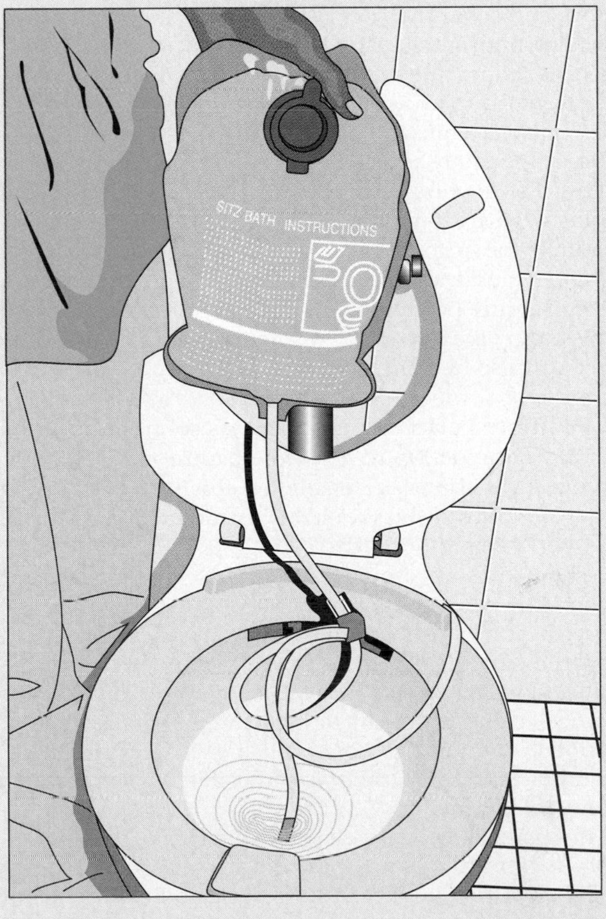

(continued)

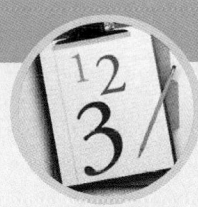

Procedure	Principle
5. Assist client with ambulating to bathroom; help with removal of perineal pad from front to back. Assist client to sit in basin.	5. Assisting ambulation minimizes risk of injury. Removing pad from front to back minimizes risk of infection transmission. Proper placement ensures effectiveness of treatment.
6. Instruct client to use clamp on tubing to regulate water flow; use robe or blankets to prevent chilling and provide for privacy. Have call bell within reach.	6. Continuous swirling water aids in reducing edema and promoting comfort. Privacy enhances self-esteem. Quick, easy access to call bell allows for prompt intervention should problems arise.
7. After 20 minutes, assist client with drying perineum and applying clean pad (holding pad by the bottom side or ends).	7. After 20 minutes, heat is no longer therapeutic because vasoconstriction occurs. Proper handling of pad prevents contamination and possible risk of infection.
8. Assist client with ambulating back to room.	8. Client may become fatigued from the procedure or lightheaded from the warm water, increasing her risk of falling.
9. Evaluate client's tolerance and response to procedure; ask client to report how she feels. Institute health teaching, such as continuing sitz baths when at home.	9. Evaluation assists with determining effectiveness of procedure and making any changes. Health teaching helps to promote continuity of care after discharge.
10. Record completion of procedure, condition of perineum, and client's condition and response.	10. Documentation provides additional means for evaluation of care and client outcomes.

larly prone to this because lochia, if allowed to dry and harden on the vulva and perineum, furnishes a bed for bacterial growth. Because the vagina lies in close proximity to the rectum, there is also always the danger that bacteria will spread from the rectum to the vagina and cause uterine infection. Interruption in skin integrity from an episiotomy also increases the client's risk for infection.

Perineal care should be done as part of the daily bath and after each voiding or bowel movement. If a woman is on bedrest during the first hour after birth, you will need to provide perineal care for her. As soon as she is ambulatory, you can instruct her to perform it herself. Perineal care should be a procedure that is easy to learn and not time consuming, so the woman can spend most of her time with her new child, not completing a complicated ritual of care.

Before beginning perineal care, wash your own hands and pull on clean gloves to prevent the risk of infection transmission. Place a plastic-covered pad under the woman's buttocks to protect the bed during the procedure. With the woman lying in a supine position, remove the perineal pad from the front to back; the direction is important in preventing the portion of the pad that has touched the rectal area from sliding forward to contaminate the vaginal opening.

Perineal care is a clean but not a sterile procedure. Agencies differ as to the cleansing that is done and the articles and solutions used. If actual washing is to be done, use a clean gauze square or a clean portion of a washcloth with soap and water for each stroke, always washing from front to back, from the pubis toward the rectum. Rinse the area in the same manner and dry.

A second common method is to spray the perineum with clear tap water from a spray bottle. Be certain that none of the solution enters the vagina, because it might be a source of contamination. The labia have a tendency to close and cover the vaginal opening, which will prevent solution from entering the vagina. Do not separate the labia; instead, allow them to perform this protective function. Spray gently to avoid splashing any blood-tinged solution on yourself (to guard against contacting body secretions). Direct the spray toward the front of the perineum and allow it to flow from front to back. If the solution is to be sprayed with the woman lying on her back, the flow will naturally be from front to back because of gravity.

It may be advantageous to have the woman turn on her side in a Sims' position to permit better visualization of the episiotomy area. In some women, better cleaning of this area can also be done in this position.

Promote Perineal Self-Care. As soon as the woman is allowed to get up to go to the bathroom (if her infant was born without an anesthetic, this is within the first hour after birth), she should be instructed in how to carry out her own perineal care.

The bathroom should have an area close to the toilet where the woman can place the equipment she needs for care: a spray bottle, sponges to dry, her clean pad, and so forth. Instruct her on how to remove the soiled perineal pad and where to dispose of it. Remind her of the importance of using any cream or medication that has been prescribed. Caution her not to flush the toilet until she is standing upright. Otherwise, the flushing water might spray the perineum.

If women are given a clear explanation of why perineal care is important, they perform it well. Self-care, however, does not eliminate your responsibility for checking the woman's perineum to ascertain its condition and the amount and type of lochia flow. By continuing with these assessments, you remain the woman's first line of defense against postpartal complications such as infection and hemorrhage.

✔ CHECKPOINT QUESTIONS

9. What is the purpose of applying ice to the perineum of a postpartal woman?
10. Name three factors related to the perineum of a postpartal client that predispose her to infection.

Nursing Diagnosis: Disturbed sleep pattern related to exhaustion from and excitement of childbirth

Outcome Identification: Client will sleep a sufficient amount to feel rested during postpartal period.

Outcome Evaluation: Client states she feels rested during postpartal period.

After birth, a woman is a paradox. She is excited. She has a baby and she wants to hold and be with this new person in her life. She wants to talk to her support person about the experience, their child, and their future. At the same time, she is exhausted and so usually falls asleep instantly.

Allow the woman to have time with her expanded family in the birthing room immediately after the baby's birth. If the father did not watch the birth for some reason, allow time for mother, father, and baby to be together as soon as possible. After this, rest should be encouraged.

Promote Rest in the Early Postpartal Period. Few women are prepared for the degree of fatigue they experience after childbirth. All procedures should be done swiftly and gently to allow as much time for sleep as possible. If a woman has discomfort from hemorrhoids, perineal stitches, or afterpains, she needs the cause of the discomfort relieved so she can rest comfortably or sleep.

Some women experience shaking chills immediately after or within a half hour of birth. This is due in part to the pressure changes in the abdomen that occur with reduction in the bulk of the uterus and temperature readjustment in response to the diaphoresis of labor. It also may result from the exhilaration they are feeling combined with exhaustion. In any event, shaking chills at this point are common. Reassure the woman of this to prevent her from attributing them to a developing cold or infection.

Covering the woman with a warm blanket, offering her a warm drink if she is not nauseated from an analgesic, and assuring her that the occurrence is normal are usually enough to make the chills transient and allow her to fall into a sound, much-needed sleep. Most women will then sleep for at least an hour.

Although a woman may choose any position to sleep, she may enjoy being able to sleep on her stomach, something she might not have been able to do during pregnancy.

Promote Rest Throughout the Puerperium. The importance of rest throughout the puerperium cannot be stressed enough. As long as the woman is in the health care facility, time for naps should be provided. Discharge instructions should include suggestions for getting adequate rest while at home. This may prove difficult for many women. They have a newborn who wakes at least twice a night and relatives and friends who come to see the baby during the day (Lee et al., 2000).

Many women do not realize how long it will take to fully return to their previous level of functioning. When families were closely knit and neighborhoods were smaller, a new mother usually had someone in her family or neighborhood to look after the baby while she napped. Today, many couples do not have family or close friends nearby. If the parents have not thought through this problem before birth, you can help them look at their situation and see what is available to them. Perhaps the woman's mother, a sister, her partner's mother, or another relative could come and stay with them for a short time, such as the first week. Perhaps the husband could take a week off from work or school to help out at home. Many employment benefit programs provide for this time. If none of these solutions seems appropriate, the couple might appreciate being given the name of a community service agency that supplies homemakers on a short-term basis. A referral to a community health agency for an early home visit is common.

The woman without support has many demands for her new role—being a mother instead of a daughter; a mother as well as a wife; a mother of three, not two. If she is overcome by sleep hunger, her judgment and sense of balance may be blurred. Extreme fatigue is associated with postpartal depression (Farrington & Ward, 2000).

Nursing Diagnosis: Risk for bathing/hygiene self-care deficit related to exhaustion from childbirth

Outcome Identification: Client will meet own self-care hygiene needs during the postpartal period.

Outcome Evaluation: Client takes daily responsibility for own hygiene. Client appears clean, dressed, and well groomed.

After childbirth, women often report that their hospital or birthing center room is being kept too warm; to prove it, they point out how heavily they are perspiring. Postpartal rooms often are kept warm so newborns will be comfortable, but the profuse perspiration the woman is experiencing normally comes from the body's attempt to regulate fluid, not from the heat of the environment.

The woman can be reassured that sweating is a normal postpartal event that helps to bring her body back to its prepregnant state. If she has profuse diaphoresis, particularly at night, she usually prefers a hospital gown to one of her own. She may need frequent gown changes to be comfortable and not become chilled.

A daily shower is refreshing. Be certain to accompany a woman for a shower on her first postpartal day because she often is more fatigued than she realizes. Standing under warm water may also make her dizzy, making it difficult for her to walk safely back to bed.

Formerly, women were not allowed to take tub baths after birth for fear that bacteria from the bath water would enter the vagina and cause infection. There appears to be little evidence that this is a real danger, so if the woman wants to bathe instead of shower, she may do so.

Nursing Diagnosis: Imbalanced nutrition, less than body requirements, related to lack of knowledge about postpartal needs

Outcome Identification: Client will ingest an adequate diet during the postpartal period.

Outcome Evaluation: Client ingests a 2200- to 2700-kcal diet and drinks 6 to 8 glasses of fluid daily.

Postpartal menu planning should include a diet of between 2200 and 2300 calories daily. Foods should be high in protein and the vitamins and minerals needed for good tissue repair. An adequate supply of roughage is important to help restore the peristaltic action of the bowel. The woman who is breastfeeding needs an additional 500 calories (a 2700-kcal diet) and an additional 500 mL of fluid (these may be from the same source) in her diet to encourage the production of high-quality breast milk. Most mothers are hungry during the immediate postpartal period and consume an adequate diet without urging.

On discharge from the health care facility, the woman needs to be instructed to continue to eat a nutritious diet. Some women become too fatigued during their first weeks at home to prepare adequate meals. Neglecting to eat properly leads to more fatigue and ultimately an even less nutritious diet.

If the woman has any prenatal vitamins or supplementary iron preparations left over from pregnancy, she should, as a rule, continue to take them until her supply is used up. If she needs further supplements, her physician or nurse-midwife will prescribe them for her either on discharge or when she returns for her postpartum checkup.

Promote Adequate Fluid Intake. The rapid diuresis and diaphoresis during the second to fifth day postpartum will ordinarily result in a weight loss of an additional 5 lb over the approximate 12 lb the woman lost at birth.

Women often feel thirsty during this period of rapid fluid loss and want additional fluid. It seems a paradox that while the body is ridding itself of unwanted fluid, it should also demand fluid. Part of this paradox stems from the woman's having had little to drink during a part of her labor. She may say immediately after birth, "I don't think I'll ever get enough to drink again." Part of the need for fluid stems from the increased amount of nitrogen being released from catabolized uterine cells. The woman needs to increase her fluid intake to rid her body of these wastes.

Some women need to be encouraged to drink adequate fluid in the first few days postpartum because they are restricting fluid in the hope of preventing their breasts from becoming engorged. Other mothers are beginning diets that they hope will bring their bodies more quickly back to their nonpregnant slim state. As mentioned previously, fluid restriction does little to thwart breast engorgement. Unless the woman is extremely obese, this is not a good time for dieting. The postpartal period is a time of rebuilding and readjusting, for which a woman needs both ample nourishment and adequate fluid intake. For this reason, encourage her to drink at least three to four 8-oz glasses of fluid a day (six to eight if breastfeeding).

Nursing Diagnosis: Risk for impaired urinary elimination or constipation related to loss of bladder and bowel sensation after childbirth

Outcome Identification: Client will remain free of any elimination problems during the postpartal period.

Outcome Evaluation: Client voids over 30 mL/h without urinary retention, beginning an hour after birth, and has a bowel movement by 4 days postpartum. No urinary incontinence noted.

Promote Urinary Elimination. Because the diuresis of the postpartal period begins almost immediately after birth, the woman's bladder begins filling almost immediately. A full bladder puts pressure on the uterus and may interfere with effective uterine contraction. An overdistended bladder may damage bladder function. (See Focus on Nursing Care Planning.)

Encourage the woman to walk to the bathroom and void at the end of the first hour postpartum. Some women have too much perineal edema to be able to void this early. Women with episiotomies may be reluctant to void because they know that acid urine against the sutures will sting. However, many women will have enough residual effect of epidural, spinal, or pudendal anesthesia at this time so that voiding is painless. Assist by providing privacy (but remain in close proximity because the woman may become dizzy if this is her first time out of bed), running water at the sink, or offering the woman a drink of water. Pouring warm tap water over the vulva, if consistent with the agency's policy for perineal care, also may help.

If the woman's bladder is distended and she is unable to void, she will need to be catheterized. Most women, however, do not have this much filling at this time. If she still has not voided by 4 to 8 hours after birth, bladder distention usually is present.

Because the perineum is edematous after birth, the vulva in postpartal women appears out of proportion. This makes it difficult to locate the urethra for urinary catheterization. Be certain that, in catheterization, you do not invade the vagina by mistake and thereby carry contamination to the denuded uterus. Occasionally, because of poor tone, the bladder in some women retains large amounts of residual urine after voiding. This urine harbors bacteria, which may cause bladder infection.

The first voiding after birth should be measured to detect if urinary retention is occurring. Whether the bladder is emptying also may be judged by measuring fundal height and position (a full bladder pushes the fundus up or to the side) or by palpating or percussing bladder prominence in the lower abdomen. If the woman is voiding less than 100 mL at a time or has a displaced uterus or a palpable bladder, her physician or nurse-midwife may order catheterization for residual urine after a voiding. Be certain you know, before catheterization, how much residual there must be before you leave the catheter in place. As a rule, if

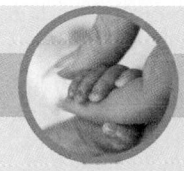

FOCUS ON *Nursing Care Planning*

A POSTPARTAL CLIENT

A client is 6 hours postpartum following birth of her fourth child. She states, "I haven't urinated since before I had the baby."

Assessment: 6 hours postpartum; labor and delivery without incident. Abdomen soft. Uterus ½ finger breadth above umbilicus, soft, and displaced to the right. Moderate lochia rubra. Midline episiotomy with intact sutures. Perineal edema present. Bladder firm on palpation above symphysis pubis. Resonant on percussion. Vital signs within acceptable parameters.

Nursing Diagnosis: Impaired urinary elimination related to perineal edema and decreased bladder tone from fetal head pressure during labor and birth

Outcome Identification: Client will void adequate amount within the next hour on her own.

Outcome Evaluation: Client states possible reason for inability to void; demonstrates measures to promote voiding; voids over 100 mL.

Interventions	Rationale
1. Assess client's overall intake, both intravenously and orally, since last voiding.	1. Assessment of overall intake provides information about the degree of bladder distention that may be occurring.
2. Assist client with ambulating to the bathroom and sitting on the commode to void.	2. Assisting with ambulation maintains safety should the client experience orthostatic hypotension from blood and fluid loss during labor and birth. Sitting on the commode allows optimal relaxation of the external sphincter and perineal muscles to facilitate voiding.
3. Run water in the sink, allow client to place her hand in warm water, and/or have client pour warm water over vulva, and encourage her to relax.	3. The sound or feel of running water coupled with relaxation can help stimulate voiding.
4. Allow client time and privacy while staying nearby.	4. Providing time and privacy allows the client some control over situation. Being nearby ensures client safety.
5. Assess amount of urine voided and reassess fundal height and position.	5. Measuring amount of urine voided and assessing fundal height and position provides evidence about the degree of bladder emptying. Retention of urine in the bladder also predisposes to infection.
6. If client is still unable to void, notify the health care provider and prepare to catheterize the client.	6. Bladder distention interferes with uterine involution and, if allowed to persist, may result in permanent loss of bladder tone.
7. Once voiding pattern is reestablished, instruct client in Kegel exercises.	7. Kegel exercises help strengthen perineal muscles.

the residual urine is over 150 mL, the catheter is left in place for 12 to 24 hours to give the bladder time to regain its normal tone and to begin to function efficiently.

Professional judgment is necessary here. A woman may report that she is out of bed and using the bathroom to void. Only a person with knowledge of the extent of the diuresis being accomplished and the amount that should be voided during this time is able to estimate whether bladder function is adequate.

Fortunately, for most women who must be catheterized, the procedure needs to be done only once after birth. After another 6 to 8 hours have passed and the bladder has filled again, some of the perineal edema has subsided, the bladder has achieved better tone, and the woman is able to void by herself if helped to the bathroom.

Because catheterization can lead to urinary infection, it should not be used indiscriminately in the postpartal period. On the other hand, it should be done before the woman's bladder is injured or the uterus is displaced and uncontracted and bleeding results.

As many as 50% of women report at least one incidence of urinary incontinence during the postpartal period resulting from poor perineal tone and sensation. Kegel exercises are helpful in strengthening perineal muscles and eliminating incontinence.

Prevent Constipation. Many women have difficulty moving their bowels during the first week of the puerperium, a condition that can be worrisome and uncomfortable.

Constipation tends to occur because of relaxation of the abdominal wall and the intestine now that it is no longer compressed by the bulky uterus. For a bowel movement, the abdominal wall must exert pressure. In its relaxed state, the pressure is not strong enough to be effective. Also, if hemorrhoids or perineal stitches are present, the woman may decline to try to move her bowels for fear of pain.

To prevent constipation, many women will have a stool softener such as docusate sodium prescribed, beginning with the first day after birth (see Focus on Pharmacology). If the woman has not moved her bowels by the third day, a mild laxative or cathartic may be ordered. There is danger in giving cathartics before the third day. The resulting increase in intestinal activity could cause uterine irritation and lead to insufficient contraction.

Early ambulation, a good diet with adequate roughage, and an adequate fluid intake all aid in preventing the problem of constipation.

Prevent Development of Hemorrhoids. The pressure of the fetal head on the rectal veins during birth tends to aggravate or produce hemorrhoids (swollen rectal veins). Some women find that the hemorrhoidal discomfort is their chief discomfort in the first few days after birth. The discomfort can be relieved by sitz baths, anesthetic sprays, witch hazel or astringent preparations, or preparations such as hydrocortisone acetate (Proctofoam). Gently replacing hemorrhoidal tissue manually may be attempted. Assuming a Sims' position several times a day aids in good venous return of the rectal area and also reduces discomfort. Increased fluid and the administration of a stool softener prevent the development of hardened stool, which can irritate hemorrhoids.

FOCUS ON PHARMACOLOGY

Docusate Sodium (Colace, Surfak)

Action: Docusate sodium is a stool softener used in the postpartal period to prevent constipation. It works by lowering the surface tension of feces, allowing water and lipids to penetrate the stool and soften it.

Pregnancy risk category: C

Dosage: 50–100 mg PO daily.

Possible adverse effects: Occasional abdominal pain and diarrhea

Nursing Implications:

- Encourage women to swallow the medication with a full glass of water or juice
- Instruct women in use of high-fiber foods to encourage elimination
- Encourage activity to promote intestinal motility

Nursing Diagnosis: Risk for ineffective peripheral tissue perfusion related to immobility and increased estrogen level

Outcome Identification: Client will experience adequate tissue perfusion during postpartal period.

Outcome Evaluation: Client demonstrates negative Homans' sign and absence of erythema or pain in calves of legs.

Assess Peripheral Circulation. To determine whether peripheral circulation is adequate, assess the thigh for skin turgor. Assess for edema at the ankle and over the tibia on the lower leg. Assess for thrombophlebitis by dorsiflexing the woman's ankle and asking her if she notices pain in her calf on that motion (**Homans' sign**). Assess also for redness in the calf area, because thrombophlebitis can be present even with a negative Homans' sign. Continue to check for adequate peripheral circulation once every 8 hours during the woman's health care facility stay. If you suspect thrombophlebitis, do not massage the area—that could cause an emboli.

Be certain to allow a woman to dangle her legs on the edge of the bed for a few minutes to prevent dizziness before she gets up the first time. Then, assist her as needed for the few steps to a nearby bathroom. Remain with her to be certain dizziness doesn't occur. After this, she may be up on her own as she wishes.

Helping the woman out of bed and assisting her to ambulate shortly after birth seem like actions that are inconsistent, given the woman's exhaustion and need for rest. However, women who ambulate quickly feel stronger and healthier by the end of their first week and have fewer bowel, bladder, and circulatory complications such as thrombophlebitis (Fig. 22-6).

Nursing Diagnosis: Pain related to primary breast engorgement

Outcome Identification: Client will experience breast pain that is at a tolerable level during postpartal period.

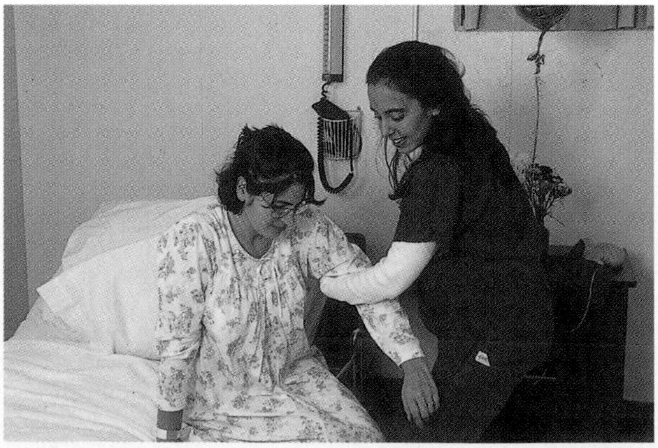

FIGURE 22.6 Ambulating postpartally helps to prevent complications.

Outcome Evaluation: Client states pain from breast engorgement is at a tolerable level.

Prevent/Alleviate Breast Engorgement. If the woman is breastfeeding, encouraging her newborn to suck at the breast is the main treatment for relief of the tenderness and soreness of primary breast engorgement (breastfeeding is discussed in Chapter 24).

Many women find the application of warm compresses or standing under a warm shower beneficial. Good support from a bra offers relief because it prevents unnecessary strain on the supporting muscles of the breasts. Good support also positions the breasts in good alignment and diminishes the amount of engorgement caused by blocked milk ducts. If the woman has not packed a bra in her suitcase, she can usually arrange to have one brought from home.

The woman who is not breastfeeding may experience similar discomfort. When little or no milk is removed from the breasts, however, the accumulation of milk inhibits further milk formation. Therefore, engorgement will subside in about 2 days. Cold compresses, applied to the breasts three or four times a day during the period of engorgement, and/or an oral analgesic provide relief. Wearing a snug-fitting bra or a commercial breast binder and avoiding nipple stimulation may help. Restriction of fluid and pumping milk from the breasts are not effective measures, and are to some degree harmful and should be avoided.

Promote Breast Hygiene. Breast care during the postpartal period is directed toward cleanliness and support. These are the same whether or not the woman is breastfeeding.

The woman should wash her breasts daily with clear water at the time of her bath or shower and then dry them with a soft towel. Soap should be avoided, because soap tends to dry and crack nipples, possibly leading to fissures and breast abscess. It is not necessary for women to wash their breasts more often than daily because excessive washing means unnecessary manipulation.

A woman who has a considerable discharge of colostrum or milk from her breasts (whether breastfeeding or not) should insert clean gauze squares or commercial nursing pads in her bra to absorb the moisture. These should be changed as often as necessary to keep the nipples dry. If nipples remain wet for any length of time, fissures may form and lead to infection.

Nursing Diagnosis: Health-seeking behaviors related to procedure for breast self-examination

Outcome Identification: Woman will voice understanding of importance of regular breast self-examination at time of discharge.

Outcome Evaluation: Woman demonstrates procedure for self-examination and states intention to perform it monthly.

Because breast tumors are a major type of neoplasm in women, women of childbearing age should know how to examine their breasts so they can check them routinely for signs of breast carcinoma. This procedure can be taught during pregnancy, but many women are not interested in hearing about cancer prevention measures at that time—the possibility of their developing cancer seems far removed from what they are doing during pregnancy, that is, creating life. In the postpartal period they are conscious of the need to remain well to raise this new child to maturity. This makes them receptive to having you review with or teach them the technique of breast self-examination.

A week after her menstrual period each month is the best time for breast self-examination because during a menstrual period or just before it, breasts may be tender, making the examination uncomfortable. The woman who is breastfeeding may not have a menstrual flow for 3 or 4 months. During this time, she should pick a day (eg, the first day of every month) to do the examination until menstrual flow "markers" return.

The technique of breast self-examination is discussed in Chapter 33. The breastfeeding woman will, of course, have a milk discharge when she squeezes her nipples as part of an examination. She may occasionally discover a distended milk gland that feels very much like a cyst or tumor. She should not worry about such distended glands unless they persist beyond two breastfeedings.

Remind women that if they do find a lump or have an abnormal nipple discharge in a breast on self-examination, they should telephone their health care provider about the finding. Also, remind the woman that most lumps found in breasts are benign. Many women do not examine their breasts because they are afraid they will find something; other women find something but are then afraid to tell anyone about it. Breast carcinoma discovered early and treated promptly (often without removal of more than the local lesion) has an excellent cure rate.

Nursing Diagnosis: Health-seeking behaviors related to woman's desire to return to prepregnant weight and appearance

Outcome Identification: Woman will demonstrate understanding of what to expect in terms of timetable for returning to prepregnant appearance after postpartal period.

Outcome Evaluation: Woman states realistic goals for return to former appearance; is able to demonstrate appropriate exercises.

After childbirth, the abdominal wall and the uterine ligaments are stretched. The abdomen pouches forward.

Wearing an abdominal binder or a girdle may help make a woman more comfortable during the first few weeks postpartum, but it does not aid, and may actually hinder, strengthening the tone of the abdominal wall. If an abdominal binder is applied for comfort in the postpartal period, it should always be applied from the top down, so that it pushes the uterus down, not up, and uterine contraction is not hampered.

The woman can best help her abdominal wall to return to good tone by using proper body mechanics and posture, getting adequate rest, and performing prescribed exercises. Exercises to strengthen the abdominal and pelvic muscles may be started with the physician's or nurse-midwife's consent as early as the first day after birth. The woman begins with easy exercises and gradually progresses to more difficult ones. She should continue these exercises until the end of the puerperium to derive the maximum benefit from them. Common abdominal and perineal strengthening exercises are described in Table 22-2. Many women find commercial abdominal exercisers helpful to fully strengthen their abdominal wall.

Teach Methods to Promote Uterine Involution. All during the postpartal period, lying on the abdomen gives support to abdominal muscles and aids involution, because it tips the uterus into its natural forward position. If this puts too much pressure on sore breasts, a small pillow under the stomach usually solves the problem.

A knee-chest position is dangerous for the woman to assume until at least the third week postpartum. In a knee-chest position, the vagina tends to open. Because the cervical os remains open to some extent until the third week, there is a danger that air will enter the vagina and the open cervix, penetrate the open blood sinuses inside the uterus, enter the circulatory system, and cause an air embolism (Cunningham et al., 2001).

It is therefore good practice for a woman to avoid this position until she returns for a postpartal examination and is assured her cervix has closed properly. Women who have used a knee-chest position during pregnancy to relieve the pressure of hemorrhoids need to be instructed that a modified Sims' position, such as they used for a rest position during pregnancy, is better for them now.

Nursing Diagnosis: Risk for ineffective sexuality patterns related to physiologic changes of postpartal period

Outcome Identification: Client will voice satisfaction in sexuality pattern after childbirth.

Outcome Evaluation: Client (if desired) states she has a satisfactory sexual relationship with her partner; demonstrates understanding of both coital and noncoital methods of sexual expression.

At one time, women were cautioned not to resume sexual relations after the birth of a baby until their medical checkup at 6 weeks. There is no apparent physiologic reason, however, to delay sexual relations this long. For most couples, therefore, coitus may be resumed as soon as lochia serosa has stopped—about 1 to 2 weeks after birth (Farrington & Ward, 2000).

Caution women that sex may be somewhat uncomfortable, however, if begun this early (Signorello et al., 2001). Tissue at an episiotomy site may be sensitive. Because vaginal epithelium is still thin, vaginal tenderness may be noticed. Use of a lubricant will help any mucosal dryness. A female-superior position can be suggested because it allows a woman to control the depth of penile penetration.

Women may already be aware that their degree of exhaustion may make them less receptive to sexual arousal than before. A woman who is breastfeeding may notice that milk is released from her nipples with sexual arousal.

Nursing Diagnosis: Risk for impaired parenting related to inadequate bonding behavior after childbirth

Outcome Identification: Parents will demonstrate adequate bonding behaviors during the postpartal period.

Outcome Evaluation: Parents hold and comfort the infant appropriately and voice positive characteristics of child.

To assess that bonding is occurring, listen to what parents say about their newborns in the immediate

TABLE 22.2 Muscle-Strengthening Exercises

EXERCISE	DESCRIPTION
Abdominal breathing	Abdominal breathing may be started on the first day postpartum, because it is a relatively easy exercise. Lying flat on her back or sitting, a woman should breathe slowly and deeply in and out 5 times, using her abdominal muscles. Check by watching her abdominal wall rise that she is actually using these muscles.
Chin-to-chest	The chin-to-chest exercise is excellent for the second day. Lying on her back with no pillow, a woman raises her head and bends her chin forward on her chest without moving any other part of her body while exhaling. She should start this gradually, repeating it no more than 5 times the first time and then increasing it to 10–15 times in succession. The exercise can be done 3 or 4 times a day. She will feel the abdominal muscles pull and tighten if she is doing it correctly.
Perineal contraction	If a woman is not already using this exercise as a means of alleviating perineal discomfort, it is a good one to add on the third day. She should tighten and relax her perineal muscles 10–25 times in succession as if she were trying to stop voiding (Kegel exercises). She will feel her perineal muscles working if she is doing it correctly.
Arm raising	Arm raising helps both the breasts and the abdomen return to good tone and is a good exercise to add on the fourth day. Lying on her back, arms at her sides, a woman moves arms out from her sides until they are perpendicular to her body. She then raises them over her body until her hands touch and lowers them slowly to her sides. She should rest a moment, then repeat the exercise 5 times.
Abdominal crunches	It is advisable to wait until the tenth or twelfth day after delivery before attempting abdominal crunches. Lying flat on her back with knees bent, a woman folds her arms across her chest and raises herself to a sitting position. This exercise expends a great deal of effort and tires a postpartal woman easily. Caution her to begin very gradually and work up slowly to doing it 10 times in a row.

postpartal period. Do they make positive statements ("I'm glad he's a boy," "She's cute") or negative ones ("I really hoped it would be a girl," "She looks like a circus clown with no hair")? First impressions may not be lasting ones. However, negative comments need to be identified so extra discussion about things such as what it feels like to have four boys can take place. If this does not occur, the family can be discharged from the agency with their needs unmet. At home, away from health care personnel who are attuned to how disappointment can interfere with parent–child interaction, parents may have great difficulty adjusting to and relating to this new child. Signs of good parent–child adaptation are shown in Box 22-2.

✔ **CHECKPOINT QUESTIONS**

11. When is the best time of the month for a woman to perform breast self-examination?
12. Why is listening to how new parents describe their newborn important?

NURSING CARE OF THE WOMAN AND FAMILY IN PREPARATION FOR DISCHARGE

The greatest need of the woman before discharge from a health care agency is education to prepare her to care for herself and her newborn at home. Women must know how to care for themselves to prevent introducing infection to the unhealed uterus or perineal suture line. They must be aware of danger signs to look for and know whom to call if they notice any of these. They must understand safe baby care. Therefore, because of shortened lengths of stay, every contact with a woman should include some teaching information. However, learning does not take place if a learner is overwhelmed and hurried. Common sense is necessary to determine when it is time to teach and when it is time to observe or listen. Observation of mother–child or parent–child interaction and evaluation of the woman's support system at home are the basis for much of the teaching.

Many women attend classes in newborn care during their pregnancies. They remember many points from these classes, but when they actually have a newborn they become worried that they will not remember enough. Many mothers say child care did not seem real during pregnancy. The postpartal period is, therefore, a time for teaching, reteaching, and offering anticipatory guidance to help in the new situations the family can expect when they go home.

During the taking-in phase of the puerperium, the woman may not show much interest in learning; she is more in need of the comfort of being taken care of. As she enters her taking-hold period, she grows increasingly receptive to advice and looks to you for the information she needs. Some nurses assume that multiparas will react negatively to child care suggestions. Multiparas are, after all, veterans of child care. If you listen carefully to a multipara, however, you will discover that a woman of two girls may feel insecure about the care of this boy. A woman whose next youngest child is 5 years old admits that in 5 years she has completely forgotten how small newborns are. She yearns to have a nurse who is comfortable with such small human beings reassure her that she is holding her new baby correctly and giving proper care. All mothers, whether primiparas or multiparas, therefore, need to be evaluated individually and helped at that point where they ask for or you find they need guidance.

BOX 22.2

SIGNS OF GOOD PARENT–CHILD ADAPTATION

Speaks of infant as desirable and attractive
Is not upset by vomiting, drooling, and the like
Holds baby warmly
Makes eye contact with infant
Plays with and soothes infant
Talks or sings to baby
Expresses confidence that infant is well
Finds physical or psychological attributes to admire about baby
Is able to discriminate between baby's signs of hunger, sleep, and so on

Group Classes

Providing group classes on bathing infants, preparing formula, breastfeeding techniques, minimizing jealousy in older children, and maintaining health in the newborn can be helpful to mothers and fathers because they can learn from other parents as well as the instructor. Be certain that a time for questions and answers is planned so the parents can apply what is being taught to their individual circumstances. Urging fathers to attend classes is helpful, because many fathers give direct child care for at least part of every day. Including the father in teaching is also important because the problems that arise with newborn care are, by their nature, family problems, and every effort should be made by nursing personnel to help both parents prepare to deal with them.

Individual Instruction

Every family needs some individual instruction in how to care for their infant and how the woman can care for herself after discharge. Rooming-in is an ideal setup for letting you observe and work with the family and the infant. How to bathe and feed the baby, how to care for the infant's cord and circumcision, a review of how much infants sleep during 24 hours, and how to fit a newborn into the family's pattern of living are topics that parents like to discuss. Teaching does not have to be formal. You can teach without lecturing by making a comment such as "Notice how large all newborns' heads seem" while you are showing the parents how to bathe the baby, or "Babies like to be bundled firmly" while you are helping dress the child or "Notice how uneven newborn respirations are." This kind of instruction saves parents many anxious moments when they are at home. Techniques for home care of the newborn are discussed in Chapter 23.

Discharge Planning

Before the postpartal family is discharged from the hospital, the woman will be given instructions by her physician or nurse-midwife concerning her care at home. These instructions differ in some aspects among different health care providers but have common points that are summarized in Table 22-3.

Before discharge from the health care agency, make sure that the woman is aware that she must return for an examination 4 to 6 weeks after birth, and that she must make an appointment to take her baby to a primary care provider for an examination at 2 to 4 weeks of age. If the woman does not have an adequate rubella antibody titer and anticipates further pregnancies, she may receive a rubella immunization before discharge.

It is important that discharge instructions for the family be given both verbally and in writing. Getting ready to go home, dressing the baby, seeing him or her in new clothes for the first time, and experiencing the thrill of realizing the baby is really theirs to take home is so exciting that oral instructions may go unheard. On the other hand, parents should not simply be handed a list of instructions. Instructions should be reviewed with the parents to make certain that they understand them.

Many health care agencies have a community liaison person, ideally a nurse, to telephone or make a home visit to mothers after discharge. This person helps the mother assess her own health and that of the baby and to answer questions from families who lose their instructions or are unable to interpret them after they have returned home.

Routinely, this type of follow up is performed within 24 to 48 hours after the client's discharge. Follow-up phone calls are completed from 2 to 7 days after discharge. Making a telephone call to or visiting a family 24 hours after discharge from a health care facility is a helpful way of evaluating whether the family is able to continue self-evaluation and infant care after discharge and is able to integrate the new infant into the family. Such visits also can reduce the number of acute care visits and rehospitalizations for newborns.

TABLE 22.3 Postpartal Discharge Instructions

AREA	INSTRUCTIONS
Work	All women should avoid heavy work (lifting or straining) for at least the first 3 weeks after birth. Women differ in their concept of heavy work, so it is a good idea to explore with the woman what she considers heavy work. If she plans to do too much, you can perhaps help her to modify her plans. It is usually advised that she doesn't return to an outside job for at least 3 weeks (better 6 weeks) not only for her own health but also for enjoyment of the early weeks with her newborn.
Rest	The woman should plan at least one rest period a day and try to get a good night's sleep. She can rest during the day when her newborn is sleeping, unless she has other children or an aged parent to care for. If she has others dependent on her, explore the possibility of a neighbor, another family member, or a person from a community health agency to relieve her.
Exercise	The woman should limit the number of stairs she climbs to one flight/day for the first week at home. Beginning the second week, if her lochial discharge is normal, she may start to increase this activity. This limitation will involve some planning on her part, especially if her washing machine is in the basement and she must wash diapers every day, or if she must go up and down stairs to check on the baby. It is probably better to arrange for a place for the baby to sleep downstairs as well as upstairs, so he or she has to be taken upstairs only at bedtime. She should continue with muscle-strengthening exercises, such as abdominal crunches.
Hygiene	The woman may take either tub baths or showers. She should continue to apply any cream or ointment as ordered for the perineal area and cleanse her perineum from front to back. Any perineal stitches will be absorbed within 10 days. She should not use vaginal douches until she returns for her postpartal checkup.
Coitus	Coitus is safe as soon as the woman's lochia has turned to alba and, if present, the episiotomy is healed (usually about the first week after birth). Vaginal cells may not be as thick as formerly because prepregnancy hormone balance has not yet completely returned. Use of a contraceptive foam or lubricating jelly will aid comfort. Be certain she knows safer sex precautions (see Box 4-2).
Contraception	If desired, the woman should begin a contraception measure with the initiation of coitus. If she wishes an IUD, this may be fitted immediately after birth or at her first postpartal checkup. Oral contraceptives are begun about 2–3 weeks after birth. A diaphragm must be refitted at a 6-week checkup. Until she returns for this checkup, an over-the-counter spermicidal jelly and condoms can provide protection.
Follow-up	The woman should notify her physician or nurse-midwife if she notices an increase, not a decrease, in lochial discharge, or if lochia serosa or lochia alba becomes lochia rubra. Delayed postpartal hemorrhage can occur in women who become extremely fatigued. Getting adequate rest during her first weeks at home will do much to prevent the possibility of this complication. Four to six weeks after birth, the woman should return to her physician or nurse-midwife for an examination. This visit is important to ensure that involution is complete and reproductive life planning, if desired, can be discussed further.

NURSING CARE OF THE WOMAN AND FAMILY AFTER DISCHARGE

Postpartal Home Visits

In today's health care climate of cost containment, most women are discharged from a health care facility 2 to 3 days after childbirth. Such a practice has the advantage of allowing the family unit to be interrupted as little as possible. The mother may rest better at home than in a strange setting, and she may eat better if she has cultural preferences for specific foods. The infant can be more quickly exposed to family routines rather than a superficial facility schedule. Early discharge, unfortunately, has the disadvantage of not allowing a new family to have the ready support of health care personnel if they have questions about the newborn or the woman's condition. Early home visits have the advantage of providing early assessment. Although helpful for everyone, home visits should always be planned, especially for high-risk newborns, including newborns who are preterm, those born with a congenital anomaly, infants of adolescent mothers, or infants of mothers who have abused drugs during pregnancy.

The purposes of a home visit for the well postpartum woman and her newborn are to help the family integrate the infant into the family structure and provide the family with additional information on newborn care they may not have been able to learn during a brief hospital stay. Such a visit also allows for physical examination of the woman and newborn and for phenylketonuria or bilirubin testing to be carried out if this was not done during the hospital stay.

Because women need to preserve their energy during the postpartal period, a home visit should be arranged at the woman's convenience. Preparation for home visiting is discussed in Chapter 16 with other aspects of home care.

Important assessments to make at a postpartal home visit are:

Pregnancy History: Were there physical factors that could have interfered with pregnancy bonding such as painful varicose veins or gestational diabetes? Were there psychosocial factors such as an unwelcome move or loss of an important support person? Ask the woman to describe her labor and birth at a home visit, both to evaluate if any complications were present and to evaluate her reaction to the event.

Newborn History: When did the baby have a physical examination and what were the findings? Is there anything about the infant the woman is concerned about? What is the baby's current intake? Is the baby sleeping at spaced intervals or constantly fretful? Is the baby voiding?

Postpartal Course: Does the woman have pain? Any concerns about her health? Is she managing to obtain adequate rest? Does she have someone she could call if she had a concern about herself or her child?

Future Plans: Will the woman be returning to work outside her home? If so, what plans has she made for child care? The woman may be unprepared for postpartal depression. Ask if she feels "blue" or extremely fatigued.

Family Assessment: How are other children adapting? Does the client have adequate help with the new baby? How are the finances?

Physical Examination of the Mother: Assess temperature, pulse, and respiratory rate to detect possible infection or excessive blood loss. Assess uterine height and consistency (by the tenth day postpartum, the uterus should no longer be palpable as an abdominal organ). Assess the perineum to be certain there are no signs of infection in episiotomy stitches and that lochia color and odor are normal. Assess breasts to see if engorgement or any sign of infection is present.

Physical Examination of the Infant: Assess temperature, heart, respiratory rate, and skin turgor. Assess the abdomen for distention. Inspect for any ecchymotic marks. Assess for full range of motion of extremities and that the child follows a moving light. Assess for jaundice. Inspect for possible diaper rash. Note that the skin around the cord is not reddened. (Assessment of the newborn is discussed further in Chapter 23.)

Follow-Up Information: Be certain that the family has made plans (or knows how to make plans) for continued care for both the infant and the mother. Be certain they have the telephone number of a health care provider they could call if they have a concern before the date of a follow-up appointment.

Visiting a new family a few days after a hospital discharge is enjoyable because most families have at least one question about their newborn they are pleased to have answered. They are always pleased to be reassured that they are parenting well.

Postpartal Examination

Every newborn should have a health maintenance visit 2 to 4 weeks after birth (see Chapter 23). Every woman should have a checkup by her physician or nurse-midwife at 4 to 6 weeks after birth (the end of the postpartal period) to assure herself and her health care provider that she is in good health and has no residual problems from childbearing.

During this examination, the woman's abdominal wall is inspected for tone. Her breasts are inspected to see that they have returned to their nonpregnant state if she is not breastfeeding, and to see that they are unfissured and free of complications if she is breastfeeding. Most important, a thorough internal examination is performed to see that involution is complete, that the ligaments and the pelvic muscle supports have returned to good functional alignment, and that any lacerations sustained during birth have healed (Table 22-4).

If a woman has hemorrhoids or varicosities as a result of the pregnancy, her physician or nurse-midwife will discuss with her whether further management of these conditions is necessary. You should discuss breast self-examination with her, as well as the necessity for a Papanicolaou (Pap) smear and a pelvic examination every year as a means of screening for cervical and uterine cancer. If the woman is over age 40, include a discussion about the need for mammogram examinations at least every other year.

TABLE 22.4 Six-Week Physical Assessment

AREA OF ASSESSMENT	DATA COLLECTION
History	Assess chief concern, family profile (support system, bonding, self-esteem, family integrity), interval history, and review of systems (urinary system for pain, frequency, or stress incontinence along with gastrointestinal tract and reproductive tract in particular). Assess maternal intake. Some new mothers are too fatigued to eat well, so they eat mainly carbohydrate snack foods or, at least, not a balanced diet.
Physical Examination	*Expected Findings*
General appearance	Alert; positive mood. If not, woman is probably still extremely fatigued
Weight	Achievement of prepregnant weight; if not, this will be her baseline postpregnant weight
Hair	Healthy, firm hair; excess loss of hair from early postpartal period has halted
Eyes	Pink and moist conjunctiva; if pallor persists, diet may be inadequate due to fatigue
Breasts	
Nursing women	Full and firm to palpation; blue veins prominent under skin; only slightly tender. No palpable nodules or lumps. If erythematous or tender, mastitis may be present. If fissures on nipples are present, the woman may need to expose her nipples to air or to apply additional cream. An occasional filled milk gland may present as a lump; reexamine after breastfeeding
Non-nursing women	Return to prepregnant size; no palpable nodules or lumps
Abdomen	Striae less prominent; linea nigra fading, muscle tone improving. No distended bowel from constipation. No distended bladder from retention. No history of pain, frequency, or blood on urination. (If no abdominal muscle tone is present, women need to increase abdominal exercises. For constipation, increase fluid and fiber. Urinary symptoms probably reflect urinary infection that needs specific treatment.)
Perineum and uterus	No lochia; cervix closed; uterus has returned to prepregnant size. Pap test is normal. Ask woman to bear down during pelvic examination to observe for uterine prolapse, rectocele, or cystocele. If involution is not complete, reason for subinvolution must be investigated
Lower extremities	Varicosities barely noticeable
Rectum	Hemorrhoids receded to prepregnant size or are no longer observable
Laboratory Report	
Laboratory values	Hct: 37%; Hb: 11–12 g/100 mL. If these are low, reassess diet; possible iron supplement may be needed Rubella antibody titer: 1:8, if low, additional immunization is recommended before a second pregnancy

Abbreviations: Hct = hematocrit; Hb = hemoglobin

The postpartal examination should be a time for the woman to discuss with you any problems she had with childbearing and any she now has with childrearing, because these are a continuum. In addition, use this time to assess for possible intimate partner abuse, because it can increase during the postpartal period (Martin et al., 2001). If reproductive life planning was not discussed immediately after birth, this visit is an opportune time for such a discussion. If the woman desires to use a diaphragm or cervical cap, these can be fitted during this examination. Subcutaneous implanted hormonal contraception (Norplant) can be inserted at this time. Additionally, encourage women who have stopped smoking during pregnancy to continue to be smoke-free (Johnson et al., 2000).

NURSING CARE OF THE POSTPARTAL WOMAN AND FAMILY WITH UNIQUE NEEDS

The Woman Who Chooses Not to Keep Her Child

Although the availability of birth control information and the increasing number of abortions being performed have reduced the number of unwanted or unplanned children, some women still may complete a pregnancy and then give up their child for adoption.

There are numerous reasons for this to occur. The woman may be unmarried or her marriage may be failing and she does not want to raise a child alone. A woman may feel her family is already complete. She may want to finish school before having a child, or she would like to pursue a career.

During pregnancy, most women decide whether they will keep their child. During labor, they express confidence in their decision, but with the actual birth of the child, they may find that their resolve wavers. A woman who was certain she was going to surrender her child for adoption may begin to change her mind. A woman who was certain she was going to keep her child could become aware for the first time of the responsibility involved and decide that the best course for the child will be adoption. In either event, a woman's feelings become confused.

For a woman who chooses not to keep her child, the long wait in the birthing room for completion of perineal repair and preparations for transfer of the baby to a nursery may seem unusually long. She may also be alone, with no partner or support person with her during this time.

Every woman has a right to see, hold, and feed her child if she wishes. The woman who is not going to keep her child may feel proud that she has produced a healthy baby. The realization that the baby is well can provide a foundation on which to build a sound future and further enhance self-esteem.

Do not attempt to change a woman's mind about keeping her child or placing her child for adoption during the postpartal period. She is extremely vulnerable to suggestion at this time, and such decisions are too long range, too important to be made at such an emotional time. Her earlier conclusions may be the sound ones. Offer nonjudgmental support. Also, be especially aware of your own feeling about this issue to avoid influencing the woman's decision-making unnecessarily.

During the taking-in phase of the puerperium, be especially careful that you do not "lead" the woman's thinking. Women enjoy having decisions made for them during this time and may ask you what you think is best. An answer such as "You're the one who has to make this decision. What are your thoughts about it?" can help her begin to think through the problem.

It is not uncommon for women who surrender their infants for adoption to experience grief reactions like those of women whose children have died. If a woman decides to surrender her child for adoption, refer her to an official adoption agency, if she has not contacted one already. An official agency gives the woman the best assurance that the parents chosen for her child will be appropriate. This assurance will help to relieve any misgivings or guilt she may have about surrendering the child and should reduce the moments of doubt that can come in future years: Is my child well cared for? Is she getting everything I could have given her?

Some women do not openly voice a wish to give up their child, but their actions demonstrate that they feel little attachment to him or her. The woman who wants to keep her baby has a tentative but eager approach to her newborn, whereas a woman who has doubts is slow to make contact, barely touching the baby even by discharge, and asking few questions about newborn care. When this happens, the hospital social service department can be of assistance in helping the woman plan the child's future. A married couple as well as a single mother may place an infant for adoption, although for some couples, family counseling may be a greater need.

It is a fallacy to assume that everything will work out once a woman and infant arrive home. The number of abused children seen in hospital emergency departments is proof of the harm that can follow when assessment to detect poor parent–child bonding is inadequate in the first few days of life.

The Woman Who Is Discharged But Whose Child Remains Hospitalized

Newborns who are ill at birth often are transported to a regional center or a neonatal intensive care nursery for care, a move that automatically separates them from their parents. Many transport teams take an instant photograph of the baby and leave it with the mother. They also leave the nursery telephone number and the name of a nurse or doctor to contact for questions or information. Most transport teams telephone the mother when they arrive at the distant hospital to assure her that the infant managed well with the stress of transport.

Maintaining communication with the nursery is important so that the parents can begin to bond with their child. Urge them to telephone the nursery at least once daily to ask about the infant. If the infant is hospitalized in the same hospital, help the mother arrange a visiting time with the infant. Transport her to the nursery so she can see and hopefully hold her child. Without this assistance, some women will not telephone or visit because they are afraid that telephoning or visiting is an imposition or inconvenience for the nursery. Assure them that their telephone calls and visits are expected (the nursery wants to encourage bonding as well as you).

Some mothers whose infant is ill at birth feel uncomfortable if a postpartal roommate is feeding her well baby. This is often a good time to arrange for a visit to the nursery or to suggest that you walk in the hallway with her to increase her amount of ambulation. Encouraging visiting in the intensive care nursery is further discussed in Chapter 26.

The Family Who Is Adopting a Child

A family who is adopting an infant may come into the hospital or birthing center to meet the new infant. Such a couple needs the same introduction to newborn care as biologic parents. Additional needs of adopting parents are discussed in Chapter 2.

✔ CHECKPOINT QUESTIONS

13. Why is it important to ask about intimate partner abuse at a 6-week checkup?
14. At a 6-week postpartum visit, how should the cervix appear?

KEY POINTS

The postpartal period or the puerperium is the 6-week period after childbirth.

The postpartal period is an important one for a family because it marks the child's introduction to the family. Women can be seen to move through an initial "taking-in" phase in which they are dependent, a "taking-hold" phase in which they manifest independence, and a "letting-go" phase in which the mother role is finally defined.

Rooming-in is the preferred health care agency arrangement for postpartal families because it allows the new family the best chance for quality interaction. The more time new parents spend with a newborn, the more likely it is that effective bonding will occur. Help parents to feel comfortable with their newborn by offering anticipatory guidance and role modeling of infant care.

"Postpartal blues" are a normal accompaniment to childbirth. Women need assurance that this is normal, and supportive care should be given until the emotion passes.

Uterine involution is the process whereby the uterus returns to its prepregnant state. A uterus decreases in size 1 fingerbreadth a day until it disappears under the pubic bone at about day 10. Lochia is the name of the vaginal flow after childbirth: the flow is lochia rubra (red) for the first 1 to 3 days; lochia serosa (pink to brown) until day 4 to 10; and lochia alba (white) until 2 to 6 weeks.

A woman is at great risk for hemorrhage in the postpartal period, so assessments done during this time are some of the most critical assessments made in nursing. Don't discount the importance of these assessments because the overall content of the postpartal period is so focused on wellness.

Lactation is the production of breast milk. Colostrum is present immediately after birth; milk forms on the third to fourth postpartal day. A feeling of fullness and firmness on this day is termed filling; if warmth and discomfort occur, it is termed *engorgement.*

Women may need various comfort measures to alleviate pain from sutures, uterine pain (afterpains), and breast tenderness. Application of cold or warmth and administration of analgesics are important nursing interventions.

Women need teaching about self-care before health care agency discharge so they can maintain self-care at home. Follow-up by a telephone call or home visit is helpful. All women should conscientiously return for a 6-week visit to be certain that their reproductive organs have returned to normal. A menstrual flow should return 6 to 10 weeks after birth in the non-breastfeeding mother, 3 to 4 months in the breastfeeding mother.

CRITICAL THINKING EXERCISES

1. You are caring for the couple that you met at the beginning of the chapter, Mike and Joan Cooper, and their baby girl. This couple needs health teaching in a number of areas. Which subject would you begin with? Why?
2. A 25-year-old woman is 1 day postpartal after giving birth to an 8-lb girl. Since she did not have an episiotomy incision, you expected that she would have little perineal discomfort. Instead, she states her perineal pain is excruciating. You notice she has hemorrhoids. You overhear her telling her husband that he is acting selfishly for paying more attention to their new daughter than to her. You observe her handing her baby roughly to her husband. How would you evaluate this family based on your observations? What additional information would you want to know before you reached a firm conclusion regarding this new family's health? What could you suggest to make the client more comfortable?
3. A woman comes for her 6-week postpartal checkup. What would you include in an assessment plan to ensure that the client has physically and emotionally adjusted well to childbirth?
4. Examine the National Health Goals related to postpartum care. Most government-sponsored money for nursing research is allotted based on these goals. What would be a possible research topic to explore pertinent to these goals that would be both fundable and advance evidence-based practice?

REFERENCES

American College of Obstetricians and Gynecologists. (2002). ACOG committee opinion: Exercise during pregnancy and the postpartum period. *Obstetrics & Gynecology, 99*(1), 171–173.

Beck, C. T. & Gable, R. K. (2001). Further validation of the postpartum Depression Screening Scale. *Nursing Research, 50*(3), 155–164.

Bridges, W. (1994). *Job shift: How to prosper in a workplace without jobs.* Menlo Park, CA: Addison-Wesley.

Cunningham, F. G., et al. (2001). *Williams obstetrics* (21st ed.). Stamford, CT: Appleton & Lange.

Department of Health and Human Services. (2000). *Healthy people 2010.* Washington, DC: Author.

Farrington, P. F. & Ward, K. (2000). Normal labor, delivery and puerperium. In J. R. Scott et al. (Eds.). *Danforth's obstetrics and gynecology* (8th ed., pp. 91–109). Philadelphia: Lippincott Williams & Wilkins.

Fiorica, J. V. (2000). The breast. In J. R. Scott et al. (Eds.). *Danforth's obstetrics and gynecology* (8th ed., pp. 631–648). Philadelphia: Lippincott Williams & Wilkins.

Harrison, J. M. (2000). Clinical physiological changes of the puerperium. *British Journal of Midwifery, 8*(8), 483–488.

Johnson, J. L., et al. (2000). Preventing smoking relapse in postpartum women. *Nursing Research, 49*(1), 44–52.

Johnson, M., Maas, M. & Moorhead, S. (2000). *Nursing outcomes classification* (2nd ed.). St. Louis: Mosby.

Karch, A. M. (2001). *Lippincott's nursing drug guide.* Philadelphia: Lippincott Williams & Wilkins.

Leathers, S. J. & Kelley, M. A. (2000). Unintended pregnancy and depressive symptoms among first-time mothers and fathers. *American Journal of Orthopsychiatry, 70*(4), 523–531.

Lee, K. A., Zaffke, M. E., & McEnany, G. (2000). Parity and sleep patterns during and after pregnancy. *Obstetrics & Gynecology, 95*(1), 14–18.

Lvoff, N. M., Lvoff, V., & Klaus, M. H. (2000). Effect of the baby-friendly initiative on infant abandonment in a Russian hospital. *Archives of Pediatrics & Adolescent Medicine, 154*(5), 474–477.

Martin, S. L., et al. (2001). Physical abuse of women before, during, and after pregnancy. *JAMA, 285*(12), 1581–1584.

McCloskey, J. & Bulechek, G. (2000). *Nursing interventions classification* (3rd ed.). St. Louis: Mosby.

Meyer, S., et al. (2001). Pelvic floor education after vaginal delivery. *Obstetrics & Gynecology, 97*(5.1), 673–677.

Milligan, R. A., et al. (2000). Breastfeeding duration among low income women, *Journal of Midwifery & Women's Health, 45*(3), 236-252.

Nel, J. T., et al. (2001). A prospective clinical and urodynamic study of bladder function during and after pregnancy. *International Urogynecology Journal & Pelvic Floor Dysfunction, 12*(1), 21-26.

Perla, L. (2002). Patient compliance and satisfaction with nursing care during delivery and recovery. *Journal of Nursing Care Quality, 16*(2), 60-66.

Rubin, R. (1977). Binding-in in the postpartum period. *Maternal Child Nursing Journal, 6*(2), 67-69.

Salonen, R., et al. (2001). Increased risks of circulatory diseases in late pregnancy and puerperium. *Epidemiology, 12*(4), 456-460.

Signorello, L. B., et al. (2001). Postpartum sexual functioning and its relationship to perineal trauma: A retrospective cohort study of primiparous women. *American Journal of Obstetrics & Gynecology, 184*(5), 881-890.

SUGGESTED READINGS

Albers, L. L. (2000). Health problems after childbirth. *Journal of Midwifery & Women's Health, 45*(1), 55-57.

Brewley, C. & Bradshaw, C. (2001). Thromboembolic disorders during pregnancy, birth and puerperium. *Midwifery Digest, 11*(1), 56-59.

Britton, H. L., Gronwaldt, V., & Britton, J. R. (2001). Maternal postpartum behaviors and mother-infant relationship during the first year of life. *Journal of Pediatrics, 138*(6), 905-909.

Da Costa, D., et al. (2000). Psychosocial correlates of prepartum and postpartum depressed mood. *Journal of Affective Disorders, 59*(1), 31-40.

Dixon, M., Booth, N., & Powell, R. (2000). Sex and relationships following childbirth: A first report from general practice of 131 couples. *British Journal of General Practice, 50*(452), 223-224.

Durik, A. M., Hyde, J. S. & Clark, R. (2000). Sequelae of cesarean and vaginal deliveries: Psychosocial outcomes for mothers and infants. *Developmental Psychology, 36*(2), 251-260.

Hayes, B. A., Muller, R., & Bradley, B. S. (2001). Perinatal depression: A randomized controlled trial of an antenatal education intervention for primiparas. *Birth, 28*(1), 28-35.

Hedin, L. W. (2000). Postpartum, also a risk period for domestic violence. *European Journal of Obstetrics, Gynecology & Reproductive Biology, 89*(1), 41-45.

Hopkinson, J. M., et al. (2000). Lactation delays postpartum bone mineral accretion and temporarily alters its regional distribution in women. *Journal of Nutrition, 130*(4), 777-783.

Koniak-Griffin, D., et al. (2000). A public health nursing early intervention program for adolescent mothers: Outcomes from pregnancy through 6 weeks postpartum. *Nursing Research, 49*(3), 130-138.

Koniak-Griffin, D. et al. (2002). Public health nursing care for adolescent mothers: Impact on infant health and selected maternal outcomes at 1 year postbirth. *Journal of Adolescent Health, 30*(1), 44-54.

Malkin, J. D., et al. (2000). Infant mortality and early postpartum discharge. *Obstetrics & Gynecology, 96*(2), 183-188.

Mandl, K. D., et al. (2000). Effect of a reduced postpartum length of stay program on primary care services use by mothers and infants. *Pediatrics, 106*(4 Suppl.), 937-941.

Matthiesen, A. S. (2001). Postpartum maternal oxytocin release by newborns: Effects of infant hand massage and sucking. *Birth, 28*(1), 13-19.

Ray, K. L. & Hodnett, E. D. (2002). Caregiver support for postpartum depression. *Cochrane Database of Systematic Reviews 1*(1).

Templeman, C. L., et al. (2000). Postpartum contraceptive use among adolescent mothers. *Obstetrics & Gynecology, 95*(5), 770-776.

CHAPTER 23

Nursing Care of the Newborn and Family

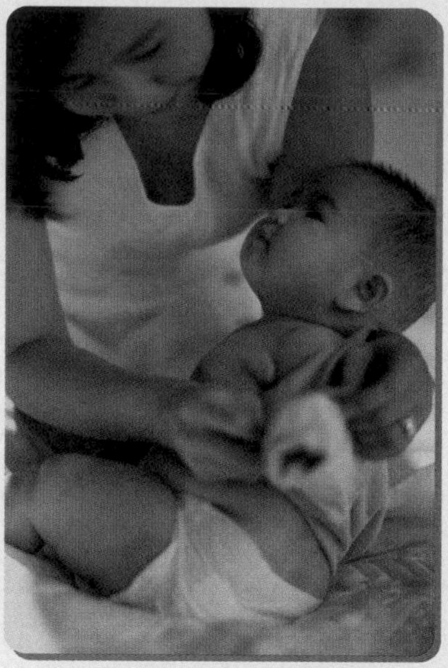

Objectives

After mastering the contents of this chapter, you should be able to:

1. Describe the characteristics of the term newborn.
2. Assess a newborn for normal growth and development.
3. Formulate nursing diagnoses related to the newborn and/or family of the newborn.
4. Identify expected outcomes for the newborn and family during this period.
5. Plan nursing care to enhance normal development of the newborn, such as ways to aid parent–child bonding.
6. Implement nursing care of the normal newborn, such as administering the first bath or instructing parents on how to care for their newborn.
7. Evaluate outcomes to determine effectiveness of nursing care and outcome achievement.
8. Identify National Health Goals related to newborns that nurses could be instrumental in helping the nation to achieve.
9. Identify areas related to newborn assessment and care that could benefit from additional nursing research or application of evidence-based practice.
10. Use critical thinking to analyze ways that the care of the term newborn can be more family centered.
11. Integrate knowledge of newborn growth and development and immediate care needs with the nursing process to achieve quality maternal and child health nursing care.

Key Terms

- **acrocyanosis**
- **caput succedaneum**
- **cavernous hemangioma**
- **central cyanosis**
- **cephalhematoma**
- **conduction**
- **convection**
- **erythema toxicum**
- **evaporation**
- **hemangioma**
- **jaundice**
- **kangaroo care**
- **kernicterus**
- **lanugo**
- **meconium**
- **milia**
- **mongolian spot**
- **natal teeth**
- **neonatal period**
- **neonate**
- **nevus flammeus**
- **physiologic jaundice**
- **pseudomenstruation**
- **radiation**
- **strawberry hemangioma**
- **subconjunctival hemorrhage**
- **thrush**
- **transitional stool**
- **vernix caseosa**

Carlotta Ruiz has just given birth to her second child, a 6-lb, 5-oz baby girl. The newborn's Apgar scores at 1 and 5 minutes were 6 and 8, respectively. Vital signs are as follows: temperature (axillary) 98.2°F (36.8°C); heart rate 136 bpm; respirations 42 breaths per minute. Further assessment reveals the newborn to be 18.5 inches in length, with a head circumference of 34 cm and chest circumference of 32 cm. After spending some time with the parents shortly after delivery, the newborn is transferred to the nursery where you'll be completing additional assessments, and giving the newborn her first bath.

Carlotta and her husband, Jose, are discussing plans for their daughter's arrival home. They live in a two-story row home and have a 3½-year-old son, Jose Jr., at home. Carlotta states, "Little Jose will be so pleased to see his new baby sister. That's all he's been talking about lately." They have much support from close family and friends. When you enter Carlotta's room, you notice that she seems a little apprehensive about caring for her new daughter. She tells you, "She's so much smaller than Jose was."

Previous chapters described the care of the pregnant woman and family during the antepartal, intrapartal, and postpartal periods. This chapter adds information about caring for the newborn and family to your knowledge base. Many profound physiologic changes occur in a newborn after birth as the newborn adjusts to extrauterine life.

After you've studied this chapter, answer the Critical Thinking Exercises at the end of the chapter, and then access the on-line study activities (http:// connection.lww.com) *to further sharpen your skills and test your knowledge.*

Newborns undergo many profound physiologic changes at the moment of birth (and, probably, psychological changes as well), because they have been released from a warm, close, dark, liquid-filled environment that has met all of their basic needs, into a chilly, unbounded, brightly lit, gravity-based, outside world.

Within minutes of being plunged into this strange environment, a newborn's body must initiate respirations and accommodate the circulatory system to extrauterine oxygenation. Within 24 hours, neurologic, renal, endocrine, gastrointestinal, and metabolic functions must be operating competently for life to be sustained.

How well a newborn makes these major adjustments depends on his or her genetic composition, the competency of the recent intrauterine environment, the care received during the labor and birth period, and the care received during the newborn or neonatal period (from birth through the first 28 days of life). National Health Goals related to the first days of life are shown in Focus on National Health Goals. Nursing plays a major role in contributing to the achievement of these goals.

Two thirds of all deaths that occur in the first year of life occur in the neonatal period. Over half occur in the first 24 hours after birth—an indication of how hazardous this time is for the infant. Close observation of the neonate for indications of distress is essential during this period (DHHS, 2000).

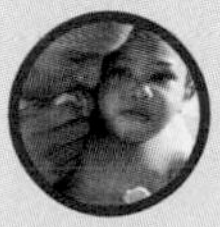

FOCUS ON NATIONAL HEALTH GOALS

A number of National Health Goals deal directly with the newborn period. These are:

- Increase to at least 75% the proportion of mothers who breastfeed their babies in the early postpartal period from a baseline of 64%.
- Increase to at least 50% the proportion of women who continue breastfeeding until their babies are 5 to 6 months old from a baseline of 29%.
- Increase the percentage of healthy full-term infants who are put to sleep on their backs from a baseline of 35% to 70%.
- Increase to at least 75% the proportion of parents and caregivers who use feeding practices that prevent baby-bottle tooth decay.
- Reduce the neonatal mortality rate to no more than 2.9 per 1000 live births from a baseline of 4.8 per 1000 live births (DHHS, 2000).

Nurses can be instrumental in helping the nation achieve these goals not only by encouraging women to begin breastfeeding but also by encouraging them to continue it through the first 6 months of life; advising parents on the advantage of placing infants on their backs to sleep and on the danger of tooth decay from letting the baby drink from a bottle of milk or juice while falling asleep; and discussing with parents who use formula the proper methods for preparation so gastrointestinal illness does not occur.

Areas that could benefit from additional nursing research include identifying the reasons why women end breastfeeding shortly after discharge from a health care agency; investigating common methods of encouraging sleep in infants other than by a bottle feeding.

NURSING PROCESS OVERVIEW

For Health Promotion of the Term Newborn

Assessment

Assessment of the newborn or **neonate** (a baby in the **neonatal period,** the first 28 days of life) includes a review of the mother's pregnancy history, physical examination of the infant, analysis of the newborn's laboratory reports such as hematocrit and blood type, if indicated, and assessment of the parent–child interaction for the beginning of bonding. Assessment begins immediately after birth and is continued at every contact during the newborn's hospital or birthing center stay, early home visits, or well-baby visits. Teaching parents to make assessments concerning their infant's temperature, respiratory rate, and overall health is crucial so they can continue to monitor their infant's health at home (see Assessing the Average Newborn).

Nursing Diagnosis
Nursing diagnoses associated with the newborn often center on the problems of establishing respirations, beginning nutrition, and assisting with parent-newborn bonding, for example:

- Ineffective airway clearance related to mucus in airway
- Ineffective thermoregulation related to heat loss from exposure in birthing room
- Imbalanced nutrition, less than body requirements, related to poor sucking reflex
- Readiness for enhanced family coping related to birth of planned infant
- Health-seeking behaviors related to newborn needs

If a minor deviation from the normal is present, such as a hemangioma, a diagnosis such as Parental fear related to hemangioma on left thigh of newborn might be relevant.

Outcome Identification and Planning
Planning nursing care must take into account the newborn's needs during this transition period and the mother's need for adequate rest during the postpartal period. Time for teaching should be adapted to the newborn's and mother's schedule. Although a woman must learn as much as possible about newborn care, she also must go home from the health setting with enough energy to practice what she has learned. Planning for newborns includes helping them regulate their temperature and growing accustomed to breast- or bottle feeding.

Implementation
A major portion of implementation in the newborn period is role modeling to help new parents grow confident with their newborn. Be aware of how closely parents observe you for guidance in child care. Conserving newborn warmth and energy to help prevent hypoglycemia and respiratory distress also is an important consideration for all interventions.

Outcome Evaluation
Evaluation of outcomes should reveal that parents are able to give beginning newborn care with confidence. Be certain that parents have made arrangements for continued health supervision for their newborn so evaluation can be continued and the family's long-term health needs can be met. Examples indicating achievement of outcomes may include the following:

- Infant establishes respirations of 30 to 60 per minute.
- Infant maintains temperature at 97.8°F to 98.6°F (36.5°C to 37°C).
- Infant breastfeeds for a minimum of 10 minutes every 3 hours.

ASSESSING the Average Newborn

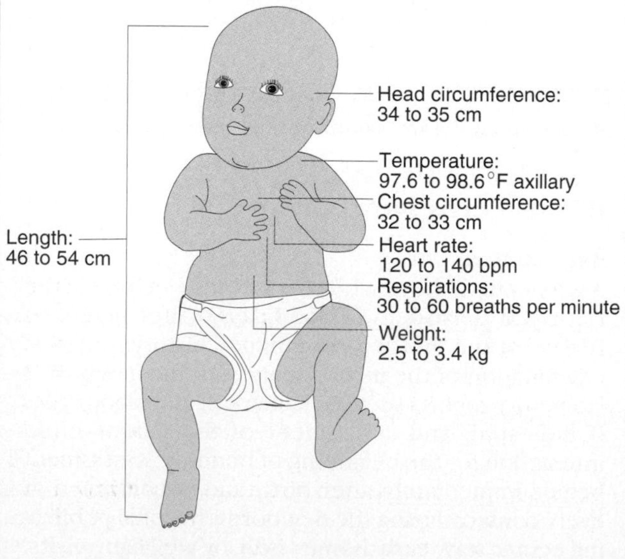

PROFILE OF THE NEWBORN

It is not unusual to hear the comment that "all newborns look alike" from people viewing a nursery full of babies. In actuality, every child is born with individual physical and personality characteristics that make him or her unique right from the start (Fig. 23-1).

Some newborns are born stocky and short, some large and bony, some thin and rangy. Some have a temperament

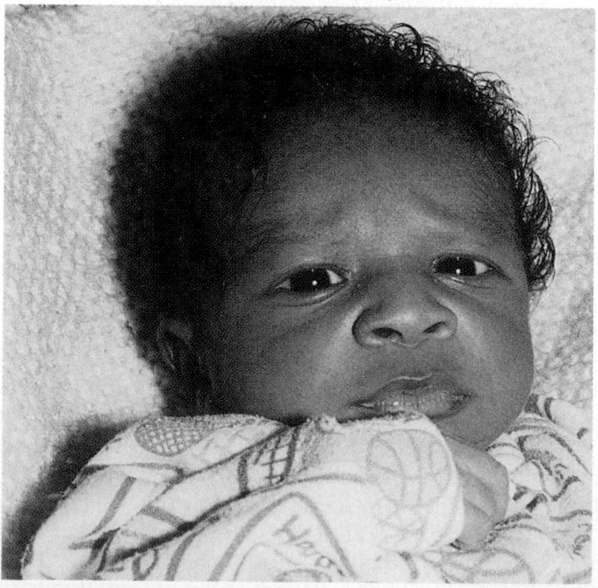

FIGURE 23.1 Personality is apparent in a newborn from the start. Note the alert, searching interest.

that causes them to feed greedily, protest procedures loudly, and respond to their parent's inexperienced handling with restlessness and spitting up. Other newborns sleep soundly, make no protest over procedures or diaper changes, and seem passive in accepting this new step in life. With experience in working with newborns, it becomes easier to differentiate newborns who are merely demonstrating the extremes of normal characteristics from those whose behavior or appearance indicates a need for more skilled care than is available in normal rooming-in surroundings.

Vital Statistics

Vital statistics for a newborn include weight, length, and head and chest circumference. The technique for obtaining these is shown in Chapter 33 with other aspects of health assessment. Be sure that all health care providers involved with newborns are aware of safety issues specific to newborn care (see Focus on Multidisciplinary Care).

Weight

The birth weight of newborns varies, depending on the racial, nutritional, intrauterine, and genetic factors that were present during conception and pregnancy. The weight in relation to the gestational age should be plotted on a standard neonatal graph, such as the one shown in Appendix E. Plotting weight this way helps identify newborns at risk because of their small size. This information also separates those who are small for their gestational age (children who have suffered intrauterine growth restriction) from pre-term infants (infants who are small only because they were born early). These first measurements also establish a baseline for future measurements.

Plotting weight in conjunction with height and head circumference is helpful in pointing out disproportionate measurements (see Appendix E). All three of these measurements should fall close to the same percentile for the same child. A newborn who falls within the fiftieth percentile for height and weight and whose head circumference is in the ninetieth percentile, for example, may have abnormal head growth. A newborn who is in the fiftieth percentile for weight and head circumference but in the third percentile for height may have a growth problem.

Second-born children generally weigh more than firstborns. Weight continues to increase with each succeeding child in a family.

The average birth weight (fiftieth percentile) for a white, mature female newborn in the United States is 3.4 kg (7.5 lb) and for a white, mature male newborn, 3.5 kg (7.7 lb). Newborns of other races weigh approximately 0.5 lb less. The arbitrary lower limit of normal for all races is 2.5 kg (5.5 lb). Birth weight exceeding 4.7 kg (10 lb) is unusual, but weights as high as 7.7 kg (17 lb) have been documented. When a newborn weighs over 4.7 kg, a maternal illness, such as diabetes mellitus, must be suspected (Cunningham et al., 2001).

The newborn loses 5 to 10% of birth weight (6 to 10 oz) during the first few days after birth. This weight loss occurs because the newborn is no longer under the influence of salt- and fluid-retaining maternal hormones. A newborn also voids and passes stool. Approximately 75 to 90% of the newborn's weight is fluid. Additional weight is lost as diuresis begins to remove a part of this high fluid load during the second to third day of life. When newborns are breastfed, intake until about the third day of life is limited by the relatively low caloric content of colostrum. If newborns are formula fed, their intake during this time is also limited. This low intake further affects weight loss because of the time needed to establish effective sucking.

After this initial loss of weight, the newborn has 1 day of stable weight. The breastfed newborn recaptures birth weight within 10 days; a formula-fed infant accomplishes this gain within 7 days. After this, the newborn will begin to gain about 2 lb/month (6 to 8 oz/week) for the first 6 months of life.

Length

The average birth length (fiftieth percentile) of a mature female neonate is 53 cm (20.9 in). For mature males, the average birth length is 54 cm (21.3 in). The lower limit of normal length is arbitrarily set at 46 cm (18 in). Although rare, babies with a length as great as 57.5 cm (23 in) have been reported (Cunningham et al., 2001).

Head Circumference

In a mature newborn, the head circumference is usually 34 to 35 cm (13.5 to 14 inches). A mature newborn with a head circumference greater than 37 cm or less than 33 cm (14.8 or 13.2 inches, respectively) should be carefully investigated for neurologic involvement, although occa-

FOCUS ON MULTIDISCIPLINARY CARE

Numerous health care personnel, such as laboratory technicians, respiratory therapists, or unlicensed assistive personnel, may be responsible for various aspects of newborn care. Be certain that they understand the need for safety at all times. For example, unlicensed assistive personnel may be responsible for weighing newborns and taking their vital signs. Be certain they are aware that even a newborn can squirm off a surface, such as a baby scale, if they do not hold a protective hand over the infant. All personnel need to be equally careful not to leave a newborn on a bed unprotected in the mother's room and to wash their hands before giving care.

Also make sure that all personnel involved in newborn care understand the importance of ensuring proper newborn identification before any task or procedure. For example, if unlicensed assistive personnel are responsible for helping discharge a newborn, be certain they understand the importance of verifying the newborn's identification before discharge and that parents have a car seat to ensure a safe trip home.

sionally a newborn will fall within these limits and still be normal. Head circumference is measured with a tape measure drawn across the center of the forehead and around the most prominent portion of the posterior head (the occiput).

Chest Circumference

The chest circumference in a term newborn is about 2 cm (0.75 to 1 in) less than head circumference. It is measured at the level of the nipples. If a large amount of breast tissue or edema of the breasts is present, this measurement will not be accurate until the edema has subsided.

Vital Signs

Temperature

The temperature of newborns is about 99°F (37.2°C) at the moment of birth, because they have been confined in an internal body organ. Their temperature falls almost immediately to below normal because of heat loss and immature temperature-regulating mechanisms. The temperature of birthing rooms, approximately 68°F to 72°F (21°C to 22°C), can add to this loss of heat.

Newborns lose heat by four separate mechanisms: convection, conduction, radiation, and evaporation (Fig. 23-2).

Convection is the flow of heat from the body surface to cooler surrounding air. The effectiveness of convection depends on the velocity of the flow (a current of air cools faster than nonmoving air). Eliminating drafts, such as from windows or air conditioners, reduces convection heat loss.

Conduction is the transfer of body heat to a cooler solid object in contact with the baby. For example, a baby placed on a cold counter or on the cold base of a warming unit would quickly lose heat to the colder metal surface. Covering surfaces with a warmed blanket or towel helps to minimize conduction heat loss.

Radiation is the transfer of body heat to a cooler solid object not in contact with the baby. A baby can lose heat by radiation to cold objects, such as a cold window surface or air conditioner. Moving the infant as far from the cold surface as possible helps reduce this heat loss.

Evaporation is loss of heat through conversion of a liquid to a vapor. Newborns are wet; therefore, they lose a great deal of heat as the amniotic fluid on their skin evaporates. To prevent this heat loss, newborns should be dried immediately. Any wet items should be removed and replaced with clean, prewarmed linens. Remember to dry a newborn's face and hair. The head, a large surface area in a newborn, can be responsible for a great amount of heat loss. Covering the hair with a cap after drying it further reduces the possibility of evaporation cooling.

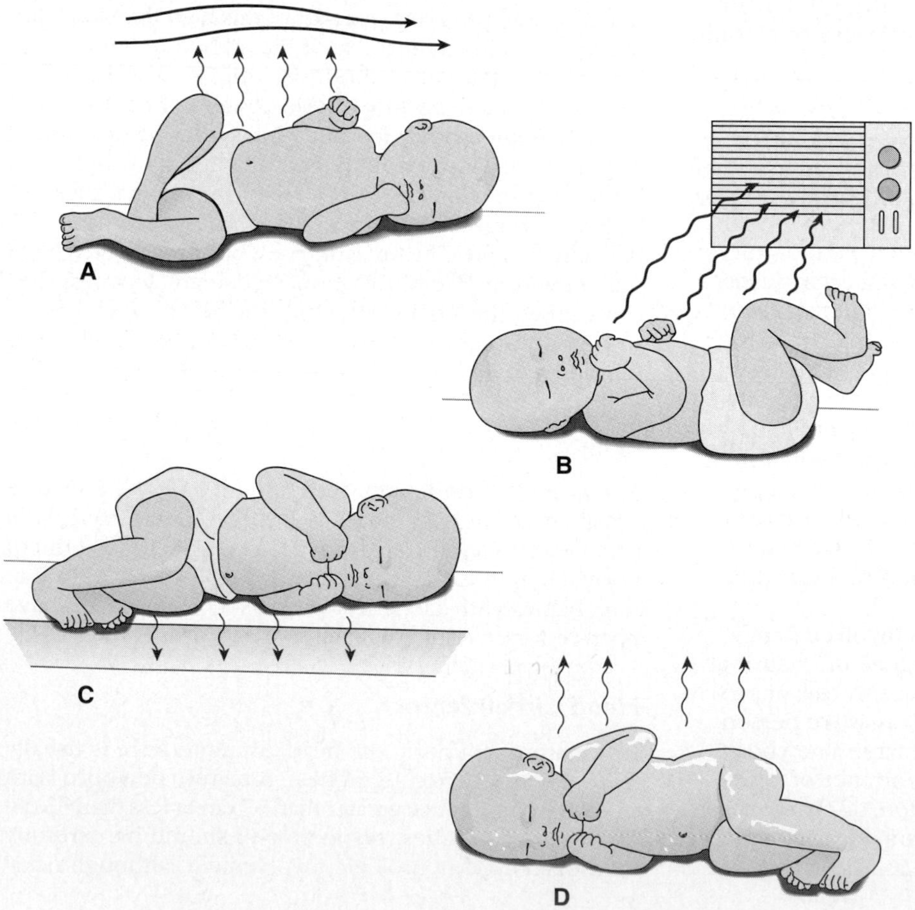

FIGURE 23.2 Heat loss in the newborn. (*A*) Convection. (*B*) Conduction. (*C*) Radiation. (*D*) Evaporation.

A newborn not only loses heat easily by the above means but also has difficulty conserving heat under any circumstance. Insulation, an efficient means of conserving heat in adults, is not effective in newborns because they have little subcutaneous fat to provide insulation. Shivering, a means of increasing metabolism and thereby providing heat in adults, is also rarely seen in newborns.

Newborns can conserve heat by constricting blood vessels. *Brown fat,* a special tissue found in mature newborns, apparently helps to conserve or produce body heat by increasing metabolism. The greatest amounts of brown fat are found in the intrascapular region, thorax, and perirenal area. It is thought to aid in controlling newborn temperature similar to temperature control in a hibernating animal. In later life, it may influence the proportion of body fat retained.

Because newborns have difficulty conserving body heat, exposure to cold can be extremely detrimental. Newborns exposed to cool air will kick and cry to increase their metabolic rate to produce more heat. This reaction, however, also increases their need for oxygen and thus increases their respiratory rate. An immature newborn with poor lung development will have trouble making such an adjustment. Newborns who cannot increase their respiratory rate in response to increased needs will be unable to deliver sufficient oxygen to their systems. The resultant anaerobic catabolism of body cells releases acid. Every newborn is born slightly acidotic. Any new buildup of acid may lead to severe, life-threatening acidosis. The newborn also becomes fatigued, placing additional strain on an already stressed cardiovascular system.

Drying and wrapping newborns and placing them in warmed cribs, or drying them and placing them under a radiant heat source, are excellent mechanical measures to help conserve heat. In addition, placing the newborn against the mother's skin and then covering the newborn also helps to transfer heat from the mother to the newborn, thus conserving heat loss (termed **kangaroo care;** Kirsten et al., 2001). All early care should be done speedily to avoid exposing the newborn unnecessarily. Any procedure during which the newborn must be uncovered (e.g., resuscitation, circumcision) should be done under a radiant heat source to prevent damaging heat loss. If chilling is prevented, a newborn's temperature stabilizes at 98.6°F (37°C) within 4 hours after birth.

In contrast to an adult, a newborn with a bacterial infection may run a subnormal temperature. Therefore, when a newborn's temperature does not stabilize shortly after birth, the cause must be investigated and corrective measures taken.

Pulse

The heart rate of a fetus in utero averages 120 to 160 beats per minute (bpm). Immediately after birth, as a newborn struggles to initiate respirations, the heart rate may be as rapid as 180 bpm. Within an hour after birth, as the newborn settles down to sleep, the heart rate stabilizes to an average of 120 to 140 bpm.

The heart rate of a newborn is often irregular because of the immaturity of the cardiac regulatory center in the medulla. Transient murmurs may result from the incomplete closure of fetal circulation shunts. During crying, the rate may rise again to 180 bpm. In addition, heart rate can decrease during sleep, ranging from 90 to 110 bpm.

The femoral pulses can be felt readily in a newborn, but the radial and temporal pulses are more difficult to palpate with any degree of accuracy. Thus, a newborn's heart rate always should be determined by listening for an apical heartbeat for a full minute. In addition, the femoral pulses also should be palpated, because their absence suggests possible coarctation (narrowing) of the aorta.

Respiration

The respiratory rate of a newborn in the first few minutes of life may be as high as 80 breaths per minute. As respiratory activity is established and maintained, the rate settles to an average of 30 to 60 breaths per minute when the child is at rest. Respiratory depth, rate, and rhythm are likely to be irregular, and short periods of apnea (without cyanosis), sometimes called *periodic respirations,* are normal. Respiration can be observed most easily by watching the movement of the abdomen, because breathing primarily involves the use of the diaphragm and abdominal muscles.

Coughing and sneezing reflexes are present at birth to clear the airway. Newborns are obligate nose-breathers and show signs of acute distress if the nostrils become obstructed. Short periods of crying, which increase the depth of respirations and aid in aerating deep portions of the lungs, are beneficial to the newborn. Long periods of crying, however, exhaust the cardiovascular system and serve no purpose. This is an important fact for parents to know.

Blood Pressure

The blood pressure of a newborn is approximately 80/46 mm Hg at birth. By the tenth day, it rises to about 100/50 mm Hg. Because blood pressure reading in the newborn is somewhat inaccurate, however, it is not routinely measured unless a cardiac anomaly is suspected. For an accurate reading, the cuff width used must be no more than two thirds the length of the upper arm or thigh. Blood pressure tends to increase with crying (and a newborn cries when disturbed and manipulated by such procedures as taking blood pressure).

A Doppler method may be used to take blood pressure (see Chapters 33 and 36). Hemodynamic monitoring is helpful when continuous assessment is necessary.

✔ CHECKPOINT QUESTIONS

1. Approximately how much weight does a newborn lose during the first few days of life?
2. What is a typical newborn head circumference?
3. What are four methods by which a newborn loses heat?

Physiologic Function

Cardiovascular System

Changes in the cardiovascular system are necessary at birth because the lungs now must oxygenate the blood that was formerly oxygenated by the placenta. When the cord is clamped, a neonate is forced to take in oxygen through the lungs. As the lungs inflate for the first time, pressure decreases in the chest generally, and in the pulmonary artery specifically (the artery leading to the lungs). The decrease in pressure in the pulmonary artery plays a role in promoting the closure of the ductus arteriosus. As pressure increases in the left side of the heart from increased blood volume, the foramen ovale closes because of the pressure against the lip of the structure (permanent closure does not occur for weeks). With the remaining fetal circulatory structures—the umbilical vein, two umbilical arteries, and the ductus venosus—no longer receiving blood, the blood within them clots, and the vessels atrophy over the next few weeks.

Figure 23-3 shows the respiratory and cardiovascular changes that occur at birth, beginning with the first breath.

The peripheral circulation of a newborn remains sluggish for at least the first 24 hours. It is common to observe cyanosis in the feet and hands (**acrocyanosis**) and for the feet to feel cold to the touch for this time.

Blood Values. A newborn's blood volume is 80 to 110 mL per kilogram of body weight, or about 300 mL. The oxygen dissociation curve is shifted to the left (the quantity of oxygen bound to hemoglobin and partial pressure of oxygen are greater in fetal blood than in the newborn's).

Because of the nature of fetal circulation, a baby is born with a high erythrocyte count, around 6 million per cubic millimeter. A newborn's hemoglobin level averages 17 to 18 g/100 mL of blood. Hematocrit level is between 45 and 50%. Capillary heel sticks may reveal a false high hematocrit or hemoglobin value because of sluggish peripheral circulation. Before obtaining the specimen, warming the extremity by wrapping it in a warm cloth increases circulation, thus improving the accuracy of this value.

Once proper lung oxygenation is established, the need for the high erythrocyte count diminishes. Therefore, within a matter of days, the erythrocyte count begins to fall. An indirect bilirubin level at birth is 1 to 4 mg/100 mL. Any increase over this amount reflects the release of bilirubin as excessive red blood cells begin their breakdown.

A newborn has an equally high white blood cell count at birth, about 15,000 to 30,000 cells/mm^3. Values as high as 40,000 cells/mm^3 may be seen if the birth was stressful. Polymorphonuclear cells (neutrophils) account for a large part of this leukocytosis, but by the end of the first month, lymphocytes become the predominant cell type. This leukocytosis is a response to the trauma of birth and is nonpathogenic; an increased white blood cell count should not be taken as evidence of infection. On the other hand, although the high white blood cell count makes infection difficult to prove in a newborn, infection must not be dismissed as a possibility if other signs of infection (e.g., pallor, respiratory difficulty, or cyanosis) are present. Blood values in the newborn are summarized in Appendix F.

Blood Coagulation. Most newborns are born with a prolonged coagulation or prothrombin time, because their blood levels of vitamin K are lower than normal. Vitamin K, synthesized through the action of intestinal flora, is necessary for the formation of factor II (prothrombin), factor VII (proconvertin), factor IX (plasma thromboplastin component), and factor X (Stuart-Prower factor). A newborn intestine is sterile at birth unless membranes were ruptured more than 24 hours before birth. Therefore, it takes about 24 hours for flora to accumulate and for vitamin K to be synthesized. Because almost all newborns can be predicted to have diminished blood coagulation ability, vitamin K (e.g., AquaMEPHYTON) is administered intramuscularly into the lateral anterior thigh, the preferred site for all injections in the newborn immediately after birth.

Respiratory System

The first breath of a newborn is initiated by a combination of cold receptors, a lowered PO_2 (PO_2 falls from 80 mm Hg to as low as 15 mm Hg), and an increased PCO_2 (PCO_2 rises as high as 70 mm Hg). A first breath requires a tremendous amount of pressure (about 40 to 70 cm H_2O). The presence of fluid in the lungs eases the surface tension on alveolar walls and makes a first breath easier. This allows the alveoli to inflate more easily than if the lung walls were dry. About a third of this fluid is forced out of the lungs by the pressure of vaginal birth. Additional fluid is quickly absorbed by lung blood vessels and lymphatics after the first breath.

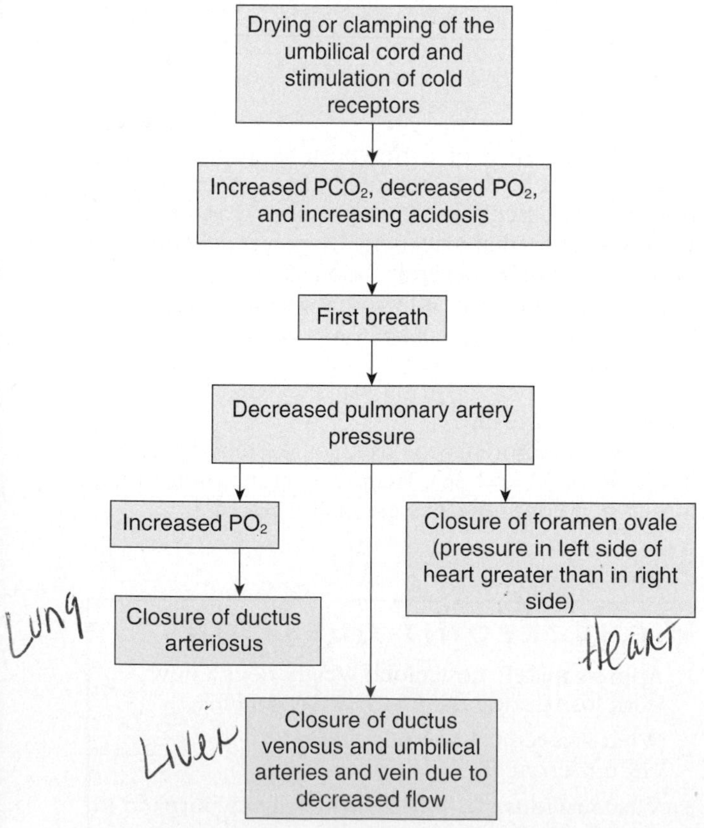

FIGURE 23.3 Circulatory events at birth.

Once the alveoli have been initially inflated, breathing becomes much easier for the baby, requiring only about 6 to 8 cm H_2O pressure. Within 10 minutes of birth, a newborn has established a good residual volume. By 10 to 12 hours of age, vital capacity is established at newborn proportions. The heart in a newborn takes up proportionately more space than in an adult, so the amount of lung expansion space available is proportionately limited.

A baby born by cesarean birth does not have as much lung fluid expelled at birth as one born vaginally, and so may have more difficulty establishing effective respiration (because excessive fluid blocks air exchange space). Newborns who are immature and whose alveoli collapse each time they exhale (because of the lack of pulmonary surfactant) have trouble establishing effective residual capacity and respirations. If the alveoli do not open well, a newborn's cardiac system is compromised, because closure of the foramen ovale and ductus arteriosus depends on free blood flow through the pulmonary artery and good oxygenation of blood. A newborn who has difficulty establishing respirations at birth should be examined closely in the postpartal period for a cardiac murmur or indication that he or she still has patent cardiac structures, especially a patent ductus arteriosus.

Gastrointestinal System

Although the gastrointestinal tract is usually sterile at birth, bacteria may be cultured from the intestinal tract in most babies within 5 hours after birth and from all babies at 24 hours of life. Most bacteria enter the tract through the newborn's mouth from airborne sources. Others may come from vaginal secretions at birth, from hospital bedding, and from contact at the breast. Accumulation of bacteria in the gastrointestinal tract is necessary for digestion and for the synthesis of vitamin K. Because milk, the infant's main diet for the first year, is low in vitamin K, this intestinal synthesis is necessary for blood coagulation.

Although a newborn's stomach holds about 60 to 90 mL, a newborn has limited ability to digest fat and starch because the pancreatic enzymes, lipase and amylase, are deficient for the first few months of life. The newborn regurgitates easily because of an immature cardiac sphincter between the stomach and esophagus. Immature liver functions may lead to lowered glucose and protein serum levels.

Stools. The first stool of the newborn, usually passed within 24 hours after birth, consists of **meconium,** a sticky, tarlike, blackish-green, odorless material formed from mucus, vernix, lanugo, hormones, and carbohydrates that accumulated during intrauterine life. A newborn who does not pass a meconium stool by 24 to 48 hours after birth should be examined for the possibility of meconium ileus, imperforate anus, or bowel obstruction.

About the second or third day of life, the newborn stool changes in color and consistency, becoming green and loose. This is termed a **transitional stool,** which may resemble diarrhea to the untrained eye. By the fourth day of life, breastfed babies pass three or four light yellow stools per day. These are sweet smelling, because breast milk is high in lactic acid, which reduces the amount of putrefactive organisms in the stool. A newborn who receives formula usually passes two or three bright yellow stools a day. These have a slightly more noticeable odor than do breastfed babies' stools.

A newborn placed under phototherapy lights to be treated for jaundice will have bright green stools because of increased bilirubin excretion. If mucus is mixed with the stool or the stool is watery and loose, a milk allergy, lactose intolerance, or some other irritant should be suspected. Newborns with bile duct obstruction will have clay-colored (gray) stools, because bile pigments do not enter the intestinal tract. Blood-flecked stools usually indicate an anal fissure. Occasionally, a newborn swallows some maternal blood during birth and will either vomit fresh blood immediately after birth or pass a tarry stool in two or more days. Maternal blood may be differentiated from fetal blood by a dipstick Apt test. If the stools remain black or tarry, intestinal bleeding should be suspected.

Urinary System

The average newborn voids within 24 hours after birth. A newborn who does not take in much fluid for the first 24 hours may void later than this, but the 24-hour point is a good general rule. Newborns who do not void within this time should be examined for the possibility of urethral stenosis or absent kidneys or ureters.

The possibility of obstruction in the urinary tract can be assessed by observing the force of the urinary stream in both male and female infants. Males should void with enough force to produce a small projected arc; females should produce a steady stream, not just continuous dribbling. Projecting urine farther than normal also may signal urethral obstruction, because it indicates urine is being forced through a narrow channel.

The kidneys of newborns do not concentrate urine well, thus the urine is usually light colored and odorless. The infant is about 6 weeks of age before much control over reabsorption of fluid in tubules and concentration of urine are evident.

A single voiding in a newborn is only about 15 mL and may be easily missed in a thick diaper. Specific gravity ranges from 1.008 to 1.010. The daily urinary output for the first 1 or 2 days is about 30 to 60 mL total. By week 1, total daily volume has risen to about 300 mL. The first voiding may be pink or dusky because of uric acid crystals that were formed in the bladder in utero. This is an innocent finding. A small amount of protein may be normally present in voidings for the first few days of life until kidney glomeruli are more fully mature. Typically, the number of voids is documented. Diapers can be weighed to determine the amount.

Immune System

Due to the difficulty forming antibodies against invading antigens until they are about 2 months of age, the newborn is prone to infection. This inability to form antibodies early also is the reason that most immunizations against childhood diseases are not given to infants younger than 2 months. The infant at birth, however, has passive antibodies (IgG) from the mother that have crossed the placenta. In most instances, these include antibodies against poliomyelitis, measles, diphtheria, pertussis, chickenpox, rubella, and tetanus. There is little natural immunity transmitted against herpes simplex. Therefore, any health care personnel with herpes simplex eruptions (cold sores) should not care for newborns until the lesions have crusted. Once this occurs, these personnel should use excellent handwashing because, without antibody protection in the infant, herpes simplex infections can become systemic or create a rapidly fatal form of the disease in the newborn (Mindel et al., 2000). Newborns are routinely administered hepatitis B vaccine during the first 12 hours after birth (AAP, 2002).

Neuromuscular System

Mature newborns demonstrate general neuromuscular function by moving their extremities, attempting to control head movement, and exhibiting a strong cry. Limpness or total absence of a muscular response to manipulation is never normal and suggests narcosis, shock, or cerebral injury. A newborn occasionally makes twitching or flailing movements of extremities in the absence of a stimulus because of the immaturity of the nervous system. A newborn at term typically demonstrates several reflexes. These reflexes can be tested with consistency by using simple maneuvers.

Blink Reflex. A blink reflex in a newborn serves the same purpose as it does in an adult, that is, to protect the eye from any object coming near it by rapid eyelid closure. It may be elicited by shining a strong light such as a flashlight or otoscope light on the eye. A sudden movement toward the eye sometimes can elicit it.

Rooting Reflex. If a newborn's cheek is brushed or stroked near the corner of the mouth, the child will turn the head in that direction. This reflex serves to help the baby find food. As the mother holds the child and allows her breast to brush the baby's cheek, the baby will turn toward the breast. The reflex disappears at about the sixth week of life. At about this time, the eyes focus steadily and a food source can be seen. Thus, the reflex is no longer needed.

Sucking Reflex. When a newborn's lips are touched, the baby makes a sucking motion. Thus, as the lips touch the mother's breast or a bottle, the baby sucks and so takes in food. The sucking reflex begins to diminish at about 6 months of age. It disappears immediately if it is never stimulated—for example, in a newborn with a tracheoesophageal fistula who is not allowed to take oral fluids. It can be maintained in such an infant by offering the child a non-nutritive sucking object such as a pacifier (after the fistula has been corrected by surgery and until oral feedings can be given).

Swallowing Reflex. The swallowing reflex in the newborn is the same as in the adult. Food that reaches the posterior portion of the tongue is automatically swallowed. Gag, cough, and sneeze reflexes also are present to maintain a clear airway in the event that normal swallowing does not keep the pharynx free of obstructing mucus.

Extrusion Reflex. A newborn will extrude any substance that is placed on the anterior portion of the tongue. This protective reflex prevents the swallowing of inedible substances. It disappears at about 4 months of age. Until then, an infant may seem to be spitting out or refusing solid food placed in the mouth.

Palmar Grasp Reflex. Newborns will grasp an object placed in their palm by closing their fingers on it (Fig. 23-4). Mature newborns grasp so strongly they can be raised from a supine position and be suspended momentarily from an examiner's fingers. The reflex disappears at about age 6 weeks to 3 months. A baby begins to grasp meaningfully at about 3 months of age.

Step (Walk)-in-Place Reflex. Newborns who are held in a vertical position with their feet touching a hard surface will take a few quick, alternating steps (Fig. 23-5). This reflex disappears by 3 months of age. By 4 months, babies can bear a good portion of their weight unhindered by this reflex.

Placing Reflex. The placing reflex is similar to the step-in-place reflex, except it is elicited by touching the anterior surface of a newborn's leg against the edge of a bassinet or table. A newborn will make a few quick lifting motions as if to step onto the table.

Plantar Grasp Reflex. When an object touches the sole of a newborn's foot at the base of the toes, the toes grasp in the same manner as the fingers do. The reflex disappears at about 8 to 9 months of age in preparation for walking. However, it may be present during sleep for a longer period.

Tonic Neck Reflex. When newborns lie on their backs, their heads usually turn to one side or the other. The arm and the leg on the side to which the head turns extend, and the opposite arm and leg contract (Fig. 23-6). If you turn a

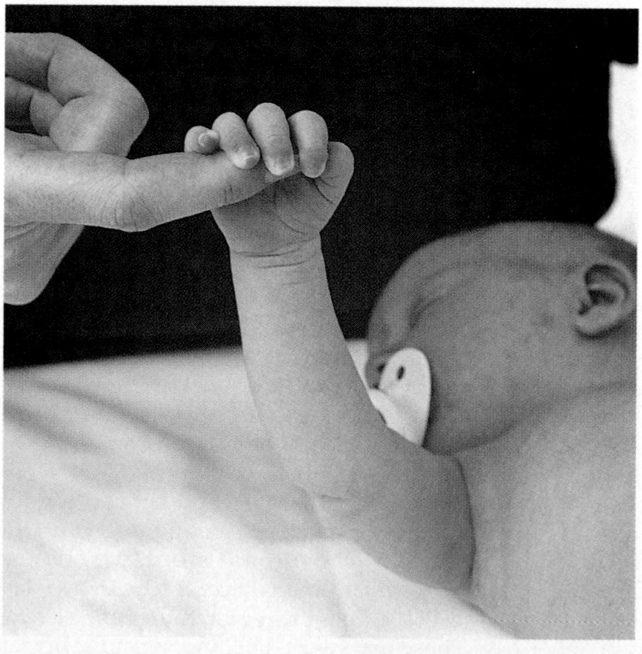

FIGURE 23.4 Palmar grasp reflex.

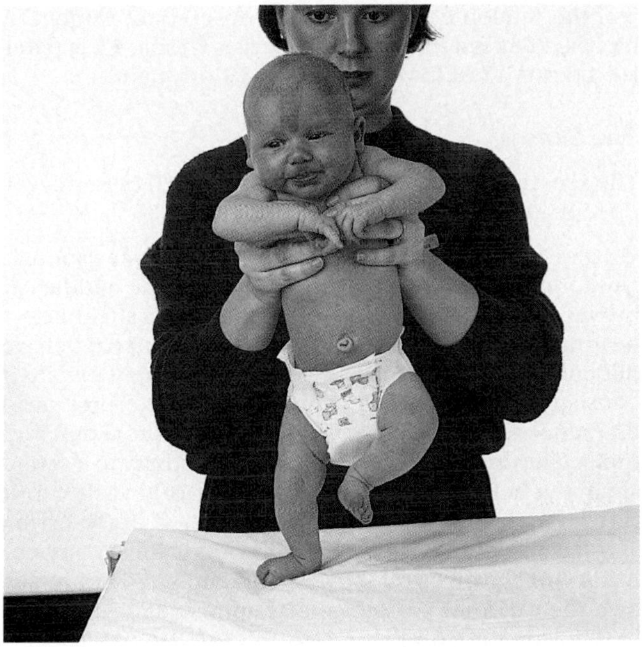

FIGURE 23.5 Step-in-place reflex.

newborn's head to the opposite side, he or she will often change the extension and contraction of legs and arms accordingly. The movement is most evident in the arms but may be observed in the legs. It is also called a boxer or fencing reflex, because the newborn's position simulates that of someone preparing to box or fence. Unlike many other reflexes, the tonic neck reflex does not appear to have a function. It does stimulate eye coordination, however, because the extended arm moves in front of the face. It may signify handedness. The reflex disappears between the second and third months of life.

Moro Reflex. A Moro (startle) reflex (Fig. 23-7) can be initiated by startling the newborn with a loud noise or by jarring the bassinet. The most accurate method of eliciting the reflex is to hold newborns in a supine position and allow their heads to drop backward an inch or so. They abduct and extend their arms and legs. Their fingers assume a typical "C" position. They then bring their arms into an embrace position and pull up their legs against their abdomen (adduction). The reflex simulates the action of someone trying to ward off an attacker, then covering up to protect himself. It is strong for the first 8 weeks of life and then fades by the end of the fourth or fifth month, when the infant can roll away from danger.

Babinski Reflex. When the side of the sole of the foot is stroked in an inverted "J" curve from the heel upward, the newborn fans the toes (positive Babinski sign; Fig. 23-8). This is in contrast to the adult, who flexes the toes. This reaction occurs because nervous system development is immature. It remains positive (toes fan) until at least 3 months of age, when it is supplanted by the down-turning or adult flexion response.

Magnet Reflex. If pressure is applied to the soles of the feet of a newborn lying in a supine position, he or she pushes back against the pressure. This and the two following reflexes are tests of spinal cord integrity.

Crossed Extension Reflex. One leg of a newborn lying supine is extended and the sole of that foot is irritated by being rubbed with a sharp object, such as a thumbnail. This causes the newborn to raise the other leg and extend it as if trying to push away the hand irritating the first leg.

Trunk Incurvation Reflex. When newborns lie in a prone position and are touched along the paravertebral area by a probing finger, they will flex their trunk and swing their pelvis toward the touch (Fig. 23-9).

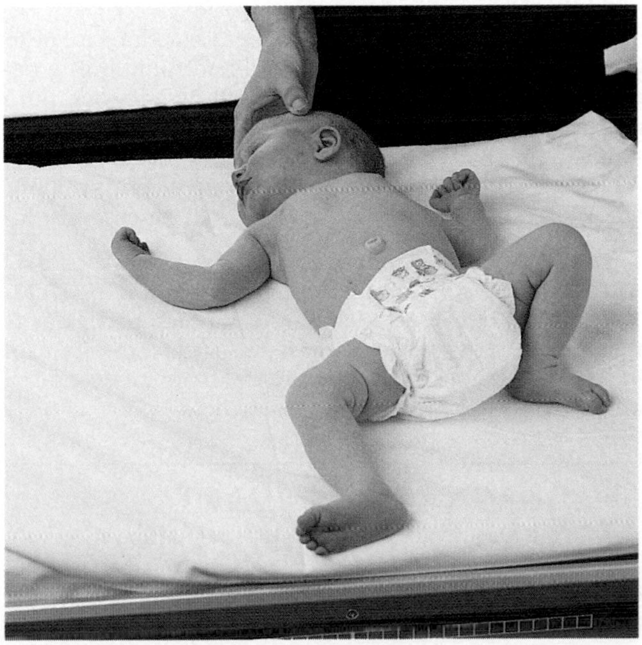

FIGURE 23.6 Tonic neck reflex.

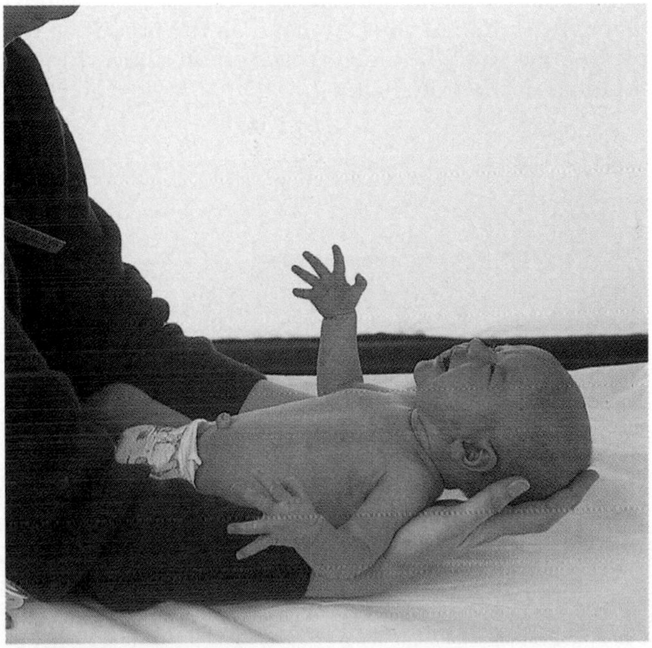

FIGURE 23.7 Moro reflex.

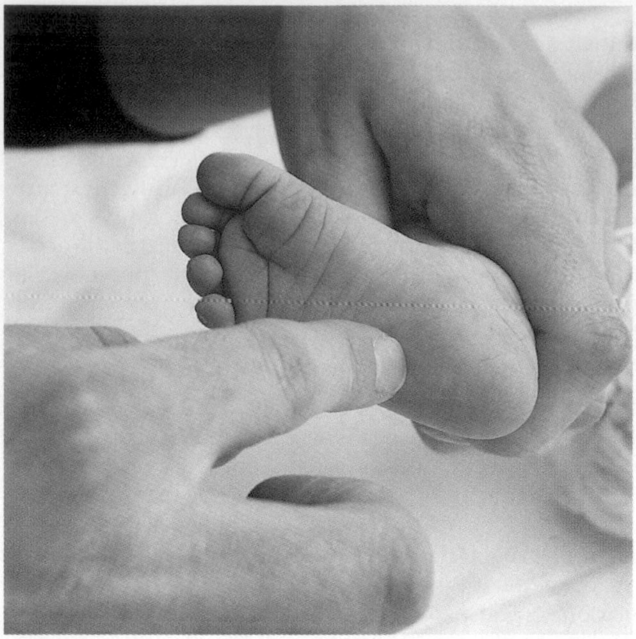

FIGURE 23.8 Babinski reflex. When the examiner moves her finger upward, the newborn's toes will fan outward.

Landau Reflex. A newborn who is held in a prone position with a hand underneath supporting the trunk should demonstrate some muscle tone. Babies may not be able to lift their head or arch their back (as they will at 3 months of age) in this position, but neither should they sag into an inverted "U" position. The latter response indicates extremely poor muscle tone, the cause of which should be investigated.

Deep Tendon Reflexes. A patellar reflex can be elicited in a newborn by tapping the patellar tendon with the tip of the finger. The lower leg will move perceptibly if the infant has an intact reflex. To elicit a biceps reflex, place the thumb of your left hand on the tendon of the biceps muscle on the inner surface of the elbow. Tap the thumb as it rests on the tendon. You are more likely to feel the tendon contract than to observe movement. A biceps reflex is a test for spinal nerves C5 and C6; a patellar reflex is a test for spinal nerves L2 through L4.

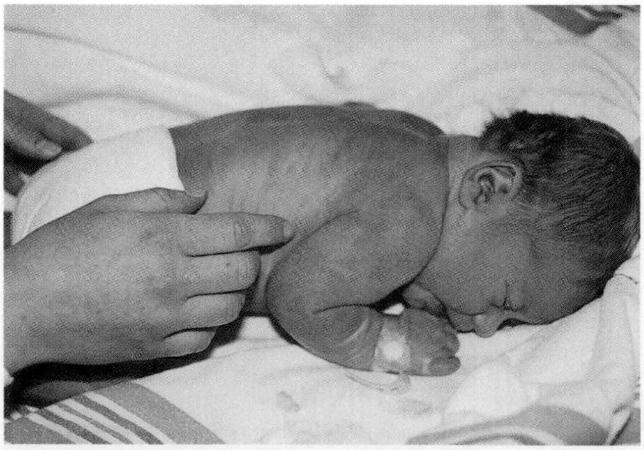

FIGURE 23.9 Trunk incurvation reflex. When the paravertebral area is stroked, the newborn flexes his or her trunk toward the direction of the stimulation.

The Senses

The senses in newborns appear to be much better developed than previously believed.

Hearing. A fetus is able to hear in utero. As soon as amniotic fluid drains or is absorbed from the middle ear by way of the eustachian tube—within hours after birth—hearing in newborns becomes acute. They appear to have difficulty locating sound, however, not turning toward it consistently. Perhaps they must learn to interpret small differences among sounds arriving at their ears at different times. They respond with generalized activity to a sound such as a bell ringing a short distance from their ear. If actively crying when the bell is rung, they will stop crying and seem to attend. Similarly, newborns calm in response to a soothing voice and startle at loud noises. They recognize their mother's voice almost immediately, as if they have heard it in utero.

Vision. Newborns see as soon as they are born and possibly have been "seeing" light and dark in utero for the last few months of pregnancy as the uterus and the abdominal wall were stretched thin. Newborns demonstrate sight at birth by blinking at a strong light (blink reflex) or following a bright light or toy a short distance with their eyes. Because they cannot follow past the midline of vision, they lose track of objects easily, so it is sometimes reported that they cannot see. They focus best on black and white objects at a distance of 9 to 12 in. A pupillary reflex is present from birth.

Touch. The sense of touch is well developed at birth. Newborns demonstrate this by quieting at a soothing touch and by positive sucking and rooting reflexes, which are elicited by touch. They also react to painful stimuli.

Taste. A newborn has the ability to discriminate taste because taste buds are developed and functioning before birth. A fetus in utero will swallow amniotic fluid more rapidly than usual if glucose is added to sweeten its taste. The swallowing decreases if a bitter flavor is added. A newborn turns away from a bitter taste such as salt but readily accepts the sweet taste of milk or glucose water.

Smell. The sense of smell is present in newborns as soon as the nose is clear of mucus and amniotic fluid. Newborns turn toward their mothers' breast partly out of recognition of the smell of breast milk and partly as a manifestation of the rooting reflex. Their ability to respond to odors can be used to document alertness.

✔ CHECKPOINT QUESTIONS

4. What factors are responsible for initiating the newborn's first breath?
5. A Moro reflex is the single best assessment of neurologic ability in a newborn. What is the best way to test this reflex?

Physiologic Adjustment to Extrauterine Life

All newborns seem to move through periods of irregular adjustment in the first 6 hours of life before their body systems stabilize. These periods were first described by Desmond in 1963 and are termed periods of reactivity (Desmond, 1963). The first phase lasts about half an hour. During this time, the baby is alert and exhibits exploring, searching activity, often making sucking sounds. Heart beat and respiratory rate are rapid. This is called the *first period of reactivity.*

Next comes a quiet *resting period.* Heartbeat and respiratory rates slow; the newborn generally sleeps for about 90 minutes. The *second period of reactivity,* between 2 and 6 hours of life, occurs when the baby wakes again, often gagging and choking on mucus that has accumulated in the mouth. He or she is again alert and responsive and interested in surroundings.

These three periods are summarized in Table 23-1. Newborns who are ill or who had difficulty at birth may not pass through these typical stages; they may never have periods of alertness or periods of quiet. Their vital signs may not fall and rise again but remain rapid; their temperature may remain subnormal. Demonstration of this typical reactivity pattern, therefore, is an indication that the baby is healthy and adjusting well to extrauterine life. The transition from one period to another is an important indicator of neurologic status.

APPEARANCE OF THE NEWBORN

Skin

General inspection of the newborn's skin reveals many characteristic findings.

Color

Most term newborns have a ruddy complexion because of the increased concentration of red blood cells in blood vessels and a decrease in the amount of subcutaneous fat, which makes the blood vessels more visible. This ruddiness fades slightly over the first month.

Cyanosis. The newborn's lips, hands, and feet are likely to appear cyanotic from immature peripheral circulation. Acrocyanosis is so prominent in some newborns that it appears as if a line is drawn across the wrist or ankle, with usual skin color on one side and blue on the other, as if some stricture were cutting off circulation. This is a normal phenomenon in the first 24 to 48 hours after birth.

Generalized mottling of the skin is common. **Central cyanosis,** or cyanosis of the trunk, however, is always a cause for concern. Central cyanosis indicates decreased oxygenation. It may be the result of a temporary respiratory obstruction or an underlying disease state.

Mucus obstructing the respiratory tract will cause sudden cyanosis and apnea in a newborn who had previously shown good color. Suctioning the mucus relieves the condition. Always suction the mouth before the nose, because suctioning the nose first may trigger a reflex gasp, possibly leading to aspiration if there is mucus in the posterior throat. Follow mouth suctioning with suction to the nose because this is the chief conduit for air in the newborn.

Hyperbilirubinemia. Hyperbilirubinemia leads to **jaundice,** or yellowing of the skin. This occurs on the second or third day of life in about 50% of all newborns as a result of the breakdown of fetal red blood cells (**physiologic jaundice**). The infant's skin and sclera of the eyes appear noticeably yellow. This occurs as the high red blood cell count built up in utero is destroyed and heme and glo-

TABLE 23.1 Periods of Reactivity: Normal Adjustment to Extrauterine Life

ASSESSMENT	FIRST PERIOD (FIRST 15–30 MIN)	RESTING PERIOD (30–120 MIN)	SECOND PERIOD (2–6 H)
Color	Acrocyanosis	Color stabilizing	Quick color changes occur with movement or crying
Temperature	Temperature begins to fall from intrauterine temperature of about 100.6°F (38.1°C)	Temperature stabilizes at about 99°F (37.2°C)	Temperature increases to 99.8°F (37.6°C)
Heart rate	Rapid, as much as 180 bpm while crying	Slowing to between 120 and 140 bpm	Wide swings in rate with activity
Respirations	Irregular; 30–90 breaths per min while crying; some nasal flaring, occasional retraction may be present	Slowing to 30–50 breaths per min; barreling of chest occurs	Becoming irregular again with activity
Activity	Alert; watching	Sleeping	Awakening
Ability to respond to stimulation	Vigorous reaction	Difficult to arouse	Becoming responsive again
Mucus	Visible in mouth	Small amount present while sleeping	Mouth full of mucus, causing gagging
Bowel sounds	Ability to be heard after first 15 min	Present	Often passage of first meconium stool

With permission from Desmond, M. N., et al. (1963). The clinical behavior of the newly born; The term baby. *Journal of Pediatrics, 62*(3), 307–309.

bin are released. Globin is a protein component that is reused by the body and is not a factor in the developing jaundice. Heme is further broken down into iron (which is also reused and therefore not involved in the jaundice) and protoporphyrin. Protoporphyrin is further broken down into indirect bilirubin. Indirect bilirubin is fat soluble and cannot be excreted by the kidneys in this state. Instead it is converted by the liver enzyme glucuronyl transferase into direct bilirubin, which is water soluble and is incorporated into stool and then excreted in feces. Many newborns have such immature liver function that indirect bilirubin cannot be converted to the direct form and, therefore, remains indirect. As long as the bilirubin remains in the circulatory system, the red coloring of the blood cells covers the yellow tint of the bilirubin. When the level of this indirect bilirubin rises above 7 mg/100 mL, however, bilirubin permeates the tissue outside the circulatory system and causes the infant to appear jaundiced.

Infants with extensive bruising (large, breech, or immature babies) must be observed carefully for jaundice. Bruising at birth leads to hemorrhage of blood into the subcutaneous tissue or skin. **Cephalhematoma,** a collection of blood under the periosteum of the skull bone, can lead to the same phenomenon. As the bruising heals and the red blood cells are hemolyzed, additional indirect bilirubin is released.

If intestinal obstruction is present and stool is not being evacuated, intestinal flora may break down bile into its basic components, leading to the release of indirect bilirubin into the bloodstream again. Early feeding of newborns promotes intestinal movement and excretion of meconium and helps prevent indirect bilirubin buildup from this source.

The level of jaundice in newborns may be judged grossly by estimating the extent to which it has progressed on the surface of the infant's body, starting in the head and spreading to the rest of the body.

Various commercial devices (transcutaneous bilirubinometry devices) are available to measure skin tone for jaundice and help in estimating jaundice levels. Although use of these devices rarely replaces serum measurements, they can be used to identify infants who need serum bilirubin determinations. Serum bilirubin is obtained by heel puncture. The technique for this is shown in Chapter 36.

There is no set level at which indirect serum bilirubin requires treatment. If the level rises above 10 to 12 mg/100 mL, treatment will usually be considered, although other factors such as age, maturity, and breastfeeding affect this. At about 20 mg/100 mL, enough indirect bilirubin has left the bloodstream that it could interfere with the chemical synthesis of brain cells, resulting in permanent cell damage, a condition termed **kernicterus.** If this occurs, permanent neurologic effects including cognitive challenge may result. Treatment for physiologic jaundice in newborns is rarely necessary except for measures such as early feeding (to speed passage of feces through the intestine and prevent reabsorption of bilirubin from the bowel). Phototherapy (exposure of the infant to light to initiate maturation of liver enzymes) may be used (see Chapter 26). If this is necessary, the incubator and light source can be moved to the mother's room so that the mother is not separated from the baby. Some infants need continued therapy after discharge, receiving phototherapy at home to prevent separation of the mother and infant.

Compared to formula-fed babies, a small proportion of breastfed babies may have more difficulty converting indirect bilirubin to direct bilirubin, because breast milk contains pregnanediol (a metabolite of progesterone), which depresses the action of glucuronyl transferase (Bertini et al., 2001). Rarely does breastfeeding cause enough jaundice to warrant therapy. The decision to stop nursing in the first 2 weeks of life must never be made lightly, because it could interfere with breast filling and the breast milk supply.

Pallor. Pallor in newborns is usually the result of anemia. Anemia may be caused by (1) excessive blood loss when the cord was cut; (2) inadequate flow of blood from the cord into the infant at birth; (3) fetal–maternal transfusion; (4) low iron stores caused by poor maternal nutrition during pregnancy; or (5) blood incompatibility in which a large number of red blood cells were hemolyzed in utero. It also may be the result of internal bleeding (the baby should be watched closely for signs of blood in stool or vomitus). Infants with central nervous system damage may appear pale and cyanotic. A gray color in newborns generally indicates infection. Twins may be born with a twin transfusion phenomenon, in which one twin is larger and has good color and the smaller twin has pallor (van Gemert et al., 2001).

Harlequin Sign. Occasionally, because of immature circulation, a newborn who has been lying on his or her side will appear red on the dependent side of the body and pale on the upper side, as if a line had been drawn down the center of the body. This is a transient phenomenon and, although startling, is of no clinical significance. The odd coloring fades immediately if the infant's position is changed or the baby kicks or cries vigorously.

Birthmarks

Several commonly occurring birthmarks can be identified in newborns. It is important to differentiate the types of hemangiomas so you neither give false reassurance to parents nor worry them unnecessarily about these lesions.

Hemangiomas. The **hemangiomas** are vascular tumors of the skin. Three types are found.

Nevus flammeus (Fig. 23-10*A*) is a macular purple or dark red lesion (sometimes called a *port-wine stain* because of its deep color) that is present at birth. These lesions generally appear on the face, although they are often found on the thighs as well. Those above the bridge of the nose tend to fade; the others are less likely to fade. Because they are level with the skin surface (macular), they can be covered by a cosmetic preparation later in life or removed surgically or by laser therapy.

Nevus flammeus lesions also occur as lighter, pink patches at the nape of the neck (*stork's beak marks;* Fig. 23-10*B*). These do not fade either, but are covered by the hairline and so are of no consequence. They occur more often in females than in males.

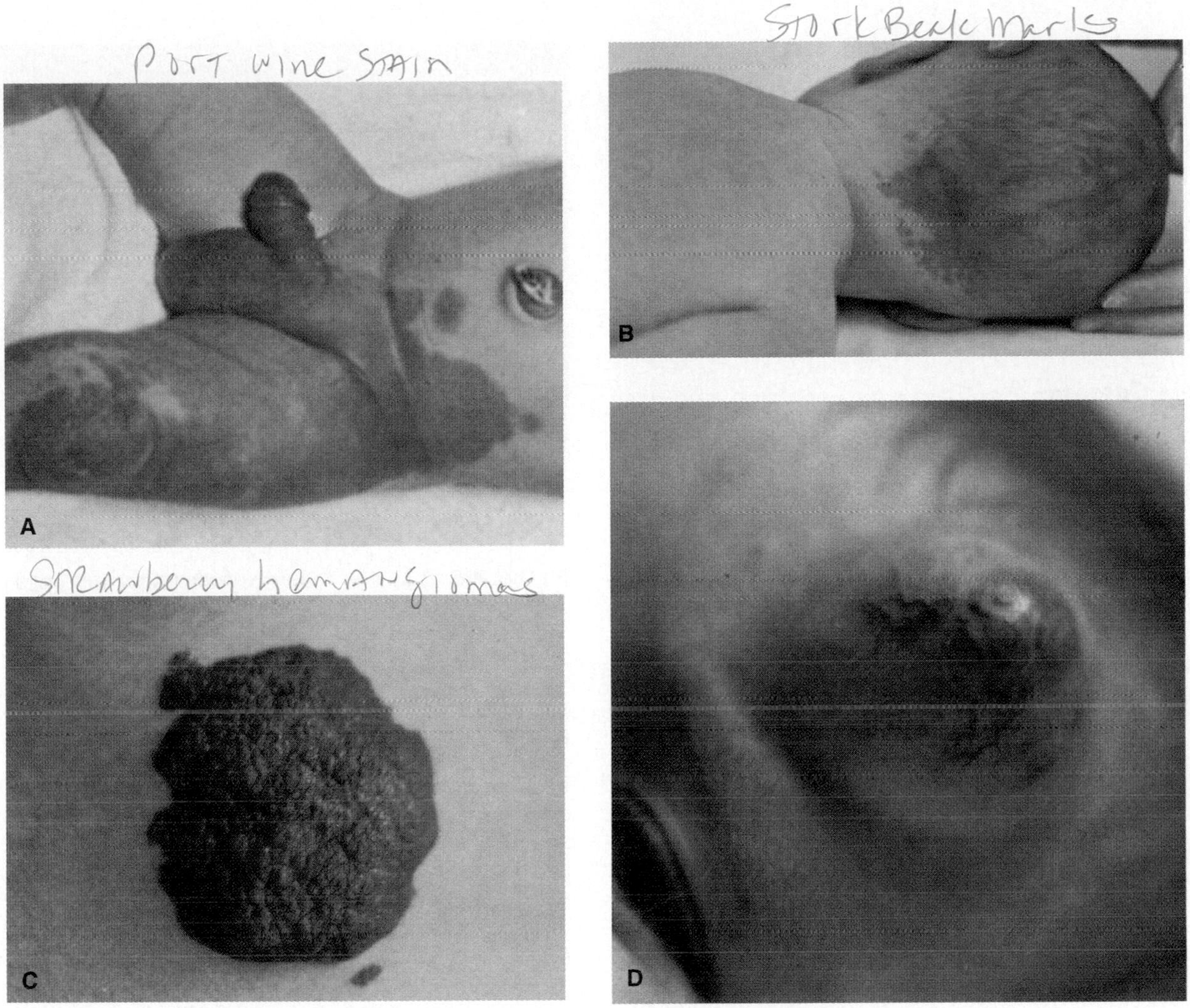

FIGURE 23.10 Types of hemangiomas found on the newborn. (*A*) Nevus flammeus (port-wine stain) formed of a plexus of newly formed capillaries in the papillary layer of the corium. It is deep red to purple, does not blanch on pressure, and does not fade with age. (*B*) Stork's beak mark, commonly occurring on nape of neck. It blanches on pressure; although it does not fade, it is not noticeable as it becomes covered by hair. (*C*) Strawberry hemangiomas consist of dilated capillaries in entire dermal and subdermal layers. They continue to enlarge after birth but usually disappear by age 10 years. (*D*) Cavernous hemangiomas consist of a communicating network of venules in subcutaneous tissue and do not fade with age.

Strawberry hemangiomas are elevated areas formed by immature capillaries and endothelial cells (Fig. 23-10*C*). Most are present at birth in the term neonate, although they may appear up to 2 weeks after birth. Typically, they are not present in the preterm infant because of the immaturity of the epidermis. Formation is associated with the high estrogen levels of pregnancy. They may continue to enlarge from their original size up to 1 year of age. After the first year, they tend to be absorbed and shrink in size. By the time the child is 7 years old, 50 to 75% of these lesions have disappeared. A child may be 10 years old before the absorption is complete. Application of hydrocortisone ointment may speed their disappearance by interfering with the binding of estrogen to its receptor sites (Dinehart et al., 2001).

Parents need to understand that the mark may grow. Otherwise, they may confuse it with cancer (a skin lesion increasing in size is one of the seven danger signals of cancer). They should also understand that the mark will disappear, so they do not think of their child as imperfect or disfigured. Surgery to remove strawberry hemangiomas is rarely recommended because it may lead to secondary infection, resulting in scarring and permanent disfigurement.

Cavernous hemangiomas (Fig. 23-10*D*) are dilated vascular spaces. They are usually raised and resemble a strawberry hemangioma in appearance. They do not disappear with time, as do strawberry hemangiomas. Subcutaneous infusions of interferon alpha 2a can be used to reduce these in size (Metry & Hebert, 2000) or they can be removed surgically. Children who have a skin lesion may have additional ones on internal organs. Blows to the abdomen, such as those from childhood games, can cause bleeding from internal hemangiomas. Children who have cavernous hemangiomas usually have their hematocrit levels assessed at health maintenance visits to evaluate for possible internal blood loss.

Mongolian Spots. **Mongolian spots** are collections of pigment cells (melanocytes) that appear as slate-gray patches across the sacrum or buttocks and possibly the arms and legs. They tend to occur in children of Asian, Southern European, or African extraction. They disappear by school age without treatment. Be sure to inform parents that these are not bruises. Otherwise, they may worry that the baby sustained a birth injury.

Vernix Caseosa

Vernix caseosa, a white, cream cheese–like substance that serves as a skin lubricant, is usually noticeable on a newborn's skin, at least in the skin folds, at birth in a term neonate. The color of the vernix should be carefully noted, because it takes on the color of the amniotic fluid. If it is yellow, the amniotic fluid was yellow from bilirubin. If it is green, meconium was present in the amniotic fluid.

Until the first bath when vernix is washed away, handle newborns with gloves to protect yourself from exposure to body fluids. Never use harsh rubbing to wash away vernix. The newborn's skin is tender, and breaks in the skin from too vigorous attempts at removal may open portals of entry for bacteria.

Lanugo

Lanugo is the fine, downy hair that covers a newborn's shoulders, back, and upper arms. It may be found also on the forehead and ears. The newborn of 37 to 39 weeks' gestational age has more lanugo than the 40-week-old infant. Postmature infants (over 42 weeks) rarely have lanugo. Lanugo is rubbed away by the friction of bedding and clothes against the newborn's skin. By age 2 weeks, it has disappeared.

Desquamation

Within 24 hours of birth, the skin of most newborns has become extremely dry. The dryness is particularly evident on the palms of the hands and soles of the feet. It may result in areas of peeling similar to those after sunburn. This is normal and needs no treatment. Parents may apply hand lotion to prevent excessive dryness if they wish.

Newborns who are postmature and have suffered intrauterine malnutrition may have extremely dry skin with a leathery appearance and cracks in the skin folds. This should be differentiated from normal desquamation.

Milia

Newborn sebaceous glands are immature. At least one pinpoint white papule (a plugged or unopened sebaceous gland) can be found on the cheek or across the bridge of the nose of every newborn. Such lesions, termed **milia** (Fig. 23-11), disappear by 2 to 4 weeks of age as the sebaceous glands mature and drain. Parents should be instructed to avoid scratching or squeezing the papules to prevent secondary infection.

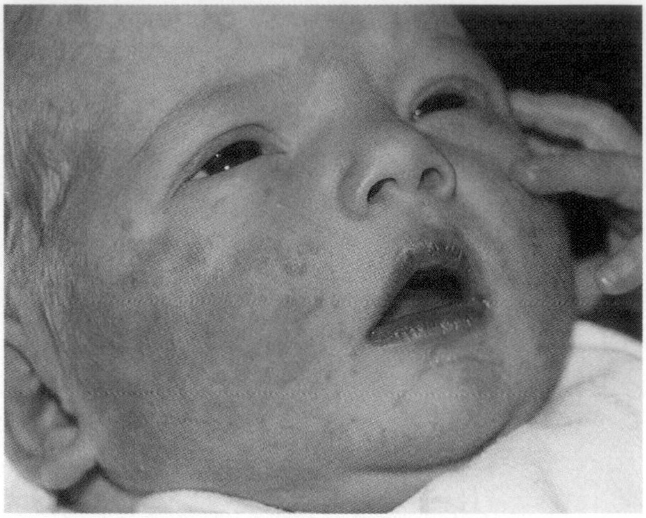

FIGURE 23.11 Milia are unopened sebaceous glands frequently found on the nose, chin, or cheeks of a newborn. One is evident here on the right check.

Erythema Toxicum

In most normal mature infants, a newborn rash called **erythema toxicum** is observed (Fig. 23-12). It usually appears in the first to fourth day of life, but may appear up to 2 weeks of age. It begins with a papule, increases in severity to become erythema by the second day, and then disappears by the third day. It is sometimes called a *flea-bite rash* because the lesions are minuscule. One of the chief characteristics of the rash is its lack of pattern. It occurs sporadically and unpredictably, and may last hours

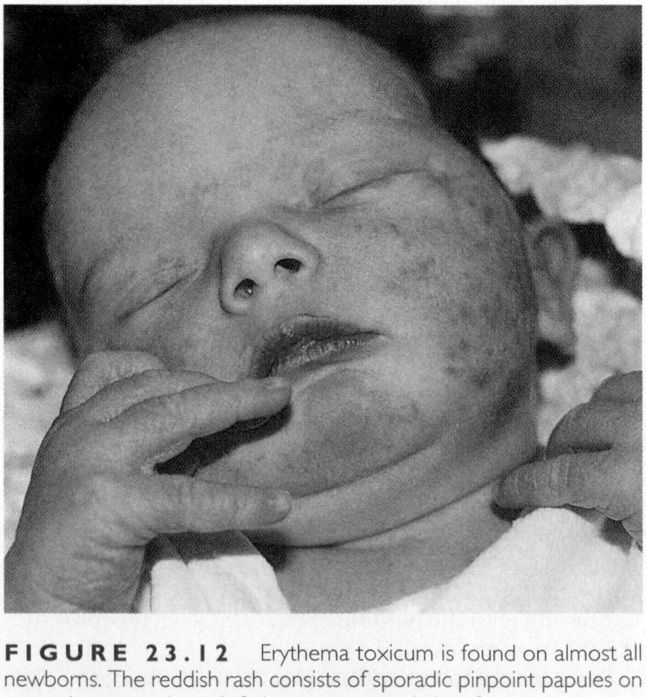

FIGURE 23.12 Erythema toxicum is found on almost all newborns. The reddish rash consists of sporadic pinpoint papules on an erythematous base. It fades spontaneously in a few days.

rather than days. It is caused by the newborn's eosinophils reacting to the environment as the immune system matures. It needs no treatment.

Forceps Marks

If forceps were used for birth, there may be a circular or linear contusion matching the rim of the blade of the forceps on the infant's cheek (Fig. 23-13). This mark disappears in 1 to 2 days along with the edema that accompanies it. The mark is the result of normal forceps use and does not denote unskilled or too vigorous application of forceps. Closely assess the facial nerve while the newborn is at rest and during crying episodes to detect any potential facial nerve compression requiring further evaluation.

Skin Turgor

Newborn skin should feel resilient if the underlying tissue is well hydrated. If a fold of the skin is grasped between the thumb and fingers, it should feel elastic. When it is released, it should fall back to form a smooth surface. If severe dehydration is present, the skin will not smooth out again but will remain in an elevated ridge. Poor turgor is seen in newborns who suffered malnutrition in utero, who have difficulty sucking at birth, or who have certain metabolic disorders, such as adrenogenital syndrome.

Head

A newborn's head appears disproportionately large because it is about one fourth of the total length; in an adult, the head is one eighth of total height. The forehead of the newborn is large and prominent. The chin appears to be receding, and it quivers easily if the infant is startled or cries. Well-nourished newborns have full-bodied hair; poorly nourished or preterm infants have thin, lifeless hair. If internal fetal monitoring was used during labor, the newborn also may exhibit a pinpoint ulcer at the point where the monitor was attached.

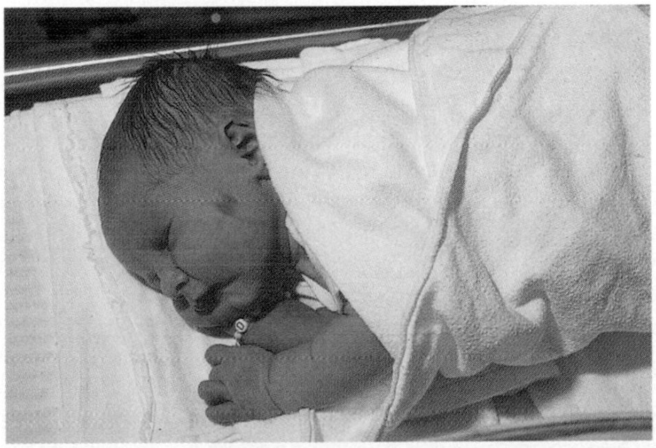

FIGURE 23.13 Forceps marks are commonly found in newborns delivered by forceps. Such marks are transient and disappear in a day or two.

Fontanelles

The fontanelles are the spaces or openings where the skull bones join. The anterior fontanelle is located at the junction of the two parietal bones and the two fused frontal bones. It is diamond shaped and measures 2 to 3 cm (0.8 to 1.2 in) in width and 3 to 4 cm (1.2 to 1.6 in) in length. The posterior fontanelle is located at the junction of the parietal bones and the occipital bone. It is triangular and measures about 1 cm (0.4 in) in length.

The anterior fontanelle will be felt as a soft spot. It should not appear indented (a sign of dehydration) or bulging (a sign of increased intracranial pressure) with the infant positioned upright at a 45° to 90°degree angle. The fontanelle may bulge if the newborn strains to pass a stool or cries vigorously. With vigorous crying, a pulse may sometimes be seen in the fontanelle. The anterior fontanelle normally closes at 12 to 18 months of age.

The posterior fontanelle is so small in some newborns that it cannot be palpated readily. The posterior fontanelle closes by the end of the second month.

Sutures

The skull *sutures,* the separating lines of the skull, may override at birth because of the extreme pressure exerted by passage through the birth canal. Overriding is a normal, transient phenomenon. When the sagittal suture between the parietal bones overrides, the fontanelles will be less perceptible than usual.

Suture lines should never appear widely separated in newborns. Wide separation denotes increased intracranial pressure from abnormal brain formation, abnormal accumulation of cerebrospinal fluid in the cranium (hydrocephalus), or an accumulation of blood from a birth injury, such as subdural hemorrhage. Fused suture lines also are abnormal and need to be confirmed with x-ray and further evaluation.

Molding

The part of the infant's head (usually the vertex) that engages the cervix molds to fit the cervix contours. After birth, this area appears prominent and asymmetric. Molding may be so extreme in the baby of a primiparous woman that the baby's head looks like a dunce cap (Fig. 23-14). The head will be restored to its normal shape within a few days of birth.

Caput Succedaneum

Caput succedaneum (Fig. 23-15*A*) is edema of the scalp at the presenting part of the head. It may involve wide areas of the head or may be the size of a large egg. The edema, which crosses the suture lines, will gradually be absorbed and disappear about the third day of life. It needs no treatment.

Cephalhematoma

A *cephalhematoma* is a collection of blood between the periosteum of the skull bone and the bone itself caused by rupture of a periosteum capillary due to the pressure

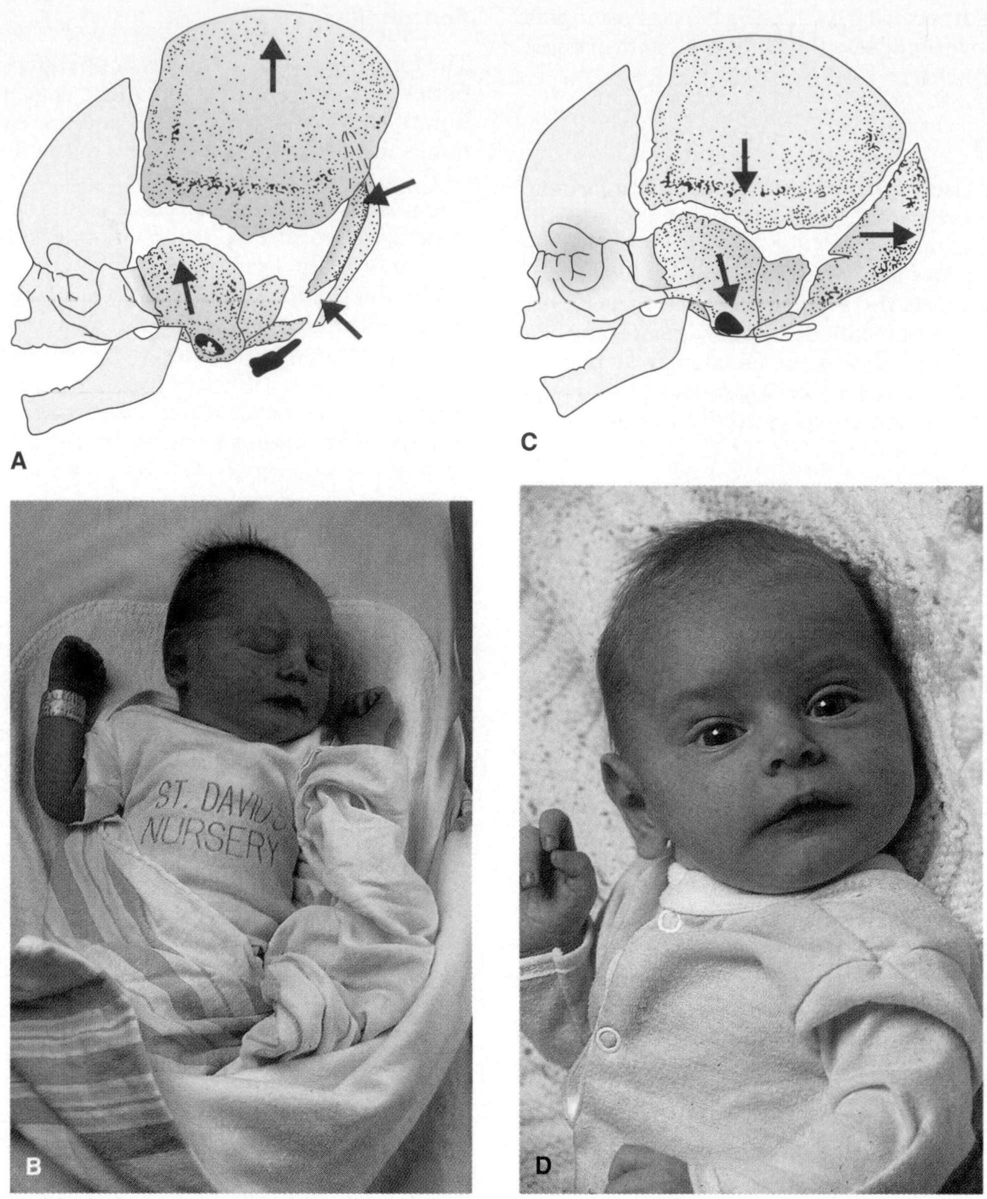

FIGURE 23.14 Molding. (*A, B*) The infant head molds to fit the birth canal more easily. On palpation, the skull sutures will be felt to be overriding. (*C, D*) The head shape returns to normal within 1 week.

of birth (Fig. 23-15*B*). It usually occurs 24 hours after birth. Although the blood loss is negligible, the swelling is generally severe and is well outlined as an egg shape. It may be discolored (black and blue) because of the presence of coagulated blood. A cephalhematoma is confined to an individual bone, so the associated swelling stops at the bone's suture line.

It often takes weeks for a cephalhematoma to be absorbed. It might appear that the blood could be aspirated to relieve the condition. However, this procedure would introduce the risk of infection and is unnecessary because the condition will subside by itself. As the blood captured in the space is broken down, a great amount of indirect bilirubin may be released, leading to jaundice.

Craniotabes

Craniotabes is a localized softening of the cranial bones. The bone is so soft that the pressure of an examining finger can indent it. The bone returns to its normal contour when the pressure is removed. The condition corrects itself without treatment after a few months.

Craniotabes is probably caused by pressure of the fetal skull against the mother's pelvic bone in utero. It is more common in firstborn infants than in infants born later, because of the lower position of the fetal head in the pelvis during the last 2 weeks of pregnancy in primiparous women. It is an example of a condition that is normal in a newborn but would be pathologic in an older child (probably the result of faulty metabolism or kidney dysfunction).

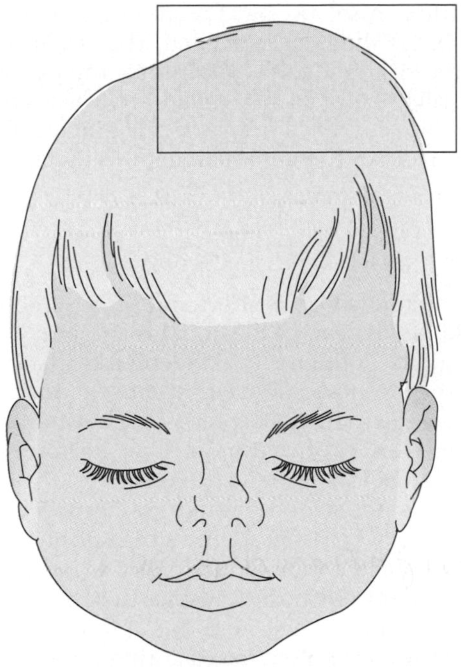

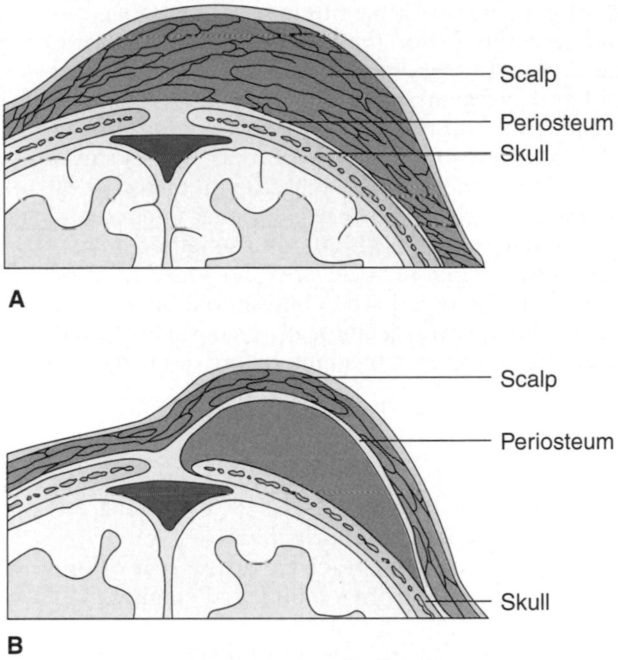

FIGURE 23.15 (*A*) Caput succedaneum. From pressure of the birth canal, an edematous area is present beneath the scalp. Note how it crosses the midline of the skull. (*B*) Cephalhematoma. A small capillary beneath the periosteum of the skull bone has ruptured, and blood has collected under the periosteum of the bone. Note how the swelling now stops at the midline. Because the blood is contained under the periosteum, it is necessarily stopped by a suture line.

WHAT IF? A new mother is holding her newborn, 2 hours old. She is inspecting the baby and says to you, "His hands and feet are cold and look blue. Is something wrong with my baby?" How should you answer?

Eyes

Newborns usually cry tearlessly because the lacrimal ducts are not fully mature until about 3 months of age. Almost without exception, the irises of the eyes of newborns are gray or blue, and the sclera may be blue due to its thinness. Infant eyes assume their permanent color between 3 and 12 months of age.

To inspect eyes, lay the infant in a supine position and lift the head. This maneuver usually causes the baby to open the eyes. The eyes should appear clear, without redness or purulent discharge. Occasionally, the administration of an antibiotic ointment such as erythromycin at birth to protect against *Chlamydia* infection as well as ophthalmia neonatorum (gonorrheal conjunctivitis) will cause a purulent discharge for the first 24 hours of life.

Pressure during birth sometimes will rupture a conjunctival capillary, resulting in a small **subconjunctival hemorrhage.** This appears as a red spot on the sclera, usually on the inner aspect of the eye, or as a red ring around the cornea. The bleeding is slight and needs no treatment. It will be completely absorbed in 2 or 3 weeks. Parents can be assured that these hemorrhages are normal variations. Otherwise they may assume that the baby is bleeding from within the eye and that vision will be impaired.

Edema is often present around the orbit or on the eyelids. This will remain for the first 2 or 3 days until the newborn's kidneys are capable of evacuating fluid efficiently.

The cornea of the eye should be round and proportionate in size to that of an adult eye. A cornea that is larger than usual may be the result of congenital glaucoma. An irregularly shaped pupil or discolored iris may denote disease (see Chapter 33). The pupil should be dark. A white pupil suggests congenital cataract.

Ears

The newborn's external ear is still not as completely formed as it will be eventually, so the pinna tends to bend easily. In the term newborn, the pinna recoils after bending.

The level of the top part of the external ear should be on a line drawn from the inner canthus to the outer canthus of the eye and back across the side of the head (see Chapter 33). Ears that are set lower than this are found in infants with certain chromosomal abnormalities, particularly trisomy 18 and 13, syndromes in which low-set ears and other physical defects are coupled with varying degrees of cognitive challenges (see Chapters 7 and 54).

Small tags of skin are sometimes found just in front of the ear. Although these may be associated with chromosomal abnormalities or kidney disease, they generally are isolated findings and are of no consequence. They can be removed by ligation immediately or when the child is a week old. A preauricular dermal sinus may be present directly in front of the ear. The area should be inspected for a pinpoint-size opening. The sinus is usually small and can be removed without consequence when a child is near school age.

Visualizing the tympanic membrane in a newborn is difficult and generally is not attempted, because amniotic fluid and flecks of vernix fill the canal and obliterate the drum and its accompanying landmarks.

A good practice is to test the newborn's hearing by ringing a bell held about 6 inches from each ear. If he or she is crying, the infant who can hear will stop momentarily. If quiet, a newborn will blink the eyes, appear to attend to the sound, and may startle. Although this method of testing is not highly accurate, a negative response (lack of response) should be noted. The child should be retested later. In many health care facilities, all newborns are tested by a standardized response to sound before discharge.

Nose

A newborn's nose may appear large for the face. As the child grows, the rest of the face will grow more than the nose, and this discrepancy will disappear.

Test for choanal atresia (blockage at the rear of the nose) by closing the newborn's mouth and compressing one naris at a time with your fingers. Note any discomfort or distress. Also record any evidence of milia.

Mouth

A newborn's mouth should open evenly when the baby cries. If one side of the mouth moves more than the other, cranial nerve injury is suggested. A newborn's tongue appears large and prominent in the mouth. Because the tongue is short, the frenulum membrane is attached close to the tip of the tongue, creating the impression that the infant is "tongue tied." At one time, it was almost routine to snip a newborn's frenulum membrane to lengthen it. Now this procedure is regarded as harmful and unnecessary, because it leaves a portal of entry for infection, risks hemorrhage because of the low level of vitamin K in most newborns, and causes feeding difficulties by making the tongue sore and irritated.

The palate of the newborn should be intact. Occasionally, one or two small round, glistening, well-circumscribed cysts (Epstein's pearls) are present on the palate, a result of the extra load of calcium that was deposited in utero. Be sure to inform the parents that these findings are insignificant and require no treatment; they disappear spontaneously in a week. A parent may be concerned about them, mistaking them for **thrush,** a *Candida* infection, which usually appears on the tongue and sides of the cheeks as white or gray patches.

All newborns have some mucus in their mouths. Newborns delivered by cesarean birth may have an increased amount of mucus. If newborns are placed on their side, the mucus drains from their mouths and gives them no distress. If their mouths are filled with so much mucus that they seem to be blowing bubbles, a tracheoesophageal fistula may be suspected. This must be determined before a child is fed; otherwise, formula can be aspirated into the lungs from the inadequately formed esophagus.

It is unusual for the newborn to have teeth, but sometimes one or two (called **natal teeth**) will have erupted. Any teeth present must be evaluated for stability. If loose, they should be extracted to prevent possible aspiration during feeding. Also, any natal teeth not covered by the gum membrane should be removed. They can loosen, increasing the risk for aspiration. Inform the parents that the baby will usually get the remaining two sets of teeth.

Small, white epithelial pearls (benign inclusion cysts) may be present on the gum margins. No therapy is necessary for these.

Neck

The neck of a newborn is short and often chubby with creased skin folds. The head should rotate freely on it. If there is rigidity of the neck, congenital torticollis from injury to the sternocleidomastoid muscle during birth should be considered (see Chapter 39). In newborns whose membranes were ruptured more than 24 hours before birth, nuchal rigidity suggests meningitis.

The neck is not strong enough to support the total weight of the newborn's head. In a sitting position, a newborn should make a momentary effort at head control. When lying prone, newborns can raise their heads slightly, usually enough to lift their nose out of mucus or spit-up formula. If they are pulled into a sitting position from a supine position, their heads will lag behind considerably. Again, however, they should make some effort to control and steady their heads as they reach the sitting position.

The trachea may be prominent on the front of the neck. The thymus gland may be enlarged because of the rapid growth of glandular tissue in comparison to the growth of other body tissues. The thymus gland triples in size by 3 years of age, remaining at that size until the child is about 10 years old. After that, its size begins to decrease. Although the thymus may appear to be bulging in the newborn, it is rarely a cause of respiratory difficulty, as was previously believed.

Chest

The chest in some infants looks small because the infant's head is large in proportion. Not until the child is 2 years of age does the chest measurement exceed that of the head.

In both female and male infants, the breasts may be engorged. Occasionally, the breasts of newborn babies secrete a thin, watery fluid popularly termed *witch's milk.* Engorgement occurs in utero as a result of the influence of the mother's hormones. As soon as the hormones are cleared from the infant's system (about a week), the engorgement and any fluid subside. Fluid should never be expressed from infant breasts. The manipulation may introduce bacteria and lead to mastitis.

The chest is as wide in the anteroposterior diameter as it is across and approximately 2 inches less in circumference than the newborn's head. The clavicles should be straight. A crepitus or actual separation on one or the other clavicle may indicate that a fracture occurred during birth and calcium is now being deposited at that point. As the area heals, a lump may be palpated from temporary calcium overgrowth. Overall, the chest should appear symmetric. Respirations are normally rapid (30 to 60 breaths per minute) but not distressed. A supernumerary nipple (usually found below and in line with the normal nipples) may be present. If so, it may be removed later for cosmetic purposes.

Retraction (drawing in of the chest wall with inspiration) should not be present. An infant with retractions (Fig. 23-16) is using such strong force to pull air into the respiratory tract that he or she pulls in the anterior chest muscle.

Because the newborn's alveoli open slowly over the first 24 to 48 hours and the baby invariably has mucus in the back of the throat, listening to lung sounds often reveals the sounds of rhonchi, the harsh, innocent sound of air passing over mucus. Abnormal sounds, such as a grunting sound, suggest respiratory distress syndrome; a high, crowing sound on inspiration suggests stridor or immature tracheal development.

Abdomen

The contour of the newborn abdomen is slightly protuberant. A scaphoid or sunken appearance may indicate missing abdominal contents or a diaphragmatic hernia. Bowel sounds should be present within an hour after birth. The edge of the liver is usually palpable 1 to 2 cm below the right costal margin. The edge of the spleen may be palpable 1 to 2 cm below the left costal margin. Tenderness is difficult to determine in a newborn. If it is extreme, however, the infant will cry, thrash about, or tense abdominal muscles to protect the abdomen as you palpate it.

For the first hour after birth, the umbilical cord appears as a white, gelatinous structure marked with the red and blue streaks of the umbilical vein and arteries. The one vein and two arteries should be counted when the cord is first cut after birth to be certain they are present. In 0.5% of deliveries (3.5% of twin deliveries), there is only a single umbilical artery, and in a third of such infants, this single artery is associated with a congenital heart anomaly; renal anomalies also may be present. Because the anomaly may not be readily apparent, any child with a single umbilical artery needs close observation and assessment until all anomalies are ruled out.

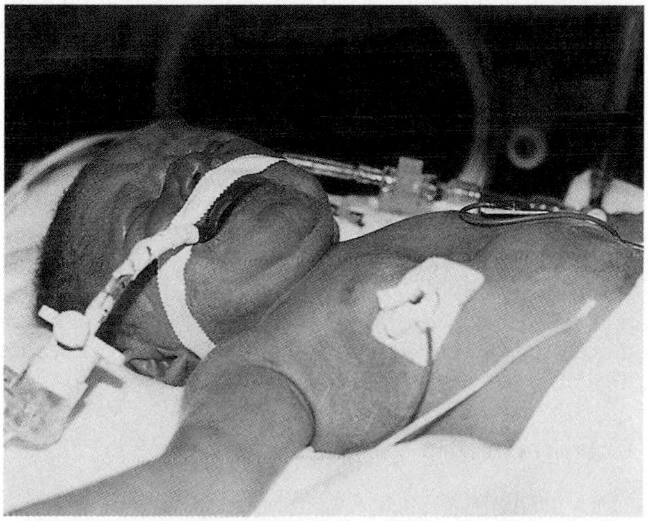

FIGURE 23.16 Sternal retractions are a sign of respiratory distress requiring immediate intervention, such as mechanical ventilation and other monitoring devices.

Inspect the cord clamp to be certain it is secure. After the first hour of life, the cord begins to dry and shrink, and turns brown like the dead end of a vine. By the second or third day, it has turned black. It breaks free by the sixth to tenth day, leaving a granulating area a few centimeters wide that heals during the following week.

There should be no bleeding at the cord site. Bleeding suggests that the cord clamp has become loosened or the cord has been tugged loose by the friction of the bedclothes. The base of the cord should appear dry. A moist or odorous cord suggests infection. If present, infection should receive immediate treatment or it may enter the newborn's bloodstream and cause septicemia. Moistness at the base of the cord also may indicate a patent urachus (a canal connecting the bladder and the umbilicus), which is draining urine at the cord site.

The base of the cord also should be inspected to ensure that no abdominal wall defects, such as an umbilical hernia, are present. If there is a fascial (abdominal wall) defect less than 2 cm in size, it will generally close on its own by school age; a defect more than 2 cm wide will probably require surgical correction. Taping or putting buttons or coins on the abdomen are home remedies that do not help defects to close. In fact, heavy taping may worsen the condition by preventing the development of good muscle tone in the abdominal wall. Tape also tends to keep the cord moist, making infection more likely than when it is dry (see Focus on Cultural Competence).

Since a newborn's voiding only demonstrates that there is at least one kidney, not that there are two, attempt to verify the presence of kidneys by deep palpation of the right and left abdomen within the first few hours after birth. After this time, the intestines fill with air, making palpation more difficult. The right kidney (at least its lower pole) can

FOCUS ON CULTURAL COMPETENCE

Although it is generally a sound policy to point out the positive aspects of a child to parents to aid parent–child bonding, in some areas of the world, such as traditional Cambodia and Laos, newborns are not given compliments this way, because it is believed to make them vulnerable to evil spirits.

In the traditional Haitian culture, infants are not named immediately, but only after a full month. In some African cultures, it is important for newborns to have an amulet (good-luck charm) tied around their neck. Respect these and leave them in place. Oiling the infant's body and placing a belly band over the umbilical cord are also common care procedures. Educate parents that leaving the cord exposed to the air helps the cord dry and reduces the possibility of infection.

Being aware of cultural variations in newborn care such as these helps you plan care that is specific and meaningful to individual parents and that can aid parent–child bonding.

usually be palpated, because it is located lower than the left; the left kidney is more difficult to locate because the intestine is bulkier on the left side, and the left kidney is higher in the retroperitoneal space. Nonetheless, try to locate it. Placing one hand behind the infant while you palpate offers a firmer base and helps when evaluating kidney size (newborn kidneys are about the size of a walnut). If a kidney feels enlarged, this suggests a polycystic kidney or pooling of urine from a urethral obstruction.

To finish abdominal assessment, elicit an abdominal reflex. Stroking each quadrant of the abdomen will cause the umbilicus to move or "wink" in that direction. This superficial abdominal reflex is a test of spinal nerves T8 through T10. The reflex may not be demonstrable in newborns until the tenth day of life.

Anogenital Area

Inspect the anus of the newborn to ensure that it is present, patent, and not covered by a membrane (imperforate anus). Test for anal patency by gently inserting the tip of your little finger, gloved and lubricated. Also note the time after birth that the infant first passes meconium. If a newborn does not do so in the first 24 hours, suspect imperforate anus or meconium ileus.

Male Genitalia

The scrotum in most male newborns is edematous and has rugae. It may be deeply pigmented in African-American or dark-skinned newborns.

Both testes should be present in the scrotum. Males with one or both undescended testicles (cryptorchidism) need further referral to establish the extent of the problem. It could be due to agenesis (absence of an organ), ectopic testes (the testes cannot enter the scrotum because the opening to the scrotal sac is closed), or undescended testes (the vas deferens or artery is too short to allow the testes to descend). Newborns with agenesis of the testes are usually referred for investigation of other anomalies because the testes arise from the same germ tissue as the kidneys (Kanemoto et al., 2002). Make a practice of pressing your nondominant hand against the inguinal ring before palpating for the testes, so they do not slip upward out of the scrotal sac as you palpate (Fig. 23-17).

The cremasteric reflex is elicited by stroking the internal side of the thigh. As the skin is stroked, the testis on that side moves perceptibly upward. This is a test for the integrity of spinal nerves T8 through T10. The response may be absent in newborns less than about 10 days old.

The penis of newborns appears small, approximately 2 cm long. If it is less than this, the newborn should be referred for evaluation by an endocrinologist. It should be inspected to see that the urethral opening is at the tip of the glans, not on the dorsal surface (epispadias) or the ventral surface (hypospadias).

The prepuce (foreskin) of the penis should be examined to be certain it is not stenosed. In most newborns, it slides back poorly from the meatal opening, so this should not be done. Although today most male newborns are circumcised, the necessity for this operation can be questioned. It is rare to find an infant who physically requires it (with a foreskin so constricted that it interferes with voiding or circulation). In addition, surgery this early in life poses the risk of hemorrhage and infection. Circumcision should not be done if hypospadias or epispadias is present, because the surgeon may want to use the foreskin as tissue in repairing these conditions (see discussion later in chapter).

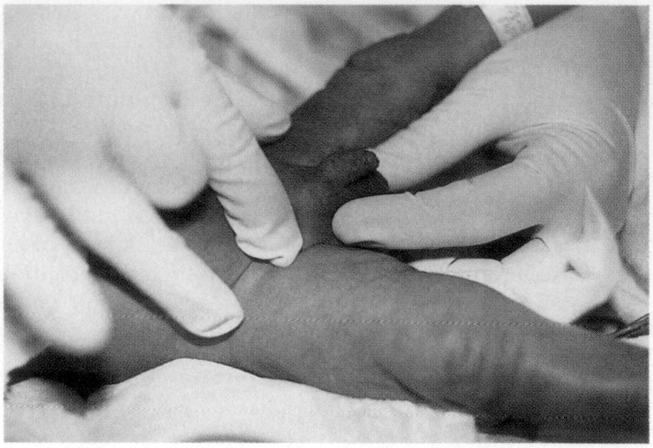

FIGURE 23.17 Pressing the nondominant hand against the inguinal ring when palpating the testes.

Female Genitalia

The vulva in female newborns may be swollen because of the effect of maternal hormones. Some newborns have a mucus vaginal secretion, which is sometimes blood-tinged (**pseudomenstruation**). Again, this is due to the action of maternal hormones. The discharge will disappear as soon as the infant's system has cleared the hormones. The discharge should not be mistaken for an infection or taken as an indication that trauma has occurred.

Back

The spine of a newborn typically appears flat in the lumbar and sacral areas. The curves seen in the adult appear only when a child is able to sit and walk. The base of the spine should be inspected carefully to be certain there is no pinpoint opening, dimpling, or sinus tract in the skin, suggestive of a dermal sinus or spinal bifida occulta.

A newborn normally assumes the position maintained in utero, with the back rounded and the arms and legs flexed on the abdomen and chest. A child who was born in a frank breech position will tend to straighten the legs at the knee and bring them up next to the face. The position of a baby presenting with a face presentation sometimes simulates opisthotonos for the first week, because the curve of the back is deeply concave.

Extremities

The arms and legs of a newborn appear short. The hands are plump and clenched into fists. Newborn fingernails are soft and smooth, and usually are long enough to extend over the fingertips. Test the upper extremities for muscle tone by unflexing the arms for approximately 5 seconds.

When you release an arm, it should return immediately to its flexed position. Hold the arms down by the sides and note their length. The fingertips should cover the proximal thigh. Unusually short arms may signify achondroplastic dwarfism. Observe for unusual curvature of the little finger and inspect the palm for a simian crease (a single palmar crease in contrast to the three creases normally seen in a palm). Although curved fingers and simian creases may occur normally, they are commonly associated with Down syndrome.

The arms and legs should move symmetrically (unless an infant is demonstrating a tonic neck reflex). An arm that hangs limp and unmoving suggests possible birth injuries, such as injury to the clavicle or the brachial or cervical plexus or fracture of a long bone. Assess for webbing (syndactyly), extra toes or fingers (polydactyly), or unusual spacing of toes, particularly between the big toes and the others (a finding in certain chromosomal disorders, although this is also a normal finding in some families). Test to see whether the toenails become blanched and refill after pressure.

Normally, the legs are bowed as well as short. The sole of the foot appears to be flat because of an extra pad of fat in the longitudinal arch. The mature newborn has many crisscrossed lines on the sole of the foot covering approximately two thirds of the foot. If these creases cover less than two thirds of the foot or are absent, suspect immaturity.

Put the ankle through a range of motion to evaluate whether the heel cord is unusually tight. Check for ankle clonus by supporting the lower leg in one hand and dorsiflexing the foot sharply two or three times by pressure on the sole of the foot with the other hand. After the dorsiflexion, one or two continued movements are normal. Rapid alternating contraction and relaxation (clonus) is abnormal, suggesting neurologic involvement. The feet of many newborns turn in (varus deviation) because of intrauterine position. This simple deviation needs no correction if the feet can be brought into the midline position by easy manipulation. When the infant begins to bear weight, the feet will align themselves. If a foot does not align readily or will not turn to a definite midline position, a talipes deformity (clubfoot) may be present. This condition needs investigation, because congenital problems of this kind are best treated in the newborn period.

With the newborn in a supine position, both legs can be flexed and abducted to such an extent (180°) that they touch or nearly touch the surface of the bed (Fig. 23-18). If the hip joint seems to lock short of this distance (160° to 170°), hip subluxation (a shallow and poorly formed acetabulum) is suggested. Test for subluxation by holding the infant's leg with the fingers on the greater and lesser trochanters and then abducting the hip; if subluxation is present, a "clunk" of the femur head striking the shallow acetabulum can be heard (Ortolani's sign). If the hip can be felt to actually slip in the socket, this is Barlow's sign. Subluxated hip may be bilateral but is usually unilateral. It is important that hip subluxation be discovered as early as possible, because correction is most successful if initiated early.

When lying on the abdomen, newborns are capable of bringing their arms and legs underneath them and raising

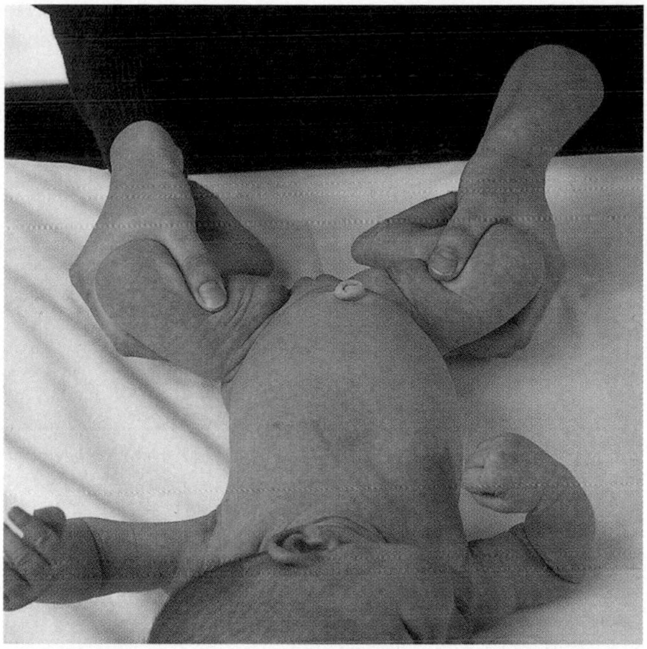

FIGURE 23.18 Hip abduction in a newborn—both hips should abduct so completely they lie almost flat against the mattress (180 degrees).

their stomach off the bed high enough for a hand to be slipped underneath. This ability helps to prevent pressure or rubbing at the cord site, since the cord site does not actually touch the bedding when in this position. The preterm newborn does not have this ability; thus, an infant's ability to do so is an indication of maturity.

✔ CHECKPOINT QUESTIONS

6. Typically, the hands and feet of newborns are blue in color during the first few hours after birth? What is this called?
7. What substance is released with red blood cell hemolysis that can be detrimental to newborn health?
8. What type of therapy does milia require?
9. What is the term for the presence of extra digits?

ASSESSMENT FOR WELL-BEING

Apgar Scoring

At 1 minute and 5 minutes after birth, newborns are observed and rated according to an Apgar score, an assessment scale used as a standard since 1958 (Apgar et al., 1958). As shown in Table 23-2, heart rate, respiratory effort, muscle tone, reflex irritability, and color are rated 0, 1, or 2; all five scores are then added. An infant whose total score is under 4 is in serious danger and needs resuscitation. A score of 4 to 6 means that the condition is guarded and a baby may need clearing of the airway and supplementary oxygen. A score of 7 to 10 is considered good, indicating that the

TABLE 23.2 Apgar Scoring Chart

	SCORE		
SIGN	0	1	2
Heart rate	Absent	Slow (<100)	>100
Respiratory effort	Absent	Slow, irregular; weak cry	Good; strong cry
Muscle tone	Flaccid	Some flexion of extremities	Well flexed
Reflex irritability:			
Response to catheter in nostril, or	No response	Grimace	Cough or sneeze
Slap to sole of foot	No response	Grimace	Cry and withdrawal of foot
Color	Blue, pale	Body normal pigment, extremities blue	Normal skin coloring

infant scored as high as 70 to 90% of infants at 1 to 5 minutes after birth (10 is the highest score possible).

The Apgar score standardizes infant evaluation and serves as a baseline for future evaluations. There is a high correlation between low 5-minute Apgar scores and mortality and morbidity, particularly neurologic morbidity (Moster et al., 2001). The following points should be considered in obtaining an Apgar rating.

Heart Rate. Auscultating the newborn heart with a stethoscope is the best way of determining heart rate; however, heart rate also may be obtained by observing and counting the pulsations of the cord at the abdomen if the cord is still uncut.

Respiratory Effort. A mature newborn usually cries spontaneously at about 30 seconds after birth. By 1 minute, he or she is maintaining regular, although rapid, respirations. Difficulty might be anticipated in a newborn whose mother received large amounts of analgesia or a general anesthetic during labor or birth (see Focus on Nursing Care Planning).

Muscle Tone. Mature newborns hold the extremities tightly flexed, simulating their intrauterine position. They should resist any effort to extend their extremities.

Reflex Irritability. One of two possible cues is used to evaluate reflex irritability: either the newborn's response to a suction catheter in the nostrils or the response to having the soles of the feet slapped. A baby whose mother was heavily sedated will probably demonstrate a low score in this category.

Color. All infants appear cyanotic at the moment of birth. They grow pink with or shortly after the first breath. The color of newborns thus corresponds to how well they are breathing. Acrocyanosis (cyanosis of the hands and feet) is so common in newborns that a score of 1 in this category can be thought of as normal.

Respiratory Evaluation

Good respiratory function obviously has the highest priority in newborn care, so assessment for it is ongoing at every newborn contact. The Silverman and Andersen index, originally devised in 1956 (Silverman & Andersen, 1956), can be used to estimate degrees of respiratory distress in newborns. For this assessment, a newborn is observed and then scored on each of five criteria (Fig. 23-19). As shown, each item is given a value of 0, 1, or 2. These values are then added. A total score of 0 indicates no respiratory distress. Scores of 4 to 6 indicate moderate distress. Scores of 7 to 10 indicate severe distress. Note that the scores of this index run opposite to those of the Apgar. In an Apgar score, a value of 7 to 10 indicates a well infant. In the Silverman and Andersen index, a value of 7 to 10 denotes a seriously distressed infant.

Physical Examination

A newborn is given a preliminary physical examination immediately after birth to detect such grossly observable conditions as meningocele, cleft lip and palate, hydrocephalus, birthmarks, congenital heart defects, imperforate anus, tracheoesophageal atresia, and bowel obstruction. This assessment may be the responsibility of the delivering physician, nurse practitioner, nurse-midwife, pediatrician, or staff nurse. This health assessment must be done quickly to prevent overexposing the newborn. Yet it must not be done so swiftly that important findings are overlooked.

The immediate birth appraisal should include auscultation of the chest for heart and respiratory sounds (perhaps already done as a part of Apgar scoring). Other procedures can be performed to rule out the common birth anomalies. Their screening importance is shown in Table 23-3. In addition, the immediate birth appraisal should include a thorough generalized inspection and tentative determination of gestational age.

Height and Weight

The newborn should be weighed nude and without a blanket in the delivery or birthing room (Fig. 23-20). Length and head, chest, and abdominal circumferences can be measured in the newborn or transitional nursery. Doing these measurements while the infant is still damp only exposes a newborn unnecessarily to chilling.

These measurements establish baselines against which all others will be compared. Thereafter, the infant is weighed

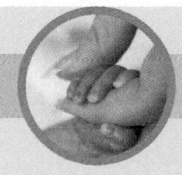

FOCUS ON *Nursing Care Planning*

A TERM NEWBORN

A 6-lb, 5-oz African-American male was born vaginally 1 hour ago. This is the parents' first child. They state, "It sounds like he has a cold. And what is this bruise on his lower back?"

Assessment: Apgar score: 7 at 1 minute; 9 at 5 minutes. Birth from LOA position. Breathed at 30 seconds after birth after administration of blow-by oxygen. Respiratory rate 74 breaths per minute with mild substernal retractions; rhonchi in upper lobes bilaterally; no grunting or nasal flaring present. Slate gray 2 × 3 cm macular area noted on sacral area. Mother attempted breastfeeding in birthing room, but newborn had difficulty sucking because of rapid respirations. Remainder of physical examination within acceptable parameters. Temperature: 97.8°F (36.6°C) at birth; 98.2°F (36.8°C) at 1 hour.

Nursing Diagnosis: Risk for ineffective airway clearance related to difficulty establishing respirations and rapid respiratory rate

Outcome Identification: Newborn will maintain patent airway with respiratory rate within acceptable parameters.

Outcome Evaluation: Respiratory rate is decreased to 30 to 60 breaths per minute; retractions, nasal flaring and grunting are absent; lungs are clear to auscultation.

Interventions	Rationale
1. Assess respiratory rate every 15 minutes for 1 hour. Report any increase in rate, retractions, or development of nasal flaring or grunting.	1. Assessment provides a baseline for evaluating changes. Increases in respiratory rate and retractions, accompanied by nasal flaring and grunting, indicate respiratory distress.
2. Position the newborn on his side with his head slightly lower than the rest of his body.	2. Positioning in this manner facilitates drainage of secretions from airway.
3. Suction mouth and then nose with bulb syringe as indicated.	3. Gentle suctioning removes secretions that may collect in these areas. Suctioning the mouth before the nose prevents possible aspiration of oral secretions.
4. Change position frequently.	4. Position changes facilitate drainage of secretions, thus enhancing lung aeration and expansion.
5. Inform the parents that the rapid respiratory rate is common in some newborns after birth because of unabsorbed lung fluid.	5. Providing information helps to allay parents' anxieties and fears.
6. Monitor newborn's temperature and keep him warm via radiant warmer. Wrap the newborn loosely in a blanket and place a cap on his head.	6. Newborns have difficulty conserving body heat. Exposure to cold increases the metabolic rate, increasing the need for oxygen and further increasing the respiratory rate.

Nursing Diagnosis: Risk for impaired parenting related to concerns about skin color variation

Outcome Identification: Parents will demonstrate positive bonding behaviors.

Outcome Evaluation: Parents identify mongolian spot as normal skin variation; demonstrate warm, accepting behaviors with the child; point out other positive attributes of their son.

(continued)

Interventions	Rationale
1. Allow parents to verbalize their concerns about the discoloration.	1. Verbalization allows a safe outlet for emotion and helps to increase the other's awareness.
2. Explain that mongolian spots are a normal variation in skin color. Inform them that no treatment is necessary and that the area usually disappears by school age.	2. Explanation as normal provides information to help allay parents' fears and concerns.
3. Point out other positive normal attributes of the newborn.	3. Pointing out other positive areas helps the parents focus attention on the unique and special qualities of their child.
4. Encourage the parents to hold, talk, touch, and explore the newborn.	4. Interaction and exploration help to promote bonding and reassure the parents that their child is normal.

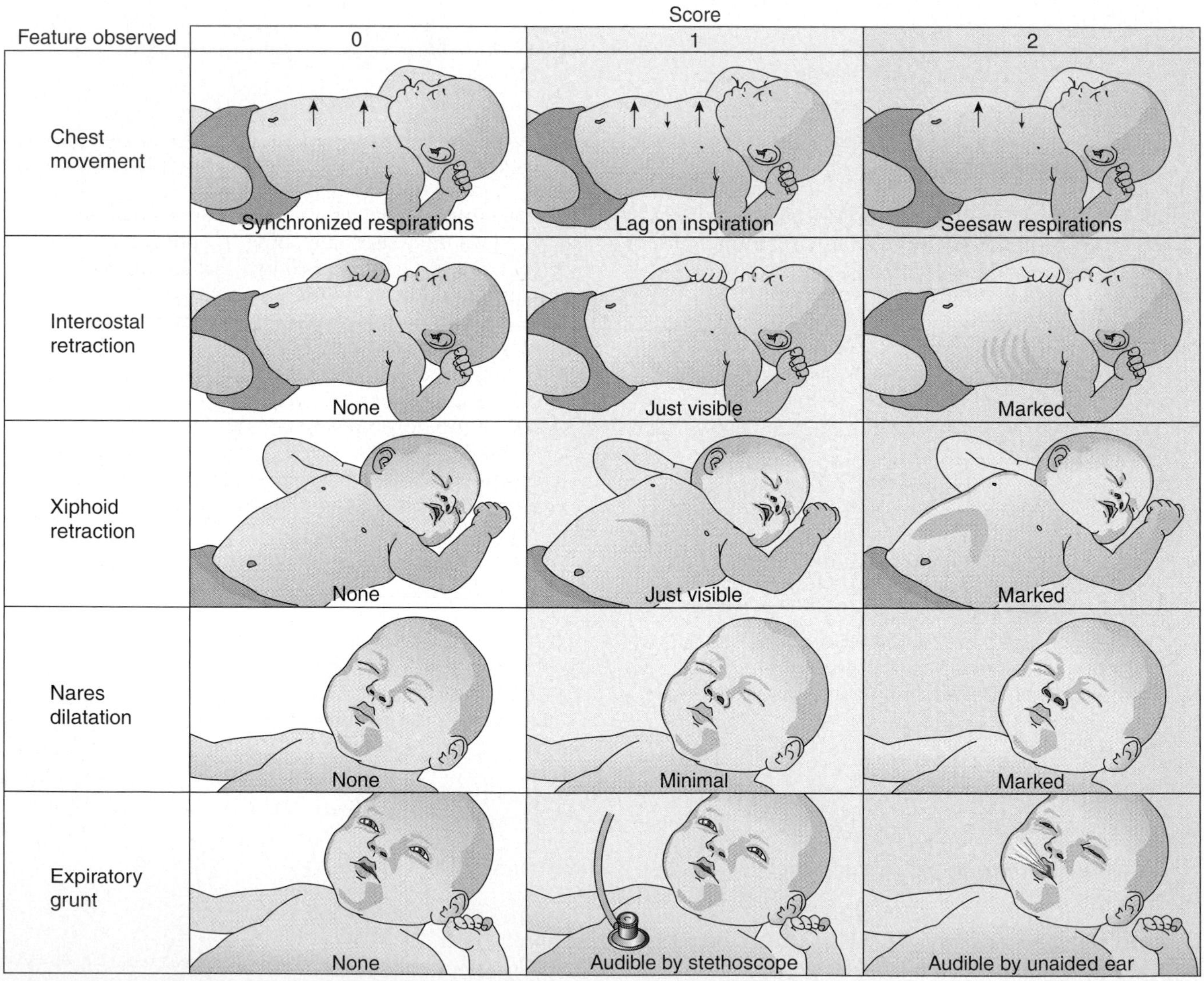

FIGURE 23.19 Grading of neonatal respiratory distress based on Silverman-Andersen index. (Silverman, W. A., & Anderson, D. H. [1956]. A controlled clinical trial of effects of water mist on obstructive respiratory signs, death rate and necroscopy findings among premature infants. *Pediatrics, 17*[4], 1–9.)

TABLE 23.3 Congenital Anomaly Appraisal

PROCEDURE	ABNORMALITIES CONSIDERED
Inquiry for hydramnios or oligohydramnios	Presence of hydramnios suggests congenital gastrointestinal obstruction. Oligohydramnios suggests genitourinary obstruction or extreme prematurity.
Appearance of abdomen	Distended abdomen suggests ascites or tumor. Empty abdomen suggests diaphragmatic hernia.
Passage of nasogastric tube (No. 8 feeding catheter) through nares into stomach	Failure to pass nasogastric tube through nares on either side establishes choanal atresia. Failure to pass it into the stomach confirms presence of esophageal atresia.
Aspiration of stomach with recording of color and amount of fluid obtained	With excess of 20 mL of fluid, or yellow fluid, duodenal or ileal atresia is suspected.
Insertion of rectal catheter	Failure to obtain meconium suggests imperforate anus or higher obstruction.
Counting of umbilical arteries	The presence of one artery suggests possible congenital urinary or cardiac anomalies or chromosomal trisomy (if other portions of examination are consistent).

With permission from Van Leeuwen, G. & Glenn, L. (1968). Screening for hidden congenital anomalies. *Pediatrics, 41*(6), 147–152. Copyright American Academy of Pediatrics, 1968.

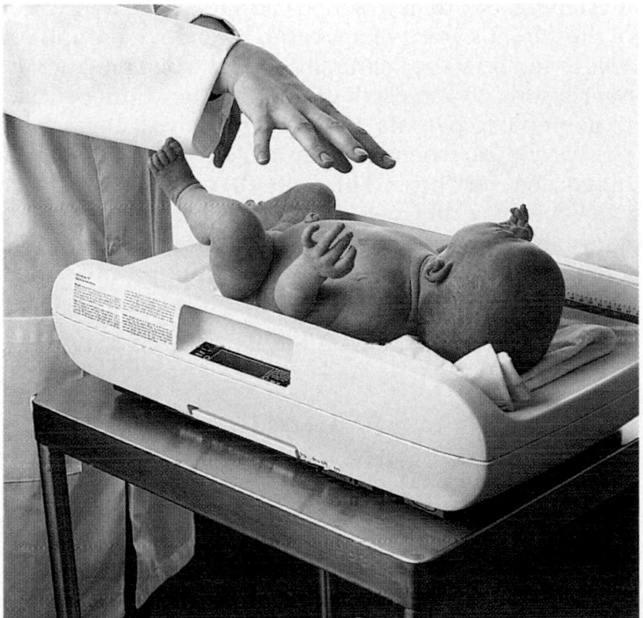

FIGURE 23.20 Weighing a newborn. Notice the protective hand held over the infant.

nude once a day at approximately the same time every day. More frequent weighing subjects the infant to unnecessary manipulation. The weight each day should be compared with that of the preceding day to be certain the infant is not losing more than the normal physiologic amount (5% to 10% of birth weight). Abnormal loss of weight may be the first indication that a newborn has an inborn error of metabolism, such as adrenogenital syndrome (salt dumping type), or is becoming dehydrated.

Laboratory Studies

On admission to a nursery or after the first hour of undisturbed rest, depending on hospital policy, newborns may have heel-stick tests for hematocrit or hemoglobin determination and hypoglycemia. Heel-sticks require a minimum of blood, and although not pain free, cause minimal trauma to the baby. In some settings, these tests are not routine but are reserved only for newborns with symptoms of anemia, polycythemia, or hypoglycemia.

Newborn anemia is difficult to detect by clinical observation. It may be caused by hypovolemia due to bleeding from placenta previa or abruptio placentae or by a cesarean birth that involved incision into the placenta. Another condition as dangerous as anemia is the presence of an excess of red blood cells (polycythemia), probably caused by excessive flow of blood into the infant from the umbilical cord. A heel-stick hematocrit reveals both of these conditions, and treatment then can be instituted. A normal hematocrit at 1 hour of life is about 50% to 55%.

Hypoglycemia may also produce few symptoms. If a blood glucose heel-stick reading is less than 40 mg/100 mL of blood (30 mg/100 mL in the first 3 days of life), it suggests hypoglycemia (Al-Ashwal, 2001). The usual protocol for this is oral glucose or infant formula given immediately to elevate the infant's blood sugar. It is important to treat hypoglycemia quickly, because if brain cells become completely depleted of glucose, brain damage can result. If the newborn exhibits symptoms of hypoglycemia (jitteriness, lethargy, seizures) in addition to the low laboratory test results, intravenous glucose probably will be prescribed. A continuous intravenous infusion of glucose may be necessary if the newborn is unable to maintain glucose levels above 40 mg/100 mL before feeding.

Assessment of Gestational Age

Specific findings on physical assessment provide evidence of a newborn's gestational age. As early as 1966, Usher et al. (1966) proposed the five criteria given in Table 23-4 as a rapid basis for evaluating gestational maturity. These are quick criteria to use for assessment of all newborns.

Dubowitz Maturity Scale

Dubowitz et al. (1970) devised a gestational rating scale that uses more extensive criteria. Newborns are observed and tested according to these criteria, and then their maturity level is rated.

All newborns appearing to be immature by Usher's criteria or who are light in weight at birth or early by dates should be assessed by means of the more definitive crite-

TABLE 23.4 Clinical Criteria for Gestational Assessment

	GESTATION AGE (WEEKS)		
FINDING	0–36	37–38	39 and Over
Sole creases	Anterior transverse crease only	Occasional creases in anterior two thirds	Sole covered with creases
Breast nodule diameter (mm)	2	4	7
Scalp hair	Fine and fuzzy	Fine and fuzzy	Coarse and silky
Ear lobe	Pliable; no cartilage	Some cartilage	Stiffened by thick cartilage
Testes and scrotum	Testes in lower canal; scrotum small; few rugae	Intermediate	Testes pendulous, scrotum full; extensive rugae

With permission from Usher, R., et al. (1966). Judgment of fetal age. *Pediatric Clinics of North America, 13*(4), 835–840.

ria. Although completing a Dubowitz assessment takes practice, it can yield important results. Using this scale can help determine whether the newborn needs immediate high-risk nursery intervention.

Ballard modified the Dubowitz scale during the 1970s and again in the 1990s (Ballard et al., 1991) to an assessment scale that can be completed in 3 to 4 minutes. The assessment consists of two portions: physical maturity and neuromuscular maturity (Fig. 23-21). The first is a series of observations about skin texture, color, lanugo, foot creases, genitalia, ear, and breast maturity. The body part is inspected and given a score of 0 to 5 as described in Figure 23-21*A*. This observation scoring should be done as soon as possible after birth, because skin assessment becomes much less reliable after 24 hours. Illustrations of mature and immature body features are shown in Chapter 26 with the discussion of the preterm infant.

To complete the second half of the examination, observe or position the baby as shown in Figure 23-21*B*. Again, the child is given numeric scores from 0 to 5.

To establish the baby's gestational age, the total score obtained (on both sections) is compared with the rating scale in Figure 23-21*C*. As can be seen by this scale, an infant with a total score of 5 is at 26 weeks' gestational age; a total score of 10 reveals a gestational age of about 28 weeks; a total score of 40 points is found in infants at term or 40 weeks' gestation.

Using such a standard method of rating maturity is helpful in detecting infants who are small for gestational age (they are light in weight but the neuromuscular and physical observation scales will be adequate for their weeks in utero), and differentiating them from those who are immature because of a miscalculated due date. An infant who is found to be less than 35 weeks' gestation requires close observation, usually in a special care nursery.

Assessment of Behavioral Capacity

Term newborns are physically active and emotionally prepared to interact with the people around them. They are people oriented from the beginning—how much so can be demonstrated by the way they immediately attune to human voices or concentrate on their mother's face (Fig. 23-22).

Brazelton Neonatal Behavioral Assessment Scale

The *Brazelton Neonatal Behavioral Assessment Scale* is a rating scale devised by Brazelton in the early 1970s (Brazelton, 1973) to evaluate the newborn's behavioral capacity or ability to respond to set stimuli. Six major categories of behavior—habituation, orientation, motor maturity, variation, self-quieting ability, and social behavior—are assessed.

To perform an assessment using the scale requires training in the different techniques to ensure that it is used consistently from one individual to another. Unlike many assessment scales, the infant is scored on best performance rather than on average performance. A total evaluation takes 20 to 30 minutes to complete.

The information supplied by this scale has provided concrete evidence that newborns are not passive, nonhearing, unseeing, unresponsive, or even all alike. An important finding from the scale is that newborns are able to quiet themselves after crying. Many of the items tested on the scale, such as how infants alert (eyes widen, head held as if listening) or orient to sound (turn toward the direction of the parent's voice or appear to listen to the sound of a voice) and how they naturally cuddle when held next to their parent, are excellent examples of newborn behavior to point out to parents. If parents perceive a newborn as passive and unresponsive, they are likely to talk or look at him or her very little. The more they know about their baby, the more they will be able to understand the baby's cues and determine and meet his or her needs. Performing a Brazelton Assessment and pointing out positive infant behavior can lead to improved parenting ability.

✔ **CHECKPOINT QUESTIONS**

10. What five areas are assessed with Apgar scoring?
11. What blood glucose value in a term newborn is suggestive of hypoglycemia?

CARE OF THE NEWBORN AT BIRTH

An island for newborn care should be provided in a delivery or birthing room apart from the equipment needed for the mother's care. Necessary equipment includes a radiant

	0	1	2	3	4	5
SKIN	gelatinous red, trans-parent	smooth pink, visible veins	superficial peeling &/or rash, few veins	cracking pale area, rare veins	parchment, deep cracking, no vessels	leathery, cracked, wrinkled
LANUGO	none	abundant	thinning	bald areas	mostly bald	
PLANTAR CREASES	no crease	faint red marks	anterior transverse crease only	creases ant. 2/3	creases cover entire sole	
BREAST	barely percept.	flat areola, no bud	stippled areola, 1–2 mm bud	raised areola, 3–4 mm bud	full areola, 5–10 mm bud	
EAR	pinna flat, stays folded	sl. curved pinna, soft with slow recoil	well-curv. pinna, soft but ready recoil	formed & firm with instant recoil	thick cartilage, ear stiff	
GENITALS Male	scrotum empty, no rugae		testes descend-ing, few rugae	testes down, good rugae	testes pendulous, deep rugae	
GENITALS Female	prominent clitoris & labia minora		majora & minora equally prominent	majora large, minora small	clitoris & minora completely covered	

A

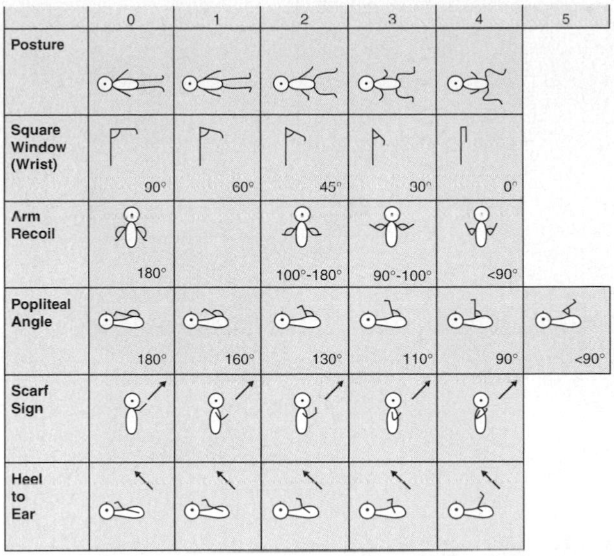

B

Score	Wks
5	26
10	28
15	30
20	32
25	34
30	36
35	38
40	40
45	42
50	44

FIGURE 23.21 Ballard's assessment of gestational age criteria. (*A*) Physical maturity assessment criteria. (*B*) Neuromuscular maturity assessment criteria. *Posture:* With infant supine and quiet, score as follows: arms and legs extended = 0; slight or moderate flexion of hips and knees = 2; legs flexed and abducted, arms slightly flexed = 3; full flexion of arms and legs = 4. *Square Window:* Flex hand at the wrist. Exert pressure sufficient to get as much flexion as possible. The angle between hypothenar eminence and anterior aspect of forearm is measured and scored. Do not rotate wrist. *Arm Recoil:* With infant supine, fully flex forearm for 5 sec, then fully extend by pulling the hands and release. Score as follows: remain extended or random movements = 0; incomplete or partial flexion = 2; brisk return to full flexion = 4. *Popliteal Angle:* With infant supine and pelvis flat on examining surface, flex leg on thigh and fully flex thigh with one hand. With the other hand, extend leg and score the angle attained according to the chart. *Scarf Sign:* With infant supine, draw infant's hand across the neck and as far across the opposite shoulder as possible. Assistance to elbow is permissible by lifting it across the body. Score according to location of the elbow: elbow reaches opposite anterior axillary line = 0; elbow between opposite anterior axillary line and midline of the thorax = 1; elbow at midline of thorax = 2; elbow does not reach midline of thorax = 3; elbow at proximal axillary line = 4. *Heel to Ear:* With infant supine, hold infant's foot with one hand and move it as near to the head as possible without forcing it. Keep pelvis flat on examining surface. (*C*) Scoring for a Ballard assessment scale. The point total from assessment is compared to the left column. The matching number in the right column reveals the infant's age in gestation weeks. (From Ballard, J. L. [1991]. New Ballard score expanded to include extremely premature infants. *Journal of Pediatrics, 119,* 417–423.)

heat table or a warmed bassinet; a warm, soft blanket; and equipment for oxygen administration, resuscitation, suction, eye care, identification, and weighing the newborn.

The philosophy of caring health care providers has always been that newborns should be handled as gently at birth as they are at any other time. The image of the obstetrician holding a newborn up by the heels and spanking to stimulate breathing has existed only in movies. It has long been accepted that holding a baby by the feet and letting the back extend fully is probably painful after the months in a flexed position in utero; a measure such as spanking is not as effective in helping a newborn breathe as gentle stimulation, such as rubbing the back.

Newborn Identification and Registration

Infant identification is important, because there always exists the possibility that a newborn may be handed to the wrong parents or, although rare, be switched or kidnapped from a health care facility. The profile of such a kidnapper is a woman who has recently lost a pregnancy or had an infant stillborn and who desires an infant very much. She often is someone familiar with hospitals; she pretends to be a volunteer or unlicensed health care worker and says she needs to take a baby out of the nursery or mother's room for a procedure. Health care agency personnel need to be alert to the potential danger for kidnapping, and not only take measures to prevent this from happening but also alert parents to the danger (Rusting, 2000; see Focus on Family Empowerment).

Identification Band

One traditional form of identification used with newborns is a plastic bracelet with permanent locks that require cutting to be removed (Fig. 23-23). A number that corresponds to the mother's hospital number, the mother's full name, and the sex, date, and time of the infant's birth are

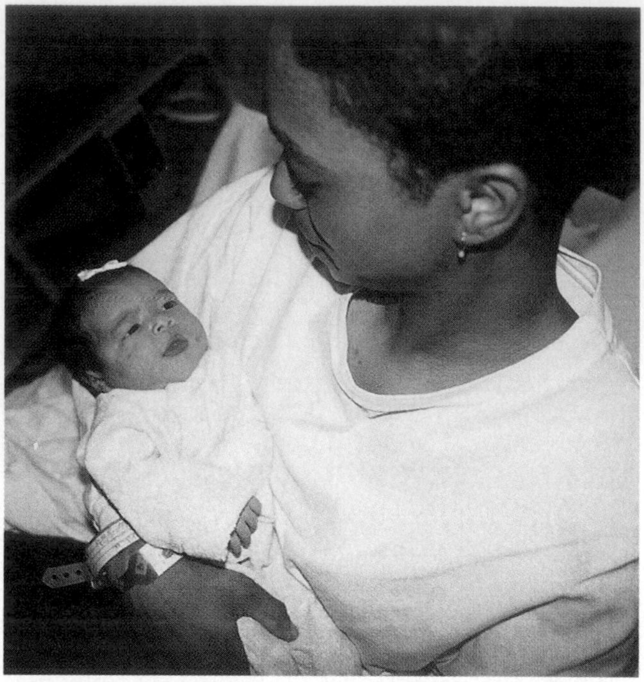

FIGURE 23.22 A newborn recognizes her parent's face.

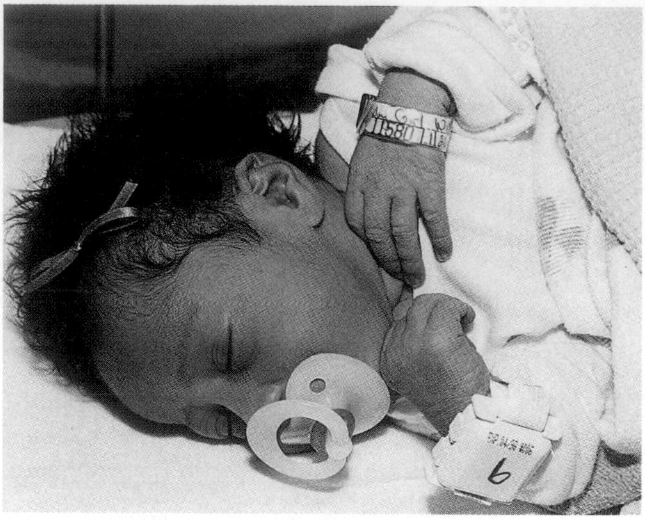

FIGURE 23.23 This newborn is wearing two types of identification bands. On her left wrist, she is wearing a traditional plastic bracelet, which includes her identification number, date of birth, sex, and mother's name. On her right wrist, she is wearing a security band, which sets off an alarm and locks exits if the infant is taken off the unit.

necessary for identification. If an identification band is attached to a newborn's arm or leg, two bands should be used. This is because a newborn's wrist and hand, as well as ankle and foot, are not too different in width, which allows the bands to slide off easily. A newer form of identification band has a built-in sensor unit that sounds an alarm, similar to those attached to clothing in department stores to stop shoplifting, if the baby is transported beyond set hospital boundaries (see Fig. 23-23).

After identification bands are attached, the infant's footprints may be taken (Fig. 23-24*A*) and thereafter kept with the baby's chart for permanent identification. If footprints will be obtained, care should be taken in securing them because they will be part of the permanent record (Fig. 23-24*B*). If footprints are required, these should be obtained in the same way for babies who are born outside the hospital when they are admitted to the hospital for follow-up care.

Birth Registration

The physician or nurse-midwife who delivered the infant must be certain a birth registration is filed with the Bureau of Vital Statistics of the state in which the infant was born. The infant's name, the mother's name, the father's name

FOCUS ON FAMILY EMPOWERMENT

Measures to Help Prevent Kidnapping From a Hospital Unit

Q. I heard such horror stories about babies being kidnapped from the hospital. How can we make sure this doesn't happen to us?

A. Although rare, this can happen. To minimize the risk, use the following as some helpful guidelines:

- Review newborn identification procedure with a nurse so you are familiar with it and can feel comfortable with the safeguards being taken.
- Check that identification bands are in place on your infant as you care for him or her. These can slide off easily over small newborn hands and feet. If a band or necklace is missing, ask a nurse to replace it immediately.
- Don't allow any person without proper hospital identification to remove your baby from your room.
- Don't leave your baby unattended in your room. Either return the baby to the nursery or have the baby accompany you if you are leaving your room to shower, for example.
- Report the presence of any suspicious person in the unit.
- Be aware that some hospitals use a microchip system embedded in identification bands that sound an alarm if a baby is removed from the unit (similar to the tag used to thwart shoplifting in department stores). If this type of band is used, be certain it is removed before hospital discharge or it will set off the alarm.

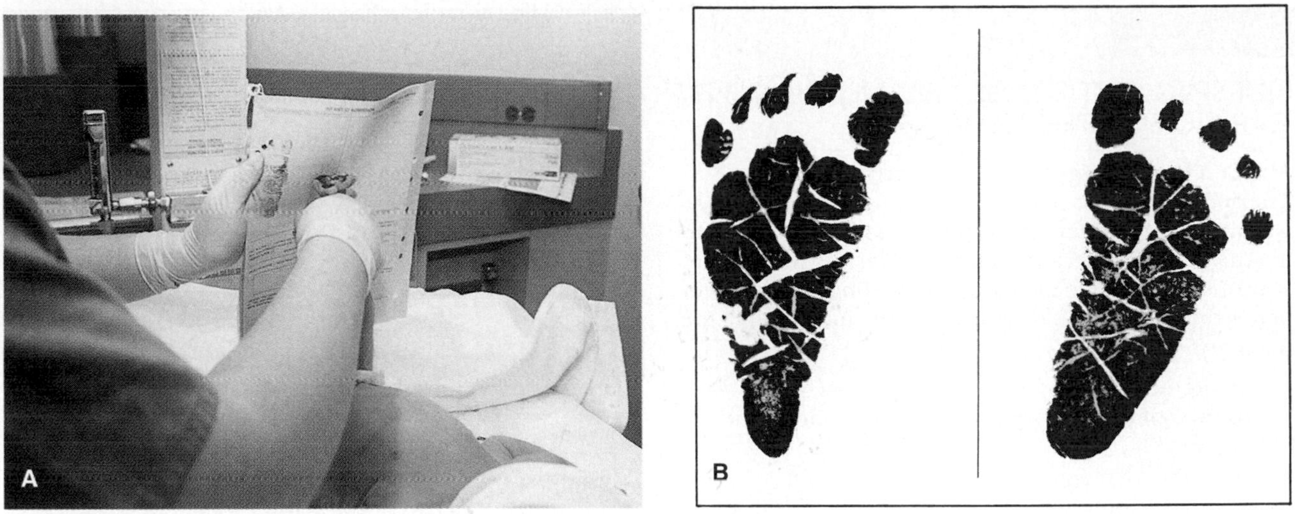

FIGURE 23.24 *(A)* Footprinting a newborn for identification. *(B)* Newborn footprints.

(if the mother chooses to reveal this), and the birth date and place must be recorded. Official birth information is important in proving eligibility for school and later for voting, passports, Social Security benefits, and so on.

Birth Record Documentation

Be certain the birth record lists the following:

- Time of birth
- Time the infant breathed
- Whether respirations were spontaneous or aided
- Apgar score at 1 and 5 minutes of life
- Whether eye prophylaxis was given
- Whether vitamin K was administered
- General condition of the infant
- Number of vessels in the umbilical cord
- Whether cultures were taken (they are taken if at some point sterile delivery technique was broken or the mother has a history of vaginal or uterine infection)
- Whether the infant (1) voided and (2) passed a stool (these are helpful if, later on, the diagnosis of bowel obstruction or absence of a kidney is considered)

Many nurses indicate a three-vessel cord with the symbol shown in Figure 23-25. Do not mistake this drawing for a "smiling face" and assume it is not important.

NURSING DIAGNOSES AND RELATED INTERVENTIONS

In most health care facilities, the delivering physician or nurse-midwife hands the newborn to the nurse moments after birth to begin care. Be certain to adhere to standard precautions when caring for newborns to avoid touching the vernix caseosa. Holding a warm, sterile blanket, grasp the infant through the blanket by placing one hand under the back and the other around a leg. Newborns are slippery because they are wet from amniotic fluid and the vernix. Box 23-1 highlights an appropriate outcome and interventions for the care of a newborn using the terminology identified by the Nursing Outcomes Classification (NOC) and Nursing Interventions Classification (NIC).

Nursing Diagnosis: Risk for ineffective thermoregulation related to newborn's transition to extrauterine environment

Outcome Identification: Newborn will establish adequate body temperature by 1 hour after birth.

Outcome Evaluation: Newborn maintains axillary temperature of 98.6°F (37°C).

Keep Newborn Warm. Gently rub infants dry so little body heat is lost by evaporation. Then swaddle them loosely with the blanket to prevent compromising respiratory effort. Lay them on their side in a warmed bassinet. Alternatively, once dried, place the newborn unwrapped on a radiant heat table. To help conserve heat, place a cap on the infant's head (Fig. 23-26) and accomplish all nursing care as quickly as possible, with minimal exposure of the newborn to chilling air. Any extensive procedures, such as resuscitation, should be done under a radiant heat source to reduce heat loss.

As soon as the infant is breathing well, ask which parent wants to hold the child and place him or her in the parent's arms. This helps conserve heat as well as encourages bonding. The period immediately after birth is an important time for parents to begin interaction. Newborns are alert (first period of activity) and respond well to their parents' first tentative touches or interaction with them. Although the temperature of newborns who are dried, wrapped, and then held by their parents immediately after birth appar-

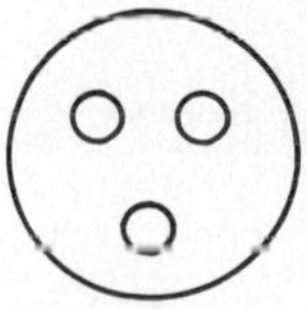

FIGURE 23.25 A chart abbreviation for a three-vessel cord.

BOX 23.1

NURSING OUTCOMES AND NURSING INTERVENTIONS CLASSIFICATION: CARING FOR THE NEWBORN

NOC: Thermoregulation, Neonate

Thermoregulation, neonate is defined as the balance among heat production, heat gain, and heat loss during the neonatal period (Johnson, Mass, & Moorhead, 2000). Some specific indicators suggesting achievement of this outcome include evidence of the following in the neonate:

- Body temperature within normal limits
- Absence of respiratory distress, restlessness, and lethargy
- Skin color changes and weight gain within accepted parameters
- Adequate hydration
- Blood glucose and bilirubin levels and acid-base balance within normal limits
- Ability to assume heat retention and heat dissipation postures as necessary

NIC: Newborn monitoring

Newborn monitoring is defined as the measurement and interpretation of physiologic status of the neonate in the first 24 hours after delivery (McCloskey & Bulechek, 2000). Some important activities involved when implementing this intervention include:

- Performing Apgar scoring at 1 and 5 minutes after birth
- Assessing color, temperature, heart rate, respiratory rate, and breathing pattern
- Assessing the neonate's ability to suck and first feeding
- Evaluating umbilical cord site
- Monitoring weight and intake and output
- Recording first voiding and bowel movement
- Monitoring for signs and symptoms of respiratory distress and hyperbilirubinemia

NIC: Newborn Care

Newborn care is defined as the management of the neonate during the transition to extrauterine life and subsequent period of stabilization (McCloskey & Bulechek, 2000). Some important activities involved when implementing this intervention include:

- Obtaining weight and measurements of length and head circumference, estimating gestational age, and comparing measurements with estimated gestational age.
- Clearing the airway of mucus and elevating the head of the mattress to promote respiratory function
- Maintaining warm body temperature with frequent monitoring, drying immediately after birth, wrapping in warm blanket, applying cap to head, and placing in isolette or under warmer as needed
- Putting the neonate to the mother's breast and monitoring sucking reflex
- Bathing neonate once temperature has stabilized
- Swaddling neonate to promote sleep and sense of security
- Providing umbilical cord site care, keeping the site dry and exposed to air
- Protecting neonate from sources of infection
- Providing a quiet, soothing environment
- Responding to cues and making eye contact when giving care

ently falls slightly lower than that of infants placed in heated cribs, their core temperature does not fall below safe limits. If a mother wishes to begin breastfeeding immediately after birth, she can be encouraged to do so.

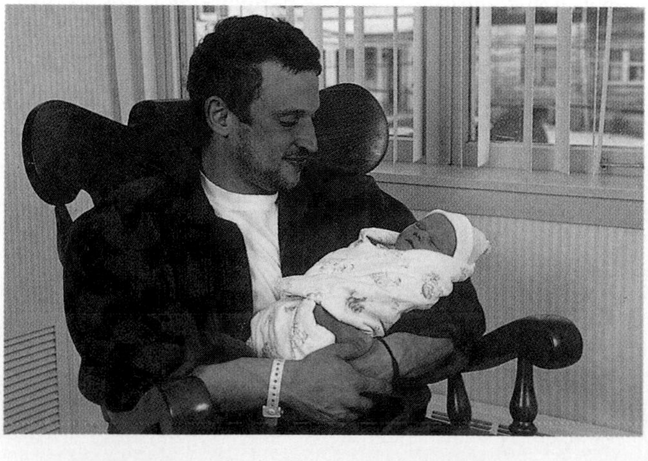

FIGURE 23.26 A newborn wrapped and capped to conserve body heat.

At the end of the first hour of life, reassess a newborn's temperature. Axillary temperatures are recommended for newborns to prevent accidental bowel perforation. If the temperature is subnormal and the baby is in a bassinet, he or she should be placed in an Isolette or under a radiant warmer for additional heat. If the temperature is normal, the newborn can be bathed quickly to remove excess vernix caseosa and blood, then dressed in a shirt and diaper, reswaddled in a snug blanket (to give the baby a familiar feeling of the tight confines of the uterus), and placed in a bassinet or returned to the mother's side.

During the first day of life, a newborn's temperature is usually taken every 4 to 8 hours. Thereafter, unless it is elevated or subnormal, or the infant appears to be in distress, once a day while in a health care facility is enough.

Nursing Diagnosis: Risk for ineffective airway clearance related to presence of mucus in mouth and nose at birth

Outcome Identification: Newborn will establish effective breathing by 5 minutes after birth.

Outcome Evaluation: The neonate maintains a respiratory rate of 30 to 60 breaths per minute without evidence of retraction or grunting.

Promote Adequate Breathing Pattern and Prevent Aspiration. Mucus should be suctioned from a newborn's mouth by a bulb syringe as soon as the head is born. As soon as the body is born, he or she should be held for a few seconds with the head slightly dependent for further drainage of secretions. It is important that mucus be removed from the mouth and pharynx before the first breath to prevent aspiration of the secretions. If an infant continues to have an accumulation of mucus in the mouth or nose after these first steps, you may need to suction further when the baby is placed under the warmer (Fig. 23-27). Use a bulb syringe or a soft, small (no. 10 or 12) catheter to suction. Vigorous suctioning should never be used. It irritates the mucous membrane and leaves portals of entry for infection. Brisk suctioning also has been associated with bradycardia in newborns owing to vagal nerve stimulation. If a bulb syringe is used, the bulb should be decompressed before being inserted in the infant's mouth or nose, or the force of decompression will push the secretions back into the pharynx or bronchi rather than remove them. When an infant is born with deeply meconium-stained amniotic fluid, it is important that the infant be both suctioned and intubated so deep tracheal suction can be accomplished before the first breath. This action helps to prevent meconium aspiration (Nelson et al., 2000).

Record the First Cry. A crying infant is a breathing infant, because the sound of crying is made by a current of air passing over the larynx. The more lusty the cry, the greater the assurance that the newborn is breathing deeply and forcefully. Vigorous crying also helps to blow off the extra carbon dioxide that makes all newborns slightly acidotic, thus helping to correct this condition. Although gentleness is necessary to make an infant's transition from intrauterine life to extrauterine life as untraumatic as possible, for the above reasons, there is no need to completely halt initial newborn crying.

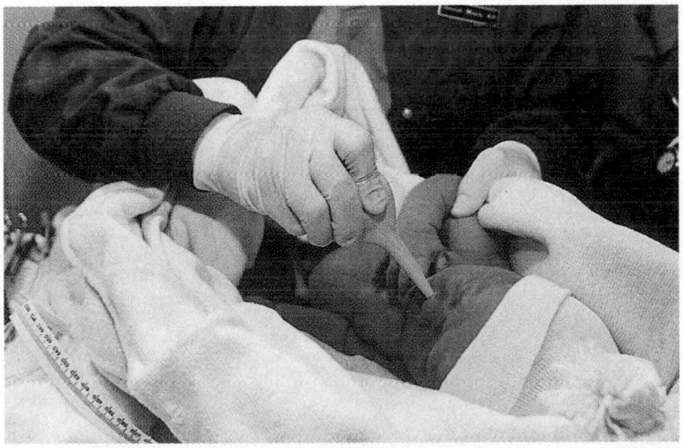

FIGURE 23.27 A newborn is suctioned by means of a bulb syringe to remove mucus from the mouth and nose. The head-down-and-to-the-side position facilitates drainage. Care is given with the infant under a radiant heat source.

It is important to note the time after birth the child first gasped and cried and whether he or she was able to maintain respirations unaided. The newborn who does not breathe spontaneously or who takes a few quick, gasping breaths but is unable to maintain respirations needs resuscitation as an emergency measure. An infant with grunting respirations needs careful observation for respiratory distress syndrome (see Chapter 26).

Nursing Diagnosis: Risk for infection related to newly clamped umbilical cord and exposure of eyes to vaginal secretions

Outcome Identification: Newborn will remain free of signs of infection during health care agency stay.

Outcome Evaluation: Area around cord is dry and free of erythema. Eyes are free of inflammation and drainage. Newborn's axillary temperature is maintained between 97.6°F and 98.6°F (36.5°C and 37°C).

Inspect and Care for Umbilical Cord. The umbilical cord pulsates for a moment after the infant is born as a last flow of blood passes from the placenta into the infant. Two clamps are then applied to the cord about 8 inches from the infant's abdomen, and the cord is cut between the clamps. Some fathers choose to do this as their responsibility. The infant cord is then clamped again by a cord clamp, such as a Hazeltine or a Kane clamp. The clamp on the maternal end of the cord should not be released after the cord is cut. Otherwise, blood still remaining in the placenta will leak out. This loss is not important, because the mother's circulation does not connect to the placenta. It is messy, however, and that is why the clamp is left in place.

Inspect the infant's cord to be certain it is clamped securely. If the clamp loosens before thrombosis obliterates the umbilical vessels, hemorrhage will result. As previously mentioned, the number of cord vessels should be counted and noted immediately after cutting the cord. Cords begin to dry almost immediately, and by the time of the infant's first thorough physical examination in the nursery, the vessels may be obscured.

Within a few minutes after the cord is cut, assess the cord for possible bleeding. Apply antibiotic ointment or triple dye as required by agency policy to help reduce infection. Until the cord falls off, at about the seventh to tenth day of life, the infant should receive a sponge bath, rather than be immersed in a tub of water. Be certain the diaper is folded below the level of the umbilical cord so that when it becomes wet, the cord does not become wet also.

It is important to remind parents to keep the cord dry until it falls off after they return home. The use of creams, lotions, and oils near the cord should be discouraged, because they tend to slow drying of the cord and invite infection. Some health care agencies recommend applying rubbing alcohol to the cord site once or twice a day to hasten drying. Others prefer that the cord be left strictly alone.

After the cord falls off, a small, pink, granulating area about a quarter of an inch in diameter may remain. This should also be left clean and dry until it has healed (about 24 to 48 more hours). If it has remained as long as a week, it may require *cautery with silver nitrate* to speed healing.

Administer Eye Care. Although the practice may shortly become obsolete (as it is in Europe), every state requires that newborns receive prophylactic eye treatment against gonorrheal conjunctivitis of the newborn. Such infections are acquired from the mother as the infant passes through the birth canal. Formerly, this procedure was done immediately after birth. Many parents today prefer to visit with the infant before the procedure to be certain the newborn can focus on them without blurry vision from ointment or drops. As long as it is completed as soon as possible after birth, either in the delivery or birthing room or on arrival in the nursery, the exact time the ointment is administered is unimportant. Silver nitrate was exclusively used for prophylaxis in the past; today, erythromycin ointment is the drug of choice. Erythromycin ointment has the advantage of eliminating not only the organism of gonorrhea but that of chlamydia as well (see Focus on Pharmacology: Erythromycin Ophthalmic Ointment).

To instill ointment, first dry the face of the newborn with a soft gauze square so the skin is not slippery. The best procedure to open a newborn's eyes is to shade them from the overhead light and open one eye at a time by pressure on the lower and upper lids. Use an individual tube or package of ointment to avoid transmitting infection from one newborn to another. With one eye open, squeeze a line of ointment along the lower conjunctival sac from the inner canthus outward, and then close the eye to allow the ointment to spread across the conjunctiva.

Crede, a German gynecologist, first proposed prophylaxis against gonorrheal conjunctivitis in 1884. For this reason, it is often referred to as the *Crede treatment* and may be listed that way on a health care agency form. Babies born outside hospitals, in homes or less orthodox settings such as the car, must have the prophylactic treatment administered on admission to the hospital.

WHAT IF? Newborns acquire eye infections during their transit through the birth canal. What if a newborn baby was born by cesarean birth? Would you still administer eye prophylaxis?

General Infection Precautions

Each infant should have his or her own bassinet. Compartments in the bassinet should hold a supply of diapers, shirts, gowns, and individual equipment for bathing and temperature taking. The sharing of equipment leads to the spread of infection. Standard precautions are necessary.

Personnel, parents, or siblings caring for newborns should wash their hands and arms to the elbows thoroughly with an antiseptic soap before handling infants. Personnel are usually required to wear cover gowns or nursery uniforms.

Personnel with infections (sore throats, upper respiratory infections, skin lesions, or gastrointestinal upsets) should be excluded from caring for mothers and infants until the condition is completely cleared. If a mother has a possible contagious illness, her newborn should be excluded from her room. An instant photograph such as a Polaroid can be taken, however, and shown to her so she can follow the baby's progress. If the infant is breastfed, the mother should manually express milk during the time the infant is excluded to maintain her milk supply; however, the milk should be discarded. The mother should resume breastfeeding as soon as it is both possible and safe.

Any baby born outside the hospital or under circumstances conducive to infection (e.g., rupture of the membranes more than 24 hours before birth) should be kept in a closed Isolette or in the mother's room until negative cultures show the newborn is free of infection. Any newborn in whom symptoms of infection develop (e.g., skin lesions, fever) should be removed to an isolation nursery or housed in the mother's room to prevent the spread of infection to other babies. There is no reason for parents not to visit a baby housed in isolation care. In fact, they may have more need to hold a baby who is isolated than the average parents, because they have an extra reason to be worried that something is wrong with the child. To visit in isolation nurseries, parents must use the same infection control techniques as staff members use.

FOCUS ON PHARMACOLOGY

Erythromycin Ophthalmic Ointment

Action: Erythromycin, an antibiotic, is effective against gonorrhea and chlamydia organisms, making it the drug of choice for eye prophylaxis at birth.

Pregnancy Risk Category: B

Dosage: 0.5–1 cm each eye

Possible Adverse Reactions: Mild irritation to conjunctiva; slight blurring of vision.

Nursing Implications

- Use a single-dose application tube.
- After gently pulling down on the newborn's lower eyelid, extrude a line of ointment the length of the lower eyelid from the inner canthus outward.
- Discard any remaining ointment to prevent it being used again.
- Close the child's eyes and count to about five.
- Wipe away any excess ointment from the child's face.
- Know that application may be delayed for an hour after birth to allow the infant to view his or her parents for the first time with the clearest vision possible.

✔ CHECKPOINT QUESTIONS

12. When should the newborn be suctioned for the first time?
13. On what day of life does the umbilical cord usually fall off?
14. What ointment is the drug of choice for eye prophylaxis?

NURSING CARE OF THE NEWBORN AND FAMILY IN THE POSTPARTAL PERIOD

A newborn should be kept in either a birthing room or a transitional nursery for optimal safety for the first few hours of life. During this period of close observation, certain principles of care always apply.

Initial Feeding

A term newborn who is to be breastfed may be fed immediately after birth. A baby who is to be formula fed may receive a first feeding at about 2 to 4 hours of age.

Both formula-fed and breastfed infants do best on a demand schedule; many need to be fed as often as every 2 hours for the first few days of life. Chapter 24 covers the elements of breastfeeding and formula feeding in detail.

Bathing

In most hospitals, newborns receive a complete bath to wash away vernix caseosa within an hour after birth. Thereafter, they are bathed once a day, although the procedure may be limited to washing only the baby's face, diaper area, and skin folds. Wear gloves when handling newborns until a first bath to avoid exposing your hands to body secretions; babies of HIV-positive mothers should be bathed immediately to decrease the possibility of HIV transmission (Kelly, 1999).

Bathing of the infant is best done by the parents under a nurse's supervision. The room should be warm (about 75°F [24°C]) to prevent chilling. Bath water should be around 98°F to 100°F (37°C to 38°C), a temperature that feels pleasantly warm to the elbow or wrist. If soap is used, it should be mild and without a hexachlorophene base. Bathing should take place before, not after, a feeding to prevent spitting up or vomiting and possible aspiration.

The equipment needed is a basin of water, soap, washcloth, towel, comb, and clean diaper and shirt. These items should be assembled beforehand, so the baby is not left exposed or unattended while the bather goes for more equipment.

Teach parents that when giving a bath, it should proceed from the cleanest to the most soiled areas of the body, that is, from the eyes and face to the trunk and extremities and, last, to the diaper area. Wipe the eyes with clear water from the inner canthus outward, using a clean portion of the washcloth for each eye to prevent spread of infection to the other eye. Wash the face with clear water to avoid skin irritation by soap, which may be used on the rest of the body.

Teach parents to wash the infant's hair daily with the bath. The easiest way to do this is, first, soap the hair with the baby lying in the bassinet, then hold the infant in one arm over the basin of water as you would a football (Fig. 23-28). Splash water from the basin against the head to rinse the hair. Dry the hair well to prevent chilling.

Each area of the baby's body should be washed, rinsed so no soap is left on the skin (soap is drying and newborns are susceptible to desquamation), and then dried. Wash the skin around the cord, taking care not to soak the cord. A wet cord remains in place longer than a dry one and furnishes a breeding ground for bacteria. Give particular care to the creases of skin, where milk tends to collect if the child spits up after feedings.

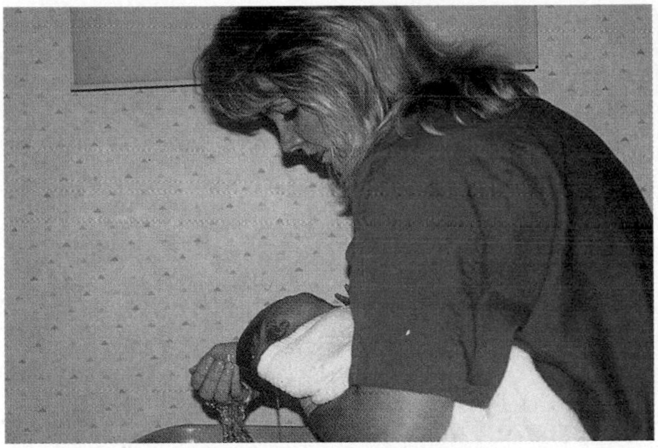

FIGURE 23.28 A football hold. Such a position supports the infant's head and back and leaves the nurse's or mother's other hand free for assembling or using equipment.

In male infants, the foreskin of the uncircumcised penis should not be forced back or constriction of the penis may result. Wash the vulva of female infants, wiping from front to back to prevent contamination of the vagina or urethra by rectal bacteria.

Most health care agencies do not apply powder or lotion to newborns because some infants are allergic to these products. In addition, many adult talcum powders contain zinc stearate, which makes talc irritating to the respiratory tract; these should always be avoided. If the newborn's skin seems extremely dry, and portals for infection are becoming apparent, a lubricant such as Nivea Oil added to the bath water or applied directly to the baby's skin should relieve the condition (Darmstadt & Dinulos, 2000).

Sleeping Position

Stress to parents that the newborn should be positioned on the back for sleeping. Sudden infant death syndrome (SIDS) is the sudden, unexplained death of an infant under 1 year of age. Although the specific cause of SIDS cannot be explained, placing the infant in a supine position has been shown to decrease the incidence of the syndrome (Gibson, 2000; Hein & Pettit, 2001; see Focus on Evidence-Based Practice).

Diaper Area Care

Preventing diaper dermatitis is a practice that parents need to start from the very beginning with their newborns (Kazaks & Lane, 2000). With each diaper change, the area should be washed with clear water and dried well. Washing the skin prevents the ammonia in urine from irritating the infant's skin and causing a diaper rash. After the cleaning, a mild ointment, such as petroleum jelly or A & D ointment, may be applied to the buttocks. The ointment keeps ammonia away from the skin and also facilitates the removal of meconium, which is sticky and tarry. Wear gloves for diaper care as part of standard precautions.

FOCUS ON EVIDENCE-BASED PRACTICE

Do Parents Follow Nurses' Instructions on Placing Newborns on Their Backs to Sleep After They Return Home?

For this study, researchers administered a questionnaire to parents or other caretakers of Sudden Infant Death Syndrome (SIDS) victims in the province of Quebec, Canada. They discovered that 157 infants died of SIDS during the time of the study. Of those 157 infants, 139 had been found sleeping prone. Most revealing was that almost half, or 64 of the infants, usually slept on their backs but had been turned or turned to the prone position before the fatal incident. In 56% of these cases, a caretaker other than the parents had laid the child down to sleep.

This is an important study for nurses because nurses are the chief people in newborn settings who talk to new parents about child care. It makes a strong point that nurses should not only emphasize the importance of placing infants to sleep on their back, but remind parents that when they use alternative caretakers, to be certain those people place the infant supine for sleeping as well. The study can provide the foundation for developing a teaching plan to ensure that parents are taught to place newborns on their backs to sleep.

Cote, A., Gerez, T., Brouillette, R. T., & Laplante, S. (2000). Circumstances leading to a change to prone sleeping in sudden infant death syndrome victims. *Pediatrics, 106*(6), E86–92.

Metabolic Screening Tests

By state law, every infant must be screened for phenylketonuria (PKU; a disease of defective protein metabolism) and hypothyroidism. This is a simple blood test in which three drops of blood from the heel are dropped onto a special filter paper. Ideally, the baby should have received formula or breast milk for 24 hours (providing an intake of phenylalanine, an essential amino acid found in milk) before the test for PKU will be accurate. If the infant has not received adequate milk before the blood sample is taken, the results may be falsely negative (a child with phenylketonuria will test as if normal). If the infant is discharged before this 24-hour period, a second screening test is necessary. Many states require other metabolic tests at birth (eg, screening for galactosemia and maple syrup urine disease) that also need filter paper blood tests.

If blood testing was not done before discharge, the parents must be made aware of this so they can schedule the tests at an ambulatory setting in 2 days' time. Always assess at the first newborn health supervision visit that this procedure was done. Like any heel stick for blood, sampling of this nature is done best by a spring-activated lancet rather than a regular lancet, so the skin incision is made as quickly and painlessly as possible. Allowing the newborn to suck on a pacifier during painful procedures may be helpful (Corbo et al., 2000).

Hepatitis B Vaccination

All newborns receive a first vaccination against hepatitis B within 12 hours after birth; a second dose is administered at 1 month and a third at 6 months. Infants whose mothers are HBsAg-positive also receive hepatitis B immune globulin (HBIG) at birth (AAP, 2002).

Vitamin K Administration

Newborns are at risk for bleeding disorders during the first week of life because their gastrointestinal tract is sterile at birth and unable to produce vitamin K, necessary for blood coagulation. Vitamin K stimulates the liver to produce factors II, VII, IX, and X. A single dose of 0.5 to 1.0 mg of vitamin K is administered intramuscularly within the first hour of life to prevent this (see Focus on Pharmacology: Vitamin K). Remember that infants born outside a hospital also should receive this important protection.

Circumcision

Circumcision is the surgical removal of the penis foreskin. In only a few males, the foreskin is so constricted (phimosis) that it obstructs the urinary meatal opening; otherwise, there are few medical indications for circumcision of the newborn male. Circumcision is performed on Jewish males on the eighth day of life as part of a religious requirement, in a ceremony called a *bris.* In the United States, from the

FOCUS ON PHARMACOLOGY

Vitamin K (Phytonadione, Aquamephyton)

Action: Vitamin K is used for the prophylaxis and treatment of hemorrhagic disease in the newborn. It is a necessary component for the production of certain coagulation factors (II, VII, IX, and X) produced by microorganisms in the intestinal tract.

Pregnancy risk category: C

Dosage: prophylaxis—0.5 to 1.0 mg IM one time immediately after birth; treatment of hemorrhagic disease—1 to 2 mg IM or SC daily.

Possible adverse reactions: Local irritation, such as pain and swelling at the site of injection.

Nursing Implications

- Anticipate the need for injection immediately after birth.
- Administer IM injection into large muscle, such as the anterolateral muscle of the newborn's thigh.
- If giving for treatment, obtain prothrombin time before administration (the single best indicator of vitamin K-dependent clotting factors).
- Assess for signs of bleeding, such as black, tarry stools, hematuria, decreased hemoglobin and hematocrit levels, and bleeding from any open wounds or base of the cord. (These would indicate that more vitamin K is necessary, because bleeding control has not been achieved.)

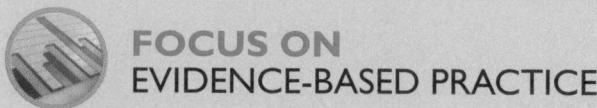

1920s to the 1960s, circumcision became so popular for aesthetic reasons that virtually all male infants were routinely circumcised at birth. The reasons supporting circumcision were easier hygiene, because the foreskin does not have to be retracted during bathing, and possibly fewer urinary tract infections. There may be an increased incidence of cervical cancer in the sexual partner of an uncircumcised male and an increased incidence of penile cancer in the male. Because the procedure does carry some risk, the American Academy of Pediatrics (AAP) does not feel that circumcision is essential. It recommends that parents be well informed about the procedure so that they can evaluate carefully whether they wish to have it performed on their sons (AAP, 1999).

Some contraindications for circumcision include congenital abnormalities such as hypospadias or epispadias, because the prepuce skin may be needed when a plastic surgeon repairs the defect. Another reason not to circumcise an infant would be a history of a bleeding tendency in the family.

The procedure should not be done immediately after birth because the infant's level of vitamin K, which would prevent hemorrhage, is at a low point, and the child would be exposed to unnecessary cold. It is best performed during the first or second day of life after the baby has synthesized enough vitamin K to reduce the chance of faulty blood coagulation. Parents may be asked to return the infant to the hospital or an ambulatory setting for the surgery. Keep in mind that some insurance plans may not reimburse for a return visit for the procedure if the newborn has been discharged.

For the procedure, the infant is placed in a supine position and restrained either manually or with a commercial swaddling board. In the past, the procedure was done without anesthesia, but today most practitioners use local or regional block anesthesia to reduce the pain as much as possible. Application of a *e*utectic *m*ixture of *l*ocal *a*nesthetics (EMLA) is also a popular choice (Taddio, 2001).

A specially designed plastic bell (Plastibell) is fitted over the end of the penis. A suture is then tied around the rim of the bell and a circle of the prepuce is cut away so that the foreskin can be easily retracted and the glans will be fully exposed (Fig. 23-29). The rim of the bell, which remains in place for about a week and then falls off by itself, protects the healing penis from sticking to the diaper. The bell also helps protect against infection and bleeding. In the past, petrolatum ointment was applied to circumcision incisions. With the bell rim in place, this is no longer necessary; however, it still may be applied if desired.

Complications that can occur include hemorrhage, infection, and urethral fistula formation. To keep the risk of these complications to a minimum, infants must be observed closely for about 2 hours after circumcision and assessed for hemorrhage. The infant should be checked for bleeding every 15 minutes for the first hour. It is also important to document the infant is voiding after the procedure.

Parents should be taught to keep the area clean and covered with petrolatum (if used) for about 3 days until healing is complete. If they see any redness or tenderness, or if the baby cries as if in constant pain, they should report it by telephone. Circumcision sites appear red but should never have a strong odor or discharge. A film of yellowish mucus often covers the glans (similar to a scab) by the second day after surgery. This should not be washed away. The yellow color is from accumulated serum, an innocent finding, and should not be mistaken for the yellow of a purulent exudate.

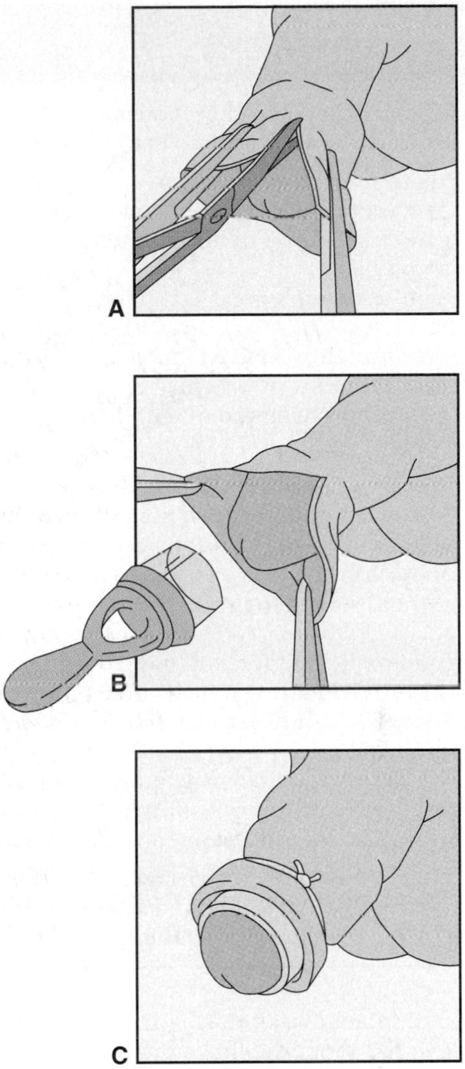

FIGURE 23.29 Technique for performing circumcision using a Plastibell. (*A*) An incision is made in the top of the foreskin. (*B*) The Plastibell is placed over the head of the penis, and the foreskin is pulled over the Plastibell. (*C*) A suture is tied around the foreskin over the tying groove in the Plastibell. Excess skin beyond the suture is trimmed away. The Plastibell falls off in 3 to 7 days. (Courtesy of Hollister Inc., Libertyville, IL.)

> **WHAT IF?** A new parent who is considering circumcision for her newborn, now 14 hours old, is undecided about what to do. How can you best counsel her to make an informed decision?

ASSESSMENT OF FAMILY'S READINESS TO CARE FOR NEWBORN AT HOME

It is important to assess how prepared each family is to care for their newborn at home (see Focus on Communication). They may need to make changes in their routine, such as shifting their usual dinner time. Sleep schedules

FOCUS ON COMMUNICATION

Mrs. Taggliono is a new mother. You notice her sitting by the side of the bed staring into her newborn's face.

Less Effective Communication

Nurse: You seem concerned. Is something wrong?
Mrs. Taggliono: Do you think she can tell how little I know about babies?
Nurse: You're doing a great job. That's the important thing.
Mrs. Taggliono: How long will it take for me to feel like a great mother?
Nurse: You're worrying too much. Relax and enjoy your new baby.

More Effective Communication

Nurse: You seem concerned. Is something wrong?
Mrs. Taggliono: Do you think she can tell how little I know about babies?
Nurse: Is there something special you feel you don't know?
Mrs. Taggliono: I don't feel anything toward her yet. Why do I keep wondering if this whole thing is real?
Nurse: Let's talk about how maternal love develops. It isn't automatic.

Most new mothers have so many questions, it is easy to dismiss a very serious question as "just another question." Resist assuring women that they will be good mothers until you are certain that you know their concern isn't something that could interfere with good mothering.

are disrupted: infants wake during the night for one or more feedings for about the first 4 months of life.

The physical environment of the home to which a newborn will be discharged is a good subject to explore with parents. Possible questions and areas to consider include the following:

- Is it an apartment or a house?
- How many flights of stairs will the mother have to climb when she takes the baby home or when she takes the baby out in a stroller?
- How many other people live in the home? Are there any pets in the home?
- Will grandparents or other persons offer support by visiting or helping with care of the child?
- Do the parents have anyone to turn to if they have questions about the baby?
- Is there a bed for the baby?
- Will the baby be sleeping alone in a room or with older children?
- Who will be the primary caregiver?
- Is there a refrigerator in which formula or breast milk can be stored?
- Is there adequate heat? An infant needs a temperature of 70°F to 75°F during the day and 60°F to 65°F at night.
- Are the windows draft free and screened to keep out insects?
- If housing is in poor condition, is there a danger that rodents might attack the baby?
- Is there a danger of lead poisoning?
- Does the mother or do the parents have a source of income? If not, what sort of referral should be made so money can be provided to care for this child?

These are not prying questions, but are a means of ascertaining whether the home is adequate and safe. All the good prenatal and postnatal care is wasted if an infant contracts pneumonia the first week home, because no one at the hospital or a birthing center took the time to ask the right questions about the home environment. If a home environment is found to be unsafe, a referral to social services may be necessary before the newborn's discharge.

NURSING DIAGNOSES AND RELATED INTERVENTIONS

Nursing Diagnosis: Health-seeking behaviors related to needs of a normal newborn after discharge from the health care facility

Outcome Identification: Parents will demonstrate a general understanding of necessary lifestyle changes and the principles of newborn care at the time of health facility discharge.

Outcome Evaluation: Parents state ways they have already altered their home and lifestyle to accommodate the newborn and indicate they are prepared for other changes; parents voice relative confidence in their ability to care for the newborn and state names of individuals within their family or community who can be resources to them when needed.

Before discharge, parents should have thought through how they are going to care for their child at home. Many parents have been mulling over these questions throughout the pregnancy, whereas others may not have addressed some or any of the important issues. Box 23-2 highlights an appropriate outcome and intervention using the terminology identified by the Nursing Outcomes Classification and Nursing Interventions Classification. Young, single mothers without family support or mothers who did not seek regular prenatal care in particular may be unprepared for the months ahead.

With all parents, try to anticipate problems that may be relevant to them. If there are other children at home, discuss if they are aware that sibling jealousy may occur. In addition, pets in the home also may cause similar problems with jealousy. Discuss with the mother who is not going to breastfeed what she will use to feed the baby until she has had time to buy formula. Most hospitals supply or sell a discharge formula kit to help parents through the first day home. Be sure parents have decided when and where they will take their newborn for health supervision. The child's identification band should be checked against the mother's one final time before discharge. This helps prevent the possibility of infants being confused or kidnapped.

Daily Care. Newborns thrive on a gentle rhythm of care, a sense of being able to anticipate what is to come

BOX 23.2

NURSING OUTCOMES AND NURSING INTERVENTIONS CLASSIFICATION: PARENTS AND THE NEONATE

NOC: Parent–infant attachment

Parent–infant attachment is defined as the behaviors demonstrating an enduring affectionate bond between parents and infant (Johnson, Maas, & Moorhead, 2000). Some specific indicators suggesting achievement of this outcome include demonstration of the following behaviors by the parents:

- Verbalizing positive feelings toward the infant.
- Holding the infant close, touching, stroking, patting, and kissing the infant
- Talking to the infant in the en face position and maintaining eye contact
- Smiling, vocalizing, and playing with the infant
- Responding to cues, consoling, and feeding the infant

Also, some specific indicators suggesting achievement of this outcome include demonstration of the following behaviors by the neonate:

- Looking at parents
- Exploring the environment
- Responding to parental cues
- Seeking proximity with the parents

NIC: Environmental Management: Attachment Process

Environmental management, attachment process is defined as manipulation of the surroundings to facilitate development of the parent–infant relationship (McCloskey & Bulechek, 2000). Some important activities involved when implementing this intervention include:

- Creating a clean, homelike environment that fosters privacy and consistency of staff
- Individualizing daily routine to meet the family's needs
- Providing comfortable seating, such as rocking chair, for parents
- Limiting the number of people in the environment, allowing for family visitation as desired
- Preventing and reducing interruptions from visitors, phone calls, and agency personnel
- Maintaining a low level of stimuli in the environment

next. Parents should decide what is the best daily at-home routine for them and their new child. There are no fixed rules. There is no set time an infant must be bathed or even a rule that requires a bath every day. All infants do not have to be in bed for the night by 8 PM. If the father works evenings, it may be important to have the baby awake at midnight so he has time to spend with the child.

Your aim in helping a mother and father plan their schedule of care is to arrive at one that:

- Offers a degree of consistency (a mother cannot expect an infant to stay awake until midnight 5 nights a week, then go to sleep at 7 PM the next)
- Appears to satisfy the infant
- Gives the parents a sense of well-being and contentment with their child

Sleep Patterns. A newborn sleeps an average of 16 hours of every 24 in the first week home and an average of 4 hours at a time. By 4 months of age, the child sleeps an average of 15 hours of every 24 and through the night.

It is exhausting for a parent who is already tired from labor and birth to have to awaken during the night to feed a newborn. Because of this, parents try various methods to induce a baby to sleep through the night much earlier than 4 months. One approach is to introduce solid food (particularly cereal) in the first weeks of life on the theory that the bulk will fill the infant's stomach for the night and therefore he or she will not wake up crying to be fed. Actually, there is no correlation between the age at which solid food is introduced and the baby's capability for sustained sleep. In fact, the newborn is not developmentally ready to deal with nonliquid food until about the end of the third month. Also, large protein molecules from solid foods pass through the newborn's immature gastrointestinal tract, becoming antigens. This may sensitize the newborn for possible allergic reactions. In addition, too-early introduction of solid foods may interfere with the desire for breast milk, decreasing the newborn's sucking and subsequently decreasing the mother's milk supply.

A baby probably wakes every 4, 5, 6, or 8 hours because of a physiologic need for fluid. Advise parents that there is no reason to try to eliminate this feeding. Knowing that their baby is not sick, that you are concerned and willing to listen to their questions, and that every other parent of a newborn is also up at night does not solve the difficulty, but it is a help.

Encourage parents to position infants on their backs. Infants should not sleep on their stomach because there is an association between this and SIDS (Hein & Petit, 2001).

Crying. Many new parents may not be prepared for the amount of time a newborn spends crying. Whenever the mother saw the baby while at the health care agency, the baby was sleeping. She woke the infant for feeding, and immediately he or she went back to sleep. Infants, however, typically cry an average of about 2 hours of every 24 for the first 7 weeks of life. The frequency seems to peak at age 6 or 7 weeks and then tapers off (Nelson et al., 2000).

Almost all infants have a period during the day when they are wide awake and invariably fussy. New parents need to recognize this as normal and not worry that their child is ill. Parents might use this fussy time for bathing or playing with the infant, arranging their schedules accordingly. Learning the infant's cues and helping the infant learn to self-quiet is important. The most typical time for wakefulness is between 6 PM and 11 PM, which, unfortunately, is when parents may be tired and least able to tolerate crying.

Whether to use pacifiers to reduce crying is a question that parents must decide for themselves, depending on how they feel about them and their infant's needs. It is rare that infants have such a need for sucking that they must have a pacifier in their mouth constantly. Discussing a few pros and cons with parents helps clarify the subject.

An infant who completes a feeding and still seems restless and discontented, who actively searches for something to put into the mouth, and who sucks on hands and clothes may need a pacifier. The major drawback of pacifiers is the problem of cleanliness. They tend to fall on the floor or sidewalk and are then put back into the infant's mouth. Wearing the pacifier on a string around the infant's neck could cause strangulation. Their use is associated with an increase in middle ear infections (Niemela et al., 2000) and early weaning with breastfeeding (Kramer et al., 2001).

Parental Concerns Related to Breathing. Some parents report that their newborns have stuffy noses or make snoring noises in their sleep and that they sneeze occasionally. Most newborns continue to have some mucus in the upper respiratory tract and posterior pharynx for up to 2 weeks after birth. The snoring noise is a result of this mucus, not a cold. Infants also breathe very irregularly for about the first month. A new parent who did not room with her child at the hospital may wake at night, notice this breathing pattern, and grow alarmed that the child is in respiratory distress. If these are the only symptoms, this is a normal newborn respiratory pattern. If the child has rhinitis (nasal discharge) or a fever, he or she needs to be seen by a health care provider, because this suggests upper respiratory infection.

Continued Health Maintenance for the Newborn. Parents do not need to continue to weigh a newborn while at home. This practice only causes worry, because weight fluctuates day by day. Parents should learn to judge an infant's state of health in terms of overall appearance, eagerness to eat, general activity, and disposition, not just weight gain (see Focus on Family Empowerment).

Make certain that parents have an appointment to visit for a first newborn assessment according to their primary care provider's schedule (2 to 6 weeks). A mother is conscientious throughout pregnancy because she wants to bring a well child into the world. Parents must now begin a health care program that will keep the child well.

Car Safety. Automobile accidents are a safety problem all during childhood. For protection, newborns should always be transported in car seats (AAP, 2001). Without this protection, if the car stops suddenly, the infant may be thrown onto the floor or, in a collision, thrown out of the car or through the windshield. In an accident, centrifugal force will cause the infant to exert a force equal to as much as 450 lb, making it impossible for a passenger to hold onto him or her. At only 30 mph, the infant may hit the dashboard with the force equal to a fall from a three-story building. If the adult holding the infant is not wearing a seat belt, the adult can be thrown against the infant and kill the child.

When purchasing a seat, parents should look at the label to be certain the seat meets federal guidelines. A local health department or Red Cross chapter should have a list of all the car seats available in a particular area and give details of their comparable features and cost. The American Academy of Pediatrics web site (*www.AAP.org*) lists these as well. Some hospitals and Red Cross chapters loan infant car seats for temporary use, such as visiting with grandparents or when first coming home from the hospital. New cars are mandated to be equipped with lower anchors and tethers for children (AAP, 2001).

The best location for a car seat is the back seat of the car. One should not be placed in a front passenger seat especially if the car has a passenger seat air bag. The force of an air bag expanding can kill an infant in the seat. While an infant is less than 21 lb or 26 inches long, the best type of car seat is an "infant-only" seat that, when properly positioned in the car, faces the back of the car (Fig. 23-30). The ideal model has a five-point harness with broad straps, which help spread the force of a collision over the chest and hips, and a shield, which cushions the head.

Parents should dress an infant in clothing with pant legs when the infant must be placed in a car seat, because the harness crotch strap must pass between the legs for a snug and correct fit. Advise parents not to use a sack sleeper or papoose bunting, nor should they wrap the baby in a bulky blanket while in the seat. To support the baby's head, parents can use a rolled-up receiving blanket, towel, or diaper on each side of the head, or purchase commercial head supports. To provide extra warmth, they can cut holes in a blanket for the harness and crotch

FOCUS ON FAMILY EMPOWERMENT
Determining If a Newborn Is Well

Q. How will we know if our newborn is well?

A. The following items are helpful to determine that your newborn is well:

- Drinks as if he or she is hungry
- Spits up a slight amount (possible) after feeding, but has no vomiting
- Moves bowels approximately three to four times per day (may be more often if breastfed), with stools that are loose or semiformed but not runny and watery
- Appears happy (although the baby has a fussy period during the day) overall and sleeps for 2 to 3 hours at a time
- Has a normal temperature
- Breathes more rapidly than an adult, but breathing is easy and not stressed
- Skin lacks appearance of a yellow or blue tone

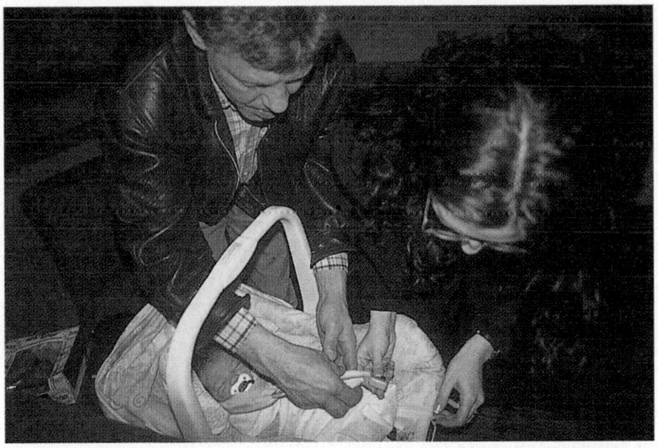

FIGURE 23.30 Most states require infants and children to ride in car seats. It is the nurse's responsibility to make sure that every parent planning to drive a child home from the health care facility is properly equipped.

straps to pass through. Teach parents how to put the blanket in the seat and pull the straps through the blanket holes. Place the baby in the seat, buckle him in, and then fold the blanket over him for warmth. Drape a second blanket over the seat if needed.

A parent should keep the seat in a backward-facing position until the child is able to sit up without support or struggles to sit up, usually when the infant weighs about 21 lb. The infant then is old enough for a toddler seat. Caution parents that plastic car seats grow extremely hot in the summer, and they should test the temperature of the surface before placing the infant in it. Stress also that it is dangerous to not use the car seat properly, such as not fastening the harness or not securing the seat belt.

✔ CHECKPOINT QUESTIONS

15. What are two metabolic screening tests required at birth?
16. What is the chief danger of male circumcision?

KEY POINTS

Converting from fetal to adult respiratory function is a major step in adaptation to extrauterine life. Newborns need particularly close observation during the first few hours of life to determine that this adaptation has been made.

Monitoring body heat is a second major problem of newborns. The temperature of the term baby's environment should be about 75°F (24°C). When procedures that require undressing the infant for an extended period are being done (eg, circumcision), a radiant heat source should be used.

Newborns may suffer hypoglycemia in the first few hours of life, because they use energy to establish respirations and maintain heat. Signs of jitteriness and a blood glucose level under 40 mg/100 mL by heel stick help to identify hypoglycemia.

Identification bands should be attached securely to the infant; careful assessment of these bands should be done before hospital discharge. To help prevent the possibility of kidnapping, be certain of the identification of anyone to whom you give a newborn.

So that parents can feel confident with newborn care, they need to hold and give care in the hospital. Encouraging them to spend as much time as possible with the newborn is a major nursing role.

CRITICAL THINKING EXERCISES

1. For the newborn described at the beginning of this chapter, outline the assessments that should be completed on admission to the nursery.
   a. How would you adapt your teaching plan for this family based on the mother's obvious apprehension?
2. You are assessing a newborn in the mother's room. What newborn reflexes would you assess with him? Suppose it is cold in the room, so you only have time to test one reflex. Which one would you test? Why?
3. You notice a macular purple (port-wine) lesion on the baby's left thigh. His parents tell you they are not concerned because they know all birthmarks fade by the time children are school age. How would you respond to the parents?
4. You discover when the family of the newborn is getting ready to go home that they have no car seat to transport the baby. What would you do? Would you ask them to stay until they arrange to rent or borrow one?
5. Examine the National Health Goals related to newborns. Most government-sponsored money for nursing research is allotted based on these goals. What would be a possible research topic to explore pertinent to these goals that would be both fundable and advance evidence-based practice?

REFERENCES

Al-Ashwal, A. (2001). Hypoglycemia in infants and children. In A. Y. Elzouki et al. (Eds.). *Textbook of clinical pediatrics.* Philadelphia: Lippincott Williams & Wilkins.

American Academy of Pediatrics. (1999). Circumcision policy statement. *Pediatrics, 103*(3), 686–693.

American Academy of Pediatrics. (2001). *2001 family shopping guide to car seats.* Available at www.aap.org/family/famshop.htm.

American Academy of Pediatrics. (2002). *2002 immunization schedule.* Washington, D.C.: Author.

Apgar, V., et al. (1958). Evaluation of the newborn infant: Second report. *Journal of the American Medical Association, 168*(2), 1985–1988.

Ballard, J. L., et al. (1991). The new Ballard Scale. *Journal of Pediatrics, 11*(4), 417-421.

Bertini, G., et al. (2001). Is breastfeeding really favoring early neonatal jaundice? *Pediatrics, 107*(3), E41-45.

Brazelton, T. B. (1973). Neonatal behavior assessment scale. *Clinics in Developmental Medicine, 50*(5), 1-15.

Corbo, M. G., et al. (2000). Nonnutritive sucking during heelstick procedures decreases behavioral distress in the newborn infant. *Biology of the Neonate, 77*(3), 162-167.

Cote, A., Gerez, T., Brouillette, R. T., & Laplante, S. (2000). Circumstances leading to a change to prone sleeping in sudden infant death syndrome victims. *Pediatrics, 106*(6), E86-92.

Cunningham, F. G., et al. (2001). *Williams obstetrics* (21st ed.). Stamford, CT: Appleton & Lange.

Darmstadt, G. L. & Dinulos, J. G. (2000). Neonatal skin care. *Pediatric Clinics of North America, 47*(4), 757-782.

Department of Health and Human Services. (2000). *Healthy people 2010.* Washington, DC: Author.

Desmond, M. N., et al. (1963). The clinical behavior of the newly born: The term infant. *Journal of Pediatrics, 62*(3), 307-309.

Dinehart, S. M., et al. (2001). Hemangiomas: Evaluation and treatment. *Dermatologic Surgery, 27*(5), 475-485.

Dubowitz, L., et al. (1970). Clinical assessment of gestational age in the newborn infant. *Journal of Pediatrics, 77*(10), 1-12.

Gibson, E., et al. (2000). Infant sleep position practices 2 years into the "back to sleep" campaign. *Clinical Pediatrics, 39*(5), 285-289.

Hein, H. A. & Pettit, S. F. (2001). Back to sleep: Good advice for parents but not for hospitals? *Pediatrics, 107*(3), 537-539.

Johnson, M., Maas, M, & Moorhead, S. (2000). *Nursing outcomes classification* (2nd ed.). St. Louis: Mosby.

Kanemoto, K., et al. (2002). The management of nonpalpable testis with combined groin exploration and transinguinal laparoscopy. *Journal of Urology, 167*(2.1), 674-676.

Kazaks, E. L. & Lane, A. T. (2000). Diaper dermatitis. *Pediatric Clinics of North America, 47*(4), 909-919.

Kelly, J. B. (1999). General care. In G. B. Avery, M. A. Fletcher, & M. G. MacDonald (Eds.). *Neonatology* (pp. 333-342). Philadelphia: Lippincott Williams & Wilkins.

Kirsten, G. F., Bergman, N. J., & Hann, F. M. (2001). Kangaroo mother care in the nursery. *Pediatric Clinics of North America, 48*(2), 443-452.

Kramer, M. S. et al. (2001). Pacifier use, early weaning, and cry/fuss behavior: A randomized controlled trial. *Journal of the American Medical Association, 286*(3), 322-326.

McCloskey, J. & Bulechek, G. (2000). *Nursing interventions classification* (3rd ed.). St. Louis: Mosby.

Metry, D. W. & Hebert, A. (2000). Benign cutaneous vascular tumors of infancy: When to worry, what to do. *Archives of Dermatology, 136*(7), 905-914.

Mindel, A. et al. (2000). Neonatal herpes prevention: A minor public health problem in some communities. *Sexually Transmitted Infections, 76*(4), 287-291.

Moster, D. et al. (2001). The association of Apgar score with subsequent death and cerebral palsy. *Journal of Pediatrics, 138*(6), 798-803.

Nelson, R. M., Stronquist, C. F., & Wyble, L. E. (2000). Newborn assessment and care. In J. R. Scott, et al. (Eds.). *Danforth's obstetrics and gynecology.* Philadelphia: Lippincott Williams & Wilkins.

Niemela, M., et al. (2000). Pacifier as a risk factor for acute otitis media: A randomized controlled trial of parental counseling. *Pediatrics, 106*(3), 483-488.

Rusting, R. R. (2000). Baby switching: An underreported problem that needs to be recognized. *Journal of Healthcare Protection Management, 17*(1), 89-100.

Silverman, W. A. & Anderson, H. (1956). A controlled clinical trial of effects of water mist on obstructive respiratory signs, death rate and necroscopy findings among premature infants. *Pediatrics, 17*(4), 1-9.

Taddio, A. (2001). Pain management for neonatal circumcision. *Paediatric Drugs, 3*(2), 101-110.

Usher, R., et al. (1966). Judgment of fetal age. *Pediatric Clinics of North America, 13*(4), 835-840.

Van Gemert, J. J. et al. (2001). Twin-twin transfusion syndrome: Etiology, severity, and rational management. *Current Opinion in Obstetrics & Gynecology, 13*(2), 193-206.

SUGGESTED READINGS

Clemons, R. M. (2000). Issues in newborn care. *Primary Care, 27*(1), 251-267.

Gartner, L. M. & Herschel, M. (2001). Jaundice and breastfeeding. *Pediatric Clinics of North America, 48*(2), 389-399.

Juberg, D. R., et al. (2001). An observational study of object mouthing behavior by young children. *Pediatrics, 107*(1), 135-142.

Kaufman, M. W., Clark, J. Y., & Castro, C. L. (2001). Neonatal circumcision: Benefits, risks and family teaching. *MCN: American Journal of Maternal Child Nursing, 26*(4), 197-201.

Lindrea, K. B. & Stainton, M. C. (2000). A case study of infant massage outcomes. *MCN: American Journal of Maternal Child Nursing, 25*(2), 95-99.

McCarthy, J. G., et al. (2002). Hemangiomas of the nasal tip. *Plastic & Reconstructive Surgery, 109*(1), 31-40.

Merewood, A. & Philipp, B. L. (2001). Implementing change: Becoming baby-friendly in an inner city hospital. *Birth, 28*(1), 36-40.

Odio, M. & Friedlander, S. F. (2000). Diaper dermatitis and advances in diaper technology. *Current Opinion in Pediatrics, 12*(4), 342-346.

Takayama, J. I., et al. (2000). Body temperature of newborns: What is normal? *Clinical Pediatrics, 39*(9), 503-510.

Willinger, M., et al. (2000). Factors associated with caregivers' choice of infant sleep position. *Journal of the American Medical Association, 283*(16), 2135-2142.

Nutritional Needs of the Newborn

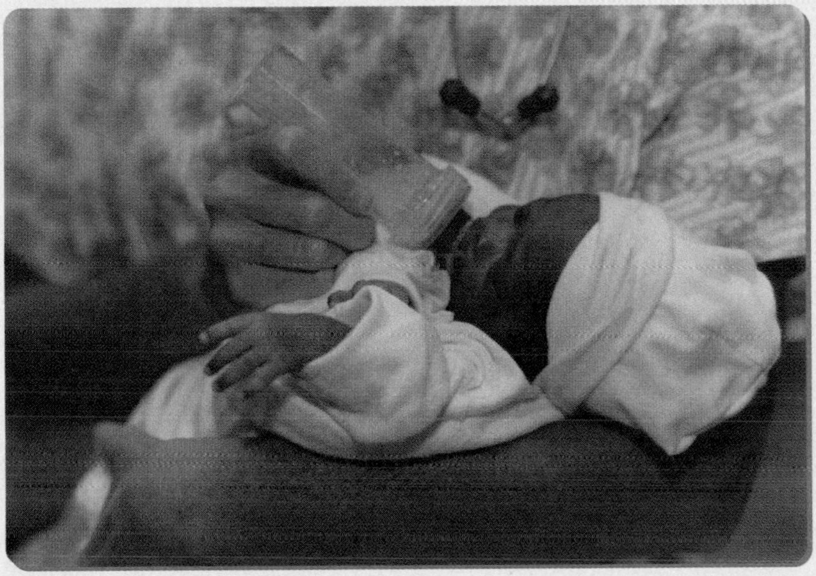

Key Terms

- areola
- bifidus factor
- colostrum
- engorgement
- foremilk
- hind milk
- interferon
- lactiferous sinuses
- lactoferrin
- let-down reflex
- lysozyme
- prolactin

Objectives

After mastering the contents of this chapter, you should be able to:

1. Describe nutritional requirements of the term newborn.
2. Assess nutritional intake of a newborn to determine adequate nutritional status.
3. Formulate nursing diagnoses related to newborn nutrition.
4. Identify outcomes for the newborn and mother related to nutrition.
5. Plan a method of infant feeding with a mother that will be satisfying for both her and the infant.
6. Implement or help parents implement feeding procedures with newborn infants.
7. Evaluate outcomes for achievement and effectiveness of care.
8. Identify National Health Goals related to newborn nutrition that nurses can be instrumental in helping the nation achieve.
9. Identify areas related to nutrition and newborns that could benefit from additional nursing research or application of evidence-based practice.
10. Use critical thinking to assist mothers with nutritional problem solving and making newborn nutrition more family-centered.
11. Integrate knowledge of normal newborn nutrition with nursing process to achieve quality maternal and child health nursing care.

Jane Smith is a new mother of a term baby girl. During the pregnancy, she and her husband, Paul, discussed feeding methods and decided on breastfeeding. Jane will be returning to work as an executive assistant after her 6-week maternity leave. She attempted to breast-feed her newborn in the birthing room with minimal success. As you offer to help her feed her baby for the second time, you notice she appears anxious. She states, "I don't know if we made the right choice. Maybe I should bottle-feed her. Then at least Paul can help and I won't have to worry about what to do when I go back to work." What suggestions would you give her?

Previous chapters described the care of the woman and family during the antepartal, intrapartal, and postpartal periods. This chapter adds information about the nutritional needs of the newborn to your knowledge base. This knowledge is important because the newborn's nutritional needs are high due to the rapid rate of growth and development. You can play a key role in educating the parents about how to provide the newborn with adequate nutrition to meet both physiologic and psychological needs.

After you've studied the chapter, answer the Critical Thinking Exercises at the end of the chapter and then access the online study activities (http://connection.lww.com) *to further sharpen your skills and test your knowledge.*

Proper nutrition is essential for optimal growth and development, especially in the first few months of life because brain growth is proceeding at such a rapid rate. Providing adequate food and nutrition for the newborn extends beyond physiologic need, however, also fulfilling important psychological needs. During feeding, the parent is close to the infant, and the baby will be particularly sensitive to the parent's demonstration of affection or lack of warmth. The infant who does not experience a warm relationship with the mother or primary caregiver may fail to thrive as surely as the one who is denied sufficient protein or calories. National Health Goals related to newborn nutrition are shown in the Focus on National Health Goals box.

FOCUS ON NATIONAL HEALTH GOALS

Two National Health Goals address nutrition of the newborn. These are:

- Increase to at least 75% from a baseline of 64% the proportion of mothers who breast-feed their babies in the early postpartum period; to at least 50%, from a baseline of 29%, the proportion who continue breast-feeding until their babies are 5 to 6 months old; and from 16% to 25% the proportion who continue breast-feeding until 1 year of age.
- Decrease the proportion of children with untreated dental decay in primary or permanent teeth from 29% to 21% (DHHS, 2000).

Nurses can be instrumental in helping the nation achieve these goals by educating women about breast-feeding during pregnancy and supporting the family during the postpartal period while the woman is breast-feeding. Home visits with postpartal families or well-child health assessments provide opportunities to advocate for continuing breast-feeding. For the woman who will formula-feed her infant, education during pregnancy should include not putting the infant to bed with a bottle of milk or juice to prevent tooth decay.

Areas that could benefit from additional nursing research include techniques parents use to initiate sleep without using a bedtime bottle; reasons women discontinue breast-feeding early in the postpartal period; and legislation or education necessary in the workplace to encourage women to continue breast-feeding after they return to work.

NURSING PROCESS OVERVIEW

For Promotion of Nutritional Health in the Newborn

Assessment

Assessment of infant nutrition begins during pregnancy with assessment of the mother's and father's attitudes and choices about infant feeding. Breast-feeding is widely accepted as the preferred method of newborn nutrition. However, if a mother chooses not to breast-feed, she must not be made to feel guilty for her choice because formula feeding can be substituted. Every person's circumstances are unique. Most importantly, parents need to feel comfortable with and confident about the feeding method they have chosen.

Teach parents how to recognize signs of hunger in a newborn, including restlessness, tense body posture, smacking lips, or tongue thrusting. Otherwise, they may wait for the infant to cry, actually a late sign of newborn hunger. Once infant feeding begins, teach a mother to assess whether the amount the infant is receiving is adequate—not by how long the newborn breast-feeds at a time or by how much formula is taken at a feeding, but by a larger measure such as whether the newborn is voiding, growing, and alert (see Assessing the Newborn for Adequate Nutrition). A bottle-fed newborn regains birthweight at about 10 days, the breast-fed infant at about 14 days.

Nursing Diagnosis

Assessment of a mother's choice regarding the method of feeding and a newborn's nutritional intake and feeding patterns may yield several important nursing diagnoses. However, it may be difficult to establish diagnoses during the first part of the newborn period because the mother and infant are still getting used

ASSESSING the Newborn for Adequate Nutrition

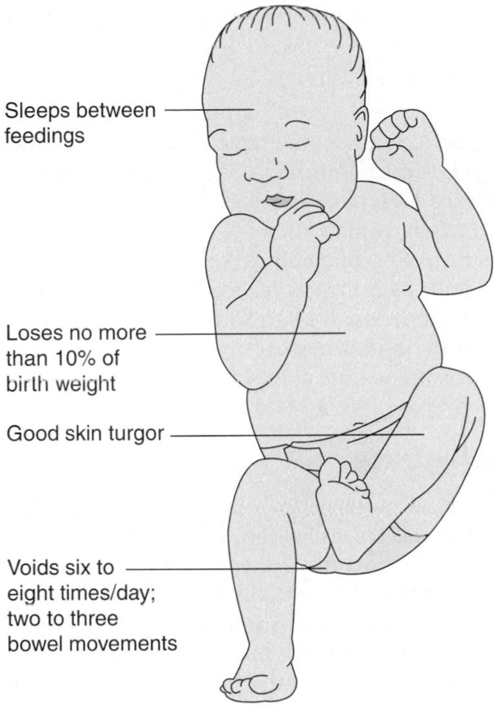

to each other. Examples of possible nursing diagnoses are:

- Effective breastfeeding related to well-prepared mother and healthy newborn
- Risk for ineffective breastfeeding related to nipple soreness
- Imbalanced nutrition, less than body requirements, related to poor newborn sucking response
- Impaired parenting related to ineffective coping secondary to father feeling resentment because the mother is breastfeeding

Outcome Identification and Planning

Planning begins while the woman is still pregnant, with the focus on providing her with the information necessary to permit an informed decision about breastfeeding or bottle-feeding. Once a decision is made, a teaching plan addressing the nutritional needs of both the woman and newborn can be developed. The woman who expects to formula-feed can purchase supplies in advance. Both can read about newborn care and plan ways to make feeding time a special one for both themselves and the baby.

Implementation

A major intervention related to newborn nutrition is supporting the mother's choice of feeding method and helping her to trust her judgment as to whether her infant is full and content and the feeding method is as natural as possible. A referral to support groups such as La Leche League (*www.lalecheleague.org*) or International Lactation Consultant Association (*www.ilca.org*) might be appropriate. In addition to sponsoring classes on breastfeeding, a helpful service of La Leche League is its hotline, through which a breastfeeding woman who is discouraged or is having difficulty can contact a member and ask for advice. "The Womanly Art of Breastfeeding," published by the League (1997), is a comprehensive and informative book for both new mothers and fathers.

When assisting a new mother with breastfeeding, remember that breast milk can carry the human immunodeficiency virus (HIV). Adhere to standard precautions when helping with manual expression of milk or disposing of used breastfeeding pads.

Outcome Evaluation

Evaluation is an important step in providing newborn nutrition. Unforeseen circumstances, such as an unsuspected milk allergy or mastitis (breast infection), may require drastic changes in desired outcomes. Help parents to understand that newborns can adapt to another feeding method if necessary. Examples suggesting achievement of outcomes related to newborn feeding might be:

- Infant breast-feeds every 2 to 3 hours; is content and sleeps between feedings.
- Newborn ingests a total of 12 oz of formula with iron every 24 hours.
- Mother states she is satisfied with chosen method of infant feeding.
- Infant voids six times daily as a measure of adequate hydration.

NUTRITIONAL ALLOWANCES FOR THE NEWBORN

Calories

Growth in the neonatal period and early infancy is more rapid than at any other period of life. Therefore, the caloric requirements exceed those at any other age. A newborn and an infant up to 2 months of age require 110 to 120 calories per kilogram of body weight (50 to 55 kcal/lb) every 24 hours to provide an adequate amount of food for maintenance and growth. After 2 months of age, the amount gradually declines until the requirement at 1 year is 100 kcal/kg, or 45 kcal/lb/day. Compare this to an adult requirement of 42 kcal/kg, or 20 kcal/lb/day.

The actual caloric requirement, of course, depends on the infant's activity level and growth rate. For example, an active infant, one who cries frequently and squirms constantly, will need more calories than one who is more passive, content to spend long hours playing quietly or just studying the environment. During growth spurts, more calories are needed to supply enough energy.

Commercial infant formulas simulate breast milk and contain about 9% to 12% of the calories as protein and 45% to 55% of the calories as lactose carbohydrate. The balance is fat, of which about 10% (4% of the calories) is linoleic acid. For information about recommended dietary allowances, see Table 24-1.

Protein

Protein, necessary for the formation of new cells, is important for the very rapid growth during infancy and the maturation and maintenance of existing cells. Thus, protein requirements are high during the newborn and infancy periods. The nutritional allowance of protein for the first 2 months of life is 2.2 g per kilogram of body weight. Both human milk and commercial formulas provide all the essential amino acids. Histidine, an amino acid that appears to be essential for infant growth but is not necessary for adult growth, is found in both milk forms.

Unaltered cow's milk is not recommended for newborns because it contains about 16% of its calories as protein, whereas human milk contains about 8%. This means that cow's milk creates such a rich solute load (the amount of urea and electrolytes that must be excreted in the urine) that a newborn's kidneys could be overwhelmed by it. In addition, the protein in cow's milk, casein, differs from that in human milk, lactalbumin, both in composition and amount. The amount of casein present in milk determines its curd tension. Thus, the curd in cow's milk is large, tough, and difficult to digest, whereas in human milk, the curd is softer and easier to digest. This is the rationale for bottle-fed infants to receive a commercial formula containing albumin rather than cow's milk. Cow's milk products, such as yogurt and cottage cheese, should not be introduced until 9 to 12 months of age for the same reason.

TABLE 24.1 Recommended Dietary Allowance for Infants

NUTRIENT	RECOMMENDED DIETARY ALLOWANCE Birth to 6 Mo	6 Mo to 1 Yr
Calories	kg × 108	kg × 98
Protein (g)	kg × 2.2	kg × 1.6
Vitamin A (μg, RE)*	375	375
Vitamin D (μg, cholecalciferol)	7.5	10
Vitamin E (mg, TE)†	3	4
Vitamin C (mg)	30	35
Folacin (μg)	25	35
Niacin (mg, NE)‡	5	6
Riboflavin (mg)	0.4	0.5
Thiamin (mg)	0.3	0.4
Vitamin B_6 (mg)	0.3	0.6
Vitamin B_{12} (μg)	0.3	0.5
Calcium (mg)	400	600
Phosphorus (mg)	300	500
Iodine (μg)	40	50
Magnesium (mg)	40	60
Zinc (mg)	5	5
Iron (mg)	6	10

*RE, retinol equivalents; †TE, tocopherol equivalents; ‡NE, niacin equivalents.

Adapted from National Research Council. (1989). *Recommended Dietary Allowances* (10th ed.). Washington, DC: National Academy Press.

Fat

Linoleic acid, an essential fatty acid necessary for growth and skin integrity in infants, is found in both human and commercial formulas. Using fat-free milk for long periods of time (when other sources of food are not being offered) can result in linoleic acid deficiency. Therefore, feeding fat-free milk as a means of controlling obesity in young infants is not the answer. In addition, fat-free milk does not contain sufficient calories (only about half as many as commercial formulas or regular milk).

Carbohydrate

Lactose, the disaccharide found in human milk and added to commercial formulas, appears to be the most easily digested of the carbohydrates. Lactose also improves calcium absorption and aids in nitrogen retention. It produces stools consisting predominantly of gram-positive rather than gram-negative bacteria. The presence of gram-positive stools decreases the possibility of gastrointestinal illness (which usually results from gram-negative organisms). Adequate lactose also allows protein to be used for building new cells rather than for calories, encouraging normal water balance and preventing abnormal metabolism of fat. Lactose intolerance, which can occur in older children, is rarely present in newborns. Thus, they use the calories provided by lactose well.

Fluid

Because their metabolic rate is high (metabolism requires water), maintaining a sufficient fluid intake in newborns is important. A newborn uses 45 to 50 kcal/kg; an adult uses 25 to 30 kcal/kg. This high rate of metabolism requires a large amount of water. In addition, the newborn's body surface area is large in relation to body mass. Thus, a baby loses a larger amount of water by evaporation than an adult does.

Water also is distributed differently in the newborn than in the adult. In a newborn, 30% to 35% of body weight is extracellular fluid; in the adult, this is approximately 20%. Consequently, loss of fluid or inadequate fluid intake quickly depletes the extracellular fluid supply, affecting as much as 35% of the newborn's fluid component. Because the kidneys of a newborn are not yet capable of fully concentrating urine, the newborn cannot conserve body water by this mechanism and must have an adequate fluid intake to prevent dehydration.

The fluid requirement for a newborn is 150 to 200 mL/kg (2.5 to 3.0 oz/lb) per 24 hours. This requirement can be supplied completely by breastfeeding or formula-feeding. Fruit juice is not recommended as a supplemental fluid because it supplies no protein and if not pasteurized can carry infectious organisms (AAP Committee on Nutrition, 2001).

Minerals

A number of minerals are particularly important to early growth.

Calcium

Calcium is an important mineral in the newborn period because of its contribution to bone growth. Because milk is high in calcium, tetany from a low calcium level seldom occurs in infants who suck well, regardless of whether they are fed human milk or commercial formula.

Iron

The term infant of a mother who had an adequate iron intake during pregnancy will be born with iron stores that, theoretically, will last for the first 3 months of life, until the newborn begins to produce adult hemoglobin. Because not all mothers' food intake is iron rich during pregnancy (and socioeconomic level is not a good criterion for judging the quality of a diet), the American Academy of Pediatrics recommends that an iron supplement be included in formula for formula-fed infants for the entire first year of life (AAP, 2000). It is unnecessary to provide iron supplementation in the breast-fed infant because breast milk usually provides an adequate amount of iron.

Fluoride

Fluoride is essential for building sound teeth and for preventing tooth decay. Because teeth grow into their primary form during pregnancy, it is important for mothers to drink fluoridated water during pregnancy. The lactating mother should continue drinking fluoridated water (although fluoride does not pass in great amounts in breast milk), and formulas should be prepared with fluoridated water. This is an essential point to remember because a mother may think she is helping her child by using bottled, "natural" water in formula rather than chlorinated (but fluoridated) water from a tap.

If a mother is breastfeeding and a source of fluoridated water is not available (the family drinks well, spring, or bottled water, or the tap water is not fluoridated), a fluoride supplement, 0.25 mg daily, may be given to the infant beginning at 6 months of age. Remind parents that too much fluoride can be detrimental or cause staining of the teeth. Doing so helps to prevent the parents from requesting unnecessary fluoride supplements (Krebs & Hambidge, 2001).

Vitamins

Vitamin additives are unnecessary for the bottle-fed infant because vitamins A, C, and D are incorporated into commercial formulas. Because vitamins are naturally included in breast milk, supplementation is not necessary for breast-fed infants either. If the newborn will not be exposed to sunlight for some reason, 400 U of vitamin D daily may be prescribed for the mother to increase this level in breast milk or given to the bottle-fed infant. Additional vitamins are not begun until the infant approaches 6 months of age.

✔ CHECKPOINT QUESTIONS

1. How many calories does a 1-month-old infant require per day?
2. Why is unaltered cow's milk difficult for newborns to digest?
3. How much of the newborn's body weight is extracellular fluid?

BREASTFEEDING

Breast milk is the preferred method of feeding a newborn because it provides numerous health benefits to both the mother and the infant; it remains the ideal nutritional source for infants through the first year of life (Sinusas & Gagliardi, 2001). Nurses can play a major role in teaching women about the benefits of breastfeeding and providing anticipatory guidance for problems that may occur. They can be instrumental in creating an atmosphere conducive to breastfeeding success in health care facilities by implementing steps such as:

- Educating all pregnant women about the benefits and management of breastfeeding
- Helping women initiate breastfeeding within half an hour of birth
- Assisting mothers to breast-feed and maintain lactation even if they should be separated from their infant
- Not giving newborns food or drink other than breast milk unless medically indicated
- Not giving pacifiers to breastfeeding infants
- Practicing rooming-in (i.e., allow mothers and infants to remain together) 24 hours a day
- Encouraging breastfeeding on demand
- Fostering the establishment of breastfeeding support groups and referring mothers to them on discharge from the birthing center or hospital

Box 24-1 highlights several outcomes and interventions related to breastfeeding using the terminology identified by the Nursing Outcomes Classification (NOC) and Nursing Interventions Classification (NIC).

Physiology of Breast Milk Production

Breast milk is formed in the acinar or alveolar cells of the mammary glands (Fig. 24-1). With the delivery of the placenta, the level of progesterone in the mother's body falls dramatically, stimulating the production of **prolactin,** an anterior pituitary hormone. Prolactin acts on the acinar cells of the mammary glands to stimulate the production of milk. In addition, when an infant sucks at

BOX 24.1

NURSING OUTCOMES AND NURSING INTERVENTIONS CLASSIFICATION: BREASTFEEDING

NOC: Knowledge: Breastfeeding

Knowledge, breastfeeding, is defined as the extent of understanding conveyed about lactation and nourishment of an infant through breast-feeding (Johnson, Maas, & Moorhead, 2000). Some specific indicators suggesting achievement of this outcome include the client's ability to describe the following:

- Benefits of breastfeeding
- Physiology of lactation, including breast milk composition, let-down process, signs of adequate milk supply, and possible passage of substances through breast milk
- Early infant hunger cues and signs of adequately nourished breastfed infant
- Proper technique for attachment, positioning, and breaking infant suction and for expressing and storing breast milk
- Nipple evaluation, including signs and symptoms of mastitis, blocked ducts, and nipple trauma
- Readiness to wean

NOC: Breastfeeding Establishment, Infant

Breastfeeding establishment, infant, is defined as the proper attachment of an infant to and sucking from the mother's breast for nourishment during the first 2 to 3 weeks (Johnson, Maas, & Moorhead, 2000). Some specific indicators suggesting achievement of this outcome include the infant's ability to demonstrate the following:

- Proper alignment, latching on, areolar grasp, areolar compression, and correct sucking and tongue placement
- Audible swallowing a minimum of 5 to 10 minutes per breast with at least 8 feedings per day
- At least 6 voidings per day with the passage of 2 or more loose yellow, seedy stools per day
- Age-appropriate weight gain
- Contentment after feeding

NOC: Breastfeeding Establishment, Maternal

Breastfeeding establishment, maternal, is defined as the maternal establishment of proper attachment of an infant to and sucking from the breast for nourishment during the first 2 to 3 weeks (Johnson, Maas, & Moorhead, 2000). Some specific indicators suggesting achievement of this outcome include the mother's ability to demonstrate the following:

- Position of comfort during feeding with support of breasts
- Identification of breast fullness prior to feeding
- Technique for let-down reflex
- Absence of nipple tenderness
- Avoidance of using artificial nipple and giving water
- Supplementation appropriate to infant's age and health status
- Ability to recognize infant hunger cues
- Appropriate techniques for hand or pump expression and proper storage
- Satisfaction with breastfeeding

NOC: Breastfeeding Maintenance

Breastfeeding maintenance is defined as the continued nourishment of an infant through breast-feeding (Johnson, Maas, & Moorhead, 2000). Some specific indicators suggesting achievement of this outcome include the demonstration of the following:

- Infant's growth and development within expected range in conjunction with family's understanding of infant's growth spurts and benefits of continued breastfeeding
- Mother's ability to safely collect and store breast milk with continuation of breast feeding on return to work or school
- Caregiver's ability to safely thaw, warm, and feed stored breast milk
- Mother's freedom from breast tenderness
- Mother's ability to recognize signs of decreased milk supply, plugged ducts, and mastitis
- Family's expression of satisfaction with available support and satisfaction with breastfeeding

NIC: Breastfeeding Assistance

Breastfeeding assistance is defined as preparing a new mother to breastfeed her infant (McCloskey & Bulechek, 2000). Some important activities involved when implementing this intervention include:

- Providing early contact opportunity between mother and infant within 2 hours after birth
- Assisting parents in identifying infant arousal cues
- Instructing mother on proper positioning and techniques
- Monitoring infant's ability to suck
- Observing infant at breast for latching on, correct positioning, audible swallowing, and suck/swallow pattern
- Encouraging mother to offer both breasts at each feeding and to allow infant to feed as long as interested
- Instructing mother on nipple care, use of breast pump if indicated, control of breast congestion with timely emptying or pumping, use of comfortable supportive nursing bra, proper storage and warming of stored breast milk, and methods for burping infant
- Teaching about normal characteristics of voiding and stool with breastfed infants
- Encouraging mother to consume a well-balanced diet with adequate fluid intake and obtain frequent rest
- Instructing mother to avoid any medications, including oral contraceptives as well as cigarettes, while breastfeeding

continued on page 675

Continued

NURSING OUTCOMES AND NURSING INTERVENTIONS CLASSIFICATION: BREASTFEEDING

- Referring parents to appropriate classes or support groups for breastfeeding, including a referral to a lactation consultant if necessary

NIC: Lactation Counseling

Lactation counseling is defined as the use of an interactive helping process to assist in maintaining successful breastfeeding (McCloskey & Bulechek, 2000). Some important activities involved when implementing this intervention include:

- Educating parents about infant feeding based on current knowledge base to allow for informed decision making
- Providing information about the advantages and disadvantages of breastfeeding, along with correcting any misconceptions, misinformation, and inaccuracies
- Supporting the mother's decision
- Referring parents to appropriate classes and support groups for breastfeeding
- Evaluating mother's understanding of infant's feeding cues
- Monitoring mother's skill with latching infant to nipple
- Instructing on recording length and frequency of feeding, infant stool and urination patterns, and infant growth spurts
- Evaluate adequacy of breast emptying at each feeding
- Demonstrating breast massage in conjunction with a discussion of its advantages for increasing milk supply
- Encouraging breast pumping between feeding sessions
- Monitoring nipple integrity, with recommendations for nipple care as appropriate
- Instructing on signs and symptoms to report to the health care provider
- Discussing signs related to readiness to wean, options for weaning, and alternative methods of feeding

the breast, nerve impulses travel from the nipple to the hypothalamus to stimulate the production of prolactin-releasing factor. This factor stimulates further active production of prolactin. Other anterior pituitary hormones, such as adrenocorticotropic hormone, thyroid-stimulating hormone, and growth hormone, probably also play a role in growth of the mammary glands and their ability to secrete milk.

Colostrum, a thin, watery, yellow fluid composed of protein, sugar, fat, water, minerals, vitamins, and maternal antibodies, is secreted by the acinar breast cells starting in the 4th month of pregnancy. For the first 3 or 4 days after birth, colostrum production continues. Because it is high in protein and fairly low in sugar and fat, colostrum is easy to digest. It also provides totally adequate nutrition for the newborn until it is replaced by transitional breast milk on the 2nd to 4th day. True or mature breast milk is produced by the 10th day.

Milk flows from the alveolar cells where it is produced through small tubules to reservoirs for milk, the **lactiferous sinuses,** behind the nipple. This constantly forming milk is called **foremilk.** Its availability depends very little on the infant's sucking at the breast. As the infant sucks at the breast, oxytocin, released from the posterior pituitary, causes the collecting sinuses of the mammary glands to contract, forcing milk forward through the nipples, thus making it available for the baby. This action is called the **let-down reflex.** A let-down reflex may also be triggered by the sound of a baby crying or thinking about the baby. New milk, called **hind milk,** is formed after the let-down reflex. Hind milk, higher in fat than foremilk, is the milk that makes the breast-fed infant grow most rapidly. Oxytocin also causes smooth muscle to contract, so when it is produced, the uterus contracts as well. As a result, the woman may feel a small tugging or cramping in her lower pelvis during the first few days of breastfeeding (Lawrence, 1999).

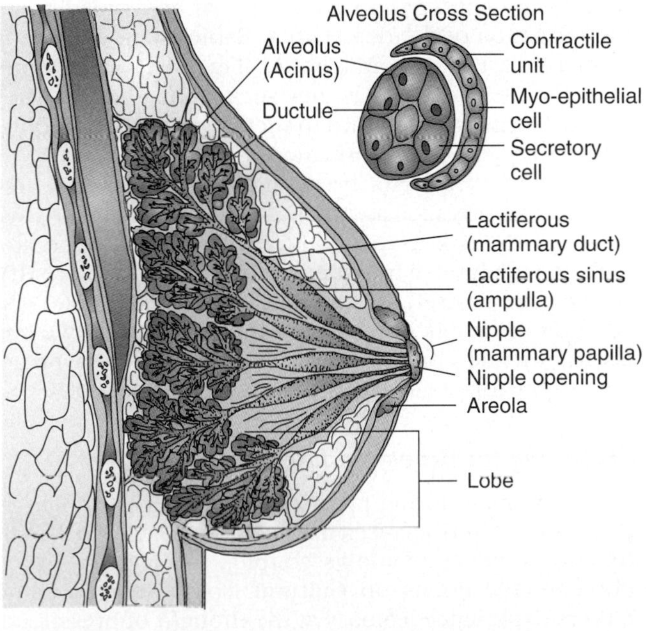

FIGURE 24.1 Anatomy of the breast.

Advantages of Breastfeeding

Little controversy exists about breastfeeding as the best nutrition for human infants, but the decision to breastfeed depends on what would please the woman the most and make her most comfortable. If she is comfortable and pleased with what she is doing, her infant will be comfortable and pleased, will enjoy being fed, and will thrive.

Breastfeeding is contraindicated in only a few circumstances, such as:

- An infant with galactosemia (such infants cannot digest the lactose in milk)
- Herpes lesions on the mother's nipples
- Mother is on a restricted-nutrient diet that prevents quality milk production
- Mother is receiving medications that are inappropriate for breastfeeding, such as lithium or methotrexate
- Maternal exposure to radioactive compounds, as could happen during thyroid testing
- Breast cancer

A number of situations call for individual planning, such as if the mother or infant is too ill for breastfeeding, the mother has undergone previous breast-reduction surgery, especially if the nipples were detached during surgery, or the mother and infant are being treated for tuberculosis.

Advantages for the Mother

A woman gains several physiologic benefits from breastfeeding, including:

1. Breastfeeding may serve a protective function in preventing breast cancer.
2. The release of oxytocin from the posterior pituitary gland aids in uterine involution.
3. Successful breastfeeding can have an empowering effect because it is a skill only women can master.

Breastfeeding also reduces the cost of feeding and preparation time. Many women feel that breastfeeding provides the best opportunity to enhance the formation of a true symbiotic bond with their child. Although this does occur readily with breastfeeding, a woman who holds her baby to bottle-feed can form this bond equally well. Some women believe that breastfeeding is a foolproof contraceptive technique. It is not: 50% of women resume ovulating by the 4th week postpartum even while breastfeeding. Some feel breastfeeding will help them lose weight gained during pregnancy. This also is not true, and women who are breastfeeding need to concentrate on eating a well-balanced diet to ensure that their milk is rich in nutrients. Some woman are reluctant to breast-feed because they fear that having to be available to feed the baby every 3 or 4 hours will tie them down. Like mothers who bottle-feed, however, they can leave a bottle (with expressed breast milk or formula) with the baby's father or a caregiver if they need to be away from the baby during a feeding.

Advantages for the Baby

Breastfeeding has major physiologic advantages for the baby. Breast milk contains secretory immunoglobulin A (IgA), which binds large molecules of foreign proteins, including viruses and bacteria, thus keeping them from being absorbed through the gastrointestinal tract into the infant. **Lactoferrin** is an iron-binding protein in breast milk that interferes with the growth of pathogenic bacteria. The enzyme **lysozyme** in breast milk apparently actively destroys bacteria by lysing (dissolving) their cell membranes, possibly increasing the effectiveness of antibodies. Leukocytes in breast milk provide protection against common respiratory infectious invaders. Macrophages, responsible for producing **interferon** (a protein that protects against viruses), interfere with virus growth. The **bifidus factor** is a specific growth-promoting factor for the bacteria *Lactobacillus bifidus.* The presence of *L. bifidus* in breast milk interferes with the colonization of pathogenic bacteria in the gastrointestinal tract, reducing the incidence of diarrhea.

In addition to these anti-infective properties, breast milk contains the ideal electrolyte and mineral composition for human infant growth. It is high in lactose, an easily digested sugar that provides ready glucose for rapid brain growth. The protein in breast milk is easily digested, and the ratio of cysteine to methionine (two amino acids) in breast milk favors rapid brain growth in early months. It contains nitrogen in compounds other than protein so that the infant receives cell-building materials from sources other than just protein.

Breast milk contains more linoleic acid, an essential amino acid for skin integrity, and less sodium, potassium, calcium, and phosphorus than do many formulas. Breast milk also has a better balance of trace elements, such as zinc, than formulas do. These levels of nutrients are enough to supply the infant's needs, yet they spare the infant's kidneys from having to process a high renal solute load of unused nutrients. Women who have a familial history of allergy are usually encouraged to breast-feed, thus eliminating the possibility of exposing the infant to cow's milk protein, which could be allergenic this early in life (Gdalevich et. al., 2001).

Breast-fed newborns appear to have less difficulty regulating calcium/phosphorus levels than those who are bottle-fed. Decreased calcium levels in the newborn may lead to tetany (muscle spasm). The increased concentration of fatty acid in commercial formulas may bind calcium in the gastrointestinal tract, increasing the danger of tetany.

A great deal of discussion about the benefits of breastfeeding has centered on the effects of breastfeeding on the formation of the dental arch. Babies suck differently from a breast than from a bottle (Fig. 24-2). Babies pull their tongue backward as they suck from a breast. They thrust their tongue forward to suck from a rubber nipple, which may lead to malformation of the dental arch.

One disadvantage of breast milk is that it may carry microorganisms such as hepatitis B and cytomegalovirus, although the risk to infants is small. HIV is carried at a high enough level in breast milk that women who are HIV positive are advised not to breast-feed (James, 2000). In addition, both illicit and prescription drugs as well as environmental contaminants can be carried via breast milk to the infant (AAP Committee on Drugs, 2001).

Preparing for Breastfeeding

Ask all women during pregnancy whether they plan to breast-feed or formula-feed their newborn. Thinking about feeding in advance allows couples to make informed choices (see Focus on Cultural Competence). Some fathers experience jealousy at the thought of breastfeeding. Early discussion of the problem can help them work

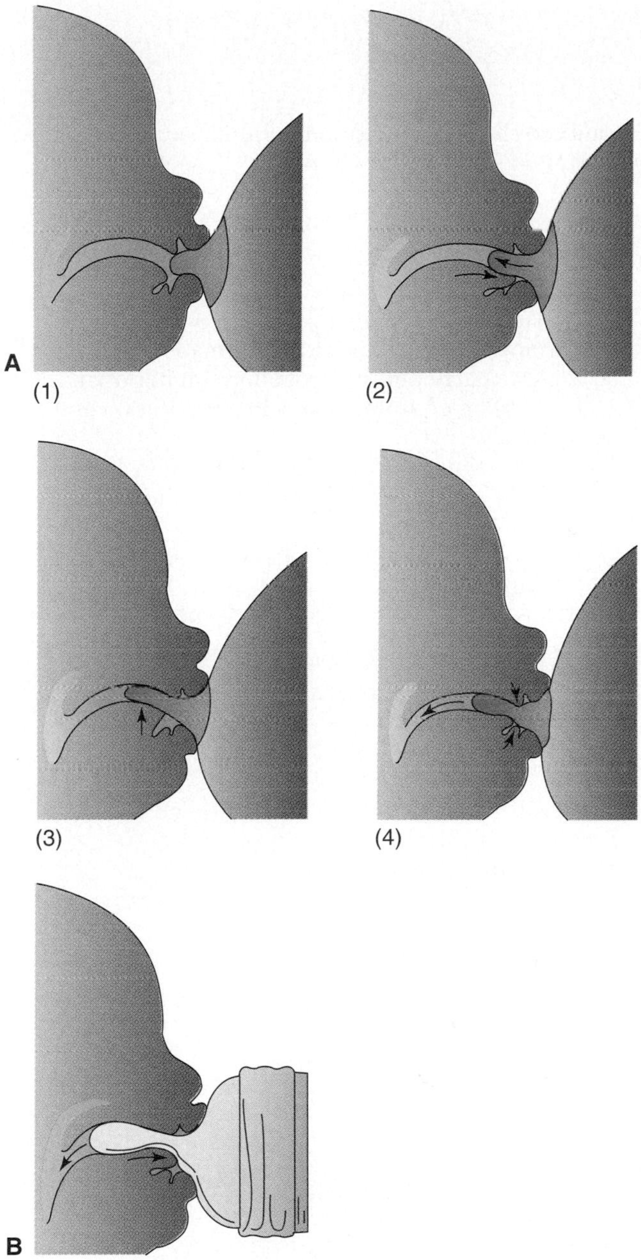

FIGURE 24.2 Differences in sucking mechanism. (*A*) The breast. (1) Lips of the infant clamp in a C-shape. The cheek muscles contract. (2) The tongue thrusts forward to grasp nipple and areola. (3) The nipple is brought against the hard palate as the tongue pulls backward, bringing the areola into the mouth. (4) The gums compress the areola, squeezing milk into the back of the throat. (*B*) Bottle-feeding. The large rubber nipple of a bottle strikes the soft palate and interferes with the action of the tongue. The tongue moves forward against the gums to control the overflow of milk into the esophagus.

through this natural sensation, with the eventual realization that parenting involves more than simply feeding the child.

Physical preparation such as nipple rolling, advised in the past as a way of making the nipples more protuberant, is no longer advised. This is unnecessary because few women have inverted or nonprotuberant nipples. Plus, oxytocin, released by this maneuver, could lead to preterm labor (nipple rolling is used to create uterine contractions for stress tests). Practicing breast massage to move the milk forward in the milk ducts (manual expression of milk) may be helpful. This can help a woman who feels hesitant about handling her breasts to grow accustomed to doing so, allowing her to assist with milk production in the first few days after birth. Manual expression consists of supporting the breast firmly, then placing the thumbs and forefinger on the opposite sides of the breast just behind the areolar margin, first pushing backward toward the chest wall and then downward until secretion begins to flow (see Nursing Procedure 24-1). During the last months of pregnancy and immediately after birth, the fluid obtained will be colostrum. By the 3rd day of infant life, milk will be obtained.

Teach women not to use soap on their breasts during pregnancy because soap tends to dry and crack nipples. The occasional woman who has inverted nipples may need to wear a nipple cup (a plastic shell) to help the nipples become more protuberant.

FOCUS ON CULTURAL COMPETENCE

Women are often the "keepers of the culture," or the main people who transmit customs to the next generation. Chief among these customs is the method for feeding newborns. If a woman comes from a family where no one has ever breastfed, she may be very interested in being a "pioneer" in her family. On the other hand, she may be more interested in following her family's tradition of formula-feeding.

How soon women want to begin breastfeeding after birth is also culturally determined. Although it is the usual practice in hospitals to begin immediately after birth, some women may believe that colostrum is not appropriate for newborns and have a cultural preference not to begin breastfeeding until milk is present, at about 3 days of age. Assessing each family individually is necessary to recognize cultural preferences such as these.

✔ CHECKPOINT QUESTIONS

4. What fluid, rather than breast milk, is produced for the first 3 to 4 days after birth?
5. How does breast milk help prevent infection in a newborn?

Beginning Breastfeeding

Breastfeeding should begin as soon after birth as possible, ideally while the woman is still in a delivery or birthing room and while the infant is in the first reactivity period.

NURSING PROCEDURE 24.1: MANUAL BREAST MILK EXPRESSION

Purpose

To assist the woman to manually express milk so she can strengthen her milk supply and supply milk for her newborn should she be separated from the newborn

Procedure	Principle
1. Explain the procedure to the client.	1. Explanations help decrease anxiety and enhance learning; they also provide information for the client to carry out the procedure on her own.
2. Assemble equipment, including a clean towel and collection container.	2. Assembling equipment aids in organization and efficiency.
3. Wash your hands and put on clean gloves; have client wash her hands.	3. Handwashing prevents the transmission of infection; use of gloves protects self and the client from possible infection.
4. Provide privacy and place the woman sitting comfortably.	4. The let-down reflex may not occur readily if the woman is tense or nervous.
5. Instruct the woman to place her right hand on her right breast, with her right thumb on the top of the breast at the outer limit of the areola and her right fingers underneath the breast. Tell the woman to press inward toward the chest wall (Fig. A).	5. Milk is expressed by pressure on the collecting ducts, not the nipple.

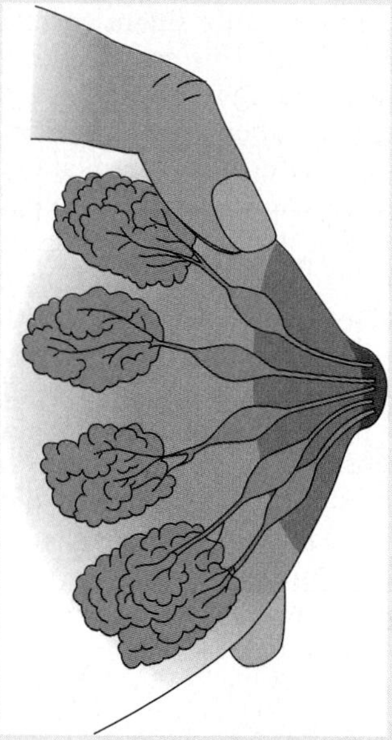

A

Procedure	Principle
6. Help the woman hold the collecting jar just under her nipple.	6. Collecting bottles should be made of plastic to preserve antibodies found in milk; having the container close by prevents waste of any breast milk that is expressed.
7. Have the woman slide her hand forward in a milking motion, causing the milk to be expressed from the nipple into an infant bottle (Fig. B).	7. Pressure on the lactiferous sinuses pushes milk forward.

(continued)

Procedure	Principle
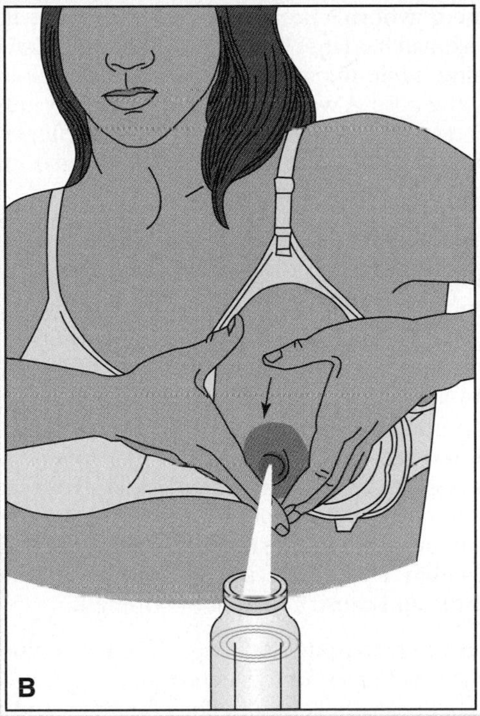	
8. Have the woman move her thumb and fingers around her breast, repeating the technique.	8. Repeating the technique ensures that all milk sinuses are emptied.
9. Caution the woman not to use excess force.	9. Excess force will damage sensitive breast tissue.
10. After collection, refrigerate milk if it will be used within 24 hours; freeze if this time is longer.	10. Breast milk spoils in the same manner as cow's milk if not protected.
11. Reinforce the woman's success with this maneuver, regardless of the amount of breast milk expressed.	11. Manual breast milk expression is an easy technique to carry out once it is learned, but it can be difficult to grasp at first. Positive reinforcement enhances progress and self-esteem.

The release of oxytocin by breastfeeding at this time begins the let-down of milk and also stimulates uterine contraction. If the woman is overly fatigued, however, trying to learn this new skill at this time may only convince her that breastfeeding is not for her.

Most women enjoy having an experienced nurse with them for a first feeding to offer suggestions. It is important that infants open their mouths wide enough so they can grasp the nipple and **areola** (the pigmented circle surrounding the nipple) when sucking. This gives them an effective sucking action and helps to empty the collecting sinuses completely. For additional feedings, an infant should be placed first at the breast at which he or she fed last in the previous feeding. This ensures that each breast is completely emptied at every other feeding. Milk forms in response to being used. If the breasts are completely emptied, they completely fill again. If half emptied, they only half fill, and, after a time, milk production will be insufficient for proper nourishment.

Because an infant sucks differently at a breast than a bottle, breast-fed infants should not be offered bottles until about 6 weeks of age. This may be true for pacifiers as well (Kloeblen & Tanner, 2001).

Prolonged Jaundice in Breastfed Infants

Jaundice may occur in as many as 15% of breastfed infants. This is because pregnanediol (a breakdown product of progesterone) in breast milk depresses the action of glucuronyl transferase, the enzyme that converts indirect bilirubin to the direct form, which is readily excreted in bile (Wagle, 2000). To prevent hyperbilirubinemia in the infant, women should feed frequently in the immediate birth period because colostrum is a natural laxative and helps promote passage of meconium and bile. Newborns who are discharged early should be observed for jaundice (Radmacher et al., 2002), although breastfeeding rarely results in a serum bilirubin level high enough to warrant therapy or require discontinuation of breastfeeding because pregnanediol remains in breast milk for only 24 to 48 hours.

NURSING DIAGNOSES AND RELATED INTERVENTIONS

In cultures where breastfeeding is practiced by almost all mothers, the technique is learned early in life by observation. In the United States, women may have had few, if any, opportunities to observe breastfeeding. Lactation consultants are health care professionals especially trained to assist women with breastfeeding. Making a referral to such a person can be extremely helpful. With managed care, fewer such specialists may be available, however, so all nurses need to be well prepared to assist with breastfeeding.

When a woman first begins breastfeeding, learning to relax is essential. If she is tense and anxious, she may have difficulty achieving a good let-down reflex, and her infant will have difficulty obtaining adequate milk. This can further lead to increasing tension and anxiety because the infant does not seem content. As a result, the infant will become hungrier and will be left even more unsatisfied, creating a vicious cycle of events. Support, adequate instruction, and reassurance from health care personnel are important in helping the woman feel secure enough to be able to relax (see Focus on Nursing Care Planning). Rooming-in allows women to sense when their infant is hungry and feed before the infant grows fatigued from crying.

Nursing Diagnosis: Health-seeking behaviors related to lack of knowledge about lactation and breastfeeding techniques

Outcome Identification: Client will voice understanding of the physiology of breastfeeding and confidence in ability to establish breastfeeding by 24 hours.

Outcome Evaluation: Woman states correct information about how lactation begins and is maintained in adequate supply; demonstrates effective positioning for baby and herself.

Provide Information Regarding Lactation and Proper Positioning Techniques. Breast milk looks like nonfat milk. It is thin and almost blue-tinged in appearance. Some women may need assurance that the color and consistency are normal; otherwise, they may think their milk is not nutritious enough (AAP Work Group on Breastfeeding, 2001).

Before breastfeeding, recommend that the woman wash her hands to be sure they are free of pathogens picked up from handling perineal pads or other sources. Washing her breasts is not necessary unless she notices caked colostrum on the nipples. When she is first attempting to breast-feed, lying on her side with a pillow under her head is a good position to assume (Fig. 24-3). This relieves fatigue for her as it allows the infant to rest on the bed. Figure 24-4 shows a sitting position with a pillow under the baby. Using the football hold with the baby supported on a pillow also may be helpful, especially if the mother underwent a cesarean birth.

Brushing the infant's cheek with a nipple stimulates the newborn's rooting reflex. The baby will then turn toward the breast. Do not try to initiate a rooting reflex by pressing the baby's face against the mother's breast: this will cause the child to turn away from the mother and toward you. Using an assessment tool such as the LATCH assessment (Table 24-2) can provide objective measures to evaluate the newborn's breastfeeding (Riordan et al., 2001).

If a woman has large breasts, the infant may have trouble breathing while nursing because breast tissue is pressed against the nose. A woman can prevent this by grasping the areolar margin between her thumb and forefinger, holding the bulk of the breast supported. This also makes the nipple more protuberant.

During the first few days of life, because they are receiving only colostrum and need the nutrients and fluid obtained by frequent sucking, babies should be fed as often as hungry (every 2 to 3 hours). Further, the more often the breasts are emptied, the more efficiently they will fill and continue to maintain a good supply of milk. Be sure the woman and all those involved in her care understand the importance of frequent breast emptying.

As important as making certain that infants grasp the areola is helping them to break away from the breast when they are through feeding. Have the mother insert a finger in the corner of the infant's mouth or pull down the infant's chin. Otherwise, the baby may pull too hard on the nipple and cause cracking or soreness.

Promote Adequate Sucking. Often, a newborn being breast-fed will drop off to sleep during the first few feedings. To stimulate milk production effectively and to ensure adequate fluid intake, help the mother attempt to keep the infant awake, urging him or her to suck. To accomplish this, advise mothers to be sure to awaken newborns fully before feeding by handling them, stroking their backs, changing their position during feeding, rubbing the arms and chest, or changing the diaper. Gently tickling the bottom of a baby's feet will also wake him or her effectively. Many women are unwilling to cause their newborns discomfort in this way to keep them awake. This reaction is a positive one because it may be one of the first signs that the woman is transferring the protectiveness toward her own body she felt during pregnancy to her newborn.

If an infant is not sucking well, the woman can use breast massage after a feeding to empty her breasts manually. This helps to ensure good milk production for the time when the infant is ready to suck.

Provide Immediate Support When Problems Arise. When handled intelligently by health care personnel, the common problems that arise with breastfeeding usually pass and seem unimportant to the mother. Otherwise, they may complicate breastfeeding, discouraging the mother from continuing. It is unfortunate if complications deter a woman from using the most natural and least complicated of all infant feeding methods.

> **WHAT IF?** What if a new mother tells you that she doesn't want to breast-feed, but her husband is insisting she do so? What would you do?

Provide Information Regarding Techniques for Burping the Breastfed Baby. Some infants seem to swallow little air when they breastfeed, whereas others swallow a great deal. As a rule, it is helpful to bubble

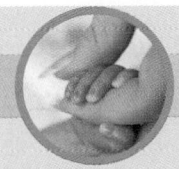

FOCUS ON *Nursing Care Planning*

A WOMAN WHO IS BREASTFEEDING FOR THE FIRST TIME

> *A new mother states, "I want to breastfeed my baby. I know it's the best choice, but I've never done it before. I'm not sure I can do it. Nothing happened when I tried right after my baby was born."*

Assessment: Mother 2 hours postpartum. Newborn had difficulty latching onto breast immediately after birth. Nipples everted without signs of redness or irritation. Breasts slightly firm. Colostrum present.

Nursing Diagnosis: Ineffective breastfeeding related to anxiety and inexperience

Outcome Identification: Client will demonstrate independence with breast-feeding by hospital discharge.

Outcome Evaluation: Client identifies ways to properly position the newborn at the breast; states newborn is latching on and sucking; feeds newborn for 10 minutes on each breast, increasing time with each session; verbalizes satisfaction and confidence with each feeding session.

Interventions	Rationale
1. Assess client's knowledge about breastfeeding and listen to her concerns. Allow time for questions.	1. Assessment provides a baseline for identifying teaching needs and building on knowledge base.
2. Explore previous exposure to breastfeeding, including any misinformation, misconceptions, or myths. Use visual aids as appropriate.	2. Exploration provides opportunities for teaching, clarifying, and correcting information. Audio-visual material enhances learning.
3. Initiate a referral to a lactation consultant.	3. Lactation consultant provides an additional source of support, encouragement, and information.
4. Assist client with attaining a comfortable position, using pillows as necessary for support.	4. Proper positioning with support aids in client relaxation prior to feeding.
5. Demonstrate various positions to hold newborn, and assist with positioning.	5. Proper positioning enhances the let-down reflex and promotes latching on. Knowledge of other positions helps to increase client self-confidence.
6. Instruct client in how to elicit rooting reflex and help newborn grasp nipple.	6. Rooting reflex assists in latching on. Nipple trauma or inadequate milk flow may occur if the newborn latches on improperly.
7. Advise client to feed newborn on one breast, starting for approximately 10 minutes, and then switch to the other side, gradually increasing the time on each breast with subsequent feedings.	7. Feeding for too short a time prevents the newborn from receiving the richer, more satisfying hindmilk.
8. Instruct client how to break suction to remove newborn from breast.	8. Proper removal prevents nipple trauma.
9. Instruct client to begin next feeding on breast newborn finished on at last feeding. Suggest client attach a safety pin to her bra on the side to begin the next feeding.	9. Alternating breasts ensures even stimulation and emptying, increasing milk supply. Safety pin acts as a reminder for the client about where to begin.
10. Continue to observe client and newborn interaction with subsequent feedings. Provide feedback and suggestions, reinforcing accomplishments and assisting with any difficulties.	10. Continued observation provides opportunities for additional teaching and feedback. Feedback and positive reinforcement promote self-confidence and learning, enhancing the success of teaching and effectiveness of breastfeeding.
11. Instruct client in care of nipples and measures to prevent problems.	11. Proper nipple care reduces the risk of problems that might interfere with breastfeeding and thus diminish client satisfaction and confidence.
12. Encourage client to wear a comfortable supportive bra at all times.	12. Well-fitting bra provides support to full breasts.
13. Advise client to drink at least 4 to 6 8-oz glasses of fluid per day.	13. Adequate fluid intake is essential to maintain an adequate milk supply.

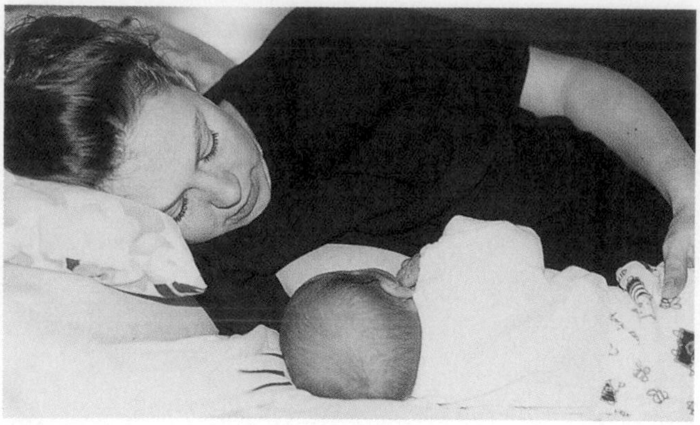

FIGURE 24.3 Side-lying position for breastfeeding.

(burp) newborns after they have emptied the first breast and again after the total feeding.

Placing the baby over one shoulder and gently patting or stroking the back is an acceptable position. This position is not always satisfactory for a small infant, who has poor head control. In addition, the parent may have difficulty supporting the baby's head and patting the back at the same time.

Holding the baby in a sitting position on the lap, then leaning the child forward against one hand, with the index finger and thumb supporting the head, is often the best position to use. This position provides head support but leaves the other hand free to pat the baby's back (Fig. 24-5). Parents usually need to be shown this method because it does not seem as natural as putting the baby against the shoulder. Lying the baby prone across the lap is another alternative position.

Nursing Diagnosis: Pain related to breast engorgement or sore nipples

Outcome Identification: Client will remain free of severe breast discomfort during early breastfeeding period.

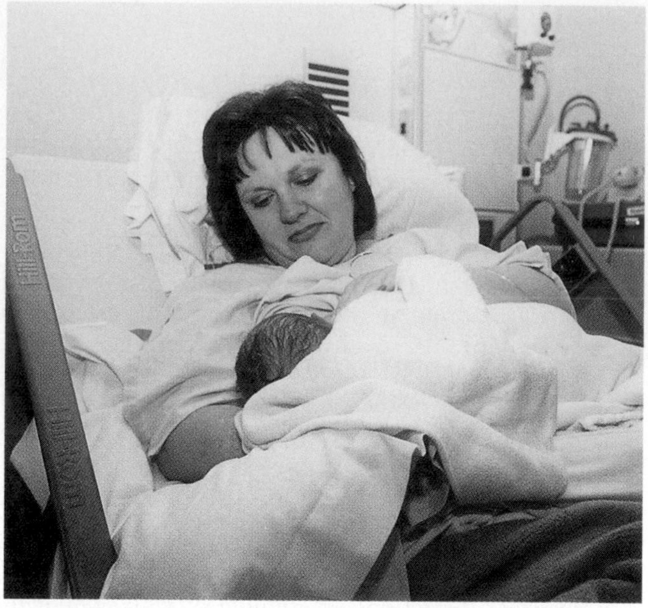

FIGURE 24.4 Sitting position for breastfeeding.

Outcome Evaluation: Client states that she is experiencing little or no discomfort; can breastfeed without undue discomfort; infant grasps nipple firmly.

On the 3rd or 4th day, when breast milk forms, some women may notice breast distention, with swelling, hardness, tenderness, and perhaps heat in their breasts. The skin appears red, tense, and shiny. This is called primary **engorgement** and is caused by vascular and lymphatic congestion arising from an increase in the blood and lymph supply to the breasts. Infants have difficulty sucking on engorged breasts because the areola is too hard to grasp (Fig. 24-6). The woman also may have difficulty breastfeeding because her breasts are very tender.

TABLE 24.2 LATCH Breastfeeding Charting System

	0	1	2
L Latch	Too sleepy or reluctant; no latch achieved	Repeated attempts; hold nipple in mouth; stimulate to suck	Grasps breast; tongue down; lips flanged; rhythmic sucking
A Audible Swallowing	None	A few with stimulation	Spontaneous and intermittent under 24 h old; spontaneous and frequent over 24 h old
T Type of Nipple	Inverted	Flat	Everted (after stimulation)
C Comfort (Breast/Nipple)	Engorged; cracked, bleeding, large blisters or bruises; severe discomfort.	Filling; reddened/small blisters or bruises; mild/moderate discomfort	Soft, nontender
H Hold (Positioning)	Full assist (staff holds infant at breast)	Minimal assist (i.e., place pillows for support, elevate head of bed); teach one side; mother does other; staff holds and then mother takes over	No assist from staff; mother able to position/hold baby by self

From Jensen, D., Wallace, S., & Kelsey, P. (1994). LATCH: A breastfeeding charting system and documentation tool. *Journal of Obstetric, Gynecologic, and Neonatal Nursing, 23*(1), 27–32.

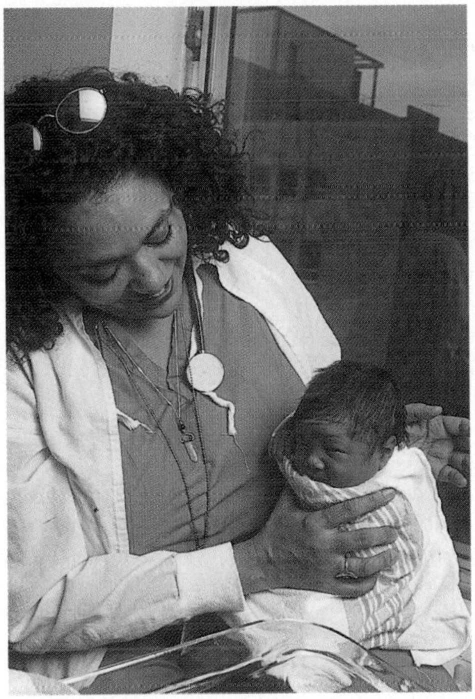

FIGURE 24.5 The nurse demonstrates a sitting position for burping a newborn. The infant's head is supported by the nurse's hand.

Prevent or Relieve Engorgement. The primary method for relieving engorgement is emptying the breasts of milk by having the infant suck more often, or at least continuing to suck as much as before. Unfortunately, sometimes, the breasts are so sore that it is difficult for a mother to continue to breast-feed unless she is given something to alleviate the pain. Some mothers find that warm packs applied for about 20 minutes before feeding afford the most relief. In addition, good breast support from a firm-fitting bra prevents a pulling, heavy feeling.

If an infant cannot grasp the nipple to suck strongly, warm packs applied to both breasts for a few minutes before feeding combined with massage to begin milk flow (e.g., standing under a shower and massaging) will often facilitate drainage and promote breast softness so the infant can suck. Manual expression or the use of a breast pump to complete emptying of the breasts after the baby has nursed can help maintain or promote a good milk supply during the period of engorgement (Fig. 24-7).

Fortunately, engorgement is a transient problem. Unfortunately, it occurs just as women are beginning to feel skilled at breastfeeding. Suddenly their breasts are swollen, hot, and tender. They may fear an infection has developed or that the baby will not get enough milk. Assure the mother that these symptoms have occurred because milk is forming, thus indicating a healthy event: that their breasts are ready to produce milk. Assure them that it is only temporary and should begin to subside 24 hours after it first becomes apparent (James, 2000).

Promote Healing of Sore Nipples. Sore nipples result from the strong sucking action of the newborn. This may be worsened by:

- Improper positioning of the infant (failure to grasp the areola as well as the nipple)
- Forcefully pulling the infant from the breast
- Allowing the infant to suck too long at a breast after it was emptied
- Permitting the nipple to remain wet from leaking milk

Normally, nipples are kept supple from the secretions of the Montgomery's tubercles. They can become sore when they are excessively dry or wet or may crack or fissure. To help prevent soreness, encourage the mother to position the baby slightly differently for each feeding. This helps prevent the same area of the areola from receiving the majority of pressure. Advise her to expose the nipples to air by leaving her bra unsnapped for 10 to 15 minutes after feeding. Some mothers use a hair dryer set on low to aid drying. Discourage the use of plastic liners that come with nursing bras, so that air is always circulating around her breasts. Applying vitamin E after air exposure may toughen the nipples and prevent further irritation.

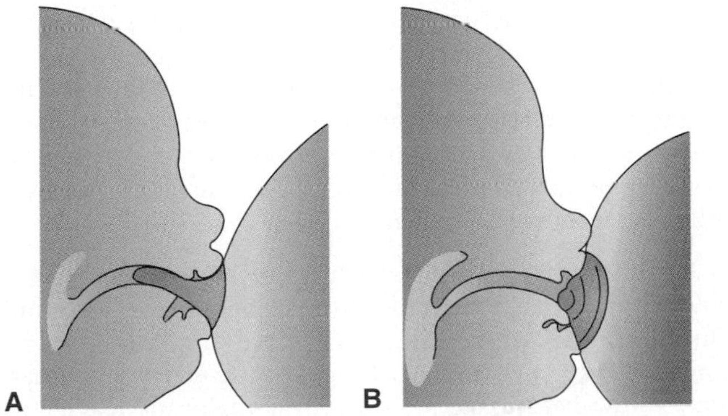

FIGURE 24.6 The problem that breast engorgement causes to breastfeeding. (*A*) When sucking at a normal breast, the infant's lips compress the areola and fit neatly against the sides of the nipple. The infant also has adequate room to breathe. (*B*) When a breast is engorged, the infant has difficulty grasping the nipple. Breathing ability is compromised.

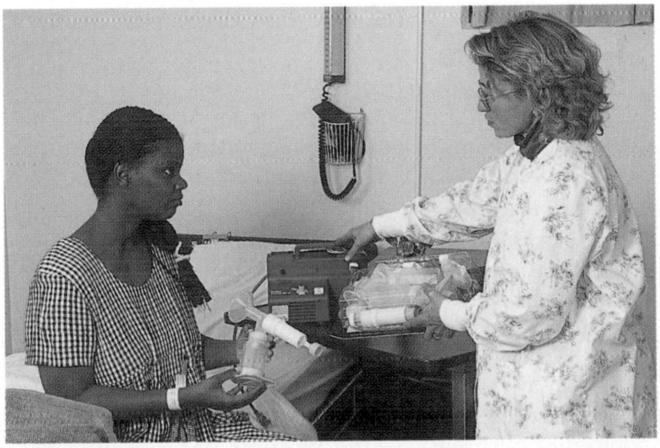

FIGURE 24.7 A nurse and mother discuss the advantages and disadvantages of an electric breast pump (shown on the table) and a manual pump (shown in the mother's hands).

If a woman's nipples are so sore that she can nurse only a short time, she should manually express milk to complete breast emptying. Advise her not to use a hand pump with sore nipples, because this may cause fissures to worsen. An electric or battery-operated pump (standard equipment in most maternity or pediatric hospitals) usually can be used because these exert less pressure on the nipples.

Sore nipples, like engorgement, are not a contraindication to breastfeeding. If steps to prevent sore nipples are followed, the problem is unlikely to become acute again.

Nursing Diagnosis: Anxiety related to inability to measure amount of food taken by baby

Outcome Identification: Client will express confidence that baby is receiving enough milk.

Outcome Evaluation: Client states that baby seems satisfied after feeding and voices confidence that baby must be getting enough milk; baby voids six to eight times per day after the first week.

Some breastfeeding mothers wonder whether the infant is getting enough to eat. They watch a woman bottle-feeding and listen to her report, "He took 3 ounces this feeding," and wish they could tell as surely that their infant's intake is adequate. Assure them that the ultimate test with either breastfeeding or bottle-feeding is that the infant seems content between feedings. During the first week of life, wetting six to eight diapers within 24 hours or no loss of more than 10% of birthweight is an acceptable criterion. After the first week, weight gain and voiding six to eight times in 24 hours are acceptable. Although the bottle-feeding mother measures the amount of formula as a way of determining this in the early weeks, soon she, too, will be using the alternative criteria: her baby is happy, voids six to eight times a day, and is gaining weight. Helping a woman to use these criteria allows her to develop confidence in her judgment to evaluate her child's health, a role that will be hers for the next 18 or more years.

Nursing Diagnosis: Deficient knowledge related to potential harm to baby of drugs taken by breastfeeding mother

Outcome Identification: Client will voice understanding by discharge that most drugs pass readily into breast milk.

Outcome Evaluation: Client states she is aware that almost all drugs taken may be found in her breast milk; voices importance of consulting physician or nurse practitioner before taking any drug.

For years, it was believed that a placental barrier protected the fetus from exposure to drugs taken by the mother. A similar protection was postulated for breast milk. It has been shown, however, that the fetus is extremely susceptible to drugs ingested by the mother. The same is true of breast-fed infants. Almost any drug may cross into the acinar cells and be secreted in breast milk. Drugs that should be avoided by breastfeeding mothers because of their documented harmful effect on infants are shown in Appendix C. The rule that a woman followed all during pregnancy, that she should take no drug unless prescribed or approved by her primary care provider, continues to apply during lactation.

Nursing Diagnosis: Effective breastfeeding related to mother's desire to provide the best nutrition for her child

Outcome Identification: Client will voice confidence in ability to breastfeed baby at home.

Outcome Evaluation: Client states that she intends to continue breastfeeding at home; voices confidence in her ability to provide adequate milk for infant; names resources for help if needed; infant exhibits adequate weight gain and elimination patterns for age.

Provide Anticipatory Guidance Regarding Potential Problems and Methods for Resolution. Common problems that can arise with breastfeeding are summarized in Table 24-3. In addition, women may ask about breastfeeding when out in public. The Focus on Evidence-Based Practice addresses this concern.

Women who do not remember to begin nursing the baby at the breast that the infant finished on the last time may find their milk supply decreasing in one breast. Although this may be easy to remember in the hospital, distractions at home may make the sequence difficult to remember. Pinning a safety pin to the bra strap on the side to start with at the next feeding is a useful way to remember.

Fatigue can be another problem upon returning home. Adequate rest periods during the day are essential. Sitting relaxed in a comfortable chair with her feet elevated, feeding her baby, and enjoying this time is an excellent way to rest.

Adequate maternal fluid intake is necessary to maintain an adequate milk supply. Women who are breastfeeding should drink at least four 8-oz glasses of fluid a day; many need to drink six glasses. They need to increase their calorie intake by about 500 calories a day (Table 24-4). A daily diet plan for a lactating woman is given in Table 24-5.

At one time, women were given a list of foods not to eat while they were breastfeeding because it was thought they caused diarrhea, constipation, or colic in infants. Today, there are no rules other than to use common sense. During lactation, a woman can eat anything that agrees with her, is taken in moderation, and to which she is not allergic.

Some women stop breastfeeding because they have no one to talk to about a problem or to give them support. A nurse working as a hospital community liaison person, community health nurse, or lactation consultant can be a valuable resource to provide answers and support.

Provide Information on the Use of Supplemental Feedings. A breastfeeding woman may leave her child during the day or evening in the care of a babysitter or another care provider, just as a bottle-feeding woman may. She can express breast milk manually and leave it in a bottle in the refrigerator or prepare a single bottle of formula for the time she is away.

Bottles used for storage should be sterilized in a dishwasher. Breast milk then may be refrigerated for 24 hours, frozen for 30 days, or placed in a deep freezer for 6 months. Commercial freezer storage bags also may be used. Using

TABLE 24.3 Common Problems of Breastfeeding

PROBLEM	CAUSE	NURSING INTERVENTIONS
Mother worries about amount of milk being taken	Mother cannot see the amount taken	Assure mother that the best way to judge amount taken is to note if infant appears content between feedings and is wetting diapers.
Infant does not suck well	Possible effect of anesthesia Infant brought to mother when not hungry Infant exhausted by crying from hunger	Adjust feeding pattern to child's needs; assure mother that effect of anesthesia is temporary. Encourage rooming-in. Encourage feeding on cue, not on demand.
Mother reports infant's stools are loose and thin	Stools normally looser and lighter in color than in formula-fed babies	Examine stools; assure mother and explain normal stool pattern and transitions.
Father feels shut out of parent–child relationship	Father does not participate in infant feeding	Show other ways of interacting with infant than through feeding.
Sore nipples	Infant not gripping entire areola Nipple kept wet	Help infant to grasp nipple correctly; expose nipple to air between feedings; aloe vera or vitamin E applied to nipples helps heal tissue.
Engorgement	Lymphatic filling as milk production begins	Encourage infant to suck normally (engorgement subsides best if infant can be encouraged to suck normally); apply warm packs to breasts or have mother take a warm shower before feeding to help soften breast tissue.

FOCUS ON EVIDENCE-BASED PRACTICE

How Comfortable Are Women With Breastfeeding in Public Places?

To answer this question, Canadian researchers recorded the perceptions of four breastfeeding and four bottle-feeding mothers about the amount and kind of attention they received while publicly feeding their babies in two separate sites: a restaurant and a shopping mall. The mothers reported that although they did feel vulnerable and had anticipated undesirable attention, in actual practice they received little attention directed at either form of infant feeding. They did receive more neutral looks from other customers during breastfeeding but no significant overtly negative attention. Mothers attributed the reasons they felt confident to breastfeed in public places were personal attributes as well as support received from other women.

Information gained from this study is interesting for nurses because women who are anticipating breastfeeding often ask whether they can breastfeed in public. Armed with the information from this study, nurses could serve as the support people mothers found important to help them with breastfeeding success.

Sheeshka, J., et al. (2001). Women's experiences breastfeeding in public places. *Journal of Human Lactation, 17*(1), 31–38.

TABLE 24.4 Recommended Daily Allowances During Lactation

NUTRIENT	DURING LACTATION
Calories (kcal)	+500
Protein (g)	6.5
Vitamin A	1,300
Vitamin D (μg)	5.0
Vitamin E (mg)	19
Vitamin K (μg)	65
Vitamin C (mg)	120
Folate (μg)	500
Niacin (mg)	17
Riboflavin (mg)	1.6
Thiamine (mg)	1.5
Vitamin B_6 (mg)	2.0
Calcium (mg)	1,000–1,200
Vitamin B_{12} (μg)	2.8
Phosphorus (mg)	700
Iodine (μg)	200
Iron (mg)	15
Magnesium (mg)	310
Zinc (mg)	19

Source: National Academy of Sciences (1989). *Recommended daily dietary allowances* (10th ed.). Washington, DC: National Academy Press.

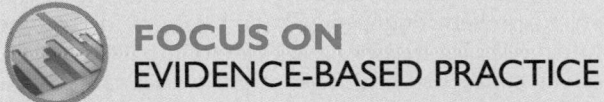

TABLE 24.5 Quantities of Food Necessary for a Lactating Woman

FOOD GROUP	QUANTITIES FOR ACTIVE NONPREGNANT WOMAN	QUANTITIES FOR LACTATING WOMAN
Meat, fowl, or fish	2 servings daily	7 servings daily
Vegetables	3 to 5 servings daily	4 servings daily
Fruits	2 to 4 servings daily	4 servings daily
Breads, cereals, rice, pasta	6 to 11 servings daily	12 servings daily
Milk	2 8-oz glasses daily	4 to 5 8-oz glasses daily
Fats, oils, sweets	Use sparingly	5 servings daily
Additional fluid	As desired	At least 2 glasses daily

Dudek, S. G. (2001). *Nutritional essentials for nursing practice.* Philadelphia: Lippincott Williams & Wilkins.

commercially prepared formula or powder formula is appropriate and convenient to replace a single feeding because one bottle at a time can be prepared.

Once breastfeeding has been established, after about 6 weeks, missing one feeding this way will not affect milk production enough to make a difference at the next feeding. Thus, there is no need for the mother to express milk manually to safeguard a supply, although she may prefer to do so to reduce tension and discomfort.

Provide Information for the Mother Who Works Outside the Home. Many women return to work while continuing to breast-feed by bringing their infant with them to their workplace. Others express breast milk for a caregiver to give by bottle while they work. Some employers have strong feelings about breastfeeding; to avoid difficulties, women should review with an employer the best way for them to continue breastfeeding (see Focus on Family Empowerment).

Provide Information on Weaning. Women breastfeed for varying lengths of time. Some do it for 1, 2, or 3 months, then wean the child from breast to bottle. Many continue until the child is 6 to 12 months of age and then wean directly to a small cup or glass. Some continue to breastfeed until the child is of toddler or preschool age (Fig. 24-8). Lengthy breastfeeding, however, may lead to nutritional deficiencies if the child is taking in a large quantity of milk at the expense of other foods (Norgate, 2001).

At any age, breastfeeding should be discontinued gradually to prevent engorgement and pain in the mother while still being satisfying for the infant. To do this, a woman should first omit one breastfeeding a day, substi-

FOCUS ON FAMILY EMPOWERMENT

Suggestions for Returning to Work While Breastfeeding

Q. I'm going to be returning to work in about 6 weeks. How can I continue to breast feed my baby?

A. Here are some suggestions for returning to work while breastfeeding:

- Some women are able to arrange for childcare near or at their worksite so they can breastfeed at lunch or during a morning or afternoon break. Discuss with your employer or your immediate work supervisor if this would be a possibility for you.
- Breastfeeding can be done in a public place such as a lounge area without undue exposure if you wear a smock-type or buttoned blouse that you lift or unfasten only as far as necessary; covering any bared breast with a shawl or towel ensures modesty.
- If you are not able to breastfeed during work hours, you will need to express milk manually at least once during the day to maintain a milk supply. You might want to rent an electric pump to keep at work. Expressed breast milk can be safely stored in the refrigerator or an iced container for 24 to 48 hours and used by your caregiver to feed the infant the next day.
- Plastic is the best type of storage container for breast milk because antibodies apparently cling to glass and will therefore be lost to the milk.
- Any reminder of a baby while you are breastfeeding may cause leaking of milk from breasts. Wear gauze pads inside your bra to prevent staining your clothing and keep an extra change of clothing at work. Pressing against your breasts with the heel of your hands may be helpful in halting leakage.
- Drink four to six 8-oz glasses of fluid during the day to ensure a high fluid intake.
- Try to arrive early at your day care center or sitter so you can breast-feed just before leaving the baby.
- Fatigue can interfere with breastfeeding. Relax and enjoy your baby during the time you are home.

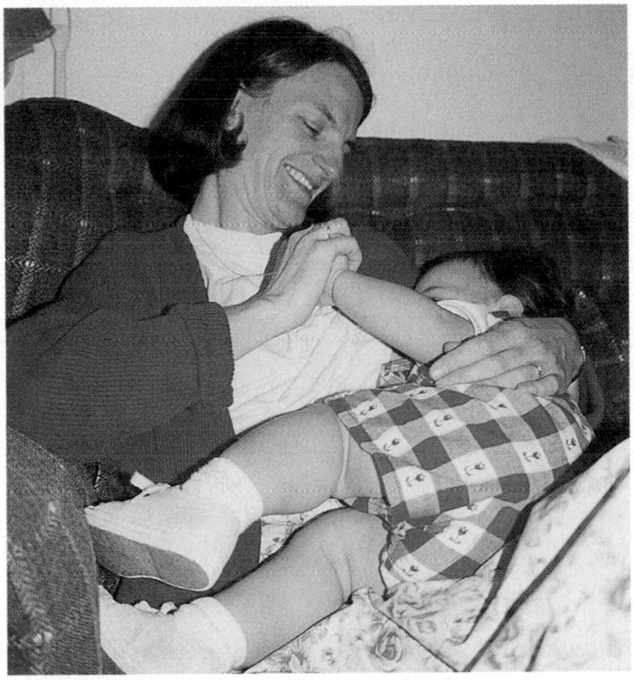

FIGURE 24.8 Some women choose to breastfeed their child beyond 1 year. Accepting various preferences is important in care planning.

tuting a bottle-feeding or milk from a glass or cup. Then she should omit two breastfeedings, then three, and so on, until the child is feeding entirely from a bottle, glass, or cup. If the breasts are not emptied by regular feedings, the resulting pressure leads to milk suppression and natural, gradual discontinuance of milk secretion. If weaned before 12 months, infants should be weaned to formula, not whole milk, so that they continue to receive the added vitamins and low solute load of formulas.

✔ CHECKPOINT QUESTIONS

6. What position is often considered the best for bubbling an infant?
7. What is an effective method for relieving the discomfort of engorgement?
8. By how much should the lactating mother increase her caloric intake during the first 6 months after birth?

FORMULA-FEEDING

Little opposition exists to the concept that breastfeeding is the best method for feeding human infants, except when a woman cannot or does not want to breastfeed. Women who develop a breast abscess may be advised not to breastfeed. Some women who are uncomfortable with the thought of exposing their breasts may not be able to hold a baby warmly and enjoy breastfeeding. Others who plan to return to work outside their home or who have older children to care for may choose not to breastfeed. Fortunately, formulas that closely resemble human milk are available for infants who will be bottle-fed, and bottle-feeding still allows women to establish a close bond with their infant. Support their choice by helping them adjust to formula-feeding (see Focus on Communication). Box 24-2 highlights an outcome and intervention related to formula-feeding using the terminology identified by the Nursing Outcomes Classification and Nursing Interventions Classification.

Preparing for Formula-Feeding

Women should use commercial formulas because they closely mimic human milk. Occasionally, an infant is allergic to the protein in infant formulas and develops diarrhea and vomiting. This can lead to such severe intestinal inflammation and irritation that the infant becomes anemic from the loss of blood and inability to absorb nutrients. In this case, the infant needs to be switched to a prescription formula.

FOCUS ON COMMUNICATION

Mrs. Morgan is a new mother who has chosen to bottle-feed her newborn. You notice on the second day after birth that she is studying the baby closely.

Less Effective Communication

Nurse: Is everything all right? You look worried.
Mrs. Morgan: I feel guilty because I'm not breastfeeding.
Nurse: Breastfeeding is better for the baby.
Mrs. Morgan: I can't. I'm going back to work next week.
Nurse: You should breastfeed. It's so much better for the baby.
Mrs. Morgan: I guess I'm not going to be a good mother.

More Effective Communication

Nurse: Is everything all right? You look worried.
Mrs. Morgan: I feel guilty because I'm not breastfeeding.
Nurse: What made you decide not to do that?
Mrs. Morgan: My job. I work as an electrician at a construction site. I can't breastfeed on a scaffold a hundred feet in the air in freezing weather.
Nurse: It sounds as if you have really thought this through. This is a good approach to mothering, and your work situation definitely seems like an exception to the rule. Infant formula may be the best option for you.
Mrs. Morgan: I'm trying to be a good mother. Thanks for the support.

Imposing your opinions on someone is not therapeutic. Allowing the woman to explain her individual situation permits the nurse to understand the woman's decision and support her with it.

BOX 24.2

NURSING OUTCOMES AND NURSING INTERVENTIONS CLASSIFICATION: FORMULA FEEDING

NOC: Knowledge: Infant Care

Knowledge, infant care, is defined as the extent of understanding conveyed about caring for a baby up to 12 months (Johnson, Maas, & Moorhead, 2000). Some specific indicators suggesting achievement of this outcome include the client's ability to describe the following:

- Nutritive versus nonnutritive sucking
- Pros and cons about feeding choices
- Infant feeding technique, including positioning, burping, and satisfaction
- Signs of problems such as dehydration

NIC: Bottle-Feeding

Bottle-feeding is defined as preparation and administration of fluids to an infant via a bottle (McCloskey & Bulechek, 2000). Some important activities involved when implementing this intervention include:

- Determining infant state prior to initiating feeding
- Warming formula to room temperature
- Holding and properly positioning infant during feeding
- Placing nipple on top of tongue
- Controlling fluid intake by regulating softness of nipple, size of hole, and size of bottle
- Encouraging sucking by stimulating rooting reflex
- Monitoring fluid intake and weight
- Instructing parents on proper equipment, preparation of bottles and formula, and formula storage
- Teaching parents proper techniques for feeding

Commercial Formulas

The contents of commercial formulas are supervised by the Food and Drug Administration. Formulas are available in three types: milk-based, soy-based, and elemental (fat, protein, and carbohydrate content is modified, such as lactose-free formula). Milk-based formulas are used for the average newborn; lactose-free formulas are used for infants with lactose intolerance or galactosemia. Soy formulas were devised for infants allergic to cow's milk protein. Today, many infants are placed on casein hydrolysate formulas, which have protein particles too small to be recognized by the immune system. Elemental formulas are used with infants with protein allergies and fat malnutrition. Milk- and soy-based and lactose-free formulas are all designed to simulate the nutritional content of breast milk. They all contain supplemental vitamins. Parents should purchase the type with added iron to ensure their newborn receives enough of this to prevent iron-deficiency anemia (Fomon, 2001). Formulas for term newborns contain 20 cal/oz when diluted according to directions. Common brands are shown in Appendix B. Parents should plan on using formula for the first full year of the infant's life. Participating in a supplemental food program such as Women, Infant, and Children (WIC) helps low-income parents afford formula.

Four separate forms of commercial formulas are available:

1. Powder that is combined with water
2. Condensed liquid that is diluted with an equal amount of water
3. Ready-to-pour type, which requires no dilution
4. Individually prepackaged and prepared bottles of formula

The powder is the least expensive. A single bottle at a time is easy to prepare by vigorous shaking. The prepackaged type does not need refrigeration or preparation (simply remove the bottle cap and it is ready), but it is the most expensive type. Cost should not be the only basis for a parent's choice, however. Tolerance of the formula by the infant and convenience for parents also are important.

Calculation of a Formula's Adequacy

To calculate the adequacy of a formula, remember these two rules of thumb:

1. The total fluid ingested for 24 hours must be sufficient to meet the child's fluid needs; 75 to 90 mL (2.5 to 3 oz) of fluid per pound of body weight per day (150 to 200 mL/kg) is needed.
2. The number of calories required per day is 50 to 55 per pound of body weight (100 to 120 kcal/kg).

If an infant is taking a commercial formula, only total fluid needs to be calculated. For example, the 7-lb infant needs 17.5 to 21 oz (7 × 2.5 to 3 oz) per day. Commercial formula contains 20 cal/oz, so this supplies 350 to 420 cal/day. This can be divided into six feedings of 3 to 3.5 oz each. A 9-lb infant would need 22.5 to 27 oz of fluid per day, supplying 450 to 540 cal/day. This will supply sufficient vitamins and minerals.

A quick rule of thumb to determine how much an infant usually takes at a feeding is to add 2 or 3 to the infant's age in months. After initially taking 0.5 to 1 oz for the first 2 days, a newborn (0 age) then takes 2 to 3 oz each feeding; a 3-month-old child, 5 to 6 oz; and a 6-month-old child, 8 oz. As infants change from six to five feedings a day (at about 4 months of age), they begin to take more at each one, keeping their total intake the same. Knowing the minimum requirements for fluid and calories per day, being able to calculate whether formula is adequate, and remembering to assess the infant's intake over 24 hours allow evaluation of the adequacy of an infant's intake.

NURSING DIAGNOSES AND RELATED INTERVENTIONS

Nursing Diagnosis: Health-seeking behaviors related to techniques of bottle-feeding

Outcome Identification: Client will verbalize knowledge of techniques of formula feeding by discharge.

Outcome Evaluation: Client accurately demonstrates proper preparation and feeding technique with her baby.

Provide Information Regarding Supplies Needed. Most parents today do not prepare a full day's supply of formula at once but prepare it bottle by bottle, as needed. They can use glass, plastic, or disposable refill bottles. Women who breastfeed and use supplemental bottles can do the same. Caution parents to keep opened cans of liquid formula covered and refrigerated, discarding any unused formula within 24 hours.

Nipples for bottles should be firm enough so that the infant sucks vigorously. A soft, flabby nipple allows a baby to suck in milk so rapidly that the need for sucking may not be satisfied. A way to judge a nipple's adequacy is to hold the bottle of milk with nipple attached upside down. The milk should come out at a rate of about one drop a second. Bottle caps to cover the nipples are helpful to keep the nipple clean when outdoors or during transport.

Provide Information Regarding Formula Preparation. Infant formula of any type must be prepared with careful attention to cleanliness to prevent pathogenic microorganisms from growing in it.

When using presterilized formula, the parent need only do the following to prepare a full day's supply of formula:

- Wash off the top of the can with warm, soapy water and rinse.
- Open the can and pour the desired amount of formula and water into each previously cleaned bottle (cleaning in a dishwasher is best).
- Put on the nipples, taking care not to handle the nipple projection.
- Place the bottle caps over the nipples and refrigerate.

To prepare a single bottle, the parent simply combines clean water and liquid or powdered formula in a bottle, caps the bottle, and shakes it to mix the ingredients.

Provide Information Regarding Feeding Techniques. Whether to warm formula is a parental decision: infants who are fed cooled formula directly from the refrigerator thrive as well as those who are fed warmed formula. Caution parents to use care when warming a bottle in a microwave oven because the milk in the center of the bottle will become hotter than that near the side. If they do use a microwave, they should shake the bottle well after microwaving it to mix the cool and warm portions and then test the temperature on their wrist before feeding.

A bottle of formula can be put into a pan of hot water, warmed in a pan of water on the stove, or placed under a faucet of running hot water. Caution parents using a pan on the stove not to allow the pan to boil dry, or the bottle of milk will burst. They also must be certain to check the temperature of the formula by allowing a drop or two to fall onto the inside of the wrist to make sure that it is not hot enough to burn the baby's mouth. Disposable bottles with plastic liners should not be heated on the stove; they tend to melt and then leak during feeding.

With any type of bottle, once it has been used, any contents remaining should be thrown away, not stored and reused. When sucking, an infant exchanges a small amount of saliva for milk. Because milk is a good growth medium for bacteria and the baby's mouth harbors many bacteria, the bacteria content in reused formula is likely to be high.

Feeding an infant is a skill that must be learned. A parent needs a comfortable chair (as does a nurse who feeds babies) and adequate time (at least half an hour) to enjoy the process and not rush the baby (Fig. 24-9). Holding the baby with the head slightly elevated reduces the danger of aspiration and retention of air bubbles. The parent should be sure that the nipple is filled and the baby is sucking milk, not air. A baby is sucking effectively if small bubbles rise in the bottle. The type of bottle used with the average baby makes no difference. A baby who develops colic (abdominal pain after feeding) may be pulling in too much air and would benefit from an angled or disposable liner bottle. Babies in the early weeks should be bubbled after every ounce of fluid taken. The technique is the same as used for breastfed infants. Some common problems that can arise with formula-feeding are summarized in Table 24-6.

WHAT IF? A new mother tells you she is going to give her baby one supplemental bottle of formula daily in addition to breastfeeding while she works. What if she tells you she isn't going to refrigerate this bottle during the day? What questions would you want to ask her to be certain this is safe for the baby?

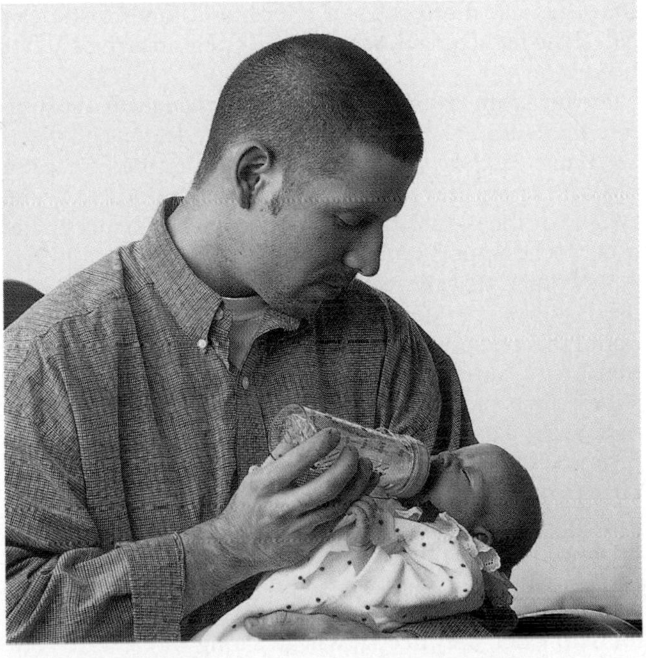

FIGURE 24.9 A newborn receives a bottle feeding from her father. Notice the en face position.

TABLE 24.6 Common Problems in Formula-Feeding

PROBLEM	POSSIBLE CAUSES	NURSING INTERVENTIONS
Infant sucks for a few minutes, then stops and cries	Either nipple is blocked and infant is unable to get milk or flow is too fast and baby has choking sensation.	Show parent how to test flow of milk from the nipple (hold bottle upside down); milk should flow from nipple at rate of about 1 drop/sec.
Infant does not bubble well after feeding	Some infants swallow little air with feeding. Parent may be handling infant too tentatively or not burping effectively.	Observe baby feeding and parent's technique of handling; rubbing newborn's back may be more effective than patting it.
Parent reports constipation	Bowel movements from formula-fed infants are not as loose as those from breast-fed infants, so parents may be concerned.	Examine stools; assure parent and explain normal stool pattern and that straining to pass stool is normal.

Remind parents not to prop up bottles, because babies are in danger of aspiration if a bottle is propped. In addition, an increased incidence of otitis media has been associated with bottle-propping because the infant's head is not upright. It also limits the amount of parent–child interaction. Also remind parents not to put a baby to bed with a bottle of formula, because this can lead to "baby bottle syndrome," or cavities of the lower teeth (see Chap. 28).

DISCHARGE PLANNING

With shortened lengths of stay in health care facilities, teaching the mother and her family is crucial. Be certain to review the mother's plans for feeding her baby just before discharge so there is time to answer any remaining questions. If this is an early discharge, check to see that a home care referral or visit has been scheduled and that the new mother has a telephone number she can call if she has a question before this person arrives at her home.

Review with women the criteria for adequate nutrition (wetting a diaper six to eight times a day, sleeping between feedings, feeding approximately 10 minutes on each breast). Supply the telephone number of the local La Leche League or the Association of Lactation Consultants or any other local support group.

Be certain that the woman has an appointment with a primary care provider for the infant or the telephone number of this person to call for an appointment. Remind her that infant nutrition is an important topic and one she should always feel free to discuss with this person at health care visits. Babies experience growth spurts during the first year at about 3 months, 6 months, and 9 months and need to be fed more frequently during these times to meet their nutritional needs. No one can anticipate all the questions or problems regarding feeding that will arise in the next few months. Empowering women to learn to make decisions regarding feeding and not to be reluctant to ask for help when they need it will go a long way toward solving these problems.

✔ CHECKPOINT QUESTIONS

9. Why is it important that a formula contain iron?
10. How much fluid would an 8-lb newborn require per day?
11. Name two physiologic risks of bottle propping.

KEY POINTS

Breastfeeding is the preferred feeding method for newborns because it supplies antibodies as well as nutrients. Urge all women at least to try breastfeeding unless they are taking a drug that would interfere with this or there is a potential for spreading a microorganism through breast milk.

Linoleic acid is an essential fatty acid necessary for growth and skin integrity that cannot be manufactured by the body. It is supplied by both infant formula and human milk but not by nonfat milk.

Both breast milk and commercial formulas contain 20 kcal/oz. A term newborn requires 120 kcal/kg/day and 160 to 200 mL/kg of fluid.

Breastfeeding mothers should be encouraged to drink fluoridated water; formula should be prepared using fluoridated water to help build strong teeth. If a newborn will not have exposure to sunlight, the breastfeeding mother may need to take a supplement of vitamin D.

Almost all drugs pass into breast milk. The breastfeeding mother must be certain not to take any medication without contacting her primary care provider for assurance regarding safety with breastfeeding.

If a baby will be bottle-fed, be certain the parents understand the potential danger of warming bottles using a microwave oven (the inner core of milk may be very hot).

Caution parents not to prop bottles. There is an increased risk for aspiration and otitis media. It also deprives infants of the pleasure of being held for feedings.

To avoid nursing bottle syndrome (cavities of the lower teeth), infants should not be put to bed with a bottle.

CRITICAL THINKING EXERCISES

1. Jane Smith is the new mother you met at the beginning of the chapter. She is unsure whether she wants to breast-feed. Analyze her learning needs. How would you address them, especially how to manage breastfeeding when she returns to work?
2. A 1-day-old newborn is being breast-fed. Her mother tells you she is unsure whether the baby is receiving enough milk. How could you assure the mother that the baby is receiving enough milk?
3. A new mother has chosen to bottle-feed her newborn. The baby's grandmother tells you she used to prepare homemade formula using evaporated milk and corn syrup. She also says that at 3 months, babies were changed to nonfat milk to keep them from gaining too much weight. How would you explain to the mother and grandmother the reasons why nonfat milk is no longer recommended for infants?
4. Examine the National Health Goals related to newborn nutrition. Most government-sponsored money for nursing research is allotted based on these goals. What would be a possible research topic to explore pertinent to these goals that would be fundable and would advance evidence-based practice?

REFERENCES

American Academy of Pediatrics Committee on Drugs. (2001). Transfer of drugs and other chemicals into human milk. *Pediatrics, 108*(30), 776–789.

American Academy of Pediatrics: Committee on Nutrition. (2000). Iron fortification of infant formulas. *Pediatrics, 104*(1), 119–123.

American Academy of Pediatrics Committee on Nutrition. (2001). The use and misuse of fruit juice in pediatrics. *Pediatrics, 107*(5), 1210–1213.

American Academy of Pediatrics Work Group on Breastfeeding. (2001). Ten steps to support parents' choice to breastfeed their baby. *Pediatric Clinics of North America, 48*(2), 533–537.

Department of Health and Human Services (2000). *Healthy people 2010.* Washington, D.C.: DHHS.

Fomon, S. J. (2001). Feeding normal infants: Rationale for recommendations. *Journal of the American Dietetic Association, 101*(9), 1002–1005.

Gdalevich, M., et al. (2001). Breastfeeding and the onset of atopic dermatitis in childhood. *Journal of the American Academy of Dermatology, 45*(4), 520–527.

James, S. D. (2000). Breastfeeding. In M. W. Schwartz (Ed.). *The 5-minute pediatric consult* (pp. 202–203). Philadelphia: Lippincott Williams & Wilkins.

Jensen, D., Wallace, S., & Kelsey, P. (1994). LATCH: A breastfeeding charting system and documentation tool. *Journal of Obstetric, Gynecologic, and Neonatal Nursing, 23*(1), 27–32.

Johnson, M., Maas, M., & Moorhead, S. (2000). *Nursing outcomes classification* (2d ed.). St. Louis: Mosby, Inc.

Kloeblen-Tanner, A. S. (2001). Pacifier use is associated with shorter breastfeeding duration among low-income women. *Pediatrics, 108*(2), 526.

Krebs, N. F., & Hambidge, M. (2001). Nutritional requirements. In W. W. Hay, A. R. Hayward, M. J. Levin, & J. M. Sondheimer (Eds.). *Current pediatric diagnosis and treatment* (15th ed.). New York: McGraw-Hill.

La Leche League International. (1997). *The womanly art of breastfeeding* (6th ed.). Schaumberg, IL: La Leche League.

Lawrence, R. A. (1999). *Breastfeeding: A guide for the medical profession.* St. Louis: Mosby.

McCloskey, J., & Bulechek, G. (2000). *Nursing interventions classification* (3d ed.). St. Louis: Mosby, Inc.

National Research Council. (1989). *Recommended dietary allowances* (10th ed.). Washington, D.C.: National Academy Press

Norgate, C. (2001). Best practice in weaning. *Nursing Times, 97*(32), 56–57.

Radmacher, P. et al. (2002). Hidden morbidity with "successful" early discharge. *Journal of Perinatology, 22*(1), 15–20.

Riordan, J., et al. (2001). Predicting breastfeeding duration using the LATCH breastfeeding assessment tool. *Journal of Human Lactation, 17*(1), 20 23.

Sheeshka, J. et al. (2001). Women's experiences breastfeeding in public places. *Journal of Human Lactation, 17*(1), 31–38.

Sinusas, K., & Gagliardi, A. (2001). Initial management of breastfeeding. *American Family Physician, 64*(6), 981–988.

Wagle, S. (2000). Breastfeeding jaundice and breast milk jaundice. In M. W. Schwartz (Ed.). *The 5-minute pediatric consult.* (pp. 204–205). Philadelphia: Lippincott Williams & Wilkins.

SUGGESTED READINGS

Belton, N. (2001). The present and future of infant nutrition. *Professional Care of Mother & Child, 11*(3, Suppl. 2), 7–9.

Bonuck, K. et al. (2002). Breastfeeding promotion interventions: Good public health and common sense. *Journal of Perinatology, 22*(1), 78–81.

Carruth, B. R., & Skinner, J. D. (2001). Mothers' sources of information about feeding their children ages 2 months to 54 months. *Journal of Nutrition Education, 33*(3), 143–147.

Forste, R., Weiss, J., & Lippincott, E. (2001). The decision to breastfeed in the United States: Does race matter? *Pediatrics, 108*(2), 291–296.

Pridham, K. F., et al. (2001). The relationship of a mother's working model of feeding to her feeding behavior. *Journal of Advanced Nursing, 35*(5), 741–750.

Nursing Care of the Woman and Family Experiencing a Postpartal Complication

CHAPTER 25

Key Terms

- endometritis
- mastitis
- peritonitis
- postpartal depression
- postpartal psychosis
- thrombophlebitis

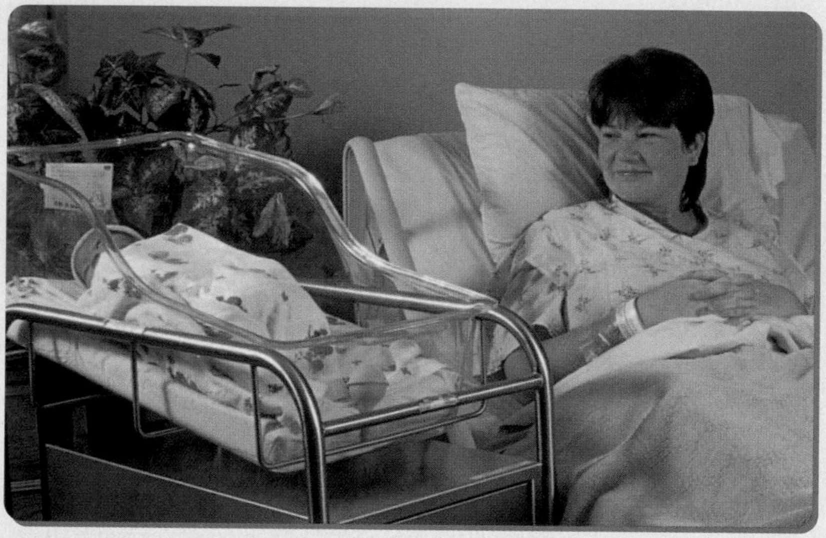

Objectives

After mastering the contents of this chapter, you should be able to:

1. Describe common deviations from the normal that can occur during the puerperium.
2. Assess the woman and her family for deviations from the normal during the puerperium.
3. Formulate nursing diagnoses related to deviations from the normal during the puerperium.
4. Identify expected outcomes of the postpartal woman experiencing a complication.
5. Plan interventions that meet the special needs of the family with a postpartal complication, such as planning for an extended hospitalization.
6. Implement nursing care when a postpartal complication such as hemorrhage, infection, hypertension of pregnancy, or postpartal psychosis develops.
7. Evaluate outcomes for achievement and effectiveness of care.
8. Identify National Health Goals related to postpartal complications that nurses can be instrumental in helping the nation achieve.
9. Identify areas related to care of women with postpartal complications that could benefit from additional nursing research or application of evidence-based practice.
10. Use critical thinking to analyze ways that promote family-centered nursing care when a postpartal complication occurs.
11. Integrate knowledge of postpartal complications with the nursing process to achieve quality maternal and child health nursing care.

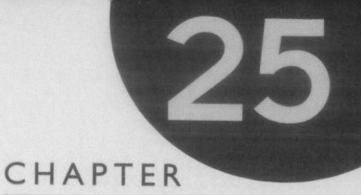

Mary Blackhawk is a 30-year-old woman who had a "textbook perfect" pregnancy. You enter her room when she is 4 hours postpartum, but because she is sleeping and appears comfortable you hesitate to awaken her. When you observe her, however, you realize that she appears pale. You obtain her vital signs and notice that her pulse is 90 beats per minute and her blood pressure is 96/50. When you fold back her bedclothes, you find her bed soaked with blood. You suspect that she is experiencing one of the most serious complications of pregnancy, postpartum hemorrhage. Yet because she was sleeping, she was totally unaware of it. What emergency measures does Ms. Blackhawk need? What should be your first action?

In a previous chapter, you learned about caring for the woman during the normal postpartal period. In this chapter, you'll add to your knowledge base information about how to care for women and their family when there is a complication during this time. This is important information because it can help protect the health of women and their family.

After you've studied the chapter, answer the Critical Thinking Exercises at the end of the chapter and then access the on-line study activities (http://connection.lww.com) *to further sharpen your skills and test your knowledge.*

Although the puerperium is usually a period of health, complications can occur. When they do, immediate intervention is essential to prevent long-term disability and interference with parent–child relationships. The Focus on National Health Goals describes National Health Goals related to this period.

A woman with a postpartal complication is at risk from three points of view: her own health, her future childbearing potential, and her ability to bond with her new infant. The family may be disrupted because of an extended hospital stay that removes the mother from other family members. Financial difficulties may arise because of the need for additional child care. Under any circumstances, pregnancy, labor, and birth create a potential crisis situation. A postpartal complication further compounds this crisis, making it more difficult for the woman and her family to manage. Fortunately, most postpartal complications are preventable, and if they do occur, the majority can be treated without too much difficulty.

FOCUS ON NATIONAL HEALTH GOALS

The postpartal period is a time when women are very susceptible to hemorrhage and thrombophlebitis, and women with a complication following childbirth may choose not to breastfeed. Two National Health Goals directly relate to this period:

- Reduce the maternal mortality rate to no more than 3.3 per 100,000 live births from a baseline of 7.1/100,000.
- Increase to at least 75% the proportion of mothers who breastfeed their babies in the early postpartal period from a baseline of 64% (DHHS, 2000).

Nurses can be instrumental in helping the nation achieve these goals by careful monitoring of uterine involution in the postpartal period and by encouraging women to breastfeed even in the face of a postpartal complication.

Areas related to complications of the postpartal period that could benefit from additional nursing research include better identification of risk factors for mastitis and endometritis; identifiable differences in women who stop breastfeeding and those who continue when a complication is present; and health teaching that is effective in preventing mastitis.

NURSING PROCESS OVERVIEW

For the Woman Experiencing a Postpartal Complication

Assessment

Assessment findings associated with a postpartal complication may be extremely subtle such as tenderness in the calf of the leg, a slight increase in pain, a slight elevation in temperature, and a slight increase in the amount of lochia (Assessing the Postpartal Woman With Complications). Because the average woman usually has no postpartal complications and the length of stay in a hospital is short, it is easy to overlook these subtle signs. Be alert to any findings that are "more than usual" because this may indicate a problem. To be certain, don't rely solely on the mother's report of perineal healing or amount of lochia. Always inspect her perineum yourself, because the report of "I feel fine" may be deceptive (she expected to have pain and so reports extreme pain as nothing out of the norm; she has no knowledge of "normal" lochia or fundal height against which to compare her own accurately).

An increased temperature exclusive of the first 24 hours after birth is an extremely serious finding. Women may try to "explain away" an increased temperature, because they know that if they have an elevated temperature they may not be allowed to go home or feed their infant. Don't be tempted to rationalize such a finding with explanations such as the room was warm, or she just had some coffee. Although these factors may make a slight difference (part of a degree) in temperature level, they do not affect it enough to account for an oral temperature over 100.4°F (38.0°C).

Nursing Diagnosis

Nursing diagnoses during this time depend on the postpartal complication. Some examples include:

- Deficient fluid volume related to increased lochia flow
- Risk for infection related to microorganism invasion of episiotomy
- Ineffective peripheral tissue perfusion related to interference with circulation from thrombophlebitis

ASSESSING the Postpartal Woman with Complications

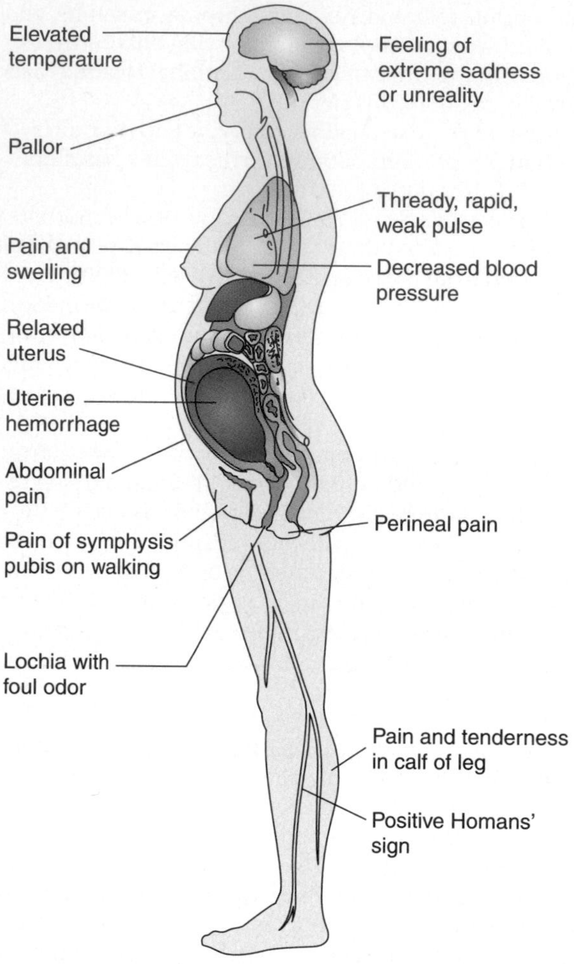

- Situational low self-esteem disturbance related to postpartal infection and inability to feed infant
- Social isolation related to precautions necessary to protect infant and others from infection transmission
- Risk for impaired parenting related to separation from infant because of infection
- Ineffective breastfeeding related to development of mastitis

Outcome Identification and Planning

Outcome identification for the woman with a postpartal complication may be particularly difficult because, although the woman wants to do everything necessary to return to health, she also does not want to allow anything to interfere with her ability to relate with her new child. During the stage of postpartal "taking-in," she may not be interested in doing things for herself; during the second stage of "taking-hold," she may not be interested in having you do procedures for her (see Chapter 22). As a rule, however, never underestimate how much a woman will undergo when preparing to care for a new child. That quality is the essence of motherhood.

When planning for the postpartal family, provide for measures that will restore the woman most quickly to health and promote contact between her, her child, and her primary support person. Infant contact is best, including physical contact such as holding and feeding. If physical contact is not possible, however, allow for frequent reports of the infant's health and preferences. During the taking-in phase, have the nursery contact the mother at least once every nursing shift to update her on the infant's status; during the taking-hold phase, encourage the mother to contact the nursery. If the infant is being cared for in another facility, ask them to supply photographs of the infant. This provides something concrete to which the woman can relate. Many mothers respond well to notes written as if they were from the child, for example, "Hi, Mom. Just a note to say hello. I'm drinking well but I miss you and can't wait for you to get better and be allowed to take care of me. Love, Kelsey Marie." Such a note serves to relieve the mother's concern for the child (she is doing well) and also helps increase the mother's self-esteem, which will promote bonding. As many as 1 woman in every 500 develops severe depression and even psychosis after childbirth (APA, 2000). The risk increases when a complication develops. A national volunteer support group offers referrals throughout the United States for women who are depressed after childbirth: Depression After Delivery (*www.Depressionafterdelivery.com*).

Implementation

Interventions for the woman with a postpartal complication should include instruction for self-care and child care (if appropriate), emphasizing the transitory nature of the complication. Continuing to review well-child care in this way helps the woman to accept her situation as temporary, reinforcing the idea that she will be able to care for the infant.

Outcome Evaluation

Evaluation of the woman with a postpartal complication should address the mother's and family's health as well as the family's ability to bond with the child. Evaluation may suggest the need for home care follow-up to assist the woman in coping with the responsibility of child care and integrating the child into the family when faced with reduced energy from illness.

Examples of outcome achievement may include the following:

- Oral temperature decreases to below 100.4°F (38.0°C).
- Lochia is free of foul odor.
- Client maintains blood pressure over 110/60 mm Hg.
- Client demonstrates bonding behaviors with infant despite separation.
- Client demonstrates warm contact with her child despite required bedrest.

POSTPARTAL HEMORRHAGE

Hemorrhage, one of the most important causes of maternal mortality associated with childbearing, poses a possible threat throughout pregnancy. It is a major potential danger in the immediate postpartal period. Traditionally, postpartal hemorrhage has been defined as *any blood loss from the uterus greater than 500 mL within a 24-hour period* (Cunningham et al., 2001). In specific agencies, the loss may not be considered hemorrhage until it reaches 1000 mL. Hemorrhage may occur either early, that is, in the first 24 hours, or late, anytime after the first 24 hours during the remaining days of the 6-week puerperium. The greatest danger of hemorrhage is in the first 24 hours because of the grossly denuded and unprotected area left after detachment of the placenta (Farrington & Ward, 2000).

There are four main causes for postpartal hemorrhage: uterine atony, lacerations, retained placental fragments, and disseminated intravascular coagulation (Fig. 25-1).

Uterine Atony

Uterine atony, or relaxation of the uterus, is the most frequent cause of postpartal hemorrhage (Cunningham et al., 2001). The uterus must remain in a contracted state after birth to allow the open vessels at the placental site to seal. Factors that predispose to poor uterine tone and an inability to maintain a contracted state are summarized in Box 25-1. When caring for a client in whom any of these conditions are present, be especially cautious in your observations and be on guard for signs of uterine bleeding. This is especially important because many postpartal clients are discharged within 48 hours after birth.

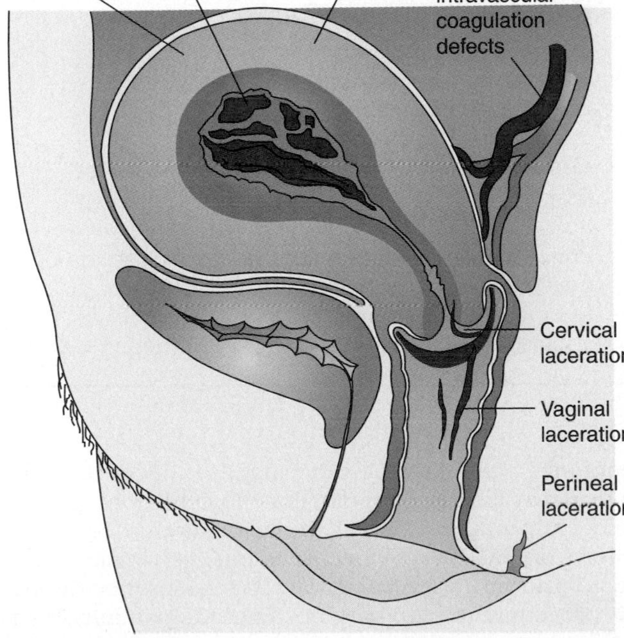

FIGURE 25.1 Common causes of postpartal hemorrhage.

BOX 25.1

CONDITIONS INCREASING A WOMAN'S RISK FOR POSTPARTAL HEMORRHAGE

Conditions That Distend the Uterus Beyond Average Capacity
Multiple gestation
Hydramnios (excessive amount of amniotic fluid)
Large baby (over 9 lb)
Presence of uterine myomas (fibroid tumors)

Conditions That Could Have Caused Cervical or Uterine Lacerations
Operative delivery
Rapid delivery

Conditions With Varied Placental Site or Attachment
Placenta previa
Placenta accreta
Premature separation of the placenta
Retained placental fragments

Conditions That Leave the Uterus Unable to Contract Readily
Deep anesthesia or analgesia
Labor initiated or assisted with an oxytocin agent
Maternal age over 30 years
High parity
Previous uterine surgery
Prolonged and difficult labor
Possible chorioamnionitis
Secondary maternal illness (e.g., anemia)
Prior history of postpartum hemorrhage
Endometritis
Prolonged use of magnesium sulfate or other tocolytic therapy

Conditions That Lead to Inadequate Blood Coagulation
Fetal death
Disseminated intravascular coagulation

Assessment

If the uterus suddenly relaxes, there will be an abrupt gush of blood from the placental site. Vaginal bleeding may be extremely large, and the client may exhibit symptoms of shock and blood loss. This may occur immediately after birth or more gradually over the first hour postpartum, as the uterus slowly becomes uncontracted. When the vaginal bleeding occurs gradually, the bleeding is seepage, not a gush of blood. Over a period of hours, however, continued seepage could be as lethal as a sudden release of blood.

It is difficult to estimate the amount of blood loss in the postpartal woman, because it is difficult to estimate the amount of blood it takes to saturate a perineal pad. A saturated perineal pad can hold between 25 and 50 mL. By counting the perineal pads saturated in given lengths of time, such as half-hour intervals, you can form a rough estimate of blood loss. Five pads saturated in half an hour is obviously a different situation from five pads saturated in 8 hours. In either situation, however, the woman will have lost close to 250 mL of blood. If either scenario is allowed to continue unattended, the woman will be in grave danger. Be sure you differentiate between *saturated* and *used* when counting pads. Weighing perineal pads before and after use and then subtracting the difference is an accurate way to measure vaginal discharge (1 g [weight] equals 1 mL [volume] of blood, because gram and milliliter are comparable measures). Always be sure to turn the woman on her side when inspecting for blood loss to be certain that large amounts are not pooling undetected beneath her. Box 25-2 highlights an appropriate outcome and intervention related to postpartum hemorrhage, using the terminology identified by the Nursing Outcomes Classification (NOC) and Nursing Interventions Classification (NIC).

Palpate a woman's fundus at frequent intervals postpartally to ascertain that the uterus is remaining in a state of contraction. This is the best measure for preventing early hemorrhage. When palpating the fundus, if you are unsure you have located it, the uterus is probably in a state of relaxation. Under normal circumstances, a well-contracted uterus is firm and easily recognized because it feels like no other abdominal structure. Frequent assessment of lochia and vital signs, particularly pulse and blood pressure, are equally important.

If the woman is losing enough blood to affect systemic circulation, she will develop signs of shock, including an increased, thready, and weak pulse; decreased blood pressure; increased and shallow respirations; pale, clammy skin; and increasing anxiety. Because the woman's circulatory system can compensate for a prolonged period of time, detecting uterine relaxation should be your first and most important assessment.

BOX 25.2

NURSING OUTCOMES AND NURSING INTERVENTIONS CLASSIFICATION: POSTPARTUM HEMORRHAGE

NOC: Circulation Status

Circulation status is defined as the extent to which blood flows unobstructed, unidirectionally, and at an appropriate pressure through large vessels of the systemic and pulmonary systems (Johnson, Maas, & Moorhead, 2000). Some specific indicators suggesting achievement of this outcome include the following:

- Vital signs, including systolic and diastolic blood pressure, pulse, and heart rate within expected ranges
- Central venous pressure and pulmonary wedge pressure within acceptable parameters
- Absence of orthostatic hypotension, abnormal heart sounds, bruits, and adventitious breath sounds
- Strong, symmetrical peripheral pulses
- Balanced 24-hour intake and output
- Cognitive status within expected range

NIC: Bleeding Reduction: Postpartum Uterus

Bleeding reduction, postpartum uterus, is defined as limiting the amount of blood loss from the postpartum uterus (McCloskey & Bulechek, 2000). Some important activities involved when implementing this intervention include:

- Providing perineal care, including observing the characteristics of lochia and weighing the amount of vaginal drainage
- Encouraging voiding and evaluating for bladder distention, catheterizing as indicated
- Monitoring vital signs frequently
- Initiating IV infusion therapy, including start of a second IV line if necessary
- Administering oxytocics as ordered
- Starting oxygen therapy via face mask
- Inserting an indwelling urinary catheter to evaluate urinary output
- Administering blood products as appropriate
- Assisting with packing the uterus, evacuating hematoma, or suturing lacerations as indicated
- Preparing for an emergency hysterectomy as needed
- Keeping the client and family informed of condition and measures being performed.

Therapeutic Management

In the event of uterine atony, the first step in controlling hemorrhage is to attempt uterine massage to encourage contraction. If the uterus cannot remain contracted, the physician or nurse-midwife probably will order a dilute intravenous infusion of oxytocin (Pitocin) to help the uterus maintain tone. Intramuscular methylergonovine (Methergine) is a second possibility (see Focus on Pharmacology, Chapter 18). Both drugs should be readily available for use in the event of postpartal hemorrhage.

The usual dosage of oxytocin is 10 to 40 U per 1000 mL of a 5% dextrose solution. When oxytocin is given intravenously, its action is immediate. However, be aware that oxytocin has a short duration of action of approximately an hour, so symptoms of uterine atony can recur quickly after administration of only a single dose.

Bimanual Massage. If fundal massage and administration of oxytocin or methylergonovine are not effective in stopping uterine bleeding, the physician or nurse-midwife may attempt bimanual compression. With this procedure, the physician or nurse-midwife inserts one hand in the vagina while pushing against the fundus through the abdominal wall with the other hand. If necessary, the woman may have a sonogram done to detect possible retained placental fragments. She may be returned to the delivery or birthing room so her uterine cavity can be explored manually. Uterine packing may be inserted during this procedure to help halt bleeding. Keep in mind that uterine manipulation is painful. Anticipate the need for analgesia or anesthesia to provide comfort.

Prostaglandin Administration. Prostaglandins promote strong, sustained uterine contractions. Prostaglandin F may be injected intramuscularly to initiate uterine contractions. Watch for nausea, diarrhea, tachycardia, and hypertension, which are possible adverse effects of prostaglandin administration (Karch, 2001).

Blood Replacement. Blood transfusion to replace blood loss with postpartal hemorrhage may be necessary. Make sure that a blood type and cross match have been done on admission of the client in labor and that blood is available. Some women may donate blood during pregnancy so they can be autotransfused if hemorrhage should occur.

Hysterectomy. Usually, the above measures are effective in halting bleeding. In the rare instances of extreme uterine atony, ligation of the uterine arteries or a hysterectomy may be necessary. These measures are done as a last resort only. Despite this emergent situation, comfort and support the woman because this is a totally unexpected outcome of childbearing for her and her support person.

After hysterectomy, the woman may want to talk about what happened, why surgery was necessary, and how she feels now that she can no longer bear children. She needs to discuss her feelings with a person who will listen quietly and help her sort through her "Why me?" feelings. She may have ambiguous feelings: she wanted to have more children (or at least have the ability to have more), but she also wanted to live. She is thankful that her life was saved, but she may feel resentful that she was left incapable of future childbearing. She may grieve for children who will not be born. If this child was born outside the hospital and the woman was brought there under emergency circumstances, she may have a need to talk about her choice of location for childbirth and her feelings. She may feel guilty that she did not choose a more controlled place for childbirth.

Open lines of communication between the couple and the staff that allow the family to vent its feelings are most helpful to the couple in this crisis. Grieving for future children who will not be born can interfere with bonding with the present child.

Nursing Interventions

The emergency measure to contract a uterus with atony is fundal massage (Nursing Procedure 25-1). Unless the uterus is extremely lacking in tone, this procedure is usually effective in causing contraction, and, after a few seconds, the uterus will assume its healthy grapefruit-like feel.

With uterine atony, even though the uterus responds well to massage, the problem may not be completely resolved. After removing your hand from the fundus, the uterus may relax and the lethal seepage may begin again. Therefore, remain with the woman after massaging the fundus to be certain that the uterus is not relaxing again. Observe her, including fundal height and consistency and lochia, closely for the next 4 hours.

In addition, include the following actions:

- Offer a bedpan or assist with ambulating to the bathroom at least every 4 hours to keep the

NURSING PROCEDURE 25.1: FUNDAL MASSAGE

Purpose

To stimulate uterine contraction, promoting uterine tone and consistency and minimizing the risk of hemorrhage.

Procedure	Principle
1. Explain the procedure to the client and provide privacy.	1. Explanations help to decrease anxiety; providing privacy enhances self esteem.
2. Ask the client to void (unless bleeding is extensive and more rapid action seems necessary).	2. An empty bladder prevents displacement of the uterus and ensures accurate assessment of uterine tone.
3. Place the client supine with her knees flexed and feet together.	3. Proper positioning enhances visualization and effectiveness of procedure.
a. Put on gloves and inspect the perineum, removing the perineal pad.	a. Gloves act as a barrier for possible infection from vaginal drainage.
b. Observe the amount and type of drainage on the pad and time since last pad change; note the appearance of any clots. Apply a new perineal pad.	b. Baseline assessment information provides information about future assessments and provides a means for evaluating the effectiveness of procedure.
4. a. Place one hand on the abdomen just above the symphysis pubis.	4. a. This location anchors the lower uterine segment.
b. Place the other hand around the top of the fundus.	b. This location helps to assess and locate the fundus and determine height.

(continued)

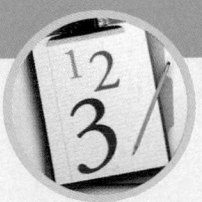

Procedure	Principle
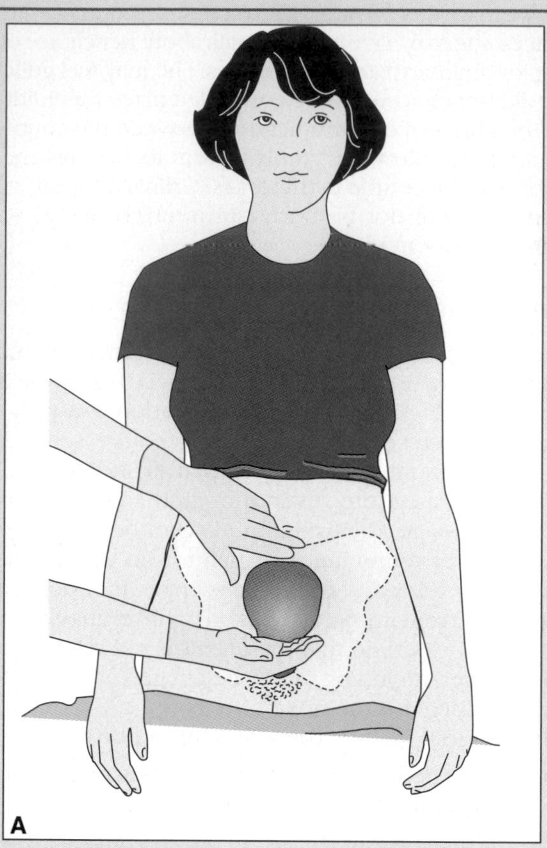	
5. Rotate the upper hand to massage the uterus until firm, being careful not to overmassage the uterus.	5. Massage should be done only when uterus is not firm, otherwise muscle fatigue and uterine relaxation may occur. Aggressive massage may lead to partial or complete uterine prolapse.
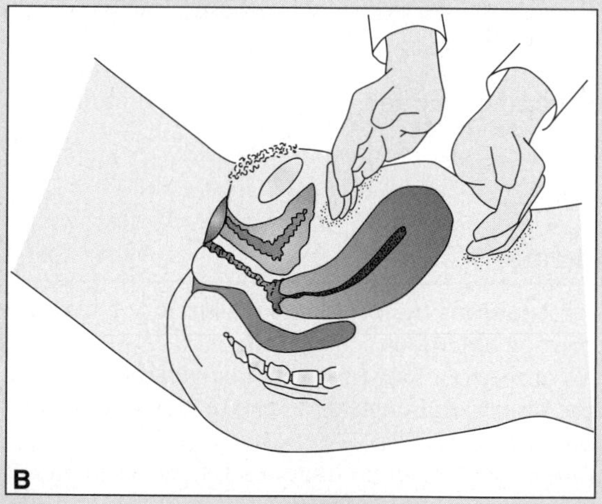	
6. When the uterus is firm, gently press the fundus between the hands using slight downward pressure against the lower hand.	6. Gently squeezing with downward pressure helps to expel blood or clots collected in the uterine cavity.
7. Observe the perineum for passage of clots and amount of bleeding.	7. This helps to assess the degree of bleeding.
8. When the uterus is again firm, cleanse the perineum, and apply a clean perineal pad. Discard gloves and soiled pads according to agency policy.	8. This helps to promote comfort and hygiene while reducing the risk for infection.
9. Document results of procedure. Continue to assess fundus and lochia according to agency policy. Notify physician or nurse-midwife if fundus does not remain firm or bleeding continues.	9. Documentation provides a means for evaluation. Continued assessment allows for early identification and prompt intervention with additional measures, such as oxytocin, to prevent hemorrhage.

woman's bladder empty. A full bladder pushes an uncontracted uterus into an even more uncontracted state. To reduce bladder pressure, insertion of a urinary catheter may be ordered.
- If a woman is experiencing respiratory distress from decreasing blood volume, administer oxygen by face mask at a rate of 4 L/minute. Position her supine to allow adequate blood flow to her brain and kidneys.
- Obtain vital signs frequently and make sure to interpret them accurately, looking for trends. For example, a continuously rising pulse rate is an ominous pattern.

In the event of slow bleeding, there is little change in pulse and blood pressure at first because of circulatory compensation. Suddenly, however, the system can compensate no more, and then the pulse rate rises rapidly. The pulse becomes weak and thready, and the blood pressure drops abruptly. The woman's skin becomes cold and clammy and she shows obvious signs of shock. Consistent frequent assessments help to detect blood loss before this point is ever reached.

When planning continuing care, remember that any woman is exhausted after birth. If a woman hemorrhages in the immediate postpartal period, her exhaustion may be intensified, possibly making her resent frequent uterine and blood pressure assessment. Explain that these measures, although disturbing, are important. Obtain vital signs as quickly and gently as possible, so the woman feels a minimum of discomfort and disruption, allowing her time to rest. Be sure that any other health care disciplines involved in caring for the woman are aware of the implications and importance of the parameters to be assessed postpartally so that these assessments are the priority (see Focus on Multidisciplinary Care).

The average woman takes the full postpartal period to regain her strength. Women who experience postpartal hemorrhage tend to have a longer than average recovery period because the physiologic exhaustion of body systems may interfere with their recovery. Iron therapy may be prescribed to ensure good hemoglobin formation. Activity level, exertion, and postpartal exercise may be restricted somewhat. Discuss with the woman the possibility of having someone stay with her at home, at least for the first week, to help with the care of her new baby and to prevent exhaustion from turning childbearing into a less than satisfying event.

Extensive blood loss is one of the precursors of postpartal infection because of the general debilitation that results. Any woman who has experienced more than a normal loss of blood should be observed closely for changes in lochia discharge. Also monitor her temperature closely in the postpartal period to detect the earliest signs of developing infection. Make sure the patient also knows how to check for normal lochia and temperature once she is discharged.

Lacerations

Small lacerations or tears of the birth canal are common and may be considered a normal consequence of childbearing. However, large lacerations are complications. They occur most often:

- With difficult or precipitate births
- In primigravidas
- With the birth of a large infant (over 9 lb)
- With the use of a lithotomy position and instruments

Either cervical, vaginal, or perineal lacerations may occur. After birth, any time the uterus is firm but bleeding persists, suspect a laceration of one of these three sites.

Cervical Lacerations

Lacerations of the cervix are usually found on the sides of the cervix near the branches of the uterine artery. If the artery is torn, the blood loss may be so great that blood gushes from the vaginal opening. Because this is arterial bleeding, the vaginal bleeding seen will be brighter red than the venous blood lost with uterine atony. Fortunately, this bleeding ordinarily occurs immediately after delivery of the placenta, when the physician or nurse-midwife is still in attendance.

Therapeutic Management. Repair of a cervical laceration is difficult, because the bleeding may be so intense that it can obstruct visualization of the area. Be certain the physician or nurse-midwife has adequate space to work, adequate sponges and suture supplies, and a good light source. The woman is not always aware of what is happening at this point, but she senses quickly that something is seriously wrong. Try to maintain an air of calm and, if possible, stand beside the woman at the head of the table. She may be worried that the extra activity in the room has something to do with her baby. Reassure her about the

FOCUS ON MULTIDISCIPLINARY CARE

Various health care personnel may be involved in caring for a woman in the postpartal period. For example, unlicensed assistive personnel may be responsible for obtaining vital signs. Be certain they are aware of the possible implications that might indicate a postpartal complication, such as a temperature over 100.4°F (38.0°C) after the first 24 hours is a danger sign of infection. Also be sure that unlicensed assistive personnel understand the rationale for precautions related to possible complications, such as no rectal temperatures in women with fourth-degree perineal lacerations. Remind them that in such a case, perineal sutures extend into the rectum and can be torn by the thermometer tip.

Alert all health care personnel to listen carefully to any statements made by the woman that might indicate a problem. Comments such as "I'm bleeding a lot," "I'm too tired to move," "I didn't think the pain after birth would be this bad," or "Why do I feel so sad?" sound simple but could indicate a report of a common complication (hemorrhage, infection, or depression). Instruct health care personnel to report these types of comments so they can be evaluated more closely.

baby's condition and inform her about the need to stay in the birthing room a little longer than expected while the doctor or nurse-midwife places additional sutures. Remember that the protective attitude women felt toward their bodies all during pregnancy is now turned toward the baby, so they are generally relieved to learn that any problem that is occurring is theirs, not the infant's.

If the cervical laceration appears to be extensive or difficult to repair, it may be necessary for the woman to be given a regional anesthetic to relax the uterine muscle and to prevent pain. Explain the need for an anesthetic and the procedures being carried out.

Vaginal Lacerations

Although rare, lacerations can also occur in the vagina. These are easier to assess because they are easier to view.

Therapeutic Management. Because vaginal tissue is friable, vaginal lacerations are harder to repair. Some oozing often follows a repair, so the vagina may be packed to maintain pressure on the suture line. An indwelling urinary catheter (Foley catheter) may be placed at the same time, because the packing causes pressure on the urethra and can interfere with voiding. If packing is inserted, document that it is in place. The physician or nurse-midwife usually removes packing after 24 to 48 hours. Ensure that the packing is removed at the designated time. Packing left in place too long tends to cause stasis and infection similar to toxic shock syndrome.

Perineal Lacerations

Lacerations of the perineum usually occur when the woman is placed in a lithotomy position for birth, because this position increases tension on the perineum. Perineal lacerations are classified in four categories, depending on the extent and depth of the tissue involved. These are shown in Table 25-1.

Therapeutic Management. Perineal lacerations are sutured and treated as an episiotomy repair. Make certain that the degree of the laceration is documented, because afterward it is often difficult to distinguish a repaired perineal laceration from an episiotomy repair on inspection. Lacerations tend to heal more slowly because the edges of the suture line are ragged. A diet high in fluid and a stool softener may be prescribed for the first week postpartum to prevent constipation and hard stools that could break the sutures. Be aware of the extent of the laceration so that you do not give any woman who has a third- or fourth-degree laceration an enema or a rectal suppository. Do not take rectal temperatures, because the hard tips of equipment could open sutures near to or including those of the rectal sphincter. Ancillary caregivers need to be informed of this, so that they understand why these measures are contraindicated. Unless a secondary complication such as infection occurs, even fourth-degree lacerations should heal without long-term dyspareunia or incontinence. However, their effect on sexual satisfaction can persist for up to 6 months (see Focus on Evidence-Based Practice).

TABLE 25.1 Classification of Perineal Lacerations

CLASSIFICATION	DESCRIPTION OF INVOLVEMENT
First degree	Vaginal mucous membrane and skin of the perineum to the fourchette
Second degree	Vagina, perineal skin, fascia, levator ani muscle, and perineal body
Third degree	Entire perineum, and reaches the external sphincter of the rectum
Fourth degree	Entire perineum, rectal sphincter, and some of the mucous membrane of the rectum

Retained Placental Fragments

Occasionally, the placenta does not deliver in its entirety. Fragments of it separate and are left behind. Because the portion retained keeps the uterus from contracting fully,

FOCUS ON EVIDENCE-BASED PRACTICE

Do Perineal Lacerations Have Long-Term Effects on Sexual Satisfaction in Women?

For this study, researchers interviewed 615 primiparous women following vaginal births. A first group had an intact perineum or only a first-degree perineal tear (211 women). A second group had second-degree trauma (336 women) and yet a third group had third- or fourth-degree perineal lacerations (68 women). Researchers found that by 6 months postpartum, one fourth of all women in the study still reported lessened sexual sensation, worsened sexual satisfaction, and lessened ability to achieve orgasm compared with similar sensations experienced before birth. Twenty-two percent reported dyspareunia. Women with a second-degree trauma were 80% more likely and women with third- or fourth-degree trauma were 270% more likely to report dyspareunia. Other factors that added to experiencing dyspareunia were breastfeeding and vacuum or forceps birth. The researchers stress the importance of efforts to minimize the extent of perineal damage from childbirth to protect against postpartum dyspareunia.

This is an important study for nurses as they are the health care providers who give support to women in labor; increased support in labor is associated with less need for operative birth procedures. It also enforces the need for encouraging good suture line care following birth, so secondary complications such as infection do not occur to prolong or worsen an already existing perineal laceration.

Signorello, L. B. et al. (2001). Postpartum sexual functioning and its relationship to perineal trauma. *American Journal of Obstetrics & Gynecology, 184*(5), 881–890.

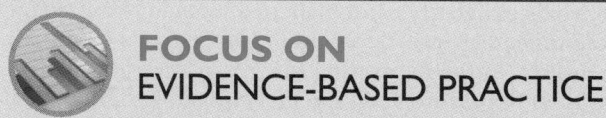

uterine bleeding occurs. Although this is most likely to happen with a succenturiate placenta—a placenta with an accessory lobe (see Chapter 21)—it can happen in any instance. Placenta accreta, a placenta that fuses with the myometrium because of an abnormal decidua basalis layer, may also be retained. Sections of this type of placenta will remain after birth and may need to be surgically incised. To detect the complication of retained placenta, every placenta should be inspected carefully after birth to see if it is complete (ACOG, 2002).

Assessment

If an undetected retained fragment is large, the bleeding will be apparent in the immediate postpartal period, because the uterus cannot contract with it in place. If the fragment is small, bleeding may not be detected until the sixth or tenth day postpartum, when the woman notices an abrupt discharge of a large amount of blood.

On examination, usually the uterus is not fully contracted. If placental tissue is still present in the woman's body, elevated serum human chorionic gonadotropin hormone (HCG) will also be present. Retained placental fragments also may be detected by sonogram.

Therapeutic Management

Removal of the placental fragment is necessary to stop bleeding. Usually, a dilatation and curettage (D&C) will be performed to remove the placental fragment. In some instances, placenta accreta may be so deeply attached it cannot be removed, requiring therapy with methotrexate to destroy the retained placental tissue. Because the hemorrhage from retained fragments may be delayed until after women are at home, instruct them to observe the color of lochia discharge and report any tendency for the discharge to change from lochia serosa or alba to rubra.

Disseminated Intravascular Coagulation

Disseminated intravascular coagulation (DIC) is a deficiency in clotting ability caused by vascular injury. It may occur in any woman in the postpartal period, but it is usually associated with women who had premature separation of the placenta, a missed early miscarriage, or fetal death in utero. This topic is discussed in Chapter 15.

Subinvolution

Subinvolution is incomplete return of the uterus to its prepregnant size and shape. With subinvolution, at a 4- or 6-week postpartal visit, the uterus is still enlarged and soft. Lochial discharge is usually still present. Subinvolution may result from a small retained placental fragment, a mild endometritis, or an accompanying problem (e.g., a myoma) that is interfering with complete contraction.

Therapeutic Management

Oral administration of methylergonovine ([Methergine] 0.2 mg four times daily) generally is prescribed to improve uterine tone and complete involution. If the uterus is tender to palpation, suggesting endometritis, an oral antibiotic also may be prescribed. Be certain that women know the normal process of involution and lochial discharge before they go home to help prevent delay in seeking health care advice. A chronic loss of blood from subinvolution will result in anemia and lack of energy, conditions that possibly could interfere with bonding.

Perineal Hematomas

A perineal hematoma is a collection of blood in the subcutaneous layer of tissue of the perineum. The overlying skin, as a rule, is intact with no noticeable trauma. Such blood collections may be caused by injury to blood vessels in the perineum during birth. They are most likely to occur after rapid spontaneous births and in women who have perineal varicosities. They may occur at an episiotomy or laceration repair site if a vein was punctured during repair. They may cause the woman acute discomfort and concern. Fortunately, they usually represent only minor bleeding.

Assessment

Perineal sutures almost always give the postpartal woman some discomfort. When a woman reports severe pain in the perineal area or a feeling of pressure between her legs, inspect the perineal area for a hematoma. If one is present, it appears as an area of purplish discoloration and obvious swelling, and may be as small as 2 cm or as much as 8 cm in diameter (Fig. 25-2). The area is tender to palpation. First, it may feel fluctuant, but as seepage into the area continues and tissue is drawn taut, it palpates as a firm globe.

Therapeutic Management

Report the presence of the hematoma, its size, and the degree of the woman's discomfort to her primary care provider. Assess the size by measuring it in centimeters with each inspection. Describing a hematoma as "large" or "small" gives little information about the actual size. Describing the lesion as 5 cm across or the size of a quarter

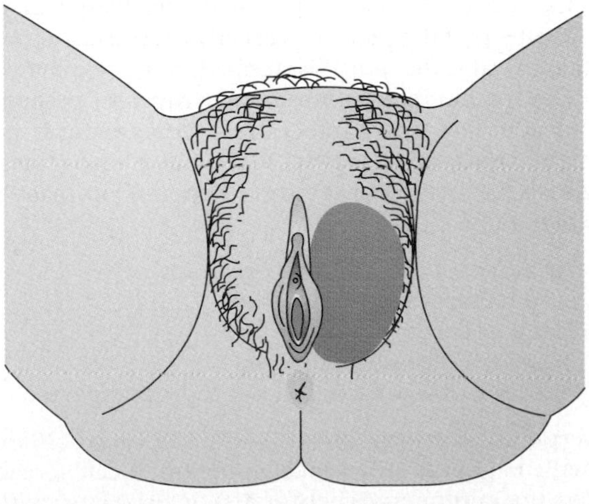

FIGURE 25.2 Appearance of a perineal hematoma from a bleeding subcutaneous vessel.

or a half dollar is more meaningful because it establishes a basis for comparison.

Administer a mild analgesic as ordered for pain relief. Applying an ice pack (covered with a towel to prevent thermal injury to the skin) may prevent further bleeding. Usually the hematoma is absorbed over the next 3 or 4 days. If the hematoma is large when discovered or continues to increase in size, the woman may have to be returned to the delivery or birthing room to have the site incised and the bleeding vessel ligated under local anesthesia.

The woman can be reassured that even though the hematoma is causing her considerable discomfort, her hospital stay probably will not be lengthened by its occurrence (unless it is extremely extensive). In most women, hematomas absorb over the next 6 weeks, causing no further difficulty. If an episiotomy incision line is opened to drain a hematoma, it may be left open and packed with gauze rather than resutured. Packing is usually removed within 24 to 48 hours. Be certain to record that this packing is in place so it can be removed before discharge or when the woman returns to an ambulatory setting. A suture line opened this way heals by tertiary intention, and thus it will heal slower than a first-degree intention suture line. Be certain the woman has clear instructions before discharge on necessary suture line care to do at home.

✔ CHECKPOINT QUESTIONS

1. What are the four major causes of postpartal hemorrhage?
2. What is the best emergency measure used to increase uterine tone?
3. What hormone level will be elevated if the woman has retained placental fragments?

PUERPERAL INFECTION

Infection of the reproductive tract is another leading cause of maternal mortality (Cunningham et al., 2001). The factors that predispose women to infection in the postpartal period are shown in Box 25-3. When caring for a woman who has any of these circumstances, be aware that the risk for postpartal infection is greatly increased.

Theoretically, the uterus is sterile during pregnancy and until the membranes rupture. After rupture, pathogens may invade. The risk of infection is even greater if tissue edema and trauma are present. When infection occurs, the prognosis for complete recovery depends on many factors, including:

- Virulence of the invading organism
- General health of the woman
- Portal of entry
- Degree of uterine involution
- Presence of lacerations in the reproductive tract

A puerperal infection is always serious because, although it usually begins as only a local infection, it can spread to involve the peritoneum (peritonitis) or circulatory system (septicemia). These conditions can be fatal in a woman already stressed from childbirth.

BOX 25.3

CONDITIONS INCREASING WOMEN'S RISK FOR POSTPARTAL INFECTION

1. Rupture of the membranes over 24 hours before birth (bacteria may have started to invade the uterus while the fetus was still in utero).
2. Placental fragments that have been retained within the uterus (the tissue necroses and serves as an excellent bed for bacterial growth).
3. Postpartal hemorrhage (the woman's general condition is weakened).
4. Pre-existing anemia (the body's defense against infection is lowered).
5. Prolonged and difficult labor, particularly instrument births (trauma to the tissue may leave lacerations or fissures for easy portals of entry for infection).
6. Internal fetal heart monitoring (contamination may have been introduced with the placement of the scalp electrode).
7. Local vaginal infection was present at the time of birth (direct spread of infection has occurred).
8. The uterus was explored after birth for a retained placenta or abnormal bleeding site (infection was introduced with exploration).

Therapeutic Management

Management for puerperal infection focuses on the use of an appropriate antibiotic after culture and sensitivity of the isolated organism. Organisms commonly cultured postpartally include group B streptococci and aerobic gram-negative bacilli such as *Escherichia coli.* Staphylococcal infections also are becoming more common. Staphylococcal infections are the cause of toxic shock syndrome, an infection similar to puerperal infection in its ability to cause death and morbidity.

NURSING DIAGNOSES AND RELATED INTERVENTIONS

Nursing Diagnosis: Risk for infection related to loss of uterine sterility with childbirth

Outcome Identification: The woman will remain free of any signs and symptoms of postpartal infection.

Outcome Evaluation: The woman's temperature remains below 100.4°F or 38°C orally, excluding the first 24 hours postpartum; lochia without foul odor.

To help prevent infection, any article such as gloves and instruments introduced into the birth canal during labor, birth, and the postpartal period should be sterile. In addition, adherence to standard precautions is essential.

Instruct the woman during the postpartal period in proper perineal care, including wiping from front to back so she does not bring *E. coli* organisms forward from the rectum. When giving perineal care, be sure to wash your hands and wear gloves. Make sure that each maternity client has her own bedpan and perineal supplies to prevent transfer of pathogens from one woman to another. Use good handwashing technique before, during, and after any client care to prevent cross-contamination.

Intravenous antibiotics usually are prescribed. Frequently used antibiotics include ampicillin, gentamicin, and third generation cephalosporins, such as cefixime (Suprax). Be certain that antibiotics are administered on time to maintain therapeutic blood levels. If women will be continuing drug therapy at home, stress that they must take the full course to prevent the infection from recurring. Be certain that women who are breastfeeding are not prescribed antibiotics incompatible with breastfeeding. Alert them to observe the infant for signs of thrush (white plaques on the tongue) or other opportunistic infection.

Nursing Diagnosis: Social isolation related to precautions necessary to protect baby and others from exposure to infectious microorganisms

Outcome Identification: Woman will demonstrate understanding of the reason for precautions and develop ways to occupy time; will demonstrate effective bonding with newborn.

Outcome Evaluation: The woman describes agency policy regarding precautions and states plans for diversional activities while in hospital; demonstrates bonding behaviors such as asking about newborn and expressing desire to see infant.

The woman with an infection may be isolated from other clients to reduce the chances that others will contract the infection.

Whether the woman who has an infection should be allowed to feed and care for her baby is always a concern on postpartal units. Most hospitals have well-defined guidelines in this area (Box 25-4). This is a time

BOX 25.4

COMMON GUIDELINES FOR THE WOMAN WITH A POSTPARTAL INFECTION

1. As a rule, the baby of a mother with an increased temperature (100.4°F [38°C]) for two consecutive 24-hour periods exclusive of the first 24 hours is kept in an isolation nursery until the cause of the infection is determined. The mother may have an upper respiratory or a gastrointestinal infection that is unrelated to childbearing but transmittable to the newborn.
2. If the cause of the fever is found to be related to childbirth but involves a closed infection, such as thrombophlebitis, when there would be no danger of the baby's contracting the disease, the mother may care for her child as long as she maintains bedrest in the prescribed position while doing so.
3. If the infection involves drainage (e.g., endometritis, perineal abscess), newborn visiting may be contraindicated. If rooming-in is continued, the mother should wash her hands thoroughly before holding the infant. She should never place the baby on the bottom bed sheet, where there may be some infected drainage from her perineal pad (furnish a clean sheet to spread over the covers).
4. Most hospitals are reluctant to return a baby to a central nursery after the baby has visited in a room where there is an infection. The hospital should provide small nurseries that may be used as isolation nurseries for these situations, or the baby can be placed in a closed Isolette in a central nursery or continue to be cared for in the mother's room.
5. If the mother has a high fever, breast milk may be deficient. With modern antimicrobial therapy, puerperal infections are limited, and the period of high fever usually will be transient. If the mother is too ill to nurse the baby during this time, or is receiving an anticoagulant or antibiotic that is passed in breast milk and would be harmful to the baby, the infant should be fed by a supplementary milk formula. The woman's breast milk should be manually expressed or pumped to maintain the production of milk so it will be available when she is again able to nurse. You may need to assist her with this, because she fatigues easily and her energy level may not be enough to support her good intentions. If it appears that the course of the infection will be long, the mother may choose to, or may be advised to, discontinue breastfeeding.
6. If it is necessary for the woman to discontinue breastfeeding, she needs to be assured that she can meet the needs of the child through bottle feeding.
7. If the woman is going to be hospitalized beyond the usual time, she may have to make arrangements for the discharge and care of the baby. She may be interested in a homemaker service or temporary foster care if she has no close friends or family. If she has older children at home, she needs to keep in close contact with them, calling them on the telephone or writing them short notes if possible. If the infant is housed in a high-risk nursery, she needs to see a photo of the newborn (a Polaroid camera should be a piece of equipment on every postpartal unit) and hear daily reports of his or her progress and well-being.

when the woman is adjusting to a new life role. It is difficult to accomplish this when things are going well. When she is segregated from others, frightened by her condition, and denied the pleasure of holding and feeding her baby, the struggle may be overwhelming. She needs friendly, understanding support from the hospital personnel who give her care. Fortunately, because modern antibiotics work quickly to reduce the possibility of contagion, periods involving separation have been reduced. Women who are breastfeeding should be encouraged to pump their breasts to maintain their milk supply if a feeding is missed.

Endometritis

Endometritis refers to an infection of the endometrium, the lining of the uterus. Bacteria gain access to the uterus through the vagina and enter the uterus either at the time of birth or during the postpartal period. Endometritis may occur with any birth, but it is associated with chorioamnionitis and cesarean birth (Farrington & Ward, 2000).

Assessment

A benign postpartal temperature elevation may occur on the first postpartal day, particularly if the woman is not drinking enough fluid. The fever of endometritis usually manifests itself on the third or fourth day postpartum, suggesting that much of the invasion occurred during labor or birth (consistent with the time it takes for infectious organisms to grow).

Normally, the white blood cell count of a postpartal woman is increased to 20,000 to 30,000/mm^3. Thus, this conventional method of detecting infection is not of great value in the puerperium. An increase in oral temperature above 100.4°F (38°C) for two consecutive 24-hour periods, excluding the first 24-hour period after birth, is defined by the Joint Committee on Maternal Welfare as a febrile condition suggesting infection (Farrington & Ward, 2000). All women with temperatures within this range should be suspected of having a postpartal infection until proven otherwise. Because many clients may be at home, any woman who feels as if she has an elevated temperature should take her temperature to be certain.

As a rule, the woman with endometritis demonstrates a rise in temperature well over 100.4°F (38°C). This rise on the third or fourth day postpartum coincides with the time breast filling occurs. Do not be led astray by attributing this elevated temperature to breast filling. Fever on the third or fourth day postpartum should be considered possible endometritis until proven otherwise.

Depending on the severity of the infection, the woman may have chills, loss of appetite, and general malaise. Most women experience some abdominal tenderness. The uterus is generally not well contracted and is painful to the touch. The woman may feel strong afterpains. Lochia will usually be dark brown and have a foul odor. It may be increased in amount because of poor uterine involution, but if the infection is accompanied by high fever, lochia may be scant or absent. Sonography may be ordered to confirm the presence of placental fragments that have become infected.

Therapeutic Management

Treatment of endometritis consists of the administration of an appropriate antibiotic, such as clindamycin (Cleocin), determined by a culture of the lochia. Be sure to obtain a culture from the vagina by a sterile swab, rather than from a perineal pad, to ensure that you are culturing the endometrial infectious organism, not an unrelated one from the pad. An oxytocic agent may be prescribed to encourage uterine contraction. The woman requires additional fluid to combat the fever. If strong afterpains and abdominal discomfort are present, she needs an analgesic for pain relief.

Place the client in Fowler's position or allow her to ambulate. These actions encourage lochia drainage by gravity and prevent pooling of infected secretions. Because the drainage is contaminated, be certain to wear gloves when helping the woman change her perineal pads. In addition, both you and the woman must use good handwashing techniques before and after handling these pads.

As with any infection, endometritis can be controlled best if it is discovered early. If you can interpret the color, quantity, and odor of lochia discharge, and the size, consistency, and tenderness of a postpartal uterus in connection with an increased temperature, you may be the first person to recognize that the problem is present. However, the client most likely will be at home when this infection occurs, so client teaching about the signs and symptoms of endometritis is essential. In addition, follow-up by a home care nurse also can help with early detection.

If the infection is limited to the endometrium, the course of infection is about 7 to 10 days. The woman may have to make arrangements for her baby's discharge before her own or help with newborn care, because her hospital stay may be extended for a few days. The client also may be discharged home on intravenous antibiotic therapy with follow-up by a home care nurse.

Endometritis can lead to tubal scarring and interference with future fertility. At a future time, if the woman desires more children, she should ask for a fertility assessment (including a hysterosalpingogram) to determine tubal patency if she has not conceived after 6 to 12 months of unprotected coitus. With mild endometritis this is usually not a problem, but the woman should be forewarned that it could occur.

Infection of the Perineum

Assessment

If a woman has a suture line on her perineum from an episiotomy or a laceration repair, a portal of entry exists for bacterial invasion. Infections of the perineum generally remain localized. They are manifested as the symptoms of any suture line infection such as pain, heat, and a feeling of pressure. The woman may or may not have an elevated temperature, depending on the systemic effect and spread of the infection.

Inspection of the suture line reveals the inflammation. One or two stitches may be sloughed away, or an area of the suture line may be open with purulent drainage present (Fig. 25-3). Notify the woman's physician or nurse-midwife of the localized symptoms and culture the

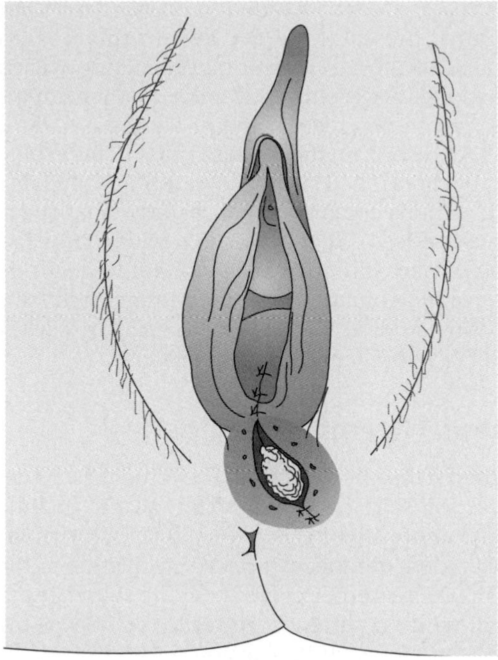

FIGURE 25.3 An infected suture line appears reddened and edematous and often contains infected secretions.

discharge by a sterile cotton-tipped applicator touched to the secretion.

Therapeutic Management

The woman's physician or nurse-midwife may choose to remove the perineal sutures to open the area and allow for drainage. Packing, such as iodoform gauze, may be placed in the open lesion to keep it open and allow drainage. Be certain the woman is aware that the packing is in place and that she knows not to dislodge the packing as she changes her perineal pad.

Typically, a systemic or topical antibiotic will be ordered even before the culture report is returned. An analgesic may be prescribed to alleviate discomfort. Sitz baths or warm compresses may be ordered to hasten drainage and cleanse the area. Remind the woman to change perineal pads frequently because they are contaminated by drainage. If left in place for a long time, they might cause vaginal contamination or reinfection. Be certain she wipes front to back after a bowel movement to prevent bringing feces forward onto the healing area.

With a local infection of this nature, a woman is usually discharged with a referral for home care follow-up because the incision site, once opened, must then heal by tertiary rather than primary intention. Infections of this nature are annoying and painful to the woman, but fortunately, with improved techniques during parturition and the puerperium, perineal infections occur only rarely. Because they are localized, there is no need to restrict a woman from caring for her infant as long as she washes her hands well before holding the newborn. Be certain not to place an infant on the bottom bed sheet of the mother's bed where he or she could contact pathogenic bacteria. Encourage the woman to ambulate and ask for analgesia as needed. Often the pain from an infected suture line can be severe, and she may decrease ambulation unless urged to continue.

Be alert to problems in the infant as a result of maternal antibiotic therapy. Assess the mouth of the infant for thrush (oral *Candida*). This occurs because a portion of the maternal antibiotic passes into breast milk and can cause an overgrowth of fungal organisms in the infant. Assess the infant for easy bruising. A decrease of microorganisms in the bowel from an antibiotic passed in breast milk may lead to insufficient vitamin K formation and consequently decreased blood-clotting ability.

WHAT IF? What if your home care client is 4 days postpartum and develops a fever of 101.5°F (41.6°C) and chills? She states that her lochia is dark brown and foul smelling. On palpation, you notice that her abdomen is very tender. What should you do next?

Peritonitis

Peritonitis, or infection of the peritoneal cavity, is usually an extension of endometritis. It is one of the gravest complications of childbearing and is a major cause of death from puerperal infection (Cunningham et al., 2001). The infection spreads through the lymphatic system or directly through the fallopian tubes or uterine wall to the peritoneal cavity. An abscess may form in the cul-de-sac of Douglas, because this is the lowest point of the peritoneal cavity and gravity causes infected material to localize there.

Assessment

The symptoms are the same as those of the surgical patient in whom a peritoneal infection develops: rigid abdomen, abdominal pain, high fever, rapid pulse, vomiting, and the appearance of being acutely ill. When assessing the abdomen of postpartal women, be sure to note not only that the uterus is well contracted but also that the remainder of the abdomen is soft. The occurrence of a rigid abdomen (guarding) is one of the first symptoms of peritonitis.

Therapeutic Management

Peritonitis is often accompanied by paralytic ileus, which requires insertion of a nasogastric tube to prevent vomiting and rest the bowel. Intravenous fluid or total parenteral nutrition may be necessary while the woman is unable to take food orally because of the intestinal paralysis. She will need analgesics for pain relief. She will be placed on large doses of antibiotics to treat the infection. Her hospital stay will be extended, but with effective antibiotic therapy, the outcome usually is good. Peritonitis may interfere with future fertility, because it leaves scarring and adhesions in the peritoneum. Adhesions formed this way may separate the fallopian tubes from the ovaries to the extent that ova can no longer easily enter the tubes.

✔ CHECKPOINT QUESTIONS

4. On what day postpartum does endometritis typically manifest itself?
5. What is the rationale for encouraging ambulation in the client with endometritis?
6. What is one of the first signs of peritonitis?

THROMBOPHLEBITIS

Phlebitis is inflammation of the lining of a blood vessel. **Thrombophlebitis** is inflammation of the lining of a blood vessel with the formation of blood clots. When thrombophlebitis occurs in the postpartal period, it is usually an extension of an endometrial infection. It occurs in the postpartal period because of:

1. Increased fibrinogen level that is still elevated from pregnancy leading to increased blood clotting
2. Dilation of lower extremity veins due to pressure of the fetal head during pregnancy and birth
3. The relative inactivity of the period or a prolonged time period in delivery or birthing room stirrups that leads to pooling, stasis, and clotting of blood in the lower extremities

Thrombophlebitis is classified as superficial vein disease (SVD) or deep vein thrombosis (DVT). Women most prone to thrombophlebitis are those with varicose veins, those who are obese, those who have had a previous thrombophlebitis, women over 30 years of age with increased parity, or those who have a high incidence of thrombophlebitis in their family (Salonen et al., 2001).

Prevention of endometritis by using good aseptic technique helps to prevent thrombophlebitis as well. Ambulation and limiting the time women remain in obstetric stirrups encourages circulation in the lower extremities, promotes venous return, and decreases the possibility of clot formation, aiding in the prevention of thrombophlebitis. Be certain that the stirrups of examining and delivery tables are well padded to prevent any sharp pressure against the calves of the legs in this position. If a woman had varicose veins during pregnancy, wearing support stockings for the first 2 weeks postpartum will help increase venous circulation and prevent stasis. If these are prescribed, be certain the woman puts them on before she rises in the morning. If she waits until she is already up and walking, venous congestion has already occurred and the stockings are less effective. Urge her to remove support stockings twice daily and assess skin underneath them for mottling or inflammation that would suggest inflammation of the veins. Additional preventive measures are summarized in Focus on Family Empowerment.

Femoral Thrombophlebitis

With femoral thrombophlebitis, the femoral, saphenous, or popliteal veins are involved. Although the inflammation site in thrombophlebitis is a vein, an accompanying arterial spasm often diminishes arterial circulation to the leg as well. This decreased circulation, along with edema, gives the leg a white or drained appearance. It was formerly believed that breast milk was going into the leg, giving it its white appearance. The condition was, therefore, formerly called *milk leg* or *phlegmasia alba dolens* (white inflammation).

Assessment

If femoral thrombophlebitis is present, it is revealed on about the tenth day after birth by an elevated temperature, chills, pain, and redness in the affected leg. The leg begins to swell below the lesion, because venous circulation is blocked at that point. The skin becomes stretched until it appears shiny and white. Homans' sign (pain in the calf on dorsiflexion of the foot) may be positive. However, keep in mind that a negative Homans' sign does not rule out obstruction. The diameter of the leg at the thigh and calf level when compared to the other side may be increased. Doppler ultrasonography or contrast venography usually is ordered to confirm the diagnosis.

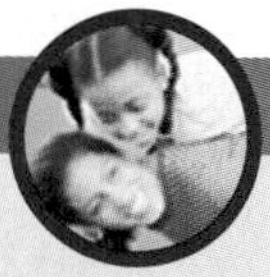

FOCUS ON FAMILY EMPOWERMENT
Preventing Thrombophlebitis

Q. I had thrombophlebitis after the birth of my first child. How can I prevent it from happening again?

A. Here are a few helpful hints for preventing thrombophlebitis:

- Ask your primary care provider if you can use a side-lying or back-lying (supine recumbent) position for birth, rather than a lithotomy position (lithotomy position can increase the tendency for pooling of blood in lower extremities).
- If you will be using a lithotomy position, ask for padding on the stirrups to prevent calf pressure.
- Don't sit with your knees bent sharply; avoid wearing constricting clothing.
- Ambulate as soon as you are able. Early ambulation is the best preventive measure. When resting in bed, wiggle your toes or do leg lifts to improve venous return.
- Ask your primary care provider if he or she recommends support stockings immediately in the postpartal period. Be certain to put these on before ambulating in the morning, before leg veins are full.

Therapeutic Management

Treatment consists of bedrest with the affected leg elevated, administration of anticoagulants, and application of moist heat. Women who have been discharged from the hospital will be cared for at home or may have to return to the hospital so that strict bedrest can be enforced. A bed cradle may be used to keep pressure of the bedclothes off the affected leg, both to decrease the sensitivity of the leg and to improve the circulation. Providing activities for the woman so she doesn't become restless helps to keep dressings in place. One way of helping the woman use her time on bedrest is to offer reading material about newborns. This activity helps a woman maintain bedrest and also educates her about infant care. Provide good back, buttocks, and heel care for the woman. Check for bed wrinkles so she does not develop a secondary problem of a pressure ulcer while on bedrest. *Never massage the affected area; this could loosen the clot, causing a pulmonary or cerebral embolism.*

Heat supplied by moist, warm compresses helps decrease inflammation. Unfortunately, this is one of the most technically difficult treatments to carry out, because dressings invariably dry or become cold after a short time. Compresses and water used in this way do not have to be sterile because, with thrombophlebitis, there is no break in the skin. Be certain to test the water temperature by dipping your inner wrist in it before soaking the dressing, to be certain that it is not too warm (because edema decreases sensation in the woman's leg, she can experience burns easily). Always cover wet, warm dressings with a plastic pad to hold in heat and moisture. In addition, a commercial pad with circulating heating coils or chemical hot packs may be positioned over the plastic to ensure the soaks stay warm. Be certain that the weight of a hot pack or pad does not rest on the leg, thereby obstructing the flow of blood.

Check the woman's bed frequently when moist compresses are used to be certain that the bed does not become wet from seeping water. For soaks to stay in place, a woman must keep her leg fairly immobile. However, be certain she doesn't interpret this as meaning she cannot turn or move about. Provide her with appropriate activities to exercise the other parts of her body and stimulate her mind.

The pain of a thrombophlebitis is usually severe enough to require administration of an analgesic. An appropriate antibiotic to reduce the initial infection will be prescribed, and often an anticoagulant (coumarin derivative or heparin) or a thrombolytic agent, such as streptokinase or urokinase, to dissolve the clot through activation of fibrinolytic precursors, and prevent further clot formation. The woman will have daily blood coagulation level determinations before administration of the anticoagulant. Depending on the drug prescribed, a baseline activated partial thromboplastin time (APTT) or prothrombin time (PT) is obtained. These will be evaluated frequently to determine the effectiveness of the drug therapy.

Heparin, an anticoagulant, can be administered by continuous intravenous infusion or intermittently by intravenous or subcutaneous injection (see Focus on Pharmacology: Heparin). If a woman will be discharged on subcutaneous therapy, be certain she has demonstrated good injection technique before discharge and understands the importance of required blood work (coagulation studies) so she schedules these appropriately. The

FOCUS ON PHARMACOLOGY

Heparin Calcium Injection (Hepalean, Liquamin Sodium)

Action: Heparin blocks the conversion of prothrombin to thrombin and fibrinogen to fibrin, decreasing clotting ability and resulting in the inhibition of thrombus and clot formation. It is used to prevent and treat thrombosis and pulmonary embolism.

Pregnancy risk category: C

Dosage: Dosage is dependent on coagulation studies. Dosage is considered therapeutic when activated partial thromboplastin time (APTT) is 1.5 to 3 times the control value. It can be given by continuous intravenous infusion or intermittent direct IV or subcutaneous injection.

Possible adverse reactions: Hemorrhage, bruising, thrombocytopenia, urticaria

Nursing Implications

- Obtain baseline coagulation studies as ordered.
- Continue to monitor APTT results and adjust dosage as ordered. Obtain 30 minutes before intermittent dosage administration or every 4 hours for continuous IV infusion.
- Anticipate use of intermittent infusion device, such as Hep-lock, to minimize the number of injections.
- Avoid any intramuscular injection of other medications because hematoma may form at injection site.
- When administering as IV infusion, do not add heparin to existing IV solutions or piggyback other drugs into heparin infusion. Use an infusion pump.
- When administering SQ, give deep, rotating injection sites; do not aspirate for blood return or massage injection site afterward; apply direct pressure to injection site after administration. Inspect injection site for signs of hematoma formation.
- Assess client for signs and symptoms of bleeding, such as oozing from the gums, nosebleeds, hematuria, or frank or occult blood in stool.
- Closely monitor client's lochia, including amount and color. Assess pad count to determine extent of vaginal bleeding.
- Institute bleeding precautions, such as use of soft toothbrush.
- Keep protamine sulfate, the antidote, readily available in case of overdose.
- Instruct client in bleeding precautions to minimize the risk of bleeding (Karch, 2001).

woman can continue to breastfeed while receiving heparin. If the woman does not wish to breastfeed, she can be switched to warfarin ([Coumadin] an oral coumarin derivative) before hospital discharge.

Commonly, the woman will have to discontinue breastfeeding during therapy with these agents as the coumarin derivative anticoagulants are passed in breast milk (see Focus on Cultural Competence). If the thrombophlebitis does not seem to be severe and the woman wants to restart breastfeeding after the course of anticoagulant (about 10 days), encourage her to manually express breast milk at the time of normal feedings to maintain a good milk supply.

Lochia will usually increase in amount in the woman who is receiving an anticoagulant. Be sure to keep a meaningful record of the amount of this discharge so it can be estimated. "Lochia serosa with scattered pinpoint clots; three perineal pads saturated in 8 hours" is far more meaningful than "large amount of lochia." Weighing perineal pads before and after use is also effective. Also assess for other possible signs of bleeding, such as bleeding gums, ecchymotic spots on the skin, or oozing from an episiotomy suture line. Protamine sulfate, the antagonist for heparin, should be readily available any time heparin is administered.

Women on anticoagulants are not normally prescribed salicylic acid (aspirin), because salicylic acid prevents blood clotting by acting as an antiplatelet agent to prevent platelet aggregation and clot formation. However, some women may be prescribed aspirin every 4 hours as a preventive measure for those at high risk for recurrent thrombophlebitis. If this is the case, be certain you do not interpret aspirin used this way as a PRN analgesic order and withhold it depending on the woman's level of pain.

With proper treatment, the acute symptoms of femoral thrombophlebitis last only a few days, but the full course of the disease takes 4 to 6 weeks before it is resolved. The affected leg may never return to its former size and may always cause discomfort after long periods of standing.

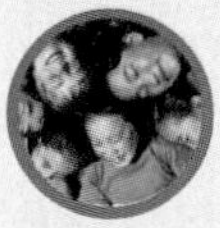

FOCUS ON CULTURAL COMPETENCE

Often, the choice to breastfeed is culturally influenced. If there is a postpartal complication that interferes with breastfeeding, the woman who feels that breastfeeding is very important can be expected to react less favorably than the woman from a culture in which formula feeding is preferred. The amount of activity that women expect to engage in after childbirth also is culturally determined. For this reason, women who assume that they will immediately return to an active lifestyle may see hospitalization for a postpartal complication as more upsetting than women who view the postpartal period as one in which they are expected to rest. Assessing each woman individually is necessary to establish the personal impact of a postpartal complication.

Pelvic Thrombophlebitis

Pelvic thrombophlebitis involves the ovarian, uterine, or hypogastric veins. It usually follows a mild endometritis. Risk factors are the same as those for femoral thrombophlebitis. Pelvic thrombophlebitis occurs later than femoral thrombophlebitis, often around the fourteenth or fifteenth day of the puerperium.

Assessment

The woman is suddenly extremely ill, with a high fever, chills, and general malaise. The infection may be so severe that it necroses the vein and results in a pelvic abscess. It can become systemic and result in a lung, kidney, or heart valve abscess.

Therapeutic Management

As with femoral thrombophlebitis, therapy involves total bedrest and administration of antibiotics and anticoagulants.

The disease runs a long course of 6 to 8 weeks. If an abscess forms, it can be located and incised by laparotomy, if necessary. Formation of an abscess is associated with a high mortality. An inflammation of this extent may leave tubal scarring and interfere with future fertility. The woman may need surgery to remove the affected vessel before attempting to become pregnant again.

Regardless of the type of thrombophlebitis, for future pregnancies, teach the client preventive measures to reduce the risk of recurrence. These measures include not wearing constricting clothing such as garters or tight stockings on her lower extremities, resting with feet elevated, and ambulating daily during pregnancy. She should be cautioned to tell the physician or nurse-midwife with her next pregnancy of the difficulty she experienced this time to ensure that extra precautions are taken to prevent thrombophlebitis.

WHAT IF? What if a client comes to the antepartal clinic for a checkup and states that she has a family history of thrombophlebitis? You notice that she also has varicose veins. What interventions should you institute now to reduce her risk of thrombophlebitis postpartally?

Pulmonary Embolus

A pulmonary embolus is obstruction of the pulmonary artery with a blood clot, usually seen as a complication of thrombophlebitis. The signs of pulmonary embolus are sudden, sharp chest pain, tachypnea, tachycardia, orthopnea (inability to breathe except in an upright position), and cyanosis (the blood clot is obstructing the pulmonary artery, thus blocking blood flow to the lungs and return to the heart). This is an emergency. The woman needs oxygen administered immediately and is at high risk for cardiopulmonary arrest. Her condition is extremely guarded until the clot is lysed or adheres to the pulmonary artery wall and is reabsorbed. Because of the seriousness of this condition, a woman with a pulmonary embolism commonly is transferred to an intensive care unit for continuing care.

> ✔ **CHECKPOINT QUESTIONS**
>
> 7. On what day postpartally would the typical signs and symptoms of femoral thrombophlebitis appear?
> 8. What drug is the antidote for heparin?

MASTITIS

Mastitis (infection of the breast) may occur as early as the seventh postpartal day or may not occur until the baby is weeks or months old (Fiorica, 2000).

The organism causing the infection usually enters through cracked and fissured nipples. Thus, measures that prevent cracked and fissured nipples also help prevent mastitis. These include:

- Making certain that the baby is positioned correctly and grasps the nipple properly, including both nipple and areola
- Releasing the baby's grasp on the nipple before removing the baby from a breast
- Washing hands between handling perineal pads and breasts
- Exposing nipples to air for at least part of every day
- Using a vitamin E ointment to soften nipples daily

If the woman has one cracked and one well nipple, encourage her to begin breastfeeding (when the infant sucks most forcefully) on the unaffected nipple.

Occasionally, the organism that causes mastitis comes from the nasal–oral cavity of the infant. In these instances, the infant has usually acquired a *Staphylococcus aureus* infection while in the hospital. Candidiasis may also be spread this way. By sucking on the nipple, the infant introduces the organisms into the milk ducts, where they proliferate (breast milk is an excellent medium for bacterial growth). This is an epidemic breast abscess; it is usually discovered that several women discharged from the hospital at the same time have similar infections.

Assessment

Mastitis is usually unilateral, although epidemic mastitis, because it originates with the infant, may be bilateral. The affected breast shows localized pain, swelling, and redness. Fever accompanies these first symptoms within hours, and breast milk becomes scant.

Therapeutic Management

The woman will be placed on a broad-spectrum antibiotic. Breastfeeding is continued, because keeping the breast emptied of milk helps to prevent growth of bacteria. Some women may find an infected breast too painful to allow the infant to suck and may prefer to express milk manually from the affected breast for 2 or 3 days until the antibiotic has taken effect and the mastitis has diminished (about 3 days). Cold or ice compresses and a good supportive bra provide much pain relief until the process improves. Warm, wet compresses may be ordered to reduce inflammation and edema.

If therapy is started as soon as symptoms are apparent, the condition runs a short course of about 2 or 3 days. If untreated, a breast infection may become a localized abscess. This may involve a large portion of the breast and rupture through the skin, with thick, purulent drainage, necessitating incision and drainage of the abscess. If an abscess forms, breastfeeding on that breast is discontinued. However, the woman is encouraged to continue to pump breast milk until the abscess has resolved to preserve breastfeeding. Some women may feel that the breast is too tender to do this. These women can be assured that formula feeding is an acceptable alternative for the child.

Neither mastitis nor breast abscess leaves any permanent breast disease. The woman can be assured that such an incident is not associated with development of breast cancer and does not interfere with future breastfeeding potential (see Focus on Nursing Care Planning).

> ✔ **CHECKPOINT QUESTIONS**
>
> 9. What are two possible sources for organisms causing mastitis?
> 10. List three typical findings of mastitis.

URINARY SYSTEM DISORDERS

Urinary Retention

Urinary retention implies inadequate bladder emptying. After childbirth, bladder sensation for voiding is decreased because of the resultant bladder edema from the pressure of birth. Unable to empty, the bladder fills to overdistention. When the woman does void, instead of emptying completely, the bladder empties only a small portion of its contents (retention with overflow). As a result, it becomes overdistended again. Bladder overdistention is potentially serious. If allowed to continue, permanent damage may occur from loss of bladder tone, leading to permanent incontinence (Nel et al., 2001).

Assessment

Urinary retention is associated with the use of anesthesia and forceps. In the postpartal woman, urinary retention with overflow may be more difficult to detect than primary or simple overdistention. With primary overdistention, the woman does not void at all. A longer-than-usual time (over 8 hours) has passed after birth or between voids. Assessment by percussion or palpation of the bladder reveals the distention.

With urinary retention and overflow, the woman is able to void. Voiding is very frequent, however, and in small amounts; her overall output is inadequate. Always measure the amount of the first voiding after birth. As a rule, if a voiding is less than 100 mL, urinary retention should be suspected.

FOCUS ON *Nursing Care Planning*

THE WOMAN WITH MASTITIS

A 26-year-old primipara, 3 weeks postpartum, calls the clinic because she has flulike symptoms, fever, and swelling and pain in her right breast. She comes to the clinic for an evaluation.

Assessment: Primipara client who gave birth vaginally 3 weeks ago and is breastfeeding. Temperature 101.1°F (38.4°C). Other vital signs within acceptable parameters. Right breast reddened and edematous, tender and warm to touch. Slight fissure noted on right nipple. A diagnosis of mastitis is made. Stated, "I don't seem to be emptying my breasts like I was, but I thought I just had the flu. It hurts so much. How can I be a good mother if I don't breastfeed my baby?"

Nursing Diagnosis: Pain related to effects of mastitis

Outcome Identification: Client will confirm she has increasing comfort.

Outcome Evaluation: Client states pain is decreasing with treatment; demonstrates measures to promote comfort. Right breast swelling, redness, and tenderness decreasing.

Interventions	Rationale
1. Apply warm compresses to right breast at visit. Instruct client in ways to apply warm moist heat, such as with a shower or warm packs, at home.	1. Moist heat promotes comfort and increases circulation to the area, decreasing inflammation and edema.
2. Encourage the client to continue breastfeeding. Advise client to completely empty the breast at each feeding. If the right breast is too sore, teach the client how to express milk either manually or with a pump.	2. Milk provides a good medium for bacterial growth. Complete emptying of breasts prevents stasis of milk and engorgement and aids in reducing the risk of further infection and pain.
3. Urge the client to breastfeed or empty breasts every 1½ to 2 hours.	3. Frequent emptying maintains lactation and aids in comfort.
4. Encourage the client to start each infant feeding on the unaffected breast.	4. Starting on the unaffected breast causes the milk ejection reflex to occur in the affected breast, promoting more efficient and complete breast emptying; it also reduces the amount of pain from forceful sucking.
5. Notify the maternal health care provider in anticipation of the need for oral antibiotic therapy.	5. Antibiotic therapy is necessary to combat the infection, aiding in the resolution of the infection and subsequent pain relief.
6. Encourage the client to wear a supportive bra.	6. A supportive bra aids in providing comfort to the edematous, inflamed breast.
7. Review breast care measures with the client.	7. Breast care measures aid in promoting the integrity of the breast, minimizing the risk of cracked or fissured nipples, and preventing mastitis.

Nursing Diagnosis: Situational low self-esteem related to feelings of inadequacy about ability to continue breastfeeding because of effects of mastitis

Outcome Identification: Client will return to previous level of satisfaction with breastfeeding.

Outcome Evaluation: Client identifies positive self attributes; identifies measures to promote comfort and effective breastfeeding; states breastfeeding is a positive experience again.

(continued)

Interventions	Rationale
1. Attempt to identify the meaning of breastfeeding to the client.	1. Identifying the meaning of breastfeeding assists in determining the impact that a diagnosis of mastitis may have on the client.
2. Encourage client to express feelings and thoughts about herself, breastfeeding, and mastitis.	2. Sharing of feelings and concerns permits a safe outlet for emotions and also aids in highlighting client's awareness of possible impact on self-esteem.
3. Review and reinforce with client positive attributes about herself.	3. Positive attributes provide a foundation for rebuilding self-esteem.
4. Clarify any misconceptions client may have about breastfeeding and mastitis. Inform client that mastitis does not result in permanent breast disease or interfere with future breastfeeding potential.	4. Misconceptions can negatively impact self-esteem. Providing information helps to alleviate possible anxiety related to any misconceptions and lack of knowledge.
5. Instruct client in measures to promote comfort and relieve pain.	5. Comfort promotion and pain relief help to minimize the effects of mastitis.
6. Assist with measures to increase independent role functioning and encourage active participation in decision making.	6. Independence and ability to perform one's role promote self-esteem; active participation enhances the feeling of control over situations.
7. Discuss possible support persons and groups. Encourage client to call the clinic with any problems, questions, or concerns.	7. Additional support can assist in reinforcing positive attributes, thus enhancing self-esteem.

Urinary retention is confirmed by catheterizing the woman immediately after a voiding. If the amount of urine left in the bladder after voiding (termed *residual*) is over 100 mL, the woman has retention above the normal amount. Typically, a physician or nurse-midwife will write an order to read "Catheterize for residual urine. If this is over 100 mL, leave indwelling catheter in place." Always use an indwelling (Foley) catheter rather than a temporary one (straight catheter) to catheterize for residual urine. This helps to minimize the risk of introducing pathogens with another catheterization, should an indwelling catheter be needed. Always use strict antiseptic technique to prevent introducing pathogenic bacteria into the sterile urinary tract and thus causing a urinary tract infection.

Catheterizing a woman during the early postpartal period may be a difficult procedure. Vulvar edema often distorts the position and appearance of the urinary meatus. Use a gentle technique, remembering that the woman's perineum is apt to feel tender to touch.

Therapeutic Management

How much urine to remove from an overdistended bladder at one time is controversial. There is a suggestion that removing more than 750 to 1000 mL of urine at any one time may create extreme pressure changes in the bladder and lower abdomen. This decreased pressure in the lower abdomen may cause blood to flow into the area, thus creating supine hypotension. There are few actual documented occurrences of this happening, however. Particularly in the postpartal period, when a bladder easily distends and the uterus is larger than normal, this shift in pressure may not be as important. Follow your health care agency policy about how much urine to remove from a full bladder at catheterization.

If an indwelling catheter will be left in place, be certain to explain the rationale for its insertion and how it works. Explain how the balloon is inflated to hold it in place. This prevents the woman from limiting her activity to try and keep it in place. Activity and ambulation help to prevent other complications, such as thrombophlebitis.

Catheterization is a procedure that has a reputation as being extremely painful. Assure the client that, as a rule, it involves only a momentary discomfort, such as a pinprick, as the catheter is inserted. Because the pain sensation of edematous tissue is decreased, the woman with extreme vulvar edema may experience only slight discomfort.

After 24 hours, the physician or nurse-midwife may order the indwelling catheter to be clamped for a short time and then removed. Encourage the woman to void by the end of 6 hours after removal of the catheter by offering fluid, administering an analgesic so she can relax, assisting her to the bathroom as necessary, and trying time-tested solutions such as running water at the sink or letting her hold her hand under warm running water. In most women, bladder and vulvar edema have decreased significantly by this time so that they are able to void without further difficulty. You may be asked to assess for residual urine again. If a woman has not voided by 8 hours after catheter removal, the physician or nurse-midwife may order reinsertion of the indwelling catheter for an additional 24 hours.

Difficulty with bladder function after childbirth is becoming less of a problem as less anesthesia and fewer forceps are used at birth, decreasing bladder and vulvar pressure. When problems do arise, it may be difficult for the woman to accept because bladder elimination is a basic step of self-care. It can be disappointing and discouraging to a woman who wants not only to be able to care for herself but to care for a new infant as well. Assure women that bladder complications are common. Usually they are present for no longer than 48 hours postpartum. They are problems that most likely will not recur.

WHAT IF? It has been approximately 7 hours since your client's delivery and she still has not voided. What should you do next?

Urinary Tract Infection

The woman who is catheterized at the time of childbirth or who is catheterized in the postpartal period is prone to developing a urinary tract infection because bacteria may be introduced into the bladder at the time of catheterization.

Assessment

When a urinary tract infection develops, the woman notices symptoms of burning on urination, possibly blood in the urine (hematuria), and a feeling of frequency or that she always has to void. The pain is so sharp on voiding that she may resist doing so, thus further compounding the problem of urinary stasis. She may have a low-grade fever and discomfort from lower abdominal pain.

A clean-catch urine specimen should be obtained from any woman with symptoms of urinary tract infection (see Chapter 10, Nursing Procedure 10-1). This can be done as an independent nursing action. So that lochial discharge does not contaminate the specimen, provide a sterile cotton ball for the woman to tuck into her vagina after perineal cleansing. Be certain to ask if the woman removed the vaginal cotton ball after the procedure; otherwise, it could cause stasis of vaginal secretions and increase the possibility of endometritis. Mark the specimen "possibly contaminated by lochia" so any blood in the specimen will not be overly interpreted by the laboratory technician.

Therapeutic Management

Although sulfa drugs are normally prescribed for urinary tract infection, they are contraindicated for breastfeeding women. Typically, therefore, a broad-spectrum antibiotic, such as amoxicillin or ampicillin, will be prescribed to treat the infection. Encourage the woman to drink large amounts of fluid (a glass every hour) to help flush the infection from her bladder. She may need an oral analgesic, such as acetaminophen (Tylenol) to reduce the pain of urination for the next few times she voids until the antibiotic begins to have an effect and the burning sensation disappears. Otherwise, because voiding is painful, she may not drink the fluid you suggest, knowing it will increase the number of times she will need to void.

Although symptoms of urinary tract infection decrease quickly, the woman will need to continue to take the prescribed antibiotic for the full 5 to 7 days to eradicate the infection completely. Once symptoms have disappeared, people often become noncompliant with medicine, particularly if a person is busy—and a woman at home with a new baby is busy. Make a chart for the woman to post on her refrigerator door as a reminder to continue taking the medication. Otherwise, bacteria in the urine will begin to multiply again, and in another week, symptoms and the active infection will recur. Be certain the woman is aware of common methods all women should use to prevent urinary tract infections, as shown in the Focus on Family Empowerment in Chapter 46.

Depending on the antibiotic prescribed, the woman may need to temporarily discontinue breastfeeding. If the antibiotic is tetracycline or a sulfonamide, check with her physician about possibly changing her antibiotic to one safe for breastfeeding, such as ampicillin. Otherwise, the client may decide to breastfeed once she is home and not take the prescribed antibiotic.

CARDIOVASCULAR SYSTEM DISORDERS

Postpartal Pregnancy-Induced Hypertension

Pregnancy-induced hypertension (PIH) is discussed in Chapter 15. Mild preexisting hypertension may increase in severity during the first few hours or days after birth. Rarely, hypertension of pregnancy develops for the first time in a woman who has had no prenatal or intranatal symptoms.

The cardinal symptoms are those of prepartal hypertension of pregnancy, namely, proteinuria, edema, and hypertension.

The treatment measures for postpartal PIH are the same as for antepartal PIH: bedrest, a quiet atmosphere, frequent monitoring of vital signs and urine output, and administration of magnesium sulfate or an antihypertensive. Antihypertensive therapy can be administered in higher doses than during pregnancy because fetal risk is no longer present. The reason the condition occurs is usually because some placenta is still present. The woman may be returned to surgery to have a D&C to be certain that all placental fragments have been removed from the uterus. After D&C, her blood pressure often falls dramatically to normal.

Seizures, if they occur postpartally, typically develop 6 to 24 hours after birth. Seizures occurring more than 72 hours after birth are probably not due to PIH but to some cause unrelated to childbearing.

Women in whom postpartal hypertension develops are bewildered by what is happening to them. If seizures occur, they are frightened to discover how little control they have over their body. They worry that one will occur after they are home while they are holding the baby. The woman can be assured that hypertension of pregnancy, although appearing late, is a condition of pregnancy. Now that she is no longer pregnant, it should not be a cause of concern. PIH may be a problem in future pregnancies, however, because women who were preeclamptic in one pregnancy may have a higher risk for it occurring in a subsequent pregnancy, especially if chronic hypertension persists.

REPRODUCTIVE SYSTEM DISORDERS

Reproductive Tract Displacement

If the support systems of the uterus are weakened because of pregnancy, the ligaments may no longer be able to maintain the uterus in its usual position or level after pregnancy.

Problems of retroflexion, anteflexion, retroversion, and anteversion or prolapse of the uterus may occur. These uterine displacement disorders may interfere with future childbearing and fertility and may cause continued pain or a feeling of lower abdominal heaviness or discomfort.

If the walls of the vagina are weakened, a cystocele (outpouching of the bladder into the vaginal wall) or a rectocele (outpouching of the rectum into the vaginal wall) may occur. These problems tend to occur most frequently in women with a high parity and after operative birth, such as forceps birth. (They are illustrated in Figure 4-8.) Surgery to repair such conditions may be necessary. If stress incontinence (involuntary voiding on exertion) occurs, Kegel exercises to strengthen perineal muscles may be helpful (Meyer et al., 2000).

Separation of the Symphysis Pubis

During pregnancy, many women feel some discomfort at the symphysis pubis because of relaxation of the joint preparatory to birth. If a fetus is unusually large or fetal position is not optimal, the ligaments of the symphysis pubis may be so stretched by birth that they actually tear.

After birth, the woman feels acute pain on turning or walking; her legs tend to rotate externally, giving her a waddling gait. A defect over the symphysis pubis can be palpated; the area is swollen and tender to touch.

Bedrest and the application of a snug pelvic binder to immobilize the joint are necessary to relieve pain and allow healing. As with all ligament injuries, a 4- to 6-week period is necessary for healing to take place (Chang & Markman, 2002). During this time, the woman may need to arrange for some type of child care at home, and must avoid heavy lifting for an extended time until healing in the ligaments is complete. She may be advised to consider a cesarean birth for any future pregnancy.

EMOTIONAL AND PSYCHOLOGICAL COMPLICATIONS OF THE PUERPERIUM

Any woman who is extremely stressed or who gives birth to an infant who in any way does not meet her expectations (e.g., the wrong sex, physically or cognitively challenged, or ill) may have difficulty bonding with the infant. Inability to bond is a postpartal complication with far-reaching implications, possibly affecting the future health of the entire family.

The Woman Whose Child Is Born With an Illness or Who Is Physically Challenged

Most women say during pregnancy that they do not care about the sex of the child as long as the child is born healthy. Therefore, they may feel cheated when this one requirement is not met. They may be angry, hurt, and disappointed. They may feel a loss of self-esteem: they have given birth to an imperfect child and so they see themselves as imperfect. A woman sometimes responds with a grief reaction, as if the child has died. This is normal, because the image of the "perfect" child she thought she was carrying *has* died.

The average woman also may have difficulty immediately after birth believing that her child is real. This difficulty is further compounded for the woman whose child is challenged in some way. She must not only grasp the fact that the baby has been born but also understand that her actual baby is different than her wished-for baby.

In most instances, parents are shown the child moments after birth, so the condition or problem can be immediately explained to them. Although a shock to couples, this allows them to face the problem with support people readily available. The physician or nurse-midwife will usually make it her responsibility to tell the parents of the defect. Be prepared to reinforce this information or review the problem. People who are under stress are not good listeners and so may need repeated explanations before they completely understand.

If possible, it is important for parents to care for the child during the postpartal period so they can touch, relate to, and "claim" the infant in as nearly normal a manner as possible. Many women wait until their support person is present to visit in an intensive care nursery so that visiting with their newborn is a family activity.

Open lines of communication between the parents and the hospital staff that allow for free discussion of feelings and fears will do much to strengthen parent–child relationships and prepare for future hospitalizations or care of the child.

The Woman Whose Child Has Died

The woman whose child dies at birth always has questions about what happened. She is likely to feel bewildered, perhaps bitter, and perhaps resentful that the hospital staff could not save the child. "Why me? Out of all the women here, why did my baby die?" She needs concerned support from health care personnel to help her cope with such a devastating loss.

Most women are interested in seeing the baby. This is generally therapeutic because it helps them begin grieving. Clean the baby, wrap the baby in an infant blanket, and bring him or her to the parents. Remain with them, but give them time to handle and inspect the child as they wish. Be familiar with the forms the mother or father will have to sign when a baby dies or is born dead. Know whether your state requires stillborn infants to be given a name and a funeral.

Other women on the unit tend to stay away from the woman whose child has died, as if what has happened to her were contagious. Friends and relatives may be equally unable to talk about the situation. Most women, therefore, want a nurse to approach them and say, "Do you want to talk about what's happened?" or "How do you feel?"

A woman whose child has died should never be placed in a room with a woman who has had a healthy child. Provide a private room to allow the woman an opportunity to grieve. Check about adjusting the visiting schedule hours. She needs her family with her to fill a portion of the void left by her loss.

The process of grieving and support necessary is further discussed in Chapter 56.

Postpartal Depression

Almost every woman notices some immediate feelings (1 to 10 days postpartum) of sadness (postpartal "blues") after childbirth. This probably occurs as a response to the anticlimactic feeling after birth and probably is related to hormonal shifts as estrogen, progesterone, and corticotropin-releasing hormone levels in her body decline (Farrington & Ward, 2000).

In a few women, these normal feelings continue beyond the immediate postpartal period. In addition to an overall feeling of sadness, the woman may notice extreme fatigue, an inability to stop crying, increased anxiety about her own or her infant's health, insecurity (unwillingness to be left alone or inability to make decisions), psychosomatic symptoms (nausea and vomiting, diarrhea), and either depressive or manic mood fluctuations. Depression that continues in this way is termed **postpartal depression** and reflects a more serious problem (APA, 2000; Table 25-2). Risk factors for postpartal depression include a history of depression, a troubled childhood, stress in the home or at work, lack of self-esteem, or lack of effective support people. Low self-esteem may be a major contributing factor. Differences between a woman wanting a pregnancy and her partner not wanting it could play a major role (Leathers & Kelley, 2000).

It is difficult to predict which women will develop postpartal depression before birth of their baby because birth can result in varied reactions; if they can be identified, pregnancy counseling may be able to prevent symptoms (Zlotnick et al., 2001). For women who have not been identified as at risk, the discovery of the problem as soon as symptoms develop is a nursing priority. The woman will need counseling and possibly antidepressant therapy to integrate the experience of childbirth into her life. This is crucial to development of a healthy maternal–infant bond, to the health of any other children in the family, and to overall family functioning. Ask at postpartal return visits and well-child visits about symptoms that would suggest this depression, and suggest an appropriate referral (see Focus on Communication).

Postpartal Psychosis

As many as 1 woman in 500 presents enough symptoms in the year after birth of a child to be considered psychiatrically ill. This statistic represents the current rate of overall mental illness (APA, 2000). Because the illness coincides with the postpartal period, it has been called **postpartal psychosis** (Cunningham et al., 2001). Rather than being a response to the physical aspects of childbearing, however, it is probably a response to the crisis of childbearing. The majority of these women will have had symptoms of mental illness before the pregnancy. If the pregnancy had not precipitated the illness, a death in the family, the loss of a husband's job, a divorce, or some other major life crisis would probably have precipitated the same recurrence (APA, 2000).

The woman usually appears exceptionally sad. By definition, psychosis exists when a person has lost contact with reality. The woman with a childbearing psychosis may deny that she has had a child and, when the child is brought to her, insist that she was never pregnant. She may voice thoughts of infanticide or that the infant is possessed. When observation tells you that a woman is not functioning in reality, you cannot improve her concept of reality by a simple measure such as explaining what a correct perception is. Her sensory input is too disturbed to comprehend this. In addition, she may interpret your attempt as threatening. She may respond with anger or become equally threatening. A psychosis is a severe mental illness that requires referral to a professional psychiatric counselor and antipsychotic medication.

While waiting for such a skilled professional to arrive, do not leave the woman alone because distorted perception might lead her to harm herself. Nor should you leave her alone with her infant.

Always keep in mind that, although rare, postpartum psychosis does exist. Remembering that childbearing can lead to this degree of mental illness helps you to put childbearing into perspective. For some people, childbearing is such a crisis in their lives that it can trigger mental illness. Certainly, it cannot be considered an everyday incident in anyone's life.

TABLE 25.2 Comparing Postpartal Blues, Depression, and Psychosis

	POSTPARTAL BLUES	POSTPARTAL DEPRESSION	POSTPARTAL PSYCHOSIS
Onset	1 to 10 days after birth	1 to 12 months after birth	Within first month after birth
Symptoms	Sadness, tears	Anxiety, feeling of loss, sadness	Delusions or hallucinations to harm infant or self
Incidence	70% of all births	10% of all births	1% to 2% of all births
Etiology (possible)	Probable hormonal changes, stress of life changes	History of previous depression, hormonal response, lack of social support	Possible activation of previous mental illness, hormonal changes, family history of bipolar disorder
Therapy	Support, empathy	Counseling	Psychotherapy, drug therapy
Nursing role	Offering compassion and understanding	Referring to counseling	Referring to counseling, safeguarding mother from injury to self or to newborn

FOCUS ON COMMUNICATION

Angie Burrows is a new mother, 48 hours postbirth, who is about to be discharged from the hospital. You notice that although her boyfriend visited with her, left some baby clothes, and then went downstairs to complete the discharge papers, Angie has made no attempt to change to street clothes or dress her new baby girl. The baby clothes her boyfriend left include a baseball-type shirt.

Less Effective Communication

Nurse: Ms. Burrows? Do you need some help with the baby?

Ms. Burrows: Are you sure I can't stay? I'm too tired to go home.

Nurse: Your insurance won't pay if you stay. [Ms. Burrows starts to cry.]

Ms. Burrows: This isn't right. I am just too tired to go home.

Nurse: It's the baby blues. If you change your mind and do need help with the baby, let me know. I'll be glad to do it for you.

More Effective Communication

Nurse: Ms. Burrows? Do you need some help with the baby?

Ms. Burrows: Are you sure I can't stay? I'm too tired to go home.

Nurse: Tell me more about that. [Ms. Burrows starts to cry.]

Ms. Burrows: I'm tired all over. It would be easier for me to kill myself than go home, try and take care of this baby myself, work full time, and still finish school.

Nurse: Is that different from how you thought things would be after you had the baby?

Ms. Burrows: I thought he'd ask me to marry him. I bet he would have if I'd had a boy instead of a girl.

Nurse: I'm worried about you going home, too.

Almost all women experience some fatigue after childbirth. As many as 75% experience a temporary feeling of sadness (baby blues). About 10%, however, develop depression severe enough to need therapy. Be sure to ask enough questions to be certain that a woman's crying is not something more serious than simple "baby blues" before discharge from a health care facility. In this way, women who have more serious problems can be referred to the proper professionals.

✔ CHECKPOINT QUESTIONS

11. Are breastfeeding women typically prescribed sulfa drugs for UTIs?
12. Do women with "baby blues" experience hallucinations?

KEY POINTS

Establishing a firm family–newborn relationship may be difficult when a woman has a postpartal complication. Investigate ways that will allow the woman to care for her baby or offer necessary support to family members so they can fulfill this role.

Hemorrhage is a major danger in the immediate postpartal period. It is defined as a loss of blood over 500 mL within a 24-hour period. The most frequent cause of postpartal hemorrhage is uterine atony. Remember that continuous limited blood loss can be as important over time as sudden, intense bleeding. With hemorrhage, administration of oxytocin may be necessary to initiate uterine tone and halt hemorrhage.

Other causes of hemorrhage include lacerations (vaginal, cervical, or perineal) and retained placental fragments. Lacerations are most apt to occur with forceps birth or with the birth of a large infant. DIC also may cause postpartum hemorrhage.

Puerperal infection is a potential complication after any birth until the denuded placental surface has healed. Retained placental fragments and the use of internal fetal heart monitoring leads are potential sources of infection.

Thrombophlebitis, an inflammation of the lining of a blood vessel, occurs most often as an extension of an endometrial infection. Therapy includes bedrest with moist heat applications and anticoagulant therapy. Never massage the leg of a woman with phlebitis or thrombophlebitis; it may cause the clot to move and become a pulmonary embolus, a possibly fatal complication.

Mastitis is infection of the breast. The symptoms include pain, swelling, and redness in a breast. Antibiotic therapy is necessary.

A woman whose child is born with a physical or cognitive challenge needs special consideration after the birth. This is obviously a time of stress, and the woman needs supportive nursing care.

Postpartal "blues" are a normal accompaniment to birth. Postpartal depression (a feeling of extreme sadness) and postpartal psychosis (an actual separation from reality) are not normal and need accurate assessment so women can receive adequate therapy for these conditions.

CRITICAL THINKING EXERCISES

1. Ms. Blackhawk, whom you met at the beginning of the chapter, was having significant vaginal

bleeding at 4 hours postpartum. Because she was sleeping, however, she was totally unaware of it. What action on your part would have prevented so much blood loss? What action would be most appropriate now?

2. A new mother, 8 hours postpartum, tells you she has frequency and burning on urination. She had a urinary tract infection during pregnancy so she recognizes the symptoms. She has some medicine left from pregnancy and tells you she will take this to cure the infection. What advice would you give her?
3. A 39-year-old client entered her pregnancy with marked varicose veins. One day postpartum, you notice red streaks on both legs along the course of the veins, and she has pain on dorsiflexion of her foot. You are concerned she is developing a thrombophlebitis. Describe a plan of care that could have reduced this risk during labor and in the immediate postpartal period.
4. Examine the National Health Goals related to postpartal complications. Most government-sponsored money for nursing research is allotted based on these goals. What would be a possible research topic to explore pertinent to these goals that would be both fundable and advance evidence-based practice?

REFERENCES

American College of Obstetricians & Gynecologists. (2002). ACOG committee opinion: Placenta accreta. *Obstetrics & Gynecology, 99*(1), 169–170.

American Psychiatric Association. (2000). *Diagnostic and statistical manual (DSM-IV).* Washington, DC: Author.

Chang, D., & Markman, B. S. (2002). Spontaneous resolution of a pubic-symphysis diastasis. *New England Journal of Medicine, 346*(1), 39–40.

Cunningham, F. G., et al. (2001). *Williams obstetrics* (21st ed.). Stamford, CT: Appleton & Lange.

Department of Health and Human Services. (2000). *Healthy people 2010.* Washington, DC: Author.

Farrington, P. F. & Ward, K. (2000). Normal labor, delivery and puerperium. In J. R. Scott, et al. (Eds.). *Danforth's obstetrics and gynecology* (8th ed., pp. 91–109). Philadelphia: Lippincott Williams & Wilkins.

Fiorica, J. V. (2000). The breast. In J. R. Scott, et al. (Eds.). *Danforth's obstetrics and gynecology* (8th ed., pp. 631–648). Philadelphia: Lippincott Williams & Wilkins.

Johnson, M., Maas, M., & Moorhead, S. (2000). *Nursing outcomes classification* (2nd ed.). St. Louis: Mosby.

Karch, A. M. (2001). *Lippincott's nursing drug guide.* Philadelphia: Lippincott Williams & Wilkins.

Leathers, S. J. & Kelley, M. A. (2000). Unintended pregnancy and depressive symptoms among first-time mothers and fathers. *American Journal of Orthopsychiatry, 70*(4), 523–531.

McCloskey, J. & Bulechek, G. (2000). *Nursing interventions classification* (3rd ed.). St. Louis: Mosby.

Meyer, S. et al. (2001). Pelvic floor education after vaginal delivery. *Obstetrics & Gynecology, 97*(5.1), 673–677.

Nel, J. T., et al. (2001). A prospective clinical and urodynamic study of bladder function during and after pregnancy. *International Urogynecology Journal & Pelvic Floor Dysfunction, 12*(1), 21–26.

Salonen, R. et al. (2001). Increased risks of circulatory diseases in late pregnancy and puerperium. *Epidemiology, 12*(4), 46–460.

Signorello, L. B. et al. (2001). Postpartum sexual functioning and its relationship to perineal trauma: A retrospective cohort study of primiparous women. *American Journal of Obstetrics & Gynecology, 184*(5), 881–890.

Zlotnick, C. et al. (2001). Postpartum depression in women receiving public assistance: Pilot study of an interpersonal-therapy-oriented group intervention. *American Journal of Psychiatry, 158*(4), 638–640.

SUGGESTED READINGS

Albers, L. L. (2000). Health problems after childbirth. *Journal of Midwifery & Women's Health, 45*(1), 55–57.

Beck, C. T. & Gable, R. K. (2001). Further validation of the postpartum Depression Screening Scale. *Nursing Research, 50*(3), 155–64.

Brewley, C. & Bradshaw, C. (2001). Thromboembolic disorders during pregnancy, birth and puerperium. *Midwifery Digest, 11*(1), 56–59.

Da Costa, D., et al. (2000). Psychosocial correlates of prepartum and postpartum depressed mood. *Journal of Affective Disorders, 59*(1), 31–40.

Durik, A. M., Hyde, J. S., & Clark, R. (2000). Sequelae of cesarean and vaginal deliveries: psychosocial outcomes for mothers and infants. *Developmental Psychology, 36*(2), 251–260.

Hayes, B. A., Muller, R., & Bradley, B. S. (2001). Perinatal depression: A randomized controlled trial of an antenatal education intervention for primiparas. *Birth, 28*(1), 28–35.

Perla, L. (2002). Patient compliance and satisfaction with nursing care during delivery and recovery. *Journal of Nursing Care Quality, 16*(2), 60–66.

Ray, K. L. & Hodnett, E. D. (2002). Caregiver support for postpartum depression. *Cochrane Database of Systematic Reviews, 1*(1).

26

CHAPTER

Nursing Care of the High-Risk Newborn and Family

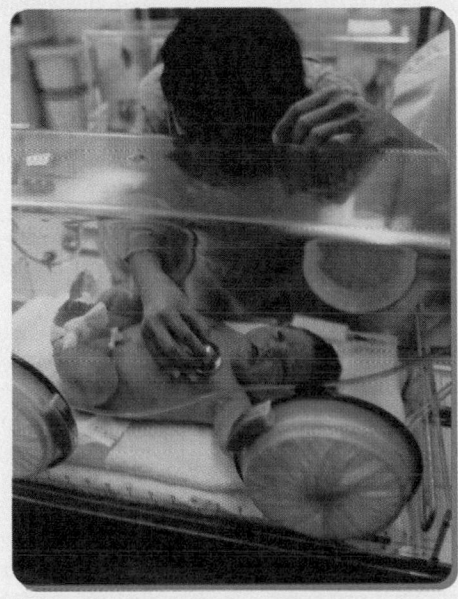

Key Terms

- apnea
- apparent life-threatening event
- appropriate for gestational age
- brown fat
- caudal regression syndrome
- cephalopelvic disproportion
- developmental care
- dysmature
- extracorporeal membrane oxygenation (ECMO)
- extremely very-low-birthweight
- fetal alcohol syndrome or exposure
- gestational age
- hemorrhagic disease of the newborn
- hydrops fetalis
- hyperbilirubinemia
- hyperglycemia
- hypocalcemia
- hypoglycemia
- intrauterine growth restriction or retardation
- kernicterus
- large for gestational age
- low-birthweight infant
- macrosomia
- ophthalmia neonatorum
- periodic respirations
- periventricular leukomalacia
- postterm infant
- postterm syndrome
- preterm infant
- primary apnea
- retinopathy of prematurity
- secondary apnea
- shoulder dystocia
- small for gestational age
- term infant
- very-low-birthwelght infant

Objectives

After mastering the contents of this chapter, you should be able to:

1. Define the following terms: small-for-gestational-age infant, term infant, large-for-gestational-age infant, preterm infant, and postterm infant and describe common illnesses that occur in these high-risk newborns.
2. Assess a high-risk newborn to determine if safe transition to extra-uterine life occurred.
3. List nursing diagnoses related to the high-risk newborn.
4. Identify appropriate outcomes for the high-risk newborn and family.
5. Plan novice-level nursing care focusing on priorities to stabilize the high-risk newborn's body systems.
6. Implement novice-level nursing care for the high-risk newborn.
7. Evaluate established outcomes to determine achievement and effectiveness of care.
8. Identify National Health Goals related to high-risk newborns that nurses could be instrumental in helping the nation to achieve.
9. Identify areas related to the care of high-risk newborns that could benefit from additional nursing research or application of evidence-based practice.
10. Use critical thinking to analyze the special crisis imposed on families when alterations of newborn development or neonatal illness occur to make nursing family-centered.
11. Integrate knowledge of the needs of the high-risk infant with nursing process to achieve quality maternal and child health nursing care.

Mr. and Mrs. Atkins had a 36-week-old, 2-lb baby boy last night after a short, 4-hour labor. The baby took a few gasping respirations at birth but then stopped breathing. He was resuscitated by the neonatal nurse practitioner and respiratory therapist and then transported to the intensive care nursery. Mr. Atkins was not present for the birth because he was out of town on business. You notice Mrs. Atkins has not visited the intensive care nursery to see her son. She also refused to sign the birth certificate because she could not decide on a name. She said, "I don't want to give him our favorite name because he might die." Mr. Atkins telephoned early this morning and acted more upset that the baby was born than relieved that the baby was receiving intensive care. You hear him ask his wife, "What did you do to cause this?" What type of help do the Atkins need to better accept what has happened?

Previous chapters described caring for the newborn who is well at birth. This chapter adds information about how to care for the newborn who is ill or has a significant variation in gestational age or weight. This is important information because learning to recognize these infants at birth and organizing care for them can be instrumental in helping protect both their present and future health.

After you've studied the chapter, answer the Critical Thinking Exercises at the end of the chapter and then access the on-line study activities (http//connection.lww.com) *to further sharpen your skills and test your knowledge of this nursing care area.*

During pregnancy, screening for risk factors that may lead to illness in the newborn is essential (see Chapter 10, Table 10-5). As described in previous chapters, maternal age (very young or older than average), concurrent disease conditions (e.g., diabetes), pregnancy complications (e.g., placenta previa), and an unhealthy maternal lifestyle (e.g., drug abuse) all signify risk potential for the newborn. In addition, the infant who is born **dysmature** (before term or postterm, or who is under- or overweight for gestational age) is also at risk for complications at birth and in the first few days of life. However, not all instances of high risk can be predicted. Even the newborn from a "perfect" pregnancy may require specialized care or develop a problem over the first few days of life necessitating special interventions. With shorter hospital lengths of stay for newborns, parents need thorough education because these problems may require rehospitalization or additional follow-up at home. National Health Goals related to the high-risk newborn are shown in Focus on National Health Goals.

Being able to predict that an infant is at high risk allows for advanced preparation so that specialized, skilled health care personnel can be present at the child's birth and perform necessary interventions, such as resuscitating the newborn who has difficulty establishing respirations. Immediate, skilled handling of any problems that occur may help to save the newborn's life and also prevent future problems, such as neurologic disorders.

FOCUS ON NATIONAL HEALTH GOALS

Preterm birth has the potential for leading to so many complications in newborns that National Health Goals were written specifically concerning it:

- Reduce low birth weight (LBW) to an incidence of no more than 5% of live births and very low birth weight (VLBW) to an incidence of no more than 0.9% of live births from baselines of 7.6% and 1.4%, respectively.
- Reduce fetal and infant deaths during the perinatal period (28 weeks of gestation to 7 days or more after birth) to 4.5/1,000 live births from a baseline of 7.5/1,000 live births.
- Reduce neonatal deaths within the first 28 days of life to 2.9/1,000 live births from a baseline of 4.8/1,000 live births.
- Reduce deaths from sudden infant death syndrome (SIDS) to 0.25/1,000 live births from a baseline of 0.72/1,000 live births (DHHS, 2000).

Nurses can be instrumental in helping the nation achieve these goals by teaching women the symptoms of preterm labor so that, ideally, birth can be delayed until infants are term. They also need to be prepared for resuscitation at birth of preterm infants and to plan developmental care that can help prevent conditions such as apnea, intraventricular hemorrhage, and periventricular leukomalacia.

Further research is needed as to how best to position infants to promote development and prevent fatigue, what measures can best prevent conditions such as intraventricular hemorrhage, and what measures can make parents feel most comfortable and allow them to interact with their infants best in neonatal intensive care units.

NURSING PROCESS OVERVIEW

For the Family of a High-Risk Newborn

Assessment

All infants should be assessed at birth for obvious congenital anomalies and **gestational age** (number of weeks they remained in utero). Both determinations can be done by the nurse who first inspects the infant. Be certain that these assessments are made with the infant under a prewarmed radiant heat warmer to safeguard against heat loss.

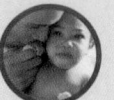

Continuing assessment of high-risk infants involves the use of instrumentation such as cardiac, apnea, and blood pressure monitoring. However, no matter how many monitors are used, they never replace the role of frequent, close, common-sense observation. Carefully evaluate comments from fellow nurses that an infant "isn't himself" or "breathes oddly." These comments, although not scientific, are the same observations that a parent who knows his or her baby well reports at health visits. A nurse who knows an infant well from having cared for the child consistently over time often senses changes before a monitor or other equipment begins to put a quantitative measurement on the factor.

Nursing Diagnosis

To establish nursing diagnoses for high-risk infants, it is important to be aware of the normal assessment parameters of this population. Nursing diagnosis generally centers on the eight priority areas of care for any newborn:

- Ineffective airway clearance related to presence of mucus or amniotic fluid in airway
- Ineffective cardiovascular tissue perfusion related to breathing difficulties
- Risk for deficient fluid volume related to insensible water loss
- Ineffective thermoregulation related to newborn status and stress from birthweight variation
- Risk for imbalanced nutrition, less than body requirements related to lack of energy for sucking
- Risk for infection related to lowered immune response in newborn
- Risk for impaired parenting related to illness in newborn at birth
- Deficient diversional activity (lack of stimulation) related to illness at birth

Outcome Identification and Planning

Be certain when establishing outcomes that they are consistent with the newborn's potential. A goal that implies complete recovery from a major illness may be unrealistic for one newborn, although completely appropriate for another. Plan individualized care that considers the newborn's developmental as well as physiologic strengths, weaknesses, and needs. This helps to ensure that parents as well as the health care team have a good understanding of the newborn's particular care priorities and potential. Include the parents in plans and interventions.

Implementation

Interventions for any high-risk newborn are best carried out by a consistent caregiver and should focus on conserving the baby's energy and providing a thermoneutral environment to prevent exhaustion and chilling. Painful procedures should be kept to a minimum to help the infant achieve a sense of comfort and balance. Parent teaching and participation with care such as bathing or feeding the infant in the nursery may help make the child seem real to them. It may also help the bonding process.

Many families of high-risk newborns will continue care of the infant at home. They may need referral to a home health care or other agency. Examples of organizations that may be helpful include:

- American Sudden Infant Death Syndrome Institute (*www.SIDS.org*)
- American Association of Premature Infants (*www.AAPI-online.org*)
- Sudden Infant Death Alliance (*www.SIDSalliance.org*)

Outcome Evaluation

High-risk newborns need long-term follow-up so that any consequences of their birth status, such as minimal neurologic injury, can be identified and arrangements for special schooling or counseling can be made for the toddler, preschool, and school years. Examples of outcomes include the following:

- Infant maintains a patent airway.
- Infant tolerates all procedures without accompanying apnea.
- Infant demonstrates growth and development appropriate for gestational age, birthweight, and condition.
- Infant maintains body temperature at 98.6°F (37.0°C) in open crib with one added blanket.
- Parents visit at least once and make three telephone calls to neonatal nursery weekly.
- Parents demonstrate positive coping skills and behaviors in response to newborn's condition.

NEWBORN PRIORITIES IN FIRST DAYS OF LIFE

All newborns have eight priority needs in the first few days of life:

1. Initiation and maintenance of respirations
2. Establishment of extrauterine circulation
3. Control of body temperature
4. Intake of adequate nourishment
5. Establishment of waste elimination
6. Prevention of infection
7. Establishment of an infant–parent relationship
8. **Developmental care,** or care that balances physiologic needs and stimulation for mental development.

These are also the priority needs of high-risk newborns. However, fulfilling these needs may require special equipment or care measures. Not all newborns will be able to achieve full wellness because of extreme insults to health at birth. Indications that the newborn is having difficulty making the transition from intrauterine to extrauterine life may be apparent during the intrapartum period, at birth, or at initial assessment using the Apgar scoring system (see Chap. 23 for an explanation of the Apgar score).

Initiating and Maintaining Respirations

Ultimately, the prognosis of the high-risk newborn depends primarily on how the first moments of life are managed. Most deaths occurring during the first 48 hours after birth result from the newborn's inability to establish or maintain adequate respirations (Department of Health and Human Services, 2000). An infant who has difficulty accomplishing effective respiratory action in the first hours of life and yet survives may experience residual neurologic dysfunction because of cerebral hypoxia. Prompt, thorough care is necessary for effective intervention.

Most infants are born with some degree of respiratory acidosis. However, this is rapidly corrected by the spontaneous onset of respirations. If respiratory activity does not begin immediately, however, respiratory acidosis will increase. The blood pH and bicarbonate buffer system will fail. Newborn defense mechanisms are inadequate to reverse the process. Therefore, the effort to establish respirations must be begun immediately after birth. By 2 minutes, the development of severe acidosis is already well under way.

Any infant who sustains some degree of asphyxia in utero, such as from cord compression, maternal anesthesia, placenta previa, or preterm separation of the placenta, may already be experiencing acidosis at birth and may have difficulty before the first 2 minutes after birth.

Resuscitation

Factors that commonly predispose infants to respiratory difficulty and thus may require resuscitation are shown in Box 26-1. If breathing is ineffective, circulatory shunts, particularly the ductus arteriosus, fail to close. Because left-side heart pressure is stronger than right-side pressure, blood circulates through a patent ductus arteriosus left to right or from the aorta to the pulmonary artery, creating ineffective pump action in the heart. Struggling to breathe and circulate blood, an infant uses available serum glucose quickly and may become hypoglycemic, thus compounding the problem.

For all these reasons, resuscitation becomes important for an infant who fails to take a first breath or has difficulty maintaining adequate respiratory movements on his or her own.

Resuscitation follows an organized process: (1) establishing and maintaining an airway, (2) expanding the lungs, and (3) initiating and maintaining effective ventilation. If respiratory depression becomes severe, the heart will fail. Resuscitation then must also include cardiac massage (American Heart Association, 2000). Box 26-2 highlights

BOX 26.1

FACTORS PREDISPOSING INFANTS TO RESPIRATORY DIFFICULTY IN THE FIRST FEW DAYS OF LIFE

Low birth weight
Maternal history of diabetes
Premature rupture of membranes
Maternal history of reserpine use
Maternal use of barbiturates or narcotics close to birth
Meconium staining
Irregularities detected by fetal heart monitor during labor
Cord prolapse
Lowered Apgar score (under 7) at 1 or 5 minutes
Postmaturity
Small for gestational age
Breech birth
Multiple birth
Chest, heart, or respiratory tract anomalies

BOX 26.2

NURSING OUTCOMES AND NURSING INTERVENTIONS CLASSIFICATION: NEONATAL RESUSCITATION

NOC: Respiratory Status, Gas Exchange

Respiratory status, gas exchange is defined as the alveolar exchange of carbon dioxide or oxygen to maintain arterial blood gas concentrations (Johnson, Maas, & Moorehead, 2000). Some specific indicators suggesting achievement of this outcome include the following:

- Uncompromised ease of breathing
- Absence of restlessness, cyanosis, and dyspnea
- Arterial blood gas values, including Po_2, Pco_2, pH, and oxygen saturation, within normal limits
- Chest x-ray findings within expected parameters

NIC: Resuscitation, Neonate

Resuscitation, neonate, is defined as the administration of emergency measures to support newborn adaptation to extrauterine life (McCloskey & Bulechek, 2000). Some important activities involved when implementing this intervention include:

- Setting up necessary equipment before birth, including testing resuscitation bag, suction, and oxygen flow to ensure proper function
- Drying with a prewarmed blanket and placing neonate under radiant warmer on back with neck slightly extended, using a rolled blanket under the shoulders to assist with correct positioning
- Suctioning nose and mouth with a bulb syringe
- Using tactile stimulation
- Inserting laryngoscope to visualize trachea and intubating to remove meconium from lower trachea if appropriate; repeating procedure until return is clear
- Monitoring heart rate and respirations
- Initiating positive-pressure ventilation for apnea or gasping
- Ventilating with properly fitting, tightly sealed resuscitation bag filled with 100% oxygen at a rate of 40 to 60 breaths per minute using 20 to 40 cm of water (for initial breaths) and 15 to 20 cm of water for subsequent pressures, continuing ventilations until adequate spontaneous respirations begin and color becomes pink
- Administering chest compressions for heart rate of less than 60 bpm or less than 80 bpm with no increase in conjunction with ongoing assessment until heart rate is greater than 80 bpm
- Auscultating breath sounds
- Inserting endotracheal tube for prolonged ventilation or poor response to bag and mask ventilation followed by auscultation of breath sounds to confirm placement
- Securing the airway
- Administering medications as ordered

appropriate outcomes and interventions using the terminology identified by the Nursing Outcomes Classification (NOC) and Nursing Interventions Classification (NIC) for neonatal resuscitation.

Airway

For the well term newborn, usually bulb syringe suction, which removes mucus and prevents aspiration of any mucus and amniotic fluid present in the mouth or nose with the first breath, is all that is necessary to help establish a clear airway (see Chap. 23).

If a newborn does not draw in a first breath spontaneously, suction the infant's mouth and nose with a bulb syringe again and rub the back to see if skin stimulation initiates respirations. Be certain the infant is dry, including the hair and head, to prevent chilling. If the newborn has to attempt to raise body temperature, this will increase the need for oxygen, which the baby cannot supply because breathing has not yet been initiated. Warmed, blow-by oxygen by face mask or positive-pressure mask may be administered.

If deeper suctioning is required, place the infant on the back and slide a folded towel or pad under the shoulders to raise them slightly so the head is in a neutral position. Slide a catheter (8F to 12F) over the infant's tongue to the back of the throat (Fig. 26-1). Do not suction for longer than 10 seconds at a time (count seconds as you suction) to avoid removing excessive air from the infant's lungs. Use a gentle touch. Bradycardia or cardiac arrhythmias can occur because of vagus stimulation (at the posterior oropharynx) from vigorous suctioning.

The infant who still makes no effort at spontaneous respirations requires immediate laryngoscopy to open the airway. Once the laryngoscope is inserted, tracheal suctioning may be performed. After deep suctioning, an endotracheal tube can be inserted and oxygen can be administered by a positive-pressure bag and mask with 100% oxygen at 40 to 60 breaths per minute.

In the first few seconds of life, a newborn this severely depressed may take several weak gasps of air and then almost immediately stop breathing; the heart rate begins to fall. This period of halted respirations is termed **primary apnea.** After 1 or 2 minutes of apnea, the infant again tries to initiate respirations with a few strong gasps. However, the child cannot maintain this effort longer than 4 or 5 minutes. After this, the respiratory effort will become weaker again and the heart rate will fall further until the infant stops the gasping effort altogether. The infant then enters a period of **secondary apnea.** Although usually a phenomenon that occurs after birth, both types of apnea may occur in utero.

During the period of the first gasps, resuscitation attempts are generally successful. Once a newborn is allowed to enter the secondary apnea period, however, resuscitation measures become difficult and may be ineffective. Because it is impossible to distinguish between the two periods simply by observation, resuscitation must always be started as if secondary apnea were occurring.

An obstetrician, pediatrician, neonatologist, anesthesiologist, or neonatal nurse practitioner skilled in laryngoscope and endotracheal tube insertion should be present at the birth of all identified high-risk infants. Laryngoscope insertion is easy in theory; in practice, the wide variation in size of infants' posterior pharynx and trachea and the emergency conditions always present make it difficult (Fig. 26-2).

Laryngoscopes are equipped with different-size blades. Size 0 or 1 is used with newborns. The endotracheal tube fits inside the laryngoscope. Infants under 1,000 g need a size 2.5-mm endotracheal tube; those over 3,000 g need a 4.0-mm tube. Because preterm infants are prone to hemorrhage owing to capillary fragility, extra care during insertion is crucial.

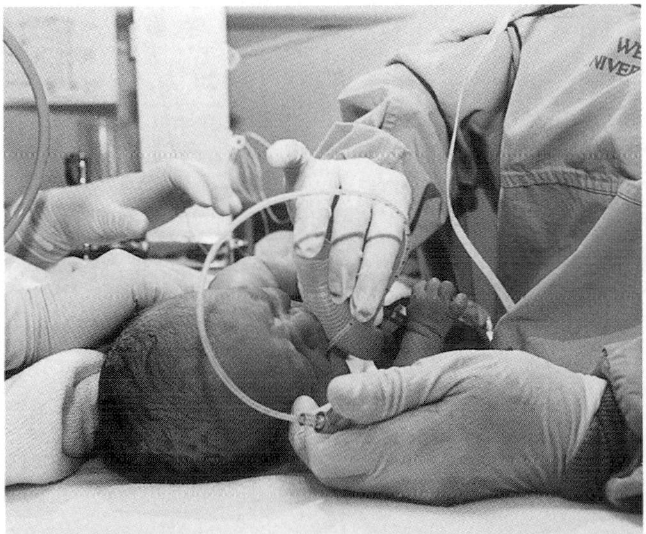

FIGURE 26.1 Suctioning a newborn with mechanical suction controlled by a finger valve. Suction is applied as the catheter is withdrawn. If the catheter is rotated as it is withdrawn, the risk of traumatizing membrane is reduced.

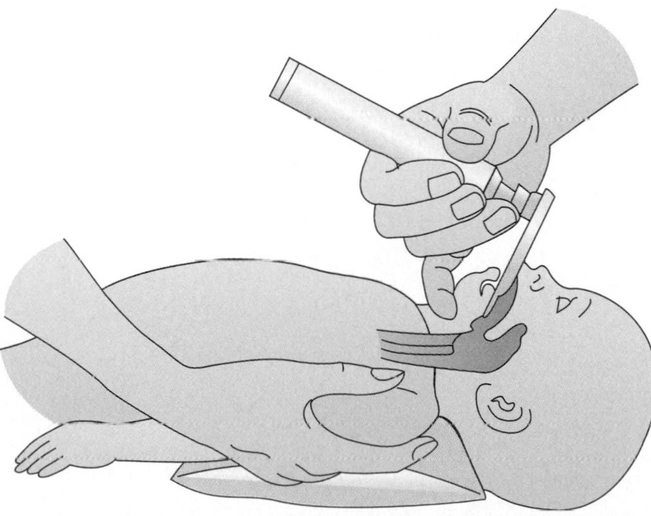

FIGURE 26.2 Intubation. Place the head in a neutral position with a towel under the shoulders. The blade of the laryngoscope is inserted to reveal the vocal cords. An endotracheal tube for ventilation is passed into the trachea, past the laryngoscope.

Lung Expansion

Once an airway has been established, the newborn's lungs need to be expanded. A well newborn inflates his or her lungs adequately with the first breath. The sound of a baby crying is proof that lung expansion is good because the vocal sounds are produced by a free flow of air over the vocal cords.

An infant who breathes spontaneously but then is unable to sustain effective respirations may need oxygen by bag and mask to aid lung expansion. The mask should cover both the mouth and the nose to be effective. It should not cover the eyes, because it can cause eye injury mechanically from the mask or drying of the cornea from oxygen administration. Administer 100% oxygen by face mask and pressure bag at a rate of 40 to 60 compressions per minute. To prevent cooling, oxygen should be administered both warmed (between 89.6° and 93.2°F, or 32° and 34°C) and humidified (60–80%).

Remember that the pressure needed to open lung alveoli for the first time is approximately 40 cm H_2O. After that, pressures of 15 to 20 cm H_2O are generally adequate to continue inflating alveoli. The pressure from anesthesia bags is controlled solely by the pressure of a hand against the bag. Other types of bags such as the AMBU bag can be set with a blow-off valve that limits the pressure in the apparatus (Fig. 26-3).

Once established, oxygen levels in the newborn must not fluctuate; lack of fluctuation helps to prevent bleeding from immature cranial vessels. In addition, no pressure above what is necessary should be used because excessive force can rupture lung alveoli. On the other hand, if adequate insufflation is not achieved, a newborn stands little chance of survival. To be certain that oxygen is reaching the lungs, auscultate the chest while simultaneously administering oxygen. In many newborns, this degree of resuscitation will initiate responsive respirations and a strong heartbeat. Color, muscle response, and reflexes will improve. Monitor the newborn's oxygen level with pulse oximetry.

If the newborn's amniotic fluid was meconium-stained, do not stimulate the infant to breathe by rubbing the back or administering air or oxygen under pressure. Doing so could push meconium down into the infant's airway, further compromising respirations. Give oxygen by mask without pressure. Wait for a laryngoscope to be passed and the trachea to be deep suctioned before oxygen under pressure is given.

As soon as a newborn has been intubated, oxygen is administered. Listen with a stethoscope to both lungs to be certain that both sides are being aerated. If air can be heard on only one side or sounds are not symmetric, the endotracheal tube is probably at the bifurcation of the trachea and blocking one of the mainstem bronchi. Drawing it back half a centimeter will usually free it and allow oxygen to flow to both lungs.

When oxygen is given under pressure to a newborn, the stomach also quickly fills with oxygen. If the resuscitation continues for over 2 minutes, inserting an orogastric tube and leaving the distal end open will help deflate the stomach and decrease the possibility that vomiting and aspiration of stomach contents will occur.

Drug Therapy

Stimulants have little place in newborn resuscitation unless an infant's respiratory depression appears to be related to the administration of a narcotic such as morphine or meperidine (Demerol) to the mother during labor. In these instances, a narcotic antagonist such as naloxone (Narcan) injected into an umbilical vessel or intramuscularly will relieve the depression (see Focus on Pharmacology: Naloxone). The dose of naloxone is determined by institutional policy but is usually 0.01 to 0.1 mg/kg body weight (Karch, 2001). However, if there is suspicion of maternal drug abuse, naloxone is

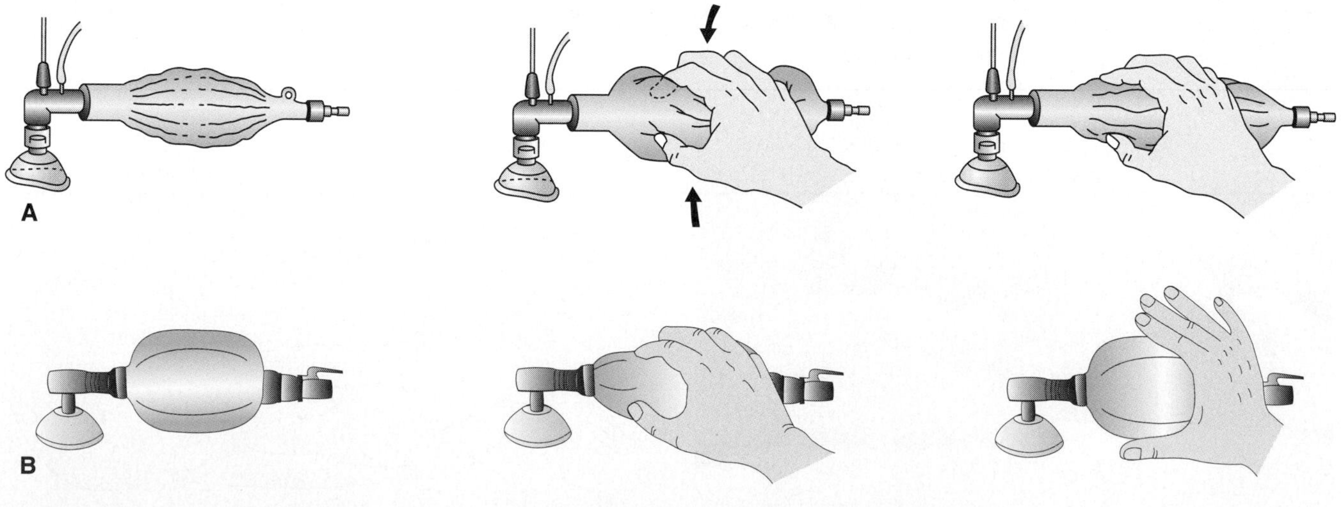

FIGURE 26.3 Types of ventilation bags used in neonatal resuscitation. (*A*) The flow-inflating (anesthesia) bag requires a compressed gas source for inflation but is able to deliver 100% oxygen. (*B*) The self-inflating (Ambu) bag remains inflated at all times and is not dependent on a compressed gas source. It is limited to delivering oxygen concentration of 40%, which is inadequate for resuscitation at birth.

FOCUS ON PHARMACOLOGY

Naloxone (Narcan)

Action: Naloxone, a pure narcotic antagonist, is administered parenterally to reverse the effects, such as respiratory depression, that may occur with opioid narcotic agents.

Pregnancy risk category: B

Dosage: Initially 0.01 mg/kg IV. Dosage may be repeated at 2- to 3-minute intervals.

Possible adverse reactions: Hypertension, irritability, tachycardia

Nursing Implications
- Assess respiratory status carefully, including rate, depth, and character of respirations.
- Anticipate the need for repeat doses.
- Maintain a patent airway at all times.
- Have emergency resuscitation equipment readily available and prepare to resuscitate if necessary.

BOX 26.3

DRUG THERAPY

Drugs commonly used in newborn resuscitation include:

Atropine: Reduces bronchial secretions, keeping the airway clear during resuscitation. Reduces vagus nerve effects, relieving bradycardia.
Calcium chloride: Increases heart contractility.
Dopamine: Increase systemic blood perfusion by increasing blood pressure through beta-agonist action.
Epinephrine: Strengthens or initiates cardiac contractions; increases heart rate and blood pressure.
Lidocaine: Counteracts ventricular arrhythmias by decreasing automaticity of ventricular cells.
Sodium bicarbonate ($NaHCO_3$) or tromethamine: Corrects metabolic acidosis. Caution: Do not give these unless ventilation is adequate or acidosis can be increased by retained CO_2.

Many preterm infants have such respiratory distress at birth that they need continued therapy, including:

Surfactant: All preterm infants weighing under 1,500 g receive surfactant administered by endotracheal tube at birth (see Focus on Pharmacology: Surfactant). Some newborns need administration of additional surfactant to prevent symptoms of respiratory distress syndrome.
Nitric oxide: Nitric oxide is a potent vascular dilator. Because it dilates the capillaries next to alveoli, it reduces the pulmonary resistance and therefore increases oxygenation.
Liquid ventilation: Liquid ventilation is the instillation of liquid fluorocarbon (Perflubron) into the lungs. It fills and clings to alveoli. Perflubron is not absorbed by the body but instead leaves the lungs by evaporation. It acts as an anti-inflammatory and can reduce oxygen toxicity and perhaps infection because bacteria cannot live in the medium. Adverse effects may be pneumothorax and mucus plugging.

not used because it can cause acute withdrawal in the neonate. In addition to naloxone, other drug therapies also may be used (see Box 26-3 and Focus on Pharmacology: Surfactant).

Ventilation Maintenance

To allow a newborn to adjust to and maintain cardiovascular changes, effective ventilation (continued respirations) must be maintained. A healthy newborn accomplishes this task on his or her own. All infants, especially those who had difficulty establishing respirations at birth, should be carefully observed in the next few hours to be certain that respirations are maintained.

An increasing respiratory rate in the newborn is often the first sign of obstruction or respiratory compromise. If the respiratory rate is increased, undress the baby's chest and look for retractions (inward sucking of the anterior chest wall on inspiration). Retractions reflect the difficulty the newborn is having in drawing in air (tugging so hard to inflate the lungs that the anterior chest muscles are drawn in).

The newborn who is having difficulty with breathing should be placed under an infant warmer and have the weight of clothing removed from the chest. Positioning the infant on the back with the head of the mattress elevated approximately 15° allows the abdominal contents to fall away from the diaphragm, affording optimal breathing space.

Keeping the infant warm is important in preventing acidosis. If secretions are accumulating in the respiratory tract, they must be suctioned. If the newborn has an endotracheal tube in place, perform tracheal suctioning. "Bagging" an infant for a minute before suctioning will improve the oxygen level and prevent it from dropping to dangerous levels during suctioning. Pulse oximetry and transcutaneous oxygen monitoring are techniques to monitor oxygen level (see Chap. 40). The cause of the respiratory distress must be determined, and appropriate interventions must be undertaken to correct the difficulty (see Chap. 40).

✔ CHECKPOINT QUESTIONS

1. If a newborn fails to spontaneously draw in a first breath, what should you do first?
2. What does a newborn's crying tell you about breathing?
3. What drug reverses the neonatal effects of a narcotic given to a mother in labor?

FOCUS ON PHARMACOLOGY

Surfactant (Survanta)

Action: Surfactant restores naturally occurring lung surfactant to improve lung compliance.

Pregnancy risk category: X

Dosage: 4 mL/kg intratracheally times four doses in first 48 hours of life

Possible adverse reactions: Transient bradycardia, rales

Nursing Implications

- Suction infant before administration.
- Assess infant's respiratory rate, rhythm, arterial blood gases, and color before administration.
- Ensure proper ET tube placement before dosing.
- Change infant's position during administration to encourage drug to flow to both lungs.
- Assess infant's respiratory rate, color, and arterial blood gases after administration.
- Do not suction ET tube for 1 hour after administration to avoid removing drug.

Establishing Extrauterine Circulation

Although establishing respirations is the usual priority at a high-risk infant's birth, lack of cardiac function may be present concurrently or may develop if respiratory function is not quickly restored. If there is no audible heartbeat, or if the cardiac rate is below 80 bpm, closed-chest massage should be started. Hold the infant with fingers supporting the back and depress the sternum with two fingers (see Chap. 41). Depress the sternum approximately ⅓ of its depth (1 or 2 cm) at a rate of 100 times per minute (American Heart Association, 2000). Lung ventilation at a rate of 30 times per minute should be continued and interspersed with the cardiac massage at a ratio of 1:3.

Continue to monitor transcutaneous oxygen or pulse oximetry to evaluate respiratory function and cardiac efficiency. If the pressure and the rate of massage are adequate, it should be possible, in addition, to palpate a femoral pulse. If heart sounds are not resumed above 80 bpm after 30 seconds of combined positive-pressure ventilation and cardiac compressions, 0.1 to 0.3 mL/kg of epinephrine (1:10,000) may be sprayed into the endotracheal tube to stimulate cardiac function (American Heart Association, 2000). Newborns who still have difficulty initiating cardiac function need to be transferred to a transitional or high-risk nursery for continuous cardiac surveillance.

Maintaining Fluid and Electrolyte Balance

After an initial resuscitation attempt, **hypoglycemia** (decreased blood glucose) may result from the effort the newborn expended to begin breathing. Assessment of serum glucose is necessary. Dehydration may result from increased insensible water loss from rapid respirations. Fluids such as Ringer's lactate or 5% dextrose in water are commonly used to maintain fluid and electrolyte levels. Electrolytes (particularly sodium and potassium) are added as necessary, depending on electrolyte analysis.

The rate of fluid administration must be carefully maintained because a high fluid intake can lead to patent ductus arteriosus or heart failure. When using a radiant warmer, there is an increase in water loss from convection and radiation. Thus, the newborn will require more fluid than if he or she were placed in a double-walled Isolette.

Urine output and urine specific gravity must also be carefully monitored. An output less than 2 mL/kg/h or a specific gravity greater than 1.015 to 1.020 suggests dehydration. Elevated specific gravity may also be caused by inappropriate antidiuretic hormone secretion or kidney failure due to a primary illness.

If an infant has hypotension without hypovolemia, a vasopressor such as dopamine may be given to increase blood pressure and improve cell perfusion. If hypovolemia is present, the cause is usually fetal blood loss from a condition such as placenta previa (see Chap. 15) or twin-to-twin transfusion. With hypovolemia, typically tachypnea, pallor, tachycardia, decreased arterial blood pressure, decreased central venous pressure, and decreased tissue perfusion of peripheral tissue, with a progressively developing metabolic acidosis, will be present. The hematocrit may be normal for some time after acute blood loss because blood cells present are in proportion to plasma. Normal saline or Ringer's lactate may be administered to increase blood volume. Control the rate carefully to prevent heart failure, patent ductus arteriosus, or intracranial hemorrhage from fluid pressure overload (Niermeyer et al., 2001).

Regulating Temperature

Any high-risk infant may have difficulty maintaining a normal temperature. In addition to stress from an illness or immaturity, the infant's body is often exposed during procedures such as resuscitation and blood drawing.

It is important to keep newborns in a neutral-temperature environment, one that is neither too hot nor too cold. Doing so places less demand on infants to maintain the minimal metabolic rate necessary for effective body functioning. If the environment is too hot, they must decrease metabolism to cool their body. If it is too cold, they must increase metabolism to warm body cells. If the infant should become chilled, this requires increased oxygen to raise the metabolic rate; without this oxygen available, body cells become hypoxic. To save oxygen for essential body functions, vasoconstriction of blood vessels occurs. If this process continues for too long, pulmonary vessels become affected and pulmonary perfusion is decreased. The infant's Po_2 level falls and Pco_2 increases. The decreased Po_2 level may open fetal right-to-left shunts again. Surfactant production may halt, which may further interfere with lung function. To supply glucose to maintain increased metabolism, the infant begins anaerobic glycolysis, which pours acid into the bloodstream. The infant becomes acidotic, and with acidosis comes the increased risk of **kernicterus** (invasion of brain cells with unconjugated bilirubin) as more bilirubin-binding sites are lost and more bilirubin is free to pass out of the bloodstream into brain cells.

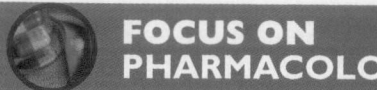

To prevent the newborn from becoming chilled after birth, wipe the infant dry, cover the head with a cap, and place him or her immediately under a prewarmed radiant warmer or in a warmed Isolette (Fig. 26-4). Air, Isolette, or radiant warmer temperatures should be kept regulated to maintain the infant's axillary temperature at 97.8°F (36.5°C). Be certain that during procedures an infant is not placed directly on cool x-ray tables, scales, or an unheated radiant warmer to prevent heat loss.

Radiant Heat Sources

Radiant heat warmers are open beds that have an overhead radiant heat source. Such units have Servocontrol probes, which when placed on the infant's skin continually monitor the infant's temperature. Abdominal skin temperature, when measured this way, should be 95.9° to 97.7°F (35.5° to 36.5°C). If the temperature falls below this level, an alarm will sound. Tape the probe or disk in place on the infant's abdomen between the umbilicus and the xiphoid process. Do not tape it under the infant or it will register a falsely high reading. Be sure it is not over the rib cage, where the thin subcutaneous tissue will not allow an accurate reading. Also do not place it over the liver, because increased metabolism may lead to falsely high readings. A plastic bridge or shield placed over the child will better preserve heat by reducing convection and radiation losses; plastic wrap placed over the infant will produce this same effect. When performing care or leaning over the infant, sometimes the heads of health care personnel can block the heat from an overhead source and keep it from reaching the baby. An additional warming pad placed under the infant may be necessary for very preterm infants or for lengthy procedures.

Isolettes

After an initial resuscitation attempt, newborns may be cared for in Isolettes (square, acrylic-sided incubators). The temperature of Isolettes varies with the amount of time portholes remain open and the temperature of the area in which the Isolette is placed. Placing it in direct sunlight or near a warm radiator can increase the internal temperature markedly. For this reason, the newborn's temperature must be checked at frequent intervals to be certain the temperature level designated is being maintained. Use of an additional acrylic shield inside the Isolette helps prevent radiation and convection heat loss when portholes are opened for care.

Similar to radiant warmers, some Isolettes have Servocontrol mechanism units that monitor the infant's temperature and automatically change the temperature of the Isolette as needed. Portholes must remain closed to keep the temperature steady.

As the infant's condition improves, weaning from an incubator may be necessary. Dress the infant as if he or

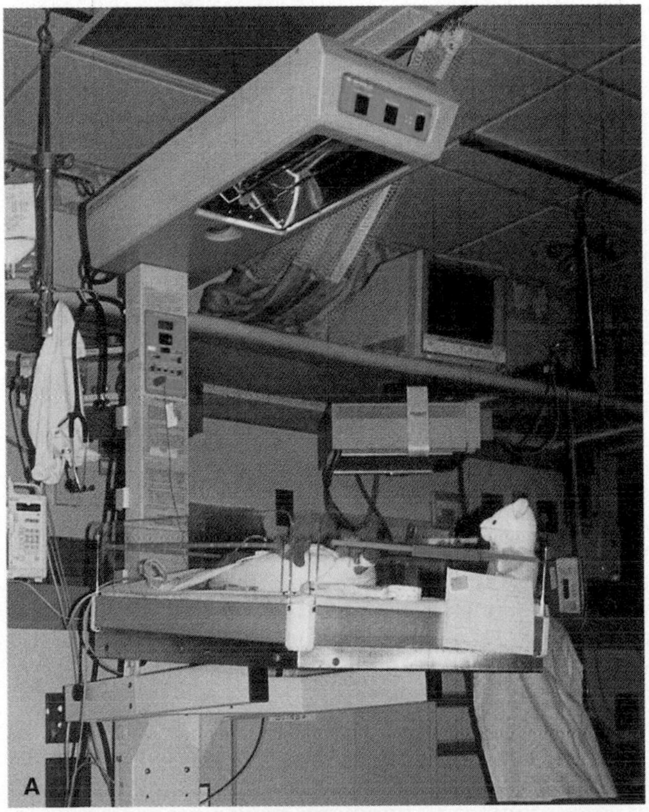

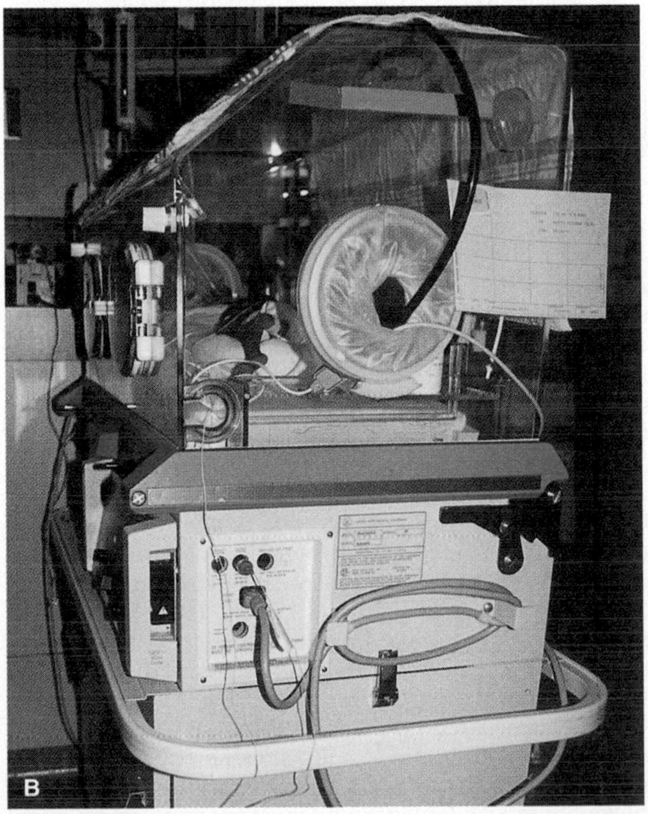

FIGURE 26.4 Neutral thermal environment. (*A*) The neonate in the intensive care bed with overhead radiant warmer can be examined periodically with ease. (*B*) Use of an incubator allows maintenance of a neutral thermal environment for neonates not requiring minute-to-minute intervention.

she were going to be in a bassinet, then set the incubator about 2°F (1.2°C) below the infant's temperature. After a half-hour, assess whether the infant is able to maintain body temperature. If so, lower the Isolette temperature another 2°F and continue until room temperature is reached. If the infant cannot maintain adequate temperature as the incubator temperature level is lowered, he or she is not yet ready for room-temperature air, and the weaning process needs to be slowed or stopped until the baby is more mature or better able to self-regulate temperature.

Kangaroo Care

Kangaroo care is the use of skin-to-skin contact to maintain body heat. The infant is undressed except for a diaper and perhaps a cap. The parent sits in a chair and holds the infant snugly against his or her chest, skin to skin (Kirsten et al., 2001). Typically, the infant and parent are placed in a quiet corner with lights dimmed. A blanket is placed over them to provide privacy. This method of care not only supplies heat but also encourages parent–child interaction (Mellien, 2001).

> **✔ CHECKPOINT QUESTIONS**
>
> 4. How far should you depress the sternum of the newborn when performing closed cardiac massage?
> 5. When using a radiant warmer, abdominal skin temperature should be maintained at what value?
> 6. What is the method of care used when the infant is placed skin to skin and chest to chest with another individual?

Establishing Adequate Nutritional Intake

An infant who experienced severe asphyxia at birth usually receives intravenous fluids until necrotizing enterocolitis (NEC) has been ruled out, as this could result from the temporary reduction in oxygen to the bowel (see Chap. 45 for a discussion of NEC). If the infant's respiratory rate remains rapid and NEC has been ruled out, gavage feeding may be necessary until the infant is older (Fig. 26-5). Preterm infants should be breast-fed if possible. If breast-feeding is not possible, the mother can manually express breast milk or use a breast pump to initiate and continue her milk supply until the infant is mature enough or otherwise ready for breast feeding. Expressed breast milk may be used in the infant's gavage feeding. Preterm infants reveal hunger by the same signs as term infants, such as rooting and crying and sucking motions. All babies who are gavage-fed need oral stimulation from nonnutritive sucking and should be supplied with a pacifier at feeding times. Exceptions are infants too immature to have a sucking reflex and infants who must not swallow air, such as those with a tracheoesophageal fistula awaiting surgery.

The techniques of gavage feeding, intravenous feeding, and gastrostomy feeding are all discussed in Chapter 36.

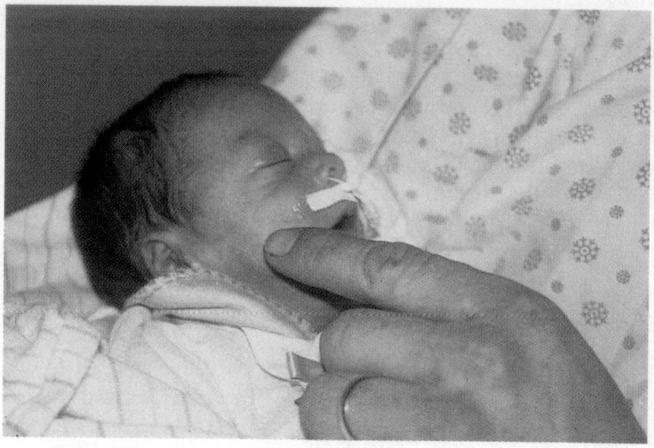

FIGURE 26.5 Infants who are ill at birth often need supplemental feedings by nasogastric or gastrostomy tube.

Establishing Waste Elimination

Although most immature infants void within 24 hours of birth, they may void later than term newborns because due to all the procedures that may be necessary for resuscitation, their blood pressure may not be adequate to fully supply their kidneys. Carefully document any voidings that occur during resuscitation. This is proof that hypotension is improving and that the kidneys are being perfused. Immature infants also may pass stool later than the term infant because meconium has not yet reached the end of the intestine by birth.

Preventing Infection

Contracting an infection would complicate a high-risk newborn's ability to adjust to extrauterine life. Infection increases metabolic oxygen demands, which the newborn may not be able to meet. In addition, infection stresses the immature immune system and already stressed defense mechanisms of the high-risk newborn. In some instances, such as preterm rupture of the membranes, it is the infection (e.g., pneumonia or skin lesions) that places the infant in a high-risk category.

Infections may have prenatal, perinatal, or postnatal causes. The most common viruses to affect infants in utero are the cytomegalovirus and toxoplasmosis viruses. An infant with either of these infections may be born with congenital anomalies (see Chap. 11). The most prevalent perinatal infections are those contracted from the vagina during birth: group B streptococcal septicemia, thrush from *Candida* infection, and herpes. Postnatal infection is most commonly spread to a newborn from health care personnel (Cunningham et al., 2001). All persons coming in contact with or caring for infants must observe good handwashing technique and standard precautions to reduce the risk of infection transmission. Health care personnel with infections have a professional and moral obligation to refrain from caring for newborns. Skin care is important to prevent skin breakdown and open portals of entry (Lund et al., 2001).

Establishing Parent–Infant Bonding

Women diagnosed as having a high-risk pregnancy should be offered a tour of a neonatal intensive care unit (NICU) so that if their infant should be admitted to an NICU, they will be more comfortable in the high-tech environment.

During resuscitation at birth, parents of the high-risk newborn should be kept informed of what is happening. They should be able to visit the special nursing unit to which the child is admitted as often as they choose, to wash and gown and hold and touch the child. This helps to make the child's birth more real to them. Should the child not survive the illness, these interactions may help make the death more real. Only when both birth and death seem real can parents begin to work through their feelings and accept these events.

All parents handle newborn babies tentatively until they have "claimed" them or have become better acquainted. It may be months before the parents of a child who has been ill since birth can handle the baby comfortably and confidently. The parents need to spend time with the infant in the intensive care nursery as the infant improves. They also need to have access to health care personnel after discharge to help them care confidently for the child at home (Bialoskurski et al., 2002).

If the infant dies, the parents often wish to see him or her. They may never have seen the infant without a myriad of equipment. Parents may need this time to reassure themselves that their newborn was a normal baby in every other way except lung function or whatever the infant's disorder. This may give them confidence to plan for other children or simply to continue their lives after such a stressful experience.

Developmental Needs

Most high-risk infants enjoy "catch-up" growth once they stabilize from the trauma of birth or whatever caused them to be classified as high risk (see Focus on Multidisciplinary Care). Parents often need support before and after their infants are discharged home to begin to view them as well and capable of doing all the things they are capable of doing. Home care visits can help parents adjust to the stress of having a high-risk infant at home.

Follow-Up of High-Risk Infants at Home

Each time the parents visit the high-risk nursery, it is important to assess their level of knowledge about their child's condition and development. Thorough education and referral to a home care agency may be necessary to help parents continue with the level of care that is required when their infant is discharged home (see Chap. 35). Before discharge, the safety of their home for the care of such a small infant needs to be evaluated. Transporting a preterm infant requires special care, including a blanket or commercial head supports, because a very small infant does not fit securely in an infant car seat (American Academy of Pediatrics, 2001).

High-Risk Infants and Child Abuse

When a child is ill or born preterm, the expected reaction of the parents would be to protect the child even more than the average child so that no further harm can result. In reality, particularly in reference to preterm children, the opposite may occur. Preterm children are at high risk for abuse (Cunningham et al., 2001). This is probably due to the separation of the child from the family at birth, which interferes with bonding. Child abuse is discussed in Chapter 55.

> ✔ **CHECKPOINT QUESTIONS**
>
> 7. How is oral stimulation provided for newborns receiving gavage feedings?
> 8. What are the two most common viruses transmitted to the newborn in utero?
> 9. Why are preterm infants at high risk for child abuse?

FOCUS ON MULTIDISCIPLINARY CARE

Many health care providers—neonatologists, physical therapists, occupational therapists, and respiratory therapists, for example—participate in the care of high-risk newborns. Additionally, unlicensed assistive personnel may be used to bottle-feed or rock and comfort infants who are growing well and are almost ready for discharge. Be certain that all health care providers are informed about things such as what each infant enjoys, how to best position the infant after feeding, and how to observe oxygen saturation levels, including what levels to report if the newborn is still being monitored. Including everyone involved in the newborn's care in this way helps to make developmental care complete.

THE NEWBORN AT RISK BECAUSE OF ALTERED GESTATIONAL AGE OR BIRTH WEIGHT

Infants are evaluated as soon as possible after birth to determine their weight and gestational age. Classification by growth charts and gestational history is important in determining the immediate health care needs of the newborn and in anticipating possible problems. Birth weight is normally plotted on a growth chart such as the Colorado (Lubchenco) Intrauterine Growth Chart (see Appendix E). Infants born after the beginning of week 38 and before week 42 of pregnancy (calculated from the first day of the last menstrual period) are classified as **term infants.** Approximately 90% of all live births are term. Infants born before term (less than the full 37th week of pregnancy) account for approximately 11% to 12% of all births and are classified **as preterm infants,** regardless of their birth weight. Infants born after the onset of week 43 of pregnancy are classified as **postterm infants** (Department of Health and Human Services, 2000).

Normally, birth weight varies for each gestational week. Infants who fall between the 10th and 90th percentiles of weight for their age regardless of gestational age are considered **appropriate for gestational age** (AGA). Infants who fall below the 10th percentile of weight for their age are considered **small for gestational age** (SGA). Those who fall above the 90th percentile in weight are considered **large for gestational age** (LGA). Infants weighing under 2,500 g are **low-birth-weight infants.** Those weighing less than 1,500 g are **very-low-birth-weight infants.** Preterm infants may be AGA, SGA, LGA, low birth weight, or very low birth weight.

Infants who are found to be preterm, postterm, SGA, LGA, low birth weight, or very low birth weight have immediate needs that are different from or more pronounced than the needs of the usual term newborn (see Focus on Cultural Competence). Each of these categories carries its own set of problems and potential risks.

The Small-for-Gestational-Age Infant

An infant is SGA if the birth weight is below the 10th percentile on an intrauterine growth curve for that age (Anderson and Hay, 2000). The infant may be born preterm (before week 38 of gestation), term (between weeks 38 and 42), or postterm (past 42 weeks). Infants who are SGA are distinctly different from infants whose weight is low but who are average for gestational age. SGA infants are small for their age because they have experienced **intrauterine growth restriction or retardation** (IUGR) or failed to grow at the expected rate in utero.

Causes

The mother's nutrition during pregnancy plays a major role in fetal growth outcome, and lack of adequate nutrition may be a major contributor to IUGR. Pregnant adolescents have a high incidence of SGA infants: The adolescent has her own nutritional and growth needs, and these, when coupled with the increased nutritional needs of pregnancy, can affect the growing fetus. However, the most common cause of IUGR is a placental anomaly: either the placenta did not obtain sufficient nutrients from the uterine arteries or it was inefficient at transporting nutrients to the fetus. Placental damage, such as partial placental separation with bleeding, limits placental function because the area of placenta that separated becomes infarcted and fibrosed, reducing the placental surface available for exchange. A developmental defect in the placenta can also prevent it from functioning properly. Women with systemic diseases that decrease blood flow to the placenta, such as severe diabetes mellitus or pregnancy-induced hypertension (both diseases where blood vessel lumens are narrowed), are at higher risk for delivering SGA babies than others. Mothers who smoke heavily or use narcotics also tend to have SGA infants (Cunningham et al., 2001).

In other instances, the placental supply of nutrients is adequate but the infant cannot use them. Infants with intrauterine infections such as rubella or toxoplasmosis may experience this. In addition, babies with chromosomal abnormalities may be SGA.

Assessment

Prenatal Assessment. The SGA infant may be detected in utero when the recorded fundal height during pregnancy becomes progressively less than expected. However, if the woman is unsure of the date of her last menstrual period, this discrepancy can be hard to substantiate. A sonogram can demonstrate the decreased size. A biophysical profile including a nonstress test, placental grading, and ultrasound examination can provide additional information on placental function. If poor placental function is apparent from such determinations, it can be predicted that the infant will do poorly during labor because periods of hypoxia during contractions could lead to neurologic damage. Cesarean birth is the birth method of choice in such circumstances.

Appearance. Generally, the infant who suffers nutritional deprivation early in pregnancy, when fetal growth consists primarily of an increase in the number of body cells, is below average in weight, length, and head circumference. The infant who suffers deprivation late in pregnancy, when growth consists primarily of an increase in cell size, may have only a reduction in weight. Regardless of when deprivation occurs, the infant has an overall wasted appearance. The child may have a small liver, which may cause difficulty regulating glucose, protein, and bilirubin levels. The infant also has poor skin turgor and generally appears to have a large head because the rest of the body is so small. Skull sutures may be widely separated from lack of normal bone growth. Hair is dull and lusterless. The abdomen may be sunken. The cord often appears dry and may be stained yellow.

In contrast, because the infant's age is more advanced than the weight implies, the child may have better-developed neurologic responses, sole creases, and ear cartilage than expected for a baby of that weight. The skull

---

FOCUS ON CULTURAL COMPETENCE

The weight of infants at birth is at least partially culturally determined. In the United States, for example, low-birth-weight infants are most apt to be born to African-American women and girls under 15 years of age (DHHS, 2000). This statistic points to a need to be aware that some women are at higher risk for giving birth to low-birth-weight infants than others are. A number of factors may contribute to this, including lack of knowledge concerning the importance of prenatal care, lack of transportation to prenatal appointments, and poor nutritional status. Assessing the particular needs of these mothers is important in preventing the problems that low-birth-weight infants experience at birth.

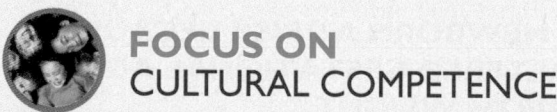

may be firmer, and the infant may seem unusually alert and active for that weight.

The SGA infant needs careful assessment for possible congenital anomalies occurring as a result of the poor nutritional intrauterine environment. Conversely, a congenital anomaly may be the cause of the poor growth by interfering with nutritional use of available substances.

Laboratory Findings. Blood studies at birth usually show a high hematocrit level (less than normal amounts of plasma in proportion to red blood cells due to lack of fluid in utero) and an increase in the total number of red blood cells (polycythemia). The increase in red blood cells is probably due to a state of anoxia during intrauterine life. The polycythemia causes increased blood viscosity, a condition that puts extra work on the heart because it is more difficult for the infant to circulate this thick blood effectively. As a consequence, acrocyanosis (blueness of the hands and feet) may be prolonged and persistently above normal. If the polycythemia is extreme, vessels may become blocked and thrombus formation can result. If the hematocrit level is more than 65% to 70%, an exchange transfusion to dilute the blood may be necessary.

Because SGA infants have decreased glycogen stores, one of the most common problems is hypoglycemia (decreased blood glucose, or a level below 40 mg/dL). Such infants may need intravenous glucose to sustain blood sugar until they are able to suck vigorously enough to take sufficient oral feedings.

NURSING DIAGNOSES AND RELATED INTERVENTIONS

Nursing Diagnosis: Ineffective breathing pattern related to underdeveloped body systems at birth

Outcome Identification: Newborn will initiate and maintain respirations at birth.

Outcome Evaluation: Newborn maintains normal respirations at a rate of 30 to 60 breaths per minute after resuscitation at birth.

Birth asphyxia is a common problem for SGA infants, both because they have underdeveloped chest muscles and because they are at risk for developing meconium aspiration syndrome due to anoxia during labor. It is believed that fetal hypoxia causes a reflex relaxation of the anal sphincter and increased intestinal movement. With gasping, the fetus draws meconium discharged into the amniotic fluid into the tracheobronchial tree. Acting as a foreign substance, it blocks airflow into the alveoli, leading to hypoxemia, acidosis, and hypercapnia. For this reason, many SGA infants require resuscitation at birth. Closely observe both respiratory rate and character in the first few hours of life. Underdeveloped chest muscles can make them unable to sustain the rapid respiratory rate of a normal newborn.

Nursing Diagnosis: Risk for ineffective thermoregulation related to lack of subcutaneous fat

Outcome Identification: Newborn will maintain body temperature within normal limits.

Outcome Evaluation: Infant's temperature is maintained at 36.5°C (97.8°F) axillary.

SGA infants are less able to control body temperature than normal newborns because they lack subcutaneous fat. A carefully controlled environment is essential to keep the infant's body temperature in a neutral zone (see Chap. 23).

Nursing Diagnosis: Risk for impaired parenting related to child's high-risk status and possible cognitive impairment from lack of nutrients in utero

Outcome Identification: Parents will demonstrate beginning bonding behavior with infant while in the hospital.

Outcome Evaluation: Parents express interest in infant and ask questions about what the child's care needs will be at home.

Although SGA infants may gain weight and appear to thrive in the first few days of life, their mental development may have been impaired because of lack of oxygen and nourishment in utero. Babies who were growing normally in utero but whose gestation was interrupted preterm (true preterm babies) usually gain weight and height so rapidly that by the end of the first year of life they are near the 50th percentile on growth charts. SGA infants, however, may always be below normal on standard growth charts. This inability to reach normal levels of growth and development may interfere with bonding because the child does not meet the parents' expectations. Eventually, it can interfere with the child's self-esteem if the child is never able to meet parental expectations.

One way to promote early parental bonding with the child is to discuss ways parents can promote the infant's development once they are at home. An SGA infant needs adequate stimulation during the infant period to reach normal growth and developmental milestones. Parents need to be encouraged to provide toys suitable for their child's chronologic age, not physical size. Because the infant tires easily in the first few weeks of life, play periods must be spaced with rest periods or hypoglycemia or apnea can occur.

> **✔ CHECKPOINT QUESTIONS**
>
> 10. What are two laboratory findings typical of an SGA newborn?
> 11. Why are SGA newborns at risk for problems with maintaining body temperature?

The Large-for-Gestational-Age Infant

An infant is LGA (also termed **macrosomia**) if the birth weight is above the 90th percentile on an intrauterine growth chart for that gestational age. Such a baby appears deceptively healthy at birth because of the weight, but a gestational age examination will reveal immature development. It is important that an LGA infant be identified immediately so that the infant is given special care appropriate to his or her gestational age rather than being treated as a term newborn.

Causes

Infants who are LGA have been subjected to an overproduction of growth hormone in utero. This happens most often to the infants of mothers with diabetes mellitus. Extreme macrosomia may occur in diabetic mothers whose condition is poorly controlled and thus demonstrate high glucose levels. Multiparous women are also prone to deliver large babies because with each succeeding pregnancy, babies tend to grow larger (Cunningham et al., 2001). Other conditions associated with LGA infants include transposition of the great vessels; Beckwith's syndrome, a rare condition characterized by overgrowth; and congenital anomalies such as omphalocele.

Assessment

A fetus is suspected of being LGA when the uterus is unusually large for the date of pregnancy. However, because a fetus lies in a flexed fetal position, he or she does not occupy significantly more space at 10 lb than at 7 lb. If a fetus does seem to be growing at an abnormally rapid rate, a sonogram can confirm the suspicion. A nonstress test to assess the placenta's ability to sustain the large fetus during labor may also be performed. The infant's lung maturity may be assessed by amniocentesis. If the infant's large size was not detected during pregnancy, it may be recognized during labor when the baby is unable to descend through the pelvic rim. Cesarean birth may be necessary because of **cephalopelvic disproportion** (i.e., the biparietal diameter is closer to 10 cm than the usual 9 cm) or **shoulder dystocia** (the wide shoulders are unable to pass through the outlet of the pelvis).

Appearance. At birth, the LGA infant may show immature reflexes and low scores on gestational age examinations in relation to his or her size. The baby may have extensive bruising or a birth injury such as a broken clavicle or Erb-Duchenne paralysis from trauma to the cervical nerves if he or she was born vaginally (see Chap. 51). Because the head is large, it may have been exposed to more than the usual amount of pressure during birth, causing a prominent caput succedaneum, cephalhematoma, or molding.

The LGA newborn requires the same cautious care necessary for a preterm infant. Specific criteria for initial or continuing assessment are shown in Table 26-1.

Cardiovascular Dysfunction. The heart rate of LGA infants should be carefully observed. Cyanosis may be a sign of transposition of the great vessels, a serious heart anomaly (see Chap. 41). Polycythemia, if present, is caused by the infant's system attempting to fully oxygenate all body tissues. Observe closely for signs of **hyperbilirubinemia** (increased serum bilirubin level), which may result from absorption of blood from bruising and polycythemia.

Hypoglycemia. An LGA infant also needs to be carefully assessed for hypoglycemia in the early hours of life because the infant uses up nutritional stores readily to sustain his or her weight. If the mother has diabetes that is poorly controlled, the infant will have an increased blood glucose level in utero, which causes the infant to produce elevated levels of insulin. After birth, these increased insulin levels will continue for up to 24 hours of life, possibly causing rebound hypoglycemia.

NURSING DIAGNOSES AND RELATED INTERVENTIONS

Nursing Diagnosis: Ineffective breathing pattern related to possible birth trauma in large-for-gestational-age newborn

Outcome Identification: Newborn will initiate and maintain respirations at birth.

Outcome Evaluation: Newborn initiates breathing at birth; maintains normal newborn respiratory rate of 30 to 60 breaths per minute.

TABLE 26.1 Important Assessment Criteria for a Large-for-Gestational-Age Infant

ASSESSMENT	RATIONALE
Skin color for ecchymosis, jaundice, and erythema	Bruising occurs with vaginal birth; jaundice may occur from breakdown of ecchymotic collections of blood; polycythemia causes ruddiness of skin.
Motion of extremities on spontaneous movement and in response to a Moro's reflex to detect clavicle fracture (crepitus or swelling may then be palpated at the fracture site) or Erb's palsy due to edema of the cervical nerve plexus	Clavicle or cervical nerve injuries may occur due to problem of birth of wider-than-normal shoulders.
A symmetry of the anterior chest or unilateral lack of movement to detect diaphragmatic paralysis from edema of the phrenic nerve	This cervical nerve may be stretched by birth of wide shoulders.
Eyes for evidence of unresponsive or dilated pupils, vomiting, bulging fontanelles, and a high-pitched cry suggestive of increased intracranial pressure	Compression of 3rd, 4th, and 6th cranial nerves by increased pressure limits eye response; other signs of increased intracranial pressure may occur.
Activities such as jitteriness, lethargy, and uncoordinated eye movements that suggest seizure activity	Seizures may be caused by increased intracranial pressure; seizures in newborns often produce only vague symptoms.

Some LGA infants have difficulty establishing respirations at birth because of birth trauma. Increased intracranial pressure from birth of the larger-than-usual head may lead to pressure on the respiratory center. This, in turn, causes a decrease in respiratory function. A diaphragmatic paralysis may occur due to cervical nerve trauma as the head is bent laterally to allow for birth of the large shoulders. This prevents active lung motion on the affected side. If the infant had to be born by cesarean birth, transient fluid can remain in the lungs and interfere with effective gas exchange. Careful observation will detect these conditions. Care of the infant with these disorders is discussed in Chapter 40.

Nursing Diagnosis: Risk for imbalanced nutrition, less than body requirements related to additional nutrients needed to maintain weight and prevent hypoglycemia

Outcome Identification: Infant will ingest adequate fluid and nutrients for growth during neonatal period.

Outcome Evaluation: Infant's weight follows percentile growth curve; skin turgor is good; specific gravity of urine is 1.003 to 1.030; serum glucose is above 40 mg/dL.

As a rule, the LGA infant needs to be breast-fed immediately to prevent hypoglycemia. The infant may need supplemental formula feedings after breast-feeding to supply enough fluid and glucose for the larger-than-normal size for the first few days. Newborns who are offered bottles often have more difficulty than others learning to breast-feed. Offer the mother and baby support to overcome this hurdle.

Do not overestimate this infant's ability to suck effectively at birth. The infant may seem as if he or she should do well with breast-feeding because the baby is already the size of a 2-month-old infant. However, the infant is an inexperienced newborn, so sucking may not be effective enough for the infant to obtain an adequate supply of milk.

Nursing Diagnosis: Risk for impaired parenting related to high-risk status of large-for-gestational-age infant

Outcome Identification: Parents demonstrate adequate bonding behavior during neonatal period.

Outcome Evaluation: Parents hold infant; speak of the child in positive terms; state accurately why the infant needs to be closely observed in postnatal period.

Parents may underestimate this infant's needs because of the child's large size. He or she seems so big and healthy; parents may be confused about why the infant needs careful watching. They may read more into the child's condition than is present (he or she must be sick in some way that they are not being told about) and so bonding does not happen as instinctively as it might. If the woman sustained a cervical or perineal tear or required a cesarean birth, she needs some time to air any resentment she may feel toward the infant. Otherwise, her perception that the infant is the cause of her additional distress may interfere with her ability to bond with the child.

An LGA infant needs the same developmental care that all other infants need. Singing or talking to the baby, stroking the child's back, and rocking the baby are all important for the large infant's development. Encourage parents to treat their baby as a fragile newborn who needs warm nurturing, not as a tough big infant who has grown past that stage. Also remind the parents that the infant's birthweight is not a correlation of the child's projected adult size. Parents may fear that the infant may grow to be a larger-than-normal adult.

✔ CHECKPOINT QUESTIONS

12. What are two reasons why a cesarean birth may be necessary for the birth of an LGA infant?
13. Why may breast-feeding be difficult for a LGA newborn?

The Preterm Infant

A preterm infant is usually defined as a live-born infant born before the end of week 37 of gestation; another criterion used is a weight of less than 2,500 g (5 lb 8 oz) at birth. Infants born after the 37th week are considered term. Infants who are born weighing 1,500 to 2,500 g are considered low-birth-weight infants; those born weighing 1,000 to 1,500 g are considered very-low-birth-weight infants. Those born weighing 500 to 1,000 g are considered **extremely-very-low-birth-weight** infants. All such infants need neonatal intensive care from the moment of birth to give them their best chance of survival without neurologic after-effects. A lack of lung surfactant makes them extremely vulnerable to respiratory distress syndrome (Whitsett et al., 2000).

The maturity of a newborn is determined by physical findings such as sole creases, skull firmness, ear cartilage, and neurologic findings that reveal gestational age, as well as the mother's report of the date of her last menstrual period and sonographic estimations of gestational age.

Preterm babies, regardless of their weight, need to be differentiated at birth from SGA babies (who also may have a low birthweight). The two conditions result from different situations and therefore will cause different problems involving adjustment to extrauterine life. A preterm infant is immature and small but well proportioned for age. Unlike the SGA infant, this baby appears to have been doing well in utero. For an unexplained reason, the trigger that initiates labor was activated too early and birth has resulted, even though the baby is immature. Preterm infants are invariably low-birthweight infants. Differentiating characteristics of SGA and preterm infants are compared in Table 26-2.

Incidence

Preterm birth occurs in approximately 7% of live births of white infants. In African-American infants, the rate is doubled to approximately 14% (Cunningham et al., 2001).

TABLE 26.2 Differences Between Small-for-Gestational-Age and Preterm Infants

CHARACTERISTIC	SMALL-FOR-GESTATIONAL-AGE INFANT	PRETERM INFANT
Gestational age	24–44 wk	Younger than 37 wk
Birthweight	Under 10th percentile	Normal for age
Congenital malformations	Strong possibility	Possibility
Pulmonary problems	Meconium aspiration, pulmonary hemorrhage, pneumothorax	Respiratory distress syndrome
Hyperbilirubinemia	Possibility	Very strong possibility
Hypoglycemia	Very strong possibility	Possibility
Intracranial hemorrhage	Strong possibility	Possibility
Apnea episodes	Possibility	Very strong possibility
Feeding problems	Most likely due to accompanying problem such as hypoglycemia	Small stomach capacity; immature sucking reflex
Weight gain in nursery	Rapid	Slow
Future retarded growth	Possibly always be under 10th percentile due to poor organ development	Not likely to be restricted in growth as "catch-up" growth occurs

When a preterm infant is recognized by a gestational age assessment by health care personnel, watch for the specific problems of prematurity such as respiratory distress syndrome, hypoglycemia, and intracranial hemorrhage.

Causes

Preterm infant deaths account for 80% to 90% of the infant mortality in the first year of life (Department of Health and Human Services, 2000). Infant mortality could be reduced dramatically if the causes of preterm birth could be discovered and corrected and all pregnancies brought to term. However, the exact cause of premature labor and early birth is rarely known.

There is a high correlation between low socioeconomic level and early termination of pregnancy. In women from middle and upper socioeconomic groups, only 4% to 8% of pregnancies are terminated early. However, in women from low socioeconomic levels, 10% to 20% end before term (Cunningham et al., 2001). The major influencing factor in these instances appears to be inadequate nutrition before and during pregnancy, as a result of either lack of money for or lack of knowledge about good nutrition. Additional factors that seem to be related to preterm birth are shown in Box 26-4. Iatrogenic causes, such as elective cesarean birth and inducement of labor according to dates rather than fetal maturity, also result in preterm births. Testing fetal maturity by amniocentesis or ultrasound is used to avoid inducing labor prematurely.

Assessment

History. Although a detailed pregnancy history may sometimes point to a potential preterm birth, the pregnancy history is often normal up to the beginning of labor.

When interviewing the mother of a preterm infant, be careful not to convey disapproval of reported pregnancy behaviors such as cigarette smoking or working a 12-hour work shift that may have contributed to preterm delivery. A woman who does these things is likely to be unaware that these actions could be detrimental to the fetus. Once the infant is born, she will need a high level of self-esteem and all of her inner resources to sustain her through the crisis. Being overburdened by guilt may be detrimental to her attempts to bond with her infant. A good answer to her direct inquiries about causes is, "No one really knows what causes prematurity."

BOX 26.4

FACTORS ASSOCIATED WITH PRETERM BIRTH

- Low socioeconomic level
- Poor nutritional status
- Lack of prenatal care
- Multiple pregnancy
- Prior previous early birth
- Race (nonwhites have a higher incidence of prematurity than whites)
- Cigarette smoking
- Age of the mother (highest incidence is in mothers younger than age 20)
- Order of birth (early termination is highest in first pregnancies and in those beyond the fourth pregnancy)
- Closely spaced pregnancies
- Abnormalities of the mother's reproductive system, such as intrauterine septum
- Infections (especially urinary tract infection)
- Obstetric complications, such as premature rupture of membranes or premature separation of the placenta
- Early induction of labor
- Elective cesarean birth

In many instances, preterm labor might have been halted had the woman been able to recognize that she was in true labor and not having Braxton-Hicks contractions. In a first labor, this can easily occur because the woman does not know what true labor feels like. Television often depicts women in labor as having agonizingly painful contractions or the opposite, simply announcing, "This is it," and then proceeding to deliver within the 30-minute show. In reality, the first-time mother does not realize that labor usually begins with subtle signs and mild contractions, not with a dramatic announcement. With preterm labor, often the woman reports not feeling well or having flulike symptoms. Because each labor proceeds differently, even a multipara may miss the early signs of labor until it is too far advanced to be reversed. Reassure the woman that it is understandable that she did not realize what was happening until cervical dilatation had occurred and labor could not be reversed.

Appearance. On gross inspection, a preterm infant appears small and underdeveloped (Fig. 26-6). The head is disproportionately large (3 cm or more greater than chest size). The skin is generally unusually ruddy because the infant has little subcutaneous fat beneath it; veins are easily noticeable, and a high degree of acrocyanosis may be present. The preterm neonate, 24 to 36 weeks, typically is covered with vernix caseosa. However, in very preterm newborns (less than 25 weeks' gestation), vernix is absent because it is not formed this early in pregnancy. Lanugo is usually extensive, covering the back, forearms, forehead, and sides of the face, because this amount is present until late in pregnancy. Both anterior and posterior fontanelles are small. There are few or no creases on the soles of the feet.

Physical findings and reflex testing are used to differentiate between term and preterm newborns (Fig. 26-7). The eyes of most preterm infants appear small. Although difficult to elicit, pupillary reaction is present. Ophthalmoscopic examination is extremely difficult and often uninformative because the vitreous humor may be hazy. The preterm infant has varying degrees of myopia (nearsightedness) because of lack of eye globe depth.

The cartilage of the ear is immature and allows the pinna to fall forward. The ears appear large in relation to the head. The level of the ears should be carefully inspected to rule out chromosomal abnormalities.

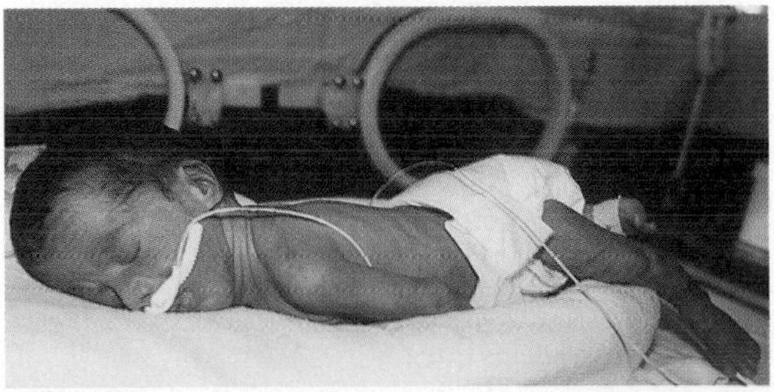

FIGURE 26.6 An immature infant. Notice the lax position of limbs due to immature muscle development.

Neurologic function in the preterm child is often difficult to evaluate. The observation of spontaneous or provoked movements may yield findings as important as reflex testing. If tested, reflexes such as sucking and swallowing will be absent if the infant's age is below 33 weeks; deep tendon reflexes such as the Achilles tendon reflex are markedly diminished. During an examination, a preterm infant is much less active than a mature infant and rarely cries. If the infant does cry, the cry is weak and high-pitched.

Laboratory Findings. Laboratory values for the preterm infant are compared with those of the term infant in Appendix F.

Potential Complications

Anemia of Prematurity. Many preterm infants develop a normochromic, normocytic anemia. Blood cells may be fragmented or irregularly shaped. The reticulocyte count is also low because the bone marrow does not increase its production until approximately 32 weeks. The infant will appear pale, may be lethargic and anorectic, and will generally fail to thrive. The fault appears to be immaturity of the hematopoietic system combined with destruction of red blood cells due to low levels of vitamin E, which normally protects red blood cells against oxidation. Excessive blood drawing for electrolyte or blood gas analysis can potentiate the problem. For this reason, keep a record of the amount of blood drawn for analysis.

Red blood cell production can be stimulated by the administration of DNA recombinant erythropoietin. In addition, the infant may need blood transfusions (to supply needed red blood cells) and vitamin E and iron provided by preterm formula (Ward & Lugo, 2000).

Kernicterus. Kernicterus is destruction of brain cells by invasion of indirect bilirubin. This invasion results from the high concentrations of indirect bilirubin in the blood from excessive breakdown of red blood cells. Preterm infants are more prone to the condition than term infants because with the acidosis that occurs from poor respiratory exchange, brain cells are more susceptible to the effect of indirect bilirubin than normally. Preterm infants also have less serum albumin available to bind indirect bilirubin and therefore inactivate its effect. Because of this, kernicterus may occur at lower levels (as low as 12 mg per 100 mL of indirect bilirubin) in these infants. It is important to monitor indirect bilirubin levels in preterm infants. If jaundice occurs, phototherapy or exchange transfusion can be started to prevent excessively high indirect bilirubin levels.

Persistent Patent Ductus Arteriosus. Because preterm infants lack surfactant, their lungs are noncompliant. It is more difficult for them to move blood from the pulmonary artery into the lungs. This condition leads to pulmonary artery hypertension, which may interfere with closure of the ductus arteriosus. Administer intravenous therapy cautiously to avoid increasing blood pressure and compounding this problem. Indomethacin may be administered to initiate closure of the patent ductus arteriosus (Flanagan et al., 2000).

A

Premature Infant | Full-term Infant

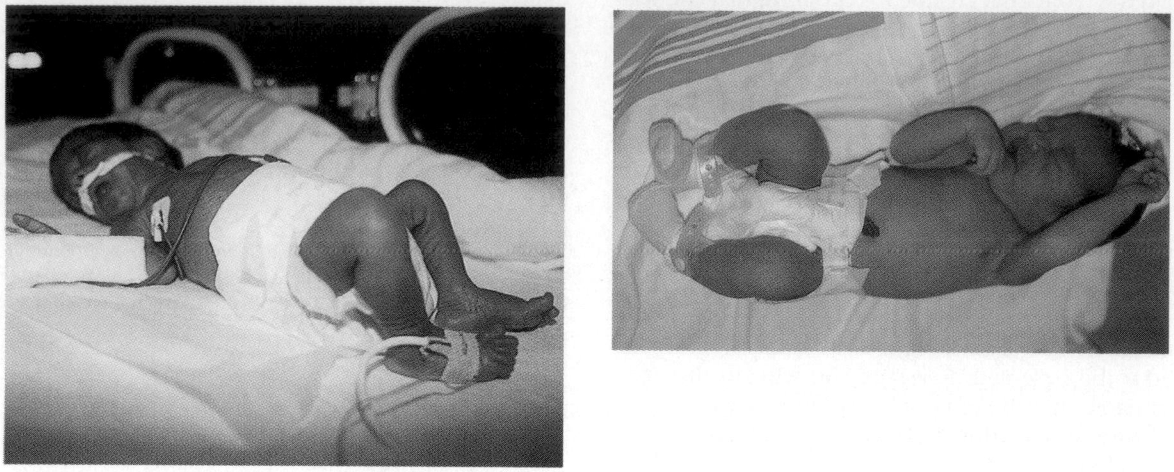

RESTING POSTURE *The premature infant is characterized by very little, if any, flexion in the upper extremities and only partial flexion of the lower extremities. The full-term infant exhibits flexion in all four extremities.*

B

Premature Infant, 28–32 Weeks | Full-term Infant

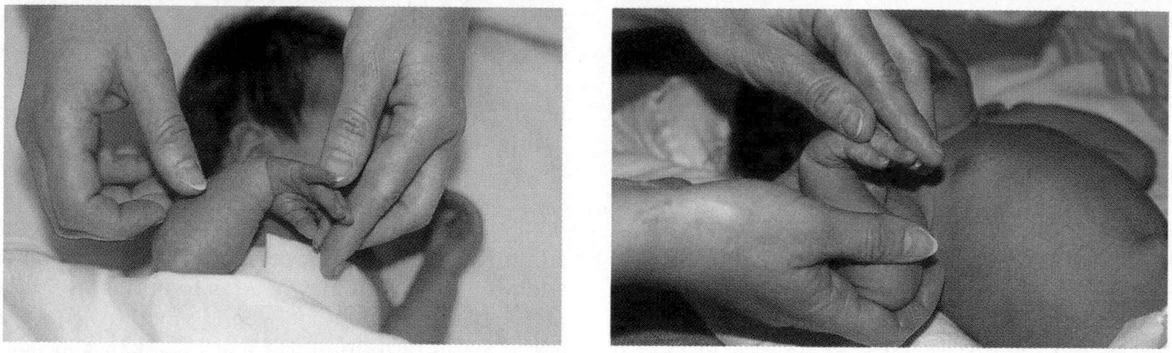

WRIST FLEXION *The wrist is flexed, applying enough pressure to get the hand as close to the forearm as possible. The angle between the hypothenar eminence and the ventral aspect of the forearm is measured. (Care must be taken not to rotate the infant's wrist.) The premature infant at 28–32 weeks' gestation will exhibit a 90° angle. With the full-term infant it is possible to flex the hand onto the arm.*

FIGURE 26.7 Examples of physical examination findings and reflex tests used to judge gestational age. (A) Resting posture. (B) Wrist flexion. *(Continued)*

Periventricular/Intraventricular Hemorrhage. Preterm infants are particularly prone to periventricular hemorrhage (bleeding into the tissue surrounding the ventricles) or intraventricular hemorrhage (bleeding into the ventricles). These conditions occur in as many as 50% of infants of very low birth weight (Bernbaum, 2000). Preterm infants have fragile capillaries and immature cerebral vascular development. This increases their susceptibility. When there is a rapid change in cerebral blood pressure, such as with hypoxia, intravenous infusion, ventilation, and pneumothorax, the capillaries rupture. The infant experiences brain anoxia beyond the rupture. Hydrocephalus may occur from bleeding into the aqueduct of Sylvius with resulting obstruction of the aqueduct. Preterm infants often have a cranial ultrasound done after the first few days of life to detect if a hemorrhage has occurred. An infant's prognosis is guarded until it can be shown that development in the infant is normal after an intracranial bleed.

Other Potential Complications. Preterm infants are particularly susceptible to a number of illnesses in the early postnatal period, including respiratory distress syndrome, apnea, retinopathy of prematurity (all discussed later in this chapter), and necrotizing enterocolitis (discussed in Chap. 45).

NURSING DIAGNOSES AND RELATED INTERVENTIONS

Because a preterm infant has few body resources, both physiologic and psychological stress must be reduced as much as possible and interventions initiated gently to prevent depletion of resources. Close observation and analysis of findings are essential to managing problems quickly.

Nursing Diagnosis: Impaired gas exchange related to immature pulmonary functioning

(Text continues on page 738)

C

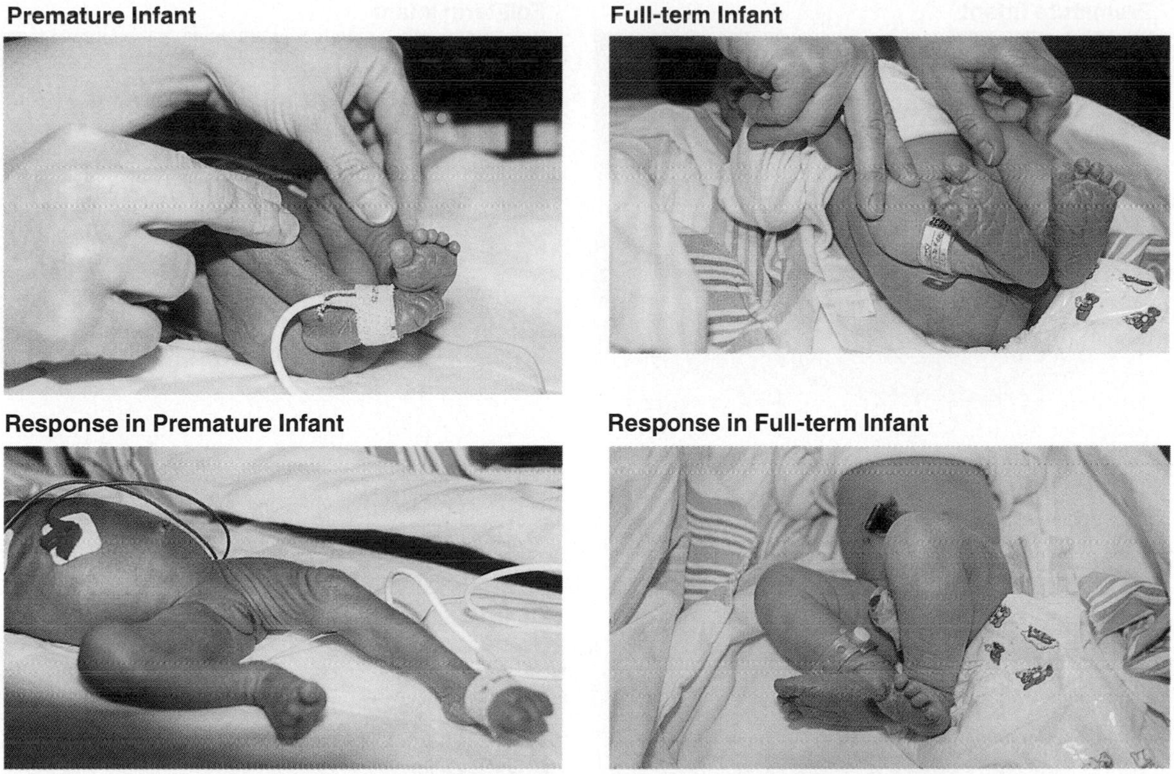

RECOIL OF EXTREMITIES *Place the infant supine. To test recoil of the legs (1) flex the legs and knees fully and hold for 5 seconds (shown in top photos). (2) extend the legs fully by pulling on the feet, (3) release. To test the arms, flex forearms and follow same procedure. In the premature infant response is minimal or absent (bottom left); in the full-term infant extremities return briskly to full flexion (bottom right).*

D

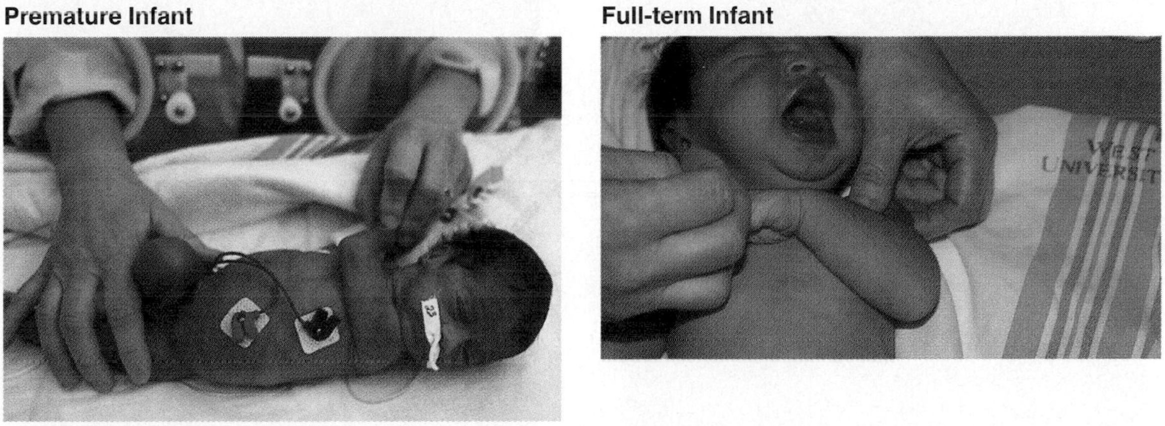

SCARF SIGN *Hold the baby supine, take the hand, and try to place it around the neck and above the opposite shoulder as far posteriorly as possible. Assist this maneuver by lifting the elbow across the body. See how far across the chest the elbow will go. In the premature infant the elbow will reach near or across the midline. In the full-term infant the elbow will not reach the midline.*

FIGURE 26.7 *(Continued)* (*C*) Recoil of extremities (legs). (*D*) Scarf sign.

E

Premature Infant **Full-term Infant**

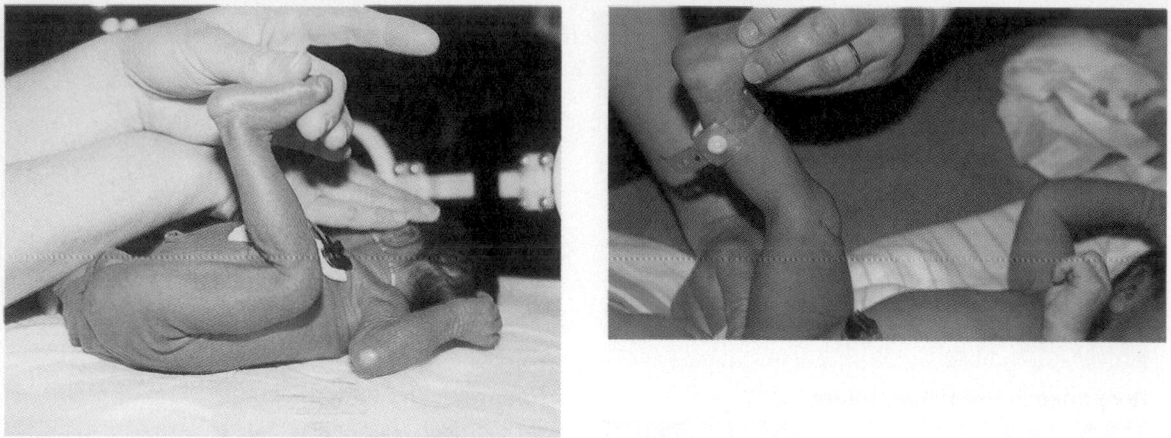

HEEL TO EAR *With the baby supine and the hips positioned flat on the bed, draw the baby's foot as near to the ear as it will go without forcing it. Observe the distance between the foot and head as well as the degree of extension at the knee. In the premature infant very little resistance will be met. In the full-term infant there will be marked resistance; it will be impossible to draw the baby's foot to the ear.*

F

Premature Infant **Full-term Infant**

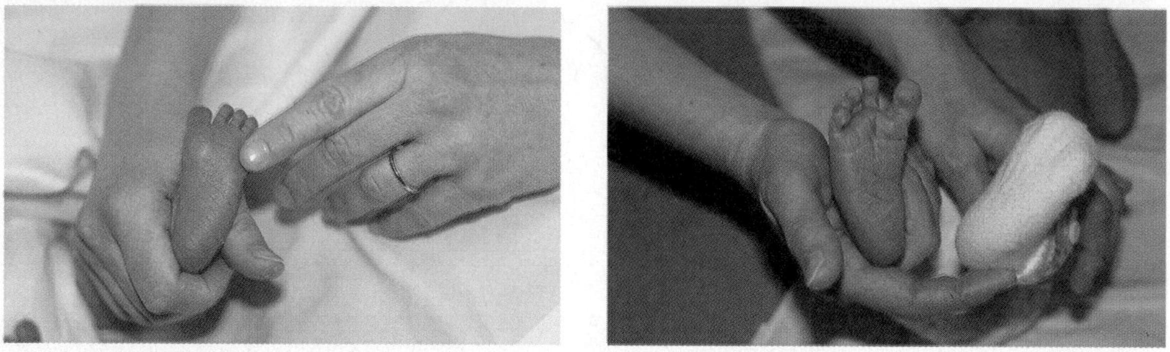

SOLE (PLANTAR) CREASES *The sole of the premature infant has very few or no creases. With the increasing gestation age, the number and depth of sole creases multiply, so that the full-term baby has creases involving the heel. (Wrinkles that occur after 24 hours of age can sometimes be confused with true creases.)*

G

Premature Infant **Full-term Infant**

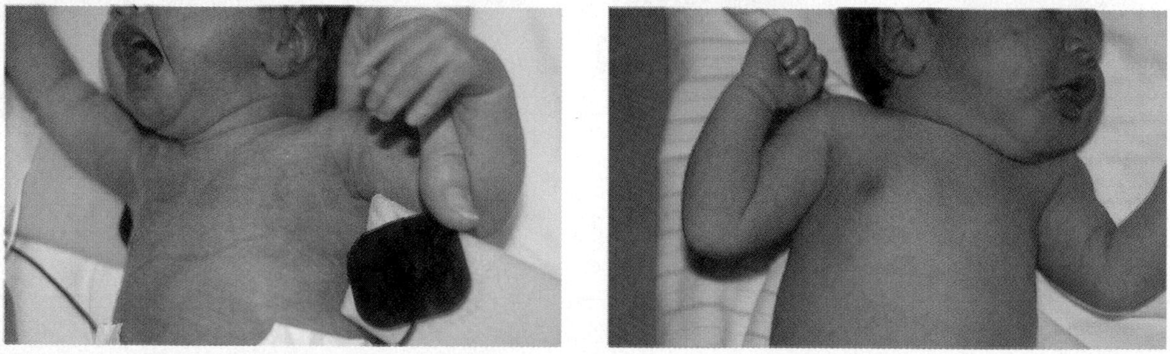

BREAST TISSUE *In infants younger than 34 weeks' gestation the areola and nipple are barely visible. After 34 weeks the areola becomes raised. Also, the infant of less than 36 weeks' gestation has no breast tissue. Breast tissue arises with increasing gestational age due to maternal hormonal stimulation. Thus, an infant of 39 to 40 weeks will have 5 to 6 mm of breast tissue, and this amount will increase with age.*

FIGURE 26.7 *(Continued)* (*E*) Heel to ear. (*F*) Plantar creases. (*G*) Breast tissue.

H

Premature Infant, 34–36 Weeks

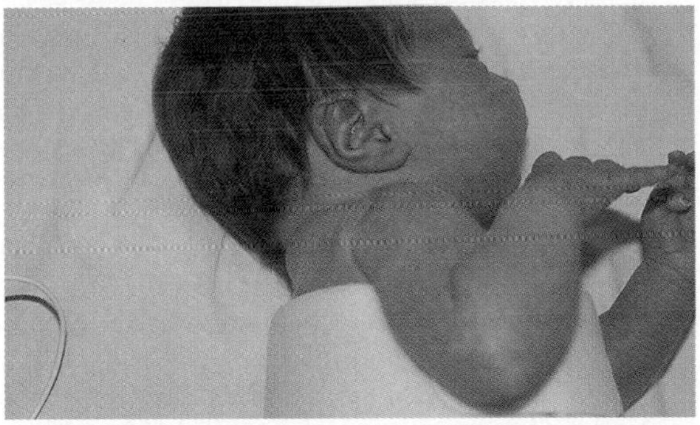

Full-term Infant

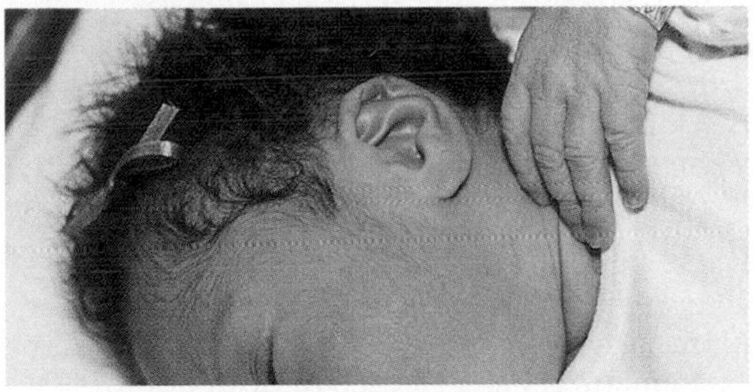

EARS *At fewer than 34 weeks' gestation infants have very flat, relatively shapeless ears. Shape develops over time so that an infant between 34 and 36 weeks has a slight incurving of the superior part of the ear; the term infant is characterized by incurving of two thirds of the pinna; and in an infant older than 39 weeks the incurving continues to the lobe. If the extremely premature infant's ear is folded over, it will stay folded. Cartilage begins to appear at approximately 32 weeks so that the ear returns slowly to its original position. In an infant of more than 40 weeks' gestation, there is enough ear cartilage so that the ear stands erect away from the head and returns quickly when folded. (When folding the ear over during examination be certain that the surrounding area is wiped clean or the ear may adhere to the vernix.)*

I

Premature Male

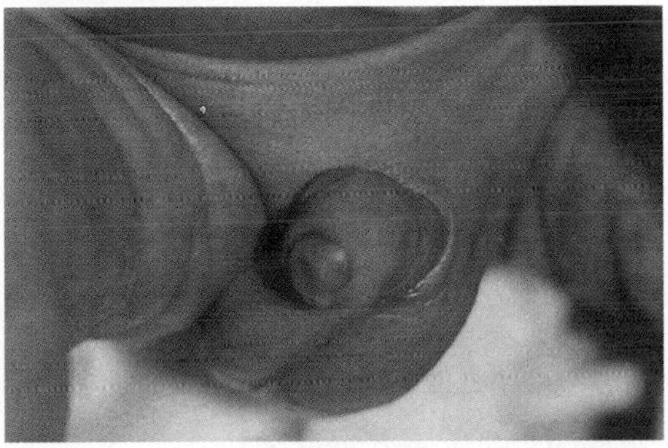

Full-term Male

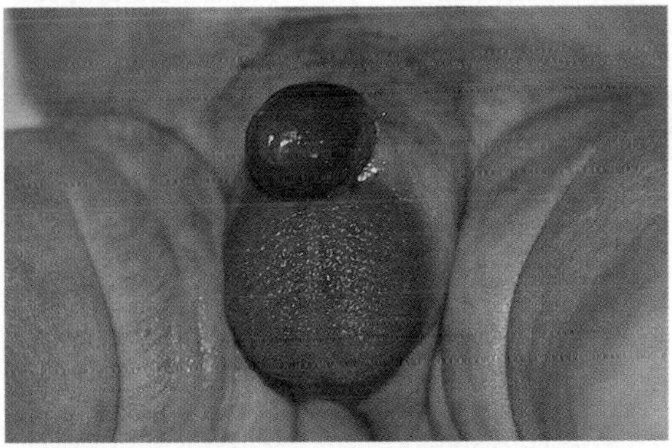

MALE GENITALIA *In the premature male the testes are very high in the inguinal canal and there are very few rugae on the scrotum. The full-term infant's testes are lower in the scrotum and many rugae have developed.*

J

Premature Female

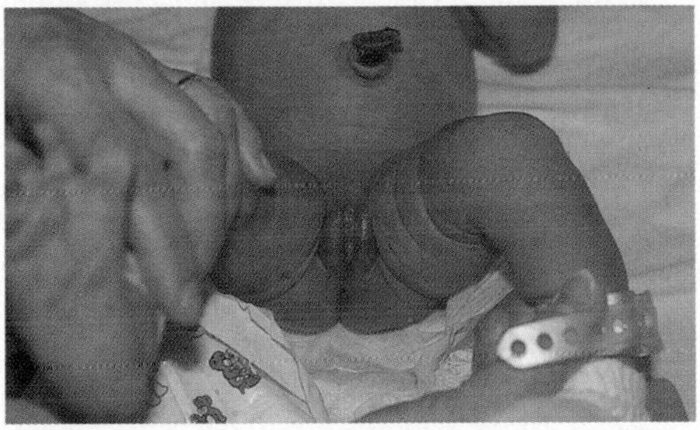

Full-term Female

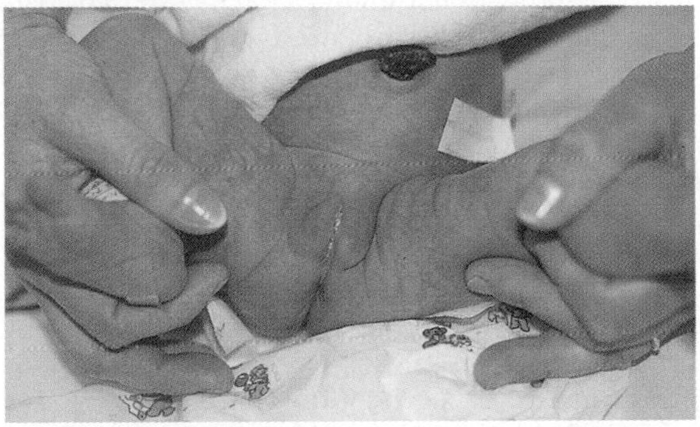

FEMALE GENITALIA *When the premature female is positioned on her back with hips abducted, the clitoris is very prominent and the labia majora are very small and widely separated. The labia minora and the clitoris are covered by the labia majora in the full-term infant.*

FIGURE 26.7 *(Continued)* (*H*) Ears. (*I*) Male genitalia. (*J*) Female genitalia.

Outcome Identification: Newborn will initiate and maintain respirations after surfactant therapy.

Outcome Evaluation: Newborn initiates breathing at birth after resuscitation; maintains normal newborn respirations of 30 to 60 breaths per minute free of assisted ventilation; exhibits oxygen saturation levels of at least 90% as evidenced by arterial blood gases (ABGs).

Preterm infants have great difficulty initiating respirations at birth because the pulmonary capillary bed is immature. Lung surfactant does not form in adequate amounts until about the 34th to 35th week of pregnancy. Thus, it may be inadequate, leading to alveolar collapse with each expiration. This requires the infant to use maximum strength to inflate the alveoli each time. Infants cannot maintain effective expirations under these conditions. In addition, because a fetus usually turns to a vertex presentation late in pregnancy, the preterm infant may still be in a breech position at birth. Breech-born infants are apt to expel meconium into the amniotic fluid. If the fetus aspirates either vaginal secretions or meconium, the respiratory problem is further compromised.

Giving the mother oxygen by mask during the birth will help provide the preterm infant with optimal oxygen saturation at birth (85%–90%). Keeping maternal analgesia and anesthesia to a minimum also offers the infant the best chance of initiating effective respirations. Cesarean birth, although it has the advantage of reducing pressure on the immature head, may lead to additional respiratory complications because of retained lung fluid.

Even term infants experience temporary respiratory acidosis. Once respirations are established, however, the condition quickly clears. Because the preterm infant is unable to initiate effective respirations as quickly as the mature infant, he or she is prone to irreversible acidosis. To prevent this, the infant must be resuscitated within 2 minutes after birth. Birthing room teams need to be prepared with preterm-size laryngoscopes, endotracheal tubes, suction catheters, and synthetic surfactant to be administered by the endotracheal tube. The infant must be kept warm during resuscitation procedures so he or she is not expending extra energy to increase the metabolic rate to maintain body temperature. All procedures must be carried out gently; the preterm infant's tissues are extremely sensitive to trauma and can be damaged or bruised easily by an oxygen mask. When blood from bruising is reabsorbed, this can lead to hyperbilirubinemia, yet another problem.

Giving 100% oxygen to preterm infants during resuscitation or to maintain respirations presents the danger of pulmonary edema and retinopathy of prematurity (blindness of prematurity; see discussion later in this chapter). The development of both of these conditions depends on saturation of the blood with oxygen (Po_2 of more than 100 mm Hg, which usually occurs when oxygen is administered at a concentration over 70%). Although the newborn's oxygen saturation level should be continually monitored, as long as an infant is cyanotic, the blood saturation level of oxygen is likely to be low.

Preterm infants may need continued oxygen administration after resuscitation to allow them to effectively maintain respirations. The soft rib cartilage of the preterm infant tends to create respiratory problems because it collapses on expiration. The accessory muscles of respiration may be underdeveloped as well, leaving the preterm infant with no backup muscles to use when he or she becomes fatigued from trying to maintain respirations.

Many preterm babies, particularly those under 32 weeks of age, have an irregular respiratory pattern (a few quick breaths, a period of 5 to 10 seconds without respiratory effort, a few quick breaths again, and so on). There is no bradycardia with this irregular pattern (sometimes termed **periodic respirations**). Although the pattern is seen in term infants as well, it seems to be intensified by immaturity and uncoordinated respiratory efforts. With true apnea, the pause in respirations is more than 20 seconds and bradycardia does occur. True apnea is discussed in more detail later in this chapter.

Nursing Diagnosis: Risk for deficient fluid volume related to insensible water loss at birth and small stomach capacity

Outcome Identification: Newborn will demonstrate intake of adequate fluid and electrolytes to meet body needs.

Outcome Evaluation: Plasma glucose is between 40 and 60 mg per 100 mL; specific gravity of urine is maintained at 1.003 to 1.030; urine output is maintained at a minimum of 1 mL/kg/h; electrolyte levels are within normal limits.

The preterm newborn has a high insensible water loss due to the large body surface compared with total body weight. The infant also is unable to concentrate urine well because of immature kidney function and thus excretes a high proportion of fluid from the body. All these factors make it important that the preterm baby receive up to 160 to 200 mL of fluid per kilogram of body weight daily (higher than the term infant).

Intravenous fluid administration typically begins within hours after birth to fulfill this fluid requirement and provide glucose to prevent hypoglycemia. Intravenous fluid should be given via a continuous infusion pump to ensure a constant infusion rate and prevent accidental overload. Intravenous sites must be checked conscientiously because if infiltration should occur, the lack of subcutaneous tissue places the preterm newborn at risk for damaged tissue. Specially designed 27-gauge needles are available for use on small veins. However, many preterm infants lack adequately sized peripheral veins for even this small a needle. Therefore, they need to receive intravenous fluid by an umbilical venous catheter. Box 26-5 highlights appropriate outcomes and interventions for a preterm neonate with an umbilical catheter using the terminology identified by the

BOX 26.5

NURSING OUTCOMES AND NURSING INTERVENTIONS CLASSIFICATION: UMBILICAL CATHETER

NOC: Tissue Integrity, Skin and Mucous Membranes

Tissue integrity, skin and mucous membranes is defined as the structural intactness and normal physiologic function of skin and mucous membranes (Johnson, Maas, & Moorhead, 2000). Some specific indicators suggesting achievement of this outcome include the following:

- Uncompromised skin intactness
- Tissue temperature, sensation, elasticity, hydration, pigmentation, color and texture within expected range
- Adequate tissue perfusion

NIC: Tube Care, Umbilical Line

Tube care, umbilical line is defined as the management of a newborn with an umbilical catheter (McCloskey & Bulechek, 2000). Some important nursing activities involved when implementing this intervention include:

- Assisting with insertion and checking position of catheter via x-ray
- Infusing medication and nutrients as ordered
- Obtaining venous or arterial pressures as indicated
- Applying antiseptic medication to umbilical stump as ordered
- Flushing catheter with heparinized solution and changing stopcock daily and prn
- Securing connections and stabilizing catheter with tape
- Cleaning outer surface and umbilical stump with alcohol as needed
- Positioning infant on back
- Applying restraints to wrists and legs with frequent range of motion to these extremities
- Observing for signs requiring catheter removal such as pulselessness, darkening of toes, hypertension, and redness around umbilicus or visible clots
- Removing the catheter as ordered followed by application of pressure or clamp to umbilicus
- Observing for hemorrhage after removal

Nursing Outcomes Classification (NOC) and Nursing Interventions Classification (NIC).

Monitor the baby's weight, urine output and specific gravity, and serum electrolytes to ensure adequate fluid intake. Too little fluid and calories may lead to dehydration and starvation, acidosis, and weight loss. Overhydration may lead to nonnutritional weight gain, pulmonary edema, and heart failure.

Most preterm infants void and pass meconium within 24 hours after birth. Measure urine output by weighing diapers rather than using urine collection bags. Disposable collection bags may lead to skin irritation and breakdown from frequent changing and leaking.

The range of urine output for the first few days of life in preterm babies is high in comparison with that of the term baby: 40 to 100 mL per kg per 24 hours, compared with 10 to 20 mL per kg per 24 hours. The specific gravity is low, rarely more than 1.012 (normal term babies may concentrate urine up to 1.030). Also, test urine for glucose and ketones. Hyperglycemia caused by the glucose infusion may lead to glucose spillage into the urine and an accompanying diuresis. If too little glucose is being supplied and body cells are using protein for metabolism, ketone bodies will appear in urine.

Blood glucose determinations every 4 to 6 hours help to determine hypoglycemia or **hyperglycemia** (increased serum glucose). Blood glucose should range between 40 and 60 mg/dL. Because of the numerous blood tests performed, be certain to keep a record of all blood drawn so the child does not become hypovolemic from the amount drawn. Check for blood in the stools to evaluate for possible bleeding from the intestinal tract. This is helpful in determining the possible cause of hypovolemia if it occurs.

Nursing Diagnosis: Risk for imbalanced nutrition, less than body requirements related to additional nutrients needed for maintenance of rapid growth, possible sucking difficulty, and small stomach

Outcome Identification: Infant will receive adequate fluid and nutrients for growth during hospitalization.

Outcome Evaluation: Infant's weight follows percentile growth curve; skin turgor is good; specific gravity of urine is maintained between 1.003 and 1.030; infant has no more than 15% weight loss in first 3 days of life and continues to gain weight after this point.

Nutrition problems arise with the preterm infant because the body is attempting to continue to maintain the rapid rate of intrauterine growth. Therefore, the preterm newborn requires a larger amount of nutrients in the diet than the mature infant does. If these nutrients are not supplied, the infant will develop **hypocalcemia** (decreased serum calcium) or azotemia (low protein level in blood). Delayed feeding and a resultant decrease in intestinal motility may also add to hyperbilirubinemia, a problem the infant already is at high risk of developing when fetal red blood cells begin to be destroyed.

Nutrition problems are compounded by the preterm infant's immature reflexes, which make swallowing and sucking difficult. In addition, the stomach's capacity is small, also possibly impeding nutrition. A distended stomach puts pressure on the diaphragm, which could lead to respiratory distress. Increased activity necessitated by ineffective sucking may increase the metabolic rate and oxygen requirements. This increases the caloric requirements even more. An immature cardiac sphincter (between the stomach and esophagus) allows regurgitation to occur readily. The lack of a cough reflex may lead the infant to aspirate regurgitated formula. Digestion and absorption of nutrients in the stomach and intestine may also be immature.

Feeding Schedule. With the early administration of intravenous fluid to prevent hypoglycemia and supply fluid, feedings may be safely delayed until the infant has stabilized his or her respiratory effort from birth. Preterm infants may be fed by total parenteral nutrition until they are stable enough for other means. Breast, gavage, or bottle feedings are begun as soon as the infant is able to tolerate them to prevent deterioration of the intestinal villi. Most preterm infants have a chest x-ray before a first feeding. The presence of air in the stomach shows that the route to the stomach is clear.

The preterm infant needs 115 to 140 calories per kilogram of body weight per day, compared with 100 to 110 needed by the term infant. Protein requirements are 3 to 3.5 g per kilogram of body weight, compared with 2.0 to 2.5 for a term newborn. Because a preterm infant has a smaller stomach capacity than a term neonate does, he or she cannot take large feedings and must be fed more frequently with smaller amounts. Feedings may be as small as 1 or 2 mL every 2 to 3 hours (Georgieff, 2000).

Gavage Feeding. The gag reflex is not intact until an infant is 32 weeks' gestation. Although a sucking reflex is present earlier, the ability to coordinate sucking and swallowing is inconsistent until approximately 34 weeks' gestation. Thus, infants born before 32 to 34 weeks' gestation and those who are ill or experiencing respiratory distress are usually started on gavage feedings. Bottle-feeding or breast-feeding is gradually introduced as they mature and their condition improves (Fig. 26-8). To avoid tiring, preterm nipples that are softer than regular nipples are used.

Preterm infants must be observed closely after both oral and gavage feeding to be certain that the filled stomach is not causing respiratory distress. Offering a pacifier during gavage feeding will help to strengthen the sucking reflex, better prepare an infant for bottle- or breastfeeding, and provide oral satisfaction. In addition, initiating and maintaining nonnutritive sucking help the newborn remember how to suck. Box 26-6 highlights an appropriate outcome and intervention addressing this topic using the terminology identified by the Nursing Outcomes Classification (NOC) and Nursing Interventions Classification (NIC).

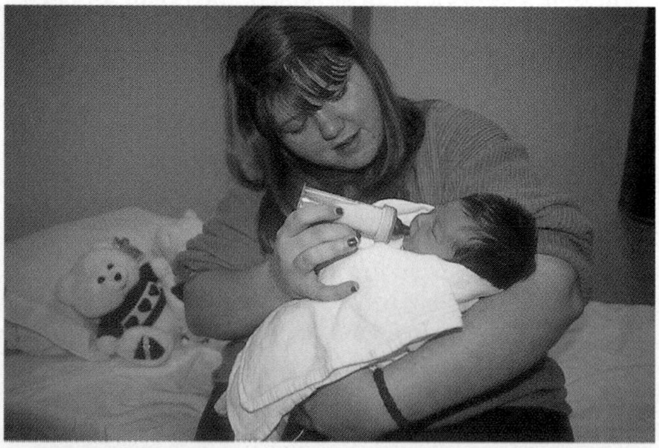

FIGURE 26.8 Feeding a preterm infant. Notice the small bottle used.

Gavage feedings may be given intermittently every few hours or continuously via tubes passed through the mouth or nose. Infants may be fed by continuous drip feedings at about 1 mL/h. This can be helpful for infants on ventilators or those who experience oxygen deprivation with han-

BOX 26.6

NURSING OUTCOMES AND NURSING INTERVENTIONS CLASSIFICATION: SUCKING AND SWALLOWING

NOC: Swallowing Status

Swallowing status is defined as the extent of safe passage of fluids and/or solids from the mouth to the stomach (Johnson, Maas, & Moorhead, 2000). Some specific indicators suggesting achievement of this outcome include the following:

- Ability to handle oral secretions
- Timely swallow reflex
- Absence of choking, coughing, or gagging
- Maintenance of gastric contents in stomach

NIC: Nonnutritive Sucking

Nonnutritive sucking is defined as the provision of sucking opportunities for the infant (McCloskey & Bulechek, 2000). Some important activities involved when implementing this intervention include:

- Selecting a smooth pacifier or pacifier substitute that is cleaned and sterilized daily, that is used only for that infant, and that meets the standards to prevent airway obstruction
- Positioning the infant to allow tongue to drop to floor of the mouth and positioning the caretaker's thumb and index finger under the infant's mandible to support the sucking reflex if necessary
- Moving the infant's tongue rhythmically with the pacifier to encourage sucking
- Rubbing the infant's cheek to stimulate the sucking reflex
- Providing a pacifier during tube feedings and for 5 minutes following the tube feeding, or at least every 4 hours if the infant is receiving total parenteral nutrition
- Rocking and holding the infant while sucking on pacifier if possible
- Informing the parents about the importance of meeting the infant's need to suck
- Encouraging a breast-feeding mother to allow nonnutritive sucking at breast after feeding is complete
- Instructing parents on alternatives to nipple sucking and the use of nonnutritive sucking

dling. As long as the infant is being gavage-fed, stomach secretions are usually aspirated, measured, and replaced before the feeding. An infant who has a stomach content of more than 2 mL just before a feeding is receiving more formula than he or she can digest in the time allowed. Feedings should not be increased but possibly even cut back to ensure better digestion and to decrease the possibility of regurgitation and aspiration. Inability to digest this way is also a symptom of necrotizing enterocolitis (see Chap. 45).

Formula. The caloric concentration of formulas used for preterm infants is usually 24 cal/oz, compared with 20 cal/oz for a term baby. Supplementing minerals such as iron, calcium, and phosphorus and electrolytes such as sodium, potassium, and chloride may be necessary, depending on the newborn's blood studies. As with a term neonate, vitamin K should be administered at birth. However, the amount administered is more often 0.5 mL instead of 1 mL because of the infant's small size. Vitamin A is important in improving healing and possibly reducing the incidence of lung disease. Vitamin E seems to be important in preventing hemolytic anemia in preterm infants.

Breast Milk. There is increasing evidence that although preterm infants grow well on the increased caloric distribution of commercial formulas, the best milk for them is breast milk. The immunologic properties of breast milk apparently play a major role in preventing neonatal necrotizing enterocolitis, a destructive intestinal disorder that often occurs in preterm babies.

The mother who wants to breast-feed can manually express breast milk for her infant's gavage feedings. If she cannot bring this in daily, the expressed breast milk can be frozen for safe transport and storage. The sodium content of breast milk in mothers whose infant has been born preterm is higher than that of milk at term. Therefore, it is better for the infant to receive his or her own mother's breast milk rather than banked milk. This high level of sodium is necessary for fluid retention in a preterm infant.

Nursing Diagnosis: Ineffective thermoregulation related to immaturity

Outcome Identification: Infant will maintain body temperature within normal limits until term age.

Outcome Evaluation: Infant's temperature is 97.6°F (36.5°C) axillary.

A preterm newborn has a great deal of difficulty maintaining body temperature because he or she has a relatively large surface area per kilogram of body weight. In addition, because the infant does not flex the body well but remains in an extended position, rapid cooling from evaporation is more likely to occur.

The preterm infant has little subcutaneous fat for insulation, and poor muscular development does not allow the child to move as actively as the older infant does to produce body heat. The preterm infant also has a limited amount of **brown fat,** the special tissue present in newborns to maintain body temperature. The infant is unable to shiver, a useful mechanism to increase body temperature; on the other hand, the child is unable to sweat and thereby reduce body temperature because of an immature central nervous system and hypothalamic control. Thus, the infant depends on the environmental temperature provided. In the delivery room, typically kept at a temperature of 62° to 68°F (16.6° to 20°C), the infant must be kept under a radiant heat warmer. A 1,500-g infant exposed to this low a temperature loses 1°C of body heat every 3 minutes if left unprotected (Baumgart et al., 2000).

Unless there are obvious abnormalities noted when the child is born, physical assessment of the infant, even weighing, should be delayed until the infant is placed in the warmth of an Isolette or under a radiant warmer with a Servocontrol.

If the infant is going to be transported to a department within the hospital, such as the x-ray department, or to a regional center for specialized care, keep the newborn warm during transport. Remember that infants lose heat by radiation. If a warmed Isolette is placed near a cold window or air conditioner, the infant will lose heat to the distant source. Also keep this in mind when transporting an infant on a cold day. The ambulance must be pulled in close to the hospital door. It and the transporting Isolette must be prewarmed. An additional heat shield or plastic wrap may be placed over an infant on a radiant warmer to help conserve heat.

Nursing Diagnosis: Risk for infection related to immature immune defenses in preterm infant

Outcome Identification: Infant will remain free of infection during hospital stay.

Outcome Evaluation: Temperature instability decreasing, being maintained at 97.6°F (36.5°C) axillary; absence of further signs and symptoms of infection such as poor growth or a reduced temperature.

The skin of the preterm baby is easily traumatized and therefore offers less resistance to infection than the skin and mucous membranes of the mature baby. In addition, the preterm infant has a lowered resistance to infection. The infant has difficulty producing phagocytes to localize infection and has a deficiency of IgM antibodies because of insufficient production. Linen and equipment used with the preterm infant must be clean to reduce the chances of infection. Staff members must be free of infection, and handwashing and gowning regulations must be strictly enforced.

✔ CHECKPOINT QUESTIONS

14. Why does acidosis clear quickly in the term newborn, but may cause irreversible problems in the preterm newborn?
15. During the first few days of life, how much urine should the preterm neonate produce?
16. How many calories are required by the preterm newborn daily?

Nursing Diagnosis: Risk for impaired parenting related to interference with parent–infant attachment resulting from hospitalization of infant at birth

Outcome Identification: Parents demonstrate adequate bonding behavior by the time of infant's discharge from the hospital.

Outcome Evaluation: Parents visit frequently and hold infant; speak of him or her in positive terms.

In the preterm infant, the first and second periods of reactivity normally observed in newborns at 1 hour and 4 hours of life (see Chap. 23) are delayed. In some infants, no period of increased activity or tachycardia may appear until 12 to 18 hours of age. If the purpose of a period of reactivity is to stimulate respiratory function, this places the preterm infant at an even greater threat of respiratory failure, because respiratory efforts may not be stimulated. A second consequence of a delayed period of reactivity is the loss of an opportunity for interaction between parents and the newborn in the early postpartal period.

At one time, a preterm infant was handled as little as possible by hospital staff to conserve the infant's energy. Parents were strictly isolated from the nursery to prevent the introduction of infection. When the child reached a "magic" weight of 4.5 or 5.5 lb, the parents were called and told that their child was ready to be discharged. Some nursery personnel offered to allow the mother to feed her infant once under supervision before the day of discharge. In other nurseries, the mother was simply handed the smallest infant she had ever seen and told to take the child home and "mother" this stranger.

Although it is extremely important to conserve the preterm infant's strength by reducing sensory stimulation as much as possible and handling the infant gently, it is now recognized that the child needs as much loving attention as possible. Rocking the infant, singing and talking to him or her, and gentle holding are measures to help the infant develop a sense of trust in people, which will enable the child to relate satisfactorily to them in the future. Holding the baby using kangaroo care (holding the infant with skin-to-skin contact) is yet another way to increase bonding. Encourage the parents to begin interacting with the infant in as normal a manner as possible (see Focus on Family Empowerment). Box 26-7 highlights appropriate outcomes and interventions using the terminology identified by the Nursing Outcomes Classification (NOC) and Nursing Interventions Classification (NIC).

Before effective bonding can be established, parents may need time to come to terms with their feelings of disappointment and guilt. A nurse can be instrumental in helping them air these feelings and develop a more positive attitude toward their preterm infant.

If the infant cannot be removed from an Isolette or radiant heat warmer, the child can still be held using kangaroo care or handled and stroked in the Isolette or warmer. Because parents are not psychologically ready for birth when the preterm baby is born, it may be more difficult for them to believe they have a child than if the baby were born at term. Encourage the mother to express breast milk for the infant if the child is too young to nurse. If a woman decides not to breast-feed, she should be encouraged to come

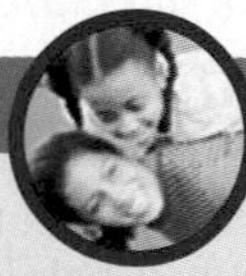

FOCUS ON FAMILY EMPOWERMENT
Guidelines for Parents of a Newborn in Intensive Care

Q. We're going to be visiting our son in the neonatal intensive care unit, but we're a little afraid. What can we do so that we're not so frightened?

A. Here are some guidelines that should be helpful:

- Learn the name of your child's primary nurse or care manager and physician. Make a point of talking to them when you visit so the information you receive is consistent and these people can get to know you.
- Discuss with your child's care manager or primary nurse the time you will usually visit so she or he can reserve this time for you. It also helps them to schedule the baby's procedures and rest times so there is time during your visits for you to hold your child and interact with him.
- Ask for explanations of any equipment or medications being used with your child so you understand the plan of care. Insist on being included in care decisions.
- If you cannot visit on any day, feel free to telephone the nursery and ask to talk to your child's primary care nurse or physician. Such telephone calls are not viewed as a bother but are welcomed as the mark of a concerned parent.
- If you planned to breast-feed, ask if you can supply expressed breast milk for your infant as soon as feedings are started. This may help to give you a feeling of having a greater part in your baby's care.
- Supply a tape recording of your voice so your baby can learn to recognize it, and a small toy for your baby's bed. These actions not only supply auditory and visual stimulation for your child but also help to give you a more "normal" feeling toward infant care.
- Use your baby's name when you talk about him (not "the baby") to help you gain a firm feeling that this is your baby, not the nursery's.
- If your child is hospitalized a distance from home, ask if transfer to a local hospital in a less technical environment at a later date will be possible.

BOX 26.7

NURSING OUTCOMES AND NURSING INTERVENTIONS CLASSIFICATION: BONDING

NOC: Parent–Infant Attachment

Parent–infant attachment is defined as the behaviors that demonstrate an enduring affectionate bond between a parent and infant (Johnson, Maas, & Moorhead, 2000). Some specific indicators suggesting achievement of this outcome include the demonstration of the following by the parents:

- Assigning specific attributes to the fetus
- Verbalizing positive feelings toward the infant
- Holding the infant close, touching, stroking, patting, kissing, and talking to the infant
- Using eye contact, smiling, and vocalizing with the infant in the en face position
- Responding to infant's cues

Indicators suggesting achievement of this outcome include the demonstration of the following by the infant:

- Responding to cues
- Seeking proximity with the parents
- Exploring the environment

NIC: Attachment Promotion

Attachment promotion is defined as the facilitation of the development of the parent–infant relationship (McCloskey & Bulechek, 2000). Some important activities to address when implementing this intervention include:

- Encouraging the parents to visit the infant frequently, touching and holding the infant, especially if infant is being transferred to another facility
- Encouraging parents to hold the infant close to the body
- Sharing information gained from the initial assessment of the newborn
- Reinforcing eye contact with the infant
- Explaining equipment used to monitor the infant
- Taking a Polaroid photo of the infant to leave with the parents before infant is transported
- Informing parents of care being given to the infant and of the behavioral characteristics that the infant exhibits while being cared for in the other facility
- Pointing out infant state changes and cues indicating responsiveness
- Reinforcing the normal aspects of infant

NIC: Kangaroo Care

Kangaroo care is defined as the promotion of closeness between parents and a physiologically stable preterm infant by preparing the parent and providing the environment for skin-to-skin contact (Johnson, Maas, & Moorhead, 2000). Some important activities to address when implementing this intervention include:

- Discussing the parents' reaction to the preterm infant and the image that they have of the infant
- Encouraging the parent to initiate infant care
- Determining if infant physiologically meets the guidelines for kangaroo care
- Preparing a quiet, draft-free environment, with parent sitting in rocking chair, wearing comfortable, open-front clothing
- Instructing how to move infant from incubator, warmer bed, or bassinet and how to manage equipment
- Positioning diaper-clad infant prone and upright on parent's chest
- Encouraging the parents to focus on infant, gently stroking and rocking as appropriate
- Encouraging use of auditory stimulation
- Supporting parents in nurturing and providing hands-on care
- Instructing parents to decrease activity when infant shows signs of overstimulation, distress, or avoidance
- Encouraging parent to let infant sleep, or breast-feed during care
- Urging parent to provide kangaroo care from 20 minutes to 3 hours at a time consistently
- Monitoring the infant's physiologic status, discontinuing kangaroo care if infant becomes compromised or agitated

into the hospital and hold the baby before and after gavage feedings or to give bottle feedings. By feeding her baby or expressing milk for the feedings, she is directly participating in the care and taking on responsibility for the infant's welfare.

If the baby is transferred to a regional center, the parents should have an opportunity to see the baby before the transfer. A photograph of the baby for them to keep is helpful in making the birth more real. Encourage them to visit as often as possible. Notes to convey messages from the baby to them can be taped to the Isolette or warmer.

On the days they cannot visit, parents can still stay in touch by telephone. By the time the baby is ready for discharge, the parents should be able to feel that they are taking home "their" baby, one who they know and are ready to love.

Parents visiting a high-risk nursery often need a great deal of attention and support from nursing personnel. Remember that although radiant warmers, Isolettes, ventilators, and monitors are familiar equipment to nurses, they are unusual and frightening to parents. A parent may want very much to touch an infant but be so afraid that touching might set off an alarm that he or she stands back with arms folded instead (Fig. 26-9).

Making parents and the baby's siblings welcome in a high-risk nursery is a major role for the nurse of

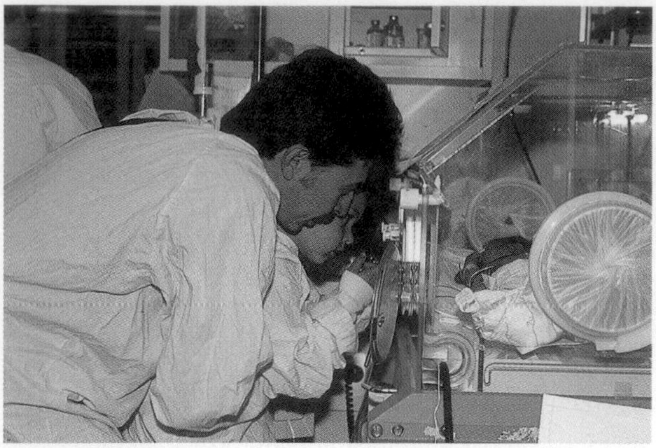

FIGURE 26.9 Families should be encouraged to visit with immature infants to establish bonding.

high-risk infants (see Focus on Communication). Be aware of any possible restrictions in sibling visitation because of infections, such as colds or fever. It is also important to make sure that siblings' immunizations are up to date and they have not been recently exposed to communicable diseases, such as chickenpox. Because preterm infants are hospitalized for long periods, parents can be baffled by receiving information from a parade of different health care professionals or a different person every time they visit. With primary nursing or case management, one nurse is the consistent caregiver who communicates the baby's nursing needs to the rest of the staff and acts as the liaison with the baby's parents.

WHAT IF? A new mother is about to visit her preterm newborn for the first time. She states, "I'm so scared. He's so tiny and frail. How can I even hold him?" How should you respond to this new mother to ease her visit?

Nursing Diagnosis: Deficient diversional activity (lack of stimulation) related to preterm infant's rest needs

Outcome Identification: Infant will receive adequate stimulation during hospitalization.

Outcome Evaluation: Infant demonstrates interaction with caregivers by attuning to faces or voices.

Preterm infants need rest to conserve energy for growth and respiratory function, to combat hypoglycemia and infection, to stabilize temperature, and to develop inner balance and attentiveness. To allow for this, procedures should be organized to maximize the amount of rest available to the infant. If this is not a coordinated effort, the infant may be awakened constantly for procedures. Recent research has shown that preterm infants may have difficulty blocking out stimuli as a result of an immature nervous system. They may react negatively by gagging, crying, splaying fingers and toes, or going limp when exposed to bright lights, noise, or too strenuous handling (Camerota and Arnold, 2000). Because these infants have little strength to move away from an unwanted stimulus, it is the caregiver's responsibility to be sensitive to these cues and move the object or noise away from the infant. Until ready to take in stimuli, the newborn may need to be shielded from noise and light as much as possible. Pain should be kept to a minimum. When the infant is ill, handling also should be kept to a minimum to preserve respiratory function.

FOCUS ON COMMUNICATION

Mrs. Atkins gave birth to a 2-lb boy at 36 weeks of pregnancy, 2 days ago. The infant has been classified as a small-for-gestational-age preterm infant. Although you told Mrs. Atkins twice that she is welcome to visit the neonatal intensive care unit (NICU), you notice on her chart that she has not yet done so.

Less Effective Communication

Nurse: Mrs. Atkins, I've noticed you haven't been to the nursery to see your son yet.
Mrs. Atkins: I'm waiting for my husband to come in.
Nurse: Will that be today?
Mrs. Atkins: Tomorrow. He's a truck driver and out on the road until then.
Nurse: Have you telephoned the nursery to ask about your son?
Mrs. Atkins: No. I'm waiting for my husband. We'll do it together.
Nurse: Okay. Let me know if there is anything else you need.

More Effective Communication

Nurse: Mrs. Atkins, I've noticed you haven't been to the nursery to see your son yet.
Mrs. Atkins: I'm waiting for my husband to come in.
Nurse: Will that be today?
Mrs. Atkins: Tomorrow. He's a truck driver and out on the road until then.
Nurse: Have you telephoned the nursery to ask about your son?
Mrs. Atkins: No. I'm waiting for my husband. We'll do it together.
Nurse: Often it's intimidating to visit or telephone a high-risk nursery. I know it is important to you to go as a family, but I hate to see you miss these first few days with your son. What if I go with you?
Mrs. Atkins: Could you? I don't want to go alone.

Visiting an NICU is intimidating for parents not only because of the high-tech equipment that surrounds their baby but because their baby often appears much smaller or sicker than they imagined. In the first scenario, the nurse assumed that waiting for the husband to come to the hospital was what was important to the mother. In the second scenario, the nurse asked enough questions to realize that another person to accompany her to the nursery was the mother's need, a need the nurse could meet.

At the same time, the infant needs planned periods of pleasing sensory stimulation. Like all newborns, preterm infants respond best to stimulation that appeals to their senses—sight, sound, and touch. A passive face, picture, or decal may be appealing for only short periods.

The view from inside an Isolette may be distorted by the acrylic dome. Most people view an infant in an Isolette from the side. Thus, the infant's face is rarely in the same line of vision as the adult (an en face position). It is important to look directly at the infant in the straightforward position so the infant is provided with the stimulation of a human face. As the infant matures, he or she should have a mobile (perhaps black and white) or a bright object placed in view. As the infant's position is changed from side to stomach to opposite side, the object should be moved to be in line with the child's vision.

An infant in a closed Isolette may be able to hear nothing but the sound of the Isolette motor. The infant may see people looking or nodding at him or her and may see their mouths moving, but he or she cannot benefit from the sound of their voices because this is obscured by the continuous hum of the motor. Provide some talk time—words spoken softly but clearly to the infant's ear—during each nursing shift to offer normal contact.

Even an infant who cannot be removed from the Isolette should not suffer from lack of touch. Gently stroking the infant's back or smoothing the back of the head should not be tiring. Transcutaneous oxygen determinations allow you to recognize when the infant is comforted by handling and when the child is growing tired. There should be time during every nursing shift for this interaction, particularly if clinical interventions with the infant include uncomfortable procedures such as suctioning or blood drawing. As soon as the infant can be out of the Isolette or removed from the warmer, he or she needs special time just to be rocked and held.

Nursing Diagnosis: Risk for disorganized infant behavior related to prematurity and environmental overstimulation

Outcome Identification: Newborn will respond and adjust positively to stimulation.

Outcome Evaluation: Newborn's vital signs remain within normal limits; demonstrates increasing ability to adapt to stimuli; demonstrates decreasing levels of irritability, crying, respiratory pauses, tachypnea, and color changes.

The amount of rest and stimulation required by preterm infants for healthy development is unknown. In the 1950s, complete bedrest and minimal handling were advocated for care; in the 1960s, stimulation by rocking or stroking was introduced. Today, developmental care (care designed to meet the specific needs of each infant) is advocated. This type of care can lead to increased weight gain and decreased crying and apnea spells in preterm infants. Box 26-8 highlights appropriate outcomes and interventions using the terminology identified by the Nursing Outcomes Classification (NOC) and Nursing Interventions Classification (NIC).

Nursing care of preterm infants must take into consideration the immaturity of their central nervous systems. Therefore, their reactions or adjustments to stimuli may be different from those of term infants. The environment of an intensive care unit is totally different from what the infant would have experienced if he or she had remained in utero until term. Based on these two premises, nursing care must be geared toward making the environment of the infant as atraumatic as possible while helping the infant adjust to new experiences with his or her limited ability.

The usual sound level of nurseries has been documented to be about 40 to 50 dB; a radio playing raises this to 60 to 65 dB. The closing of portholes or tapping on the sides of Isolettes raises the sound level inside them to 80 dB or more. Other abnormal stimuli are bright lights for 24 hours a day, frequent handling, and painful procedures.

When a preterm infant is stressed, behaviors such as respiratory pauses, tachypnea, color changes, tremors, sighing, flaccidity, finger splaying, and gaze averting occur. Such behaviors should alert a caregiver that the environment has become too stimulating and needs to be modified. Activities such as dimming the lights or covering an Isolette, turning the infant to the side and containing his body with rolled towels, offering nonnutritive sucking, and maintaining a "quiet hour" to reduce sound are all ways to reduce stimuli.

Nursing Diagnosis: Parental health-seeking behaviors related to preterm infant's needs for health maintenance

Outcome Identification: Parents will express confidence in routine follow-up health care at time of hospital discharge.

Outcome Evaluation: Parents describe schedule for basic immunizations and health assessments and state who will provide ongoing health care.

Discharge from an NICU is a major transition for parents as well as the infant. Before discharge from a health care facility, the parents of a preterm infant need to learn and practice any special methods of care necessary for their infant and interventions to help maximize their child's development. Some parents tend to overprotect preterm infants, such as not allowing visitors or not taking the infant outside. Let the parents know that this is not necessary. Doing so does not alleviate the problem, but it may help make the parents feel normal in light of their concern.

Ongoing health maintenance of the preterm infant follows the usual pattern of well-child care. Basic immunizations are given according to the chronologic age of the infant. In many communities, neonatal intensive care nurseries maintain their own well-child conferences for infants who were hospitalized there. This allows for long-term follow-up

BOX 26.8

NURSING OUTCOMES AND NURSING INTERVENTIONS CLASSIFICATION: DEVELOPMENTAL CARE

NOC: Child Development (various age determinations)

Child development is defined as the milestones of physical, cognitive, and psychosocial progression by specific age determinations, such as 2 months, 4 months, 6 months, 12 months, 2 years, and so on (Johnson, Maas, & Moorhead, 2000). Some specific indicators suggesting achievement of this outcome for the child at 2 months of age include the following:

- Closed posterior fontanelle
- Ability to lift head, neck, and upper chest with support on forearms when prone
- Frequently open hands
- Fading of grasp reflex
- Demonstration of interest in auditory and visual stimuli
- Smiling
- Evidence of pleasure in interactions, especially with primary caregivers

NIC: Developmental Care

Developmental care is defined as structuring the environment to provide care in response to the behavioral cues and states of the preterm infant (McCloskey & Bulechek, 2000). Some important activities associated with implementing this intervention include:

- Providing space on the unit and at the bedside for the parents
- Supplying accurate, factual information about the infant's condition, treatment, and needs
- Informing parents about developmental concerns and issues
- Assisting parents to become acquainted with their infant
- Teaching parents to recognize cues and states
- Demonstrating infant capabilities and how to elicit infant's visual and auditory attention
- Pointing out infant's self-regulatory activities
- Providing time-out when infant exhibits signs of stress
- Providing boundaries to maintain flexion of extremities while still allowing room for extension and supports to maintain positioning
- Monitoring stimuli, decreasing environmental ambient light and environmental noise
- Positioning incubator away from noise sources
- Timing infant care and feeding around sleep/wake cycle
- Clustering care to promote longest possible sleep interval and energy conservation
- Using slow, gentle movements when handling, feeding, or caring for the newborn
- Promoting parent participation in feeding, including use of nonnutritive sucking
- Establishing consistency and predictable routines
- Providing stimulation using tape-recorded instrumental music, mobiles, massage, rocking, and touch as appropriate

studies on the effect of oxygen or drug therapy and continuity of care. Many parents prefer bringing their infant back to such a facility rather than establishing a new network of health care because they have already established trust and confidence in that health care team. This often also increases their self-esteem because they hear the staff's delight in the progress made by the child. However, preterm infants can be followed by any health care provider.

When plotting the height and weight of preterm infants, remember to account for early birth on the growth chart by double charting—that is, plotting the child's weight and height according to the chronologic age (a pattern that probably in the early months places the child below the 10th percentile). Then, in another color, plot the height and weight according to the infant's "setback" or adjusted age, or the age the infant would be if he or she had been born at term. A preterm baby typically gains "catch-up" weight in the first 6 months of life, so by age 1 year the baby reaches over the 10th percentile on a growth chart without accounting for a setback age.

Evaluate growth and development of the infant by the same manner. A preterm infant can be expected to meet first-year milestones not at the chronologic age but at the setback age. Also evaluate the parents' transition to having the neonate at home.

At health promotion visits, ask if the parents are:

- Beginning to feel more comfortable with the infant
- Able to allow the child to stay with a babysitter or another family member
- Experiencing less of the shock of having such a fragile infant
- Beginning to incorporate the infant normally into their family life
- Making plans beyond the immediate newborn period

✔ CHECKPOINT QUESTIONS

17. What are signs that a preterm infant is overly stressed?
18. At what age are first immunizations such as polio vaccine given to a preterm infant?

The Postterm Infant

A postterm infant is one born after the 42nd week of a pregnancy. Most nurse-midwives and obstetricians recommend inducing labor at 2 weeks postterm to avoid postterm births. However, when gestational age has been miscalculated or if for some other reason labor is not induced until week 43 of pregnancy or after, the pregnancy may result in a postterm infant.

An infant who stays in utero past week 42 of pregnancy is at special risk because a placenta appears to function effectively for only 40 weeks. After this time, it seems to lose its ability to carry nutrients effectively to the fetus. The fetus who remains in utero with a failing placenta may die or develop **postterm syndrome.** Infants with this syndrome have many of the characteristics of the SGA infant: dry, cracked, almost leather-like skin from lack of fluid, and absence of vernix. They may be lightweight from a recent weight loss that occurred because of the poor placental function. The amount of amniotic fluid may be less at birth than normal, and it may be meconium-stained. Fingernails have grown well beyond the end of the fingertips. Such infants may demonstrate an alertness much more like a 2-week-old baby than a newborn (Alexander et al., 2001).

When a pregnancy becomes postterm, a sonogram may be obtained to measure the biparietal diameter of the fetus. A nonstress test or complete biophysical profile (see Chap. 8) may be done to establish whether the placenta is still functioning adequately. Cesarean birth may be indicated if a nonstress test reveals that compromised placental functioning may occur during labor.

At birth, the postterm baby is likely to have difficulty establishing respirations, especially if meconium aspiration occurred. In the first hours of life, hypoglycemia may develop owing to insufficient stores of glycogen, which were used for nourishment in the last weeks of intrauterine life. Subcutaneous fat levels may also be low, having been used up in utero. Therefore, temperature regulation may be difficult. Protect the infant from chilling at birth or during transport. Polycythemia may be present from decreased oxygenation in the final weeks. The hematocrit may be elevated because of the polycythemia and dehydration, which lowers the circulating plasma level.

Any woman is anxious when she does not have her baby on her due date. She becomes extremely anxious and perhaps angry when it is determined that her baby is postterm. It may seem to her that if the baby stayed so long in utero, he or she should be extra healthy and strong. Why, then, is the baby being transferred for special care? She may also feel guilty for not providing well for the infant in the last few weeks of pregnancy.

The mother needs to spend time with her newborn to assure herself that although birth did not occur at the predicted time, the baby should do well with appropriate interventions to control possible hypoglycemia or meconium aspiration. All postterm infants need follow-up care until at least school age to track their developmental abilities. The lack of nutrients and oxygen in utero may have left them with neurologic symptoms that will not become apparent until they attempt fine motor tasks.

ILLNESS IN THE NEWBORN

Respiratory Distress Syndrome

Respiratory distress syndrome (RDS) of the newborn, formerly termed *hyaline membrane disease,* most often occurs in preterm infants, infants of diabetic mothers, infants born by cesarean birth, or those who for any reason have decreased blood perfusion of the lungs. The pathologic feature of RDS is a hyaline-like (fibrous) membrane comprising products formed from an exudate of the infant's blood that lines the terminal bronchioles, alveolar ducts, and alveoli. This membrane prevents exchange of oxygen and carbon dioxide at the alveolar-capillary membrane. The cause of RDS is a low level or absence of surfactant, the phospholipid that normally lines the alveoli and reduces surface tension on expiration to keep the alveoli from collapsing on expiration.

As many as 30% of low-birth-weight infants and as many as 50% of very-low-birth-weight infants are susceptible to this complication (Whitsett et al., 2000). Other newborns who are more prone than others to develop this condition include those born by cesarean birth, those with meconium-stained amniotic fluid, and those with infection.

Pathophysiology

High pressure is required to fill the lungs with air for the first time and overcome the pressure of lung fluid. It takes a pressure between 40 and 70 cm H_2O to inspire a first breath but only 15 to 20 cm H_2O to maintain quiet, continued breathing. If alveoli collapse with each expiration, as happens when surfactant is deficient, however, it continues to take forceful inspiration to inflate them.

Even very immature infants release a bolus of surfactant at birth into their lungs from the stress of birth. However, with deficient surfactant, areas of hypoinflation occur and pulmonary resistance is increased. Blood then shunts through the foramen ovale and the ductus arteriosus as it did during fetal life. The lungs are poorly perfused, affecting gas exchange. As a result, the production of surfactant decreases even further.

The poor oxygen exchange leads to tissue hypoxia, which causes the release of lactic acid. This, combined with the increasing carbon dioxide level resulting from the formation of the hyaline membrane on the alveolar surface, leads to severe acidosis. Acidosis causes vasoconstriction, and decreased pulmonary perfusion from vasoconstriction further limits surfactant production.

With decreased surfactant production, the ability to stop alveoli from collapsing with each expiration becomes impaired. This vicious cycle continues until the oxygen-carbon dioxide exchange in the alveoli is no longer adequate to sustain life without ventilator support.

Assessment

Most infants who develop RDS had difficulty initiating respirations at birth. After resuscitation, they appear to have a period of hours or a day when they are free of symptoms because of an initial release of surfactant. During this time, subtle signs may appear:

- Low body temperature
- Nasal flaring
- Sternal and subcostal retractions
- Tachypnea (more than 60 respirations per minute)
- Cyanotic mucous membranes

Within several hours, expiratory grunting, which indicates a prolonged expiratory time, becomes apparent. The sound is a compensatory mechanism from closure of the glottis. This mechanism increases the pressure in the alveoli on expiration, helps to keep the alveoli from collapsing, and makes oxygen exchange more complete. Even with this attempt at better oxygen exchange, however, as the disease progresses infants become cyanotic and their Po_2 and oxygen saturation levels fall on room air. On auscultation, there may be fine rales and diminished breath sounds because of poor air entry. As distress increases, the infant may exhibit the following:

- Seesaw respirations (on inspiration, the anterior chest wall retracts and the abdomen protrudes; on expiration, the sternum rises)
- Heart failure, evidenced by decreased urine output and edema of the extremities
- Pale gray skin
- Periods of apnea
- Bradycardia
- Pneumothorax

The diagnosis of RDS is made on the clinical signs of grunting, cyanosis in room air, tachypnea, nasal flaring, retractions, and shock. A chest x-ray film will reveal a diffuse pattern of radiopaque areas that look like ground glass (haziness). Blood gas studies (taken from an umbilical vessel catheter) will reveal respiratory acidosis. A beta-hemolytic, group B streptococcal infection may mimic RDS. This infection is so severe in newborns that the insult to the lungs is intense enough to stop surfactant production. Cultures of blood, cerebrospinal fluid, and skin may be obtained to rule out this condition. An antibiotic (penicillin or ampicillin) and an aminoglycoside (gentamicin or kanamycin) may be started while culture reports are pending.

Therapeutic Management

RDS can be largely prevented by the administration of surfactant through an endotracheal tube at birth for the infant at risk because of low gestational age.

Surfactant Replacement. As a preventive measure, synthetic surfactant is sprayed into the lungs by a syringe or catheter through an endotracheal tube at birth while the infant is first positioned with the head held upright and then tilted downward. The infant is suctioned before surfactant administration. It is important that the infant's airway not be suctioned for as long a period as possible after administration to avoid suctioning the drug away. Although there are almost no unfavorable reactions to surfactant administration, some, such as mucus plugging from the solution, do occur. The infant who is receiving surfactant and then is placed on a ventilator needs close observation because lung expansion can improve rapidly. Anticipate the need to adjust ventilator settings to prevent excessive lung pressure.

Oxygen Administration. Administration of oxygen is necessary to maintain correct Po_2 and pH levels. Continuous positive airway pressure (CPAP) or assisted ventilation with positive end-expiratory pressure (PEEP) will exert pressure on the alveoli at the end of expiration and keep the alveoli from collapsing. This greatly improves oxygen exchange. A possible complication of oxygen therapy in the very immature or very ill infant is retinopathy of prematurity (see discussion later in chapter) or bronchopulmonary dysplasia (see Chap. 40).

Ventilation. Normally, on a ventilator, inspiration is shorter than expiration, or there is an inspiratory/expiratory ratio (I/E ratio) of 1:2. It is difficult to deliver enough oxygen to stiff, noncompliant lungs in this usual ratio without forcing the air into the lungs at such a high pressure and rapid rate that a pneumothorax becomes a constant fear. Infant ventilators are available with a reversed I/E ratio (2:1). These are pressure-cycled, which controls the force with which air is delivered. High-frequency, oscillatory, and jet ventilation are other methods of introducing oxygen to infants with noncompliant lungs. These systems maintain airway pressure and then intermittently "jet" or oscillate at a rapid rate (400 to 600 times a minute) an additional amount of air to inflate alveoli.

Complications of any type of ventilation are possible, such as pneumothorax and impaired cardiac output because of decreased flow through the pulmonary artery from lung pressure. There is also a possible risk of increased intracranial and arterial pressure and hemorrhage. Limiting fluid intake may help to decrease pulmonary artery pressure.

Indomethacin may be used to cause closure of the patent ductus arteriosus, thus making ventilation more efficient. Indomethacin, however, has been associated with adverse effects such as decreased renal function, decreased platelet count, and gastric irritation. Carefully monitor urine output and observe for bleeding, especially at blood puncture sites.

Additional Therapy. Yet another method of increasing pulmonary blood flow is by using muscle relaxants. Pancuronium (Pavulon) is administered intravenously to the point of abolishing spontaneous respiratory action. Doing so allows mechanical ventilation to be accomplished at lower pressures because there is no normal muscle resistance to overcome. The possibility of pneumothorax is reduced while Po_2 is increased. Obviously an infant who has no spontaneous respiratory function because of drug administration needs critical observation and frequent arterial blood gas analysis because he or she totally depends on caregivers at this point (Cools & Offringa, 2000).

The effects of pancuronium decrease as the life of the drug expires; its effects can be interrupted by the administration of atropine or injectable neostigmine methylsulfate (Prostigmin Methylsulfate Injectable).

When pancuronium is being administered, both atropine and Prostigmin should be immediately available. The infant's plan of care should be specially marked to show that pancuronium therapy is being used so that in the event of a power failure, manual ventilatory assistance can be begun immediately.

Some infants are maintained on **extracorporeal membrane oxygenation** (ECMO) to ensure adequate oxygenation (Hintz et al., 2000). Other therapies include liquid ventilation or administration of perfluorocarbons and inhalation of nitric oxide.

> **WHAT IF?** What if while you were caring for an infant who was ventilator-dependent and receiving pancuronium, a power failure occurred? What would be your first actions?

Extracorporeal Membrane Oxygenation. ECMO was first developed as a means of oxygenating blood during cardiac surgery. Its current use has expanded to the management of chronic severe hypoxemia in newborns with illnesses such as meconium aspiration, RDS, pneumonia, and diaphragmatic hernia. It is used also for near-drowning victims or infants with severe lung infection (Hintz et al., 2000). Blood is removed by gravity using a venous catheter advanced into the right atrium of the heart. The blood circulates from the catheter to the ECMO machine, where it is oxygenated and rewarmed. It is then returned to the infant's aortic arch by a catheter advanced through the carotid artery. ECMO is typically used for 4 to 7 days. ECMO has many potential complications, chief of which is intracranial hemorrhage, possibly from the anticoagulation therapy that is necessary to prevent thromboembolism. Constant nursing care is required for the child receiving ECMO to ensure the child's blood volume remains adequate, bleeding does not occur, and adequate oxygen is being supplied to the body tissues.

Liquid Ventilation. Liquid ventilation involves the use of perfluorocarbons, substances used in industry to assess for leakage in pipes. When oxygen is bubbled through it, perfluorocarbons pick up and carry the oxygen with them. When perfluorocarbons are introduced into lungs that inflate poorly because they are deficient in surfactant, or in lungs damaged by trauma or disease, the weight of the fluid, which is heavy compared with air, helps to distend the lung. As the liquid moves into the lung, oxygen is carried along with it; as the liquid spreads over all lung surfaces, an exchange of oxygen occurs. The administration of liquid ventilation is effective in delivering oxygen and surfactant to newborns' lungs. (Chappell et al., 2001).

Nitric Oxide. An additional measure that can help to oxygenate newborn lungs is the administration of nitric oxide. This causes pulmonary vasodilation and can be very helpful to increase blood flow to the alveoli when persistent pulmonary hypertension is present (Ward and Lugo, 2000).

Supportive Care. The infant with RDS needs specialized intensive care. The infant must be kept warm because cooling increases acidosis in all newborns, and for the newborn with RDS it may increase to lethal levels. Keeping the infant warm also reduces the metabolic oxygen demand. Provide hydration and nutrition with intravenous fluids, glucose, or gavage feeding because the respiratory effort makes the infant too exhausted to suck (see Focus on Nursing Care Planning).

Prevention

RDS rarely occurs in mature infants. Dating a pregnancy by sonogram or the lecithin/sphingomyelin ratio of amniotic fluid is an important way to be certain that an infant born by cesarean birth or induced is mature enough that RDS is not apt to occur. If the level of lecithin in surfactant exceeds that of sphingomyelin by 2:1, the lungs are mature and RDS is not likely to occur.

Using tocolytic agents such as terbutaline helps to prevent preterm births. Because steroids appear to quicken the formation of lecithin production pathways, it may be possible to prevent RDS in infants by administering two injections of a glucocorticosteroid, such as betamethasone, to the mother at 12 and 24 hours before birth. This is most effective when given between weeks 24 and 34 of pregnancy. Unfortunately, there is often no warning that preterm birth is imminent until hours before birth. Because the steroid does not take effect before 24 to 48 hours, some labors and births will progress too rapidly for this preventive measure to be effective.

> ✔ **CHECKPOINT QUESTIONS**
>
> 19. What is the underlying cause of respiratory distress syndrome?
> 20. What is the rationale for administering pancuronium to infants on ventilators?

Transient Tachypnea of the Newborn

At birth, a newborn may have a rapid rate of respiration, up to 80 breaths per minute when crying. Within 1 hour, however, this rapid rate slows to between 30 and 60 breaths per minute. In about 10 in 1,000 live births, the respiratory rate remains at a high level, between 80 and 120 breaths per minute (Whitsett et al., 2000). The infant does not appear to be in a great deal of distress, aside from the tiring effort of breathing so rapidly. He or she has mild retractions but not marked cyanosis. Mild hypoxia and hypercapnia may be present. Feeding is difficult because the child cannot suck and breathe this rapidly at the same time. A chest x-ray reveals some fluid in the central lung, but aeration is adequate.

Transient tachypnea appears to result from slow absorption of lung fluid. It may reflect a slight decrease in production of phosphatidyl glycerol or mature surfactant. These factors limit the amount of alveolar surface area available to the infant for oxygen exchange. Thus, the infant must increase the respiratory rate and depth to better use the surface available. Transient tachypnea occurs more often in infants who are born by cesarean birth, in infants whose mothers received extensive fluid administration during labor, and in preterm infants. Infants born by cesarean birth are probably more prone to develop this form of respiratory distress because the thoracic cavity is not

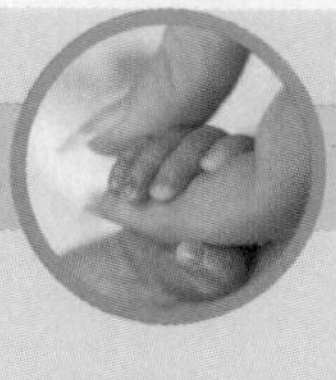

FOCUS ON *Nursing Care Planning*

A NEWBORN WITH RESPIRATORY DISTRESS SYNDROME

A preterm, small-for-gestational-age newborn, born at 29 weeks' gestation and transported to the neonatal intensive care unit (NICU) at a major urban medical center 50 miles away, is diagnosed with respiratory distress syndrome.

Assessment: Newborn, 5 hours old, delivered vaginally. Difficulty establishing respirations at birth. Temperature 97.2°F (36.2°C). Bradycardic and tachypneic with grunting respirations. Sternal and subcostal retractions present. Skin pale and somewhat cyanotic. Chest x-ray with ground-glass appearance. Arterial blood gases (ABGs) reveal respiratory acidosis. Endotracheal (ET) intubation, mechanical ventilation, supplemental oxygen, and intravenous fluid therapy initiated. Parents briefly saw newborn immediately after birth. Husband with mother who will be discharged tomorrow from the community hospital. Voicing concerns about the newborn's condition.

Nursing Diagnosis: Impaired gas exchange related to immaturity of the newborn's lungs and diminished surfactant

Outcome Identification: Newborn will demonstrate signs of improved gas exchange within 24 hours.

Outcome Evaluation: Vital signs within acceptable parameters. Temperature maintained at 97.7°F (36.5°C). Absence of cyanosis; diminished retractions; ABG values within acceptable parameters.

Interventions	Rationale
1. Assess newborn's respiratory status closely and note any signs and symptoms of increasing respiratory distress. Assess respiratory rate, depth, and rhythm; auscultate lung sounds; evaluate ABG results and skin color.	1. Assessment provides a baseline for future comparisons. Signs and symptoms of increasing respiratory distress are ominous.
2. Maintain endotracheal tube, mechanical ventilation, and supplemental warm humidified oxygen. Assess oxygen saturation levels via pulse oximetry. Anticipate the need for CPAP or PEEP.	2. The ET tube maintains a patent airway. Mechanical ventilation assists with delivering necessary air to the lungs. Using warm, humidified oxygen prevents cold stress and drying of mucous membranes. Oxygen saturation levels provide information about tissue oxygenation. CPAP and PEEP exert pressure on alveoli at end expiration, preventing alveolar collapse.
3. Prepare to administer surfactant via ET.	3. Surfactant restores the naturally occurring lung surfactant to improve lung compliance.
4. Change the newborn's position during administration and refrain from suctioning the ET tube for up to 1 hour following administration.	4. Position changes enhance drug delivery to both lungs. Suctioning would remove the drug from its intended site.
5. Continue to assess the newborn's respiratory status closely. Adjust ventilator settings as indicated based on assessment findings.	5. Continued assessment is necessary to evaluate the effectiveness of drug therapy and for early detection of possible adverse effects. Surfactant can improve lung function rapidly. Too-high ventilator settings may cause pneumothorax.
6. Anticipate administration of indomethacin and pancuronium.	6. Indomethacin causes closure of a patent ductus arteriosus, making ventilation more effective. Pancuronium is a neuromuscular blocker that helps to prevent the neonate from "fighting" the ventilator.

(continued)

Interventions	Rationale
7. Maintain a neutral thermal environment and minimize physical activity.	7. Neutral thermal environment minimizes the risk of cold stress, which increases metabolic demands for oxygen. Physical activity increases metabolic oxygen demands.
8. Suction the ET tube as necessary.	8. Suctioning ensures a patent airway. Surfactant, although relatively safe, can cause mucous plugging.
9. Plan nursing care to allow for frequent rest periods and attempt to anticipate the newborn's needs. Handle the newborn gently and slowly.	9. Anticipating needs and providing rest minimize oxygen demands.
10. Continue frequent monitoring of all aspects of the newborn's respiratory status for changes.	10. Frequent follow-up assessments provide information about the newborn's status and allow for early detection and prompt intervention should health status deteriorate.

Nursing Diagnosis: Risk for imbalanced nutrition, less than body requirements related to immaturity and increased nutrient needs associated with effects of respiratory distress syndrome and its treatments

Outcome Identification: Newborn will ingest sufficient nutrients to support recovery and growth.

Outcome Evaluation: Newborn exhibits weight gain of at least 0.5 oz/day with caloric intake of 110 to 150 cal/kg/day. Urine output within appropriate parameters for weight.

Interventions	Rationale
1. Obtain daily weight.	1. Daily weights are a reliable indicator of hydration and nutritional status.
2. Administer nutrition via enteral feedings with breast milk supplemented with high-calorie formula. Anticipate the need for total parenteral nutrition.	2. Additional nutrients are necessary for optimal growth and development because the stress of respiratory distress syndrome and its associated treatments can result in increased caloric expenditure greater than the intake. Total parenteral nutrition may be necessary to meet these additional needs.
3. Provide a means, such as a pacifier, for nonnutritive sucking.	3. Nonnutritive sucking meets the newborn's need for sucking and also offers some comfort.
4. Maintain intravenous fluid infusions as ordered. Monitor intake and output closely.	4. Intravenous fluid provides additional fluid, glucose, and electrolytes to meet increased nutritional needs. Intake and output provides indicators of the newborn's fluid status.
5. Assess blood glucose levels every 4 hours by heel stick.	5. Glucose is a source of energy. Monitoring glucose levels helps to determine if sufficient energy is available to meet the newborn's metabolic needs.

Nursing Diagnosis: Risk for impaired parent–infant attachment related to physical separation from the newborn and high-risk status

Outcome Identification: Parents will exhibit positive attachment behaviors toward the newborn.

Outcome Evaluation: Parents hold infant close and make eye contact; verbalize positive feelings about the newborn; telephone NICU every day; participate in newborn's care when visiting.

(continued)

Interventions	Rationale
1. Telephone the parents and inform them of the newborn's condition.	1. Telephoning initiates the relationship between the parents and the newborn's caregivers.
2. Encourage the parents to telephone the NICU as often as they desire to check on the status of their baby.	2. Frequent phone calls may assist in alleviating some of the parental anxiety and concern.
3. Encourage the parents to verbalize their concerns and feelings and to ask questions.	3. Sharing of feelings and concerns and asking questions permit a safe outlet for expression and open lines of communication, fostering trust.
4. Provide time for the parents to cry and grieve if appropriate.	4. Allowing the parents time to grieve may be necessary before attachment can occur.
5. Invite parents to see and touch the newborn during visits and to spend as much time as possible with the newborn. Guide the parents in activities such as skin-to-skin contact, touching through the portholes of the Isolette, and basic caregiving.	5. Seeing, touching, and caring promote attachment. Guidance in activities helps to alleviate anxiety.
6. Suggest parents bring in a mobile or toy to keep near newborn.	6. A mobile or toy provides visual stimulation and promotes feelings of participation in the newborn's care.
7. Investigate possible community resources available for the parents, such as transportation, lodging, or finances.	7. Community resources provide additional support in areas of need.

compressed by the force of vaginal birth; thus, less lung fluid is expelled than normally.

Close observation of the newborn is the priority. Watch carefully to see that the increased effort is not tiring. Also watch for beginning signs of a more serious disorder, because a rapid respiratory rate is often the first sign of respiratory obstruction. Oxygen administration may be necessary. Transient tachypnea of the newborn peaks in intensity at approximately 36 hours of life and then begins to fade. Typically, by 72 hours of life, it spontaneously fades as the lung fluid is absorbed and respiratory activity becomes effective (Whitsett et al., 2000).

Meconium Aspiration Syndrome

Meconium is present in the fetal bowel as early as 10 weeks' gestation. An infant with hypoxia in utero experiences a vagal reflex relaxation of the rectal sphincter, which releases meconium into the amniotic fluid. Babies born breech may expel meconium into the amniotic fluid from pressure on the buttocks. In both instances, the appearance of the fluid at birth is green to greenish black from the staining. Meconium staining occurs in approximately 10% to 12% of all pregnancies (Whitsett et al., 2000). It does not tend to occur in extremely-low-birth-weight infants because the substance has not passed far enough in the bowel for it to be at the rectum in these infants.

An infant may aspirate meconium either in utero or with the first breath after birth. Meconium can cause severe respiratory distress in three ways: it can bring about inflammation of bronchioles because it is a foreign substance; it can block small bronchioles by mechanical plugging; and it can cause a decrease in surfactant production through lung cell trauma. Hypoxemia, carbon dioxide retention, and intrapulmonary and extrapulmonary shunting occur. A secondary infection of injured tissue may lead to pneumonia.

Assessment

Infants with meconium-stained amniotic fluid may have difficulty establishing respirations at birth (those who were not born breech have had a hypoxic episode in utero to cause the meconium to be in the amniotic fluid). The Apgar score is apt to be low. Almost immediately, tachypnea, retractions, and cyanosis occur.

With meconium-stained amniotic fluid, the infant should be suctioned with a bulb syringe or catheter while at the perineum, before the delivery of the shoulders, to avoid meconium aspiration. The infant should be intubated and meconium should be suctioned from the trachea and bronchi as soon as the infant is born. Do not administer oxygen under pressure (bag and mask) until the infant has been intubated and suctioned, so that the pressure of the oxygen does not drive small plugs of meconium farther down into the lungs, worsening the irritation and obstruction. After the initiation of respirations, the infant's respiratory rate may remain elevated (tachypnea); coarse bronchial sounds may be heard on auscultation. The infant may continue to have retractions because the inflammation of bronchi tends to trap air in the alveoli. This may cause enlargement of the anteroposterior diameter of the chest (barrel chest). Blood gases will reveal a poor gas exchange, evidenced by a decreased Po_2 and an increased Pco_2. A chest x-ray will show bilateral coarse infiltrates in the lung, with spaces of hyperaeration (a peculiar honeycomb effect). The diaphragm will be pushed downward.

Therapeutic Management

Intrapartally, amniotransfusion may be used to dilute the amount of meconium in amniotic fluid and reduce the risk of aspiration. After tracheal suction, infants may be treated with oxygen administration and assisted ventilation. Antibiotic therapy may be used to forestall the development of pneumonia as a secondary problem. Lung tissue is fairly noncompliant after meconium aspiration, which may necessitate high inspiratory pressure. This can cause pneumothorax or pneumomediastinum. Infants must be observed closely for signs of trapping air in the alveoli, because the alveoli can expand only so far and then will rupture, sending air into the pleural space.

Because of increased pulmonary resistance, the ductus arteriosus may remain open, causing blood to shunt from the pulmonary artery into the aorta, compromising cardiac efficiency and increasing hypoxia. Observe the infant closely for signs of heart failure (e.g., increased heart rate or respiratory distress). Maintain a temperature-neutral environment to prevent increasing the metabolic oxygen demands. Some infants will be maintained on ECMO to ensure adequate oxygenation.

Chest physiotherapy with clapping and vibration may be helpful to encourage removal of remnants of meconium from the lungs (see Chap. 40).

Apnea

Apnea is a pause in respirations longer than 20 seconds with accompanying bradycardia. Beginning cyanosis also may be present. Many preterm infants have periods of apnea as a result of fatigue or the immaturity of their respiratory mechanisms. Babies with secondary stresses, such as infection, hyperbilirubinemia, hypoglycemia, or hypothermia, tend to have a high incidence of apnea (Cunningham et al., 2001).

Gently shaking an infant or flicking the sole of the foot often stimulates the baby to breathe again, almost as if the child needed to be reminded to maintain this function. If an infant does not respond to these simple measures, resuscitation is necessary.

Closely observe all newborns, but especially preterm ones, to detect these apneic episodes. Apnea monitors that record respiratory movements are invaluable tools to detect failing respiration and sound a warning that an infant needs attention. An infant with frequent or difficult-to-correct episodes may be placed on a ventilator to provide respiratory coordination until he or she is more mature.

To help prevent episodes of apnea, maintain a neutral thermal environment and use gentle handling to avoid excessive fatigue. Always suction gently to minimize nasopharyngeal irritation, which can cause bradycardia due to vagal stimulation. Using indwelling nasogastric tubes rather than intermittent ones can also reduce the amount of vagal stimulation. After feeding, observe an infant carefully because the full stomach can put pressure on the diaphragm. Careful burping also helps to reduce this effect. Never take rectal temperatures in infants prone to apnea; the resulting vagal stimulation can reduce the heart rate (bradycardia), which can lead to apnea. Theophylline or caffeine sodium benzoate may be administered to stimulate respirations. The mechanism by which these drugs reduce the incidence of apneic episodes is unclear, but they appear to increase an infant's sensitivity to carbon dioxide, ensuring better respiratory function. Infants who have had an apneic episode severe enough to require resuscitation are at a high risk for sudden infant death syndrome (SIDS). Such infants may be discharged home with a monitoring device to be used for 2 to 6 months.

✔ **CHECKPOINT QUESTIONS**

21. How early in gestation is meconium present in the fetal bowel?
22. What treatment may be used intrapartally to reduce the risk of meconium aspiration?

Sudden Infant Death Syndrome

SIDS is a sudden unexplained death in infancy (Hunt, 2000). It tends to occur at a higher-than-usual rate in the infants of adolescent mothers, infants of closely spaced pregnancies, and underweight infants and preterm infants. Also prone to SIDS are infants with bronchopulmonary dysplasia, twins, siblings of another child with SIDS, Native American infants, Alaskan native infants, economically disadvantaged black infants, and infants of narcotic-dependent mothers. The peak age of incidence is 2 to 4 months of age (Hunt, 2000).

Although the cause of SIDS is unknown, a number of theories about its cause have been postulated. In addition to prolonged but unexplained apnea, other possible contributing factors may include:

- Viral respiratory or botulism infection
- Pulmonary edema
- Brain stem abnormalities
- Neurotransmitter deficiencies
- Heart rate abnormalities
- Distorted familial breathing patterns
- Decreased arousal responses
- Possible lack of surfactant in alveoli
- Sleeping prone (respiratory muscles are restricted)

Typically, affected infants are well nourished. Parents report that the infant may have had a slight head cold. After being put to bed at night or for a nap, the infant is found dead a few hours later. Infants who die this way do not appear to make any sound as they die, which indicates that they die with laryngospasm. Although many infants are found with blood-flecked sputum or vomitus in their mouths or on the bedclothes, this seems to occur as the result of death, not as its cause. An autopsy often reveals petechiae in the lungs and mild inflammation and congestion in the respiratory tract. However, these symptoms are not severe enough to cause sudden death. It is clear that these children do not suffocate from bedclothes or choke from overfeeding, underfeeding, or crying. Since the American Academy of Pediatrics' recommendation to always put newborns to sleep on their back or side, the incidence of SIDS has declined dramatically (Gibson et al., 2000).

Parents have a difficult time accepting the death of a child, especially when it happens so suddenly. In discussing the child, they often use both the past and present tense as if they are not yet aware of the death. Many parents experience a period of somatic symptoms that occur with acute grief, such as nausea, stomach pain, or vertigo. Parents should be counseled by a nurse or someone else trained in counseling at the time of the infant's death; it helps if they can talk to this same person periodically for however long it takes to resolve their grief. Some supportive organizations are listed at the beginning of the chapter.

Autopsy reports should be given to parents as soon as they are available (if toxicology tests are included in the autopsy, results will not be available for weeks). Reading the report that their child died an unexplained death can help to reassure them that the death was not their fault. They need this assurance if they are to plan for other children. If there are older children in the family, they also need assurance that SIDS is a disease of infants and that the strange phenomenon that invaded their home and killed a younger brother or sister will not also kill them. If they wished the infant dead, as all children wish siblings were dead on some days, reassure them that their wishes are not that powerful and that they did not cause the baby's death.

When another child is born, the parents can be expected to become extremely frightened at any sign of illness in the child. They need support to see them through the first few months of the second child's life, particularly past the point at which the first child died. Some parents need support to view a second child as an individual child and not as a replacement for the one who died.

Often the sibling of a SIDS infant is screened using a sleep study as a precaution within the first 2 weeks of life. Depending on the parents' level of anxiety, the sibling may receive this screening before hospital discharge. The sibling may then be placed on apnea monitoring pending the results of the sleep study.

Apparent Life-Threatening Event

Some infants have been discovered cyanotic and limp in their beds but have survived after mouth-to-mouth resuscitation by parents. An episode of this kind is called an **apparent life-threatening event** (Gray et al., 1999). For these children as well as for preterm infants with a tendency toward apnea or the siblings of a child who died from SIDS, apnea monitoring is available. An alarm sounds when the neonate experiences a period of apnea of 20 seconds or more or a decreased heart rate below 80 bpm (Fig. 26-10). If parents are going to use an apnea monitor at home, make certain they will be able to hear it in all parts of the house or apartment. Usually the alarm is not loud enough to be heard in the basement from an upstairs bedroom. Caution them about household noises such as a loud television, radio, vacuum cleaner, or hair dryer that may interfere with hearing the alarm. Be sure they know how to apply and reposition the leads and that they are comfortable enough with the monitor to see past it to the child. In addition, parents of high-risk infants should be taught cardiopulmonary resuscitation before the infant is discharged from the hospital (Fig. 26-11).

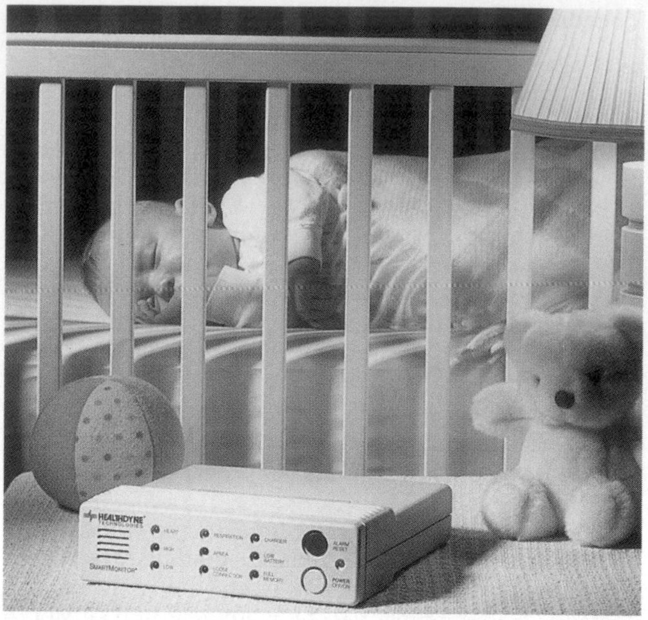

FIGURE 26.10 An apnea monitor for home monitoring.

Caring for a child at home on an apnea monitor may be extremely stressful for the parents and their relationship. Parents often have trouble finding a competent babysitter. These parents can benefit from a community or home care referral so they have a second opinion as to how well they are managing, as well as a listening ear to discuss the strain of having to be constantly alert for a sound that means their infant has stopped breathing. Having someone periodically review with them what steps to take should the alarm sound (jiggle the baby, begin mouth-to-mouth resuscitation, call the emergency squad) can be very comforting. These parents are under a tremendous strain. This may be accentuated by a lack of sleep at night because many parents report that they are always listening for an alarm. Because SIDS is a baffling disease, these parents may live in fear of it until their child reaches at least 1 year of age.

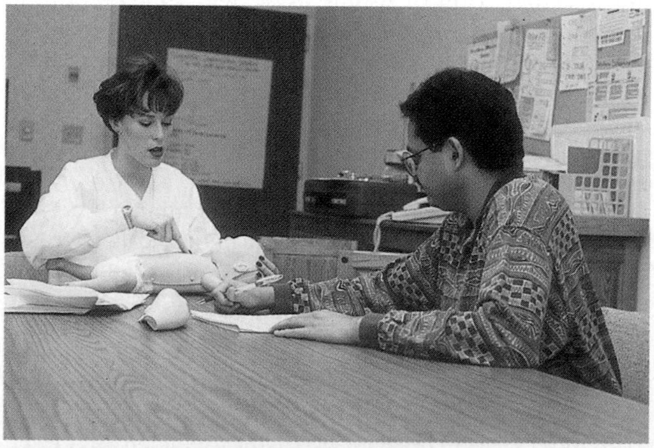

FIGURE 26.11 Parents of infants with respiratory disorders at birth need to learn resuscitation before the infant is discharged from the hospital. Here a nurse teaches the technique using a doll.

Periventricular Leukomalacia

Periventricular leukomalacia (PVL) is abnormal formation of the white matter of the brain (Hill & Volpe, 2000). It is caused by an ischemic episode that interferes with circulation to a portion of the brain. Phagocytes and macrophages invade the area to clear away necrotic tissue. What is left is an area in the white matter of the brain that is revealed on a sonogram as a hollow space. PVL occurs most frequently in preterm infants who experience cerebral ischemia. Once the condition has occurred, there is no therapy. Infants may die of the original insult; they may be left with long-term effects such as learning disabilities. Any action to reduce environmental stimuli or sudden shifts in cerebral blood flow, such as avoiding rapid fluid infusions or sudden noises, is important in preventing PVL and limiting the long-term effects of prematurity.

✔ CHECKPOINT QUESTIONS

23. What is the peak age of incidence for SIDS?
24. When does the alarm sound on an apnea monitor?

Hyperbilirubinemia

In the newborn, hyperbilirubinemia (an elevated level of bilirubin in the blood) results from destruction of red blood cells by either a normal physiologic process (see Chap. 23) or the abnormal destruction of red blood cells.

Hemolytic Disease of the Newborn

The term "hemolytic" is derived from the Latin for destruction (lysis) of red blood cells. In the past, hemolytic disease of the newborn was most often caused by an Rh blood type incompatibility. Because prevention of Rh antibody formation has been available for almost 40 years, the disorder is now most often caused by an ABO incompatibility. In both instances, the mother builds antibodies against the infant's red blood cells, leading to hemolysis (destruction) of the cells. The destruction of red blood cells causes severe anemia and hyperbilirubinemia. Prevention of the condition begins in pregnancy, as discussed in Chapter 15.

Rh Incompatibility

Theoretically, no direct connection exists between the fetal and maternal circulation, and no fetal blood cells enter the maternal circulation. In actuality, occasional placental villi break and a drop or two of fetal blood does enter the maternal circulation. If the mother's blood type is Rh (D) negative and the fetal blood type is Rh positive (contains the D antigen), the introduction of fetal blood causes sensitization to occur, and the mother begins to form antibodies against the D antigen. Few antibodies form this way, however. Most form in the mother's bloodstream in the first 72 hours after birth because there is an active exchange of fetal–maternal blood as placental villi loosen and the placenta is delivered. After this sensitization, in a second pregnancy, there will be a high level of antibody D circulating in the mother's bloodstream, which acts to destroy the fetal red blood cells early in the pregnancy if the fetus is Rh positive. By the end of a second pregnancy, a fetus can be severely compromised by the action of these antibodies crossing the placenta and destroying red blood cells. Some infants require intrauterine transfusions to combat red cell destruction. Preterm labor may be induced to remove the fetus from the destructive maternal environment.

ABO Incompatibility

In most instances of ABO incompatibility, the maternal blood type is O and the fetal blood type is A; it may also occur when the fetus has type B or AB blood. A reaction in an infant with type B blood is often the most serious.

Hemolysis can become a problem with a first pregnancy in which there is an ABO incompatibility. The antibodies to A and B cell types are naturally occurring antibodies, which are present from birth in individuals whose red cells lack these antigens. Unlike the antibodies formed against the Rh D factor, these antibodies are of the large (IgM) class and do not cross the placenta. The infant of an ABO incompatibility, therefore, is not born anemic, as is the Rh-sensitized child. Hemolysis of the blood begins with birth, when blood and antibodies are exchanged during the mixing of maternal and fetal blood as the placenta is loosened and may continue for up to 2 weeks of age.

Assessment

Interestingly, preterm infants do not seem to be affected by ABO incompatibility. This may be because the receptor sites for anti-A or anti-B antibodies do not appear on red cells until late in fetal life. Even in the mature newborn, the direct Coombs' test may be only weakly positive because of the few anti-A or anti-B sites present. The reticulocyte count (immature or newly formed red blood cells) is usually elevated as the infant attempts to replace destroyed cells.

Rh incompatibility of the newborn can be predicted by finding a rising anti-Rh titer or a rising level of antibodies (indirect Coombs' test) in the mother during pregnancy. It can be confirmed by detecting antibodies on the fetal erythrocytes in cord blood (positive direct Coombs' test) by percutaneous umbilical blood sampling (see Chap. 8) or at birth. The mother in this situation will always have Rh-negative blood (dd), and the baby will be Rh positive (DD or Dd).

With Rh incompatibility, the infant may not appear pale at birth despite the red cell destruction that has occurred in utero. This is because the accelerated production of red cells during the last few months in utero compensates to some degree for the destruction. The liver and spleen may be enlarged from an attempt to destroy damaged new blood cells. If the number of red cells has decreased, the blood in the vascular circulation may be hypotonic to interstitial fluid; fluid shifts from the lower to higher isotonic pressure by the law of osmosis, causing extreme edema. Finally, the severe anemia results in heart failure.

Hydrops fetalis is an old term for the appearance of a severely involved infant at birth. Hydrops refers to the edema, and fetalis refers to the lethal state. The infant does not appear jaundiced because the maternal circulation has evacuated the rising indirect bilirubin level. With birth, progressive jaundice, usually occurring within the first 24 hours of life, indicates in both Rh and ABO incompatibility that a hemolytic process is at work. The indirect bilirubin level rises rapidly as red blood cells are destroyed and indirect bilirubin is released. Indirect bilirubin is fat-soluble and cannot be excreted from the body. Under normal circumstances, the liver enzyme glucuronyl transferase converts indirect bilirubin to direct bilirubin. Direct bilirubin is water-soluble and combines with bile for excretion from the body with feces. In preterm infants or those with extreme hemolysis, the liver is unable to convert bilirubin, which is why jaundice becomes so extreme.

Pregnanediol, the breakdown product of progesterone, can interfere with the conjugation of indirect bilirubin. It is excreted in breast milk until the high levels of progesterone that were present during pregnancy are decreased, usually by 24 to 48 hours. Breast-fed babies, therefore, may evidence more jaundice than bottle-fed babies.

Normally, cord blood has an indirect bilirubin level of 0 to 3 mg/100 mL. An increasing indirect bilirubin level is dangerous because if the level rises above 20 mg/dL in a term infant or 12 mg/dL in a preterm infant, brain damage from kernicterus (invasion of bilirubin into brain cells) can occur. Meanwhile, the infant needs to use glucose stores to maintain metabolism in the presence of anemia. This can cause a progressive hypoglycemia, compounding the initial problem. A decrease in hemoglobin during the first week of life to a level less than that of cord blood is a later indication of blood loss or hemolysis.

Therapeutic Management

Initiation of early feeding, use of phototherapy, and exchange transfusion all may be immediate measures necessary to reduce indirect bilirubin levels in the infant affected by ABO or Rh incompatibility. In newborns with severe hemolytic disease, the hemoglobin concentration may continue to drop during the first 6 months of life or their bone marrow may fail to increase production of erythrocytes in response to continuing hemolysis. If this occurs, the infant may need an additional blood transfusion to correct this late anemia. Therapy with erythropoietin to stimulate red blood cell production is also possible.

Initiation of Early Feeding. Bilirubin is removed from the body by being incorporated into feces. Therefore, the sooner bowel elimination begins, the sooner bilirubin removal begins. Early feeding (either breast milk or formula), therefore, stimulates bowel peristalsis and accomplishes this.

Phototherapy. An infant's liver processes little bilirubin in utero because the mother's circulation does this for the infant. With birth, exposure to light apparently triggers the liver to assume this function. Additional light appears to speed the conversion potential of the liver. Phototherapy is the light technique that is most often used. In phototherapy, the infant is continuously exposed to specialized light such as quartz halogen, cool white daylight, or special blue fluorescent light. The lights are placed 12 to 30 inches above the newborn. Specialized fiberoptic light systems incorporated into a fiberoptic blanket also have been developed and are ideal for home care (Maisels, 2000). The infant is undressed except for the diaper so that as much skin surface as possible is exposed to the light (Fig. 26-12).

Term newborns are generally scheduled for phototherapy when the total serum bilirubin level rises to 15 mg/dL at 25 to 28 hours of age (Maisels, 2000).

Although the long-term effects have not yet been studied, there appears to be minimal risk to the infant from phototherapy, provided the infant's eyes remain covered and dehydration from increased insensitive water loss does not occur.

Continuous exposure to bright lights this way may be harmful to the newborn's retina, so the infant's eyes must always be covered while under bilirubin lights. Eye dressings or cotton balls can be firmly secured in place by an additional dressing. The infant must be checked frequently to be certain the dressings have not slipped or are causing corneal irritation. A constant concern is that suffocation from eye patches could occur.

The stools of an infant under bilirubin lights are often bright green because of the excessive bilirubin that is excreted as the result of the therapy. They are also frequently loose and may be irritating to skin. Urine may be dark-colored from urobilinogen formation. Assess skin turgor and intake and output to ensure that dehydration is not occurring. Monitor axillary temperature to prevent the infant from overheating under the bright lights.

An infant receiving phototherapy should be removed from under the lights for feeding so that he or she continues to have interaction with the mother. In addition, supplemental feedings with additional formula may be recommended to prevent dehydration. Remove the eye patches during the time the infant is with the mother to

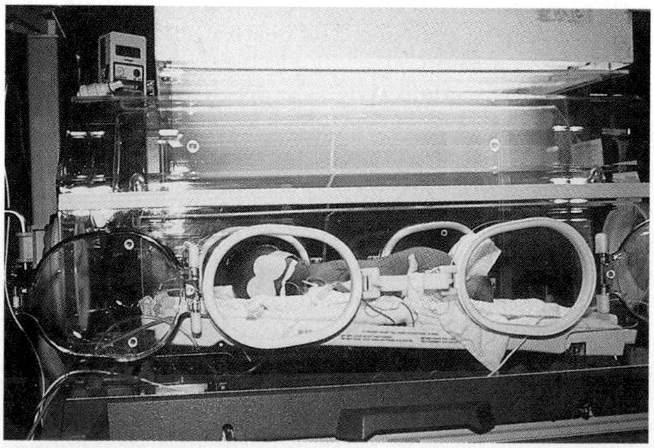

FIGURE 26.12 A newborn receiving phototherapy is undressed except for a diaper so that he receives maximum exposure to the lights. His eyes are covered snugly to protect them from the bright light.

give the infant a period of visual stimulation. To prevent a lengthy hospital stay, infants may be discharged and continue therapy at home.

Parents need an explanation of the rationale for phototherapy. Isolettes are automatically associated with seriously ill infants, but the use of lights does not seem scientific (almost a home remedy). Parents can easily be confused by the two interventions, one seemingly serious and the other seemingly not serious at all.

WHAT IF? What if the parents of an infant who is receiving phototherapy ask you if she is receiving enough stimulation? How would you answer them?

Home Phototherapy. Home phototherapy allows for uninterrupted contact between the parents and the newborn and therefore has the potential to aid bonding. The parents must understand the importance of the therapy, the lights must be a full 12 inches away from the infant to prevent burning, the infant must continuously wear eye patches and a diaper during phototherapy to protect the retinas and the ovaries or testes, and bilirubin levels should be assessed approximately every 12 hours. Home phototherapy is primarily used for decreasing physiologic jaundice rather than that associated with blood incompatibility.

The infant should have the eye patches removed when away from the lights for feeding for a period of visual stimulation and interaction. The point at which infants are most apt to dislodge eye patches is when they cry as they wake for a feeding. Urge parents not to allow an infant under bilirubin lights to cry for a sustained period to avoid having this happen.

The infant's progress can be measured daily by a transcutaneous bilirubinometer, a hand-held fiberoptic light placed against the infant's skin. The intensity of the yellow color of the skin is measured by the meter, and a numeric level of bilirubin is calculated (Fischbach, 2000).

A newer innovation for hyperbilirubinemia management is the phototherapy blanket, a fiberoptic blanket that is wrapped around the baby. Light generated by the blanket has the same effect on bilirubin levels as banks of overhead lights. The advantages of a blanket are that the infant can be held for long periods without interrupting the phototherapy, and eye patches are unnecessary (see Focus on Family Empowerment).

Exchange Transfusion. Intensive phototherapy in conjunction with hydration and close monitoring of serum bilirubin levels is the preferred method of treatment. However, despite these measures, if bilirubin levels are rapidly rising, exchange transfusion may be necessary. Before the procedure, the baby's stomach is aspirated to minimize the risk of aspiration from the manipulation involved.

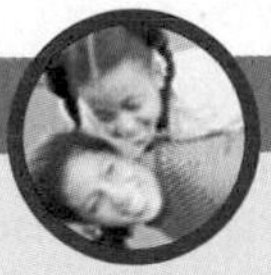

FOCUS ON FAMILY EMPOWERMENT

Home Phototherapy Blanket

Q. The doctor has ordered a special blanket for us to use at home to help with our baby's jaundice. What should we do to ensure that we use the blanket correctly and effectively?

A. Use the guidelines below to ensure the effectiveness of the home phototherapy blanket:

- Be aware that a home care nurse will assist you in setting up and using the equipment. The nurse will also obtain daily blood specimens to check your infant's bilirubin levels.
- Take your infant's temperature every 8 hours throughout the course of therapy. Because the blanket being used does not provide heat, changes in temperature may indicate a problem, such as an infection.
- Monitor your infant's urine output. Keep track of the number of diapers she wets.
- Also monitor your infant's bowel movements. She may have loose, green-tinged bowel movements as the bilirubin begins to break down. Keep the skin clean and dry to prevent irritation.
- With feedings, keep track of the amount (if bottle-feeding) or length (if breast-feeding) of feeding and the frequency of feedings. Usually, the infant receiving phototherapy should be fed approximately every 3 hours.
- Supplement formula or breast milk with glucose water unless you are told otherwise. The infant needs additional fluids during this time.
- When placing the child in the blanket device, be sure the fabric side goes against the infant's skin, with the lower portion on the outside of the baby's diaper. Be sure to fold the diaper down below the baby's navel in front and as far as possible in back so as much of the skin as possible is exposed to the light.
- Do not wrap the baby too tightly. Leave a space about the size of two fingers between the panel and the baby's skin.
- Don't be afraid to pick up the baby at any time and hold her. You can rock, cuddle, or feed her. Be careful not to walk around with the baby wrapped in the blanket, because you could trip on the cord and fall, injuring yourself or the baby.
- Call your pediatric care provider if you find any of the following: refusal of feedings, persistent temperature control problems, fewer than five wet diapers in 24 hours, pronounced change in the child's level of activity, or vomiting of entire feedings.

The umbilical vein is catheterized as the site for transfusion. The procedure involves alternatively withdrawing small amounts (2–10 mL) of the infant's blood and then replacing it with equal amounts of donor blood. The blood is exchanged slowly to prevent alternating hypovolemia and hypervolemia. Thus, an exchange transfusion is a lengthy procedure of 1 to 3 hours. An automatic pump can perform this exhausting repeated ritual. At the end of the procedure, using the last specimen of blood withdrawn, hematocrit, bilirubin, electrolytes (especially calcium), glucose determination, and blood culture are taken. Exchange transfusion may need to be repeated because additional unconjugated bilirubin from tissue moves into the circulation after the initial exchange.

The therapy may be used for any condition that leads to hyperbilirubinemia or polycythemia. When used as therapy for blood incompatibility, it removes approximately 85% of sensitized red cells. It reduces the serum concentration of indirect bilirubin and often prevents heart failure in infants. Because indirect bilirubin levels rise at relatively predictable levels, standards for performing exchange transfusion depend on the indirect bilirubin concentration, and transfusion is used when this level exceeds:

- 5 mg per 100 mL at birth
- 10 mg per 100 mL at age 8 hours
- 12 mg per 100 mL at age 16 hours
- 15 mg per 100 mL at 24 hours

It also may be used if serum bilirubin is rising more than 0.5 mg/h in infants with Rh incompatibility or 1.0 mg/h in infants with ABO incompatibility.

Keep the newborn warm during the procedure to prevent energy expenditure to maintain body temperature. Maintain the blood being given at room temperature, or shock from the cold insult can result. Use only commercial blood warmers to warm blood, not hot towels or a radiant heat warmer, which can destroy red cells.

Albumin may be administered 1 to 2 hours before the procedure to increase the number of bilirubin binding sites and to increase the efficiency of the transfusion. Be extremely careful to monitor the rate of flow of the albumin transfusion, because rapid flow of such a viscous fluid can quickly overburden the infant's heart. The type of blood used for transfusion is O Rh-negative blood, even though the infant's blood type is positive; if Rh-positive or type A or B blood were given, the maternal antibodies that entered the infant's circulation would destroy this blood also, and the transfusion would be ineffective. If the baby is transported to a regional center for the exchange transfusion, a sample of the mother's blood must accompany the infant, so cross-matching on the mother's serum can be done there. An amount equal to twice the blood volume (average is 86 mL/kg) is used because this quantity will ensure an exchange of erythrocytes that is 85% to 90% effective.

During the transfusion, carefully monitor the newborn's heart rate, respirations, and blood pressure.

Because blood stored for transfusion contains acid-citrate-dextrose (ACD), added to blood as an anticoagulant, which can lower blood calcium levels and cause acidosis, calcium gluconate is given through the exchange catheter after each 100 mL of blood. If citrate-phosphate-dextrose is used as a preservative, hyperglycemia may occur during the transfusion from the dextrose in the preservative. This is followed by overproduction of insulin and hypoglycemia. If heparinized blood is used, the heparin content may interfere with clotting after the transfusion. In addition, because of its relatively low glucose concentration, it may also lead to hypoglycemia. Administering protamine sulfate aids in the metabolism of heparin and restoration of clotting ability.

After the transfusion, closely observe for umbilical vessel bleeding. Redness or inflammation of the cord suggests infection. Report any changes in vital signs. In addition, the infant needs a blood glucose determination at 1 hour after the procedure. Monitor bilirubin levels for 2 or 3 days after the transfusion to ensure that the level of bilirubin is not rising again and that no further transfusion is necessary. Erythropoietin may be administered to increase new blood cell growth and prevent extended anemia.

✔ CHECKPOINT QUESTIONS

25. What are the maternal and fetal blood types most commonly associated with ABO incompatibility?
26. What is the most common method used for treating hyperbilirubinemia in the newborn?

Hemorrhagic Disease of the Newborn

Hemorrhagic disease of the newborn results from a deficiency of vitamin K. Vitamin K is essential for the formation of prothrombin by the liver. Lack of it causes decreased prothrombin function and impaired blood coagulation. Vitamin K is formed by the action of bacteria in the intestine. Because the intestinal tract of a newborn is sterile at birth, the infant forms minimal amounts of vitamin K until normal intestinal tract flora are established at about 24 hours of age. Babies born to mothers receiving anticonvulsive medication are at high risk for the condition because many of these medications interfere with vitamin K formation. Administering vitamin K intramuscularly to these mothers before delivery can help to protect the child (Doyle et al., 2000).

Newborns with vitamin K deficiency show petechiae from superficial bleeding into the skin. They may have conjunctival, mucous membrane, or retinal hemorrhage. They may vomit fresh blood or pass black, tarry stools because of bleeding into the gastrointestinal tract.

Distinguishing between tarry stools and normal meconium stools is difficult in the first 1 or 2 days of life by simple observation. However, if the infant's stool does not change as it should from greenish-black (meconium) to the yellow color of a bottle-fed or breast-fed baby, or if the stool color changes normally and then becomes black again, gastrointestinal bleeding should be suspected. Check for the presence of blood in the stool (a guaiac test).

Such bleeding generally occurs on day 2 to day 5 of life, when the available prothrombin is at its lowest level. The prothrombin time will be prolonged; the coagulation time may be normal or prolonged.

Hemorrhagic disease of the newborn can be prevented by the intramuscular administration of 1 mg of vitamin K to all newborns immediately after birth. Make certain that infants who were born in unusual circumstances, such as those born outside the hospital, are given vitamin K on their admission to the hospital nursery. Also double-check that infants whose birth involved an emergency, such as maternal hemorrhage or failure of the newborn to breathe spontaneously, have received it.

The infant who develops hemorrhagic disease of the newborn is treated with vitamin K, given intravenously or intramuscularly. If bleeding is severe, the infant may need a transfusion of fresh, whole blood to increase the prothrombin level immediately.

Handle the infant with this disease extremely gently to prevent further bleeding, because he or she bruises easily from heavy pressure. Subdural hemorrhage may occur, making hemorrhagic disease a serious and potentially fatal disorder (Hill & Volpe, 2000).

Twin-to-Twin Transfusion

Twin-to-twin transfusion is a phenomenon that can occur if twins are monozygotic (identical; share the same placenta) and if abnormal arteriovenous shunts occur that direct more blood to one twin than the other. The process occurs in as many as one third of all identical twin pregnancies. However, enough blood is exchanged to be clinically important in only 15% of such pregnancies (van Gemert et al., 2001). The result of this shift of blood leads to anemia in the donor twin and polycythemia in the receiving twin. The anemic twin may also be SGA because of the lack of nutrients or oxygen for growth. This same SGA twin will be prone to hypoglycemia from lack of glucose stores. He or she will appear pale next to the polycythemic twin, who is prone to hyperbilirubinemia as the excessive red blood cell level is broken down.

Twin-to-twin transfusion can be identified in utero by sonogram: one twin is noticeably larger than the other. All identical twins should have hemoglobin determinations done at birth and the results should be compared. A difference of more than 5.0 g per 100 mL is enough to suggest that a transfusion has occurred. Each twin needs therapy as indicated by the extent of the blood distribution. The donor twin may need a transfusion to establish a functioning blood level; the recipient twin may need an exchange transfusion to reduce the polycythemia and viscosity of the blood.

Necrotizing Enterocolitis

Necrotizing enterocolitis develops in approximately 5% of all infants in intensive care nurseries. The bowel develops necrotic patches, interfering with digestion and possibly leading to a paralytic ileus. Perforation and peritonitis may follow. NEC may occur as a complication of exchange transfusion. The disorder is discussed in Chapter 45.

Retinopathy of Prematurity

Retinopathy of prematurity (ROP), an acquired ocular disease that leads to partial or total blindness in children, is due to vasoconstriction of immature retinal blood vessels. It was first recognized as an eye disorder in 1942, but only later was a high concentration of oxygen established as the causative agent (Isenberg, 2000). Immature retinal blood vessels constrict when exposed to high oxygen concentrations. In addition, endothelial cells in the layer of nerve fibers in the periphery of the retina proliferate, leading to retinal detachment and blindness. Infants who are most immature and most ill (and consequently receive the most oxygen) are at highest risk.

The preterm infant who is receiving oxygen must have blood Po_2 levels monitored by pulse oximeter, transcutaneous oxygen saturation, or blood gas monitoring. Keeping blood Po_2 levels within normal limits lowers the risk. With blood Po_2 levels rising to more than 100 mm Hg, the danger of the disease increases greatly.

In the past, once ROP occurred, there was no reversing it. Today, cryosurgery or laser therapy may be effective in preserving sight. A person experienced in recognizing ROP should examine the eyes of all low-birthweight newborns and those who have received oxygen therapy before discharge from the nursery and again at age 4 to 6 weeks of age to detect any occurrence of the syndrome.

✔ **CHECKPOINT QUESTIONS**

27. On which day after birth does bleeding from hemorrhagic disease of the newborn typically occur?
28. What is the cause of retinopathy of prematurity?

THE NEWBORN AT RISK BECAUSE OF MATERNAL INFECTION OR ILLNESS

Maternal Infection

Newborns are susceptible to infection at birth because their ability to produce antibodies is immature. A newborn who appears ill at birth or becomes ill shortly after birth is usually screened by a TORSCH assay, which tests for the presence of antibodies to toxoplasmosis, rubella, syphilis, cytomegalovirus, and herpes organisms. The effect on the mother from these disorders is discussed in Chapter 11.

Beta-Hemolytic, Group B Streptococcal Infection

The major cause of infection in newborn infants is the beta-hemolytic, group B streptococcal organism (GBS; Freij & McCracken, 2000). This gram-positive bacterium is a natural inhabitant of the female genital tract. Between 50 and 300 infants in every 1,000 live births display a positive culture for this organism. It may be spread from baby to baby if good handwashing technique is not used in handling newborns. If a mother is determined to be positive for GBS during late pregnancy, ampicillin administered intravenously at 28 weeks and again during labor helps to reduce the possibility of newborn exposure.

Assessment. The newborn may not exhibit any signs and symptoms of infection. Typically, the newborn at risk, such as one born after prolonged rupture of membranes or if the mother's vaginal culture is positive for GBS, will be screened for infection with a blood culture.

Colonization by GBS can result in an early-onset or a late-onset illness. With the early-onset form, symptoms of pneumonia become apparent within the first day of life and may include the following: tachypnea; apnea; symptoms of shock such as decreased urine output, extreme paleness, or hypotonia; and chest x-ray almost indistinguishable from that of respiratory distress syndrome (a ground-glass appearance). Pneumonia may develop so rapidly that as many as 20% of infants who contract the infection die within 24 hours of birth.

A late-onset type occurs at 2 to 4 weeks of age; instead of pneumonia being the infection focus, meningitis tends to occur. Typical signs and symptoms include lethargy, fever, loss of appetite, and bulging fontanelles from increased intracranial pressure as meningitis develops. Mortality from the late-onset type is not as high as from the early onset form (15% vs. 20%), but neurologic consequences occur in up to 50% of infants who survive (Cunningham et al., 2001).

Therapeutic Management. If the newborn displays signs and symptoms or a blood screening test is positive, antibiotics are administered. Gentamicin, ampicillin, and penicillin are all effective against GBS infections.

Parents may have difficulty understanding how their infant could suddenly become this ill. They may need a great deal of support in caring for the infant. This is even more important if the newborn survives the infection but is left neurologically challenged. In the future, immunization of all women of child-bearing age against streptococcal B organisms could decrease the incidence of newborns infected at birth.

Congenital Rubella

The rubella virus is capable of causing extensive congenital fetal malformations if the mother is infected during the first trimester of pregnancy. Although childhood immunization programs have greatly decreased the incidence of this infection, in urban areas of the United States, as many as 10% to 20% of women of childbearing age are still susceptible to rubella (Department of Health and Human Services, 2000). During pregnancy, women should be assessed for this susceptibility by blood sampling for an antibody titer. A titer of less than 1:8 indicates a woman is susceptible.

The greatest risk to an embryo from the rubella virus is during weeks 2 to 6 of intrauterine life, when body organs are first forming. The frequency of malformations is approximately 50% if the virus invasion occurs during these early weeks.

Assessment. The classic symptoms of the rubella syndrome include thrombocytopenia, cataracts, heart disease, deafness, microcephaly, and motor and cognitive impairment.

Thrombocytopenia is manifested by purpura, red-purple macula with a "blueberry muffin" appearance. The diagnosis is confirmed by identifying IgM antibodies against rubella in the infant's serum at birth. IgM antibodies do not cross the placenta, so they cannot have come from the mother; they must have been produced by the fetus in response to invasion by the rubella antigen.

Therapeutic Management. Treatment is symptomatic, depending on the congenital defects present. Live rubella virus may be cultured from nasopharyngeal secretions of affected infants at birth. At age 1 year, approximately 10% of these infants are still shedding live virus. Follow contact precautions when caring for this newborn initially and any time he or she is readmitted to the hospital until 1 year of age, unless nasopharyngeal and urine cultures are negative after 3 months of age. Susceptible pregnant women also should avoid contact with these newborns. All women in the postpartal period who have low rubella titers should be identified and offered a rubella vaccine to ensure that rubella infection does not occur with a future pregnancy. Women cannot be immunized during pregnancy because the vaccine used contains a live virus.

Ophthalmia Neonatorum

Ophthalmia neonatorum is an eye infection that occurs at birth or during the first month. The most common causative organisms include *Neisseria gonorrhoeae* or *Chlamydia trachomatis.* The infant contracts the organism during vaginal birth. *N. gonorrhoeae* infection is an extremely serious form of conjunctivitis. If left untreated, the infection progresses to corneal ulceration and destruction, resulting in opacity of the cornea and severe vision impairment.

Assessment. Ophthalmia neonatorum is generally bilateral. The conjunctivae become fiery red, with thick pus. The eyelids are edematous. Although this usually occurs on day 1 to day 4 of life, it should be considered as a possibility when conjunctivitis occurs in infants younger than 30 days.

Prevention. The prophylactic instillation of erythromycin ointment into the eyes of newborns prevents both gonococcal and chlamydial conjunctivitis. In the past, eye prophylaxis was given immediately after birth so it was never forgotten. Now it is customary to delay administration of ointment until after the first reactivity period so the child can see the parents clearly during this important attachment period. This makes it easy to forget administration, so use some type of a checklist as a reminder of this important prophylaxis. Infants born outside the hospital also need prophylaxis to prevent ophthalmia neonatorum, the same as infants born in a delivery or birthing room.

Therapeutic Management. Therapy is individualized depending on the organism cultured from the exudate. If gonococci are identified, intravenous ceftriaxone (Rocephin) and penicillin are effective drugs. If chlamydia is identified, an ophthalmic solution of erythromycin is used.

Use standard and contact precautions when caring for this newborn. In addition to systemic antibiotic therapy, the eyes are irrigated with sterile saline solution to clear the copious discharge. When irrigating eyes, use a sterile medicine dropper or bulb syringe, and use barrier protection, including goggles. The solution should be at room temperature. Direct the stream of the irrigation fluid laterally so it does not enter and contaminate the other eye.

The mother of the infected infant needs treatment for gonorrhea or chlamydia, before fallopian tube sterility or pelvic inflammatory disease results. Sexual contacts of the mother should be treated also, so the spread of the disease can be halted. With either infection, parents can be assured that with early diagnosis and treatment the prognosis for normal eyesight in the child is good.

Hepatitis B Virus Infection

The hepatitis B virus (HBV) can be transmitted to the newborn through contact with infected vaginal blood at birth when the mother is positive for the virus (HBsAg+). Hepatitis B is a destructive illness: 70% to 90% of infected infants become chronic carriers of the virus. A number of these newborns will develop liver cancer later in life (Cunningham et al., 2001).

To reduce the possibility of HBsAg being spread to newborns in the future, infants are now routinely vaccinated at birth. If the mother is identified as HBsAg+, the infant is also administered immune serum globulin (HBIG) within 12 hours of birth to decrease the possibility of infection. The infant should be bathed as soon as possible after birth to remove HBV-infected blood and secretions. Gentle suctioning is necessary to avoid possible trauma to the mucous membrane, which could allow HBV invasion. Although the virus is transmitted in breast milk, once immune globulin has been administered, women may breastfeed without risk to the infant. Hepatitis B is further discussed in Chapter 45 because it also occurs in older children.

Generalized Herpesvirus Infection

A herpes simplex virus type 2 (HSV-2) infection, most prevalent among women with multiple sexual partners, can be contracted by a fetus across the placenta if the mother has a primary infection during pregnancy. More often, however, the virus is contracted from the vaginal secretions from the mother who has active herpetic vulvovaginitis at the time of birth. Between 15% and 30% of women of childbearing age demonstrate antibodies to this virus or have the potential to have active lesions during labor (Chatterjee et al., 2001).

Assessment. If the infection was acquired during pregnancy, an infant may be born with vesicles covering the skin. The long-term prognosis of the child is guarded, because severe neurologic damage may have occurred simultaneously. If infants acquire the infection at birth, at approximately day 4 to day 7 of life they show a loss of appetite, perhaps a low-grade fever, and lethargy. Stomatitis (ulcers of the mouth) or a few vesicles on the skin appear. Herpes vesicles are always clustered, pinpoint in size, and surrounded by a reddened base. After the vesicles appear, infants become extremely ill. They develop dyspnea, jaundice, purpura, convulsions, and shock. Death may occur within hours or days. Between 25% and 70% of newborns who survive acquired generalized herpesvirus infections have permanent central nervous system sequelae.

To confirm the diagnosis, cultures are obtained from representative vesicles as well as the nose, throat, anus, and umbilical cord. Blood serum is analyzed for IgM antibodies.

Therapeutic Management. Acyclovir (Zovirax), a drug that inhibits viral deoxyribonucleic acid synthesis, is effective in combating this overwhelming infection. Prevention, however, is the newborn's best protection. Women with active herpetic vulvar lesions are often delivered by cesarean rather than vaginal birth to minimize the newborn's exposure. Infants with an infection should be separated from other infants. Although transmission from this source is rare, women with herpes lesions on their face (herpes simplex or cold sores) should not feed or hold their newborns until lesions are crusted and no longer contagious. Health care personnel who have herpes simplex infections must not care for newborn infants until the lesions are crusted. Although herpes simplex lesions are probably caused by herpesvirus type 1, limiting contact does not seem excessive in light of the severity of HSV-2 disease. A woman who is separated from her newborn at birth needs to view the infant from the nursery window and participate in planning care for the infant to aid bonding.

Human Immunodeficiency Virus Infection

Human immunodeficiency virus (HIV) infection and acquired immunodeficiency syndrome (AIDS) can be caused by placental transfer or direct contact with maternal blood during birth. The care of the infant with this infection is discussed in Chapter 42.

✔ **CHECKPOINT QUESTIONS**

29. Which organism is the major cause of neonatal infections?
30. What drug may be use to treat generalized herpesvirus type 2 infection in newborns?

The Infant of a Diabetic Mother

The infant of a diabetic mother whose illness was poorly controlled during pregnancy is typically longer and weighs more than other babies (macrosomia). The baby also has a greater chance of having a congenital anomaly such as a cardiac defect, as if hyperglycemia were teratogenic to the rapidly growing fetus. **Caudal regression syndrome** (hypoplasia of the lower extremities) is a syndrome that occurs almost exclusively in such infants.

Most such babies have a cushingoid (fat and puffy) appearance. They tend to be lethargic or limp in the first days of life as a result of hyperglycemia. The macrosomia results from overstimulation of pituitary growth hormone during pregnancy and extra fat deposits created by high levels of insulin during pregnancy. The infant's large size is deceptive, however: such babies are often immature.

Their lungs, especially, may be immature. RDS occurs frequently in these infants because they may be born preterm or even at term, possibly because lecithin pathways do not mature as rapidly in them. High fetal insulin secretion during pregnancy to counteract the hyperglycemia may interfere with cortisol release. This blocks the formation of lecithin and prevents lung maturity. A term frequently used for these infants is "fragile giant."

An infant of a diabetic mother loses a greater proportion of weight in the first few days of life than does the average newborn because of the loss of the extra fluid accumulated. Observe the infant closely to be certain that this large weight loss actually represents a loss of extra fluid and that dehydration is not occurring.

Complications

If infants are macrosomic, there is greater chance of birth injury, especially shoulder and neck injury. Typically cesarean birth is necessary to avoid cephalopelvic disproportion. Immediately after birth, the infant tends to be hyperglycemic because the mother was slightly hyperglycemic during pregnancy, causing excessive glucose to diffuse across the placenta. The fetal pancreas responds to this higher glucose level with islet cell hypertrophy, resulting in matching high insulin levels. After birth, the infant's glucose level begins to fall because the mother's circulation is no longer supplying glucose. The overproduction of insulin causes the development of severe hypoglycemia. Hyperbilirubinemia also may occur in these infants because, if immature, they cannot effectively clear bilirubin from their system. Hypocalcemia also frequently develops because parathyroid hormone levels are lower in these infants due to hypomagnesemia from excessive renal losses of magnesium (see Chap. 48).

The infant born to a woman with diabetes and extensive blood vessel involvement may be SGA because of poor placental perfusion. The problems of hypoglycemia, hypocalcemia, and hyperbilirubinemia remain the same.

Therapeutic Management

Hypoglycemia is defined as a serum glucose level of less than 40 mg/dL in a newborn (Cunningham et al., 2001). To avoid the serum glucose level from falling this low, infants of diabetic mothers are fed early with formula or administered a continuous infusion of glucose. It is important that the child not be given only a bolus of glucose; otherwise, rebound hypoglycemia (accentuating the problem) may occur. Some infants of diabetic mothers have a smaller-than-usual left colon, apparently another effect of intrauterine hyperglycemia, which limits the amount of oral feedings they can take in their first days of life. Signs of an inadequate colon include vomiting or abdominal distention after the first few feedings. Careful monitoring for normal bowel movements is important.

The Infant of a Drug-Dependent Mother

Infants of drug-dependent women tend to be SGA. If the mother is dependent on a drug, the infant will show withdrawal symptoms (neonatal abstinence syndrome) shortly after birth (see Assessing the Newborn of a Drug-Addicted Mother). These include:

- Irritability
- Disturbed sleep patterns
- Constant movement, possibly leading to abrasions on their elbows, knees, or nose
- Tremors
- Frequent sneezing
- Shrill, high-pitched cry
- Possible hyperreflexia and clonus (neuromuscular irritability)
- Convulsions
- Tachypnea (rapid respirations), possibly so severe that it leads to hyperventilation and alkalosis
- Vomiting and diarrhea, leading to large fluid losses and secondary dehydration

Specific tools may be used to quantify and assess the infant's status. These tools are often called neonatal abstinence scoring tools.

In newborns experiencing opiate withdrawal, symptoms usually begin 24 to 48 hours after birth, but in

ASSESSING the Newborn of a Drug-Addicted Mother

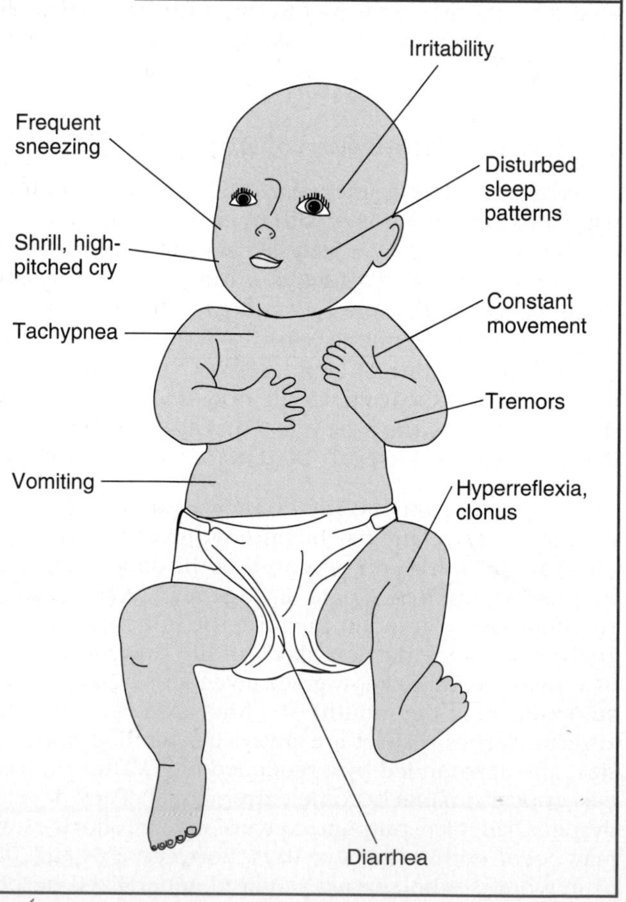

some cases they may not appear for up to 10 days. Generally they last approximately 2 weeks, but in some infants mild symptoms may appear for up to 6 months. In heroin-addicted neonates, the symptoms begin within the first 2 weeks of life, with an average onset of approximately 72 hours. The symptoms may last 8 to 16 weeks or longer. In methadone-addicted newborns, withdrawal begins later and lasts longer than heroin withdrawal. The onset varies. The newborn may exhibit signs and symptoms beginning at 24 to 28 hours, or the newborn may have early symptoms, improve, then have these symptoms reappear at 2 to 4 weeks of age. A newborn may exhibit no signs and symptoms until he or she is 2 to 3 weeks old.

There is no predictable withdrawal sequence noted for the cocaine-addicted neonate. Whether cocaine causes long-term effects varies with different studies, but factors such as maladaptive coping behaviors appear to be present in such newborns (Singer et al., 2001).

Narcotic metabolites or quinine (heroin is often mixed with quinine) may be obtained from an infant's urine in the first hour after birth. These products are quickly cleared from the body, however, so by the time symptoms become severe, detection of narcotic substances may no longer be possible.

Infants of drug-dependent women usually seem most comfortable when firmly swaddled. They should be kept in an environment free from excessive stimuli (a small isolation nursery, not a large, noisy one). Some quiet best if the room is darkened. Many infants of heroin-addicted women suck vigorously and continuously and seem to find comfort and quiet if given a pacifier. Infants of methadone- and cocaine-addicted women may have extremely poor sucking ability and may have difficulty getting enough fluid intake unless gavage-fed.

Specific therapy for an infant is individualized according to the nature and severity of the symptoms. Maintenance of electrolyte and fluid balance is essential. If the infant has vomiting or diarrhea, intravenous administration of fluid may be indicated. The drugs used to counteract withdrawal symptoms include paregoric, phenobarbital, methadone, chlorpromazine (Thorazine), and diazepam (Valium). These are typically used if the neonatal abstinence scoring system average score is elevated on three successive occasions and nursing interventions do not reduce the score. An infant should not be breast-fed to avoid passing narcotics in breast milk to the child.

Once an infant has been identified as having been exposed to drugs in utero, the mother needs treatment for withdrawal symptoms and follow-up care as much as the infant. In addition, evaluation is necessary to determine before discharge whether an environment that allowed for drug abuse will be safe for an infant. Infants who are exposed to drugs in utero may have long-term neurologic problems.

The Infant With Fetal Alcohol Syndrome

Alcohol crosses the placenta in the same concentration as is present in the maternal bloodstream. This results in **fetal alcohol exposure** and **fetal alcohol syndrome.** Fetal alcohol syndrome appears in 2 per 1,000 newborns (Gardner, 2000). Documenting fetal alcohol exposure is more difficult. Because it is unknown if there is a safe threshold of alcohol ingestion during pregnancy, all pregnant women are advised to avoid alcohol intake to prevent any teratogenic effects on their newborn.

The newborn with fetal alcohol syndrome has a number of possible problems at birth. Characteristics that mark the syndrome include pre- and postnatal growth restriction; central nervous system involvement such as cognitive challenge, microcephaly, and cerebral palsy; and facial features such as short palpebral fissures and a thin upper lip. During the neonatal period, the infant may be tremulous, fidgety, and irritable and may demonstrate a weak sucking reflex. Sleep disturbances are common, with the baby tending to be either always awake or always asleep, depending on the mother's alcohol level close to birth.

The most serious long-term effect is cognitive challenge. Behavior problems such as hyperactivity may occur in school-age children. Growth deficiencies may remain through life. The infant needs follow-up so any future problems can be discovered. The mother needs follow-up to see if she can reduce her alcohol intake for better overall health.

✔ CHECKPOINT QUESTIONS

31. Why are infants of diabetic mothers fed early?
32. What is the average time of onset for withdrawal symptoms for the heroin-addicted neonate?
33. Name two characteristic facial features of the newborn with fetal alcohol syndrome.

KEY POINTS

Priorities for infants born with special needs, such as preterm or postterm infants, are the same as for term infants: initiation and maintenance of respirations, establishment of extrauterine circulation, control of body temperature, intake of adequate nourishment, establishment of waste elimination, establishment of an infant–parent relationship, prevention of infection, and provision of developmental care for mental and social development.

Many high-risk infants need resuscitation at birth. Prompt action with such measures as warmth, oxygen, intubation, and suctioning are needed.

A small-for-gestational-age infant is one whose birthweight is below the 10th percentile on an intrauterine growth curve for that age infant. The infant could be preterm, term, or postterm.

Small-for-gestational-age infants have difficulty maintaining body warmth because of low f and may develop hypoglycemia from low glucose stores.

A large-for-gestational-age infant is one whose birthweight is above the 90th percentile on an intrauterine growth chart for that gestational age. The infant could be born preterm, term, or postterm.

Large-for-gestational-age infants tend to be infants of diabetic mothers; they are particularly prone to hypoglycemia or birth trauma.

A preterm infant is one born before 37 weeks of gestation. Preterm infants have particular problems with respiratory function, anemia, jaundice, persistent patent ductus arteriosus, and intracranial hemorrhage. Infants who are born weighing 1,500 to 2,500 g are also termed low-birth-weight infants; those born weighing 1,000 to 1,500 g are very-low-birth-weight infants; those born weighing between 500 and 1,000 g are extremely very-low-birth-weight infants. All such infants need intensive care from the moment of birth to give them their best chance of survival without neurologic after-effects caused by their being so critically close to the age of viability.

A postterm infant is one who has remained in utero past week 42 of pregnancy. Postterm infants have particular problems with establishing respirations, meconium aspiration, hypoglycemia, temperature regulation, and polycythemia.

Respiratory distress syndrome commonly occurs in preterm infants from a deficiency or lack of surfactant in the alveoli. Without surfactant, the alveoli collapse on expiration and require extreme force for reinflation. Primary therapy is synthetic surfactant replacement at birth by endotracheal tube insufflation, followed by oxygen and ventilatory support.

Transient tachypnea of the newborn is a temporary condition caused by slow absorption of lung fluid at birth. Close observation of the infant is necessary until the fluid is absorbed and respirations slow to a normal rate.

Meconium aspiration syndrome occurs from the infant inhaling meconium-stained amniotic fluid during birth. Meconium is irritating to the airway and may lead to both airway spasm and pneumonia. Infants need oxygen, ventilatory support, and possibly an antibiotic until the effects of the insult to the airway subside. It is important that they are suctioned before oxygen administration under pressure to prevent meconium being forced further into their lungs.

Apnea is a pause in respirations longer than 20 seconds, with accompanying bradycardia. It tends to occur in preterm infants who have secondary stresses such as infection, hyperbilirubinemia, hypoglycemia, or hypothermia. Apnea monitors are used to detect this, and infants who are high risk for this are discharged home on a home monitoring program.

Sudden infant death syndrome is the sudden, unexplained death of an infant. It is associated with infants sleeping on their stomachs (prone) and infants who were born preterm. An important preventive measure is advising parents to position their infant on the back for sleeping.

Hyperbilirubinemia results from the destruction of red blood cells, due either to a normal physiologic response or an abnormal destruction of the red blood cells. Hemolytic disease of the newborn is destruction of red blood cells from Rh or ABO incompatibility. The administration of RHIG (Rh antibodies) to Rh-negative mothers during pregnancy and after the birth of an Rh-positive infant to an Rh-negative mother has greatly reduced the incidence of the condition. Affected infants are jaundiced from release of bilirubin from injured red blood cells. Phototherapy or exchange transfusion is used to prevent kernicterus (deposition of bilirubin in brain cells, causing destruction of the cells).

Hemorrhagic disease of the newborn is a lack of clotting ability resulting from a deficiency of vitamin K at birth. Prevention is by injection of vitamin K to all infants at birth.

Retinopathy of prematurity is destruction of the retina due to exposure of immature retinal capillaries to oxygen. Monitoring oxygen saturation via arterial blood gases is an important preventive measure.

Severe infections that may be seen in newborns include streptococcal group B pneumonia, hepatitis B infection, ophthalmia neonatorum (gonococcal and chlamydial conjunctivitis), and herpesvirus infection. Assessing newborns for symptoms of these infections is an important nursing responsibility.

Infants of diabetic women and those of drug-abusing women are at high risk at birth for further complications. Both need careful assessment for respiratory distress and hypoglycemia.

CRITICAL THINKING EXERCISES

1. The Atkinses are the family you met at the beginning of the chapter. Mrs. Atkins doesn't want to visit or "waste my favorite name" on her new baby because the baby might die. How would you advise her?
2. A client, at 30 weeks' gestation, is in preterm labor. Based on your knowledge of gestational development, you know her child will be at high

risk for the development of respiratory distress syndrome. How would you explain to her why her baby will be at high risk for this?
3. Retinopathy of prematurity is an example of a disease that is caused by the therapy given the infant. Elaborate on the measures you can take to safeguard infants against this disorder.
4. Infants who are cared for in neonatal nurseries may need either reduced stimulation because they fatigue so easily or increased stimulation because their stay in the nursery will be so extended. Develop a plan for each instance to demonstrate your understanding of the effects of sensory deprivation and stimulation in this situation.
5. Examine the National Health Goals related to high-risk newborns. Most government-sponsored money for nursing research is allotted based on these goals. What would be a possible research topic to explore pertinent to these goals that would be fundable and would advance evidence-based practice?

REFERENCES

Alexander, J. M., McIntire, D. D., & Leveno, K. J. (2001). Prolonged pregnancy: Induction of labor and cesarean births. *Obstetrics & Gynecology, 97*(6), 911–915.

American Academy of Pediatrics. (2001). 2001 family shopping guide to car seats (*www.aap.org/family/famshop.htm*)

American Heart Association. (2000). Newborn resuscitation. *Circulation, 102*(1), 343–346.

Anderson, M. S., & Hay, W. W. (2000). Intrauterine growth restriction and the small-for-gestational age infant. In Avery, G. B., Fletcher, M. A., & MacDonald, M. G. (Eds.). *Neonatology* (5th ed., pp. 411–444). Philadelphia: Lippincott Williams & Wilkins.

Baumgart, S., Harrasch, S. C., & Touch, S. M. (2000) Thermal regulation. In Avery, G. B., Fletcher, M. A., & MacDonald, M. G. (Eds.). *Neonatology* (5th ed., pp. 395–408). Philadelphia: Lippincott Williams & Wilkins.

Bernbaum, J. C. (2000). Medical care after discharge. In Avery, G. B., Fletcher, M. A., & MacDonald, M. G. (Eds.). *Neonatology* (5th ed., pp. 1463–1497). Philadelphia: Lippincott Williams & Wilkins.

Bialoskurski, M. M., Cox, C. L. & Wiggins, R. D. (2002). The relationship between maternal needs and priorities in a neonatal intensive care environment. *Journal of Advanced Nursing, 37*(1), 62–69.

Camerota, A. J., & Arnold, J. H. (2000). Anesthesia and analgesia. In Avery, G. B., Fletcher, M. A., & MacDonald, M. G. (Eds.). *Neonatology* (5th ed., pp. 1447–1459). Philadelphia: Lippincott Williams & Wilkins.

Chappell, S. E. et al. (2001). A comparison of surfactant delivery with conventional mechanical ventilation and partial liquid ventilation in meconium aspiration injury. *Respiratory Medicine, 95*(7), 612–617.

Chatterjee, A., et al. (2001). Severe intrauterine herpes simplex disease with placentitis in a newborn of a mother with recurrent genital infection at delivery. *Journal of Perinatology, 21*(8), 559–564.

Cools, R., & Offringa, M. (2000). Neuromuscular paralysis for newborn infants receiving mechanical ventilation. *Cochrane Database of Systematic Reviews* (4), CD002773.

Cunningham, F. G., et al. (2001). *Williams' obstetrics* (21st ed.). Stamford, CT: Appleton & Lange.

Department of Health and Human Services. (2000). *Healthy people, 2010.* Washington, DC: DHHS.

Doyle, J. J., et al. (2000). Hematology. In Avery, G. B., Fletcher, M. A., & MacDonald, M. G. (Eds.). *Neonatology* (5th ed., pp. 1045–1086). Philadelphia: Lippincott Williams & Wilkins.

Fischbach, F. (2001). *A manual of laboratory and diagnostic tests* (5th ed.). Philadelphia: Lippincott Williams & Wilkins.

Flanagan, M. F., et al. (2000). Cardiac disease. In Avery, G. B., Fletcher, M. A., & MacDonald, M. G. (Eds.). *Neonatology* (5th ed., pp. 577–646). Philadelphia: Lippincott Williams & Wilkins.

Freij, B. J., & McCracken, G. H. (2000). Acute infections. In Avery, G. B., Fletcher, M. A., & MacDonald, M. G. (Eds.). *Neonatology* (5th ed., pp. 1189–1225). Philadelphia: Lippincott Williams & Wilkins.

Gardner, J. (2000). Living with a child with fetal alcohol syndrome. *MCN: American Journal of Maternal Child Nursing, 25*(5), 252–257.

Georgieff, M. K. (2000). Nutrition. In Avery, G. B., Fletcher, M. A., & MacDonald, M. G. (Eds.). *Neonatology* (5th ed., pp. 363–394). Philadelphia: Lippincott Williams & Wilkins.

Gibson, E., et al. (2000). Infant sleep position practices 2 years into the "back to sleep" campaign. *Clinical Pediatrics, 39*(5), 285–289.

Gray, C., Davies, F. & Molyneux, E. (1999). Apparent life-threatening events presenting to a pediatric emergency department. *Pediatric Emergency Care, 15* (3), 195–199.

Hill, A., & Volpe, J. J. (2000). Neurological and neuromuscular disorders. In Avery, G. B., Fletcher, M. A., & MacDonald, M. G. (Eds.). *Neonatology* (5th ed., pp. 1231–1252). Philadelphia: Lippincott Williams & Wilkins.

Hintz, S. R., et al. (2000). Decreased use of neonatal extracorporeal membrane oxygenation (ECMO): How new treatment modalities have affected ECMO utilization. *Pediatrics, 106*(6), 1339–1343.

Hunt, C. E. (2000). Sudden infant death syndrome. In Avery, G. B., Fletcher, M. A., & MacDonald, M. G. (Eds.). *Neonatology* (5th ed., pp. 533–555). Philadelphia: Lippincott Williams & Wilkins.

Isenberg, S. J. (2000). Eye disorders. In Avery, G. B., Fletcher, M. A., & MacDonald, M. G. (Eds.). *Neonatology* (5th ed., pp. 1285–1300). Philadelphia: Lippincott Williams & Wilkins.

Johnson, M., Maas, M., & Moorhead, S. (2000). *Nursing outcomes classification* (2d ed.). St. Louis: Mosby, Inc.

Karch, A. M. (2001). *Lippincott's nursing drug guide.* Philadelphia: Lippincott Williams & Wilkins.

Kirsten, G. F., Bergman, N. J., & Hann, F. M. (2001). Kangaroo mother care in the nursery. *Pediatric Clinics of North America, 48*(2), 443–352.

Lund, C. H., et al. (2001). Neonatal skin care: Clinical outcomes of the AWHONN/NANN evidence-based clinical practice guideline. *Journal of Obstetric, Gynecologic & Neonatal Nursing, 30*(1), 41–47.

Maisels, M. J. (2001). Phototherapy—traditional and nontraditional. *Journal of Perinatology, 21*(S1), 93–107.

McCloskey, J., & Bulechek, G. (2000). *Nursing interventions classification* (3d ed.). St. Louis: Mosby, Inc.

Mellien, A. C. (2001). Incubators versus mothers' arms: Body temperature conservation in very-low-birth-weight premature infants. *Journal of Obstetric, Gynecologic and Neonatal Nursing, 30*(2), 157–164.

Niermeyer, S. et al. Resuscitation of newborns. *Annals of Emergency Medicine, 37*(4S), 110–125.

Singer, L. T., et al. (2001). Developmental outcomes and environmental correlates of very low birthweight, cocaine-exposed infants. *Early Human Development, 64*(2), 91–103.

van Gemert, J. J., et al. (2001). Twin-twin transfusion syndrome: etiology, severity, and rational management. *Current Opinion in Obstetrics & Gynecology, 13*(2), 193–206.

Ward, R. M., & Lugo, R. A. (2000). Drug therapy in the newborn. In Avery, G. B., Fletcher, M. A., & MacDonald, M. G. (Eds.). *Neonatology* (5th ed., pp. 1263–1398). Philadelphia: Lippincott Williams & Wilkins.

Whitsett, J. A., et al. (2000). Acute respiratory disorders. In Avery, G. B., Fletcher, M. A., & MacDonald, M. G. (Eds.). *Neonatology* (5th ed., pp. 485–508). Philadelphia: Lippincott Williams & Wilkins.

ABC XYZ SUGGESTED READINGS

Callister, L. C. (2001). Culturally competent care of women and newborns: Knowledge, attitude, and skills. *Journal of Obstetric, Gynecologic & Neonatal Nursing, 30*(2), 209–215.

Chatfield, J. (2001). ACOG issues guidelines on fetal macrosomia. *American Family Physician, 64*(1), 169–170.

Coles, C. D., et al. (2000). Early identification of risk for effects of prenatal alcohol exposure. *Journal of Studies on Alcohol, 61*(4), 607–616.

Fuloria, M., & Kreiter, S. (2002). The newborn examination. *American Family Physician, 65*(2). 265–270.

Heaman, M. I., et al. (2001). Reducing the preterm birth rate: A population health strategy. *Journal of Obstetric, Gynecologic, & Neonatal Nursing, 30*(1), 20–24.

Hogan, D. P., & Park, J. M. (2000). Family factors and social support in the developmental outcomes of very low-birth weight children. *Clinics in Perinatology, 27*(2), 433–459.

Kelly, J. J., et al. (2000). The drug epidemic: Effects on newborn infants and health resource consumption at a tertiary perinatal centre. *Journal of Paediatrics & Child Health, 36*(3), 262–264.

O'Shea, T. M., & Dammann, O. (2000). Antecedents of cerebral palsy in very low-birth weight infants. *Clinics in Obstetrics & Gynecology,* 285–302.

Powderly, K. (2001). Ethical and legal issues in perinatal HIV. *Clinical Obstetrics & Gynecology, 44*(2), 300–311.

Ruiz, R. J., et al. (2001). Specialized care for twin gestations: Improving newborn outcomes and reducing costs. *Journal of Obstetric, Gynecologic, & Neonatal Nursing, 30*(1), 52–57.

Warner, B. B., Keily, J. L., & Donovan, E. F. (2000). Multiple births and outcome. *Clinics in Perinatology, 27*(2), 347–362.

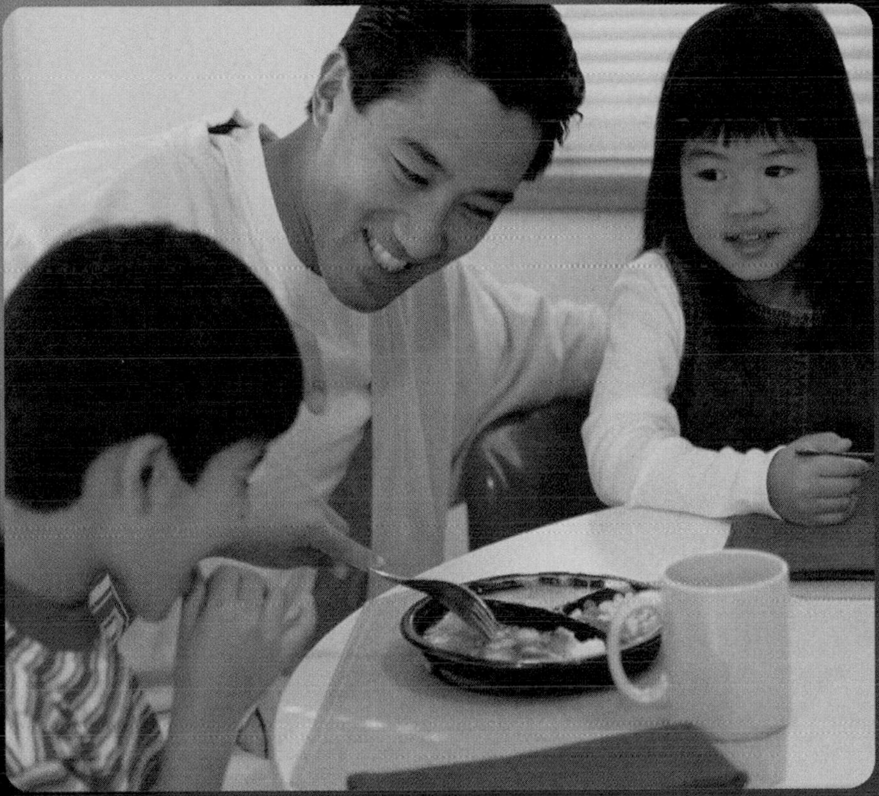

The Nursing Role in Health Promotion for the Childrearing Family

UNIT VI

Principles of Growth and Development

CHAPTER 27

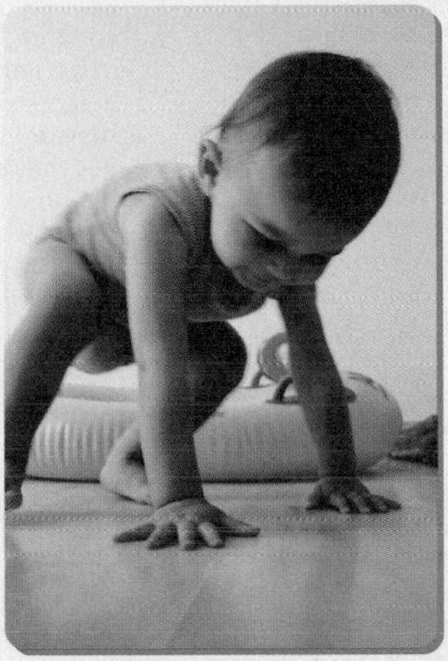

Key Terms

- abstract thought
- accommodation
- adaptability
- approach
- assimilation
- attention span
- autonomy versus shame
- centering
- cognitive development
- concrete operational thought
- conservation
- conventional development
- development
- developmental milestones
- developmental task
- distractibility
- egocentrism
- formal operational thought
- growth
- identity versus role confusion
- industry versus inferiority
- initiative versus guilt
- intuitive thought
- libido
- macronutrient
- maturation
- micronutrient
- mood quality
- permanence
- postconventional development
- preoperational thought
- prereligious stage
- reversibility
- rhythmicity
- role fantasy
- schemas
- sensorimotor stage
- temperament
- theory
- threshold of response
- trust versus mistrust

Objectives

After mastering the contents of this chapter, you should be able to:

1. Describe principles of growth and development and developmental stages according to major theorists.
2. Assess a child to determine the stage of development he or she has reached.
3. Formulate nursing diagnoses that address wellness as well as both a potential for and an actual delay in growth and development.
4. Identify expected outcomes for nursing goals for a growing child.
5. Plan nursing interventions to assist a child in achieving and maintaining normal growth and development.
6. Implement nursing actions such as providing age-appropriate play materials to support normal growth and development patterns.
7. Evaluate outcomes to be certain that nursing goals related to growth and development have been achieved.
8. Identify National Health Goals related to growth and development that nurses can be instrumental in helping the nation to achieve.
9. Identify areas of nursing care related to growth and development that could benefit from additional nursing research or application of evidence-based practice.
10. Use critical thinking to analyze factors that influence growth and development and family-centered ways to strengthen paths to achieving a new developmental stage.
11. Integrate knowledge of growth and development with nursing process to achieve quality maternal and child health nursing care.

John Olson is a 4-year-old boy you see at an ambulatory care visit. At 4 months of age, John was taken away from his mother because she was not caring for him adequately. He was then moved back and forth among 12 different foster homes until he was finally adopted at age three and a half. His adoptive parents, who have cared for him for 6 months, tell you they find him cold and unloving, unable to respond to them. They ask you what they can do to change this. How has John's background contributed to his behavior? What stage of psychosocial development does he not seem to have achieved? How could his parents help him?

Previous chapters discussed childbearing and what an important time the first year can be in a child's life. This chapter adds information about growth and development that is important for all the continuing years of the child's life. This is important information because nurses are directly responsible for assessing the growth and development of children.

After you've studied the chapter, answer the Critical Thinking Exercises at the end of the chapter and then access the on-line study activities (http://connection.lww.com) *to further sharpen your skills and test your knowledge.*

All children pass through predictable stages of growth and development as they mature. Understanding the stage of development a child has reached is important, because parents often will ask a nurse what to expect from their child regarding his or her developmental progress. Health care visits provide opportunities not only to assess present growth and development but also to supply anticipatory guidance on the topic (Thomas, 2002).

For these reasons, learning about growth and development is essential to the establishment of complete and effective nursing care plans for children. This chapter addresses the most important factors to assess for each age group. Later chapters supply detailed descriptions of individual age groups. National Health Goals related to growth and development are presented in the Focus on National Health Goals box.

FOCUS ON NATIONAL HEALTH GOALS

National Health Goals that address growth or development of children include the following:

- Reduce growth retardation among low-income children aged 5 and younger to less than 5% from a baseline of 8%. Growth retardation is defined as height-for-age below the fifth percentile on a standard growth chart.
- Reduce the occurrence of developmental disabilities in children, including mental retardation, from a baseline of 131/100,000 to a target of 124/100,000.
- Reduce the proportion of children and adolescents who are overweight or obese from a baseline of 11% to 5% (DHHS, 2000).

Recognizing normal growth and development patterns for children helps in determining if children are following normal development and when referrals are needed. Nursing research topics that could add information in this area are: Are there differences between urban and rural children in the way they approach childhood problems? How do characteristics of temperament affect the way children respond to hospitalization? What are specific ways that the environment of children influences health? What can nurses do to help reduce the obesity epidemic in children?

NURSING PROCESS OVERVIEW

For Promotion of Normal Growth and Development

Assessment

Height and weight should be measured and plotted on a standard growth chart for children at all health care visits. History taking and observation should focus on whether **developmental milestones** (major markers of normal development) have been met. A 24-hour recall history for nutritional intake, sleep, and a description of school and play behaviors should also be documented. Periodic screening tests (i.e., the Denver II, vision tests, and audiometry screening) should be scheduled at standard times, as discussed in Chapter 33. For the most accurate assessment, be certain to account for illness, sleepiness, fatigue, or "bad days" (a day on which the child did not test well). The developmental stage that children have reached is assessed through observation and careful listening to how they describe themselves, not how their parents describe them, and what specific activities they can accomplish (Fig. 27-1).

Nursing Diagnosis

When assessment is completed, a child profile is devised. Based on this profile, needs and problems are identified. Nursing diagnoses most frequently used in this area include:

- Risk for delayed growth and development related to lack of age-appropriate toys and activities
- Delayed growth and development related to prolonged illness
- Readiness for enhanced family coping related to parent's seeking information about child's growth and development
- Health-seeking behaviors related to appropriate stimulation for infants
- Imbalanced nutrition, less than body requirements, related to parental knowledge deficit regarding child's protein need
- Deficient knowledge related to potential long-term effects of obesity in school-age child

Outcome Identification and Planning

To provide holistic nursing care, consider all aspects of the child's health—physical, emotional, cultural,

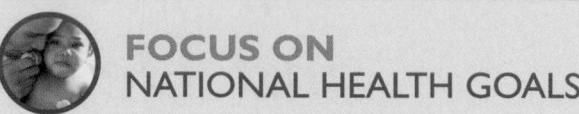

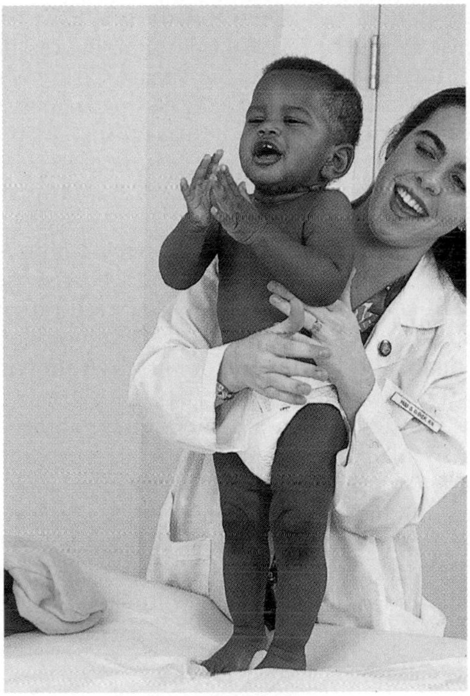

FIGURE 27.1 Growth and development are assessed by both observation and specific testing. Here a 12-month-old demonstrates mastery of well-coordinated and intentional hand movements.

cognitive, spiritual, nutritional, and social—and remember that each child's developmental progress is unique. A child cannot be forced to achieve milestones faster than his or her own timetable will allow. However, through anticipatory guidance a child can be encouraged to reach his or her maximum developmental potential, and outcomes for this should be established. Nurses can play an important role in offering guidance to both the child and family on ways to encourage child development and preparing children for new experiences.

Planning includes the child's family even when the child is no longer completely dependent on it; however, be certain to consider privacy issues for adolescents. To develop psychosocially, children continue to need emotional support from loved ones, just as they need nutritional support to grow physically. Parents of a child with a developmental delay may use denial as a protective mechanism for a long time. This means that planning may have to be centered first on helping parents accept what is happening; plans for the child may have to be delayed until the parents are convinced that a problem exists.

Implementation

Interventions to foster growth and development include encouraging age-appropriate self-care in the child and suggesting age-appropriate toys or activities to parents. It may be necessary to help parents accept a child's delayed growth or motivate a child to reach his or her upper limits. Role modeling is an important ongoing intervention with both children and families. Modeling, for example, can demonstrate that problem solving is a more effective approach to life's challenges than acting out.

Outcome Evaluation

Evaluation for specific growth and developmental milestones (see Chaps. 28 through 32) must be ongoing to be accurate and useful, because many children do not test well on any given day until school age. Ongoing evaluation is necessary also because it provides an opportunity for early detection of various problems. If a child has difficulty achieving one developmental task, he or she may have difficulty with the next as well. Evaluation must also be comprehensive. If a developmental task involves only gross motor function, it may not be apparent that something is wrong with the child's fine motor function until the child is asked to perform fine motor tasks in school. The following are examples of outcome criteria that might be developed:

- Child, by 5 years of age, expresses less negativism at next clinic visit.
- At 9-month checkup, parents describe how they have made a safe space in their home for their infant to crawl so he is not confined to the playpen.
- Parents list tasks they believe are appropriate for a 6-year-old child by next office visit.
- Parents state how they are beginning to phase out high-carbohydrate, nonnutritive snacks for their preschooler.

IMPORTANCE OF KNOWLEDGE ABOUT GROWTH AND DEVELOPMENT TO THE ROLE OF THE NURSE

Information about growth and development is important in all phases of childcare.

Health Promotion and Illness Prevention

Determining a child's developmental stage is often the primary focus of a health interview. For instance, during her child's 24-month checkup, a mother might ask if it is normal that her child cannot yet pedal a tricycle. This question, or any other questions about a child's developmental progress, cannot be answered without a full understanding of the average ranges.

In addition to reassurance that their child is doing well, parents also need periodic anticipatory guidance regarding their child's development. For example, it would be important to discuss additional home safety with a parent when a child is approaching the age for creeping. Parents should be cautioned to think about fencing open stairways and clearing cleaning compounds out of bottom cupboards. Parents of a child who is almost 1 year old will appreciate being cautioned that the child's appetite may decrease during the coming year; armed with this knowledge, they will not interpret the child's rejection of food as the beginning of a feeding problem but will see it as a usual step of development. The parent of a child approaching puberty generally welcomes a discussion on how to prepare a child for this growth phase.

Anticipatory guidance must be offered at the appropriate time, or it will be useless. Information given too early is forgotten by the time it is needed. If it is given too late, the parents may have already addressed (or ignored) the issues, possibly not in the most growth-enhancing way for the child. To be able to supply anticipatory guidance this way at the appropriate time or to plan nursing care to meet the needs of children and families, you must be able to recognize the predictable stages of growth and development, from newborn to young adult, through which each child passes.

Health Restoration and Maintenance

It is also essential to consider developmental stages when caring for a sick child or one having surgery. Preparing a 5-year-old child for surgery, for example, would be ineffective unless you know how much a 5-year-old child can be expected to comprehend and assess if the child will understand things such as the fact that an anesthetic is a gas, what a surgeon is, and what stitches are. Understanding the child's developmental stage helps in choosing the right words. It is just as important to keep developmental stages in mind when teaching parents; for example, evaluate whether an oral form of medicine is appropriate for a child if the child is too young to coordinate tongue and throat muscles.

Physical growth is another important factor to consider, because disease affects children differently at various stages of growth. A 12-year-old child who has fractured a long bone, for example, has a potentially more serious fracture than an 8-year-old child who fractures the identical bone. The 8-year-old child must metabolize enough calcium to meet two major needs: healing the fracture site and maintaining healthy bone cells. The 12-year-old child, who is undergoing a period of rapid growth, must meet three needs: his or her body must supply not only enough calcium for healing and maintaining existing healthy bone cells but also an additional amount for rapid bone growth. If the child does not take in adequate calcium during the healing period to supply the extra amount for growth, the affected limb may be left shorter than its mate. Extra calcium will be needed so that no permanent disability will result.

PRINCIPLES OF GROWTH AND DEVELOPMENT

Growing up is a complex phenomenon because of the many interrelated facets involved. Children do not merely grow taller and heavier as they get older; maturing also involves growth in their ability to perform skills, to think, to relate to people, and to trust or have confidence in themselves.

The terms "growth" and "development" are occasionally used interchangeably, but they are different. **Growth** is generally used to denote an increase in physical size or a quantitative change. Growth in weight is measured in pounds or kilograms; growth in height is measured in inches or centimeters. **Development** is used to denote an increase in skill or the ability to function (a qualitative change). Development can be measured by observing a child's ability to perform specific tasks (e.g., how well the child picks up small objects such as raisins), by recording the parent's description of the child's progress, or by using standardized tests such as the Denver II. **Maturation** is a synonym for development.

Psychosexual development is a specific type of development that refers to developing instincts or sensual pleasure (Freudian theory). Psychosocial development refers to Erikson's stages of personality development. Moral development is the ability to know right from wrong and to apply these to real-life situations.

Cognitive development refers to the ability to learn or understand from experience, to acquire and retain knowledge, to respond to a new situation, and to solve problems (intelligence; see the section below on Piaget's theory of cognitive development). It is measured by intelligence tests and by observing the child's ability to function effectively in his or her environment.

Patterns

Neither physical growth nor aspects of maturation occur haphazardly; several principles govern this process (Box 27-1). As shown in Figure 27-2, general growth (i.e., growth of respiratory, digestive, renal, musculoskeletal, and circulatory tissue) proceeds fairly smoothly during childhood. Certain body tissues, however, mature more rapidly than others. Neurologic tissue (spinal cord and brain) grows so rapidly the first 2 years that the brain reaches mature proportions by 2 to 5 years. Lymphoid tissue (e.g., spleen, thymus, lymph nodes, and tonsillar tissue) also grows rapidly during infancy and childhood to protect the child against infection. The spleen is usually palpable 1 or 2 cm in preschool children, and in 5-year-olds, tonsillar tissue has already reached its peak size (about twice that of an adult). On assessment, younger school-age children appear to have large tonsils and thymus glands because of this early growth of lymphoid tissue (the back of their throat seems to be "all tonsils" but will soon decrease in size again). In contrast, the reproductive organs (i.e., genital tissue) show little growth until puberty.

✔ CHECKPOINT QUESTIONS

1. What is the difference between the terms "growth" and "development"?
2. Which body systems grow most rapidly during early childhood?

FACTORS INFLUENCING GROWTH AND DEVELOPMENT

Genetic inheritance and environmental influences are the two primary factors in determining a child's pattern of growth and development. Temperament is an example of

BOX 27.1

PRINCIPLES OF GROWTH AND DEVELOPMENT

Principle	Example
Growth and development are continuous processes from conception until death.	Although there are highs and lows in terms of the rate at which growth and development proceed, at all times a child is growing new cells and learning new skills. An example of how the rate of growth changes is a comparison between that of the first year and later in life. An infant triples birthweight and increases height by 50% during the first year of life. If this tremendous growth rate were to continue, the 5-yr-old child, ready to begin school, would weigh 1,600 lb and be 12 ft 6 in tall.
Growth and development proceed in an orderly sequence.	Growth in height occurs in only one sequence—from smaller to larger. Development also proceeds in a predictable order. For example, the majority of children sit before they creep, creep before they stand, stand before they walk, and walk before they run. Occasionally, a child will skip a stage (or pass through it so quickly that the parents do not observe the stage). Occasionally, a child will progress in a different order, but most children follow a predictable sequence of growth and development.
Different children pass through the predictable stages at different rates.	All stages of development have a range of time rather than a certain point at which they are usually accomplished. Two children may pass through the motor sequence at such different rates, for example, that one begins walking at 9 mo, another only at 14 mo. Both are developing normally. They are both following the predictable sequence; they are merely developing at different rates.
All body systems do not develop at the same rate.	Certain body tissues mature more rapidly than others. For example, neurologic tissue experiences its peak growth during the first year of life, whereas genital tissue grows little until puberty.
Development is cephalocaudal.	*Cephalo* is a Greek word meaning "head"; *caudal* means "tail." Development proceeds from head to tail. A newborn can lift only the head off the bed when he or she lies in a prone position. By age 2 mo, the infant can lift the head and chest off the bed; by 4 mo, the head, chest, and part of the abdomen; by 5 mo, the infant has enough control to turn over; by 9 mo, he or she can control the legs enough to crawl; and by 1 yr, the child can stand upright and perhaps walk. Motor development has proceeded in a cephalocaudal order—from the head to the lower extremities.
Development proceeds from proximal to distal body parts.	This principle is closely related to cephalocaudal development. It can best be illustrated by tracing the progress of upper extremity development. A newborn makes little use of the arms or hands. Any movement, except to put a thumb in the mouth, is a flailing motion. By age 3 or 4 mo, the infant has enough arm control to support the upper body weight on the forearms, and the infant can coordinate the hand to scoop up objects. By 10 mo, the infant can coordinate the arm and thumb and index fingers sufficiently well to use a pincerlike grasp or be able to pick up an object as fine as a piece of breakfast cereal on a high-chair tray.
Development proceeds from gross to refined skills.	This principle parallels the preceding one. Because the child is able to control distal body parts such as fingers, he or she is able to perform fine motor skills (a 3-yr-old colors best with a large crayon; a 12-yr-old can write with a fine pen).
There is an optimum time for initiation of experiences or learning.	A child cannot learn tasks until his or her nervous system is mature enough to allow that particular learning. A child cannot learn to sit, for example, no matter how much the child's parents have him or her practice, until the nervous system has matured enough to allow back control. Children who are not given the opportunity to learn developmental tasks at the appropriate or "target" times for that task may have more difficulty than the usual child learning the task later on. A child who is confined to a body cast at 12 mo, the time the child would normally learn to walk, may take a long time to learn this skill once free of the cast at, say, age 2 yrs. The child has passed the time of optimal learning for that particular skill.
Neonatal reflexes must be lost before development can proceed.	An infant cannot grasp with skill until the grasp reflex has faded nor stand steadily until the walking reflex has faded. Neonatal reflexes are replaced by purposeful movements.
A great deal of skill and behavior is learned by practice.	Infants practice over and over taking a first step before they accomplish this securely. If children fall behind in growth and development because of illness, they are capable of "catch-up" growth to bring them equal again with their age group.

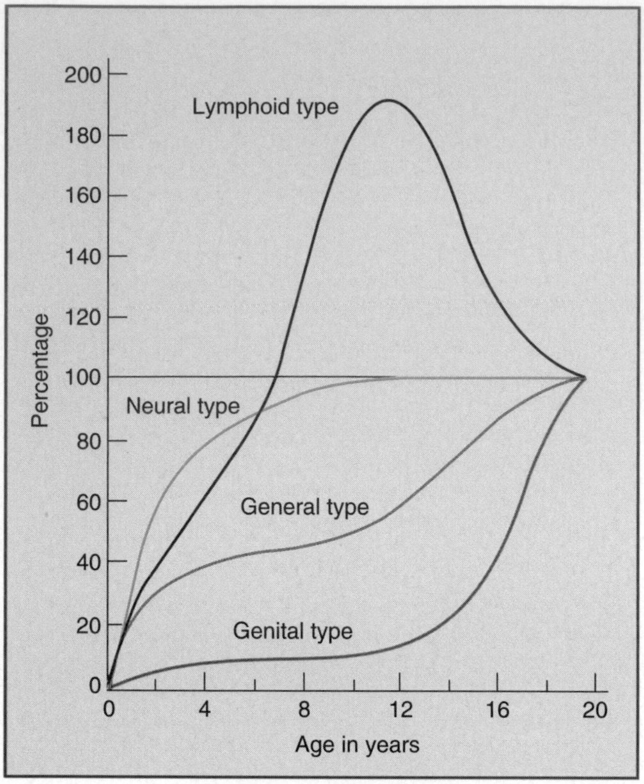

FIGURE 27.2 Main types of postnatal growth of various body tissue types. (Redrawn from Scammon, R. E. [1930]. The measurement of the body in childhood. In Harris, J. A., et al. [Eds.]. *The measurement of man,* pp. 214–226. Minneapolis: University of Minnesota Press, with permission.)

genetic influence. Nutrition is an environmental influence. A unique combination of these factors determines how each child grows and matures.

Genetics

From the moment of conception when a sperm and ovum fuse, the basic genetic makeup of an individual is cast. Although each child is unique, certain gender-related characteristics will influence normal growth and development. In addition to physical characteristics such as eye color and height potential, inheritance determines other characteristics such as learning style and temperament. An individual may also inherit a genetic defect, which may result in disability or illness at birth or later in life.

Gender

On the average, girls are born lighter (by an ounce or two) and shorter (by an inch or two) than boys. Boys tend to keep this height and weight advantage until prepuberty, at which time girls surge ahead because they begin their puberty growth spurt 6 months to 1 year earlier than boys. By the end of puberty (14 to 16 years), boys again tend to be taller and heavier than girls. This difference in growth patterns is reflected in the different growth charts used for boys and girls (see Appendix E).

Health

A child who inherits a genetically transmitted disease may not grow as rapidly or develop as fully as the healthy child, depending on the type of illness and the therapy or care available for the disease. Before insulin was discovered in 1922, for example, children with type 1 diabetes mellitus were left physically challenged; many of them died. Currently, with good health supervision and insulin therapy, the effects of the disease can be minimized so children with diabetes thrive and grow normally.

Intelligence

Children with high intelligence do not generally grow faster physically than other children, but they do tend to advance faster in skills. Occasionally, a child of high intelligence will fall behind in physical skills because he or she spends time with books or mental games rather than with games that develop motor skills and so does not receive practice in these areas.

Temperament

Temperament can be defined as the usual reaction pattern of an individual, or an individual's characteristic manner of thinking, behaving, or reacting to stimuli in the environment (Chess & Thomas, 1995). Unlike cognitive or moral development, temperament is not developed by stages but is an inborn characteristic (see Focus on Evidence-Based Practice).

It is important to explore the concept of temperament with parents at child health assessments. Understanding that children are not all alike—some adapt quickly to new situations and others adapt slowly, and some react intensely and some passively—will help parents to better understand their child and therefore to care for the child more constructively.

Reaction Patterns

In assessing the temperament of a child, Chess and Thomas have identified nine separate characteristics that define reactivity patterns. Each child's pattern is made up of these individual elements.

Activity Level. The level of activity among children differs widely. Some babies are constantly on the go and rarely quiet. They wiggle and squirm in their crib as early as 2 weeks of age. Parents put such children to sleep in one end of a crib and find them in the other end an hour later; such children will not stay seated in bathtubs and refuse to be confined in playpens. Other babies, by contrast, move little, stay where they are placed, and appear to take in their environment in a quieter, more docile way. Both patterns are normal; they merely reflect two extremes of motor activity, one characteristic of temperament.

Rhythmicity. A child who has **rhythmicity** manifests a regular rhythm in physiologic functions. Even as infants, such children tend to wake up at the same time each morning, are hungry at regular 4-hour periods, nap the same

FOCUS ON EVIDENCE-BASED PRACTICE

Does Temperament Influence Adolescent Behavior? Temperament is an inborn characteristic that continues throughout life. To assess if temperament influences alcohol use by adolescents, researchers held structured interviews with 438 adolescents aged 12 to 18 years and their parents. Results of the study showed that for both genders of adolescents, difficult temperament was a significant predictor of alcohol use as well as being negatively related to the quality of parent–adolescent relationships (adolescents with a difficult temperament had poor relationships with their parents compared with adolescents with easy temperaments). The researchers suggest that alcohol abuse prevention and treatment programs for adolescents should consider the role of basic temperamental characteristics as a key for the development of alcohol abuse and the possibility that the parent–adolescent relationship quality may be a key point to begin interventions.

This is an interesting study for nurses because it documents that temperament is a long-term characteristic, not a fleeting one of preschool children. Knowing this should alert you to the importance of educating parents about temperament so they understand better why children differ in their response to new situations or ability to persist at tasks.

Neighbors, B. D., et al. (2000). Difficult temperament, parental relationships and adolescent alcohol use disorder symptoms. *Journal of Child & Adolescent Substance Abuse, 10*(1), 69–86.

time every day, and have a bowel movement the same time every day. They are predictable and easy to care for in that their parents learn early what to expect from them. On the other end of the scale are infants with an irregular rhythmicity. They rarely awaken at the same time 2 days in a row. They may go a long time without eating one day and the next day appear hungry almost immediately after a feeding. Such children may be difficult to care for because it is not easy to plan a schedule for them, and parents must constantly adapt their own routines to the child's.

Approach. **Approach** refers to a child's response on initial contact with a new stimulus. Some children approach new situations in an unruffled manner. They smile and "talk" to strangers and accept a first feeding or a new food without spitting up or fussing. They explore new toys without apprehension. Other infants demonstrate withdrawal rather than approach to new situations. They cry at the sight of strangers, new toys, and new foods; they fuss the first time they are placed in a bathtub. They are difficult to take on vacation or to meet a new childcare provider because they react so fearfully to new situations.

Adaptability. **Adaptability** is the ability to change one's reaction to stimuli over time. Infants who are adaptable change their first reaction to situations without exhibiting extreme distress. The first time such children are placed in a bathtub they might protest loudly, for example, but by the third time they sit splashing happily. This is in contrast to infants who cry for months whenever they are put into a bathtub or who cannot seem to accustom themselves to a new bed, new playpen, or new caregiver.

Intensity of Reaction. Some children react to situations with their whole being. They cry loudly, thrash their arms, and begin temper tantrums when their diapers are wet, when they are hungry, and when their parents leave them. Others rarely demonstrate such overt symptoms of anger or have a mild or low-intensity reaction to stress.

Distractibility. Children who are easily distracted or who can easily shift their attention to a new situation (**distractibility**) can be easily managed. As infants, they are diverted and calmed by a pacifier. If they are crying over the loss of a toy, they can be appeased by the offer of a new one. Other children cannot be distracted; their parents may describe them as stubborn, willful, or unwilling to compromise because they persistently return to an activity.

Attention Span and Persistence. **Attention span** is the ability to remain interested in a project or activity. Like other aspects of temperament, it varies among infants. Some play by themselves with one toy for 1 hour; others spend no more than 1 or 2 minutes with each toy. The degree of persistence also varies. Some infants keep trying to perform an activity even when they fail time after time; others stop trying after one unsuccessful attempt.

Threshold of Response. The **threshold of response** is the intensity level of stimulation that is necessary to evoke a reaction. Children with a low threshold need little stimulation; those with a high threshold need intense stimulation before they demonstrate a change in behavior.

Mood Quality. The child who is always happy and laughing can be said to have a positive **mood quality.** Obviously, this can make a major difference in the parents' enjoyment of a child. Parents are bound to spend more time with him or her than parents whose child has a negative mood quality.

Nursing Implications Regarding Temperament

Three categories of temperament are shown in Box 27-2. Children who have a normal activity level and regular rhythmicity, who approach and adapt to new situations easily, and who have a long attention span, a high level of persistence, and a positive mood quality are "ideal" or "easy" children to care for, from a parent's point of view. Highly active infants are much more difficult for new parents to learn to care for, especially if they demonstrate irregular physiologic rhythms, withdrawal rather than approach, and little ability to adapt. They require more planning and creative distraction measures.

It is useful to talk to parents about their child's reactivity patterns at health maintenance visits because these patterns tend to persist. The way children will react in the future depends a great deal on their current pattern of behavior. The child who withdraws from rather than

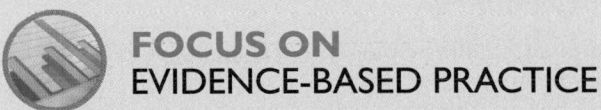

BOX 27.2

CATEGORIES OF TEMPERAMENT

The Easy Child

Children are rated as "easy to care for" if they have a predictable rhythmicity, approach and adapt to new situations readily, have a mild to moderate intensity of reaction, and have an overall positive mood quality. Most children, 40% to 50%, are rated by their parents as being in this category.

The Difficult Child

Children are "difficult" if they are irregular in habits, have a negative mood quality, and withdraw rather than approach new situations. Only about 10% of children fall into this category.

Slow-to-Warm-Up Child

Children fall into this category if they are overall fairly inactive; respond only mildly and adapt slowly to new situations, and have a general negative mood. About 15% of children display this pattern. When discussing this temperament with parents, try to use positive terms such as "ways to find a healthy fit for your child" rather than stressing ways the child is hard to manage.

approaches a first toy, for example, may react in the same way to toilet training or starting day care. The parents of such children will need to focus on preparing them for new activities more than will the parents of children who approach new situations easily. Those who are aware that their baby shies away from new experiences such as baths and new foods will be able to take it in stride when the child is slow to adapt to a Head Start program at age 4 years; they will know it is simply their child's method of coping.

Bring these characteristics to parents' attention, because understanding the child is the beginning of accepting and respecting him or her as an individual and is essential for successful child-rearing.

Notice a child's temperamental characteristics when he or she is admitted to a hospital so that you can anticipate the child's reactions to procedures or pain. For example, a child with a mild reactivity pattern may not show a great deal of response to even acute pain, but a child with an intense pattern may react as strongly to minor discomfort as to major pain, making it difficult to evaluate the true level of pain the child is experiencing.

Carey and McDevitt (1994) developed an Infant Temperament Questionnaire that can be used as a screening tool for temperament in infants; it is described in Chapter 33 with other assessment tools. Carey and colleagues have also developed temperament scales for other age groups.

WHAT IF? What if a father tells you his son rarely plays long at any activity, yet he screamed loudly when the father took a toy gun away from him and could not be distracted by another toy no matter how the father tried? Is he describing a child who is easy to manage or difficult to manage?

Environment

Although children cannot grow taller than their genetically programmed height potential allows, their adult height may be considerably less than genetic potential if the environment hinders their growth in some way. For example, the child may receive inadequate nutrition because of the family's low socioeconomic status; the caregiver may lack skills or not give the child enough attention; or the child may have a chronic illness. Many illnesses lower children's appetite; others, such as certain endocrine disorders, directly alter the growth rate.

Environmental influences, however, are not always detrimental. For example, children with phenylketonuria, an inherited metabolic disease, can achieve normal growth and development despite their genetic makeup if their diet (a part of the environment) is properly regulated. The following environmental influences are those most likely to affect growth and development.

Socioeconomic Level

Because health care and good nutrition both cost money, children born into families of low socioeconomic means may not receive adequate health supervision or good nutrition. Poor health supervision can leave them without immunization against measles or other childhood illnesses and thus vulnerable to diseases that could cause permanent neurologic damage if complications occur.

Parent–Child Relationship

Children who are loved thrive better than those who are not. Either parent or a nonparent caregiver may serve as the primary caregiver or form the primary parent–child love relationship. It is the quality of time spent with children, not the amount of time, that is important. Loss of love from a primary caregiver, as might occur with the death of a parent, or interruption of parental contact through prolonged hospitalizations, divorce, or inadequate parental love, can interfere with a child's desire to eat, improve, and advance. Cultural norms within the family also play a role in determining when a child is expected to achieve particular developmental milestones (see Focus on Cultural Competence).

Ordinal Position in the Family

The position of a child in the family (first-born child, middle child, youngest child, only child) and the size of the family have some bearing on the child's growth and development. An only child or the oldest child in a family generally excels in language development because conversations are mainly with adults. Children learn by watching other children, however, so that a firstborn or only child, who has no example to watch, may not excel in other skills, such as toilet training at an early age.

Health

Diseases that come from environmental sources can have as strong an influence on growth and development as genetically inherited diseases. Infants cared for in neonatal

FOCUS ON CULTURAL COMPETENCE

Not all nations foster the growth and development of children in the same manner, in part because of cultural variations. In some countries, the predominant theory of child-rearing is protective nurturing. Children are not rushed into new experiences like toilet training or beginning school. In others, it is customary to treat children in a harsh, strict manner, using shame or corporal punishment for discipline. Praising children for learning a new skill may be viewed as unnecessary or actually harmful, because this could result in a child being subject to evil forces.

Childhood in the United States covers a relatively long time period. In other countries, childhood is short because girls are asked to assume domestic responsibilities early in life and outside or farm work is required early for boys. In Asian cultures, an infant's personality is thought to depend not so much on genetic or environmental influences but on the year and time of birth.

What foods children receive depends very much on culture. Vegetables such as jicama and chayote, for example, may not even be recognized by children in the northeast United States but are very popular with those in the Southwest.

Asking questions such as, "What do you do when the baby cries?" "What kind of things do you think a 2-year-old should be able to do?" "What do you do when your 4-year-old misbehaves?" can help isolate cultural differences.

Recognizing that such cultural variations exist helps in planning care that is specific to a particular child and family.

intensive care units may develop some decrease in hearing because of the overstimulation of sound, an example of health being directly influenced by the environment. Children who have residual heart impairment as a result of rheumatic fever might be limited in their ability to play an active sport. The eventual degree of disability will depend not only on the damage caused by the actual disease but also on the attitudes of the people around the child—how disabled they believe the child is and how they treat the child. Treating a child as if he or she were sick or vulnerable to sickness is referred to as vulnerable child syndrome (Green & Solnit, 1964). These attitudes are an influence of environment on the child's development. Fortunately, if an illness does not last long, the child may well achieve "catch-up" growth afterward.

Nutrition

In the past 20 years, nutrition has become a major focus of health promotion and disease prevention in the United States because the quality of a child's nutrition during the growing years (including prenatally) has a major influence on his or her health and stature (Alaimo et al., 2001). Poor maternal nutrition may limit the growth and intelligence potential of the child from the moment of birth. Children whose own diets lack essential nutrients show inadequate physical growth. A lack of energy and stamina prevents children from learning at their best intellectual level. As many as 50% of American children are obese today (Erickson et al., 2000). Children who eat too many carbohydrates and become obese may develop motor skills more slowly than other children because physical movement is more tiring for them. Obese children are sometimes taunted by their playmates and may become loners or have difficulty relating to their peers because of depression about their weight (von Kries et al., 2000).

Nutrition also plays a vital role in the body's susceptibility to disease because poor nutrition limits the body's ability to resist infection. Lack of calcium could leave a child prone to rickets, a disease that affects growth by causing shortening or bowing of long bones. Lack of vitamins can lead to visual impairments and poor healing.

Poor nutrition also plays a major role in the development of chronic illness. Of the eight leading causes of death in adults, six have been linked to dietary excesses: heart disease, cancer, cerebrovascular disease, diabetes mellitus, cirrhosis, and arteriosclerosis. It is clear, too, that dietary habits have a cumulative effect; for instance, although heart disease is not one of the top causes of death in children, the arterial changes that cause it begin in childhood. Increased consumption of food and alcohol, decreased levels of exercise, and smoking all lead to a greater incidence of these diet-related diseases in adult life. Establishing healthy eating patterns early in life can contribute to better health in the adult years.

Food Guide Pyramid Guidelines for a Healthy Diet

Basic guidelines for a healthy diet have been outlined by a variety of governmental groups, including the U.S. Department of Agriculture (USDA), and the U.S. Department of Health and Human Services. In 1992, a food guide pyramid was developed by the USDA to illustrate these guidelines. The food guide pyramid suggests a range of daily servings from each major food group. It is also designed to emphasize variety, moderation, and balance. Table 27-1 lists recommended servings for children from the five pyramid food groups. In addition, good nutrition in children should follow a number of "healthy eating" guidelines.

Eat a Variety of Foods. Choices from all food pyramid groups—dairy, meat and poultry, fruits, vegetables, cereals and grains—should be included in the diet every day. It is also important to vary choices within each group and recognize that not all foods within a group are nutritionally equivalent.

Balance the Food You Eat With Physical Activity—Maintain or Improve Your Weight. Although the tendency for obesity may be inherited, being overweight in early life may also play a role. Parents need to be certain that children receive all the nutrients they need for the substantial growth they are undergoing (including a percentage of fat, because this is important for myelination

TABLE 27.1 Servings of the Five Pyramid Food Groups for Children

GROUP	FOODS	RECOMMENDED DAILY AMOUNTS: Children 2–6 yrs	RECOMMENDED DAILY AMOUNTS: Older Children	MAJOR NUTRIENTS PROVIDED
Bread, cereals, rice, pasta	Whole-grain and enriched	6 servings	6–11 servings	Thiamin, niacin, riboflavin (if enriched); iron (if enriched); incomplete protein, carbohydrates
Vegetable	Vegetables (yellow and green)	3 servings	3–5 servings	Vitamin A, iron, calcium, carbohydrates (include vitamin A source at least every other day)
Fruit	Fruit	2 servings	2–4 servings	Vitamin C (include vitamin C daily); carbohydrates
Milk, yogurt, cheese	Whole milk and other milk products except butter	2 servings	2–3 servings	Calcium, phosphorus, complete protein, riboflavin, niacin, vitamin D (if vitamin D–fortified milk used), fats
Meat, poultry, fish	Muscle meats (veal, beef, pork) dry beans, eggs; fish; poultry	2 servings	2–3 servings	Complete protein, iron, thiamin, riboflavin, niacin, vitamin B_{12}, fats
Fats, oils, sweets	Candy, cake, fried foods	Use sparingly	Use sparingly	Essential fatty acids, carbohydrates

Data from Saltos, E. (1999). Adapting the food guide pyramid for children: Defining the target audience. *Family Economics and Nutrition Review, 12*(3+4), 3–17.

of nerves); at the same time, it is important that they not be overfed. Balancing a lifestyle of physical activity with sound nutrition prevents obesity best.

Choose a Diet With Plenty of Grain Products, Vegetables, and Fruits. Foods with starch and fiber are more beneficial for gastrointestinal function than more processed foods. Fiber, in particular, has been linked to the lowered incidence of a variety of illnesses such as constipation. Fiber can be included as early as during preschool years in the form of whole-grain cereals and raw fruits such as apples.

Choose a Diet Low in Fat, Saturated Fat, and Cholesterol. The American diet has changed substantially over the past 10 years to reflect this important goal. Many adults now consume low-fat diets, substituting nonfat milk for whole milk, decreasing their consumption of eggs and other high-cholesterol sources, and reducing their consumption of meat. Fat intake does not need to be restricted for the first 2 years of life. Thereafter, fat intake can be tailored to meet the guidelines of 30% total intake for both children and adults. Some foods now contain Olestra, a synthetic fat. It should not be used by children (or should be used sparingly) until further study is completed because of the danger of fat-soluble vitamins being excreted with the product.

Choose a Diet Moderate in Sugars. Too much sugar in the diet can contribute to both dental caries and obesity. Refined sugar such as that used in soft drinks, prepared foods, candy, and chocolate represents "empty" calories: it is high in calories yet provides no essential nutrients. Although children need adequate carbohydrate for energy, families can give their children a good start by preventing excessive sugar intake.

Choose a Diet Moderate in Salt and Sodium. The taste for salt is acquired. If unsalted or only lightly salted solid food is offered to infants, they do not develop a desire for heavily salted foods. It is helpful to assess the diet of school-age children and check whether they are eating a diet heavier in salt than necessary because of many salty after-school snacks.

If You Drink Alcoholic Beverages, Do So in Moderation. Adolescents are at increased risk for establishing unhealthy patterns of alcohol use. Educating them on the importance of healthy nutrition for growth is as important as educating them about the long-term consequences of alcohol use (see Chap. 32).

Components of a Healthy Diet

Eating a variety of foods from all five pyramid food groups in moderation is a way of guaranteeing the intake of a balanced diet of proteins, carbohydrates, fats, vitamins, and minerals (Fig. 27-3).

Protein. Protein is the major component of bones, skin, hair, and muscle and is responsible for a wide variety of essential functions in the body. Because it is essential for growth, protein intake is crucial for children. Complete proteins contain all amino acids; incomplete proteins do not. Mixing these two types of protein (pasta and beans, for example) is a common dietary practice.

Carbohydrate. Carbohydrates are the main and preferred fuel of the body to supply energy, which is essential to the functioning of most body systems, the neurologic system in particular. This is why carbohydrates are so important to infants and toddlers, whose brain cells are actively growing. Starches, as a rule, supply sustained

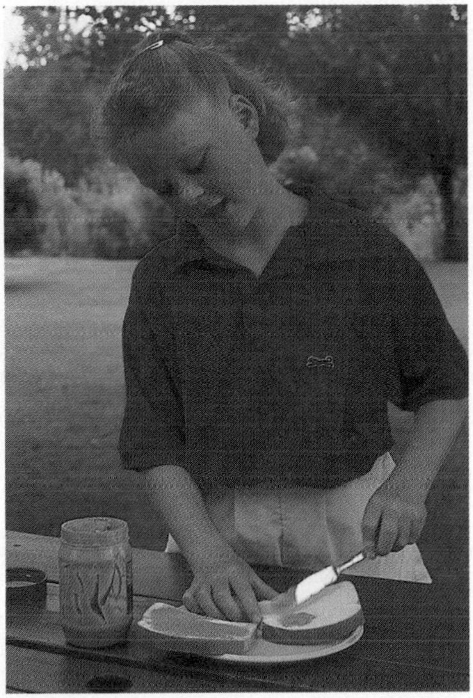

FIGURE 27.3 Good nutritional habits developed early in life provide a child with a health advantage.

energy; sugar supplies an immediate but short-term source of energy.

Fat. Dietary fat is also a source of energy to the body. It can be an immediate energy source or can be stored if not used, then released when energy is required. Some fat deposits also serve as insulating material for subcutaneous tissues; in infants, fats are necessary to assure myelination of nerve fibers.

Vitamins. Vitamins are organic compounds that are essential for specific metabolic actions in cells. They do not produce energy but are essential in order for cells to be able to do so. For children, the sources of fat-soluble vitamins (A, D, K, and E) are mainly fortified dairy products, fortified cereals, and plant oils or fish oils. Such vitamins can leave the gastrointestinal tract only by being absorbed with fat molecules. Once absorbed, they are used by the cells for growth and function or are stored in the liver and fat cells for later use. Because fat-soluble vitamins can be stored by the body, an infant or child may ingest too many of them, although overdosing usually occurs from supplements rather than dietary sources. Water-soluble vitamins (B complex and C) are not stored well in the body, so they must be taken daily to maintain effective levels in the blood. Sources and functions of essential vitamins and results of their deficiency are summarized in Table 27-2.

Minerals. Minerals are necessary to build new cells and regulate body processes (e.g., fluid and electrolyte balance, nerve transmission, muscle contraction). Minerals such as calcium are crucial to bone development and childhood growth. Therefore, they are vital to the health of a growing infant or child. Minerals are classified according to the amounts needed daily. If more than 100 mg is needed daily, a mineral is a **macronutrient,** or major mineral. If the amount needed is less than 100 mg, it is a **micronutrient,** or minor mineral. Trace minerals refer to those needed in only extremely small amounts. Sources and functions of various minerals and results of their deficiency are listed in Table 27-3.

Promoting Adequate Nutritional Intake in Vegetarian Diets

Increasing numbers of adults of child-rearing age are vegetarians; therefore, many children will eat such diets during their years of most rapid growth. Although a balanced vegetarian diet can be sufficient during childhood, careful assessment and family education are necessary to ensure that it is adequate for growth.

There are four main types of vegetarian diets:

- A lacto-ovo-vegetarian diet includes dairy products ("lacto"), eggs ("ovo"), and plants (vegetables, fruits and grains).
- An ovovegetarian diet includes eggs but excludes dairy products.
- A lactovegetarian diet includes dairy products but excludes eggs.
- A vegan diet excludes all animal products and thus consists of vegetables, fruits, and grains.

The first three types of diets are usually described as vegetarian diets. The vegan diet is most restrictive, and referral to a dietitian is recommended to ensure that children receive adequate nutrients. A fifth type of vegetarian diet is a macrobiotic diet, which falls between vegetarian and vegan diets. Its main sources of protein are grains, seeds, and nuts, but small quantities of egg, fish, and wild game can be added. Macrobiotic diets have different levels of restrictions. In the 1960s, a popular Far Eastern version consisted only of cereal and restricted fluid; it was so restricted that it caused death from starvation and nutrient inadequacy (and created a bad reputation for macrobiotic diets). This strict level is rarely seen currently; more lenient macrobiotic diets are adequate for children.

Families may select vegetarian diets for many reasons:

- Economic: vegetables and grains are less expensive than animal food.
- Ecologic: if everyone ate lower on the food chain, world hunger could be reduced.
- Medical or health-related: avoiding animal foods stops the ingestion of hormones and chemicals used in meat production and probably lowers serum cholesterol, thereby reducing the frequency of atherosclerosis and obesity; avoiding red meat may reduce the likelihood of developing intestinal cancer. Because of the association between saturated fat and bowel cancer and atherosclerosis, the number of families avoiding red meat will probably increase in the future.
- Philosophical: belief that killing animals for food is unnecessary
- Religious: many practicing Hindus and Seventh-Day Adventists are vegetarians.

TABLE 27.2 Vitamins Essential for Health

VITAMIN	SELECTED DIETARY SOURCES	FUNCTION IN BODY	RESULTS OF DEFICIENCY
*Fat-Soluble**			
A (retinol)	Liver, carrots, spinach	Important for night vision and corneal integrity and growth	Keratinization of the eye (xerophthalmia) and blindness
D	Egg yolk, margarine, salmon, fortified milk, fortified cereals	Regulates absorption of calcium and phosphorus for bone growth	Rickets (bone deformity) in growing children
E	Margarine, corn oil, peanuts (not for children <3 yrs)	An antioxidant that protects red blood cells from destruction by oxygen	In immature infants, severe anemia from destruction of red blood cells
K	Cabbage, spinach, pork. Best source: Green leafy vegetables	Aids blood clotting (synthesis of prothrombin)	Bleeding from lack of sufficient clotting action
Water-Soluble			
B complex:			
Thiamin	Wheat germ, yeast, pork	Important for use of glucose in cells	Beriberi, a disease that causes nerve paralysis
Riboflavin	Beef, chicken, liver, avocados, milk	Breaks down fatty acids and amino acids for energy	Red swollen tongue, inflamed eyes, fissures of lips
Niacin	Peanuts, rice bran, liver	Converts glucose to energy, involved in carbohydrate, protein, and fat metabolism	Pellagra (diarrhea, mental confusion, dermatitis, death)
B_6 (pyridoxine)	Liver, herring, salmon, chicken, fish, pork, eggs	Metabolizes amino acids and glucose	Neuritis, depression, nausea, vomiting
B_{12} (cobalamin)	Lamb, beef kidney, egg yolk, animal products	Blood formation; DNA and RNA synthesis; myelin formation; carbohydrate, protein, and fat metabolism	Macrocytic, megaloblastic anemia (large, nonfunctioning red blood cells)
Folic acid (folacin)	Liver, asparagus, bran	Red and white blood cell structure	Poor red cell formation
C (ascorbic acid)	Broccoli, collards, citrus fruit	Collagen structure, antioxidant	Scurvy (weakness, easy bleeding, joint pain)

*All fat-soluble vitamins can be absorbed only in the presence of lipids and can be transported only in the presence of protein.

To promote adequate nutritional intake in vegetarian diets, parents must have some training in nutrition and essential nutrients.

Protein. Lacto-ovo-vegetarian, ovovegetarian, and lactovegetarian diets provide all of the essential amino acids for growth (both eggs and dairy products provide complete proteins). Vegan diets can also supply essential amino acids, but from different sources. Complementary proteins include cereal and legume combinations such as peanut butter and wheat bread, corn and lima beans, pasta and beans, corn tortillas and beans, or chickpeas and sesame seeds. Complementary proteins do not have to be eaten at the same time, as long as varied plant proteins are consumed over the course of the day.

Calcium. Dairy products such as milk and cheese supply calcium as well as protein. When these are not eaten, calcium must be obtained from other sources, such as green leafy vegetables (e.g., broccoli) or grain products such as calcium-fortified tofu or soy flour.

Iron. Meats are the best sources of iron. With meat omitted from a diet, iron must be included from foods such as legumes, whole grains, fortified cereals, dark-green leafy vegetables, or dried fruits. Vitamin C enhances the duodenal absorption of iron found in plants, so eating fruits and vegetables rich in vitamin C (e.g., tomatoes and broccoli) aids iron absorption.

Vitamins. Vitamin B_{12} is unique among vitamins because it is present only in animal products. This includes eggs and milk. Children who totally omit animal sources need to supplement this vitamin daily. Reliable supplements of B_{12} include vitamin supplements or fortified foods such as commercial breakfast cereals, soy beverages, and some brands of nutritional yeast.

Riboflavin is normally supplied by fortified milk. However, it may be supplied by soy milk, vegetables, or brewer's yeast, all of which contain all the B vitamins except B_{12}. Thus, it is usually present in a vegetarian diet daily without additional supplementation. Good sources of riboflavin in vegan diets are whole and enriched grains and cereals, nuts, and dark-green leafy vegetables.

Vitamin D is necessary for calcium and phosphorus metabolism and is normally supplied in fortified milk. It is not present in plant foods, and therefore it must be sup-

TABLE 27.3 Minerals Essential for Health

MINERAL	SELECTED DIETARY SOURCES	FUNCTION IN BODY	RESULTS OF DEFICIENCY OR EXCESS
Macronutrients			
Calcium	Milk, hard cheese	Formation of bone and teeth; muscle contractility	Improper bone growth and maintenance shown by diseases such as rickets in children
Phosphorus	Milk, meats	Formation of bone and teeth; used in cell structure; aids use of glucose	Deficiency unlikely as long as calcium and protein needs are met
Sodium	Table salt	Regulates fluid volume and pH	Deficiency rare but excess leads to hypertension in genetically determined individuals
Chloride	Table salt	Formation of hydrochloric acid; regulates body fluid with sodium	Deficiency rare except with vomiting, which causes loss of hydrochloric acid
Potassium	Meats, dried fruits	Major cation of cells; essential for electrical conduction in muscle and therefore in heart action	Deficiency leading to muscle weakness and heart irritability; occurs in people taking diuretics, because potassium is excreted with urine
Sulfur	Milk, meat, eggs	Essential for protein formation and cell growth	Deficiency rare as long as protein intake is adequate
Magnesium	Cocoa, nuts, green leafy vegetables	Relaxation of muscles after contraction	Deficiency leads to muscle contraction
Micronutrients			
Iodine	Seafood, dairy, iodized salt	Formation of thyroxine and regulation of metabolic rate	Reduced basal metabolic rate and goiter (enlarged thyroid gland)
Iron	Meats, fish, dried fruits, nuts, fortified cereals	Formation of hemoglobin; transport of oxygen to body cells	Deficiency leads to microcytic (small) and hypochromic (pale) red blood cells (iron-deficiency anemia); excess leads to infiltration of tissue (hemosiderosis)
Copper	Nuts, raisins, legumes	Formation of collagen and nerve fiber	Anemia, neutropenia, and severe bone demineralization
Fluoride	Fluoridated water	Reduces dental caries and demineralization from bone	Dental caries
Zinc	Meat, eggs, seafood	Formation of eyes, male reproductive organs, insulin, and taste sensation	Diabetes-like symptoms due to decreased insulin production; poor taste sensation leading to poor food intake
Manganese	Nuts, grains, legumes	Formation of enzymes	Deficiency unlikely
Molybdenum	Organ meats, grains	Mobilizes iron in body	Deficiency apparently unknown
Cobalt	Many sources	Formation of red blood cells in bone marrow	Deficiency rare as long as animal food sources are ingested
Selenium	Seafood, kidney, liver	Immunoglobin formation and prevention of oxidation of cells	Deficiency unknown
Chromium	Meat, cheese, grains	Glucose metabolism	Deficiency seen only in severe malnutrition
Silicon	Many sources	Aids growth of connective tissue and bone	Retarded growth and bone deformity
Nickel	Many sources	Duplication of growth of cells	Has not been determined to be essential for health in humans
Vanadium	Many sources	Lipid metabolism	Has not been determined to be essential for health in humans
Tin	Many sources	Blood formation	Has not been determined to be essential for health in humans

plemented in a vegan or ovovegetarian diet by vitamin D drops or tablets. Exposure to sunshine is an inadequate source (Dudek, 2001).

Minerals. Zinc is present primarily in animal foods but is also present in brewer's yeast, nuts, and wheat germ. Iodine is supplied normally by seafood or iodized table salt. In a vegan or vegetarian diet, it can be supplied by seaweed and iodized table salt. Many families add a small amount of powdered kelp (a seaweed) to food two or three times a week to ensure an adequate iodine intake.

Total Calories. Plant foods have fewer total calories than meats. Therefore, one serving of nuts and one serving of legumes are recommended in place of two meat servings. All other recommended serving sizes for various caloric level patterns are the same as those presented in the food guide pyramid (see Appendix K).

WHAT IF? What if the mother of a 2-year-old tells you she cannot afford to buy meats, explaining that she can get more food for the family if she purchases mostly pasta and cereals? How would you help her plan meals that are low in cost but high in nutritional value?

THEORIES OF DEVELOPMENT

A **theory** is a systematic statement of principles that provides a framework for explaining some phenomenon. Developmental theories provide road maps for explaining human development.

A **developmental task** is a skill or a growth responsibility arising at a particular time in an individual's life, the achievement of which will provide a foundation for the accomplishment of future tasks. It is not so much chronological age as the completion of developmental tasks that defines whether a child has passed from one developmental stage of childhood to another. For example, children are not toddlers just because they are 1 year plus 1 day old; they become toddlers when they have passed through the developmental stage of infancy. For reference, however, childhood is generally divided into the periods shown in Table 27-4.

A number of theories have been proposed to describe how children grow emotionally, psychologically, and intellectually as they pass through these different periods. Sociocultural theories stress the importance of environment on growth and development. Learning theory proposes that children are blank pages that can be shaped by learning (Horowitz, 1994). Epigenetic theories stress that genes are the true basis for growth and development. Previously discounted as too simplistic, epigenetic theories are being revised based on new knowledge about genes that is available through the National Genome Project, which will map all the body's genes, and the realization that human cloning is possible (Davis et al., 2000). Still other theories deal mainly with negative aspects of childrearing that can cause mental illness in children, either immediately or later, when the child reaches adulthood (Freud). Erikson discusses the positive aspects necessary for normal growth and for development of a mentally healthy and productive adult.

TABLE 27.4 Basic Divisions of Childhood

STAGE	AGE PERIOD
Neonate	First 28 days of life
Infant	1 mo–1 yr
Toddler	1–3 yr
Preschooler	3–5 yr
School-age child	6–12 yr
Adolescent	13–20 yr

Freud's Psychoanalytic Theory

Sigmund Freud (1856–1939), an Austrian neurologist and the founder of psychoanalysis, offered the first real theory of personality development (Berger, 2001). Freud based his theory of development on his observations of mentally disturbed adults. He described adult behavior as being the result of instinctual drives that have a primarily sexual nature (**libido**) from within the person and the conflicts that develop between these instincts (represented in the individual as the id), reality (the ego), and society (the superego). He described child development as being a series of psychosexual stages in which the child's sexual gratification becomes focused on a particular body site. Freud's stages of childhood are summarized in Table 27-5.

Infant

Freud termed the infant period the "oral phase" because infants are so interested in oral stimulation or pleasure during this time (Berger, 2001). According to this theory, infants suck for enjoyment or relief of tension, as well as for nourishment.

Toddler

Freud described the toddler period as the "anal phase." Toddlers' interests widen, and their main focus is on the anal region. Elimination takes on new importance. Children find pleasure in both the retention of feces and defecation. This anal interest is part of toddlers' self-discovery, a way of exerting independence, and thus probably accounts for some of the difficulties parents may experience in toilet-training children of this age.

Preschooler

During the preschool period, children's pleasure zone appears to shift from the anal to the genital area. Freud called this period the "phallic phase." Masturbation is common during this phase. Children may also show exhibitionism, suggesting they hope this will lead to increased knowledge of the two sexes.

School-Age Child

Freud saw the school-age period as being a "latent phase," a time in which children's libido appears to be diverted into concrete thinking. He saw no developments

TABLE 27.5 Summary of Freud's and Erikson's Theories of Personality Development

	FREUD'S STAGES OF CHILDHOOD		ERIKSON'S STAGES OF CHILDHOOD	
	Psychosexual Stage	***Nursing Implications***	***Developmental Task***	***Nursing Implications***
Infant	Oral stage: Child explores the world by using mouth, especially the tongue.	Provide oral stimulation by giving pacifiers; do not discourage thumb-sucking. Breastfeeding may provide more stimulation than formula feeding because it requires the infant to expend more energy.	Developmental task is to form a sense of trust versus mistrust. Child learns to love and be loved.	Provide a primary caregiver. Provide experiences that add to security, such as soft sounds and touch. Provide visual stimulation for active child involvement.
Toddler	Anal stage: Child learns to control urination and defecation.	Help children achieve bowel and bladder control without undue emphasis on its importance. If at all possible, continue bowel and bladder training while child is hospitalized.	Developmental task is to form a sense of autonomy versus shame. Child learns to be independent and make decisions for self.	Provide opportunities for decision making, such as offering choices of clothes to wear or toys to play with. Praise for ability to make decisions rather than judging correctness of any one decision.
Preschooler	Phallic stage: Child learns sexual identity through awareness of genital area.	Accept child's sexual interest, such as fondling his or her own genitals, as a normal area of exploration. Help parents answer child's questions about birth or sexual differences.	Developmental task is to form a sense of initiative versus guilt. Child learns how to do things (basic problem solving) and that doing things is desirable.	Provide opportunities for exploring new places or activities. Allow play to include activities involving water, clay (for modeling), or finger paint.
School-age child	Latent stage: Child's personality development appears to be nonactive or dormant.	Help the child have positive experiences so his or her self-esteem continues to grow and the child prepares for the conflicts of adolescence.	Developmental task is to form a sense of industry versus inferiority. Child learns how to do things well.	Provide opportunities such as allowing child to assemble and complete a short project so that child feels rewarded for accomplishment.
Adolescent	Genital stage: Adolescent develops sexual maturity and learns to establish satisfactory relationships with the opposite sex.	Provide appropriate opportunities for the child to relate with opposite sex; allow child to verbalize feelings about new relationships.	Developmental task is to form a sense of identity versus role confusion. Adolescents learn who they are and what kind of person they will be by adjusting to a new body image, seeking emancipation from parents, choosing a vocation, and determining a value system.	Provide opportunities for the adolescent to discuss feelings about events important to him or her. Offer support and praise for decision making.

Adapted from Erikson, E. H. (1993). *Childhood and society.* New York: W.W. Norton; and Freud, S. (1962). *Three essays on the theory of sexuality.* New York: Hearst Corporation, with permission.

as obvious as those in earlier periods appearing during this time.

Adolescent

The adolescent period is termed the "genital phase." Freudian theory considers the main events of this period to be the establishment of new sexual aims and the finding of new love objects.

Criticisms of Freud's Theory

To construct his theory, Freud relied on his knowledge of people with mental illness or looked at things that people should do to avoid becoming mentally ill. This "looking at illness" rather than "looking at wellness" perspective limits the applicability of the theory as a promotion of health measure, although the behaviors he discussed are as applicable as ever.

Erikson's Theory of Psychosocial Development

Erik Erikson (1902–1996) was trained in psychoanalytic theory but later developed his own theory of psychosocial development that stresses the importance of culture and society in development of the personality (Erikson, 1993). One of the main tenets of his theory, that a person's social view of himself or herself is more important than instinctual drives in determining behavior, allows for a more optimistic view of the possibilities for human growth. Where Freud looked at ways that mental illness develops, Erikson looked at actions that lead to mental health. Erikson describes eight developmental stages covering the entire life span. At each stage, there is a conflict between two opposing forces. According to Erikson, the successful resolution of each conflict, or accomplishment of the developmental task of that stage, allows the individual to go on to the next phase of development. Table 27-5 shows Erikson's developmental stages through adolescence. Young adulthood and middle age, stages important in childbearing and childrearing, are discussed below.

Infant

According to Erikson, the developmental task for infants is learning **trust versus mistrust** (other terms might be learning confidence or learning to love). Infants whose needs are met when those needs arise, whose discomforts are quickly removed, who are cuddled, played with, and talked to, come to view the world as a safe place and people as helpful and dependable. However, when their care is inconsistent, inadequate, or rejecting, it fosters a basic mistrust: infants become fearful and suspicious of the world and of people. Like a burned child who avoids fire, emotionally burned children may shun the potential pain of further emotional involvement and carry this attitude through later stages of development. Such children can be "stuck" emotionally at this stage, although they continue to grow and develop in other ways.

Fortunately, because not all children achieve developmental tasks readily, each task need not be resolved once and for all the first time it arises. The problem of trust versus mistrust, for example, is not resolved forever during the first year of life but arises again at each successive stage of development. Children who enter school with a sense of mistrust may come to trust a teacher with whom they form a close relationship; given this second chance, children may overcome early mistrust. On the other hand, children who come through infancy with a vital sense of trust intact may still have a sense of mistrust activated at a later stage if their parents are divorced or separate under unpleasant circumstances.

Toddler

Erikson defines the development task of the toddler age as learning **autonomy versus shame** or doubt. Autonomy (self-government or independence) builds on children's new motor and mental abilities. Children take pride in new accomplishments and want to do everything independently, whether it is pulling the wrapper off a piece of candy, selecting a vitamin tablet out of the bottle, flushing the toilet, or replying, "No!" If parents recognize that toddlers need to do what they are capable of doing, at their own pace and in their own time, then children will develop a sense of being able to control their muscles and impulses. When caregivers are impatient and do everything for them, however, this enforces a sense of shame and doubt. If children are never allowed to do things they want to do, they will eventually doubt their ability to do them; they will stop trying and cannot do them. If children leave this stage with less autonomy than shame or doubt, they can be disabled in their attempts to achieve independence and may lack confidence in their abilities to achieve well into adolescence and adulthood (Fig. 27-4).

Preschooler

Erikson defines the developmental task of the preschool period as learning **initiative versus guilt.** Learning initiative is learning how to do things. Children can initiate motor activities of various sorts on their own and no longer merely respond to or imitate the actions of other children or of their parents. The same is true for language and fantasy activities.

Whether children leave this stage with a sense of initiative outweighing a sense of guilt depends largely on how parents respond to self-initiated activities. When children are given much freedom and opportunity to initiate motor play such as running, bike riding, sliding, and wrestling or are exposed to such play materials as finger paints, sand, water, and modeling clay, their sense of initiative is reinforced. Initiative is also encouraged when parents answer the child's questions (intellectual initiative) and do not inhibit fantasy or play activity. If children are made to feel that their motor activity is bad (perhaps in a small apartment or a hospital), that their questions are a nuisance, and that their play is silly and stupid, they may develop a sense of guilt over self-initiated activities that will persist in later life. Those who do not develop initiative may later have limited brainstorming and problem-

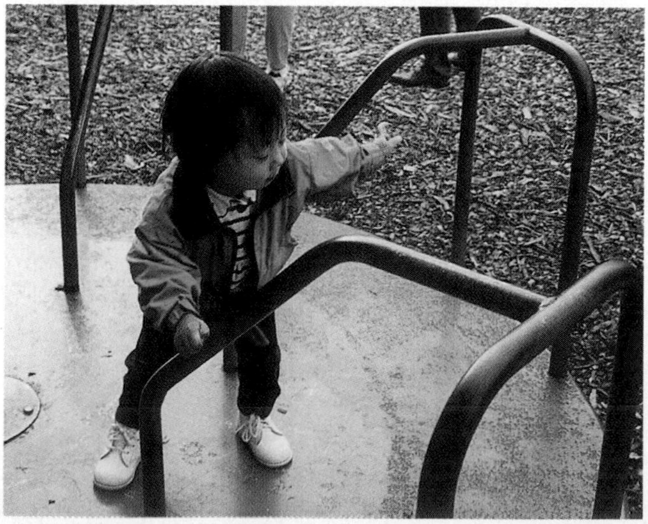

FIGURE 27.4 A toddler enjoys active, independent exploration as part of building a sense of autonomy.

solving skills; they may wait for clues or guidance from others before acting.

WHAT IF? What if a father does not allow his preschool daughter Jill to play freely because he demands an orderly household? What if she begins to show signs of poor initiative? How would you counsel this parent?

School-Age Child

Erikson states that the developmental task of the school-age period is to develop **industry versus inferiority,** or accomplishment rather than inferiority. During the preschool period, children were learning initiative—how to do something. Now, children are interested in learning how to do things well. When they are absorbed in a project, children ask, "Am I doing a good job? Am I doing this right?" When they are encouraged in their efforts to do practical tasks or make practical things and are praised and rewarded for the finished results, their sense of industry grows (Fig. 27-5). Parents who see their children's efforts at making and doing things as merely "mischief" or who don't show appreciation for their children's work may cause them to develop a sense of inferiority rather than pride and accomplishment.

During the elementary school years, a child's world grows to include the school and community environment, and success or failure in those settings can have a lasting impact. Children with an intelligence quotient of 80 or 90 (slightly below normal), for example, may have a particularly traumatic school experience, even when their sense of industry is rewarded and encouraged at home. Their learning style may be so different from the average child's that they cannot compete with children of average ability; they experience repeated failures in their efforts to learn, reinforcing their sense of inferiority. On the other hand, children whose sense of industry has been destroyed at home may have it revitalized at school through the efforts of a committed teacher. A nurse can also fulfill this role.

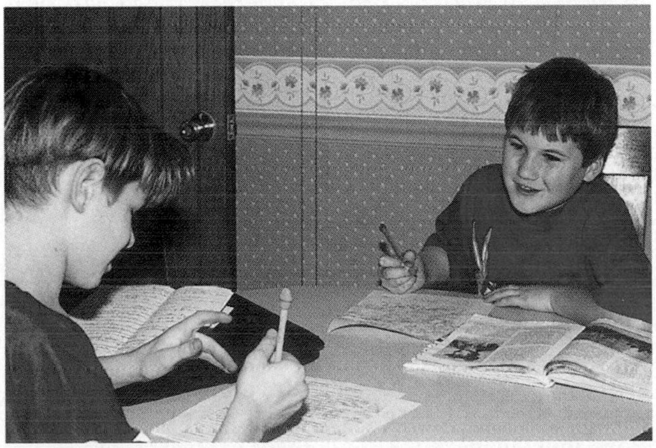

FIGURE 27.5 School-age children develop their sense of industry by working on projects that result in a feeling of accomplishment.

Adolescent

Erikson believes that the new interpersonal dimension that emerges during adolescence is a sense of **identity versus role confusion.** To achieve this, adolescents must bring together everything they have learned about themselves as a son or daughter, an athlete, a friend, a fast-food cook, a student, a scout, and so on, and integrate these different images of themselves into a whole that makes sense. If adolescents cannot do so, they are left with role confusion; that is, they are unsure what kind of person they are and are uncertain what they can do or what kind of person they can become. Some adolescents seek a negative identity: even being identified as a drug abuser or runaway may be preferable to no identity at all.

Young Adult

The developmental crisis of the young adult is achieving a sense of intimacy versus isolation. Intimacy is the ability to relate well with other people, not only with members of the opposite sex but also with one's own sex to form long-lasting friendships.

People need a strong sense of identity before they can reach out fully and offer deep friendship or love. Because there is always the risk of being rejected or hurt when offering love or friendship, individuals cannot offer it if they do not have confidence that they can cope with rejection. Women without a sense of intimacy may have more difficulty than others accepting a pregnancy and beginning to love a newborn child.

Middle Age

The developmental task of middle age is to establish a sense of generativity versus stagnation; people extend their concern from just themselves and their families to the community and the world. They may become politically active, work to solve environmental problems, or participate in far-reaching community or world-based decisions.

People with a sense of generativity are self-confident and better able to juggle their various lives (mother, soccer coach, church member, teacher, political party chairperson, gourmet cook). People without this sense become stagnated or self-absorbed. Those who have devoted themselves to only one role are more likely to find themselves at the end of middle age with a narrow perspective and lack of ability to cope with change. Women without a sense of generativity may have more difficulty than others accepting a late-in-life pregnancy and a new role of childbearing and childrearing.

Criticisms of Erikson's Theory

Erikson's main contribution to human development was the creation of stages so that development can be broken down into separate phases for study. A criticism of his theory is that life does not occur in easily divided stages, and trying to divide it that way can create superficial divisions.

✔ **CHECKPOINT QUESTIONS**

3. Freud's use of the term "libido" is often misunderstood. What did he mean by this word?
4. A toddler answers almost all questions asked him with a resounding "no." Erikson would have said the child was working through which developmental task?
5. To gain a sense of initiative, what is the best type of toy or activity for a preschooler?
6. What is the developmental task of the adolescent?

Piaget's Theory of Cognitive Development

Jean Piaget (1896–1980), a Swiss psychologist, introduced concepts of cognitive development that are similar to those of both Freud and Erikson and yet separate from each. Piaget defined four stages of cognitive development; within each stage are finer units or **schemas.** Each period is an advance over the previous one. To progress from one period to the next, the child reorganizes his or her thinking processes to bring them closer to reality (Piaget, 1952). Piaget's stages of cognitive development are summarized in Table 27-6.

Infant

Piaget refers to the infant stage as the **sensorimotor stage.** Sensorimotor intelligence is practical intelligence, because words and symbols for thinking and problem solving are not yet available at this early age. At the beginning of infancy, babies relate to the world through the senses, using only reflex behavior. As infants progress through this stage (which includes the schemas of primary and secondary circular reactions and coordination of secondary reactions, as defined in Table 27-6), they learn the basic concept that people are entities separate from objects. Piaget uses the term "primary" to refer to activities related to the child's own body and the term "circulatory reaction" to show that repetition of behavior occurs (the infant accidentally brings his or her thumb to the mouth, enjoys the sensation of sucking, and so repeats it).

The term "secondary" refers to activities that are separate from the child's body. An example of secondary schema learning is when a baby hits a mobile, notices that this makes it move, and so hits it again. During this secondary schema, infants also learn that objects in the environment—bottle, blocks, bed, or even a parent—are permanent and continue to exist even though they are out of sight or changed in some way. For example:

- Infants will search for a block hidden by a blanket, knowing the block still exists.
- Infants will know that a parent remains the same person whether dressed in a robe and slippers or pants and a T-shirt.
- Infants play peek-a-boo because they realize that the person playing with them exists behind their hands.
- Infants learn that they are a separate entity from objects. They learn where their body stops and their bed, playthings, or parent begins.

A great deal of the mouthing and handling of objects by infants and the delight of watching a caregiver appear is part of primary and secondary schemas and discovering permanence. The world begins to make sense and the developmental task of achieving trust falls into place when the concept of **permanence** has been learned (infants know their parents exist and will return to them). Gaining a concept of permanence also contributes to "eighth-month anxiety," a stage in which infants continue to cry for their parents because they know their parents still exist even when out of sight.

During the final phase of the infant year (coordination of secondary reactions), infants begin to demonstrate goal-directed behavior. After noticing that hitting a mobile makes it move, infants then reach for and hit a music box nearby, in this way actively seeking new experiences. It is important that infants have stimulating objects around for exploring so that experimenting and learning can proceed in this way.

Toddler

The toddler period is one of transition as children complete the final stages of the sensorimotor period (defined in Table 27-6 as tertiary circular reaction and invention of new means) and begin to develop some cognitive skills of the preoperative period, such as symbolic thought and egocentric thinking. In the tertiary circular reaction schema, children use trial and error to discover new characteristics of objects and events. Toddlers sitting in a high chair and dropping objects over the edge of the tray are exploring both permanence and the different actions of toys. During the schema of "invention of new means," children are able to think through actions or mentally project the solution to a problem. If given a box, children will investigate how the top of the box can be removed; if given a second box, even one that varies in shape, children can foresee how the top can be removed. Toddlers following a ball that has rolled under a coffee table no longer have to follow the ball's path to retrieve it but can project where it rolled and walk around the coffee table to find it again.

During the period of **preoperational thought,** children relearn on a conceptual level some of the lessons they mastered as infants at the sensorimotor level, before having language. Now, children are able to use symbols to represent objects. However, they cannot view one object as necessarily being different from another. On a walk through a department store, for example, children do not know whether they are seeing a succession of toys or if the same ones keep reappearing. They draw conclusions only from obvious facts they see: Daddy is shaving; therefore he must be going to work, because he went to work after he shaved yesterday. This type of faulty reasoning (prelogical reasoning) will lead children to wrong conclusions and will make their judgment faulty as well.

How children think has many implications for nursing. If you made John's bed yesterday and then he went to surgery, he may cry at the sight of you approaching with

TABLE 27.6 Piaget's Stages of Cognitive Development

STAGE OF DEVELOPMENT	AGE SPAN	NURSING IMPLICATIONS
Sensorimotor		
Neonatal reflex	1 mo	Stimuli are assimilated into beginning mental images. Behavior entirely reflexive.
Primary circular reaction	1–4 mo	Hand–mouth and ear–eye coordination develop. Infant spends much time looking at objects and separating self from them. Beginning intention of behavior is present (the infant brings thumb to mouth for a purpose: to suck it). Enjoyable activity for this period: a rattle or tape of parent's voice.
Secondary circular reaction	4–8 mo	Infant learns to initiate, recognize, and repeat pleasurable experiences from environment. Memory traces are present; infant anticipates familiar events (a parent coming near him will pick him up). Good toy for this period: mirror; good game: peek-a-boo.
Coordination of secondary reactions	8–12 mo	Infant can plan activities to attain specific goals. Perceives that others can cause activity and that activities of own body are separate from activity of objects. Can search for and retrieve toy that disappears from view. Recognizes shapes and sizes of familiar objects. Because of increased sense of separateness, infant experiences separation anxiety when primary caregiver leaves. Good toy for this period: nesting toys (i.e., colored boxes).
Tertiary circular reaction	12–18 mo	Child is able to experiment to discover new properties of objects and events. Capable of space perception and time perception as well as permanence. Objects outside self are understood as causes of actions. Good game for this period: throw and retrieve.
Invention of new means through mental combinations	18–24 mo	Transitional phase to the preoperational thought period. Uses memory and imitation to act. Can solve basic problems, foresee maneuvers that will succeed or fail. Good toys for this period: those with several uses, such as blocks, colored plastic rings.
Preoperational Thought	2–7 yr	Thought becomes more symbolic; can arrive at answers mentally instead of through physical attempt. Comprehends simple abstractions but thinking is basically concrete and literal. Child is egocentric (unable to see the viewpoint of another). Displays static thinking (inability to remember what he or she started to talk about so that at the end of a sentence the child is talking about another topic). Concept of time is now, and concept of distance is only as far as he or she can see. Centering or focusing on a single aspect of an object causes distorted reasoning. No awareness of reversibility (for every action there is an opposite action) is present. Unable to state cause–effect relationships, categories, or abstractions. Good toy for this period: items that require imagination, such as modeling clay.
Concrete Operational Thought	7–12 yr	Concrete operations includes systematic reasoning. Uses memory to learn broad concepts (fruit) and subgroups of concepts (apples, oranges). Classifications involve sorting objects according to attributes such as color; seriation, in which objects are ordered according to increasing or decreasing measures such as weight; multiplication, in which objects are simultaneously classified and seriated using weight. Child is aware of reversibility, an opposite operation or continuation of reasoning back to a starting point (follows a route through a maze and then reverses steps). Understands conservation, sees constancy despite transformation (mass or quantity remains the same even if it changes shape or position). Good activity for this period: collecting and classifying natural objects such as native plants, sea shells, etc. Expose child to other viewpoints by asking questions such as, "How do you think you'd feel if you were a nurse and had to tell a boy to stay in bed?"
Formal Operational Thought	12 yr	Can solve hypothetical problems with scientific reasoning; understands causality and can deal with the past, present, and future. Adult or mature thought. Good activity for this period: "talk time" to sort through attitudes and opinions.

From Piaget, J. (1961). *The growth of logical thinking from childhood to adolescence.* New York: Basic Books, with permission.

clean sheets today, thinking he will have to go to surgery again.

Preschooler

Piaget sees preschool children as moving on to a substage of preoperational thought termed **intuitive thought.** During this time, children tend to look at an object and see only one of its characteristics (referred to as **centering**). For example, they see that a banana is yellow but do not notice that it is also long. Centering is noticeable when children are learning about medicine (they observe that it tastes bitter, but cannot understand that it is also good for them).

Centering contributes to the preschooler's lack of **conservation** (the ability to discern truth, even though physical properties change) or **reversibility** (ability to retrace steps). For example, if preschoolers see beads being poured from one glass into another glass that is taller and thinner, they will only notice one changing characteristic. They might say that there are now more beads in the second glass (because the level has risen), or that there are fewer beads (because the second glass is narrower), even when told that no beads have been added or removed. When the beads are poured back into the first glass, they still will not understand that the number of beads is unchanged. This immature perception leads children, as it did during the toddler period, to make faulty conclusions. It takes more years of development for children to learn that when thought processes (i.e., they know the number of beads did not change) and perceptions conflict, thought processes are more trustworthy.

Preschool thinking is also influenced by **role fantasy,** or how children would like something to turn out. Children use **assimilation** (taking in information and changing it to fit their existing ideas). For example, because a child wants to go outside and play, he or she says that the outside wants him or her to come and play. Children believe that wishes are as real as facts, that dreams are as real as daytime happenings. They perceive animals and even inanimate objects as being capable of thought and feeling (saying that the dog took the doll because the dog was feeling sad). This is often called magical thinking. Later, children learn **accommodation** (i.e., they change their ideas to fit reality rather than the reverse). **Egocentrism,** or perceiving that one's thoughts and needs are better or more important than those of others, is also strong during this period. Preschoolers cannot believe that not everyone knows facts they know; if asked, "What is your name?" they may reply, "Don't you know my name?" Children define objects mainly in relation to themselves, so that a spoon is "what I eat with," not just a curved metal object.

School-Age Child

Piaget viewed school age as a period during which **concrete operational thought** begins. School-age children can discover concrete solutions to everyday problems and recognize cause-and-effect relationships. By understanding that beads do not change in number just because they are poured from one glass to another, children have grasped the concept of conservation. Conservation of numbers is learned as early as age 7 years, conservation of quantity at age 7 or 8 years, conservation of weight at age 9 years, and conservation of volume at age 11 years. Reasoning during school age tends to be inductive, proceeding from specific to general. Thus, school-age children can reason that a toy they are holding is broken, that the toy is made of plastic, and that all plastic toys break easily.

Adolescent

Piaget sees adolescence as the time when cognition achieves its final form, that of **formal operational thought.** When this stage is reached, adolescents are capable of thinking in terms of possibility—what could be (**abstract thought**)—rather than being limited to thinking about what already is (concrete thought). This makes it possible for adolescents to use scientific reasoning.

Criticisms of Piaget's Theory

Piaget has been criticized because he used only a small sample of subjects (his own children) to develop his theory. Because children today begin activities to learn reading much earlier than they did at the time the theory was devised, the age groups and "norms" may no longer be relevant. Learning computer use at an early age may change both the rate and type of cognitive development.

Kohlberg's Theory of Moral Development

Lawrence Kohlberg (1927–1987), a psychologist, studied the reasoning ability of boys and, based on Piaget's development stages, developed a theory on moral reasoning, or the way that children gain knowledge of right and wrong.

Children pass through stages of moral development as well as cognitive and psychosocial development. These stages as described by Kohlberg (1984) are summarized in Table 27-7. Recognizing these stages can help identify how a child may feel about an illness (e.g., whether the child thinks it is fair that he is ill). Recognizing moral reasoning also helps determine whether children can be depended on to carry out self-care activities such as administering their own medicine (i.e., whether the child has internalized standards of conduct so he or she does not "cheat" when away from external control). Moral stages closely approximate cognitive stages of development, because a child must be able to think abstractly (be able to conceptualize an idea without a concrete picture) before being able to understand how rules apply, even when no one is there to enforce them.

Infant

The infant period is a **prereligious stage.** Infants have little concept of any motivating force beyond that of their parents. Infants learn that when they do certain actions, parents give affection and approval; for other actions, parents scold and label the behavior as "bad." To support this stage of development, it is important for caregivers to praise the infant for doing what he or she is asked to do. Caregivers should also know that the average infant is trying hard to please; if an infant falls short of doing this, it

TABLE 27.7 Kohlberg's Stages of Moral Development

AGE (YEAR)	STAGE	DESCRIPTION	NURSING IMPLICATIONS
Preconventional (Level I)			
2–3	1	Punishment/obedience orientation ("heteronomous morality"). Child does right because a parent tells him or her to and to avoid punishment.	Child needs help to determine what are right actions. Give clear instructions to avoid confusion.
4–7	2	Individualism. Instrumental purpose and exchange. Carries out actions to satisfy own needs rather than society's. Will do something for another if that person does something for the child.	Child is unable to recognize that like situations require like actions. Unable to take responsibility for self-care, because meeting own needs interferes with this.
Conventional (Level II)			
7–10	3	Orientation to interpersonal relations of mutuality. Child follows rules because of a need to be a "good" person in own eyes and eyes of others.	Child enjoys helping others because this is "nice" behavior. Allow child to help with bed making and other like activities. Praise for desired behavior such as sharing.
10–12	4	Maintenance of social order, fixed rules and authority. Child finds following rules satisfying. Follows rules of authority figures as well as parents in an effort to keep the "system" working.	Child often asks what are the rules and is something "right." May have difficulty modifying a procedure because one method may not be "right." Follows self-care measures only if someone is there to enforce them.
Postconventional (Level III)			
Older than 12	5	Social contract, utilitarian law-making perspectives. Follows standards of society for the good of all people.	An adolescent can be responsible for self-care because he or she views this as a standard of adult behavior.
	6	Universal ethical principle orientation. Follows internalized standards of conduct.	Many adults do not reach this level of moral development.

From Kohlberg, L. (1984). *The psychology of moral development.* New York: Harper & Row, with permission.

is probably due to immature development rather than any effort to displease.

The development of trust is important in moral development because infants who have developed a sound sense of trust can better develop a spiritual orientation in future years and thus be bound by a moral conscience (they can trust in a spiritual being as well as humans around them).

Toddler

Toddlers begin to formulate a sense of right and wrong, but their reason for doing right is centered most strongly in "mother or father says so" rather than in any spiritual or societal motivation. Kohlberg refers to this as a punishment obedience orientation (the child is good because a parent says the child must be, not because it is "right" to be good).

Toddlers may not obey requests from people other than their parents because they do not view their authority as being at the same level as their parents' authority. While providing nursing care, it might be necessary to ask a parent to reinforce instructions to be certain the toddler will follow them.

Preschooler

Preschoolers tend to do good out of self-interest rather than out of true intent to do good or because of a strong spiritual motivation. When asked why it is wrong to steal from a neighbor, for example, the preschooler will answer, "Because my mother says it's wrong." Children at this age imitate what they see, so if they see less-than-perfect role models, they may copy those wrong actions and assume those actions are correct. Preschoolers have great difficulty knowing what rules apply to new situations because they cannot judge whether a previously learned principle of right or wrong can be applied to this new situation. Because of egocentrism, a preschooler will do things for others only in return for things done for him or her. This means it may be necessary to remind the child of actions taken on his or her behalf or trade off actions (e.g., "Lie still now for me while I change your dressing and I'll read you a story when I'm through").

School-Age Child

School-age children enter a stage of moral development termed **conventional development,** the level at which many adults function. Young school-age children adhere to a phase of development termed the "nice girl, nice boy" stage. Children engage in actions that are "nice" or "fair" rather than necessarily right. Sharing, for example, is "nice." Taking turns is "fair." Stealing is not. Young school-age children may lie about their actions to disguise that they have been involved in an action that is not "nice."

When asked why it is wrong to steal from a neighbor, the school-age child most often answers, "Because it's not nice or fair" because they have learned about community resources, or "The police will arrest you." School-age children may have difficulty following self-care measures reliably when out of a nurse's or parent's sight because they feel it is necessary to obey rules only when the rules can be clearly enforced.

Adolescent

As adolescents become capable of abstract thought, they become capable of internalizing standards of conduct (they do what they think is right regardless of whether they have social rules or anyone is watching). This is termed **postconventional development** and is the mature form of moral reasoning. In this stage, if asked why it is wrong to steal from a neighbor, the adolescent will answer, "Because it deprives the neighbor of possessions he or she has earned." Adolescents can carry out self-care measures even when someone else is not present because they can understand not only the importance of the measures to themselves but also the principle that certain things should be done simply because they are right. Many adolescents do not enter this phase of development, however, and as adults they continue to act like school-age children, doing right things only when obvious authority or set rules are present.

Criticisms of Kohlberg's Theory

Kohlberg's theory is being challenged as being male-oriented because his original research was conducted entirely with boys. Carol Gilligan (1982) has suggested that girls do not score well on Kohlberg's scale because, being more concerned with relationships than boys are, they make moral decisions based on individual circumstances.

✔ CHECKPOINT QUESTIONS

7. If a preschool child tells you that his broken leg wants to get better, what type of thinking is he using?
8. Suppose the same child tells you that he knows all nurses wear white and because you are not wearing white, you cannot be a nurse. What type of thought process is he using?
9. Why is the stage of moral reasoning of the school-age child often termed the "nice" or "fair" stage?
10. What is a common criticism of Kohlberg's theory of moral development?

KEY POINTS

Knowledge of growth and development is important in health promotion and illness prevention because it lays the basis for assessment and anticipatory guidance.

Genetic factors that influence growth and development are gender, race and nationality, intelligence, and health.

Environmental influences include quality of nutrition, socioeconomic level, parent–child relationship, ordinal position in the family, and environmental health.

To meet growth and development needs, children need to follow basic guidelines for a healthy diet, such as eating a variety of foods; maintaining ideal weight; avoiding too much saturated fat and cholesterol; eating foods with adequate starch and fiber; and avoiding too much sugar, the same as adults.

Temperament is a child's characteristic manner of thinking, behaving, or reacting. Helping parents understand the effect of temperament is a nursing role.

Common theories of development are Freud's psychoanalytic theory and Erikson's theory of psychosocial development. Both of these theories describe specific tasks that children must complete at each stage of development in order to become a well-adapted adult.

Piaget's theory of cognitive development describes ways that children learn. Kohlberg advanced a theory of moral development, or how children use moral reasoning to solve problems they face.

Although growth and development occur in known patterns, their rate varies from child to child. Caution parents not to be concerned because two siblings are different as long as they both fit within usual parameters.

CRITICAL THINKING EXERCISES

1. John is the 4-year-old boy you met at the beginning of the chapter. He had lived in many foster homes before he was recently adopted. His parents state that they find him cold and unloving. What developmental task was John unable to complete because of these frequent moves at such a young age? What are actions his new parents could take to try to strengthen this developmental task at this point?
2. A mother describes her two children as "totally different." One is shy and quiet and agreeable, and one is aggressive and persistent. What characteristic is she describing? Which child does she probably view as easier to care for? What anticipatory guidance could you give her to help her better understand these differences in her children?
3. The parents of a 2-year-old say they want their child to achieve well in life. They ask you what specific steps they should take to foster high achievement in their child. What advice would you give them?

4. Children who are hospitalized for long periods may fall behind in development. What specific measures could you take to promote developmental growth and encourage a sense of autonomy in a hospitalized 2-year-old? To promote a sense of industry in a hospitalized 10-year-old?
5. Examine the National Health Goals related to growth and development of children. Most government-sponsored money for nursing research is allotted based on these goals. What would be a possible research topic to explore pertinent to these goals that would be fundable and would advance evidence-based practice?

REFERENCES

Alaimo, K., et al. (2001). Low family income and food insufficiency in relation to overweight in U.S. children: Is there a paradox? *Archives of Pediatrics & Adolescent Medicine, 155*(10), 1161–1167.

Berger, K. S. (2001). *The developing person through the life span.* New York: Worth Publishers.

Carey, W. B., & McDevitt, S. C. (1994). *Prevention and early intervention: Individual differences as risk factors for the mental health of children.* New York: Brunner/Mazel.

Chess, S., & Thomas, A. (1995). *Temperament in clinical practice.* New York: Guilford Publications.

Davis, J., Krasnewich, D., & Puck, J. M. (2000). Genetic testing and screening in pediatric populations. *Nursing Clinics of North America, 35*(3), 643–651.

Department of Health and Human Services. (2000). *Healthy people 2010.* Washington, D.C.: DHHS.

Dudek, S. G. (2001). *Nutrition handbook for nursing practice.* Philadelphia: Lippincott Williams & Wilkins.

Erickson, S. J., et al. (2000). Are overweight children unhappy? Body mass index, depressive symptoms, and overweight concerns in elementary school children. *Archives of Pediatrics & Adolescent Medicine, 154*(9), 931–935.

Erikson, E. H. (1993). *Childhood and society.* New York: W.W. Norton.

Gilligan, C. (1982). *In a different voice: Psychological theory and women's development.* Cambridge, Mass.: Harvard University Press.

Green, M. & Solnit, A. (1964). Reactions to the threatened loss of a child: A vulnerable child syndrome. *Pediatrics, 34*(8), 58–62.

Horowitz, F. D. (1994). John B. Watson's legacy: learning and environment. In D. Ross, et al. (eds.). *A century of developmental psychology.* Washington, D.C.: American Psychological Association.

Kohlberg, L. (1984). *The psychology of moral development.* New York: Harper & Row.

Neighbors, B. D., et al. (2000). Difficult temperament, parental relationships and adolescent alcohol use disorder symptoms. *Journal of Child & Adolescent Substance Abuse, 10*(1), 69–86.

Piaget, J. (1952). *The origins of intelligence in children.* New York: International Universities Press.

Thomas, D. O. (2002). Special considerations for pediatric triage in the emergency department. *Nursing Clinics of North America, 37*(1), 145–159.

von Kries, R., et al. (2000). Does breast-feeding protect against childhood obesity? *Advances in Experimental Medicine & Biology, 478*(1), 29–39.

SUGGESTED READINGS

Balling, K., & McCubbin, M. (2001). Hospitalized children with chronic illness: Parental caregiving needs and valuing parental expertise. *Journal of Pediatric Nursing, 16*(2), 110–119.

Beilin, H., & Fireman, G. (1999). The foundation of Piaget's theories: Mental and physical action. *Advances in Child Development & Behavior, 27*(3), 221–246.

Blackwell, P. L. (2000). The influence of touch on child development: Implications for intervention. *Infants & Young Children, 13*(1), 25–39.

Butler, G. A., & Thompson, L. S. (2000). Building skills for child advocacy. *Journal of Pediatric Nursing, 15*(5), 323–325.

Hunter, A. J. (2001). A cross-cultural comparison of resilience in adolescents. *Journal of Pediatric Nursing, 16*(3), 172–179.

Morris, B. H., et al. (2002). Patterns of physical and neurologic development in preterm children. *Journal of Perinatology, 22*(1), 31–36.

Munsen, R. B. (2001). Children and puberty. *Journal of Pediatric Nursing, 16*(1), 66–67.

Nesdale, D., & Flesser, D. (2001). Social identity and the development of children's group attitudes. *Child Development, 72*(2), 506–517.

Qayumi, S. (2001). Piaget and his role in problem-based learning. *Journal of Investigative Surgery, 14*(2), 63–65.

Rushforth, H. (1999). Practitioner review: Communicating with hospitalized children: Review and application of research pertaining to children's understanding of health and illness. *Journal of Child Psychology & Psychiatry & Allied Disciplines, 40*(5), 683–691.

Saltos, E. (1999). Adapting the food guide pyramid for children: Defining the target audience. *Family Economics and Nutrition Review, 12*(3&4), 3–17.

Ziegert, D. I., et al. (2001). Longitudinal study of young children's responses to challenging achievement situations. *Child Development, 72*(2), 609–624.

28

CHAPTER

The Family With an Infant

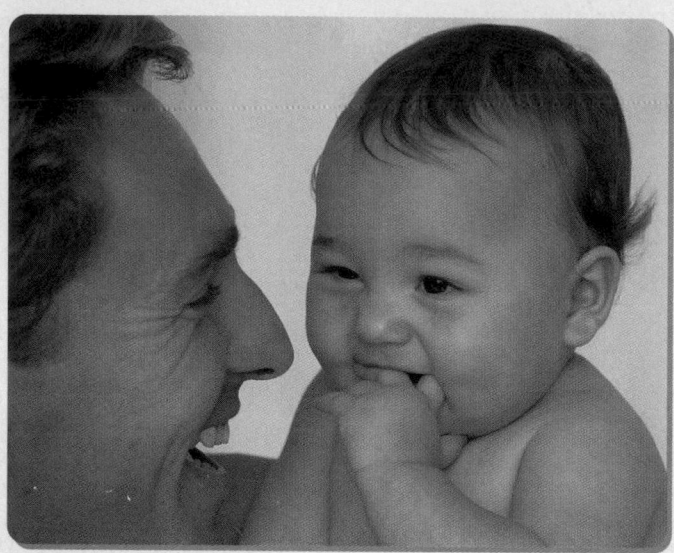

Key Terms

- baby-bottle syndrome
- binocular vision
- coordination of secondary schema
- deciduous teeth
- eighth-month anxiety
- extrusion reflex
- fine motor development
- gross motor development
- hand regard
- Landau reflex
- natal teeth
- neck-righting reflex
- neonatal teeth
- object permanence
- parachute reaction
- pincer grasp
- prehensile ability
- primary circular reaction
- seborrhea
- secondary circular reaction
- social smile
- thumb opposition
- ventral suspension

Objectives

After mastering the contents of this chapter, you should be able to:

1. Describe normal infant growth and development and associated parental concerns.
2. Assess an infant for normal growth and development milestones.
3. Formulate nursing diagnoses related to infant growth and development and associated parental concerns.
4. Identify outcomes to promote optimal infant growth and development and health.
5. Plan nursing care to meet the infant's growth and development needs.
6. Implement nursing care related to normal growth and development of the infant.
7. Evaluate outcomes for achievement of optimal growth and development and effectiveness of care.
8. Identify National Health Goals related to infant growth and development that nurses can be instrumental in helping the nation achieve.
9. Identify areas related to nursing care of the infant that could benefit from additional nursing research or application of evidenced-based practice.
10. Use critical thinking to analyze methods of care for the infant to be certain care is family-centered.
11. Integrate knowledge of infant growth and development with nursing process to achieve quality maternal and child health nursing care.

You meet Mrs. Simpson at a pediatric clinic when she brings in her 2-month-old son, Bryan. She looks tired. She tells you that she feels exhausted because her baby is "awake all night, crying constantly." She stopped breastfeeding and changed him to formula to see if that would help, but it didn't. She tells you his bowel movements are normal. When you weigh Bryan, you find that he is gaining weight well. When you talk to him, he demonstrates a social smile. What condition common to early infancy might Mrs. Simpson be describing? Is this normal infant behavior? What factors might be playing a role? What suggestions could you make to help her enjoy caring for Bryan more?

Previous chapters described the newborn and the capabilities with which children are born. This chapter adds information about the dramatic changes, both physical and psychosocial, that occur during the first year. This is important information because it builds a base for care and health teaching for the age group.

After you've studied the chapter, answer the Critical Thinking Exercises at the end of the chapter and then access the on-line study activities (http://connection.lww.com) *to further sharpen your skills and test your knowledge.*

Traditionally, infancy is designated as the period of time from 1 month to 1 year of age. This year is one of rapid growth and development, with the infant tripling his or her birthweight and increasing length by 50%. In these important months, the infant undergoes such rapid development that parents sometimes believe their baby looks different and demonstrates new abilities each day. During this period, the baby's senses sharpen and, with the process of attachment to primary caregivers, he or she forms a first social relationship. Because of the growth and learning potential, this first year is a crucial one. Without proper nutrition, the baby will not grow and physically thrive, and without the proper stimulation and nurturing care by consistent caregivers, the infant may not develop a healthy interest in life or a feeling of security essential for future development (Goldson & Hagerman, 2001).

As a result, infant health promotion has been the subject of much concern. National Health Goals addressing this important developmental stage are highlighted in the Focus on National Health Goals box.

Infants are usually seen at health care facilities for health maintenance at least six times during the first year. Although infant health care visits are scheduled less frequently than formerly, a standard schedule is for 2-week, 2-month, 4-month, 6-month, and 12-month visits (AAP, 2001). These visits are as important for the parents as they are for the infant because they provide an opportunity for parents to ask questions about their child's growth pattern and developmental progress. They also provide opportunities for health care providers to assess for potential problems. Anticipatory guidance offered at these visits can help parents prepare for the rapid changes that mark the first year of life. When appropriate, encouraging parents to join clubs or networking groups helps to increase their knowledge base and confidence level.

FOCUS ON NATIONAL HEALTH GOALS

A number of National Health Goals focus on promotion of health during the infant year. These are:

- Increase the proportion of mothers who breastfeed until 1 year of age from 16% to 25%.
- Increase to at least 75% the proportion of parents and caregivers who use feeding practices that prevent baby bottle tooth decay. Special target population: parents and caregivers with less than high school educations.
- Reduce fetal and infant deaths from 7.5/1,000 to 4.5/1,000.
- Increase the use of child restraints from 92% to 100%.
- Increase the percentage of healthy full-term infants who are put down to sleep on their backs from 35% to 70%.
- Increase to at least 90% the proportion of infants who receive all recommended immunizations for the infant at appropriate intervals (DHHS, 2000).

Nurses can be instrumental in helping the nation achieve these goals by educating parents about the importance of not putting an infant to bed with a bottle of milk or juice, the use of infant car seats, and continuing breastfeeding for a full year. A number of areas related to these topics that could benefit from additional nursing research include: effective ways that mothers can comfort an infant in a car seat without removing the infant from the seat; characteristics of programs that are successful in promoting breastfeeding; and effective ways to teach about immunizations so parents secure those required for infants.

Table 28-1 details the usual procedures at infant health maintenance visits. First-year immunizations (see Focus on Evidence-Based Practice) and any risks associated with these are discussed in Chapter 33 and listed in Appendix J.

NURSING PROCESS OVERVIEW

For Healthy Development of the Infant

Assessment

Nursing assessment of the infant should begin by interviewing the primary caregiver. Important areas to discuss include nutrition, growth patterns, and development. The infant's height, weight, and head circumference are important indicators of growth and should be measured and plotted on standard growth charts. These charts represent average growth and are used to determine if the baby's growth is falling within the same relative percentile at each checkup.

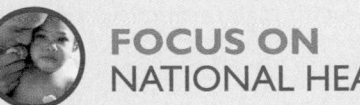

TABLE 28.1 Health Maintenance Schedule, Infant Period

AREA OF FOCUS	METHODS	FREQUENCY
Assessment		
Developmental milestones	History, observation	Every visit
	Denver Developmental Screening Test (DDST II)	At 3 months and 1 year
Growth milestones	Height, weight, head circumference plotted on standard growth chart; physical examination	Every visit
Nutritional adequacy	History, observation	Every visit
Parent/child relationship	History, observation	Every visit
Sleep positioning counseling	Discussion of placing infants on back to sleep	Every visit up to 9 months
Injury and violence counseling	Discussion of safety measures to take with infants	Every visit
Vision and hearing screening	Observation and history	Every visit
Dental health	History, physical examination	Every visit after teeth erupt
Anemia	Hematocrit, hemoglobin	9- or 12-month visit
Lead screening	Finger stick	9- or 12-month visit
Tuberculosis screening	PPD test	12-month visit
Immunizations	Review of history and health record; teaching caregiver about any risks and side effects; administering immunization in accordance with health care agency policies	
Diphtheria, pertussis, tetanus (DPT)		2-, 4-, & 6-month visits
Haemophilus influenzae type B (HiB)		2-, 4-, & 6-month visits
Inactivated poliomyelitis		2-, 4-, & 6-month visits
Pneumococcal		2, 4, & 6-month visits
Hepatitis B		Birth, 2-month, & 12-month visits

For more information about typical assessment findings, see Assessing the Average Infant.

Physical assessment of the infant must be done quickly yet thoroughly because the baby can tire or become hungry, making it difficult to judge his or her overall behavior and temperament. The primary caregiver should be present to make the child comfortable. Using a calm, unhurried approach helps the infant feel safe enough to accept your interventions.

Nursing Diagnosis

Much of your assessment of the infant and family will focus on basic needs such as sleep, nutrition, and activity and the parents' adjustment to their new role. Possible nursing diagnoses might include:

- Ineffective breast-feeding related to maternal fatigue
- Deficient knowledge related to normal infant growth and development
- Imbalanced nutrition, less than body requirements, related to difficulty sucking
- Health-seeking behaviors related to adjusting to parenthood
- Delayed growth and development related to lack of stimulating environment
- Risk for impaired parenting related to long hospitalization of infant
- Readiness for enhanced family coping related to increased financial support
- Disturbed sleep pattern (maternal) related to baby's need to nurse every 2 hours
- Social isolation (maternal) related to stress of caring for infant and lack of adequate social support
- Ineffective role performance related to new responsibilities within the family

Outcome Identification and Planning

Outcomes established for infant care must be realistic. Parents of infants, especially first-time parents, must do a lot of adjusting, and this takes time. Try to suggest activities that can be easily incorporated into the family's lifestyle. If your assessment data indicate that a child needs more exposure to language and you know that both parents work during the day, for example, you might suggest that the parents ask their child's caretaker to increase vocalization around the child. Encourage parents to spend a certain amount of time each evening reading or reciting nursery rhymes to their baby. Doing so helps infants learn language.

Implementation

One of the most important interventions of the infant period is teaching new parents about normal growth and development milestones, such as the age range for rolling over or reaching for objects. Whenever possible, this information should be anticipatory so parents are prepared for changes and developments before they occur.

FOCUS ON EVIDENCE-BASED PRACTICE

What Factors Influence Whether Infants Receive Immunizations or Not?

To answer this question, researchers interviewed 369 mother/infant pairs selected from District of Columbia hospitals at 3 to 7 months and again at 7 to 12 months after the baby's birth. Results of interviews showed that at 3 months of age, 75% of infants were current with immunizations. By 7 months, however, this percentage had fallen to 41%. Factors that were associated with parents obtaining immunizations were enrollment in a Women, Infants and Children (WIC) nutrition program during pregnancy, intention to breastfeed, and presence of the infant's grandmother in the household. Factors that were associated with babies being fully immunized at 7 months included lower birth order, maternal employment, and low perceived barriers to immunization.

This is an important study for nurses because nurses are the health care professionals who frequently remind mothers of the importance of immunizations, help enroll women in WIC programs, and monitor whether infants obtain immunizations. Particularly important in this study is the finding that employed women sought more immunizations for their infants than those who were unemployed. It implies that lack of time to secure immunizations is not a factor in failure to obtain immunizations for infants.

Brenner, R. A., et al. (2001). Prevalence and predictors of immunization among inner-city infants. *Pediatrics, 108*(3), 661-670.

Outcome Evaluation

Outcomes established for care should be evaluated at each visit to detect changes in growth and development. Help parents understand that the total developmental profile, not a single element, provides the most important description of their child. Variation is the rule rather than the exception, so a 2-month variation from the average during the infant year is considered normal. Many 4-month-old infants, for example, have mastered most of the 4-month skills and some of the 5-month skills, yet they may still be at a 3-month level on one or two other criteria.

Examples suggesting achievement of outcomes may include the following:

- Mother states she feels fatigued but able to cope with sleep disturbance from night waking.
- Parents state five actions they are taking daily to encourage bonding.
- Father states both he and spouse are adjusting to new roles as parents.
- Parents verbalize appropriate techniques to stimulate infant.
- Infant demonstrates age-appropriate growth and development.
- Infant exhibits weight, height, and head and chest circumference within acceptable norms.

GROWTH AND DEVELOPMENT OF THE INFANT

Infants rapidly grow both in size and in their ability to perform tasks.

Physical Growth

The physiologic changes that occur in the infant year reflect the increasing maturity and growth of body organs.

Weight

As a rule, most infants double their birthweight at 4 to 6 months and triple it by 1 year. During the first 6 months, infants typically average a weight gain of 2 lb per month. During the second 6 months, weight gain is approximately 1 lb per month. The average 1-year-old boy weighs 10 kg (22 lb); the average girl weighs 9.5 kg (21 lb). The infant's weight, however, is relevant only when plotted on a standard growth chart and compared to that child's own growth curve (see Appendix E).

Height

The infant increases in height during the first year by 50%, or grows from the average birth length of 20 in to about 30 in (50.8 cm to 76.2 cm). Height, like weight, is best assessed if it is plotted on a standard growth chart. Infant growth is most apparent in the trunk during the early months. During the second half of the first year, it becomes more apparent as lengthening of the legs. At the end of the first year, the child's legs may still appear disproportionately short, however, and perhaps bowed. For accuracy, an infant should be measured lying supine on a measuring board (see Nursing Procedure 33-1).

Head Circumference

Head circumference increases rapidly during the infant period, reflecting rapid brain growth. By the end of the first year, the brain has already reached two thirds of its adult size.

Some infants' heads appear asymmetric until the second half of the first year. This may occur from always being placed in one sleeping position, causing the skull bones to flatten on that side. Suggest to the parents that they place the infant on the back to sleep and prone when playing. This head distortion gradually corrects itself as the child sleeps less and spends more time with the head in an erect position. Persistence of asymmetry may suggest that the infant is not receiving enough stimulation or is spending the majority of time lying in bed.

Body Proportion

Body proportion changes during the first year from that of a newborn to a more typical infant appearance. The mandible becomes more prominent as bone grows. By

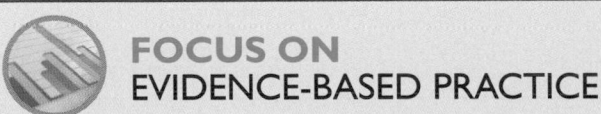

ASSESSING the Average Infant

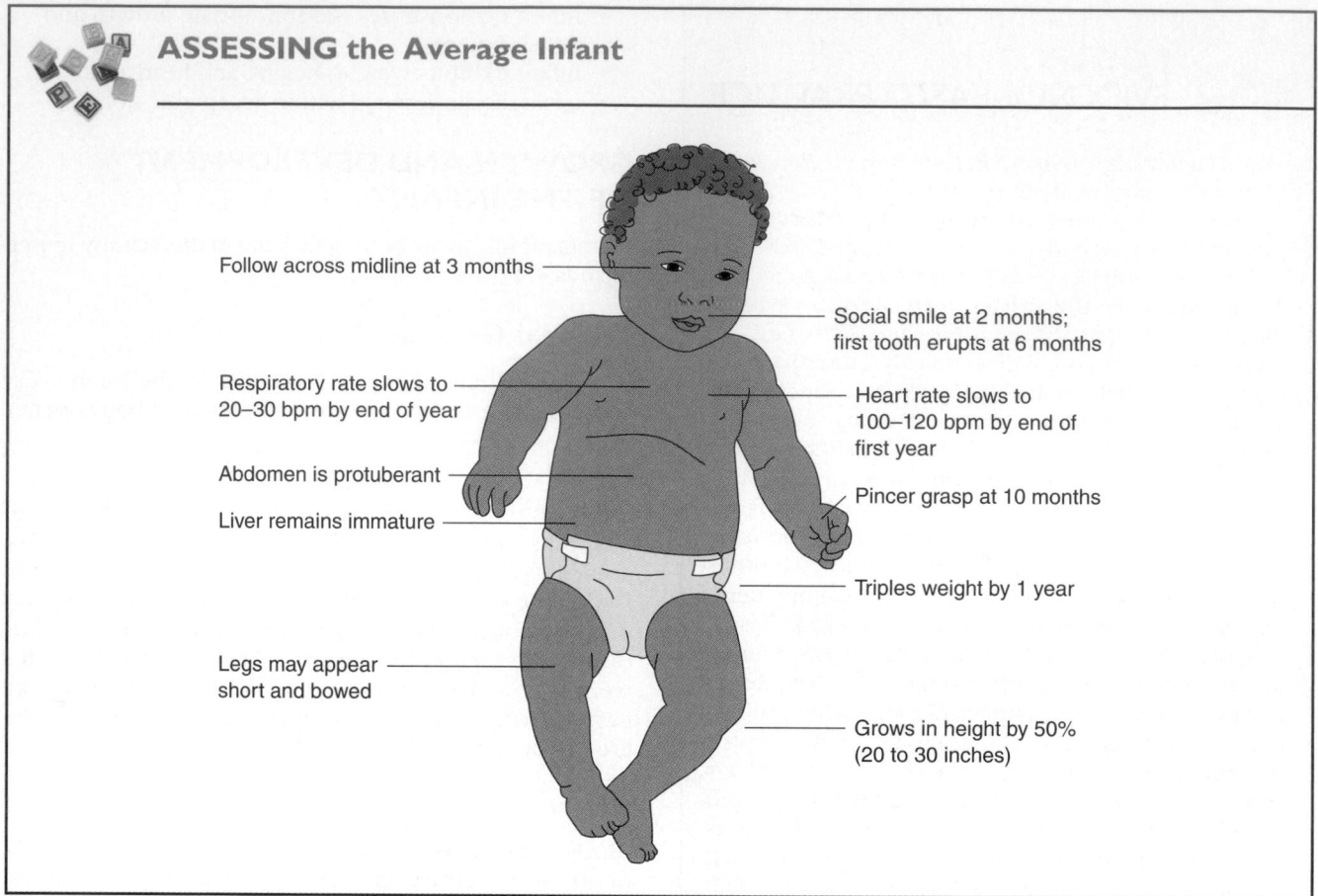

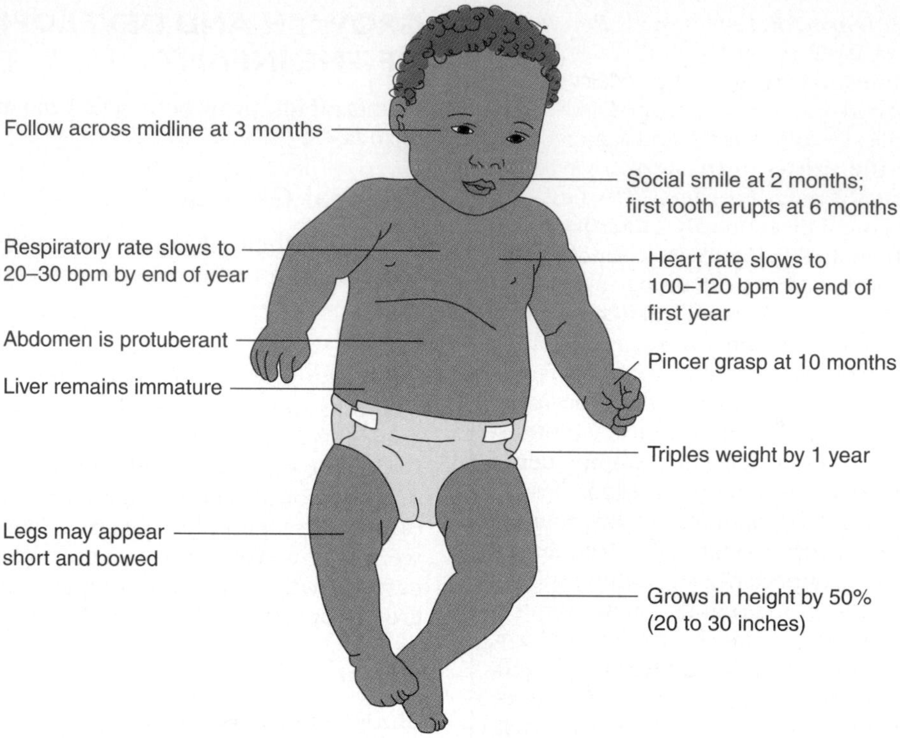
Follow across midline at 3 months
Social smile at 2 months; first tooth erupts at 6 months
Respiratory rate slows to 20–30 bpm by end of year
Heart rate slows to 100–120 bpm by end of first year
Abdomen is protuberant
Pincer grasp at 10 months
Liver remains immature
Triples weight by 1 year
Legs may appear short and bowed
Grows in height by 50% (20 to 30 inches)

the end of the infant period, the lower jaw is prominent and remains that way throughout life.

The circumference of the chest is generally less than that of the head at birth by about 2 cm. It is even with the head circumference in some infants as early as 6 months and in most by 12 months. The abdomen remains protuberant until the child has been walking well for some time, generally well into the toddler period. Cervical, thoracic, and lumbar vertebral curves develop as infants hold up their head, sit, and walk.

Lengthening of the lower extremities during the last 6 months of infancy readies the child for walking and often changes the appearance from "baby-like" to "toddler-like."

Body Systems

In the cardiovascular system, heart rate slows from 120 to 160 bpm to 100 to 120 bpm by the end of the first year. The heart continues to occupy a little over one-half the width of the chest. Pulse rate may begin to slow with inhalation (sinus arrhythmia), but this does not become marked until preschool age. That the heart is becoming more efficient is shown by the decreasing pulse rate and a slightly elevated blood pressure (from an average of 80/40 to 100/60 mm Hg).

Infants are prone to develop a physiologic anemia at 2 to 3 months of age. Anemia occurs because this is the time when many fetal red blood cells are destroyed (the life of a red cell is 4 months) and new cells are not yet being produced in adequate replacement numbers. Hemoglobin in an infant becomes totally converted from fetal to adult hemoglobin at 5 to 6 months of age. Infants experience a second decrease in serum iron levels at 6 to 9 months as the last of iron stores established in utero are used.

The respiratory rate of the infant slows from 30 to 60 breaths/min to 20 to 30 breaths/min by the end of the first year. Because the lumen (tubal cavity) of the respiratory tract remains small and mucous production by the tract is still inefficient, upper respiratory infections occur readily and tend to be potentially more severe than in adults.

At birth, the gastrointestinal tract is immature in its ability to digest food and mechanically move it along. These functions mature gradually during the infant year. Although the ability to digest protein is present and effective at birth, the amount of amylase, necessary for the digestion of complex carbohydrates, is deficient until approximately the third month. Lipase, necessary for the digestion of saturated fat, is decreased in amount during the entire first year.

The liver of the infant remains immature, possibly causing inadequate conjugation of drugs (if a drug should be necessary for treatment of illness) and inefficient formation of carbohydrate, protein, and vitamins for storage. Until age 3 or 4 months, an **extrusion reflex** (food placed on the infant's tongue is thrust forward and out of the mouth) prevents some infants from eating effectively. Drinking from a cup can be possible as early as 4 months with parental control of the fluid flow. The infant may be able to independently drink from a cup by age 8 or 10 months.

The immune system becomes functional by at least 2 months of age; the infant is able to produce both IgG and IgM antibodies by 1 year of age. The levels of other immunoglobulins (IgA, IgE, and IgD) are not plentiful until preschool age, the underlying rationale for protecting infants from infection.

The ability to adjust to cold is mature by age 6 months. By this age, an infant can shiver in response to cold (which increases muscle activity and provides warmth) and has developed additional adipose tissue that serves as insulation. The amount of brown fat, which protected the newborn from cold, decreases during the first year.

The kidneys remain immature and not as efficient at eliminating body wastes as in the adult. The endocrine system remains particularly immature in response to pituitary stimulation, such as adrenocorticotropic hormone, or insulin production from the pancreas. Without these hormones functioning effectively, an infant cannot react to stress efficiently.

Although the fluid in body compartments shifts to some extent, extracellular fluid accounts for approximately 35% of the infant's body weight and intracellular fluid accounts for approximately 40% at the end of the first year, in contrast to adult proportions of 20% and 40%, respectively. This proportional difference increases the infant's susceptibility to dehydration from illnesses, such as diarrhea, in which a large amount of body fluid is lost.

Teeth

The first baby tooth (typically a central incisor) usually erupts at age 6 months, followed by a new one monthly. However, teething patterns can vary greatly among children. Figure 28-1 illustrates the approximate ages of baby tooth eruption by tooth type.

Some newborns (about 1 in 2,000) may be born with teeth (called **natal teeth**) or have teeth erupt in the first 4 weeks of life (called **neonatal teeth**). The mandibular central incisors (see Fig. 28-1) are the teeth most frequently involved in this early growth. In most children, natal or neonatal teeth are deciduous. They are fixed firmly and should not be removed because no other teeth will grow to replace them until the permanent teeth erupt at age 6 or 7. **Deciduous teeth** (temporary or baby teeth) are also essential for protecting the growth of the dental arch. Natal and neonatal teeth may also be supernumerary (extra) teeth. Supernumerary teeth may be membranous and thus be reabsorbed. If they are loosely attached, these teeth must be removed before they loosen spontaneously and are aspirated by the infant.

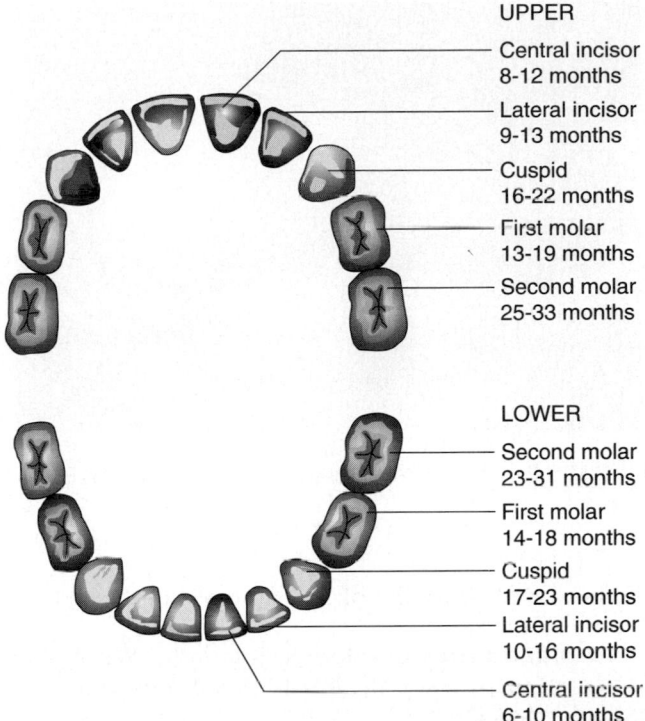

> ✔ **CHECKPOINT QUESTIONS**
>
> 1. What is the typical range for heart rate in infants by the end of the first year?
> 2. Why is an infant more prone to dehydration from illness?

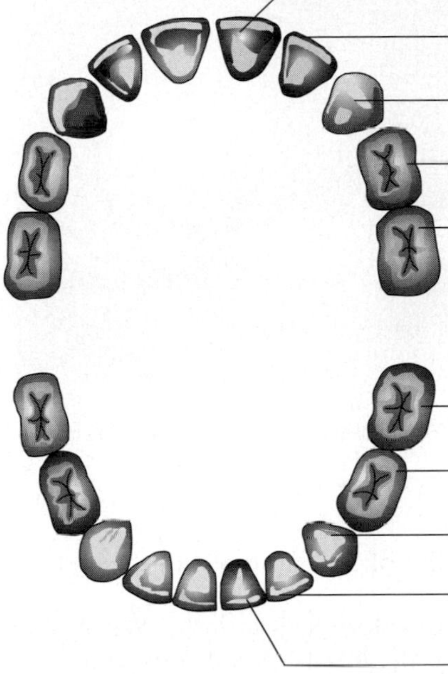

FIGURE 28.1 Eruption pattern of deciduous teeth.

Motor Development

The average infant progresses through systematic motor growth during the first year that strongly reflects the principles of cephalocaudal development and gross to fine motor development. Control proceeds from head to trunk to lower extremities in a progressive, predictable sequence. Different infants accomplish different tasks at different ages; the ages given here are only averages.

To assess motor development, the infant should be evaluated in two major areas. The first is **gross motor development** (ability to accomplish large body movements). The second is **fine motor development,** which is measured by observing or testing **prehensile ability** (ability to coordinate hand movements).

Gross Motor Development

To evaluate gross motor development, an infant is observed in four positions: ventral suspension, prone, sitting, and standing.

Ventral Suspension Position. **Ventral suspension** refers to the infant's appearance when held in midair on a horizontal plane, supported by a hand under the abdomen (Fig. 28-2A). In this position, the newborn allows the head to hang down with little effort at control. A 1-month-old child lifts the head momentarily, then drops it again. He or she may flex the elbows, extend the hips, and flex the knees. Two-month-old children hold their heads in the same plane as the rest of their body, a major advance in muscle control. The 3-month-old child lifts and maintains

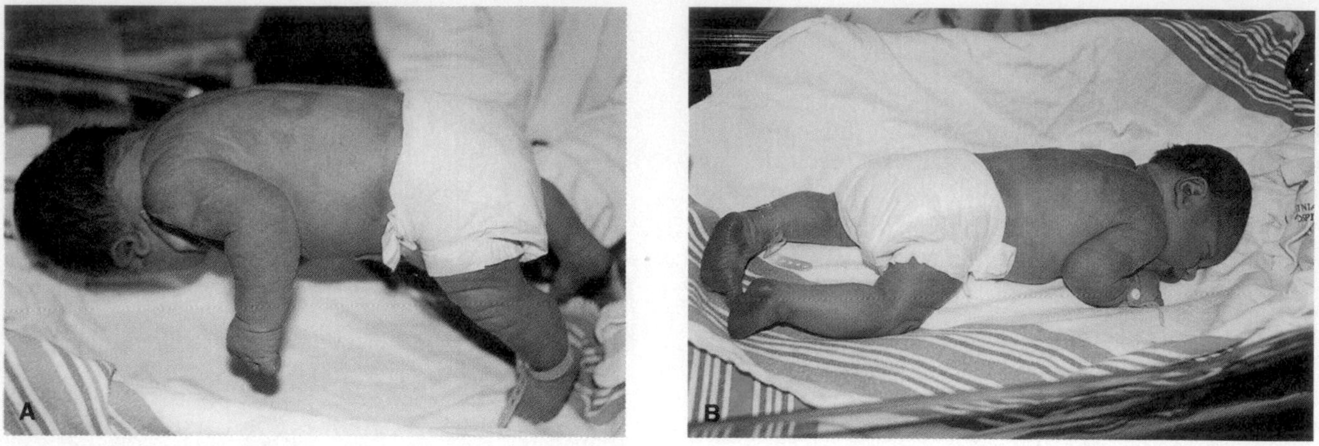

FIGURE 28.2 (*A*) Ventral suspension position. (*B*) Prone position.

the head well above the plane of the rest of the body in ventral suspension.

A **Landau reflex** develops at 3 months. When held in ventral suspension, the infant's head, legs, and spine extend. When the head is depressed, the hips, knees, and elbows flex. This reflex continues to be present in most infants during the second 6 months of life, but then it becomes increasingly difficult to demonstrate. A child with motor weakness, cerebral palsy, or other neuromuscular defect will not be able to demonstrate the reflex.

At 6 to 9 months, an infant demonstrates a **parachute reaction** from a ventral suspension position. When infants are suddenly lowered toward an examining table from ventral suspension, the arms extend as if to protect themselves from falling. In children with hemiplegia, the response is noticeable only on the unaffected side. Children with cerebral palsy do not demonstrate this response because when in this position, they have extreme flexion activity.

Prone Position. When lying on their stomach, newborns can turn their head to move it out of a position where breathing is impaired, but they cannot hold it raised (see Fig. 28-2*B*). By 1 month of age, infants lift their head and turn it easily to the side. They still tend to keep the knees tucked under the abdomen as they did as a newborn. Two-month-old infants can raise their head and maintain the position, but they cannot raise their chest high enough to look around yet. Their head is still held facing downward.

The 3-month-old child lifts the head and shoulders well off the table and looks around when prone. The pelvis is flat on the table, no longer elevated. Some children can turn from a prone to a side-lying position at this age.

Four-month-old children lift the chest off the bed and look around actively, turning the head from side to side. They can turn from front to back. The first time, this tends to occur as an extension of lifting the chest combined with the **neck-righting reflex,** which begins at this age. When the infant turns the head to the side, the shoulders, trunk, and pelvis turn in that direction, too. This reflex causes the baby to lose his or her balance and roll sideways when lifting the head up. The baby is frightened by the sudden feeling of rolling free and probably cries. After this happens a few more times, however, the baby begins to delight in this new accomplishment. Most babies turn front to back first and then, 1 month later, back to front. When taking a health history, ask which way the child turned first. Those with spasticity may turn first in the opposite direction. This is not necessarily an indication of spasticity, however, because some healthy babies turn back to front first.

A 5-month-old child rests his or her weight on the forearms when prone. The infant can turn completely over, front to back and back to front. At 6 months, infants rest their weight on their hands with extended arms. They can raise their chest and the upper part of their abdomen off the table.

By 9 months, the child can creep from the prone position. Creeping is a new skill, advanced from hitching (the infant slides along the floor) that he or she may have been doing. Creeping means the child has the abdomen off the floor and moves one hand and one leg and then the other hand and leg, using the knees on the floor to locomote (Fig. 28-3).

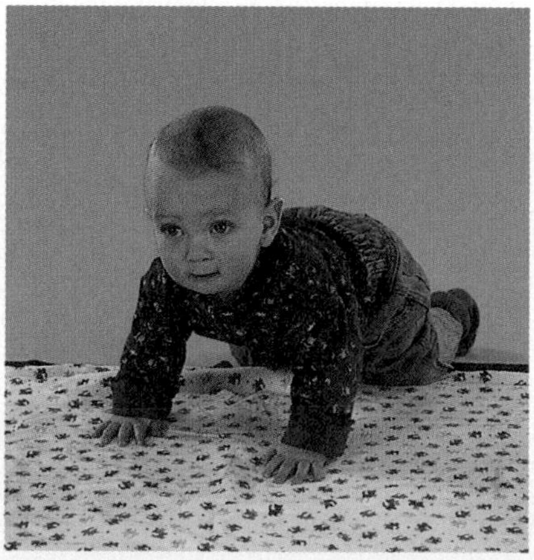

FIGURE 28.3 Creeping. The older infant moves forward, carrying his torso above and parallel to the floor.

Sitting Position. When placed on his or her back and then pulled to a sitting position, the 1-month-old child has gross head lag as in the first days of life (Fig. 28-4). In a sitting position, the back is rounded and the infant demonstrates only momentary head control. The 2-month-old child can hold his or her head fairly steady when sitting up, although it does tend to bob forward. The infant at this age still has head lag when pulled to a sitting position.

The 3-month-old child has only slight head lag when pulled to a sitting position. A 4-month-old child reaches an important milestone by no longer demonstrating head lag when pulled to a sitting position.

A 5-month-old child can be seen to straighten his or her back when held or propped in a sitting position. By 6 months, children sit momentarily without support. They anticipate being picked up and reach up with their hands from this position. Some parents expect a child this age to sit securely and are worried because the sitting posture is still extremely shaky. However, it is more common for the 6-month-old child to have only a limited ability to sit independently (Fig. 28-5). Six-month-old children often sit with their legs spread and their arms stiffened between them, hands on the floor, as a prop. Infants are capable of movement by hitching or sliding backward from this position. Parents should know that an infant this young is capable of moving from one spot to another in this way, so they are prepared for this and can prevent accidents.

A 7-month-old child sits alone, but only when the hands are held forward for balance. An 8-month-old child can sit securely without additional support (Fig. 28-6). This is a major milestone in development that should always be considered in assessment. Children with delayed mental or motor development may not accomplish this step at this time.

At 9 months, infants sit so steadily that they can lean forward and regain their balance. They may still lose their balance if they lean sideways, a skill that is not achieved for another month.

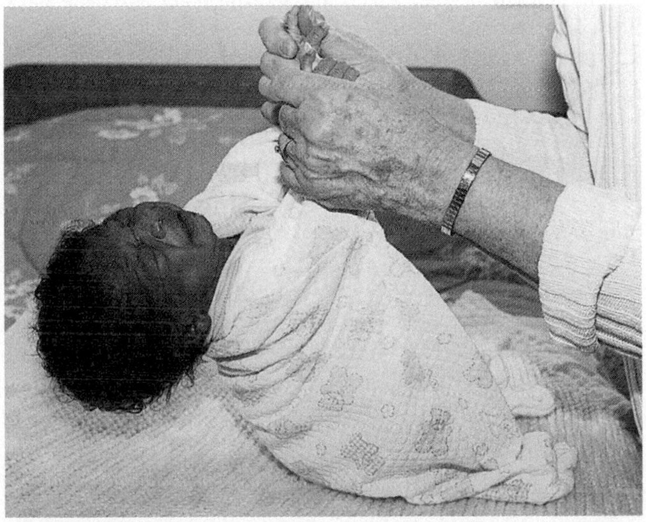

FIGURE 28.4 An infant is pulled to a sitting position to demonstrate head lag. Notice how evident this is in the very young infant.

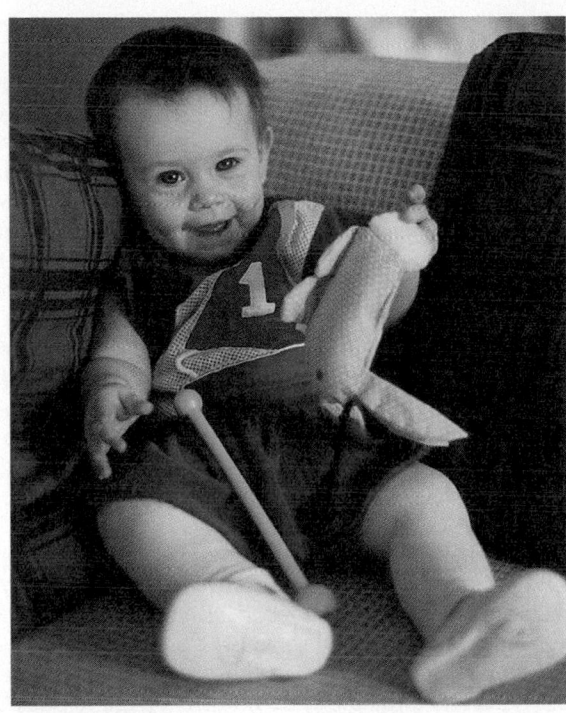

FIGURE 28.5 A 6-month-old infant sitting. Notice how she is propped with pillows to maintain the position.

Standing Position. A newborn stepping reflex can still be demonstrated at 1 month of age. In a standing position, the infant's knees and hips flex rather than support more than momentary weight. A 2-month-old child, when held in a standing position, holds his or her head up with the same show of support as in a sitting position. The stepping reflex

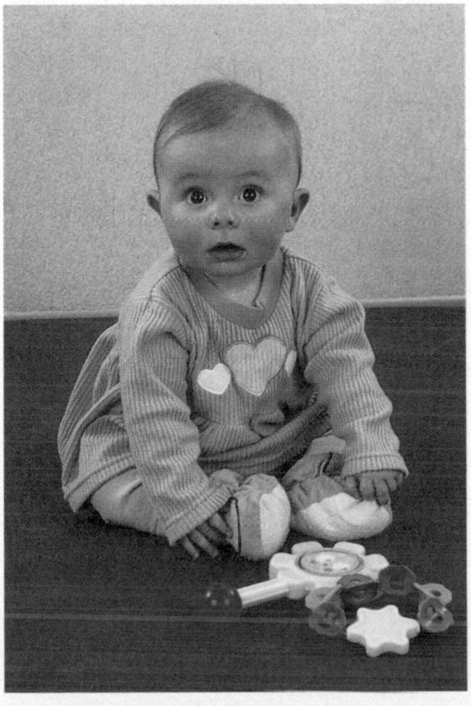

FIGURE 28.6 At 8 months the infant sits independently.

is still present. At 3 months, infants begin to try to support part of their weight. The stepping reflex begins to fade.

At 4 months, infants make an attempt to sustain their weight actively on their legs. They are successful at doing this because the stepping reflex has faded.

The 5-month-old child continues the ability to sustain a portion of his or her weight. The tonic neck reflex should be extinguished, and the Moro reflex is fading. By 6 months, infants support nearly their full weight when in a standing position. A 7-month-old child bounces with enjoyment in a standing position.

The 9-month-old child can stand holding onto a coffee table if he or she is placed in that position. Some 9-month-old children can pull up to that position. Ten-month-old children can pull themselves to a standing position by holding onto the side of a playpen or a low table, but they cannot let themselves down again as yet.

At around 11 months, the child learns to "cruise" or move about the crib or room by holding onto objects such as the crib rails, chairs, walls, and low tables (Fig. 28-7). At 12 months, a child stands alone at least momentarily. Some parents expect their child to walk at this time and are disappointed to see him or her not moving but merely standing. A child has until about 22 months of age to walk and still be within the normal limit, however (Fig. 28-8).

✔ CHECKPOINT QUESTIONS

3. What four positions are used to evaluate gross motor development?
4. By what age would you expect an infant to sit securely without support?

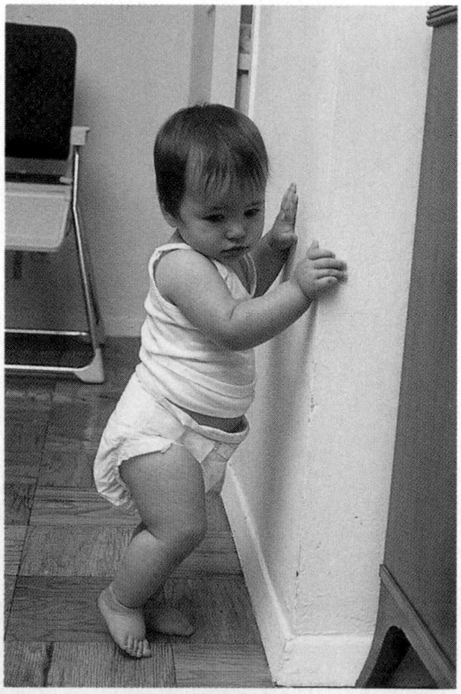

FIGURE 28.7 An 11-month-old child cruising along the walls. Further childproofing of the house will be necessary to keep the infant safe.

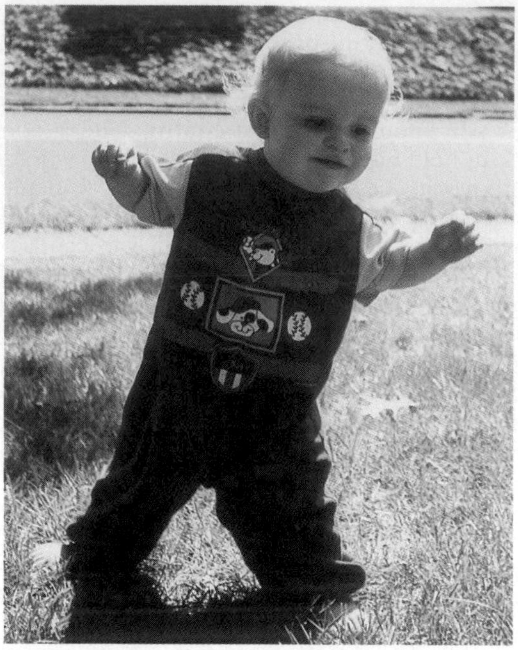

FIGURE 28.8 There is a wide variation in the age at which walking is first accomplished, typically ranging from 8 to 15 months. Here a child has mastered it by 1 year.

Fine Motor Development

One-month-old infants still have a strong grasp reflex and so hold their hands in fists so tightly it is difficult to extend the fingers. As the grasp reflex begins to fade, the 2-month-old child will hold an object for a few minutes before dropping it. The hands are held open, not closed in fists.

At 3 months, infants reach for attractive objects in front of them. Their grasp is unpracticed, however, so they usually miss them. Inform parents that this is part of normal development. Otherwise, they may think the child is nearsighted or farsighted or has poor coordination.

By 4 months, infants bring their hands together and pull at their clothes. They will shake a rattle placed in their hand for a long time. **Thumb opposition** (ability to bring the thumb and fingers together) is beginning, but the motion is a scooping or raking one, not a picking-up one, and is not very accurate. The infant is limited to handling large objects (Fig. 28-9). Palmar and plantar grasp reflexes have disappeared.

The 5-month-old child can accept an object that is handed to him or her and grasp it with the whole hand. He or she can reach and pick up an object without its being offered and often plays with his or her toes as objects. Fisting that persists beyond 5 months suggests a delay in motor development. Unilateral fisting suggests hemiparesis or paralysis on that side.

By 6 months, grasping has advanced to a point where the child can hold objects in both hands. Infants at this age will drop one toy when a second one is offered for the same hand. They can hold a spoon and start to feed themselves (with much spilling). Moro, palmar grasp, and the tonic neck reflex have completely faded. A Moro reflex that persists beyond this point should arouse grave suspicion of neurologic disease.

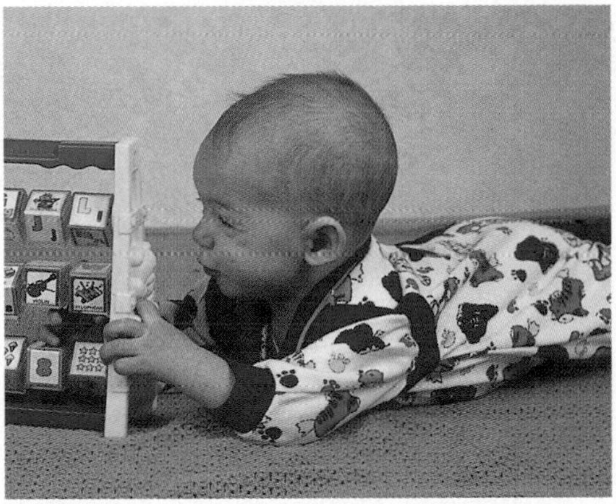

FIGURE 28.9 By age 4 months, the infant is able to manipulate large objects.

The 7-month-old child can transfer a toy from one hand to the other. He or she holds a first object when a second one is offered. By 8 months, random reaching and ineffective grasping have disappeared as a result of advanced eye–hand coordination.

A major milestone of 10 months is the ability to bring the thumb and first finger together in a **pincer grasp** (Fig. 28-10). This enables the child to pick up small objects such as crumbs or pieces of cereal from a highchair tray. The infant uses one finger to point to objects. He or she offers toys to people but then cannot release them.

At 12 months, infants can draw a semistraight line with a crayon. They enjoy putting objects such as small blocks in containers and taking them out again. They can hold a cup and spoon to feed themselves fairly well (if they have been allowed to practice) and can take off socks and push their hands into sleeves (again, if they have been allowed to practice). They can offer toys and release them.

WHAT IF? What if a 10-month-old infant can pick up very small articles such as marbles? How would achievement of this milestone affect the infant's safety?

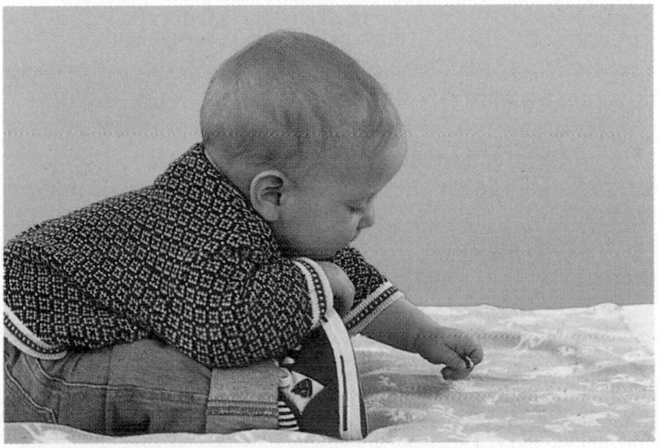

FIGURE 28.10 An infant almost ready to demonstrate a pincer grasp.

Developmental Milestones

In addition to the gross and fine motor skills that are developing at this time, language and play behavior also mark major milestones in the first year of life. Motor and cognitive development and play throughout this year are summarized in Table 28-2.

Language Development

A child begins to make small, cooing (dovelike) sounds by the end of the first month. The 2-month-old child differentiates a cry. For example, caregivers can distinguish a cry that means "hungry" from one that means "wet" or from one that means "lonely." This is an important milestone in development for an infant and in marking how far a parent has progressed in the task of learning the infant's cues. A first-time parent has more difficulty making the distinction in crying than one who has experienced this before. The infant's ability to make throaty, gurgling, or cooing sounds also increases at this time.

In response to a nodding, smiling face or a friendly tone of voice, the 3-month-old child will squeal with pleasure. This is an important step in development because the baby becomes even more fun to be with. Parents spend increased time with infants at this age, not just to care for them but because they enjoy their company.

By 4 months, infants are very "talkative," cooing, babbling, and gurgling when spoken to. They definitely laugh out loud. By 5 months, an infant says some simple vowel sounds (for example, "goo-goo" and "gah-gah"). At 6 months, infants learn the art of imitating. They may imitate a parent's cough, for example, or say "Oh!" as a way of attracting attention.

The amount of talking infants do increases at 7 months. They can imitate vowel sounds well (for example, "oh-oh," "ah-ah," and "oo-oo"). By 9 months, the infant usually speaks a first word: "da-da" or "ba-ba." Occasionally a mother may need reassurance that "da-da" for daddy is an easier syllable to pronounce than "ma-ma" for mommy. German mothers report that the first word their babies say is "da," which means "here" in German. By 10 months, the infant masters another word such as "bye-bye" or "no." At 12 months, infants can generally say two words besides "ma-ma" and "da-da;" they use those two words with meaning.

Play

Parents often ask what toy their child would enjoy. Because they can fix their eyes on an object, 1-month-old children are interested in watching a mobile over their crib or playpen. Mobiles should be black and white or brightly colored and light enough in weight so they move when someone walks by. They should face down toward the infant, not sideways toward the adults standing beside the crib. Musical mobiles provide extra stimulation. One-month-old children spend a great deal of time watching the parent's face, appearing to enjoy this activity so much that the face may become their favorite "toy." Help parents understand that they are not spoiling their infants by sitting and holding them for long periods of time. Parents

TABLE 28.2 Summary of Infant Growth and Development

MONTH	MOTOR DEVELOPMENT	FINE MOTOR DEVELOPMENT	SOCIALIZATION AND LANGUAGE	PLAY
0–1	Largely reflex	Keeps hands fisted; able to follow object to midline		Enjoys watching face of primary caregiver, listening to soothing sounds
2	Holds head up when prone	Has social smile	Makes cooing sounds; differentiates cry	Enjoys bright-colored mobiles
3	Holds head and chest up when prone	Follows object past midline	Laughs out loud	Spends time looking at hands or uses them as toy during the month (hand regard)
4	Grasp, stepping, tonic neck reflexes are fading			Needs space to turn
5	Turns front to back; no longer has head lag when pulled upright; bears partial weight on feet when held upright			Handles rattles well
6	Turns both ways; Moro reflex fading	Uses palmar grasp	May say vowel sounds (*oh-oh*)	Enjoys bathtub toys, rubber ring for teething
7	Reaches out in anticipation of being picked up; first tooth (central incisor) erupts; sits unsteadily (still needs support)	Transfers objects hand to hand	Shows beginning fear of strangers	Likes objects that are good size for transferring
8	Sits securely without support		Has peaked fear of strangers (ability to tell known from unknown people)	Enjoys manipulation, rattles and toys of different textures
9	Creeps or crawls (abdomen off floor)		Says first word (*da-da*)	Needs space for creeping
10	Pulls self to standing	Uses pincer grasp (thumb and finger) to pick up small objects		Plays games like patty-cake and peek-a-boo
11	"Cruises" (walks with support)			"Cruises"
12	Stands alone; some infants take first step	Holds cup and spoon well; helps to dress (pushes arm into sleeve)	Says two words plus *ma-ma* and *da-da*	Likes toys that fit inside each other (pots and pans); nursery rhymes; will like pull toys as soon as walking

will enjoy recalling such calm moments later, when they are stacking blocks, winding up toys, or playing table games with their growing child.

Hearing is a second sense that is a source of pleasure for the child in early infancy. Even a newborn "listens" to the sound of a music box or a musical rattle. He or she stirs and seems apprehensive at the sound of a raucous rattle.

Two-month-old infants will hold light, small rattles for a short period of time and then drop them. They are very attuned to mobiles or cradle gyms strung across their crib. They continue to spend a great deal of time just watching the people around them.

Three-month-old children can handle small blocks or small rattles. Four-month-old children need a playpen or a sheet spread on the floor so they have an opportunity to exercise their new skill of rolling over. Rolling over is so intriguing it may serve as a "toy" for the entire month.

Five-month-old infants are ready for a variety of objects to handle, such as plastic rings, blocks, squeeze toys, clothespins, rattles, and plastic keys. All these should be small enough that the infant can lift them with one hand, yet big enough that the baby cannot possibly swallow them.

A 6-month-old child can sit steadily enough to be ready for bathtub toys such as rubber ducks or plastic boats. Because they are starting to teethe, infants enjoy a teething ring to chew on at this time.

Because 7-month-old children can transfer toys, they are interested in items such as blocks, rattles, or plastic keys that are small enough to be used for this. As their mobility increases, they begin to be more interested in brightly colored balls or toys that previously rolled out of reach.

Eight-month-old children are sensitive to differences in texture. They enjoy having toys that have different feels to them, such as velvet, fur, fuzzy, smooth, or rough items.

The 9-month-old infant needs the experience of creeping. This means time out of a crib or playpen so there is room to maneuver. Many 9-month-olds begin to enjoy toys that go inside one another, such as a nest of blocks or rings of assorted sizes that fit on a center post. Some are more interested in pots and pans that stack rather than toys.

By 10 months, infants are ready for peek-a-boo and will spend a long time playing the game with their hands or with a cloth over their head that they can reach and remove. They can clap and are also ready to play patty-cake. These games have a positive value, just as laughing out loud did for the 3-month-old child. They make the baby feel like an active part of the household. A family feeling begins to grow as the baby can participate in active games.

At 11 months, children have learned to cruise or walk along low tables by holding on. They often find this so absorbing that they spend little time doing anything else during the month.

Twelve-month-old infants enjoy putting things in and taking things out of containers. They like little boxes that fit inside one another or dropping objects such as blocks into a cardboard box. As soon as they can walk, they will be interested in pull toys. A lot of time may be spent listening to someone saying nursery rhymes or listening to music.

✔ CHECKPOINT QUESTIONS

5. At what month should an infant be able to pick up small objects using a pincer grasp?
6. How many words would a typical 12-month-old infant use?

Development of Senses

Like other facets of development, maturation of the senses proceeds step by step during the infant year.

Vision

One-month-old infants regard an object in the midline of their vision (directly in front of themselves) as it is brought into close proximity, about 18 in (46 cm) away. They follow it a short distance, but not across the midline as yet. They study or regard a human face with a fixed stare. Two-month-old infants focus well (from about age 6 weeks) and follow objects with the eyes (although still not past the midline). Ability to follow and focus this way is a major milestone in development, indicating that the infant has achieved **binocular vision,** or the ability to fuse two images into one (Fig. 28-11).

Three-month-old infants typically hold their hands in front of their face and study their fingers for long periods of time (**hand regard**). Blind children also demonstrate this phenomenon, however, so it may not be so much a test of vision as of cognitive or exploratory development.

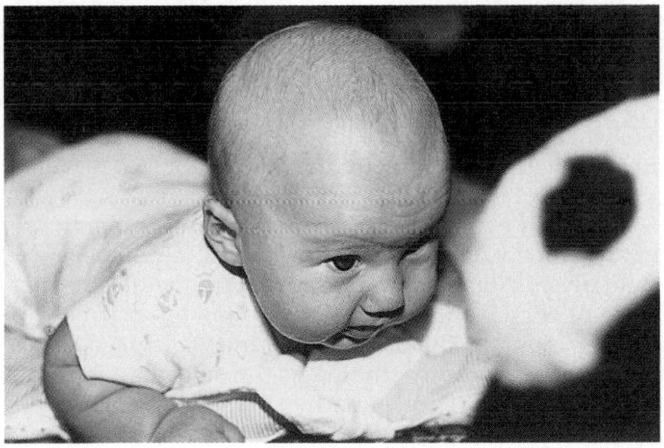

FIGURE 28.11 The 2-month-old infant focuses steadily and lifts her head up while prone. Note her interest in the stuffed panda bear.

Four-month-old infants recognize familiar objects, such as a frequently seen bottle, rattle, or toy animal. They follow their parents' movements with their eyes eagerly. At 6 months, infants are capable of organized depth perception. This increases the accuracy of their reach for objects as they begin to perceive distances accurately. Up until 6 months of age, infants may experience difficulty in establishing eye coordination. After this age, however, an infant whose eyes still "cross" should be examined by a physician.

Seven-month-old children pat their image in a mirror. Their depth perception has matured to the extent that they can perform such tasks as transferring toys from hand to hand. By 10 months, the infant looks under a towel or around a corner for a concealed object (beginning of **object permanence**).

Hearing

Hearing is demonstrated by the 1-month-old child who quiets momentarily at a distinctive sound such as a bell or a squeaky rubber toy. Hearing awareness becomes so acute by 2 months of age that infants will listen or stop an activity at the sound of spoken words. Many 3-month-old infants turn their heads to attempt to locate a sound. At 4 months of age, infants hear a distinctive sound and turn toward the sound and look in that direction.

By 5 months of age, infants demonstrate that they can localize sounds downward and to the side, by turning the head and looking down. Six-month-olds have progressed to being able to locate sounds made above them. By 10 months, infants can recognize their name and listen acutely when spoken to. By 12 months, infants can easily locate sounds in any direction and turn toward it. A vocabulary of two words plus "ma-ma" and "da-da" also demonstrates that the infant can hear.

Emotional Development

Socialization, or learning how to interact with others, is an extensive phenomenon. One-month-old infants show that they can differentiate between faces and other objects by studying a face or the picture of a face longer than other objects. They quiet best and eat best for the person who has been their primary caregiver.

When an interested person nods and smiles at a 6-month-old infant, the infant smiles in return. This is a **social smile** and is a definite response to the interaction, not the faint, quick "smile" that younger infants, even newborns, demonstrate. It is a major milestone for assessing a number of areas, most notably vision, motor control, and intelligence. Mentally challenged children or children with spasticity may not demonstrate a social smile until much later.

By 3 months, infants demonstrate increased social awareness by readily smiling at the sight of a parent's face (Fig. 28-12). Three-month-old infants laugh out loud at the sight of a funny face.

By 4 months, when a person who has been playing with and entertaining an infant leaves, the infant is likely to cry to show he or she enjoyed the interaction. Infants at this age recognize their primary caregiver and prefer that person's presence to others. By 5 months, infants may show displeasure when an object is taken away from them. This is a step beyond showing displeasure when a person leaves. The infant can be counted on to laugh at seeing a funny face.

By 6 months, infants are increasingly aware of the difference between people who regularly care for them and strangers. They may begin to draw back from unfamiliar people. Seven-month-old infants begin to show obvious fear of strangers. They may cry when taken from their parent, attempt to cling to him or her, and reach out to be taken back. Parents may view this as a bad trait or a regression in socialization. Help them appreciate that it is actually a big step forward, because it shows that infants can differentiate between persons and know the difference between those they trust and those they do not know.

Fear of strangers appears to reach its height during the eighth month, so much so that this phenomenon is often termed **eighth-month anxiety,** or stranger anxiety. An infant at the height of this phase will not go willingly from a parent's arms to a nurse's. Taking a few minutes to talk to the child and parent first is time well spent.

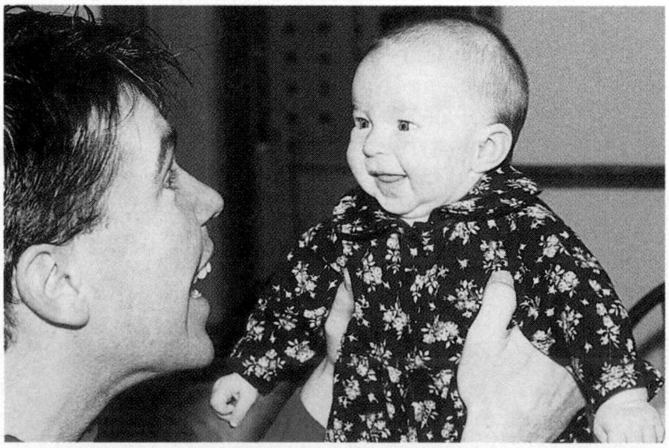

FIGURE 28.12 A 3-month-old smiles delightedly at her father's happy face. This indicates that the child has developed increased social awareness.

Nine-month-old infants are very aware of changes in tone of voice. They will cry when scolded, not because they understand what is being said but because they sense their parent's displeasure.

By 12 months, most children have overcome their fear of strangers and are alert and responsive again when approached. They like to play interactive nursery rhymes and rhythm games and "dance" with others. They like being at the table for meals and joining in family activities.

✔ CHECKPOINT QUESTIONS

7. What does the ability to focus and follow objects with the eyes indicate?
8. At what age do infants demonstrate a social smile?
9. When does an infant typically exhibit stranger anxiety?

Cognitive Development

In the first month of life, an infant mainly uses simple reflex activity. There is little evidence that infants at this age see themselves as separate from their environment. However, this does not mean they cannot respond actively or interact with people. They are very people-oriented from within moments after birth.

Primary Circular Reaction

By the third month of life, the child enters a cognitive stage identified by Piaget (1966) as **primary circular reaction.** During this time, the infant explores objects by grasping them with the hands or by mouthing them (Fig. 28-13).

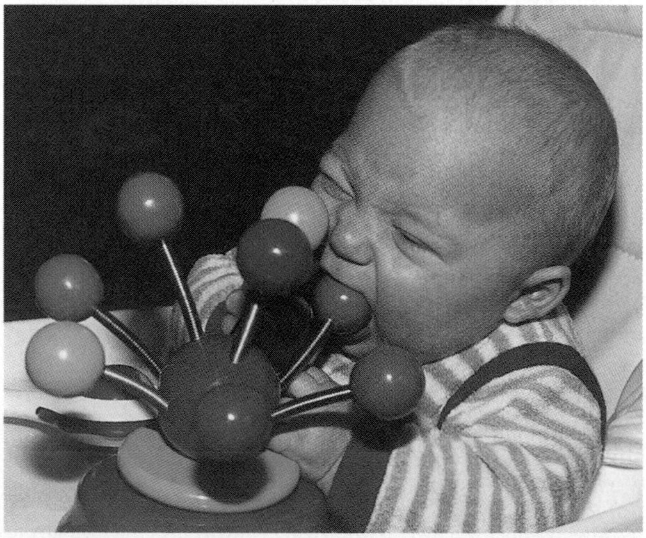

FIGURE 28.13 Mouthing of objects or fingers is a method by which an infant explores the world. This also helps the infant to separate self from environment.

At this stage, infants appear to be unaware of what actions they can cause or what actions occur independently. For example, if an infant's hand should accidentally strike a mobile across the crib, the infant appears to enjoy watching the brightly colored birds move in front of him, but makes no attempt to hit the mobile again because he does not realize that his hand caused the movement.

Secondary Circular Reaction

At about 6 months of age (cognitive development has wide variation), infants pass into a stage that Piaget (1966) called **secondary circular reaction.** During this time, they can grasp the idea that their actions can initiate pleasurable sensations. Now when infants reach for a mobile above the crib, hit it, and watch it move, they realize that their hand initiated the motion, and so hit it again.

Infants are still unaware of the permanence of objects by the end of this stage. For example, if an object is hidden from vision (a baby drops it from her hand or it is hidden by a blanket), the infant will not search for it. Gone is gone. If any part of the object is exposed, the infant can visualize the whole object and will reach to obtain it.

Coordination of Secondary Schema

Infants of 10 months discover object permanence, or become aware that an object out of sight still exists. Infants are ready for peek-a-boo once they have gained the concept of permanence. They know their parent still exists even when hiding behind a hand or blanket and wait excitedly for the parent to reappear. If a baby drops a piece of breakfast cereal or a spoon from a highchair tray, although it is out of sight, the infant knows it still exists and will reach for it. Piaget (1966) called this stage of cognitive development **coordination of secondary schema.**

As infants reach 1 year of age, they are capable of reproducing interesting events (they accidentally hit a mobile once; it moves; they hit it again) and producing new events. They drop objects from a highchair or playpen and watch where they fall or roll. This is a frustrating activity for caregivers because it involves a great deal of reaching and picking up. It is an important activity for infants, however, because it conforms to their awareness of the permanence of objects and how they are able to control events in their world.

✔ CHECKPOINT QUESTIONS

10. When would an infant be ready to play peek-a-boo?
11. When an infant mouths an object, appearing unaware of what actions he or she can cause or what actions occur independently, which cognitive stage is he is she displaying?
12. What does it mean when an infant develops object permanence?

THE NURSING ROLE IN HEALTH PROMOTION OF THE INFANT AND FAMILY

The nursing role with infants is wide-ranging because infants are so dependent on their caregivers for safety, learning, and emotional development.

Promoting Achievement of Developmental Task: Trust Versus Mistrust

Erikson (1993) proposed that the developmental task of the infant period is to form a sense of trust. When the infant is hungry, a parent feeds and makes him or her comfortable again. When the infant is wet, a parent changes him or her and the infant is dry again. When the infant is cold, a parent holds and warms him or her. By this process, infants learn to trust that when they have a need or are in distress, a person will come and meet that need.

A synonym for trust in this connotation is love. By the way that infants are handled, fed, talked to, and held, they learn to love and recognize that they are loved. Infants who have numerous caregivers, who may be fed one day on a rigid schedule and the next only when they are hungry, who sometimes are treated roughly and sometimes gently, can have difficulty learning to trust anyone. If infants cannot trust, they cannot enjoy deeply satisfying interactions with others and can have difficulty trusting themselves or experiencing high self-esteem. They may have difficulty establishing close relationships as adults.

It is important for people to establish the ability to love, or trust, early in life because development is sequential. If the first developmental step is inadequate, this inadequacy can pervade all future steps. The end result can be adults unable to instill a sense of trust in their own children, and thus the inadequacy is perpetuated from generation to generation.

How do parents (or a nurse) encourage a sense of trust in an infant? Trust arises primarily from a sense of confidence that one knows what is coming next. This does not mean that parents should set up a rigid schedule of care for a child. It does imply establishing some schedule; for example, breakfast, bath, playtime, nap, lunch, walk outside, quiet playtime, dinner, story, and bedtime. This gentle rhythm of care gives infants a sense of being able to predict what is going to happen and feel that life has some consistency. All little children thrive on routine; for example, the same story read over and over again, the same bedtime rituals, the same spoon every day for lunch. Infancy is not too early for children to learn family traditions that will help them feel secure in the world as they grow. Some parents have difficulty accepting routine as important to a child. They may be so tired of the work treadmill that they want to raise their children as free spirits. Do not discourage this philosophy; however, suggest a few modifications to instill some order into infants' lives.

As important to an infant as the rhythm of care is that the care be given largely by one person (Fig. 28-14). This person can be the mother, father, grandparent, a conscientious babysitter, a foster parent, or anyone who can give consistent care. For infants ill at birth who are hospitalized for months, this person is often a primary nurse or case

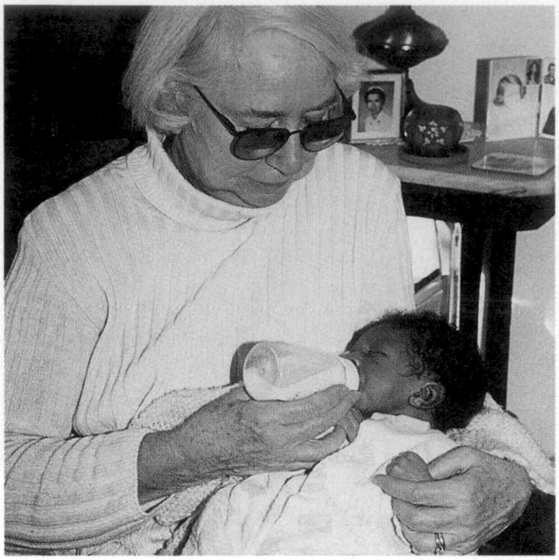

FIGURE 28.14 An infant's sense of trust develops through warm interpersonal relationships. Here a foster parent and child develop a bond during feeding.

manager. Women who work outside their home during the first year of a baby's life (at least 90% of women today) should try to arrange for one person to care for the child while they are away from home or choose a day care center that will provide a consistent caregiver. They should discuss their methods of childcare with alternative caregivers to prevent disrupting the infant's routine. When a child is admitted to a hospital, document and use this information.

Parents should make sure that the caretaker will actively interact with the child to provide a sense of trust. Passively caring for infants—not talking to them or touching or stroking them while feeding or changing them—amounts to not being with them. Caregivers may have to be encouraged not to feel self-conscious talking to a baby who does not talk back. Pointing out the importance of such interactions and role modeling them while caring for children help caregivers to use this type of stimulation as they care for the baby's physical needs. An increasing number of parents are installing video cameras to make sure the caretaker is actively talking to the baby and helping to instill a sense of trust in the child. Nursing actions designed to help the ill infant develop a sense of trust are detailed in Table 28-3.

Promoting Infant Safety

Accidents are a leading cause of death in children from 1 month through 24 years of age. They are second only to acute infections as a cause of acute morbidity and physician visits (Battan & Dart, 2001).

Most accidents in infancy occur because parents either underestimate or overestimate the child's ability. Nursing interventions that help parents become sensitive to their infant's developmental progress help to establish sound parent–child relationships and provide anticipatory guidance for the child's safety (see Focus on Family Empowerment). Box 28-1 highlights an appropriate outcome and intervention related to infant safety using the terminology identified by the Nursing Outcomes Classification (NOC) and Nursing Interventions Classification (NIC).

TABLE 28.3 Ways for Nurses to Help an Ill Infant Develop a Sense of Trust

AREA OF CARE	NURSING ACTIONS
Nutrition	Encourage mothers to breast-feed if possible; provide privacy and support as necessary.
	Hold the infant no matter what feeding method is used (gavage, total parenteral, oral, enteral). If this is not possible, hold infants for a time after or between feedings so they receive holding equal to what they would ordinarily receive.
	If infant feeding is not oral, provide a pacifier (medical condition considered) five or six times daily for sucking pleasure.
	Hold and comfort after an episode of vomiting, usually not noticeably disturbing to infants.
Dressing change	Use nonallergenic tape to avoid irritation while applied and pain when removed.
	Use a minimum of tape so the least amount has to be pulled free from sensitive skin (consider using stockinette, rolled gauze, or Kling gauze to hold a bandage in place rather than tape).
	To prevent chilling, be certain irrigation solutions are warm. Minimize exposure of the child during dressing changes to conserve warmth.
	Restrain only those body parts necessary for security.
	Talk to the infant. Hearing an explanation of what you are doing is comforting, not for the meaning of the words but for the nonthreatening tone of your voice.
Medicine administration	Flavor oral medicine to disguise disagreeable taste (being careful not to increase the amount to beyond what the child will take readily). Offer a drink of flavorful fluid afterward to counter medicinal taste.
	Never administer medicine in an infant's formula to prevent changing the formula's taste.
	Comfort the infant after injections or intravenous insertion by holding and rocking, or give immediately to a parent for this. Check intravenous sites frequently (every 30 min) for swelling to prevent infiltration and pain. Hold and play with infants despite tubing and restraints.

(continued)

TABLE 28.3 Ways for Nurses to Help an Ill Infant Develop a Sense of Trust *(Continued)*

AREA OF CARE	NURSING ACTIONS
Rest	Encourage parents to sit and hold infants; infants sleep in a parent's arms as soundly as they do in bed.
	Rock infants to sleep if this is comforting. If contagion is not a problem, bring the crib to the nursing desk where the infant can see you until he or she falls asleep.
	Always wake infants gently, because it is frightening (for anyone) to be awakened by a stranger.
	If bedrest is necessary, check for irritated elbows, heels, and knees from the infant's skin rubbing against sheets; protect with long sleeves or pants.
Hygiene	Check the temperature of bath water for comfort and to prevent chilling.
	Change diapers frequently to reduce discomfort from irritation.
	To avoid caries and prevent pain, begin toothbrushing with first tooth.
Pain	Hold and comfort an infant in pain.
	Do not ask parents to hold a child during a painful procedure; it is difficult for them to see their child in pain. Allow them to comfort the child afterward.
	Reduce painful procedures to a minimum; combine blood drawing so only one puncture is necessary for many tests, etc.
Stimulation	Talk to infants while you care for them so they come to know you.
	Remember that infants focus longest on a human face.
	Provide a crib mirror or a mobile, because visual stimulation is satisfying to an infant.
	If no mobile is available, create one from a wire coat hanger, string, or strips of adhesive tape and objects that will suspend easily and are light enough to move from motion of the crib or an air current (colored paper, cotton balls, colored tongue blades). For safety, hang the mobile high enough for the infant to see but not reach.
	During the second half of the 1st year, remember that infants need to try to crawl. Put a pad or sheet on the floor and encourage the infant to come to you or to explore on his or her own while you stand by to offer reassurance (this is almost impossible to accomplish in a crib).

Aspiration Prevention

Aspiration is always a potential threat to infants. Round, cylindrical objects are more dangerous than square or flexible objects in this regard. A 1-in (3.2-cm) cylinder, such as a carrot or hot dog, is particularly dangerous because it can totally obstruct the infant's airway. A deflated balloon can be sucked into the mouth, obstructing the airway in the same way. Educate parents who feed their infant formula not to prop bottles. By doing this, they are overestimating their infant's ability to push the bottle away, sit up, turn the head to the side, cough, and clear the airway if milk should flow too rapidly into the mouth and the infant begins to aspirate.

Other instances of aspiration occur because parents underestimate their infant's ability to grasp and place objects in their mouth. Newborns' grasp and sucking reflexes automatically cause them to react this way. Even a newborn can wiggle to a new position to reach an attractive object such as a teddy bear with small button eyes. Caution parents to be certain that nothing comes within the infant's reach that would not be safe to put into the mouth. Using clothing without decorative buttons, and checking toys and rattles to ensure that they have no small parts that could snap off or fall out are good steps for parents to follow. A test of whether a toy could be dangerous if the infant puts it inside the mouth is whether it fits inside a toilet paper roll. If it does, it is small enough to be aspirated. When solid foods are introduced, encourage parents to offer small pieces of hot dogs or grapes, not large chunks. Children under about 5 years should not be offered popcorn or peanuts because of this danger of aspiration.

As infants become more adept at handling toys, parents should check toys again for loose pieces or parts. If parents are going to offer an infant a pacifier, they should use ones that have a one-piece construction with a flange large enough to keep it from completely entering the child's mouth (Fig. 28-15).

Fall Prevention

Falls are a second major cause of infant accidents. As a preventive measure, no infant, beginning with the newborn, should be left unattended on a raised surface. Normal wiggling can bring a baby to the edge of a bed, couch, or table top, resulting in a fall.

Teach parents to be prepared for their infant to roll over by 2 months of age. From that time on, they must be vigilant not to leave the baby unattended on a changing table or counter. If the child sleeps in a crib, the mattress should be lowered to its bottom position so the height of the side rails increases; rails should be 2⅜ inches apart, narrow enough so the child cannot put his or her head between them. Two months is about the maximum length of time infants can safely sleep in a bassinet; they need the protection of a crib and high siderails before they can turn over.

All of these safety precautions apply to the hospital environment as well as to the home. Be sure crib sides are

FOCUS ON FAMILY EMPOWERMENT
Accident Prevention Measures for Infants

Q. How can we make sure that our infant stays safe?

A. Here are some tips to help prevent specific types of accidents:

Potential Accident	*Prevention Measures*
General	Know the whereabouts of infants at all times.
	Be aware that the frequency of accidents is increased when parents are under stress. Take special precautions at these times.
	Choose babysitters carefully and explain and enforce all precautions when sitters are in charge.
Aspiration	Be certain any object that an infant can grasp and bring to the mouth is either safe to eat or too big to fit in the mouth. Do not feed an infant foods such as popcorn or peanuts, because these are easily aspirated. Store baby products such as powder out of infant's reach; powder is high risk for aspiration.
	Inspect toys and pacifiers for small parts that could be aspirated if broken off; don't make homemade pacifiers.
Falls	Never leave the infant on an unprotected surface, such as a bed or couch, even if the child is in an infant seat.
	Place a gate at the top and bottom of stairways; do not allow an infant to walk with a sharp object in the hands or mouth (it could pierce the throat in a fall).
	Raise crib rails and make sure they are locked before walking away from crib.
	Do not leave a child unattended in a highchair; avoid using an infant walker.
Motor vehicle	Never transport unless the infant is buckled into an infant car seat in the back seat of the car. Don't place an infant seat in the front passenger side if the car has an air bag. Be aware of the proper technique for placing an infant in a car seat.
	Do not be distracted by an infant while driving.
	Do not leave an infant unattended in a parked car (can become dehydrated from excess heat, move gear shift, or be abducted).
Suffocation	Allow no plastic bags within infant's reach.
	Do not use pillows in a crib.
	Store unused appliances such as refrigerators or stoves with the doors removed.
	Buy a crib that is approved for safety (spacing of rails is not over $2\frac{3}{8}$ in [6 cm] apart).
	Remove constricting clothing such as a bib from neck at bedtime.
Drowning	Do not leave infants alone in a bathtub or unsupervised near water (even buckets of cleaning water).
Animal bites	Do not allow the infant to approach a strange dog; supervise play with family pets.
Poisoning	Never present medication as a candy.
	Buy medications in containers with safety caps; put away immediately after use.
	Never take medication in front of infants. Place all medication and poisons in locked cabinets or overhead shelves.
	Never leave medication in a pocket or handbag.
	Use no lead-based paint in any area of the home.
	Hang plants or set on high surfaces.
	Post telephone number of the poison control center by the telephone.
Burns	Test warmth of formula and food before feeding (use extra precaution with microwave warming).
	Do not smoke or drink hot liquids while holding or caring for infant.
	Buy flame-retardant clothing for infants.
	Use a sunscreen on a child over 6 months when out in direct or indirect sunlight; limit the child's sun exposure to less than $\frac{1}{2}$ h at a time.
	Turn handles of pans toward back of stove.
	Use a cool-mist, not a hot-mist, vaporizer; remain in room to monitor so child cannot reach vaporizer. Keep a screen in front of a fireplace or heater.
	Monitor infants carefully near candles.
	Do not leave infants unsupervised near hot-water faucets.
	Do not allow infants to blow out matches (don't teach children that fire is fun).
	Keep electric wires and cords out of reach; cover electrical outlets with safety plugs.

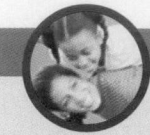

BOX 28.1

NURSING OUTCOMES AND NURSING INTERVENTIONS CLASSIFICATION: INFANT SAFETY

NOC: Knowledge, Child Safety

Knowledge, child safety, is defined as the extent of understanding conveyed about safely caring for a child (Johnson, Maas, & Moorhead, 2000). Some specific indicators suggesting achievement of this outcome include the parent's ability to describe the following:

- Appropriate activities for child's developmental level
- Drowning hazards and measures to prevent drowning
- Measures to prevent electrical shock, choking, falls, and burns
- First aid techniques and CPR, including demonstration
- Proper surveillance of activities

NIC: Teaching, Infant Safety

Teaching, infant safety, is defined as instruction on safety during the first year of life (McCloskey & Bulechek, 2000). Some important activities involved when implementing this intervention include instructing the parent/caregiver in the following at:

0 to 3 months

- Using carseat
- Putting infant to sleep on back
- Maintaining all equipment such as swings, strollers in proper working condition
- Checking temperature of formula and bath water
- Keeping pets at a safe distance
- Never shaking, tossing, or swinging infant in air

4 to 6 months

- Avoiding use of walkers or jumpers
- Never leaving infant unattended in tub
- Using a safe highchair
- Feeling only soft or mashed foods
- Removing small objects from infant's reach

7 to 9 months

- Avoiding sources of lead poisoning
- Providing barriers to potentially dangerous areas
- Supervising infant's activity at all times

10 to 12 months

- Providing protection from glass furniture, sharp edges, and appliances
- Storing all cleaning supplies out of infant's reach
- Using childproof latches on cupboards
- Preventing infant's access to upper-story windows, balconies, and stairs
- Selecting toys according to manufacturer's age recommendations
- Ensuring barriers to pools, hot tubs, ponds, and all containers with liquid

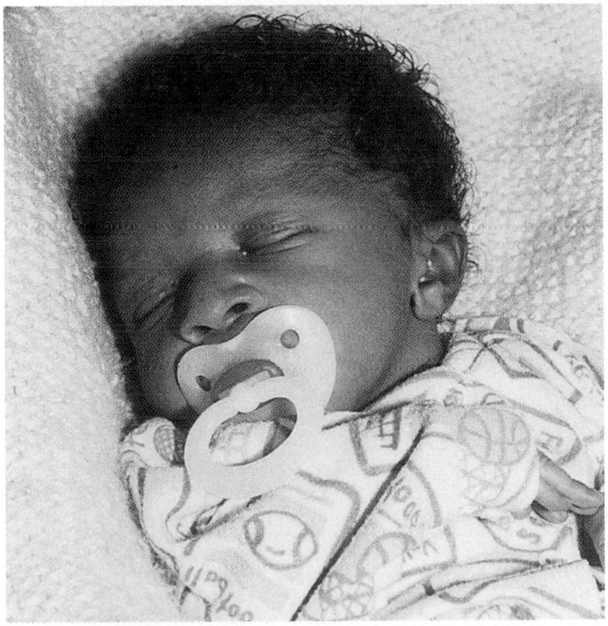

FIGURE 28.15 Many infants enjoy sucking on a pacifier to help them fall asleep. Notice the one-piece construction and large flange.

raised and secure before you walk away from a crib, even for just a moment. Also ensure that the space between the mattress and headboard is small enough that the infant's head could not become trapped. Make sure that cords from nursing call bells or safety pins are out of the infant's reach.

Car Safety

Teaching car safety for infants (as well as for the whole family) is a vital preventive health measure. The use of car seats for newborns is discussed in Chapter 23. Car seats should continue to be used without interruption through the preschool age, or until the child reaches 40 to 60 lb. If parents are firm about keeping an infant in a car seat even when he or she gets fussy or impatient, the child will eventually become more comfortable in the seat than outside it. Infants up to 20 lb should be placed in rear-facing seats in the back seat because an inflating front-seat airbag could suffocate the infant (AAP Committee on Safety, 2001).

Safety with Siblings

As infants become more fun to play with at about 3 months, older brothers and sisters grow more interested in interacting with them. You may need to remind parents that children under 5 years of age, as a group, are not responsible enough or knowledgeable enough about infants to be left unattended with them. They might introduce an unsafe toy or engage in play that is too rough for the infant. Some preschoolers may be so jealous of a new baby that they will physically harm the infant if left alone.

Bathing and Swimming Safety

As babies begin to develop good back support, many parents begin to bathe them in an adult tub. Caution parents never to leave an infant unattended in a tub, even when propped up out of the water or sitting in a bath ring or bath seat. Normal wiggling can easily cause the baby to slip down under the water. This applies to the hospital setting as well.

Many communities offer infant swim programs for babies as young as 6 months. If their child is enrolled in one of these programs, parents may become overconfident about the infant's ability to operate safely in water. Because children can dog-paddle momentarily in a swimming pool does not mean they can sustain that position for any length of time in a bathtub or pool (AAP Committee on Injury and Poison Prevention and Committee on Sports Medicine and Fitness, 2000). Being able to swim momentarily may cause children to lose their instinctive fear of water and thus be in more danger when around water than children who are still naturally more cautious. Such programs may also spread microorganisms because infants this age are not yet toilet-trained (CDC, 2001).

Childproofing

When infants begin teething at 5 to 6 months, they seek to chew on any object within reach to lessen gum line pain. Remind parents to check for possible sources of lead paint, such as painted cribs, playpen rails, or windowsills. Paints safe for baby furniture should be marked "Safe for use on surfaces that might be chewed by children." If the infant is going to be allowed to play on the floor, parents should move furniture in front of electrical fixtures or buy protective caps for the outlets. Infants are especially fascinated by the holes and will probe them with (often wet) fingers. Parents may need to install safety gates at the top and bottom of stairways.

Urge parents to move all potentially poisonous substances from bottom cupboards and store them well out of their infant's reach. Infants of any age should not be left unattended in carriages, highchairs, grocery shopping carts, or strollers. Baby walkers are extremely dangerous because infants can maneuver them near stairways and fall the length of the stairway.

When infants begin creeping, remind parents to recheck bottom cupboards and stairways for safety. When the child begins to walk, higher areas, such as coffee tables, should be cleared of dangerous items. In a hospital setting, assess low counter areas for dangerous objects. Do not leave possibly dangerous supplies in an infant's room.

By 10 months, achievement of a pincer grasp makes infants able to pick up very small objects. Remind parents to check play areas or areas such as table tops for pins or other sharp objects that could be swallowed. Some of the infant's toys are now also 10 months old and need to be checked to be certain they are still intact and safe.

Children who can walk may venture into the street or a swimming pool if not carefully supervised (Fig. 28-16). Although they seem very independent and able to take care of themselves, their judgment about what is dangerous is immature. In a hospital setting, a 12-month-old child can wander onto an elevator, out of the hospital, or into a laboratory area, or fall down a flight of stairs if not supervised.

> ✔ **CHECKPOINT QUESTIONS**
>
> 13. How do parents instill trust in an infant?
> 14. What are two of the most frequent types of accidents in infants?
> 15. For how long is it safe for an infant to sleep in a bassinet?

Promoting Nutritional Health of the Infant

The best food for the infant during the first 12 months of life (and the only food necessary for the first 6 months) is breast milk (see Chap. 24). With breastfeeding, as long as the mother is ingesting an adequate diet, no additional supplements such as iron or vitamins are necessary, except for fluoride if it is not included in the water supply. If infants will not be exposed to sunshine, vitamin D may also be prescribed. How long mothers continue to breast-feed is an individual choice, although it

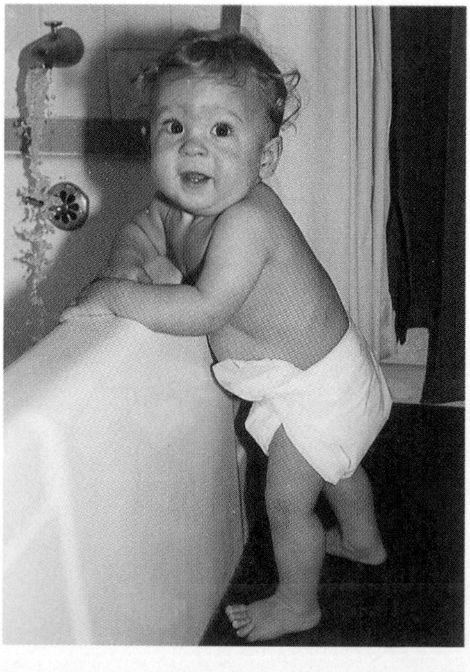

FIGURE 28.16 Once locomotion begins, the extended range of activities brings the infant in contact with potentially dangerous places or objects unless the house is childproofed. The bathroom is an important place to childproof.

is recommended through the entire first year (Bonuck et al., 2002). Prolonged breastfeeding into the preschool period is not usually recommended because it may impair the child's growth.

For infants whose mothers choose not to breastfeed, a commercial iron-fortified formula may be used (see Appendix B). As with breast-feeding, supplementation is unnecessary with commercial formula unless the water supply does not contain fluoride. Infants who are changed to cow's milk before 1 year of age (a practice that is not recommended because the protein in cow's milk is difficult for the infant to digest) should receive a supplementary form of vitamin C and iron to make up for the deficiency of these components. The use of cow's milk may lead to such intestinal irritation that slight but continuous gastrointestinal bleeding occurs, resulting in anemia. Box 28-2 highlights an outcome and intervention related to infant nutrition using the terminology identified by the NOC and NIC.

Recommended Daily Dietary Allowances for the Infant

Because children's nutritional needs vary from infancy through adolescence, the recommended allowances of calories, protein, vitamins, and minerals also vary with each period of development.

The entire first year of life is one of extreme rapid growth, so a high-protein, high-calorie intake is needed. Calorie allowances can be reduced during the year from a level of 120 per kilogram of body weight at birth to approximately 100 per kilogram of body weight at the end of the first year. The number of calories must be gradually reduced during the first year; otherwise, babies tend to become overweight.

Although heredity plays a role, a baby who is overweight during the first year of life is more likely to become an obese adult than one whose weight is within normal limits. Breastfed infants gain less weight than those who are formula-fed (von Kries et al., 2000). Overfeeding in early life may produce large numbers of excess fat cells (adipocytes) used to store fat. Because these cells are permanent and remain filled with fat, once they are present, weight regulation can become difficult throughout life.

Introduction of Solid Food

From a nutritional standpoint, a normal full-term infant can thrive on a commercial iron-fortified formula or breast milk without the addition of any solid food until age 6 months. Delaying solid food until this time helps prevent overwhelming the infant's kidneys with a heavy solute load. It also may delay the development of food allergies in susceptible infants. Most parents are eager to begin feeding their infant solid food, hoping that this will help the child sleep through the night. Some parents do begin food before age 6 months without apparent ill effects, possibly because much of the food is probably not processed by the gastrointestinal tract, passing through undigested due to the immaturity of the digestive system and decreased amylase and lipase secretion (Krebs & Hambridge, 2001).

BOX 28.2

NURSING OUTCOMES AND NURSING INTERVENTIONS CLASSIFICATION: INFANT NUTRITION

NOC: Knowledge, Diet

Knowledge, diet, is defined as the extent of understanding conveyed about diet (Johnson, Maas, & Moorhead, 2000). Some specific indicators suggesting achievement of this outcome include the parent's ability to:

- Describe recommendations for infant intake, including foods allowed and not allowed
- Select appropriate foods

NIC: Teaching, Infant Nutrition

Teaching, infant nutrition, is defined as instruction on nutrition and feeding practices during the first year of life (McCloskey & Bulechek, 2000). Some important activities involved when implementing this intervention include instructing the parent/caregiver in the following at:

0 to 3 months
- Feeding only breast milk or formula for first year
- Always holding infant when feeding and never propping bottle when feeding
- Limiting water intake to ½ oz to 1 oz at a time
- Avoiding use of honey or corn syrup
- Allowing non-nutritive sucking

4 to 6 months
- Introducing solid foods without added salt or sugar and iron-fortified cereal, one food at a time
- Avoiding use of juice or sweetened drinks
- Feeding from a spoon only

7 to 9 months
- Introducing finger foods and cup when infant is able to sit up
- Having infant join family at mealtimes
- Allowing self-feeding, with observation to prevent choking
- Offering fluids after solids
- Introducing limited amounts of diluted juice in a cup
- Avoiding sugary desserts and soda

10 to 12 months
- Offering 3 meals and healthy snacks
- Beginning to wean from bottle and beginning table foods
- Avoiding fruit drinks and flavored milk
- Allowing infant to feed self with spoon

FOCUS ON FAMILY EMPOWERMENT
Tips to Help Introduce Solid Foods to Infants

Q. When and how should I begin to feed my baby solid foods?

A. Infants typically are ready for solid food at approximately 6 months of age. Use these guidelines to help when you start feeding your infant solid foods:

- Introduce one food at a time, waiting 5 to 7 days between new items.
- Introduce the food before formula or breast-feeding when the infant is hungry.
- Introduce small amounts of a new food (1 or 2 tsp) at a time.
- Respect infant food preferences; a child cannot be expected to like all new tastes equally well.
- Use only minimal to no salt and sugar on solid foods to minimize the number of additives.
- Remember that the extrusion reflex is present for the first 4 to 6 months of life, so any food placed on an infant's tongue will be pushed forward.
- To prevent aspiration, *do not* place food in bottles with formula.
- Introduce foods with a positive, "You'll like this" attitude.

Generally speaking, infants are physiologically ready for solid food when they are taking more than 32 oz (960 mL) of formula a day and do not seem satisfied, or are nursing vigorously every 3 to 4 hours and do not seem satisfied. Infants are not ready to digest complex starches until amylase is present in saliva at approximately 2 to 3 months. Biting movements begin at approximately 3 months. Chewing movements do not begin until 7 to 9 months. Thus, foods that require chewing should not be given until this age (see Focus on Family Empowerment).

Loss of Extrusion Reflex

When anything is placed on the anterior third of the newborn's tongue, it is automatically extruded or thrust out of the mouth by the tongue (extrusion reflex; Fig. 28-17). This is a life-saving reflex because it prevents infants from swallowing or aspirating foreign objects that touch the mouth. Infants extrude food when a spoonful of it is placed on the tongue in the same way. The reflex fades at 3 to 4 months. Until this time, it may be difficult to get a child to eat solids.

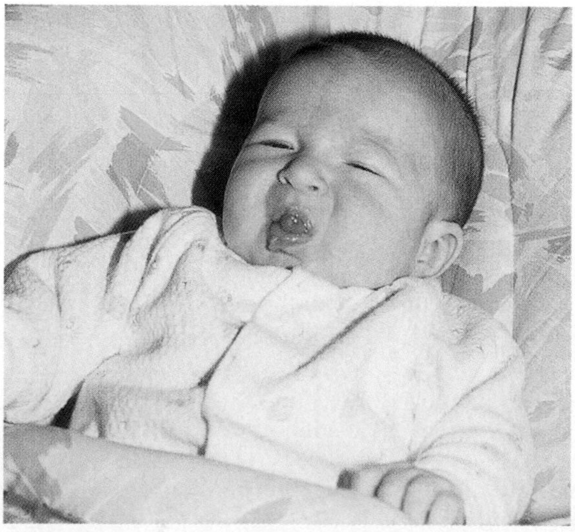

FIGURE 28.17 A 3-month-old baby demonstrates an extrusion reflex. Caution parents not to interpret this action as a food dislike but recognize it as the reflex action that it is.

Techniques for Feeding Solid Food

Table 28-4 shows the usual times and patterns for introducing solid food. Teach parents to offer new foods one at a time and allow the child to eat that item for about 1 week before introducing another new food. This system helps parents to detect possible food allergy. For example, if they start egg yolk on Monday and by Tuesday evening the child is breathing noisily or has a rash, they could suspect that the child is allergic to eggs. If two new foods had been started on Monday, it would be hard to know which one was suspect. Introducing foods one at a time also helps to establish a sense of trust in infants, because it minimizes the number of new experiences in any one day.

It is best for the first solid food feeding if the infant is held in the parent's arms as if for bottle-feeding or breastfeeding. This reduces the newness of the experience and minimizes the amount of stress associated with it. Some infants accept new experiences of this type readily, whereas other infants resist heartily. If an infant does not take readily to solid food, advise parents to wait a few days and then try again. Remind them that this is not a contest to see whose child takes cereal, vegetables, or fruit first.

Babies have distinct taste preferences even at young ages and may spit out a food because they do not like the taste. Even after the extrusion reflex has faded (at approximately 4 months), infants may appear to be spitting out food, because they have never experienced anything but liquid. This is because infants drink from a bottle or breast by pressing their tongue and the nipple against their hard palate. When an infant tries to eat solid food using the same technique, it appears that the child is spitting it out with the tongue. A parent who knows an infant's cues will be able to distinguish taste preferences from inadequate management of solid food. The Focus on Family Empow-

TABLE 28.4 Suggested Schedule for Introduction of Solid Foods

AGE (mo)	FOOD TO INTRODUCE*	RATIONALE
5–6	Iron-fortified infant cereal mixed with breast milk, orange juice, or formula	Aids in preventing iron-deficiency anemia; the least allergenic type of food; an easily digested food
7	Vegetables	Good source of vitamin A; adds new texture and flavors to diet
8	Fruit	Best source of vitamin C, good source of vitamin A; adds new texture and flavors to diet
9	Meat	Good source of protein, iron, and B vitamins
10	Egg yolk	Good source of iron

*Wheat, tomatoes, oranges, fish, and egg white should be omitted if there are allergies in the family, because these foods are most likely to cause allergies.

erment earlier in the chapter lists pointers to help make the introduction of solid foods a positive experience.

Quantities and Types of Food

Infants take different quantities of food according to their preferences and needs. A newborn's stomach can hold approximately 2 tablespoons (30 mL). At 1 month, the stomach can hold approximately 2 tablespoons (30 mL). At 1 year, the stomach can hold approximately 1 cup (240 mL). For this reason, when they begin eating solid food, infants rarely take more than 2 tablespoons (30 mL) at a time.

Cereal. The first food generally given to infants is infant cereal fortified with B vitamins and iron. These are precooked, fine dry powders to which orange juice, expressed breast milk, or infant formula is added. Orange juice is a good liquid to add because the iron in the cereal is absorbed best from an acid medium, which the orange juice supplies.

Initially, cereal should be mixed with enough fluid to make the mixture fairly liquid. As the infant adjusts to eating food from a spoon, parents can gradually thicken it. Adding sugar to cereal is unnecessary. Extra sugar in the diet can lead to diarrhea in young infants and beginning caries in older infants.

Fortified cereal costs no more than unfortified cereal, so remind parents to buy the fortified product. The first cereal introduced is usually rice cereal, because fewer children are allergic to rice products than to wheat and corn products. Usually, it is offered twice a day, morning and evening. Once the child has taken rice cereal for 1 week, another kind may be tried.

Some parents mix cereal with the infant's formula and give it to the child from a bottle. Caution parents to avoid this practice because (1) it is necessary to cut a larger hole in the bottle nipple for the cereal and milk mixture to flow freely, and there is a danger that the infant may aspirate if too big a hole is cut; (2) there is a real danger of aspiration if the parent then uses that nipple for formula without cereal added; and (3) it denies the child the opportunity of learning to eat from a spoon and experiencing different food tastes and textures.

Infant cereal is so rich in iron that parents should continue feeding it at least through the first year. Ideally, children should eat infant cereal until age 3 or 4 years, as few popularly advertised products can match the nutrients of fortified infant cereal.

Vegetables and Fruit. Because their iron content is generally higher than that of fruits, vegetables are usually the second food added to the diet (at approximately 7 months of age). Parents who have a blender, strainer, or grinder can prepare their own. They simply cook a vegetable and then blend or strain it so it does not have to be chewed. Caution parents not to add butter or salt to the preparation, because infants have difficulty digesting fats until almost the end of the first year, and the added salt is unnecessary. Additional sugar is also unnecessary. By filling ice-cube trays with the blended vegetables, parents can make a 1-week supply and defrost a cube at a time. An ice cube is approximately 1 oz, or one-fourth the size of a jar of baby food.

If parents use commercial baby food, they should feed it from a dish rather than directly from the jar. This is because if the spoon carries salivary enzymes from the infant's mouth to the food, the enzymes will liquefy what remains in the jar. Also, there is danger of transferring bacteria (principally streptococci) from the infant's mouth to the jar. Then, if the parent keeps the jar for another feeding in the next 24 hours, bacteria will multiply rapidly because the contents serve as a culture medium. Baby food jars should be refrigerated once they are opened, and manufacturers recommend that they be used no later than 48 hours after they have been opened.

When vegetables are added to the diet, they are usually offered at the noon meal. Remind parents to offer both green and yellow vegetables. Help them to remember that their own dislike of a particular vegetable does not mean their child will feel the same way about it. If they convey distaste for the food, the child will pick up on the feeling and will not like the vegetable either.

Fruit is usually offered 1 month after beginning vegetables (at approximately age 8 months). It can be given in addition to cereal for breakfast and dinner. Raw mashed banana is easy to prepare with just a fork; peaches are easily prepared in a blender. As with vegetables, parents should offer a selection so the infant is exposed to different tastes and textures.

Meat and Eggs. Meat is usually introduced at 9 months. Parents can grind a portion of the meat they have prepared for their own meal so it is tender, or they can use commercially prepared products. If they use commercial baby meat, urge them to use the plain meat products, not vegetable and meat dinners, because these contain mostly vegetables. Chicken has the advantage of being low in cholesterol, but this is not a priority with infants. Beef and pork have more iron than chicken, so encourage parents to offer these more frequently than chicken. When meat is added to the infant's diet, it is usually added as part of the evening meal in place of cereal.

Egg yolks are offered by 10 months of age. Egg yolks contain the bulk of the iron content of eggs; the white contains the bulk of protein. Egg yolk alone should be given at first, because the protein of the egg white can lead to allergy or can be difficult for the infant to digest. Eggs may be prepared by hard-boiling (then adding a little formula or breast milk to the mashed yolk to make it more liquid) or purchased as commercial baby food. Soft-boiling or poaching is not usually recommended, because Salmonella, the chief offending microorganism in eggs, may not be killed by these methods. Also, cooking makes protein easier to digest.

Table Food. With the introduction of solid food, encourage parents to establish a three-meal-a-day pattern, if that is the family's lifestyle, and to have the infant join the family at the table. Generally, encourage parents to use homemade foods rather than relying on commercially prepared junior foods, although commercial foods are now prepared without excessive additives and are convenient for parents who have little preparation time. Mashed potatoes or peas and cut-up meatloaf are examples of table foods that infants older than age 6 months like to eat and busy parents can prepare quickly. If hot dogs are offered, caution parents to cut them into small bite-size portions; otherwise, they can be aspirated. As infants begin teething, they enjoy dried bread, teething biscuits, or zwieback.

Some infants are too distracted by the activity at a family table to eat well. Parents may find that these children eat more if they are fed first and then allowed to have a small amount to "feed themselves" or a cracker to chew on while just sitting at the table and being with the family.

Remind parents that highchairs are one of the most dangerous pieces of baby equipment they own. Urge them always to fasten the restraint and never leave an infant unattended in a highchair, because even a 6-month-old can squirm out of a chair with little effort. Nurses must also keep this in mind when feeding infants in a hospital setting.

A child who adapts to change poorly may have difficulty accepting the first solid food and may have difficulty with each new food. The parents may need support to remember that the child is not conducting this struggle out of a desire for conflict but because this is a characteristic of temperament. Giving food to others is interpreted by many as giving love, so refusing food is equated with refusing love. Help parents to understand that this is not what is happening. Refusing a teaspoonful of carrots is refusing a teaspoonful of carrots, nothing more.

Most infants, however, eat hungrily. Thus, feeding problems generally are reported more frequently as a second-year or toddler problem than as an infant concern. If an infant does refuse to eat, ask the parents what foods they are offering. Have them list exactly the types and amounts of foods the child ate the day before (a 24-hour dietary recall history). It may be apparent that enough is being eaten in a day's time and that the parents' expectations are unrealistic for the child's size and age.

If intake is inadequate and the child is, indeed, a fussy eater, ask about the parents' methods of feeding. For example, ask if they are offering a bottle first and then infant food. Infants generally accept the new experience of eating from a spoon when they are hungry, not when their stomach is full. On the other hand, some babies, particularly those with an intense temperament, may be so hungry at mealtime that they cannot tolerate the frustration of spoon-feeding until some of their hunger is relieved. They may need to drink 2 or 3 oz of formula or nurse at the breast for a few minutes before they will eat a spoonful of food.

An infant who is fatigued or overstimulated may not eat well. Providing a quiet environment away from older brothers or sisters before mealtime may solve this problem.

Encourage parents not to force infants to eat if they do not seem hungry. Healthy, happy infants will be hungry at mealtime and will eat. Those who refuse a meal may be tired, distracted, or perhaps ill. Forcing only leads to regurgitation or, if they are ill, vomiting. It also can result in feeding problems or a situation in which infants refuse to eat altogether. Infants who are eating and not thriving or not eating and therefore not thriving should be examined to determine the cause. Causes include metabolic disorders and failure to thrive (see Chaps. 48 and 55).

WHAT IF? What if a parent tells you she always insists that her infant finish everything she puts on his plate so he doesn't waste food? Is always cleaning a plate a good or bad habit for parents to enforce? Why or why not?

Establishment of Healthy Eating Patterns

Some parents may need reminding that there are no hard-and-fast rules for infant feeding. The rules are only guidelines based on what seems to work well with most infants. Encourage them to individualize their approach according to the cues their child is giving them for readiness.

Weaning

Infants are capable of approximating their lips to a cup so that they can drink effectively from one at about 9 months of age. The sucking reflex begins to diminish in intensity between ages 6 and 9 months, which makes this the time to consider weaning.

To wean from formula or breast milk, the mother chooses one feeding a day and then begins offering fluid by the new method at that feeding. She should choose a time of day that is not the infant's fussy period; other than that, the time is immaterial. After approximately 1 week, when the infant has become acclimated to the one change, the mother changes a second feeding. Should an illness such as an upper respiratory infection occur or should the child have teething discomfort, there will be setbacks, so no set number of weeks should be prescribed to complete weaning. Infants usually need more fluid during hot weather than cold weather because of increased perspiration. Thus, it may be more difficult to begin weaning during the summer.

Self-Feeding

At approximately 6 months of age, infants become interested in handling a spoon and beginning to feed themselves. Their coordination, unfortunately, has not developed enough for them to use a spoon without a great deal of spilling, so they are much more adept at feeding themselves with their fingers (Fig. 28-18). Parents concerned with neatness can spread newspapers, a plastic tablecloth, or a towel on the floor around the highchair to catch most of the dropped food, and then let the child practice. When an infant becomes fatigued or frustrated by attempts at self-feeding, a parent can then quietly help without making an issue of it. Parents who insist on continuing to spoon-feed past the time the infant wants to feed himself or herself can cause the infant to balk and eat nothing. Often, a compromise is helpful. If a parent gives the infant a spoon, the child can poke at a cereal dish with it while the parent continues to offer him or her bites from a second spoon. In this way, the child is "in charge" of the feeding yet receptive to taking food from the parent.

When infants no longer attempt to feed themselves at a meal but merely begin to play with their food by squeezing it through their fingers or dabbing it in their hair, it is time to end the meal. This behavior indicates that they have had enough.

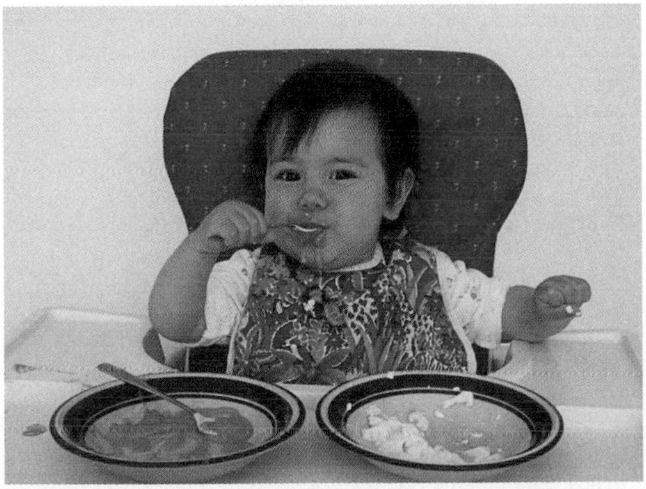

FIGURE 28.18 Self-feeding is not always a neat process for an infant.

Adequate Intake With a Vegetarian Diet

The infant eating a vegetarian diet should continue to be breastfed or ingest an iron-fortified, balanced, commercial formula for the entire first year. If a milk allergy is present, a soy-based formula can be used. When solid foods are added at 6 months, an assortment of foods should be provided, including vegetables such as avocados, potatoes, and broccoli; fruits such as apples, prunes (high in iron), and bananas; infant cereal; tofu; wheat germ; legumes; brewer's yeast; and synthetic vitamin D. Feeding a fortified cereal through the first year will ensure that iron stores are built. If the diet is to include dairy products, these can be added toward the end of the first year as usual.

Because vegetarian diets are high in fiber, they may cause infants to have more frequent and looser-than-normal bowel movements. Teach parents to change diapers frequently to avoid skin irritation. Using less fibrous, more concentrated forms of protein, such as tofu and powdered nuts rather than cereal mixtures, can minimize this problem.

A sound vegetarian diet can be easily designed for the older infant who prefers finger foods, because many vegetables, fruits, and grains (e.g., pieces of oranges, peaches, tomatoes, and crackers) are easily eaten this way (Messina & Mangels, 2001).

✔ CHECKPOINT QUESTIONS

16. At what age are solid foods usually introduced?
17. What is usually the first solid food given to infants?
18. How long should breast-feeding be continued?

Promoting Sensory Stimulation

Vision

Teach parents that they should make a point of initiating eye-to-eye contact with newborns right from the beginning as a method of stimulating vision as well as promoting socialization.

Most parents are aware that infants enjoy mobiles and also a crib mirror (Fig. 28-19). Occasionally they may overdo the amount of visual stimulation, overwhelming their infant with too many patterns and objects dangling above the crib. Ask parents to consider how all these trappings must appear from the infant's view.

In a hospital environment, assess that an infant is receiving visual stimulation. Add or reduce objects as appropriate. If the child's movement is restricted in any way, move the position of the mobile from time to time. Photos of family members brought from home or pictures drawn by older brothers or sisters can be posted near the infant's crib. Ask the parents if there are any items from home that the infant would normally see during the course of the day while being fed, changed, or bathed. It may be possible to bring these into the hospital for visual stimulation.

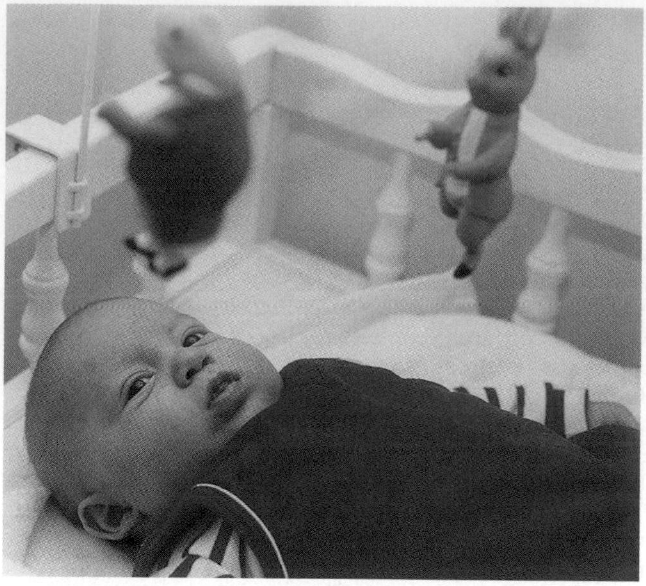

FIGURE 28.19 A 2-month-old infant enjoys watching a simple mobile.

Hearing

Infants appear to enjoy soft, musical sounds or soft, cooing voices; they are startled by harsh, raucous rattles or loud bangs. Parents should choose for the infant's first toys ones that make these types of welcoming sounds. Tape recordings of maternal heart sounds can be soothing to very young infants. For the hospitalized infant, an audiotape of family voices might be a soothing reminder of their presence. Encourage parents to read to their child daily from the beginning of life through the early school-age years, not only because the sound of the parent's voice is comforting but also because this increases language development dramatically (see Focus on Communication).

Touch

An infant needs to be touched so he or she experiences skin-to-skin contact. Clothes should feel comfortable and soft rather than rough; diapers should be dry rather than wet. Teach parents to handle infants with assurance and gentleness. Remind parents that right now their child is a baby; he or she will have time enough to become a strong man or woman later.

Because premature infants need to be kept warm while being held, parents may be advised to cuddle an infant next to their bare chest ("kangaroo care"). This is also effective with term infants as a way of promoting close physical contact (see Focus on Cultural Competence).

Taste

Infants demonstrate that they have an acute sense of taste by turning away from or spitting out a taste they do not enjoy. Urge parents to make mealtime a time for fostering

FOCUS ON COMMUNICATION

Mrs. Simpson is the mother of a 2-month-old child. You listen to her while she dresses her son after a clinic visit.

Less Effective Communication

Mrs. Simpson: Don't move. And take your thumb out of your mouth. I have to put on your sweater. All right. Let's go.

Mrs. Ortello is also the mother of a 2-month-old child. You listen to her as she dresses her son as well.

More Effective Communication

Mrs. Ortello: We're going bye-bye. First, we're getting dressed. Next, we'll pick up Daddy. Then we're going shopping. Remember shopping? That's when you ride in the red car seat while I buy things. I hope you have my shopping gene because we do a lot of shopping. This is your yellow sweater Aunt Mary gave you. Remember her? The funny lady we visited yesterday? The one who said you were cute except that you have no hair? Okay. We're ready. As soon as I put on my coat, we'll go.

These two women's approaches to talking to their children differ because the second mother seems to understand and appreciate that infants enjoy the sound of a parent's voice. In the first scenario, the mother is only giving instructions. Which infant might you anticipate will develop the largest vocabulary? Which one will be more aware of the names of colors sooner? Nurses can be instrumental in assisting parents with more effective communication techniques such as this.

FOCUS ON CULTURAL COMPETENCE

Childrearing practices during the first year vary from country to country. One difference is in the way mothers carry their infants. Many mothers tend to carry infants in their arms and put them down to work. Native American mothers, in contrast, may use a papoose board; South American women may carry the infant in a shoulder sling or on their hip. These positions allow the woman to continue to work while holding the infant close.

The amount of infant bathing that is done is also inconsistent across cultures. In the United States, most infants are bathed daily. In colder climates or countries where clean water is not readily available, however, infant bathing is very limited. The use of diapers varies also. In hot climates, infants are often not diapered. Being aware of these cultural differences leads to better understanding of the reasons for an individual woman's particular method of childrearing.

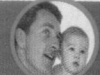

trust as well as supplying nutrition by being certain that feedings are done at the infant's pace and the amount offered fits the child's needs and not the parent's idea of how much should be eaten.

Smell

Infants can smell accurately within 1 or 2 hours after birth. They respond to an irritating smell by drawing back from it. They appear to enjoy pleasant odors and learn early in life to identify the familiar smell of breast milk. Teach parents to be alert to substances that cause sneezing when sprayed into the air, such as room deodorizers or cleaning compounds, and to keep irritating odors out of the child's environment.

Promoting Infant Development in Daily Activities

In the first year, caring for the infant—feeding, bathing, dressing, and so forth—occupies what may seem like nearly all of the parents' waking hours. Worrying about their infant's sleep patterns may take up the rest of their time, often because the parents are not getting enough sleep themselves. All of these basic care-related activities provide important opportunities for caregivers and infants to get to know one another and to become used to each other's personalities and patterns. Nurses play a key role in teaching parents about these activities and stressing their importance. Box 28-3 highlights an outcome and intervention related to infant care using the terminology identified by the NOC and NIC.

Bathing

Except in very hot weather, an infant does not need a bath every day. If a parent is tired and would not enjoy bath time or if some days are just too rushed, a complete bath can be omitted, with only the infant's face, hands, and diaper area washed. Some infants do need their head and scalp washed frequently (every day or every other day) to prevent **seborrhea,** a scaly scalp condition often called cradle cap. If seborrhea lesions do develop, they adhere to the scalp in yellow, crusty patches. The skin beneath them may be slightly erythematous. The patches can be softened by oiling the scalp with mineral oil or petroleum jelly and leaving it on overnight. The crusts can then be removed by shampooing the hair the next morning. A soft toothbrush or fine-toothed comb can be used to help remove crusts.

Bath time should be fun for an infant and can serve many functions other than just the obvious one of cleanliness (Fig. 28-20). Especially during the second half of the first year, a child enjoys poking at soap bubbles on the surface of the water or playing with bath toys. Bathtime also helps an infant learn different textures and sensations and provides an opportunity to exercise and kick, as well as a good opportunity for a parent to touch and communicate with the child.

BOX 28.3

NURSING OUTCOMES AND NURSING INTERVENTIONS CLASSIFICATION: INFANT CARE

NOC: Knowledge, Infant

Knowledge, infant, is defined as the extent of understanding conveyed about caring for a baby up to 12 months (Johnson, Maas, & Moorhead, 2000). Some specific indicators suggesting achievement of this outcome include the parent's ability to describe the following:

- Normal infant characteristics and development
- Proper holding and positioning
- Infant safety measures
- Feeding choices and techniques
- Signs of problems such as dehydration or jaundice
- Infant bathing, diapering, cord care, temperature taking, sleep-wake patterns, communication, stimulation methods, and relaxation techniques
- Family adjustments to addition of infant
- Considerations when choosing a childcare provider
- Community resources for infant care

NIC: Parent Education, Infant

Parent education, infant, is defined as instruction on nurturing and physical care needed during the first year of life (McCloskey & Bulechek, 2000). Some important activities involved when implementing this intervention include the following:

- Determining parents' knowledge and readiness to learn, along with continued monitoring of learning needs
- Providing anticipatory guidance about developmental changes and behavioral characteristics
- Assisting with ways to integrate infant into family system
- Teaching parents skills to care for infant, including formula preparation and selection, use of pacifiers, addition of solid foods to diet, fluoride supplementation, dentition, oral hygiene, elimination patterns, and sleep patterns
- Demonstrating ways to stimulate infant's development
- Encouraging holding, cuddling, massaging, touching, talking, reading, playing, and providing pleasurable auditory and visual stimulation
- Providing examples of appropriate toys
- Assisting with interpreting infant cues
- Demonstrating infant's abilities and strengths, quieting techniques
- Monitoring parents' skill in recognizing infant's needs and reinforcing caregiver role behaviors
- Providing information about safety needs in the home and car

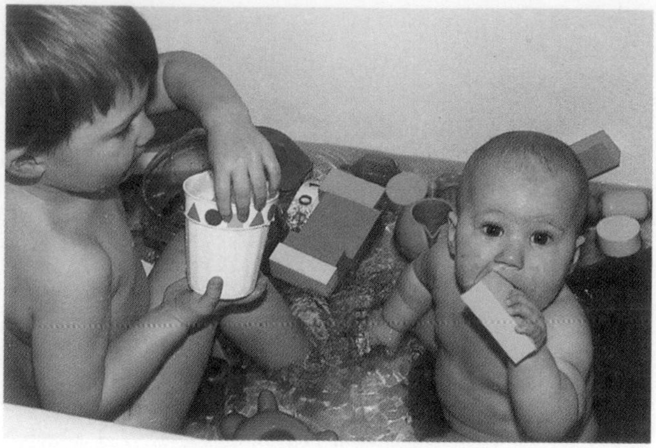

FIGURE 28.20 An 8-month-old enjoys bathtime with his big brother, while his parents carefully watch.

Diaper-Area Care

The most effective means of promoting good diaper-area hygiene is to change diapers frequently, about every 2 to 4 hours. However, it is rarely good practice to interrupt the child's sleep to change diapers. If an infant develops a rash from sleeping in wet diapers, air drying or sleeping without a diaper may be a solution.

At each diaper change, the parents should wash the skin with clear water or with a commercial alcohol-free diaper wipe (and perfume-free if the infant has sensitive skin), then pat or allow to air dry. Routinely using an ointment such as Desitin or A & D ointment to keep urine and feces away from the infant's skin is good prophylaxis. Parents do not need to use baby powder. If they choose to, advise them to sprinkle the powder on their hands first, and then apply it to the infant's skin. Caution them not to shake the powder on the infant, to reduce the possibility of aspiration. The container should be placed out of the infant's reach afterward.

Care of Teeth

It is well accepted that exposing developing teeth to fluoride is one of the most effective ways to promote healthy tooth formation and prevent tooth decay. The most important time for children to receive fluoride is between 6 months and 12 years of age. A water level of 0.6 ppm fluoride is recommended because this is the level that protects tooth enamel yet does not lead to staining of teeth. In communities where the water supply does not provide enough fluoride, the use of an oral fluoride supplement beginning at 6 months or the use of fluoride toothpaste or rinses after tooth eruption is recommended (AAP, 2001).

Teach parents to ask about the presence of fluoride in the drinking water in their community and help them to determine what, if any, supplementation is necessary. Breast-fed infants do not receive a great deal of fluoride from breast milk, so it may be recommended that they receive fluoride drops once a day. Teach parents to begin "brushing" even before teeth erupt by rubbing a soft washcloth over the gum pads. This eliminates plaque and reduces the presence of bacteria, creating a clean environment for the arrival of the first teeth. Once teeth erupt, all surfaces should be brushed with a soft brush or washcloth once or twice a day. Children lack the coordination to brush effectively until they are school-age, so parents must be responsible for this activity well past infancy. Toothpaste is not necessary for the infant, because it is the scrubbing that removes the plaque.

The initial dental checkup should be made by 2 years of age; checkups should continue at 6-month intervals throughout adulthood.

Dressing

Parents should choose clothing for infants that is easy to launder and simply constructed, so that dressing and undressing are not a struggle. Infants enjoy kicking and making gross body movements, so their clothing should not be binding. When they begin to creep, they need long pants to protect their knees. Until they begin to walk, they need only soft-soled shoes or merely socks or booties to keep their feet warm. Even when they begin walking, the soles of their shoes need only be firm enough to protect their feet against rough surfaces. Extremely hard soles and high ankle sides are unnecessary.

Sleep

Sleep needs and habits vary greatly among infants, but most require 10 to 12 hours of sleep at night and one or several naps during the day. Parents are usually advised to let the baby sleep in a separate space rather than in their bed so the parents do not awaken at every toss and squeak. Doing so allows infants to learn to quiet themselves and go back to sleep should they awaken briefly. This may help prevent sleep problems such as night waking in the future. Caution parents not to place pillows in an infant's bed to avoid suffocation. Always place an infant on his or her back to sleep because this position markedly reduces the incidence of sudden infant death syndrome (SIDS; Thilo & Rosenberg, 2001). See Chapter 26 for further discussion.

Exercise

Infants benefit from outings in a carriage or stroller because sunlight provides a natural source of vitamin D. In hot weather, parents need to protect the infant from sunburn by exposing the child to the sun for only very short periods, beginning with 3 to 5 minutes the first day, a little more the next day, and so on up to 15 to 20 minutes at a time. The sun is most intense between 10 AM and 3 PM, so early mornings and late afternoons are the best times for infants to be outside. These short time spans are necessary because the use of sunscreen is not recommended in children until they are at least 6 months old.

Toward the end of the first year, infants need space to crawl and then to walk, such as in an enclosed outdoor play space. In addition to providing fresh air, going for leisurely walks while pointing out the sights of the world—trees, birds, dogs, houses, neighbors—helps children develop language.

Parents can judge how much outdoor clothing to put on an infant by how much they need themselves. If the adult needs a winter coat, the infant will need a snowsuit; sweaters may be adequate for both; if the adult needs no outer clothing, the infant probably doesn't either.

It is not necessary to enroll infants in formal exercise programs for them to secure adequate exercise. Such programs may put unusual strain on muscles and tendons. Infants using infant walkers must be closely supervised, because they can be injured if they maneuver the walker too near a stairway and fall.

Promoting Healthy Family Functioning

A primary task of parents during the infant year is to learn to interpret their infant's cues to decipher his or her needs. It is helpful if they can learn early on to perceive the infant as a separate individual with his or her own needs. This becomes an easier task by 2 months, when infants can indicate by their particular cry whether they are feeling cold, hungry, wet, or lonely. Parents spend a great deal of time with their infant in these first months, which gives them the opportunity to learn and recognize nonverbal cues and to become aware of their baby's needs.

Parental Concerns and Problems Related to Normal Infant Development

Some of the difficulties that parents have in evaluating the health of infants are shown in Table 28-5. New parents may need reassurance and answers to questions about childcare procedures or health during the infant period because they have not yet learned their child's cues. However, the need for reassurance may be just as great in experienced parents. The unique characteristics of each child require some adjustment from parents.

Teething

Most infants have little difficulty with teething, but some appear very distressed. Generally, the gums are sore and tender before a new tooth breaks the surface. As soon as the tooth is through, the tenderness passes.

Because of this pain, infants can be resistant to chewing for a day or two and be slightly cranky, possibly because they are a little hungry from not eating as much as usual. High fever, seizures, vomiting or diarrhea, and earache are never normal signs of teething. An infant with any of these symptoms has an underlying infection or disease process requiring further evaluation.

Many over-the-counter medicines are sold for teething pain. As a rule, their use should be discouraged if they contain benzocaine, a topical anesthetic, because if applied too far back in the throat, this could interfere with the gag reflex. Acetaminophen (Tylenol), 10 to 15 mg/kg every 4 hours, up to four times a day, may be used for this discomfort. Always encourage the parents to check with the infant's health care provider before giving any over-the-counter drug this way. Teething rings that can be placed in the refrigerator provide soothing coolness against the tender gums. An infant who is teething will place almost any object in the mouth, so parents must screen articles within the baby's reach to be sure they are edible or safe to chew on.

Thumb Sucking

Sucking is a surprisingly strong need, so strong that sonograms demonstrate fetal thumb sucking in utero. Many infants begin to suck a thumb or finger at about 3 months of age and continue the habit through the first few years of life. The sucking reflex peaks at 6 to 8 months, whereas thumb sucking peaks at about 18 months.

Parents can be assured that thumb sucking is normal and does not deform the jaw line as long as it stops by school age. It does not cause "baby talk" or any of the other symptoms commonly attributed to it. The best approach is to be certain the infant has adequate sucking pleasure and then to ignore thumb sucking. Making an issue of it rarely causes the child to stop; if anything, it usually intensifies and prolongs it.

Use of Pacifiers

Whether to use pacifiers is a question that parents must settle for themselves, depending on how they feel about them and their infant's needs. Infants rarely have such a

TABLE 28.5 Common Difficulties Parents Experience in Evaluating the Health of Infants

DIFFICULTY	SUGGESTIONS FOR IMPROVING ASSESSMENT
Evaluating pain	Infants manifest pain by fussiness. They can reveal arm and leg pain by immobility of the body part; ear pain by brushing or tugging at the ear; stomach pain by pulling up the legs against the abdomen.
Evaluating degree of reduced activity	Lack of interest in smiling or interaction is an important observation. Increased sleeping or lying supine with legs nonflexed (frog-legged) as if exhausted is important.
Evaluating infant temperature	All parents should learn how to take an axillary or tympanic temperature so they can report a specific degree of fever rather than a subjective finding, such as "feels hot."
Evaluating amount of vomiting or diarrhea	Knowing the number of times vomiting and/or diarrhea has occurred is important. Estimating amount in comparisons with what the child has eaten is helpful as well as estimating an amount (a cupful, etc.). Knowing whether diapers are "soaked" or "stained" with stools is important in estimating amount. Caution parents that vomiting and diarrhea are always serious in infants.

need for sucking that they must have a pacifier in their mouth constantly. Discussing a few pros and cons with the parents clarifies the subject.

An infant who completes a feeding and still seems restless and discontent, who actively searches for something to put into the mouth, and who sucks on hands and clothes may need a pacifier. Babies who have colic crave sucking and enjoy pacifiers because their abdomen hurts, and they interpret this as a hunger sensation. If the child is formula-fed, the parents should check the nipples to be certain that the holes are small and the rubber is sturdy, so that the infant can suck hard enough to derive pleasure. If the nipples are satisfactory, parents could offer a pacifier after feeding for more sucking. Theoretically, the child whose sucking needs are met in infancy will not crave as much oral stimulation later in life and is less likely to become a pencil chewer, cigarette smoker, nail biter, or the like.

The use of pacifiers has been associated with an increased incidence of otitis media (Warren et al., 2001). A major drawback of pacifiers is the problem of cleanliness. They tend to fall on the floor or sidewalk and are then put back into the infant's mouth. If not well constructed, they may come apart and be aspirated. Hanging the pacifier on a string around the infant's neck could cause strangulation.

Parents should attempt to wean the child from a pacifier any time after 3 months of age and certainly during the time that the sucking reflex is fading at 6 to 9 months. Weaning after this age is difficult because the pacifier becomes a comfort mechanism, like a warm blanket or fuzzy toy to which a child may cling.

Head Banging

Some infants rhythmically bang their heads against the bars of a crib for a period of time before falling asleep. This is distressing behavior for parents. Besides fearing that children will hurt themselves, some parents may have heard that blind children or those with mental illness do this and worry that their child is ill in some way.

Head banging in this limited fashion—beginning during the second half of the first year of life and continuing through to the preschool period, associated with naptime or bedtime, and lasting under 15 minutes—can be considered normal. Children use this measure to relax and fall asleep. Investigating stress factors operating in the house may be helpful. If some of them can be relieved (e.g., parents' overestimation of the child's development, marital discord, illness in another family member), the head banging may decrease, or it may have already become such a strong habit that it will persist for months or even years.

Advise parents to pad the rails of cribs so infants cannot hurt themselves, and reassure them that this is a normal mechanism for relief of tension in children of this age. No therapy should be necessary. Excessive head banging done to the exclusion of normal development or activity, or head banging past the preschool period, suggests a pathologic basis, and such children need a referral for counseling and further evaluation.

Sleep Problems

Sleep problems develop in early infancy because of colic or because an otherwise healthy infant takes longer than usual to adjust to sleeping through the night. Breast-fed babies tend to wake more often than those who are formula-fed because breast milk is more easily digested and so infants become hungry sooner. In late infancy, the problem of waking at night and remaining awake for an hour or more becomes common. Although the infant may be content and not cry during this time, parents are reluctant to sleep while the child is awake and thus parents may become extremely fatigued. This is an increasing concern because more and more families today consist of two wage-earning parents; there is no time for parents to nap during the day to make up for sleep lost at night. Suggestions for eliminating or at least coping with night waking are (1) delay bedtime by 1 hour; (2) shorten an afternoon sleep period; (3) do not respond immediately to infants at night so that they may have time to fall back to sleep on their own; and (4) provide soft toys or music to allow infants to play quietly alone during this wakeful time. Reassuring parents that infants take varying lengths of time to adjust to night sleeping is helpful in assuring them their child is normal. Suggesting that parents use the time they are awake at night (e.g., solve a problem at work, plan a shopping list) may help them view the situation as a constructive time rather than a problem.

Constipation

Breastfed infants are rarely constipated because their stools tend to be loose. Constipation may occur in formula-fed infants if their diet is deficient in fluid. This can be corrected simply with the addition of more fluid.

Some parents misinterpret the normal pushing movements of a newborn to be constipation. When infants defecate, their faces do turn red, and they grimace and grunt. As long as stools are not hard and contain no evidence of fresh blood (as might occur with a rectal fissure), this is normal infant behavior.

If constipation persists beyond 5 or 6 months of age, encourage parents to check with the infant's health care provider about measures to relieve this. Adding foods with bulk, such as fruits or vegetables, and increasing fluid intake generally relieves the problem. Apple juice (3 or 4 oz) or prune juice (0.5 to 1 oz daily) may be given as a temporary measure.

All infants with a history of constipation for more than 1 week should be examined for an anal fissure or tight anal sphincter. Softening stools and thereby relieving the pain of defecation often solves the problem and helps the fissure to heal. If an unusually tight anal sphincter exists, parents will be given instructions to manually dilate the sphincter two or three times daily until it dilates sufficiently. Hirschsprung's disease (aganglionic megacolon, or lack of nerve innervation to a portion of the colon) may be manifested early in life as constipation. If no stool is present in the rectum of a constipated infant on rectal examination, this disease is suggested (Mascarenhas, 2000). A careful history must then be taken to assess for other symptoms of Hirschsprung's disease: ribbonlike stools, bouts of diarrhea, and a distended abdomen (see Chap. 45).

Chronic constipation also may occur in children with congenital hypothyroidism (decreased functioning of the thyroid gland). Therefore, an infant with constipation also should be carefully observed for characteristic signs of hypothyroidism, such as lethargy, protruding tongue, and failure to meet developmental milestones (see Chap. 48). Infants with either Hirschsprung's disease or hypothyroidism need therapy to correct the disorder.

Loose Stools

Many new parents are unfamiliar with the consistency or color of normal newborn stools, so they mistakenly report normal stooling as diarrhea. Stools of breastfed infants are generally softer than those of formula-fed infants. If a mother takes a laxative while breastfeeding, the infant's stools may be very loose. The infant who is formula-fed may have loose stools if the formula is not diluted properly.

Occasionally, loose stools may begin with the introduction of solid food, such as fruit. Malabsorption syndrome (celiac disease), or inability to digest fat, may manifest itself first by loose stools and a distended abdomen and deficiency of fat-soluble vitamins (see Chap. 45).

When talking to a parent about loose stools, ask about the duration of the loose stools, the number of stools per day, their color and consistency, and whether there is any mucus or blood in them. Is there associated fever, cramping, or vomiting? Does the infant continue to eat well? Appear well? Seem to be thriving? Is the infant wetting at least six diapers daily?

Infants with associated signs and symptoms such as fever, cramping, vomiting, loss of appetite, a decrease in voiding, and weight loss should be examined by a health care provider because this suggests an infectious process. Dehydration occurs rapidly in a small infant who is not eating and is losing body fluid through loose stools.

Colic

Colic is paroxysmal abdominal pain that generally occurs in infants under 3 months of age (McGlaughlin, 2000). The infant cries loudly and pulls the legs up against the abdomen. The infant's face becomes red and flushed, the fists clench, and the abdomen is tense. If offered a bottle, the infant will suck vigorously for a few minutes as if starved, then stop as another wave of intestinal pain occurs.

The cause of colic is unclear. It may occur in susceptible infants from overfeeding or from swallowing too much air while feeding. Formula-fed babies are more likely to have colic than breastfed babies, possibly because they swallow more air while drinking (Carey, 2000).

Although infants continue to thrive despite colic, the condition should not be dismissed as unimportant. It is a distressing and frightening problem for parents because the infant not only appears to be in acute pain, but the distress persists for hours, usually into the middle of the night, so that no one in the family gets adequate rest. This is a difficult beginning to a parent–child relationship, which needs to be strong and binding for the parents to enjoy parenting and for the infant to thrive in their care.

Take a thorough history of the infant with signs of colic because intestinal obstruction or infection may mimic an attack of colic and be misinterpreted by the casual interviewer. Ask parents about the duration of the problem and its frequency; it usually lasts up to 3 hours a day and occurs at least 3 days every week. Ask what happens just before the attack (e.g., if it occurs after feeding), and ask the parent to describe the attack itself and associated symptoms. Document the number and type of bowel movements, because bowel movements are not abnormal with colic. Constipation; narrow, ribbonlike stools; and the presence of blood or mucus in the stool suggest other problems. A family medical history is important to obtain because allergy to milk may simulate colic.

Determine the baby's feeding pattern: breastfed or bottle-fed; if bottle-fed, ask about the type of formula and how it is prepared. Ask parents how they are feeding the baby and whether they are burping the infant adequately after feeding. Are they holding the baby firmly upright so air bubbles can rise? For the breastfed baby, a change in maternal diet (e.g., avoiding "gassy" foods) might be helpful to reduce or limit colicky periods. It may be helpful to recommend that both breast- and formula-fed infants receive small, frequent feedings to prevent distention and discomfort. Offering a pacifier may be comforting.

Some recommend placing a hot water bottle on the infant's stomach for comfort, but this should be discouraged. A basic rule for any abdominal discomfort is to avoid heat in case appendicitis is developing. This is highly unlikely in so young an infant, but parents will remember they once used heat and may use it again when the child is older. Hot water bottles and heating pads also might burn the delicate skin of infants.

Changing formula bottles to the type with disposable bags that collapse as the baby sucks may help minimize the amount of air swallowed. Taking infants for car rides is often reported as being helpful in soothing colicky babies. Some music boxes simulate the sound of a heartbeat, which also may be helpful.

It is important to think of colic as a family problem or else a vicious circle may gradually begin. The infant cries and the parents become tense and unsure of themselves. The infant senses the tension and develops more colic. Help parents plan relief time from infant care to relieve their stress level and prevent this cycle.

In most infants, colic disappears almost magically at 3 months of age, probably because it becomes easier to digest food and the infant maintains a more upright position by this time, which allows less gas to form (see Focus on Nursing Care Planning).

Spitting Up

Almost all infants spit up, although formula-fed babies appear to do it more than breastfed babies. Parents who did not handle their infant much in the health care facility where the child was born may discover spitting up

FOCUS ON *Nursing Care Planning*

AN INFANT WITH COLIC

The parents bring their 2-month-old son in for a routine health maintenance visit. Their major concern is what to do about his crying at night.

Assessment: Well-proportioned 2-month-old boy. Height and weight at 50th percentile on growth chart. Bottle feeding with intake of approximately 4 oz of commercial formula every 4 hours. Experiencing 2 or 3 soft yellow bowel movements daily. "He's been crying every night lately from about 6 P.M. till 2 A.M. His face gets red, and he pulls his legs up against his belly. I give him a bottle, he sucks for a few minutes like he's starving, and then stops and starts to cry, pulling his legs up again. We've tried everything but my husband and I are exhausted. We're at the end of our rope." Physical examination within normal limits. Diagnosis of colic is made.

Nursing Diagnosis: Compromised family coping related to difficulty managing infant crying episodes

Outcome Identification: Parents will demonstrate positive coping measures by the end of 1 week.

Outcome Evaluation: Parents state increased feelings of control over situation; identify measures for stress reduction

Interventions	Rationale
1. Educate the parents about the common characteristics of colic, including duration, timing, and intensity of crying, and bottle-feeding as a possible factor in the presence of normal stool passage.	1. Education promotes better understanding of the problem, alleviating some of the stress and anxiety associated with it.
2. Reassure parents that they are not the cause of the child's discomfort.	2. Parents may feel guilty if they are unable to soothe their child. Reassurance that the problem is not their fault can aid in objective problem solving.
3. Caution parents that crying in infants produces frustration in adults. Help the parents plan constructive ways to deal with the crying.	3. Acknowledging their frustration helps to validate their feelings. A plan of action provides opportunities to regain some control over the situation.
4. Help the parents devise some respite time.	4. Time away can help relieve feelings of frustration and tension.
5. Urge the parents to call the health care provider for suggestions if they need further help. Explain that colic generally resolves by 3 months of age.	5. Support from health care providers can aid in coping. Knowing that colic is usually a time-limited problem provides the parents with the knowledge that there is an end in sight.

Nursing Diagnosis: Health-seeking behaviors related to appropriate measures for colic relief

Outcome Identification: Parents will verbalize increased confidence in caring for infant within 1 week.

Outcome Evaluation: Parents state that infant appears playful after feeding; sleeps at least for some period between 6 P.M. and 2 A.M.

(continued)

Interventions	Rationale
1. Support parents in attempts to allow infant to cry for short periods (e.g., 5 to 10 minutes) before comforting.	1. Infants can learn self-quieting abilities to comfort themselves.
2. Have parents relate steps used to prepare formula and demonstrate bottle-feeding and burping techniques. Review methods for proper formula preparation, bottle holding, and burping.	2. Proper techniques can minimize the amount of air swallowed during feeding and possible subsequent development of intestinal gas.
3. Advise parents to feed the infant in a quiet environment.	3. Quiet environmental surroundings are soothing to the infant.
4. Recommend small, frequent feedings.	4. Small, frequent feedings prevent distention and discomfort.
5. Instruct parents to place the infant in an infant seat or upright position for ½ hour after feeding, gently rock or rub the infant's back or abdomen, use music boxes, or take the infant for a ride in the car.	5. An upright position prevents distention. The other measures provide comfort and are soothing to the infant.
6. Suggest the use of a pacifier.	6. Sucking on a pacifier may increase peristalsis and promote passage of gas through the intestine.
7. Advise parents to contact the health care provider if these measures are ineffective. Anticipate the need for possible pharmacologic therapy.	7. Medications to reduce colic symptoms should be given to an infant only under the direction of a health care provider.

only after they take the baby home. They may interpret this as vomiting or think the infant is developing an infection. Ask them to describe carefully what they mean by "spitting up." How long has the baby been doing it? How frequently? What is the appearance of the spit-up milk? Almost all milk that is spit up smells at least faintly sour, but it should not contain blood or bile.

The baby who spits up a mouthful of milk (rolling down the chin) two or three times a day (or sometimes after every meal) is experiencing normal, early-infancy spitting up. Associated signs such as diarrhea, abdominal cramps, fever, cough, cold, or loss of activity suggest illness. If the infant is spitting up so forcefully that the milk is projected 3 or 4 feet away, it may be beginning pyloric stenosis (an abnormally tight valve between the stomach and duodenum), which requires surgical intervention. If the spitting up is a large amount with each feeding, parents may be describing gastroesophageal reflux, in which a lax cardiac sphincter and esophagus allow regurgitation of gastric contents into the esophagus. This also requires medical attention (see Chap. 45).

Burping the baby thoroughly after a feeding often limits spitting up. Parents may try sitting the infant in an infant chair for half an hour after feeding. Changing formulas generally is of little value. Reassure parents that spitting up decreases in amount as the baby becomes better at coordinating his or her swallowing and digestive processes (the cardiac sphincter matures). In the meantime, a bib can protect the baby's clothing and the parent. After a few months, the child will naturally stay in an upright position longer, and gravity will help to correct the problem.

Diaper Dermatitis

Some infants have such sensitive skin that diaper dermatitis (diaper rash) is a problem from the first few days of life. It occurs for a number of reasons.

When parents do not change the child's diaper frequently, feces are left in contact with skin, and irritation may result in the perianal area. Urine that is left in diapers too long breaks down into ammonia, a chemical that is extremely irritating to infant skin. Ammonia dermatitis of this type is generally a problem in the second half of the first year of life, when the infant is producing a larger quantity of urine than before. For some infants, however, it is a problem from the first week.

Frequent diaper changing, applying A & D or Desitin ointment, and exposing the diaper area to air may relieve the problem. Some infants may have to sleep without diapers at night to control the problem.

Whenever the entire diaper area is erythematous and irritated so that the outline of the diaper on the skin can be identified, one must suspect an allergy to the material in the diaper or to laundry products if a commercially washed or home-washed diaper is being used. Changing the brand or type of diaper or washing solution usually alleviates the problem.

If a diaper area is covered with lesions that are bright red, with or without oozing, last longer than 3 days, and appear as red pinpoint lesions, suspect a fungal (monilial or candidiasis) infection. This is discussed in Chapter 43.

Miliaria

Miliaria, or prickly heat rash, occurs most often in warm weather or when babies are overdressed or sleep in overheated rooms. Clusters of pinpoint, reddened papules with occasional vesicles and pustules surrounded by erythema usually appear on the neck first and may spread upward to around the ear and onto the face or down onto the trunk.

Bathing the infant twice a day during hot weather, particularly if a small amount of baking soda is added to the bath water, may improve the rash. Eliminating sweating by reducing the amount of clothing on the infant or lowering the room temperature should bring almost immediate improvement and prevent further eruption.

Baby-Bottle Syndrome

Putting an infant to bed with a bottle can result in aspiration or decay of all the upper teeth and the lower posterior teeth (Thilo & Rosenberg, 2001; Fig. 28-21). Decay occurs because while the infant sleeps, liquid from the propped bottle continuously soaks the upper front teeth and lower back teeth (the lower front teeth are protected by the tongue). The problem, called **baby-bottle syndrome,** is most serious when the bottle is filled with sugar water, formula, milk, or fruit juice. The carbohydrate in these solutions ferments to organic acids that demineralize the tooth enamel until it decays.

To prevent this problem, advise parents never to put their baby to bed with a bottle. If parents insist that the bottle is necessary, encourage them to fill it with water and use a nipple with a smaller hole to prevent the baby from receiving a large amount of fluid. If the baby refuses to drink anything but milk, the parents might dilute the milk with water more and more each night until the bottle is down to water only.

Obesity in Infants

Obesity in infants is defined as a weight greater than the 90th to 95th percentile on a standardized height/weight chart. Obesity occurs when there is an increase in the number of fat cells due to excessive calorie intake. Preventing obesity in infants is important because the extra fat cells formed at this time are likely to remain through childhood and even into adulthood. If the child becomes obese because of overingesting milk, iron-deficiency anemia may also be present because of the low iron content of both breast and commercial milk. Once infant obesity begins, it is difficult to reverse, so prevention is the key (von Kries et. al., 2000).

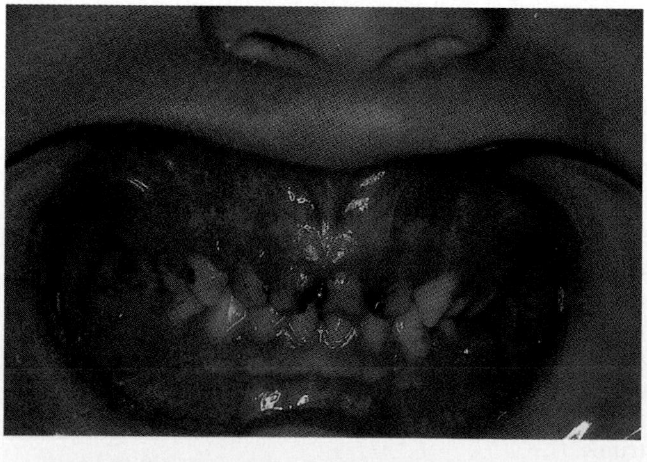

FIGURE 28.21 Baby-bottle syndrome. Notice the extensive decay in the upper teeth.

Overfeeding in infancy often occurs because parents were taught to eat everything on their plate, and they continue to instill this concept in their children. This appears to be the case most often with formula-fed infants whose parents urge them to empty their bottle or finish a cereal serving. It can occur any time parents automatically feed an infant when the child cries, rather than investigating what the cry might really mean. An infant should take no more than 32 oz of formula daily. When solid food is introduced, a bottle of water can be substituted for formula at one feeding. Nonfat milk should not be given because it contains so little fat that essential fatty acid requirements may not be sufficient to ensure cell growth.

Another way to help prevent obesity is to add a source of fiber, such as whole-grain cereal and raw fruit, to the infant's diet. These prolong the stomach-emptying time and can thus help reduce food intake. Caution parents about giving obese infants foods with high amounts of refined sugars, such as pudding, cake, cookies, and candy. Encourage parents to learn more about balanced nutrition and to provide this for their entire family.

Concerns of the Family With a Cognitively or Physically Challenged or Chronically Ill Infant

An infant born with a cognitive or physical challenge or an illness is usually hospitalized immediately after birth for diagnosis and treatment. This may result in delayed bonding because the newborn is separated from the parents during this time. Encourage the parents to visit regularly to help form a strong parent—child attachment. If parents cannot visit, urge them to telephone the hospital as frequently as they can to inquire about their child. In addition, nurses can supply Polaroid photographs of the infant for parents to take home.

Many of the developmental events of the infant year (social smile, laughing out loud, reaching for an object, uttering the first word, sitting, talking) are activities that encourage parent-child interaction because they make an infant fun to be with and naturally make a parent want to spend more time with the child. Children who are cognitively challenged may not reach these milestones. Children who are physically challenged may be unable to achieve them as well if they cannot reach up and pat their mother's face or hold out arms to be picked up by a father. If children cannot interact with the parents in these ways, the parents may find themselves equally unable to interact with the children. If infants leave the hospital with a cast or other equipment such as a ventilator for care, parents may be so concerned with these items that they cannot initiate normal singing and playing activities with their children.

To encourage a good parent-child relationship, point out the positive things the infant can do. Perhaps the child's facial expression says, "Pick me up," even though he doesn't reach up with his hands; perhaps his eyes follow his mother's actions even though he can't yet call to her.

Helping parents to interact more fully with their infants helps to build a sense of trust in the infant. Without a sense of trust, children have difficulty expressing themselves to others; they may not believe that they are lovable or that people would want to interact with them. Physically challenged individuals, no matter what their ages, need people around them to give them help at whatever point they cannot meet their own needs. It is unfortunate when a physically challenged child cannot reach out for help because he or she does not have a sense of trust.

Infants who are cognitively or physically challenged or chronically ill experience the same health and growth problems as other infants. Parents may be reluctant to bring up these concerns at health care visits because they believe such problems pale in comparison to the primary illness or condition. When taking the health histories of children with chronic or longstanding medical problems, ask the parents about secondary concerns. "What about everyday things? Any problems there?" Treat these concerns seriously, so parents can feel confident about bringing them to your attention at health care visits. Also mention that they are part of normal infant development so parents can begin to view their child apart from his or her illness.

Teething pain, discomfort from diaper rash, and colic are all potential problems in infancy and may occur even more frequently in babies with other illnesses. For instance, parents may not want to "bother" an ill infant with physical care as often as they would a well child (e.g., before homes were well-heated, bathing an ill infant could cause extensive chilling, and many people still believe that bathing is not appropriate for ill children). Colic may occur because parents are reluctant to tire ill infants by burping them after a feeding. Parents' attention may be so focused on the primary health problem rather than on everyday concerns, such as diaper care, that diaper dermatitis occurs. The bowel movements of physically disabled or chronically ill children may be looser than normal because of a liquid diet or medicine. Their urine may be more concentrated because of reduced intake. These conditions may lead to diaper rash. Offering anticipatory guidance to parents can go a long way toward helping them meet the needs of their infants.

Nutrition and the Cognitively or Physically Challenged Infant

Nutrition is often a concern for infants who are born physically challenged or are ill at birth. Infants who have fevers because of illness have increased metabolic needs and require more calories than normal. To compound the problem, ill children may become too fatigued to take adequate feedings. If any degree of neurologic involvement exists, sucking and swallowing reflexes may not be coordinated. With gastrointestinal involvement, feeding may be impossible.

To ensure adequate calorie and protein intake, infants may need to be maintained on nasogastric tube or gastrostomy feedings, or total parenteral nutrition. These methods limit the amount of sucking that is possible. Because sucking provides pleasure as well as satisfying thirst, this is a major loss. Provide the infant with non-nutritive sucking experiences if possible to fill this need.

Infants who are ill for a long time may not eat solid foods eagerly once they are introduced because they are not hungry enough to be interested in a new eating method. Help parents to experiment with different foods to find a taste that does appeal to ill children, or teach them to limit foods to only those the child appears to like most from all five food groups.

✔ CHECKPOINT QUESTIONS

19. What is the cause of colic?
20. What is baby-bottle syndrome?
21. Can infants who are physically challenged develop a sense of trust?

KEY POINTS

The infant period is from 1 month to 12 months. Children typically double their birthweight at 4 to 6 months and triple it at 1 year.

Infants develop their first tooth at about 6 months; by 12 months, they have six to eight teeth.

Important gross motor milestones during the infant year are lifting the chest off a bed at 2 months, sitting at 6 to 8 months, creeping at 9 months, "cruising" at 10 to 11 months, and walking at 12 months.

Important fine motor accomplishments are the ability to pass an object from one hand to the other (7 months) and a pincer grasp (10 months).

Important milestones of language development during the first year are differentiating a cry (2 months), making simple vowel sounds (5 to 6 months), and saying two words besides ma-ma and da-da (12 months). The more infants are spoken to, the easier it is for them to acquire language.

Providing infants with proper toys for play helps development. All infant toys need to be checked to be sure they are too large to be aspirated.

Important milestones of vision development are the ability to follow a moving object past the midline (3 months), and ability to focus securely without eyes crossing (6 months).

According to Erikson, the developmental task of the infant year is the development of a sense of trust versus mistrust.

Infants must be protected from aspiration of small objects and falls. A skill an infant cannot accomplish one day, such as crawling, may be accomplished the next.

Solid food is generally introduced into the infant's diet at 5 to 6 months of age. Before infants can eat solid food, they must lose their extrusion reflex.

Common concerns related to infant development include teething, thumb sucking, use of pacifiers, sleep problems, constipation, colic, diaper dermatitis, baby-bottle syndrome (decayed teeth from sucking on a bottle of formula while they sleep), and obesity. Nurses play a key role in teaching parents about these problems and measures to deal with them.

Remember that parent–infant attachment is critical to mental health. Urge parents to continue to give as much care as possible to sick infants to maintain this important relationship.

CRITICAL THINKING EXERCISES

1. Bryan, the 2-month-old boy you met at the beginning of the chapter, was diagnosed as having colic. What are common suggestions you could make to his parents to help reduce his discomfort and crying?
2. A 3-month-old child will be hospitalized for several months out of state because of severe burns. What steps could you, her nurse, take to foster a sense of trust in her in light of this extensive separation from her parents?
3. The mother of a 10-month-old boy tells you that he is "into everything." What questions would you want to ask to assess whether the infant's house is safe for him? Develop a teaching plan for the parents that addresses this boy's safety needs.
4. A 1-month-old infant is going to be followed in your health maintenance setting. Describe the immunization schedule you would discuss with her father as recommended for the first year.
5. The father of a 4-month-old child tells you his son spits out all the solid food he tries to feed him. What advice would you give him?
6. Examine the National Health Goals related to infant health. Most government-sponsored money for nursing research is allotted based on these goals. What would be a possible research topic to explore pertinent to these goals that would be fundable and would advance evidence-based practice?

REFERENCES

American Academy of Pediatrics. (2001). *Recommendations for using fluoride to prevent and control dental caries in the United States*, Washington, DC: AAP.

American Academy of Pediatrics Committee on Practice & Ambulatory Medicine. (2001). *Recommendations for preventive pediatric health care*. Washington, DC: AAP.

American Academy of Pediatrics Committee on Safety. (2001). *Children and car seats.* New York: AAP.

American Academy of Pediatrics Committee on Injury and Poison Prevention and Committee on Sports Medicine and Fitness. (2000). Swimming programs for infants and toddlers. *Pediatrics, 105*(4,1), 868–870.

Battan, F. K., & Dart, R. C. (2001). Emergencies and injuries. In W. W. Hay, A. R. Hayward, M. J. Levin, & J. M. Sondheimer (Eds.). *Current pediatric diagnosis and treatment* (15th ed.). New York: McGraw-Hill.

Bonuck, K. et al. (2002). Breast-feeding promotion interventions: Good public health and economic sense. *Journal of Perinatology, 22*(1), 78–81.

Brenner, R. A., et al. (2001). Prevalence and predictors of immunization among inner-city infants. *Pediatrics, 108*(3), 661–670.

Carey, W. B. (2000). Colic. In M. W. Schwartz (Ed.). *The 5-minute pediatric consult* (pp. 264–265). Philadelphia: Lippincott Williams & Wilkins.

Centers for Disease Control. (2001). Protracted outbreaks of cryptosporidiosis associated with swimming pool use. *Morbidity and Mortality Weekly Report, 50*(20), 406–410.

Department of Health and Human Services. (2000). *Healthy people 2010.* Washington, D.C.: DHHS.

Erikson, E. (1993). *Childhood and society* (3rd ed.). New York: W.W. Norton.

Goldson, E., & Hagerman, R. J. (2001). Normal development. In W. W. Hay, A. R. Hayward, M. J. Levin, & J. M. Sondheimer (Eds.). *Current pediatric diagnosis and treatment* (15th ed.). New York: McGraw-Hill.

Johnson, M., Maas, M., & Moorhead, S. (2000). *Nursing outcomes classification* (2nd ed.). St. Louis: Mosby.

Krebs, N. F. & Hambridge, K. M. (2001). Normal childhood nutrition and its disorders. In W. W. Hay, A. R. Hayward, M. J. Levin, & J. M. Sondheimer (Eds.). *Current pediatric diagnosis and treatment* (15th ed.). New York: McGraw-Hill.

Mascarenhas, M. R. (2000). Constipation. In M. W. Schwartz (Ed.). *The 5-minute pediatric consult* (pp. 280–281). Philadelphia: Lippincott Williams & Wilkins.

McCloskey, J., & Bulechek, G. (2000). *Nursing interventions classification* (3rd ed.). St. Louis: Mosby.

McGlaughlin, A. (2000). Learning curve: Babies who cry persistently: Responses and prevention. *Nursing Times, 96*(11), 47–48.

Messina, V., & Mangels, A. R. (2001). Considerations in planning vegan diets in infants. *Journal of the American Diabetic Association, 101*(6), 661–669.

Piaget, J. (1966). *The origins of intelligence in children.* New York: International University Press.

Thilo, E. H., & Rosenberg, A. A. (2001). The newborn infant. In W. W. Hay, A. R. Hayward, M. J. Levin, & J. M. Sondheimer (Eds.). *Current pediatric diagnosis and treatment* (15th ed.). New York: McGraw-Hill.

von Kries, R., et al. (2000). Does breast-feeding protect against childhood obesity? *Advances in Experimental Medicine and Biology, 478*(1), 29–39.

Warren, J. J., et al. (2001). Pacifier use and the occurrence of otitis media in the first year of life. *Pediatric Dentistry, 23*(2), 103–107.

SUGGESTED READINGS

Akin, F., et al. (2001). Effects of breathable disposable diapers: Reduced prevalence of *Candida* and common diaper dermatitis. *Pediatric Dermatology, 18*(4), 282-290.

Aldous, M. B. (1999). Nutritional issues for infants and toddlers. *Pediatric Annals, 28*(2), 101-105.

American Academy of Pediatrics Committee on Drugs. (2001). Transfer of drugs and other chemicals into human milk. *Pediatrics, 108*(3), 776-789.

American Academy of Pediatrics Work Group on Breastfeeding. (2001). Ten steps to support parents' choice to breastfeed their baby. *Pediatric Clinics of North America, 48*(2), 533-537.

Belton, N. (2001). The present and future of infant nutrition. *Professional Care of Mother and Child, 11*(3), 7-8.

Blackwell, P. B. & Baker, B. M. Estimating communication competence of infants and toddlers. *Journal of Pediatric Health Care, 16*(1), 29-35.

Blackwell, P. L. (2000). The influence of touch on child development: Implications for intervention. *Infants and Young Children, 13*(1), 25-39.

Butler, G. A., & Thompson, L. S. (2000). Building skills for child advocacy. *Journal of Pediatric Nursing, 15*(5), 323-325.

Carruth, B. R., & Skinner, J. E. (2001). Mother's sources of information about feeding their children ages 2 months to 54 months. *Journal of Nutrition Education, 33*(3), 143-147.

Foote, J. M., & Dutcher, M. E. (2000). Nutrition and feeding. *Pediatric Basics, 88*(2), 13-15.

Hiscock, H., & Wake, M. (2001). Infant sleep problems and postnatal depression: A community-based study. *Pediatrics, 107*(6), 1317-1322.

James, S. D. (2000). Breastfeeding. In M. W. Schwartz (Ed.). *The 5-minute pediatric consult* (pp. 202-203). Philadelphia: Lippincott Williams & Wilkins.

Lawrence, R. A. (1999). *Breastfeeding: A guide for the medical profession.* St. Louis: Mosby.

Long, T., & Johnson, M. (2001). Living and coping with excessive infantile crying. *Journal of Advanced Nursing, 34*(2), 155-162.

Norgate, C. (2001). Best practice in weaning. *Nursing Times, 97*(32), 56-57.

Wilson, M. E., et al. (2000). Family dynamics, parental-fetal attachment, and infant temperament. *Journal of Advanced Nursing, 31*(1), 204-210.

The Family With a Toddler

CHAPTER 29

Key Terms

- **assimilation**
- **autonomy**
- **deferred imitation**
- **discipline**
- **lordosis**
- **parallel play**
- **preoperational thought**
- **punishment**
- **tertiary circular reaction stage**

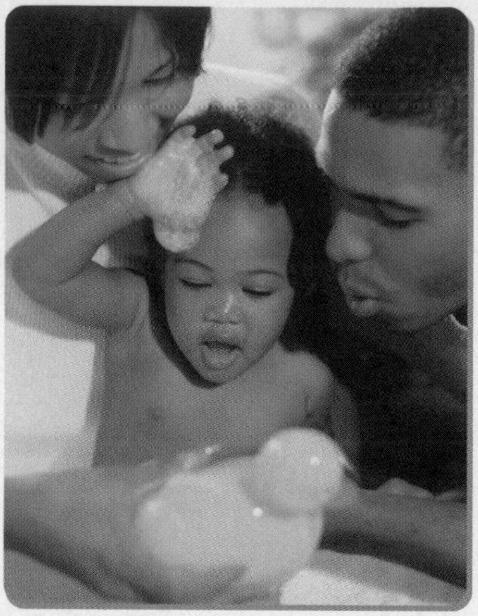

Objectives

After mastering the contents of this chapter, you should be able to:

1. Describe normal growth and development of the toddler period as well as common parental concerns.
2. Assess a toddler for normal growth and development milestones.
3. Formulate nursing diagnoses related to toddler growth and development or parental concerns regarding development.
4. Identify expected outcomes for nursing care of the toddler.
5. Plan nursing care to meet the toddler's growth and development needs, such as anticipatory guidance to prevent problems such as sleep disturbances, temper tantrums, or inappropriate toilet training practices.
6. Implement nursing care to promote normal growth and development of the toddler, such as discussing toddler developmental milestones with parents.
7. Evaluate goal outcomes established for care to be certain nursing goals associated with growth and development have been achieved.
8. Identify National Health Goals related to the toddler age group that nurses can be instrumental in helping the nation to achieve.
9. Identify areas related to care of the toddler that could benefit from additional nursing research or application of evidence-based practice.
10. Use critical thinking to analyze methods of care for the toddler to be certain care is family-centered.
11. Integrate knowledge of toddler growth and development with nursing process to achieve quality maternal and child health nursing care.

Jason is a 2.5-year-old boy you see at a pediatric clinic. His mother tells you he has changed completely in the last 6 months from an easy-to-care-for baby into a "monster" who refuses to do anything she asks. The only word he says anymore is "no." She tells you this has changed parenting from "fun" to "a real chore." What advice could you give to help Jason's mother regain a positive relationship with her toddler?

The previous chapter discussed the infant and the abilities children develop in the first year. This chapter adds information about the dramatic changes, both physical and psychosocial, that occur during the toddler years. This is important information because it builds a base for care and health teaching for the age group.

After you've studied the chapter, answer the Critical Thinking Exercises at the end of the chapter and then access the on-line study activities (http://connection.lww.com) *to further sharpen your skills and test your knowledge.*

FOCUS ON NATIONAL HEALTH GOALS

A number of National Health Goals relate specifically to safety during the toddler years. These are:

- Increase use of child restraints in children 4 years and under from 92% to 100%.
- Reduce deaths caused by poisonings from 6.8/100,000 to 1.5/100,000 (DHHS, 2000).

Nurses can be instrumental in helping the nation achieve these goals by continuing to educate parents about the importance of using car seats and child-proofing their homes against poisoning.

Areas that could benefit from additional nursing research are exploring methods parents can use to keep their toddlers entertained while in automobiles, and identifying specific home situations in which poisoning is apt to occur.

In the toddler period, usually considered to be from age 1 to 3 years, enormous changes take place in the child and, consequently, in the family. During the toddler period, children accomplish a wide array of developmental tasks and change from largely immobile and preverbal infants, who are dependent on caregivers for the fulfillment of most needs, to walking, talking young children with a growing sense of autonomy and independence. Parents must also grow during this period. Their task is to support their child's growing independence with patience and sensitivity and to learn methods for handling the child's frustrations that arise from the quest for autonomy. This chapter provides an overview of normal growth and development of the child and family through the toddler period, covering, in particular, those areas to assess at routine health maintenance visits. Because healthy children and families are constantly being challenged by the process of normal development, parents often have questions about how to guide their children in different situations. This chapter, then, also provides guidelines useful in helping parents cope with special needs and concerns relevant to this age. National Health Goals related to the toddler age group are shown in the Focus on National Health Goals box.

NURSING PROCESS OVERVIEW

For Healthy Development of the Toddler

Assessment

Whether a child is seen for a routine checkup or has come to a health care center because of a specific health concern, assessment begins with taking a careful health history. Asking parents about the toddler's ability to carry out activities of daily living offers assessment information on his or her developmental progress as well as important clues about the child–parent relationship.

Careful observation is another crucial element of nursing assessment of the toddler. This is because parents may become so emotionally involved in a health concern that they may not describe it with complete objectivity. On the other hand, parents see their children daily and so are the best source of information and opinion on when a child seems to be acting "out of sorts" or different (a typical sign that a child may not be feeling well). Table 29-1 provides some guidelines to help parents evaluate illness at this age. For more information about typical assessment findings, see Assessing the Average Toddler.

Nursing Diagnosis

Nursing diagnoses related to normal growth and development of toddlers usually focus on the parents' eagerness to learn more about the parameters of normal growth and development or issues of safety or care. Examples are:

- Health-seeking behaviors related to normal toddler development
- Deficient knowledge related to method of toilet training
- Risk for injury related to impulsiveness of toddler
- Interrupted family process related to need for close supervision of 2-year-old
- Readiness for enhanced family coping related to parents' ability to adjust to new needs of child
- Readiness for enhanced parenting related to increased awareness for poison prevention
- Disturbed sleep pattern related to lack of bedtime routine

Outcome Identification and Planning

To help parents resolve a concern during the toddler period, focus largely on family education and anticipatory guidance. Urge them to establish realistic goals and outcomes so they can meet the rapidly changing needs of the toddler and learn to cope with typical toddler behaviors. Otherwise, parents can expect too much of a toddler and grow frustrated instead of enjoying being a parent of a child this age.

TABLE 29.1 Parental Difficulties in Evaluating Illness in Toddlers

PROBLEM	GUIDELINES FOR PARENTS
Evaluating seriousness of illness	Toddlers typically answer "No" to almost all questions. A question such as "Does your arm hurt?" may bring a "No" response even if the arm does hurt. Observing children for indications of illness (holding an arm stiffly, rubbing abdomen, crying when they void) is more helpful. Many toddlers do not know the words to describe a feeling of nausea or a sore throat. They reveal these symptoms by not eating. If the child is normally a light eater, as many are, it is difficult for a parent to appreciate these signs.
Differentiating tiredness from illness	Toddlers tend to whine or sleep when they are either tired or ill. Reviewing the child's day and activity often helps to evaluate what is happening. If the child is not tired (it is not nap or bedtime), or there is not a break in usual routine, crying and whining or temper tantrums suggest illness.
Evaluating nutritional intake	Toddlers are normally fussy eaters compared to infants. Evaluating children as to whether they are active and growing is better than assessing any one day's food intake. Check weekly intake history.
Age-specific diseases to be aware of	The toddler period is an important age to assess speech development; children should be further evaluated if they cannot use simple sentences composed of a noun and verb ("me go") by 2 years of age. As children begin to walk, they should be observed for abnormal gait. Osteomyelitis (bone infection) occurs with a high frequency in toddlers; symptoms of limping, swollen joints, or arm or leg pain should be regarded as serious until ruled otherwise. Toddlers contract 10–12 mild upper respiratory infections a year. Otitis media (middle ear infection) may occur as a complication of these. The child with an upper respiratory infection who suddenly develops a high fever and pulls or manipulates ears should be seen by a physician. Children who attend day care programs have a high incidence of hepatitis A, *Giardia,* and *Shigella* infections. Teach parents to report jaundice or diarrhea promptly to a health care provider to detect these infections.

ASSESSING the Average Toddler

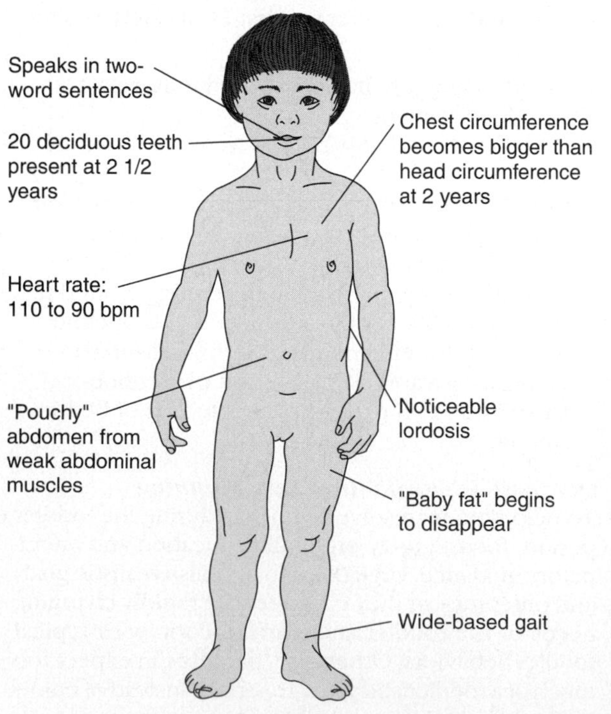
Speaks in two-word sentences
20 deciduous teeth present at 2 1/2 years
Chest circumference becomes bigger than head circumference at 2 years
Heart rate: 110 to 90 bpm
"Pouchy" abdomen from weak abdominal muscles
Noticeable lordosis
"Baby fat" begins to disappear
Wide-based gait

Implementation

When teaching about typical toddler behavior, teach parents that a good rule is to think of the toddler as a visitor from a foreign land who wants to participate in everything the family is doing, but doesn't know the customs or the language. Helping a toddler learn customs and language is much the same phenomenon.

Teach parents how to approach a current problem, and encourage them to learn adequate methods for resolving similar situations in the future. If parents do not learn methods that can be applied throughout the child's growing years, they may win battles but lose wars. For instance, parents may have found that promising their child a treat when she is in the middle of a temper tantrum will stop the tantrum, but it will certainly not prevent other tantrums from occurring in the future (and, in fact, may encourage them). Health visits are opportunities to provide parents with guidance on healthy coping techniques. In addition, demonstrating good communication skills with toddlers can serve as a model for healthy communication behavior with families (see Focus on Communication).

Outcome Evaluation

Care goals must be evaluated frequently during the toddler period because children learn so many new skills during this time that their abilities and associated parental concerns can change from day to day. Examples of outcome criteria that might be established are:

FOCUS ON COMMUNICATION

Ms. Matthis has brought her 2½-year-old son, Jake, to the clinic for a health maintenance visit. Jake is rambunctious and uncooperative. Ms. Matthis is obviously frustrated.

Less Effective Communication

Nurse: Come on, Jake, sit quietly so I can hear your heartbeat.
Jake: No!
Mom: Jake, listen to the nurse.
Jake: No!
Nurse: If you promise to sit still, I'll let you play with the stethoscope.
Jake: Okay.
Jake plays with the stethoscope.
Mom: Jake, now it's time to give the stethoscope back to the nurse.
Jake: No.
Nurse: There are other children waiting to see me. I really must listen to your heart now.

Mom takes the stethoscope from Jake. Jake starts crying.

Mom: Jake, if you stop crying and sit still, I'll take you for ice cream on our way home.
Jake: (whimpering a bit) Okay.
Mom to Nurse: Sometimes he can be so difficult.
Nurse: Oh, those terrible twos!

More Effective Communication

Nurse: Jake, I need to listen to your heart so you must be very quiet. Would you rather sit quietly on the chair or the table?
Jake: The table.
Nurse: All right, Jake, jump up.
Jake climbs onto the table and starts to fidget.
Mom: Jake, sit still for the nurse.
Jake: No!
Nurse: If you'd like, you can play with the stethoscope for a few seconds. Do you want to listen to your mom's heart or my heart?
Jake: Mom's.
Nurse: Great, now we will both be very quiet so you can hear.

Jake listens to his mom's heart.

Nurse: Good, now it's my turn.
Jake: Okay. (Jake hands back the stethoscope.)
Mom to Nurse: How did you get him to listen so well? At home he never listens. It can be so frustrating.
Nurse: Yes, this can be a frustrating period. By giving Jake choices, you can help him feel more in control without having to directly challenge your authority.

Toddlerhood can be a challenging and frustrating time for parents. You can teach parents effective communication skills to help toddlers assert their independence, while allowing parents to maintain discipline. It is important to show parents that offering choices rather than bribes is far more effective and long-lasting in modifying the toddler's behavior. In the first scenario, the nurse and mother both bribe Jake. Jake finally does what they want, but the situation is still frustrating, and his behavior change will not likely be long-lasting. In the second scenario, the nurse demonstrates how to better communicate by asking questions. The situation is much more enjoyable for everyone.

- Parents state child is maintaining a consistent bedtime routine within 2 weeks.
- Parents state they have childproofed the home by putting a lock on household products cupboard by next clinic visit.
- Grandmother states she has modified usual activities to conserve strength to care for toddler granddaughter by 1 week.

NURSING ASSESSMENT OF GROWTH AND DEVELOPMENT OF THE TODDLER

Assessment of the toddler should center on the child's physical growth and skill development.

Physical Growth

While toddlers are making great strides developmentally, their physical growth actually begins to slow.

Weight, Height, and Head Circumference

Plot weight and height on a standard growth chart at each health care visit (see Appendix E) to determine if progress is normal for each individual child. A child gains only about 5 to 6 lb (2.5 kg) and 5 in (12 cm) a year during the toddler period. Subcutaneous tissue, or baby fat, begins to disappear toward the end of the second year as the child changes from a plump baby into a leaner, more muscular little girl or boy. The toddler's appetite decreases accordingly, yet adequate intake of all nutrients is essential to meeting the toddler's energy needs (Berger, 2001).

Head circumference equals chest circumference at 6 months to 1 year of age. At 2 years, chest circumference is greater than that of the head. Head circumference increases only about 2 cm during the second year compared to about 12 cm during the first year.

Body Contour

Toddlers tend to have a prominent abdomen—a pouchy belly—because although they are walking, their abdominal muscles are not yet strong enough to support abdominal contents as well as they will later (Fig. 29-1*A*). They also have a forward curve of the spine at the sacral area (**lordosis**). As they walk longer, this will correct itself naturally. Toddlers waddle or walk with a wide stance (see Fig. 29-1*B*). This stance seems to increase the lordotic curve, but it keeps them on their feet.

Body Systems

Body systems continue to mature during this time:

- Respirations slow slightly but continue to be mainly abdominal.
- The heart rate slows from 110 to 90 bpm; blood pressure increases to about 99/64 mm Hg.
- The brain develops to about 90% of its adult size.
- In the respiratory system, the lumens of vessels increase progressively so the threat of lower respiratory infection is lower.
- Stomach capacity increases to the point that the child can eat three meals a day.
- Stomach secretions become more acid; therefore, gastrointestinal infections also become less common.
- Control of the urinary and anal sphincters becomes possible with complete myelination of the spinal cord.
- IgG and IgM antibody production becomes mature at 2 years of age. The passive immunity effects from intrauterine life are no longer operative.

Teeth

Eight new teeth (the canines and the first molars) erupt during the second year. All 20 deciduous teeth are generally present by 2.5 to 3 years of age (Kaplan & Love, 2001).

✔ CHECKPOINT QUESTIONS

1. You notice that a 2-year-old has a prominent lordosis (forward curve) of the spine. Is this an expected finding?
2. Why do toddlers have distended abdomens?

Developmental Milestones

The developmental milestones of the toddler years are less numerous but no less dramatic than those of the infant year, because this is a period of slow and steady, not sudden, growth. Toddler development is influenced to some extent by the amount of social contact and the number of opportunities children have to explore and experience new degrees of independence. It is strongly influenced by individual readiness; when children are developmentally ready for a new skill, they will acquire it. Table 29-2 highlights growth and development milestones of gross and fine motor, language, and play development of the toddler years.

Language Development

Toddlerhood is a critical time for language development. To master language, children need to practice talking. A child who is 2 years old and does not talk in two-word, noun–verb simple sentences should be examined to assess the cause. This is beyond a point of normal development.

A word that is used frequently by toddlers and that is a manifestation of their developing autonomy is "no."

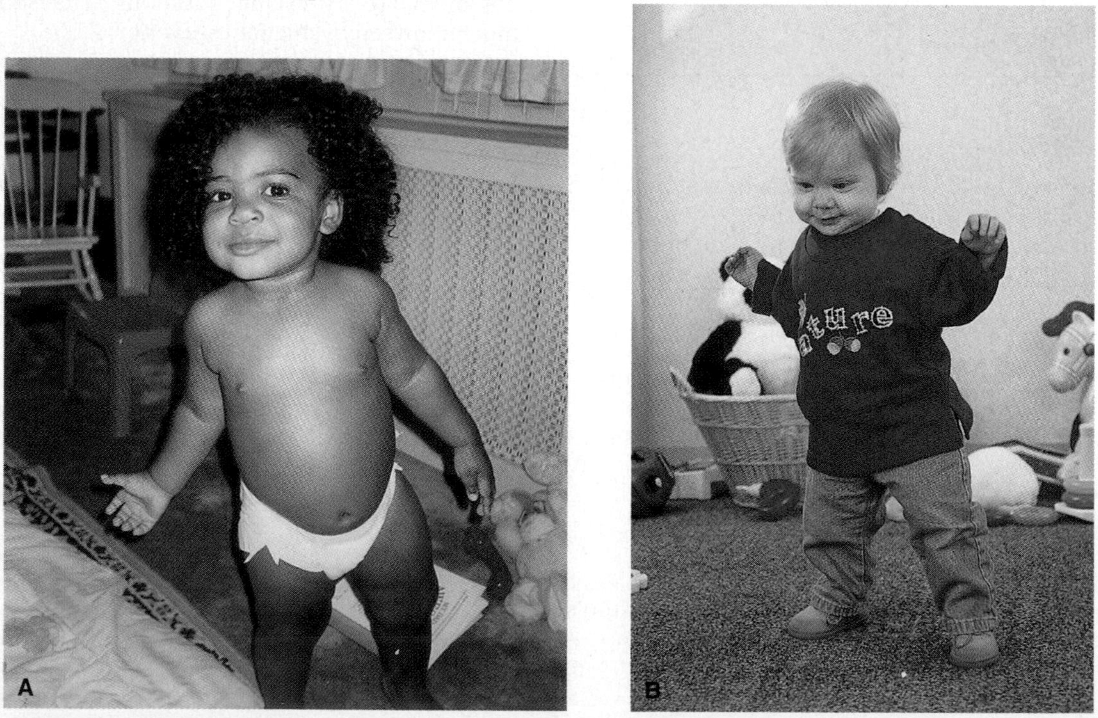

FIGURE 29.1 Physical characteristics of toddlers. (*A*) Toddlers typically have a prominent abdomen. (*B*) Toddlers typically walk with an unsteady gait for better stability.

TABLE 29.2 Milestones of Toddler Growth and Development

AGE (MONTHS)	FINE MOTOR	GROSS MOTOR	LANGUAGE	PLAY
15	Puts small pellets into small bottles. Scribbles voluntarily with a pencil or crayon. Holds a spoon well but may still turn it upside down on the way to mouth	Walks alone well; can seat self in chair; can creep upstairs	4–6 words	Can stack 2 blocks; enjoys being read to; drops toys for adult to recover (exploring sense of permanence)
18	No longer rotates a spoon to bring it to mouth	Can run and jump in place. Can walk up and down stairs holding onto a person's hand or railing. Typically places both feet on one step before advancing.	7–20 words, uses jargoning; names 1 body part	Imitates household chores, dusting, etc.; begins parallel play (playing beside not with another child)
24	Can open doors by turning doorknobs, unscrew lids	Walks up stairs alone still using both feet on same step at same time	50 words, 2-word sentences (noun-pronoun and verb), such as "Daddy go," "me come"	Parallel play evident
30	Makes simple lines or strokes for crosses with a pencil	Can jump down from chairs	Verbal language increasing steadily. Knows full name; can name 1 color and holds up fingers to show age	Spends time playing house, imitating parents' actions; play is "rough-housing" or active

Toddlers may use the word to mean they are refusing a task, or they do not understand it, or they may only be practicing a sound that they have noticed has potent effects on those around them.

To learn other words, children need exposure to conversation and need to be read to often. Language develops most quickly if children grasp the use of language and if parents respect what they have to say. Always answering the child's questions is a good way to do this. Answers for toddlers should be simple and brief because children have a short attention span.

Urge parents to encourage language development by naming objects as they play with their child (ball, block, music box, doll) or when they give their toddler something ("Here is your drink of water," "Let's put on these pajamas," and so on). This helps children grasp that words are not meaningless sounds; they apply to people and objects and have uses.

Some toddlers do not develop language readily because they are not called on to use it. When they point at an object, for example, someone hands it to them; when they climb into their highchair, someone places a meal in front of them. In other families, an older child may speak for a younger one. To assess whether parents are encouraging language development, ask them what happens when the child wants something. Do they provide opportunities for the child to ask for things before they supply them? Children should not be made to name an object before they can have it (because their vocabulary is so limited, the objects they could have would be restricted to 10 or fewer), but parents can reinforce language by rewording a question; for example, "You want the ball?" Reading aloud strengthens vocabulary in the same way. Reading the exact words in a book is not as important to toddlers as pointing to the pictures that accompany them. For example, Jane threw the ball ("See Jane throwing the ball?") or the dog ran away with the ball ("Look, that dog took the ball!").

The child who is very active may use fewer words than the child who is less active. The first child is too busy doing things to describe what he or she is doing; another child may be too busy obtaining objects to ask for many things. Such a child probably has a large unexpressed vocabulary; that is, the child understands more words (comprehensive vocabulary) than can be expressed (expressive vocabulary).

Because children learn language from imitating what they hear, they will speak like those around them. If they are spoken to in baby talk, their enunciation of words may be poor; if they hear examples of bad grammar, they will not use good grammar. Remind parents that pronouns are difficult for children to use correctly; many children are 3.5 or 4 years of age before they can separate the different uses of I, me, him, and her. Bilingual children interchange words from both languages.

Emotional Development

Developmental Task: Autonomy Versus Shame or Doubt. According to Erikson (1993), the developmental task of the toddler period is to learn a sense of autonomy or independence. Toddlers who do not develop a sense of autonomy may manifest feelings of shame or doubt. Children who have learned to trust themselves and others during the infant year are better prepared to do this than those who cannot trust themselves or others.

To develop a sense of **autonomy** is to develop a sense of independence. Children who are constantly told not to try things because they will hurt themselves may be left with a stronger sense of doubt than confidence at the end of the toddler period. Children who are made to feel that it is wrong to be independent may leave the toddler period with a stronger sense of shame than autonomy. A healthy level of autonomy is achieved when parents are able to encourage independence while still maintaining consistently sound rules for safety.

Infants appear to have difficulty differentiating between their bodies and those of others; they think of their bodies as extensions of their parents or their primary caregivers. When infants approach toddlerhood, they begin to make the differentiation. As they recognize that they are separate individuals, they realize they do not always have to do what others want them to do. From this realization comes the reputation toddlers have for being negativistic, obstinate, and difficult to manage.

This reputation is little deserved, however, and exists largely because parents misinterpret children's cues. For example, a child's refusal to accept help putting on shoes may be seen by a parent as disobedience, whereas the child may see this as insisting on performing an act he or she can do independently—a positive expression of autonomy.

Socialization. Once toddlers are walking well, they become resistant to sitting in laps and being cuddled. This is not lack of a desire for socialization but a function of being independent. Fifteen-month-old children are still enthusiastic about interacting with people, providing those people are willing to follow the toddlers where they want to go.

By 18 months, toddlers imitate the things they see a parent doing, such as "study" or "sweep," so they seek out parents to observe and initiate interactions. By 2 or more years, children become aware of gender differences and may point to other children and identify them as "boy" or "girl."

Play Behavior. All during the toddler period, children play beside the children next to them, not with them. This side-by-side play (often called **parallel play**) is not unfriendly but is a normal developmental sequence that occurs during the toddler period (Fig. 29-2). Caution parents that if two toddlers are going to play side by side, they must provide duplicate toys or an argument over one toy is likely to occur.

The toys toddlers enjoy most are those they can play with by themselves and that require action. Trucks they can make go, squeaky frogs they can squeeze, waddling ducks they can pull, horses they can ride, pegs they can pound, blocks they can stack, and a toy telephone they can talk on are all favorites. These are all toys children can control, giving them a sense of power in manipulation, an expression of autonomy (Fig. 29-3).

Some parents are not prepared for this change of play habits in their child. They wonder why a child who used to play quietly in her crib is now more interested in banging trucks together. However, they need only watch a toddler tug a pull toy, stop to see if it is following, walk again, and stop and look to see if it is still following to understand the feeling of accomplishment involved in manipulating toys.

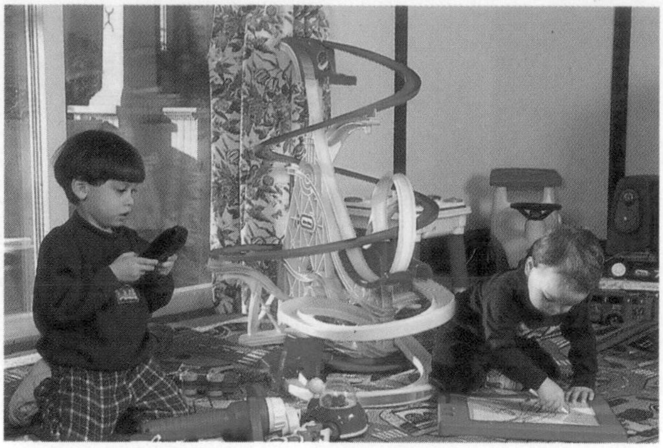

FIGURE 29.2 Toddlers play beside but not with other children (parallel play).

Fifteen-month-old children are still in a put-in, take-out stage, so they continue to enjoy stacks of boxes or balls that fit inside each other. They enjoy throwing toys out of a playpen or from a highchair tray as long as someone will pick them up and return them again and again.

The 18-month-old child enjoys pull toys. Toys should be strong enough to take a great deal of abuse, because there are many things in the world toddlers do not recognize or know about. This causes them to use toys in ways other than those for which they were designed. (Whereas the infant sat and softly stroked a stuffed cat, the toddler picks it up by the tail and swings it, pounds it, or pulls at it.) Parents should not correct children about the way a toy is being used as long as it appears to give satisfaction. If toddlers find a toy frustrating because they are holding or using it incorrectly, showing them the right way will ease frustration.

By age 2, toddlers begin to spend time imitating adult actions in their play; for example, wrapping a doll and putting it to bed, "setting the table," or "driving the car." They use fewer toys than before; imitating actions they see

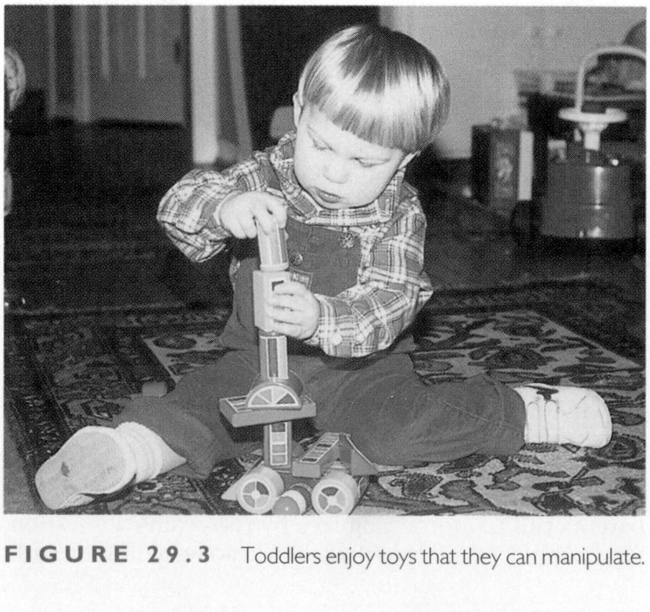

FIGURE 29.3 Toddlers enjoy toys that they can manipulate.

parents doing has replaced them. Both boys and girls begin to like rough-housing and spend at least part of every day in this very active, stimulating type of play (Fig. 29-4). Encourage parents to schedule this type of play outdoors, where vases or other prized possessions cannot be broken. Because of this rough activity, most toddlers have at least one black-and-blue mark on their legs at all times from tripping over their feet while trying to run too fast or jumping or bumping into a chair or doorway. The child who feels a need for active play is unable to sit down and eat, fall asleep, or play quiet games. When this happens, it is good to explore with the parents the amount of outside or rough-housing time the child has each day. A trip in a stroller is not the same kind of activity as walking and running. Stroller walks are good because they provide fresh air and sunshine, but the child must also have opportunities to engage in strenuous activity.

Cognitive Development

The toddler enters the fifth and sixth stages of sensorimotor thought (Table 29-3). Piaget referred to stage 5 (between 12 and 18 months) as a **tertiary circular reaction stage,** describing the toddler in this stage as "a little scientist" because of the child's interest in trying to discover new ways to handle objects or new results that different actions can achieve (Piaget, 1969). For instance, by trial and error, toddlers discover that cats do not like baths and that cookies on the center of a table can be reached by crawling up onto the table or pulling on the tablecloth. Obviously, this type of investigating can lead to errors or injury. Toddlers have also advanced beyond what they could do as infants in terms of dropping objects and watching where they roll. As infants, to retrieve an article that rolled under a chair, they would crawl under the chair along the same path the object took. Many children at 15 months are able to follow a different path (walk in back of the chair) to obtain the object. This results from increased awareness that the object is permanent and, even if it follows a different direction from the one the child must take, it will be there to retrieve.

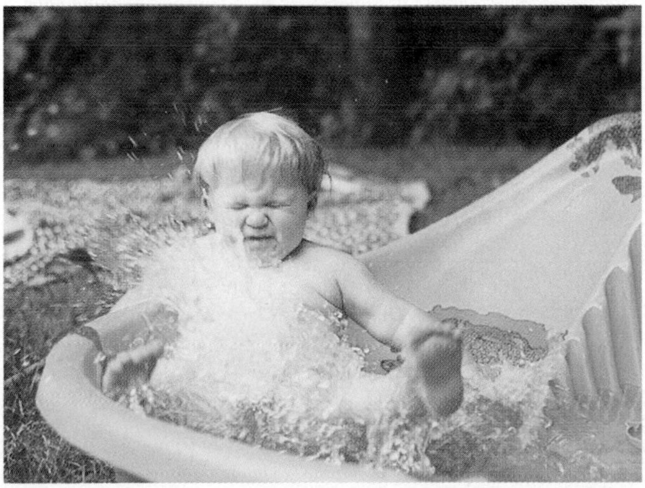

FIGURE 29.4 Toddlers usually enjoy rough and tumble play.

TABLE 29.3 Cognitive and Psychosocial Development of the Toddler

AGE IN MONTHS	STAGE	TASK
Cognitive		
12–18	Sensorimotor 5	Child experiments by trial and error methods
18–24	Sensorimotor 6	Can pretend and use deferred imitation; object permanence is complete
24	Preoperational thought	Able to use assimilation or change situation to fit thoughts
Psychosocial		
24–36	Autonomy vs. shame or guilt	Learn independence and the beginning of problem solving

From Piaget, J. (1969). *The theory of stages in cognitive development.* New York: McGraw-Hill; and Erikson, E. H. (1993). *Childhood and society.* New York: W.W. Norton; with permission.

By stage 6 (between 18 and 24 months), toddlers are able to try out various actions mentally rather than having to actually perform them—the beginning of problem solving or symbolic thought. Children at this stage are also able to remember an action and imitate it later (**deferred imitation**); they can do such things as pretend to drive a car or put a baby to sleep. Object permanence is complete.

At the end of the toddler period, children enter a second major period of cognitive development: **preoperational thought.** During this period, children deal much more constructively with symbols than they did while still in the sensorimotor period of cognition. They begin to use a process termed **assimilation.** Because they are not able to change their thoughts to fit a situation, they learn to change the situation (or how they perceive it) to fit their thoughts. This ability is what causes toddlers to use toys in the "wrong" way. For example, if they are given a toy hammer, instead of pounding with it, they might shake it to see if it rattles, using the toy in a way that they had previously played (the child has changed the toy's use to fit his or her thoughts, or used assimilation).

> ✔ **CHECKPOINT QUESTIONS**
>
> 3. What type of sentence should the 2-year-old have mastered?
> 4. What is the typical type of play pattern enjoyed by toddlers?

PLANNING AND IMPLEMENTATION FOR HEALTH PROMOTION OF THE TODDLER AND FAMILY

Toddlers tend to develop many upper respiratory and ear infections but otherwise come to a health care facility most often for health maintenance visits (recommended at 15,

18, and 24 months) and the immunizations important at these times. These visits allow a nurse to focus on health promotion and provide an opportunity for early detection of any growth and development delays. Table 29-4 lists specific areas to assess during these visits.

Routine health maintenance visits also provide an opportunity to help parents through the normal crises of the toddler period. Ways to encourage parents to promote the healthy development of independence in their toddler include listening carefully to their concerns, asking questions that will help to separate the objective circumstances surrounding a problem from the parents' possible emotional biases, and providing guidelines for how to handle specific problems.

Promoting Toddler Safety

Accidents are the major cause of death in children of all ages. Accidental ingestions (poisoning) are the type of accidents that occur most frequently in toddlers. Although these can involve medicine, they most often occur from ingestion of cleaning products. Aspiration or ingestion of small objects such as watch or hearing aid batteries, pencil erasers, or crayons is also a major danger for children of this age. Urge parents to childproof the house by putting all poisonous products, drugs, and small objects out of reach by the time the infant is crawling, and certainly by the time an infant is walking (see Chap. 28). Box 29-1 highlights an appropriate outcome and intervention using the ter-

TABLE 29.4 Health Maintenance Schedule, Toddler Period

AREA OF FOCUS	METHODS	FREQUENCY
Developmental milestones	History, observation	Every visit
	Formal Denver Developmental Screening Test (DDST II)	18th-month visit
Growth milestones	Height, weight plotted on standard growth chart; physical examination	Every visit
Nutrition	History, observation; height/weight information	Every visit
Parent–child relationship	History, observation	Every visit
Behavior problems	History, observation	Every visit
Vision and hearing defects	History, observation	Every visit
Dental health	History, physical examination; first dental appointment	Every visit; first at 24 months
Anemia	Hematocrit/hemoglobin	24th-month visit
Lead screening	Whole blood lead level	Depending on risk level; 24-month visit
Tuberculosis	PPD test	Depending on prevalence in community
Urinalysis	Clean-catch urine	24th-month visit
Immunizations		
Measles, mumps and rubella	Check history and past records; inform caregiver about any risks and side effects.	12th- or 15th-month visit
Haemophilus influenzae type B (HiB)	Administer immunization in accordance with health care agency policies	12th- or 15th-month visit
Diphtheria, tetanus, and pertussis; inactivated poliomyelitis		15th- or 18th-month visit
Varicella vaccine		12th- or 18th-month visit
Anticipatory Guidance		
Toddler care	Active listening and health teaching	Every visit
Expected growth and developmental milestones before next visit		Every visit
Poison and accident prevention	Provide syrup of ipecac to be used in case of poisoning; counseling. Provide telephone number and location of nearest poison control center.	Every visit
Problem Solving		
Any problems expressed by caregiver during course of the visit	Active listening and health teaching regarding temper tantrums, toilet training, negativity	Every visit

BOX 29.1

NURSING OUTCOMES AND NURSING INTERVENTIONS CLASSIFICATION: TODDLER SAFETY

NOC: Knowledge, Child Safety

Knowledge, child safety, is defined as the extent of understanding conveyed about safely caring for a child (Johnson, Maas, & Moorhead, 2000). Some specific indicators suggesting achievement of this outcome include the parents' ability to describe the following:

- Appropriate activities for the child's developmental level
- Drowning hazards and preventive measures
- Use of bicycle helmets
- First aid techniques and CPR (including demonstration)
- Methods to prevent playground accidents
- Proper surveillance of outdoor activities
- Teaching about stranger awareness

NIC: Teaching, Toddler Safety

Teaching, toddler safety, is defined as instruction on safety during the second and third years of life (McCloskey & Bulechek, 2000). Some important activities involved when implementing this intervention include instructing the parent/caregiver in the following at:

13 to 18 months

- Supervising child outdoors
- Educating child about dangers of throwing, hitting, safe ways to interact with pets
- Preventing access to electrical outlets, cords, and appliances or tools
- Securing gates and doors
- Maintaining water heater temperature at 120° to 130°F

19 to 24 months

- Using car seat according to manufacturer's instructions
- Instructing child on street dangers
- Storing all chemicals, cleaners, and personal care products out of child's reach
- Ensuring multiple barriers to pools and hot tubs

25 to 36 months

- Instructing child on dangers of weapons and fires, and also how to get help when feeling scared or in danger
- Selecting toys according to manufacturer's recommendations
- Storing matches and lighters out of child's reach
- Supervising child when near swimming pool, ponds, or hot tubs
- Instructing child about stranger danger and good touch/bad touch
- Using appropriate helmet for bike riding
- Supervising child closely when in public settings

minology identified by the Nursing Outcomes Classification (NOC) and Nursing Interventions Classification (NIC).

Other accidents common to toddlers include motor vehicle accidents, burns, falls, and playground injuries. These occur because a toddler's motor ability jumps ahead of his or her judgment. Toddlers can walk surely and swiftly enough so that if they are left outside to play, they can very quickly travel a block away. Because they have no judgment concerning moving cars, they must never be left outside unsupervised. To prevent serious injury, parents must be alert and know what their toddler is doing at all times. Until children weigh 40 to 60 lb, they need a toddler-size car seat for safety in automobiles (Fig. 29-5). They should be placed in the back seat if the car has a passenger seat airbag (AAP Committee on Safety, 2001). They need to wear a helmet as soon as they begin riding a tricycle. Parents should remove drawstrings from hooded clothing to prevent strangulation. Focus on Evidence-Based Practice discusses a study related to preventable accidents.

Some 15-month-old children can climb over the side rails of their cribs and enjoy exploring the house early in the morning before anyone else is awake. Parents might have to move the child to a regular bed with a side rail as early as 15 months to keep him or her from falling when climbing out of the crib. A safety gate on the door of the room is another way to keep the toddler contained and safe.

As the child reaches 2 years of age and begins to imitate housework or repairing the car, parents must be sure the child does not use real cleaning compounds or sharp tools. Focus on Family Empowerment summarizes accident prevention measures to encourage parents to take with their toddler.

Lead Screening

All children between the ages of 6 months and 6 years who live in communities with houses built before 1950 should be tested periodically for the presence of too much lead in the body (lead poisoning). Lead poisoning is caused by eating, chewing, or sucking on objects such as windowsills, paint chips, or furniture that are covered with lead-based paint. Although federal law has prohibited the use of lead

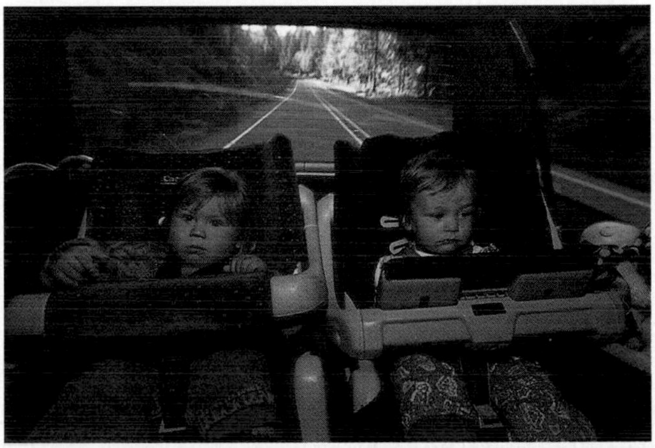

FIGURE 29.5 Toddlers should use a car seat for safety while riding in an automobile.

FOCUS ON EVIDENCE-BASED PRACTICE

Do Young Mothers Realize the Toddler Age Is One Prone to Accidents?

About 30,000 children in the United States die each year from preventable accidents. To see if young mothers were aware that injury prevention is an important part of their role, researchers interviewed 17 first-time adolescent mothers about what they thought were important aspects of parenting, and if they knew usual causes of injury and strategies to prevent injuries in young children. Results showed that no mother spontaneously identified injury prevention as an important part of mothering. More than half of parents believed that injuries were not preventable. In addition, mothers identified a limited number of strategies they could take to prevent injury. None of them reported that they had discussed injury presentation with their child's pediatrician. The researchers concluded injury prevention is an important area to discuss with young mothers.

This is an important study for nurses because nurses are the health care providers who provide health information on normal growth and development, including accident prevention, to parents. Knowing that young mothers do not see accident prevention as a large part of their role identifies an area of health education for teaching.

Murphy, L. M. B. (2001). Adolescent mothers' beliefs about parenting and injury prevention: Results of a focus group. *Journal of Pediatric Health Care, 15*(4), 194–199.

in the manufacture of interior and exterior paints since the mid-1970s, many older houses still contain lead paint. Additional sources of lead poisoning can include:

- Soil around the exterior of the house and potentially contaminated food grown there
- Dust or fumes created by home renovation
- Pottery made with lead glazes
- Colored print in newspapers
- Old water pipes
- Lead-based gasoline—children who live in high-traffic areas are at high risk for contamination by lead fumes
- Lead dust brought home on the clothing of parents who work with lead products

A diet high in fat and low in calcium, magnesium, iron, zinc, and copper may increase the absorption of lead.

Because lead is toxic to body tissue, lead poisoning can cause serious damage to the brain and nervous system, kidneys, and red blood cells. High levels may result in seizures, cognitive challenges, coma, and even death. Levels as low as 10 to 15 μg/dL can cause learning and behavioral problems (Kaplan & Love, 2001).

Symptoms of lead poisoning include irritability, headaches, fatigue, and abdominal pain. Often, however, there are no symptoms, which is why periodic blood screening is essential. The American Academy of Pediatrics Committee on Practice and Ambulatory Medicine (2001) recommends screening for all children between the ages of 9 and 12 months and again at 24 months. A small amount of blood taken by a finger prick is analyzed. A positive result (over 10 μg/dL) must be confirmed by further testing.

Promoting Nutritional Health of the Toddler

Because growth slows abruptly after the first year of life, the toddler's appetite is smaller than the infant's. Children who ate hungrily 2 months earlier will now sit and play with their food. If feeding problems begin, it is often because parents are unaware that their toddler's appetite has decreased and food consumption is less. Because the actual amount of food eaten daily varies from one child to another, parents should place a small amount of food on a plate and allow the child to eat it and ask for more rather than serve a large portion that the child cannot finish. One tablespoonful of each food served is a good start. Also, cleaning a plate gives the child a feeling of independent functioning, whereas leaving food uneaten may suggest to the child that parents expected something more. It is important to educate parents while the child is still an infant that this decline in food intake will occur so they will not be concerned when it happens (Krebs & Hambridge, 2001). Box 29-2 highlights an appropriate outcome and intervention using the terminology identified by NOC and NIC.

Toddlers insist on feeding themselves and will resist eating if a parent insists on feeding them. A child may react to repeated attempts by refusing to eat at all. Allowing self-feeding is a major way to strengthen independence in a toddler. At the same time, toddlers may insist on the same type of food over and over because of the sense of security this offers. Offering finger foods and allowing a choice between two types of food helps promote independence. Nutritious finger foods that toddlers enjoy include pieces of chicken, slices of banana, pieces of cheese, and crackers.

Toddlers usually do not like food that is "mixed up" such as casseroles (except maybe spaghetti); they often prefer that different foods do not touch one another on their plate. Frequently they eat all of one item before going on to another. They often prefer brightly colored foods to bland colors. They imitate what their parents eat (Fisher et al., 2002).

Recommended Daily Dietary Allowances

Parents may become frustrated when trying to provide adequate nutrition for their toddler because of the toddler's varying and unpredictable appetite and food preferences. Although the toddler's daily food consumption may vary greatly, energy needs are generally met when sufficient food is supplied in a positive environment. Children ages 1 to 3 years should consume 1,300 kcal daily. Protein and carbohydrate needs are often easily met during the toddler period; diets high in sugar should be avoided. Fats should generally not be restricted for children under 2 years old; however, children over 2 years old should consume no more than 30% of total daily calories from fat. Adequate calcium and phosphorus intake is important for bone

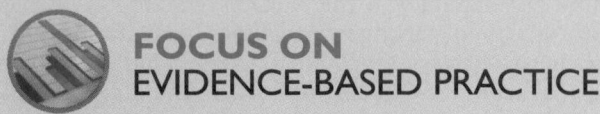

FOCUS ON FAMILY EMPOWERMENT

Common Safety Measures to Prevent Accidents During the Toddler Years

Q. My toddler is constantly on the go. How can I keep him safe?

A. Accident prevention needs to be ongoing while your child is a toddler. Try the following precautions:

Potential Accident	*Prevention Measure*
Motor vehicles	Maintain child in car seat; do not be distracted from safe driving by a child in a car.
	Do not allow child to play outside unsupervised. Do not allow child to operate electronic garage doors.
	Supervise toddler who is too young to be left alone on a tricycle.
	Teach safety with pedaling toys (look before crossing driveways; do not cross streets) but do not expect that toddler will obey these rules at all times (in other words, stay close by).
Falls	Keep house windows closed or keep secure screens in place.
	Place gates at top and bottom of stairs. Supervise at playgrounds.
	Do not allow child to walk with sharp object in hand or mouth.
	Raise crib rails and check to make sure they are locked before walking away from crib.
Aspiration	Examine toys for small parts that could be aspirated; remove toys that appear dangerous.
	Do not feed toddler popcorn, peanuts, etc.; urge children not to eat while running. Do not leave toddler alone with a balloon.
Drowning	Do not leave toddler alone in a bathtub or near water (including buckets of cleaning water and washing machines).
Animal bites	Do not allow toddler to approach strange dogs.
	Supervise child's play with family pets.
Poisoning	Never present medication as candy. Buy medications with childproof caps; put away immediately after use.
	Never take medication in front of child.
	Place all medication and poisons in locked cabinets or overhead shelves where child cannot reach them.
	Never leave medication in parents' purse or pocket, where child can reach it.
	Always store food or substances in their original containers.
	Know the names of house plants and find out if they are poisonous. (Call regional poison control center for information.)
	Hang plants or set them on high surfaces beyond toddler's grasp.
	Post telephone number of nearest poison control center by the telephone.
	In all first-aid boxes, maintain supply of syrup of ipecac, an emetic, with proper instructions for administering if poisoning should occur. Never administer ipecac without medical authorization, because it is contraindicated in the treatment of some poisonous ingestions.
Burns	Buy flame-retardant clothing.
	Cook on the back burners of stove if possible and turn handles of pots toward back of stove to prevent toddler from reaching up and pulling them down.
	Use cool-mist vaporizer rather than steam vaporizer or remain in room when vaporizer is operating so child is not tempted to play with it.
	Keep screen in front of fireplace or heater.
	Monitor toddlers carefully when they are near lit candles.
	Do not leave toddlers unsupervised near hot-water faucets.
	Check temperature setting for hot-water heater and turn down thermostat if it is over 125°F.
	Do not leave coffee/tea pots on a table where child can reach them.
	Never drink hot beverages when a child is sitting on your lap or playing within reach.
	Do not allow toddlers to blow out matches (teach that fire is not fun); store matches out of reach.
	Keep electric wires and cords out of toddler's reach; cover electrical outlets with safety plugs.
General	Know whereabouts of toddlers at all times. Toddlers can climb onto chairs, stools, etc., that they could not manage before; can turn door knobs and go places they could not go before.
	Be aware that the frequency of accidents increases when the family is under stress and therefore less attentive to children. Special precautions must be taken at these times.
	Be aware some children are more active, curious, and impulsive and therefore more vulnerable to accidents than others.

BOX 29.2

NURSING OUTCOMES AND NURSING INTERVENTIONS CLASSIFICATION: TODDLER NUTRITION

NOC: Knowledge, Diet

Knowledge, diet, is defined as the extent of understanding conveyed about diet (Johnson, Maas, & Moorhead, 2000). Some specific indicators suggesting achievement of this outcome include the parents' ability to:

- Describe recommendations for infant intake, including foods allowed and not allowed
- Select appropriate foods
- Plan appropriate meals using diet guidelines

NIC: Teaching, Toddler Nutrition

Teaching, toddler nutrition, is defined as instruction on nutrition and feeding practices during the first years of life (McCloskey & Bulechek, 2000). Some important activities involved when implementing this intervention include instructing the parent/caregiver in the following at:

13 to 18 months

- Discontinuation of bottle feeding
- Offering of textured solids as small portions and frequent feedings
- Continued use of spoon and self-feeding
- Avoidance of force feeding
- Use of healthy snacks

19 to 24 months

- Use of drinking water for thirst
- Limitation of fluids before meals
- Inclusion of foods high in iron and protein
- Regularity of meal times
- Discontinuation of bottle feeding

25 to 36 months

- Healthy food choices for the child, including raw and cooked vegetables, healthy snacks between meals, foods from all food groups, and iron-fortified cereals
- Use of small portions
- Creative food preparation for the picky eater
- Limitation of fat content in foods
- Avoidance of high-sugar cereals
- Child participation in food preparation
- Avoidance of food as a reward

mineralization. Milk should be whole milk until age 2 years, after which 2% milk can be introduced (Dudek, 2001). Parents should limit diluted fruit juices; these supply few calories or minerals (AAP Committee on Nutrition, 2001).

Promoting Adequate Intake With a Vegetarian Diet

Vegetarian diets are adequate for toddlers if parents are well informed about needed vitamins and minerals. A vegetarian diet can be easily designed for the toddler who prefers finger foods, because many vegetables, fruits, and grains (e.g., pieces of oranges, peaches, raisins, chickpeas, tomatoes, and crackers) are easily eaten this way. The use of fortified soy milk prevents fluid, protein, B_{12}, and calcium deficiencies.

✔ **CHECKPOINT QUESTIONS**

5. What is the most common source of lead poisoning in toddlers?
6. Should fat be restricted in the diet of a child under age 2?

Promoting Toddler Development in Daily Activities

The toddler's new independence and developing abilities in self-care, such as dressing, eating, and to a limited extent hygiene, present special challenges for parents. Learning how to promote autonomy yet maintain a safe, healthful environment is a major goal for the family.

Dressing

By the end of the toddler period, most children can put on their own socks, underpants, and undershirt (Fig. 29-6). Some may also be able to pull on slacks, pullover shirts (the sleeves of a shirt often confuse the toddler), or simple dresses. Parents may be reluctant to encourage toddlers to dress themselves. It is often much easier and quicker to put their clothes on for them, and the toddler who is dressed by parents will (usually) be wearing clothes in the correct way. When toddlers dress themselves, they invariably put shoes on the wrong feet and shirt and pants on backwards. Encourage parents to give up perfection for the benefit of the child's developing sense of autonomy. If children end up with underpants or shirt on backwards, in most instances it does not make that much difference, and toddlers are not likely to feel independent and confident if their attempts at dressing are criticized. If the parents feel they must change the child's clothes, they should begin

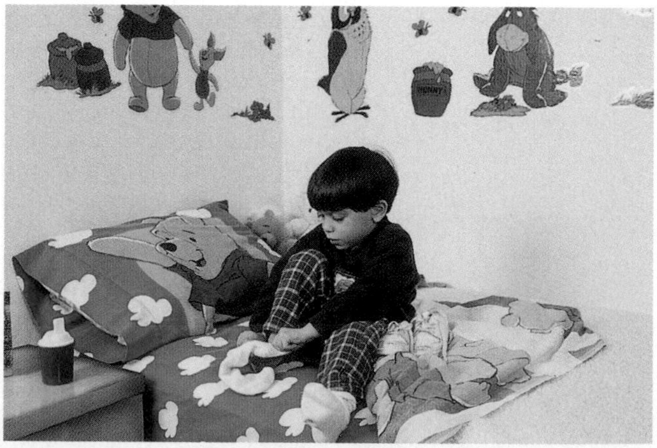

FIGURE 29.6 Getting dressed by himself is a fun morning activity for this older toddler.

with a positive statement, such as "You did a good job," before making the switch.

During a health assessment, ask parents if their child can put on any clothing. Parents who allow this name those items the child can manage. Parents who do not allow self-dressing will probably describe the daily battle they have about dressing: "She puts up such a fuss, I don't think she will ever do it on her own." These parents may need help to understand the situation: the child may be resisting because she wants to dress herself. Don't judge how much independent exploration parents encourage by what they do in a physician's office or pediatric clinic. In these settings, they may dress the child quickly to show the child that the examination is over, or they may simply be in a hurry to get home.

As soon as children are up on their feet and walking, they need shoe soles that are firm enough to provide protection from rough surfaces. However, toddlers do not need extremely firm or ankle-high shoes. Because the toddler's arches are still developing, it is better for the arches to provide foot support rather than having it provided by shoes. Sneakers are an ideal toddler shoe because the soles are hard enough for rough surfaces and arch support is limited.

Sleep

The amount of sleep children need gradually decreases as they grow older. They may begin the toddler period napping twice a day and sleeping 12 hours each night, and end it with one nap a day and only 8 hours' sleep at night. Parents who are not aware that the need for sleep declines at this time may view a child's disinterest in sleeping as a problem. A parent's insistence that the child get more sleep may lead to sleeping problems or refusal to sleep at all. If the child cannot fall asleep at night, maybe it is time to omit or shorten an afternoon nap. If a child is so short-tempered at dinnertime that eating is impossible, perhaps the child needs two naps a day.

Toddlers naturally fall asleep when they are tired. They may begin to resist naps, however, as well as nighttime sleep because they are aware for the first time that activities go on while they sleep, and they do not want to miss anything. Parents need to be sure that when they say, "We'll do this after naptime," they wait until then to do it. Otherwise, the child may be reluctant to nap the next day for fear of missing another activity. Also, parents must be sure that older siblings do not point out to the toddler all the exciting things the toddler missed while napping.

Other toddlers resist naptime as part of their developing negativism. Parents might minimize this by including a nap as part of lunchtime routine, not as a separate activity: the child always goes from the table directly to bed. The parent can state simply, "It's naptime now," and then give a secondary choice: "Do you want to sleep with your teddy bear or your rag doll?" Toward the end of the toddler period, when children are ready to omit their afternoon naps, they may be agreeable to a "shoes-off" or quiet-play period until they begin to attend school full time.

As with any other activity of this period, the toddler loves a bedtime routine: bath, pajamas, a story, toothbrushing, being tucked into bed, having a drink of water, choosing a toy to sleep with, and turning out the lights. Parents must be careful, however, that a child does not maneuver them into such a long procedure that sleep is delayed considerably past the time initially set. Although toddlers need to be independent, they also need a feeling of security. Just as adults like to know there are guardrails along steep mountain roads, toddlers must be sure that parents are firm, consistent people who can be counted on to be reliable.

Many toddlers are ready to be moved out of a crib into a youth bed or regular bed with protective side rails or a chair strategically placed beside it by the end of the toddler period. Moving children to a more grown-up bed is usually preferable to forcing them to sleep in a crib if they no longer feel they should be there. Either the child will not fall asleep in the crib or he or she will scale the side rails and perhaps fall.

Parents should stress that sleeping in a regular bed does not give children the right to get in and out of bed as they choose. Some toddlers do well if they are allowed to sleep in a regular bed and a folding gate is placed across the door to their room. This arrangement gives them a feeling of independence but still keeps them safe. When first moved to a bed without side rails, many children are found sleeping on the floor of the room in the morning. There is no harm in this unless it is cold or drafty. Dressing the child in warm pajamas or putting a blanket on the floor might be solutions to help parents accept this behavior.

Bathing

The time for a toddler's bath should depend on the parents' and the child's wishes and schedule. Some parents prefer to bathe a toddler before the evening meal because it has a quieting effect and prepares the child for eating; others prefer to give it at bedtime because it has a relaxing effect and helps the child sleep. The time, however, is not as important as the attempt to establish a sense of routine, a sense that life has order. Learning to be independent is sometimes frightening, and there is security in knowing that certain events are predictable.

Toddlers usually enjoy bathtime, and parents should make an effort to make it fun by providing a toy, such as a rubber duck, boat, or plastic fish. Bathtime is usually so enjoyable for toddlers that parents can use it as a recreational activity or something to do on a rainy day when they can find nothing else to interest the child. Remind parents that although toddlers can sit well in a bathtub, it is still not safe to leave them there unsupervised. They might slip and get their head under water or reach and turn on the hot-water faucet and scald themselves.

Care of Teeth

Between-meal snacks are important for growing children. Encourage parents to offer fruit (bananas, pieces of apple, orange slices) or protein foods (cheese or pieces of chicken) rather than more traditional high-carbohydrate items for snacks. Such foods not only are nutritious but also reduce dental decay by limiting exposure of the child's teeth to carbohydrate. Calcium (found in large amounts in milk, cheese, and yogurt) is especially important to the development of strong teeth. In addition, children should continue to drink fluoridated water, if it is available, so that all new teeth form with cavity-resistant enamel.

Toddlers should have a toothbrush they recognize as their own. Toward the end of the toddler period, they can begin to do the brushing themselves under supervision (almost all children need some supervision until about age 8). Remind parents that it is better for a child to brush thoroughly once a day, probably at bedtime, than to do it poorly many times a day. After brushing, parents should use dental floss to clean between the child's teeth and to remove plaque.

Urge parents to schedule a first visit to a dentist skilled in pediatric dental care by 2.5 years of age for assessment of dentition. Parents can prepare their child for this first and subsequent visits by reading a story about a dentist visit, maintaining a positive attitude about the visit, avoiding the use of frightening words like "drill" or "shot," and answering their child's questions honestly without going into too much detail.

Promoting Healthy Family Functioning

Learning self-reliance is the primary goal of the child during the toddler period. Because of this, some parents who enjoyed caring for their child as an infant may find it difficult to have their authority challenged by a toddler. Help parents to understand that their responses to these attempts at independence are crucial to the healthy development of their child. Although the child still needs firm limits to feel secure, a child must be given some room to make independent decisions in areas that the parents feel they do not necessarily need to control. An outside person, such as a nurse, can provide an important perspective on this issue.

If parents punish the child excessively at each move toward independence, he or she will not fight them indefinitely. Instead, the child will begin to feel guilty for wanting to do things independently. Adults without a sense of autonomy feel this way about independent thought. These people may follow orders well, but when the job calls for a new program or function, they cannot reach into unknown areas without a great deal of consultation and help.

You may need to caution some parents not to begin to function at the same level as their toddler. An easy reaction to a toddler's refusal to allow a parent to help is, "You won't let me help you with this, so I won't do anything for you." This is a defense mechanism that prevents parents from feeling rejected. Teach parents that refusing to accept help is not refusing to accept love. Refusing to let mother put on a shoe is an instance of refusing to let mother put on a shoe, nothing more.

At bedtime, naptime, or anytime they are tired, toddlers may become much more like their old selves, wanting to sit on a parent's lap and be rocked or picked up and carried. This does not signal babyish behavior or regression in the toddler; it is a natural state between infant and preschool ages.

Parental Concerns Associated With the Toddler Period

Parental concerns of the toddler period usually arise because of a conflict over autonomy.

Toilet Training

Toilet training is one of the biggest tasks the toddler must achieve. There are many theories concerning toilet training, and understanding the procedure thus becomes one of the biggest tasks of this period for parents. Most first-time parents ask when to start, when the training should be completed, and how to go about it. The answer is that toilet training is an individualized task for each child. It should begin and be completed according to a child's ability to accomplish it, not according to a set schedule. When it is started can be culturally determined (see Focus on Cultural Competence).

Before children can begin to be toilet trained, they must have reached three important developmental levels, one physiologic and the other two cognitive:

1. They must have control of rectal and urethral sphincters.
2. They must have a cognitive understanding of what it means to hold urine and stools until they can release them at a certain place and time.
3. They must have a desire to delay immediate gratification for a more socially accepted action.

Because physiologic development is cephalocaudal, the rectal and urethral sphincters are not mature enough for control in most children until at least the end of the first year, when tracts of the spinal cord are myelinated to the anal level. A good way for a parent to know that a child's development has reached this point is to wait until the child can walk well independently.

Toilet training need not start this early, however, because cognitively and socially, many children do not understand what is being asked of them until they are 2 or even 3 years old. The markers of readiness are subtle, but as a rule children are ready for toilet training not only when they can understand what their parents want them to do but also when they begin to be uncomfortable in wet diapers. They demonstrate this by pulling or tugging at soiled

FOCUS ON CULTURAL COMPETENCE

In the United States, toilet training is usually introduced during the toddler period. Like so many other aspects of childrearing, the time when parents begin these activities is culturally determined. In other countries, toilet training may be started as soon as the child can sit, at about 6 months. Although praise is used in the United States as a common means of encouraging toddlers to learn new tasks, other cultures believe praise will bring a child harm by releasing evil spirits. Strategies of shame or strict discipline are used instead. Being aware that childrearing practices are not consistent across the world is a help in understanding why parents approach childrearing problems differently and why childrearing advice must be individualized.

diapers; they may bring a parent a clean diaper after they have soiled so that they can be changed (Fig. 29-7).

Teach parents not to underestimate the difficulty of the task that they expect their child to achieve. Infants live by a pleasure principle: they want what they want when they want it. Before they can complete toilet training, children must be able to give up an immediate pleasure—relieving themselves whenever they have the urge—to gain other pleasure later on—improved physical comfort and another step in growing up. For tips on how to potty train a toddler, see Focus on Family Empowerment.

Some toddlers smear or play with feces, often at about the same time that toilet training is started. This occurs because they have become aware of body excretions but have no adult values toward them; stools are little different from the clay that they play with. This activity can be minimized by providing toddlers with play substances of similar texture and by changing diapers immediately after defecation. Teach parents to accept this behavior for what it is: enjoyment of the body and of the self, and the discovery of a new substance. After a child is fully toilet trained, this activity rarely persists.

✔ CHECKPOINT QUESTIONS

7. What is a physical milestone that alerts you a child is physically ready for toilet training?
8. Are toddlers old enough to be left alone in a bathtub?

Ritualistic Behavior

Although toddlers spend a great deal of time every day investigating new ways to do things and doing things they have never done before, they also enjoy ritualistic patterns. They will use only "their" spoon at mealtime, only "their" washcloth at bath time. They will not go outside unless mother or father locates their favorite cap.

The child who seems to need an excessive number of objects to cling to or an excessive number of routines, however, may be trying to say, "I need more guidelines, more rules. Don't let me be quite so independent."

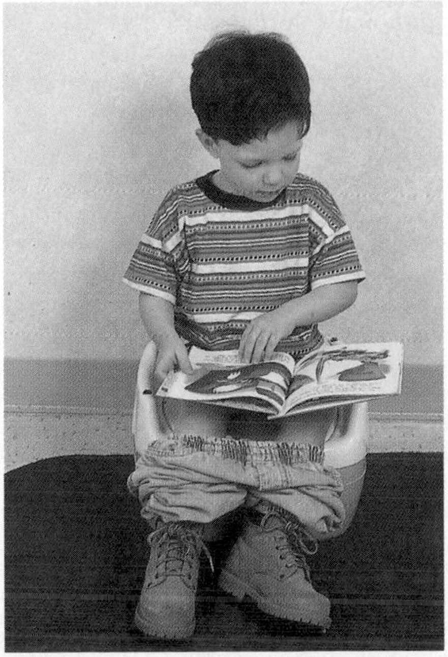

FIGURE 29.7 Toddlers are interested in toilet training as an expression of autonomy.

Negativism

As part of establishing their identities as separate individuals, toddlers typically go through a period of extreme negativism. They do not want to do anything that a parent wants them to do. Their reply to every request is a very definite "no."

It is easy for parents to believe their authority is being questioned when this happens and to worry that the child is becoming so disrespectful that he or she will have difficulty getting along in the world. They can be baffled by the extreme change from a happy, cooperative infant who lived to please them to this irritating, uncooperative child. They may need some help to realize that this is not only a normal phenomenon of toddlerhood but also a positive stage in development. This change indicates that toddlers are learning that they are separate individuals with separate needs. It is important that toddlers do this if they are to grow up to be persons who are independent and able to take care of their own needs and desires.

Parents who went away from home for the first time to college or camp might remember that they behaved similarly. They may recall that they rarely slept or ate sensibly; they tried, in effect, to break every rule that their parents used to enforce on them. Most regained their equilibrium in time to find a midpoint between irresponsible independence and common sense. If parents can recall such circumstances, they will become aware that this behavior in their toddler is not specific to the age but to the first feeling of independence. They can also remember that they meant no vindictiveness by their behavior, so they can realize that the child means none. This understanding can help to put the child's "no" in perspective.

Extreme negativism passes after it runs its course. The more parents try to make children obey them, the more children are likely to resist. Some long-term parent–child interaction problems begin during this period because parents insist on being obeyed totally or are inconsistent in their approach.

A toddler's "no" can best be eliminated by limiting the number of questions asked of the child. A father does not really mean, for example, "Are you ready for dinner?" He means, "Come to the table. It's dinnertime." A mother asks, "Will you come take a bath now?" She means, "It's time for your bath." Making a statement instead of asking a question can avoid a great many negative responses.

A toddler needs experience in making choices, however. To provide the opportunity to do this, a parent might give a secondary choice. "No" is not allowed for the major task, so the parent states, "It's bathtime now" but then says, "Do you want to take your duck or your toy boat into the tub with you?" Other examples are, "It's lunchtime. Do you want to use a big or little plate?" or "It's time to go shopping. Do you want to wear your jacket or your sweater?"

FOCUS ON FAMILY EMPOWERMENT
How to Potty Train a Toddler

Q. How can I tell if my 2-year-old is ready for toilet training? And if she is, how do I start?

A. Try the following suggestions:

1. Plan 1 or 2 weeks of "readiness" activities, which will help your child realize that the task of toilet training is a step toward being grown. If your child feels that toilet training is something only toddlers do, she may react with extreme negativism. Readiness activities may include showing your child that other family members use the toilet; making it clear that bigger people customarily leave urine and feces in the toilet, without suggesting that these materials are dirty or distasteful; and introducing training pants and showing your child that bigger people wear underpants too.
2. Check that training pants pull down readily and that slacks are free of complicated buttons or grippers; otherwise, your child will have accidents because she cannot undress quickly enough.
3. Purchase either a potty chair that sits on the floor or an infant seat that is placed on the regular toilet. The potty chair is low and potentially less frightening to a child, but it must be emptied and cleaned after each use. If you choose an infant seat, place a footstool in front of the toilet so your child has some support for her feet.
4. Put your child on the potty chair or toilet at regular intervals (e.g., when the child wakes up in the morning, after breakfast, during midmorning, before lunch, after lunch).
5. Praise your child if she does urinate or defecate. Remind her to wash her hands.
6. Be careful not to flush the toilet while the child is sitting on it. Two-year-old children are unable to realize that they will not be flushed away and may become frightened. Encourage your child to flush the toilet independently after you have helped her get cleaned and redressed.
7. Do not allow the child to remain on the potty chair for much longer than 10 minutes (less than that if she is resistant). Also, do not allow your child to use the chair to eat or as a play table so she doesn't become confused as to its purpose.
8. If your child is not ready or does not successfully use the potty on a continual basis, have her return to diapers for a short period. Be careful not to make your child feel as if this represents failure. Be careful not to equate "good" with being dry and "bad" with being wet. Continue with readiness activities. Reintroduce training pants and attempt toilet training again when your child seems more ready.
9. Some toddlers have difficulty remaining dry at night until they are 3 to 4 years old. Do not pressure your child to accomplish nighttime dryness, but assume that she is doing the best she can do. Put the child into diapers for the night by explaining (not punitively) that it is hard to keep dry during the night. After your child has been dry during the daytime for about 1 month, you may begin to leave the child in training pants.
10. Do not wake the child during the night and carry her to the bathroom to void. This system may keep her dry during the night, but it does not help her stay dry for long periods of time. It may even prolong nighttime wetness because it conditions her to void every 4 hours or so instead of retaining urine for 12 hours while she sleeps.

Although this solution is simple, it is one that parents may not arrive at themselves because finding a solution is always more difficult for the person in the middle of a problem than for an objective observer. Once they are helped to practice this approach, however, parents usually find it helpful in smoothing out the friction caused by the negativism of the toddler period.

WHAT IF? What if you ask a toddler you are caring for to take her medicine and she says, "No"? Was this a good approach?

Discipline

Some parents ask during the last part of the infant year or the early toddler period when they should start to discipline their child, or when toddlers are old enough that it is all right to punish them. Remind parents that discipline and punishment are not interchangeable terms. **Discipline** means setting rules or road signs so children know what is expected of them. **Punishment** is a consequence that results from a breakdown in discipline, from the child's disregard of the rules that were learned.

Parents should begin to instill some sense of discipline early in life because part of it involves setting safety limits and protecting others or property. Their child must stay away from the fireplace or heater; she must not go in the street; she must not hit other children, for example. Enforcing limits, however, arises out of the day-to-day interaction with the child, out of the rhythm of childcare, not out of a set procedure such as, "Today, I'm going to teach discipline." Two general rules to follow are (1) parents need to be consistent, and (2) rules are learned best if correct behavior is praised rather than wrong behavior punished.

"Timeout" is a technique of helping children learn that actions have consequences. To use "timeout" effectively, parents first need to be certain their children understand the rule they are trying to enforce: "If you hit your brother, you'll have timeout," etc. Parents should give one warning. If the child repeats the behavior, parents select an area that is nonstimulating, such as a corner of a room or a hallway. The child is directed to go immediately to the "timeout" space. The child then sits there for a specified period of time. If the child cries or shows any other disruptive behavior, the timeout period doesn't begin until there is quiet. When the child is quiet, the time period begins. When the specified time period has passed, the child can return to the family. A guide as to how long children should remain in their "timeout" chair is 1 minute per year of age. Using a timer, such as one for the stove that rings when time is up, lets children know when they can return to the family.

Separation Anxiety

As discussed in Chapter 35, fear of being separated from parents begins at about 6 months of age and persists throughout the preschool period. This universal fear of this age group is known as separation anxiety. For this reason, toddlers have difficulty accepting being separated from their primary caregiver to spend the day at a day care center or if they or their primary caregiver are hospitalized. Chapter 35 discusses nursing responsibility for care of toddlers in the hospital as well as the reactions of toddlers to the separation caused by hospitalization and the methods used to minimize these reactions.

Parents may ask what they can do about this problem. They believe they have a right to leave the child in a babysitter's or center's care, but how can they tolerate the crying at the door? Most toddlers react best to separation if a regular babysitter is employed or the day care center is one with consistent caregivers. Many are more comfortable if they are cared for in their own home. It helps if they have fair warning that they will have a babysitter. For example, they might be told, "Mommy is fixing dinner early because Mommy and Daddy are going to visit some friends tonight. Marsha is going to come and babysit for you. She'll put you to bed. When you wake up in the morning, Mommy and Daddy will be here again."

No matter how well prepared toddlers are, they may cry when the babysitter actually appears or may greet the babysitter warmly only to cry when the parents reach for their coats. It helps if parents say goodbye firmly, repeat the explanation that they will be there when the child wakes in the morning, and then leave. Prolonged goodbyes only lead to more crying. Sneaking out prevents crying and may ease the parents' guilt, but it should be discouraged because it can strengthen fear of abandonment. This applies to hospital visits as well.

> ✔ **CHECKPOINT QUESTIONS**
>
> 9. How can parents minimize the toddler's extreme negativism?
> 10. What is meant by "timeout"?

Temper Tantrums

Almost every toddler has a temper tantrum at one time or another. The child may kick, scream, stamp feet, shout, "No, no, no," lie on the floor, flail arms and legs, and bang the head against the floor. Children may even hold their breath until they become cyanotic and slump to the floor. When this happens, the child has a distended chest (a halt after inspiration), often air-filled cheeks, and increasing distress as the child's body registers oxygen want. This is harmless breath holding; ignoring it will make it ineffective and the child will give it up. True breath holding is a neurologic problem in which the child appears to "forget" to breathe or halts breathing after expiration, usually at the peak of anger. A third type is associated with seizures; with this, the cessation of breathing occurs as part of generalized seizure activity (see Chap. 49). Guidelines that are helpful in differentiating simple breath holding from neurologic disorders are shown in Table 29-5.

Temper tantrums are a natural consequence of toddlers' development. Toddlers are independent enough to know what they want, but they do not have the vocabulary or the wisdom to express their feelings in a more socially acceptable way. For example, temper tantrums occur most often when children are tired, just before naptime or bedtime, or during a long shopping trip or visit. The tantrums are often a response to an unrealistic request by a parent: asking a child to comb his hair before he is coordinated enough to do so, asking her to pick up her toys before she has a feeling of family responsibility, or asking him to share before he can understand what is wanted. Also, they may occur if parents are saying "no" too frequently with regard to such things as touching the coffee table, getting dirty, using a spoon, or running and jumping; thus, the child feels constantly thwarted. A tantrum may be a response to difficulty making choices or decisions or to pressure from activities such as toilet training. Such a child needs to express feelings in some way and does so with temper tantrums. These episodes are taxing for the parents; they are also energy-consuming for the child (Stein et al., 2001).

Nurses can assess the tantrums and the parents' reactions in an effort to help families find ways to manage temper tantrums (Box 29-3). Probably the best approach is for parents to tell the child simply that they disapprove of the tantrum and then ignore it. They might say, "I'll be in the bedroom. When you're done kicking, you come into the bedroom, too." Children who are left alone in the kitchen will usually not continue a tantrum but will stop after 1 or 2 minutes and rejoin their parents. Parents should then accept the child warmly and proceed as if the tantrum had not occurred. This same approach works well for nurses caring for hospitalized toddlers.

NURSING DIAGNOSES AND RELATED INTERVENTIONS

Nursing Diagnosis: Risk for compromised family coping related to toddler behavior

Outcome Identification: Family will demonstrate better methods for coping with temper tantrums.

Outcome Evaluation: Family states temper tantrums occur less than two times daily.

TABLE 29.5 Differentiating Temper Tantrums, Breath Holding, and Seizures

ASSESSMENT	TEMPER TANTRUMS	BREATH HOLDING	SEIZURES
Provocation	Usually provoked—parent can state a reason for it (she asked toddler to come to dinner, but he wanted to finish an activity)	Usually provoked; child very angry; child breathes out and forgets to breathe in	Not provoked
Appearance of cyanosis	Child holds breath, becomes cyanotic, then slumps to floor	Child breathes out, becomes cyanotic, then slumps to floor	Child slumps to floor first, then becomes cyanotic

BOX 29.3

HELPING PARENTS MANAGE A TODDLER'S TEMPER TANTRUM

Explore with the parents the reasons for the behavior:

- Do tantrums always occur just before bedtime? If so, the parents might schedule an earlier bedtime or an afternoon nap.
- Do tantrums occur every time the parent goes shopping? If so, perhaps it would help to schedule two shorter trips each week rather than one long one.
- Do tantrums occur whenever the parent asks the child to do something? If so, investigate whether the child is being asked to perform age-appropriate tasks.
- Do tantrums occur in response to decision making? If so, parents may have to limit the number of choices they are asking of the child.

After determining which circumstances generally lead to temper tantrums, ask parents to describe the behavior:

- Does it sound like a tantrum or something more?
- Is there a possibility a parent is mistaking seizure activity for temper tantrums?
- Could a parent be confusing neurologic breath holding with a temper tantrum?

Assess what the parents do when the child has a tantrum:

- Do the parents give either material or emotional bribes (e.g., "Come and get a cookie," or "Stop and I'll give you a kiss"). This method is rarely effective. If they accede to the child's wishes, the child is generally encouraged to have more tantrums because they are so successful.
- Do the parents punish the child? Toddlers have a right to express opinions; they need to be guided to learn a more controlled and mature way of expressing them.
- Do parents demonstrate adult behavior in managing a toddler's temper tantrums? For example, if the child shouts or kicks, does the parent respond, "I can shout as loud as you. I can kick as hard as you"? Instead of showing the child a better way to express feelings, this reinforces the way the child is responding.

Helping parents to correct problems early may limit the number of tantrums they must deal with; it will not prevent them, however, because parents cannot anticipate all the circumstances that will cause this reaction. In fact, parents should not feel they must prevent all of them; they are, after all, parents, not mind readers (see Focus on Nursing Care Planning). As the child matures, increases his or her vocabulary, and is capable of better responses to stress situations, tantrums begin to fade by themselves.

WHAT IF? What if a toddler you are caring for in the hospital has a temper tantrum in the middle of a busy hallway? Would you ignore it, or move the child to a quieter place?

Sibling Rivalry

Sibling rivalry, or jealousy of younger siblings, can occur during the toddler period. It is discussed in Chapter 30 with concerns of the preschool child.

Concerns of the Family With a Physically Challenged or Chronically Ill Toddler

It may be difficult for children with handicaps to achieve a sense of autonomy or independence because they will never be totally independent. It is important for these children to develop as strong a sense of autonomy as possible so they see themselves as independent and work to become increasingly self-sufficient as they grow older. It takes courage for an adult to do such things as move a wheelchair through a busy airport or a concert crowd. Nursing actions designed to help the challenged or chronically ill child develop a sense of autonomy are outlined in Table 29-6. Most important are actions to support the family. If a toddler has physical limitations, he or she may be unable to explore freely or may not have the physical ability to pound and manipulate toys as the average toddler does.

The toddler with a long-term illness or who is physically challenged can be expected to exhibit normal toddler behaviors, such as temper tantrums, and to have normal outlooks, such as negativism. Parents whose child is uncoordinated or has a neurologic disease may mistake temper tantrums for seizure activity. Investigate such activity carefully, and explain to parents the difference between the two. Parents may also mistake particular toddlers' insistence on having their own way as a manifestation of illness. Remind these parents that the behavior is more often an indication of age and development rather than of illness so they can respond firmly.

The mother of a 2-year-old boy brings the child in for a health maintenance visit. She states, "I just don't know how to handle his temper tantrums."

FOCUS ON *Nursing Care Planning*

A TODDLER WITH TEMPER TANTRUMS

Assessment: Well-nourished 2-year-old boy. Physical findings within normal limits. Mother reports the child is having temper tantrums at least 20 times a day. "He throws himself on the floor and pounds his head and fists." Mother unable to describe any precipitating factors for the tantrums. She states, "He seems to have them just when I start to do something. I could be playing with him one minute, and then I get up to do something, like answer the phone or start dinner, and then he starts." Mother reports picking up the child immediately because she fears he will hurt himself. "I just don't know what to do anymore."

Nursing Diagnosis: Health-seeking behaviors related to measures for handling and reducing the number of temper tantrums

Outcome Identification: Mother demonstrates measures to manage temper tantrums within 2 weeks.

Outcome Evaluation: Child demonstrates a decrease in the number of tantrums to less than 4 per day. Mother identifies measures to manage tantrums, reports tantrums have decreased in number by the end of 1 week.

Interventions	Rationale
1. Review events surrounding the temper tantrum episodes, asking the mother to describe the events before, during, and after the tantrum. Explore possible reasons for the behavior.	1. Description of events provides helpful information, including possible contributory factors for the tantrums, providing a baseline for identifying possible strategies to limit them.
2. Assess the child for possible neurologic and cognitive problems. If present, refer to appropriate health care provider.	2. Parents may mistakenly interpret problems such as seizures or motor tics as tantrum activity. Further assessment of the toddler helps to rule these out as possible causes.
3. Review normal toddler growth and development, explaining that some temper tantrums during this period are natural occurrences.	3. Information about normal toddler growth and development provides a foundation for further teaching and instruction.
4. Inform the mother that children rarely hurt themselves during tantrums and that they are the child's way of expressing his needs and feelings.	4. Increased knowledge about the underlying reasons for, and minimal risk of injury during, tantrums helps to alleviate some of the mother's anxiety about the situation, thus helping her to view the episodes more objectively.
5. Discuss with the mother ways to offer secondary choices to the child.	5. Offering secondary choices provides the child with options, reducing his feelings of frustration and enhancing his sense of control and independence. Secondary choices also provide a means for the mother to prevent tantrums.
6. Work with the mother to develop actions to try (e.g., ignoring the tantrum, telling the child she disapproves of the behavior, or beginning timeout). Encourage the mother to avoid picking up the child and only to do so if there is actual danger of injury.	6. These actions provide concrete methods for dealing with tantrums, enhancing the possibility for the child to better express his feelings. Picking up the child each time only serves to reinforce the behavior.
7. Assist the mother with setting up a routine for spending consistent time with the child engaging in an enjoyable activity each day.	7. Routine planning with a consistent activity helps to reassure the child and reinforce positive behaviors.
8. Instruct the mother to keep a diary of the child's behavior and measures used during the next week. Set up an appointment for a telephone conference with the mother next week to review the diary and discuss the child's behavior.	8. Keeping a diary and reviewing it over the telephone aids in evaluating the child's behavior and effectiveness of the methods used. Follow-up telephone call also provides an additional opportunity for feedback, teaching, and support.

TABLE 29.6 Nursing Interventions to Help the Physically Challenged or Chronically Ill Child Develop a Sense of Autonomy

AREA	NURSING ACTION
Nutrition	A special diet may limit typical finger foods. Use imagination to offer other foods not usually eaten this way as finger foods. Allow child to help pour liquid diet for a tube feeding. Toddlers are frightened by vomiting because they have no control over it. Check for possibility of nausea; toddlers have no way to express this other than by not eating.
Dressing changes	The child can hold pieces of tape or put tape in place to maintain sense of control. The child can remove an old bandage if it is not contaminated. Allow the child to view his or her incision and watch dressing changes; explaining each step of a procedure as you perform it helps the child maintain control.
	Restrain only those body parts necessary during a procedure to allow the child a sense of control.
	Remove all supplies after a procedure, or the child may "redo" the dressing.
Medication	Allow children no choice as to whether a medicine will be taken. Do allow a child to choose a "chaser," such as milk or juice, after oral medicine. Do not ask a toddler to indicate a choice of site for an injection or intravenous insertion; this is too advanced a decision for a toddler to handle.
Rest	Locate or create a ritual for bedtime (put child into bed, tuck him in, say, "Goodnight, Bobby." Tuck in bear. Say, "Goodnight, Bear"). Allow a choice of toy or cover but not a choice of bedtime or naptime hour.
Hygiene	Allow the child a choice of bathtub toy or clothing. Allow the child to wash face and hands to gain control of the situation.
	Allow the child to put toothpaste on a brush, but you should brush or "touch up" teeth afterward to ensure that all plaque has been removed.
Pain	Encourage a child to express pain ("Say 'ouch' when I pull off the tape").
	Help channel the child's self-expression to what is acceptable (e.g., the child may shout but may not kick).
Stimulation	Provide a toddler with a toy that can be manipulated, such as boxes that fit inside one another and can be taken out again, trucks that can be pushed, and pegs that can be pounded. In a health care setting, items can usually be found that fit together (boxes from central supply or plastic vials from the pharmacy). Another action toy: buy a non-latex balloon and tie it to the crib side to be used as a punching bag; another one tied to the foot of the crib can serve as a leg exerciser.
Elimination	A child who is toilet trained needs to be encouraged to use a potty chair or toilet during an illness. Help children with ureter or bowel stomas to help with changing bags so they are as independent in bowel function as possible.

Toilet training is difficult for a child who is hospitalized at periodic intervals, as success usually requires a consistent caregiver; in addition, hospitalization can result in regressive behaviors. If a chronically ill child also has difficulty with ambulation, soiling accidents may occur beyond the usual age for them because the toddler's neurologic development is not sufficient or because of inability to reach the bathroom easily.

Children who survive a long-term illness are sometimes referred to as medically fragile or vulnerable children (Green & Solnit, 1964). Some parents tend to protect and shelter such a child, and you may have to remind them that even though chronically ill, a toddler will demand independence and has the right to explore. A child who uses a lower-extremity prosthesis, for example, might prefer to crawl somewhere rather than wait for help to put the prosthesis in place. Although this degree of independence is good, parents may have to limit how it is expressed so the child will learn how to use the prosthesis (for example, they could make a rule that the child must use the prosthesis to walk but can choose whether to use a spoon when eating).

Nutrition and the Physically Challenged or Chronically Ill Toddler

Toddlers need experience feeding themselves if at all possible. Help parents accept the accidents that occur with self-feeding, particularly if the child has difficulty with coordination; suggest finger foods if possible.

If on a special diet, children may not be allowed to eat finger foods; if they are tube fed, they receive no experience with finger foods at all. For these toddlers, parents should try to provide other, comparable experiences in independence, such as letting them choose where they prefer to eat or what food they would like to eat first.

✔ CHECKPOINT QUESTIONS

11. What is the best way to manage toddler temper tantrums?
12. What type of foods best encourage autonomy?

KEY POINTS

Erikson's developmental task for the toddler period is to form a sense of autonomy or independence versus shame or doubt.

Toddlers make great strides forward in development, but their physical growth slows.

- A critical milestone of toddler development is being able to form two-word sentences by 2 years of age.
- Toddlers are capable of preoperational thought or are able to deal much more constructively with symbols than they could while still infants.
- Important aspects of care are promoting toddler safety, including screening for lead poisoning; promoting toddler development, such as promoting daily activities; and healthy family functioning.
- Toddler appetites decrease from those of the infant, so children eat proportionally less than they did as infants.
- Common concerns of parents during the toddler period are toilet training, ritualistic behavior, negativism, temper tantrums, discipline, and separation anxiety.
- Promoting autonomy in the child who is physically challenged or chronically ill calls for creative planning, because there may be many tasks that must be done for the child to be certain they are done safely.

CRITICAL THINKING EXERCISES

1. Jason is the toddler you met at the beginning of the chapter. His mother told you he refuses to do anything she tells him to do. What are three questions you would want to ask his mother to help her explore the problem?
2. A parent tells you that her toddler eats "almost nothing." What is the best way to evaluate if the child's intake is adequate? Why does the intake of toddlers decrease from what it was during the infant year?
3. The mother of a 2-year-old tells you her toddler has at least three temper tantrums a day. She asks you how to deal with these when they happen while shopping. What would you advise?
4. Many working mothers are concerned that toilet training will be especially difficult because their child has two or three caregivers every day. What suggestions could you offer to make toilet training easier under these circumstances?
5. Examine the National Health Goals related to toddler health. Most government-sponsored money for nursing research is allotted based on these goals. What would be a possible research topic to explore pertinent to these goals that would be fundable and would advance evidence-based practice?

REFERENCES

American Academy of Pediatrics Committee on Nutrition. (2001). The use and misuse of fruit juice in pediatrics. *Pediatrics, 107*(5), 1210–1213.

American Academy of Pediatrics Committee on Practice and Ambulatory Medicine. (2001). *Recommendations for preventive pediatric health care.* Washington, D.C.: AAP.

American Academy of Pediatrics Committee on Safety. (2001). *Seat belt safety and children.* Washington, D.C.: AAP.

Berger, K. S. (2001). *The developing person through the life span* (5th ed.). New York: Worth Publishing.

Department of Health and Human Services. (2000). *Healthy people 2010.* Washington, D.C.: DHHS.

Erikson, E. H. (1993). *Childhood and society.* New York: W.W. Norton.

Dudek, S. G. (2001). *Nutrition: Essentials for nursing practice.* Philadelphia: Lippincott Williams & Wilkins.

Fisher, J. O. et al. (2002). Parental influences on young girls' fruit and vegetable, micronutrient, and fat intake. *Journal of the American Dietetic Association, 102*(1), 58–64.

Green, M., & Solnit, A. (1964). Reactions to the threatened loss of a child: A vulnerable child syndrome. *Pediatrics, 34*(1), 58–64.

Johnson, M., Maas, M., & Moorhead, S. (2000). *Nursing outcomes classification* (2nd ed.). St. Louis: Mosby.

Kaplan, D. W., & Love, K. A. (2001). Growth & development. In W. W. Hay, A. R. Hayward, M. J. Levin, & J. M. Sondheimer (Eds.). *Current pediatric diagnosis and treatment* (15th ed.). New York: McGraw-Hill.

Krebs, N. F., & Hambridge, K. M. (2001). Normal childhood nutrition and its disorders. In W. W. Hay, A. R. Hayward, M. J. Levin, & J. M. Sondheimer (Eds.). *Current pediatric diagnosis and treatment* (15th ed.). New York: McGraw-Hill.

McCloskey, J., & Bulechek, G. (2000). *Nursing interventions classification* (3d ed.). St. Louis: Mosby.

Murphy, L. M. B. (2001). Adolescent mothers' beliefs about parenting and injury prevention: Results of a focus group. *Journal of Pediatric Health Care, 15*(4), 194–199.

Piaget, J. (1969). *The theory of stages in cognitive development.* New York: McGraw-Hill.

Stein, M. T., et al. (2001). Temper tantrums, impulsivity, and aggression in a preschool-aged boy. *Journal of Developmental & Behavioral Pediatrics, 22*(2), S23–S28.

SUGGESTED READINGS

Bjorkqvist, K., & Osterman, K. (2001). At what age do children learn to discriminate between act and actor? *Perceptual & Motor Skills, 92*(1), 171–176.

Blackwell, P. L. (2000). The influence of touch on child development: Implications for intervention. *Infants & Young Children, 13*(1), 25–39.

Dobrez, D., et al. (2001). Estimating the cost of developmental and behavioral screening of preschool children in general pediatric practice. *Pediatrics, 108*(4), 913–922.

Gazi, M. A. (2001). Management of penile toilet seat injury. *Canadian Journal of Urology, 8*(3), 1293–1294.

Halpert, E. (2000). On lying and the lie of a toddler. *Psychoanalytic Quarterly, 69*(4), 659–675.

Kawauchi, A., et al. (2001). Follow-up study of bedwetting from 3 to 5 years of age. *Urology, 58*(5), 772–776.

Monsen, R. B. (2001). Giving children control and toilet training. *Journal of Pediatric Nursing, 16*(95), 375–376.

Rhodes, C. (2000). Effective management of daytime wetting. *Paediatric Nursing, 12*(2), 14–17.

Thomas, D. O. (2002). Special considerations for pediatric triage in the emergency department. *Nursing Clinics of North America, 37*(1), 145–159.

Ziegert, D. I., et al. (2001). Longitudinal study of young children's responses to challenging achievement situations. *Child Development, 72*(2), 609–624.

30

CHAPTER

The Family With a Preschooler

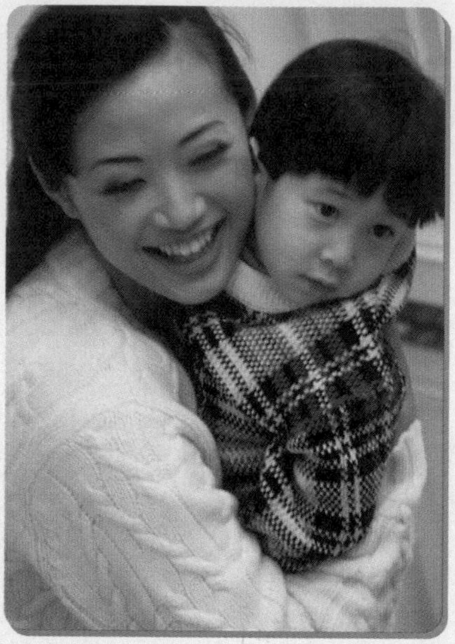

Key Terms

- broken fluency
- bruxism
- conservation
- ectomorphic body build
- Electra complex
- endomorphic body build
- genu valgus
- intuitional thought
- Oedipus complex
- secondary stuttering

Objectives

After mastering the contents of this chapter, you should be able to:

1. Describe normal growth and development as well as common parental concerns of the preschool period.
2. Assess a preschooler for normal growth and developmental milestones.
3. Formulate nursing diagnoses related to preschool growth and development and common parental concerns.
4. Identify expected outcomes for nursing care of the toddler.
5. Plan nursing care to meet the preschooler's growth and development needs, such as planning age-appropriate play activities.
6. Implement nursing care related to normal growth and development of the preschooler, such as preparing a preschooler for an invasive procedure.
7. Evaluate outcome criteria established for care to be certain normal growth and development goals have been achieved.
8. Identify National Health Goals related to the preschool period that nurses can be instrumental in helping the nation to achieve.
9. Identify areas related to care of the preschool-age child that could benefit from additional nursing research or application of evidence-based practice.
10. Use critical thinking to analyze additional ways in which growth and development problems of the preschool child can be prevented and care can be family-centered.
11. Integrate knowledge of preschool growth and development with nursing process to achieve quality maternal and child health nursing care.

Terry is a 3-year-old girl. Her mother tells you that Terry plays and talks constantly with an imaginary friend named Emma. She makes up stories about events that can't possibly be true. When corrected, Terry stutters so badly no one can understand her. Is Terry's mother describing typical preschool behavior, or does Terry need a referral to a child guidance counselor?

The previous chapter described the toddler and the abilities children develop during that period. This chapter adds information about the changes, both physical and psychosocial, that occur during the preschool years. This is important information because it builds a base for care and health teaching for the age group.

After you've studied the chapter, answer the Critical Thinking Exercises at the end of the chapter and then access the on-line study activities (http://connection.lww.com) *to further sharpen your skills and test your knowledge.*

The preschool period traditionally includes ages 3, 4, and 5 years. Although physical growth slows considerably during this period, personality and cognitive growth are substantial. This is also an important period of growth for parents. They may be unsure about how much independence and responsibility for self-care they should give their preschooler. Most children of this age want to do things for themselves—choose their own clothing and dress by themselves, feed themselves completely, wash their own hair, and so forth. As a result, parents of a preschooler may find their child dressed in one red and one green sock, going to school with unwashed ears, or trying to eat soup with a fork. They need reassurance that this behavior is typical and helps the child develop more initiative and control of life. They may also need some guidance in separating those tasks that a preschooler can accomplish independently from those that still require some adult supervision. Sensible limits must be set so children do not harm themselves or others while participating in all the interesting experiences available to them. The Focus on National Health Goals box lists National Health Goals related to the period.

FOCUS ON NATIONAL HEALTH GOALS

A number of National Health Goals are designed to target the preschool population:

- Increase use of helmets by bicyclists.
- Reduce infectious diarrhea by at least 25% among children in licensed childcare centers.
- Reduce acute middle ear infections among children age 4 and younger, as measured by days of restricted activity or school absenteeism.
- Increase the use of child auto restraints in children age 4 and under from 92% to 100%.
- Reduce deaths caused by poisoning from 6.8/100,000 to 1.5/100,000 (DHHS, 2000).

Nurses can be instrumental in helping the nation achieve these goals by serving as consultants at day care and preschool settings to be certain that protection from the spread of infectious diseases in these settings is provided and by urging parents to fit their children with helmets before beginning bicycle riding and to protect against poisoning.

A number of questions could benefit from additional nursing research, such as: What practices seem most effective in reducing the spread of infection in day care or preschool settings? What are the barriers to parents buying helmets for this age child? What proportion of parents know the signs and symptoms of common illnesses their child might contract in a childcare or preschool setting?

NURSING PROCESS OVERVIEW

For Healthy Development of the Preschooler

Assessment

Regular assessment of the preschooler includes obtaining a health history and performing both a physical and developmental evaluation (see Assessing the Average Preschooler). Preschoolers speak very little during a health assessment; they may even revert to baby talk or babyish actions such as thumb sucking if they find a health visit stressful. A history that details their usual performance level is therefore very important for accurate evaluation.

Assess the child's weight and height according to standard growth charts (see Appendix E). Keep in mind that these charts are based on average weights and heights of white American children, and that children from other ethnic or cultural backgrounds may not follow these norms. For instance, Asian children are often seen at the low end of the charts; children with exceptionally tall parents tend to fall at the higher ranges. Also assess the child for general appearance. Does the child appear to be alert? Happy? Active? Healthy? (Colds are frequent in all children; the average preschooler may have 6 to 12 a year.) Ask whether the child is able to attend a half-day session at a preschool or day care center without becoming exhausted. Are the teeth free of cavities? Is the gait symmetrical?

Nursing Diagnosis

A wellness-oriented nursing diagnosis used in health promotion of the preschooler is:

- Health-seeking behaviors related to developmental expectations

Other nursing diagnoses that relate to the developmental stage of the preschooler include:

- Risk for injury related to increased independence outside the home
- Delayed growth and development related to frequent illness
- Risk for poisoning related to maturational age of child

ASSESSING the Average Preschooler

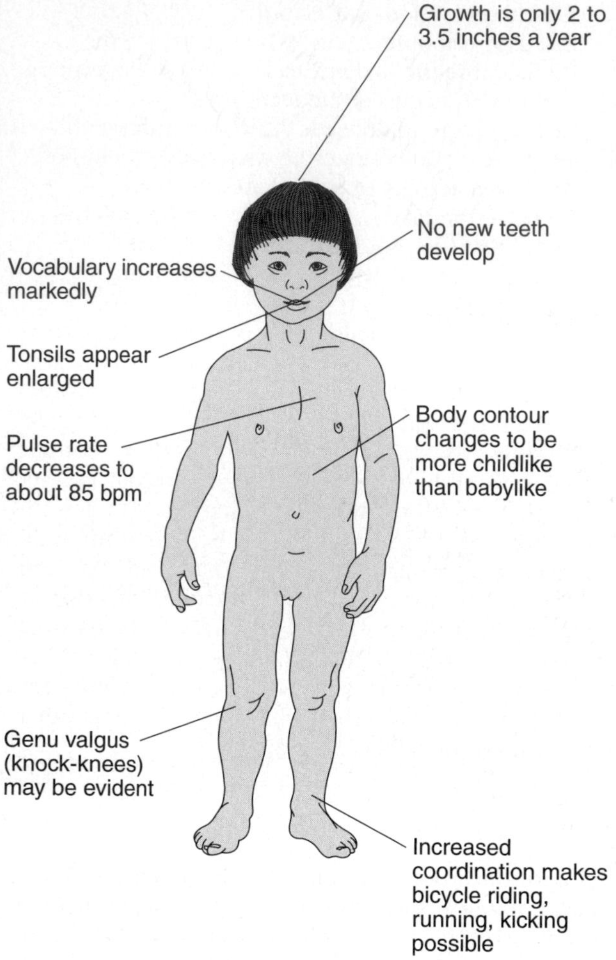
Growth is only 2 to 3.5 inches a year
No new teeth develop
Vocabulary increases markedly
Tonsils appear enlarged
Pulse rate decreases to about 85 bpm
Body contour changes to be more childlike than babylike
Genu valgus (knock-knees) may be evident
Increased coordination makes bicycle riding, running, kicking possible

- Parental anxiety related to lack of understanding of childhood development

Outcome Identification and Planning
Planning and establishing expected outcomes for care of the preschooler often begin with establishing a schedule for discussing normal preschool development with the parents (this should be done at all health maintenance visits). For many parents, this is a difficult time because the child is at an in-between stage: no longer an infant, although not yet ready for formal school. Planning for accident prevention is very important as the child begins to have experiences away from home. It is equally important to plan opportunities for adventurous activities, messy play, and independent decision making. When asking parents to incorporate adventurous activities or messy material into a preschooler's play, you may be asking them to do something they don't personally enjoy. Most parents successfully initiate activities with a child if they believe they are important, but some are able to do this better than others. Allowing children choices may also be difficult for parents because they want to protect their children from making errors.

Implementation
Preschool children imitate moods as well as actions. An important nursing intervention, then, is role playing a mood or attitude you would like a child to learn. To project an attitude toward health assessment as an enjoyable activity, you might suggest preschoolers participate by listening to their heart. Accident prevention is also best taught by role modeling (a parent always crosses streets at the corner and doesn't start the car until seatbelts are in place).

Outcome Evaluation
Evaluation of expected outcomes should be continuous and frequent. Because growth during this period is more cognitive and emotional than physical, parents may report little growth. Evaluating specific areas helps them to see that progress has occurred. Examples of expected outcomes might be:

- Child states importance of holding parent's hand while crossing streets.
- Parent states realistic expectations of 3-year-old's motor ability by next visit.
- Mother reports she has prepared 4-year-old for new baby by next visit.

NURSING ASSESSMENT OF GROWTH AND DEVELOPMENT OF THE PRESCHOOLER

Assessment of preschoolers needs to include physical, cognitive, and developmental growth.

Physical Growth

A definite change in body contour occurs during the preschool years. The wide-legged gait, prominent lordosis, and protuberant abdomen of the toddler change to slimmer, taller, and much more childlike proportions. Contour changes are so definite that future body type—**ectomorphic** (slim body build) or **endomorphic** (large body build)—becomes apparent. Handedness begins to be obvious. A major step forward is the child's ability to learn extended language, which is affected not only by motor but also by cognitive development. Children of this age who are exposed to more than one language or who live in a bilingual family have a unique opportunity to master two languages with relative ease because of this increased cognitive ability.

Lymphatic tissue begins to increase in size, particularly the tonsils, and levels of IgG and IgA antibodies increase. These changes tend to make preschool illnesses more localized (an upper respiratory infection remains localized to the nose with little systemic fever).

Physiologic splitting of heart sounds may be present for the first time on auscultation; innocent heart murmurs may also be heard for the first time. This type of murmur occurs owing to the changing size of the heart in reference to the thorax. The anteroposterior and transverse diameters of the chest reach adult proportions. Pulse rate decreases to about 85 bpm; blood pressure holds at about 100/60 mm Hg.

The bladder is easily palpable above the symphysis pubis; voiding is frequent enough (9 or 10 times a day) that play is interrupted, and accidents may occur if the child becomes absorbed in an activity.

The child who earlier in life had an indeterminate longitudinal arch in the foot generally demonstrates a well-formed arch now. Muscles are noticeably stronger and make activities such as gymnastics possible. Many children at the beginning of the period exhibit **genu valgus** (knock-knees); this disappears with increased skeletal growth at the end of the preschool period.

Weight, Height, and Head Circumference

Weight gain is slight during the preschool years. The average child gains only about 4.5 lb (2 kg) a year. Appetite remains as it was during the toddler years, which is considerably less than some parents would like or expect. Parents may bring their preschooler to the health care facility because they fear their child is losing weight. When the child's weight is plotted on a growth chart, however, it becomes evident that he or she is indeed putting on some weight; what parents are noticing is the age-appropriate change in body shape from rounded to slim.

Height gain is also minimal during this period: only 2 to 3.5 inches (6 to 8 cm) a year on average. Head circumference is not routinely measured at physical assessments on children over 2 years of age (see Appendix E for averages).

Teeth

Children generally have all 20 of their deciduous teeth by 3 years of age. Rarely do new teeth erupt during the preschool period (Kaplan & Love, 2001).

> **✔ CHECKPOINT QUESTIONS**
>
> 1. Are gains in height and weight dramatic during the preschool period?
> 2. How many new teeth usually develop during this time?

Developmental Milestones

Each year during the preschool period marks a major step forward in gross motor, fine motor, and language development. Play activities change focus as the preschooler learns new skills and understands more about the world (Fig. 30-1). Table 30-1 summarizes the major milestones of the period.

Language Development

A 3-year-old child has a vocabulary of about 900 words. These are used to ask questions constantly, mostly "how" and "why" questions, such as "Why is snow cold? How do worms hear? What does your tongue do?" A child needs simple answers to such questions so curiosity, vocabulary building, and questioning are encouraged, and also because the depth of the child's understanding is often deceptive. For example, if a parent tells a child that shoes should go on with the buckles on the outside, the child may seem to understand but may return in a few minutes to ask, "Why do I have to go outside to put on my shoes?" Words with double and triple meanings can be truly confounding to children of this age. Four- and 5-year-old children continue to ask many questions. They enjoy participating in mealtime conversation and can describe something from their day in great detail (see Focus on Cultural Competence). Preschoolers imitate language exactly, so if they hear less-than-perfect language, this is the language pattern they adopt. They may imitate and use "bathroom language" if not corrected because of the attention from adults this generates.

Preschoolers are egocentric, so they define objects in relation to themselves (a key is not a metal object but "what I use to open a door," and a car is not a means of transportation but "what Mom uses to take me to school").

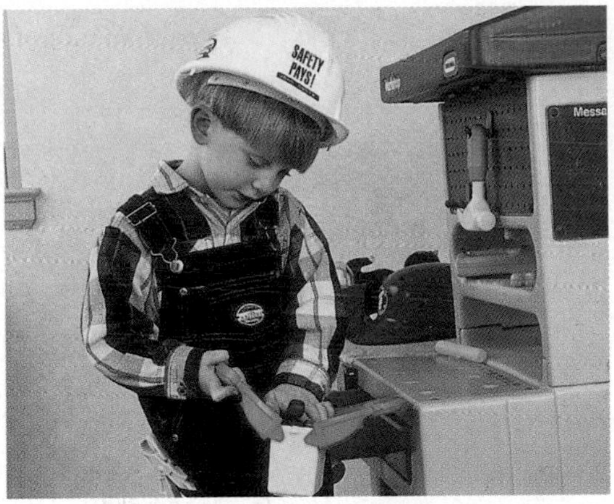

FIGURE 30.1 Preschoolers enjoy meaningful play and like to imitate the roles of adults, as they learn about the world around them.

Play

Preschoolers do not need many toys. Their imaginations are keener than they will be at any other time in their lives, so they enjoy games that use imitation, such as playing house. They imitate what they see parents doing: eating meals, mowing the lawn, cleaning the house, arguing, and so forth. They pretend to be teachers, cowboys, firefighters, and store clerks. Many preschoolers have imaginary friends as a normal part of having an active imagination. These often exist until children formally begin school.

Four- and 5-year-olds divide their time between roughhousing and imitative play. Five-year-olds are also interested in group games that they have learned in kindergarten or preschool.

Emotional Development

Children change a great deal in their ability to understand the world and how they relate to people during the preschool years.

TABLE 30.1 Summary of Preschool Growth and Development

AGE (YRS)	FINE MOTOR	GROSS MOTOR	LANGUAGE	PLAY
3	Undresses self; stacks tower of blocks; draws a cross	Runs; alternates feet on stairs; rides tricycle; stands on one foot	Vocabulary of 900 words	Able to take turns; very imaginative
4	Can do simple buttons	Constantly in motion; jumps; skips	Vocabulary of 1,500 words	Pretending is major activity
5	Draws a 6-part man; can lace shoes	Throws overhand	Vocabulary of 2,100 words	Likes games with numbers or letters

Developmental Task: Initiative Versus Guilt

The developmental task for the preschool-age child is to achieve a sense of initiative (Erikson, 1993). The child with a well-developed sense of initiative has discovered that learning about new things is fun.

If children are criticized or punished for attempts at initiative, they develop a sense of guilt for wanting to try new activities or have new experiences. Those who leave the preschool period with guilt may carry it with them into new situations, such as starting elementary school. They may even have difficulty later in life making decisions about everything from changing jobs to choosing an apartment, because they cannot envision that they are capable of solving associated problems.

To gain a sense of initiative, preschoolers need exposure to a wide variety of experiences and play materials so they can learn as much about the world as possible. They are ready to reach outside their homes for new experiences, such as a trip to the zoo or an amusement park (Fig. 30-2). They are interested in seeing new places, and especially enjoy going with the family on vacation. These types of experiences lead to increased vocabulary; for instance, at the zoo, preschoolers not only learn words such as giraffe, elephant, and bear, but they learn to transfer them from abstract concepts to the objects to which they relate.

Urge parents to provide play materials that encourage creative play, such as finger paints, soapy water to splash or blow into bubbles, mud to make pies, sand to build castles, and modeling clay or homemade dough to mold into figures or make into pretend cookies. These are messy activities, and many parents cannot let a child indulge in them more than once a week, but any experience with free-form play is helpful.

Preschoolers tend to have such active imaginations that they need little guidance in this type of play. They smear both hands into clay or finger paint and create instinctively. Urge parents to support this kind of play and not try to take it over. If a parent draws a tree with finger paint, for example, and says, "Now you draw one," a child may decide it is no fun to finger paint because he knows that his tree will not look as good as his parent's. As he is not ready for competition, he will drop out of the activity rather than be shown up as inferior.

Preschoolers may make nothing recognizable out of clay or finger paint, preferring simply to handle the medium. As long as they enjoy the feel of the material, they do not need to make anything. Pressure to make things is not fun and can discourage their interest in learning.

Imitation. Preschoolers need free rein to imitate the roles of the people around them. Again, role playing should be fun and does not have to be accurate. If a boy is pretending to be a police officer and is busy putting out fires, or a firefighter and is stopping playmates from

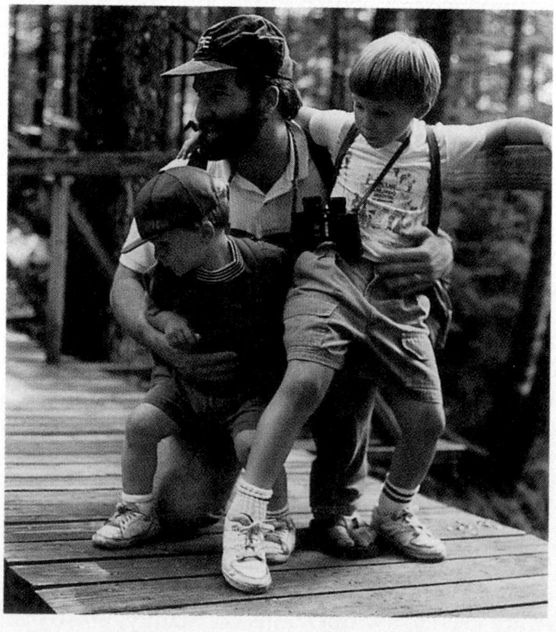

FIGURE 30.2 Preschoolers like exposure to new events and places. Here a 3-year-old is eager to explore the woods during a hike with the family.

FOCUS ON CULTURAL COMPETENCE

Whether children are allowed to ask questions or not is culturally determined. In a society in which children are expected to be seen and not heard, a preschool child may not have the same expressive vocabulary as a child who has been encouraged to ask questions. Recognition that differences among cultures can affect levels of development means that assessment must be individualized and meaningful in terms of the cultural milieu.

speeding, the fact that he is freely imitating a role is more important than getting the role absolutely correct. If a parent is concerned that the child should separate these two roles accurately, it is usually best not to stop the play to do so. Rather, the next time they are driving past the fire station, the parent could explain that this is where firefighters work, and they put out fires, or that the police station is where police officers work, and they make certain that people drive safely.

Children generally imitate activities they see their parents performing at home. A young girl will set the table for breakfast, eat with her "husband," help clean off the table, and leave for work. A young boy might cook, pretend to feed a doll, and put the doll to bed as he has seen his father do with a younger sister. In addition to learning what activities adults carry out at home, preschoolers should also be introduced to their parents' work environments. Such visits not only provide a visual context for the parent's job but also let the child learn such words as photocopier, cash register, and fax machine.

Today, as many as 90% of mothers of childbearing age work outside the home at least part time. Remind a mother to introduce her preschooler to her "other" self—lawyer, secretary, or telephone repair person—in the same way the child is exposed to the father's work side.

Fantasy. Toddlers cannot differentiate between fantasy and reality; they believe cartoon characters are real. Preschoolers begin to make this differentiation. They may become so intense about a fantasy role, however, that they are afraid they have lost their own identity and that they have become "stuck" in their fantasies. Such intense involvement in play is part of "magical thinking," or believing that thoughts and wishes come true.

Parents sometimes strengthen this feeling without realizing it: they (and you) need to be careful in this regard. A preschooler, for example, may pretend that she is a white rabbit. Her mother walks into the room, is aware of the game, and decides to participate. She says, "That's strange, I don't see Cindy anywhere. All I see is a white rabbit." Then she leaves the room. Cindy may be frightened that she has actually become a white rabbit. She worries that her mother will not want her to live in the house any more. A better response for the mother would be to support the imitation—this is age-appropriate behavior and a good way of exploring roles—while helping the child maintain a difference between pretend and real. She might say, "What a nice white rabbit you're pretending to be," thus supporting the fantasy and yet reassuring the child that she is still herself.

In a health care setting, it is particularly important that you let children know they are still recognizable. When examining the ears of a girl who tells you she is a rabbit, comment that her ears are all better again, rather than play to the make-believe with remarks about long, furry rabbit ears.

Oedipus and Electra Complexes

Although the development of Oedipus and Electra complexes may have been overstated by Freud because of gender biases, many children do appear to manifest such behavior. An **Oedipus complex** refers to the strong emotional attachment of a preschool boy to his mother; an **Electra complex** is the attachment of a preschool girl to her father. Each child competes with the same-sex parent for the love and attention of the other parent. Parents who are not prepared for this behavior may feel hurt or rejected. For example, a daughter prefers to sit beside her father at the table or in the car; she asks her father to tuck her in at night. She is "Daddy's girl." The mother may feel left out of the family interaction when this happens. On the other hand, a boy will ask his mother for favors. He wants to sit beside her, to have her read to him, and to tuck him in for the night, and the father may feel left out (Berger, 2001).

Parents can be reassured that this phenomenon of competition and romance in preschoolers is normal. Parents may need help in handling feelings of jealousy and anger, particularly if the child is vocal in expressing feelings toward a parent. It is difficult for a mother to reply calmly to a 3-year-old daughter who is shouting at her, "I hate you! I only love Daddy!" By understanding the motivation behind such a statement, the parent may be able to calmly react by stating, "Well, I don't like to be shouted at, but I still love you."

Gender Roles

Preschoolers need exposure to an adult of the opposite gender so they can become familiar with opposite gender roles. Encourage single parents to plan opportunities for their children to spend some time with adults other than themselves, such as a grandparent, a friend, an aunt, or an uncle, for this exposure. A nursery school teacher may serve as this person. Because most nursery school teachers are women, the mother may have to look elsewhere to find an adult male role model. If a child is hospitalized during the preschool period, a male nurse could help fill this role.

Children's gender-typical actions are strengthened by parents, strangers, nursery school teachers, other family members, and other children. Parents who do not want their child to grow up as they did, with a fixed role as a result of gender stereotyping, should be aware that they reinforce such attitudes by their actions as well as by their words. For example, a father may tell his son that it is important for both boys and girls to do housework, but if the father will not do dishes he is teaching the child that managing a household is not a man's job.

Socialization

Because 3-year-olds are capable of sharing, they play with other children their age much more agreeably than do toddlers, which is why the preschool period is a sensitive and critical time for socialization. Children who are exposed to other playmates have an easier time learning to relate to people than those raised in an environment where they never see other children of the same age (Fig. 30-3).

Although 4-year-olds continue to enjoy play groups, they may become involved in arguments more than they did at age 3, especially as they become more certain of their role in the group. This development, like so many others, may make parents worry that a child is regressing.

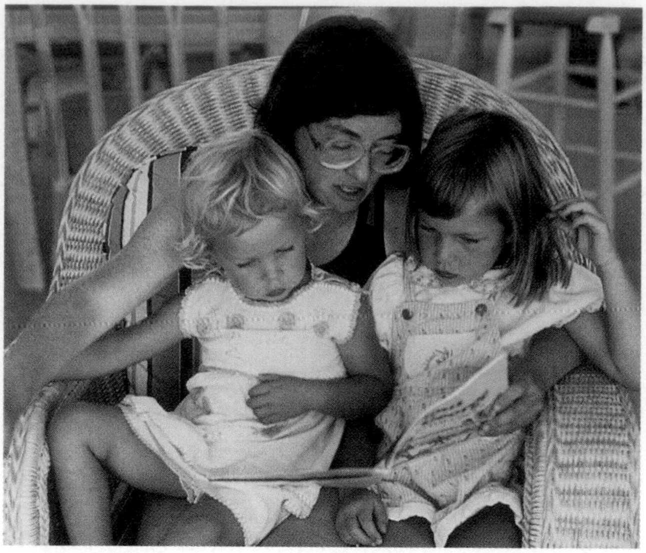

FIGURE 30.3 Preschoolers are interested in sharing activities with other children, such as listening to a story.

However, it is really forward movement, involving some testing and identification of their group role.

Five-year-olds begin to develop "best" friendships, perhaps on the basis of who they walk to school with or who lives closest to them. The elementary rule that an odd number of children don't play well together pertains to children at this age. Two or four will play; three or five will quarrel.

Cognitive Development

At age 3 years, cognitive development according to Piaget is still preoperational (Piaget, 1969). Although children during this period do enter a second phase called **intuitional thought,** they lack the insight to view themselves as others see them or put themselves in another's place. Because preschoolers cannot make this kind of mental substitution, they feel they are always right. This causes them to argue with the forcefulness that comes from believing they are 100% correct. This is an important point to remember when explaining procedures to preschoolers. They cannot see your side of the situation; they cannot hurry because you must have something done by 10 o'clock; they cannot hold still just because you want them to.

Also, preschoolers are not yet aware of the property of **conservation.** This means that if they have two balls of clay of equal size, but one is squashed flatter and wider than the other, preschoolers will insist that the flatter one is bigger (because it is wider) or that the intact one is bigger (because it is taller). They cannot see that only the form, not the amount, has changed. This inability to appreciate conservation has implications for nurses working with preschoolers. Preschoolers will not be able to comprehend that a procedure done two separate ways is the same procedure. Thus, if the nurse before you told a child to turn on his right side and then his left side while his bed was made, you may have to allow him to turn those same ways.

✔ CHECKPOINT QUESTIONS

3. How many words does a 3-year-old typically have in his or her vocabulary?
4. How might children who do not develop a sense of initiative react in a new situation?

Moral and Spiritual Development

Children of preschool age determine right from wrong based on their parents' rules. They have little understanding of the rationale for these rules or even whether the rules are consistent. If asked the question, "Why is it wrong for you to steal from your neighbor's house?" the average preschooler answers, "Because my mother says it's wrong." When pressed further, the preschooler justifies that conviction with, "It just is, that's all."

Because preschoolers depend on their parents to supply rules for them, when faced with a new situation they have difficulty seeing that the rules they know may also apply to a new situation.

WHAT IF? What if a preschooler understands the rule "Don't steal from stores"? Would he also understand "Don't steal from a hospital"?

Preschoolers begin to have an elemental concept of God if they have been provided some form of religious training. Belief in an outside force aids in the development of conscience (Kohlberg, 1984); however, preschoolers tend to do good out of self-interest rather than because of strong spiritual motivation. Children this age enjoy the security of religious holidays, prayers, and grace said before meals because these rituals can offer them the same reassurance and security that a familiar nursery rhyme read over and over does.

PLANNING AND IMPLEMENTATION FOR HEALTH PROMOTION OF THE PRESCHOOLER AND FAMILY

Preschoolers are old enough to begin to take responsibility for their own actions. The preschooler's safety, nutritional health, daily activities, and family functioning are all affected by this increased responsibility. Box 30-1 highlights appropriate outcomes and interventions using the terminology identified by the Nursing Outcomes Classification (NOC) and Nursing Interventions Classification (NIC).

Promoting Preschooler Safety

As preschoolers broaden their horizons, safety issues increase. By age 4, children may project an attitude of independence and the ability to take care of their own needs. Part of this is pseudo-independence; however, they still need supervision to be certain they do not injure themselves or other children while rough-housing and to ensure they do not stray too far from home. Their interest

BOX 30.1

NURSING OUTCOMES AND NURSING INTERVENTIONS CLASSIFICATION: PRESCHOOLER DEVELOPMENT

NOC: Child Development, 2, 3, 4, 5 Years

Child development is defined as the milestones of physical, cognitive, and psychosocial progression by 2, 3, 4, and 5 years of age (Johnson, Maas, & Moorhead, 2000). Some specific indicators suggesting achievement of this outcome include the child's ability to demonstrate the following at:

2 years
- Walking, including walking backward and up and down stairs one step at a time
- Kicking and throwing a ball
- Stacking 5 or 6 blocks
- Following two-step commands
- Using two- or three-word phrases
- Listening to stories and looking at pictures
- Imitating adults
- Participating in parallel play

3 years
- Balancing on one foot
- Dressing self
- Pedaling a riding toy
- Controlling daytime bladder and bowel elimination
- Engaging in magical thinking
- Beginning cooperative play
- Using three- or four-word sentences
- Giving own first name and age

4 years
- Walking, climbing, jumping, and running
- Riding a tricycle or bicycle with training wheels
- Building a tower of 10 blocks
- Drawing a person with 3 parts
- Using short paragraphs with sentences of 4 or 5 words
- Distinguishing fantasy from reality
- Giving first and last name
- Singing a song

5 years
- Walking, climbing, and running with coordination
- Dressing self independently
- Drawing a person with head, body, arms, and legs
- Copying a triangle or square
- Counting using fingers
- Speaking in short paragraphs, with recognition of most alphabet letters
- Giving own address and phone number
- Following rules of interactive peer games

NIC: Development Enhancement, Child

Developmental enhancement, child, is defined as the facilitating or teaching of parents/caregivers to facilitate optimal gross motor, language, cognitive, social, and emotional growth of preschool and school-age children (McCloskey & Bulechek, 2000). Some important activities involved when implementing this intervention include:

- Building a trusting relationship, including one-on-one interaction with the child
- Identifying special needs and adaptations as needed
- Teaching caregivers about normal developmental milestones and associated behaviors
- Facilitating caregivers' contact with community resources and support groups
- Encouraging child interaction with others, including sharing and taking turns and fostering of cooperation
- Assisting child with learning self-help skills
- Offering age-appropriate toys
- Providing activities to foster exercise and development, such as time on playground and material for building and drawing, puzzles, and manipulating shapes
- Teaching child to write name and recognize first letter of name
- Telling and reading stories
- Providing structured and consistent behavior management, redirecting attention when necessary

NIC: Parent Education, Childrearing Family

Parent education, childrearing family, is defined as assisting parents to understand and promote the physical, psychological, and social growth and development of their toddler, preschooler, or school-age child/children (McCloskey & Bulechek, 2000). Some important activities involved when implementing this intervention include:

- Teaching normal physiologic, emotional, and behavioral characteristics of the child
- Identifying appropriate developmental task for the child
- Facilitating discussion of methods of discipline
- Reviewing child's nutritional requirements, dental hygiene needs, grooming needs, safety issues, anger management, and expression of feelings
- Informing of community resources
- Encouraging use of different childrearing strategies
- Role-playing techniques and communication skills
- Referring to support groups or parenting classes as indicated

in learning adult roles may lead them into exploring the blades of a lawn mover or an electric saw. They must be reminded repeatedly of automobile safety. A preschooler's thought "I want to play with Mary across the street" can be so quick and so intense that the child will run into the middle of the street before remembering the rules "Watch out for cars" or "Don't cross the street."

Because preschoolers imitate adult roles so well, they may imitate taking medicine if they see family members doing so. A good rule for parents is never to take medicine in front of children. Safety points for the preschool period are summarized in Focus on Family Empowerment.

Keeping Children Safe, Strong, and Free

The preschool years are not too early a time to educate children about the potential threat of harm from strangers or even how to address bullying behavior from people (children or adults) they know. This includes:

- Warning a child never to talk with or accept rides from strangers.
- Teaching a child how to call for help in an emergency (yelling or running to a designated neighbor's house if outside, or dialing 911 if near a phone).
- Describing what police officers look like and expressing that police officers can help in an emergency situation.
- Explaining that if children or adults ask them to keep secrets about anything that has made them uncomfortable, they should tell their parents or another trusted adult, even if they have promised to keep the secret.

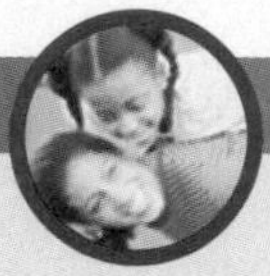

FOCUS ON FAMILY EMPOWERMENT

Common Safety Measures to Prevent Accidents During the Preschool Years

Q. My preschooler is so active! How can I keep her safe?

A. Try these tips:

Possible Accident	*Prevention Measure*
Motor vehicles	Keep child in car seat; do not be distracted by child while driving.
	Do not allow preschooler to play outside unsupervised.
	Do not allow preschooler to operate electronic garage door opener.
	Teach safety with tricycle (look before crossing driveways; do not cross streets).
	Teach child to always hold hands with a grownup before crossing a street.
	Teach parking lot safety (hold hands with grownup; do not run behind cars that are backing up).
	Children should wear helmets when riding bicycles.
Falls	Supervise preschooler at playgrounds.
	Remove drawstrings from hooded clothing.
	Help child to judge safe distances for jumping or safe heights for climbing.
Drowning	Do not leave child alone in bathtub or near water.
	Teach beginning swimming.
Animal bites	Do not allow child to approach strange dogs.
	Supervise child's play with family pets.
Poisoning	Never present medication as a candy.
	Never take medication in front of a child.
	Never store food or substances in containers other than their own.
	Post telephone number of local poison control center by the telephone.
	Stock each first-aid box with syrup of ipecac, with proper instructions for administration.
	Teach child that medication is a serious substance and not for play.
Burns	Buy flame-retardant clothing.
	Turn handles of saucepans toward back of stove.
	Store matches in closed containers.
	Do not allow preschooler to help light birthday candles, fireplaces, etc. (fire is not fun or a "treat").
	Keep screen in front of a fireplace or heater.
Community safety	Teach preschooler that not all people are friends ("Do not talk to strangers or take candy from strangers").
	Define a stranger as someone the child does not know, not someone odd-looking.
	Teach child to say "no" to people whose touching he does not enjoy, including family members. (When a child is sexually abused, the offender is usually a family member or close family friend.)
General	Know whereabouts of preschooler at all times.
	Be aware that frequency of accidents is increased when parents are under stress. Special precautions must be taken at these times.
	Some children are more active, curious, and impulsive and therefore more vulnerable to accidents than others.

- Explaining that bullying behavior from other children is not to be tolerated but reported so they can receive help managing it.

It is often difficult for parents to impart this type of information to a preschooler because parents can't imagine their children will ever be in situations in which they will need the information, nor do they want to terrify their children about the world around them. However, if the information is presented in a calm yet serious manner, children can begin to use it to build safe habits that will help them later when they are old enough to walk home from school alone or play with their friends, unsupervised, at a public playground (AAP, 2001).

WHAT IF? What if a preschooler tells you she knows not to leave preschool with anyone who is strange? Is that the same as knowing not to leave with a stranger?

Motor Vehicle and Bicycle Safety

With more and more cars being equipped with front-seat air bags, make certain that parents safely buckle preschoolers into car seats in the back seat (AAP Committee on Safety, 2001). Many preschoolers outgrow their first car seats during this period (when they reach 40 lb) and need to graduate to a booster-type seat. The shoulder harness should be carefully positioned so it does not go across the child's face or throat. Remind parents that preschoolers can unhook seat belts without difficulty. Parents must stress the important role of seat belts in preventing injury in accidents.

Preschool is also the right age to promote bicycle safety. Head injuries are a major cause of death and injury to preschoolers, and bicycle accidents are among the major causes of such injuries. Some parents may have already purchased a helmet for their child when he or she was a toddler and riding in a bicycle seat. Once children begin riding independently, however, they definitely need a safety helmet approved for children their age and size. Encourage parents who ride bicycles to demonstrate safe riding habits by wearing helmets as well. A parent who routinely wears a helmet may well be the most compelling reason for the preschooler to wear one.

Promoting Nutritional Health of the Preschooler

Like the toddler period, the preschool years are not a time of fast growth, so the child is not likely to have a ravenous appetite. Offering small servings of food is still a good idea, so the child is not overwhelmed and is allowed the successful feeling of cleaning a plate and asking for more.

Most children are hungry after preschool and enjoy a snack when they arrive home. Because sugary foods may dull a child's appetite for dinner, urge parents to make the snack nutritious (fruit, cheese, or milk rather than cookies and a soft drink).

Teach parents to make mealtime a happy and enjoyable part of the day for everyone. Some preschool children learn to eat as quickly as possible (and thus incompletely) to escape from the table before something unpleasant happens, such as an argument that they know is brewing. Initiative, or learning how to do things, can be strengthened by allowing a child to prepare simple foods, such as making a sandwich or spreading jelly on toast.

Recommended Daily Dietary Allowances

Parents need to select foods for a preschooler based on the food pyramid, making sure to offer a variety. Preschoolers may not eat a great deal of meat. Many parents ask whether their preschooler needs to take supplementary vitamins. As long as the child is eating foods from all pyramid food groups and meets the criteria for a healthy child (i.e., alert and active, with height and weight within normal averages), additional vitamins are unnecessary.

If parents do give vitamins, they must remember that the child will undoubtedly view the vitamin as candy rather than medicine because of the attractive shapes and colors of preschool vitamins, so they must store them out of reach. Caution parents not to give more vitamins than the recommended daily amount, because poisoning from high doses of fat-soluble vitamins and iron can result (Krebs & Hambridge, 2001).

Promoting Nutritional Health With a Vegetarian Diet

A vegetarian diet is usually colorful and therefore appeals to preschoolers. Many vegetables, fruits, and grains are also good snack foods and so are convenient for the child who eats frequently during the day.

If vegetarian diets are deficient in any aspects, they usually lack calcium, vitamin B_{12}, and vitamin D. Check to see that the child is ingesting a variety of calcium sources (green leafy vegetables, milk products). Vitamin D is found in fortified cereals and milk. Vitamin B_{12} is found almost exclusively in animal products, so the child may need a supplemental source of this (Dudek, 2001).

✔ CHECKPOINT QUESTIONS

5. Do preschoolers need to wear helmets when riding bicycles?
6. Are preschool vitamin supplements necessary for all children?

Promoting Development of the Preschooler in Daily Activities

The preschooler has often mastered the basic skills needed for most self-care activities, including feeding, dressing, washing (with supervision), and toothbrushing (again, with supervision).

Dressing

Many 3-year-olds and most 4-year-olds can dress themselves except for difficult buttons, although there may be a conflict over what the child will wear. Preschoolers prefer bright colors or prints and may select items that do not match. As with other preschool activities, however, children need the experience of choosing their own clothes. One way for parents to solve the problem of mismatching is to fold together shirts and pants that go together so the child sees them as a set rather than individual pieces. If children insist on wearing mismatched clothes, parents should make no apologies for their appearance. A simple statement such as "Mark chose his own clothes today" explains the situation. Anyone who understands preschoolers knows that the experience children gain in being able to select their own clothing is worth more than a perfect appearance by adult standards.

Sleep

Many toddlers going through a negative phase resist taking naps no matter how tired they are. Preschoolers, on the other hand, are more aware of their needs; when they are tired, they often curl up on a couch or soft chair and fall asleep. Many, particularly those who attend afternoon childcare or preschool, give up afternoon naps. Encourage parents to learn whether the school requires children to take a nap or not. If they rest there, the child may have some difficulty getting to sleep at the usual bedtime established at home.

Children in this age group may also refuse to go to sleep because of fear of the dark. Night waking from nightmares or night terrors reaches its peak. Preschoolers may need a night light, although they did not need one before. A helpful suggestion for parents is to maintain enjoyable activities and continue bedtime routines to reduce stress before bedtime.

Exercise

The preschool period is an active phase, so children receive a great deal of exercise. Rough-housing is a good way of getting rid of tension and should be allowed as long as it does not become destructive. In addition, preschoolers love time-honored games such as ring-around-the-rosy, London Bridge, or other more structured games that they were not ready for as toddlers.

Bathing

Preschoolers can wash and dry their hands perfectly adequately if the faucet is regulated for them (so they do not scald themselves with hot water). Children this age are not paragons of neatness, however, and may clean their hands at the expense of a bathroom towel. When possible, parents should turn down the temperature of the water heater to under 120°F to help prevent scalds.

Although preschoolers certainly sit well in bathtubs, they should still not be left unsupervised at bathtime. They may decide to add more hot water and scald themselves or to practice swimming and slip and be unable to get their head out of the water. Some girls develop vulvar irritation (and perhaps bladder infection) from exposure to products such as bubble bath. Preschoolers do not clean their fingernails or ears well, so these areas often need "touching up" by a parent or older sibling.

Hair washing can be a problem. The preschooler is too heavy for a parent to hold over the sink to rinse his or her hair. Children also cannot close their eyes well enough or long enough (because they insist on opening them to see whether the parent is finished) to keep soap out while they have their hair rinsed in an upright position. Hanging a mobile over the tub so they have a reason to look up and using a nonirritating shampoo are good suggestions.

Because preschoolers like to imitate adults, they begin to be interested in taking showers rather than baths if they see their parents doing this. Although children may not get too clean the few times they try showering, parents do not usually have to be concerned because most preschoolers shower only a few times, then return to tub soaking, which allows them to play with bath toys.

Care of Teeth

If independent toothbrushing was not started as a daily practice during the infant or toddler years, it should be started during the preschool years. The child should continue to drink fluoridated water or receive a prescribed oral fluoride supplement if fluoride is not provided in the water supply (AAP Committee on Practice and Ambulatory Medicine, 2001).

One good toothbrushing period a day is often more effective than more frequent half-hearted brushings. Although many preschoolers do well brushing their own teeth, parents must check that all tooth surfaces are cleaned. They should floss the teeth, because this is a skill beyond a preschooler's motor ability.

Toothbrushing is generally well accepted by preschoolers because it imitates adults. Electric or battery-operated toothbrushes are favorites because of the adult responsibility involved in handling them. Children must be supervised when using an electric toothbrush, however, and must be taught not to use it or any other electrical appliance near a basin of water.

Encouraging children to eat apples, carrots, celery, chicken, or cheese for snacks rather than candy or sweets is yet another way to attempt to prevent tooth decay. If a child is allowed to chew gum, it should be the sugar-free variety.

Children should have made a first visit to a dentist by age 2.5 years for evaluation of tooth formation. Because this visit usually shows no cavities, this should have been a pain-free experience, so the child should not fear the dentist, and the idea that dentists like to help rather than hurt should have been implanted. If parents did not take the child for this visit previously, it should be done during the preschool period.

Deciduous teeth must be preserved to protect the dental arch. If teeth have to be pulled as a result of disease, the permanent teeth can drift out of position or the jaw may not grow enough to accommodate them.

Night Grinding. **Bruxism,** or grinding the teeth at night (usually during sleep), is a habit of many young children. Teeth grinding may be a way of "letting go," similar to body rocking, that children do for a short time each night to release tensions and allow themselves to fall asleep. Children who grind their teeth extensively may have greater-than-average anxiety. Children with cerebral palsy may do it because of the spasticity of jaw muscles. If the grinding is extensive, the crowns of the teeth can become abraded. The condition may advance to such an extent that the tooth nerves are exposed. If the problem seems to stem from anxiety, identifying and relieving the source of the anxiety are essential for treatment. If some damage is evident, refer the family to a pedodontist so the teeth can be evaluated, repaired (capped), and conserved.

Promoting Healthy Family Functioning

Some parents who enjoyed maintaining a rhythm of care for an infant and allowed for ritualistic behavior of a toddler may have difficulty being the parents of a preschooler because more flexibility and creativity are required. Others come into their own as the parents of a preschooler; they delight in encouraging imaginative games and play.

A major parental role during this time is to encourage vocabulary development. One way to do this is to read aloud to the child; another is to answer questions so the child sees language as an organized system of communication. Answering a preschooler's questions is often difficult because the questions are frequently philosophical; for example, "Why is grass green?" The child may listen to an explanation of chlorophyll but then repeat the question, regardless of the clarity of the explanation, because the parent underestimated the extent of the question: the child did not want to know what makes grass green, but why, philosophically, it is not red or blue or yellow. The obvious answer to that is, "I don't know." Many parents, however, have trouble making such an admission to a child. Those who are confident can give this answer without feeling threatened. Parents who are less sure of themselves may feel extremely uncomfortable when they do not know the answers to a 4-year-old's questions (see Focus on Communication).

Discipline

Preschoolers have definite opinions on things such as what they want to eat, where they want to go, and what they want to wear. This may bring them into opposition with their parents. It is important for parents to guide a child through these struggles without discouraging the child's right to have an opinion. "Timeout" is a good technique to correct behavior for parents to continue through the preschool years (see Chap. 29). This technique allows parents to discipline without using physical punishment and allows the child to learn a new way of behavior without extreme stress.

Parental Concerns Associated With the Preschool Period

Common Health Problems of the Preschooler

The mortality of children during the preschool years is low and becoming lower every year as more infectious diseases are preventable. This results in the major cause of death being automobile accidents, followed by poisoning and falls (DHHS, 2000).

FOCUS ON COMMUNICATION

Mr. Edwards is the father of a preschooler, Darryl. You overhear him talking to his son while they wait for a well-child visit.

Less Effective Communication

Darryl: Why are we waiting?
Mr. Edwards: It's how things work here.
Darryl: Why?
Mr. Edwards: I have no idea.
Darryl: Why is that girl here? Is she sick?
Mr. Edwards: I have no idea.
Darryl: When are we going home?
Mr. Edwards: I have no idea.
Darryl: What's that girl's name?
Mr. Edwards: I have no idea.

More Effective Communication

Darryl: Why are we waiting?
Mr. Edwards: It's how things work here.
Darryl: Why?
Mr. Edwards: People have to take turns. We're waiting for our turn.
Darryl: Why is that girl here? Is she sick?
Mr. Edwards: She might be. Some children are here because they're sick and some are just in for a checkup like you.
Darryl: When are we going home?
Mr. Edwards: As soon as the nurse practitioner checks you over.
Darryl: What's that girl's name?
Mr. Edwards: I don't know. Do you want to ask her?

Preschoolers ask 300 to 400 questions a day as they explore their world. In the first scenario, Mr. Edwards tries to discourage questions by offering almost no answers. In the second scenario, when he tries to answer the child's questions, the father is not only supplying information, he is also helping the child build vocabulary. Because preschoolers ask so many questions, you may have to encourage parents to continue to answer questions this way. Otherwise, discouraging questions can become the method of interaction.

In contrast, the number of minor illnesses, such as colds, ear infections, and flu symptoms, in preschoolers is exceptionally high, more than that of any other age. Children who live in homes in which parents smoke have a higher incidence of ear (otitis media) and respiratory infections than others. Children who attend childcare or preschool programs also have an increased incidence of respiratory infections and gastrointestinal disturbances (such as vomiting and diarrhea).

This may be the parents' first experience with other than a transient illness in their child. Many parents may find it even more difficult to cope with the parade of constant minor colds. Thus, stress may arise between parent and child, an almost monthly battle of "Stay indoors until your cold is better," conflict over childcare, or frequent whining and clinging behavior because the child's stomach is upset. Such illnesses may cause parents to perceive a child as sickly or not able to cope with everyday life. Whereas parents encouraged independence before, they may now begin to overprotect (to shelter to too great a degree). Give reassurance that frequent minor illnesses are common in preschoolers. As parents become more experienced in handling these conditions, their perception of whether an illness is a problem will change.

Table 30-2 shows the usual health maintenance schedule for preschoolers. Table 30-3 lists problems that parents may have in evaluating a preschooler's illness.

Common Fears of the Preschooler

Because preschoolers' imagination is so active, it can lead to a number of fears. Fears of the dark, mutilation, and separation or abandonment are all very real to the preschooler.

Fear of the Dark. The tendency to fear the dark is an example of a fear heightened by the child's vivid imagination: a stuffed toy by daylight becomes a threatening monster in the dark. Children awaken screaming because of a nightmare. They may be reluctant to go to bed or to go back to sleep by themselves unless a light is left on.

If parents are prepared for this fear and understand that it is a phase of growth, they will be better able to cope with it. It is generally helpful if they monitor the stimuli their children are exposed to, especially around bedtime. This includes television, adult discussions, and frightening stories. Parents are sometimes reluctant to leave a child's light on at night because they do not want to cater to the fear. Burning a dim night light, however, can solve the problem and costs only pennies. Children who awake terrified and screaming need reassurance that they are safe, that whatever was chasing them was a dream and is not in their room. They may require an understanding adult to sit on their bed until they can fall back to sleep again (Fig. 30-4). Most preschoolers do not remember in the morning that they had such a dream; they remember for a lifetime that they received comfort when they needed it.

If parents take sensible precautions against fear of the dark or nightmares and a child continues to have this kind of disturbance every night, it may be a reaction to undue stress. In these instances, the source of the stress should be investigated. Giving sleep medication to counteract the sleep disturbance does not help solve the basic problem, so this is rarely recommended. Fear of the dark can become intensified in a hospital setting and requires careful planning to relieve.

Fear of Mutilation. Fear of mutilation is also significant during the preschool age, as revealed by the intense

TABLE 30.2 Health Maintenance Schedule, Preschool Period

AREA OF FOCUS	METHODS	FREQUENCY
Assessment		
Developmental milestones	History, observation	Every visit
	Formal Denver Developmental Screening Test (DDST II)	Before start of school
Growth milestones	Height, weight plotted on standard growth chart; physical examination	Every visit
Hypertension	Blood pressure	Every visit
Nutrition	History, observation; height/weight information	Every visit
Parent–child relationship	History, observation	Every visit
Behavior problems	History, observation	Every visit
Vision and hearing defects	History, observation	Every visit
	Formal Preschool E and audiometer testing	Before start of school
Dental health	History, physical examination	Every visit
Tuberculosis	PPD test (if there are high-risk factors)	Before start of school
Immunizations		
Diphtheria, pertussis, and tetanus	Check history and past records; inform caregiver about any risks and side effects; administer immunization in accordance with health care agency policies	Before start of school
MMR	MMR #2	Before start of school
Poliomyelitis (inactivated)	IVP #4	Before start of school
Anticipatory Guidance		
Preschool care	Active listening and health teaching	Every visit
Expected growth and developmental milestones before next visit	Active listening and health teaching	Every visit
Accident prevention	Counseling about street and personal safety	Every visit
Any problems expressed by caregiver during course of the visit	Active listening and health teaching regarding temper tantrums, toilet training	Every visit

TABLE 30.3 Parental Difficulties Evaluating Illness in the Preschool Child

DIFFICULTY	HELPFUL SUGGESTIONS FOR PARENTS
Evaluating seriousness of illness or condition	Preschoolers are eager to please and tend to answer all questions such as, "Does your stomach hurt?" with a yes. Observing the child for signs of illness—refusing to eat, holding an arm stiffly having to go to the bathroom frequently—is often more productive as an evaluation technique.
Evaluating bowel and bladder problems	Preschoolers are independent in toilet habits for the first time, so parents do not have diaper contents to evaluate. Frequent trips to the bathroom, rubbing the abdomen, and holding genitals are the usual signs of bowel or bladder dysfunction.
Evaluating nutritional intake	Preschoolers begin to eat away from home at friends' houses or at childcare, or to stay overnight with grandparents, so parents do not observe daily food intake as accurately as before. Observing whether the child is growing and active is better than monitoring any one day's food intake.
Evaluating bedwetting	Many preschoolers continue to have occasional enuresis at night until school age. If other signs are present—pain, low-grade fever, listlessness—the child should have a urine culture, as persistent bedwetting can indicate a low-grade urinary tract infection.
Evaluating activity vs. hyperactivity	Many lay magazines have articles on hyperactivity in children. Parents often wonder whether their active child is truly hyperactive. As a rule of thumb, if a child can sit through a meal (when he is hungry), watch a half-hour television show (that is his favorite), or sit still while his favorite story is read to him, he is not hyperactive.
Age-specific diseases to be aware of	Preschool age is a time for vision and hearing assessment. For the first time, the child is able to be tested by a standard chart or by audiometry.
	Urinary tract infections tend to occur with a high frequency in preschool-age girls.
	Language assessment should be done if the child is not able to make wants known by complete, articulated sentences by age 3 (exceptions are transposing *w* for *r* and broken fluency: "I want-want-want to go").

reaction of a preschooler to even a simple injury such as falling and scraping a knee. The child cries afterward not only from the pain but also from the sight of the injury. Part of this fear arises because preschoolers do not know which body parts are essential and which ones—like an inch of scraped skin—can be easily replaced. Boys develop a fear of castration because developmentally they are more in tune with their body parts and they are starting to identify with the same-sex parent as they go through the Oedipal phase. Preschoolers worry that if blood is taken out of their bodies, all of their blood will leak out. They often lift a bandage to peek at an incision or cut to see if their body "stuff" is flowing out. They dislike invasive procedures, such as needlesticks, rectal temperature assessment, otoscopic examination, or having a nasogastric tube passed into their stomach, for the same reason. They need good explanations of the limits of health care procedures (e.g., a tympanic thermometer does not hurt, a finger prick heals quickly) in order to feel safe.

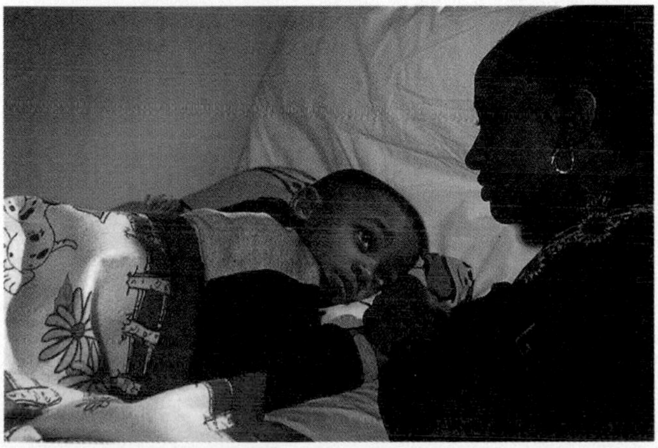

FIGURE 30.4 Having mom close by after a bad dream is a comfort to the preschooler.

Fear of Separation or Abandonment. Fear of separation continues to be a major concern for preschoolers. For some children, it intensifies because their keen imagination allows them to believe they are being deserted when they are not. Their sense of time is still so distorted that they are not comforted by assurances such as, "Mommy will pick you up from preschool at noon." Their sense of distance is also limited, so making a statement such as "I work only a block away" is not reassuring. Relating time and space to something the child knows, such as meals, television shows, or a friend's house, is most effective. For example, stating, "Mommy will pick you up from preschool after you have had your snack" or showing the child the work site might be more comforting (see Focus on Nursing Care Planning).

Caution parents to be sensitive to such fears when they talk about missing children or if they have their preschooler's fingerprints taken for identification. A child whose chief fear is that he will be abandoned or kidnapped might not hear that fingerprints are being taken to keep him safe, only that someone might take him away from his parents.

A hospital admission or going to a new school often brings a child's fear of separation to the forefront. Help parents thoroughly prepare preschoolers for these experiences so they can survive them in sound mental health.

FOCUS ON *Nursing Care Planning*

A PRESCHOOLER WITH FEARS

A 3½-year-old girl is brought to the office by her father, who is concerned about his daughter's crying at day care.

Assessment: 3½-year-old girl within normal limits for height, weight, and development. While talking with her, the child states, "My daddy left me at school and I was all by myself. I missed my daddy. I didn't think he was coming back." Child currently enrolled in morning nursery school program followed by day care for the remainder of the day until father picks child up after work. Single-parent household. Father works full time. Older sibling, 8 years of age, in school til 3:30 P.M. and then in after-school program until father picks him up after work.

Nursing Diagnosis: Fear related to separation and abandonment during preschool period

Outcome Identification: Child will demonstrate a decrease in the number of crying episodes at day care by end of 1 month.

Outcome Evaluation: Child verbalizes fear. Father demonstrates measures to minimize child's fears; reports crying episodes at school have decreased by 2 weeks.

Interventions	Rationale
1. Explore with the child further about her feelings, nursery school, and day care.	1. Exploration provides valuable clues to understanding the child's behavior and developing possible strategies for dealing with this behavior.
2. Review with the father the typical fears experienced by the preschooler, including those of separation and abandonment.	2. Knowledge of normal growth and development helps to reduce the father's anxiety about the behavior and possible causes.
3. Assist the father with identifying behaviors indicative of the child's fears. Instruct the father in measures to help reduce fears, such as being honest with the child and reinforcing the time that he will return.	3. Instruction aids in providing the father with concrete suggestions for identifying and addressing the problem.
4. Encourage the father to talk with the nursery school and day care staff about the problems and methods to decrease the child's fear.	4. Discussion with the care providers helps to reinforce the measures used by the father, providing consistency and thereby helping to minimize the child's fears.
5. Have the father reassure the child that he will pick her up every day at school and that he will call if he's running late. Encourage the child to tell her father what she's feeling as much as possible.	5. Reassurance helps to reduce the child's fears. Verbalization helps to increase the child's and father awareness of the situation.
6. Encourage the father to set up a special time for himself and his daughter, possibly in the evening or on the weekends, and to adhere to this time consistently.	6. Special time for the father and his daughter enhances the parent–child relationship. Consistently adhering to this time helps to foster a sense of trust and security in the child.
7. Arrange for a follow-up telephone call within 2 weeks.	7. Follow-up provides additional support and means for evaluating the effectiveness of the methods used.

✔ CHECKPOINT QUESTIONS

7. Why might a preschooler grind her teeth at night?
8. When leaving a preschooler with a babysitter, how might a parent minimize the child's fear of separation?

Behavior Variations

A combination of a keen imagination and immature reasoning results in common behavior variations in preschoolers.

Telling Tall Tales. Stretching stories to make them seem more interesting is a phenomenon frequently encountered in this age group. After a trip to the zoo, for example, if you ask a child of this age, "What happened today?" the child perceives that you want something exciting to have happened, so he or she might answer, "A bear jumped out of his cage and ate up the boy next to me." This is not lying, but merely supplying an expected answer. Caution parents not to encourage this kind of storytelling, and instead help the child separate fact from fiction by saying, "That's a good story, but now tell me what really happened." This conveys the idea that the child has not told the truth, yet does not squash imagination or initiative.

Imaginary Friends. Many preschoolers have an imaginary friend who plays with them. They tell a parent to "wait for Eric" or "set a place at the table for Lucy." Although imaginary friends are a normal, creative part of the preschool years and can be invented by children who are surrounded by real playmates as well as by those who have few friends, parents may find them disconcerting. If so, ask parents to make sure their child has exposure to real playmates. As long as imaginary playmates don't take center stage in children's minds and prevent them from socializing with other children, they should not pose a problem and often leave as quickly as they came. In the meantime, they may provide an outlet for the child to express innermost feelings or serve as a handy scapegoat for behavior about which the child has some conflict.

Parents can help their preschooler separate fact from fantasy by saying, "I know Eric isn't real, but if you want to pretend, I'll set a place for him." This response helps the child to understand what is real and what is fantasy without restricting the child's imagination or creativity.

Difficulty Sharing. Sharing is a concept that first comes to be understood around the age of 3 years. Before this, children engage in parallel play (two children need two toys and two spaces to play, because they cannot pass one toy back and forth or play together). Around 3 years of age, children begin to understand that some things are theirs, some belong to others, and some can belong to both. For the first time, they can stand in line to wait for a drink, take turns using a shovel at a sandbox, and share a box of crayons. Sharing does not come easily, however; children who are ill or under stress have even greater difficulty with it.

Preschoolers must have experience in learning property rights: "This is my private drawer and no one touches what is in it except me." "That is your dresser top, and no one touches the things on it but you." "A shovel is ours and can be used by everyone playing in the sandpile." Defining limits and exposing children to these three categories (mine, yours, ours) helps them figure out which objects belong to which category.

Most parents become concerned if their child does not share readily. They can be reassured that sharing is a difficult concept to grasp and that, as with most skills, preschoolers need practice to understand and learn it.

Regression. Some preschoolers, generally in relation to stress, revert to behavior they previously outgrew, such as thumb sucking, negativism, loss of bladder control, and inability to separate from their parents. Although the stress that causes this may take many forms, it is usually the result of such things as a new baby in the family, a new school experience, seeing frightening and graphic television news, stress in the home from financial or other problems, marital difficulties, or separation caused by hospitalization.

Help parents understand that regression in these circumstances is normal, and the child's thumb sucking is little different from the parents' reaction to stress (smoking many cigarettes, nail biting, overeating), to make it easier for them to accept and understand. Obviously, removing the stress is the best way to help the child discontinue this behavior. The stresses mentioned, however, are not easily removed. New babies cannot be returned, irreparable marriages cannot be patched together, frightening news happens every day, and hospitalizations do occur.

Techniques for minimizing the stress of hospitalization for preschoolers are discussed in Chapter 35. Children's reactions to severe and prolonged stress are discussed in Chapter 54. Children undergoing less severe stress must be assured that although situations are changing, the important aspects of their life—that someone still loves them and will continue to take care of them—are not. Thumb sucking or other manifestations of stress are best ignored; calling them to the child's attention merely causes more stress, because it makes the child aware that he or she is not pleasing parents, in addition to experiencing the primary stress.

Sibling Rivalry. Jealousy of a brother or sister may first become evident during the preschool period, partly because this is the first time that children have enough vocabulary to express how they feel (know a name to call) and partly because preschoolers are more aware of family roles and how responsibilities at home are divided. For many children, this is also the time when a new brother or sister is born.

A firstborn child is rarely allowed the privileges of a second child. The parents are untried, unsure of how far they should let the child venture or what level of responsibility the child can accept. This makes the firstborn serve as the "trial run" for all the children who come after. This phenomenon can lead to sibling rivalry, because children as young as preschool can sense that a younger sibling is allowed behavior that is not tolerated in them. They are little appeased by the explanation, "Leslie is a baby."

To help them feel secure and promote their self-esteem, supplying preschoolers with a private drawer or box for their things that parents or other children do not touch can be helpful. This can help defend their possessions against younger children who do not appreciate their property rights.

Preparing for a New Sibling

Introduction of a new sibling is such a major happening that parents need to take special steps to be certain their preschooler will be prepared. There is no rule as to when this preparation should begin, but it should be before the time when the child begins to feel the difference the new baby will make. This is perhaps when the mother first begins to look pregnant. It is certainly before parents begin to make physical preparations for the new child. It is always less frightening for a child of any age to understand why things are happening, no matter how distasteful they may be, than to hear people whispering or having parents obviously evading the issue. The unknown is something to fear, whereas a definite event can be faced and conquered.

Help parents not to underestimate the significance of a bed to a preschool child. It is security, consistency, and "home." If the preschooler has been sleeping in a crib that is to be used for the baby, it is usually best if he or she is moved to a bed about 3 months in advance of the birth. The parents might explain, "It's time to sleep in a new bed now because you're a big boy." The fact that he is growing up is a better reason for such a move than because a new brother or sister wants the old bed. The latter is a direct route to sibling rivalry and jealousy.

If children are to start preschool or childcare, they should do so either before the baby is born or 2 or 3 months afterward, if possible. That way, children can perceive starting school as a result of maturity and not of being pushed out of the house by the new child.

If the mother will be hospitalized for the birth, she should be certain the child is prepared for this separation in advance as well. The mother is likely to go to the hospital during the night, and the child cannot be expected to be happy about the arrival of a new sibling when he or she wakes in the morning to find mommy gone. Some communities offer preparation for birth classes for preschoolers, the same as for parents, or include children in adult preparation courses to help them master this new experience.

Encourage women to maintain contact with their preschooler during the short time they are hospitalized for birth. Some preschoolers may react very coldly to their mothers, turning their head away and refusing to come to them after even a few days' separation. This is a reaction not to the new baby but to the separation, the same phenomenon that may occur when a child returns home after being hospitalized (see Chap. 35).

Ask pregnant women or couples what kind of preparation they are making for their older children; ask the mother of a new baby how everything is working out. Most parents find that the problem of jealousy is bigger than they anticipated and welcome a few suggestions about how to provide more time for their preschooler during the day and which activities a preschooler would especially enjoy (Fig. 30-5; see Focus on Family Empowerment).

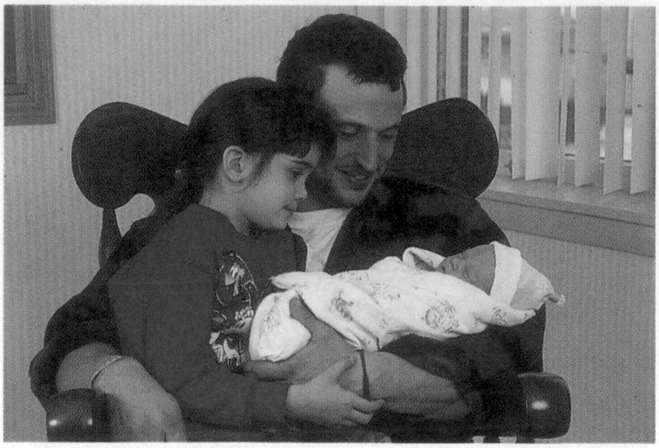

FIGURE 30.5 A preschooler greets a new baby sister. She feels special as dad explains how important it is to be a big sister.

> **✔ CHECKPOINT QUESTIONS**
>
> 9. If a child has an imaginary friend, is this "normal" development?
> 10. Would you recommend that visitors who come to see a new baby bring a gift for a preschooler as well?

Sex Education

Children during the preschool age become acutely aware of the difference between boys and girls, possibly because it is a normal progression in development, possibly

FOCUS ON FAMILY EMPOWERMENT
Suggestions to Help Minimize Sibling Rivalry

Q. My 3-year-old is jealous of his new sister and she's only hours old. How can I reduce sibling jealousy?

A. This isn't a simple problem, but the following suggestions might help:

- After returning home from the hospital, devote attention to your preschooler and spend some special time together after the baby has gone to bed.
- When friends and family visit, encourage them to spend time with the preschooler as well as the baby. If they bring gifts for the baby, it is often wise for them to bring a small present for the preschooler as well.
- So that your preschooler doesn't come to expect gifts (promoting sibling rivalry), teach him to help open the baby's gifts and explain to him that it is the baby's birthday and on his birthday he will receive gifts, too.
- Don't ask your preschooler a question such as, "Do you like your new sister?" It is better to express feelings of empathy such as, "New babies cry a lot. It's hard to get used to that, isn't it?"
- Provide special time for your preschooler during each day, so that when you say, "Mother and Daddy love you just the same," it seems real. This might be a quiet time for talking or reading.
- While feeding the baby, read or tell a story to the preschooler. Some children enjoy feeding a doll while a parent feeds the baby or giving a doll a bath while the baby has one.

because this may be the first time in their lives they are exposed to the genitalia of the opposite sex. They watch while a new brother or sister has diapers changed, they see other children using the bathroom at a preschool, or they see a parent nude.

Preschoolers' questions about genital organs are simple and fact finding; for example, "Why does James look like that?" or "How does Jasmine pee?" Explanations should be just as simple: "Boys look different from girls. The different part is called a penis." It is important for parents not to convey that these body parts are never to be talked about; parents should leave an open line of communication for sexual questions. Occasionally, girls attempt to void standing up as they have seen boys doing; boys may try sitting down to void.

Preschoolers may engage in masturbation while watching TV or being read to or before they fall asleep at night. The frequency may increase under stress, as does thumb sucking. If observing the child doing this bothers parents, suggest that they explain to the child that certain things are done in some places but not in others. Children can relate to this kind of direction without feeling inhibited, just as they can accept the fact that they use a bathroom in private or eat only at the table. Calling unnecessary attention to the act can increase anxiety and cause increased, not decreased, activity.

An important part of sex education for preschoolers is teaching them to avoid sexual abuse, such as not allowing anyone to touch their body unless they agree it is all right (see Chap. 31, Box 31-1). Because children are taught this, remember to ask permission before giving nursing care that involves touching.

Because this may be the time a new brother or sister comes into the family, it is also the most likely time for questions such as, "Where do babies come from?" Because the child is asking a simple fact-finding question, parents usually find that a simple, factual answer is best: "Babies grow in a special place in a mother's body called a uterus." Saying "uterus" rather than "tummy" prevents children from envisioning babies and food all mixed together in their mother's stomach (Fig. 30-6).

It is so natural for preschoolers to ask about where babies come from that those who do not ask are exceptions. Preschoolers who don't ask may be reticent because they sense from a preliminary exploratory question that the subject is closed. A parent could introduce the subject by visiting a new baby in the neighborhood with the child or pointing out a neighbor who is pregnant. The birth of kittens or puppies can also offer the chance to introduce the subject. If the new baby will be born at a birthing center or at home, many parents allow preschoolers to watch the birth. Encourage parents to prepare children well for this experience, or else the sight of their mother in pain and the wonder of birth can be overwhelming for them.

Preschool children generally do not ask how babies get inside mothers to start growing or how babies get out at the end of the process. Should they ask, a suitable explanation might be, "When a woman and a man love each other and decide they want a baby, the man plants a seed inside the woman. The man's seed and the woman's seed grow together in the special place inside the mother into a new baby." Some parents prefer to say, "God plants a seed." This

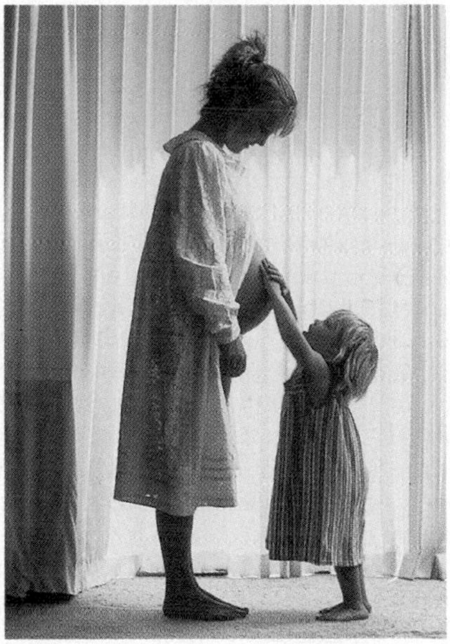

FIGURE 30.6 Preschool children are interested in learning where babies grow and have beginning sexual awareness.

answer may leave preschool boys feeling cheated that men have such a little role in this wondrous process. Perhaps a compromise statement would be, "God helps the man plant a seed." If preschoolers ask how the baby gets out, an answer might be, "The woman goes to the hospital and the doctor or nurse helps the baby get out from the vagina."

Many new books for children explain where babies come from, including descriptions of sexual relations and orgasm. These are helpful for parents to read to the child to increase understanding.

Choosing a Preschool or Childcare Center

The terms "childcare center," "preschool," and "nursery school" are often used interchangeably, so parents cannot depend on the name of a school to define its structure. Traditionally, the main purpose of a childcare center is to provide childcare while parents work or are otherwise occupied. The preschool or nursery school is dedicated to stimulating children's sense of creativity and initiative and introducing them to new experiences and social contacts they would not ordinarily receive at home. Head Start programs and many modern childcare centers fulfill both functions. A school or childcare experience is helpful for preschoolers as peer exposure appears to have a positive effect on social development (see Focus on Evidence-Based Practice). Children who have learned to be comfortable in a group approach school comfortably and ready to learn; children who have played only infrequently in groups during the preschool age are forced into this new situation in kindergarten or first grade. They may be so busy adjusting to this gross concept that they are left behind in finer components.

If there are other 3- or 4-year-old children in the neighborhood with whom the child has almost daily contact, and if a parent can supervise organized play dates and projects (providing peer interaction, in which working together is the key), a preschool program may not be nec-

FOCUS ON EVIDENCE-BASED PRACTICE

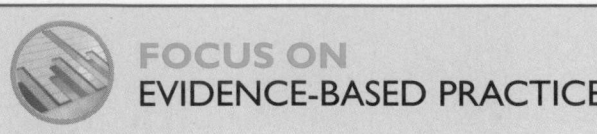

Is Childcare Good for Preschool Children?

Although parents need to use childcare for young children so they can continue to work outside their home or attend school, they may wonder whether childcare is good for their children. To answer this question, researchers reviewed randomized controlled trials of nonparental childcare for preschool children under 5 years of age. Results showed that childcare experiences had positive effects on children, such as increasing children's IQ, as well as beneficial effects on development and school achievement. Also identified were positive effects on mothers' education, employment, and interaction with their children. Long-term effects that may occur are increased economic status and decreased criminal behavior.

This is an important study for nurses because nurses are often the health care providers asked by parents if a childcare center would be appropriate for their child so they can work outside their home or attend school. Knowing that childcare can have positive effects on children can lend strength to advice.

Zoritch, B., Roberts, I., & Oakley, A. (2001). Day care for preschool children. *The Cochrane Library (Oxford), 4*(1), online.

essary. On the other hand, if all the neighborhood children are either older or younger or there is only one other child available to play with during the day, a preschool experience will probably be beneficial. Parents with large families point out that their child gets ample exposure to groups, that every meal is a "group session." This is not a peer group, however. Older siblings give in to the 3- or 4-year-old child, and younger siblings are not capable of peer competition. This situation does not offer the same experience that preschool does.

Parents need to investigate preschools or childcare centers carefully before they enroll their child. Guidelines to aid parents in this assessment are shown in Table 30-4.

To continue to evaluate their child's school experience, urge parents to make a habit of asking children what happened at school, what they learned, and the names of new friends. For the remainder of the growing years, school will have important effects on the child's development. Parents need to take an active role in providing input into education to influence what and how their child learns.

Childcare centers are often blamed for the spread of infectious disease among the 5-and-under population because bringing together children from many different homes to one setting each day does increase the risk of spreading contagious disease. Preschoolers may develop frequent upper respiratory infections or gastrointestinal illnesses from an early school setting. Outbreaks of cytomegalovirus and human parvovirus (fifth disease) make working in such centers a particular hazard to pregnant women. To prevent the spread of infection, parents should teach children to wash their hands frequently and cover their mouths when coughing. Childcare centers where infants as well as older children are enrolled need to take special precautions against hepatitis A infection, as this can be spread by caregivers' not washing their hands or the changing table after changing diapers. The disease may be subclinical in the preschooler, but other members of the preschooler's family may develop overt symptoms as the illness spreads through the family.

Preparing the Child for School

At the end of the preschool period, children begin a formal school experience. Parents may wonder whether their child is old enough for this, especially if the child's birthday is in the late summer or early fall. Parents should discuss their concern with school officials to determine whether the child should be registered for kindergarten or delayed for a year. As school involves a great deal of children's time and influences their future greatly, parents need to take time to prepare preschoolers well for the experience.

Essential to this preparation is the parents' attitude. If school is always discussed as something to look forward to, as an adventure that will be satisfying and rewarding, a child will view it from early on as a positive experience. If school is presented as a punishment ("Wait until you get into first grade—your teacher will make you sit up and behave"), there can be little delight in anticipating it.

If a child was not attending preschool, some parents may have to change their child's daily routine a few months in advance of beginning school to accustom the child to waking earlier and going to bed earlier. School has so many new components that it is wise to try to eliminate as many distractions like this as possible.

If the child is to ride a bus to school, a parent might take the child on a municipal bus as an introduction to this form of transportation. If the child is to walk, a trial walk is in order. In either instance, safety should be stressed: "Don't walk behind the bus because the driver can't see you" and "Wait for the crossing guard to help you cross streets."

If the child will be required to take a lunch to school, the parent can introduce this new experience by preparing a bagged lunch at home some noon. If the child is to purchase lunch at school, the parent can play "cafeteria" at home by serving a meal buffet-style and letting the child practice walking from one dish to another to select food.

Some kindergartens suggest that children know how to tie their shoes, name basic colors, and print their name before they begin. Parents should familiarize themselves with any such suggestions from the school, but the wisdom of requiring these skills can be questioned. Identifying colors should be established by this age, but some children are not coordinated enough at 4.5 years to tie their shoes or print. A better contribution for parents to make toward their children's achievement in school is to instill in their children the concept that learning is fun and that they will not always be able to do all the things that other children can do, but trying to do their individual best is what is important. Trying to make children complete fine motor tasks for which they are not developmentally prepared does not instill that concept.

For children to do well in a formal school setting, they must be able to follow instructions and sit at a table and

TABLE 30.4 Questions to Use in Evaluating Childcare Centers

QUESTION	FINDING
Management	
How long has the center been in operation?	Length of operation does not necessarily indicate quality, but it allows you to locate other parents who have used the center to ask about their experience there.
Is the center licensed, registered, approved, or inspected by the appropriate agency?	Ask in your local community what agency has the responsibility for licensing childcare centers. If not licensed, its quality is suspect.
What are the qualifications of staff members?	If staff members are teachers, more learning activities will be provided; staff should be qualified to perform cardiopulmonary resuscitation.
Is there a fast turnover rate of staff?	A fast turnover rate means little continuity of care will be provided (and probably suggests dissatisfaction with center administration).
What is the child–staff ratio?	A ratio of 3 or 4 children to 1 staff member provides time for quality interaction.
What is the center's policy on parental visits?	Parents should be able to drop in at any time. Be wary of facilities that restrict parental visiting in any way.
Physical Environment	
Is there adequate space in the center?	There should be opportunities for rough-and-tumble and imaginative play and naptime as well as table activities.
Does the space appear safe?	Stairways should be fenced. No paint should be peeling.
Can children get in and out of the building easily?	A first-floor plan is safest. Fire exits should be well marked. An evacuation plan should be practiced.
Is there a safe play area for children outside?	Find out how often children are taken outside (once or twice a day) or only occasionally for "outings."
Is there a quiet place for naps?	Ask if a child can nap if tired or has to wait until a set naptime.
Can the bathroom be reached easily?	Both potty chairs and small toilet seats should be available.
If food is provided, does it meet preschool recommendations?	Food should meet RDA recommendations.
Is there adequate refrigeration?	Food poisoning is a concern without refrigeration.
Staff Philosophy	
Are the workers warm and affectionate toward the children?	Watch how they greet children. They should ask questions and listen to answers.
Do caretakers spend more of their time performing janitorial tasks (cleaning) and reprimanding children, or can they devote their time to the children?	It is best if cleaning staff is separate from care staff.
Is each child assigned to a particular caregiver on a continuing basis?	Ask staff to describe their care pattern; if this is not planned, little continuity of care results.
Are the children provided stimulating toys and equipment?	Imaginative items, such as a puppet theater, finger paint, and water play, should be included.
How do the staff discipline children? Do they yell or treat the children roughly?	The method should reflect the parents' philosophy. Staff should be able to talk to children calmly without raising their voices in anger.
Is there a planned curriculum?	There should be specific individualized goals the staff hopes to accomplish.
Can the child pursue an individual interest?	Play or learning activities should be individualized.
Health Care Protocols	
How does the center care for an ill child?	There should be access to a nurse. Staff should be able to evaluate for illness. They should know actions to take in an emergency.
What precautions does the staff take to prevent spread of infection?	Counter where diapers are changed should be wiped with a disinfectant; tissues and handwashing facilities should be present.
Does the center follow good sanitary practices?	Be sure the center requires waterproof disposable diapers to minimize contamination of the environment and other children, and separates diaper-changing areas from other activities, especially anything related to food handling. Observe adult caregivers changing diapers. Do they wash hands after each change?
Under what conditions are children not allowed to attend the center?	A center should have a very specific policy on what illness symptoms require a child to be kept home—and they should enforce this policy strictly. For instance, runny nose may be acceptable, but a fever is not; children with chickenpox should be kept at home until the scabs are healed over. Talk to parents whose children have been at the center long enough to have experienced some illnesses, and find out what the family did and how the center responded.
Children's Behavior	
Do the children appear happy and relaxed?	Observe for at least 1 morning.
Do they rush to greet any new visitors?	This could be a sign of boredom with their center's activities and a strong need for adult attention.

chair for a short work period. When some parents examine their child's day, they are surprised how few instructions they give the child to follow in a day. They put on their coats, pick up their toys, and lead them to the table for dinner. Similarly, they never encourage their child to spend any time in a chair, which is something the child will do for at least short periods in school. Coloring at a table rather than on the floor will introduce this situation without any problem.

Finally, going to school is a form of separation and a new experience if the child has not attended childcare or preschool, so parents must make preparations for this. It might be good to arrange to have the child stay with another caregiver for part of a day. Staying at school can then be compared with that event.

These are minimum preparations parents can complete to ready their child for school. Caution both parents and children that no matter how hard they try, not everything can be anticipated; school will bring some new happenings no one predicted. If the child has been led to believe that learning is fun and new experiences are enjoyable (creating a strong sense of initiative), these unpredictable instances can be accepted as fun. The concept that new experiences are enjoyable will prepare the child not only for a first day at school but for thousands of profitable days and experiences ahead.

Broken Fluency and Swearing

Developing language is such a complicated process that children from 2 to 6 years of age typically have some speech difficulty that parents may interpret as stuttering. The child may begin to repeat words or syllables, saying, "I-I-I want a n-n-new spoon-spoon-spoon." This is called **broken fluency** (repetition and prolongation of sounds, syllables, and words). It is often referred to as **secondary stuttering** because the child begins to speak without this problem and then, during the preschool years, develops it. Unlike the adult who stutters, the child is unaware that he or she is not being fluent unless it is called to his or her attention. It is a part of normal development and, if accepted as such, will pass. The parent who knows a chronic stutterer, however, or who was a chronic stutterer at one time may react to this normal broken fluency of the preschooler in a more emotional way than the problem deserves. It is resolved most quickly if parents follow a few simple rules (see Focus on Family Empowerment). If the child becomes conscious of a disrupted speech pattern, it is less likely that the problem will correct itself.

Many preschoolers imitate their parents or older children in the family so well during this time that they incorporate swear words into their vocabularies. Parents may have to be reminded that the child does not understand what the words mean; he or she has simply heard them, just as he or she has heard hundreds of other words and decided to use them. Correction should be unemotional; for example, "That's not a word we like to hear you use. When you're angry, why don't you say 'fudge' (or whatever)?" The correcting is no different from that involved when the child uses poor grammar. If parents become emotional, the child realizes the value of such words and may continue using them to get attention.

Concerns of the Family With a Physically Challenged or Chronically Ill Preschooler

Learning how to do things when you have physical limitations can be frustrating. Being unable to understand how to do things because of physical or mental limitations can be even more so. To learn problem solving, however, is part of developing a sense of initiative. A preschooler with a disability such as cerebral palsy has a greater need for problem-solving skills than the average child, because even simple procedures such as eating or getting dressed can be difficult if a physical challenge limits the options.

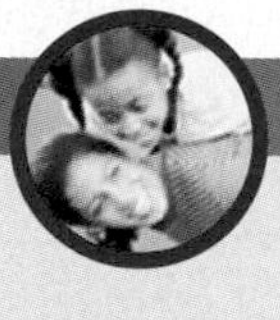

FOCUS ON FAMILY EMPOWERMENT
Suggestions to Help Stuttering in the Preschool Child

Q. My 4-year-old son stutters. What can I do to stop this?

A. What sounds like stuttering in a preschooler is often broken fluency. Helpful tips to improve fluency are:

- Do not discuss in the child's presence the difficulty he is having with speech. Do not label him a "stutterer." This makes him conscious of his speech patterns and compounds the problem. If you have to think about every word you say, it is difficult not to have difficulty speaking.
- Listen with patience to what the child is saying. Do not interrupt or fill in a word for him. Do not tell him to speak more slowly or to start over. These actions make the child conscious of his speech, and his broken fluency increases.
- Talk to him in a calm, simple way. It is difficult for the child to keep up with adult speech. If adults talk slowly to him, he sees no need to rush and so speaks more clearly.
- Protect space for him to talk if there are other children in the family. Rushing to say something before a second child interrupts is the same as rushing to conform to adult speech.
- Do not force the child to speak if he does not want to. Do not ask him to recite or sing for strangers.
- Do not reward him for fluent speech or punish him for nonfluent speech. Broken fluency is a developmental stage in language formation, not an indication of regression or a chronic speech pattern.

Physically challenged or chronically ill preschoolers should attend a preschool program if at all possible. Many of the learning activities that preschoolers enjoy, such as playing with paint, clay, or soap bubbles, are messy. If the child must remain in bed, parents might not offer these types of experiences. A large tray of dry oatmeal or other breakfast cereal with sand shovels or cars and trucks is a good substitute activity for such a child. Although not necessarily neat, these substances (which are available even in a hospital setting) can be swept away easily at the finish of play. Table 30-5 lists the nursing actions that aid a chronically challenged child to solve problems and develop a sense of initiative.

Nutrition and the Physically Challenged or Chronically Ill Preschooler

Experiences with eating help to reinforce a sense of initiative in preschoolers. Chronically ill preschoolers who are limited in the foods they can eat (e.g., they have to maintain a diet of soft foods) or in their ability to help with food preparation may miss this reinforcement. If their appetite is diminished because of illness to the point where they take little or nothing orally, it is still important that they continue to join the family at meals. In most households, this is a time for socialization, and preschoolers are ripe for the learning that goes with this type of daily interaction. Encourage parents to include the ill child in family meals and other social occasions whenever possible.

✔ CHECKPOINT QUESTIONS

11. How should parents react to their preschooler if he begins to masturbate while watching television?
12. What types of illness are frequent in preschoolers attending a childcare center?
13. Is broken fluency true stuttering?

KEY POINTS

Although preschoolers grow only slightly and gain just a little weight, they seem much taller than when they were toddlers because their contour changes to more childlike proportions.

TABLE 30.5 Nursing Actions That Encourage a Sense of Initiative in the Physically Challenged or Chronically Ill Preschooler

CONSIDERATION	NURSING ACTIONS
Nutrition	Serving toast or sandwiches cut into animal shapes with cookie cutters, cereal in the form of alphabet characters, or food arranged on a plate to make a face appeals to the imagination and may make a preschooler more interested in food.
	Respect child's food preferences.
Dressing change	Allow preschooler to measure and cut tape or draw a face on it.
	Allow child to see incision site. Explain steps of dressing change as you work to reduce unknowns and areas of fear.
	Provide extra bandages to put on a doll so child can see that bandages themselves are not to be feared.
Medicine	Allow child to choose a chaser such as juice or milk after oral medicine.
	Choosing site for injection or intravenous line is too advanced for the preschooler; do not allow such choices.
Rest	Provide a light in the room or bring child's bed into hallway so fear of the dark is reduced and child can deal with only reality problems.
	Identify sounds the preschooler might hear in the hospital, such as an air conditioner turning on.
Hygiene	Allow child to choose bathtub toys, clothing.
	Allow child to wash own hands and face.
	Allow child to splash in water as a play activity as well as for cleanliness.
Pain	Encourage preschooler to express pain.
	Allow child to handle syringe or suction catheter, and give "shots" or suction to a doll to alleviate anger or fear.
	Encourage child to ask for analgesic if necessary.
Stimulation	Guessing games encourage a sense of initiative. Draw a dog or a house and ask child to close his or her eyes when you add one more detail to the drawing, such as an ear or a chimney; ask child to identify new item. Reverse the game and ask child what you erased from the drawing, or allow child to do own drawing.
	Provide manipulative toys, such as finger paint, soapy water, clay, or dry cereal to use as sand.
	Allow preschooler to accompany you to other departments as a way of teaching more about the hospital.
	Use "Simon Says" games not only for socialization but also to urge treatments, such as deep-breathing exercises.
	Encourage use of playroom for socialization.
	Encourage child to interact with family by drawing pictures for siblings or telephoning home.

Erikson's developmental task for the preschool period is to gain a sense of initiative or learn how to do things. Play materials ideal for this age group are those that stimulate creativity, such as modeling clay or colored markers.

Promoting childhood safety is a major role because preschoolers' active imaginations can lead them into dangerous situations.

Appetite is not large because this is not a rapid growth time. Preschoolers are interested in helping with food preparation.

Common parental concerns during the preschool period are with broken fluency, imaginary friends, difficulty sharing, and sibling rivalry.

Preschool is often the time when a new sibling is born. Good preparation for this is necessary to prevent intense sibling rivalry.

Preschoolers have a number of universal fears, including fear of the dark, mutilation, and abandonment. All care provided for this age group must include active measures to reduce these fears as much as possible.

Preschoolers are still operating at a cognitive level that prevents them from understanding conservation (objects have not changed substance although they have changed appearance). This means they need an explanation, for example, of how they will be the same person postoperatively as they were preoperatively.

Preschoolers are self-centered (egocentric). This makes it difficult for them to share and view someone else's side of a problem. They need good explanations of how a procedure will benefit them before they can agree to it.

Many preschoolers begin preschool programs or childcare. Late in the preschool period, they may be enrolled in kindergarten. Parents often appreciate guidance in how to orient their children to these new experiences.

Preschoolers who are physically challenged or who have chronic illnesses may have difficulty achieving a sense of initiative, because they may be limited in their ability to participate in activities that stimulate initiative. They may need special playtimes set aside for stimulation and learning.

CRITICAL THINKING EXERCISES

1. Terry is the 3-year-old girl you met at the beginning of the chapter. Terry's mother was concerned because Terry told exaggerated stories about events at her preschool. How would you recommend her mother handle this?
2. Many children these days are raised as vegetarians. Is this an adequate diet for a preschooler? What are simple foods preschoolers can help prepare to build a sense of initiative and interest in food?
3. A 3-year-old is starting childcare because his mother is returning to work. What suggestions could you make to his mother about choosing a safe setting? How should she prepare her son for the experience?
4. The parents of a preschooler tell you that their daughter keeps the entire family awake at night because she is so afraid of the dark. Formulate a plan of action to enable her family to help her sleep.
5. The mother of a 4-year-old boy whom you see in a well-child conference tells you she cannot stand messy activities. What activities could you suggest to the mother that would stimulate a sense of initiative without being messy?
6. Examine the National Health Goals related to preschoolers. Most government-sponsored money for nursing research is allotted based on these goals. What would be a possible research topic to explore pertinent to these goals that would be fundable and would advance evidence-based practice?

REFERENCES

American Academy of Pediatrics. (2001). *Communication with children about disasters.* Washington, D.C.: AAP.

American Academy of Pediatrics Committee on Practice and Ambulatory Medicine. (2001). *Recommendations for preventive pediatric health care.* Washington, D.C.: AAP.

American Academy of Pediatrics Committee on Safety. (2001). *Seat belt safety and children.* Washington, D.C.: AAP.

Ball, T. M. et al. (2002). Influence of attendance at day care on the common cold from birth through 13 years of age. *Archives of Pediatrics & Adolescent Medicine, 156*(2), 121–126.

Berger, K. S. (2001). *The developing person through the life span* (5th ed.). New York: Worth Publishing.

Department of Health and Human Services. (2000). *Healthy people 2010.* Washington, D.C.: DHHS.

Dudek, S. G. (2001). *Nutrition: Essentials for nursing practice.* Philadelphia: Lippincott Williams & Wilkins.

Erikson, E. H. (1963). *Childhood and society.* New York: W.W. Norton.

Johnson, M., Maas, M., & Moorhead, S. (2000). *Nursing outcomes classification* (2d ed.). St. Louis: Mosby, Inc.

Kaplan, D. W., & Love, K. A. (2001). Growth and development. In W. W. Hay, A. R. Hayward, M. J. Levin, & J. M. Sondheimer (Eds.). *Current pediatric diagnosis and treatment* (15th ed.). New York: McGraw-Hill.

Kohlberg, L. (1984). *The psychology of moral development.* New York: Harper & Row.

Krebs, N. F., & Hambridge, K. M. (2001). Normal childhood nutrition and its disorders. In W. W. Hay, A. R. Hayward, M. J. Levin, & J. M. Sondheimer (Eds.). *Current pediatric diagnosis and treatment* (15th ed.). New York: McGraw-Hill.

McCloskey, J., & Bulechek, G. (2000). *Nursing interventions classification* (3d ed.). St. Louis: Mosby Inc.
Piaget, J. (1969). *The theory of stages in cognitive development.* New York: McGraw-Hill.
Zoritch B. et al. (2001). Day care for preschool children. *The Cochrane Library* (Oxford), *4*(1).

ABC XYZ SUGGESTED READINGS

American Academy of Pediatrics Committee on Nutrition. (2001). The use and misuse of fruit juice in pediatrics. *Pediatrics, 107*(5), 1210-1213.
Bar-on, M. E. (2000). The effects of television on child health: Implications and recommendations. *Archives of Disease in Childhood, 83*(4), 289-292.
Bjorkqvist, K., & Osterman, K. (2001). At what age do children learn to discriminate between act and actor? *Perceptual & Motor Skills, 92*(1), 171-176.
Committee on Sports Medicine and Fitness/Committee on School Health, American Academy of Pediatrics. (2001). Organized sports for children and preadolescents. *Pediatrics, 107*(6), 1459-1462.
Dobrez, D., et al. (2001). Estimating the cost of developmental and behavioral screening of preschool children in general pediatric practice. *Pediatrics, 108*(4), 913-922.
Finn, K. et al. (2002). Factors associated with physical activity in preschool children. *Journal of Pediatrics, 140*(1), 81-85.
Foote, J. M., & Dutcher, M. E. (2000). Nutrition and feeding. *Pediatric Basics, 88*(2), 13-15.
Gazi, M. A. (2001). Management of penile toilet seat injury. *Canadian Journal of Urology, 8*(3), 1293-1294.
Green, M., & Solnit, A. (1964). Reactions to the threatened loss of a child: A vulnerable child syndrome. *Pediatrics, 34*(1), 58-64.
Hockman, C. S. (2000). Growth and development. *Pediatric Basics, 88*(2), 22-30.
Hetherington, P. T. (2000). Caring for multiple-birth families. *Pediatric Basics, 88*(2), 5-12.
Kinsman, A. M., & Wildman, B. G. (2001). Mother and child perceptions of child functioning: Relationship to maternal distress. *Family Process, 40*(2), 163-172.
Lemery, K. S., et al. (1999). Developmental models of infant and childhood temperament. *Developmental Psychology, 35*(1), 189-204.
Stein, M. T., et al. (2001). Temper tantrums, impulsivity, and aggression in a preschool-aged boy. *Journal of Developmental & Behavioral Pediatrics, 22*(2), S23-S28.

The Family With a School-Age Child

31

CHAPTER

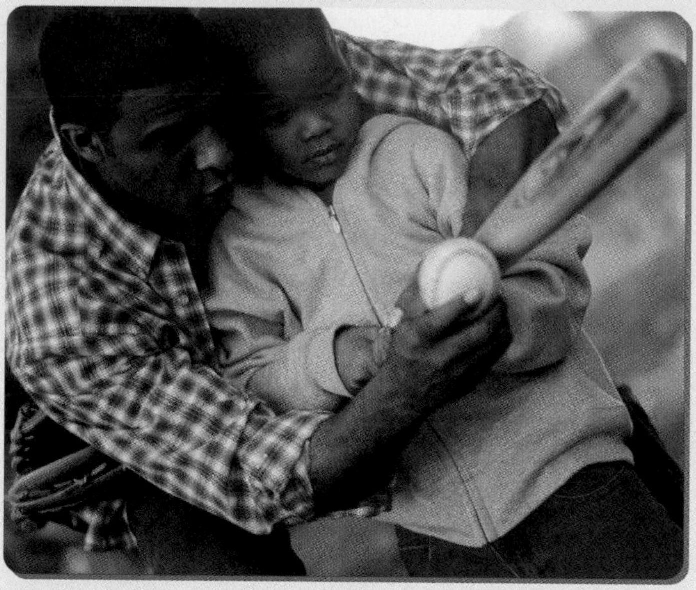

Key Terms

- accommodation
- caries
- class inclusion
- conservation
- decentering
- inclusion
- latchkey children
- malocclusion
- nocturnal emissions
- preconventional reasoning

Objectives

After mastering the contents of this chapter, you should be able to:

1. Describe the normal growth and development pattern and common parental concerns of the school-age period.
2. Assess a school-age child for normal growth and development milestones.
3. Formulate nursing diagnoses for the family of a school-age child.
4. Identify expected outcomes based on health assessment findings.
5. Plan anticipatory guidance to prevent problems of growth and development in the school-age child (e.g., teaching about normal puberty).
6. Implement nursing care to help achieve normal growth and development of the school-age child, such as counseling parents about helping their child adjust to a new school.
7. Evaluate outcome criteria to be certain that goals of care have been achieved.
8. Identify National Health Goals related to the school-age child that nurses can be instrumental in helping the nation achieve.
9. Identify areas related to care of school-age children that could benefit from additional nursing research or application of evidence-based practice.
10. Use critical thinking to analyze ways in which the care of the school-age child can be more family-centered.
11. Integrate knowledge of school-age growth and development with the nursing process to achieve quality maternal and child health nursing care.

Shelly Lewis is a 6-year-old girl who recently started first grade. Her mother tells you that although Shelly says she likes school, she has developed a lot of nervous habits such as nail biting since school started. Her mother asks you if this is normal. How would you advise her?

The previous chapter discussed the preschooler and the abilities children develop in these years. This chapter adds information about the dramatic changes, both physical and psychosocial, that occur during the school-age years. This is important information because it builds a base for care and health teaching for the age group.

After you've studied the chapter, answer the Critical Thinking Exercises at the end of the chapter and then access the on-line study activities (http://connection.lww.com) *to further sharpen your skills and test your knowledge.*

The term "school age" commonly refers to children between the ages of 6 and 12. Although these years represent a time of slow physical growth, cognitive growth and developmental growth proceed at rapid rates. Because of this, there are many differences among children from one year to the next. For example, 7- and 10-year-old children have very different needs and outlooks, as do 11- and 12-year-old children. Always assess children as individuals to understand the particular developmental needs of each child based on what developmental status he or she has achieved, not on what stage you think he or she should have reached.

The school-age period is usually the first time that children begin to make truly independent judgments. This may create some conflicts with parents if they are not prepared for this. Unlike the infant or toddler, whose progress is marked by obvious new abilities and skills (e.g., ability to sit up or roll over; ability to speak a full sentence), the development of the school-age child is more subtle and may be marked by mood swings; what the child enjoys on one occasion may not be acceptable on the next. For instance, a child may ask his parents for a guitar and lessons, but then after the family invests in these, he may quickly lose interest in music. Children of school age are also more influenced by the attitudes of their friends than previously. They may choose not to do something that was previously enjoyable because no friends are interested in that activity. Parents who make too much of these likes and dislikes may find themselves engaged in unnecessary conflicts with their child. The Focus on National Health Goals box lists National Health Goals related to the school-age period.

FOCUS ON NATIONAL HEALTH GOALS

A number of National Health Goals address the health of the school-age population:

- Increase the proportion of public and private schools that require daily physical education for all students from a baseline of 17% to a target of 25%.
- Reduce deaths caused by motor vehicle accidents to no more than 9.2 per 100,000 children from a baseline of 15.6 per 100,000.
- Reduce the proportion of children who have dental caries (in permanent or primary teeth) to no more than 11% from a baseline of 18%.
- Increase use of safety belts in automobiles from 69% to 92%.
- Increase use of helmets by bicyclists (DHHS, 2000).

Nurses can be instrumental in helping the nation achieve these goals by urging children to begin and maintain a consistent exercise program, brush teeth and go for dental checkups regularly, and follow safety rules both in and around automobiles. Additional nursing research that would be helpful includes: What is the ideal exercise program that is interesting enough to children that it will hold their attention for a long span of time? What are effective ways to teach street safety to children in the early school years? What strategies are most effective in helping school-age children brush teeth daily?

NURSING PROCESS OVERVIEW

For Healthy Development of the School-Age Child

Assessment

Use both history and physical examination to assess growth and development of the school-age child. Include questions about school activities and progress in the history. School-age children are interested and able to contribute to their own health history; it is useful to interview children 10 years or older at least in part without their parents being present. During the physical examination, show your respect for the child's adult-level modesty by having him or her use a cover gown.

Parents of school-age children often mention behavioral issues or conflicts during yearly health visits. Some parents feel they are losing contact with their children during these years. This can cause them to misinterpret a normal change in behavior, especially if they are not prepared for what to expect from their child. Other parents may consider children who behave differently from their siblings as "abnormal" when they are just expressing their own personality.

When problems are discussed in the health care setting, take the history from the parent and also allow the child to express the problem. It may be necessary to obtain the opinion of school personnel (with the parents' permission) regarding the problem or even just determine whether school personnel feel a problem exists. In some instances, a counselor's opinion may be necessary. If the problem is related to a medical condition, its effect on the family should also be assessed, because the illness of a child affects the functioning of the entire family unit.

Nursing Diagnosis

Common nursing diagnoses pertinent to growth and development during the school-age period include:

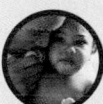

- Health-seeking behaviors related to normal school-age growth and development
- Readiness for enhanced parenting related to improved family living conditions
- Anxiety related to slow growth pattern of child
- Risk for injury related to deficient parental knowledge about safety precautions for a school-age child

Outcome Identification and Planning

When identifying expected outcomes and planning care, keep in mind the school-age child's tendency to enjoy small or short-term projects rather than long, involved ones. A child with diabetes, for example, in her early school years may gain a feeling of achievement by learning to assess her own serum glucose level, but she may have difficulty continuing glucose assessment on a long-term basis.

Behavior problems need to be well defined before outcomes are identified and interventions planned. Often, it is enough for parents to accept the problem as one consistent with normal growth and development.

Implementation

School-age children are interested in learning about adult roles, so this means they will watch you to see your attitude as well as your actions in a given situation. When giving care, keep in mind that children this age feel more comfortable knowing the "hows" and "whys" of actions. They may not cooperate with a procedure until they are given a satisfactory explanation of why it must be done.

Outcome Evaluation

Yearly health visits covering both physical and psychosocial development are important at this age. It may be useful for parents to look back at problems identified at the last visit and discuss if and how they were resolved. Often, some problems and conflicts fade away without anyone really noticing. As some problems recede, however, others may emerge. At times, the same concerns of parents and the child may appear to be unresolved at each visit. Make sure no underlying problem exists that prevents resolution. Examples of outcome criteria are:

- Parent states he will allow child to make own decisions about how to spend allowance.
- Parent states she reads to child daily.
- Child states he understands his growth is normal, even though he is the shortest boy in his eighth-grade class.
- Child does not sustain injury from sports activities during summer.

NURSING ASSESSMENT OF GROWTH AND DEVELOPMENT OF THE SCHOOL-AGE CHILD

As school age is a relatively long time span, children grow and develop extensively during this period.

Physical Growth

School-age children grow slowly but steadily. Their annual average weight gain is approximately 3 to 5 lb (1.3 to 2.2 kg); the increase in height is 1 to 2 inches (2.5 to 5 cm). Children who did not lose the lordosis and knock-kneed appearance of toddlers during the preschool period lose these now. Posture becomes more erect.

By age 10 years, brain growth is complete, so fine motor coordination becomes refined. As the eye globe reaches its final shape at about this same time, an adult vision level is achieved. If the eruption of permanent teeth and growth of the jaw do not correlate with final head growth, malocclusion with teeth malalignment may result.

The immunoglobulins IgG and IgA reach adult levels, and lymphatic tissue continues to grow up until about age 9. The resulting abundance of tonsillar and adenoid tissue in the early school years is often mistaken for disease during respiratory illness. It may also result in temporary conduction deafness from eustachian tube obstruction until this tissue recedes normally. The appendix is also lined with lymphatic tissue, and swelling of this tissue in the narrow tube can lead to trapped fecal material and inflammation (appendicitis) in the early school-age child. Frontal sinuses develop at about age 6 years, and sinus headache becomes a possibility (before then, headache in children is rarely caused by a sinus infection).

The left ventricle of the heart enlarges to be strong enough to pump blood to the growing body. Innocent heart murmurs may become apparent due to the extra blood crossing heart valves. The pulse rate decreases to 70 to 80 bpm; blood pressure rises to about 112/60 mm Hg. Maturation of the respiratory system leads to increased oxygen–carbon dioxide exchange, which increases exertion ability and stamina (Berger, 2001).

Sexual Maturation

At a set point in brain maturity, the hypothalamus transmits an enzyme to the anterior pituitary gland to begin production of gonadotropic hormones, which activate changes in testes and ovaries and produce puberty. Hormone changes that occur with puberty are discussed in Chapter 4. Table 31-1 describes the usual order for secondary sex characteristics.

Timing of the onset of puberty changes varies widely, between 10 and 14 years of age. The length of time until sexual maturity also varies. Sexual maturation in girls occurs between 12 and 18 years; in boys, between 14 and 20. Puberty is occurring increasingly earlier, however, and, in a class of 10-year-old sixth graders, it is not unusual to discover that more than half of the girls are already menstruating. Therefore, to be effective, sex education must be introduced as part of the school curriculum in grade school, not in middle school or high school.

✔ CHECKPOINT QUESTIONS

1. Why is appendicitis apt to occur in early school-age children?
2. Why do sinus headaches first occur at early school age?

TABLE 31.1 Chronologic Development of Secondary Sex Characteristics

AGE (YR)	BOYS	GIRLS
9–11	Prepubertal weight gain occurs.	Breasts: elevation of papilla with breast bud formation; areolar diameter enlarges.
11–12	Sparse growth of straight, downy, slightly pigmented hair at base of penis.	Straight hair along the labia. Vaginal epithelium becomes cornified.
	Scrotum becoming textured; growth of penis and testes begins.	pH of vaginal secretions acid; slight mucous vaginal discharge present.
	Sebaceous gland secretion increases.	Sebaceous gland secretion increases.
	Perspiration increases.	Perspiration increases.
		Dramatic growth spurt.
12–13	Pubic hair present across pubis.	Pubic hair grows darker; spreads over entire pubis.
	Penis lengthens.	Breasts enlarge, still no protrusion of nipples.
	Dramatic linear growth spurt.	Axillary hair present.
	Breast enlargement occurs.	Menarche occurs.

Sexual and Physical Concerns

Changes in physical appearance lead to problems and worries for both children and their parents. School age is a time for parents to discuss with children the physical changes and the sexual responsibility they require. This is also the time to reinforce previous teaching with children that their body is their own, to be used only in the way they choose. Specific measures for children to help prevent sexual abuse are discussed later in the chapter. School nurses can play a major role in this type of education as well.

In both sexes, puberty brings changes in the sebaceous glands. Under the influence of androgen, glands become more active, setting the stage for acne (see Chap. 32). Vasomotor instability commonly leads to blushing; perspiration increases (Kaplan & Love, 2001).

Concerns of Girls. Prepubertal girls are usually taller, by about 2 inches (5 cm) or more, than preadolescent boys because their typical growth spurt begins earlier. In a culture in which boys are expected to be taller than girls, this can cause concern for girls. Sometimes a girl notices the change in her pelvic contour when she tries on a skirt or dress from the year before and realizes her hips are becoming broader. She may misinterpret this finding as a gain in weight and attempt a crash diet. She can be reassured that broad bone structure of the hips is part of an adult female profile.

Girls are usually conscious of breast development. A girl who is developing ahead of her peers may tend to slouch or wear loose clothing to hide her breast development. Another girl studies herself in front of the mirror and wonders whether her breasts are going to develop enough. Breast development is not always symmetrical, and it is not unusual for a girl to have breasts of slightly different sizes. After the condition has been checked during a physical examination, she can be reassured that this development is normal—that one breast is not filled with a tumor to make it bigger or the other diseased in some way to make it smaller. Supernumerary (additional) nipples may darken or increase in size at puberty. Be sure girls understand that a supernumerary nipple is affected by the hormones in her body in the same way as other breast tissue, so these changes are normal.

Early preparation for menstruation is important preparation for future childbearing and for the girl's concept of herself as a woman (see Focus on Communication). A girl who is told that menstruation is a normal function that occurs every month in all healthy women has a different attitude toward her body than the girl who wakes up one morning to find blood on her pajamas and is told bluntly, "You'd better get used to that. You'll have to put up with it for the rest of your life." In the first instance, the girl can trust her body: it is doing what every woman's body does. In the second instance, she feels that her body is beyond her control. How can she accept and enjoy growing up if it involves something so unpredictable? In addition to an explanation of the reason for menstrual flow, girls need an explanation of good hygiene and reassurance that they can bathe, shower, and swim during their periods. They can use either sanitary napkins or tampons; if they use tampons, they must take precautions to avoid toxic shock syndrome (see Chap. 47).

Girls also need to know that vaginal secretions will appear. If this is not explained, a girl may fear needlessly that she has an infection. Explain that any secretions that cause vulvar irritation should be evaluated at a health care facility, because this does suggest infection.

Most girls have some menstrual irregularity during the first year or two after menarche (the start of menstruation). This occurs primarily because a girl's cycles are anovulatory at first. With maturity and the onset of ovulation, the cycle becomes more regular.

Menstrual irregularity may be a significant concern for preadolescents. A girl may fear that irregular periods indicate a hormone imbalance, and she may worry about her future ability to conceive, or she may be ill informed about how conception occurs and fear that irregularity of her periods means she is pregnant. Some other causes of irregular periods are malnourishment and obesity. Emotions can also affect menstruation. If irregularity continues beyond the first year, a careful history of the girl's school, social, and home adjustment should be taken. (Dysmenorrhea, or painful menstruation, is discussed in Chap. 47.)

FOCUS ON COMMUNICATION

Barbara is a 12-year-old girl who comes to the nurse's office at her school.

Less Effective Communication

Nurse: Hello, Barbara. What can I do for you?
Barbara: I'm having cramps.
Nurse: Are you having your period?
Barbara: No. I haven't started them yet.
Nurse: Describe your cramps to me.
Barbara: Both my sisters started their periods when they were 10.
Nurse: Are you sick to your stomach?
Barbara: I'm the only girl in my gym class who doesn't have her period yet.
Nurse: Let's talk about the cramps. What do you think is causing those?
Barbara: They're not really bad. I'll go back to class.

More Effective Communication

Nurse: Hello, Barbara. What can I do for you?
Barbara: I'm having cramps.
Nurse: Are you having your period?
Barbara: No. I haven't started them yet.
Nurse: Describe your cramps to me.
Barbara: Both my sisters started their periods when they were 10.
Nurse: Are you sick to your stomach?
Barbara: I'm the only girl in my gym class who doesn't have her period yet.
Nurse: You sound as if you're more worried about that than what you came in for.
Barbara: I need to know if I'm all right.
Nurse: Let's talk about that.

In the past, when topics such as menstruation were discussed only in whispers and neither television nor magazines advertised sanitary pads or medicine for menstrual discomfort, most 12-year-old children had little idea about what to expect at puberty. Today, with this information readily available to the public, it is easy to forget that preadolescents, because they may not read magazines or watch adult television shows, still may not know much about what to expect at puberty. Be aware that almost all prepubescent girls are concerned about puberty changes. Through effective communication and listening, you can help them talk about their problems and concerns.

Girls need to know when their periods will occur so they can get used to this new phenomenon and learn to trust their bodies. A girl in college can explain matter-of-factly that she prefers not to go to the beach today because she has her period and does not want to use tampons, but for a preadolescent, this topic is too sophisticated and too emotionally charged to discuss openly. She wants to be able to plan activities to avoid having to make such explanations.

For a nominal charge, manufacturers of sanitary napkins will mail an introductory kit of their products, together with well-illustrated, factual booklets, to introduce girls to menstruation. Such kits are useful if they supplement a parent's or a nurse's discussion, but they should not take the place of individual attention.

Concerns of Boys. Boys who are not prepared for the physical changes of puberty worry about them in the same way that girls do. Just as girls are keenly aware of breast development, boys are aware of increasing genital size. If they do not know that testicular development precedes penis growth, they can worry that their growth is inadequate. Men tend to measure their manliness by penis size, so a boy who develops late may feel inferior.

Hypertrophy of breast tissue (gynecomastia) can occur in prepuberty, most often in stocky or heavy boys. A youth with this condition may be concerned that a breast tumor is present or be embarrassed about growing breasts. He can be reassured that this is a transitory phenomenon and, although it makes him self-conscious, will fade as soon as his male hormones become more mature and active.

Some boys are also concerned because although they have pubic hair, they cannot yet grow a beard or do not have chest hair—outward, easily recognized signs of maturity. You can assure them that pubic hair normally appears first and that chest and facial hair may not grow until several years later.

As seminal fluid is produced, boys begin to notice ejaculation during sleep, termed **nocturnal emissions.** Preadolescent boys may believe the old myth that loss of seminal fluid is debilitating; also, boys may have heard the term "premature ejaculation" and worry that this is a forewarning of a problem in years to come. Both are fallacies.

Teeth

Deciduous teeth are lost and permanent teeth erupt during the school-age period (Fig. 31-1). The average child gains 28 teeth between 6 and 12 years of age: the central and lateral incisors; first, second, and third cuspids; and first and second molars (Fig. 31-2).

Developmental Milestones

Gross Motor Development

School-age development is summarized in Table 31-2. At the beginning of the school-age period (age 6), children endlessly jump, tumble, skip, and hop. They have enough coordination to walk a straight line. Many can ride a bicycle. They can skip rope with practice. A 7-year-old appears quiet compared with a rough-and-tumble 6-year-old. Seven-year-olds usually have enough accuracy in jumping to play hopscotch and to skip rope well. Gender differences usually begin to manifest in play: there are "girl games," such as dressing dolls, and "boy games," such as pretending to be pirates.

The movements of 8-year-olds are more graceful than those of younger children, although as their arms and legs grow, they may stumble on furniture or spill milk and food. They ride a bicycle well and enjoy sports such as gymnastics, soccer, and hockey.

Nine-year-olds are on the go constantly, as if they always have a deadline to meet. They have enough eye–hand coordination to enjoy baseball, basketball, and volleyball.

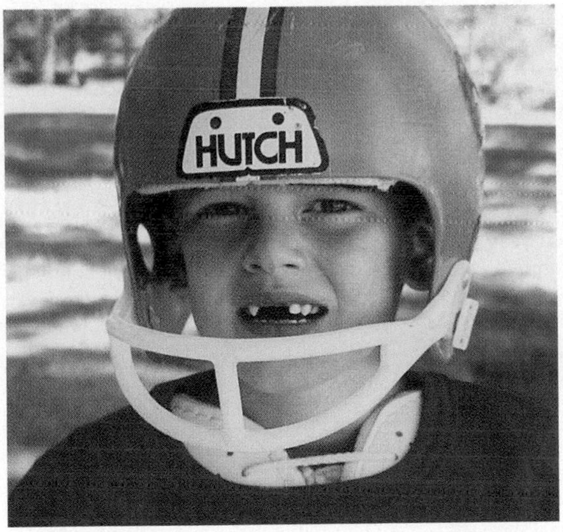

FIGURE 31.1 Early-school-age children typically have a missing upper incisor as deciduous teeth are replaced by permanent teeth.

By 10 years of age, they are more interested in perfecting their athletic skills than previously.

At age 11, many children feel awkward because of their growth spurt and thus do less well at sports. This deficiency may bother the ones who see sports as the key to popularity or self-esteem. They may drop out of sports activities at this time rather than look ungainly in their attempts. Their energy is then channeled into constant motion: drumming fingers and tapping pencils or feet.

Twelve-year-olds plunge into activities with intensity and concentration. They often enjoy participating in sports events for charities (e.g., walk-a-thons). They may be refreshingly cooperative around the house, able to handle a great deal of responsibility and complete given tasks.

Fine Motor Development

Six-year-olds can easily tie their shoelaces. They can cut and paste well and draw a person with good detail. They can print, although they may routinely reverse letters. Seven-

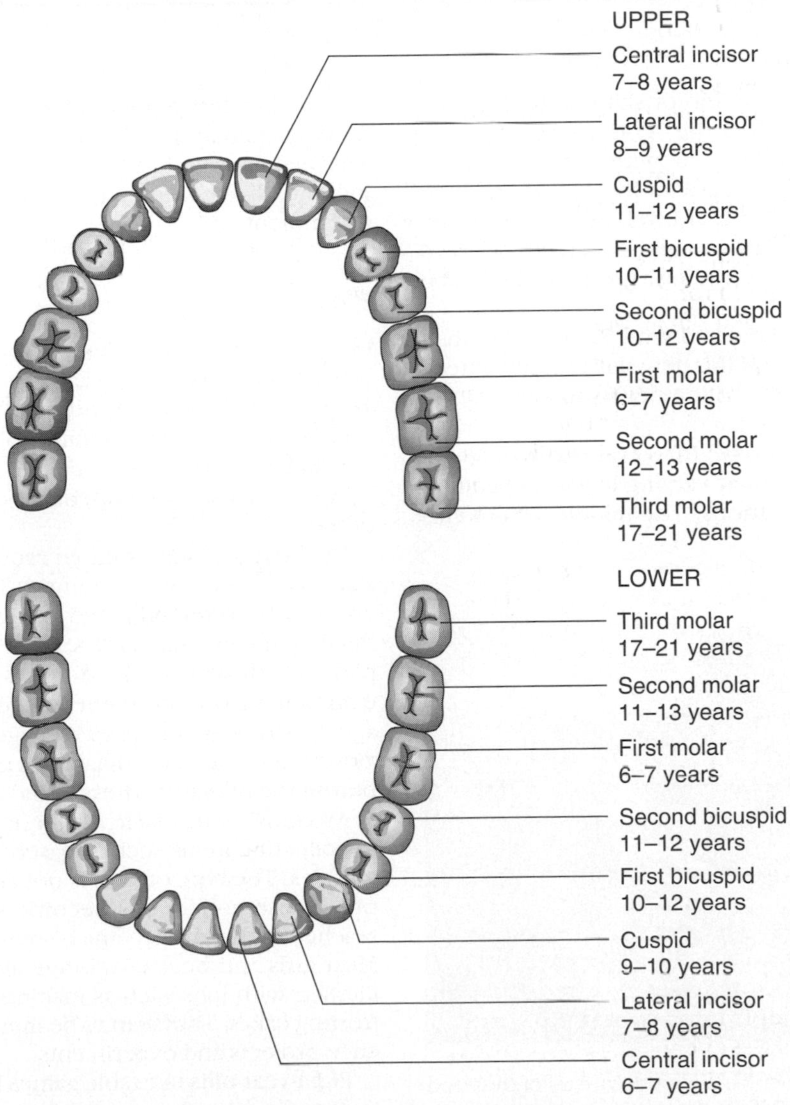

FIGURE 31.2 Eruption pattern of permanent teeth.

TABLE 31.2 Summary of School-Age Development

AGE (YR)	PHYSICAL DEVELOPMENT	PSYCHOSOCIAL AND COGNITIVE DEVELOPMENT
6	A year of constant motion; skipping is a new skill; first molars erupt.	First-grade teacher becomes authority figure; adjustment to all-day school may be difficult and lead to nervous manifestations of fingernail biting, etc. Defines words by their use: a key is to unlock a door, not a metal object.
7	Central incisors erupt; difference between sexes becomes apparent in play (video games vs. dolls); spends time in quiet play.	A quiet year; striving for perfection leads to this year being called an *eraser* year. Conservation (water poured from tall container to a wide, flat one is the same amount of water) is learned; can tell time; can make simple change.
8	Coordination definitely improved; playing with gang becomes important; eyes become fully developed.	"Best friends" develop; whispering and giggling begin; can write as well as print; understands concepts of past, present, and future.
9	All activities done with gang.	Gang age; a 9-year-old club is formed to spite someone, has secret codes, is all boy or all girl; gangs disband and reform quickly.
10	Coordination improves.	Ready for camp away from home; collecting age; likes rules; ready for competitive games.
11	Active, but awkward and ungainly.	Insecure with members of opposite sex; repeats off-color jokes.
12	Coordination improves.	A sense of humor is present; is social and cooperative.

year-olds concentrate on fine motor skills more than previously. This has been called the "eraser year" because children are never quite content with what they have done. They set too high a standard for themselves and then have difficulty performing at that level. By 7 years of age, children's eyes are developed enough so that they can read regular-size type. This makes reading a greater pleasure and school more enjoyable (Fig. 31-3).

Eight-year-olds learn to read and write script rather than print. They enjoy showing off this new skill in cards, letters, or projects. By age 9, their writing begins to look mature and less awkward.

Older school-age children begin to evaluate their teachers' ability and can perform at varying levels, depending on each teacher's expectations. The middle school curriculum involves more challenging science and mathematics courses than previously and includes good literature. This may be a child's first exposure to reading as a fulfilling and worthwhile experience rather than just as an assignment.

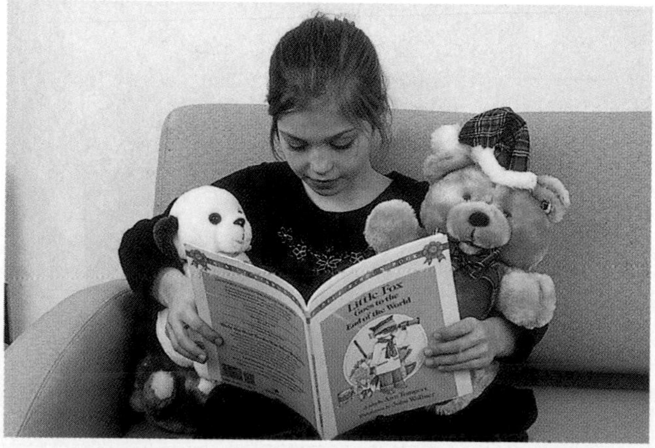

FIGURE 31.3 One of the biggest discoveries of childhood is that reading and writing are fun. Reading and writing are activities that can help a child pass the hours of illness.

Play

Play continues to be rough; however, when children discover reading as an enjoyable activity that opens doors to other worlds, they will begin to spend quiet time with books. Many children spend hours playing increasingly challenging video games, an activity that can either foster a healthy sense of competition or create isolation from others.

By 7 years of age, children require more props for play than when they were younger. To be a police officer, a 7-year-old needs a badge and gun, whereas before a pointed finger sufficed. This is the start of a decline in imaginative play, which will continue unless the child receives adequate stimulation and is encouraged to use imagination. By age 7, girls begin to prefer teenage dolls if they didn't previously, and their coordination is good enough for them to button the miniature dresses and pull on the tiny boots.

Around 7 years of age, children also develop an interest in collecting items such as baseball cards, dolls, rocks, or marbles. The type of item is not as important as the quantity. These collections become structured as the child reaches 8 years of age; time is spent sorting and cataloging. Most girls and boys of this age also enjoy helping in the kitchen with jobs such as making cookies and salads and frosting cakes. They start to be more involved in simple science projects and experiments.

Eight-year-olds like table games but hate to lose, so they tend to avoid competitive games. They may change the rules in the middle of the game to keep from losing.

Many children of 8 or 9 enter a phase of reading comic books. These can be read quickly, so they complement a sense of industry, the developmental task of the school-age years. If parents forbid comic-book reading, the child may read the comics under the covers at night or at other children's houses. Parents would do better to set good reading examples and patiently wait out the child's acute interest in comic books. Their child is reading and will eventually seek other types of books as well.

Nine-year-olds play hard. They wake in the morning, squeeze in some activity before school, and plan something the moment they arrive home. They have difficulty going to bed at night because they want to play just one more game. Play is rough; children are not as interested in perfecting their skills as they will be in another year. Some parents or coaches expect children of this age to be more interested in perfecting their skills, so conflict often arises.

Many schools begin music lessons for children at about 9 years of age. Children do well if others in their group are taking similar lessons. Talent for music or art becomes evident, and children respond with new interest in school or wherever they are exposed to these arts.

Many 10-year-olds spend most of their time playing handheld or television remote-control games. Boys and girls play separately at age 10, although interest in the opposite sex is apparent. Boys show off as girls pass their group; girls talk loudly or giggle at the sight of a familiar boy. Girls become more interested in the way they look and dress. They may feel old enough for stockings and lipstick. Slumber parties and camp-outs become increasingly popular. The children talk, giggle, and rough-house into the middle of the night.

In the 10th year, children are interested in rules and fairness. Before this time, they gave younger children breaks in games, allowing extra turns or hints. Now they strictly enforce rules (Fig. 31-4). Club activities become structured, with a president, a secretary, and rules of order.

Eleven- and 12-year-old children enjoy dancing to popular music and playing table games and are accommodating enough to be able to play with younger siblings who need the rules modified to their advantage. Time with friends is often spent just talking. If older school-age children use their bedroom as a place to meet with friends, they become more interested in seeing that it is picked up. Twelve-year-olds typically like to do jobs such as raking leaves or babysitting for money. Both boys and girls seem to feel that they are on the verge of something great and anxiously wait to turn 13 and become a teenager.

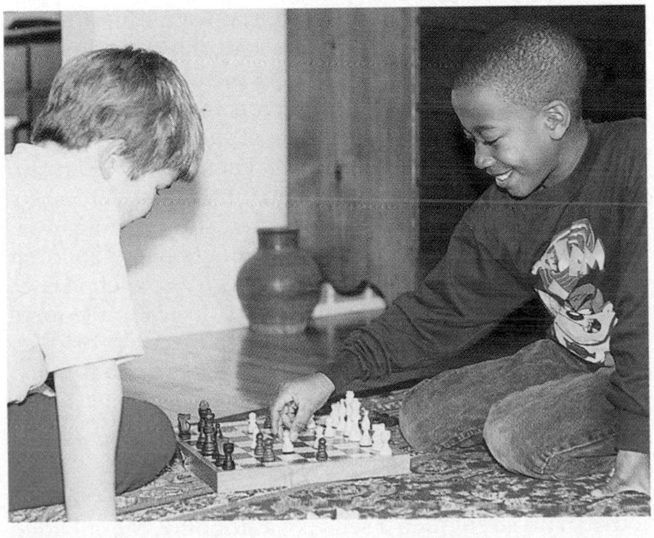

FIGURE 31.4 By 10 years of age children are ready for competition. These two children enjoy a game of chess.

✔ CHECKPOINT QUESTIONS

3. Do supernumerary nipples enlarge with puberty?
4. At what age do boys begin to experience nocturnal emissions?

Language Development

Six-year-olds talk in full sentences, using language easily and with meaning. They no longer sound as though talking is an experiment but appear to have incorporated language permanently. They still define objects by their use: a key is to unlock a door; a fork is to eat with.

Most 7-year-olds can tell the time in hours, but they may have trouble with concepts such as half past and quarter to, especially with the prevalence of digital clocks and watches. They know the months of the year and can name the months in which holidays fall. They can add and subtract and make simple change (if they have had experience), so they can go to the store and make simple purchases. Much of a child's talk is concerned with these con- cepts as he or she practices them and shows them off for family or friends.

As children discover "dirty" jokes at about age 9, they like to tell them to friends or try to understand those told by adults. They use swear words to express anger or just to show other children they are growing up. They may have a short period of intense fascination with "bathroom language," as they did during preschool years. As before, parents should make it clear that they find such language unacceptable and refrain from using it themselves in their child's presence.

By 12 years of age, a sense of humor is apparent. Twelve-year-olds can carry on an adult conversation, although stories are limited because of their lack of experience.

Emotional Development

Ideally, children enter the school-age period with the ability to trust others and with a sense of respect for their own worth. They can accomplish small tasks independently because they want to be independent (a sense of autonomy). They should have practiced or mimicked adult roles and had the opportunity to explore at preschool or other social environments. At the same time, they should have learned to share, to have discovered that learning is fun and an adventure, and to have learned that doing things is more important and more rewarding than watching things being done (a sense of initiative).

Developmental Task: Industry Versus Inferiority

During the early school years, children attempt to master yet another developmental step: learning a sense of industry or accomplishment (Erikson, 1993). If gaining a sense of initiative can be defined as learning how to do things, then gaining a sense of industry is learning how to do things well.

If children are prevented from achieving a sense of industry or do not receive rewards for accomplishment, they can develop a feeling of inferiority or become convinced that they cannot do things that they actually can do. These children will have difficulty tackling new situations later in life (new job, new school, new responsibility) because they cannot envision how they could be successful in handling them. This can result in frustration in school or work activities.

The questions a preschool child asks reflect curiosity, such as "how," "why," and "what." During the early school years, children concentrate their questions on the "how" of tasks: "Is this the right way to do this?" "Am I making this right?" "Is this good?" Often the school-age child will comment, "I can't do anything right" because his or her craft project does not look perfect or falls short of expectations. School-age children need reassurance that they are doing things correctly. This reassurance is best if it comes frequently rather than infrequently after long waits.

The best type of book for school-age children has many short chapters; children feel a sense of accomplishment when they finish each chapter, rather than having to wait until the end of the book. Small chores that can be completed quickly also give this type of reward. Children can survey their finished work and see that they have done a good job. A child may dislike vacuuming, for instance, because the rug may not look very different when the task is complete. Picking up the scattered contents of a toy box, however, is a more obvious task that clearly makes a difference in the appearance of the room.

Hobbies and projects also are enjoyed best if they are small and can be finished within a short time. Most school-age children, for example, prefer putting together two or three fairly simple model-car kits to assembling one extremely complicated kit. The three kits offer three rewards; the involved one delays the reward so long that the child may become bored and never complete it. With adolescence will come more respect for quality. Children will realize that if they want the better model, they will have to spend the extra energy and attention—quality products involve quality work (Fig. 31-5).

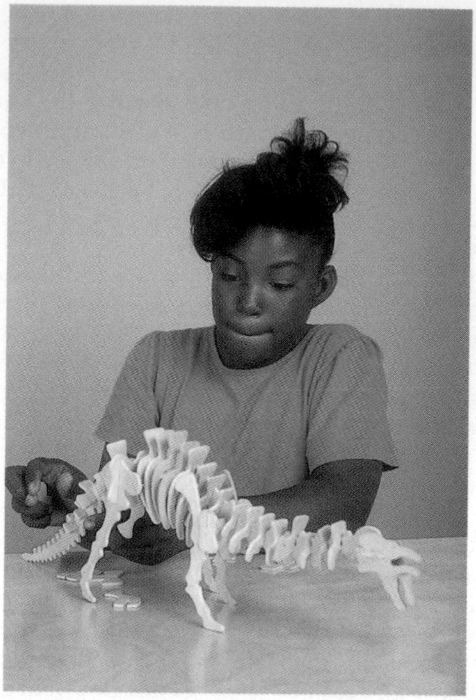

FIGURE 31.5 Assembling this simple model in a short time helps the school-age child gain a sense of industry.

Home as a Setting to Learn Industry. Parents of a school-age child need to take a step forward in development along with their child. For the first time, they realize that their child is dependent on role models other than themselves. Parents who enjoyed fostering imagination in a preschooler may feel frustrated when the school-age child begins to conform to rules and insists on the "right way" to do things. They may feel they have failed to encourage the child's creativity, but conformity is vital to children at this age. It is how they learn more about their world's rules.

Eight- or 9-year-olds begin to spend more and more time with their peers and less time with their family. They forget to do household chores they once enjoyed, such as setting the table or cleaning the garage, or they may do the work sloppily so they have more time with their friends. Although this may seem like a regression in behavior, it is actually a step of independence away from the parents and into the larger world, a developmental task that will help them become emotionally mature. This is an example of a new role the child is trying out, one of many he or she will try in the process of reaching maturity, when he will eventually find a "right-fit" role.

School As a Setting to Learn Industry. Adjusting to and achieving in school are two of the major tasks for this age group. Ideally, a child's teacher will think of learning as fun and will encourage the child to plunge into new experiences. Unfortunately, parents must monitor teachers and school activities to make sure their children are being led this way while not being pushed too hard.

Schools are increasingly assuming responsibility for education about sex, safety, avoidance of substances of abuse, and preparation for family living. These discussions are generally superficial, however, and if the classes are large, they may raise more questions than they can answer. Although learning these skills with peers helps children learn other people's opinions in these areas, such classes should not replace parental teaching. If given adequate encouragement and preparation by health care providers, most parents will be eager to maintain such responsibility.

Structured Activities. Girl Scouts, Boy Scouts, Campfire Girls, and 4-H clubs are respected school-age activities. If the local chapters are well run by leaders who understand children's needs, they can provide hours of constructive activity and strengthen a sense of autonomy. Merit badge systems are geared to the needs of school-age children, offering small but frequent rewards. As with school activities, parents should determine the worth of each organization for their individual child.

Urge parents to evaluate competitive sports programs as well. Before children can compete successfully, they must be able to lose a game without feeling devastated; in other words, to be able to say, "I lost because I played badly," not "I lost because I am a bad person." Children do not usually develop sufficient ego strength to do this until they are about 10 years old.

Another problem to consider with organized contact sports is the possibility of athletic injuries. Encourage parents to consider their child's maturity and the risk of athletic injuries (see Chap. 51) before they decide whether team competition is right for their child. Box 31-1 highlights appropriate outcomes and interventions using the terminology identified by the Nursing Outcomes Classification (NOC) and Nursing Interventions Classification (NIC).

Problem Solving. An important part of developing a sense of industry is learning how to solve problems. Parents and teachers can help children develop this skill by encouraging practice. When the child asks, "Is this the right way to do this?" the parent can say, "Let's talk about possible ways of doing it."

The world depends on machinery, so mishaps and breakdowns (and therefore sudden changes) do occur. The child who can create an indoor playhouse with a card table and blanket when it is too wet or cold to use an outdoor playhouse will be able, as an adult, to find another solution to a data distribution problem when a computer malfunctions. This attitude of optimism rather than pessimism produces adults who rarely say, "It can't be done." Just as important, it leaves these adults with confidence and a sense of pride, feeling good about themselves because they have control of their environment and abilities.

Learning to Live With Others. School-age children are sometimes so interested in tasks and in accomplishing physical projects that they forget they must work with people to achieve these goals. A good time to urge children to learn compassion and thoughtfulness toward others is during the early school years, when children are first exposed to large groups of other youngsters. Writing thank-you letters and shoveling an older neighbor's sidewalk are examples of activities that can help children develop empathy toward others.

Learning to give a present without receiving one in return or doing a favor without expecting a reward is also a part of this process, and this can be taught by example. Children should see their parents doing such things with an attitude not of "What will I get?" but "What can I contribute?"

Children may show empathy toward others as early as 20 months, but cognitively they cannot relate others' experiences to their own until about 6 years of age. Therefore, it is usually ineffective to lecture a child by saying, "That was cruel to call Mary names." The child may feel she had every right to do so. A better technique is to ask the child to put herself in Mary's place for a minute and imagine how she would feel if she were Mary. The school-age child will generally be able to do this and understand why name-calling hurts and makes children feel rejected. Following this, a simple statement like, "It doesn't feel good to be called names, does it?" may suffice.

BOX 31.1

NURSING OUTCOMES AND NURSING INTERVENTIONS CLASSIFICATION: SPORTS INJURIES

NOC: Safety Behavior, Personal

Safety behavior, personal, is defined as individual or caregiver efforts to control behaviors that might cause physical injury (Johnson, Maas, & Moorhead, 2000). Some specific indicators suggesting achievement of this outcome include the child's demonstration of the following:

- Balanced periods of sleep and rest with activity
- Appropriate use of helmets, seat or safety belts, and clothing for activity
- Correct use of protective devices
- Avoidance of recreational drugs, including tobacco, and high-risk behaviors

NIC: Sports-Injury Prevention, Youth

Sports-injury prevention, youth, is defined as reducing the risk of sports-related injury in young athletes (McCloskey & Bulechek, 2000). Some important activities involved when implementing this intervention include:

- Encouraging general fitness, modification of game rules based on age and ability of participants, and appropriate matching of competitors by age, weight, and stage of physical maturation
- Monitoring adherence to recommended training guidelines, compliance with safety rules, field of play for safety conditions, and proper use and condition of safety equipment
- Assisting child in selection of sport that is a good fit with interests and abilities that will promote life-long fitness behaviors
- Assisting parents and coaches in setting realistic goals for participation
- Monitoring sports physicals and return of athletes to participation following injury
- Encouraging the use of warm-up and cool-down exercises and relaxation and coping strategies
- Teaching child and family about measures to prevent injuries and signs and symptoms of overuse injuries, dehydration, heat exhaustion, use of performance-enhancing drugs, eating disorders, and stress
- Arranging for coaches and personnel to obtain annual CPR and first aid training
- Encouraging parents to be involved in child's sports programs
- Advocating for the health of young athletes

Socialization

Six-year-old children play in groups, but when they are tired or under added stress, they prefer one-to-one contact. In a first-grade classroom, students compete actively for a few minutes of special time with the teacher. At the end of a day, they enjoy time spent individually with parents. You may have to remind parents that this is not babyish behavior but that of a typical 6-year-old.

Seven-year-olds are increasingly aware of family roles and responsibility. Promises must be kept, because 7-year-olds view them as definite, firm commitments. These children tattle because they have a strong sense of justice. This tattling may dissolve play groups quickly.

Eight-year-olds actively seek the company of other children. Most 8-year-old girls have a close girlfriend; boys have a close boyfriend. Girls begin to whisper among themselves, annoying parents and teachers.

Nine-year-olds take the values of their peer group very seriously. They are much more interested in how other children dress than in what their parents say is proper. This is typically the gang age because children form clubs, usually "spite clubs." This means if there are four girls on the block, three form a club and exclude the fourth. The reason for exclusion is often unclear; it might be that the fourth child has a chronic disease, that she has more or less money than the others, that she was at the dentist's the day the club was formed, or simply that the club cannot exist unless there is someone to exclude. Such clubs typically have a secret password and secret meeting place. Membership is generally all girls or all boys. If an excluded child does not react badly to being shut out, the club will probably disband after a few days because its purpose is lost. The next day, the excluded member may meet with two others and snub a different child. Parents have to be careful not to intervene with this type of play, because loyalties shift quickly. The child they defend today may be the excluded one tomorrow.

Nine-year-olds are ready for activities away from home, such as a week at camp. They can take care of their own needs and are mature enough to be separated from their parents for this length of time. Going to camp before this age usually results in homesickness and can be a negative introduction to being away from home.

Although 10-year-olds enjoy groups, they also enjoy privacy. They like having their own bedroom or at least their own dresser, where they can store a collection and know it is free from parents' or siblings' eyes. One of the best gifts for a 10-year-old is a box that locks.

Girls become increasingly interested in boys and vice versa by 11 years of age. Favorite activities are mixed-sex rather than single-sex ones. Children of this age are particularly insecure, however, and girls tend to dance with girls while boys talk together in corners. Better socialization patterns need not be rushed. Just as infants crawl before they walk, so 11-year-olds must attempt many awkward and uncomfortable social experiences before they become comfortable forming relationships with the opposite sex.

Twelve-year-olds feel more comfortable in social situations than they did the year before. Boys experience erections on small provocation and may feel uncomfortable being pushed into boy–girl situations until they know how to control their bodies better. As some children develop faster than others, every group has some that are almost adolescent and some that are still children, making social interests sometimes difficult.

✔ **CHECKPOINT QUESTIONS**

5. What are the characteristics of a 9-year-old gang?
6. Why are Boy Scouts and Girl Scouts still popular organizations?

Cognitive Development

The period from 5 to 7 years of age is a transitional stage when children undergo a shift from the preoperational thought they used as preschoolers to concrete operational thought, or the ability to reason through any problem that they can actually visualize (Piaget, 1969; Fig. 31-6).

Children can use concrete operational thought because they learn several new concepts, such as:

- **Decentering,** the ability to project the self into other people's situations and see the world from their viewpoint rather than focusing only on their own view
- **Accommodation,** the ability to adapt thought processes to fit what is perceived (i.e., understanding that there can be more than one reason for other people's actions). The preschooler might expect to see the same nurse in the morning that he or she had in the evening; the school-age child can understand that different nurses work different shifts.
- **Conservation,** the ability to appreciate that a change in shape does not necessarily mean a change in size. If you pour 30 mL of cough medicine from a thin glass to a wide one, the preschooler will say that one glass holds more than the other; the school-age child will say both glasses hold an equal amount.
- **Class inclusion,** the ability to understand that objects can belong to more than one classification. The preschooler can categorize items in only one way (e.g., stones and shells are found at the beach); the school-age child can categorize them in many

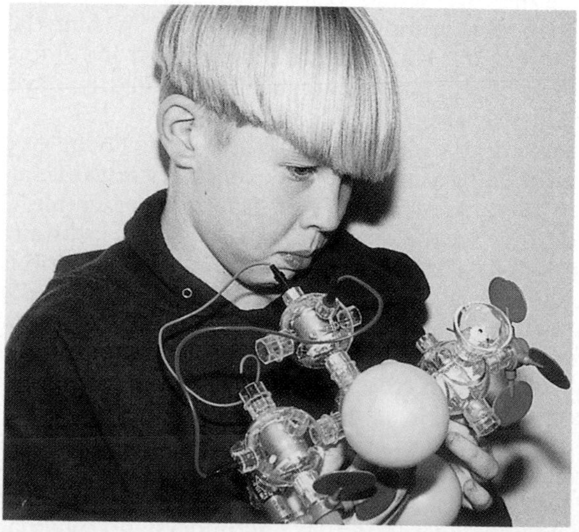

FIGURE 31.6 School-age children learn concrete operational thought or concentrate on phenomena they can actually see occurring.

ways (e.g., stones and shells can be differentiated by shapes, sizes, and textures).

These cognitive developments lead to some of the typical changes and characteristics of the school-age period. Decentering enables the school-age child to feel compassion for others, which was not possible in younger years. Because he or she understands conservation, the school-age child is not fooled by perceptions as often as before; thus, sibling arguments over food (your piece of pie is bigger than mine, his glass of cola is bigger than mine) decrease during the school-age years. The ability to classify objects leads to the collecting activities of the school-age period. Class inclusion is also necessary for learning mathematics and reading, systems that categorize numbers and words.

WHAT IF? You make a child's hospital bed one day and then give him an injection. What if the next day the child starts to cry while you're making the bed? The lack of what cognitive process led him to believe your action would be the same the second day?

Moral and Spiritual Development

School-age children begin to mature in terms of moral development as they enter a stage of **preconventional reasoning,** sometimes as early as 5 years of age (Kohlberg, 1984). During this stage, if asked, "Why is it wrong to steal from your neighbor?" school-age children will answer, "The police say it's wrong," or "Because if you do, you'll go to jail." They concentrate on "niceness" or "fairness" and cannot see yet that stealing hurts their neighbor, the highest level of moral reasoning.

School-age children begin to learn about the rituals and meaning behind their religious practice, so that the distinction between right and wrong becomes more important to them than it was when they were preschoolers. Parent role modeling is also important. Remember that school-age children are rule-oriented; when they pray, they may expect their God to follow rules also (if you are good and pray for something, you should receive it). This makes children of this age confused if a prayer is not immediately answered. Because they are still limited in their ability to understand others' views, they may interpret something as being right because it is good for them, not because it is right for humanity as a whole.

PLANNING AND IMPLEMENTATION FOR HEALTH PROMOTION OF THE SCHOOL-AGE CHILD AND FAMILY

Promoting School-Age Safety

School-age children are ready for time on their own without direct adult supervision. Many children as young as 8 or 9 stay by themselves after school (see the section on latchkey children later in this chapter). A child is generally ready for this type of experience if he or she can reliably follow instructions (don't use the fireplace; don't open the door) and can occupy himself or herself for an hour's time. As with adults, accidents tend to occur when children are under stress. Be certain that school-agers know to use seatbelts in cars and bicycle safety around cars (AAP Committee on Safety, 2001). The Focus on Family Empowerment lists common measures helpful in preventing accidents in this age group.

Sexual abuse is an unfortunate and all-too-common hazard for children. Teaching points to help children avoid sexual abuse are summarized in Box 31-2 (see also Chap. 55).

✔ CHECKPOINT QUESTIONS

7. What cognitive skill allows children to find collecting so interesting?
8. Why are school-age children so interested in "fairness"?

Promoting Nutritional Health of the School-Age Child

Most school-age children have good appetites, although any meal is influenced by the day's activity. If the child had a full day of activities, he or she may come to the dinner table ready to eat anything. If the day was full of frustration—the child received a poor mark in school, had an argument with a friend, or has a big game to think about—he or she may pick and poke at the food. This is no different from the way adults feel at times, and should be respected (Krebs & Hambridge, 2001).

Establishing Healthy Eating Patterns

School-age children need breakfast to provide enough energy to get them through active mornings at school. They eat best if parents get up in the morning with their children to prepare breakfast and eat some themselves. Children react badly to the instruction, "Do as I say, not as I do."

Many children qualify for a free or reduced-price school lunch and breakfast. A government-regulated school lunch (type A) provides milk (8 oz), protein (2 oz), one starch serving, vegetable (3/4 cup), and fruit (3/4 cup). Serving sizes vary according to age to provide one third of a child's recommended allowances for a day (Fig. 31-7). Check that children are actually eating school lunches, not trading items they do not want, so they receive the full benefit of the program.

If children take a packed lunch to school, urge parents to allow them some say in what type of meal it is to be, because packed lunches become tedious for everyone after a while. Whether they take lunch or buy it at school, school-age children should know some elementary facts of nutrition so they do not trade a sandwich for cake or choose only desserts from the cafeteria. Ideally, children should receive guidance from school personnel, but this often is impossible in a busy lunchroom. Health care personnel, therefore, should play an active role in nutrition education at health maintenance visits.

FOCUS ON FAMILY EMPOWERMENT

Common Safety Measures to Prevent Accidents During the School Years

Q. My schoolager is constantly on the go. How can I keep her free from accidents?

A. Putting preventive steps in place is the key.

Accident	*Preventive Measure*
Motor vehicle accidents	Encourage children to use seat belts in a car; role model their use.
	Teach street-crossing safety; stress that streets are no place for rough-housing, pushing, or shoving.
	Teach bicycle safety, including advice not to take "passengers" on a bicycle and to use a helmet.
	Teach parking lot and school bus safety (do not walk in back of parked cars, wait for crossing guard, etc.).
Community	Avoid areas specifically unsafe, such as train yards, grain silos, back alleys.
	Do not go with strangers (parents can establish a code word with child; child does not leave school with anyone who does not know the word).
	Children should say "no" to anyone who touches them whom they do not wish to do so, including family members (most sexual abuse is by a family member, not a stranger).
Burns	Teach safety with candles, matches, campfires—fire is not fun. Teach safety with beginning cooking skills (remember to include microwave oven safety, such as closing firmly before turning on oven; not using metal containers). Teach safety with sun exposure—use sun block.
	Do not climb electric poles.
Falls	Teach that rough-housing on fences, climbing on roofs, etc., is hazardous.
	Teach skateboard, scooter, and skating safety.
Sports injuries	Teach that wearing appropriate equipment for sports (face masks for hockey; mouthpiece and cup for football; helmet for bicycle riding, skateboarding, or in-line skating; batting helmets for baseball) is not babyish but smart.
	Stress not to play to a point of exhaustion or in a sport beyond physical capability (no pitching baseball or toe ballet for an early grade-school child).
	Use trampolines only with adult supervision to avoid serious neck injury.
	For late school-age, teach rules of safer sex (use of condoms; inspecting partner, etc.).
Drowning	Teach how to swim; dares and rough-housing when diving or swimming are not appropriate. Do not swim beyond limits of capabilities.
Drugs	Help your child avoid all recreational drugs and take prescription medicine only as directed. Avoid tobacco and alcohol.
Firearms	Teach safe firearm use. Keep firearms in locked cabinets with bullets separate from gun.
General	School-age children should keep adults informed as to where they are and what they are doing.
	Be aware that the frequency of accidents increases when parents are under stress and therefore less attentive. Special precautions must be taken at these times.
	Some children are more active, curious, and impulsive and therefore more vulnerable to accidents than others.

Most children are hungry after school and enjoy a snack when they arrive home. Because sugary foods may dull a child's appetite for dinner, urge parents to make the snack nutritious: fruit, cheese, or milk, rather than cookies and a soft drink.

Teach parents to make every attempt to make mealtime a happy and enjoyable part of the day for everyone. Some school-age children learn to eat as quickly as possible (and thus incompletely) to escape from the table before something unpleasant happens, such as an argument that they know is brewing.

WHAT IF? What if, as a preschooler, a child liked spinach, but as a 7-year-old he is told by his friends that no one likes spinach? Do you think the child will start to refuse spinach?

Fostering Industry

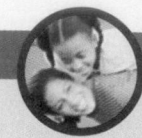

As a part of fostering industry, school-age children usually enjoy helping to plan meals. They can prepare foods such as instant pudding, Jello, salads, scrambled eggs, and sand-

BOX 31.2

TEACHING POINTS TO HELP CHILDREN AVOID SEXUAL ABUSE

1. Your body is your property and you can decide who looks at it or touches it.
2. Secrets are fun things to keep. If a person asks you not to tell about something that was done to you that you didn't like, it's not a secret. It's all right to tell about it.
3. Don't go anywhere with a stranger (a stranger is someone you do not know, not someone "strange"). Don't be fooled by people asking you to give them directions or to go with them because your mother is sick or hurt.
4. Being touched by someone you like is a good feeling. You don't have to allow anyone to touch you in a way you don't like. Don't allow yourself to be left alone with a person you are uncomfortable with because he or she touches you in a way you don't like.
5. A "private part" is the part of you a bathing suit touches. If anyone asks you to show them a private part or touches a private part, tell them to stop, and tell someone else.
6. If the person you tell doesn't believe you, keep telling people until someone believes you.

wiches. They may eat meals that they have planned or prepared more willingly than ones that are just set in front of them.

Most parents would like children to develop better table manners. Because they are in a hurry to finish eating, school-age children tend to gulp their food. Many meals are interrupted by spilled milk. As children become teenagers and are more aware of the impression they make on others, manners often improve dramatically. It is some comfort for parents to know that children usually display better table manners in other people's homes than in their own.

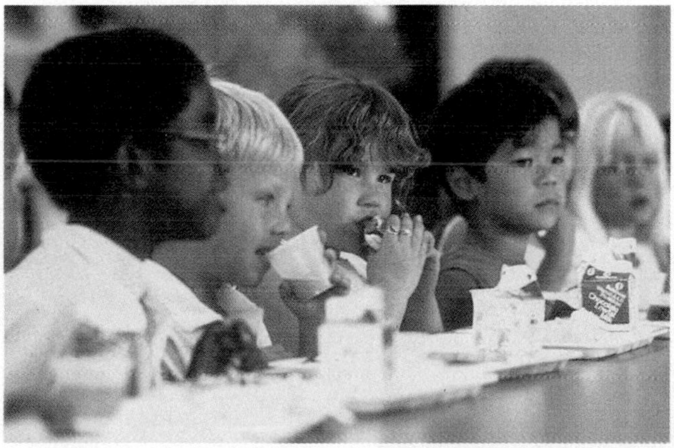

FIGURE 31.7 School lunch programs provide nutritious meals to help school-age children meet recommended daily allowances.

Recommended Daily Dietary Allowances

Nutrition is a major area of focus for health promotion of the school-age child. Although parents may have less to say about what the school-age child eats, it is important that the increasing energy requirements that come with this age (often in spurts) are met daily with foods of high nutritional value.

During the late school years, the recommended daily dietary allowances begin to be separated into categories for girls and boys because boys require more calories and other nutrients at this time. Because school-age children typically dislike vegetables, their intake may be deficient in fiber. Both girls and boys require more iron in prepuberty than they did between the ages of 7 and 10. Adequate calcium and fluoride intake remains important to ensure good teeth.

Promoting Nutritional Health With a Vegetarian Diet

School-age children who are raised in vegetarian homes need to learn aspects of vegetarian nutrition if they are going to eat in a school cafeteria. Unfortunately, many school lunch programs offer mainly milk and meat or cheese foods, such as sloppy joe sandwiches, macaroni and cheese, or pizza. This forces children who are vegetarians to carry packed lunches with foods such as cucumber, tomato, or peanut butter sandwiches on whole-grain bread; hot soups; salads; vegetable sticks; and fruit. When eating at a friend's house, they need to notify the host that they eat a special diet or to choose correctly from foods they are served.

A potential problem to assess with vegetarian school-age children is whether they are obtaining enough protein and calcium so they are prepared for the rapid growth spurt of puberty. Foods high in calcium are green, leafy vegetables (e.g., spinach and turnip greens), prunes, nuts, enriched bread, and cereals. Soybeans, legumes, nuts, grains, and immature seeds (e.g., green beans, lima beans, and corn) are relatively high in protein. As with any individual on a vegetarian diet, children may need a vitamin B_{12} supplement. Encourage outside activities for sun exposure to increase vitamin D. Iron may need to be supplemented, especially if girls have heavy menstrual flows (Dudek, 2001).

Promoting Development of the School-Age Child in Daily Activities

With life centered on school activities and friends, the school-age child still needs parental guidance for most daily activities, because the habits and lifestyle patterns gained during this period will form the basis for healthy (or unhealthy) patterns of living later in life. Figure 31-8 shows a day in the life of a family with school-age children. Along with nutritional needs, areas of concern for the school-age child and family include dressing, sleep needs, exercise, hygiene, and dental care.

FIGURE 31-8.

A day in the life of a family with young children.

7:00 AM: The family sits down to a healthy breakfast. Claudia helps Laura with the butter.

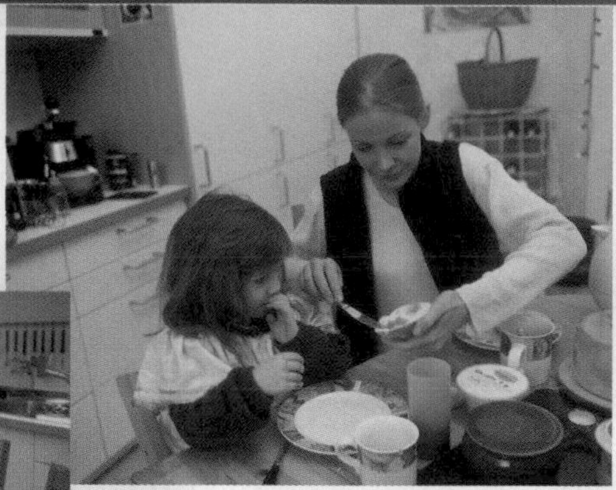

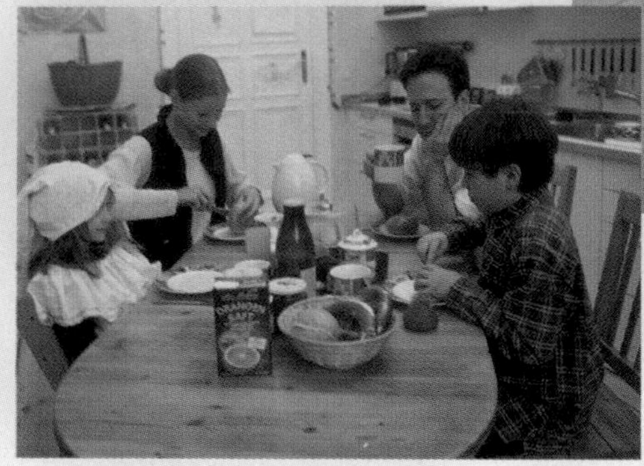

7:30 AM: John walks Marc to school, emphasizing safety when crossing the street.

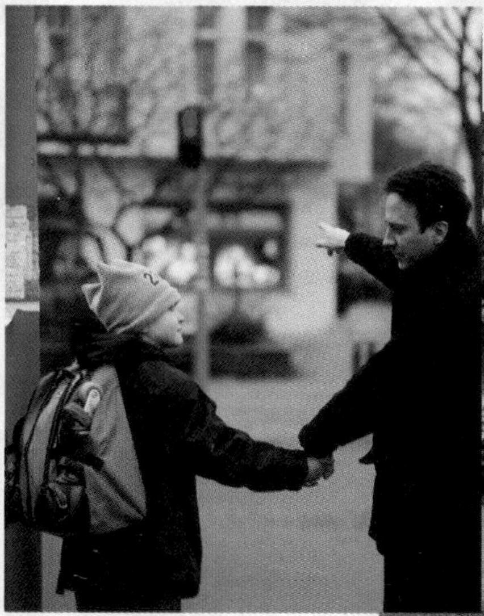

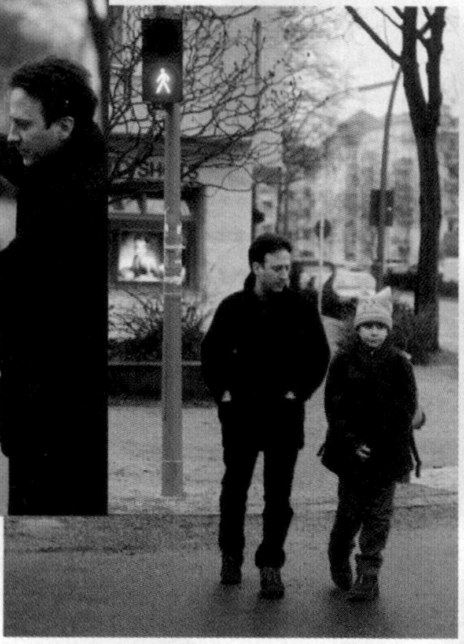

10:00 AM: Claudia and Laura bake a cake for the night's dessert. Four-year-old Laura enjoys practicing adult roles.

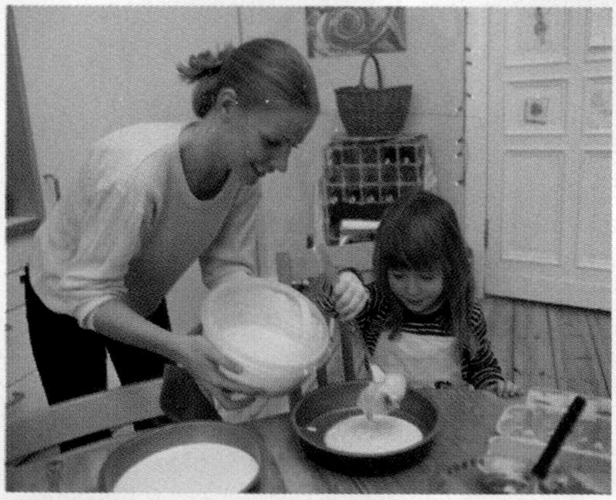

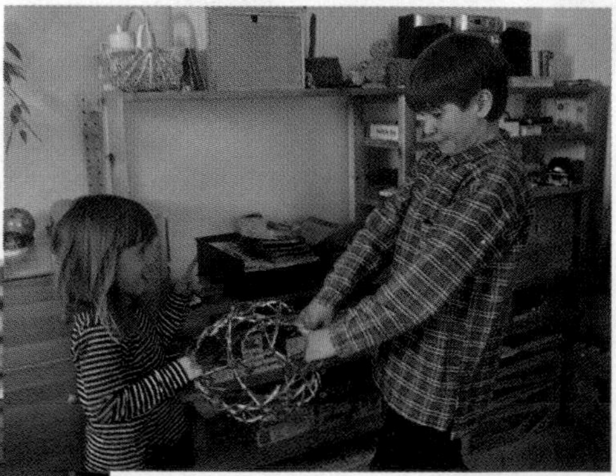

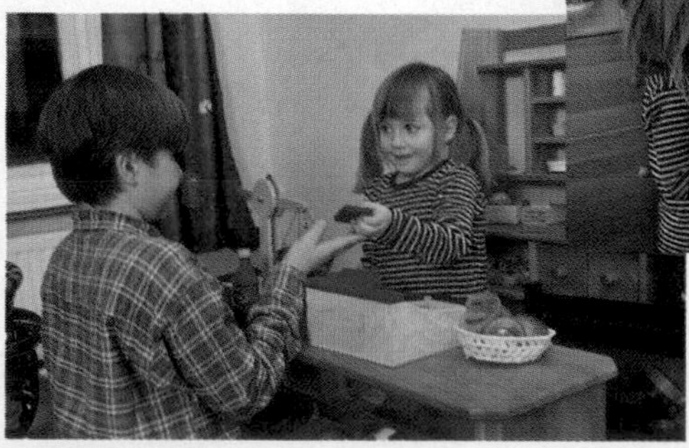

3:00 PM: Marc and Laura play together after Marc gets home from school. Their cooperative play is punctuated by an occasional fight.

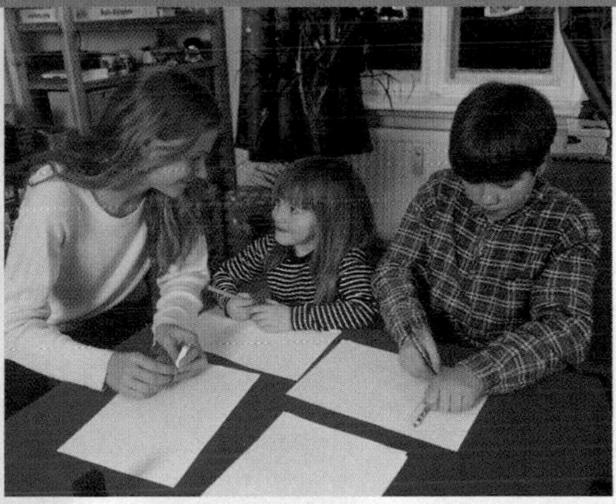

4:00 PM: Claudia helps Marc with his homework. Laura likes to draw alongside her big brother.

5:00 PM: The family greets John as he comes home from work.

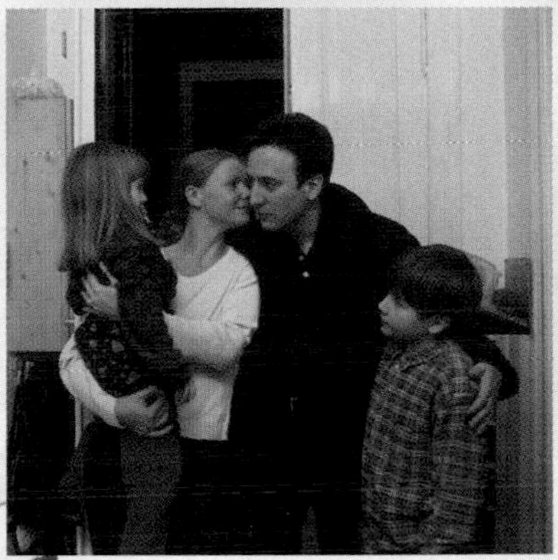

5:30 PM: John and Mark go rollerblading before dinner. John makes sure Marc's protective gear is in place.

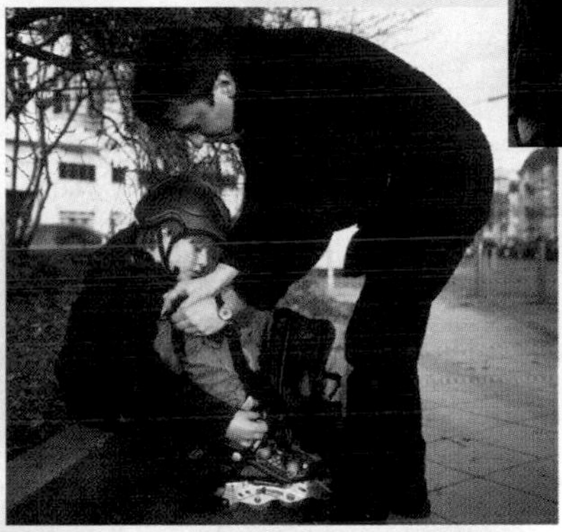

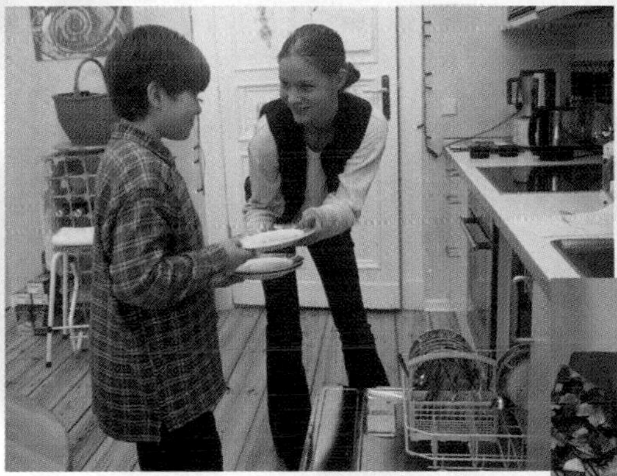

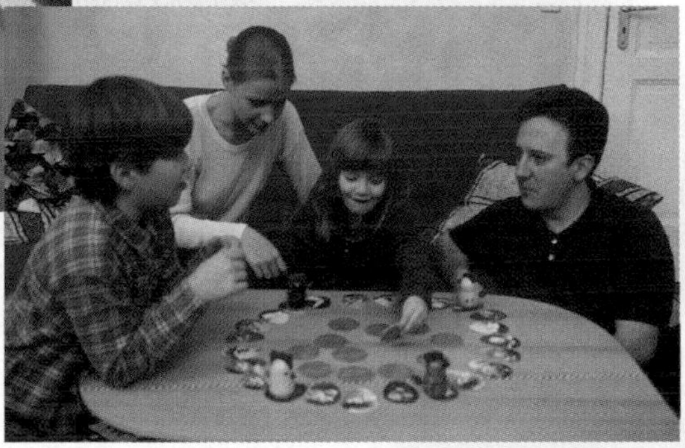

7:00 PM: After dinner, Marc helps with the dishes; then the family spends time together playing a game.

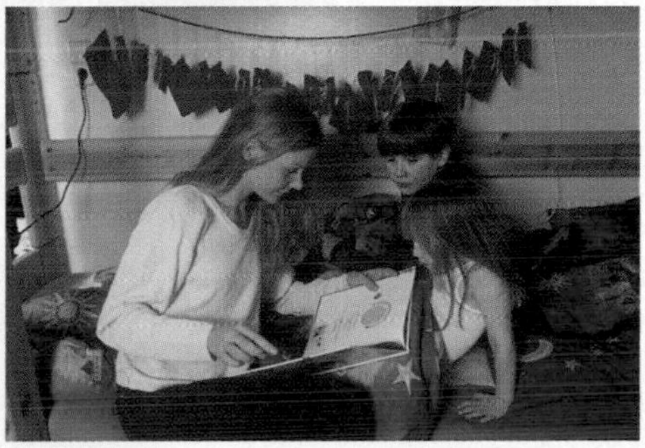

8:30 PM: Time to get ready for bed! Claudia helps the kids clean up and brush their teeth. And there's always time to read them a story.

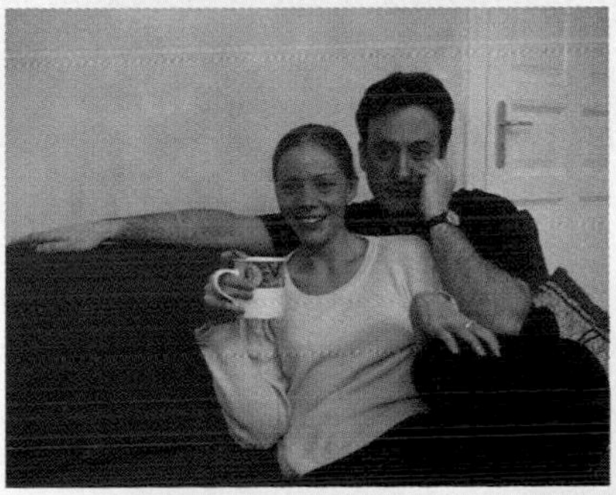

9:00 PM: John and Claudia relax together at the end of the day.

Dress

Although school-age children can fully dress themselves, they are not as good at taking care of their clothes until later in the school-age years. This is the right age, however (if not started already), to teach children the importance of caring for their own belongings. School-age children have definite opinions about clothing styles, often based on the likes of their friends rather than the preferences of their parents. Insisting that a child dress differently from classmates is unfair and even cruel. A child who wears different clothing may become the object of exclusion from a school club or group. In schools with a gang culture, children may not be able to wear a certain color or style or will be mistaken for a gang member. Many schools require uniforms to avoid this problem.

Sleep

Sleep needs vary among individual children. Younger school-agers generally require 10 to 12 hours of sleep each night, and older ones require about 8 to 10 hours. Most 6-year-olds are too old for naps but do require a quiet time after school to get them through the remainder of the day. Nighttime terrors may continue during the early school years and may actually increase during the first-grade year as the child reacts to the stress of beginning school.

During the early school years, many children enjoy a quiet talk or a reading time at bedtime. At about age 9, when friends become more important, children generally are ready to give up pre-bedtime talks with parents. Some parents react strongly to this change and feel rejected. They may need some help to take at face value their child's statement, "I'm tired. I'd rather go to sleep."

Exercise

School-age children need daily exercise. Although they go to school all day, they do not automatically receive much exercise because school is basically a sit-down activity. Children who are bussed to and from school may therefore return home without having spent much time in active exercise.

Exercise need not involve organized sports. It can come from neighborhood games, walking with parents, or bicycle riding. As children enter preadolescence, those with poor coordination may become reluctant to exercise. Urge them to participate in some daily exercise, or else obesity, or osteoporosis later in life, can result (Leonard & Zemel, 2002).

Hygiene

Children of 6 or 7 years of age still need help in regulating the bath water temperature and in cleaning their ears and fingernails. By age 8, children are generally capable of bathing themselves but may not do it well because they are too busy to take the time or because they do not find bathing as important as their parents do.

Both boys and girls become interested in showering as they approach their teens. This can be encouraged as perspiration increases with puberty, along with sebaceous gland activity. When girls begin to menstruate, they may be afraid to take baths or wash their hair during their period if they have heard that this is not safe. They need information on the importance and safety of good hygiene during their menses. Boys who are uncircumcised may develop inflammation under the foreskin from increased secretions if they do not wash regularly.

Care of Teeth

With proper dental care, the average child today can expect to grow up cavity-free. To ensure that this happens, school-age children should visit a dentist at least twice yearly for a checkup, cleaning, and possibly a fluoride treatment to strengthen and harden the tooth enamel (Fig. 31-9). Some children develop a fear of dentists and, if the dentist hurts them, want to avoid going at all. The advantage of frequent visits is that if cavities are filled when they are small, the drilling required is minimal and little pain is involved. If cavities are not treated promptly in this way but are allowed to grow large, the drilling hurts, causing these children to refuse to go back to the dentist. More large cavities then grow, and a vicious circle develops. Pedodontists specialize in caring for children's teeth and understand the developmental level of their patients. Children who tend to develop caries might be encouraged to visit a pedodontist if one is available and affordable.

School-age children have to be reminded to brush their teeth daily. If brushing becomes an area of conflict for the family, brushing well once a day may be more effective than brushing more often but doing an inadequate job. For effective brushing, the child should use a soft toothbrush, fluoride-based toothpaste, and dental floss to clean between teeth to help remove plaque.

Snacks are best limited to high-protein foods such as chicken and cheese rather than candy. Fruits, vegetables, and cereals fortified with minerals and vitamins can all be fun after-school snacks for school-agers. If the child does eat candy, a type that is eaten quickly and dissolves quickly, such as a plain chocolate bar, is better than slowly dissolving or sticky candy, which stays in contact with the teeth longer.

Promoting Healthy Family Functioning

At 6 years of age, most children have passed through a preschool phase of attraction for the parent of the opposite sex and identify again with the parent of the same sex (Freud, 1962). Children from one-parent homes, or those with a parent who has difficulty being a good role model, may need help in finding a suitable adult to serve as this important person in their life.

To their parents' annoyance, many 6-year-olds often quote their teacher as the final authority on all subjects. This may be the first time the parents see someone surpassing them in their child's eyes, and accepting the situation can be painful. Children also cite their friends as guides for behavior: "Mary Jane doesn't have to go to bed until 10 o'clock," or "Carlos' mother lets him go to the movies every Saturday." Parents may require help to realize that these remarks are a normal consequence of being exposed to other adults and children. A simple statement such as, "There are all kinds of ways to do things, but in

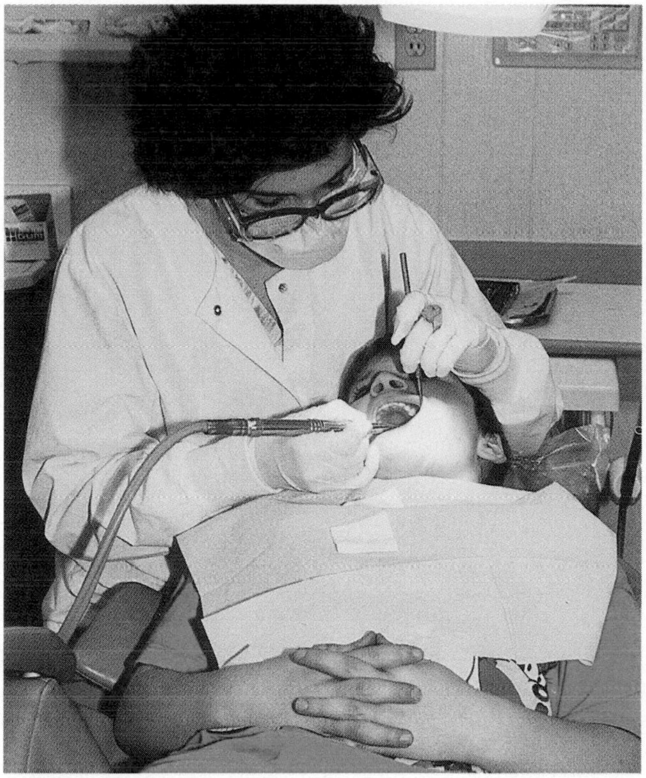

FIGURE 31.9 Dental caries are the number-one health problem in school-age children. Children need to be taught dental health measures and encouraged to visit a dentist twice a year.

our house, the rule is this" shows no criticism of Carlos' or Mary Jane's family, yet conveys a special "our house" feeling and offers security to the child.

Parents often must be reminded that even the simplest tasks of everyday life require repeated practice before they can be accomplished well. The way parents correct children as they learn these tasks can influence the children's opinions of themselves and their ability to continue learning. "Putting all the silverware in a pile is one way of putting it away; another way would be to divide spoons, forks, and knives separately" is always preferable to "What a silly way to put away silverware!" Comments such as, "Can't you do anything right?" or "Why don't you ever do what I say?" should be avoided because children will rise only to the level expected of them. Children who are constantly told that they are stupid, thoughtless, bad, or ill behaved may begin to act that way to conform to the parents' expectations.

If parents have difficulty telling what a child's completed project is supposed to be, the time-honored "Tell me about it" is preferable to "What is it?" It is good for parents to find a redeeming characteristic in a project, no matter how shakily put together it is: "I like the bright color you painted it" or "That must have been fun to make." Displaying and using children's gifts are part of having school-age children in a family. A finger painting hung on the refrigerator door will enhance, not detract from, the most elegant home. The best-dressed woman looks even more radiant wearing her child's necklace made of macaroni on a string. Both examples are gestures of love, which goes well with everything.

In talking to parents of school-age children, good questions to ask to estimate the degree of interaction that occurs in the home and whether the parents are strengthening the child's sense of accomplishment are:

- How do you correct John when he does something wrong?
- Do you display his school projects?
- Does he have chores that are his to accomplish?

✔ CHECKPOINT QUESTIONS

9. A type A school lunch supplies what portion of a child's RDA?
10. If children attend school every day, do they need additional exercise?

Common Health Problems of the School-Age Period

Children in their early school years have one of the lowest rates of death and serious illness of any age group. The two leading causes of death are accidents and cancer. Minor illnesses are largely due to dental caries, gastrointestinal disturbances, and upper respiratory infections.

Table 31-3 shows the usual health maintenance pattern for the school-age child (AAP Committee on Practice, 2001). Table 31-4 lists problems that parents may have in evaluating illness in school-age children. Many communities are establishing school-based community health care clinics to improve the health care available for school-age children.

Dental Caries

Caries (cavities) are progressive, destructive lesions or decalcification of the tooth enamel and dentine. When the pH of the tooth surface drops to 5.6 or below (which happens after children eat readily fermented carbohydrates, such as table sugar), acid microorganisms (acidogenic lactobacilli and aciduric streptococci) found in dental plaque attack the organic cementing medium of teeth and destroy it. Plaque tends to accumulate in deep grooves of the teeth and contact areas between teeth, making these areas most susceptible to dental decay. The enamel on primary teeth is thinner than on permanent teeth, making them more susceptible to destruction. The distance from the enamel to the pulp is shorter also, so destruction of the tooth nerve can occur quickly. Neglected caries result in poor chewing and therefore poor digestion, abscess and pain, and sometimes osteomyelitis (bone infection).

As stated earlier, dental caries are largely preventable with proper brushing and use of fluoridated water or fluoride application. When caries do occur, it is important that they be treated quickly, and the child's dental hygiene practices should be evaluated and improved if necessary. Most important, children must believe that they have a stake in the health or disease of their teeth so they willingly undertake the self-care measures necessary to ensure healthy teeth, with parental support rather than parental command.

TABLE 31.3 Health Maintenance Schedule, School Age Period

AREA OF FOCUS	METHODS	FREQUENCY
Assessment		
Developmental milestones	History, observation	Every visit
Growth milestones	Height, weight plotted on standard growth chart; physical examination	Every visit
Hypertension	Blood pressure	Every visit
Nutrition	History, observation; height/weight information	Every visit
Parent–child relationship	History, observation	Every visit
Behavior or school problems	History, observation	Every visit
Vision and hearing disorders	History, observation	Every visit
	Formal Snellen or Titmus testing	At 7–8 yr and 10–12 yr
	Audiometer testing	At 6 yr and 10–12 yr
Dental health	History, physical examination	Every visit
Scoliosis	Physical examination	Yearly after age 8 yr
Thyroid	Physical examination, history	Every visit after age 10 yr
Tuberculosis	PPD	Depending on prevalence of tuberculosis in community
Bacteriuria	Clean-catch urine	At 6–7 yr
Anemia	Hematocrit/hemoglobin	At 11–12 yr
Immunizations		
Rubeola, mumps, and rubella	Check history and past records; inform caregiver about any risks and side-effects; administer immunization in accordance with health care agency policies.	At 4–6 yr (MMR2)
Hepatitis B		If not administered in infancy or three injections were not completed
Td		At 11–12 yr if at least 5 yr have elapsed since last DTP, DTaP, DT
Varicella		At any age after 1 yr if not previously immunized or at 11–12 yr if lacking reliable history of chickenpox
Anticipatory Guidance		
School-age care	Active listening and health teaching	Every visit
Expected growth and developmental milestones before next visit	Active listening and health teaching	Every visit
Accident prevention	Counseling about street and personal safety	Every visit
Problem Solving		
Any problems expressed by caregiver during course of the visit	Active listening and health teaching regarding cigarette smoking, drug abuse, sex education, school adjustment	Every visit

Malocclusion

The upper jaw in children matures rapidly in early childhood along with skull growth; the lower jaw forms more slowly, which forces teeth to make a prolonged series of changes until they reach their final adult alignment and position. Good tooth occlusion, in which the upper teeth overlap the lower teeth by a small amount and teeth are evenly spaced and in good alignment, is necessary for optimal formation of teeth, health of the supporting tissue, optimal speech development, and what most people view as a pleasant physical appearance for high self-esteem. **Malocclusion** (a deviation from the normal) may be congenital and related to conditions such as cleft palate, a small lower jaw, or familial traits tending toward malocclusion. The condition can result from constant mouth breathing or abnormal tongue position (tongue thrusting). Thumb sucking appears to have little role in malocclusion as long as the thumb sucking does not persist past the time of eruption of the permanent front teeth (6 to 7 years). The loss of teeth due to extraction or accident may lead to malocclusion if not properly treated to maintain alignment.

Malocclusion may be either crossbite (sideways) or anterior or posterior. Children with a malocclusion should be evaluated by an orthodontist to see if orthodontic braces or other therapy is necessary. The time to begin correction varies with the extent of the malocclusion and the jaw size. Braces are expensive and painful when they are first applied

TABLE 31.4 Parental Difficulties Evaluating Illness in the School-Age Child

DIFFICULTY	HELPFUL SUGGESTIONS FOR PARENTS
Evaluating seriousness of illness	For the first time, a school-age child may view illness as a way to avoid unpleasant activities (school, a coach who asks too much, household chores). Evaluating whether the child has symptoms when he is asked to do something he likes to do often reveals the difference between exaggeration and an ill child (too sick to eat spinach, not too sick to eat ice cream; too sick to go to school, not too sick to go ice skating). If the child uses symptoms of illness as a means of avoiding situations, parents must evaluate what it is that the child wants so badly to avoid and see if some change should be made in expectations.
Evaluating nutritional intake	Many school-age children eat lunch at school; they may spend weekends away from home and weeks away at camp. As with all ages, noting whether they are growing and active is better than monitoring any one day's food intake.
Evaluating puberty changes	There is a wide variation in the time that secondary sex characteristics occur (9–17 yr for girls; 10–18 yr for boys). Children should be examined if and when they or their parents are concerned that pubertal changes are delayed.
Age-specific diseases to be aware of	School age is a time to evaluate vision; children normally develop vision changes as maturity of the eye globe increases. Squinting, rubbing eyes, or poor marks in school may be signs of poor vision.
	Streptococcal sore throats occur with a high frequency in early-school-age children. Those with sore throats should be examined by a health care provider to prevent complications, such as glomerulonephritis or rheumatic fever, from developing. Girls, in particular, must be evaluated for scoliosis (curvature of the spine). Parents detect this by noticing that the girl's skirts hang unevenly or bra straps are uneven.
	Parents may need to be cautioned that vomiting or headache in the morning that passes fairly quickly (at about the same time the school bus leaves) may be a symptom of school phobia, but physical examination is in order because these are also symptoms of other conditions.
	Absence seizures, a neurologic condition that typically arises in school-age years, can be confused with behavior problems if observation is not thorough (see Chap. 49).
	Attention deficit hyperactivity disorder (ADHD) (see Chap. 54) can also lead to behavior or inattention disorders.

and at periodic visits when they are tightened to maintain pressure for further straightening. Some children develop mild, shallow ulcerations (canker sores) of the buccal membrane from friction of metal wires. Rubbing the offending wire with dental wax dulls the surface and gives relief. Oral acetaminophen or Ora-Jel (an over-the-counter drug) rubbed on the ulceration also gives relief. Children who wear braces need to have their teeth assessed frequently to see that they are brushing properly around the braces (a Water Pik is often recommended for thorough cleaning) and that they are using dental floss to remove plaque from around wires.

After the removal of braces, many children must wear retainers to maintain the correction the braces achieved. Although braces are wired into place, retainers are not. Wearing a retainer can prove troublesome for a child if it must be removed when eating (e.g., in the school cafeteria or in a restaurant). Show appropriate sympathy and help children problem-solve if they are bothered by the appearance of braces or wearing a retainer. For instance, if removing the retainer in front of friends is embarrassing for a child, perhaps it could be removed in the bathroom before going to the cafeteria each day. Braces and retainers have become a common feature of life for children of school age. Most children will find some comfort in not being the only one to suffer this indignity and, once used to their own appliances, experience little reluctance in letting their classmates see them.

Concerns and Problems of the School-Age Period

One of the most important disorders of the school age period is attention deficit hyperactivity disorder (ADHD) because it interferes so dramatically with school progress (see Chap. 54). Other problems concern language, fears, and responsibility.

NURSING DIAGNOSES AND RELATED INTERVENTIONS

Nursing Diagnosis: Parental anxiety related to behavior of school-age child

Outcome Identification: Parent will voice that he feels less anxious by next health supervision visit.

Outcome Evaluation: Parent states that undesired behavior has decreased in frequency; parent feels less stress about child's health or future.

Problems Associated With Language Development

The common speech problem of the preschool years is broken fluency; the most common problem of the school-age child is articulation. The child has difficulty pronouncing *s, z, th, l, r,* and *w* or substitutes *w* for *r* ("west" instead of "rest") or *r* for *l* ("radies" instead of "ladies"). This is most noticeable during the first and second grades; it usually disappears by the third grade. Unless it persists, speech therapy for this normal developmental stage is not necessary.

Common Fears and Anxieties of the School-Age Child

Anxiety Related to Beginning School. Adjusting to grade school is a big task for 6-year-olds. Even if they attended preschool, grade school is different: the rules are firmer, and the elective feeling ("If I don't like it, I can quit") is gone. School is for keeps until age 16 or longer, a time span that is difficult for the child to imagine. Whereas preschool learning was carried out through fun activities, part of every day in grade school involves obvious work (see Focus on Nursing Care Planning).

Because school is an adjustment, a health assessment of all school-age children should include an inquiry about progress in school. You can obtain information by asking the parent, "How is Susan doing in school?" followed by a second question, "How does her teacher say she is doing?" If there is a discrepancy between the answers, the situation bears study. The answer to the first question reveals the parent's attitude toward the child's progress. The answer to the second may indicate that the child is having trouble adjusting to a structured school environment. Some parents have to alter their expectations to conform to their child's actual ability. This can be difficult.

One of the biggest tasks of the first year of school is learning to read. It is best if parents have prepared children for this by reading to them since infancy, pointing to the words and pictures as they go along. This helps children to realize that sentences flow from left to right and that the words, not the pictures, tell the story. The Focus on Family Empowerment offers some useful hints to help parents encourage reading in their young school-age child.

Many first-graders are capable of mature action at school but appear less mature when they return home. Their pseudo-sophistication of the day is gone. They may bite their nails, suck their thumb, or talk baby talk. Some develop tics (irregular movements of isolated muscle groups), such as wrinkling the forehead, shrugging the shoulders, twisting the mouth, coughing, clearing the throat, or frequently blinking or rolling the eyes. Such movements may occasionally be confused with seizure activity. Tics, however, disappear during sleep and occur mainly when the child is subjected to stress or anxiety. Scolding, nagging, threatening, or punishing does not stop either tics or nail biting; it invariably makes these problems worse. Methods such as using bad-flavored nail polish and restraining the child's hands to prevent nail biting are also ineffective.

These behaviors stop when the underlying stress is discovered and alleviated. Urge parents to spend some time with the child after school or in the evening so the child continues to feel secure in the family and does not feel pushed out by being sent to school. If such behavior manifestations persist despite attempts to eliminate their cause, the family might benefit from formal counseling.

School Phobia. School phobia is fear of attending school. It is a type of "social phobia" similar to agoraphobia (fear of going outside the home). Children who resist attending school this way may develop physical signs of illness, such as vomiting, diarrhea, headache, or abdominal pain on school days. This lasts until after the school bus has left or the child is allowed to stay home for the day. The cause of this resistance to school must be determined before it can be cured. A second type of school phobia

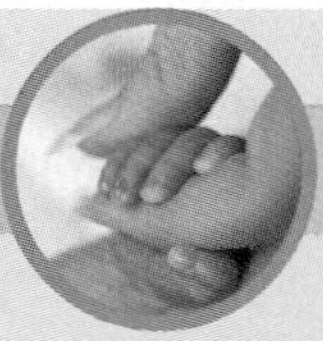

FOCUS ON *Nursing Care Planning*

A SCHOOL-AGED CHILD STARTING KINDERGARTEN

A 6-year-old girl is brought to the clinic for a checkup in preparation for starting school in the fall.

Assessment: 6-year-old girl within normal limits for height, weight, and development. Currently attending afternoon nursery school 5 days a week. Her mother states, "She's been attending this school for the last 2 years. In the fall, she'll be going to a new school for a full day." Child observed to be restless in chair during conversation with mother about the new school. When asked, child says, "I don't want to go to a new school. I want to stay in my old school with all my friends."

Nursing Diagnosis: Anxiety related to beginning a new school in the fall

Outcome Identification: The child will exhibit signs of increased comfort about new school experience.

Outcome Evaluation: Child verbalizes positive statements about new school; voices desire to visit school and meet teachers; exhibits age-appropriate coping behaviors.

(continued)

Interventions	Rationale
1. Assess the child for her thoughts and feelings about current nursery school routine, including teachers, friends, and activities.	1. Assessment provides information about the child's school experience and possible clues for the child's anxiety, providing a baseline for future strategies and teaching.
2. Explore with the child's mother her views on the child's experiences in her current school and expectations for the new school.	2. Exploration with the mother provides additional clues to understanding the child's anxieties and serves as a means for identifying possible stressors that may be affecting the child.
3. Talk with the child about what she thinks the new school will be like, acknowledging her anxieties and providing feedback to clarify any misconceptions.	3. Talking with the child allows her to share feelings and concerns openly and safely, possibly increasing the child's awareness of them and their impact on her. Acknowledging the child's anxiety validates her feelings. Providing feedback helps to correct any misinformation.
4. Encourage the mother to contact the school district to arrange for a visit to the school with her daughter.	4. Visiting the school provides the child with exposure to the new environment, preparing her for the actual experience.
5. Have the mother arrange for a follow-up visit to the school with her daughter to meet the teachers and spend time observing and being part of the classroom experience.	5. Spending time with the teachers and class allows the child to actively participate in the experience, helping to alleviate feelings of the unknown and to increase feelings of control.
6. Urge the mother to contact the parents of another child who is currently attending the school to act as the daughter's "buddy."	6. Having a buddy helps to minimize the feelings of isolation and loneliness.
7. Arrange for a follow-up clinic appointment within 1 month with the mother and daughter.	7. A return visit aids in evaluating the child's level of anxiety and in determining the effectiveness of the suggestions.

occurs as a result of fear of separation from parents. The child may be overly dependent on the parents or may be reluctant to leave home because of worry that younger siblings will usurp the parents' affection. The anxiety of separation may also result because the parent is overprotective of the child or is the one having the most difficulty separating.

A particular child may be reacting to a situation such as a harsh teacher, having to shower in gym class, or facing a class bully every day. In these instances, the child's fear

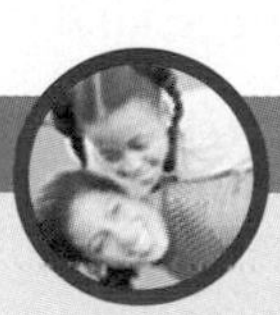

FOCUS ON FAMILY EMPOWERMENT
Tips to Help Make Reading More Enjoyable for Your Child

Q. I want my child to enjoy reading. How can I encourage this?

A. Integrating reading into a total lifestyle is the best approach.

- Read yourself to set an example, so your child associates learning to read with adult activity. If you spend most of your free time watching television, your child will think reading is mainly for children and assume that it is not important.
- Make reading more fun by encouraging the practical use of reading. Ask your child to read recipes while you cook or to read road signs during a car trip.
- Play a treasure hunt game in which you hide a small object, such as a favorite toy, then write simple clues on slips of paper—"Look under a lamp," then, under the lamp, "Look in a book," and so on until your child has been led to the hidden object. Such games help your child see reading as an important means of obtaining information. Your child can develop writing skills by playing the same game for you to follow.
- Suggest to relatives that a gift certificate from a book store would be a good present. Let your child browse the store to select the book.
- Talk about books the child has read—what was good or what was bad or what he or she learned.
- Read a book together as a pre-bedtime family activity.

may be well grounded. Counseling may help the child manage the situation better. If not, parents can attempt to have the child transferred to another classroom or perhaps excused from a disliked situation such as showering to stop the school resistance. Because the problem of school phobia is usually only partly the child's, the entire family generally requires counseling to resolve the issue. As a rule, once it has been established that the child is free of any illness and the resistance stems from separation anxiety, the child should continue to attend school. Reinforcement by parents should prevent the development of problems such as school failure, peer ridicule, or a pattern of avoiding difficulties. The child may benefit from a gradual program of school involvement, such as walking to school but not going in for one day, then going to school but staying for only 1 hour the next day, then staying for half a day, and so on, until the child can stay all day every day. Give support to parents so they can treat the child's illness symptoms matter-of-factly (a great deal of reassurance that these symptoms are not major will be necessary) so they can take the child firmly to the bus or to the classroom.

Managing school phobia requires coordination among the school, school nurse, and health care provider who diagnoses the problem. A nurse is the ideal person to coordinate such efforts and to help the parents allow the child some independence not only in going to school but in other activities. A few children have such difficulty they require psychiatric therapy to resolve their difficulties with school.

Latchkey Children

Latchkey children are schoolchildren who are without adult supervision for part of each weekday. The term alludes to the fact that they generally carry a key so they can let themselves into their home after school.

Latchkey children have become a prominent concern because in as many as 90% of families today in the United States, both parents work at least part-time outside the home. Few parents have work hours so flexible that they can always be at home when the child leaves for or returns from school. Extended family members who once watched children after school are often working as well or may no longer be close at hand; many communities are no longer close-knit enough to have neighbors who can be depended on to help out with informal childcare.

A major concern is that latchkey children can feel lonely or have an increased tendency to have accidents, delinquent behavior, alcohol and beginning drug abuse, and decreased school performance from lack of adult supervision. For children who feel safe in their community, however, a short period of independence every day may actually be beneficial, because it encourages problem solving in self-care.

Suggestions for parents whose children must spend time alone before or after school are shown in Box 31-3. Many communities offer special after-school programs for such children. Nurses are in a position to educate parents about such services so their children can feel both safe and stimulated creatively during this time. Boy Scouts of America and the Council of Campfire Girls are examples of organizations that offer programs to help children adjust to being home alone. Many communities are organizing hotline numbers that a child who is alone can call if a problem arises. At health visits, assess whether parents and the child appear to have a problem with or are uncomfortable about after-school arrangements. For the child who is extremely fearful or impulsive or who finds problem solving difficult, time alone after school may not be appropriate. Determine the individual circumstances, and recommend changes when possible.

✔ CHECKPOINT QUESTIONS

11. If children eat candy, what is the best type for them to eat in terms of preventing caries?
12. Should children with school (social) phobia be encouraged to attend school?

Sex Education

It is important that school-age children be educated about pubertal changes and responsible sexual practices so they are well prepared for these. Also, preteens should have adults they can turn to for answers to questions about sex. Ideally, these should be their parents, but because sex is an emotionally charged topic, some parents may be extremely uncomfortable discussing it with their children. As a result, health care personnel often become resource persons.

The American Academy of Pediatrics recommends that sex education be incorporated into health education throughout the school years in a manner that is appropriate to age and development (AAP Committee on Practice, 2001). Topics to teach and discuss in a sex education course for both preadolescent boys and girls include:

- Reproductive organ function
- Secondary sexual characteristics, so children will know what is going on in their bodies
- Physiology of reproduction, so they understand what menstruation is and why it occurs
- Male sexual functioning, including why the production of increased amounts of seminal fluid leads to nocturnal emissions
- Explanation of the physiology of pregnancy and the possibility that comes with sexual maturity for unplanned or unwanted pregnancies
- Birth control measures and the principles of safer sex (see Chap. 5)
- Social and moral implications of sexual maturity

A sex education course that includes films and discussions is helpful but never answers all of a preteen's questions. (Most youngsters would rather avoid asking a question than risk appearing ignorant in front of their peers.) Handing children booklets or showing films with the words, "If you have any questions after you've read (or watched) this, come and ask me" is equally ineffective because it implies that they should have no questions. Parents or health educators need to watch films or read booklets with children to show that they are truly available to answer questions.

BOX 31.3

TIPS FOR LATCHKEY CHILDREN AND PARENTS

Safety Teaching for Children

Always lock doors and never show keys to others or indicate that they stay home alone.

When answering the telephone, say a parent is busy, not absent from home.

Have a plan in event they lose their key (stay with a neighbor, etc.).

Don't go into the house if the door is open or a window is broken.

Learn fire safety (practice a fire drill from all rooms of the house).

Check in with parents by telephone when they first arrive home from school.

Identify a caller before opening the door. Agree on a secret code word; child should not open the door or go with a person unless the person knows the word.

Learn how to change light bulbs safely if it will be dark before parents return home. If appropriate, teach child how to change fuses or reset circuit-breaker switches.

Learn how to report a fire and telephone police (practice this with the child).

Safety Responsibilities for Parents

Prepare a safety kit and keep it filled; include a flashlight in case of a power failure so children do not need to light candles.

Plan after-school snacks that do not require cooking to prevent burns.

Keep firearms locked, with the key in a place unknown to child. Instruct in firearm safety.

Keep a list of emergency telephone numbers (including parents' work numbers) by the telephone.

Arrange with a neighbor who is usually home during the late afternoon for children to stay there in an emergency.

If an older child will be watching a younger one, be certain both children understand the rules laid down and the degree of responsibility expected.

Be certain children understand that rules that apply during other times (never swim alone; do not play by the railroad tracks) also apply during independent time.

Parental Actions to Prevent Loneliness

Urge children to telephone a parent when they get home to touch base (be sure children have parents' work telephone numbers).

Be certain to make additional time available after work so children can describe their day.

Each morning help children plan an activity for that day so they have something purposeful to look forward to during time alone.

Allow special privileges such as listening to music that other members of the family do not like as well; allow extra television hours during this time.

Consider a pet. Even a caged animal, such as a hamster or a bird, offers companionship in a quiet house.

Call children if there will be a delay in arriving home; unexpected time alone is very frightening.

Leave messages on the refrigerator or in the bathroom that just say hi.

Leave a tape- or video-recorded message for children to play (make sure it is not full of tasks to do, but is a welcoming message).

Encourage children to read; fictional characters serve as friends as well as help to pass time.

Urge children to network with other latchkey children as to how they use time effectively; talking on the telephone or e-mailing another child reduces loneliness for both.

Parental Actions to Increase Socialization

Help children plan after-school activities such as joining a science club for one afternoon a week.

Explore sports programs at school or in the community, as these often are held after school.

Explore childcare programs at the school the child attends, a public library, or a church or synagogue.

Network with other parents or ask for flex time so child supervision can be alternated after school.

Be sure children have opportunities to socialize with friends on weekends or on days when either parent is home.

Parental Actions to Increase Self-Esteem

Praise children for the ability to take care of themselves for short time intervals (rather than scold that there are cracker crumbs on the carpet).

Walk with children through the empty house and together identify sounds (the click of the furnace turning on, the refrigerator starting to defrost, etc.), so they can determine the cause of sounds when home alone and not be frightened.

Help children to view quiet time as beneficial time in which they can do some things more efficiently than at noisy times (e.g., homework).

Do not allow children to use the latchkey role to provoke parental guilt. Allow children to have some say in family spending so they can see how their time alone (which allows both parents to work) contributes to family unity and progress.

Stealing

During early school age, most children go through a period in which they steal loose change from their mother's purse or father's dresser. This usually happens at around 7 years of age, when children are first learning how to make change and discovering the importance of money. Stealing occurs because although the child is gaining an appreciation for money, this appreciation is not yet balanced by strong moral principles.

Parents should explore the reason for the stealing:

- Do other children on the block receive an allowance and so have money for small items?
- Did the child make a bet that must be paid?
- Is the child buying a bully's friendship by purchasing gum or candy for that child?
- Does the child view money as security?

As a rule, early childhood stealing is best handled without a great deal of emotion. The child should be told that the money is missing. The importance of property rights should be reviewed: mother's and father's money is theirs; the child's money is the child's; they are not interchangeable. Youngsters who continue to steal past 9 years of age may require counseling because they should have progressed beyond this normal developmental step by this age.

Some shoplifting occurs with early school-agers, but the major problem with this arises during preadolescence. Some of this happens for the same reason that past generations tipped over outhouses or untied the preacher's horse and buggy: it is a public act of rebellion against authority, a "coming of age" ritual. In most instances, it occurs because of peer pressure (e.g., when the child believes he must have a certain type of clothing to belong to the "in" crowd). It can also be an initiation ritual for a gang.

WHAT IF? What if a child understands that stealing from a neighbor is wrong? Will he also understand that stealing from a large department store or taking things from a health clinic is wrong?

Shoplifting must be taken seriously by parents because it is a punishable crime, not a prank. Just as money missing from a purse should not be ignored, shoplifting should be confronted immediately to prevent the child who succeeds once from taking something even bigger the second time. The child should be asked how he or she came to possess the article and should not be allowed to use it. The child should then be denied access to stores until he or she demonstrates more responsibility. A child who shoplifts more than once may need counseling; it reflects more than simple confusion about property rights.

As an overall principle, parents must set good examples if they expect their child to be honest. If one parent takes money from the other without permission, neither should be surprised to find their child attempting to do the same. If a parent changes price tags or unwraps items and eats them without paying for them in the supermarket, he or she cannot expect the child to do otherwise.

Violence or Terrorism

Children basically view their world as safe, so it is a shock to them when violence such as a school shooting or international terrorists enter their lives. A number of organizations have proposed guidelines on how to help children deal with terrorism. The AAP (2001) recommends that parents:

- Assure children that they are safe; the violence is isolated to another part of the world and they are out of danger.
- Assure children that the parents are actively involved in keeping them safe.
- Observe for signs of stress such as sleep disturbances, fatigue, lack of pleasure in activities, or signs of beginning substance abuse.
- Not allow children or adolescents to view footage of traumatic events over and over, as this decreases the ability to feel safe.
- Watch news programs with their children so they can explain that the situation portrayed is not near them and that the child is safe.
- Explain that there are bad people in the world, and bad people do bad things, but help children to appreciate that not all people in a particular group or who look a particular way are bad. Lashing out at people who resemble them only causes more harm.
- Prepare a family disaster plan, including such things as bottled water, blankets, toiletries, pet supplies, appropriate clothing, and flashlights and information such as what immunizations their children have had (particularly tetanus) and, if a child is ill, a history of medical needs or care.
- Designate a "rally point" where they will meet if separated by a disaster or evacuation.

Some parents may be resistant to talk to their children about a disaster plan for the family, believing that these preparations will frighten children unnecessarily, but such preparations should have the major effect of increasing a feeling of safety, not decreasing it (Bishop & Rankin, 2001).

Bullying

A frequent reason that school-agers cite for feeling so violent that they turn guns on fellow classmates is that they were ridiculed or bullied to the point they could no longer take such abuse (Espelage et al., 2001). Why do some children become bullies and some become victims? Traits commonly associated with school-age bullies are:

- Advanced physical size and strength for their age
- Aggressive temperament (both male and female)
- Parents who are indifferent
- Parents who are permissive with an aggressive child
- Parents who typically resort to physical punishment
- Presence of a child who is a "natural victim" (underweight, small, anxious, insecure, cautious, or sensitive, with low self-esteem)

Suggestions for school personnel to deal with bullies are:

- Supervise recreation periods closely.
- Intervene immediately to stop bullying.

- Talk to both bully and victim privately and insist that if such behavior does not stop, both school and parents will become involved.
- Therapy may be needed to correct bullying behavior if it is ingrained (Dacey & Travers, 1999).

Recreational Drug Use

Once considered a college or high school problem, illegal drugs are available to children as early as elementary school and certainly by the time they reach the seventh and eighth grades. Because alcohol and inhalants are available in so many homes and often can be purchased in small stores without proof of age, these are the commonly abused drugs of this age group. Cocaine is becoming increasingly easy for children to obtain.

The use of hard drugs and alcohol and ways to encourage children to avoid their use are discussed in Chapter 32. Inhalants that are easily available to school-age children, and so may be abused by them, are airplane glue (toluene) and household spray products. Children do not become physically addicted to glue but do become psychologically dependent on it. To achieve the desired effect, they drop quantities of the glue into a paper bag, then sniff the fumes and experience a feeling of exhilaration or giddiness. This may seem a harmless procedure, but in high concentrations the fumes can cause extensive liver damage or pulmonary edema that can be fatal. Inhalants such as cooking spray or computer keyboard cleaner give this same effect. Because these products contain Freon, they can cause severe respiratory and cardiac irregularity.

Parents should suspect glue sniffing or some other form of recreational drug use if their child regularly appears irritable, inattentive, or drowsy. School health personnel should be aware of the increase in this practice among students and look for warning signs.

Abuse of steroids to improve muscle mass can be found in children as young as sixth grade. Counsel children against this because abuse of steroids leads to cardiovascular irregularities, uncontrollable aggressiveness, and possible cancer in later life (AAP Committee on Sports, 2001).

Cigarette smoking also begins in school-age children. With the sure knowledge that cigarette smoking plays a large part in the development of lung cancer and other serious respiratory illnesses, many parents assume that their children will know not to start. Smoking is considered by children to be an adult activity, so adopting the habit can be considered to be a giant step on the road to adulthood. Although the amount of cigarette advertising targeting young people as consumers has decreased, school-age children should be taught to recognize advertising manipulation aimed at them. Caution children against experimenting with smokeless tobacco, which can lead to mouth and throat cancer. Children may try this after seeing professional athletes using it.

To discourage use of tobacco by school-agers, health care professionals and parents need to be role models of excellent health behaviors in hopes that children will follow these good examples.

Children of Alcoholic Parents

As many as one in five children live with an alcoholic parent (AACAP, 2001). Such children are at greater risk for having emotional problems. Alcoholism may have a genetic cause, so children of alcoholics are more likely to become alcoholics (Obot et al., 2001). Immediate problems that can occur with children of alcoholics are:

- A feeling of guilt that the child is the cause of the parent's drinking
- Constant worry that the alcoholic parent will become sick or die, leaving the child; at the same time, fear of violence from the alcoholic parent and a wish that the parent would leave
- A feeling of shame that prevents the child from inviting friends home or asking for help
- Decreased ability to trust adults because the parent has been unreliable so many times
- Concern because the alcoholic parent's behavior is so erratic that no regular schedule of bedtime and meals exists
- Anger at the alcoholic parent for drinking and at the nonalcoholic parent for not doing more to correct things
- Helplessness to change the situation

Such fears may be revealed by failing marks in school, withdrawal from friends or social activities, and delinquent behavior such as stealing. With adolescence may come depression, suicidal thoughts, or abuse of drugs or alcohol. School nurses are in an excellent position to identify such children, monitor their school progress, and refer them to organizations such as Al-Anon or Alateen (*www.al-anon-alateen.org*) for support.

Obesity

As many as 50% of school-age children are obese by body-mass index guidelines for ideal weight. Some of these children have been overweight since infancy; their prepubertal natural weight gain makes them obese. Children with an endomorphic build (a natural tendency to accumulate body fat) are more likely to be obese at any time of life than those with a mesomorphic (normal) or ectomorphic (slender) build. Many families rely on fast-food meals several times a week, and such foods tend to be high in calories and fat and can lead to obesity. Children of obese parents are also inclined to obesity; perhaps genetic influences have some bearing. If parents ingest a diet full of excessive calories, the child is encouraged to eat similarly; thus, environmental factors also play a role.

Obese children begin to develop many of the same health problems as obese adults, such as hypertension and an elevated total cholesterol level, with possible atherosclerosis. They also may be ridiculed for their size and be unable to participate on sports teams. This is strong evidence for the need for active measures to help preteens regulate their weight (Sahota et al., 2001).

Those who become so obese that friends leave them out of activities or who cannot play sports because they tire quickly may develop such a poor self-image that they have little motivation for self-improvement. A weight-reduction program for school-age children that emphasizes long-term lifestyle changes is best. Such programs should contain three aspects.

1. Intake of about 1,200 calories (no more than 30% as fat)
2. An active exercise program
3. A counseling program to discuss aspects such as self-image and motivation to reduce weight

Total caloric intake cannot be reduced too drastically because children need calories to form new body tissue for continued growth. If carbohydrate intake is restricted too greatly, protein is broken down for body energy and a negative nitrogen balance is produced. Caution children not to try faddish high-protein diets (as most adults should not), because those diets do not supply enough carbohydrates and may produce a heavy renal solute load (the breakdown product of proteins) for the kidneys. It helps if children aim to lose 5 lb over a short time rather than 50 lb over a year. This short-term goal coincides better with the task of developing industry.

Surgical techniques such as an intestinal bypass are obviously extreme measures and inappropriate for children. Obese children might request one, however, in an attempt to avoid the not insignificant difficulty of long-term weight loss.

NURSING DIAGNOSES AND RELATED INTERVENTIONS

Nursing Diagnosis: Noncompliance with weight reduction plan related to lack of motivation to reduce weight

Outcome Identification: Child will demonstrate understanding and importance of weight loss and regular exercise to her own health by 1 month and state plan for losing weight.

Outcome Evaluation: Child states reasonable weight loss and exercise goals; discusses feelings with nurse about being overweight and reactions from schoolmates; expresses positive feelings about self-worth.

Motivating preteens to lose weight can be difficult because they often have little regard for what will happen to them in the future. They are not upset when told that obese people do not live as long as slimmer persons and have more heart attacks. They do, however, have a great respect for adults who are sympathetic to their problems. They are also aware that slim children are usually the most popular, and they wish they could look that way. They follow better dietary regimens, therefore, if they are asked to do so by a respected adult, such as a nurse, or if they fear being left out of social interactions.

Overweight school-age children often do well if a dieters' club is formed. They are not too young to participate in formal weight control organizations. Having tangible support from other group members helps them follow tedious and monotonous nutrition patterns. Behavior modification can be useful in teaching children how to eat in a healthier manner.

As a way of increasing daily activity, preadolescents do well with formal exercise classes because they enjoy the support from other children. In addition, encourage them to increase informal exercise, such as walking to and from school. Encourage coaches of childhood sports to accept obese children as part of a team, not because they will necessarily benefit the team, but because the exercise will benefit the children. Exercise burns up calories, and if children's daylight hours are filled with activities and friends, they have less time to eat.

Lifestyle change is the ultimate goal for the entire family, because obesity is usually a family problem. Rather than preparing special meals for just the obese child, the entire family probably needs to eat in a healthier manner. Because preadolescents do not generally prepare their own food, the person in the home who prepares meals requires as much information on the planned weight loss as the child. The old concepts that used to hold ("A clean plate is good; how can you leave food when people in other countries are starving?") may have to be changed so children and other family members reduce their intake appropriately. The importance of exercise should also be reflected in the home. Family members should not only encourage the obese child to exercise but also should partake in some form of daily activity themselves. There is some danger in pointing out to preadolescents that they are terribly overweight because some children become so obsessed with losing weight that they become bulimic or anorexic (see Chap. 32; Hsu et al., 2001). Stressing that children "become healthier" or "improve stamina" may be better advice than talking about dieting.

Concerns of the Physically Challenged or Chronically Ill School-Age Child

One of the biggest problems facing a school-age child with a long-term illness or physical challenge is time lost from school. This threatens not only academic achievement but also the child's relationships with his or her peers. It may make him or her the "odd person out" with respect to making friends or joining gangs. Whether children are confined to the home or hospitalized, helping them to keep in contact with friends by telephone, e-mail, or letters can help foster the socialization that is important to continued development. Encourage parents (or school friends) to obtain schoolwork, and help these children with their homework so they can progress with learning at a usual pace and continue to build self-esteem.

Most children with physical or cognitive challenges attend regular schools and classes (**inclusion**) because federal law (PL 99-457) stipulates that all children must receive equal education in the least restrictive situation possible. Placement in classrooms is determined by a committee in each school system. You may need to advocate for a child with such a committee to demonstrate, for example, that although the child is wheelchair challenged or needs continuous oxygen, he or she can participate in a regular classroom setting; or that a child would benefit from a period each day with a special resource teacher. It may be necessary to meet with a school nurse, teacher, or the child's classmates (with the parents' permission) to increase their understanding and acceptance of the child's illness (see Focus on Evidence-Based Practice).

Children with physical or cognitive challenges should be assigned household chores just like other children their age and should participate in activities, such as Girl or Boy Scouts, in which accomplishment is encouraged. It is important for such children to develop a sense of industry or accomplishment so they can persevere in measures that will help them to be as independent as possible (Fig. 31-10).

When you are caring for a school-age child who is chronically ill or physically challenged, choose short-term activities that can be completed independently, as with all school-age children. Conversely, be careful not to insult a child with tasks that are obviously not age-appropriate. Table 31-5 describes some nursing actions that can help to foster a sense of industry in children who are physically challenged.

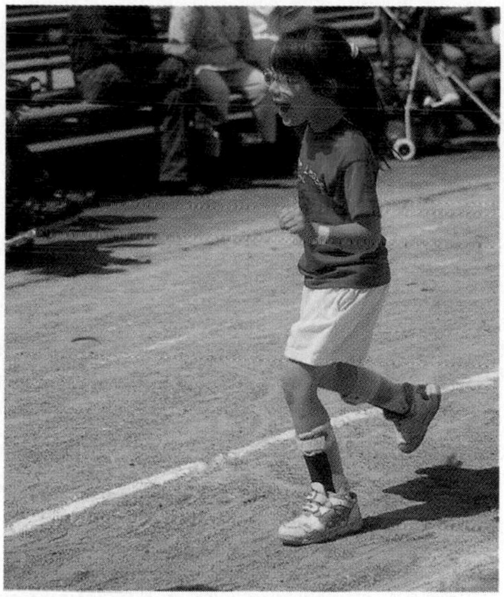

FIGURE 31.10 A school-age child who is physically challenged is elated at the finish line. This accomplishment goes far toward her developing a sense of industry.

Nutrition and the Challenged School-Age Child

Food preparation and dishwashing time are times for socializing in most households. The school-age child who cannot be involved in these activities because of a physical challenge needs extra time during the day to make up for these lost socializing experiences, such as a specific hour set aside for talking or sharing a project that can be accomplished in one sitting.

When eating in cafeterias or at a friend's home, a child who must eat a special diet is usually tempted to select the same food as everyone else rather than limit what he or she chooses. The child may decline invitations rather than admit to requiring a special diet or needing help with eating. Ask at health care visits if any of these problems are present. Help children with special diets to plan ways they could be comfortable in social food-based settings (e.g., bringing a party snack that is easily eaten and appropriate for the child, or politely declining particular foods). Help children who are hospitalized to select a diet that is enjoyable as well as nutritious.

FOCUS ON EVIDENCE-BASED PRACTICE

Should Cognitively Challenged Children Be Mainstreamed Into School Classrooms?

Most studies on the worth of including children into regular classrooms center on the ability of children to achieve in such settings. In this study, a researcher looked instead at the quality of friendships that mainstreaming allowed children to achieve. Participants included 121 students who were cognitively challenged in special education schools, 189 students who were cognitively challenged in self-contained mainstreamed schools, and 265 students who were not cognitively challenged. Results of the study showed that students in special schools had fewer friends than students with like cognitive challenges in mainstreamed schools. Overall, the students in special schools responded more passively than others and reported feeling lonelier than students in the other groups.

This is an interesting study for nurses because school nurses are instrumental in helping to place students in special or mainstreamed classrooms. Nurses in ambulatory settings are often asked for their opinion on whether mainstreaming is helpful for children who are cognitively challenged. Knowing that such a school placement can lead to increased friendships could be a helpful aspect for counseling parents.

Heiman, T. (2000). Friendship quality among children in three educational settings. *Journal of Intellectual & Developmental Disability, 25*(1), 1-12.

✔ CHECKPOINT QUESTIONS

13. What is a common household product frequently abused by school-agers?
14. Are bullies always boys?

KEY POINTS

School-age children mature slowly but steadily. Their average annual weight gain is 3 to 5 lb; their increase in height is 1 to 2 inches.

At about age 10, children begin to develop secondary sex characteristics. Preparation for this helps them accept these changes positively.

Deciduous teeth are lost and permanent teeth erupt during the school-age period.

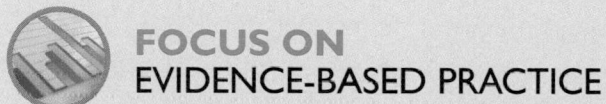

TABLE 31.5 Nursing Actions That Encourage a Sense of Industry in the Physically Challenged or Chronically Ill School-Age Child

CATEGORY	ACTIONS
Nutrition	Allow choices of food and respect food preferences.
	Provide small food servings that child can finish, encouraging sense of accomplishment.
Dressing	Allow child to make out requisitions for supplies.
	Ask for suggestions as to how bulky the child wants dressing, where to apply tape.
Medicine	Teach child name and action of medicine.
	Encourage child to keep track of medication times by clock or record.
	Child may feel more in control of injections or intravenous insertions if allowed to choose the site from among options offered.
	Allow child to choose oral medicine form (capsules or liquid) if possible.
Rest	Establish clear rules for rest periods (reading or watching television is all right; playing a game is not, etc.).
Hygiene	Respect modesty of school-age child at an adult level.
	Allow as much choice as possible (e.g., own clothing, timing of self-care).
Pain	Encourage child to express and rate pain.
	Encourage child to use distraction techniques, such as counting backward from 100 or imagery, during episodes of pain.
	Explain source and cause of pain to give child sense of mastery.
Stimulation	Encourage school work.
	Encourage activity that ends in a product (putting together a picture puzzle rather than listening to a CD).
	Encourage paper-and-pencil games, such as connect the dots, tic tac toe.
	Card games provide social interaction and also encourage simple addition skills (make a deck from paper if one is not available).
	Don't suggest competition games for children less than age 10 yr.
	Encourage using playroom for socialization.
	Encourage child to keep in contact with school friends by telephoning or writing notes to them.

Erikson's developmental task for the school-age period is to gain a sense of industry, or how to do things well.

Common health problems during the school-age period include minor respiratory and gastrointestinal infections as well as dental caries and malocclusion.

Common parental concerns about the school-age child are language development, fears and anxieties, and behavior problems such as stealing and using recreational drugs.

As many as 90% of parents of school-age children are dual-earner families. This means many school-age children return home before their parents. Counseling families on ways to turn this independent time alone into a positive experience is a nursing responsibility.

Children in a concrete stage of operational thought are limited to understanding concepts they can actually see. When health teaching, use concrete examples (actually let them hold a syringe, don't just talk about it) to increase their understanding.

School-age children thrive on rules. It is confusing for them when rules are changed (medicine will now be taken four rather than three times a day) unless they have a clear explanation of why the change is occurring.

School-age children are looking for good adult role models; it is hard for them to feel confidence in an adult who isn't honest with them or who fails to live up to their expectations by not following through on promises.

School-age children with a family tendency toward obesity may become overweight. Helping the family learn a healthier lifestyle is important.

CRITICAL THINKING EXERCISES

1. Shelly is the 6-year-old you met at the beginning of the chapter. Her mother told you that she has developed many nervous habits since she started school. She asks you if this is normal. How would you answer? What suggestions would you make to her mother regarding this?
2. School-age children can develop obesity because of excessive nutritional intake, lack of exercise, and inheritance or family factors. What can parents do to help prevent this from happening? What is a

possible consequence of telling school-age children that they are overweight?

3. A 12-year-old boy is confined to a wheelchair because of muscular dystrophy. Why might developing a sense of industry be particularly difficult for him? What suggestions could you make to encourage this?
4. A number of children in the school where you are the school nurse are vegetarians. They have difficulty finding nonmeat choices to pack as school lunches. What would you suggest to them?
5. Examine the National Health Goals related to school-age children. Most government-sponsored money for nursing research is allotted based on these goals. What would be a possible research topic to explore pertinent to these goals that would be fundable and would advance evidence-based practice?

ABC XYZ REFERENCES

American Academy of Child & Adolescent Psychiatry. (2001). *Fact sheet: Children of alcoholics.* Washington, D.C: Author.

American Academy of Pediatrics. (2001). *Communication with children about disasters.* Washington, D.C.: AAP

American Academy of Pediatrics Committee on Practice and Ambulatory Medicine. (2001). *Recommendations for preventive pediatric health care.* Washington, D.C.: AAP.

American Academy of Pediatrics Committee on Safety. (2001). *Seatbelt safety and children.* Washington, D.C.: AAP.

American Academy of Pediatrics, Committee on Sports Medicine and Fitness/Committee on School Health. (2001). Organized sports for children and preadolescents. *Pediatrics, 107*(6), 1459–1462.

Berger, K. S. (2001). *The developing person through the life span* (5th ed.). New York: Worth Publishing.

Bishop, V., & Rankin, W. W. (2001). Children affected by violence. *Journal of Pediatric Nursing, 16*(5), 377–3778.

Dacey, J. S., & Travers, J. F. (1999). Human development across the life span (4th ed.). New York: McGraw-Hill.

Department of Health and Human Services. (2000). *Healthy people 2010.* Washington, D.C.: DHHS.

Dudek, S. G. (2001). *Nutrition: Essentials for nursing practice.* Philadelphia: Lippincott Williams & Wilkins.

Erikson, E. H. (1993). *Childhood and society.* New York: W.W. Norton.

Espelage, D. L., Bosworth, K., & Simon, T. R. (2001). Short-term stability and prospective correlates of bullying in middle-school students: An examination of potential demographic, psychosocial, and environmental influences. *Violence & Victims, 16* (4), 411–426.

Freud, S. (1962). *Three essays on the theory of sexuality.* New York: Hearst Corporation.

Heiman, T. (2000). Friendship quality among children in three educational settings. *Journal of Intellectual & Developmental Disability, 25*(1), 1–12.

Hsu, L. K. et al. (2001). Cognitive therapy, nutritional therapy and their combination in the treatment of bulimia nervosa. *Psychological Medicine, 31*(5), 871–879.

Johnson, M., Maas, M., & Moorhead, S. (2000). *Nursing outcomes classification* (2d ed.). St. Louis: Mosby, Inc.

Kaplan, D. W., & Love, K. A. (2001). Growth and development. In W. W. Hay, A. R. Hayward, M. J. Levin, & J. M. Sondheimer, J. M. (Eds.). *Current pediatric diagnosis and treatment* (15th ed.). New York: McGraw-Hill.

Kohlberg, L. (1984). *The psychology of moral development.* New York: Harper & Row.

Krebs, N. F., & Hambridge, K. M. (2001). Normal childhood nutrition & its disorders. In W. W. Hay, A. R. Hayward, M. J. Levin, & J. M. Sondheimer, J. M. (Eds.). *Current pediatric diagnosis and treatment* (15th ed.). New York: McGraw-Hill.

Leonard, M. B. & Zemel, B. S. (2002). Current concepts in pediatric bone disease. *Pediatric clinics of North America, 49*(1), 143–173.

McCloskey, J., & Bulechek, G. (2000). *Nursing interventions classification* (3d ed.). St. Louis: Mosby, Inc.

Obot, I. S., Wagner, F. A., & Anthony, J. C. (2001). Early onset and recent drug use among children of parents with alcohol problems. *Drug & Alcohol Dependence, 65*(1), 1–8.

Piaget, J. (1969). *The theory of stages in cognitive development.* New York: McGraw-Hill.

Sahota, P., et al. (2001). Randomized controlled trial of primary school-based intervention to reduce risk factors for obesity. *British Medical Journal, 323* (7320): 1029–1032.

ABC XYZ SUGGESTED READINGS

American Academy of Pediatrics, Committee on Public Education. (2002). Media violence. *Pediatrics, 108*(5), 1222–1226.

Balling, K., & McCubbin, M. (2001). Hospitalized children with chronic illness: Parental caregiving needs and valuing parental expertise. *Journal of Pediatric Nursing, 16*(2), 110–119.

Butler, G. A., & Thompson, L. S. (2000). Building skills for child advocacy. *Journal of Pediatric Nursing, 15*(5), 323–325.

Hewitt, M., et al. (2001). Evaluation of "Sun-Safe": A health education resource for primary schools. *Health Education Research, 16*(5), 623–633.

Munsen, R. B. (2001). Children and puberty. *Journal of Pediatric Nursing, 16*(1), 66–67.

Nesdale, D., & Flesser, D. (2001). Social identity and the development of children's group attitudes. *Child Development, 72*(2), 506–517.

Perez-Rodrigo, C., et al. (2001). The school setting: An opportunity for the implementation of dietary guidelines. *Public Health Nutrition, 4*(2B), 717–724.

Qayumi, S. (2001). Piaget and his role in problem-based learning. *Journal of Investigative Surgery, 14*(2), 63–65.

Saltos, E. (1999). Adapting the food guide pyramid for children: Defining the target audience. *Family Economics and Nutrition Review, 12*(3&4), 3–17.

Thomas, D. O. (2002). Special considerations for pediatric triage in the emergency department. *Nursing Clinics of North America, 37*(1), 145–159.

Ziegert, D. I., et al. (2001). Longitudinal study of young children's responses to challenging achievement situations. *Child Development, 72*(2), 609–624.

32

CHAPTER

The Family With an Adolescent

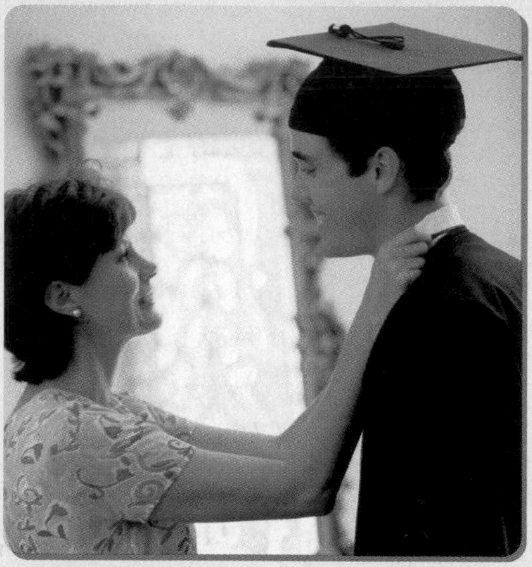

Key Terms

- adolescence
- comedones
- formal operations
- glycogen loading
- identity
- puberty
- role confusion
- stalking
- substance abuse

Objectives

After mastering the contents of this chapter, you should be able to:

1. Describe the normal growth and development pattern and common parental concerns of the adolescent period.
2. Assess adolescents for normal growth and development milestones.
3. Formulate nursing diagnoses for the family of an adolescent.
4. Identify expected outcomes based on health assessment findings.
5. Plan nursing care related to growth and development concerns of the adolescent, such as planning health teaching necessary to accept pubertal changes.
6. Implement nursing care related to growth and development or special needs of the adolescent, such as organizing a discussion group on ways to prevent drug abuse.
7. Evaluate expected outcomes to be certain that nursing care was comprehensive.
8. Identify National Health Goals related to the adolescent that nurses could be instrumental in helping the nation to achieve.
9. Identify areas related to care of adolescents that could benefit from additional nursing research or application of evidence-based practice.
10. Use critical thinking to analyze ways in which care of the adolescent could be more family centered.
11. Integrate knowledge of adolescent growth and development with nursing process to achieve quality maternal and child health nursing care.

Raul is a 16-year-old boy you see at an adolescent clinic. His chief concern is a head cold. His parents tell you Raul seemed depressed for a long time after his girlfriend broke up with him but now seems happy again. They are pleased to see him maturing so much that he recently gave away his collection of model airplanes to a young neighbor. You mention to Raul that a decongestant would probably make him feel better. He asks you how many pills it would take to kill someone, then jokes that he was kidding. His parents tell you Raul has been joking about killing himself a lot lately.

The physician in the clinic prescribes a decongestant and suggests Raul return in 6 months. Did Raul have some needs that were not met by his clinic visit?

The previous chapter discussed school-age children and the capabilities children develop during that time period. This chapter adds information about the changes, both physical and psychosocial, that occur during the adolescent years. This is important information because it builds a base for care and health teaching for the age group.

After you've studied the chapter, answer the Critical Thinking Exercises at the end of the chapter and then access the on-line study activities (http://connection.lww.com) *to further sharpen your skills and test your knowledge.*

Adolescence is the time period between 13 years and 18 to 20 years, a time period that serves as a transition period between childhood and adulthood. It can be divided into an early period (13 to 14 years), a middle period (15 to 16 years), and a late period (17 to 20 years). During all periods, adolescence is defined not so much by chronologic age as by physiologic, psychological, and sociologic factors. The drastic change in physical appearance and the change in expectations of others (especially parents) may lead to both emotional and physical health problems.

Adolescents invariably feel a sense of pressure throughout this period. They want to work but are too young for a full-time job. They are mature in some respects but still young in others. For example, the adolescent's sexual interests are awakening, yet personal or parental pressures often discourage sexual exploration. This duality causes a major dilemma for the adolescent, leading to many of the growth and developmental concerns of the age.

There is such a strong adolescent subculture today that parents may feel from the minute their child enters the teenage years that all communication stops. Parents may expect difficulty controlling the child or understanding teenage values, as though entering this period locks the adolescent into a shell or pulls down a curtain between child and parents. This can become a self-fulfilling prophecy, whereby the parents actually cause the communication breakdown. At other times, communication problems can begin when a teenager refuses to respect parents' opinions or stops asking for them. Many of the problems adolescents bring to health care personnel arise from this communication impasse, no matter how it started. They often come to health care facilities with many misconceptions, seeking adult help and guidance. National Health Goals related to adolescence are shown in Focus on National Health Goals.

FOCUS ON NATIONAL HEALTH GOALS

Health teaching in the adolescent years is important, because healthy habits begun at this time can influence health over a lifetime. For this reason, a number of National Health Goals relate to adolescent health:

- Reduce the number of adolescents who are overweight or obese to a prevalence of no more than 5% from a baseline of 11%.
- Reduce tobacco use by adolescents to 16% from a baseline of 35%.
- Reduce smokeless tobacco use by adolescents to no more than 1% from a baseline of 8%.
- Reduce deaths caused by alcohol-related motor vehicle accidents to no more than 18% among people ages 15 to 24 from a baseline of 21.5%.
- Reduce the rate of suicide attempts by adolescents to no more than 1% from a baseline of 2.6%.
- Increase to 35% the proportion of adolescents who exercise regularly from a baseline of 22% (DHHS, 2000).

Nurses can be instrumental in helping the nation achieve these goals by educating adolescents against the use of cigarettes, smokeless tobacco, alcohol, drug abuse, and acts of violence, and by acting as support people for adolescents during times of crisis to help prevent suicide. Areas in which additional knowledge is needed that could benefit from additional nursing research are identifying effective programs that reduce the use of smokeless tobacco or cigarette smoking, documenting the best actions for nurses to take in emergency rooms when adolescents are admitted after suicide attempts, and constructing rapid surveys to identify adolescents who are abusing drugs.

NURSING PROCESS OVERVIEW

For Healthy Development of the Adolescent

Assessment

Parents rarely bring adolescents for health maintenance visits, and adolescents generally don't come to health care facilities on their own unless they are ill. Unless adolescents need a physical examination for athletic clearance, these children are usually not seen for health assessments as often as they were when younger. When adolescents are accompanied by their parents at health visits, it is best to obtain a health history separately from parents to promote independence and responsibility for self-care. When performing physical examinations on adolescents, be aware that they may be very self-conscious. They also need health assurance and appreciate comments such as "Your hair has a nice, healthy feel," or "This is an accessory nipple. Have you ever wondered about it?"

so they can learn more about their rapidly changing bodies (see Focus on Cultural Competence).

Nursing Diagnosis

Frequently used nursing diagnoses related to adolescents and their families are:

- Health-seeking behaviors related to normal growth and development
- Low self-esteem related to facial acne
- Anxiety related to concerns about normal growth and development
- Risk for injury related to peer pressure to use alcohol and drugs
- Readiness for enhanced parenting related to increased knowledge of teenage years

Outcome Identification and Planning

When planning with adolescents, respect the fact that they have a desire to exert independence and do things their own way. This means that they are not likely to adhere to a plan of care that disrupts their lifestyle or makes them appear different from others their age. Including them in planning is essential so the plan will be accepted. Establishing a contract (e.g., the adolescent agrees to take medication daily) may be the most effective means to reach a mutual understanding.

Adolescents are very present oriented, so a program that provides immediate results, such as increased respiratory function, will be carried out well. Conversely, a regimen oriented toward the future, with long-term goals such as preventing hypertension, may not be as successful. This does not mean that it is not important to teach adolescents about the necessity of reducing future health risks—by eating well, *not* smoking, and generally taking care of their bodies—but that information will be best accepted if geared as much as possible to specific, short-term benefits to their health.

FOCUS ON CULTURAL COMPETENCE

In the United States, as in most developed countries, adolescence covers a long time span. In developing countries, in contrast, adolescence tends to be much shorter because children must take full-time jobs to help support their families early in life. Socioeconomic factors definitely influence the length of adolescence across all cultures. Recognizing that adolescents may have differing responsibilities and life experiences based on cultural expectations can be useful when making an assessment. In a family in which an adolescent is expected to begin working full-time or to marry at an early age, you may need to include factors such as occupational hazards or the effects of job, family, and financial stress on the adolescent. Readiness for childbearing is also important.

Teaching by peers is another effective way to motivate teens. Organizing peer support groups this way can be a major activity of school nurses.

Implementation

Adolescents do poorly with tasks that someone else tells them they *must* do. If they help to plan tasks, however, they can carry them out successfully. Adolescents have little patience with adults who do not demonstrate the behavior they are being asked to achieve; a parent or nurse who smokes and asks an adolescent not to smoke will probably not be successful. Evaluate how an intervention appears from the adolescent's standpoint before initiating instructions.

Organizations that address some of the concerns of adolescence and may be of use for possible referral are.

American Association of Suicidology (*www.suicidology.org*)
Partnership for a Drug-Free America (*www.drugfreeamerica.org*)
Al-Anon/Alateen (*www.alateen.com*)
Planned Parenthood Federation of America, Inc. (*www.plannedparenthood.org*)
Sexual Information and Education Council of the United States (SIECUS) (*www.siecus.org*)

Outcome Evaluation

Evaluation of outcomes should include not only whether desired outcomes have been achieved but whether adolescents are pleased with their accomplishments. Individuals will have difficulty accomplishing desired goals as adults unless they have high self-esteem that includes feeling secure in body image.

The following are examples of outcome criteria that might be established:

- Client states she is able to feel good about herself even though she is the shortest girl in her class.
- Client states he has not consumed alcohol in 2 weeks.
- Parents voice that they feel more confident about their ability to parent an adolescent.
- Client states she feels high self-esteem despite persistent facial acne.

NURSING ASSESSMENT OF GROWTH AND DEVELOPMENT OF THE ADOLESCENT

Adolescents both grow rapidly and mature dramatically during this period.

Physical Growth

The major milestones of development in the adolescent period are the onset of puberty and the cessation of body growth. Between these milestones, physiologic growth and development of adult coordination occur. At first, the gain in physical growth is mostly in weight, leading to the stocky, slightly obese appearance of prepubescence; later comes the thin, gangly appearance of late adolescence.

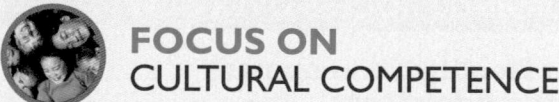

Most girls are 1 to 2 inches (2.4 to 5 cm) taller than boys coming into adolescence and generally stop growing within 3 years from menarche. Thus, those girls who start menstruating at 10 years of age may reach their adult height by age 13.

Boys grow about 4 to 12 inches (10 to 30 cm) in height and gain 15 to 65 lb (7 to 30 kg) during adolescence. Girls grow 2 to 8 inches (5 to 20 cm) in height and gain 15 to 55 lb (7 to 25 kg). Growth stops with closure of the epiphyseal lines of long bones. This occurs at about 16 or 17 years of age in females and about 18 to 20 years of age in males.

The increase in body size does not occur in all organ systems at the same rate. For example, the skeletal system grows faster than the muscles, and muscle mass increases more rapidly than heart size. These differences in growth rates make adolescents appear long-legged and awkward during a rapid growth spurt, because their extremities elongate first, followed by trunk growth. Both sexes may lack coordination. A 13-year-old child, for example, typically reaches to pick up a glass of milk at the dinner table and spills it, having reached beyond it because the arm is longer than the child realized.

Because the heart and lungs increase in size more slowly than the rest of the body, blood flow and oxygen availability are reduced. Thus, adolescents may have insufficient energy and become fatigued trying to do the various activities that interest them. Pulse rate and respiratory rate decrease slightly (to 70 bpm and 20 breaths/min, respectively), and blood pressure increases slightly (to 120/70 mmHg), reaching adult levels by late adolescence. With adulthood, blood pressure becomes slightly higher in males than females because more force is necessary to distribute blood to the larger male body mass.

All during adolescence, androgen stimulates sebaceous glands to extreme activity, sometimes resulting in acne, a common adolescent skin problem. Apocrine sweat glands (glands present in the axillae and genital area) form shortly after puberty. Apocrine sweat glands produce a strong odor in response to emotional stimulation. Therefore, adolescents begin to notice they must shower or bathe more frequently than they once did in order to be free of body odor.

Teeth

Adolescents gain their second molars at about 13 years of age and their third molars (wisdom teeth) between 18 and 21 years of age. Third molars may erupt as early as 14 to 15 years of age. The jaw reaches adult size only toward the end of adolescence. As a result, adolescents whose third molars erupt before the lengthening of the jaw is complete may experience pain and may need these molars extracted because they do not fit their jawline.

Puberty

Adolescence is the physiologic period between the beginning of puberty and the cessation of bodily growth. **Puberty** is the stage at which the individual first becomes capable of sexual reproduction. A girl has entered puberty when she begins to menstruate; a boy enters puberty when he begins to produce spermatozoa. These events usually occur between ages 11 and 14 years (Berger, 2001).

Secondary Sex Changes

Secondary sex characteristics (eg, body hair configuration and breast growth) distinguish the sexes from each other but play no direct part in reproduction. The secondary sex characteristics that begin in the late school-age period (see Chapter 31) continue to develop during adolescence. The typical stages of sexual maturation are shown in Table 32-1.

Sexual maturity in males and females is classified according to Tanner stages, named after the original researcher on sexual maturity (Tanner, 1962). Stages of female sexual development are shown in Figure 32-1; stages of male genital growth are shown in Figure 32-2.

TABLE 32.1 Sexual Maturation in Adolescents

AGE (YR)	MALES	FEMALES
13–15	Growth spurt continuing; pubic hair abundant and curly; testes, scrotum, and penis enlarging further; axillary hair present; facial hair fine and downy; voice changes happening with annoying frequency	Pubic hair thick and curly, triangular in distribution, breast areola and papilla form secondary mound; menstruation is ovulatory, making pregnancy possible
15–16	Genitalia adult; pubic hair abundant and curly; scrotum dark and heavily rugated; facial and body hair present; sperm production mature	Pubic hair curly and abundant (adult); may extend onto medial aspect of thighs; breast tissue adult and nipples protrude; areolas no longer project as separate ridges from breasts; may have some degree of facial acne
16–17	Pubic hair curly and abundant (adult), may extend along medial aspect of thighs; testes, scrotum, and penis adult in size; may have some degree of facial acne; gynecomastia (enlarged breast tissue), if present, fades	End of skeletal growth
17–18	End of skeletal growth	

Tanner, J. M. (1962). *Growth at adolescence* (2nd ed.). Oxford: Blackwell.

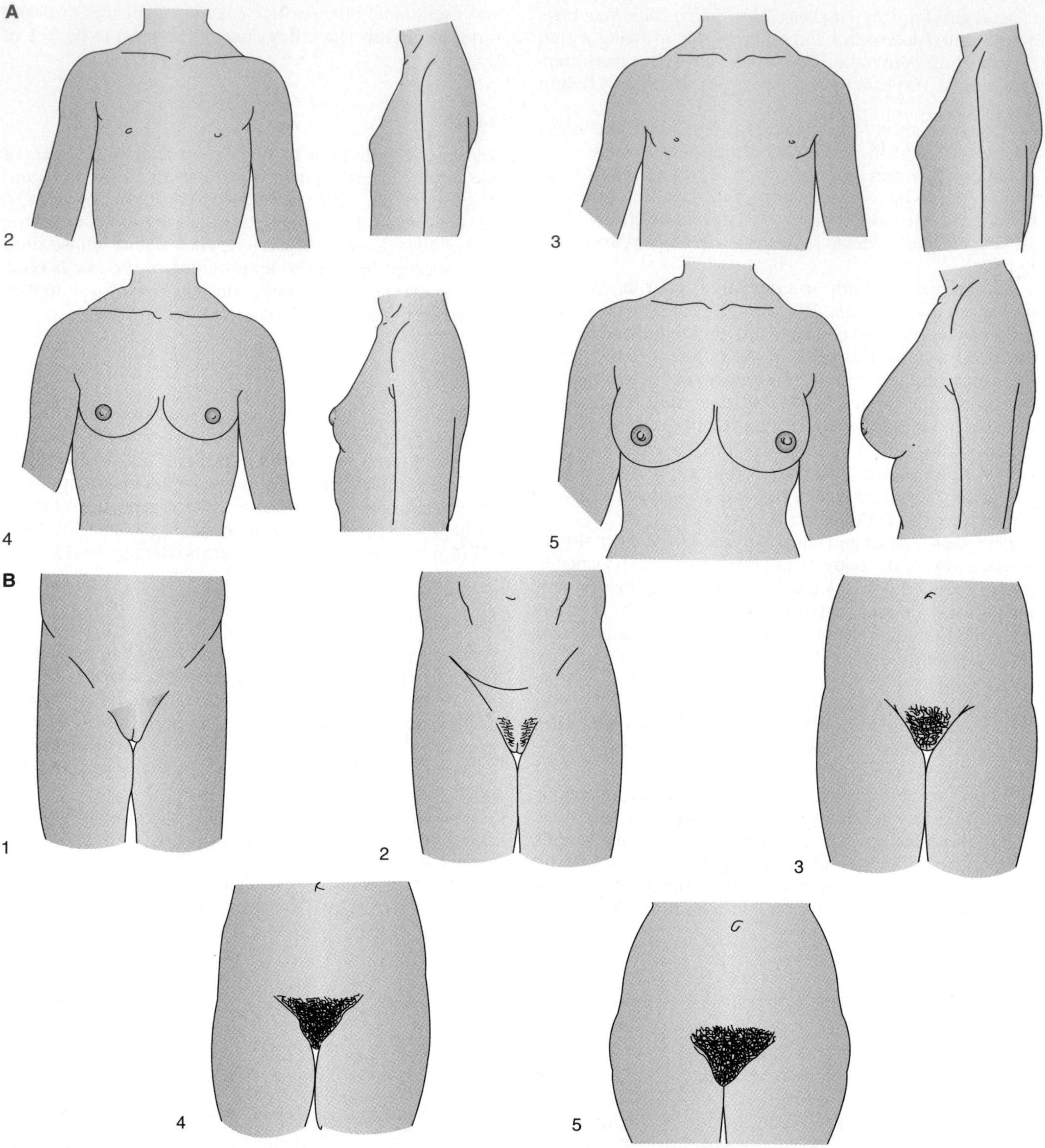

FIGURE 32.1 (*A*) Female breast development. *Sex maturity rating 1* (not shown): prepubertal; elevation of papilla only. *Sex maturity rating 2:* breast buds appear; areola is slightly widened and projects as small mound. *Sex maturity rating 3:* enlargement of the entire breast with no protrusion of the papilla or the nipple. *Sex maturity rating 4:* enlargement of the breast and projection of areola and papilla as a secondary mound. *Sex maturity rating 5:* adult configuration of the breast with protrusion of the nipple; areola no longer projects separately from remainder of breast. (*B*) Female pubic hair development. *Sex maturity rating 1:* prepubertal; no pubic hair. *Sex maturity rating 2:* straight hair extends along the labia and, between rating 2 and 3, begins on the pubis. *Sex maturity rating 3:* Pubic hair increased in quantity, darker, and present in the typical female triangle but in smaller quantity. *Sex maturity rating 4:* pubic hair more dense, curled, and adult in distribution but less abundant. *Sex maturity rating 5:* abundant, adult-type pattern; hair may extend onto the medial part of the thighs. (Adapted from Tanner, J. M. [1962]. *Growth at adolescence* [2nd ed.]. Oxford: Blackwell.)

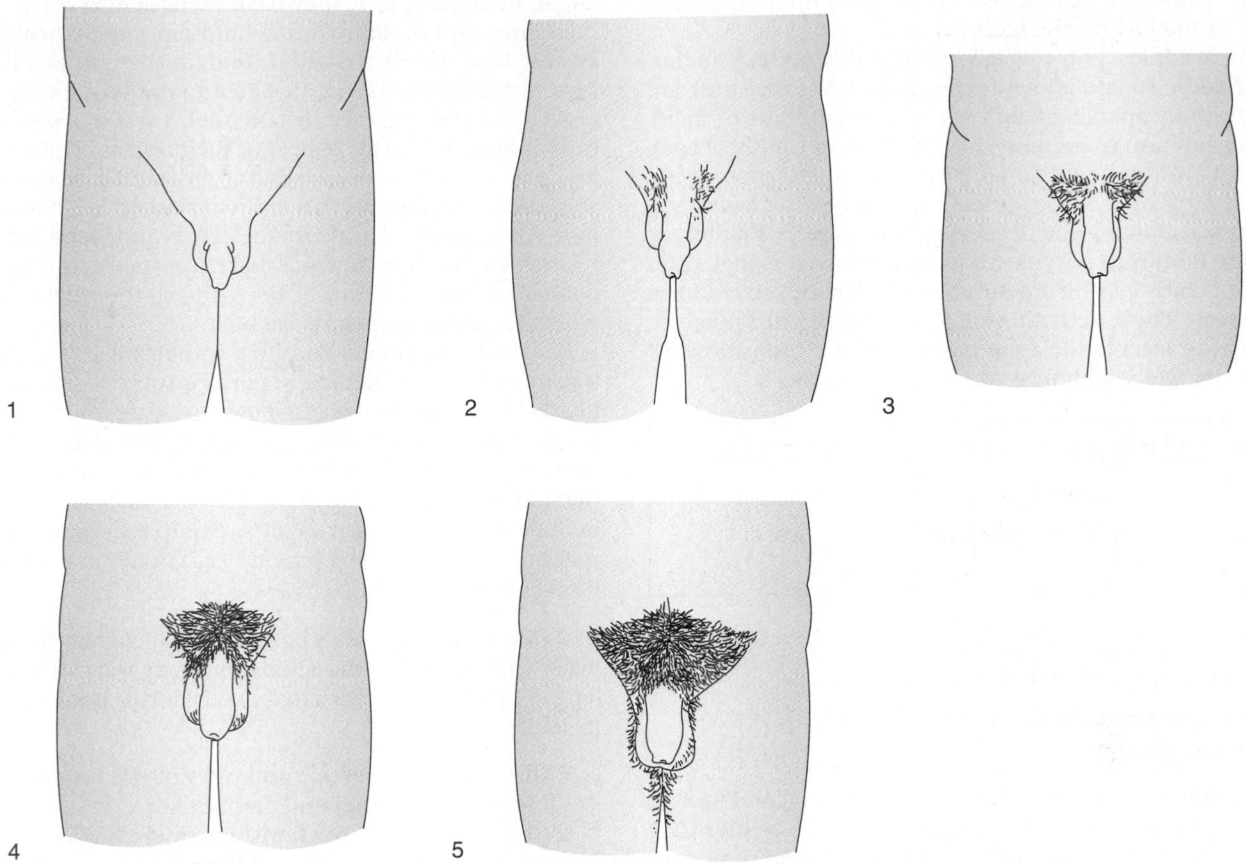

FIGURE 32.2 Male genital and pubic hair development. Ratings for pubic hair and for genital development can differ in a typical boy at any given time, since pubic hair and genitalia do not necessarily develop at the same rate. *Sex maturity rating 1:* prepubertal; no pubic hair; genitalia unchanged from early childhood. *Sex maturity rating 2;* light, downy hair develops laterally and later becomes dark; penis and testes may be slightly larger; scrotum becoming more textured. *Sex maturity rating 3:* pubic hair has extended across the pubis, testes and scrotum are further enlarged; penis is larger, especially in length. *Sex maturity rating 4:* more abundant pubic hair with curling; genitalia resemble those of an adult; glans has become larger and broader, scrotum is darker. *Sex maturity rating 5:* adult quantity and pattern of pubic hair, with hair present along inner borders of thighs; testes and scrotum are adult in size. (Adapted from Tanner, J. M. [1962]. *Growth at adolescence* [2nd ed.]. Oxford: Blackwell.)

Developmental Milestones

Thirteen-year-old children are beyond the age of spending time in any form of childhood play. Both sexes do spend a great deal of time playing sports. Team (or school) loyalty is intense, and following a coach's instructions becomes mandatory. This attitude is similar to the loyalty that 6-year-old children show toward their first-grade teacher.

Young adolescents who do not have the physical ability to compete successfully in sports usually avoid these activities. Urge parents to encourage youngsters to play sports for their own health and well-being and the companionship involved, even though they do not excel. If not successful at sports, the young adolescent needs a sympathetic person to listen to frustrations and to be encouraged to try other activities in which they may excel, such as science, music, or art. Overuse injuries from athletics occur in early adolescence until adolescents learn more about their limits and begin to respect the advice of adults on being well prepared and trained for sports participation.

Most adolescents spend a great deal of time just talking with peers as social interaction. Some parents disapprove of the number of hours spent in this activity, afraid their children are wasting important time, or at least exchanging a great deal of trivial conversation. For the adolescent, however, talking is no more a waste of time than was imaginative play as a preschooler. It is a major way to learn about the world.

Fifteen-year-old children may spend a great deal of time in their room or, if they do not have a room of their own, in a quiet corner of the home away from traffic and conversation areas. If they cannot find privacy somewhere in the house, they tend to spend time elsewhere.

Beginning at age 16, most adolescents want part-time jobs to earn money. Such jobs can teach young persons how to work with others, accept responsibility, and spend money wisely.

When families were larger, each older child had responsibility for a younger sibling and baby care was a natural activity. With small nuclear families, many adolescents have never had the responsibility of caring for anyone younger than themselves. For their own sake and that of the children they care for, adolescents who plan to babysit should learn some basic rules of child care and safety.

Many schools or Red Cross organizations offer courses in babysitting just for the teenager.

Many adolescents engage in charitable endeavors during middle to late adolescence. They learn that they are strong and capable enough not only to take care of themselves but also to help less fortunate people in their community. Adolescents do well organizing and supervising swimming or gym programs for physically challenged children, cooking and delivering food to older shut-ins, or raising money to purchase equipment for a hospital. High school clubs may be organized to send money to children overseas. These activities fulfill the adolescent's need for satisfying interaction with others and are indications of maturity and willingness to accept adult roles.

> **✔ CHECKPOINT QUESTIONS**
>
> 1. Why does growth stop during adolescence?
> 2. What glands are responsible for adolescent body odor?

Emotional Development

Developmental Task: Identity Versus Role Confusion

According to Erikson (1993), the developmental task in early and midadolescence is to form a sense of **identity,** that is, to decide who they are and what kind of person they will be. In late adolescence, the task is to form a sense of intimacy or form close relationships with persons of the opposite as well as the same sex. It is the concentration on these two tasks that leads to typical adolescent behavior. The four main areas in which adolescents must make gains to successfully achieve a sense of identity are:

1. Accepting their changed body image
2. Establishing a value system or what kind of person they want to be
3. Making a career decision
4. Becoming emancipated from their parents

If young persons do not achieve a sense of identity, they develop a sense of **role confusion** or can have little idea what kind of person they are (Erikson, 1993). This can lead to their having difficulty achieving effectively as adults, because they are unable, for example, to decide what stand to take on a particular issue or how to approach new challenges or situations. Some adolescents may become delinquent or exhibit acting-out (attention-getting) behavior, because they believe it is better to be socially unacceptable than to be nobody at all. Those who do not develop a sense of intimacy at the end of adolescence have difficulty forming long-term relationships.

Body Image. Adolescents who developed a strong sense of industry during their school-age years have learned to solve problems and are best equipped to adjust to their new body image. Nurses who care for adolescents can do much to educate them about their bodies and help them to accept the changes that mark maturity. Some adolescents, for example, are disappointed with their final height; they had hoped to be 6 ft in height and are only 5 ft, 6 inches tall. In other instances, they have seen themselves as ugly ducklings and dreamt they would emerge as beautiful swans. They are depressed to find, at the end of adolescence, that they have not turned into the image they fantasized. Adolescents are usually their own worst critics, never pleased with any aspect of their bodies. Those with low self-esteem may need parental or health care provider support to understand that a person's worth is based on more than physical appearance. They may need help to realize that the characteristics that make someone creative, compassionate, and fun to be with are the qualities on which lasting relationships are built.

Help parents understand how important it is for adolescents to have immediate successes such as making the high school basketball team or having a date for the senior prom. Parental comments, such as "When you're older, these things won't be so important," are not likely to erase the hurt that comes from being 16 years old and not being included in such major events. Compassionate understanding ("It's hard to be left out") is a better communication technique.

Self-Esteem. Like body image, self-esteem may undergo major changes during the adolescent years and can be challenged by *all* the changes that occur during adolescence, including:

- Changes in one's body and physiologic functioning
- Changes in feelings and emotional focus
- Changes in social relationships (including relationships with both family and friends)
- Changes in family and school expectations

All of these factors can have an effect on the adolescent's feelings about himself or herself, sometimes resulting in crisis.

In recent years, a number of researchers have looked at the differences in the way boys and girls handle these emotional crises of adolescence. Several researchers have proposed that adolescence is a period of particular crisis for girls who are trying to find a place in a male-dominated society. The psychologist Carol Gilligan and her colleagues interviewed more than 500 girls between the ages of 7 and 16 over a 5-year period and found that many girls who, at age 11, were feisty, confident, and eager to speak their minds, became, by early adolescence, hesitant to voice their opinions aloud, having pushed their earlier resistance "underground" (Gilligan, 1982). Gilligan ties this change to a growing realization among girls during adolescence that their forthrightness may not be appealing to boys; they begin to self-censor, hoping to become more popular. At the same time, girls are expected to grow up and to value independent and academic (or athletic) success over close relationships, a situation that conflicts with the girl's need to maintain personal connections. This scenario presents a double-edged sword for the developing adolescent whose concern with relationships is not valued by others and who can no longer necessarily rely on her former outspokenness to get across her concerns and opinions.

Although the turmoil of adolescence can be just as confusing to boys as it is to girls, Gilligan hypothesizes that there may be less pressure on boys, who may have already learned to be competitive, independent, and separated from feelings. Gilligan describes the rearing of boys as including separation from emotions and feelings at an earlier age, whereas girls are encouraged to maintain their concern for people throughout their childhood. Girls are thus at risk for more conflicting feelings throughout adolescence.

Parents can help their adolescent girls deal with these conflicts by encouraging them to maintain their honesty and forthrightness. According to Gilligan, however, this option puts the adolescent at risk for criticism from other adults. The cost of going underground, by repressing one's views and feelings, may, however, be higher. Long-term psychological problems, notably eating disorders, which by some statistics are said to affect as many as one in five women in the United States, may be one unfortunate result of such repression.

Value System. Adolescents develop values through talking to peers. They also need an attentive adult ear, someone who will listen to their fears, hopes, dreams, and the pressure they feel to be somebody, the pressure of wanting to do something and yet not knowing what or how.

In early adolescence, girls tend to band together with girls and boys with boys. They dress identically with other members of the group: jeans and sweatshirts, special jackets, or whatever the fashion may be. On the surface, this makes adolescents appear to be losing their identities rather than finding them (Figure 32-3). Adolescents who are considered to be different for whatever reason (e.g., they are overweight or they come from a different socioeconomic, racial, or cultural background) often are excluded from groups in the same way that they were from clubs as 9-year-olds. This behavior may seem immature, but, like banding together, it is a necessary way for adolescents to establish a sense of identity. They know they are like the rest of the group because they dress, talk, and think the same way and go to the same places. They also know they are not like the excluded member. Knowing who they are *not* is one step in discovering who they are.

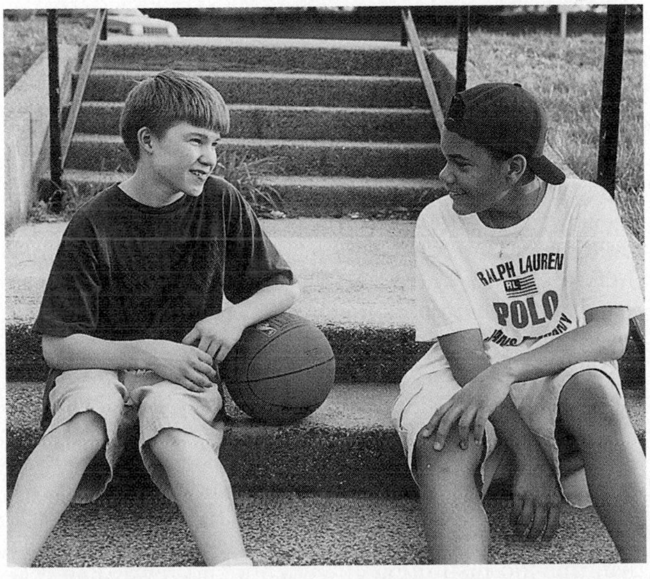

FIGURE 32.3 Adolescents have a need to interact with peers to learn more about themselves and others.

Helping adolescents to appreciate it is not fair to exclude others on the basis of superficial characteristics helps them move more quickly through this stage.

Some parents may be concerned about an early adolescent's lack of interest in the opposite sex. Occasionally, they worry about an intensely close girl-girl or boy-boy relationship. Teach parents that adolescents must feel secure and pleased with their own sex before they can relate comfortably to the opposite sex.

Career Decisions. Part of the feeling of knowing what kind of person you are is knowing what kind of job you can do. Because of the varieties of opportunities available, making a career decision can be difficult.

Many adolescents are encouraged to wait until they have been in college for 2 years before choosing a major. This delay may be an advantage because of the wide range of available options. It delays settling on a concrete goal until about 20 years of age, however, and therefore puts off a choice that strengthens the adolescent's sense of identity. Some school-age children do poorly in school during preadolescence, but, as adolescents, show increased interest in learning as they select a job field at the high school level and come to see education as relevant to their future.

Emancipation From Parents. Emancipation from parents can become a major issue during the middle and late adolescent years for two reasons. Some parents may not yet be ready for their child to be totally independent, and some adolescents may not yet be sure that they want to be on their own. They may fight bitterly for a right—for example, to stay out until midnight or later on a weekend—then never use the privilege once they have gained it. Winning the battle was more important than exercising the newly won right.

In some instances, the closer the tie that adolescents feel with their parents, the more severe is their struggle. Because they love and feel loved, severing bonds is difficult. As long as parents are reasonable in their restrictions, the amount of noise being made is proof that the ties are strong and that separation or emancipation is not easy.

Encourage parents to give adolescents more freedom (e.g., allowing them to buy their own clothes, use their own judgment about allotting time for studying, choose their friends, join clubs, or choose after-school activities); at the same time, help parents continue to place some restrictions on adolescent behavior (e.g., "You must drive the car safely or you can't use it," "You must continue to take responsibility for household chores," "We must know where you go after school."). These are not unreasonable rules and actually help adolescents accept the responsibility that must come with independence.

Help parents make emancipation a gradual reeling-out process. Some parents err on one side or the other, either by neglecting to let out the line at all until adolescents, feeling trapped, have no other choice but to break free and swim away; or letting it all out at once, leaving adolescents to flounder because they cannot yet swim effectively on their own.

In some instances, friction and misunderstandings arise because the parents had such traumatic experiences as adolescents that they fear seeing their children reach this stage. Their own experiences may cause them to react so strongly that they are unable to discuss anything with their children. Adolescents then often feel they have offended the parents in some way. They do not understand that the parental attitudes are based not on anything they may have done, but on old, unresolved conflicts that are being brought to the surface. In other instances, parents may view adolescent growth as threatening. Seeing their adolescent grow up may make them feel old or, if a marriage is not strong, fear that once their child becomes independent they no longer need to stay together. They may strive to keep their child immature (thus producing conflict) in an effort to keep these thoughts from entering the corners of their minds.

Both parents and adolescents may need help to understand that emancipation does not mean severance but a change in a relationship. People who are independent of one another can have even better relationships than those who are dependent on one another. This step is actually no different from the one children accomplished when they grew from infants to toddlers, when they changed from wanting to be held and rocked to wanting to run. If parents can think of it in this light, they will gain a better perspective and may begin to see that they will continue to like their children as independent adults.

By the time children are 18 years of age, they have survived leaving high school. They are in college or have found a beginning job and have begun to manage their own lives, perhaps even their own apartment. They are like swimmers who have discovered that the water is not as cold as they thought it would be.

Many 18-year-old adolescents so enjoy their new independence that they find it difficult to understand why adulthood is thought to be challenging. A little more maturity will help them to realize that initial success as an independent young adult does not necessarily guarantee additional success, that beginning adult life may be far easier than the years ahead.

Sense of Intimacy. Once adolescents have achieved a sense of identity in early or midadolescence, they are ready to work on a second development task, that of achieving a sense of intimacy (Erikson, 1993). The ability to form intimate relationships is strongly correlated with the sense of trust, the first developmental task in infancy. Infants who are unable to form a sense of trust may be unable to relate to others on a deep enough level to form lasting and close relationships as adults. Conversely, adults unable to gain a sense of intimacy may be unable to foster a sense of trust in an infant.

Some adolescents require help from parents or other adults to differentiate between sound relationships and those that are based only on sexual attraction. Never do adolescents need an adult to listen to them more than when they are struggling with the heart-rending feelings of young love or wondering whether a particular love relationship is temporary or lasting. It helps to put this into perspective if parents or health care personnel who counsel adolescents remember that first love is such an intense emotion, it physically hurts.

Some parents may not be able simply to listen without interjecting their own opinions, because they worry that love between adolescents may involve a sexual relationship. Parents should feel an obligation to inform their children of their feelings about adolescent sexual relationships. They also should be realistically aware that some adolescents will not follow their advice. Rates of teenage pregnancy and sexually transmitted diseases, including human immunodeficiency virus (HIV), are high and still rising. If parents suspect that their adolescent is sexually active, they must make sure their child is knowledgeable about safer sex practices (see Box 4-3 for guidelines regarding safer sex; see Chapter 17 for a discussion of adolescent pregnancy).

Some adolescents may believe that intense sexual yearnings or peer pressure can only be alleviated by a sexual act. They can be reassured that they are pleasant people to be with because of the many fine qualities they possess and that sexual intercourse can be delayed until two persons have come to know these qualities in each other and have made a mutual commitment based on a deeper level than simply physical passion.

Intimacy involves this deeper level of relationships or developing a sense of compassion or concern for other persons. It means being able to discern when words will hurt, when a companion is unhappy and needs encouragement, or when a friend is floundering and needs support.

In our busy modern society in which adolescents can engage in such a variety of activities, they may need help learning how to project themselves into another person's situation and to ask themselves how the world looks from that position. This ability, *empathy*, is feeling for another or a developed sense of intimacy in its finest form.

✔ CHECKPOINT QUESTIONS

3. What are the four tasks adolescents must achieve to gain a sense of identity?
4. Why do early adolescents often dress and act alike?
5. What should parents do if they suspect their adolescent is sexually active?

Socialization

Early teenagers may feel more full of self-doubt than self-confidence. They want to look grown up, but they still look like children. The voices of most boys have not yet dependably deepened; thus, they cannot trust their voices to carry the serious tone they wish to convey. Most girls' bodies have not yet fully developed; they may look at themselves in a mirror and compare their profiles with those of girls in popular magazines and feel inadequate.

Both male and female 13-year-old adolescents tend to be loud and boisterous, particularly when peers of the opposite sex whose attention they would like to attract are nearby. They are impulsive and very much like 2-year-old children in that they want what they want immediately, not when it is convenient for others.

Many 13-year-old adolescents fall "in love." At this age, however, they may spend more time longing for someone than they do instituting an in-depth and rewarding relationship. They have too little experience with life, too limited a frame of reference yet to know how to offer a deep commitment to another or accept one from that person.

Fourteen-year-old adolescents are often quieter and more introspective than they were the year before. They are becoming used to their changing bodies, have more confidence in themselves, and feel more self-esteem.

Adolescents watch adults carefully during this period, searching for good role models with whom they can identify. They usually have a hero—a film star, writer, scientist, doctor, or athlete—whom they want to grow up to be like. Fourteen-year-old adolescents often form a friendship with an older adolescent of the same sex, trying to imitate that person in everything from thoughts to clothing. If the older adolescent has dropped out of school or plays a particular sport, the younger person may express a wish to drop out or train for the idealized sport too.

Idolization of famous people or older adolescents fades as adolescents become more interested in forming reciprocal friendships. Attachments to older adolescents are often severed abruptly and painfully as the older teenagers make it clear they are more interested in being with people their own age. Rejection by an older member of a pair forces the younger member to turn to own-age friends and ends the intense hero worship so typical of early adolescence.

Most 15-year-old adolescents fall in love five or six times a year. However, many are sexually attracted because of physical appearance, not because of inner qualities or characteristics that are necessarily compatible with their own. Because infatuation is fleeting, it can lead to extremely intense but brief attachments that fade once the two young people discover that they really have little in common. However, falling in love this often does not mean their feelings are any less strong or that they feel any less pain when the relationship ends (Fig. 32-4).

By age 16, boys are becoming sexually mature (although they continue to grow taller until about 18 years of age). Both sexes are better able to trust their bodies than they were the year before. By age 17, they tend to be quieter and thoughtful about interactions. They have left behind the childish behaviors they used in early adolescence—shoving and punching—to get the attention of the opposite sex.

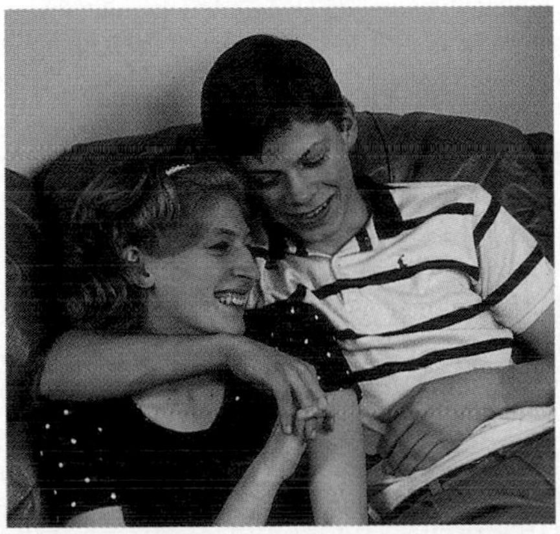

FIGURE 32.4 Although love can be fleeting, adolescents may feel intensely for each another.

Cognitive Development

The final stage of cognitive development, the stage of **formal operations,** begins at age 12 or 13 years and grows in depth over the adolescent years (Piaget, 1969). This step involves the ability to think in abstract terms and use the scientific method to arrive at conclusions. The problems that adolescents are asked to solve in school depend on this type of thought (eg, a boy rowing upstream at 5 miles per hour against a current of 2 miles per hour will go how far in 1 hour?). Problem solving in any situation depends on the ability to think abstractly and logically.

With the ability to use scientific thought, adolescents can plan their future. They can create a hypothesis (What if I go to college? What if I don't go to college?) and think through the probable consequences. Thinking abstractly is what allows adolescents to project themselves into the minds of others and imagine how others view them or their actions (display compassion).

Moral and Spiritual Development

Because adolescents enlarge their thought processes to include formal reasoning, they are able to respond to the question, "Why is it wrong to steal from your neighbor's house?" with "It would hurt my neighbor by requiring him to spend money to replace what I stole," rather than with the immature response of the school-age child, "The police will punish me." Some adolescents, however, may have difficulty envisioning a department store or a large corporation as capable of suffering economic loss from stealing, a concept that may contribute to the frequent practice of petty shoplifting at this age.

Almost all adolescents question the existence of God and any religious practices they have been taught (Kohlberg, 1984). This questioning is a natural part of forming a sense of identity and establishing a value system at a time in life when they draw away from their families.

> ✔ **CHECKPOINT QUESTIONS**
>
> 6. What is the final stage of cognitive development?
> 7. Why doesn't formal reasoning protect adolescents from shoplifting?

PLANNING AND IMPLEMENTATION FOR HEALTH PROMOTION OF THE ADOLESCENT AND FAMILY

Promoting Adolescent Safety

Accidents, most commonly those involving motor vehicles, are the leading cause of death among adolescents. Although teenagers are at the peak of physical and sensorimotor functioning, their need to rebel against authority or to gain attention leads them to take foolish chances while driving, such as speeding or driving while intoxicated.

In the interest of the adolescent's safety and that of others, parents need to have the courage to insist on emotional maturity rather than age as the qualification for obtaining a driver's license. Encourage adolescents to take driver education courses to learn not only the techniques of driving but also a sense of responsibility toward others. The use of seat belts should be mandatory. Adolescents tend to dismiss seat belts as childish, and they need convincing that it is only sensible to use every precaution available when in a motor vehicle.

Equally dangerous for adolescents are motorcycles, motorbikes, and motor scooters, which are appealing because of their low cost and convenience in parking. Both drivers and riders should wear safety helmets to prevent head injury; long pants to prevent leg burns from exhaust pipes; and full body covering to prevent abrasions in case of an accident. Adolescents who choose these forms of transportation should be as familiar with safety rules as automobile drivers. They should be prevented from driving motorcycles or scooters until they are emotionally mature enough to use sound driving judgment.

Drowning is another chief accident of adolescence, even though it is largely preventable. Teaching all children to swim is not the only preventive measure, because some drownings occur when good swimmers go beyond their capabilities on dares or in hopes of impressing friends. Teaching water safety, such as not swimming alone or when tired, is as important as teaching the mechanics of swimming.

The second most common cause of death in adolescents is homicide, related to the easy accessibility of guns to teenagers. Gang violence and the desire to protect themselves from this add to this problem. Accidental gunshot injuries increase in early adolescence, often for the same reason that drowning increases: youngsters want to impress friends. Some teenagers play gunshot Russian roulette to prove to their friends that they are courageous. Both water and firearm safety must be taught creatively to adolescents by encouraging problem solving rather than lecturing, because they tend to rebel against such lectures or claim that they have heard it all before.

Athletic injuries tend to occur during adolescence because of the vigorous level of competition that occurs. In early adolescence, overuse injuries result from poor conditioning. Athletic injuries are discussed in Chapter 51. Health teaching measures to prevent accidents and athletic injuries are summarized in Focus on Family Empowerment.

Promoting Nutritional Health for the Adolescent

Adolescents experience so much growth that they may always feel hungry (Fig. 32-5). If adolescents' eating habits are unsupervised, they will tend to eat faddish or quick snack foods rather than more nutritionally sound ones. Some adolescents may turn away from the five pyramid food groups to eat great quantities of sweets, soft drinks, or empty-calorie snacks, which leaves them poorly nourished despite the large intake. One form of rebellion is to refuse to eat foods parents believe are good for them. Parents who stock their kitchens with more nutritious foods, always keeping plenty of milk, and healthy snacks such as fruit and vegetables on hand, and who are willing to meet their adolescents halfway in terms of food preferences (e.g., serving pizza once a week) will be more certain their child is eating nutritious foods during the day. Giving the adolescent some responsibility for food planning or meals (eg, making dinner every Wednesday night) may teach some important lessons about nutrition without conflict.

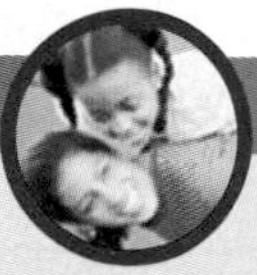

FOCUS ON FAMILY EMPOWERMENT

Measures to Prevent Accidents in Adolescents

Q. My adolescent doesn't always use mature judgment. How can I keep her safe from accidents?

A. Teach the following points:

Accident	*Health Teaching Measure*
Motor vehicle	Use a seat belt whether as a driver or passenger. Do not drink alcohol while driving, and refuse to ride with anyone who has been drinking. Wear helmet and long trousers as driver or passenger on a motorcycle. Accepting dares has no place in safe driving. Take a driver education course to learn safe driving habits for both two-wheel and four-wheel vehicles.
Firearms	Always consider all guns loaded and potentially lethal. Learn safe gun handling before attempting to clean a gun or hunt.
Drowning	Learn how to swim. Follow safe water rules, such as never swimming alone, no diving into shallow end of swimming pools, no hyperventilating before swimming under water, no swimming beyond own limit. Taking dares has no place in water safety.
Sports	Use protective equipment, such as face masks for hockey, pads for football. Do not attempt participation beyond physical limits. Careful preparation for sports through training is essential to safety. Recognize and set own limit for sports participation.

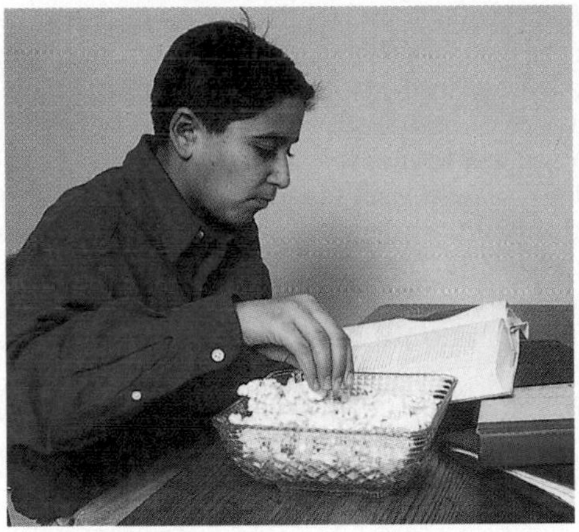

FIGURE 32.5 Adolescents experience rapid physical growth; typically, they are always hungry.

Adolescents who are slightly obese because of prepubertal changes may begin low-calorie or starvation diets to lose excess weight. Some develop eating disorders such as bulimia or anorexia nervosa (see Chapter 54). A weight-loss diet may be appropriate during adolescence, but it must be supervised to ensure that the adolescent consumes sufficient calories and nutrients for growth. For example, many adolescents omit breads and cereals entirely to lose weight rather than just reducing the amounts they consume. Diets such as these may be deficient in thiamine and riboflavin.

Recommended Daily Dietary Allowances

An adolescent needs an increased number of calories to maintain a rapid period of growth. As shown in Appendix E, males grow more than females during this period. One of the most important things adolescents can learn is that just filling their stomachs will not provide adequate nutrition. Foods that supply the necessary carbohydrates, vitamins, protein, and minerals are essential.

The nutrients that are most apt to be deficient in both male and female adolescent diets are iron, calcium, and zinc. Large amounts of iron are necessary to meet expanding blood volume requirements. Females require a high iron intake not only because of increasing blood volume but also because iron begins to be lost with menstruation. Girls with a heavy menstrual flow (menorrhagia) may need to take an additional iron supplement to prevent iron-deficiency anemia (see Chapter 44). Increased calcium is necessary for rapid skeletal growth. Good intake during adolescence is important to "stockpile" calcium to prevent osteoporosis later in life (Dudek, 2001). Zinc is necessary for sexual maturation and final body growth. Good sources of iron are meat and green vegetables; calcium is abundant in milk and milk products; meat and milk are also high in zinc.

Promoting Nutritional Health With a Varied Diet

Vegetarian Diets. Because vegetables generally contain fewer calories than meat, adolescents need to consume large amounts of them to achieve an adequate caloric intake with a vegetarian diet. Textured vegetable protein can be purchased and added to meals to increase the amount of protein supplied and help meet adolescent growth needs. Some adolescents may find it difficult to follow a vegetarian diet because it makes them different from their peers and limits foods they can eat at parties or at school, such as pizza, meat tortillas, or hot dogs. Whether to continue to follow this type of diet is a decision the adolescent must make as part of achieving a sense of identity. Be certain that adolescent vegetarians are following a sound diet and not only eating fruits and vegetables as a way to lose weight (Kolasa, Poehlman & Peery, 2000).

Glycogen Loading. Athletes need more carbohydrate or energy than do people who do not engage in strenuous activity, and the source of carbohydrate that best sustains athletes comes from the breakdown of glycogen because this supplies slow steady release of glucose. **Glycogen loading** is a procedure used to ensure there is adequate glycogen to sustain energy through an athletic event. Several days before a sports event, athletes lower their carbohydrate intake and exercise heavily to deplete muscle glycogen stores. They then switch to a diet high in carbohydrate. With the renewed carbohydrate intake, muscle glycogen is stored at approximately twice the usual level ready to supply twice the glucose for sustained energy. The effects of frequent glycogen loading are unknown, and it is not recommended for adolescents. As a rule, the goals of nutrition that are best for everyone, such as eating a well-balanced diet, are also the best rules for athletes, rather than diets that interfere with carbohydrate, fluid, or fat intake.

Promoting Development of the Adolescent in Daily Activities

Maintaining adequate nutrition to support rapid adolescent growth is essential to continued healthy development, as discussed above. Maintaining adequate sleep, hygiene, and exercise are also important and should become the adolescent's responsibility rather than the parents'. Parents can, however, encourage adolescents to engage in healthy patterns of living—primarily through role modeling.

Dress and Hygiene

Adolescents are capable of total self-care, and, because of their body awareness, they may even be overly conscientious about personal hygiene and appearance. They often wash their hair every day, but then grow dissatisfied because their hair has lost so much natural oil that it is dull and stringy. Both sexes try many types of shampoo, deodorant, breath fresheners, and toothpaste. They may take seriously (without admitting it) the content of ads showing toothpastes or deodorants helping to win an attractive person or instant success. Remember this when caring for hospitalized adolescents. Providing time for self-care, such as shampooing hair, is important to include in an adolescent's nursing care plan.

Adolescents are acutely aware of what their peers are wearing. When adolescents cannot trust or are disappointed in their bodies, it is very reassuring to be dressed exactly like everyone else. When they first begin to work, many adolescents spend their first paychecks entirely on clothing. This seems inappropriate to many parents; they want their child to learn to spend money on more lasting items or to show an interest in saving. Adolescents may have to mature fully, however, before they discover that the real person shows through the clothing.

Remembering how important clothing is for adolescents also helps you plan care for them during a hospitalization. Most teenagers seem to improve markedly when allowed to wear their own clothing rather than a hospital gown.

Care of Teeth

Adolescents are generally very conscientious about toothbrushing because of a fear of developing bad breath. They should continue to use a fluoride paste rather than a brand advertised as providing white teeth. They tend to snack a great deal, so their teeth are always exposed to bacterial erosion. Some may develop cavities for the first time during this period. Those individuals with braces must be extremely conscientious in toothbrushing to prevent plaque buildup on tooth surfaces.

Sleep

Although it is widely believed that adults need 8 h of sleep a night, some need more and others can adjust to considerably less. Protein synthesis occurs most readily during sleep. Because of this, adolescents need proportionately more sleep than school-age children to support the growth spurt during this time that demands the formation of so many new cells. In addition, because this is a stress period similar to first grade, adolescents may sleep restlessly as their mind reworks the day's tensions; sleep may not leave them feeling refreshed.

Many adolescents attempt to get by with too little sleep, because they are constantly busy and because staying up late is a symbol of the adult status they long for. Frequent lack of sleep can lead to chronic fatigue. Adolescents admitted to a hospital for even a minor illness may sleep as if exhausted for the day to make up for a chronic lack of sleep.

✔ CHECKPOINT QUESTIONS

8. What is the leading cause of death among adolescents?
9. What three minerals are most apt to be deficient in an adolescent diet?
10. Do adolescents need more or less sleep than school-age children?

Exercise

Adolescents need exercise every day to maintain muscle tone and to provide an outlet for tension. Although they are constantly on the go, they often receive little real exercise. They ride a bus to school, sit for classes, sit at a mall after school and talk to friends, sit and watch a basketball game in the evening. They have put in a full day from 7:00 in the morning until 11:00 at night, yet they have had little exercise compared with the amount they used to get when they came home from school and played tag or hide-and-seek for several hours before dinner. Adolescents who have had an injury and must learn an activity such as crutch walking should do muscle-strengthening exercises at first, just as adults must.

Adolescents who are involved in structured athletic activities do receive daily exercise. If they have not participated in competitive sports before, however, they may need advice on increasing exercise gradually so they do not overdo and consequently develop muscle sprains or other injuries.

WHAT IF? What if an adolescent who previously maintained a daily exercise program is hospitalized? In what ways could such a program be continued?

THE NURSING ROLE IN HEALTH PROMOTION OF THE ADOLESCENT AND FAMILY

Promoting Healthy Family Functioning

Early adolescents may have many disagreements with parents that stem partly from wanting more independence and partly from being so disappointed in their bodies. It is frustrating for children to be told by parents that they are too old to behave in a certain manner when they still don't feel or look older. At other times, just when they begin to accept their maturing appearance, parents tell them they are too young to do something. It may be helpful to counsel parents to appreciate that, although it is not easy to live with a teenager, it is equally difficult to be the teenager. Box 32-1 highlights an appropriate outcome and interventions using the terminology identified by the Nursing Outcomes Classification (NOC) and Nursing Interventions Classification (NIC).

When a child reaches about age 15, parent–child friction tends to reach a peak. By age 15, adolescents have discovered from careful observation that most adults are far from perfect. The teachers they previously thought of as all-knowing are revealed to have very human shortcomings: they may not be able to answer every question; some may make it clear they do not have time for questions. Even a favorite coach may be discovered to be imperfect. School marks may slump as a reflection of this "fallen angel" syndrome.

Adolescents find even more fault in their parents and wonder how they can exist with their outdated ideas. They have trouble respecting parents who are so obviously imperfect. These adolescents may follow health advice poorly because they view health care personnel in the same light.

By the time they are 16 years old, adolescents generally become more willing to listen and to talk about problems. As a result, they may learn that adults are not as inadequate as they previously thought. Their parents, for example,

BOX 32.1

NURSING OUTCOMES AND NURSING INTERVENTIONS CLASSIFICATION: ADOLESCENT DEVELOPMENT

NOC: Child Development, Adolescence (12 to 17 years)

Child development, adolescence is defined as the miles of physical, cognitive, and psychosocial progression between 12 and 17 years of age (Johnson, Maas & Moorhead, 2000). Some specific indicators suggesting achievement of this outcome include the adolescent's ability to demonstrate the following:

- Practice of good health habits including responsible sexual behaviors and avoidance of alcohol, tobacco, and drugs
- Expression of comfort with own sexual identity
- Use of social interaction and conflict resolution skills
- Maintenance of good peer relationships with same and opposite gender
- Capacity for intimacy
- Increasing levels of autonomy including description of personal value system
- Use of formal operational thinking
- Development of academic goals
- School performance according to level of ability

NIC: Developmental Enhancement, Adolescent

Developmental enhancement, adolescent is defined as facilitating optimal physical, cognitive, social, and emotional growth of individuals during the transition from childhood to adulthood (McCloskey & Bulechek, 2000). Some important activities involved when implementing this intervention include:

- Encouraging active adolescent involvement in own health care decisions
- Screening for health problems
- Providing appropriate immunizations as needed
- Promoting personal hygiene and grooming, healthy diet, regular participation in safe exercise program, responsible sexual behavior including contraception as indicated, vehicle safety
- Enhancing communication and assertiveness skills
- Facilitating a sense of responsibility for self and others
- Encouraging nonviolent responses to conflict resolution, goal setting, social relationship development and maintenance, participation in school, and extracurricular and community activities
- Initiating referrals for counseling as needed

NIC: Parent Education, Adolescent

Parent education, adolescent is defined as assisting parents to understand and help their adolescent children (McCloskey & Bulechek, 2000). Some important activities involved when implementing this intervention include:

- Discussing earlier parent–child relationships and own parental discipline when parents were teenagers
- Teaching normal physiologic, emotional, and cognitive characteristics of adolescents
- Identifying normal adolescent developmental tasks and commonly used adolescent defense mechanisms
- Addressing effects of adolescent cognitive development on information processing and decision making
- Describing importance of power and control issues
- Teaching parents appropriate communication skills
- Discussing effects of adolescent separation from parents on spousal relationships
- Sharing strategies for managing adolescent's perception of parental rejection
- Identifying measures to assist adolescent to manage anger
- Teaching parents how to use conflict for mutual understanding and family growth
- Role-playing strategies for family conflict management
- Discussing limit setting including appropriate strategies
- Teaching use of reality and consequences as means to manage adolescent behavior

may not be exactly the kind of persons these adolescents might wish they were, but, generally, 16-year-old children can understand that adults are this way because they are, after all, only human. This changed perception does not mean that the adolescent of 16 is calm and quiet, free of parent–child discord. Adolescents may comprehend how hard it was for parents to get where they are, but they may not understand, for example, why they themselves are not allowed to stay out beyond midnight on weekends.

Seventeen-year-old adolescents who have stayed in school are usually high school seniors, and, for most, this year is likely to be stormy. Looking ahead to leaving a school system with which they have been involved since they were very young may give some 17-year-old adolescents a feeling of losing security. Even if going away to college or beginning a full-time job seems exciting, it may also be an unwelcome change from the people and routines that they feel so comfortable with to new contacts and new regulations that appear strange and even hostile.

The ambivalence that such feelings create makes 17-year-old adolescents difficult to understand. They like to see parents perpetuating family traditions: a vacation in an old familiar place, the house decorated for a holiday in the same way, or the traditional birthday meal. Parents should appreciate that clinging to security this way is not the step backward it may seem. Instead, this behavior may be the preliminary working through to a time of separation that will be a major milestone in growing up.

To prove that they are old enough to leave high school and to enter into a more mature college or work world, adolescents may experiment with drugs or alcohol, sometimes interpreting their use as the mark of being an adult.

Common Health Problems of the Adolescent

A health maintenance schedule for the adolescent period and the assessments to be included at visits are shown in Table 32-2 (American Academy of Pediatrics [AAP], 2001).

Hypertension

Hypertension is present if blood pressure is above the 95th percentile, or 127/81 mmHg for 16-year-old girls; 131/81 for 16-year-old boys for two consecutive readings in different settings (see Appendix G). Adolescents who are obese, are African American, eat a diet high in salt, or have a family history of hypertension are most susceptible to developing the disease. Prevention and management of hypertension are discussed in Chapter 41. All children over 3 years of age should have their blood pressure taken routinely at health assessments to detect this. This is particularly true for adolescents (AAP, 2001).

Poor Posture

Many adolescents demonstrate poor posture, a tendency to round shoulders and a shambling, slouchy walk. This is due in part to the imbalance of growth, the skeletal system growing a little more rapidly than the muscles attached to it. Poor posture particularly seems to develop in adolescents who reach adult height before their peers. They slouch to appear no taller than anyone around them. Girls,

TABLE 32.2 Health Maintenance Schedule, Adolescent Period

AREA OF FOCUS	METHODS	FREQUENCY
Assessment		
Developmental milestones	History, observation	Every visit
Growth milestones	Height, weight plotted on standard growth chart; physical examination	Every visit
Hypertension	Blood pressure	Every visit
Nutrition	History, observation; height/weight information	Every visit
Hypercholesterolemia	Total cholesterol and triglycerides	During adolescence for children with family members with the disorder
Parent–child relationship	History, observation	Every visit
Behavior or school problems	History, observation	Every visit
Vision and hearing disorders	History, observation	Every visit
	Formal Snellen or Titmus testing	At 15 and 18 years
	Audiometer testing	At 15 and 18 years
Dental health	History, physical examination	Every visit
Scoliosis	Physical examination	Every visit to 16 years
Thyroid	Physical examination, history	Every visit
Tuberculosis	PPD test	Depending on prevalence of tuberculosis in community
Bacteriuria	Dipstick	Annually if sexually active
Anemia	Hematocrit or hemoglobin	Annually for menstruating females
Cervical or vaginal cancer	Pap test, pelvic examination	Every 1 to 3 years for sexually active females
Sexually transmitted diseases	History, observation	Every visit if sexually active
Immunizations		
Tetanus & diphtheria (Td)	Check history and past records; inform caregiver about any risks and side effects; administer vaccine in accordance with health care agency policies	At 10 years since last booster
Hepatitis B, MMR and varicella		If not previously immunized
Anticipatory Guidance		
Adolescent care including violence and nutrition counseling	Active listening and health teaching	Every visit
Expected growth and developmental milestones before next visit	Active listening and health teaching	Every visit
Injury prevention	Counseling about street and personal safety	Every visit
Problem Solving		
Any problems expressed by caregiver during visit	Active listening and health teaching regarding cigarette smoking, drug abuse, school adjustment	Every visit

especially, may slouch so as not to appear taller than boys in the belief that males will only date females shorter than themselves. Girls may also slouch to diminish the appearance of their breast size if they are developing more rapidly than their friends.

Urge children of both sexes to use good posture during these rapid-growth years. Tall adolescents of both sexes are generally picked out by basketball or track coaches and thus may have the incentive, if properly guided, to maintain good posture. Assess posture at all adolescent health appraisals to detect the difference between normal posture and the beginning of scoliosis (lateral curvature of the spine; see Chaps. 33 and 51).

Body Piercing and Tattoos

Body piercing and tattoos are becoming a mark of adolescence. Both sexes have ears, lips, chins, navels and breasts pierced and filled with earrings, or tattoos applied to arms, legs, or their central body. These acts have become a way for adolescents to make a statement (I am different from you). Be certain they know the symptoms of infection at a piercing or tattoo site (redness, warmness, drainage, swelling, mild pain) and to report these to a health care provider if they occur. Caution them that sharing needles for piercing or tattooing carries the same risk as sharing needles for intravenous drug therapy.

Fatigue

So many adolescents comment that they feel fatigued to some degree that this can be considered normal for the age group. Because fatigue may be a beginning symptom of disease, however, it is important that it be investigated as a legitimate concern and not underestimated. The adolescent's diet, sleep patterns, and activity schedules should be assessed, because all can contribute greatly to fatigue. Take a careful history, noting when the fatigue began. A short period of extreme tiredness is more likely to suggest disease than a long, ill-defined report of always feeling tired.

If an adolescent's sleep and diet appear to be adequate, the activity schedule is reasonable (in an attempt to be popular, some adolescents take on a schedule that would exhaust three people) and physical assessment suggests no illness, then the fatigue may be of emotional origin. It can be a means of avoiding school, avoiding conflict with parents (when children appear ill, parents are more sympathetic), or avoiding social situations. Those who are understimulated by school may develop fatigue as a sign of boredom.

Blood tests may be indicated to rule out anemia and the infection that is so common in adolescents, infectious mononucleosis (see Chap. 43). If these are normal, teenagers can be assured that they are healthy and offered guidance to solve the problem with better diet, more sleep, fewer activities, and development of better problem-solving techniques to relieve tensions.

Menstrual Irregularities

Menstrual irregularities can be a major health concern of adolescent girls as they learn to adjust to their individual body cycles. Chapter 47 discusses these problems in detail.

Acne

Acne is a self-limiting inflammatory disease that involves the sebaceous glands that empty into hair shafts (the pilosebaceous unit) mainly of the face and shoulders. It is the most common skin disorder of adolescence, occurring slightly more frequently in boys than girls. The peak age for the lesions to occur in girls is 14 to 17 years; for boys, 16 to 19 years. Although not proven, genetic factors may play a part in their development. Cigarette smoking may also increase the number of inflammatory lesions.

Before the rapid increase in androgen secretion with puberty, the sebaceous glands that enter into hair follicles are small and relatively inactive, so acne is nonexistent. Changes associated with puberty cause acne to develop:

- As androgen levels rise in both sexes, sebaceous glands become active.
- Abnormal keratinization (cell growth) of the lining of the ducts occurs; this overgrowth obstructs the ducts.
- The output of sebum increases. Sebum is largely composed of lipids, mainly triglycerides.
- If all of the material formed cannot be eliminated to the skin surface due to the narrow gland ducts, the glands enlarge, and trapped sebum causes whiteheads, or closed **comedones**.
- As trapped sebum darkens from accumulation of melanin and oxidation of the fatty acid component on exposure to air, blackheads, or open comedones, form.
- Bacteria (generally, *Propionibacterium acnes*) lodge and thrive in the retained secretions, forming papules.
- Leakage of free fatty acid from triglycerides causes a dermal inflammatory reaction.
- If glands rupture, sebum is extruded into adjacent skin, which produces reddened inflammatory cysts.

Acne is categorized as mild (comedones are present), moderate (papules and pustules are also present), or severe (cysts are present). The most common locations of acne lesions are the face, neck, back, upper arms, and chest (Fig. 32-6). Flare-ups are associated with emotional stress, menstrual periods, or the use of greasy hair creams or makeup that can further plug gland ducts (Stoll et al., 2001). Lesions are less noticeable in summer months, probably because of increased exposure to the sun, which increases epidermic peeling, and the reduction of stress, possibly as a result of being out of school.

Assessment. Always ask adolescents at health assessments if they are troubled with acne and to what extent it interferes with their self-image. Inspect for facial, chest, and back lesions on physical examination.

Therapeutic Management. The goal of therapy is threefold: (1) decrease sebum formation, (2) prevent comedones, and (3) control bacterial proliferation.

External Medication. Medications that are applied externally peel away the superficial skin layer to prevent sebum plugs from forming and are sufficient if only comedones are present. The most frequently used over-the-counter medications contain benzoyl peroxide. A common

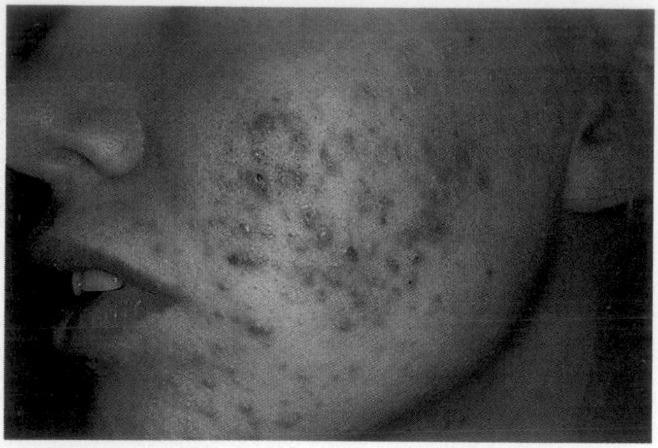

FIGURE 32.6 Facial acne in an adolescent.

prescription medication is tretinoin (Retin-A cream). This reduces keratin formation and plugging of ducts. Caution adolescents using a vitamin A cream to avoid prolonged sun exposure or to use a sunblock of SPF 15 or higher, because the preparation makes their skin more susceptible than usual to ultraviolet rays. Caution adolescents also that, for the first week or two of therapy, peeling or oxidizing may make the complexion actually appear worse rather than better. Topical antibiotic creams such as erythromycin and clindamycin may be prescribed to reduce the bacterial level on skin, but usually only after oxidizing agents have not succeeded; these creams may sensitize adolescents unnecessarily to antibiotics.

Systemic Medication. In pustular and cystic acne, systemic (oral) antibiotics are helpful. Tetracycline (500 mg twice daily the first week, then tapered to 250 mg daily for maintenance) is effective against the anaerobic bacteria that break down sebum to form irritating acids. Improvement is not generally seen for 2 weeks, so you may need to support adolescents to continue to take the medication during the waiting period. Without noticeable improvement, adolescents have a tendency to continue taking the higher dose or even increase the dose, hoping to initiate an effect. Tetracycline is not prescribed for children under age 12, because it can cause permanent staining of teeth and possibly interfere with growth of long bones. Because tetracycline may interfere with oral contraceptives, adolescent girls should use another method of birth control while on the antibiotic. Tetracycline should not be given to females who may be pregnant, because it causes faulty bone growth in a fetus (Karch, 2001).

Because food impairs the absorption of tetracycline, the drug should be taken on an empty stomach (2 h before or after eating). Adolescents must be certain of the date of expiration of the drug; outdated tetracycline breaks down into an extremely toxic composition. Females taking systemic antibiotics for long periods of time become very susceptible to developing candidal vaginitis and must be instructed about the symptoms of this: a white, pruritic vaginal discharge. Alternative antibiotics prescribed are erythromycin, minocycline, or clindamycin. Although these drugs avoid the complications of tetracycline, they may not produce the same results.

Isotretinoin (Accutane), a form of vitamin A, is an extremely effective oral drug for reducing sebum production and abnormal keratinization of gland ducts; it is prescribed for cystic acne (Honein et al., 2001; see Focus on Pharmacology).

Other Treatment Methods. If inflammatory reactions from acne are extreme, a corticosteroid such as prednisone or a nonsteroidal anti-inflammatory drug (NSAID) may be prescribed. Steroids must be used with caution in growing adolescents, because they can lead to stunted growth. Cortisone may be injected directly into cystic lesions to reduce them rapidly. This type of injection may reduce keloid formation, which is why it is usually reserved for adolescents who are prone to this permanent form of scarring.

Estrogen, alone or in combination with progesterone, suppresses sebaceous gland activity and is, therefore,

FOCUS ON PHARMACOLOGY

Isotretinoin (Accutane)

Action: Isotretinoin is a vitamin metabolite, which reduces sebum secretion.

Pregnancy Classification: X

Dosage: 0.5–2 mg/kg PO per day for a course of 15 to 20 weeks.

Possible adverse reactions: Nausea, vomiting, abdominal pain, skin fragility, dry skin, pruritus, rash, lethargy, insomnia, fatigue, headache, epistaxis, dry nose, dry mouth, cheilitis, eye irritation, conjunctivitis, elevated sedimentation rate, hypertriglyceridemia, white cells in urine, proteinuria, hematuria

Nursing Implications

- Drug is highly teratogenic (destructive to fetal growth). Girls should have a pregnancy test before treatment to be certain they are not pregnant. Suggest girls use a form of birth control to prevent pregnancy while on the drug and for 1 month afterward.
- Serum levels of both triglycerides and cholesterol and liver function studies should be obtained because both triglycerides and cholesterol serum are raised by the drug.
- Drug is extremely drying to skin; caution adolescents to discontinue all other acne medications during therapy to reduce this effect.
- Caution adolescents to continue to avoid sunlight or use a sunblock. If eyes become too dry, the use of contact lenses may need to be discontinued.
- Advise adolescents to take drug with meals to avoid gastric irritation.
- Adolescents with severe headache or visual disturbances should report these symptoms and the medication should be discontinued.
- Advise adolescents not to donate blood while taking the drug because of potential damage to the fetus of a recipient.

useful therapy in some girls. However, Isotretinoin is more often prescribed instead of estrogen for two reasons: (1) high estrogen levels tend to close epiphyseal centers of long bones causing bone growth to stop; (2) long-term therapy does have dangerous side effects, including embolism and thrombophlebitis.

Although acne may be treated, some degree of scarring may result. Laser therapy is a follow-up possibility to reduce the effect of scarring.

NURSING DIAGNOSES AND RELATED INTERVENTIONS

Nursing Diagnosis: Risk for low self-esteem related to development of acne during adolescence and lack of knowledge regarding treatment possibilities

Outcome Identification: Adolescent will express positive self-evaluation by next health maintenance visit.

Outcome Evaluation: Adolescent verbalizes positive aspects of self; states that acne does not affect positive self-image; or, if client admits to feelings of negative self-esteem, is able to discuss feelings and concerns about condition with nurse; describes ways to prevent or reduce acne outbreaks and states realistic short- and long-term goals of treatment.

It is important to respect what acne means to the adolescent. The actual extent of the condition often is not as important as an adolescent's feelings about it. When one's face is constantly covered by red marks, it is extremely difficult for an individual to feel good about oneself (see Focus on Nursing Care Planning).

When carrying out interventions, remember that acne is a potentially destructive disease that, if left untreated, can cause irreparable physical and emotional scarring. Therefore, parents and adolescents should be advised to seek medical treatment rather than self-medicate if the condition is severe. At the

FOCUS ON *Nursing Care Planning*

AN ADOLESCENT WITH ACNE

A 15-year-old male comes to the clinic for his yearly health maintenance visit. He states, "Look at my skin. It's horrible!"

Assessment: 15-year-old male with history of acne for the last 6 months. Reports washing his face approximately 5 to 6 times a day with abrasive soap and covering lesions with cocoa butter cream twice a day. "I don't eat chocolate. And even with all this, my skin is getting worse instead of better. I dread going to school, and forget about getting my picture taken. My mom says to just wait it out." Physical examination reveals scattered pustules and comedones on forehead and face, very prominent on nose and both cheeks. Two lesions on right cheek with large erythematous base and tender to touch. Remainder of physical examination unremarkable.

Nursing Diagnosis: Knowledge deficit related to cause and treatment for acne

Outcome Identification: Adolescent will verbalize accurate information about acne.

Outcome Evaluation: Adolescent states causes of acne; identifies measures for prevention and treatment; demonstrates appropriate skin care measures.

Interventions	Rationale
1. Assess adolescent's understanding of acne and its causes.	1. Obtaining a baseline knowledge assessment provides a foundation on which to build future teaching strategies.
2. Review the structure and function of the skin and sebaceous glands and development of acne. Clarify any misconceptions.	2. Reviewing and clarifying aids in learning and strengthening understanding.
3. Discuss treatment options available. Refer to dermatologic health care provider for evaluation and treatment.	3. Discussion provides the adolescent with information about the numerous treatment options available for acne, providing him with the opportunity for making informed decisions, thereby enhancing control over the situation.

(continued)

Interventions	Rationale
4. Instruct adolescent in measures to prevent and control acne, including twice-daily washing with mild soap and water; a healthy, well-balanced diet; avoidance of picking or squeezing lesions; and avoidance of greasy or oily skin preparations.	4. Daily washing removes irritating fatty acids; excessive washing can rupture glands and exacerbate acne. A healthy, well-balanced diet is essential for overall good health. Picking or squeezing lesions ruptures glands and spreads sebum. Greasy or oily skin preparations can plug gland ducts, increasing comedone formation.
5. Review treatment program prescribed. Assist adolescent with setting up a schedule for prescribed therapy. Caution adolescent that results of therapy are not immediate.	5. Reviewing the program aids in the adolescent's understanding, thus helping to promote compliance, which is essential for successful treatment.
6. Arrange for a follow-up visit in 2 weeks.	6. A follow-up visit allows time for evaluation, feedback, review of compliance, and further teaching.

Nursing Diagnosis: Self-esteem disturbance related to appearance from acne

Outcome Identification: Adolescent will verbalize positive feelings about himself by next health care visit.

Outcome Evaluation: Adolescent states impact of acne on appearance and feelings of self-esteem; actively discusses feelings and concerns; participates actively in care and treatment; reports some degree of control over the situation.

Interventions	Rationale
1. Attempt to identify the meaning of his appearance and acne to the adolescent.	1. Identifying the meaning assists in determining the degree of its possible effect on the client.
2. Encourage the adolescent to express feelings and thoughts about self, appearance, and acne.	2. Sharing of feelings and concerns permits a safe outlet for emotions and also aids in highlighting client's awareness of possible impact on self-esteem.
3. Review and reinforce with the adolescent positive attributes about self.	3. Positive attributes provide a foundation for rebuilding self-esteem.
4. Clarify any misconceptions he may have about acne.	4. Misconceptions can negatively impact self-esteem.
5. Assist with measures to prevent and control acne, encouraging independent role functioning and active participation in decision making.	5. Independence and ability to perform one's role promotes self-esteem; active participation enhances the feeling of control over situations.
6. Provide ample time for questions and concerns.	6. Providing time for questions and concerns helps clarify information, individualize information, and promote a feeling of control and trust.

same time, overconcern may lead to undue self-consciousness that affects performance in school and establishment of social relationships. Health teaching measures for the prevention and treatment of acne are summarized in Focus on Family Empowerment.

Obesity

Most overweight adolescents have obese parents, suggesting that both inheritance and environment may play a part in the development of obesity; the majority of such adolescents continue to be obese as adults. It can be difficult for adolescents to learn to like themselves (achieve a sense of identity) if they do not like their reflection in a mirror. It is equally difficult if they are always excluded from groups because of their weight. Some adolescents may be unaware that their food intake is excessive, because they have been told that they need excess nutrients for healthy adolescent growth and everyone in their family eats large portions. They may state that their friends are overweight but their own weight is all right, even though they are considerably overweight (Rand & Resnick, 2000). Health teaching with these adolescents needs to begin with a discussion of "normal" weight.

A reducing diet of fewer than 1,400 to 1,600 calories per day can rarely be tolerated by adolescents. Such a diet would provide insufficient protein and be deficient in vitamins. If adolescents eat a diet that is too low in protein for any length of time, they can develop an inadequate nitrogen balance, which can seriously impair their growth. They generally can adhere to a diet of 1,800 calories per day (Krebs & Hambridge, 2001).

FOCUS ON FAMILY EMPOWERMENT
Guidelines for the Prevention and Treatment of Acne

Q. I'm 16 and have had acne for the last 3 months. How can I make this go away?

A. Most adolescents have some acne. Try the following suggestions:

1. Diet does not influence the development of acne lesions. Eat a healthy, well-balanced diet for good general health.
2. Do not pick or squeeze acne lesions, which ruptures glands and spreads sebum into the skin, increasing symptoms. The times you are most likely to do this are during periods of stress, such as when you are taking a test. When you find your hand on your face, distract yourself with some other motion, such as interlocking your fingers.
3. Makeup, greasy hair preparations, or tight sweatbands can plug ducts of glands and increase comedone formation. Avoid these, if possible. Using medicated makeup both covers and helps lesions heal.
4. Topical acne preparations work by unplugging glands. You must use them consistently to make them effective. Plan enough time in the morning before school and a time in the evening to apply these. Post a chart by your bathroom mirror to remind yourself.
5. Washing daily to remove irritating fatty acids is helpful. Excessive washing is not necessary to prevent lesion formation. Excessive washing can actually harm healing by rupturing glands.
6. Oral medications work by reducing sebum secretions or preventing bacterial invasion. These only work if you take them conscientiously. Make a chart to post in your bathroom or kitchen to remind yourself to take these, also. Remember that tetracycline must be taken on an empty stomach or it is not effective.
7. If you are taking oral vitamin A (Accutane), do not take another source of vitamin A in a tablet. Accutane is very harmful to fetal growth. Take measures to prevent pregnancy while taking the drug and for 1 month afterward. If you should become pregnant while taking the drug, stop taking it immediately and notify your physician.
8. Both topical and oral vitamin A make your skin very sensitive to sunlight. Avoid long exposures to sunlight, or you will sunburn readily.
9. No acne medication works immediately. While you are waiting for lesions to heal, keep yourself occupied with a new activity (join a school club, try dancing lessons). When your skin is clear once more, these experiences will help make you an interesting person as well as one with clear skin.

NURSING DIAGNOSES AND RELATED INTERVENTIONS

Nursing Diagnosis: Ineffective individual coping by overeating related to stresses of adolescent period that have led to obesity

Outcome Identification: Adolescent will determine cause of stress and demonstrate healthy ways of dealing with it by 1 month.

Outcome Evaluation: Adolescent identifies stressful situations in life that lead to overeating; describes ways to avoid those situations or methods for coping with them.

Adolescents who are overweight because of stress need support until their pleasure in eating diminishes and their satisfaction with themselves as a "new" person or their friends' satisfaction with them can sustain them. They may have to visit a health care facility once or twice a week for encouragement and praise for their efforts. National weight control organizations are good if other adolescents also attend the meetings. They are ineffective if all the other members are adults because adolescents generally cannot relate to adult problems. It is important that the adolescent's self-esteem is maintained or the adolescent may switch to binge eating or such severe dieting that the opposite—extreme weight loss—occurs.

In addition to reducing calories consumed, encourage activities that use up calories, such as swimming or participation in gym classes and other school activities. Adolescents could perhaps walk to school rather than ride, or walk the dog for three blocks rather than one. These activities are generally preferable to formal exercises, such as sit-ups and push-ups, which can be viewed as punishment.

Adolescents who continually cope with stress by overeating rarely succeed in losing weight. They may require psychological counseling rather than diet counseling if they are to develop a more mature emotional response. Behavior modification is sometimes successful with adolescents as a means of helping them lose weight, but it is rarely recommended for obesity alone. If the obesity is causing serious body image problems, lowered self-esteem, and depression, behavior modification might be suggested (see Chapter 34).

Measures to help adolescents decrease overeating include:

- Making a detailed log of the amount they eat, the time, and the circumstances (including how they

felt while they were eating) and then changing those circumstances
- Always eating in one place (the kitchen table) instead of while walking home from school or watching television
- Slowing the process of eating by counting mouthfuls, putting the fork down beside the plate between bites; and being served food on small plates so helpings look larger

These measures may be of little use, however, unless they are combined with a suitable diet and adequate activities. Despite all these interventions, weight reduction may not always be effective with adolescents. For some, a more realistic goal might be to prevent additional weight gain until they reach adulthood.

Concerns Regarding Sexuality and Sexual Activity

Because of increasing exposure to and acceptance of premarital sexual relations in society, more adolescents than ever before engage in sexual intercourse. Because of this, as part of routine health assessment of adolescents and preadolescents, you should ask if they are sexually active.

Adolescents are usually interested in discussing this matter with a health care provider because they are concerned that they are exposing themselves to HIV infection or other sexually transmitted diseases and to pregnancy. At the same time, it is a difficult topic for them to discuss. Some adolescents may feel trapped into engaging in sex even though they are unwilling, because they perceive it as a way of having friends. Counseling can help them improve their perspective and learn how to say no. In contrast, some would like to be sexually active but are not, because they believe myths: early sexual relations will drain their strength and make them poor athletes; having sex too early in life will stretch the vagina and make sexual relations later on unenjoyable. Unless these falsehoods are explored through discussion, the adolescents who believe them may never be comfortable with sexual relationships.

Sometimes adolescents use a mild cold or a mild acne condition as a reason to come to a health care facility, where they hope that someone will stumble onto their real concern of sexual activity. After asking adolescents at health maintenance visits if they are sexually active, ask if they have any questions or problems they want to discuss with you about this. Ask if they are interested in learning more about contraception. Be certain they are practicing safer sex measures (see Chapter 4 and Box 4-3). Overall guidelines on counseling the adolescent with respect to sexual activity are summarized in Box 32-2.

Be certain to provide information on date rape and rape prevention as well, because adolescents are in a high-risk age group for date rape (Box 32-3; see also Chapter 52). Caution adolescents about the dangers of flunitrazepam (Rohypnol), a benzodiazepine, which is readily available. It is colorless, odorless, and tasteless, so, if it can be dropped into a drink, it can remain undetected. The effects are drowsiness, impaired motor skills, and amnesia (Karch, 2001). Adolescents who are seen for sexual assault who appear intoxicated or have amnesia for the event should be suspected of unknowingly ingesting flunitrazepam. In these instances, a urine specimen should be analyzed for the drug's metabolites. If a clinic does not have the ability to do this type of test, the manufacturer of the drug (Hoffmann-LaRoche Inc.) will assess for the drug.

BOX 32.2

HEALTH TEACHING GUIDELINES FOR ADOLESCENTS REGARDING SEXUALITY

1. It is your choice whether to participate in sexual relations. Do not be influenced by friends who may be exaggerating stories to impress you or who ask you for involvement you do not want. When you say no, be firm and clear about your wishes.
2. Pregnancy can occur with *any* sexual encounter unless you use some prevention to avoid it. Be direct with a sexual partner in discussing abstinence or birth control measures.
3. Sexual relations neither add to nor detract from your physical strength or general wellness.
4. The mark of an adult sexual relation is that the activity is pleasurable to both partners. If a sexual partner is not interested in your enjoyment as well as his or her own, you should reconsider the relationship.
5. There is no "normal" mode of sexual expression. Any activity that is pleasurable to both partners is normal.
6. Learn about safer sex techniques. Practice them (see Box 4-3).

Stalking

Stalking refers to the repetitive, intrusive, and unwanted actions directed at an individual to gain the individual's attention or evoke fear. The usual stalker is a male who stalks a female who has rejected him. Stalkers instill fear into their victims by the constant and threatening pursuit. In some instances, the stalker can resort to attacking the victim and even murder if further rejected.

Stalking behavior can begin in adolescents; adolescent girls may become victims (Davis & Frieze, 2000). It is difficult to prevent stalking because adolescents cannot evaluate when they first begin a relationship how it will end. Measures to help avoid being stalked are the same as those for avoiding rape, such as don't put themselves in positions where they will be vulnerable to being alone with a stalker, and report stalking to law enforcement officers so they can obtain a restraining order to prevent the stalker from any longer coming near them.

BOX 32.3

HEALTH TEACHING GUIDELINES FOR THE PREVENTION OF RAPE IN ADOLESCENTS

Home

1. Do not advertise that you stay alone while a parent works or is on vacation.
2. Ask for identification from meter readers or repairmen before admitting them into the home.
3. Insist on adequate lighting for hallways in an apartment building or around your own home.
4. Have your house key in your hand when you approach your door; do not stand fumbling for it by the doorway.
5. Keep your doors and windows locked when you are alone at home.

Car

1. Avoid isolated parking places; park near a building or in a lot with a parking attendant.
2. Lock your car when waiting in it and after parking it.
3. Look in the back seat before unlocking and entering your car.
4. Have your car key ready when you approach your car; do not stand fumbling for it.

Work or School

1. Do not enter an elevator with a stranger.
2. Lock the outside door, and do not admit people you do not know when working alone at night.
3. Ask for security protection to walk out to your car.
4. When going to and from school or work after dark, walk in the street rather than next to shrubs or dark buildings.

Dates

1. Be clear with your date that when you say no, you mean no.
2. Limit alcohol use because this can lead to risk-taking behavior.
3. Make it clear that you consider date rape the same as any rape and you would press charges.
4. Rohypnol is a sedative, known as a "date rape" drug. Do not date any individual who brags that he knows how to obtain it or use it.

Personal Actions

1. Do not wear chains around your neck that could be used to strangle you.
2. Learn self-defense; scratch the attacker to obtain skin and blood specimens under fingernails.
3. Be aware that an attacker could take any weapon away and use it on you; use caution carrying a weapon or Mace.
4. Fight or struggle cautiously to prevent harm to you beyond the rape itself. Actions such as kicking or gouging eyes may not be effective and may cause more violence.
5. If an attack occurs, observe the attacker's appearance as carefully as possible. Note identifying characteristics, such as a birthmark, scar, tattoo, words, or manner of speech, to be able to identify the individual later.
6. Press charges in court to make rape a crime of extreme magnitude and as an opportunity to fight back.
7. Work to provide rape prevention information and a united front against rape in your community.

✔ CHECKPOINT QUESTIONS

11. What type of infection are girls who take tetracycline for acne apt to develop?
12. What is the danger of a very low caloric diet for obese adolescents?
13. What are the effects of Rohypnol?

Concerns Regarding Substance Abuse

Substance abuse refers to the use of chemicals to improve a mental state or induce euphoria. This is so common among adolescents that as many as nearly 50% of high school seniors report having experimented with some form of drug. Drug use occurs in adolescence from a desire to expand consciousness or to feel more confident and mature; it also can be a response to peer pressure or a form of adolescent rebellion (see Focus on Evidence-Based Practice). This type of rebellion is more emotionally charged than acts such as staying out late or wearing clothes other than those approved by parents, because it is not only harmful but also illegal. Stages of substance abuse that have been identified are shown in Table 32-3.

Types of Abused Substances

Drugs that adolescents abuse are those that they can obtain on limited budgets and through limited contacts. They may take sedatives or pain medication prescribed for another family member or a pet. Many adolescents have a family member who is taking a pain medication, such as morphine, because of cancer therapy. Adolescents who steal these can easily overdose. Methylphenidate (Ritalin) is a drug frequently prescribed for attention deficit hyperactivity disorder. Prescribed as an oral drug, when Ritalin tablets are crushed and injected intravenously, they offer a feeling of giddiness and extreme well-being. Unfortunately, because they do not completely dissolve, the resultant small particles remaining in the bloodstream can result in pulmonary embolus or emphysema. Every house has a number of inhalants such as a spray-type oil for cooking or gas, butane, or lighter fluid that can also be abused

FOCUS ON EVIDENCE-BASED PRACTICE

Why Is Substance Abuse Attractive to Adolescents? Substance abuse can result in both immediate and long-term health risks. Knowing this, why do adolescents begin or continue substance abuse?

To see why adolescents use illicit drugs, researchers asked a sample of 364 adolescents who had used either alcohol, marijuana, amphetamines, ecstasy, LSD, or cocaine about their drug use habits. Results of this study showed that the most popular reason for using drugs was to relax (96%), become intoxicated (96%), keep awake at night while socializing (95%), enhance an activity (88%), and alleviate a depressed mood (86%).

This is an important study for nurses because nurses are often the health care professionals who conduct classes for adolescents on substance abuse. Knowing why drugs are appealing to adolescents can guide nurses in designing classes that will be most relevant and therefore, hopefully, most effective with this age group.

Boys, A., Marsen, J., & Strang, J. (2001). Understanding reasons for drug use amongst young people: A functional perspective. *Health Education Research, 16*(4), 457–469.

by adolescents. Abuse of inhalants can lead to cardiac failure even on a first use (Kurtzman et al., 2001).

Tobacco. Although it is well documented that cigarette smoking leads to increased cardiovascular and respiratory illnesses by middle age, as many as 20% of adolescents still smoke cigarettes. Adolescents usually begin smoking because the habit conveys a stamp of maturity; it may be viewed as especially desirable by those who are having difficulty demonstrating maturity in other areas. One of the strongest determinants of whether adolescents will begin smoking is whether their friends smoke. Although at one time proportionately more males than females smoked, adolescent girls now are the population most likely to begin smoking. As cigar smoking becomes more popular with adults, it also is becoming more popular with adolescents.

Most school systems have extensive programs as early as grade school that caution children against cigarette smoking. Unfortunately, the ultimate danger of illness or death in middle age is not a strong threat to young persons who are interested only in the present (Corbett, 2001).

More effective, therefore, might be campaigns that point out that cigarette smoking causes foul-smelling hair, clothes, and breath and thus detracts from physical appearance. Helping adolescents find other methods to demonstrate their maturity, such as allowing them opportunities for increased decision making, and emphasizing that being able not to smoke is a sign of true maturity may also be effective.

Remember that adolescents are very reluctant to follow instructions that are given from a "do as I say, not as I do" standpoint. Nurses who smoke, therefore, will have extreme difficulty launching an effective campaign against the habit with adolescents (Higgs et al., 2000).

Stopping smoking is especially difficult during periods of stress or inactivity. Trying to introduce such an action during exam week or the first week of summer vacation is not good planning. During an illness is also a bad time, unless not feeling well has reduced the urge to smoke. A return visit for follow-up and health maintenance care might be a better time to introduce the topic.

Adolescents can be urged to quit cigarette smoking through enrolling in a formal cigarette withdrawal program. Nicotine gum and nicotine patches have both been successfully used with adolescents.

Another source of nicotine that school-age children and adolescents may abuse is "smokeless tobacco," or chewing tobacco. Many baseball players use this form of tobacco, and adolescents who admire them may be particularly drawn to this tobacco source. Although chewing tobacco does not have the potential dangers of smoking tobacco in relation to lung disease, it can lead to lip and mouth cancer. It can be just as habit forming as cigarette tobacco.

TABLE 32.3 Stages of Substance Abuse

STAGE	NAME	CHARACTERISTICS
0	Preabuse	Curious about drugs, need for peer acceptance; anger or boredom
1	Experimentation	Learning the high; little behavior change except lying; commonly used drugs: tobacco, alcohol, and marijuana; use is confined to social situations on weekends in the company of others, with others supplying the drugs.
2	Early regular use	Adolescent actively seeks the drug-induced mood swing; drugs are no longer just on social occasion but to relieve everyday stress. Use is frequent and may be solitary, regularly on weekends and occasionally on weekdays. Adolescent has his or her own supply. Drugs used include stimulants, sedatives, and inhalants. Behavior changes include change in dress, friends, deteriorating school performance, mood swings, lying, and stealing.
3	Late regular use	Dependent on substance of abuse; deteriorating behavior, fighting, lying, stealing, prostitution; often depressed, suicidal ideation, self-destructive or risk-taking behaviors
4	End stage	Substance use to avoid dysphoria; withdrawal; continued deterioration of behavior and mental state

Muramoto, M. L., & Leshan, L. (1993). Adolescent substance abuse. *Primary Care, 20*(3), 141–144.

Alcohol. As many as 90% of high school seniors report having used alcohol. Despite the fact that its use is correlated with motor vehicle accidents, homicide, and suicide in adolescents, alcohol does not carry the stigma of many other drugs. Some parents are actually relieved when they realize that their child's strange behavior on returning home from a party is caused by drunkenness and not illegal drugs. Alcohol use cannot be taken lightly, because it is linked to diseases such as cirrhosis, cognitive challenge, and destructive behaviors such as driving while intoxicated, addiction, depression, and vulnerability to date rape.

Environment has a definite role in the use of alcohol. Heredity may play a part in whether the adolescent becomes addicted (Enoch & Goldman, 1999). Parents should be certain to set good examples for adolescents in the use of the drug and not drink indiscriminately.

Most adolescents will admit they use alcohol if asked two specific questions: (1) Do you think you have a drinking problem? and (2) When was your last drink? Adolescents who answer yes to the first and "within the last 24 hours" to the second need further assessment.

Once adolescents face the fact that they are alcohol dependent, organizations such as Alcoholics Anonymous are invaluable in helping them to stop drinking. Encourage the remainder of the family to join Al-Anon, the organization for families of alcoholics, so both children and families can restructure their lives to find satisfaction without the use of alcohol.

Many adolescents are not primary alcohol abusers but are the children of alcoholic parents. Make an effort to identify this group of children as well, not only to prevent them from becoming users of alcohol, but to help them build self-esteem and coping abilities for the difficulties they face living in a disorganized household.

Anabolic Steroid Abuse. Steroids are derivatives of the natural hormone, testosterone. Common names are stanozolol, an oral compound, and testosterone propionate, an injectable form. Adolescents take steroids (obtained illegally) with the thought that they will enhance lean body mass and muscular development and so improve their athletic ability or appearance. Steroids also have the side effects of euphoria and lessened fatigue, which make them doubly appealing (Midgley, Heather & Davies, 2001).

To obtain maximum effects, teenagers may take up to 30 times the therapeutic dose. This leads to adverse effects, such as early closure of the epiphyseal line of long bones, acne, elevated triglycerides, hypertension, aggressiveness, possibly psychosis, and abnormal liver function and perhaps liver cancer.

Students using steroids need to be identified so they can be cautioned that the use of such drugs is illegal in sports competition as well as being detrimental to their health. There is also concern that the use of such drugs serves as a gateway to additional drug use. If needles are shared, this can lead to hepatitis B or HIV infection.

Marijuana. Marijuana (widely known as *pot* or *grass*) is derived from the leaves and stems of the Indian hemp plant, *Cannabis sativa.* It is generally rolled into cigarettes ("joints" or "reefers") and smoked, although it can be mixed with food or sniffed. Scraping the resin from the flowering leaves produces a much stronger substance called hashish. *Sinsemilla* is a seedless form that is even more potent.

Breakdown products of marijuana are not readily eliminated from the body but remain in the fatty cells of the brain. This residue results in synaptic gaps that can delay electrical brain waves and memory storage. Physical and psychological effects of all forms of marijuana are euphoria and a sense of well-being, temporary impairment of coordination or motor activities, altered sensory perceptions, rapid mood swings, altered self-image, decreased attention span, and loss of memory for recent events (up to 1 h time). Withdrawal symptoms include irritability, drowsiness, and cravings for high-carbohydrate snacks.

Long-term side effects include pulmonary disorders such as sinusitis, bronchitis, emphysema, and perhaps lung cancer (these can develop after only 1 year of continual use compared with 20 years of use for cigarette smoking), and lack of sperm formation or infertility in males.

Despite its known dangers, marijuana is the most commonly used illicit substance, next to alcohol, in adolescents. Help adolescents realize that marijuana is more than an amusing leisure activity or a way to relieve stress so they can put its use into true perspective (Copeland, Swift & Rees, 2001).

Amphetamines. The amphetamines are a group of drugs sometimes used in the treatment of hyperactivity and narcolepsy, among other central nervous system disorders. They are easily manufactured in "meth labs" in people's homes so are readily available to adolescents. Amphetamines are called *uppers* or *speed* because they give the user a false sense of well-being, alertness, or self-esteem. A newer, stronger form that produces intense symptoms is known as *ice.* Some of the side effects that can occur are aggressive or demanding behavior, paranoia, and extreme restlessness. Because amphetamines suppress the appetite, adolescents may lose weight or eat only sporadically while taking them. Their use without a prescription is illegal (Baldwin, 2000).

Cocaine. It is difficult to document how many adolescents use cocaine, but estimates range from 3% to 9%. Common street names for cocaine are *snow* and *white lady,* because it is supplied as a fine, white powder that can be inhaled or injected. A stronger form, called *crack,* is manufactured by heating cocaine powder with baking soda and water. This preparation process is dangerous in itself because it involves using volatile solvents that can ignite or explode. The resulting crack, often called *free-base* or *rock,* is so strong it can cause immediate cardiac and respiratory arrhythmias.

Cocaine that is inhaled or smoked is absorbed through the mucous membrane into the bloodstream. After absorption, blood levels rise rapidly for the first 20 min, peak at 60 min, and then decline over the next 3 h. Although a toxic dose of cocaine is usually considered to be 600 to 700 mg, toxicity has been reported with as low as 20 mg (a single line).

Cocaine produces the physical effects of increased pulse and respiration rates, increased temperature, increased blood pressure, and decreased appetite. It can be a major cause of cardiovascular arrest in young adults (Hahn & Hoffman, 2001). Psychological effects produced are euphoria, excitement and restlessness, increased sociability, and possible hallucinations.

Toxic symptoms include seizures, tachyarrhythmias, tachypnea, hypertension, increased deep tendon reflexes, decreased response to stimuli, nausea and vomiting, abdominal pain, headaches, and chills and fever.

Cocaine is rarely ingested orally, but occasionally adolescents swallow it when trying to hide a supply from parents or school personnel. Gastric acid destroys the action of cocaine so that it is potentially harmless when swallowed this way. Cocaine has been swallowed in plastic pouches with the idea that it will pass harmlessly through the gastrointestinal tract packaged this way and be recovered later in stool. However, if peristaltic action in the intestine causes the bag to break, the cocaine is absorbed into the bloodstream at toxic levels. This can lead to sudden cardiac and respiratory arrest.

Teach adolescents that, although cocaine sniffing may be fascinating and offer temporary pleasure and relief from stress, it also causes psychological dependency and is potentially extremely dangerous because of its cardiac and respiratory effects. Chronic inhalation of cocaine can cause ulceration in the mucous membranes of the nose, and injection of the substance exposes the adolescent to the risk of HIV/acquired immunodeficiency syndrome (AIDS), hepatitis, and other diseases contracted through contaminated equipment.

Hallucinogens. Examples of hallucinogenic drugs are lysergic acid diethylamide (LSD), dimethyltryptamine (DMT), 2,5-dimethoxy-4-methamphetamine (STP), phencyclidine hydrochloride (PCP), and methaqualone (Quaalude). The use of LSD has increased substantially since the 1960s when it first became popular among young people, because it is a drug that can be manufactured by an informed adolescent in a "kitchen lab."

These drugs cause bizarre mind reactions such as distortions in vision, smell, or hearing. Adolescents report seeing colors more vividly than they have ever seen before, hearing sounds so clear they cause physical pain, and perceiving themselves as being totally impervious to harm.

The effect of such drugs can be extremely pleasurable (described as a "good trip") or extremely terrifying (a "bad trip"). Recurrences or flashbacks of drug-induced experiences may, unfortunately, recur at unpredictable times and in unexpected places. Such flashbacks are not only disconcerting but can be dangerous, especially if they occur while a person is driving a motor vehicle; they can be so frightening that some users believe they are becoming mentally deranged.

It is illegal to produce, sell, or possess hallucinogens in the United States. A hallucinogen related to mescaline, MDMA (known as *ecstasy*), was previously used by some psychotherapists to make patients more receptive to therapy. It has been added to Schedule I of the Controlled Substances Act because it was found to cause brain damage, and it is now illegal as all others (Arria et al., 2002).

Opiates. Opiates are drugs such as heroin, meperidine (Demerol), and morphine. At one time, they were not typically used by adolescents because they are expensive, but now they are gaining popularity among teens.

Opiates can be extremely dangerous because of their tendency to decrease respiratory rate. Addiction to opiates can cause such a physiologic craving that adolescents, like adults, will steal, defraud, turn to prostitution, or resort to whatever method available to secure enough money to buy a day's supply. In addition to the direct danger of opiates, adolescents who use them risk the danger of contracting HIV/AIDS and hepatitis B infection if they share contaminated needles. "Snorting" heroin can lead to acute cerebral vascular accident and death.

Methadone or LAAM (levo-methadylacetate) programs may be prescribed to help adolescents wean themselves from opiates. The users report to a center every day and receive an oral dose of methadone, which fulfills the same physiologic need as heroin. Methadone is a narcotic itself, but, because adolescents do not have to pay for it, they no longer have to steal or prostitute themselves to obtain it. It allows them to continue in school or hold a job and become productive citizens. Caution them that methadone overdose can occur the same as with any narcotic (Green et al., 2000). After a time, LAAM is gradually substituted for methadone. The advantage of LAAM over methadone is that its effect lasts longer—72 h rather than 24 h—so less frequent administration is necessary.

Assessment of Substance Abuse

If adolescents trust health care personnel who are giving them care, they will generally admit that they have engaged in drug experimentation (see Focus on Communication). Some common findings on the health history that suggest an adolescent is abusing some substance are:

- Failure to complete assignments in school
- Demonstration of poor reasoning ability
- Decreased school attendance
- Frequent mood swings
- Deteriorating physical appearance
- Recent change in peer group
- Expressed negative perceptions of parents

These are not necessarily diagnostic findings, however, because they can also be part of an adolescent's search for identity. Substance abuse can be strongly suspected in an adolescent who is hospitalized for hepatitis B or who is HIV positive and overly anxious to leave a facility, as well as one who appears to receive no benefit from the usual analgesic agents. General physical symptoms that indicate drug abuse are summarized in Table 32-4.

NURSING DIAGNOSES AND RELATED INTERVENTIONS

Nursing Diagnosis: Risk for injury related to the use of alcohol or illegal chemical substances

Outcome Identification: Adolescent will refrain from chemical experimentation by 1 month's time.

Outcome Evaluation: Adolescent states that he is not experimenting with drugs; can demonstrate a way to respond to peers who encourage such use; shows no evidence of drug use (such as lethargy, confusion, positive urine drug screen, or parental suspicion).

FOCUS ON COMMUNICATION

Brenda is an adolescent girl you see in an adolescent clinic.

Less Effective Communication

Nurse: Here's a pamphlet about adolescents and drug use. I hope you haven't been using any.
Brenda: No problem.
Nurse: Drugs can be really harmful. It takes an absolutely stupid person to do them.
Brenda: No problem.
Nurse: I want you to feel free to talk to me if you have been or are thinking about experimenting with drugs.
Brenda: No problem.
Nurse: Have you been doing any?
Brenda: No problem.

More Effective Communication

Nurse: Here's a pamphlet about adolescents and drug use. I hope you haven't been using any.
Brenda: No problem.
Nurse: Sometimes it's difficult for children to talk to parents or other adults about such things.
Brenda: No problem.
Nurse: I want you to feel free to talk to me if you have been or are thinking about experimenting with drugs.
Brenda: No problem.
Nurse: Have you been doing any?
Brenda: No problem.

Brenda answered with the same response in both conversations. Do you think she meant the same thing in both conversations? Was the nurse wise to announce that only stupid people use drugs and then ask if Brenda was using any?

In addition to any physical damage that substance abuse may cause, one of the greatest dangers of early drug experimentation is that it affects the adolescent's ability to solve problems, with a consequent delay in maturity. The adolescent may cling to peers to shield drug use and stay away from adults they are afraid might detect it, removing themselves from exposure to adult role models. It is important to help adolescents plan ways that they can feel satisfaction in life without substance use, such as how to feel secure enough to interact with others without relying on cocaine or marijuana, or how to accomplish activities to increase self-esteem so alcohol is not needed.

When establishing outcomes with adolescents who are chemically dependent, remember that it is difficult for them to appreciate how much they depend on a drug until they try to stop using it. A goal of not using a drug for 24 h at a time may be the only one possible at first.

Caution adolescents against substance abuse in the same way you would caution about the unwise use of motor vehicles or swimming beyond personal limits. Scare stories (soft drugs automatically lead to hard drugs, marijuana rots your brain, drug addicts are sex perverts) cloud the issue and make adolescents dismiss all advice given them about drugs as worthless.

To maintain a realistic approach to the problem, health care personnel and parents should counsel (not lecture) that substance abuse is both illegal and harmful but also remember how difficult it is for adolescents to say no to peer pressure. Important teaching points to preventing substance abuse are summarized in Box 32-4.

Therapeutic communities or 24-hour facilities in which adolescents can live while they recover from chemical dependency may be necessary for some adolescents. The aim of all these programs is to increase adolescents' sense of self-esteem, improve problem-solving ability, realign them with society's values, and increase their self-awareness so they can function normally without the aid of abusive substances. Unfortunately, campaigns against substance abuse for adolescents have not been very successful, so the problem continues. Adolescents who are no longer chemically dependent should be evaluated by a history and physical examination at all health care visits because, if the circumstances that initially caused them to become chemically dependent are repeated, they may return to a dependency pattern. A continuing relationship with health care personnel not only allows time for this evaluation but also provides concrete role models of nonchemical, productive behavior.

✔ CHECKPOINT QUESTIONS

14. What organization is used for referral to children of alcoholics?
15. What facial changes might you find in an adolescent using cocaine?

Concerns Regarding Attempted Suicide

Suicide is deliberate self-injury with the intent to end one's life. Successful suicide occurs more frequently in males than in females, although more females apparently attempt suicide than males (about 8:1). Adolescent suicides are attempted most often in the spring or the fall, reflecting school stress at these times of year, and between 3 pm and midnight, reflecting depression that increases with the dark. Suicide is so common in adolescents that it ranks third as a cause of death in the 15- to 19-year-old group. This statistic may actually be underestimated because some well-meaning coroners or physicians may report these deaths as accidents to spare the family additional pain.

Some automobile or hiking accidents may be attempts at self-destruction; in addition, some homicides may be caused by deliberately provoking another person in the hope of being killed. Incest, abuse, increased chemical dependency, marital instability in the family, and poor problem-solving ability are reasons that may lead an adolescent to the decision that death may be easier than coping with overwhelming problems. Drug and alcohol use

TABLE 32.4 Symptoms to Help Identify Drug Abusers

DRUGS USED	SYMPTOMS OF USE	DANGERS
Glue	Violence, drunken appearance, dreamy or blank expression Glue smears on clothing or fingers; tubes of glue, paper bags in possession	Lung, brain, or liver damage; death through suffocation or choking; anemia
Heroin, morphine, codeine	Stupor, drowsiness, needle marks on body, watery eyes, loss of appetite, bloodstains on shirt sleeve, runny nose Needle or hypodermic syringe, cotton, tourniquet string, burnt bottle caps or spoons, glassine envelopes in possession	Death from overdose; addiction; liver and other infections due to unsterile needles
Cough medicine containing codeine and opium	Drunken appearance, lack of coordination, confusion, excessive itching Empty bottle of cough medicine in possession	Addiction
Marijuana	Sleepiness, wandering mind, enlarged pupils, lack of coordination Strong odor of burnt leaves, small seeds in pocket lining, cigarette paper, discolored fingers	Psychological dependence
Hallucinogens (LSD, DMT, PCP)	Severe hallucinations, feelings of detachment, incoherent speech, cold hands and feet, laughing and crying, vomiting Possession of cube sugar with discoloration in center, strong body odor	Suicidal tendencies, unpredictable behavior; chronic exposure may have neurologic effects
Stimulants (amphetamine, cocaine)	Aggressive behavior, giggling, silliness, rapid speech, confused thinking, no appetite, extreme fatigue, dry mouth, shakiness, insomnia Pills or capsules of varying colors in possession; absence of nasal hair; possession of a glass pipe	Death from overdose; hallucinations; psychosis
Depressants (barbiturates, alcohol)	Drowsiness, stupor, dullness, slurred speech, drunken appearance, vomiting Pills or capsules of varying colors in possession; odor of alcohol on breath	Death or unconsciousness from overdose; addiction; seizures from withdrawal

BOX 32.4

HEALTH TEACHING GUIDELINES FOR THE PREVENTION OF SUBSTANCE ABUSE IN ADOLESCENTS

1. All chemicals are harmful to the body, at least to some extent (alcohol, for example, causes liver disease).
2. Relying on drugs to give you courage to solve problems (or help to forget you have problems) prevents you from learning to handle life situations and maturing.
3. The bottom line of drug abuse is that you have the final say: you are the only one who can stop chemical dependency from happening.
4. Whether a drug is inhaled, swallowed, or injected, it still is absorbed and enters your body.
5. Despite their social acceptability, alcohol and nicotine are drugs. A month of daily use of either can make you addicted.

may contribute to suicide by further impairing judgment (King, 2001).

Some degree of depression is present in most adolescents, because they are not only losing their parents at this time as they grow apart from them, they are also losing their carefree childhood. If school failure or loss of a friend or in a competition is superimposed on an existing depression, the pressure may be great enough to cause some adolescents to attempt suicide. Some other reasons for attempting suicide include anger with others, trying to get even, and manipulation (psychological blackmail) as a way of having one's needs met. Loss of a parent, of a girlfriend or boyfriend, of a community, or of self-esteem are all significant, which can serve as the trigger to suicide. Because some adolescents may be unable to believe that a parent was at fault in the case of divorce or that the death of a parent could not have been prevented, they believe, instead, that they somehow caused the parent to leave or to die. The loss of a girlfriend or boyfriend is particularly significant because it involves two types of loss: friendship and self-esteem. Rejection from a peer group, sports team, or school club may cause a similar loss of self-esteem.

Assessment

Adolescents need to have thorough physical examination at health maintenance visits to assure them they are in good physical health. Assess for signs of depression such as anorexia, insomnia, excessive fatigue, or weight loss. In younger adolescents, depression may be manifested by behavior problems such as disobedience, temper tantrums, truancy, and running away from home. Self-destructive behavior or accident proneness may be noted. Difficulties in school; acting out with chemicals, alcohol, or sexual promiscuity; or trouble with legal authorities may be further clues. Occasionally, depressed adolescents find it so hard to be alone that they seek constant activity as a means of escape. In contrast, others may withdraw from contact with other persons and become completely isolated. Either behavior may be detected through assessment of activity and interaction levels.

Adolescents who attempt suicide fall into no one category, although many tend to be loners or to have difficulty expressing their feelings to others and, therefore, do not receive emotional support from friends. Others are "perfect" students. The stress of trying to achieve continually at this level, however, is the trigger that provokes suicide. Gay and lesbian youth appear to have higher levels of suicide than others. Assess for these lifestyles as well.

If another member of a family or a close friend has committed suicide, the chance that an adolescent will do so is greater than usual, as adolescents see suicide as a method of coping and use it. The anniversary of a family member's suicide is an emotional time and may be especially difficult for an adolescent; wishing to join the dead family member appears attractive. When one adolescent in a high school commits suicide, there is a good chance that another will take similar action soon afterward. Adolescent suicide rates may actually reach epidemic proportions after a popular student's suicide.

Because suicide usually reflects a problem in family interaction, family assessment is helpful. A thorough family history may reveal conflict with one or both parents. Many adolescents express a desire to get even with them. "They'll be sorry when I'm dead" is frequently expressed. School friends may often be aware that an adolescent is contemplating suicide before the parents. Caution parents not to discount reports of friends who tell them they are concerned about their child. Close to the chosen time of suicide, some adolescents may demonstrate characteristic behaviors that show they are making preparations to end their life. Teach family and friends the typical danger signs (see Focus on Family Empowerment).

After an actual suicide attempt, ask enough questions on a health history so you know whether the adolescent made a detailed suicide plan. For example, a young person who took four aspirins and left the empty aspirin container conspicuously on the kitchen counter just before the mother was due to arrive home from work is more likely to be only crying for help; the one who took 100 aspirins and hid the container under the bed just after the mother left for 8 h of work is making a serious attempt. You may be the first person in a health care facility to realize that an adolescent talking about suicide is not "just talking" (it is a fallacy that people who talk about suicide do not attempt it) but has a definite, well-thought-out plan to accomplish it. The adolescent who has been admitted to a hospital unit after a serious aborted suicide attempt may formulate a new plan that will be successful the next time unless some action is taken and the adolescent's life can be changed in some way.

NURSING DIAGNOSES AND RELATED INTERVENTIONS

Nursing Diagnosis: Risk for violence, self-directed, related to symptoms of depression or expressed desire to hurt oneself

Outcome Identification: Client will not harm self; will demonstrate other means of solving problems by 1 week's time.

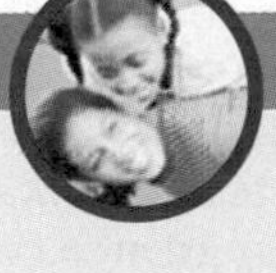

FOCUS ON FAMILY EMPOWERMENT
Suicide Warning Signs

Q. Our neighbor's son recently committed suicide. What are warning signs of this to look for in our son?

A. The following are commonly seen clues:

- Giving away prized possessions
- Organ donation questions, such as "How do you leave your body to a medical school?"
- Sudden, unexplained elevation of mood. Mood elevation may indicate that the individual has reached a decision about the suicide and feels relief.
- Accident proneness, carelessness, and death wishes
- A statement such as "This is the last time you will see me."
- Decrease in verbal communication
- Withdrawal from peer activities or previously enjoyed events
- Previous attempt (80% of all completed suicides have been preceded by a failed attempt)
- Preference for art, music, and literature with themes of death
- Recent increase in interpersonal conflict with significant others
- Running away from home
- Inquiring about the hereafter
- Asking for information (supposedly for a friend) about suicide prevention and intervention
- Almost any sustained deviation from the normal pattern of behavior

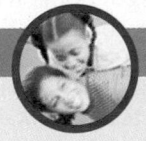

Outcome Evaluation: Client expresses feelings of depression to health care providers or other adults; states that she will contact support person should the desire to commit suicide become overwhelming.

Crisis intervention for adolescents who are contemplating suicide includes trying to alleviate their pain and depression and counseling them in an effort to help them change their perspective on the value of life. Be aware that establishing outcomes with adolescents who are contemplating suicide or who have made an attempt will be difficult because they are often too depressed to come up with an alternative solution to their problems (their goal is to kill themselves, not solve problems).

Try to find out the things in life that are still important to them; build a plan that will help them see that life is worth living enough to work through problems. Show them that no one can change everything, but everyone can make one or two changes that will make a difference. After these small changes are made, a domino effect can be created to change more and more of one's circumstances.

Because adolescents resort to suicide as a method of solving problems, helping them in this area is a prime intervention strategy. Ask them "what would happen if" questions. Suppose you did fail a course, what would happen? Are there ways you can reverse the finality of the problem? (Talk to a teacher about make-up assignments? Ask a friend for help in reviewing material? Buy a review book that will help in studying?) Do not count on everyone being willing to help. A high school teacher may feel that to be asked to do outside tutoring is an imposition, and for you to advise adolescents to seek this kind of help will only add to their depression if the teacher refuses. You may have to make these contacts yourself (with the adolescent's permission) because, generally, persons who are depressed have difficulty initiating this type of action because they do not believe that anyone cares about them.

A general measure is to help adolescents speak honestly about thoughts of suicide and the problems that have led them to thinking death is a solution. Most problems begin to seem manageable if they can be put into words in this way. It is important not to underestimate an adolescent's determination to end his or her life. In most instances, the adolescent needs referral to a consultant well versed in suicide prevention to improve self-image and offer alternative solutions to problems.

For the adolescent's safety, a period of observation in a hospital setting is desirable after a suicide attempt to prevent the individual from inflicting personal injury and to allow him or her to be evaluated in a neutral setting, away from the stress that precipitated the attempt. This can take place in an adolescent service rather than a psychiatric service.

Antidepressant medicine alone, a therapy used with depressed adults, may be of little value in treating depressed children and adolescents. Continuing evaluation by both history taking and physical examination is necessary, because the young person who has attempted suicide may attempt it again if support people and better problem-solving ability are not available at another time.

Concerns Regarding Runaways

A *runaway* is commonly defined as an adolescent between the ages of 10 and 17 years who has been absent from home at least overnight without permission of parent or guardian. The frequency of running away for adolescents may be as high as one in eight. Fortunately, most do not go far or stay away long (under 1 week); about 1 in 20 adolescent runaways stays away as long as 1 year; some never return home. Runaway adolescents are most likely to be from low- or high-income families. Unemployment, alcoholism, sexual abuse, attempted suicide, and poverty are frequent characteristics. They are slightly more likely to be male than female (Rew, Taylor-Seehafer & Fitzgerald, 2001).

Assessment

Running away is usually preceded by an argument with parents that is often the last straw after a number of long-term disagreements. Other reasons may be personal concerns such as loneliness, pregnancy, and problems with friends, school, or the police. Incest can also be a precipitating cause, as can other parental abuse. A school history often reveals frequent truancy, failing grades, possible drug use, and runaway behavior by friends. It is a sad fact that some adolescents are "throw-aways" or cannot remain at home because they have been rejected by their families (Steele & O'Keefe, 2001).

Common health reasons for which runaway adolescents are seen at health care facilities are sexually transmitted diseases, including HIV/AIDS, rape, pregnancy, substance abuse, hepatitis, and vaginitis. They also have a high incidence of suicide attempts. When caring for adolescents with these concerns, be certain to secure a thorough history so the fact that they are no longer living at home will not be missed. To obtain a complete history, be nonjudgmental in questioning. Revealing that you are shocked by the report that he or she has slept overnight on a park bench for 2 months, has been robbed, or steals to obtain money will prevent you from learning even greater concerns, such as having a sexually transmitted disease, being pregnant, or using drugs. Ask if they want to return home. Many adolescent runaways want to but do not know how to take the first step back toward their parents.

NURSING DIAGNOSES AND RELATED INTERVENTIONS

Nursing Diagnosis: Ineffective individual coping related to stress of adolescent period and inadequate family resources

Outcome Identification: Adolescent will demonstrate adequate coping mechanisms by 1 month's time.

Outcome Evaluation: Adolescent states that stress level at home is manageable; is able to describe how he can use family and community resources to help solve problems and aid in a crisis.

Adolescents may run away because they are unable to solve a problem in any other way; therefore, setting goals with them may be difficult. A short-term goal to stay home through a holiday rather than a long-term one of finishing high school may be all you can achieve.

Because adolescent runaways lack references for jobs and do not necessarily qualify for public assistance programs, they generally have no sound source of income. Both males and females may resort to prostitution to support themselves, or they may resort to stealing. Police consider them to be juvenile delinquents and are required to return them to their homes if discovered. If they leave home again, they may be sentenced to an institution for care; unfortunately, these facilities are often crowded and may not have the means to meet adolescent needs other than food and clothing.

Try to imagine yourself in adolescent runaways' circumstances to ascertain whether your health instructions are sensible for their lifestyle. Giving them instructions to eat a high-protein diet or iron-rich foods, for example, may be ludicrous. They may not have a source of running water, and thus washing or changing a dressing may be difficult. They may have no way to pay for health care, making it impossible to obtain a prescription medication, so giving them a sample of a drug is often more practical. They may not have means of transportation so are unable to return to a health care facility for frequent follow-up visits. Meet as many of the runaway's needs as possible, therefore, at one visit. Remember that many runaways have associated school failure and may be poor readers; discuss the information with them when giving them a pamphlet.

Be certain that runaway adolescents are familiar with the national Youth Crisis Hotline, which they can telephone day or night when they want to return home. The phone number is 1-800-448-4663 (1-800-HIT HOME). Remember also that they are runaways because, for some reason, their home was intolerable. Although they agree to return home, they may not remain there unless circumstances can be changed.

Nursing Diagnosis: Impaired parenting related to inability of family to adjust to adolescent needs

Outcome Identification: Family will demonstrate increased ability to make necessary adjustments for family living within 1 month.

Outcome Evaluation: Parents list definite changes they have made in family life to better accommodate an adolescent, such as providing increased privacy or using "contracting" with adolescent.

In some instances, it is impossible for a family to reestablish itself after a child has run away because the family is dysfunctional (incest or abuse has occurred). In other instances, family life can be modified to welcome the runaway adolescent back home.

So that parents and the adolescent can learn to communicate better, it is helpful to insist that they establish ground rules for communication (shouting or threats are not allowed; no subject is too difficult to be discussed calmly; no emotion or feeling is to be called "foolish"). Once ground rules are laid, parents and the adolescent should meet to discuss how difficult it is to be an adolescent and how equally difficult it is to be the parent of an adolescent; in the past, they became so engaged in arguing that they did not appreciate the other side of the controversy.

Helping parents and adolescents establish a contract for behavior can be effective (for the right to have her own private room, the adolescent can't do drugs; for the right to stay overnight at a friend's house on Friday, she must eat with the family all other nights, for example). Contracting is effective with adolescents, but it does carry the responsibility for parents of being certain that they are abiding with their half of the contract (not invading the private room) and of being prepared to enforce the contract. Some families benefit by calling on a mediator (a relative, a close friend, a minister or rabbi) to listen to both sides of an issue and make a ruling.

WHAT IF? What if, after a fair trial of trying to make adjustments, parents are still unable to maintain a functional home life? What other arrangements would you help them make for safe care of the adolescent?

Unique Concerns of the Family With a Physically Challenged or Chronically Ill Adolescent

Achieving a sense of identity may be difficult for adolescents who have spent much of their life with an illness or other challenge. It is vital, however, for such individuals to learn to look past their particular condition to their real selves. For example, a 16-year-old girl in a wheelchair must perceive herself as a teenager who is normal intellectually, is a good conversationalist, has a good sense of humor, enjoys watching football, and only incidentally is in a wheelchair.

Some of the biggest problems of chronically ill adolescents are likely to be difficulties in being as independent as they would like, achieving in school, and establishing intimate relationships. Those who cannot learn to drive when their friends are learning to do so, who are not invited to dances and parties, or who are too hesitant to ask someone to go with them, may feel acute losses of self-esteem. Moreover, the loss of many hours of school due to illness or frequent hospitalization may result in the inability to pursue a desired career, at least without a delay. Adolescence may be the first time these children realize that certain occupations or opportunities, such as a military career, may be closed to them. As they prepare to leave the security of a familiar school system, it may be the first time they examine just how they will be able to function on their own. Some may come to realize that they will never be able to do so completely independently.

TABLE 32.5 Nursing Actions That Encourage a Sense of Identity in the Physically Challenged or Chronically Ill Adolescent

CATEGORY	ACTIONS
Nutrition	If adolescent is on special diet, discuss role of his or her food preferences with dietitian (hot dogs, pizza, etc.).
	Respect food preferences.
Dressing change	Allow adolescent to order supplies.
	Ask for suggestions as to final appearance of dressing.
	If soaks are included, have adolescent time the treatment.
	Allow adolescent to choose time for dressing change.
Medicine	Offering the adolescent a choice of site for injection or intravenous insertion encourages a sense of control.
	Teach name, action, and possible side effects of medicine.
Rest	Contract with adolescent for time and length of rest periods.
Hygiene	Respect modesty of the adolescent as being at adult level.
	Contract with adolescent for extent of self-care (will give own bath and make bed, not medicate self).
Pain	Encourage adolescent to express pain; teach distraction technique for sharp pain, such as deep breathing, counting backward from 100.
	Encourage adolescent to ask for analgesics as needed.
Stimulation	Provide tapes of favorite music with earphones.
	Provide a radio for adolescent to listen to talk show to foster active involvement.
	Encourage school work, crossword puzzles (you may need to help adolescents divide school assignments so they do not become overly fatigued and frustrated).
	Provide cards for games to increase socialization (make or have the adolescent make a card deck from pieces of paper if one is not available).
	Encourage adolescents to network with one another.
	Encourage adolescents to keep in contact with school friends through telephoning or writing notes to them.

Chronic hospitalization or realization that they will never be free of symptoms can cause depression in adolescents, placing them at high risk for substance abuse or suicide. Helping these adolescents realize that even completely well people must compromise life decisions for other reasons (eg, lack of money, lack of ability or qualifications, extra personal responsibilities) helps them feel they are not so different from others. This type of guidance can be time consuming, but sometimes the fact that an adult was willing to make this time commitment with them is enough to give these adolescents the self-esteem they need to alter aspirations and plans and find a future role that is consistent with their capabilities. Nursing actions that encourage a sense of identity in the adolescent with a long-term illness or who is physically challenged are summarized in Table 32-5.

Nutrition and the Chronically Ill Adolescent

Adolescents who are not fully mobile must be aware of their total calorie intake, or as growth needs decline at the end of adolescence they can become obese. They should also be knowledgeable about good nutrition, so they can participate in meal planning, an action that helps them feel a sense of control over this area of their life. Assess how often they have a chance to eat at fast-food restaurants; although this is not a source of excellent nutrition, eating there occasionally provides an important social experience and a chance to be like their peers.

✔ CHECKPOINT QUESTIONS

16. Why is a happy mood a sign of potential suicide?
17. Why don't runaways want to return home?

KEY POINTS

The major milestones of development in the adolescent period are the onset of puberty and the cessation of body growth. Between these milestones, physical growth is rapid although the development of adult coordination and thought processes is slow.

The development of secondary sex characteristics is completed during adolescence. These are rated according to Tanner stages.

The developmental task of the adolescent according to Erikson is to establish independence from parents through gaining a sense of identity versus role confusion. Adolescents, therefore, usually respond best to health care personnel who respect their attempts at independence and allow them as many choices as possible in care.

Adolescents reach a point of cognitive development termed *formal operational thought.* With this gained, they are able to think in abstract terms and use the scientific method to arrive at conclusions.

Adolescents need to consume adequate calories and especially protein, iron, calcium, and zinc to meet their increased growth needs.

To appear older than they are, some adolescents present an assured, "I know that" attitude. To be effective, health teaching may have to be introduced with "I know you know this, so I'll just review it" approach that allows the adolescent to maintain a mature front, while gaining additional information.

Being an adolescent is difficult in today's world. Be aware that, to reduce stress, some adolescents begin to use abusive substances. Asking about an adolescent's drug experiences, if any, during a health assessment is not intruding on privacy; it is conducting safe health interviewing.

Promoting adolescent safety is an important nursing role. Motor vehicle accidents, homicide, and suicide are leading causes of death in this age group.

Common health problems in the adolescent are sometimes minor and include poor posture, fatigue, or acne; they can also be serious, such as beginning hypertension, substance abuse, and suicide. Identifying these problems and referring the adolescent for help are important nursing actions.

CRITICAL THINKING EXERCISES

1. Raul is the 16-year-old boy you met at the beginning of the chapter. His parents tell you he was depressed after the loss of a girlfriend but now is suddenly happy. He has been collecting baseball cards since he was 8. Recently, he gave his collection away to a neighbor boy because he "wouldn't need them where he's going." Why might you be concerned about him? What additional questions might you ask him? If you learned he is about to leave to be an exchange student in England, how would this affect your assessment of the situation?
2. A 15-year-old boy whom you meet in an ambulatory clinic tells you during history taking that he does not smoke, but you smell cigarette smoke on his clothing. Although he says he doesn't use drugs, a number of blue and white capsules fall out of his shirt pocket when he unbuttons his shirt. What questions would you ask to determine if he is smoking cigarettes or using drugs? Describe your next action if he does admit he is not only heavily into drugs but does not intend to stop using them.
3. A shy, quiet, 14-year-old girl you care for in a hospital setting tells you she is concerned because she has not menstruated yet. This is making her feel "left out" at school. How would you counsel her? What if she were 16 and had the same concern?
4. A 17-year-old boy you meet at an adolescent clinic tells you he is on a "pizza only" diet. What suggestions would you want to make about what kind of pizza to eat?
5. Examine the National Health Goals related to adolescents. Most government-sponsored money for nursing research is allotted based on these goals. What would be a possible research topic to explore pertinent to these goals that would both be fundable and would advance evidence-based practice?

REFERENCES

American Academy of Pediatrics Committee on Practice and Ambulatory Medicine. (2001). Recommendations for preventive pediatric health care. Washington, DC: AAP.

Arria, A. M. et al. (2002). Ecstasy use among club rave attendees. *Archives of Pediatrics & Adolescent Medicine, 156*(3), 295-296.

Baldwin, S. (2000). Speed kills: Amphetamines, children and nurses. *Nursing Ethics, 7*(6), 535-537.

Berger, K. S. (2001). *The developing person through the life span* (5th ed). New York: Worth Publishing.

Boys, A., Marsen, J., & Strang, J. (2001). Understanding reasons for drug use amongst young people: A functional perspective. *Health Education Research, 16*(4), 457-469.

Copeland, J., Swift, W., & Rees, V. (2001). Clinical profile of participants in a brief intervention program for cannabis use disorder. *Journal of Substance Abuse Treatment, 20*(1), 45-52.

Corbett, K. K. (2001). Susceptibility of youth to tobacco: A social ecological framework for prevention. *Respiration Physiology, 128*(1), 103-118.

Davis, K. E., & Frieze, I. H. (2000). Research on stalking: What do we know and where do we go? *Violence & Victims, 15*(4), 473-487.

Department of Health and Human Services. (2000). *Healthy people 2010.* Washington, DC: DHHS.

Dudek, S. G. (2001). *Nutrition: Essentials for nursing practice.* Philadelphia: Lippincott Williams & Wilkins.

Enoch, M. A., & Goldman, D. (1999). Genetics of alcoholism and substance abuse. *Psychiatric Clinics of North America, 22*(2), 289-299.

Erikson, E. H. (1993). *Childhood and society.* New York: W.W. Norton.

Gilligan, C. et al. (1982). *In a different voice: Psychological theory and women's development.* Cambridge, MA: Harvard University Press.

Green, H., et al. (2000). Methadone maintenance programs: A two-edged sword? *American Journal of Forensic Medicine & Pathology, 21*(4), 359-361.

Hahn, J., & Hoffman, R. S. (2001). Cocaine use and acute myocardial infarction. *Emergency Medicine Clinics of North America, 19*(2), 493-510.

Higgs, P. E., et al. (2000). Evaluation of a self-directed smoking prevention and cessation program. *Pediatric Nursing, 26*(2), 150–155.

Honein, M. A., et al. (2001). Continued occurrence of Accutane-exposed pregnancies. *Teratology, 64*(3), 142–147.

Johnson, M., Maas, M., & Moorhead, S. (2000). *Nursing outcomes classification* (2nd ed.). St. Louis: Mosby.

Kaplan, D. W., & Love, K. A. (2001). Growth & development, In W. W. Hay, A. R. Hayward, M. J. Levin & J. M. Sondheimer (Eds.). *Current pediatric diagnosis & treatment* (15th ed.). New York: McGraw-Hill.

Karch, A. M. (2001). *Lippincott's nursing drug guide*. Philadelphia: Lippincott Williams & Wilkins.

King, K. A. (2001). Developing a comprehensive school suicide prevention program. *Journal of School Health, 71*(4), 132–137.

Kohlberg, L. (1984). *The psychology of moral development.* New York: Harper & Row.

Kolasa, K. M., Poehlman, G. S., & Peery, A. I. (2000). Is a vegetarian diet healthy for kids? *Patient Care for the Nurse Practitioner, 3*(3), 61–75.

Krebs, N. F., & Hambridge, K. M. (2001). Normal childhood nutrition and its disorders. In W. W. Hay, A. R. Hayward, M. J. Levin & J. M. Sondheimer (Eds.). *Current pediatric diagnosis & treatment* (15th ed.). New York: McGraw-Hill.

Kurtzman, T. L., Otsuka, K. N., & Wahl, R. A. (2001). Inhalant abuse by adolescents. *Journal of Adolescent Health, 28*(3), 170–180.

McCloskey, J., & Bulechek, G. (2000). *Nursing interventions classification* (3rd ed.). St. Louis: Mosby.

Midgley, S. J., Heather, N., & Davies, J. B. (2001). Levels of aggression among a group of anabolic-androgenic steroid users. *Medicine, Science & the Law, 41*(4), 309–314.

Piaget, J. (1969). *The theory of stages in cognitive development.* New York: McGraw-Hill.

Rand, C. S., & Resnick, J. L. (2000). The "good enough" body size as judged by people of varying age and weight. *Obesity Research, 8*(4), 309–316.

Rew, L., Taylor-Seehafer, M., & Fitzgerald, M. L. (2001). Sexual abuse, alcohol and other drug use, and suicidal behaviors in homeless adolescents. *Issues in Comprehensive Pediatric Nursing, 24*(4), 225–240.

Steele, R. W., & O'Keefe, M. A. (2001). A program description of health care interventions for homeless teenagers. *Clinical Pediatrics, 40*(5), 259–263.

Stoll, S., et al. (2001). The effect of the menstrual cycle on acne. *Journal of the American Academy of Dermatology, 45*(6), 957–960.

Tanner, J. M. (1962). *Growth at adolescence* (2nd ed.). Oxford: Blackwell.

SUGGESTED READINGS

Degenhardt, L., Hall, W., & Lynskey, M. (2001). The relationship between cannabis use and other substance use in the general population. *Drug & Alcohol Dependence, 64*(3), 319–327.

Kiess, W., et al. (2001). Clinical aspects of obesity in childhood and adolescence: Diagnosis, treatment and prevention. *International Journal of Obesity, 25*(1), S75–S79.

Krowchuk, D. P., & Lucky, A. W. (2001). Managing adolescent acne. *Adolescent Medicine, 12*(2), 355–374.

Obot, I. S., Wagner, F. A., & Anthony, J. C. (2001). Early onset and recent drug use among children of parents with alcohol problems. *Drug & Alcohol Dependence, 65*(1), 1–8.

Seguire, M., & Chalmers, K. I. (2000). Late adolescent female smoking. *Journal of Advanced Nursing, 31*(6), 1422–1429.

Smith, J. A. (2001). The impact of skin disease on the quality of life of adolescents. *Adolescent Medicine, 12*(2), 343–353.

Somers, C. L., & Fahlman, M. M. (2001). Effectiveness of the "Baby Think it Over" teen pregnancy prevention program. *Journal of School Health, 71*(5), 188–195.

Spear, B. A. (2002). Adolescent growth and development. *Journal of the American Dietetic Association, 102*(35), 23–29.

Wichstrom, L., & Pedersen, W. (2001). Use of anabolic-androgenic steroids in adolescence: Winning, looking good or being bad? *Journal of Studies on Alcohol, 62*(1), 5–13.

Zimmer-Gembeck, M. J., et al. (2001). Contraceptive dispensing and selection in school-based health centers. *Journal of Adolescent Health, 29*(3), 177–185.

33

CHAPTER

Child Health Assessment

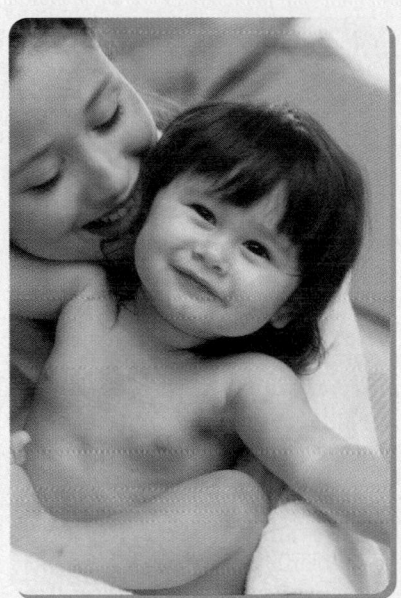

Key Terms

- antitoxins
- audiogram
- auscultation
- bruit
- chief concern
- conjunctivitis
- deep tendon reflexes
- diaphragmatic excursion
- epispadias
- esotropia
- exotropia
- gamma globulin
- geographic tongue
- hordeolum
- hydrocele
- hypospadias
- immune serum
- inspection
- intelligence
- intercostal spaces
- kwashiorkor
- palpatlon
- percussion
- physiologic splitting
- point of maximum impulse
- ptosis
- retractions
- review of systems
- sinus arrhythmia
- strabismus
- temperament
- toxoid
- turgor
- varicocele

Objectives

After mastering the contents of this chapter, you should be able to:

1. State the purposes for health assessment in children of all ages.
2. Assess a child and family by health interview, physical examination, and development screening.
3. Formulate nursing diagnoses based on health assessment findings.
4. Identify expected outcomes based on health assessment findings.
5. Plan nursing care based on health assessment findings such as informing parents of health deviations.
6. Implement nursing care such as conducting an age-appropriate health interview or physical examination by modifying techniques based on the child's age.
7. Evaluate outcomes for achievement.
8. Identify National Health Goals related to health assessment of children that nurses can be instrumental in helping the nation to achieve.
9. Identify areas related to health assessment of children that could benefit from additional nursing research or application of evidence-based practice.
10. Use critical thinking to analyze ways that health assessment skills can be incorporated into nursing care procedures.
11. Integrate nursing process with knowledge of health assessment to achieve quality maternal and child health nursing care.

Terry is a 5-year-old boy you meet in an ambulatory clinic. His father has brought him for a health assessment before he begins kindergarten. His father is worried that Terry doesn't see well because he always sits very close to the television. Terry's mother didn't want to bring him for a preschool assessment because she doesn't want glasses prescribed for him. What questions would you want to ask Terry? What screening tests for vision would be best for this 5-year-old child?

Previous chapters described the normal growth and development of children. This chapter adds information about techniques for assessing the health of children, including history taking, physical examination, related screening procedures for hearing, vision, and development, and immunizations. This is important information because it builds a base for care and health teaching for differing age groups.

After you've studied the chapter, answer the Critical Thinking Exercises at the end of the chapter and then access the on-line study activities (http://connection.lww.com) *to further sharpen your skills and test your knowledge.*

ASSESSING the Child Overview

History
- → Demographic data
- → Chief concern
- → History of chief concern
- → Health and family profile
- → Past health history
- → Family health history
- → Review of systems

Physical examination
- → General appearance
- → Vital signs

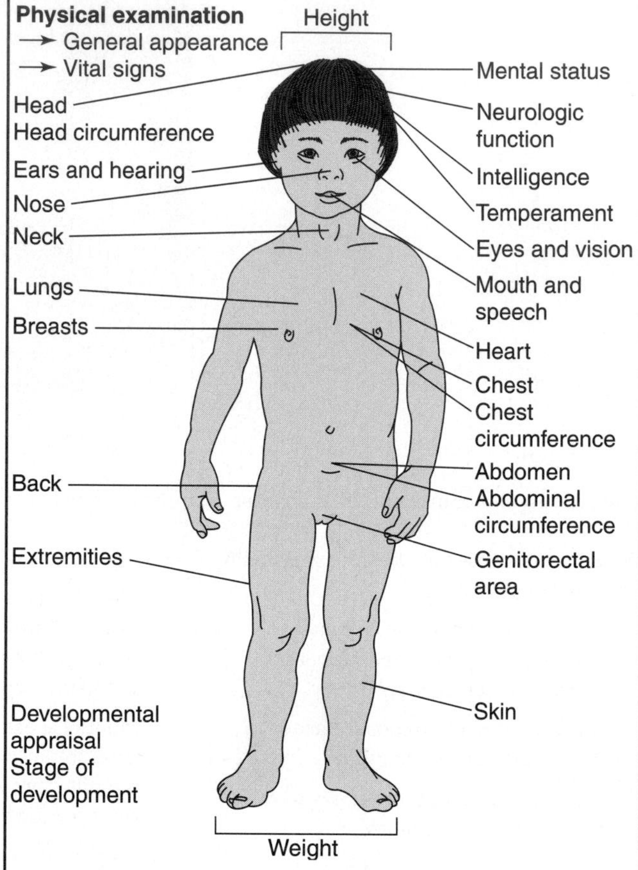

Nursing assessment is not only the first step in the nursing process, but also the fundamental means by which a nurse establishes and maintains contact with a child and family. Child health assessment is especially important as an opportunity to provide families with information about health promotion, signs of health and illness, and expected developmental progress in children. This anticipatory guidance can have a long-lasting positive impact on the health of the child and family.

Effective assessment for the maternal–child population first requires you to be familiar with health maintenance standards and usual findings, because this knowledge is essential to the ability to recognize illness. Most health screening procedures are performed in ambulatory settings (e.g., well-child conferences, physicians' offices, health maintenance organizations, community clinics, and schools), but they can be used to evaluate children in all settings.

Sometimes it is necessary to complete just a partial history or a partial physical examination, such as when a child is referred for vision examination. This chapter, however, covers all aspects of physical examination so that, when necessary, a complete examination can be performed (see Assessing the Child: Overview). Procedures specific to a particular illness appear in later chapters with the illness they detect. The Focus on National Health Goals box lists goals related to health assessment.

NURSING PROCESS OVERVIEW

For Health Assessment of the Child and Family

Assessment

Health assessment of children can be a positive, educational experience for the child and family if time is taken to listen carefully to a family's concerns and responses to questions. Never rush either an interview or a physical examination. Be sure the child has time to familiarize himself or herself with the environment and equipment that will be used.

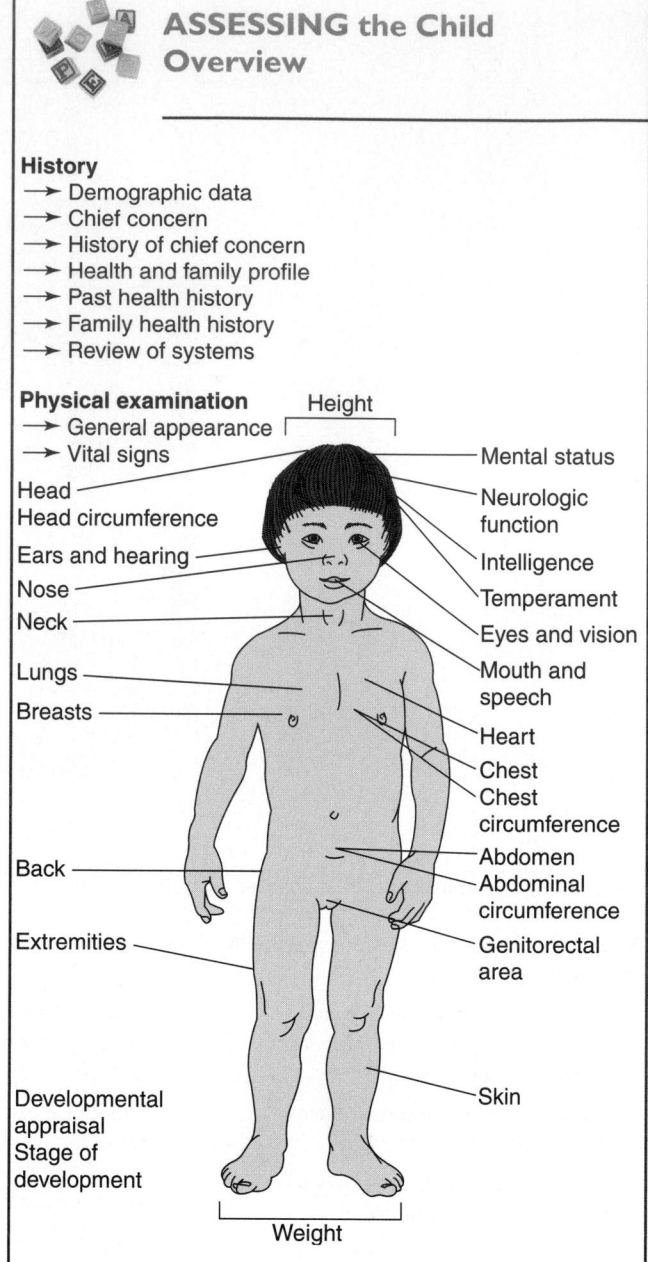

Obtaining health histories and performing physical examinations can be done independently or as part of a total preventive health care program for the child. The recommendations for standard preventive pediatric health care for the United States are shown in Table 33-1.

Nursing Diagnosis

Health assessment provides the data used to identify potential problems and serves as the basis for the establishment of nursing diagnoses. Be certain not to overlook diagnoses that accentuate the healthy functioning of the child and family, even when diagnoses

(text continues on page 942)

TABLE 33.1 Recommendations for Preventive Pediatric Health Care

Each child and family is unique; therefore, these Recommendations for Preventive Pediatric Health Care are designed for the care of children who are receiving competent parenting, have no manifestations of any important health problems, and are growing and developing in satisfactory fashion. Additional visits may become necessary if circumstances suggest variations from normal.

These guidelines represent a consensus by the Committee on Practice and Ambulatory Medicine in consultation with national committees and sections of the American Academy of Pediatrics. The Committee emphasizes the great importance of continuity of care in comprehensive health supervision and the need to avoid fragmentation of care.

	INFANCY[4]									EARLY CHILDHOOD[4]				
Age[5]	**Prenatal**[1]	**Newborn**[2]	**2–4d**[3]	**By 1mo**	**2mo**	**4mo**	**6mo**	**9mo**	**12mo**	**15mo**	**18mo**	**24mo**	**3y**	**4y**
History														
Initial/Interval	•	•	•	•	•	•	•	•	•	•	•	•	•	•
Measurements														
Height and Weight		•	•	•	•	•	•	•	•	•	•	•	•	•
Head Circumference		•	•	•	•	•	•	•	•	•	•	•		
Blood Pressure													•	•
Sensory Screening														
Vision		S	S	S	S	S	S	S	S	S	S	S	O[6]	O
Hearing		O[7]	S	S	S	S	S	S	S	S	S	S	S	O
Developmental/Behavioral Assessment[8]		•	•	•	•	•	•	•	•	•	•	•	•	•
Physical Examination[9]		•	•	•	•	•	•	•	•	•	•	•	•	•
Procedures-General[10]														
Hereditary/Metabolic Screening[11]		←	•	→										
Immunization[12]		•	•	•	•	•	•	•	•	•	•	•	•	•
Hematocrit or Hemoglobin[13]								• →	→	*	*	*	*	*
Urinalysis														
Procedures-Patients at Risk														
Lead Screening[16]								* →	→			*		
Tuberculin Test[17]									*	*	*	*	*	
Cholesterol Screening[18]												*	*	*
STD Screening[19]														
Pelvic Exam[20]														
Anticipatory Guidance[21]	•	•	•	•	•	•	•	•	•	•	•	•	•	•
Injury Prevention[22]	•	•	•	•	•	•	•	•	•	•	•	•	•	•
Violence Prevention[23]	•	•	•	•	•	•	•	•	•	•	•	•	•	•
Sleep Positioning Counseling[24]	•	•	•	•	•	•	•							
Nutrition Counseling[25]	•	•	•	•	•	•	•	•	•	•	•	•	•	•
Dental Referral[26]									←	←	←	←	•	

(continued)

TABLE 33.1 Recommendations for Preventive Pediatric Health Care *(Continued)*

	MIDDLE CHILDHOOD[4]				ADOLESCENCE[4]										
Age[5]	**5y**	**6y**	**8y**	**10y**	**11y**	**12y**	**13y**	**14y**	**15y**	**16y**	**17y**	**18y**	**19y**	**20y**	**21y**
History															
Initial/Interval	•	•	•	•	•	•	•	•	•	•	•	•	•	•	•
Measurements															
Height and Weight	•	•	•	•	•	•	•	•	•	•	•	•	•	•	•
Head Circumference															
Blood Pressure	•	•	•	•	•	•	•	•	•	•	•	•	•	•	•
Sensory Screening															
Vision	O	O	O	O	S	O	S	S	O	S	S	O	S	S	S
Hearing	O	O	O	O	S	O	S	S	O	S	S	O	S	S	S
Developmental/Behavioral Assessment[8]	•	•	•	•	•	•	•	•	•	•	•	•	•	•	•
Physical Examination[9]	•	•	•	•	•	•	•	•	•	•	•	•	•	•	•
Procedures-General[10]															
Hereditary/Metabolic Screening[11]															
Immunization[12]	•	•	•	•	•	•	•	•	•	•	•	•	•	•	•
Hematocrit or Hemoglobin[13]	*				←		•[14]								→
Urinalysis	•				←					•[15]					→
Procedures-Patients at Risk															
Lead Screening[16]															
Tuberculin Test[17]	*	*	*	*	*	*	*	*	*	*	*	*	*	*	*
Cholesterol Screening[18]	*	*	*	*	*	*	*	*	*	*	*	*	*	*	*
STD Screening[19]					*	*	*	*	*	*	*	*	*	*	*
Pelvic Exam[20]					*	*	*	*	*	*	*	*	← *[20]	*	→ *
Anticipatory Guidance[21]	•	•	•	•	•	•	•	•	•	•	•	•	•	•	•
Injury Prevention[22]	•	•	•	•	•	•	•	•	•	•	•	•	•	•	•
Violence Prevention[23]	•	•	•	•	•	•	•	•	•	•	•	•	•	•	•
Sleep Positioning Counseling[24]															
Nutrition Counseling[25]	•	•	•	•	•	•	•	•	•	•	•	•	•	•	•
Dental Referral[26]															

Key: • = to be performed; * = to be performed for patients at risk
S = subjective, by history; O = objective, by a standard testing method
←•→ = the range during which a service may be provided, with the dot indicating the preferred age.

From American Academy of Pediatrics (2000). *Policy statement recommendations for preventive health care* (RE9939), *105*[03], March, p. 645, with permission.

1. A prenatal visit is recommended for parents who are at high risk, for first-time parents, and for those who request a conference. The prenatal visit should include anticipatory guidance, pertinent medical history, and a discussion of benefits of breastfeeding and planned method of feeding per AAP statement "The Prenatal Visit" (1996).
2. Every infant should have a newborn evaluation after birth. Breastfeeding should be encouraged and instruction and support offered. Every breastfeeding infant should have an evaluation 48–72 hours after discharge from the hospital to include weight, formal breastfeeding evaluation, encouragement, and instruction as recommended in the AAP statement "Breastfeeding and the Use of Human Milk" (1997).
3. For newborns discharged in less than 48 hours after delivery per AAP statement "Hospital Stay for Healthy Term Newborns" (1995).
4. Developmental, psychosocial and chronic disease issues for children and adolescents may require frequent counseling and treatment visits separate from preventive care visits.
5. If a child comes under care for the first time at any point on the schedule, or if any items are not accomplished at the suggested age, the schedule should be brought up to date at the earliest possible time.
6. If the patient is uncooperative, rescreen within 6 months.
7. All newborns should be screened per the AAP Task Force on Newborn and Infant Hearing statement, "Newborn and Infant Hearing Loss: Detection and Intervention" (1999).
8. By history and appropriate physical examination: if suspicious, by specific objective developmental testing. Parenting skills should be fostered at every visit.
9. At each visit, a complete physical examination is essential, with infant totally unclothed, older child undressed and suitably draped.
10. These may be modified, depending upon entry point into schedule and individual need.
11. Metabolic screening (eg, thyroid, hemoglobinopathies, PKU, galactosemia) should be done according to state law.
12. Schedule(s) per the Committee on Infectious Diseases, published annually in the January edition of *Pediatrics*. Every visit should be an opportunity to update and complete a child's immunizations.
13. See AAP *Pediatric Nutrition Handbook* (1998) for a discussion of universal and selective screening options. Consider earlier screening for high-risk infants (eg premature infants and low birth weight infants). See also "Recommendations to Prevent and Control Iron Deficiency in the United States". *MMWR.* 1998;47 (RR-3): 1-29.
14. All menstruating adolescents should be screened annually.
15. Conduct dipstick urinalysis for leukocytes annually for sexually active male and female adolescents.
16. For children at risk of lead exposure consult the AAP statement "Screening for Elevated Blood Levels" (1998). Additionally, screening should be done in accordance with state law where applicable.
17. TB testing per recommendations of the Committee on Infectious Diseases, published in the current edition of *Red Book: Report of the Committee on Infectious Diseases.* Testing should be done upon recognition of high-risk factors.
18. Cholesterol screening for high-risk patients per AAP statement "Cholesterol in Childhood" (1998). If family history cannot be ascertained and other risk factors are present, screening should be at the discretion of the physician.
19. All sexually active patients should be screened for sexually transmitted diseases (STDs).
20. All sexually active females should have a pelvic examination. A pelvic examination and routine pap smear should be offered as part of preventive health maintenance between the ages of 18 and 21 years.
21. Age-appropriate discussion and counseling should be an integral part of each visit for care per the AAP *Guidelines for Health Supervision III* (1998).
22. From birth to age 12, refer to the AAP injury prevention program (TIPP–MS 534) as described in *A Guide to Safety Counseling in Office Practice* (1994).
23. Violence prevention and management for all patients per AAP Statement "The Role of the Pediatrician in Youth Violence Prevention in Clinical Practice and at the Community Level" (1999).
24. Parents and caregivers should be advised to place healthy infants on their backs when putting them to sleep. Side positioning is a reasonable alternative but carries a slightly higher risk of SIDS. Consult the AAP statement "Changing Concepts of Sudden Infant Death Syndrome: Implications for Infant Sleeping Environment and Sleep Position" (2000).
25. Age-appropriate nutrition counseling should be an integral part of each visit per the AAP *Handbook of Nutrition* (1998).
26. Earlier initial dental examinations may be appropriate for some children. Subsequent examinations as prescribed by dentist.

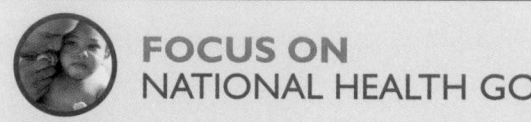

FOCUS ON NATIONAL HEALTH GOALS

A number of National Health Goals relate directly to health assessment of children. These are:

- Increase the proportion of territories and states that have service systems for children with special health care needs from a baseline of 15% to a target of 100%.
- Increase the proportion of children and youth, 17 years of age and younger, who have a specific source of ongoing care from a baseline of 93% to a target of 97%.
- Achieve and maintain effective vaccination coverage levels for universally recommended vaccines among young children from baselines of 84% (DTaP); 87% (hepatitis B); 91% (polio); 43% (varicella); and 92% (MMR) to a target level of 90% (DHHS, 2000).

Nurses can be instrumental in helping the nation to achieve these goals by participating actively in health assessment and conscientiously screening for and administering vaccines. Nursing research that might add more information in this area would include techniques that can be used to orient preschoolers quickly to a health care setting, effective techniques for eliciting health interview information from adolescents, and methods to help parents better record or remember what immunizations their children have received.

that address specific problems have been identified. These wellness diagnoses are crucial components of the entire assessment picture and often provide an avenue for addressing identified problems. For instance, the nursing diagnosis of "Impaired social interaction related to lack of self-esteem secondary to disability" would be appropriate for a 4-year-old child confined to a wheelchair who, according to the parents, feels uncomfortable when around other children. If the parents have difficulty adapting to their child's disability but are eager to accept advice from health care experts on how to provide the most stimulating environment for their child, the diagnosis of "Readiness for enhanced family coping" would also be appropriate. Using both these diagnoses allows the development of a plan of care that takes the best advantage of this family's strengths.

Outcome Identification and Planning

Nursing diagnoses serve as the basis for identifying outcomes. Health promotion and illness prevention are vital parts of this process. Help parents plan for their child's next developmental stage; keep them aware of important safety measures and other ways to keep children well. Remind them about immunizations needed in the future and make sure they know when to schedule the next health visit.

Implementation

Health interviewing and physical examination both require a great deal of skill, skill that can be perfected only through practice. To perfect skills and judgment with children of different ages, take advantage of every opportunity to practice interviewing and physical examination techniques.

Outcome Evaluation

Health assessment of children is an ongoing process that does not end when the first database is obtained. Data must be added at all future interactions so the database remains current and meaningful. Examples suggesting achievement of outcomes would include:

- Parents state they are satisfied with child's motor development immediately after health examination.
- Child states she is aware that her vision needs correction after Snellen test.
- Parents state they will continue to assess child's growth by weighing child weekly.

HEALTH HISTORY: ESTABLISHING A DATABASE

The assessment of a young child begins with an interview of the child's parents. An adolescent or preadolescent may choose to be interviewed without the parents present, although many preadolescents and adolescents still prefer to have a parent with them as support.

The purpose of a health interview is to gather information that will direct physical or laboratory examinations to complete a thorough health evaluation. An extensive interview elicits facts such as parental problems in childrearing or detection of future health problems. It lays a foundation for health education and health promotion. A number of important principles of child health interviewing are reviewed below.

Interview Setting

An interview is best conducted in a private room with all parties seated comfortably (Fig. 33-1); if not seated, a health care provider appears rushed and can't interact at eye level. During the interview, call the parents by their names. This lets them know that their input and opinions about how their child is developing are valued. A question such as, "Does John sit up yet, Mr. Wiser?" is far more personal and a better form than, "Does baby sit up yet?" As children grow they are able to speak and answer questions directly.

Types of Questions Asked

The phrasing of questions varies depending on the type of answer desired. Closed-ended and open-ended questions are two types of effective questions; compound, expansive, and leading questions, on the other hand, are three types of questions to avoid.

Closed-Ended Question

This simplest form of question asks directly for a fact: "Does John walk yet?" "Did you take John's temperature?" This is an effective type of question if a particular point is

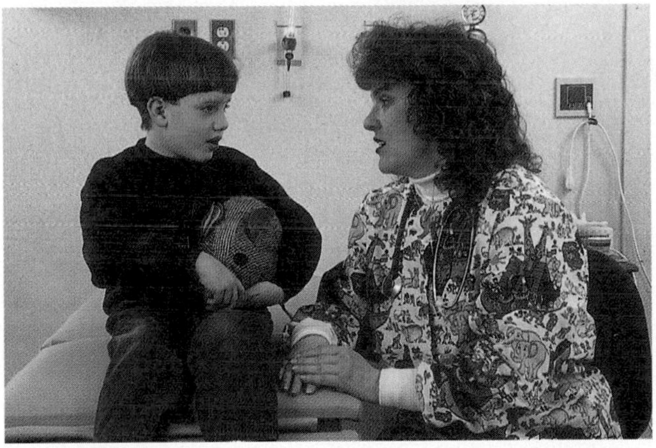

FIGURE 33.1 Maintaining good eye contact and allowing children to be as active a part as possible in the assessment process are important.

being sought. It is limited in scope, however, because the response usually will be only a yes or no, with no further elaboration.

Open-Ended Question

An open-ended question allows the parent to elaborate. In contrast to the closed-ended question "Did you take John's temperature?" the question "What did you do for John?" is open-ended. The parent answers with a listing of all the things he or she did: took John's temperature, had him lie on the couch, gave him extra fluid, and so on. It is important to ask open-ended questions with school-age children and adolescents so they are encouraged to describe a problem fully.

Compound Question

Compound questions are confusing and should be avoided because the information they elicit is often inaccurate and must be followed by a clarifying question. An example is, "Did John have nausea and vomiting?" The parent answers yes, but it still is not known whether John had vomiting and nausea, just vomiting, or just nausea.

Expansive Question

This is an open-ended question gone wrong because it is too broad to answer. "What can you tell me about John?" leaves a parent wondering where to start. "How has John been since his last visit?" limits the question and makes it answerable.

Leading Question

A leading question supplies its own answer and thus should be avoided. "John has had all his immunizations, hasn't he?" implies that John should have had them and that the parent is somehow a poor caregiver if he or she answers that question any way but yes. The penalty for such an exchange could be a child left vulnerable to disease.

Health Interview

Data gathering for an initial health assessment can be divided into nine categories:

1. Introduction and explanation
2. Demographic data
3. Chief concern
4. History of chief concern
5. Health and family profile
6. Day history
7. Past health history, including the pregnancy history
8. Family health history
9. Review of systems

At return visits, the categories used generally include introduction and explanation, chief concern, health and family profile, interval history, and day history.

While conducting a health interview, be certain to make a transition statement before shifting from one part of an interview to another. Without a transition, a parent could be left wondering what importance the questions have, possibly misinterpreting their significance. For instance, if a parent has been providing information on the family's hospital insurance policy and, without a transition statement, is asked whether the child has been vomiting, a parent may think that the child needs hospitalization when that is not the intent at all. A statement such as, "Before we talk about Jane's current symptoms, let me ask you some general questions about your family as a whole," is an example of a good transition statement.

Introduction and Explanation

As a matter of courtesy, parents and the child should be told to whom they are talking and about what topics they will be talking. "Hello, Ms. Wiser, I'm Janet Dickson, a nurse here in the One Day Surgery Department. I'd like to talk to you about John this morning" is an example of a suitable introduction. Because some families have never had the benefit of in-depth health care, it is also helpful to include a statement about the subjects that will be discussed during the interview. For example, a statement such as, "So that I can get a picture of John's overall health, I'll be asking you questions about why you've brought him here today, your pregnancy with him, concerns you've had in the past, and questions about your typical day with John," would be appropriate. The parent begins to concentrate on those areas because he or she realizes that health care providers in this setting are interested not just in John's health that particular day, but in his total health (see Focus on Cultural Competence).

Demographic Data

To begin collecting demographic data, it is important to identify the client. Information such as the client's name, address, and gender and the person who provided information should be included. To provide culturally competent care and make provisions for special needs, the child's culture, ethnicity, place of birth, religious or spiritual practices, and primary and secondary language should

FOCUS ON CULTURAL COMPETENCE

Health assessment of children is a skill that is learned with practice. Successful interviewing depends on respecting cultural variations. Whether people establish eye contact with an interviewer, for example, is a characteristic that is culturally determined. In Vietnam, touching the head of a child during physical assessment is thought to be harmful because the head is considered to be the seat of the soul.

Findings and techniques in children also differ depending on racial and ethnic characteristics. Assessing for cyanosis, for example, is more difficult in dark-skinned than in fair-skinned children (mucous membrane is the best place to detect this). Because height and weight charts are standardized on middle-class white children, measurements of children who do not fit this description may not plot well on these charts.

Recognizing that people hold differing cultural expectations and characteristics can help in establishing rapport with children and their families and help make health assessment more meaningful.

FOCUS ON COMMUNICATION

Keoto Weigel is a 13-year-old girl you see at an ambulatory clinic. She has frequency and burning on urination. Her mother accompanies her.

Less Effective Communication

Nurse: Hello, Keoto. What's the reason you've come into the clinic today?
Mrs. Weigel: It hurts when she urinates.
Nurse: How long ago did that start, Keoto?
Mrs. Weigel: She started complaining about it yesterday.
Nurse: Has she had any blood in her urine?
Mrs. Weigel: She hasn't said anything about that. The important thing is the pain.
Nurse: Okay. I'm sure we need a urine specimen for culture. Let's get that to get started here.

More Effective Communication

Nurse: Hello, Keoto. What's the reason you've come into the clinic today?
Mrs. Weigel: It hurts when she urinates.
Nurse: Let's let Keoto answer for herself, Mrs. Weigel. Tell me what you think is the problem, Keoto.
Keoto: It hurts when I go to the bathroom.
Nurse: How long ago did that start, Keoto?
Mrs. Weigel: She started complaining about it last night.
Nurse: Keoto? When do *you* think it started?
Keoto: About an hour after I came in from my date last night.
Nurse: Have you had any blood in your urine?
Mrs. Weigel: She hasn't said anything about that.
Nurse: Keoto? Have you noticed your urine is red or dark brown?
Keoto: I had bright blood last night.
Nurse: Let me take you down to the lavatory and explain about a urine specimen. While we're there, I'd like to ask you some more questions about last night.

At about 10 years of age, children are able to supply much of a health history by themselves. As children become teenagers, it is increasingly important for them to do this because they may not have shared a total history with a parent. In the above scenario, for example, when the child is asked directly for information, she supplied more than when her history was given by the mother. Some urinary tract infections occur in girls after their first sexual relations. It would be important to ask Keoto if she is sexually active (what her date last night included), not only to document the probable cause of the urinary tract infection, but also to be certain she is knowledgeable about pregnancy prevention and safer sex practices.

also be identified. Ask if older children have a Social Security number.

In addition, it is important to identify the child's primary caregiver. If the parents are divorced or deceased, it is especially important to identify who has custody of the child and who has the right to sign the consent for health care treatment.

Chief Concern

After gathering demographic data, begin data collection with the reason the parents have brought the child to the health care agency: the **chief concern.** This is what parents are most concerned about, and it is important that they get this immediate concern off their mind early in the interview. An effective way to elicit this information is to ask an open-ended question such as, "Why did you bring John to the clinic today, Ms. Wiser?" Such an opening allows the parent freedom to answer in a number of areas of concern: physical, emotional, nutritional, and developmental. If asked, "How is John feeling today?" or "Is John ill?" the parent is left to think about only physical aspects and may not voice his or her biggest concern: John's teething difficulty or his frequent temper tantrums. For more details on eliciting information about children's chief concern, see Focus on Communication.

History of Chief Concern

Once the parent has voiced this chief concern, ask him or her to describe at least six aspects of the problem:

1. Duration
2. Intensity
3. Frequency
4. Description
5. Associated symptoms
6. Actions taken

In discussing duration, it is important to know when the child was last well to determine when he or she became ill.

For example, on Saturday morning, John began having long crying periods. On Monday night, he developed a fever. On Tuesday afternoon, his mother brought him into the clinic for a checkup. The parent states that John vomited three times Monday morning and thinks this was caused by teething. Unless the parent is asked when John was last well, she may pinpoint Monday as the beginning of the illness (the vomiting) when actually it was Saturday (the crying).

In this example, the intensity of the illness refers to the kind of vomiting the child is having. Is it drooling, spitting up, or actual vomiting? The description is the amount (a cupful? a mouthful?) and color (whether it contains blood, bile, or mucus). Associated symptoms might include fever, abdominal pain, difficulty eating, or signs of respiratory illness. A good question to use to obtain this information is, "Is John ill in any other way?"

It is important to know the parent's actions for a number of reasons. First, it is important to know whether anything a parent has been doing has been making the illness worse (e.g., offering a great deal of fluid to replace that vomited and by doing so causing more vomiting; using a home remedy or alternative therapy). It also reveals what the parent has previously tried but found ineffective. Telling a parent to give the child two tablets of acetaminophen (Tylenol) every 4 hours for fever if the parent has already done that and the fever has not improved would be unproductive. This information also reveals the parent's response to caring for an ill child. A parent who says, "I tucked him into bed and gave him a little tea to drink" is different from one who replies, "Nothing. I fall all apart when my child is ill." If the child is going to return home under the parents' care, the second parent in the example will need more instructions and support before he or she leaves the health care setting than the first parent does.

Obtaining information about the chief concern puts the parent's observations in proper perspective. In the previous example, the parent is probably not describing teething difficulty (teething does not cause vomiting); more likely, the child has a viral gastroenteritis. Unless the problem is investigated, it is easy to accept the parent's statement at face value as a teething problem without appreciating its full significance.

During this phase of the interview, it is also important to gather information about related or other health concerns. After the chief concern is documented, ask another open-ended question to elicit additional information: "Is there anything else that worries you about John?" Now the parent might want to talk about John's temper tantrums. Unless asked about a second problem, the parent will go home with the first problem cared for but the second one still not addressed. When the parent arrives home and John begins stomping his feet in the car, unwilling to go into the house, she will begin to feel the health care John received was less than adequate because she did not receive help with this concern.

Do not assume that parents will always reveal their worst fears in the initial minute of an interview: it can be frightening to put these fears into words. As long as a concern is hanging as a nebulous thought in the mind, it is easy to tell oneself that it may not be true. Only when a parent voices the thought ("Do you think that John is retarded?" "Do you think this is leukemia?" "Could this be inherited?") does the fear become real. Before parents dare to speak openly this way, they must trust health care providers not to treat their statement lightly. For this reason, it is helpful to repeat the question about a second concern at the very end of the interview.

✔ CHECKPOINT QUESTIONS

1. What type of interview question supplies its own answer?
2. What are six areas to explore regarding a chief concern?

Health and Family Profile

Before pursuing the past history or development of a child, it is important to understand something about the circumstances in which the child lives. A good introduction to a health and family profile is a sentence such as, "Before we talk about any past illnesses or happenings with John, let me ask you some questions about John's health and your family as a whole."

Important information concerning the child's current health status includes:

- Who is the child's primary health care provider?
- How often is the child seen for routine health examinations? Are the child's immunizations up to date?
- Can you describe the child's general state of health? How does this compare to the child's health 1 and 5 years ago (if appropriate)?
- Does the child have any known allergies?
- Does the child have a chronic illness or disability?
- Is the child taking any prescription medications? Over-the-counter medications? Home or folk remedies, such as herbal remedies?
- Is the child undergoing any treatments?

Important information concerning the family includes:

- Is the parent married, single, or divorced?
- Is the family nuclear or extended?
- How many children are in the family?
- What are the family's current living arrangements?
- What are the parents' occupations? (This helps establish the family's socioeconomic level and means of family support.)
- If both parents work, how do they manage child care?

Obtaining a health and family profile is sometimes delayed by medical interviewers until the end of the interview, when, theoretically, a parent or child is more comfortable and will answer these personal questions more readily. However, by following a nursing model and obtaining the information earlier in the interview, the health care practitioner can better assess the child and evaluate data.

Day History

The child's current skills, sleep patterns, hygiene practices, eating habits, and interactions with the family can all be elicited by asking the parent to describe a typical day. Day histories are fun to obtain because most parents are eager to describe their day with their child. Information gained this way is surprisingly rich and pertinent, much more so than if parents are just asked how their child sleeps, eats, or plays.

Begin by asking, "Was yesterday a fairly typical day for John?" (The parent says yes, it was.) "Would you describe for me all that John did yesterday, beginning with when he woke up?" Some parents do this in great detail; with others, it is necessary to backtrack for particular details: "What did he eat for breakfast? Does he use a fork and spoon? Does he sit in a high chair or on your lap?"

Play. Play, the work of children, reveals a great deal about the child's development and overall well-being. Important questions to ask about play include:

- Is John kept in a playpen or allowed room to run?
- What is John's favorite toy?
- Does he play active, chasing games or engage in quiet, pretending types of activities?
- Do you (the parent) spend time reading to the child?
- Do you (the parent) play with him or let him play by himself? (This allows for an estimation of the quality of interaction during the day.)

Sleep. Every child needs adequate rest for healthy growth and development. Poor sleep patterns can often reveal a psychosocial or physical health problem. Important questions regarding sleep include:

- When the child sleeps, how long does he sleep?
- Is falling asleep a problem?
- Where does he sleep? Does he have night terrors?
- Does he sleepwalk?
- Does he wet his bed (depending on whether the child is toilet-trained)?

Hygiene. Good hygiene practices promote healthy teeth, gums, and skin, prevent infections, and improve self-esteem. Poor hygiene may reflect neglect, depression, drug abuse, or low socioeconomic status. Important questions regarding hygiene include:

- How much self-care does the child do?
- Does the child take baths or showers?
- Does the child brush his teeth? How often? Does he or she floss regularly? (Responses depend on the age of the child.)
- Does the child wash his hands before snacks and meals?
- Has there been a recent change in hygiene practices?

Nutrition. Nutritional assessment is an important portion of a health assessment because it influences health so strongly (Carney & Meguid, 2002). Characteristics of a nutritionally healthy child that can be revealed by assessment are summarized in Table 33-2. Food and nutrient intake risk factors are summarized in Box 33-1.

Taking a history of a child's food intake can help determine whether there are any foods missing in a typical meal plan or whether any quantities seem inadequate or excessive. Be certain to assess not only the quantity of food taken but the quality as well (e.g., for the infant, cereal should be iron-fortified).

To do this, ask parents to describe a typical day (24-hour recall), listing what the child ate for each meal and between meals as well. With an older child, the 24-hour recall can be a joint parent–child venture. Providing this history can be difficult when the child consumes some meals at home and others at day care or school. It may be necessary to ask for a weekend history to get a complete picture.

When assessing the adolescent, take a 24-hour recall nutritional history without a parent present, if possible. In front of a parent, adolescents may add nutritional foods to a food intake history or leave out foods they have eaten (e.g., milkshakes, potato chips, or pizza) to avoid a lecture later; on the other hand, they may leave out healthy items or add less desirable ones because they may enjoy the obvious parental disapproval, indicative of their rebellion against adult authority.

After taking a history of the child's food intake, determine whether the child is receiving foods that comply with the recommendations of the food guide pyramid. If

TABLE 33.2 Physical Signs of Adequate Nutrition

ASSESSMENT	FINDING
Overall impression	Alert, with good energy level; positive mood
Hair	Shiny, strong, with good body
Eyes	Good eyesight, particularly at night; conjunctiva moist and pink
Mouth	No cavities in teeth; no swollen or inflamed gingivae; no cracks or fissures at corners of mouth; mucous membrane moist and pink; tongue smooth and nontender
Neck	Normal contour of thyroid gland
Skin	Smooth; normal color and turgor; no ecchymotic or petechial areas present
Extremities	Normal muscle mass and circumference; normal strength and mobility; no edema present; no tender joints; normal reflexes; legs not bowed
Gastrointestinal	No diarrhea or constipation present
Finger and toenails	Smooth, pink; not cracked or broken
Height and weight	Within normal limits on growth chart
Blood pressure	Normal for age

BOX 33.1

FOOD AND NUTRIENT INTAKE RISK FACTORS

History or evidence of any of the following may pose a potential nutritional risk:

- Intake less or greater than standard for age, calories, protein, or activity
- Intake less or greater than standard for nutrients (i.e., vitamins and minerals)
- Unusual food habits, such as pica, faddism, and meal skipping
- Inappropriate use of supplements (vitamins, minerals, fortified food products)
- A physician's order for NPO or a clear liquid diet for more than 3 days without enteral or parenteral nutrition
- Inadequate transitional feeding, enteral support, or parenteral support
- Minimal or no intake from a major food group
- Fluid intake less than output
- Eating disorders such as bulimia or feeding disorders
- Food allergies
- Restricted diet

whole food groups are absent or grossly inadequate, the follow-up evaluation should include a food frequency record as a double-check to see if 24-hour recall was truly representative of a usual day. Remember that children do not have to eat food from all groups every meal, as long as they eat from them every day. If parents think in terms of days rather than meals, they may exert less pressure on a child at each meal (Carruth & Skinner, 2000).

WHAT IF? What if an adolescent tells you he eats a hamburger with lettuce, onion, and tomatoes on a bun, french fries, and a chocolate milkshake every night for dinner? Does this adhere to the recommendations of the food guide pyramid?

Be sure to consider the role of food preferences and cultural, lifestyle, and financial variations when assessing food intake. The number of meals eaten at home versus outside the home, the form and content of traditional meals cooked at home, and the pattern of meals should all be considered. Any religious dietary restrictions should also be determined (see Focus on Cultural Competence). Do not appear critical of a child's diet. If you convey dismay at erratic eating habits, parents or older children (especially adolescents) may begin to fabricate the food history to make it seem more acceptable.

Past Health History

For a past health history, ask whether the child ever had any serious illnesses. Parents do not generally think of childhood diseases such as measles, chickenpox, and

FOCUS ON CULTURAL COMPETENCE

In addition to personal likes and dislikes, nutritional practices are culturally determined. Children whose religions prevent them from eating meat, for example, most likely will be vegetarians. Some families prepare food with many spices, whereas others prepare food blandly. Some families use corn as a dietary staple, some rice, and some potatoes or wheat. Lactose intolerance prohibits many Asian children from drinking milk. The main meal of the day is also culturally determined: for some families this is the noon meal; for others it is the evening meal. Assessment is always necessary to understand the meaning of food to a particular family.

mumps as serious illnesses; inquire about these separately. Also inquire about the child's immunization history and whether the immunizations are up to date for the child's age. (See the discussion of immunizations later in this chapter.) Has the child had any accidents? Any surgery? Parents may not think of a tonsillectomy as surgery because there were no stitches; ask about that separately. Did the child ever ingest anything that was inedible or harmful? Has the child been hospitalized for any reason? How many times has the child been seen in an emergency room? These last questions provide information about the degree of adult supervision, and possibly clues to abuse.

Information about the outcome of past illnesses is as important to obtain as information about the illnesses themselves. If the child had otitis media (middle ear infection) at age 2 years and received an antibiotic and recovered without complications, the parent has every reason to be confident that the child will get better from a present illness also; the parent has confidence in health care personnel. If the child had an allergic reaction to the antibiotic or was left with a hearing difficulty from the previous illness, the parent may distrust the care being given to the child now; he or she may not follow instructions well, thinking that nothing works anyway. Or the parents may need extra support to follow instructions. This is important information for planning care.

When parents report a past health concern or outcome, be sure to ask for details and record the responses. This can help to minimize inaccurate data and ensure that the present and future care of the child is appropriate. For example, some parents believe that their child is allergic to an antibiotic because while the child was taking the drug he or she developed diarrhea. There is a strong possibility that the diarrhea was associated with the reason for taking the antibiotic, not with the drug itself. In this example, you would want to ask about specific symptoms and record what the parent says about allergies so the person who prescribes medication for the child can decide whether a true allergy exists.

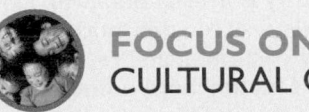

The health of children is affected by their mother's health during pregnancy. For children under age 5 years, therefore, a pregnancy history is usually obtained. Document which pregnancy this was for the mother. Were there complications in any past pregnancies? Abortions or miscarriages? Stillbirths? Children born prematurely? A history of the pregnancy of the child being assessed can begin with a question such as, "How was your pregnancy with John?" This allows the mother to answer in physical and emotional areas. After exploring details mentioned by the mother, ask about specific events that are known to occur with pregnancy, such as:

- Did the mother have any complications such as bleeding, falls, swelling of hands and feet, high blood pressure, or unusual weight gain?
- Did she take any medication?
- Were any x-ray films taken?
- Did she smoke cigarettes, drink alcohol, or use recreational drugs?
- Did the pregnancy end early or late?

Because life contingencies such as loss of finances or illness in the family during a pregnancy may affect a parent's ability to form a bond with a child, the emotional experiences of a woman during pregnancy are also important to obtain. Ask if the parents planned the pregnancy. A question such as, "A lot of pregnancies come as a sort of surprise. Is that how it was with John?" or "Some unmarried women want to have children and some don't. How was it with you?" lets parents know you accept any answer they give.

Next, review labor and delivery. Questions to ask may include:

- How long was labor? Was it what the woman expected it to be?
- Were there any complications? Was the birth vaginal or cesarean?
- Was anesthesia used for birth?
- Was the baby born vertex (head-first) or breech?

Ask about the health of the child at birth as well. Questions to ask may include:

- Did the baby cry right away?
- Did the infant need special procedures or equipment either at birth or in the nursery?
- Was there cyanosis or jaundice?
- Did the infant go to a regular nursery?
- Was the infant discharged from the hospital with the mother?
- How did the parents feel about having a boy or girl?
- How did it feel for them to be new parents?

Family Health History

Because some diseases are inherited or familial, it is important to know which ones occur in a family. Ask if any family member has heart disease (childhood or adult type), kidney disease, a congenital anomaly, seizures, mental retardation, mental illness, diabetes (type 1 or 2), tuberculosis, a sexually transmitted disease, or allergies. Keep in mind that events may have been misinterpreted and reports may be inaccurate, so it is important to ask for details and record what is said about specific familial health problems and outcomes.

Review of Systems

The last step in a health interview is a summary of body symptoms or a **review of systems.** Once more, make certain to introduce this part of the history with a transition statement. Otherwise a parent may think that the local problem (vomiting) he or she has been describing suggests other problems. For example, a statement, such as, "I'd like to ask about different parts of John's body, from his head down to his toes, just to be certain I don't miss anything" provides a transition.

Although the important items to be covered in a review of systems differ according to the age of the child, a basic list is shown in Box 33-2.

A review of systems covers a lot of ground, but it generally takes no more than 5 minutes. However, do not rush through the questions so quickly that the parent does not have time to answer or begins to believe this part of the interview is only an unimportant exercise ("Has John ever had nausea-vomiting-diarrhea-painful joints-broken bones?") All the questions are important. If the child shows any of the symptoms described, an entirely new area needs to be explored.

Conclusion

A health history should close with one last open-ended question: "Is there anything more about John that we should know?" or "Is there anything I didn't mention that you want to ask about?" A parent may have been reluctant to bring up something earlier. Asking this final question gives the parent a final opportunity to do this.

✔ CHECKPOINT QUESTIONS

3. What are the important areas to consider when obtaining a day history?
4. Why is it important to ask for a family health history?
5. What question should be asked at the end of every interview?

PHYSICAL ASSESSMENT

Physical assessment is one of the most frequently practiced skills of a nurse. The scope and extent of pediatric physical assessment vary, like health interviewing, depending on the circumstances of each health visit. Sometimes only a single segment is required to obtain the information needed. For example, if a child has a gastrointestinal disorder, assessment might be only a brief, multisystem examination concentrating on the gastrointestinal system (i.e., mouth, abdomen, and rectum) and fluid status (i.e., skin turgor, lips, and mucous membranes). At a first health care encounter, however, children usually receive a complete physical examination. Mastery of physical examination techniques is essential to incorporating physical assessment data into the assessment step of the nursing process.

BOX 33.2

REVIEW OF SYSTEMS

The following questions provide a guide when completing the review of systems:

Neuropsychiatric symptoms: Has the child ever had seizures? Head injury? Attention problems? Depression? Aggressive behavior? Has the parent ever had such difficulty rousing the child that the parent believed the child was unconscious? Have there been any problems with suspected substance abuse?

Eyes: Has the child had difficulty with eyes not focusing? Eye infection? Does the parent have any reason to believe that the child does not see well? Does the child wear eyeglasses? Contacts?

Ears: Ear infections? Drainage from the ears? Ear aches? Tubes in ears? Any infection from piercing? Reason to believe the child does not hear well?

Nose: Frequent drainage or cold symptoms? Difficulty breathing? Nosebleeds?

Mouth: Difficulty with teeth or teething? Mouth infections? Has the child seen a dentist (if older than age 2 years)? Does the child chew tobacco?

Throat: Throat infections? Difficulty swallowing?

Neck: Masses or swelling? Stiffness? Does the child hold his or her head straight? (Torticollis or wry neck will make the child hold the head crookedly; children with poor vision also may cock their heads to the side to try to see better.)

Chest: Is breast development in girls appropriate for age? For adolescent girls over 14 years and Tanner stage V, ask about breast self-examination.

Lungs: Breathing problems? Infections? Pneumonia? Asthma? Does the child smoke any substance?

Heart: Has a physician ever said there was difficulty? What exactly was said?

Gastrointestinal system: Has there been an eating problem? Frequent nausea? Vomiting? (Ask separately from nausea; children with pyloric stenosis [obstruction of the pyloric opening of the stomach] have vomiting but no nausea; children with a brain tumor may also have vomiting but no nausea; pregnant teenagers may have nausea but not vomiting.) Diarrhea? Any constipation? Is the child toilet-trained? Any difficulty with this?

Genitourinary system: Pain or burning on urination? Blood in urine? Does the child have a good urine stream? If a girl is age 10 years or older, has she started menstruation? Any problems with menstruation? If an adolescent male, has he begun testicular self-examination? If an adolescent, is the child sexually active? Using contraception? Want more information on contraception? Ever had an STD? (To protect privacy, it is essential to ask the adolescent, not the parents, questions regarding sexuality.)

Extremities: Painful or swollen joints? Broken bones? Muscle sprains? Is the parent pleased with the child's coordination?

Skin: Rashes? Lesions such as warts?

Immunizations: What immunizations has the child received to date?

Purpose and Techniques

The actual process of physical examination involves four separate techniques:

1. Inspection
2. Palpation
3. Percussion
4. Auscultation

These techniques are usually carried out in the above order in each area of the body except the abdomen (auscultation should follow inspection and precede palpation of the abdomen, because handling the abdomen may obliterate bowel sounds). **Inspection** is used to determine whether there is redness or swelling or any break in the skin. **Palpation** yields information on warmth and edema; **percussion** helps determine the consistency of tissue beneath the surface area, and **auscultation** reveals the presence of sound (Box 33-3). The findings from these techniques strengthen or validate history findings and help determine whether a problem requires immediate action.

Use physical examination to complement the questions asked when a parent describes some symptom a child is experiencing. If a parent says he or she thinks the child has pain, for example, ask about the duration, intensity, frequency, associated symptoms, and any action or activity that precipitates the pain. Then examine the area for signs of inflammation and palpate for tenderness.

Effective use of physical assessment skills takes practice. Palpating an abdomen, for example, is a simple procedure; recognizing abdominal pathology through palpation is a more complicated skill. It is difficult to distinguish between normal liver tissue and a distended liver, for example, until both these conditions have been felt many times.

Equipment, Setting, and Approach

When performing a complete physical assessment, you'll need the following equipment: a thermometer, a stethoscope, a tongue depressor, an ophthalmoscope, an otoscope, a sphygmomanometer, a tape measure, a tuning fork, a reflex (percussion) hammer, rubber gloves, and perhaps a client drape or drawsheet. Nurses who work in community settings or clients' homes must be sure to carry any equipment that may be needed with them.

Examining body parts such as the mouth or an open lesion exposes the hands to body fluids. As part of infection control precautions, wear gloves as appropriate during the examination. During a complete physical examination, every part of the child's body should be exposed for

BOX 33.3

TECHNIQUES OF PHYSICAL EXAMINATION

Inspection is examining a child or adolescent initially with your eyes or nose, being alert to visual indications or odors that may point to a health problem.

Palpation is examining by touch and can be either light or deep touch. Use light palpation before deep palpation so the child or adolescent does not tense muscles and make light palpation difficult. The tips of your fingers are most sensitive to texture, vibration, consistency, and contour; the back of your hand is most sensitive to warmth. *If a child has a sensitive or painful body part, palpate that area last.* Otherwise, the child may be unwilling to allow you to touch other parts for fear he or she will experience additional pain.

Percussion is the assessment of a body structure by determining the sound you hear in response to striking the part with an examining finger and then interpreting the sound. Dense body areas such as bone have a dull, flat sound; those filled with air, such as lungs, are resonant. If an organ is stretched (a distended bladder), it has a hyperresonant or low and hollow sound. An organ stretched to an even greater point of distention has a tympanic or extremely hollow, ringing sound.

Auscultation is listening to sounds that are either discernible to the ear (wheezing or heavy breathing) or, as in most cases, made louder by means of a stethoscope. Always listen for four qualities of sound: duration, frequency, intensity (loudness), and pitch (high or low).

inspection. To protect against chilling and to provide for modesty, expose body parts individually and only for the amount of time necessary for the examination. Use a client gown or a drawsheet as a drape as necessary.

Be certain the temperature in an examining room is comfortable, and provide privacy. Paper table covers should be changed between children to avoid possible spread of illness.

People have the right not to have another person touch their body unless they permit them to do so. It is essential, therefore, to inform children that it is necessary to touch them for a physical examination, and tell them what is happening at each step during a physical examination so they know when they will be touched (e.g., "Next I will look at your throat"). If some action will cause discomfort, such as deep palpation of the abdomen, offer fair warning: "You'll feel pressure for a minute." Such explanations are also psychologically reassuring because they prevent surprises.

Assume that adolescents will cooperate in placing themselves in whatever position is required to inspect body parts unless they are short of breath or in some other way unable to comply. Small children may not cooperate and may need to be restrained during an examination of body parts such as the nose, throat, and ears. This is done to enable an examiner to see well and also to ensure that the instrument used will not accidentally injure the child. As a rule, do not ask parents to restrain during any procedure in which the child will be hurt; parents are best used as protectors and comforters. However, because a physical examination is rarely associated with pain or hurt, parental participation is helpful. Some procedures, such as ear examination, do require a strong restraining hand, and this can be frightening to children. Urge parents to do this with a positive approach such as, "I'll help you keep your hand still."

Variations for Age and Developmental Stage

Techniques of physical examination must be tailored to the age and developmental stage of the individual being assessed (Table 33-3). Expected findings also depend on the child's age and developmental stage.

Newborn

All newborns receive a physical examination immediately after birth and again after the first 24 hours of life. When examining newborns, remember that maintaining body temperature is one of the newborn's most difficult tasks. Cover body areas that are not being directly examined. Take axillary or tympanic temperatures to prevent rupture of rectal mucosa. Assess the heart rate apically because peripheral pulses are too faint to be counted accurately. Be certain to take femoral pulses in newborns to rule out coarctation of the aorta. Include newborn reflexes, head circumference, and an assessment of gestational age (see Chap. 23) as routine parts of the examination. Do not take blood pressure because this value is unreliable in the newborn.

Infant

Infants are usually examined most effectively if a parent holds them during most of the examination. Use an "isn't this fun?" or "this is a game" approach. As a rule, assess heart and lung function first; intrusive procedures such as ear and throat assessment should be done last so the infant does not cry and complicate the remainder of the examination. Blood pressure is still not taken routinely. Include assessment of newborn reflexes until age 6 months; continue to take the heart rate apically and the temperature in the axilla or by tympanic membrane. Measure head circumference for a full year.

Toward the end of the first year, children become fearful of strangers. Taking an extra minute to become well acquainted with the infant at the beginning of the examination helps to counteract this problem.

Toddler and Preschooler

Both toddlers and preschoolers may be afraid of examining equipment. To alleviate their fears, let them handle items such as stethoscopes, otoscopes, and blood pressure cuffs (Fig. 33-2). Leave intrusive procedures such as assessment

TABLE 33.3 Techniques of Physical Examination Based on Child's Age

AGE	TECHNIQUES
Newborn	Undress only the body part being examined or use a radiant heat warmer to conserve heat (be certain all body parts are exposed during examination). Examine heart and respiratory systems first before the newborn cries, then follow head-to-toe procedure, performing all manipulative procedures such as throat and eyes last. Examine newborn with parents present, using this assessment time to teach them about normal appearance and development.
Infant	As with newborns, begin examination with heart and respiratory assessment, then follow head-to-toe procedure, performing all manipulative procedures such as throat and ears last. Begin examination while parent holds infant in arms or lap to calm the child. Talk to the infant as you proceed; infants calm to sound of your voice or the feeling tone that you radiate as much as they do to what you actually say. A positive tone ("This is like a game") therefore often brings better cooperation than a strict, businesslike approach. Infants older than 3 mo like to handle tongue blades. They can be distracted by brightly colored toys while you listen to their heart or lungs. They cooperate best if a parent holds them for major portion of examination. Offering a bottle of water or pacifier may be necessary during heart assessment.
Toddler	Allow toddler to handle equipment; include games, such as blowing out otoscope light, to relax child. Ask parent to remove clothing or allow child to do it independently. Use head-to-toe procedure; leave uncomfortable procedures such as throat and ear examination for last.
Preschooler	Use games such as "Simon Says" to ease child's fright. Ask child to undress; do not remove underpants. Keep in mind that preschoolers are extremely threatened by intrusive procedures. Thus, they are frightened of examining instruments. Allow them to handle instruments before use. Assure them that instruments do not hurt. Children up to school age often need to be restrained for ear and throat examination because they grow fearful about procedures performed on a part of the body they cannot see (ears) or about a throat examination that may be uncomfortable.
School-age child	Ask whether child wants parent present or not. Proceed with head-to-toe assessment; leave genitalia for last. Allow child to undress except for underpants; supply gown. Explain equipment and reasons for procedures. Teach whys and hows of procedures.
Adolescent	Ask if the adolescent wants parent present or not. Teach adolescent about good health care during examination. Comment on body parts as you examine them: "Your heart sounds good," "Ears look fine." Sometimes an adolescent is so concerned with a part of his or her body (a supernumerary nipple, for example) that he or she is unable to voice this concern. A comment such as, "This is a supernumerary (extra) nipple. Does it ever worry you that you have that?" may help the adolescent to talk about what has indeed been a concern for years. Use head-to-toe procedure; leave genitalia for last. Include health teaching on breast and testicular self-examination.

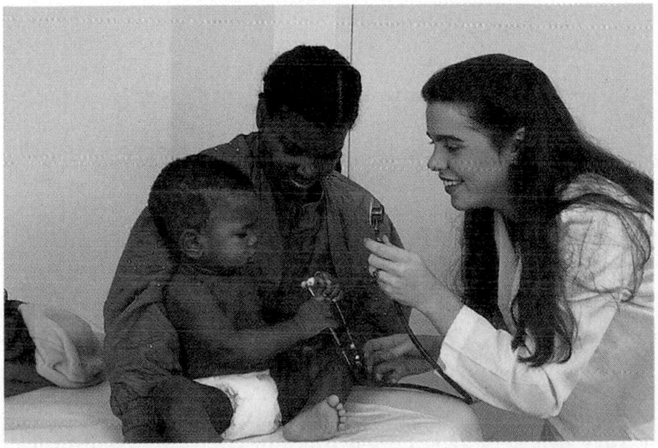

FIGURE 33.2 Children need the opportunity to play with examining equipment so they become more familiar with and less frightened by it.

of the genitalia, ears, and throat until last. Give generous praise for cooperation (anything short of hysterical screaming or kicking is good cooperation for intrusive procedures in this age group). Focus on Family Empowerment describes ways parents can prepare young children for assessment.

Begin to include blood pressure as part of routine assessment at age 3 years; taking an oral temperature by an electronic thermometer can also begin at this age. Before beginning an examination, establish a good rapport with the child's parents, because children this age sense parental trust or suspicion.

School-Age Child and Adolescent

Some children of this age may still be unaware of what a physical examination includes and whether it will cause discomfort. Offer good explanations so they are not frightened by the unknown. Provide older children with a choice

FOCUS ON FAMILY EMPOWERMENT
Suggestions for Preparing a Child for a Health Assessment

Q. How can I best prepare my son for a preschool health exam?

A. Here are some suggestions to help prepare a child for a health assessment:

- Promote the attitude that a health visit will be a positive experience.
- Bring a comfort item from home (favorite doll or toy).
- Never threaten the child that if he is not good, a doctor or nurse will punish him.
- Review with your son what he can expect during an assessment (a health care provider will ask some questions of his parent; she or he will then look at the child's head, hands, etc.).
- If a child has been taught not to let strangers touch his body (as he should have been taught), reassure your son that it is all right for the health care provider to examine him.
- Dress your son in clothing that is easy to remove and replace so you can quickly dress him after an examination. This is a way of assuring him that the examination is over.

about having a parent with them during the examination. Some may enjoy having a parent with them; others may resent their presence. Adolescents are often worried about some normal physical finding such as a mole or supernumerary (extra) nipple. Make a habit of commenting on such findings—"This is a mole on your hand; that's normal"—as both a means of reassurance and health teaching.

Remember that school-age children and adolescents are particularly modest. Respect this by careful use of gowns or drapes. Begin to include teaching for breast and testicular self-examination when appropriate (usually age 14 and Tanner 5 stage for girls; age 13 for boys).

✔ CHECKPOINT QUESTIONS

6. What four techniques are used in physical assessment?
7. At what age is blood pressure included as a routine procedure?

COMPONENTS OF PHYSICAL EXAMINATION

A physical examination may be done in any order, but traditionally the order proceeds from head to toe, examining each body part thoroughly before moving on to the next. With infants and young children, however, it is easiest to begin with the heart and lungs; this is because if the infant cries, findings in these areas become difficult to assess over the sound of crying.

Presented here are the components of a routine or general physical assessment. If abnormalities are discovered during an examination, further assessment is necessary. A complete neurologic examination, for example, is not routine and thus is not included here (see Chap. 49 for details on neurologic examination). It is important to recognize what a "general" physical examination of this nature entails so you can interpret the extent of assessment that a child has received when the parent states, "He had a routine physical."

Vital Sign Assessment

Vital signs refer to temperature, pulse, respiration, blood pressure, or the state of vital bodily functions (e.g., heart and lung function, metabolic rate, and comfort level). Because of the important information they provide, measurements of these signs are recorded not only with complete physical examinations but in many other instances of care (see Focus on Multidisciplinary Care). Techniques of these measurements and the nursing responsibilities that accompany them are discussed in Chapter 36.

General Appearance

Physical examination begins with inspection of general appearance to form an overall impression of the child's health and well-being and to pinpoint specific body areas that will need detailed assessment (Fig. 33-3). Assess such areas as:

- Does the child appear well or ill overall?
- Is the child's height and weight proportional?
- Does the child appear well nourished?
- What is the child's color: pale? yellow (jaundiced)? cyanotic (blue)?

FOCUS ON MULTIDISCIPLINARY CARE

Many health care disciplines such as physical therapists or nutritionists also perform physical examinations or health interviews. Be certain they are aware of how to care for any examining equipment used. Also reinforce the need that they report any conversation they have with the child or parents during this time, because this can be interpreted by the parents as history taking. If parents interpret it this way, they may not repeat some of this information, assuming that it has been recorded and is now known by all health care personnel.

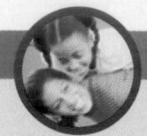

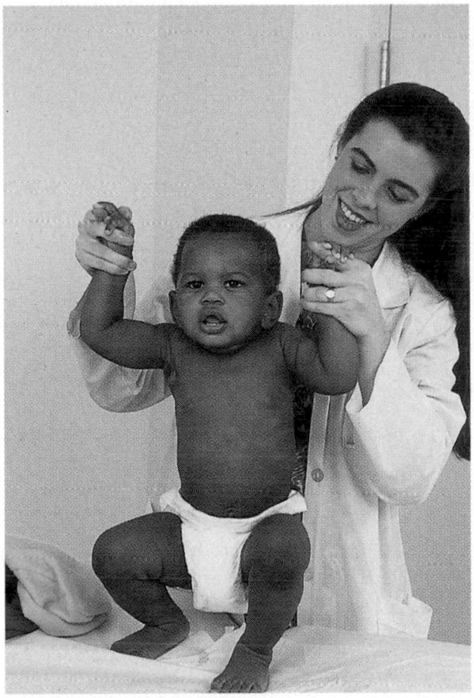

FIGURE 33.3 General appearance assessment reveals that this child is well proportioned and active.

- Is posture normal? (Children who are in pain often assume an abnormal posture for relief.)
- What is the child's hygiene level?
- Are lesions or symptoms of a specific illness present?
- Are there any significant body odors (Table 33-4)?
- Does the child appear relaxed or distressed? Lethargic or active?
- Is breathing easy or distressed?

Mental Status Assessment

A mental status assessment is also made early in an examination as a complement to general appearance information. As with general appearance, additional information is gained on mental status throughout the entire examination.

Begin by assessing the child's level of consciousness: Is the child alert? Able to respond to questions easily? Assess orientation, or awareness of person, place, and time (awareness of who they are, where they are, and the date). Assess the appropriateness of behavior and mood: for example, is the child hostile, frightened, or relaxed? At some point in the examination of children above preschool age, ask questions that test recent memory and distant memory.

Body Measurements

Body measurements are important determinants of health in children because with chronic illness the body expends so many nutrients combating the destructive process of the disease that normal height and weight cannot be maintained. Conversely, overweight (obesity) may be the cause of illnesses such as heart and lung disease later in life. Obesity has become such a health problem that as many as 50% of children in the United States are currently overweight (Davis et al., 2000).

TABLE 33.4 Significant Body Odors

SOURCE OF ODOR	POSSIBLE CAUSE
Breath	
Alcohol	Possible recent ingestion (important if coma or neurologic symptoms are present as cause of abnormal functioning)
Camphor	Mothball ingestion
Halitosis (bad breath)	Poor dental hygiene, lung infection; foreign body in respiratory tract
Burnt rope	Marijuana use
Sweet	Acidosis (seen in a child in diabetic coma)
Body	
Stale urine	Incontinence; poor kidney functioning leading to uremia; infrequently changed diapers; neglect
Sweat	Possible implication of unusual fatigue recently, or that child has not maintained usual hygiene regimen
"Spoiled fruit"	Wound infection
Sweet	*Pseudomonas* infection
Urine	
Maple syrup	Protein metabolic condition
Musty or mousy	Phenylketonuria or a protein metabolism disorder
Ammonia	Urinary tract infection or poor hydration leading to concentrated urine
Stool	
Putrid	Fat in stool from inadequate absorption

Height

In children, height is as good a determinant of health and normal nutrition as weight is. To accurately measure the height of infants and older children, see Nursing Procedure 33-1: Measuring the Child's Height.

Plot height measurements for children on a standard graph the same as for weight. Height and weight should follow the same percentiles. Remember that height/weight charts have been standardized for typical American children, so there will be variations among children from different cultural backgrounds. The important thing to look for is a consistency of measurements over time (always at the same percentile).

Weight

Until they can stand well, infants are weighed on a sitting or infant scale. Because diapers can be heavy in proportion to total body weight, infants are weighed nude. Always keep a protective hand over an infant on an infant scale (hovering but not touching, as infants squirm readily and there is danger of them falling; Fig. 33-4A). Cover both infant scales and adult scales with scale paper before weighing to prevent spread of infection from one child to another.

NURSING PROCEDURE 33.1: MEASURING THE CHILD'S HEIGHT

Purpose
To assess for optimal growth.

Plan	Principle
Infant	
1. Until they can stand securely (at approximately age 2 years), measure infants lying down on a measuring frame or an examining table.	1. Promotes accuracy.
2. Align the infant's head snugly against the top bar of the frame and ask an assistant to secure it there. Parents can help you restrain infants for height measurements because it is a painless procedure.	2. Provides a starting point for measurement.
3. Straighten the infant's body (Figure *A*).	3. Straightens knees to ensure accuracy. Knees are difficult to straighten in infants because they always keep them flexed.

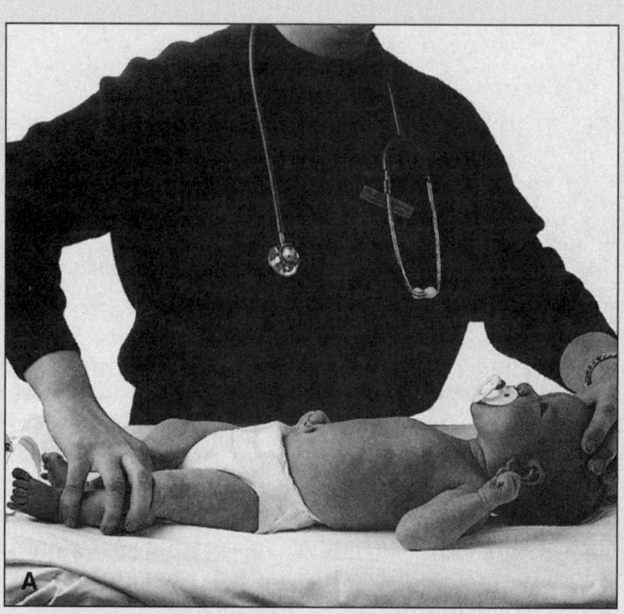

Plan	Principle
4. Hold the infant's feet in a vertical position. Bring the foot board up snugly against the bottom of the foot.	4. Completes measurement.
5. If an examining table is used, mark the spots at the top of the child's head and bottom of feet and then measure between the marks.	5. Provides for an alternative approach.
6. Plot height measurements on a standard graph.	6. Allows for interpretation of findings.
Older Child	
1. Have the child remove his or her shoes.	1. Promotes accuracy.
2. Have the child stand straight with his or her head held level.	2. Puts the child in the proper position for accurate measurement.
3. Align the measuring bar of a standing scale with the top of the head.	3. Determines the measurement.
4. If a scale with a measuring bar is not available, place a flat object such as a clipboard on the	4. Provides for an alternative approach.

(continued)

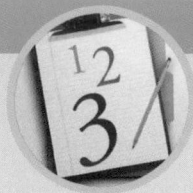

Plan	Principle
child's head in a horizontal position and read the height at the point at which the object touches a measuring tape on the back of the scale or a flat wall surface (Figure *B*).	
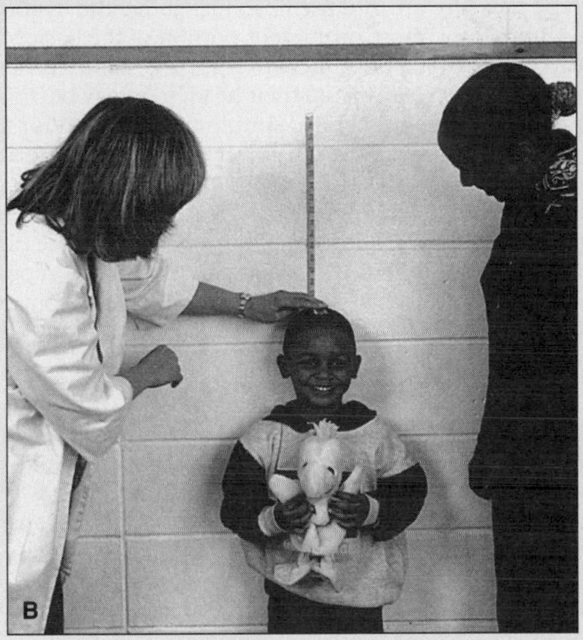	
5. Plot height measurements on a standard graph.	5. Allows for interpretation of findings.

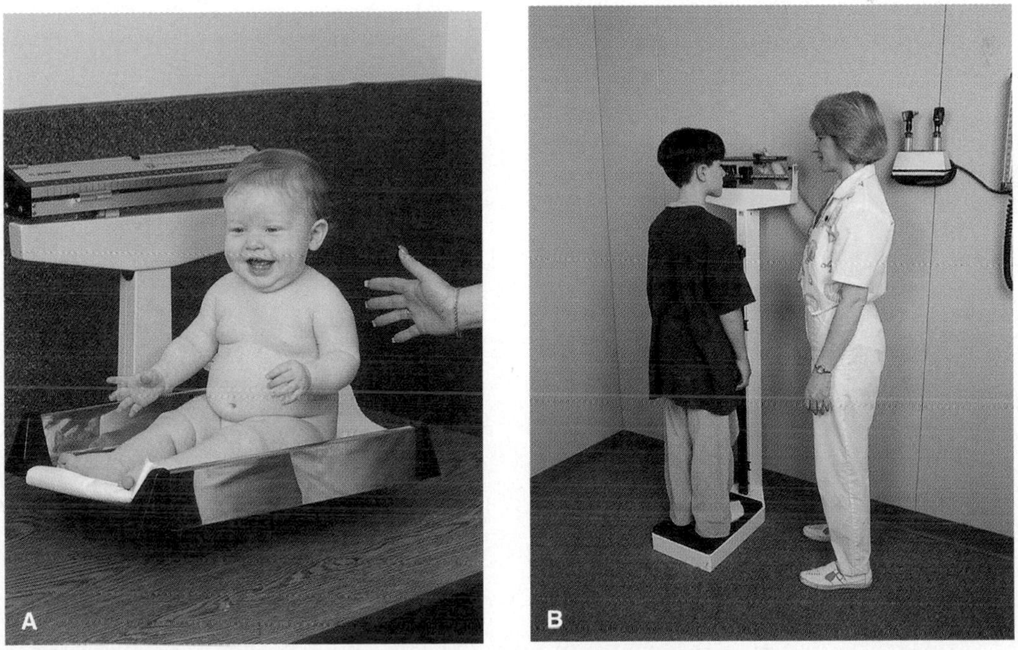

FIGURE 33.4 (*A*) Weighing an infant. Note the protective hand to ensure the infant's safety. (*B*) Weighing an older child.

Children older than age 2 years are weighed on standing scales, in street clothes (no shoes), or, if in a hospital, in a gown or robe (Fig. 33-4*B*). If children are going to have serial weights (weighed every day or several times a day), it is important that they wear the same clothing every time they are weighed so any discrepancy in weight is truly a difference in body weight and not a weight change due to more or less clothing. Take the weight at the same time each day (preferably before breakfast) on the same scale for greatest accuracy.

Most children and their parents want to know their weight. To convert from kilograms to pounds, multiply the kilogram amount by 2.2 (50 kg × 2.2 = 110 lb).

To assess whether weight is average for height, compare the child's weight with a standardized height/weight graph. Child and infant values of these are shown in Appendix E for easy reference. In the standardized scale for children, all weights between the 10th and 90th percentiles are considered normal (statistically, a range of weights that includes two standard deviations from the mean or the 50th percentile). As important as the fact that a child's weight falls between the 10th and 90th percentile on a growth chart is that over time the weight follows one of the percentile curves—in other words, that the child is not at the 80th percentile the first time he or she is weighed and a month later at the 40th percentile, for example. Although both readings are within the normal range, they reflect a weight loss that needs investigation. Gaining weight in the same way could be equally serious. A child is defined as having a "failure to thrive" syndrome (medical diagnosis) if height or weight drops below the third percentile on a standardized growth chart. Any height or weight in this category definitely needs to be reported so its cause can be investigated.

Another method to determine whether the child's weight is consistent with height is to compute the body mass index (BMI). Table 33-5 describes the formula used to calculate BMI and the implications of the values obtained (see also Appendix E).

WHAT IF? What if a 14-year-old girl weighs 93 lb? Would you be concerned? What if 6 months earlier she had weighed 110 lb and a year earlier she had weighed 105 lb?

TABLE 33.5 Body Mass Index Findings

To calculate the body mass index (BMI), divide the child's weight in kilograms by the square of the child's height in meters:

$$\frac{\text{Body weight in kg}}{(\text{Height in meters})^2} = \text{BMI}$$

BMI	IMPLICATION
Below 18.5	Underweight
18.5 to 24.9	Normal
25.0 to 29.9	Overweight
Over 30	Obese

Head Circumference

Head circumference is measured at birth and routinely on physical assessment until age 1 year (many health care agencies measure routinely until age 2 years). Head growth occurs because the brain is growing, so head circumference is an important determinant of brain growth and potential neurologic function. The measurement is made by placing a tape measure around the head just above the eyebrows and around the most prominent portion of the back of the head, the occipital prominence (Fig. 33-5). Babies generally push any object away from their head, so it may be difficult to carry out this otherwise simple procedure. Plot measurements on a standardized graph (Appendix E). Head circumference should correlate with the child's length (e.g., if length is in the 40th percentile, head circumference also should be). If measurements of head circumference plot at different percentiles over time, this should be reported because it implies that brain or skull growth is in some way abnormal and needs investigation.

Chest and Abdominal Circumference

Measurements of chest and abdominal circumference are not done routinely, but only when specific pathology warrants. The measurement of chest circumference is made at the nipple line; the measurement of abdominal circumference is made at the level of the umbilicus.

Skin

Skin is assessed in conjunction with the examination of each body region. Assess the following:

- Temperature
- Color

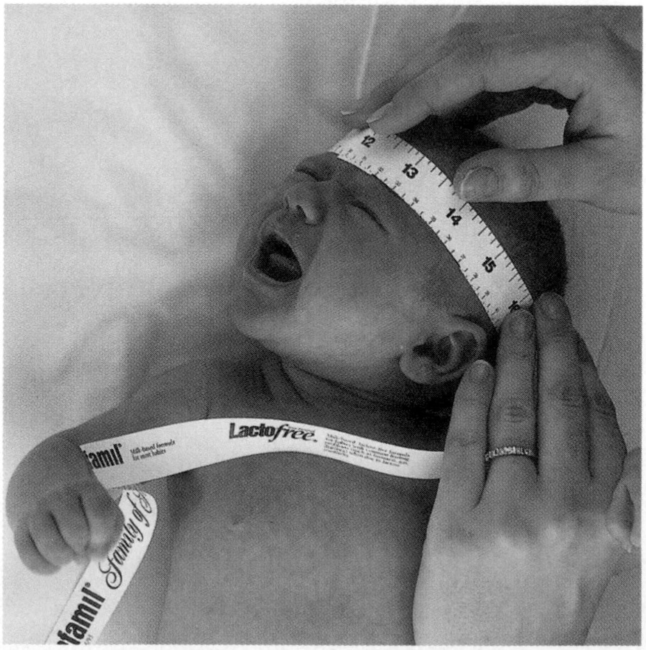

FIGURE 33.5 Measuring head circumference. The measuring tape passes just above the eyebrows and around the prominent posterior aspect of the head.

- Texture
- **Turgor** (amount of fluid in body tissue; Fig. 33-6)
- Presence of any lesions

Table 33-6 summarizes various other findings that may be detected. Be certain to examine the child's total skin surface at some time during an examination. As necessary, remove and replace adhesive bandages and other dressings that could hide important findings. Be sure that there is adequate lighting, especially when assessing dark-skinned children.

Newborn and Infant

Newborns may appear ruddy because their layer of subcutaneous fat is thin and the intense redness of their blood circulation is visible. Erythema toxicum (newborn rash) may be present. Birthmarks (hemangiomas, mongolian spots, or nevi) may be present. After the first few days of life, a diaper rash may be present.

Toddler, Preschooler, and School-Age Child

Many children this age have minor lesions from mosquito bites or from flea bites if they own a pet. They also typically have a number of ecchymotic spots on their lower extremities from bumping into objects during active play. Ecchymotic spots on upper extremities suggest a blood coagulation problem. Be certain in evaluating ecchymotic spots on all age children to consider the possibility of child abuse (Muscari, 2001).

Adolescent

Acne lesions on the face or back are usually present in the adolescent. Lesions or rashes caused by allergies to cosmetics also may be seen. If the child has a tattoo or body piercing, assess the site for inflammation to reveal beginning infection.

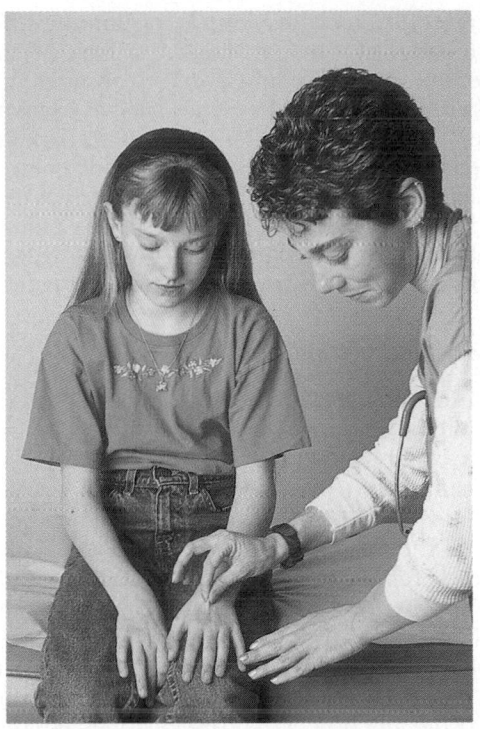

FIGURE 33.6 Assessing skin turgor. If the ridge of tissue does not immediately return to place, this suggests that the child is poorly hydrated.

Head

To examine the head, slide a hand over the skull, assessing for irregular configurations or tenderness. Most children have a prominent occipital outgrowth; do not mistake this natural head contour for an abnormality. Assess the texture and cleanliness of the hair. Children who are well nourished usually have hair of good texture; poorly nourished

TABLE 33.6 Skin Findings in Children That Suggest Illness

FINDING	INDICATION
Central bluish color	Cyanosis from decreased respiratory function or cyanotic heart disease. Acrocyanosis (blue hands and feet) is normal in newborn for first 48 hours.
White color	Edema (accumulated subcutaneous fluid is stretching the skin)
Pale color	Anemia or decreased circulation to a body part
Reddened area	Local inflammation or increased systemic temperature
Linear abrasion	Scratch marks from local irritation from an insect bite, or allergic reaction
Ecchymoses (black and blue marks)	Recent injury to skin
Petechiae (pinpoint blood marks)	Blood dyscrasia (poor clotting ability)
Yellow color	Jaundice from increased bilirubin in subcutaneous tissue; carotenemia (excess carotene in skin)
Moistness	Excess perspiration from elevated temperature
Localized cold temperature	Decreased circulation to particular body part
Warm temperature	Local irritation or elevated systemic temperature
Poor turgor	Dehydration
Rash	Infectious childhood illness, excessive heat, allergy

children tend to have dry, brittle, or limp hair. If hair is exceptionally oily, it may suggest a lack of adequate hygiene, possibly from fatigue due to an unidentified illness. If a serious protein deficiency such as **kwashiorkor** is present, the hair becomes striped with dark and light color; dark hair forms during periods of good protein intake and the light color forms during periods of protein deficit. Patches of hair loss (alopecia) suggest a fungal infection (tinea capitis), child abuse, or a possible drug reaction (chemotherapy will cause total hair loss, not patches).

Newborn and Infant

In the newborn, the head usually shows molding (an elongated shape due to pressure against the cervix before birth). A caput succedaneum or cephalhematoma from the pressure of birth may be present (see Chap. 23). Skull suture lines may be palpable. In both newborns and infants, sit the child upright and palpate the skull for the presence of fontanelles (the places where the skull bones fuse). The anterior fontanelle is at the junction of the two parietal bones and the two fused frontal bones. It is diamond-shaped and measures 2 to 3 cm (0.8–1.2 in) in width and 3 to 4 cm (1.2–1.6 in) in length. The posterior fontanelle is at the junction of the parietal bones and the occipital bone. It is triangular and measures approximately 1 cm (0.5 in) in length (see Fig. 18-2).

With the infant sitting, fontanelles should be felt as soft spots but should not appear indented (a sign of dehydration) or bulging (a sign of increased intracranial pressure). When an infant cries, cerebral pressure increases. Thus, with crying, fontanelles will feel tense, and sometimes even the fluctuation of a pulse is present. The anterior fontanelle normally closes at age 12 to 18 months and the posterior fontanelle by the end of age 2 months. Therefore, these should not be palpable after these times. The closing of fontanelles too early or too late may be an indication of decreased or increased brain or ventricle growth.

A scalp problem commonly encountered in infants is seborrhea (scaling, greasy-appearing, salmon-colored patches). This is referred to by parents as "cradle cap." Increasing the frequency of hair washing to once a day typically reduces this problem.

Toddler, Preschooler, and School-Age Child

Examine the hair of children who attend school or day care carefully for small white-yellow, sand-sized particles attached to hair strands—the eggs (nits) of pediculi (head lice). Nits cling and cannot be readily removed from hair by running fingers the length of the hair. The child may have recent scratch marks on the scalp and generally states that the scalp feels itchy. Pediculi spread easily in school-age children due to the sharing of combs and towels in school.

Also examine the scalp carefully for round circular areas (perhaps weeping in the center, crusting and scaling on the edges) that would suggest tinea capitis (ringworm, a fungal infection). Like pediculi, fungal infections are spread readily among school-age children; a prescription medication is necessary to cure the condition (see Chap. 43).

Adolescent

Adolescents may streak their hair with dye or arrange it in a way that requires gel, hair extensions, or use of a curling iron. Inspect to see that their scalp and hair are healthy underneath the styling.

Eyes

Observe the eyes for symmetry and signs of frequent blinking, crusting, squinting, or rubbing. Observe lids and lashes for redness (erythema), which suggests infection. Common infections include **conjunctivitis** ("pink eye," an infection of the thin conjunctiva that covers the eye) or a **hordeolum** or sty (an infection of the gland that lubricates an eyelash). Both conditions require an antibiotic for therapy (see Chap. 50).

Assess the location of eyes in relation to the nose (not unusually wide- or narrow-spaced) and the relationship of the globe to the socket (neither sunken nor protruding from the socket [exophthalmos]). Abnormalities in these areas occur in chromosomal or metabolic illnesses such as hyperthyroidism. Inspect the sclera of the eye for spots of hemorrhage (called subconjunctival hemorrhage) or yellowing. African-American children often have a slight yellowing of the sclera and small black spots on the sclera; do not mistake these for abnormal findings. Assess that no sclera shows above the pupil (if it does, this is termed a sunset sign, an indication of increased intracranial pressure).

Palpate each eye globe with the eyelid closed to assess for tenseness, a finding suggesting glaucoma (rare in children). Determine whether the eyelids completely close (edema or neurologic illnesses may make eyelids too short to do this) when the child shuts the eyes. Also determine whether the lids retract far enough so they do not obscure vision when the child opens the eyes. When a lid obscures vision, a condition termed **ptosis,** it generally denotes neurologic involvement. The difference in Western and Eastern eye creases is shown in Figure 33-7.

Examine the inner lining of the lower eyelid (the conjunctiva) by pulling the lid down slightly with a fingertip. Here, the mucous membrane should appear pink and moist. In children with anemia, it often appears pale; with allergy or infection, it may appear unusually red and irritated. Do not initiate a blink reflex by touching the cornea with a wisp of cotton, as can be done in adults; this is momentarily painful and frightening to children.

In addition, observe whether the eyes appear to be in good alignment. **Strabismus** refers to eyes that are not evenly aligned. If an eye is always turning in, the condition is called **esotropia;** if it always turns out, **exotropia.** Two screening procedures for straight eye alignment include a Hirschberg's test and a cover test. During a Hirschberg's test, the light of an otoscope should reflect evenly off both pupils if they are in equal alignment (Fig. 33-8).

To perform a cover test (Fig. 33-9), follow these steps:

- Have the child fix his or her vision on an attractive object approximately 4 ft in front of the child.

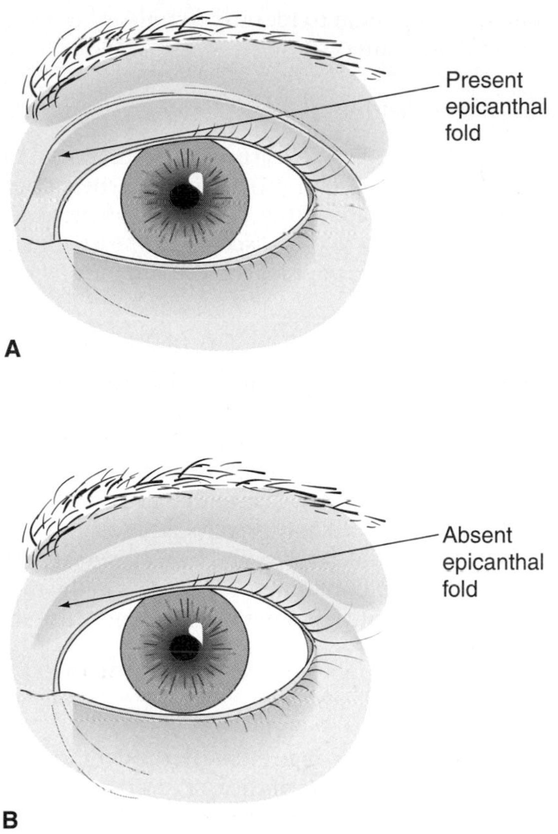

FIGURE 33.7 Differences in eye formation. (*A*) Western. (*B*) Eastern. The extra inner fold of tissue is an epicanthal fold.

- Hold a 3 × 5-in card over the left eye for a count of five. If any degree of strabismus is present, the eye will wander to its misaligned position while covered.
- Remove the card and observe the eye for movement.
- As the child again fixes his or her vision on the specified object in front, the eye will move back into line, thus revealing the misalignment.
- Repeat the process with the right eye.

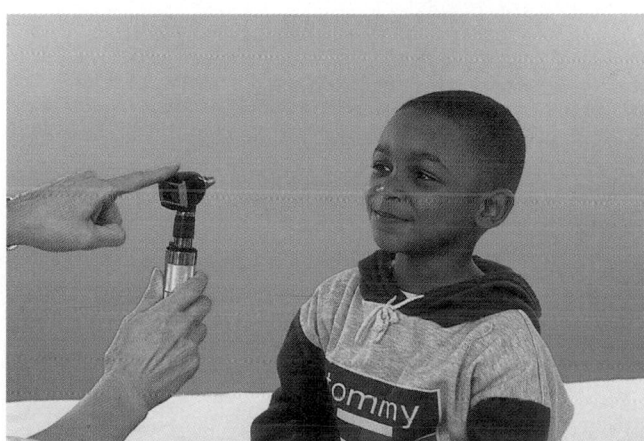

FIGURE 33.8 Testing of good eye alignment by Hirschberg's test. The child is asked to look directly at the light of the otoscope. The light reflex on the pupils of both eyes will be equal if the eyes are in straight alignment.

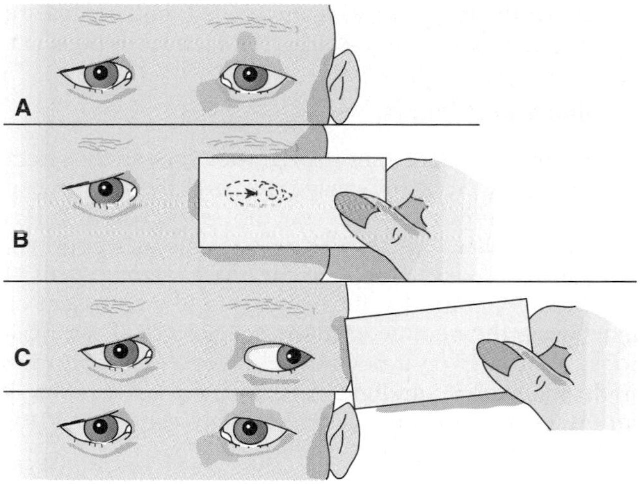

FIGURE 33.9 Cover test. (*A*) The child's eyes appear to be in good alignment. (*B*) The left eye is covered for 5 seconds. (*C*) When the card is removed, the left eye is seen to move perceptibly back to good alignment. This movement indicates that it "drifted" into a deviant position while covered, that is, that an exophoria (misalignment) is present.

Some children, particularly preschoolers who have wide epicanthic folds, may appear, at a quick glance, to show misalignment. A cover test is helpful in these children. There is no eye movement after removal of the card because there is no misalignment present, only the temporary appearance of misalignment. Reasons for true misalignment are discussed in Chapter 50.

Test the eyes for their ability to focus in all fields of vision by following these steps:

- Ask the child to follow a moving light (or catch the attention of an infant with a moving light) while holding the child's chin stationary.
- Move the light out to the side, then up, then down.
- Cross to the opposite side and move it up and down.
- Bring the light back to the midline and observe whether the child's eyes converge (follow the light to the nose) as the light moves in toward the nose. Infants under age 3 months cannot follow past the midline; the eyes of children under school age do not converge well.

Observe if the pupil constricts (reduces in size) in response to a light, an indication that the third cranial nerve is intact. It is best to approach the child's eye from the forehead so the light suddenly appears on the pupil rather than advancing toward the child slowly. This makes the pupil constrict more dramatically. This should occur in response to a light shining directly on a pupil (direct constriction); when one pupil constricts, this will also occur in the opposite eye (consensual constriction). Record that pupils are equal in size and react to light as "PERL" (pupils equivalent, react to light). If the pupil converges (moves to follow a light in toward the nose), this is charted as "PEARL" or "PERLA" (pupils equal, react to light, accommodate).

For a final step, shine a flashlight or ophthalmoscope light into the pupil. A red reflex should appear. This is evidence that the retina is intact and the lens and cornea are clear (no tumor, cataract, scarring, or infection is present).

Newborn and Infant

Newborns often have a small, bright-red spot on the sclera (a subconjunctival hemorrhage) because the pressure of birth has ruptured a small conjunctival blood vessel. This is normal and will fade in 7 to 10 days as the blood is absorbed.

Infants can easily be tested for a red reflex, but until they are age 3 months, they cannot follow an object or light across the midline or follow a light into all six positions of gaze. Even a newborn, however, can follow a bright light to the midline. Assessing for a red reflex is important because a congenital cataract can lead to loss of central vision if not discovered.

Toddler and Preschooler

Most young children are reluctant to let someone look into their eyes. Explaining what will happen during an eye examination is effective in reducing the child's anxiety about this part of the assessment.

School-Age Child and Adolescent

Many older children wear contact lenses (a red reflex is visible with a contact lens in place); some may be nervous about having their eyes examined because they know they should be wearing prescribed eyeglasses but have not done so because they do not like their appearance. Observe carefully for pupillary appearance and ability to constrict in adolescents as a sign of drug abuse. Many adolescent girls are anemic and so have pale conjunctiva.

> ✔ **CHECKPOINT QUESTIONS**
>
> 8. On a standardized scale, what range of weight is considered normal for children?
> 9. What factors should be assessed during an examination of the skin?
> 10. How is a red reflex elicited?

Nose

Observe the nose for flaring of the nostrils (a sign of need for oxygen). Using an otoscope light, observe the mucous membrane of the nose for color (it should be pink; pale suggests allergies, redness suggests infection). Note and describe any discharge. Document that the septum is in the midline (displaced septa such as those that occur after facial injuries can interfere with respiration and make nasal intubation in emergencies difficult). Gently press one nostril closed and ask the child to inhale; repeat on the opposite side to ensure that both sides of the nose are patent (i.e., that no choanal atresia or no membrane obstructing the posterior nares exists). Sinuses do not fully develop until about age 6 years. For children 6 years or older, palpate the areas over the frontal and maxillary sinuses for tenderness, a symptom of sinus infection. Assess the sense of smell in school-age children and adolescents by asking them to identify a familiar odor such as chocolate or an orange.

Newborn and Infant

Infants are obligate nose breathers. They cannot coordinate mouth breathing, so they become disturbed when the nose is temporarily blocked to check for patency; do this only momentarily to avoid discomfort. Most newborns have milia (small white papules) on the surface of the nose.

Older Children

Many children, preschool age and older, have upper respiratory infections that cause reddened nasal mucous membranes and a purulent discharge. In contrast, allergies cause a clear discharge and pale mucous membranes. Children who have dry mucosa due to dry air (which leads to cracking and nosebleed) may be reluctant to allow inspection of their nose. Adolescents who sniff cocaine lose nasal hair and may have excoriations or abscesses in the mucous membrane. If the child has a nasal ring, inspect the site for redness or drainage.

Ears

Observe ears for proper alignment. In the average child, a line from the inner canthus of the eye to the outer canthus and then to the ear will touch the top of the pinna of the ear (Fig. 33-10). Ears set lower than this are associated with chromosomal disorders such as trisomy 13. Observe the opening to the ear canal for any discharge. Touch the pinna and watch for evidence of pain (a sign of external canal infections). Observe the area immediately in front of the ear for a dermal sinus or a skin tag (a finding that is usually innocent but may be associated with kidney abnormalities). Observe the ear lobes for redness or drainage from infected pierced earring sites.

To examine the ear canal, follow these steps:

- Straighten the ear canal by pulling the pinna gently down and back in the child under age 2 years and up and back in the older child.

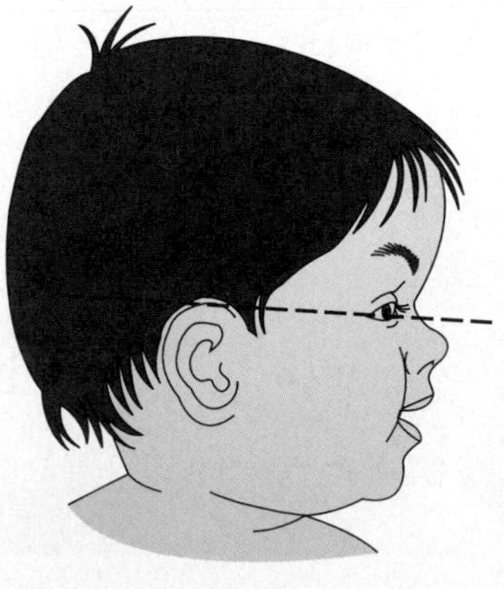

FIGURE 33.10 Normal ear alignment. When a line is drawn from the inner canthus through the outer canthus to the ear, the top of the ear pinna should meet the line. Abnormal ear alignment is associated with certain chromosomal abnormalities.

- Select an otoscope tip. Otoscope tip sizes vary; use the smallest size possible that still gives adequate visibility.
- With the ear canal held straight, insert an otoscope tip into the external canal.
- Rest the instrument on a hand, not on the child's head (Fig. 33-11). In this position, the otoscope will move with the child, avoiding the danger that the plastic tip will scratch the canal if the child should move his or her head suddenly.
- Inspect the sides of the ear canal and locate landmarks on the surface of the tympanic membrane.

The outline of the malleus of the inner ear through the translucent membrane is a key landmark to visualize (Fig. 33-12). The color of the membrane is pinkish gray; if the tension of the membrane is normal, a cone of light (the light reflex) should be present in one of the lower corners (at either the 5 o'clock or 7 o'clock position).

Although many children have wax (cerumen) in their ear canals, appearing as a dark-brown, glistening substance, viewing the tympanic membrane past the wax is almost always possible. If a middle ear infection is suspected, it will be necessary to visualize the entire eardrum. If ear wax occludes visualization, it will need to be cleaned away.

If ear infection is present, the tympanic membrane appears reddened and often bulges forward so the malleus is no longer discernible and the cone of light is absent. If there is fluid in the middle ear, it may be possible to see bubbles of air through the membrane. With chronic middle ear disease (serous otitis media), the tympanic membrane may be retracted, the malleus is extremely prominent, and the cone of light is again missing. If the membrane has been torn from trauma or rupture, the jagged edge and opening to the middle ear are discernible. Inspect also for any ulcerated areas that could be a cholesteatoma or an ingrowing tumor (see Chap. 50).

The mobility of the eardrum can be tested by injecting a column of air into the ear canal against the drum by a pneumatic attachment on the otoscope that looks like the bulb of a blood pressure cuff (Fig. 33-13). A normal drum is freely mobile and can be seen to move with pressure on

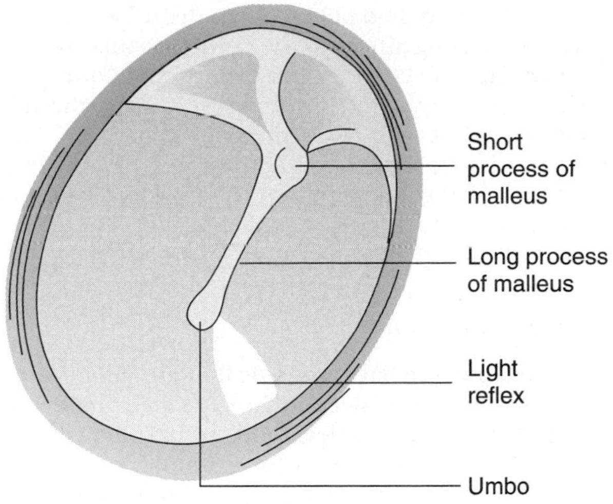

FIGURE 33.12 A tympanic membrane as viewed with an otoscope.

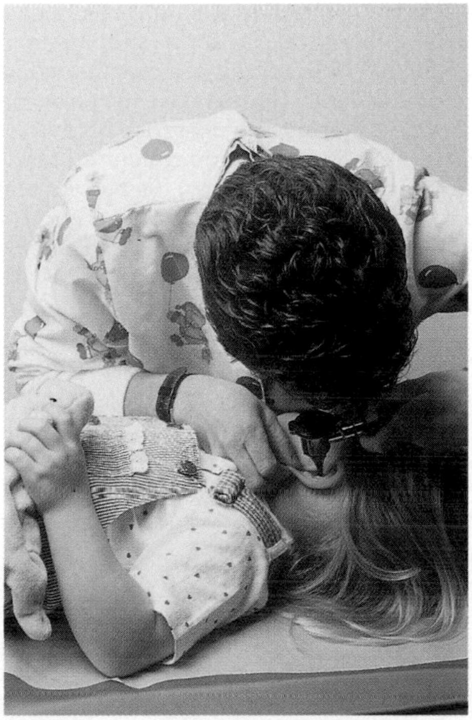

FIGURE 33.11 Otoscopic examination. Note how the nurse's hand rests between the otoscope and the child's head. Should the child move suddenly, no injury to the tympanic membrane will be sustained with this technique because the otoscope will move along with the child's head.

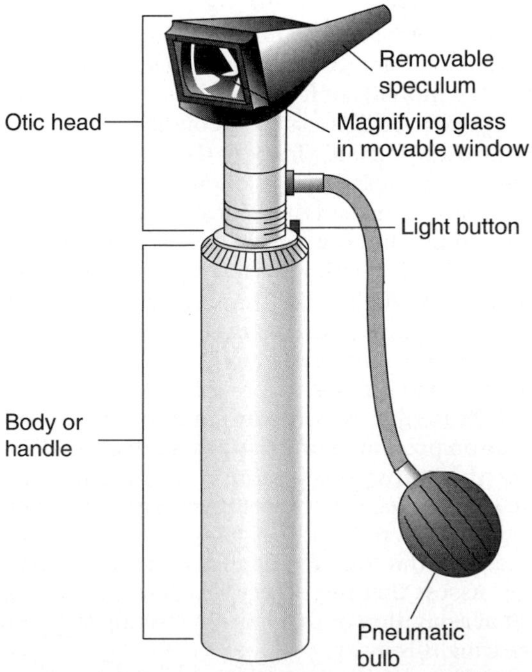

FIGURE 33.13 Otoscope with pneumatic attachment.

the bulb; one with fluid behind it has decreased mobility. Before introducing air, warn the child that this "tickles."

Finally, appraise hearing. Appraisal can be done grossly in older children by assessing their response to questions. Distract an infant with a toy; then make a sound behind the infant's back, out of peripheral vision, and watch for the response. Hearing infants will show some noticeable reaction, although they have difficulty looking directly toward or locating the sound until 4 months of age.

Newborn and Infant

Many newborns still have amniotic fluid or vernix caseosa in their ear canal, so inspecting the ear canal is ineffective. Be certain to assess for ear level and normal pinna contour. Assess gross hearing ability—for example, by watching the infant startle to a sudden sound or quiet to the calming effect of quiet talking.

Older Children

Middle ear infection (otitis media) is a common childhood illness. This causes the ear to be painful when examined. An external ear infection (often called swimmer's ear) causes any movement of the pinna to be painful. For these reasons and because children are told many times never to put anything into their ears, they usually resist ear examinations. Explaining what is happening helps to allay any fears. Beginning with preschool age, children may have myringotomy tubes (small circular plastic tubes placed into the tympanic membrane) to relieve chronic fluid collected in the middle ear. Inspect that the area surrounding the tube is not inflamed and the tube is not merely lying in the external canal and no longer inserted into the membrane (see Chap. 50).

Mouth

Assess the external appearance of the lips, looking for symmetry and color. Ask the child to smile and frown to evaluate the mobility of facial muscles. Count the number of teeth present and assess their condition (number missing or cavities present). Inspect the gum line (gingivae) for redness, tenderness, and edema, symptoms of periodontal disease. Inspect the buccal membrane and palate for color (pink) and the presence of any lesions. Ask the child to stick out the tongue and assess for midline position and no fasciculations (trembling). Inspect the area under the tongue for lesions in school-age children and adolescents who smoke or chew tobacco because this is the most common first site for oral cancer.

A child's tongue is normally smooth and moist. With dehydration present, it often appears roughened and dry. **Geographic tongue** is a term for the rough-appearing tongue surface that often accompanies general symptoms of illness such as fever; it may also occur normally. If the child has had the tongue pierced, inspect for redness at the site. Assess that the object is secure so there is little chance of aspiration or that it is not striking tooth enamel and wearing this away.

Inspect the uvula to be certain it is in the midline. Use a tongue blade to press down and forward on the back of the tongue (Fig. 33-14). The epiglottis can usually be observed with the tongue depressed. Observe for abnormal enlargement, palatine redness, or drainage of tonsils. Although tonsillar tissue differs greatly in size, it should not be reddened or have pus in the crypts (indentations). After initiating the gag reflex in an infant to view the back of the throat, always turn the infant's head to the side so he or she does not choke on any saliva that accumulated in the mouth during the throat examination. Infants are less able to manage this than adults are.

It is important not to depress the tongue of any child who is suspected to have epiglottitis or whose glottis is inflamed. If a swollen, inflamed epiglottis rises with the pressure of a tongue blade, it can obstruct the respiratory tract so completely that the child is immediately unable to breathe. Symptoms of this condition are a sore throat, drooling, fever, difficulty with respiration, dysphagia, and a barking cough.

Newborn and Infant

Many newborns have considerable mucus in their mouths because they are less able to handle swallowing due to immature muscle coordination. If a newborn has teeth, evaluate them for stability; if loose, they need to be removed to prevent aspiration. Assess for white patches that do not scrape away from the buccal membrane or tongue (thrush), a frequent but abnormal finding in infants.

Older Children

Tonsillar tissue in children reaches its maximum growth at early school age, making many preschool children appear to be "all tonsils." As long as the tissue does not appear reddened or tender, it can be assumed to be normal for the age. Many children have irregular, pale-pink, elevated projections on the posterior pharynx as a normal finding. A stream of mucopurulent discharge in the posterior pharynx is not unusual if an upper respiratory infection and a "postnasal" flow of secretions are present. For the child with orthodontic appliances such as braces, assess carefully for pinpoint ulcers to be certain the wires are not causing undue discomfort or infection.

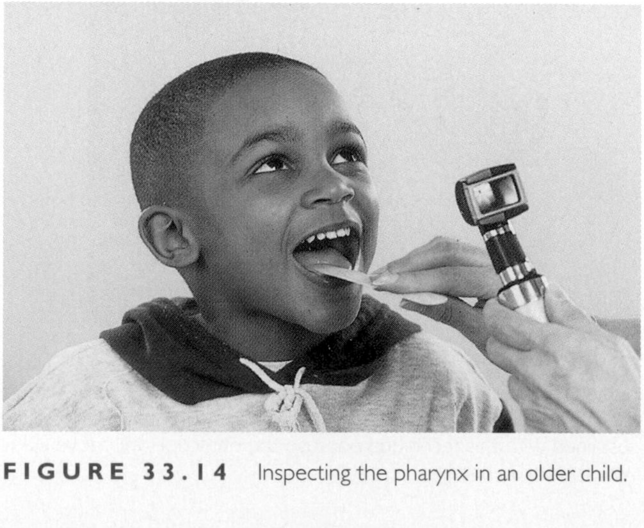

FIGURE 33.14 Inspecting the pharynx in an older child.

Cavities appear as dark-brown areas on the tooth enamel. Many school-age children or adolescents have at least one present.

Neck

Assess the neck for symmetry (the trachea should be in the midline; any deviation suggests lung pathology). Observe the outline of the thyroid gland (barely noticeable before puberty because it is obscured by the sternocleidomastoid muscle) on the anterior neck. Palpate the area in front of the ear (location of the parotid gland) and smooth a hand over the location of lymph nodes at the sides of the neck and under the chin to palpate for swelling. Figure 33-15 shows the location of lymph node chains of the head and neck. Because children have so many upper respiratory infections, a few nodes that are freely movable, about the size of peas, are often present. Commonly, preauricular and postauricular nodes are palpable after ear infections, and postoccipital nodes are palpable after a scalp infection. Submental nodes generally denote a tooth abscess. Palpable submaxillary, anterior, and posterior cervical nodes follow throat infections.

Ask the child to move the head (or move it for the child) through flexion (touch chin to chest) and extension (raise chin as high as possible), and turn it right and left (rotation) to see that the child does this easily. Pain on forward flexion is an important sign of neurologic (meningeal) irritation.

Newborn and Infant

With infants, the ability to control the head should be assessed. Lay the infant supine and pull the child to a sitting position. Babies younger than age 4 months will let their heads lag backward as they are pulled up; they right their heads only as they reach a sitting position. After age 4 months, infants should bring their head up with them (no head lag) if their neuromuscular coordination is adequate for their age. This simple but important test yields information about overall neuromuscular control.

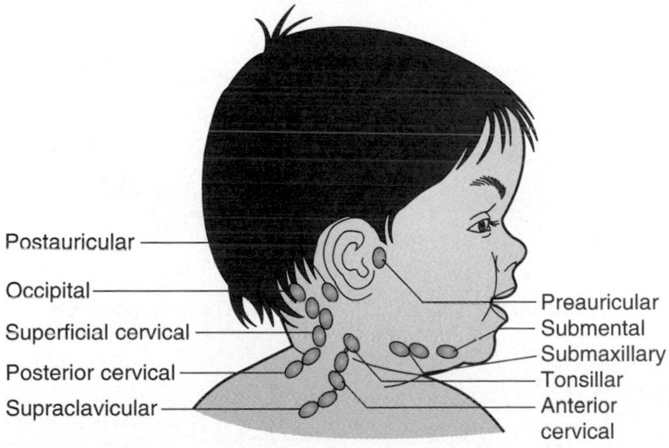

FIGURE 33.15 Location of lymph node chains in the head and neck.

Adolescent

In adolescents, palpate the thyroid gland for symmetry and possible nodes. To do this, press on the right side of the gland, causing it to be more prominent on the left side. Then palpate the left half to discern any irregularities (areas of hardness). Repeat on the right side. A finding of a thyroid node needs to be investigated. It may be only an innocent transient cyst, or it may be the first indication of thyroid malignancy. Many adolescents have some increase in the size of the thyroid at puberty; this hypertrophy should not be accompanied by any nodes.

Chest

For ease in specifying the location of chest pathology, the chest is divided into sections by imaginary lines drawn through the midclavicle, midmammary, and midsternum points on the front; the midaxilla on the side; and the midscapula on the back. Pathology is described in terms of these lines (e.g., abnormal lung sound heard at left mid-axillary line). Other helpful means of locating pathology is by the suprasternal notch, the ribs, and the spaces between them (**intercostal spaces**). Intercostal spaces are numbered according to the ribs immediately above them (Fig. 33-16). Inspect both front and back surfaces of the chest for symmetry of appearance and motion. An infant with a diaphragmatic hernia (intestine herniated into the chest cavity) may have a chest enlarged on that side. An infant with atelectasis (collapsed lung) may have a chest that is smaller on the affected side. If a child has an enlarged heart, the left side of the chest may appear larger. Inspect for **retractions** or indentation of intercostal spaces or the suprasternal and substernal areas that reflect difficult respirations. Assess the proportion of anteroposterior to lateral diameter (normally 1:2). Children with chronic lung disease develop a broad (barrel) chest or one more rounded than normal. This and other chest abnormalities are shown in Figure 33-17.

Breasts

The degree of breast assessment depends on the child's age and development. As part of a normal breast assessment, inspect and palpate the breasts of all children to detect any deformities or abnormalities.

Newborn

Both male and female newborns may have breast edema from the influence of maternal hormones. A few drops of clear fluid may even be present from the nipples. This is normal. Document if a supernumerary nipple is present for baseline data.

School-Age Child and Adolescent

Breast examination should be done routinely on all children past puberty. This is also the time when girls should begin breast self-examination. If a girl younger than 8 years is beginning breast development, precocious puberty (see Chap. 48) should be suspected. Many preadolescent boys

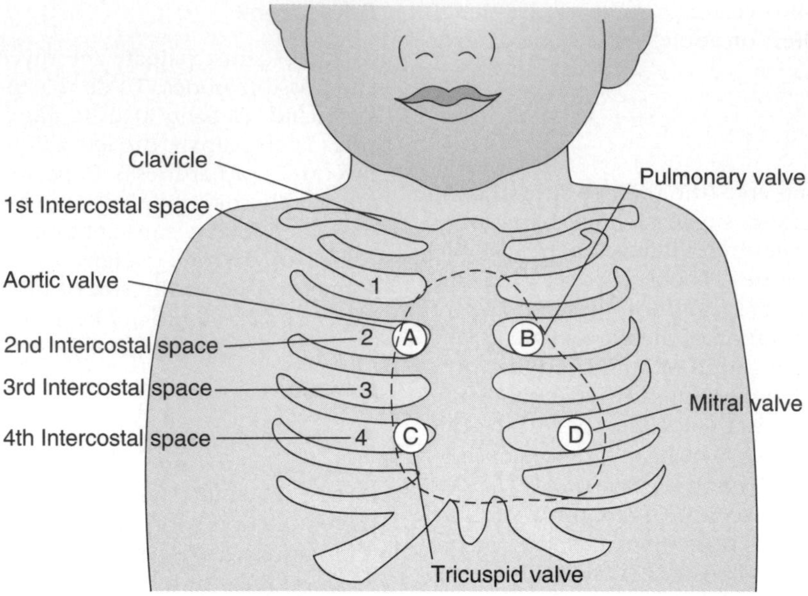

FIGURE 33.16 Intercostal (between rib) spaces are numbered according to the ribs immediately above them. The points (*A*, *B*, *C*, and *D*) to which the sounds of the heart valves radiate or where the sounds can be heard best are the listening posts of the heart.

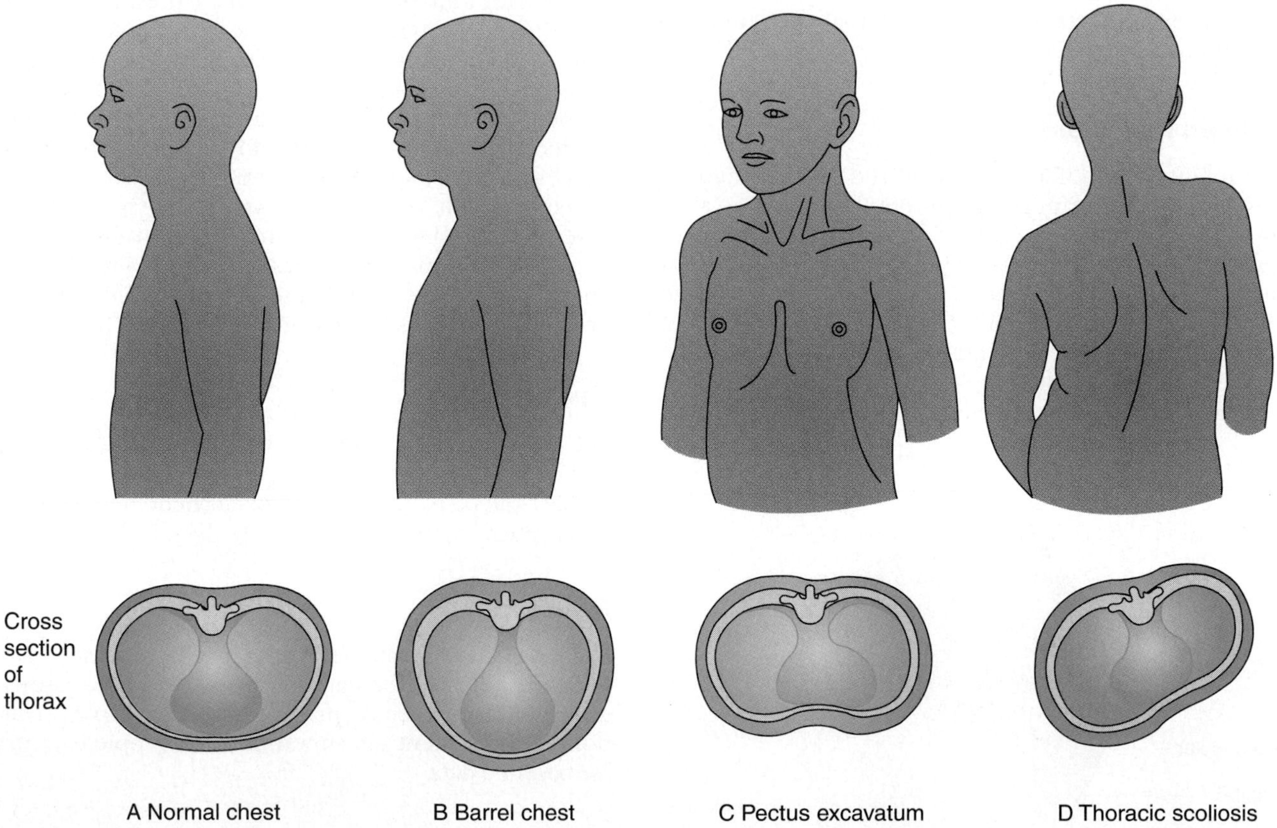

FIGURE 33.17 Chest contours that can be assessed by inspection. (*A*) Normal chest. (*B*) Barrel chest. (*C*) Funnel chest (pectus excavatum). (*D*) Thoracic kyphoscoliosis.

develop hypertrophy of breast tissue due to increased hormonal influences (gynecomastia); they are generally concerned and need reassurance that this is normal for their age and will fade as soon as androgen becomes their dominant hormone. Adolescent girls may be concerned their breast tissue is inadequate or that breast growth is uneven. They need assurance that not all women have completely symmetric breasts.

Inspection of breast tissue is easiest if the child sits on the examining table, arms at the sides, with both breasts exposed. Inspect for symmetry. It is normal and not unusual for a girl to have breasts of slightly unequal size.

Inspect breasts for edema, erythema, wrinkling, retraction, or dimpling of the skin; all suggest that a tumor is growing in deeper layers of the tissue. Erythema occurs from inflammation due to abnormal, rapidly growing tissue; edema results from the blockage of lymph channels due to tumor pressure. Breast edema makes the skin appear not only swollen but pitted (an orange-peel effect). Note any nipple discharge or "pulled" nipple placement as another way to detect edema.

With the girl's arms at her sides to take pressure off breast tissue, palpate well into each axilla (because breast tissue extends this far), and also palpate to assess axillary lymph nodes. Normally, no nodes should be felt. Ask the girl to lie down; place a folded towel under her near shoulder. Palpate the near breast with her lying down with her arm raised and placed under her head because this spreads out breast tissue; begin at the nipple and palpate outward in a circular motion. The lower edge of each breast feels hard; do not mistake this or rib prominences underneath for a tumor.

Girls age 14 years or older (or at the point that they have developed breasts) should inspect their own breasts monthly on the day after the end of their menstrual period. This time not only serves as a marking point but is a time when hormonal influences on breast tissue are at a low ebb, so breast tissue is not swollen or tender. The American Cancer Society's technique of breast self-examination is shown in Focus on Family Empowerment. A health examination is a good time to have the adolescent perform a breast-self examination so she can be given feedback on the technique.

> ✔ **CHECKPOINT QUESTIONS**
>
> 11. What is the rule of thumb for determining normal ear level?
> 12. When is it important not to elicit a gag reflex?
> 13. What signs suggest that a tumor is growing in the deeper layers of breast tissue?

Lungs

Assess the rate of respirations and whether respirations are easy and relaxed or if accessory muscles are necessary for effective ventilation. Palpate over lung areas for vibrations caused by difficult respirations.

On the anterior chest, lung tissue extends from above the clavicles to the sixth or eighth rib. On the posterior chest, lung tissue is as low as the 10th to 12th thoracic vertebra. The right lung has three lobes; the left, only two. It is important when assessing lung tissue to attempt to evaluate all five lobes because lung disease can be specific for a lobe or involve the entire lung.

Next, percuss over lung tissue. Normal lung sounds in older children are resonant; normal lung sounds in infants and younger children are hyperresonant due to the thinness of the chest walls; overexpanded lungs sound hyperresonant in older children; and lungs filled with fluid sound dull in older children and less resonant in younger children. The lower anterior lobe of the right lung will sound dull because the liver covers it on the anterior surface below the fourth or fifth intercostal space. The space over the heart will also sound dull.

Diaphragmatic expanse (the distance the diaphragm descends with inhalation) is an estimate of lung volume. To establish this:

- Ask the child to take in a deep breath and hold it.
- Percuss downward to locate the bottom of the lungs (the percussion note changes from resonant to flat at this point).
- Ask the child to expire fully and momentarily hold that position.
- Percuss upward to locate the expired or empty lung position (the percussion note changes from flat to resonant).

The difference between these two points is the **diaphragmatic excursion.**

Auscultate breath sounds by listening with the diaphragm of a stethoscope over each lung lobe while the child inhales and exhales (preferably with his or her mouth open). Listen both anteriorly and posteriorly; compare the left side with the right side for equal findings. Normal breath sounds are slightly longer on inspiration than expiration. Consider whether there are any abnormal sounds. Table 33-7 describes normal breath sounds and transmitted airway sounds as well as adventitious sounds that, if heard, might reflect illness.

Newborn and Infant

Infants cannot breathe in and out on request. Try to listen to breath sounds early in an examination, because the breath sounds are difficult to hear clearly over the sound of crying.

Heart

Heart assessment begins with visual inspection to see if there is a point on the chest where the heartbeat can be observed. This point represents the location of the left ventricle or the point where the apical heartbeat can be heard best. In children younger than age 7 years, this point is generally lateral to the nipple line and at the fourth intercostal space. In children older than age 4 years, it is at the nipple line or just medial to it and at the fifth intercostal space. This point is termed the **point of maximum impulse** (PMI) and is observable in approximately 50% of children.

FOCUS ON FAMILY EMPOWERMENT

Breast Self-Examination

Q. How often should I examine my breasts? And what is the best way to do it?

A. Follow these steps each month on the day after your menstrual period ends:

Step 1. Inspect

(A) In front of a mirror, look for any change in the size or shape of the breast, puckering or dimpling of the skin, or changes in the nipple.

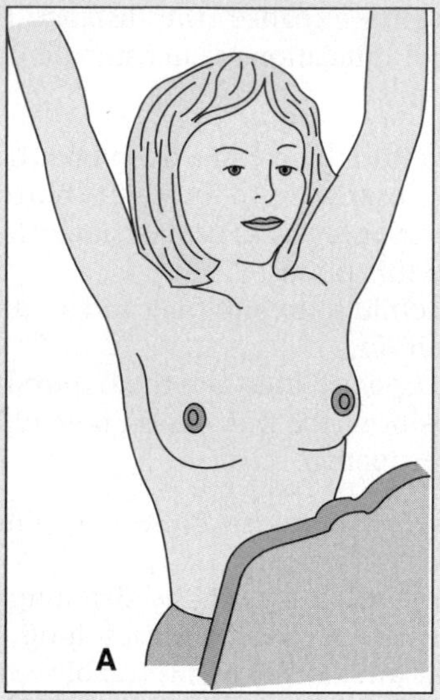

(B) Inspect in three positions: (1) with arms relaxed at sides, (2) with arms held overhead, and (3) with hands on hips, pressing in to contract the chest muscles. Turn from side to side to view all areas.

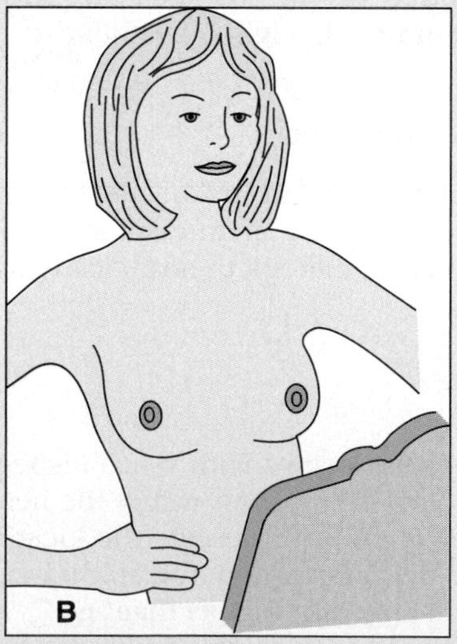

(C) Nipple examination: Gently squeeze the nipple of each breast between thumb and index finger to check for discharge.

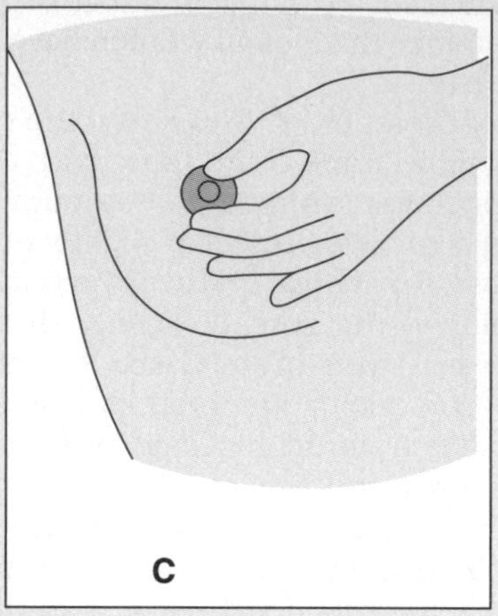

Step 2. Palpate or feel

(D) In shower or bath, fingers will glide over wet, soapy skin, making it easier to feel changes in the breast. Check the breast for a lump, knot, tenderness, or change in the consistency of normal tissue. To examine your right breast, put your right hand behind your head. With the pads of your fingers of your left hand held flat and together, gently press on the breast tissue using small circular motions. Imagine the breast as the face of a clock. Beginning at the top (12 o'clock position), make a circle around the outer area of the breast. Move in one fingerwidth; continue in smaller and smaller circles until you have reached the nipple. Cover all areas including the breast tissue leading to the axilla. Repeat the procedure for the left breast. At the lower border of each breast, a ridge of firm tissue may be felt. This is normal.

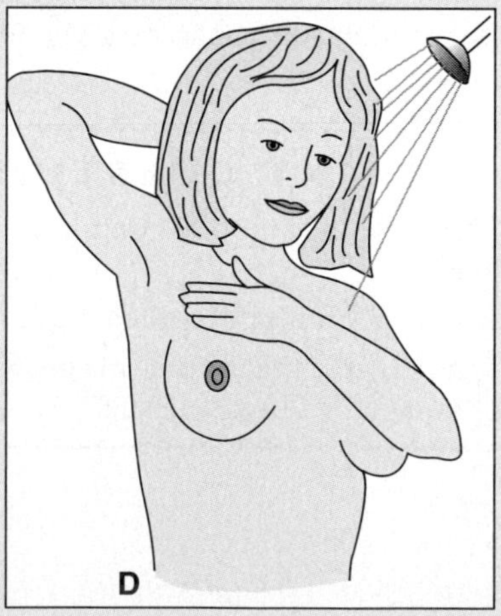

(E) Underarm examination. Examine the left underarm area with your arm held loosely at your side. Cup the fingers of the opposite hand and insert them high

(continued)

into the underarm area. Draw fingers down slowly, pressing in a circular pattern, covering all areas. Reverse the procedure for the right underarm.

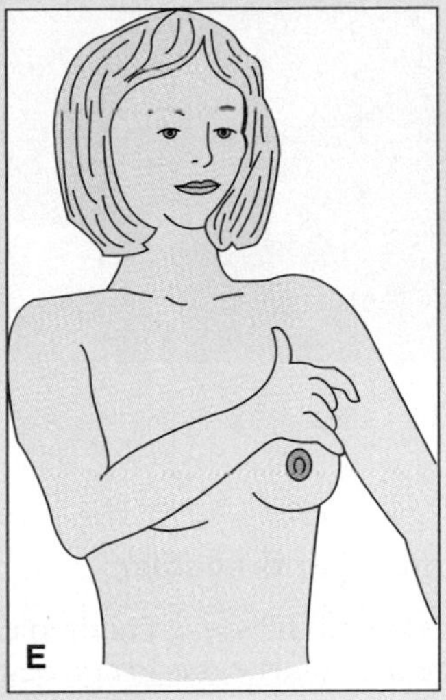

(F) Lying down. While lying flat, place a small pillow or folded towel under the right shoulder. Examine the right breast using the same circular motion as was used in the shower. Cover all areas. Repeat this procedure for the left breast. Press firmly but gently while examining your breast, rolling the tissue between your fingers and the chest wall.

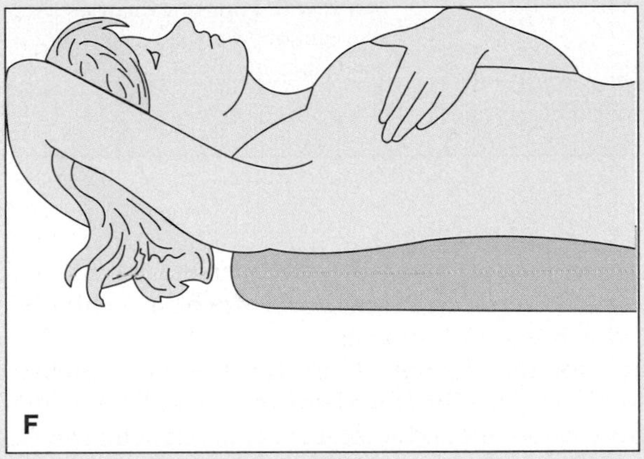

(Courtesy of the American Cancer Society, New York State Division, Inc. East Syracuse, New York.)

Percuss the left side of the chest to discern the left side of the heart. Percussing in from the axilla, the sound will become dull as the heart is identified. A heart that is located farther to the left than usual suggests enlargement. Normally, the percussion note changes from resonant (percussing over lung) to flat (percussing over heart) midway between the midaxillary and midmammary line.

Heart Sounds

To hear heart sounds, auscultate at four main points. Although these are not the anatomic locations of heart valves, they are the listening points to which the sounds of the valves radiate and can be heard best (see Fig. 33-16).

- The mitral valve is heard best at the fourth or fifth left intercostal space at the nipple line.
- The tricuspid is heard best near the base of the sternum (fourth or fifth right intercostal space).
- The pulmonary valve is heard best at the second left intercostal space.
- The aortic valve is heard best at the second right intercostal space.

Table 33-8 describes normal and abnormal heart sounds that may be heard on auscultation. Abnormal sounds are heard best if the diaphragm of the stethoscope is used first, followed by the bell of the stethoscope.

To understand heart sounds, recall heart physiology. The first sound heard (S_1) is that of the mitral and tricuspid valves closing and the ventricles contracting (described as a "lub" sound). The second sound (described as a "dub"; S_2) is made by the closure of the aortic and pulmonary valves and atrial contraction. The first sound is generally

TABLE 33.7 Breath Sounds Heard on Auscultation

SOUND	CHARACTERISTICS
Vesicular	Soft, low-pitched, heard over periphery of lungs, inspiration longer than expiration. Normal.
Bronchovesicular	Soft, medium-pitched, heard over major bronchi; inspiration equals expiration. Normal.
Bronchial	Loud, high-pitched, heard over trachea; expiration longer than inspiration. Normal.
Rhonchi	Snoring sound made by air moving through mucus in bronchi. Normal.
Rales (also called crackles)	Crackling or crinkling sound (like cellophane) made by air moving through fluid in alveoli. Abnormal.
Wheezing	Whistling on expiration made by air being pushed through narrowed bronchi. Abnormal; seen in children with asthma or foreign body obstruction.
Stridor	Crowing or rooster-like sound made by air being pulled through a constricted larynx. Abnormal; seen in children with upper respiratory obstruction.

TABLE 33.8 Heart Sounds Heard on Auscultation

SOUND	CAUSE
S_1 (first heart sound)	Closure of tricuspid and mitral valves with beginning of ventricular contraction (systole)
S_2 (second heart sound)	Closure of pulmonary and aortic valves with beginning of atrial contraction (diastole)
S_3 (third heart sound)	Rapid ventricular filling
S_4 (fourth heart sound)	Abnormal filling of ventricles

longer and lower-pitched than the second sound. It is louder than the second sound over the heart ventricles; otherwise, it is slightly quieter.

Listen for the rhythm of the heart sounds. Rhythm should be regular. **Sinus arrhythmia** is a phenomenon that most school-age and adolescent children demonstrate. Although it sounds abnormal, it is not. In sinus arrhythmia, a marked heart rate increase occurs as the child inspires and a marked decrease in heart rate is noted as the child expires. Ask the child to hold his or her breath, and the rhythm of the heart remains the same.

With inspiration and the normal resulting increase of pressure in the lungs, the pulmonary valve tends to close slightly later than the aortic valve. This is termed **physiologic splitting** and is heard as "lub d-dub." As long as this is associated with inspiration, it is a normal finding. Fixed splitting implies that there is always difficulty with the pulmonary valve closing and suggests pathology.

At times, a distinct third heart sound (S_3) may be heard due to rapid filling of the ventricles. Although this is not necessarily a serious finding, further investigation is warranted. The presence of a fourth heart sound (S_4) generally signifies heart pathology because this sound (a gallop rhythm) is caused by abnormal filling of the ventricles.

Listen to the heart in all areas; assess rate and compare this to the child's age to determine if it is a normal rate (Fig. 33-18). A heart murmur is caused by the sound of blood flowing with difficulty or in a different pathway within the heart (sounds like a swishing sound) and can be either innocent (functional) or pathogenic (organic). If a heart is pumping with abnormal force, there may be a palpable vibration termed a thrill on the chest wall. Palpate the precordium (area over the heart) for evidence of this (feels like a cat purring) or a heave (a definite outward chest movement), which also denotes a struggling heart. On hearing or palpating any accessory heart sounds or movements, try to describe them with reference to Table 33-9.

All unusual heart sounds need further identification and investigation of their cause. The skills of listening to and identifying normal and abnormal heart sounds require considerable practice. Determining the cause of an abnormal heart sound requires a cardiac specialist. Determining that an abnormal sound exists, however, and securing proper referral is an important nursing role.

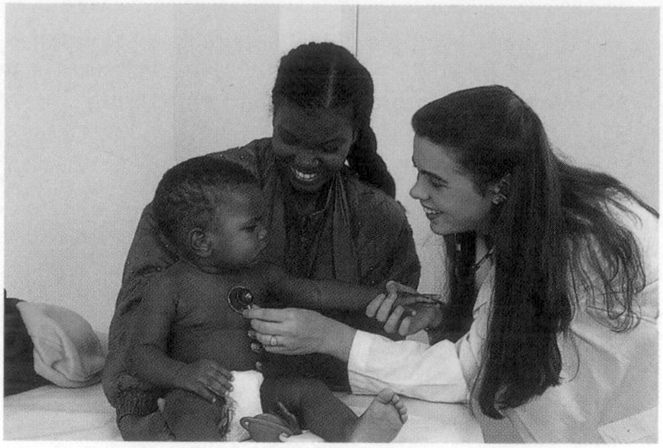

FIGURE 33.18 Auscultating heart sounds.

Newborn, Infant, and Toddler

Listen to heart sounds in young children early in an examination, before the child begins to cry, because it is almost impossible to evaluate heart sounds over the sound of crying. Allowing a parent to hold a child while doing this helps reduce fear.

School-Age Child and Adolescent

Listen carefully for sounds of murmurs in children of school age and older. Refer them to a physician for further evaluation if any abnormalities are detected. Parents are always frightened by an unusual heart sound; unless the child has other symptoms, they can be assured that most murmurs are generally innocent (functional) and caused only by the normal flow of blood across valves.

Abdomen

The abdomen is divided anatomically into four quadrants. The quadrants and the organs that lie within them are shown in Figure 33-19. To assess the abdomen, first inspect the surface for symmetry and contour. It will be slightly protuberant in infants and scaphoid in older children. Note any skin lesions or scars.

Auscultate the abdomen for bowel sounds before palpating, because palpating may alter bowel movement (peristalsis) and therefore disturb bowel sounds. Bowel sounds can normally be heard in all quadrants of the abdomen. They are high "pinging" sounds that occur normally at intervals of approximately 5 to 10 seconds. Since these sounds are high-pitched, they may be heard best with the bell of a stethoscope. If a bowel is distended, the sounds occur more frequently; if the bowel is blocked so that there is no movement of contents, the sounds will be absent below the obstruction. Listen for 3 to 5 minutes before concluding that no bowel sounds are present.

Listen along the middle of the abdomen over the aorta for irregular sounds. A **bruit** is a swishing or blowing sound that occurs if there is an outpouching of the aorta (an aneurysm), a condition that can be congenital, although it usually occurs with aging.

TABLE 33.9 Description of Accessory Heart Sounds

ASSESSMENT	INFORMATION TO BE GATHERED
Location	At which listening post is the sound most distinct?
Quality	Can sound be described as blowing, rubbing, rasping, musical?
Intensity	*Murmurs* are graded according to the following criteria:
	Grade 6: So loud it can be heard with stethoscope not touching the chest wall; has a thrill (palpable vibration).
	Grade 5: Very loud but must touch stethoscope to chest to hear; has a thrill.
	Grade 4: Loud; may or may not have a thrill.
	Grade 3: Moderately loud; no thrill.
	Grade 2: Quiet but easily discernible.
	Grade 1: Very quiet; difficult to hear.
Timing	When in relation to S_1 and S_2 did you hear it? A sound superimposed between S_1 and S_2 is a *systolic murmur;* one between S_2 and the next S_1 is a *diastolic murmur.* Innocent murmurs (functional, denoting no pathology) are usually systolic, although there are exceptions to this; pathologic murmurs are more likely to be diastolic.
Pitch	Can the sound be described as high- or low-pitched?
Radiation and thrills	Is there an accompanying thrill? Does sound radiate so it can be heard at another location, such as back of chest?

Palpate the abdomen in a systematic manner to include all four quadrants. First palpate lightly, then deeply. Ascertain whether any area is tender by watching the child's face while palpating; observe for guarding or the child tensing the abdominal muscles to keep anyone from pressing deeply at that point. If the child has indicated that any portion of the abdomen is tender, begin assessment at the farthest point and work toward the tender area. If no tenderness is present, the order of palpation is unimportant as long as it is thorough. Note any hard areas or masses. If a tender area is detected, attempt to elicit rebound tenderness to determine its cause. To do this, press in on the abdomen, then lift your hand suddenly. This causes internal organs to vibrate. More pain with the vibration than with the original pressure is diagnostic of appendicitis.

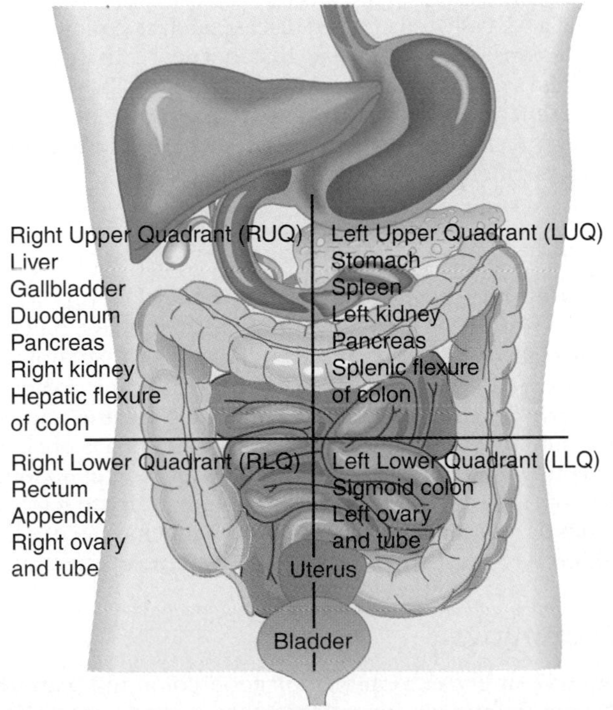

FIGURE 33.19 Quadrants of the abdomen and underlying structures.

By palpating from the right lower quadrant to the right upper quadrant, the hand will bump against the lower edge of the liver 1 to 2 cm below the right ribs. On the left side, the lower edge of the spleen may be discernible in the same way. A liver or spleen larger than this is suggestive of disease. Palpate the umbilicus to try to identify the presence of an umbilical hernia. A fascial ring at the umbilicus of more than 2 cm in diameter in an infant denotes a ring of fascia larger than will normally close spontaneously; when this is present, the child will generally need surgery to prevent an umbilical hernia. Liver, spleen, and bladder size can all be documented further by percussion.

Newborn and Infant

Kidneys may be located by deep abdominal palpation in newborns and infants. The right kidney is slightly lower than the left and thus is easiest to locate. The optimal time to palpate the kidney of a newborn is during the first few hours of life, before the bowels begin to fill with air and obscure palpation. To palpate the kidneys:

- Place a hand under the infant's back just below the 12th rib.
- Press upward.
- Place the other hand on that side of the abdomen just below the umbilicus.
- Press deeply.

- Locate the kidney, which can be felt as a firm mass approximately the size of a walnut between the hands.

Preschooler and School-Age Child

Children's abdomens at this age are often "ticklish," and children may tense or guard their abdominal muscles when touched, making it difficult to palpate. Distract the child by asking a question about home or school, or let the child put his or her hand under the examiner's to help relax (Fig. 33-20).

Genitorectal Area

In both sexes, the rectum should be inspected for any protruding hemorrhoidal tissue (rare in children) or fissures. Fissures may signify chronic constipation, intra-abdominal pressure, or sexual abuse.

Female Genitalia

Inspection of the external female genitalia and assessment of femoral nodes are included in every complete health assessment. An external examination consists of inspecting for Tanner stage of hair growth and configuration (an inverted triangle) and inspection of external genitalia (i.e., clitoris, labia majora, and labia minora) for normal contours. Look for signs of discharge or irritation. A vaginal discharge or fourchette tear in a young child may be an indication of sexual abuse (Gully et al., 2000). A pelvic examination is usually scheduled at the time the girl becomes sexually active or at age 18 (AAP, 2000). Internal pelvic examination is discussed in Chapter 10.

Male Genitalia

Inspection of male genitalia consists of observing:

- The distribution and Tanner stage of hair, which has a diamond-shape pattern
- The penis for lesions

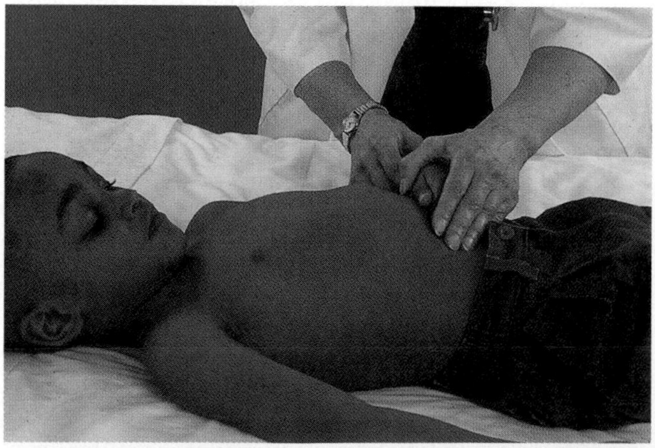

FIGURE 33.20 Decrease ticklishness during abdominal palpation by placing the child's hand under yours.

- Appearance and placement of the urethral opening, which should be slitlike and centered at the penis tip. Children with repeated urinary tract infections develop scarring of the meatal opening, making it small and round.
- The ability of the foreskin to retract if the boy is uncircumcised. Phimosis exists when the foreskin of a child older than 6 to 12 months is too tight to retract.

Hypospadias is a term for a urethral opening located on the inferior or ventral (under) surface of the penis; **epispadias** denotes a urethral opening on the superior or dorsal (upper) surface. Both these conditions need to be identified. If more than a slight deviation is present, repair is usually initiated before school age because such a urethral placement may interfere with fertility and self-image if not corrected.

Inspect the scrotum for size and the presence of testes. In most boys, the left testicle is slightly lower than the right, so the scrotum does not appear truly symmetric. Palpate to check that testes are both present by placing one hand over the top of the scrotum at the inguinal ring and then palpating the testis on that side (see Fig. 23-18). This hand position prevents the testis from slipping up into the inguinal ring and appearing to be absent on palpation. Any swelling or mass in the scrotum needs to be identified. The most likely cause of such a condition is a **hydrocele,** or a fluid-filled sac, but it could represent a serious finding such as testicular cancer in adolescents. Hydroceles can be transilluminated: when a flashlight is held in back of the scrotum, the fluid-filled cyst glows. A **varicocele** (enlarged veins of the epididymis) may be palpated. These are not important findings in young boys, but they may interfere with fertility in later life.

Assess the urethral meatus for any discharge that could reveal a sexually transmitted disease such as gonorrhea or any lesions that would suggest herpes 2 infection or syphilis (see Chap. 47). Beginning at puberty, boys should be taught to do testicular palpation every month. The technique for this is shown in the Focus on Family Empowerment: Testicular Self-Examination.

Inguinal Hernia

To assess for the presence of an inguinal hernia in an infant, simply observe the groin area for any bulging (especially while the infant is crying). In a school-age child or adolescent, with the child standing, place a fingertip against the inguinal ring in the groin area and ask the child to cough. If the tendency for a hernia is present, coughing tightens abdominal muscles and forces abdominal contents to bulge against the finger. Palpate femoral nodes (located in the groin and on the inner surface of the upper thigh) for any swelling, which suggests infection.

Extremities

Observe upper extremities for good color and warmth. Inspect fingernails for color, contour, and shape. Normally, nails are pink, smooth, and convex. They should feel hard to touch and not brittle so they do not break

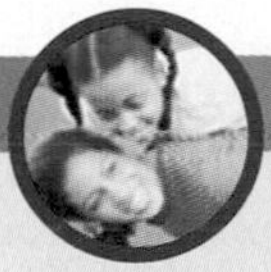

FOCUS ON FAMILY EMPOWERMENT
Testicular Self-Examination

Q. The doctor said that I should check my testicles. How do I do that, and how often should I do it?

A. Starting in your adolescent years, you need to perform testicular self-examination. Follow these guidelines:

- Select a certain day each month (first day, last day, and so forth) to perform the examination.
- Perform the examination in or immediately after a shower, because that is when scrotal skin is most relaxed.
- Gently roll each testicle between your thumb and fingers, feeling for any hard lumps or nodules, change in consistency, or difference in size.
- If you notice any of these changes, call your doctor.
- Also feel for the epididymis, found at the rear of the testes. It should feel like a strong cord.
- Remember that for most males, one testicle is slightly larger than the other and hangs a little lower in the scrotal sac.

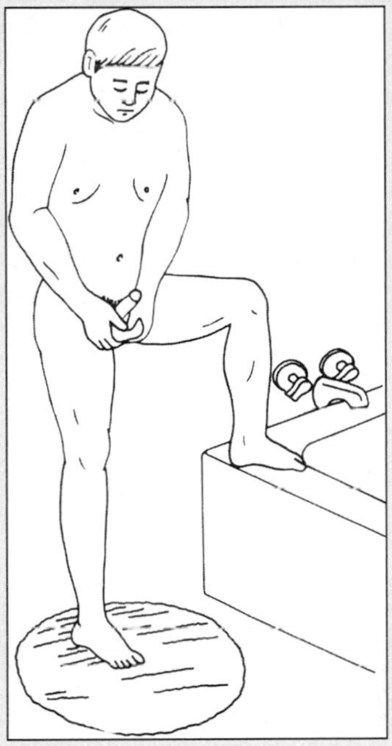

readily. Signs of bitten fingernails in the school-age child may reflect a high level of stress. Darker-skinned children's nails are more deeply pigmented. A blue or purple tinge denotes cyanosis; a yellow tinge is jaundice. Children who have decreased respiratory function or heart disease develop clubbed fingers (Fig. 33-21); children with endocarditis often have characteristic linear hemorrhages under the nails. Iron deficiency anemia may cause extremely concave surfaces (spoon-shaped). Press against a fingernail, release the pressure, and time the refilling interval (should be under 5 seconds). Count the fingers and check for webbing between fingers. Examine for the pattern of fingerprints. Distinctive dermatoglyphics are present on fingertips from the third month of intrauterine life; these are unique to every person but show patterns of circular grooves. Abnormal fingerprints may occur with chromosomal anomalies. Check for normal palmar creases. Children with chromosomal abnormalities often have one central palm crease (a simian line) on each hand rather than the normal three. Check the wrist, elbow, and shoulder joints for movement and normal range of motion; palpate joints for swelling or warmth. Palpate to be certain that no lymph nodes are present in the antecubital space; palpate to check that the radial pulse is present.

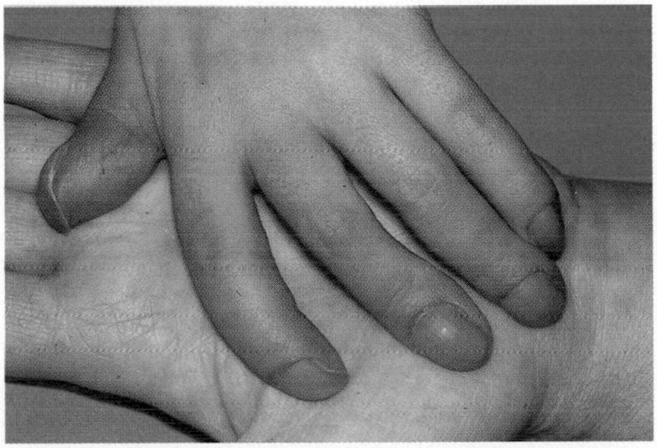

FIGURE 33.21 Clubbed fingers are a sign of cyanosis from heart or respiratory disease.

Inspect the lower extremities for color and warmth. Count the toes and check for webbing between toes. Check the ankle, knee, and hip joints for normal range of motion. Check for developmental hip dysplasia in infants by attempting to abduct fully the hip (see Fig. 23-19). Palpate to ensure that no enlarged lymph nodes are present in the groin or popliteal areas and that femoral pulses are present and equal bilaterally. Ask the older child to walk, and observe for ease of gait, limping, or any foot displacement such as toeing in or out. Toddlers typically walk with a wide-based gait; they walk best if allowed to walk toward their parent (a safe action) rather than away. Many adolescents are self-conscious and slouch or amble rather than presenting their true, natural gait. Children who limp need further evaluation. The limp can be due to something simple such as a blister on the foot from wearing new shoes to a serious hip or bone condition (Gunner & Scott, 2001).

Back

Inspect the back for symmetry and the spinal column for any deviation. Inspect the base of the spine for a dermal sinus (a pinpoint opening) or for a tuft of hair or a hemangioma that might reveal a spina bifida occulta (a defect of the bony structure of the canal). Inspect also for any dimpling that might denote a dermal cyst (pilonidal cyst). This is an innocent finding unless it becomes infected or connects to deeper tissue layers. Assess for tenderness along the spinal column by palpating each vertebra.

Routine assessment of the school-age child over 12 years and the adolescent includes a scoliosis (sideways curvature of the spine) screening (Yawn & Yawn, 2000). Nursing Procedure 33-2: Scoliosis Screening details the steps to follow for a scoliosis screen. (See Chap. 51 for more details on scoliosis.)

Neurologic Function

A full neurologic examination takes at least 20 minutes to complete, so it is not included in a routine physical examination. It is important, however, to assess for deep tendon reflexes (such as triceps, biceps, patellar, and Achilles reflexes) to test for motor and sensory function and balance and coordination. Techniques for eliciting **deep tendon reflexes** are shown in Figure 33-22. Grade reflexes according to the scale in Table 33-10. The biceps reflex tests the fifth and sixth cervical nerves; the triceps reflex tests the seventh and eighth cervical nerves; the patellar reflex tests the second, third, and fourth lumbar; and the Achilles reflex tests the first and second sacral. Test the sole of the foot for a Babinski reflex (see Fig. 23-8). This will demonstrate a fanning of the toes in an infant younger than age 3 months and a downward reflex of the toes

NURSING PROCEDURE 33.2: SCOLIOSIS SCREENING

Purpose
To assess for scoliosis.

Plan	Principle
1. Have the child remove clothing, except for undergarments. Ask the child to stand up straight, with his or her feet together and arms at sides. Observe the child from a posterior view.	1. Promotes optimal view of back.
2. Inspect for unequal shoulder or hip level, prominence of one scapula, or a curved spinal column (Figure *A*).	2. Denotes signs of spinal curvature.

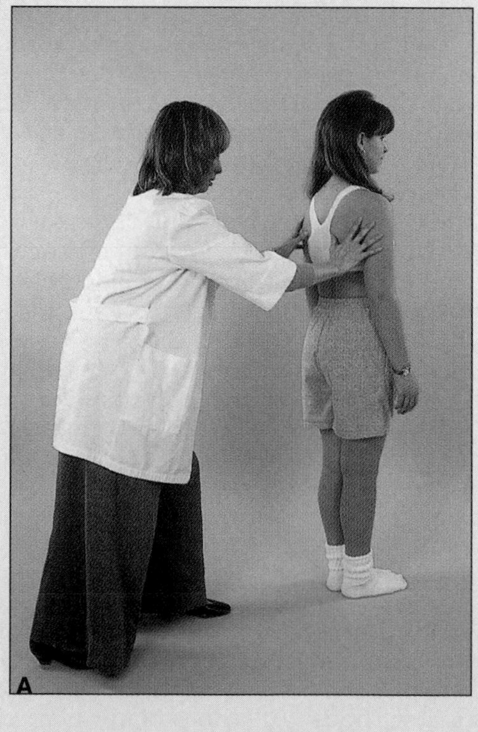
A

(continued)

Plan	Principle
Ask yourself the following questions: • Is one shoulder higher than the other? • Is one shoulder blade more prominent than the other? • Does one hip seem higher or more prominent than the other? • Does the child seem to lean to one side? • Does the spinal column appear curved?	
3. Compare the level of the elbows in relation to the iliac crests. Be sure the arms are hanging down at the sides. Ask yourself the following questions: • Is the distance between one arm and body greater than on the other side? • Are the elbows uneven? • Do the elbows fall at the level of the crest or closer to the crest on the one side? (Normally the elbows fall above the iliac crest.)	3. Helps to determine uneven posture because it will affect level of elbows.
4. Ask the child to bend over and touch his or her toes while you continue to observe the back (Figure *B*).	4. Provides evidence of spinal rotation. As the child bends, the rotation of the spine accompanying scoliosis becomes more prominent.

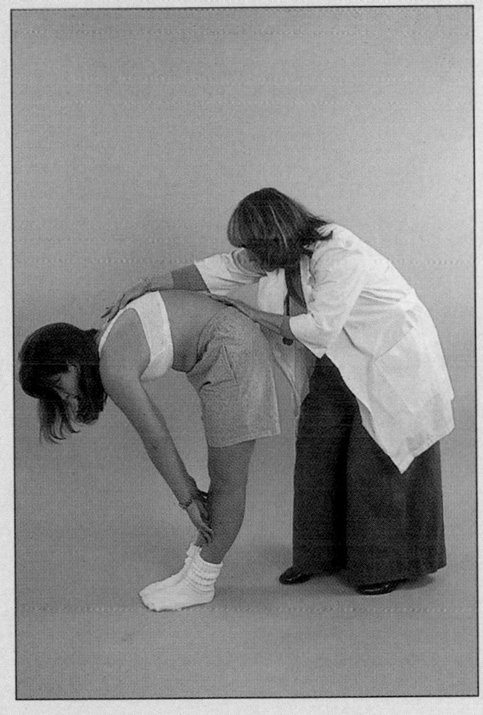

B

Plan	Principle
Ask yourself the following questions: • Is there a hump in the back? • Does the spinal column appear to curve? • Is one shoulder blade more prominent than the other?	
5. Refer the child to a physician for further examination if the answer to any of the above questions is yes.	5. Provides for proper referral.
6. Educate the child to inform parents or health care providers if signs of scoliosis, such as a skirt hanging unevenly, or bra straps that need to be adjusted, begin to develop.	6. Encourages health promotion.

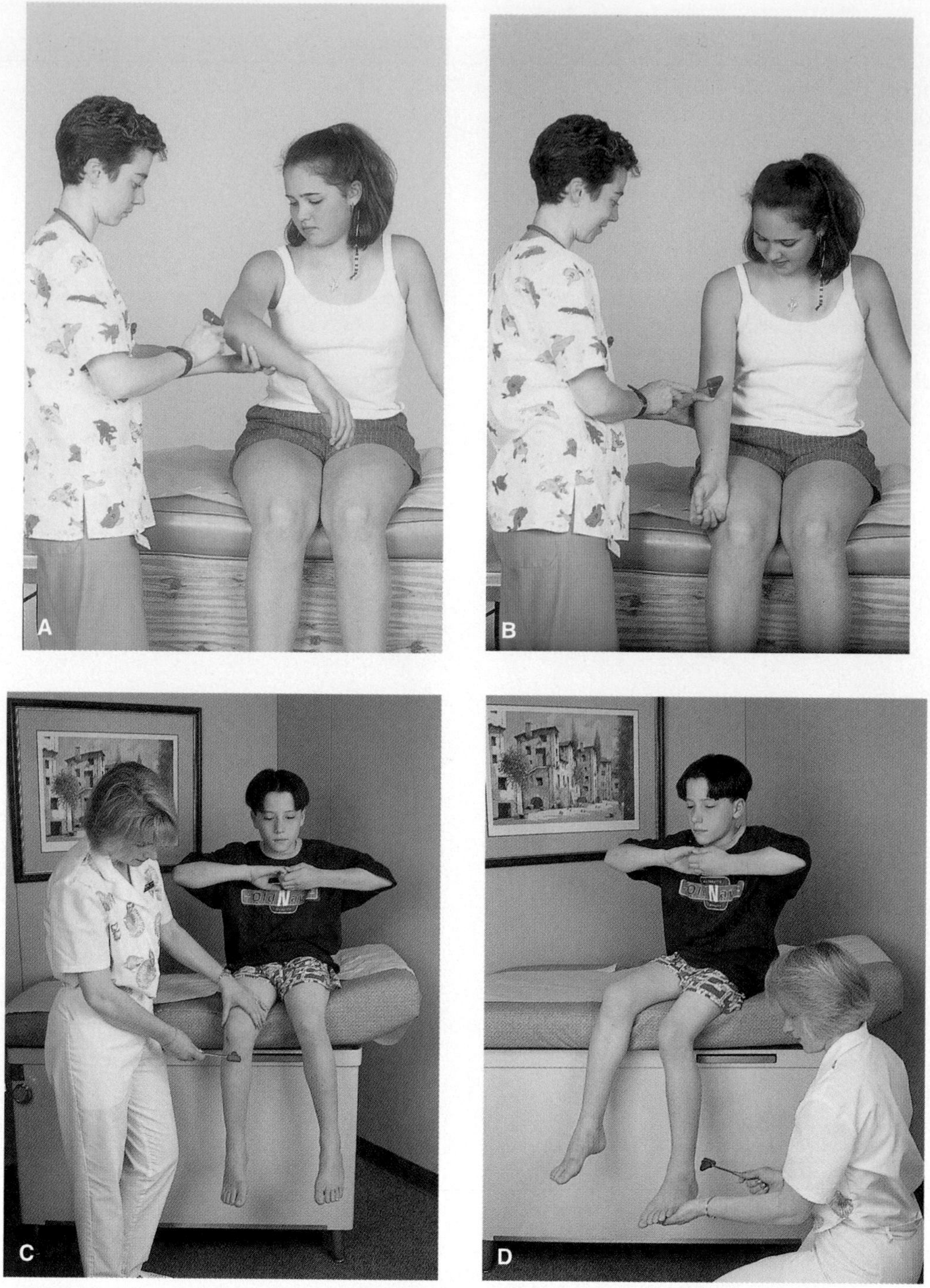

FIGURE 33.22 Deep tendon reflexes. (*A*) Triceps reflex. The triceps tendon is struck. The forearm will move perceptibly if the reflex is elicited. (*B*) Biceps reflex. The examiner's thumb is placed over the biceps tendon. The reflex hammer actually strikes the examiner's thumb. The examiner will feel the child's forearm move when the reflex is elicited. (*C*) Patellar reflex. (*D*) Achilles reflex. In both *C* and *D*, the child grasps his hands together and pulls as a means of distracting him away from what the nurse is testing. This helps to decrease muscle tension, facilitate the reflex arc, and elicit more accurate results.

beyond age 3 months. (Some normal infants demonstrate a flaring Babinski response until age 2 years; in the absence of other neurologic findings, this is not significant.)

Test for superficial reflexes: abdominal reflexes in both sexes, cremasteric reflex in boys. An abdominal reflex is elicited by lightly stroking each quadrant of the abdomen. Normally, the umbilicus moves perceptibly toward the stroke. Presence of the reflex indicates integrity of the 10th thoracic nerve and the first lumbar nerve of the spinal cord. A cremasteric reflex is elicited by stroking the medial

TABLE 33.10 Grading of Deep Tendon Reflexes

GRADE	INTERPRETATION
4+	Hyperactive; extremely marked reaction; abnormal
3+	Stronger than average but within normal range
2+	Average response
1+	Less than average response but within normal range
0	No response; abnormal

aspect of the thigh in boys. The testes move perceptibly upward. The presence of this reflex indicates integrity of the first and second lumbar nerves.

Motor and Sensory Function

Test general facial nerve function by asking the child to make a face. The child's ability to grasp with the hands and push against a surface with the feet establishes general motor ability. Recall whether gait was adequate when the child was observed walking to assess for balance and coordination.

To test sensory function, ask the child to close the eyes and identify the location where he or she is touched at six points (at least) on different body parts.

✔ CHECKPOINT QUESTIONS

14. At what place is the pulmonary heart valve heard best in a child?
15. At what age should routine scoliosis screening begin?

VISION ASSESSMENT

Assessing vision is an important part of physical assessment because good vision is so important to development. The extent of testing depends on the age of the child.

Any child with congenital anomalies, low birthweight, or fetal alcohol syndrome is at risk for eye abnormalities, as is a child who received oxygen at birth. During an assessment, if you notice an unreported injury or infection or signs of neglected vision, make a special note. Because the average parent is careful of a child's eyes, these findings may be indicative of child neglect.

Vision Screening

Routine vision screening is usually begun at 3 years of age. Common vision screening indicators and techniques for children of different ages are summarized in Table 33-11. Parents can provide important clues to possible problems: listen carefully any time a parent expresses concern about or questions a child's ability to see well.

TABLE 33.11 Common Vision Screening Indicators and Procedures

AGE	COMMON TEST
Newborn	General appearance*
	Ability to follow moving object to midline; focus steadily on an object at 10–12 in
Infant and toddler	General appearance*
	Ability to follow light past midline
3 yr–school age	General appearance*
	Random dot E for stereopsis (depth perception)
	Allen cards or preschool E chart for visual acuity
	Ishihara's plates for color awareness
School age–adult	General appearance*
	Snellen's test for visual acuity

* Note redness, blinking, squinting, crusting, and so forth.

Newborn and Infant

A parent's description of a child's activity may give clues to vision problems. Ask the parents if the infant's eyes follow them as they move around the room. Does the infant who is older than 6 weeks return their smile? Do the parents have any reason to think the child has difficulty seeing?

Newborns should be able to focus on a moving object such as a finger and follow it to the midline. Infants see black and white objects better than they do colored objects. They seem to see objects that are closest to them (a distance of about 19 cm [8–10 in]; Nelson et al., 2000).

Toddler and Preschooler

Ask the parents of an older infant, toddler, or preschooler if their child does any of the following:

- Rubs his or her eyes, blinks frequently, squints, or frowns
- Covers one eye to look at objects
- Tilts the head to see things better
- Stumbles over objects in the path
- Holds books and toys extremely close or extremely far away to look at them

Asking whether children sit close to a television set is meaningless because almost all children do that if allowed.

School-Age Child and Adolescent

Ask the parents if their child does any of the following:

- Reports frequent headaches
- Does poorly with classwork
- Avoids sports that require long-distance vision, such as baseball or softball
- Avoids watching movies
- Skips over words when reading aloud

- Reports blurriness or double vision
- Has reddened conjunctivae or drainage from the eyes
- Blinks at bright light

Techniques of Vision Testing

Vision is tested by asking the child to read an eye chart. All children need good orientation to such testing so they can appreciate that this is not a test in the usual sense of the word; otherwise, they may be unusually anxious or try to pass it by cheating. Vision testing needs to be started in the preschool period so that children with amblyopia (lazy eye; see Chap. 50) or a potentially serious vision disorder can be identified while the condition is still correctable (Simon & Kaw, 2000; Eibschitz-Tsimhoni et al., 2000).

Snellen Chart

As soon as children can identify letters of the alphabet (early school age), their vision can be tested at a health checkup by using a Snellen eye chart. This chart is standardized, so set procedures must be followed when using it to test vision (see Nursing Procedure 33-3: Snellen Eye Chart Assessment).

NURSING PROCEDURE 33.3: SNELLEN EYE CHART ASSESSMENT

Purpose
To assess vision.

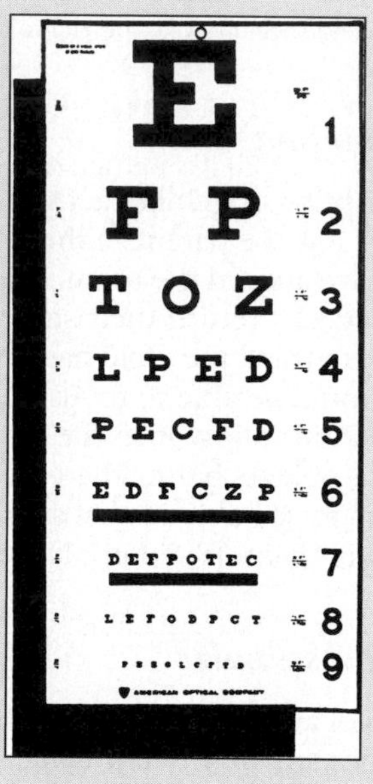

Plan	Principle
1. Hang the chart so the 20-ft line is at the child's eye level.	1. The child who has to look up or down must look farther than the child who is looking straight across at the chart. A possible solution to avoid moving the chart is to have smaller children stand and taller children sit. To accommodate children in wheelchairs, the chart needs to be lowered (or else have all children sit for the test).
2. Provide a good light for the chart and place it so there is no glare. A light intensity of 20 foot-candles is recommended.	2. Appropriate lighting provides for optimal test conditions.
3. Measure a distance of 20 ft from the chart. Mark the floor at this point with a piece of masking tape or other similar mark. For younger children, it is helpful to cut out paper footprints and paste them to the floor with the *heels* of the footprints touching the 20-ft line. If the child sits in a chair, the back legs of the chair should touch the 20-ft line.	3. Twenty feet is the optimal distance from the chart for testing.

(continued)

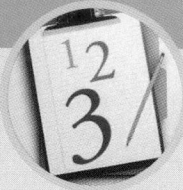

Plan	Principle
4. Provide an individual 3 × 5-in card (to cover the eye not being tested) for each child who is examined.	4. Covering the other eye allows for one eye to be tested at a time.
5. If the child wears glasses, screen while he or she is wearing the glasses. If a child has forgotten to bring glasses, defer the screening until the child can bring the glasses. Do not screen the child first without glasses and then with them, because this forces the child to strain to read the chart.	5. Testing with corrective lenses screens for corrected eyesight. After squinting, a child may have difficulty readjusting to reading with glasses, and this makes the prescription appear too weak or too strong.
6. To begin testing, tell the child to stand with his or her shoes on the footprints (heels against the line); keep both eyes open; and cover the left eye with the occluding card. Be certain the child does not press the card against the eye (instead, the edge of the card should rest across the child's nose).	6. Covering the eye not being tested provides optimal test conditions. Pressure will cause blurred vision when the child removes the card to test that eye.
7. Begin at the 40-ft line of the chart and, using a pointer or pencil, point to each symbol on the line from left to right (the order in which children are taught to read). If the child reads a majority of symbols in a line, he or she sees the line satisfactorily.	7. Starting at the 40-ft line is the standardized testing procedure.
8. If the child "passes" the 40-ft line, have the child read the 30- and 20-ft lines or the last line the child can read. Record the last line read. If the child fails to read the 40-ft line satisfactorily, then begin at the top of the chart and move downward to identify the last line the child can read. Record this reading. Because the 200-ft, 100-ft, and 70-ft lines have so few symbols, the child must read all the symbols on them to have read satisfactorily.	8. Moving to the 30-ft line or less reflects use of standardized testing procedure.
9. Visual acuity is always stated as a fraction. The top number is the distance in feet the child stands from the chart (always 20). The bottom of the fraction represents the last line the child read correctly. The adult with good (average) vision can read the 20-ft line from 20 ft away and thus is said to have 20/20 vision.	9. Using a fraction for visual acuity is the standardized reporting procedure.
10. It is important to test the eyes separately, then together. For example, Tony reads all the symbols on the 40-ft line with his right eye; he misses three out of four on the 30-ft line. His visual acuity for his right eye is 20 (the distance from the chart) over 40 (the last line he read correctly). With his left eye, Tony reads the 40-ft, 30-ft, and 20-ft lines correctly. His vision in that eye is 20/20. With both eyes, Tony reads the 40-ft, 30-ft, and 20-ft lines correctly. His visual acuity for both eyes is 20/20.	10. If only this last reading were taken, the right eye weakness (a symptom of amblyopia or "lazy eye") would be missed.
11. Observe the child for straining or squinting as he or she reads the chart.	11. By squinting and changing the shape of the eyeball, a child can improve his or her vision and will score higher. The child will appear to see better than he or she actually does in everyday situations.

Preschool E Chart

Between age 3 years and the age they can read the alphabet, children can have their vision tested by using a preschool E chart (Fig. 33-23). This chart is also helpful in testing children who are cognitively challenged or those who speak a foreign language. The procedure is similar to that of the standard Snellen chart:

1. The child stands 20 ft from the chart. The child should read first with the right eye, then with the left, then both eyes, as with standard testing.

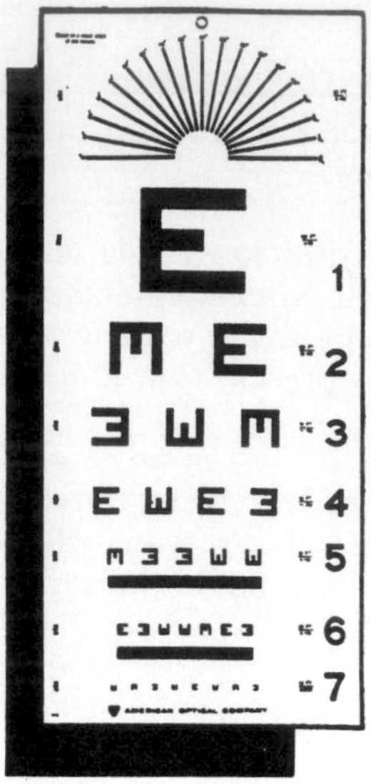

FIGURE 33.23 Astigmatic and preschool E chart. (From the American Optical Corporation, with permission.)

Young children do not understand the importance of not pressing the card against their eye or of not peeking, so a second person is often needed to hold the occluder card for children of this age.
2. It is helpful to compare the E with a table with three legs and ask the child which way the legs of the table point. Children age 3 years are familiar with tables, but Es are strange symbols. Tell the child to point with the entire arm and hand in the direction the legs point so you do not confuse the hand motion.
3. Begin at the 40-ft line, as with the standard Snellen chart, and work downward until the child passes all lines or cannot read the majority of symbols on a line.

National Association for the Prevention of Blindness Home Test

A home eye test is available from the National Association for the Prevention of Blindness for parents to use to test children age 3 to 6 years at home. It is similar to the preschool E chart except that it is smaller and the child stands only 10 ft away. The test can help alert parents that a child needs a professional eye examination. It can be given or suggested to parents whose child is tired or for some other reason has not tested well in a health care facility.

Allen Cards

Preschool children may be tested with Allen cards, which consist of pictures of common objects such as a horse and rider, car, house, and birthday cake. These are shown to the child at a 15-ft distance, and the child is asked to identify the pictures (proof that the child sees them). Be certain the child has time to examine the cards before the test so he or she knows the names of the objects.

Stycar Cards

For this test, the child is given cards with nine letters: H, C, O, L, U, T, X, V, and A. The child holds up the card that matches the one pointed to on a chart.

Titmus Vision Tester

Another useful method for testing the vision of children is the Titmus Vision Tester. This is the same instrument used by many motor vehicle license offices. As the child looks into the eyepieces of the machine, alphabet letters or preschool Es are projected onto a well-lighted screen for the child to identify. Closed vision testers such as the Titmus have an advantage over wall charts in that the child is less easily distracted during testing. Also, because the child cannot see the vision chart beforehand, he or she cannot memorize the letters.

Color Vision Discrimination Testing

The inability to discern colors is a sex-linked recessive characteristic that tends to occur in males rather than in females, although females carry the gene for the disorder. All male children should be screened once for the disorder during their early school years.

To test a child for color awareness, ask the child to identify the colored stripes at the top of a Snellen eye chart or show the child a series of colored diagrams (Ishihara's plates). With the latter, a person with color vision can see hidden figures, but people with red-green or yellow-blue color vision deficits cannot. Detecting color vision deficit in children is important because many educational materials depend on the ability to identify color. In addition, certain occupations are closed to people who cannot identify colors. Even such a simple childhood pleasure as riding a bicycle safely on city streets depends on being able to distinguish colors, such as red from green on a traffic light.

Vision Referrals

Screen children twice before referring them to a physician for corrective eye care. Some children do not perform well on eye tests because they are easily distracted or do not know their alphabet as well as they pretend. For example, they may say that they do not see a letter when they really mean they do not know or remember its name. Testing twice helps eliminate or identify this type of misleading result.

After a second screening, generally children require a vision referral for the following:

- Preschool children who have 20/50 vision in one or both eyes
- Children in kindergarten or later who have 20/40 vision or worse in one or both eyes
- Any child with a two-line difference between the eyes, which might be the beginning of amblyopia
- Any child who states or shows symptoms of visual disturbance

HEARING ASSESSMENT

A thorough health assessment should include an evaluation of hearing, including both history and observation, because good hearing is necessary for the development of age-appropriate skills. When taking an auditory history, be certain to ask the accompanying adult or parent an overall question such as, "Do you have any reason to believe Lucy doesn't hear as well as she should?" Parents and grandparents are usually attuned to hearing difficulty in children and may be suspicious of it in advance of its official detection.

Auditory Screening

Routine screening for adequate hearing levels is usually begun at 3 years of age. This requires knowledge of the technique and use of an audiometer. It requires a quiet, undistracted setting.

Newborn and Infant

Certain infants who are at risk should be screened at birth. These may include any of the following conditions:

- History of childhood hearing impairment in the family
- Perinatal infection, such as cytomegalovirus, rubella, herpes, toxoplasmosis, or syphilis
- Anatomic malformations involving the head or neck
- Birthweight less than 1,500 g
- Hyperbilirubinemia at a level exceeding indication for exchange transfusion
- Bacterial meningitis, especially when caused by *Haemophilus influenzae*
- Severe birth asphyxia: infants with an Apgar score of 0 to 3, those who failed to breathe spontaneously within 10 minutes of birth, or those with hypotonia persisting to 2 hours of age

If a newborn's hearing is assessed, it usually is done through simple response testing (observing whether an infant stirs or responds to a sound made or delivered to the child with a commercial device; Erenberg, 1999). It can also be done by brain stem auditory-evoked response (BAER) testing. For this method, an earphone is placed on the infant and an electrode is attached to the scalp. When sound is transmitted to the child's ear through the earphone, the electrical potential created as the sound is processed by the brain stem is read by the scalp electrode, processed by a microcomputer, and plotted on a graph. This type of testing may be used at any age and is even successful for children who are comatose or anesthetized. Smaller units using transient evoked otoacoustic emissions (TEOAE) are also available. With these, a click stimulus delivered to a normal ear produces an echo from the cochlea. This can be detected by a miniature microphone to reveal even minor hearing loss. Although newborn hearing screening can lead to false-positive results because many infants of this age are still sleepy from birth analgesia, repeating the test usually decreases the incidence of false-positive results (Clemens & Davis, 2001).

Older Children

Older children who are at risk for hearing loss are those who have been exposed to loud noises, were of low birthweight, have congenital anomalies, have a repaired cleft palate, or have had repeated ear infections. During history taking, ask children if they ever worry that they have difficulty hearing. Ask them how they are doing in school. Some children with a minimum hearing impairment are considered to have behavioral problems in school because they do not follow directions or appear not to be following the teacher's discussion when in fact they may be unable to hear what is being said. Be certain not to confuse difficulty hearing with shyness or recalcitrance in answering. Children with an ear infection (otitis media) or allergies should be tested after the fluids in their ears clear because their hearing may be temporarily affected by these conditions. Cerumen in the ear canal has not been documented to substantially decrease hearing.

Principles of Audiometric Assessment

Frequency

Sound is the result of vibration; frequency is the number of vibrations a sound creates per second. When frequency is increased, the pitch of the sound increases. For audiometric testing, frequency is measured in Hertz units. Normal speech sounds fall into a narrow range, 500 to 2,000 Hz. To function adequately and speak effectively, a child must be able to hear in this range. Children are tested for a wider frequency range than this, from 500 to 6,000 Hz, on a routine screening assessment.

Loudness

Decibels are an expression of the intensity of loudness of a sound (or vigor of the vibrations). A decibel level of 0 dB is the softest sound that can be heard. Normal conversation is approximately 50 to 60 dB. The sound level at which inner ear damage can occur is about 90 dB. Sound levels of 140 dB are so intense they actually cause pain. Screening audiometry is done at 25 dB.

Hearing Loss

Table 33-12 lists levels of hearing loss. The inability of a child to hear sounds softer than 30 dB indicates the child will have some difficulty hearing normal instructions and questions. If a child is unable to hear sounds softer than 50 dB, the child misses most normal conversation and cannot hope to achieve in a regular classroom environment. The hearing loss is severe. The child will be speech challenged because he or she does not hear normal speech sounds.

If a child can hear all frequencies at the 25-dB level, he or she has passed an audiometric screening check. If the child fails to hear two or more frequencies at 25 dB, in either or both ears, the child has failed a screening audiometry test and should be referred to a physician or an otologist. An **audiogram** is a record of audiometric testing. Figure 33-24 shows an audiogram of a child with normal

TABLE 33.12 Levels of Hearing Loss

HEARING LOSS (DB LEVEL)	HEARING LEVEL PRESENT
Slight (less than 30)	Inability to hear whispered words or faint speech
	No speech challenge present
	Possible lack of awareness of hearing difficulty
	Achievement in school and home is attained by leaning forward, speaking loudly
Mild (30–50)	Beginning speech challenge possibly present
	Difficulty hearing if not facing speaker; some difficulty with normal conversation
Moderate (55–70)	Speech challenge present, possibly requiring speech therapy
	Difficulty with normal conversation
Severe (70–90)	Difficulty with any but nearby loud voice
	Vowels easier to hear than consonants
	Speech therapy required for clear speech. Possible ability to still hear loud sounds such as jets or whistle of train.
Profound (more than 90)	Almost no sound heard

hearing in the right ear (the child heard all frequencies at the 20-dB level) but an inability to hear sounds softer than 45 dB in the left ear at frequencies of 1,000, 2,000, and 4,000 Hz.

Acoustic Impedance Testing

Acoustic impedance testing is based on the principle that sound entering the ear canal meets resistance at the tympanic membrane. If the middle ear is functioning normally, there will be a symmetric pattern of resistance on a tympanogram printout. If the middle ear is functioning abnormally, the level of resistance will be greater or less than normal, so the pattern will be abnormal.

Acoustic impedance testing is performed by audiologists. For the assessment, the ear to be tested is plugged with a rubber disc. Sound is then administered to the ear through the center of the disc. The resistance met at the eardrum is registered and recorded as a graph. Tympanograms are inaccurate in children younger than age 7 months because the tympanic membrane is too compliant under that age to register normal impedance.

Conduction Loss Testing

Although not very accurate, both the Rinne and the Weber tests can be used to help determine the cause of hearing loss in older children (Box 33-4).

✔ CHECKPOINT QUESTIONS

16. What type of eye chart would be best to use for cognitively challenged or non-English-speaking children?
17. What is the decibel level of normal conversation?

SPEECH ASSESSMENT

Speech problems are directly related to hearing problems: the child who does not hear will make preliminary babbling sounds but then will not develop intelligible speech because he or she is unable to hear and repeat sounds. Speech difficulties may also be related to:

- Motor development (e.g., the child cannot control tongue and facial muscles well enough to form proper words)
- Cognitive development (e.g., the cognitively challenged child does not grasp the concept of speech or word use until later than normal, or possibly not at all)
- Cultural influences (e.g., the parents speak two languages, making it difficult for the child to accurately learn and articulate either language)

Speech screening begins by asking the child a few simple questions to determine his or her language pattern. Parents are also asked if they have noticed any difficulties with their child's pronunciation or comprehension. Standardized tests, such as the Denver Articulation Screening Examination (DASE), may also be administered.

Denver Articulation Screening Examination

Assessing for language development is double assessment in that it assesses for both cognitive and hearing ability. The DASE is designed to detect significant developmental delays and normal variations in the acquisition of speech sounds. Because it is a standardized test, its directions must be followed carefully. The test is useful only with English-speaking children.

Administration

For the test, explain that the child will need to repeat some words he or she hears. Give enough examples so the child will understand what he or she is to do: "When I say 'boat,' then you say 'boat.' " When you are certain that the child understands the directions, say each of the 22 words shown on the DASE form (Fig. 33-25A). Convey the impression that there are no right or wrong answers. Give the child approval for responding and following directions correctly, no matter how inaccurately the child repeats the word.

Scoring

The DASE is designed for use with children between ages 2.5 and 6 years. In scoring, consider the child's age to be the closest previous age shown on the percentile rank

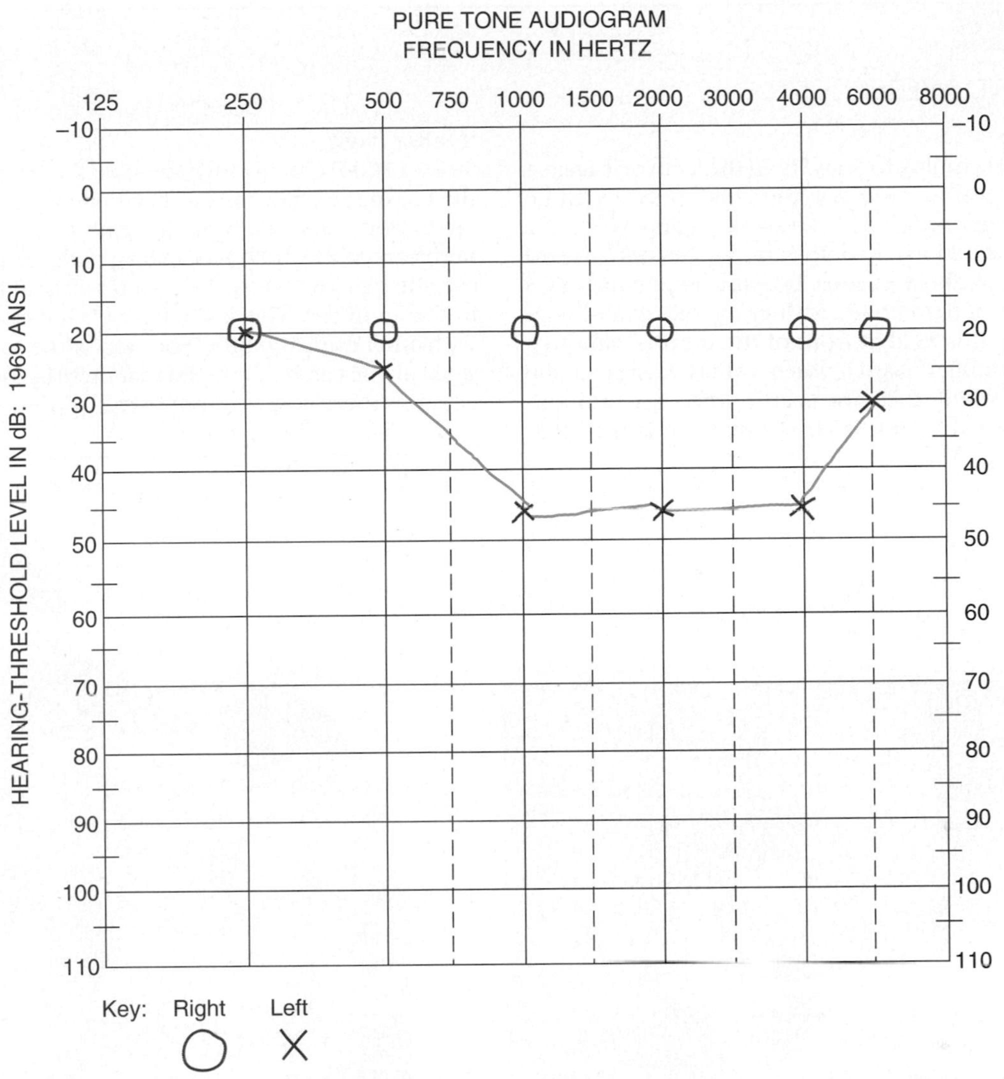

FIGURE 33.24 An audiogram done as a screening procedure. Notice that hearing is normal in the right ear (all frequencies are heard at the 20-dB level). In the left ear there is hearing loss (the frequencies 1000, 2000, and 4000 Hz are heard only at the 45-dB level). (Courtesy of Dr. H. Schill, Speech Pathology and Audiology Department, Boston University.)

chart (see Fig. 33-25*B*). Score the child's pronunciation of the underlined sounds or blends in each word on the test form. A perfect raw score is 30 correctly articulated sounds. Match this raw score on the percentile rank chart with the column representing the child's age. The number at which the raw score line and the age column meet is the percentile rank of the child (how the child compares with other children of that age). Percentiles shown above the heavy line are abnormal; those below the line are normal. For example, a 3-year-old who says only 12 sounds correctly ranks in the 9th percentile (abnormal ranking); the 3-year-old who scores 20 sounds correctly ranks in the 58th percentile (normal ranking).

In addition to determining the percentile ranking, rate the child's spontaneous speech in terms of intelligibility as 1, easy to understand; 2, understandable half the time; 3, not understandable; or 4, cannot evaluate (e.g., the child does not speak in sentences or phrases during the contact with the child). Score intelligibility according to the chart in Figure 33-25*B*. For a final score, rate the child's total test result (normal or abnormal on the DASE or intelligibility).

Children who score abnormally on this screening test should be retested in 2 weeks. If they still score abnormally, they should be referred for complete speech evaluation.

DEVELOPMENTAL APPRAISAL

It would be ideal if children demonstrated all the developmental skills of which they are capable every time they are asked to demonstrate them. Rarely, however, do they accomplish this feat. Infants may become hungry, sleepy, or upset during testing. Older children may become shy. A portion of developmental information on almost all health assessments, therefore, must be elicited by history taking.

BOX 33.4

RINNE AND WEBER TESTS

Rinne Test

Strike a 500-Hz tuning fork and hold the stem of it against the child's mastoid bone. Ask the child to say when he or she no longer hears the tuning fork ringing. When the child says it is no longer audible, move the fork forward so it is at the auditory meatus. Because air conduction is normally better than bone conduction, the child should hear it when it is held in front of the meatus, although he or she no longer heard it when it was held against the bone. If the child does not hear it when it is brought forward, then the child's air conduction is probably reduced.

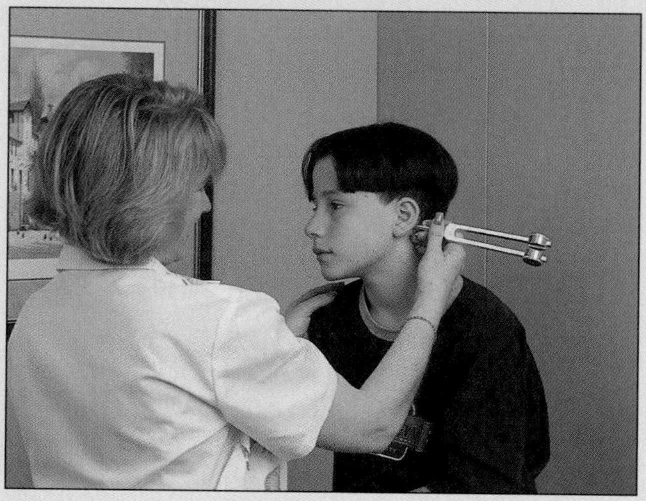

Weber Test

Strike a 500-Hz tuning fork and hold the stem of it against the top of the child's head. The child with normal hearing in both ears will hear the sound equally well with both ears. If the child has an air conduction loss in one ear, the child will hear the sound better in that ear than in the good ear. The test must be used in conjunction with other evaluation tools because if the sound is intensified in one ear, it may mean that there is no hearing perception (there is nerve loss) in the opposite ear.

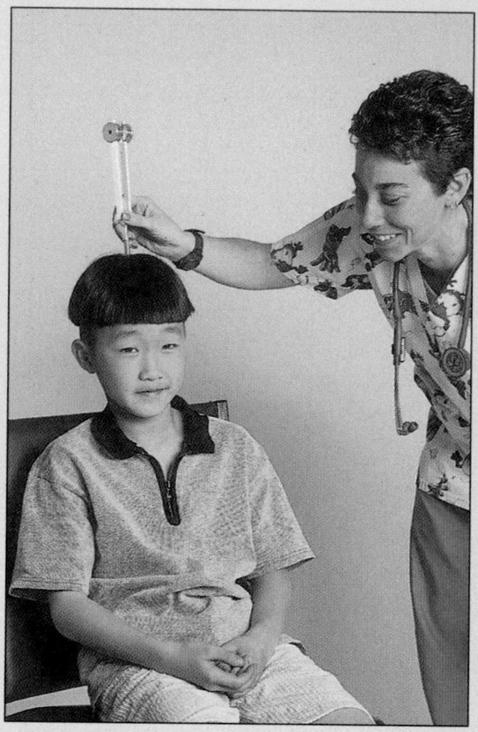

All previous developmental milestones must be obtained this way.

Developmental History

Many parents keep careful records of their first child's development, a less careful record of their second, a scanty record of the third, and so on. Most of this information must, therefore, be obtained by recall.

Parents may not be able to recall the month during which a skill was first demonstrated. It is often helpful to ask them to try to remember in terms of holidays or seasons. For example, they may not know at which month the infant first used a pincer grasp (grasped cleanly with index finger and thumb) but do recall the way the child pinched the ear of the family dog at a summer picnic.

If parents seem to have no recall at all of developmental milestones that are important for the child's present evaluation, suggest that they ask other family members or look through family photographs to jog their memories and then call with as much information as they can gather.

In addition to getting the parents' description of the skills a child has mastered, it is often helpful to watch the child perform skills and rate him or her according to standard criteria.

Denver Developmental Screening Test

The Denver Developmental Screening Test (DDST; Denver II) is the most widely used tool to assess development and has been recently revised (Frankenburg, 1994; see Appendix H). The DDST detects developmental delays during infancy and preschool years. Four main categories of development are rated:

1. Personal-social
2. Fine motor-adaptive

DENVER ARTICULATION SCREENING EXAM
for children 2 1/2 to 6 years of age

Instructions: Have child repeat each word after you. Circle the underlined sounds that he pronounces correctly. Total correct sounds is the Raw Score. Use charts on reverse side to score results.

NAME

HOSP. NO.

ADDRESS

Date: ______ Child's Age: ______ Examiner: ______ Raw Score: ______
Percentile: ______ Intelligibility: ______ Result: ______

1. table	6. zipper	11. sock	16. wagon	21. leaf
2. shirt	7. grapes	12. vacuum	17. gum	22. carrot
3. door	8. flag	13. yarn	18. house	
4. trunk	9. thumb	14. mother	19. pencil	
5. jumping	10. toothbrush	15. twinkle	20. fish	

Intelligibility: (circle one) 1. Easy to understand 2. Understandable 1/2 the time. 3. Not understandable 4. Can't evaluate

Comments:

Date: ______ Child's Age: ______ Examiner: ______ Raw Score ______
Percentile: ______ Intelligibility: ______ Result: ______

1. table	6. zipper	11. sock	16. wagon	21. leaf
2. shirt	7. grapes	12. vacuum	17. gum	22. carrot
3. door	8. flag	13. yarn	18. house	
4. trunk	9. thumb	14. mother	19. pencil	
5. jumping	10. toothbrush	15. twinkle	20. fish	

Intelligibility: (circle one) 1. Easy to understand 2. Understandable 1/2 the time. 3. Not understandable 4. Can't evaluate

Comments:

Date: ______ Child's Age: ______ Examiner: ______ Raw Score ______
Percentile: ______ Intelligibility: ______ Result: ______

1. table	6. zipper	11. sock	16. wagon	21. leaf
2. shirt	7. grapes	12. vacuum	17. gum	22. carrot
3. door	8. flag	13. yarn	18. house	
4. trunk	9. thumb	14. mother	19. pencil	
5. jumping	10. toothbrush	15. twinkle	20. fish	

Intelligibility: (circle one) 1. Easy to understand 2. Understandable 1/2 the time. 3. Not understandable 4. Can't evaluate

Comments:

A

FIGURE 33.25 Denver Articulation Screening Exam (DASE). (*A*) Test form. (*B*) Percentile rank form. (Reprinted by permission. Copyright 1971 by Amelia F. Drumwright, University of Colorado Medical Center, Denver, CO.) *(continued)*

3. Language
4. Gross motor skills

Administration

The Denver II ideally should be completed when the child is approximately age 3 months or 4 months, again at age 10 months, and again at age 3 years. It is a supplement to the developmental evaluation by history that should be a part of every well-child assessment.

The materials to administer the test must be purchased as a kit. They include a skein of red wool, a box of raisins, a small bottle, a bell, a rattle with a narrow handle, a tennis ball, ten 1-in brightly colored blocks, a small plastic doll, a toy baby bottle, a plastic cup, and a pencil.

Although administration of the Denver II is not difficult, it should not be attempted except by health care providers trained specifically in its procedures and interpretation. This precaution is necessary to ensure the validity of its developmental norms. Periodic retraining and proficiency testing are recommended to sustain a high degree of accuracy in administration.

The parent should be told before administration that this is not a test of intelligence but of the child's level of

To score DASE words: Note Raw Score for child's performance. Match raw score line (extreme left of chart) with column representing child's age (to the closest previous age group). Where raw score line and age column meet number in that square denotes percentile rank of child's performance when compared to other children that age. Percentiles above heavy line are ABNORMAL percentiles, below heavy line are NORMAL.

PERCENTILE RANK

Raw Score	2.5 yr.	3.0	3.5	4.0	4.5	5.0	5.5	6 years
2	1							
3	2							
4	5							
5	9							
6	16							
7	23							
8	31	2						
9	37	4	1					
10	42	6	2					
11	48	7	4					
12	54	9	6	1	1			
13	58	12	9	2	3	1	1	
14	62	17	11	5	4	2	2	
15	68	23	15	9	5	3	2	
16	75	31	19	12	5	4	3	
17	79	38	25	15	6	6	4	
18	83	46	31	19	8	7	4	
19	86	51	38	24	10	9	5	1
20	89	58	45	30	12	11	7	3
21	92	65	52	36	15	15	9	4
22	94	72	58	43	18	19	12	5
23	96	77	63	50	22	24	15	7
24	97	82	70	58	29	29	20	15
25	99	87	78	66	36	34	26	17
26	99	91	84	75	46	43	34	24
27		94	89	82	57	54	44	34
28		96	94	88	70	68	59	47
29		98	98	94	84	84	77	68
30		100	100	100	100	100	100	100

To Score intelligibility:

	NORMAL	ABNORMAL
2 1/2 years	Understandable 1/2 the time, or, "easy"	Not Understandable
3 years and older	Easy to understand	Understandable 1/2 time Not understandable

Test Result: 1. NORMAL on Dase and Intelligibility = NORMAL

2. ABNORMAL on Dase and/or Intelligibility = ABNORMAL

* If abnormal on initial screening rescreen within 2 weeks. If abnormal again child should be referred for complete speech evaluation.

B

FIGURE 33.25 *Continued*

development. The child's inability to perform a task that most children of the same age can accomplish indicates a delay in that area. Further evaluation is then needed to determine the reason for this delay.

Scoring

The child is scored P (passed), F (failed), R (refused), or N.O. (no opportunity) on each item by reference to guidelines in the instruction manual. Each item is represented on the test form (see Appendix H) by a bar showing the ages by which 25%, 50%, 75%, and 90% of children normally have mastered that item. The left end of the bar is the 25% mark; the tick mark at the top of the bar, 50%; the left end of the colored (gray) area, 75%; and the right end of the bar, 90%. Looking at the form, notice, for example, the item "plays pat-a-cake" in the area of personal-social development. With this item, 25% of children show the trait at age 7 months, 50% between ages 9 and 10 months, 75% between ages 10 and 11 months, and 90% by ages 11 to 12 months. Interpretation of performance is detailed in the manual.

Prescreening Test

A Denver Prescreening Developmental Questionnaire (R-PDQII) is available in addition to the Denver II. The PDQII is designed to identify children who require further testing with a full Denver II. It is a questionnaire completed by the parents addressing 10 developmental items. A child who scores 8 out of 10 or fewer should be retested in approximately 2 weeks. If the initial score is under 6 or the retest score is 8 or below, the child should have a full DDST.

INTELLIGENCE

Children must learn many important concepts or ideas such as near, far, here, there, number sequences, how to judge time intervals, how to reason and solve problems, and how to judge weight before they can function effectively in the world.

This type of learning—gaining concepts—is called cognitive learning and is measured by intelligence tests. **Intelligence** can be defined as an ability to think abstractly, to adjust to new situations, and to profit from experience. Almost everyone has had his or her intelligence quotient (IQ) rated at some point in a school career. Although intelligence tests are not part of routine health appraisals, it is helpful to be familiar with those that are used for childhood measurements because these findings are helpful in evaluating children's development.

The IQ is the ratio of mental age as measured by an intelligence test to chronologic age. The formula is as follows:

$$\frac{\text{Mental age}}{\text{Chronological age}} \times 100 = \text{IQ}$$

A child aged 9 years old (chronologic age) who passes all the items on an intelligence test that an average 9-year-old child passes would be scored as follows:

$$\frac{9\ (\text{Mental age})}{9\ (\text{Chronological age})} \times 100 = 100\ (\text{the child's IQ})$$

If a child passes no more items than the average 5-year-old child would, the IQ would be scored as:

$$\frac{5\ (\text{Mental age})}{9\ (\text{Chronological age})} \times 100 = 55$$

If a child passed all the items that a 12-year-old child normally passes, the IQ would be scored as:

$$\frac{12\ (\text{Mental age})}{9\ (\text{Chronological age})} \times 100 = 133$$

Children may score poorly on intelligence tests because of test anxiety. Cultural bias and past experience can also affect how they score. Therefore, labeling children by IQ and classifying them into divisions is often unfair and must be done with considerable thought and study.

It is difficult to test young children with any degree of accuracy because they lack the ability to complete tasks in the areas used for scoring intelligence tests: comprehension, imagination, reasoning, memory, and vocabulary. The most common tests used with infants include the Cattell Infant Intelligence Scale, the Bayley Mental Scale, and the Gesell Developmental Schedule. These tests rely heavily on perceptual and motor skills as rating devices.

The two most frequently used tests for older children are the Wechsler Intelligence Scale for Children and the Stanford-Binet test. All schoolchildren take one of these tests during the primary school grades. The results are made available to child health teams if they can demonstrate to school officials that such information is necessary for total health care or planning. If the information is unavailable, the child can be referred to a psychologist or a psychological testing clinic for assessment.

Goodenough-Harris Drawing Test

A child's drawing can reveal information on developmental or emotional problems. A Goodenough-Harris Drawing Test is a quick intelligence measurement that can be administered without special training (Goodenough, 1926). Give a child between ages 3 and 10 years a pencil and paper and ask the child to draw a person. Urge the child to draw it carefully in the best way he or she knows how and to take enough time to do it well (Box 33-5).

The child receives one point for each of the items in the drawing listed in Box 33-5. For each four points scored, 1 year is added to a base age of 3 years to get the child's mental age. The picture shown in Box 33-5 was drawn by a 4.5-year-old child: it received eight points. The child's IQ level is

$$\frac{5.0}{4.5} \times 100 = 111$$

Scores on the test are reasonably reliable, correlating well with a Stanford-Binet test, although results may not be as reliable with children who are mentally ill. A child who scores significantly lower than his or her chronologic age (after allowing for fatigue, illness, strange surroundings, nervousness, physical ability to use a pencil, and previous practice using a pencil and paper) should be referred for more refined testing.

TEMPERAMENT

Temperament refers to a child's innate behavioral characteristics, such as activity level, rhythmicity, tendency to approach or withdraw, and adaptability to situations (see Chap. 27). A child with an "easy" temperament is generally adaptable and easy to care for; a child with a "difficult" temperament, in contrast, will almost automatically create childrearing concerns. Helping parents to assess their children's temperament helps them, in turn, to recognize their children's uniqueness and to anticipate and ideally prevent personality conflicts as a child grows older and expresses identified reactions to situations. If a behavior or parent–child interaction problem is already present, a nursing assessment can be useful to determine whether temperament is a factor in the problem and to assist parents with constructive solutions (Thomas & Chess, 1977).

One instrument that is helpful in evaluating temperament is the Carey-McDevitt Infant Temperament Questionnaire (Carey & McDevitt, 1978). This consists of 95 responses and can be answered by a parent in approximately 25 minutes. General categories center on the child's responses to feeding, sleeping, soiling and wetting, dressing, bathing, and diapering, as well as to people and new situations.

Give the questionnaire to parents when their infant is between ages 4 and 8 months (before this, temperament

BOX 33.5

GOODENOUGH-HARRIS DRAWING TEST

Score one point for each characteristic listed below that is present on drawing. For every four points, 1 year is added to a base mental age of 3 years.

1. Head present
2. Legs present
3. Arms present

4a. Trunk present
 b. Length of trunk greater than breadth
 c. Shoulders indicated
5a. Both arms and legs attached to trunk
 b. Legs attached to trunk; arms attached to trunk at correct point
6a. Neck present
 b. Neck outline continuous with head, trunk, or both
7a. Eyes present
 b. Nose present
 c. Mouth present
 d. Nose and mouth in two dimensions, two lips shown
 e. Nostrils indicated
8a. Hair shown
 b. Hair nontransparent, over more than circumference
9a. Clothing present
 b. Two articles of clothing nontransparent
 c. No transparencies, both sleeves and trousers shown
 d. Four or more articles of clothing definitely indicated
 e. Costume complete, without incongruities
10a. Fingers shown
 b. Correct number of fingers shown
 c. Fingers in two dimensions, length greater than breadth, angle less than 180°
 d. Opposition of thumb shown
 e. Hand shown distinct from fingers or arms
11a. Arm joint shown, either elbow, shoulder, or both
 b. Leg joint shown, either knee, hip, or both
12a. Head in proportion
 b. Arms in proportion
 c. Legs in proportion
 d. Feet in proportion
 e. Both arms and legs in two dimensions
13. Heel shown
14a. Firm lines without overlapping at junctions
 b. Firm lines with correct joining
 c. Head outline more than circle
 d. Trunk outline more than circle
 e. Outline of arms and legs without narrowing at point of junction with body
 f. Features symmetric, correct position
15a. Ears present
 b. Ears in correct position and proportion
16a. Eye detail: brow and lashes shown
 b. Eye detail: pupil shown
 c. Eye detail: proportion correct
 d. Eye detail: glance directed to front in profile drawing
17a. Both chin and forehead present
 b. Projection of chin shown

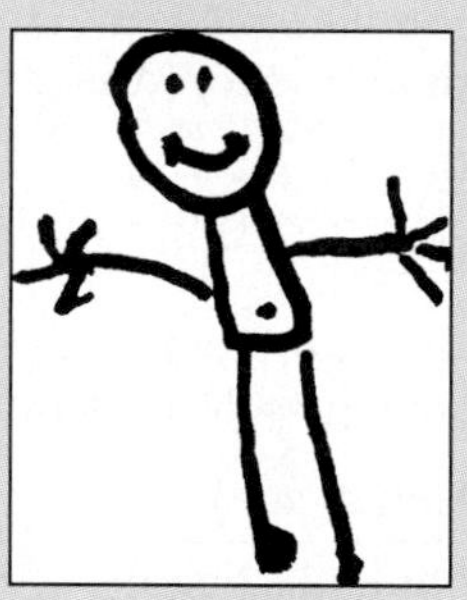

An 8-point drawing

From Goodenough, F.L. (1926). ***Measurement of intelligence by drawings.*** New York: World Book Company, with permission.

is not developed enough to be evident). The parent reads each behavioral description and then selects the option that most accurately describes the child. If an item does not apply at all, the parent crosses it out. Finally, the parent is asked to describe general impressions of the child's temperament, activity level, positive and negative moods, and distractibility.

When scored, a child can be categorized into one of four groups:

1. Difficult: arrhythmic, withdrawing, low in adaptability, intense, and negative in mood
2. Slow to warm up: inactive, low in approach and adaptability, and negative in mood
3. Intermediate: some characteristics of both groups
4. Easy: rhythmic, approaching, adaptable, mild, and positive in mood

IMMUNIZATIONS

One of the most important health promotion measures for children is to ensure that their immunization status is up to date (McPhillips & Marcuse, 2001). Routine immunization schedules call for children to receive immunity against a number of dangerous infections, including measles, mumps, rubella, diphtheria, tetanus, pertussis, hepatitis B, poliomyelitis, pneumococcal pneumonia, *H. influenzae* meningitis, and varicella (chickenpox). New influenza vaccines are developed yearly to help high-risk clients (e.g., infants, elderly people, and immunosuppressed individuals) ward off influenza viruses. Research continues on the development of vaccines to combat other diseases, including HIV (see Focus on Cultural Competence).

Teach parents about the need for children to be immunized and the need to be able to describe the record of immunizations that their child has received. If gaps occur in the child's immunizations, remind the child's primary care provider about this lack in protection and prepare to administer the necessary vaccines.

Parents need to understand that although diseases such as measles and mumps are referred to as common childhood illnesses, they are serious diseases, leading to complications such as pneumonia and encephalitis. When children develop these common communicable diseases, they need to be seen by a primary health care provider to minimize the risk for these complications.

Types of Immunizations

Immunizations or vaccines are the solutions used to immunize children to provide artificially acquired active or passive immunity. Box 33-6 reviews active and passive immunity.

Vaccines are prepared in a number of forms. Attenuated vaccines are made from live organisms that have been reduced in virulence to a point where they will not cause active disease but will ensure a good antibody response. Because they are strong and effective solutions, a single dose usually provides a good degree of active immunity.

Because some bacteria, such as diphtheria, cause disease by producing a toxin, the vaccine against such a disease, a **toxoid,** is actually an extract of the toxin with reduced virulence. The antibodies for toxin-producing bacteria are **antitoxins.** A solution given for passive immunity against diphtheria is an antitoxin.

Gamma globulin is serum obtained from the pooled blood of many people. Because it combines the serum of many people, it probably has antibody protection against measles, rubella, poliomyelitis, varicella, and hepatitis B, among many other infectious diseases. It offers artificially acquired passive immunity.

Immune serums are also available against specific diseases such as diphtheria, tetanus, the pit viper snake, black widow spider, and respiratory syncytial virus. Like general immune globulin, these provide passive immunity.

BOX 33.6

ACTIVE VERSUS PASSIVE IMMUNITY

Immunity, the ability to combat a particular antigen, may be either active or passive.

Active Immunity. When a child produces antibodies after the natural invasion of a pathogen (the child has measles, for example), the child is said to have *naturally acquired active immunity.* Active antibodies (or the child's ability to produce antibiotics rapidly should the specific antigen [measles] invade again) last a lifetime. When pathogens are artificially injected into the child by immunization, the child receives *artificially acquired active immunity.* If the specific antigen should enter again, antibodies are produced against the pathogen that are just as lasting as those produced in naturally acquired active immunity.

Passive Immunity. IgG antibodies that a woman possesses either through immunization or through having had a disease are transferred across the placenta to a fetus in utero. Because the fetus does not make these antibodies but merely receives them, this is termed *naturally acquired passive immunity.* Passive immunity lasts only months. Some antibodies transferred across the placenta may have slightly longer lifetimes than this. For example, measles antibodies have been isolated up to age 1 year, and that is why measles immunization must be delayed until age 15 months (AAP, 2002).

When children are exposed to a disease against which they have no antibodies, antibodies made synthetically or obtained from animal serum may be injected into the child to give rapid immunity (*artificially acquired passive immunity*). Like naturally acquired passive antibodies, these last only approximately 6 weeks. A child who is susceptible to tetanus, for example, would receive tetanus antibodies after a stab wound.

FOCUS ON CULTURAL COMPETENCE

Some cultures are much more aware of the role of communicable disease in childhood illnesses than others and thus advocate for all children to be immunized against these disorders. Even if awareness about the danger of disease spread exists, however, it doesn't mean that all people in a community are conscientious about having their children immunized. Other factors such as cost and convenience and ethical beliefs are also important.

Some religious groups, such as the Amish, discourage immunizations. In these communities, the prevalence of illnesses such as measles can rise to high numbers. Being aware that immunization rates are not consistent from place to place aids in understanding the importance of planning health education and health surveillance based on individual community needs.

Available Vaccines

The American Academy of Pediatrics issues specific recommendations for childhood immunization. These recommendations are shown in Appendix J.

Diphtheria, Tetanus, Pertussis (DTaP) Vaccines

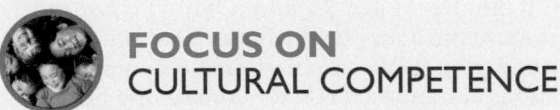

Diphtheria, tetanus toxoid, and acellular pertussis (whooping cough) vaccines are supplied in a single vial as DTaP and given in one intramuscular injection. It is recommended that children receive a primary series of four immunizations with the vaccine (2, 4, 6, and 15 to 18 months). A booster is then given between ages 4 and 6 years, or before entry into school. Diphtheria and tetanus toxoid (Td vaccine) is given at 11 to 12 years, then every 10 years thereafter to keep tetanus immunization current.

In the past, a great deal of controversy arose about the safety of the diphtheria-tetanus-pertussis vaccine, most of it directed at the pertussis component. Severe reactions, such as high fever, persistent crying, and rarely seizures, were reported. For this reason, the former DTP vaccine has been modified to DTaP or contains a less reactive pertussis component. Side effects can still include drowsiness, fretfulness, low-grade fever, and redness and pain at the injection site.

Some parents, after hearing about reactions to the former vaccine, refuse immunizations for their children. This is their right. However, children who are not immunized against pertussis (unless there is a medical or moral contraindication) may be refused admittance to preschool or beginning school programs. Parents should be informed of this when they refuse to sign consent for immunization.

Pertussis vaccination is contraindicated in children who have a progressive or unstable neurologic disorder or who have had a severe allergic reaction to pertussis in a previous DTP vaccination. If pertussis immunization is contraindicated, the DT, or diphtheria-tetanus vaccine, is substituted.

Pertussis vaccine is not generally given after age 6 because the side effects of the vaccine may be more common in older children. Diphtheria toxoid used is the adult or more diluted form.

Polio Vaccines

Oral polio vaccine (OPV) and inactivated polio vaccine (IPV) contain all three strains of poliovirus and are both available for use in the United States. The inactivated form of polio vaccine (Salk vaccine or IPV) is preferred for routine immunization.

IPV is administered in a primary series of three doses and given along with DTaP at 2, 4, and 6 to 18 months of age. A fourth booster dose is given between the ages of 4 and 6 years, before school entry (AAP, 2002).

Measles, Mumps, Rubella (MMR) Vaccines

Measles-mumps-rubella vaccine is furnished in one vial and routinely administered as a single injection. A first dose is given around the time of the 15-month checkup. A second dose of MMR is generally given between the ages of 4 to 6 years or, if the child did not receive the 4- to 6-year dose, at 11 to 12 years. Although MMR may be given as early as 12 months, it is usually recommended that the vaccine not be administered to children younger than age 15 months because children receive a great deal of passive immunity to this disease from their mothers across the placenta. Until this passive immunity has faded, the injected vaccine will be neutralized by passive antibodies and no immunity will result. For the same reason, children who have recently received immune globulin or other blood products that contain antibodies should defer the MMR for 3 months because the passively acquired antibodies could interfere with the child's immune response to the vaccine.

Side effects of the vaccine include transient rashes and a fever, which may begin 5 to 12 days after vaccination and last several days. Adverse reactions include joint pain, low-grade fever, rash, and lymphadenopathy 5 to 12 days after vaccination.

Children should be skin-tested for tuberculosis before measles vaccine administration because measles virus can cause tuberculosis to become systemic. Tuberculosis skin tests may show false-negative reactions if given shortly after measles immunization (a child who has active tuberculosis will be wrongly identified as not having it).

Formerly, there was a concern that the administration of the MMR vaccine was associated with the development of autism in children, as symptoms of autism often begin to be apparent during the second year or close to the time of MMR vaccine administration. Further research has shown there to be no causal relationship between the vaccine and autism, dispelling this fear (Farrington et al., 2001). Parents may ask about this, however, and refuse to have their child immunized against MMR on the possibility that the association exists.

Hepatitis Vaccine

The vaccine for hepatitis B (HBV) is recommended for all infants in the United States. Three doses are required. Those born of HBsAg-negative mothers should receive the first dose in the newborn period or by age 2 months, a second dose 1 month after the first dose, and a third dose 2 months later but not before 6 months of age. Those infants born of HBsAg-positive mothers receive hepatitis B immune globulin within 12 hours of birth plus HBV. A second dose of HBV is recommended at 1 to 2 months and a third dose at 6 months. If the mother's HBsAg status is unknown, infants should receive the vaccine within 12 hours of birth, the second dose at 1 month of age, and the third dose at 6 months of age. Children who did not receive the vaccine at birth may begin the series at any well-child visit. In addition, HBV immunization is recommended for populations at increased risk for contracting hepatitis B infection, including (but not limited to) health care workers with significant exposure to blood, clients receiving hemodialysis, those with hemophilia and others receiving clotting factor concentrates, illicit injectable drug users, and sexually active individuals with multiple sexual partners.

Currently, the American Academy of Pediatrics does not recommend the use of hepatitis A vaccination for children in the United States. In undeveloped countries, where the incidence of the disease is considerably higher, hepatitis A vaccine is combined with hepatitis B vaccine. It is anticipated that in the future, U.S. children will also receive this combined vaccine (Van Damme and Van der Wielen, 2001).

H. influenzae Type B Vaccines

H. influenzae type b conjugate vaccine (Hib) protects against *H. influenzae* bacteria, a major cause of meningitis in children. You may need to explain the difference between *H. influenzae* (a bacteria) and influenza virus, so that parents do not think a "flu shot" protects against this. Several formulations of this vaccine are available, and three of them are currently licensed for use in infancy. Depending on the individual vaccine, they are administered in a two-dose (at age 2 and 4 months) or a three-dose regimen (at 2, 4, and 16 months). Local reactions include tenderness at the injection site. Systemic reactions such as crying and fever may occur (AAP, 2002).

Varicella Vaccine

Varicella (chickenpox) vaccine was a difficult vaccine to develop because of the complex structure of the herpes-zoster virus. It is an important vaccine because once a generation of children has been successfully immunized, it will mark the end of common childhood diseases. Infants may receive varicella vaccine at any visit after their first birthday (usually scheduled at 12 to 18 months). Those who lack a reliable history of chickenpox should be immunized during the 11- to 12-year visit. Children 13 years of age or older should receive two doses, at least 1 month apart.

Pneumococcal Pneumonia Vaccine

The pneumococcal vaccine is recommended for all children at 2 to 23 months. It is especially recommended for children (and adults) who would be prone to a pneumococcal infection (those with pulmonary or cardiac disease, those without a spleen, those who are immunosuppressed; Poland, 2001). The vaccine is admitted as a single injection and provides protection for 6 to 10 years (AAP, 2002).

Lyme Disease Vaccine

Lyme disease is a serious and debilitating infection caused by *Borrelia burgdorferi* and transmitted by the bite of a deer tick. A vaccine to guard against it is available for high-risk populations such as workers who maintain power lines and hunters. Although the initial trials are favorable, it has not yet been approved for children under 15 years of age (Rahn, 2001).

Influenza Vaccine

Influenza is caused by A, B, or C retroviruses, which mutate so easily that it has been impossible to design a vaccine that is effective for more than one year. Susceptible individuals, including children who have chronic pulmonary or cardiovascular disorders or are immunosuppressed, should receive a yearly injection of the vaccine (Altemeier, 2000).

Anthrax and Smallpox Vaccines

Anthrax is a potentially fatal disease caused by a gram-positive spore-forming anthracis bacillus spread by farm animal feces. It is extremely rare, but parents may ask about a vaccine for it because of the threat of biologic warfare associated with terrorism. A vaccine is available for people in high-risk occupations, such as hunters, taxidermists, or veterinarians; it is not recommended for children.

Smallpox is an extremely infectious disease caused by the smallpox virus and transmitted by direct or indirect contact. Smallpox vaccination has not been required in the United States for over 30 years because the disease is theoretically extinct across the world. Like anthrax, parents may ask about vaccination for it because it is a disease associated with biologic warfare and terrorism. Both a vaccine (active artificial immunity) and passive artificial immunity are available should a child be exposed to the virus.

Administration of Immunizations

Assess well children at health maintenance visits and assess the immunization status of ill children at clinic or hospital admission to identify those who need their immunizations updated. Keep in mind that children who are seriously ill should not receive immunizations. However, a slight upper respiratory tract infection (a stuffy nose with no fever) is not a contraindication. So many infants and preschoolers have common cold symptoms (the average toddler has 10–12 colds a year) that if children are not immunized at health maintenance visits when they have slight cold symptoms, they may never receive basic immunizations.

Because children with chronic illness may be hospitalized when an injection is due, such children often fall behind schedule. Children who miss the scheduled time for an immunization do not have the series started over but are simply continued where they left off.

Primary care providers may choose to alter the sequence of immunization schedules if specific infections are prevalent at the time. For example, measles vaccine might be given on a first health maintenance visit (providing a child is older than age 12 months) if an epidemic were currently underway in the community.

Children who are immunosuppressed, receiving corticosteroids, or receiving chemotherapy or radiation therapy should not receive live virus vaccines. The live attenuated viruses such as measles, rubella, oral polio (OPV), and mumps also must not be given to girls who are pregnant because these vaccines could cross the placenta, causing actual disease in the fetus. Before traveling internationally, parents should consult their local public health service.

WHAT IF? What if a parent tells you she has moved so often she doesn't know what immunizations her child has had, but she knows he has never received a full series of anything. What would you do? Should the child have everything repeated?

When preparing to administer an immunization, be sure to follow the manufacturer's recommendations for storage and handling of vaccines (e.g., whether to expose to light or whether to refrigerate). Failure to follow these precautions may significantly reduce the potency and effectiveness of vaccines.

Although measles, mumps, and rubella vaccines are prepared from chick embryo cultures, egg sensitivities are not likely to occur because egg albumin and yolk components of the egg are absent from the culture. Children with egg allergy should have their allergist's permission for immunization, however, to rule out the possibility of a hypersensitivity reaction.

Parental Education

A major reason that parents do not bring children for routine immunizations is that they do not know what is required or have misconceptions about immunity (Sporton & Francis, 2001). Fully inform parents and, when old enough, children about what immunizations are needed, what is being given, and what side effects may be expected (see Focus on Evidence-Based Practice). Because children may develop a low-grade fever after immunization, counsel parents that they may need to give acetaminophen (Tylenol) or children's ibuprofen for a fever of more than 101°F (38.4°C).

Parents should report any untoward symptoms of immunization, such as high fever. Unfavorable reactions are most likely to occur within a few hours or days of administration. With live attenuated virus vaccines, viruses can multiply, so reactions may occur up to 30 days later. With rubella vaccine, a reaction (serum sickness) may occur up to 60 days later.

Record the date, type of vaccine, vaccine manufacturer, lot number, and name and address of the vaccine provider so that if a vaccine reaction should occur, the instance can be investigated. Make a copy of the child's immunization record and urge parents to keep such records at home as well. They will need this information to admit their child to school and in the event of an epidemic of a particular disease. They will need to know their child's record of tetanus immunization if the child should receive a puncture wound so that the correct therapy can be given.

FOCUS ON EVIDENCE-BASED PRACTICE

Do Parents Understand the Importance of Immunizations?

To answer this question, 1,600 parents of children 6 years of age or younger were asked about immunizations by telephone. The child's health care providers were cited as the most important source of information on immunizations, and 87% stated that they thought immunization was an extremely important action that parents can take to keep children well. Parents also believed that the child's immune system could be weakened by too many immunizations; 23% believed that children receive more vaccines than are good for them.

This is an important study for nurses because it reveals how important nurses' opinions are to parents. It also predicts that parents may have increasing difficulty accepting new vaccines if hepatitis A or another vaccine is added to the current recommendations. Nurses can apply this research to develop specific teaching plans about the importance of immunizations, thereby helping to dispel any misconceptions that parents may have about immunizations.

Gellin, B.G., Maibach, E. W., & Marcuse, E.K. (2000). Do parents understand immunizations? *Pediatrics, 106*(5), 1097–1102.

CONCLUDING A HEALTH ASSESSMENT

At every health maintenance visit, the parents and the child, if the child is old enough to understand, should be informed of any available results of screening procedures performed. After learning the results, some parents may require counseling to assist them with health or behavior concerns.

Ask parents if they have any other remaining questions. If the health assessment revealed some health concerns and follow-up procedures are planned, be certain that the parents understand the reason for the upcoming tests. Suggest to parents that follow-up phone calls are welcome after they return home from a health assessment so additional questions can be answered. Provide parents with the best hours to call so someone will be available to answer questions for them.

✔ CHECKPOINT QUESTIONS

18. At what ages do children typically receive the DTaP immunization?
19. When is the immunization for varicella usually given?

KEY POINTS

Health assessment always causes some degree of apprehension for both parents and children because of worry that some illness will be detected. Giving reassurance of wellness during examinations helps to alleviate this worry.

A health history is an important part of a health assessment. The purpose is to gather information that will supplement physical or laboratory examinations to provide a more thorough health evaluation.

The parts of a complete health history consist of introduction, chief concern, present health, family profile, history of past illnesses, day history, family health history, and review of systems.

Physical examination consists of four techniques: inspection, palpation, percussion, and auscultation. Techniques and approaches must be varied according to the child's age.

Be certain to use examining instruments safely (supporting an otoscope base so that if the child moves, the otoscope moves with the child). Be certain that young children are not left unsupervised on an examining table or they could fall.

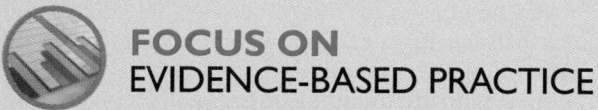

The components of a physical examination are vital sign assessment; general appearance; mental status assessment; body measurements; and assessment of head, eyes, nose, ears, mouth, neck, chest, breasts, lungs, heart, abdomen, rectogenital area, extremities, back, and neurologic function.

Adolescent girls can be taught breast self-examination and boys testicular self-examination at the time of a health appraisal.

Vision assessment consists of asking children to read a standardized chart such as a Snellen Chart, cover testing, or color discrimination assessment.

Hearing assessment consists of such assessments as audiometric testing and a Rinne and Weber test.

Development is an important part of total assessment. The Denver Developmental Screening Test (Denver II) and the Denver Articulation Screening Examination are specific development tests.

The Goodenough-Harris Drawing Test correlates well with intelligence quotient (IQ) and is an easy test to administer to children between the ages of 3 and 10 years.

Temperament refers to a child's innate behavioral characteristics, such as activity level, rhythmicity, and tendency to approach or withdraw and adapt to situations. Assessing this can help parents to better understand behavior in their child.

Assessment of immunization status is included as part of a health assessment. Childhood immunizations are a major safeguard for children against common illnesses.

CRITICAL THINKING EXERCISES

1. Terry is the 5-year-old boy you met at the beginning of the chapter. His father has brought him to your ambulatory clinic for a preschool checkup because he is worried that he needs glasses (he sits so close to the television set). His mother was reluctant to bring him because she doesn't want him to be prescribed glasses. What questions on history would be important to ask the father or Terry? What type of eye chart would you use with Terry to assess his vision?
2. A 2-year-old child being seen in a health maintenance clinic for well-child care is very resistant to being examined. What techniques would you use to help the toddler adjust better to a physical examination?
3. Children may cheat on vision and hearing tests because they do not understand the importance of them. What are techniques to use to keep children from doing this with these assessments?
4. Children should be completely undressed for physical examinations, and all body surfaces should be inspected. What would be your response if a parent said she did not want to undress a child? What if she did not want to remove a Band-Aid from a child's hand?
5. Joey, age 10 years, will be spending the next year in India. His mother knows that he will need vaccines such as cholera that aren't normally required in the United States. She asks you if he will need boosters of his required vaccines as well. How would you advise her?
6. Examine the National Health Goals related to health assessment. Most government-sponsored money for nursing research is allotted based on these goals. What would be a possible research topic to explore pertinent to these goals that would be fundable and would advance evidence-based practice?

REFERENCES

Altemeier, W. A. (2000). Children and influenza outbreaks. *Pediatric Annals, 29* (11), 670–671.

American Academy of Pediatrics. (2000). *Policy statement recommendations for preventive health care* (RE9939), 105(03), 645. New York: AAP.

American Academy of Pediatrics. (2002). *2002 immunization schedules.* New York: AAP.

Carey, W. B., & McDevitt, S. C. (1978). Revision of the infant temperament questionnaire. *Pediatrics, 61*(4), 735–739.

Carney, D. E. & Meguid, M. M. (2002). Current concepts in nutritional assessment. *Archives of Surgery, 137*(1), 42–45.

Carruth, B. R., & Skinner, J. D. (2000). Revisiting the picky eater phenomenon: Neophobic behaviors of young children. *Journal of the American College of Nutrition, 19*(6), 771–780.

Clemens, C. J., & Davis, S. A. (2001). Minimizing false-positives in universal newborn hearing screening: A simple solution. *Pediatrics, 107*(3), E29.

Davis, S. P., Northington, L., & Kolar, K. (2000). Cultural considerations for treatment of childhood obesity. *Journal of Cultural Diversity, 7*(4), 128–132.

Department of Health and Human Services. (2000). *Healthy people, 2010.* Washington, D.C.; DHHS.

Eibschitz-Tsimhoni, M., et al. (2000). Early screening for amblyogenic risk factors lowers the prevalence and severity of amblyopia. *Journal of AAPOS: American Association for Pediatric Ophthalmology & Strabismus, 4*(4), 194–199.

Erenberg, S. (1999). Automated auditory brainstem response testing for universal newborn hearing screening. *Otolaryngologic Clinics of North America, 32*(6), 999–1007.

Farrington, C. P., Miller, E., & Taylor, B. (2001). MMR and autism: Further evidence against a causal association. *Vaccine, 19*(27), 3632–3635.

Frankenburg, W. K. (1994). Preventing developmental delays: Is developmental screening sufficient? *Pediatrics, 93*(4), 586–589.

Gellin, B. G., Maibach, E. W., & Marcuse, E. K. (2000). Do parents understand immunizations? A national telephone survey. *Pediatrics, 106*(5), 1097–1102.

Goodenough, F. L. (1926). *Measurement of intelligence by drawings.* New York: World Book Company.

Gully, K. J., et al. (2000). The child sexual abuse experience and the child sexual abuse medical examination. *Journal of Child Sexual Abuse, 9*(10), 15–27.

Gunner, B., & Scott, A. C. (2001). Evaluation of a child with a limp. *Journal of Pediatric Health Care, 15*(1), 38–40.
McPhillips, H., & Marcuse, E. K. (2001). Vaccine safety. *Current Problems in Pediatrics, 31*(4), 91–121.
Muscari, M. E. (2001). *Advanced pediatric clinical assessment.* Philadelphia: Lippincott Williams & Wilkins.
Nelson, R. M., et al. (2000). Newborn assessment and care. In Scott, J. R., et al. (Eds.). *Danforth's obstetrics and gynecology* (8th ed, pp. 131–142). Philadelphia: Lippincott Williams & Wilkins.
Poland, G. A. (2001). The prevention of pneumococcal disease by vaccines: Promises and challenges. *Infectious Disease Clinics of North America, 15*(1), 97–122.
Rahn, D. W. (2001). Lyme vaccine: Issues and controversies. *Infectious Disease Clinics of North America, 15*(1), 171–187.
Simon, J. W., & Kaw, P. (2001). Commonly missed diagnoses in the childhood eye examination. *American Family Physician, 64*(4), 623–628.
Sporton, R. K., & Francis, S. A. (2001). Choosing not to immunize: Are parents making informed decisions? *Family Practice, 18*(2), 181–188.
Thomas, A., & Chess, S. (1977). *Temperament and development.* New York: Brunner/Mazel.
Van Damme, P., & Van der Wielen, M. (2001). Combining hepatitis A and B vaccination in children and adolescents. *Vaccine, 19*(17–19), 2407–2412.
Yawn, B. P., & Yawn, R. A. (2000). The estimated cost of school scoliosis screening. *Spine, 25*(18), 2387–2391.

SUGGESTED READINGS

Agnew, P. S., & Raducanu, Y. (2000). An algorithmic approach to evaluation of the flatfoot: Avoidance of pitfalls. *Clinics in Podiatric Medicine & Surgery, 17*(3), 383–396.
Bettler, J., & Roberts, K. E. (2000). Nutrition assessment of the critically ill child. *AACN Clinical Issues: Advanced Practice in Acute & Critical Care, 11*(4), 498–506.
Cale, C. M. & Klein, N. J. (2002). The link between rotavirus vaccination and intussusception: Implications for vaccine strategies. *Gut, 50*(1), 11–12.
Davis, T. C., et al. Childhood vaccine risk/benefit communication in private practice office settings: A national survey. *Pediatrics, 107*(2), E17.
Ebell, M. H., et al. (2000). Does this patient have strep throat? *JAMA: Journal of the American Medical Association, 284*(22), 2912–2918.
Gross, G. J., & Howard, M. (2001). Mothers' decision-making processes regarding health care for their children. *Public Health Nursing, 18*(3), 157–168.
Mayer, B. W., & Burns, P. (2000). Differential diagnosis of abuse injuries in infants and young children. *Nurse Practitioner, 25*(10), 15–21.
Narrigan, D. (2000). Newborn hearing screening update for midwifery practice. *Journal of Midwifery & Women's Health, 45*(5), 368–377.
Perry, D. F., & Ireys, H. T. (2001). Maternal perceptions of pediatric providers for children with chronic illnesses. *Maternal & Child Health Journal, 5*(1), 15–20.
Peter, G., & Gardner, P. (2001). Standards for immunization practice for vaccines in children and adults. *Infectious Disease Clinics of North America, 15*(1), 9–19.
Shields, S. R. (2000). Managing eye disease in primary care: How to screen for occult disease. *Postgraduate Medicine, 108*(5), 69–72.
Stewart, C. E. (2000). Not just a sore throat. *Emergency Medical Services, 29*(7) 56–61.
Wilson, T. (2000). Factors influencing the immunization status of children in a rural setting. *Journal of Pediatric Health Care, 14*(3), 117–121.

34

CHAPTER

Communication and Teaching With Children and Families

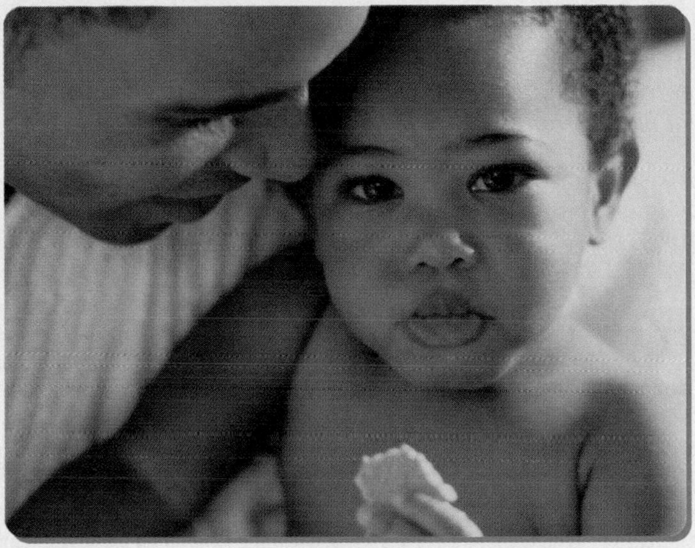

Key Terms

- affective learning
- behavior modification
- clarifying
- cognitive learning
- communication
- demonstration
- empathy
- feedback
- focusing
- health fairs
- nontherapeutic communication
- paraphrasing
- perception checking
- positive reinforcement
- psychomotor learning
- redemonstration
- reflecting
- teaching plan
- therapeutic communication

Objectives

After mastering the contents of this chapter, you should be able to:

1. Describe principles of effective communication and teaching and learning as they relate to health teaching with children.
2. Assess children for their ability to communicate and readiness to learn.
3. State nursing diagnoses related to communication and health teaching with children.
4. Identify expected outcomes for a specific child based on the child's age, developmental maturity, emotional needs, and communication or learning style.
5. Plan nursing care based on utilization of communication and health teaching priorities.
6. Implement health teaching (e.g., devising a puppet show) using principles of effective communication and teaching–learning.
7. Evaluate outcome criteria to be certain that outcomes established for care have been achieved.
8. Identify National Health Goals related to communication and teaching and children that nurses could be instrumental in helping the nation achieve.
9. Identify areas of care related to effective communication or health teaching of children that could benefit from additional nursing research or application of evidence-based nursing practice.
10. Use critical thinking to analyze ways that therapeutic communication and health teaching can be further incorporated into the nursing care of children and families to make it family centered.
11. Integrate knowledge of effective communication and teaching–learning with the nursing process to achieve quality maternal and child health nursing care.

Bill is a 3-year-old boy who is scheduled for repair of syndactyly (webbed fingers) next week. One of his favorite activities is coloring. His mother tells you she is concerned that Bill will be hard to entertain after surgery because the large pressure bandage he will have afterward will prevent him from coloring with that hand. "I don't even want to begin to talk to him about surgery," she tells you. How would you help her? What would be a good strategy for teaching about this type of surgery to a 3-year-old child?

Previous chapters discussed normal growth and development and how children's understanding increases with age. This chapter adds information about techniques for effective communication and health teaching with children. This is important information because it builds a base for disease prevention and health promotion for the age group.

After you've studied the chapter, answer the Critical Thinking Exercises at the end of the chapter and then access the on-line study activities (http://connection.lww.com) *to further sharpen your skills and test your knowledge.*

Communication and health teaching are independent nursing actions that accompany all nursing care. They are probably the most frequently used interventions for nurses working with childbearing and childrearing families for whom health promotion is such a priority. Education is a prime method for empowering families to assume responsibility for their own health. It is as important as any intervention for families experiencing some type of illness or injury; it is especially important when preparing a child for surgery or some other medical procedure. New areas that require teaching are constantly arising as the health care environment continues to change.

Communication can be formal or informal. Health teaching may be offered to an individual or to a group of children with similar learning needs. It is offered both formally (e.g., teaching a group of preschoolers about hospitalization) and informally (e.g., when a nurse assures a parent that his or her child is getting enough nutrition, even though the child snacks rather than sits down to regular meals). The same principles of effective teaching and learning apply whether teaching is informal or formal, or offered to an individual or to a group. National Health Goals regarding health teaching and children are shown in Focus on National Health Goals.

FOCUS ON NATIONAL HEALTH GOALS

A number of National Health Goals address good communication or health teaching, because it is such an important mechanism of preventive health care. These include:

- Increase the proportion of middle, junior high, and senior high schools that provide school health education to prevent: unintentional injuries, violence, suicide, tobacco use and addiction, alcohol and other drug use, unintended pregnancy, HIV/AIDS and STD infection, unhealthy dietary patterns, inadequate physical activity and environmental health problems from a baseline of 28% to 70%.
- Increase the proportion of the nation's elementary, middle, junior high, and senior high schools that have a nurse-to-student ratio of at least 1:750 from 28% to 50%.
- Increase the proportion of local health departments that have established culturally appropriate and linguistically competent community health promotion and disease prevention programs from 35% to 50% (DHHS, 2000).

Nurses can be instrumental in helping the nation achieve these goals by consulting with schools and health care organizations to develop health teaching programs and by teaching such programs. Areas that could benefit from nursing research include ways in which busy health care providers can better incorporate health teaching into care; what special techniques are needed to be certain that underserved populations are addressed; and whether different teaching techniques are necessary for material with immediate application than for material for long-term care.

NURSING PROCESS OVERVIEW

For Health Teaching With Children

Assessment

Neither communication nor health teaching can be effectively accomplished unless they are placed within the context of the nursing process. Learner needs and characteristics, teacher characteristics, available support people, and level of content are all factors that will affect learning or whether communication is received so they must be assessed to formulate nursing diagnoses that clearly state the specific health needs that teaching will address (see Assessing the Child's Learning and Communication Capabilities).

Nursing Diagnosis

The following are examples of common nursing diagnoses related to communication or health teaching:

- Impaired verbal communication related to use of Russian as primary language
- Deficient knowledge related to importance of taking medicine daily
- Health-seeking behaviors related to ways to improve the child's nutritional intake
- Impaired verbal communication related to placement of endotracheal tube
- Anxiety related to perceived amount of material needed to be learned for home care of child

Outcome Identification and Planning

After formulation of a nursing diagnosis, an individualized plan for communication or teaching is constructed. A plan should detail not only what is to be communicated or learned but also methods as to how

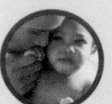

ASSESSING the Child's Learning and Communication Capabilities

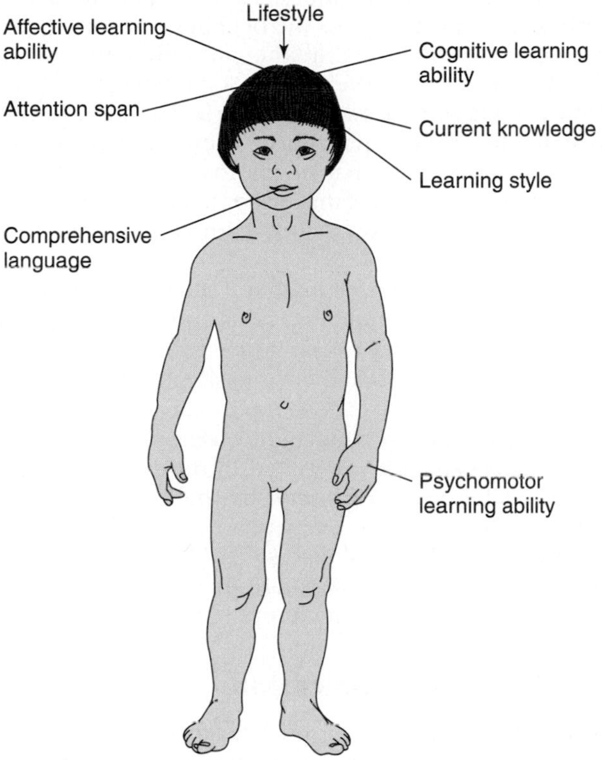

this will be evaluated. The most effective way to ensure that the expected outcomes are achieved is to ask the child or family to join in planning. Be certain that outcomes are concrete and measurable (not "Child will discuss general aspects of his disease," but "Child will list three steps to prevent disease").

Implementation

The step of implementation involves the actual communication or teaching. Teaching children is not always easy and requires practice and knowledge of a child's particular developmental level.

Outcome Evaluation

As a final step of communication or teaching, what was communicated or learned must be evaluated. A new plan may need to be developed to continue teaching if communication or learning was less than optimal. Examples of outcome criteria are:

- Child demonstrates self-injection of insulin.
- Child effectively demonstrates anger by language rather than punching wall.
- Child lists foods to include in a high-protein diet.
- Family demonstrates improved communication techniques by next clinic visit.
- Parents demonstrate effective cardiopulmonary resuscitation technique at home visit.

COMMUNICATION

Communication is the exchange of ideas between two or more persons. It can be verbal, using words, or nonverbal, using actions such as touch or eye contact or a remote system such as mail or e-mail. It is an important process in care of children because it can make or break an effective relationship (Kiehl & Wink, 2000). Communication, as a process, can be divided into two major categories: nontherapeutic (casual, everyday conversation) and therapeutic (helpful and constructive interchanges).

Nontherapeutic Communication

Nontherapeutic communication is identified by its lack of structure or planning (i.e., it lacks deliberate purpose other than socializing). Dinner conversation is an example of nontherapeutic communication.

Therapeutic Communication

Therapeutic communication is an interaction between two people that is planned (you deliberately intend to determine the true way a child feels), has structure (you use specific wording techniques that will encourage the response that you expect to elicit), and is helpful and constructive (at the end of the exchange you will know much more about the child than you did at the beginning, and the child hopefully also knows more about himself).

In some instances, there is no cure for a child you care for—no surgery, no medication, no pain relief. If you practice therapeutic communication, however, you still have something to offer these children: support by your words or a nonverbal communication such as touch. This is often the most valued, most appreciated, and most helpful aspect of all the care you offer.

Components of Good Communication

Communication can be broken down and diagrammed according to its essential component: the encoder, the code, the decoder, and response or feedback (Fig. 34-1).

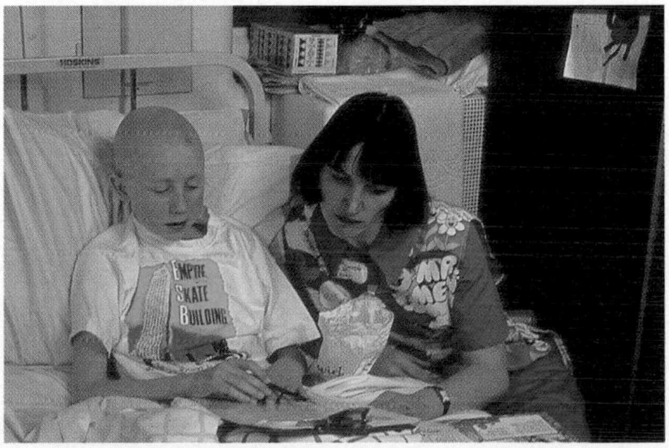

FIGURE 34.1 Health teaching is an interactive process, in which both the teacher and the learner share in the learning experience.

The Encoder

The encoder is the person who originates a message. Such a person desires to share a thought or feeling with someone else. They mold this thought into a form suitable for transferring to another person (a code). Communication can be ineffective if the person omits cognitive processing or speaks without thinking, chooses the wrong words for the message or accompanies the spoken words with a facial expression, tone of voice or gesture inappropriate for the message.

The Code

The code is the message that is conveyed, as well as the medium or system used to convey it. Although this usually involves a simple spoken system, messages can also be conveyed by a painting, poem, novel, Morse code, Braille, computer, television, radio, audiotape, movie projector, or telephone. Communication is often ineffective because a person chooses the wrong medium for a message (e.g., delivering a lecture with many technical words when a drawing with carefully labeled parts would have made the message much clearer, or e-mailing when confronting a person directly would have been more effective).

The Decoder

The receiver (decoder) of the message not only receives it (hears it, reads it, views it) but interprets or decodes it (cognitive processing). Messages are interpreted in light of the receiver's store of knowledge. They may be misinterpreted if a receiver's store of knowledge is too different from that of the sender. Messages may also be misinterpreted if the receiver misses part of the transmission, such as the wink accompanying the spoken words that would have let him know the sender was joking. Under stress, children tend to narrow their ability to receive information to a small area of concern. When you are dealing with children who are extremely anxious, you may find that, although you gave excellent instructions (both sender and message component of communication were adequate), they did not "hear" you (did not receive or could not interpret the message because of anxiety).

Feedback or Response

Feedback is the reply that the decoder returns to the sender to acknowledge that the message has been received and interpreted. This could be a spoken statement, a nod of the head, a facial grimace, or the sudden slamming of a telephone receiver. With feedback, the roles of sender and receiver become reversed and another communication cycle is begun. Communication can be ineffective if children do not offer feedback at all (the message was either not understood or not acknowledged) or offer feedback before the message is fully interpreted (acting before thinking). When you are caring for children with sensory challenges such as vision or hearing difficulties, you may have to change your usual feedback mechanisms in order to be understood, because a nod of the head or quiet response may not be received.

The Development of Language

Development of language involves not only physically being able to form and voice words but comprehension of what they mean and how they are used. One of the first responses an infant makes at birth is to communicate. A first cry is important because it means that the infant is breathing well. It also announces to the parents that the birth is real and stimulates the beginning of parent–child interaction. Early in life, infants not only cry, they kick their legs and thrash their arms. Some new parents may comment that their newborns have bad tempers because their infant seems very angry. They are actually commenting on the way that newborns respond with their total body to stimuli. Infants discontinue gesturing wildly with every need as soon as they learn a more refined communication system.

By age 2, children have mastered language well enough to put two-word sentences (a noun and a verb) together. By preschool age, they not only have a vocabulary of about 900 words, but can code them into simple jokes or stories.

School-age children enlarge their ability to communicate from largely spoken language to use of e-mail on computers. They can write poetry and, by the end of the period, show an adult sense of humor by the jokes they create. Adolescents progress to a new phase in which they appropriate new words ("cool" and so forth). This form of communication helps them separate their world from adults and keep their adolescent culture separate.

Levels of Communication

Every conversation that you engage in does not (and should not) have the same depth level. Throughout a day, a person may use as many as five levels, from clichés to peak communication.

First-Level: Cliché Conversation

Cliché conversation is pleasant chatting (comments such as, "Have a nice day") between people who think that their relationship will not extend beyond a superficial level. It is important when meeting a child for the first time that you introduce yourself with not only your name but your position and function (a student nurse who is going to take care of you; a nurse who will be visiting you in your home). This information leads the family to move the conversation from the cliché level to a more meaningful one.

Second Level: Fact Reporting

Fact reporting is simply stating facts about oneself ("I'm 12; I'm in sixth grade"). Fact reporting is necessary for you to understand children but it does not tell you anything about their feelings or needs. Children can move from this level to a higher level of communication only when they feel that they can trust you with more information.

Third Level: Shared Personal Ideas and Judgments

When children know you well they are able to share ideas ("I always wanted to be an astronaut") and judgments "This is too hard for me; I need to learn a different way.").

This level of communication exposes them to loss of self-esteem if their views are not respected. It is the level that is the beginning of therapeutic interactions.

Fourth Level: Shared Feelings

It is difficult to share feelings until you truly trust one another, because feelings are tenuous, fragile concepts, easily destroyed and crushed by incpt or uncaring comments. Listen carefully for an expression of feeling from children ("It's terrible to be always sick"). These admissions are telling you much more than how they experience their world; they represent trust in you, and the depth of the relationship that they have established with you.

Fifth Level: Peak Communication

The fifth level of communication is a sense of oneness, or being able to know what the other person is experiencing without it actually being voiced. It sometimes occurs spontaneously in high-intensity situations but generally arises out of long-term relationships. For example, you notice that a parent sits soundlessly beside her daughter's bedside for hours at a time. When she leaves, the daughter says, "She makes me feel so much better when she's here." It would be easy to view this mother as nonsupportive (she says almost nothing during the time she's there), but by using fifth-level communication, she has given her daughter more comfort than other visitors who talk the entire time they visit.

Nonverbal Communication

What children communicate nonverbally is at least as important as the words they actually voice. Nonverbal communication can be especially important in areas such as intensive care units when many children are unable to speak because of endotracheal tubes and ventilators. Nonverbal communication can be expressed in a variety of ways.

Distance

Although it is affected by cultural and personal variables, the distance at which you position yourself from others may indicate your feelings toward them or the type of conversation you want to have. People generally consider the space directly surrounding them (up to 18 inches) as *intimate* space, to be crossed only by people who know them well or with whom they are comfortable having close body contact. Sometimes, you will notice in a heated discussion that one person moves aggressively into this space and the other automatically steps back to protect it.

Any time you touch a child, you violate this space; if children allow you to do this without protest, it means they see you as safe, protective, and helpful.

The space between 18 inches to 4 feet is sensed by most people as *personal* space. This is the distance that people stand apart from each other for usual conversation. It is a comfortable hand-shaking distance. When you stand by the side of a crib or bed or sit next to a person at home, you are within this space. It is a concerned, I-care-about-you distance, but does not invade intimate space.

The distance between 4 feet and 12 feet is *social* space, the distance used to conduct business or teach a class. Conversation spoken at this distance is readily heard by others. Do not use social space to ask a personal question. If you ask a child "How are you feeling?" as you pass in a hallway, for example, they will probably answer, "Fine, thank you," the programmed reply almost everyone is taught in early childhood. In contrast, if you ask that same question from a personal or intimate distance, providing privacy, the answer might be, "I'm scared I'm never going home again."

Distance beyond 12 feet is *public* space. To communicate from this distance, you need to shout; privacy is not respected at all. Waving to a friend in a hallway or across a parking lot is an example of public space communication. Most people perceive speaking on the telephone or using e-mail as either social or personal space. The tone of voice and the words used help to differentiate which area they consider it to be. A message such as, "Have I got news for you!" suggests social space. "Can you keep a secret?" brings it into intimate space.

Genuineness

Genuineness is a quality of projecting sincerity or being yourself. Children have difficulty trusting you and, therefore, cannot move to a deep relationship with you if you change your behavior from one day to the next (e.g., from maximum patience to short-tempered), because they have to spend energy every day testing to see who you are that day. The way to achieve a feeling of genuineness is not to try to be what you are not. The insecurity that comes from pretending manifests itself as negative feelings such as aggressiveness or a bored attitude.

Warmth

Warmth is an innate quality, and some people manifest it more spontaneously than others. Basic ways in which warmth is demonstrated are direct eye contact, use of a gentle tone of voice, listening attentively, approaching the child within a comfortable space of 1 to 4 feet (closer may be threatening; farther away may be distancing), and using touch appropriately. Warmth is a quality that you display best when you know another person well. Any action that helps you to know a person better (taking a health history, talking about school or family, or how a child feels about a present situation) not only lets you plan care but allows you to become increasingly comfortable with the child and deepen your relationship.

Empathy

Empathy is the ability to put yourself in another's place and experience a feeling as that person is experiencing it. People who are capable of empathy are the best support people because they can anticipate a child's reactions or fears. At first, it seems that empathy would require you to have experienced all the situations that children experience. This is not necessarily true, however, because you understand the common emotion of all situations in other ways. If you have hoped for something very strongly and then not attained it, loved someone and not had that emotion returned, lost someone or something that was so important to you that you felt actual pain, you can feel empathy for children who have received a disappointing diagnosis or who are unhappy for other reasons you have never experienced. Feeling empathy can be emotionally draining because, when you assume another person's emotions, you experience them at the same depth. Nurses who are capable of empathy should surround themselves with good support people so they have refueling resources when they need them.

Gestures

Children vary a great deal in the gestures they use to accompany their spoken words. Although this is culturally influenced, it is also an individual trait. Be careful not to assess emotion only by a child's gestures; some children wave their arms wildly describing an everyday occurrence; others would use that degree of expression only when in extreme distress. Be aware that your own gestures are always being read by children. A statement that you approve of something is contradicted by placing your arms across your chest in a disapproving, stern manner.

Body Posture and Gait

Children who feel good about themselves usually assume an upright body posture and walk rapidly and surely; those who are depressed tend to slouch and move more slowly and timidly; those who are threatened tend to either draw back or act aggressively. Children who are in agreement with you usually maintain eye contact with you as you speak to them. Very depressed or insecure children do not do that (they feel too inferior), nor do children who are very angry. Children from some cultures do not meet your gaze because it is not culturally appropriate.

Facial expression is an important accompanying gesture. Clenched teeth, frowns, and smiles are easily interpreted by everyone. The degree of pain a child is experiencing may be more evident by facial expression than words.

General Appearance

The way children dress often suggests the importance of what they are saying; the tone they use to speak reveals the intensity of a message. Children who have good self-esteem tend to maintain good body hygiene and care about their appearance. Those who are depressed may not feel that the effort involved in grooming is worthwhile. Personal hygiene varies, however, and it is difficult to assess it on your first contact with a child. What you see as ill kempt may be neat and trim for that particular child; what you think of as well groomed may be comparatively sloppy for that child.

Be aware that your impression of how children dress registers very strongly on your subconscious. Do not let an unconscious dislike for a mode of dress of some child (body piercing or a turban) cause you to draw back. Preparing to give nursing care is not the same kind of activity as evaluating whether you wish to invite someone to dinner.

Touch

Touch is the most intimate and meaningful of nonverbal techniques. When words are inadequate, touch rarely is. Learn to use touch such as clapping a child's shoulder or squeezing a hand to accompany reassuring words or in place of words as a strong support signal (I'm here; I understand; it's all right to be afraid). On the other hand, be aware that some children enjoy being touched more than others. Due to individual preferences or cultural variations, some children do not like you to use this nonverbal signal with them. Assess individually for the appropriateness of using touch.

Use of Humor

Some people have a natural knack for finding humor in any situation; others do not instinctively have this quality and must cultivate it. Those who are able to laugh at their own mistakes are usually nice people to have around, because their laughter at themselves suggests that, when you make a mistake, they will be able to accept it the same way (or at least not be angry about it).

Be careful of the use of humor with children who are fatigued or ill, however. They may be looking for a firm support person to be with them more than one who is amusing. You can often measure a child's progress by noting the first time after a procedure that the child responds to you with a humorous statement. Remember, though, that laughter and joking can also be signs of increasing anxiety. Evaluate the use of humor to be certain a child really finds a situation amusing.

Use of Drawings

A useful nonverbal technique to learn how children feel about a frightening experience is to ask them to draw a picture of what happened or a picture of themselves. A child hospitalized for heart surgery might draw her heart prominently. Surely she realizes that she cannot survive if something happens to such an important body part.

A child's use of color may be a clue as to mood (happy children tend to use bright colors; depressed children use black or dark colors). A child with good self-esteem usually fills the full page with a drawing; one with less crowds a drawing into a corner. These observations are quite variable, however; a child may have had only a black crayon with which to color or may be saving the rest of the paper for a second drawing.

Use of Music

The type of music to which children prefer to listen often conveys their mood. The better they feel about themselves, the more likely they are to choose music that has a lively quality; if they are sad, they often choose a quieter, more comforting type. Children enjoy repetition, however, so may play the same music over and over, independent of their mood.

Techniques That Encourage Therapeutic Communication

Several techniques are effective in deepening communication patterns and relationships. These techniques can be learned if they are not a spontaneous part of your present communication pattern.

Attentive Listening

The importance of attentive listening cannot be overstressed. Making it clear that you are concentrating on what another is saying by such a motion as nodding indicates that you have respect for a child and value what is being said. A child who feels valued is much more likely to confide feelings and concerns than one who senses that you consider him not important. (See Focus on Family Empowerment.)

Open-Ended Questions

A pointed or direct question asks for a specific task; it implies that all you are interested in hearing about is that one fact. An example of a direct question is, "Do you take Tylenol when you have a headache?" An open-ended question is not limited to a simple answer but invites a wide variety of responses because it is so comprehensive (e.g., "Tell me what you do when you have a headache"). The child might answer by describing not only the amount of analgesic she takes but using a cold towel, going home from school, and closing her eyes to stop the pain. Three or four times more information has been elicited.

Open-ended questions are not effective if the topic is difficult for a child to describe (a preschooler has difficulty responding even yes or no; a paragraph of material would be impossible) or if the child is naturally shy or defensive about the subject (he knows that he has not been doing the things you told him to do and would rather not admit it).

Most communication is a combination of direct and open-ended questions. Listen carefully the next time you ask someone to explain something to see if you make use of mostly direct (information-limiting) questions or open-ended (information-expanding) ones.

Reflecting

Reflecting is another technique, like attentive listening, that is so simple that its importance is easy to discount. Reflecting is restating the last word or phrase a child has said when there is a pause in the communication. A child says, "I'm worried," and then stops. You repeat the last word. "Worried?" The child, assured that you are listening and interested, will generally enlarge on the first statement: "I'm worried I won't make the football team this year." Older school-age children may not respond well to reflection; they may see it as imitating them, not information seeking.

Clarifying

Clarifying consists of repeating statements others have made so you and they can be certain you understood them. This is particularly helpful if a child has been describing a set of symptoms or series of actions. You would clarify such a statement by saying, "Let me see if I understand this. You said that you always get the pain first in your stomach. Then it spreads to your chest." If you are not quoting correctly, the child will interrupt and restate the problem: "No, the chest pain comes first."

Paraphrasing

Paraphrasing is restating what children have said not only to assure them that you have heard correctly (as in clarifying) but to help them explain what they have been trying to say. In clarifying, you repeat a child's exact words; in paraphrasing, you retain the meaning of the words but repeat them in a clearer or more condensed form. The child says, for example, "I don't talk about my problems with my parents." A paraphrasing statement might be, "You're telling me that you and your parents haven't discussed home care. Is that right?" Ask for confirmation that

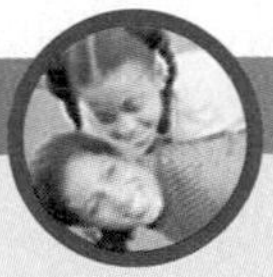

FOCUS ON FAMILY EMPOWERMENT

Listening to Children

Q. My children tell me I don't listen to them. How can I be a better listener?

A. Try the following tips:

1. Stop talking. You cannot listen if you are talking.
2. Look and act interested. Don't read or write while they talk. Listen to understand rather than to reply.
3. Remove distractions. Do not doodle, tap, or shuffle papers. Would it be quieter if you turned off the television?
4. Empathize. Try to put yourself in your children's place so you can see their point of view.
5. Be patient. Allow plenty of time. Do not interrupt. Do not edge toward the door or walk away.
6. Hold your temper. An angry person gets the wrong meaning from words.
7. Hold argument or criticism. This puts children on the defensive. They may stop talking or get angry.
8. Ask questions. This is proof that you have been listening.
9. Stop talking. This is the first and last because all other suggestions depend on it.

your interpretation is correct; otherwise, you may find yourself putting words in children's mouths.

When the topic is embarrassing or emotionally charged (an adolescent discussing sexual orientation), the child might use such vague terms that the explanation becomes difficult to follow. Paraphrasing using basic terms would let him know not only that you understand him but that, if he can describe the problem better with such words than with medical terminology, it is acceptable to you.

Perception Checking

Perception checking documents a feeling or emotion reported to you. This makes it a step deeper than paraphrasing. In paraphrasing, you document a statement or fact; in perception checking, you document a feeling or emotion. The child says, "I'm not at all worried about surgery. I know a lot of kids have the same thing done every day. I mean, what could happen? " You say, "You're telling me that you're not worried, but the number of times you've said it make me wonder if you really are worried. Are you?"

Always ask for validation that your perception is correct so you do not put ideas into a child's mind. As a rule, children are not ready to deal with emotions until they can admit that they are experiencing them. When you bring an emotion out on the table this way, it allows them to confront it and deal with it for the first time. They may lose their reluctance to admit other worries because you have implied that worrying is acceptable.

Focusing

Focusing helps children to center on a subject that you suspect is causing them anxiety because they comment about it indirectly or else completely avoid it. It is done by repeating something that they said ("You mentioned that you feel tired all the time") or by mentioning the avoided topic ("You haven't said a word about how you feel about this surgery. Is that a problem?"). Once a subject is brought up for discussion, most children respond to it. As long as it can be avoided, however, they cannot face the problem and begin to solve it.

Supportive Statements

Supportive statements let children know that you accept their behavior or at least appreciate that they have dealt well with unfortunate circumstances. For example, an adolescent says, "My girlfriend dumped me while I was in the hospital." Not only was such an experience undoubtedly difficult for the adolescent at the time, but talking about it revives his hurt and anger. Such a statement deserves a reply such as, "That must be hard on you." The adolescent will take this response to mean that you want to discuss the topic and, encouraged by your empathy, may elaborate on it as it still affects him.

Silence

If you ask a question and a child does not respond immediately, it is natural to ask another question, or perhaps change the subject, assuming the child is not interested. This is a social custom that allows you to back off so you do not put someone into the awkward position of having to discuss a sensitive topic. Silence, however, is an effective therapeutic technique. If you ask an emotion-laden question ("Are you worried?") and the child does not answer immediately, allow a period of silence to pass. Because you do not hurry to fill in the silence, the child is likely to respond by hurrying an answer (to fill in the silence): when this happens, the answer is usually spontaneous and often open and uninhibited. In other instances, a child may answer the question deliberately and cautiously and, because you have provided a period of time to answer, offer additional information.

Do not overdo silence, however, either by the number of times you use it or the length of time you allow it to extend. In this era of constant noise, many individuals are extremely uncomfortable with silence. Too much silence can indicate to a child that you are not interested enough to keep the conversation going.

Factors That Can Interfere With Effective Communication With Children

Because so much of nursing care is influenced by verbal communication, it is important to avoid miscalculations in communication and to recognize common situations in which meanings can be distorted.

Age and Developmental Level

Age and developmental levels are important to communication ability because they influence vocabulary so greatly (Kaiser et al., 2001). A 3-year-old child may not have the vocabulary to explain the way her knee feels (she has heard the word "ache" but only in connection with headache; she does not know that knees can ache as well). Early school-age children have difficulty describing the blurring that they experience as they focus on a blackboard with less than perfect eyesight, because this is the way they have always seen. The ability to describe inner feelings such as anger, sadness, and fear comes only with adolescence.

Intellectual Level

Intellectual level, like age, affects vocabulary and ability both to encode and decode messages. It influences the number of languages a child speaks, reading ability, and the depth of explanation that a child is capable of understanding.

Physical Factors

Physical factors such as speech impairments and hearing or vision challenges interfere with the transmission and reception of messages. When children are distracted by such sensations as fatigue or pain, they may have reduced ability to transmit or receive messages correctly.

Technical Terminology

Adults have heard common medical words so usually have little difficulty understanding an explanation of one. Children, in contrast, understand few medical words. Listen to explanations you give them to be sure that you would have understood that explanation at their age.

Inattentive Listening

No one likes to talk to someone who does not appear to be listening or responding. Good listening, like speaking, is not passive but active. Be aware that your body posture reveals to a great extent whether you are listening (sitting, not standing, to convey that you are not on the run; leaning forward, not backward; stooping to meet a child's level). Nodding, maintaining eye contact, and stopping all other activities are strong indicators that you are attuned to what is being said. In some instances, it is necessary to repeat a part of what the child said, interject an appropriate "uh-huh" or "m-m-m," or make a direct statement ("I'm listening. Go on.") to indicate that you are listening. Be certain when you are listening to your tenth or twentieth child on any given day that you do not exhibit "end-of-the day" behavior. To be therapeutic, you have to give everyone's concerns the same alert attention.

Showing Disapproval

Children do not come for health care to be criticized; they come to learn more about how to stay well or recover from illness. If you criticize them, they may not reveal their main problem to you because they do not want you to react in the same way you did to their preliminary statements.

Suppose a child says, "I never drink milk. That's for babies." Knowing that milk is an important source of calcium, you respond, "That's not right. You should drink at least two glasses a day." This discourages the adolescent from telling you any more about eating habits (she doesn't eat much protein either, but you miss this information because she will not expose herself to your criticism again).

Be aware that nonverbal disapproval (frowning, sighing) can be just as detrimental as spoken disapproval. On the other hand, this does not mean that you should show approval of wrong actions. Merely listen to them with no action or comment and make a mental note. At the end of your interaction, introduce the change in behavior that you wish to see ("Let's plan some ways you can include more calcium with your meals without drinking milk").

Not Showing Approval When Warranted

Every student has had the experience of completing a difficult assignment and receiving only criticism from a teacher—no comment that, aside from the part that was not satisfactory, the rest of the assignment was done well. This is because the instructor assumed that the student would do a good job; no reward was given for meeting minimum criteria. From the other side of the desk, however, it would have been satisfying—and offered motivation to continue to do well—to have heard the words "good job."

When discussing health care problems with children, it is easy to forget that what you accept as standard behavior may take a great deal of effort for an ill child to accomplish (coughing and deep breathing after surgery seems simple but is actually very difficult to do because it is so painful). Giving children praise for what they do well encourages them to tell you more about themselves and to try other things. If a topic is difficult for them to talk about, saying that you appreciate that it is a sensitive topic helps them continue to discuss it.

Being Defensive

In the same way that children who request health care do not enjoy being criticized, neither does the average health care provider. If a child makes a critical remark, therefore, it is easy to respond with a defensive or protective comment rather than a therapeutic one. An adolescent might say, "We have to wait so long here, this is a really dumb clinic." It is easy to reply, "Don't say that. This is a good clinic." This type of response implies that any complaint is out of line. Try to respond instead with a supportive comment such as, "I know it makes a long day for you." No health care agency is so perfect that there is nothing to criticize.

Cliché Advice

Cliché advice (advice given from a formula, not individualized to the situation) is meaningless because it is too general to be helpful. Statements such as "Rome wasn't built in a day" and "You have to walk before you can run" are examples of this kind of advice. Each child considers his or her problem unique and resents being given advice that could apply to everyone.

Topping Off

Topping off is minimizing a child's views by telling a better story. A child tells you, for example, that he has a headache; you say, "You should feel the one I have." A child says she has a problem; you say, "You want to know what problems really are? Come and work here." This implies to children that their problems are inconsequential. They will not be likely to tell you any more about themselves after such responses.

Communication Situations That Require Special Skills

Some communication situations require special skills in addition to usual therapeutic communication techniques to promote understanding.

The Shy Child

The amount of verbal communication children use varies culturally and individually. Some children talk excessively when they are nervous; those who are shy may stop talking completely. Children who are verbal reach out to secure the help they need from others by talking; shy individuals are more likely to have their needs go unrecognized. It is difficult to assess how shy children feel when they are reluctant to communicate about such things as whether they are really psychologically ready for surgery or if they really understand the long-term effect a disease is going to have. If they do not give you much verbal feedback, the tendency is to believe that they do not have a concern. That leaves them without support people when they most need them.

Fortunately, in most instances, once children realize that they really know you and can trust you, shyness fades. A therapeutic response, therefore, is not to leave them alone but to maintain an active relationship despite the lack of feedback. This does not necessarily involve talking to children but may involve checking on them frequently, remaining in the room while a physician completes an examination, helping with the adhesive strip after a technician draws a blood sample, or sitting with them for a few minutes while a medication takes effect.

The Angry Child

It is difficult to work with angry children because you feel yourself being pulled into their anger. The typical response at hearing an angry outburst is to imitate it (a child is radiating anger as tight-lipped silence, and you say nothing; he or she shouts at you, and you shout back). This is not therapeutic, however. Make a point of not allowing yourself to be drawn into children's anger that way, while acknowledging that it is all right to be angry. Help them to focus anger if at all possible so they can better understand it and begin to deal with it.

To encourage focusing, ask a child to detail what it is he or she is angry about. An adolescent who feels angry at the entire health care delivery system is highly frustrated because he cannot begin to handle the whole bureaucracy; establishing that what he is really angry about is one nurse's action builds a base for resolving the problem. If a child uses silence as a method of maintaining anger, suggesting possible reasons for the anger may be helpful ("I know Doctor Smith was just talking to you. Are you angry about something she said?" or, "I know you were asking about crutch walking before. Does it have something to do with that?"). Once the subject is out in the open, few children can resist describing the extent of or reason for their anger. Be aware, too, that, when you ask someone to explain why they are angry, you ask for the emotion and the distress that go with it to be expressed as well. Even if you are the object of the anger, you are committed to listening to the child's views.

Helping the child focus anger this way moves them toward a constructive solution (focusing anger at the physical therapy department seems justified, but swearing at you, not eating dinner, or shouting at a parent does not). If necessary, censor the way that the anger is expressed, not the right to be angry. Keep anger from affecting you by reacting to the explanation not the tone or force of it. Keep any response on your part a tone gentler and quieter than that used toward you.

The Demanding Child

Nursing has few equals in job satisfaction (provided that salary and other working conditions are adequate) because the majority of people you care for are grateful for everything you do for them. It can be upsetting to discover a particular child who is not grateful for or even satisfied with anything you do. This type of child is also easy to back away from or avoid.

Demanding behavior generally stems from insecurity or fear (so afraid that something will happen to them while you are out of the room that they constantly find more for you to do to keep you there, or so afraid of unplanned events that they structure things so that nothing unexpected can happen). Give more of yourself, not less, to counteract this response. When you have proven that you are dependably there for them, children do not feel so insecure, and the need to be demanding usually fades. Withdrawing may increase the child's insecurity and the demanding behavior. Ask instead, "Is there anything else I can do for you?" not, "Haven't I already done enough?"

The Sexually Aggressive Adolescent

Sexually aggressive behavior stems from the same cause as every other aggressive and demanding behavior: insecurity. It may be pronounced in adolescents who worry that illness or surgery will interfere with sexual function. Adolescents with this degree of insecurity may benefit from counseling to help them channel coping responses into more socially acceptable behaviors. Be sure that they have factual information as to the extent or effect of their illness. Set limits, as necessary, to make giving care acceptable to you. Always censor the action, not the adolescent. Be aware that sexually aggressive behavior occurs in both males and females.

The Child Who Speaks Another Language

It is not unusual in any nursing care setting to encounter children who have a different primary language from yours; in other instances, children's speech may be limited or difficult to understand because of an accent, dialect, or speech impairment; some children may speak your same language but their use of words is so different from yours that the words have different meanings.

Most children who speak another language have a support person who can serve as a interpreter. Anticipate the instructions you will need to give the child (cough, deep breathe, save urine, and so forth) and ask the interpreter to write them out in the child's language. Post them conspicuously in the room or the child's care plan so that everyone giving care can be familiar with them.

Most health care facilities have a list of people who serve as translators as needed; many times, you can contact such a person by telephone to ask for a specific word you want to know. In the event that you have to give instructions and no translator is present, do not be self-conscious about using hand gestures or drawing a picture to express the action that you want (a child lying in bed, an arrow pointing to a chair, and a child sitting in a chair for, "I'm going to help you get out of bed." Allow children ample paper and a clipboard to draw pictures to show what they want to tell you. Supply pictures for preschool children so they can select the one they want.

Everyone has a tendency to shout at children who speak a different language as if loudness will increase understanding. When using an interpreter, be certain to speak slowly and use common words that can be translated literally. "I need to stick Mary's arm for blood" could be interpreted literally to mean putting a stick in the child's arm.

The Unconscious Child

Hearing is the last sense lost with unconsciousness and the first sense regained with consciousness. Always be aware that children who do not respond to you may be able to hear and interpret anything you say. Never say anything to unconscious children or within their hearing, therefore, that you would not say if they were fully alert. Continue to use nonverbal communication such as touch to help convey your message.

The Hearing-Challenged Child

When communicating with hearing-challenged children, check whether they use a hearing aid; if so, be certain that it is turned on. Face them when you speak so they can follow your lip movements. Use hand gestures as necessary to convey your message, or write out instructions. If you have difficulty understanding what they are trying to say, ask them to write it if they're old enough. Use common sense about how loud to raise your voice to facilitate communication. As a rule, at the point that privacy is lost, it is time to resort to written words or sign language. Children who use sign language to communicate have a right to have an interpreter present to facilitate communication the same as children who do not use English as their primary language.

The Vision-Challenged Child

When speaking to children who are challenged visually, do not rely on nonverbal communication techniques such as hand gestures. A statement such as, "Take a piece of gauze about this long," without an accompanying hand gesture showing the length you mean is meaningless. Never touch children who cannot see you without speaking to them first so that you do not startle them.

Process Recording

Process recording is a method to examine how effective you are at therapeutic communication. After your next interaction with a child, take a few minutes and write down in the left hand column of a sheet of paper, a statement made to you by a child. In the middle column, write what you thought on hearing the statement. In a third column, write your response. Try to record both statements and responses verbatim or as close to the actual words used as possible. The average person can recall about 3 min of communication accurately this way.

Next, examine your responses to each statement. "Did I encourage the child to tell me more or did I block communication by my response? Were my responses supportive or critical or trite? Did I use open-ended questions or closed, direct ones? Did I check perceptions or did I just assume that I understood correctly what was told me?" (Box 34-1).

BOX 34.1

PROCESS RECORDING

The following is a record of an interaction between a nursing student and Barry Sandoz, a 15-year-old boy who is hospitalized. Barry has been diagnosed as having a peptic ulcer.

What Client Said and Did	What I Thought and Felt	What I Said and Did
	I felt anxious meeting a new patient, although I thought he'd be friendly because he was so close to my age.	I walked into his room and said, "Good morning."
He was sitting up in bed holding his hands on his abdomen. He said, "Get me something for this pain," without even looking at me.	I felt attacked. As if he thought I should have done something sooner, but I had just arrived.	I asked, "What kind of pain are you having?"
He said, "I need a student nurse like a hole in the head. Isn't there anyone else around?"	Now, I really felt attacked.	I said, "I can get you something for pain. I just need to know what kind of pain you have."
He said, "Hydrochloric acid is carving a hole into my stomach. Is that enough explanation for you to get me something?"	I felt angry that he insisted on putting me down so.	I said, "It certainly is. And I appreciate that if I had pain like that I would not want to answer questions either."
		I left to find my instructor and get him something for pain. I returned in 15 minutes and said, "I have an injection for you."

continued on page 1004

Continued

PROCESS RECORDING

He asked, "Did you have to take so long to do that?"	I was getting really angry.	I said nothing. I just checked his ID band and gave him the injection.
He asked, "Now could you get me my purple pill?"	I was angry at his demanding tone and threatened because I didn't even know what he meant by his "purple pill."	I said, "I'll have to check your medication sheet."
He said, "Any chance you could do that in a hurry?"	Even more angry.	I said, "Are you always so demanding?"
He turned on his side so his back was to me, clenched his teeth, and pushed his hands into his abdomen again.	I realized that my criticism was unfair because he was in pain. But it was too late to take it back.	I said, "I'm sorry. I know you're uncomfortable."
He shouted, "I am not uncomfortable! I am having my stomach ripped out! Could you help me out in any decent way with that?"	I realized I was in over my head. I thought I'd limit any further interaction so he couldn't make me angry again.	I said nothing. I just left to check on whether he could have any other medicine. I returned (quickly as I could) with Prilosec (his purple pill).
He asked, "Do you know if Dr. M. is still in surgery?"	Threatened again; I didn't even know how to find that out.	I said, "I can find out for you."
He said, "Hand me that book on the chair over there, before you go, will you?"	Trying to concentrate on not being angry at his demanding tone, yet I had medicine I had to give safely.	I said, "Let me see your ID band again first."
He turned his wrist over so I couldn't read his ID.	I thought: I am tired of him demanding things and getting the book was not as important as what I was doing.	I said nothing.
He said, "If I don't get to that book today, I might as well cash it in."	Getting angry again, but also "hearing" what he had said for the first time.	I said, "Cash it in?"
He said, "Don't you think I ought to? I can't go back to school with pain like this. Wouldn't dying be better than failing out?"		I was surprised how one quick response on my part had brought out so much emotion. I also knew I was in over my head again, (but in a nice way).

Evaluation

My overall interaction with Barry would have been better if I hadn't been caught so off guard in the beginning by assuming that he was going to be someone who had a lot in common with me (student–student, close age-group). His initial response to me seemed so much more intense because I had stereotyped him that way.

My responses to him were adequate up to the point that I became angry. I should have answered his comment, "Do you always take so long to do something?" with a supportive one such as, "I know it's hard to be in pain." (I heard a nurse answer that question for a client with, "Believe it or not, sometimes I take longer," and all of us laughed. I think the client felt good about being able to appreciate something funny, but I'm glad I didn't try humor here. Silence was inadequate but at least not irritating).

If I had been more sensitive to what Barry was saying (and less angry), I would have noticed that after I gave the injection he became nicer to me (asking if I could get him his Prilosec, not just demanding it). I was too angry to notice his change in behavior though, so I cut off his preliminary attempt to interact with me by criticizing him ("Are you always so demanding?") My supportive statement ("I'm sorry; I know you're uncomfortable") was ineffective after the criticism.

In the final interaction, I was so concerned with my own needs (get my work done) that I completely missed what he said about why the book was important to him. Fortunately, at the last minute, I got my mind off my problem and onto his and was able to produce a therapeutic response for him. He shouldn't have had to describe something with the impact of driving a truck over me before he caught my attention, though. Better listening (and thinking while I'm listening) would make me hear better and be more helpful sooner in this type of interaction.

✔ CHECKPOINT QUESTIONS

1. What is the difference between paraphrasing and perception checking?
2. What is the first step in being a good listener?

HEALTH TEACHING IN A CHANGING HEALTH CARE ENVIRONMENT

In the past, when children were admitted to hospitals well in advance of surgery and remained in the hospital after surgery or therapy until they were almost totally well, there was a wide window of time for effective health teaching. Today, with many children never admitted to hospitals, surgery conducted as a 1-day experience, and early discharge after all procedures, the window for teaching has narrowed. Nurses must use more creative approaches to achieve the same results in these short time spans.

Children's sophistication about learning techniques has also changed. When children are exposed to a diet of clever animation on television or in movies, a simple lecture on good nutrition seems dull and uninteresting. Children who are adept at arcade or computer games where dexterity is the requirement may find handling a syringe or feeding tube not a challenging feat. Assess each child individually to be certain what they expect to learn, what is their individual learning style, and what teaching techniques would suit them best before beginning.

TABLE 34.1 Principles of Teaching

PRINCIPLE	RATIONALE
Know the subject.	To effectively teach children, you must be able not only to present material but also to answer questions about it. Children's questions can be as probing as an adult's and they can often be more frequent, because children are used to asking questions of a teacher or a parent.
Know the audience.	Children vary a great deal in cognitive development depending on their age group. To teach preschoolers about health, you might choose to teach how to brush teeth using puppets as a teaching aid. The same clever puppet and tooth-brushing presentation likely would not be well received among adolescents.
Know yourself.	Analyze which teaching techniques (lecture, role playing, small group discussion, audiovisual aids) fit your teaching style. Using techniques that are comfortable allows teaching to be most effective.
Assess individual learning styles.	Most children respond well to visual images (seeing a demonstration or drawing) to complement learning. Assessing individual learning styles helps to meet each child's best way of learning.
Define expected outcomes.	Expected outcomes serve as guidelines to help you select from all you know about a subject that part which is most pertinent to an individual child. They should be realistic, measurable, and mutually established. Instruction on how to walk using crutches for an early school-age child would include how to carry school books while using crutches; for an adolescent, instruction would include how to board a city bus so he or she could get to and from a part-time job.
Provide an environment conducive for learning.	Children are easily distracted from learning because of so many new experiences in their world. Divide material into segments to keep teaching sessions short; avoid competing factors such as television or mealtime.
Be consistent.	Nothing is more confusing to a person learning something for the first time than to be told two different ways to do it. Choose one method that should work best for a child and then consistently stress that method. After a child has learned the one method, then suggest alternative methods if the child is interested.
Be honest.	Abstract concepts such as "little white lies" cannot be understood by children younger than adolescents.
Recognize that actions teach as much as or sometimes more than verbal statements.	Children watch facial expressions and nonverbal gestures as much as they listen. Be certain that a nonverbal statement is not contradicting a verbal one.
Teach from the simple to the complex.	Fundamentals must be grasped before extensive learning can proceed. Many children have little idea of body anatomy. Often you need to begin with the basics; when these are mastered, you can proceed to teach about a disease condition.
Teach principles.	Teaching children the principle behind why they are doing something gives them reason to do it. It expands learning in that it allows children to modify and change to an alternative method as long as the principle is fulfilled.
Emphasize what the child should do; mention, but do not emphasize what the child should not do.	Teaching from a positive standpoint makes learning more enjoyable. Because health care information should last a lifetime, thinking of it in a positive way makes it applicable to lifetime use. However, children need to know both the do's and don'ts regarding health issues.
Include evaluation as a final step.	The only way to determine the effectiveness of teaching is to test or evaluate if learning has occurred. Structure the time and method of evaluation when first establishing a teaching plan.

THE ART OF TEACHING

Teaching is more than presenting information; it is presenting information to increase someone's knowledge or insight. Before teaching can be considered effective, learning has to have occurred. Conversely, before learning occurs, teaching must have occurred in some form. Common principles of teaching are summarized in Table 34-1.

The Teacher–Learner Relationship

Effective teaching and learning depend a great deal on the teacher–learner relationship. An equal partnership encourages learning more readily than a relationship in which the teacher maintains ultimate control and authority. As a teacher, you can only influence an individual to learn; you cannot force learning. A teacher–learner relationship based on mutual sharing empowers and motivates an individual to learn. To foster mutual sharing in the learning process, first negotiate with the learner to establish learning needs and goals. Allow this negotiation to continue throughout the entire learning process as needs and goals change. Next, focus on the whole person by considering the learner's cognitive and developmental abilities, values, beliefs, feelings, experiences, and learning style. Finally, the teacher–learner relationship should be interactive (see Fig. 34-1). The teacher and learner should both actively participate in the process and modify the teaching plan as they learn from one another.

THE ART OF LEARNING

Learning is a two-step process involving both the acquisition of knowledge and a change in behavior based on the new knowledge. Learning has not really occurred unless the change in behavior is measurable. For example, a parent teaching a child about the need to brush teeth daily must not only elicit the child's statement that daily brushing is important but also watch that the child is, in fact, brushing her teeth every day. If the topic is abstract, such as helping a child change a concept about a chronic illness, change can still be measured (the child not only talks about the illness but also begins to take action to prevent complications). Principles of learning are summarized in Table 34-2.

Types of Learning

There are many types of learning. Learning the mathematical formula necessary to change pounds to kilograms, for example, is different from learning how to fill a syringe. Learning to be kind to a brother with a chronic illness is yet another type. Before teaching can begin, it is important to analyze the type of learning desired. This will help in setting goals and designing teaching strategies.

Cognitive Learning

Cognitive learning involves a change in the individual's level of understanding or knowledge. Learning the princi-

TABLE 34.2 Principles of Learning

PRINCIPLE	RATIONALE
Learning occurs best when child is ready to learn.	Interferences with learning may be physical (eg, pain or hunger) or psychological (eg, fear or anxiety). The first time a child is told that he or she must inject insulin daily, for example, the child may be too anxious to learn about it.
Learning occurs most quickly if a child can see how the new information will benefit him or her.	Sixteen-year-old children learn how to drive a car quickly because they grasp readily that being able to drive will immediately enlarge their world. Children are not ready to learn insulin injections until they can see an advantage of giving them. Make a habit of including the benefit of learning in the introduction of learning.
Learning occurs best if rewards, not penalties, are offered.	Notice the amount of shoulder patting and back slapping that high school coaches engage in (rewarding by praise). Giving positive reinforcement immediately like this makes it more effective than if such reinforcement is delayed. If you must criticize the way a task was done, first compliment children on some aspect they did well and then explain the part that needs improvement. This increases self-esteem and allows children to feel good enough about themselves so that they can accept the criticism. Never be reluctant to praise in public; always criticize in private.
Children learn best by actively participating in learning.	Active participation requires involvement in learning. Ask questions to involve participation; allow children to touch and handle equipment to increase participation.
Learning occurs best in a nonstressful and accepting environment.	No one wants to take a chance redemonstrating a procedure or asking a question if they believe that actions or opinions will not be respected. People do learn from "top sergeants," but the learning experience has so many unpleasant memories attached to it that they may not retain the learning. Health teaching is too important to be presented in a way that will lead to its being quickly discarded.
Children learn best those things that hold a particular interest for them.	Everyone is more interested in something than others. A child with diabetes mellitus who enjoys dancing might be most interested in learning regulation of insulin for exercise; a child anxious to leave for college might be most interested in selecting a diabetic diet from a cafeteria.
Learning ability plateaus.	Children learn to the point of saturation; learning and interest in learning halt at that point and do not continue until the material learned is thoroughly digested and understood. Wait until information is processed, and, at that point, the child will be interested once more.

ple behind why a particular medicine must be injected into a muscle, as opposed to subcutaneous tissue, is cognitive learning. Cognitive learning requires adequate development, intelligence, and attention span. It can be gained through exposure to any teaching technique but is usually learned through lecture, reading, and audiovisual aids. Techniques for teaching when cognitive learning is the goal must be based on the learner's cognitive ability. During the school-age years, learning capability is concrete (children have difficulty picturing body parts functioning unless they actually see them doing this); during the adolescent years, it becomes possible to learn abstract concepts and children can accept that liver enzymes are released with liver damage even though they never see that occur (Piaget, 1969).

Psychomotor Learning

Psychomotor learning requires a change in a person's ability to perform a skill. Learning to hold a syringe, draw up medicine, and inject it into muscle is an example of psychomotor learning. Acquiring psychomotor skills depends on muscle and neurologic coordination. It is mastered best through demonstration and redemonstration.

Affective Learning

Affective learning involves a change in a person's attitude. It is the most difficult area in which to bring about change. To successfully teach a child the reason for and the skill of giving a self-injection, for example, may be easy; teaching the child to *like* giving a self-injection may never be possible. The goal could be that the child will *value* the procedure because it will prevent him from developing hyperglycemia. Affective learning is gained best though role modeling, role playing, or shared-experience discussion.

✔ **CHECKPOINT QUESTIONS**

3. What change in health care has dramatically changed health teaching?
4. What are three types of learning?

Influence of Age and Stage on Ability to Learn

Learning ability varies a great deal depending on children's stage of development and the past experiences they have had in the specific area of learning (Osborne, 2001).

Infant

An infant learns by exploring the environment with his or her senses (psychomotor learning). An infant learns best from his or her primary caregiver because that is whom the infant most wants to please. Few health care points are taught at this age. Any that are taught must be presented not as a structured activity but as a game or an amusing or attractive activity for the child. A parent could teach an infant to exercise a leg by showing the child how to kick a balloon tied to a crib rail or rolling a ball and encouraging the child to move and creep after it, for example.

Toddler

Children during the toddler period are developing a sense of autonomy (ie, learning to be independent; Erikson, 1993). Trying to teach a 2 year-old child a new activity such as eating a new food or brushing his or her teeth may be met with a sharp "No!" as the child exerts this new independence. The retort does not mean that the activity is not appealing to the child, but merely that the child is aware that he does not have to do everything he is told. Toddlers also sometimes resist a change in routine because they need rituals to feel secure. If an activity will allow the child to increase a level of independent functioning, he or she will usually learn it rapidly. Teaching activities such as exercise or deep breathing by having a child imitate the action is an effective teaching method because it presents the activity as a game (so there is nothing to be resisted). Parents can be instrumental in maintaining a new skill the child has learned by incorporating it into a daily routine or a ritual.

Preschooler

Preschool children are interested in learning, because developing a sense of initiative is the main developmental task of the period. Provided that instructions are geared to their small vocabularies, they "soak up" new methods of doing things. Because they are so imaginative and uninhibited, they have few reservations about the "right" way to do things. They will experiment with trial-and-error methods. They will both watch eagerly and freely redemonstrate a skill. They ask many questions about equipment and procedures. Keep explanations short and words simple; a preschooler's attention span rarely exceeds 5 min (see Focus on Evidence-Based Practice).

Remember that, in terms of cognitive development, preschool children "center" or are able to learn only one characteristic of an object. This may limit their ability to learn all aspects of care or more than one method of doing something on any one day (Piaget, 1969).

Preschoolers tend to be frightened of intrusive procedures (eg, rectal temperature taking, bladder catheterization, or nasopharyngeal suction). They typically remove adhesive bandages minutes after application to check on the condition of the skin underneath (that it has not disappeared); they worry that any blood removed is the last they have. Teaching this type of procedure or explaining to the child why it is necessary calls for clear explanations and praise for learning. Use dolls or puppets to help the child visualize details whenever possible (Fig. 34-2).

Parents are often most aware what technique will best motivate their preschooler. Often, this begins with reading or telling a story about the problem.

School-Age Child

School-age children enjoy short projects that offer an immediate reward. Therefore, they learn best if a procedure is broken down into different stages and presented as sep-

FOCUS ON
EVIDENCE-BASED PRACTICE

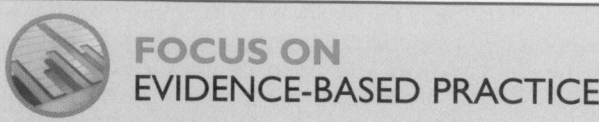

How Old Are Children Before You Could Expect Them to Learn Health or Safety Information?

To answer this question, 308 preschool children (133 boys and 175 girls), ranging in age from 28 to 80 months (2 to 6½ years) were asked to answer 50 questions about health or safety. Ninety-seven percent of the children older than age 3 years were able to complete the entire questionnaire. The children's mean score on the questionnaire was 37 (out of a possible 50). Results of the survey revealed that items related to safety were learned first by children followed by those related to hygiene, health promotion, and nutrition. The researchers concluded that preschoolers are ready and willing learners of health and safety information.

This is an interesting study for nurses because nurses are often the health care providers who teach safety and health information to preschoolers in childcare or nursery school settings or in the hospital when children are ill. Knowing that children this age are ready learners helps in planning these types of program.

Mobley, C. E., & Evashevski, J. (2000). Evaluating health and safety knowledge of preschoolers: Assessing their early start to being health smart. *Journal of Pediatric Health Care, 14*(4), 160–165.

arate short procedures rather than one long one. They enjoy games; playing "Simon Says" may be an effective way to have a child learn deep breathing, for example.

School-age children are used to learning things and accept learning a new procedure or new information as just another experience in a busy day. The "staying power" of school-age children is notoriously short, however; the ability to continue to perform at the level taught tends to decrease sharply if learning is not reinforced. Be certain that a backup person in the home knows the health care information as well as the child so the person can reinforce it or carry out a procedure of care if necessary.

Toward the end of the school-age period, children become interested in doing only those things that their friends are also doing. The child may interpret as unreasonable a request to do something after school (come home and take a medication) that is different from what all his or her friends are doing (e.g., stopping at the playground). Modify a teaching plan as necessary to help the child fit what he or she must learn into a school and social schedule, or else the teaching will be short-lived (Humphries, 2002).

As part of moral development, school-age children thrive on rules or the "right way" to do things (Kohlberg, 1984). Be certain that, if two or more people are going to be involved in teaching, they are consistent in their approach. It is frustrating for a school-age child not to have a "right way" to do something.

Parents who have been supervising their child's school learning through checking homework easily assume a role in supervising health learning also. Parents who haven't been monitoring learning previously may need support to fulfill this role.

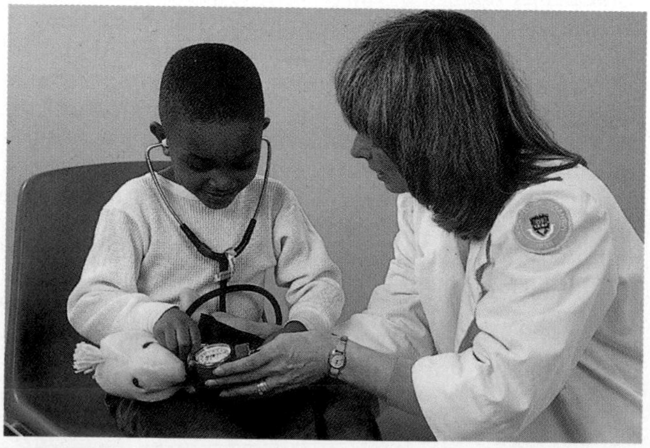

FIGURE 34.2 Teaching with dolls can help to make intrusive procedure seem less frightening for the preschooler.

Adolescent

Adolescents, struggling for identity, like to learn things separately from their parents. They can be responsible for their own self-care as a rule; if they understand how the new actions they have been taught will directly benefit them, unlike school-age children, they will continue to carry those actions out conscientiously. Adolescents have a strong need to be exactly like their friends, however; they rarely continue any action that makes them different or conspicuous in front of their friends. They focus best on things they can do rather than on things they cannot.

Remember that adolescents are present oriented; they learn procedures and new information best if they can see how it will immediately benefit them. They learn poorly if the only benefit of new information presented to them occurs at some future date. Rotating insulin injection sites, for example, prevents "pockmark" formations (*lipoatrophy*) in the skin when the person reaches approximately 30 years of age. Given this information, an adolescent tends not to rotate injection sites because the benefit is not relevant to him or her at the moment. An explanation such as "Rotating injection sites will ensure insulin absorption and allow you to play basketball this semester" (an equally true statement) is a better adolescent motivator.

For the first time, adolescents are able to think abstractly or use scientific reasoning. This means they can create hypotheses ("what if" questions) and think through what will be consequences from an action (Piaget, 1969). This allows them to understand the principle of what they are being taught and enforces the reason for the learning. Parents may find they are not as effective with teaching their child as they were when the child was younger. They may need to accept "stepping aside" until a phase of adolescent rebellion passes.

DEVELOPING AND IMPLEMENTING A TEACHING PLAN

A **teaching plan** is a design of the content to be taught and the teaching–learning techniques to be used. The first step in developing a teaching plan consists of assessing the child's current level of knowledge, ability, and motivation to learn new knowledge.

Areas of Assessment

Important areas for assessment include the child's current level of understanding; cognitive, physical, psychosocial aspects; and how the new knowledge will meld with the child's and family's lifestyle.

Language Level

Assessing language development includes assessing both the child's spoken vocabulary (how well the child speaks) and comprehensive vocabulary (how many words the child understands). Most children have a comprehensive vocabulary well above their speaking one or can understand words they do not use. Assess also "family vocabulary" or specific words the family uses. Be aware that, if English is not a child's primary language, comprehensive vocabulary may not be greater than spoken vocabulary in the second language. Additional pictures, drawings, or diagrams may be necessary to convey meaning.

Child's Current Knowledge

Assessing how much a child currently knows about the health area in question helps to establish the needs and goals of the teaching plan (Hall-Long, Schell & Corrigan, 2001). Current knowledge is, in part, developmentally based and, in part, experience based. Parents can tell you if a young child has had experience with the subject area. Some school-age children have had excellent anatomy and health classes as part of their science curriculum and are well aware of a topic. Other children may have lived with a family member with an illness and may already know what home care problems occur with that particular illness; on the other hand, what they know about the illness may be accompanied by so many misconceptions that they need a great deal of teaching to prevent being hampered by half-truths or unnecessary restraints. A helpful method of assessment, which promotes mutual sharing in the learning process, is asking children to list what they know about the health area on one side of a piece of paper and what they want to know more about on the opposite side. Young children can be asked to draw pictures of themselves, of someone with their illness, or of a good thing to do to keep well, to reveal this type of information.

Child's Intellectual Capability

Intellectual capability, in many instances, can be inferred from developmental milestones (eg, spoke in two-word sentences at 2 years) or from educational level (ie, attends the age-appropriate class in school). However, most children regress at least slightly with illness; what one would normally expect from a 10-year-old child may be impossible for an *ill* 10-year-old child. Children with chronic illnesses may not have met developmental milestones because of their lack of experiences, not because they do not have the cognitive ability to learn.

Child's Physical Capabilities

If a procedure that requires a certain level of psychomotor skill, such as medicine injection, will be necessary for care, assess children's physical ability to perform the procedure. If this is not present, the procedure will be frustrating because you are asking children to perform skills above their capabilities. Assess vision and hearing ability and right- or left-hand dominance as well; these are important considerations for determining not only whether children can accomplish procedures but also how the material will be presented.

Child's Psychological or Emotional Capabilities

To learn best, children need some motivation to learn or to appreciate how their life will be improved through learning this new skill. It may be difficult for a young child to grasp this concept. Some children are too ill, feel too exhausted, or have too much pain to be ready for learning until these factors can be alleviated. With early hospital discharge, a great deal of health education may be delayed until a child has returned home.

Children, like adults, may have difficulty learning about aspects of their care that they find distasteful. A child who uses food as comfort, for example, may have trouble learning about a restrictive diet because it conflicts with the way the child views food. A child with urinary or bowel disorders may have difficulty learning about these body parts if they view them as "dirty" or distasteful. School-age and adolescent children may have difficulty discussing and asking questions about a reproductive tract illness not only because they lack knowledge of the subject but also because they sense sexual functioning is not an "open" topic in their family.

Children with low self-esteem are less capable of learning self-care than others. For some children, it may be necessary to plan ways to increase self-esteem first before planning active teaching.

Child's Sociocultural Values

Different cultures have different values about what good health means. If a child from a family that values sports develops an illness that impairs her ability to run, for example, the family might consider the disability overwhelming. If the family believes that being able to write and read well are the cues to succeeding in life, the physical leg impairment might not be viewed as being that important. Study each family individually to determine which aspect of health will be most important to emphasize when teaching (see Focus on Cultural Competence).

An important aspect of culture is whether children are raised in an environment where they are urged to be

FOCUS ON CULTURAL COMPETENCE

Cultural differences between a teacher and a learner can complicate techniques and evaluation of the effectiveness of health teaching. Even when language is not a barrier, the way children show that they are listening or comprehending may vary from culture to culture. Looking directly at a speaker, for example, is considered disrespectful in many Asian countries. A traditional "OK" sign in Spain is interpreted as a vulgar one, not a positive one. In South Africa or some Middle Eastern countries, a "thumbs up" sign is insulting. In India, the way people shake their head to express yes and no can be opposite those used in the United States.

Being aware of these cultural differences is important when planning health teaching for diverse cultural groups so that neither teaching nor reactions to teaching are misinterpreted.

active participants in learning (allowed a lot of "hands-on" experimentation) or whether they are encouraged to be "watchers." Male/female roles also are culturally determined. This means a girl from a female-passive culture might not be enthusiastic about learning a self-care procedure because self-care is not expected of her. How long children are expected to be children (carefree, no responsibility) also varies culture to culture. In a family where children are expected to be out working and contributing to the family income by age 15, a child might have a very different attitude toward learning a self-care activity than the same-age child in a family where children are expected to remain noncontributing family members until after college (at least 21 years of age).

Child's Attention Span

The attention span of children and the capability to comprehend concepts and perform psychomotor skills differ a great deal depending on individuality and age. In general, the younger the child, the shorter the attention span (under school age, 5 min is all that can be expected). This means you must use more "attention-getting" teaching to hold attention. Think about the clever puppet shows or animation children are exposed to today. Teaching that is not accompanied by these attention-holding techniques needs to be very short to be effective.

Child's Lifestyle

Lifestyle refers to the common pattern of a child's life. For example, a child who attends school daily and returns home every day at 3:00 PM has a fairly consistent lifestyle. A busy adolescent who works, participates in several clubs, and socializes on the weekends may have a varied pattern of activity every day.

Knowing family patterns helps to plan the timing of such activities as medication administration or exercise or meal times. If both parents work during the day and do not return home until 6:00 PM, medication may have to be administered after this time; exercises may have to be supervised in the evening, not the morning. A family that goes camping every weekend will need to plan ways to carry out a health routine at remote camp sites.

Child's Learning Style

Some children learn well from oral descriptions. Others have to see a statement in print before they can fully comprehend it. Still others are visually oriented: if they see a picture or a diagram, they grasp the explanation almost immediately. These different learning styles vary from child to child. Few children are aware of their own learning style, so they are unable to explain what it is. After caring for them for a time, it becomes easier to detect the way children learn best. Tailor a teaching plan to a learning style for the most effective learning situation.

✔ CHECKPOINT QUESTIONS

5. What age group is concerned with "concrete" learning?
6. What factors may affect a child's emotional readiness to learn?
7. What is the typical attention span of a preschooler?

Formulating the Plan

Formulating a teaching plan begins with establishing expected outcomes and techniques of teaching. It may need to include communication strategies for parents as well as children (Scott et al., 2001).

Identifying Personal Strengths and Limitations

When formulating a teaching plan, be honest about your capabilities. If you feel uncomfortable teaching a child about surgery with clever puppets dressed in surgical scrub suits, it might be better to avoid this approach; in the wrong hands, such a method can sound so flat that the child is left feeling more frightened by the presentation than comforted. The use of humor can be effective in teaching health care. Consider whether this is a teaching strength for you. Attempting to use a teaching method that is uncomfortable can cause children to interpret apparent insecurity as evidence that there is something wrong with them, not with the method.

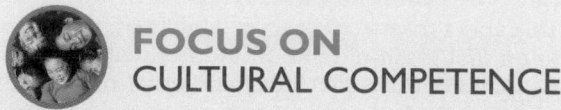

Some health teaching involves giving instructions in areas of care that may be personally embarrassing (instructing a member of the opposite sex how to obtain a clean-catch urine specimen, for example). Proceeding blindly may not result in effective teaching, because the child may be so embarrassed by your discomfort that he or she cannot concentrate on the instructions. In doing this type of teaching, nothing serves as well (as in any client contact) as honesty. Admit to the child or adolescent that you are not used to giving this type of instruction. This approach will probably evoke a response from the adolescent that he or she is not used to having anyone talk about it. Once you have found common ground (this is not the most comfortable discussion for either of you), there is a basis for effective health teaching. Honesty also allows a child to know that your discomfort is not from lack of knowledge on the subject (the child can trust what is being said) and not the child's fault (the subject, not the child, is the disturbing factor).

Preparing Expected Outcomes

Planning outcomes is most effective when they are planned collaboratively with the child and family. They should reflect the type of learning desired: cognitive, psychomotor, or affective. They should help to establish both content and time guidelines. They should be consistent with both the child's cognitive ability to learn and the time frame it will take to learn. It is unnecessary (and often overwhelming) for a child to learn everything about his or her illness in the first day or week after the diagnosis. Likewise, information on how to stay well does not need to be presented in one setting. In many instances, it is effective to teach only part of the information needed; another nurse in another setting such as an ambulatory clinic or in the child's home can teach the remainder. For best results, state outcomes as behavioral objectives or as the activity the child is expected to demonstrate when the child has learned the new knowledge—not "Tim understands the importance of deep breathing exercises daily" but "Tim does deep breathing exercises daily."

Identifying Teaching Formats

Teaching techniques vary with the content to be covered, teacher–learner characteristics and environment for teaching.

Formal Versus Informal Teaching. Both formal and informal teaching may be a part of health education. Careful assessment is necessary to determine which format would be the best technique for a given situation. An example of formal teaching would be conducting a class on healthy eating as part of a health education course. An example of informal teaching would be explaining to a child who refuses to eat that he needs to at least drink something because his body needs more fluids to get better. Sometimes informal teaching occurs so spontaneously that it is easy to be unaware of it. It may occur, for example, in response to a question such as "How long will I have to take this medicine?" If a nurse answers, "For 2 weeks," that is just answering a question. If the nurse says, "For 2 weeks because . . .," that is teaching.

Be careful not to equate informal teaching with disorganized, or unnecessary, teaching. It is just as important as formal teaching; it is just communicated in a less structured way. Informal teaching requires that teaching and learning principles (ie, know the subject, recognize individual learning styles, provide an effective environment, limit time span, and so forth) are followed, just as with more formal teaching. Table 34-3 lists ways to incorporate informal teaching into care.

Group Versus Individual Teaching. Although most health teaching is done on an individual basis, teaching

TABLE 34.3 Ways to Incorporate Informal Teaching Into Care

ACTIVITY	TYPE OF TEACHING
Medication administration	Children as young as early school age should know the type and action and any expected side effects of all medication they are taking. Present medicine not by saying, "Here is your pill" but "Here is your [name of medication], medicine to help your temperature come back to normal. After you take this, you might feel yourself start to sweat. That means it's working."
Vital sign measurement	When taking vital signs such as blood pressure, temperature, and pulse, tell children what normal levels are: "Your blood pressure is 100/70. That's normal." If the child is in a high-risk category for hypertension, add some prevention measures to teaching.
Any procedure	Always tell children the purpose and principle of procedures, not "You need to drink a lot of fluid," but "You need to drink a lot of fluid because . . ."
Dressing changes	Dressing changes provide an opportunity to teach the danger of introducing infection into an open wound. The parents or child may not change this dressing, but they will apply many adhesive bandages to small cuts and will benefit from teaching.
Mealtime	Provide information about nutrition: "I know you're not hungry enough to eat the entire sandwich, but could you try the meat? Meat is high in protein and that's important for healing."
Hygiene	Emphasize the necessity of good perineal hygiene to decrease the possibility of urinary tract infection.
Physical assessment	Explain aspects of self-breast or self-testicular examination and describe "normal" findings as both education and reassurance.
Positioning	Teach the hazards of immobility and how change of position and ambulation increase circulation and respiratory function.
Sleep	Teach that sleep is a healing therapy and should not be considered a waste of time.
Bowel elimination	Teach children that elimination patterns vary; occasional variations in their elimination patterns are normal.

groups of children is common in some situations. Individual instruction more directly addresses the child's unique needs; however, group teaching can meet individual needs while adding depth to learning as children discuss information within the group. For many children, hearing that they are not the only person with their problem is comforting. Hearing another child discuss how to solve a problem may be more meaningful than hearing the same information from an adult. Peer learning not only improves knowledge but may improve attitude and motivation to learn.

Consider the following important guidelines when group teaching:

1. Assess for common interests and goals in order for information to appeal to as many in the group as possible.
2. Be certain all members of a group can see and hear all others.
3. Encourage all members of the group to participate in discussions by calling on them if necessary.
4. Limit any one person from dominating the group by a statement such as "That's a good point, Reneé. Has anyone else had a similar experience?"
5. Avoid competition in the group. No one is always right; no one is always wrong.
6. Ask group members to evaluate the experience afterward to be sure it met the group's needs.

Home Versus Institutional Teaching. Health teaching is just as important in the home as it is in a health care agency, school, or community setting. Teaching in the health care agency may focus on immediate acute care concerns. Teaching in the school may focus on topics such as basic health promotion and hygiene, reproductive and sex education, and drug prevention. Teaching in the home may focus on medication regimens, dressing changes, or measures to prevent complications of a particular illness. It may also involve helping a child and parents adapt a procedure to the home setting, such as accommodating a wheelchair at home. Be certain that parents have obtained the necessary supplies for the procedure they need to learn for home teaching.

Teaching in the home offers the advantage of being able to assess the child's environment, interactions with other family members, and overall family functioning. This may yield data that prove useful to further planning and implementation of care. It may also provide an opportunity to include other family members—siblings, grandparents, and so forth—in the teaching plan, which will strengthen the impact of teaching and ensure that all family members understand procedures in the same way.

Always include evaluation as a step of teaching in all settings so you can feel confident that learning occurred.

WHAT IF? What if an adolescent needs to begin a lower calorie nutrition pattern? Would you need to teach the adolescent, the person who prepares the food, or the person who buys the food?

Determining Teaching Strategies

Because children's knowledge base, capabilities, learning styles, and attention spans vary, strategies of teaching are most effective when they are intermixed and when they are selected in response to the individual situation and child to be taught. The more interactive the method, the better (Hewitt et al., 2001).

Lecture. Lecture (or directly explaining information) is the most efficient and time-saving method of offering information to both individual children and to groups. A lecture, however, does not allow for participation, and it is effective only in short, well-structured time spans. It is rarely effective for children who are not yet school age.

Demonstration. **Demonstration** is actually performing a procedure such as a dressing change or instillation of eye drops so the child can see clearly how the procedure should be done. Do not demonstrate a procedure unless you have all the necessary equipment. If you stop in the middle of a demonstration to say, "Be sure to use a sterile syringe, not what I'm using," the poor technique demonstrated may be the lesson learned, not the good technique. The purpose of demonstration is to show how the procedure actually is done; having to imagine steps is little different from reading about it. School-age children, because of their stage of cognitive development (concrete operations), learn best by demonstration.

Redemonstration. To determine if a child has truly grasped a demonstration, ask the child to redemonstrate, or exactly imitate the procedure (Fig. 34-3). **Redemonstration** is best if it immediately follows demonstration. Praise the effort to redemonstrate even if the redemonstration is not of the quality desired. No one likes to be put on the spot, and children may be unwilling to expose themselves again by a second demonstration if criticized.

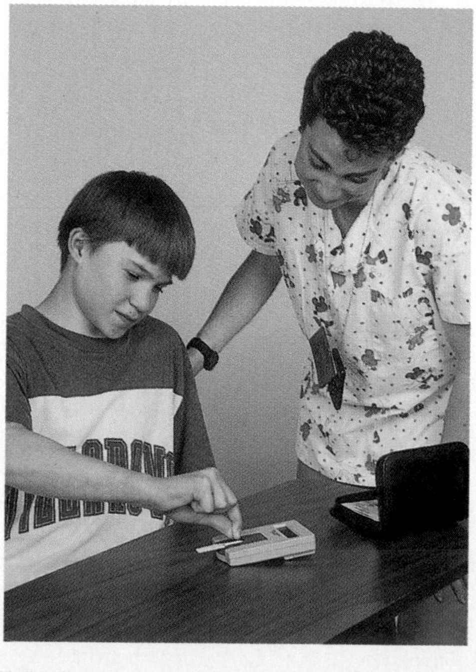

FIGURE 34.3 An adolescent redemonstrates blood glucose monitoring.

Be aware that there are many different ways to do almost everything. Children do not have to follow the motions exactly, as long as their technique accomplishes the same goal. An effective way to correct a wrong action is to say, "That's one way of doing that; most children, however, find it easier to. . . ." This type of criticism is nonthreatening because it acknowledges the child's effort in a positive way before offering a correction.

Discussion. Discussion is a shared learning experience in which children ask questions about particular concerns and these are answered based on their individual circumstances, or children are asked questions about some problem, such as how they anticipate managing some aspect of care, and together the problem is solved. At the beginning of health education, children tend to ask few questions because they do not know enough about an illness or health issue to anticipate concerns. As their knowledge increases, so does their ability to project and modify information to fit their own lifestyle. Remember that children tend to think in the present. A problem that will arise tomorrow is usually more important to a child than one that can be predicted to arise repeatedly in years to come. School-age and adolescent children enjoy discussion.

Role Modeling. Role modeling is demonstrating a certain attitude or behavior that you want the child to learn. Be certain when health teaching to not only present facts but also radiate a positive attitude. Showing frustration at getting a bubble out of medicine in a syringe demonstrates, for example, that giving injections is frustrating; a bored attitude toward nutrition instructions implies that nutrition information is boring. The child picks up the role modeling cues more readily than the spoken message. Role modeling is an important technique used to teach new parents newborn care; as they watch a nurse hold, comfort, and talk to their newborn, they quickly learn to model these behaviors.

Behavior Modification. Typically, learning occurs best with **positive reinforcement** (a child tries to understand a new procedure, is praised for the effort, and tries even harder). **Behavior modification** is a term used for a system aimed at *erasing* some form of behavior that interferes with health functioning. It was originally designed to help people who are cognitively challenged erase socially unacceptable behavior; currently, it has many uses, including such concerns as controlling disruptive classroom behavior. The basic premise of behavior modification is that the child is rewarded for healthful behavior, whereas unhealthful behavior is ignored or unrewarded. For example, a cognitively challenged child may have a socially unacceptable habit of constantly rocking back and forth. The child is not scolded or criticized for rocking, but the action is ignored. On the other hand, preferred behavior (sitting for 15 min without rocking) is praised. As another example, a child might be ignored while biting her fingernails, then praised for not biting them for an hour. Children respond best to behavior modification if, in addition to praise, they receive a tangible reward such as a star on a chart or an extra privilege of some sort for good behavior.

A behavior modification program must be discussed with the child before it is begun, because no behavior can be modified, just as no new behavior can be learned, until the child truly wants a change to occur. It might be necessary to ask older children to sign a learning contract to be certain that both teacher and learner agree on the method to be used. Many older children are able to use self-rewards to reinforce a behavior modification program (e.g., rewarding themselves with playing a video game or going to a movie for an afternoon of efficient studying or an hour of doing breathing exercises).

Behavior modification is a technique that must be used with common sense and concern so children are not being manipulated more than they are being helped to achieve a more healthful lifestyle. It is a legitimate device to use in helping a child with attention deficit hyperactivity disorder sit still long enough to eat a meal or learn in school. It can be helpful in encouraging children to do as much self-care as possible.

Some experts suggest that trying to modify beliefs or values by behavior modification is unethical and a reason that behavior modification is often criticized as a learning technique. However, some behavior changes also require a change in values to be effective and long-term. For example, a child's behavior of talking back to parents can be extinguished by ignoring or not responding to the behavior, and praising polite communication. At the same time, this method teaches the child to value improved communication and parental approval in order to meet his or her needs.

✔ CHECKPOINT QUESTIONS

8. Which is best—informal or formal teaching?
9. What are the benefits of peer learning?
10. Is it ethical to use behavior modification technique in an attempt to change values?

Selecting Teaching Tools

Teaching tools are the mechanical devices used to present content. They vary based on content, teacher–learner characteristics, and environment.

Visual Aids. "A picture is worth a thousand words" is not an idle quotation but a realistic one. Because small children know little about their bodies or where body organs are located, using visual aids such as drawings or photographs of anatomy can be very helpful. Figure 34-4 shows internal abdominal contents as an example of such a drawing. You could use such an illustration to show a preschooler how food moves through the body. Figure 34-5 is an example of a good tool to use while naming body parts. Pointing to a figure drawing and saying, "This is the part of your tummy the doctor will fix," is less threatening than actually pointing to the child's abdomen. Clarifying body parts this way is important, because young children may have no clear understanding of where a body part such as a hand ends and an arm begins.

Do not be afraid to draw a picture of a heart, a kidney, a bladder, or any other organ to make a point about anatomic structure. Children are more interested in understanding procedures or the reason for a health maintenance measure than criticizing your artwork (they likely do not

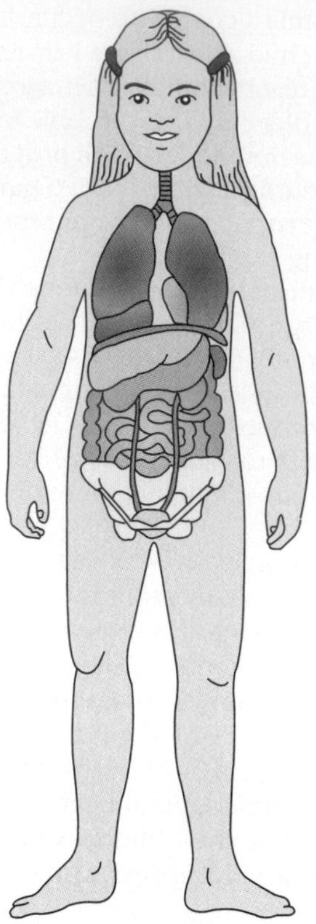

FIGURE 34.4 Anatomic drawings are helpful to illustrate basic health education topics as well as health care procedures.

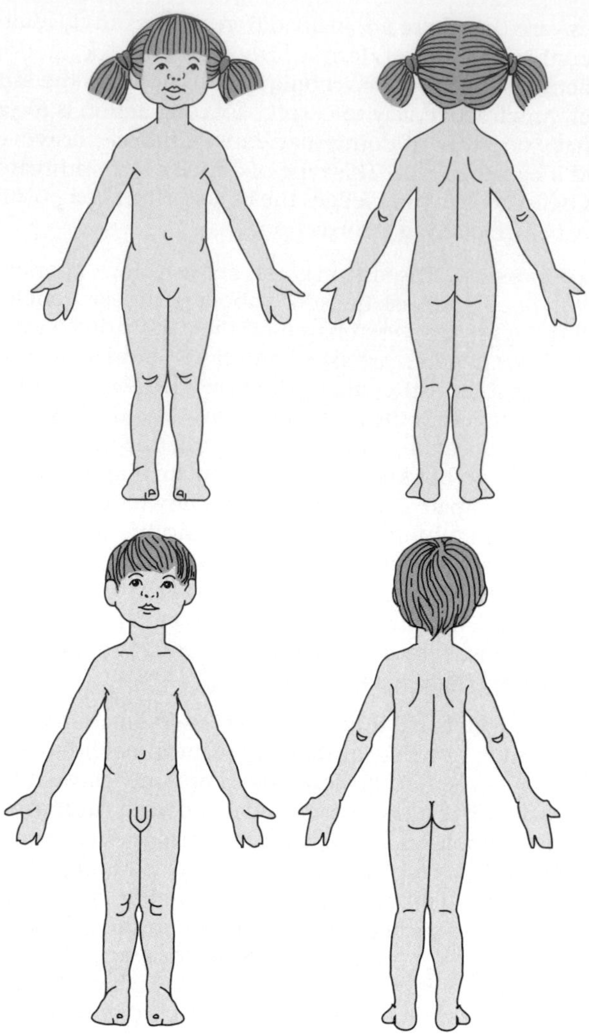

FIGURE 34.5 Simple line drawings such as these can be used to explain to a child exactly what part of his or her body will be "fixed" in surgery. For many children, having this pointed out on a drawing seems much less intrusive than having it pointed to on their own bodies.

know anatomy well enough to be able to tell if a drawing is distorted).

Pamphlets. *Pamphlets* are helpful teaching aids with school-age children and adolescents because they usually contain brief, easily understood information and are often cleverly illustrated with cartoon characters to make them enjoyable. Be certain to read any pamphlet before offering it to children to be certain that the information included in it is accurate. Medical advances are made so quickly that a 1-year-old pamphlet may contain a gross inaccuracy in the light of subsequent knowledge.

If a pamphlet has some statements in it that are inaccurate or that do not apply to the child, do not simply cross out the information that would be contradictory before offering it (most children deliberately read what they have been told not to); take the time to explain why it doesn't apply. Also, do not be misled into believing that because someone is given a clever pamphlet, they will necessarily read it and learn from it. Sit with a school-age child and read the pamphlet together; talk with an adolescent about the pamphlet's contents later to ensure it has been read.

Learning Games. For memorizing certain kinds of information, such as what foods are high or low in potassium or sodium, the use of flash cards is a helpful learning action. Many children enjoy playing trivia-type board games. Instead of the usual categories of information, make up new cards with a question such as "Where is insulin produced in your body?" If the child can answer the question correctly, he or she advances a designated number of spaces on the board. Children learn information quickly this way because the reward for learning is so immediate. Having parents play the game with their child educates the parents at the same time.

Word scrambles are easy games to develop. Crossword puzzles are fairly easy to design; one might be developed to address the activities that are important for a child to do after surgery.

Videotapes, Slides, and Films. Many health care agencies, homes, schools and community centers have videotape or DVD playback equipment or projectors that can be used to show a short tape or slide presentation as part of a health education program. Most households have VCRs or DVD players so tapes or disks can be sent home for families to view. As with pamphlets, view the material first before showing it; be certain to check that the vocabulary used is appropriate for an individual child or family.

Puppets and Dolls. Many children are shy about talking with strangers; this shyness, in addition to their con-

FOCUS ON COMMUNICATION

Bill is a 3-year-old boy scheduled for a syndactyly (webbed fingers) repair next week. You speak with him through a puppet at a clinic visit to assess his understanding of the surgery.

Less Effective Communication

Nurse: Hello. Could you tell me what the little boy named Bill is going to have done in surgery?
Bill: His fingers got sick when he was born.
Nurse: When is he having them fixed?
Bill: The day after we go to church.
Nurse: Will it hurt?
Bill: No. His fingers are going to sleep.
Nurse: Will he have a big bandage afterward?
Bill: So he can't see how his fingers got cut.
Nurse: Okay. Thank you for talking to me. I'll see you Monday.

More Effective Communication

Nurse: Hello. Could you tell me what the little boy named Bill is going to have done in surgery?
Bill: His fingers got sick when he was born.
Nurse: When is he having them fixed?
Bill: The day after we go to church.
Nurse: Will it hurt?
Bill: No. His fingers are going to sleep.
Nurse: Will he have a big bandage afterward?
Bill: So he can't see how his fingers got cut.
Nurse: What does that mean? Cut?
Bill: Cut so they're not there any more.
Nurse: Why do you think that's going to happen?
Bill: I think he's been bad.

The two scenarios above are good examples of what asking children about what they expect to happen in surgery can reveal. When asked what he means by cut, it becomes obvious that Bill needs additional teaching, probably using a drawing to illustrate what will be done. After surgery, when his fingers are covered by a pressure dressing so he can't see them, he will need additional reassurance that his fingers are still intact underneath.

cern about what will happen to them, may make it difficult for them to discuss or explain what they know about their health, illness, or intended surgery. However, they may be able to open up to an uncritical puppet or doll (see Focus on Communication). Preschool children are particularly receptive to puppets and dolls because they can believe the puppet or doll is actually talking to them.

Teaching preschool children about what to expect from a hospital experience is often taught by using a series of puppets to represent different hospital personnel such as a surgeon, a nurse, and a nurse's assistant. Children can practice giving the doll "shots" or submitting it to the procedures that they will experience (see Chapter 35 for a discussion of therapeutic play). It's best if the doll is made of rubber or cloth so the child can easily manipulate it.

Mass Media. Television and radio are examples of effective mass media that reach many children on topics about self-help or self-care health. Consulting on the topics to present or helping develop material used in health messages can be an important role for nurses. Messages originated for these media must be attention-getting and brief to compete with the programs and commercial messages that precede or follow them.

Computers. Many children learn to solve problems by computers as early as preschool through exposure to computers at home or child care. Using a computer application to answer questions about an illness is effective because this type of activity can be both entertaining and informative for children.

Health Fairs. **Health fairs** are displays presenting health-related information to large numbers of people. They are effective with children if they encourage active participation through easily visualized displays or playing computer games.

Preparing Teaching Supplies

To avoid having to reorganize equipment or instructions each time a procedure is taught, put together a basket or box of supplies that contains all the information and equipment needed to teach a particular task. This helps ensure that teaching is organized and is economical in that everyone on a hospital unit is not opening new equipment for demonstrations. It also helps to ensure that everyone is teaching the same information. Nothing is more confusing to anyone learning a new skill than to be taught two different principles for doing it or two different techniques.

Implementing the Plan

Health teaching can begin immediately and flow easily if goals have been developed well and strategies for teaching have been designed carefully.

Resource People

Many health care agencies, including home care agencies, have specific people who are available for health teaching about specific subjects (e.g., diabetes, stomal care, or respiratory exercises in the hospital or home setting; drug prevention in a community setting). Using such people is helpful because they know all the "tricks of the trade" for teaching that particular subject.

Some children do not learn well from such designated teachers because they see them infrequently, whereas they see their primary nurse daily. Some parents react badly to the thought that it takes an expert to tell them about the care needed (if care is so complicated, how can they possibly learn it?). Health teaching is a part of nursing care, and it is unfair to parents to be told that their questions cannot be answered until the following day when the appropriate person is available to answer them. Coordinating teaching with other health care professionals or specialists helps ensure it will be consistent (see Focus on Multidisciplinary Care).

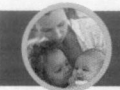

FOCUS ON MULTIDISCIPLINARY CARE

Children who are hospitalized or receiving health care at home can interact with, and receive health instructions from a multitude of health care providers. Based on different aspects of care, these different health care providers can offer conflicting health advice. Nurses can serve as coordinators to be certain that information offered is consistent or gaps in teaching do not occur.

Unlicensed assistive personnel can be assigned to review hospital admission or surgery preparation procedures for children and their parents in ambulatory clinics. They can review home care instructions for children with long-term illness at clinic visits to be certain that children are continuing to practice respiratory exercises or follow a special diet. Be certain to review with them the information they need to cover so you can be assured their information is accurate. Be sure they include some type of evaluation measures in teaching so you (and they) can be certain that learning occurred.

Parent Education

With very young children, parents as well as children need teaching. It is good practice with all children to be certain that at least one adult in the household has the necessary information or can perform the required skill as well as the child. Let the child choose this person. The individual who everyone assumes is a child's chief support person may not be the person the child perceives as the most reliable choice and, therefore, not the one the child wants as a health care backup. This person, when identified, needs as much information as the child does about why the health measure is important.

WHAT IF? What if a preschooler refuses to tell you whether she has pain because you are a "stranger" and she doesn't talk to strangers? What would you do?

Evaluating the Effectiveness of Teaching

Evaluation, or assessing whether teaching has been effective, is the final step in teaching. Evaluation occurs not only after the teaching plan has been implemented but throughout the entire learning process. This ongoing evaluation helps the teacher and learner modify the teaching plan to better meet the changing needs of the child.

There is some advantage in asking children questions before and after teaching to prove that teaching was effective and the child has safely learned a new health care measure. Demonstration of a change of behavior or attitude, however, is the real proof that learning has occurred.

HEALTH TEACHING FOR THE SURGICAL EXPERIENCE

Teaching to prepare a child for surgery is an example of teaching that requires planning for several stages of learn-

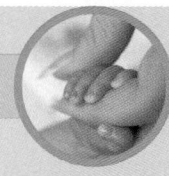

FOCUS ON *Nursing Care Planning*

A PRESCHOOLER UNDERGOING SURGERY

Kim, a preschooler, is admitted to your unit for 1-day surgery.

Assessment: Kim is a 3-year-old girl admitted to the hospital for revision of scar tissue on her right hand from a burn she accidentally received as an infant. She can't fully open her right hand or hold a crayon securely because of a scar contraction. She is frightened of surgery despite preparation by her parents for the experience. When nervous or frightened, she has a habit of biting the scar tissue on her hand; she has done this constantly since admission.

Nursing Diagnosis: Deficient knowledge related to what to expect in surgery

Teaching Points: Child is shy with strangers; mother states that she learns best by "hands on" experiences; "cocks head" when puzzled. Also learns best from her mother rather than her father (father tends to be authoritarian).

Cognitive Learning to be Taught: Why surgery is necessary.
Psychomotor Skills to be Taught: To keep hand in elevated position after surgery.
Affective Aspects to be Taught: Accepts surgery as a positive experience.

Outcome Identification: Child will voice that she feels prepared for surgery.

Outcome Evaluation: Child voices expected outcomes of surgery. Demonstrates a minimum of nervous behaviors such as biting hand, can play "Simon Says" and describe how pain will be relieved by "special button" (patient-controlled analgesia).

(continued)

Interventions	Rationale
1. Assess Kim's and parents' knowledge of surgery.	1. Establish a baseline so teaching is not repeated or gaps are left unmet.
2. Assess Kim's cognitive level.	2. Understanding the child's ability to learn helps you devise a teaching plan that will best meet child's needs.
3. Using puppets, teach that hand must be washed for surgery and that Kim will be NPO, will ride in cart, will have intravenous line, and will have patient-controlled analgesia after surgery, and so forth.	3. Puppets provide an excellent prop for teaching children Kim's age.
4. Introduce dressing and the way hand will be suspended postoperatively by letting Kim dress and suspend doll's hand.	4. Therapeutic play provides an excellent medium for teaching and learning with toddlers and preschoolers.
5. Introduce postoperative hand exercises she will need to do by playing, "Simon Says."	5. Games are another appealing way to keep the preschooler interested and motivated.
6. Introduce the fact that Kim will have pain after surgery but that it can be relieved by a "special button" on her intravenous line.	6. Preparing a child for postoperative procedures and how pain will be relieved before surgery (when the child still feels well) can help reduce the amount of learning the child needs to accomplish after surgery, when she doesn't feel well.
7. Ask mother to reinforce preparation.	7. Kim learns best from mother; mother's reinforcement could help Kim go into the operation viewing it as a helping experience, not because Kim has to.

ing (see Focus on Nursing Care Planning). The child and the child's parents often feel anxious about the surgery and its results, so teaching must first address this anxiety. Do not downplay the family's fears but allow the child and family caregivers an opportunity to express their concerns as part of the teaching–learning process.

Assessing Current Level of Knowledge

Many children's surgeries are done on an ambulatory or 1-day basis. Before admission, discuss with parents the preparation they have made for this experience and what specifically they have told the child about what will happen. It is good to ask also whether the child's concerns about the experience seem more or less than parents had anticipated. Ask if there has been an unpleasant surgery or hospitalization in the family that the child might have heard discussed. Has the child seen anything recently on a medical show on television that might have been upsetting? Using puppets, dolls, or a play telephone is a helpful way to assess younger children's level of knowledge.

Formulating and Implementing the Plan

It is best to prepare a child for surgery or hospitalization in stages because it is difficult for a child to absorb everything at once. However, contact before surgery may be limited to only one office or clinic visit, so time constraints can force information to be more compacted.

Be certain to discuss preparations for surgery such as coming for blood work and not eating the morning of surgery. If the child will have general anesthesia, it is important to emphasize that anesthetized sleep is "special" sleep. Otherwise, toddlers or preschoolers may be reluctant to fall asleep after surgery for fear that people will come and do strange things to them. Do not say a child will be "put to sleep." Dogs and cats that are put to sleep are not seen again. To help prepare younger children for surgery, a doll could be used: its abdomen washed, an injection given to make it sleepy, and a hospital gown put on. It could be carried to a cart made from a cardboard box. After saying goodbye to its parents, the doll could be wheeled to surgery by a puppet nurse.

The surgery procedure should be discussed but minimized in play. "After you're sleeping, the doctor will fix your tummy. You won't feel anything the doctor is doing because of the special sleep. When you wake up, you'll be in a room called a recovery room where you'll stay until you're wide awake." Be honest concerning pain: "Your tummy will feel sore afterward, but I'll give you something to make it feel better" is a fair statement.

It is important for children to be alerted that nurses and doctors in surgery and perhaps the x-ray department dress differently from those they are used to seeing. Stress particularly that nurses and doctors in surgery wear surgical masks. Assure toddlers and preschoolers that the persons behind the masks are doctors and nurses, some of whom the child has probably already met.

It is good to mention recovery rooms, because this may be an area that parents neglected to mention. In fact, parents may not be aware that, in some institutions, they will not be allowed in the recovery room and may have promised the child, "When you wake up, I will be there." Clarify the parents' misconceptions about recovery rooms, and reiterate that children will get to see their parents back in their own room once they are fully awake. This makes the parents' preparation correct and saves the child from feeling deceived.

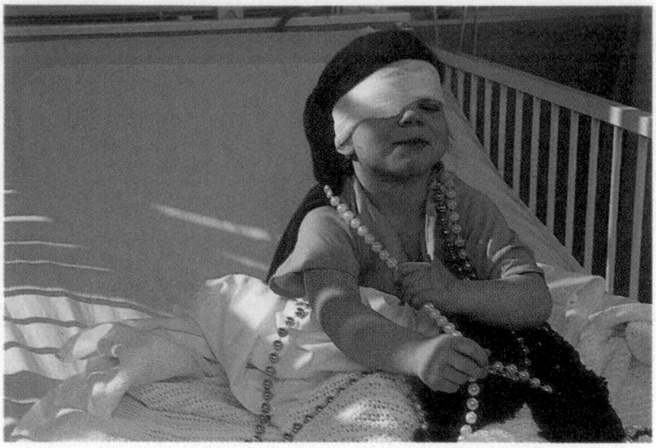

FIGURE 34.6 Pretending to be a pirate helps this young child prepare for having to wear an eye patch after surgery.

Explain postsurgery items, such as the use of oxygen, monitors, bedpans, bandages, or intravenous equipment. Playing a game or furnishing a doll with such equipment is especially helpful in preparing younger children (Fig. 34-6). This prevents preschoolers from feeling overwhelmed by being taken to an intensive care unit and shown actual monitors and respirators. After surgery, be certain to evaluate whether a child's preparation was adequate, both to document that the experience was as trauma free as it could be and to gain expertise in teaching children.

✔ CHECKPOINT QUESTIONS

11. Is playing board games a good teaching strategy for school-age children?
12. Do children listen to mass media messages on television?

KEY POINTS

Communication is the exchange of ideas between two or more persons. It can be verbal or nonverbal.

Therapeutic communication is a planned interaction, has structure, and is constructive. Nontherapeutic communication lacks deliberate purpose other than socializing.

Successful communication requires an encoder, a code, a decoder, and feedback or response.

Levels of communication range from (1) cliché, (2) fact reporting, (3) shared ideas, (4) shared feelings, and (5) a sense of knowing what another wants without it needing to be voiced.

Typical methods of nonverbal communication are: using distance, gestures, body posture and gait, touch, use of drawings, and empathy.

Techniques that encourage therapeutic communication are: attentive listening, open-ended questions, reflecting, clarifying, paraphrasing, perception checking, focusing supportive statements, and silence.

Some situations require special communication techniques such as interacting with demanding or shy children, children who are visually or hearing challenged, or children who speak another language.

Children's cognitive development must be evaluated to ensure that material being presented can be easily comprehended. Preschoolers, for example, are egocentric so are only able to see situations from their standpoint, not others'. School-age children are concrete thinkers. They learn best what they can see and touch and handle. Adolescents can grasp abstract concepts.

Establishing a teacher–learner relationship based on mutual input and setting expected outcomes is an effective way to meet the unique needs and goals of the child and family.

There are three types of learning: cognitive, psychomotor, and affective. For something to be learned well, all of these areas must be involved.

To individualize a teaching program for a child, assess the child's attention span, cognitive or intellectual capability, lifestyle, learning style, and your own teaching strengths and limitations.

In many instances, there is a great deal of material that a child must learn about an illness. If taught all at once, however, this could be overwhelming. If possible, divide material into lessons that must be taught immediately and lessons that can be taught at spaced return health visits.

The format and strategies of teaching used with children vary depending on the child's age and developmental level. Various types to consider are: formal versus informal, single or group teaching, lecture, discussion, and role playing.

Behavior modification is a special technique aimed at erasing some form of behavior that interferes with good health.

Remember that children are present oriented. They learn information that they can see will immediately benefit them more easily than information that has future benefits.

Children are learning many other things besides health information every day. This may make the retention of information not as great as you would like. You may need to schedule frequent reviews and updates to keep information current.

CRITICAL THINKING EXERCISES

1. Bill is the preschooler you met at the beginning of the chapter. He will be having surgery in a week for bilateral syndactyly (webbed fingers). His mother asks you how to prepare him for this. What suggestions would you make? The child will be left with a noticeable scar and some lack of function after surgery, so he cannot be reassured that everything will be all right. How will this affect your teaching?
2. What if a 12-year-old child with lactose intolerance tells you, "Don't tell me anything about foods I can't eat. I've heard it all." You say, "Heard it all?" She says, "Don't repeat what I said. That really bugs me." You know that she needs to learn more about not eating milk products so she can eat safely at school. What would you do?
3. A 10-year-old child with asthma has to learn how to monitor his medication needs by using a peak flow meter at least once daily. How would you teach this skill? Suppose he states that he has no intention of learning how to read the meter because his mother can do it for him. Would your teaching plan be different?
4. An adolescent who has familial hypercholesterolemia is prescribed a low-cholesterol diet. What teaching techniques would be especially effective in introducing a new nutrition pattern to him? His mother has to learn this, too. Would you teach her any differently?
5. Examine the National Health Goals related to health education and children. Most government-sponsored money for nursing research is allotted based on these goals. What would be a possible research topic to explore pertinent to these goals that would both be fundable and would advance evidence-based practice?

REFERENCES

Department of Health and Human Services. (2000). *Healthy people 2010.* Washington, DC: DHHS.

Erikson, E. H. (1993). *Childhood and society.* New York: W.W. Norton.

Hall-Long, B. A., Schell, K., & Corrigan, V. (2001). Youth safety education and injury prevention program. *Pediatric Nursing, 27*(2), 141–148.

Hewitt, M., et al. (2001). Evaluation of 'Sun-safe': A health education resource for primary schools. *Health Education Research, 16*(5), 623–633.

Humphries, J. (2002). The school health nurse and health education in the classroom. *Nursing standard, 16*(17), 42–45.

Kaiser, A. P., et al. (2001). Supporting communication in young children with developmental disabilities. *Mental Retardation & Developmental Disabilities Research Reviews, 7*(2), 143–150.

Kiehl, E. M., & Wink, D. M. (2000). Nursing students as change agents and problem solvers in the community: Community-based nursing education in practice. *Nursing & Health Care Perspectives, 21*(6), 293–297.

Kohlberg, L. (1984). *The psychology of moral development.* New York: Harper & Row.

Mobley, C. E., & Evashevski, J. (2000). Evaluating health and safety knowledge of preschoolers: Assessing their early start to being health smart. *Journal of Pediatric Health Care, 14*(4), 160–165.

Osborne, H. (2001). In other words . . . start where they are: Communicating with children and their families about health and illness. *On-Call, 4*(3), 46–47.

Piaget, J. (1969). *The origins of intelligence in children.* New York: International Universities Press.

Scott, J. T., et al. (2001). Communicating with children and adolescents about their cancer. *Cochrane Database System Review, 1,* CD002969.

SUGGESTED READINGS

Betz, C. L. (2000). The continual challenge of empowering children and families. *Journal of Pediatric Nursing: Nursing Care of Children & Families, 15*(2), 61–62.

Blackwell, P. B. & Baker, B. M. (2002). Estimating communication competence of infants and toddlers. *Journal of Pediatric Health Care, 16*(1), 19–35.

Boyd, J. R. (2001). A process for delivering bad news: Supporting families when a child is diagnosed. *Journal of Neuroscience Nursing, 33*(1), 14–20.

Ely, B. (2001). Pediatric nurses' pain management practice: Barriers to change. *Pediatric Nursing, 27*(4), 473–480.

Evans, D., et al. (2001). Can children teach their parents about asthma? *Health Education & Behavior, 28*(4), 500–511.

Gresham, L. S., et al. (2001). Partnering for injury prevention: Evaluation of a curriculum-based intervention program among elementary school children. *Journal of Pediatric Nursing: Nursing Care of Children & Families, 16*(2), 79–84.

Lassman, J. (2001). Pedestrian safety: Teaching points and resources for ED nurses educating the community. *Journal of Emergency Nursing, 27*(4), 360–363.

McCaffery, M., & Pasero, C. L. (1999). How can we improve the way we perform our pain assessments to meet the needs of patients from diverse cultures? *American Journal of Nursing, 99*(8), 18–22.

Simons, J., Franck, L., & Roberson, E. (2001). Parent involvement in children's pain care: Views of parents and nurses. *Journal of Advanced Nursing, 36*(4), 591–599.

Sydnor-Greenberg, N., & Dokken, D. L. (2001). Communication in healthcare: Thoughts on the child's perspective. *Journal of Child & Family Nursing, 4*(3), 225–230.

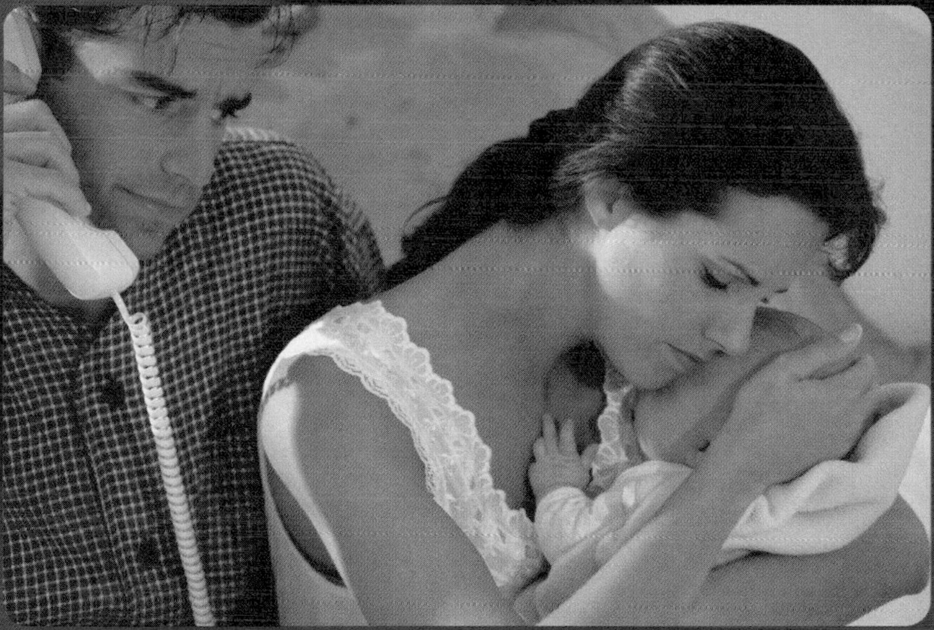

The Nursing Role in Supporting the Health of Ill Children and Their Families

UNIT VII

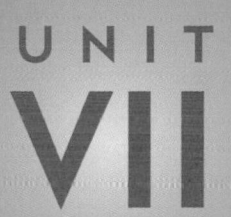

Nursing Care of the Ill Child and Family

35

CHAPTER

Key Terms

- calorie counting
- case management nursing
- direct care
- home care
- hospice care
- indirect care
- nonrapid eye movement (NREM) sleep
- play therapy
- primary nursing
- rapid eye movement (REM) sleep
- sensory deprivation
- sensory overload
- skilled home care
- sleep deprivation
- therapeutic play

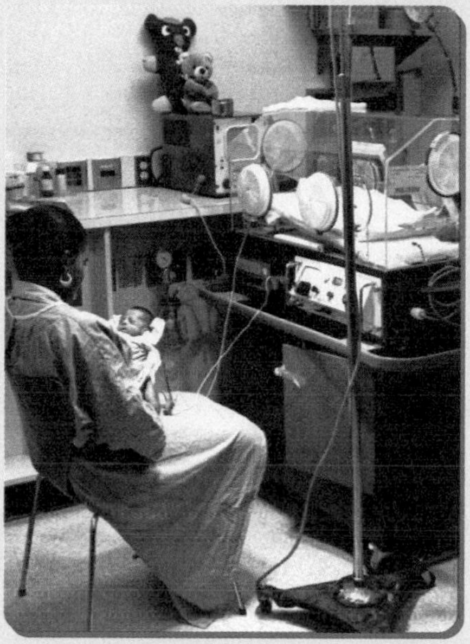

Objectives

After mastering the contents of this chapter, you should be able to:

1. Describe the meaning of illness and home care, ambulatory, and in-hospital experiences to children.
2. Assess the impact of an illness, especially one requiring a hospital stay, on a child.
3. Formulate nursing diagnoses related to the stress of illness in children.
4. Establish expected outcomes for the ill child.
5. Plan nursing care to reduce the stress of illness, such as helping parents plan for hospitalization or home care.
6. Implement measures such as orientation, education, and therapeutic play to reduce the stress of illness.
7. Evaluate outcomes for achievement and effectiveness of care for the ill child.
8. Identify National Health Goals related to hospitalization or health care that nurses can be instrumental in helping the nation to achieve.
9. Identify areas related to illness in children that could benefit from additional nursing research or application of evidence-based practice.
10. Use critical thinking to analyze ways in which illness care can be made more family-centered and less traumatic for children.
11. Integrate knowledge about the child's response to illness with the nursing process to achieve quality maternal and child health nursing care.

Becky is a 7-year-old who burned her foot in a campfire accident. She is going to be admitted to the hospital for 1-day surgery to have the wound debrided. Becky's parents tell you that Becky "hasn't been herself" since the injury. She has reverted to temper tantrums and sulking, more like a 4-year-old than one of early school age. Even though she has been told that eating meat is important because it provides protein for healing, she refuses to eat anything but Jello or soup. In the admission suite of the hospital, she picked up a doll and twisted its leg off. "What can I do with her?" her mother asks you. "How can we get our old daughter back again?"

Becky is obviously showing some effects of her accident. What type of additional explanation might be helpful to her? What advice would you give her mother to help her better prepare Becky for the upcoming debridement procedure?

Previous chapters described the normal growth and development of children and their special needs at each stage of development. This chapter adds information about the additional needs of children when they become ill. This is important information because it builds a base for nursing care and health teaching.

After you've studied the chapter, answer the Critical Thinking Exercises at the end of the chapter and then access the on-line study activities (http://connection.lww.com) *to further sharpen your skills and test your knowledge.*

FOCUS ON NATIONAL HEALTH GOALS

Illness can be a major stress to children and thus a major threat to mental health. Two National Health Goals address the mental health of children:

- Increase the proportion of children with mental health problems who receive treatment.
- Increase the number of states and territories that have an operational mental health plan that addresses cultural competence (DHHS, 2000).

Helping with assessment of children's stress level and reducing the stress of hospitalization or health care are ways that nurses can help the nation achieve these goals. Areas where additional nursing research or evidence-based practice could aid understanding are: What measures do parents want taken to be able to feel most comfortable in a hospital setting; what are the deterrents to therapeutic play on hospital units and how could these be removed; and are there additional contributions nurses could make to shorten hospital stays for children?

Illnesses that require the attention of health care professionals are outside the usual occurrences of childhood, so most children typically have little knowledge about them. Helping a child and family prepare for or adjust to such an experience is a fundamental nursing role. This role goes well beyond providing information on what to expect throughout an illness. National Health Goals related to children and illness are shown in the Focus on National Health Goals box.

Nurses can work to provide orientation programs before hospital admissions and advocate for more open parental visiting and overnight stay policies whenever these are not already in effect. In addition, nurses can help families provide a therapeutic environment for care of the ill child in the home. For individual families, nurses can perform a number of interventions that promote comfort, safety, security, and continued growth and development. Play is one of the more powerful tools available to a nurse working toward this objective.

NURSING PROCESS OVERVIEW

For the Ill Child

When children become ill, many of their needs, such as those for nutrition, play, and family support, change. If a child will need long-term home care or hospitalization, the entire family will find their priorities needs changing. Unless these changing needs are examined, recognized, and met, a child may achieve physical wellness again but not mental or emotional health. The family may be left severely incapacitated. Identifying additional needs this way and putting in place necessary services or interventions is an important nursing role.

Assessment

Assessment for the ill child begins with an interview of the child and parents to identify ways they think the illness will change their lives. This could include a wide range of situations such as increased expenses, changes in schedules to visit or stay with a hospitalized child, the need for one parent to take a leave from work to care for an ill child at home, the need to schedule frequent ambulatory visits, consultation to handle body image changes, and the need to arrange for child care for other children. Because these needs change as the course of an illness changes, assessment must be ongoing (see Assessing the Child for Effects of Illness).

Nursing Diagnosis

Nursing diagnoses vary greatly depending on the extent of a child's illness, the care needed, and the age of the child. Those often used with families of children seen in ambulatory settings include:

- Health-seeking behaviors related to lack of knowledge regarding illness
- Anxiety related to pending hospital admission
- Risk for social isolation related to planned hospitalization

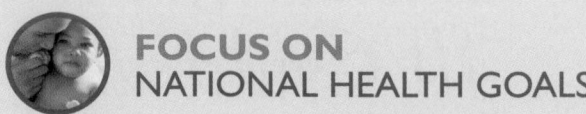

Nursing diagnoses established for children in the home are the same as those that would be established with the same findings in a health care facility. Often, however, because of the increased participation of the family necessary for home care, nursing diag-

ASSESSING the Child for Effects of Illness

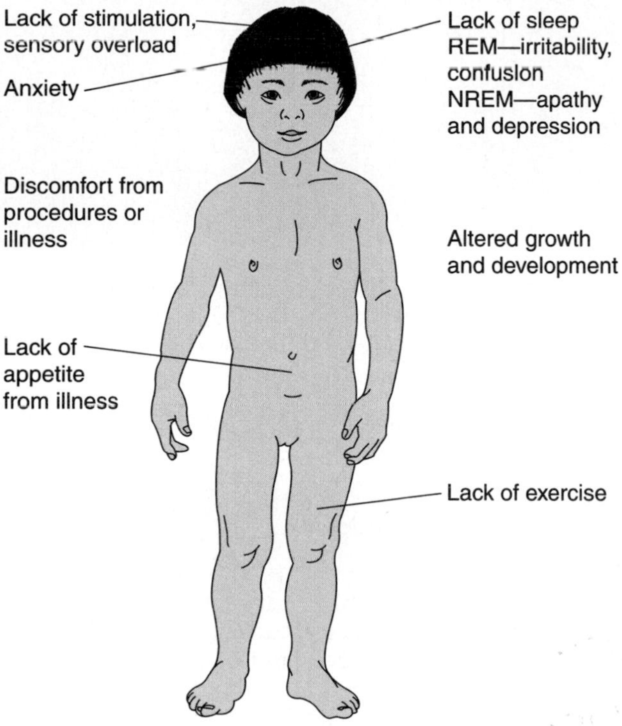

noses are more family-oriented. Home care can place a heavy burden on the family. The stress of being responsible for an ill child's daily health status can have a negative impact on a parent's self-esteem or a couple's marital relationship, or it can prevent parents from spending time with their other children. Examples of possible nursing diagnoses include:

- Readiness for enhanced family coping related to increased time together because of home care
- Health-seeking behaviors related to skills needed to continue home care
- Risk for delayed growth and development related to lack of usual childhood activities
- Interrupted family processes related to dependence of ill child
- Disabled family coping related to changes in family routine brought about by home care needs of ill child

Outcome Identification and Planning

Planning for the care of an ill child requires consideration of all aspects of a child's and family's life: financial, social, and personal.

Implementation

Five hazards that may occur with all illnesses include (1) experiencing harm or injury, such as physical discomfort, pain, mutilation, and death; (2) being separated from routines, parents, peers, and respected adults; (3) facing the unknown (new and strange sights and sounds and happenings); (4) facing uncertain limits (unclear definition of acceptable and expected behavior); and (5) experiencing a loss of control (loss of competence or loss of the ability to make decisions).

Awareness of these potential problems is important to guard against those that are preventable and to reduce the child's anxiety associated with those that cannot be prevented (such as facing new sights and sounds). Discussing these hazards with older children is important so that implementations to reduce their impact can be tailored to each individual child. Reading to the child, role playing, and puppetry are all useful techniques for easing the younger child's experience. Be certain that the techniques used are appropriate not only to the child's age but also to his or her individual learning style.

Nursing interventions for home care often involve teaching family members how to give care. This may include encouraging members to voice the frustration they feel at being constantly confined at home or what they perceive to be a lack of progress in their child's condition. If the child has a terminal illness, parents need support to express their grief. They can also grow discouraged because the work they are accomplishing is making the child comfortable but not preventing death.

Outcome Evaluation

Evaluation of outcomes for ill children should include specific measures such as whether discomfort was kept to a minimum during the experience. Indicators to evaluate outcomes that are long term should include whether the child was able to return to his or her usual behavior after the experience. The following are examples suggesting achievement of outcomes regarding a hospital experience:

- Parents state that their level of anxiety regarding hospitalization of their infant is now at a tolerable level.
- Parents have effectively changed work schedules to be able to stay with the child in the hospital.
- Social isolation of toddler is minimized through case manager nursing assignment.

Because a home setting is less structured than a health care facility setting, evaluation will show that some goals for care are more difficult to accomplish in the home; for the same reason, because there is more room for innovation at home, some goals will be more easily accomplished. Examples suggesting achievement of outcomes in the home setting might include:

- Parents state that they have been able to make adjustments to accommodate care of ill child at home.
- Child states he or she enjoys respite care in hospice setting one weekend a month.

- Parents state they are actively trying to supply adequate growth experiences for siblings in light of home care of oldest child.

THE MEANING OF ILLNESS TO CHILDREN

The response of children to illness depends on their cognitive development, past experiences, and level of knowledge. From early school age, children generally know quite a bit about the workings of their major body parts. As general guidelines, early grade-school children are usually able to name the function of the heart, lungs, and stomach. They may not be able to do that for the kidneys or bladder. This lack of information may reflect the difficulty some parents have in discussing elimination with their children.

Younger children may think the cause of illness is magical (no one knows where it comes from) or that it occurs as a consequence of breaking a rule (e.g., walking in the rain or eating candy after school). With this perspective, they can think that getting well again is possible only if they follow another set of rules, such as staying in bed and taking medicine. By fourth grade, children are generally aware of the role that germs play in illness but may be fooled by thinking that all illness is caused by germs. Because of this, they may see a passive role for themselves in getting well, because illness comes from outside influences. At about eighth grade, children are able to voice an understanding that illness can occur from several causes, such as being susceptible to chickenpox because they did not get the vaccine and played with a child who had chickenpox. Once they accept this, they can take an active role in getting better. These concepts parallel cognitive development (see Chap. 27).

Knowing how children of each age view illness affects the planning of nursing care, influencing how explanations should be worded. For example, saying that you are going to "stick" the child for blood work could be interpreted by a young child as meaning that you are actually going to put a stick in him or her. Saying that the child will receive a dye for a test can be interpreted as the child will "die" during the procedure. Children who think illness comes as punishment for breaking rules can interpret nursing procedures (e.g., taking a rectal temperature or giving an injection) as punishment. They can be confused about explanations of procedures because some words sound alike or have double meanings (e.g., "drawing" as in making a picture vs. drawing blood). Because of these distorted perceptions, explanations of procedures do not always relieve children's stress.

Differences in Responses of Children and Adults to Illness

Keeping in mind that children are not just small adults is important when evaluating how children react to illness, perceive an illness, or react to health care (Fig. 35-1). Their body images, as evidenced in their drawings, are different from those of adults. They can have difficulty telling which body parts are indispensable and which are not (this is why it is wise to talk to preschool and early school-age children about "fixing" body parts, such as tonsils, rather than "taking them out").

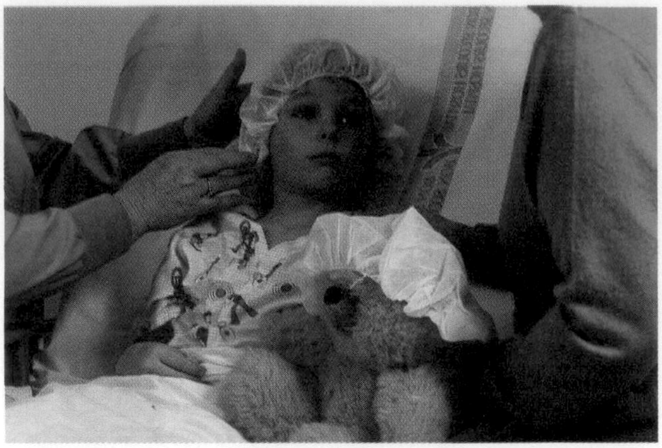

FIGURE 35.1 Illness is potentially traumatic because of the unknown and pain and discomfort that may be involved. Children need extra attention and reassurance to calm their fears.

Inability to Communicate

Very young children do not have the vocabulary to describe symptoms. Headache is an example of a symptom that children younger than 5 years have a great deal of difficulty describing. Dizziness and nausea can be equally bewildering because children this age do not know the words to express these phenomena.

By the time they reach school age, most children can describe symptoms with accuracy. They may intensify their concerns, however, if they believe that someone expects symptoms to be more serious. They may minimize symptoms if they are afraid illness will interfere with an activity.

Determine a child's symptoms as much by observation as by the child's report. The crying, whining preschooler who is "just not herself" probably has a symptom she cannot describe. The school-age child who guards her abdomen (keeps abdominal muscles rigid) is in pain just as clearly as the child who verbalizes the source of discomfort. Keen, astute observations are necessary to ascertain the extent of a child's illness at any given time.

Inability to Monitor Own Care and Manage Fear

Adults who are ill often ask about medications prescribed for them or procedures they are scheduled to undergo. For example, if a hospitalized man knows he is to receive a diuretic three times a day and by 10 AM has not been given it, he usually reminds someone of the oversight. School-age and younger children are unable to monitor their own care this way because they may not know which medicine or procedures they are to receive. If they do know, they may be confused about time. In addition, children have fears that adults do not have. The infant, for example, fears separation above all else; the toddler and preschooler fear such things as separation, the dark, the unknown, intrusive procedures, and mutilation of body parts. The school-age child and adolescent are concerned about the loss of body parts, loss of life, and loss of friends. Adults have fears also, but most have learned to cope with them. Children in a strange environment (such as a hospital) require more support and active intervention to cope with their stress and fears (LaMontegue et al., 2000).

Nutritional Needs

In addition to psychological differences, there are major physiologic differences in the way illness affects children compared with adults. This is because children have different physiologic needs and respond to imbalances in different ways.

Children need more nutrients (calories, protein, minerals, and vitamins) per pound of body weight than adults, for example, because their basic metabolic rate is faster, and they must take in not only enough to maintain body tissues but also enough to allow for growth. The infant requires 120 kcal per kilogram of body weight per day; the adult requires only 30 to 35. An ill child who must limit food intake because of nausea or vomiting, therefore, may require hospitalization that would be unnecessary for an adult under the same circumstances.

Fluid and Electrolyte Balance

In the adult, extracellular water (in plasma and outside body cells) composes approximately 23% of total body water; in a newborn, extracellular water is closer to 40%. This means that an infant does not have as much water stored in the cells as an adult does and thus is more likely to lose a devastating amount of body water with diarrhea or vomiting. Because of this, there is no such thing as "only diarrhea" or "simple diarrhea" in a child younger than 1 year. The full implications of both vomiting and diarrhea are discussed in Chapter 45.

Systemic Response to Illness

Because their bodies are immature, young children tend to respond to disease systemically rather than locally. The child with pneumonia, for example, may be brought to an emergency room not because of a cough (although the child has one) but because of accompanying systemic symptoms such as fever, vomiting, and diarrhea. Nausea and vomiting, in fact, occur so frequently in children with any type of illness that these symptoms do not have the diagnostic value they have in adults. Systemic reactions can delay diagnosis and therapy and cause increased fluid and nutrient loss, circumstances that compound an initial illness and can result in hospitalization.

Age-Specific Diseases

Because of their growth requirement and their immaturity, children are susceptible to some diseases that do not affect adults. For example, because infants are growing, a lack of vitamin D will cause rickets, but this same lack does not affect adults. Most adults have achieved immunity to common infectious diseases; children, however, are susceptible to childhood diseases such as measles, mumps, and chickenpox because of lack of immunity. Children younger than 5 years who have a high temperature may respond with generalized seizures (febrile seizures), a phenomenon that rarely occurs after this age. Children younger than 1 year of age are subject to iron-deficiency anemia because fetal red blood cells are destroyed after birth and are replaced by mature red blood cells very slowly.

> ✔ **CHECKPOINT QUESTIONS**
>
> 1. How well do school-age children understand the workings of major body parts?
> 2. Why are newborns more likely to lose a devastating amount of body fluid with diarrhea or vomiting?

CARE OF THE ILL CHILD AND FAMILY IN THE HOSPITAL

Based on the theory that hospitalization can be an unnecessary stress to children, only those who cannot successfully be managed on an ambulatory basis are now admitted to the hospital. This was not always true. For example, most children with head injuries automatically stayed overnight for observation. Currently, unless a child is unconscious or shows other signs of neurologic injury, he or she is sent home to be observed by parents for signs of increased intracranial pressure. This policy requires that time be spent in teaching parents skills such as how to take a pulse or evaluate consciousness. Teaching them requires patience because parents under stress can have difficulty comprehending instructions. However, because psychological trauma as well as excessive health care costs are prevented by allowing a child to return home, it is important teaching.

Instead of being admitted to the hospital, many children will have procedures such as tonsillectomy done on an ambulatory or outpatient basis. This prevents the major problem of separation anxiety. However, it does not necessarily reduce parents' or children's anxiety about the procedure. Some parents actually feel less confident and more anxious with ambulatory procedures than they did with in-hospital admissions because they sense that their responsibility for preparation and follow-up care will be significantly greater. They often comment that the system is not as good as when children were admitted and that this change is a result of cost containment by insurance companies. Although it is true that short hospital stays reduce cost, it is helpful to inform parents that ambulatory or outpatient procedures are as safe as those performed with hospital admissions and that ambulatory procedures are scheduled to prevent separation as well as contain cost.

Preparing the Ill Child and Family for Hospitalization

Many childhood illnesses such as febrile seizures, appendicitis, poisonings, and asthma attacks strike suddenly, making advance preparation for hospital admission impossible. However, when hospitalization is planned ahead of time, for orthopedic or second-stage surgeries, for example, preparation is possible. As a rule, parents eagerly seek guidance from nurses on what and how much to tell their children about an anticipated admission. The preparation a parent makes for a child obviously varies according to the child's age and individual experience. No matter what the child's age, however, parents should be encouraged to convey a positive attitude. Statements such as, "They'll make you behave in the hospital" or "Wait until you have to stay in bed all day" should be avoided.

Children can worry unnecessarily if they are told about their approaching hospitalization too far in advance. Conversely, few things are more frightening for children than to hear conversation halt as they enter a room or to hear adults spelling out unknown words. As a rule, therefore, children between 2 and 7 years of age should be told about a scheduled ambulatory or inpatient hospitalization as many days before the procedure as the child's age in years. For example, a 2-year-old should be informed 2 days before hospitalization; a 4-year-old, 4 days before; and so forth. Children older than 7 years should be told as soon as the parents are aware of it.

On the day of admission, it is important for you to discuss the preparations to ensure that the child and family accurately understand the child's condition and upcoming procedures. Based on that, you can provide further health teaching and clear up any misunderstandings (see Focus on Communication).

NURSING DIAGNOSES AND RELATED INTERVENTIONS

Nursing Diagnosis: Deficient knowledge related to preparation for hospitalization

Outcome Identification: Parents and child will be prepared for hospital experience at a level appropriate to child's age and development by day of hospital admission.

Outcome Evaluation: Parents and child both state they feel prepared for hospitalization; child has brought some personal items important to self. Child describes with accuracy and detail appropriate to age the reason for hospital stay; asks questions and expresses feelings appropriate to age about hospitalization with health care providers.

Preparing Family Caregivers. Parents experience anxiety about a child's hospitalization as well as the child (Foley, 2000). Therefore, planning for hospitalization should begin as soon as the parents know that hospitalization will be necessary. Some parents, however, may be so concerned about the reason for hospitalization that they are unable to begin this type of preparation until they are better prepared themselves. Easing parental anxiety regarding illness and hospitalization is particularly important because infants and children can keenly sense a parent's stress. No amount or type of preparation for children will be effective if they react to their parents' unspoken tension. Even though parents may say, "Don't worry, everything will be all right," a child will sense if parents really do not believe that everything will be all right, a situation that may hamper recovery.

FOCUS ON COMMUNICATION

Gregory is a 4-year-old you are going to admit to the ambulatory surgical unit for an elective tonsillectomy. His mother and he arrive together on the unit.

Less Effective Communication

Nurse: Hello, Gregory. How are you?
Gregory: Good.
Nurse: Do you know why you're coming into the hospital?
Mrs. Miller: We've talked about surgery. He knows that's why he's here.
Nurse: Did you bring a favorite toy, Gregory?
Gregory: I brought a book to color.
Nurse: You sound ready. Let's get you admitted.

More Effective Communication

Nurse: Hello, Gregory. How are you?
Gregory: Good.
Nurse: Do you know why you're coming into the hospital?
Mrs. Miller: We've talked about surgery. He knows that's why he's here.
Nurse: Tell me why you're here, Gregory.
Gregory: To read a book. I brought a book.
Nurse: Let's talk about everything you told him, Mrs. Miller, about surgery.
Mrs. Miller: I've told him he'll be super sick. I still remember feeling like I was going to die when I had mine out.
Nurse: Let's take some time and talk about a few other things.

The above poor communication example happened because the nurse assumed that when the parent said she had prepared her son, she had prepared him in the same way that the nurse would have. The communication improved when the nurse stopped assuming about the level of preparation and asked direct questions of the mother and child about what they knew.

As part of preparation, parents should ask questions about the hospitalization so they become as familiar as possible with what will happen. If they are well informed in this way, they will (at least theoretically) have as low an anxiety level as possible. If they arrive at a hospital unit with questions unanswered, fill in gaps immediately.

Advise parents to ask about things such as what diagnostic procedures will be necessary, how long the hospital stay will be, and what kind of dressings or other equipment will be used. If you are practicing in a doctor's office or clinic where surgery or a hospital admission is first proposed, become familiar with these facts to serve as the parents' backup informant. Many parents ask a nurse for their main information or ask to have the physician's explanation clarified to be certain they have understood it correctly. An organization that offers helpful information on hospitalization of children is the National Association of Child Care Professionals (*www.NACCP.org*).

Preparing the Infant. Because an infant cannot understand explanations of surgery or treatments, preparation is minimal. Special items such as a favorite toy, blanket, or pacifier should be packed. These objects provide a special kind of security for which there is no substitute.

A primary caregiver should consider spending a great deal of time in the hospital with an infant. For rooming in, he or she needs to make plans for older children or a spouse ahead of time. If the parent cannot arrange to room-in, make plans to have a consistent nurse assigned to the infant. This can help decrease parental anxiety and minimize separation anxiety in the infant.

Preparing the Toddler and Preschooler. Three chief fears of the toddler or preschooler are fear of the unknown, fear of abandonment or separation, and fear of mutilation. These children, therefore, need preparation clearly aimed at alleviating these fears. Bringing a favorite toy or personal item such as a blanket can help. Referred to as transitional objects, these items are symbols of the longed-for return home. Some parents buy a new toy to replace the child's favorite one because they feel ashamed of a teddy bear with one ear or one eye missing. A new bear may mean nothing to the child, however, and clinging to it may not offer comfort.

When making hospital beds or changing the paper on examining tables, watch for ragged blankets and threadbare stuffed animals; these can cling to sheets and could be easily discarded. Throw nothing away without first asking the child or parent if it is all right. What looks like a useless alphabet block may be extremely important to the child.

When children are admitted in an emergency, they rarely have toys with them. In these instances, suggest that a parent give the child a familiar object, such as the parent's wallet (money and papers removed) or a sweater. The child will hold these in the same way as a favorite toy. The child's outside shoes can serve this same purpose if the parents leave them with the child.

WHAT IF? What if a parent brought pots and pans as son's favorite play items? Would you suggest she bring a better toy?

A number of helpful books about hospitalization are available for parents to read with children and also learn more about children's health care. These can be obtained from local bookstores, libraries, or Internet book sites, or by writing directly to the publishers (Box 35-1). A parent could read one of these books to a child, adapting the story to include information specific to the child. Some books fail to orient children well to hospitalization because they are too sweet (as if the child were going to a picnic rather than a hospital). Other may omit pertinent facts, such as that surgery will involve some pain (stress that the child will be given medicine so that the pain will go away) or that when bedrest is required, the child will have to use a bedpan. Using a bedpan is difficult for toddlers and preschoolers to accept because they may have been toilet-trained only recently and have been told repeatedly that they must use only the bathroom.

BOX 35.1

BOOKS ON HOSPITALIZATION FOR CHILDREN

Bridwell, N. (1998). *Clifford Visits the Hospital.* New York: Scholastic Publishers. (Grades pre-K–3)
Civardi, A. (1994). *Going to the Hospital.* Tulsa, OK: EDC Publications. (Infant-preschool)
Dooley, V. (1996). *Tubes in My Ears: My Trip to the Hospital.* Greenvale, NY: Mondo Publishing. (Grades K–3)
Duncan, D. (1994). *When Molly Was in the Hospital: A Book for Brothers and Sisters of Hospitalized Children* (Minimed Series Vol. 1). Windsor, CA: Rayve Productions. (Grades K–4)
Ganz, P., & Scofield, T. (1996). *Life Isn't Always a Day at the Beach: A Book for All Children Whose Lives Are Affected by Cancer.* Lincoln: High Five Publishing. (Grades K–6)
Hautzig, D. (1985). *A Visit to the Sesame Street Hospital (Please Read to Me).* New York: Random House. (Grades K–3)
Jennings, S., et al. (2000). *Franklin Goes to the Hospital.* New York: Scholastic Publishers. (Grades pre-K–3)
Krall, C. B., & Jim, J. M. (1987). *Fat Dog's First Visit: A Child's View of the Hospital.* Atlanta: Pritchett & Hull Associates. (Preschool)
Rey, H. A. (1976). *Curious George Goes to the Hospital.* Boston: Houghton Mifflin Co. (Grades 2–3)
Rogers, F. (1997). *Going to the Hospital.* New York: PaperStar Publishers. (Grades K–3)

Because the imagination of preschoolers is at a peak, role playing also is an effective means of preparing a child of this age for a new experience. To do this, a parent could encourage the child to play hospital with dolls, or the parent might act out a hospitalization experience. For example, the child changes into pajamas and gets into bed. The parent acts out a physical examination, a meal in bed, a bedpan (a round cake pan simulates this), or anesthesia administration (a strainer can be used for an induction mask). At the end of the session, the parent should stress that when the child's tummy or throat is better, he or she will change back to street clothes and come home. Remind parents that it is always better to use the word "fix" rather than "cut" when talking about surgery with young children, because "cut" automatically suggests pain and mutilation.

Preparing the School-Age Child and Adolescent. School-aged children enjoy reading, so books about surgery and hospitalization would be helpful. Also, both school-age children and adolescents need factual explanations of what will happen during such an experience. This also includes what will not happen: for example, surgery will require a small abdominal incision, but it will not create a scar that will show when wearing a bathing suit.

Many community hospitals sponsor hospital orientation programs for children's groups or school groups in which hospitalization is discussed. These programs are beneficial because they lay a foundation for all children about what to expect in a hospitalization; then, if they must be admitted on an emergency basis, they may not be so frightened. Programs are offered by nurses at the hospital or on visits to children's groups or schools (Fig. 35-2). Box 35-2 provides guidelines for setting up hospital tours or discussions for early school-age children.

Be sure that parents have the necessary factual information themselves so that they can provide accurate and appropriate explanations to school-age children. If they do not know the answer to a question, caution them that the best response is simply, "I don't know" rather than a guess. This prevents a child from feeling betrayed when the real answer is different. At approximately 9 years of age, when children first begin to understand the full meaning of death, parents need to be especially careful to explain that an anesthetic causes a "special sleep," not that the child is "put to sleep." Animals who are "put to sleep" are not seen again. Talking to another child who has undergone the same experience and come through it intact also is helpful to prepare school-age children and adolescents for hospitalization. Although parents cannot usually supply such a person in advance, on admission to the hospital, a visit to a recovering patient is often possible and is a constructive way to give reassurance.

If hospitalization is to be more than 1 week long, a parent must think about continuing the child's schooling. Advise the parents to ask the physician at what point the child will be able to do homework. Many school systems provide tutors; children's hospitals often have their own teachers from the local school system to carry out this service.

Preparing the Child of a Different Cultural Background. Perhaps the most important aspect to consider when preparing a child from a different cultural background for hospitalization is that it is your customs that seem different to the child and family. Ask enough questions and practice good listening skills to gain information about the particular needs of a child and family. When cultural differences do exist, be prepared to act as a liaison between the family and the health care team. If language is a problem, a translator may be necessary in this preparation phase. Provide the opportunity for parents to voice their fears and ask questions at the time of hospitalization or treatment. When families speak a different language or are unfamiliar with hospital routine, allow more time and more opportunities for discussion and communication.

BOX 35.2

GUIDELINES FOR CONDUCTING HOSPITAL TOURS WITH EARLY SCHOOL-AGE CHILDREN

1. Keep groups small (about 10 children per group) so individual reactions to the presentations can be assessed.
2. Allow or encourage parents to join the tour so their anxiety about the hospital can also be relieved.
3. Conduct the tour for only 20 to 30 minutes to meet the short attention span of children.
4. Use an indirect method to present various aspects of a hospital, such as puppets, films, or a slide show, to decrease anxiety.
5. Present the features of a hospital in a nonthreatening environment, such as the hospital playroom. Avoid the emergency room, ICUs, or operating rooms while touring, because these are anxiety-producing areas for children. Talk about these areas by using slides or photographs instead.
6. Present explanations about hospitalization in concrete terms and at the child's level of understanding. Include only what the child will see, hear, and feel.
7. Avoid dwelling on unpleasant and threatening events or intrusive procedures, such as blood drawing or anesthesia, that may create anxiety.
8. Allow children opportunities to ask questions.
9. Allow children opportunities to play with dolls and hospital equipment, both to decrease anxiety and satisfy curiosity.

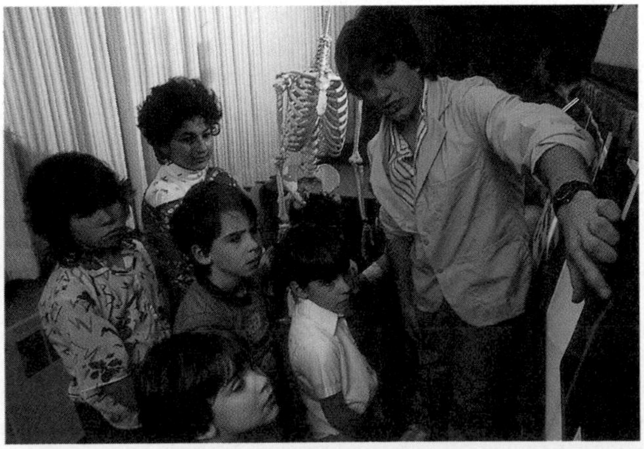

FIGURE 35.2 Children learn what to expect from hospitalization during a prehospital program.

Preparing the Physically Challenged or Chronically Ill Child. Physically challenged or chronically ill children frequently come to ambulatory health care settings for care; they often are admitted to a hospital for care, possibly remaining in a hospital for extended visits and continuing care at home. Think through ways in which a new hospitalization or visit will be like past ones and other ways in which it will be different to determine how best to prepare a child. Help children to maintain contact with their families and school friends during a long hospitalization or home care experience by encouraging telephone calls, e-mails, letters, and open visiting.

Admitting the Ill Child and Family

Whether an ambulatory or inpatient hospital unit admission, children and parents need to be admitted as a single entity to encourage the parents to feel they are true partners in care. A child coming to a hospital for an elective admission generally arrives at a reception area, where significant factual information is obtained, such as name, age, address, and hospital insurance coverage. The child and parents are then brought to the hospital unit. Remember that first impressions count. If parents are left standing at the desk while nurses chat, they can easily feel that no one appreciates their concern and that possibly their child will not receive optimal care. It is true that at certain times on a children's unit all nurses may be busy finishing the treatments for other children before they can take the time to admit a new child. Even so, one nurse should take the time to introduce himself or herself and find a comfortable place for the family to wait until someone is available. When introducing yourself to children, stoop down so that your face is level with the child's face (Fig. 35-3). Call the child by name or ask for a nickname. Calling all children "honey" or "pumpkin" can cause a child to worry that he or she has been confused with another child.

On admission to a health care facility, all children should have an armband attached giving their name and hospital chart number. Because their hands are not much larger than their wrists and their feet are not much larger in diameter than their ankles, neonates (infants younger than 1 month of age) often need two bands in place as an extra safeguard. If a band falls off, never tape it to the crib or bedside stand. This is not adequate protection. If an infant is placed in the wrong crib by mistake, he or she may be given a medicine that is lethal before the mistake is realized.

Assessment on Admission

Assess each child's level of preparation for a hospitalization on admission to the facility. Be aware of not only what the child describes orally but also what facial expressions or nervous manifestations may be indicating.

Interview parents on hospital admission for a nursing history to obtain the information needed to plan nursing care (Chap. 33 describes a full child database interview history). Many hospitals have information checklists for parents to bring with them. Obtaining information in this way is highly efficient, but it may not be as satisfying to worried parents as hearing a nurse taking a few minutes to ask questions personally or specifically review the completed form. The information that is necessary to obtain about a child is shown in Table 35-1. It is included in the child's plan of care as a vital step of assessment.

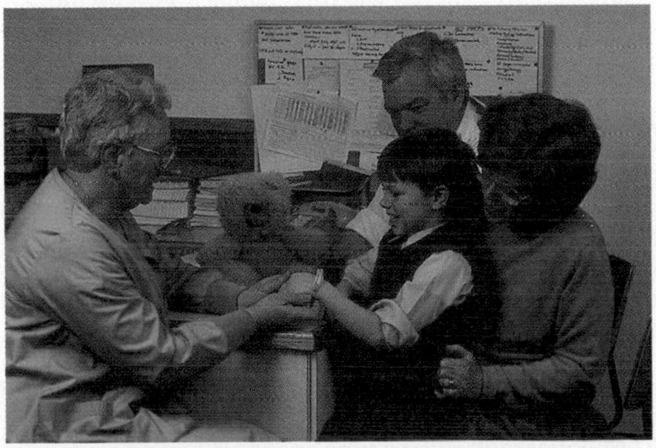

FIGURE 35.3 A child is admitted to a hospital unit. Notice how the nurse greets the child at the child's own level.

Make a note of any medication or food allergy on the child's plan of care and, if pertinent, post this information by the child's bed because unlike an adult, a child cannot call these things to the attention of health care personnel when food or medication is offered.

Take and record the child's temperature, pulse, and respirations. Measure height and weight to determine overall growth and to allow for determination of surface area, the measurement on which medication dosage is calculated. Whether blood pressure needs to be taken depends on the age (usually in children over 3 years of age) and condition of the child. Obtain a specimen for urinalysis as another routine procedure. Be sure to explain all equipment used and allow the child to touch and handle it as much as possible to help reduce anxiety.

Inspect for gross motor ability when weighing the child and measuring height. Listen for language ability (although children in strange situations may say nothing). Perform a physical examination (see Chap. 33) to gain the information necessary for nursing diagnoses and planning.

The way that children deal with hospitalization is based on the same factors that determine how they deal with any crisis: perception of the event, support people available, and effectiveness of past coping experiences or skills. After assessment, analyze whether a child's coping ability will be enough to balance the hazards of inpatient or ambulatory care hospitalization.

NURSING DIAGNOSES AND RELATED INTERVENTIONS

Nursing Diagnosis: Parental and child anxiety related to the need for child's hospitalization

Outcome Identification: Parents and child will demonstrate reduced anxiety through understanding of child's condition and treatment plan by 1 day.

Outcome Evaluation: Parents and child state accurately the reason for child's hospital admission and therapy child will receive; state that although worried, they feel confident they can manage their anxiety.

To help reduce family anxiety regarding hospitalization, be certain that the family is oriented to a hospital stay before admission by discussing the need for hospitalization and what they can except when the hospitalization is first suggested to them in an ambulatory care setting. When children are admitted for emergency care, this type of orientation must be completed immediately, as soon as their physical needs are met. Whether children are admitted for an ambulatory care admission or are being hospitalized for a potentially longer stay, be certain that parents and the child are oriented to the unit, the personnel who will be caring for them, and the usual routine.

On admission, parents and the child need basic information about the child's condition. If the diagnosis is uncertain, what steps are being taken to con-

TABLE 35.1 Information Necessary for the Child's Plan of Care on Admission

AREA OF INFORMATION	SPECIFIC KNOWLEDGE
Chief concern	Determine what the parents' understanding is of why the child is being admitted. (This view may differ widely from the physician's view regarding the reason the child is being admitted.) What has the child been told about the reason for hospitalization?
Family profile	Obtain child's name and birthday. Who lives at home (include pets)? Ask about parents' occupation and education levels. Who is the child's primary caregiver? Have there been any disruptive happenings lately in the child's life, such as a move or a divorce, that would make the child particularly insecure at this time? Will a parent be staying with the child? If parents are separated or divorced, what will arrangements be? Who has legal authority to sign medical permission?
Past experience with illness or separation	Ask about previous hospital experiences and how the child feels about them. Has there been a recent hospitalization for anyone in the family that resulted in a bad outcome? Has the child been away from the parents before? Overnight at a grandparent's? Summer camp? What is the child's past experience with taking medicine? Has the child swallowed pills before? Does the child have any known allergies to food or medications? (Document these by asking for exact symptoms and happenings.)
Daily routines	Ask about the child's regular bedtime and sleep times. Does the child nap? Does the child have a bedtime ritual? What type of bed does he or she sleep in? Does the child sleep with a favorite toy or blanket? What is his or her bathtime routine? Does the child brush his or her own teeth and hair or need help? What words does the child use for voiding and defecating? Is the child completely toilet-trained? If a preschooler, is the child accustomed to using a potty chair or toilet? Does the child have enuresis (bedwetting)? What is the child's usual meal plan? Are there foods the child does not eat? What is the child's favorite toy? Does he or she have it with him or her? What are the child's favorite games and hobbies or interests? Are there television programs the parents especially like the child to see or not see?
Developmental survey	Ascertain the child's developmental level. Does child feed self? Use a spoon, cup, bottle? Dress self? If school age, what grade in school?
Special information	Obtain any special information about the child that would make him or her more comfortable in the hospital.

firm one? It helps if these steps are named specifically: for instance, blood work, radiographic studies, observation, recording of vital signs, or calling in a consultant. What is the tentative plan for the child? Complete bedrest or infection control procedures until the results of blood work or cultures are back? Special diet? Special procedures? If the primary care provider physician has written no orders as yet, be honest: "The specific plan of care isn't written yet. I'll let you know as soon as I'm sure what it will be." Although this answer does not provide the family with information, it does tell them that you appreciate how difficult and bewildering it is when a child is admitted to a health care facility.

For an emergency admission, parents may have little understanding of the child's condition or the treatment plan. Conversely, someone might have taken a great deal of time to explain what was happening while the child was being cared for in the emergency room or brought to the unit (see Focus on Multidisciplinary Care). To determine their knowledge level, ask parents if they have any questions about their child's condition or the course of treatment that they want to discuss with the inpatient facility's health care team.

If parents must leave rather than remain with a child, be certain they see the child's room before they leave. This is important in convincing the child that the parents will know where they can find him or her when they return. If there are other children in the room, introduce the new child to them. Let children wear their own clothes if possible rather than changing to hospital gowns.

Promoting a Positive Hospital Stay

Promoting a positive hospital stay is important to the health of both children and their families. Several nursing actions are important to make the difference between a successful and an unsuccessful hospital experience.

Minimizing Length of Hospital Stay

Hospitalization should be limited to the shortest time possible. At one time, all children having tonsillectomies and herniorrhaphies were admitted at least overnight. Currently, these types of surgeries can be performed early in the morning, and after a short recovery period the child returns home.

Be certain that diagnostic procedures are scheduled for the child's, not the hospital's, convenience so that no child stays in a hospital longer than is necessary. Pressure from concerned nurses who insist on having a voice in policies can make a big difference in a department's willingness to cooperate with scheduling.

FOCUS ON MULTIDISCIPLINARY CARE

Many different disciplines typically are involved when a child is admitted to the hospital. This means that coordinating care with these disciplines (for example, occupational or physical therapists, surgery department personnel, nutritionists, and respiratory therapists) is necessary so that the child's hospital stay is both as short and as atraumatic as possible.

In addition to the various health professionals, unlicensed assistive personnel can play a major role in helping families and children adjust to an illness. They often serve as the people who escort a child and parents from the admissions department of a hospital to a care unit. They may be included on a home health care team to give simple care, such as hygiene or range-of-motion exercises. Be certain that such personnel are aware that few things are as confusing to parents and the child as receiving conflicting information and, because children's conditions vary, what is true for one child is not automatically true for all children with that same illness. This means that when they don't know the answer to a question, a simple "I don't know, but I'll find that out for you" is always superior to guessing at an answer. This achieves what parents want (to be well informed) and yet prevents them from receiving confusing information.

Providing Continuity of Care

To ensure that children are exposed to as few substitute care people as possible and to maintain the consistency and quality of care, nursing assignments should be made so that one nurse gives as much care to the same child as possible (**primary nursing** or **case management nursing;** Fig. 35-4). These staffing patterns allow one nurse to admit the child, take the nursing history, establish nursing diagnoses, set goals for care in cooperation with the parents and the child, and evaluate progress toward achieving goals. It allows children to have one main nurse to whom to relate. It allows parents to establish meaningful contact with hospital staff and maintains continuity of care planning and implementation.

Decreasing Separation Anxiety

It is difficult to explain the meaning that a primary caregiver has for a child, but the intensity of the relationship can be demonstrated. As early as 4 months of age, an infant registers disapproval if his or her primary caregiver walks away. As early as 5 months of age, the infant registers anxiety when strangers are present or when people other than the usual caregiver pick up the infant. The infant fixes his or her eyes on the stranger, becomes restless, perhaps thrashes arms or legs, and begins to cry. This activity peaks at approximately 8 months of age and is commonly called 8-month anxiety. It is a developmental milestone that shows the infant is able to distinguish the primary caregiver from other persons. It also means that a child has reached a stage in emotional development at which he or she reacts poorly to separation or to the threat of it.

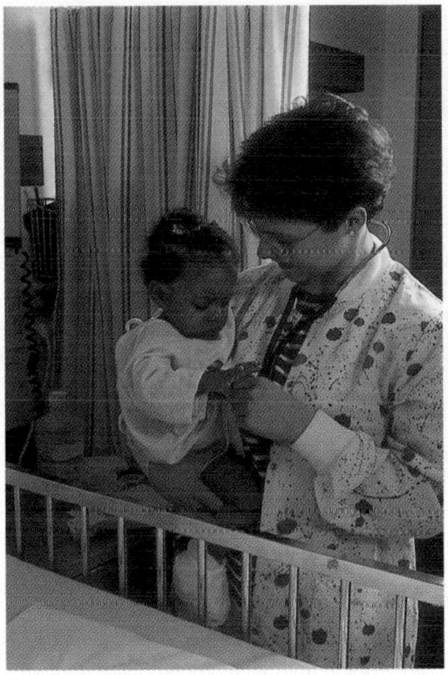

FIGURE 35.4 Each hospitalized child should have one nurse who is "hers" to minimize the effect of separation from parents (primary care nursing).

Toddlers and preschoolers can be as affected by separation as infants can. In some instances, they express their feelings better, louder, and longer than infants. Although many toddlers and preschoolers attend day care and have had prior experiences with separation, others may have had only limited experiences. Being hospitalized may be the first time they are away from parents in a strange setting or away from home overnight. If this is so, many preschoolers may wonder whether they will ever live with their parents again. Problems of separation are especially intense in younger children because they do not understand time. Statements such as, "Mom will visit again tomorrow" or "Dad will be here by 6 o'clock" are meaningless to children younger than 5 years of age because they do not know what either tomorrow or 6 o'clock means.

School-age children and adolescents react better than younger children to the separation imposed by hospitalization because they have experiences with which to compare it. They have been to school for whole days; perhaps they have stayed with a grandparent or a friend overnight; they may have been to camp. This can make hospitalization a time for developing self-esteem and confidence in their ability to be independent. Even in light of this, ill school-age children and adolescents may still feel anxious about being separated from their parents. They appreciate their parents' presence and need reassurance that their parents support and love them.

Remember that parents may have an equally difficult time being separated from children. You may need to spend time with them assuring them that their child will receive good care at all times, even when they are absent.

To appreciate why preventing separation is so important, it is helpful to review the research that provided the foundation for this method of care.

Spitz (1945) was one of the first researchers to document the effects of separation on children. He observed children in a penal nursery and in a foundling home who were separated from their mothers for both short and long periods, documenting how poorly children responded to separation from their parents. Bowlby (1966) conducted additional studies after World War II. Building on Spitz's and Bowlby's work, Robertson (1958) studied the effect of hospitalization on children and supplied labels for separation effects (Table 35-2). Although defined 50 years ago, these are still applicable to children today (Partis, 2000).

Effects of hospitalization can be so severe that they can be compared to posttraumatic stress disorder, the development of characteristic symptoms following exposure to an extremely traumatic situation. Children who develop this condition demonstrate persistent symptoms of anxiety such as difficulty falling asleep, irritability, outbursts of anger, difficulty concentrating or completing tasks, or stomachaches and headaches. They re-experience the traumatic event happening over and over through dreams or flashbacks (APA, 2000).

Despite the best preparation, not all of these effects of hospitalization can be prevented (Daviss et al., 2000). Reducing the ill effects of separation and hospitalization to the extent possible should be a high priority for health care providers. Nurses can play a major role in this on both direct care and management levels (see Focus on Evidence-Based Practice).

NURSING DIAGNOSES AND RELATED INTERVENTIONS

Nursing Diagnosis: Anxiety of child related to separation during hospitalization

Outcome Identification: Child will demonstrate little evidence of separation anxiety during hospitalization.

Outcome Evaluation: Child actively relates to hospital personnel and hospital routine in ways appropriate to child's age and stage of development.

Promoting Open Parent Visiting. When possible, children younger than 5 years should have their primary caregiver room-in with them when they are in the hospital (Fig. 35-5). Children younger than 10 to 12 years continue to enjoy the feeling of security that this provides. This policy is expensive for a hospital because a bed or cot must be provided for this person as well as for the child, and despite the presence of this person, no reduction in nursing staff is possible. In many instances, because so much parental education is needed, requirements for health care personnel actually increase. However, such policies greatly reduce symptoms of separation anxiety.

Not all parents can stay in the hospital continuously. Mothers and fathers who cannot stay may need help in smoothing the transition of their coming or going. For example, when a toddler first sees his parents after being separated, his reaction might be to ignore them (a sign of despair). This is a defense mechanism: "I won't show

TABLE 35.2 Stages of Separation Anxiety

STAGE	MANIFESTATIONS
Protest	The child cries loudly and demandingly; rejects any attempts to be comforted by nurse or substitute primary caregivers.
Despair	The child becomes less active and cries monotonously or wails in a state of mourning; may turn away from parent's approach; often lies on abdomen, facial expression flat; may lose weight and develop insomnia; loses developmental skills; prone to minor ailments such as upper respiratory infections; IQ will measure lower than previous measurement.
Denial	The child is silent, face expressionless; represses feelings for absent caregiver to protect self; deterioration in developmental milestones is apparent; may respond quickly but superficially to all caregivers; may have difficulty forming close relationships later in life.

FOCUS ON EVIDENCE-BASED PRACTICE

Do Children Suffer Posttraumatic Stress Reactions After Hospitalization?

For this study, 48 children aged 7 to 17 years of age who had been hospitalized for accidental injuries were interviewed 1 month after discharge and evaluated to see if they showed signs of posttraumatic stress disorder. Their parents were given a questionnaire asking them about their child's actions since they returned home. Results of the study revealed that a total of 12.5% of children demonstrated full symptoms of posttraumatic stress disorder at the time of follow-up; an additional 16.7% had partial symptoms of the syndrome. The development of posttraumatic stress disorder was associated with high levels of acute distress on the part of the parent or child and prior psychopathology in the child. The researchers concluded that it is relatively common for symptoms of posttraumatic syndrome to be present for 1 month or more after children are hospitalized for injuries.

This is an important study for nurses because nurses are the people who are directly involved in spending time with parents of ill children to reduce their stress and that of their children. The study suggests that the more effective nurses can be in stress reduction while the child is in the hospital, the less apt the child is to have long-term consequences from the hospitalization or illness. The information from this study provides an additional foundation for implementing stress-reduction strategies for ill children and their families.

Daviss, W. B., et. al. (2000). Predicting posttraumatic stress after hospitalization for pediatric injury. *Journal of the American Academy of Child & Adolescent Psychiatry, 39*(5), 576–583.

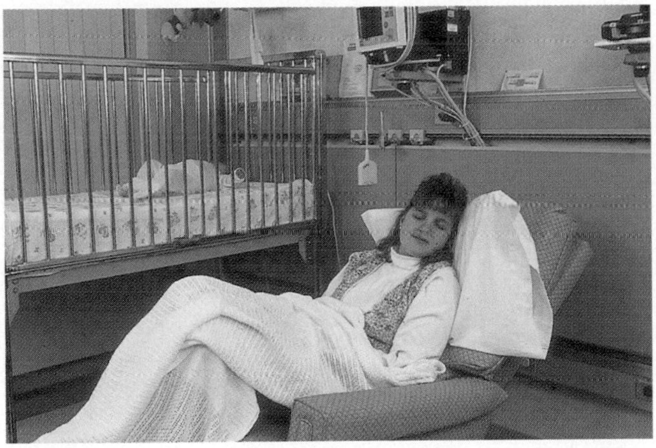

FIGURE 35.5 Rooming-in helps alleviate separation anxiety for both the child and caregiver.

them that I love them until they show me that they love me; that way I won't be hurt again." The parents' reaction to being treated this way may be anger. If this makes the parents go and play with a child in the next bed—a "well, be that way then" reaction—the toddler's worst fears are fulfilled: his parents do not love him any more. However, if the parents speak to the child for a few minutes or try to interest him in a toy, the child will generally reach out to be comforted. Educate them to do this.

Parents often need help in saying goodbye when it is time to leave a child to eat a meal or go home for the night (if the parent is not sleeping in). Assure parents that although someone will not be in the child's room every minute while they are gone, he or she will be well cared for. When the parents of an infant are leaving, go into the room a few minutes before the parents leave and hold or play with the infant. Help a parent to say once, "I have to go now," and then go. Prolonged departures only delay the process and do not reduce the amount of crying that may occur. After parents leave, infants may cry until they fall asleep from exhaustion. Hold and rock them, letting them know that they will be safe.

If the parents of a toddler or preschooler have to leave, urge them first to give a warning that they will soon have to go: "I will have to leave in a minute to fix dinner." When the time to go has come, the parent should say firmly that he or she must go and explain when he or she will return. Time for a preschooler is best measured in terms of events rather than clock hours. Time periods, such as, "I'll be back after you've eaten supper," "after you wake up tomorrow," or "after nap time" gives the child a concrete event by which to measure time. Like infants, toddlers need someone with them when their parents leave; they like to be held or played with so that they know they are not alone.

When parents leave a school-age child or adolescent, urge them to provide definite times when they will return and to leave suggestions for activities the child could do to occupy the time ("Why don't you finish your book? Start your homework and I'll check it when I come back."). Remind them it is more comforting to say specifically, "I will be back around 9 tomorrow morning" rather than, "I will be back sometime tomorrow."

Providing Opportunities for Parents to Participate in Child's Care. Participating in their child's care can make the parents feel more in control, thereby reducing anxiety. Therefore, encourage parents to give as much care as possible during a hospital stay, such as bathing or feeding the child, giving oral medicine, helping with procedures such as warm soaks, or checking that the child is awake from anesthesia. Most parents are eager to help and do so spontaneously. Be certain they receive proper instruction on the tasks they will be able to do. Be sure that parents who change diapers or feed children know whether the number of diaper changes or the amount of food intake needs to be recorded; ask them to report when they do these things or write them down on a flow sheet attached to the child's door or crib.

Occasionally parents may be reluctant to give care for fear of being judged inadequate. Assure them that they are the persons from whom their child would most like to receive care. A parent may point out that he or she is paying for nursing care and so wants nurses to give the child's care. This type of parent will usually soften if approached professionally and assured that nurses are willing to help but for the best interests of the child, the parent is the better caregiver.

Children may be apprehensive about undergoing a procedure without a parent present. There is rarely any reason a parent cannot accompany a child into a treatment room to help with undressing, measuring weight and height, and taking a temperature or accompanying a child to another department for a sonogram or blood work. Most importantly, the mother or father can comfort the child in these strange surroundings.

Although helping with procedures can strengthen the parent–child relationship, remind parents that their most important role is being parents. Sitting and rocking or reading to the child and just being there will be their best role in minimizing the adverse effects of hospitalization. When a child is to have surgery, it may be especially difficult for parents to separate from their child so the child can leave for the operating room. Helping them do this is an important part of preoperative nursing care (Voepel-Lewis et al., 2000; Fennell, 1999).

Supporting Sibling and Grandparent Visitations. Sibling visitation refers to a policy of allowing the brothers and sisters of hospitalized children to visit. Allowing this alleviates loneliness on both sides and helps prevent other children at home from imagining that the ill child is sicker than is true. It helps the ill child continue to feel part of the family and allows grandparents to offer much-needed support. Siblings who visit need to be free of communicable disease. Nurses may need to help parents divide their time between the ill child and siblings during a visit (short, frequent visits may be better for young children than long, sustained ones). Before a visit, ensure that the ill child's room is safe for younger children's visits (e.g., no poisonous substances or electric wires within reach).

Minimizing Negative Effects of Procedures. Ill children often undergo numerous diagnostic and therapeutic procedures. Such procedures can cause pain, fear, and anxiety for the child. Details related to specific procedures are discussed in Chapter 36. General guidelines to make any procedure less painful or frightening are discussed in the following sections.

NURSING DIAGNOSES AND RELATED INTERVENTIONS

Nursing Diagnosis: Fear or anxiety related to diagnostic or therapeutic procedure

Outcome Identification: Child will state fear or anxiety is kept at a tolerable level.

Outcome Evaluation: Child voices satisfaction with comfort measures; describes how he or she participated in a procedure.

Reducing or Eliminating Pain. Some pain and discomfort is unavoidable in association with health care. Limit this whenever possible by, for instance, advocating for the use of intermittent infusion devices such as heparin locks (see Chap. 37) to eliminate multiple punctures for intravenous medication or blood sampling, administering ample analgesia, including alternative therapy techniques such as distraction or imagery, providing traditional comforts such as a change of clothing or position, reading to the child, and planning a special project. Children do not always express discomfort as freely as adults; therefore, closer assessment may be necessary to reveal how they feel. Because pain increases with anxiety, reducing a child's anxiety with good preparation and encouraging a sense of control can also help to eliminate discomfort (see Chap. 38).

Maintaining the Bed as a Safe Area. To assure children that their bed is an area that is safe, all painful procedures should be done in a treatment room, away from the child's bed. Be sure that this rule is not broken, because only one painful experience at the bedside can be enough to significantly increase a child's anxiety. This rule should include finger sticks for blood work; although done quickly, they cause pain and stress. In addition, dressing changes, although not necessarily painful, can cause worry and so should be done in a treatment room, not at the child's bedside.

Helping Children to Maintain Control. Events are always more frightening if they appear to be beyond our control. Explaining to children what will happen (i.e., what they will feel or what they will see) and helping them to make choices whenever possible limit this type of fear because these actions offer a sense of control (Fig. 35-6). In almost any procedure, there is some choice a child can make (use a straw to drink or not, decide what size of tape to use on a bandage, or walk one way in the hall or the other). Letting a child participate in signing a consent form can be an additional way to help the child maintain control.

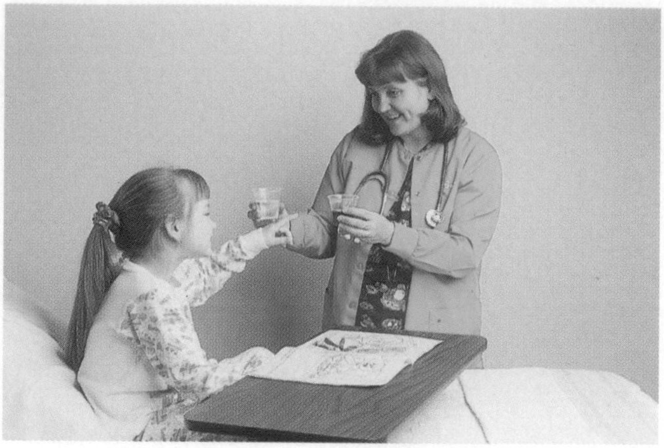

FIGURE 35.6 Children should be included in procedures whenever possible as a way of maintaining control. Here, a nurse gives the child a choice of fluids to drink with her medication.

Providing Adequate Play Facilities

Play is the medium through which children learn. To continue development during hospitalization, children need to be able to play as normally as possible, no matter how long their stay. Children's hospital units should have a playroom or play space in which children can feel secure and in which they know that they will not be hurt. No medical procedures, not even painless ones, should be performed in this area. Children who are in bed need toys or crafts with them there. In addition, because hospitalization is a traumatic experience, children need the opportunity to express their feelings through therapeutic play (Price et al., 2002). The uses of play and guidelines for providing therapeutic play are discussed later in this chapter.

Setting Limits on Behavior

Setting limits on behavior can help promote a positive hospital stay because it can help to provide a sense of security and safety for the child. The average child is motivated to follow instructions and rules and demonstrate good behavior during a hospital stay because he or she wants to get well again and return home as soon as possible. The occasional child who misbehaves in a hospital setting usually does so because he or she lacks a clear understanding of what is expected or is demonstrating that his or her personal needs have not been recognized and met.

A child who needs frequent reminders to stop running in the hallway, for example, is probably bored with staying in a room. Providing more activities (playing a game with the child) or allowing more structured exercise (letting the child accompany a nursing aide to take a blood specimen to a laboratory) can prevent further unsafe activity.

Children who refuse to cooperate for procedures generally do so out of fear of the unknown rather than deliberate misbehavior. The better prepared a child is for such a procedure, therefore, the better the child is apt to accept it. For potentially painful procedures such as a bone marrow aspiration, lumbar puncture, blood sampling, or cast removal, any behavior short of hysterical screaming can be considered "good" behavior.

If limit setting is necessary, such as with a child who hits or bites other children, confer with parents about the need for limit setting and what measures they would suggest. Gain their cooperation and approval. Using "time out" periods or removing the child to a nonstimulating area for a short time is an effective measure. Be certain the child understands the rules (if the child bites or hits, he or she will have to sit alone for a designated period). The next time the child misbehaves, give one warning that the behavior is against the rules; if the behavior does not improve, take the child to the "time out" spot. If the child is disruptive, begin timing the period from when the child quiets down. When the child has been quiet for the specified duration (usually 1 minute per year of age), he or she can leave the "time out" place and rejoin activities.

Discharge Planning

Discharge planning is an important link between hospital and home.

NURSING DIAGNOSES AND RELATED INTERVENTIONS

Nursing Diagnosis: Parental health-seeking behaviors related to care for child at home after hospital discharge

Outcome Identification: Parents will demonstrate ability to care for child at home before discharge.

Outcome Evaluation: Parents state accurately the care their child will need at home; describe and demonstrate any procedures they will need to perform with child.

Many children, particularly those having surgery, are hospitalized for only a few hours; as soon as they are able to take and retain fluid and have voided once, they are discharged. This represents such a short time frame that preparation for discharge must start even before they are admitted to the hospital.

If a child has been admitted on an inpatient basis, preparation for discharge should begin on the day of admission. If some procedures will need to be done later at home, allow parents to perform them in the hospital so that they can become comfortable with the techniques and discover any problems while help is still available. Urge parents to think through problems they might have with the procedures at home. Suppose a parent will be doing warm sterile soaks to an open lesion at home. How does he or she sterilize water? Where can the parent buy dressings? Can the parent afford them? What can he or she use to keep the soaks warm for 20 minutes? What suggestions would be helpful to give the parent for keeping the child quiet and content for 20 minutes, so that the child does not move a great deal and knock off the dressing? These are real problems that must be worked out before a parent can perform the procedure at home. Do not leave this kind of instruction until the last day, because then there will not be time left to solve such problems.

Discharge planners can be indispensable in helping ready parents for home care. In a general hospital setting, however, if the discharge planner is unfamiliar with specific procedures (or children), he or she may not be helpful on a practical level. Some parents require follow-up help in their homes that can be provided by a community or home health care nurse. Do not leave the full responsibility for teaching to these nurses, however. Teach the parents what they must do on the first day they are at home before further help arrives. Be certain that they know the person to contact if plans do not work out as anticipated and that they have a definite return appointment for follow-up care.

Many preschool children manifest behavior problems such as thumb-sucking, bed wetting, temper tantrums, and nightmares after returning home from a hospital stay; school-age children may manifest these behaviors to a lesser extent. Parents can be assured that these behaviors are part of the child's normal response to hospitalization. These behaviors do not happen because the child has been "spoiled" by the hospital staff or by the parents during the illness but because the experience was too intense for the child to handle, even with all the precautions taken to prevent stress. As children realize that they are safely back home and the experience is over, these behavior reactions become less frequent and eventually disappear.

✔ CHECKPOINT QUESTIONS

3. What is a good technique for preparing preschool children for hospitalization?
4. Why is it important to obtain height and weight measurements on hospital admission?
5. According to Robertson, what is the first stage of separation anxiety?

CARE OF THE ILL CHILD AND FAMILY IN THE HOME

Home care is care of children in their own home, provided by or supervised through a certified home health care or community health care agency.

In recent years, the need for home health care services has grown substantially. Acute care or postsurgical clients, including children, often require regular home nursing visits through a rehabilitation period. Children with chronic conditions such as bronchial pulmonary dysphasia, cystic fibrosis, and childhood cancer are cared for at home rather than in hospital settings when at all possible. Many children with terminal diseases are cared for at home (**hospice care**).

Several factors have contributed to the success of the home as a health care setting. Technological advances have made it possible for potentially complicated procedures, such as the administration of total parenteral nutrition and ventilation therapy, to be performed safely at home. There is also a strong economic incentive to provide care in the home (it is less costly for health care plans). Perhaps the greatest benefit of home care for children is the opportunity it brings to include the entire family in health care planning and the ability to focus not only on a specific health problem but also on promoting healthy behaviors for the entire family.

Several types of agencies and services help to meet the growing demands for home health care. Home care agencies, which may be free-standing or allied with a health care facility, provide services from a wide variety of disciplines such as nurses, therapists, and physicians. Specialized services such as providing supplies for total parenteral nutrition, oxygen therapy, or laboratory analysis may be furnished by special service companies. Voluntary agencies often provide services such as transportation, vans to carry children to and from health care agency assessments, or respite care so parents can have a break from continual care.

Be certain that parents whose child is admitted to a home care program know what their responsibilities will be, when home care personnel will visit, any modifications of their home that need to be made, and the dates and times of return visits to a health care facility. Be certain that parents have a telephone number that they can call if they have questions about care or their child's condition.

Advantages of Home Care

Although home care of children is not without drawbacks, it has two clear advantages: reduced cost and increased comfort and support.

Reduced Cost

As with adults, in most instances, it is less costly to care for a child at home than in a hospital setting. If the child does not need one-on-one nursing care, home care achieves cost containment. However, cost containment must be weighed against the safety and quality of care. Because not all home settings are safe for care and not all parents have the commitment necessary for home care, it is not an alternative for all families. In addition, although home care is cost-effective for health care agencies, it may not be cost-effective for the family. Costs that health insurance would have paid for, such as dressings and medications, had the child been hospitalized may no longer be covered once the child is transferred to home care.

Comfort and Support

Unlike a child who is separated from family and friends in a hospital facility, a child being taken care of at home has these people nearby. For children who are acutely but not terminally ill, this extra emotional support may not be as immediately important as physical care. For those who are chronically ill or dying, being close to their family and friends may be the most important aspect of their care. For these children, home care is ideal.

Disadvantages of Home Care

There are some disadvantages to home care that make it a poor option for some families. Sometimes the physical care required (for example, tracheal suctioning or a complicated medication regimen) can be overwhelming. The financial strain of at least one parent being needed at home full-time and, therefore, not earning an income, the social isolation this creates for the parent, and the disruption of normal family life are other major disadvantages that can outweigh the benefits of home care.

Assessing the Ill Child in the Home

Nursing assessment of the child at home is similar to assessment of the child in a hospital or other health care facility. Being in the home may actually make it easier to obtain data on the family and family functioning. If an in-depth history or physical examination is necessary, be sure to provide the same level of privacy for the child that he or she would be provided in a clinic or hospital. To do this, it may be necessary to find a room or space that is quiet and free from the distractions of normal family activity.

Often, nursing responsibility includes determining whether a child should be cared for at home. This type of assessment begins with investigation to determine whether the child's condition is compatible with home care as well as whether the family is capable of handling the stress of home care. Ongoing assessment of the suitability of the home environment and overall family functioning is necessary for continued health care. Even though health care providers have initially established that the family is able to provide home care for the child, the situation may change: the child's condition may require more monitoring than originally believed, the demands may be too great for the family to bear, or family composition may change, making a responsible caregiver no longer available. Important aspects to be included in an assessment are described in the following sections.

Identifying the Primary Care Provider

Begin assessment by identifying the child's primary caregiver. Although traditionally this was the mother, in today's families, if a father works more flexible hours, he may be the parent best able to give the bulk of care. In some homes, a grandparent or an older sibling will be the person primarily responsible for care. Arrange to include this person in planning and problem solving because this person knows best what strategy of care will be most effective with the child, as well as what strategy will be most appropriate in light of the physical layout of the home and the family's financial ability and lifestyle.

Determining Knowledge Level of Family

Before a child can be cared for at home, teaching will be required so that the family understands the child's illness and principles of care. A teaching plan for the family should include the things to be learned immediately and additional care measures that will need to be taught as the child's condition changes.

Identifying Available Resources

The term "resources" refers not only to material objects (e.g., hospital bed, portable oxygen, or glucometer) but also to whether family members are able to deal with the chronic stress of fatiguing, around-the-clock nursing care.

Assess physical surroundings, such as: Is there adequate floor space for a hospital bed, oxygen equipment, and so forth? Is a fire company nearby, able to respond in case cardiopulmonary resuscitation (CPR) is needed? Is a power backup resource available to power needed equipment if a blackout should occur? Does the family have a telephone? Could the child be evacuated easily in case of a fire? Does the family have available transport to a health care facility for follow-up care? Table 35-3 lists additional assessments to make, depending on the age of the child.

Determining Current Level of Family Functioning

The family that is supportive of all family members and provides an environment conducive to each member's continued growth and development is more likely to be able to manage home care than a family that has a history of ineffective or destructive coping strategies—that is, a family in which parents have unrealistic expectations of family members, one with a history of abusive relationships, or one that is coping ineffectively with other stressors in their lives. Even a family that appears to be functioning well, however, may be so adversely affected by the stress of home care that its members' ability to be successful with home care is limited. For example, the loss of employment income, resentment over missed promotions, or cramped living space could put the family at risk for ineffective coping. Consider not only the family's current status but also how it will be affected in the future when determining the advisability of home care. Remember that every family operates differently and handles stress in different ways. Events that may seem overwhelming for a visiting health care provider may actually be easy for the family to handle. Conversely, problems that seem minor could be disruptive enough to affect the family's ability to provide adequate care for their child at home (see Focus on Cultural Competence).

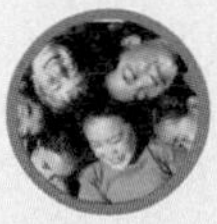

FOCUS ON CULTURAL COMPETENCE

Whether home care is successful or not can be influenced by male–female roles. In a family in which men and women share responsibility, for example, care tasks as well as time away from the stress of home care can be distributed equally. In contrast, in cultures in which the male is dominant and child care is strictly delegated to the woman, women can become exhausted from trying to keep house, prepare meals, care for other children, and give total care to a medically fragile child at the same time.

Evaluating families individually is important to see what the family's usual child-rearing practices are as well as how care is given during illness.

Planning and Implementing Care

Nursing in the community requires a great deal of independent judgment because neither a nursing supervisor nor an attending physician is on the premises to offer advice. It also calls for creativity in adjusting procedures to the confines of a home and the lifestyle of the family. In addition, it requires nurses to be assertive enough to help a family secure adequate funding and resources for home care.

Care at home may include **direct care,** in which a nurse remains in continual attendance or visits frequently and actually administers care, or **indirect care,** in which a nurse plans and supervises care given by others, such as home health care aides or the parents. Nursing care is considered **skilled home care** if it includes physician-prescribed procedures such as dressing changes, admin-

TABLE 35.3 Assessment Criteria for Home Care by Age Group

AGE	POINTS TO ASSESS
All age groups	Are there adequate three-pronged plugs for the care equipment needed? If oxygen will be used, is there a sign to omit smoking in the room? Is the oxygen away from a fireplace, gas space heater, or stove? Does the family know not to light candles near oxygen in a power failure or for a birthday? Is there adequate space for supplies? If a special diet is necessary, does the person who will cook have adequate knowledge of food preparation? Do caregivers know the emergency call system procedure in their community? How to reorder supplies? Has the power company been notified if an electrical appliance is necessary for life support? What would be the caregiver's actions in a power failure? What emergency steps should the caregiver take if the child is suddenly worse? Is there a smoke detector in the child's room?
Infant	Is there a suitable sleeping place? Do side rails of a crib lock securely? Can the infant be heard from the parents' room at night? Is there a functioning refrigerator if formula will be used? Is there protection from mosquitoes? Is the home free of rodents that might attack a small infant?
Toddler and preschooler	Is there a safe area for play free from stairs and poisoning possibilities? Are there screens or locks on windows to prevent child from crawling onto a ledge? Is there provision for stimulation and learning activities?
School-age child and adolescent	What is the provision for schooling (possibly an intercom with a regular classroom or home tutor)? Is peer interaction possible? If adolescent is self-medicating, will reminder sheets or some other reminder system be necessary?

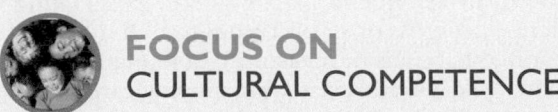

istration of drugs, health teaching, and observation of the client's progress or status through such measures as monitoring vital signs or measuring fluid intake and output. In many instances, classifying nursing care as skilled or not determines whether it will be paid for by third-party reimbursement.

Although home care interventions vary depending on the child's physical condition and stage of illness, nursing interventions such as teaching family members how to give care and encouraging them when they become frustrated remain a priority.

NURSING DIAGNOSES AND RELATED INTERVENTIONS

Nursing Diagnosis: Interrupted family process related to stress of caring for ill child at home

Outcome Identification: Parents will be able to keep family intact and functioning as a unit and successfully manage home care.

Outcome Evaluation: Parents state they feel able to manage home care; family meets weekly to discuss problems and share accomplishments.

Providing a Therapeutic Environment. For home care to be successful, the home must be one that is able to accommodate and adapt to the health care needs of the child. Modifications may be necessary.

Children cared for at home often require a room similar to that provided in a health care agency. Be sure that the house is properly equipped or that medical equipment brought into the home can be accommodated (Fig. 35-7). Hospital beds can be rented from medical supply companies. If a family cannot afford one, they can elevate a house bed on wooden or concrete blocks. Many home mattresses are not firm; a piece of plywood slid under the mattress improves firmness. A cardboard box or additional pillows can be placed under the mattress to elevate the head of a regular bed to a gatch position. Bed trays can be purchased at any department store or made from a heavy cardboard box.

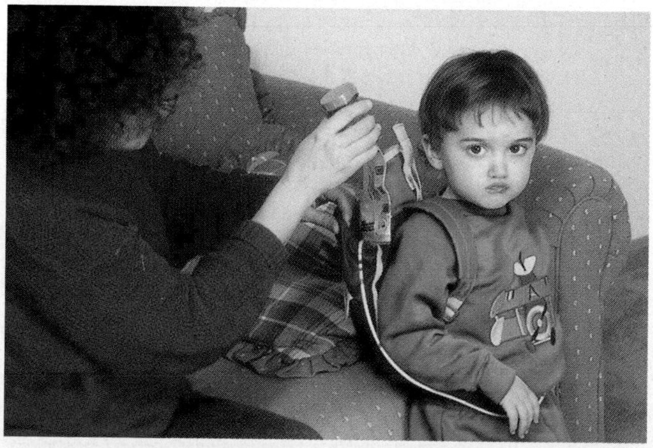

FIGURE 35.7 Procedures at home need to be modified to adjust to the setting. Here a young boy uses a backpack to carry an ambulatory bag for his gastrostomy tube feeding.

If a child is confined to a wheelchair, parents need to consider what adaptations of their home will be necessary. A local carpenter can build a ramp across the house steps to allow wheelchair access. Unless the child will be using a motorized wheelchair, the ramp should have a railing for the child to grasp to pull the chair upward or to stop the wheelchair from moving down too fast; the child then can enter and leave the house independently. Wheelchair lifts or elevators can be purchased and mounted alongside house steps, but they are usually more expensive.

Because it is difficult to move a wheelchair across a high-pile carpet, covering the carpet with plastic is helpful. Throw rugs usually have to be removed lest they become tangled in the wheelchair. Placing furniture along the walls allows increased safe turning space for a wheelchair.

It is impossible to reach high shelves from a wheelchair. To encourage the child to help with meal preparation in the kitchen, urge parents to move supplies that the child will use often, such as boxes of cereal, to a lower cabinet. A pair of tongs can help the child reach supplies in upper cupboards. If the counter is too high to prepare foods, placing a board across the wheelchair arms provides a workspace. If a stove has controls at the back, it is difficult for a person in a wheelchair to use. Caution parents that if the child attempts to reach across a hot burner to reach the controls, he or she could be badly burned. A microwave oven placed on a low table can be a solution that allows a child to warm up meals and prepare snacks independently.

Installing a safety rail by the toilet in the bathroom helps the child to transfer from wheelchair to toilet. A chair placed in the bathtub alongside safety rails allows the child to transfer to the bathtub.

Federal law mandates that all public buildings provide easy access for people in wheelchairs or using walkers. In some towns, buildings may not be equipped this way because no one has ever asked for the service before. Urge parents to contact their city council if a problem exists. Advocate for children if the parents' approach is met with less-than-prompt action so that the child (and other people who use wheelchairs) will have access to facilities such as the public library, zoo, museums, and shopping malls.

Promoting Healthy Family Functioning. Although many families are good candidates for home care, they continue to need helpful advice to adapt constructively to the crisis of illness and home management. The stress and problems that can occur from being responsible for an ill child can lower parents' self-esteem. The time involved can harm their marital relationship or prevent parents from spending time with other children. Physical care requirements can disrupt the normal family routines and shift the focus of attention onto the ill child and away from other children in the family (Fig. 35-8). The needs of the parents may also be neglected (see Focus on Nursing Care Planning).

Help these families by promoting communication and encouraging family members to identify and share their feelings about the new situation at home. Encourage members to voice the frustration they feel at being constantly confined at home or what they perceive to be a lack of progress in their child's condition. If the child has a ter-

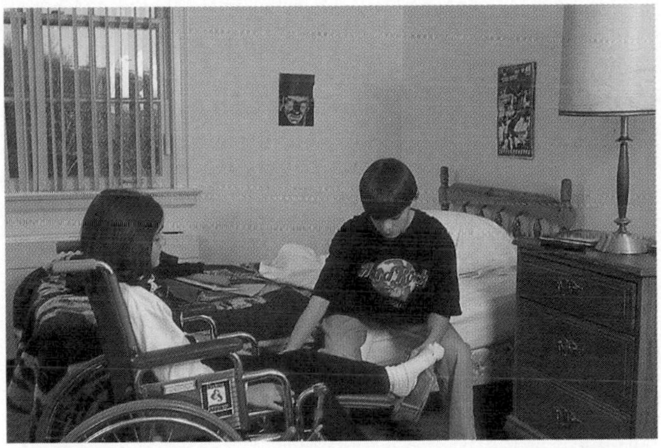

FIGURE 35.8 Home care of a child is family care. Here a brother helps his sister settle into her wheelchair.

minal illness, support parents to express their grief and not grow discouraged, because the work they are accomplishing is making the child comfortable before death. Continued successful coping will require that the family acknowledge and take seriously the impact of home care on each family member and work together to solve identified problems. They may need to renegotiate roles and responsibilities within the family or seek outside help.

When the family is not functioning well at the beginning of home care or does not adjust to the child's illness, nursing measures to support family functioning become even more important. A family whose coping strategies are maladaptive and ineffective may not be able to care for a sick family member at home for long.

> **✔ CHECKPOINT QUESTIONS**
>
> 6. As a rule, is home care more or less cost-effective than hospital care?
> 7. How can you modify a bed at home to make it simulate a gatched bed?

NURSING RESPONSIBILITIES FOR CARE OF THE ILL CHILD AND FAMILY

Nursing responsibilities will vary, naturally, with the type, extent, and seriousness of a child's illness, age, care setting, and individual circumstances. A number of responsibilities, however, such as promotion of normal growth and development, sleep, stimulation, and play, cross all ages and phases of care. Chapter 36 discusses specific responsibilities related to diagnostic tests or interventions. Chapter 38 discusses the important role of promoting comfort in the ill child.

Promoting Growth and Development of the Ill Child

It is easy for children to fall behind in growth and development because of an illness unless health care providers monitor for this.

NURSING DIAGNOSES AND RELATED INTERVENTIONS

Nursing Diagnosis: Risk for delayed growth and development related to effects of illness

Outcome Identification: Child will demonstrate increased growth and development during illness.

Outcome Evaluation: Child, depending on age and stage of development, demonstrates only limited signs of regression to previous stage; is able to continue doing the things he or she most recently accomplished.

Illness represents a crisis event. In a crisis state, children, like adults, are susceptible to change and growth with only the slightest intervention. Without intervention, they are likely to be overwhelmed.

Promoting Growth and Development of the Infant. To promote optimal growth and development, try to change the infant's normal routine as little as possible. This provides security to the child and encourages the development of trust. When admitting an infant to a hospital, ask parents what type of bed the child normally sleeps in. A child who is used to sleeping in a bassinet may feel loose and insecure in a large crib. Such a child should be swaddled in a receiving blanket in a large crib to offer the close, bound feeling of a smaller sleeping area.

Also, attempt to change the infant's diet as little as possible. Unless the child is diagnosed with failure to thrive or is obviously underweight, illness is not an ideal period in which to introduce new foods or formula. Unless their physical condition warrants a change, infants who breastfeed should continue to do so for as many feedings as possible. Expressed breast milk can be given by bottle to the child when the mother is not available. Overall, because infants cannot begin to understand the strange feelings accompanying illness, they need increased swaddling and comforting. As their condition improves, they need to be provided stimulation and play opportunities.

Promoting Growth and Development of the Ill Toddler and Preschooler. Because illness can limit autonomy and prevent children from learning how to do new things, it is important to find opportunities to promote both autonomy in toddlers and initiative in preschoolers. Urge parents to encourage children to make choices about their care whenever possible. For example, coloring in a medication schedule is the kind of task that helps to encourage initiative in a preschooler.

If admitted to the hospital, toddlers and preschoolers who are not used to sleeping in cribs may resent being put in a crib unless the reason is explained to them ("All our beds here have side rails"). Watch toddlers closely to be certain that they do not climb over crib rails to get out of bed. A child who does try may be safer in a bed than a crib.

As with infants, illness is a poor time to change the eating habits of toddlers and preschoolers. Because children of this age insist on self-feeding, they generally do poorly eating in bed and often do better sitting at low tables. Many child-care units in hospitals organize tables for toddlers and preschoolers to eat together. Some children do

(text continues on page 1044)

FOCUS ON *Nursing Care Planning*

A 3-month-old infant receiving continuous mechanical ventilation and intermittent gastrostomy tube feedings is being cared for at home.

CARE OF THE FAMILY WITH A VENTILATOR-DEPENDENT INFANT AT HOME

Assessment: 3-month-old boy delivered at 28 weeks' gestation and diagnosed with respiratory distress syndrome requiring mechanical ventilation. Unable to be weaned from ventilator satisfactorily. Discharged home with continuous mechanical ventilation and intermittent gastrostomy feedings. Height and weight currently at 25th percentile.

Infant lives with parents and 4-year-old sibling. Mother is primary caretaker during the day while father works; father is primary caretaker at night while mother works. Parents demonstrate ability to provide ventilator care and gastrostomy tube feeding and care with minimal assistance. Home care follow-up scheduled three times per week.

During visit today, father was present; stated, "I'm working from home today." Infant was lying in crib. Father demonstrated limited eye contact and difficulty soothing infant when crying.

Mother reports that she and husband are managing adequately at present but voices apprehension at continuing such close health surveillance for an extended time: "It seems like all we do is care for these tubes. We're slaves to these machines." Mother also concerned because she never has time for 4-year-old daughter: "She might as well be an orphan."

Nursing Diagnosis: Caregiver role strain related to continuous care needs of the ill infant and family demands

Outcome Identification: Parents will demonstrate positive adjustment to care of ill infant.

Outcome Evaluation: Parents verbalize frustrations related to caregiving responsibilities; identify sources of support and ways to spend time with each other and older child; develop a plan for help; report an increase in control over the situation.

Interventions	Rationale
1. Explore with the parents their views about their current lifestyle, including work and social responsibilities, parenting, and caregiver obligations.	1. Exploration provides baseline information for identifying the parents' needs, beliefs, and responsibilities and the impact of the child's illness on their life.
2. Allow the parents time to verbalize their feelings, needs, and concerns and discuss the family's plans and goals. Offer realistic feedback.	2. Verbalization of feelings permits a safe outlet for emotions and helps to increase the other person's awareness of the situation. Discussion with realistic feedback promotes sharing and working toward common attainable goals, thus promoting family cohesiveness.
3. Review each parent's daily routine. Investigate any at-home leisure activities and outside social activities.	3. Daily routine provides insight into the situation. Investigation of leisure activities provides additional clues about family functioning.
4. Reinforce with parents their caregiving behaviors thus far in light of the difficulties. Emphasize the positive aspects of the situation and what can be controlled.	4. Positive reinforcement and emphasizing the positive and controllable aspects aid in coping, promote a sense of accomplishment, and enhance self-esteem.
5. Arrange for a home health aide to assist with caregiving and household tasks at least once a week.	5. A home health aide provides additional support for the family and helps to share care responsibilities, thus alleviating some of the burden felt by the parents.

Interventions	Rationale
6. Inform the parents of different services and resources available. Assist them with identifying those that would be most helpful, and initiate referrals as appropriate.	6. Services and resources aid in providing additional support and respite specific to the family's needs.
7. Assist parents with ways to obtain information and support. Encourage parents to respond to offers for help. Role-play possible scenarios.	7. Parents with an ill child often have difficulty asking for and seeking help. Assistance in this area enhances coping and provides much-needed support. Role playing is an effective teaching method.
8. Encourage the parents to give themselves permission to enjoy themselves. Discuss the need for spending time with each other as a couple, time with their older child, and also time as a family.	8. Permission to enjoy themselves and to take time together helps to enhance the couple's relationship and promote health. Allowing time with the older child and as a family promotes the growth and development of all family members.
9. Work with the parents to develop a plan that includes additional time with the older child, such as reading a book or playing a game while the infant is sleeping.	9. The older child needs stimulation for optimal growth and development. Working with the parents promotes active participation and helps turn their focus away from the ill child in a positive way.
10. Discuss ways to assist the older child to adapt to the situation. Include the older child in care of the ill infant and decisions as appropriate. Encourage the parents to maintain routines for the older child as much as possible.	10. Including the child helps promote family cohesiveness and reduces the older child's feelings of being alone and less important. Maintaining routines provides consistency for the older child and helps to minimize the child's exposure to the stress of change.
11. Encourage the parents to call the agency's office with any concerns or questions.	11. Availability of a contact person and phone number provides additional support for the parents.

Nursing Diagnosis: Delayed growth and development related to stress and complexity of the infant's care regimen and inadequate stimulation

Outcome Identification: Infant will exhibit developmentally age-appropriate behaviors.

Outcome Evaluation: Child smiles when spoken to; demonstrates age-appropriate developmental milestones; responds to parents' voices and touch. Parents identify ways to stimulate the ill infant; demonstrate appropriate responses to infant's cues.

Interventions	Rationale
1. Assess the parents' understanding about infant growth and development. Assess the infant for age-appropriate behaviors.	1. Determining the parents' knowledge level provides a foundation for future teaching strategies. Infant assessment provides a baseline for evaluation.
2. Review typical infant growth and development and need for stimulation. Clarify any misconceptions.	2. Reviewing and clarifying aids in learning and strengthening understanding.
3. Encourage the parents to initiate eye-to-eye contact with the infant and touch him gently when providing care.	3. Eye-to-eye contact and touch promote sensory stimulation and development of trust.
4. Recommend the use of a crib mirror or simple mobile.	4. Crib mirror or simple mobile provides visual stimulation. However, too much stimulation can overwhelm the infant.
5. Suggest the use of soft music or voices when the infant is resting or sleeping. If possible, have the parents place the infant's crib as far away from the mechanical ventilator as possible.	5. Soft music or voices promote auditory stimulation while also providing a soothing environment. Too much environmental stimuli, such as from the noise of the ventilator, can overtax the infant, leading to disorganized behaviors.

Interventions	Rationale
6. Encourage the parents to hold and cuddle the infant while performing gastrostomy feedings and to spend some time after the feeding just holding and rocking the infant.	6. Holding, cuddling, and rocking help to develop the infant's sense of trust.
7. Suggest the use of a pacifier if appropriate.	7. Use of a pacifier helps to meet the infant's non-nutritive sucking needs.
8. Monitor the infant's responses to stimulation. Explain to the parents the effects of excessive environmental stress on the infant. Review with them the signs of stress in their infant. Assist them with exposing the infant to one stimulus at a time and interpreting these cues.	8. Infants can become overwhelmed with too many stimuli, increasing their energy expenditure and interfering with their self-regulatory abilities.
9. Instruct the parents in the infant's need for adequate rest and sleep. Work with them to develop a plan of care that includes time for rest, sleep, and stimulation.	9. All infants need sleep for optimal growth and development. The child exposed to the stress of illness and repeated procedures and treatments needs additional rest. Providing a balance of rest and activity minimizes the risk for overwhelming the infant while promoting opportunities for optimal growth and development. Infant rest time also provides the parents with time for rest or other activities.
10. Suggest that the parents include the older child in one aspect of infant stimulation.	10. Including the older child, yet limiting the involvement, allows the child to actively participate, promotes the child's feelings of self-esteem, and helps to enhance the sibling relationship.

well at these tables, but others are too distracted by the activity and the noise and may need a separate low table by their bed to eat well.

Illness is also a poor time to begin toilet-training, even if it is appropriate to the child's age. If the parents have already begun toilet-training, continue it with as normal a routine as possible.

Promoting Growth and Development of the Ill School-Age Child. School-age children need to continue to work on a sense of industry while ill. This means learning more about how and why things are done. Explain to them about specific procedures and involve them as much as possible in planning their care to help foster a sense of industry.

Remember that children who are ill are not at their best and so may not act as mature as usual. This means that a 7-year-old whose parents describe him as very mature may seem to function at the level of a 5-year-old. Children of any age should not be held to their chronologic age when they are ill. In a hospital, school-age children enjoy sharing a room with another child close in age so they can play games together. School-age children do well with competition when they are healthy but often do poorly with competition when they are ill. They may revert to experiences that they would normally dismiss as too young for them.

School-age children and adolescents should continue schooling if they are ill for a long time, provided their condition will allow it. Because it is age-appropriate, ill children do well with school activities or working with a tutor. It is such a normal, everyday activity that it provides security in an otherwise insecure situation. It also reassures them that they are expected to get better and to return to school when this is over.

During the times the child will not be attending school, working on projects such as needlecraft, helping plan family menus, writing for brochures about the place the family plans to visit on vacation next year, and viewing videotapes on science or nature are activities that not only help pass the time but also encourage learning. School-age children also are developing moral responsibility and can find comfort in spiritual practices. Ways to assist with spiritual needs are shown in Table 35-4.

Encourage school-age children to carry out self-care and, if cared for at home, to contribute to the household routines, such as helping with dishes and picking up after themselves, as much as they are able. This not only takes some burden off caregivers but also makes the child feel like an intrinsic part of the family.

Promoting Growth and Development of the Ill Adolescent. The adolescent who is struggling to develop a sense of identity may find it very difficult to be ill because limitations imposed by the illness change the concept of identity. Help adolescents to continue to participate in as many activities as they did before as possible to help them feel that their world is not totally changing. Encourage them to maintain self-care activities and good hygiene practices to help preserve their self-esteem.

Illness can be difficult for adolescents also because peer relationships are so important to them. They may miss being chosen for a school play, a sports team, or competing for a scholarship. A girlfriend or boyfriend may fall in love with somebody else while the adolescent is away.

TABLE 35.4 Nursing Interventions To Meet Children's Spiritual Needs

ACTION	IMPLEMENTATION
Prayers	School-age children may be learning and saying prayers. Ask on hospital admission whether a child says grace with meals or a prayer at bedtime. Write it on the plan of care so that nurses can help with this. Remember that saying grace also applies to unconventional meals, such as a tube feeding. Bedtime prayers may be especially important by lending security in a strange environment.
Religious services	Many children of school age and older enjoy attending a religious service in a hospital chapel. Include time for this in the plan of care and be certain that transportation by wheelchair or cart is available.
Visits from clergy	Many school-age children and adolescents enjoy an active recreation or social program at a church facility when well. They enjoy a visit from clergy when they are ill, not so much for its religious importance as for support from a respected adult. Free the child's time as necessary for such visits.
Religious articles	A child's parent may wish to attach a religious article to the child's clothing or pillow or to post it over the bed. Be careful when changing linen that you do not throw away such articles. Mark their presence and importance on the plan of care.

This makes them feel excluded and hurt. For these reasons, it is important for them to have visitors from their peer group, just as much as infants need visits from parents. For example, giving hospitalized adolescents prepaid telephone cards to use to contact friends is an easy way for them to maintain contact with individuals who are important to them.

Adolescents appreciate being hospitalized in a special adolescent unit or at least in rooms free of childish decor. Hospital units should be organized with the same considerations for visiting parents as other children's units; parents should be able to stay overnight if they and the adolescent wish. Anxiety and pain of separation are not limited to the under-13 set. Because parents often do not remain overnight with them, adolescents appreciate knowing that their parents are concerned about their welfare and that they are getting well. They also enjoy being separated from their parents (assuming everything is going all right).

Often adolescents convey a blasé attitude toward procedures: having radiographs taken is nothing; surgery is a cinch; or a cast change is a snap. Listen carefully to make certain that adolescents really feel this way. They may be trying to convince themselves that a procedure is harmless. Adolescents are extremely worried about their body parts. Make sure they know what is going to happen in surgery and in other departments such as radiology. It is easy to assume from their attitude that they know more than they do.

✔ CHECKPOINT QUESTION

8. How can you promote a sense of trust in the ill infant, a sense of autonomy in the ill toddler, a sense of initiative in the ill preschooler, a sense of industry in the ill school-ager, and a sense of identity in the ill adolescent?

PROMOTING NUTRITIONAL HEALTH OF THE ILL CHILD

Nursing responsibilities related to nutrition for ill children include maintaining optimal nutritional status in the face of illness or treatment that interferes with adequate intake; correcting nutritional deficiencies or otherwise aiding children and families to follow the nutritional care plan devised by the health care team; and educating the child and family regarding specific nutritional needs as well as overall sound nutritional health. Specific procedures for promoting nutrition such as measuring fluid intake and output and providing enteral feedings, gastrostomy tube feedings, and total parenteral nutrition are discussed in Chapter 36.

NURSING DIAGNOSES AND RELATED INTERVENTIONS

Nursing Diagnosis: Risk for imbalanced nutrition, less than body requirements related to lack of appetite

Outcome Identification: Child will continue to follow weight percentile or stay at same weight level throughout illness.

Outcome Evaluation: Child maintains skin turgor and age- and size-determined weight pattern; ingests 80% of prescribed diet daily.

An acute illness in children, such as pneumonia, is often accompanied by a loss of appetite; gastrointestinal illnesses often cause nausea and vomiting. Because most acute illnesses last only a few days, there is no need for children to eat more than a small amount during this time as long as they can drink fluid. Trying to force them to eat only increases nausea and vomiting, which increases the possibility of creating an electrolyte imbalance. When an illness lasts for more than a few days, however, providing adequate nutrition becomes increasingly important because children need nutrients not only to repair ill or diseased tissue but also to maintain normal childhood growth.

Important points to address when planning nutrition for ill children are summarized in Table 35-5. Children who are hospitalized often tolerate hospital-prepared food, which can be repetitious and bland, better than adults do. Provided that it is the kind of food they like, such as hot dogs and hamburgers, it appeals to children more than the elaborate dishes with spices and sauces preferred by adults. Children

TABLE 35.5 Areas to Consider When Planning Nutrition for Ill Children

AREA	IMPORTANCE
Meaning of food	Early in life, infants learn to associate eating with being held and loved; if they cannot eat for some reason (e.g., nothing by mouth for surgery), they may view the restriction as punishment or restriction of love.
Opportunity for socialization	Mealtime is often a time of the day when children socialize with other family members; they may feel lonely eating alone and consequently may have a poor appetite.
Level of stress	Children under stress may either feel a loss of appetite or experience a need to snack frequently; planning is necessary to see that children maintain adequate intake if not hungry and that their snacks are nutritious.
Custom	Custom is important: for example, many children like foods served separately and resist eating them if mixed into a casserole.
Culture	Most children eat best foods with which they are familiar; in many instances, parents can bring in favorite foods from home to provide culturally preferred items.
Environment	Hunger is associated with the sight and sounds of food; many children are normally in the kitchen while meals are being prepared; they may not be hungry when food is served to them without their having seen and smelled it being prepared.

who are receiving care at home need as much nursing supervision of their diet as those in health care agencies do (possibly more) because they may not have a dietitian planning meals to ensure adequate nutrition. Assess not only the quantity but also the quality of food to ensure that intake is optimal.

Encouraging Fluid Intake. Increasing oral fluid intake has traditionally been termed "forcing fluid." It is better to avoid this term with children, though, because they can interpret the instruction to mean someone is physically about to force them to swallow fluid. A physician's order should state in detail the amount of fluid a child is to receive during 24 hours, because the amount differs so much for different ages. The following are some practical guidelines for encouraging fluid intake:

- Offer small, full glasses frequently rather than half-full larger glasses; children are mid-school age before they evaluate the amount of fluid in a container rather than the size of the container.
- Determine the child's favorite fluid, and then offer it.
- Try changes of temperature in fluid offered (hot cocoa, then cold juice, then hot soup) for variety. Broth can be a nice change of liquid (many commercial types are quick to prepare, but be aware of their high sodium content).
- Keep in mind that popsicles and Jello are fluids (Fig. 35-9).
- Know that children can drink more of a clear fluid (ginger ale, water) than a thicker fluid (milk shakes or cream soups), because thicker fluids are absorbed from the stomach more slowly.
- Use soothing beverages such as Kool-Aid, Snapple, or milk for children with mouth lesions. They may be unable to drink fruit juices because the acid content stings their mouths; carbonated beverages may also cause discomfort.
- Because ice melts to one-half its volume, count a glass of ice chips as only a half-full glass of fluid.
- Unless contraindicated, let children drink fluids with a straw; this is a novelty to many who do not normally use these and encourages intake.
- Introduce a game, such as "Simon Says" (Simon says, "Drink") or one in which a child takes turns and with each turn takes a drink.

Encouraging Food Intake. **Calorie counting,** as the name implies, involves counting the number of calories that children ingest in 1 day. To do this, list all the foods that a child eats during each 24-hour period, being certain to include snacks, candy, or gum. A dietitian then will analyze the list and determine the caloric intake. Be certain that you describe the types of food and amounts (not "some toast," but "half a slice of whole wheat toast"). Be sure that everyone caring for the child is aware that

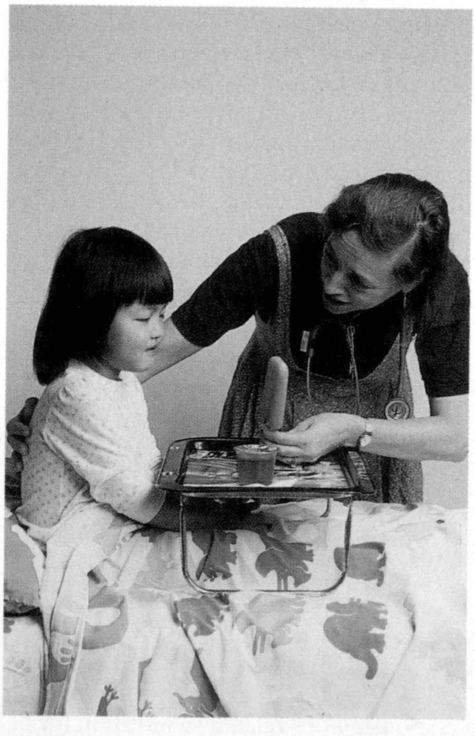

FIGURE 35.9 The nurse offers this young child a popsicle, which is a good source of fluid.

calories are being counted so that they also record this information accurately.

PROMOTING SAFETY FOR THE ILL CHILD

A prime consideration of nursing interventions is to keep the child safe during illness care.

NURSING DIAGNOSES AND RELATED INTERVENTIONS

Nursing Diagnosis: Risk for injury related to procedures or therapy necessary for care

Outcome Identification: The child will not sustain any injury or accident during illness.

Outcome Evaluation: Child remains free of injuries and accidents, such as a fall from bed or injury from medical equipment.

Promoting safety for children is a responsibility for all health care providers. Care of the ill or physically challenged child at home includes assessing the safety of the house and providing family teaching. It also includes making provisions for emergencies. For example, a family may need to install a counter-level telephone so a child in a wheelchair can call for emergency help. They might need to make a plan for how to evacuate the ill child in an emergency. Safety on a children's unit or clinic is the responsibility of everyone, from the administrator of the institution to part-time health care personnel. To make the child health care environment a safer place, follow these steps:

- Always be sure of the location of all children in your care.
- Ensure that doors or gates are provided near stairways or elevators.
- Ensure that back doors of health care facilities have working alarms to prevent children from going out and strangers from coming in.
- Be sure that windows are covered by screens or guards so that children cannot climb up on sills and fall out.
- Check that side rails of beds and cribs are in good repair and raised appropriately.
- Always raise bedside rails after a child has received preoperative or sedative medication.
- Test a crib rail after it is raised to ensure that the lock has caught and that the rail will remain raised.
- Push bedside tables or stands away from cribs so that a child cannot climb over the railing and use the stand as a step down.
- Be sure that crib caps are provided for small children to prevent them from climbing out of bed.
- Fasten the seat belt restraint for infants in high chairs. Never leave an infant in a high chair (at home or in a hospital) without someone close enough to reach the child if he or she should fall from the chair.
- Ensure that electrical cords or appliances such as electric hair dryers are not used in bathrooms, where they will come in contact with water.
- Be careful of the placement of TV/call cords or venetian blind cords so they cannot lead to strangulation.
- Never leave children younger than 5 years alone in a bathtub because they can turn on the hot water and scald themselves or slip under the water and drown.
- Never leave equipment or items that would be harmful to eat within the reach of children.
- Adhere to all fire precaution measures.
- Closely follow standard precautions to prevent the spread of infections.

Promoting Fire Safety. Fire precautions both in the home and in the hospital unit are essential in preserving the safety of ill or disabled children. Adults can usually take responsibility for removing themselves from a burning structure; children depend on care providers. Ensure that there is a plan of action in case of a fire and that everyone in the home, in the clinic, or on the unit knows it. To be certain a home is safe, a smoke detector on each floor is a wise precaution. A downstairs bedroom is not only safest in case of a fire but also allows the child more self-care ability. Fire departments supply free decals for the bedroom windows of children or those who are physically challenged. Encourage parents to contact their local fire departments for this safety measure.

Electrical equipment such as respiratory and cardiac monitors, radiant heat warmers, special-care equipment, and even electrical thermometers are often used in the care of children. Do not use equipment with frayed cords or equipment that is not properly grounded. Plugs should be three-pronged for extra safety; do not overload circuits with additional plugs. Electrical outlets should have safety caps to cover them when they are not in use so that toddlers cannot poke objects into them and electrocute themselves.

Adhering to Standard Precautions. In every health care setting, closely follow standard precautions to protect the ill child, family, and staff from infections. Because of a compromised immune system, ill children may be more susceptible to repeat or secondary infections than usual. Proper handwashing techniques, disposal of tissues and waste materials, and efforts to minimize exposure to other ill children or adults are all effective methods to decrease the risk of infection. For more details, see Chapter 43.

> ✔ **CHECKPOINT QUESTIONS**
>
> 9. Do young children accept large or smaller glasses of fluid better?
> 10. What measures should be taken to ensure that a hospital crib is safe?

PROMOTING ADEQUATE SLEEP FOR THE ILL CHILD

Ill children need adequate rest and sleep so that their body tissues can effectively use nutrients for repair, and normal growth can continue. Children may not sleep well when they are ill because of discomfort, pain, administration of medications, or intensified symptoms of chronic sleep problems. They may not sleep well in a hospital because it is a strange setting; they may have to undergo so many procedures that they do not nap or rest as much as usual. Children who are recovering from trauma such as injuries from a car accident or burns may be unable to sleep for fear the accident will happen again. They may suffer sleep deprivation in the same way as a child who is frequently awakened for procedures during the night. Encourage parents to stay with these children for support and comfort.

Sleep Patterns

Sleep is influenced by anxiety level, state of health, habit, medication, and environment at the time of sleep. Stages of sleep are summarized in Table 35-6. Figure 35-10*A* shows the pattern of normal sleep. As a sleep cycle begins, a child first enters **nonrapid eye movement (NREM) sleep.** This type of sleep occurs in up to 80% of total sleep time. As a child falls deeper and deeper asleep, he or she passes from stage I to stages II, III, and IV of NREM sleep over a period of 20 to 30 minutes. **Rapid eye movement (REM) sleep** follows. In infants, most of sleep time is REM sleep, whereas young adults have the least. The sleep pattern of a child who is awakened frequently during the night for procedures would resemble that shown in Figure 35-10*B*.

The purpose of NREM sleep is rest and restoration of the body; it keeps body cells functioning and healthy. During the periods of stage III and IV NREM sleep, the secretion of growth hormone (somatotropic hormone) from the pituitary is at its highest level. Growth hormone is necessary for protein synthesis and growth of new cells and for repair and maintenance of all cells. Corticosteroids and adrenaline from the adrenal gland, which are instrumental in the catabolism or breakdown of cells, are at their lowest levels. This balance of hormones is the ideal combination for protein synthesis and cell growth and repair.

The purpose of REM sleep is less clear. The rapid eye movements may serve to coordinate binocular vision. Dreams that occur during this time apparently serve as a release of tension or help to integrate new knowledge and experience with old in the brain's memory system. During REM sleep, vital signs rise to near-normal levels. These periods of REM sleep interspersed with NREM sleep may be a fail-safe measure to prevent vital signs from falling too low during sleep.

Sleep Deprivation

Children who do not receive enough sleep can suffer **sleep deprivation** just as adults do. After approximately 4 days of poor sleep, they show difficulty in concentrating and experience episodes of disorientation and misperception. They are generally irritable and can manifest feelings of persecution and marked physical fatigue.

If the sleep loss is mainly REM deprivation, children mainly show symptoms of irritability and difficulty concentrating. Lack of stage IV NREM sleep tends to cause apathy and depression and can slow recovery. This is the same phenomenon that can happen in adolescents if they are studying for exams, or in younger children during illness if they are awakened frequently for treatments.

TABLE 35.6 Stages of Sleep in Children

STAGE	DESCRIPTION	NURSING IMPLICATIONS
NREM		
I	A feeling of drifting or falling. Often described as twilight sleep. Temperature and heart rate decrease slightly; EEG waves show peaked, frequent waves (alpha waves).	A child can be roused easily from this early sleep by the slightest noise or even the silent presence of another person in the room. Reduce noise level in room to promote sleep.
II	Sleep deepens. Temperature and heart rate decrease slightly more.	It is more difficult to wake a child from sleep when this point has been reached
III	Sleep deepens still further. An EEG tracing reveals mixed spindle and delta (slow) waves. Temperature and heart rate decrease further. This period lasts about 10 min.	It is very difficult to wake a child from stage III sleep. Use patience to wake a child fully to offer medicine.
IV	Approximately 20 to 30 min after beginning to fall asleep, a child enters stage IV sleep. Respirations are slow and deep, temperature and heart rate slow even more, and blood pressure decreases; EEG shows delta (slow, steady) waves. A child remains at a stage IV sleep level for approximately 30 min, then progresses back through stages III and II until he or she then passes into a phase of REM sleep.	A child will be confused and unable to orient himself/herself readily if awakened from stage IV sleep. Use patience until a child is fully awake, particularly if asking a question.
REM	Eyes move in rapid, involuntary motions. Respirations are irregular; body turnings, movements, and penile erections may occur. Lasts 10 to 30 min and then a new sleep cycle with NREM sleep begins.	Dreaming occurs during REM sleep. Although the child appears to be close to waking because of the active eye movements, he or she is really very soundly asleep. A child may wake afraid and crying, disturbed by a frightening dream.

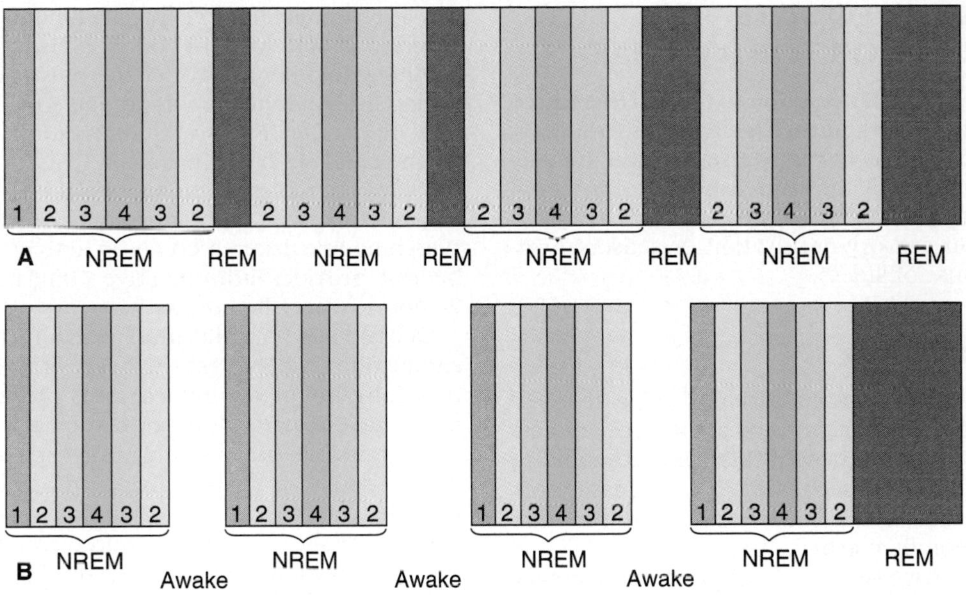

FIGURE 35.10 Sleep patterns. (*A*) Normal sleep pattern. Notice how the periods of REM sleep increase in length during the last half of the night. (*B*) The sleep pattern of a child who has been awakened frequently during the night. Notice how little REM sleep is present.

NURSING DIAGNOSES AND RELATED INTERVENTIONS

Nursing Diagnosis: Disturbed sleep pattern related to timing of medication, discomfort, or sleep disorder

Outcome Identification: Child will maintain regular sleep pattern during illness.

Outcome Evaluation: Child sleeps through the night without interruption (when therapeutic regimen allows); is alert and active during the day; is able to take nap during the day if that is part of usual sleep schedule.

Because sleep is important for ill children, parents and health care providers need to take some special steps to ensure that children are able to sleep during an illness. Being certain that children are free of pain and worry is key. Measures such as maintaining a usual routine (bath, changing to nightclothes, nighttime story, prayers) are also important. Providing an atmosphere conducive to sleep (lights out, quiet surroundings, reassuring support people) is also helpful. Children who are bored with bedrest may catnap constantly during the day and then be wide awake at night. Providing more interesting activities for them during the day can help.

Managing Chronic Sleep Problems. Some children may have chronic sleep problems such as night terrors, nocturnal enuresis, somnambulism (sleepwalking), sleep talking, and sleep apnea. These sleep problems may intensify with illness and increase sleep deprivation in ill children.

Somnambulism is a common sleep problem in children. It apparently occurs during NREM sleep, probably during the deepest part of stage IV. It is frightening for children to wake and realize that they have been sleepwalking. They are confused because they are waking from such a deep stage of sleep. Sleepwalking can be especially dangerous when a child is ill because, while getting out of bed, the child could dislodge intravenous tubing or oxygen equipment. It is untrue that sleepwalkers should not be wakened; instead, wake them gently, help them get reoriented, and then return them to bed after being reassured that they are safe. Be certain that side rails are raised on the bed of a child who tends to sleepwalk. In a hospital, it may be necessary to move a child's bed out into the hallway at night near the nurse's desk if a parent will not be sleeping over, so the child can be observed for sleepwalking.

Sleeptalking seems to occur during REM sleep. Dreaming of some frightening or puzzling situation, a child calls out a name or instruction such as, "Stop!" Because illness is a stressful situation that increases anxiety, sleeptalking may occur at an increased rate during this time. It is unnecessary to wake a child who is sleeptalking unless the child is thrashing about and would dislodge equipment such as intravenous tubing. Because sleeptalking usually results from a frightening dream, waking the child gently, however, is comforting. Parents may need to be assured that sleeptalking is harmless and will probably subside when their child is well again.

Some children are prone to night terrors, or wake screaming approximately 20 minutes after they fall asleep. The condition tends to be familial. Waking them and comforting them helps everyone in the house return to sleep. In the morning, children rarely remember the incident.

Sleep apnea is the cessation of respirations during sleep for 20 seconds or more. It tends to occur more frequently in obese children. It is a possible cause of sudden infant death syndrome (see Chap. 40). Infants who are diagnosed with this condition are prescribed respiratory monitors to evaluate their breathing pattern and warn against any cessation of respirations.

PROMOTING ADEQUATE STIMULATION FOR THE ILL CHILD

Children are in constant interaction with both their internal environment (body) and their external environment (surroundings) by means of the five senses and the central nervous system. Thus, they can respond to changes in environment and by so doing meet basic needs. They can experience either sensory deprivation or sensory overstimulation because of illness.

Sensory Deprivation

Sensory deprivation is the condition of being deprived of, or lacking, adequate sensory, social, physical, or cognitive stimulation. Children with this condition tend to lose the ability to make decisions and become easily confused and depressed. Some children are more prone to sensory deprivation than others.

Ill children may have sensory deprivation because they are confined to their homes or hospital rooms and their varied activities such as school, sports, and clubs are replaced with hours of watching television or playing video games. Parental interaction may be compromised because of the stress of illness or separation imposed by hospitalization. When parental interaction is poor, children generally receive less-than-normal cognitive stimulation. Such children need a warm, reassuring relationship with health care personnel and cognitive stimulation to develop normally.

Children with hearing or visual deficits are prone to sensory deprivation. Children with forms of sensory nerve loss or who are receiving chemotherapy may lose their sense of touch, taste, or proprioception (sense of where they are in space). After losing these forms of perception, children may also draw back from interacting with other people because they are self-conscious about the loss, and thus they may be deprived of social and cognitive stimulation. Techniques for interacting with sensory-deprived children are discussed in Chapter 50.

Some children receive medication to lessen awareness of the stimulating factors in their environment. To ensure that they do not suffer sensory deprivation, give them definite orientation measures, such as always mentioning the time of day and the day of the week in conversations with them. At the same time, they often must have overly stimulating factors reduced, such as the number of visitors, so that perceptions can be interpreted clearly.

NURSING DIAGNOSES AND RELATED INTERVENTIONS

Nursing Diagnosis: Deficient diversional activity related to lack of appropriate toys and peers

Outcome Identification: Child will receive age-appropriate stimulation while ill.

Outcome Evaluation: Child demonstrates alert and interested attitude toward self-care and play activities.

Providing Stimulation for Children on Bedrest. Children on bedrest are unable to secure materials for cognitive stimulation by themselves or to participate in physical stimulation, except to a limited degree. A room where walls and windows offer no visual appeal and therapeutic equipment provides the only sound offers them little sensory stimulation. If no one comes into the room, they may suffer from social deprivation. When possible, let the child sit in a wheelchair. This will provide some mobility and transportation to a place of interest, such as near a window or, in the hospital, near the nursing desk. Watching television, a common activity for children on bedrest, provides little cognitive stimulation after the first 24 hours, when the novelty has worn off.

Occasionally, a child must remain in bed to reduce stimulation (e.g., to rest the heart or to increase kidney function), but generally bedrest is prescribed mainly to inactivate one part of the body, such as a fractured bone. When possible, other stimulation, such as a favorite toy, games, books, or simply talking with someone, must be provided for the child to maintain physical bedrest; otherwise, he or she will become bored and irritable and will thrash and turn instead of lying still (Fig. 35-11).

If the child's bedroom is away from the main home activities, encourage family members to include the ill child in as many family activities as possible—bring the television set into the child's bedroom so the entire family gathers there, or set up a card table in the room so everyone can eat there—or encourage the child to join the rest of the family for activities by resting on the couch in the living room, a lounge chair in the backyard, or sitting in the kitchen. This principle applies to hospitalized children as well. To more easily interact, a toddler may rest in a parent's lap rather than in a bed.

Providing Stimulation for Children on Transmission-Based Precautions. Children who are placed on transmission-based precautions because of the possibility of contagious illness may experience severe sensory deprivation if everyone who enters the room must wear a gown and mask or if the number of visitors is kept to a minimum. If gloves are part of precautions, the child can experience a significant loss of skin-to-skin contact. Transmission-based precautions are discussed in Chapter 43. Careful planning must be done to ensure that a child who is isolated this way is not psychologically isolated and that

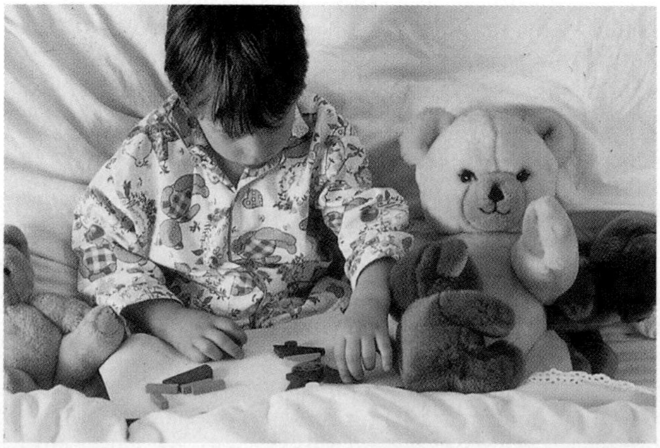

FIGURE 35.11 Children on bedrest need stimulation. Here, a young child enjoys putting together a puzzle.

every possible measure is performed to maintain sensory, social, physical, and cognitive stimulation. For example, try to visit with a child at times in addition to those times in which procedures are performed; place the bed so the child can see out of the room; encourage him or her to telephone friends; make posters for walls; and encourage interactive play such as electronic games. For ideas on providing stimulation to children in specific age groups, refer to Chapters 28 to 32.

Sensory Overload

Sensory overload, in contrast to deprivation, occurs when a child receives more stimulation than he or she can tolerate or process. Children with sensory overload react similarly to those with sensory deprivation (i.e., they are confused, unable to make decisions, and severely fatigued). Sometimes it is difficult to determine the cause of these symptoms (whether they are caused by sensory deprivation or overload) unless assessed carefully.

The lights in intensive care units (ICUs), for example, are never turned out. Although children may find this comforting, excessive stimulation also may result. In addition to constant light, there is excessive sound (e.g., whir of machines, buzzing of ventilators, ringing of alarms, or mix of voices in consultation). Most ICUs have no windows because the wall space is used for monitoring equipment; therefore, night and day are not easily distinguished. It is easy for a child to become confused about time and place in such a setting. For children who are cared for at home, for example, in a family room where people talk constantly, the television is always on, and activity never ceases, sensory overload may also occur. An important nursing role is reducing sensory stimulation attributable to overload. Orient children to the time of day by making frequent references to it and by providing calendars and clocks. If necessary, provide eye covers or ear plugs to reduce stimulation.

✔ CHECKPOINT QUESTIONS

11. During what stage of sleep does sleepwalking occur?
12. What are symptoms of sensory deprivation?

PROMOTING PLAY FOR THE ILL CHILD

Play, often described as the work of children, is an invaluable component of child health care. Providing a space and opportunity for play can help a child feel more comfortable and allow for an important release of energy for a child who is confined to a room or bed. Play also may be used to help assess a child's level of knowledge and feelings about his or her condition so that more individualized nursing care can be planned. Depending on the child's age, play can also be a useful tool in health teaching (see Chap. 34).

Defining play is not a simple task, because play activities vary greatly from child to child and among different age, cultural, and socioeconomic groups (see Focus on Cultural Competence). A common definition is that play is any voluntary activity engaged in for the purpose of enjoyment. If a child views an activity as enjoyment, therefore, no matter what it is and whether it would be fun or not for an adult, it is play.

FOCUS ON CULTURAL COMPETENCE

Although play is a universal activity of children, not all parents realize how important it is to children. Also, play activities vary greatly depending on cultural and socioeconomic circumstances. However, more and more parents are becoming aware of the value of reading to young children, and many bring favorite books to the hospital along with games and teddy bears. Encourage parents also to bring toys that a young child can manipulate independently to encourage independent play time or to allow parents the time to talk with the child's health care team about progress.

When a child does not understand English and that is the language of health care providers, games such as stacking blocks or building with Tinkertoys can be played despite communication difficulty. Playing tapes or records of well-loved children's songs can also be effective, because the child doesn't need to be able to understand the words to enjoy the music or clap with the rhythm.

Play is clearly the means by which children develop increasing cognitive, psychomotor, and social capabilities. Touching a soft rabbit, passing colored blocks from one hand to the other, pounding with a plastic hammer, feeding a doll, and playing board games are all ways in which children are exposed to and learn about different textures and colors, experience the feeling of possessing and owning, and learn about competition, winning, and losing. A soft toy tells the child more clearly than can be described that this is what the word "soft" means. Colored blocks show him or her how parts can join to make a whole, how things stacked too high will fall (there are limits one cannot go beyond), and that practice makes perfect. As the child talks with playmates during play, he or she develops both language and social skills. The repetitive acts involved in most games encourage the development of musculoskeletal skills. Play is not something a child does when he or she has nothing else to do; it is something the child *has* to do. During illness, it provides a feeling of security because it is an activity that has continuity with everyday life.

The manner in which children play differs as they mature. Types of play and the age groups in which these types are seen most frequently are shown in Focus on Family Empowerment.

Assessing Child Health Through Play

Children who are acutely ill do not play or play very little. They do not have the strength, the attention span, or the interest in activities that are required for play. They con-

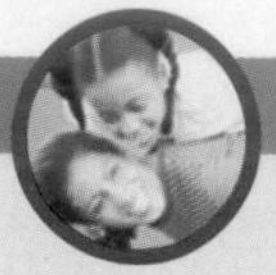

FOCUS ON FAMILY EMPOWERMENT
Understanding Different Play Types

Q. My child doesn't like toys as much as the boxes they come in. What's normal for children and play?

A. Children play differently at different ages. Examples of typical play patterns include:

TYPE OF PLAY/AGE	DESCRIPTION	EXAMPLE
Observation/Infant	Child watches particular play intently, although not actively engaged in it.	Watching a mobile
Parallel/Toddler	Two children play side by side but seldom attempt to interact with each other.	Playing separately with similar push toy
Associative/Preschooler	Children play together in a similar activity; there is little organization of responsibilities	Engaging in typical backyard play
Cooperative/School-age	Children play with an organized structure or compete for desired goal or outcome.	Playing organized games with rules

tinue, however, to enjoy being read to, and they find comfort in holding a favorite toy even if they do not actively manipulate it. Once children are over the acute phase of an illness, interest in play usually returns. Whether a child is spontaneously playing, then, is a good index of health. The toys a child uses at play are a good indication of his or her growth and development level and emotional state.

The average parent knows a child's play preferences and his or her current favorite game or toy. Asking for this information helps to assess the child's developmental level and whether it is age-appropriate. It also helps to assess the quality of parenting (if parents view play as important or are familiar with the child's activities).

Providing Play in Ambulatory Settings

Children in ambulatory departments are under a great deal of stress. They sit in a waiting room and glance fearfully at the door that leads to the examining room. They hear children crying beyond the door and wait in terror for what lies in store for them when it is their turn.

Most parents know that when their child is coming to a hospital to be admitted, they should pack the child's favorite toy. Often they do not think of an ambulatory visit as a sufficiently threatening circumstance to warrant bringing a favorite toy, however, so the child has nothing to play with. Having a parent sit beside them is so comforting that they may ignore or hesitate moving 4 feet away to get toys furnished by the health care facility unless they are urged to do so.

Ambulatory departments should be stocked with toys that can be played with quickly and by single children. The departments should have low tables and chairs so that a parent can come to a table to play with a child. Examining rooms should have toys also—they may be needed to distract a child while a procedure such as an ear examination is performed, and because the wait in an examining room may be as long as the wait in a waiting room. Well siblings who accompany a parent and sick child to the facility should have toys to distract them as well so that the parent can concentrate on the ailing child. Some hospitals furnish computer games for older children for this reason. Specific examples of ways that play can be used in an ambulatory care setting are shown in Table 35-7.

Providing Play in the Hospital

Ideally, all hospital units in which children are cared for should have play space big enough for most of the children on the unit. There should be enough space to accommodate children who are not fully ambulatory, such as

TABLE 35.7 Ways to Incorporate Play Into Ambulatory Nursing Care

NURSING CARE	PLAY ACTIVITY
Aid with physical assessment	Distract child's attention with puppet during respiratory and cardiac assessment.
	Play "Simon Says" to encourage child to take deep breaths for respiratory assessment.
	Allow child to listen to own heart with stethoscope.
	Play "Follow the Leader" to assess gait.
	Draw a face on the tongue blade used to assess throat.
	Show child how to "blow out" the otoscope light.
	Draw child's outline on the table examining paper and give it to him or her to take home to color.
Health teaching	Use puppets as teacher.
	Create word scrambles or crossword puzzles.

those with casts or wheelchairs (Fig. 35-12). Tables for board games and play materials such as crayons and paints should be available. Children can release a great deal of anger or tension by splashing water, squeezing or pouring sand, or smearing finger paint.

Provide school-age children with a game such as shuffleboard or sand bags to toss for tension relief and competition. Adolescents enjoy table tennis and pool tables. A great deal of "play" in older school-age children and adolescents centers around conversation with peers.

Children who are hospitalized for 1 week or more may enjoy putting on a puppet show or playing school, store, or house. A corner of a playroom should be devoted to this kind of imaginative play: a structure that will serve as a store front, puppet stage, house, or school, and dolls, cribs, empty food boxes and cans, and puppets should be provided. Large blocks, 6 × 12 inches, are available for playrooms so that such structures can be built and rebuilt each day. For ill children, the blocks must be made of cardboard, not wood, because ill children tire easily when lifting heavier wood blocks. Table 35-8 lists games that require no equipment other than that readily available on a nursing unit for children who have brought nothing of their own to play with or who have grown bored with existing games.

Providing play equipment and supervision for a recreational play program in most instances is economically feasible through donations and volunteers. Generally toys for a playroom can be secured through donations from clubs in the community. For safety reasons, children need to be supervised while they play. Because they do not feel well in a hospital or are shy in these different surroundings, they usually enjoy having a concerned adult to watch over them and suggest new activities. Such adults may be volunteers. Supervision is an excellent after-school activity for members of a future nurses' association. Ideally, child life or play specialists fill such roles.

If play supervisors are unavailable through other sources, the nursing staff must free such personnel as necessary to lead play activities. This shows that play is important—for example, that supervising finger painting is as important a duty for assistive personnel as straightening beds, or that organizing a puppet show for long-term clients is as important as giving a bed bath. A clear sign that the nurses on a particular children's unit understand little about their young patients' needs is a locked playroom door and the explanation, "We have no one to staff it."

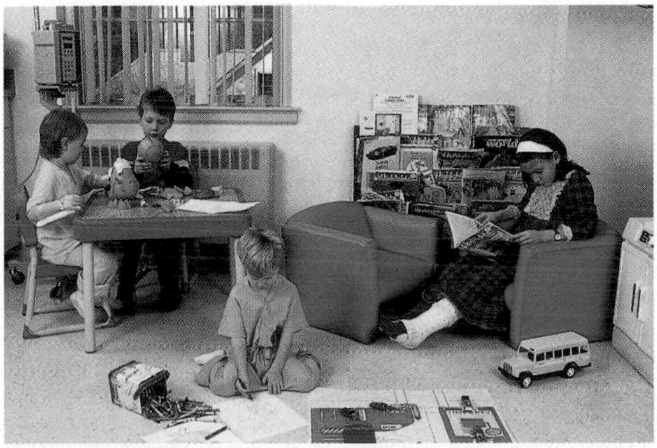

FIGURE 35.12 Children enjoying themselves in a hospital playroom, which is spacious and well equipped with age-appropriate toys and activities.

Providing Play for Children on Bedrest

Children who are on bedrest, at home or in a hospital, need to have play periods built into their day. The length of time for play and the toys individual children can play with depend on their age and physical and emotional states. Play activities for children on bedrest are shown in Table 35-9.

Infants need toys in their cribs, such as mobiles, blocks, soft toys, and rattles. They also need to be out of cribs, sitting on a parent's or a nurse's lap, or sitting in strollers or swings. As soon as they are able, they need some time on the floor (with a sheet under them) to practice crawling or walking. At age 3 months, when an infant discovers the hands, those are his or her "toys." For a child learning to crawl or "cruise" or walk, that activity is his or her toy or interest for the month.

Toddlers need put-in and take-out types of toys such as blocks that can be repeatedly dropped into a bottle or that can be stacked to play with in bed. They enjoy listening to tapes of songs and nursery rhymes. Toddlers are in constant motion. They need to be out of bed as much as their physical condition allows, playing with take-apart, put-together, or pull-and-push toys. Preschoolers need creative materials such as modeling clay or sand. School-age children need quiet games such as books or crayons or markers by their bedside. While in bed, they enjoy radios, compact disk players, or tapes. Most activities for hospitalized children must be short-term projects because children are called away for treatments or procedures, and because when they are ill their attention span is shorter than usual. Short-term projects always appeal to the school-age child because they help this age child achieve a sense of industry.

Television watching is a nonparticipant activity, so it is not the best activity for children. Watching favorite tapes on a VCR is better. There is some value in watching nature programs or "after-school specials" on television that depict school-age children in real-life situations coping with problems common to many of their peers. Encouraging parents or friends to watch a game show with a school-age child and help the child guess the solution to a puzzle or watch "Sesame Street" with a preschooler makes the activity a participatory one. Watching a soap opera with an adolescent and then discussing the people and their problems can also turn television watching into active participation.

Safety With Play

Be certain to screen all toys for safety. They should be washable, with no sharp edges and no small parts that could be swallowed or aspirated. A cylinder 1 inch in diameter, such as a rubber hot dog, is the most dangerous size for a toy because it totally occludes the trachea if it is aspirated. A toy smaller than this would cause only partial

TABLE 35.8 Games and Activities Using Materials Available on a Nursing Unit

AGE	ACTIVITY
Infant	Make a mobile from roller gauze and tongue blades to hang over a crib. Ask the pharmacy or central supply for different-size boxes to use for put-in, take-out toys. (Do not use round vials from pharmacy; if accidentally aspirated, these can completely occlude the airway.) Blow up a glove as a balloon; draw a smiling face on it with a marker. Hang it out of infant's reach. Play "patty cake," "so big," "peek-a-boo."
Toddler	Ask central supply for boxes to use as blocks for stacking. Tie roller gauze to a glove box for a pull toy. Sing or recite familiar nursery rhymes such as "Peter, Peter, Pumpkin Eater."
Preschool	Play "Simon says" or "Mother, may I?" Draw a picture of a dog; ask child to close eyes; add an additional feature to the dog; ask child to guess the added part, repeat until a full picture is drawn. Make a puppet from a lunch bag or draw a face on your hand with a marker. Cut out a picture from a newspaper or a magazine (or draw a picture); cut it into large puzzle pieces. Pour breakfast cereal into a basin; furnish boxes to pour and spoons to dig. Furnish chart paper and a magic marker for coloring. Make modeling clay from 1 cup salt, ½ cup flour, ½ cup water from diet kitchen. Play "Ring-Around-the-Rosey" or "London Bridge."
School-age	Play "I Spy" or charades. Make a deck of cards to play "Go Fish" or "Old Maid"; invent cards such as Nicholas Nurse, Doctor Dolittle, Irene Intern, Polly Patient. Play "Hangman." Furnish scale or table paper and a marker for a huge drawing or sign. Hide an object in the child's room and have the child look for it (have the child name places for you to look if the child cannot be out of bed).
Adolescent	Color squares on a chart form to make a checker board. Have adolescent make a deck of cards to use for "Hearts" or "Rummy." Compete to see how many words the adolescent can make from the letters in his or her name. Compete to guess whether the next person to enter the room will be a man or woman, next car to go by window will be red or black, and so forth. Compete to see who can name the most episodes of "Star Trek" or "The Brady Bunch."

obstruction; something larger could not be inhaled into the trachea. As a rule, if a toy can fit through the center of a toilet tissue tube, it is too small.

Be certain that toys offered will not lead children into danger. Tossing a ball to a toddler on bedrest is generally a safe activity. One who has a large cast in place, however, might lean over to retrieve a dropped ball and fall out of bed. Chasing a ball could lead to collisions with door frames or oxygen equipment.

If children become bored with a toy because it is not stimulating enough or they have had it for too long a time, they may begin to use the toy in an unsafe way. After a toddler grows tired of stacking blocks, for example, he or she may begin to throw them. Children who normally play safely with modeling clay but who are on a restricted diet may eat it because they are hungry. Knowing where children are and what activity they are engaged in at all times is the best prevention against unsafe play.

For the child cared for at home, parents may need to purchase new toys. This is especially true if the bulk of the toys they furnished previously were for outside play such as balls or Rollerblades or skateboards. Because of an illness, they may now need to provide more "sit down" toys such as markers, puzzles, or board games.

✔ **CHECKPOINT QUESTIONS**

13. What can you or a parent do to make television watching more interactive?
14. What is the most dangerous size for a toy?

Child Life Programs

Child life programs are incorporated into all major children's hospitals and are an integral feature of child health care (Webster, 2000). As part of a child life program, a child life specialist offers children the opportunity to re-enact and thereby master the anxiety associated with illness. Through therapeutic play, child life specialists provide programs that prepare children for hospitalization, and once hospitalized, prepare children for surgery or for procedures that could be painful. They consult with parents about good toys to choose for home care. These specialists help children air their frustration about painful or intrusive procedures, prevent social isolation of children by means of an active recreation program, and ensure that the total health care environment is conducive to children's well-being.

TABLE 35.9 Play Activities for Children on Bedrest

CARE MEASURE	PLAY ACTIVITIES
Bathing	Allow child to play in bath water with water toys. Play a game such as "I Spy" while giving a bed bath.
Encouraging fluid	Hold a "tea party" for a preschooler and drink "tea" with important but imaginary guests. Play a board game with a school-age child in which each turn starts with taking a drink. Draw a circle and let child color in a section each time he or she drinks until the circle is full. Play "Simon Says," in which Simon says, "Drink."
Deep breathing exercises	Have child blow soap bubbles in a glass of soapy water with a straw. Have child blow a cotton ball across the surface of a bedside table. Play "Simon Says," in which Simon says, "Take a deep breath." Allow the child to score points for reaching a high number on an incentive spirometer.
Muscle-strengthening exercises	Have child throw bean bags or large wads of paper (computer waste) at a wastebasket. Play "Simon Says," in which Simon says, "Raise your arms," and so forth. Have child throw and catch a ball. Have child squeeze and mold modeling clay. Encourage child to kick balloon suspended near foot of bed. Help a preschooler pretend he or she is a butterfly, airplane, and so forth.
Procedure such as blood transfusion	Save a favorite game or activity only for these times.
Health teaching	Use puppets as teacher. Make up board games, word scrambles, and crossword puzzles.

Such a program not only aids in promoting children's mental health but also leads to more cooperative responses of children to treatments or procedures. It is complementary to play programs initiated by nurses.

Therapeutic Play

Any occurrence almost automatically becomes less threatening when a person can talk about it. Many children are unable to talk about what is happening to them during illness because of fear or because their vocabulary is so limited that they are unable to describe their feelings.

Because play is the language of children, children who have difficulty voicing their thoughts in words can often speak clearly through play. **Play therapy** is a psychoanalytic technique used by psychiatrists to help children understand their feelings and thoughts and motivations better. In play therapy, the therapist attempts to interpret the child's verbal and nonverbal cues. Interpreting nonverbal cues and helping the child understand them this way requires the skill of a psychiatric nurse-clinician or others with specialized training. **Therapeutic play** is a play technique that can be used by nurses to better understand children's feelings and thoughts (Ellis, 2000). For therapeutic play, only the child's verbal cues are used as responses. Box 35-3 highlights an appropriate outcome and intervention using the terminology identified by the Nursing Outcomes Classification (NOC) and Nursing Interventions Classifications (NIC).

Therapeutic play can be divided into three types:

1. Energy release
2. Dramatic play
3. Creative play

Energy Release

Children release anxiety by pounding, hitting, running, punching, or shouting. Furnishing children with materials that allow them to do these things helps them release anxiety. Toddlers pound pegs with a plastic hammer or pretend to cut wood with a toy saw. Other examples include giving modeling clay to a preschooler (an anxious child often pounds it flat; a relaxed child, however, will build it into shapes) or tying a balloon to an overbed trapeze for a school-age child or adolescent to punch.

Dramatic Play

Dramatic play is acting out an anxiety situation. It is most effective with preschool children because they are at the peak of imagination. During illness, the situations about which children need to express feelings are illness-related, and therefore the equipment needed for therapeutic play is common health care equipment: dolls, doll beds, play stethoscopes, intravenous equipment, syringes, masks, and gowns. Puppets of doctors, nurses, mothers, fathers, and children help young children express their feelings. Anatomically correct dolls are used to help children describe their feelings about sexual abuse.

It is good to have a play session with a child near the beginning of his or her illness to see whether the child communicates any fears concerning this experience through play. This initial session also serves as a way of preparing the child for events that will occur during the illness (Fig. 35-13). Repeat a play session after any painful or traumatic procedure such as surgery so that the child can express new feelings. A list of procedures that fall into this category is shown in Table 35-10. If such play ses-

BOX 35.3

NURSING OUTCOMES AND NURSING INTERVENTIONS CLASSIFICATION: PLAY

NOC: Play Participation

Play participation is defined as the use of activities as needed for enjoyment, entertainment, and development by children (Johnson, Maas, & Moorhead, 2000). Some specific indicators suggesting achievement of this outcome include the following behaviors by the child:

- Participating in appropriate play
- Expressing emotions and enjoyment
- Using social and physical skills and imagination
- Using role playing

NIC: Therapeutic Play

Therapeutic play is defined as the purposeful and directive use of toys or other materials to assist children in communicating their perception and knowledge of their world and to help gain mastery of their environment (McCloskey & Bulechek, 2000). Some important activities involved when implementing this intervention include:

- Providing a quiet, interruption-free environment for a sufficient amount of time
- Communicating the purpose of the play session to the child and parents
- Providing safe, developmentally appropriate, stimulating, creative play equipment, including real or simulated hospital or medical equipment
- Encouraging manipulation of equipment and sharing of feelings, knowledge, and perceptions
- Monitoring child's reactions and anxiety level throughout session
- Identifying misconceptions or fears through comments made
- Continuing play sessions on regular basis as appropriate

sions reveal fears, a child should be scheduled for other play sessions, perhaps one daily.

Furnish children with a wide range of equipment and then let them choose those items with which they wish to play. Children invariably choose a piece of equipment that has been used with them. They poke at a doll with a syringe or enjoy giving it a "shot." They wrap the doll in bandages or put tubes into its mouth or stomach, acting out things that were done to them or that they saw done to other children on a nursing unit or at a clinic visit or that they fear will be done to them. Play should be nondirective (let the child proceed at his or her own pace, choosing freely what equipment to play with and what he or she wants to do with the equipment). As a child works through an experience this way, the experience becomes less fearful and the child masters increased control of it.

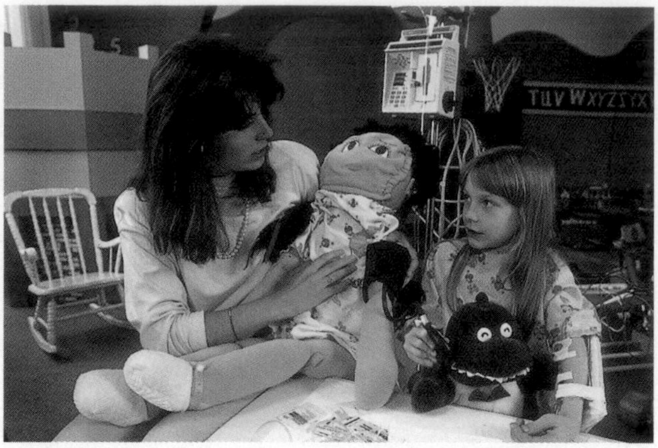

FIGURE 35.13 Therapeutic play allows children the opportunity to voice their fears of illness and procedures.

Observe for children who may be using equipment in an unusual way, such as hitting dolls with stethoscopes or poking them in the eye with a thermometer (suggesting they are confused about the purpose of such equipment). Such behavior alerts health care providers to the importance of explaining the purpose of equipment to children. Listen to what children say as they play. A comment such as, "I'm giving shots to all the bad dolls" suggests the child thinks injections are punishment. It would be important to stress the next time the child needs an injection that medicine is to make the child feel well again. A comment such as, "This doll is going to surgery, so you won't have her anymore" could suggest that the child thinks she will not return from surgery (she may have heard a family member describe someone who died after surgery and is asking for reassurance that such a thing is not going to happen to her). Do not be surprised about the force with which children insert nasogastric tubes into dolls. In part, this reflects how they perceive these procedures, but it also represents energy or anxiety release, in the way that pounding or hitting releases anger.

To better understand how the child feels, repeat what the child says verbally: "You're giving the bad dolls shots?" or ask the child to tell you more about what he or she said: "Do you think that's the only kind of children who get shots? Bad children?" Don't rush to reassure ("Don't worry, that isn't going to happen to you"). Quick reassurance rather than being reassuring tells the child that he or she should not ask any more questions or that the topic is not open for discussion.

Sometimes even children who seem well prepared may be taken by surprise during a procedure. For example, 7-year-old Tanya, seen in an ambulatory setting for a diagnostic workup after a urinary tract infection, showed little interest in dolls and syringes and tubing in the playroom. She had been prepared by her mother for the experience and seemed to understand what would happen during her x-ray procedure. After returning from the x-ray room, where she had a voiding cystourethrogram, however, she was obviously upset. Her nurse brought her a rag doll, a doctor and a nurse figure, a play x-ray machine, and some

TABLE 35.10 Therapeutic Play Techniques for Children After Procedures

PROCEDURE	PLAY ACTIVITY (PROVIDE A DOLL AND . . .)
Radiograph	Table and box labeled "x-ray machine"; children sometimes worry that x-rays have injured them, just as laser rays in science fiction shows do.
Blood drawing	Syringe, alcohol wipes, tourniquet, or finger lancets; remember that finger sticks are as frightening for children as are needles.
Clean-catch urine	Alcohol wipes and a collection cup; children are often more embarrassed by urine collection than adults realize.
Intravenous therapy	Intravenous tubing, as well as restraints and armboard; some children are as angry about being restrained as having the needle inserted.
Endoscopy such as bronchoscopy, cystoscopy	Catheters or a penlight to simulate a scope
Scans	Intravenous fluid and tubing, because scans usually require the intravenous injection of isotopes
Bone marrow	Alcohol wipes, syringe
EEG, EKG	Electrode leads that attach to a box; children might be afraid of these procedures because of their fear of electricity.
Surgery	An anesthesia mask and a blunt kitchen knife; watch and listen for where the child cuts and how he or she describes the experience.
Dental examination	Suction catheter, a penlight to simulate a drill, and a 4 × 4 piece of plastic to simulate a dental dam; some children are angered by the use of plastic in their mouth.
Dressing changes	Gauze and adhesive tape
Cast application or removal	Provide plaster to soak and apply; simulate a cast cutter with an electric razor or hair dryer.
Nasogastric tube insertion, enema, catheterization	Appropriate tubes
Temperature assessment	Thermometer

tubing that could simulate a urinary catheter and encouraged Tanya to play with them. Tanya picked up the girl doll and put her under the x-ray machine. She imitated the doctor doll shouting, "Pee in front of everybody!" Tanya's mother had not realized that she would have to void during a cystourethrogram and so had not prepared her for that. Tanya felt betrayed by not being really prepared for this embarrassing situation. Her play brought her emotion out in the open, where it could be talked about and handled. When Tanya was scheduled the next day for ureteral reflux surgery, her parent was alerted to make the preparation absolutely thorough.

Children older than 9 or 10 years find playing with dolls too childish to be of benefit. They enjoy handling syringes, however, and being able to see and handle such equipment as nasogastric tubes in advance of their being placed. Active handling helps to eliminate fear because it identifies exactly what the child has to face; it meets their concrete-level learning needs.

Creative Play

Some children are too angry to be able to act out their feelings through dramatic play. However, they may be able to draw a picture that expresses their emotions or conveys the extent of their knowledge. To encourage this, give a child a blank paper and crayons or markers. If a child seems reluctant to draw something spontaneously, suggest a topic: "Why don't you draw a picture of yourself?"

Some children are so concerned with particular parts of their bodies that when asked to draw pictures of themselves, they draw only the body parts about which they are worried. Such a child generally is saying that he or she needs to talk about that part of the body, to be given reassurance that it is going to be all right. Figure 35-14*A* shows a picture drawn by a 9-year-old who was admitted to the hospital for 1-day surgery for debridement of a campfire burn on her left foot. She stated on admission that she was being admitted to have the burn on her foot "cleaned out." This sounds like a child who understands what debridement involves. Note, however, that the figure she drew has no left leg. One has to wonder whether she was concerned that she was going to surgery to have more than debridement. After the word "debridement" was explained to her, she drew the picture in Figure 35-14*B*. The child in the drawing now has a left and a right leg, the left leg covered by a bandage. Through a drawing, this child was able to say something she could not express without this help.

Many ill children draw pictures that reflect punitive images: a boy or girl tied to a bed or shut behind bars, or doctors and nurses frowning at them, obviously unhappy with them. Such children may need assurance that they are not being punished; they need to stay in bed or are being cared for by doctors and nurses to be made well (Fig. 35-15). Other children draw pictures that are symbolic of death: airplanes crashing, boats sinking, buildings on fire, children in graveyards. They need assurance that they will not die.

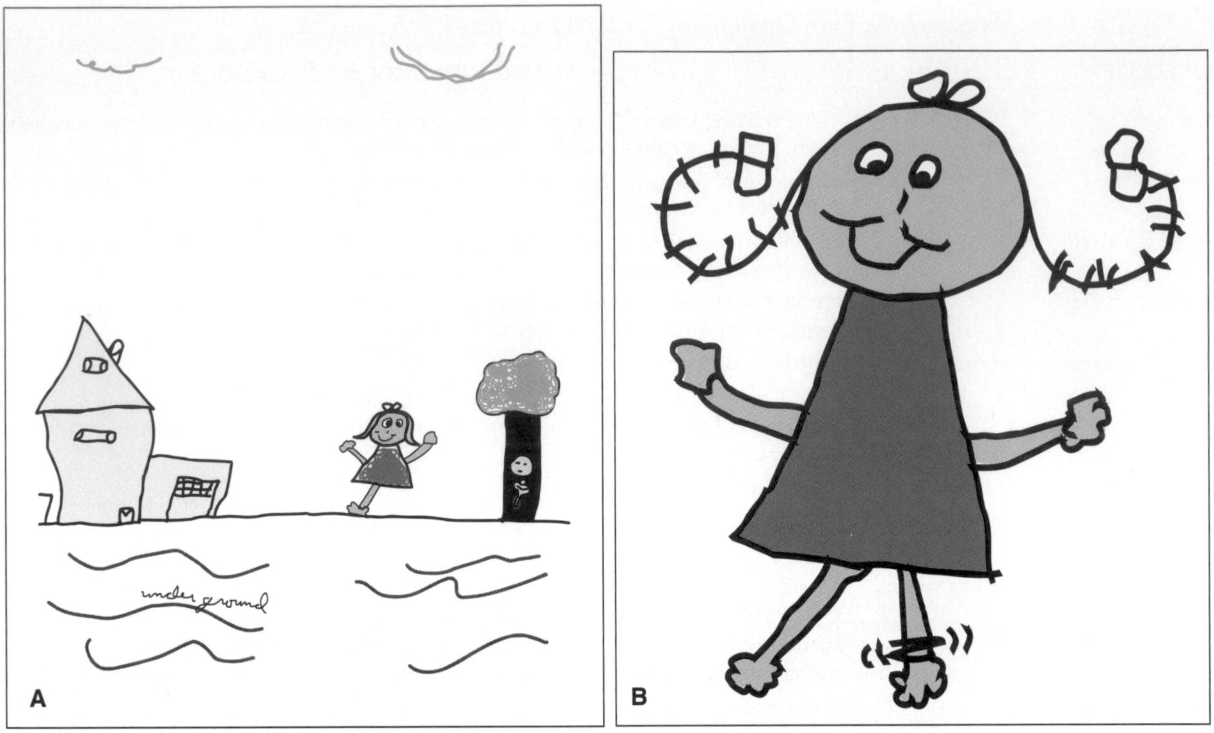

FIGURE 35.14 (*A*) Children who are concerned about body parts may draw pictures with that part missing or exaggerated. Note the missing left leg here. (*B*) After reassurance that her leg will be all right, the girl who did the drawing in *A* now draws a girl with two legs.

Other concerns such as fear of abandonment and loss of independence may also be manifested in drawings. For example, preschoolers may draw a child in one corner of a picture and an adult in a far corner. They may comment that the parent cannot find the little child because she's gone to the hospital. They need to be reassured that their parents know where they will be and will visit them each day after work.

Older school-age children and adolescents may not be interested in drawing but can be interested in making a list of procedures or experiences they like and dislike. Examine the dislike list for procedures such as "shots" or "chemo." Mark the nursing care plan for nurses to take special time to explain these procedures and to offer special support when they must be done.

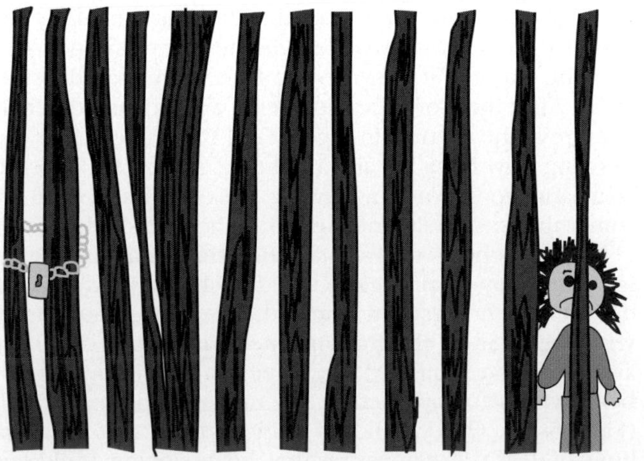

FIGURE 35.15 A picture drawn by a hospitalized child. Note the prison-like appearance of the crib. (Courtesy of Rita Crever.)

Guidelines for Conducting Therapeutic Play

Use common sense when conducting therapeutic play. Be certain not to interpret a child's black and gloomy drawing as meaning the child is depressed when a black marker was the only one available. Many children 4 to 5 years of age draw a person lacking many body parts because that is the best human form they can draw.

WHAT IF? What if a 3-year-old draws a purple person with only three body parts? Would this worry you? Why or why not?

Remember, too, that all children occasionally treat dolls badly. A 2-year-old pounding and banging a rag doll may not be expressing anger toward the doll image at all, but may be intent on discovering the feel of a new texture and is unaware for the moment that the object is a doll.

A conference with health care team members, including a psychologist or a psychiatric nurse specialist, may be called for if a child continues to express mutilating behavior after normal reassurance. Guidelines for conducting therapeutic play are summarized in Box 35-4.

✔ CHECKPOINT QUESTIONS

15. What is therapeutic play?
16. Would you initiate therapeutic play before or after surgery?

BOX 35.4

GUIDELINES FOR THERAPEUTIC PLAY

1. Allow a child to choose the articles with which he or she wants to play (something may be too frightening for a child to play with immediately; he or she needs time to work up to the activity).
2. Provide the materials specific to the child's experiences of which you, the nurse, are aware (e.g., nasogastric tube, syringe, or bandages), but do not supply only those things; a child may have misunderstandings and fears of situations you cannot know about.
3. Allow play to be unstructured; let the child use the materials however he or she wishes. If a child seems uninterested in materials, initiate play with him or her (e.g., give a doll an injection) to see if this reduces his or her anxiety enough to be able to handle items.
4. If a child cannot manipulate materials himself or herself (due to such things as a cast or traction), ask the child what he or she would like you to do with it.
5. Reflect only what the child expresses (verbal expression).
6. Do not criticize play; this inhibits further expression.
7. Use a therapeutic response—not "Don't worry, that won't happen," but "Are you worried that could happen?"
8. Ask children to describe paintings, not "That's a good picture of yourself," but "Tell me about your picture."
9. Do not be reluctant to use real equipment (e.g., real catheters and blood lancets). Handling real equipment best helps to reduce stress.
10. Supervise therapeutic play, because some equipment could cause an accident (and therapeutically responding to the child's comments is necessary).

KEY POINTS

Illness may be more traumatic for children than for adults because of their inability to communicate and monitor their own care and because they have different nutrition, fluid, and electrolyte needs. The stress of hospitalization can be so acute that it can result in posttraumatic stress syndrome.

Separation from parents because of hospitalization can have permanent psychological effects on children. Methods to reduce this include keeping hospital stays as brief as possible, promoting open parent and sibling visiting, and providing primary or case management nursing.

Currently, many medical procedures can be done on an ambulatory basis. Advocating for care to be done in such settings is a nursing responsibility.

The presence of parents during health care can help reduce trauma to children. Making parents as welcome as possible makes it possible for them to room-in. Include the parents in both the planning and the implementation of care. Parents reinfect children with fear if their own fear is not reduced.

Preschoolers may have the most difficult time during hospitalization because they have so many fears. Preparation and promotion of therapeutic play are essential to reduce trauma to a tolerable level.

Because hospitalizations currently are so brief, parents need good discharge instructions to continue to care for children safely at home. Providing clear instructions and danger signs for parents to watch for is a nursing responsibility.

Home care is increasing as a way of providing care to chronically ill children. It has the advantages of being cost-effective and providing meaningful comfort and support to the child. Disadvantages are that parents can become fatigued, the loss of a job for the primary caregiver can cause financial hardship, and social isolation and disruption of normal home life may occur.

Not all homes are ideal for home care. Assess that a primary care provider is present; the family is knowledgeable about the care necessary; necessary resources are available; and safety features such as a smoke detector, a safe area for oxygen storage, and a safe refrigerator for food or medicine are present.

Home care can be exhausting for parents. Be certain that they devise a schedule of care that allows them enough rest. Advocate for medicine or treatment schedules that allow for administering medications during the day rather than a schedule that requires medication administration at night.

Parents may need respite care to continue to be effective care providers, just as professionals need time off. Help parents to take turns giving care so that each has some free time during a week.

CRITICAL THINKING QUESTIONS

1. Becky is the 7-year-old you met at the beginning of the chapter. Her foot was burned in a campfire accident. Since then she has refused to eat anything but Jello or soup. In the hospital playroom, she picked up a doll and tore off its leg. Her mother asked you why her daughter is acting this way. What suggestions would you make to her?

The burn occurred because Becky was left momentarily unsupervised by a campfire. Is there a possibility her mother may not be acting her usual self because of guilt over the injury?
2. A 3-year-old has had emergency surgery while on vacation with her single mother. Her mother has to return home because of work responsibilities, so the 3-year-old will have no family with her for a week. What measures would you take to help make hospitalization and separation less traumatic for her?
3. A 14-year-old will be cared for at home after orthopedic surgery. She is concerned that because her home stay will be lengthy she will be cut off from her friends for a long time. What suggestions could you make to help her maintain contact with friends? Her parents state that they are exhausted because of the necessity for round-the-clock care. What suggestions could you make to them to make care easier?
4. Examine the National Health Goals related to children and hospitalization. Most government-sponsored money for nursing research is allotted based on these goals. What would be a possible research topic to explore pertinent to these goals that would be fundable and would advance evidence-based practice?

REFERENCES

American Psychiatric Association. (2000). *Diagnostic and statistical manual (DSM-IV)*. New York: APA.
Bowlby, J., et al. (1966). *Maternal care and mental health*. New York: Schocken Books.
Daviss, W. B., et al. (2000). Predicting posttraumatic stress after hospitalization for pediatric injury. *Journal of the American Academy of Child & Adolescent Psychiatry, 39*(5), 576–583.
Department of Health and Human Services (2000). *Healthy people, 2010*. Washington, DC: DHHS.
Ellis, J. (2000). Games without frontiers . . . therapeutic play. *Nursing Times, 96*(26), 32–33.
Fennell, M. E. (1999). Parents in the OR? You bet! *RN, 62*(12), 38–40.
Foley, J. (2000). The effects of hospitalisation on children. *Nursing Review, 18*(1), 4–5.
Johnson, M., Maas, M., & Moorhead, S. (2000). *Nursing outcomes classification* (2nd ed.). St. Louis: Mosby, Inc.
LaMontague, L. L., et al. (2000). Effects of surgery type and attention focus on children's coping. *Nursing Research, 49*(5), 245–252.
McCloskey, J., & Bulechek, G. (2000). *Nursing interventions classification* (3rd ed.). St. Louis: Mosby, Inc.
Partis, M. (2000). Focus: children. Bowlby's attachment theory: Implications for health visiting. *British Journal of Community Nursing, 5*(10), 499–503.
Price, D., et al. (2002). Preparation for renal biopsy: A play package. *Paediatric Nursing, 12*(2), 38–39.
Robertson, J. (1958). *Young children in hospitals*. London: Tavistock.
Spitz, R. A. (1945). Hospitalism: An inquiry into the genesis of psychiatric conditions in early childhood. *Psychoanalytic Study of the Child, 1*(3), 53–59.
Voepel-Lewis, T., et al. (2000). Separation and induction behavior in children: Are parents good predictors? *Journal of Perianesthesia Nursing, 15* (1), 6–11.
Webster, A. (2000). The facilitating role of the play specialist. *Paediatric Nursing, 12*(7), 24–27.

SUGGESTED READINGS

Boyd, J. R. (2001). A process for delivering bad news: Supporting families when a child is diagnosed. *Journal of Neuroscience Nursing, 33*(1), 14–20.
Kane, J. R., & Primomo, M. (2001). Alleviating the suffering of seriously ill children. *American Journal of Hospice & Palliative Care, 18*(3), 161–169.
Keenan, H. T., et al. (2002). Social factors associated with prolonged hospitalization among diabetic children. *Pediatrics, 109*(1), 40–44.
Kolk, A. M., et al. (2000). Preparing children for venipuncture. *Child: Care, Health & Development, 26*(3), 251–260.
Narayanasamy, A., & Owens, J. (2001). A critical incident study of nurses' responses to the spiritual needs of their patients. *Journal of Advanced Nursing, 33*(4), 446–455.
Parker, J. D., & Schoendorf, K. C. (2000). Variation in hospital discharges for ambulatory care-sensitive conditions among children. *Pediatrics, 106*(4S), 942–948.
Perry, D. F., & Ireys, H. T. (2001). Maternal perceptions of pediatric providers for children with chronic illnesses. *Maternal & Child Heath Journal, 5*(1), 15–20.
Prensner, J. D., et al. (2001). Music therapy for assistance with pain and anxiety management in burn treatment. *Journal of Burn Care & Rehabilitation, 22*(1), 83–88.
Schaffer, P., et al. (2000). Revision of a parent satisfaction survey based on the parent perspective. *Journal of Pediatric Nursing, 15*(6), 373–377.
Woodring, B. C. (2000). Family matters: If you have taught—have the child and family learned? *Pediatric Nursing, 26*(5), 505–509.
Yule, W. (2001). Posttraumatic stress disorder in the general population and in children. *Journal of Clinical Psychiatry, 62* (17S), 23–28.

36 CHAPTER

Nursing Care of the Child Undergoing Diagnostic Techniques and Other Therapeutic Modalities

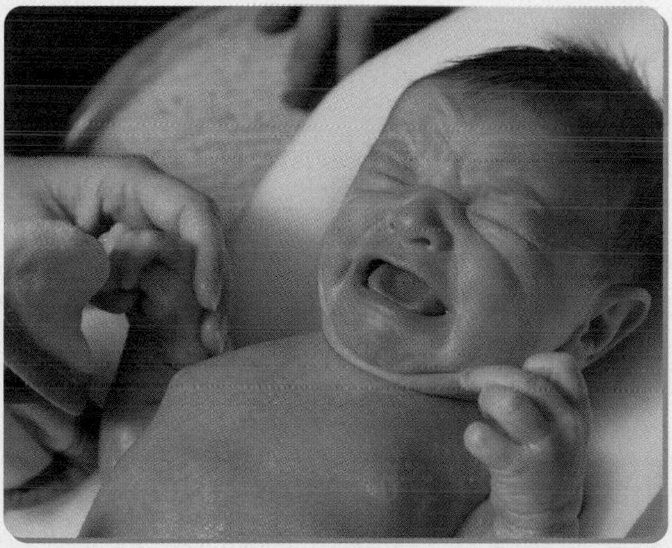

Key Terms

- **aspiration studies**
- **barium contrast studies**
- **bronchoscopy**
- **clean-catch urine specimen**
- **colonoscopy**
- **computed tomography (CT)**
- **electrical impulse studies**
- **endoscopy**
- **gavage feedings**
- **magnetic resonance imaging (MRI)**
- **positron emission tomography (PET)**
- **radiopharmaceutical**
- **single photon emission computed tomography (SPECT)**
- **total parenteral nutrition (TPN)**
- **ultrasound**

Objectives

After mastering the contents of this chapter, you should be able to:

1. Describe common nursing interventions used in the health care of children to aid diagnosis and therapy.
2. Assess children as to developmental stage and knowledge level before beginning diagnostic or therapeutic procedures or other nursing interventions.
3. Formulate nursing diagnoses related to common diagnostic or therapeutic procedures used with children.
4. Identify outcomes for the child undergoing a diagnostic or therapeutic procedure.
5. Plan nursing interventions to aid in diagnosis or therapy for children.
6. Implement nursing interventions relevant to diagnostic or therapeutic procedures.
7. Evaluate outcomes related to diagnostic and therapeutic procedures for achievement.
8. Identify National Health Goals related to diagnostic and therapeutic procedures for children that nurses could be instrumental in helping the nation achieve.
9. Identify areas related to nursing procedures with children that could benefit from additional nursing research or application of evidence-based practice.
10. Use critical thinking to analyze ways that diagnostic and therapeutic procedures can be modified to meet the needs of children of all ages.
11. Integrate knowledge of common diagnostic and therapeutic procedures with nursing process to achieve quality maternal and child health nursing.

Wally is a preschooler who is scheduled to have a magnetic resonance imaging (MRI) study for a possible head injury. "How can I agree to this?" his mother asks you. "He's afraid of the dark. How can I allow him to be wheeled into a long dark machine that way?" How would you explain MRI to Wally to make the procedure more acceptable to him?

Previous chapters described the growth and development of well children. This chapter adds information about how to care for children when they become ill. This is important information because it builds a base for care and health teaching.

After you've studied the chapter, answer the Critical Thinking Exercises at the end of the chapter and then access the on-line study activities (http://connection.lww.com) *to further sharpen your skills and test your knowledge.*

Illness can be particularly stressful if many diagnostic and therapeutic procedures are necessary for care. In today's health care climate, there is less time for teaching and preparation than once available, so good planning and follow-through are essential. Chapter 35 described measures to make the experience of illness a more positive one. Health teaching, discussed in Chapter 34, is a cornerstone in this process. However, everything that nurses do with and for ill children will have a major influence on the child's progress toward health as well as on the child's and family's perception of professional health care and the ability to carry out healthful practices in the future.

Many nursing actions offer an opportunity to accomplish several goals. Supporting the child and family during a diagnostic procedure, for instance, not only can aid in efficient diagnosis but also may help establish a trusting relationship between the family and health care providers that will make all future interactions more successful. This chapter describes the most common diagnostic and therapeutic techniques used in the care of ill children, including modifications needed to make these procedures safe and reduce associated stress, depending on the child's age and outlook. National Health Goals that address this area of child health practice are shown in the Focus on National Health Goals box.

FOCUS ON NATIONAL HEALTH GOALS

A key component for minimizing the threat of hospitalizations and procedures for children, and thus maximizing safety, is to limit the length of time children spend in the hospital. A number of National Health Goals address reducing the length of time that children spend in hospitals. One example is:

- Reduce hospital rates for children with pediatric asthma to 17 per 10,000 from a baseline of 23 per 10,000.

A major role of health care providers is to keep children free from disease so that they receive a minimum of procedures. A National Health Goal also addresses this:

- Increase the proportion of persons appropriately counseled about health behaviors (DHHS, 2000).

Nurses can be instrumental in helping the nation achieve these goals by providing health counseling to aid in preventing children from becoming ill and subsequently requiring hospitalization.

Areas related to these goals that could benefit from additional nursing research and application of evidence-based practice include determining what teaching techniques are most effective in keeping children well; what methods are efficient to ensure that children's hospitalizations are as short as possible; and what techniques or supplies are most satisfactory to children when procedures are performed.

NURSING PROCESS OVERVIEW

For the Child Undergoing Diagnostic or Therapeutic Procedures

Assessment

Before performing procedures such as assisting with a diagnostic test or collecting laboratory specimens, first carefully evaluate the child's age and developmental stage, as well as any special needs the child may have. Even the most common and painless procedures produce a certain amount of stress for the child and parents. During complex diagnostic procedures, this stress level is almost certain to increase. Unfamiliar doctors and nurses, high-tech supplies and equipment, and strange surroundings all add up to a frightening experience for most adults; imagine how frightening they can seem to children!

Assess the child's level of anxiety associated with unfamiliar equipment, circumstances, and surroundings as well as the child's knowledge concerning a technique before initiating a procedure or beginning health teaching. It may be possible to increase cooperation by acknowledging and respecting the child's past experience with similar procedures.

Nursing Diagnosis

Common nursing diagnoses related to diagnostic and therapeutic procedures are as varied as the procedures and environment but include:

- Fear related to new and strange surroundings of the procedure room
- Pain related to lumbar puncture
- Deficient knowledge related to technique for 24-hour urine collection
- Deficient diversionary activity related to lack of appropriate toys in required setting
- Imbalanced nutrition, less than body requirements related to lack of familiar foods
- Risk for injury related to a biopsy procedure

Outcome Identification and Planning

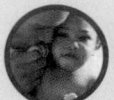

Illness in itself creates anxiety in the child; unless the child is helped to feel comfortable and safe, every procedure can result in even more stress. An important nursing goal is to perform interventions with the least degree of anxiety possible. To achieve this goal, plan specific ways to prepare children in advance. Planning should include the best way to explain the procedure to a particular child and also how to ensure that the child is not overwhelmed by the number of diagnostic or therapeutic procedures performed in any one day. With small children, it may make more sense to stagger ambulatory diagnostic tests over a number of days to preserve the child's coping ability. Conversely, some older children (and parents) do better if they can complete all necessary tests in 1 day, so that they do not have to anticipate more testing over a long period. Use nursing judgment and data from periodic assessments to help primary care providers determine the type of schedule that is in the child's and family's best interest.

Implementation

Whether assisting with a procedure or performing a therapeutic intervention, it is necessary to function in several roles at the same time: performing (or assisting with) the procedure, providing active support to the child and parents, and observing and then documenting the child's reactions. Providing support is a major role, and there are many ways to do this, such as holding a child's hand or placing a hand on the parent's shoulder. Playing a distracting game with an older child can also be helpful. Important observations to be made include signs of discomfort, changes in vital signs, or other signals of distress such as pallor or dizziness. Maintain a flowsheet of observations during a procedure. After a procedure, the procedure, the child's reaction, and specimens obtained can then be documented accurately and efficiently in the child's record.

As a final follow-through step, think of therapeutic play techniques to introduce that would be helpful in relieving stress caused by the procedure.

Outcome Evaluation

Evaluating outcomes related to diagnostic and therapeutic procedures helps not only in determining the effect of the procedure but also in planning, should other procedures be required. Recording that a particular child who did not appear nervous during a procedure later admitted to being "more scared than I've ever been before," for example, can help another nurse provide reassurance to this child, even when the child is masking his emotions the next time. Examples suggesting achievement of outcomes might include:

- Child says she is able to cope with further bone marrow aspiration.
- Child lists steps to take to collect 24-hour urine at home.
- Child participates in 1 hour of active play daily.
- Child eats a minimum of 1,000 calories per day.
- Child experiences minimal loss of blood (less than 10 mL) during diagnostic procedure.
- Parent outlines plan to use alternative therapies to reduce the child's anxiety.

NURSING RESPONSIBILITIES WITH DIAGNOSTIC AND THERAPEUTIC TECHNIQUES

Responsibilities of the nurse in assisting with procedures performed on children include the following:

- Helping to obtain consent as needed
- Explaining the procedure to the child and his or her parents to prepare them psychologically
- Scheduling the procedure
- Preparing the child physically and psychologically
- Obtaining equipment for the procedure and ensuring adherence to standard precautions
- Accompanying the child to the treatment room or hospital department where the procedure will be performed
- Providing support during the procedure
- Assessing the child's response to the procedure
- Providing care to the child and specimens obtained once the procedure is completed
- Overseeing or cooperating with other health care disciplines to ensure the safety and efficacy of all procedures (see Focus on Multidisciplinary Care)

Obtaining Consent

Consent to perform a procedure must be obtained if the procedure carries any risk that would not be present if it were not performed. For a parent to sign a consent form, he or she must be informed about the content of the procedure and the risks of having or not having it performed. Although actually obtaining this is the physician's responsibility, seeing that it is obtained is a nursing responsibility. Acting as an advocate for the family if they do not understand the consent, procedure, or risk is also an important nursing role. Be certain that the rights of emancipated minors are respected and that in single-parent families, the custodial parent has given the permission.

Explaining Procedures

To be able to explain procedures clearly and answer questions about them appropriately, it is important to see as many procedures performed as possible. Asking a child

FOCUS ON MULTIDISCIPLINARY CARE

Health care professionals from other disciplines, such as nutritionists, physical therapists, and respiratory therapists, often participate with diagnostic or therapeutic procedures. Offer to provide additional support and guidance to them when explaining procedures to children as many times as needed to gain children's cooperation. Also, encourage the various professionals to spend time with the parents to ensure that the parents understand the procedure, reminding them that children cannot relax until their parents are also relaxed.

after any procedure what sensations he or she experienced not only helps the child work through a possibly frightening situation (often called debriefing) but it also increases your knowledge of common procedures.

As a general guide, a child needs a detailed description of the procedure, such as, "I'll clean your finger. You will feel a small pinprick . . .", and an explanation of the following:

- Why the procedure is performed—for example, "The doctor needs to look at your blood to see why you're so sick."
- Where the procedure will be done—for instance, the x-ray department or a treatment room
- Any unusual sensations to be expected during the procedure—for example, alcohol for cleaning skin will feel cold
- Any pain involved—for instance, "The needle will sting, although I'll put some cream on first to dull the feeling."
- Any strange equipment used—for instance, a large x-ray machine
- The approximate length of time the procedure will take
- Any special care after the procedure—for example, "You will need to lie quietly for 15 minutes afterward."

Use age-appropriate language when explaining procedures. Be careful not to use words that might be confusing during an explanation, such as "transducer" or "electrode," without defining them. Try to associate the procedure with something with which the child is already familiar and comfortable (e.g., an x-ray machine is "a big camera"). Try not to use the word "test" in explanations because school-age children associate the word "test" with a pass/fail situation. This can make them unduly worried after a procedure about whether they have "passed" it.

If you are unfamiliar with what a procedure entails, do not guess. Nothing is more confusing to a child or parents than being told two different versions of something. Most technical personnel will take the time to describe important information that a child should know about a study or procedure, because having a well-informed patient makes their job easier. Be certain that parents also receive an explanation of the procedure. A child has difficulty relaxing if parents are still anxious because they do not understand what is going to happen. Encourage parents to stay with the child during most procedures, because they can be extremely helpful in reducing a procedure's threatening aspects (Boyd, 2001).

Scheduling

Most diagnostic procedures are scheduled on an ambulatory basis. Try to arrange for the child to have time for meals and some free play time between procedures. If food or fluid must be restricted for procedures, monitor the child's degree of discomfort and physiologic needs related to this; advocate as necessary for a time lapse between examinations or improved coordination in scheduling to decrease the time spent without food or fluid.

Preparing the Child and Family Physically and Psychologically

Physical preparation varies depending on what procedure is to be performed. In many instances, preparing a child for an examination (e.g., barium enema) involves another procedure (a saline enema), so physical preparation becomes education for the real examination. In all instances, be certain to explain both the preparative and actual procedures. Appropriate explanations aid in reducing anxiety and fear.

For many procedures, especially those that may be painful, such as a bronchoscopy, conscious sedation may be used. Conscious sedation refers to the depressed level of consciousness induced by the intravenous administration of a sedative such as diazepam (Valium) in combination with a narcotic such as morphine sulfate. About 60 minutes before the procedure, children may be given oral chloral hydrate both to relieve apprehension and make them feel sleepy.

While under conscious sedation, children are able to maintain their ability to breathe independently and also respond appropriately to verbal commands such as to lift their head. This type of sedation is used in both ambulatory and inpatient settings. Before conscious sedation is begun, emergency equipment, including respiratory and pharmacologic measures, must be readily available. The child's level of consciousness and ability to respond, heart rate, respiratory rate, blood pressure, and oxygen saturation are monitored during the procedure. Using conscious sedation is very effective to allow children to accept a potentially painful procedure emotionally and physically. Be certain that a child is prepared both for the diagnostic procedure and the use of conscious sedation (Rodriguez & Jordan, 2002).

Accompanying the Child

If a procedure will be done at another site rather than the primary care clinic or hospital unit with which a child is comfortable, ideally a nurse who the child knows should accompany the child to the other department and remain with the child for the procedure, or at least until the child has met a primary person who will be with him or her during the assessment. Older children do well without being accompanied as long as they have been introduced in advance to the new person who will give them care. A parent who can accompany a child is of invaluable help.

Before leaving the patient unit or clinic, have the child void for comfort unless this is a contraindication to the procedure. Check for any medication or specific assessment procedures such as a blood pressure recording that should be given or done before leaving the unit for another department, in case the child is away from the primary unit for an extended time. If the child is an inpatient, check also that the identification band is securely in place and readily visible despite any intravenous equipment. If there will be a considerable wait in another department, ask the child if he or she would like to engage in some activity during a wait, such as a playing a game or reading a book. Hallways can be cool. Provide adequate blankets for comfort, especially for infants. Always use cart straps and side rails for safety.

Providing Support

Children do well with diagnostic and evaluative procedures as long as they have adequate support from a concerned provider or parent. Provide this both verbally (explain what is going to happen; assure a child that he or she is sitting still effectively) and nonverbally (a hand on the arm or a nearby presence).

Modifying Procedures According to the Child's Age and Developmental Stage

A child's age and potential understanding of procedures must be considered when planning the number and order of tests and the way they are performed.

The Infant

The number of painful or uncomfortable procedures done on infants should be kept to a minimum to avoid interfering with the infant's developing a sense of trust. Parents should be allowed to accompany their child to hospital departments and remain during procedures to offer support. Some parents may ask to hold their child during a procedure that causes pain, but do not ask parents to restrain the child during such a procedure. Their role should be a supportive and comforting one.

Infants need to be picked up and comforted after procedures (a child of any age likes a hug or honest compliment for cooperation). Be aware that both obtaining blood specimens (which can deplete blood stores) and x-rays (which are possibly harmful to bone marrow) should be kept to a minimum in infants. Help parents understand why these procedures are being limited so they do not think that their infant's care is being compromised by so few diagnostic procedures.

The Toddler and Preschooler

Toddlers and preschoolers resist any diagnostic testing that involves any degree of discomfort or pain or that is unfamiliar. Give children of this age short explanations of what to expect, close to the time of the procedure so that little time can be spent worrying over it.

The School-Age Child and Adolescent

School-age children are interested in the theory and reason for procedures. Often they can be persuaded to cooperate for a procedure by being promised a look at their x-ray or laboratory report afterward. Be careful to ensure that viewing the results is actually possible when promising children; otherwise, it can be difficult to obtain any further cooperation. Adolescents may project an air of maturity or sophistication beyond their years to remain in control of themselves in the face of frightening procedures. Do not be misled into thinking a child this age would not appreciate an explanation or a comforting hand on a shoulder during a procedure.

> **WHAT IF?** What if an adolescent who was scheduled for a series of diagnostic tests said, "I'm not a kid, you know," and refused to listen when you started to explain a procedure? Later, he acted angry because he had been "tricked" into having the procedure. How could you give explanations to him without offending him? What do you think is the basis for his actions?

Promoting Safety During Procedures

Safety is an important component of all patient care. When your patient is a child, there is an even greater concern for safety. Children's immaturity, which makes them unable to form mature judgments, leaves them vulnerable to harm unless their caretakers give special consideration to promoting safety.

NURSING DIAGNOSES AND RELATED INTERVENTIONS

Nursing Diagnosis: Risk for injury related to diagnostic procedures

Outcome Identification: The child will not sustain any injury during series of diagnostic procedures.

Outcome Evaluation: Child remains free of injury from diagnostic equipment.

Children require special precautions to ensure their safety during procedures. As a basic safety measure, before giving any food or performing any procedure, look at the identification armband. If an armband must be removed because it interferes with an intravenous infusion site, cut it away but immediately anchor it to another extremity with adhesive tape. Ask the admissions department to provide a new armband as soon as possible. Do not leave the old one off while waiting for a replacement band. This leaves the child susceptible to the danger of mistaken identity during the waiting period.

Because of their natural curiosity, children tend to fuss with equipment to see what will happen if they turn a knob or spin a dial. They need close monitoring while procedures are performed to ensure that they do not touch any buttons or in other ways accidentally harm themselves. After a procedure, be sure to remove all equipment from a room. Children may pick up scissors or forceps left at bedsides and incur eye injuries; they may drink antiseptics left at bedsides and poison themselves. Cleaning agents such as alcohol or povidone-iodine are potential poisoning sources; syringes and needles can cause puncture injuries. Young children can choke on small objects such as needle covers.

Use of Restraints

A restraint is used to keep a child safe during a procedure. It must always be used with care, because if improperly applied or used, it can cause more harm than help (Mohr & Mohr, 2000). Children may have difficulty distinguishing between restraint and punishment, so restraint should never be used more often or for any time longer than necessary. Parents must be given careful explanations about why their child has a restraint in place—for example, because of a particular danger of this procedure, it is safer for their child.

Check restraints every 15 minutes to see that they are not occluding circulation; remove them every hour so that the body part can be exercised (provided the exercise does not dislodge a device or interfere with a treatment). No part of the child's body other than that which is necessary should be restrained. When a child has a scalp vein infusion in place, such as for injection of a radioactive isotope for a nuclear medicine scan, the child's arms may need to be immobilized so that he or she does not touch the infusion. The trunk may be immobilized so that the child does not turn. The child's lower extremities may not have to be restrained, however, so he or she can still actively kick and exercise them. When a nurse or a parent is with the child, in most instances, all restraints can be removed.

Several types of restraints may be used to secure the child during a procedure or to prevent the child from touching equipment. The various types of restraints are shown in Table 36-1 and Figure 36-1.

Providing Care After Procedures

After a procedure, assess how well a child reacted to it by both observation and history. Allowing children to explain what happened helps them retrace the procedure in their mind so they can conquer the fear of it. Fill in gaps in information as necessary to improve a child's perception of the procedure. Providing therapeutic play is another measure to reduce anxiety (see Chap. 35).

Be certain that tissue samples obtained after a procedure such as bone marrow aspiration are sent to the proper department for analysis as soon as possible. Guard against specimens being dropped or improperly labeled; children do not have extra body fluids such as blood to sacrifice for additional specimen collection.

If conscious sedation was used, be sure that children are awake before they are discharged home or return to an inpatient hospital unit. Using a postanesthesia score sheet such as shown in Figure 36-2 is an effective method to rate recovery from anesthesia.

Children can be discharged as soon as 30 minutes after conscious sedation if the airway is patent and respiratory status is stable (no retraction, stridor, or wheezing); oxygen has not been needed for at least 15 minutes; oxygen saturation is 95% or greater in room air; and the child is awake and reactive, has adequate circulation and normal blood pressure, has heart and respiratory rates appropriate for age, and is reasonably free of pain (Tolia et al., 2000).

Parents often have questions about what care the child will need after they return home. Tips for parents are highlighted in the Focus on Family Empowerment box.

> **✔ CHECKPOINT QUESTIONS**
>
> 1. Why is it better not to talk about diagnostic procedures as "tests" with school-aged children?
> 2. When should a mummy restraint be used?

COMMON DIAGNOSTIC PROCEDURES

Diagnostic and therapeutic procedures used with children vary widely, depending on a child's condition and age. As in adults, blood, urine, and stool studies are commonly used. These are discussed under techniques of specimen collection. Respiratory illnesses require special procedures. These are discussed in Chapter 40. Biopsies (surgical procedures to remove tissue for examination) are discussed in Chapter 53. Stress testing is discussed in Chapter 41. More common diagnostic procedures are discussed in the following sections.

Electrical Impulse Studies

Electrical impulse studies are those that include electrical conduction. Children need special preparation for studies such as electrocardiograms (ECGs; Fig. 36-3) or electroencephalograms (EEGs) because they have been warned not to play with electric wires and may worry about being burned or electrocuted. They can be reassured that the electricity passes from their body to the machine, not the other way around; except for electromyelograms, children can be assured that these tests are painless. Electrodes are attached to the body by paste, which is easily removable (Tipple, 2000). If possible, give the child a portion of the test strip afterward as a souvenir.

Radiologic Studies

A variety of radiologic studies are used to inspect internal body tissues. These range from the simple x-ray to the more complicated computed tomography (CT) scan or dye contrast study.

Flat-Plate X-Rays

As a rule, children accept radiographs well because an x-ray machine can be compared with a camera, an instrument with which they are familiar (Fig. 36-4). Caution children that although you or a parent may be able to accompany them to the x-ray department, you will not be allowed to stay in the room while the picture is actually taken. If it is necessary for you to remain in the room to restrain a child, do not do this without lead apron and lead glove protection. Such protection is also necessary for portable x-rays taken by a child's or infant's bedside.

Dye Contrast Studies

To visualize a body cavity, some type of radiopaque dye may be swallowed or injected into the cavity and then examined on x-ray. **Barium contrast studies,** for example, are used to observe the outline of the gastrointestinal tract. Barium may be swallowed to outline the upper gastrointestinal tract or instilled by enema to outline the lower portion. Caution the child that barium, even if flavored, does not taste terribly good. In studies such as an intravenous pyelogram (IVP), dye is injected intravenously; as it circulates to the kidneys, an x-ray is taken. Children must be thoroughly prepared for dye contrast procedures. Because iodine is incorporated in most of the radiopaque material, be sure to check whether the child is allergic to iodine. At the time of

TABLE 36.1 Safety Restraints

TYPE OF RESTRAINT	PURPOSE	METHOD
Wheelchairs and carts	Promote safety while transporting children to and from a procedure. Remind children to stay in a wheelchair while being transported. Prevent children from rolling off a cart while being transported.	For a wheelchair, use a vest restraint. Attach straps to the frame of the wheelchair with enough slack so the child has some mobility. For a cart, fasten a restraining belt and raise the side rails. Even with restraints in place, never leave a child unattended in hallways outside departments in a wheelchair or on a cart. Not only is this unsafe because the child may attempt to get down from the cart or wheelchair, but the anxiety of waiting in a strange department for a procedure is too acute for him or her to handle.
Clove-hitch restraints	Secure one arm or leg for a procedure, such as an intravenous infusion (see Chap. 37).	Use disposable restraints, gauze, or soft muslin tape. Soft muslin tape "gives" a little if the child exerts pressure against it so it will not pull too tight and reduce circulation or cause pain. Tie the restraint as shown in Figure 36-1*A*. If a child struggles against restraints, fold several layers of soft gauze around the wrist or ankle under the restraint. Secure the restraint to the underpart of the bed. Never tie restraints to side rails: when a side rail is lowered, it will jerk the child's arm or leg and possibly cause an injury. Release arm and leg restraints whenever someone can be with the child to keep the limb in the desired position.
Jacket restraints	Restrain children younger than 6 months in a supine position. (This method is not effective with older children because they are too active: they maneuver so much that they may squirm out of the jacket or put so much pressure on the trachea that they suffocate.)	Fasten the ties at the back of the jacket. Tie strips attached to the sides of the jacket under the mattress to keep the child in one position (see Fig. 36-1*B*).
Elbow restraints	Prevent children from touching the head or face—for example, during scalp vein infusion or after cleft lip or cleft palate repair.	Use a double-layered piece of soft muslin, which has pockets wide enough to fit tongue depressors. Place pockets vertically. Wrap the restraint around the child's arm. Secure the restraint with ties, tape, or pins (see Fig. 36-1*C*). It may be necessary to pin the restraint to the child's undershirt to prevent slippage. If *No-No sleeves*, a commercial elbow restraint, is used, slip the *No-No sleeves* up over the infant's arms and secure it by the Velcro strips (see Fig. 36-1*D*). The baby should wear a long-sleeved infant shirt under the sleeves to prevent irritation. Observe the child to be certain the sleeves are not too tight and interfere with circulation.
Mummy restraints	Temporarily immobilize young children for a procedure involving the head, neck, or throat—for example, during insertion of a nasogastric tube or drawing blood.	Use this only for the duration of the procedure because it is a total body restraint. Follow the steps shown in Figure 36-1*E*. If the child is exceptionally strong, a few safety pins can be used to hold the restraint even more firmly. For the infant who needs continuous observation for respiratory function, fold the mummy restraint so the chest is exposed. For newborns or infants, use a "Papoose Board," commercial restraints used in this same way as full or mummy restraints (see Fig. 36-1*F*).

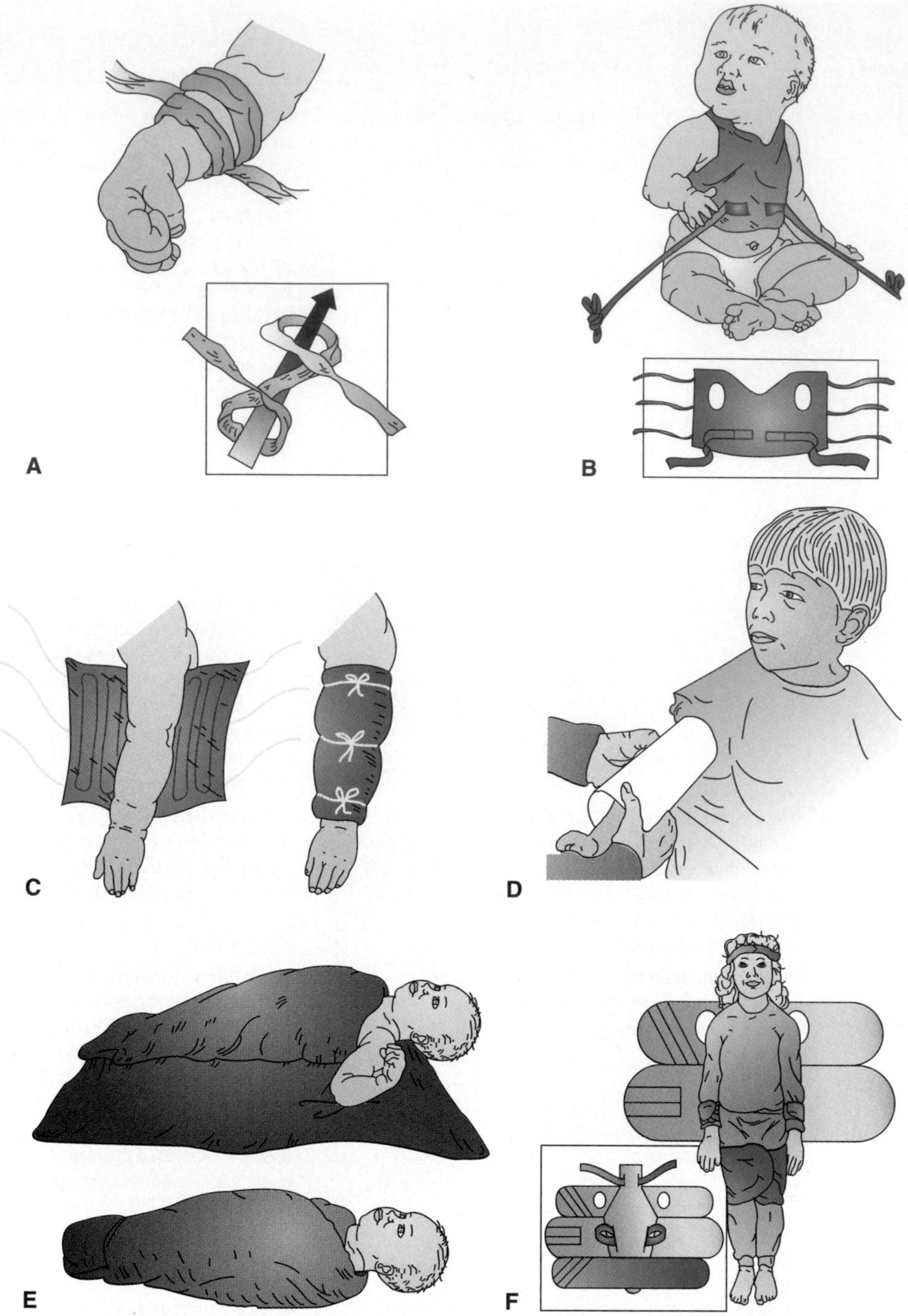

A B C D E F

FIGURE 36.1 (*A*) Clove hitch restraint. (*B*) Jacket restraint. (*C*) Elbow restraint. (*D*) No-no sleeve or commercial elbow restraint. (*E*) Mummy restraint. (*F*) Papoose board.

an intravenous injection for such a study, the child may feel a hot flush, a sensation that can be frightening if the child is unprepared for it. Try not to use the word "dye" while describing the procedure to prevent a young child from worrying he or she will be dyed like a colored egg or will "die." Use "medicine" instead.

Children easily grow bored with this type of procedure because of the time involved waiting for the dye to reach the specific organ to be studied. Have the child take along an activity to make the time pass faster. If a child is not allowed to eat for the duration of a long procedure, be certain that he or she receives supervision or else, not realizing the importance of this, the child may decide to snack. Ensure that parents understand that the child will not be "radiating" x-rays or radioactivity after the procedure, so they will not be afraid to hold the child closely for comfort.

Computed Tomography

Computed tomography (CT) is an x-ray procedure in which many views of an organ or body part are made to represent what the organ would look like if it were cut

Activity:	Description:	Score:
Activity	Able to move four extremities	2
	Able to move two extremities	1
	Able to move no extremities	0
Respiration	Regular, able to deep breathe/cough	2
	Dyspnea, limited and obstructed breathing	1
	Apneic	0
Circulation	BP within 20 mm Hg of preprocedure	2
	BP within 20–25 mm Hg of preprocedure	1
	BP 25 mm Hg above preprocedure level	0
Level of consciousness	Awake, alert	5
	Drowsy, but easily aroused	4
	Stupor, aroused by vigorous stimuli	2
	Responds to pain only	1
	No response to pain	0
Skin color	Pink, warm, dry	2
	Pale, dusky, blotchy, clammy	1
	Cyanotic, diaphoretic, cold	0
Ambulation	Ambulates with minimum help	5
	Ambulates with minimum support	4
	Unable to ambulate	2

FIGURE 36.2 Post-Anesthesia Recovery Score. A passing score is at least 10 with a level of consciousness score no lower than 4. (From Tolia, V., et al. [2000]. Sedation for pediatric endoscopic procedures. *Journal of Pediatric Gastroenterology and Nutrition, 30*[5], 477–485.)

into thin slices. As with any x-ray, dense structures appear white and less dense structures appear gray to black on the films.

The procedure may require injection of an iodine-based contrast medium. If a radioisotope is added, the study is referred to as **positron emission tomography (PET)** or **single photon emission computerized tomography (SPECT).**

Because a CT scan involves so many films, it is a lengthy procedure. The machinery is complex, large, and potentially frightening (Fig. 36-5*A*). Children must lie still during the long procedure to avoid creating shadows on the film.

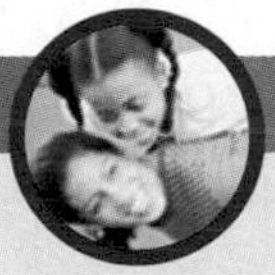

FOCUS ON FAMILY EMPOWERMENT

After Conscious Sedation

Q. My daughter received conscious sedation for a diagnostic procedure. What special care will she need when I get her home?

A. Here are some tips to help you when you get your daughter home:

- Keep in mind that most children sleep after leaving the ambulatory care facility or hospital. Some are sleepy for the remainder of the day.
- Don't allow the child to walk alone for at least 4 hours. The child may feel suddenly dizzy and fall without warning.
- Wait until getting home to give the child something to eat or drink to avoid car sickness. Conscious sedation may cause children to feel nauseated more easily than usual.
- For the first 12 hours after awaking, don't ask the child to do any activity that requires alertness, coordination, or balance, such as riding a bicycle, swimming, or doing homework. The sedative can affect the child's coordination and balance.
- Remember that the child may forget things readily for the rest of the day. This forgetfulness should go away after a night's sleep.
- Keep in mind that a sedative may cause children to behave in unexpected ways, such as losing self-control or becoming very emotional. By the next day, the child's behavior should return to normal.
- Give infants clear liquids (water, apple juice, tea) after getting home. Wait approximately 30 minutes to make sure the child does not choke or vomit. Then milk, formula, or other foods may be given.
- Do not allow children to drink until they can hold a cup without help to make sure they are awake enough to keep from choking. Wait approximately 30 minutes. If there is no vomiting or choking, the child can have the foods he or she usually eats.
- Call your primary care provider if the child has recurrent vomiting or if any of the effects above last for more than 12 hours or if the child has pain.

Tolia, V., et al. (2000). Sedation for pediatric endoscopic procedures. *Journal of Pediatric Gastroenterology & Nutrition, 30*(5), 477–485.

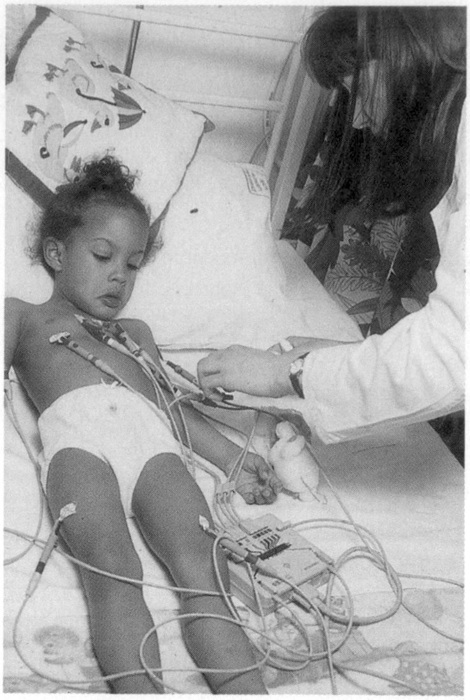

FIGURE 36.3 Administering an ECG. Children can be assured that this is a painless procedure.

To help them to lie still for an extended period, they may be given a sedative such as chloral hydrate before the procedure, which makes them sleepy. Conscious sedation, the state of depressed consciousness obtained by intravenous analgesia therapy, also may be used. Parents need reassurance that although the radiation exposure from CT scans occurs over a long period, such low doses are used that the actual exposure is less than during a regular x-ray.

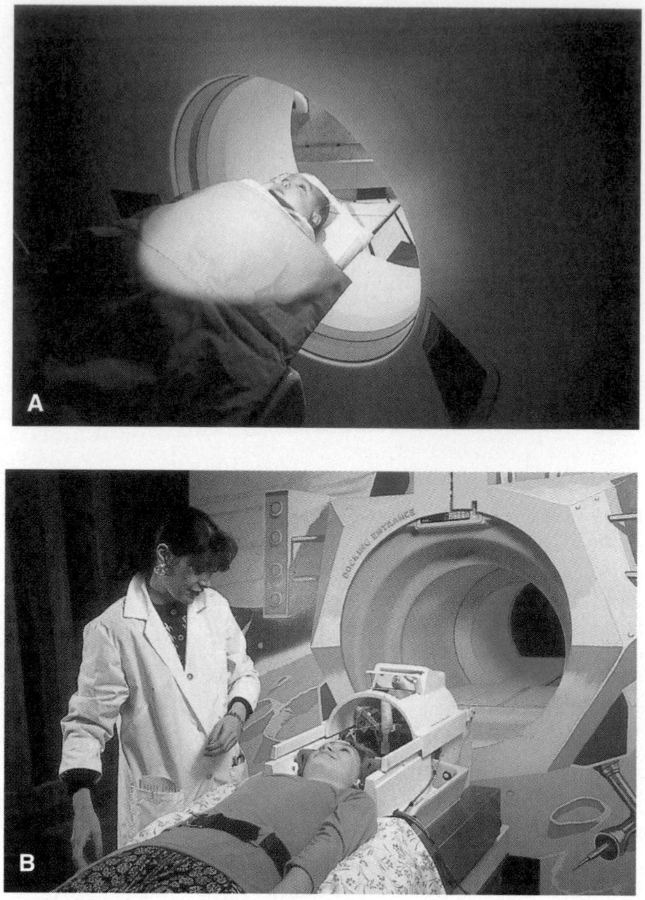

FIGURE 36.5 Some procedures are potentially frightening because of the size of the machinery used. (*A*) A CT scanner. (*B*) An MRI scanner.

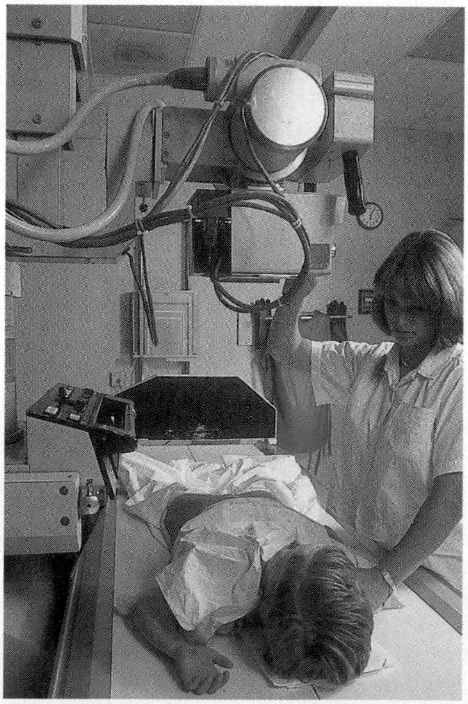

FIGURE 36.4 Positioning of a child for an x-ray.

Magnetic Resonance Imaging

Magnetic resonance imaging (MRI) combines a magnetic field, radiofrequency, and computer technology to produce diagnostic images to aid in the diagnosis of disorders such as the cause of hip pain (White et al., 2001). The child lies on a moving pallet that is pushed into the core of the machine—the magnet (see Fig. 36-5*B*). When the magnetic field surrounding the child is turned on, it causes tissue atoms to line up in a parallel fashion. As radio waves are turned on and off, the atoms change position. This change is sensed and converted into a visual display on a computer screen.

The procedure has an advantage over x-ray in that it has no apparent ill effects, it can reveal astonishingly clear structural defects in soft tissue, and if a contrast medium is required, it is not iodine-based, so the danger of a reaction is minimal. Because metal may deflect the magnetic waves, children with a metal prosthesis or metal dental braces may be poor candidates for the procedure. Hairpins and eye makeup (which often has a metallic base), watches, or other jewelry should be removed. Be certain a child's hospital gown does not have a metal snap at the neckline.

When the radio waves are turned on and off during the procedure, a booming noise occurs. Prepare children for this sound (often compared with the sound of drums) as well as the feeling of claustrophobia that they may experience. Because the procedure may take up to 45 minutes, some children need a sedative or conscious sedation so they can lie quietly for the duration of the procedure. Newer, more open MRI machines are being developed to alleviate the feeling of claustrophobia associated with the procedure.

Ultrasound

Ultrasound is a painless procedure in which pictures of internal tissue and organs, such as the appendix, are produced by sound waves (Emil et al., 2001). Because it is noninvasive, children accept ultrasound easily and may even enjoy watching the oscilloscope screen during the procedure. The transducer that is used on the body surface to pick up internal images can be compared to a television camera (Fig. 36-6). Explain to parents that ultrasound is not an x-ray and appears to have no long-term effects. Tell the child that a clear gel will be applied to the skin over the body part to be studied to aid sound conduction. Also warn them that the gel can feel cold and sticky.

Nuclear Medicine Studies

Radiopharmaceuticals are radioactive-combined substances that, when given orally or by injection, flow to designated body organs. When a scintillation machine (a form of Geiger counter) is passed over the organ where the radiopharmaceutical has collected, the pattern of the collected material outlines the organ; the pattern can be produced as a screen image or a photograph.

Parents may worry that a child will be harmed by such exposure to a radioactive substance. Inform them that the dose of radiation in these studies is no greater than that used for a diagnostic x-ray, so this is not a danger. Tagged iodine (iodine-131) is frequently the medium used for such studies. Iodine will go immediately to the thyroid gland when injected intravenously, with the result being that enough concentrated radioactivity could accumulate to destroy the thyroid gland. For this reason, a blocking agent such as potassium perchlorate that prevents thyroid gland accumulation may be given prior to the test. This prevents the radioactive substance from concentrating in the thyroid, thereby protecting the gland. Always check whether a blocking agent is required before transporting a child to the nuclear medicine department.

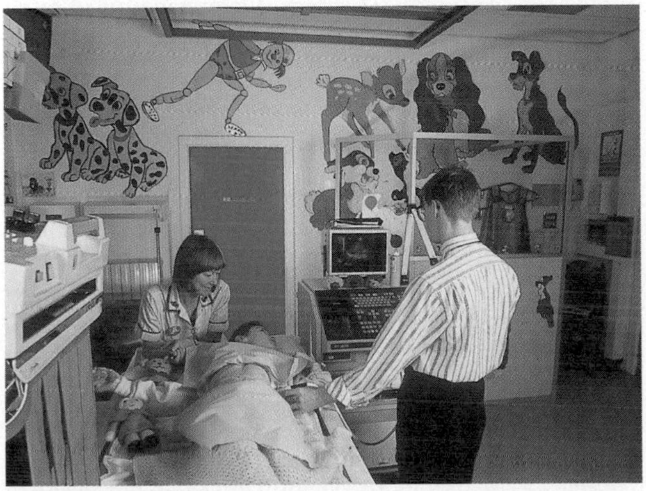

FIGURE 36.6 Sonography can be potentially frightening for children. Seeing the image on the television screen helps to relieve their fright.

Direct Visualization Procedures

Direct visualization procedures involve the observation of an internal body cavity by way of a thin tube inserted through a body surface opening. Types of direct visualization include **endoscopy,** in which an endoscope is passed through the mouth to examine the gastrointestinal tract; **bronchoscopy,** in which a bronchoscope is passed through the nose or mouth to observe the larynx, trachea, bronchi, and alveoli; and **colonoscopy,** in which a colonoscope is passed through the anus to examine the rectum or colon.

Endoscopy

Endoscopy has become a common method of diagnosis for gastrointestinal disorders in children. When first developed, endoscopes were straight, stiff, metal instruments, which limited their use. Currently, endoscopes are fiberoptic (using a flexible, easily maneuvered, brightly lit tube), so these examinations are more common and not as uncomfortable as before.

The procedure is often frightening, however. A child can easily understand an explanation of the procedure (the physician will extend the child's head and pass a tube down into the child's stomach for direct observation), but the child is uncomfortable at the thought of someone doing it. Children are placed on nothing by mouth (NPO) status for about 4 hours before the procedure. They may need a sedative or conscious sedation so they can lie quietly for the time needed. Good support during the procedure is also important (Fig. 36-7). Ask whether the child can have a

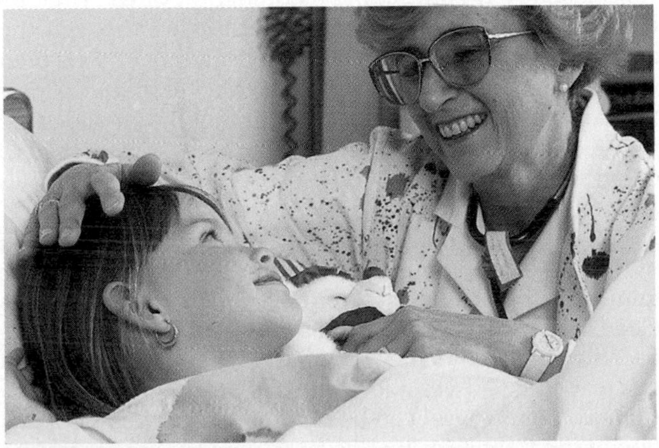

FIGURE 36.7 Here a nurse provides support to a child before undergoing an endoscopy.

Polaroid photo taken during the procedure to keep as a souvenir. Endoscopy is also used as an emergency measure to remove objects such as quarters or safety pins swallowed by children.

After an endoscopy study, edema may occur from the pressure of the scope on the esophagus and pharynx. Aftercare consists of close assessment to see that edema is not interfering with a vital function such as respiration or causing discomfort. After the procedure, be sure to check for return of the gag reflex before offering any fluid to drink. Also observe the child closely the first time that he or she drinks after the procedure to ensure that the gag reflex is intact despite throat edema from the procedure or the effect of a local pharyngeal anesthetic that may have been sprayed into the throat before the procedure.

Bronchoscopy

Bronchoscopy is the direct visualization of the larynx, trachea, and bronchi through a lit, flexible, fiberoptic tube (a bronchofiberscope). The procedure is used with children who have aspirated a foreign object such as a peanut or to take culture and biopsy specimens. Before the procedure, the child may be given atropine by injection to reduce bronchial secretions and encourage bronchial relaxation. Typically the throat is sprayed with a local pharyngeal anesthetic to numb the area. Because the procedure can be frightening and thus make it difficult for the child to cooperate, a sedative or conscious sedation usually is administered. Any manipulation of the airway has the potential to cause increased bronchial secretions and edema, leading to narrowing of the airway. Therefore, closely observe the child's respiratory function and airway for at least 4 hours after the procedure. An ice bag applied to the neck often helps reduce the possibility of edema and relieve throat discomfort. Assess for the presence of a gag reflex before offering any oral fluids to the child after the procedure. Also, observe children carefully the first time they drink after the procedure to be certain their gag reflex is intact.

Colonoscopy

Colonoscopy is endoscopic examination of the large intestine with a flexible fiberscope inserted through the anus and advanced as far as the ileocecal valve. Air is then infused to expand the bowel walls. The technique allows the colon walls to be visualized, and if abnormalities are found, photographs can be taken for analysis. It is used to diagnose inflammatory bowel disease or obtain biopsies if a malignancy is suspected.

Before the procedure, children are given a clear liquid diet for about 24 hours. Then they are given an isotonic saline laxative that causes fluid diarrhea so their bowel is clean for the procedure. It can be difficult for younger children to drink as much of the laxative solution as is needed to clear their bowel completely of stool. Playing games such as "Simon Says" can be helpful to gain their cooperation. If the laxative cannot be taken, a saline enema may be necessary. Conscious sedation is used during the procedure to reduce discomfort.

If done on an ambulatory basis, children are discharged about 2 hours after the procedure (keep them NPO during that time to allow the bowel to have a brief rest). Children may pass a great deal of flatus in the first 12 hours because of the air introduced during the procedure. Be certain parents have instructions on what to observe for after they return home: abdominal pain, blood in stool, weakness, paleness, or signs of bowel bleeding. Even with conscious sedation, colonoscopies are difficult procedures for children to accept. Give generous praise afterward for their cooperation with the preparation for the procedure and the actual procedure.

Aspiration Studies

Aspiration studies (removal of body fluids by such techniques as lumbar puncture or bone marrow aspiration) are always frightening procedures; often just looking at the size of the needle is frightening. A child may need a sedative or conscious sedation so that he or she can lie quietly. Support and restrain the child by talking and using touch as appropriate. Assess for bleeding at the puncture site after the procedure and apply pressure as needed to halt bleeding completely (see Chaps. 44 and 49).

✔ CHECKPOINT QUESTIONS

3. Why do most children have a blocking agent administered before a procedure with radioactive iodine?
4. What is the difference between endoscopy and bronchoscopy?

MEASUREMENT OF VITAL SIGNS

Vital signs for children need to be recorded both conscientiously and with knowledge of the underlying condition so that they can be analyzed meaningfully (DeNicola et al., 2001). Vital sign values differ according to the size and age of children. Appendix G shows the average pulse rates, respiration rates, and blood pressures for children of different ages.

Pulse Rate

As children grow older, the heart rate slows and the range of normal values narrows. If possible, measure a child's pulse rate at rest. An apical pulse (listening at the heart apex through a stethoscope) is taken in children younger than 1 year because their radial (wrist) pulse is too faint to palpate accurately. In an infant, the point of maximum intensity, or the point on the chest wall where the heartbeat can be heard most distinctly, is just above and outside the left nipple (just lateral to the midclavicular line at the third or fourth intercostal space). This point gradually becomes more medial and slightly lower up to the age of 7 years. By 7 years of age it is at the fourth or fifth interspace at the midclavicular line. For greatest accuracy, count the pulse rate for 1 full minute.

Respiratory Rate

Respirations also should be measured before an infant is disturbed because the respiratory rate increases with crying. Take this while the child is sitting in the parent's lap or lying quietly in a crib before lowering the side rail. Infants tend to breathe with their abdominal muscles; therefore, it is as accurate to take respirations by counting movements of the abdomen as it is to count chest movements. Again, for greatest accuracy, respirations should be counted for 1 full minute.

Temperature

Normal temperature values in children are the same as in adults: axillary, 97.6°F (36.5°C); oral or tympanic, 98.6°F (37.0°C); and rectal, 99.6°F (37.6°C). Thermometers that assess tympanic membrane temperature are ideal for assessment in children because they register within 2 seconds and therefore cause less fear in the child because he or she does not have to be restrained for long (Fig. 36-8*A*). However, tympanic membrane temperatures may not be most effective for newborns (see Focus on Evidence-Based Practice).

Newborns should always have their temperature taken by the axillary or tympanic membrane method because of the danger of damaging their rectal mucosa with a rectal thermometer (see Fig. 36-8*B*). Because preschoolers generally fear intrusive procedures, consider taking axillary or tympanic temperatures in children until 4 years of age (Saxena et al., 2001).

For a tympanic temperature recording, insert the tip of the tympanic thermometer gently into the child's ear canal. Straighten the ear canal by pulling down on the earlobe in a child younger than age 3 and pulling up on the child older than age 3. This directs the sensor beam toward the center of the tympanic membrane and not the sides of the canal. Tympanic membrane temperature is not affected by the presence of ear wax. It gives consistently accurate results (Houlder, 2000; see Focus on Evidence-Based Practice). By 4 years of age, children are usually old enough to close their mouth sufficiently for oral temperature recording by an electronic thermometer.

For an axillary recording, place the tip of an electronic thermometer in the axilla and hold the child's arm down to the side to keep the thermometer firmly in place until it registers. For the rare occasions when a rectal temperature must be taken, insert a thermometer only to the length of the bulb (½ inch) in infants and not over 1 inch in older children, and hold it in place for 5 minutes.

FOCUS ON EVIDENCE-BASED PRACTICE

Which Temperature Recording Method Is Best to Use With Newborns?

To answer this question, nurse researchers compared the accuracy and cost of four types of temperature assessment tools: digital disposable, electronic, tympanic membrane, and glass mercury thermometers. One hundred and eighty-four newborns between 1 and 168 hours of age were included in the study. Temperatures were obtained at either an axillary or left tympanic membrane site with the infant either in an open crib, under a radiant warmer, or in the mother's arms.

Results of the study revealed that the measurements taken by the electronic, glass, and digital thermometers were highly correlated. Despite its convenience, the tympanic membrane thermometer recording had a low correlation. Although tympanic thermometers are recognized as being the most cost efficient, the researchers suggest that tympanic thermometers may not be the method of choice for recording accurate temperatures in healthy newborn infants.

This is an important study for nurses because they may need to advocate for the use of electronic or digital thermometers when assessing temperatures in newborns to ensure the most accurate data.

Sganga, A., Wallace, R., Kiehl, E., Irving, T., & Witter, L. (2000). A comparison of four methods of normal newborn temperature measurement. *MCN: The American Journal of Maternal/Child Nursing, 25*(2), 76–79.

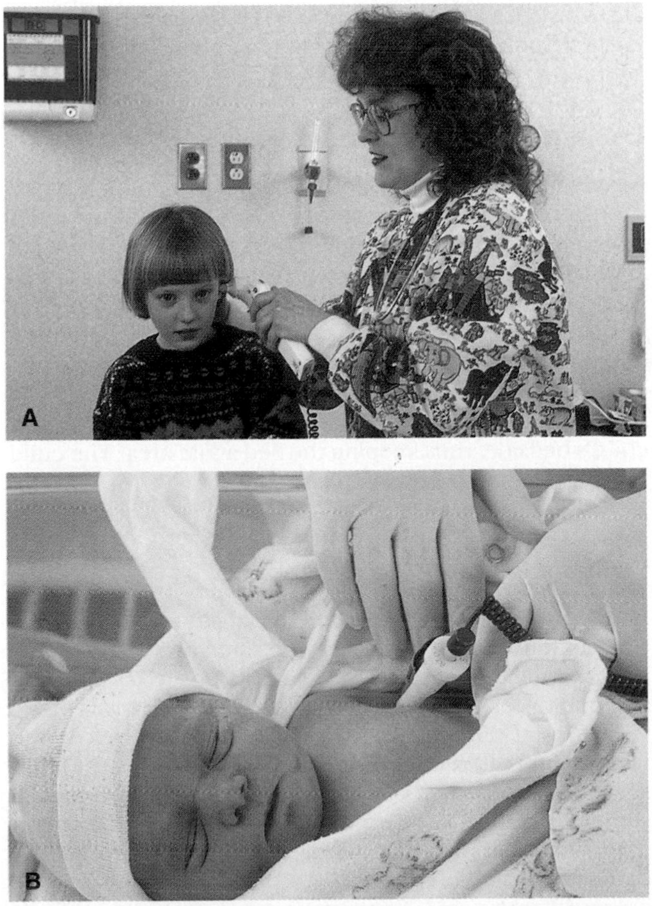

FIGURE 36.8 Temperature taking. (*A*) Tympanic membrane temperature. (*B*) Axillary temperature.

Blood Pressure

Blood pressure should be included in the routine physical assessment of all children older than 3 years of age. Offer a good explanation of the procedure, especially to young children, because wrapping their arm and applying pressure can be frightening if they are not prepared for it.

Blood pressure is difficult to measure in infants because of mechanical problems. The cuff used should be no more than two-thirds and not less than one-half the length of the upper arm; a wider cuff (larger bladder size) gives a lower reading and a narrower cuff gives a higher reading (Fig. 36-9). Therefore, Doppler ultrasound blood pressure recording is especially effective with infants. This technique bounces high-frequency sound waves off body parts; the rate and pitch at which they return depends on the density of the body part that is struck. If a Doppler lead is placed over an artery, either the movement of the blood (pulse wave) or its tension (blood pressure) can be registered in a digital readout or monitor print. Dopplers can be adapted to broadcast the sound of the pulse waves for auscultatory assessment.

Electronic blood pressure recording is most helpful when a continuous assessment is necessary, but it can be used for a single recording. Watching the digital readout numbers is interesting for preschoolers. Direct measurement (intra-arterial monitoring by an indwelling catheter into the radial or femoral artery) is used with children who are critically ill. This technique is reviewed in Chapter 41.

Systolic pressure in children is read as the manometer pressure is being lowered, at the moment that sound first appears. The point at which the sound disappears is considered the diastolic pressure in children (Kay et al., 2001).

Blood pressure can be obtained by wrapping the cuff over the thigh and palpating or auscultating the popliteal pulse (posterior knee). In infants younger than 1 year, the thigh and arm blood pressure should be equal. In children older than 1 year, the systolic pressure in the thigh tends to be 10 to 40 mm Hg higher, while diastolic pressure remains the same. If the thigh blood pressure reading is lower than that in the arm, suspect coarctation of the aorta or an interference with circulation to the lower extremities.

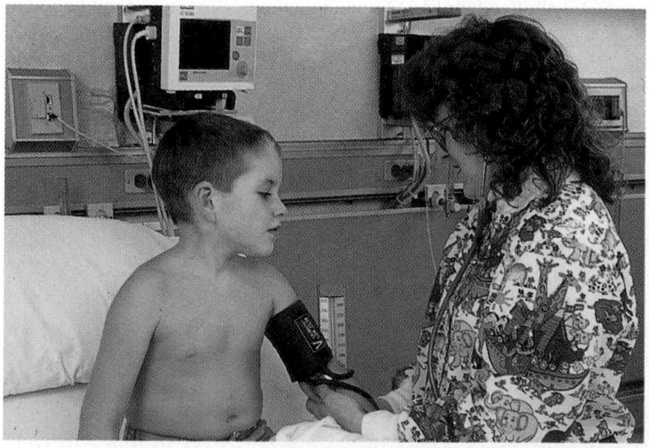

FIGURE 36.9 Measurement of blood pressure is essential during routine health assessments and before diagnostic or therapeutic procedures. Here a nurse assesses the child's blood pressure in preparation for a procedure.

When assessing blood pressure, be certain to pay attention to the pulse pressure—the difference between systolic and diastolic readings. Both unusually wide (more than 50 mm Hg) and narrow (less than 10 mm Hg) ranges may suggest congenital heart disease. An abnormally narrow pulse pressure, for instance, is a sign of aortic stenosis. An abnormally low diastolic pressure (causing a wide pulse pressure) occurs with patent ductus arteriosus.

✔ CHECKPOINT QUESTIONS

5. What is the ideal size of a blood pressure cuff for an infant?
6. How long does it take for a tympanic thermometer to register?

SPECIMEN COLLECTION

The collection of body fluids, secretions, and excretions is a collaborative nursing function essential to the complete assessment of a child. Elements of these fluids can be measured by a variety of means and compared with baseline standards of health. Findings may be used to help diagnose an illness, evaluate the progress of a particular condition, or evaluate a child's response to therapy. As with all procedures, use of standard precautions is essential when obtaining, transporting, and discarding or storing specimens.

Obtaining Blood Specimens

Never underestimate how frightening obtaining a blood specimen can be to children. For many children, any experience of losing blood has been from a nosebleed or a cut knee, which they remember as causing discomfort or pain. They have had injections for immunizations also, so they know that injections sting. Putting the two experiences together makes having blood drawn an extremely frightening procedure. For this reason, blood specimens should always be obtained from somewhere other than at the child's bedside, thus keeping the bed a safe area. The child also needs good preparation and support.

Venipuncture

Even for very small infants, the usual sites for venipuncture (entrance into a vein) are the same as for adults: the superficial veins of the dorsal surface of the hand or the antecubital fossa. In a few instances, the jugular or femoral vein is used (Fig. 36-10). Apply EMLA cream before the venipuncture to reduce pain (see Chap. 38). Give the child a simple explanation of what will be done: "I need to take some blood from your hand. First, I'll put some cream on your skin. Then in a little while, I'll come back to get the blood and you won't even feel a pinprick because of the cream." Let the child know you understand how difficult it is to agree to the procedure. A statement such as, "No one likes to have blood taken; I'm going to do this as

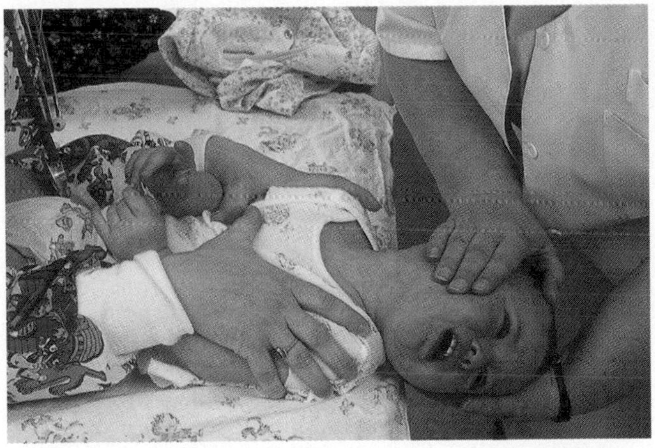

FIGURE 36.10 Positioning for jugular venipuncture. The infant's head is held sideways over the edge of the table by one nurse, while his body is restrained by a second nurse.

quickly as possible" is always a better approach than, "Be a big girl" or "Come on, show me how much of a big boy you can be." The second approach shames a child who is unable to hold still. Try not to use the phrase "drawing blood." This sounds as if an activity with crayons is being proposed, not a procedure with some discomfort (see Focus on Communication).

Preschoolers may have to be restrained for blood sampling, because no matter how cooperative or brave they might be initially, the minute they see the needle, they are too overwhelmed with fear to hold still.

FOCUS ON COMMUNICATION

T.J. is a 4-year-old you meet in an ambulatory care clinic. He's coloring a picture when you approach him to obtain a blood specimen for electrolyte levels.

Less Effective Communication
Nurse: Hi, T.J. Is it all right if I draw some blood?
T.J.: Okay.
Nurse: Hold out your arm for me.
T.J.: Are you drawing on me?
Nurse: I'm going to wipe off your arm, then prick your skin. T.J. begins crying.
T.J.'s Mother: He thought you meant you were going to play with him.

More Effective Communication
Nurse: Hi, T.J. Because you're not feeling well, I need to take some blood from your arm.

The nurse in the first scenario makes two mistakes in introducing a procedure: making the activity seem like a game and also asking for permission to carry it out. In the second scenario, the nurse takes a little more time to both explain what she needs to do and why it is important. It's easy to forget that what a word means to you may not be interpreted the same way by a young child.

Capillary Puncture

Capillary blood is often obtained for glucose and hematocrit determinations by a fingertip or a heel puncture. The technique for this is described in Nursing Procedure 36-1. For fingertip punctures, be certain to use the side of the finger, not the center, to reduce discomfort afterward; for heel punctures, use the lateral aspect of the heel to avoid striking the medial plantar artery or the periosteum of the bone. Apply EMLA cream prior to the procedure to reduce discomfort.

Obtaining Urine Specimens

Depending on the type of test required, urine may be collected with a usual voiding, after the external meatus has been cleaned (a clean-catch specimen), by catheterization, or by suprapubic aspiration. The test may require a single specimen or collection of all voidings in a 24-hour period.

Routine Urinalysis

Routine urinalysis requires a single voiding specimen. The term "urinalysis" refers to assessment for appearance, glucose, specific gravity, and microscopic analysis of urine. Specimens for this must be collected in clean containers to prevent contamination by additives.

The Infant or Toddler. A child who has not been toilet-trained cannot be expected to urinate on command, so it is necessary to attach a collecting device to a girl's perineum or a boy's penis and scrotum to collect the child's next voiding. Be certain to wash and dry the site where the collecting device will be attached to ensure good adherence (Fig. 36-11*A*). If an infant attempts to loosen the collector, cover the device with a diaper to keep it out of reach. Otherwise, leave it visible so that it can be observed for voiding. Offer the child something to drink. Most infants void shortly after a feeding, so if the collector is applied just before a regular feeding, voiding will probably result soon afterward. Remove the collector as soon as the infant voids and transfer the specimen to a specimen cup by clipping a bottom corner of the bag.

Urine may be aspirated from diapers for tests such as specific gravity, dipstick protein, pH, or glucose. This does not pull enough lint into the specimen to change its specific gravity (see Fig. 36-11*B*). With disposable diapers, urine tends to be pulled into the diaper and is best available for testing if the diaper is torn apart. Placing cotton balls inside the diaper can be a help because they can be squeezed for additional urine. Although not an ideal method for urine collection, urine extracted from a disposable diaper can be analyzed for bacteria for urinary tract infections. Be sure to note on the laboratory form how the urine specimen was collected.

The Preschooler or School-Age Child. It may be difficult to obtain routine urine specimens from preschoolers or toilet-trained toddlers because they can void only when they feel a definite urge to do so, not on command. Another problem is language. It is not unprofessional to use words such as "pee-pee" if this is what the child will understand. Provide a potty chair if one is available; if not, put a urine collection cap device on a toilet. A generally

NURSING PROCEDURE 36.1: TECHNIQUE FOR FINGERTIP OR HEEL CAPILLARY PUNCTURE

Purpose
To obtain a blood sample from a peripheral capillary.

Procedure	Principle
1. Wash your hands; identify child; explain procedure to child.	1. Prevents spread of microorganisms from you to child. Promotes safety and well-being.
2. Assess status of puncture site.	2. Site must be warm and free of lesions.
3. Analyze appropriateness of procedure; adjust plan to individual circumstances.	3. Nursing care is always individualized based on professional judgment of client need.
4. Plan and give health teaching and preparation information as necessary.	4. Health teaching and preparation is an independent nursing action always included in care.
5. Assemble necessary equipment: gloves, alcohol swab, lancet, collecting capillary blood tube, dry compress or cotton ball, adhesive bandage.	5. Organization and preparation help conserve energy and maximize efficiency.
6. Assess the temperature of the selected site. Fingertips and heels must be warm. Warm by holding finger or heel in your hand for a moment or two. Warming heels or fingers by immersing them in warm water or covering with a warm compress is not advised.	6. Although warmth helps to dilate vessels and allows blood to flow more freely, warm water methods increase the flow of blood so much that values become comparable with arterial, not venous, values.
7. Select the exact puncture site: sides of tip of finger; right or left of medial artery of heel (see figure below). Allow child to choose finger if appropriate.	7. Using the child's nondominant hand avoids the child from having to use the tender finger on dominant hand afterward. Allowing choices adds to child's feelings of control and self-esteem.

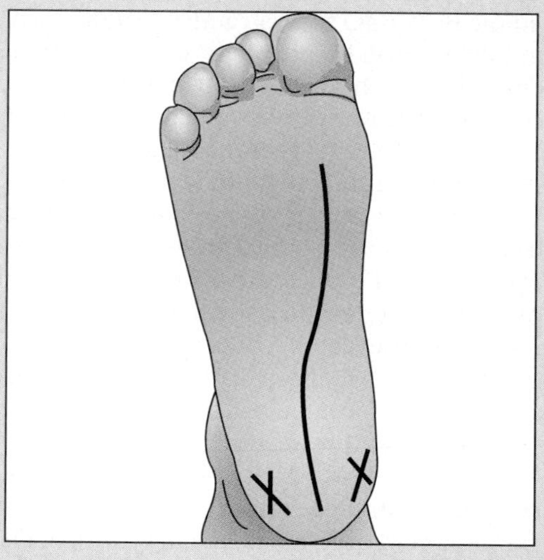

Procedure	Principle
8. Apply gloves. Swab site with alcohol and allow to dry. Puncture with a quick thrusting movement; wipe away first drop of blood with dry cotton ball.	8. Allowing the alcohol to dry prevents burning from the puncture. Wiping away first drop prevents contamination or dilution of the specimen.
9. Hold heel or finger lower than proximal extremity; touch capillary tube to blood drop and tip to encourage flow. Do not squeeze tissue around site.	9. Capillary action will quickly fill the collecting tube; squeezing causes tissue injury.
10. After filling required number of blood tubes, apply dry compress to site; apply adhesive bandage.	10. Applying dry compress to site halts bleeding.
11. Label specimen appropriately and send to proper laboratory for analysis.	11. Labeling and prompt transport ensure continuity of care.
12. Evaluate effectiveness, efficiency, cost, safety, and comfort aspects of procedure; record procedure and child's reaction.	12. Evaluation determines effectiveness of care. Documentation provides evidence of nursing care and the child's status.

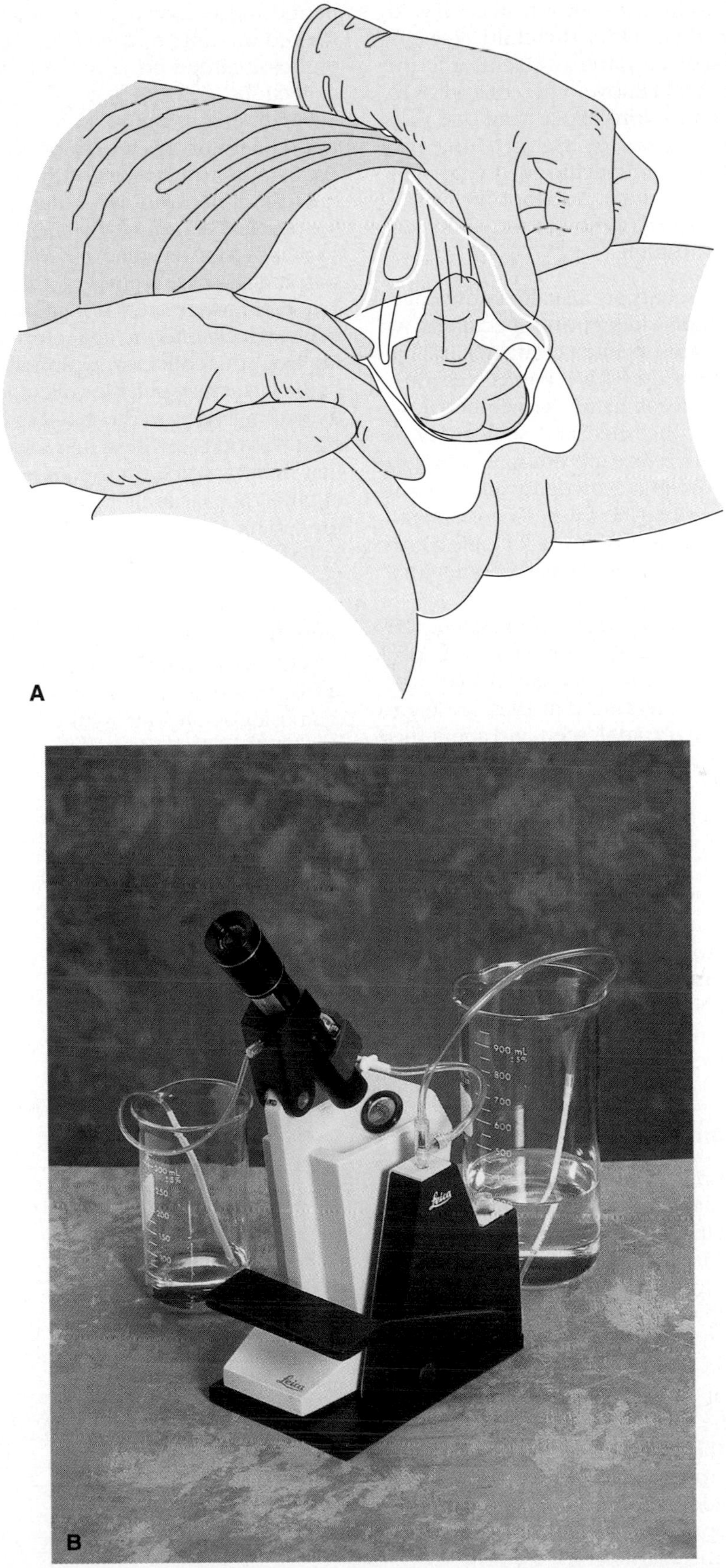

FIGURE 36.11 (*A*) Urine collector for infants. The trick to making the collector adhere is to be certain that the child's skin is dry. (*B*) Testing specific gravity of urine with a refractometer. The advantage of this is that only one drop of urine is required.

successful approach with a child this age is to act as if voiding is not a difficult procedure. Offer the child a glass of water or other fluid, and ask a parent to reinforce the request to void so that the child knows a parent approves. Do not encourage children to drink more than one glass of fluid to induce voiding, however, or else their urine production may be so diluted that the specific gravity, protein, and glucose levels will be inaccurate. A school-age child is usually able to void when asked, although the child may find it more difficult than the adult.

The Adolescent. Adolescents are usually knowledgeable and cooperative about providing urine specimens. As with adults, give them a clean specimen container and tell them what is needed. Unless they have voided recently, they usually are able to void on command. Remember, however, that adolescents are concerned and self-conscious about body functions and therefore are often reluctant to carry a urine specimen through a crowded waiting room or reception desk area. They may be too self-conscious to void if they know someone is nearby—just outside a curtain, for example. Send them to a nearby bathroom with a closed door, or leave the area to give them privacy.

Some adolescents are suspicious that a urine specimen is being requested for drug testing. Providing a good explanation of its actual purpose relieves this fear. Adolescent girls may be embarrassed to mention that they are menstruating. Be sure to question the adolescent girl about this so that the presence of any red blood cells in a urine specimen can be explained.

To avoid having a urine specimen contaminated by menstrual blood (which changes the specific gravity, protein, and red blood cell analysis), ask the girl who is menstruating to wash her perineum well with soap and water and rinse and dry it to remove menstrual blood. Next, supply a sterile cotton ball for her to insert gently into her vagina just before voiding (and remove again following voiding). Mark the specimen "possibly contaminated by menstrual blood" even though it does not appear discolored, because red blood cells may be present microscopically.

Twenty-Four-Hour Urine Specimens

Although urinalysis of a single urine specimen will indicate the presence of substances such as protein or glucose, a 24-hour urine specimen is necessary to determine the quantitative amount of many substances or how much of a substance is excreted during a day (quantitative analysis). To begin a 24-hour urine collection, ask the child to void (with an infant, attach a collecting bag and wait for the child to void). This specimen (the discard specimen) is then thrown away so that a specific time for the ensuing collection is known. If the urine collection was started early in the morning and this first specimen was counted as part of the collection, the urine collected during the next 24 hours would include urine that had been forming all night, resulting in an approximately 32-hour collection period that would distort the analysis.

Record the start of the collection period as the time of the discarded urine. Save all urine voided for the next 24 hours and place it in one collection bottle. Have the child void (or watch for an infant to void) at the end of the 24-hour period and add the final specimen to the collection bottle. Record the time of the collection as being from the time of the discarded urine to the final specimen added to the collection.

For an infant, use a 24-hour urine collector. A collector will adhere for this length of time only if the child's perineum is thoroughly dry at the time of application. Apply tincture of benzoin or a commercial product to toughen the perineal skin and make the skin somewhat tacky. Doing so helps to ensure that the collector firmly adheres to the skin and also eases removal of the collector. Place an infant in a semi-Fowler's position, if possible, to encourage urine to flow freely into the collector. Make certain that the tubing from the collector is pinned out of the infant's reach or the infant may pull the collector free. It may be necessary to place a diaper on the infant to keep the apparatus out of sight. Provide activities; make sure the parents understand that they can pick up the infant and hold him or her during this time, as long as they take care not to kink or pull the tubing.

To keep the bacterial count to a minimum, 24-hour collections are generally kept on ice or poured into a container that is then refrigerated during the 24-hour period until they are transported to the laboratory for analysis.

With active infants, fitting them with a colostomy bag applied to cover the urinary meatus may be more effective than using a collector with tubing (Fig. 36-12). Puncture a small hole in the corner of the top of the bag. Insert a small feeding tube through this into the bottom of the bag. When the child voids, attach a syringe to the feeding tube and aspirate the urine. Transfer the specimen to the collection bottle. This type of urine collector has an advantage in that it allows the child to be ambulatory. For the active toddler, this collector may be the only type that is acceptable to the child.

Clean-Catch Specimens

A **clean-catch urine specimen** is ordered when a urine culture for bacteria is desired. The objective of the specimen is to obtain urine that is uncontaminated by external

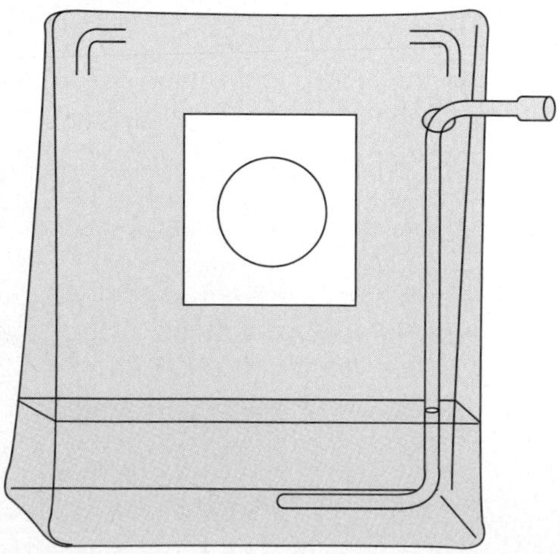

FIGURE 36.12 A 24-hour urine collector made from a colostomy bag. When the infant voids the bag fills with urine, which can be aspirated from the bag by the inserted feeding tube.

organisms that would increase the organism count of the urine. This type of specimen requires that the urinary meatus and the surrounding structures be cleaned before voiding. Specimens used for protein or blood analysis may be ordered as clean-catch specimens because this careful cleaning also reduces the possibility that vaginal or foreskin secretions, which contain protein or blood, would be added to the specimen.

The technique for obtaining a clean-catch urine specimen from an older child is the same as that for an adult (see Nursing Procedure 10-1). Some modifications are necessary for the young child or infant, as it is not always possible to obtain a midstream urine specimen from young children. To collect a specimen from a young child, ask the child to void into a sterile emesis basin or sterile container attached to a toilet or potty seat. Then dip a sterile container into the urine stream to obtain the specimen. If the child voids only a small amount, send that in the sterile container, marked "not midstream." To collect a specimen from an infant, wash the genitalia and apply a sterile urine collector. If the infant does not void within 2 hours, remove the collecting bag and recleanse the perineum or penis because some microorganisms will have collected after this period of time. After the area is recleansed, then reapply a new sterile bag. Again, mark the specimen as "not midstream" for laboratory purposes.

Clean-catch urine specimens have a major advantage over catheterized specimens: they are not intrusive, so they carry no risk of introducing a bladder infection. If clean-catch specimens are obtained with care, they practically eliminate the need for catheterization. A clean-catch specimen with a bacterial colony count of more than 100,000 per mL is considered a positive specimen, or evidence that a urinary tract infection exists. Specimens that appear clear, not cloudy, are probably not infected (Bulloch et al., 2000).

It is almost impossible for young girls to wash their perineum thoroughly because they cannot see it well, so they usually need assistance. Young boys also must be assisted to wash until they have enough coordination to do it themselves. Be aware that this is embarrassing for children. Ask a parent to confirm for the child that the procedure is all right, because they have been told not to let adults touch this part of their body.

To be certain that school-agers and adolescents understand the procedure, have them repeat the instructions given to them; then send them to a nearby bathroom to carry out the procedure by themselves.

Suprapubic Aspiration

Suprapubic aspiration involves the withdrawal of urine by insertion of a sterile needle into the bladder through the anterior wall of the abdomen. It is used to obtain urine for culture in infants who cannot void on command. It is a procedure usually done by physicians, although nurse practitioners or nurses in specialty units may perform it. The steps for this procedure are as follows:

1. The anterior abdominal wall is cleaned with an antiseptic.
2. The urinary meatus is blocked by gloved finger pressure, confining urine in the bladder.
3. A needle is inserted just above the pubis into the bladder.
4. Urine is aspirated through the needle into a sterile syringe.

Although suprapubic aspiration for urine appears complicated, it is not. The bladder is the most anterior of abdominal organs and, when distended with urine, is easily accessible just under the abdominal wall (Fig. 36-13). Because the needle can cause a bladder spasm, however, it can produce sharp discomfort. Parents may not have heard of this procedure and may wonder why their child had urine drawn by needle and syringe instead of by catheter. The method is used because theoretically the risk of bladder infection from needle insertion is less than that from catheter insertion.

Catheterization

Bladder catheterization is accomplished most easily in children up to school age if a small (no. 5 or no. 8) feeding tube is used instead of a urinary catheter. This thin tube passes readily through the meatus of even an infant. Before beginning catheterization, be certain to observe the perineum of females to locate the urinary meatus. It is not as readily observable in infants and young children as it is in adult women. Cleanse the perineum or penis well before inserting the tube to reduce the risk of infection (Langley et al., 2001).

Catheterization is an invasive procedure, so all children must be prepared in advance. Caution children that the catheter will sting for an instant as it is inserted and they

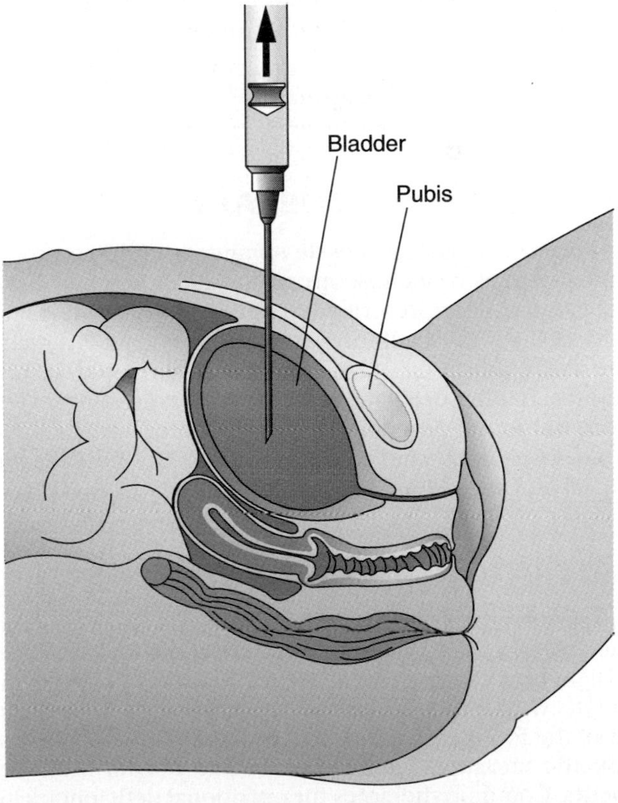

FIGURE 36.13 A suprapubic aspiration. The full bladder is easily accessible by an abdominal puncture.

will have to lie still until the urine specimen is obtained. They need both support to submit to the procedure and praise afterward for their cooperation. Preschool boys may need assurance that the procedure has no long-term consequences to reduce their fear of castration.

Obtaining Stool Specimens

Obtain stool specimens from children who are toilet-trained by asking them to use a potty seat or by placing a collector cap device on a toilet. For effective communication, be certain to know the word the child uses for stool. Transfer the specimen to a collection cup with tongue blades. To obtain a specimen from a child who is not toilet-trained, scrape stool from a diaper using tongue blades and place it in a stool collection cup. Some stool specimens need a preservative added to the container. If it is important to keep urine from contaminating the stool specimen, place a separate urine collector bag on the infant.

Be certain that stool specimens are sent to the laboratory promptly so that they do not dry and have to be collected a second time, because they are difficult to obtain. If the stool specimen is for ova and parasites, see that it arrives in the laboratory in less than 1 hour. Do not refrigerate ova and parasite specimens because refrigeration destroys the organisms to be analyzed.

✔ CHECKPOINT QUESTIONS

7. What are two appropriate sites for obtaining a capillary blood sample in children?
8. When collecting a 24-hour urine specimen, you should time the collection from what point?
9. Why is pressure to the urinary meatus applied during suprapubic aspiration?

HOT AND COLD THERAPY

Children who sustain muscle sprains or undergo procedures such as bronchoscopy or tonsillectomy may have cold applications prescribed to prevent inflammation and edema (Fig. 36-14). If inflammation or edema is already present, application of heat may be prescribed to help it resolve. It is important to implement measures to prevent both burns and boredom in the child during treatments. Guidelines for hot and cold applications are shown in the Focus on Family Empowerment box.

NUTRITIONAL CARE

Because almost all illnesses affect children's nutritional and fluid balance, assessment of these areas sheds a great deal of light on a child's general health. Nutritional assessment begins with asking a child or parent for a 24-hour recall of all the foods eaten during that time, followed by more specific measures such as intake and output measurements. Common therapies for nutritional deficiencies include enteral feeding, gastrostomy, and total parenteral nutrition (TPN).

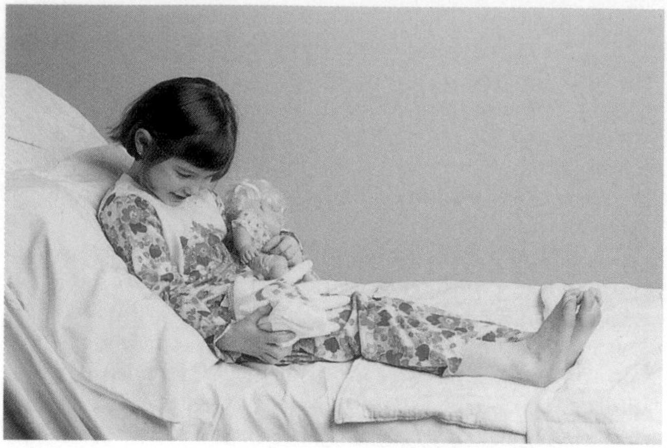

FIGURE 36.14 A rubber glove used as an ice pack. A face drawn on it helps to make it seem friendlier.

NURSING DIAGNOSES AND RELATED INTERVENTIONS

Nursing Diagnosis: Risk for imbalanced nutrition, less than body requirements related to chronic illness

Outcome Identification: Child will ingest a diet adequate for nutritional needs during illness.

Outcome Evaluation: Skin turgor is good; no signs of dehydration are present; child gains a minimum of 1 pound weekly as evidence of nutritional needs being met.

Measure Fluid Intake and Output

Fluid is an essential element of nutrition because of the water supplied and because it can also be a source of calories and vitamins. To document fluid balance, some children may have fluid intake and output measured and recorded. This is especially true for children with vomiting, diarrhea, burns, hemorrhage, dehydration, cardiac and kidney disease, draining wounds, gastrointestinal suction, edema, and diuretic or intravenous therapy.

Intake

Estimating the intake of infants who are formula-fed is simply a matter of estimating the kind and amount of fluids that were swallowed. Intake in breast-fed infants is merely recorded as "breast-fed." If it is necessary to estimate the amount more closely than this, the infant can be weighed before and after a feeding. The difference in weight in grams is the number of milliliters of breast milk ingested. This measurement is not very accurate, however, because if the child voided or had a bowel movement, weight would be affected by these losses.

With preschool children, be certain to record fluids ingested during snacks, because children this age usually have many during the day. At approximately 10 years of age, children can be depended on to record their own intake as long as they have a list of how many milliliters are contained in each glass or cup they use (an average cup

FOCUS ON FAMILY EMPOWERMENT
Guidelines for Hot and Cold Applications With Children

Q. I need to apply cold compresses to my child's leg. What should I do?

A. When applying any type of hot or cold therapy such as cold or warm compresses, use the following guidelines:

- Apply neither heat nor cold for longer than 20 minutes unless prescribed otherwise, because after this time, the vasoconstriction caused by cold and the vasodilatation caused by heat is reversed.
- When using electrical sources of heat with toddlers and preschoolers, never make a game of plugging in and pulling out the apparatus that makes the light come on or a dial glow. Otherwise, the child may play with it after you leave.
- Supply a special activity for a child to enjoy while a hot or cold application is in place (playing a board game or reading a story to the child) so that the procedure is not viewed as a chore but as a pleasant time to look forward to because of the accompanying enjoyable activity.
- Put tape on the gauge of an electric appliance at the point where you want it so that a child cannot change the setting.
- Always test the warmth of solutions or heat sources with your inner wrist or dorsal surface of your hand before applying them to the child, to be certain they are not too hot.
- Do not apply ice packs or ice directly to the skin. Cover the pack or ice with a towel or other cover to prevent frostbite and cell damage from cold.
- Be cautious about heat or cold applications with a child who is receiving an analgesic because the child's perception of heat or cold may be reduced, and he or she could easily be burned.

is 150 mL; a glass, 180 mL). Be certain to check that they remember that soup, flavored frozen ice such as Popsicles, and sherbet are liquids and should be counted.

Output

Diapers can be readily used as a method of measuring urine output. Weigh the diaper before it is placed on the infant and record this weight conspicuously (mark it on the front of the plastic covering with a ballpoint pen). Reweigh the diaper after it is wet and subtract the difference to determine the amount of urine present. This difference will be in grams. Because 1 g = 1 mL, the amount can be recorded in milliliters. In infants who have liquid stools, it is difficult to separate stool from urine because these blend together in a diaper. Separate urine from stool by applying a urine collector; check it frequently for filling.

Girls often void along with bowel movements when they use a toilet, which means that a urine specimen is easily lost. To separate urine from bowel movements, teach older children to void first.

Provide Enteral Feedings

Enteral feedings, also called nasogastric tube feedings, are a common means of supplying adequate nutrition to an infant who is unable to suck or tires too easily when sucking, or to an older child who cannot eat. Enteral feedings have the advantage over parenteral nutrition of preserving the stomach mucosa and decreasing the risk of intravenous infection (Irving et al., 2000). In infants, such feedings are traditionally called **gavage feedings** (see Nursing Procedure 36-2 and Table 36-2).

Whether enteral catheters should be passed through the nares or the mouth is controversial. Orogastric insertion allows for easier breathing because the nose is not blocked (Asfaw et al., 2000). Because newborns are nose breathers, it seems reasonable that passing the catheter through the mouth in this size infant will lead to less distress than passing it through the nose. Orogastric insertion can also decrease the possibility of striking the vagal nerve and causing bradycardia. If the tube is to be left in place, however, it may be passed through a nostril. For the older child, insertion through a nostril is more comfortable.

Children are generally offered bolus or intermittent feedings rather than continuous infusions to more closely mimic a normal feeding pattern. Children with long-term neurologic disabilities may have enteral tubes left in place for continuous feedings administered by an enteric feeding pump. Give mouth care at least twice a day to older children who are receiving nasogastric tube feedings; otherwise, their mouths become dry and ulcers can form.

Provide Gastrostomy Tube Feedings

Children may have gastrostomy tubes inserted for feeding. Gastrostomy tube feedings may be necessary for children who cannot swallow or those with esophageal atresia, severe gastroesophageal reflux, or esophageal stricture. With the use of regional anesthesia, the tube is inserted through a puncture wound in the abdominal wall into the stomach (Fig. 36-15). The tube used in children is usually an indwelling urinary catheter (Foley catheter) rather than a true gastrostomy tube. This is because a Foley catheter can be removed easily and changed should it become plugged. In addition, the balloon is small enough not to obscure and fill the small stomach space.

As with nasogastric feedings, gastrostomy feedings should be at room temperature to prevent chilling. Before a feeding, elevate the child's upper trunk 30 to 40 degrees so the fluid will remain in the stomach and not flow upward into the esophagus, possibly causing aspiration. Do

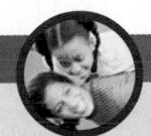

NURSING PROCEDURE 36.2: INITIATING AN ENTERAL FEEDING FOR AN INFANT

Purpose

To supply nutrition by an enteral tube.

Procedure	Principle
1. Loosely swaddle the infant using a mummy restraint.	1. Mummy restraints effectively contain arms and legs without causing any unwarranted pressure on the infant.
2. Measure the space from the bridge of the infant's nose to the earlobe to a point halfway between the xiphoid process and the umbilicus using a no. 8 or no. 10 feeding tube. If the infant is older than 1 year of age, measure from the bridge of the nose to the earlobe to the xiphoid process.	2. Measuring the tube ensures that it will be long enough to enter the stomach. If a tube is passed too far, it will curl and end up in the esophagus; if not passed far enough, it will also be in the esophagus. Both situations could lead to aspiration of the feeding.

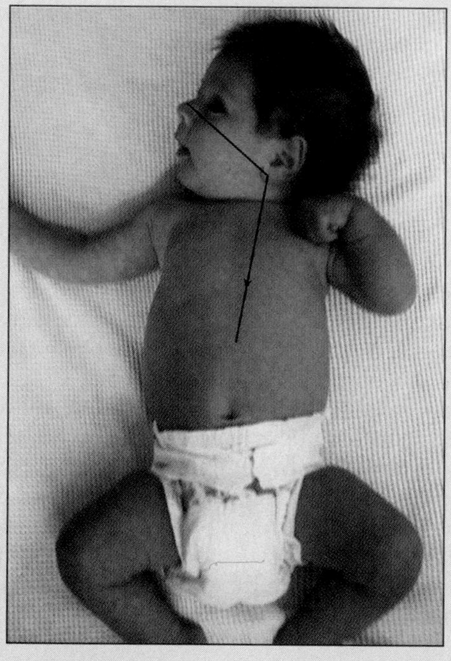

Procedure	Principle
3. Mark the tube at the measured point with a small clamp or piece of tape. Lubricate the tip of the catheter with water.	3. Lubrication helps the tube pass through the esophagus without trauma. An oil lubricant is never used because although the tube is going to be passed into the stomach, occasionally it can accidentally pass into the trachea. Oil left in the trachea could lead to lipoid pneumonia, a complication an infant already burdened with a disease may not be able to tolerate.
4. Pass the catheter with gentle pressure to the point of the clamp or tape. If the catheter is inadvertently passed into the trachea rather than the esophagus, the infant usually will cough and become dyspneic. If this happens, withdraw and replace the catheter.	4. Using gentle pressure helps to ensure comfort and safety.
5. Assess the catheter for position (that it is not in the trachea) before administering a feeding (see Table 36-2).	5. Assessing for proper placement helps to ensure that the feeding will enter the stomach, not the infant's respiratory tract.

(continued)

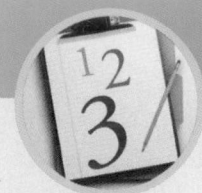

Procedure	Principle
6. Aspirate stomach contents for amount. If the amount aspirated is small (a few milliliters), merely replace it at the beginning of the feeding. If large (large is determined by a physician's order), replace it through the tubing, and reduce the amount of the feeding by that amount.	6. Assessing stomach content amount aids in determining if the previous feeding was absorbed. Replacing stomach secretions rather than discarding them helps prevent electrolyte loss.
7. After being certain that the catheter is in the stomach, attach a syringe or special feeding funnel to the tube. Elevate the infant's head and chest slightly to encourage fluid to flow downward into the stomach.	7. Elevating the infant's upper body allows the feeding to flow by gravity.
8. Add the specific kind and amount of feeding prescribed to the syringe or funnel and allow it to flow by gravity into the infant's stomach. Don't elevate the syringe end of the tube more than 12 inches above the infant's abdomen (see figure below).	8. Excessive elevation can cause the feeding to flow too quickly, filling the esophagus and increasing the risk for aspiration. Hurrying feedings by using the plunger of the syringe or a bulb attachment for more pressure also can lead to aspiration.

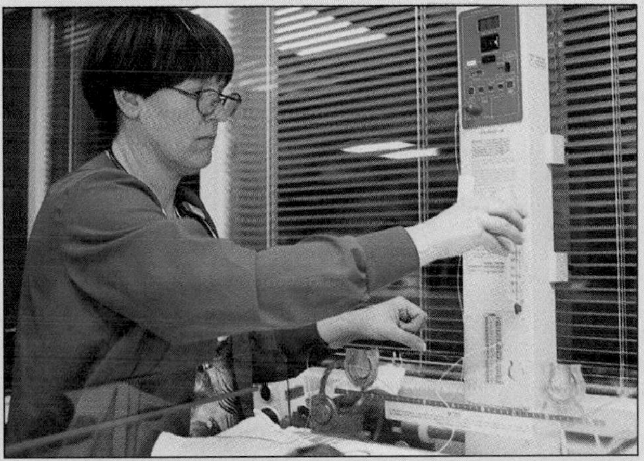

Procedure	Principle
9. Offer a pacifier (nonnutrient sucking) during the feeding if the infant appears to enjoy this.	9. Nonnutrient sucking can help satisfy the infant's normal need to suck, which would otherwise go unsatisfied with gavage feedings.
10. When the feeding has passed through the tube, reclamp the tube securely and gently and rapidly withdraw it.	10. Clamping the tube before it is withdrawn is important to prevent any milk remaining in the tube from flowing out as the tube is removed, thereby reducing the risk of aspiration.
11. If the tube is to remain in place, flush it with 1 to 5 mL of clear water and cap it.	11. Flushing a tube helps prevent clogging and plugging of the tube with the feeding solution. Capping a tube helps to prevent air and bacteria from entering.
12. If the tube is to be left in place, tape it below the nose and to the cheek. Do not tape it to the forehead.	12. Taping a tube to the forehead can put pressure on the anterior naris, leading to ulceration.
13. Bubble the baby after an enteral feeding as you would after a bottle or breast feeding. If a parent is present, encourage him or her to do this.	13. Bubbling helps in preventing air accumulation and regurgitation of feeding. Encouraging parental participation aids in promoting close contact, which is essential to the baby's development.
14. Unswaddle and place the infant on the right side with the head slightly elevated or hold and rock the infant in this position.	14. Placing on the right side helps the feeding solution enter the pyloric valve, promoting stomach emptying.
15. Assess that the infant appears comfortable. If a parent observed the procedure, answer any questions or concerns.	15. Assessing the infant after the feeding aids in outcome evaluation. Helping parents feel comfortable with alternative feeding methods can help increase their self-esteem and promote bonding with the infant.

TABLE 36.2 Methods to Determine Proper Gavage Tube Placement

METHOD	CONSIDERATIONS
Attach syringe to the tube and aspirate stomach contents. Test for pH (below 7 is acid).	In most instances, stomach contents aspirated this way are returned to the stomach before the feeding; in small infants, the amount of stomach contents is subtracted from the prescribed amount of feeding; because stomach contents are highly acid, discarding them at each feeding can lead to alkalosis.
Inject 5 mL air into the gavage tube and listen over the stomach with a stethoscope to the sound of injected air.	The injected air is heard as a whistling or growling sound; do not use an adult-size stethoscope on small infants to listen for it; the diaphragm of the stethoscope will be partially over lung, and where one is hearing the air injection is unknown.

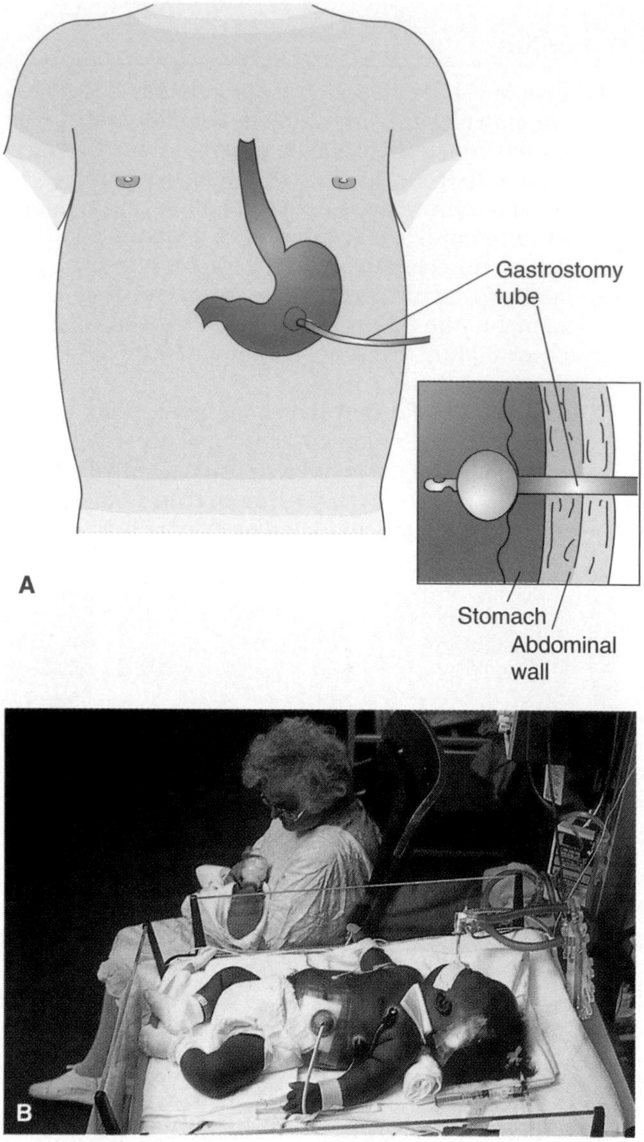

FIGURE 36.15 Children who are ill often need supplemental feeding by nasogastric or gastrostomy tube feedings. (*A*) Internal placement of a gastrostomy tube. (*B*) An infant with a gastrostomy tube in place.

this by holding an infant in the lap or placing him or her in an infant seat. For an older child, use pillows or elevate the head of the bed. Use a syringe to aspirate the tube for any stomach residual. After noting the amount, replace this fluid. To administer the feeding, attach a syringe to the tube and allow the specified amount to flow by gravity only (to prevent reflux and possible aspiration).

After the feeding, flush the tube with a specified amount of clear water to clear it of the feeding solution. Following esophageal surgery, suspend the unclamped tube in an elevated position. Leaving the tube unclamped and elevated ensures that if the child should vomit, vomitus will be evacuated from the stomach by the tube rather than through the esophagus. If a tube is left elevated and unclamped, cover it with a clean piece of porous gauze to prevent bacteria from entering it. Keep the child's head elevated for at least 1 hour after a feeding.

Infants who are fed by gastrostomy tube miss the pleasure of sucking. Offer a pacifier to suck on during the procedure. Talk or sing to the child as if the feeding were being given orally.

The biggest problem with gastrostomy tubes is that often they do not fit snugly, and formula or gastric secretions can leak around the tube onto the abdominal skin. These secretions are irritating because of their high hydrochloric acid content. Consult a wound ostomy continence nurse specialist for wound care. Often commercially available skin protectants can be placed around the tube to protect the skin. One method of helping to provide a snug fit for the tube is to place a soft nipple used with premature infants (enlarge the nipple opening slightly) over the catheter (nipple tip up) so the base of the nipple fits against the skin protectant. Tape the tube to the nipple at the tip, which brings the balloon of the tube up against the stomach wall and prevents leakage. Tape the nipple to the skin and skin protectant securely using nonadhesive tape. Clean the skin around the nipple daily with a product such as half-strength hydrogen peroxide; change the skin protectant as directed by the manufacturer's instructions. At the time of the change, expose the skin to air for approximately 1 hour.

A major complication associated with the use of a gastrostomy tube is that it can move into the duodenum through the pyloric sphincter and cause obstruction. Observe and report any vomiting, abdominal distention, or brown or green tube drainage (duodenal secretions that would suggest the tube has moved). Testing residual aspiration fluid to see that it is acid is a guarantee that the tube is in the stomach (stomach secretions are acid; duodenal secretions are alkaline). Putting a mark on the tube with an indelible pen just above the nipple lets you check that the tube has not migrated into the stomach but is remaining securely in place.

Tubes are replaced approximately every 6 weeks. To replace a tube, deflate the catheter balloon by withdrawing the water in it and then gently pull the tube free. Insert a clean catheter into the stomach opening approximately 1 inch beyond the balloon; inflate the balloon with 2 to 4 mL water. Attach a nipple and tape in place.

Most children receiving gastrostomy feedings will have the tube in place for an extended time. Teach the parents how to feed their child this way, how to remove and to replace a tube, and the danger signs to watch for (e.g., vomiting, abdominal discomfort, or skin excoriation). Help parents to see this as an alternative way of feeding, not a totally different one. Be certain that they are comfortable with the procedure before the child is discharged from the hospital, so that they can feed the child by this method. Reinforce with them the understanding that it does not hurt the child to have the tube replaced or to have pressure put against the tube, so that they need not worry about holding the child snugly. Many children on long-term gastrostomy feedings have gastrostomy buttons implanted for easier stomach access (Fig. 36-16). For feeding, a catheter is inserted through the device; it is removed following the feeding. With this in place, only a small access device is visible, not a large bulky tube.

Percutaneous endoscopic gastrostomy (PEG) tubes are feeding tubes that are passed using endoscopy through the esophagus into the stomach and then pulled through a stab wound to the outside of the abdominal wall. The tube is then held in place by an external restraining disc. Although tubes may be passed as far as the jejunum by this same method, such tubes bypass normal stomach digestion rather than support it, so are much less used in children. The overall use of such tubes is limited because a small child's esophagus may not be wide enough to insert the tube by this route.

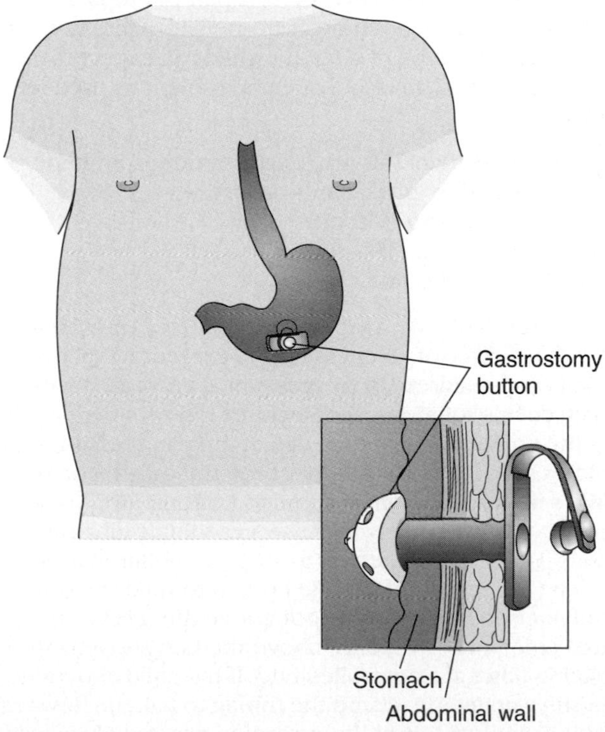

FIGURE 36.16 Placement of a gastrostomy button

WHAT IF? What if a parent wants to take her child with a gastrostomy tube in place to a restaurant so the child learns about "eating out." Would you agree with her that this is a good idea?

Provide Total Parenteral Nutrition

NURSING DIAGNOSES AND RELATED INTERVENTIONS

Nursing Diagnosis: Imbalanced nutrition, less than body requirements related to malabsorption of nutrients

Outcome Identification: Child will receive adequate nutrients for physiologic needs during course of illness.

Outcome Evaluation: Skin turgor is good; no signs of dehydration are present; child loses no weight during therapy; intestinal cramps and distention lessen.

Total parenteral nutrition (TPN) has become one of the most important therapies for children who have illnesses such as gastrointestinal or respiratory conditions that prevent proper absorption of basic caloric or fluid requirements. Traditional intravenous therapy contains fluid, electrolytes, and sugars but not protein and fat, which are essential for the maintenance and growth of body tissues. With TPN, all of a child's nutritional needs can be met by a concentrated hypertonic solution of intravenous therapy containing glucose, vitamins, electrolytes, trace minerals, and protein. An intralipid solution (emulsified fat able to be administered intravenously) given once or twice per week supplies needed fatty acids. Children with chronic diarrhea or vomiting, bowel obstruction, anorexia, or extreme immaturity are examples of children who benefit greatly from TPN.

Solutions may be administered via a central intravenous access site or via a peripherally inserted central venous catheter (PICC). If a central access site is chosen, a catheter is inserted through the right external jugular vein into the superior vena cava or directly into the subclavian vein under strict aseptic conditions (see Chap. 37). The catheter is secured at the site of insertion with sutures and covered with a sterile dressing to help reduce bacterial contamination. A major vein of this type is chosen to avoid inflammation reactions and resulting venous thrombosis from the high-caloric and high-osmotic fluid that will be infused.

TPN solution is prepared in a pharmacy under sterile conditions according to prescription. A millipore filter, which removes small particles present in the solution that might cause an embolus to form, is inserted into the tubing. The solution should be administered by means of a constant infusion pump so that the rate can be governed. If the rate should fall behind, do not increase it the next hour to make up the amount of fluid. Serious cardiovascular overload may result because of the concentrated fluid being administered.

Infection is a major danger of TPN because the solution is a perfect medium for the growth of bacteria or *Candida* organisms. The dressing over the insertion site and the intravenous tubing are changed every 1 to 2 days to avoid infection; the tubing should not be used for drawing blood or for adding medications (unless a double-barreled tube is used), because either process may introduce infection. Sterile technique is required in changing bottles of solution so that the tubing is not contaminated. Some health care facilities require nurses to wear both masks and gloves while doing this to avoid airborne and direct contamination. Fewer restrictions are necessary for home care. The insertion site should be inspected at the time of the dressing change for indications of local infection, such as redness, tenderness, or discharge.

A second major problem that can occur with TPN is dehydration. A TPN solution contains approximately twice the amount of glucose normally administered in an intravenous solution to ensure that the amino acids in the solution will be used for protein synthesis, not for energy. Dehydration may occur as the body tries to reduce the amount of glucose recognized by the kidneys as excessive by excreting it (the same phenomenon that leads to high urine output in persons with diabetes mellitus). When TPN is begun, urine should be tested for glucose and for specific gravity with each voiding. If two or more consecutive samples indicate a 3^+ or 4^+ glucose level, either the rate of the infusion or the amount of glucose in the solution should be decreased or insulin should be added to the solution to counteract the excess glucose. Generally, decreasing the concentration of glucose and then gradually increasing it again allows the child's body to adjust to the glucose overload.

After the first few days of TPN, a rebound effect (the child's body produces increased insulin) may cause hypoglycemia. A urine sample that suddenly is negative for glucose after several serial specimens have been highly positive is therefore not necessarily an encouraging sign; rather, it may be a warning that the child's glucose level is dangerously low. The TPN solution should not be discontinued abruptly but gradually tapered, or a glucose rebound effect will also occur. If a TPN catheter should be accidentally pulled out by a child, the child must be immediately assessed for hemorrhage from the insertion site and closely observed in the next few hours for signs of hypoglycemia (i.e., lethargy, incoordination, fidgeting, or seizures). Parents need to be alerted to these concerns for safe home care.

Remember that to a child, eating is more than a means of receiving nourishment; it is also a means of receiving comfort and love. Even though children are able to voice the reason they must have TPN and appear to understand that they are receiving all the needed nutrients, they still may miss eating food and the natural social interaction that comes with it. While in the hospital, they may be upset by the smell of food from a hospital unit kitchen or by the fact that playmates have to leave to eat a meal. Finding an activity for the child to do while other children eat (e.g., helping to check supplies on the emergency cart or stamping laboratory slips) may be helpful in supplying the interaction the child misses. Ask whether the child can be allowed chewing gum or occasional hard candy for chewing and taste sensations. Tooth brushing twice a day is necessary to keep the oral mucous membrane healthy because the child is not chewing. An infant needs sucking pleasure from a pacifier.

Many children on long-term TPN are cared for by parents at home. Careful coordination with the home care agency is necessary to ensure that parents are familiar with the system and know how to obtain TPN fluid so the child's care continues safely. Parents need to arrange for special time each day with the child to make up for the time normally spent interacting at meals.

✔ CHECKPOINT QUESTIONS

10. How do you measure the correct length for a feeding tube in an infant?
11. Why might dehydration occur with TPN therapy?

ASSISTANCE WITH ELIMINATION

Two aspects of intestinal elimination that require special care are administration of enemas and ostomy care.

Administering Enemas

Enemas are rarely used with children unless they are therapy for Hirschsprung's disease or a part of preparation for surgery or a radiologic study. If an enema is necessary, offer a careful explanation of what the child can expect to experience. The usual amounts of enema solutions used are as follows:

Infant: Less than 250 mL (exact amount should be stipulated by physician's order)
Preschooler: 250–350 mL
School-age child: 300–500 mL
Adolescent: 500 mL

For an infant, use a small, soft catheter (no. 10 to 12 French) in place of an enema tip to prevent rectal trauma. Infants and children up to ages 3 or 4 years are unable to retain enema solutions, so they must rest on a bedpan during the procedure. Pad the edge of the pan so that it is not cold or sharp. Place a pillow under the infant's or young child's upper body for positioning and comfort. Lubricate the catheter generously with a water-soluble lubricant and insert it only 2 to 3 inches (5–7 cm) in children and only 1 inch (2.5 cm) in infants. Be certain to hold the solution container no more than 1 foot above the level of the sigmoid colon (12–15 inches above the bed surface) so the solution flows at a controlled rate. If the child experiences intestinal cramping, clamp the tubing to halt the flow temporarily and wait until the cramping passes before instilling any more fluid. An older child can be asked to take a deep breath to help the cramping sensation pass. The amount of solution used in infants is so small that this is not usually a problem. If the enema solution is to be retained, such as an oil solution, hold the child's buttocks together for about a count of 10 after administration.

Until late school age, children cannot retain an enema as adults can (rarely more than 5–10 minutes). For this reason, be certain the bathroom the child will use is available before administering the enema.

Commercial enemas, such as Fleet enemas, are not routinely administered to children younger than 2 years because of the harsh action of the sodium biphosphate and sodium phosphate they contain. Tap water is not used because it is not isotonic and causes rapid fluid shifts of water in body compartments, leading to possible water intoxication. Normal saline (0.9% sodium chloride) is the usual solution. It can be made by parents at home by adding 1 teaspoonful of salt to 1 pint (500 mL) of water.

After enema administration, praise the child for cooperating. Allow a preschooler an opportunity for therapeutic play, because this is a frightening procedure for a child of this age.

Providing Ostomy Care

An ostomy is an opening of the bowel on the surface of the abdomen. Ostomies in newborns are created to relieve bowel obstruction caused by conditions such as ileal atresia, necrotizing enterocolitis, and imperforate anus. In older children they are constructed for conditions such as inflammatory bowel syndrome. If an ostomy is created in the ileum (an ileostomy), the stoma is located on the right side of the abdomen and drains liquid stool, which is extremely irritating to the skin because of the digestive enzymes it contains. If an ostomy is created in the sigmoid portion of the bowel (colostomy), the stoma is on the left lower abdomen and passes normally formed stool (Fig. 36-17).

An ileostomy requires the use of a collecting ostomy appliance to contain acid stool and prevent excoriation of the abdominal skin. Older children also may use an appliance with a colostomy. For an infant colostomy, parents may choose (with support and advice) whether to use an appliance.

Two basic problems commonly arise when using an ostomy appliance with an infant: it may be difficult to locate one small enough to contain liquid drainage without leaking; and the skin under the appliance may become extremely irritated. Consulting with a Wound, Ostomy, Continence nurse specialist (WOCN) can be helpful. Clear plastic colostomy bags without a ring can often be cut more easily to fit the size of the stoma and the contour and size of an infant's abdomen than a ring type. A commercial skin sealant is helpful to harden the skin surrounding the stoma. Apply according to the brand directions and fan to dry. If a spray is used, protect the infant's face so that he or she does not inhale the solution. Apply the chosen stoma collection appliance. Tuck it inside the diaper to help keep the infant from pulling it loose.

Check the appliance or bag for collecting stool at least every 4 hours. To protect the underlying skin, do not remove a self-adhering bag if it is full, but drain collected stool from the bottom of the appliance into a basin or paper cup for disposal. To reduce odor, flush the appliance bag with a warm water and soap solution, using a bulb-type syringe (an Asepto syringe), and rinse with clear water. Change the bag no more frequently than the point at which leakage occurs (perhaps as long as 1 week) to reduce skin irritation. To remove a bag that was placed with a sealant, be certain to use the designated solvent to prevent pulling or harming underlying skin. Then wash the solvent away with soap and water or it will become an irritant itself. Because most infants enjoy tub bathing, a long, soaking bath is also an excellent way to loosen an appliance.

If an appliance or bag is not used, stool will be discharged onto the abdomen three or four times a day (no different than a usual newborn or infant stool pattern). To care for a colostomy without using an appliance, wash and dry the stoma and surrounding skin area well. Follow the agency's protocol for skin care, such as applying karaya powder, an ointment such as Desitin, or a skin protectant

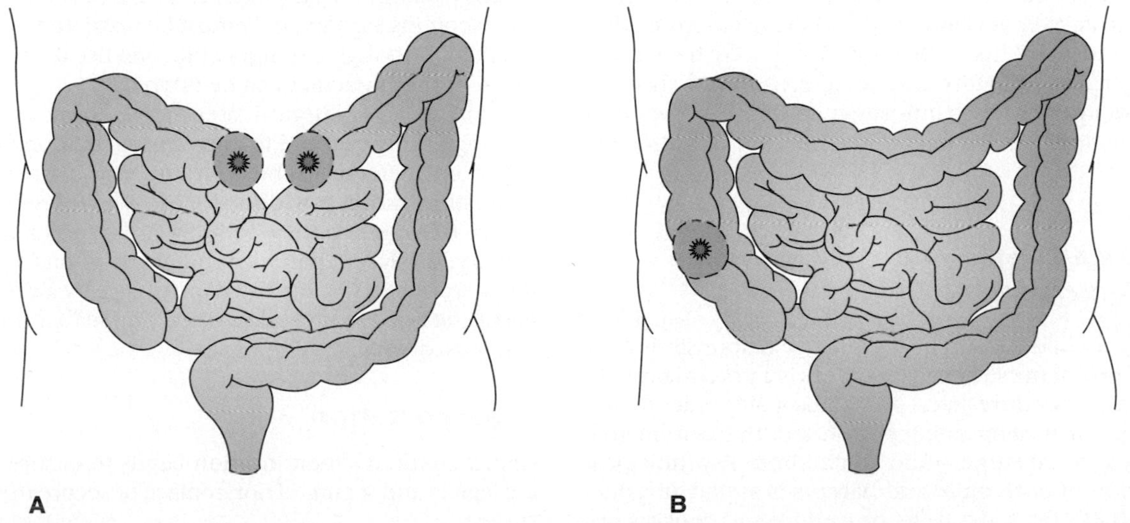

FIGURE 36.17 Different sites for ostomies. (*A*) A double-barrel colostomy. (*B*) A single-barrel colostomy.

to protect the skin. Apply ample absorbent gauze (fluffed) and an absorbent pad. Secure in place with nonadhesive tape or a binder. Check the dressing approximately every 4 hours. Remove and replace it when soiled, washing the skin well and applying new powder or ointment as necessary. Without an appliance in place, stool is kept from touching the skin only by the protection of the ointment and frequent changing of the dressing. Turning an infant from side to side after every feeding may be helpful in keeping stool from flowing continuously to one side. Leaving the abdominal skin exposed to air for at least 1 hour per day also helps healing.

Stress to parents that caring for an infant with an ostomy is little different from usual. All parents must change their infant's diapers frequently and clean the diaper area. Stress that the stoma has no nerves, so a parent can feel free to wash it without hurting the child and that compression against the stoma will not cause the child pain. These explanations may help the parents feel comfortable placing the infant on his or her abdomen or holding the infant closely against their body for comfort.

Colostomies are rarely irrigated in children. On occasion, to prepare a child for second-stage abdominal surgery, irrigation of the "blind-end" bowel (bowel between the rectum and colostomy) of a double-barreled colostomy may be ordered daily to keep it lubricated and to maintain bowel tone. The exact amount of fluid to be used should be specified by the physician. Typically, the amount is small, approximately 40 to 100 mL in infants. Normal saline (0.9% sodium chloride) should be used in place of tap water, which could lead to water intoxication because it is not isotonic.

Children who have had a colostomy since infancy adapt well to it because they have never known another method of defecation. Parents should begin toilet-training for urine control at the usual time. In contrast, school-age children often have a great deal of difficulty adjusting to a colostomy. Encourage children to perform self-care as fully and as soon as possible so they can be independent. Preschool children usually benefit from therapeutic play that helps them work through their feelings. Provide some time for older children to discuss concerns about being accepted by others and how to answer questions about a colostomy from other children. Adolescents with a colostomy may have questions regarding sexuality and need reassurance that this should not interfere with intimate relationships. They may appreciate open discussion of how they see this affecting their life.

PREPARATION OF A CHILD FOR SURGERY

Preparing a child for surgery is a major responsibility for the child health nurse because surgery is a potentially very frightening procedure. Such preparation differs according to the type of surgery being performed, but certain activities apply to all surgery and all children. Psychological preparation of both child and parents is aimed at reducing the child's fears about the procedure and consists primarily of providing health teaching and opportunities for therapeutic play. Physical preparation includes providing for restrictions on food and fluid intake before surgery, preparing the incision site on the child's skin, and arranging for transportation of the child to surgery. Because many children's surgical procedures are done on an ambulatory basis, preparation must also include informing the parents about the details of the preparation techniques, the surgery, and the postoperative period and the steps they must take toward preparation.

Emotional Preparation

Preparing a child emotionally for surgery requires minimizing fears common to all children (e.g., fear of separation, fear of mutilation, or fear of death). This can be accomplished by telling the child about the procedure and describing any specific equipment and techniques that will be used, such as anesthesia, eye bandages, nasogastric tubes, sutures, or special aftercare. A teaching plan is essential for explaining all of these features of surgery to the child (see Chap. 34). Be certain that preparation is appropriate to the child's age. More children undergoing surgery receive a general anesthetic, rather than a local or regional anesthetic as might be used with adults, because this minimizes their fears of intrusive or mutilating procedures, and because children who are not yet adolescent are not mature enough to cooperate adequately during surgery.

Physical Preparation

Most children will be placed on nothing by mouth (NPO) status for surgery. The length of the time the child will remain NPO depends on the child's age. Adolescents and school-age children may be restricted from taking food or fluid from midnight until the time of surgery the following morning; but if infants younger than 6 months were held NPO for as long a time as this, they would be taken to surgery in dehydration. Therefore, infants younger than 6 months may be kept NPO for as little as 4 hours. At the end of the 4 hours, as the infant becomes hungry, he or she will begin to cry and fuss for fluid. Parents need an explanation that infants who vomit during surgery because of recent feedings may aspirate; therefore, even though they are becoming hungry, they must be restricted from ingesting fluid. Although a hungry child will usually not suck on one for long, a pacifier can be offered.

Preparation of surgical sites varies. In most instances, shaving of the area and final cleansing are done in a holding room adjacent to the operating room after the child is anesthetized. A povidone-iodine wash may be ordered before transport to the operating room for some types of surgery. Washing a particular body part in this manner can be interpreted as an intrusive procedure by a preschooler. He or she needs a great deal of assurance that the solution being used will not sting.

Transportation

Check children's identification bands to ensure that they are legible and secure. If not, replace or secure them before surgery.

Immediately before transport, remove barrettes and bobby pins from the child's hair and check the mouth for loose teeth (particularly in children ages 6, 7, and 8 years, who are losing their central and lateral incisors) or for dental appliances. It is rare to find a child with full dentures but not uncommon to find a post or screw-in tooth that may have to be removed before surgery or a retainer used to maintain an orthodontic correction after brace removal. Teeth braces do not need to be removed. Make certain the anesthesiologist knows about any loose teeth before an airway for surgery is inserted (a loose tooth could be knocked totally free and aspirated during the procedure).

For some children, having to give up their own pajamas or their bedroom slippers or outside shoes to change to a hospital gown is a terrifying moment. Giving up underpants is a step that many preschool and early school-age children cannot tolerate, so many children are allowed to wear their own pajamas or clothes until they are under an anesthetic.

In ambulatory settings, children may walk to surgery. If they will ride in a cart, this should have been introduced during preparation. Be sure to fasten a restraining strap for safety (presented with, "Here's your seat belt; it's just like going in a car."). Preschoolers may enjoy taking a favorite toy or blanket to surgery with them. Ideally, they should be allowed to keep this with them until they are under an anesthetic. Parents should be allowed to accompany their children to the operating suite. Some parents can accompany their child into an anesthesiologist's induction room; for others, this is inappropriate or too anxiety-producing. A nurse whom the child knows should accompany the child to the operating room and remain there until the child is under the anesthetic, if possible. Even if the child has been well prepared for the surgical experience and the change in personnel on arrival to the surgical suite, saying goodbye to parents at the door of the surgical suite and the actual sight of strange personnel can lead to high levels of anxiety and fear.

Although it may not be cost-effective to have a staff nurse wait with a child until he or she is under an anesthetic, the nurse's wait will probably not be long if the child has been called for surgery when the surgical suite is almost ready. The psychological benefit of a familiar nurse's comforting presence is very important.

POSTOPERATIVE WOUND CARE

Children frequently have a dressing or bandage in place to cover a surgical incision or sutured laceration. Such dressings differ from adult dressings in terms of material, size, and methods used to secure them. Keeping a dressing dry to avoid introducing infection to the wound in infants and toddlers who are not toilet-trained can be a major problem. In many instances after surgery, collodion (a clear substance similar to nail polish) or other commercially available "wound glues" are used to cover the incision (Charters, 2000). Applied to a suture line to serve as the dressing, these products keep the suture line from coming in contact with urine or feces. Since these materials are clear, they allow good visualization of the healing surface. Assure parents that such a covering is adequate and actually preferable if the incision is in the groin, such as a hernia repair.

If a gauze dressing is used, it can be covered with plastic, securely held in place with nonadhesive, waterproof tape. Be certain when cutting plastic to cover a dressing not to leave an extra piece behind in the crib; the child could pull it over his or her head and suffocate.

Occlusive dressings (hydrogel sheets, hydrocolloids, or polyurethane films) are dressings especially designed to provide a healing surface over a wound. These need to be applied and removed according to each product's directions.

Infants and young children usually have skin that is too sensitive for adhesive tape to be used to secure dressings. Use nonadhesive tape (silk or paper) instead or secure a dressing with a nonadhering bandage (Kling) or roller gauze. Young children, as a rule, find bandages comforting and accept them as a "badge of courage," displaying them proudly. Apply adhesive bandages (Band-Aids) generously after venipuncture or finger punctures for this reason. Preschool children have little concept of how long it takes healing to occur. They are often surprised that their incision or wound has not yet healed the day after surgery. Preschoolers are often worried that a part of their body under a dressing is missing and find it reassuring to see that the body part is still there (they may pull a dressing away to do this). It is better to know what something is like than to worry about the unknown. Therefore, do not discourage children from looking at their incision during dressing changes. Even if the area looks raw and unhealed, it may look better than what the child has envisioned was under the dressing. Teach parents and children how to continue wound dressings when they return home. As many as 15% of children receiving home care have wounds that need continuing dressings and care (Pieper et al., 2000).

ELEVATED TEMPERATURE REDUCTION IN CHILDREN

NURSING DIAGNOSES AND RELATED INTERVENTIONS

Nursing Diagnosis: Risk for hyperthermia related to illness affecting temperature regulation, medications, or surgery

Outcome Identification: Child's temperature will return to normal with appropriate interventions within 2 hours.

Outcome Evaluation: Child's temperature is 98.6°F (37°C) orally.

Many illnesses cause elevated temperatures. Because the temperature-regulating mechanism in children is immature, fever tends to be more marked in them than in adults and may even be out of proportion to the seriousness or extent of the disease. An increased temperature occurs because the child's temperature-regulating point (set point) has been elevated. The temperature cannot be reduced until the set point returns (or is returned) to normal. An important nursing intervention with infants and young children is helping to reduce high temperatures, or giving a parent instructions on how to reduce the temperature at home.

Acetaminophen (Tylenol) is an excellent antipyretic (i.e., it acts to reduce the temperature set point), and it is the drug most often prescribed to reduce fever in children (see Focus on Pharmacology: Acetaminophen). Children's ibuprofen is also effective (see Focus on Pharmacology: Ibuprofen).

Parents often do not give enough of an antipyretic such as acetaminophen to be effective because they are afraid the child will have a bad reaction to it. Encourage them to give the full dose every 4 hours, up to five doses a day, until their child's temperature is reduced. Conversely, caution them not to give too much or a severe overdose with liver or kidney toxicity can occur (Karch, 2001). An antipyretic is generally ordered for any child whose oral or tympanic temperature is more than 101°F (38.4°C) or whose rectal temperature is more than 102°F (39.0°C). Caution parents not to give acetylsalicylic acid (aspirin) to children with fever because aspirin is associated with Reye's syndrome (see Chap. 49).

Teach parents that fever is actually a body protection measure, and unless it is exceptionally high (more than 106°F [41.1°C]), it does no specific harm. In fact, there is some evidence that fever may be of value in helping to combat infection, because it aids in destroying microorganisms. In addition to antipyretic administration, dress children with fever in lightweight clothing, such as summer pajamas. Remove all clothing but the diaper from an infant. Many parents dress febrile children warmly in flannel nightgowns to keep them from "getting a chill." This increases the child's temperature and does not prevent the shaking, trembling reaction that comes with high fever. Placing a cool cloth (not ice) on the child's forehead feels comforting. Sponging children to lower the temperature is no longer recommended because it can lead to extreme chilling and shock to an immature nervous system and has little advantage over the use of oral antipyretics (Purssell, 2000).

FOCUS ON PHARMACOLOGY

Acetaminophen (Tylenol)

Action: Used for moderate temperature elevation or pain; does not have anti-inflammatory properties

Pregnancy risk category: B

Dosage: Oral: 10–15 mg/kg every 4–6 hours as needed; may repeat 4 or 5 times per day; do not exceed 5 doses in 24 hours

Possible adverse effects: Elevated liver enzymes, jaundice, rash

Nursing Implications

- Caution parents that drug can cause severe liver toxicity with overdose.
- Educate parents not to administer a larger dose or more frequently than prescribed.
- Encourage parents to increase the child's fluid intake to aid in reducing fever.

FOCUS ON PHARMACOLOGY

Ibuprofen (Advil, Pediaprofen)

Action: Used to reduce inflammation, fever, and mild to moderate pain

Pregnancy risk category: B; D if used in last trimester

Dosage: (for fever or pain) 5–10 mg/kg every 6–8 hours; do not exceed 40 mg in 24 hours

Possible adverse effects: Gastric upset, headache, dizziness, nausea, occult blood loss, prolonged bleeding, peptic ulceration

Nursing Implications

- Use with caution in children with gastrointestinal irritation.
- Drug can cause renal failure if child becomes dehydrated; encourage fluid intake.
- Administer with food or drink to minimize gastrointestinal irritation.

✔ CHECKPOINT QUESTIONS

12. How far should an enema catheter be inserted in an infant?
13. Would you recommend a parent give aspirin or acetaminophen for a child's fever?

KEY POINTS

Preparing children for procedures reduces anxiety. Prepare a child and parents by trying to relate a procedure to something the child is already familiar with, such as comparing an x-ray machine to a camera.

Include parents in both the planning and implementation of care. Parents reinfect children with fear if their own fear is uncontrolled. Give explanations on two levels. "I'm going to change the dressing on her suture line" for a parent; "I'm going to put a clean bandage on your tummy" for the child.

Reduce painful procedures to the minimum number possible (combine blood sampling procedures, if possible).

Perform any procedures that will cause pain in a treatment room or away from the child's bedside so the bed remains a safe place.

Perform treatments without chilling or exposure. Even small children expect modesty to be respected.

Allow the child to voice anger or fear of a procedure. Provide therapeutic play after a procedure to help reduce these reactions.

Identify a child well before a procedure; children do not monitor their own care as do adults.

Children enjoy adults who are secure in their actions. Practice as necessary the steps of a procedure before you begin so you demonstrate confidence and skill.

Once you have announced that a procedure needs to be done, proceed to do it; waiting for something to happen is often as stressful as actually having it done.

Involve children in procedures because this gives them a sense of control. Allow a child to examine electrodes or apply lubricant for electrode contact. Give the child a portion of an ECG strip as a badge of courage after the procedure, or let the child apply his or her own adhesive bandage.

Praise children for cooperation even if none was visibly obvious. For painful procedures, any behavior short of hysterical screaming counts as cooperation.

Following the use of conscious sedation, observe children carefully until they are fully awake. Check for the return of the child's gag reflex before offering any fluids to minimize the risk of aspiration.

Help make feeding by a route such as a gastrostomy tube as close to normal as possible by talking to the child to simulate mealtime conversation and socialization.

CRITICAL THINKING EXERCISES

1. Wally is the 4-year-old you met at the beginning of the chapter who is frightened of dark places. He is scheduled to have an MRI of his head done, which means he will be wheeled into a huge, dark, hollow tube. How would you prepare him for this?
2. An infant who has had three seizures is scheduled to have a CT scan done with dye injected. The mother asks you to assure her that her son will not have a reaction to the dye. How will you answer her?
3. An infant who had bowel surgery at birth and now has a temporary colostomy is ready for hospital discharge. His grandmother will be caring for him two mornings a week while his mother attends school. The grandmother tells you that she cannot imagine how she will care for an infant with a colostomy. What could you do to try to make her feel more comfortable with the baby's care? Will his care really be much different from that for other newborns?
4. Examine the national health goals related to health care of children. Most government-sponsored money for nursing research is allotted based on these goals. What would be a possible research topic to explore pertinent to these goals that would be fundable and would advance evidence-based practice?

REFERENCES

Asfaw, M., Miles, A., & Caplan, D. B. (2000). Orogastric enteral feeding: An alternative feeding access. *Nutrition in Clinical Practice, 15*(2), 91-93.

Boyd, J. R. (2001). A process for delivering bad news: Supporting families when a child is diagnosed. *Journal of Neuroscience Nursing, 33*(1), 14-20.

Bulloch, B., et al. (2000). Can urine clarity exclude the diagnosis of urinary tract infection? *Pediatrics, 106*(5), E60-E65.

Charters, A. (2000). Wound glue: A comparative study of tissue adhesives. *Accident & Emergency Nursing, 8*(4), 223-227.

Department of Health and Human Services (2000). *Healthy people, 2010.* Washington, DC: DHHS.

DeNicola, L. K., et al. (2001). Noninvasive monitoring in the pediatric intensive care unit. *Pediatric Clinics of North America, 48*(3), 573-588.

Emil, S., et al. (2001). Clinical versus sonographic evaluation of acute appendicitis in children: A comparison of patient characteristics and outcomes. *Journal of Pediatric Surgery, 36*(5), 780-783.

Houlder, L. C. (2000). Evidence-based practice: The accuracy and reliability of tympanic thermometry compared to rectal and axillary sites in young children. *Pediatric Nursing, 26*(3), 311-314.

Irving, S. Y., et al. (2000). Nutrition for the critically ill child: enteral and parenteral support. *AACN Clinical Issues: Advanced Practice in Acute & Critical Care, 11*(4), 541-558.

Karch, A. M. (2001). *Lippincott's nursing drug guide.* Philadelphia: Lippincott Williams & Wilkins.

Kay, J. D., Sinaiko, A. R., & Daniels, S. (2001). Pediatric hypertensions. *American Heart Journal, 142*(3), 422-432.

Langley, J. M., et al. (2001). Unique epidemiology of nosocomial urinary tract infection in children. *American Journal of Infection Control, 29*(2), 94-98.

Mohr, W. K., & Mohr, B. D. (2000). Mechanisms of injury and death proximal to restraint use. *Archives of Psychiatric Nursing, 14*(6), 285-295.

Pieper, B., et al. (2000). Prevalence and types of wounds among children receiving care in the home. *Ostomy Wound Management, 46*(4), 36-42.

Purssell, E. (2000). Physical treatment of fever. *Archives of Disease in Childhood, 82*(3), 238-239.

Rodriguez, E. & Jordan, R. (2002) Contemporary trends in pediatric sedation and analgesia. *Emergency Clinics of North America, 20*(1), 199-222.

Saxena, A. K., et al. (2001). Application criteria for infrared ear thermometers in pediatric surgery. *Technology & Health Care, 9*(3), 281-285.

Sganga, A., Wallace, R., Kiehl, E., Irving, T., & Witter, L. (2000). A comparison of four methods of normal newborn temperature measurement. *MCN: The American Journal of Maternal/Child Nursing, 25*(2), 76-79.

Tipple, M. A. (2000). Usefulness of the electrocardiogram in diagnosing mechanisms of tachycardia. *Pediatric Cardiology, 21*(6), 516-521.

Tolia, V., et al. (2000). Sedation for pediatric endoscopic procedures. *Journal of Pediatric Gastroenterology & Nutrition, 30*(5), 477-485.

White, P. M., et al. (2001). Magnetic resonance imaging as the primary imaging modality in children presenting with acute non-traumatic hip pain. *Emergency Medical Journal, 18*(1), 25-29.

SUGGESTED READINGS

Anderson, C. (2000). Enteral feeding: A change in practice. *Journal of Child Health Care, 4*(4), 160-162.

Bachur, R., & Harper, M. B. (2001). Reliability of the urinalysis for predicting urinary tract infections in young febrile children. *Archives of Pediatric Adolescent Medicine, 155*(1), 60-63.

Carney, D. E. & Meguid, M. M. (2002). Current concepts in nutritional assessment. *Archives of Surgery, 137*(1), 42-45.

Casey, G. (2000). Fever management in children. *Nursing Standard, 14*(40), 36-42.

Foley, J. (2000). The effects of hospitalisation on children. *Nursing Review, 18*(1), 4-5.

Gharpure, V., et al. (2000). Indicators of postpyloric feeding tube placement in children. *Critical Care Medicine, 28*(8), 2962-2966.

LaMontagne, L. L., Hepworth, J. T., & Cohen, F. (2000). Effects of surgery type and attention focus on children's coping. *Nursing Research, 49*(5), 245-252.

Mayoral, C. E., et al. (2000). Alternating antipyretics; Is this an alternative? *Pediatrics, 105*(5), 1009-1012.

Woodring, B. C. (2000). Family matters: If you have taught—have the child and family learned? *Pediatric Nursing, 26*(5), 505-509.

CHAPTER 37

Nursing Care of the Child Undergoing Medication Administration and Intravenous Therapy

Key Terms

- **absorption**
- **distribution**
- **excretion**
- **Intracath**
- **intermittent infusion devices**
- **metabolism**
- **pharmacokinetics**
- **vascular access port**

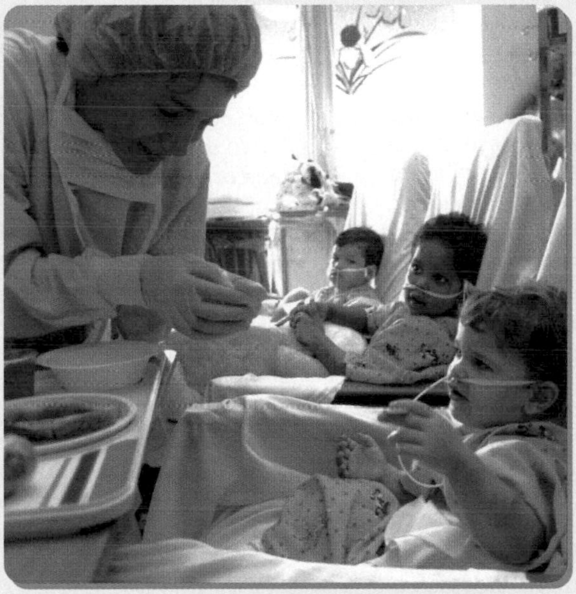

Objectives

After mastering the contents of this chapter, you should be able to:

1. Describe common methods of medication and intravenous therapy used in the health care of children.
2. Assess the developmental stage and knowledge level of children and adolescents before beginning medication or intravenous therapy.
3. Formulate nursing diagnoses related to medication or intravenous therapy with children.
4. Identify expected outcomes for children receiving medication or intravenous therapy.
5. Plan nursing interventions to aid in making medicine and intravenous therapy maximally effective.
6. Implement nursing interventions concerned with medication and intravenous therapy and children.
7. Evaluate outcomes related to medication and intravenous therapy with children.
8. Identify National Health Goals related to medication or intravenous therapy that nurses could be instrumental in helping the nation to achieve.
9. Identify areas related to medication or intravenous therapy with children that could benefit from additional nursing research or application of evidence-based practice.
10. Use critical thinking to analyze ways that medicine or intravenous therapy can be modified to meet the needs of children of all ages.
11. Integrate knowledge of medication and intravenous therapy with nursing process to achieve quality maternal and child health nursing.

Terry is a 2-year-old who has been prescribed prednisone 5 mg PO three times a day. When you give her a first pill to swallow, she spits it out. She does the same when you repeat with a second pill. Her mother tells you Terry can't swallow pills. Her father tells you, "You'll have to give her the medicine intravenously." What would you do? How would you gain Terry's cooperation?

Previous chapters described the difficulty children may have adjusting to illness and also diagnostic and therapeutic procedures that are frequently used with children. This chapter adds information about techniques for administering medication and intravenous therapy to children. This is important information as almost all illnesses today involve some form of medicine or intravenous administration.

After you've studied the chapter, answer to the Critical Thinking Exercises at the end of the chapter and then access the on-line study activities (http://connection.lww.com) *to further sharpen your skills and test your knowledge.*

Most adults have little difficulty understanding that taking medicine will be important to relieve whatever symptoms they are experiencing from their illness. Because children do not necessarily have this same level of understanding, they may resist taking medicine until its importance is thoroughly explained to them and the medication is given to them by a method that best meets their preference. Many children do not have enough coordination to swallow oral medicine until they are 6 or 7 years of age. This can make taking oral medication difficult. Almost all children fear intrusive procedures. Thus, accepting medication given by the rectal, nasal, intramuscular, or intravenous route may be very frightening. Because children range in size from 7 pounds to 150 pounds for late adolescents, there is no "standard" dose of medicine. This makes determining a correct dose difficult for health care providers. In addition, children cannot report adverse effects of medicine as accurately as adults. Therefore, determining if side effects or adverse effects are occurring is also more difficult. All these things make medicine administration for children one of the most difficult and challenging interventions in nursing. National Health Goals that address this area of child health practice are shown in the Focus on National Health Goals box.

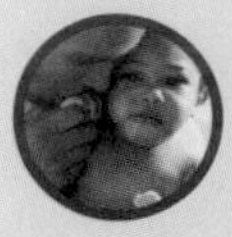

FOCUS ON NATIONAL HEALTH GOALS

When administering medicine to children or teaching children and parents how to take medicine, remember that medicines can be as dangerous in overdoses as they are helpful in the correct doses. They can be ineffective if the doses are inadequate or not taken. Poisoning and drug abuse are addressed by the following national health goals:

- Reduce childhood poisonings from a baseline of 348/100,000 population to a target of 292/100,000 population.
- Increase the proportion of adolescents not using alcohol or any illicit drug during the past month from a baseline of 79% of adolescents to a target of 89%.
- Reduce the amount of steroid use among adolescents in the past year from a baseline of 1.5% to 0.4% (DHHS, 2000).

Nurses can be instrumental in helping the nation achieve these goals by educating parents about safe drug storage (locked in elevated cabinets) and teaching children and parents about effective nonpharmacologic ways to relieve stress or anxiety to help reduce drug dependence.

Areas related to these goals that could benefit from additional nursing research to strengthen evidence-based practice would include studies on the most effective ways to teach parents about safe drug storage, the phenomenon that drug poisoning increases when families are under stress, and effective ways to impart information to adolescents about the seriousness of drug abuse and its possible consequences.

NURSING PROCESS OVERVIEW

For the Child Needing Medication/Intravenous Therapy

Assessment

Because children vary so greatly in size and individual need, medication administration to children begins with assessment of the child's height and weight so that a correct dose of medicine can be calculated based on the child's surface area. Also crucial to assessment is the child's developmental age. This is important to determine the child's ability to swallow oral medicine or to plan the best site for an intramuscular or intravenous injection. Be sure to include an assessment of the child's past experience with taking medicine to help predict what his or her response to medicine administration might be. Assess the child's chronological age and cognitive level to aid in planning the most appropriate level of explanation that will be needed. Also inquire about the family's cultural beliefs and attitudes toward medications, including use of herbal or folk remedies (see Focus on Cultural Competence). Following the medicine administration, careful observation is necessary to determine if the medication is having its desired effect and if any unwanted or adverse effects are occurring.

Nursing Diagnosis

Common nursing diagnoses related to medicine administration can vary widely. Some examples may include:

- Disturbed sleep pattern related to timing of medication administration
- Deficient knowledge related to action and side effects of medicine

FOCUS ON CULTURAL COMPETENCE

People's attitude about the worth or wisdom of medicine is not consistent across cultures. Not all families, therefore, can be expected to accept medicine administration as enthusiastically as others; some families believe that an herb or home remedy actually will be preferable. Thus, they accept a prescription but then do not obtain the medicine or administer it. Some families give herbal remedies in addition to a prescribed medicine that can duplicate or counteract the medicine's effect. Keep in mind, too, that without health insurance, medicine is expensive (Feinberg et al., 2002).

As an intrinsic part of health histories, ask if a child takes any type of herbal or home remedy for an illness. When you give the parents a prescription, ask them if they think they will have any difficulty with obtaining or giving it or assessing for the medicine's effect (after you explain the action of the medicine), or returning for a follow-up appointment to evaluate the medicine's effect. Such questions allow the parents to say that they have questions about the medicine or are uncertain whether they should give it or not because of a cultural belief.

- Fear related to intravenous administration of medicine
- Rash related to side effect of medicine
- Health-seeking behaviors by parent related to desire to learn more about different types of medicine available for child's illness

Outcome Identification and Planning

Planning for medicine administration for children involves the same safe rules of administration as those for adults: right medicine, right child, right dose, right route, right time, and right patient instruction. Extra consideration is necessary at each step because determining the right form and route of the medicine (liquid or capsule, oral or intramuscular, for example) can vary widely. Establishing that the dose is accurate for that size child can involve recalculating the dose using a nomogram that shows body surface area. The schedule for administration must be not only one that is effective for the drug's action but also one that will not interfere with school activities, eating, or sleep.

WHAT IF? What if a parent tells you that her child's school has a "no drug" policy, so her child is unable to independently take even a prescription drug in school? How would you advise her?

Explanation of what effects the child can expect from the medicine is necessary. Be certain that this explanation is given at an age-appropriate level and is consistent with any prior explanation a parent or other health care provider has given. A helpful Internet site to recommend to parents for information on general medicine administration and tips on how to read medicine labels is the American Academy of Pediatrics site (*www.aap.org/family/medication.htm*).

Correct patient identification is critical. In the hospital setting, the best way to identify all children before administering medicine is to check the armband; in an ambulatory care setting, ask a parent to confirm the child's identification.

Implementation

Medicine interventions with children include both administering medicine to ill children and teaching parents and children how to continue to take the medicine when at home (approximately 5% of children take medicine while at school; McCarthy et al., 2000). As long as a child is uncomfortable or has definite disease symptoms, parents tend to give medicine conscientiously. However, when symptoms fade, the child returns to school, and the family returns to its busy everyday schedule, it is easy for parents to forget to continue to give medicine. This can leave children open to a recurrence of the condition or symptoms, such as pain or recurrent infections, because the organisms causing the illness were only suppressed, not killed. Therefore, helping parents fill out administration schedules to post in a readily visible location, such as on the refrigerator or bathroom mirror, can be as important an act as explaining the drug's action to help ensure that all doses of medicine will be given.

Outcome Evaluation

Outcomes associated with medication administration should ensure that the child received the medicine as prescribed and that the medicine had the desired effect. Specific examples suggesting outcome achievement may include:

- Child states she understands that she must continue to take thyroid hormone for a lifetime.
- Parents list the adverse effects of the drug and state the telephone number they will call if adverse symptoms occur.
- Adolescent describes an administration program that includes four doses daily but allows time for sports activities after school.

MEDICATION ADMINISTRATION

Medications in children are given by a variety of routes: orally, intranasally, transdermally, topically, rectally, and via injection (such as intramuscularly, intravenously, or epidurally) or inhalation. Epidural administration is described in Chapter 38. Inhalation techniques are discussed in Chapter 40.

Safe medication administration is a priority in child health nursing because "children" vary from 7-lb newborns to 150-lb 18-year-olds. This wide weight range, combined with the relative immaturity of body systems in children, means that there is rarely a "standard" pediatric dosage of a particular drug. Each dose must be calculated individually. To administer drugs safely, it is important to have a good understanding of **pharmacokinetics** (the way a drug is absorbed, distributed throughout the body, metabolized, inactivated, and excreted). Each drug, each dose, and each child must be carefully and individually evaluated to ensure that the six rights of medicine administration—right medicine, right client, right dose, right route, right time, and right client instruction—are provided.

Pharmacokinetics in Children

The four basic processes of absorption, distribution, metabolism and excretion determine the intensity and duration of a drug's action. The immaturity of body systems in children (and especially in newborns) plays a major role in drug action throughout each of these processes.

Absorption

Drug **absorption** (transfer of the drug from its point of entry in the body into the bloodstream) is influenced by the route of administration as well as by the concentration and acidity of a drug. Some routes of administration in children are limited and thus are not used. For example, children younger than school age usually cannot hold tablets under their tongue for sublingual administration. In addition, the smaller muscle size of young children limits sites for intramuscular injection. Small children may inadvertently pull off transdermal patches because they do not understand that this is a drug. Gastrointestinal absorption may be immature at birth, so oral absorption in newborns may be reduced. Vomiting and diarrhea, frequent symptoms of childhood illnesses, interfere with absorption because drugs do not remain in the gastrointestinal tract long enough to be absorbed.

Distribution

Distribution refers to the movement of the drug through the bloodstream to the specific site of action. Many drugs are distributed bound to serum albumin (manufactured by the liver). This binding action limits the amount of free drug in the circulation, thereby providing protection against toxic levels of the drug. As free drug is used, the bound drug is released to maintain a therapeutic level. Newborns have sluggish peripheral circulation, so distribution in infants this young may be affected. Any child with cardiovascular disease also may have limited distribution of drugs. Newborns with immature liver function may not have enough serum albumin to transport drugs readily. This is particularly true if elevated bilirubin is present, because bilirubin is also carried by serum albumin. Bound to serum albumin this way, bilirubin is harmless. In free form, however, it can leave the bloodstream and enter other body tissues. If it enters the brain cells, it destroys their ability to function (kernicterus). If a newborn who has a high level of bilirubin from destruction of fetal hemoglobin receives a drug such as sulfonamide that competes for albumin-binding sites, a large quantity of bilirubin may be left unbound, and the infant may develop kernicterus.

Metabolism

Metabolism involves the conversion of the drug into an active form (biotransformation) or an inactive form (inactivation). Because a child's basic metabolic rate is faster than that of an adult, certain drugs are metabolized more rapidly in children. This means that the drug must be administered more frequently to a child to maintain effective drug levels. Some drugs, such as the salicylates and chloramphenicol, are metabolized directly by liver enzymes. Because liver enzymes are not fully developed in newborns, these drugs cannot be metabolized and will reach toxic levels rapidly. Older children with liver disease who have impaired liver enzymes also have decreased ability to inactivate drugs.

Excretion

The **excretion** (elimination of raw drug or drug metabolites, a process that largely prevents properly administered drugs from becoming toxic) of drugs is potentially limited until the age of 12 months, when kidney function becomes mature. If a child has kidney disease, excretion potential is limited at any age. A few drugs are excreted in bile (e.g., digitoxin). In the newborn with sluggish bile formation, excretion of these drugs is questionable. Monitoring intake and output is important in children receiving drugs to be certain that urine excretion or an outlet for drug metabolites is adequate.

Adverse Drug Reactions in Children

Children respond to drugs in much the same way as adults, but they may experience unique or exaggerated side effects because of immature liver function or rapid metabolism during periods of rapid growth. The newborn may suffer adverse effects from drugs administered to (or taken by) the mother prenatally or from drugs taken by the breast-feeding mother.

Safe Storage of Drugs

Since young children do not appreciate that overdoses of medicine can be serious and even fatal, they may help themselves to additional medicine or, mistaking its pleasant taste for candy, inadvertently poison themselves. Children may use medicine in a suicide attempt. Adolescents can deliberately take extra doses of drugs such as steroids or pain medicine for effect. Oxycodone (OxyContin), for example, is a pain reliever that is frequently prescribed for adolescents and also frequently abused by them (Spake, 2001).

In a health care setting, medicine must be kept in safe places. On an adult unit, for example, a medication cart can be left in the middle of a hallway or in a patient room while the phone is answered or another activity is performed. However, on a children's unit, this would be inappropriate. Children such as toddlers walking past such a cart could easily remove a handful of pills poisonous to them. For the same reason, medicine should never be left on a bedside table for a child to take later if the child is temporarily playing a game or taking a shower. A nearby toddler could take the medicine first.

When teaching parents about administering medicine at home, stress that they need to keep the drug in a safe place. In most homes, this is in a locked medicine cabinet or drawer above the height that the child could reach.

Remind parents that most childhood poisonings occur when the family is under stress. During these times, usual procedures such as locking away a drug may be forgotten. Therefore, reinforce the need for taking special precautions to lock medications at these times of added stress. Also be sure to review with parents that they should never pour or prepare medicine in the dark. Because almost all medicine bottles dispensed from local pharmacies look and feel the same, it is easy to pour the wrong liquid, extract the wrong pills, or read the bottle instructions incorrectly without adequate light.

Determination of Correct Dosage

The correct dosage of most drugs for children is based on body surface area, using a nomogram such as the one shown in Figure 37-1. To calculate surface area using such a chart, find the child's height in the left-hand column (e.g., 40 cm); next, find the child's weight in the right-hand column (e.g., 20 kg). Hold a ruler or straightedge to connect the two points. The mark at which the ruler crosses the center column is the child's body surface area (0.38 m^2 in the example). Obtaining and recording height and weight measurements at health visits or on hospital admission (or as frequently as daily during an admission) is important to supply this information for dose calculation.

Before administering any medication to a child, confirm that the dose ordered is correct for the child's weight or body surface. Every pediatric unit or clinic should have a drug reference, such as the *Physicians' Desk Reference,* for this purpose. Remember that there are always exceptions to a rule. For example, a child with a gunshot wound may receive more than the usual dose of antibiotics because the risk of infection is very high. A 3-year-old weighing only as

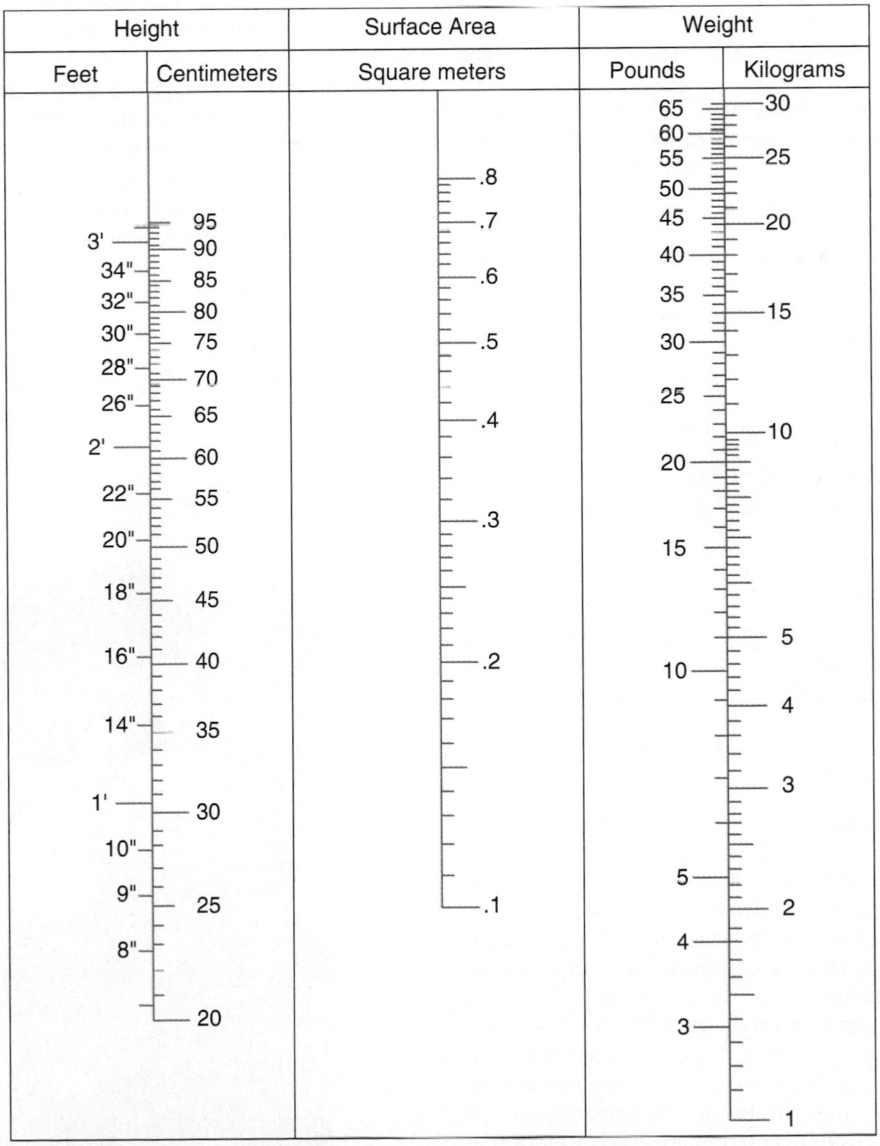

FIGURE 37.1 A nomogram to estimate body surface area. To use such a chart, draw a line from the child's height to the child's weight. The point at which it crosses the middle line is the child's surface area.

much as a 1-year-old would receive a dose of an antibiotic consistent with that given to a 1-year-old (not the child's actual age) because of small body size. Because of such exceptions, an ordered dose that does not conform to the standard dose may not be incorrect. The dose must be rechecked for accuracy with the prescribing physician or nurse practitioner, however, before it is administered. Preventing medication errors in children is a serious nursing responsibility (Cox et al., 2001). In one study, most medication errors occurred at the stage of drug ordering; intravenous medications were a common drug group in which errors occurred (Kaushal et al., 2001).

Although most medication currently is supplied in unit doses, child health nurses may still need to calculate fractional dosages. By verifying drug dosages, nurses serve as children's first line of defense against dosage error.

Identification of the Child

Children cannot be depended on to give their correct names before drugs are administered. Therefore, identification bands must be checked before medicine is offered. Anxious to please, a preschooler will answer the question, "Are you Johnny Jones?" with "yes." The child may also agree with any other name proposed. A school-age child who is anxious to avoid taking any medicine may deny that he or she is the person whose name is called. To prevent these types of errors, never ask children their names for identification. Instead, read their identification arm bands and compare them with the medication sheet or medical record. In ambulatory care settings or homes, ask a parent to confirm the child's identity.

✔ CHECKPOINT QUESTIONS

1. Why might newborns have more difficulty with drug distribution than older infants or children?
2. How would you use a nomogram to calculate a child's body surface area?
3. What is the best way to identify a child before giving a medication?

Oral Administration

Children younger than 9 years old often have difficulty swallowing tablets. For children younger than 3 years of age, this is virtually impossible. Most oral medication for young children, therefore, is furnished in liquid form.

In infants, oral medication can be given with a medicine dropper or a unit dose syringe (without a needle). Gently restrain the child's arms and head by holding the child against your body. Never give medicine with the child lying completely flat; otherwise, the child may choke and aspirate. If the child is crying, he or she actively opens the mouth. If not, gently open the mouth by pressing on the child's chin. Press the bulb of the medicine dropper or use the plunger of the syringe to gently allow the fluid to flow slowly into the side of the child's mouth. The end of the syringe or dropper should rest at the side of the infant's mouth to help prevent aspiration (some infants prefer to suck the contents of the syringe into their mouth) (Fig. 37-2). An infant also may be given fluid from a small glass or spoon. Allow the fluid to flow a little at a time so that the child has time to swallow between small sips.

Because firm pressure is used with the infant, he or she may be frightened afterward. Take time to sit and comfort the child or let a parent do this. This action is as important as checking the correct dosage of the drug. Protecting a child's mental health is as important as protecting physical health.

Preschoolers and early school-agers respond well to rewards such as stickers that they can paste into a book each time they take their medicine. For older children, hand them the glass of medicine as if they are expected to take it. Offer a "chaser" if necessary and not contraindicated (see Focus on Communication). If children have difficulty swallowing tablets, the tablets can be crushed and added to a teaspoonful of applesauce or a flavored syrup. If pills are not to be chewed (capsules or enteric-coated tablets), the child must be instructed not to chew them. Some children are old enough to swallow tablets but have never done it before. To teach a child how to swallow them, it is often easier to use small bits of ice for practice; they melt rapidly and do not stick in the back of the throat or esophagus. Have the child put the ice on the back of the tongue, take a sip of water, and swallow the water. Praise the child on learning this new skill.

Another useful technique to help a child to swallow pills is to push them into a spoonful of ice cream or pudding. Children tend not to chew this type of food; rather, they swallow it along with the pill. If using this technique, push the pill into the ice cream or pudding in front of the child.

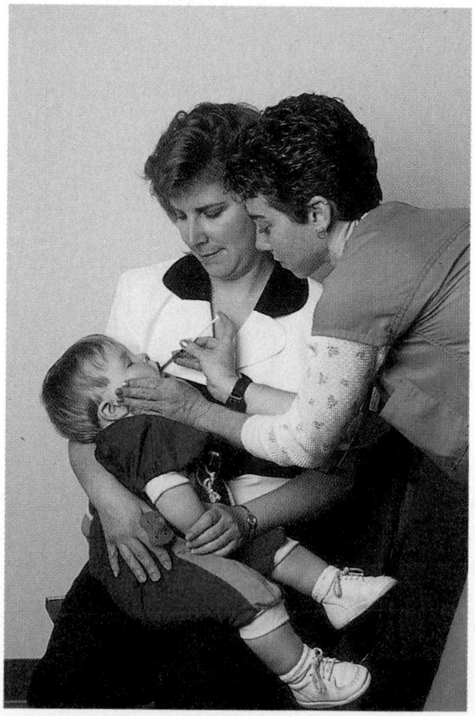

FIGURE 37.2 To administer oral medicine with a syringe, place the medicine at the side of the child's mouth.

FOCUS ON COMMUNICATION

You have a prescription for acetaminophen (Tylenol) for an 8-year-old who has a fever and sore throat. You approach the child to give the two tablets.

Less Effective Communication

Nurse: I have your medicine, Nicole. Swallow these for me?

Child: No. My throat is too sore.

Nurse: If you don't swallow them, I'll put them into a shot and give it that way. And that will really hurt.

Child: My throat is sore so I'd rather get a shot.

Nurse: Well, I can't do that. Tylenol doesn't come that way.

Child: Then I'm not going to take it.

More Effective Communication

Nurse: I have your medicine, Nicole. Swallow these for me.

Child: No. My throat is too sore.

Nurse: That's why I want you to swallow them. They'll take away the soreness.

Child: My throat is so sore I'd rather get a shot.

Nurse: I know. But this medicine needs to be swallowed. Do you want a drink of orange juice or soda pop to drink after it?

Child: Soda pop.

Nurse: Okay. Take a big swallow and it'll be gone.

The nurse in the first scenario makes two important medication administration errors: first, he asked the child if she would swallow the tablets rather than telling her to swallow them; second, he threatened the child; even worse, he threatened with a measure he could not enforce (acetaminophen doesn't come in an injectable form). When the child refuses the request and contradicts his threat, he is left powerless. A better approach is shown in the second scenario: here, the nurse explains the advantage of taking the medicine and conveys that he expects the child to be cooperative. Allowing a secondary choice, such as done above, offers children a sense of control but does not allow them to say no to the primary request.

The method is not to hide the pill, but to help the child learn to swallow medicine.

WHAT IF? What if a parent tells you that her preschooler is such a "picky eater" that he rarely eats a full meal? When should she give a medicine that should be taken with a meal?

A number of guidelines are helpful to remember when administering oral medication to children or teaching parents how to give medicine at home (see Focus on Family Empowerment). Be sure that the parents understand the correct dosage to be given (see Focus on Evidence-Based Practice).

Intranasal Administration

Having someone drop medicine into the nose is uncomfortable. Explain to the child that you understand this, but that the medicine is important because it will help the child get better. Inform the child of the procedure: "I'm going to place two drops of medicine into your nose. Then I want you to sniff for me [demonstrate]. Then I'll put two drops into the other side of your nose and I want you to sniff again."

Place the child on his or her back. A school-age child could extend the head over the side of the bed so that it is lower than the trunk. Preschoolers generally are too frightened by this strange position and do better with a pillow under their shoulders so that their head extends over the pillow and rests downward. An infant generally must be restrained in a mummy restraint for nose drop administration (see Chap. 36 for a discussion of appropriate restraints).

Drop the appropriate number of drops into one nostril. Turn the child's head to the side—to the left after the left nostril, to the right after the right nostril—so that the medicine stays in the nose longer. If the child is a preschooler or older, ask him or her to further sniff the medicine. Have the child remain in the head-flat position for at least 1 minute to let the medicine come in contact with the mucous membrane of the nose. If the child gets up immediately, the medicine will flow out and will be less effective.

Give the child high praise even if he or she did not cooperate at all. Praise tells the child you understand how hard it was to remain still.

More and more medicines today are provided as liquids to be sprayed into the nostrils. Children over about age 6 can do this independently but need to be introduced to the technique. Acknowledge that spraying a liquid into the nose is uncomfortable because it tickles or causes a sneezing sensation. Have the child sit or stand upright, hold the spray bottle upright with the tip just inside one side of the nose, and gently squeeze the spray bottle. In most instances the child should then tip the head to the side (the right side for the right nostril, the left side for the left nostril) or sniff, depending on the bottle instructions, for best absorption. The medicine administration is then repeated for the second nostril. Stress that although this form of medication administration seems simple and "fun," drugs are well absorbed across the nasal mucosa. This route is an effective means of drug administration and can be a route for important and even life-sustaining drugs.

Ophthalmic Administration

Ophthalmic administration involves administering medication via eye drops into the conjunctival sac of the eye. This type of administration is uncomfortable and frightening to children because they have been warned many times never to put anything into their eyes. Also, children know that getting something in the eye, such as dust, which has probably happened at some point, can be painful. As a result, infants and preschoolers generally must be restrained in a mummy restraint for eye drop administration. Always explain what you are going to do and that

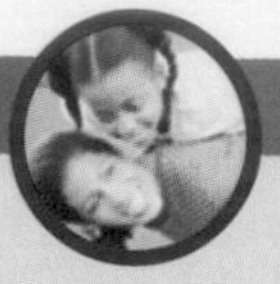

FOCUS ON FAMILY EMPOWERMENT
Guidelines for Administering Oral Medication

Q. My children fight me anytime they need to be given medicine. How can I get my children to take medicine without a battle?

A. Use the following guidelines to help make this task a bit easier:

- Do not say, "*Can* you drink this for me?" If an adult seems unsure whether a child can do it, the child may develop grave doubts himself.
- Do not say, "*Will* you drink this for me?" This leaves the child the opportunity to say no and creates the awkward position of having to admit that the child really does not have a choice in the matter; the child *must* take the medicine.
- State firmly, "It's time for you to drink your medicine now." Give the child a secondary choice that allows a sense of control: "It is time to drink your medicine now; do you want a drink of milk or water to swallow after it?" is a suitable choice, assuming both milk and water are compatible with the medication.
- Never refer to medicine as candy. Children may swallow medicine in fatal amounts when they think it is candy. (When everyone's back is turned, they help themselves to more "candy.")
- Do not bribe children to take medicine. Bribing may work for one dose, but when a second dose is due, the child will ask for a bigger bribe; for a third dose, an even bigger one. At some point (generally reached quickly), it is impossible to supply such large bribes and therefore it is impossible to enforce the rules.
- Do not threaten. Statements such as, "Take this quickly or I'll make it into a shot" cannot be followed through. The child calls the bluff (many medicines do not come in a form that can be injected intramuscularly), and once more the child is in control. A statement such as, "Take this or I'll call your doctor" is unfair (the physician has been made the villain) and ultimately undermines authority (it is obvious a person must not have much power or he or she would not need help).
- Do not lie about the taste of medicine. Children expect honesty from adults. If in doubt about the taste, taste it (with the obvious exception of drugs such as digitoxin). Most children's medicines are artificially flavored with raspberry, orange, or cherry syrup so do not taste bad.
- If a medicine tastes bitter, mix it with a spoonful of strained applesauce or a teaspoonful of flavored syrup. Do not mix medicine with a full jar of baby food because the child will then have to eat the entire jar of food to get all of the medicine. As a rule, encourage children to take medicine straight, then follow it with a pleasant-tasting drink to take away any bitter taste.
- If a medicine is supplied in tablet form, crush or dissolve it in water and mix it with syrup or applesauce for a better taste if appropriate. Be certain before removing the particles from a capsule that the medicine will work properly when not in capsule form: some are encapsulated to keep them from dissolving in the stomach and to bring them into the intestine, where they have their therapeutic effect. The same precaution must be followed when handling enteric-coated tablets.
- Never leave medicine by a child's bed for the child to take "in a minute" or "after your shower." The child may become involved with another activity "in a minute" and will not take it, or when he or she is not looking, a smaller child could find the medicine appealing and swallow it.

the medicine does not hurt (assuming that this is true). Place the child on the back. Open the eyes of infants and preschoolers by gently but firmly pressing on the lower lid with the thumb and on the upper lid with the index finger. A school-age child or adolescent will open his or her eyes cooperatively but may need to have a hand rested on the eyelid to keep an eye open long enough for the drug to be administered (Fig. 37-3). Be sure that your fingernails are short to avoid inadvertently scratching the child's cornea.

Drop the correct number of drops of medication into the conjunctiva of the lower lid. Allow the eyelid to close. Avoid placing the drops directly on the cornea because that may be painful. To prevent the conjunctiva from drying, do not hold the eyelids apart any longer than is necessary. After the child has blinked two or three times, allow the child to get up. Praise the child for his or her cooperation even if cooperation was not evident.

Otic Administration

Administering otic medications, primarily ear drops into the ear canal, is difficult for children to accept because they have been told not to put anything into their ears. Ear drops are generally administered for earache, which is sharp, excruciating pain. A child may worry that having medicine put into the ear will make the pain worse. Also, he or she cannot watch what is happening. Plus, the odd sensation of drops of fluid running into an ear can cause a tickling sensation that can add to the discomfort. Assuming that you have been honest with the child up to this point, remind the child of the following: "Remember how I told you that

FOCUS ON EVIDENCE-BASED PRACTICE

Are Household Teaspoons an Accurate Method for Parents to Use to Measure Liquid Medicines?

It is well known that although household teaspoons are supposed to hold 5 mL of liquid, many of them commonly hold more or less. For this study, 130 parents in the waiting area of primary care clinics were interviewed as to what they commonly used to measure liquid medications at home. They were then shown seven liquid dosing devices and asked which they owned or had ever used. They were next observed and scored on their ability to measure liquid medicine and interpret dosing instructions such as would be written on a typical prescription or medicine bottle. Results showed that parents most often used a household teaspoon to measure liquid medications at home. Common errors that occurred when parents demonstrated their measuring techniques were misinterpreting instructions, confusing teaspoons and tablespoons, and misreading a dosage chart when a child's weight for age was not in line with usual instructions.

This is an important study for nurses because nurses play a primary role in providing the majority of instructions about medicine administration. In addition, they also are the first-line persons who help to resolve administration concerns for parents. This study reinforces and supports the need for education to ensure that parents understand the difference between tablespoons and teaspoons and other measuring devices. It also supports the use of commercial 5-mL teaspoon measurement devices or oral dosing syringes as important measuring devices. Considering that a parent or child may inadvertently be measuring liquid medicine inaccurately should be considered if a drug seems to be having a decreased effect or side effects different from those anticipated.

Madlon-Kay, D. J., & Mosch, F. S. (2000). Liquid medication dosing errors. *Journal of Family Practice, 49*(8), 741–744.

the injection would hurt a little? Well, if this would hurt, I'd tell you now, too. But this doesn't hurt." Remind the child that ear drops can feel funny, as if someone were tickling the ear.

Place the child on the back, in a mummy restraint if necessary. Turn the head to one side (Fig. 37-4). The slant of the ear canal in children is shown in Chapter 50. If the child is younger than 3 years, straighten the external ear canal by pulling the pinna down and back. If the child is older than 3 years, pull the pinna of the ear up and back. Drop the specified number of drops into the ear canal. Hold the child's head in the sideways position for at least 1 minute to ensure that the medication fills the entire ear canal. Ear drops must always be used at room temperature or warmed slightly. Cold fluid, such as medication taken from a refrigerator, causes pain and may cause severe vertigo as it touches the tympanic membrane. Praise the child for cooperation after the procedure.

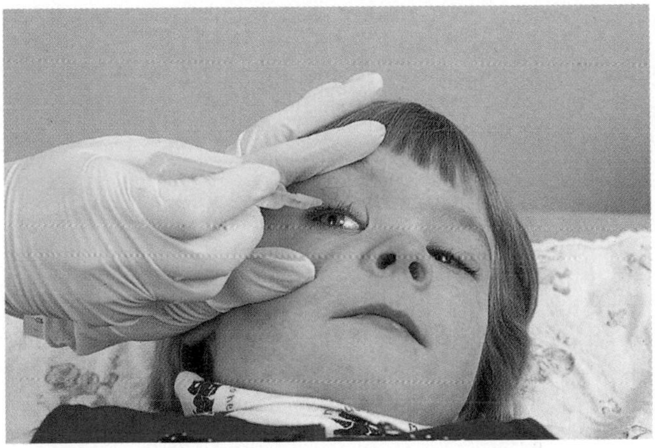

FIGURE 37.3 Administering eye drops.

✔ CHECKPOINT QUESTIONS

4. What would be an effective way to teach young children to swallow pills?
5. In what part of the eye should eye drops be instilled?
6. At what temperature should ear drops be given?

Rectal Administration

A good route for administering medication to children is by rectal insertion, because this allows the drug to be absorbed across the mucous membrane of the intestine. However, parents rate this as the least desirable method for administering medications (Seth et al., 2000). Some medications are given by rectal suppository; a few are given by retention enema.

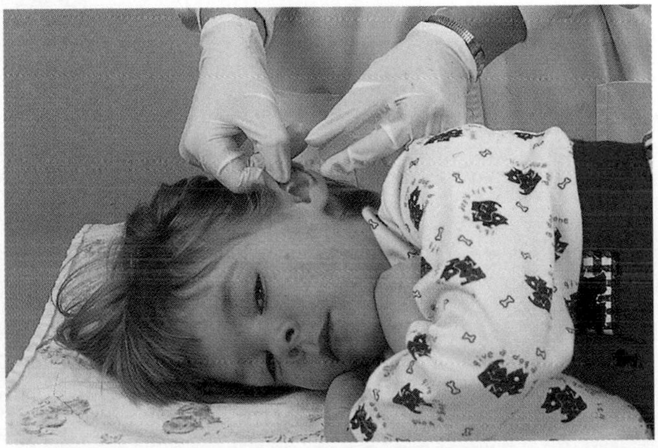

FIGURE 37.4 Administering ear drops. For the child over 3 years old, the pinna of the ear is pulled up and back.

Because the child cannot see what is happening, he or she can be easily frightened by this procedure. Show the child the medication so that he or she can be certain it is not an injection. Having been honest with the child up to this point will be helpful again: "If it were anything else, I would tell you so."

Use a glove and insert a well-lubricated suppository gently but quickly beyond the rectal sphincters (approximately a half-inch or as far as the first knuckle of the little finger for infants, and approximately 1 inch or as far as the first knuckle of the index finger for older children). Withdraw the finger and press the child's buttocks together firmly for a count of approximately 10, until the child's urge to evacuate the suppository passes. If a suppository is not prelubricated, dip the tip of it into a water-soluble lubricant such as K-Y jelly before insertion.

If the medication is to be administered by enema to a young child, use the usual enema technique, but with as small an amount as possible so the child can retain it. Press the child's buttocks firmly together for approximately 15 seconds after administering the enema or a child will expel the solution and the medicine will be lost. Using a distraction technique, such as asking the child to count backward or saying the alphabet backward, can also help a defecation reflex to pass. Invasive procedures are particularly threatening to the preschooler. Give lavish praise for cooperation.

Transdermal Administration

A number of medicines are available by transdermal patch, because absorption of drugs through the skin can be yet another effective and pain-free route for administration. Be certain that the child's skin is dry and intact at the site where the patch will be applied. Always apply patches over the trunk or major muscle, not on distal extremities, for best absorption. Assess the skin under the patch every time a patch is changed to be certain that the site is not irritated. Change the site every time a new patch is applied to decrease the possibility of irritation to the skin.

Young children tend to remove transdermal patches the same as they do Band-Aids because of normal curiosity about what could be underneath. Putting clothes on the young child immediately so the patch is hidden and out of sight is helpful. Also ensure that patches applied to children wearing diapers are not placed where a leaking diaper could wet the patch and irritate the skin or dilute the medicine absorption.

Intramuscular and Subcutaneous Administration

Intramuscular (IM) injections are rarely prescribed for children because children do not have sufficient muscle mass for easy deposition of medication, and IM injections are often painful. For IM injections in infants, the mandatory site for administration is the vastus lateralis muscle of the anterior thigh (Fig. 37-5). Be certain to use the lateral aspect rather than the extremely tender medial portion, where an injection would cause more pain. Using the gluteal muscle in children younger than 1 year is extremely hazardous. The muscle is not well developed until the child walks, so the sciatic nerve occupies a larger portion of the area than later on and could become permanently damaged by gluteal injections. Figure 37-5 shows an effective restraining technique for giving injections to infants. In older children, as in adults, the deltoid muscle (Fig. 37-6*A*) or a ventrogluteal site (see Fig. 37-6*B*) may be used.

Never give injections to children who are sleeping in the hope that they will not wake up and notice what is happening. They will wake terrified at being attacked. Instead, always give a short explanation: "I have some medicine for

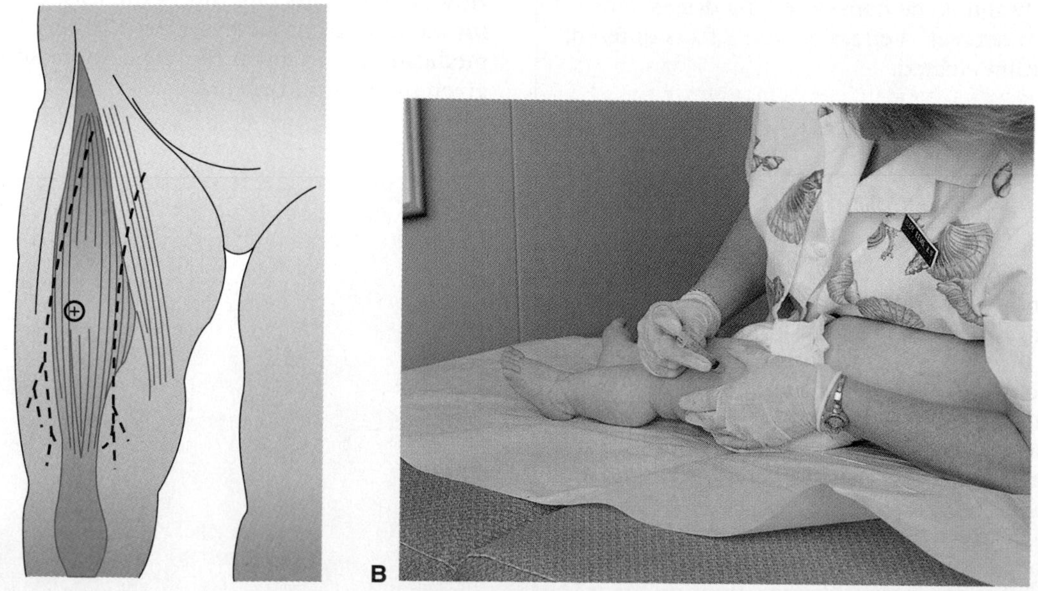

A B

FIGURE 37.5 (*A*) For infants under walking age, use the vastus lateralis muscle for intramuscular injections. (*B*) Technique for administering an intramuscular injection to an infant. Note the way the nurse uses her body to restrain and stabilize the infant.

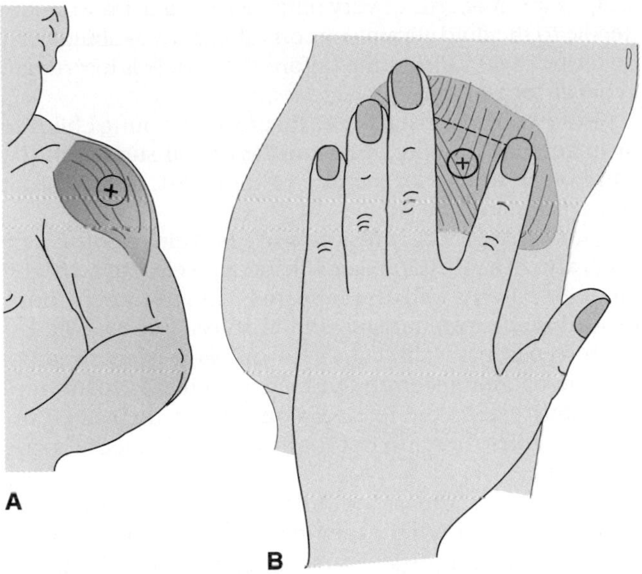

A

B

FIGURE 37.6 Sites for intramuscular injection. (A) In older children, the deltoid muscle is an acceptable site. (B) A ventrogluteal site may also be used in older children. Place the heel of the hand on the greater trochanter and the index finger angled toward the child's anterosuperior iliac crest, spreading the middle finger along the crest posteriorly. The triangle formed by the space between the index and middle fingers is the correct site.

you, Lynn. I'm going to put it into your leg. The injection will sting for a second just like a pinprick. Then it will be over." Be honest about the pain involved; try to describe it accurately so that the child knows it has limits (a small amount of pain for a short time). To reduce pain further, ask for a prescription for EMLA cream, which is applied an hour before the injection (see Chap. 38). Most children react well to injections if it is acknowledged that even with analgesia cream application, injections can still hurt.

After explaining the drug's purpose, do not delay giving the injection further by trying to distract the child or convince him or her it will not be bad. The suspense that the child feels caused by waiting during this time is worse than the actual injection. Give the injection quickly but always use good technique. Remember to aspirate (if indicated). Quickness counts, but safety is your priority. Massage the area briefly after the injection to ensure absorption of the medication, but remember that the rubbing may be as painful as the actual injection.

Statements such as, "Don't cry" are not therapeutic. If the child hurts, he or she should be allowed to cry. Tell them they can say "ouch" or yell or scream when the needle is inserted. They will appreciate being given approval to vent their feelings this way.

If necessary, ask for help in restraining a child when giving an injection, because having an extra pair of hands available may ensure safe administration. School-age children, however, may be proud that they are able to lie still. Being restrained would shame them. Be certain to hold and comfort the young child after all painful procedures, or let a parent do this. Record the site of an IM injection as well as the medication injected, so that sites can be rotated for better absorption.

✔ CHECKPOINT QUESTIONS

7. How far should a rectal suppository be inserted in an infant?
8. What special precautions are necessary when using transdermal patches in small children?
9. What is the preferred administration site for an intramuscular injection in an infant?

INTRAVENOUS THERAPY

Intravenous (IV) therapy is the quickest and most effective means of administering fluid or medicine to the ill infant and child and, as such, is a relatively common pediatric therapy (Shin et al., 2001). It has several major uses, including maintenance of fluid and electrolyte balance; an avenue to bring drugs quickly up to therapeutic levels in the body; and nutritional support. IV fluid may be infused into a peripheral vein, a central venous access device, or a peripherally inserted central venous catheter. The amount, type, and rate of IV fluids for children are prescribed carefully to prevent fluid overload.

Determining Fluid and Caloric Needs of the Child

It is important that IV fluid administered to children and infants is isotonic (exerts the same osmotic pressure as their bloodstream). Using isotonic fluid does not cause a pressure gradient that would lead to fluid shifting into the interstitial tissue, as would happen if the IV fluid were hypotonic, or fluid shifting from interstitial tissue into their bloodstream, as would happen if the IV fluid were hypertonic. Lactated Ringer's and 0.9% normal saline are two isotonic IV fluids commonly used with children. Normal saline 0.45% is a hypotonic solution that may be used with children who are dehydrated to restore blood volume quickly. Dextrose 5% in 0.9% sodium chloride is an example of a hypertonic solution that might be used to cause fluid to shift into the bloodstream and relieve cerebral edema.

It is important to understand the principles of IV therapy, including the fluid and caloric needs of the child (which differ significantly from those of the adult) to act as a second level of protection against overhydration or underhydration. A easy formula that can be used to calculate water need in children is as follows: for every 100 kcal expended in metabolism, the child must replace 115 mL water, 3 mEq sodium, and 2 mEq potassium.

Table 37-1 shows a method of calculating caloric expenditure. Fluids administered using this table should contain 25 mEq sodium and 20 mEq potassium per liter and 5% dextrose. Common IV solutions and oral electrolyte formulas used with infants (Pedialyte and Lytren) contain these proportions. According to Table 37-1, a child weighing 45 kg would have a caloric expenditure of 2,000 Kcal. Therefore, the child would need 2,300 mL of a maintenance solution containing 5% dextrose, 25 mEq sodium, and 20 mEq potassium per liter. A flow rate would be calculated for this amount (2,300 mL fluid in 24 hours = 95 mL/h).

TABLE 37.1 A Method to Calculate Caloric Expenditure

BODY WEIGHT	CALORIC EXPENDITURE PER 24 H
Up to 10 kg	100 kcal/kg
11–20 kg	1000 kcal + 50 kcal/kg for each kg more than 10 kg
More than 20 kg	1500 kcal + 20 kcal/kg for each kg more than 20 kg

From Siegel, N. J., Carpenter, T., & Gaudio, K. M. (1999). The pathophysiology of body fluids. In Oski, F. A., et al. *Principles and practice of pediatrics.* Philadelphia: Lippincott Williams & Wilkins.

Obtaining Venous Access

The needle size for IV therapy varies depending on the solution and the rate at which it will be administered. Commonly used catheter sizes include 22-gauge, 24-gauge, and 25-gauge (in newborns). "Butterfly" needles are metal needles with an extra flange of plastic added on both sides of the needle hub to give the person beginning the infusion a wider surface to grasp, thereby guiding needle placement better. Butterflies are also termed scalp vein needles because they were originally designed for entrance into infant scalp veins. A length of very narrow tubing leads from the needle to the fluid administration tubing. This tubing must be flushed with IV solution before the needle is inserted to avoid an air embolus.

Sites frequently used for IV insertion in young children or infants include the veins on the dorsal surface of the hand or on the flexor surface of the wrist. Leg and foot veins also may be used.

Another site for IV infusion is a scalp vein over the temporal area. An infusion placed in a scalp vein can be frightening to parents because it seems a much more serious procedure than an infusion administered into an arm. Explain to parents that scalp vein infusion is an effective method of administering fluid or medicine in infants and ultimately causes the least discomfort for their child because needles there do not infiltrate readily (see Nursing Procedure 37-1).

Preschoolers and older children often express some preference as to where they want an infusion inserted. Offer a choice, if possible, or suggest the nondominant hand. Act as the child's advocate and see that his or her wishes are respected.

Children who have IV infusions for long periods may require the placement of an **Intracath** (a slim, pliable catheter threaded into a vein). This type of device is advantageous because it cannot be dislodged as easily as a normally inserted IV needle. Therefore, the child can usually move about more freely.

NURSING PROCEDURE 37.1: INITIATING A SCALP VEIN INFUSION

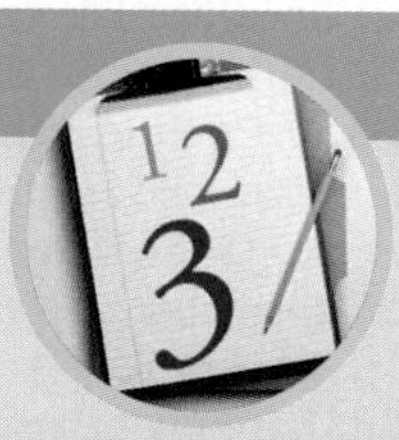

Purpose
To initiate a scalp vein infusion.

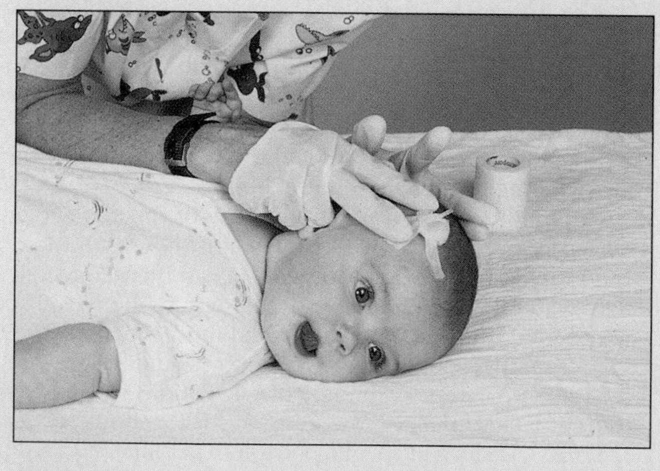

Plan	Principle
1. Adequately restrain the infant, using a mummy restraint.	1. Restraining the infant promotes safety. Mummy restraints are useful because it is physically exhausting to try to hold the infant's arms and legs still.

(continued)

Procedure	Principle
2. Press the child's head to the side and hold it firmly in that position, one hand on the occiput, the other securing the front of the head. Be certain that the hand resting over the child's face does not obstruct the child's breathing.	2. This positions the child without interfering with respirations.
3. Lather the site over the temporal bone with a cleaning solution.	3. The cleaning solution reduces the possibility of infection.
4. Carefully shave the hair. Assure parents that the hair will grow in quickly after the procedure. Ask parents if they want to save the clippings of hair if it is their child's first haircut.	4. Hair removal allows a clear view of the insertion site and possibly reduces the risk of infection.
5. Apply EMLA cream to chosen site. After 60 minutes, place a rubber band around the infant's head at the level of the forehead.	5. A tourniquet is needed to dilate scalp veins. EMLA cream decreases discomfort but takes time to anesthetize the site.
6. Wash the shaved area with an antiseptic solution.	6. Washing the scalp further reduces the possibility of infection.
7. Insert a special small scalp vein needle or polytetrafluoroethylene (Teflon) catheter. Scalp vein needles have protruding plastic "wings" (often referred to as butterflies) on the sides to allow easy manipulation.	7. Use of an appropriate insertion device establishes a fluid route.
8. Continue to hold the infant firmly until the needle is securely taped in place, and until satisfied that the infusion is running well.	8. Securing the infant and device ensures an effective insertion site.
9. Cover the infusion needle with a piece of gauze (a plastic protector taped onto the site provides additional protection).	9. Covering the site keeps the infant from brushing the needle out of place when he or she turns the head.
10. If necessary, pin the shirt sleeves to the sides of the diaper or use a trunk or jacket restraint for an infant who is old enough to turn over.	10. Pinning the shirt keeps the infant from brushing at the site. Using restraints prevents the infant from turning over.
11. Spend some time comforting the child, talking and smiling at him or her, and lightly touching and stroking. Many infants enjoy sucking a pacifier after painful procedures; being held and rocked is the best comfort.	11. The infant may be frightened by the pinprick of the needle insertion, as well as by having been held so firmly for a length of time.

For all children (including adolescents), IV infusions must be secured in place with an armboard. Although children may say that they will be careful not to move their arms, without an armboard it is easy to move unintentionally to turn off the television set or reach for something falling off the bed and accidentally dislodge the needle. Tape a board to the arm of an older child with the words, "This is just to remind you to keep your arm still"—an explanation more acceptable than if the child thinks you doubt his or her ability to hold the hand still.

Determining Rate and Amount of Fluid Administration

Because children's hearts and circulatory systems are smaller than those in adults, IV fluid must flow at a slower rate. If administered at an adult rate, the child's cardiovascular system would quickly become overloaded. Automatic rate flow infusion pumps facilitate the infusion of potent medications. They should be mandatory for small children because they regulate the flow accurately to a few drops per minute (Fig. 37-7). Overloading of IV fluid in infants and children can also be prevented by use of fluid chambers, devices that allow only 50 to 100 mL of fluid into the drip chamber at a time. Even if the pump fails, with these in place, only the amount in the drip chamber will be allowed to enter the child's circulation, not the entire contents of the bag suspended above the child's head.

A third fluid safety measure is the use of a minidropper, a device that reduces the size of the drop in the control chamber to 60 drops per mL (usually there are 10–15 drops per mL). With a normal dropper in place, an infusion regulated to administer 30 mL/h drips at a rate of 7 or 8 drops per minute and is therefore difficult to regulate. With a minidropper in place, the drops are smaller; the same infusion (still providing the same amount of fluid per hour) drops at 30 drops per minute. This flow is easier to regulate and provides more accurate IV administration.

Keeping a careful record of both the rate and amount of IV fluid administered is important. At least once an hour, record the type and amount of fluid; the rate of flow

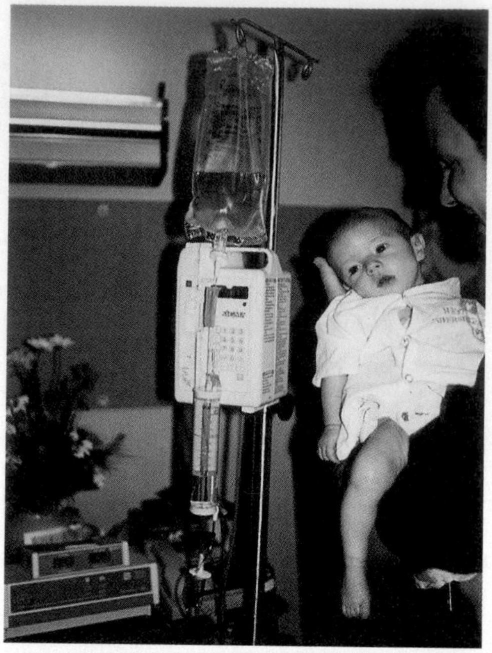

FIGURE 37.7 An infusion pump and calibrated infusion chamber are safety features used with children's intravenous infusions.

FOCUS ON MULTIDISCIPLINARY CARE

Because the majority of medication for children is given intravenously today, many children have continuous intravenous infusions in place. This means that all health care professionals need to be aware of the importance of these lines and take precautions not to disrupt them when assisting the child with such activities as physical, respiratory, or occupational exercises. Offer to explain the importance of such lines or to offer assistance to protect them as needed. When children are transported to another area of the hospital, such as the x-ray department, you or another health care provider may need to accompany the child to ensure that the intravenous line is not dislodged and continues to function.

(including the number of drops per minute); and, for a cross-check, the amount of fluid remaining in the bag. Signs of fluid overload are those of congestive heart failure: increased pulse rate and blood pressure. As the heart fails from excessive fluid, blood pressure falls and signs of edema develop. Be on guard for changes in vital signs such as these when children are receiving IV fluids. In addition, assess the specific gravity of urine at least every 4 hours to detect extremely dilute urine (specific gravity under 1.003) or to determine whether the child is excreting a large quantity of fluid in an effort to reduce circulating volume.

It is difficult for children to lie still and wait for an infusion to finish. They need to be provided with activities and allowed out of bed as much as possible. Infants and preschoolers may have to have their other arm restrained to keep them from playing with the infusion needle. Infants who receive total fluids by IV infusion generally enjoy sucking on a pacifier to fulfill their oral needs. Be sure all personnel involved in the child's care understand the importance of the IV therapy (see Focus on Multidisciplinary Care).

Parents and children often have numerous questions about IV therapy. These questions and appropriate answers are highlighted in Box 37-1.

Medication Administration

Medication may be added to an IV line as a small, one-time administration (bolus) or by piggyback or longer infusions.

To administer medicine by a bolus technique, clamp the IV tubing above the medicine port provided in the IV line; clean the port with alcohol; insert the syringe and needle

BOX 37.1

GENERAL CONSIDERATIONS FOR INTRAVENOUS THERAPY

Parents and children often want to know about intravenous therapy. Some of the typical questions that you may hear include (answers are provided in parentheses):

- Will the insertion hurt? (Yes, but only as the needle is inserted; after that the infusion will be pain-free.)
- How long will the infusion be necessary? (Estimate a time interval depending on the medicine and fluid prescription, but add that the time interval can vary depending on the effect of the medicine or fluid.)
- Isn't there another way to administer the same medicine? (Explain how intravenous administration allows medicine to reach the bloodstream immediately so is the method of choice when immediate effect is important; also, some medications can only be given intravenously.)
- What can the child do during the infusion? (Any activity that will not interfere with the infusion. If a child will have medicine administration daily, help the parents and child plan a special activity such as play a board game, listen to special music, or watch a favorite TV program, an activity reserved for only that time. This changes the IV infusion from a dreaded activity to a "can't wait for" activity.)
- Will it hurt when the needle is removed? (No, although taking off the tape that holds the needle in place may cause some discomfort.)

filled with the prescribed medicine into the port; and inject the medicine slowly and gently based on the manufacturer's instructions. Once the medication has been given, remove the syringe and needle and reopen the IV line immediately to allow the IV solution to flush the medicine into the child.

As with any medication administration, be certain to identify the child beforehand. Also ensure that the drug to be injected is compatible with the IV fluid being infused.

For a piggyback infusion of medicine, medication is provided by the pharmacy and prepared and diluted in small IV fluid plastic bags. Depending on the type of IV equipment in use by the health care agency, to begin a piggyback infusion, hang the piggyback bag, clean the medicine port on the IV line, and insert the piggyback system into the port. Lower the level of the main infusion bag and adjust the flow rate to that desired to allow the piggyback system to operate. As soon as the piggyback bag has emptied, elevate the maintenance bag of fluid again and assess that the IV line is flowing well and at the proper rate.

Children accept piggyback administrations of fluid well because it seems no different from receiving maintenance IV fluid. Older children can take an active role in alerting health care providers that the total medication amount has infused and it is time to return to maintenance fluid.

Using Intermittent Infusion Devices

Intermittent infusion devices, or heparin locks, are devices that maintain open venous access for medicine administration while allowing children to be free of IV tubing so that they can be out of bed and more active (Fig. 37-8). The vessels of the back of the hand are generally chosen as the IV site. Scalp vein tubing is used and capped at the end with a specially designed rubber stopper or a commercial trap. The tubing is filled with a dilute solution of heparin or normal saline through the rubber stopper and flushed again with solution every 2 to 8 hours (depending on hospital policy) to keep it patent. IV medication can be added as needed. The tubing and stopper must be firmly secured to the wrist, and an armboard is taped in place to remind the child to protect the site from inadvertent trauma.

Children who are hospitalized or receiving home care for a long time and who need only IV medication, not additional fluid, are good candidates for such devices. Heparin locks also can be used with children when frequent venous blood samples are required. If blood is drawn from the already inserted tubing, the child is pricked only once (when the device is originally placed) no matter how many samples are drawn. Similar devices may be inserted into arteries when arterial blood is required—for example, for the child who is having blood gases monitored frequently.

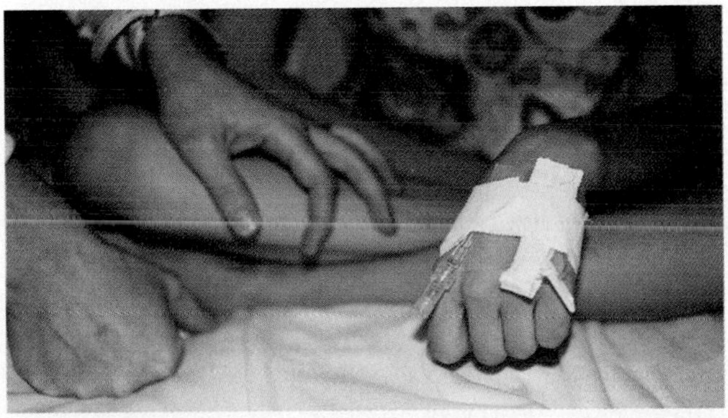

FIGURE 37.8 An intermittent infusion device (heparin lock) in place. Advocating for this type of apparatus minimizes pain.

Using Central Venous Access Catheters and Devices

Venous access for long-term IV therapy can be gained by insertion of a catheter into the vena cava just outside the right atrium; the catheter exits the chest just under the clavicle (Racadio et al., 2001; Fig. 37-9). Typical catheters used in this way include Broviac, Hickman, and Groshong catheters. Such catheters have a wrinkle-resistant fabric (Dacron) cuff that adheres to the subcutaneous tissue and helps to seal the catheter in place and keep infection out. These catheters can be used to administer bolus or continuous infusions of medications and fluid. Care of the catheters (depending on agency policy) consists of daily or weekly changes of dressings over the exit site and periodic irrigation with heparin or saline to ensure patency.

Such catheters are advantageous because discomfort from further skin punctures is avoided. However, one disadvantage is that the catheter could become snagged on something and accidentally be pulled out. If this happens, it is an emergency because the child could lose an appreciable amount of blood from the point of entrance into a vein as major as the vena cava. Unless there is a waterproof dressing covering the insertion site, children with central venous catheters in place are usually not allowed to swim or take showers, to avoid infection.

Vascular access ports (VAPs; infusion ports that can be implanted) are small plastic devices that are implanted under the skin, usually on the anterior chest just under the clavicle, for long-term fluid or medication administration via bolus or continuous administration (see Fig. 37-9*D*). A small catheter threads from the port internally into a central vein. Common brands include Port-A-Cath, Infus-A-Port, and Groshong Venous Port. Blood samples can be removed or medication can be injected following skin cleansing by a puncture through the chest skin into the port. Although this device requires a skin puncture (causes pain), it may be well accepted by children because it is not as visible as a central venous catheter, no dressing is required, and it allows a full range of activities such as showering and swimming. Be certain when accessing these ports to use only the needle supplied by the manufacturer because a regular needle tends to "core" or remove a small circle of the membrane over the port and destroy the integrity of the device. Use EMLA cream to decrease discomfort as necessary.

Children also may have peripherally inserted central catheters (PICC lines) for therapy; these are advantageous because they can remain in place for up to 4 months without being changed (Racadio et al., 2001). These catheters are inserted into an arm vein (usually at the antecubital space into the median, cephalic, or basilic vein) and advanced until the tip rests in the superior vena cava. If a

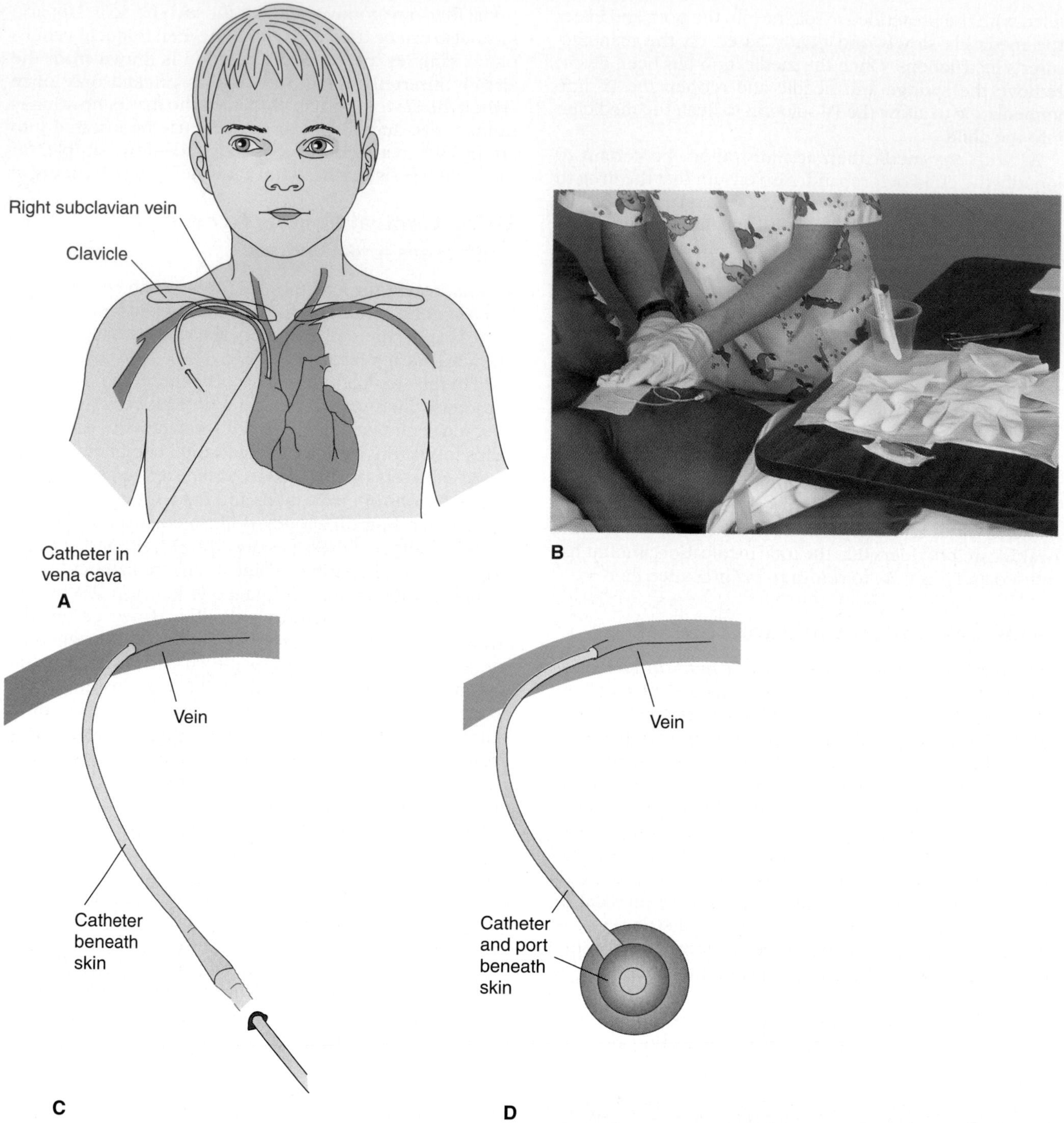

FIGURE 37.9 (*A*) Insertion site for placement of a central venous catheter for intravenous infusion. (*B*) Changing a dressing for a central venous catheter. (*C*) Central venous catheter beneath the skin. (*D*) A vascular access port (VAP) device beneath the skin.

shorter catheter is used, the tip will rest closer to the head of the clavicle (a midline insertion).

Drugs commonly administered include antibiotics and analgesics. After medication is administered, the line is flushed with a solution such as normal saline. The dressing over the insertion site is changed according to agency policy.

Many parents seem more comfortable with this type of insertion than with a central venous catheter because it appears so much more like a routine IV. Newborns can have a catheter inserted into an umbilical vessel, with fluid and medications being administered by that route (see Chap. 26).

All central venous access systems have the potential to cause thromboses because they partially occlude a vein (Glaser et al., 2001). In addition, the dressing must be changed using strict aseptic technique to prevent infection (Colomb et al., 2000; Chiang & Baskin, 2000).

Using an Infusion Pump

An infusion pump delivers a continuous infusion of a drug by the constant forward movement of a plunger of a medicine-filled syringe to inject the medicine into subcutaneous tissue. The tissue site chosen is usually the abdomen, as this both protects the pump and allows it to be out of sight. Insulin (see Chap. 48) and heparin are two drugs often prescribed to be infused by infusion pumps today. Based on the success of this infusion technique for long-term drug administration, the system likely will be more frequently used in the future.

For administration, a syringe is filled with medicine and a small tube with the needle attached at the distal end is attached to the hub of the syringe. The syringe is then clamped to the pump and the skin site is cleaned with alcohol and the needle inserted at a 45-degree angle (usual subcutaneous insertion technique). As soon as the needle is taped in place, the pump is turned on.

The insertion site should be changed every 1 to 2 days to reduce the possibility of infection. The pump should be removed to shower (the syringe, tubing, and needle can be left taped in place). For swimming or tub bathing, the entire pump, syringe, tubing, and needle should be removed. If used with children who are not yet toilet-trained, it is important to keep the pump and insertion site away from an area that could be soiled with urine or stool.

Older children, like adults, can be worried at first that the pump will fail to operate, so they check it often to be certain the syringe is emptying. With small children, cover the pump with clothing to prevent them from touching the pump.

Administering an Intraosseous Infusion

Intraosseous infusion is the infusion of fluid into the bone marrow cavity of a long bone, usually the distal or proximal tibia, the distal femur, or the iliac crest. Because the bone marrow communicates directly with the circulatory system, the time at which fluid reaches the bloodstream when administered this way is the same as if it were administered IV. All fluids that can be administered IV, including whole blood or medication, can also be administered by this route.

Intraosseous infusion is used in an emergency when it is difficult to establish usual IV access or in a child with such extensive burns that the usual sites for IV infusion are not available. Intraosseous infusion is a temporary measure until a usual route of administration can be obtained because of the danger of osteomyelitis, a devastating infection with long-term effects to bone marrow. It must be initiated with sterile technique, and if continued for an extended time, the infusion point is rotated about every 2 to 3 days to minimize the risk of infection.

Intraosseous infusion is painful as the needle enters the bone marrow cavity and again at the time of the bone marrow aspiration. Prepare the child for this and offer support.

The following are steps used to initiate an intraosseous infusion:

1. The skin over the chosen site is cleaned with povidone-iodine and anesthetized with a local anesthetic.
2. A small incision is made into the skin with a scalpel blade.
3. A large hypodermic or bone marrow needle is inserted through the incision into the cavity of the bone.
4. To ensure that the needle tip has reached the bone marrow cavity, a syringe is attached to the needle and aspirated for bone marrow.
5. If bone marrow is obtained, the syringe is removed and intravenous tubing, including a filter and the fluid to be administered, is attached to the needle and opened to a gravity flow.
6. A dressing with additional iodine is then applied over the needle site.
7. A restraint is applied to the leg to help the child hold the leg still.

Tubing must be changed about every 48 hours and the dressing over the site must be changed about every 24 hours—again, to reduce the possibility of infection. Assess for a distal pulse and adequate temperature and color of the leg every hour during the length of the infusion to ensure adequate circulation to the extremity. If the needle should become dislodged, symptoms of circulatory impairment or pain and taut skin over the site occur.

Occasionally during fluid administration, a bone chip or thick marrow will occlude an intraosseous needle and slow the infusion. If this occurs, a stylet passed through the needle clears it and allows for continued fluid administration.

Administering a Subcutaneous (Hypodermoclysis) Infusion

Before safe IV infusion was perfected with infants, fluid was given to them subcutaneously (perfusing fluid into subcutaneous skin layers by an IV infusion set). The technique is still appropriate for children with blood disorders who receive a medication to remove stored iron from their body by this route. Sites used for hypodermoclysis generally include the pectoral region, the back, or the anterolateral aspects of the thighs. The IV needle is inserted into the subcutaneous layer of the skin and the infusion apparatus is opened. The rate is governed by the rate of absorption by the subcutaneous layer of skin; it is not a set rate.

✔ CHECKPOINT QUESTIONS

10. What are three safety devices for the administration of intravenous fluid in children?
11. When are intraosseous transfusions used?
12. When are hypodermoclysis infusions used?

KEY POINTS

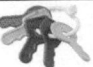

The effectiveness of medicines varies depending on the pharmacokinetics (absorption, distribution, metabolism, excretion) of the drug.

The principles of safe medicine administration for adults also apply to children: right medicine, right client, right dose, right route, right time and right patient instructions.

The correct drug dose in children is usually calculated according to the child's body surface area, determined by use of a nomogram.

Use adequate restraints when giving medicine to be certain that the child will allow the medicine to be given and will not inadvertently harm himself or herself in the process.

Teach parents safe actions for giving medicine at home so children continue to receive accurate doses after hospital discharge.

In children, the majority of medications are given orally or intravenously to avoid the pain of intramuscular injections.

IV therapy may be administered peripherally or via a central venous access site. The scalp vein is a common IV site used for infants.

An intraosseous infusion is used in an emergency when it is difficult to establish usual IV access or in a child with such extensive burns that the usual sites for IV infusion are not available.

CRITICAL THINKING EXERCISES

1. Terry is the 2-year-old you met at the beginning of the chapter who has never learned how to swallow pills. How would you handle this problem? What would you do to teach her how to do this?
2. Suppose you know that a 4-year-old is so frightened of injections that she screams at the sight of any kind of needle. You have to begin an intravenous infusion on her. What steps would you take to help her overcome her fear?
3. Suppose a school-ager tells you that she doesn't believe in introducing any "foreign" substance into her body so she doesn't intend to take an antibiotic for her infected foot. Would there be a way to change her decision? How would you counsel her?
4. Examine the National Health Goals related to medicine administration and children. Most government-sponsored money for nursing research is allotted based on these goals. What would be a possible research topic to explore pertinent to these goals that would be fundable and would advance evidence-based practice?

REFERENCES

Chiang, V. W., & Baskin, M. N. (2000). Uses and complications of central venous catheters inserted in a pediatric emergency department. *Pediatric Emergency Care, 16*(4), 230–232.

Colomb, V., et al. (2000). Central venous catheter-related infections in children on long-term home parenteral nutrition: Incidence and risk factors. *Clinical Nutrition, 19*(5), 355–359.

Cox, M., D'Amato, S., & Tillotson, D. J. (2001). Reducing medication errors. *American Journal of Medical Quality, 16*(3), 81–86.

Department of Health and Human Services. (2000). *Healthy people, 2010.* Washington DC: DHHS.

Feinberg, E., et al. (2002). Family income and the impact of a children's health insurance program. *Pediatrics, 109*(2), E29–E32.

Glaser, D. W., et al. (2001). Catheter-related thrombosis in children with cancer. *Journal of Pediatrics, 138*(2), 255–259.

Kaushal, R., et al. (2001). Medication errors and adverse drug events in pediatric inpatients. *Journal of the American Medical Association, 285*(16), 2114–2120.

Madlon-Kay, D. J., & Mosch, F. S. (2000). Liquid medication dosing errors. *Journal of Family Practice, 49*(8), 741–744.

McCarthy, A. M., Kelly, M. W., & Reed, D. (2000). Medication administration practices of school nurses. *Journal of School Health, 70*(9), 371–376.

Racadio, J. M., et al. (2001). Pediatric peripherally inserted central catheters complication rates related to catheter tip location. *Pediatrics, 107*(2), E28–E32.

Seth, N., et al. (2000). Parental opinions regarding the route of administration of analgesic medication in children. *Paediatric Anaesthesia, 10*(5), 537–544.

Shin, D., et al. (2001). Postoperative pain management using intravenous patient-controlled analgesia for pediatric patients. *Journal of Craniofacial Surgery, 12*(2), 129–133.

Spake, A. (2001). "Not an appropriate use". Did the makers of OxyContin push too hard? *US News & World Report, 131*(1), 26.

SUGGESTED READINGS

Engelhardt, T., & Crawford, M. (2001). Sublingual morphine may be a suitable alternative for pain control in children in the postoperative period. *Paediatric Anaesthesia, 11*(1), 81–83.

Foley, J. (2000). The effects of hospitalisation on children. *Nursing Review, 18*(1), 4–5.

Li, S. F., Lacher, B., & Crain, E. F. (2000). Acetaminophen and ibuprofen dosing by parents. *Pediatric Emergency Care, 16*(6), 394–397.

Lorenz, J. M., et al. (2001). Radiologic placement of implantable chest ports in pediatric patients. *American Journal of Roentgenology, 176*(4), 991–994.

Marino, B. L., et al. (2000). Prevalence of errors in a pediatric hospital medication system. *Outcomes Management for Nursing Practice, 4*(3), 129–135.

Nicholls, J. (2000). Prescribing issues: Paediatric prescribing: the principles and pitfalls. *Community Nurse, 6*(4), 55–56.

Nielsen, L., & Martin, S. A. (2001). Cardiac polypharmacy: Caring for the child postoperatively. *American Journal of Nursing, 101*(5), 34–41.

Rodriquez, E., & Jordan, R. (2002). Contemporary trends in pediatric sedation and analgesia. *Emergency Medical Clinics of North America, 20*(1), 199–222.

Woodring, B. C. (2000). Family matters: If you have taught—have the child and family learned? *Pediatric Nursing, 26*(5), 505–509.

38

CHAPTER

Pain Management in Children

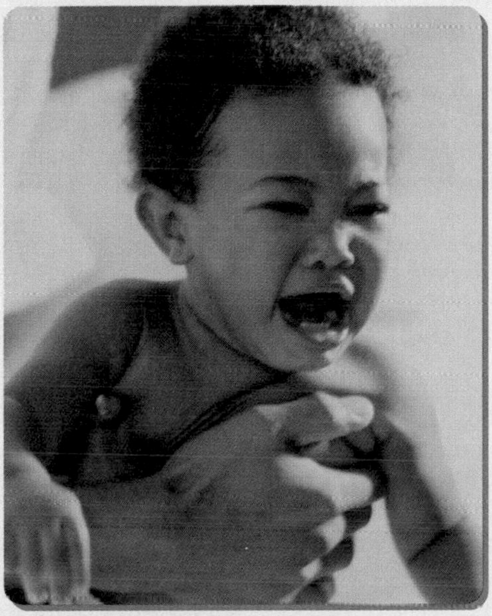

Key Terms

- acute pain
- conscious sedation
- chronic pain
- cutaneous pain
- distraction
- epidural analgesia
- gate control theory
- nociceptors
- pain
- pain threshold
- pain tolerance
- patient-controlled analgesia
- referred pain
- somatic pain
- substitution of meaning
- thought stopping
- transcutaneous electrical nerve stimulation
- visceral pain

Objectives

After mastering the contents of this chapter, you should be able to:

1. Describe the major methods and techniques of pain management in children.
2. Assess a child as to whether pain management is needed or adequate.
3. Formulate nursing diagnoses for children with pain.
4. Identify expected outcomes for children with pain.
5. Plan nursing care for children with pain.
6. Implement nursing care related to the child with pain.
7. Evaluate outcomes for achievement and effectiveness of care.
8. Identify National Health Goals related to children with pain that nurses could be instrumental in helping the nation to achieve.
9. Identify areas related to care of children with pain that could benefit from additional nursing research or application of evidence-based practice.
10. Use critical thinking to analyze ways that nursing care for a child with pain could be more family-centered.
11. Integrate knowledge of pain in children with nursing process to achieve quality maternal and child health nursing care.

Robin is a 3-year-old girl who is admitted to your hospital unit for a severe burn of her hand. When seen in the emergency room, she was screaming with pain. She received intravenous morphine for pain relief. Now, an hour later, her mother asks you if Robin can have additional morphine. "She's not having pain yet," her mother tells you, "but I want her to have something before the pain comes back." Is this mother's assessment of her child's pain apt to be accurate? Would anticipating pain in this way be the best intervention for Robin?

Previous chapters described the growth and development of children. This chapter adds information about the management of pain in children. This is important information because it builds a base for care and health teaching in a crucial area.

After you've studied the chapter, answer the Critical Thinking Exercises at the end of the chapter and then access the on-line study activities (http://connection.lww.com) *to further sharpen your skills and test your knowledge.*

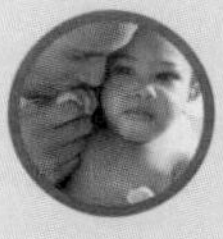

FOCUS ON NATIONAL HEALTH GOALS

Although National Health Goals do not speak directly to alleviation of pain in children, many of the goals speak to reducing unintentional accidents, and unintentional accidents are a major source of pain in children. Some of these objectives are:

- Increase use of automobile safety belts and infant safety seats to 100% for children under age 4 from a baseline of 92%.
- Increase the use of helmets to at least 79% of motorcyclists from a baseline of 67%.
- Increase the number of states with laws requiring bicycle helmets for riders under the age of 15 from 10 states to all states.
- Increase the presence of functional smoke detectors to 100% in all inhabited residential dwellings from a baseline of 88%.
- Reduce hospital emergency department visits for nonfatal dog bite injuries to 114/100,000 of the population from a baseline of 151/100,000 (DHHS, 2000).

Nurses can be instrumental in helping the nation to reduce children's pain by teaching about the importance of using safety belts and bicycle helmets. As primary care providers, they can lead the effort to be certain that children and parents receive counseling on safety precautions. Additional nursing research that is needed in the area of pain relief concerns what is the best way for children to rate pain and what nonpharmacologic measures work best with different age groups.

Pain is a difficult concept to define because it is experienced so differently by different people. It's important to remember that it is subjective (experienced by the person), not objective (able to be determined by observation). Children who are cognitively challenged or from another culture may have difficulty describing pain (Hennequin et al., 2000; McCaffery & Pasero, 1999). McCaffery's classic description of pain (McCaffery & Pasero, 1997) is the one most useful with children: "The sensation of pain is whatever the person experiencing it says it is, and it exists whenever he or she says it does."

For children, pain is not only a hurting sensation, but it can be a confusing one because they did not anticipate the pain, cannot explain its presence, and cannot always understand its cause. In addition, preschoolers and younger children lack an understanding of time, which makes it difficult to explain when the pain will go away. Children may feel frustrated because no one is able to prevent pain or give them relief. Because children may have difficulty describing pain in a manner that adults are able to understand, it is difficult to assess the extent of their discomfort (Zarbock, 2000). Both helping children describe the type and extent of pain they are feeling and performing active interventions to relieve pain are important nursing roles. Assessing for pain is so important that it can be considered the fifth vital sign.

The National Health Goals do not address pain relief in children directly. However, they do address the reduction of unintentional injury, which is a major source of pain in children. These goals are shown in the Focus on National Health Goals box.

NURSING PROCESS OVERVIEW

For the Child With Pain

Assessment

Children, like adults, experience pain differently depending on the type and cause, their temperament, their previous experience with pain, and their expectation of relief. Infants and young children cannot verbalize what they are feeling and thus have the most trouble communicating how they feel.

Beginning with preschool age, children are able to indicate where they feel pain and can learn to express the degree of pain through a system such as comparing it to a number of poker chips or drawings of faces. Older school-age children and adolescents can be asked to rate their pain on a scale of 1 to 10. Be aware that children may be reluctant to admit pain because they are trying to be brave. Some may be reluctant to say they have pain because they are afraid the "shot" they will receive to relieve it will cause more pain. As a rule, including assessment of pain level along with vital sign measurement is an efficient way to ensure that pain is assessed (the fifth vital sign). Let children know that admitting to having pain is necessary to obtain adequate relief. Common findings in the child with pain are shown in Assessing a Child With Pain.

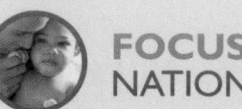

Parents often are unclear what role they should assume in pain management. Frequently parents believe that the nurses are the experts and will automatically treat their child's pain. Nurses, on the other hand, may assume that parents will speak up if their child is in pain. How pain will be assessed, the par-

ASSESSING a Child With Pain

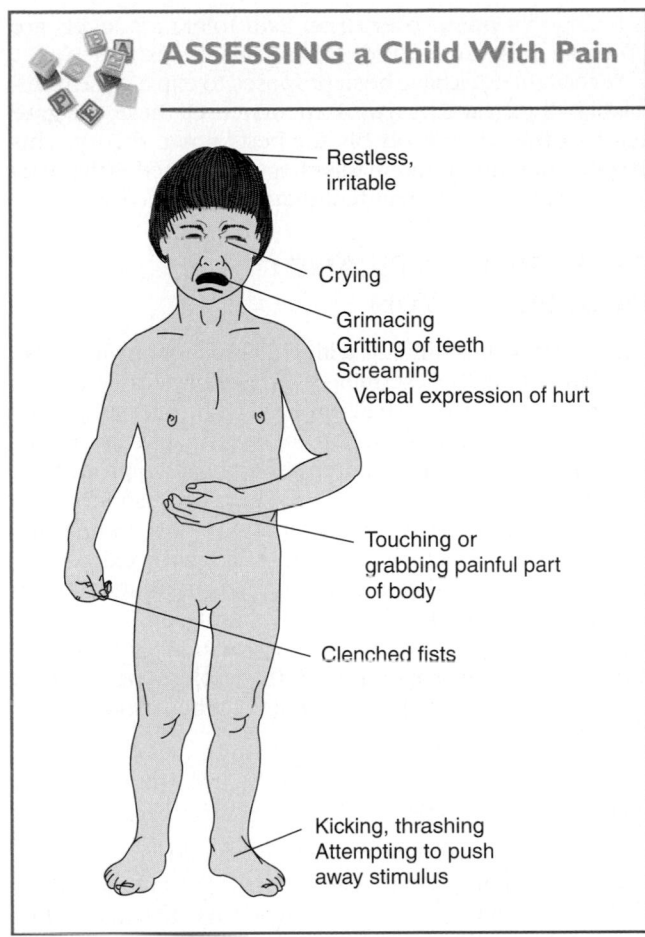

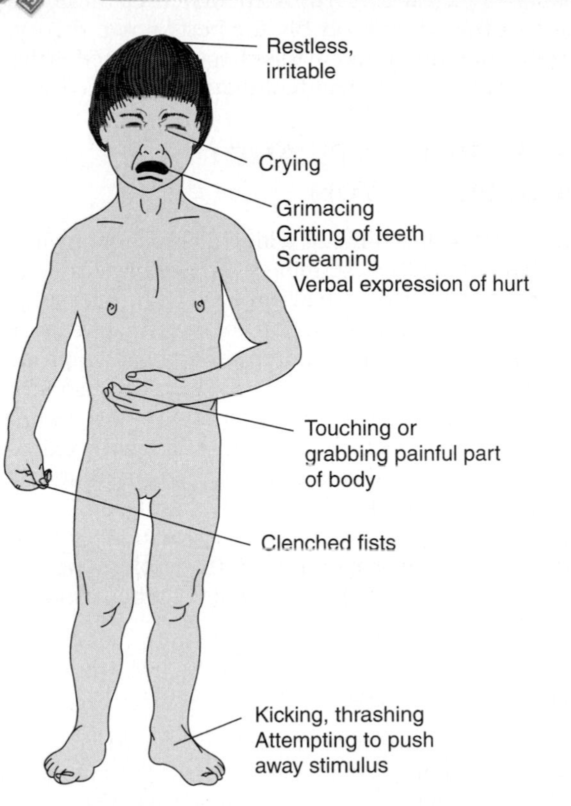

ents' role, and what is available for pain relief should be discussed clearly and openly so these misunderstandings do not occur.

Nursing Diagnosis

Nursing diagnoses for children with pain focus not only on the pain but also on the stress or fear that having pain produces. Young children have a very difficult time separating pain and anxiety. Nursing diagnoses that might be used with children with pain include:

- Pain related to frequent invasive procedures
- Fear related to anticipation of painful procedures
- Disturbed sleep pattern related to chronic pain
- Anxiety related to planned dressing changes

Outcome Identification and Planning

The mark of efficient pain control is to anticipate when pain will occur and plan interventions to prevent it rather than let it occur and then relieve it. Three common reasons that nurses may not provide adequate pain relief to children are: a belief that infants and young children do not experience pain, a fear of addiction to pain relief medications, and a fear of causing respiratory depression. Infants and young children do experience pain, and there is no confirmation that children will become addicted to pain medication or that opiates cause greater respiratory depression in children than in adults. Although the use of opiates can lead to dependency, this is very different from addiction and can addressed with a weaning regimen as needed.

Implementation

Implementation for pain relief includes choosing the best method of pain relief for each child. All persons involved in the child's care need to be aware of the signs and symptoms of pain and ways to help the child manage the pain (see Focus on Multidisciplinary Care). If a child is reluctant to admit that he or she has pain because of the fear of injections, advocate for an oral form of medication or an intermittent intravenous (IV) infusion device such as a heparin lock or patient-controlled analgesia (PCA) as appropriate options. Many parents are unsure about the safety of using strong analgesics for pain relief. Therefore, educating parents about the need for pain relief and taking actions to involve them in the assessment and evaluation process are essential. Planning and assisting with complementary therapies is yet another area to consider (Buckle, 2001).

Outcome Evaluation

Evaluation is a key aspect of managing pain because no one pain relief measure is effective for everyone.

FOCUS ON MULTIDISCIPLINARY CARE

Many health care professionals such as laboratory technicians, physicians, and x-ray or endoscopic assistants are called on to perform some procedures with a child that could cause pain. Assist these individuals to schedule procedures at times that a child can be administered optimal pain relief.

Also, teach other health care personnel involved with the child's care how to look for signs and symptoms of a child's pain during procedures so they can advocate for pain relief measures. Be certain they realize that it is healthy for children to express fear and pain. Advise them not to use such statements as, "Be a big boy" or "Stop crying," but say instead, "It's all right to cry. I know it hurts." Teaching nonpharmacologic techniques to children such as thought stopping can be time-consuming. Once instructed in them, other disciplines can reinforce these techniques with the child and parents. Caution them to review the technique with children before procedures for best results.

Unlicensed assistive personnel are often called on to restrain children during procedures. Be sure that they understand when and to what degree the child should be restrained. In many cases, the use of restraints or holding the child down increases the child's anxiety, panic, and combative response. If the child is unable to hold still despite trying to elicit his or her cooperation, sedation should be considered. If a procedure goes poorly for the child the first time, an even stronger negative response can be expected from the child at a later procedure.

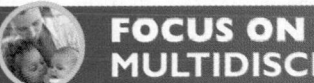

For example, when a child has pain and is given an analgesic, it is essential to determine whether the drug was effective. Look for nonverbal clues, assess vital signs, and listen to the child's statements about pain. Based on these findings, the techniques of pain management may need to be modified or increased. A new technique may need to be added to the regimen so the child receives maximum pain relief.

Possible examples indicating successful achievement of outcomes may include:

- Child states pain is at a tolerable level.
- Adolescent says she has managed her fear through imagery.
- Child describes ways he will help to reduce pain when it returns.
- Child resumes age-appropriate behaviors.

PHYSIOLOGY OF PAIN

As in adults, pain in children occurs for one of four reasons: reduced oxygen in tissues from impaired circulation, pressure on tissue, external injury, or overstretching of body cavities with fluid or air. The stimuli causing pain are not always visible or measurable. In addition, anxiety can lead to increased pain regardless of the physical stimuli.

Pain conduction consists of four major steps: transduction (sensing the pain sensation), transmission (routing the pain sensation to the spinal cord), perception (the brain interprets the sensation as pain), and modulation.

Transduction begins in the peripheral nerves when a mechanical, thermal, or chemical stimulus activates **nociceptors,** a specialized group of sensory receptors. A number of neurotransmitters are involved in conducting pain (namely, substance P). Sharp pain impulses are conducted by both A-alpha and A-beta fibers (large fibers that are myelinated and conduct the response at a rapid rate). Light pressure and vibration are conducted by A-delta fibers, fibers that are smaller and thus conduct at a slower rate. C fibers are still smaller and conduct at an even slower rate.

Pain impulses join central nervous system (CNS) fibers in the dorsal horn of the spinal cord. Here the impulses are projected upward to the brain, where they will be perceived as pain. **Acute pain** is sharp pain. It generally occurs abruptly after an injury. Paper cuts are examples of lacerations that cause acute pain. **Chronic pain** is pain that lasts for a prolonged period (often defined as 6 months). Acute pain usually causes extreme distress and anxiety; chronic pain can lead to depression (Hunfeld et al., 2001).

Cutaneous pain is pain that arises from superficial structures such as the skin and mucous membrane. A paper cut is an example. **Somatic pain** is pain that originates from deep body structures such as muscles or blood vessels. The pain of a sprained ankle is somatic pain. **Visceral pain** involves sensations that arise from internal organs such as the intestines. Appendix pain is considered visceral pain. **Referred pain** is pain that is perceived at a site distant from its point of origin. Right lower lobe pneumonia is often first thought to be abdominal pain because it is referred to the abdomen.

The **pain threshold** refers to the point at which a person first feels pain. This varies greatly and is probably most influenced by heredity. All people also have a point above which they are not willing to bear any additional pain. This is a person's **pain tolerance.** Pain tolerance levels are probably most affected by cultural influences.

Several theories have been proposed to explain the transmission of pain and the pain experience. Of these, the **gate control theory** is probably the best-known theory. This theory is described later in this chapter and used as the basis for the pain management techniques discussed here.

ASSESSING TYPE AND DEGREE OF PAIN

Pain assessment is difficult with children, not only because they have difficulty describing it but also because some will suffer with pain rather than report it. Using only subjective measures such as observation to assess pain can be misleading because some children mask their symptoms and thus do not appear to be in pain. They may distract themselves by methods such as concentrating on play. Some children may sleep, not from comfort but from the exhaustion caused by pain. Cultural differences also influence how pain is expressed (see Focus on Cultural Competence).

Pain assessment techniques vary widely from assessment of the nonverbal infant to the adolescent. Keep in mind the child's developmental level when assessing for pain.

The Infant

In the past, it was believed that infants do not feel pain because of incomplete myelinization of peripheral nerves. This is no longer believed, because myelinization is not necessary for pain perception.

A second argument against needing to provide pain relief to infants is that they have no memory. It can be shown, however, that physiologic changes do occur with pain, so even with a lack of memory, it is clear that pain is experienced. In all ages, including premature infants, pain

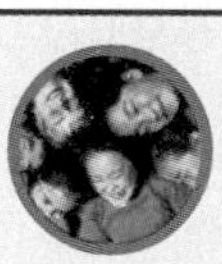

FOCUS ON CULTURAL COMPETENCE

Because pain is an individual sensation, it can be experienced totally differently by different children. In South American countries, for example, pain may be expressed very openly and freely. In Asian or northern European countries, children are expected to be more stoic about pain. In China, children may not accept something offered for pain relief until it has been offered twice. Because the expression of pain is culturally determined this way, two children having the same degree of pain may express it very differently.

Additionally, a child's perception of the situation influences his or her response to a situation independent of the intensity of the stimulus. Therefore, a child experiencing a procedure less intrusive than another child's may still describe the degree of pain as more intense, based on his or her perception. Assessment for pain must be individualized.

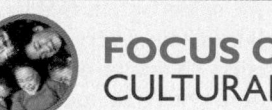

has been shown to have the potential for serious physical harm. Because they are preverbal, assessing pain in infants is especially difficult. Observing for cues such as diffuse body movement; tears; a high-pitched, sharp, harsh cry; stiff posture; lack of play; and fisting can all be helpful (Rouzan, 2001). Even newborns instinctively guard a body part by holding an extremity still or tensing the abdomen. Perhaps the chief mark of pain in infants is that when pain is present, they cannot be comforted completely. Preterm neonates may not be able to organize a distress response to cue a health care provider to the presence of pain. When working with infants of this age, be sensitive to situations that could cause pain. Be alert for subtle alterations in facial expression, such as eyes squeezed shut or a quivering chin, that might signal pain.

The Toddler and Preschooler

Determining when and how much pain is present continues to be difficult with toddlers and preschoolers because they may not have a word in their limited vocabularies to describe it. They may have difficulty comparing it to past pain (is it better or worse) because they have had little experience with past pain. Words such as "sharp," "nagging," or "aching" have no meaning in relation to pain until the child has experienced each type. Parents may have encouraged children this age to refer to pain as "my boo-boo" or some other word instead of "pain." To assess such a child's pain accurately, use the child's term or teach the child that "pain" is the same as "boo-boo." For some toddlers, pain is such a strange sensation that, aside from crying in response to it, they may react aggressively (pounding and rocking) as if to fight it off. They also may avoid being touched or held.

Preschool children can describe that they have pain but continue to have difficulty describing the intensity. They are able to begin to use comforting mechanisms, such as gritting teeth, pressing a hand against a forehead, pulling on their ear, holding their throat, rubbing an arm, or grimacing, to control or express pain. Some preschoolers do not think to mention they have pain because they believe it is something to be expected or, due to their egocentric thinking, may assume adults are already aware of their pain. They may think the pain is punishment for some act, so this is what they deserve. They also can believe that, if they admit to pain, they will receive an injection, a circumstance seen as worse than the original pain. It is sometimes difficult to comfort children this age during painful procedures because they do not yet have a perception of time. Soothing statements such as, "It's only for a minute" are not comforting to the preschooler who does not know how long that is.

For all young children who cannot fully verbalize their pain state, carefully examine their behavior. In addition to behaviors already discussed, young children may regress or become very withdrawn when in pain. Ask yourself, "What would this child normally be doing (for example, playing, eating, sleeping)?" Deviations from usual behavior may, in the absence of any other verbal description, be signs that the child is in pain. Input from parents on how their child usually behaves also is very valuable. Keep in mind that any procedure or condition that would normally cause pain in an adult will cause pain in a child. In a nonverbal child, a trial dose of analgesia may be used. You can then evaluate behavior changes after the dose is given. The child who resumes his or her usual behavior after analgesia was probably in pain before it.

The School-Age Child and Adolescent

Children who think concretely (preadolescents) can have difficulty envisioning that a word like "sharp" applies both to knives and to the feeling in their abdomen. Thus, they continue to have difficulty describing pain. They may assume that because a nurse is an authority figure, the nurse knows they have pain. They may be in middle school before they are able to understand how to use a pain rating scale or that the scale intensifies from left to right. Doing some preassessment work with them, such as giving them 10 different-sized triangles and asking them to arrange them from smallest to largest, is a good way to evaluate if they understand incremental measurements. The child who can arrange triangles this way understands the concept of least to most. Once children have grasped this concept, they are able to describe pain intensity in a very measurable way. A scale of 1 to 5 can be used in younger children.

Adolescents commonly use adult mechanisms for controlling pain. Some are more stoic in the face of pain than adults, trying to avoid the stereotypes of "cry-baby" or "chicken." This makes assessing for body motions such as clenched hands, clenched teeth, rapid breathing, and guarding of body parts that might indicate pain not as helpful as they may be in adults. Some children of school age will regress with pain (e.g., talking baby-talk or lying in a fetal position). Children this age can understand that if pain will last only an instant, such as with an injection, it can be controlled through nonpharmacologic activities such as distraction techniques.

> ✔ **CHECKPOINT QUESTIONS**
>
> 1. What are frequent physiologic findings that indicate pain in infants?
> 2. What if a toddler uses the word "oowie" for pain? Should you use his word or insist he learn the word "pain"?

PAIN ASSESSMENT

The techniques of pain assessment vary depending on the age of the child and the type and extent of pain. Although monitoring for physiologic findings such as a change in pulse or blood pressure may give some indication that the child is under stress, these are not the most dependable indicators of pain. Common fallacies about pain in children are shown in Table 38-1. Because pain is a subjective finding, once children can speak, asking them to tell you about their pain (self-reporting on a pain rating scale) is the most accurate method for assessment.

A variety of pain rating scales have been devised for use with children. None has been proven to be consistently better than the others, mainly because both children and the type of pain they can be experiencing vary so much. As a rule, pick one scale to use with a child and then use it consistently for the child rather than asking the child to adapt to different assessment techniques. Be sure to fol-

TABLE 38.1 Common Fallacies About Pain in Children

FALLACY	FACT
Nurses can accurately estimate children's pain from physical appearance or activity.	Nurses commonly underestimate children's pain when they do not rely on children's self-reports.
Young children, particularly newborns, do not feel pain.	Newborns and children do feel pain.
A child who resumes usual activity or sleeps cannot be in pain.	Some children distract themselves with play or music while in pain. They may sleep from exhaustion from the pain.
Because of the possible adverse effects, narcotic analgesics are too dangerous for young children.	Narcotics can be used safely with children, including low-birth-weight infants.
Experiencing pain will not harm an infant or young child.	Newborns with pain can become cyanotic and bradycardic; no one knows the psychological stress of pain at this age.
If a child denies he or she is feeling pain, you should believe him or her.	Children may deny pain to avoid a procedure, such as an injection, which they view as more painful. They may be afraid, fearing that they are being punished, or believe others know how they feel.

low the individual instructions for that scale (see Focus on Communication).

Pain Experience Inventory

The Pain Experience Inventory is a tool consisting of eight questions for children and eight questions for the child's parents. It is designed to elicit the terms the child uses to denote pain and what actions the child thinks will best alleviate the pain. Such a form can be used when a child is admitted to an acute care facility or on an initial home care visit (Box 38-1). If possible, it should be used before the child has pain.

CRIES Neonatal Postoperative Pain Measurement Scale

The CRIES inventory is a 10-point scale on which five physiologic and behavioral variables frequently associated with neonatal pain can be assessed and rated:

- Amount and type of crying
- Need for oxygen administration
- Increased vital signs
- Facial expression
- Sleeplessness (Krechel & Bildner, 1995)

Each area is scored from 0 to 2, and then a total score is obtained (Table 38-2). On the scale, infants with a score of 4 or more are most likely to be in pain and need pain management interventions to reduce discomfort. The scale cannot be used with infants who are intubated or paralyzed for ventilatory assistance because they would have no score for cry, and because their faces are obscured, they would not be able to be rated for facial expression.

FLACC Pain Assessment Tool

The FLACC Pain Assessment Tool (Merkel et al., 1997) is a scale by which health care providers can rate a child's pain when the child cannot give input. It incorporates five types

FOCUS ON COMMUNICATION

Faye Harvey is a 4-year-old girl who has just returned from tonsillectomy surgery. You know this type of surgery is painful, so you want to assess her level of pain.

Less Effective Communication
Nurse: Faye? How are you feeling?
Mrs. Harvey: Her throat is too sore to talk.
Nurse: I'm going to show you some faces, Faye. Just point to the one that looks the way you feel. If you point to a sad one, I'll get you a shot to take away your pain.
Faye: (Points to the first face—the "no pain" face.)
Nurse: No pain? Good. That's probably because your anesthetic is still working.

More Effective Communication
Nurse: Faye? How are you feeling?
Mrs. Harvey: Her throat is too sore to talk.
Nurse: Faye? Remember the faces we looked at this morning before surgery? I want you to use them to tell me how you feel. This one means "no hurt." This one means "the most hurt you could have." Point to the one that shows how much hurt you have.
Faye: (Points to the middle face—the "moderate pain" face.)

It is important when using pain rating scales to introduce them to children before surgery or before they will have pain from procedures so that both the pain and the rating tool are not new to the child all at once. It is important also to give the correct instructions for standardized assessment tools, or the results will not be accurate. Mentioning a "shot for pain" can cause children not to report pain because they imagine that the injection will cause even more pain rather than relieving pain.

BOX 38.1

PAIN EXPERIENCE INVENTORY

Questions for Child

Tell me what pain is.
Tell me about the hurt you have had before.
What do you do when you hurt?
Do you tell others when you hurt?
What do you want others to do for you when you hurt?
What don't you want others to do for you when you hurt?
What helps the most to take away your hurt?
Is there anything special that you would like me to know about you when you hurt? (If yes, have child describe.)

Questions for Parents

Describe any pain your child has had before.
How does your child usually react to pain?
Does your child tell you or others when he/she is hurting?
How do you know when your child is in pain?
What do you do for your child when he/she is hurting?
What does your child do for himself/herself when he/she is hurting?
Which of these actions work best to decrease or take away your child's pain?
Is there anything special that you would like me to know about your child and pain? (If yes, have parents describe.)

Hester, N.O., & Barcus, C.S. (1986). Assessment and management of pain in children. *Pediatrics: Nursing Update, 1*(14), 2. Princeton, NJ: Continuing Professional Education Center, Inc.

of behaviors usually seen with pain: facial expression, leg movement, activity, cry, and consolability. Data indicate that the scale is reliable and valid. Because the child does not provide active input, the child may experience a loss of the self-control that can come from active participation.

Poker Chip Tool

The Poker Chip Tool (Hester & Barcus, 1986) uses four red poker chips placed in a horizontal line in front of the child. It can be used with children as young as 4 years of age, provided the child can count or has some concept of numbers. To use the tool, tell the child, "These are pieces of hurt." Beginning at the chip nearest the child's left side and ending at the one nearest the child's right side, point to the chips and say, "This is a little bit of hurt, this is a little more hurt, this is more hurt, and this [the fourth chip] is the most hurt you could ever have." Then ask the child, "How many pieces of hurt do you have right now?" Children without pain will reply that they do not have any, so do not give children an option for zero hurt. Clarify the child's answer by a follow-up question such as, "Oh, you have a little hurt? Tell me about the hurt." This is an effective tool for young children because the poker chips are concrete items (Fig. 38-1).

FACES Pain Rating Scale

This scale consists of six cartoon like faces ranging from smiling to tearful. Explain to the child that each face corresponds to a person who has no hurt up to a lot of hurt. Use the words under each face to describe the amount of pain. Ask the child to choose the face that best describes his or her own pain (Wong & Baker, 1996). Record the number under the face the child chooses. Children as young as 3 years can use this scale. This scale appeals to health care providers because it is cute. However, it is not as concrete a measure as the Poker Chip Tool and therefore may not be as effective with all children (Fig. 38-2).

TABLE 38.2 CRIES Neonatal Postoperative Pain Measurement Scale

	INFANT'S SCORE		
ASSESSMENT	*0*	*1*	*2*
Crying	No	High-pitched	Inconsolable
Oxygen required for saturation above 95%	No	>30%	>30%
Increased vital signs	Heart rate and blood pressure within 10% of preoperative values	Heart rate or blood pressure 11–20% higher than preoperative value	Heart rate or blood pressure 21% or more above preoperative value
Expression	None	Grimace	Grimace/grunt
Sleepless	No	Waking at frequent intervals	Constantly awake
Total infant score			

Krechel, S.W., & Bildner, J. (1995). CRIES: A new neonatal postoperative pain management score. *Pediatric Anesthesia, 5*(1), 53.

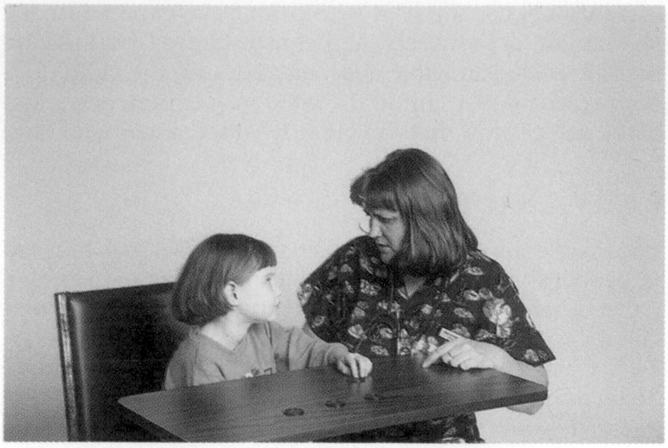

FIGURE 38.1 The child points to the poker chip indicating the degree of pain she is experiencing.

Oucher Pain Rating Scale

The Oucher (Beyer et al., 1992) scale consists of six photographs of children's faces representing "no hurt" to "biggest hurt you could ever have." Also included is a vertical scale with numbers from 0 to 100. To use the photograph portion, point to each photograph and explain what each means: the first photograph from the bottom (0) is "no hurt"; the next (photograph 2) means "a little hurt"; the next (photograph 3) means "a little more hurt"; the next (photograph 4) means "even more hurt"; the next (photograph 5) is "pretty much or a lot of hurt"; and the top photograph (photograph 6) is the "biggest hurt you could ever have."

To use the scale portion, point to each section of the scale and explain what it means: 0 means "no hurt"; 1 to 29 means "a little hurt"; 30 to 69 means "middle hurt"; 70 to 99 means "big hurt"; and 100 means "the biggest hurt you could ever have." Ask the child to point to the section of the scale that represents his or her level of hurt. Children as young as 3 can use the tool by pointing to the photograph that best describes their level of pain. If the child can count to 100 by ones and understands the concept of increasing value, the numbered scale can be used. The Oucher scale has Caucasian, African-American, and Hispanic-American versions. Allow children to select the version they want to use or present the version that most closely matches the cultural characteristics of the child.

Numerical or Visual Analog Scale

A numerical or visual analog scale (Fig. 38-3) uses a line with end points marked "0 = no pain" on the left and "10 = worst pain" on the right. Divisions along the line are marked in units from 1 to 9. Explain to children that the left end of the line (the 0) means a person feels no pain. At the other end is a 10, which means a person feels the worst pain possible. The numbers 1 to 9 in the middle are for "a little pain" to "a lot of pain." Ask children to choose a number that best describes their pain. As soon as they can count and have a concept of numbers, children can use a numerical scale. Be certain to show school-age children the scale; don't just say score your pain from 0 to 10. Until children reach late adolescence, they use concrete thought processes and may need the help of seeing the line to rate their pain accurately.

Adolescent Pediatric Pain Tool

The Adolescent Pediatric Pain Tool (APPT) combines a visual activity and a numerical scale (Savedra et al., 1992). On one half of the form (Fig. 38-4) is an outline figure showing the anterior and posterior view of a child. The child is asked to color in the areas as big or as small as the place where the pain is on the figures to show where he or she has pain. On the right side of the form, the child rates the pain in reference to "no pain," "little pain," "medium pain," "large pain," and "worst possible pain." For a third activity, children are asked to point to or circle as many words as possible on the form that describe their pain (words such as horrible, pounding, cutting, and stinging). The scale is suggested for use in children 8 through 17 years.

Many school-age children need help reading and interpreting the multitude of words that describe pain. This is a useful tool for involving parents to talk with the child about his or her pain. Reading the words together helps the child examine the type, location, and level of pain he or she is experiencing. It also helps parents to better understand what their child is experiencing.

Logs and Diaries

Having the child keep a log or diary in which he or she notes when pain occurs and self-rates the pain each time it occurs is useful for assessing a child with chronic but intermittent pain. Examining such a diary can provide direction for pain management. For example, if it shows that the child always awakens with pain in the morning, the child needs longer-acting analgesia at bedtime; if the pain is worse during weekends spent at a grandparent's

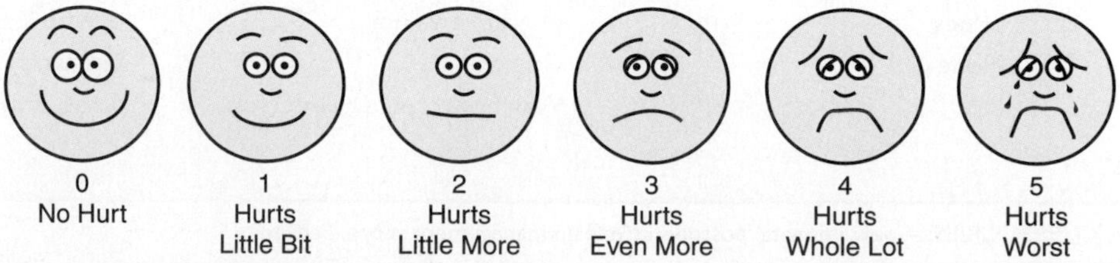
0
No Hurt
1
Hurts
Little Bit
2
Hurts
Little More
3
Hurts
Even More
4
Hurts
Whole Lot
5
Hurts
Worst

FIGURE 38.2 The FACES pain rating scale. (*Whaley and Wong's essentials of pediatric nursing*, ed. 5, 1997, p. 1216. Copyright by Mosby-Year Book, Inc. Reprinted by permission.)

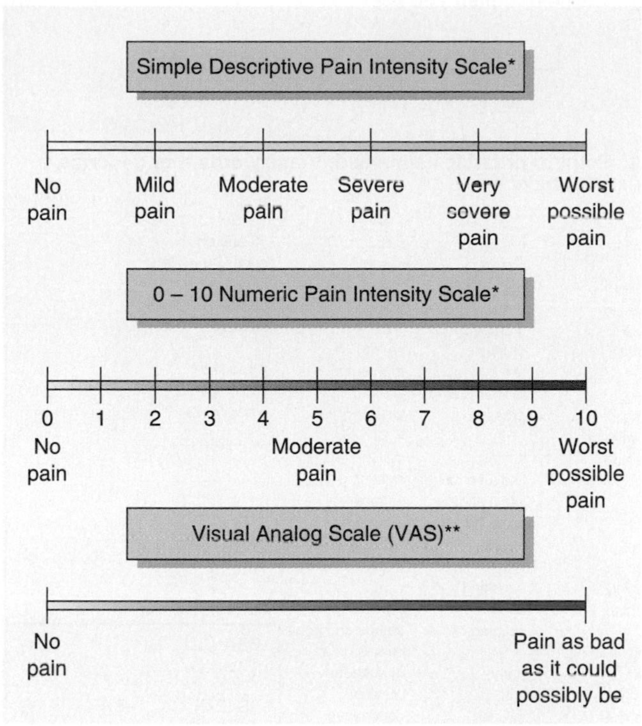

* If used as a graphic rating scale, a 10-cm baseline is recommended.

** A 10-cm baseline is recommended for VAS scales.

FIGURE 38.3 Numerical and visual analog scales.

house, then something different may be happening in that setting than at home.

WHAT IF? What if a child completely colored in the figures on the Adolescent Pediatric Pain Tool? Would you assess that the child has pain all over? Explain why or why not. If not, what might account for this?

PAIN MANAGEMENT

Pain management techniques vary greatly depending on the age of a child and the degree and type of pain present. Many health care agencies employ nurses specially prepared in pain management to serve on an interdisciplinary team of health care providers, including physicians, anesthesiologists, patient advocates, and wound therapy nurses, to plan individual pain management programs for children. In the past, children frequently were not prescribed potent analgesics because of the fear that the drugs commonly used, such as morphine, would decrease their respiratory rate to an unsafe level. Children who had adequate analgesia prescribed may not have received it because a nurse was overly concerned about causing respiratory distress. Today, it is recognized that if the dosage of an opiate such as morphine is based on the child's size, there is no more danger of respiratory depression in children than in adults. Therefore, after checking that the correct dosage has been prescribed, opiates can be given with confidence to decrease pain without untoward effects. A good rule for determining whether children need pain relief for a procedure is to remember that if the procedure would cause pain in an adult, it will also cause pain in a child. Often a combination of nonpharmacologic and pharmacologic methods is most effective (see Focus on Nursing Care Planning).

Children with chronic pain or pain not relieved with standard approaches may benefit from a referral to a pain management specialist. Relief of frequent pain episodes or prolonged pain may require intense, consistent assessment and intervention, which is difficult to achieve in an acute care setting or during infrequent office visits. Whatever tools are used for assessment, the staff should become very familiar and comfortable with their use. It is important that pain be assessed in an organized and consistent manner so relief and interventions do not vary based on the health care provider. General measures to alleviate pain that are helpful to parents as well as health care providers are summarized in the Focus on Family Empowerment box. These guidelines are based primarily on the gate control theory described below.

The gate control theory of pain (Melzack & Wall, 1965) attempts to explain how pain impulses travel between a site of injury and the brain, where the impulse is actually registered as pain. This theory envisions that gating mechanisms in the substantia gelatinosa of the dorsal horn of the spinal cord, when activated, are capable of halting an impulse at that level of the cord. This prevents the pain impulse from being received at the brain level and interpreted as pain. Gating mechanisms can be stimulated by three techniques: cutaneous stimulation, distraction, and anxiety reduction.

Cutaneous stimulation has an effect because when peripheral nerves next to an injury site are stimulated, the ability of the A-delta or C-fiber nerve fibers at the injury site to transmit pain impulses appears to decrease. Rubbing an injured part such as a stubbed toe or applying heat or cold to the site is an effective maneuver to suppress pain because it activates these nearby fibers. This technique is especially effective with children because the rubbing is not only comforting from a physical standpoint but also conveys psychological warmth.

Distraction allows the cells of the brain stem that register an impulse as pain to be preoccupied with other stimuli so the pain impulse cannot register. Having a child focus on an action or a thought is a common form of distraction (Fig. 38-5). Telling a child to say "ouch" while an injection is administered is the simplest use of this technique.

Pain impulses are perceived more quickly if anxiety is also present. Therefore, attempt to reduce the child's anxiety as much as possible. Teaching a school-age child about what to expect with a procedure is one method. As well as knowing when something is going to happen, children also should know when nothing is going to happen. Being told that a clinic visit will not involve painful procedures allows a child to relax and feel less anxiety.

The effectiveness of gate control theory techniques varies with the child's age, ability to cooperate, degree of pain, and time allowed for learning and applying the techniques. Because memory may influence the sensation of pain (expecting to have pain produces anxiety, which increases pain), these techniques are best taught to children before they begin to have pain. In all instances, children should know to use them just before or at the moment they first feel the pain. If they wait until the pain is intense, the

CODE ______________

DATE ______________

Adolescent and Pediatric Pain Tool(APPT)

1. INSTRUCTIONS

Color in the areas on these drawings to show where you have pain. Make the marks as big or as small as the place where the pain is.

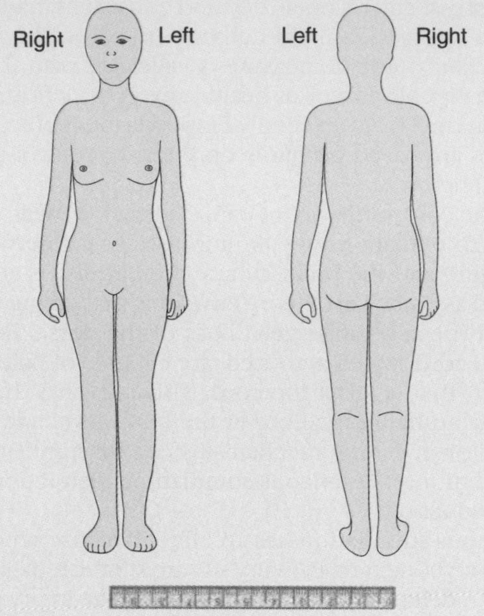

2. Place a straight, up and down mark on this line to show how much pain you have.

No pain — Little pain — Medium pain — Large pain — Worst possible pain

3. Point to or circle as many of these words that describe your pain

1	5	10	15
annoying	blistering	awful	off and on
bad	burning	deadly	once in a while
horrible	hot	dying	sneaks up
miserable	6	killing	sometimes
terrible	cramping	11	steady
uncomfortable	crushing	crying	
2	like a pinch	frightening	If you like
aching	pinching	screaming	you may add
hurting	pressure	terrifying	other words:
like an ache	7	12	______________
like a hurt	itching	dizzy	______________
sore	like a scratch	sickening	______________
3	like a sting	suffocating	
beating	scratching	13	
hitting	stinging	never goes away	
pounding	8	uncontrollable	
punching	shocking	14	
throbbing	shooting	always	
4	splitting	comes and goes	
bitting	9	comes on all of	
cutting	numb	a sudden	
like a pin	stiff	constant	
like a sharp knife	swollen	continuous	
pin like	tight	forever	
sharp			
stabbing			

For office use only

BSA: ________
IS: ________

#S (2-9) ____/37= ____ %
#A (10-12)____/11= ____ %
#E (1,13) ____/8= ____ %
#T (14,15)____/11= ____ %

Total ____/67= ____%

FIGURE 38.4 Adolescent Pediatric Pain Tool (APPT). (Savedra, M.C., Tesler, M.D., Holzemer, W.L. & Ward, J.A. [1992]. *Adolescent pediatric pain tool: User's manual.* San Francisco: University of California–San Francisco.)

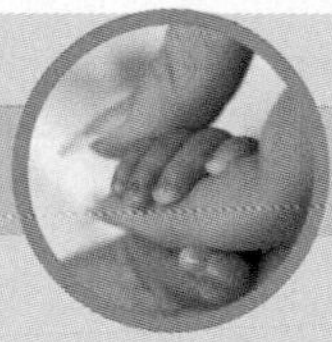

FOCUS ON *Nursing Care Planning*

THE CHILD REQUIRING PAIN MANAGEMENT

A 5-year-old is scheduled for a bone marrow aspiration to rule out the possibility of a hematologic disorder.

Assessment: 5-year-old female with a history of frequent nosebleeds, petechiae, and bruising is admitted for diagnostic testing. This is the child's first experience with hospitalization. Parents at bedside talking with child. Bone marrow aspiration scheduled in 3 hours. Child upset and crying, "Why do I have to have this test? It's gonna hurt so much."

Nursing Diagnosis: Anxiety related to fear of the unknown, lack of experience with previous testing, and anticipation of painful procedure

Outcome Identification: Child will express feelings and concerns verbally and through play.

Outcome Evaluation: Child talks openly about the test; identifies the reason for the test; exhibits age-appropriate coping behaviors; relates options for minimizing pain.

Interventions	Rationale
1. Assess the child's understanding about the reason for the bone marrow aspiration. Explore with the child her thoughts and feelings about it.	1. Assessment and exploration reveal information about the child, her knowledge base, and possible clues to her anxiety, providing a foundation on which to build future strategies and teaching.
2. Talk with the child about what she thinks the test will be like, acknowledging her anxieties and providing feedback to clarify misconceptions.	2. Talking with the child allows her to share her feelings and concerns openly and safely. Acknowledging her anxieties validates her feelings. Feedback helps correct misinformation.
3. Explain the procedure to the child at the appropriate age level. Incorporate the use of play materials and role playing.	3. Explanations that also include play aid in the child's learning and understanding. Role playing can be an effective technique for preparing children for new and unfamiliar experiences.
4. Inform the child about various techniques, both nonpharmacologic and pharmacologic, for pain control. Allow the child to practice nonpharmacologic methods. Include the parents in these practice sessions.	4. Information about pain relief measures may help to alleviate some of the child's anxiety about the hurt. Practice helps the child become proficient with the technique, thereby enhancing its effectiveness.
5. Introduce the child to the pain assessment tool to be used, such as the Poker Chip Tool or Oucher Pain Rating Scale.	5. Introducing the child to the tool prior to the onset of pain minimizes the anxiety associated with a new experience and increases the tool's usefulness and accuracy in determining the child's pain level.

Nursing Diagnosis: Pain related to invasive procedure of bone marrow aspiration

Outcome Identification: Child will verbalize that pain is within tolerable limits.

Outcome Evaluation: Child states pain is controlled; identifies pain as no higher than one with Poker Chip Tool or Oucher Pain Rating Scale; exhibits few to no nonverbal indicators of pain.

Interventions	Rationale
1. Apply EMLA cream to intended aspiration site and cover with an occlusive dressing 1 hour before scheduled procedure.	1. EMLA cream is a topical analgesic cream that acts to anesthetize the skin. An occlusive dressing enhances absorption and tissue penetration.
2. Anticipate the need for possible conscious sedation. If ordered, prepare the child for its use. Administer analgesic as ordered. Anticipate the use of intravenous route if child will receive conscious sedation.	2. A bone marrow aspiration is painful. If the child experiences pain, analgesia is necessary for relief. Conscious sedation results in a pain-free, sedated state that leaves the child's protective reflexes intact. Preparation for this technique helps to minimize the child's anxiety and fears.
3. Assess the child's pain immediately prior to the procedure using the appropriate tool.	3. Pain assessment prior to the procedure provides a baseline for evaluation.
4. Just prior to the procedure, remove the occlusive dressing and wipe away the EMLA cream. Look for reddened or blanched skin.	4. Removal prior to the procedure is necessary to cleanse skin. Reddened or blanched skin indicates that the drug has been effective.
5. Warn the child of the possible feeling of pressure with needle insertion and of sharp pain with aspiration. Encourage the child to use guided imagery.	5. Anticipatory knowledge of events and feelings helps to prepare the child and aids in coping.
6. After the procedure, assess the child's pain and compare to baseline.	6. Assessment and comparison to baseline identifies the child's level of pain postprocedure.
7. Engage the child in quiet activities for the first hour after the procedure.	7. The child is at risk for bleeding from the puncture site. Quiet activities reduce the risk for bleeding and also provide distraction.
8. Provide opportunities for therapeutic play with a doll and syringe.	8. Therapeutic play helps the child express her feelings now that the procedure is completed.

FOCUS ON FAMILY EMPOWERMENT
Relieving Pain

Q. How can we make sure that our daughter gets relief from her pain?

A. Here are some ways to offer additional pain relief:

- Administer pain medication before pain becomes intense to help prevent pain rather than just relieve it. If the child is in the hospital, inform the staff if one approach works or doesn't work.
- Let the child know it is important to try to take the pain away and that you will work with the child to relieve it. Use a positive approach: "This medicine will take away the pain," not "Let's see if this works or not."
- Never just give an analgesic. Make the child comfortable, such as straightening the sheets or offering a backrub.
- Ask your child about measures she thinks will be helpful, such as an additional pillow, the television turned on, a favorite toy nearby.
- Help your child talk about and describe the pain. This can help to make it more concrete and not as psychologically frightening.
- Relieve anxiety about other phases of life, if possible. Relaxation reduces muscle strain and tension that add to pain.
- Offer support to your child. Pain never seems as bad when a support person is present. Reassuring your child that she is loved and you will be there for her can be very comforting.

pain may be so distracting that they cannot concentrate on using the technique. Children who were able to use a distraction technique in the past but can no longer do so need to be evaluated for what is changing. Is it their ability to cope with the pain, or is the pain increasing in intensity? Contrary to common belief, familiarity with procedures does not necessarily lessen either the fear or the pain experienced (see Focus on Evidence-Based Practice).

NONPHARMACOLOGIC PAIN MANAGEMENT

The techniques described below are considered nonpharmacologic pain relief measures. In addition, they also fit under the umbrella of alternative and complementary therapies.

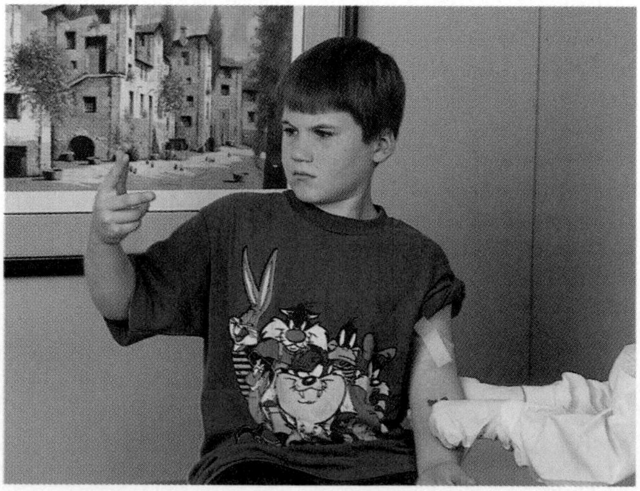

FIGURE 38.5 A child using distraction as a pain management technique.

Substitution of Meaning or Imagery

Substitution of meaning or guided imagery is a distraction technique to help the child place another meaning (a nonpainful one) on a painful procedure. This technique works well with quick, simple procedures such as venipunctures (Sparks, 2001). Children are often more adept at this than adults because their imagination is less inhibited. Success with this technique requires practice, so it has limited application in an acute care setting. A venipuncture, for example, could be viewed as a silver rocket probing the moon to transport specimens back to earth or a submarine diving under the water to escape torpedoes just in time. Be certain a child thinks of a specific image. Help him or her elaborate on the image to make it more concrete each time it is used so the child's mind stays on the image (what color is the rocket ship? Are there stripes on the sides? What does the pilot look like?).

When helping parents teach a distraction technique to their child, be certain they don't interpret distraction as just talking to the child or suggesting a video game to divert attention. Although this is distraction, simple distraction like this will allow pain to break through.

Thought Stopping

Thought stopping is a technique whereby children are taught to stop anxious thoughts by substituting a positive or relaxing thought. As with imagery, this technique also requires a great deal of practice before using it in the actual situation. Anticipatory anxiety is a negative force because it increases the pain experience during a procedure and makes the time before it full of anxiety also. For this technique, help the child to think of a set of positive factors about the approaching feared procedure. For a bone marrow aspiration, for example, this might include, "It doesn't take long; the doctor and nurse who do it are helping me; it's important to help me get better." Next, tell the

FOCUS ON EVIDENCE-BASED PRACTICE

Is Distraction an Effective Method to Reduce Injection Pain in Preschool Children? Are Nurses Who Care for Children as Knowledgeable as They Could Be About Pain Management in Children?

To answer this first question, 105 preschool children (53 girls and 52 boys) were randomly assigned to receive touch, bubble-blowing, or usual care before a DPT immunization injection. They were then asked to rate the degree of pain they experienced on an Oucher scale. Results showed that both forms of distraction (touch or bubble-blowing) significantly reduced pain perception of the injection.

To answer the second question, 274 pediatric nurses from a large hospital were administered a questionnaire asking about their knowledge and attitude toward children's pain. Nurses surveyed were able to answer 66% of the questions correctly. Those with a master's degree scored significantly higher than others. Hematology/oncology nurses and nurses from intensive care units and the emergency room also scored significantly higher than nurses from other patient care units. The researcher concluded that there are gaps in nurses' pain management knowledge regarding both pharmacologic and nonpharmacologic pain strategies.

These are important studies for nurses because they provide evidence of an area of nursing education that has gaps and also suggest an innovative, inexpensive, nonpharmacologic method of distraction (bubble-blowing) that can be effective in reducing children's perceptions of pain. Bubble-blowing is a technique that could be recommended to parents to use at home as well as on inpatient units for procedures such as venipuncture.

Sparks, L. (2001). Taking the "ouch" out of injections for children. Using distraction to decrease pain. *MCN: American Journal of Maternal Child Nursing, 26*(2), 72–78; Manworren, R.C.B. (2000). Pediatric nurses' knowledge and attitudes survey regarding pain. *Pediatric Nursing, 26*(6), 610–614.

child that whenever he or she starts to think about the impending procedure, he or she should stop whatever he or she is doing and recite the list of positive thoughts to himself or herself if others are present or out loud if the child is alone or important support people are present. The child can then return to the activity. Every time the anxious thoughts appear, however, the child should stop and recite the exercise.

Thought stopping is an effective technique because it allows children to feel in control of their thoughts, which is different from merely saying, "Don't think about it." This technique does not suppress thoughts; rather, it changes them into positive ones. The secret is for the child to use the technique every time the disturbing, anxious thought appears even if, at first, such thoughts crowd in as frequently as every few minutes.

Hypnosis

Hypnosis is not a common pain management technique with children but can be very effective when a child is properly trained in the technique. For best results, the child needs to train with a therapist before anticipated pain, so at the time of the pain, the child can use a trance-like state to avoid sensing pain (Liossi & Hatira, 1999).

Aromatherapy and Essential Oils

Aromatherapy is based on the principle that the sense of smell plays a significant role in overall health. When an essential oil is inhaled, its molecules are transported via the olfactory system to the limbic system in the brain. The brain responds to particular aromas with emotional responses. When applied externally, the oils are absorbed by the skin and then carried throughout the body (Marks, 2000). When a drop of an oil (for instance, lavender) is placed on the skin, you should be able to taste it within 15 seconds. Essential oils may be able to penetrate cell walls and transport nutrients or oxygen to the inside of cells. Jasmine and lavender are oils thought to be responsible for relieving pain.

Magnet Therapy

Magnet therapy is based on the belief that magnets can control or shift body energy lines to restore health or relieve pain. Magnets can be applied as jewelry or sewn into clothing or shoes. Copper also is believed to have pain-relieving ability and is often incorporated into rings and bracelets for this reason.

Music Therapy

Music therapy is the use of music for calming or improving well-being (Prensner et al., 2001). It can help to relieve pain because it can be so relaxing. Children may "blast" music not because they enjoy hearing it that loud but are feeling great pain and trying to use music to "blast" it out of their bodies.

Yoga and Meditation

Yoga, a term derived from the Sanskrit word for union, involves a series of exercises that were originally designed to bring people who practice it closer to God. It offers a significant variety of proven health benefits, such as increasing the efficiency of the heart, slowing the respiratory rate, improving fitness, lowering blood pressure, promoting relaxation, reducing stress, and allaying anxiety. Exercises consist of deep-breathing exercises, body postures to stretch and strengthen muscles, and meditation to focus the mind and relax the body. Yoga may be helpful in reducing pain through its ability to relax the body and possibly through the release of endorphins that may occur (Marks, 2000).

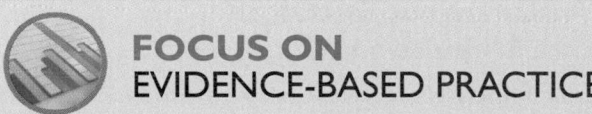

Acupuncture

Acupuncture is healing by insertion of needles into critical positions (meridian lines) in the body to achieve pain relief. Although almost painless, children can be very afraid of acupuncture at first because of the site of the needles. This level of stress can make it an unattractive option as a method of pain management for children. Children who consent to having it done, however, particularly those with chronic pain, report that the overall process is pleasant and the method offers good pain relief (Kemper et al., 2000).

Crystal or Gemstone Therapy

Some believe that gemstones or crystals have healing powers, which are magnified when they are positioned around the body. If these are being used, be careful when changing bedding or rearranging equipment in the child's room. In addition, respect the position of these stones because the child may feel they may lose their pain-relieving powers if placed in a different position (Marks, 2000).

Herbal Therapies

Parents may believe that specific herbs are helpful in relieving pain for their child and in general improving the child's health. Some examples include chamomile tea (inflammation reduction); garlic (anti-inflammatory; anticancer); ginger (nausea or vomiting reduction); goldenrod (urinary tract inflammation reduction); or St. John's wort (antidepressant) (Cirigliano, 2000). Always ask when taking health histories if a child is being given any herbs, both to be informed about common herbs and to be certain that they are complementing, not interfering with, a pain medication.

Biofeedback

Biofeedback is based on the belief that people can regulate internal events such as heart rate and pain response. A biofeedback apparatus is used to measure muscle tone or the child's ability to relax. Biofeedback can be effective with adolescents but is less effective with school-age and younger children because they resist the biofeedback information or cannot concentrate for long enough for training to be effective. Children who want to use biofeedback need to attend a number of sessions to condition themselves to regulate their pain response.

Therapeutic Touch and Massage

Therapeutic touch is the use of touch to provide comfort and relieve pain. It is based on the concept that the body contains energy fields; when plentiful they lead to health, but when they are in lesser supply ill health results. Proponents believe that it is possible to redirect the energy fields to increase the release of endorphins. Therapeutic touch may serve as a form of distraction.

Transcutaneous Electrical Nerve Stimulation

Transcutaneous electrical nerve stimulation (TENS) involves applying small electrodes to the dermatones that supply the body portion where pain is experienced. When children sense pain, they push a button on a control box, which then delivers a small electrical current to the skin. The principle underlying this technique is the same as rubbing an injured part: the current interferes with the transmission of the pain impulse across small nerve fibers.

TENS can be used to manage either acute or chronic pain. Some children (and parents) dislike TENS therapy because they are afraid or nervous about the electric current. Assure them that the current is a very mild one and will not harm the child. TENS is not recommended if the child is incontinent or has a wound that is likely to cause the electrodes to get wet.

Heat or Cold Application

Cold reduces pain by constricting capillaries and therefore reducing vessel permeability and edema at an injured site. After the first 24 hours of an injury, applying heat may be more helpful because this dilates capillaries, increases blood flow to the area, and again helps reduce edema.

✔ CHECKPOINT QUESTIONS

3. Why does a technique such as imagery work well for children to reduce the sensation of pain?
4. How do the techniques of thought stopping and substitution of meaning differ?

PHARMACOLOGIC PAIN RELIEF

Pharmacologic pain relief refers to the administration of a wide variety of analgesic medications. Many children need analgesic agents in addition to nonpharmacologic techniques for pain relief, especially for acute pain. Medications can be applied topically or given orally, intramuscularly, intravenously, or by epidural injection. As a rule, intramuscularly administered analgesia should be avoided if possible because children dislike injections. Be certain that children understand that it is acceptable to ask for medication for pain; they may not know they can unless this is stressed by health care providers (Pederson et al., 2000).

Topical Anesthetic Cream

To reduce the pain of procedures such as venipuncture, lumbar puncture, and bone marrow aspiration, a local anesthetic cream (EMLA, consisting of lidocaine and prilocaine) or a solution of lidocaine and epinephrine is available (Singer & Stark, 2001). EMLA is available by prescription from local pharmacies. Anesthetic solutions are most frequently used in the emergency department by anesthesiologists.

EMLA cream is applied to the skin and covered with an occlusive dressing, such as Tegaderm or plastic wrap. To be most effective, it must be applied at least 1 hour before an expected procedure (see Focus on Pharmacology). Parents can apply EMLA cream at home before bringing a child to a clinic visit for a procedure such as bone marrow aspiration (Fig. 38-6). Caution them not to allow the child to remove the dressing and eat the cream (it could anesthetize the gag reflex). It also is potentially dangerous if rubbed into the eyes. EMLA, the more frequently used cream, has changed procedures such as blood drawing from painful ones to procedures to which children can submit without experiencing pain. A disadvantage of EMLA cream is that a procedure must be anticipated by at least 1 hour for the medication to be effective. However, it can be applied up to 3 hours before a procedure and still be effective. A number of research studies have been conducted to evaluate its efficiency in reducing the pain of circumcision at birth, and it has been shown to be efficient and safe for this use (Joyce et al., 2001).

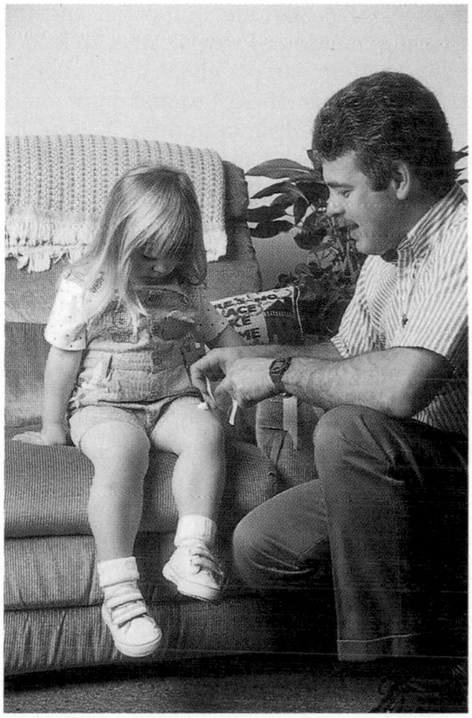

FIGURE 38.6 A father applies EMLA cream at home prior to a painful procedure.

FOCUS ON PHARMACOLOGY

EMLA Cream

Action: EMLA is a topical analgesic cream containing lidocaine and prilocaine. It acts to anesthetize skin before potentially painful procedures.

Pregnancy risk category: B

Dosage: Dollop of cream to intended skin site for at least 1 hour before procedure (2–3 hours before deeper procedures such as lumbar puncture or bone marrow aspiration)

Possible adverse reactions: Hypersensitivity

Nursing Implications

- Explain to the child that the cream will help take the hurt away.
- Apply a dollop of cream to the intended site and cover with a transparent occlusive dressing at least 1 hour before the procedure. Do not spread cream or rub it in.
- If the cream is to be applied at home, instruct the parents how to apply the cream and the occlusive dressing. Suggest that the parents use plastic wrap, such as Saran wrap, for the occlusive dressing.
- Instruct the child not to touch the dressing while it is in place. If necessary, cover the occlusive dressing with an opaque material to prevent the child from touching or playing with the dressing.
- Just before the procedure, remove the dressing and then wipe the skin to remove cream.
- Observe the skin. Look for reddened or blanched skin, which indicates that the drug has penetrated the skin.
- Do not use the drug for a child with a known history of sensitivity or allergy to local anesthetics such as lidocaine.
- The drug is not approved for use in infants under 1 month of age.

WHAT IF? What if a child is scheduled to have a bone marrow aspiration at 10 AM and, to prepare for this, you apply EMLA cream at 9 AM, but the surgeon who is going to do the aspiration arrives early? Would you ask the surgeon to wait for the hour, or explain to the child that the cream isn't going to work?

Oral Analgesia

Oral analgesia is advantageous because it is cost-effective and relatively easy to administer. Analgesia can be adequately achieved if dosing is correct. Many analgesics can be prepared as elixirs or suppositories for children unable to swallow pills.

Over-the-counter analgesics, such as acetaminophen (Tylenol), are flavored to make them taste good. Caution parents about this. Reinforce with them the need for proper storage (locked or out of the child's reach). Otherwise, children may help themselves to more when the parent leaves the room. Toxicity from too-frequent or overly large doses of acetaminophen can lead to severe liver damage in children. Never refer to medicine as "candy."

Nonsteroidal anti-inflammatory drugs (NSAIDs) are excellent for reducing the pain that accompanies inflammation in injuries such as sprained ankles or rheumatic conditions. They also are effective in reducing bone pain.

Examples of NSAIDs include ibuprofen and naproxen. Long-term administration of any NSAID can lead to severe gastric irritation. Help parents giving any analgesia around the clock for a number of days to make out a medication sheet to hang on their refrigerator door. This both reminds them when the next dose is due and alerts them not to give the drug doses too close together.

Children should not receive acetylsalicylic acid (aspirin) for routine pain relief, especially in the presence of flu-like symptoms, because there is an association between aspirin administration and the development of Reye's syndrome (see Chap. 49).

For managing severe or acute pain, such as postoperative pain or the pain of a sickle-cell crisis, opioids, such as morphine, codeine, and hydromorphone (Dilaudid), are the drugs of choice. Codeine is often given in combination with acetaminophen. Because this class of drugs is also referred to as narcotics, parents may be reluctant to give their children these medications, concerned that their child will become addicted. Acknowledge their concern and reassure them that the risk for addiction is remote. Reinforce that the main concern is supplying adequate pain relief for their child.

Intramuscular Injection

Few analgesics for children are given by intramuscular injection. This route is associated with pain on administration and also produces great fear in children. It is also associated with a number of risks, including uneven absorption, unpredictable onset of action, and nerve and tissue damage. Other routes should be used whenever possible.

> ✔ **CHECKPOINT QUESTIONS**
>
> 5. Can a child's pain management program include both nonpharmacologic and pharmacologic methods?
> 6. Why is the intramuscular route infrequently used to administer analgesia to children?

Intravenous Administration

IV administration of analgesia, the most rapid-acting route, is the method of choice in emergency situations, in the child with acute pain, and in the child requiring frequent doses of analgesia but in whom the gastrointestinal tract cannot be used. Common opioids given by this route include morphine, fentanyl and hydromorphone (Dilaudid). They can be given by bolus injection or by continuous infusion. If doses will be added periodically to an IV line, advocate for the use of an intermittent infusion device (a heparin lock) to avoid repeated venipunctures with each new dose.

If a child's pain is frequent or constant, continuous IV administration may be used. When the child is able to take medications by mouth, oral forms of analgesics should be administered. It is important that when changing from IV to oral medications, equianalgesic doses be used. As-needed (prn) dosing should be avoided because it leads to inconsistent administration.

All opioids have the potential to decrease respiratory rate. Other side effects include nausea, pruritus, vasodilatation, cough suppression, and constipation. If toxicity with opioids should occur, naloxone (Narcan) can be administered to counteract the effects.

Hydromorphone is eight to ten times stronger than morphine but very similar to morphine in action. Fentanyl has a shorter duration of action than morphine. Side effects of pruritus and vasodilatation are less. These features make it an ideal drug to use for short, painful procedures, such as debriding a burn or inserting a chest tube to relieve a pneumothorax.

Patient-Controlled Analgesia

Patient-controlled analgesia (PCA) is a form of administration that allows a child to self-administer IV boluses of medication, usually opioids, with a medication pump (see also Chap. 19). Children as young as 5 or 6 years may be able to assess when they need a bolus of medicine and press the button on the pump that will deliver the new dose to an established IV line. Parents or a nurse can administer a new dose to children younger than this. Morphine is a common analgesic used for PCA administration (Shin et al., 2001). The pump is set with a lock-out time so that after each dose the pump will not release further medication even if the button is pushed again. Thus, a child cannot overmedicate himself or herself. If the pain is constant, a continuous infusion should be used so pain relief is not lost while the child is sleeping. The pump can still be programmed for bolus dosing to cover episodes of increased pain.

Conscious Sedation

Conscious sedation refers to a state of depressed consciousness obtained by IV analgesia therapy. The technique allows the child to be both pain-free and sedated for a procedure. Unlike with general anesthesia, protective reflexes are left intact and the child can respond to instructions during the procedure. The technique is used for procedures such as extensive wound care; bone marrow aspiration, which is potentially very painful; magnetic resonance imaging, which requires a child to lie still for a long period of time; and endoscopy, which is both potentially frightening and requires the child to lie still for a period of time (Tolia et al., 2000). In many health care settings, conscious sedation is administered and monitored by nurses specially prepared in the technique (Fig. 38-7). Drugs commonly used for conscious sedation include a combination of pentobarbital sodium (Nembutal), which produces sedation, and midazolam and fentanyl, which provide relief of both anxiety and pain and depress the child's memory of the event.

Intranasal Administration

Midazolam (Versed) is a short-acting adjuvant sedative that can be administered intranasally by nasal drops or nasal spray (Hansen et al., 2001) or administered IV as described above. It may be used for sedation before surgery and procedures such as nuclear medicine scan-

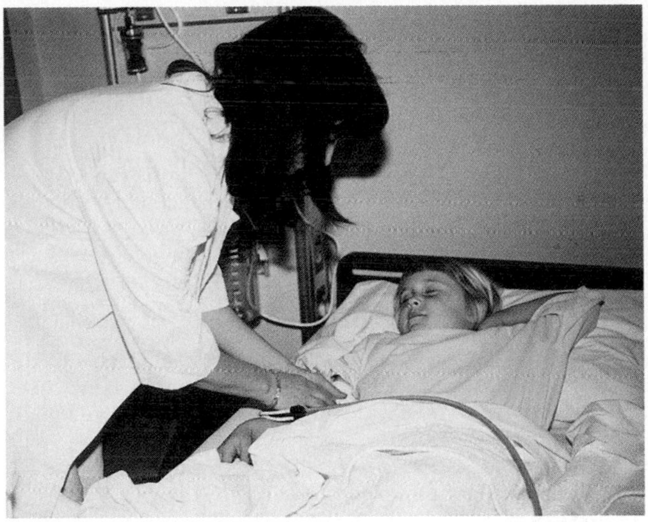

FIGURE 38.7 The nurse monitors the vital signs of a child who has received conscious sedation.

ning. Because it has a very short duration of action, it may require readministration. Because midazolam has no analgesic action, analgesia, such as with morphine, should be added if the procedure is painful.

Local Anesthesia Injection

Local anesthetics stop pain transmission by blocking nerve conduction of the impulse. Children can receive local anesthetic injections, such as lidocaine, before procedures such as bone marrow aspiration and peritoneal dialysis. For many children, the sight of the anesthetic needle is so frightening that they cannot listen to the assurance that the momentary needle stick of the anesthetic will prevent further pain. The use of EMLA cream before the injection relieves the needle stick pain and allows the anesthetic to numb the deeper tissues.

Epidural Analgesia

Epidural analgesia, injection of an analgesic agent into the epidural space just outside the spinal canal, can be used to provide analgesia to the lower body for 12 to 24 hours. An opioid, often combined with a long-acting anesthetic, is instilled continuously or administered intermittently. Opiate receptors in the spinal cord are affected directly, providing analgesia without the undesirable effects that would occur when opiate receptors in the brain are affected. Children who have spinal fusion or chest surgery, for example, may have an epidural catheter inserted in the operating room and continue to receive analgesia by this method (Aram et al., 2001). This is a very effective route of analgesia in the postoperative child in the first few days.

Some parents may be reluctant to allow this type of analgesia because they equate it with spinal anesthesia, which can be followed by severe headaches. Assure them that an epidural needle does not enter the cerebrospinal fluid, so spinal headaches are rare.

ONGOING PAIN RELIEF

Be certain children who begin a pain management program in a health care setting are provided with support and follow-up pain management. Otherwise, lack of pain relief at home can be overwhelming (Zarbock, 2000).

Oral analgesia in the home setting may be needed. Parents need instruction on dosing, administration, frequency, and expected outcomes and level of relief. Provide them with the name and number of a health care professional whom they can call about pain management. Earlier discharge and the increased use of outpatient surgery necessitate adequate pain management in the home setting (Swallow et al., 2000).

✔ CHECKPOINT QUESTIONS

7. What is the effect of conscious sedation?
8. Why are spinal headaches not associated with epidural analgesia?

KEY POINTS

- Many children and infants are undermedicated for pain relief because of common misperceptions by health care personnel, such as that infants do not feel or remember pain.
- Inviting parents and the child, if preschool age or older, to participate in assessment and pain management is an important aspect of pain therapy.
- Pain in children is best assessed by means of a standardized self-report tool such as the Poker Chip or FACES tool. Without self-report forms, both nurses and parents may underestimate children's pain. Nurses should choose tools and become very familiar with their use.
- Many children benefit from a combination of nonpharmacologic and pharmacologic methods of pain management.
- Many nonpharmacologic pain relief measures such as imagery, distraction, and TENS are based on the gate control theory of pain management.
- Few analgesics are administered intramuscularly to children. IV administration is the method of choice for the child with acute pain. Patient-controlled analgesia, commonly used to administer morphine, can be used effectively with children.
- Conscious sedation is useful for short procedures. Protective reflexes are left intact, and the child is able to respond to instructions during the procedure.

CRITICAL THINKING EXERCISES

1. Robin is the 3 year-old girl you met at the beginning of the chapter. She was given IV morphine in the emergency room an hour ago for a burn on her

hand. Her mother asks you now if Robin can have some more, not because her pain has returned, but because the mother wants to give it before the pain comes back. Is this mother's assessment of her child's pain apt to be accurate? Would this be the best intervention for Robin?

2. A 6-year-old girl is scheduled for daily debridement of a pressure ulcer, a very painful procedure. She screams before the procedure begins. What type of pain management should be used? How should the child's anxiety be addressed?
3. A fellow nurse tells you that she does not use self-report tools with children; she feels they take the place of her nursing judgment. You like to use rating scales. How would you justify your view? What types of approaches could be used to change staff behavior about pain management?
4. Examine the National Health Goals related to pain management in children. Most government-sponsored money for nursing research is allotted based on these goals. What would be a possible research topic to explore pertinent to these goals that would be fundable and would advance evidence-based practice?

REFERENCES

Aram, L., et al. (2001). Tunneled epidural catheters for prolonged analgesia in pediatric patients. *Anesthesia & Analgesia, 92*(6), 1432–1438.

Beyer, J., Denyes, M., & Villarruel, A. (1992). The creation, validation, and continuing development of the Oucher: A measure of pain intensity in children. *Journal of Pediatric Nursing, 7*(5), 335–339.

Buckle, J. (2001). The role of aromatherapy in nursing care. *Nursing Clinics of North America, 36*(1), 57–72.

Cirigliano, M. D. (2000). Herbal treatments in practice. In Schwartz, M. W. *The 5-minute pediatric consult* (2nd ed., pp. 907–915). Philadelphia: Lippincott Williams & Wilkins.

Department of Health and Human Services. (2000). *Healthy people, 2010.* Washington, D.C.: DHHS.

Hansen, S. L., et al. (2001). A retrospective study on the effectiveness of intranasal midazolam in pediatric burn patients. *Journal of Burn Care & Rehabilitation, 22*(1), 6–8.

Hennequin, M., Morin, C., & Feine, J. S. (2000). Pain expression and stimulus localisation in individuals with Down's syndrome. *Lancet, 356*(9245), 1882–1887.

Hester, N. O., & Barcus, C. S. (1986). Assessment and management of pain in children. *Pediatrics: Nursing Update, 1*(14), 2–6.

Hunfeld, J. A., et al. (2001). Chronic pain and its impact on quality of life in adolescents and their families. *Journal of Pediatric Psychology, 26*(3), 145–153.

Joyce, B. A., Keck, J. F., & Gerkensmeyer, J. (2001). Evaluation of pain management interventions for neonatal circumcision pain. *Journal of Pediatric Health Care, 15*(3), 105–114.

Kemper, K. J., et al. (2000). On pins and needles? Pediatric pain patients' experience with acupuncture. *Pediatrics, 105*(4.2), 941–947.

Krechel, S. W., & Bildner, J. (1995). CRIES: A new neonatal postoperative pain measurement score. *Paediatric Anesthesia, 5*(1), 53–57.

Liossi, C., & Hatira, P. (1999). Clinical hypnosis versus cognitive behavioral training for pain management with pediatric cancer patients. *International Journal of Clinical & Experimental Hypnosis, 47*(2), 104–116.

Manworren, R. C. B. (2000). Pediatric nurses' knowledge and attitudes survey regarding pain. *Pediatric Nursing, 26*(6), 610–614.

Marks, G. K. (2000). Alternative therapies. In Nichols, F. H., & Humenick, S. S. (Eds.). *Childbirth education: Practice, research and theory* (2d ed., pp. 376–398). Philadelphia: Saunders.

McCaffery, M., & Pasero, C. L. (1997). Pain ratings: The fifth vital sign. *American Journal of Nursing, 97*(2), 15–19.

McCaffery, M., & Pasero, C. L. (1999). How can we improve the way we perform our pain assessments to meet the needs of patients from diverse cultures? *American Journal of Nursing, 99*(8), 18–22.

Melzack, R., & Wall, P. (1965). Pain mechanisms: A new theory. *Science, 150*(4), 971–976.

Merkel, S. I., et al. (1997). The FLACC: A behavioral scale for scoring postoperative pain in young children. *Pediatric Nursing, 23*(3), 293–298.

Pederson, C., Parran, L., & Harbaugh, B. (2000). Children's perceptions of pain during 3 weeks of bone marrow transplant experience. *Journal of Pediatric Oncology Nursing, 17*(1), 22–32.

Prensner, J. D., et al. (2001). Music therapy for assistance with pain and anxiety management in burn treatment. *Journal of Burn Care & Rehabilitation, 22*(1), 83–88.

Rodriquez, E., & Jordan, R. (2002). Contemporary trends in pediatric sedation and analgesia. *Emergency Medicine Clinics of North America, 20*(1), 199–222.

Rouzan, I. A. (2001). An analysis of research and clinical practice in neonatal pain management. *Journal of the American Academy of Nurse Practitioners, 13*(2), 57–60.

Savedra, M. C., Tesler, M. D., Holzemer, W. L., & Ward, J. (1992). *Adolescent pediatric pain tool: User's manual.* San Francisco: University of California, San Francisco.

Shin, D., et al. (2001). Postoperative pain management using intravenous patient-controlled analgesia for pediatric patients. *Journal of Craniofacial Surgery, 12*(2), 129–133.

Singer, A. J., & Stark, M. J. (2001). LET verses EMLA for pretreating lacerations: A randomized trial. *Academic Emergency Medicine, 8*(3), 223–230.

Sparks, L. (2001). Taking the "ouch" out of injections for children. Using distraction to decrease pain. *MCN: American Journal of Maternal Child Nursing, 26*(2), 72–78.

Swallow, J., Briggs, M., & Semple, P. (2000). Pain at home: Children's experience of tonsillectomy. *Journal of Child Health Care, 4*(3), 93–98.

Tolia, V., et al. (2000). Sedation for pediatric endoscopic procedures. *Journal of Pediatric Gastroenterology & Nutrition, 30*(5), 477–485.

Wong, D., & Baker, C. (1996). *Reference manual for the Wong-Baker FACES pain rating scale.* Duarte, CA: CHNMC.

Zarbock, S. F. (2000). Pediatric pain assessment. *Home Care Provider, 5*(5), 181-184.

SUGGESTED READINGS

Anie, K. A., & Green, J. (2000). Psychological therapies for sickle cell disease and pain. *Cochrane Database of Systematic Reviews* (3), CD001916.

Byrne, A., Morton, J. & Salmon, P. (2001). Defending against patients' pain: A qualitative analysis of nurses' responses to children's postoperative pain. *Journal of Psychosomatic Research, 50*(2), 69-76.

Field, T. (2002). Massage therapy. *Medical Clinics of North America, 86*(1), 163-171.

Hellsten, M. B. (2000). All the king's horses and all the king's men: Pain management from hospital to home. *Journal of Pediatric Oncology Nursing, 17*(3), 149-159.

Kane, J. R. & Primomo, M. (2001). Alleviating the suffering of seriously ill children. *American Journal of Hospice & Palliative Care, 18*(3), 161-169.

Kolk, A. M., et al. (2000). Preparing children for venipuncture. *Child: Care, Health & Development, 26*(3), 251-260.

Lal, M. E., et al. (2001). Comparison of EMLA cream versus placebo in children receiving distraction therapy for venipuncture. *Acta Paediatrica, 90*(2), 154-159.

Owens, M. R., et al. (2000). A pilot program to evaluate pain assessment skills of hospice nurses. *American Journal of Hospice & Palliative Care, 17*(1), 44-48.

Sarrell, E. H., et al. (2001). Efficacy of naturopathic extracts in the management of ear pain associated with acute otitis media. *Archives of Pediatric & Adolescent Medicine, 155*(7), 796-799.

Squire, S. J., Kirchhoff, K. T., & Hissong, K. (2000). Comparing two methods of topical anesthesia used before intravenous cannulation in pediatric patients. *Journal of Pediatric Health Care, 14*(2), 68-72.

Zernikow, B., & Lindena, B. (2001). Long-acting morphine for pain control in paediatric oncology. *Medical & Pediatric Oncology, 36*(4), 451-458.

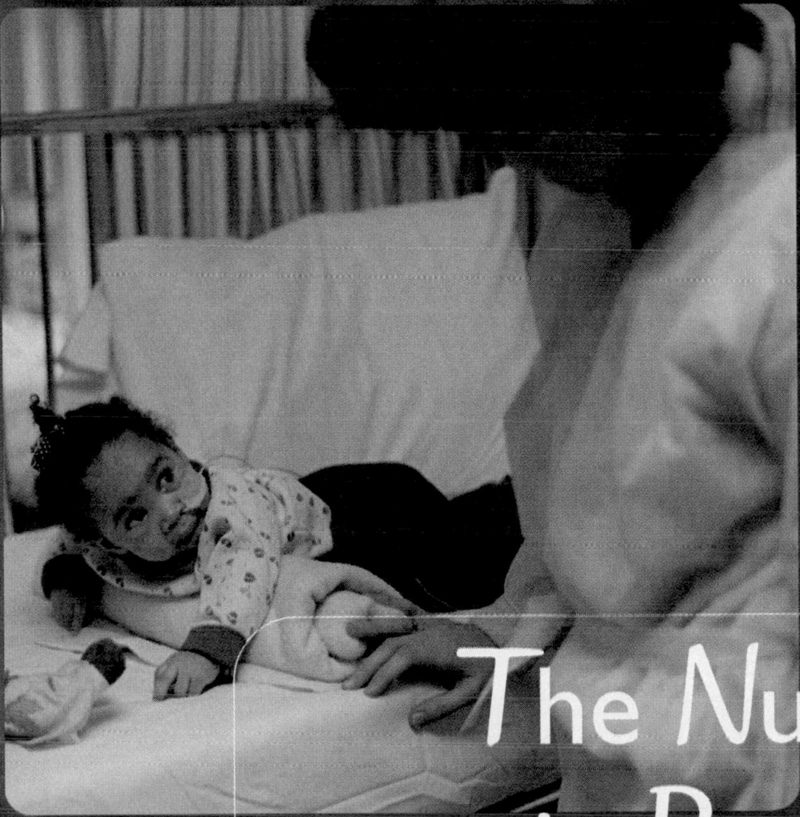

The Nursing Role in Restoring and Maintaining the Health of Children and Families With Physiologic Disorders

UNIT VIII

39

CHAPTER

Nursing Care of the Child Born With a Physical Developmental Disorder

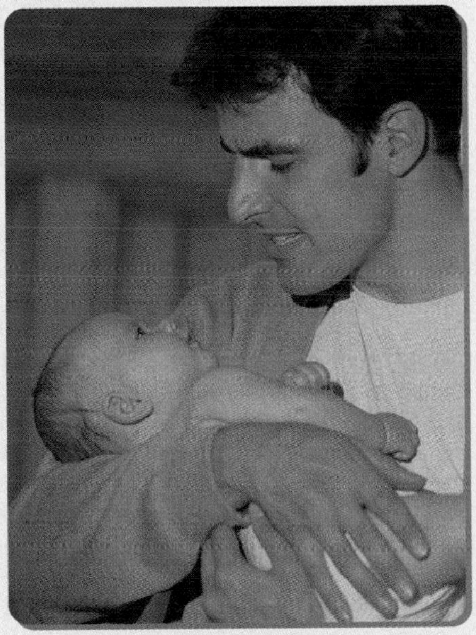

Key Terms

- ankyloglossia
- atresia
- cleft lip
- cleft palate
- developmental hip dysplasia
- fistula
- frenulum
- hydrocephalus
- meconium plug
- omphalocele
- polydactyly
- spina bifida
- stenosis
- syndactyly
- transillumination
- volvulus

Objectives

After mastering the contents of this chapter, you should be able to:

1. Describe common physical developmental birth disorders.
2. Assess a newborn who is born physically challenged.
3. Develop nursing diagnoses for the child born with a physical developmental disorder.
4. Establish outcomes to meet the needs of the child with a physical developmental disorder.
5. Plan nursing care to meet the established outcomes of care for the child born with a physical developmental disorder.
6. Carry out nursing interventions for care of children born with physical developmental disorders, such as preventing infection in the child with spina bifida.
7. Evaluate outcomes to determine achievement and effectiveness of care.
8. Identify National Health Goals related to children born physically challenged that nurses could be instrumental in helping the nation achieve.
9. Identify areas related to developmentally challenged infants that could benefit by additional nursing research or application of evidence-based practice.
10. Use critical thinking to analyze the impact of a developmentally challenged child on the family and propose ways to make care more family-centered.
11. Integrate knowledge of congenital physical anomalies with the nursing process to achieve quality maternal and child health nursing care.

Mrs. Sparrow is a 29-year-old woman whose baby was admitted to the intensive care unit because of a diaphragmatic hernia. Mrs. Sparrow is obviously upset over the diagnosis. She asks you why the intestine would have herniated into the chest. If the diaphragm is incomplete, does it mean the baby has other incomplete parts as well? Most important, could this have happened from the cough medicine she took during pregnancy? How would you answer Mrs. Sparrow? What type of advice would be most helpful to her?

Previous chapters described the importance of assessing all infants at birth. This chapter adds information about common congenital anomalies, structural disturbances, and genetic disorders that may occur in children. This information is important both as the basis for newborn assessment and as the basis for health teaching for parents.

After you've studied the chapter, answer the Critical Thinking Exercises at the end of the chapter and then access the on-line study activities (http://connection.lww.com) *to further sharpen your skills and test your knowledge.*

Few things, other than maternal hemorrhage during delivery, can change the usually expectant, joyous tone of a birthing room faster than the birth of a baby with a physical developmental disorder. Physicians or nurse-midwives, who are used to saying "perfect boy" or "beautiful girl" and holding up the infant for the parents' first glance, are suddenly without words. The nurse is in the same predicament. Words of congratulations hang unsaid in the air.

When a child is born with an apparent physical developmental defect, nurses play a major role in supporting and educating the parents, helping them to move forward from this point. Some disorders are easily repaired; others require surgery but the prognosis is good; some disorders, however, represent serious, even life-threatening problems for the infant, and long-term, financially draining responsibilities for the parents. This chapter covers the physical congenital disorders that are apparent at birth or soon after. Such disorders primarily involve the gastro-intestinal, neurologic, and skeletal systems. Congenital disorders of the cardiovascular system, which also represent life-threatening problems for the infant, are addressed in Chapter 41. National Health Goals related to children with congenital anomalies are shown in the Focus on National Health Goals box.

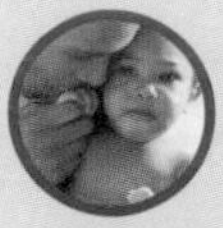

FOCUS ON NATIONAL HEALTH GOALS

Many congenital anomalies, such as cleft lip, omphalocele, and neural tube disorders, can be detected during intrauterine life. The following National Health Goals address the importance of early identification and therapy:

- Reduce the occurrence of developmental disabilities by 5%.
- Reduce the occurrence of spina bifida and other neural tube defects by 50%.
- Increase the proportion of pregnancies begun with an optimum folic acid level from a baseline of 21% to a target level of 80%.
- Increase the proportion of territories and states that have service systems for children with special health care needs to 100% from a baseline of 15% (DHHS, 2000).

Nurses can be instrumental in helping the nation achieve these goals by ensuring that women obtain prenatal care and receive comprehensive therapy after diagnosis.

Additional nursing research in this area is needed concerning what factors determine which women will continue their pregnancy after a congenital anomaly is discovered in their fetus; how far it is reasonable to ask parents to travel for follow-up care for a newborn; the measures parents feel were most helpful to them at the time of a fetal or newborn anomaly diagnosis; and the most effective way to inform all women about the importance of folic acid during pregnancy.

NURSING PROCESS OVERVIEW

For Care of the Physically Challenged Child

Assessment

Nursing assessment of the physically challenged newborn, focuses on determining the infant's immediate physiologic needs required to sustain life and the parents' immediate emotional needs to promote bonding between child and parents. Evaluate how the anomaly affects the infant's eight primary needs:

- Establishment and maintenance of adequate respiration
- Establishment of extrauterine circulation
- Establishment of body temperature control
- Ability to take in adequate nourishment
- Establishment of waste elimination
- Prevention of infection
- Development of an infant–parent bond
- Exposure to adequate stimulation

The parents' response to the diagnosis of a congenital defect must also be assessed. Anomalies that affect the child's appearance may have the most immediate effect on the parents' ability to establish a positive feeling about their child. It is important, however, not to jump to conclusions about parents' responses. Assessment of the family's verbal and nonverbal responses must be as thorough and objective as assessment of the infant's health status.

Nursing Diagnosis

Many nursing diagnoses established for children who are physically challenged address the effect on body function, including the child's primary needs, and also on family interaction. The following diagnoses are examples:

- Imbalanced nutrition, less than body requirements, related to inability to take in adequate nutrition secondary to physical defect

- Impaired physical mobility related to congenital anomaly
- Risk for impaired parenting related to birth of child with anomaly
- Anticipatory grieving (parental) related to loss of "perfect" child

Outcome Identification and Planning

Nurses play an important role in providing care to high-risk infants at birth and guarding their health until a team arrives to transport the infant to a high-risk nursery (Wright, 2000). When establishing outcomes and planning care, be certain to consider both the short- and long-term needs of the newborn and how these needs may affect the family. Also consider the family's resources, both emotional and financial, and devise a plan of care with these in mind. A parent or parents with supportive family members nearby may be able to accept the limits of a child's disorder and turn their attention to the planned treatment regimen or care priorities sooner than those without close friends or relatives to whom they can turn for comfort and support. For the latter, you may need to act not only as a source of information and support but also as a sounding board and advocate until the parents can begin to develop positive coping mechanisms that will help them come to terms with this unexpected turn of events. Referrals for support groups may also be beneficial, allowing parents to learn that they are not alone in this situation.

Implementation

Nursing interventions for the newborn who is physically challenged include immediate life-sustaining measures such as providing for adequate intake of nutrients when a disorder prevents the infant from sucking. Educating the parents regarding pre- and posttreatment procedures and encouraging them to hold, touch, and talk with their baby are especially important to the future emotional well-being of the child and family.

Parents may suffer a loss of self-esteem with the child's birth, feeling as if the baby is proof that something in the combination of their genes or the prenatal environment they provided was inadequate (see Focus on Cultural Competence). They need to hear positive comments about themselves and need to be given support until they can realize that by caring for the child they are accomplishing more, not less, than other couples.

Parents can be expected to move through the same stages of grief as those whose child has died at birth. Chapter 56 describes those stages and helpful nursing interventions in more detail.

Parents are acutely aware of what people think of their child. They watch closely how the nurse or other health care providers handle their baby to see if he or she is giving as much attention to their baby as to other babies (see Focus on Multidisciplinary Care). It is important for the baby who is born with a physical developmental disorder, and for the parents' acceptance of their child, to treat the child in the same manner as any other child—for example, rocking the baby after feeding and cooing and talking to the baby as much as with the other babies. Otherwise, parents may think that if a professional finds their child distasteful, how will they dare show the child to their

FOCUS ON CULTURAL COMPETENCE

The cause of most congenital anomalies is unknown, although they probably arise from a combination of environmental and genetic factors. Still, many people persist in believing that infants with congenital anomalies are born to people less deserving than others or to those who have sinned or have been looked on by someone with envy during pregnancy. Eating raisins during pregnancy causes brown spots and strawberries cause hemangiomas are beliefs that still proliferate.

The way that parents carry infants may contribute to the formation of hip dysplasia. Infants who are carried straddled on their parents' hips the way Latin American mothers carry their infants may have less hip dysplasia than those carried with their legs consistently brought together, such as Native American infants carried by swaddling boards.

New parents need a chance to talk about why they believe their child's disorder occurred, to relieve their guilt that they were the cause and to allow them to regain sufficient self-esteem to be able to raise a child with a congenital disorder.

Ensuring that women ingest a folic acid supplement during pregnancy has decreased the incidence of ventral and dorsal nonclosure disorders. Teaching women from all cultures that taking this important supplement before and during pregnancy is a major nursing responsibility.

FOCUS ON MULTIDISCIPLINARY CARE

Many health care providers are involved in the rehabilitation teams necessary for the comprehensive care of infants born with physical developmental disorders. Remind all care providers that consistency in care is vital. Reinforce the need for rocking, cooing, and gentle talking with the infant as appropriate. In addition, ensure that they are aware of the need for close monitoring of the child during the time that they are providing care. Also, be certain that all nursing team members can recognize danger signs in the newborn and infant, such as failure to pass meconium, bile-colored vomitus, and abdominal distention, because these are frequently associated with some of the most common anomalies.

family and friends? If a nurse is able to look past the anomaly to the whole child, however, they begin to do so, too. Through positive role modeling, you can set the stage for healthy parent–child inter-action every time you handle an infant born with a physical developmental disorder.

Parents may also need the assistance of support groups and community organizations. The following organizations may be helpful sources of support for parents:

National Easter Seal Society (*www.easter-seals.org*)
Spina Bifida Association of America (*www.sbaa.org*)
March of Dimes Birth Defects Foundation (*www.modimes.org*)
American Cleft Palate/Craniofacial Association (*www.cleftline.org*)

Outcome Evaluation

Evaluation should focus on outcomes established for the child's physical health and developmental needs, as well as the family's ability to cope with whatever special care and growth needs the child may have in the future. Be sure parents have numbers to call for questions, follow-up care, and support.

Evidence suggesting achievement of the outcomes may include:

- Child is ambulatory with walker by 2 years of age.
- Parent describes positive features of child by 2 weeks.
- Parents say they accept talipes anomaly as a correctable condition by 1 month.

RESPONSIBILITIES OF THE NURSE AT THE BIRTH OF AN INFANT BORN PHYSICALLY CHALLENGED

Most physicians and nurse-midwives believe that relating the news of congenital physical anomalies to parents is their responsibility. However, because the physician or nurse-midwife must deliver the placenta and suture the perineum if an episiotomy was used for birth, if a neonatal specialist is not immediately available, many minutes may pass before this person is ready to make a second inspection of the baby, assess the extent of the disorder from the physical symptoms present, and tell the parents about the baby's condition and prognosis. This delay affects the parents in two ways: It leaves them believing for that time either that they gave birth to a perfect child among people who do not share their enthusiasm, or they have just given birth to a child so deformed that all the professionals in the room find it too horrible to even talk to them. Because parents are aware of the atmosphere in a birthing room, the second response is by far more likely. In terms of parent–child interaction, this response is unhealthy. Parents may begin anticipatory grieving for what they believe is a severely deformed child. Even when they are told later that the defect is not extensive and is easily correctable, and that as soon as the correction is made the child will be fine, the anticipatory grief reaction may be hard to stop. They may continue to cut themselves off emotionally from the child.

For this reason, nurses need to be familiar with the most frequently encountered physical anomalies so that as the person who at that moment in the birth process is most free for patient education, they explain the problem to parents. In other instances, nurses serve as back- up informants to answer the parents' questions after being told by a primary provider that their child has been born less than perfect. It is probably best to explain to parents what the disorder consists of and what is the usual prognosis before showing the baby to them. Parents may find it hard to look at an infant with a cleft lip or palate or exposed abdominal contents and also listen. Their minds are so consumed with the visual image their eyes are sending them, so unlike the child they had imagined, that they cannot hear. For example, a typical explanation would be:

"Your baby's upper lip isn't completely formed. That's called a cleft lip. Your doctor will call one of the plastic surgeons here to look at your baby. This is a problem that can be repaired so well surgically that you'll barely be able to tell your baby had this problem. I'll bring the baby over so you can see her. Remember when you look at her that this can be repaired. She seems perfect in every other way."

These statements define and limit the problem for the parents. They also give them direction about where and how they should proceed in beginning to seek help for their child.

GASTROINTESTINAL SYSTEM DEVELOPMENTAL DISORDERS

Many of the most common congenital anomalies involve the gastrointestinal system because the gastrointestinal tract forms first as a solid tube, then undergoes canalization. If this subsequent canalization does not occur, a blockage or obstruction will occur. Other disorders of the tract, such as cleft lip and cleft palate, are the results of midline closure failure extremely early in intrauterine life. All of these disorders can interfere with or delay breast-feeding. Thus, you may need to reinforce the mother's resolve to breastfeed as appropriate to aid in her success with this method of feeding (Black & Highlander, 2000).

Ankyloglossia (Tongue-Tie)

Ankyloglossia is an abnormal restriction of the tongue caused by an abnormally tight frenulum. Normally, the **frenulum,** the membrane attached to the lower anterior tip of the tongue, is short and near the tip of the tongue. As the anterior portion of the tongue grows, the frenulum becomes located farther back. In most instances, the tongue is normal at birth; it just seems short to parents who are unaware of a newborn's appearance. This condition rarely causes speech difficulty or destructive pressure on gingival tissue. If it does, then surgical release may be performed.

Showing parents other newborns or photographs of normal tongues is helpful in convincing them that a short frenulum is normal. Explore with them why they are concerned. Is there a child in the family with a speech defect or a cleft lip and palate? Do the parents need assurance in any other way that their child is all right?

Thyroglossal Cyst

A thyroglossal cyst arises from an embryogenic fault that leaves a cyst formed at the base of the tongue that drains through a fistula open to the anterior surface of the neck. This condition may occur as a dominantly inherited trait. The cyst may involve the hyoid bone (the bone at the anterior surface of the neck at the root of the tongue) or may contain aberrant thyroid gland tissue. As the cyst fills with fluid, swelling and obstruction can lead to respiratory difficulty. If infected, the cyst appears swollen and reddened, with drainage of mucus or pus from the anterior neck (Nicollas et al., 2000).

Surgical removal of the cyst is performed to avoid future infection of the space or, if thyroid tissue is present, the possibility of carcinoma later in life (Tradati et al., 2000). Observe infants closely in the immediate postoperative period for respiratory distress, because the operative area will develop some nearby edema. Position infants on their sides so secretions drain freely from their mouths. Intravenous fluid therapy is given after surgery until the edema at the incision recedes somewhat and swallowing is safe once more (approximately 24 hours). If the mother is breast-feeding during this time, encourage her to express her milk manually to preserve her milk supply. Observe infants closely the first time they take fluid orally to be certain they do not aspirate. Be certain parents feed them before they are discharged from the surgical unit to ensure that they can see the infant is swallowing safely. This is important to their development of confidence in themselves as parents and their ability to feed the infant at home in a relaxed and comfortable way.

Cleft Lip and Palate

The fusion of the maxillary and median nasal processes normally occurs between weeks 5 and 8 of intrauterine life. In infants with **cleft lip,** the fusion fails in varying degrees, with the defect ranging from a small notch in the upper lip to a total separation of the lip and facial structure up into the floor of the nose. Upper teeth and gingiva may be absent. The nose is generally flattened because the incomplete fusion of the upper lip has allowed it to expand in a horizontal dimension (see Fig. 7-12). The deviation may be unilateral or bilateral. Cleft lip is more prevalent among boys than girls. It occurs at a rate of approximately 1 in every 700 live births (Carmin-Dillon & Low, 2000).

Cleft lip occurs as a familial tendency or most likely occurs from the transmission of multiple genes. It is twice as prevalent in the Japanese population and occurs rarely in African Americans. Formation may be aided by teratogenic factors present during weeks 5 to 8 of intrauterine life, such as a viral infection (Curtin, 2000) or deficiency of folic acid (Loffredo et al., 2001). Parents of a child with a cleft lip should be referred for genetic counseling to ensure they understand that future children are at a greater risk than usual for this problem.

The palatal process closes at approximately weeks 9 to 12 of intrauterine life. A **cleft palate,** an opening of the palate, is usually on the midline and may involve just the anterior hard palate, the posterior soft palate, or both (Fig. 39-1). It may be a separate anomaly, but as a rule it

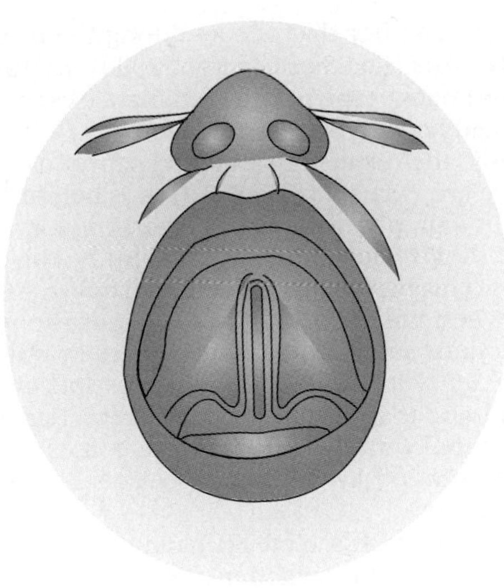

FIGURE 39.1 Appearance of a cleft palate. Both the hard and soft palate are involved.

occurs in conjunction with a cleft lip. As a single entity, it tends to occur more frequently in girls than boys. Like cleft lip, it appears to be the result of polygenic inheritance or environmental influences. In connection with cleft lip, the incidence is approximately 1 in every 1,000 births. As a single entity, it occurs in approximately 1 in every 2,000 births (Carmin-Dillon & Low, 2000).

Assessment

Cleft lip is readily apparent on inspection at birth. Cleft palate can be determined by depressing the tongue with a tongue blade. This reveals the total palate and the extent of a cleft palate. Be sure to have good lighting to visualize the palate clearly. Because cleft palate is a component of many syndromes, a child with a cleft palate must be assessed for other congenital anomalies that would suggest it is only one of a combination of problems.

Therapeutic Management

Cleft lip may be detected by sonogram while the infant is in utero. Although not usually attempted, the condition can even be repaired by fetal surgery at this early time. In most children, the disorder is not discovered until birth. A cleft lip is repaired surgically shortly after birth, sometimes at the time of the initial hospital stay and sometimes between 2 and 10 weeks. Because the deviation of the lip interferes with nutrition, infants may be a better surgical risk at birth than they are after a month or more of poor nourishment. Early repair also helps infants experience the pleasure of sucking as soon as possible. It is equally important from a psychological standpoint that these disorders be repaired early. Parents may find it extremely difficult to bond with an infant whose face is deformed in this way. This is not a sign of a "bad" parent, but reality and a problem that requires intervention. A revision of the original repair may be necessary when the child reaches 4 to 6 years of age.

The repair of cleft palate is usually postponed until the child is 6 to 18 months old to allow the anatomic change in the palate contour that occurs during the first year of life to take place (Letcher-Glembo, 2000). Repairs made before this change (the palate arch increases) may be ineffective and have to be repeated.

Currently, the results of surgical repair of cleft lip and cleft palate are excellent (Fig. 39-2). It is helpful to show parents photographs of babies with good repairs to assure them that their child's outcome can also be this successful. The older term for this condition, harelip, should not be used when talking with parents about the problem. Before modern surgical techniques were available, children were left with large lip scars, gross speech impediments, and a poor appearance after surgery. Harelip tends to be associated with these negative outcomes rather than with the current positive outlook (see Focus on Evidence-Based Practice).

Some infants with a cleft lip have an accompanying deviated nasal septum, which may need to be repaired in later years for good air exchange. Because palate repair narrows the upper dental arch or because the original cleft may have involved the dental arch, there may be less space in the upper jaw for the eruption of teeth, causing poor tooth alignment. These children need follow-up treatment by a pedodontist or a dentist skilled in children's dental problems so that as the child grows, extractions or realignment of teeth can be done as indicated.

NURSING DIAGNOSES AND RELATED INTERVENTIONS

Nursing Diagnosis: Risk for imbalanced nutrition, less than body requirements, related to feeding problems caused by cleft lip or palate

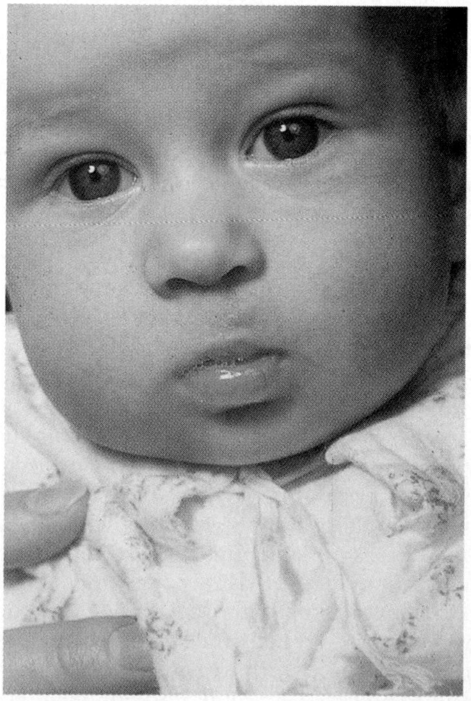

FIGURE 39.2 Infant showing surgical repair of cleft lip. Parents can be encouraged that the results of cleft lip repair are generally excellent.

FOCUS ON EVIDENCE-BASED PRACTICE

What Information Do Parents of Newborns Born With Cleft Lip or Palate Want to Know?

For this study, a questionnaire asking questions about diagnosis, prognosis, management, home care, and psychosocial issues was administered to parents whose child had been born in the last 6 years with either a cleft lip or palate or both. Parents were asked to rank how "critical" it would have been for the person first talking with them about their child's condition/care to have discussed these issues during the first day of their child's life. Parents rated feeding and learning to identify illness in their baby as their highest priorities. They also wanted to know that their baby was not in pain. Ninety-five percent of them wanted to be shown all normal aspects of their baby's exam, and 87% wanted to be assured that the child's disorder was not their fault. Hearing the health care provider use proper terminology to describe the abnormal findings was also important.

This is an important study for nurses because it documents how important talking to a health care provider about their child's disorder in the child's first day of life is to parents. Since nurses frequently are the health care providers assuming this role, the study provides direction and guidance to the important topics for discussion. Of particular importance is the finding that parents wanted to be told that their child was not in pain. This could be such a common assumption by people familiar with the disorder that it is information easy to neglect.

Young, J.L., et al. (2001). What information do parents of newborns with cleft lip, palate, or both want to know? *Cleft Palate-Craniofacial Journal, 38*(1), 55–58.

Outcome Identification: Child will demonstrate adequate nutritional intake during preoperative interval.

Outcome Evaluation: Child ingests an adequate diet of 50 kcal/lb (110 kcal/kg) in 24 hours; weight is maintained within 10% of birth weight.

Preoperative Period. Before a cleft lip or palate is repaired, feeding the infant is a problem because the infant has difficulty maintaining suction. In addition, it is important that the child does not aspirate.

It may be possible for an infant with a cleft lip to breast-feed, because the bulk of the mother's breast tends to form a seal against the defective upper lip. Although the baby needs the enjoyment of sucking, some surgeons do not want the baby to breast-feed or suck on a nipple before surgical correction of the defect to avoid any local bruising of tissue. Therefore, the best feeding method for the child with cleft lip may be to support the baby in an upright position and feed the infant gently using a commercial cleft lip nipple. A Breck feeder, an apparatus similar to a bulb syringe, or a Haberman feeder may be used (Fig. 39-3). If the surgical repair will be done immediately, the mother will be able to breast-feed as early as 7 to 10 days after surgery. Teach her how to pump or manually express breast milk to maintain a milk supply for this time. If surgery will be delayed for 1 month, she will need to decide whether she wants to continue to express milk for this long a period of time; continuing support and encouragement from the nursing staff are important.

Ensure that the infant with a cleft lip is bubbled well after feeding because of the tendency to swallow air caused by the inability to grasp a nipple or syringe edge securely with the mouth. If the cleft extends to the nares, the infant will breathe through the mouth; the infant's mucous membranes and lips can become dry. Offering small sips of fluid between feedings may help to keep the mucous membranes moist and prevent cracks and fissures that could lead to infection.

Infants with cleft palate cannot suck effectively either, because pressing their tongue or a nipple against the roof of their mouth could force milk up into their pharynx, subsequently leading to aspiration. The most successful method for feeding this infant, then, like the child with cleft lip, is to use a commercial cleft palate nipple with an extra flange of rubber to close the roof of the mouth. The nipple can be used with a plastic bottle that can be squeezed gently to increase the flow of the feeding to the infant's mouth to compensate for poor sucking. A Breck feeder may also be used.

If surgery is delayed beyond age 6 months or the time solid food is introduced, teach parents to be certain that any food offered is soft. Particles of coarse food could invade the nasopharynx and cause aspiration. Infants whose surgery is delayed to this point can be fitted with a plastic palate guard to form a synthetic palate and help prevent this.

Postoperative Period. After surgery for both cleft lip and palate, the infant is kept on NPO status for approximately 4 hours. The infant is introduced to liquids (plain water) at the end of this time. Begin the process gradually to prevent vomiting.

It is important that no tension is placed on a lip suture line. Avoiding tension helps to keep sutures from pulling apart and leaving a large scar. During this immediate postoperative period, the infant is usually fed using a specialized feeder because bottle- or breast-feeding is contraindicated.

After palate surgery, liquids are generally continued for the first 3 or 4 days, and then a soft diet is given until healing is complete. Ask the parents what fluids the child prefers so they will be available after surgery.

After a cleft palate repair, when the child begins eating soft food, he or she should not use a spoon, because the child will invariably put it against the roof of the mouth and possibly disrupt sutures. If being fed evokes an intense reaction, it is better to leave the child on a liquid diet, including milkshakes or concentrated formulas, until the sutures are removed. Be certain milk is not included in the first fluids offered because milk curds tend to adhere to the suture line. After a feeding, offer the child clear water to rinse the suture line and keep it as clean as possible.

Nursing Diagnosis: Risk for ineffective airway clearance related to oral surgery

Outcome Identification: Child's airway will remain patent.

Outcome Evaluation: Child's respiratory rate is 20 to 30 respirations per minute without retractions or obvious distress.

Because of the local edema that occurs after cleft lip or palate surgery, observe children closely in the immediate postoperative period for respiratory distress. Before surgery, the infant with a cleft lip breathed through the mouth. After surgery, the infant now has to breathe through the nose, possibly adding to respiratory difficulty. Generally, however, this is not a problem because newborns normally are strict nose-breathers.

Infants may need suction to remove mucus, blood, and unswallowed saliva. When performing suctioning, be gentle and do not touch the suture line with the catheter. After cleft lip surgery, do not lie infants on their abdomen. Doing so puts pressure on the

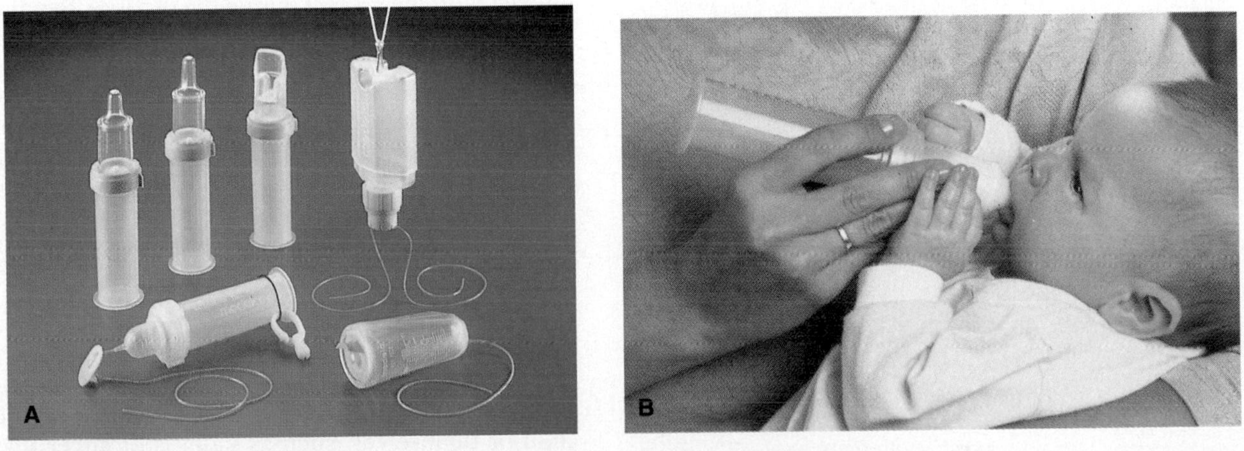

FIGURE 39.3 (A) Specialty feeding devices used for infants with cleft lip and cleft palate. (B) An infant uses a Haberman Feeder™

suture line, possibly tearing it. Position them on their side or, as soon as awake, in an infant chair.

Nursing Diagnosis: Impaired tissue integrity at incision line related to cleft lip/cleft palate surgery

Outcome Identification: Child's incision will heal without signs or symptoms of infection or trauma.

Outcome Evaluation: Incision line appears clean and intact and free of erythema or drainage during postoperative period.

After cleft lip surgery, the suture line is held in close approximation by a Logan bar (a wire bow taped to both cheeks; Fig. 39-4) or an adhesive bandage such as a Band-Aid simulating a bar that approximates the incision line but does not cover the incision. Assess the Logan bar or Band-Aid-simulated bar after each feeding or cleaning of the suture line to be certain that it is secure and continues to protect the suture line from tension. If possible, do not allow the infant to cry, because crying increases tension on the sutures. To help avoid crying, try to anticipate the infant's needs. Have formula ready to feed on demand—do not wait until after the infant is awake and crying. Help the parents use whatever measures, such as rocking, carrying, or holding, that are necessary to make the infant feel secure and comfortable. The baby also will need to be bubbled well after a feeding because there is a tendency to swallow more air than the average infant does. This tendency is due to the nonsucking method of feeding used.

Nothing hard or sharp must come in contact with a recent cleft suture line. Observe infants after palate repair carefully to be certain that they do not put toys with sharp edges into their mouths. They should not use a straw to drink, nor should they brush their own teeth—they will certainly brush the suture line accidentally. Keep elbow restraints in place as necessary so they do not put their fingers in their mouth and poke or pull at the sutures. Most children run their tongues over their sutures because of the odd feeling in the roofs of their mouths, and most children this age do not respond to a caution not to do this. Because this often occurs when children have nothing to think about, help the parents provide diversional activities such as reading or singing to them.

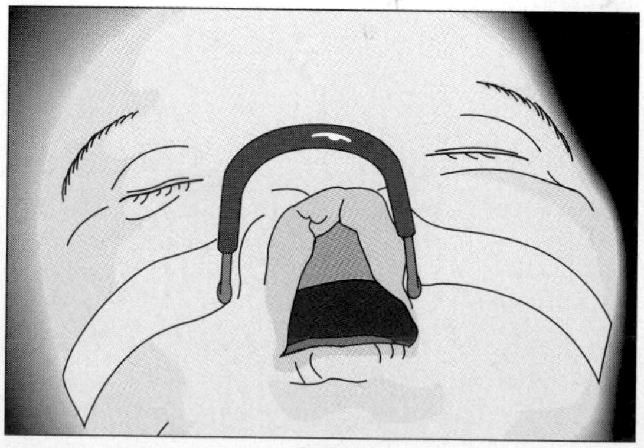

FIGURE 39.4 A Logan bar is an apparatus that may be used to protect the surgical incision for a cleft lip repair.

Acetaminophen (Tylenol) may be prescribed to keep children comfortable. Be certain parents are aware of the correct dosage and time schedule for administration. Also ensure that parents can demonstrate measures to protect the suture line at home until healing is complete.

Nursing Diagnosis: Risk for infection related to surgical incision

Outcome Identification: Infant will remain free of infection during postoperative period.

Outcome Evaluation: Infant's temperature is below 98.6°F (37°C) axillary; incision site is clean, dry, and intact without erythema or foul drainage.

Infection, and subsequent scarring, may result if crusts from serous drainage are allowed to form on a cleft lip suture line. Most surgeons prescribe cleaning the suture line with sterile water, sterile saline, or 50% hydrogen peroxide in sterile water used with sterile cotton-tipped applicators after every feeding or whenever the normal serum that forms on suture lines accumulates. Use a smooth, gentle, rolling motion to apply the solution. Do not rub, because this can loosen sutures. If hydrogen peroxide is used, it will foam as it reacts with the protein particles at the suture line. Rinse the area with sterile water afterward. Gently dry the suture line with a dry sterile cotton-tipped applicator. Remember that the infant has sutures on the inside of the lip that need the same meticulous care as those visible on the outside.

Nursing Diagnosis: Risk for impaired parenting related to the birth of an infant who is physically challenged

Outcome Identification: Parents will demonstrate acceptance of infant by 48 hours after surgery.

Outcome Evaluation: Parents state a belief in a positive outcome for child; they demonstrate positive coping behaviors, evidenced by holding and helping with infant care.

To promote bonding, parents need to hold and interact with their infant during the preoperative and postoperative period. Caution them that the incision line will appear swollen in the immediate postoperative period. Reassure them that this appearance will improve over time. As soon as the child's sutures have been removed, the infant may be bottle-fed (with an ordinary bottle) or breast-fed. Caution both the breast-feeding mother (who has been maintaining her milk supply through expression) and the formula-feeding mother that because the infant has never sucked before, he or she will need time to learn, just as a newborn does.

Notice whether the parents look at their baby's face while feeding the baby. Help them to understand that any negative feelings directed toward the child or themselves, such as sadness or anger that their baby was born this way, are normal. This does not instantly make them feel better about what has happened, but the knowledge that what they are experiencing is normal can help them begin to deal with such emotions. Many communities have support groups for parents of children born with a cleft lip or palate. Referral to these groups can be helpful.

Nursing Diagnosis: Risk for situational low self-esteem related to facial surgery

Outcome Identification: Child will demonstrate age-appropriate self-esteem.

Outcome Evaluation: Child participates in normal childhood activities that involve contact with other people; states activities he or she enjoys at health care visits; demonstrates age-appropriate developmental milestones.

If a scar remains after cleft lip surgery, the child may need some help in adjusting to it. Reinforce the child's positive attributes, stressing that the scar is only one small aspect of who he or she is. As children reach adolescence, the inheritance pattern of cleft lip may need to be reviewed so adolescents are informed of the possible risk of transmission to their own children.

Nursing Diagnosis: Risk for infection (ear) related to altered slope of eustachian tube with cleft palate surgery

Outcome Identification: Child experiences few to no middle ear infections during childhood.

Outcome Evaluation: Parents state possible signs and symptoms of ear infection and state importance of early treatment; parents list signs of hearing loss and appropriate agencies for support and guidance.

Changing the contour of the palate when it is repaired also changes the slope of the eustachian tube to the middle ear. This can lead to a high incidence of middle ear infection (otitis media) because organisms are more readily able to reach this area. Review the signs of infection (e.g., fever, pain, pulling on the ear, or discharge from the ear) with parents of children with a cleft palate. Also remind them of the importance of reporting pharyngeal infection to their primary care provider promptly so it can be treated before the infection spreads to the middle ear. Because the eustachian tube may remain partially closed owing to its changed position, serous otitis media (accumulation of fluid in the middle ear) also tends to occur more frequently in these children than in others (Letcher-Glembo, 2000). Myringotomy tubes may be inserted at the time of palate repair to drain middle ear fluid and help protect hearing (Carmin-Dillon & Low, 2000). Be certain that parents understand the need for routine screening for hearing loss during childhood, because this is a common first-noticed sign of serous otitis media.

Nursing Diagnosis: Risk for impaired verbal communication related to cleft palate

Outcome Identification: Child will communicate clearly enough to make needs known by 2 years.

Outcome Evaluation: Family members voice satisfaction with child's speech; developmental milestone of clearly articulated two-word sentences by age 2 years is met.

Infants with a cleft palate will begin to make speech sounds at the normal time (age 2 months), although their speech may be guttural and harsh. At age 9 months, when other children begin to say meaningful words ("bye-bye," "mama," "dada"), assuming the cleft palate is still unrepaired, their sounds will be unclear. Some parents try to discourage their baby from talking, thinking that if he or she does not talk until after the cleft palate repair is made, a speech impediment will not develop. Speech occurs at a specified developmental time, however, and despite the unfused palate should be encouraged at these age-appropriate times. The child with a cleft palate can enunciate vowel sounds with the most clarity, so these are the sounds a parent should encourage the child to voice. Words such as "me," "they," "no," "mama," "home," "moon," "rain," "yell," and "row" are words consisting largely of vowel sounds and thus can be enunciated by the child before the cleft palate repair.

Almost all children with cleft palates continue to have accompanying speech problems after the repair. The soft palate must function for the child to pronounce "p" and "b" sounds. If cleft palate surgery is going to be delayed much past age 2 years (as might happen if the child has other congenital anomalies, such as heart disease), a plastic prosthesis to cover the palate defect may be prescribed. This allows the child to articulate more normally.

If the child learned to speak with a speech impediment before the repair, he or she generally continues to speak this way after repair. Children do not spontaneously outgrow bad speech patterns. Speech training by a speech therapist then will be necessary. Commonly used exercises that children are asked to perform include blowing games, such as blowing a feather or a table tennis ball (a blowing motion is what is required to pronounce "p" and "b").

✔ CHECKPOINT QUESTIONS

1. In which sex is cleft lip more prevalent?
2. After a cleft palate repair, why should the use of a drinking straw be avoided?
3. Before surgery for a cleft lip, why is feeding the infant typically problematic?

Pierre Robin Syndrome

The Pierre Robin syndrome is a triad of micrognathia (small mandible), cleft palate, and glossoptosis (a tongue malpositioned downward). It is an example of cleft palate occurring as only one disorder in a syndrome of others. Children may have associated disorders of congenital glaucoma, cataracts, or cardiac disorders. They need thorough physical and genetic assessments to be certain that none of these associated disorders is present (St-Hilaire & Buchbinder, 2000).

All infants with Pierre Robin syndrome need to be observed carefully to be certain they are free of airway obstruction. They may need frequent nasopharyngeal suction to remove unswallowed saliva. Beginning at birth, children with this syndrome are apt to have episodes in which they have difficulty breathing because, due to the small jaw, their tongue is too large for their mouth. This causes it to drop backward and obstruct the airway. This is most noticeable when they are lying in a supine position. Unlike well infants, no infant with this syndrome should be placed in a supine position to sleep; they are in grave danger of anoxia if left in this position. A side-lying or prone position is recommended. Occasionally, infants have extensive airway obstruction; attaching a suture to the anterior aspect of the tongue and pulling it forward is used to provide relief. This position is maintained by attaching the suture to the mucous membrane of the lower lip (creating an artificial tongue-tied condition).

Parents need instructions to feed these infants with the same care and concern given all children with cleft palate. A gastrostomy tube or button may be inserted to relieve feeding difficulty (see Chap. 36). As the child grows older, the jaw will grow somewhat, although the mandible will always be small. Growth, coupled with a repair of the cleft palate, will decrease the respiratory problems.

Parents of the child with Pierre Robin syndrome take on a great deal of responsibility when first assuming the infant's care. Ensure that the parents have the name and number of a health care provider they can call when they have questions. Many of these parents grow exhausted during the first few weeks of the child's life, afraid they may fall soundly asleep at night and miss their child having respiratory difficulty. As their confidence grows in their ability to provide care, this problem lessens, but it may be months or even years before a high level of confidence is achieved.

Tracheoesophageal Atresia and Fistula

Between weeks 4 and 8 of intrauterine life, the laryngotracheal groove develops into the larynx, trachea, and beginning lung tissue. The esophageal lumen is formed parallel to this. A number of anomalies may occur if the trachea and esophagus are affected by some teratogen that does not allow the esophagus and trachea to separate normally.

Esophageal atresia is an obstruction of the esophagus. Often a **fistula** (opening) occurs between the closed esophagus and the trachea. The five usual types of esophageal atresia that occur are:

1. The esophagus ends in a blind pouch; there is a tracheoesophageal fistula between the distal part of the esophagus and the trachea (Fig. 39-5*A*).
2. The esophagus ends in a blind pouch; there is no connection to the trachea (see Fig. 39-5*B*).
3. A fistula is present between an otherwise normal esophagus and trachea (see Fig. 39-5*C*).
4. The esophagus ends in a blind pouch. A fistula connects the blind pouch of the proximal esophagus to the trachea (see Fig. 39-5*D*).
5. There is a blind end portion of the esophagus. Fistulas are present between both widely spaced segments of the esophagus and the trachea (see Fig. 39-5*E*).

These are serious disorders because during a feeding, milk can fill the blind esophagus and overflow into the trachea, or a fistula can allow milk to enter the trachea, resulting in aspiration. The incidence of tracheoesophageal fistula is approximately 1 in 3,000 live births (Rescorla, 2001).

Assessment

Tracheoesophageal atresia must be ruled out in any infant born to a woman with hydramnios (excessive amniotic fluid). Normally, a fetus swallows amniotic fluid during intrauterine life. However, the fetus with a tracheoesophageal atresia cannot swallow, so the amount of amniotic fluid may thus become abnormally large. Many infants are born preterm because of the accompanying hydramnios, compounding the problem with immaturity. The

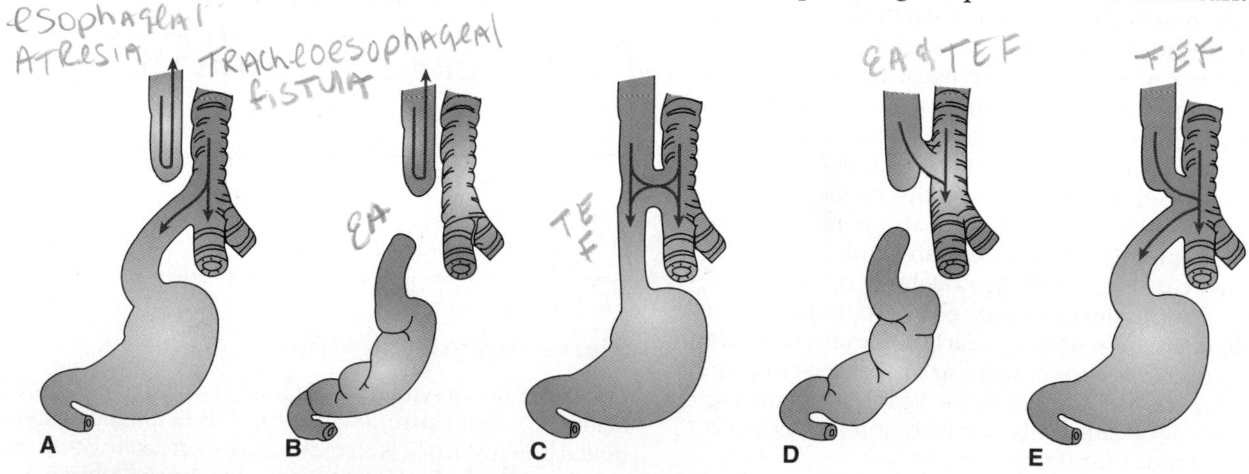

FIGURE 39.5 Esophageal atresia and tracheoesophageal fistula. (*A*) In the most frequent type of esophageal atresia, the esophagus ends in a blind pouch. The trachea communicates by a fistula with the lower esophagus and stomach (approximately 90% of infants with the defect have this type). (*B*) Both upper and lower segments end in blind pouches (5% to 8% of infants with the defect have this type). (*C*) Both upper and lower segments communicate with the trachea (2% to 3% of infants with the defect have this type). (*D*) Very rarely, the upper segment ends in a blind pouch and communicates by a fistula to the trachea, or (*E*) a fistula connects to both upper and lower segments of the esophagus.

infant needs to be examined carefully for other congenital anomalies that could have occurred from the teratogenic effect at the same week in gestation that caused the tracheoesophageal fistula, such as vertebral, anorectal, and renal disorders (VATER syndrome).

Diagnosing a tracheoesophageal fistula before an infant is fed is important. Otherwise, the infant will cough, become cyanotic, and have obvious difficulty breathing as fluid is aspirated. A newborn who has so much mucus in the mouth that he or she appears to be blowing bubbles should be suspected of having tracheoesophageal fistula. The condition can be diagnosed with certainty if a catheter cannot be passed through the infant's esophagus to the stomach and stomach contents cannot be aspirated. Use of a firm catheter is necessary because a soft one will curl in a blind-end esophagus and appear to have passed. If a radiopaque catheter is used, it can be demonstrated coiled in the blind end of the esophagus on x-ray. A flat-plate x-ray of the abdomen also may reveal a stomach distended with the air that is passing from the trachea into the esophagus and stomach. Either a barium swallow or a bronchial endoscopy examination will reveal the blind-end esophagus and fistula.

Therapeutic Management

Emergency surgery for the infant with tracheoesophageal fistula is essential to prevent the development of pneumonia from leakage of stomach secretions into the lungs or dehydration or an electrolyte imbalance from lack of oral intake. A gastrostomy may be performed (under local anesthesia) and the tube allowed to drain by gravity to keep the stomach empty of secretions and prevent reflux into the lungs. Upper right lobe pneumonia from aspiration is one of the major complications of this disorder. Thus, antibiotics also may be prescribed to prevent this complication.

Surgery consists of closing the fistula and anastomosing the esophageal segments. It may be necessary to complete the surgery in different stages and to use a portion of the colon to complete the anastomosis if the esophageal segments are far apart from each other. Observe infants closely at postoperative days 7 to 10, when sutures dissolve, because leaks occurring at anastomosis sites can occur at this time. If this occurs, fluid and air leak out into the chest cavity, and pneumothorax (collapse of the lung) can occur.

In some infants, some stenosis or stricture at the anastomosis site remains. In this case, esophageal dilatation at periodic intervals to keep the repaired esophagus fully patent may be necessary. Gastroesophageal reflux may also occur after a repair if the esophagus is left shorter than usual. This can lead to recurrent fistula formation from the presence of stomach acid in the esophagus.

The ultimate prognosis for children with this disorder will depend on the extent of the repair necessary, the condition of the child at the time of surgery, and the presence or absence of other congenital anomalies. If surgery can be performed on the child before pneumonia develops and the defect is amenable to surgical correction, the prognosis is good. However, the mortality rate for the condition remains high because of the presence of other congenital disorders and low birthweight that often accompany the tracheal abnormality.

NURSING DIAGNOSES AND RELATED INTERVENTIONS

Outcomes established for the child with tracheoesophageal fistula must be realistic in terms of the extent of the disorder, the timing of anticipated surgery, and the stage of grief or readiness for decision making and planning that the parents have reached.

Nursing Diagnosis: Risk for imbalanced nutrition, less than body requirements, related to inability for oral intake

Outcome Identification: Child will ingest adequate nutrition during course of therapy.

Outcome Evaluation: Child maintains weight within 10% of birth weight; maintains weight in same percentile on growth curve.

Before surgery, because oral fluid cannot be given until the esophagus is repaired, intravenous therapy or total parenteral nutrition can supply fluid and calories to the infant. This is continued for a time after surgery until the possibility of vomiting from the anesthetic is decreased. Then the infant may be fed orally, may be continued on total parenteral nutrition, or may be started on gastrostomy feedings, depending on whether the surgery was able to be completed in one stage or not. Early introduction of fluid may help to ensure patency of the esophagus because it helps to decrease adhesion formation from the anastomosis and allows the infant the enjoyment and practice of sucking. The formula ordered for a gastrostomy feeding should be introduced into the tube slowly and allowed to run by gravity, never by pressure, to prevent it from entering the esophagus and putting pressure on the suture line. After the feeding, the end of the tube should be elevated, covered by sterile gauze, and kept in that position. It should not be clamped. In this way, air introduced during the feeding will bubble from the tube and not enter the esophagus and pass the fresh suture line. This also helps to ensure that if the infant should vomit the feeding, the vomitus will be projected into the gastrostomy tube and not contaminate the fresh sutures. Most newborns enjoy sucking a pacifier during gastrostomy feedings for sucking pleasure. If the mother wishes to breastfeed, she can manually express breast milk for the gastrostomy feedings.

If the child is to return home to await a second-stage operation, the gastrostomy tube will be left in place for a month or two. Therefore, parents must learn how to do gastrostomy feedings. Be certain that the parents know to continue usual infant care, such as holding or talking to the infant.

Nursing Diagnosis: Risk for infection related to aspiration or seepage of stomach secretions into lungs

Outcome Identification: Child will remain free of infection during course of therapy.

Outcome Evaluation: Child's temperature remains below 98.6°F (37°C) axillary; absence of rales on auscultation.

Preoperative Care. Before surgery, position the infant upright or on the right side to prevent gastric juice from entering the lungs from the fistula. Because the infant cannot swallow mucus, frequent oropharyngeal suctioning is necessary. A catheter may be passed into the blind-end esophagus and attached to low continuous or intermittent suction to keep this segment of the esophagus from filling with fluid and causing aspiration. Irrigation of the catheter may be necessary to keep it patent, because mucus tends to dry and plug it.

If surgery will be delayed, the infant may have a cervical esophagostomy (the distal end of the blind esophagus is brought to the surface just over the sternum so that mucus can drain). Use absorbent gauze around the opening to absorb moisture and prevent excoriation of the skin. Apply a protective ointment liberally to protect skin. A consult by a wound, ostomy, and continence therapy nurse may be needed to prevent further skin irritation.

Keeping the infant under a radiant heat warmer with a high-humidity oxygen source helps to maintain body heat and liquefy bronchial secretions. Try to keep the infant from crying as much as possible. Doing so prevents air from entering the stomach from the trachea, distending the stomach, and causing vomiting with aspiration into the lungs. A pacifier may help relax the baby and also satisfy a sucking need.

Postoperative Care. After surgery, the infant will have one or two chest tubes in place because the chest cavity was entered for the repair. The posterior tube drains collecting fluid; the anterior tube allows air to leave the chest space, re-expanding the lung. Care of the child with chest tubes is discussed in Chapter 41.

In the first few days after surgery, observe the infant closely for respiratory distress. Continue to suction the child as ordered because mucus tends to accumulate in the pharynx from surgical trauma. Suctioning must be done only shallowly, however, to prevent the suction catheter from touching the suture line in the esophagus. Turn the child frequently to discourage fluid from accumulating in the lungs. Humidified oxygen helps to keep respiratory secretions moist. Keep an infant laryngoscope and endotracheal tube readily available at the bedside in case extreme edema develops, increasing the infant's risk for airway obstruction.

Nursing Diagnosis: Risk for impaired skin integrity related to gastrostomy tube insertion site

Outcome Identification: Child's skin will remain intact during course of therapy.

Outcome Evaluation: Child's skin remains clean and dry without erythema.

Gastric secretions, which are highly acidic, may leak onto the skin from the gastrostomy site, leading to skin irritation. Protect the skin by using a cream or commercial skin protector system. Consulting with a wound, ostomy, and continence therapy nurse can be helpful to reduce the possibility of further skin irritation.

Omphalocele

An **omphalocele** is a protrusion of abdominal contents through the abdominal wall at the point of the junction of the umbilical cord and abdomen (Fig. 39-6). The herniated organs are usually the intestines, but they may include stomach and liver. They are usually covered and contained by a thin transparent layer of peritoneum. At approximately weeks 6 to 8 of intrauterine life, the fetal abdominal contents are extruded from the abdomen into the base of the umbilical cord. At 7 to 10 weeks, the intestine returns to the abdomen. Omphalocele occurs when the abdominal contents fail to return to the abdomen.

Assessment

The incidence of omphalocele is as rare as 1 in 5,000 live births. Thirty percent to 60% of infants have accompanying disorders that also were caused by the teratogenic insult that prevented normal intestinal growth (Rescorla, 2001). Many omphaloceles are diagnosed by prenatal sonogram. If not, the presence of omphalocele is obvious on inspection at birth. When an omphalocele is identified in utero, cesarean birth may be performed. However, if this is the only disorder, vaginal birth is considered safe (How et al., 2000). Be sure to document the omphalocele's general appearance and its size in centimeters at birth to demonstrate its extent and appearance (Fuloria & Kreiter, 2002).

Therapeutic Management

Most infants will have immediate surgery to replace the bowel before the thin peritoneal membrane ruptures or becomes infected. If the omphalocele is large, infants may be managed by topical application of a solution such as silver sulfadiazine to prevent infection of the sac, followed by delayed surgical closure. During surgery it is often difficult to replace the entire bowel because the abdomen, which did not need to grow to accommodate the abdominal contents, is smaller than usual. If the total bowel were replaced into this small abdomen, respiratory distress might result from the pressure of the visceral bulk on the diaphragm and lungs. For this reason, after surgery,

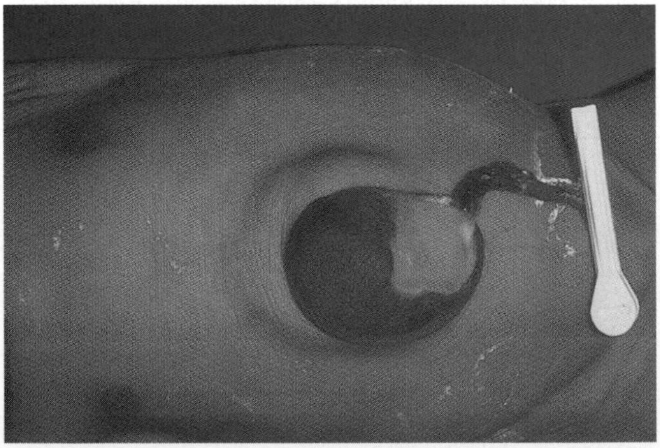

FIGURE 39.6 Omphalocele. This large example seen at birth contains intestine and liver.

the bowel may be contained by a Silastic pouch suspended over the infant's bed. Over the next 5 to 10 days, this is decreased in size as more bowel is gradually returned to the abdomen (Vanamo, 2000). During this time, the infant can be fed by total parenteral nutrition to supply nutrients and keep the bowel from filling.

NURSING DIAGNOSES AND RELATED INTERVENTIONS

Outcomes established must be realistic in terms of the extent of the disorder, the timing of anticipated surgery, and the stage of grief or readiness for decision making and planning that the parents have reached. Omphalocele is a shock to parents; it is a condition that is obviously severe and yet one that is generally unknown.

Nursing Diagnosis: Risk for infection related to exposed abdominal contents

Outcome Identification: Child remains free of infection until repair is complete.

Outcome Evaluation: Child's temperature is below 98.6°F (37°C) axillary; skin surrounding omphalocele is clean, dry, and intact, without erythema or foul drainage.

Before surgery, it is important that the lining of peritoneum covering the omphalocele not be ruptured or allowed to dry out and crack. Otherwise, infection and malrotation of the uncontained intestine can occur, complicating the surgical repair. Exposure of intestine to air also causes a rapid loss of body heat. Therefore, immediately place the baby in a warmed isolette. Do not leave infants under a radiant heat source because this will quickly dry the exposed bowel. To keep the sac moist, cover it with either sterile saline-soaked gauze or a sterile plastic bowel bag until surgery. Because of the large amount of exposed intestinal surface, the saline used must be at body temperature to prevent lowering body temperature.

The prognosis for a final successful surgical repair is good. Except for a large abdominal scar, the child who had an omphalocele will be the child originally envisioned by his or her parents. If the size of the scar is a problem for the child in later life, plastic surgery can reduce its appearance.

Nursing Diagnosis: Risk for imbalanced nutrition, less than body requirements, related to exposed abdominal contents

Outcome Identification: Child's nutritional intake will be adequate for needs during course of treatment.

Outcome Evaluation: Child's weight remains within 10% of birth weight; skin turgor is good; specific gravity of urine is 1.003 to 1.030.

A nasogastric tube is inserted to prevent intestinal distention, which would enlarge the bowel lumen, making it more difficult to replace. An infant must not be fed orally or suck on a pacifier until the bowel repair is complete. Doing so would distend the exposed bowel with food or air and make its return to the abdomen more difficult. Some infants have an accompanying **volvulus** (a twisting of the bowel causing obstruction), which is another reason to omit oral feedings. After surgery, the infant is maintained on total parenteral nutrition. Once the final stage of bowel repair is completed, a normal infant diet can be introduced gradually. Observe infants carefully for signs of obstruction (e.g., abdominal distention, constipation or diarrhea, or vomiting) when they begin oral feedings.

Infants with omphalocele will be hospitalized or receive home care for a long time (a minimum of 1 or 2 months) waiting for a second-stage or even a third-stage operation, depending on the extent of bowel involved. If the infant is hospitalized, encourage parents to visit frequently. Also be sure that the infant has age-appropriate toys available for stimulation.

Parents can become distressed that their child's operation is being done in such small stages. Offer support to help them accept that this treatment method is the best way to manage this type of intestinal disorder.

✔ CHECKPOINT QUESTIONS

4. What is the chief danger associated with a tracheoesophageal fistula?
5. What is the most important consideration in the care of the child with an omphalocele at birth?

Gastroschisis

Gastroschisis is a condition similar to omphalocele, except that the abdominal wall defect is a distance from the umbilicus and abdominal organs are not contained by peritoneal membrane but rather spill freely from the abdomen (Rescorla, 2001). A greater amount of intestinal content tends to herniate, which increases the potential for volvulus and obstruction. The surgical procedure is the same as that for omphalocele. Children with gastroschisis often have decreased bowel mobility, and even after surgical correction they may have difficulty with absorption of nutrients and passage of stool. Long-term follow-up may be necessary to ensure that nutrition and elimination are adequate (Kitchanan et al., 2000).

Intestinal Obstruction

If canalization of the intestine does not occur in utero at some point in the bowel, an **atresia** (complete closure) or **stenosis** (narrowing) of the fetal bowel can occur. The most common site is the duodenum.

Obstruction may occur because the mesentery of the bowel twists as the bowel re-enters the abdomen (after being contained in the base of the umbilical cord early in intrauterine life) or from the looseness of the intestine in the abdomen of the neonate (this continues to be a problem for the first 6 months of life). Obstruction also can occur because of thicker-than-usual meconium formation, blocking the lumen.

Assessment

Intestinal obstruction may be anticipated if the mother had hydramnios during pregnancy (amniotic fluid could not be absorbed effectively by the fetus) or if more than 30 mL of stomach contents can be aspirated from the newborn stomach by catheter and syringe at birth (fluid is not passing freely through the tract). If the obstruction is not revealed by either of these findings, then symptoms of intestinal obstruction in the neonate are the same as at any other time in life: the infant passes no meconium or may pass one stool (meconium that formed below the obstruction) and then halt; the abdomen becomes distended and tender. As the effect of the obstruction progresses, the infant will vomit. Remember that many neonates spit up feedings when burped. This rapid ejection of milk smells barely sour. True vomiting is usually sour-smelling (stomach acid has acted on it) and occurs spontaneously without coughing or back-patting.

Obstructions are rare above the ampulla of Vater, the junction of the bile duct with the duodenum, so vomitus will be bile-stained (greenish). Because meconium is black, vomitus may also be dark. Bowel sounds increase with obstruction owing to the increased peristaltic action as the intestine attempts to push stool pass the point of obstruction. Waves of peristalsis may be apparent across the abdomen. The infant may evidence pain by crying—hard, forceful, indignant crying—and by pulling the legs up against the abdomen. The child's respiratory rate will increase as the diaphragm is pushed up against the lungs and lung capacity decreases. An abdominal flat-plate x-ray or sonogram will reveal no air below the level of obstruction in the intestines. A barium swallow or barium enema x-ray film may be used to reveal the position of the obstruction (Mulberg, 2000).

WHAT IF? What if a nursing assistant tells you that a baby born with meconium staining 2 days ago is spitting up green mucus? Would it be safe to assume the nursing assistant is reporting meconium-stained mucus? Is there a possibility she is reporting a baby vomiting bile-stained emesis?

Therapeutic Management

If bowel obstruction is established, an orogastric or nasogastric tube is inserted and then attached to low suction or left open to the air to prevent further gastrointestinal distention from swallowed air (see Chap. 36). Always use low intermittent suction with decompression tubes in neonates. Pressure greater than this can irritate and ulcerate the stomach lining.

Intravenous therapy is necessary to restore fluid, and immediate surgery is scheduled because bowel obstruction is an emergency that must be treated before dehydration, electrolyte imbalance, or aspiration of vomitus occurs.

Repair of the obstruction (with the exception of meconium plug syndrome) is accomplished through an abdominal incision. The area of stenosis or atresia is removed, and the bowel is anastomosed. If the repair is anatomically difficult or the infant has other anomalies that interfere with overall health, a temporary colostomy may be constructed and the infant discharged to home care, with surgery rescheduled for age 3 to 6 months. Care of the child with a colostomy is discussed in Chapter 36. The final surgical procedure will restore the child to full health unless a large portion of the bowel had to be removed, which would have an impact on nutrient absorption.

NURSING DIAGNOSES AND RELATED INTERVENTIONS

Nursing Diagnosis: Risk for deficient fluid volume related to vomiting

Outcome Identification: Infant will demonstrate signs of a normal circulating fluid volume during course of therapy.

Outcome Evaluation: Child's skin turgor is good; pulse rate is 100 to 120 bpm; no further vomiting occurs; urine output is at least 30 mL/h.

Once an obstruction is suspected, the infant must be kept NPO to prevent the bowel from filling, thus compounding the problem, and to prevent vomiting and aspiration. Vomiting in neonates is always serious, not only because aspiration may occur but also because infants lose fluid rapidly, which results in dehydration. They also lose chloride (a component of the hydrochloric acid found in the stomach contents), leading to metabolic alkalosis. The body attempts to compensate for the loss of chloride by excreting potassium, which can cause infants to become hypokalemic quickly. Keeping the infant NPO, restoring fluid by intravenous therapy, and monitoring laboratory values for electrolyte balance until surgery can be scheduled are crucial.

Meconium Plug Syndrome

A **meconium plug** is an extremely hard portion of meconium that has completely blocked the intestinal lumen, causing bowel obstruction. The cause is unknown but probably reflects normal variations of meconium consistency. Meconium plugs usually form in the lower end of the bowel because this meconium formed early in intrauterine life and has the best chance to become dry and obstruct the bowel lumen.

Assessment

Because the obstruction is low in the intestinal tract, signs of obstruction such as abdominal distention and vomiting do not occur for at least 24 hours. Typically, the infant will be identified first as an infant who has had no meconium passage and is past 24 hours of age. A gentle rectal examination may reveal the presence of hardened stool, although the plug may be too high up in the bowel to be palpated. An x-ray or sonogram may reveal distended air-filled loops of bowel up to the point of obstruction. A barium enema study not only may reveal the level of obstruction but also may be therapeutic in loosening the plug.

Therapeutic Management

The administration of saline enemas (never use tap water in newborns because it leads to water intoxication) may cause enough peristalsis to expel the plug. Instillation of acetylcysteine (Mucomyst) with diatrizoate (Hypaque) rectally may be prescribed to dissolve the plug. Gastrografin, a highly osmotic radiographic substance, can be administered as an enema. The substance pulls fluid into the bowel because of its low osmotic pressure, allowing the stool to soften so that it will pass (Rescorla, 2001).

Once the thickened portion of meconium has been passed, the infant should have no further difficulty and, over the next several hours, may pass a great amount of stool. The infant must be observed for further passage of meconium (should occur at least once daily) over the next 3 days, however, to be certain that additional plugs do not exist farther up in the bowel. If an infant is going to be discharged before this time, instruct the parents on the importance of observing for meconium and also about telephoning their primary care provider should the infant have no further bowel movements while at home.

Occasionally, a neonate passes a small plug of hardened meconium—hard enough that it would have caused an obstruction except that it is so small—in the first 1 or 2 days of life. Be certain to record and report such a finding, because the infant will need close observation for continued defecation, the same as for the infant who actually had an obstruction, to be certain that the infant does not have another larger and truly obstructing plug higher in the bowel.

Assess the family history of a newborn who has a meconium plug for cystic fibrosis, a recessively inherited disorder, or aganglionic megacolon, a polygenic inherited disorder. Both of these disorders may present with absence of meconium. Hypothyroidism is another disorder that may present with constipation or hardened stool in newborns. Additional signs of hypothyroidism include a large protruding tongue, lethargy, or subnormal body temperature. Hypothyroid screening is done along with phenylketonuria screening. Be certain this blood test is obtained in any newborn with a meconium plug.

Meconium Ileus

Meconium ileus (obstruction of the intestinal lumen by hardened meconium) is a specific phenomenon that occurs almost exclusively in infants with cystic fibrosis (Flores-Arroyo, 2000). With cystic fibrosis, the enzyme that moistens and makes all body fluids free-flowing is absent. All body fluids are therefore thick and tenacious. Cystic fibrosis (see Chap. 40) is most often thought of as a lung disorder, because the most severe manifestation of tenacious secretions is in the lung; tenacious lung fluid leads to stasis and infection and alveolar obstruction that reduces air exchange. Intestinal and pancreatic secretions are affected also, however, and this may be signaled at birth by hardened obstructive meconium at the ileus level from lack of pancreatic trypsin secretion (meconium ileus). This will lead to the usual symptoms of bowel obstruction: no meconium passage, abdominal distention, and vomiting of bile-stained fluid. If the obstruction is too high for enemas to reduce it, the bowel must be incised and the hardened meconium surgically removed. The infant must be further assessed for cystic fibrosis in the following months.

✔ CHECKPOINT QUESTIONS

6. Why is low intermittent nasogastric suction for decompression used for the newborn?
7. Where is the most common site for intestinal obstruction in the infant?

Diaphragmatic Hernia

A diaphragmatic hernia is a protrusion of an abdominal organ (usually the stomach or intestine) through a defect in the diaphragm into the chest cavity. This usually occurs on the left side, causing cardiac displacement to the right side of the chest and collapse of the left lung. It occurs in approximately 1 in 3,000 live births. There is no difference between male and female incidence (Rescorla, 2001).

Early in intrauterine life, the chest and abdominal cavity are one; at approximately week 8 of growth, the diaphragm forms to divide them. If it does not form completely, the intestines can herniate through the diaphragm opening into the chest cavity (Fig. 39-7).

Assessment

Diaphragmatic hernia is occasionally detected in utero by sonogram (Bustillo & Kravitz, 2000). If extreme, surgery to remove the bowel from the chest can be attempted by fetoscopy while the fetus is still in utero. More often, however, the condition is diagnosed at birth. Newborns with a diaphragmatic hernia will have respiratory difficulty from the time of birth, because at least one of the lobes of their lungs is unable to expand satisfactorily (and may not have formed fully). They may also have cyanosis and intercostal

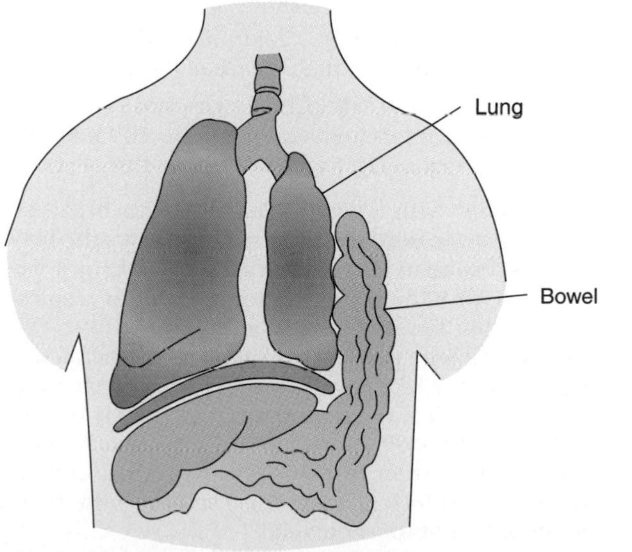

FIGURE 39.7 Diaphragmatic hernia. The bowel loop in the chest compresses the heart and lung on that side.

or subcostal retractions. Their abdomen generally appears sunken because it is not as filled as in the normal newborn. Breath sounds will be absent on the affected side of the chest cavity. These infants have a potential for developing persistent pulmonary hypertension because the blood is unable to perfuse readily through the unexpanded lung. This leads to right-to-left shunting through the foramen ovale in the heart and also causes the ductus arteriosus to remain patent. One condition, then, has led to another, and heart involvement complicates an already complicated lung picture. The mechanics of right-to-left heart shunts are further discussed in Chapter 41.

Therapeutic Management

Unfortunately, the mortality rate of children with diaphragmatic hernia ranges from 25% to 50%, with death often due to associated anomalies of the heart, lung, and intestine (Rescorla, 2000).

Treatment is emergency surgical repair of the diaphragm and replacement of the herniated intestine. Such a repair usually requires a thoracic incision and the placement of chest tubes. If the defect in the diaphragm is large, an insoluble polymer (Teflon) patch may be used in reconstruction. The repair is complicated if there is not enough room in the abdomen for the intestine to be returned. In these infants, the abdominal incision may not be closed but left open to allow the intestine to protrude abdominally. It is covered by silicone elastomer (Silastic) and left to be closed at a later date after the abdomen has grown.

Over the next week, the compressed lung (if it is normal) will gradually expand and begin to function. If it is hypoplastic from the pressure of the intestine in utero, it will not expand; it will be removed at the time of surgery.

NURSING DIAGNOSES AND RELATED INTERVENTIONS

Nursing Diagnosis: Risk for ineffective airway clearance related to displaced bowel

Outcome Identification: Child will exhibit adequate respiratory function through course of therapy.

Outcome Evaluation: Child's respiration rate is 30 to 50 breaths per minute; Po is 60 to 100 mm Hg; Pco is 30 to 35 mm Hg; lungs are clear to auscultation.

The infant with a diaphragmatic hernia breathes better with the head elevated, which allows the herniated intestine to fall back as far as possible into the abdomen, providing a maximum amount of respiratory space in the chest. Positioning the infant so the compressed lung is down also allows the unaffected lung to expand most completely. A nasogastric tube or a gastrostomy tube is inserted immediately to prevent distention of the herniated intestine, which would cause further respiratory difficulty. Be certain only low intermittent suction is used to avoid injuring the lining of the stomach.

After surgery, the infant also is kept in a semi-Fowler's position in an infant chair to keep pressure of the replaced intestine off the repaired diaphragm. Keep the infant in a warmed humidified environment to encourage lung fluid drainage. Suction as necessary. Chest physiotherapy may be ordered to ensure that lung secretions do not pool and to prevent pneumonia. Positive-pressure ventilation may be ordered to increase lung expansion, although this pressure is kept to a minimum to prevent tearing the undeveloped or previously unopened lung tissue. Maintaining arterial oxygen (Po_2) at a high level of 100 mm Hg and the Pco_2 at a low level of 30 to 35 mm Hg may help to prevent arterial vasoconstriction of the hypoplastic lung, thereby improving lung function.

Infants with diaphragmatic hernia are critically ill. They may be treated with nitric oxide or maintained on extracorporeal membrane oxygenation (ECMO; a heart–lung machine) after surgery until lung tissue is able to function (Rescorla, 2001; see Chaps. 26 and 41).

Nursing Diagnosis: Risk for imbalanced nutrition, less than body requirements, related to NPO status

Outcome Identification: Child will receive adequate nutritional intake during course of therapy.

Outcome Evaluation: Child's skin turgor is good; weight is maintained within 10% of birth weight or between a percentile curve on growth chart.

Infants diagnosed with diaphragmatic hernia are kept NPO, because filling of the intestine with food or activating peristaltic motion will further impair lung function. If the infant is fed, he or she may vomit because of twisting and obstruction of the herniated bowel.

After surgery, to prevent pressure on the suture line in the diaphragm by a full stomach and bowel, nutrition will be supplied intravenously, such as with total parenteral nutrition. When starting oral feedings, be certain to bubble the infant well after feeding to reduce the amount of swallowed air and limit bowel pressure against the diaphragm.

Umbilical Hernia

An umbilical hernia is a protrusion of a portion of the intestine through the umbilical ring, muscle, and fascia surrounding the umbilical cord. This creates a bulging protrusion under the skin at the umbilicus. It is rarely noticeable at birth while the cord is still present but becomes increasingly noticeable at health care visits during the first year.

Umbilical hernias occur most frequently in African-American children and more often in girls than in boys. The structure is generally 1 to 2 cm (½ to 1 inch) in diameter but may be as big as an orange when children cry or strain (Blanchard et al., 2000). The size of the protruding mass is not as important as the size of the fascial ring through which the intestine protrudes. If this fascial ring is less than 2 cm, closure will usually occur spontaneously and no repair of the defect will be necessary. If the defect is more than 2 cm, surgery for repair will generally be indicated to prevent intestinal obstruction or bowel strangulation. This usually is done when the child is 1 to 2 years of age.

Some parents believe that holding an umbilical hernia in place by using "belly bands" or taping a silver dollar over the area will help to reduce the hernia. These actions can actually lead to bowel strangulation and should be avoided.

Surgery is generally accomplished on an ambulatory outpatient basis. The child returns from surgery with a pressure dressing, which remains in place until the sutures are well healed. Remind parents to sponge-bathe the child until they return for a postoperative visit and the dressing is removed.

Imperforate Anus

Imperforate anus (Fig. 39-8) is stricture of the anus. In week 7 of intrauterine life, the upper bowel elongates to pouch and combine with a pouch invaginating from the perineum. These two sections of bowel meet, the membranes between them are absorbed, and the bowel is then patent to the outside. If this motion toward each other does not occur or if the membrane between the two surfaces does not dissolve, imperforate anus occurs. The defect can be relatively minor, requiring just surgical incision of the persistent membrane, or much more severe, involving sections of the bowel that are many inches apart with no anus. There may be an accompanying fistula to the bladder in boys and to the vagina in girls, further complicating a surgical repair. The problem occurs in approximately 1 in 5,000 live births, more commonly in boys than girls. Imperforate anus may occur as an additional complication of spinal cord defects, because both the external anal canal and the spinal cord arise from the same germ tissue layer (Telega, 2000).

Assessment

Inspection of the perineum may reveal no anus is present or may be unhelpful because the anus appears normal because the condition is so far inside that it is missed on simple inspection. Occasionally, the condition may be revealed because a membrane filled with black meconium can be seen protruding from the anus. A "wink" reflex (touching the skin near the rectum should make it contract) will not be present if sensory nerve endings in the rectum are not intact. If these methods fail to detect the condition, it can be discovered in a newborn by the inability to insert a rubber catheter into the rectum. No stool will be passed, and abdominal distention will become evident. An x-ray or sonogram will reveal the defect if the infant is held in a head-down position to allow swallowed air to rise to the end of the blind pouch of the bowel. This method is also helpful to estimate the distance the intestine is separated from the perineum.

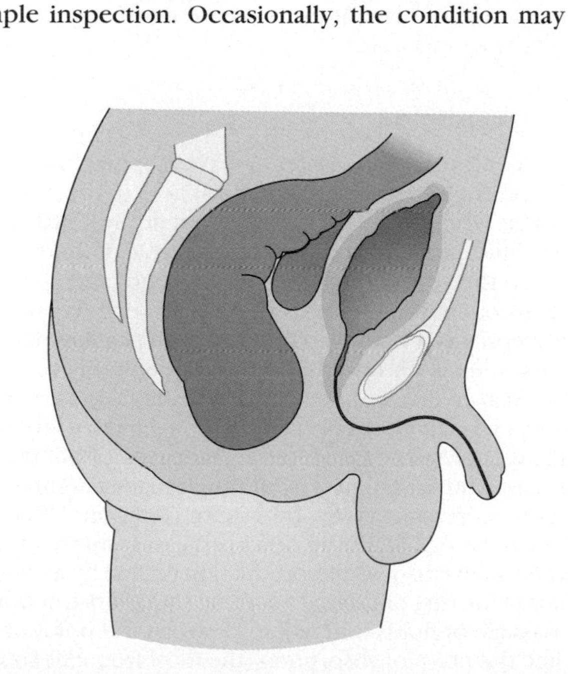

FIGURE 39.8 Imperforate anus. The lower bowel ends in a blind pouch.

Formerly, when all newborns stayed in the hospital 3 to 4 days after birth, imperforate anus was always discovered. When infants failed to pass stools after the first 24 hours, the reason was investigated. Currently, because newborns are discharged from health care facilities at 2 or 3 days or even a few hours after birth, possibly no one will notice that an infant has not passed a stool in that time. For an infant born in a birthing center or at home, follow-up must include assessment of whether the infant is defecating. Collect a urine specimen on infants with imperforate anus so it can be examined for the presence of meconium to help determine whether the child has a rectal-bladder fistula. Placing a urine collector bag over the vagina in girls may reveal a meconium-stained discharge or a rectovaginal fistula.

Therapeutic Management

The degree of difficulty in repairing an imperforate anus depends on the extent of the problem. If the rectum ends close to the perineum (below or at the level of the levator ani muscle) and the anal sphincter is formed, repair involves simple anastomosis of the separated bowel segments. The repair becomes complicated if the end of the rectum is at a distance from the perineum (above the levator ani muscle) or the anal sphincter exists only in an underdeveloped form. All repairs are complicated if a fistula to the bladder or urethra is present. If the repair will be extensive, the surgeon may create a temporary colostomy, anticipating final repair when the infant is somewhat older (6 to 12 months). For a successful repair, it is unnecessary for an internal rectal sphincter to be present as long as the subrectal muscle is judged to be intact.

NURSING DIAGNOSES AND RELATED INTERVENTIONS

Nursing Diagnosis: Imbalanced nutrition, less than body requirements, related to bowel obstruction and inability for oral intake

Outcome Identification: Child will receive adequate nutritional intake during course of therapy.

Outcome Evaluation: Child's weight remains within 10% of birth weight or is maintained on a percentile curve on a growth chart; skin turgor is good.

Preoperative Care. Before surgery, keep the infant NPO to avoid further bowel distention. A nasogastric tube attached to low intermittent suction for decompression will be inserted to relieve vomiting and prevent pressure on other abdominal organs or the diaphragm from the distended intestine. Intravenous therapy will be started to maintain fluid and electrolyte balance.

Postoperative Care. The newborn will return from surgery with a nasogastric tube still in place. When bowel sounds are present and the nasogastric tube is removed, small oral feedings, first of glucose water or formula or breast milk, are begun.

Some infants, who are scheduled for repair in a second-stage operation and who have a temporary colostomy, are not permitted high-residue foods to lessen the bulk of stools. Although this is rarely a problem with infants because their diet naturally is a low-residue one, do not assume that parents know what low residue means. Examples include rice cereal and strained fruits and vegetables. They should avoid unrefined rice and grains, vegetables with fibers, or fruits with peels.

Nursing Diagnosis: Impaired tissue integrity at rectum related to surgical incision

Outcome Identification: Surgical incision will heal without damage to sutures or new tissue by day 7.

Outcome Evaluation: Incision line is free of erythema or drainage by day 7 after surgery.

If a rectal repair was completed, remember there is a fresh suture line at the rectum. Take axillary or tympanic temperatures rather than rectal temperatures. Place a sign above the infant's crib so that anyone taking temperatures does not inadvertently take a rectal temperature. Infants should have no enemas, suppositories, or any other intrusive rectal procedures. They may be given a stool softener daily to keep the stool from becoming hard and tearing the healing suture line. Clean the suture line well after bowel movements by irrigating it with normal saline. Placing a diaper under, not on, the infant may be helpful so bowel movements can be cleansed away as soon as they occur. Do not place the infant on the abdomen because, in this position, newborns tend to pull their knees under them, causing tension in the perineal area. A side-lying position is best.

The infant may need rectal dilatation done once or twice a day for a few months after surgery to ensure proper patency of the rectal sphincter. Review this technique (gently inserting a lubricated cot-covered finger into the rectum) with the parents and document that they are able to perform this procedure before the child is discharged. Be certain they also understand the importance of the procedure. The best surgical repair could end in failure if constriction occurs because the parents do not follow up with this procedure. If infants are to be discharged with a prescription for a daily stool softener, be certain parents understand why this is also important and have a plan for remembering the correct times and dosage.

Nursing Diagnosis: Risk for impaired parenting related to difficulty in bonding with infant ill from birth

Outcome Identification: Parents will demonstrate adequate bonding behavior during course of therapy.

Outcome Evaluation: Parents hold and comfort infant; describe positive characteristics of infant.

An imperforate anus may be a difficult anomaly for a parent to accept because it deals with a body area that they may not feel comfortable discussing. If it involves a temporary (or permanent) colostomy, learning to care for their infant may be difficult. For these reasons, parents need a great deal of support following the diagnosis. If a final surgical repair is successful, they can be assured their child will have normal bowel function thereafter. If a final repair could not be surgically achieved, they have the even harder task of caring for a child with a permanent ostomy. They can be assured that children who always have ostomies accept these well as they grow older, because they have never known any other method of defecation (see Chap. 36 for a discussion of care priorities for the child with an ostomy).

✔ CHECKPOINT QUESTIONS

8. Before surgery, what is the best way to position an infant who has a diaphragmatic hernia?
9. What is the danger of taping a coin on a newborn's umbilicus to reduce an umbilical hernia?
10. What technique is important for parents to perform after surgical repair of an imperforate anus?

NERVOUS SYSTEM DEVELOPMENTAL DISORDERS

The most frequently seen developmental disorders of the nervous system at birth include abnormal accumulation of cerebrospinal fluid (hydrocephalus), which has several causes, and abnormalities associated with neural tube closure (meningocele).

Hydrocephalus

Hydrocephalus is an excess of cerebrospinal fluid (CSF) in the ventricles and subarachnoid spaces of the brain. In the infant whose cranial sutures are not firmly knitted, this excess fluid causes enlargement of the head. If fluid passes between the ventricles and the spinal cord, the disorder is called communicating hydrocephalus or extraventricular hydrocephalus. If there is a block to such passage of fluid, the disorder is an obstructive hydrocephalus or intraventricular hydrocephalus. Hydrocephalus is also classified as to whether it occurs at birth (congenital) or from an incident later in life (acquired). The cause of congenital hydrocephalus is unknown, although maternal infection such as toxoplasmosis may be a factor (Bingham, 2000).

An excess of CSF in the newborn can result from one of three main reasons: overproduction of fluid by a choroid plexus in the first or second ventricle (rare); obstruction of the passage of fluid somewhere between the point of origin and the point of absorption (the most frequent cause); or interference with the absorption of the fluid from the subarachnoid space.

Overproduction is most frequently caused by a tumor in the choroid plexus. Obstruction generally occurs as a congenital atresia, usually along the narrow aqueduct of Sylvius leading to the third ventricle. Other common sites include the foramina of Magendie and Luschka, the openings that allow fluid to leave the fourth ventricle. In an older child, infections such as meningitis or encephalitis may leave adhesions that lead to obstruction. Hemorrhage from trauma or a growing tumor also may obstruct the passage of CSF. An Arnold-Chiari deformity (elongation of the lower brain stem and displacement of the fourth ventricle into the upper cervical canal) is yet another cause. Interference with absorption can occur if a portion of the subarachnoid membrane is removed or after extensive subarachnoid hemorrhage when portions of the membrane absorption surface become obscured.

Assessment

Hydrocephalus occurs at an incidence of approximately 3 to 4 per 1,000 live births (Harvey & Lidder Jackson, 2000). When an obstruction is present, the excessive fluid accumulates and dilates the system above the point of obstruction. If the atresia is in the aqueduct of Sylvius, the first, second, and third ventricles will dilate. If it is at the exit from the fourth ventricle, all ventricles will dilate. Symptoms may develop rapidly or slowly, depending on the extent of the atresia.

Although hydrocephalus may be present prenatally and can sometimes be detected on sonogram, it generally is not evident during pregnancy or even at birth because of intrauterine pressure, but it becomes evident in the first few weeks or months of life. The fontanelles widen and appear tense, the suture lines on the skull separate, and the head diameter enlarges. As the fluid accumulation continues, the scalp becomes shiny and scalp veins become prominent. The brow bulges in a typical appearance (bossing), and the eyes become "sunset eyes" (the sclera shows above the iris because of upper lid retraction). Infants show symptoms of increased intracranial pressure, such as decreased pulse and respirations, increased temperature and blood pressure, hyperactive reflexes, strabismus, and optic atrophy. They may become either irritable or lethargic, and they fail to thrive. They may have a typical shrill, high-pitched cry (see Assessing the Infant With Hydrocephalus).

ASSESSING the Infant With Hydrocephalus

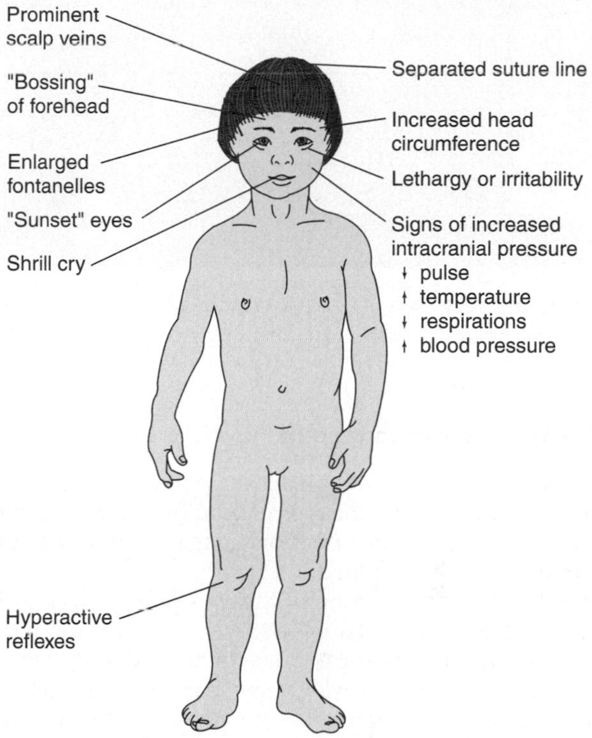

Treatment is most effective when the disorder is recognized early, because once intracranial pressure becomes so acute that brain tissue is damaged and motor or mental deterioration results, the best shunting procedure cannot replace and repair the damage to the brain cells. Assisting with detection of hydrocephalus is an important role for nurses in ambulatory child health settings. All children under age 2 years should have their head circumference recorded and plotted on an appropriate growth chart at health care visits, so a child whose head is growing abnormally can be detected.

Measure the head circumference of all infants within an hour of birth and again before discharge from the health care facility to establish a baseline. Older children who have suffered head trauma severe enough to be seen in a medical facility should have their head circumference noted at the time of the accident; if other symptoms of increased intracranial pressure appear, head circumference can be added meaningfully to the store of information available concerning the child's condition.

In addition to the general enlargement of the head, note any asymmetry that is occurring, because this may suggest the point of obstruction. A skull that is enlarging anteriorly with a shallow posterior fossa, for example, suggests that the obstruction is in the aqueduct or third ventricle.

The infant's motor function becomes impaired as the head enlarges, because of both neurologic impairment and atrophy caused by the inability to move such a heavy head. However, as long as a child has more than 1 cm of cerebral tissue present, motor function often is not impaired. Even with an extremely enlarged head, children's intelligence may remain normal, although fine motor development may be affected.

Hydrocephalus can be demonstrated by sonogram, computed tomography, and magnetic resonance imaging. A skull x-ray film will reveal the separating sutures and thinning of the skull bones. **Transillumination** (holding a bright light such as a flashlight or a specialized light [a Chun gun] against the skull with the child in a darkened room) will reveal a skull filled with fluid rather than solid brain substance (Fig. 39-9). If the hydrocephalus is a noncommunicating type, dye inserted into a ventricle through the anterior fontanelle will not appear in CSF obtained from a lumbar puncture.

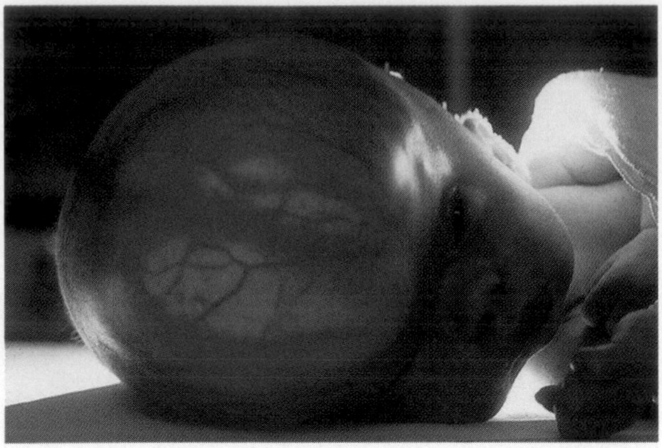

FIGURE 39.9 An infant with hydrocephalus. Transillumination reveals a fluid-filled skull.

Therapeutic Management

The treatment of hydrocephalus depends on its cause and extent. If the hydrocephaly is caused by overproduction of fluid, acetazolamide (Diamox) may be ordered to promote the excretion of fluid.

Destruction of a portion of the choroid plexus may be attempted by ventricular endoscopy, or if a tumor in that area is responsible for the overproduction of fluid, removal of the tumor should provide a solution. Hydrocephalus is usually caused by obstruction, however, so the treatment usually involves laser surgery to reopen the route of flow or bypassing the point of obstruction by shunting the fluid to another point of absorption.

As ventricular endoscopy is perfected, and obstructions in the third or fourth ventricle can be relieved, the next generation of children with hydrocephalus may not need artificial shunting (Broggi et al., 2000). Children today may still undergo a shunting procedure, and you may care for many older children or adults who have shunts in place. A shunting procedure involves threading a polyethylene catheter under the skin from the ventricles to the peritoneum (Fig. 39-10). Fluid drains and is absorbed across the peritoneal membrane and into the body circulation. This type of shunt has to be replaced as the child grows and it becomes too short. It may become enclosed in a fold of peritoneum and become obstructed.

The prognosis for infants with hydrocephalus is improving every day, as shunting and surgical procedures become more common and more effective (see Focus on Communication). The ultimate prognosis for the child depends on whether brain damage occurred before shunting or surgery and, if a shunt is in place, whether the parents are able to recognize when it needs replacing to reduce the possibility of increased intracranial pressure.

NURSING DIAGNOSES AND RELATED INTERVENTIONS

Nutrition and parent–child bonding are two major concerns for the infant with hydrocephalus. The Focus on Nursing Care Planning illustrates these and

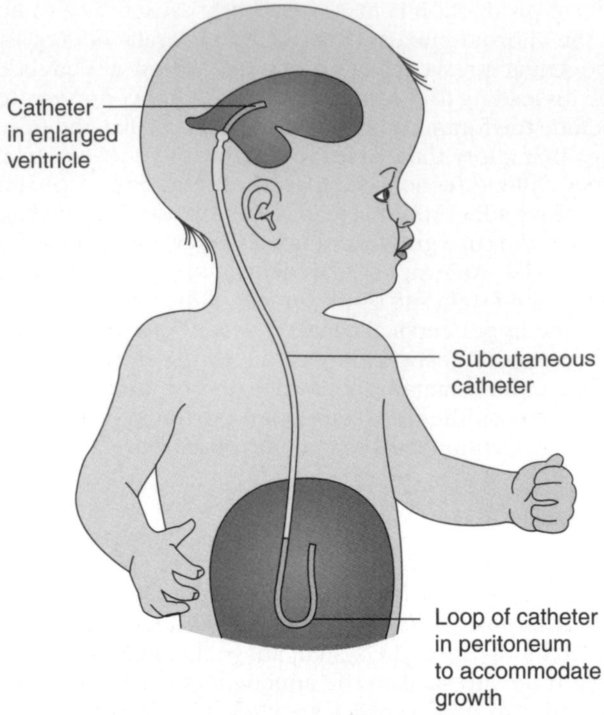

FIGURE 39.10 A ventriculoperitoneal shunt removes excessive cerebrospinal fluid from the ventricles and shunts it to the peritoneum. A one-way valve is present in the tubing behind the ear.

other concerns, as do the following important nursing diagnoses:

Nursing Diagnosis: Risk for ineffective cerebral tissue perfusion related to increased intracranial pressure

Outcome Identification: Child will remain free of signs of increased intracranial pressure during childhood.

Outcome Evaluation: Child shows no increased temperature and blood pressure, or decreased pulse rate, decreased respiratory rate, or decreased level of consciousness; PERLA; muscle strength equal and strong bilaterally; head circumference is maintained at age-appropriate level.

After a shunt is inserted, the infant's bed is usually left flat or raised only about 30 degrees so the head remains level with the body. If the child's head is raised excessively, CSF may flow too rapidly and decompression may occur too rapidly, leading to possible tearing of cerebral arteries.

A valve in the shunt is inserted to open when CSF has accumulated to the extent that pressure has increased (Drake et al., 2000). It closes when enough fluid has drained to reduce the pressure. The surgeon who performed the shunting procedure will write specific orders about how often the infant is to be turned and to what side after surgery. Often infants are not turned to lie on the side with the shunt to prevent putting pressure on the valve, which might cause it to open and rapidly decompress.

FOCUS ON COMMUNICATION

Mr. Marlow's son was born with hydrocephalus. The infant is scheduled to have a ventriculoperitoneal shunt inserted this afternoon. You talk with Mr. Marlow before surgery.

Less Effective Communication
Nurse: Is there anything I can explain to you about your son's surgery, Mr. Marlow?
Mr. Marlow: No. I just want to see him back here with a smaller head.
Nurse: The shunt won't actually make his head smaller. Its purpose is to keep his head from growing any larger.
Mr. Marlow: What is the chance that he'll die in surgery?
Nurse: All surgery has a risk, certainly, but he should do well.
Mr. Marlow: But there is a chance he'll die in surgery?
Nurse: You're worrying over nothing. Why don't you relax and go for coffee until he gets back?

More Effective Communication
Nurse: Is there anything I can explain to you about your son's surgery, Mr. Marlow?
Mr. Marlow: No. I just want to see him back here with a smaller head.
Nurse: The shunt won't actually make his head smaller. Its purpose is to keep his head from growing any larger.
Mr. Marlow: What is the chance that he'll die in surgery?
Nurse: All surgery has a risk, certainly, but he should do well.
Mr. Marlow: But there is a chance he'll die in surgery?
Nurse: You sound more worried than I'd expect. Is there something specific you're worried about?
Mr. Marlow: I'd like him to die in surgery. How are we going to take care of a child with such a deformed head?
Nurse: I can't give you a simple answer for that. Let's sit down and talk about this some more.

Because surgical procedures are so safe today and the results of surgery for newborns are so successful, it is easy to begin to think of these disorders as more inconvenient than serious: the infant, after all, will grow up with only a few minor problems. To a parent, however, the difference between a child born with one of these conditions and the "perfect" child the parent envisioned can be great. Careful listening is necessary to appreciate the extent of a parent's understanding of the problem. Handling a problem by giving quick reassurance, as in the first scenario above, can lead to missing a parent's concern. Better listening, as in the second scenario, reveals the true problem.

Assess for signs of increased intracranial pressure after surgery: tense fontanelles, increasing head circumference, irritability or lethargy, decreased level of consciousness, poor sucking, vomiting, an increase in blood pressure (difficult to measure accurately in infants unless Doppler instrumentation is used), increasing temperature, and a decrease in pulse and respiratory rates (see Chap. 49 for a neurologic assessment). Also assess for symptoms of infection (i.e., increased temperature, increased pulse rate, general malaise, and signs of meningitis such as a stiff neck and marked irritability) (see Focus on Family Empowerment). Be certain the child receives adequate pain management to minimize any upset, because crying elevates CSF pressure.

Nursing Diagnosis: Risk for imbalanced nutrition, less than body requirements, related to increased intracranial pressure

Outcome Identification: Child will ingest adequate nutritional intake after shunt placement.

Outcome Evaluation: Child's weight remains within 5th to 95th percentile on height/weight chart; no vomiting occurs.

Because an abdominal incision is involved to thread the catheter into the peritoneum, most children have a nasogastric tube placed during surgery. Keep them NPO until bowel sounds return and the tube can be removed. Introduce fluid gradually in small quantities after removal of the tube. Vomiting that results from the introduction of fluid too soon after any surgery causes increased intracranial pressure.

Like other infants, infants with hydrocephalus should be held when being fed if possible. Be certain to support their heads well when moving them to avoid strain on their neck. Hold their head with the whole palm, not just the fingertips, because the skull is thinned to some degree and could actually be punctured with a stiff, forceful touch. Urge parents to use a rocking chair with an armrest to provide support for their arm while feeding the infant. Otherwise, the infant's head can be so heavy that they may not want to spend as much time holding the infant after the feeding as they might spend otherwise. No contraindications for breast-feeding exist. Help breast-feeding mothers to find a comfortable position for feeding so that they can be successful with this.

Note how the child sucks. Increased intracranial pressure may be noted first because of poor or ineffective sucking. Vomiting after feeding, without nausea (difficult to detect in a small infant), is also a sign of increased intracranial pressure.

Observe for constipation, because straining while passing stool causes increased intracranial pressure. This is not usually a problem of infants who are totally breast- or formula-fed. However, it can be a problem when children return for shunt replacement at an older age. Urge parents to increase fluid and roughage in the diet as a preventive measure.

FOCUS ON *Nursing Care Planning*

A CHILD WITH HYDROCEPHALUS

A 3-month-old infant with hydrocephalus is admitted to an acute care facility for insertion of a ventriculo-peritoneal shunt.

Assessment: 3-month-old infant whose head circumference has continued to increase since birth. Head circumference at birth was normal (40th percentile); increased to 60th percentile at 6 weeks of age and now increased to 80th percentile. Mother reports being placed on bedrest late in pregnancy for elevated blood pressure. Gave birth vaginally without problems at 39 weeks. Newborn's Apgar score 9/10. Mother noted infant had increasing irritability and lethargy over the last few weeks.

On examination, infant's head is enlarged, with widened and tense anterior fontanelle. Scalp veins prominent. Eyes appear sunset. Parents report two episodes of forceful vomiting yesterday. "His cry is so high-pitched and shrill, and he hasn't been feeding well lately." Mother is breast-feeding. Cerebral perfusion pressure: 55 mm Hg. Blood pressure 100/40; pulse 100 bpm; respirations 16. Afebrile. Parents asking many questions about the surgery. "The doctor said he has to put in a shunt. That'll fix everything, right?"

Nursing Diagnosis: Risk for ineffective cerebral tissue perfusion related to increased intracranial pressure from hydrocephalus

Outcome Identification: Infant will exhibit signs of adequate cerebral tissue perfusion prior to surgery.

Outcome Evaluation: Infant's vital signs are within age-appropriate parameters; head circumference is maintained at current level; infant responds to auditory stimuli. CPP is above 50 mm Hg.

Interventions	Rationale
1. Assess infant's neurologic status closely, including response to sound, behavior, pupillary response, and motor and sensory function. Watch for increasing irritability or lethargy.	1. Assessment of infant's neurologic status provides a baseline for evaluating changes, allowing early identification and prompt intervention. Irritability and lethargy are signs of increasing intracranial pressure.
2. Measure and record head circumference every 4 hours. Assess anterior fontanelle for tenseness and bulging.	2. Head circumference, if increasing, or a tense, bulging fontanelle indicates accumulating cerebrospinal fluid and increased intracranial pressure.
3. Position the infant with the head of the bed elevated 15° to 30° and prevent hyperextension, flexion, or rotation of the head. Record cerebral perfusion pressure.	3. Elevating the head of the bed before surgery facilitates venous return, helping to reduce intracranial pressure. Cerebral perfusion pressure reveals extent of intracranial pressure.
4. Monitor vital signs frequently, every 1 to 2 hours.	4. Changes in vital signs, such as increased blood pressure, increased temperature, decreased respiratory rate, and decreased pulse rate, are clues to increasing intracranial pressure.
5. Administer oxygen as ordered. Have emergency equipment readily available.	5. Increased intracranial pressure can cause brain stem compression, which could result in respiratory or cardiac failure.
6. Monitor intake and output closely. Administer osmotic diuretic and corticosteroids as ordered.	6. Adequate hydration is necessary to ensure renal function. Overhydration may increase intracranial pressure. Osmotic diuretics act to pull water from the edematous tissue, decreasing intracranial pressure. Corticosteroids aid in reducing cerebral edema and thus intracranial pressure.
7. Anticipate the need for a ventricular tap should the infant's condition begin to deteriorate.	7. A ventricular tap removes excess cerebrospinal fluid, thus decreasing intracranial pressure.

(continued)

Nursing Diagnosis: Risk for imbalanced nutrition, less than body requirements, related to vomiting episodes and difficulty feeding secondary to increased intracranial pressure

Outcome Identification: Infant will exhibit signs of adequate nutrition.

Outcome Evaluation: Infant's weight remains within age-acceptable parameters; skin turgor is good; intake and output within normal limits; episodes of vomiting decrease; infant ingests adequate calories from breast-feeding.

Interventions	Rationale
1. Encourage mother to breast-feed infant if possible.	1. Breast milk is considered the optimal nutrition for an infant.
2. Assist mother with positioning the infant properly, supporting the head without flexion or hyperextension during feeding.	2. Breast-feeding promotes parent–child interaction and bonding. Proper positioning is important for latching on and also preventing neck vein compression, which could increase intracranial pressure.
3. Administer intravenous fluids as ordered. Assess intake and output closely. Check skin turgor and urine specific gravity every 4 hours.	3. Intake and output, skin turgor, and urine specific gravity provide valuable clues about the infant's hydration status and aid in identifying possible problems with fluid excess or overload.
4. Obtain daily weights.	4. Weight is a reliable indicator of overall fluid status.
5. If vomiting occurs, have the mother attempt to refeed the infant.	5. Refeeding helps maintain adequate fluid and nutritional intake.
6. If vomiting continues, anticipate the need for enteral or total parenteral nutrition.	6. Alternative methods may be necessary to ensure optimal nutrient intake if the infant is unable to tolerate oral feedings.

Nursing Diagnosis: Deficient parental knowledge related to hydrocephalus and shunt insertion

Outcome Identification: Parents will express accurate information about their infant's condition and scheduled procedure.

Outcome Evaluation: Parents describe hydrocephalus and how it affects their infant; identify measures used to treat the condition; state realistic expectations about their infant following shunt insertion.

Interventions	Rationale
1. Assess the parents' understanding of hydrocephalus and treatment measures.	1. Obtaining a baseline knowledge assessment provides a foundation on which to build future teaching strategies.
2. Review the structure and function of the brain and how hydrocephalus develops. Clarify any misconceptions.	2. Reviewing and clarifying aid in learning and strengthening understanding.
3. Provide ample time for questions and concerns.	3. Providing time for questions and concerns helps to clarify information, individualize teaching, and promote a feeling of trust and control.
4. Review with the parents what the physician has told them about the shunt insertion procedure, including why it is necessary, and what parents might expect to see after the surgery.	4. Review and reinforcement help to prepare the parents for events both before and after the surgery, thereby helping to minimize their anxiety.
5. Instruct parents about the appearance and care of their infant after surgery, including the need for follow-up visits, monitoring for infection, and providing stimulation.	5. Instruction helps to prepare the parents for what will be required of them.
6. Assist parents with caring for the child as much as possible; offer positive reinforcement frequently.	6. Caring for the child promotes active participation and parent–infant bonding. Positive reinforcement enhances self-esteem and aids in coping.
7. Refer parents to support group of other parents of children with hydrocephalus. Anticipate the need for home care following discharge.	7. Support groups of other parents in similar situations promote sharing, decrease feelings of isolation and loneliness, and provide opportunities for further learning. Follow-up home care provides continuing support, guidance, and education.

FOCUS ON FAMILY EMPOWERMENT

Caring for a Child With a Ventriculoperitoneal Shunt

Q. Our son had a shunt inserted to treat his hydrocephalus. How should we take care of him?

A. Here are some helpful things to remember:

- Observe for signs of increased intracranial pressure, such as drowsiness, vomiting, headache, irritability, and anorexia.
- Observe the pump site daily for any sign of swelling or redness.
- Have your child sleep with his head slightly elevated at night to help ensure fluid flow through the tube. Do not allow your child to fall asleep with his head hanging over the side of a couch or bed.
- Do not allow your child to become constipated, because hard stool might press against and obstruct the shunt. Encourage fruit, vegetables, cereal, and a generous amount of fluid in his diet.
- Do not call attention to the pump behind your child's ear; teach him not to touch the pump when he's nervous or as an attention-getting action.
- Be certain your child wears a helmet for tricycle and bicycle riding (as should all children) to avoid injury to the shunt. Otherwise, there are no special precautions that need to be taken for normal play.
- If your child develops signs of infection such as an increased temperature, telephone your primary care provider. Also remind the person that your child has a shunt in place. This is probably a simple infection of childhood but could indicate an infected shunt.
- Be certain to keep your regularly scheduled health assessment visits. As your child grows taller, the shunt will eventually need to be replaced for proper functioning.

Nursing Diagnosis: Risk for impaired skin integrity related to weight and immobility of head

Outcome Identification: Child's skin will remain intact during course of illness.

Outcome Evaluation: Child's skin remains clean, dry, and intact, without signs of erythema or ulceration.

The head of the infant with hydrocephalus can become so heavy that it cannot be moved freely. If the skin of the head stretches thin, skin breakdown can occur on the pressure points. Wash the child's head daily and change the position of the head approximately every 2 hours so that no portion of the head rests against the mattress for a long period. A synthetic sheepskin pad or an air, water, or alternating air mattress may help to relieve pressure points. If a Kling or stockinette bandage is used to hold a surgical head dressing in place, place a piece of gauze or cotton behind the child's ear before the bandage is applied to prevent skin surfaces from touching and becoming excoriated. Observe that the bandage does not become wet from backward-draining oral secretions or shunt leakage.

Nursing Diagnosis: Deficient knowledge related to home care needs of child with hydrocephalus

Outcome Identification: Parents will demonstrate understanding of shunt placement and voice confidence in their ability to care for child by hospital discharge.

Outcome Evaluation: Parents state fears regarding ability to provide care; state signs of increased intracranial pressure for which to watch; demonstrate competence in shunt care.

Caring for a child with a shunt in place is a continuing responsibility for parents. If parents do not seem to be asking many questions about the child's care after surgery, do not assume this is because they are taking the child's care in stride. They may be too frightened or not understand neuroanatomy enough to ask questions. An opening such as, "Most parents are a little nervous when they think about taking a child home with a shunt in place; do you feel that way?" gives them an opportunity to admit how they feel. For many people, being able to talk about a problem suddenly brings it down to manageable size. Talking about how nervous they feel about the responsibility will not immediately make them more comfortable with the child's care. However, it does provide them with a starting point. Assure them that the health care providers caring for their child are interested in helping and supporting them.

If a valve has been inserted in the shunt, it can be palpated below the skin just behind the ear. Help parents stress to their child that this strange object is not to be felt continually. A child nervously fidgeting with a pressure pump can inadvertently evacuate CSF from the ventricles at a dangerously rapid rate.

Before an infant is discharged after surgery, be certain the parents have ample opportunity to feed and provide care so they can be comfortable and feel that they "know" their infant. Because irritability, lethargy, vomiting, and a change in the baby's cry are signs of increased intracranial pressure, the parents need to report these symptoms immediately to their primary care provider. Before parents can report a change in the infant's disposition in this way, they must know the infant well. A referral for home care follow-up may be appropriate to offer further support.

Nursing Diagnosis: Risk for delayed growth and development related to potential neurologic challenge

Outcome Identification: Child will achieve developmental growth to the maximum of potential.

Outcome Evaluation: Child demonstrates regular observable growth and achieves age-appropriate developmental milestones.

Although children may have mild learning or motor problems, the cognitive functioning of a child with hydrocephalus may remain intact despite extreme thinning of the brain cortex (Ding, 2001). Therefore, after a shunting procedure, although the head may remain larger than normal, intelligence may be normal. Like all children, children with hydrocephalus need stimulation: they need to be talked to, smiled at, played with. If the child's head is enlarged, turning it to look at things can be difficult. It may be necessary to reposition mobiles or pictures so the child receives adequate visual stimulation. Role-model talking and singing to the child to help parents include these actions in their care.

At the time of discharge, be certain parents have the telephone number of the person they should call if they have a question or concern about the child's condition or care, and a referral for home care follow-up, if appropriate. They also need an appointment for the child's first checkup. Be sure they understand that infection of the shunt is a possibility and a severe complication because it can lead to meningitis. If this should occur, the infant will show signs of increased intracranial pressure as well as those of infection. In addition to being hospitalized, receiving the usual treatment for meningitis (see Chap. 49), and receiving intravenous antibiotics, the child may have an extraventricular shunt placed to promote drainage. This allows antibiotics to be administered directly to the cerebral fluid and ensures that infected CSF is not draining to the peritoneal cavity, where it could cause peritonitis.

As the child reaches preschool and school age, parents need to confer with the school nurse to make the nurse aware that the child has a shunt in place and that the child may need special head protection, if necessary, for sports activities.

✔ **CHECKPOINT QUESTIONS**

11. What changes in vital signs occur with increased intracranial pressure?
12. After a shunting procedure, how should the infant's bed be positioned?

Neural Tube Disorders

Because the neural tube forms in utero first as a flat plate and then molds to form the brain and spinal cord, it is susceptible to malformation. The term **spina bifida** (Latin for "divided spine") is most often used as a collective term for all spinal cord disorders, but there are well-defined degrees of spina bifida involvement, and not all neural tube disorders involve the spinal cord. All these disorders, however, occur because of lack of fusion of the posterior surface of the embryo in early intrauterine life. They can be compared with cleft palate or cleft lip—these are also closure defects.

The incidence of neural tube disorders has fallen dramatically in recent years, from 3/1,000 to 0.6/1,000. Such disorders may occur as a polygenic inheritance pattern, but poor nutrition, especially a diet deficient in folic acid, appears to be a major contributing factor. As a result, pregnant women are advised to ingest 0.4 mg folic acid daily to help prevent these disorders (Department of Health and Human Services [DHHS], 2000). The risk of bearing a second child with a neural tube defect once one child is born with such a defect increases to as much as 1 in 20. Therefore, women who have had a child with a neural tube disorder are advised to ingest 4 mg of folic acid (DHHS, 2000). Also, women who have had one child with a spinal cord defect are advised to have a maternal serum assay or amniocentesis of alpha-fetoprotein (AFP) levels to determine if such a defect is present in a second pregnancy (levels will be abnormally increased if there is an open spinal lesion). Serum assessment is done at week 15 of pregnancy, when AFP reaches its peak concentration. AFP level testing is a routine test in many prenatal settings. If the result is elevated, an amniocentesis will be done to assess the level of AFP in amniotic fluid. A sonogram is also helpful to determine the presence of the disorder (see Chap. 10 for further discussion of these prenatal assessments).

Types of Defects

Anencephaly. Anencephaly is absence of the cerebral hemispheres. It occurs when the upper end of the neural tube fails to close in early intrauterine life. It is revealed by an elevated level of AFP in maternal serum or on amniocentesis and confirmed by sonogram.

Infants with anencephaly may have difficulty in labor because the underdeveloped head does not engage the cervix well. Many such infants present in a breech position. On visual inspection at birth, the disorder is obvious (Fig. 39-11). Children cannot survive with this disorder because they have no cerebral function. Because the respiratory and cardiac centers are located in the intact medulla, however, they may survive for a number of days after birth.

When the condition is discovered prenatally, parents are offered the option of abortion. An ethical problem has arisen in a number of instances when parents, aware that the child cannot survive, elect to carry the infant to term so the organs can be used for transplant. Nurses need to think through their feelings about caring for such infants, because it can be difficult to give care to a child who will most likely die or who has been born only to help others live.

Microcephaly. Microcephaly is a disorder in which brain growth is so slow that it falls more than three standard deviations below normal on growth charts. The cause might be a defect in brain development associated with an intrauterine infection such as rubella, cytomegalovirus, or toxoplasmosis. Microcephaly may also result from severe malnutrition or anoxia in early infancy.

The prognosis for a normal life is guarded in children with microcephaly and depends on the extent of restriction of brain growth and on the cause. Generally the infant is cognitively challenged because of the lack of functioning

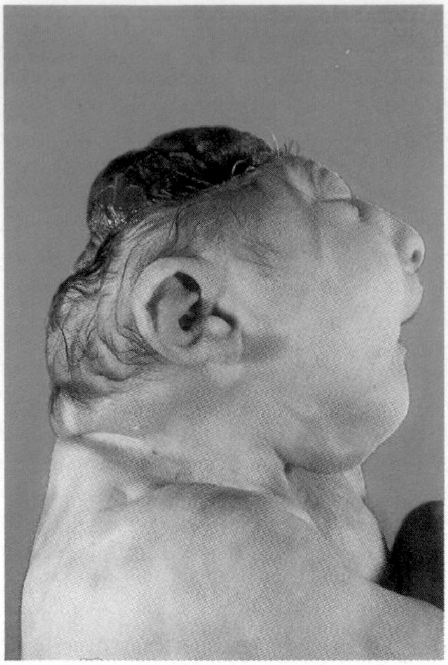

FIGURE 39.11 An infant with anencephaly.

brain tissue. True microcephaly must be differentiated from craniosynostosis (normal brain growth but premature fusion of the cranial sutures), which also causes decreased head circumference. Infants with craniosynostosis have abnormally closed fontanelles and often show bulging (bossing of the forehead and signs of increased intracranial pressure). With surgery, craniosynostosis can be relieved and brain growth will be normal.

Spina Bifida Occulta. Spina bifida occulta occurs when the posterior laminae of the vertebrae fail to fuse. This occurs most commonly at the fifth lumbar or first sacral level but may occur at any point along the spinal canal. The normal spinal cord is shown in Figure 39-12*A*. The disorder may be noticeable as a dimpling at the point of poor fusion; abnormal tufts of hair may be present (see Fig. 39-12*B*). Simple spina bifida occulta is a benign defect; it occurs as frequently as in one of every four children.

The term "spina bifida" is often used wrongly to denote all spinal cord anomalies. Because of this wrong usage, parents, when told that their child has a spina bifida occulta, may interpret this as meaning that the child has an extremely serious defect. Health professionals should use the terms correctly to reduce any confusion.

Meningocele. If the meninges covering the spinal cord herniate through unformed vertebrae, a meningocele occurs. The anomaly appears as a protruding mass, usually approximately the size of an orange, at the center of the back (see Fig. 39-12*C*). It generally occurs in the lumbar region, although it might be present anywhere along the spinal canal. The protrusion may be covered by a layer of skin or only the clear dura mater.

Myelomeningocele. In a myelomeningocele, the spinal cord and the meninges protrude through the vertebrae defect the same as with a meningocele. The difference is that the spinal cord ends at the point of the defect, so motor and sensory function is absent beyond this point (see Fig. 39-12*D*). Because this results in lower motor neuron damage, the child will have flaccidity and lack of sensation of the lower extremities and loss of bowel and bladder control. The infant's legs are lax, and he or she does not move them; urine and stools continually dribble because of lack of sphincter control. Children often have accompanying talipes (clubfoot) disorders and developmental hip dysplasia. Hydrocephalus accompanies myelomeningocele in as many as 80% of infants due to the lack of a subarachnoid membrane; the higher the myelomeningocele occurs on the cord, the more likely hydrocephalus will accompany it (Dlugos, 2000). It is generally difficult to tell from visual appearance whether the disorder is myelomeningocele or the simpler meningocele (Fig. 39-13).

Encephalocele. An encephalocele is a cranial meningocele or myelomeningocele. The defect occurs most often in the occipital area of the skull but may occur as a nasal or nasopharyngeal defect. Encephaloceles generally are covered fully by skin, but they may be open or covered only by the dura. It is difficult to tell from the size of the encephalocele how much brain tissue is trapped in the defect. Transillumination of the sac will reveal solid substance or fluid in

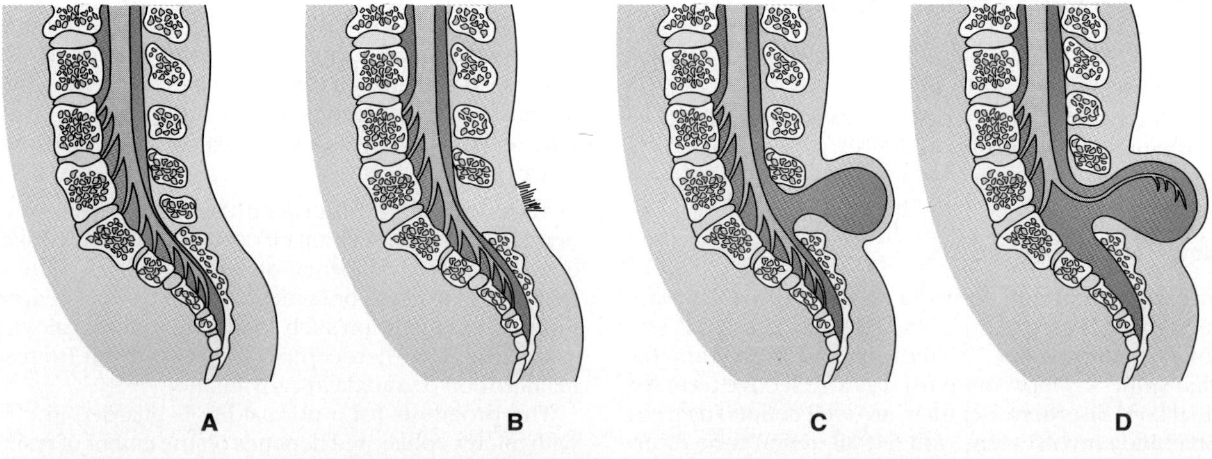

FIGURE 39.12 Degrees of spinal cord anomalies. (*A*) Normal spinal cord. (*B*) Spina bifida occulta. (*C*) Meningocele. (*D*) Myelomeningocele.

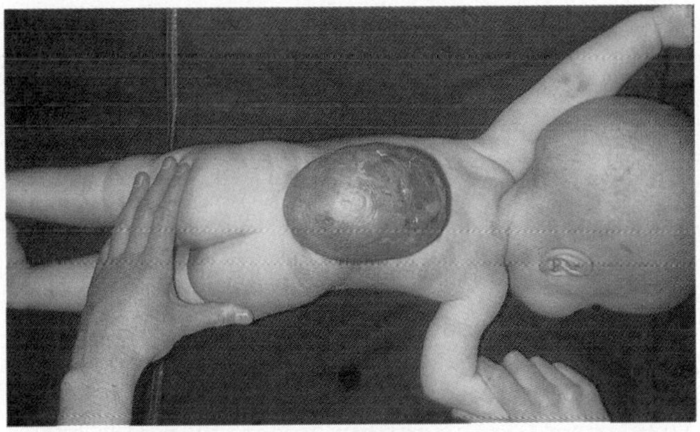

FIGURE 39.13 A myelomeningocele. The infant also has hydrocephaly and a subluxated hip.

the sac. X-ray or sonography will reveal the size of the skull defect.

Assessment

Neural tube defects may be discovered during intrauterine life by sonography, fetoscopy, amniocentesis (discovery of increased AFP in amniotic fluid), or analysis of AFP in maternal serum. When infants are detected as having meningocele or myelomeningocele, they may be born by cesarean birth to avoid pressure and injury to the spinal cord. Observe and record whether an infant born with a neural tube disorder has spontaneous movement of the lower extremities. Also assess the nature and pattern of voiding and defecation. A normal infant appears to be "always wet" from voiding but actually voids in amounts of approximately 30 mL and then is dry for 2 or 3 hours before voiding again. An infant without sphincter control voids continually. This pattern is the same for defecation. Observing these features aids in differentiating between meningocele and myelomeningocele. Differentiation can be further established by sonography.

Therapeutic Management

Children with spina bifida occulta need no immediate surgical correction. The parents should be made aware of its existence, however, so they are not surprised when someone points it out to them later. Some children may eventually need surgery to prevent vertebral deterioration due to the unbalanced spinal column.

Treatment for a meningocele, myelomeningocele, or encephalocele involves surgery to replace the contents that are replaceable and to close the skin defect to prevent infection. The child with myelomeningocele will continue to have paralysis of the lower extremities and loss of bowel and bladder function after surgery because the absent lower cord cannot be replaced. Table 39-1 provides a classification of motor function ability according to the location of the spinal cord disruption. In the past, surgery for neural tube disorders was done only after the infant had survived the newborn period. Currently, it is done as soon after birth as possible (usually within 24 to 48 hours) so infection through the exposed meninges does not occur. Parents need to be cautioned that the surgery is not without risk and that brain defects accompanying an encephalocele may limit the child's cognitive potential.

TABLE 39.1 Motor Function Ability in Myelomeningocele

SPINAL CORD LESION	RESULTANT EFFECTS
T6–12	Complete flaccid paralysis of the lower extremities; weakened abdominal and trunk musculature in higher lesions; kyphosis and scoliosis common; ambulation with maximal support
L1–2	Hip flexion present; paraplegia, ambulation with maximal support
L3–4	Hip flexion, adduction, and knee extension present; hip dislocation common; some control of hip and knee movement possible; ambulation with moderate support
L5	Hip flexion, adduction, and varying degrees of abduction; knee extension and weak knee flexion; paralysis of the lower legs and feet; ambulation with moderate support
S1–2	As above, with preservation of some foot and ankle movement; ambulation with minimal support
S3	Mild loss of intrinsic foot muscular function possible; ambulation without support

The prognosis depends on the extent of the disorder. The loss of meninges by surgery may limit the rate of absorption of CSF. This may lead to a buildup in amount, resulting in hydrocephalus. Parents need a great deal of support to care for a child with a myelomeningocele because their child has multiple challenges. Referral to a community support group can be helpful.

WHAT IF? What if a parent tells you he wants to let his newborn die rather than undergo palliative surgery to close a neural tube disorder? Whose rights should be honored, the parents' or the child's, and how should these rights be determined? What would be your role?

NURSING DIAGNOSES AND RELATED INTERVENTIONS: IMMEDIATE CONCERNS

Although parents of an infant with a myelomeningocele were told before surgery that their child's spinal disorder is a type that means motor and sensory function are absent in the child's lower extremities, parents do not necessarily hear this information. Only after surgery do they begin to comprehend what the extent of the condition will be. When the child is discharged from the hospital, be certain the parents understand what the next step in follow-up care will be. This prevents them from feeling deserted when they most need support—the time when they first begin to appreciate what this problem will mean to them in the coming years, and what it will mean to the child throughout life.

Nursing Diagnosis: Risk for infection related to rupture or bacterial invasion of the neural tube sac

Outcome Identification: Child will not develop an infection before surgery.

Outcome Evaluation: The neural tube sac remains intact; the child's axillary temperature remains below 98.6°F (37°C).

If the exposed meningeal sac is allowed to dry, it can crack, allowing CSF to drain and microorganisms to enter. Pressure on the protruding mass also can rupture the sac, leading to quick decompression of the CSF (which can lead to herniation of the brain stem into the spinal cord and interference with respiratory and cardiac centers) and possibly to infection (meningitis). Such pressure may also force CSF from the sac into the spinal column, increasing intracranial pressure. Therefore, it is crucial to prevent drying of and pressure on the exposed membrane.

Preoperative Positioning. Before surgery, use sterile gloves and sterile linens when caring for the infant. Position infants carefully to prevent pressure on the exposed meninges, either in a prone position or supported on their side. When they are on their side, use a rolled blanket or diaper placed behind their upper back (above the defect) and a separate one behind their lower back (below the defect). This way, no pressure will be exerted on the lesion, and the infant will be protected from rolling backward onto it. Placing infants on their abdomen has the added advantage of keeping the flow of feces and urine away from the defect as well as keeping the lesion free from pressure. A folded towel under the abdomen helps to flex the infant's hips, reduce pressure on the sac, and ensure good leg position. If an infant is on his or her side, putting a folded diaper between the legs prevents skin surfaces from touching and rubbing (and also helps to keep the hips from internally rotating). Always notice the position of the infant's legs. If they are paralyzed because of lack of motor control, the infant cannot move and straighten them to a comfortable position.

Placing a piece of plastic or sturdy plastic wrap below the meningocele on the child's back like an apron and taping it in place is another method of preventing feces from touching the open lesion. A sterile wet compress of saline, antiseptic, or antibiotic gauze over the lesion may be used to keep the sac moist. Rather than remove this to wet it again and risk rupturing the sac, merely add additional fluid.

Although no pressure should be exerted on the open lesion by a top sheet, make certain that the child is adequately warm. The presence of the sac adds to the amount of body surface area exposed, thus increasing heat loss. He or she may need to be kept in an isolette to maintain body heat if a large area of the back cannot be covered. Use caution when placing the infant under a radiant heat source for warmth because radiant heat can dry the lesion and cause cracking. Any seepage of clear fluid from the defect should be reported promptly, because this is probably escaping CSF. Checking any leakage for evidence of glucose will confirm the fluid is CSF fluid (urine or mucus will not test positive for glucose).

Postoperative Care. After surgery, a child is again placed on the abdomen until the skin incision has healed (about 7 days). The same careful precautions against allowing urine or feces to touch the incision area are necessary.

Nursing Diagnosis: Risk for imbalanced nutrition, less than body requirements, related to difficulty assuming normal feeding position

Outcome Identification: Infant will take in adequate nutrition during period of healing.

Outcome Evaluation: Infant's skin turgor is good; weight is maintained within 10% of birth weight; specific gravity of urine remains between 1.003 and 1.030.

To maintain nutrition, help the parents to hold the infant in as normal a feeding position as possible. Make certain that a supporting arm does not press against the lesion. Remind the parents that when bubbling the infant, they should not pat the back over the defect. If the defect is large and the risk in picking up the infant is too great, the infant may be fed while lying on his or her side in bed or prone on a specialized bed frame. Raise the infant's head slightly by slipping a folded diaper under it. Stroke the head, arms, or upper back while the infant sucks to give the child the same comfort and assurance at feeding time as a baby receives while being held. Talk to the infant and let him or her know that someone is nearby to care for him or her. The infant may enjoy a pacifier after feeding, because he or she does not experience the same enjoyment of sucking while feeding that would be experienced if he could be held and cuddled. All new parents have some difficulty getting comfortable with feeding an infant. Parents who must feed their child in an unusual position or with the infant on a support frame will have even more difficulty. Role-model a warm, comforting parental role so the parents begin to form a positive parent–child interaction.

Children with increased intracranial pressure tend to suck poorly. If this complication develops after surgery, breast-feeding may be difficult. Parents need a realistic explanation of the treatment planned for the child so they can decide whether to continue breast-feeding. If it is necessary to forgo breast-feeding for this child, assure parents that the child will thrive on commercial formula.

Nursing Diagnosis: Risk for ineffective cerebral tissue perfusion related to increased intracranial pressure

Outcome Identification: Infant will remain free of symptoms of compression from increased intracranial pressure or an increase in skull circumference during childhood.

Outcome Evaluation: Infant's head circumference remains within present percentile on growth chart; signs and symptoms of increased intracranial pressure are absent.

Preoperative Care. Increasing head size from poor absorption of CSF (hydrocephalus) is a complication of neural tube disorders. To detect increased head size (development of hydrocephalus), measure head circumference once daily (or more frequently if ordered) in the preoperative period. Head circumference measurements are accurate only if the tape measure is placed on the same points of the child's head each time. Placing an indelible or ballpoint pen mark on the forehead just above the eyebrows and at the most prominent point of the occiput allows different people to measure the head during the day and yet be sure that they all measure at the same point.

Postoperative Care. Children may develop hydrocephalus after surgery, probably because of interference with subarachnoid absorption of CSF. The shortening of the meninges creates an Arnold-Chiari disorder (see below) or traction of the hindbrain into the spinal cord. The child must be observed frequently for signs of increased intracranial pressure such as changes in vital signs, neurologic signs such as pupillary changes, or an increase in head circumference or bulging fontanelles, as well as behavioral changes such as irritability or lethargy.

Nursing Diagnosis: Risk for impaired skin integrity related to required prone positioning

Outcome Identification: Infant will not experience disruption in skin integrity during preoperative or postoperative period.

Outcome Evaluation: Infant's skin remains intact, without erythema or ulceration.

Preserving skin integrity is a major problem before surgery because the constant prone position puts pressure on the infant's knees and elbows. Laying the infant on a synthetic sheepskin helps reduce friction; after surgery, use paper tape or stockinette for dressing changes or place protective dressings such as Stomahesive on the skin under the area where the tape will touch. Change diapers frequently to prevent excessive contact of acid urine with skin. If hydrocephalus has developed, the head will be heavy and pressure areas at the temples can occur if the head is not repositioned every 2 hours.

NURSING DIAGNOSES AND RELATED INTERVENTIONS: LONG-TERM CONCERNS

Nursing Diagnosis: Impaired physical mobility related to neural tube disorder

Outcome Identification: Child will be mobile within the limits of nerve involvement after surgery.

Outcome Evaluation: Child ambulates with the least amount of accessory equipment possible.

Help parents begin to plan stimulation and activities for the infant that he or she can accomplish with limited mobility. Encourage them to take the infant to the places a child would normally accompany parents—relatives' homes, shopping, the zoo, and so forth. Encouraging the child to be as independent as possible will help him or her to lead as normal a life as possible (Fig. 39-14).

Parents will need to perform passive exercises to prevent muscle atrophy and formation of contractures if a child has impaired lower extremity motor control. The child may need leg braces to help maintain good alignment and enable walking with crutches. Parents are generally anxious to do something for their child and follow routines of passive exercises well if they are given sufficient support for their accomplishments at health care visits. As the child grows older, tendon transplants or osteotomy may be necessary to prevent contractures and poor bone alignment. Because these children have no sensation in their lower extremities, parents must make a routine of inspecting the child's lower extremities and buttocks daily for any area of irritation or possible infection. Teach children as they grow older to do this themselves. When children are using a wheelchair, be certain they press with their arms on the armrests to raise their buttocks off the wheelchair seat at least once every hour. This will help provide adequate circulation to the lower extremities.

Nursing Diagnosis: Risk for impaired elimination related to neural tube disorder

Outcome Identification: Child will achieve a satisfactory method of elimination by school age.

Outcome Evaluation: Child demonstrates ability to independently manage bowel and bladder elimination.

To ensure bladder emptying, the intermittent clean urinary catheterization technique is taught to parents. As the child reaches school age, he or she can learn this technique and be taught clean self-catheterization

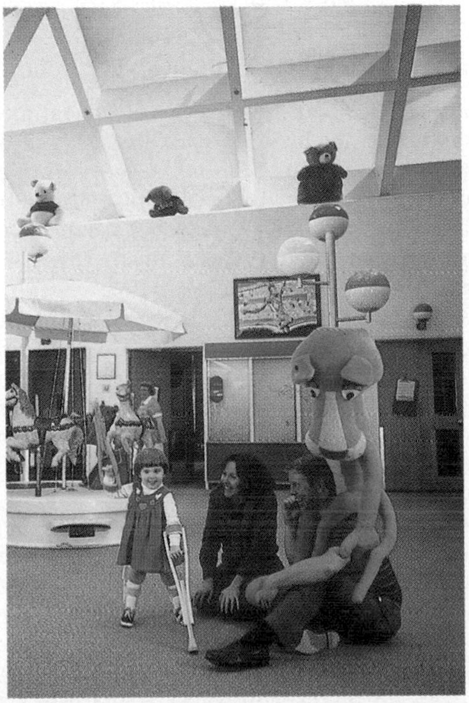

FIGURE 39.14 A child born with a neural tube disorder demonstrates her ability to walk using braces and a crutch.

(inserting a clean catheter through the urethra into the bladder every 4 hours to drain urine from the bladder; see Focus on Family Empowerment). Caution parents that because the catheters are latex, the child may develop a latex sensitivity. Prescription of a drug such as oxybutynin chloride (Ditropan) may improve bladder capacity (see Focus on Pharmacology). Artificial bladder sphincters may be placed to help establish continence. In some children, a continent urinary reservoir or ureterosigmoidostomy (see Chap. 46) is constructed to bypass the nonfunctioning bladder. However, children who are begun on intermittent clean catheterization from birth require less bladder augmentation procedures than those who are not.

Arnold-Chiari Deformity (Chiari II Malformation)

The Arnold-Chiari deformity is caused by overgrowth of the neural tube in weeks 16 to 20 of fetal life. The specific anomaly is a projection of the cerebellum, medulla oblongata, and fourth ventricle into the cervical canal. This causes the upper cervical spinal cord to jackknife backward, obstructing CSF flow and causing hydrocephalus. A lumbosacral myelomeningocele is also present in approximately 50% of children with this anomaly (Nickel, 2000).

The prognosis for the child with an Arnold-Chiari malformation depends on the extent of the defect and the surgical procedure possible. Because of the upper motor neuron involvement, gagging and swallowing reflexes may be absent, increasing the risk for tracheal aspiration.

> **✔ CHECKPOINT QUESTIONS**
>
> 13. Why must a meningocele sac be kept moist?
> 14. When is surgery performed to repair a neural tube defect?

SKELETAL DEVELOPMENTAL DISORDERS

Several steps compromising fetal physical development result in skeletal disorders in the newborn.

Absent or Malformed Extremities

Congenital skeletal disorders may result from unknown reasons, such as maternal drug ingestion, virus invasion during pregnancy, or amniotic band formation in utero. If a child is born with a bone deformity, record a careful

---

FOCUS ON FAMILY EMPOWERMENT

Instructions For Self-Catheterization (Female)

Q. The doctor said that I need to learn to catheterize myself. My parents used to do this. Now, how should I do this?

A. Here are some helpful guidelines to follow:

1. Remember that the purpose of self-catheterization is to keep the bladder empty by using clean technique and frequent emptying so microorganisms do not have time to grow in urine in the bladder. It is important that you always use clean equipment and that you self-catheterize at least every 4 hours to accomplish this.
2. Always carry your self-catheterization equipment with you (a plastic bag containing a clean catheter and water-soluble lubricant). This enables you to stay longer away from home if you wish. If you will be using a public lavatory, you might want to include a presoaped washcloth rather than have to use rough paper towels.
3. To begin self-catheterization, wash your hands in warm, soapy water. This reduces the chance that you will introduce germs from your hands into the bladder.
4. Next wash your private area (perineum) with a clean washcloth and warm, soapy water. Rinse the washcloth and wash again with clear water. This reduces the chance that germs on your skin will be pushed into the bladder.
5. Coat a clean catheter with a water-soluble lubricant. This reduces friction and makes the catheter slide into the bladder easily.
6. Use one hand to spread the lips of the perineum so the bladder entrance is exposed. Locate the urinary meatus and gently but quickly insert the catheter approximately 1 inch. Urine should begin to flow immediately through the catheter. Let this drain into the toilet.
7. When urine stops flowing, gently remove the catheter. Clean the catheter with soap and water, rinse with clear water, and replace in the plastic bag with the lubricant.
8. Examine your schedule at the beginning of each day and plan ways that you will be able to use a bathroom or school lavatory every 4 hours.
9. Be certain that on special days (e.g., school trips or vacation) you do not forget the importance of self-catheterization.
10. Ask your parents to telephone your health care provider if urine is ever blood-tinged, smells foul, or is cloudy rather than clear; if you have pain in your abdomen or lower back; or if you have an elevated temperature. These may be symptoms of a urinary tract infection.

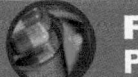

FOCUS ON PHARMACOLOGY

Oxybutynin Chloride (Ditropan)

Action: Oxybutynin is an anticholinergic, urinary antispasmodic that relaxes smooth muscle to relieve symptoms of bladder instability associated with neurogenic bladder.

Pregnancy risk category: C

Dosage: 5 mg orally, b.i.d.

Possible adverse effects: Drowsiness, dizziness, blurred vision, decreased sweating

Nursing Implications

- Advise the parents to give or the child to take the medication exactly as prescribed.
- Alert the parents about the need for frequent bladder examinations during treatment to document the drug's effect.
- Ask the child to report drowsiness or blurred vision. Caution the child not to attempt activities that require balance while taking the drug.
- Caution the child and parents that with decreased sweating, body temperature can rise. Encourage the parents to keep the child's environment cool and avoid high temperatures.

pregnancy history. In most instances, however, the cause of the anomaly cannot be established. Children born without an extremity or with a malformed extremity can be fitted with a prosthesis early in life. In most instances, children will have better function if the malformed portion of an extremity is amputated before a prosthesis is fitted. This is a difficult decision for parents to make because it is one that they cannot undo later. They need assurance that arms that appear like seal flippers, for example, will not later grow to become normal. A well-fitted prosthesis that a child learns to use at an early age will provide more function and allow a more normal childhood and adult life than if the original deformity is left unchanged (Fig. 39-15). Lower extremity prostheses are fitted as early as age 6 months (so an infant will learn to stand at the normal time). Upper extremity prostheses are fitted this early also, so an infant will handle and explore objects readily.

Introducing a prosthesis early also prevents a child from adjusting to a missing extremity, such as writing with the feet or sliding across a floor rather than walking. Children can become so proficient at these adjustments that later in life they do not see the advantage of a prosthesis and refuse to use one. Although these self-adjustments may be cute in infants, in the long run they greatly limit the child's potential.

Children who are born with an absent extremity may need help not only in mastering the use of a prosthesis but also in mastering a positive body image of themselves as whole. Learning to use a hand prosthesis takes weeks to months. Help parents think of interesting activities when introducing the prosthesis so the child uses a prosthesis to accomplish something rather than feeling he or she is only

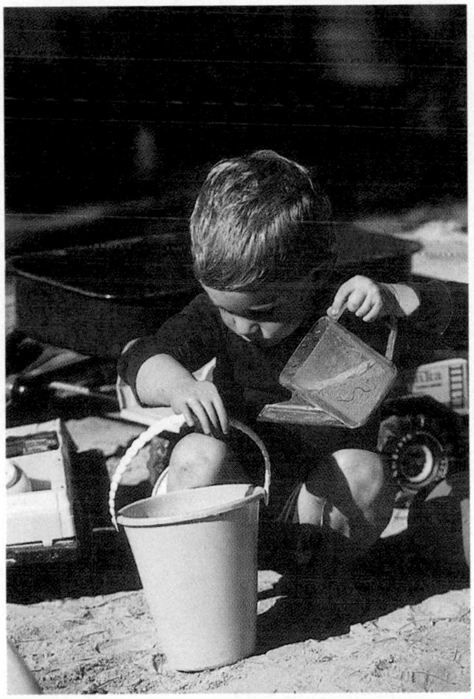

FIGURE 39.15 A young child learns to use a hand prosthesis during play.

performing a ritual. Gait training for use of lower extremity prostheses begins with the use of parallel bars and proceeds to independent walking and mastery of steps.

If possible, in the newborn period, introduce parents to the rehabilitation team who will be following their child. Further steps then will be outlined for them to help move them past the helplessness they may feel to more positive action. Visiting with a child who uses a prosthesis well can be a great help in convincing parents that their child can lead a normal life. Children with a congenital extremity loss do not grieve over the lost extremity as do adults or older children, which means they are often better prepared to move quickly to rehabilitation.

Finger Conditions

Polydactyly is the presence of one or more additional fingers (Bromley et al., 2000). When an entire finger forms, the supernumerary finger is usually amputated in infancy or early childhood. These extra fingers are often just cartilage or skin tags, and removal is simple and cosmetically sound. In **syndactyly** (two fingers are fused), the fusion is usually caused by a simple webbing (Fig. 39-16); separation of the fingers into two sound and cosmetically appealing ones is usually successful. In other instances, the bones of the fingers are also fused, and the cosmetic appearance and function of fingers cannot be fully reconstructed.

These hand anomalies are always upsetting to parents (one of the first things that new parents do is count the fingers and toes of newborns). They may need time to air their feelings and concerns. They need reassurance at health maintenance visits throughout the child's development that he or she is normal in other ways so they can accept and help the child develop self-esteem. Children

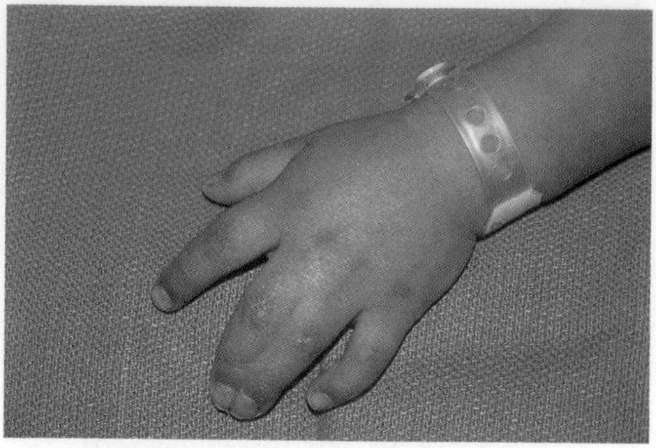

FIGURE 39.16 Syndactyly.

need this same type of assurance so they can think of themselves as well people.

Pectus Deviations

Pectus excavatum is an indentation of the lower portion of the sternum. Children usually are born with this condition, but they may also develop it after chronic obstructive lung disease or rickets. As a result, lung volume decreases and the heart is displaced to the left. This condition can be repaired for cosmetic reasons or to expand lung volume (Molik et al., 2001). With pectus carinatum, the sternum is displaced anteriorly, increasing the anterior-posterior diameter of the chest. This condition also can be repaired for physiologic or cosmetic reasons.

Torticollis (Wry Neck)

Torticollis is a term derived from *tortus* (twisted) and *collum* (neck). Torticollis (wry neck) occurs as a congenital anomaly when the sternocleidomastoid muscle is injured and bleeds during birth. This tends to occur in newborns with wide shoulders when pressure is exerted on the head to deliver the shoulder. The infant holds the head tilted to the side of the muscle involved; the chin rotates to the opposite side. The injury may not be noticeable in the newborn and may become evident only as the original hemorrhage recedes and fibrous contraction occurs at age 1 to 2 months. A thick mass over the muscle can be palpated.

Parents need to begin passive stretching exercises and encouraging the infant to look in the direction of the affected muscle. Parents could encourage this by holding the child to feed in such a position that the child must look in the desired direction. Placing a mobile on the child's crib to encourage the child to look toward the affected side also is helpful. The parents should speak to and hand the child objects always from the affected side to make the child look that way.

If manual stretching is begun early and consistently by the parents, further treatment usually is not necessary (Cheng et al., 2001). Parents need to understand that these actions are important therapy and not just games. The exercises seem so simple that parents may neglect to take them seriously. In the few instances in which simple exercises are not effective and the condition still exists at 1 year of age, surgical correction followed by a neck immobilizer will be necessary. If extreme injury to the muscle occurred, torticollis can lead to the continued elevation of one shoulder. Although a rare complication, this has the potential to lead to scoliosis later in life.

Parents may ask about the use of botulism (Botox) injections, because adults who develop spastic torticollis may receive this type of treatment (Yin et al., 2000). This type of treatment is not recommended for children.

Craniosynostosis

Craniosynostosis is premature closure of the sutures of the skull. This may occur in utero or early in infancy because of rickets or irregularities of calcium or phosphate metabolism; it also may occur without any known cause. It occurs more often in boys than girls.

This condition needs to be detected early because premature closure of the suture line will seal the skull closed and compromise brain growth. When the sagittal suture line closes prematurely, the child's head tends to grow anteriorly and posteriorly. If the coronal suture line fuses early, the orbits of the eyes become misshapen, and the increased intracranial pressure may lead to exophthalmos, nystagmus, papilledema, strabismus, and atrophy of the optic nerve with consequent loss of vision. Premature closure of the coronal suture line is associated with syndactyly. Therefore, closely observe all infants with syndactyly for head circumference. Also assess all infants with craniosynostosis for syndactyly. Cardiac anomalies, choanal atresias, or defects of elbows and knee joints are also associated with craniosynostosis.

Measure head circumference on all children age 2 years or younger at health maintenance visits and compare these measurements with normal head circumference charts. The posterior fontanelle normally closes at age 2 months, the anterior fontanelle at age 12 to 18 months. Children whose fontanelles close before these typical times need continued assessment to ensure that craniosynostosis is not developing.

Craniosynostosis is diagnosed by x-ray or sonogram, which reveals the fused suture line. If the suture line is the sagittal one, treatment may involve only careful observation; if the coronal suture line is involved, it will need to be surgically opened to prevent brain compression (Marentette & Kim, 2001).

Achondroplasia

Achondroplasia (chondrodystrophia) is a failure of bone growth inherited as a dominant trait. This involves a defect in cartilage production in utero. The epiphyseal plate of long bones cannot produce adequate cartilage for longitudinal bone growth, which results in both arms and legs becoming stunted.

Because the bones of the cranium are of membranous origin, they continue to grow normally. Children's heads will therefore appear unusually large in contrast to the extremities. The forehead is prominent and the bridge of the nose is flattened. Because this is a cartilage, not a brain, problem, intelligence generally is normal. Children's trunks are of near-normal size, but a thoracic kyphosis (outward curve) and lumbar lordosis (inward curve) of the spine may develop.

Achondroplasia can be diagnosed in utero or at birth by comparing the length of extremities to the normal length (in the average child, the arms can be extended to the distance of the midthigh) or by x-ray, which will reveal characteristic abnormally flaring epiphyseal lines. People with achondroplasia rarely reach a height of more than 4 feet 6 inches (140 cm). Women with this condition will have difficulty with childbearing because of a small pelvis, generally necessitating a cesarean birth.

Children with achondroplasia become aware of their appearance as early as the preschool years. They are apt to become acutely aware of their appearance during school age, when they realize they are different from the other children. Children may be prescribed growth hormone to increase their ultimate height (Kanaka-Gantenbein, 2001), but this is not always successful. Ideally, such children have parents who have adjusted well to their own short stature and therefore have developed good self-esteem and can implant these qualities in their child.

The child nearing reproductive age must be informed that, as with all dominantly inherited disorders, there is a high probability that any children will inherit the disorder. Adolescence may be a particularly difficult time for these children as they realize that occupational and reproductive options may be limited for them. Continued guidance or counseling can help them to emerge from this period with feelings of high self-esteem in themselves as adults.

Talipes Deformities

Talipes is a Latin word formed from the words *talus* (ankle) and *pes* (foot). The talipes deformities are ankle–foot disorders, popularly called clubfoot. The term "clubfoot" implies permanent crippling to many people, so avoid using this term when discussing talipes deformities with parents. With the orthopedic correction techniques currently available, correction should leave the child with fairly normal foot position. However, shoe size may vary as much as two shoe sizes, and the child may have asymmetry of leg length.

Approximately 1 in every 1,000 children is born with a talipes deformity, occurring more often in boys than girls. It probably is inherited as a polygenic pattern. It usually occurs as a unilateral problem (Davidson, 2000).

Some newborns have a pseudo-talipes deformity that has developed because of their intrauterine position. In these infants, the foot looks to be turned in but can be brought into a straight position by manipulation. In a true defect, the foot cannot be properly aligned without further intervention. Be certain to demonstrate to parents that if a pseudo-deformity is present, the foot can easily be brought into line or is not deformed. Otherwise, the first time parents fit booties or shoes on the infant, they will notice this and worry that the foot is misshapen.

A true talipes deformity can be one of four separate types: plantarflexion (an equinus or "horsefoot" position, with the foot lower than the heel); dorsiflexion (the heel is held lower than the foot or the anterior foot is flexed toward the anterior leg); varus deviation (the foot turns in); or valgus deviation (the foot turns out). Most children with talipes deformities have a combination of these conditions or have an equinovarus (Fig. 39-17*A*) or a calcaneovalgus deformity (a child walks on the heel with the foot everted).

Assessment

The earlier a true deformity is recognized, the better the correction will be. Make a habit of straightening all newborn feet to the midline as part of initial assessment to detect this defect.

Therapeutic Management

Correction is achieved best if it is begun in the newborn period. A cast is applied while the foot is placed in an overcorrected position. Although the deformity involves the ankle, the cast extends above the knee to ensure firm correction (see Fig. 39-17*B*). (Care of the child in a cast is discussed in Chap. 51.) Because talipes casts are high on the leg, change diapers frequently to prevent a wet diaper from touching the cast and causing it to become soaked with urine or meconium. Review with parents how to

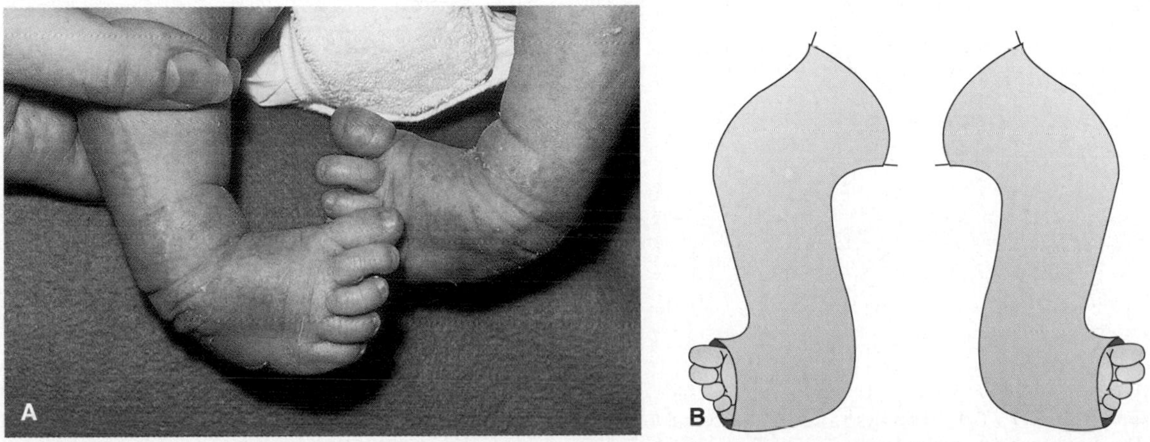

FIGURE 39.17 (*A*) Talipes equinovarus. (*B*) Casts for bilateral equinovarus.

check the infant's toes for coldness or blueness and how to blanch a toenail bed and watch it turn pink to assess for good circulation. Because a newborn is unable to report pain except by generalized crying, crying episodes in the infant must be evaluated carefully. Such crying may be due to colic, hunger, or wet diapers; it might also be due to the tingling feeling of circulatory compression (as when a foot is "asleep" from too tight a cast).

Infants grow so rapidly in the neonatal period that casts for talipes deformities must be changed almost every 1 or 2 weeks. If a mother has a complication of childbirth or is exhausted from childbirth (depression due to the child having been born congenitally challenged may manifest itself as exhaustion), be certain she knows to make arrangements for another family member to bring the infant to the hospital for cast changes.

After approximately 6 weeks (the time varies depending on the extent of the problem), the final cast is removed. After this, parents may need to perform passive foot exercises such as putting the infant's foot and ankle through a full range of motion several times a day for several months. These seem like simple maneuvers, but be sure to stress their importance to the parents; otherwise, they are easy exercises to omit when people's lives are busy. The infant may have to sleep in Denis Browne splints (shoes attached to a metal bar to maintain position) or high-top shoes at night for a few more months.

Although a successful correction cannot be guaranteed, the prognosis for a full correction is good. For children who do not achieve correction by casting, surgery is an option to achieve a final correction.

✔ **CHECKPOINT QUESTIONS**

15. What is the name of the condition when two fingers are fused?
16. What is an important care measure to teach parents of the child with a torticollis?

Developmental Hip Dysplasia

Developmental hip dysplasia (often referred to as congenital hip dysplasia) is improper formation and function of the hip socket. It may be evident as subluxation or dislocation of the head of the femur (Fig. 39-18).

With this disorder, the acetabulum of the pelvis is flattened or shallow. This prevents the head of the femur from remaining in the acetabulum and rotating adequately. In a subluxated hip, the femur "rides up" because of the flat acetabulum; in a dislocated hip, the femur rides so far up that it actually leaves the acetabulum. Why the defect occurs is unknown, but it may be from a polygenic inheritance pattern. It may also occur from a uterine position that causes less-than-usual pressure of the femur head on the acetabulum.

Developmental hip dysplasia occurs most often in children of Mediterranean ancestry. It is found six times more frequently in girls than in boys, possibly because the hips are normally more flaring in females and possibly because the maternal hormone relaxin causes the pelvic ligaments to be more relaxed. Thus, the femur does not press as

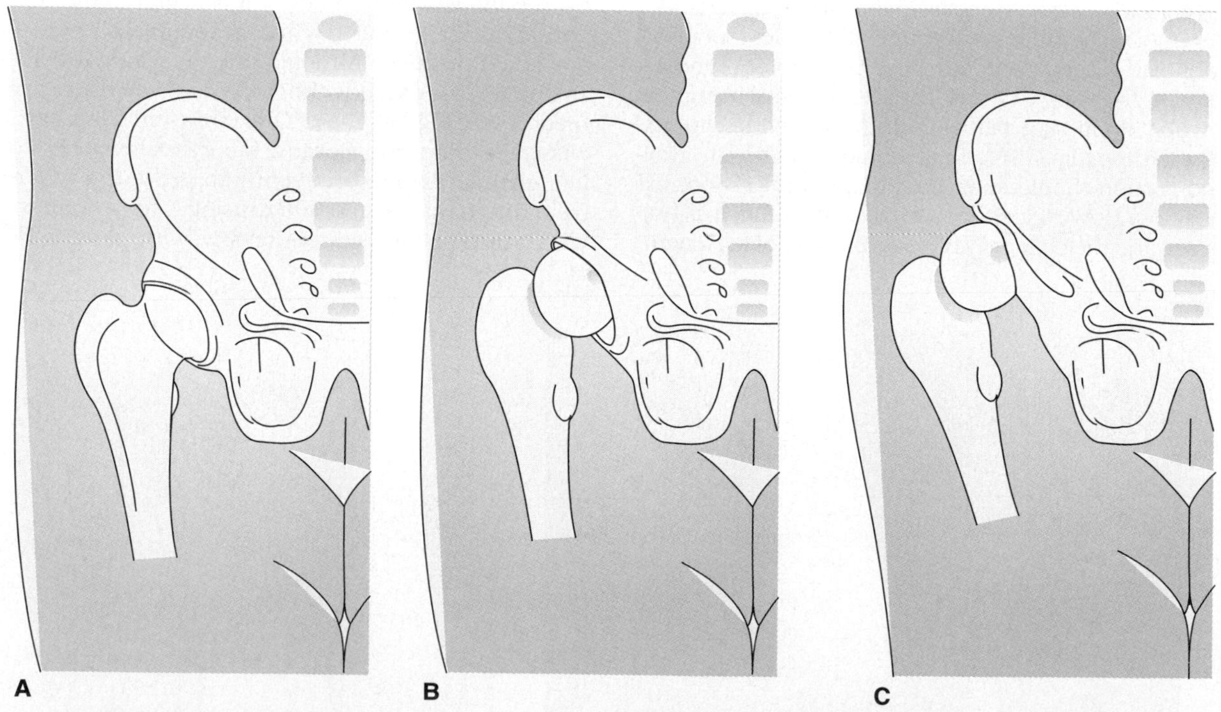

FIGURE 39.18 Hip dysplasia. (*A*) A normal femur head and acetabulum. (*B*) A subluxated hip. The femur head is "riding high" in the shallow acetabulum. (*C*) A dislocated hip. The femur head is not engaged in the shallow acetabulum.

effectively into the acetabulum during intrauterine life, deepening the space. Involvement usually is unilateral (Keenan, 2000). Sociocultural methods of childrearing, such as the way infants are carried, may promote or decrease the extent of the involvement (see the Focus on Cultural Competence earlier in this chapter).

Assessment

Detecting developmental hip dysplasia in the newborn is important because the longer the condition goes undetected, the more difficult it is to correct. Sometimes the affected leg may appear slightly shorter than the normal one because the femur head rides so high in the socket. This is most noticeable when the child is lying supine and the thighs are flexed to a 90-degree angle toward the abdomen. One knee will appear to be lower than the other (Fig. 39-19*A*). An unequal number of skin folds may be present on the posterior thighs (see Fig. 39-19*B*). This finding is unreliable, however, because some infants with normal hips have an uneven number of posterior thigh skin folds. Subluxated or dislocated hips are best assessed by noting whether the hips abduct (see Nursing Procedure 39-1).

In some infants, the hip abducts properly at a newborn assessment, but at the time of the health maintenance visit at approximately age 4 to 6 weeks, a secondary shortening of the adductor muscles will have occurred, and the disorder will be evident. Hip dysplasia is difficult to detect at birth in an infant who was born from a footling or frank breech presentation because the knees are stiff and do not flex readily. Always assess hip function in these infants at each health maintenance visit. Tight adductor muscles occur in children with cerebral palsy, so this disorder must be ruled out. An x-ray, sonogram, or magnetic resonance imaging scan will reveal the shallow acetabulum and a more lateral placement of the femur head than is ordinarily seen.

Therapeutic Management

Correction of subluxated and dislocated hips involves positioning the hip into a flexed, abducted (externally rotated) position to press the femur head against the acetabulum and cause it to deepen its contour by the pressure. Splints, halters, or casts may be used. If the child is older, traction is used first to bring the femur head into good position with the acetabulum. The small number of children who do not achieve correction by these methods will have surgery and a pin inserted to stabilize the hip.

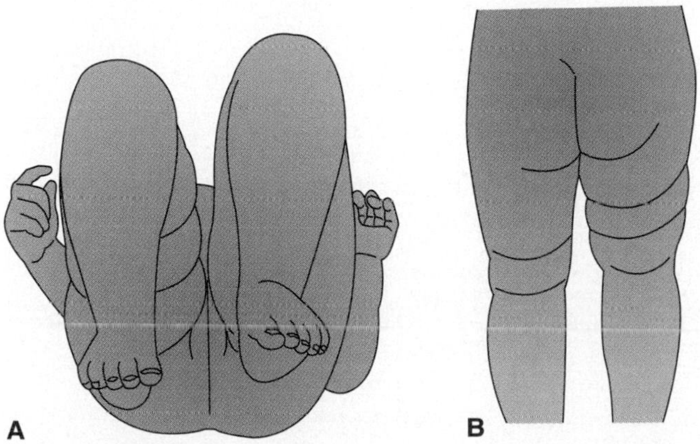

FIGURE 39.19 Signs of developmental dysplasia. (*A*) With child in a supine position, the right knee on the side of the subluxation appears lower than the left because of malposition of the femur head. (*B*) Asymmetry of skin folds and prominence of the trochanter on the right side.

NURSING DIAGNOSES AND RELATED INTERVENTIONS

Nursing Diagnosis: Deficient parental knowledge related to splint, halter, or cast correction for hip dysplasia

Outcome Identification: Parents will demonstrate increased knowledge of the care of the child in a splint, halter, or cast by discharge from the health care agency.

Outcome Evaluation: Parents verbalize correct technique for and correctly demonstrate application and removal of splint or halter device and care of device or cast.

Multiple Diapers or Splints. Often splint correction (to hold the legs in a frog-leg, or abducted, externally rotated position) is begun during the newborn's initial hospital stay by placing two or three diapers on the infant. The extra bulk of cloth between the child's legs effectively separates and spreads them. Many brands of disposable diapers are cut narrow between the legs; thus, they do not offer this much bulk and will not work as well as cloth diapers do.

A Frejka splint is made of plastic and buckles onto the child like a huge confining diaper (Fig. 39-20*A*). Parents need to keep the splint in place at all times, except when changing diapers or bathing the infant. Although firm pressure may be needed to abduct the hip to place the splint correctly, forcible abduction is to be avoided because this might compromise the blood supply to the leg or the femur head.

Having a splint in place continually can lead to a severe diaper rash. Remind parents of good diaper area care: change diapers frequently and wash the area with clear water after voiding or defecation, and apply an ointment such as A & D Ointment, Vaseline, or Desitin at each diaper change. Padding the edges of the brace with an additional diaper can increase comfort and decrease irritation. Teach parents to swaddle babies tightly because this action is comforting. Be certain, however, these parents understand that bringing the child's legs together with a tight swaddling blanket will not be good for their infant. Some Native American parents still use a swaddling board for their child. Be sure these parents know not to straighten the child's legs while swaddling with a board.

Pavlik Harness. A Pavlik harness is an adjustable chest halter that abducts the legs. It is the method of choice for long-term therapy because it reduces the time interval for therapy to 3 to 4 weeks and simplifies care (see Fig. 39-20*B*). Soft plastic stirrups (booties) with quick-fastening closures such as Velcro attach to leg extension straps and

NURSING PROCEDURE 39.1: ASSESSING ORTOLANI'S AND BARLOW'S SIGNS

Purpose

To assist in detecting developmental hip dysplasia

Procedure	Principle
1. Lay the infant supine and flex the knees to 90° at the hips.	1. Proper positioning ensures accurate results.
2. Place your middle fingers over the greater trochanter of the femur and your thumb on the internal side of the thigh over the lesser trochanter.	2. Placing your fingers in this way allows for abduction of the hips.

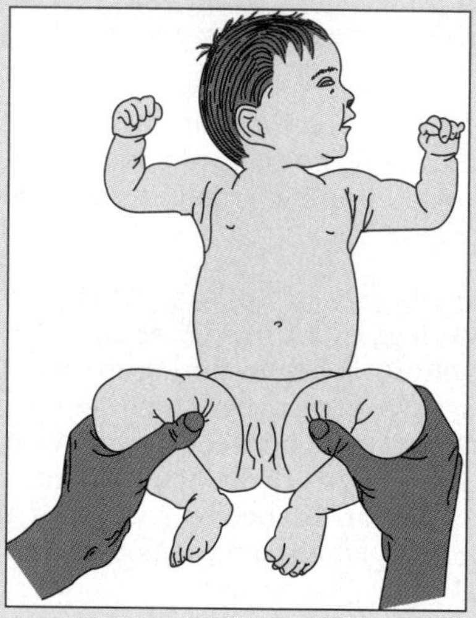

Procedure	Principle
3. Abduct the hips while applying upward pressure over the greater trochanter, and listen for a clicking sound.	3. Normally, no sound is heard. A clicking or clunking sound is a positive Ortolani's sign and occurs when the femoral head re-enters the acetabulum.
4. Next, with your fingers in the same position, and holding the hips and knees at 90° flexion, apply a backward pressure (down and laterally) and adduct the hips. Note any feeling of the femoral head slipping.	4. Normally, the hip joint is stable. A feeling of the femur head slipping out of the socket posterolaterally is a positive Barlow's sign indicative of hip instability associated with developmental hip dysplasia.

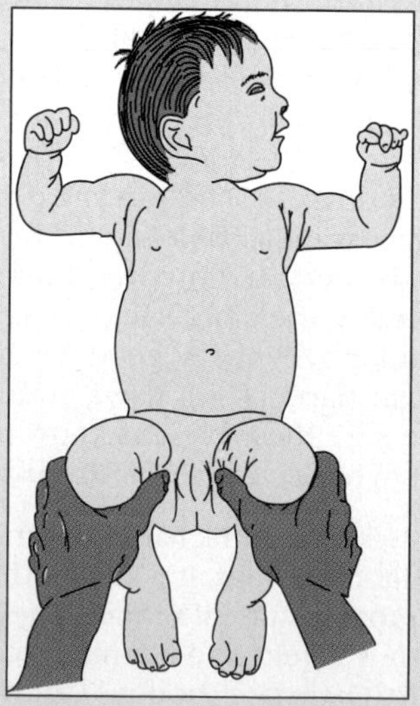

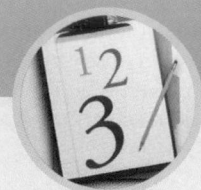

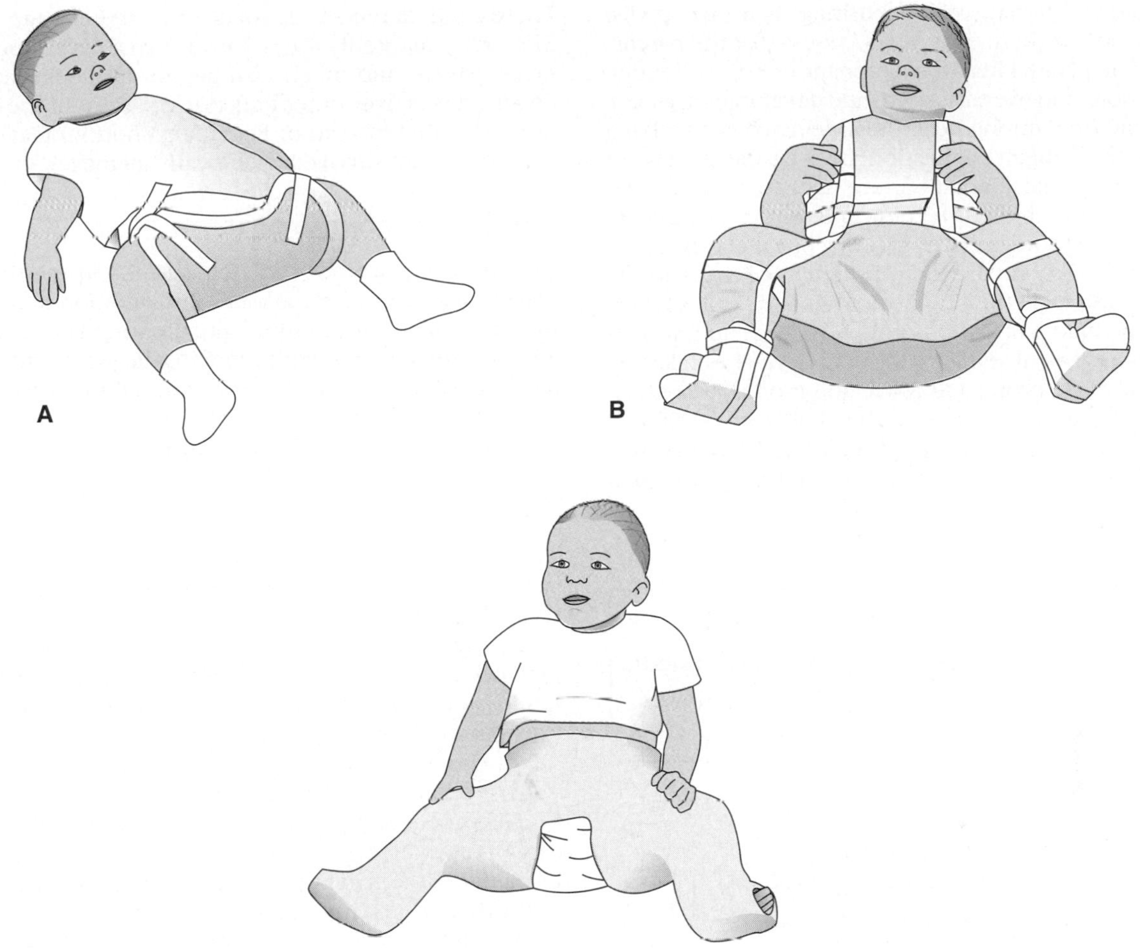

FIGURE 39.20 (*A*) Hip abduction splint (Frejka splint) holds the hips in an abduction position, forcing the femur head into the acetabulum. (*B*) A Pavlik harness. (*C*) A hip abduction cast for correction of subluxation of the hip.

hold the hips flexed, abducted, and externally rotated. Instruct parents to lie the infant supine, grasp the infant's thighs and abduct them to place the femoral head into the acetabulum, and then apply the harness. The harness is then worn continually except for bathing. Advise the parents to assess the skin under the straps daily for irritation or redness.

A Pavlik harness is advantageous because it does not show under a shirt and long trousers and promotes gentle reduction of the hip. However, if a hip is completely dislocated, a Pavlik harness may not be firm enough to hold the hips in the proper position. In addition, the harness will be ineffective if parents remove it more frequently than keeping it applied.

Spica Cast. If a hip is fully dislocated or the subluxation is severe, the infant may be placed immediately in a frog-leg cast or a spica cast to maintain an externally rotated hip position. The child may first be placed in Bryant's traction for a week to better position the hip. The hip is then placed in an abducted position and a large hip spica cast or an A-line cast is applied (see Fig. 39-20*C*). These casts are heavy and are so wide that dressing infants or sitting them in an infant car seat or bassinet can be difficult. Be certain parents have a car seat that can be modified to accommodate a large cast. Newborns are unable to report that a cast is causing circulatory constriction, so they need to be assessed hourly for circulation to the extremities for the first 24 hours the cast is in place and daily thereafter. Teach parents how to do this type of neurovascular assessment (check temperature and circulation in toes) before they take an infant home from the hospital so they can prevent circulatory compression from a rapidly growing limb outgrowing a cast. Casts will be changed but maintained for 6 to 9 months.

General Care Guidelines. No matter what type of therapy is used—double-diapering, splint, harness, or cast—surgery may still be necessary for a final correction. Making parents aware of this from the start prevents them from thinking that their child's condition is so serious that the usual methods of treatment failed. It helps them from becoming discouraged or dissatisfied with health care. It also helps them to accept from the beginning that this condition is a long-term care concern. Some children will be 2 years old before the final cast or harness is removed.

The child and parents will be visiting their orthopedist frequently during these early years. Assess that the parents also schedule general health maintenance visits for routine immunizations and overall growth and development assessment. Spend time during health maintenance visits talking with them about infant stimulation. Because the child is not fully mobile, special adaptations are necessary. Teach parents to hold their child for feeding and to rock and cuddle the infant, even though a large cast or a brace may be bulky and awkward. Teach parents to bring experiences to the infant because the child cannot crawl and walk toward interesting objects in the environment. A child's wagon makes for convenient and fun transportation. The child may also be able to lie prone and move about on a large skateboard. Many parents worry that the child who is still in a large cast at the normal age for walking (12 months) will never learn to walk. They can be assured that this is not a problem; when the cast is removed, the child will quickly catch up on this developmental step.

✔ **CHECKPOINT QUESTIONS**

17. How is developmental hip dysplasia best assessed?
18. To correct developmental hip dysplasia, how should the affected hip be positioned?

COMMON CHROMOSOMAL DISORDERS THAT RESULT IN PHYSICAL OR COGNITIVE DEVELOPMENTAL DISORDERS

A number of chromosomal disorders may be apparent at birth on physical assessment. The most common disorders revealed this way are nondisjunction syndromes. All have the potential to cause physical and cognitive challenges. (Care of the child who is cognitively challenged is discussed in Chap. 54.)

Trisomy 13 Syndrome

Trisomy 13 syndrome (Patau's syndrome; 47XX13+ or 47Xy13+) is a condition in which children have an extra chromosome 13. Children with this disorder are severely cognitively challenged. The incidence of this disorder is low, approximately 0.45 per 1,000 live births (Matthews, 1999). Common findings include midline disorders such as microcephaly with abnormalities of the forebrain and forehead; eyes that are smaller than normal (microphthalmia) or absent; cleft lip and palate; low-set ears; heart defects, particularly ventricular septal defects; and abnormal genitalia. Most of these children do not survive past early childhood.

Trisomy 18 Syndrome

Children with trisomy 18 syndrome (47XX18+ or 47Xy18+) have three number 18 chromosomes. They also are severely cognitively challenged. The incidence of this disorder is approximately 0.25 per 1,000 live births (Matthews, 1999). These children tend to be small for gestational age at birth. They have markedly low-set ears, a small jaw, congenital heart defects, and misshapen fingers and toes (the index finger crosses over other fingers). The soles of the feet are often rounded instead of flat (rocker-bottom feet). These children do not survive beyond early infancy.

Cri du Chat Syndrome

Cri du chat syndrome (46XX5q– or 46Xy5q–) is the result of a short arm on chromosome 5. In addition to an abnormal cry, which sounds more like the sound of a cat's than a human infant's cry, children with the syndrome tend to have a small head, wide-set eyes, and a downward slant to the palpebral fissure of the eye. They are severely cognitively challenged (Baird et al., 2001).

Turner's Syndrome

The child with Turner's syndrome (gonadal dysgenesis; 45XO) has only one functional X chromosome. The child is short. The hairline at the nape of the neck is low-set, and the neck may appear to be webbed and short. The newborn may have appreciable edema of the hands and feet and a number of congenital anomalies, most frequently coarctation (stricture) of the aorta and kidney disorders. The child has only streak (small and nonfunctional) gonads, so that with the exception of pubic hair, secondary sex characteristics do not develop at puberty. Females with this disorder cannot reproduce because of limited ovarian function. The incidence of the syndrome is approximately 1 per 1,000 live births (Ranke & Saenger, 2001).

Although children with Turner's syndrome may be cognitively challenged, more commonly intelligence is normal. Some children may have learning disabilities.

Growth hormone can be helpful to achieve additional height. If treatment with estrogen is begun at approximately 13 years, secondary sex characteristics will appear. If girls continue taking estrogen for 3 out of every 4 weeks, they will have withdrawal bleeding that results in a menstrual flow. This flow, however, does not correct the problem of sterility. The gonadal tissue is scant and inadequate for ovulation because of the basic chromosomal aberration.

Klinefelter's Syndrome

Infants with Klinefelter's syndrome are boys with an XXY chromosome pattern (47XXY) (Boone et al., 2001). The incidence is about 1 in 1,000 live births. Characteristics of the syndrome may not be noticeable at birth. At puberty, the child does not develop secondary sex characteristics. The testes are small and produce ineffective sperm. Boys with the disorder tend to develop gynecomastia (increased breast size). The syndrome may be associated with an increased risk of developing male breast cancer.

Fragile X Syndrome

Fragile X syndrome is an X-linked pattern of inheritance in which one long arm of an X chromosome is weakened. The incidence is about 1 in 1,000 live births. It is the most common cause of cognitive challenge in boys (Hagerman, 2000).

Before puberty, boys with fragile X syndrome typically have maladaptive behaviors such as hyperactivity and autism. They have reduced intellectual functioning, with marked deficits in speech and arithmetic. They may be identified by the presence of a large head, a long face with a high forehead, a prominent lower jaw, and large protruding ears. Hyperextensive joints and cardiac disorders may also be present. After puberty, enlarged testicles may become evident. Affected individuals are fertile and can reproduce.

Carrier females may show some evidence of the physical and cognitive characteristics. Although intellectual function of children with the syndrome cannot be improved, both folic acid and phenothiazine administration may improve symptoms of poor concentration and impulsivity.

Down Syndrome (Trisomy 21)

Trisomy 21 (47XX21+ or 47Xy21+), the most frequently occurring chromosomal abnormality, is seen as frequently as 1 in 800 live births. The syndrome occurs most frequently in the pregnancies of women who are over 35 years of age (the incidence is as high as 1 in 100 live births for these women). Paternal age (over 55) may also contribute to the increased incidence (Chung, 2000).

The physical features of children with Down syndrome are so marked that fetal diagnosis is possible by sonogram in utero. The nose is broad and flat, the eyelids have an extra fold of tissue at the inner canthus (an epicanthal fold), and the palpebral fissure (opening between the eyelids) tends to slant laterally upward. The iris of the eye may have white specks in it, called Brushfield's spots. Even in the newborn, the tongue may protrude from the mouth because the oral cavity is smaller than normal. The back of the head is flat; the neck is short, and an extra pad of fat at the base of the head causes the skin there to be so loose it can be lifted up (like a puppy's neck). The ears may be low-set. Muscle tone is poor, giving the baby a rag-doll appearance. This can be so lax that when the child lies supine, the child's toe can be touched against the nose (not possible in the average mature newborn). The fingers of many children with Down syndrome are short and thick, and the little finger is often curved inward. There may be a wide space between the first and second toes and the first and second fingers. The palm of the hand shows a peculiar crease (a simian line) or a horizontal palm crease rather than the normal three creases in the palm.

Children with Down syndrome usually have some degree of cognitive challenge, but the degree can range from that of less involvement (IQ 50 to 70) to one requiring total care (IQ less than 20). The degree of cognitive challenge is not evident at birth. Those with near-average IQs may represent mosaic chromosomal patterns. The fact that the brain is not developing well is shown by a head size that is generally under the 10th to 20th percentile.

In addition to the above difficulties, children with Down syndrome appear to have altered immune function, making them prone to upper respiratory infections. Congenital heart diseases, especially atrioventricular defects, stenosis or atresia of the duodenum, strabismus, and cataract disorders also are common. For unknown reasons, acute lymphocytic leukemia occurs approximately 20 times more frequently in children with Down syndrome than in the healthy population. Even if children are born without an accompanying disorder such as heart disease, their lifespan generally is only 50 to 60 years, as aging seems to occur faster than normally (Nehring & Vessey, 2000).

Children with Down syndrome need to be exposed to early educational and play opportunities (see Chap. 54). Because they are prone to infections, sensible precautions such as using good handwashing technique should always be taken when caring for them. The enlarged tongue may interfere with swallowing and cause choking unless the child is fed slowly.

As with all newborns, children with Down syndrome need physical examination at birth so that the genetic disorder can be detected and counseling and support for parents can begin.

✔ CHECKPOINT QUESTIONS

19. What feature of Turner's syndrome affects the child's reproductive capacity?
20. How are the muscles of children with Down syndrome typically characterized?

KEY POINTS

Learning about the way that a child will be physically challenged early on helps the parents and child adjust to it. Advocate for parents by helping them obtain as much information as they need about the condition.

Parent–infant bonding is often difficult to establish when the child is hospitalized at birth. Assess family relationships at health maintenance visits to see that bonding is occurring.

Cleft lip and palate result from the failure of the maxillary process to fuse in intrauterine life. Surgical repair is possible early in life, with a good prognosis for both these conditions.

Tracheoesophageal atresia and fistula occur from failure of the trachea and esophagus to divide appropriately in intrauterine life. Surgical intervention often needs to be completed in several procedures.

Omphalocele is the protrusion of abdominal contents through the abdominal wall at birth, protected only by a peritoneal membrane. When the membrane is not present, this is called gastroschisis. Although several stages of repair are often necessary, surgical correction has a good outcome.

Intestinal obstruction can result from atresia (complete closure) or stenosis (narrowing) of a part of the bowel. Correction is surgical removal of the narrowed bowel portion.

A meconium plug occurs when an extremely hard portion of meconium blocks the lumen of the intestine. Infants with meconium plug syndrome need to be observed for continuing bowel function and may have a sweat test done for cystic fibrosis, because a meconium plug is often a symptom of this.

Diaphragmatic hernia occurs when the abdominal organs protrude through a defect in the diaphragm into the chest cavity. This prevents the lungs from fully expanding at birth. These infants are critically ill at birth and need extensive surgical correction.

Imperforate anus is stricture of the anus, resulting in inability to pass stool. The infant may have a temporary colostomy done before a final surgical correction.

Physical developmental disorders of the nervous system include hydrocephalus (excess CSF in the ventricles) and spina bifida (incomplete closure of the spinal cord). Infants with hydrocephalus need surgery to relieve a ventricular obstruction or have a shunt implanted from their ventricles to the peritoneal cavity to remove excess CSF. Children with myelomeningocele, the most severe form of spinal cord defect, face permanent loss of lower neuron function that requires continued rehabilitation.

Absent or malformed extremities may range from absence of a finger to absence of an entire limb. Children may need physical therapy and teaching on how to use a prosthesis to have full function.

Developmental hip dysplasia is the improper formation and function of the hip socket; talipes deformities are foot and ankle deformities. Children may need extensive bracing and casting to correct these disorders.

Common nondisjunction genetic disorders that cause physical developmental concerns include Down syndrome (trisomy 21), trisomy 13 syndrome, trisomy 18 syndrome, Turner's syndrome, and Klinefelter's syndrome. Most of the children affected by these disorders are cognitively challenged.

CRITICAL THINKING EXERCISES

1. Mrs. Sparrow is the mother of the child with a diaphragmatic hernia you met at the beginning of the chapter. She asked you what caused the condition. Now she asks you why everyone is telling her that a diaphragmatic hernia is an emergency. She thought a simple hernia repair could be done later when the child is older. How would you explain this to her?
2. You are in the birthing room when a child with various developmental disorders, including an omphalocele and a cleft palate, is born. The neonatal nurse practitioner who examines the baby tells you she thinks the baby has trisomy 18 syndrome. The mother becomes upset when she is told the omphalocele repair will result in an abdominal scar because she wants her daughter to be a model when she grows up. How would you respond to the mother? Will her daughter be able to be this?
3. A newborn who has been diagnosed with a tracheoesophageal fistula is awaiting transport to an intensive care nursery. What assessments would be important? How would you explain this disorder to his parents? What position would you place the child in while awaiting transport?
4. You notice that the 16-year-old mother of a child born with a cleft lip is obviously upset at the child's appearance. She doesn't want to feed the baby and voices the thought of placing her for adoption. In contrast, the child's father, age 22, handles the baby warmly and asks questions about surgery. No grandparents visit. What interventions would you want to begin with this family?
5. Examine the National Health Goals related to physically challenged newborns. Most government-sponsored money for nursing research is allotted based on these goals. What would be a possible research topic to explore pertinent to these goals that would be fundable and would advance evidence-based practice?

REFERENCES

Baird, S. M., et al. (2001). Young children with Cri-du-chat: Genetic, developmental and behavioral profiles. *Infant-Toddler Intervention: The Transdisciplinary Journal, 11*(1), 1–14.

Bingham, P. M. (2000). Hydrocephalus. In Schwartz, M. W. (Ed.). *The 5-minute pediatric consult* (pp. 444–445). Philadelphia: Lippincott Williams & Wilkins.

Black, K. A., & Hylander, M. A. (2000). Breast-feeding the high-risk infant: Implications for midwifery management. *Journal of Midwifery & Women's Health, 45*(3), 238–245.

Blanchard, H., et al. (2000). Repair of the huge umbilical hernia in black children. *Journal of Pediatric Surgery, 35*(5), 696–698.

Boone, K. B., et al. (2001). Neuropsychological profiles of adults with Klinefelter syndrome. *Journal of the International Neuropsychological Society,* 7(4), 446–456.

Broggi, G., et al. (2000). Image-guided neuroendoscopy for third ventriculostomy. *Acta Neurochirurgica, 142*(8), 893–898.

Bromley, B., et al. (2000). Isolated polydactyly: Prenatal diagnosis and perinatal outcome. *Prenatal Diagnosis, 20*(11), 905–908.

Bustillo, M., & Kravitz R. M. (2000). Diaphragmatic hernia. In Schwartz, M. W. (Ed.). *The 5-minute pediatric consult* (pp. 324-325). Philadelphia: Lippincott Williams & Wilkins.

Carmin-Dillon, C. A., & Low, D. W. (2000). Cleft lip and palate. In Schwartz, M. W. (Ed.). *The 5-minute pediatric consult* (pp. 256–257). Philadelphia: Lippincott Williams & Wilkins.

Cheng, J. C., et al. (2001). Clinical determinants of the outcome of manual stretching in the treatment of congenital muscular torticollis in infants. *Journal of Bone & Joint Surgery, 83A*(5), 679–687.

Chung, E. K. (2000). Down (trisomy 21) syndrome. In Schwartz, M. W. (Ed.). *The 5-minute pediatric consult* (pp. 336–337). Philadelphia: Lippincott Williams & Wilkins.

Curtin, G. (2000). Cleft lip and palate. In Jackson, P. L., & Vessey, J. A. *Primary care of the child with a chronic condition* (3d ed., pp. 331–351). St. Louis: Mosby.

Davidson, R. S. (2000). Clubfoot. In Schwartz, M. W. (Ed.). *The 5-minute pediatric consult* (pp. 258–259). Philadelphia: Lippincott Williams & Wilkins.

Department of Health and Human Services. (2000). *Healthy people, 2010.* Washington, D.C.: DHHS.

Ding, Y., et al. (2001). Impaired motor learning in children with hydrocephalus. *Pediatric Neurosurgery, 34*(4), 182–189.

Dlugos, D. J. (2000). Neural tube defects. In Schwartz, M. W. (Ed.). *The 5-minute pediatric consult* (pp. 568–569). Philadelphia: Lippincott Williams & Wilkins.

Drake, J. M., et al. (2000). CSF shunts 50 years on: Past, present and future. *Child's Nervous System, 16*(10–11), 800–804.

Flores-Arroyo, H. L. (2000). Cystic fibrosis. In Schwartz, M. W. (Ed.). *The 5-minute pediatric consult* (pp. 304–305). Philadelphia: Lippincott Williams & Wilkins.

Fuloria, M. & Kreiter, S. (2002). The newborn evaluation. *American Family Physician, 65*(2), 265–270.

Hagerman, R. J. (2000). Fragile X syndrome. In Jackson, P. L., & Vessey, J. A. *Primary care of the child with a chronic condition* (3d ed., pp. 495–513). St. Louis: Mosby.

Harvey, J. & Lidder Jackson, P. (2000). Hydrocephalus. In Jackson, P. L., & Vessey, J. A. *Primary care of the child with a chronic condition* (3d ed., pp. 560–582). St. Louis: Mosby.

How, H. Y., et al. (2000). Is vaginal delivery preferable to elective cesarean delivery in fetuses with a known ventral wall defect? *American Journal of Obstetrics & Gynecology, 182*(6), 1527–1534.

Kanaka-Gantenbein, C. (2001). Present status of the use of growth hormone in short children with bone diseases. *Journal of Pediatric Endocrinology, 14*(1), 17–26.

Keenan, G. F. (2000). Developmental dysplasia of the hip. In Schwartz, M. W. (Ed.). *The 5-minute pediatric consult* (pp. 314–315). Philadelphia: Lippincott Williams & Wilkins.

Kitchanan, S., et al. (2000). Neonatal outcome of gastroschisis and exomphalos: A 10-year review. *Journal of Paediatrics & Child Health, 36*(5), 428–430.

Letcher-Glembo, L. (2000). Craniofacial disorders. In Nickel, R. E., & Desch, L. W. *The physician's guide to caring for children with disabilities and chronic conditions* (pp. 477–512). Baltimore: Paul H. Brooks Publishing Co.

Loffredo, L. C., et al. (2001). Oral clefts and vitamin supplementation. *Cleft Palate-Craniofacial Journal, 38*(1), 76–83.

Marentette, L. J., & Kim, J. Y. (2001). Correction of non-syndromal craniosynostosis. *Facial Plastic Surgery Clinics of North America, 9*(1), 93–99.

Matthews, A. L. (1999). Chromosomal abnormalities: Trisomy 18, trisomy 13, deletions, and microdeletions. *Journal of Perinatal & Neonatal Nursing, 13*(2), 59–75.

Molik, K. A., et al. (2001). Pectus excavatum repair: Experience with standard and minimal invasive techniques. *Journal of Pediatric Surgery, 36*(2), 324–328.

Mulberg, A. E. (2000). Intestinal obstruction. In Schwartz, M. W. (Ed.). *The 5-minute pediatric consult* (pp. 482–483). Philadelphia: Lippincott Williams & Wilkins.

Nehring, W. M., & Vessey, J. A. (2000). Down syndrome. In Jackson, P. L., & Vessey, J. A. *Primary care of the child with a chronic condition* (3d ed., pp 445–474). St. Louis: Mosby.

Nickel, R. E. (2000). Meningocele and related neural tube defects. In Nickel, R. E., & Desch, L. W. *The physician's guide to caring for children with disabilities and chronic conditions* (pp. 425–428). Baltimore: Paul H. Brooks Publishing Co.

Nicollas, R., et al. (2000). Congenital cysts and fistulas of the neck. *International Journal of Pediatric Otorhinolaryngology, 55*(2), 117–124.

Ranke, M. B., & Saenger, P. (2001). Turner's syndrome. *Lancet, 358*(9278), 309–314.

Rescorla, F. J. (2001). Surgical emergencies in the newborn. In Polin, R. A., Yoder, M. C., & Burg, F. D. *Workbook in practical neonatology* (3rd ed., pp. 423–459). Philadelphia: Saunders.

St-Hilaire, H., & Buchbinder, D. (2000). Maxillofacial pathology and management of Pierre Robin sequence. *Otolaryngologic Clinics of North America, 33*(6), 1241–1256.

Telega, G. (2000). Imperforate anus. In Schwartz, M. W. (Ed.). The 5-minute pediatric consult (pp. 466–467). Philadelphia: Lippincott Williams & Wilkins.

Tradati, N., et al. (2000). Papillary carcinoma in thyroglossal duct remnants. *Oncology Reports, 7*(6), 1349–1353.

Vanamo K. (2000). Silo reduction of giant omphalocele and gastroschisis utilizing continuous controlled pressure. *Pediatric Surgery International, 16*(7), 536–537.

Wright, J. D. (2000). Before the transport team arrives: Neonatal stabilization. *Journal of Perinatal & Neonatal Nursing, 13*(4), 87–107.

Yin, S. et al. (2001). Clinical application of botulinum toxin in otolaryngology, head and neck practice. *Journal of the Louisiana State Medical Society, 153*(2), 92–97.

Young, J. L. et al. (2001). What information do parents of newborns with cleft lip, palate or both want to know? *Cleft Palate/Craniofacial Journal, 38*(1), 55–58.

SUGGESTED READINGS

Bellah, R. (2001). Ultrasound in pediatric musculoskeletal disease: Techniques and applications. *Radiologic Clinics of North America, 39*(4), 597–618.

Cheng, J. C. et al. (2000). The clinical presentation and outcome of treatment of congenital muscular torticollis in infants. *Journal of Pediatric Surgery, 35*(7), 1091–1096.

Clemons, R. M. (2000). Issues in newborn care. *Primary Care, 27*(1), 251–267.

Del Bigio, M. R. (2001). Future directions for therapy of childhood hydrocephalus: A view from the laboratory. *Pediatric Neurosurgery, 34*(4), 172–181.

Enepekides, D. J. (2001). Management of congenital anomalies of the neck. *Facial Plastic Surgery Clinics of North America, 9*(1), 131–145.

Hubbard, A. M. (2001). Imaging of pediatric hip disorders. *Radiologic Clinics of North America, 39*(4), 721–732.

Johnston, I., & Teo, C. (2000). Disorders of CSF hydrodynamics. *Child's Nervous System, 16*(10–11), 776–799.

McCollough, M. & Sharieff, G. O. (2002). Common complaints in the first 30 days of life. *Emergency Medicine Clinics of North America, 20*(1), 27–48.

O'Connell, R., & Bradfield, L. (1999). Neonatal surgery: Are operating rooms always necessary? A practical guide to surgery within the NICU. *Journal of Neonatal Nursing, 5*(2), 8–12.

Reynolds, M. (2000). Abdominal wall defects in infants with very low birth weight. *Seminars in Pediatric Surgery, 9*(2), 88–90.

Saenger, P., et al. (2001). Recommendations for the diagnosis and management of Turner syndrome. *Journal of Clinical Endocrinology & Metabolism, 86*(7), 3061–3069.

Van Riper, M. (2000). Family variables associated with well-being in siblings of children with Down syndrome. *Journal of Family Nursing, 6*(3), 267–286.

CHAPTER 40

Nursing Care of the Child With a Respiratory Disorder

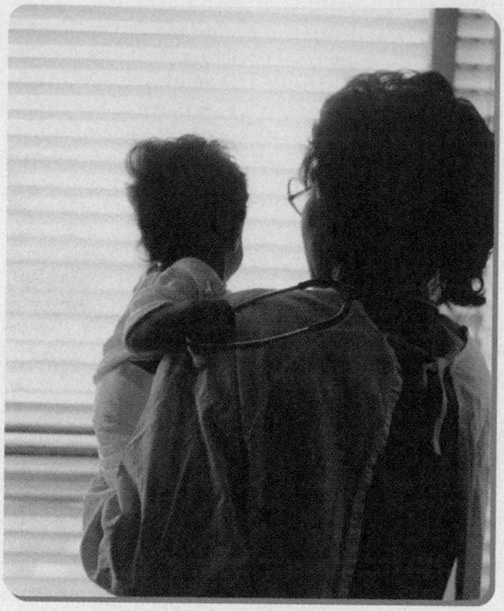

Key Terms

- adventitious sounds
- aspiration
- atelectasis
- crackles
- clubbing
- cyanosis
- expiration
- hypoxemia
- hypoxia
- inspiration
- paroxysmal coughing
- percussion
- pneumothorax
- rales
- retraction
- steatorrhea
- stridor
- tachypnea
- tracheostomy
- tracheotomy
- vibration
- wheezing

Objectives

After mastering the contents of this chapter, you should be able to:

1. Describe common respiratory illnesses in children.
2. Assess the child with a respiratory illness.
3. Formulate a nursing diagnosis related to respiratory illness in children.
4. Identify outcomes that address the priority needs of the child with a respiratory illness.
5. Plan nursing care for the child with a respiratory illness.
6. Implement nursing care for the child with a respiratory illness.
7. Evaluate outcomes for achievement and effectiveness of care.
8. Identify National Health Goals related to children with respiratory disorders that nurses could be instrumental in helping the nation achieve.
9. Identify areas related to care of children with respiratory disorders that could benefit from additional nursing research or application of evidence-based practice.
10. Use critical thinking to analyze ways that nursing care for a child with a respiratory illness could be more family-centered.
11. Integrate knowledge of respiratory illness in children with nursing process to achieve quality maternal and child health nursing care.

Michael is a 5-year-old who is seen in the emergency department. He was brought in by his nanny because he was coughing and obviously short of breath. He has such loud wheezing you can hear it without a stethoscope. "I can't breathe!" Michael shouts at you. "Help him!" the nanny shouts. "If he dies, everyone will say it's my fault!" What emergency care does Michael need? What about Michael's action would lead you to believe his airway is not yet completely obstructed?

Previous chapters described the growth and development of well children. This chapter adds information about the dramatic changes, both physical and psychosocial, that occur when children develop respiratory disorders. This is important information because it builds a base for care and health teaching.

After you've studied the chapter, answer the Critical Thinking Exercises at the end of the chapter and then access the on-line study activities (http://connection.lww.com) *to further sharpen your skills and test your knowledge.*

Respiratory disorders are among the most frequent causes of illness and hospitalization in children. Overall, respiratory dysfunction in children tends to be more serious than in adults because the lumens in the child's respiratory tract are smaller and therefore more likely to become obstructed with disease. Because respiratory disorders range from minor illnesses such as a simple upper respiratory tract infection to life-threatening lower respiratory tract diseases, such as pneumonia, and because the level of acuity can change quickly, respiratory disorders are often difficult for parents to evaluate. Both the child and parents need a great deal of nursing support when disease interferes with the function of breathing, because even very young children can panic when breathing becomes labored. Early diagnosis and treatment are essential in preventing a minor problem from turning into a more serious one.

Because respiratory disorders are such a frequent cause of childhood illness and hospitalization, National Health Goals have been established for children with respiratory illnesses. These are shown in the Focus on National Health Goals box.

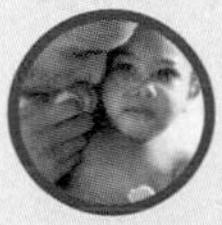

FOCUS ON NATIONAL HEALTH GOALS

A number of National Health Goals focus on respiratory illness in children:

- Reduce tobacco use by adolescents from a baseline of 35% to a target of 21%.
- Reduce invasive pneumococcal infections in children under age 5 years from a baseline of 76/100,000 to a target of 46/100,000.
- Reduce tuberculosis from a baseline of 6.8/100,000 cases yearly to a target level of 1.0/100,000.
- Reduce indoor allergen levels such as dust mites.
- Increase or maintain the number of territories or states that monitor diseases such as asthma that can be caused by exposure to environmental hazards from a baseline of 6 to 25.
- Reduce asthma deaths in children aged 5 to 14 years from a baseline of 3.3/million to a target level of 1.0/million.
- Reduce hospital emergency department visits for children with asthma under the age of 5 years from 150/10,000 to 80/10,000 (DHHS, 2000).

Nurses can be instrumental in helping the nation achieve these goals by teaching children to avoid beginning cigarette smoking, teaching programs to help children with asthma learn ways of increasing activity and steps to take to reduce the severity of an attack, and reminding parents to come for child health maintenance visits so that children can receive pneumococcal immunization or screening for tuberculosis as appropriate.

Additional nursing research is needed about the accuracy of parents in self-reading and interpreting tuberculosis screening tests; motivations for children to keep participating in asthma exercise programs; and information required by new parents to better manage respiratory illness in infants and young children.

NURSING PROCESS OVERVIEW

For the Child With a Respiratory Disorder

Assessment

Respiratory illness can begin at birth when a newborn has difficulty initiating a first breath or establishing regular respirations. Rating a newborn using the Apgar score can help to quickly identify the newborn who may be experiencing respiratory difficulty at this early stage.

As a nurse in a well-child clinic or health maintenance organization, you are often the first health care provider to talk to a parent about a child's respiratory illness. It is important to establish both the onset and duration of the problem so that its seriousness can be determined. Infants who cannot finish a bottle feeding because of exhaustion or rapid breathing or children who cannot run with other children because they do not have enough breath, for example, should be suspected of having a chronic respiratory disorder. An episode of acute coughing is suggestive of an acute respiratory disorder.

The child admitted to the hospital with a respiratory disorder is usually in an acute stage of the illness. The child's condition may worsen rapidly in the first few hours until a prescribed medication, such as an antibiotic or bronchodilator, begins to take effect. Nursing assessment that a child is developing tachypnea or retractions may be the first indication of a child's worsening condition.

Nursing Diagnosis

Nursing diagnoses established for the child with a respiratory disorder focus both on the alteration in mechanisms of breathing and on the emotional distress such problems can create. "Ineffective airway clearance" is a common diagnostic category used in this area. The problem may be related to any one of a variety of factors, such as ineffective cough, fatigue, weakness, viscous secretions, pain, aspiration of a foreign body, or lack of knowledge about the importance of coughing.

The diagnostic categories "Impaired gas exchange" and "Ineffective breathing pattern" also may be used, although because the nurse does not generally prescribe definitive treatment for these problems (except when caused by hyperventilation), it may be more appropriate for a nursing diagnosis to focus on the effects of impaired gas exchange or ineffective breathing on daily activities and psychosocial health (Carpenito, 2001). Additional nursing diagnoses include the following:

- Activity intolerance related to insufficient oxygenation
- Fatigue related to impaired gas exchange
- Fear related to inability to breathe without effort
- Impaired social interaction related to difficulty in keeping up with physical activities of peers
- Deficient knowledge related to need for continued treatment

Outcome Identification and Planning

If a child is experiencing an acute respiratory problem, the outcomes and plan of care will focus on supporting the child and family through prescribed therapy and keeping parents informed about their child's health status and response to treatment. Often the treatment period for respiratory illness is prolonged, so parents of children with chronic conditions need to learn how to continue therapy at home. Helping parents to plan programs of exercise and teaching chest physiotherapy and the actions of prescribed medications are important nursing activities. Parents also need to understand that their approach to these programs must change as their child grows older. With an infant, they simply need to perform the prescribed procedures. A game might be a good way to get a toddler or preschooler to perform a procedure ("Simon says, cough. Simon says, take five deep breaths"). Parents need to plan exercise programs for school-age children around the school day. Otherwise, parents may have difficulty carrying out the program or may be able to carry it out only sporadically. If they include other family members, such as older siblings (within reason) or grandparents, in a respiratory therapy program, this may help to diffuse the burden of care and also to unite the family in working toward a common goal.

Implementation

Collaborative nursing interventions in the care of the child with respiratory dysfunction include suctioning to remove respiratory secretions, administering oxygen, and providing humidification and expectorant therapy to help children maintain clear airways. Some of the most important nursing interventions in this area are independent nursing functions: placing a child in an upright position to help her cough more effectively; providing an interesting game to teach the child the importance of strengthening chest muscles; supporting a child and family through the anxiety created when a child is not breathing normally; and teaching parents of the child with chronic respiratory dysfunction the basics of percussion or chest physiotherapy techniques. All of these interventions require sound nursing judgment and skill.

Referring parents and children to community resources and organizations for support is also a key nursing function. Some organizations to recommend as support to parents of the child with a respiratory disorder include:

American Lung Association (*www.lungusa.org*)
National Easter Seal Society (*www.easter-seals.org*)
National Asthma Education and Prevention Program (*www.nhlbi.nih.gov*)
Asthma & Allergy Foundation of America (*www.aaga.org*)
Cystic Fibrosis Foundation (*www.cff.org*)

Outcome Evaluation

An acute respiratory illness such as pneumonia is extremely frightening for parents. After the child has recovered, talk with the parents to determine whether they have come to terms with their fear and are able to treat the child as a well child again. Otherwise, overprotection of the child by the parents may result in a well but dependent child. This pattern is one that nursing evaluation can help to prevent.

Outcomes for the child with chronic respiratory disease will change as the child grows and develops. No matter what the specific concerns are, however, evaluation should always include examination of how well the child individually and the family as a whole have adapted to managing the limitations imposed by the disorder while maintaining a lifestyle that fosters growth and development for all family members.

Examples indicating achievement of outcomes may include the following:

- Infant maintains respiratory rate of at least 20 breaths/min.
- Child describes a reduced program of school activities he will maintain to reduce fatigue.
- Child's Po_2 is maintained at 80 to 100 mm Hg in room air.
- Child lists steps she will take if breathing becomes impaired while at school.
- Parents demonstrate correct techniques for performing respiratory treatments at home.

ANATOMY AND PHYSIOLOGY OF THE RESPIRATORY SYSTEM

The respiratory system is usually separated into two divisions for discussion: the upper respiratory tract, composed of the nose, paranasal sinuses, pharynx, larynx, and epiglottis; and the lower tract, composed of the bronchi, bronchioles, and lungs. Through inspiration, the respiratory system delivers warmed and moistened air to the alveoli; transports oxygen across the alveolar membrane to hemoglobin-laden red blood cells; and allows carbon dioxide to diffuse from red blood cells back into the alveoli. Through expiration, carbon dioxide-filled air is discharged to the outside. Levels of oxygen and carbon dioxide in the lungs, blood, and body cells are shown in Figure 40-1.

The respiratory center is located in the medulla of the brain. Peripheral receptors located in the aortic arch and carotid arteries sense diminished Po_2 levels. Central respiratory receptors in the medulla sense increased Pco_2 levels along with body acidity, temperature, and blood pressure. An inhibitory center in the pons halts inspiratory impulses before the lungs become overextended. Depth of respiration is influenced by proprioceptors located in the lung periphery that register lung fullness. Often children with chronic lung disease such as cystic fibrosis have adapted so well to a chronically high Pco_2 level that central receptor sites no longer register this as abnormal. In these instances, the main stimulus for respiration is a low oxygen level. In such children, administering high levels of oxygen may be dangerous because it alleviates oxygen want and their main respiratory stimulus.

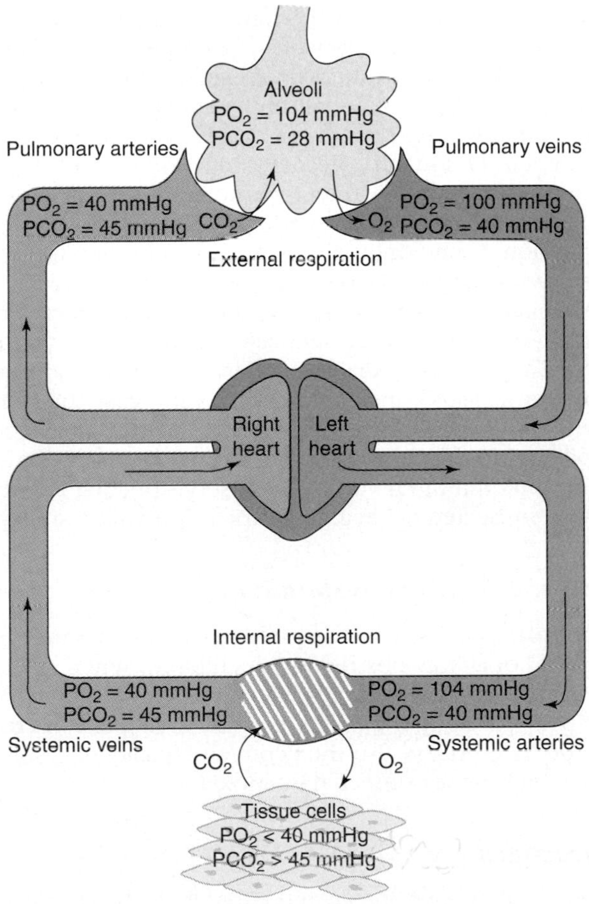

FIGURE 40.1 Partial pressure of gas (mm Hg) as measured in peripheral and systemic circulation. Because of the differences in partial pressure of the gases in the different areas, O_2 moves from alveoli to pulmonary capillaries (i.e., the gas moves from the area of greater concentration to one of a lesser concentration). When it reaches the tissue capillaries, O_2 partial pressure in cells is less, so O_2 goes into the tissues and CO_2 moves out.

Respiratory Tract Differences in Children

Embryologic development of the respiratory tract is discussed in Chapter 8. The ethmoidal and maxillary sinuses are present at birth; the frontal sinuses (those sinuses most frequently involved in sinus infection) and the sphenoidal sinuses do not develop until 6 to 8 years of age. Due to rapid growth of lymphoid tissue, tonsillar tissue is normally enlarged in early school-age children.

Respiratory mucus functions as a cleaning agent by moving invading organisms or other particles out of the lungs. However, newborns produce little respiratory mucus, which makes them more susceptible to respiratory infection than older children. Excessive production of mucus in children up to 2 years of age can readily lead to obstruction because the bronchial lumens are smaller in a child of this age.

After 2 years of age, the right bronchus is noticeably shorter, wider, and more vertical than the left. For this reason, inhaled foreign bodies more often lodge in the right bronchus. Infants use their abdominal muscles to inhale. The change to thoracic breathing begins at 2 to 3 years of age and is complete at 7 years. Because accessory muscles are used more in children than adults, weakness of these muscles from disease may more easily result in respiratory failure in children than in adults.

In infants, the walls of the airways have less cartilage than in older children and adults and thus are more likely to collapse after expiration. An advantage of immature development is that a lessened amount of smooth muscle in the airway means that an infant does not develop bronchospasm as readily as an older child or adult. Therefore, **wheezing** (the sound of air being pushed through constricted bronchioles) may not be a prominent finding in infants even when the lumen of the airway is severely compromised.

✔ CHECKPOINT QUESTIONS

1. Which sinuses do not develop until approximately age 6 years?
2. Where would you anticipate that an inhaled foreign body would lodge in a 4-year-old?

ASSESSING RESPIRATORY ILLNESS IN CHILDREN

Assessment of respiratory illness in children includes an interview, physical examination, and laboratory testing. If the child is in acute distress, the interview and health history may cover only the most important details: when the child first became ill and what symptoms are present. It is important, however, to get as accurate a picture as possible, because the problem could be the result of a variety of circumstances (see Assessing the Child for Signs and Symptoms of Respiratory Dysfunction).

Symptoms of **hypoxemia** (deficient oxygenation of the blood), for example, are often insidious. Peripheral vasoconstriction (a mechanism to save the available oxygen for central life-sustaining body organs) leads to a pale appearance. Tachypnea and tachycardia (efforts to oxygenate bet-

ASSESSING the Child for Signs and Symptoms of Respiratory Dysfunction

History

Chief concern: Cough, rapid respirations, noisy breathing, rhinitis, reddened sore throat, lethargy, cyanosis, difficulty sucking, fever.

Past medical history: Poor weight gain, difficulty with respirations at birth; prematurity.

Family history: History of family member with asthma; other family members with respiratory infection.

Physical examination

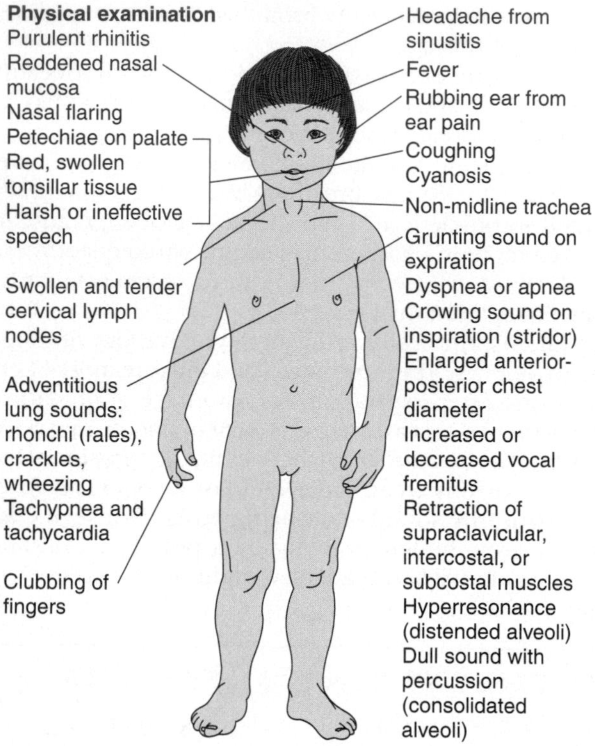

FOCUS ON CULTURAL COMPETENCE

Upper respiratory illnesses occur universally, making them a concern of parents the world over. Home remedies for such illnesses vary greatly, however. Hanging garlic around a child's neck is a frequent therapy in Mediterranean countries. "Cupping" or applying pressure to the back to "draw out" an infection (which leaves read circular ecchymotic marks on the child's back) also may be used. It is important to respect these remedies. Although the therapeutic value of these remedies may not be proven, it is important to the nurse–patient and nurse–family relationships to respect family traditions.

ter), anxiety, and confusion (caused by limited cerebral perfusion) may occur. A poor feeding pattern may be one of the first signs noted in the infant because an infant cannot suck and breathe rapidly at the same time. Cardiac arrhythmia may occur because of inadequate cardiac tissue perfusion.

Physical Assessment

Physical assessment of the child with a respiratory disorder includes observation of presenting symptoms such as cough, cyanosis, or pallor, as well as evaluation of respirations and lung sounds. While assessing the child, be alert for cultural factors such as home remedies that may have been used (see Focus on Cultural Competence). Lung sounds are best heard if an infant or child is not crying. Spending time comforting the child to stop crying is time well spent.

Cough

A cough reflex is initiated by stimulation of the nerves of the respiratory tract mucosa by the presence of dust, chemicals, mucus, or inflammation. The sound of coughing is caused by rapid expiration past the glottis. Coughing is a useful procedure to clear excess mucus or foreign bodies from the respiratory tract. It becomes harmful and needs suppression only when there is no mucus or debris to be expelled and the amount of coughing becomes exhausting. This might occur with respiratory tract inflammation. **Paroxysmal coughing** refers to series of expiratory coughs after a deep inspiration. Commonly, this occurs in children with pertussis (whooping cough) or those who have aspirated.

Although helpful in removing mucus, coughing increases chest pressure and may decrease venous return to the heart. This lowers cardiac output and can lead to fainting (syncope). Paroxysmal coughing may increase the pressure in the central venous circulation to such an extent that bleeding into the central nervous system results. Because young children often vomit after a series of coughs, they may be suspected of having a gastric disturbance initially.

Rate and Depth of Respirations

Tachypnea (an increased respiratory rate) often is the first indicator of airway obstruction in children. When assessing respiratory rate, particularly in infants, try to count the rate before waking the infant, because crying distorts respiratory rate. Assess also the depth and quality of respiration, which are also affected by anoxia.

Retractions

When children must inspire more forcefully than normally to inflate their lungs because of an airway obstruction or stiff, noncompliant lungs, such as that which occurs in newborns with pulmonary dysplasia, intrapleural pressure is decreased to the point that the nonrigid parts of the chest (the intercostal spaces) draw inward, creating **retractions** (Fig. 40-2). Retractions occur more often in the newborn and infant than in the older child because the intercostal

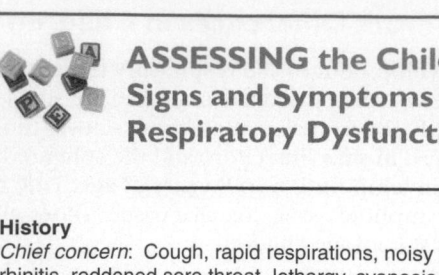

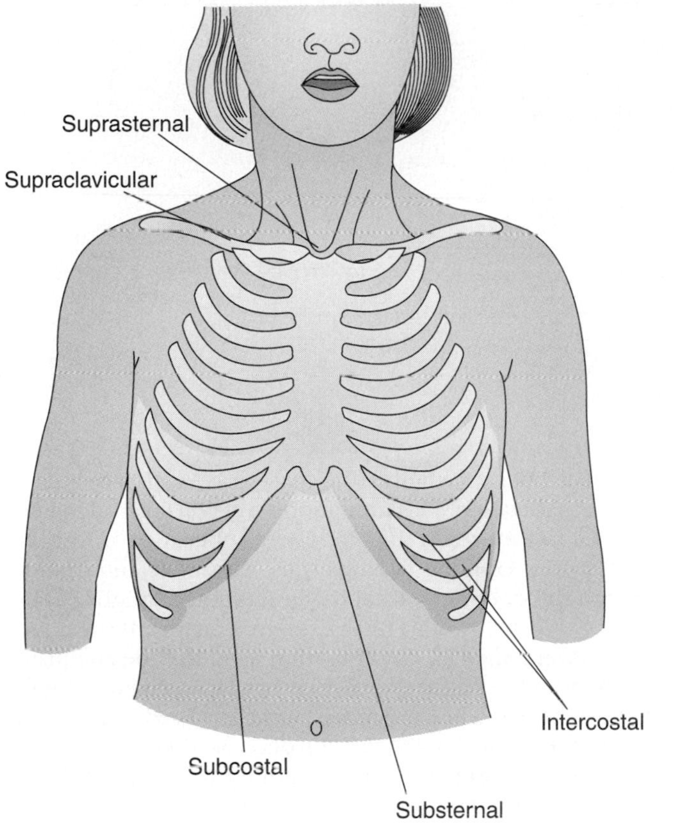

FIGURE 40.2 Sites of respiratory retraction.

tissues are weaker and less developed in the younger child. Retraction of upper chest muscles (supraclavicular or suprasternal) suggests upper airway obstruction; retraction of intercostal or subcostal muscles suggests lower airway obstruction.

Restlessness

When children or infants have difficulty securing adequate oxygenation (**hypoxia**), they become anxious and restless. In infants, restlessness coupled with tachypnea may be one of the first signs of airway obstruction. Be careful not to interpret the excessive movements of infants with respiratory distress as a sign that they are improving; anxious, restless stirring may be their only way of signaling that their respiratory obstruction is becoming acute.

Cyanosis

Cyanosis (a blue tinge to the skin) indicates hypoxia. It becomes apparent when the Po_2 is under 40 mm Hg or the level of unoxygenated hemoglobin increases to over 3 g/100 mL (because incompletely oxygenated red blood cells in the circulation are what give blood a dark color). If children have a low red blood cell count, cyanosis may not be apparent because there are not enough red blood cells to give the arterial blood its color. This occurs at hemoglobin levels below 5 g/100 mL. The degree of cyanosis present, therefore, is not always an accurate indication of the degree of airway difficulty.

As the Po_2 drops and cyanosis results, children increase their respiratory effort in an attempt to supply more oxygen to the tissues. When they do this, the difference in pressure between the intralumen of a not yet fully developed trachea and the surrounding tissue becomes so great that the trachea may collapse, compounding the obstruction problem. When children have accompanying peripheral vasoconstriction caused by shock, cyanosis of the extremities may or may not be apparent.

Clubbing of Fingers

Children with chronic respiratory illnesses often develop **clubbing** of the fingers, a change in the angle between the fingernail and nailbed because of increased capillary growth in the fingertips (Fig. 40-3). The increased capillary growth occurs as the body attempts to supply more oxygen routes (more capillaries) to distal body cells.

Adventitious Sounds

Normal breath sounds are reviewed in Chapter 33. **Adventitious sounds** (extra or abnormal breathing sounds) are caused by pathologic conditions and can be heard on lung assessment in children with respiratory disorders. On chest auscultation, the inspiratory sound is normally softer and longer than the expiratory sound. This is referred to as vesicular breathing. If you listen over the trachea, this pattern in terms of the length of **inspiration** (breathing in) and **expiration** (breathing out) is reversed. This is bronchial or tubular breathing. If you hear bronchial breath sounds in the periphery of the lungs, where normally you would expect to hear a vesicular pattern, it indicates that gas exchange in peripheral alveoli is being compromised (such as happens in pneumonia), and you are listening to transmitted tracheal sounds.

Accessory sounds of respiration result from the vibrations produced as air is forced past obstructions such as mucus. If the obstruction is in the nose or pharynx, the noise produced is a snoring sound (rhonchi). If the obstruction is at the base of the tongue or in the larynx, you will hear a harsh, strident sound on inspiration. This is laryngeal stridor. It is often most marked when the child is in a supine position and less marked when the child sits upright. If the obstruction is in the lower trachea or bronchioles, it is most noticeable on expiration; the sound that resembles a whistle (wheezing) is an expiratory sound. If the alveoli become fluid-filled, fine crackling sounds (**rales**) are heard. Diminished or absent breath sounds occur when the alveoli are so fluid-filled that little or no air can enter them.

Chest Diameters

With chronic obstructive lung disease, children may be unable to exhale completely, allowing air to be chronically trapped in lung alveoli (hyperinflation). This produces an elongated anteroposterior diameter, sometimes termed a pigeon breast. There is an accompanying tympanic or hyperresonant (loud and hollow) sound heard on percussion over lung spaces.

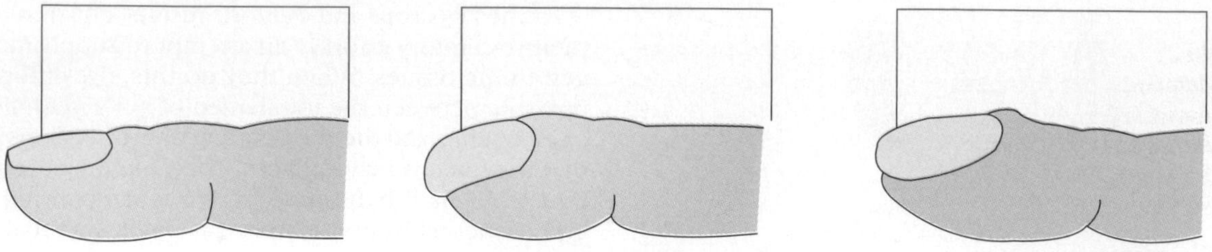

FIGURE 40.3 Clubbing of the fingers. (*Left*) The angle between the nail and digit is normally about 20 degrees in a child. (*Center*) Flattened angle represents early stage of clubbing. (*Right*) In advanced clubbing, the nail is rounded over the end of the finger. Note also that the distal phalanx is bulbous and of greater depth than the proximal portion of the finger (interphalangeal depth).

✔ CHECKPOINT QUESTIONS

3. What manifestation is often the first indication of airway obstruction?
4. When is wheezing usually heard?

Laboratory Tests

A number of laboratory tests can be used to confirm or rule out the presence of a respiratory problem and to help identify the cause and severity of the problem. These include analysis of arterial blood gases, nasopharyngeal culture, sputum analysis, and sweat chloride analysis. The sweat chloride test, which is used in the diagnosis of cystic fibrosis (CF), is discussed along with that disorder later in this chapter. The other tests are described in the following sections.

Blood Gas Analysis

Blood gas analysis is an invasive method for determining the effectiveness of ventilation and acid–base status. The normal values of arterial blood gases are shown in Table 40-1.

Blood gas analysis provides important information about oxygenation of the blood. Values may indicate not only whether the arterial partial pressure of oxygen (Po_2) is adequate but also whether the oxygen saturation of hemoglobin is adequate. This saturation level will fall if adequate oxygen cannot reach the bloodstream because of respiratory distress or if the hemoglobin is defective and cannot carry a full complement of oxygen (such as might occur with sickle cell anemia or thalassemia major). If the child has a severe anemia, the saturation level may be adequate (95% to 100%), but body cells may not be receiving enough oxygen because of the limited number of red blood cells present. With increased Pco_2 or decreased Po_2, a low pH, or decreased temperature, the ability of hemoglobin to accept oxygen diminishes.

Pco_2 measures the efficiency of ventilation. In children who are hypoventilating, it will be increased because they cannot blow off CO_2; in children who are hyperventilating, it will be decreased because they are blowing off too much. When children cannot evacuate accumulated CO_2 because of an obstruction or hypoventilation, the partial pressure of CO_2 in the arterial blood rises as the concentration of carbonic acid (formed when carbon dioxide dissolves in plasma) rises. This leads to acidosis (a decrease in serum pH or an increase in acidity).

If respiratory distress is incomplete, the body can compensate for developing acidity for a long time by increasing kidney tubular reabsorption of bicarbonate. When respiratory distress is relieved (by removal of an obstruction or by assisted ventilation), the amount of bicarbonate present

TABLE 40.1 Blood Gas Values

MEASURE	DEFINITION	NORMAL VALUE	CLINICAL SIGNIFICANCE
Po_2	Partial pressure of oxygen in arterial blood	80–100 mm Hg	Decreased if child cannot inspire adequately
Pco_2	Partial pressure of carbon dioxide in arterial blood	35–45 mm Hg	Increased if child cannot expire adequately
O_2 saturation	The percentage of hemoglobin carrying oxygen	95%–100%	Decreased if O_2 cannot reach red blood cells, if unoxygenated cells are being mixed with oxygenated ones, or if hemoglobin is defective
pH	The hydrogen ion concentration of blood	7.35–7.45	Decreased if CO_2 is being retained as carbonic acid in blood
HCO_3	The bicarbonate concentration in blood	22–26 mEq/L	Decreased in compensated respiratory alkalosis; increased in respiratory alkalosis
Base excess	Bicarbonate available for buffering	−2.5 or +2.5 mEq/L	(+) = alkaline excess (−) = alkaline deficit

in the bloodstream may exceed the amount of acid produced, and the child's condition may change to alkalosis. With alkalosis, the respiratory rate decreases as a means to conserve CO_2. As a result, periods of apnea may occur. Children require close observation during this time, including frequent blood gas and electrolyte determinations to ensure prompt treatment to reverse these changes when they occur. Respiratory alkalosis and respiratory acidosis are compared in Table 40-2. Box 40-1 shows steps for evaluating arterial blood gases.

To analyze blood gases, arterial blood rather than venous blood must be used (arterial blood will reflect how well the lungs are oxygenating the blood, whereas venous blood will reflect only the metabolism of the particular extremity from which the blood was drawn). In the young infant, the temporal artery may be used as a site; in newborns, an umbilical artery catheter can be used. In older children, the radial artery is the site of choice because of the collateral circulation present at the wrist. (If clotting should occur in the radial artery, the hand would still be well nourished by collateral circulation; see the Allen test in Box 40-2.)

For an arterial blood gas assessment, a specimen is withdrawn into a heparinized syringe (to prevent clotting). After any arterial puncture, always firmly compress the site. Otherwise, blood from the punctured vessel can seep into subcutaneous tissue, possibly causing a large hematoma and obscuring the site for further assessment. If frequent specimen collections are required, an arterial catheter, inserted either peripherally or centrally, may be used. Doing so allows frequent specimen collections without the trauma of additional punctures. Be sure to apply dressings over the area where an arterial catheter exits the skin to help prevent a young child from fussing or playing with the site. Soft restraints, such as an elbow or hand restraint, may be needed to keep the child from dislodging the catheter.

In small infants, when it is impossible to obtain arterial blood directly, heel or finger sticks may be used. If the heel or finger is warmed for about 20 minutes in warm water before the procedure, local blood flow increases so much that the blood gas levels of the capillaries approach those of arteries (Bell & Oh, 1999).

Be certain to note the use of oxygen, if any, and its liter flow on laboratory slips for arterial blood gas assessments. Also include a notation about the site from which the specimen was obtained. While they are being transported to the laboratory, arterial blood gas specimens should be kept on ice to ensure accurate results (CO_2 levels decline in room air).

The oxygen saturation of hemoglobin also can be obtained noninvasively using pulse oximetry and transcutaneous oxygen monitoring.

Pulse Oximetry. Pulse oximetry is a continuous, noninvasive technique for measuring oxygen saturation. For the measurement, a sensor and a photodetector are placed around a vascular bed, most often a finger in a child or a foot in an infant (Fig. 40-4). Infrared light is directed through the finger from the sensor to the photodetector. Because hemoglobin absorbs light waves differently when it is bound to oxygen than when it is not, the oximeter can detect the degree of oxygen saturation (Sao_2) in the hemoglobin.

Oxygen saturation is closely aligned with Po_2 (Fig. 40-5). When Sao_2 is 95%, the Po_2 is within the normal range of 80 to 100 mm Hg. When Sao_2 has fallen to 90%, the Po_2 is 60 mm Hg. An easy rule to remember concerning the relationship between Sao_2 and Po_2 is the 60 to 30, 90 to 60 rule: when Sao_2 is 60, Po_2 is 30; when Sao_2 is 90, Po_2 is 60. Any reading under 90, therefore, is cause for concern.

An advantage of pulse oximetry is that it is noninvasive. A second advantage is that the continuous monitoring provided by a pulse oximeter allows you to modify your care appropriately. If an oxygen level should begin to fall while you are handling an infant, for example, you could immediately stop care until the infant's Po_2 again returns to normal. A disadvantage is that the sensor is small and must be checked frequently to see that it remains in place. Excess light in a room may distort the reading. Therefore, the sensor may need to be covered with a blanket in a neonatal

TABLE 40.2 Comparison of Respiratory Alkalosis and Respiratory Acidosis

ACID–BASE CONDITION	CAUSE	FINDINGS
Respiratory alkalosis	Hyperventilation	Rapid, deep breathing Confusion, unconsciousness Elevated plasma pH (above 7.45) Elevated urine pH (above 7) Decreased Pco_2 (below 40 mm Hg) Plasma bicarbonate –Initially normal –Compensated: below 20 mEq/L Base excess: 0 or a negative reading such as −4
Respiratory acidosis	Hypoventilation trapping carbon dioxide in alveoli	Shallow breathing; inability to expire freely Confusion, disorientation Decreased plasma pH (below 7.35) Decreased urine pH (below 6) Elevated Pco_2 (over 40 mm Hg) Plasma bicarbonate –Initially normal –Compensated: above 25 mEq/L Base excess: 0 or a positive reading such as +4

BOX 40.1

QUICK ASSESSMENT OF ABGs

Use a systematic format to assess ABGs quickly:

1. Evaluate the pH: Normally, pH falls between 7.35 and 7.45. A pH below 7.35 denotes acidemia; one above 7.45 reflects alkalemia. If the patient has more than one acid-base imbalance at work, the pH identifies the process in control.
2. Evaluate PCO_2: The partial pressure of arterial CO_2 (PCO_2) normally ranges between 35 and 45 mm Hg. A PCO_2 greater than 45 mm Hg indicates ventilatory failure and respiratory acidosis from CO_2 accumulation. A PCO_2 less than 35 mm Hg indicates alveolar hyperventilation and respiratory alkalosis.
3. Evaluate HCO_3: A bicarbonate (HCO_3^-) less than 22 mEq/L or a base excess (BE) less than −2 mEq/L denotes metabolic acidosis. A bicarbonate level greater than 26 mEq/L or a BE greater than 2 mEq/L reflects metabolic alkalosis. If the two measurements conflict, the BE is the better indicator of metabolic status.
4. Determine which is the primary and which is the compensating disorder: Often, two acid-base imbalances coincide; one is primary, the other is the body's attempt to return the pH to normal. When both the PCO_2 and the HCO_3^- are abnormal, one denotes the primary acid-base disorder and the other denotes the compensating disorder.
   a. To decide which is which, check the pH. *Only a process of acidosis can make the pH acidic; only a process of alkalosis can make the pH alkaline.* For example, if steps 2 and 3 indicate that the patient has respiratory acidosis and metabolic alkalosis and the pH is 7.25, the primary disorder must be respiratory acidosis. The remaining disorder is compensating for the primary problem.
   b. When pH rises (becomes alkalotic), PCO_2 decreases in amount (will be below 35 mm Hg). When pH decreases (becomes acidotic), PCO_2 increases (will be above 45 mm Hg). When an opposite problem exists this way (pH increased; PCO_2 decreased), the problem is respiratory in origin.
   c. pH and HCO_3 normally move in the same direction (when pH is elevated, HCO_3 is elevated). When these two measurements correspond this way (pH decreased, HCO_3 decreased), then the cause of the problem is metabolic in origin.
   d. Three states of compensation are possible: *noncompensation,* reflected in an alteration of only PCO_2 or HCO_3^-; *partial compensation,* in which both PCO_2 and HCO_3^- are abnormal and, because compensation is incomplete, the pH is also abnormal; and *complete compensation,* in which both PCO_2 and HCO_3^- are abnormal but, because compensation is complete, the pH is normal. To identify the primary disorder when compensation is complete, consider a pH between 7.35 and 7.40 indicative of primary acidosis and a pH between 7.40 and 7.45 indicative of primary alkalosis.
5. Evaluate oxygenation: Normally PO_2 remains between 80 and 100 mm Hg. A PO_2 between 60 and 80 mm Hg reflects mild hypoxemia; between 40 and 60 mm Hg, moderate hypoxemia; and below 40 mm Hg, severe hypoxemia.
6. Interpret the findings: Your final analysis should include the degree of compensation, the primary disorder, and the oxygenation status; for example, "partially compensated respiratory acidosis with moderate hypoxemia."

BOX 40.2

ALLEN TEST

Before obtaining an ABG from the radial artery, it is important to establish that the child has collateral circulation to the hand. Otherwise, the needle puncture may block the artery and block blood flow to the hand.

To prove that there is collateral circulation, compress both the radial and ulnar arteries on the inner side of the wrist and elevate the hand until color disappears. Release the pressure over the ulnar artery and observe for a color change in the hand. If the hand does not pinken (proof the blood has flowed into the hand), the radial artery on that wrist should not be used for catheter insertion.

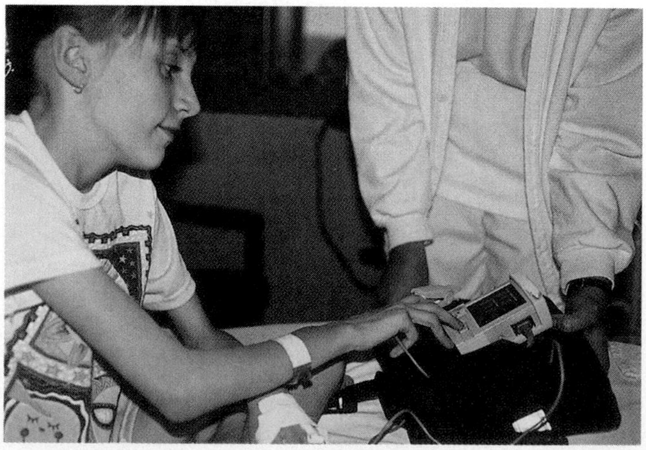

FIGURE 40.4 The older school-aged child participates in her care by checking her oxygen saturation level.

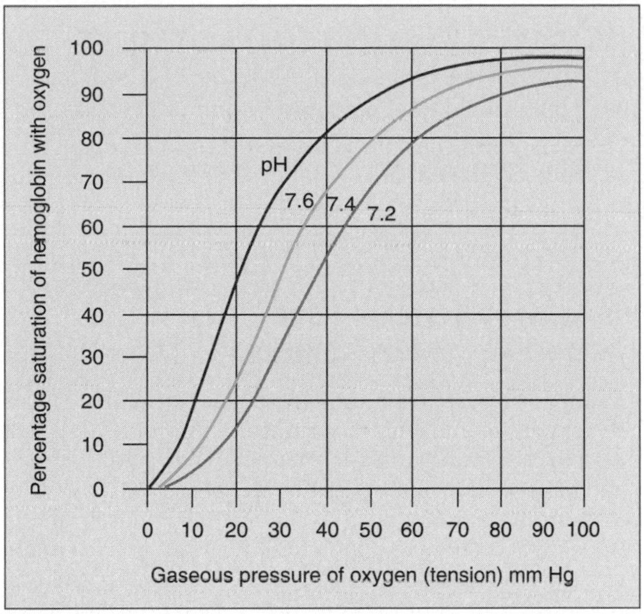

FIGURE 40.5 Oxyhemoglobin dissociation curve.

intensive care unit or brightly lit nursery for readings to be accurate. Young children also tend to remove the sensors just as they frequently remove adhesive bandages from their fingers.

Transcutaneous Oxygen Monitoring. Transcutaneous monitoring is another means of continuous, noninvasive measurement of oxygen saturation. For the determination, electrodes heated to 44°C are attached to an infant's chest. The heat causes vasodilation underneath the skin and brings the peripheral arterial blood to the surface to be read for oxygen content. This is converted to mm Hg for a monitor readout. The oxygen saturation level read by this method correlates with intra-arterial Po_2, the same as with pulse oximetry. Transcutaneous monitoring has a disadvantage compared with pulse oximetry because the probe position needs to be changed every 3 to 4 hours to prevent a burn to the skin, and sensor recalibration is necessary with each position change.

Nasopharyngeal Culture

When done efficiently, nasopharyngeal cultures cause little discomfort. However, most children are terribly frightened by having something placed in their noses or throats and may resist accordingly. Firm, calm support during the procedure is essential. Nose and throat cultures can reveal only the organisms present in the upper respiratory tract. As a result, they may not show organisms causing a lower respiratory tract infection. A throat culture will miss pathogenic organisms if the culture tip is not touched to the infected aspect of the pharynx.

Respiratory Syncytial Virus Nasal Washings

Nasal washings are obtained to diagnose an infection by the respiratory syncytial virus (RSV). For this, the child is placed in the supine position, and 1 to 2 mL sterile normal saline is dropped with a sterile needleless syringe into one nostril. The nose is then aspirated using a small, sterile bulb syringe. The secretions removed are placed in a sterile container to be sent to the laboratory for analysis. Nasal washings are even more uncomfortable for children than nasal swabbing and are potentially frightening because of the saline that is instilled. Provide comfort to the child afterward and assure the child the specimen collection is over.

Sputum Analysis

Because they cannot raise sputum with a cough, sputum collection is rarely feasible in children younger than school age. Older children, however, are able to cough and raise sputum. Teach them exactly what you want (a specimen of what they are coughing up, not just clearing from the back of their throat) and then ask them to breathe in and out several times and then cough deeply.

Diagnostic Procedures

A number of diagnostic procedures commonly are used to identify respiratory disorders in children. Many of these procedures are also used with adults, with modifications to account for the physical and developmental differences of children. Bronchoscopy (visualization of the bronchi through a bronchoscope) is discussed in Chapter 36. Radiologic examination (chest x-ray and bronchography) and pulmonary function testing are discussed in the following sections.

Chest X-Ray

Chest x-ray films will show areas of infiltration or consolidation in the lungs; if a foreign body is opaque, an x-ray study will show its location. Chest x-ray films are more difficult to obtain in infants than in older children, because infants cannot take a breath and hold it when instructed. It is therefore difficult to picture the lungs at their most expanded position. Computed tomography (CT) scans may be ordered for children with chronic lung disease because this technique can best mark disease progress.

Bronchography

On a chest radiograph, the air-filled larynx, trachea, and major bronchi are revealed. Any obstruction or distortion in the organs will be apparent. For further definition of structures, a radiopaque solution may be introduced into the respiratory tract by an ultrasonic nebulizer or by a catheter inserted into the trachea before the x-ray study is performed. Children may require conscious sedation for this because nebulization can be frightening. Afterward, children may have an increase in mucus production from bronchial irritation by the procedure. Observe them carefully after such a procedure for possible respiratory obstruction from accumulating mucus.

Pulmonary Function Studies

The process of ventilation, or the work of breathing, involves three main forces: (1) an inertial force that must be overcome to change the speed and direction of air when the lungs change from exhalation to inhalation, or vice versa; (2) an elastic force to help the lungs expand with inhalation and "snap back" with exhalation; and (3) the flow resistance force or resistance to the movement of air through the bronchial tree that must be overcome. Flow resistance must be at a minimum for best ventilation. It becomes increased when the bronchioles are narrowed or plugged with mucus. Pulmonary function tests measure the forces of inertia, elasticity, and flow resistance.

The alveoli of the lungs are never completely empty at the end of expiration because the bronchioles collapse, trapping air in the alveoli. In contrast, alveoli are never completely filled on inspiration because their potential for expansion exceeds that necessary for good respiratory function. Children with obstructive lung diseases such as asthma or cystic fibrosis have some difficulty moving air into the lungs, but they have even more difficulty moving air out of the lungs. Even if they can expire the same amount of air as the average child, they will expire it over a longer period. Children with restrictive ventilatory disorders, such as neuromuscular disorders, will have equal difficulty with inspiration and expiration.

A number of lung capacity studies can be done to determine the degree of obstruction or restricted ventilation ability. For these studies, the child breathes into a spirometer, a device that records air exchange, or a computerized vital capacity chamber.

Children younger than 4 years of age are usually unable to participate in pulmonary function tests because these tests require their cooperation. All children need good preparation and teaching for these tests because they must breathe forcefully through the mouth into a mouthpiece on cue. Some tests require that the nose be closed by a clamp or clip or an assistant's hand while the child blows out. This can be a frightening feeling for children with respiratory disease. They may need some trial runs to assure themselves that they can breathe with the clamp in place. Without good orientation to the equipment, they may become so anxious about their performance that they may develop tachypnea or fail to inhale or exhale at their full capacity, thus skewing the test results.

Common pulmonary function tests are outlined in Table 40-3. The results of pulmonary function studies help determine the nature and extent of a child's respiratory problem and the best methods for achieving more effective ventilation.

✔ CHECKPOINT QUESTIONS

5. What are two noninvasive methods used for measuring oxyhemoglobin saturation?
6. What term is used to denote the amount of air inhaled and exhaled in a normal respiratory movement?

HEALTH PROMOTION AND RISK MANAGEMENT

A number of ways to promote respiratory health are available for parents and children. The common cold is the most common respiratory disorder seen in children. Children as young as toddlers can be taught to help avoid spreading colds through their family by washing their hands, properly disposing of tissues, and covering the mouth while coughing. These measures need to be stressed again with school-age children to help prevent them from contracting or spreading germs through their schoolroom. The incidence of *Haemophilus influenzae* type B, the cause of bronchiolitis, can be reduced by ensuring that children receive their routine immunizations against this (HIB vaccine). Children with chronic respiratory illnesses also should receive the pneumococcal vaccine and a yearly influenza vaccine. Parents of the child with asthma can take major steps to reduce exacerbations by environmental control. Reducing respiratory irritation by reducing secondary smoke can help prevent asthma, upper respiratory infections, and otitis media.

THERAPEUTIC TECHNIQUES USED IN THE TREATMENT OF RESPIRATORY ILLNESS IN CHILDREN

The primary goal of nursing interventions in the care of children with respiratory disorders is to maintain or reestablish the airway to help ensure adequate oxygen to the blood. Often this includes interventions aimed at liquefying and removing mucus secretions so they do not clog the bronchial pathways. Such clogging prevents adequate oxygenation and contributes to the development of bronchial and alveolar infections.

TABLE 40.3 Pulmonary Function Tests

TEST	MEASUREMENT	CLINICAL IMPLICATIONS
Vital capacity (VC)	The maximum amount of air expelled after a maximum inspiration	Decreased if bronchial lumens are narrowed or obstructed
Tidal volume (TV)	The amount of air inhaled and exhaled in a normal respiratory movement	Decreased if bronchial lumens are constricted
Residual volume	The amount of air remaining in the lungs after a maximum expiration	Increased if there is air trapping in alveoli, as in obstructive lung disease
Functional residual capacity (FRC)	The volume of air remaining in the lungs after a normal expiration	Increased if ability to breathe out is impaired
Forced expiratory volume (FEV)	The amount of air expired in 1 sec	Decreased in obstructive disease that prevents free expiration

Expectorant Therapy

Any irritation of the respiratory tract causes the production of large amounts of mucus. The amount produced can become so great that the natural mechanisms for clearing it (coughing and upward cilia action) are no longer adequate. If a child is breathing rapidly because of respiratory distress, the frequent passage of air over the mucus tends to dry it and make it more viscid, compounding the removal problem (Ford, 2001). A number of measures may be employed to liquefy and raise mucus.

Liquefying Agents

Pharmacologic agents (expectorants) such as guaifenesin (Robitussin), given orally, are designed to liquefy mucus in the trachea and bronchi. Instilling saline nose drops or using saline nasal sprays can be effective in moistening and loosening dried mucus in the nose.

Humidification

Humidification is the provision of moisture to the airway. Common methods of delivering moisture include vaporizers and nebulizers.

Vaporizers. Vaporizers emit a stream of air moistened by fine droplets of water into a room, providing either a cool or a warm mist to the entire room. Caution parents when using warm mist that a serious scald burn can result if children accidentally pull a vaporizer over on themselves. To avoid this type of accident, they should be certain the vaporizer is never placed within reach of the child. Although cool mist can create a clammy atmosphere in a room, this can be advantageous for the child who also has a fever, helping to cool and moisten the whole environment. Caution parents to clean vaporizers thoroughly after use to prevent the growth of *Pseudomonas* or other organisms.

Nebulizers. Nebulizers are mechanical devices that provide a stream of moistened air directly into the respiratory tract. Most are hand-held masks that fit over the nose and mouth and are attached to an electrical pump as a power source (Fig. 40-6). Ultrasonic nebulization delivers such minuscule droplets into the respiratory tract that even the smallest bronchioles can be moistened. Nebulizers also serve as an important means for the delivery of respiratory tract medications. Drugs such as antibiotics or bronchodilators can be combined with the nebulized mist.

Many children find nebulizer treatments uncomfortable because the feeling of the mist in their upper respiratory tract can be frightening or irritating. Assure them that aerosol administration is the most effective route for moisture and medication to reach and cause an effect in the respiratory tract.

During aerosol medication administration, watch carefully for signs of both local tracheal or bronchial effect (spasm or edema) that might result from airway irritation and systemic symptoms that might result from absorption of a medication by the membrane.

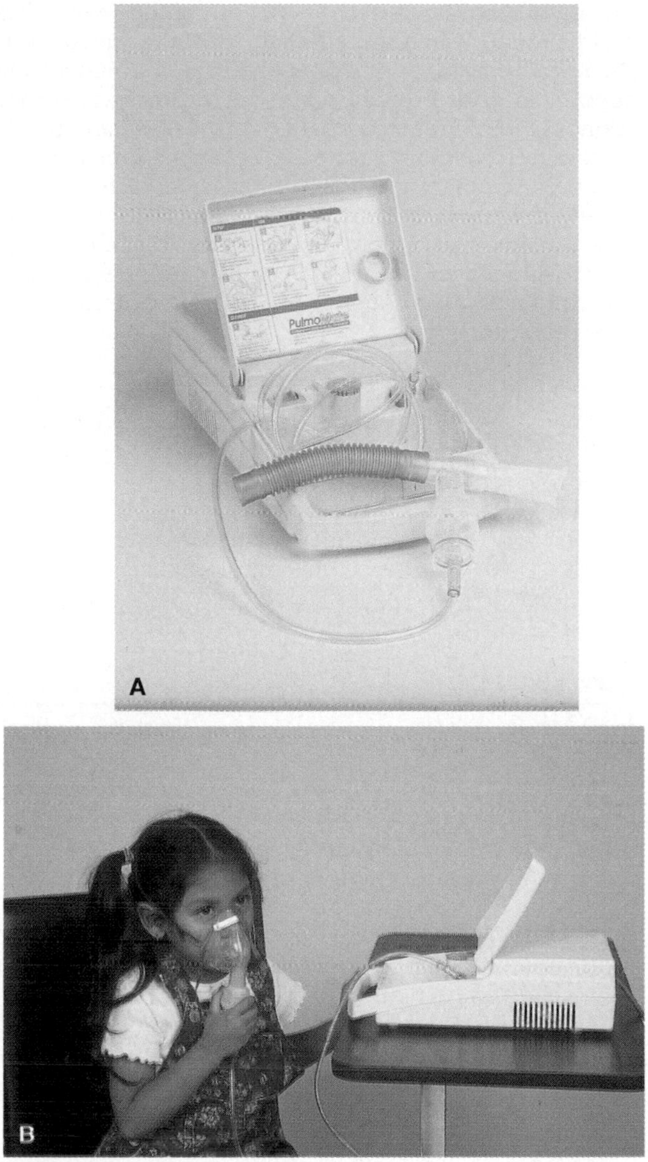

FIGURE 40.6 (A) Ultrasonic nebulizer. (B) Child using a nebulizer.

Coughing

As a rule, encourage coughing rather than suppressing it in children because it is an effective method of raising mucus. Changing a child's position and suggesting mild exercise and deep breathing are helpful techniques to initiate coughing. If a cough is caused by mucus dripping from the nose because of nasal congestion, a decongestant such as pseudoephedrine (Sudafed) will best halt the draining mucus and therefore the cough. Caution parents not to give adult cough syrups to children. A number of these contain codeine in doses too great for children.

Chest Physiotherapy

Simply changing a child's position helps mucus to move, initiate a cough reflex, and be expelled. When the child is positioned so the chest is lower than the abdomen, gravity aids in the removal of mucus from the lower lobes and bronchi. When the child sits upright, gravity aids drainage from the upper lobes and bronchi. When lying supine, anterior bronchi drain; when prone, posterior bronchi drain. Frequent changes of position are important, therefore, to prevent pools of mucus from forming in a certain lung area. If a child has a localized mucus problem, lying predominantly in one position can encourage drainage of that lung segment. When the child is repositioned and the mucus drains into new bronchi, the child will often cough from irritation caused by this new drainage.

Three techniques are involved with chest physiotherapy (CPT) to loosen mucus for expectoration: postural drainage, percussion, and vibration. Each technique can be used alone, but they are usually more effective at moving mucus toward the mainstem bronchus when performed together.

CPT is best scheduled before meals or at least an hour after a meal so that the subsequent coughing does not cause vomiting. Techniques are summarized in Nursing Procedure 40-1 and described below. Limit CPT to approximately 30 minutes each time, because these techniques can be tiring. Modifications in the techniques or shorten-

NURSING PROCEDURE 40.1: CHEST PHYSIOTHERAPY

Purpose

To encourage the loosening and raising of mucus from the respiratory tract through the use of postural gravity drainage and percussion (clapping) and vibrating techniques.

Procedure	Principle
1. Wash your hands; identify child; explain procedure to child.	1. Handwashing prevents spread of microorganisms. Explaining the procedure beforehand promotes child's understanding and compliance and helps to minimize anxiety.
2. Assess child as to status; analyze appropriateness of procedure; modify plan as necessary.	2. Chest physiotherapy is physically exhausting; can increase intracranial pressure when head is lowered in dependent position. Wait 1 h after meals to avoid inducing vomiting with coughing.
3. Assemble supplies: pillow or slant board, disposable tissues (sputum cup if specimen for culture is desired); percussion device (if infant); nebulizer with correct fluid and medicine if prescribed.	3. Organizing care increases efficiency and helps prevent tiring child. Nebulization before postural drainage may be prescribed to promote bronchodilation, dilute mucus, and aid mobility of secretions.
4. Select a drainage position (see Fig. 40-7). Position child appropriately but comfortably. Auscultate and percuss lung area for baseline determinations.	4. Positions aid in the gravity drainage of secretions.
5. Use percussion and clapping technique (see figure) for 1–2 min and vibrate during 4 or 5 exhalations the section of chest indicated for the position. Observe child closely for respiratory distress. 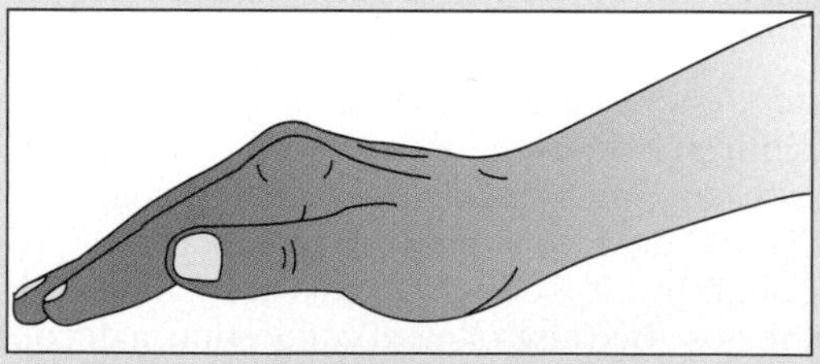	5. Percussion and vibration loosen bronchial mucus and allow it to be coughed from the respiratory tract. As mucus moves, it may plug a bronchus; observe for cyanosis, tachypnea, dyspnea, and violent coughing as signs of this.
6. Ask child to deep breathe and cough to raise secretions. Auscultate lung section to ascertain clearing of secretions.	6. Coughing also helps move secretions.
7. Reposition; percuss and vibrate the chest areas in additional drainage positions as prescribed. Continue to observe for signs of respiratory distress. Provide rest as necessary between positions.	7. Position changes allow for loosening and drainage in other lung segments. Child may grow tired after repeated percussion/vibration.

(continued)

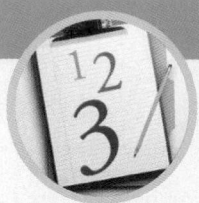

Procedure	Principle
8. At finish of prescribed positions, return child to bed. Provide mouthwash if desired (and age-appropriate); discard used tissues.	8. Coughed sputum may taste unpleasant. Use standard precautions to avoid touching soiled tissues.
9. Evaluate effectiveness, cost, comfort, and safety of procedure. Plan health teaching as necessary, such as benefits of procedure.	9. Evaluation allows for determining effectiveness of the procedure and need for modifications for future treatments. Health teaching is an independent nursing action always included in nursing care.
10. Record procedure, description of sputum raised, and child's reaction to procedure. If sputum specimen is obtained, send to laboratory for analysis.	10. Documentation provides evidence of nursing care, child's status, and effectiveness of interventions.

ing of the time periods may be necessary, depending on the child's ability to tolerate the position changes and the techniques.

Common postural drainage positions for the infant are shown in Figure 40-7. An infant may be positioned on your lap, whereas a slant board or other surface is needed for postural drainage with an older child. Not all positions are tolerated well. Be ready to modify the positions used depending on the child's condition and tolerance.

Use a cupped or curved palm against the chest to perform **percussion** (cupping). This technique causes a loud, thumping noise that sounds as if it hurts, but you can assure parents that it does not. In infants and some small children, a specialized device, a nipple, or a small oxygen mask may be used (Fig. 40-8). These devices concentrate the motion and may increase the amount of mucus removed.

Vibration is done by pressing a vibrating hand against a child's chest during exhalation. Like percussion, it mechanically loosens and helps move tenacious secretions upward. Vibration also may be accomplished by a mechanical vibrator or a vibrating vest.

Position the child so that the lobe of the lung to be drained is in a superior position. Because percussing or vibrating is exhausting, the child may not have all lobes drained at each session. For example, before breakfast, the upper right and the left upper and lower lobes might be done; before lunch, the right lower lobe and right middle lobe might be done; before supper or at bedtime, the upper and lower lobe on both sides might be done.

After each position, ask the child to cough. Children cough best if you demonstrate the proper technique by taking a deep breath, blowing it out, taking a deep breath, blowing that out, taking a deep breath, and coughing. The irritation of mucus in the major airway by the third breath makes a cough happen almost spontaneously.

Formerly, CPT was done in hospital settings by respiratory therapists. However, in today's health care climate of managed care, nurses are now often required to both perform CPT and teach it to parents. One or both parents may need to learn the technique before their child is discharged so that it can be continued at home.

WHAT IF? What if a preschooler refuses to cough? How could you get him to cough?

Mucus-Clearing Device

A mucus-clearing device (a Flutter device) can be used to aid in the removal of mucus. This device looks like a small plastic pipe. A stainless-steel ball inside the device moves when the child breathes out, causing vibrations in the lungs (Fig. 40-9). This vibration helps loosen mucus so that it can be moved up the airway and expectorated. This device is used most frequently with children who have cystic fibrosis to help remove mucus from the lungs.

Therapy to Improve Oxygenation

Oxygen Administration

Oxygen administration elevates the arterial saturation level by supplying more oxygen to the respiratory tract. Oxygen may be delivered to infants by flooding an isolette or by using a plastic hood. Plastic oxygen hoods are tight-fitting enclosures that can keep oxygen concentration at nearly 100% (Fig. 40-10). Check that the hood fits snugly over the infant's head, making sure that it does not rub against the infant's neck, chin, or shoulders. Be sure that the gas does not blow directly into the infant's face.

A nasal catheter or nasal prongs can be used for older children. These provide a concentration of approximately 50% with an oxygen flow of 4 L/min. Most children do not like nasal prongs because they are intrusive. Assess their nostrils carefully when using prongs. The pressure of prongs can cause areas of necrosis, particularly on the nasal septum.

A snug-fitting oxygen mask is another method for supplying nearly 100% oxygen (Fig. 40-11). However, masks are often not well tolerated by children. If necessary, let them hold a mask rather than strapping it in place to allow them more control.

Regardless of the delivery method used, oxygen must be administered warmed and moistened. Without proper humidification, oxygen dries mucous membranes and thickens secretions. Oxygen, like any other drug, requires careful administration and follow-up assessment. If concentrations are too low, oxygen is not therapeutic; in concentrations greater than those desired, oxygen can be toxic. If newborns are subjected to oxygen concentrations over 100 mm Hg for an extended time, retinopathy of prematurity can occur (see Chap. 26). In any child, administering

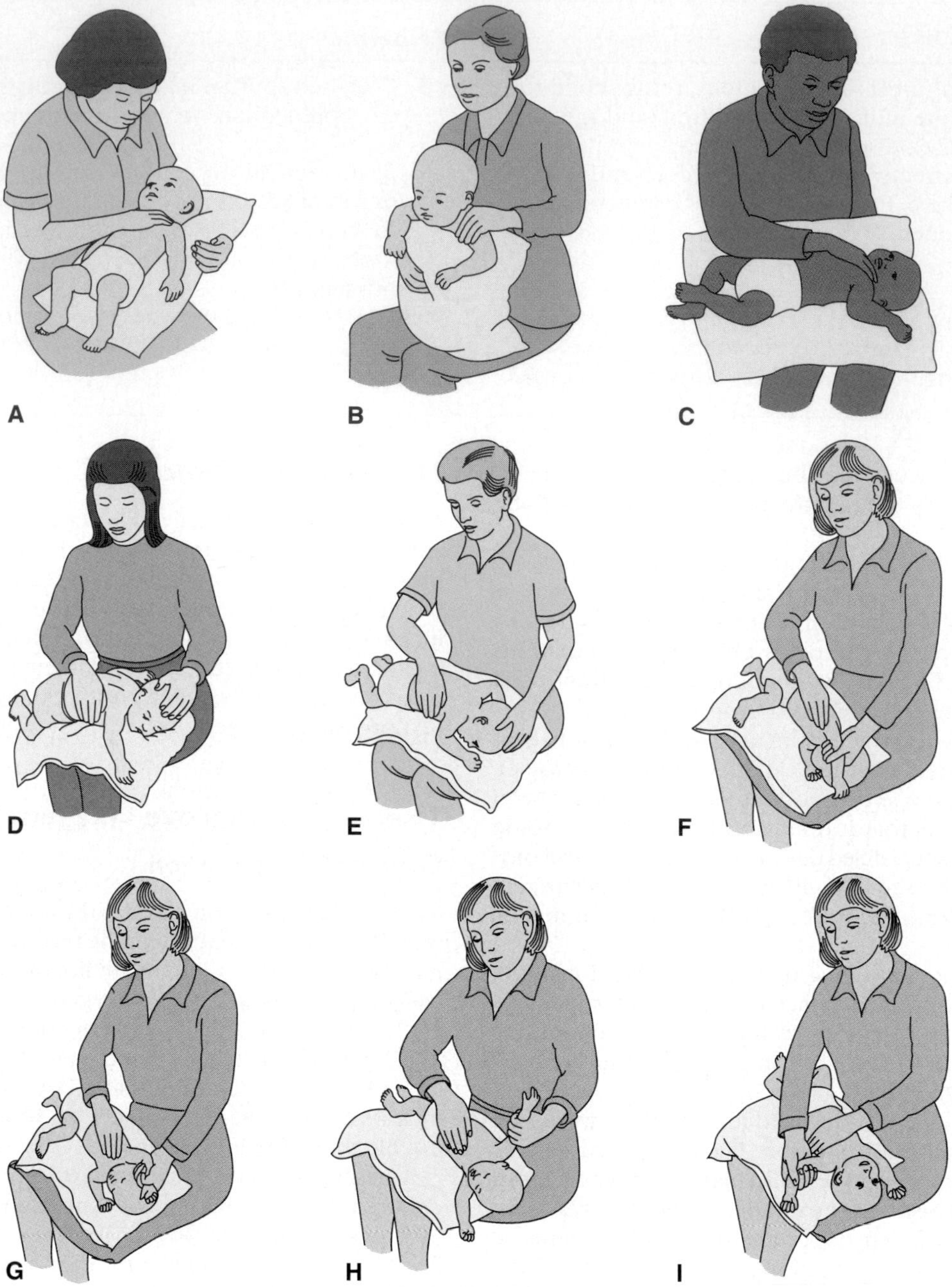

FIGURE 40.7 Positions for bronchial drainage for major segments of all lobes in infants. This procedure is most readily performed with the infant in your lap, with your hand on the chest over the area to be cupped or vibrated. (*A*) Apical segment of left upper lobe. (*B*) Posterior segment of left upper lobe. (*C*) Anterior segment of left upper lobe. (*D*) Superior segment of right lower lobe. (*E*) Posterior basal segment of right lower lobe. (*F*) Lateral basal segment of right lower lobe. (*G*) Anterior basal segment of right lower lobe. (*H*) Medial and lateral segments of right middle lobe. (*I*) Lingular segments (superior and inferior) of left upper lobe.

oxygen concentrations of 70% to 80% for an extended period may lead to a thickening of the lung alveoli and a loss of lung pliancy (oxygen toxicity or bronchopulmonary dysplasia). For these reasons, oxygen should not be given in high concentrations for long periods unless adequate facilities for blood gas analysis are available.

When caring for any child with any form of oxygen equipment, be sure that you follow good safety rules. Because oxygen supports combustion, keep open flames away from oxygen and minimize the risks of sparks. Since oxygen is humidified, oxygen equipment is a good source of microbial contaminants. Change equipment according to your agency's policy, but at least once a week to keep bacterial counts within safe limits. Monitor and record the child's oxygen saturation level via pulse oximetry or transcutaneous pulse oximetry as indicated. Be sure to obtain arterial blood gas measurements with any change in condition or oxygen flow (see Focus on Multidisciplinary Care).

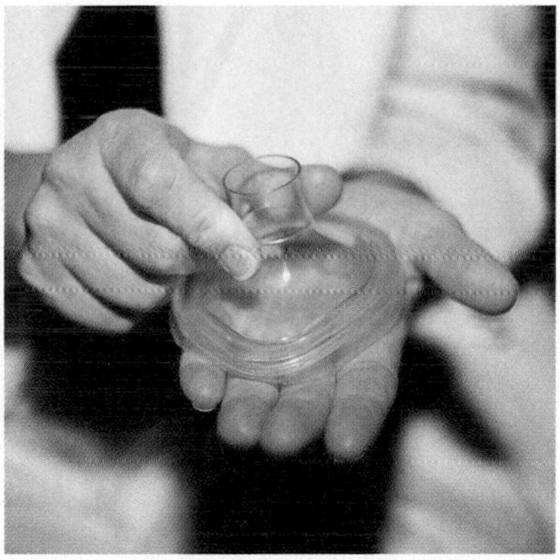

FIGURE 40.8 Alternative percussion device. To assist with percussing an infant or small child, a nipple or mask such as that from a manual resuscitation bag may be used.

Pharmacologic Therapy

Children notice difficulty with exchange of air when the airway becomes obstructed because of unusual mucus production, bronchoconstriction, or inflammation. A number of drugs may be used in children to reverse these processes. Nasal sprays such as normal saline can be administered to moisten and loosen nasal secretions. Antihistamines given by this route can reduce mucus production and thereby enlarge the airway. Decongestants cause vasoconstriction, leading to shrinkage of the mucous membranes. Expectorants such as guaifenesin (Robitussin) help to raise mucus. Most of these agents also cause drowsiness, so the dose must be regulated, especially in adolescents who will be driving automobiles. Bronchodilators such as albuterol (Ventolin), terbutaline (Brethine), and levalbuterol (Xopenex) are used to open the lower airway. Antibiotics may be given intravenously, intramuscularly, orally, or inhaled through nebulization to reduce infection and limit purulent mucus and inflammation. Corticosteroids taken either orally or by inhalation enlarge the airway by reducing further inflammation.

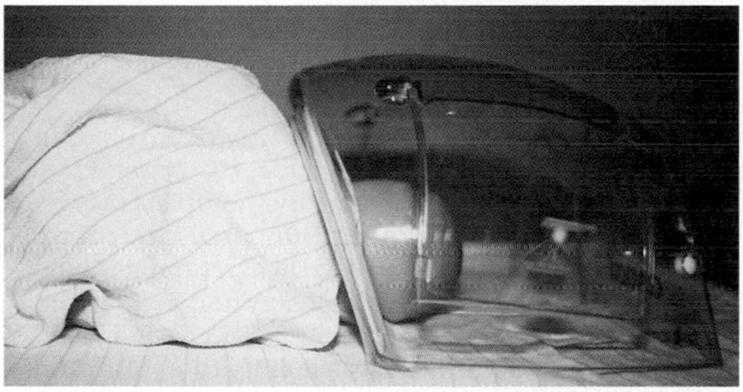

FIGURE 40.10 Oxygen hood for an infant.

Metered-Dose Inhalers. A metered-dose inhaler (MDI) is a hand-held device that provides a route for medication administration directly to the respiratory tract. The child inhales while pressing a trigger on the apparatus. Small children may need a spacer device attached to the apparatus, a plastic extension tube or chamber that helps better coordinate inhalation with the medication delivery. For successful use, children need to follow these six general rules: shake the canister, exhale deeply, activate the inhaler as they begin to inhale, take a long slow inhalation, and

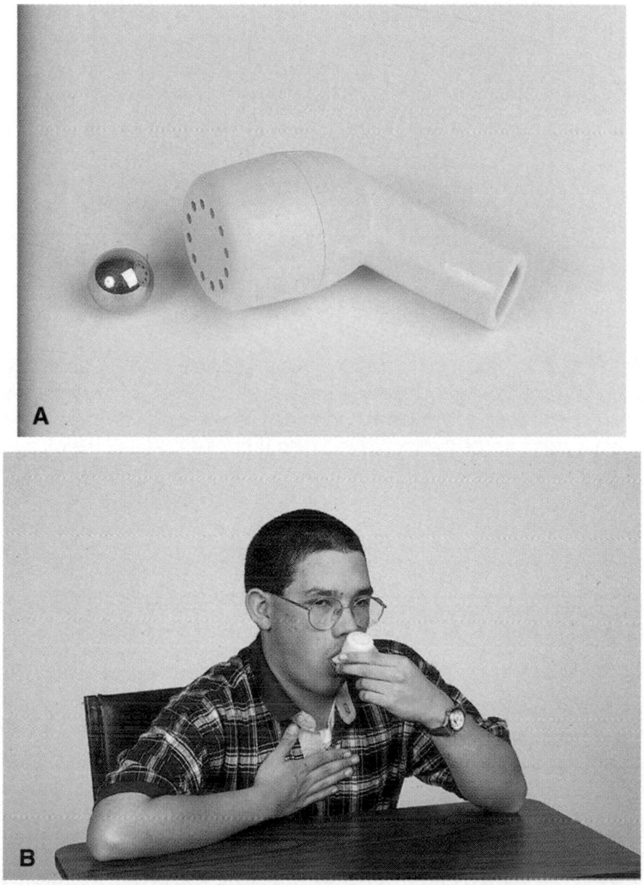

FIGURE 40.9 (*A*) Flutter device. The metal ball (shown) is enclosed in the chamber and causes the vibration. (*B*) Adolescent using flutter device.

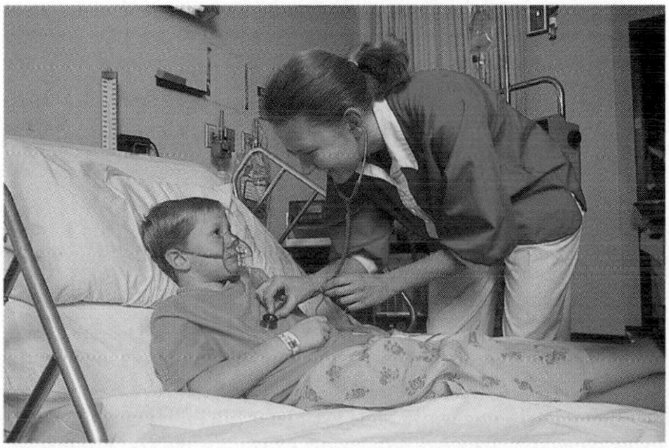

FIGURE 40.11 A nurse assesses a child's lungs while he receives oxygen therapy via a mask.

FOCUS ON MULTIDISCIPLINARY CARE

Numerous health care personnel may be involved in caring for children with respiratory disorders. Physical, occupational, or respiratory therapists may be involved in performing chest physiotherapy. Nutritionists may be directly involved in determining liquid oral feedings or total parenteral nutrition for children who experience respiratory distress when eating solid food. Respiratory therapists can help to explain and set up oxygen administration systems. Thorough communication among all involved is key.

When oxygen is being used, review oxygen safety measures with all disciplines involved and reinforce the concept that oxygen supports combustion. Providing a birthday cake with lit candles, for example, might seem like a nice idea but could be very hazardous, even fatal, because of the risk for an explosion.

When unlicensed assistive personnel give care, be certain they understand the importance of not allowing a child with a respiratory disorder to grow fatigued during care. Instruct them in the need to maintain oxygen therapy as ordered and to watch oxygen saturation levels (if pulse oximetry is attached), reporting any changes in oxygen saturation levels below specified values.

then hold their breath for 5 to 10 seconds. They should take only one puff at a time with a 1-minute wait between puffs (Karch, 2001).

Incentive Spirometry

Incentive spirometers are devices to encourage children to inhale deeply to aerate the lungs fully or move mucus. Although manufactured in different configurations, a common type consists of a hollow plastic tube containing a brightly colored ball or dome-shaped disk that will rise in the tube when a child inhales through the attached mouthpiece and tubing. The deeper the inhalation, the higher the ball rises in the tube.

Children need instruction on how to use this type of device, because their first impression is that they should blow out against the mouthpiece rather than inhale (Fig. 40-12*A*). Incentive spirometry is effective with children because the device and procedure resemble a game more than an actual treatment.

Breathing Techniques

Some children need exercises prescribed to help them better inflate alveoli or more fully empty alveoli. Blowing a piece of cotton or a plastic ball across a table, blowing through a straw, or blowing out with the lips pursed are effective techniques (see Fig. 40-12*B*). Yet another method for increasing aeration is to ask the child to blow up a balloon, which requires the child to take a deep inhalation. For best results, make these activities a game or contest rather than an exercise.

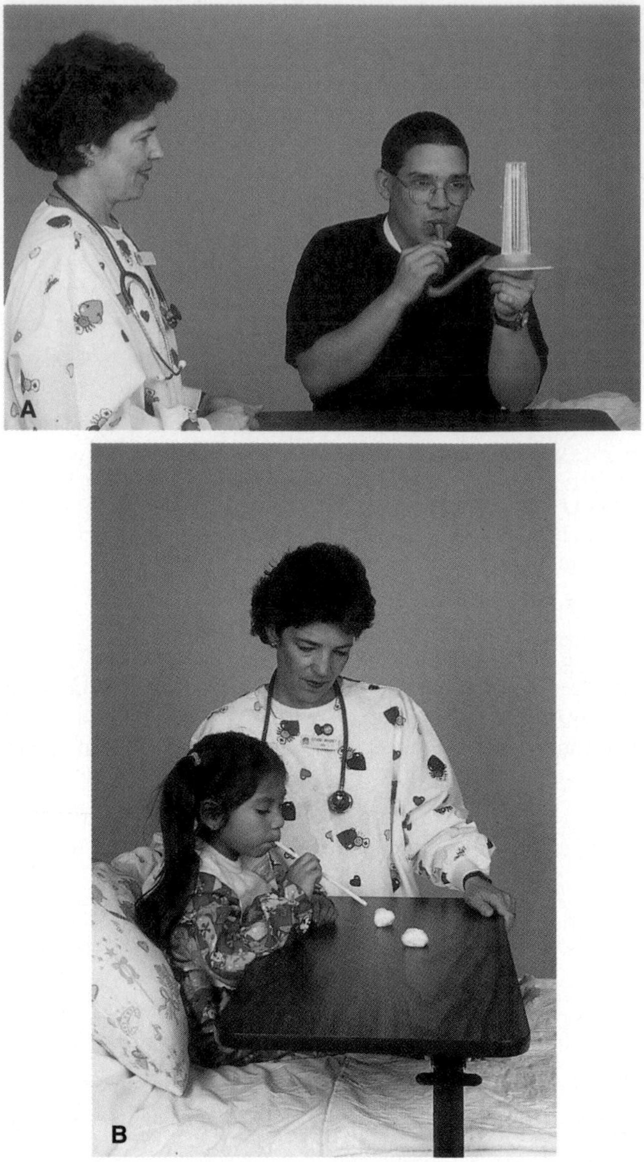

FIGURE 40.12 (*A*) Incentive spirometry is an appealing method to encourage children to aerate their lungs. (*B*) Encouraging children to take a deep breath and try to blow a cotton ball across the table is also an entertaining way to help them fully expand their lungs.

✔ CHECKPOINT QUESTIONS

7. Why do children find nebulizers uncomfortable?
8. What is the chief point to teach children about using incentive spirometers?

Tracheostomy

A **tracheostomy** involves an opening into the trachea to create an artificial airway to relieve respiratory obstruction that has occurred above that point. The procedure to create the airway is a **tracheotomy;** the resultant airway is the tracheostomy. Tracheostomies also may be used as a route for suctioning mucus when accumulating mucus causes lower airway obstruction. A tracheostomy eliminates the warming and filtering action of the nose and pharynx, making children more susceptible to infection. For these reasons, endotracheal intubation, not tracheostomy, has become the method of choice to relieve airway obstruction. The exception to this is obstruction in the pharynx, because it is often impossible to pass an endotracheal tube beyond obstruction at this point.

Emergency Intubation. Few medical emergencies are as frightening to a child or parents as an acute obstruction of a child's upper airway requiring a tracheotomy or endotracheal intubation. The child suddenly becomes limp and breathless, with his or her color changing quickly from pink to pale, followed by systemic cyanosis. Tracheotomies are done more easily on a treatment room table than on a bed or crib, so it is generally best to carry the child immediately to a treatment room. If the child cannot be moved quickly, however, because of accessory equipment, no time should be lost in transport. For tracheotomy, the cricoid cartilage of the trachea is swabbed with an antiseptic; if readily available, a local anesthetic may be injected into the cartilage ring. (This is not necessary in the unconscious child.) An incision is made just under the ring of cartilage and a tracheostomy tube with its obturator in place is inserted into the opening (Fig. 40-13*A*). When the obturator is removed, the child is able to breathe through the hollow tracheostomy tube. Have suction equipment available for immediate use to clear any blood caused by the incision (this is minimal) and any obstructing mucus from the trachea.

The color change in children after tracheostomy is usually dramatic. They inhale deeply a number of times through the tube, and color returns to normal. A few sutures may be necessary at the tube insertion site to halt bleeding or to reduce the size of the incision so the tube fits snugly.

As children begin to breathe normally and, if unconscious, regain consciousness, they often thrash and push at people around them, both from oxygen deficit and from fright. They call for a parent but can make no sound, adding to their fright. Assure the child that everything is all right, even though he or she cannot speak (see Fig. 40-13*B*). A school-age child can understand a simple explanation; for example, "You cannot speak right now because of the tube in your throat." As soon as the child's respirations are even and he or she is no longer experiencing acute respiratory distress, show the child that by placing a finger over the tracheostomy tube, air will again flow past the larynx and he or she can speak. If this causes the child to become short

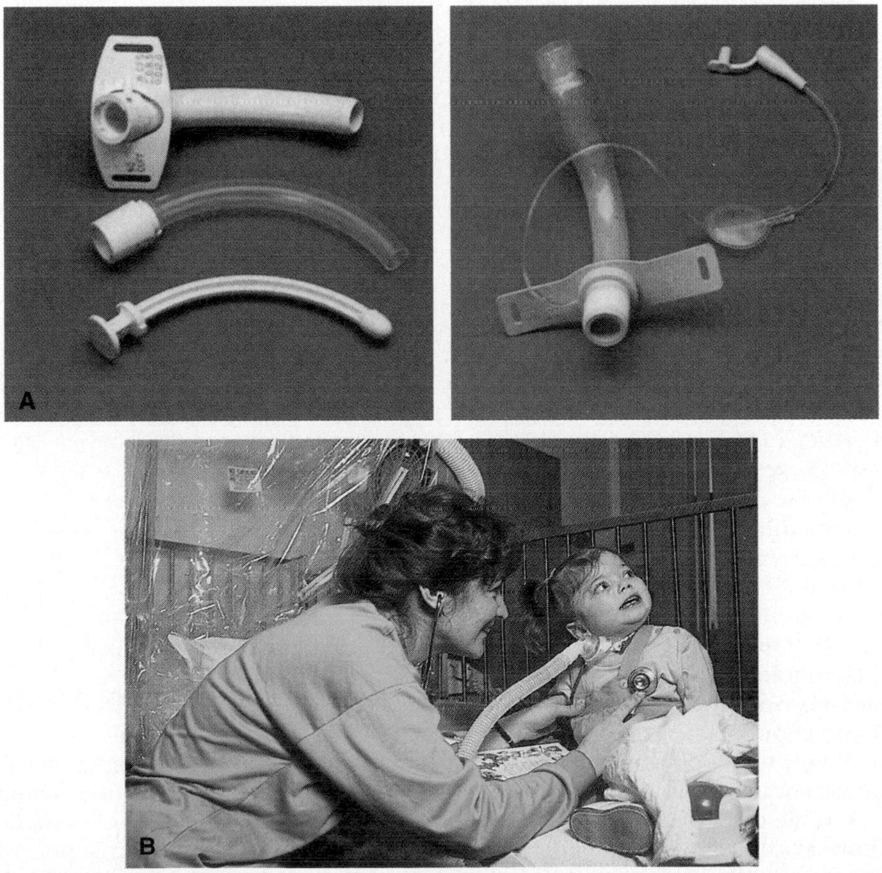

FIGURE 40.13 (*A*) Tracheostomy tubes: (*left*) a plastic tube, inner cannula, and obturator; (*right*) a plastic, cuffed tube. (*B*) A nurse interacts with a child receiving oxygen by a tracheostomy.

of breath, supply a paper and pencil or chalkboard for communication.

Be certain that parents understand why the tube is in place. Assure them that it is a temporary measure (provided this is true). Let them see the child as soon as possible after the procedure to assure themselves that their child is again all right. Children have difficulty relaxing enough to accept this strange new way of breathing until their parents can relax and accept it. Some children hyperventilate, not because of respiratory difficulty, but because of their fear.

Suctioning Technique. Most tracheostomy tubes used with children today are plastic. They do not include an inner cannula that would require removal and regular cleaning. Most children, however, do require frequent suctioning (perhaps as often as every 15 minutes) to keep the airway free of mucus. Use sterile technique to prevent introducing infection, and suction gently yet thoroughly. Ineffective suctioning does not remove obstructive mucus; because of irritation, it can actually cause more mucus to form. Be certain you know how deeply to suction. Some children need to be suctioned only the length of the tracheostomy tube so that the catheter does not touch and irritate the tracheal mucosa. Others need to be deeply suctioned to reduce the possibility that mucus will become so copious or so thickened that it obstructs the trachea.

Tracheostomy suctioning technique is shown in Nursing Procedure 40-2. Because suctioning removes air as well as secretions from the trachea, children may become oxygen-deprived during the procedure. Preoxygenating them by "bagging" or administering oxygen for approximately 5 minutes before the procedure helps reduce this problem.

Young children may need to wear elbow restraints while being suctioned to keep their hands away from the catheter. In addition, restraints may be necessary at all times when they are alone to prevent them from fussing with the tracheostomy tube and accidentally removing it.

Frequently check on children with tracheostomies to assess for possible respiratory difficulty. Make certain to spend time playing with them or just sitting and rocking them so that they come to think of you in ways other than as the person who comes to suction them. If parents are unable to stay with the child, assure them that you check on their child more frequently than what would be necessary for suctioning alone, so they can feel confident that if the child should have another episode of acute obstruction,

NURSING PROCEDURE 40.2: TRACHEOSTOMY SUCTION

Purpose
To remove mucus from the trachea.

Procedure	Principle
1. Wash hands; identify child; explain procedure to child.	1. Handwashing minimizes the risk for spread of microorganisms; explaining the procedure helps to encourage cooperation and minimize anxiety.
2. Assess child, especially breath sounds; analyze appropriateness of procedure. Plan ways to modify care based on individual circumstances.	2. Assessment prior to procedure provides a baseline for future evaluation. Modifications enhance individualization of nursing care based on client need.
3. Assemble supplies: suction source and tubing, sterile suction catheter (#12 or 14F) or sterile suction kit, sterile gloves, bottle of sterile normal saline, sterile medicine dropper or syringe, manual resuscitator. Plan method to keep child from touching sterile catheter (placing a restraint, distraction, or asking assistance from another nurse).	3. Organizing supplies will increase efficiency of procedure.
4. Open the bottle of sterile normal saline and suction catheter or kit. Pour a small amount of saline solution into disposable container included in kit. Prepare syringe or dropper with small amount of sterile normal saline; put on sterile gloves.	4. Sterile technique is important to prevent introducing microorganisms.
5. Hold suction catheter with one gloved hand, suction tubing with other gloved hand, and attach tubing to sterile catheter; dip tip of catheter into normal saline and suction a small amount through catheter.	5. Proper handling of equipment using sterile technique reduces the risk of contamination because once a sterile glove touches suction tubing, it is no longer sterile. Using sterile normal saline to suction through the catheter and tubing ensures patency.

(continued)

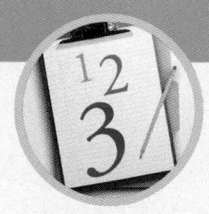

Procedure	Principle
6. If necessary, instruct assistant to hyperoxygenate child with manual resuscitator. 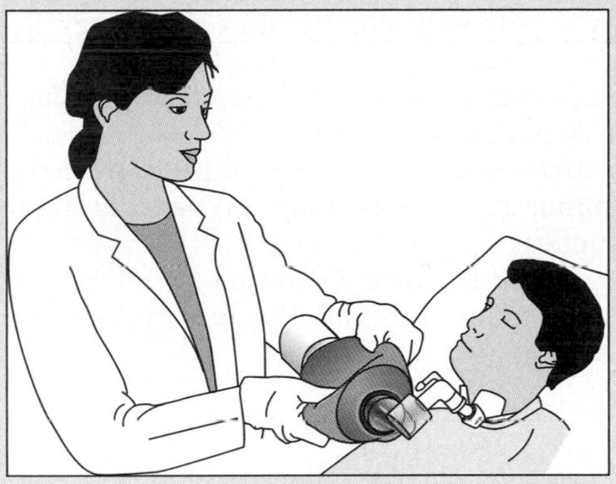	6. Hyperoxygenation prevents child from developing hypoxia during suctioning.
7. Hold your breath; introduce sterile catheter into tracheostomy tube to desired length. Apply suction for 5 to 10 sec and gently withdraw, rotating gently. 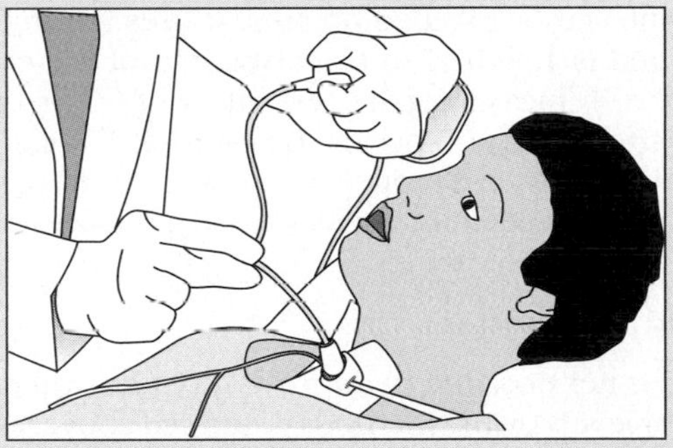	7. Holding your breath helps you not to suction longer than is comfortable. Applying suction only on withdrawal allows the catheter to pass freely without irritating the trachea and prevents over-suctioning. Prolonged suctioning longer than 10 sec can cause hypoxia.
8. Rinse catheter by dipping tip in normal saline and applying suction.	8. Rinsing catheter ensures that it remains patent.
9. Repeat procedure until airway sounds clear. Be careful not to suction longer than necessary.	9. Suctioning is fatiguing to children. Extended suctioning can lead to airway irritation and further mucus production.
10. Assess effectiveness and efficiency of procedure; plan teaching such as importance of procedure to parents; document procedure.	10. Comparing initial baseline assessments with post-procedure status provides information about effectiveness of the procedure. Teaching is an important independent nursing care activity for the child and parents.
11. Comfort child; remain with child for support. Provide opportunities for therapeutic play.	11. Suctioning is frightening; offering support and comfort after all such procedures helps to decrease fears and anxieties.

someone will be nearby. If the tracheostomy tube is to be left in place after discharge from the hospital, teach the parents how to care for it at home.

Tracheostomy tubes are held in place by cloth ties that fasten at the back of the child's neck. Change ties when they become soiled or loose, and check them frequently to be certain they remain tied. Children can fuss with and untie such things, whereas adults may not. Assess that the ties fit snugly but allow for one finger to be inserted underneath them so they don't rub and cause pain. For preschoolers or younger children, it is a good idea to cover the tracheostomy opening with a gauze square tied to the child's neck like a bib while they eat. This prevents crumbs or spilled liquids from entering the tracheostomy opening. Do not give children small toys that could fit into the lumen of the tube and cause obstruction (see Focus on Family Empowerment).

Each child is considered individually as to when it is time to remove a tracheostomy tube. Tubes are generally sealed off partially by adhesive tape or a commercial occlusion

FOCUS ON FAMILY EMPOWERMENT

Preventing Aspiration in the Child With a Tracheostomy

Q. How can we prevent something from falling into our child's tracheostomy?

A. Use the following to help prevent aspiration:

- Use a bib tied loosely over the tracheostomy when your child is eating to prevent food from entering the tube.
- Avoid buying toys with small parts that could be removed and dropped into the tube.
- Inspect stuffed toys to be certain they don't shed (fur could enter the tube).
- Supervise play with other children to be certain they don't place anything in the tube.
- Stay with your child in a bathtub to be certain water doesn't splash into the tube.
- Keep sprays such as perfume or room fresheners to a minimum, because they can be irritating to the trachea.
- Avoid cold air because it can cause tracheal spasm (cover the child's throat with a loose cotton scarf when out in cold weather).

device for a day or two before removal; then they are completely occluded (but not removed) for another day. This provides a weaning period where suctioning is still possible if it is needed. Occasionally, children cough so forcefully that they dislodge a tracheostomy tube. You might be with a child when this occurs, or you might walk into the room and find the tube lying beside the child on the bedclothes. As long as a child is not in distress, this is not an emergency, because the incision site usually does not close completely to occlude the tracheal opening when a tube is dislodged. Keep a new tube and inserter (obturator) at the bedside in case replacement is necessary. Slide the obturator into the tube and gently replace it in the tracheal opening. Remove the obturator and secure the new tube in place. If you do this quickly yet calmly, the average child is not alarmed and so will not protest. If, however, a child senses your excitement or if you indicate that something is terribly wrong, a child may begin to cry and turn away, making it difficult to replace the tube without assistance.

✔ CHECKPOINT QUESTIONS

9. Why is it necessary to wear gloves when suctioning a tracheostomy?
10. What is a good method to keep crumbs out of a tracheostomy while a child eats?

Endotracheal Intubation

Endotracheal intubation (nasal or oral intubation) is the preferred means of bypassing upper airway obstruction and allowing free entry of air to the trachea. However, since intubation tubes cause edema and local irritation, they cannot be left in place as a permanent solution. As with tracheostomies, children cannot speak while intubated. Supply those old enough to write with a pencil and paper for effective communication. Preschoolers can point to pictures to indicate what they need. Providing simple drawings or photos (a drink, a straw, a blanket, the television turned on, a urinal) to make needs known is helpful. Endotracheal tubes are held in place by being taped to the face. Make sure that tubes are carefully secured, because children can easily dislodge them. As much as possible, limit the number of tape changes to protect the skin on the child's cheeks.

A capnometer is a device that measures the amount of CO_2 in inhaled or exhaled breaths. It uses infrared technology and is attached to the distal end of the endotracheal tube. By measuring the percentage of CO_2 in expired air, the arterial CO_2 (PCO_2) can be estimated. A capnometer, used this way, can reduce the number of arterial punctures that are needed for arterial blood gas analysis.

Assisted Ventilation

When it is not possible to improve oxygen saturation to sufficient levels by the methods described above, assisted ventilation may be necessary. Positive-pressure machines deliver moistened or nebulized air or oxygen to the lungs under enough pressure and with appropriate timing to produce artificial, periodical inflation of alveoli; they rely on the elastic recoil of the lungs to empty the alveoli.

Depending on the type of ventilator, the inspiration-expiration cycle is determined by a timed interval, a volume limit, or a pressure limit, depending on the child's condition. Ventilators can supply high tidal volumes at a low frequency rate or low tidal volumes at rates as high as 200 to 300 breaths/min. Hyperinflation of lungs can occur with high-frequency ventilation because there is not enough time for expiration to occur. For this reason, some high-frequency ventilators are set so air is sucked out of the lungs rather than depending on the normal elastic recoil of the lungs. Some commonly used terms associated with ventilator therapy are presented in Table 40-4.

Children who need respiratory assistance are frightened. A great many fight ventilators or refuse to lie quietly and let the ventilator breathe for them. Pancuronium (Pavulon) may be administered intravenously to a point of abolishing spontaneous respiratory action to overcome resistance and allow mechanical ventilation to be accomplished at lower pressures because without normal respiratory action, there is no normal muscle resistance to overcome (see Focus on Pharmacology). Clearly, a child who receives pancuronium has no spontaneous respiratory function and needs critical

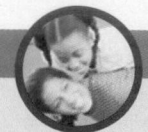

TABLE 40.4 Terms Commonly Used With Ventilator Therapy

TERM	DEFINITION	CLINICAL APPLICATION
IMV	Intermittent mandatory ventilation	Number of mandatory breaths the ventilator will deliver each hour. A child may breathe most of the time without assistance, but a set (mandatory) number of breaths per minute is delivered to ensure adequate lung expansion and oxygenation.
PEEP	Positive end-expiratory pressure	Pressure delivered to lungs at the end of each expiration to keep alveoli from collapsing on expiration and to ensure adequate oxygenation
Sigh	A deep inhalation delivered by the ventilator	Method used to fully inflate the lungs a number of times each minute
CPAP	Continuous positive airway pressure	A constant pressure exerted on the alveoli to keep them from collapsing on expiration
FiO_2	Concentration of oxygen the child is receiving (inspiring)	A child on oxygen therapy will have an FiO_2 from 22% to 100%

FOCUS ON PHARMACOLOGY

Pancuronium Bromide (Pavulon)

Action: Pancuronium is a neuromuscular blocking agent that relaxes skeletal muscles during assisted mechanical ventilation or endotracheal intubation.

Pregnancy risk category: C

Dosage: 0.03–0.04 mg/kg intravenously initially, then 0.03–0.1 mg/kg intravenously, repeated every 30 to 60 minutes as needed.

Possible adverse effects: Prolonged dose-related apnea; tachycardia, excessive salivation, and sweating.

Nursing Implications

- Keep in mind that the child's respiratory muscles do not function after administration; maintain assisted ventilation.
- Know that the drug peaks in approximately 2 to 3 minutes and lasts approximately 1 hour (longer in children with poor renal perfusion).
- Remember that the drug does not alter state of consciousness. Anticipate the need for sedation or analgesia for procedures.
- Keep equipment for emergency resuscitation (Ambu bag) at bedside in case of a power or mechanical ventilator failure.
- Be sure to explain all events and procedures to the child; even though the respiratory muscles may be paralyzed, the child can still hear. Also encourage the parents to talk to the child when they visit.
- Be prepared to reverse the effects of the drug by administering atropine and neostigmine methylsulfate (Prostigmin).
- Monitor all physiologic parameters, including vital signs, heart rate, and blood pressure. Obtain electrolyte levels as ordered, because electrolyte imbalances can potentiate neuromuscular effects.

observation and frequent arterial blood analysis because he or she depends totally on caregivers at that point.

Mechanical ventilation for a prolonged period requires that children either have a tracheotomy performed or have an endotracheal tube passed (Fig. 40-14). A cuffed tube is used with ventilators so the seal at the trachea is airtight. Infants need a nasogastric tube inserted to prevent stomach distention from air entering the esophagus. Providing adequate nutrition may be difficult for children on ventilators. Enteric (nasogastric) feedings or total parenteral nutrition solves this problem. Providing a balance of rest, stimulation, and assurance for the child is a challenge for nursing personnel and parents.

Once children become accustomed to assisted ventilation, it can be difficult to discontinue a device, even when there is no longer a clinical indication for it. This is most pronounced in adolescents, who are aware of the role of oxygen and proper ventilation for life function. You may need to provide a number of trial periods free of the ventilator with someone remaining close by them, so that they can be assured that if they do have difficulty breathing, someone is standing by to help. Many children are too afraid to fall asleep on the first night off a ventilator unless someone is with them and has assured them that they will be there through the night.

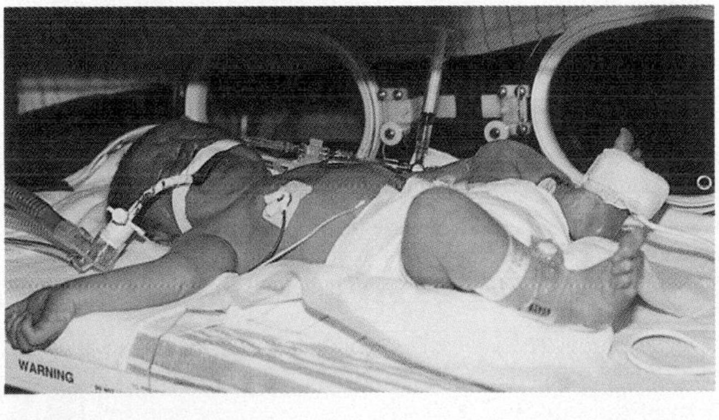

FIGURE 40.14 An infant with an endotracheal tube receiving assisted ventilation.

Lung Transplantation

Lung transplantation is a possibility for children with a chronic respiratory illness such as cystic fibrosis. Lung transplantation may involve a single lung or it can be done in conjunction with heart transplantation if chronic respiratory disease has caused ventricular hypertrophy.

As with any organ transplantation, children need immunosuppression therapy with drugs such as cyclosporine or azathioprine (Imuran) following lung transplant to decrease cell-mediated immunity. Although this level of immunosuppression is the key to successful transplantation, it also makes post-transplant children susceptible to fungal, bacterial, and viral lung infections. In addition, families experience a tremendous psychosocial toll as they wait to see whether the new transplant will be rejected (Kurland & Orenstein, 2001). Children may need to have chest physiotherapy or use a portable spirometry device daily to help mobilize secretions resulting from loss of nerve innervation or a reaction to accumulating mucus in the transplanted lung.

✔ CHECKPOINT QUESTIONS

11. What device is used to measure the amount of carbon dioxide in exhaled air when the child is intubated?
12. What drug is sometimes used to abolish spontaneous respiratory activity to allow lower pressures for mechanical ventilation?

DISORDERS OF THE UPPER RESPIRATORY TRACT

The upper respiratory tract warms, humidifies, and filters the air that enters the body (Fig. 40-15). As such, the structures of the upper respiratory tract constantly come into contact with a barrage of foreign organisms, including pathogens, that can lead to airway irritation and illness. Congenital malformations of respiratory structures also cause some upper respiratory tract disorders.

Choanal Atresia

Choanal atresia is congenital obstruction of the posterior nares by an obstructing membrane or bony growth, preventing a newborn from drawing air through the nose and down into the nasopharynx. It may be either unilateral or bilateral.

Newborns up to approximately 3 months of age are naturally nose-breathers. Infants with choanal atresia, therefore, develop signs of respiratory distress at birth or immediately after they quiet for the first time and attempt to breathe through the nose. Passing a soft no. 8 or 10 French catheter through the posterior nares to the stomach is a part of birthing room procedure in many health care facilities. If such a catheter will not pass bilaterally, the diagnosis of choanal atresia is confirmed immediately at birth.

Choanal atresia can also be assessed by holding the newborn's mouth closed, then gently compressing first one nostril, then the other. If atresia is present, infants will struggle as they experience air hunger when their mouth is

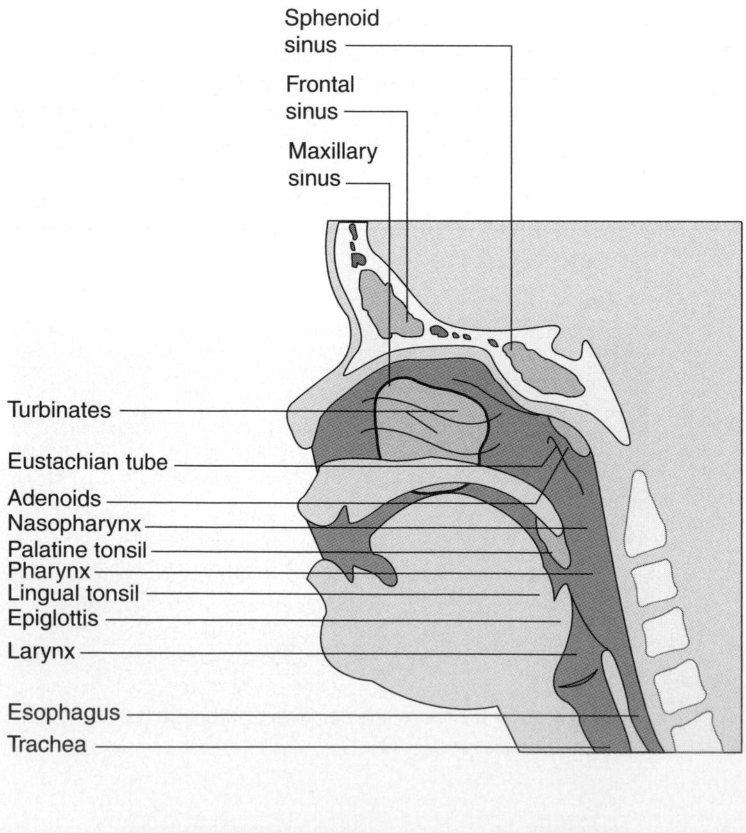

FIGURE 40.15 Structures of the upper respiratory tract.

closed. Their color improves when they open their mouth to cry. Atresia is also suggested if infants struggle and become cyanotic at feedings because they cannot suck and breathe through the mouth simultaneously.

The treatment for choanal atresia is either local piercing of the obstructing membrane or surgical removal of the bony growth. Because infants with choanal atresia have such difficulty with feeding, they may receive intravenous fluid to maintain their glucose and fluid level until surgery can be performed. Some infants may need an oral airway inserted so they can continue to breathe through their mouths. Following surgery, children have no further difficulty or symptoms.

Acute Nasopharyngitis (Common Cold)

The common cold is the most frequent infectious disease in children. Toddlers have an average of 10 to 12 colds a year. School-age children and adolescents have as many as four or five yearly. The incubation period is typically 2 to 3 days. Most occur in the fall and winter.

Acute nasopharyngitis (the common cold) is caused by one of several viruses, most predominantly by rhinovirus, coxsackie virus, respiratory syncytial virus, adenovirus, and parainfluenza and influenza viruses. Children are exposed to colds at school or while playing with other children. If they are in ill health from some other cause, or if their immune system is compromised, they are more susceptible to the cold viruses than others are. Although difficult to prove, stress factors also appear to play a role.

Assessment

Symptoms begin with nasal congestion, a watery rhinitis, and a low-grade fever. The mucous membrane of the nose becomes edematous and inflamed, constricting airway space and causing difficulty breathing. Posterior rhinitis, plus local irritation, leads to pharyngitis. Upper airway secretions that drain into the trachea lead to a cough. Cervical lymph nodes may be swollen and palpable. The process lasts about a week and then symptoms fade. In some children, a thick, purulent nasal discharge occurs because bacteria such as streptococci invade the irritated nasal mucous membrane and cause a secondary purulent infection.

Infants can be critically ill yet not develop a fever because their temperature-regulating system is still immature. With the common cold, they often develop a fever elevated out of proportion to the symptoms, possibly as high as 102° to 104°F (38.8° to 40°C). Infants also may develop secondary symptoms, such as vomiting and diarrhea, as a general response. Because they cannot suck and breathe through the mouth at the same time, they refuse feedings. This can lead to dehydration. Older children rarely develop as high a fever, rarely above 102°F (38.8°C). Because older children can breathe through the mouth, nasal congestion does not seem as acute.

Therapeutic Management

There is no specific treatment for a common cold. Because it is caused by a virus, antibiotics are not effective unless a secondary bacterial invasion has occurred (Levin & Weinberg, 2001). If a child has a fever, it should be controlled by an antipyretic such as acetaminophen (Tylenol) or children's ibuprofen (Motrin). It is important for parents to understand that these drugs are effective only in controlling fever symptoms, but they do not reduce congestion or "cure" the cold. Therefore, they should not be given unless the child has a fever, generally defined as an oral temperature over 101°F (38.4°C). Remind parents that children younger than 18 years should not be given acetylsalicylic acid (aspirin) because this is associated with the development of Reye's syndrome, a potentially fatal disorder (see Chap. 49).

If infants have difficulty nursing because of nasal congestion, saline nose drops or nasal spray may be prescribed to liquefy nasal secretions and help them drain. Removing nasal mucus via a bulb syringe before feedings allows infants to breathe more freely and thus be able to suck more efficiently. Caution parents that if they use a bulb syringe, they must compress the bulb first, then insert it into the child's nostril. If they insert the bulb syringe first, then depress the bulb, they will actually push secretions further back into the nose, causing increased obstruction.

There is little proof that oral decongestants relieve congestion to an appreciable degree with the common cold. Most parents believe that these products give relief, however, and feel better if one is prescribed for the child. It is not good policy to suppress the cough of a common cold, because a cough raises secretions, preventing pooling of secretions and consequent infection. Guaifenesin is an example of a drug that loosens secretions but does not suppress a cough. Parents may use a cool mist vaporizer to help loosen nasal secretions. The efficiency of home vaporizers is questionable, however, and safe use of a vaporizer, including proper cleaning, must be stressed or it can serve as a reservoir for infection.

NURSING DIAGNOSES AND RELATED INTERVENTIONS

Nursing Diagnosis: Parental health-seeking behaviors related to management of child's cold

Outcome Identification: Parents will demonstrate knowledge of what is and what is not helpful in the treatment of a cold by end of health visit.

Outcome Evaluation: Parents state intention to use cool mist vaporizer to loosen secretions, to encourage oral fluid, to administer an antipyretic to reduce fever, and to avoid cough medicine.

Care of the child with a cold is primarily supportive until the infection runs its course. Children with a cold often show a loss of appetite. They may prefer simple liquids to solid food for the first few days of the illness. Parents generally ask whether children should remain on bed rest. Children characteristically restrict their activity when ill. With acute cold symptoms, children may naturally curl up on the couch and sleep. One of the best ways that parents can judge when children are improving is to note that they have begun to increase their activity or are "acting like themselves" again.

Because the symptoms in infants are so out of proportion to the seriousness of the disorder, parents may need assurance that a cold in an infant is only a cold and nothing more. A possible complication of a cold is otitis media (middle ear infection). Instruct parents about this possibility and the necessity to report symptoms suggestive of this infection (e.g., sudden elevated temperature and ear pain). If otitis media occurs, a child needs antibiotics and further evaluation to protect against hearing impairment.

Pharyngitis

Pharyngitis is infection and inflammation of the throat. The peak incidence occurs between 4 and 7 years of age. It may be either bacterial or viral in origin. It may occur as a result of a chronic allergy in which there is constant postnasal discharge that results in secondary irritation. At least a slight pharyngitis usually accompanies a common cold.

Viral Pharyngitis

If the causative agent of the pharyngitis is a virus, the symptoms are generally mild: a sore throat, fever, and general malaise. On physical assessment, regional lymph nodes may be noticeably enlarged. Erythema will be present in the back of the pharynx and the palatine arch. Laboratory studies will indicate an increased white blood cell count.

If the inflammation is mild, children rarely need more than an oral analgesic such as acetaminophen or ibuprofen for comfort. Warm heat applied to the external neck area using a warm towel or heating pad also can be soothing. By school age, children are capable of gargling with a solution such as warm water to relieve the pain. Before this age, children tend to swallow the solution unless the procedure is well explained and demonstrated to them.

Because children's throats feel so sore, they often prefer liquid to solid food. Infants, especially, must be observed closely until the inflammation and tenderness diminish to be certain that they take in sufficient fluid to prevent dehydration (McCartney & Bagarazzi, 2000).

Streptococcal Pharyngitis

Group A beta-hemolytic streptococcus is the organism most frequently involved in bacterial pharyngitis in children. All streptococcal infections must be taken seriously because they can lead to cardiac and kidney damage from an autoimmune process.

Assessment. Streptococcal infections generally appear more severe than viral infections. The fact that the symptoms are mild, however, does not rule out streptococcal infection. With a streptococcal pharyngitis, the back of the throat and palatine tonsils are usually markedly erythematous (bright red); the tonsils are enlarged and there may be a white exudate in the tonsillar crypts. Petechiae may be present on the palate. The child typically appears ill with a high fever, an extremely sore throat, difficulty swallowing, and overall lethargy. Temperature is usually elevated to as high as 104°F (40°C). The child often has a headache. Swollen abdominal lymph nodes may cause abdominal pain. A throat culture, often completed as a quick office procedure, confirms the presence of the *Streptococcus* bacteria.

Therapeutic Management. Treatment consists of a full 10-day course of an oral antibiotic such as penicillin V or a single injection of benzathine penicillin G. Cephalosporins or broad-spectrum macrolides such as erythromycin may be prescribed if resistant organisms are known to be in the community (Ogle & Anderson, 2001). Help parents understand the importance of completing the full 10 days of therapy. The prolonged treatment is necessary to ensure that the streptococci are eradicated completely. If not, children may develop a hypersensitivity or autoimmune reaction to group A streptococci that results in rheumatic fever (although the chance of rheumatic fever occurring is probably as low as 1%) and glomerulonephritis.

Symptoms of acute glomerulonephritis (blood and protein in urine) appear in 1 to 2 weeks after the pharyngitis. For this reason, 2 weeks after treatment, children are asked to return to the health care facility with a urine specimen to be examined for protein so that developing acute glomerulonephritis can be detected.

To ensure that the child receives the full antibiotic course, help parents make a reminder sheet to place on a cabinet or refrigerator door. In addition, instruct parents about measures for rest, relief of throat pain, and maintaining hydration, the same actions as for a common cold. Because it is impossible for parents to discriminate between a pharyngitis caused by a virus (and needing no therapy other than comfort measures) and a streptococcal pharyngitis (needing definite therapy to prevent life-threatening illnesses), a child with pharyngitis always should be examined by health care personnel.

Retropharyngeal Abscess

In infants, the lymph nodes that drain the nasopharynx are located behind the posterior pharynx wall. These nodes may become infected in an infant following an acute nasopharyngitis or pharyngitis. Since these nodes disappear by preschool age, the problem is usually limited to young infants.

Assessment. Typically, infants have an upper respiratory tract infection or sore throat for a few days. Suddenly, they refuse to eat. They develop a high fever and may drool because they are unable to swallow saliva past the obstruction in their throat. They "snore" with respirations as the pharynx becomes further occluded. To allow themselves more breathing space, they may hyperextend the head, a very unusual position for infants.

Physical assessment reveals enlargement of the regional lymph nodes. The mass in the posterior pharynx may not be visible if it is below the point of vision. An ultrasound or x-ray study using a swallowed contrast medium will reveal the bulging tissue in the pharynx. Laboratory studies will reveal leukocytosis.

Therapeutic Management. Because the most frequent cause of retropharyngeal abscess is group A beta-hemolytic streptococcus, benzathine penicillin G or penicillin V is effective. As a result of their poor swallowing, infants' mouths may need to be suctioned to remove secretions. Be careful not to touch the suction catheter to the posterior pharynx because this might rupture the abscess, possibly leading to aspiration of the abscess contents (producing respiratory obstruction or a pneumonia caused by the aspirated purulent material). Blood vessels invade some retropharyngeal abscesses, so that rupture of the structure also could lead to profuse bleeding (dangerous to the child because of the loss of blood from major arteries such as the carotid artery and because the blood could be aspirated).

Place infants in a side-lying position to allow difficult-to-swallow mouth secretions to drain forward. Limit oral intake to fluids. A hard food such as a toast crust (a food often recommended for teething) could rupture the abscess with its hard edges.

Although some postpharyngeal abscesses resolve on their own, some need to be incised by a surgeon to promote drainage. This is done with the child in a Trendelenburg position so that drainage from the abscess can be suctioned away to prevent aspiration. After surgery, maintain the child in a Trendelenburg or a side position to encourage further drainage and prevent aspiration. Monitor vital signs closely. Increased respiratory rate suggests airway obstruction. Observe any drainage from infants' mouths to detect fresh bleeding. Frequent swallowing is also a sign of postpharyngeal bleeding.

Oral fluid is introduced as soon as the swallowing and gag reflexes are intact after surgery. Although the throat is undoubtedly still sore, most infants suck eagerly and need supplemental intravenous fluid administration following surgery for only a short time.

On admission parents may be thoroughly frightened by the extent of the child's symptoms (gurgling or snoring sound, high temperature, dyspnea). Allow parents to handle infants and care for them while overnight in the hospital to help them allay their fears and regain confidence in their parental roles.

✔ CHECKPOINT QUESTIONS

13. When would the child with choanal atresia typically develop signs of respiratory distress?
14. Why are infants not prescribed acetylsalicylic acid (aspirin) for the pain of pharyngitis?

Tonsillitis

Tonsillitis is the term commonly used to refer to infection and inflammation of the palatine tonsils. Adenitis refers to infection and inflammation of the adenoid (pharyngeal) tonsils.

Tonsillar tissue is lymphoid tissue that filters pathogenic organisms from the head and neck area. The palatine tonsils are located on both sides of the pharynx; the adenoids are in the nasopharynx. Tubal tonsils are located at the entrance to the eustachian tubes. Lingual tonsils are located at the base of the tongue. All of the tonsils, referred to collectively as Waldeyer's ring, are easily infected because of the bacteria that pass through or are screened through them with lymph.

Assessment

Infection of the palatine tonsils presents with all of the symptoms of a severe pharyngitis. Children drool because their throat is too sore for them to swallow saliva. They may describe swallowing as so painful that it feels as if they are swallowing bits of metal or glass. In addition, they usually have a high fever and are lethargic. Tonsillar tissue appears bright red and may be so enlarged that the two areas of palatine tonsillar tissue meet in the midline. Pus can be detected on or expelled from the crypts of the tonsils.

In addition to fever, lethargy, pharyngeal pain, and edema, the symptoms of adenoidal tissue infection also include a nasal quality of speech, mouth breathing, difficulty hearing, and perhaps halitosis or sleep apnea. The mouth breathing, change in speech, and apnea result from the postpharyngeal obstruction by the enlarged tissue. The difficulty with hearing occurs because of eustachian tube obstruction. Long-term obstruction this way can further cause either serous and acute otitis media (middle ear infection).

Tonsillitis occurs most commonly in school-age children. The responsible organism is identified by a throat culture. In children younger than 3 years of age, the cause is often viral. In school-age children, the organism is generally a group A beta-hemolytic streptococcus.

Therapeutic Management

Therapy for bacterial tonsillitis includes an antipyretic for fever, an analgesic for pain, and a full 10-day course of an antibiotic such as penicillin. If the cause is viral, no therapy other than comfort or fever reduction strategies is necessary. Although the pain of the infection will subside a day or two after the antibiotic administration is begun, remind parents that children need the full 10-day course of antibiotic to eradicate streptococci completely from the back of the throat. After a tonsillar infection, tonsillar tissue may remain hypertrophied, or it may atrophy and appear smaller than what it previously was.

Tonsillectomy. Tonsillectomy is removal of the palatine tonsils. Adenoidectomy is removal of the pharyngeal tonsils. In the past, tonsillectomy was a common procedure after tonsillitis. Today, tonsillectomy is not recommended unless all other measures to prevent frequent infections prove ineffective. Tonsillar tissue is removed by ligating the tonsil or by laser surgery. Because sutures are not placed, the chance for hemorrhage after this type of surgery is higher than after surgery involving a closed incision. The danger of aspiration of blood at the time of surgery and the danger of a general anesthetic compound the risk.

Chronic tonsillitis is about the only reason for removal of palatine tonsils. Adenoids may be removed if they are so hypertrophied that they are causing obstruction or sleep apnea. At one time, adenoids and palatine tonsils were always removed together; today, depending on the symptoms and the extent of hypertrophy and infection, children may have a tonsillectomy, an adenoidectomy, or both.

Tonsillectomy or adenoidectomy is never done while the organs are infected, because an operation at such a time might spread pathogenic organisms into the bloodstream, causing septicemia. Parents often ask why an operation to remove tonsils must be delayed until the child is well again. They think that as long as the tonsils are sore, they should be immediately removed. Help them understand why this is not possible and why it is safer to schedule surgery for a later date. Most parents report an improvement in their child's general health and performance after surgery.

NURSING DIAGNOSES AND RELATED INTERVENTIONS

Nursing Diagnosis: Risk for deficit fluid volume related to blood loss from surgery

Outcome Identification: Child will maintain adequate fluid volume balance postoperatively.

Outcome Evaluation: Child's pulse and blood pressure are normal for age group; there is absence of extensive bleeding; intake and output are within acceptable parameters.

Tonsillectomies are done as ambulatory or 1-day surgery following completion of a complete history and physical examination and laboratory tests, including bleeding and clotting times, complete blood count, and urinalysis. Teach parents to use common sense in their child's care during the week before hospital admission so that the child does not have a cold or recurrent tonsillitis at the time planned for surgery. An important aspect of immediate assessment on the day of surgery is to observe for loose teeth that could be dislodged during surgery and aspirated. If loose teeth are present, mark this on the front of the child's chart and report it to the anesthesiologist.

After surgery, observe vital signs carefully to make certain that the child is not bleeding from the denuded surgical area. Place the child on the side or abdomen with a pillow under the chest so that the head is lower than the chest. This allows blood and unswallowed saliva to drain from the child's mouth rather than back to the pharynx, where it might be aspirated (Fig. 40-16).

If hemorrhage occurs after tonsillectomy, it can be acute and intense. Because children will swallow any blood that is oozing from the surgical site, a child can be bleeding heavily and yet little blood is apparent. To detect bleeding, assess for subtle signs of hemorrhage, such as an increasing pulse or respiratory rate, frequent swallowing, throat clearing, or a feeling of anxiety. A child's first line of defense against hemorrhage is a nurse who recognizes these subtle signs of bleeding before the bleeding is so intense that signs of shock occur.

If you find that the surgical site is bleeding, elevate the child's head and turn him or her on the side to reduce vascular pressure on the operative site while continuing to prevent obstruction. Use a good light to inspect the posterior throat. Have a dental mirror available so that the child's surgeon can thoroughly inspect the bleeding area. If the surgical area is bleeding heavily, the child may need to be returned to surgery for a suture or two to halt bleeding.

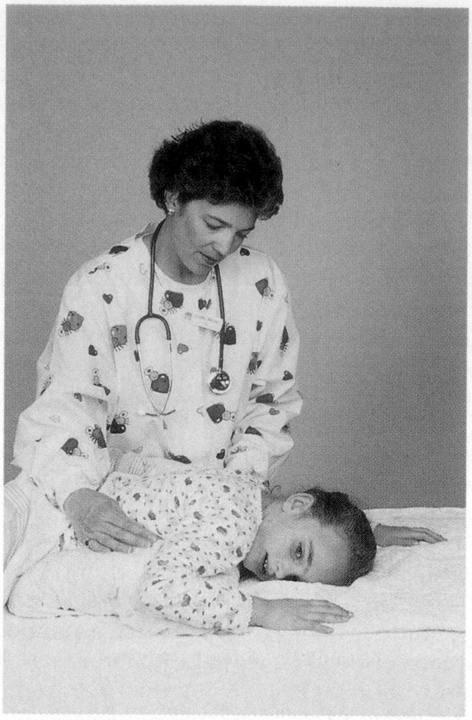

FIGURE 40.16 Positioning a child after tonsillectomy. The pillow under the chest helps secretions flow out of the mouth.

The most dangerous periods for the child after a tonsillectomy are the first 24 hours, when the clots covering the denuded surgical area are forming, and days 5 to 7, when the clots begin to lyse or dissolve. If new granulation tissue is not yet present when the clots dissolve, hemorrhage from the denuded surface can occur.

If children have no complications from surgery, are able to swallow fluids, and have voided, they are discharged later the same day of surgery. Parents need careful instruction concerning the danger signs to watch for in children during their first day home (frequent swallowing, clearing the throat, increasing restlessness). They are usually advised to restrict their child's activity (no gymnastics, swimming) until after the seventh day, when firm healing should have taken place. The child needs a return appointment to a health care facility approximately 2 weeks after surgery for follow-up assessment that the surgical area has healed without complication.

Nursing Diagnosis: Pain related to surgical procedure

Outcome Identification: Child's discomfort will be limited to a tolerable level.

Outcome Evaluation: Child states that level of pain is tolerable.

Tonsillectomy is an uncomfortable and painful procedure for children. Be sure they receive good preparation for the procedure and for the sensations they will experience afterward. Although tonsils are removed, it is better to talk about tonsils being "fixed" rather than taken out; children may be extremely frightened to know that a body part will be removed, however small it is.

Children's throats are extremely sore following a tonsillectomy. Liquid analgesics are better tolerated than pills or tablets because they are easier to swallow. Rectal administration is a possibility for very young children. Occasionally, a child may require intravenous pain relief.

Most children are thirsty immediately after surgery, and drinking is helpful because swallowing fluid causes active pharyngeal movement, increasing the blood supply to the area and reducing edema and pain. Children commonly are promised by well-meaning people that they can have all the ice cream they want after a tonsillectomy. However, because it forms tenacious secretions that are difficult to swallow, it is not a food of choice. Offer instead frequent sips of clear liquid, Popsicles, or ice chips. Avoid acid juices because these sting the denuded tissue. Carbonated beverages also can irritate the area unless they stand for a time to become "flat." Avoid red fluid such as Kool-Aid, which if vomited can be mistaken for swallowed blood.

Children can be gradually advanced to a soft diet including foods such as gelatin, mashed potatoes, soups, and cooked fruits after 24 to 48 hours. They should continue to eat only soft foods for the first week (no toast crusts or other foods that could cause pharyngeal irritation if not chewed well). Be certain that parents know the telephone number they should call (clinic, hospital, or pediatrician) if they have a question or concern about the child's condition or care. Caution parents that some children develop a mild earache after tonsillectomy for the first week, probably caused by shifting pressure on the eustachian tube.

Epistaxis

Epistaxis (nosebleed) is extremely common in children and usually occurs from trauma, such as picking at the nose, from falling, or from being hit on the nose by another child. In older homes that lack humidification, the hot dry environment makes children's mucous membranes dry, uncomfortable, and susceptible to cracking and bleeding. In all children, epistaxis tends to occur during respiratory illnesses. It also may occur after strenuous exercise, and it is associated with a number of systemic diseases, such as rheumatic fever, scarlet fever, measles, or varicella infection (chickenpox). It can occur with nasal polyps, sinusitis, or allergic rhinitis. Some families show a familial predisposition.

Nosebleeds are always frightening because of the visible bleeding and a choking sensation if blood should run down the back of the nasopharynx. The fear is generally out of proportion to the seriousness of the bleeding.

Keep children with nosebleeds in an upright position with their head tilted slightly forward to minimize the amount of blood pressure in nasal vessels and to keep blood moving forward, not back into the nasopharynx. Apply pressure to the sides of the nose with your fingers (Fig. 40-17). Make every effort to quiet the child and to help him or her stop crying, because crying increases pressure in the blood vessels of the head and prolongs bleeding. If these simple measures do not control the bleeding, epinephrine (1:1,000) may be applied to the bleeding site to constrict blood vessels. A nasal pack may be necessary to provide continued pressure (Osterhoudt, 2000).

Teach parents that every child has occasional nosebleeds. Chronic nasal bleeding, however, should be investigated to rule out a systemic disease or blood disorder.

WHAT IF? What if a father tells you his child has "nosebleeds that just will not stop"? How would you advise him to position the child?

Sinusitis

Sinusitis is rare in children younger than 6 years of age because the frontal sinuses do not develop fully until age 6 (Chung, 2000). It occurs as a secondary infection in older children when streptococcal, staphylococcal, or *H. influenzae* organisms spread from the nasal cavity. Children develop a fever, a purulent nasal discharge, headache, and tenderness over the affected sinus. A nose and throat culture will identify the infectious organism.

Treatment for acute sinusitis consists of an antipyretic for fever, an analgesic for pain, and an antibiotic for the specific organism involved. Oxymetazoline hydrochloride (Afrin), supplied as nose drops or a nasal spray, shrinks the edematous mucous membranes and allows infected ma-

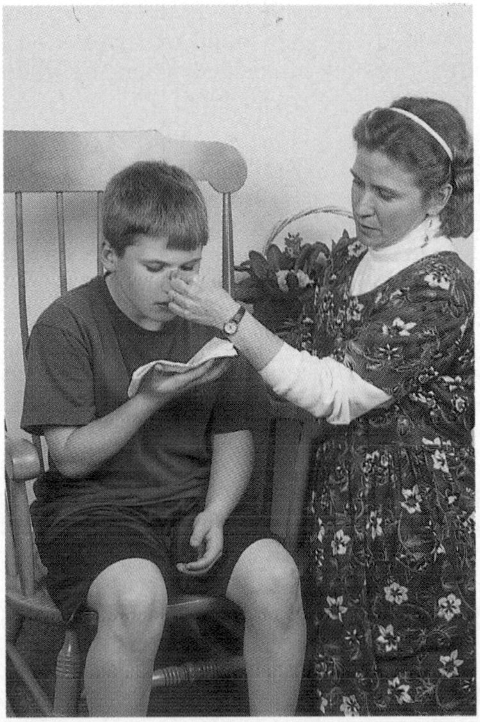

FIGURE 40.17 Emergency therapy for a nosebleed is to tilt the head slightly forward and apply pressure to the sides of the nose.

terial to drain from the sinuses. To avoid a rebound effect, nasal sprays should be used for only 3 days at a time; otherwise, they actually cause more nasal congestion than was present originally. Some children need acetaminophen (Tylenol) for pain. Warm compresses to the sinus area may encourage drainage and relieve pain.

Sinusitis is considered by many adults to be a minor illness. It needs to be treated, however, because it can have serious complications if the infection spreads from the sinuses to invade the facial bone (osteomyelitis) or the middle ear (otitis media). Chronic sinusitis can interfere with school and social interactions because of the constant pain.

Laryngitis

Laryngitis is inflammation of the larynx. It results in brassy, hoarse voice sounds or inability to make audible voice sounds. It may occur as a complication of pharyngitis or from excessive use of the voice, as in shouting or loud cheering. Laryngitis is as annoying for children as it is for adults. Sips of fluid (either warm or cold, whichever feels best) offer relief from the annoying tickling sensation often present. The most effective measure, however, is for the child to rest the voice for at least 24 hours, until inflammation subsides. For infants with laryngitis, attempt to meet their needs before they have to cry for things. Simply caution older children not to speak. Provide them with a paper and pencil or chalkboard for communication.

Congenital Laryngomalacia

Congenital laryngomalacia means that an infant's laryngeal structure is weaker than normal and collapses more than usual on inspiration. This produces laryngeal **stridor** (a high-pitched crowing sound on inspiration) present from birth, possibly intensified when the infant is in a supine position or when sucking.

Assessment

The infant's sternum and intercostal spaces may retract on inspiration because of the increased effort needed to pull air into the trachea past the collapsed cartilage rings. Many infants with this condition must stop sucking frequently during a feeding to maintain adequate ventilation and to rest from their respiratory effort, which is exhausting.

Therapeutic Management

When parents wake at night and listen in a quiet house to the sound of stridor, it seems unbearably loud. This makes it difficult for them to believe that it is safe for them to care for the infant at home.

Most children with congenital laryngomalacia need no routine therapy other than to have parents feed them slowly, providing rest periods as needed. The condition improves as infants mature because cartilage in the larynx becomes stronger at about 1 year of age. Many parents sleep at night with the child's crib next to their bed or with one hand resting on the infant's chest so they can be assured during the night that the child is continuing to breathe. At health care visits, assess whether the parents are receiving enough sleep at night and are not becoming too exhausted to be able to continue their daily activities. Showing them a weight chart that demonstrates that their child is growing and thriving despite this problem can be reassuring.

Teach parents about the importance of bringing the child for early care if signs of an upper respiratory tract infection develop. If not, laryngeal collapse will be even more intense during these times, and complete obstruction of the trachea could occur. Any time stridor becomes more intense, advise parents to have the infant seen by their primary care provider, because generally this indicates beginning obstruction and probably the beginning of an upper respiratory tract infection. As parents become more accustomed to the sound their infant makes while breathing, they will become astute reporters of change in the infant's condition; listen to them carefully when they report a change to prevent overlooking this important information.

✔ CHECKPOINT QUESTIONS

15. Which tonsils are typically involved with tonsillitis?
16. What subtle signs best reveal post-tonsillectomy bleeding?
17. What is the most effective treatment for laryngitis?

Croup (Laryngotracheobronchitis)

Croup (inflammation of the larynx, trachea, and major bronchi) is one of the most frightening diseases of early childhood for both parents and children. In children between 6 months and 3 years of age, the cause of croup is usually a viral infection such as parainfluenza virus. In children between ages 3 and 6 years, it most often occurs from parainfluenza virus type I. In previous years, the most common cause was *H. influenzae.* However, since immunization against this organism has been included in a routine immunization series, the incidence of croup has declined by 90% (Phillips, 2000).

Assessment

With croup, children typically have only a mild upper respiratory tract infection at bedtime. Temperature is normal or only mildly elevated. During the night, they develop a barking cough (croupy cough), inspiratory stridor, and marked retractions. They wake in extreme respiratory distress. The larynx, trachea, and major bronchi are all inflamed. These severe symptoms typically last a number of hours and then, except for a rattling cough, subside by morning. Symptoms may recur the following night. Cyanosis is rarely present, but the danger of glottal obstruction from the laryngeal inflammation is very real. Pulse oximetry and transcutaneous CO_2 monitors are helpful measures to document whether hypoxemia is occurring (Wright et al., 2002).

Therapeutic Management

One emergency method of relieving croup symptoms is for a parent to run the shower or hot water tap in a bathroom until the room fills with steam, then keep the child in this warm, moist environment. If this does not relieve symptoms, instruct the parents to bring the child to an emergency department for further evaluation and care. When a child is seen at the emergency room, cool moist air with a corticosteroid such as dexamethasone, or racemic epinephrine, given by nebulizer, can reduce inflammation and produce effective bronchodilation to open the airway (Phillips, 2000). Intravenous therapy may be prescribed to keep the child well hydrated. Maintain accurate intake and output records and test urine specific gravity to ensure that hydration remains adequate.

NURSING DIAGNOSES AND RELATED INTERVENTIONS

Nursing Diagnosis: Ineffective airway clearance related to edema and constriction of airway

Outcome Identification: Child will demonstrate adequate airway clearance by 1 hour.

Outcome Evaluation: Respiratory rate is below 22 breaths/min; no cyanosis is present; Po_2 is 80 to 100 mm Hg; Sao_2 is over 95%.

Attach a sensor for pulse oximetry monitoring and remain constantly with the child, not only to observe closely for increasing respiratory distress but also to reduce anxiety. Take vital signs as often as every 15 minutes, because extreme restlessness and thrashing, increased stridor, increased heart and respiratory rates, and cyanosis are symptoms of oxygen deprivation. In some children, it is difficult to distinguish between fright from the newness of the experience (and their sense of their parents' fright) and the anxiety that comes from oxygen deprivation. Keep a continuous record of vital signs and activity as a way to demonstrate increasing respiratory rate and restlessness. Arterial blood gases may be obtained to assess for sufficient oxygenation if pulse oximetry is not being used. A tracheostomy or endotracheal intubation along with oxygen therapy may be necessary if symptoms do not diminish. (It is difficult to intubate children with croup because of the severe respiratory tract edema.)

Laryngospasm with total occlusion of the airway can occur when a child's gag reflex is elicited or when the child is crying. Therefore, do not elicit a gag reflex in any child with a croupy, barking cough, and provide comfort to prevent crying.

Croup is a frightening disease for parents because their child is suddenly ill with severe symptoms. When the severe symptoms disappear by morning, parents may feel foolish that they rushed to a hospital with the child in the middle of the night. Assure them that their judgment was correct. When they brought the child in, he or she was seriously ill. Parents may be reluctant to see their child discharged in the morning until they are convinced that he or she is now well enough to go home.

WHAT IF? What if a child who had loud stridor suddenly has no stridor present? Would you be relieved (his condition must be improving) or worried (his airway may be so blocked that not enough air is entering to make the sound of stridor)? How should you respond?

Epiglottitis

Epiglottitis is inflammation of the epiglottis (the flap of tissue that covers the opening to the larynx to keep out food and fluid during swallowing). Although it occurs rarely, inflammation of the epiglottis creates an emergency situation because the swollen epiglottis is unable to rise and allow the airway to open. It occurs most frequently in children from 2 to about 7 years of age (Bagarazzi, 2000).

Epiglottitis can be either bacterial or viral in origin. *H. influenzae* type B has been replaced as the most common bacterial cause of the disorder by pneumococci, streptococci, or staphylococci. Echovirus and respiratory syncytial virus also can cause the disorder.

Assessment

Symptoms begin as those of a mild upper respiratory tract infection. After 1 or 2 days, as inflammation spreads to the epiglottis, the child suddenly develops severe inspiratory stridor, a high fever, hoarseness, and a very sore throat. The child may have such difficulty swallowing that he or she drools saliva. The child may protrude the tongue to increase free movement in the pharynx.

If a child's gag reflex is stimulated with a tongue blade, the swollen and inflamed epiglottis rises in the back of the throat as a cherry-red structure. It can be so edematous, however, that the gagging procedure causes complete obstruction of the glottis and respiratory failure. Therefore, in children with symptoms of epiglottitis (dysphagia, inspiratory stridor, fever, and hoarseness), ***never attempt to visualize the epiglottis directly with a tongue blade or obtain a throat culture*** unless a means of providing an artificial airway, such as tracheostomy or endotracheal intubation, is readily available. This is important for the nurse who functions in an expanded role and performs physical assessments and routinely elicits gag reflexes.

With epiglottitis, laboratory studies will show leukocytosis (20,000 to 30,000 mm^3), with the proportion of neutrophils increased. A blood culture to evaluate for septicemia and arterial blood gases to evaluate respiratory sufficiency may be ordered. However, because excessive crying can precipitate entrapment of the epiglottis and obstruction, such tests may be delayed in preference to a lateral neck x-ray film or sonogram, which will show the enlarged epiglottis. Do not allow a child with possible epiglottitis to go to these departments accompanied only by parents or a nursing aide, in case obstruction occurs in the x-ray or sonograph room.

Therapeutic Management

Children need moist air to reduce the epiglottal inflammation. If cyanosis is present, they need oxygen. An antibiotic, such as a second-generation cephalosporin (e.g., cefuroxime), may be prescribed until a throat culture indicates a specific antibiotic drug. Being unable to swallow, children need intravenous fluid therapy to maintain hydration. They may need a prophylactic tracheostomy or endotracheal intubation to prevent total obstruction. It is often difficult to intubate children with epiglottitis because the tube cannot be passed beyond the edematous epiglottis. After antibiotic therapy, the epiglottal inflammation recedes rapidly. By 12 to 24 hours, it has reduced in size enough that the airway may be removed. Antibiotic administration will continue for a full 7 to 10 days. Siblings of the ill child may be prescribed prophylactic antibiotic therapy to prevent them from developing the same symptoms.

Initially, the symptoms of epiglottitis are not unlike those of croup. As a result, parents may not realize the extent of the occlusion in their child, especially if the child has had croup on other occasions. They may question why a prophylactic tracheostomy was necessary this time when it was not used when the child had croup. Explain to them the difference between the two diseases (Table 40-5).

Some infants with epiglottitis die because obstruction occurs before a tracheotomy can be accomplished. If this should happen, parents need to be assured that they could not realize the seriousness of their child's symptoms. They may become overcautious, bringing other children to health care settings repeatedly for symptoms that are obviously not serious. These parents need time to regain confidence in themselves as parents and in their ability to judge a child's health again.

Aspiration

Aspiration (inhalation of a foreign object into the airway) occurs most frequently with infants and toddlers. When a child aspirates a foreign object, the immediate reaction is choking and hard, forceful coughing. Usually, this dislodges the object. However, if the airway becomes so obstructed that coughing is impossible (no sound with cough), or if there are signs of increased respiratory difficulty accompanied by stridor, some intervention is essential. A series of Heimlich subdiaphragmatic abdominal thrusts are recommended for children, the same as for adults. This recommendation does not extend to infants, however, because of the great risk of rupturing the liver (American Heart Association, 2000).

For the Heimlich maneuver, stand behind the child and place a fist just under the child's diaphragm (a point immediately below the anterior rib cage). Embrace the child, grip your fist with your other hand, and pull back and up with a rapid thrust. The pressure created by this action of pushing up on the diaphragm forces the aspirated material out of the trachea (Larsen et al., 2001; Fig. 40-18).

If a child is lying on his or her back at the time of the aspiration, stand at the head of the bed or table, place your hands in the same position as described above, and exert the same inward and upward thrust. A Heimlich maneuver may cause the child to vomit as well as expel an aspirated object. Turn the child's head to the side to prevent aspiration of vomitus.

For infants, use back thrusts to dislodge an aspirated object. Turn the infant prone over your arm and administer up to five quick back blows forcefully between the infant's shoulder blades, using the heel of the hand (Fig. 40-19*A*). If the object is not expelled, turn the infant while carefully supporting the head and neck and hold the infant in a supine position draped over your thigh. Be sure to keep the infant's head lower than his or her chest. Provide up to five quick downward thrusts in the lower third of the sternum (see Fig. 40-19*B;* American Heart Association, 2000). This is generally enough to dislodge the foreign object. However, if this does not occur, rescue breathing may then be attempted.

Bronchial Obstruction

The right main bronchus is straighter and has a larger lumen than the left bronchus in children older than 2 years of age. For this reason, an aspirated foreign object that is

TABLE 40.5 Comparison of Laryngotracheobronchitis (Croup) and Epiglottitis

ASSESSMENT	LARYNGOTRACHEOBRONCHITIS	EPIGLOTTITIS
Causative organism	Usually viral	Usually pneumococci or streptococci
Usual age of child	6 mo–3 yr	3–6 yr
Seasonal occurrence	Late fall and winter	None
Onset pattern	Preceded by upper respiratory infection; cough becomes worse at night	Preceded by upper respiratory infection; suddenly very ill
Presence of fever	Low grade	Elevated to about 103°F
Appearance	Retractions and stridor; prolonged inspiratory phase of respirations; not very ill-appearing	Drooling; very ill-appearing; neck hyperextended to breathe. (Do not attempt to view enlarged epiglottis, or immediate airway obstruction can occur.)
Cough	Sharp, barking	Muffled cough
Radiographic findings	Lateral neck radiograph showing subglottal narrowing	Lateral neck radiograph showing enlarged epiglottis
Possible complications	Asphyxia due to subglottic obstruction	Asphyxia due to supraglottic obstruction

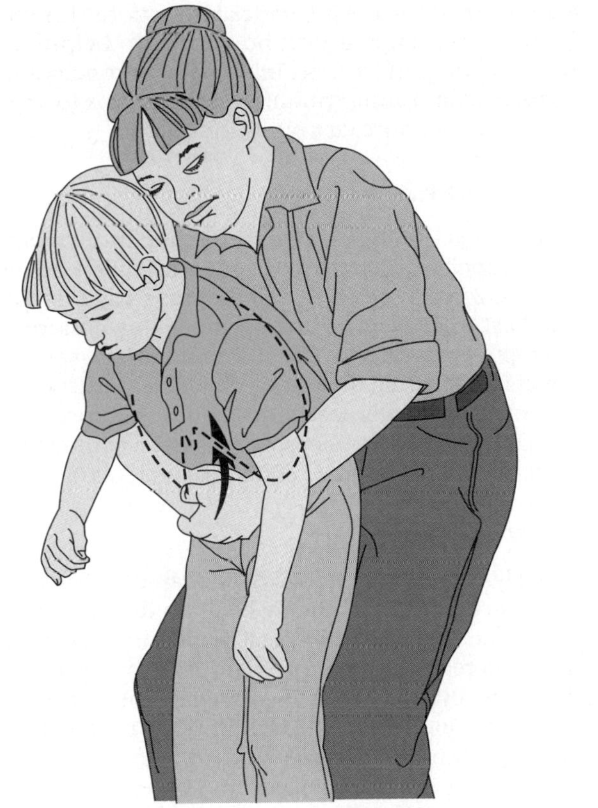

FIGURE 40.18 Heimlich maneuver on a school-age child.

not large enough to obstruct the trachea may lodge in the right bronchus, obstructing a portion or all of the right lung. The alveoli distal to the obstruction will collapse as the air remaining in them becomes absorbed (**atelectasis**), or hyperinflation and pneumothorax may occur if the foreign body serves as a ball valve, allowing air to enter but not leave the alveoli.

Assessment

After aspirating a small foreign body, the child generally begins to cough violently and may become dyspneic. Hemoptysis, fever, purulent sputum, and leukocytosis will result if the object scratches the airway or infection develops. Localized wheezing (a high whistling sound on expiration made by air passing through the narrowed lumen) may occur. Because this is localized, it is different from the generalized wheezing of a child with asthma.

A chest x-ray will reveal the presence of a radiopaque object. Objects most frequently aspirated include bones, popcorn, nuts, and coins. As a rule, nuts or popcorn should not be given to children younger than school age. In addition to these objects being frequently aspirated, they also are coated with oil, and as they swell with moisture in the respiratory tract, they cause not only obstruction but also lipid pneumonia, a persistent type of pneumonia. Foreign bodies that are inhaled this deeply are rarely coughed up spontaneously, despite the severe coughing that ensues. Because objects such as bones and nuts cannot be visualized well on x-ray film, an x-ray study may be inconclusive. Objects can be identified and removed by bronchoscopy.

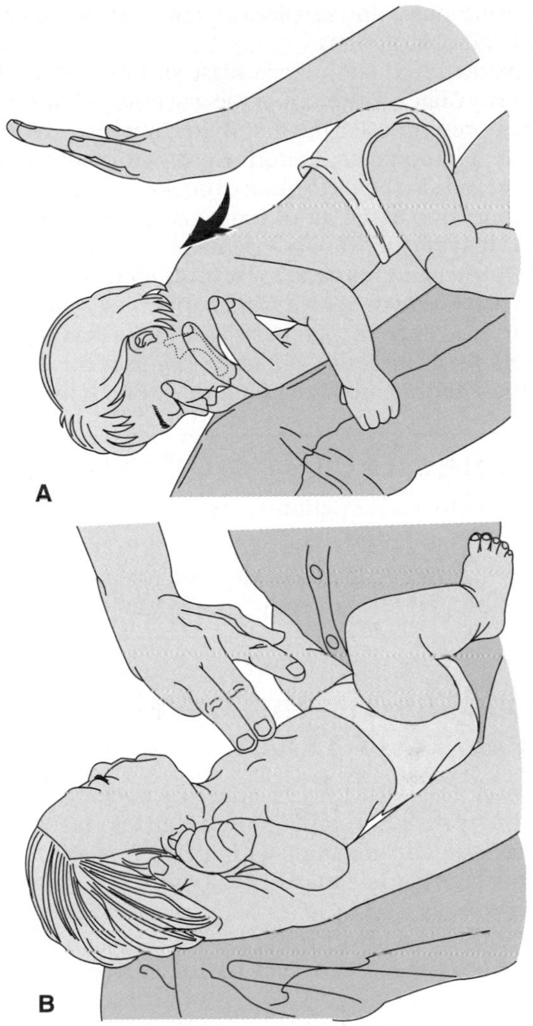

A

B

FIGURE 40.19 Back blows (*A*) and chest thrusts (*B*) to relieve complete foreign body airway obstruction in an infant. (From American Heart Association. [2000]. *Resuscitation in the newborn.* Dallas, TX: AHA.)

Therapeutic Management

Children who are seen in emergency departments because of this type of aspirated foreign body are in distress from pain and are choking and coughing. Their parents are frightened by the degree of distress. Parents may feel bad about having offered the child (or allowing the child to reach) a food such as a peanut. Children need quick orientation to the treatment environment, as they move from the emergency department to x-ray and then possibly to surgery or a treatment room. If possible, allow the parents to go with them as appropriate. Throughout, be vigilant in observing the child for coughing up the foreign body or developing increasing respiratory distress.

A bronchoscopy may be necessary to remove the foreign body. Children are often given conscious sedation for the procedure. (For details of a bronchoscopy procedure and conscious sedation, see Chap. 36.) After bronchoscopy, assess the child closely for signs of bronchial edema and airway obstruction secondary to mucus accumulation from bronchus manipulation. Obtain frequent vital signs (increasing pulse and respiratory rate suggests increased edema and obstruction).

Keep the child NPO for at least an hour after a bronchoscopy. Check for return of the gag reflex. Once the gag reflex is present, offer the first fluid cautiously to prevent possible additional aspiration. Cool fluid may feel more soothing and also helps to reduce the soreness in the throat. Breathing cool, moist air or having an external ice collar applied may further reduce edema.

Obviously, parents need to be cautioned about the dangers of aspiration to keep it from happening again. Do not lecture, however. A parent whose child has just been through this experience already recognizes the danger of aspiration and the need to be more careful in the future.

✔ CHECKPOINT QUESTIONS

18. If a child has epiglottitis, what should you never attempt?
19. What two maneuvers are used to dislodge an aspirated foreign body in an infant?

DISORDERS OF THE LOWER RESPIRATORY TRACT

The structures of the lower respiratory tract are subject to infection by the same pathogens that attack the upper respiratory tract. Inflammation and infection of the lungs, or pneumonia, is particularly troublesome: it occurs in various forms and is caused by several organisms. Other illnesses that occur in the lower respiratory tract, such as asthma and cystic fibrosis, can lead to secondary pneumonia infections.

Bronchitis

Bronchitis, or inflammation of the major bronchi and trachea, is one of the more common illnesses affecting preschool and school-age children. It is characterized by fever and cough, usually in conjunction with nasal congestion. Causative agents include the influenza viruses, adenovirus, and *Mycoplasma pneumoniae,* among others.

Assessment

The child usually has a mild upper respiratory tract infection for 1 or 2 days; the child then develops a fever and a dry, hacking cough that is hoarse and mildly productive in older children. The cough is serious enough to wake the child from sleep. These symptoms may last for a week, with full recovery sometimes taking as long as 2 weeks (Larsen et al., 2001).

On auscultation, rhonchi and coarse **crackles** (the sound of rales) can be heard. A chest x-ray will reveal diffuse alveolar hyperinflation and some markings at the hilus of the lung.

Therapeutic Management

Therapy is aimed at relieving respiratory symptoms, reducing fever, and maintaining adequate hydration. An antibiotic is prescribed for bacterial infections. If mucus is viscid, an expectorant may be needed to help the child raise it. It is important that children with bronchitis cough to raise accumulating sputum. Cough syrups to suppress the cough, therefore, are rarely indicated.

Bronchiolitis

Bronchiolitis is inflammation of the fine bronchioles and small bronchi. It occurs most often in children younger than age 2 years, peaking at 6 months of age. Incidence is highest in the winter and spring. Many children who develop asthma later in life have numerous instances of bronchiolitis during their first year of life. Viruses, such as adenovirus, parainfluenza virus, and respiratory syncytial virus (RSV), in particular, appear to be the pathogens most responsible for this illness (Hakonarson, 2000).

Assessment

Typically, infants have 1 or 2 days of an upper respiratory tract infection, then suddenly begin to demonstrate nasal flaring, intercostal and subcostal retractions on inspiration, and an increased respiratory rate. They may have a mild fever, leukocytosis, and an increased erythrocyte sedimentation rate, indicating the amount of bronchial inflammation present. Both mucus and inflammation block the small bronchioles, so air can no longer enter or leave alveoli freely. Most infants develop alveolar hyperinflation because air enters more easily than it leaves inflamed, narrowed bronchioles. The expiratory phase of respiration is prolonged, and wheezing may be present. After initial hyperinflation, areas of atelectasis may occur as alveoli are blocked and the air they contain is absorbed. Tachycardia and cyanosis develop from hypoxia. Infants soon become exhausted from the rapid respirations. A chest x-ray may show pulmonary infiltrates caused by a secondary infection or collapse of alveoli (atelectasis). Pulse oximetry shows low oxygen saturation. A throat culture will identify the offending organism.

Therapeutic Management

For children with less severe symptoms, antipyretics, adequate hydration, and maintaining a watchful eye for progression to more serious illness is all that is necessary. Hospitalization is warranted for children in severe distress (e.g., if the infant is tachypneic, has marked retractions, seems listless, or has a history of poor fluid intake).

Antibiotics are not commonly used in the treatment of bronchiolitis, because bacteria are rarely a causative factor. Children with chronic pulmonary disease may receive anti-RSV immunoglobulin if RSV was identified as the causative agent.

Children need humidified oxygen to counteract hypoxemia and adequate hydration to keep respiratory membranes moist. Nebulized bronchodilators and steroids may be used. Some children need ventilatory assistance to achieve adequate ventilation. They all need to be carefully observed because, if RSV is the cause, apnea may occur. In some infants, extracorporeal membrane oxygenation (the same as that used for heart surgery) is necessary to maintain adequate oxygenation.

Infants are usually positioned in a semi-Fowler's position to facilitate breathing, although some appear to be more comfortable on their abdomen. The prone position may allow the weight of the body to help empty the chest more completely on expiration. Feeding is often a problem because infants tire easily and therefore cannot finish a feeding. Intravenous fluids may be given for the first 1 or 2 days of illness to eliminate the need for oral feeding.

NURSING DIAGNOSES AND RELATED INTERVENTIONS

Nursing Diagnosis: Parental anxiety related to respiratory distress in child

Outcome Identification: Parents will demonstrate reduced anxiety regarding child's illness by 24 hours.

Outcome Evaluation: Parents state that their anxiety level is tolerable as signs and symptoms of disease decrease.

Be certain that parents receive a good explanation of their child's condition. Most parents are aware of bronchi but are unfamiliar with the word "bronchiole." This leaves them unsure about how a simple cold has become so severe. They wonder whether they should have sought medical attention sooner. This may cause them to lose confidence in themselves as parents. Assure them that bronchiolitis begins as only a cold and that it was impossible to know that this cold would take a more serious turn.

The acute phase of bronchiolitis lasts 2 or 3 days. After this time, the child's condition improves rapidly. Although mortality from bronchiolitis is less than 1%, it is a serious disorder of infancy; without treatment, a larger number of infants certainly would die (Hakonarson, 2000).

Asthma

Asthma, an immediate hypersensitivity (type I) response (see Chap. 42), is the most common chronic illness in children, accounting for many days of absenteeism from school and many hospital admissions each year. It tends to occur initially before age 5 years, although in these early years it may be diagnosed as frequent occurrences of bronchiolitis rather than asthma (Table 40-6). The condition may be intermittent, with symptom-free periods, or chronic, with continuous symptoms.

Asthma tends to occur in children with atopy or those with a tendency to react with hypersensitivity to allergens. Mast cells release histamine and leukotrienes that result in diffuse obstructive and restrictive airway disease because of inflammation, bronchoconstriction, and increased mucus production. Severe bronchoconstriction can occur because of exposure to cold air or irritating odors, such as turpentine or smog, as well as inhalation of a known allergen. Air pollutants such as cigarette smoke may lower the threshold for hypersensitivity reactions and worsen the condition. Most children with asthma can be shown to have sensitization to inhalant antigens such as pollens, molds, or house dust. Food also may be involved. Although there may be a seasonal factor responsible for the child's symptoms, most children have multiple sensitivities and are affected all year long.

Mechanism of Disease

Asthma primarily affects the small airways and involves three separate processes: bronchospasm, inflammation of bronchial mucosa, and increased bronchial secretions (mucus). All three processes act to reduce the size of the airway lumen, leading to acute respiratory distress. Bronchial constriction occurs because of stimulation of the parasympathetic nervous system (cholinergic mediated system), which initiates smooth muscle constriction. Inflammation occurs because of mast cell activation to release leukotrienes, histamine, and prostaglandins. These cause

TABLE 40.6 Comparison of Bronchiolitis, Pneumonia, and Asthma

ASSESSMENT	BRONCHIOLITIS	PNEUMONIA	ASTHMA
Cause	Usually respiratory syncytial virus	Possibly bacterial (pneumococcal, or *H. influenzae*), viral, or mycoplasmal; possibly secondary to aspiration	Hypersensitivity type I immune response
Age of child	Under 2 yr	All through childhood	Onset 1–5 yr
Onset pattern	Follows an upper respiratory infection	Follows an upper respiratory infection	Follows initiation by an allergen
Appearance	Fatigued, anxious, shallow respirations, increasing anteroposterior diameter of chest	Fatigued, anxious, shallow respirations	Wheezing, exhausted, frightened
Cough	Paroxysmal, dry	Productive, harsh cough	Paroxysmal, with thick mucus production
Fever	Low grade	Elevated	None
Auscultatory sounds	Barely audible breath sounds, crackles, expiratory wheezing	Decreased breath sounds, crackles	Wheezing

bronchoconstriction and mucus production. Once viewed as a long-term, poorly controlled disorder, newer therapy makes this a reversible or manageable disorder (Chedevergne et al., 2000).

Assessment

The word asthma is derived from the Greek word for panting. Typically, after exposure to an allergen or trigger, an episode begins with a dry cough, often at night as bronchoconstriction begins. Because bronchioles are normally larger in lumen on inspiration than expiration even with bronchoconstriction, children may inhale normally or have little difficulty. They develop increasing difficulty exhaling as it becomes more and more difficult to force air through the narrowed lumen of the inflamed bronchioles filled with mucus. This causes the dyspnea and the wheezing (the sound caused by air being pushed forcibly through obstructed bronchioles) typically associated with this disorder. Remember that wheezing is heard primarily on expiration. However, when severe, wheezing may be heard on inspiration as well. If the child coughs up mucus, it is generally copious and may contain white casts bearing the shape of the bronchi from which it was dislodged.

History. Assessment should include a thorough history of the development of the child's symptoms—for example, what the child was doing at the time of the attack, and what actions were taken by the parents or child to decrease or arrest the symptoms. When an acute attack has passed, ask the parent or child to describe the home environment, including any pets, the child's bedroom, outdoor play space, classroom environment, and type of heating in the house to see whether more environmental control could reduce future occurrences.

Physical Assessment. A physical assessment includes examining for the specific symptoms of asthma. Cyanosis may be present. On auscultation, wheezing typically is heard on expiration. In many children, this initial wheezing is so loud that it can be heard without a stethoscope. In others, it is evident only by auscultation. Asthma affects all lobes of the lungs, so although the wheezing may be more prominent in one lobe than in another, it is generally audible in all lung fields. Audible wheezing in only one lobe suggests that only one bronchus is plugged, which suggests that a foreign body such as a peanut is more likely responsible, rather than asthma.

Bronchospasm leads to CO_2 trapping and retention; thus, arterial oxygen saturation monitored by a pulse oximeter may be decreased because of the inability to fully aerate the lungs. The child is often frightened because of an acute feeling of suffocation. A peak flow meter shows decreased ability to exhale. The eosinophil count is elevated.

The lungs are hyperresonant to percussion (i.e., they make a louder, hollower noise on percussion than usual) because of pockets of trapped air behind clogged bronchi. In normal respiration, the inspiration phase of breathing is longer than the expiration phase. During an attack of asthma, children must work so hard to exhale that the expiration phase becomes longer than the inspiration phase. Time the two phases to demonstrate this. Also observe for retractions, because children use intercostal accessory muscles to achieve full breaths.

As constriction becomes acute, the sound of wheezing may decrease because so little air is able to leave the alveoli. Hypoxemia and possibly cyanosis will become severe. When blood gases show an increased P_{CO_2} level and the sound of wheezing suddenly stops, respiratory failure is imminent.

During attacks, children with asthma are generally more comfortable in a sitting or standing position rather than lying down. If seated in a chair, they lean forward and raise their shoulders to give themselves more breathing space. Do not urge children to "lie down and relax." This causes severe anxiety and increased difficulty in breathing. Children who do agree to lie down are either at the end of an attack and so beginning to feel less threatened by the dyspnea or are so exhausted by the paroxysms of coughing that they no longer have the strength to sit upright.

Over time, as the child has many bouts of asthma, he or she may develop a shield-like or barrel-shaped chest from constant overinflation of air in alveoli. Clubbing of the fingers (from the growth of excess capillaries initiated when polycythemia is sensed because of poor tissue oxygenation in distal parts) may be noticeable. If the child has been treated for a long period with steroids, growth may be stunted.

Pulmonary Function Studies

Good pulmonary function depends on good ventilation (both drawing adequate air into the lungs and expelling it again), adequate transfer of gases across the alveolar capillary membranes, and adequate volume and distribution of pulmonary capillary blood flow. In children with asthma, the vital capacity may be low or the capacity may be normal but, because of narrowed bronchioles as a result of bronchospasm, the expiratory rate may be abnormally long (more than 10 seconds rather than the normal 2 or 3 seconds). If the child has atelectasis, the vital capacity will be low because of air absorption behind bronchial plugging. When a vital capacity test is abnormal, the child may have it repeated after an inhalation treatment. A gross measure of vital capacity is to ask a child to blow out a match. A child with an average vital capacity should be able to do this when the match is held at 6 inches.

Peak Expiratory Flow Rate Monitoring. Children with asthma often use a home peak flow meter daily to measure gross changes in peak expiratory flow over time. This can help in planning an appropriate therapeutic regimen (Fig. 40-20). Children with asthma should be able to tell you their usual reading and personal best score.

To use a peak flow meter, a child places the indicator at the bottom of the numbered scale, and takes a deep breath. He or she places the meter in the mouth and blows out as hard and fast as possible. He or she then repeats this two more times and records the highest number achieved as the peak flow meter result. During a 2-week period when the child feels well, this should be done daily. The highest number achieved during this time is recorded as the child's personal best.

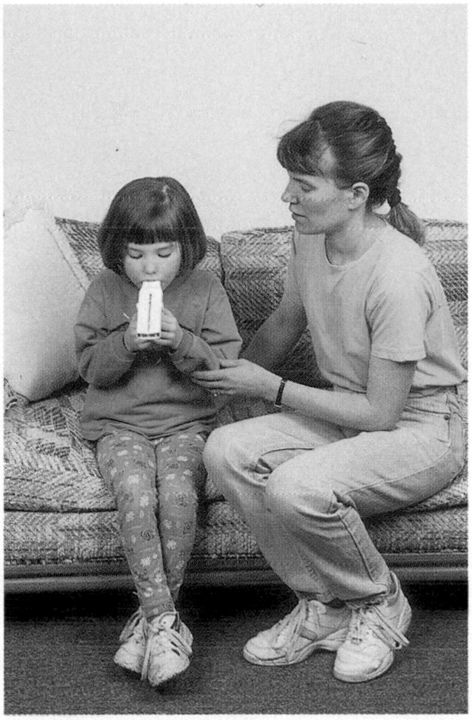

FIGURE 40.20 Children with any chronic illness require periodic evaluation and sometimes home monitoring. Here a child with asthma practices using a home peak flow meter to track her peak expiratory flow readings on a daily basis.

Children are assigned zones to rate their expiratory compliance:

- Green zone (80% to 100% of their personal best) means no asthma symptoms are present, and they should take their routine medications.
- Yellow zone (50% to 80% of personal best) signals caution. An episode of asthma may be beginning.
- Red zone (below 50% of personal best) indicates an asthma episode is beginning. The child should immediately take an inhaled beta-2-agonist and then repeat the peak flow assessment. If the second reading is not in the green zone, the parent should alert the child's primary care provider.

Therapeutic Management

Therapy for children with asthma involves planning for the three goals of all allergic disorders: avoidance of the allergen by environmental control; skin testing and hyposensitization to identified allergens; and relief of symptoms by pharmacologic agents.

The child with mild but persistent asthma usually is prescribed an inhaled anti-inflammatory corticosteroid such as fluticasone (Flovent) daily. If the child needs to supplement the primary therapy this way on a daily basis, additional long-term control therapy may be necessary.

Children who have moderate persistent symptoms usually are prescribed an inhaled anti-inflammatory corticosteroid daily and a long-acting bronchodilator at bedtime. Children who have severe persistent asthma symptoms take a high dose of both an oral corticosteroid and an inhaled corticosteroid daily as well as a long-acting bronchodilator at bedtime. In addition, children are prescribed a short-acting beta-2-agonist bronchodilator, such as albuterol or terbutaline, to use if an attack should begin (see Focus on Pharmacology: Albuterol Sulfate). Cromolyn sodium is a mast cell stabilizer given by a nebulizer or metered-dose inhaler that can prevent bronchoconstriction and thereby prevent the symptoms of asthma (see Focus on Pharmacology: Cromolyn Sodium). It is not effective once symptoms have begun.

Another group of drugs used in the treatment of asthma are leukotriene receptor antagonists such as Montelukast (Singulair). This drug is used for prophylaxis and chronic treatment of asthma in children over the age of 6 years. It is not effective in an acute attack.

If children are to receive medication by nebulizer or inhaler, be certain that they learn to use these wisely. It is easy to take this type of medication lightly (the belief that it is "not really medicine" because it is not swallowed). As

FOCUS ON PHARMACOLOGY

Albuterol Sulfate (Proventil, Ventolin)

Action: Albuterol is a beta-2-adrenergic agonist that acts selectively to cause bronchodilation and vasodilation for relief of bronchospasm.

Pregnancy risk category: C

Dosage: Orally, 2 or 4 mg 3 or 4 times daily not to exceed 32 mg/day in children older than 14 years; 2 mg 3 or 4 times daily not to exceed 24 mg/day in children ages 6 to 14 years; 0.1 mg/kg 3 times daily not to exceed 2 mg, gradually increasing to 0.2 mg/kg 3 times daily not to exceed 4 mg in children ages 2 to 6 years. By inhalation, 2 puffs every 4 to 6 hours in children 12 years of age and older or 2.5 mg (0.5 mL of 0.5% solution diluted with 2.5 mL of 0.9% sodium chloride) or 3 mL of 0.083% solution 3 or 4 times daily.

Possible adverse effects: Restlessness, apprehension, anxiety, fear, nausea, cardiac arrhythmias, paradoxical airway resistance with repeated, excessive use of inhalation preparations, sweating, pallor, and flushing.

Nursing Implications

- Instruct parents and child in method to administer drug. Teach child and parents about use and care of nebulized solution or metered-dose inhaler and spacer devices if ordered.
- Caution child and parents not to exceed the number of ordered puffs to prevent possible tolerance to drug.
- If more than one inhalation is ordered, advise child to wait 1 to 2 minutes before taking the second puff.
- If the child is also receiving an inhaled corticosteroid, advise the child and parents to have the child use the albuterol first to open the airways and then wait approximately 5 minutes before using the corticosteroid, to maximize its effectiveness.

FOCUS ON PHARMACOLOGY

Cromolyn Sodium (Intal)

Action: Cromolyn is a mast cell inhibitor that acts to inhibit the release of histamine and slow-releasing substance of anaphylaxis, and leukotriene, thus decreasing the overall allergic response. In asthma, it is used prophylactically to prevent severe bronchospasms.

Pregnancy risk category: B

Dosage: Initially, 20 mg inhaled (via spinhaler inhalant or as nebulized solution) 4 times daily at regular intervals; one ampule orally 4 times daily one-half hour before meals and at bedtime (not recommended for use in children under the age of 5 years)

Possible adverse effects: Dizziness, headache, nausea, dry and irritated throat, cough, nasal congestion, epistaxis, sneezing

Nursing Implications

- Instruct parents and child that this drug is not effective in an acute attack.
- Caution child and parents to take the drug exactly as prescribed and to continue other agents, such as bronchodilators.
- Instruct child and parents in the use of metered-dose inhaler or nebulizer for administration of cromolyn.
- If the oral form is prescribed, instruct parents to open the ampule and pour the contents into a glass of water and to wait for the medication to dissolve. Caution parents not to substitute the oral form for the inhalant form and vice versa.
- Instruct parents and child to watch for a possible recurrence of asthma symptoms if dosage is decreased.
- Know that this drug is only given once the acute episode is over and the child's airway is clear to prevent a further episode.
- Caution child and parents not to exceed the number of ordered puffs via inhaler to prevent possible tolerance to drug.
- If more than one inhalation is ordered, advise child to wait 1 to 2 minutes before taking the second puff.
- If the child is also receiving an inhaled bronchodilator, advise the child and parents to have the child use the bronchodilator first to open the airways and then wait approximately 5 minutes before using the cromolyn, to maximize its effectiveness.

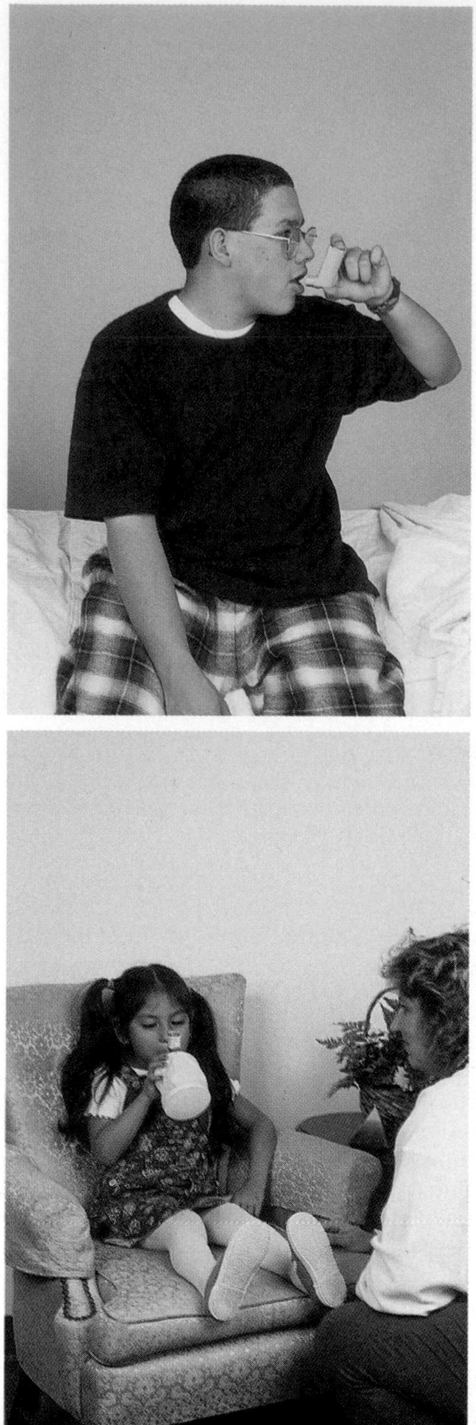

A

B

FIGURE 40.21 (*A*) Many children with asthma use a metered dose inhaler to administer a bronchodilator to themselves. Be certain children respect such medicine as medicine and thus use sensible precautions. (*B*) Younger children need a "spacer" with inhalers so they do not need to correlate administration with inhalation.

a result, overdose from constant use of nebulizers or metered-dose inhalers can occur. Metered-dose inhalers require that the child trigger the inhaler at the same time he or she breathes in (Fig. 40-21*A*). Because it is difficult for children younger than approximately 12 years to do this, placing a spacer tube between the inhaler and the mouthpiece eliminates this problem (see Fig. 40-21*B*).

Dehydration occurs rapidly in children during an asthma attack from decreased oral intake (children stop drinking because they are coughing, or coughing makes them vomit and parents stop offering fluid) and the increased insensible loss that occurs from tachypnea. Dehydration may contribute to increased mucus plugging and further airway obstruction. Encourage children to continue to drink fluids (ask about favorite beverages and offer small sips of them). Avoid milk or milk products because they cause thick mucus and difficulty swallowing. In an emergency setting, an intravenous line is established to supply continuous fluid therapy and provide a route for emergency drug administration.

NURSING DIAGNOSES AND RELATED INTERVENTIONS

Nursing Diagnosis: Fear related to sudden onset of asthma attack

Outcome Identification: Parents and child will demonstrate ability to manage sudden attacks within 1 month.

Outcome Evaluation: Parents and child express confidence in their ability to prevent attacks and handle any that occur.

Asthma is a frightening disease. At the time it is diagnosed, parents may have already gone through a long period of wondering what was wrong with their child. After diagnosis, parents may be afraid to allow children to attend school for fear that they will have an attack while away from them. They may be afraid to leave them alone with baby-sitters or even relatives so that they may have evenings to themselves or enjoy a vacation. Help parents find a middle ground: to allow a child enough freedom for growth and development while still being certain that he or she is safe. Taking steps to slow breathing, better emptying alveoli through pursed-lip breathing, and administering medications to prevent symptoms are key measures to teach. Children can have long periods without attacks. When a new one occurs after a long absence, it is almost as frightening as the original attack because everything seems so new again.

Nursing Diagnosis: Health-seeking behaviors related to prevention of and treatment for asthma attacks

Outcome Identification: Parents and child within 1 month will demonstrate understanding of ways to prevent attacks and measures to manage attacks when they occur.

Outcome Evaluation: Parents and child accurately state triggers that cause an attack; child correctly demonstrates breathing exercises, use of inhaler, and peak expiratory flow meter.

Children need to learn how to avoid possible triggers through environmental control. (For more information about controlling triggers in the home, see Chap. 42.) If foods are a trigger, children need to learn to be responsible for their own diets so they can avoid these foods. Children as young as age 6 years can learn the foods they cannot eat and take responsibility for telling a friend's parent if at a birthday party or a schoolteacher that they must not eat certain foods. They must learn to use a metered-dose inhaler or nebulizer if prescribed. At the same time, they must not become inhaler-dependent or carry the inhaler with them constantly, afraid to go anywhere without it. This will invariably result in their using the inhaler much more often than is necessary.

To prevent children with asthma from losing chest mobility and to decrease their tendency to develop a barrel chest, they may be taught a number of breathing or mobility exercises to do daily at home. Such exercises are aimed at increasing expiratory function (diaphragmatic or side expansion breathing). Recommended activities include bending side to side, bending forward and touching the left foot with the right hand, and swinging the arms rhythmically in front of the body like a windmill. These exercises can be incorporated into a bedtime or after-school routine. Parents (and nurses) who do mobility exercises with children find that the exercises help to reduce abdominal size, because they tighten abdominal muscles as well. Using an incentive spirometer daily is another method to exercise the lungs and keep chest muscles supple.

The prognosis in children who develop asthma is good if they adhere to their treatment regimen. Children do not outgrow asthma, although most of them may become symptom-free as adults, probably because the lumens of major airways enlarge with adulthood.

When informing parents of these facts, be certain not to convey the impression that asthma is a disease that is outgrown. Although asthma may not always last into adulthood, the need for careful environmental control, conscientious administration of medication, and hyposensitization, if indicated, during childhood should not be diminished.

Status Asthmaticus

Under ordinary circumstances, an asthma attack responds readily to the aerosol administration of a bronchodilator such as albuterol, terbutaline, or levalbuterol (Xopenex). When children fail to respond and an attack continues, they are in status asthmaticus. This is an extreme emergency because if the attack cannot be relieved, the child may die of heart failure caused by the combination of exhaustion, atelectasis, and respiratory acidosis from bronchial plugging.

Assessment

A child with status asthmaticus is in acute respiratory distress. Both heart rate and respiratory rate are elevated. Sao_2 and Po_2 levels are low; Pco_2 levels are elevated because bronchi are so constricted that the child cannot exhale, resulting in CO_2 accumulation. The rising Pco_2 level rapidly leads to acidosis. In contrast to the loud wheezing heard in children initially with asthmatic attacks, children with status asthmaticus may have so little air able to pass in or out of their lungs that breath sounds are limited. Pulse oximetry will reveal the poor oxygenation (Carpenter et al., 2001).

Status asthmaticus is often initiated by pulmonary infection, which acts as the triggering mechanism for the prolonged attack. If this occurs, obtain cultures from coughed sputum, and be prepared to administer a broad-spectrum antibiotic until the cultures are returned. Be sure the sputum obtained for culture is coughed from deep in the respiratory tract and not just from the back of the throat.

Therapeutic Management

By definition, the child in status asthmaticus has failed to respond to first-line therapy. Continuous nebulization with an inhaled beta-2-agonist and intravenous corticosteroids may be necessary to reduce symptoms. The Po_2 level usually is maintained at more than 90 mm Hg with oxygen administration. This is best given by face mask or nasal prongs. These methods supply good oxygen concentrations and yet leave the child unobscured for easy observation. To prevent drying of pulmonary secretions, always give oxygen with humidification. Oxygen is best administered at a concentration of 30% to 40%, not 100%. If concentrations greater than 40% are needed, a Venturi mask that allows for rebreathing may be used. Some children in severe status asthmaticus have such a carbon dioxide buildup (because they cannot exhale properly) that they develop carbon dioxide narcosis with no stimulation for inhalation. The child's respiratory stimulus, therefore, is hypoxia, or lack of oxygen. If 100% oxygen were administered, the oxygen lack would disappear, and respirations would cease. The idea "if a little is good, a lot is better" does not apply here. After it has been ascertained that the child is not in acidosis (from blood gas and pH studies), oxygen levels may be increased, but for initial therapy, keep the level at 40%.

After an acute stage of status asthmaticus, children need increased fluid to keep airway secretions moist. Drinking tends to aggravate coughing, so they are unlikely to drink; as a result, they are often dehydrated on admission to the hospital. An intravenous infusion such as 5% glucose in 0.45 saline is started to supply fluid. If the child is able to drink, do not offer cold fluids because these tend to aggravate bronchospasm. Also, ask parents if they have given any cough suppressants. As a rule, as long as children can continue to cough up mucus, they are not in serious danger. When they stop coughing up mucus, thick plugs form that may lead to pneumonia, atelectasis, and further acidosis. Loss of cough and no wheezing is, therefore, an ominous sign. Monitor intake and output; measure the specific gravity of urine. Under stress, antidiuretic hormone is released, so fluid retention and overhydration may occur.

An increasing Pco_2 level is a danger sign because it indicates the degree of hypoventilation. In severe attacks, endotracheal intubation and mechanical ventilation may be necessary to maintain effective respirations.

✔ CHECKPOINT QUESTIONS

20. When is bronchiolitis most commonly seen?
21. What is the most common presenting symptom in a child with asthma?
22. What is the chief medication given for an acute asthma attack?

Bronchiectasis

Bronchiectasis is chronic dilatation of the bronchi. It may follow pneumonia, aspiration of a foreign body, pertussis, or asthma. It is often associated with cystic fibrosis (Larsen et al., 2001).

Children develop a chronic cough with mucopurulent sputum. Young infants may have accompanying wheezing or stridor. If a large area of lung is involved, children may have cyanosis. As the disease becomes chronic, children develop symptoms of chronic lung disease, such as clubbing of the fingers and easy fatigability. Their physical growth may become restricted. Their chest may become enlarged from overinflation of alveoli caused by the air trapped behind inflamed bronchi.

Chest physiotherapy may be necessary to raise the tenacious sputum. An antibiotic will be necessary if infection is present. The cause of the bronchiectasis must be identified and relieved before the chronic process can be relieved. Surgery to remove the affected lung portion may be necessary.

Pneumonia

Pneumonia, inflammation of the alveoli, occurs at a rate of 2 to 4 children in 100. It may be of bacterial origin (pneumococcal, streptococcal, staphylococcal, or chlamydial) or viral origin, such as respiratory syncytial virus (RSV). Aspiration of lipid or hydrocarbon substances also causes pneumonia. Pneumonia is the most common pulmonary cause of death in infants younger than 48 hours of age. It occurs most often in late winter and early spring. Newborns who are born more than 24 hours after rupture of the amniotic membranes and those who aspirated amniotic fluid or meconium during birth are particularly prone to developing pneumonia in their first few days of life (Thilo & Rosenberg, 2001). When it is known that the membranes have been ruptured for more than 24 hours before birth, prophylactic broad-spectrum antibiotics may be given to prevent pneumonia. Differences between bronchiolitis, pneumonia, and asthma are summarized in Table 40-6. *Pneumocystis carinii* pneumonia, the type seen almost exclusively with human immunodeficiency syndrome, is discussed in Chapter 42.

Pneumococcal Pneumonia

The onset of pneumococcal pneumonia is generally abrupt and follows an upper respiratory tract infection. In infants, pneumonia tends to remain bronchopneumonia with poor consolidation (infiltration of exudate into the alveoli). In older children, pneumonia may localize in a single lobe, and consolidation may occur. With this, children may have blood-tinged sputum as exudative serum and red blood cells invade the alveoli. After 24 to 48 hours, the alveoli are no longer filled with red blood cells and serum but fibrin, leukocytes, and pneumococci. At this point, the child's cough no longer raises blood-tinged sputum but thick purulent material.

Assessment. Children develop a high fever, nasal flaring, retractions, chest pain, chills, and dyspnea. Some children report the pain as being abdominal. The fever with pneumococcal pneumonia may rise so fast that a child has a febrile convulsion (see Chap. 49).

Children with pneumococcal pneumonia appear acutely ill. Tachypnea and tachycardia develop. Because lung space is filled with exudate, respiratory function is diminished. Breath sounds become bronchial (sound transmitted from the trachea) because air no longer or only poorly enters fluid-filled alveoli. Crackles (rales) may be present as a result of the fluid. Dullness on percussion over a lobe indicates that consolidation has occurred. Chest radiographs will show lung consolidation in older children and patchy diffusion in young children. Laboratory studies will indicate leukocytosis (Silver, 2000).

Therapeutic Management. Before antibiotic therapy was available for pneumonia, it was almost always a fatal disease, especially in infants, so parents may be more worried about a child's condition than is warranted (see Focus on Communication).

FOCUS ON COMMUNICATION

B. J. is a 2-year-old who has been admitted to your hospital unit with pneumonia. His mother called home to tell the grandmother about the diagnosis. Since she returned from the telephone, Mrs. Silver seems tearful and visibly upset.

Less Effective Communication

Nurse: Is something wrong, Mrs. Silver? You seem upset.
Mrs. Silver: I am. I didn't realize pneumonia was so serious until I talked to my mother.
Nurse: Because it's serious is why B. J.'s been admitted to the hospital.
Mrs. Silver: She told me my brother had pneumonia when he was a baby. Is this oxygen? My mother said to check B. J.'s getting oxygen.
Nurse: It sure is. He's also going to get an antibiotic. Why don't you stay with him while I get the equipment for that?

More Effective Communication

Nurse: Is something wrong, Mrs. Silver? You seem upset.
Mrs. Silver: I am. I didn't realize pneumonia was so serious until I talked to my mother.
Nurse: Because it's serious is why B. J.'s been admitted to the hospital.
Mrs. Silver: She told me my brother had pneumonia when he was a baby. Is this oxygen? My mother said to check B.J.'s getting oxygen.
Nurse: Let's talk about everything your mother told you about pneumonia. Because the treatment has changed so much, what happened years ago isn't the same as what happens now.

Before the advent of antibiotics, a diagnosis of pneumonia in a young child was almost automatically a fatal diagnosis. Ask enough questions of parents today to be certain they understand that their child's prognosis, although serious, is not the fatal diagnosis of years ago.

Therapy for pneumococcal pneumonia is antibiotics. Either ampicillin or a third-generation cephalosporin is effective against pneumococci. Amoxicillin-clavulanate (Augmentin) also may be prescribed for penicillin-resistant organisms. Children need rest to prevent exhaustion. Plan nursing care carefully to conserve the child's strength. At the same time, turn and reposition the child frequently to avoid pooling of secretions. Intravenous therapy may be necessary to supply fluid, especially in infants, because infants tire so readily with sucking that they cannot achieve a good oral intake. They may need an antipyretic such as acetaminophen to reduce fever (Silver, 2000). (See Focus on Nursing Care Planning.)

Humidified oxygen may be necessary to alleviate labored breathing and prevent hypoxemia. Assess oxygen saturation levels frequently via pulse oximetry. Chest physiotherapy encourages the movement of mucus and prevents obstruction. Older children may need to be encouraged to cough so that secretions do not pool and become further infected.

After pneumonia, children usually have a period of at least a week when they tire easily and need frequent, small feedings. Parents need to be cautioned that this is an expected outcome and not a complication in itself. Children with chronic illness, those who have had a splenectomy, or those who are immunocompromised should receive a pneumococcal vaccine to prevent pneumococcal pneumonia.

Chlamydial Pneumonia

Chlamydia trachomatis pneumonia is most often seen in newborns up to 12 weeks of age as the chlamydial organism is contracted from the mother during birth. Symptoms usually begin gradually with nasal congestion and a sharp cough; infants fail to gain back their birthweight. Symptoms progress to tachypnea, with wheezing and crackles audible on auscultation. Laboratory assessment will show an elevated level of immunoglobulin IgG and IgM antibodies, peripheral eosinophilia, and a specific antibody to *C. trachomatis.* Such an infection is treated with a macrolide antibiotic such as erythromycin with good results (Nachajon, 2000).

Viral Pneumonia

Viral pneumonia is generally caused by the viruses of upper respiratory tract infection: the RSVs, myxoviruses, or adenoviruses. Symptoms begin as an upper respiratory tract infection. After a day or two, additional symptoms such as a low-grade fever, nonproductive cough, and tachypnea begin. There may be diminished breath sounds and fine crackles on chest auscultation. RSV may cause apnea. Chest radiographs will show diffuse infiltrated areas.

Because this is a viral infection, antibiotic therapy usually is not effective. The child needs rest and, possibly, an antipyretic for the fever; intravenous fluid may be necessary if the child becomes exhausted from feeding or is dehydrated and refusing fluids. After recovery from the acute phase of illness, the child will have a week or two of lethargy or lack of energy, as occurs with bacterial pneumonia. Parents may be confused because their child is not

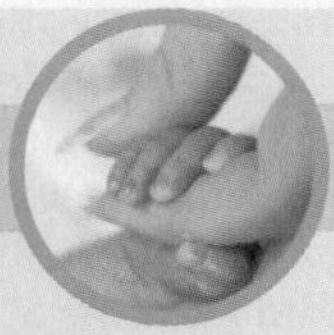

FOCUS ON *Nursing Care Planning*

A CHILD HOSPITALIZED WITH PNEUMONIA

A 3-year-old brought to the emergency department by his parents is admitted to the hospital with a diagnosis of pneumococcal pneumonia. His parents state, "He just had a cold but now he's coughing up thick yellow mucus."

Assessment: 3-year-old male within age-acceptable parameters for height and weight. Child is diaphoretic and pale. Tympanic temperature, 102.2°F (39.0°C); pulse, 146; respirations, 40. Nasal flaring and intercostal retractions noted. Lungs with decreased breath sounds. Scattered crackles auscultated and dullness to percussion noted in right upper and middle lobes. Productive cough with thick purulent sputum. Child reports difficulty breathing. Mother states, "He hasn't been drinking much because of his coughing. And all he seems to want to do is lie on the couch."

Chest x-ray reveals patchy diffusion; white blood cell count reveals leukocytosis. Unable to obtain sputum specimen for culture.

Nursing Diagnosis: Ineffective breathing pattern related to physiologic effects of pneumonia

Outcome Identification: Child will exhibit signs and symptoms of adequate ventilation.

Outcome Evaluation: Respiratory rate, oxygen saturation, and arterial blood gas levels are within age-acceptable parameters without the use of supplemental oxygen. Lungs are clear to auscultation. Child states breathing is easier; demonstrates measures to improve ventilation and ease the work of breathing.

Interventions	Rationale
1. Administer supplemental, humidified oxygen via face mask at prescribed rate. Obtain arterial blood gases (ABGs) as ordered and monitor oxygen saturation levels via pulse oximetry.	1. Supplemental, humidified oxygen aids in improving ventilation without drying the mucous membranes and in minimizing the risk for hypoxemia. ABGs and pulse oximetry provide objective evidence of the child's tissue oxygenation.
2. Assess vital signs and respiratory status, including lung sounds, initially every 1 to 2 hours and then according to institution's policy.	2. Frequent assessment of vital signs and respiratory status provides information about any improvement or deterioration in the child's condition.
3. Administer antibiotic therapy, such as ampicillin, as ordered.	3. Ampicillin is effective against pneumococci.
4. Place the child in a semi-Fowler's to high Fowler's position. Reposition the child frequently.	4. An upright position facilitates breathing and promotes optimal lung expansion by relieving diaphragmatic pressure. Frequent repositioning prevents pooling and stasis of secretions.
5. Perform chest physiotherapy as ordered.	5. Chest physiotherapy helps to mobilize secretions to prevent mucous plugging and aids in expectoration.
6. Use play to encourage the child to cough, deep breathe, and use incentive spirometry every 1 to 2 hours. Involve the parents in these activities.	6. Coughing, deep breathing, and incentive spirometry help to maximize ventilation. Play helps to enhance the child's participation. Involving the parents promotes active participation in the child's care.
7. Assist the child and parents with measures to relax.	7. Anxiety and stress increase the child's oxygen demands. Assisting the parents to relax also helps to minimize the effect of the parents' anxiety on the child.

(continued)

Nursing Diagnosis: Risk for deficient fluid volume related to diminished oral intake and increased insensible fluid losses secondary to tachypnea, diaphoresis, and fever

Outcome Identification: The child will exhibit signs and symptoms of adequate fluid balance.

Outcome Evaluation: Skin turgor is good. Intake and output, urine specific gravity, laboratory studies, and weight remain within age-appropriate parameters.

Interventions	Rationale
1. Obtain baseline weight and monitor daily.	1. Weight is an accurate indicator of fluid balance.
2. Administer intravenous fluid therapy at prescribed rate, using an infusion pump or controller.	2. Intravenous fluid therapy assists in replacing fluid losses, especially when there is difficulty with ingesting appropriate amounts of oral fluid. Using a pump or controller ensures an accurate flow rate, minimizing the risk for fluid overload.
3. Offer the child sips of fluid frequently. Try different forms of fluid such as gelatin, Popsicles, or fruit bars based on the child's likes. Incorporate the use of play to encourage the child to drink, such as taking a sip or spoonful of gelatin each time after his turn in a game. Involve the parents in these activities.	3. Oral fluid intake is necessary for replacement. Different forms of fluid may be more appealing to the child and enhance his intake. Using games and play are effective methods for encouraging fluid intake in a child. Involving the parents promotes active participation in the child's care.
4. Institute measures to control fever, such as administering acetaminophen as ordered and dressing child in lightweight clothing.	4. Reducing fever aids in reducing insensible fluid loss.
5. Monitor intake and output, urine specific gravity, urine and serum electrolytes, blood urea nitrogen, creatinine, and osmolality.	5. Intake and output and urine specific gravity are reliable indicators of fluid balance. Fluid loss can result in dehydration, leading to decreased renal function and ability to eliminate wastes.

Nursing Diagnosis: Activity intolerance related to effects of pneumonia and tachypnea

Outcome Identification: Child will exhibit a return to preillness activity level.

Outcome Evaluation: Child's oxygen saturation level and vital signs are within age-acceptable parameters with activity. Child participates in self-care activities with minimal to no reports of difficulty breathing.

Interventions	Rationale
1. Provide a balance of activity with rest periods. Cluster nursing care to prevent overexertion.	1. Activity increases myocardial oxygen demand, further compromising respiratory function.
2. Continue to administer supplemental oxygen and monitor vital signs, oxygen saturation levels, and breathing difficulties before and after any activity.	2. Oxygen is necessary for adequate tissue perfusion. A decrease in oxygen saturation levels or vital signs or increasing difficulty breathing in response to activity indicates an increase in oxygen demand that the child is not able to meet.
3. Provide small, frequent meals.	3. Eating requires energy expenditure. Small, frequent meals prevent overtiring, which could further compromise respiratory function and also interfere with nutrition.

(continued)

Interventions	Rationale
4. As the pneumonia resolves, gradually allow an increase in activity, such as self-care activities, getting out of bed to a chair, and ambulation, using oxygen saturation levels as a guide.	4. Gradual increase in activity within acceptable oxygen saturation levels minimizes the risk for further respiratory compromise.
5. Provide frequent support and contact with the child and family.	5. Frequent contact and support helps to alleviate anxiety, which increases the child's oxygen demands.

receiving an antibiotic, despite the diagnosis being pneumonia. They need an explanation of the difference between viral and bacterial infections so they can understand their child's therapy and plan of care.

Mycoplasmal Pneumonia

The Mycoplasma organisms are similar to yet larger than viruses. Mycoplasmal pneumonia occurs more frequently in older children (over 5 years) and more often during the winter.

The symptoms of mycoplasmal pneumonia make it difficult to differentiate from other pneumonias. The child has a fever and a cough and feels ill. Cervical lymph nodes are enlarged. The child may have a persistent rhinitis.

Mycoplasmal organisms generally are sensitive to erythromycin or tetracycline. Erythromycin is the preferred drug for children younger than 8 years of age, because tetracycline tends to stain teeth brown and possibly stunt long bone growth (Karch, 2001).

Lipid Pneumonia

Lipid pneumonia is caused by the aspiration of oily or lipid substances. It is much less common than it once was because children are not given oil-based tonics, such as castor oil or cod liver oil, as they were in the past. Today it is most often caused by aspirated oily foreign bodies such as peanuts or popcorn. A proliferative inflammatory response occurs when lung lipases act on the aspirated oil. This may be followed by diffuse fibrosis of the bronchi or alveoli. The area then becomes secondarily infected.

A child may have an initial coughing spell at the time of aspiration. A period follows during which the child is symptomless; then a chronic cough, dyspnea, and general respiratory distress occur. A chest radiograph shows densities at the affected site.

Antibiotic therapy is ineffective unless a secondary bacterial infection has occurred. Surgical resection of a lung portion may be done to remove a lobe or segment if the pneumonitis does not heal by itself.

Hydrocarbon Pneumonia

A number of common household products such as furniture polish, cleaning fluids, turpentine, kerosene, gasoline, lighter fluid, and insect sprays have hydrocarbon bases. These products are a common cause of childhood poisonings and result in hydrocarbon pneumonia.

Assessment. Children who swallow a hydrocarbon-based product usually exhibit gastrointestinal symptoms such as nausea and vomiting. Next, they become drowsy because of inhalation of the vapors of the substance and may develop a cough as vapors from the stomach rise and are inhaled. As bronchial edema occurs from irritation and inflammation, respirations become increased and dyspneic.

Physical assessment shows an increased percussion sound caused by the presence of air trapped in the alveoli beyond the point of inflammation. Crackles may be heard as air passes through collected mucus. Because air is unable to reach and inflate the alveoli fully, breath sounds may be diminished.

Therapeutic Management. Hydrocarbon aspiration may occur when children initially swallow the fluid. If they are given an emetic to induce vomiting, they may aspirate at the time of vomiting. This is why vomiting is never induced if a child has swallowed a hydrocarbon. Parents should telephone a poison control center to ask for advice before inducing vomiting if they do not know the substance ingested or are unsure whether it was a hydrocarbon. Gastric lavage may be done by health care personnel with great care to remove the substance from the stomach.

The child is usually admitted to a hospital observation unit for a short time. Obtain vital signs and observe the child's general appearance carefully for evidence of increased respiratory tract obstruction or increasing drowsiness or other symptoms of central nervous system involvement from central nervous system intoxication. Cool, moist air administered by a nebulizer with supplemental oxygen may be ordered to decrease lung inflammation. If febrile, the child needs an antipyretic. Frequent changes of position will prevent pooling of secretions, which could lead to a secondary infection. Chest physiotherapy will help to move secretions and reduce areas of stasis.

The initial inflammation reaction from hydrocarbon aspiration may lead to such occlusion that emphysema (pocketing of air in alveoli) occurs, causing rupture of the alveoli into the pleural space, with consequent pneumothorax and atelectasis.

Often, children who swallow a household cleaner or other substance are aware that they should not have been handling substances kept under the sink. As a result, they cannot help but interpret the hospitalization, blood drawing, and other uncomfortable procedures as punishments for their action. They may benefit from therapeutic play with puppets or dolls that will help alleviate their guilt and anger at being "punished" so severely.

Hydrocarbon pneumonia is slow to resolve (Battan & Dart, 2001). After the illness, reinforce the need with parents to keep poisons in a safe place. They need a listening ear so they can explain that they did not mean this to happen and were unaware of the dangers of these everyday household products.

Atelectasis

Atelectasis is the collapse of lung alveoli. It may occur in children as a primary or secondary condition.

Primary Atelectasis

Primary atelectasis occurs in newborns who do not breathe with enough respiratory strength at birth to inflate lung tissue or whose alveoli are so immature or so lacking in surfactant that they cannot expand. This is seen most commonly in immature infants or in infants with central nervous system damage. It may occur if infants have mucus or meconium plugs in the trachea.

When atelectasis occurs, the newborn's respirations become irregular, with nasal flaring and apnea. After a few minutes, a respiratory grunt and cyanosis may occur. The sound of a respiratory grunt is caused by the newborn's glottis closing on expiration. At first, this is a helpful action because pressure in the respiratory tract increases, forcing more air into the alveoli for better inflation. As the infant tires, hypoxemia increases and the infant becomes hypotonic and flaccid. The Apgar score is invariably low.

As infants cry or are administered oxygen, more alveoli become aerated and cyanosis may decrease. The cause of the atelectasis must be established so that therapy directed to the specific cause can be initiated.

Secondary Atelectasis

Secondary atelectasis occurs in children when they have a respiratory tract obstruction that prevents air from entering a portion of the alveoli. As the residual air in the alveoli is absorbed, the alveoli collapse. The causes of obstruction in children include mucus plugs that may occur with chronic respiratory disease or aspiration of foreign objects. In some children, atelectasis occurs because of pressure on lung tissue from outside forces, such as compression from a diaphragmatic hernia, scoliosis, or enlarged thoracic lymph nodes (Fig. 40-22).

The signs of secondary atelectasis depend on the degree of collapse. Asymmetry of the chest may be noticed. Breath sounds on the affected side are decreased. If the process is extensive, tachypnea and cyanosis are present. A chest radiograph will show the collapsed lung (a "white-out").

Children with atelectasis are prone to secondary infection because mucus, which provides a good medium for bacteria, continues to be secreted.

Therapeutic Management

Atelectasis caused by inspiration of a foreign object will not be relieved until the object is removed by bronchoscopy. Atelectasis caused by a mucus plug will resolve when the plug resolves or is moved or expectorated. Children may need assisted ventilation to maintain adequate respiratory function until this time.

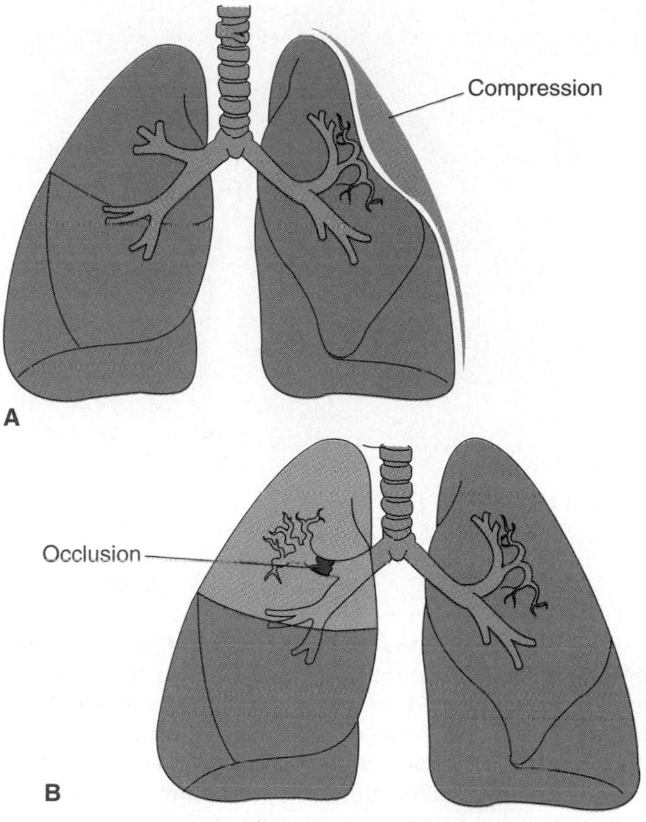

FIGURE 40.22 (*A*) Atelectasis caused by compression of lung tissue. (*B*) Atelectasis caused by obstruction.

Make certain that the chest of a child with atelectasis is kept free from pressure so that lung expansion is as full as possible (to allow as much breathing space as possible). If restraints are being used to keep an infant positioned, make certain that body restraints are not crossing the chest area and interfering with chest expansion. Check clothing to be certain that it is loose and nonbinding. Make certain that the child's arms are not positioned across the chest, where their weight could interfere with deep inspiration.

A semi-Fowler's position generally allows for the best lung expansion because it lowers abdominal contents. Increase the humidity of the child's environment to prevent further bronchial plugging; suction and chest physiotherapy may be necessary to keep the respiratory tract clear and free of mucus. Observe closely for increased respirations or cyanosis. Atelectasis is a serious disorder that must be considered as a possibility in all children with respiratory distress.

Pneumothorax

Pneumothorax is the presence of atmospheric air in the pleural space; its presence causes the alveoli of the lungs to collapse (Kravitz, 2000; Fig. 40-23). Pneumothorax in children usually occurs when air seeps from ruptured alveoli and collects in the pleural cavity. It also can occur when external puncture wounds allow air to enter the chest.

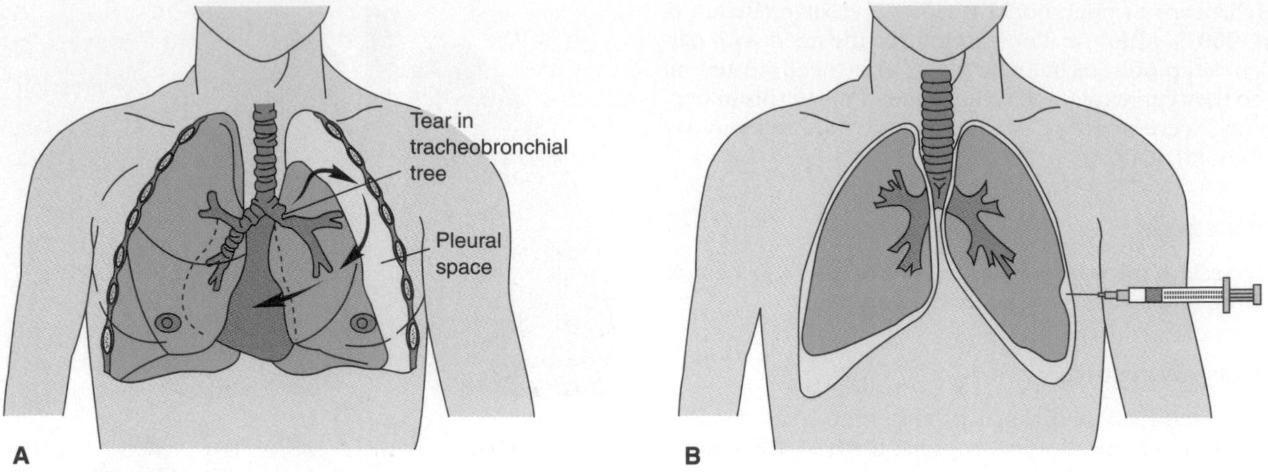

FIGURE 40.23 (*A*) Pneumothorax. A tear in the tracheobronchial tree has caused air to move into the pleural space; the lung collapses and the mediastinum shifts to the unaffected side. (*B*) Aspiration of air from the pleural space allows lung to reexpand after a pneumothorax.

Pneumothorax occurs in approximately 1% of newborns, probably due to rupture of the alveoli from the extreme intrathoracic pressure needed to initiate the first inspiration. The infant develops tachypnea, grunting respirations, flaring of the nares, and cyanosis. Auscultation reveals absent or decreased breath sounds on the affected side. Percussion may not be revealing, despite the hollow air space; the sound may be hyperresonant. A more revealing sign may be the shift of the apical pulse (mediastinal shift) away from the site of the pneumothorax and the resulting atelectasis. A chest film will show the darkened area of the air-filled pleural space.

Children need oxygen therapy to relieve respiratory distress. A thoracotomy catheter or needle may be placed in the pleural space and low-pressure suction with water-seal drainage applied to remove accumulated air. In most children with pneumothorax, symptoms are relieved within 24 hours after suction is begun. The use of water-seal drainage with children is discussed in Chapter 41.

If the air in the pleural space is from a puncture wound such as a stab wound, the chest wound must be covered immediately by an impervious material, such as petrolatum gauze, to prevent further air from entering. In an emergency, the impervious object can be your gloved hand.

Pneumothorax is always a potentially serious respiratory problem. The extent of the symptoms and the outcome will depend on the cause of entry of air into the pleural space.

✔ CHECKPOINT QUESTIONS

23. Which children should receive a vaccine to prevent pneumococcal pneumonia?
24. What position is best to aid lung expansion?

Bronchopulmonary Dysplasia

Bronchopulmonary dysplasia (BPD) is chronic pulmonary involvement that occurs in 10% to 40% of infants who are treated for acute respiratory distress in the first days of life. The condition is thought to occur from a combination of surfactant deficiency (decreased from lung trauma), barotrauma (lung damage from ventilator pressure), oxygen toxicity (from high levels needed to counteract the original respiratory distress), and continuing inflammation. The condition most often occurs in infants who received mechanical ventilation for respiratory distress syndrome.

Infants with the syndrome develop tachypnea, retractions, nasal flaring, tachycardia, oxygen dependence, and abnormal radiographic findings that show areas of overinflation and atelectasis. On auscultation, decreased air movement can be detected. Although some infants are left ventilator-dependent (see Focus on Evidence-Based Practice), administration of a corticosteroid and a bronchodilator greatly reduces inflammation and improves respirations (Larsen et al., 2001).

Tuberculosis

Tuberculosis is a highly contagious pulmonary disease. The causative agent is *Mycobacterium tuberculosis* (tubercle bacillus). The mode of transmission is inhalation of infected droplets. The incubation period is 2 to 10 weeks (Larsen et al., 2001).

Children generally contract this disease from someone in the immediate family. When any member of a family contracts tuberculosis, all family members must be tested (a Mantoux skin test) to screen for the disease. In some children, the contact is not known, and the disease is first detected when symptoms appear. Children who are homeless or severely impoverished tend to be more susceptible than other children are. Children with chronic illness or malnutrition are more susceptible than healthier children because of their overall susceptibility to infection.

When *M. tuberculosis* invades the child's lung, there is primary inflammation. The child develops a slight cough. Leukocytes and lymphocytes invade the area, effectively walling off the primary infection. The wall surrounding the bacteria calcifies and confines the organism permanently. This development of a primary focus is the most usual form

FOCUS ON EVIDENCE-BASED PRACTICE

What Is the Quality of Life of Ventilator-Assisted Children?

For many children, ventilator therapy is used only during a very short stage of critical illness. For others, especially those with conditions such as bronchopulmonary dysplasia or spinal cord injuries, they will be ventilator-dependent for a lifetime. To examine the quality of life of ventilator-dependent children, researchers interviewed 38 ventilator-dependent children and their parents. Of the 38 children, although older children were significantly less satisfied with their daily activities than younger children, 79% felt they were satisfied or very satisfied with how they spent their time each day. Seventy-seven percent were rated as having an excellent or good emotional adjustment to their need for mechanical ventilation. A surprising result is the opinions of ventilator-dependent adolescents and their parents were in agreement as to the adolescent's emotional status or adjustment to mechanical ventilation.

This is an important study for nurses because nurses are frequently the individuals whom parents first ask: How will we be able to cope with this? when they realize their child will be ventilator-dependent. Knowing that the majority of children and parents feel that ventilator-dependent life is rated as satisfactory can help nurses make forward thinking future plans.

Lumeng, J. C., Warschausky, S. A., Nelson, V. S., & Augenstein, K. (2001). The quality of life of ventilator-assisted children. *Pediatric Rehabilitation, 4*(1), 21–27.

of tuberculosis in children. If a child is in poor health or does not have adequate calcium intake for the body to confine the infection, tuberculosis may spread to other lung areas or to other parts of the body. If the bacteria are not confined as a primary focus, miliary tuberculosis develops. The child develops anorexia, weight loss, night sweats, and low-grade fever. Other body sites that may be affected are bones and joints, lymph nodes, kidneys, and the subarachnoid space (tuberculous meningitis).

Assessment

The diagnosis of tuberculosis is suggested by the history of a recent contact. All children should have a tuberculin test as part of basic preventive health care at 9 to 12 months of age, and yearly thereafter if they live in an area in which there is a high risk of tuberculosis. The test should not be done immediately after measles immunization or the test will read falsely negative (a child with tuberculosis will be considered free of the disease). Also, the measles vaccine can cause a primary tuberculosis focus to become miliary; thus, it is important to have a negative tuberculin result before administering this vaccine.

For a Mantoux test, also called a purified protein derivative (PPD) test, 5 units of protein derivative vaccine is injected intradermally. A health care professional inspects the area in 72 hours and notes the reaction. A positive reaction (the formation of 5 to 15 mm of reddened induration) indicates that the child has been exposed to tuberculosis (has developed a sensitivity to the foreign products of the tuberculosis organism; Fishbach, 2001). Children with positive reactions need follow-up care, such as a chest radiograph, to ascertain the importance of the reaction; that is, whether a current infection exists. Skin testing should not be done on children who are known to have had tuberculosis. Such a child will have such an intense reaction that the skin at the site of the test may slough off and necrose.

To confirm a diagnosis of active disease, sputum may be analyzed. Make certain that the child understands that you want him or her to expectorate mucus raised from the lungs, not just from the back of the throat. Have the child demonstrate a deep cough to you so that you can be sure you are both talking about the same thing. Infants and children younger than 5 years do not raise sputum but swallow it. In young children, therefore, gastric lavage may be necessary to obtain the sputum specimen (because tuberculosis bacteria are acid-fast, they are not destroyed by gastric secretions). Schedule this test early in the morning before the child eats. This prevents vomiting and allows for the collection of large numbers of organisms because the child has been coughing sputum and swallowing it all night. To collect the specimen, a nasogastric tube is passed either nasally or orally. The stomach contents are aspirated and placed in a sterile container for laboratory processing. Analysis is generally done for 3 consecutive days because individual specimens may not contain organisms.

Having a large tube passed into the stomach is uncomfortable, and the concept itself is frightening. Offer support during the procedure. Encourage children to express their feelings about the procedure afterward. They may enjoy playing with a plastic catheter and a doll into which a tube can be inserted. It is revealing to see the force and the anger they use to insert the tube into the doll. This helps you to understand how they envision the procedure being done to them.

In the early course of tuberculosis, because the initial focus of the tuberculosis is so small, it may not be evident on a chest radiograph. As local inflammation occurs, however, cloudiness in the inflamed area will be noticeable on the film, as will calcification as it occurs.

Children who have primary tuberculosis are not infectious because they have a minimal pulmonary lesion and little or no cough. They need not be isolated. As soon as drug therapy has been started and clinical symptoms have disappeared, children can return to regular activities, including school. Therapy will be continued, however, for up to 18 months.

Before drug therapy was available, a diagnosis of tuberculosis meant a hospital stay of approximately a year. Parents who believe that tuberculosis is still treated this way will need assurance that it is all right for their child to return home and attend regular school as soon as he or she starts taking the medication.

Therapeutic Management

A number of medications are effective against tuberculosis. Isoniazid (INH) is the drug of choice for therapy. INH may lead to peripheral neurologic symptoms if pyridoxine (vitamin B) is not administered concurrently. Rifampin is often used in combination with INH. Para-aminosalicylic acid (PAS) is bacteriostatic to *M. tuberculosis* and for a long time served as the mainstay of therapy. However, PAS administration may lead to such gastrointestinal disturbances in children that it is not used as much as in the past. If it is prescribed, it should be administered after meals, never on an empty stomach.

Ethambutol is used with older children. It must be used with caution with infants because one side effect is optic neuritis; the inability to do adequate eye examinations in children under school age to discover this side effect can make ethambutol unsafe for long-term use.

In addition to drug therapy, children should receive a diet high in protein, calcium, and pyridoxine, especially if INH is being used, to wall off organisms in lung tissue.

A major concern in tuberculosis therapy is that the tuberculosis organism is becoming resistant to commonly used drugs. Children should have periodic chest radiographs for the rest of their life to make certain that the disease does not become active later. A woman who had tuberculosis as a child must tell her primary care provider when she becomes pregnant; lung changes that occur in pregnancy as a result of the pressure of the growing uterus against the lungs can break down calcifications and reactivate tuberculosis. Children who develop another chronic disease that interferes with appetite and, therefore, with calcium intake have a high risk of reactivation of calcium-contained tuberculosis.

Because children will be taking medicine for a long time, they need periodic health care visits to evaluate the extent of drug compliance. Assess that they receive regular childhood immunizations so that they do not contract a second disease until they have fully recovered from tuberculosis. It is most important to prevent pertussis (whooping cough) because the paroxysmal cough caused by this illness could easily reactivate tuberculosis lesions.

The bacille Calmette-Guerin (BCG) vaccine is available against tuberculosis, but it is not used routinely in the United States. A skin test will be strongly positive after effective BCG vaccination. For this reason, most people advocate placing children on prophylactic INH when there is known tuberculosis in the home rather than vaccinating them against tuberculosis. As long as a repeat PPD test remains negative, you know that they are disease-free. After BCG vaccine is administered, the value of skin testing is lost.

Cystic Fibrosis (CF)

Children with CF have a generalized dysfunction of the exocrine glands. Mucus secretions of the body, particularly in the pancreas and the lungs, have difficulty flowing through gland ducts. There is also a marked electrolyte change in the secretions of the sweat glands (chloride concentration of sweat is two to five times above normal). The cause of the disorder is an abnormality of the long arm of chromosome 7. This results in the inability to transport small molecules across cell membranes; this leads to dehydration of epithelial cells in the airway and pancreas and dried secretions.

The disorder is inherited as an autosomal recessive trait. It occurs in approximately 1 in 2,500 live births. It occurs most commonly in whites, rarely in blacks and Asians. Although the disease can be fatal in early life, as many as 50% of children now live to be more than 30 years of age. With the availability of lung transplants, full life expectancy is possible. Because the gene that causes the disorder can be isolated, chorionic villi sampling or amniocentesis can be done early in pregnancy to detect fetuses who have the disease. In the future, it is expected that gene therapy will be available to reverse the effect of the involved gene.

Boys with CF may not be able to reproduce because they have persistent plugging and blocking of the vas deferens from tenacious seminal fluid. Girls may have such thick cervical secretions that sperm penetration is limited. In this case, artificial insemination or in vitro fertilization can be accomplished if they desire to become pregnant.

Pancreas Involvement

The acinar cells of the pancreas normally produce lipase, trypsin, and amylase, enzymes that flow into the duodenum to digest fat, protein, and carbohydrate. With CF, these enzyme secretions become so thickened that they plug the ducts; eventually, there is such back-pressure on the acinar cells that they become atrophied and are then no longer capable of producing the enzymes. The islets of Langerhans and insulin production are little influenced by this process until late in the disease because they have endocrine (ductless) activity.

Without pancreatic enzymes in the duodenum, children are unable to digest fat, protein, and some sugars. The child's stools are large, bulky, and greasy (**steatorrhea**). The intestinal flora increases because of the undigested food; this, when combined with the fat in the stool, gives the stool an extremely foul odor, often compared to that of a cat's stool. The bulk of feces in the intestine leads to a protuberant abdomen. Because children are benefiting from only about 50% of the food they ingest, they show signs of malnutrition—emaciated extremities and loose, flabby folds of skin on their buttocks. The fat-soluble vitamins, particularly A, D, and E, cannot be absorbed because fat is not absorbed, so children develop symptoms of low levels of these vitamins. These four symptoms—malnutrition, protuberant abdomen, steatorrhea, and fat-soluble vitamin deficiencies—are the same four symptoms that are part of celiac disease (malabsorption syndrome), so they are referred to as the celiac syndrome (see Chap. 45).

The meconium in a newborn is normally thick and tenacious. In approximately 10% of children with CF, it may be so thick, because pancreatic enzymes are lacking, that it obstructs the intestine (meconium ileus). The newborn develops abdominal distention with no passage of stool. Meconium ileus should be suspected in any infant who does not pass a stool by 24 hours of life. Rectal prolapse from straining to evacuate hard stool is another common finding in infants with CF.

Lung Involvement

Pockets of infection begin in pooled thick secretions of the bronchial tree, obstructing the bronchioles. The organisms most frequently cultured from lung secretions in children with CF are *Staphylococcus aureus, Pseudomonas aeruginosa,* and *H. influenzae.* Secondary emphysema (overinflated alveoli) occurs because the air cannot be pushed past the thick mucus on expiration, when all bronchi are narrower than they are on inspiration. Bronchiectasis and pneumonia occur. Atelectasis occurs as a result of complete absorption of air from alveoli behind blocked bronchioles. The child's fingers become clubbed because of the inadequate peripheral tissue perfusion. The anterior-posterior diameter of the chest becomes enlarged. Respiratory acidosis may develop because obstruction interferes with the ability to exhale carbon dioxide.

Sweat Gland Involvement

Although the sweat glands themselves do not appear to be changed in structure, the electrolyte composition of perspiration is changed. In children with CF, the level of chloride to sodium is increased two to five times above normal. Some parents report that they knew their newborn had the disease before they had laboratory tests done because when they kissed their child, they could taste such strong salt in the perspiration.

Assessment

CF is diagnosed by the history and the combination of the abnormal concentration of chloride in sweat, the absence of pancreatic enzymes in the duodenum, the presence of immunoreactive trypsinogen in the blood, and pulmonary involvement.

CF may be suspected in a newborn when he or she loses the normal amount of weight at birth (5% to 10% of birthweight), but then, because the infant cannot make use of the fat in milk, does not gain it back at the usual time of 7 to 10 days and perhaps not until 4 to 6 weeks of age. Nurses are the individuals who often weigh babies and may be the first to detect this lack of weight gain. In addition, at birth, meconium may be so tenacious that the baby has intestinal obstruction (meconium ileus) and so is unable to pass stool. All babies with meconium ileus should be tested for CF. This can be done by analysis of serum immunoreactive trypsin (IRT) in the stool. This is elevated in newborns with the disease because of obstruction in the pancreas as early as during fetal life.

Children may be seen in a health care setting at about 1 month of age because of a feeding problem. Using only about 50% of their intake because of their poor digestive function, they are always hungry. This causes them to eat so ravenously that they tend to swallow air. This is manifested as colic or abdominal distention and vomiting. Stools are large, bulky, and greasy and may be loose and frequent. The appearance of the stools is an important finding because children with simple colic do not show changes in stool consistency this way.

Children may be seen by health care providers between 4 and 6 months of age because of frequent respiratory infections, a chronic cough, and failure to gain weight. Even at this early stage of the disease, wheezing and rhonchi may be heard on chest auscultation.

By the time the child with CF is a preschooler, a cough is a prominent finding. On percussion, the chest is hyperresonant, reflecting the emphysema present. Crackles and rhonchi are heard. Clubbing of the fingers may already be apparent. It is rare for a child to go undiagnosed beyond this time because the symptoms of the illness have become so persistent and evident.

Sweat Testing. A sweat test is a test for the chloride content of sweat. Although this may be done as early as the first days of life, the test may be delayed until 6 to 8 weeks of age because newborns do not sweat a great deal, and interpretation of the early tests may not be accurate.

For a sweat test, pilocarpine (a cholinergic drug that stimulates sweat gland activity) is dropped onto a gauze square. This is placed on the child's forearm, and copper electrodes are connected to it. A small electrical current is then applied to carry the pilocarpine into the skin. Because the electrical current is of such low intensity, it should be painless. After the application of the electrical current, the area on the arm is washed with water and dried, and a filter paper is applied to collect the sweat that forms. The filter paper must be lifted by forceps rather than by the examiner's fingers, because the sweat from the examiner's skin could transfer to the paper and make the test analysis inaccurate.

A normal concentration of chloride in sweat is 20 mEq/L. A level of more than 60 mEq/L chloride in children is diagnostic of CF. Values between 50 and 60 mEq/L are suggestive of the disease and call for a repeat of the test.

Duodenal Analysis. Analysis of duodenal secretions for detection of pancreatic enzymes is done by passing a nasogastric tube into the duodenum and then aspirating secretions for analysis. This test may take a considerable amount of time because the tube is allowed to pass through the pylorus and into the duodenum by natural peristaltic action. You can tell a tube has passed from the stomach into the duodenum by aspirating secretions from the tube and testing them for pH. Stomach secretions are acid (pH less than 7.0); duodenal secretions are alkaline (pH more than 7.0). The initial insertion of the tube typically is frightening to children because they may choke and gag as it passes the pharynx. Children, however, are generally surprised that once the initial insertion is done, the tube is not uncomfortable. They need a great deal of support during the procedure, however, because it is so unusual for them and initially so uncomfortable. Duodenal analysis may also be done by endoscopy; for this, children usually receive conscious sedation (Tolia et al., 2000).

The secretions removed from the duodenum are sent to the laboratory for analysis of trypsin content, the easiest pancreatic enzyme to assay. Keep the secretions cold during transport. They should be analyzed immediately for accurate results.

Stool Analysis. Stool may be collected and analyzed for fat content, although description of the large greasy appearance may be all that is necessary.

Pulmonary Testing. A chest radiograph generally confirms the pulmonary involvement (pockets of emphysema and perhaps beginning pneumonia infiltration). Pulmonary function tests may be done to determine if atelectasis and emphysema are present.

Therapeutic Management

Therapy for children with CF consists of measures to reduce the involvement of the pancreas, lungs, and sweat glands.

> ## FOCUS ON PHARMACOLOGY
>
> **Pancrelipase (Cotazym)**
>
> *Action:* Pancrelipase is an enzyme replacement used for children with cystic fibrosis.
>
> *Pregnancy risk category:* C
>
> *Dosage:* 2,000 U orally per meal (children 6 months to 1 year of age); 4,000 to 8,000 U orally with each meal and 4,000 U with snacks (children 1 to 6 years of age); 4,000 to 12,000 U orally with each meal and with snacks
>
> *Possible adverse effects:* Nausea, abdominal cramps, diarrhea, hypersensitivity
>
> *Nursing Implications*
> - Administer the drug before or with meals and snacks. Instruct parents and child in the same.
> - Caution child and parents to avoid inhaling powder or spilling it on the hands because it may irritate the skin or mucous membranes.
> - Do not crush or let the child chew the enteric form of the drug.
> - Instruct the child and parents about possible adverse effects and encourage them to contact the health care provider should any become severe.

NURSING DIAGNOSES AND RELATED INTERVENTIONS

Nursing Diagnosis: Imbalanced nutrition, less than body requirements, related to inability to digest fat

Outcome Identification: Child will absorb an adequate nutritional amount daily.

Outcome Evaluation: Child's height and weight follow percentile growth curves; quantity of stool decreases; signs and symptoms of vitamin deficiency are absent.

Children with CF are placed on a high-calorie, high-protein, moderate-fat diet. Water-miscible forms of vitamins A, D, and E are supplemented. During the hot months of the year, extra salt may be added to food to replace that lost though perspiration. Medium-chain triglycerides are used with the diet because these are more readily digested than other oils.

Generally, infants with CF cannot be totally breastfed because there is not enough protein in breast milk for them (they need large amounts because they cannot make use of all the protein they ingest). Breastfeeding with supplementary formula is required. Some of these children, unfortunately, are initially diagnosed as having a milk allergy and are treated by being placed on a soybean formula. This does not contain enough protein either, and their malnutrition increases greatly while they are taking this formula. A high-protein formula, such as Probana, is generally recommended.

Children with CF have a ravenous appetite and eat well. Before each meal or snack, they need to take a synthetic pancreatic enzyme, pancreatic lipase (Cotazym or Pancrease), to replace the enzyme they cannot produce (see Focus on Pharmacology). These synthetic enzymes are supplied in large capsules that must be opened for young children because they cannot swallow such a big capsule; infants, in particular, may not have enough gastric acids to dissolve the capsule. The powder from the capsule is then added to a small amount (no more than a teaspoonful) of food. It should not be added to hot food, or a large portion of enzyme activity will be destroyed. Also, it must not be added to the infant's bottle of formula, because the infant may not drink the entire bottle and therefore will not receive the total benefit of the enzyme. When children are taking a synthetic source of pancreatic enzyme this way, the size of stools and the accompanying foul odor decreases. Children begin to gain weight. In adolescence, children may have a great deal of difficulty eating enough to maintain weight, even with enzyme therapy, because their growth spurt requires so many additional calories.

If children with CF become overheated, they begin to lose excessive sodium and chloride through perspiration and become dehydrated. Caution parents to keep their house temperature at 72°F or below and to offer water frequently. They also need to supervise outside play to guard against overexertion or heat exposure.

Nursing Diagnosis: Ineffective airway clearance related to inability to clear mucus from the respiratory tract

Outcome Identification: Child's airway will remain patent during course of illness.

Outcome Evaluation: Child's temperature is below 100.4°F (38.0°C); Po_2 is 80 to 90 mm Hg; Pco_2 is less than 40 mm Hg.

Unfortunately, the pulmonary effects of CF progress despite supplementation with pancreatic enzyme; infection from plugged airways is always a possibility. Therefore, it is important to try to keep bronchial secretions as moist and freely flowing as possible so they can drain from the bronchial tree. This is done by frequent nebulization or aerosol therapy followed by chest physiotherapy.

Humidified Oxygen. Oxygen is supplied to children by mask, prongs, ventilators, or nebulizers and rarely by tent. Mist can be supplied by an ultrasonic compressor and delivered through a nebulizer mask, which makes the droplet size so small that the mist reaches the smallest bronchial spaces.

Aerosol Therapy. Three or four times a day, children may be given aerosol therapy by means of a nebulizer to provide antibiotics or bronchodilators. Antibiotics are specifically determined by culture. A mucolytic, such as acetylcysteine (Mucomyst), can be added to the mist to aid in diluting and liquefying secretions. The cough will become loose and productive after using aerosol therapy. Provide a box of tissues so the child can cough up these loose secretions. Observe the child to ensure that he or she can cough and keep the airway clear. Never give cough syrups to suppress a cough, because getting secretions out is essential for air exchange and to prevent infection. Likewise, question an order for codeine as an analgesic, because codeine suppresses the cough reflex.

Chest Physiotherapy. Because the bronchial secretions with CF are so tenacious, even with liquefaction by mist or aerosol therapy, children may be unable to raise them. To aid drainage of secretions, children need chest physiotherapy frequently, approximately three or four times a day.

Activity. Children with CF need to maintain their usual activities as much as possible. When in bed, they need frequent position changes so that, at various times of the day, all lobes of their lungs will be encouraged to drain by being in a superior position. Therefore, they should alternately lie on either side, on the abdomen, and on the back. They should sit up part of the day to drain the upper lobes. This change in position also helps to prevent skin breakdown over bony prominences, and it helps to aerate the lungs by furnishing some activity for them.

Frequent Observation. Observe children with CF frequently because their condition can change rapidly. If a portion of a lung becomes obstructed from a plug of mucus, they can quickly experience respiratory difficulty. The right side of the heart tends to enlarge in children with chronic respiratory disease because the congestion in the lungs increases pressure in the pulmonary artery and the right ventricle. After a period of stress or exercise, children may begin to show signs of cardiac failure because their already enlarged heart cannot compensate any further.

Respiratory Hygiene. The sputum that a child coughs up may have a disagreeable taste or odor. Offer frequent mouth care, toothbrushing, and a good-tasting mouthwash to make the mouth feel fresh.

Adequate Rest and Comfort. Any child who has compromised lung function has a degree of dyspnea that leads to exhaustion. To counteract this, provide periods of rest during the day, but do not group too many activities or procedures together all at once, as this could exhaust the child. Plan a rest period before meals so that the child is not too tired to eat. Also plan for a long rest period before chest physiotherapy so that the child will be able to tolerate it better. Achieving a balance between allowing periods of rest and yet not doing all procedures at once is not an easy task.

Growth and Development. Children need to be exposed to as many normal life experiences as possible. This may be difficult because it is important not to tire the child out or expose him or her to crowds of people (possibly increasing the risk for infection). Assist the parents with planning age-appropriate activities with the child.

Nursing Diagnosis: Risk for impaired skin integrity related to acid stools

Outcome Identification: Child's skin will remain intact during course of illness.

Outcome Evaluation: Child does not exhibit areas of erythema or ulceration; rectal prolapse is not present.

Until children are regulated on pancreatic enzymes, the stool is particularly irritating because of its high fat content. Children who are not toilet-trained need to have their diapers changed immediately after they wet or pass stool so that they do not develop skin irritation and breakdown in the diaper area.

After a bowel movement, check the rectum for rectal prolapse. Because of weak musculature of the rectal area, this is a common complication. A prolapse of rectal mucosa appears as a bright-red mass protruding from the anal sphincter. This mucosa must be replaced promptly before its blood supply is compromised. Place the child on the slant board used for chest physiotherapy with the head lower than the buttocks; then, with a lubricated, gloved hand, gently replace the prolapsed rectal mass. Afterward, compress the buttocks together to maintain gentle pressure on the anus for a few minutes. This is much less of a problem in children who are receiving pancreatic enzymes than in those who are not, because the incidence of rectal prolapse decreases with better nutrition.

Nursing Diagnosis: Risk for compromised family coping, related to chronic illness in a child

Outcome Identification: Family members demonstrate an adequate level of coping ability during course of illness.

Outcome Evaluation: Family members state they have adequate resources to cope with current circumstances.

The parents of children with CF are asked to assume a great deal of responsibility for care of their child. Begin discharge planning when a child is first admitted to a hospital in terms of what changes need to be made at home to accommodate the child's homecoming and to familiarize parents with the necessary care measures. For example, many children with this disorder sleep with oxygen by cannula at night when they are at home. Thus, parents need to be taught the functions of oxygen and how to regulate the flow. This type of learning is most effective if a little is taught every day (for example, "Could you turn the oxygen on for me, Mrs. Smith? I'm ready to tuck Brian in to sleep" rather than a sit-down, let-me-tell-you-how-oxygen-works lecture given close to the day of discharge). Teach parents how to do chest physiotherapy the same way.

The family will have to think through how the care of this child will affect their home life. They are going to be spending a great deal of time caring for the child, so they will need to balance work, care of the child, and care of the rest of the family. Many parents become fatigued after the first week of having the child at home because they are afraid to fall soundly asleep at night for fear of not hearing the child call if he or she should be in distress. As they grow more confident in their ability to evaluate the child's condition before bedtime, their apprehension will lessen, but real confidence may not come for months, even years. This may always be a problem for some parents.

Be sure that the parents have the telephone number of the health care provider they should call if they feel overwhelmed. Encourage parents to join a support group, so that there are other people available to understand and to whom they can voice their concerns. At these times, one of the most important needs they have is to verbalize to someone what it feels like to be the parent of a child with CF, including feelings of guilt they may be experiencing because the disease is inherited.

Children should attend regular school if at all possible so they are provided with the socialization experiences with other children. If this is not possible, a home tutor can be arranged for them. Urge children to participate to the extent that they can in physical fitness activities in school or with friends. Make out a reminder sheet as necessary so that they can remember to take pancreatic enzyme with them if they are going to be eating lunch in the school cafeteria or outside the home.

Ensure that children with CF receive periodic health assessment and routine childhood immunizations. It is not unusual for children with a chronic disease to fall behind in routine check-ups and immunizations because they are hospitalized at the times these are routinely done. It is particularly important that children with CF receive the pertussis and measles vaccines, because these two infections cause severe respiratory complications. Children also should receive influenza, meningococcal, and pneumococcal vaccines.

As children with CF reach adolescence, they are candidates for lung transplants. Some of these are done as lower lobe transplants from a living donor. People who donate a single lobe in this manner report that they feel little loss of lung capacity afterward (Cohen & Starnes, 2001). A lung transplant is advantageous for children with CF because the new lung does not possess the defective gene that caused mucus to be so thick. Lifespan can greatly improve.

✔ CHECKPOINT QUESTIONS

25. What term is used to describe tuberculosis that has spread to other parts of the body?
26. What result of a sweat test would be diagnostic for CF?

KEY POINTS

Respiratory tract disorders tend to occur more frequently in children than adults, because the lumens of bronchi are narrow and obstruction and infection can occur more easily.

Infants with respiratory illness need extremely close observation because they cannot describe oxygen deprivation. Young children do not comprehend the fact that oxygen supports combustion. Observe them more frequently than adults to be certain that no flames, such as birthday candles, are brought within 10 feet of an oxygen source.

Acute nasopharyngitis (common cold) is the most common infectious disease in children. There is no specific therapy for a cold other than comfort measures.

Tonsillitis is infection and inflammation of the palatine tonsils. Adenitis is infection and inflammation of the adenoid tonsils. Children with recurring infections may have their tonsils surgically removed.

Laryngotracheobronchitis (croup) is inflammation of the larynx, trachea, and major bronchi. Epiglottitis is inflammation of the epiglottis. Both of these conditions can cause severe impairment of the airway. Children with epiglottitis should never be assessed for a gag reflex with a tongue blade because the elevated epiglottis can completely occlude the airway.

Bronchitis is inflammation of the major bronchi and trachea. Bronchiolitis is inflammation of the fine bronchioles. They are caused by bacterial or viral invasion.

Respiratory syncytial virus infection is an infection that accounts for the majority of lower respiratory infections in young children. Infants with RSV infections must be observed closely because they are prone to apnea.

Asthma, a type I hypersensitivity reaction, is a diffuse and obstructive airway disease with wheezing as the most common symptom. Newer drugs such as leukotriene receptor antagonists and careful environmental control have aided in the management of this disorder.

Pneumonia may occur from a variety of organisms (viral, pneumococcal, chlamydial, mycoplasmal, lipid, and hydrocarbon). Except for viral pneumonia, children need specific antibiotics, depending on the organism present.

Tuberculosis is a lung infection that is growing in incidence, with some strains becoming very resistant to the usual therapy. The entire family needs drug therapy if one member develops a primary lesion.

Cystic fibrosis is a disease in which there is generalized dysfunction of the exocrine glands. This results in malabsorption and tenacious pulmonary secretions, leading to infection and pneumonia. Lung transplantation can be used to replace the diseased lung tissue and improve the child's lifespan.

CRITICAL THINKING EXERCISES

1. Michael is the 5-year-old you met at the beginning of the chapter. His nanny brought him to the emergency room because his respirations were rapid and he was wheezing. He is diagnosed as having asthma. Both he and his nanny shouted instructions at you. What about Michael's actions would lead you to believe his airway is not yet extremely constricted? Would you encourage him to lie down and rest? What emergency care does Michael need?
2. A 3-year-old has a permanent tracheostomy tube in place. Her parents are going to enroll her in a preschool center. What precautions would you want to review with the parents to keep this experience safe?
3. A 10-year-old has just returned from tonsillectomy surgery. What observations would be most important to make? Why is the 7th day after tonsillectomy surgery a particularly important day for close observation?
4. The parents of a 16-year-old with CF want to take her on an extended vacation in the Caribbean. What anticipatory guidance would you give the adolescent and her parents?
5. Examine the National Health Goals related to respiratory disorders. Most government-sponsored money for nursing research is allotted based on these goals. What would be a possible research topic to explore pertinent to these goals that would be fundable and would advance evidence-based practice?

REFERENCES

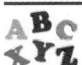

American Heart Association. (2000). Newborn resuscitation. *Circulation, 102*(1), 343–346.

Bagarazzi, M. (2000). Epiglottitis. In Schwartz, M. W. (Ed.). *The 5-minute pediatric consult* (pp. 354–355). Philadelphia: Lippincott Williams & Wilkins.

Battan, F. K., & Dart, R. C. (2001). Management of specific common poisonings. In W. W. Hay, A. R. Hayward, M. J. Levin, & J. M. Sondheimer (Eds.). *Current pediatric diagnosis and treatment* (15th ed.). New York: McGraw-Hill.

Bell, E. F., & Oh, W. (1999). Fluid and electrolyte management. In Avery, G. B, Fletcher, M. A., & MacDonald, M. G. *Neonatology* (5th ed., pp. 345–361). Philadelphia: Lippincott Williams & Wilkins.

Carpenito, L. (2001). *Nursing diagnosis: Application to clinical practice* (9th ed.). Philadelphia: Lippincott Williams & Wilkins.

Carpenter, T. C., et al. (2001). Critical care. In W. W. Hay, A. R. Hayward, M. J. Levin, & J. M. Sondheimer (Eds.). *Current pediatric diagnosis and treatment* (15th ed.). New York: McGraw-Hill.

Chedevergne, F., et al. (2000). The role of inflammation in childhood asthma. *Archives of Disease in Childhood, 82*(2S), 116–119.

Chung, E. K. (2000). Sinusitis. In Schwartz, M. W. (Ed.). *The 5-minute pediatric consult* (pp. 758–759). Philadelphia: Lippincott Williams & Wilkins.

Cohen, R. G., & Starnes, V. A. (2001). Living donor lung transplantation. *World Journal of Surgery, 25*(2), 244–250.

Department of Health and Human Services. (2000). *Healthy people 2010*. Washington, DC: DHHS.

Fischbach, F. (2001). *A manual of laboratory and diagnostic tests* (6th ed.). Philadelphia: Lippincott Williams & Wilkins.

Hakonarson, H. (2000). Bronchiolitis. In Schwartz, M. W. (Ed.). *The 5-minute pediatric consult* (pp. 208–209). Philadelphia: Lippincott Williams & Wilkins.

Karch, A. M. (2001). *Lippincott's nursing drug guide*. Philadelphia: Lippincott Williams & Wilkins.

Kravitz, R. M. (2000). Pneumothorax. In Schwartz, M. W. (Ed.). *The 5-minute pediatric consult* (pp. 636–637). Philadelphia: Lippincott Williams & Wilkins.

Kurland, G., & Orenstein, D. M. (2001). Lung transplantation and cystic fibrosis: The psychosocial toll. *Pediatrics, 107*(6), 1419–1420.

Larsen, G. L., et al. (2001). Acquired disorders of the intrathoracic airways. In W. W. Hay, A. R. Hayward, M. J. Levin, & J. M. Sondheimer (Eds.). *Current pediatric diagnosis and treatment* (15th ed.). New York: McGraw-Hill.

Levin, M. J., & Weinberg, A. (2001). Infections: Viral and rickettsial. In W. W. Hay, A. R. Hayward, M. J. Levin, & J. M. Sondheimer (Eds.). *Current pediatric diagnosis and treatment* (15th ed.). New York: McGraw-Hill.

Lumeng, J. C. et al. (2001). The quality of life of ventilator-assisted children. *Pediatric Rehabilitation, 4*(1), 21–27.

Macartney, K. K., & Bagarazzi, M. L. (2000). Pharyngitis. In Schwartz, M. W. (Ed.). *The 5-minute pediatric consult* (pp. 622–623). Philadelphia: Lippincott Williams & Wilkins.

Nachajon, R. V. (2000). Tracheomalacia/laryngomalacia. In Schwartz, M. W. (Ed.). *The 5-minute pediatric consult* (pp. 832–833). Philadelphia: Lippincott Williams & Wilkins.

Ogle, J. W., & Anderson, M. S. (2001). Infections: Bacterial and spirochetal. In W. W. Hay, A. R. Hayward, M. J. Levin, & J. M. Sondheimer (Eds.). *Current pediatric diagnosis and treatment* (15th ed.). New York: McGraw-Hill.

Osterhoudt, K. C. (2000). Nosebleeds (epistaxis). In Schwartz, M. W. (Ed.). *The 5-minute pediatric consult* (pp. 578–579). Philadelphia: Lippincott Williams & Wilkins.

Phillips, S. C. (2000). Croup (laryngotracheobronchitis). In Schwartz, M. W. (Ed.). *The 5-minute pediatric consult* (pp. 292–293). Philadelphia: Lippincott Williams & Wilkins.

Silver, D. L. (2000). Bacterial pneumonia. In Schwartz, M. W. (Ed.). *The 5-minute pediatric consult* (pp. 634–635). Philadelphia: Lippincott Williams & Wilkins.

Thilo, E. H., & Rosenberg, A. A. (2001). The newborn infant. In W. W. Hay, A. R. Hayward, M. J. Levin, & J. M. Sondheimer (Eds.). *Current pediatric diagnosis and treatment* (15th ed.). New York: McGraw-Hill.

Tolia, V. et al. (2000). Sedation for pediatric endoscopic procedures. *Journal of Pediatric Gastroenterology & Nutrition, 30*(5). 477–485.

Wright, R. B., et al. (2002). New approaches to respiratory infections in children: Bronchitis and croup. *Emergency Medicine Clinics of North America, 20*(1), 93–114.

SUGGESTED READINGS

Harwell, J. I., & Brown, R. B. (2000). The drug-resistant pneumococcus: Clinical relevance, therapy and prevention. *Chest, 117*(2), 530–541.

Ishimine, P. (2001). Assessment and management of pediatric upper-airway emergencies. *Journal of Emergency Medical Services, 26*(5), 56–73.

Lerou, P. (2001). Lower respiratory tract infections in children. *Current Opinion in Pediatrics, 13*(2), 200–206.

London, S. J., et al. (2001). Family history and the risk of early-onset persistent, early-onset transient, and late-onset asthma. *Epidemiology, 12*(5), 577–583.

Marco, T., et al. (2000). Home intravenous antibiotics for cystic fibrosis. Cochrane Database of Systematic Reviews CD001917.

Mattila, P. S., et al. (2001). Causes of tonsillar disease and frequency of tonsillectomy operations. *Archives of Otolaryngology: Head & Neck Surgery, 127*(1), 37–44.

Principi, N., et al. (2001). Role of *Mycoplasma pneumoniae* and *Chlamydia pneumoniae* in children with community-acquired lower respiratory tract infections. *Clinical Infectious Diseases, 32*(9), 1281–1289.

Shapiro, G. G. & Stout, J. W. (2002). Childhood asthma in the United States: Urban issues. *Pediatric Pulmonary, 33*(1), 47–55.

Swingler, G. H., Hussey, G. D., & Zwarenstein, M. (2000). Duration of illness in ambulatory children diagnosed with bronchiolitis. *Archives of Pediatrics & Adolescent Medicine, 154*(10), 997–1000.

Yankaskas, J. R., & Aris, R. (2000). Outpatient care of the cystic fibrosis patient after lung transplantation. *Current Opinion in Pulmonary Medicine, 6*(6), 551–557.

41

CHAPTER

Nursing Care of the Child With a Cardiovascular Disorder

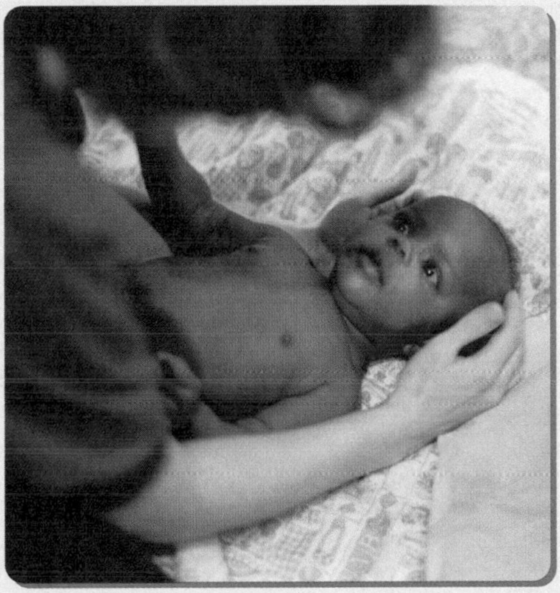

Key Terms

- acyanotic heart disease
- afterload
- balloon angioplasty
- cardiac catheterization
- congestive heart failure
- contractility
- cyanosis
- cyanotic heart disease
- diastole
- echocardiography
- electrocardiogram
- fluoroscopy
- innocent heart murmur
- left-to-right shunt
- organic heart murmur
- phonocardiogram
- polycythemia
- postcardiac surgery syndrome
- postperfusion syndrome
- preload
- right-to-left shunt
- systole
- vasculitis

Objectives

After mastering the contents of this chapter, you should be able to:

1. Describe the common cardiovascular disorders of childhood.
2. Assess a child with a cardiovascular dysfunction.
3. Formulate nursing diagnoses for the child with a cardiovascular disorder.
4. Establish appropriate outcomes based on the priority needs of the child with a cardiovascular disorder.
5. Plan nursing care for the child with a cardiovascular disorder.
6. Implement nursing care for the child with a cardiovascular disorder.
7. Evaluate outcomes for achievement and effectiveness of care.
8. Identify National Health Goals related to cardiovascular disorders and children that nurses could be instrumental in helping the nation achieve.
9. Identify areas related to the care of children with cardiovascular problems that could benefit from additional nursing research or application of evidence-based practice.
10. Use critical thinking to analyze ways that nursing care of children with cardiovascular disorders could be more family-centered.
11. Integrate knowledge of cardiovascular disorders with nursing process to achieve quality maternal and child health nursing care.

Megan is a newborn who was born with tetralogy of Fallot. By 1 hour of age, she developed rapid respirations, tachycardia, and cyanosis. An echocardiogram revealed the typical four structural defects of the syndrome. Megan's parents will be taking her home for a month to await cardiac surgery. They tell you their doctor told them to "watch her carefully" during that time. "What does that mean?" they ask you. Will they be able to take her outside in a stroller? Should she sleep in their bedroom? Exactly what should they watch for? What advice would you give them?

Previous chapters described the growth and development of well children. This chapter adds information about the child who is ill with heart disease and the stress that such a serious diagnosis places on a family. This is important information because it builds a base for care and health teaching for children with these disorders.

After you've studied the chapter, answer the Critical Thinking Exercises at the end of the chapter and then access the on-line study activities (http://connection.lww.com) *to further sharpen your skills and test your knowledge.*

The cardiovascular system, the body system on which all other systems depend, consists of the heart, which acts as a reliable pump; the blood, which provides the fluid and cells for transport; and the blood vessels, which provide the means and routes for transport throughout the body. The regular pumping of the heart propels oxygen and needed nutrients through the bloodstream to cells and allows waste products to be removed from cells and transported to the lungs or kidneys for excretion. The cardiovascular system also transports regulatory materials such as hormones, enzymes, and antibodies to the body systems. It can adapt to changing body needs by adjusting the rate and force of heart pumping, modifying the size of the blood vessels, and altering the volume and composition of the blood.

Most cardiovascular disorders in children occur as a result of a congenital anomaly; either the heart has developed inadequately in utero, or the heart cannot adapt to extrauterine life for some reason. Open-heart surgery often is the only treatment that will correct the primary congenital problem. Children also may experience acquired cardiovascular disorders, such as rheumatic fever or Kawasaki disease. All these disorders can lead to heart failure or infection or inadequate heart function.

Cardiovascular disorders are frightening for children and adults alike. Even small children realize the importance of the heart in sustaining life, and they recognize the seriousness of any illness that undermines the heart's activity. For the families of children who are experiencing a cardiovascular disease, understanding the functioning of the heart and circulation is an important first step toward coping with the illness. Cardiac disorders are a major focus of health promotion and disease prevention measures in both adults and children. National Health Goals related to cardiovascular illness and children are shown in Focus on National Health Goals box.

FOCUS ON NATIONAL HEALTH GOALS

Cardiovascular illness is a major health problem in adults. However, the illness and its effects can be prevented or at least minimized by instituting measures early in childhood. A number of National Health Goals address ways children should modify nutrition or exercise to achieve cardiovascular health:

- Increase to at least 85% from a baseline of 65% the proportion of children and adolescents ages 5 through 17 who engage in vigorous physical activity that promotes the development and maintenance of cardiorespiratory fitness 3 or more days per week, for 20 or more minutes per occasion.
- Increase the proportion of persons aged 2 years and older who consume less than 10% of calories from saturated fat from a baseline of 75% to a target level of 36%.
- Reduce the proportion of children and adolescents who are overweight or obese from a baseline of 11% to a target level of 5% (DHHS, 2000).

Nurses can be instrumental in helping the nation achieve these goals by educating parents and children about the importance of reducing obesity and planning exercise and nutrition programs for sound cardiovascular health. It is equally important for nurses to caution parents not to begin reduced-fat diets until their children are 2 years old to allow for myelination of nerve cells.

Nursing research is needed to determine what weight loss programs are the most effective for children, what reduced-fat foods make the best finger foods for preschoolers, what snacks schools could provide in snack machines that would have a reduced fat content and would also be eaten by children, and how to increase physical activity in adolescents who do not participate in any type of organized sport or exercise program.

NURSING PROCESS OVERVIEW

For Care of the Child With a Cardiovascular Disorder

Assessment

Assessment of the child with a cardiovascular disorder includes both careful history taking and physical examination, because many of the signs and symptoms of heart disease in children are subtle. A variety of diagnostic studies may be used to confirm the diagnosis and prepare for surgery. Teaching and providing psychological support to children and their families are two major responsibilities of nurses throughout the assessment process.

Nursing Diagnosis

Examples of nursing diagnoses established for children with heart disease may include the following:

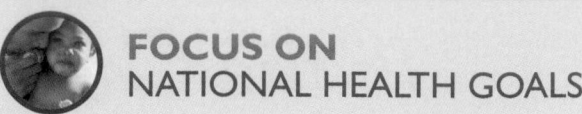

- Decreased cardiac output related to congenital structural defect
- Ineffective tissue perfusion related to inadequate cardiac output
- Deficient knowledge related to care of the child pre- and postoperatively
- Fear related to lack of knowledge about child's disease
- Interrupted family processes related to stresses of the diagnosis and care responsibilities
- Ineffective coping related to lack of adequate support
- Impaired parenting related to inability to bond with critically ill newborn

If the concerns in the latter three diagnoses are not identified when the child is ill, they may continue long after the child is treated and returns home.

If the child will be undergoing surgery or cardiac catheterization, nursing diagnoses will focus on the psychological needs of the child and family for preparation and postprocedure care in addition to physical concerns after the procedure (e.g., Hypothermia related to cooling during surgery, conscious sedation during cardiac catheterization).

Outcome Identification and Planning

Nursing planning is essential to help parents and children understand heart anatomy, thereby establishing a sound knowledge base for them to understand the necessity for diagnostic testing. Additional teaching is necessary to prepare the parents and children for procedures or surgery and recovery at home. Teaching parents to conscientiously administer cardiac medications is another area where planning plays an important role. Part of this planning includes establishing appropriate outcomes to help the child and parents, now and in the future (e.g., coping with their present fears and caring for the child at home).

Implementation

Nursing interventions in the care of the child with a cardiovascular disorder include teaching, providing an opportunity for children and their families to express fears about the child's illness and treatment plan, providing physiologic and psychological support such as comfort measures after surgery, and caring for the child in cardiac failure (see Focus on Evidence-Based Practice). An equally important role is teaching prevention of heart disease. Measures such as promoting nonsmoking and exercise, maintaining an appropriate weight, and eating a low-fat diet are discussed in Chapter 31 with care of the school-age child. For additional help, parents may wish to contact the American Heart Association (*www.AHA.org*) for educational materials and family support groups in their area.

FOCUS ON EVIDENCE-BASED PRACTICE

Do Children Understand What Is the Cause of Their Heart Disease?

For this study, interviews were conducted with 63 children or adolescents, 7 to 18 years of age, identified as having a variety of heart ailments. As a part of the interview, participants were asked how much they understood about their heart disease. Results showed that only 30% of children had a good understanding of their illness; as many as 77% did not know the medical name of their condition and 33% had a wrong or poor understanding of their illness. Which children understood their condition and which did not was not related to age, sex, or the nature of the heart disease. Reasons suggested for this poor understanding were inadequate knowledge of normal anatomy and physiology, inadvertent use of jargon and overly technical explanations by cardiac specialists, and a tendency for patients and parents to forget a large proportion of what they were told because of their stress level. Subtle developmental delays in children from chronic anoxia may also contribute to poor knowledge retention. The researchers concluded that health care providers should take better steps to ensure that children understand the nature of their heart condition, both to enlarge their own knowledge and so they can give accurate health history information to future health care providers.

This is an important study for nurses because nurses are often the primary people who "back up" or clarify information given to children and parents about cardiac disease. Knowing that this is an area where more information may be needed serves as an alert to ensure that such clarifying sessions are important and can aid the understanding of children and parents about heart disease.

Veldtman, G.R., et al. (2000). Illness understanding in children and adolescents with heart disease. *Heart, 84*(4), 395–397.

Outcome Evaluation

Outcome evaluation should be both long term and short term for the child and family. It is important for families to receive adequate support during procedures and treatment. Once treatment is completed, and even if long-term care is necessary, evaluating the family's ability to think of their child not in terms of illness but in terms of wellness is also key. Provide the opportunity for parents to express their concerns about their child at follow-up visits to help address any misconceptions about the child's future.

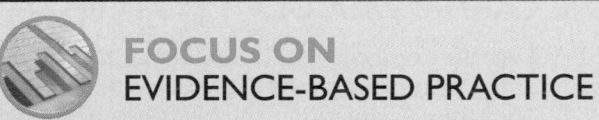

Examples suggesting achievement of outcomes may include the following:

- Child's heart rate remains within accepted parameters for age.
- Child demonstrates age-appropriate coping skills related to diagnosis and possible surgery.
- Parents demonstrate competence with procedures required for care of the child.
- Parents exhibit positive coping skills related to the child's diagnosis and required care to foster optimal growth and development in the child.
- Parents verbalize positive aspects about the child.

THE CARDIOVASCULAR SYSTEM

Embryologic development of the heart is described in Chapter 8. Cardiac adaptations at birth are described in Chapter 23. After these adaptations, the heart can be thought of as consisting of two pumps: the right side pumps blood to the lungs, where it is oxygenated before returning to the left side of the heart; the left side pumps the oxygenated blood to the peripheral tissues through systemic arteries. After supplying nutrients and collecting wastes, the blood returns through the veins to the right side of the heart, where the cycle begins again. Contraction of the chambers is termed **systole;** relaxation is termed **diastole.** Normal heart anatomy is reviewed in Figure 41-1.

Most heart disease in children occurs because embryonic structures did not close at birth or the heart formed inappropriately. For example, a septal defect between the right and left sides of the heart may remain open. Because pressure and volume on the left side of the heart are greater than on the right side, blood will flow through the connective structure left to right, or from the area of stronger heart action to the area of weaker heart action, compromising function (Sondheimer et al., 2001*a*).

Cardiac output (CO) is the volume of blood pumped by the ventricles each minute. It is calculated by multiplying stroke volume (the volume of blood a ventricle ejects during systole) by the heart rate (beats per minute). CO is affected by three main factors: preload, contractility, and afterload. **Preload** is the volume of blood in the ventricles at the end of diastole (the point just before contraction). **Afterload** refers to the resistance against which the ventricles must pump. **Contractility,** the ability of the ventricles to stretch, refers to the force of contraction generated by the myocardial muscle. The Frank-Starling law predicts that the stroke volume can be increased by increasing the stretch of the fibers. Excessive stretch, however, results in a decrease in CO. Much of the therapy of heart disease is aimed at reducing preload and afterload and increasing contractility.

ASSESSMENT OF HEART DISORDERS IN CHILDREN

The assessment of heart disease in children begins with a thorough history and a physical assessment. More specific diagnostic studies, such as electrocardiography or echocardiography, are ordered as indicated. Because all children with heart disorders have an increased risk of poor tissue perfusion, which may affect growth and development, developmental testing also is incorporated into the assessment.

History

As a result of technological advances in prenatal health care, such as prenatal ultrasound, which shows poor heart action or a distended heart, heart disease is being recognized earlier than it had been in previous years. However, even with these advances, heart disease may not be detected before birth. In the newborn period, because the newborn heart rate is so rapid that extra sounds of abnormal circulation cannot be heard, heart disease still may not be detected. Because of relatively high pulmonary resistance, defects of the septum may not be readily apparent at birth. The infant may be brought to a primary care setting at 1 week of age by parents because the child is having difficulty feeding. Infants with heart disease gen-

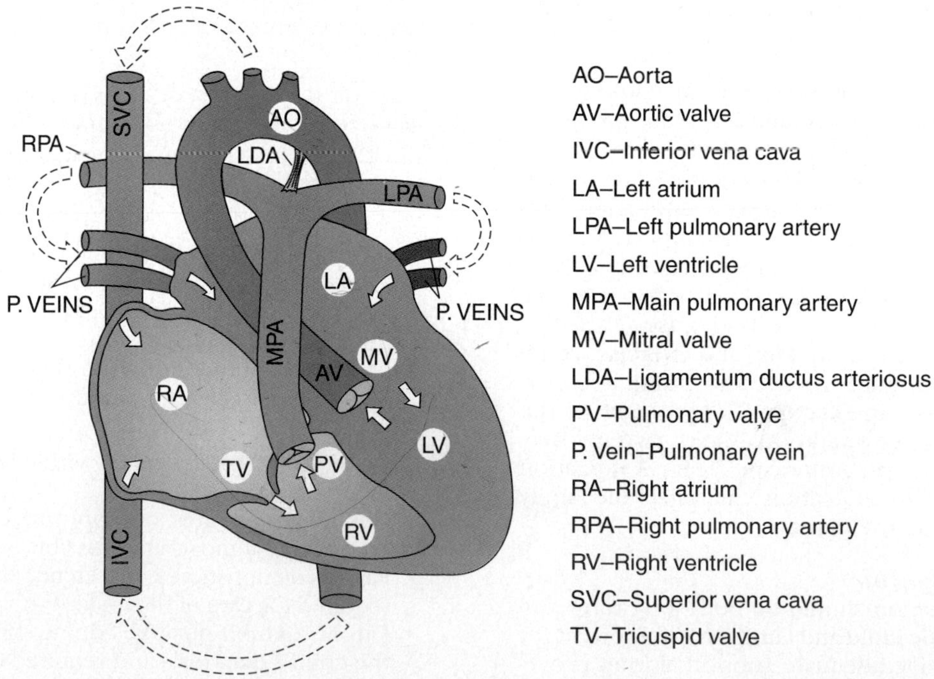

FIGURE 41.1 Anatomy of the normal heart.

erally have tachycardia and tachypnea. The infant who is breathing rapidly has to stop sucking on the bottle or breast frequently to breathe. The infant who is easily fatigued because of ineffective heart action has to stop sucking to rest before finishing a feeding.

The history should include a thorough pregnancy history to try to determine whether an intrauterine insult may have led to poor fetal formation. Cardiac anomalies can occur as a result of an infection such as toxoplasmosis, cytomegalovirus, or rubella during intrauterine life. Also ask if the mother took any medication during pregnancy, if nutrition was adequate, or whether she was exposed to any radiation, because these may also contribute to congenital heart disorders.

Older children with heart disease are easily fatigued. When obtaining the history, ask how much activity it takes before the child becomes tired: an hour of strenuous play? a short walk? Be sure parents are not confusing sedentary activities (the child who prefers to sit and read) with activities that are the result of fatigue (e.g., coming home from school and falling asleep day after day).

Ask about the child's usual position when resting. Some infants with congenital heart disease prefer a knee–chest position, whereas older children often voluntarily squat. These positions trap blood in the lower extremities because of the sharp bend at the knee and hip, allowing the child to oxygenate the blood remaining in the upper body more fully and easily. Also ask about frequency of infections, because children with heart disease have a higher incidence of lower respiratory tract infections than do other children (Sondheimer et al., 2001*a*). Children with left-to-right shunts tend to perspire excessively because of sympathetic nerve stimulation. Is there an indication of this? Urine is produced only when cardiac function is adequate to perfuse the kidneys. Ask if the infant is wetting diapers or if the older child is voiding normally. Edema from retained fluid is a late sign of heart disease in children. If it does occur, periorbital edema generally occurs first. **Cyanosis** (a blue tinge to the skin) may occur if a shunt allows deoxygenated blood to enter the arterial system. Such infants generally fail to thrive and are below normal height and weight on a standard growth chart. Children with coarctation of the aorta who have high blood pressure in the head and upper extremities have a history of nosebleeds and headaches. Because of corresponding low blood pressure in the lower extremities, such children may have pain in the legs on running (reported as "growing pains").

Some congenital heart disorders, such as atrial septal defects, may have a polygenic inheritance pattern. Ask if other family members have heart disease. Also be alert for other disorders such as cognitive impairment and renal disease, because cardiac anomalies often occur in conjunction with other disorders (Harris, 2000).

Physical Assessment

Physical assessment of the child with a suspected heart disorder begins with measuring height and weight and comparing these findings against standard growth charts. A thorough physical examination should then be done, with particular emphasis on certain body parts or systems (see Assessing the Child With a Cardiovascular Disorder).

ASSESSING the Child With a Cardiovascular Disorder

History

Chief concern: fatigue, cyanosis, frequent upper respiratory infections, feeding difficulty, poor weight gain, growth failure

Past medical history: infection during pregnancy; difficulty with resuscitation at birth

Family medical history: Other members with heart disorders

Physical examination

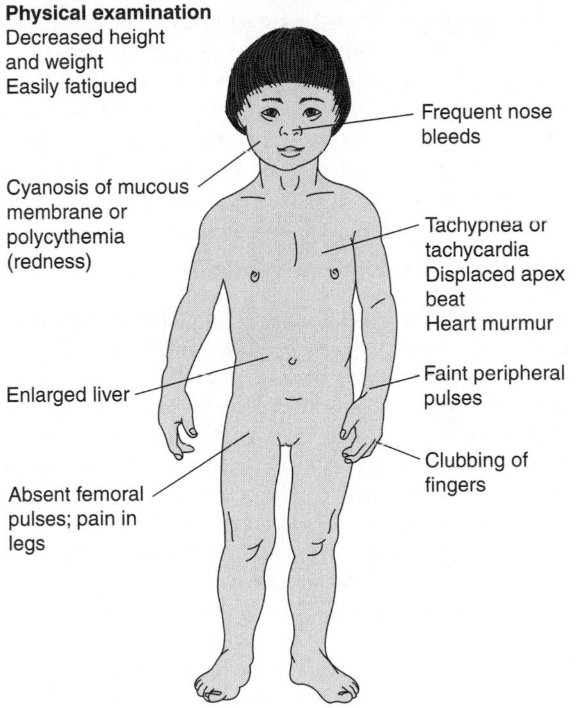

Because a major part of the physical assessment will include inspection, palpation, and auscultation of the chest for heart function, it is best if the child is relaxed and not crying. Provide age-appropriate toys that can distract the child readily. Provide a bottle of glucose water in case an infant grows hungry. Play with the child before the examination so he or she is acquainted with you.

General Appearance

Inspect the toes and fingers (particularly the thumbs) for clubbing and color. If you press on a fingernail, it will blanch white and then quickly return to pink in a child with good circulation and oxygenation. In a child with poor tissue perfusion, the pink color returns slowly (more than 5 seconds). Inspect the mucous membranes of the mouth for color and evidence of cyanosis.

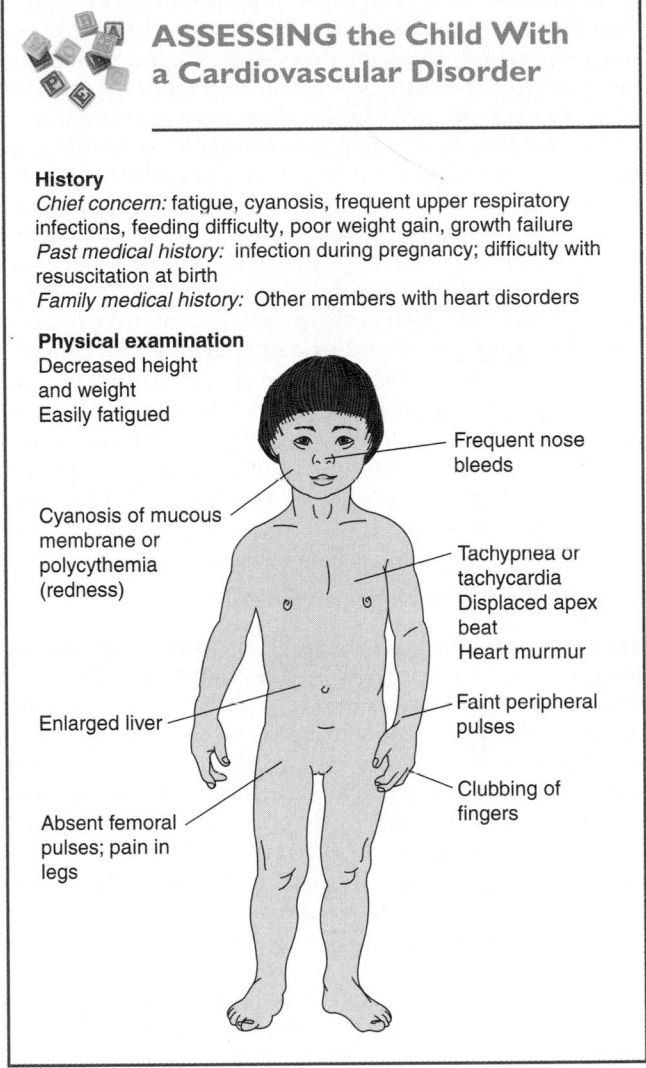

Cyanosis can best be recognized in the tongue and mucous membrane of the newborn. However, if the hemoglobin is reduced below 4 to 6 g/100 mL, cyanosis may not be evident because severe anemia masks it. Cyanosis persisting for over 20 minutes after birth (except for

acrocyanosis) suggests serious cardiopulmonary dysfunction. If the cyanosis increases with crying, cardiac dysfunction is suggested, implying that the child cannot meet the increased circulatory demands. If the cyanosis decreases with crying, pulmonary dysfunction is suggested because crying deepens respirations and aerates more lung tissue. Because cyanosis is difficult to detect in darker-skinned individuals, inspect the buccal membrane to detect cyanosis.

A ruddy complexion may be present in some children with heart disease because the body overproduces red blood cells (**polycythemia**) in an attempt to better oxygenate body cells. Also observe for lethargy and rapid respirations, symptoms that the heart is an ineffective pump.

Inspection of the chest may reveal a prominence of the left side and an obvious heart movement (apex beat, or point of maximum impulse). If a chest is extremely flat, loud innocent murmurs, accentuated heart sounds, and palpable cardiac activity may be very noticeable because of the proximity of the heart to the chest wall.

Pulse, Blood Pressure, and Respirations

The techniques for assessing pulse and blood pressure are described in Chapter 36. Normal findings for children of different ages are shown in Appendix G. Abnormal pulse patterns that tend to occur in children with heart disorders are shown in Table 41-1. Tachycardia is a pulse rate more than 160 bpm in an infant and more than 100 bpm at 3 years of age. An increase in pulse rate over these standards needs further investigation. Tachycardia is particularly significant if it persists during sleep, when the possibility of excitement is removed.

Murmurs of no significance are termed functional, insignificant, or innocent murmurs. In discussing such murmurs with parents, the term **innocent heart murmur** is best to use because it most clearly describes that the sound heard is not important. Using this term also helps to reassure parents that this is nothing to worry about. Such murmurs probably reflect a normal variation of vibration in the heart or pulmonary artery. They may become more pronounced during febrile illness, anxiety, or pregnancy. Hence, they may become audible for the first time at a hospital admission or with a sick-child visit.

Although innocent murmurs are of no consequence, parents need to be told when their child has an innocent murmur because this finding will undoubtedly be discovered again at a future health assessment. Teach parents that although an innocent murmur is present, it is not a sign of any heart disease. Activities need not be restricted, and the child will require no more frequent health appraisals than other children. Also teach parents that innocent murmurs do not turn into serious murmurs; otherwise, some parents can view them as a prelude to heart disease. At future health assessments, parents may need to be reassured again that the murmur is innocent.

If a murmur occurs as the result of heart disease or a congenital defect, it is termed an **organic heart murmur.** The characteristics of innocent and organic murmurs are compared in Table 41-2.

Describe any murmur that you hear according to the following: its position in the cardiac cycle (e.g., early systolic, midsystolic, late diastolic); duration; quality (blowing, rasping, rumbling); pitch; intensity; location (where heard best; the point of maximum intensity); presence of a thrill (a palpable purring sensation); and the response of the murmur to exercise or change of position. The intensity, or loudness, of the murmur is graded according to the standard criteria shown in Table 33-9.

> ✔ **CHECKPOINT QUESTIONS**
>
> 1. What two signs are typically present in infants with heart disease?
> 2. What term is used to denote a murmur resulting from heart disease?

Diagnostic Tests

The diagnostic studies performed on a child with suspected heart disease vary with the specific lesion suspected.

Electrocardiogram

An **electrocardiogram** (ECG) is a written record of the electrical voltages generated by the contracting heart. It provides information about heart rate, rhythm, state of

TABLE 41.1 Abnormal Pulse Patterns

PULSE PATTERN	DESCRIPTION
Water hammer	Very forceful and bounding pulse (Corrigan's pulse); capillary pulsations possibly apparent even in the fingernails; suggestive of cardiac insufficiency, as in patent ductus arteriosus
Pulsus alternans	A pulse of one strong beat and one weak beat; suggestive of myocardial weakness
Dicrotic	A double radial pulse for every apical beat; symptomatic of aortic stenosis
Thready	Weak and usually rapid pulse; suggestive of ineffective heart action

TABLE 41.2 Comparison of Innocent and Organic Murmurs

CHARACTERISTIC	INNOCENT	ORGANIC
Timing	Systolic	Systolic or diastolic
Duration	Short	Longer
Quality	Soft, musical	Harsh, blowing
Intensity	Soft	Loud
Position in which heard	Usually supine positions	Heard in all positions
Affected by exercise	Yes	No

the myocardium, presence or absence of hypertrophy (thickening of the heart walls), ischemia or necrosis due to inadequate cardiac circulation, and abnormalities of conduction. It also can provide information about the presence or effect of various drugs and electrolyte imbalances.

On an ECG waveform tracing, an upward pattern indicates a positive voltage, whereas a downward pattern indicates a negative voltage. The heartbeat is initiated by the sinoatrial (SA) node in the right atrial wall near the entrance of the superior vena cava. From the SA node, the electrical impulse spreads over the atria, reaching the atrioventricular (AV) node in the lower right atrium. From there, it spreads through the AV bundle (bundle of His) and the Purkinje fibers to the wall and septum of the ventricles. At the point that the ventricles have filled, the electrical flow has reached a peak, causing the ventricles to contract.

A normal ECG consists of an atrial wave (the P wave, denoting atrial depolarization), a brief hesitation before the AV node is activated, then the prominent ventricular peak (the QRS spike), another brief hesitation, and then a large slow wave caused by ventricular recovery (the T wave, denoting repolarization), and often an incompletely understood additional slow wave (the U wave; Fig. 41-2). A longer-than-normal P wave suggests that the atria are hypertrophied and it is taking longer than usual for the electrical conduction to spread over the atria. A lengthened PR interval suggests that there is difficulty in coordination between the SA and AV nodes (first-degree heart block). A heightened R wave indicates that ventricular hypertrophy is present. An R wave that is decreased in height means that the ventricles cannot contract fully, as happens if they are surrounded by fluid (pericarditis). Elongation of the T wave occurs in hyperkalemia; depression of the T wave is associated with anoxia; depression of the ST segment is associated with abnormal calcium levels.

Radiography

Radiographic (x-ray) examination furnishes an accurate picture of the heart size and the contour and size of the heart chambers. It can reveal fluid collecting in the lungs or pulmonary artery from cardiac failure. It also can be used to confirm the placement of pacemaker leads. In a posteroanterior view (in children over 1 year of age), if the cardiac width is more than half the chest width, the heart is unusually enlarged. In infants, the more horizontal position of the heart increases this ratio to more than half.

In addition to a chest x-ray, an upper gastrointestinal (UGI) series may be done. The esophagus is so closely related to cardiac chambers that when it is visualized with barium, it can help define cardiovascular structures. Even with this technique, interpretation of atrial or ventricular hypertrophy in infants and children by radiographic means is difficult. X-ray findings are therefore usually complemented by an ECG, a more sensitive and accurate measure of ventricular enlargement.

Fluoroscopy, a form of radiography, provides a permanent motion-picture record of important information about the size and configuration of the heart and great vessels, lungs, thoracic cage, and diaphragm. Because prolonged observation is necessary to record this information, special precautions must be taken to protect the child and health care personnel from radiation.

In radioangiocardiography, a radioactive substance such as technetium is injected intravenously into the bloodstream. As the substance circulates through the heart, it may be traced and recorded on videotape. The procedure involves a low dose of radiation and may be used to demonstrate, in particular, septal shunts.

Generalized angiography, or instillation of dye followed by radiographs, has little value in demonstrating pediatric heart defects. Selective angiocardiography, however, performed as part of a cardiac catheterization, allows identification of specific abnormalities if followed by serial x-ray films. After a contrast medium has been introduced into a specific heart chamber, closed-circuit video equipment records the fluoroscopy pictures. Angiocardiography is not without hazard: deaths have been reported from sensitivity to the dye used, cardiac arrhythmias, and pulmonary edema.

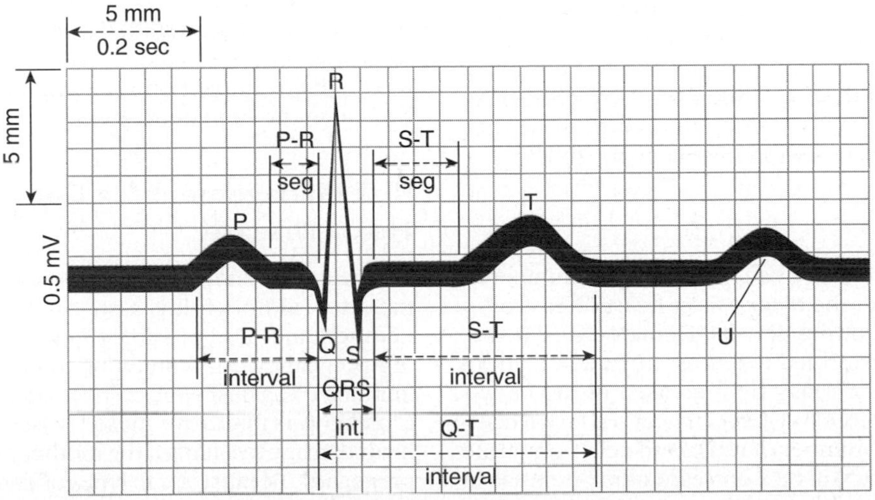

FIGURE 41.2 A normal ECG configuration.

Echocardiography

Echocardiography, or ultrasound cardiography, has become the primary diagnostic test for heart disease (Sondheimer et al., 2001*a*). High-frequency sound waves, directed toward the heart, are used to locate and study the movement and dimensions of cardiac structures, such as the size of chambers, thickness of walls, relationship of major vessels to chambers, and the thickness, motion, and pressure gradients of the valves. This technique is referred to as M-mode, a single beam that reveals chamber contractility; two-dimensional, a technique used to reveal chamber and vessel size; and Doppler technique, which reveals the velocity of blood flow. Remind parents that echocardiography does not use x-rays; thus, it can be repeated at frequent intervals without exposing children to the possible risk of radiation. It may be done using a transesophageal probe to better reveal heart chambers. Fetal echocardiography can reveal heart anomalies as early as 18 weeks into a pregnancy. This can alert staff to be prepared with immediate resuscitation or other needed equipment at the baby's birth (Danford, 2000).

Phonocardiography and Magnetic Resonance Imaging

A **phonocardiogram** is a diagram of heart sounds translated into electrical energy by a microphone placed on the child's chest and then recorded as a diagrammatic representation of heart sounds. The technique can measure the timing of heart sounds that occur too quickly or at too high or too low a sound frequency for the human ear to detect by direct auscultation. Magnetic resonance imaging (MRI) may also be used to evaluate heart structure or size or blood flow.

Exercise Testing

Exercise tests using treadmill walking to demonstrate that the pulmonary circulation can increase to meet the increased respiratory demands of exercise may be performed with children, although these tests are not used as extensively with children as they are with adults. With children who have heart defects that obstruct the flow of blood to the lungs (such as pulmonary stenosis), accommodation to exercise is not possible, and the child will evidence exertional dyspnea. Such tests are difficult to perform successfully with young children because they require the child's cooperation (Karila et al., 2001).

Laboratory Tests

Children with heart disease usually undergo a number of blood tests to support the diagnosis of heart disease or to rule out anemia or clotting defects. Hematocrit or hemoglobin studies are performed to assess the rate of erythrocyte production, which may be increased in the body's attempt to produce more oxygen-carrying red blood cells. If the increase in the number of red blood cells is extreme (polycythemia), there will be a corresponding increase in blood volume and possibly an increase in blood viscosity. Newborns are normally slightly polycythemic. In a newborn, polycythemia may be defined as a hemoglobin level over 25 g/100 mL or a hematocrit level over 70%. In an older child, polycythemia may be defined as a hemoglobin level over 16 g/100 mL or a hematocrit level over 55%. An elevated erythrocyte sedimentation rate (ESR) denotes inflammation and is useful in documenting that an inflammatory process, such as occurs with rheumatic fever, Kawasaki disease, or myocarditis, is present.

Blood gas levels also are determined. To test for this, infants may be given 100% oxygen for 15 minutes. If an infant still has a Po_2 less than 150 mm Hg after this time, a shunt directing deoxygenated blood into oxygenated blood can be suspected. Oxygen saturation levels also are assessed; children with a deoxygenated to oxygenated shunt have a lower-than-normal oxygen saturation level in arterial blood. Normally, arterial blood oxygen saturation is 95% to 100%; oxygen saturation is under 92% when venous arterial shunts are present.

Before cardiac catheterization or surgery, blood clotting must be assessed. Expect prothrombin and partial thromboplastin times and platelet count studies to be completed before the procedure. Some children with polycythemia from heart disease have an associated reduced platelet count (thrombocytopenia). Because platelet formation is necessary for blood coagulation, the platelet count must be corrected before cardiac surgery.

In children with heart failure, a serum sodium level is obtained to ensure that an increased sodium level is not compounding edema. All children receiving diuretics should have serum potassium levels determined because diuretics tend to deplete the body of potassium. Low serum potassium levels potentiate the effect of cardiac glycosides, such as digoxin. Thus, serum potassium levels must also be obtained in children receiving these medications.

HEALTH PROMOTION AND RISK MANAGEMENT

Cardiac disease prevention in adults has received extensive attention in the health literature. Because the risk factors that lead to adult heart disease such as obesity, high cholesterol serum levels, and lack of consistent exercise involve health habits that begin in childhood, prevention of cardiac disease has shifted from an adult to a child focus. Early interventions to reduce risk factors in early life should have a major impact on reducing the incidence of heart disease in the next generation.

Risk Management for Congenital Heart Disease

The cause of congenital heart disease often cannot be documented, although it is associated with familial patterns of inheritance and possible triggers such as infection during pregnancy. All women of childbearing age should be immunized against rubella (German measles) and varicella (chickenpox) because these viruses are known to cause heart damage to a fetus if the mother contracts them during pregnancy. Because some types of congenital heart defects have a familial incidence, parents who have a family member born with a heart defect need to alert their primary care provider so other children can be carefully screened prenatally and at birth for the possibility of a similar defect. The incidence of a child being born with a cardiac defect is as high as 15% in these families (Sondheimer et al., 2001a).

Risk Management for Acquired Heart Disease

Acquired heart diseases in children that have identified risk factors include rheumatic fever, hypertension, and hyperlipidemia. Rheumatic fever is an autoimmune response that follows a group A beta-hemolytic streptococcal infection. Ensuring that all parents know that children with streptococcal infections from otitis media, streptococcal pharyngitis, and impetigo should receive adequate antibiotic therapy is essential for disease prevention (Ogle & Anderson, 2001).

Although hypertension (elevated blood pressure) occurs mainly because of a genetic predisposition, a high intake of sodium (such as that in table salt), lack of exercise, and obesity increase the chances of developing the disorder in susceptible children by the time they reach late childhood (Kay et al., 2001). If infants are never introduced to high-sodium foods, perhaps by the time they are selecting their own meals they may continue to eat a diet prudent in sodium amount, helping to prevent the development of hypertension in later life. For this reason, baby food manufacturers have stopped adding salt and monosodium glutamate to infant food. Urging school-age children and adolescents to reduce their intake of canned soups, cheese, lunch meats, and hot dogs, all foods with high sodium content, can reduce salt intake in these age groups. School nurses can play an important role in this effort by monitoring the foods served daily in school cafeterias and advocating for more nutritious menus. Beginning when a child is 3 years of age, blood pressure should be included as part of routine assessment to detect hypertension as early as possible.

A diet high in saturated fat has been implicated in the development of hypercholesterolemia and hyperlipidemia. It is important that fat intake not be restricted in infants because they need fat and the calories that it provides for brain growth. School-age children and adolescents, however, should reduce their fat intake to 30% of total calories (the same recommendation as for adults). The use of vegetable oils in place of saturated fat should begin when children begin solid food. Children from high-risk families (a family member has had an early myocardial infarction) should be regularly screened for elevated cholesterol and triglyceride levels beginning at about 3 years of age. Children with cholesterol values above 170 mg/dL should receive nutritional counseling and instruction about a regular exercise program to enhance their health.

✔ CHECKPOINT QUESTIONS

3. How do blood tests help in the diagnosis of heart disease?
4. At what age should routine blood pressure screening begin?

NURSING CARE OF THE CHILD WITH A HEART DISORDER

Most parents have many questions about how to care for a child with heart disease. Encourage parents to handle and feed their newborn in the hospital so they can feel secure in caring for him or her at home. Encourage them to learn as much as possible about their child's disorder. Be certain they recognize that not all children with congenital heart disease have the same disease or need the same degree of restriction. If this is not made clear to parents, they may unnecessarily limit the child's activity, assuming that because another child was told not to do some activity, their child should not do it either.

NURSING DIAGNOSES AND RELATED INTERVENTIONS

Nursing Diagnosis: Parental health-seeking behaviors related to desire to be informed about child's disorder

Outcome Identification: Parents will demonstrate a full understanding of child's illness and treatment plan before discharge.

Outcome Evaluation: Parents accurately state the nature of the illness and unique needs of their child; are able to name primary care providers who will follow child's progress; state they will telephone if they have any questions.

Provide Information About Care. Parents generally ask whether it is safe to let the baby cry. If the infant has a cardiac disorder such as tetralogy of Fallot in which cyanotic spells tend to develop, the baby should not be allowed to cry for long periods of time (no baby should). However, crying for a few minutes while a parent warms formula or fully awakens at night will, as a rule, not harm the baby.

Another common question is, "Does our child need special nutrition?" As with all newborns, breast-feeding is the preferred method of feeding. Salt is only rarely restricted during this period because infants need sodium to regulate water balance. Because anemia stresses the heart, infants are generally given an iron supplement, either with formula or separately, to prevent iron deficiency anemia during the first year. Like all infants, they should receive supplemental vitamins with formula or when breast-feeding is stopped. Because some infants with congenital heart disease tire readily, frequent small feedings during the day rather than the usual pattern of feedings every 3 to 4 hours may be necessary. If the child is an extremely poor eater, a high-calorie formula or enteral or gastrostomy feedings may be necessary.

"How much activity can we allow the baby?" The answer to this question depends on the type and extent of the heart disorder. As a rule, infants or young children naturally limit their own activity. Parents may need guidance, however, in setting limits on activity. Roughhousing with infants, such as tossing them up in the air and watching them squeal and laugh, or playing games such as chasing a ball may not be advised. Encourage parents to observe the infant carefully to learn to recognize the first signs of respiratory distress and the point at which the child's activity is beginning to exceed his or her tolerance. Caution parents to observe the child carefully and thoughtfully as new activities are introduced and new interests are gained, so the child's activity is limited to what the heart can accommodate.

"What do we do if he becomes ill?" Although children with congenital heart disorders are usually seen by a cardiologist for health supervision, it is important that they are also seen by health care personnel who can ensure that they are receiving normal childhood immunizations and health guidance. As a rule, infants with heart disorders need prompt treatment for minor illnesses. The fever that accompanies a cold, for instance, can increase the metabolic rate of a child who has a severe congenital heart defect to beyond the point at which the child's heart can compensate. Dehydration must be avoided in children with polycythemia or the polycythemia may become so severe that clotting or thrombophlebitis may result. It is also important that infections be treated vigorously so infectious endocarditis does not develop.

Children with congenital heart defects or rheumatic fever need prophylactic antibiotic therapy before they have oral surgery (tooth extractions or tonsils removed). Streptococcal organisms generally present in the mouth can lead to infectious endocarditis if the organisms enter the bloodstream during surgery. It is a good rule for parents to ask that their children be given prophylactic antibiotics before they visit the dentist at all, because they cannot always anticipate what procedures the dentist will do at any one visit. Oral penicillin is the preferred prophylactic antibiotic; erythromycin can be used for a child sensitive to penicillin. Some parents need reassurance that their child will not become immune to penicillin if it is taken this way over long periods. Children with congenital heart disease should receive routine immunizations and be considered for pneumonia and influenza vaccines.

Review Steps for Follow-Up Care and Emergencies. Before parents leave the hospital with a newborn who has a congenital heart disorder, be certain they have the name and number of the person to call if they have a question regarding their infant's health (their primary care provider and an emergency telephone number as a back-up). Review with them the steps to take if their child should become cyanotic, such as placing him or her in a knee–chest position. Be certain they have an appointment for a first health assessment. This helps to reassure them that the responsibility of caring for this child is not being placed solely on their shoulders but will be shared by concerned health care personnel. In many instances, parents are first-time parents. If they are unsure whether their child is in distress or ill, urge them to err on the side of caution by bringing the child to the primary care setting. Everyone who cares for infants or children with heart disease appreciates the responsibility that parents feel and the difficulty they can have in making health judgments about their child.

Most parents feel relieved to know that they can have home follow-up. In addition to providing opportunities for child and family assessment, a home visit allows parents to discuss the sometimes frightening responsibility they feel and to obtain a second opinion of their child's health. Teach cardiopulmonary resuscitation (CPR) and how to activate their community's emergency medical system (EMS). It may be reassuring for the parents to visit their closest EMS station so that they know the staff is acquainted with their child should an emergency call be necessary.

✔ **CHECKPOINT QUESTIONS**

5. Why is an iron supplement prescribed for an infant with congenital heart disease?
6. What is the rationale for prophylactic antibiotic administration before oral surgery for the child with heart disease?

The Child Undergoing Cardiac Catheterization

Cardiac catheterization, a procedure in which a small radiopaque catheter is passed through a major vein in the arm, leg, or neck into the heart to secure blood samples or inject dye, helps to evaluate cardiac function. Diagnostic cardiac catheterization is used to help diagnose specific heart defects in anticipation of surgery. Interventional cardiac catheterization is used to correct an abnormality, such as dilating a narrowed valve by the use of a balloon catheter or other device. With both types, the pressure of blood flow in any heart chamber and total cardiac output can be evaluated. Blood specimens can be obtained to determine oxygen saturation levels, or a contrast dye can be injected for angiography. Electrodes can be introduced to record electrical activity and diagnose arrhythmias.

This procedure may be done as ambulatory or 1-day surgery using conscious sedation. Children must have a recent chest x-ray, ECG, and electrolyte levels and blood must be typed and cross-matched before the procedure. Take and record pedal pulses for a baseline assessment. Also measure and record height and weight. This information is used to determine catheter size. Because it is vital that the vessel site chosen for catheterization not be infected at the time of catheterization (or obscured by a hematoma), do not draw blood specimens from the projected catheterization entry site before the procedure. Generally, children scheduled for the procedure are kept NPO for 2 to 4 hours beforehand to reduce the danger of vomiting and aspiration during the procedure.

In the cardiac catheterization room, ECG and pulse oximetry leads are attached. The site for catheterization is locally anesthetized with EMLA cream or intradermal lidocaine, and a catheter is threaded through a large-bore needle inserted into the site. The specific vessel used differs according to the technique being planned. In neonates, an umbilical artery can be catheterized. For right-side heart catheterization, a right femoral vein or a vein in the antecubital fossa usually is used. Left-side heart catheterization can be performed using either a venous or an arterial approach. If done by the arterial route, a catheter is inserted into either the femoral or brachial artery. If a venous route is used, the catheter is inserted into the right femoral vein. Under fluoroscopy, the catheter is advanced to the right atrium and through the heart septum. Once the catheter is in a selected heart chamber, radiopaque dye is injected to outline the heart configuration (Fig. 41-3).

Cardiac catheterization has a mortality rate of under 0.1% when done as an elective procedure and approximately 2% when performed in a severely distressed child (Sondheimer et al., 2001*b*). Arrhythmias may occur during passage of the catheter through heart chambers or during the injection of contrast media. Such arrhythmias generally are transitory or stop abruptly with withdrawal of the catheter. Inadvertent perforation of the heart may occur during passage of the catheter. Other complications include bleeding from the insertion site (secondary to heparin introduced into the catheter to reduce the possibility of clot formation) and thrombophlebitis (from platelet aggregation due to irritation by the catheter, a foreign body). Because cardiac catheterization is necessary for a cardiac surgeon to visualize and plan a cardiac repair, the key to making cardiac surgery safe, the benefit of the procedure outweighs the risks.

NURSING DIAGNOSIS AND RELATED INTERVENTIONS: PREPROCEDURE PHASE

Nursing Diagnosis: Anxiety related to lack of knowledge about cardiac catheterization procedure

Outcome Identification: Parents and child will demonstrate reduced anxiety with increased knowledge before procedure; will express confidence about need for and outcome of procedure.

Outcome Evaluation: Parents and child (when possible) state goal of procedure and reasons for preparation and aftercare measures; state that anxiety is less after teaching.

Because most cardiac catheterizations are done with children under conscious sedation, they may need more information about what is going to happen during this procedure than they will need for cardiac surgery, when they will be anesthetized. Provide explanations about the procedure for the child with the parents present, if possible. This allows parents to help reinforce the information. After this explanation, provide parents with a more detailed explanation of the procedure and allow time to ask any questions they do not want to ask in the child's presence.

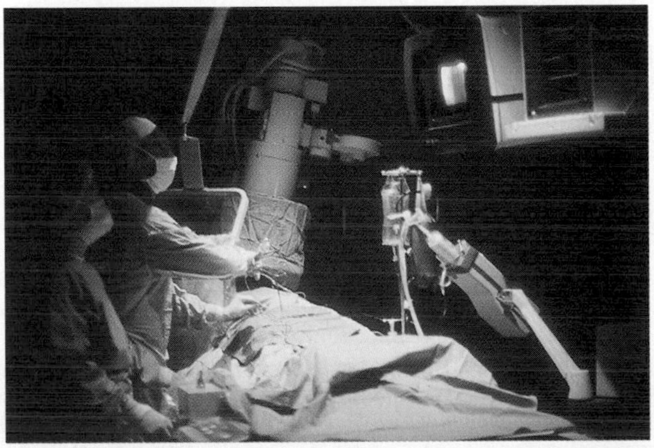

FIGURE 41.3 A child undergoing a cardiac catheterization.

Parents often need a review of heart anatomy. Although the cardiologist may have already done this, many parents appreciate reinforcement and review of this information. Show them the pathway the catheter will take during the procedure.

Be aware that consenting to a cardiac catheterization experience arouses the realization that cardiac surgery may be necessary. As a result, parents may be so concerned with what the procedure may reveal that they cannot listen well to preprocedure explanations. Allow them to accompany their child to the catheterization room and, if possible and appropriate, to remain there for support during the procedure if they choose.

Review with the child what he or she will see in the catheterization room. Small children can become overwhelmed by seeing the actual equipment. Therefore, try building a facsimile room out of small cardboard boxes (representing the x-ray machine, the fluoroscopy screen, the ECG machine, and so forth). A puppet or small doll can serve as the patient in the miniature room. Dress the puppets in surgery suits and masks like those worn by cardiac catheterization personnel and act out what the child can expect to happen. Older children prefer a tour of the cardiac catheterization area and the opportunity to meet the personnel.

If children have never seen ECG leads or restraints before, let them touch and feel the equipment. Caution them that the procedure may be as long as 3 to 4 hours and that they will need to lie still during this time. Help them master imagery or another stress-reduction technique to help reduce apprehension.

Do not underestimate what children know about the heart's purpose and function; even preschoolers know that the heart is vital to the body. Reassure them that the doctors are only taking a look at their heart, not cutting it or removing any part of it.

Teach children of all ages that when the catheter is inserted, it will not hurt. Warn them that they may feel a momentary speeding up of the heart, a feeling that is uncomfortable. When dye is inserted, they may feel a stinging sensation. Do not use the word "dye," which young children may misinterpret as "die." Instead, say "medicine." Caution them that the lights will be turned off after the medicine is injected so the doctor can watch the medicine on a television screen (fluoroscopy) as it passes through the heart. Let children know that after the procedure, a pressure dressing will be placed over the catheter insertion site to reduce the risk of bleeding. They will need to keep that extremity flat and unbent to prevent the dressing from loosening.

NURSING DIAGNOSES AND RELATED INTERVENTIONS: POSTPROCEDURE PHASE

Nursing Diagnosis: Risk for ineffective cardiopulmonary and peripheral tissue perfusion related to cardiac catheterization

Outcome Identification: Child will maintain adequate tissue perfusion during the recovery period.

Outcome Evaluation: Child's vital signs are within normal limits; absence of arrhythmia; absence of bleeding or hematoma formation at catheterization site; pedal pulse is present distal to catheterization site.

When the child returns from the procedure, assess the pressure dressing over the catheterization site to see that it is snug and intact and that no bleeding is present. Instruct the child not to bend the hip (if the femoral site was used) or the elbow (if the brachial site was used) to keep the pressure dressing secure and to prevent hematoma formation. This is particularly important when an artery was used for catheterization; a loose dressing on an artery will cause a large blood loss in a very short time. Palpate pulses and assess color, temperature, and circulation (blanch the toe or fingernail and watch to see that it turns pink again readily) distal to the insertion site to ensure that blood flow in the extremity is unobstructed. If there is bleeding at the insertion site, apply firm, continuous pressure and notify the physician who performed the procedure immediately.

Children often appreciate being asked to describe their experience afterward. Saying out loud how frightened they were—by the x-ray machine being pushed in over them or by the thought of a tube going all the way into their heart—helps alleviate their fear and allows better acceptance of the procedure. Praise them for their cooperation during a very stressful experience.

Keep the child flat in bed for 2 to 3 hours until he or she is completely awake from conscious sedation. This helps to prevent oozing at the insertion site and postural hypotension, which may occur when the child rises suddenly after lying flat while under sedation for a long period. In the immediate postcatheterization period, the blood pressure may be 10% to 15% lower than the precatheterization level because of the hypotensive effect of the radiopaque dye.

Cardiac arrhythmias and bradycardia may be present from the mechanical action of the catheter having touched the conduction nodes of the heart. Assess pulse, blood pressure, and respirations at frequent intervals (about every 15 minutes) for the first several hours. Monitor the pulse for a full minute to aid in recognizing abnormalities. Be alert for signs of possible arrhythmias. Small children cannot describe the odd feeling that accompanies an arrhythmia. Older children might describe it as the heart "fluttering" or "skipping beats." Therefore, be alert for signs of increasing anxiety in the child after a catheterization; this may be the child's way of reporting these feelings.

Infants may need IV fluid during the procedure and for several hours afterward to prevent dehydration that results from being NPO for a period of time. If the infant is polycythemic, IV fluid helps minimize the risk of vessel thrombi. Regulate IV fluid carefully to prevent heart failure from fluid overload.

The adverse effects of cardiac catheterization may be manifested by spells of apnea, sternal retractions, or dyspnea. If oxygen was administered during the catheterization procedure, it may be continued for a period of time after the procedure to reduce the stress of respirations. Like arrhythmias, dyspnea, bradycardia, and blood pressure anomalies may be transient, but all should be reported so they can be evaluated.

Nursing Diagnosis: Risk for infection related to presence of cardiac catheterization incision site

Outcome Identification: The child will remain free of signs and symptoms of infection after the procedure.

Outcome Procedure: The child's temperature is less than 100.4°F (38.0°C) axillary; the catheter insertion site is free of erythema or drainage.

If the dressing is over the femoral artery or vein, keep it clean of stool and urine. Waterproofing the dressing with plastic may be necessary. Assess temperature immediately after the procedure to determine a baseline. Some children have a transient elevation in temperature already due to physiologic dehydration as a result of having been NPO or as a reaction to the dye. Others have slightly subnormal temperature readings from lying in a cool procedure room for a lengthy period. This below-normal body temperature quickly compromises respiratory and heart action because, to raise body temperature, infants must increase their metabolic rate. This requires rapid breathing and increased heart action, which can lead to exhaustion. Infants may need to be placed under radiant heat warmers to help regain and maintain normal body temperature and also to allow accurate temperature determinations.

Also check the insertion site for signs of infection, because any opening in the skin is a portal of entry for bacteria. Alert parents to observe the catheter insertion site daily for redness. Most parents are advised to monitor their child's temperature daily for about 3 days and to omit tub baths and strenuous exercise for their child for 2 to 3 days to aid healing.

✔ CHECKPOINT QUESTIONS

7. What sensation might the child feel when a cardiac catheter is inserted?
8. Why might a child develop cardiac arrhythmias after cardiac catheterization?

The Child Undergoing Cardiac Surgery

Open-heart surgery is made possible by the use of cardiopulmonary bypass or extracorporeal membrane oxygenation (ECMO). For this, the venous return to the heart is diverted from the right atrium or inferior and superior vena cava to a heart–lung machine, where it is artificially oxygenated. It is returned to the body's arterial system by way of the aorta, bypassing the heart. The heart, practically bloodless, now can be opened and operated on. Blood returns to the coronary and pulmonary capillary beds under pressure from the aorta so that even though blood bypasses the heart, it still receives an adequate blood supply for self-maintenance during the bypass procedure. During surgery, hypothermia (reducing the child's body temperature to 68° to 79°F [20° to 26°C]) is used to reduce the child's metabolic needs and slow the heart rate. If extreme hypothermia is used (59° to 68°F [15° to 20°C]), usually in an infant, the body temperature drops so low that the heart stops beating and the surgeon can work in a quiet and bloodless field. Very ill infants may be maintained by ECMO by the same technique after surgery (Morrow, 2000).

Preoperative Care

Before surgery, obtain vital signs (blood pressure, temperature, pulse, and respirations) to establish a baseline. Count pulse and respiratory rates for a full minute for accuracy. Some children may need baseline pulse determinations done at several pulse points or blood pressures of both upper and lower extremities. Before obtaining a blood pressure, have the child rest for about 15 minutes and take the recording with the child lying down. Record height and weight, because these parameters are necessary for the estimation of blood volume for the heart–lung machine and for medication dosages. Weighing also is helpful in estimating blood loss or edema after surgery. Children who are receiving digoxin usually have their dose withheld 24 hours before surgery because cardiac surgery may cause arrhythmias in the presence of cardiac glycosides.

The immediate surgical preparation of children varies from one institution to another but usually includes preparing the skin site. The skin over the surgical incision area is scrubbed with an antiseptic solution to ensure as clean a surgical field as possible. Most children and parents are startled to learn that cardiac surgery may be performed through the sternal bone, not over the left side of the chest, and may question the area being prepared for the incision. An enema also may be given to keep children from straining to pass stool in the immediate postoperative period and thus placing additional strain on the heart.

NURSING DIAGNOSES AND RELATED INTERVENTIONS: PREOPERATIVE PHASE

Nursing Diagnosis: Deficient knowledge related to cardiac surgery and its outcome

Outcome Identification: Parents and child will demonstrate increased knowledge before procedure and confidence in their health care team.

Outcome Evaluation: Parents and child accurately state the reason for surgery and expected outcome.

Bringing a child to the hospital for cardiac surgery is a large responsibility for parents. They want their child to be made well, but they are aware that there is a definite risk from this surgery. They may have been protecting and guarding their child for months or years, and they feel no less protective the morning of surgery. For this reason, parents of children being readied for cardiac surgery may watch preoperative procedures more carefully than usual. Review with them what they already know about the surgery to correct any misconceptions and inform them what laboratory tests will be scheduled. Prepare them for the amount of equipment that will surround their child after surgery such as cardiac monitors, oxygen and IV equipment, chest tubes, and a ventilator. Parents usually appreciate visiting the intensive care unit (ICU) where their child will go after surgery. Be certain that they have an opportunity to meet the ICU staff, especially if these nurses are not the same ones who are caring for the child preoperatively.

Prepare Child for Surgery and Postoperative Care. It is best if the child is prepared for surgery with the parents present. This allows parents the opportunity to reinforce your teaching and shows the child that his or her parents approve and feel secure with these surgery plans. Parents will then need additional time to discuss the surgical procedure with you and ask questions they might not have wished to ask in the presence of their child.

Do not underestimate how much children understand about the importance of their heart or the seriousness of this surgery (Fig. 41-4). Remember when caring for them preoperatively (or any time) not to make careless remarks. For example, statements such as, "These syringes never work right" (when all you mean is that you prefer another brand) or "Amy [an ICU nurse] is a real clown" (when you mean she is not only a competent nurse but has a good sense of humor besides) could be interpreted by anxious parents or children to mean a child is in less-than-competent hands. Because many children having cardiac surgery have had previous cardiac catheterizations, talking to them about

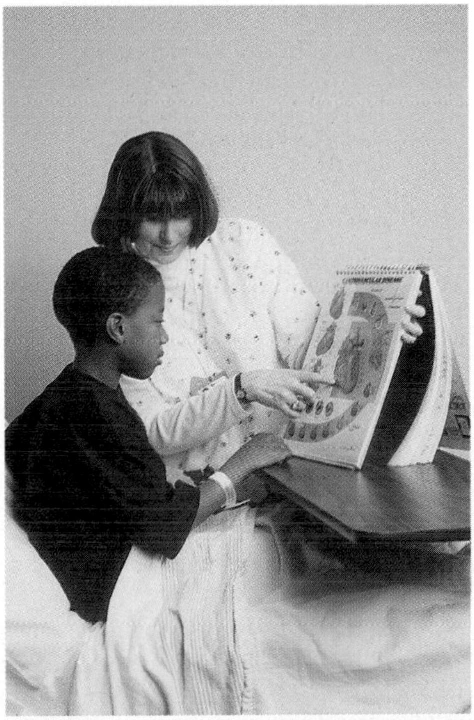

FIGURE 41.4 Orientation for cardiac surgery includes time for talking and learning more about the heart.

their previous hospitalization experiences is helpful. Talking will reveal the things they fear the most this time. Any misconceptions they have about past experiences can then be discussed and clarified.

Both parents and children may have questions about the difference between cardiac catheterization and cardiac surgery. One important difference is that children are sedated but awake for the former but anesthetized for the latter. For some children, knowing that they will be asleep is more reassuring; for others, it is more frightening. When they were awake, they knew that they were all right; asleep, how can they know? Encourage them to express these feelings so they can receive reassurance that anesthetized sleep is a special sleep from which they will have no difficulty waking. Meeting the anesthesiologist and receiving reassurance directly from him or her that they will be watched over while they are asleep is often helpful.

As with cardiac catheterization, it may help to make models of the equipment that will surround the child postoperatively. Parents and older children can be taken to the ICU where they will return after surgery and be shown the actual equipment and setting.

After surgery, the child will need to cough and deep-breathe and use incentive spirometry to help the lungs expand. Introduce these exercises preoperatively to let the child know what will be expected. Familiarize children with chest tubes. Caution both children and parents that chest tubes must stay in place until it is time for them to be removed. If children want to turn over with tubes in place, they need to ask for help to prevent the tubes from being dislodged. Caution parents that a chest-tube drainage reservoir must remain below the level of the child's chest and must not be raised for any reason. If children are not familiar with ECG leads, introduce them to these as part of the preoperative preparation. Comparing these tubes or leads to being "hooked up" like an astronaut is often appealing to children. In addition, introduce children to the form of oxygen therapy they will receive after surgery (mask, cannula, or ventilator). Orienting children to oxygen equipment is discussed in Chapter 40.

Postoperative Care

After surgery and before leaving the operating room, an x-ray film is taken and the child is weighed. Future estimates of lung expansion and weight will be checked against these two measurements.

NURSING DIAGNOSES AND RELATED INTERVENTIONS: POSTOPERATIVE PHASE

Nursing Diagnosis: Risk for ineffective cardiopulmonary tissue perfusion related to cardiac surgery

Outcome Identification: Child will maintain adequate tissue perfusion during the recovery period.

Outcome Evaluation: Vital signs are within normal limits; central venous pressure (CVP) or pulmonary artery wedge pressure is within acceptable parameters.

Taking accurate vital signs, as often as every 15 minutes, is essential in the immediate postoperative period. Continuous cardiac monitoring and assisted ventilation with endotracheal intubation also are usually necessary. Blood pressure will probably be monitored directly by means of an intra-arterial catheter or indirectly with an automated blood pressure recording device. Hemodynamic monitoring by way of a pulmonary artery or central venous catheter reveals information on chamber pressures and oxygen saturation (Fig. 41-5).

Adequate voiding after surgery indicates that the kidneys are receiving adequate circulation. An indwelling urinary (Foley) catheter is usually inserted at the time of surgery so urine output can be carefully recorded postoperatively (it should be 1 mL/kg/hour). Be certain to mark the amount of urine drainage present when children first return from surgery so that lack of or diminished urinary output will not be missed or misinterpreted. Individual samples may be tested for specific gravity and pH. A specific gravity below 1.010 implies that the kidneys are not concentrating urine well, perhaps because of the stress of surgery. The pH should remain slightly acid; however, extreme acidity may indicate respiratory acidosis from poor pulmonary perfusion.

Carefully record all IV fluid administered to the child after heart surgery. Fluid overload can pose a severe threat to the heart during the immediate postoperative period. Use an infusion control device to regulate the amount and rate of infusion.

Laboratory tests such as arterial blood gases (PO_2 and PCO_2), hemoglobin, hematocrit, clotting time, and electrolytes (particularly sodium and potassium) will be monitored closely to assess cardiac and pulmonary function postoperatively. Oxygen saturation

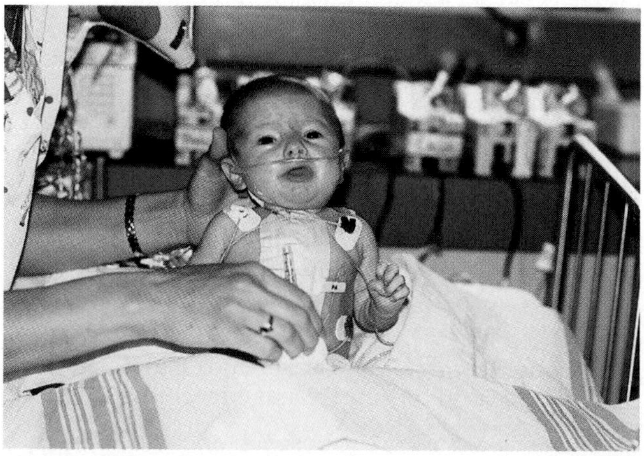

FIGURE 41.5 Because children typically have a myriad of wires and tubes attached to monitors, pumps, and equipment, parents need to be prepared for how their child will look after cardiac surgery. As the child's condition improves, the equipment is discontinued. Here, an infant is 2 days post-cardiac surgery. Note his level of alertness and the use of only a few monitoring devices and equipment.

levels may be monitored by pulse oximetry or transcutaneous oxygen monitoring. A drug such as dopamine may be administered to improve cardiac output (Carpenter et al., 2001).

Central Venous Pressure Monitoring. CVP may be recorded by inserting a catheter into a brachial, jugular, or subclavian vein, and ultimately into the right atrium (Fig. 41-6). CVP is an excellent way to evaluate the child's fluid volume status. CVP will rise with heart failure, indicating that the heart cannot handle the blood arriving at the atria.

Pulmonary Artery Pressure Monitoring. To assess the pressure in the left side of the heart parallel to CVP measurement, a multilumen pulmonary artery catheter, such as a Swan-Ganz catheter, is threaded through the venous circulation through the right side of the heart and into the pulmonary artery. The pressure, registered there as a waveform on a cardiac monitor, reflects both the resistance of the lungs to the passage of blood (pulmonary artery resistance) and the ability of the left side of the heart to handle the circulating fluid volume. Such catheters must be kept from clotting with frequent irrigations of heparin or with a constant infusion system. When withdrawing blood specimen samples from the catheter, make sure that no air is allowed to enter, because this would immediately flow into the left side of the heart and possibly to a cerebral artery as an embolus.

Nursing Diagnosis: Impaired gas exchange related to unexpanded lung space and collection of lung excretions

Outcome Identification: Child will demonstrate adequate respiratory function during the recovery period.

Outcome Evaluation: Child's respiratory rate remains within age-appropriate parameters; absence of crackles (rales) or other adventitious breath sounds; chest tubes function normally.

Measures to Prevent the Pooling of Secretions in the Lungs. Suction as necessary while the child is receiving ventilatory assistance to prevent pooling of secretions in the respiratory tract. As soon as the endotracheal tube and ventilator are removed, encourage the child to cough and deep-breathe or use an incentive spirometer at hourly intervals to help mobilize secretions. Although the child may have practiced such procedures preoperatively, he or she may have difficulty carrying them out now because coughing or deep-breathing can be very painful, especially without continuous pain relief. To minimize the pain, administer the prescribed analgesia or alert the child to use the PCA pump 10 to 15 minutes before it is time to deep-breathe. For optimal effectiveness, demonstrating this technique again, sometimes deep-breathing with the child, may be necessary. Chest physiotherapy with percussion and vibration may be prescribed to keep lung secretions mobile. Be certain that parents understand that games such as blowing cotton balls or blowing up a balloon are not really games but important exercises to help achieve lung expansion. Otherwise, they may interpret these exercises as too tiring for the child and discourage them.

Most children have two thoracotomy chest tubes inserted following surgery. The upper tube drains air to aid lung re-expansion and the lower one drains fluid to encourage lung expansion and decrease the possibility of infection. These tubes are connected to a water-seal drainage apparatus (a Pleur-Evac; Fig. 41-7).

Pleur-Evacs consist of three chambers, one to collect drainage, one to furnish a water seal, and one that can be

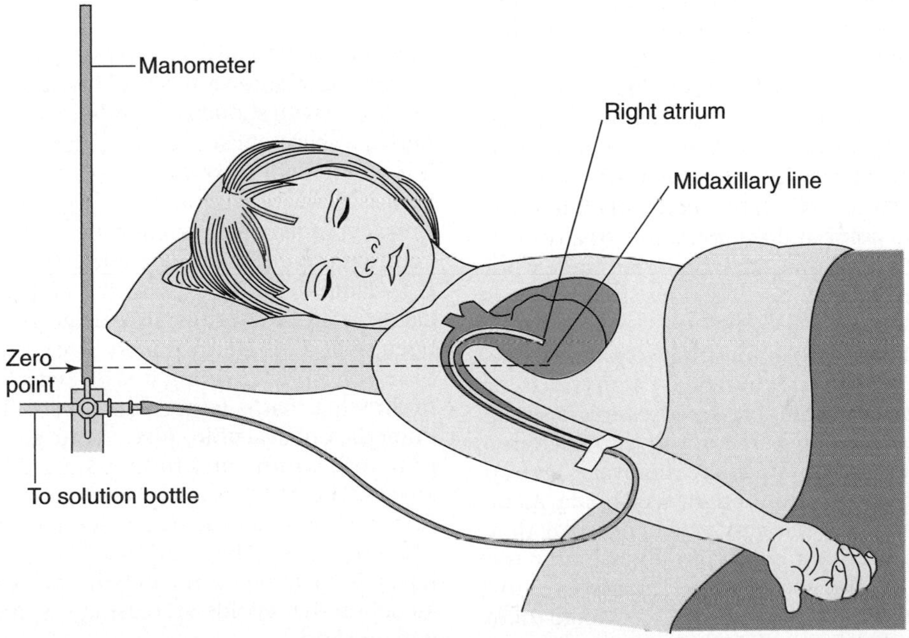

FIGURE 41.6 A CVP catheter may be inserted after cardiac surgery to monitor fluid volume. The zero point on the scale is at the level of the right atrium.

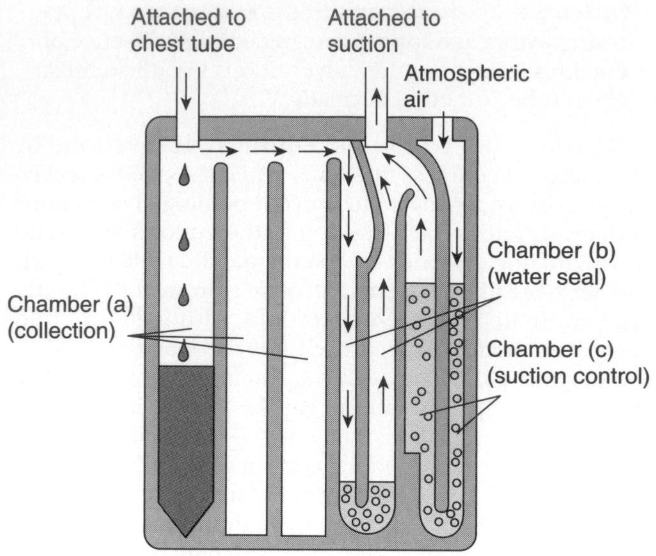

FIGURE 41.7 Pleur-Evac system for chest tube drainage.

attached to suction. A thoracotomy tube connects to the first drainage compartment. Because of the water seal, atmospheric air cannot enter the tube and flow back to the pleural space. Note how much drainage is occurring and if the level of fluid fluctuates (proof that the apparatus is airtight). On the third or fourth postoperative day, the fluctuation will cease, indicating that the lungs are fully expanded. Then it is time for the tubes to be removed.

Maintain the child in a semi-Fowler's position. Thoracotomy tubes drain best in this position and often there is less dyspnea as well because the chest is elevated and the abdominal contents do not press on the lungs. Keep thoracotomy chest tube drainage systems below the level of the child's chest so that fluid does not flow back into the pleural space. Check that tube connections are secure and that the Pleur-Evac is not cracked or broken. Otherwise, air can enter the chest cavity and collapse the lungs (pneumothorax; see Focus on Multidisciplinary Care).

Mark the fluid level in the collecting chamber immediately after surgery. Continue to mark the level of fluid in the drainage chamber every hour so the hourly amount of drainage can be determined (approximately 5 mL/kg/hour). Also note the color and the presence of any clots in the drainage. Drainage fluid may be blood-tinged but should not contain fresh blood. If it does, this suggests active bleeding.

A chest x-ray confirms that full lung expansion has returned. The tubes are then removed by a physician or nurse practitioner while an impervious dressing is simultaneously applied to the puncture wound. Provide emotional support during thoracotomy tube removal. Children know these tubes are important for their well-being. Aside from worrying about the momentary pain of removal, they may believe that something bad will happen after the tubes are removed. Do not change any dressings over former thoracotomy tube sites (lifting them to change them could allow air to enter).

Occasionally, despite being cautioned not to, children turn so suddenly after surgery that they pull a thoracotomy tube out accidentally. This creates an emergency situation because air rushing into the child's chest can cause a pneumothorax with sudden dyspnea, tachycardia, cyanosis, and perhaps sharp chest pain. If a tube is only loosened or air is leaking slowly through a connection, the symptoms may be less dramatic and include restlessness and apprehension accompanying gradually increasing dyspnea. If the air entering the chest is the result of air leaking into the tubing, clamp the tube close to the child's chest with a large clamp to prevent further air leakage. If the tube actually has been pulled out, immediately close the puncture wound to the chest by covering it with petrolatum gauze, a type of dressing that is impervious to air. If such gauze is not immediately available, place your gloved hand over the puncture wound and hold it snugly in place until help arrives. The child may need emergency oxygen administration to counteract the decreased amount of air exchange space he or she has left as a result of partial lung collapse. Remaining calm will help the child to remain calm, an action that avoids increasing respiratory rate and oxygen demand.

Nursing Diagnosis: Risk for infection related to surgical incision and tube sites

FOCUS ON MULTIDISCIPLINARY CARE

Many health care personnel are involved in caring for the child with cardiac disease. A physical or occupational therapist might plan an exercise program; a nutritionist might design a diet of small frequent feedings; radiologic and echocardiographic physicians and technicians will take and interpret many diagnostic studies; a cardiac catheterization or surgery team, including a surgeon, may design and perform surgery; intensive care nurses will design pre- and postoperative care plans; ambulatory, community health, and school nurses will plan care during the initial screening and postoperative periods. Be certain that all the disciplines that are providing care are aware that these children tire easily. Remind them that even simple activities, such as sucking on a bottle, can be tiring so they do not persist with an activity beyond the child's tolerance. Also remind them to check with you about what games seem too tiring for them to play. Open lines of communication among all team members are crucial.

If the child has thoracotomy chest tubes in place, instruct all personnel never to raise the drainage system above the level of the child's chest. Otherwise, drainage fluid will flow backward into the child's chest. Be sure to tell them to check the connections of the tubes, which should be sealed with extra adhesive tape, and to inform you if they seem loose or not airtight. Make sure the drainage system container is marked, "Do Not Empty." Emptying the container allows air to enter the system and can cause dangerous problems, such as a pneumothorax.

Outcome Identification: Child will remain free of signs and symptoms of postoperative infection.

Outcome Evaluation: Child's temperature remains at or below 100.4°F (38.0°C) axillary; incision site is clean, dry, and without evidence of erythema or foul drainage.

Some children begin a prophylactic course of a broad-spectrum antibiotic before surgery. If so, this will be continued for 24 to 48 hours postoperatively. Frequently monitor temperature postoperatively to assess for infection. Frequently assess the dressing of the surgical incision and the points of insertion of the thoracotomy tubes for drainage and erythema. Use strict aseptic technique when changing the incisional dressing to avoid introducing pathogens.

Nursing Diagnosis: Hypothermia related to cooling during surgery

Outcome Identification: Child's temperature will return to normal by 4 hours after surgery.

Outcome Evaluation: Child's temperature is above 96.8°F (36.0°C) axillary. Capillary refill is less than 5 seconds.

If hypothermia was induced for surgery, the child's temperature may be low postoperatively and a hyperthermia blanket, warm blankets, or radiant heat may be necessary to elevate the temperature to normal. Alternatively, the child's temperature may be above normal because of an inflammatory response to hypothermia. Unless infection is developing, these temperature readings will gradually return to normal in a few days.

Nursing Diagnosis: Risk for excess or deficient fluid volume related to fluid shifts accompanying cardiac surgery

Outcome Identification: Child will remain free of signs and symptoms of fluid volume excess or deficit during the recovery period.

Outcome Evaluation: Child maintains weight; skin turgor is good; central venous pressure or pulmonary artery pressure is within acceptable parameters.

Children tend to develop hypervolemia after cardiac surgery because of increased production of aldosterone by the adrenal glands and an increase in antidiuretic hormone secretion by the pituitary gland in response to stress. Also, if cardiopulmonary bypass was used, some fluid may have been shifted from the intravascular system to the interstitial spaces during surgery. After surgery, this fluid returns by osmosis to the vessels, increasing hypervolemia. On the other hand, the child may have experienced excessive bleeding because of the heparin used during surgery and may subsequently develop hypovolemia.

Monitor central venous or pulmonary artery pressure to evaluate the child's hemodynamic status. Monitor IV fluid administration carefully to prevent fluid overload. Typically, oral fluid intake is withheld for at least the first 24 hours after surgery. Once bowel sounds have returned, oral fluids can be introduced gradually.

Nursing Diagnosis: Parental anxiety related to lack of knowledge of postoperative routine and exercises

Outcome Identification: Family members demonstrate adaptive coping behaviors during the recovery period.

Outcome Evaluation: Family members accurately state plans for child's postoperative recovery; relate less anxiety after teaching and support.

Most children recover quickly from heart surgery. Passive range-of-motion exercises may be prescribed the day of surgery. By 24 hours, children are out of bed and ambulating. Encourage parents to do whatever they want to for their child's care during this period. It is difficult for them to accept the fact that the surgery is over and their child is now a well child (or will be at the end of the recovery period).

Offering the child sips of water or helping him or her take a bath (under supervision) helps parents see that the child is returning to usual activities and doing well. Be certain that in the midst of the postoperative excitement, the child receives adequate rest the first postoperative days. You may need to monitor and regulate visits by staff and outside visitors to make sure the child is undisturbed for sustained rest periods. Urge parents to read to children or play music for them as a way to provide quiet rest periods. Caution parents not to pick up an infant under the arms because this pulls on the chest incision. Show them how to lift an infant by placing their hands under the shoulders and buttocks instead.

Once the immediate postoperative period has passed, the child will be moved from the ICU to a routine patient unit. This may be a difficult move for both the child and the parents because they have developed confidence in the ICU staff and are reluctant to entrust themselves to new personnel (even if the patient unit is the one to which the child was initially admitted before surgery). It helps the transition if the regular nursing staff visits the child daily in the ICU. Generally, place children returning from the ICU in a room near the nursing station, and place the bed so it can be easily seen from the hallway. Although you are not providing the constant attendance that the child received in the ICU, you can show that you are very observant and aware of individual needs. Stopping to look in every time you pass the room reassures the family that you are always close by. Allow parents an opportunity to voice their concern over the change in personnel and surroundings. Accepting this change can help prepare them for the day of hospital discharge, when they will be observing and caring for their child on their own.

At hospital discharge, parents need clear explanations of the activities in which the child will and will not be able to participate. Be sure that they have an appointment for a checkup for the child and the telephone number they should call if they have any questions regarding the child's care. The protectiveness they felt for the child before surgery does not diminish instantly, even though surgery has been completed. They may find themselves saying, "Don't run" for months after the child has been allowed full activity. They may appreciate being referred to a community health nurse so they have a listening ear for their concerns, which may include feeling they are not as important to their child as they were when the child was ill. Reinforce the need for continued parental supervision and guidance (see Focus on Communication).

Complications

A number of complications can arise after cardiac surgery because of the use of cardiopulmonary bypass and the extent of the surgery. The first of these is hemorrhage, because heparin is used to prevent blood coagulation during the cardiopulmonary bypass. Although protamine sulfate (the antidote for heparin) is administered IV immediately after surgery, some heparin is still present in the child's system. Monitor the child's coagulation time and vital signs and observe thoracotomy tube drainage to identify early signs of bleeding.

Shock, another possible complication, is manifested by hypotension, oliguria, acidosis, and cyanosis. It may result from hypovolemia or cardiac tamponade (bleeding into the heart muscle or pericardium, interfering with the heart's ability to contract forcibly), or it may be a reaction to prolonged extracorporeal perfusion. It is treated according to individual needs, including plasma volume expanders, continued mechanical ventilation, and perhaps a return to surgery to stop the bleeding. Heart block or arrhythmias may occur as the result of edema or trauma compromising the effectiveness of the bundle of His. An artificial pacemaker may be inserted to correct these problems. If the child had congestive heart disease before surgery, this may persist for a week or more after surgery. If it occurs as a new entity, it suggests that the surgery has caused a stricture to circulation at some point, causing either the right or left side of the heart to become overwhelmed. Measures for treating postoperative congestive heart failure are the same as those in children who have this syndrome from any cause. Neurologic symptoms, also a possible complication, may occur if the child experienced hypoxia during surgery.

A **postcardiac surgery syndrome** may develop at the end of the first postoperative week. This is a febrile illness with pericarditis and pleurisy that appears to be a benign inflammatory response to the surgical procedure. Anti-inflammatory therapy and bedrest reduce the symptoms. The symptoms may recur months after surgery.

FOCUS ON COMMUNICATION

Jerry is an 8-year-old boy who is being discharged after cardiac surgery. You stop at his room to give discharge instructions to his mother.

Less Effective Communication

Nurse: Good morning, Mrs. Carver. Let me review a few instructions with you.

Mrs. Carver: The most important thing you can tell me is how to keep Jerry on bedrest.

Nurse: It will be important for him not to overdo it for about a week. Most children still have enough chest pain, however, that they automatically reduce their activity.

Mrs. Carver: He's always been active. Before surgery, he spent a long time playing Frisbee with his dog. It'll be hard to keep him from doing that.

Nurse: His appetite should be back to normal in a few days. Check back with the clinic if it doesn't improve.

Mrs. Carver: That could be a problem. He never eats well when he's in bed.

Nurse: Jerry will need to continue to take digoxin until he returns for his checkup in 1 week. Do you have any questions about his dose?

Mrs. Carver: No. It's hard to get him to cooperate, though, when he's unhappy about having to stay in bed all the time.

Nurse: You'll need to check the incision daily and report any redness or increasing pain.

Mrs. Carver: I can do that. The thing I'll have trouble with is keeping him on bedrest.

Nurse: Like I said, children generally limit their own activity. That shouldn't be a problem. Wait here, now, until I call transportation to take you downstairs.

More Effective Communication

Nurse: Good morning, Mrs. Carver. Let me review a few instructions with you.

Mrs. Carver: The most important thing you can tell me is how to keep Jerry on bedrest.

Nurse: It will be important for him not to overdo it for about a week, but he doesn't have to stay on bedrest.

Mrs. Carver: It's hard to get him to cooperate, though, especially when he's unhappy about staying in bed all the time.

Nurse: Mrs. Carver, let me review. Jerry doesn't have to stay in bed all the time.

Mrs. Carver: He's always been active. But staying in bed will be tough. Before, he spent a long time playing Frisbee with his dog. It'll be hard to keep him from doing that.

Nurse: You've mentioned bedrest several times. Jerry doesn't have to stay on bedrest. He just needs to avoid overdoing it for about the first week. Let's talk about what activities he can do.

Because cardiac surgery is such serious surgery, most parents assume that it will take their child a very long time to recover from it. In the above scenarios, the mother has overestimated the time it will take her child to return to normal activities. Only when really listening to what the mother is saying, rather than just continuing to review discharge instructions, does the nurse recognize that the mother has not heard the first instruction—let the child return to activities at as near normal a level as possible.

Postperfusion syndrome may occur 3 to 12 weeks after surgery. The child develops a fever, splenomegaly, general malaise, and a maculopapular rash. Hepatomegaly also may be present. The white blood count reveals a leukocytosis, with lymphocytes as the predominant cell type. Such a reaction is usually caused by a cytomegalovirus infection contracted from the donor blood used in the cardiopulmonary bypass machine. The illness runs a short course, with no permanent effect.

✔ **CHECKPOINT QUESTIONS**

9. Should children cough and deep-breathe after cardiac surgery? Why or why not?
10. Why might a child develop hypervolemia after cardiac surgery?
11. When is postperfusion syndrome most apt to occur?

The Child With an Artificial Valve Replacement

A number of congenital heart anomalies, such as aortic stenosis, and diseases such as rheumatic fever or Kawasaki syndrome can require artificial heart valve replacement. Valve replacement is technically more complicated in children than adults because children's hearts are smaller. Because children have a longer life expectancy than adults, valve durability also is a prime consideration. In addition, the advantage of the long-term anticoagulation therapy necessary to prevent clots from forming at the valve site must be weighed against the problem of extensive bleeding from normal childhood accidents.

Formerly, artificial valves were obtained from pig (porcine) or cow (bovine), synthetic material (prosthetic), or human donors (homografts). Today, most valves implanted are made of synthetic materials because these provide the best long-term replacement (Smolens & Bolling, 2001). After surgery to place an artificial valve, the child is given either anticoagulation or antiplatelet therapy to prevent thrombosis formation at the valve implantation site. The drugs prescribed most commonly for anticoagulation therapy are heparin or warfarin sodium (Coumadin). Antiplatelet therapy also may be used, most often acetylsalicylic acid (aspirin) and dipyridamole (Persantine). Aspirin decreases platelet aggregation; dipyridamole decreases platelet adhesiveness. The dosage for these drugs must be periodically monitored by blood analysis to ensure that they remain adequate as the child grows.

In addition, the child generally is prescribed prophylactic antibiotic therapy to guard against endocarditis. If the child should develop a bacterial infection, organisms tend to cluster and colonize at the valve site. Additional therapy is prescribed if the child is scheduled for dental work or any other invasive procedure.

Adolescent girls need counseling about avoiding pregnancy because the artificial valve may be unable to accommodate the increased blood volume associated with pregnancy and support the adolescent's growth as well. In addition, because warfarin is teratogenic, any girl contemplating pregnancy needs to be changed to a heparin regimen before conception. Girls with artificial valves in place should not use an estrogen-based birth control pill, because this can increase blood coagulation and possibly lead to thrombi. They also should not use an intrauterine device (IUD) because an IUD may cause an increased rate of pelvic inflammatory disease, which could spread to the valve site.

Hemolytic anemia may occur as a complication of artificial valve replacement. The extreme turbulence of blood through the prosthetic valve apparently results in breakage of red blood cells. Blood replacement may be necessary if the hemolytic process persists.

The Child Undergoing Cardiac Transplant

Children who have a hypoplastic left ventricle or extensive cardiomyopathy from any cause are candidates for heart transplantation. The procedure is highly successful. Over 2,000 transplants have been performed, and the average half-life of transplanted hearts is 15 years (Laks et al., 2001).

After removal from the donor, the transplant heart is perfused with a balanced electrolyte solution and chilled immediately. It can be maintained this way for 2 to 3 hours before being transplanted using cardiopulmonary bypass technique. For the procedure, the aorta of the child who will be receiving the heart is cross-clamped, and the original heart is removed except for the upper portion of the right atrium, which contains the SA node. Once the new heart is transplanted and the major cardiac vessels are reattached, intrathoracic hemodynamic monitoring lines and ventricle pacing wires are implanted. Transplanted hearts can beat normally except for autonomic nervous system control. This means the transplanted heart varies its rate in response to the amount of blood arriving at it rather than by nervous system control. An ECG will show two P waves (one from the residual original heart and one from the donor heart) because both SA nodes are intact.

Postoperative care is similar to that for any child undergoing cardiac surgery. The child has the same potential problems: decreased cardiac output, impaired gas exchange, risk for infection, imbalanced nutrition, and ineffective family coping. Children are prone to arrhythmias because of possible injury to the SA node during transport or transplant.

Although a long-term consequence of cardiac transplantation is severe atherosclerosis, apparently as a result of inflammation, rejection of the transplant is the number-one cause of death in cardiac transplant patients. An antithymocyte antibody preparation and drugs such as cyclosporine A, prednisone, and azathioprine are commonly used for immunosuppression in an attempt to reduce the risk of rejection. However, rejection still can occur in hyperacute, acute, or chronic forms. Hyperacute rejection occurs immediately and is manifested by coronary thrombosis. Acute rejection occurs in about 7 days and is manifested by low-grade fever, tachycardia, and ECG changes. Cardiac catheterization is performed a week after transplant to obtain a biopsy sample from the heart muscle to evaluate for signs of acute rejection (tissue necrosis will have started to occur). Long-term or chronic rejection may begin at about a year. At any point that rejection is beginning, additional antithymocyte globulin (ATG) or monoclonal antibodies to CD3T-lymphocytes (OKT-3) may be infused to help stop the process.

Once past the rejection period, most children adjust well to cardiac transplant. They can participate in normal growth and development activities after the procedure. Depending on the specific protocol, they return to the transplant center about once yearly for a repeat cardiac catheterization and evaluation of progress.

The Child With a Pacemaker

A child whose heart has ineffective SA node function or has difficulty in transmitting impulses from the SA node to the ventricles may have an artificial pacemaker inserted to control the heartbeat by stimulating the ventricles electronically. The pacing system consists of two components: a pulse generator that contains the battery and programmed instructions, and wire leads that connect to the heart. Most leads placed in children are an epicardial type and are attached to the epicardium (the outside wall of the heart) by suture. The generator is placed under the skin in the subxiphoid or mid- or lower abdomen. Heart defects that will need pacing can be detected during intrauterine life by fetal monitoring. In these children, pacemakers can be implanted as soon as they are born.

Commonly, the type of pacemaker and its functions are denoted by either a three- or five-letter code. With the three-letter system, the first letter identifies the chamber paced, the second the chamber sensed, and the third the pacemaker's response to the intrinsic activity of the heart. If a fourth letter is used, it denotes whether rate modulation is possible; a fifth letter denotes whether anti-tachyarrhythmia function, such as the ability to produce a shock to defibrillate, is possible (Cohen et al., 2001). For example, a pacemaker that is set to pace the ventricle, sense the ventricle, and be inhibited (cannot modify the rate and does not respond as long as the heart initiates a normal beat) is a VVI pacemaker.

Teach the parents of the child with a pacemaker how to take the child's pulse accurately. They will need to do this daily at home and report any alterations in the pulse rate to their primary care provider until it is certain that the paced rate is appropriate. They also will need to telephone the health care center periodically and transmit a recording of the child's heart action to the center by means of a telephone attachment to ensure that the paced rate remains accurate.

Some parents stay awake at night worrying that the pacemaker batteries will suddenly stop operating and the child will die. Because of this, they may be afraid to take vacations or allow the child to go away to camp. How long a pacemaker battery lasts depends on the percentage of time pacing is needed (continuous or intermittent), the battery energy output in amplitude (the amount of battery voltage needed to create each pacing impulse), and the pulse width (the length of time the impulse is being delivered). With usual pacemaker parameters, such as an intermittent pattern, low amplitude, and narrow pulse width, a battery can last up to 15 years. In all instances, parents can be reassured that pacemaker batteries lose power slowly, not abruptly. They will have ample time to recognize weakening batteries through signs in their child such as dizziness, fatigue, fainting, or a slow pulse rate and arrange to have the pacemaker replaced before the child's heart would fail.

Occasionally, pacemaker leads in the right ventricle of infants lie in such close proximity to the diaphragm that they stimulate the diaphragm to contract with each ventricular contraction. This causes constant hiccupping. If this occurs, the leads may need a position adjustment. Another problem with infants is that there is not room to implant the generator deeply, so it can trigger airport security systems.

Help parents learn to evaluate whether toys are safe. As a rule, magnets should be avoided. Toys that emit an electrical current can interfere with a pacemaker's operation and thus are not recommended. Also question the use of MRI (which involves the use of magnets) or electrocautery (which involves the use of electricity) with these children.

✔ CHECKPOINT QUESTIONS

12. After an artificial valve replacement, what drugs are most commonly prescribed for anticoagulation?
13. When do signs and symptoms of acute rejection after cardiac transplantation most frequently occur?

CONGENITAL HEART DISEASE

About 8% of term newborns are born with a congenital cardiovascular abnormality (Sondheimer et al., 2001*a*). This rate is even higher in preterm infants. Overall, these defects affect equal numbers of male and female infants, but specific defects show a tendency toward sex differences. Patent ductus arteriosus and atrial septal defect, for example, are found more commonly in girls. Conditions such as valvular aortic stenosis, coarctation of the aorta, tetralogy of Fallot, and transposition of the great vessels occur more often in boys.

The usual cause of congenital heart disease is failure of a heart structure to progress beyond an early stage of embryonic development. Maternal rubella is known to lead to defects such as patent ductus arteriosus, pulmonary or aortic stenosis, atrial or ventricular septal defects, or pulmonary stenosis. Atrial and ventricular septal defects tend to be familial. If a parent has an aortic stenosis, atrial septal defect, ventricular septal defect, or pulmonic stenosis, the incidence of this occurring also in the child is 10% to 15% (Sondheimer et al., 2001a).

Classification

Formerly, congenital heart disease was classified based on the physical sign of cyanosis, classifying these disorders as either cyanotic or acyanotic defects.

Acyanotic heart disease involves heart or circulatory anomalies that involve either a stricture to the flow of blood or a shunt that moves blood from the arterial to the venous system (oxygenated to unoxygenated blood, or **left-to-right shunts**). These disorders cause the heart to function as an ineffective pump and make the child prone to heart failure. **Cyanotic heart disease** occurs when blood is shunted from the venous to the arterial system as a result of abnormal communication between the two (deoxygenated blood to oxygenated blood; **right-to-left shunt**). Although helpful, this classification system led to difficulties because children with acyanotic heart disease can develop cyanosis, and children with cyanotic disease may not exhibit cyanosis until they are seriously ill.

To solve this problem, another classification system has been established that addresses the hemodynamic and blood flow patterns of the defects, allowing a more uniform and predictable set of signs and symptoms. As identified by this system, the four classifications include disorders with:

- Increased pulmonary blood flow
- Obstruction to blood flow (out of the heart)
- Mixed blood flow (oxygenated and deoxygenated blood mixing in the heart or great vessels)
- Decreased pulmonary blood flow

Defects With Increased Pulmonary Blood Flow

Congenital heart disease associated with increased pulmonary blood flow involves blood flow from the left side of the heart, which is under greater pressure, to the right side of the heart, which is under less pressure, through some abnormal opening or connection between the two systems or the great arteries. Defects of this type include ventricular septal defect (VSD), atrial septal defect (ASD), atrioventricular canal (AVC) defect, and patent ductus arteriosus (PDA).

Ventricular Septal Defect

VSDs are the most common congenital cardiac defects. They account for about 30% of all cases of congenital heart disease, or about 3 in every 1,000 live births (Sondheimer et al., 2001a). With this defect, an opening is present in the septum between the two ventricles. Because pressure in the left ventricle is greater than that in the right ventricle, blood will shunt from left to right across the septum (an acyanotic defect). This impairs the effort of the heart because blood that should go into the aorta and out to the body is shunted back into the pulmonary circulation, resulting in right ventricular hypertrophy and increased pressure on the pulmonary artery (Fig. 41-8).

Assessment. A VSD may not be evident at birth. With incomplete opening of the alveoli, there is still high pulmonary artery resistance, causing little blood to be shunted through the defect. At about 4 to 8 weeks of age, the infant begins to demonstrate easy fatigue, and a loud, harsh pansystolic murmur becomes evident along the left sternal border at the third or fourth interspace. This typical murmur is generally widely transmitted. A thrill also may be palpable. The diagnosis of VSD is based on examination by echocardiography with color flow Doppler or MRI, which reveals right ventricular hypertrophy and possibly pulmonary artery dilatation from the increased blood flow. An ECG will reveal right ventricular and pulmonary artery hypertrophy.

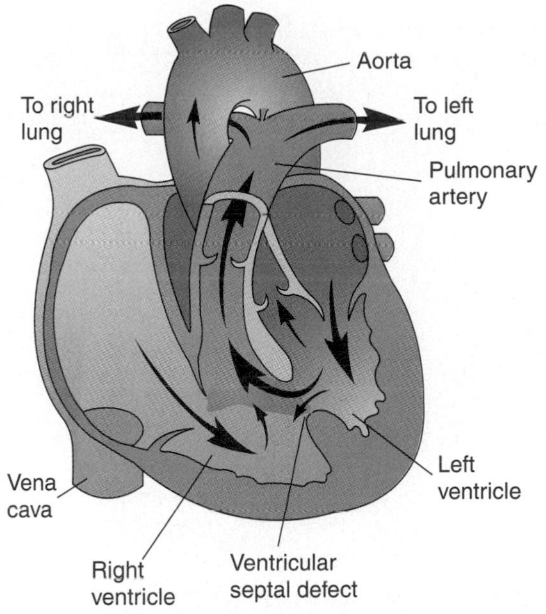

FIGURE 41.8 A ventricular septal defect.

Therapeutic Management. Up to 85% of VSDs are so small that they close spontaneously (Sondheimer et al., 2001a). Those that are moderate in size can be closed by interventional cardiac catheterization. Larger ones (over 3 mm) require open-heart surgery done before 2 years of age to prevent pulmonary artery hypertension. Closure is important because if the defect is left open, infectious endocarditis and cardiac failure can result. If surgery is performed, after cardiopulmonary bypass, the edges of the opening are approximated and sutured. If the defect is exceptionally large, a Silastic or Dacron patch is sutured into place to occlude the space. With time, septal tissue grows across the synthetic patch and knits it firmly into place.

Surgery requires the use of extracorporeal circulation and a quiet heart. Postoperatively, be alert for arrhythmia because edema in the septum may interfere with ventricular conduction. Children may receive prophylactic antibiotics to prevent bacterial endocarditis for 6 months afterward. If there are no complications, children can expect a normal quality of life.

Atrial Septal Defect

An ASD is an abnormal communication between the two atria, allowing blood to shift from the left to the right atrium (an acyanotic defect). It is twice as common in girls as boys (Sondheimer et al., 2001a). Blood flow is from left to right (oxygenated to deoxygenated) because of the stronger contraction of the left side of the heart. This causes an increase in the volume in the right side of the heart and generally results in ventricular hypertrophy and increased pulmonary artery blood flow (Fig. 41-9). There are two types of ASDs: ostium primum (ASD1), where the opening is at the lower end of the septum, and ostium secundum (ASD2), where the opening is near the center of the septum. ASD2 defects may be asymptomatic.

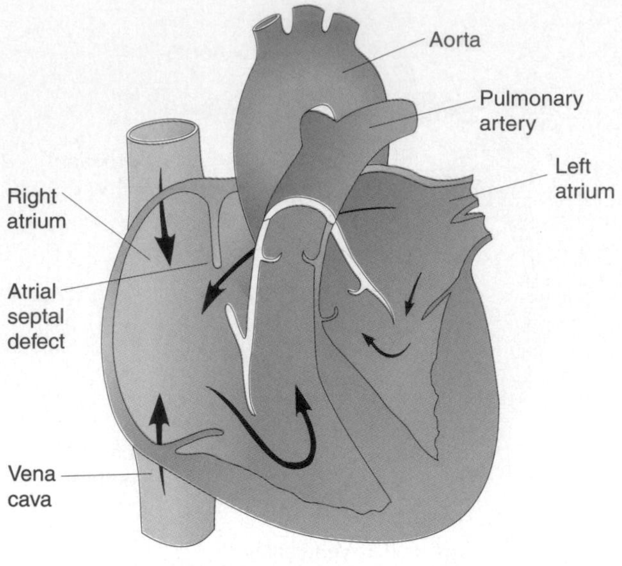

FIGURE 41.9 Atrial septal defect.

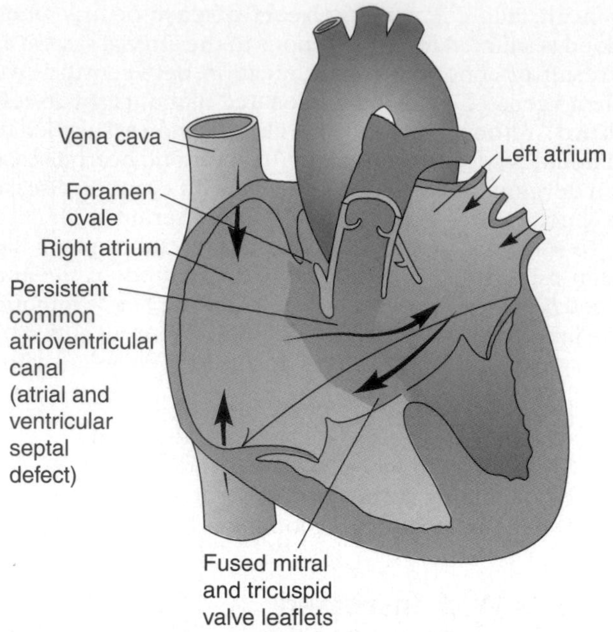

FIGURE 41.10 Atrioventricular canal defect.

Assessment. A harsh systolic murmur is heard over the second or third interspace (the pulmonic area) because of the extra amount of blood crossing the pulmonic valve. As the volume of blood causes the pulmonic valve to close consistently later than the aortic valve, the second heart sound will be split (fixed splitting). Such a sound is almost always diagnostic of ASD.

Echocardiography with color flow Doppler will generally reveal the enlarged right side of the heart and the increased pulmonary circulation. Cardiac catheterization, although rarely needed for diagnosis, would reveal the separation in the atrial septum and the increased oxygen saturation in the right atrium (Mosca et al., 2001).

Therapeutic Management. Surgery to close the defect is done electively between 1 and 3 years of age. Closure is important because without it, the child is at risk for infectious endocarditis and eventual heart failure. It is particularly important that ASDs be repaired in girls, because they can cause emboli during pregnancy. Management is by open-heart surgery or interventional cardiac catheterization. For surgery, after a cardiopulmonary bypass, the edges of the opening are approximated and sutured. As with VSDs, if the defect is large, a Silastic or Dacron patch may be sutured into place to occlude the space. Postoperatively, carefully observe the child for arrhythmias in case edema of the right atrium interferes with SA node function. With uncomplicated surgery, children can expect a normal quality of life (Sondheimer et al., 2001*a*).

Atrioventricular Canal Defect

AVC, also called an endocardial cushion defect, results from incomplete fusion of the endocardial cushion or in the septum of the heart at the junction of the atria and the ventricles (Fig. 41-10). Usually there is a low ASD continuous with a high VSD and distortion of the mitral and tricuspid valves. Although blood flow is generally left to right, blood may flow between all four heart chambers. Although rare in the general population, about one fourth of children with trisomy 21 (Down syndrome) who have heart disease have this type of congenital cardiac defect (Sondheimer et al., 2001*a*). It leads to the same symptoms as other atrial septal defects (i.e., right ventricular hypertrophy, increased pulmonary blood flow, and fixed S2 splitting). An ECG often will reveal first-degree heart block as impulse conduction is halted before the AV node. Echocardiography will confirm the diagnosis. Pulmonary artery banding may be done palliatively in selected infants. However, surgery is always necessary for a final repair because these defects are too large to close spontaneously. Because surgery may involve a valve repair as well as a septal repair, mitral and tricuspid insufficiency from poor valve function may occur at a later date. Postoperatively, closely observe children for jaundice resulting from red blood cell destruction from the newly constructed valves. Both prophylactic anticoagulation and antibiotic therapy may be necessary postoperatively, but with these drugs, the quality of life will be good.

Patent Ductus Arteriosus

The ductus arteriosus is an accessory fetal structure that connects the pulmonary artery to the aorta. If it fails to close at birth (closure should begin with the first breath, but complete closure may not occur until 3 months of age), blood will shunt from the aorta (oxygenated blood) to the pulmonary artery (deoxygenated blood) because of the increased pressure in the aorta. The shunted blood returns to the left atrium of the heart, passes to the left ventricle, out to the aorta, and again to the pulmonary artery (Fig. 41-11). This causes right ventricle hypertrophy and increased pressure in the pulmonary circulation from the extra shunted blood. The defect accounts

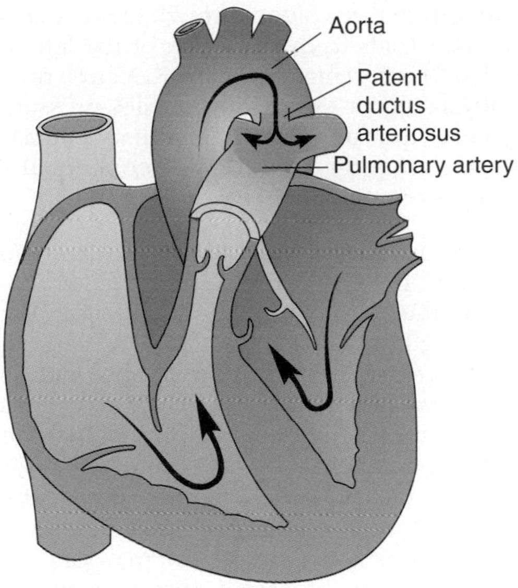

FIGURE 41.11 Patent ductus arteriosus.

for about 10% of all cases of congenital heart disease (Sondheimer et al., 2001*a*).

Assessment. PDAs are twice as common in girls as boys and occur at a higher incidence at higher altitudes. In preterm infants, the incidence may be as high as 20% to 60% (Sondheimer et al., 2001a). On physical examination, the child usually has a wide pulse pressure (the difference between systolic and diastolic blood pressures). The diastolic pressure, a measure of peripheral resistance, is low because of the shunt or runoff of blood, which reduces resistance. A typical continuous (systolic and diastolic) "machinery" murmur will be heard at the upper left sternal border or under the left clavicle in older children. In newborns, the murmur may not be quite so characteristic, perhaps a short grade II or III harsh systolic sound. An ECG is generally normal, although it may demonstrate ventricle enlargement if the shunt is large. Echocardiography provides good visualization of the open vessel. Cardiac catheterization is generally not necessary for diagnosis but may be performed to rule out associated defects.

Therapeutic Management. One reason that the ductus arteriosus remains open in fetal life is stimulation by prostaglandins, particularly PGE, from the placenta and the low oxygen level of fetal blood. After birth, when the PGE level falls and the oxygen level increases, the ductus arteriosus is stimulated to close. Medical management for the preterm infant may consist of the administration of oral or IV indomethacin, a prostaglandin inhibitor (Mosca et al., 2001). This lowers the PGE level and leads to ductus closure. The drug can be repeated as many as three times 12 to 24 hours apart. Assess for possible side effects of indomethacin therapy, including reduced glomerular filtration, impaired platelet aggregation, and diminished gastrointestinal and cerebral blood flow (see Focus on Pharmacology: Indomethacin).

If medical management fails to bring about closure of the ductus arteriosus, the defect can be closed by insertion of Dacron-coated stainless-steel coils by interventional cardiac catheterization when the child is age 6 months to 1 year. Exceptionally large defects can be closed surgically by ductal ligation. This involves major surgery because opening the chest (thoracotomy) and manipulating the great vessels is necessary. However, it is not open-heart surgery and so does not involve the use of extracorporeal circulation. Rather, it may be performed using only three small thoracotomy incisions on the chest. If surgery is not done by one of these techniques, the child is at risk for heart failure from the increased amount of blood pouring back into the pulmonary artery and infectious endocarditis developing from the recirculating blood and potential stasis in the pulmonary artery.

FOCUS ON PHARMACOLOGY

Indomethacin (Indocin)

Action: Indomethacin is a nonsteroidal anti-inflammatory agent that inhibits prostaglandin synthesis, although its exact mechanism of action is unknown.

Pregnancy risk category: B (D in third trimester)

Dosage: 0.2 mg/kg intravenously for the first dose, followed by 0.1 mg/kg (if child is less than 48 hours old), 0.2 mg/kg (if child is 2 to 7 days old), or 0.25 mg/kg (if child is over 7 days old) for second and third doses given at 12- to 24-hour intervals.

Possible adverse effects: Headache, dizziness, somnolence, nausea, gastrointestinal bleeding, constipation, rash, apnea, and increased bleeding problems

Nursing Implications

- Administer reconstituted solution intravenously over 5 to 10 seconds.
- Space doses at specified intervals.
- Educate the parents about the rationale for using the drug.
- Observe the child closely for possible adverse effects. Check the infusion site carefully for signs of oozing or bleeding indicative of impaired clotting. Also assess vomitus or urine for bleeding.

Defects with Obstruction to Blood Flow

A number of congenital anomalies cause the blood flow to be obstructed because of narrowing of a vessel or a valve. Pressure is increased before the narrowing and decreased after the narrowing. These are problematic defects in that they prohibit enough blood from reaching its intended site, the lungs or the rest of the body; they threaten to overwhelm the heart because of back-pressure. Obstructive defects include pulmonary stenosis, aortic stenosis, and coarctation of the aorta.

Pulmonary Stenosis

Pulmonary stenosis is a narrowing of the pulmonary valve or the pulmonary artery just distal to the valve (Fig. 41-12). It accounts for 10% of congenital heart anomalies

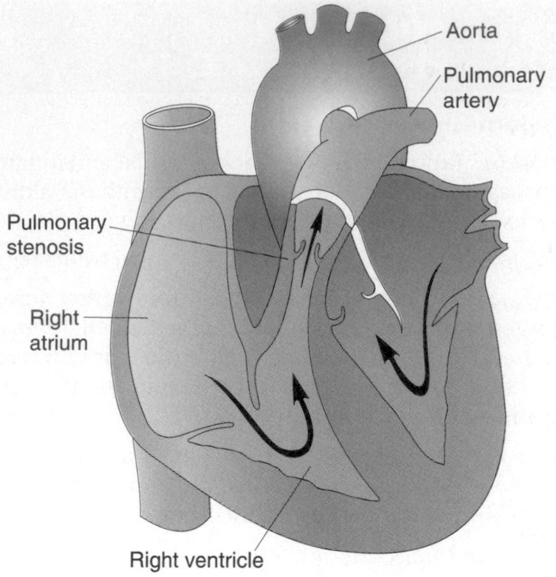

FIGURE 41.12 Pulmonary stenosis.

(Sondheimer et al., 2001*a*). Inability of the right ventricle to evacuate blood by way of the pulmonary artery because of the obstruction may lead to right ventricular hypertrophy.

Assessment. Infants with pulmonary stenosis may be asymptomatic or have signs of mild (right-sided) heart failure. If the narrowing is severe, cyanosis may be present from lack of blood flow to the lungs for oxygenation or right-to-left shunting across the foramen ovale. A typical systolic ejection murmur, grade IV or V crescendo-decrescendo in quality, will be heard, which is loudest at the upper left sternal border but may radiate to the suprasternal notch. A thrill may be present in the upper left sternal area or at the suprasternal notch. The second heart sound may be widely split because of late closure of the pulmonary valve. An ECG or echocardiography will reveal right ventricular hypertrophy. Cardiac catheterization is rarely necessary for diagnosis but is used for interventional enlargement of the stenosed valve.

Therapeutic Management. The management of the defect depends on the severity of the stenosis and the child's age. **Balloon angioplasty** by way of cardiac catheterization is the procedure of choice. With this procedure, a catheter with an uninflated balloon at its tip is inserted and passed through the heart into the stenosed valve. As the balloon is inflated, it breaks valve adhesions and relieves the stenosis. Following the procedure, although children may always have a residual heart murmur, they can expect a normal lifespan and quality of life.

Aortic Stenosis

Stenosis, or stricture, of the aortic valve prevents blood from passing freely from the left ventricle of the heart into the aorta. It causes increased pressure in the heart as the heart attempts to force blood through the strictured valve and therefore leads to hypertrophy of the left ventricle (Fig. 41-13). If left ventricular failure occurs, pressure in the left atrium increases, resulting in back-pressure in pulmonary veins and subsequent pulmonary edema. Aortic stenosis accounts for about 7% of congenital cardiac abnormalities (Sondheimer et al., 2001a).

Assessment. Most children with aortic stenosis are asymptomatic, but physical assessment generally reveals a typical murmur, a rough systolic sound heard loudest in the second right interspace (the aortic space). The murmur may be transmitted to the right shoulder, clavicle, and up the vessels of the neck; it may also be transmitted to the heart's apex. A thrill may be present, particularly at the suprasternal notch. If severe, decreased cardiac output evidenced by faint pulses, hypotension, tachycardia, and inability to suck for long periods may be present. When the child is active, he or she may develop chest pain similar to angina. Sudden death can occur when the amount of oxygen needed by the heart muscle on exertion far exceeds what is available because of the aortic stenosis.

ECG or echocardiography will reveal left ventricular hypertrophy. Cardiac catheterization is rarely necessary unless interventional therapy by this route is planned.

Therapeutic Management. Stabilization with a beta-blocker or calcium channel blocker may be necessary to reduce cardiac hypertrophy before the defect is corrected. Balloon valvuloplasty is the surgical treatment of choice. Surgery that involves dividing the stenotic valve or dilating an accompanying constrictive aortic ring can be used for severe defects. Such a repair may lead to aortic valve insufficiency in later life, at which time further surgery may be needed. Some children will need artificial valve replacement for correction. If a prosthetic

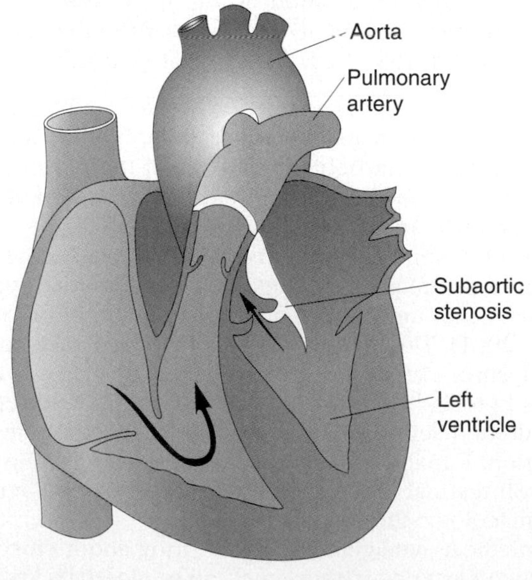

FIGURE 41.13 Aortic stenosis.

valve is used, children generally continue to receive anticoagulation or antiplatelet therapy and antibiotic prophylaxis against endocarditis. In addition, children need exercise testing before participating in competitive sports.

Coarctation of the Aorta

Coarctation of the aorta, a narrowing of the lumen of the aorta due to a constricting band (Fig. 41-14), accounts for about 6% of cases of congenital heart disease (Sondheimer et al., 2001a). It occurs more frequently in boys than in girls and is the leading cause of congestive heart failure in the first few months of life. There are two locations in which this commonly occurs. The first is termed preductal, or the constriction exists between the subclavian artery and the ductus arteriosus. The second is postductal, in which the constriction is distal to the ductus arteriosus.

Because it is difficult for blood to pass through the narrowed lumen of the aorta, pressure increases proximal to the coarctation and decreases distal to it. This results in increased blood pressure in the heart and upper portions of the body as pressure in the subclavian artery increases. Elevated upper body blood pressure produces headache and vertigo. Because a child under 3 years of age cannot describe these sensations, exceptional irritability may be the main clue that these symptoms are present. Epistaxis (nosebleed) and cerebrovascular accident, an event not generally associated with children, can occur from this dangerously elevated blood pressure.

Assessment. If the coarctation is slight, absence of palpable femoral pulses may be the only symptom. Children who have an obstruction proximal to the left subclavian artery may have absent brachial pulses as well. Therefore, include evaluation of femoral pulses in all initial newborn assessments and admission inspections to newborn nurseries. As children with coarctation of the aorta grow older, they may experience leg pain on exertion secondary to the diminished blood supply to the lower extremities. Because collateral circulation is necessary to allow blood to flow around the constriction, collateral arteries enlarge and may be seen on the ribs as obvious nodules as the child grows older.

The diagnosis of coarctation of the aorta may be made on the grounds of the history and physical assessment. On examination, the blood pressure in the arms will be at least 20 mm Hg higher than in the legs, a reversal of the normal pattern. Echocardiography, ECG, MRI, or radiographic examination of older children will reveal left-sided heart enlargement from back-pressure and also notching of the ribs from the enlarged collateral vessels. Occasionally, a murmur is present that is variable in position, intensity, and character. The most frequent type is a soft or moderately loud systolic murmur, especially prominent at the base of the heart and transmitted to the left interscapular area. The absence of a murmur, however, does not rule out coarctation of the aorta.

Therapeutic Management. Management of coarctation of the aorta is by interventional angiography (a balloon catheter) or surgery. With surgery, the narrowed portion of the aorta is removed, and the new ends of the aorta are anastomosed (Mosca et al., 2001). A graft of transplanted subclavian artery may be necessary if the narrowed section is so extensive that an anastomosis cannot be accomplished readily.

Many infants with coarctation of the aorta require therapy with digoxin and diuretics before surgery can be performed. This drug therapy aims to reduce the severity of the congestive heart failure.

Planning a time for correction of the condition is important. It would be ideal if children could achieve the greater part of their adult height before surgical correction to prevent a strain on the incision line as they grow. At the same time, in terms of self-image, correction is best done before children begin to think of themselves as chronically ill or before they develop a complication, such as chronic hypertension. Girls must have the defect repaired before child-bearing age, or the extra blood volume during pregnancy can cause heart failure. Therefore, surgical repair is usually scheduled by 2 years of age. If the surgery is successful, without complications, the child can expect to live a normal life. After surgery, abdominal vessels receive more blood than they did previously. This may result in abdominal pain or generalized abdominal discomfort, but this is a short-term problem. Some children continue to have elevated upper body hypertension after the repair. They need continued treatment with antihypertensive agents. Some children require repeat balloon angioplasty at adolescence to re-enlarge the aortic lumen.

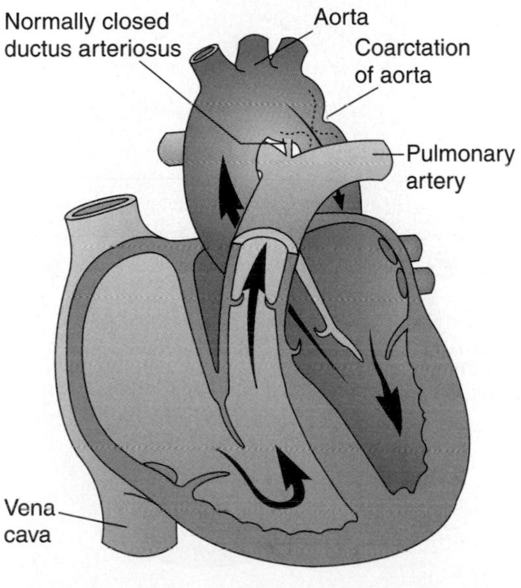

FIGURE 41.14 Coarctation of the aorta.

> ✔ **CHECKPOINT QUESTIONS**
>
> 14. In which direction does blood shunt in a child with an atrial septal defect?
> 15. What drug is used to treat patent ductus arteriosus?

Defects with Mixed Blood Flow

Mixed defects are cardiac anomalies that involve mixing of blood from the pulmonary and systemic circulation in the heart chambers. This mixing results in a relative deoxygenation of systemic blood flow, although cyanosis is not always visible. Mixed defects include transposition of the great arteries, total anomalous pulmonary venous return, truncus arteriosus, and hypoplastic left heart syndrome.

Transposition of the Great Arteries

In transposition of the great arteries, the aorta arises from the right ventricle instead of the left, and the pulmonary artery arises from the left ventricle instead of the right. Blood enters the heart from the vena cava to the right atrium, then flows to the right ventricle, and goes out into the aorta to the body completely deoxygenated. It reenters the heart from the pulmonary veins, goes to the left atrium, left ventricle, and out the pulmonary artery to the lungs to be oxygenated, and returns to the left atrium, a second closed circulatory system (Fig. 41-15). This severe a defect is incompatible with life. In most instances, atrial and ventricular septal defects occur in connection with this transposition, making the entire heart one mixed circulatory system. It tends to occur in large newborns (9 to 10 lb) and occurs more often in boys than in girls. This disorder accounts for about 5% of congenital heart anomalies (Sondheimer et al., 2001a).

Assessment. Infants with this defect are usually cyanotic from birth. There may be no murmur, or there may be various murmurs, depending on the shunting of blood through atrial or ventricular defects or through the ductus arteriosus, which usually remains open. Echocardiography generally reveals an enlarged heart. An ECG may or may not reveal heart changes. Cardiac catheterization will reveal the low oxygen saturation resulting from the mixing of blood in the heart chambers.

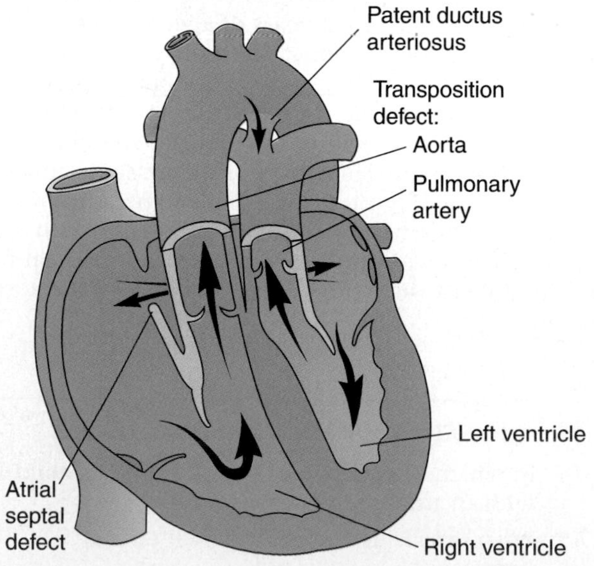

FIGURE 41.15 Transposition of the great vessels.

Therapeutic Management. If no septal defect exists or if the defect is too small to allow enough mixing of blood to sustain life, PGE will be administered to keep the ductus arteriosus patent. A balloon atrial septal pull-through operation will then be done in the infant's first few days. With this procedure, at cardiac catheterization, a deflated balloon catheter is passed from the right atrium through the foramen ovale into the left atrium. The balloon is then inflated, and the catheter is drawn back into the right atrium. This enlarges the opening of the foramen ovale and creates an artificial ASD.

Surgical correction of transposition of the great vessels, done at 1 week to 3 months of age, involves an arterial switch procedure in which the major vessels are actually switched in position. The child will be transported to a major center for the surgery and care as soon as the defect is diagnosed. Survival following surgery is as high as 95%.

Total Anomalous Pulmonary Venous Return

In this disorder, the pulmonary veins return to the right atrium or the superior vena cava instead of to the left atrium as they normally would. For blood to reach the systemic circulation, it must shunt across a patent foramen ovale or a PDA (Fig. 41-16). This defect accounts for only 2% of all congenital heart disorders (Sondheimer et al., 2001a). An absent spleen is often associated with this disorder. These infants are mildly cyanotic and tire easily. If the ductus closes or the septal defect is small, cyanosis increases in amount; right-sided heart failure ensues.

Surgery involves reimplanting the pulmonary veins into the left atrium. Until this can be carried out, a balloon atrial septal pull-through procedure may be necessary to enlarge a small foramen ovale. The child may be main-

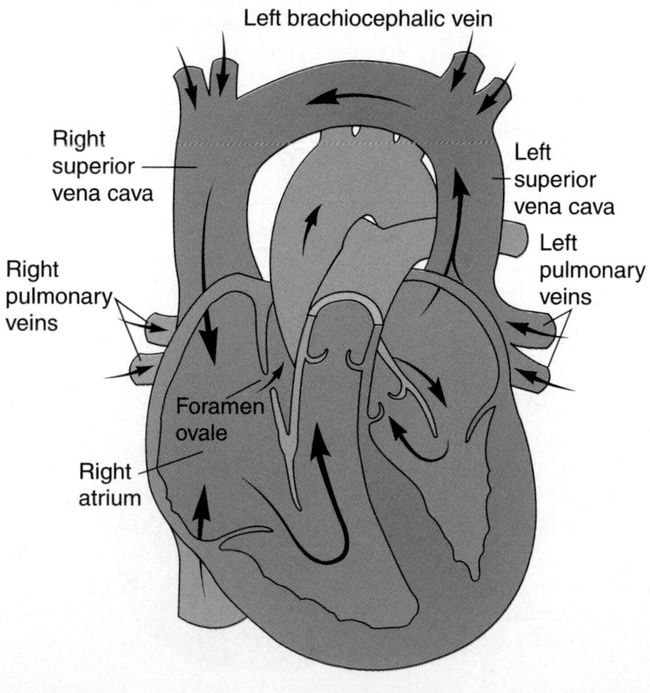

FIGURE 41.16 Total anomalous pulmonary venous return.

tained on a continuous IV infusion containing PGE to help keep the ductus arteriosus open (Thilo & Rosenberg, 2001).

Truncus Arteriosus

In truncus arteriosus, a rare defect (approximately 1% of initial cardiac lesions), one major artery or "trunk" arises from the left and right ventricles in place of a separate aorta and pulmonary artery (Fig. 41-17). There is usually an accompanying VSD. The child is cyanotic and may have a typical VSD murmur. Repair involves restructuring the common trunk to create separate vessels (Sondheimer et al., 2001a). Some children need a second procedure by school age as the graft inserted to separate the aorta and pulmonary artery is outgrown.

Hypoplastic Left Heart Syndrome

In hypoplastic left heart syndrome, a rare defect accounting for only 1% to 3% of cases of congenital heart disease, the left ventricle is nonfunctional. There may be accompanying mitral or aortic valve atresia. The nonfunctioning left ventricle lacks adequate strength to pump blood into the systemic circulation. This causes the right ventricle to hypertrophy as it tries to maintain the entire heart action (Sondheimer et al., 2001*a*). Mild to moderate cyanosis develops as deoxygenated blood is shunted across the foramen ovale because of the greater pressure on the right. Echocardiography effectively diagnoses this condition. Prostaglandin therapy to maintain a PDA will be started to increase blood to the aorta. Inhaled nitrogen may be prescribed to decrease Po_2, an action that increases pulmonary resistance and allows the right heart to shift more blood into the left heart and aorta. Attempts at surgery have limited success with this syndrome, although a great deal of research is being done in this area and a two- or three-stage procedure (restructuring of the heart) is possible. Heart transplant is the ultimate answer for prolonging the child's life, but the number of donor hearts available for newborns is limited (Mosca et al., 2001).

Defects With Decreased Pulmonary Blood Flow

Defects with decreased pulmonary blood flow involve some type of obstruction to pulmonary blood flow. Because of the obstruction, pressure increases in the right side of the heart. If an ASD or VSD also is present, deoxygenated blood shunts from the right to the left. This results in deoxygenated blood invading the systemic circulation. Common defects include tricuspid atresia and tetralogy of Fallot.

Tricuspid Atresia

Tricuspid atresia is an extremely serious disorder because, as the name implies, the tricuspid valve is completely closed, allowing no blood to flow from the right atrium to the right ventricle. Instead, blood crosses through the patent foramen ovale into the left atrium, bypassing the lungs and the step of oxygenation. It reaches the lungs for oxygenation by being shunted back through a PDA (Fig. 41-18). As long as the foramen ovale and ductus arteriosus remain open, the child can obtain adequate oxygenation. At the point they close, however, the infant will develop extreme cyanosis, tachycardia, and dyspnea. An IV infusion of PGE is started to ensure that the ductus remains open. Surgery consists of the construction of a vena cava-to-pulmonary artery shunt, which deflects more blood to the lungs, or a Fontan procedure (sometimes termed a Glenn Shunt baffle), which restructures the right side of the heart.

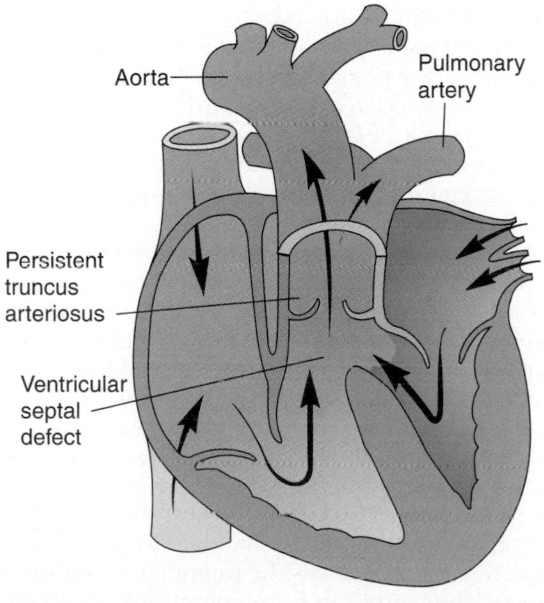

FIGURE 41.17 Truncus arteriosus.

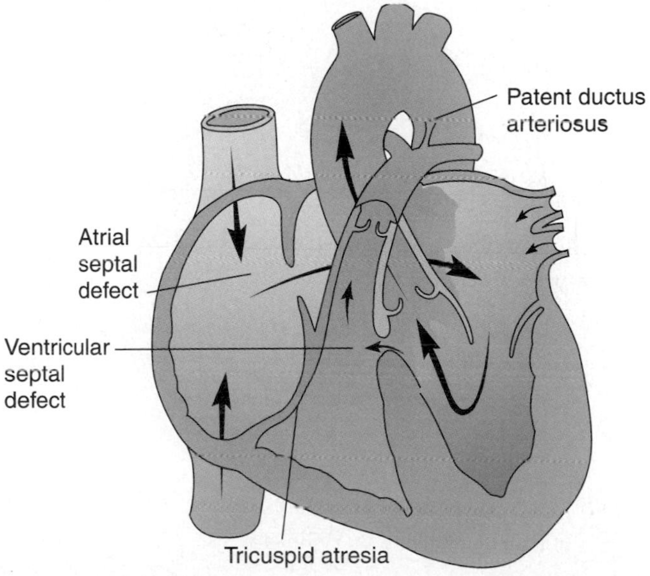

FIGURE 41.18 Tricuspid atresia.

Tetralogy of Fallot

Tetralogy of Fallot, one of the first types of congenital heart disease described, occurs in about 10% of children with congenital cardiac disease (Sondheimer et al., 2001a). It is called a tetralogy because four anomalies are present: pulmonary stenosis, VSD (usually large), dextroposition (overriding) of the aorta, and hypertrophy of the right ventricle. Because of the pulmonary stenosis, pressure builds up in the right side of the heart. Blood then shunts from this area of increased pressure into the left ventricle and the overriding aorta. The extra effort involved to force blood through the stenosed pulmonary artery causes the fourth deformity, hypertrophy of the right ventricle (Fig. 41-19). As many as 15% of children with this disorder show a deletion abnormality of chromosome 22 (22q11) or the disorder results from a documented chromosome disorder (Sondheimer et al., 2001a).

Assessment. Although this is an extremely serious form of heart disease, newborns may not exhibit a high degree of cyanosis immediately after birth. As they become more active, however, their skin acquires a bluish tint as cyanosis begins. Polycythemia (increase in the number of red blood cells) occurs as the body attempts to provide enough red blood cells to supply oxygen to all body parts. This is a potential danger because the increased concentration of red blood cells causes the blood to become too thick (increased viscosity), and clots in blood vessels may occur, with complications of thrombophlebitis, embolism, or cerebrovascular accident.

If the condition is not corrected, the child generally develops severe dyspnea, growth restriction, and clubbing of the fingers. He or she tends to assume a squatting or a knee-chest position when resting, a position that other children rarely assume. Squatting gives physiologic relief to an overstressed heart by trapping blood in the lower extremities. Unfortunately, this position can leave an insufficient amount of total circulating blood for the body to oxygenate and deliver to major body organs.

Children may develop syncope (fainting) and hypoxic episodes (sometimes called tet spells) caused by decreased blood and oxygen supply to the brain. These usually follow prolonged crying or exertion. A cognitive challenge may develop for the same reason.

Tetralogy of Fallot is diagnosed based on the history and physical symptoms, laboratory results, echocardiography, ECG, and cardiac catheterization. A loud, harsh, widely transmitted murmur or a soft, scratchy, localized systolic murmur in the left second, third, or fourth parasternal interspace may be present. It is so widely transmitted that it is often heard as well in the left clavicular area or posteriorly, in the interscapular space. Splitting of the second heart sound rarely occurs with tetralogy of Fallot because blood is forced through the shunt; the pulmonic valve does not, therefore, close later than the aortic valve.

Echocardiography and ECG both show the enlarged chamber of the right side of the heart. Echocardiography also shows the decrease in the size of the pulmonary artery and the reduced blood flow through the lungs. Cardiac catheterization and angiography will permit a definitive evaluation of the extent of the defect, particularly the pulmonary stenosis and the VSD. Laboratory findings reveal polycythemia, increased hemoglobin, hematocrit, and total red blood cell count and reduced oxygen saturation.

> **WHAT IF?** What if you noticed that a school-age child always sits with his knees drawn up tightly against his chest? Would this be a concern for you? Why or why not?

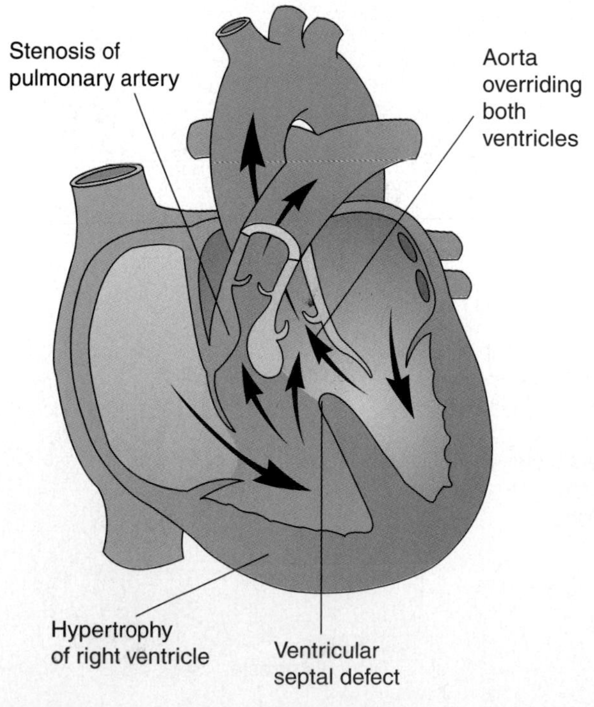

FIGURE 41.19 Tetralogy of Fallot.

Therapeutic Management. Final management of tetralogy of Fallot is surgical to correct the heart defects, done at 1 to 2 years of age. If infants overexert themselves during the waiting period, this leaves them without enough oxygen for body cells (hypoxic episodes). If a baby begins to have a hypoxic episode, administering oxygen, placing him or her in a knee-chest position (to trap blood in the lower extremities), and administering morphine sulfate generally reduces symptoms. If not, propranolol (Inderal, a beta-blocker) may be prescribed orally to aid vessel dilation. A temporary or palliative surgical repair, called the Blalock-Taussig procedure, can create a shunt between the aorta and the pulmonary artery (thereby creating a ductus arteriosus). This will allow blood to leave the aorta and enter the pulmonary artery, oxygenate in the lungs, and return to the left side of the heart, the aorta, and the body. Because the subclavian artery is used in a Blalock-Taussig procedure, the child will not have a palpable pulse in the right arm afterward. For this reason, blood pressure and venipunctures should be avoided in the affected arm.

A full repair that relieves the pulmonary stenosis, VSD, and overriding aorta can be accomplished (a Brock procedure). Postoperatively, observe for arrhythmias, which may result from ventricular septal repair, edema, and conduction interference.

✔ CHECKPOINT QUESTIONS

16. With total anomalous pulmonary venous connection, how does blood reach the left side of the heart?
17. What four defects are present with tetralogy of Fallot?

ACQUIRED HEART DISEASE

The most commonly acquired heart disease in children is **congestive heart failure** (CHF), which usually occurs as a result of a congenital heart disorder or a disease such as rheumatic fever, Kawasaki disease, or infectious endocarditis.

Congestive Heart Failure

CHF results when the myocardium of the heart cannot pump and circulate enough blood to supply oxygen and nutrients to body cells. Blood pools in the heart (excessive preload) or in the pulmonary or venous systems. This may result from a congenital defect that lessens the effectiveness of the heart's pumping action, or it may occur after cardiac surgery or rheumatic fever, when the myocardium is weakened. Severe anemia, hypocalcemia, and myocarditis may contribute to the heart's inability to function effectively. CHF is most apt to occur in children under 1 year of age (Sondheimer et al., 2001b).

The heart can compensate in several ways to move blood forward and attempt to increase cardiac output. The muscle fibers can lengthen, causing the ventricles to enlarge and handle more blood with each heart stroke (ventricular hypertrophy). The number of beats per minute can also increase. As long as these mechanisms allow for adequate cardiac output, the signs of heart failure are not apparent. However, the heart's capacity for compensation is limited, particularly in infants, an age group in which hypertrophy is restricted. Eventually, in children of all ages, the heart can no longer compensate and becomes overwhelmed by the amount of blood present, which cannot be pushed forward effectively.

As blood flow to the kidneys decreases, the glomerular filtration rate slows, resulting in stimulation of the renin-angiotensin system, which causes fluid and sodium retention. Aldosterone secretion by the adrenal glands further promotes sodium retention in an attempt to increase blood flow to the kidneys. Antidiuretic hormone secretion by the pituitary is also increased to help retain fluid. Sympathetic nervous system stimulation causes the frequently seen symptoms of excessive sweating and pallor.

Assessment

One of the first signs of CHF is tachycardia as the heart attempts to beat faster to move blood forward more effectively; this is quickly followed by tachypnea. When a child has primary right heart failure, increased venous pressure and hepatomegaly (enlarged liver) occur from back-pressure in the portal circulation. The child may feel irritable and restless from the abdominal pain caused by the liver distention. Lower extremity edema, usually a primary sign in adults, is often a late sign of heart failure in children (see Assessing the Child With Heart Failure).

With left-sided heart failure, blood accumulates in the pulmonary system. Dyspnea is usually the dominant symptom, especially when the child lies in a supine position (orthopnea; due to increased pulmonary congestion). The child may have crackles (rales) and may produce bloody sputum on coughing (from lung capillaries broken under increased pulmonary blood pressure). The child may appear cyanotic from interference with gas exchange in the alveoli, which begin to fill with fluid (pulmonary edema). Left-sided heart failure can ultimately lead to right-sided heart failure as extensive pressure in the pulmonary system prevents blood from leaving the right ventricle (Balaguru et al., 2000).

ASSESSING the Child With Heart Failure

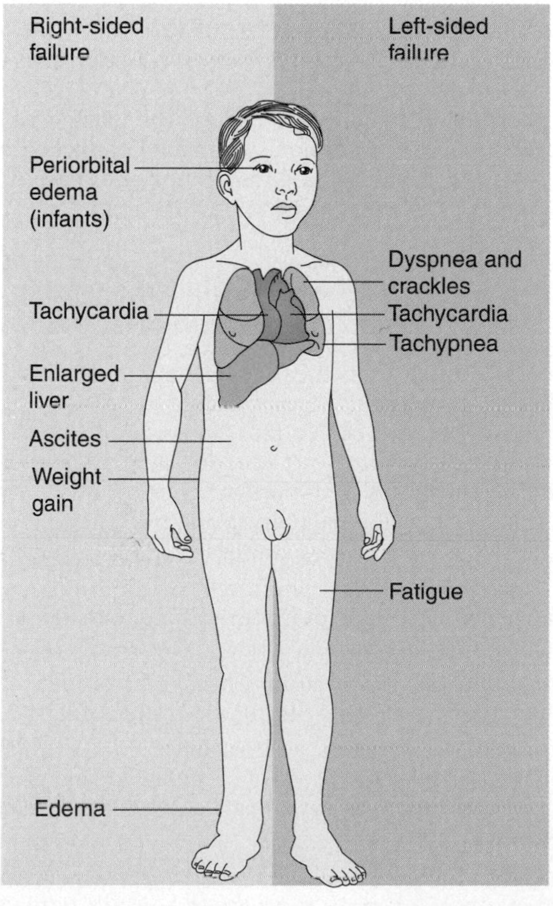

In an infant, heart failure is often difficult to detect because it presents with very subtle signs. The infant becomes breathless from rapid respirations, tires easily, and has difficulty feeding because of the exhaustion and dyspnea present. Often the infant becomes diaphoretic from the effort of feeding. If edema is present, it is generalized rather than dependent and often is first noticed as periorbital edema. An abrupt gain in weight may be the most obvious indication. On physical examination, the infant will have an enlarged liver (a liver palpable more than 2 cm below the right costal margin) and may have ascites.

The apical heartbeat is displaced laterally and downward. As a rule of thumb, if the width of the heart is more than half the width of the chest (in a child over 1 year of age), the heart is enlarged. In addition, a galloping heart rhythm or an accentuated third heart sound may be heard because of the sudden distention of the ventricle during the rapid filling phase. Tachycardia and tachypnea are present. Heart failure may be confirmed by echocardiography, which reveals the enlarged heart. Ventricular hypertrophy can be confirmed by ECG.

Therapeutic Management

The therapeutic management of heart failure consists of reducing the workload of the heart by measures such as evacuating the accumulated fluid (reduces preload) with diuretics, slowing the heart rate and strengthening cardiac function (increases contractility) by administering an inotropic (heart-strengthening) drug, and reducing afterload with vasodilators.

Commonly used diuretics include furosemide (Lasix) and spironolactone (Aldactone). The most common drug used to increase contractility and slow tachycardia is digoxin. Drugs that decrease afterload include hydralazine, an arteriolar vasodilator; nifedipine, a calcium channel blocker; nitroprusside, a direct-acting vasodilator; and captopril, an angiotensin-converting enzyme (ACE) inhibitor.

NURSING DIAGNOSES AND RELATED INTERVENTIONS

Be certain that outcomes established for care of the child with congestive heart disease are realistic and individualized for each child. Interventions focus on helping to support heart function and helping parents deal with this crisis until the child's body regains resources to again maintain strong heart action (see Focus on Nursing Care Planning).

Nursing Diagnosis: Ineffective cardiopulmonary and peripheral tissue perfusion related to inadequate heart function

Outcome Identification: Child will maintain adequate tissue perfusion during the course of illness.

Outcome Evaluation: Child's pulse, blood pressure, and respiratory rate are within acceptable parameters for age group; abnormal heart sounds, edema, and ascites are absent.

Provide for Rest Periods. Rest, a major aspect of care for the child with heart failure, reduces metabolic rate, decreasing myocardial and body oxygen demand. Most children with heart failure feel more comfortable in a semi-Fowler's position than in a supine position. This chest-elevated position lowers the abdominal contents, enlarging the thoracic cavity and allowing for easier, more comfortable lung expansion. Babies are most comfortable in an infant seat, which supports them in a semi-Fowler's position. Sedation, such as with morphine, may be necessary to encourage bedrest in some children. Most children with heart failure, however, automatically limit their activity, so the need for sedation must be considered on an individual basis.

Organize nursing care to allow periods of sustained rest. At the same time, do not attempt to perform too many procedures at once or you will exhaust the child. Be certain that both you and the child's parents understand how much rest the child is to have each day. The term "complete bedrest" is often loosely used and has different meanings to different people. Does it mean that the child may eat by herself or must be fed? Does it mean bathroom privileges or not? Playtime or not? Unless children are exceptionally exhausted, most children need to be entertained or played with to remain on bedrest. Activities such as watching television, being read to, or listening to music can quiet a child and promote better rest than if the child is expected to rest quietly without any diversion.

Provide Oxygen as Necessary. If the child has dyspnea, hypoxemia, or cyanosis, supplemental oxygen by way of hood, mask, or nasal prongs is usually necessary. Monitor oxygen saturation levels with pulse oximetry. Assess the nostrils of the child receiving oxygen with nasal prongs every 4 hours to prevent possible pressure and subsequent irritation and breakdown on the nostrils (this is a major problem in newborns). For a child with heart failure, it is a strain to be submitted to strange, frightening equipment. Orient the child to oxygen equipment before it is brought to the bedside. Children generally experience such relief from dyspnea when they are receiving oxygen that their apprehension over its use quickly disappears.

Administer Drugs as Ordered to Strengthen Heart Action. Digoxin is a cardiac glycoside made from digitalis, which acts directly on the heart to increase the contractility of the myocardium (and the force of contraction). It also slows the ventricular response in atrial arrhythmias. Digoxin is a potent drug, so doses must be prepared with extreme accuracy. For safest administration, digoxin should be prescribed with the dose designated in both milligrams and milliliters. When this is done, the milligram dose can be checked against the milliliter dose to be certain that the decimal point of the milligram dose has not been inadvertently misplaced (i.e., 0.03 mg, not 0.3 mg). Digoxin may also be ordered in micrograms (μg; e.g., 0.02 mg equals 20 μg). Digoxin preparations are administered intravenously first in a large dose (the digitalizing dose). Six to 8 hours later, one fourth of the initial dose is given; another one-fourth dose is given again in 6 to 8 hours. An ECG and serum digoxin level are generally obtained before the second or third dose of digoxin is administered to assess the adequacy of the dose. Following this, maintenance doses are given once daily. For children under 10 years of age, the dose could be divided into two and given at 12-hour intervals.

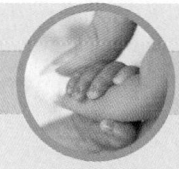

FOCUS ON *Nursing Care Planning*

A CHILD WITH HEART FAILURE

A 7-year-old girl is brought to the emergency department by her parents. Her mother says, "She's been so tired lately. She seems to get out of breath just walking around the house."

Assessment: A 7-year-old girl with a history of rheumatic fever approximately 6 weeks ago. Pale, tachycardic, and dyspneic. Afebrile; pulse 110 bpm; respirations 36. Oxygen saturation via pulse oximetry 80 mm Hg. Apical heart rate displaced down and laterally. S3 heart sound noted. Lungs with harsh rhonchi and rales (sound of crackles) on auscultation. Generalized edema with hepatomegaly. A diagnosis of heart failure is made.

Nursing Diagnosis: Ineffective cardiopulmonary tissue perfusion related to impaired cardiac function and increased cardiac workload

Outcome Identification: Child will exhibit signs and symptoms of adequate cardiopulmonary tissue perfusion.

Outcome Evaluation: Child's vital signs are within age-acceptable parameters; skin color pink and warm; verbalizes a decrease in dyspnea. Absence of S3 heart sound; oxygen saturation more than 95 mm Hg. Lungs clear to auscultation.

Interventions	Rationale
1. Administer supplemental oxygen as ordered.	1. Supplemental oxygen enhances tissue perfusion without increasing the child's metabolic oxygen demands.
2. Elevate the head of the bed 30° to 60° or have the child sit upright.	2. Elevating the head of the bed relieves pressure on the diaphragm, enhancing lung expansion. Upright position redistributes blood to dependent areas, decreasing venous return to the heart.
3. Assess vital signs including heart rate, pulse, and respirations. Auscultate heart and lung sounds.	3. Vital signs and heart and lung sounds are important indicators of overall heart function.
4. Monitor arterial blood gas values and oxygen saturation levels via pulse oximetry.	4. Arterial blood gases and pulse oximetry provide information about the status of tissue oxygenation.
5. Institute continuous cardiac monitoring as ordered.	5. Continuous cardiac monitoring provides objective evidence of cardiac function, including changes indicative of ischemia.
6. Remove any constricting clothing from the chest.	6. Constricting clothing interferes with chest expansion.
7. Limit procedures to those that are necessary and provide adequate rest periods.	7. Activity increases metabolic and myocardial oxygen demands, further impairing cardiopulmonary tissue perfusion.
8. Administer medications, such as digoxin and diuretics, as ordered. Assess apical pulse prior to digoxin administration. Obtain serum digoxin levels as ordered.	8. Digoxin improves myocardial contractility. Diuretics reduce fluid overload. Too rapid or too slow a heart rate may indicate digoxin toxicity. Measuring serum digoxin levels aids in evaluating the effectiveness of therapy and preventing digoxin toxicity.

Nursing Diagnosis: Excess fluid volume related to impaired cardiac contractility and venous congestion

Outcome Identification: Child will demonstrate signs and symptoms of adequate fluid balance.

Outcome Evaluation: Child states breathing is easier. Urine output, urine specific gravity, and weight are within age-acceptable parameters. Lungs clear to auscultation.

(continued)

Interventions	Rationale
1. Obtain baseline weight and monitor at least daily.	1. Weight is an accurate indicator of fluid balance.
2. Administer diuretics, such as furosemide, as ordered.	2. Diuretics reduce edema from the pulmonary vasculature, thus reducing afterload.
3. Obtain serum electrolyte levels and monitor results on an ongoing basis. Assess for signs and symptoms of hypokalemia.	3. Electrolytes such as potassium are lost as large amounts of fluid are lost. With furosemide, potassium is lost, placing the child at risk for hypokalemia.
4. Monitor intake and output and urine specific gravity. Administer intravenous fluid therapy if ordered, using an infusion pump or controller.	4. Intake and output and specific gravity are reliable indicators of fluid balance. Using an infusion pump or controller ensures an accurate flow rate, thus minimizing the risk of additional fluid overload.
5. Assess lung sounds every 4 hours. Monitor for reports of increasing dyspnea or difficulty breathing. Change the child's position every 2 hours.	5. Increasing respiratory distress and adventitious lung sounds are indicative of fluid overload. Position changes help mobilize pulmonary secretions.

Nursing Diagnosis: Activity intolerance related to effects of heart failure and dyspnea

Outcome Identification: Child will demonstrate a gradual increase in activity level.

Outcome Evaluation: Child's oxygen saturation level and vital signs are within age-acceptable parameters with activity. Child participates in self-care activities with minimal to no dyspnea.

Interventions	Rationale
1. Provide a balance of activity with rest periods. Cluster nursing care to prevent overexertion.	1. Activity increases myocardial oxygen demand, further compromising cardiac function.
2. Continue to administer supplemental oxygen and monitor vital signs, oxygen saturation levels, and dyspnea before and after any activity.	2. Oxygen is necessary for adequate tissue perfusion. A decrease in oxygen saturation levels or vital signs and increasing dyspnea in response to activity indicate an increase in myocardial oxygen demand that the child is not able to meet.
3. Provide small, frequent meals.	3. Eating requires energy expenditure. Small, frequent meals prevent overtiring, which could further compromise heart function and also interfere with nutrition.
4. As heart failure resolves, gradually allow an increase in activity, such as self-care activities, getting out of bed to the chair, and ambulation, using oxygen saturation levels as a guide.	4. Gradual increase in activity within acceptable oxygen saturation level minimizes the risk for further cardiac compromise.
5. Provide frequent support and contact with the child and family.	5. Frequent contact and support help to alleviate anxiety, which increases myocardial oxygen demands.

Before administering a dose of digoxin, obtain the child's apical pulse. As a rule, the pulse rate should be above 100 bpm in infants and above 70 bpm in older children. When effective, digoxin improves the strength of the heart's contraction, improving kidney perfusion. Diuresis begins and relieves any edema present. Changes in ECG (a lengthening of the PR interval or a depression of the ST segment) confirm that digitalization has taken place.

The "window" between effective digitalization and digoxin toxicity is very narrow. Monitor serum digoxin levels closely as ordered. Symptoms of toxicity include anorexia, nausea and vomiting, dizziness, diarrhea, headache, and arrhythmia.

Many children are discharged on long-term administration of digoxin (Lanoxin). If parents will be administering the digoxin after their child's discharge from the hospital, be certain they understand the drug's correct dosage and frequency of administration. Help them choose a specific time for administration to which they can adhere faithfully. Make out a reminder sheet to aid compliance. Instructions for home administration of digoxin are given in the Focus on Family Empowerment.

Diuretics such as furosemide (Lasix) may be administered to decrease pulmonary edema, thus reducing afterload. This choice appears to be more effective than restricting salt and fluid in young children. Daily weights are a good way to gauge the diuretic's effectiveness. Be certain that children are weighed at the same time, with the same scale, in the same clothing (or nude) every day so measurements are accurate and any weight loss can be noted easily. As large quantities of fluid can be lost through diuretics, so can potassium, which could lead to hypokalemia (low serum potassium levels). For these reasons, monitor urine output and serum electrolyte levels, including the potassium level. Normal urine output is 1 to 2 mL/kg/hour. If hypokalemia occurs, the risk for digoxin toxicity increases. Hydrochlorothiazide (HCTZ) is a typical diuretic used for long-term therapy. Because HCTZ, a thiazide diuretic, also promotes potassium excretion, a diet high in potassium and perhaps oral potassium supplementation may be prescribed to maintain potassium levels. Liquid potassium is irritating to the gastrointestinal tract and should be given mixed with fruit juice.

WHAT IF? What if a child you are caring for vomits a digoxin dose immediately after you give it to him? Would you repeat the dose?

Nursing Diagnosis: Risk for imbalanced nutrition, less than body requirements, related to fatigue

Outcome Identification: Child will ingest adequate nutritional intake during the course of illness.

Outcome Evaluation: Child maintains percentile curve on growth chart; skin turgor is good.

Maintaining proper nutrition may be a problem for children with heart failure because they tire easily. Eating six to eight small meals daily is often less tiring than eating three large meals. Smaller meals also prevent the child's stomach from pressing upward on the diaphragm and compromising an enlarged heart. Sucking is hard work, so infants may need to drink smaller amounts frequently to maintain an adequate fluid intake or receive a higher-calorie formula to allow for adequate calories without added fluid volume. Using soft "preemie" nipples may be helpful because they make sucking easier. If the infant is breast-fed, the mother may need to consult a lactation consultant to coordinate a program of frequent feedings or supplemental bottle feedings.

Nursing Diagnosis: Fear related to child's ill appearance and possible disease outcome

Outcome Identification: Parents and child will demonstrate improved psychological comfort.

Outcome Evaluation: Parents and child openly discuss fears and concerns, actively question, and express confidence in treatment plan and health care team.

Children with heart failure are usually aware of the seriousness of their condition. They learn this from the frequent procedures and visits by cardiologists and from the exhaustion they feel because their heart is not working well. They may lie stiffly in bed, afraid to move, afraid to burden their already overtaxed heart with even simple activities such as turning pages in a book. Offer reassurance that although their heart is a little behind in its action, the oxygen and medication they are receiving are helping. Reassure them that people are checking on them frequently, observing them closely in between as well as during procedures. Give them time to talk and use play to express their fears.

Parents of a child with heart failure need the same reassurance (provided, of course, the statements are true). They are as frightened by what the physician has told them as by their child's obviously ill appearance. It is often helpful to point out subtle signs of improvement in their child that they may not notice on their own, such as a slower heart rate or slower, less distressed respirations.

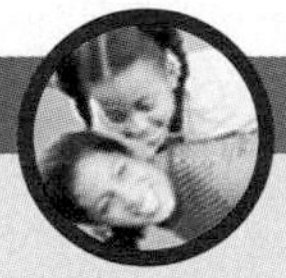

FOCUS ON FAMILY EMPOWERMENT

Giving Digoxin Safely at Home

Q. The doctor has prescribed our son digoxin to take at home. Are there special kinds of things we should do?

A. Use the guidelines below to ensure safe digoxin administration at home:

- Always assess an apical pulse before administration; do not administer the drug if your child's heart rate is below 100 bpm (or as specifically instructed as he grows older).
- Always use the same measuring device (spoon or dropper) each time so the dose given remains consistent.
- Do not change the amount or timing of the dose without specific instructions from your primary care provider.
- If you omit a single dose, give the next dose on time as prescribed.
- If you omit more than one dose, telephone your primary care provider for further instructions.
- Give digoxin 1 hour before or 2 hours after feeding to avoid a dose being lost with spitting up.
- If a dose is vomited, do not repeat the dose. Give the next dose at the scheduled time. If the child vomits the next dose, call your primary care provider.
- Notify your primary care provider if the child vomits more than once each day, because vomiting is a sign of digoxin overdose (toxicity).
- Notify your primary care provider if administration of the medicine or the timing of the dose is difficult for your lifestyle.

If the child will be cared for at home, review CPR techniques to be certain parents know what to do in an emergency. Be certain they have a follow-up appointment scheduled and a telephone number they can call if they have any concerns about their child's condition.

> ✔ **CHECKPOINT QUESTIONS**
>
> 18. What is the most common drug given to a child with heart failure to strengthen heart contractility?
> 19. A child with heart failure is receiving furosemide. For what should you be alert?

Persistent Pulmonary Hypertension

Persistent pulmonary hypertension (PPH) results when the pulmonary vascular resistance present at birth because of unopened alveoli fails to fall to normal after the birth and alveoli open. The disorder occurs most often in full-term infants who have experienced perinatal asphyxia from conditions such as meconium aspiration, respiratory distress syndrome, or intrauterine infection.

PPH occurs because hypoxia and acidosis from respiratory difficulty cause vasoconstriction of the pulmonary artery. The infant develops tachypnea. Pulse oximetry shows a low Po_2 from inability of blood to perfuse the lungs because of the pulmonary artery constriction. The resulting hypoxia and acidosis cause even greater vasoconstriction of the pulmonary artery. An echocardiogram slows right-to-left shunting across the patent ductus or foramen ovale.

Treatment consists of supportive therapy such as oxygen, high-frequency oscillatory ventilation, IV glucose to provide calories, antibiotics to combat infection, medications to reduce pulmonary resistance, and other drugs, such as low-dose dopamine, to elevate systemic blood pressure. Sodium bicarbonate may be necessary to relieve acidosis to help reverse pulmonary vasoconstriction. Inhaled nitric oxide may be administered to promote pulmonary vasodilatation. Infants who do not respond to these usual measures may require ECMO to allow the lungs to rest until adequate pulmonary vasodilatation and the return of alveoli perfusion can be achieved.

PPH is a serious threat to newborns, both because of the original insult from respiratory distress that produced the syndrome and the prolonged therapy course. Because of this, a newborn may be left with neurologic damage from severe hypoxia and inadequate brain cell oxygen perfusion (Thilo & Rosenberg, 2001).

Rheumatic Fever

Rheumatic fever is an autoimmune disease that occurs as a reaction to a group A beta-hemolytic streptococcal infection. Inflammation from the immune response leads to fibrin deposits on the endocardium and valves, in particular the mitral valve, and in the major body joints. The disease often follows an attack of pharyngitis, tonsillitis, scarlet fever, "strep throat," or impetigo, because the organism common to these infections is a group A beta-hemolytic streptococcus. In 95% of children with acute rheumatic fever, there is an elevation of one or more antistreptococcal antibodies, an indication of a recent streptococcal infection (Sondheimer et al., 2001b).

Although the incidence of rheumatic fever has declined greatly in recent years, the disease has not been eradicated, and in some areas the incidence is rising. It occurs most often in children 6 to 15 years of age, with a peak incidence at 8 years. It is seen most often in poor, crowded urban areas. Because children do not develop immunity to streptococcal infections, streptococcal infections recur; rheumatic fever also recurs (Carapetis & Currie, 2001).

The symptoms of the original infection subside in a few days with or without antimicrobial therapy. Children appear well again. After 1 to 3 weeks, however, if the child was not treated with an appropriate antibiotic for the original infection, the onset of rheumatic fever symptoms can begin. Because nurses are the primary people who advise parents when to seek health care and how to comply with medicine administration, nurses have contributed greatly to the decline of this disorder.

Assessment

The signs and symptoms of rheumatic fever are divided into major and minor symptoms according to the Jones criteria (see Assessing the Child With Rheumatic Fever). Of these, the heart involvement is the most serious. The child usually has a systolic murmur indicative of mitral insufficiency and prolonged PR and QT intervals on ECG due to inflammation and slowing of impulse conduction. Chorea (sudden involuntary movement of the limbs) is the most striking symptom. This loss of voluntary muscle control occurs most often in children between 7 and 14 years of age (very rarely after age 20). It occurs more frequently in girls than boys (Sondheimer et al., 2001b). Dysfunctional speech from chorea may be demonstrated by asking the child to count rapidly. Children with chorea begin with clear speech, but then suddenly the sounds become garbled or they are unable to speak for several seconds. If asked to protrude the tongue, children are unable to keep from making undulating, jerky movements. If asked to extend their arms in front of them, they soon hyperextend their wrists and fingers. Hand grasp may be weak or may consist of spasmodic contractions and relaxation. If asked to smile, the facial expression may change rapidly from a "Cheshire cat" grin to a flat, expressionless affect or grimace. Erythema marginatum, a macular rash found predominantly on the trunk, and subcutaneous nodules, painless lumps on tendon sheaths by the joints (a sign of polyarthritis), are additional manifestations. Large joints become swollen and tender. Important laboratory findings include the presence of an antibody antistreptococci titer (ASO) and an increased ESR and C-reactive protein levels (Fischbach, 2001).

Therapeutic Management

The course of rheumatic fever is 6 to 8 weeks. Children are maintained on bedrest only during the acute phase of illness or until CHF is not present and the ESR decreases, and the C-reactive protein level and pulse rate return to normal. Bedrest guidelines are based on the degree of carditis present, ranging from 1 week to 6 months. Because pulse rate

ASSESSING the Child With Rheumatic Fever

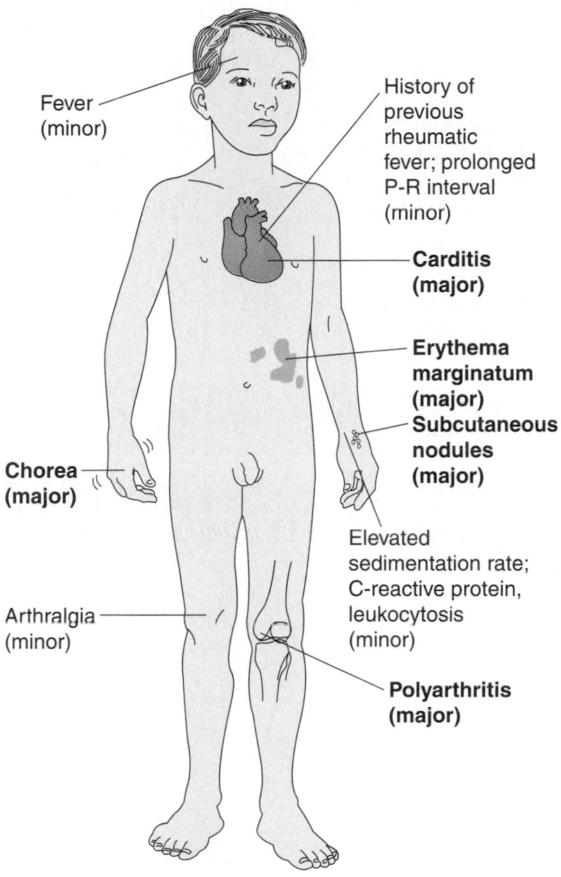

is a valuable sign of improvement, monitoring vital signs is essential during the acute phase. Obtaining an apical pulse for a full minute is preferred. It may be ordered when the child is asleep as well as when the child is awake to measure the effect of activity on the pulse rate.

A course of penicillin therapy or a single intramuscular injection of benzathine penicillin is used to eliminate group-A beta-hemolytic streptococci completely from the child's body. Erythromycin is used for children sensitive to penicillin. Oral acetylsalicylic acid (aspirin) or ibuprofen is prescribed to reduce inflammation and joint pain. Observe for symptoms of aspirin toxicity such as tinnitus, nausea, vomiting, headache, and blurred vision, which may result from the high dosage given. If the aspirin dosage interferes with prothrombin synthesis, purpura may result. Corticosteroids are prescribed to reduce inflammation for children who are not responding to salicylate therapy alone. Possible side effects of corticosteroid therapy include hirsutism, a round moon face (Cushing's syndrome), and an increased susceptibility to infection.

Phenobarbital is effective in reducing the purposeless movements of chorea. If heart failure is present, measures to reduce heart failure such as digoxin and diuretics will be prescribed.

The prognosis for the child with rheumatic fever depends on the extent of myocardial involvement. Valve destruction from formation of Aschoff's bodies (fibrin deposits) may result in permanent valve dysfunction, especially of the mitral valve. With severe myocarditis the heart dilates and, when it cannot maintain this compensation, eventually fails to contract effectively. Children may be left with mitral valve insufficiency, which is especially hazardous for girls, because this may lead to heart failure during pregnancy. Some children need mitral valve replacement to restore heart function. Usually, there are no residual effects from joint or chorea involvement.

NURSING DIAGNOSES AND RELATED INTERVENTIONS

Nursing Diagnosis: Risk for noncompliance with drug therapy related to knowledge deficit about importance of long-term therapy

Outcome Identification: Child will maintain prophylaxis against reinfection for prescribed interval.

Outcome Evaluation: Child takes oral penicillin daily; absence of symptoms of throat infection; vital signs within age-acceptable parameters.

Prevent Initial Attacks. The incidence of rheumatic fever can be greatly reduced by eliminating streptococci from entering the upper respiratory tract. After mild cases of streptococcal pharyngitis, rheumatic fever occurs in about 0.3% of children. After severe streptococcal infections, the attack rate may be as high as 1% to 3% (Sondheimer et al., 2001b). Amoxicillin or penicillin is used to eliminate streptococci from the upper respiratory tract. To be effective, a drug level must be maintained for 10 to 14 days. Erythromycin is used in children sensitive to penicillin; it, too, must be continued for at least 10 days. One intramuscular injection of a long-acting penicillin, such as benzathine penicillin (Bicillin), should be used with children when there is a question whether the parent will give, or the child will take, the full course of oral penicillin. Be sure to repeat prescription instructions for parents in ambulatory settings so they understand how often and how much of a drug is to be given and the need to give the drug for the full 10 to 14 days. Usually the child's symptoms will fade before then, and if the parents are not cautioned about the importance of this, they may give the drug only for 2 or 3 days and then discontinue it.

Prevent Recurrent Attacks. Children who have had rheumatic fever must be prevented from contracting the disease again to prevent valve damage occurring a second time. To do this, they must take prophylactic antibiotic therapy for at least 5 years after the initial attack, or until they are 18 years of age. If some valve involvement is present, many physicians advocate maintaining the child on penicillin indefinitely. Penicillin may be prescribed as monthly injections of benzathine penicillin G or daily oral doses of aqueous penicillin (penicillin V).

Additional prophylactic measures should be instituted when dental or tonsillar surgery is planned, because most children have streptococci in their throats. With an open incision in the mouth, the risk of streptococcal invasion of the bloodstream increases.

Nursing Diagnosis: Situational low self-esteem related to choreal movements secondary to rheumatic fever

Outcome Identification: Child will express confidence in self and transitory nature of the chorea; will continue with major part of self-care during the course of illness.

Outcome Evaluation: Child expresses frustration with inability to control movements; continues to feed and dress self with help as needed.

Children may have difficulty feeding themselves because of chorea. They may also be emotionally unstable and cry easily. Emphasize the transitory nature of the chorea; stress that it is frustrating to have to be fed and to be unable to use your hands meaningfully, but that this lack of coordination will pass without permanent effects. If chorea is present, provide toys and games for children that do not require fine coordination, because it may be frustrating to try to do something such as move checkers or chessmen on a board (a typical low-activity game). Children with chorea who are on bedrest may need to have the bedrails padded so they do not injure themselves from thrashing movements.

Kawasaki Disease

Kawasaki disease (mucocutaneous lymph node syndrome) is a febrile, multisystem disorder that occurs almost exclusively in children before the age of puberty. Peak incidence is in boys under 4 years of age. There is a higher incidence in late winter and spring. **Vasculitis** (inflammation of blood vessels) is the principal (and life-threatening) finding, leading to formation of aneurysm and myocardial infarction (Nasr et al., 2001).

The cause of Kawasaki disease is unknown, but it apparently develops in genetically predisposed individuals after exposure to an as-yet-unidentified infectious agent. After the infection (perhaps an upper respiratory infection), altered immune function occurs. An increase in antibody production creates circulating immune (antibody–antigen) complexes that bind to the vascular endothelium and cause inflammation. The inflammation of blood vessels leads to aneurysms, platelet accumulation and the formation of thrombi or obstruction in the heart and blood vessels.

Assessment

Kawasaki disease begins with an acute phase (stage I) of high fever (102° to 104°F [39.0° to 40.0°C]) that does not respond to antipyretics (see Assessing the Child With Kawasaki Disease). The child acts lethargic or irritable and may have reddened and swollen hands and feet. Soon the bulbar mucous membranes of the eyes become inflamed (conjunctivitis) and the child develops a "strawberry" tongue and red, cracked lips. A variety of rashes occur, often confined to the diaper area. Cervical lymph nodes become enlarged. As internal lymph nodes swell, children may develop abdominal pain, anorexia, and diarrhea. Joints may swell and redden, simulating an arthritic process. White blood cell count and ESR are both elevated.

At about 10 days after onset, a subacute phase begins. The skin desquamates, particularly on the palms and soles of the feet. The platelet count rises. This increases the possibility of clotting and perhaps necrosis of distant body cells that are not receiving adequate blood, particularly in the fingertips. Aneurysms may form in coronary arteries. Symptoms may lead to sudden death from accumulating thrombi or rupture of the aneurysm, making this the most dangerous phase for the child.

ASSESSING the Child With Kawasaki Disease

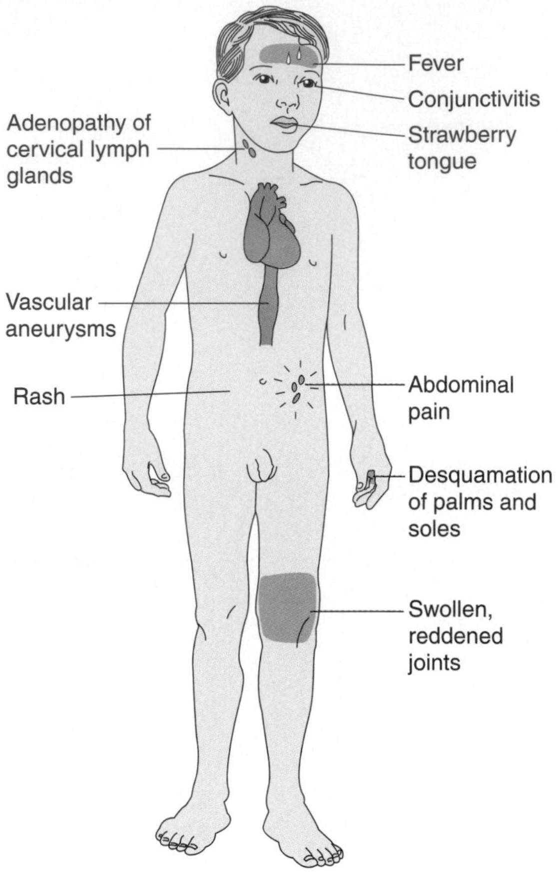

The convalescent phase (stage II) begins at about the 25th day and lasts until 40 days. Stage III lasts from 40 days until the ESR returns to normal. To be diagnosed with Kawasaki disease, a child must manifest fever and four of the typical symptoms shown in Box 41-1, plus echocardiographic confirmation of artery disease. Children are followed by sequential echocardiograms to monitor for possible development of aneurysms.

Therapeutic Management

The administration of acetylsalicylic acid (aspirin) or ibuprofen decreases inflammation and blocks platelet aggregation. Abciximab is a platelet receptor inhibitor specific for Kawasaki disease (Williams et al., 2002). IV immune globulin can also be administered to reduce the immune response. Steroids, which may increase aneurysm

BOX 41.1

CRITERIA FOR DIAGNOSIS OF KAWASAKI DISEASE

1. Fever of 5 or more days
2. Bilateral congestion of ocular conjunctivae
3. Changes of the mucous membrane of the upper respiratory tract, such as reddened pharynx; red, dry, fissured lips; or protuberance of tongue papillae ("strawberry" tongue)
4. Changes of the peripheral extremities, such as peripheral edema, peripheral erythema, desquamation of palms and soles
5. Rash, primarily truncal and polymorphous
6. Cervical lymph node swelling

formation, are contraindicated. If the child is left with coronary artery disease from stenosis of the coronary arteries, coronary artery bypass surgery may be necessary in the future.

WHAT IF? What if a child with Kawasaki disease has ibuprofen ordered every 4 hours but tells you she no longer has pain or fever? Should you continue to give it?

NURSING DIAGNOSES AND RELATED INTERVENTIONS

Nursing Diagnosis: Risk for ineffective peripheral tissue perfusion related to inflammation of blood vessels

Outcome Identification: Child will maintain adequate tissue perfusion during the course of illness.

Outcome Evaluation: Child's pulse, blood pressure, and respiratory rate are within age-acceptable parameters; capillary filling time is less than 5 seconds.

Observe the child for signs of heart failure such as tachycardia, dyspnea, crackles (rales), and edema. Inspect the extremities for color and palpate for warmth and capillary filling in toes and fingers to evaluate peripheral tissue perfusion. If the child is developing myocarditis, be alert for chest pain, arrhythmias, and ECG changes. All these are findings that need to be reported and documented.

Nursing Diagnosis: Pain related to swelling of lymph nodes and inflammation of joints

Outcome Identification: Child will experience a tolerable level of pain during the course of illness.

Outcome Evaluation: Child states that level of pain is tolerable.

A child with Kawasaki disease is uncomfortable from the joint involvement, edema, pruritic rash, abdominal discomfort, and the frequent blood sampling necessary to monitor the platelet count. The high fever can lead to dry, cracked lips. Ibuprofen, administered for its anti-inflammatory action, helps reduce both the pain and itchiness (which is a low level of pain). Provide additional comfort measures such as rocking and holding, and reassure the child that these measures are being done to relieve pain. Protect edematous areas from pressure; make certain clothing is not constricting and irritating areas of rash. Applying lip balm protects lips from drying and cracking.

Because the fever remains high, offer extra fluid to help maintain hydration and reduce mouth tenderness; keep the child free of heavy blankets or clothing and prevent overexertion. Monitor IV fluid to prevent fluid overload.

Children with Kawasaki disease lose their appetite and generally eat poorly because of the systemic illness and mouth soreness from cracks and fissures. Carefully monitor and record the child's intake and output. Encourage the child to continue brushing his or her teeth (use a soft toothbrush or a padded tongue blade), even though the oral mucous membrane is tender. Soft, nonirritating food such as gelatin (Jello) may be better tolerated than food that requires chewing and acidic fluids, such as orange juice, that might sting. Observe for possible signs of gastrointestinal obstruction, such as vomiting. Most children with Kawasaki disease can expect to recover fully. However, a few children may need cardiac bypass surgery to treat aneurysms that developed in the coronary arteries (Sondheimer et al., 2001b).

Endocarditis

Endocarditis is inflammation and infection of the endocardium or valves of the heart. It may occur in the child without heart disease but more commonly occurs as a complication of congenital heart disease such as tetralogy of Fallot, VSD, or coarctation of the aorta. The infection is generally caused by streptococci of the viridans type, although staphylococcal or fungal organisms may be at fault. The streptococcal infection tends to invade the body at a time of oral surgery, such as with dental extractions. It also can enter from a urinary infection or a skin infection, such as impetigo. As the disease progresses, vegetation composed of bacteria, fibrin, and blood appears on the endocardium of the valves and heart chambers. This tends to occur more commonly on the left side of the heart, although if a heart defect is present the erosion begins at the site of the defect. Over a period of time, the invading process destroys the endocardial lining of the heart. Underlying muscle and valves may also be affected (Sondheimer et al., 2001*b*).

Assessment

The onset of the illness is insidious. Children often look pale, with anorexia and weight loss. Arthralgia, malaise, chills, or periods of sweating, especially at night, may occur. As the vegetative process begins to erode the heart's valves, significant murmurs are audible. Signs of heart failure appear. Petechiae of the conjunctiva or oral mucosa or hemorrhages of the fingernails or toenails (that simulate a splinter inserted under the nail) may be present. The child may notice left upper quadrant pain from infarction of the spleen; on physical assessment, the spleen may be enlarged. Laboratory studies may reveal proteinuria or hematuria; a normochromic, normocytic anemia may be present. There may be leukocytosis and an increased ESR. An echocardiogram shows vegetative growths on the heart valves. The diagnosis may be confirmed by a blood culture that reveals the presence of the invading organism.

Therapeutic Management

All children with congenital heart disease and those who have had rheumatic fever should have prophylactic administration of an antibiotic before ear, nose, throat, tonsil, or mouth surgery (and before childbirth) to prevent infectious endocarditis. If it occurs, the prognosis in children treated with intensive antibiotics is good. Therapy is directed toward the underlying infection and also includes supportive measures to reduce heart failure. Because the invading organism is generally streptococcus, a penicillinase-resistant penicillin such as nafcillin (Unipen) is prescribed and given IV through a central venous access device. Giving the drug into a large vessel allows quick dilution and distribution. Children need long-term follow-up care to be certain that the invading organism is eliminated and the disease process has halted. Prognosis is good unless an embolus from the vegetations on the valves causes a complication such as renal occlusion or cerebrovascular accident.

✔ CHECKPOINT QUESTIONS

20. What organism is usually responsible for rheumatic fever?
21. During the first stage of Kawasaki disease, what is the primary manifestation?
22. What is an important preventive measure for endocarditis?

Arrhythmias

Children have fewer cardiac arrhythmias than adults do, but the number of these is increasing as more and more children survive cardiac surgery for congenital heart disease but are left with a cardiac arrhythmia. Better means of monitoring cardiac rhythm patterns through Holter monitors has also made detection of cardiac arrhythmia easier. Most children show normal sinus arrhythmia or a slowing of the heart rate during inspiration (increased lung size slows lung perfusion, putting enough back-pressure on the heart to slow the heartbeat), with resumption of the normal rate on expiration.

Ventricular tachycardia and atrial fibrillation are syndromes that occur because of multiple or abnormal initiation of the heartbeat and can occur following surgery for congenital heart disease. These can cause episodes of syncope, palpitations, and exercise intolerance. If bradycardia occurs, it can be treated with a drug such as atropine to counteract vagal stimulation; digoxin is commonly used for decreasing and strengthening the heart rate if needed. A few children may require pacemakers to maintain a steady heart rhythm.

Radiofrequency ablation is a nonsurgical transvenous catheter technique that can permanently disrupt an abnormal arrhythmia focus. A technique once reserved for adults, this can now be used even for infants (Sondheimer et al., 2001b).

Hypertension

Although primary hypertension may occur in children, it usually occurs as a secondary manifestation of another disease such as a kidney disorder. It has a higher incidence among black children than other ethnic groups and occurs in about 1% of schoolchildren and adolescents (Kay et al., 2001; see Focus on Cultural Competence).

It is difficult to define hypertension in children because normal blood pressure varies with the age of the child. A systolic pressure reading above the 95th percentile for a given age may be used as a practical criterion.

Assessment

Beginning at 3 years of age, blood pressure should be included as a part of routine assessment. Normal blood pressure and the technique of blood pressure recording in children are discussed in Chapter 33. To ensure accuracy, be sure the child is relaxed, after at least 1 or 2 minutes of rest, before taking a blood pressure. When children are discovered on routine physical assessments to have hypertension, the reading should be repeated at a successive visit to confirm that the abnormal reading was not a reaction to the stress of the examination or some other emotional event of that day. Only when the blood pressure is still elevated on a third occasion is hypertension diagnosed.

When a child has hypertension, a number of additional studies are performed to discover underlying disease conditions. The most common diseases associated with hypertension in children are renal and cardiac disease (coarctation of the aorta), Cushing's syndrome, primary hyperaldosteronism, adrenogenital syndrome, pheochromocytoma (a tumor of the adrenal gland), and brain tumor. If blood pressure is elevated, record blood pressure in lower extremities and upper extremities to rule out coarctation of the aorta (which results in low pressure in the lower extremities). Obtain a urine specimen for

FOCUS ON CULTURAL COMPETENCE

Hypertension, hypercholesterolemia, and congenital heart disorders occur at higher incidences in some adolescents than others because there is a tendency for these disorders to be familial. Hypertension, for example, occurs at a higher incidence in African Americans than in other groups. Nurses have a responsibility to educate adolescents about the importance of maintaining a sensible sodium intake and reducing saturated fat and cholesterol intake, in an attempt to minimize these familial disorders. Be knowledgeable about cultural preferences in foods when planning preventive health care.

analysis of microalbuminuria, a finding that accompanies hypertension. If red blood cells are present in urine, this suggests glomerulonephritis. White blood cells suggest pyelonephritis. Children should have a funduscopic examination to determine the presence of papilledema or spasm, or hemorrhage of the retinal arteries from the consistently elevated blood pressure. If papilledema is present, children need immediate care to prevent optic nerve damage. Further studies to rule out adrenal or renal disease may be ordered if these preliminary assessment procedures do not reveal a cause for the hypertension.

Therapeutic Management

Therapy for hypertension depends on the underlying primary disease. Although the underlying disease conditions that lead to hypertension are serious disorders, they are also ones that can respond to therapy. Thus hypertension must not be dismissed lightly.

If essential hypertension (elevated blood pressure for no identifiable reason) is present and a child is obese, he or she is placed on a reducing diet and urged to increase the level of exercise. Salt intake is rarely limited, but it may be if intake has been excessive; girls are advised not to use oral contraceptives, which elevate blood pressure. Unfortunately, because mild hypertension gives children few symptoms, often they do not adhere to nutritional suggestions or suggested exercise programs. For these children, a single medication such as an angiotensin-converting enzyme (ACE) inhibitor (e.g., captopril [Capoten]) may be prescribed.

A diuretic such as furosemide (Lasix) or vasodilators such as hydralazine (Apresoline) may also be added. Because few symptoms are present, many children do not adhere to their medication regimen and need continued counseling at health care visits (Kay et al., 2001).

Educate children with hypertension and their parents about its long-term effects (increased risk of heart and blood vessel disease). Only if they understand these long-term consequences of elevated blood pressure can they see the benefits of taking medication today.

Dyslipidemia

Dyslipidemia (increased lipids in blood serum) can involve cholesterol or triglycerides. Risk factors include familial hypercholesterolemia, a dominantly inherited disease occurring in 5% to 25% of children; obesity; a sedentary lifestyle; and a high-fat diet. For this reason, all children of parents with premature coronary artery disease (disease before the age of 55) or a family history of hypercholesterolemia (parents with blood cholesterol level higher than 200 mg/dL or low-density lipoprotein [LDL] above 130 mg/dL) should be screened for total serum cholesterol, because there is an association between total cholesterol and LDL and the incidence of coronary artery disease. This is particularly important if the child smokes, is obese, or has a sedentary lifestyle (Sondheimer et al., 2001b).

Acceptable levels of total cholesterol and LDL are less than 170 mg/dL and less than 110 mg/dL, respectively. Levels are borderline if they are 170 to 199 mg/dL and 110 to 129 mg/dL. They are high if over 200 mg/dL and 130 mg/dL.

If the total triglyceride, cholesterol, or LDL level is found to be elevated, the child's diet should be regulated in an attempt to lower these levels. Exercise also should be increased. Adolescents may be placed on the American Heart Association's step-one diets (total fat no more than 30% of calories; cholesterol less than 300 mg/day) to attempt to bring them into adulthood with sound nutritional habits. Children rarely are placed on low-fat diets because they need calories for growth. Use of low-fat diets in infants under 2 years of age is even less common because fat is needed for myelinization of nerves. When the child becomes an adolescent and the diet has not been effective, one of the many cholesterol-reducing agents such as cholestyramine (Questran) may be prescribed. These reduce the cholesterol level by binding bile acids and decreasing their reabsorption. Side effects of these drugs include large, bulky stools and possible gastrointestinal discomfort. If this therapy is ineffective, an HMG-CoA inhibitor such as lovastatin (Mevacor) may be prescribed.

Because hypercholesterolemia has no symptoms, it is difficult to motivate children to continue a special diet and take medication. They need continued counseling at health care visits or they will not be compliant (Sondheimer et al., 2001b).

Cardiomyopathy

The term "cardiomyopathy" refers to a structural or functional abnormality of the ventricular myocardium that occurs following an adenovirus, cytomegalovirus, or HIV/AIDS infection and results in severe dilation of the left or both ventricles. This impairs systolic function and leads to heart failure. Idiopathic dilated cardiomyopathy (IDC) is a rare form that presents before 2 years of age, usually after a viral respiratory or gastrointestinal illness.

In the older child, symptoms appear gradually. Physical examination reveals an ill-appearing child with severe respiratory distress. Peripheral pulses are weak and blood pressure is decreased. Pulsus alternans is a common finding. The liver is enlarged from backflow pressure. A chest x-ray, echocardiogram, and ECG all reveal the enlarged heart.

Therapy is directed at controlling the heart failure by bedrest, fluid restriction, and pharmacologic agents to decrease the cardiac load, improve myocardial contractility, and decrease afterload. Immune globulin may help reverse the process. If the child fails to respond to medical therapy, the prognosis is poor unless the child is eligible for cardiac transplantation.

✔ CHECKPOINT QUESTIONS

23. What criterion is used to determine hypertension in children of any age?
24. What levels of cholesterol and LDL are considered acceptable for children?
25. What is the most frequent effect of cardiomyopathy?

CARDIOPULMONARY ARREST

Children with heart disease are at high risk for cardiopulmonary arrest, although this may occur for other reasons such as airway obstruction, trauma, anaphylactic reactions, central nervous system depression, drowning, or electrocution. Management of cardiopulmonary arrest may vary according to the cause of the arrest and the age of the patient, but the basic considerations are the same.

Many health care facilities and public buildings provide automated external defibrillators (AEDs) for use in cardiac resuscitation. Nurses who respond to emergencies need to familiarize themselves with this equipment as well as CPR technique (Berg et al., 2001).

Assessment

Respiratory failure is the most frequent cause of cardiac arrest because anoxia in the heart muscle quickly leads to cardiac arrest. When this occurs, no audible heart sounds or pulses can be obtained. No blood pressure can be recorded (don't waste time trying to obtain one). If a cardiac monitor was attached before the arrest, it will show no ECG complex. This is a helpful assessment if available, but again do not waste time attaching monitor leads if they are not already in place. It is better to err on the side of unnecessary resuscitation. The outcome for the child will depend to a great extent on the speed with which resuscitation is begun. The steps for resuscitation can be remembered as "ABCs" (airway, breathing, and circulation).

Airway

The first step in resuscitation is to shake the child and call the child's name to verify that that child is not just sleeping soundly. If the child does not respond to this action, call for help. Turn the child onto his or her back and open the mouth. Tip the child's head backward slightly to a neutral position or place a rolled towel or other fairly firm object under the neck to hyperextend the head slightly (a "sniffing" position). Do not overextend the neck, however, or you will occlude, not clear, the airway (American Heart Association [AHA], 2001).

Breathing

Emergency equipment such as an Ambu bag should be readily available at all health care settings so that mouth-to-mouth resuscitation is not necessary. If no breathing bag is available, use a protective one-way valve mask for mouth-to-mouth resuscitation to protect yourself from body secretions.

For small infants, place the bag mask over the infant's mouth and nose, creating a seal. For large infants and children, make a bag-to-mouth seal, pinching the child's nose tightly with the thumb and forefingers. Provide two slow breaths (1 to 1.5 seconds per breath). It may be necessary to adjust the head-tilt chin position to obtain optimal airway patency (although this should not be done if neck or spine trauma is suspected; AHA, 2001).

If oxygen is available, attach it to the resuscitation bag, running at a rate of about 4 L/min. However, do not wait for oxygen if it is not available. Room air contains an oxygen content of about 21%, so additional oxygen is helpful but not necessary for resuscitation.

Observe the child's chest with each of the breaths you administer to see if it rises. If it does not, the airway is obstructed and air cannot reach the lungs. Perform back blows and chest thrusts for an infant or abdominal thrusts for a child to help relieve the obstruction. Continued breaths should be at the rate of normal respirations (20/min) in both infants and older children. When respiratory arrest has occurred and mechanical ventilation is anticipated, the child needs to be intubated to provide an open airway, as discussed in Chapter 40.

Circulation

After the two ventilations, feel for a carotid pulse (in an infant, the brachial pulse) or assess for other signs of circulation, such as adequate color (Fig. 41-20). People who are inexperienced in evaluating pulses should not take more than 10 seconds to attempt this (AHA, 2001). It is better to use the carotid than the peripheral pulse as an indicator of cardiac function in older children, because with shock, the peripheral pulses may be absent while the heart is still beating. The carotid pulse is also the easiest to assess from your position near the child's head. In an infant, however, the neck may be too chubby for you to easily palpate the carotid pulses.

If you feel no pulse, begin chest compression. In a newborn, enough pressure will be generated by two fingers pressed on the midsternum about a fingerbreadth below the nipple line to a depth of 0.5 to 1 inch (Fig. 41-21). Midsternal compression is used with newborns and infants to prevent excessive pressure on the ribs and the possibility of breaking either a rib or the xiphoid process (which then might puncture the heart or liver). In the older child, you need to apply the heel of your palm over the sternum (measure one or two fingerbreadths up from the sternal-costal notch and place the palm there and compress 1 to 1.5 inches (Fig. 41-22). Compress the chest at a rate of 100 bpm in both infants and older children (AHA, 2001).

Breathing and cardiac compression must be carried out concurrently but not exactly at the same time. If there are two people available for resuscitation, one can adminis-

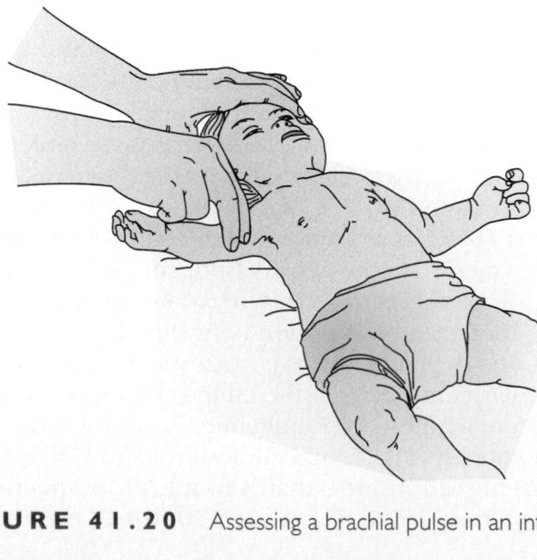

FIGURE 41.20 Assessing a brachial pulse in an infant.

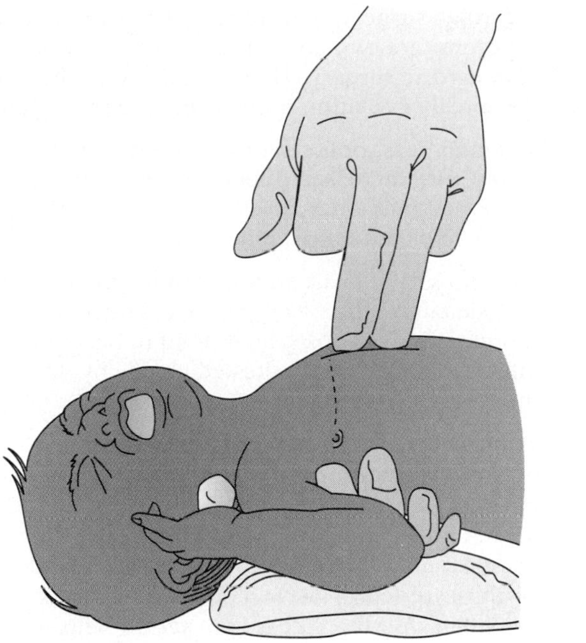

FIGURE 41.21 With cardiac resuscitation in a newborn or infant, chest compression is best done by pressing two fingers on the midsternum. Notice the slight extension of the infant's head to maintain a patent airway.

ter breaths to the child while the other compresses the chest. If you are by yourself, you must do both. For infants, administer one breath, then compress the chest five times; administer another breath, then compress the chest five more times, and so forth. This 1:5 ratio of ventilations to compressions will effectively ventilate and circulate blood. For older children, use a 2:15 ratio. Be certain that you release the pressure on the chest between compressions; this allows the heart to fill more readily. Do not lift your fingers or hands off the chest, however, because doing so requires time spent to properly reposition them. Also make sure to maintain a patent airway by using the head-tilt chin lift using the hand not performing the compressions. If the attempt is successful, the child's color will improve (especially the oral mucous membrane, which is readily visible) and the carotid pulse will become palpable. If two rescuers are working, continue to use a 1:5 ratio of ventilations to compressions in the infant and children less than 8 years of age or a 2:15 ratio in the older child. A 2:15 ratio reduces the number of times compressions must be interrupted (Cummins & Hazinski, 2000).

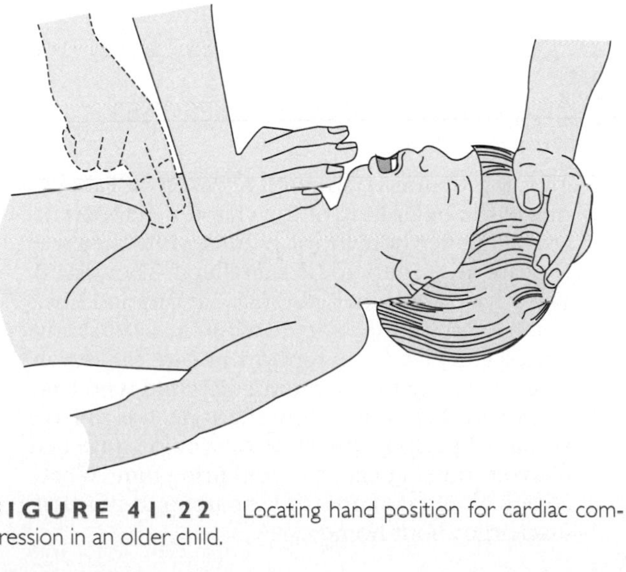

FIGURE 41.22 Locating hand position for cardiac compression in an older child.

These three techniques (clearing the airway, ventilating the lungs, and circulating blood by cardiac compression) will provide adequate oxygenation to major body organs for several minutes until additional personnel arrive who can initiate further resuscitation measures. The outcome of these secondary measures depends on how well and promptly the initial measures were performed.

Secondary Measures

IV access must be accomplished for drug administration. If this is not possible in about a minute's time span, an intraosseous catheter should be inserted. Drugs administered through an intraosseous route reach the circulation as rapidly as IV administration because of the rich blood supply in bone. Drugs such as epinephrine, lidocaine, and atropine also may be given by way of an endotracheal tube. An endotracheal dose is calculated by multiplying the IV dose by 2 or 3. The drug is then diluted with normal saline, administered by a catheter inserted deeply into the tube, and followed by an additional 1 or 2 mL of normal saline and several positive-pressure breaths.

A number of drugs are helpful in resuscitation procedures and should be available on a pediatric emergency resuscitation cart. These may include:

- Atropine: Reduces bronchial secretions, keeping the airway clear during resuscitation attempts. It also reduces vagus nerve effects, relieving bradycardia.
- Calcium chloride: Increases heart contractility. A contraindication to its use is the presence of digitalis toxicity.
- Epinephrine: Strengthens or initiates cardiac contractions; increases heart rate and blood pressure; bronchodilates.
- Adenosine: Relieves arrhythmias.
- Bretylium tosylate: Like lidocaine, counteracts ventricular arrhythmias.
- Dopamine: Increases cardiac output. It acts on alpha-receptors to cause vasoconstriction.
- Dobutamine: Acts as a direct-acting beta-agonist that increases contractility and heart rate.
- Lidocaine: Counteracts ventricular arrhythmias.

Psychological Support

A cardiopulmonary arrest is an acute emergency, and everyone who arrives at the scene should know what course of action to take. Even after heart action has been initiated, ventricular fibrillation may occur, requiring defibrillation. As soon as the child begins to respond to resuscitation, be aware that he or she begins to hear. The child is obviously frightened by the number of people and all the equipment surrounding him or her, such as cardiac monitor leads, IV tubing, and possibly an endotracheal tube. The child may have vivid memories of frightening body sensations just before going into cardiac arrest. The child may regain consciousness struggling and fighting. Assure the child that everyone is there to help him or her. It is extremely frightening for parents to see their child suddenly cease breathing. Although it is comforting to see emergency personnel arrive promptly and efficiently, parents are frightened to realize their child is ill enough to need such skilled personnel. Assist, inform, and comfort the child's parents.

Provide specific information on the child's condition as soon as it is available, and update the parents often. Allow them to see the child as soon as possible after the resuscitation attempt is complete to assure themselves that the child is breathing and has heart function. Be certain that they know that follow-up procedures such as ECG monitoring or blood-gas measurements are being undertaken to prevent another emergency. Offer support to help them begin grieving if the child does not survive.

✔ CHECKPOINT QUESTIONS

26. What is the most frequent cause of cardiac arrest in children?
27. What is the ratio of ventilations to compressions used for resuscitating an infant?

KEY POINTS

Cardiovascular disorders in children may be either structural, such as congenital heart disease, or acquired, such as Kawasaki disease or rheumatic fever. Assessment of children with heart disease includes history and physical examination. Echocardiogram, MRI, and cardiac catheterization are procedures used frequently for diagnosis.

Children with cardiac disease may fall behind in developmental progress because they do not have the energy to play usual childhood games. Help parents to think of games that are intellectually or developmentally stimulating without being physically exhausting.

Limiting saturated fat intake and following a consistent exercise program are important strategies for children to prevent heart disease in later life.

A number of therapies are available for children with cardiac disease. For example, children born with a septal defect undergo open-heart surgical repairs; those with hypoplastic left heart syndrome may undergo cardiac transplant. Children born with ineffective SA node function may have pacemakers implanted to improve heart function.

The families of children undergoing cardiac surgery need a great deal of support so they can cope well enough with this major event to be a support.

Postcardiac surgery syndrome and postperfusion syndrome are two complications that may occur after cardiac surgery. They are related to the extracorporeal circulation used during the procedure.

Congenital heart defects are classified as those associated with increased pulmonary blood flow, decreased pulmonary blood flow, obstruction to blood flow, and mixed blood flow.

Common signs of heart failure seen in children include tachycardia, tachypnea, enlarged liver, dyspnea, and cyanosis. Signs tend to be subtle in infants and may be manifested chiefly by difficulty in feeding from exhaustion and dyspnea.

Rheumatic fever is an autoimmune disease that occurs after a group-A beta-hemolytic streptococcal infection. Common signs and symptoms include fever, chorea, arthralgia, polyarthritis, erythema marginatum, subcutaneous nodules, and an elevated erythrocyte sedimentation rate. Taking prophylactic penicillin after the illness until age 18 helps prevent further recurrence and cardiac involvement. Some children with congenital heart disease may also need this same protective routine.

Kawasaki disease results from altered immune function. An inflammation of blood vessels leads to platelet aggregation and formation of thrombi and aneurysms.

Infectious endocarditis is infection of the endocardium of the heart. It may be a complication of congenital heart disease.

Hypertension in children usually occurs as a result of a secondary disorder. A diet that is moderate in cholesterol content along with regular exercise and maintenance of a weight proportional to height can help prevent this condition.

Children with heart disease are at high risk for cardiopulmonary arrest. Nurses and parents need to know how to perform cardiopulmonary resuscitation to be prepared for this emergency.

CRITICAL THINKING EXERCISES

1. Megan is the newborn with tetralogy of Fallot you met at the beginning of the chapter. Her parents are taking her home for a month while they wait for cardiac surgery to be scheduled. They asked you what "watch her carefully" means and how much exercise they should allow her. What advice would you give them for how to care for Megan?
2. You are caring for a 6-month-old child who has heart failure. His most important need is to have sustained periods of rest. How would you schedule your nursing care to avoid tiring him? What advice would you give to his parents at hospital discharge about home care?

3. A 10-year-old girl is recovering from rheumatic fever. She lives during the week with her mother and visits her father on the weekends. She will need to continue to take penicillin daily for the next 8 years. What steps would you take to ensure compliance over this long period of time?
4. Examine the National Health Goals related to cardiovascular disorders. Most government-sponsored money for nursing research is allotted based on these goals. What would be a possible research topic to explore that would be fundable and would advance evidence-based practice?

REFERENCES

American Heart Association. (2001). *Pediatric advanced life support.* Dallas, TX: Author.

Balaguru, D., et al. (2000). Management of heart failure in children. *Current Problems in Pediatrics, 30*(1), 1–35.

Berg, R. A., et al. (2001). Chest compressions and basic life support-defibrillation. *Annals of Emergency Medicine, 37*(4), S26–S35.

Carapetis, J. R., & Currie, B. J. (2001). Rheumatic fever in a high incidence population. *Archives of Disease in Childhood, 85*(3), 223–227.

Carpenter, T. C., et al. (2001). Critical care. In W. W. Hay, A. R. Hayward, M. J. Levin, & J. M. Sondheimer (Eds.). *Current pediatric diagnosis and treatment* (15th ed.). New York: McGraw-Hill.

Cohen, M. I., et al. (2001). Epicardial pacemaker implantation and follow-up in patients with a single ventricle after the Fontan operation. *Journal of Thoracic & Cardiovascular Surgery, 121*(4), 804–811.

Cummins, R. O., & Hazinski, M. F. (2000). The most important changes in the International ECC and CPR Guidelines 2000. *Circulation, 102*(8), S371–S376.

Danford, D. A. (2000). Effective use of the consultant, laboratory testing, and echocardiography for the pediatric patient with heart murmur. *Pediatric Annals, 29*(8), 482–488.

Department of Health and Human Services (2000). *Healthy people, 2010.* Washington, D.C.: DHHS.

Fischbach, F. (2001). *A manual of laboratory and diagnostic tests* (5th ed.). Philadelphia: Lippincott Williams & Wilkins.

Harris, G. D. (2000). Heart disease in children. *Primary Care, 27*(3), 767–784.

Karila, C., et al. (2001). Cardiopulmonary exercise testing in children: An individualized protocol for workload increase. *Chest, 120*(1), 81–87.

Kay, J. D., et al. (2001). Pediatric hypertension. *American Heart Journal, 142*(3), 422–432.

Laks, H., et al. (2001). Heart transplantation in the young and elderly. *Heart Failure Reviews, 6*(3), 221–226.

Morrow, W. R. (2000). The new world of pediatric cardiology. *Pediatric Annals, 29*(8), 464–466.

Mosca, R. S., et al. (2001). Congenital heart disease and cardiac tumors. In L. J. Greenfield. *Surgery: Scientific principles and practice.* Philadelphia: Lippincott Williams & Wilkins.

Nasr, et al. (2001). Kawasaki disease: An update. *Clinical & Experimental Dermatology, 26*(1), 6–12.

Ogle, W. & Anderson, M. S. (2001). Bacterial infections. In W. W. Hay, A. R. Hayward, J. J. Levin, & J. M. Sondheimer (Eds.). *Current pediatric diagnosis and treatment* (15th ed.). New York: McGraw-Hill.

Smolens, I. A., & Bolling, S. F. (2001). Valvular heart disease. In L. J. Greenfield. *Surgery: Scientific principles and practice.* Philadelphia: Lippincott Williams & Wilkins.

Sondheimer, M., et al. (2001a). Congenital heart disease. In W. W. Hay, A. R. Hayward, M. J. Levin, & J. M. Sondheimer (Eds.). *Current pediatric diagnosis and treatment* (15th ed.). New York: McGraw-Hill.

Sondheimer, M., et al. (2001b). Acquired heart disease. In W. W. Hay, A. R. Hayward, M. J. Levin, & J. M. Sondheimer (Eds.). *Current pediatric diagnosis and treatment* (15th ed.). New York: McGraw-Hill.

Thilo, E. H., & Rosenberg, A. A. (2001). Cardiac problems in the newborn infant. In W. W. Hay, A. R. Hayward, M. J. Levin, & J. M. Sondheimer (Eds.). *Current pediatric diagnosis and treatment* (15th ed.). New York: McGraw-Hill.

Veldtman, G. R., et al. (2000). Illness understanding in children and adolescents with heart disease. *Heart, 84*(4), 395–397.

Williams, R. V., et al. (2002). Does Abciximab enhance regression of coronary aneurysms resulting from Kawasaki disease? *Pediatrics, 109*(1), E4–E6.

SUGGESTED READINGS

Adrogue, H. E., & Sinaiko, A. R. (2001). Prevalence of hypertension in junior high school-aged children. *American Journal of Hypertension, 14*(5.1), 412–414.

Chang, A. C. (2000). Pediatric cardiac intensive care: Current state of the art and beyond the millennium. *Current Opinion in Pediatrics, 12*(3), 238–246.

Erickson, C. C., & Jones, C. S. (2000). Pediatric sudden cardiac death. *Pediatric Annals, 29*(8), 509–518.

Hirata, S. et al. (2002). Long-term consequences of Kawasaki disease among first-year high school students. *Archives of Pediatrics & Adolescent Medicine, 156*(1), 77–80.

Lewin, M. B. (2000). The genetic basis of congenital heart disease. *Pediatric Annals, 29*(8), 469–481.

McConnell, M. E., Adkins, S. B., & Hannon, D. W. (1999). Heart murmurs in pediatric patients. *American Family Physician, 60*(2), 558–565.

McCrindle, B. W. (2000). Screening and management of hyperlipidemia in children. *Pediatric Annals, 29*(8), 500–508.

Oechslin, E. N., et al. (2000). Mode of death in adults with congenital heart disease. *American Journal of Cardiology, 86*(10), 1111–1116.

Pedra, C. A., et al. (2000). Transcatheter closure of atrial septal defects using the Cardio-Seal implant. *Heart, 84*(3), 320–326.

Somerville, J. (2001). Grown-up congenital heart disease. *Thoracic & Cardiovascular Surgeon, 49*(1), 21–26.

Walters, H. L. (2000). Congenital cardiac surgical strategies and outcomes: HEARTS. *Pediatric Annals, 29*(8), 489–499.

CHAPTER 42

Nursing Care of the Child With an Immune Disorder

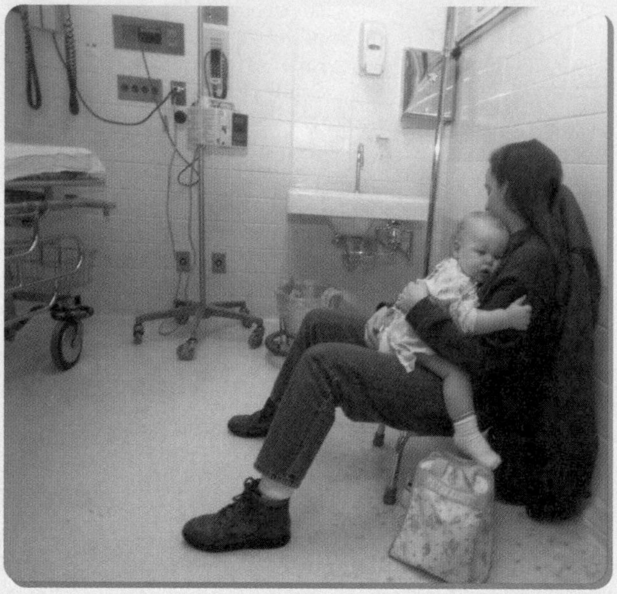

Key Terms

- allergen
- anaphylaxis
- angioedema
- antigen
- autoimmunity
- B lymphocyte
- cell-mediated immunity
- chemotaxis
- complement
- contact dermatitis
- cytotoxic response
- cytotoxic T cells
- delayed hypersensitivity
- environmental control
- hapten formation
- helper T cells
- humoral immunity
- hypersensitivity response
- hyposensitization
- immune response
- immunity
- immunocompetent cells
- immunogen
- immunoglobulins
- lymphokines
- lysis
- macrophage
- memory cell
- phagocytosis
- plasma cell
- suppressor T cells
- T lymphocyte
- tolerance
- urticaria

Objectives

After mastering the contents of this chapter, you should be able to:

1. Describe the immune process as it relates to childhood illness.
2. Assess the child with a disorder of the immune system.
3. Formulate nursing diagnoses for the child with a disorder of the immune system.
4. Establish outcomes for the child with a disorder of the immune system.
5. Plan nursing care pertinent to the child with an immune system disorder.
6. Implement nursing care for the child with an immune disorder.
7. Evaluate outcomes for achievement and effectiveness of care of the child with an immune disorder.
8. Identify National Health Goals related to immune disorders and children that nurses could be instrumental in helping the nation achieve.
9. Identify areas related to care of the child with an immune disorder that could benefit from additional nursing research or application of evidence-based practice.
10. Use critical thinking to analyze ways that nursing care for the child with an immune disorder can be more family-centered.
11. Integrate knowledge of immune disorders and the nursing process to achieve quality maternal and child health nursing care.

Dexter Goodenough is a 6-year-old boy you see in an ambulatory setting. His eyes are reddened and watering, and his nose is draining a clear discharge. His mother tells you he is constantly listless and other children make fun of him because of his appearance. His grades are "terrible" because the minute he gets to school, his symptoms begin. Dexter is diagnosed as having atopic rhinitis (hay fever). "Thank heavens," his mother exclaims. "I thought he had something serious. What a relief to know it's only an allergy."

In light of the effect this condition is having on Dexter's life, is this "only" an allergy? What additional information would you want his mother to know about the condition? Knowing this problem is worse at school, what environmental control measures would you want to suggest for Dexter?

Previous chapters described normal growth and development of children. This chapter adds information about the dramatic changes, both physical and psychosocial, that occur when a child is born with or develops a disorder of the immune system. This is important information because it builds a base for care and health teaching for children with these diseases.

After you've studied the chapter, answer the Critical Thinking Exercises at the end of the chapter and then access the on-line study activities (http://connection.lww.com) *to further sharpen your skills and test your knowledge.*

The immune system consists of a complex network of cells interacting to protect the body against invasion by foreign substances. The study of the immune system has grown immensely over the past several years, and almost every day brings a new finding. More diseases are being attributed at least in part to a malfunctioning of the immune system, all of which makes an understanding of how the immune system works in health and disease essential for safe nursing care.

Disorders of the immune system include deficiencies of immune substances and function that affect the body's ability to ward off infection (immunodeficiency disorders); abnormal and excessive immune response to foreign substances (hypersensitivity disorders, or allergies); and abnormal and excessive immune response to self (autoimmune disorders). Immunodeficiencies and examples of allergic disorders are described in this chapter. Autoimmune disorders, which include a wide range of illnesses affecting many body systems, are addressed in the chapters that discuss the affected system (e.g., rheumatoid arthritis, which affects the joints, is discussed in Chap. 51).

Immune disorders in children are a focus of much research and study because they may hold the key to understanding why major illnesses such as HIV/AIDS and possibly cancer occur. National Health Goals related to immune disorders and children are shown in the Focus on National Health Goals box.

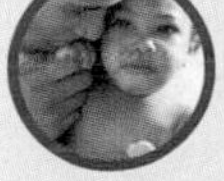

FOCUS ON NATIONAL HEALTH GOALS

Of the immunologic disorders, human immunodeficiency virus (HIV) is the most serious, not only because it is still ultimately fatal but also because its spread has been so difficult to stop. A number of National Health Goals address this problem:

- Increase to at least 95% from a baseline of 85% the proportion of adolescents who abstain from sexual intercourse or use condoms if sexually active.
- Reduce occupational needlestick injuries among health care workers from a baseline of 600,000/year to 420,000/year, a 30% improvement.
- Reduce AIDS among adolescents and adults from a baseline of 19.5 new cases/100,000 of the population to a target level of 1.0/100,000.
- Reduce new cases of perinatally acquired HIV infection.
- Increase the proportion of middle, junior high, and senior high schools that provide education on HIV/AIDS from a baseline of 65% to a target level of 90% (DHHS, 2000).

Nurses can be instrumental in helping the nation achieve these goals by initiating educational programs for children that include educating children and adolescents about the way HIV is transmitted (sexual relations and unclean intravenous needles) and protective measures they can take to avoid contracting the disease (using safer sex practices and not using intravenous drugs).

Nursing research that could add helpful information to the area includes research that attempts to answer questions such as: How can parents of school-age children be persuaded that safer sex practices should be part of usual school-age health awareness curricula? What methods work best to educate adolescents about the danger of unprotected sex?

NURSING PROCESS OVERVIEW

For the Child With an Immune Disorder

Assessment

The immune system provides protection for the body from invading organisms (antigens). A deficiency of **immunocompetent cells** (cells capable of resisting foreign invaders) or alteration in their function may limit this protection. Assessment focuses on analysis of blood components, particularly the white blood cells, to determine exactly what components are altered, missing, or not functioning properly. When the immune system reacts excessively or inappropriately to the invasion of certain antigens, a thorough history and analysis of presenting symptoms are usually the best way to identify the problem and develop appropriate interventions (see Assessing the Child With an Immune Disorder).

Nursing Diagnosis

Risk for infection related to altered immune response is the most relevant diagnosis associated with immune dysfunction. Nursing diagnoses for children experiencing allergic responses focus on their particular allergic symptoms. These may include:

- Situational low self-esteem related to effects of contact dermatitis
- Ineffective breathing pattern related to bronchospasm of anaphylaxis
- Anxiety related to continued allergic response
- Powerlessness related to difficulty determining cause of allergy
- Risk for delayed growth and development related to chronicity of HIV/AIDS

Outcome Identification and Planning

Outcome identification and planning for the child with an immune disorder focuses both on present and future concerns. Relief of immediate symptoms is the first priority. This is followed by planning for long-term care and prevention of problems. Looking into possible organizations for information or support could be key.

Implementation

A major nursing intervention in the care of children with immune disorders is client and family teaching. The family of the child with an immunodeficiency may need help in identifying ways to keep a child from contracting life-threatening infections while at the same time providing enough stimulation and social contact to promote normal growth and development. A similar teaching goal must be established for the child with a chronic allergic disorder. Parents need to learn ways to help their child avoid triggers or situations that provoke allergy, but they must not keep the child so isolated or fearful that the child misses out on important experiences. A referral to informational and support organizations such as those listed below may be helpful:

Asthma and Allergy Foundation of America (*www.aafa.org*)
Elizabeth Glaser Pediatric AIDS Foundation (*www.pedaids.org*)
Eczema Association for Science and Education (*www.eczema-assn.org*)

Outcome Evaluation

Examples suggesting achievement of outcomes may include the following:

- Child voices high self-esteem even if contact dermatitis rash has not completely faded.
- Child's respiratory rate is reduced to 20 breaths per minute with minimal wheezing.
- Child and parents state they can cope with their present level of anxiety.
- Child lists three actions she takes daily to help feel a greater sense of control.
- Child demonstrates achievement of developmental milestones within age-acceptable parameters.

Because the field of immunology is continually evolving, theories about immune diseases and associated treatments may change from visit to visit. Be certain that parents are kept abreast of new developments in the field, especially those that will affect their ability to provide an environment that is safest for their child.

ASSESSING the Child With an Immune Disorder

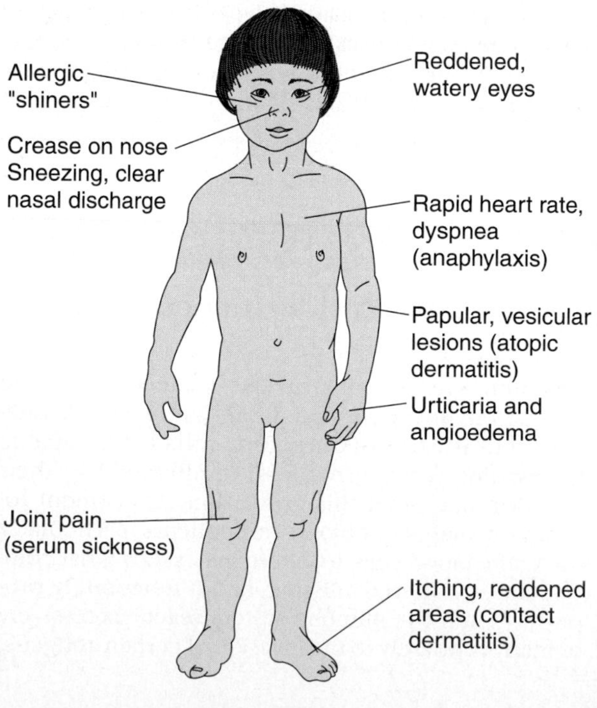

THE IMMUNE SYSTEM

The immune system functions to protect the body from invasion by foreign substances by several mechanisms. First, body surfaces such as the skin, cilia, and mucous membranes act as physical protective barriers. When an invading pathogen does get through this barrier, the process of **phagocytosis** (destruction of invaders) begins. **Macrophages** (mature white blood cells) engulf, ingest, and neutralize the pathogen. At the same time, an inflammatory response creates vascular and cellular changes that help to rid the body of dead tissue and the inactivated antigens. The immune system maintains cells ready to attack this way whenever necessary, directing the efforts of macrophages and supplementing the inflammatory response as necessary. It also singles out specific antigens for interactions (antibody–antigen reactions). This immune response not only furnishes immediate protection but also creates a template for how to destroy that particular antigen again in the future.

Immune Response

The **immune response** is the body's action plan devised to combat invading organisms or substances by leukocyte and antibody activity. An **antigen** is any foreign substance (molecule) capable of stimulating an immune response. Most antigens are proteins, but other large molecules such as polysaccharides may also function as antigens. Penicillin, although not antigenic by itself, may become antigenic when it combines with a higher-weight molecule, usually a protein (a process called **hapten formation,** which explains why penicillin reactions occur). If an antigen is one that can be readily destroyed by an immune response, and **immunity** (the ability to destroy like antigens) results, the antigen may be referred to as a simple **immunogen.** If, in the course of the immune response, mediating substances are released that cause tissue injury and allergic symptoms, the antigen is termed an **allergen.** Allergens may enter the body through a variety of routes. They may be ingested (e.g., foods such as eggs or wheat), inhaled (e.g., pollen, dust, or mold spores), injected (e.g., drugs), or absorbed across the skin or mucous membranes (e.g., poison ivy).

Immune System Organs and Cells

The organs of the immune system consist of the lymph nodes, bone marrow, thymus, spleen, and tonsils. Bone marrow produces lymphocytes, which are divided into B lymphocytes and T lymphocytes. Lymphocytes, after being produced, travel throughout the lymphoid system and are stored in the lymph nodes and spleen. T and B lymphocytes recognize invading organisms and provide for attack of specific antigens (Fig. 42-1).

B Lymphocytes

Originating in the bone marrow (the reason for their name), the **B lymphocytes** develop into plasma cells and memory cells when exposed to antigens. **Plasma cells** secrete large quantities of immunoglobulins or antibodies, which bind to and destroy specific antigens (termed **humoral immunity**). When an antibody is formed in response to a particular antigen this way, it is specific to that antigen. An antibody against the pertussis antigen, for instance, will not have any effect on the tetanus antigen. **Memory cells** are responsible for retaining the formula or ability to produce specific **immunoglobulins.** Immunoglobulins are classified as IgG, IgA, IgM, and IgE. Those involved in immunity are IgG, IgA, and IgM. IgM reaches adult levels at approximately age 1 year, IgG at age 4 years, and IgA at adolescence. IgE is primarily responsible for allergic or hypersensitivity responses. It is present at proportions capable of extreme response early in infancy. The functions of the immunoglobulins are summarized in Table 42-1.

T Lymphocytes

T lymphocytes account for 70% to 80% of blood lymphocytes and are responsible for cell-mediated immunity. They are also produced by the bone marrow but mature under the influence of the thymus gland (hence the term T cells). When mature, T lymphocytes leave the thymus to enter specific body regions (thymus-dependent zones), mostly in the lymph nodes and spleen; there they react specifically to viruses, fungi, and parasites, but have an effect on all antigens. T cells can be differentiated into three subtypes.

The first type, **cytotoxic (killer) T cells,** are phagocytic T lymphocytes that have the specific feature of binding to the surface of antigens and directly destroying the cell

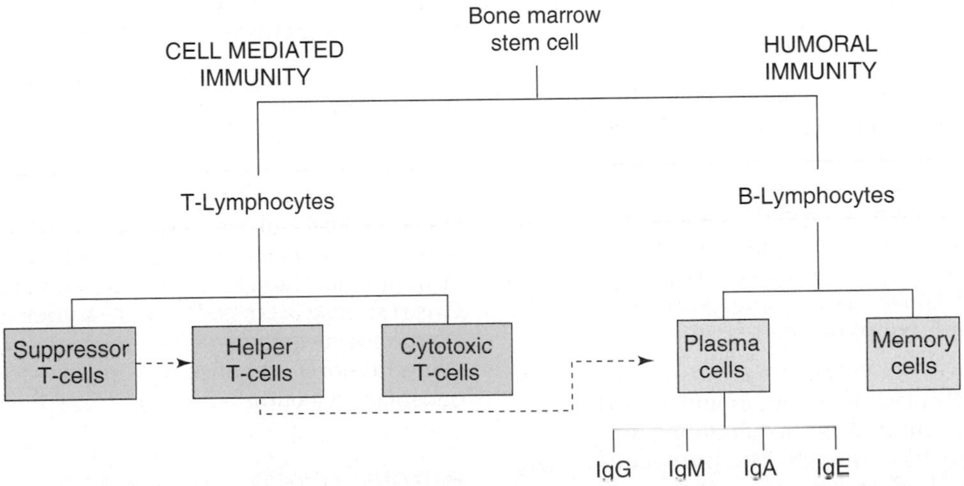

FIGURE 42.1 Lymphocyte production. From the bone marrow stem cell, T- and B-lymphocytes are formed. T-lymphocyte action leads to cell-mediated immunity. B-lymphocyte action results in humoral immunity.

TABLE 42.1 Location and Function of Immunoglobulins

IMMUNOGLOBULIN	DESCRIPTION
IgM	Effective in agglutinating antigen as well as lysing cell walls; discovered early in the course of an infection in the bloodstream
IgG	Most frequently occurring antibody in plasma; during secondary response, it is the major immunoglobulin to be synthesized; it freely diffuses into extravascular spaces to contact antigens; in prenatal life, it diffuses across the placenta to supply passive immune protection to the fetus and until the infant can effectively produce immunoglobulins; it has the major responsibility for neutralizing bacterial toxins and in activating phagocytosis (destruction of bacteria)
IgA	Found in external body secretions such as saliva, sweat, tears, mucus, bile, and colostrum; provides defense against pathogens on exposed surfaces, especially those of the gastrointestinal tract and respiratory tract, apparently by preventing adherence of pathogens to mucosal cells
IgD	Found in plasma; may be the receptor that binds antigens to lymphocyte surfaces
IgE	Involved in immediate hypersensitivity reactions; exists bound to mast cells on tissue surfaces; when contacted by an antigen, cellular granules are released; associated with allergy and parasitic infections

membrane and therefore the cell. As a part of this process, cytotoxic cells secrete **lymphokines,** a substance that contains or prevents migration of antigens and calls other lymphocytes into the area. Interferon is an example of a lymphokine important in preventing viral spread and helping to call leukocytes into the area (the property of **chemotaxis**).

The second type, **helper T cells** (CD4 cells), stimulate B lymphocytes to divide and mature into plasma cells and begin secretion of immunoglobulins. IgA antibody response depends on stimulation by helper T cells. Helper T cells can be identified in blood because of specific markers on their surface. Analysis of these (CD4 counts) is an important assessment of the competency of the immune system.

The third type, **suppressor T cells,** are T cells that reduce the production of immunoglobulins against a specific antigen and prevent their overproduction.

Types of Immunity

The action of B and T lymphocytes leads to two different types of immunity: humoral and cell-mediated immunity.

Humoral Immunity

Humoral immunity refers to immunity created by antibody production or B-lymphocyte involvement. Helper T cells recognize the antigen and cause activation of B lymphocytes (possibly by an intermediary macrophage). The specific B lymphocytes differentiate into plasma cells and begin secretion of specific immunoglobulins to mark the antigen for destruction (Fig. 42-2). A few antigens (e.g., *Escherichia coli*) are capable of activating B-lymphocyte response without recognition by T lymphocytes.

Primary Response. The first time a specific antigen enters the body, B-cell differentiation and growth begin. Within 6 days, IgM antibodies specific to the antigen can be measured in the bloodstream. The production of IgM antibodies peaks at 14 days and then declines until, within a few weeks, there are few present. At approximately day 10, IgG production begins and remains high for several weeks (Fig. 42-3).

Secondary Response. When a specific antigen enters the body a second or additional time, antibody production begins immediately because of memory cells. The type of immunoglobulin mainly produced in a secondary response is IgG (see Fig. 42-3).

Complement Activation. **Complement** comprises 20 different proteins that are normally nonfunctional molecules; however, when activated by antigen–antibody contact, these molecules begin a cascade response that leads to increased vascular permeability, smooth muscle contraction, chemotaxis ("calling" leukocytes into the area), phagocytosis, and **lysis** (killing) of the foreign antigen. The affected area feels warm and looks reddened and swollen, indicating an inflammatory reaction. Although an inflammatory reaction causes some local injury to tissue around the antigen, it is helpful overall because it produces an environment harmful to the antigen. Complement reactions that persist beyond the usual time for resolution (2 to 3 days) may be responsible for many of the autoimmune disorders.

Cell-Mediated Immunity

Cell-mediated immunity is the type of immune response due to T-lymphocyte activity. Cytotoxic T cells attack and directly destroy invading antigens through the release of chemical compounds on the antigen membrane, injection of a toxin directly into the antigen, or secretion of lymphokines. A wheal and flare response occurs due to accumulation of lymphocytes around small blood vessels, resulting in minor destruction to blood vessels (see Fig. 42-2). This response is termed delayed **hypersensitivity** if the T-lymphocyte activity occurs solely without an accompanying humoral response. It is this response that causes transplant rejection.

Autoimmunity

Autoimmunity results from an inability to distinguish self from nonself, causing the immune system to carry out immune responses against normal cells and tissue. Auto-

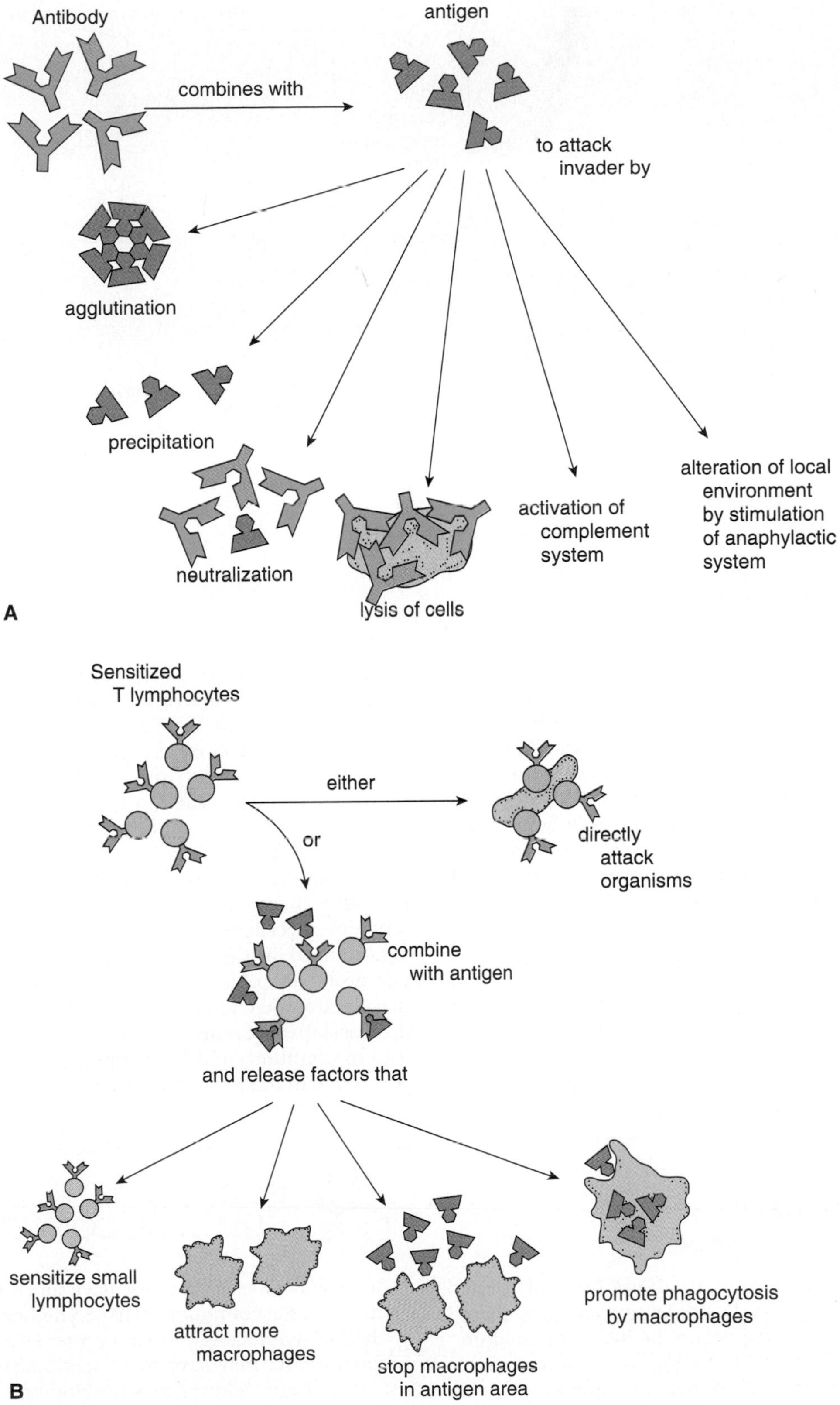

FIGURE 42.2 Mechanism of immunity response. (A) Humoral immunity. (B) Cell-mediated immunity.

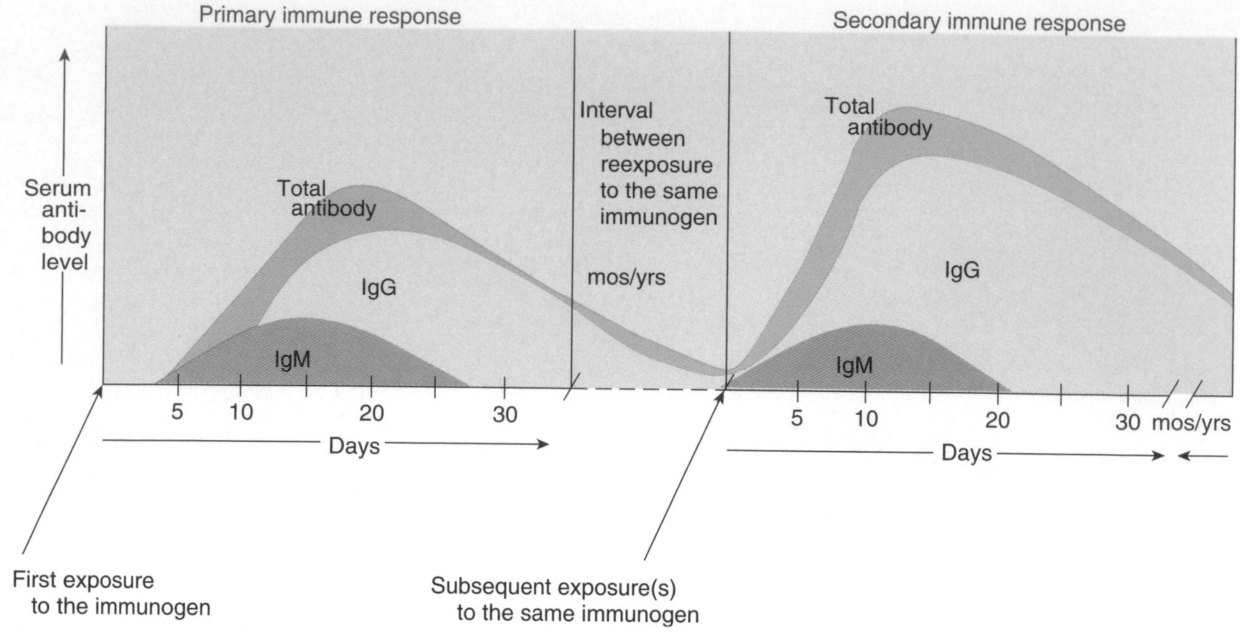

FIGURE 42.3 Primary and secondary humoral responses. IgM is the first immunoglobulin to appear in the serum.

immune responses may be organ-specific (i.e., limited to one organ), as in Hashimoto's disease (see Chap. 48) or generalized and systemic (not organ-specific), as in rheumatoid arthritis and systemic lupus erythematosus (see Chap. 46). There is currently much research oriented toward the study of autoimmune responses and their possible implication in a wide variety of disorders, including multiple sclerosis and rheumatoid arthritis. Autoimmune disorders occur at a greater rate in some families than in others and in girls and women (Rote, 2002).

> ✔ **CHECKPOINT QUESTIONS**
>
> 1. What type of white blood cell is responsible for engulfing, ingesting, and neutralizing a pathogen?
> 2. What are the two types of lymphocytes produced by the bone marrow?

HEALTH PROMOTION AND RISK MANAGEMENT

As many as 15% of children have some form of allergy (Boguniewicz & Leung, 2001). Preventing allergies, therefore, could have a major impact on the health of children. Early prevention can begin with encouraging women to breast-feed. Urging parents to delay the introduction of solid food until at least after 6 months of age can also delay exposure to foreign proteins. In families with a tendency for allergies (atopic families), parents can be encouraged to begin environmental control measures before their children are born (buying stuffed toys with synthetic filling only and removing dust collectors such as venetian blinds and shag rugs; see Focus on Cultural Competence).

Health promotion is also important to prevent HIV/AIDS. Teaching children safer sex practices is an important part of this. All health care providers can help prevent the spread of HIV/AIDS by using standard precautions. The parents of children with immune deficiencies may need to be reminded periodically to take measures to keep their children free of disease (keep immunizations updated, seek help immediately for infections).

Allergies are a type of disorder that typically cause chronic rather than acute symptoms. For this reason, children who develop allergies often need to be encouraged to be vigilant in taking their medicine. For the same reason, once parents begin a child on an immunotherapy program, they may need to be encouraged to continue it. It helps if children and their parents understand how allergic reactions lead to symptoms and how important it is for children to play a role in their own therapy.

> **FOCUS ON CULTURAL COMPETENCE**
>
> Because families with atopy have more allergies than others, some communities have a higher incidence of children with allergies than others. As a result, these communities may have more services and specialists to treat these children, thus developing a "community culture" of allergy acceptance and treatment. Children typically may leave school early for immunotherapy. School cafeterias commonly offer allergy-free foods. In other communities where fewer children have allergies, a child with an allergy is viewed as unique or not typical and needs additional support.

If parents are going to prepare allergy-free foods, be sure that they consider the child's likes and dislikes and think through the child's weekly intake to ensure that he or she receives all essential nutrients. If a child eats at school or has a meal prepared every day at a child care center, remind parents to make sure that the center, babysitter, or school dietitian is aware of the child's allergies. If a child is allergic to wheat products and cannot eat bread, preparing a bag lunch for school may be a difficult daily problem that only good planning can eliminate.

If a child's allergies involve pollen sensitivities, planning activities such as vacations at a time when the pollen count is low may make the vacation more pleasant for the family. If desensitization against a pollen is necessary, assist parents in planning to start desensitization so it will be effective by the time the pollen count of the offending allergen rises.

Although it is probably impossible to keep children with atopic allergies free of reactions and manifestations of allergies, parents who know of familial allergy patterns can take some preventive steps in this direction.

In families with allergies, infants should be breast-fed if possible. Parents should delay beginning solid food until 6 months of age and should introduce foods singly so food allergies can be detected and offending foods eliminated. Parents should omit eggs and chocolate for the first year. Environmental control begins when the parents choose furniture for the child's room, such as eliminating wool blankets, choosing toys carefully, and keeping the room free of dust. Teach parents to use a minimum of washing compounds so that children are exposed to as few chemical products as possible. Pets should not be introduced into the house. Avoiding spray products such as perfumes and air fresheners and discontinuing cigarette smoking also help.

These are sensible rules for parents to follow beforehand, rather than waiting for a child to develop allergic rhinitis or atopic dermatitis and then having to put more extreme measures into effect.

IMMUNODEFICIENCY DISORDERS

The immune system is a complex, interlocking network of cells with specific functions. When any one portion is not functioning adequately, an immunodeficiency results. The entire system may fail in its goal of protecting the body from invading organisms. The immunodeficiency disorder may be primary (congenital) or acquired (secondary to viral invasion or exposure to a toxic substance).

Primary (Congenital) Immunodeficiency

Children with primary congenital immunodeficiencies are born without an essential immune substance or function or with inadequate amounts of immune substances. Usually these deficiencies become apparent relatively early in life. However, it may take a few months for B-lymphocyte deficiencies to produce symptoms, because a newborn is born with enough maternal IgG (which crosses the placenta during pregnancy) to supply protection for approximately the first 6 months of life. It is important for parents and children to understand that primary disorders are not the same as acquired immunodeficiency syndrome (AIDS).

B-Lymphocyte Deficiencies

B-lymphocyte deficiencies create abnormally low levels of immunoglobulins either selectively (as in an IgA deficiency) or totally, which is referred to as hypogammaglobulinemia or agammaglobulinemia (Rudy, 2000).

Hypogammaglobulinemia. Hypogammaglobulinemia is an inherited X-linked recessive defect in the maturation of B lymphocytes that results in abnormally low levels of all immunoglobulins. At approximately 6 months of age, at the point passively transferred maternal antibodies fade, male infants begin to show susceptibility to bacterial infections, developing frequent respiratory, digestive, and throat infections. Autoimmune diseases such as rheumatoid arthritis and systemic lupus erythematosus may occur in later life. Cellular or T-lymphocyte response remains adequate, allowing the child to resist viral, fungal, and parasitic infections (Rudy, 2000).

This deficiency is treated with monthly intravenous immune globulin (IVIG) injections to supply immunoglobulins (Schwartz, 2000). Bone marrow transplantation may be successful in restoring immune competency. Parents and children, as they grow older, need to be taught the importance of recognizing infection early. Also help them set up a schedule for IVIG injections so these are not forgotten.

Common Variable Immunoglobulin Deficiencies. The most common disorder in this group is deficiency of IgA in surface secretions. The overall level of B lymphocytes is normal, but IgA production is reduced or absent, perhaps due to an increase of IgA suppressor cells or a defect in T-helper cells important for IgA synthesis. Without IgA, infection of surfaces exposed to the external environment and normally protected by mucus becomes common. Sinusitis, upper respiratory tract illness, and inflammatory bowel disease are apt to occur. There are associated atopic diseases (allergies) because without IgA on the surface mucosa, many more antigens than usual enter the body, permitting more antigens to interact with IgE and produce allergic symptoms. Chronic irritation due to these large numbers of antigens predispose exposed tissue to malignant transformation, so malignancy of the respiratory, gastrointestinal, and lymphoid systems occurs more readily. There is an increased risk that an antibody will cross-react with a self-antigen to cause autoimmune illness, so systemic lupus erythematosus and rheumatoid arthritis also occur at increased rates. IgA deficiency can occur as a secondary type due to treatment with phenytoin (an anticonvulsant) and penicillamine (a copper chelating agent). IVIG contains little IgA, so therapy with this does not greatly reduce symptoms. Because prevention, not treatment, is the key, parents need to be conscientious about preventing infections and perhaps administering prophylactic antibiotics to prevent respiratory infections (Smith, 2000).

T-Lymphocyte Deficiencies

T-lymphocyte immunodeficiencies involve inadequate numbers or inadequate functioning of one or more types of T lymphocytes; this affects cell-mediated immunity and also, because of helper T-lymphocyte function, possibly humoral immunity. DiGeorge anomaly (which includes failure of the thymus to develop) and chronic mucocutaneous candidiasis are two disorders caused by T-lymphocyte deficiency or malfunction.

Combined T- and B-Lymphocyte Deficiency

Severe combined immunodeficiency syndrome (SCIDS) is the most frequently seen disorder characterized by an absence or reduction of both humoral and cell-mediated immunity. SCIDS occurs as either an X-linked or autosomal recessive disorder. It is caused by a developmental abnormality (sometimes but not always related to the absence of a particular enzyme), which prevents the formation of T lymphocytes (a stem cell abnormality). This, in turn, prevents the maturation of both T and B lymphocytes. Children cannot respond to antigen invasion, and no antibodies are produced. Stem cell transplantation has proven to be an effective treatment for this disorder (Horwitz, 2000).

Secondary (Acquired) Immunodeficiency

Secondary immunodeficiency, or loss of immune system response, can occur from factors such as severe systemic infection, cancer, renal disease, radiation therapy, severe stress, malnutrition, immunosuppressive therapy, and aging. There can be complete or partial loss of both B- and T-lymphocyte response.

Stress appears to alter the immune response by stimulating the release of corticosteroids from the adrenal gland. This suppresses the inflammatory response by inhibiting macrophage action. Immunosuppressive drugs, such as prednisone, and radiation act to limit or destroy rapidly growing cells. Because both T and B lymphocytes are rapidly growing and dividing cells, they are killed by these drugs or radiation. Extreme infection can result in a decreased immune response because it exhausts the body's continued ability to combat infection.

Malnutrition decreases immunity because rapidly growing cells need protein for synthesis; renal disease with protein loss will also deplete the amount of protein available for new lymphocyte production.

Acquired Immunodeficiency Syndrome (HIV/AIDS)

AIDS is an acquired immunodeficiency caused by the RNA human immunodeficiency retrovirus HIV (McFarland, 2001). The virus has at least two divisions, HIV-1 and HIV-2, with a variety of further subtypes. It is contracted through blood and body secretions. The virus acts by attacking the lymphoreticular system, in particular CD4-bearing helper T lymphocytes. The virus enters and replicates in these lymphocytes and, in the process, destroys them. There is no defense against the virus, so it remains in the body for life. This results in loss of CD4 lymphocytes and the ability to initiate an effective B-lymphocyte response. The final result is that the immune response and the ability to screen and remove malignant cells from the body are lost. Because B-lymphocyte or humoral immune function, which initiates the production of antibodies, is affected, antibody formation will be decreased (hypogammaglobulinemia). When monocytes and macrophages become affected as well, the person with HIV infection cannot resist normal infection and is susceptible to opportunistic ones such as fungal infections.

Transmission. Pediatric HIV/AIDS accounts for only 1% to 2% of total AIDS cases (Boguniewicz & Leung, 2001). HIV/AIDS infection is spread by exposure to blood and other body secretions through sexual contact, sharing of contaminated needles for injection, transfusion of contaminated blood or blood products, perinatally from mother to fetus/newborn, and through breast-feeding. A few children have acquired the infection through sexual abuse.

Although decreasing in incidence, transmission of HIV/AIDS from mother to child by placental spread is still the most common reason for childhood HIV/AIDS in the United States. This transmission can occur during pregnancy, at birth, and possibly during breast-feeding. Transmission by this route has declined 80% since HIV-positive women have been prescribed zidovudine during pregnancy (McFarland, 2000).

In the past, many children with hemophilia, because they receive so many blood product transfusions, received contaminated blood and were infected. This source of transmission now almost never occurs. HIV is not transmitted by animals or through usual casual contact, such as shaking hands or kissing, or in households, day care centers, or schools. The increasing rate of sexual activity and the rapidly rising incidence of sexually transmitted diseases among adolescents are making this group vulnerable to growing rates of HIV/AIDS (Merchant & Keshavarz, 2001).

Assessment. HIV has a long incubation period of about 10 years in adults. This disorder appears to progress more rapidly in children and infants who receive the virus through placental transmission and do not receive treatment. These individuals are usually HIV-positive by 6 months and develop clinical signs by 1 to 3 years of age. Children who receive the virus from another source usually convert to HIV positivity by 2 to 6 weeks, or at least by 6 months after exposure. During this preconversion time, the child may have poor resistance to infection, such as fever, swollen lymph nodes, respiratory tract infections, and thrush.

All infants born to infected mothers test positive for antibodies to the virus at birth because of passive antibody transmission. This persists for about 18 months. The disease is diagnosed, therefore, by recovery of the HIV antigen in children under this age and antibodies to the virus in children over this age. Tests for detection of the antigen are termed PCR (polymerase chain reaction) tests; those for the antibody are termed ELISA (enzyme-linked immunosorbent assay) and Western blot confirmation. CD4 counts are used to document the disease status and predict disease progression. Normal counts vary according to age because the lymphocyte count normally varies by age. Table 42-2 shows the use of Centers for Disease Control & Prevention (CDC) guidelines and CD4 counts to determine disease progress. Severe suppression indicates a condition serious enough to cause life-threatening infections (Nielsen & Bryson, 2000).

The CDC classification of HIV/AIDS in children has three categories:

TABLE 42.2 CD4 Cell Counts Related to Progress of Disease in Children

	AGE OF CHILD		
	Under 12 Months	**1–5 Years**	**6–12 Years**
No evidence of suppression	1,500 cells/μL	1,000 cells/μL	500 cells/μL
Evidence of moderate suppression	750–1,499 cells/μL	500–999 cells/μL	200–499 cells/μL
Severe suppression	750 cells/μL	500 cells/μL	200 cells/μL

(Centers for Disease Control. [1997]. 1997 USPHS/IDSA guidelines for prevention of opportunistic infections in persons infected with HIV. *Morbidity and Mortality Weekly Report, 46*[12], 1.)

- Category A, Mildly Symptomatic: two or more symptoms such as enlarged lymph nodes, liver, or spleen, or recurrent or persistent upper respiratory infections, sinusitis, or otitis media.
- Category B, Moderately Symptomatic: more serious illnesses such as oropharyngeal candidiasis, bacterial meningitis, pneumonia, or sepsis, cardiomyopathy, cytomegalovirus infection, hepatitis, herpes simplex virus (HSV) bronchitis, pneumonitis, or esophagitis, herpes zoster (shingles), lymphoid interstitial pneumonia (LIP), pulmonary lymphoid hyperplasia complex, or toxoplasmosis.
- Category C, Severely Symptomatic: serious bacterial infections such as septicemia, pneumonia, meningitis, bone or joint infection, or abscess of an internal organ or body cavity; candidiasis (esophageal or pulmonary), encephalopathy, herpes simplex lasting over 1 month, histoplasmosis, lymphoma, tuberculosis, Mycobacterium or *Pneumocystis carinii* pneumonia. Unlike adults, children rarely develop Kaposi's sarcoma (CDC, 2001).

Therapeutic Management. Because of the success of zidovudine administration during the pregnancy of HIV-positive women, many fewer infants are born with HIV today. Those who are born with a perinatal infection, once thought to have a short life expectancy, now have an opportunity for long-term survival. To accomplish this, therapy involves a complex regimen of nutritional supplements to prevent weight loss, vaccines to prevent infections, and antiviral and antibacterial agents to combat the HIV virus and opportunistic infections (Merchant & Keshavarz, 2000).

NURSING DIAGNOSES AND RELATED INTERVENTIONS

Nursing Diagnosis: Risk for infection related to decreased immune function

Outcome Identification: Child will remain free of infection.

Outcome Evaluation: Child's temperature is within normal parameters; no cough or skin lesions are present.

Children with HIV/AIDS and their families must maintain strict personal hygiene (e.g., frequent handwashing) and avoid close contact between the child and anyone who has a respiratory infection to try to prevent the child from contracting dangerous opportunistic infections. When infections do occur, antibiotic and antifungal treatment should be prompt and aggressive.

Combating the infection requires specific antiretroviral medications to prevent progressive deterioration of the immune system and to provide prophylactic measures against opportunistic infections. Three classes of drugs are the mainstay of therapy: nucleoside reverse transcriptase inhibitors (NRTIs), nonnucleoside reverse transcriptase inhibitors (NNRTIs), and protease inhibitors:

- NRTIs are drugs designed to block production of viral DNA, limiting the ability of the virus to infect cells. Zidovudine is an example of this type drug (see Focus on Pharmacology).
- NNRTIs also inhibit the DNA synthesis of viruses but act at different sites on the viral enzyme. Nevirapine and efavirenz are examples.
- Protease inhibitors stop the ability of the virus to produce protease, limiting metastasis. Amprenavir, nelfinavir, and ritonavir are examples of protease inhibitors used with children.

The CDC has recommended that children be prescribed a regimen involving multiple drugs, such as one protease inhibitor plus two NRTIs (CDC, 2001).

Many children are given prophylactic therapy for *P. carinii* pneumonia (trimethoprim/sulfamethoxazole [TMP-SMZ]) beginning at 6 months of age. Children with HIV/AIDS are more susceptible to tuberculosis than other children (Zumla et al., 2000). If the child develops tuberculosis, a combination of antituberculosis drugs, such as isoniazid or rifampin, is used. Preventing tuberculosis is becoming more difficult because strains of tuberculosis have become resistant to the usual drugs.

Children should receive routine immunizations with the killed virus vaccines (all except oral polio and varicella vaccines) according to the usual schedule. If they are exposed to varicella, intravenous varicella zoster immune globulin (VZIG) is prescribed in an attempt to prevent this disease. Yearly influenza vaccinations should begin at 6 months of age. Children should receive pneumococcal vaccine at 2 years of age.

Nursing Diagnosis: Risk for compromised family coping related to diagnosis of HIV/AIDS in child

FOCUS ON PHARMACOLOGY

Zidovudine (ZDV)

Action: Zidovudine is a thymidine analog that inhibits the replication of some retroviruses, including HIV.

Pregnancy risk category: C

Dosage: 2 mg/kg every 6 h to infants born to HIV-positive mothers, starting within 12 h of birth to 6 wk of age. 180 mg/m^2 (720 mg/m^2/dose) orally or intravenously every 6 h to children ages 3 mo to 12 y (dosage not to exceed 200 mg every 6 h)

Possible adverse reactions: Nausea, loss of appetite, change in taste, paresthesia, headache, fever, agranulocytopenia, and rash

Nursing Implications

- When administering the drug intravenously, infuse the drug over 60 min to avoid too rapid an infusion.
- Administer the drug around the clock for maximum effectiveness.
- Monitor blood studies frequently for changes.
- Advise child to eat frequent small meals to counteract change in taste and loss of appetite.
- If the child experiences paresthesias, institute safety precautions and instruct the child and parents in measures to prevent injury related to loss of feeling.
- Caution child and parents that ZDV does not reduce the risk of HIV transmission, except placentally. Reinforce hygiene and infection control measures.

Outcome Identification: Family will demonstrate ability to care for child and maintain family functioning within 1 month.

Outcome Evaluation: Parents state ability to continue providing child's physical care; identify outside resources for help with care and decision making.

The diagnosis of HIV/AIDS in an infant or child can prove devastating for a family. When the disease is transmitted maternally, this diagnosis may be the first indication of the existence of HIV/AIDS in the mother; as such, this signals tremendous stress for the whole family. If the child contracted HIV/AIDS from a contaminated blood transfusion or organ donation (rare with current protocols for donor screening), the family can feel so betrayed and angry that they are unwilling to cooperate with health care providers who, in their minds, are responsible for their child's illness. In any case, the family's coping skills, even if they were previously healthy, are sure to be compromised. Siblings may feel left out of the family circle because of the many health care appointments needed for the ill child. They may fear contracting the disease themselves. One of the first nursing priorities in the care of such a family should be to help the family re-establish their previous level of functioning so they can turn their attention to their child's emotional and physical care needs and to their own needs as well (Bartlett, 2002).

Physical care requirements for the child with HIV/AIDS may be extensive, depending on the child's symptoms and disease progression. No matter what the child's physical needs, however, love and emotional support are essential to his or her well-being and psychological health. Parents or caregivers need extensive support, education, and anticipatory guidance from nurses and other members of the health care team. Encourage parents to seek medical care for their child at the first sign of illness or infection to prevent unnecessary hospitalization and pain.

✔ CHECKPOINT QUESTIONS

3. What is the transmission method by which most children acquire HIV/AIDS?
4. Why are many HIV-positive children prescribed prophylactic TMP-SMZ?

ALLERGY

Allergic diseases occur as a result of an abnormal antigen-antibody response. Approximately 3 in every 15 children suffer from some form of allergy (Smith, 2000). Allergic symptoms can be chronic and minor, such as those that occur with seasonal rhinitis, or acute and severe, as in an anaphylactic reaction. They can disrupt a child's life and development and the life of the family. When the cause of an allergic response is difficult to pinpoint, the child and parents often become frustrated. Even when the child has a known allergy, symptoms can vary from minor to acute without warning, ultimately disrupting family functioning.

Hypersensitivity

The underlying cause of all allergic disorders appears to be an excessive antigen–antibody response when the invading organism is an allergen rather than a simple immunogen. This is termed a type I response or a hypersensitivity response when it happens immediately. It can also occur as a type II, III, or IV response (Table 42-3). Types I, II, and III are mediated by antibodies (humoral response), whereas type IV is mediated by the T lymphocytes (cell-mediated response).

Type I: Anaphylaxis

With a type I allergic response, IgE receptor antibodies attached to the surface of mast cells bind to IgE antibodies responding to the presence of an antigen. Mast cells are specialized cells found lining blood vessels and in connective tissue, the mucous membranes, and skin. The IgE immunoglobulin triggers them to release intracellular granules. These contain histamine, leukotrienes, a slow-reacting substance of anaphylaxis (SRS-A), and chemotactic substances (substances to draw leukocytes into the area). Histamine and leukotrienes cause peripheral vasodilation and permeability of blood vessels. This leads to vascular congestion and edema. SRS-A causes extreme bronchial constriction and reduced vasodilation and permeability. **Anaphylaxis** is an acute reaction characterized

TABLE 42.3 Classification of Hypersensitivity Reactions

TYPE	INVOLVED CELL	MECHANISM	EFFECT
I Anaphylaxis	IgE	IgE attached to surface of mast cell triggers release of intracellular granules from mast cells on contact with antigens	Allergies, asthma, atopic dermatitis, anaphylaxis
II Cytotoxic	IgG or IgM	Antigen–antibody reaction leading to antigen destruction; complement is activated	Hemolytic anemia, transfusion reaction, erythroblastosis fetalis
III Immune complex disease	IgG or IgE	Antigen–antibody complexes precipitate; complement is activated, leading to inflammatory response	Rheumatoid arthritis, systemic lupus erythematosus
IV Delayed	T lymphocyte	T cells combine with antigen to induce inflammatory reactions by direct cell involvement or release of lymphokines	Contact dermatitis, transplant graft reaction

by extreme vasodilation that leads to circulatory shock and extreme bronchoconstriction that decreases the airway lumens.

Type II: Cytotoxic Response

In a **cytotoxic** (cell-destroying) **response,** cells are detected as foreign and immunoglobulins directly attack and destroy them without harming surrounding tissue. Foreign red blood cells that are introduced to an Rh-negative woman by a Rh-positive fetus are destroyed by this process (see Chap. 26). Tumor cells may be destroyed by this process. Why this immune response fails when malignant cells begin to proliferate is not understood. Current research is attempting to devise ways to activate the natural immune response as a method of destroying malignant cells. Care of the child with a malignancy (neoplasm) is discussed in Chapter 53.

Type III: Immune Complex

A type III response is an IgG- or IgE-mediated antigen–antibody complex reaction that involves complement and initiates the inflammatory response. Complement reactions that persist beyond the usual inhibition may serve as the basis for many of the autoimmune illnesses, such as glomerulonephritis and systemic lupus erythematosus (Frank, 2000; see Chap. 46). Serum sickness also occurs as a result of a type III response.

Type IV: Cell-Mediated Hypersensitivity

In a **delayed hypersensitivity** response, T lymphocytes react with antigens and release lymphokines to call macrophages into the area. An inflammatory response occurs that helps to destroy the foreign tissue. A Mantoux or purified protein derivative (PPD) tuberculin test is an example of this. Redness and induration of the site do not begin initially but only after approximately 12 hours from the injection. The reaction peaks in 24 to 72 hours (a delayed response).

Contact dermatitis is another example of a delayed hypersensitivity response. Certain substances, such as cosmetics, household products, or cured leather, alter the protein of skin cells so that they become an antigen, or the foreign substance combines with the protein (hapten formation) to become an antigenic protein. Lymphocytes and macrophages infiltrate the area and attempt to destroy the offending protein. Redness and vesicles may occur, and pruritus may be intense.

Assessment of Allergy in Children

History

Taking a health history of a child with an allergy can be time-consuming because many factors must be considered. A family history is important because there are familial tendencies with allergic diseases. Also, the exact symptoms of the allergy are important in helping to identify the allergen—rhinitis is probably due to an airborne antigen; urticaria (swelling and itching) is often caused by ingested antigens; and contact dermatitis (often a rash) must be from something that contacts the skin in that area. The time of the year that the allergy occurs also may give a clue to its cause. If the child's allergy exists all year, the antigen must be one that is present all year (house dust mites, pet dander, or a common food). If it occurs in the spring, it may be due to a tree pollen; in summer, a grass pollen; if it occurs just in August, ragweed is a prime suspect as the offending antigen (see Focus on Evidence-Based Practice).

Many symptoms of allergy are vague, described as "colds all winter," "itching," or "runny nose." Listen carefully: even though no one symptom is acute, together such symptoms can interfere with a child's comfort, school experience, and long-term health (see Focus on Multidisciplinary Care). Having the parents and the child keep a chart of when symptoms are worse and better often helps identify a specific allergen. Children with allergic rhinitis (hay fever), for example, have more symptoms on a windy day and fewer after a rainstorm (the rain washes pollen out of the air). Children are often poor reporters because they cannot remember clearly whether they had the same rhinitis and watery eye symptoms last summer as they do this summer. A record that details when symptoms start—for example, on arising, or only after the child reaches school—also can help identify an allergen.

FOCUS ON EVIDENCE-BASED PRACTICE

What Is the Most Common Allergen Found in Homes?

The usual answer to this question is the mites found in house dust. To see if this is true in inner-city homes, researchers reviewed the medical records of 196 children from 5 months to 16 years of age who had undergone skin testing for allergies to see if they had positive IgE skin reactions to cockroach allergen. Results of the chart review revealed that of the 63 children in the study younger than 4 years of age, 15 (23%) had cockroach allergen sensitivity; only 8 children (12%) were skin test positive for dust mite allergy. Nine of the children were sensitized only to cockroach allergen, not dust mites. The researchers concluded that cockroach allergy sensitivity begins early in life and may be just as important as house dust mite allergy in young inner-city children.

This is an interesting study for nurses because nurses are often the health care providers responsible for obtaining health histories on children in health care facilities. It suggests that if a child has symptoms of allergy or asthma and lives in an inner city, be sure to ask about the home environment and the possible presence of cockroaches. Nurses can use this study as a basis for designing appropriate allergy history tools to ensure that in addition to the questions usually asked about environmental control, questions about insects such as cockroaches in the home are addressed.

Alp, H., et al. (2001). Cockroach allergy appears early in life in inner-city children with recurrent wheezing. *Annals of Allergy, Asthma & Immunology, 86*(1), 51-54.

FOCUS ON MULTIDISCIPLINARY CARE

Various health care personnel assist with the care of children and families in acute care and ambulatory settings. For example, unlicensed assistive personnel often take children's vital signs, or laboratory technicians obtain specimens for laboratory testing. While interacting with the children and their families, they often talk to the parents about the reason the child is being seen. In many instances, a child's allergic symptoms are not the reason the child is being seen or treated. These symptoms are a major concern for the parents and child, however. Teach personnel to report these secondary concerns to primary health care providers so therapy for them can be instituted. In addition, be sure all personnel understand the importance of using standard precautions, especially when caring for the child with HIV/AIDS.

Laboratory Testing

Few laboratory tests are helpful in establishing a diagnosis of allergy. A determination of IgE serum antibodies can be made. Most children with an allergy have an increased eosinophil count. Five percent or more of eosinophils on a differential count, or an eosinophil count of 250 or more cells per cubic millimeter, is significant. Another main cause of an increased eosinophil count is invasion by ova or parasites. Thus, a stool specimen for ova and parasites is generally collected to rule out these problems as the cause of the increased eosinophil count. A radioallergosorbent test (RAST) may be ordered. This is an indirect radioimmunoassay in which the child's serum IgE is allowed to react with specific allergens impregnated in laboratory disks.

Skin Testing

Skin testing is done to detect the presence of IgE in the skin, or to isolate an antigen (allergen) to which the IgE is responding or to which a child is sensitive. When an allergen is introduced into the child's skin and the child is sensitive to that allergen, a wheal or flare response appears at the site of the test. This is due to the release of histamine, which leads to local vasodilation. Because this reaction appears quickly, the test should be read in 20 minutes. Systemic or aerosol administration of an antihistamine will inhibit the flare response, so the child should not receive these drugs for 8 hours before skin testing. Corticosteroid therapy does not affect immediate skin reactivity and so may be continued during skin testing.

Skin testing may be done by applying a patch or using a scratch or an intracutaneous injection technique. Patch testing has become the method of choice because it is painless and more efficient. For the child with rare allergies not typically provided by commercial patches, scratch or intracutaneous testing still may be necessary. Scratch testing is done by placing a drop of allergen solution on the skin, then scratching through the drop of liquid with a sterile needle. A relatively concentrated extract of allergen must be used for scratch testing because little allergen enters the child's skin.

Intracutaneous injections are done by injecting a small amount of a solution of allergen below the epidermis of the skin. This is usually done on the forearm so that if a sensitivity reaction does occur, a tourniquet can be applied proximal to the test site to prevent further absorption of the antigen. If the categories to be tested are extensive, the back can be used. Solutions used for intracutaneous injections are more dilute than those used for scratch testing (1 : 500 dilution compared with 1:5 for scratch testing). This means that the allergen extracts are not interchangeable from a group prepared for scratch testing to a group prepared for intracutaneous injections (or vice versa).

Because intracutaneous injections are given just below the epidermal layer of skin, they are almost painless. This is the same phenomenon as passing a needle or pin under the top layer of skin of a fingertip, a trick every school-age child does at least once to the horror of friends. The child needs a great deal of support for this type of skin testing, however, because it looks as if it will be painful, and the sight of a needle is frightening.

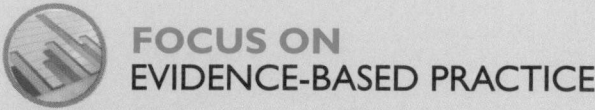

After all forms of skin testing, if the child is allergic to the test solution, a wheal and erythema (redness) will occur at the test site (Fig. 42-4). The size of the reaction is measured and graded as 1+ to 4+ or as slight, moderate, or marked. The allergens chosen for skin testing depend on the child's symptoms. Few children need more than 30 test media tried. This is because most allergies are worse at certain times of the year, and only those allergens prevalent at that time of year need to be evaluated.

Have a syringe filled with 1 mL epinephrine (Adrenalin) 1:1,000 on hand to counteract an unexpected anaphylactic reaction from skin testing. Epinephrine is given subcutaneously in doses of 0.01 mg/kg, up to 0.5 mg. Children should stay in the health care setting for at least 30 minutes after skin testing so they are there when such a reaction is most apt to occur.

Skin testing with food extracts is largely ineffective. Food allergies are best identified by eliminating a suspected food from the diet and observing whether there is an improvement in symptoms. After a time of improvement, the food is reintroduced. If it is one to which the child is allergic, symptoms will return with its reintroduction ("rechallenging").

Therapeutic Management

No matter what the symptoms of a child's allergy, there are three goals for therapy: reduce the child's exposure to the allergen, hyposensitize the child to produce a state of increased clinical **tolerance** (a state of not responding) to the allergen, and modify the child's response to the allergen with a pharmacologic agent.

Reducing the child's exposure to the allergen is possible when the offending allergen is a drug, food, or irritant. Reducing exposure is much more difficult when the child is found to be allergic to allergens such as molds, dust, feathers, or other substances found almost everywhere.

Environmental Control

Environmental control means removal of as many common allergens as possible from the child's environment. Common measures of environmental control are shown in Table 42-4 and the Focus on Family Empowerment. Some parents carry out instructions to reduce potential allergens in their house without difficulty, but for others the process seems too involved to undertake. Help parents understand that environmental control can make a great deal of difference in their child's symptoms (see Focus on Communication). If environmental control is effective with the child, this is preferable to hyposensitization, which involves many visits to the doctor and many injections.

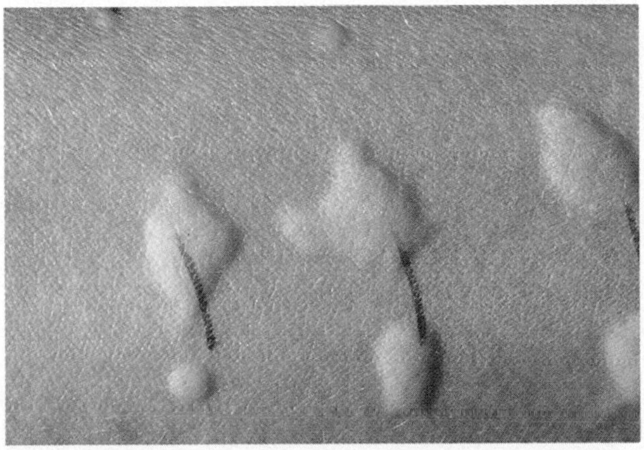

FIGURE 42.4 Allergy skin testing. Note the positive reactions.

Hyposensitization

Hyposensitization, or immunotherapy, is done when the child's allergy symptoms cannot be controlled by avoidance of the allergen or conventional drug therapy. It is expensive and may not be successful. It is usually considered only after environmental control has been tried.

Hyposensitization works by increasing the plasma concentration of IgG antibodies. IgG acts to prevent or block IgE antibodies from coming in contact with the allergen. After specific allergens have been recognized with skin testing, small amounts of the allergy extract (dilute enough to be clinically subreactive) are injected subcutaneously at 3- to 5-day intervals. The dose of antigen is increased in strength each time until a peak concentration is reached. The peak dose corresponds to the greatest strength that does not give clinical symptoms after injection. After hyposensitization has been achieved, the child then needs periodic injections every 3 to 4 weeks to maintain hyposensitization to this allergen. If a child is going to have an anaphylactic reaction to the injected allergen, it generally occurs within 30 minutes after the injection. Therefore, always have the child wait in the health care setting for 30 minutes after the injection before going home.

Immunotherapy is generally continued for 2 to 3 years because the longer it is used, the longer the period of relief from symptoms after it is stopped. Be certain that parents know at the beginning of therapy that this therapy will not "cure" their child. It will make the child symptom-free or will decrease symptoms for a length of time, however, and it may delay a disease such as hay fever (allergic rhinitis) from turning into asthma. Be certain children have adequate preparation for the procedure. Help them understand the importance of returning for additional injections.

A newer technique of immunotherapy is the sublingual administration of chosen allergen solutions (Pajno et al., 2000). SLIT (sublingual immunotherapy) is administered for an equal length of time as injection therapy, but SLIT has the advantage of being painless while producing equal results.

Pharmacologic Therapy

A number of pharmacologic preparations can be used to reduce the symptoms of childhood allergies. Like hyposensitization procedures, these drugs do not change the sensitivity to allergens; they only relieve the symptoms.

Antihistamines block histamine release and as a result control itching, sneezing, and rhinorrhea. Diphenhydramine hydrochloride (Benadryl) is a prototype of this drug class (see Focus on Pharmacology). It is effective but causes

TABLE 42.4 Common Measures for Environmental Control of Allergens

AREA OF CONCERN	MEASURES	RATIONALE
Child's bedroom	Encase mattress and pillow in sturdy plastic.	Reduces dust and dust mites
	Cover the zipper of plastic pillow and mattress case with adhesive tape.	Keeps dust confined
	Use blankets or quilts made of or stuffed with smooth, synthetic material; avoid wool.	Minimizes dust; wool is a good dust collector or may be an allergen itself
	Take down any ornamental items, such as a bed canopy.	Prevents dust collection
	Remove stuffed chairs and replace with wooden ones.	Removes dust collectors
	Remove venetian blinds and curtains that need to be dry-cleaned; replace with easily laundered types.	Removes dust collectors
	Remove stuffed toys unless filled with synthetic material.	Removes dust collectors and possible sources of allergens
	Remove aquariums and plants.	Removes mold spores
	Clean closet so it contains only currently used items.	Eliminates dust collectors
	Remove any fur or woolen items from child's wardrobe.	Removes possible allergens
Living room	Remove all carpets. If a rug is necessary, replace an animal hair pad with a foam rubber one.	Avoids containers for dust collection
	Provide a wooden chair for sitting.	Provides space free from allergens
	Vacuum frequently.	Minimizes dust collection
	Use linoleum or plastic laminate surface on carpet if child sits on the floor.	Provides space free from allergens
	Discourage child from lying on rug.	Reduces exposure to allergens
Bathroom	Use nonscented toilet paper, soaps, cleaners.	Minimizes exposure to potential irritants
School room	Have child sit away from blackboard, caged animals, or fish tanks.	Minimizes exposure to chalk, mold spores, and animal dander, which are allergens
	Keep locker free of collectibles	Reduces dust collection
General	Purchase a dehumidifier; add compounds to paint to decrease mold spores.	Reduces mold spores
	Use HEPA filters on furnaces, vacuums.	Filters air of possible allergens
	Do not keep a pet.	Reduces exposure to animal dander
	Dust daily with a moist cloth.	Controls dust better than dry dusting

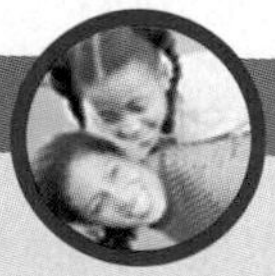

FOCUS ON FAMILY EMPOWERMENT
Avoiding Secondary Smoke

Q. Neither my husband nor I smoke, but some of our relatives and friends do. How can we keep our infant free from secondary smoke?

A. Use the following guidelines to help avoid secondary smoke:

- Declare your home a smoke-free zone.
- If family members smoke, ask them to smoke outside.
- If at a restaurant, ask to sit in a no-smoking area, or visit only smoke-free restaurants.
- If staying at a hotel, ask for a nonsmoking room.
- Don't be reluctant to ask people around your child at a social gathering to stop smoking.
- Encourage your friends or family members who smoke to take quit-smoking courses (for their own benefit as well as yours).

FOCUS ON COMMUNICATION

The Bryants are a couple who have been instructed on environmental control measures because their daughter, Pamela, has severe allergic rhinitis. Despite this, Pamela's symptoms have not improved. You meet with them to confirm that they are carrying out these measures.

Less Effective Communication

Nurse: Have you made the changes around your house that we discussed to reduce dust?
Mrs. Bryant: As many as we can.
Nurse: What about Pam's bedroom? Do you have the mattress covered? Any frilly curtains down? Anything wool taken out?
Mrs. Bryant: I've done everything I can.
Nurse: In the living room, it's important she has a protected floor space. Also that she doesn't sit in overstuffed chairs.
Mrs. Bryant: I've done everything I can.
Nurse: Okay, you sound in good shape. It's puzzling, though, why, in the face of all you've done, Pam's symptoms haven't improved.

More Effective Communication

Nurse: Have you made the changes around your house that we discussed to reduce dust?
Mrs. Bryant: As many as we can.
Nurse: What about Pam's bedroom? Do you have the mattress covered? Any frilly curtains down? Any stuffed animals taken out?
Mrs. Bryant: I've done everything I can.
Nurse: It's puzzling why Pam's symptoms haven't improved. Why don't you tell me exactly what steps you've taken?
Mrs. Bryant: I covered the mattress. I had to leave the curtains up because they match the rug and canopy on the bed. I took out a lot of the toys, but I left the stuffed bears because they match the wallpaper.
Nurse: Let's review again what environmental control means and the effect it can have on reducing Pam's symptoms.

The above scenarios are examples of what can happen when nurses assume that what they mean by a term is also what a parent means by the same term. In this instance, by taking the parent's statement that she has done everything possible to mean she has done everything that needs to be done, the nurse makes an incorrect assumption. Following up by asking the parents to be more specific reveals better information.

severe drowsiness. Second- and third-generation antihistamines, such as cetirizine (Zyrtec) and loratadine (Claritin), cause less drowsiness and provide a longer effect.

Decongestants, such as pseudoephedrine (Sudafed), decrease nasal edema and can help enlarge breathing space. Intranasal corticosteroids reduce inflammation, producing a similar effect as for decongestants. Intranasal cromolyn can be used prophylactically to prevent symptoms.

FOCUS ON PHARMACOLOGY

Diphenhydramine Hydrochloride (Benadryl)

Action: Diphenhydramine is a first-generation antihistamine that acts to block the effects of histamine at H_1 receptor sites, resulting in relief of symptoms associated with histamine release disorders such as allergic rhinitis.

Pregnancy risk category: B

Dosage: 12.5 to 25 mg t.i.d. to q.i.d. or 5 mg/kg/day or 150 mg/m^2/day orally (in children weighing over 10 kg [20 lb]) up to a maximum dose of 300 mg/day

Possible adverse reactions: Drowsiness, dizziness, sedation, epigastric distress, dry mouth, thickening of bronchial secretions, hypotension

Nursing Implications

- Administer drug with food if gastrointestinal upset occurs.
- Use a humidifier to keep nasal mucosa moist.
- Be alert for drowsiness, which may interfere with school or sports performance; notify the health care provider for possible change in dosage or drug.
- Encourage the child to suck on sugarless lozenges to combat dry mouth.
- Notify health care provider if child develops a lower respiratory tract disorder. Antihistamines should not be used when secretions need to be kept moist to enhance expectoration.
- Do not use this drug if the child has glucose-6-phosphate dehydrogenase deficiency. Severe hemolysis may occur.

✔ CHECKPOINT QUESTIONS

5. What type of hypersensitivity reaction initiates contact dermatitis?
6. What test is used to isolate an allergen to which a child is sensitive?

COMMON IMMUNE REACTIONS

Anaphylactic Shock

Anaphylactic shock is an immediate, life-threatening, type I hypersensitivity reaction that occurs after exposure to an allergen in a previously sensitized child. Within minutes of antigen invasion (being stung by an insect or receiving an injection of a drug to which a child has been sensitized), symptoms begin.

Assessment

Initially, the child may become nauseated, with vomiting and diarrhea, because of the sudden increase in gastrointestinal secretions produced by the stimulation of histamine. This is followed by urticaria and angioedema. Bronchospasm is so severe the child becomes dyspneic and hypoxemic. Continued bronchospasm leads to hypoxia and possibly cyanosis. As blood vessels dilate, the blood pressure and pulse rate may fall. Seizures and death may follow as soon as 10 minutes after the allergen was introduced into the child's body (Boguniewicz & Leung, 2001).

It is sometimes difficult to distinguish anaphylactic shock from fainting (syncope). Children, as a rule, do not faint after an injection or a bee sting. Syncope rarely occurs if a person is lying prone, so if the reaction occurred while the child was lying on the treatment table, it is most likely that the reaction is anaphylactic. With syncope, although the child falls and is momentarily unconscious, the pulse and blood pressure remain normal. The child appears pale and may have intense perspiration, but he or she can be roused readily after breathing amyl nitrite (smelling salts). The child with an anaphylactic reaction cannot be roused this way.

FOCUS ON PHARMACOLOGY

Epinephrine Hydrochloride (Adrenalin)

Action: Epinephrine is a sympathomimetic drug that acts on both alpha- and beta-receptor sites of sympathetic receptor cells to cause increased blood pressure and heart rate. It also relaxes the smooth muscles of the bronchi. It is used to counteract the symptoms of anaphylaxis.

Pregnancy risk category: C

Dosage: 0.01 mg/kg or 0.3 mL/m^2 of a 1 : 1,000 solution subcutaneously every 20 min or more often if needed for 4 h, not to exceed 0.5 mL (0.5 mg) in a single dose (for children and infants); 0.005 mL/kg (0.025 mg/kg) subcutaneously of a 1 : 200 suspension (in infants and children 1 mo to 1 y)

Possible adverse reactions: Anxiety, restlessness, headache, nausea, arrhythmias, hypertension, palpitations, pallor

Nursing Implications

- Be sure to calculate the drug dosage and check the solution strength carefully; solution is available in different concentrations, and epinephrine is a very potent drug.
- Obtain blood pressure, pulse, and respirations and auscultate breath sounds before and immediately after administration. Assess the child for signs indicating resolution of anaphylaxis.
- Rotate injection sites to prevent necrosis.
- Have a rapidly acting alpha-adrenergic blocking agent or vasodilator readily available in case of hypertensive reaction; have a beta-adrenergic blocking agent readily available in case of arrhythmias.
- Protect the drug from light and heat. Use only solutions that are clear and colorless.

Therapeutic Management

Preventing anaphylaxis is as important as knowing how to respond when it occurs. Before giving drugs that are known to have a high incidence of anaphylactic reactions (e.g., penicillin, aspirin, or antitoxin serums), be certain to ask parents if the child has ever had a reaction to the drug before. If in doubt, withhold the drug until its safety can be confirmed. Check the child's chart to be certain that no prior reactions are noted. People who have hypersensitivity reactions to any injectable substance should wear a bracelet or necklace identifying the drugs to which they are allergic. Some children object to this safety measure because they do not want to look conspicuous, but assure them that this is important. Generally, children who have hypersensitivity reactions to insect stings are advised to undergo hyposensitization therapy.

Epinephrine is the drug of choice to treat anaphylaxis (see Focus on Pharmacology). Additional emergency interventions for anaphylactic shock are summarized in Box 42-1. If anaphylaxis follows an injection or an insect sting, give the epinephrine in the opposite arm. Place a tourniquet on the extremity of the allergenic injection or sting proximal to the injection site to prevent further absorption of the allergen. Release the tourniquet every 15 minutes.

If a sensitized child receives an injection or is stung by an insect while at home, parents must know the proper procedure to follow so they can give their child immediate help. In place of a tourniquet, they can apply ice to the injection or sting site to slow absorption. If the child is prescribed an antihistamine, they should give that. Then the parents should notify an emergency squad that their child is having a severe reaction. Caution them not to attempt to give an oral medication if the child is comatose. Parents may purchase an emergency kit (e.g., Ana-Kit), an insect sting treatment kit that contains measured doses of epinephrine (often in a device called an EpiPen, which injects the epinephrine; see Focus on Family Empowerment) and an antihistamine.

Evaluation of the child after an anaphylactic reaction involves not only a physical examination but also evaluation to help the child avoid such a serious reaction from occurring again. This involves health teaching about the substance that caused the reaction and related substances that could have the same effect.

Urticaria and Angioedema

Urticaria, or hives, refers to flat wheals surrounded by erythema arising from the chorion layer of skin; they are intensely pruritic (often described as a burning sensation). Elevations may occur so close together they tend to coalesce (blend together). Urticaria occurs from a type I or immediate hypersensitivity reaction created by the release of histamine from an antibody–antigen reaction, similar to but of lesser intensity than anaphylaxis. In chronic urticaria, no causative allergen may be found. There is dilatation of capillaries and venules with increased permeability.

Angioedema is edema of the skin and subcutaneous tissue. This occurs most frequently on the eyelids, hands, feet, genitalia, and lips—areas where skin is loosely bound by subcutaneous tissue. Angioedema can be distinguished from other edemas because it is not dependent, is generally asymmetrically distributed, and usually occurs with

BOX 42.1

EMERGENCY MEASURES FOR ANAPHYLACTIC SHOCK

Anaphylaxis is an emergency, and fast action is necessary.

- Position the child with head even with the body to counteract hypotension.
- Administer aqueous epinephrine (Adrenalin) 1:1,000 subcutaneously at a dosage of 0.01 mg per kilogram of body weight up to 0.5 mg. This relieves laryngeal edema and severe bronchospasm.
- Administer nebulized bronchodilators such as albuterol to halt wheezing.
- If hypoxia is present, administer oxygen by mask or nasal cannula.
- Notify the cardiac arrest team because both respiratory and cardiac arrest may occur.
- Anticipate use of diphenhydramine (Benadryl) IM or IV as a secondary medication, particularly if urticaria (itching and swelling) is present.
- Anticipate the need for an IV fluid line as a route for a vasopressor such as dopamine and fluid to help restore blood pressure.
- If the child is experiencing seizures, prepare to administer phenobarbital or diazepam.
- Be prepared to administer corticosteroids as second-line drugs. Corticosteroids do not act immediately but reduce inflammation, which is necessary. IV methylprednisolone is a typical drug given.
- Keep the child and family members calm; anxiety adds to bronchospasm and decreases breathing ability.

urticaria. In severe angioedema, the larynx may be involved. This is serious because laryngeal edema may lead to airway obstruction and subsequently asphyxiation and death.

The allergens that most frequently cause urticaria and angioedema include drugs, foods, and insect stings. Exposure to hot or cold can also cause these reactions. The cause of the reaction should be identified so it can be avoided in the future. Although hot and cold exposure is a rare cause, children with this form must be identified because if they swim in cold water, the sudden release of histamine could cause dizziness so severe that they could drown. Therapy for urticaria or angioedema is subcutaneous epinephrine or an oral antihistamine.

Serum Sickness

Serum sickness is a type III hypersensitivity response of the body to a foreign serum antigen or drug. Examples of foreign sera given to children include tetanus antitoxin, diphtheria antitoxin, and rabies antiserum. These are obtained from horse serum. Children may experience a serum sickness reaction to a drug (e.g., penicillin), but this is rare.

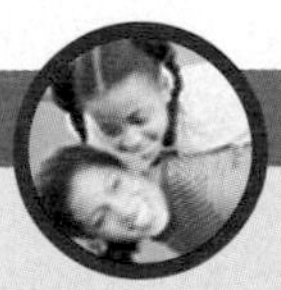

FOCUS ON FAMILY EMPOWERMENT

Guidelines for Using an EpiPen

Q. If my child is stung by a bee, I'm supposed to inject epinephrine. How do I do that?

A. It's important that you think about this in advance, because at the moment your child is stung, it will be an emergency situation.

- Purchase an EpiPen, a commercial syringe with a designated dose of epinephrine for use in emergencies.
- If necessary, purchase additional EpiPens so you have one at home, provide one for your child's school, and maybe keep one in your car to avoid having to remember to carry a single one with you.
- Store EpiPens at room temperature; don't refrigerate.
- Inspect the color of the solution in the EpiPen once a month; replace it if it is cloudy or discolored.
- If your child is stung, remove the gray safety cap from the device and wipe the outer fleshy portion of your child's thigh with an alcohol wipe.
- Place the EpiPen against the thigh until the device activates, injecting the solution into your child's thigh. If necessary, you can place the device on top of your child's clothing. The needle is long enough to pass through the clothing and into your child's skin.
- Be careful before injecting that you are holding the EpiPen with the needle toward your child. If not, you will accidentally inject your own thumb (a serious circumstance, as the dose of epinephrine could seriously injure your thumb).
- Keep in mind that the EpiPen is designed so that not all the solution in the pen will be ejected. Do not try to give the remainder of the solution.
- Remember that epinephrine will control symptoms for about 20 minutes. After administering the dose, therefore, call 911 for transportation assistance or transport your child to an emergency facility for further care.

Assessment

Symptoms of serum sickness begin 7 to 12 days after the serum injection. If the child has received the same type of foreign serum previously, some symptoms may occur as early as 1 to 5 days. Children notice itching, edema, and erythema at the injection site. There is generalized urticaria (hives) with or without angioedema (generalized edema). Erythematous maculopapular rashes, erythema multiforme (a generalized macular eruption with dark red papules), or purpura (hemorrhage into the skin) may result.

Urticaria with pruritus is usually present. There may be fever and arthralgia (joint pain). Lymphadenopathy may be present, especially of the regional nodes near the site of the injection. The child may have weight gain, nausea, vomiting, and abdominal pain. In more extreme instances, the child's nervous system may be involved and optic neuritis, stupor, and coma may occur. If edema is severe, laryngeal edema will become the paramount symptom that needs treatment (Salerno, 2000).

Therapeutic Management

Serum sickness lasts days or weeks. In its usual form (i.e., urticaria, edema, arthralgia, or pruritus), the treatment is only symptomatic because the condition will improve by itself with time. However, an antihistamine such as diphenhydramine (Benadryl) or epinephrine may be helpful in relieving symptoms. Acetylsalicylic acid (aspirin) or a nonsteroidal antiinflammatory drug (NSAID) such as ibuprofen (Motrin) may be necessary to relieve the fever and joint pain.

Like anaphylactic reactions, serum sickness reactions are frightening to the child and parents. Parents need an explanation of why the reaction occurred (their child has a low threshold of sensitization to this particular substance), that it was not anyone's fault, and that it did not occur from administration of the wrong compound (assuming that proper precautions to ascertain sensitivity to the solution were taken before the incident). Because serum sickness mimics so many other diseases, parents need reassurance that it is not arthritis (the arthralgia may make them think it is) and that their child will not have long-term effects from it.

The child should not receive the foreign serum or drug that was responsible for this primary occurrence of serum sickness again. Otherwise, if administered again, the manifestation of the reaction may be anaphylaxis. The child should wear a bracelet or necklace stating the solutions to which he or she is hypersensitive. Children should have their immunizations (and records) kept current so there is never a need to give sera such as tetanus or diphtheria antitoxins.

> **✔ CHECKPOINT QUESTIONS**
>
> 7. What is the first-line drug to treat anaphylaxis?
> 8. In what areas of the body does angioedema occur?

ATOPIC DISORDERS

Individuals with atopy are prone to all allergic responses. Three disorders occur most frequently in atopic individuals: hay fever (allergic rhinitis), eczema (atopic dermatitis), and asthma (see Chap. 40). Although these diseases show a familial tendency, different family members may have different symptoms. In one family, for example, the father may have allergic rhinitis, one child may have asthma, and another may have atopic dermatitis.

The gene responsible for an immune response is located chromosomally near the human leukocyte antigen that is responsible for graft rejection. In certain children, a tendency for sensitivity to antigens or abnormality of this gene is apparently inherited. These children have a higher-than-normal production of IgE antibody that makes them more responsive to allergens than other people. However, there is also a strong environmental component to these diseases. Children whose parents smoke have twice the incidence of atopic disorders compared with children of parents who do not smoke.

Allergic Rhinitis

Allergic rhinitis is caused by a type I or immediate hypersensitivity immune response. It occurs in 10% to 15% of children (Boguniewcz & Leung, 2001).

Assessment

Common symptoms of allergic rhinitis include sneezing, nasal engorgement, and a profuse watery nasal discharge. The eyes may water. The conjunctivae of the eyes may be pruritic, often with a distinctive pebbly appearance. Children may constantly rub their noses in an upward motion, termed an allergic salute. Over a long period, rubbing the nose this way leads to a horizontal crease across the tip of the nose, called an allergic crease. Because of congestion in the nose, there tends to be back-pressure to the blood circulation around the eye orbit, which leads to blackened areas under the eyes, termed allergic shiners (Fig. 42-5). The mucous membrane of the nose is generally paler than normal. It may be edematous, adding to nasal congestion.

Children older than 6 years (when frontal sinuses develop) may report a full frontal headache. This becomes more marked with adolescence. Some children feel exhausted and lethargic and cannot function well in school. Recurrent otitis media may occur due to the swollen pharyngeal tissue (eustachian tubes are blocked to the middle ear). A smear of the nasal discharge will reveal an increased eosinophil count (more than 10% of the white cell count). RAST analysis may reveal the offending allergens.

The allergens that cause allergic rhinitis are generally pollens or molds rather than foods or drugs. Many of these children are brought to a health care setting during peak pollen months because parents think they have a "summer cold." However, with an upper respiratory infection, the mucous membrane of the nose is more apt to be reddened than pale, and the secretions draining from the nose are apt to be thick white or yellow rather than the thin, watery secretions of allergic rhinitis. Children with an upper res-

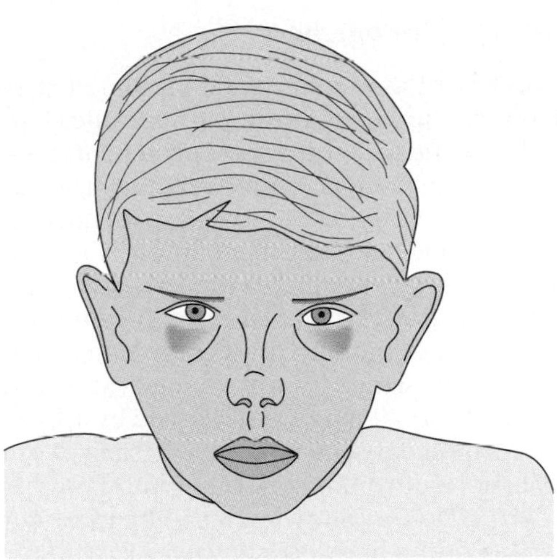

FIGURE 42.5 Back pressure to the blood circulation around the eye orbit from allergic rhinitis may lead to dark areas under the eyes (allergic shiners). The frequent rubbing of the nose in an upward direction can lead to a peculiar horizontal crease (Dennie's line).

piratory infection often have a fever; children with allergic rhinitis do not. With an upper respiratory infection, a sore throat and cervical adenopathy may be present, but these are rare with allergic rhinitis.

Therapeutic Management

Allergic rhinitis is managed by avoidance of allergens, use of pharmacologic agents (antihistamines, leukotriene inhibitors, or corticosteroids), or immunotherapy. Parents usually ask how sick children should be before they need to see an allergist about skin testing and definite treatment (an expensive, time-consuming, and potentially painful procedure). Individual circumstances dictate the direction of treatment. As a rule, a child whose symptoms are increasing in intensity, who has associated lower respiratory tract involvement, or whose condition interferes with activities in which he or she wants to participate needs definitive testing and treatment. Others can be managed by environmental control and medications to reduce symptoms.

Intranasal corticosteroids are effective in reducing symptoms in most children. Caution children and parents that antihistamines tend to cause sleepiness. Assess if this will interfere with schoolwork. Be certain that parents understand that if nasal antihistamine sprays are given for more than 3 days, a rebound effect may occur (the nasal mucosa becomes more edematous rather than less edematous). If symptoms are so severe that they interfere with the child's ability to function in school, skin testing to locate individual allergens may be prescribed. Once identified, hyposensitization therapy against the responsible allergens can be initiated.

Avoidance of allergens is rather ineffective with allergic rhinitis. If children always show symptoms at one particular time of the year, parents may be able to carry out environmental control for that period of the year. Some children with allergic rhinitis are more comfortable in air-conditioned buildings; others have strong symptoms in the presence of air conditioning (probably accounting for the high incidence of headaches that occur at school; Galant & Wilkinson, 2001).

Allergic rhinitis is often considered a minor illness by parents, something that children will grow out of. However, for children who have the condition, it may not be a minor illness and it may keep them from interacting with other children during certain months because they dread going outside and initiating symptoms. Help parents understand the importance of avoiding allergens and the need for conscientious administration of intranasal corticosteroids or antihistamines to minimize symptoms.

Perennial Allergic Rhinitis

Allergic rhinitis becomes perennial (year-round) when the allergen is one that is capable of affecting the child year-round, such as house dust mites or pet hair. Although the child's symptoms may not result in the obvious distress associated with seasonal allergic rhinitis, the child needs treatment just as much because the symptoms occur constantly. Because the agent that causes perennial allergic rhinitis is often house dust, environmental control plays a big role in the control of the disorder. Serous otitis media may be a serious consequence of perennial allergic rhinitis (see Chap. 50).

Atopic Dermatitis (Infantile Eczema)

Atopic dermatitis is primarily a disease of infants, beginning as early as the second month of life and possibly lasting until age 2 to 3 years. Apparently, it is primarily related to a food allergy because it tends to occur more often in formula-fed infants than in breast-fed infants and more frequently if infants are fed solid food before 6 months. Sweating, heat, tight clothing, and contact irritants such as soap increase the pruritus. Symptoms may be more annoying in the winter, when additional irritating clothing is present, with marked improvement in the summer.

Assessment

With infantile atopic dermatitis, capillary permeability increases, causing a loss of serous fluid out into the tissues. Children develop papular and vesicular skin eruptions with surrounding erythema. The vesicles rupture and exude yellow, sticky secretions that form crusts on the skin as they dry. Because the lesions are extremely pruritic, the child scratches and further irritates the lesions, causing linear excoriations. Secondary infections of open lesions may then occur. As the infected lesions heal, the skin becomes depigmented and lichenified (shiny), and dry, flaky scales form. If secondary infection occurs, local lymph nodes will be swollen. The child may have a low-grade fever. An increased eosinophil count revealing that the condition is allergy-based will be present in blood serum.

The common sites for lesions include the scalp and forehead, the cheeks, neck, behind the ears, and the extensor surfaces of the extremities (Fig. 42-6). The palms of the hands and the soles of the feet are uninvolved. Because the lesions are uncomfortable, children with infantile atopic

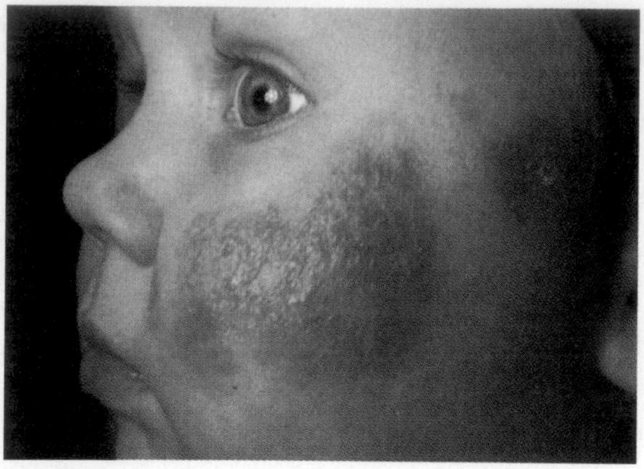

FIGURE 42.6 Infant with atopic dermatitis.

dermatitis may be overly fussy and irritable. They may not eat well due to this discomfort.

Although infantile atopic dermatitis is generally diagnosed while taking the family history (considering other allergic individuals in the family) and noticing the characteristic lesions and their patterns, it is sometimes difficult to distinguish it from seborrheic dermatitis (cradle cap; see Chap. 23). The findings in seborrheic dermatitis and infantile atopic dermatitis are compared in Table 42-5. Seborrheic dermatitis is a fairly benign condition of infants, requiring little treatment other than frequent shampooing of the hair and soaking the lesions in mineral oil and combing them away. A child with infantile atopic dermatitis, on the other hand, will not respond to these measures but must be referred for additional treatment. Also, children with infantile atopic dermatitis should have a repeat test for phenylketonuria (PKU) done because children with PKU often have atopic dermatitis.

Skin testing is ineffective because the allergen causing infantile atopic dermatitis is often a food allergen. However, it may also be caused by pollens, dust, or mold spores. For this reason, skin testing may be attempted to isolate a causative allergen.

Therapeutic Management

The treatment of atopic dermatitis is aimed at reducing the amount of allergen exposure, if such allergens can be identified. The most likely foods to which infants are allergic are milk, eggs, wheat, chocolate, fish, tomatoes, and peanuts. The use of elimination diets to identify food allergens is discussed later in this chapter. A second major consideration in treatment is aimed at reducing pruritus so children do not irritate lesions and cause secondary infections by scratching. Hydrating the skin by bathing or applying wet dressings (wet with tap water or Burow's solution) for 15 to 20 minutes, followed by application of a hydrating emollient such as petroleum jelly (Vaseline) or vegetable shortening (Crisco), is helpful (Boguniewicz & Leung, 2001). Do not allow infants to become chilled if a large portion of the body is to be covered with wet dressings. A stockinette dressing with holes cut out for the eyes, nose, and mouth pulled over the head will hold wet dressings in place on the face and neck. To prevent corneal irritation, be careful that such dressings do not come in contact with the eyes.

Some infants need an antihistamine to reduce itching. Topical steroids such as 1% hydrocortisone cream do a great deal to relieve the discomfort and appearance of lesions by reducing the inflammation and pruritus. If the lesions are dry, a corticosteroid ointment is most effective. If moist, a lotion may be most effective. Applying the cream or lotion and then covering the area with an occlusive dressing such as plastic wrap overnight may speed the healing process. If the lesions are secondarily infected, hydrocortisone mixed with an antibiotic (generally neomycin) and a suitable base is prescribed. Caution parents not to discontinue application of cortisone cream abruptly. Although absorption with topical application is limited, some does occur. This reduces adrenal gland functioning. If the cream is discontinued abruptly, the infant's adrenal response (ability to produce epinephrine) in an emergency might be limited. Also caution the parents not to overuse the cortisone cream. More is not better and may increase the risk of systemic absorption.

TABLE 42.5 Comparison of Seborrheic Dermatitis and Atopic Dermatitis

FINDING	SEBORRHEIC DERMATITIS	ATOPIC DERMATITIS
Age at onset	0–6 months	2–6 months
Length of disease	Rarely 1 year	2–3 years
Mood of child	Happy; parents happy	Irritable; parents tired
Location of lesions	Scalp, behind ears, near umbilicus	Cheeks, extensor surfaces, some flexor surfaces
Types of lesions	Salmon-colored erythematous lesions with greasy scales	Papulovesicular erythematous lesions with weeping and crusting
Itching	No	Severe
Depigmentation	No	Yes
Lichenification	No	Yes
White dermographism	No	Yes
Eosinophilia	No nasal mucus or blood eosinophilia	Nasal mucus or blood eosinophilia
IgE serum levels	Low	High

NURSING DIAGNOSES AND RELATED INTERVENTIONS

Nursing Diagnosis: Risk for impaired parenting related to feelings of inadequacy secondary to infant's chronic atopic dermatitis

Outcome Identification: Parents will demonstrate positive attachment behaviors throughout course of illness.

Outcome Evaluation: Parents express confidence in their ability to follow recommended therapy; express positive aspects of infant; hold infant close and smile and talk to infant.

Parents of children with infantile atopic dermatitis need a great deal of support through the course of the disease because children can be irritable from the constant pruritus. No matter how hard parents try, they cannot seem to make them happy. Parents need a listening ear so they can vent these concerns and maintain their self-esteem as parents. Support groups also can help meet this need.

Nursing Diagnosis: Impaired skin integrity related to infantile atopic dermatitis

Outcome Identification: Infant will demonstrate improved skin appearance by 2 weeks.

Outcome Evaluation: Infant does not scratch lesions; parents state infant is less irritable and easier to care for. Lesions show signs of healing.

When lesions begin to heal, a skin emollient and moisturizer, such as Eucerin, or baths with a substance to lubricate the skin, such as Alpha-Keri, are prescribed to prevent excessive skin dryness. The infant should soak in the bath with the lubricant for approximately 15 minutes, then be patted, not rubbed, dry so the lesions are not aggravated. Caution parents not to use soap because it can be drying.

Suggest that parents trim the infant's fingernails short or cover his or her hands with cotton socks to prevent scratching. Exposure to the herpes virus can cause a generalized reaction. Caution parents to screen babysitters or alert child care personnel with active herpes lesions not to care for their infants while atopic dermatitis is active.

In most infants, the lesions of infantile atopic dermatitis clear by the time the child is 3 years old. Unless secondary infection with scarring results, the skin surface will not be marked. Many of these children go on to develop other allergies, however, as they grow older. In the preschool years, the child's parents may report that the child has "one cold after another" (allergic rhinitis). By early school years, the child may show signs of asthma (see Chap. 40).

Atopic Dermatitis in the Older Child

Atopic dermatitis in the older child may occur at any age, but frequently it occurs at puberty or late adolescence. Atopic dermatitis that occurs at these later ages is prominent on the flexor surface of the extremities and on the dorsal surfaces of the wrists and ankles. It often occurs in the eyebrows; if the child scratches the lesions, the child may be left with scant eyebrows. Depigmentation or hyperpigmentation is usually present, and lichenification is marked. The fingernails often have a glossy sheen from the buffing action of constant rubbing and scratching. In some children, an itch–scratch cycle in response to stress may lead to an exacerbation of symptoms. For example, a child begins to feel pressured in school or upset because he or she is left out of the neighborhood group of children. The child rubs his or her skin, a nervous, comforting mannerism, and the rubbing or scratching leads to irritation of lesions. Then the lesions itch, and the child scratches vigorously because of discomfort. The more the child scratches, the worse the lesions become; the more lesions there are, the more the child scratches, and so on.

WHAT IF? What if a school-age child's atopic dermatitis is worse every December and every June at the end of school semesters? What might you suspect as the cause of an itch–scratch cycle at this time?

Therapeutic Management

Atopic dermatitis is a difficult disease for older children. Because they can see that the scratching leads to depigmentation or lichenification, they know they should stop scratching to keep the disorder under control. The itching is so intense, however, that they wake at night scratching and cannot stop. Adolescents are acutely aware of their appearance, so this is an especially difficult illness for them. Suggest they not use soap or use only a prescription soap to prevent skin drying. They should avoid swimming in chlorinated pools. Encourage other summer sports if possible. If children are required to swim in school, encourage them to shower well to remove chlorine from the skin and apply a skin emollient and moisturizer such as Eucerin after swimming. After a period of activity in which sweating occurs, suggest that the child take a shower to remove perspiration, which is irritating to skin. Avoiding tight clothing at the flexor portions of the extremities may also help. Caution children not to use medication intended for acne cover-up on atopic dermatitis lesions because these medications are designed to dry the skin.

Medical treatment is basically the same as for the infant with atopic dermatitis: keeping the skin hydrated and identifying allergens and any psychological problems that are initiating an itch–scratch cycle. Application of hydrocortisone cream can make a big difference in helping lesions improve (see Focus on Nursing Care Planning).

Evaluation for the older child with atopic dermatitis should include evaluating how well the lesions are healing and also how well the child is adjusting to school and family. A child who enters adulthood with poor self-esteem because of a chronic allergic disorder during childhood will probably have difficulty achieving a high level of wellness.

✔ CHECKPOINT QUESTIONS

9. What is the probable cause of atopic dermatitis in infants?
10. In the older child, what body parts are typically affected by atopic dermatitis?

FOCUS ON *Nursing Care Planning*

AN OLDER CHILD WITH ATOPIC DERMATITIS

A 13-year-old girl comes to the clinic reporting severe itching on her arms and ankles. "These sores are so ugly, but I just can't stop scratching."

Assessment: 13-year-old girl with papular and vesicular lesions with erythematous base noted on flexor surfaces of both arms and dorsal aspect of both ankles. Four lesions on arms with yellow exudate. Some hyperpigmentation and lichenification present. Nails glossy. States she has pruritus followed by scratching, followed by increased pruritus with more scratching. She states, "Sometimes it wakes me up at night." During interview, client states, "It's a good thing that I didn't make cheerleader even though all my friends did. How could I wear that outfit with these ugly things?" When questioned further, client reported being upset about not becoming a cheerleader. Itching and lesions started shortly after.

Nursing Diagnosis: Situational low self-esteem related to feelings of inadequacy and embarrassment

Outcome Identification: Client will verbalize positive feelings about herself.

Outcome Evaluation: Client states impact of lesions and not becoming cheerleader on appearance and self-esteem; actively discusses feelings and concerns; participates actively in care measures; reports some degree of control over the itching.

Interventions	Rationale
1. Attempt to identify the meaning of making cheerleader, her appearance, and presence of lesions.	1. Identifying the meaning of making cheerleader, appearance, and lesions assists in determining the degree of impact that a diagnosis of atopic dermatitis may have on the client.
2. Encourage client to express feelings and thoughts about herself, her appearance, and not becoming a cheerleader.	2. Sharing of feelings and concerns permits a safe outlet for emotions and also aids in highlighting client's awareness of possible impact on self-esteem.
3. Review and reinforce with client positive attributes about self.	3. Positive attributes provide a foundation for rebuilding self-esteem.
4. Clarify any misconceptions client may have about her appearance or the lesions. Inform client that with treatment the lesions will heal.	4. Misconceptions can reduce self-esteem. Providing information helps to alleviate possible anxiety related to any misconceptions and lack of knowledge.
5. Instruct client in measures to promote comfort, relieve itching, and promote healing.	5. Comfort promotion helps to minimize the effects of the lesions.
6. Assist with measures to increase independent role functioning and encourage active participation in decision making.	6. Independence and ability to perform one's role promote self-esteem; active participation enhances the feeling of control over situations.
7. Assist client with finding an appropriate alternative activity to cheerleading.	7. An alternative activity provides the client with a sense of accomplishment, helping to promote self-esteem.

Nursing Diagnosis: Impaired skin integrity related to lesions resulting from itching and scratching

Outcome Identification: Client will exhibit signs of healing lesions within 2 weeks.

Outcome Evaluation: Lesions are decreased in number, becoming pale without exudate. No new lesions are present. Client reports diminished itching with no scratching; demonstrates appropriate skin care measures.

(continued)

Interventions	Rationale
1. Assess the lesions for number, color, location, distribution, and drainage.	1. Assessment provides a baseline for evaluating the effectiveness of interventions.
2. Encourage the client to refrain from scratching.	2. Scratching lesions perpetuates the itch-scratch cycle, possibly leading to additional lesion formation and possible infection.
3. Instruct client in measures to decrease the itching, such as cool moist compresses, light patting rather than scratching, and distraction techniques.	3. Reducing the itch minimizes the risk for further scratching and subsequent lesion formation.
4. Teach client how to apply wet dressings and topical corticosteroids with nighttime occlusive dressings.	4. Wet dressings help to hydrate the skin and decrease pruritus. Topical corticosteroids reduce inflammation. Occlusive dressings may speed the healing process.
5. Advise client to avoid commercial soaps and to use a prescription soap only when washing.	5. Soap dries the skin, increasing the possibility for itching.
6. Encourage the client to shower after swimming in chlorinated pools and after any activities that cause perspiration. Suggest use of an emollient moisturizer afterward.	6. Chlorine is drying to the skin. Sweat irritates the skin. An emollient adds moisture to the skin, decreasing the risk for irritation.
7. Urge the client to avoid tight clothing over affected areas.	7. Tight clothing interferes with the evaporation of moisture, increasing the risk for further irritation.
8. Arrange for a follow-up appointment in 2 weeks.	8. Follow-up appointment allows for evaluation of the client's progress and reinstruction if necessary.

DRUG AND FOOD ALLERGIES

Drug Allergies

One of the hazards of giving any medication is the danger that a child may experience a reaction to it or exhibit allergic symptoms. Because reactions to drugs differ, it is important to be familiar with whether a child is showing symptoms of an allergic reaction, a toxic reaction, or a known side effect to a drug.

A toxic reaction is one that occurs when a child has received too much of a drug. Side effects of drugs are those that are known to occur in addition to a therapeutic effect. When an allergic effect occurs, unpredictable symptoms occur. The drug itself may not be an allergen, but when the drug combines with body protein, it becomes an allergen. This is why allergic responses occur not with the initial administration of a drug but only after the protein interaction (hapten formation or sensitivity) has occurred. When drugs are applied to skin or mucous membrane, the chance of a drug allergy is highest. With the exception of acetylsalicylic acid (aspirin), allergy occurs rarely to orally administered drugs. Children with atopic diseases appear to be most prone to allergic drug reactions, although anyone can have such a reaction.

Reactions to drugs differ, but skin manifestations seen frequently include urticaria, angioedema, allergic contact dermatitis, pruritus, and purpura. Respiratory symptoms include wheezing or rhinitis. There may be thrombocytopenia and hemolytic anemia. Anaphylactic shock and serum sickness may occur. Children with a known drug allergy should wear a medical identification bracelet indicating the drug to which they are sensitive (Huang, 2000).

Drugs used in children that are frequently involved in allergic reactions include parenteral penicillin and vaccines. In most instances, just discontinuing the drug and never again administering the vaccine is the only therapy needed. If urticaria or serum sickness occurs, an antihistamine (such as diphenhydramine hydrochloride [Benadryl]) is needed to relieve the symptoms. If anaphylaxis results, the treatment would be the same as for any anaphylaxis.

Food Allergies

Food allergies manifest themselves differently from one child to another, but urticaria, angioedema, pruritus, stomach pain, colic, cramps, diarrhea, respiratory symptoms, and atopic dermatitis are common symptoms.

A symptom such as urticaria begins to manifest itself only minutes after an offending food is eaten. Other symptoms may be delayed, making the offending food difficult to recognize. Whole protein is probably the cause of immediate reactions, whereas delayed reactions are the result of a sensitivity to some protein breakdown product.

Skin testing is unreliable with food allergies because it is done with whole protein extracts. Delayed reactions, therefore, will not be detected this way. The most common foods that cause immediate allergy symptoms include egg white, fish and other seafood, berries, and nuts. Delayed food reactions are commonly caused by cereals (wheat and corn), milk, chocolate, pork, legumes, white potatoes, beef, food additives and colorings, and oranges. If children are allergic to milk, they are probably allergic to milk products as well. Children who are allergic to eggs often cannot eat any foods that contain egg, such as pudding or baked goods (Burks, 2000).

Assessment

Young children cannot describe why they do not enjoy eating because they do not know the word for "headache," "stomachache," or "itchiness," but they tend to avoid the foods that affect them. This gives them a reputation of being "fussy eaters." This is not diagnostic of food allergies, however, because children may refuse to eat foods as a form of toddler rebellion or may be reported as fussy eaters because parents are expecting them to eat more than their small size requires.

Encouraging the child or parents to keep a food diary or a record of everything the child eats each day often is the best way to spot offending foods. They should note the presence of symptoms, if any. A food that is found on lists when symptoms were few, but not on days when the child is in distress, is not an offending food. A food that appears only on "bad days," however, can be strongly suspected as an allergen.

An elimination diet is another method that can be used to detect food allergens. For this, parents feed the child only foods that rarely cause allergy, such as rice, lamb, carrots, peas, and sweet potatoes, for about 7 days. Then they add, one by one, at 2- to 3-day intervals, foods that are suspected of causing allergy. When a food is introduced this way, the child must be encouraged to eat a lot of it that day. If symptoms occur, the food is then eliminated from the child's meals on a permanent basis. If no symptoms occur, the child can continue to eat the food.

Therapeutic Management

The treatment of food allergy is to eliminate offending foods from the child's diet. This is relatively easy to do if there are only a few offending foods, but it becomes difficult when the foods are great in number or, like milk, wheat, or eggs, are found in many products. Parents should become careful shoppers, reading labels carefully to be certain that the foods they are buying do not contain products to which their child is sensitive. Help school-age children learn to choose foods they can safely eat at the school cafeteria or at summer camp.

Milk Allergy

The true incidence of milk allergy is probably not as high as the number of diagnoses made. Milk allergy is typified by failure to gain weight, diarrhea, perhaps vomiting, and abdominal pain. These symptoms may also occur in a gastroenteritis infection. Some infants with colic (characterized by abdominal pain, no change in stools, and no failure to gain weight) or those with lactase deficiency (they cannot ingest the lactose in milk) may also be incorrectly diagnosed as having a milk allergy. If milk allergy is suspected, children are given a casein hydrolysate formula. When this is done, symptoms are relieved dramatically. To establish whether the cause of the problem was truly a milk allergy, milk should be reintroduced at a later date. If the problem was a true milk allergy, signs will recur at this reintroduction to milk.

STINGING INSECT ALLERGY

Children may have severe hypersensitivity reactions to stings from bees, wasps, hornets, or yellow jackets. Although a serum sickness reaction may occur, the usual reaction to these stings is an immediate type I hypersensitivity reaction (anaphylaxis). The peak season for insect stings is summer, and more boys than girls have allergic reactions to insect stings (Bahna, 2000).

Assessment

The first time a child is stung, the total reaction is probably only local edema at the site. The second time, generalized urticaria, pruritus, and edema may develop. The third time, symptoms may progress to wheezing and dyspnea. The next time, the reaction could be so severe that shock and death result. The progression of symptoms may be slower than this (involving 10 to 12 stings); if the stings are received close together (1 or 2 days apart, or even 3 weeks apart), the progression to fatal symptoms may occur as early as the second or third exposure.

The time interval between the fatal sting and death is extremely short, approximately 10 minutes. For this reason, these children must be identified and given medication to combat shock immediately (there is no time to transport them for emergency care).

Therapeutic Management

The best way to protect children with allergies to stinging insects is to begin hyposensitization against insect stings after the first reaction. An extract of wasp, yellow jacket, hornet, and honeybee accomplishes this.

The child who has not been hyposensitized must be treated immediately after the sting. This can be done by subcutaneous injection of epinephrine, which will give rapid relief (EpiPens are available for self-injection; see the Focus on Family Empowerment earlier in this chapter). If the child is going on a hiking or camping expedition away from parents, caution parents that the child will need to learn to administer this to himself or herself, or be certain that a responsible adult accompanying the child will be able to do it. Someone at school should be given the responsibility of administering this if the child is stung during recess or an outside gym period. If a school nurse is in attendance, this certainly is his or her job. In schools where there is no full-time nurse, another person must be designated and taught how to give the injection. If the child has antihistamine medication in addition to epinephrine, this should be given also. Ice applied to the site minimizes the amount of venom absorbed. The child should then be transported to the nearest hospital in case additional epinephrine is needed (the effectiveness of the initial injection will last only approximately 20 minutes).

Teach children who are allergic to stinging insects not to wear scented preparations such as hair spray, deodorants, lotions, or perfume because these attract bees and wasps. They should not go outside barefoot because bees are often found in ground cover. They should not be assigned household chores such as mowing the lawn or weeding the garden, actions that might stir up bees. Because insects tend to cluster around garbage containers, taking out the trash is also an inappropriate chore for these children. Encourage the child to refrain from drinking from open soda cans at picnics and outside activities; bees and wasps are drawn to the sugar in the soda, and the child may be unaware that an insect has entered the open can. Caution the child to have a fast-acting insecticide handy when out of doors to use on flying insects (Klinek, 2000).

CONTACT DERMATITIS

Contact dermatitis is an example of a delayed or type IV hypersensitivity response; it is a reaction to skin contact with an allergen (a substance irritating only to the child with prior sensitization). The first reaction is generally erythema, followed by intensely pruritic papules and then vesicles. The allergen causing the irritation is often suggested by the part of the child's body that is affected. For example, dermatitis from a diaper-washing compound appears in the diaper area. Allergy to cosmetics appears on the face. Oozing at the site of pierced ears suggests an allergy to the nickel used in earring posts. Poison ivy appears on the hands and arms where the child brushed against the plant (Fig. 42-7). Many children as well as health care providers are developing reactions to latex gloves (Charous et al., 2002). Footwear, because of the chemicals used to tan leather, is also a frequent offender.

WHAT IF? What if an adolescent who is allergic to leather develops an erythematous, pruritic area on his right buttock? What would be a likely object causing the irritation? How would you help determine the cause?

Assessment

Patch testing may be used to identify contact dermatitis allergens. A child should not take a corticosteroid at the time of patch testing because these drugs reduce delayed hypersensitivity reactions. However, the child may take antihistamines or sympathomimetic drugs because these do not interfere with delayed reactions. After 48 hours, the patches are removed and the reactions are graded 1+ to 4+, the same as in regular skin testing.

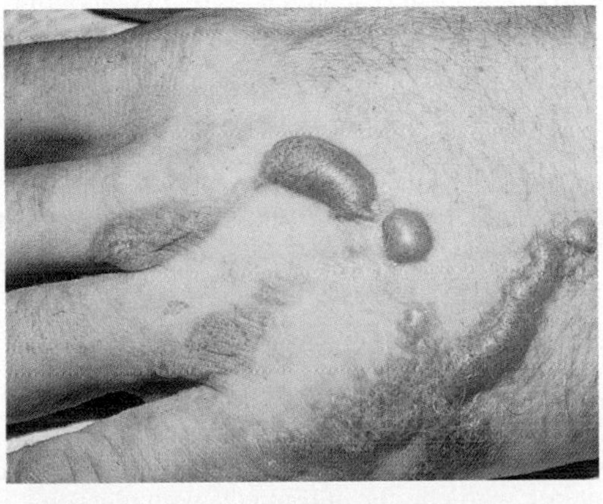

FIGURE 42.7 Poison ivy on a child's hand.

Therapeutic Management

Treatment for contact dermatitis consists of removing the identified allergen from the child's environment. In children, this is generally not difficult to do. In adults, because allergens are often job-related, this is much more difficult.

Dressings wet with water, saline, or Burow's solution relieve itching. Calamine or Caladryl lotion is a standby that is also generally effective. Hydrocortisone lotions or creams reduce itching and also promote healing. Baths with baking soda or oatmeal in the water may be helpful if a large area of the body is involved. Some children need a sedative to relieve their discomfort during the period of intense pruritus.

✔ CHECKPOINT QUESTIONS

11. How is a food allergy usually treated?
12. What type of testing is used to identify the allergen of contact dermatitis?

KEY POINTS

An antigen is a foreign substance capable of stimulating an immune response. The immune system protects the body from invasion by foreign substances.

Humoral immunity refers to immunity created by antibody production. B lymphocytes are involved in this type of reaction. Cell-mediated immunity refers to T-lymphocyte involvement.

Autoimmunity results from an inability to distinguish self from nonself, causing the immune system to carry out immune responses against normal cells.

Immunodeficiency disorders can be primary, such as B-lymphocyte and T-lymphocyte deficiencies, or secondary, such as acquired immunodeficiency syndrome (AIDS). HIV/AIDS is spread by the retrovirus HIV through blood and body secretions. Conscientious use of standard precautions is essential to prevent transmission.

Allergic disorders occur as a result of an abnormal antigen–antibody response. As many as 15% of children have some form of allergy.

Immune disorders, as a category, are long-term disorders, and children must participate in their own care to remain well (e.g., avoiding allergens, conscientiously taking an antihistamine). Involving children from the start helps them play an active role in their own care.

Anaphylactic shock is an acute type I hypersensitivity reaction characterized by extreme vasodilation and bronchoconstriction. If action is not taken immediately, the reaction can be fatal.

Environmental control refers to ways to reduce the number of allergens to which children are exposed. Hyposensitization is a method to increase the plasma concentration of IgG antibodies to prevent or block IgE antibody formation and allergic symptoms.

Atopic disorders include allergic rhinitis (hay fever), atopic dermatitis, and asthma.

Promoting breast-feeding and delaying the introduction of solid foods until at least age 6 months may be prime interventions to help prevent food allergies in allergy-prone families.

CRITICAL THINKING EXERCISES

1. Dexter, the boy you met at the beginning of the chapter, was diagnosed as having allergic rhinitis. His symptoms start when he arrives at school. Knowing this problem is worse at school, what environmental control measures would you want to suggest for Dexter?
2. An infant you see has atopic dermatitis (infantile eczema). Almost her entire face is covered with weeping, crusting lesions. Her forehead is lined with scratch marks. Her mother is obviously exhausted. She tells you her baby never sleeps because of the constant itching. What suggestions could you make to the mother to help make her infant more comfortable? What would you suggest she do for herself?
3. A 4-year-old child has a primary B-lymphocyte immune deficiency. His teacher calls you because she is afraid to have him in her classroom because he will spread the HIV virus to classmates. What would you want to explain to the child's teacher about immune deficiency disorders?
4. Examine the National Health Goals related to immune disorders in children. Most government-sponsored money for nursing research is allotted based on these goals. What would be a possible research topic to explore pertinent to these goals that would be fundable and would advance evidence-based practice?

REFERENCES

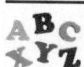

Alp, H. et al. (2001). Cockroach allergy appears early in life in inner-city children with recurrent wheezing. *Annals of Allergy, Asthma & Immunology, 86*(1), 51–54.

Bahna, S. L. (2000). Insect sting allergy: A matter of life and death. *Pediatric Annals, 29*(12), 753–759.

Bartlett, J. A. (2002). Addressing the challenges of adherence. *Journal of Acquired Immune Deficiency Syndromes, 29*(2), S2–S10.

Boguniewicz, M., & Leung, D. Y. M. (2001). Major allergic disorders seen in pediatric practice. In W. W. Hay, A. R. Hayward, M. J. Levin, & J. M. Sondheimer (Eds.). *Current pediatric diagnosis and treatment* (15th ed.). New York: McGraw-Hill.

Burks, W. (2000). Diagnosis of allergic reactions to food. *Pediatric Annals, 29*(12), 744–752.

Centers for Disease Control & Prevention (2001). *HIV/AIDS recommendations.* Washington, DC: CDC.

Charous, B. L. et al. (2002). Natural rubber latex allergy after 12 years: Recommendations and perspectives. *Journal of Allergy & Clinical Immunology, 109*(1), 31–34.

Department of Health and Human Services (2000). *Healthy people, 2010.* Washington, D.C.: DHHS.

Frank, M. M. (2000). Complement deficiencies. *Pediatric Clinics of North America, 47*(6), 1339–1354.

Galant, S. P., & Wilkinson, R. (2001). Clinical prescribing of allergic rhinitis medication in the preschool and young school-age child: What are the options? *Biodrugs, 15*(7), 453–463.

Horwitz, M. E. (2000). Stem-cell transplantation for inherited immunodeficiency disorders. *Pediatric Clinics of North America, 47*(6), 1371–1387.

Huang, S. (2000). Drug allergy in children. *Pediatric Annals, 29*(12), 760–767.

Klinek, M. M. (2000). Insect sting reactions. In M. W. Schwartz (Ed.). *The 5-minute pediatric consult* (pp. 480–481). Philadelphia: Lippincott Williams & Wilkins.

McFarland, E. J. (2001). Human immunodeficiency virus (HIV) infection. In W. W. Hay, A. R. Hayward, M. J. Levin, & J. M. Sondheimer (Eds.). *Current pediatric diagnosis and treatment* (15th ed.). New York: McGraw-Hill.

Merchant, R. C., & Keshavarz, R. (2001). Human immunodeficiency virus postexposure prophylaxis for adolescents and children. *Pediatrics, 108*(2), 38–45.

Nielsen, K., & Bryson, Y. J. (2000). Diagnosis of HIV infection in children. *Pediatric Clinics of North America, 47*(1), 39–63.

Pajno, G. B., et al. (2000). Clinical and immunologic effects of long-term sublingual immunotherapy in asthmatic children sensitized to mites: A double-blind, placebo-controlled study. *Allergy, 55*(9), 842–849.

Rote, N. S. (2002). Immunity. In K. L. McCance & S. E. Huether. *Pathophysiology* (4th ed.). St. Louis: Mosby.

Rudy, B. J. (2000). Immune deficiency. In M. W. Schwartz (Ed.). *The 5-minute pediatric consult* (pp. 462–463). Philadelphia: Lippincott Williams & Wilkins.

Salerno, D. (2000). Serum sickness. In M. W. Schwartz (Ed.). *The 5-minute pediatric consult* (pp. 744–745). Philadelphia: Lippincott Williams & Wilkins.

Schwartz, S. A. (2000). Intravenous immunoglobulin treatment of immunodeficiency disorders. *Pediatric Clinics of North America, 47*(6), 1355–1369.

Smith, C. A. (2000). The allergic child. In M. W. Schwartz (Ed.). *The 5-minute pediatric consult* (pp. 8–9). Philadelphia: Lippincott Williams & Wilkins.

Zumla, A. et al. (2000). Impact of HIV infection on tuberculosis. *Postgraduate Medical Journal, 76*(895), 259–268.

SUGGESTED READINGS

Alles, R., et al. (2001). The prevalence of atopic disorders in children with chronic otitis media with effusion. *Pediatric Allergy & Immunology, 12*(2), 102–106.

Curtis, J. (2000). Insect sting anaphylaxis. *Pediatrics in Review, 21*(8), 256–261.

Downs, S. H., et al. (2001). Continued increase in the prevalence of asthma and atopy. *Archives of Disease in Childhood, 84*(1), 20–23.

Elder, M. E. (2000). T-cell immunodeficiencies. *Pediatric Clinics of North America, 47*(6), 1253–1274.

Fields-Gardner, C., & Ayoob, K. T. (2000). Nutrition intervention in the care of persons with human immunodeficiency virus infection. *Journal of the American Dietetic Association, 100*(6), 708-717.

Fiocchi, A., et al. (2001). Severe anaphylaxis induced by latex as a contaminant of plastic balls in play pits. *Journal of Allergy & Clinical Immunology, 108*(2), 298–300.

Gaudreau, J. M. (2000). The challenge of making the school environment safe for children with food allergies. *Journal of School Nursing, 16*(2), 5–10.

Gunther, K. P., et al. (2000). Allergic reactions to latex in myelodysplasia. A review of the literature. *Journal of Pediatric Orthopaedics, 9*(3), 180–184.

Lack, G. (2001). Pediatric allergic rhinitis and comorbid disorders. *Journal of Allergy & Clinical Immunology, 108*(1 Suppl), S9–S15.

Meltzer, E. O. (2001). Quality of life in adults and children with allergic rhinitis. *Journal of Allergy and Clinical Immunology, 108*(1), S45–S53.

Nelson, E. (2001). The miseries of passive smoking. *Human & Experimental Toxicology, 20*(2), 61–83.

Scadding, G. K. (2001). Corticosteroids in the treatment of pediatric allergic rhinitis. *Journal of Allergy & Clinical Immunology, 108*(1 Suppl), S59–S64.

Solomon, W. R. (1999). Nasal allergy: More than sneezing and a runny nose. *Contemporary Pediatrics, 16*(8), 114–122.

Sorensen, R. U., & Moore, C. (2000). Antibody deficiency syndromes. *Pediatric Clinics of North America, 47*(6), 1225–1252.

Weber, R W. (2002). Atopic persons sensitive to cat dander. *Annals of Allergy, Asthma & Immunology, 88*(1), 4–6.

Ylitalo, L., et al. (2000). Natural rubber latex allergy in children: A follow-up study. *Clinical & Experimental Allergy, 30*(11), 1611-1617..

43

CHAPTER

Nursing Care of the Child With an Infectious Disorder

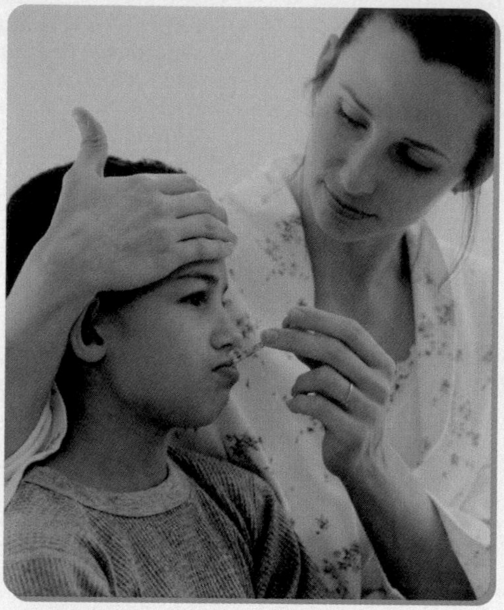

Key Terms

- catarrhal stage
- chain of infection
- complement
- convalescent period
- enanthem
- exanthem
- exotoxin
- fomites
- incubation period
- interferon
- Koplik's spots
- means of transmission
- portal of entry
- portal of exit
- prodromal period
- reservoir
- septicemia
- susceptible host

Objectives

After mastering the contents of this chapter, you should be able to:

1. Describe the causes and course of common infectious disorders of childhood.
2. Assess the child with an infectious disorder.
3. Formulate nursing diagnoses for the child with an infectious disorder.
4. Establish outcomes for the care of a child with an infectious disorder.
5. Plan nursing care for the child with an infectious disorder.
6. Implement nursing care specific to the child with an infectious disorder.
7. Evaluate outcomes for achievement and effectiveness of care for the child with an infectious disorder.
8. Identify National Health Goals related to infectious disorders in children that nurses could be instrumental in helping the nation achieve.
9. Identify areas of nursing care related to children with infectious disease that could benefit from additional nursing research or application of evidence-based practice.
10. Use critical thinking to analyze ways that care of the child with an infectious disorder could be more family-centered.
11. Integrate knowledge of infectious diseases and nursing process to achieve quality maternal and child health nursing care.

Marty, a 10-year-old boy, was admitted to the hospital for appendicitis. The morning after surgery, his chest was covered by a very itchy, red, macular rash. By afternoon, some of the lesions had turned to papules. By the next morning, the lesions had changed to vesicles, and a number were crusting. Marty was diagnosed as having chickenpox. "How could this have happened?" his mother asks you. "I thought that he was too old to get this. That's why I didn't get him the vaccine." What advice would you give his mother? Is it likely that Marty contracted this while he was in the hospital, or before he was admitted? What action would you recommend to help reduce the itching?

Previous chapters described growth and development of well children. This chapter adds information about the dramatic changes, both physical and psychosocial, that can occur when children contract an infectious disorder. This is important information because it builds a base for care and health teaching.

After you've studied the chapter, answer the Critical Thinking Exercises at the end of the chapter and then access the on-line study activities (www.connection.lww.com) *to further sharpen your skills and test your knowledge.*

Despite the number of preventive measures available, infectious disease remains a leading cause of morbidity in children (Ogle & Anderson, 2001). Nurses play a key role in educating parents and the public about common childhood infectious disorders and appropriate preventive steps. They must be able to identify the symptoms of common infectious diseases of childhood, because nurses are often the first to see evidence of infection. For example, a school nurse is asked to be an expert on screening children for potentially communicable infections such as impetigo or tinea capitis (ringworm). In health care settings, nurses often perform triage, identifying children who must be seen immediately, those who can wait to be seen, and those who should not stay in a waiting room with other children because they may have an infectious disorder. Occasionally, children admitted to an inpatient unit develop diarrhea soon after admission. It is vital that a nurse quickly recognize that this could be contagious so other children in the hospital, especially those who are immunosuppressed, can be protected.

Several National Health Goals related to the prevention of infectious disorders in children have been developed. These are shown in the Focus on National Health Goals box.

FOCUS ON NATIONAL HEALTH GOALS

Several National Health Goals address the prevention and reduction of occurrence of infectious diseases. Examples of these include the following:

- Reduce Lyme disease from a baseline of 17.4 new cases/100,000 to a target of 9.7 new cases/100,000 population.
- Reduce hospital-acquired central-line-associated bloodstream infection of people in intensive care units from 5.3/1,000 days stay to 4.8/1,000 days stay.
- Achieve and maintain effective vaccination coverage levels for universally recommended vaccines among young children such as varicella vaccine from a baseline of 43% to a target level of 90% (DHHS, 2000).

Nurses can be instrumental in helping the nation achieve these goals by educating parents about the importance of immunizations and ways to avoid diseases such as Lyme disease. They can be instrumental in helping prevent the spread of infection in hospital units by adhering to infection control precautions.

Nursing research that could increase understanding in this area includes studies aimed at answering questions such as: What precautions can summer camps or camp sites take to discourage children from petting wild animals or being exposed to ticks? What information do parents need to help them obtain full immunizations for children? What orientation do new staff nurses need to help them learn or better follow infection prevention techniques?

NURSING PROCESS OVERVIEW

For the Child With an Infectious Disorder

Assessment

Many infectious diseases begin subtly. Parents report symptoms such as, "he doesn't act like himself" or "she's so listless." Assessing the Child With Common Signs and Symptoms of Infectious Disorders highlights important information to obtain with the history and physical examination.

Many childhood infectious diseases involve an **exanthem** (a rash). Rashes can be difficult to identify, so it is important to obtain as full a description and history of the rash as possible.

Nursing Diagnosis

Nursing diagnoses for children with infectious disorders may include:

- Pain related to pruritus from skin lesions
- Impaired skin integrity related to rash, pruritus, and scratching
- Risk for infection related to presence of infective organism in sibling

Additional diagnoses when children must be separated from others to prevent infection transmission may include:

- Social isolation related to precautions required to prevent infection transmission
- Deficient diversional activity related to activity restriction and precautions to prevent disease transmission

Outcome Identification and Planning

When establishing outcomes for care, include those that help parents deal with the current infection and

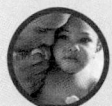

ASSESSING the Child With Common Signs and Symptoms of Infectious Disorders

History

Chief concern: Does child have a fever, general malaise, vomiting, or diarrhea? Was child recently exposed to someone with an infection?

Past medical history: Are child's immunizations current?

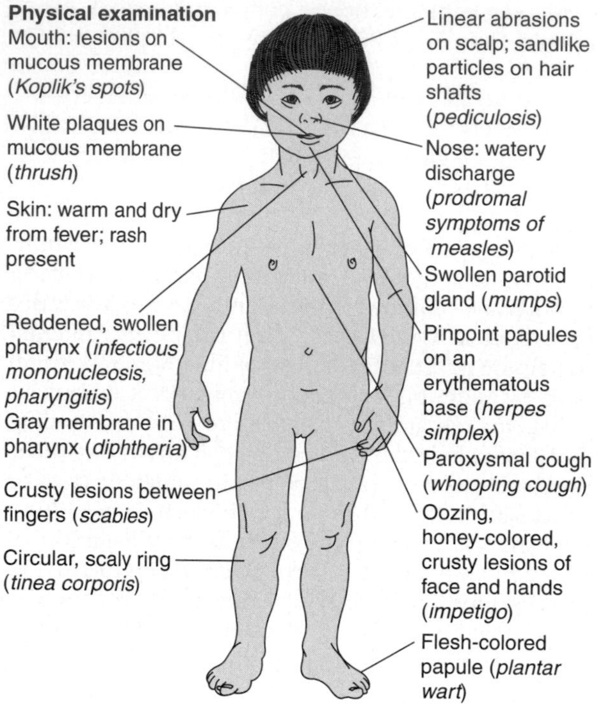

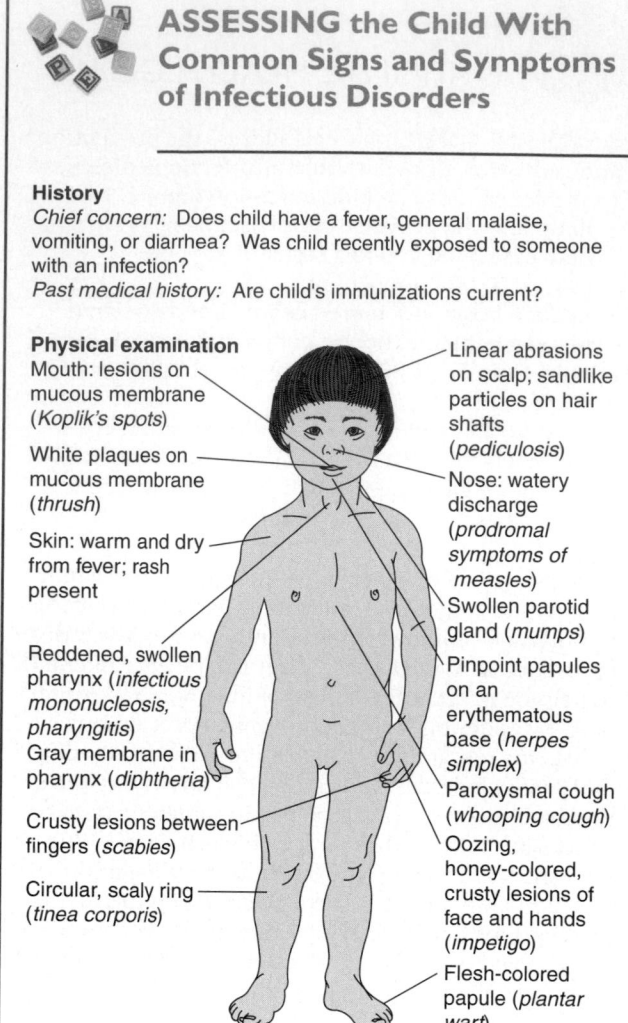

also prevent another infection (e.g., teaching about necessary infection control precautions and immunizations). Parents often ask about communicability to their other children and to the infected child's playmates or schoolmates. Planning care for a child who requires restrictions to prevent transmission requires thoughtful consideration to prevent boredom.

Implementation

Nursing responsibilities when caring for the child with an infectious disorder depend on the setting in which the child is seen. Often, a child will not be brought into a clinic if the disease can be easily identified over the phone. Counseling parents about techniques to relieve the irritation of rashes and other symptoms of infectious illness must be addressed, often over the telephone. Administering antibiotics and being alert for potential adverse effects are other major nursing responsibilities. Two organizations helpful for referral are:

National Foundation for Infectious Diseases (*www.NFID.org*)

National Center for Infectious Disease (*www.cdc.gov*)

Outcome Evaluation

Evaluation of outcomes for the child with an infectious disease should determine whether the child is returning to wellness and whether the child and family have learned more about ways to prevent infectious diseases. If one member of the family is receiving steroid therapy or has an immune system dysfunction, prevention of transmission takes on even greater importance.

Examples indicating achievement of outcomes may include:

- Child states pain from pruritus and skin lesions is at tolerable level.
- Sibling remains free of signs and symptoms of infectious disorder.
- Parent names activities he has planned to provide diversional activities.

THE INFECTIOUS PROCESS

Pathogens are organisms that cause disease. They can be classified into five types of microorganisms: viruses, bacteria, rickettsiae, helminths, and fungi. The properties of these organisms are discussed in conjunction with the common diseases they cause.

Stages of Infectious Disease

Infectious diseases follow certain stages during which the communicability (ability to be spread to others) or severity of the illness can be predicted (Fig. 43-1). The **incubation period** is the time between the invasion of an organism and the onset of symptoms of infection. During this time, microorganisms grow and multiply. The incubation period varies depending on the pathogen. A common interval is 7 to 10 days, but it can be longer. The incubation period for tetanus, for example, is 2 to 21 days.

Systemic infections usually have a **prodromal period,** or a time between the beginning of nonspecific symptoms and specific symptoms. Nonspecific symptoms include lethargy, low-grade fever, fatigue, and malaise. During

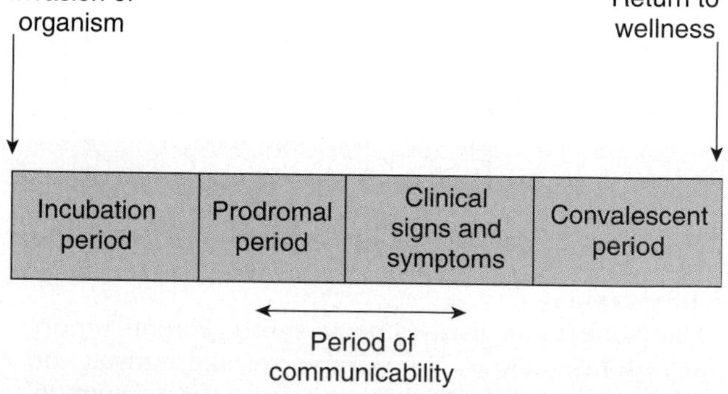

FIGURE 43.1 Time frame for infectious diseases. Period of communicability is the time during which the disease can be transmitted to other people.

a prodromal period, infectious diseases spread readily through communities to any susceptible individuals. Children are infectious (capable of spreading the microorganisms to others) during this time, and because their symptoms are so vague they do not generally take any precautions against spreading disease. Prodromal stages are generally short, ranging from hours to a few days.

Illness is the stage during which specific symptoms are evident. Most illnesses have local symptoms related to the body organ affected and also systemic symptoms that affect the entire body, such as fever, increased white blood cell count, or headache. Many childhood infections have an accompanying rash on the skin (exanthem) or mucous membrane (**enanthem**).

The **convalescent period** is the interval between when symptoms begin to fade and the child returns to full wellness. Because fatigue is often an accompanying symptom of infection, the convalescent period, or the time until full energy is restored, is often longer than anticipated.

Chain of Infection

Chain of infection refers to the method by which organisms are spread and enter a new individual to cause disease. An important method of preventing infection is to break the chain of infection. Nurses are instrumental in teaching parents how to prevent the spread of infection in homes and how to carry out safe practices so infection does not spread in health care facilities.

Reservoir

The **reservoir** is the container or place in which organisms grow and reproduce. The source of a human pathogen could be another human with the disease, a human carrying the disease, soil, or an animal or insect. Immunizations are helpful in limiting the use of children as reservoirs for organism growth.

Portal of Exit

The **portal of exit** is the method by which organisms leave an infected child's body to be spread to others. This could be by upper respiratory excretions, feces, vomitus, saliva, urine, vaginal secretions, blood, or lesion secretions (Table 43-1). To break a chain of infection at this point, follow good aseptic technique and prescribed transmission-based precautions such as wearing a gown, gloves, or mask as appropriate. Teach parents good handwashing technique after the use of a bathroom or after handling diapers. Supply an adequate number of disposable tissues so droplet or airborne spread can be limited.

Means of Transmission

The **means of transmission** of pathogens can be by direct or indirect contact, by **fomites** (i.e., inanimate objects such as soil, food, water, bedding, towels, combs, or drinking glasses) or by insects, rats, or other vermin (vectors). Direct contact implies body-to-body touching. Sexually transmitted diseases (STDs) and skin disorders are spread this way. The most common means of indirect contact is the spread of mouth and nose secretions (droplet infection) through talking, sneezing, coughing, breathing, and kissing. Some droplets containing pathogenic organisms are spread immediately to another individual in this way. Some droplets fall to the ground, where the organisms dry and then are spread by dust. If small, the organisms become suspended in the air (airborne transmission) and can infect people from a distance. Common respiratory tract infections, for example, are spread by indirect contact.

TABLE 43.1 Methods by Which Infections Spread

PORTAL OF EXIT	MEANS OF TRANSMISSION	PORTAL OF ENTRY	PREVENTION MEASURES
Blood	Arthropod vectors	Injection into the bloodstream	Decreasing vector incidence
	Blood sampling		Careful handling of blood sampling equipment
	Transfusion		Screening of transfused blood for organisms such as human immunodeficiency virus (HIV) or hepatitis B
Respiratory secretions	Airborne droplets	Respiratory tract	Wearing mask
	Fomites		Droplet precautions
			Airborne precautions
			Handwashing
Feces	Water, food	Gastrointestinal tract	Handwashing before eating, after using bathroom or handling diapers
	Fomites		
	Vectors such as flies		
Exudate from lesions	Direct contact	Skin, mucous membranes	Contact precautions
	Contact with soiled dressings		Self-screening for sexual contacts
			Gloves

Head lice (tinea capitis) can be spread by a fomite such as a comb if it is passed from one child to another. Soil constantly contains some anaerobic organisms (those that grow without oxygen), such as tetanus bacilli. When a child receives a puncture wound, such as from stepping on a rusty nail, some dirt may be left in the closed wound, and tetanus bacilli contained in the soil can begin to multiply in the closed area. Staphylococcal gastrointestinal disorders can be caused by improperly refrigerated food. Insects carry and spread rickettsial diseases. To break a chain of infection at this point, use transmission-based precautions as appropriate and wash hands before, between, and after client care. Also teach parents and children good handwashing technique.

Portal of Entry

The **portal of entry** through which a pathogen can enter a child's body can be by inhalation, ingestion, or breaks in the skin such as bites, abrasions, and burns. To break a chain of infection at this point, teach children to wash their hands after sneezing or coughing and before eating and after using the bathroom. Teach girls to wipe their perineum from front to back after defecating or voiding to prevent organisms from spreading from the rectum to the urethra. Teach parents to wash cuts and abrasions before bandaging them.

Susceptible Host

For infection to occur, a child must be susceptible to the infection (**susceptible host**). Certain characteristics make some individuals more prone to infection than others. These include:

- Age—infection occurs most readily in the very young and the very old
- Gender—girls, for example, have more urinary tract infections than boys
- Virulence—some organisms are stronger than others or cause disease more readily
- Body defenses present—physical, chemical, and immune responses all protect against foreign invaders

Immune Response to Organisms

When a foreign organism (antigen) is identified, it can be destroyed by the phagocytic (cell-engulfing) action of white blood cells or by activation of the body's immune system. Phagocytes are white blood cells that are capable of cell destruction. The cells chiefly responsible for this function are neutrophils. Monocytes serve as backup cells for phagocytosis. The action of white blood cells is summarized in Table 43-2.

The action of phagocytes on organisms produces pus (remnants of the organisms, phagocytes, and destroyed tissue). Children and parents alike may need a review of the purpose of pus because they think its presence indicates that an infection is becoming worse. More likely, it indicates that phagocytosis is occurring and the infection is resolving.

If bacteria escape the action of the phagocytes, they enter the blood and lymph systems and are transmitted to other body locations, activating the immune system. Pathogenic organisms in the bloodstream create **septicemia,** which is always a serious development because it means that the organism is being spread systemically.

With activation of the immune system, B lymphocytes (humoral immunity) and T lymphocytes (cell-mediated immunity) are produced. B lymphocytes form antibodies specific to offending antigens that either actively destroy cells or activate **complement,** a special body protein that is capable of lysing cells (see Chap. 42).

T lymphocytes (thymus-dependent) can destroy antigens by direct contact and release of lymphokines. An example of a lymphokine is **interferon,** a substance that prevents cells from being host to more than one virus at a time. This is why it is rare to see a child with two viral diseases at the same time, although it is not impossible to see a child with both a virus and a bacterial disease (e.g.,

TABLE 43.2 Types and Functions of White Blood Cells (Leukocytes)

TYPE	PERCENTAGE OF TOTAL COUNT	ORIGIN	FUNCTION
Granular Forms			
Neutrophils	60 at birth 33 at 2 y 60 thereafter	Bone marrow	Active in acute bacterial infections
Eosinophils	1–4	Bone marrow	Increased in parasitic infection
Basophils	0.0–0.5	Bone marrow	Increased with inflammation
Nongranular Forms			
Lymphocytes	30 at birth 50 at 2 y 30 thereafter	Bone marrow Divides into B cells and T cells	Direct reaction with antigens (T lymphocytes—centered in thymus gland); antibody production by B lymphocytes against antigens
Monocytes	5–10	Bone marrow	Backup for neutrophils in acute infection; macrophages are mature form

scarlet fever and a common cold) at the same time. This is also why two virus vaccines are not given to a child at the same time unless they are specially designed to be given together (such as measles, mumps, and rubella). (See Chap. 42 for a more detailed discussion of the immune response and Chap. 33 for a discussion of immunizations.)

✔ CHECKPOINT QUESTIONS

1. What are the four stages of infectious disorders?
2. What are the five components of the chain of infection?

HEALTH PROMOTION AND RISK MANAGEMENT

Prevention of infectious diseases begins with being certain that all children are in general good health. Adequate nutrition is important to provide protein and vitamins to supply adequate white blood cells so both phagocytic and antibody-producing B lymphocytes are available to destroy invading organisms.

A second important step is to be certain that all parents are aware of the need for their children to be immunized. Nurses need to ensure that immunizations are offered to children at well-child and many illness health care visits (see Chap. 33 for a discussion of immunizations, and see Focus on Cultural Competence).

FOCUS ON CULTURAL COMPETENCE

The responsibility expected of parents and children to help prevent the spread of communicable diseases differs from country to country and varies among cultures. In the United States, both federal and state governments have taken an active role in preventing infectious disease spread by requiring children to have immunizations against the most common illnesses. Parents are expected to obtain such immunizations for children by school age. Schools and school nurses, as the school system's front-line health officers, take an active role in enforcing these regulations. Community health nurses are instrumental in administering immunizations and counseling families on how to prevent the spread of disease in their home.

War-torn countries have a great deal of difficulty maintaining this same level of disease prevention. Remember when caring for children newly arrived from another country that the child may not have the same level of immunization as usually seen. This opens an important area of health teaching as the parents may not be aware of the importance of immunizations, which ones are required, or what community services are available to supply these.

It is important that parents also understand that although diseases such as scarlet fever, chicken pox, and mumps are referred to as common childhood illnesses, they have the potential to be serious illnesses, leading to complications such as pneumonia and encephalitis. When children develop these common communicable diseases, they need to be seen by a primary health care provider to minimize the risk for these complications.

Preventing the Spread of Infections

Nosocomial infections, or infections that are contracted while in the hospital, represent a major threat to hospitalized children. The overall rate of nosocomial, or hospital-acquired, infection in children ranges from 0% in low-risk settings to 23% in high-risk settings such as intensive care units (Sax et al., 2001). Children younger than 2 years, children with a nutritional deficit, those who are immunosuppressed, those who have indwelling vascular lines or catheters, those receiving multiple antibiotic therapy, or those who remain in the hospital for longer than 72 hours are at highest risk for contracting a nosocomial infection. Nurses provide a line of defense against infection by adhering to strict aseptic techniques, such as frequent and thorough handwashing, and by following protective transmission-based precautions when indicated. Nurses and other health care providers must also take precautions to protect themselves from acquiring communicable diseases (see Focus on Evidence-Based Practice), including HIV and hepatitis, by adhering to standard precautions recommended by the Centers for Disease Control (CDC). Box 43-1 and Appendix I summarize standard precautions and transmission-based infection control precautions.

CARING FOR THE CHILD WITH AN INFECTIOUS DISEASE

NURSING DIAGNOSES AND RELATED INTERVENTIONS

Nursing Diagnosis: Pain related to pruritus from skin lesions

Outcome Identification: Child reports pain is within tolerable limits during course of illness.

Outcome Evaluation: Child states he is more comfortable; reports less itching; is not seen scratching rash; no signs of excessive scratching or bleeding present.

Providing comfort for the pruritus of skin lesions is important for many childhood infections. No matter what agent is causing the disease, a rash tends to be extremely itchy and uncomfortable. Fortunately, a number of simple remedies are available for reducing the discomfort. Because pruritus is a minimal form of pain, an analgesic, such as acetaminophen (Tylenol), may be helpful to reduce discomfort. An antihistamine, such as diphenhydramine hydrochloride (Benadryl), is extremely helpful. Calamine lotion is a nonprescription lotion that is cooling and soothing and often helps to relieve itching. Colloidal baths, such as baking soda or oatmeal (approximately 1 cup

FOCUS ON EVIDENCE-BASED PRACTICE

Are Nurses Who Care for Young Children More Susceptible to Contracting Infections Than Others?

Over a million people (mostly women) are employed as out-of-home child care providers in the United States. To discover whether these people are more prone to contracting infections than others, a researcher completed a literature review of infections commonly seen in preschool children. Results revealed that child care providers are more apt to contract cytomegalovirus, parovirus B19 (fifth disease), giardiasis, shigellosis, hepatitis A, and fungal infections. The researcher recommended that handwashing and overall good hygiene are important measures for child care workers to use to prevent infection while working in these settings.

This is an important study for nurses because nurses are often employed in child care settings. They have major roles in caring for children at both ambulatory and in-service health care facilities. Performing good handwashing between diaper changes and washing diaper-changing counters between use are excellent prevention measures that nurses in these settings can use to help prevent these infections, which are most often spread by contact with feces. Nurses could use the information from this study to design an infection control plan to minimize the risk of exposure to these infections in the child care setting.

Cordell, R. L. (2001). The risk of infectious diseases among child care providers. *Journal of the American Medical Women's Association, 56*(3), 109–12.

to 3 inches of bath water), are soothing for some children. Warn parents to take precautions to prevent clogging the drain if oatmeal is used. Caution parents to use only lukewarm water, not hot, because heat usually increases the sensation of itching. Bathing serves two purposes: it can be soothing and also distracting. The child, especially a preschooler, may splash for 15 to 20 minutes in a bathtub without noticing the discomfort of a rash.

Some parents bundle up children with rashes, believing that the extra clothing brings out the rash, and that if a rash does not come out, it will go in and affect a child's heart or brain. In reality, bundling up only serves to make a rash more uncomfortable and probably increases any accompanying fever. Instead, dress the child in light cotton clothing. Remove wool blankets from the bed. Cut the child's fingernails short so scratching will not open up lesions, causing secondary infection. Placing cotton gloves on the child, especially at night, may help. Comfort measures for relieving the discomfort of rashes are summarized in the Focus on Family Empowerment.

None of these measures is foolproof. Some may provide great relief to some children and little or none to others. Regardless of whether they offer direct relief, they do give a parent a constructive and comforting activity to carry out, providing parents with an opportunity to soothe their children and themselves.

Most infectious diseases also involve fever. Measures to combat fever in children are discussed in Chapter 36.

Nursing Diagnosis: Social isolation related to required activity restrictions associated with precautions to prevent transmission

Outcome Identification: Child will participate in activities to keep self occupied.

Outcome Evaluation: Child states reasons for restrictions; expresses interest in activities proposed by nurses or parents.

A child who is restricted from others because of infection control precautions can begin to feel lonely and depressed unless stimulation and social needs are also met.

Children easily associate isolation and restriction with being punished. In a hospital setting, make as few trips as possible in and out of the room to limit the possibility of pathogen spread; on the other hand, do not make care visits seem hurried. If there is a procedure scheduled at 9:00 AM and another at 9:30 AM, stay in the room rather than leave and return again, if possible. Use the time to read a story to the child, play a card game, or talk about how strange and lonely it feels to be separated from other people.

When the child is hospitalized and requires transmission-based infection control precautions, parents must follow these precautions just as all hospital personnel do. Many parents can feel so self-conscious about having to gown and wash that they may stay away rather than visit. Remember that when children are admitted to a hospital, parents may not hear all of what is being said to them during admission because of their anxiety. If the gowning technique is explained on admission, therefore, do not expect parents to remember the next day what was said. Explain techniques again as many times as necessary.

Parents may be reluctant to give children who require transmission-based precautions their favorite toy, thinking that the hospital will insist on destroying it after the precautions are discontinued. Few pathogens exist that are not destroyed by exposure to sunlight, and few articles are available that cannot be further gas-sterilized to ensure that pathogens have been removed. Check the rooms of children requiring transmission-based precautions for favorite toys, therefore, the same as in all rooms. Never leave children in a room before checking that they have a toy to play with or an activity that will keep them busy for the length of time the child will be alone. Deficient diversional activity related to the monotony of confinement is a nursing diagnosis associated with transmission-based precautions. See Chapter 35 for a discussion of interventions that can be used to promote adequate stimulation for the child requiring transmission-based precautions.

BOX 43.1

STANDARD AND TRANSMISSION-BASED PRECAUTIONS FOR INFECTION CONTROL

To reduce the risk of disease transmission in the health care setting:

1. Wash hands immediately with soap and water before and after examining patients and after any contact with blood, body fluids, and contaminated items—whether or not gloves were worn. Use of a plain, non-antimicrobial soap is recommended.
2. Wear clean, nonsterile gloves anytime there is contact with blood, body fluids, mucous membrane, and broken skin. Change gloves between tasks or procedures on the same patient. Before going to another patient, remove gloves promptly and wash hands immediately and then put on new gloves.
3. Wear a mask, protective eyewear, and gown during any patient care activity when splashes or sprays of body fluids are likely. Remove the soiled gown as soon as possible and wash hands.
4. Handle needles and other sharp instruments safely. Do not recap needles. Make sure contaminated nondisposable equipment is not reused with another patient until it has been cleaned, disinfected, and sterilized properly. Dispose of nonreusable needles, syringes, and other sharp patient care instruments in puncture-resistant containers.
5. Routinely clean and disinfect frequently touched surfaces including beds, bedrails, examination tables, and bedside tables.
6. Do not touch linens soiled with blood or body fluids with bare hands. Use plastic bags to transport soiled linen.
7. Place a patient whose blood or body fluids are likely to contaminate surfaces or other patients in an isolation room or area.
8. Minimize the use of invasive procedures to avoid the potential for injury and accidental exposure. Use oral rather than injectable medications whenever possible.
9. When a specific diagnosis is made, find out how the disease is transmitted. Use precautions according to the transmission risk.

Airborne Precautions

Airborne precautions reduce the risk of small-particle organisms being transmitted through the air. Microorganisms carried by this route can be carried widely. If airborne transmission is possible:

1. Place the patient in an isolation room that is not air-conditioned or where air is not circulated to the rest of the health care facility. Make sure the room has a door that can be closed.
2. Wear a HEPA or other biosafety mask when working with the patient and in the patient's room.
3. Limit movement of the patient from the room to other areas. Place a surgical mask on the patient who must be moved.

Droplet Precautions

Droplet precautions reduce the risk of pathogens being spread through large-particle droplet contact by acts such as coughing, sneezing, and talking or through procedures such as suctioning or bronchoscopy. Large droplets do not remain suspended in the air for long periods and generally travel only short distances, so close proximity is required for spread of disease. If droplet transmission is possible:

1. Place the patient in an isolation room.
2. Wear a HEPA or other biosafety mask when working with the patient.
3. Limit movement of the patient from the room to other areas. If the patient must be moved, place a surgical mask on the patient.

Contact Precautions

Contact precautions reduce the risk of transmission of pathogens by direct contact such as skin-to-skin contact (shaking hands) or indirect contact through an intermediate object such as a comb or soiled dressing. If contact transmission is possible:

1. Place the patient in an isolation room and limit access.
2. Wear gloves during contact with patient and with infectious body fluids or contaminated items. Reinforce handwashing throughout the health facility.
3. Wear two layers of protective clothing.
4. Limit movement of the patient from the isolation room to other areas.
5. Avoid sharing equipment between patients. Designate equipment for each patient, if supplies allow. If sharing equipment is unavoidable, clean and disinfect it before use with the next patient.

Centers for Disease Control. (2002). *Recommendations for isolation precautions in hospitals.* Washington, DC: CDC.

FOCUS ON FAMILY EMPOWERMENT

Relieving the Itch of a Rash

Q. Our son says that his rash is so itchy. What can we do to help him?

A. Itching is a very uncomfortable sensation. Use the following to help relieve the itch of a rash:

- Dress your child in light cotton clothing so overheating and perspiration do not occur. Perspiration can make itching worse.
- Avoid wool clothing, because this can irritate skin and increase itching.
- Offer adequate fluid to maintain good hydration, because dry skin increases discomfort.
- Keep your child's fingernails short to avoid injury to the skin from scratching.
- Teach your child to press on an itchy area rather than scratching to relieve discomfort; cold cloths applied to an area can also be helpful.
- Administer an analgesic such as acetaminophen as needed for comfort.
- Adding a few teaspoonfuls of baking soda to bath water can be soothing. Use lukewarm rather than hot water.
- Keep in mind that some children need an antihistamine such as diphenhydramine (Benadryl) to reduce itching. Ask your primary care provider about using it.

✔ CHECKPOINT QUESTIONS

3. What are the three categories of transmission-based precautions?
4. How might children interpret the restrictions necessary because of infection control precautions?

VIRAL INFECTIONS

Viruses are the smallest infectious agents known, so small they cannot be seen through an ordinary microscope. They are not true cells because they contain either ribonucleic acid (RNA) or deoxyribonucleic acid (DNA), but not both. Because they are incomplete, viruses increase in number by replication inside bacteria, plant, animal, or human cells using the biochemical products of living cells to function. Although a body cell may not be outwardly altered by a virus invasion, it could fail to function or die because of lysis or rupture. Symptoms usually do not become apparent until many cells have been interrupted in this way. Some viruses are capable of invading only specific cells. The Epstein-Barr virus, for example, invades only B lymphocytes, HIV viruses invade CD4 T lymphocytes, and influenza viruses affect specific receptor sites in tracheal cells.

Viral Exanthems

The majority of childhood exanthems (rashes) are caused by viruses, and each of these diseases has specific symptoms, characteristic lesions, and a specific distribution or pattern to the rash that allows it to be identified (Figs. 43-2 and 43-3).

Exanthem Subitum (Roseola Infantum)

- Causative agent: Human herpesvirus 6 (HHV-6)
- Incubation period: Approximately 10 days
- Period of communicability: During febrile period
- Mode of transmission: Unknown
- Immunity: Contracting the disease offers lasting natural immunity; no artificial immunity is available.

Assessment. Roseola is a disease whose symptoms appear more severe than the disease actually is. It generally occurs in children ages 6 months to 3 years, mainly in the spring and fall, although it can occur any time of the year. The first symptom is a high fever (104° to 105°F [40.0° to 40.6°C]). Infants may be irritable and anorexic but rarely appear as ill as this high fever suggests. They usually remain playful and alert. The pharynx may be slightly inflamed. The occipital, cervical, and postauricular lymph nodes may be enlarged. The white blood count is usually decreased, with the proportion of lymphocytes present increased (75% to 85%; Bell, 2000).

After 3 or 4 days, the fever falls abruptly and a distinctive rash appears (see Fig. 43-3). The lesions are discrete, rose-pink macules approximately 2 to 3 mm in size. They fade on pressure and occur most prominently on the trunk. The rash resembles that of rubella or measles, but it is darker in color, and children have no accompanying coryza (cold symptoms), conjunctivitis, or cough. Because it occurs mainly on the child's trunk, parents may report it as a heat rash. The rash lasts 1 to 2 days. The diagnosis of roseola is based on the physical signs and symptoms. The hallmark of roseola is the appearance of a rash immediately after the sharp decline in fever.

Therapeutic Management. Treatment focuses on measures to reduce the discomfort of the rash and fever. The fever will respond to acetaminophen (Tylenol) or ibuprofen (Motrin), but after 4 hours is apt to rise again to the high level. The most frequent complication of roseola is a febrile seizure with the onset of the disease because the temperature rises so rapidly. Management of this type of seizure is discussed in Chapter 49. If the infant develops this exanthem in the hospital, follow standard precautions.

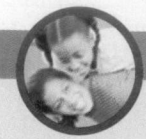

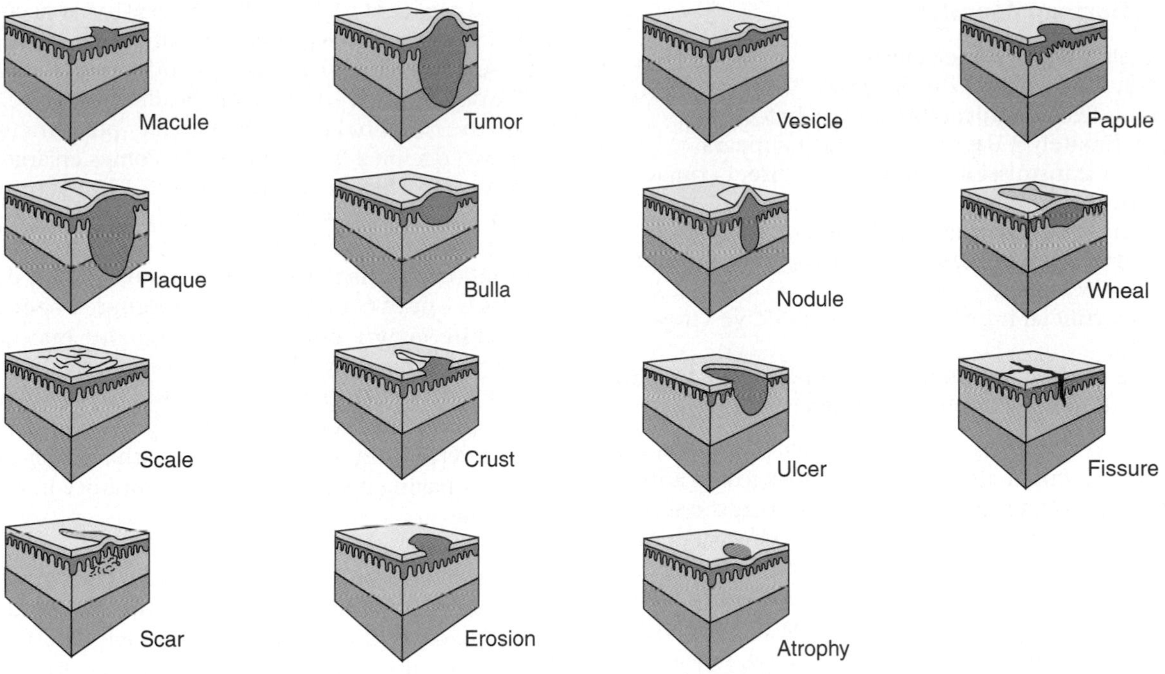

FIGURE 43.2 Primary and secondary skin lesions and their characteristics.

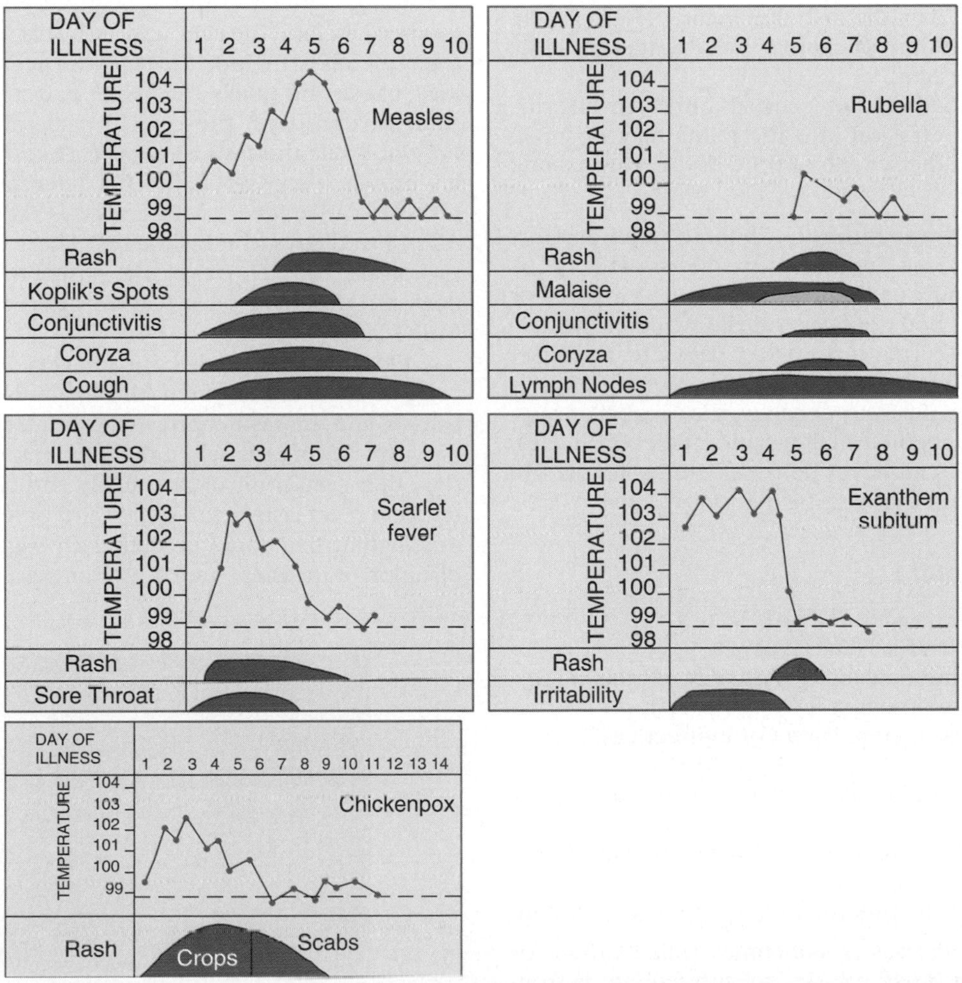

FIGURE 43.3 Differences between five acute exanthems characterized by rash.

Rubella (German Measles)

- Causative agent: Rubella virus
- Incubation period: 14 to 21 days
- Period of communicability: 7 days before to approximately 5 days after the rash appears
- Mode of transmission: Direct and indirect contact with droplets
- Immunity: Contracting the disease offers lasting natural immunity; a high rubella titer reveals infection has occurred.
- Active artificial immunity: Attenuated live virus vaccine
- Passive artificial immunity: Immune serum globulin is considered for pregnant women

Assessment. Rubella is a disease rarely seen today but when it does occur, it affects older school-age and adolescent children; it occurs most commonly during the spring. The symptoms begin with a 1- to 5-day prodromal period, during which children have a low-grade fever, headache, malaise, anorexia, mild conjunctivitis, possibly a sore throat, a mild cough, and lymphadenopathy. The nodes most noticeably affected are the suboccipital, postauricular, and cervical nodes.

After the 1 to 5 days of prodromal signs, a discrete pink-red maculopapular rash (see Fig. 43-3) begins first on the face, then spreads downward to the trunk and extremities. On the third day, the rash disappears. There is generally no desquamation (peeling); if present, it is primarily fine flaking of the skin.

Fever with rubella is not marked, although arthritis (joint pain) with effusion into the joints may occur in some children on the second or third day, lasting as long as 5 to 10 days.

Therapeutic Management. Children need comfort measures for the rash and an antipyretic such as acetaminophen (Tylenol) or ibuprofen (Motrin) for fever or joint pain. If the child develops rubella while in the hospital, follow droplet precautions for 7 days after the onset of the rash in addition to standard precautions.

If rubella occurs during pregnancy, it is capable of causing extensive congenital malformation (see Chap. 26). Because of this, it can never be considered a simple disease. It is important that girls be immunized against it.

Measles (Rubeola)

- Causative agent: Measles virus
- Incubation period: 10 to 12 days
- Period of communicability: Fifth day of incubation period through the first few days of rash
- Mode of transmission: Direct or indirect contact with droplets
- Immunity: Contracting the disease offers lasting natural immunity
- Active artificial immunity: Attenuated live measles vaccine
- Passive artificial immunity: Immune serum globulin

Assessment. Measles is sometimes called brown or black, regular, or 7-day measles to differentiate it from rubella (German, or 3-day, measles). Like rubella, it is rarely seen today except for periodic outbreaks that occur in the underimmunized college-age population. The incidence of the disease is highest in the winter and spring (Bell, 2000b).

The disease has a 10- to 11-day prodromal period, during which the lymphoid tissue, particularly postauricular, cervical, and occipital lymph nodes, becomes enlarged. Children develop a high fever (103° to 104°F [39.5° to 40.0°C]) and malaise. By the second day of the prodromal period, coryza (rhinitis and a sore throat), conjunctivitis with photophobia (sensitivity to light), and a cough develop. **Koplik's spots** (small, irregular, bright-red spots with a blue-white center point) appear on the buccal membrane. Unfortunately, the coryza of measles is indistinguishable from that of a common cold (nasal congestion, a mucopurulent discharge, and a deep brassy, bronchial cough). As a result, many children with measles are diagnosed as having a simple upper respiratory infection at this point.

Koplik's spots distinguish the disease because none of the other exanthems has this finding. They appear first on the buccal membrane opposite the molars and then extend to cover the entire buccal surface (Fig. 43-4). The raised base of the spots may coalesce so that the blue-white centers stand out as grains of salt on the erythematous membrane.

By the fourth day of fever, the rash appears. This deep-red maculopapular eruption begins at the hairline of the forehead, behind the ears, and at the back of the neck and then spreads to include the face, the neck, upper extremities, trunk, and finally the lower extremities (Fig. 43-5). After several days, the typical rash turns from red to brown. While the rash is red, it fades on pressure; when it is brown, it does not fade. This differentiates it from the rash of scarlet fever, which always fades on pressure. After 5 to 6 days, the rash fades. There is a fine desquamation after this. However, the skin of the hands and feet does not desquamate, a feature again differentiating it from scarlet fever.

Children with measles appear very ill because their cough is loud and frequent, the coryza is acute, the fever is high, and the rash is pruritic. Fortunately, on the third or fourth day of rash, when the temperature begins to fall, the other symptoms clear quickly and children feel better. Fever that lasts beyond the third or fourth day of rash or coughing that continues generally suggests that a complication of measles, such as pneumonia, has occurred.

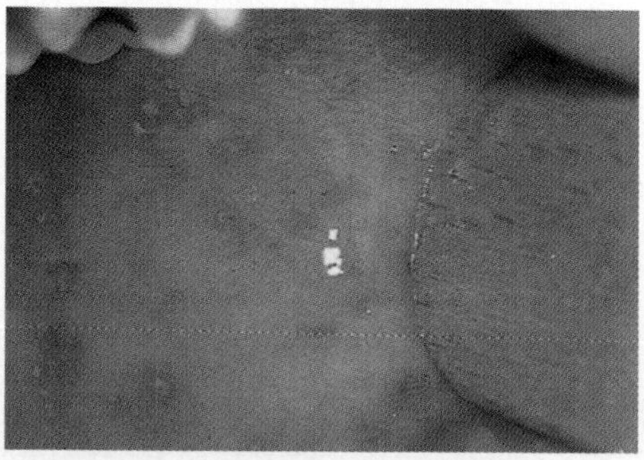

FIGURE 43.4 Koplik's spots on the oral mucous membrane.

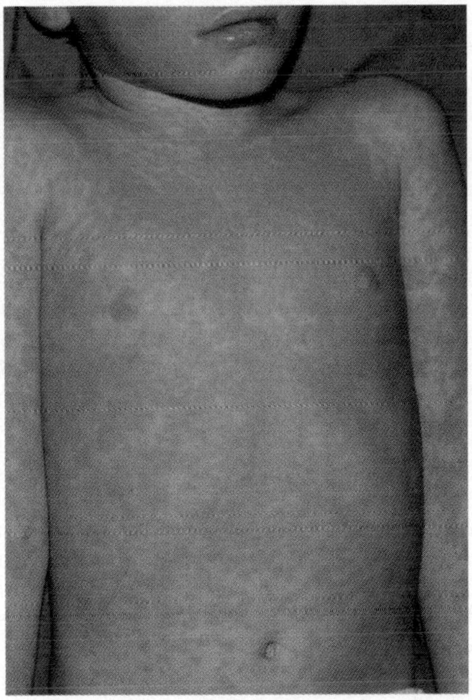

FIGURE 43.5 The typical rash of measles on a child's upper body.

Therapeutic Management. Children with measles need comfort measures for the rash and an antipyretic for the fever. The coryza, which does not respond to decongestants, fortunately lasts only a few days. The child's skin below the nose may become excoriated from the constant nasal drainage. Applying a lubricating jelly or an emollient (A and D ointment) to the area may help prevent excoriation. The child may need a cough suppressant to control the cough; otherwise, the throat can become painful from frequent irritation. Because children with measles have photophobia, it is painful for them to look at bright lights; thus, it may be painful for them to watch television. They are often more comfortable with the shades or curtains drawn or wearing dark glasses, so these measures should be instituted. Children need to be seen by a health care provider because the complications of measles include otitis media (middle ear infection), pneumonia, airway obstruction, and acute encephalitis. If the child is hospitalized, follow airborne precautions for the duration of the illness in addition to standard precautions.

Chickenpox (Varicella)

- Causative agent: Varicella-zoster virus
- Incubation period: 10 to 21 days
- Period of communicability: 1 day before the rash to 5 to 6 days after its appearance, when all the vesicles have crusted
- Mode of transmission: Highly contagious; spread by direct or indirect contact of saliva or vesicles
- Immunity: Contracting the disease offers lasting natural immunity to chickenpox; because the same virus causes herpes zoster, it may be reactivated at a later time as herpes zoster.
- Active artificial immunity: Attenuated live virus vaccine.
- Passive artificial immunity: There is little passive placental immunity to chickenpox. Children who are immunosuppressed, such as those with leukemia or HIV/AIDS, or those who are being treated with corticosteroids are given varicella-zoster immune globulin (VZIG). This may prevent or modify chickenpox if given within 72 hours of exposure.

Assessment. Chickenpox is another common childhood infection that is decreasing in incidence because of required immunization. The population most prone to it are those who have not been immunized, such as older children and college students. The disease is marked by a low-grade fever, malaise, and, in 24 hours, the appearance of a rash (see Fig. 43-3). The lesion begins as a maculae, then progresses rapidly within 6 to 8 hours to a papule, then a vesicle that first becomes umbilicated and then forms a crust. Each lesion is approximately 2 to 3 mm in diameter and is surrounded by an erythematous area. When the first crop of lesions appears, the child's temperature may rise markedly to 104° or 105°F (40.0° or 40.6°C).

Most of the chickenpox lesions are found on the trunk, although the face, scalp, palate, and neck also may be involved. They appear in approximately three separate series or crops, with each new lesion moving through progressive stages (Fig. 43-6). At one time, all four stages of lesions (macule, papule, vesicle, and crust) are present.

Therapeutic Management. If the scab from crusting is allowed to fall off naturally and lesions do not become secondarily infected, no scarring results. Scabs removed prematurely may leave a white, round, slightly indented

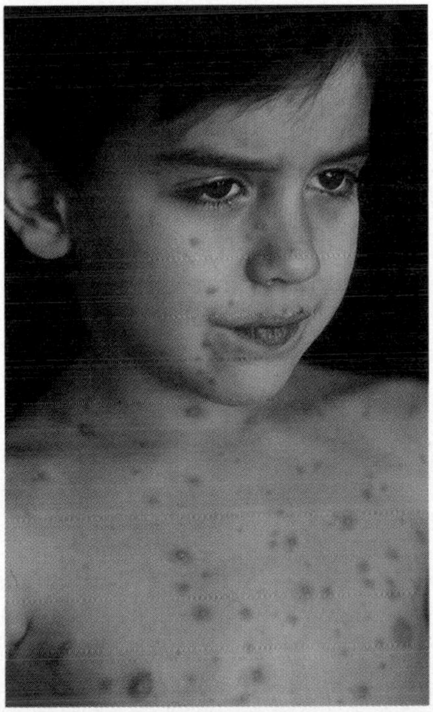

FIGURE 43.6 An older school-age boy with varicella.

scar at the site. Because it is important that children not scratch and remove scabs, although the rash of chickenpox is extremely pruritic, preventing scratching becomes a difficult problem for parents. A prescribed antihistamine usually helps to reduce the itchiness to a bearable level, and an antipyretic will counteract the high fever. Acyclovir may be prescribed to reduce the number of lesions and shorten the course of the illness (Watson, 2000). The development of Reye's syndrome has been associated with aspirin use during varicella and influenza virus illness (see Chap. 49). Caution parents when treating all childhood exanthems to avoid aspirin and to use acetaminophen to control fever instead.

If the child is hospitalized, follow airborne and contact precautions until all lesions are crusted, in addition to standard precautions. Children may return to school as soon as all the lesions are crusted (the crusts are not infectious). Complications include secondary infections of the lesions, pneumonia, and encephalitis.

Herpes Zoster

Herpes zoster is caused by the varicella-zoster virus, the same virus as chickenpox. Apparently, the first time children are invaded by the virus, they have symptoms of chickenpox. Thereafter, herpes zoster symptoms may appear due to reactivation of a latent virus or possibly due to a second or third exposure. Herpes zoster tends to occur in older children or young adults, although it can occur at any age.

The first manifestations are pruritus and cutaneous vesicular lesions on erythematous bases that follow the distributions of the lumbar and thoracic nerves (usually on the trunk, face, or upper back) and cause deep nagging pain (Fig. 43-7).

Treatment for herpes zoster includes measures to reduce pruritus and analgesia for pain. Acyclovir, which inhibits viral DNA synthesis, may be effective in limiting the disease. VZIG may minimize symptoms.

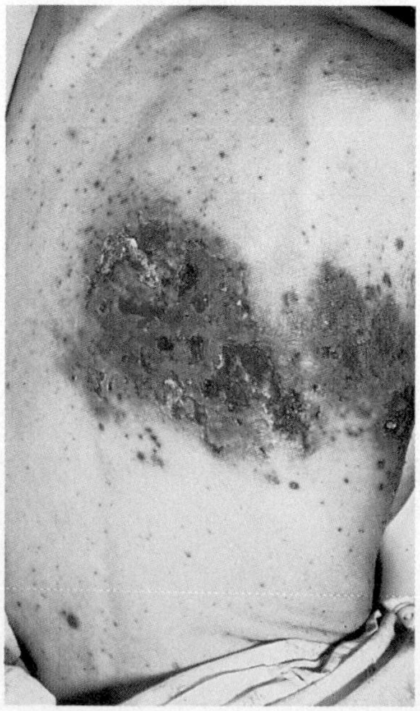

FIGURE 43.7 Herpes zoster on a child's lower back.

Smallpox (Variola)

- Causative agent: Smallpox virus
- Incubation period: 7 to 17 days
- Period of communicability: From onset of rash until all crusts have been shed
- Mode of transmission: Direct or indirect contact
- Immunity: Lasting natural immunity after contracting the disease
- Active artificial immunity: No longer recommended
- Passive artificial immunity: Vaccinia immune globulin (VIG)

Smallpox is a disease that has been extinct in the world since 1995. However, health care providers need to be able to recognize symptoms of it because viruses, colonies of which are stored in various laboratories throughout the world, could be used as an agent of biologic terrorism.

The disease has a 3- to 4-day prodromal period of chills, fever, headache, and vomiting. The child looks extremely ill and exhausted. On day 3 or 4, a rash and high fever appear. The lesions, most prominent on the distal extremities and face, begin as macules, then progress to papules, vesicles, and pustules, eventually crusting over a 10- to 14-day period.

Although the lesions of smallpox resemble those of chickenpox, they can be differentiated by the appearance of the pustular stage (not seen with chickenpox) and the fact that they arise as one crop of lesions and all progress at the same rate (chickenpox occurs in stages). The crusts of chickenpox are not contagious, but the crusts of smallpox are (Henderson, 2002).

Smallpox is a serious illness because it has a mortality rate as high as 50% and can be spread readily from an infected person to another. Children are treated with an antibiotic to prevent secondary infection of lesions. They may need oxygen or other measures to support respiratory function and measures such as a cardiac glycoside to support cardiac function.

Erythema Infectiosum ("Fifth Disease")

- Causative agent: Parvovirus B19
- Incubation period: 6 to 14 days
- Period of communicability: Uncertain
- Mode of transmission: Droplet
- Immunity: None

Assessment. Erythema infectiosum (the fifth important childhood exanthem) occurs most often in children ages 2 to 12 years. The first phase includes fever, headache, and malaise. A week later, a rash, which erupts in three stages, appears. It is intensely red and appears first on the face. The lesions are maculopapular and coalesce on the cheeks to form a "slapped face" appearance (Fig. 43-8). The facial lesions fade in 1 to 120 days.

A day after the facial lesions appear, a rash appears on the extensor surfaces of the extremities. One day later, it invades the flexor surfaces and the trunk. These lesions last for 1 week or more. When they fade, they fade from

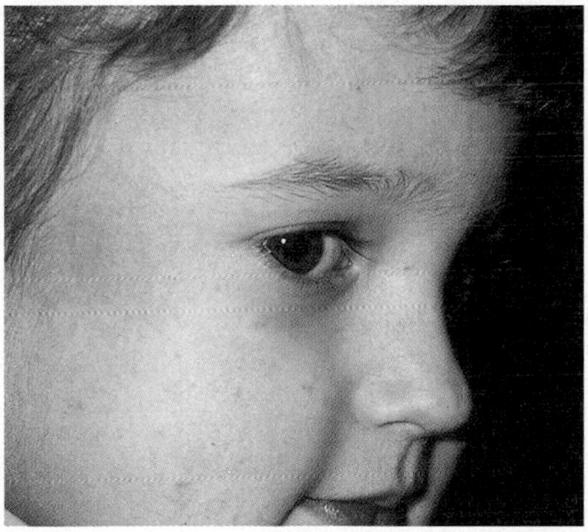

FIGURE 43.8 The rash of Fifth disease.

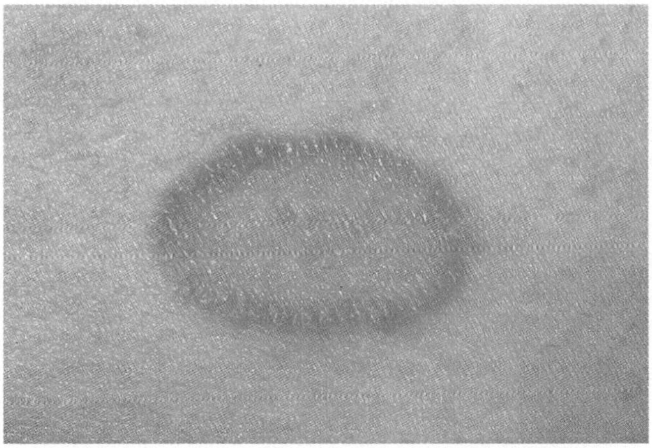

FIGURE 43.9 The "herald patch" of pityriasis rosea.

the center outward, giving the lesions a lacelike appearance. After the rash has faded, it may reappear if precipitated by skin irritation such as trauma, sunlight, hot, or cold. Some children develop a persistent arthritis.

Therapeutic Management. Treatment is typically supportive with antipyretics and analgesics. Children also may need comfort measures for the rash (see Focus on Family Empowerment earlier in this chapter). There are no known complications of fifth disease for the child; it is teratogenic for a fetus, however, so children with this disorder should avoid contact with pregnant women. Use droplet precautions in a hospital. Children can return to school as soon as the rash appears because they are no longer infectious at this point (Hanson, 2001).

Pityriasis Rosea

- Causative agent: Probably a virus
- Incubation period: Unknown
- Period of communicability: Unknown
- Mode of transmission: Unknown
- Immunity: Apparently none

Pityriasis rosea occurs in school-age and older children. Children may have a short, mild prodromal period of fever and sore throat. A herald patch, an erythematous round lesion with a scaly border, usually appearing on the trunk, is the first obvious lesion (Fig. 43-9). Approximately 1 week after the appearance of the herald patch, a generalized rash of papules, vesicles, or urticaria appears. This is generally also confined to the trunk. It follows skin lines, giving it the unique configuration of a Christmas tree.

The rash lasts 6 to 8 weeks. It is pruritic and, because it lasts so long, is particularly worrisome to children and parents. Because the lesions, particularly the herald patch, are scaly at the edges, they are often confused with tinea corporis (ringworm). Treatment is limited to oral antihistamines and other comfort measures for rash.

Pityriasis rosea appears to have no sequelae or complications; in fact, it is difficult to demonstrate in what manner it is infectious. It is a baffling rash of childhood but should be differentiated from serious (severe) exanthems (Nelson & Stone, 2000).

✔ CHECKPOINT QUESTIONS

5. What is the relationship between the rash and fever in roseola infantum?
6. What is the first sign typically noticed by the parents of a child with rubella?
7. What assessment finding is characteristic of rubeola?
8. What are the four stages of chickenpox lesions?

Enteroviruses

There are three main types of enteroviruses: echoviruses (33 subdivisions), coxsackievirus A (24 subdivisions) and coxsackievirus B (6 types), and polioviruses (3 subdivisions).

Echovirus Infections

The echoviruses are responsible for a number of childhood diseases, including aseptic meningitis, diarrhea, acute respiratory illness, and maculopapular rashes. Such infections are usually benign and self-limiting. Treatment is aimed toward supportive measures. If the child is hospitalized, follow contact precautions for the duration of the illness, in addition to standard precautions.

Coxsackievirus Infections

The coxsackievirus groups are responsible, like the echovirus groups, for a variety of diseases. One of the most frequently found diseases of children caused by coxsackievirus A is herpangina. With herpangina, children have an abrupt elevation of temperature, up to 104° or 105°F (40.0° or 40.6°C) for 1 to 4 days. Anorexia, difficulty swallowing, sore throat, and vomiting may be present. Children may have headaches and abdominal pain. Small lesions, generally discrete grayish vesicles, pinpoint in size, appear on the tonsillar fauces, soft palate, and uvula. They may be present elsewhere in the mouth or throat as well. The lesions gradually change to shallow ulcers surrounded by a red areola. They disappear within a few days after the temperature returns to normal. There are generally no complications.

Children need to be maintained on soft or liquid foods while their mouth and throat are sore. They may need an antipyretic for the fever. If the child is hospitalized, follow contact precautions for the duration of the illness, in addition to standard precautions.

Poliovirus Infections: Poliomyelitis (Infantile Paralysis)

- Causative agent: Poliovirus
- Incubation period: 7 to 14 days
- Period of communicability: Greatest shortly before and after onset of symptoms when virus is present in the throat and feces (1 to 6 weeks)
- Mode of transmission: Direct and indirect contact
- Immunity: Contracting the disease causes active immunity against the one strain of virus causing the illness.
- Active artificial immunity: Inactivated polio virus vaccine (IPV)
- Passive artificial immunity: None

Poliomyelitis, no longer seen in the United States, may be caused by any of the three strains of poliovirus, the rationale for immunizing children with the trivalent (three-strain) vaccine. Poliomyelitis does occur in other parts of the world. Thus, a concern of world health is that the level of poliomyelitis immunization in war-torn countries will fall so low that a worldwide epidemic could occur (Tangermann et al., 2000).

Assessment. The poliovirus enters the child's gastrointestinal tract, where it multiplies and produces symptoms such as fever, headache, nausea, vomiting, or abdominal pain. Moderate pain of the neck, back, and legs soon develops. The cerebrospinal fluid shows increased protein and lymphocytes.

These initial symptoms are followed by intense pain and tremors of the extremities and then paralysis, occurring either immediately or over a period of 1 to 7 days as the virus invades the central nervous system. Kernig's sign, a test for meningeal irritation, is positive. Children demonstrate a tripod sign—when sitting on the floor or on an examining table, they cannot sit without placing both the arms and hands behind them to brace themselves. Their deep tendon reflexes are hyperactive at first and then diminish as the central nervous system is fully invaded. Laryngeal paralysis makes swallowing or talking difficult, and respiratory paralysis halts respiration.

Therapeutic Management. Treatment for poliomyelitis is bedrest with analgesia and moist hot packs to relieve pain. Polio is such a crippling disease in its severest form that children must receive immunization against it. If the respiratory muscles are involved, long-term ventilation is necessary. Survivors tend to develop progressive muscle atrophy (postpoliomyelitis muscular atrophy syndrome) in late adulthood, further reducing their ability to be self-sufficient (Chasens & Umlauf, 2000).

Viral Infections of the Integumentary System

Viral infections of the skin include the herpes infections and warts (verrucae).

Herpesvirus Infections

Herpesviruses are responsible for a number of infections in children.

- Causative agent: Herpes simplex or herpes type 1 or type 2 virus
- Incubation period: 2 to 12 days
- Period of communicability: Greatest early in the course of the infection
- Mode of transmission: Direct contact
- Immunity: Immunity to a primary herpes response is gained after one incident. There is no immunity to recurrent herpes infections because the virus lies dormant in the body until it is activated by stress, sun exposure, fever, other illness, or menstruation.

When children are first invaded by a herpesvirus, they have no antibodies against the virus, so a primary form of the disease such as herpetic gingivostomatitis occurs. The virus remains latent in the neurons of local sensory ganglia, or children become permanent carriers of the herpes simplex virus (Levin & Weinberg, 2001).

Acute Herpetic Gingivostomatitis. Acute herpetic gingivostomatitis is the most common form of herpes simplex invasion in children. It is an example of the primary, not the recurrent, response. It occurs in children ages 1 to 4 years. Children have a high fever (104° to 105°F [40.0° to 40.6°C]), are restless, and have anorexia and a sore mouth. Their gumline is swollen and reddened and bleeds easily. White plaques or shallow ulcers with red areolae appear on the buccal mucosa, tongue, palate, and perhaps on the tonsillar fauces. The anterior cervical lymph nodes are enlarged and tender. The disease runs its course in 5 to 7 days (Gould, 2000). Use contact precautions.

Children need an antipyretic to reduce fever. They also need soft, acid-free foods that they can eat with minimum irritation or abrasion. Popsicles are soothing against inflamed mucous membranes. Oral acyclovir helps with healing.

Children with gingivostomatitis are often very ill. Do not dismiss this as just a reaction to herpes simplex. It can become very serious if children's mouths are so sore that they cannot swallow readily and they become malnourished and dehydrated.

Herpes Simplex (Herpes Labialis). Herpes simplex infection, popularly known as a cold sore or fever blister, represents the recurrent form of a type 1 herpesvirus invasion that has remained dormant in the ganglia of the trigeminal or fifth cranial nerve. Herpes simplex typically appears as clusters of painful, grouped vesicles on the lips or skin surrounding the mouth. After 2 or 3 days, vesicles crust, then gradually dry. Keeping lesions dry helps them to fade sooner, but keeping them lubricated with an ointment reduces pain. Application of topical acyclovir or administration of oral acyclovir reduces pain and increases healing. Children feel conspicuous about the appearance of herpes simplex lesions. They may need counseling to assure them that the lesions are not as obvious to others as they imagine.

Acute Herpetic Vulvovaginitis (Genital Herpes). Genital herpes is caused by the herpesvirus type 2, which remains dormant in the ganglia of the sacral nerves. Because this form is spread primarily by sexual contact, it is discussed in Chapter 47 with other STDs.

Eczema Herpeticum. Children with atopic dermatitis (infantile eczema) may have a generalized reaction if they contract a herpes infection. They develop a fever as high as 104° to 105°F (40.0° to 40.6°C), irritability, and crops of vesicles that erupt at the sites of eczematous skin lesions. Lesions may occur at different times during the disease course of 7 to 9 days. Generally by day 10, all lesions are crusted.

In children with severe eczema, the number of lesions that appear may be extreme. Enough body fluid can be lost through the oozing of the vesicles to cause serious fluid loss. Pain can be intense. The extent of the involvement can make children gravely ill.

Warts (Verrucae)

Warts, one of the most common dermatologic diseases in children, are caused by the papilloma virus. This virus has an incubation period of 1 to 6 months. The mode of transmission is unknown, but it is probably by direct contact (Kim, 2000).

Warts are flesh-colored, dirty-appearing papules. They generally occur on the dorsal surface of the hands, although they may occur anywhere. Plantar warts appear on the soles of the feet and are painful when children walk. They may be differentiated from calluses in that they obliterate skin lines as they grow, whereas calluses do not.

Warts on the hands or the face are generally removed if they are cosmetically unattractive to children. Plantar warts may have to be removed because of the discomfort they cause. Parents can use over-the-counter wart-removing preparations, such as Compound W, to dissolve them. Application of 40% salicylic acid may be prescribed to remove plantar warts. Carbon dioxide snow, liquid nitrogen, electrodesiccation, and curettage are also effective for removal, but these methods are painful and rarely necessary.

Children need reassurance that people do not catch warts from frogs or toads and even if left without any treatment, warts will eventually fade by themselves after about 24 months.

Viruses Causing Central Nervous System Diseases

Viruses are responsible for causing a number of central nervous system disorders. Both encephalitis and meningitis may be caused by several viruses of the arbovirus group or by certain bacteria. These are discussed in Chapter 49. Rabies is discussed here.

Rabies

- Causative agent: Rabies virus
- Incubation period: 2 to 6 weeks, possibly as long as 12 months
- Period of communicability: 3 to 5 days before the onset of symptoms through the course of the disease
- Mode of transmission: The bite of rabid animals; rarely through saliva from infected animals being transferred to open lesions on a child's skin
- Immunity: Contracting the disease apparently offers active immunity, but few people have ever survived the illness to verify this.
- Active artificial immunity: Human diploid cell rabies vaccine
- Passive artificial immunity: Rabies immune globulin (RIG)

Any warm-blooded animal can contract rabies. Wild animals, such as skunks, squirrels, raccoons, and bats, constitute the most important sources of infection from rabies in the United States. However, children receive more bites and, therefore, more treatments for rabies from bites of dogs or cats. Bites of rodents are seldom found to be rabid. Bites from other children are not rabid, although therapy is required because such bites usually contain streptococci. In the animal infected with rabies, the virus can be cultured from the central nervous system, saliva, urine, lymph, and blood. When a child is bitten by an infected animal, the virus migrates from the bite area to the child's central nervous system. Cranial nerve and spinal cord nuclei become acutely damaged. Negri bodies (cytoplasmic inclusion bodies) can be isolated from nerve cells.

Assessment. The diagnosis of rabies is established largely from the history of an animal bite and the clinical symptoms. After the long incubation period of the virus, children begin to show prodromal signs of malaise, fever, anorexia, nausea, sore throat, drowsiness, irritability, and restlessness. They may notice numbness or hyperesthesia at the area of the bite and along the course of the involved nerves. The white blood cell count will show slight leukocytosis. The cerebrospinal fluid is usually normal, with perhaps only a slight elevation in protein and cells. As the symptoms increase, there is high fever, anxiety, and hyperexcitability. Involuntary twitching movements and generalized seizures may occur. When children try to drink, there are violent contractions of the muscles of the mouth. They may drool saliva rather than swallow it because swallowing is extremely painful. These two phenomena give the disease its popular name, hydrophobia ("water-fear").

As symptoms progress, children become comatose, with possible total body paralysis. Peripheral vascular collapse and death follow quickly in only 5 or 6 days. Postmortem examination will reveal the diagnostic Negri bodies in brain cells.

Therapeutic Management. Once the disease process begins, rabies is invariably fatal. The key is preventing the active process. All children who receive an animal bite should be seen by a primary care provider to evaluate the circumstances surrounding the bite and to decide whether to begin rabies prevention measures. The decision to treat must be made immediately if treatment is to be effective.

Taking a history of the incident to determine the type of animal is of primary importance. Most children are sure they know the type of animal if it was a dog; they may be unsure if it was a wild animal. Do not lead children into naming an animal just to please. If asked, "Was it a skunk? A raccoon? A squirrel?" the child may choose an animal name because he or she thinks that is the answer expected. Instead, ask the child to describe the animal; from that description, establish the kind of animal that bit the child. It helps in rural health facilities to have a picture book of animals handy so that preschoolers in particular can identify the animal that bit them. A rabid animal usually does not act normally. It runs blindly, often staggering; it may dribble saliva rather than swallow it. It is easy to assess whether a household pet is acting this way. It is sometimes difficult to assess the actions of a wild animal because the fear it experiences at being trapped or cornered may make it run about frantically.

An unprovoked attack is highly suggestive that the animal is rabid, rather than if the bite happens during a provoked attack. Let children know that they will not be punished if they were provoking an animal so they feel free to say so. Statements such as "I was only hugging him or feeding him" may sound innocent but may have constituted a provoked attack to the animal.

The kind of wound that the child receives also is instrumental in deciding whether to begin treatment. A bite mark is much more serious than a scratch from an animal's claws. The immunization status of the animal should be checked if available. An animal that has been properly immunized against rabies will rarely transmit the virus. Whether rabies exists in the community at the time of the attack will also influence the decision. If there have been no other reported instances in domestic animals, the chance that this dog bite is serious in terms of rabies is lower than if other dogs with rabies have been reported in the area.

Inspect the wound carefully to see whether it was caused by teeth marks or scratch marks. Wash the wound well with soap and water and a suitable antiseptic. If puncture wounds are present, the wound must not be sutured and closed, because tetanus (organisms that are anaerobic and grow in deep, closed wounds, where oxygen does not reach) can develop in the wound. The animal that caused the bite should be located if possible and then confined for 5 to 10 days. If it develops any signs of rabies during this period, it will be destroyed and the brain examined for evidence of rabies. Domestic animals are not destroyed unless they show signs of rabies; if people are unaware of this, they may resist surrendering an animal for observation.

If the animal is found to be rabid, children receive both rabies vaccine and antirabies serum (RIG). This applies also if the animal escapes and its condition is unknown (it is assumed to be rabid). A portion of the dose is injected into the wound site and the remainder is given intramuscularly (Dibs, 2000).

It may seem contradictory to give an active immunization serum (administering antigen to children) when they have received an animal bite (which administers antigen to them). This is done because the rabies virus has a long incubation period before antibody production is stimulated; administering RIG provides antibodies against the rabies virus immediately. Administering rabies vaccine allows the child to begin additional antibody formation so by the time the rabies virus from the bite begins to have an effect (2 to 6 weeks after the bite), the child has developed sufficient antibodies to combat it and prevent the illness.

Other Viral Infections

Mumps (Epidemic Parotitis)

- Causative agent: Mumps virus
- Incubation period: 14 to 21 days
- Period of communicability: Shortly before and after onset of parotitis
- Mode of transmission: Direct or indirect contact
- Immunity: Contracting the disease gives lasting natural immunity
- Active artificial immunity: Attenuated live mumps vaccine
- Passive artificial immunity: Mumps immune globulin

Assessment. Mumps is now a rare disease due to successful immunization programs. It is most likely to be seen in adolescents who have not been immunized. If the disease occurs, it begins with fever, headache, anorexia, and malaise. Within 24 hours, an "earache" occurs. When the child points to the site of the pain, however, he or she points not to the ear, but to the jaw line just in front of the ear lobe. Chewing movements aggravate the pain. By the next day, the parotid gland (located just in front of the ear lobe) is swollen and tender. As the parotid gland swells, typically lasting for 1 to 6 days, it displaces the ear upward and backward. Boys also may develop testicular pain and swelling (orchitis).

It is often difficult to differentiate mumps from submaxillary adenitis (swelling of lymph nodes). The best method of differentiation is to place a hand along the child's jaw line. If the major amount of swelling is above the hand, it is probably mumps. If the largest amount of swelling is below the hand line, it is probably adenitis (Fig. 43-10).

Therapeutic Management. Because chewing movements are so painful, children may need soft or liquid foods until the major portion of the swelling recedes. It is also more difficult for them to swallow sour foods than sweet ones. They may need an analgesic for pain and an antipyretic for fever. If the child is hospitalized, follow droplet precautions in addition to standard precautions. Children should not return to school until 9 days after the onset of parotid swelling (Tsarouhas, 2000a).

One attack of mumps gives lasting immunity. Some parents report that the child had mumps only on one side 1 year ago, so they are afraid he or she will develop mumps on the opposite side in the future. If a child appears to have had mumps twice, the diagnosis was probably confused with cervical adenitis one of the two times.

Mumps is a potentially serious illness because a number of serious complications can arise. If mumps orchitis develops, it is generally unilateral. A single testis swells rapidly and is painful and tender. When the fever declines,

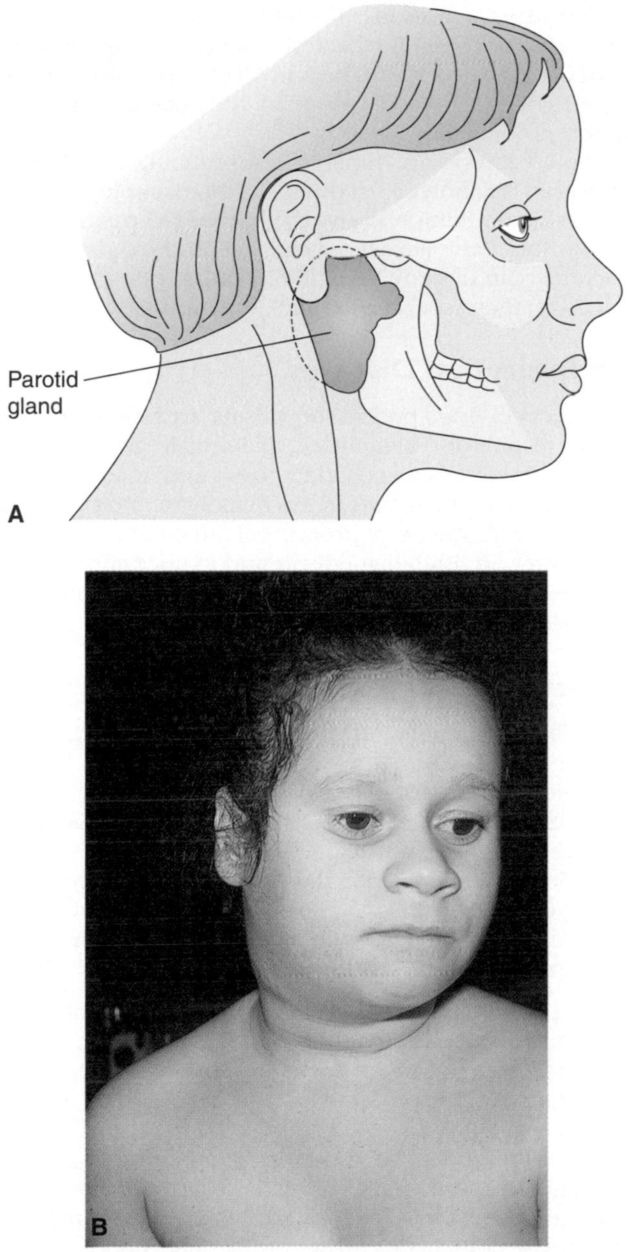

FIGURE 43.10 Infectious parotitis. (*A*) The parotid gland is located just in front of the ear. (*B*) A boy with parotitis (mumps).

testicular swelling also decreases, although the tenderness may exist for weeks. Atrophy of the testis may result. The chance that mumps orchitis will lead to complete sterility is exaggerated, however (Tsarouhas, 2000a).

The complication of meningoencephalitis occurs in a few children. Severe permanent hearing impairment is a rare complication that may occur because of neuritis of the auditory nerve.

Infectious Mononucleosis

- Causative agent: Epstein-Barr virus
- Incubation period: Unknown; probably 2 to 8 weeks
- Period of communicability: Unknown; probably only during acute illness
- Mode of transmission: Direct and indirect contact
- Immunity: One episode apparently gives lasting immunity. No vaccination is available.

Infectious mononucleosis is also known as glandular fever or, because it was first discovered as a disease that is transferred readily from one person to another by kissing, the kissing disease. It occurs most commonly in adolescents and young adults, although it may occur in any age child (Papesch & Watkins, 2001).

Assessment. The beginning symptoms include chills, fever, headache, anorexia, and malaise. Children develop lymphadenopathy and a severe sore throat. The fever is generally high (103°F [39.5°C]) and lasts approximately 6 days.

The cervical lymph nodes, most markedly affected, are firm and tender. The tonsils feel painful and are enlarged and erythematous. A thick, white membrane may cover the tonsils (Fig. 43-11), and often petechiae appear on the palate. If the mesenteric lymph nodes enlarge, children may experience abdominal pain so sharp it simulates appendicitis. The spleen enlarges, placing the child at risk for spontaneous rupture. Hepatitis, skin manifestations (e.g., a maculopapular eruption similar to the rash of rubella), pneumonitis, and central nervous system involvement (e.g., encephalitis, meningitis, or polyneuritis) may occur.

Lymphocytosis, with lymphocytes representing more than 50% of the total white blood cell count, occurs. Of these lymphocytes, a significant number (>20%) are atypical; they are larger-than-normal, mature lymphocytes, and their nuclei are somewhat less dense. A serologic test, known as the heterophil antibody test, is based on the fact that the antibody produced in infectious mononucleosis will agglutinate sheep red blood cells. A technique known as the monospot test has also been developed, using horse red blood cells. This test can be performed in minutes. A positive test, along with the increased number of atypical lymphocytes apparent on a blood slide, confirms the diagnosis of infectious mononucleosis. Epstein-Barr virus antibodies can be recovered from blood serum for a final diagnosis.

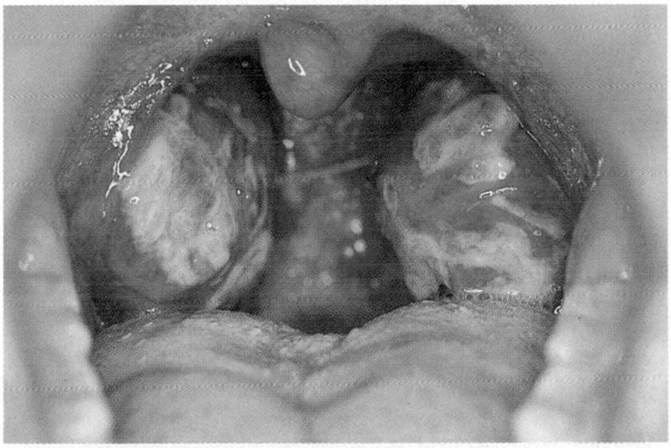

FIGURE 43.11 Appearance of the tonsils in a child with infectious mononucleosis. Note the degree of erythema, enlargement, and purulent covering.

Therapeutic Management. Children with infectious mononucleosis need bedrest during the acute stage of the illness (7 to 10 days) because with the splenomegaly there is a danger of spleen rupture with any trauma to that area. If the child is hospitalized, follow standard precautions. Be careful in helping children with this disease turn in bed so that no pressure is placed over the splenic area. When palpating the spleen, do so gently to avoid inadvertent rupture.

Teach children and parents the importance of maintaining a good fluid intake despite the sore throat. Cool, nonacidic fluids are often tolerated best.

Children may notice weakness and general fatigue for up to 6 weeks after the illness. Caution them to avoid contact sports as long as the spleen is enlarged (Burroughs, 2000). Because infectious mononucleosis occurs primarily in young adults, it may interrupt school or career plans. Help these young adults to voice their frustration with this illness. Offer support to help them through this unexpected interruption in their life.

Hantavirus Pulmonary Syndrome Infection

The hantavirus is a member of the arbovirus group. The virus infects small rodents and perhaps cats who have eaten mice. In the Far East, the virus produces an illness marked by extreme purpura from thrombocytopenia and severe gastrointestinal symptoms. In 1993, an outbreak of severe illness from a previously undiscovered hantavirus occurred in the United States; major symptoms included fever, muscle aches, thrombocytopenia, gastrointestinal symptoms, and hypotension. Death occurred from rapid progressive pulmonary edema (Ramos et al., 2001). Although the mortality from this particular hantavirus infection has been high (about 75%), treatment with the antiviral agent ribavirin may be effective.

> ✔ **CHECKPOINT QUESTIONS**
>
> 9. Where is the swelling of mumps typically located?
> 10. For the child with infectious mononucleosis, why must abdominal palpation be performed gently?

BACTERIAL INFECTIONS

Bacteria reproduce by fission, in which one cell enlarges and duplicates itself, then divides into two equal parts. They are usually single-celled organisms occurring in three main shapes: spheres (cocci), rods (bacilli), and spirals (spirochetes). Bacteria are independent, living organisms. They have a nucleus, cytoplasm, and a cell wall, and they contain both DNA and RNA.

Bacteria are most commonly observed under a microscope after being fixed to a slide by heating followed by staining. Bacteria that stain violet are gram-positive organisms; those that stain red are gram-negative organisms. Those that cannot be decolorized with acid after being stained are acid-fast. As some bacteria grow, they produce **exotoxins,** or poisons. If this happens, disease symptoms arise not from the bacteria themselves but from the effect of these toxins on the body. Tetanus, botulism, and diphtheria are diseases caused by the systemic spread of toxins produced by bacteria.

Some bacteria are capable of producing enzymes as they grow. Hemolytic streptococci, for example, produce streptokinase, which allows the bacteria to pass through blood clots. Penicillinase, an enzyme produced by certain bacteria, can destroy penicillin. Natural penicillin is ineffective, therefore, against such organisms.

Streptococcal Diseases

Streptococci, gram-positive organisms, are found normally in the respiratory, alimentary, and female genital tracts. Most severe diseases in children result from infection with *Streptococcus pyogenes* (beta-hemolytic streptococci, group A). Streptococcal pharyngeal infection is discussed in Chapter 40. Rheumatic fever and glomerulonephritis, conditions that may result as an autoimmune response, are discussed in Chapters 41 and 46, respectively.

Scarlet Fever

- Causative agent: Beta-hemolytic streptococci, group A
- Incubation period: 2 to 5 days
- Period of communicability: Greatest during acute phase of respiratory illness; 1 to 7 days
- Mode of transmission: Direct contact and large droplets
- Immunity: One episode of disease gives lasting immunity to scarlet fever toxin.

Assessment. Scarlet fever occurs most commonly in the 6- to 12-year-old age group, although it may be seen in preschoolers. The incidence is highest in temperate climates, and the disease occurs usually in late winter or early spring.

The symptoms of scarlet fever begin abruptly and are those of a streptococcal pharyngitis: fever, sore throat, perhaps headache, chills, and malaise. As the beta-hemolytic, group A streptococcus grows in the child's body, it produces a number of toxins; erythrogenic toxin is the one responsible for the rash of scarlet fever. The rash appears 12 to 48 hours after the onset of the pharyngeal symptoms (see Fig. 43-3). The fever is high (103° to 104°F [39.5° to 40.0°C]) on the first day of throat symptoms and again on the day the rash appears, and then gradually returns to normal. The pulse rate may be increased out of proportion to the fever.

The rash of scarlet fever is both enanthematous and exanthematous (on both mucous membrane and skin). The tonsils are inflamed and enlarged and usually covered with white exudate. The uvula and pharynx are beefy red. The palate is usually covered with erythematous punctiform (pinpoint) lesions and perhaps scattered petechiae. The tongue, during the first 2 days of the illness, is white and appears furry. By day 3, papillae enlarge and protrude through the white coat, giving the tongue a "white strawberry" appearance. By day 4 or 5, the white coat disappears and the prominent papillae of the tongue give it a "red strawberry" appearance. A "strawberry tongue" is distinctive for scarlet fever and helps to differentiate the disease from other rashes.

The skin rash has red, pinpoint lesions that blanch on pressure. Lesions are densest on the trunk and in skin folds. Few lesions appear on the face. The area around the mouth tends to be abnormally pale (circumoral pallor). There are areas of hyperpigmentation in the folds of the joints (Pastia's sign). The rash persists for approximately 1 week. It desquamates, with large areas of skin peeling off in fine flakes. A throat culture reveals streptococci.

Therapeutic Management. Children with scarlet fever usually appear ill. They need a soft or liquid diet for a few days until their throat soreness has diminished. They may need an analgesic and antipyretic, such as acetaminophen (Tylenol) or children's ibuprofen (Motrin) for pain and fever. The rash of scarlet fever tends to be pruritic, so comfort measures are necessary. Because the underlying cause of the illness is a streptococcal infection, a 10-day course of penicillin is prescribed (Bagarazzi & Cohen, 2000). Caution parents to give the full amount prescribed for the full course to prevent the complications of beta-hemolytic, group A streptococcal infections (acute glomerulonephritis or rheumatic fever). If the child is hospitalized, follow droplet precautions until 24 hours after therapy is started, in addition to standard precautions (see Focus on Nursing Care Planning).

Children who receive penicillin may not develop the typical extreme rash and obviously do not have as severe a

FOCUS ON *Nursing Care Planning*

THE HOSPITALIZED CHILD WITH SCARLET FEVER

A 7-year-old girl who is hospitalized following abdominal surgery develops a fever of 103°F (39.5°C) and a red, macular rash on her chest and abdomen on her second postoperative day. She states, "My throat hurts."

Assessment: Macular, pinpoint erythematous rash on abdomen, groin folds, and chest. Lesions blanch with pressure. Groin fold areas hyperpigmented. "This rash itches so much it hurts." Child scratching lesions constantly. Uvula and pharynx beefy red. Tonsils inflamed and enlarged with white exudate. Pinpoint lesions with two or three scattered petechiae noted on palate. Tongue white and furry. Throat culture positive for streptococcus. Other physical examination findings within normal limits for postoperative course. A diagnosis of scarlet fever is made. Child upset and crying. "I wish my mommy were here to stay with me. I'm all by myself. I can't even go to the playroom." Mother is single parent with two smaller children, ages 4 years and 1 year, at home. Usually visits once a day in the late afternoon.

Nursing Diagnosis: Social isolation related to required restrictions associated with infection control precautions

Outcome Identification: Child will participate in stimulating activities while hospitalized.

Outcome Evaluation: Child states reason for restrictions; identifies time when restrictions will be lifted; expresses interest in activities proposed.

Interventions	Rationale
1. Explain the reasons for restrictions and infection control precautions. Inform child that restrictions will be necessary for 24 hours. Institute droplet precautions.	1. Child may associate precautions and restrictions with feelings of being punished. Explanations help to increase understanding and decrease anxiety about unfamiliar events. Information about duration of restrictions provides the child with an end point to work toward. Droplet precautions are followed until 24 hours after the initiation of therapy, minimizing the time required for the child to be restricted and separated from others.
2. Allow the child to see caregivers' faces before putting on necessary barriers such as masks prior to entering the room.	2. Being able to identify the person coming into the room helps to minimize the child's anxieties about strangers and the unknown.

(continued)

Interventions	Rationale
3. Visit the child frequently, at least every hour, and provide her with opportunities for therapeutic play.	3. Frequent visits help to decrease feelings of being alone. Therapeutic play helps the child deal with feelings associated with her condition.
4. Plan age-appropriate activities that the child can engage in with health care personnel and when alone.	4. Participation in age-appropriate activities fosters growth and development. Joint activities help to decrease feelings of loneliness. Solo activities help to occupy time when child is alone.
5. Encourage the child to talk about how she feels about being separated from others.	5. Talking with the child allows her to share feelings and concerns openly and safely, possibly increasing the child's awareness of them and helping to diminish feelings of loneliness.
6. Encourage the child and mother to telephone each other if possible throughout the day.	6. Telephone contact helps to increase feelings of safety and security.
7. Encourage the child's mother to bring in the child's favorite toy.	7. Having a favorite toy nearby provides the child with a sense of security.
8. Begin antibiotic therapy (Penicillin V) as ordered.	8. Penicillin is effective for group A beta-hemolytic streptococcus.

Nursing Diagnosis: Pain related to pruritus from the skin lesions and sore throat

Outcome Identification: Child will report pain is within tolerable levels.

Outcome Evaluation: Child states she is comfortable; reports itching is less severe; is not observed scratching lesions. Absence of further irritation or excoriation.

Interventions	Rationale
1. Administer analgesics and antihistamines as ordered.	1. Analgesics act to decrease pain. Antihistamines act to block histamine release associated with the inflammatory process.
2. Apply calamine lotion or use colloidal baths in lukewarm water as indicated.	2. Calamine lotion and colloidal baths help soothe the skin and decrease itching. Heat causes vasodilation and increases the sensation of itching.
3. Instruct the child to press on the itchy area rather than scratch.	3. Pressing on the area may help to diminish the itching sensation without further irritation and possible subsequent skin breakdown from excessive scratching.
4. Apply cool compresses to the area. Encourage the child to participate with applying the dressings.	4. Cool compresses cause vasoconstriction, decrease inflammation, and help soothe the itching sensation. Participation by the child provides a purposeful activity and helps to promote a feeling of control.
5. Provide diversional activities.	5. Diversional activities help to focus the child's attention on other things than the itch.
6. Dress the child in cool, lightweight, cotton clothing.	6. Appropriate clothing allows for evaporation of perspiration and heat. Perspiration and overheating worsen itching, further irritating the skin.
7. Provide frequent fluids with a soft or liquid diet.	7. Adequate fluid intake is important to prevent skin dryness, which increases discomfort. A soft or liquid diet is less irritating to the child's sore throat.
8. Cut the child's fingernails short and use cotton gloves as necessary.	8. Keeping fingernails short and using cotton gloves help to minimize the risk for injury from excessive scratching.

systemic illness as those who do not receive penicillin. As a result, scarlet fever is currently popularly termed scarlatina (a small, scarlet rash). Caution parents that regardless of the name, the consequences can be grave and penicillin therapy is necessary.

Impetigo

- Causative agent: Beta-hemolytic streptococcus, group A (nonbullous); *Staphylococcus aureus* (bullous)
- Incubation period: 2 to 5 days
- Period of communicability: From outbreak of lesions until lesions are healed
- Mode of transmission: Direct contact with lesions
- Immunity: None

Impetigo is only mildly infectious because it seems to be transmitted only by direct contact. It is not uncommon to see several children in a family with identical lesions, however. Parents may be upset at being told their child has impetigo because at one time the lesions (dirty and crusty-appearing) were associated with poor hygiene.

WHAT IF? What if a parent insists that her child cannot have impetigo because she knows that it occurs only in children who are not kept clean, and both her child and home are very clean? How would you explain why her child has impetigo?

Assessment. Impetigo is a superficial infection of the skin. It begins as a single papulovesicular lesion surrounded by localized erythema. As more vesicles appear, they become purulent, ooze, and form honey-colored crusts (Fig. 43-12). They are found most commonly on the face and extremities. They are often seen as secondary infections of insect bites or in children who have pierced ears. If there are a number of lesions, children may have local adenopathy.

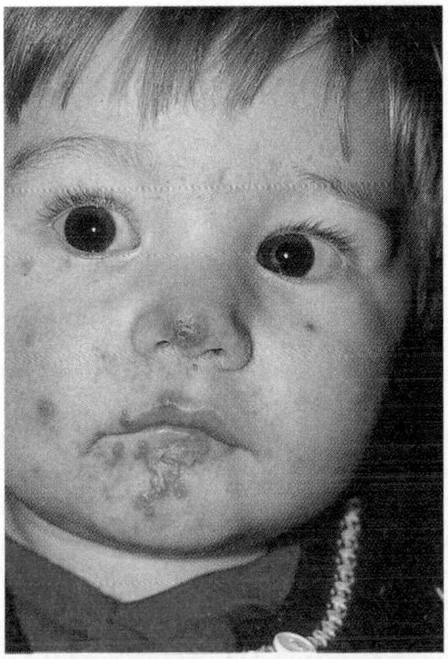

FIGURE 43.12 Impetigo in a toddler. Note the honey-colored crust appearance of some of the lesions.

Therapeutic Management. Treatment is oral administration of penicillin or erythromycin or the application of mupirocin (Bactroban) ointment for 7 to 10 days (see Focus on Pharmacology; Foster, 2000). The lesions heal most quickly if a parent or the child washes the crusts daily with soap and water.

Although rare, complications of rheumatic fever or acute glomerulonephritis may occur after impetigo, as they may after other streptococcal infections. If the child develops impetigo while in the hospital, follow contact precautions until 24 hours after initiation of therapy.

Cat-Scratch Disease

- Causative agent: *Bartonella henselae* bacteria
- Incubation period: 3 to 10 days
- Period of communicability: Unknown
- Mode of transmission: Bite or scratch from a cat or kitten
- Immunity: One episode of disease gives lasting immunity; no passive artificial immunity

Cat-scratch disease occurs most commonly in preschool children because children at that age play roughly with cats or pick them up against their will and thus receive scratches. At the time the child contracts the disease, the cat does not appear ill.

FOCUS ON PHARMACOLOGY

Mupirocin (Bactroban)

Action: Mupirocin is a topical antibiotic treatment for impetigo caused by *Staphylococcus aureus* and *Streptococcus pyogenes.*

Pregnancy risk category: B

Dosage: Small amount applied three times a day to the affected areas for 10 days

Possible adverse effects: Erythema, dry skin, pruritus, burning, stinging

Nursing Implications

- Advise parents to wash the lesions with soap and water and pat dry before applying ointment to soften crusts for better absorption.
- Caution parents that causative organisms are infectious by direct contact. Instruct them to wash their own hands before and after applying the ointment.
- Urge parents to continue to use the ointment to ensure eradication of the causative germs. The lesions may begin to improve before 10 days have elapsed.
- Instruct the parents to use caution when applying the ointment around the eyes. Ointment is irritating to the eyes.
- Teach the parents about the signs and symptoms of secondary fungal infection that may occur and to notify a health care provider should any occur.

The first symptom for the child is a single skin papule or pustule that lasts 1 to 3 weeks. Approximately 2 weeks after the scratch, severe local lymphadenopathy develops. The nodes most markedly involved are those of the head, neck, and axilla. The node enlargement generally lasts 2 to 3 months. In some children, there is node suppuration (a node breaks open to the skin and drains sterile pus).

Some children have a low-grade fever and malaise. Occasionally, central nervous system involvement, such as encephalitis or meningitis, occurs. A positive reaction to a skin test of cat-scratch disease antigen is present. This, along with the history of a cat scratch and the aspiration of sterile pus from enlarged lymph nodes, is diagnostic. Treatment is symptomatic, although an antibiotic may be prescribed to help shorten the course of the disease (Conrad, 2001). Children may need an analgesic for painful adenopathy. Aspiration of involved nodes may be necessary to relieve pain.

Parents may ask if the cat should be destroyed. Because an attack of cat-scratch disease gives lifetime immunity and fewer than 10% of children scratched by the same cat contract cat-scratch disease, there is no need to destroy the cat for an act it saw as defending its safety.

Staphylococcal Infections

Staphylococcal organisms are gram-positive. Colonies of staphylococci are normally found on the skin, so they are generally the organisms involved in skin infections (pyodermas). Because the organisms grow rapidly in cream foods that are not well refrigerated, such as potato salad or cream pies, they are often the organisms involved in food poisoning episodes during the summer. Food poisoning produces gastrointestinal symptoms (see Chap. 45).

Furunculosis (Boils)

A furuncle is a staphylococcal infection of the hair follicle. A yellow pustule forms at the site. There is localized redness, pain, and edema of the surrounding skin. Urge children not to rupture these lesions but rather to allow them to run their self-limiting course so the infection is not spread to surrounding tissue and does not become a cellulitis.

Cellulitis

Cellulitis is a staphylococcal inflammation of the deeper layers of skin. It occurs generally on the extremities or face, or surrounding wounds. The skin feels warm and is edematous and reddened. Cellulitis is treated with a systemic antibiotic. Warm soaks relieve pain and inflammation.

Scalded Skin Disease

Scalded skin disease (Ritter's disease) is a staphylococcal infection seen primarily in newborns. Children develop rough-textured skin and general erythema. Large bullae (vesicles), filled with clear fluid, form. The epidermis separates from children in large sheets, leaving a red, glistening, scalded-looking surface. Children need intensive intravenous antibiotic therapy to survive this extreme infection (Conway & Bagarazzi, 2000).

✔ CHECKPOINT QUESTIONS

11. What organism is responsible for scarlet fever?
12. What organisms are often involved in food poisoning episodes during the summer?

Other Bacterial Infections

Diphtheria

- Causative agent: *Corynebacterium diphtheriae* (Klebs-Löffler bacillus)
- Incubation period: 2 to 6 days
- Period of communicability: Rarely more than 2 weeks to 4 weeks in untreated persons; 1 to 2 days in patients treated with antibiotics
- Mode of transmission: Direct or indirect contact
- Immunity: Contracting the disease gives lasting natural immunity
- Active artificial immunity: Diphtheria toxin given as part of DTaP vaccine
- Passive artificial immunity: Diphtheria antitoxin

Assessment. When diphtheria bacilli invade and grow in the nasopharynx of children, they produce an exotoxin (a potent protein poison) that causes massive cell necrosis and inflammation. The necrosing material lends itself well to the growth of the bacilli, so the bacilli reproduce rapidly. The inflammation and necrosing cells form a characteristic gray membrane on the nasopharynx. This may extend up into the nose and down into the major bronchi, causing a purulent nasal discharge and a brassy cough. The toxin is absorbed from the membrane surface and spread systemically by the bloodstream to affect the major organs, such as the heart and nervous system. If untreated, myocarditis with heart failure and conduction disturbances may occur. Central nervous system involvement can include severe neuritis with paralysis of the diaphragm and pharyngeal and laryngeal muscles. The diagnosis of diphtheria is made based on clinical appearance and on a throat culture, which reveals the presence of the bacilli.

Therapeutic Management. Treatment involves intravenous administration of antitoxin in large doses. In addition, children are given penicillin or erythromycin intravenously. Complete bedrest is crucial during the acute stage of the illness. Droplet precautions must be followed until cultures are negative. Children need careful observation at all times to prevent airway obstruction. If obstruction occurs, endotracheal intubation may be necessary.

Because the diphtheria vaccine is included in routine immunizations for infants, diphtheria is almost extinct in the United States. However, isolated instances do occur, and when they do, prompt recognition and treatment are necessary (Ogle & Anderson, 2001).

Whooping Cough (Pertussis)

- Causative agent: *Bordetella pertussis*
- Incubation period: 5 to 21 days
- Mode of transmission: Direct or indirect contact
- Period of communicability: Greatest in catarrhal (respiratory illness) stage

- Immunity: Contracting the disease offers lasting natural immunity
- Active artificial immunity: Pertussis vaccine given as part of DTaP vaccine
- Passive artificial immunity: Pertussis immune serum globulin

Pertussis is a serious disease of childhood, but because of required immunizations, it is rarely seen today. Those most susceptible are children who were not immunized. A previous vaccine had possible side effects that led parents to refuse immunization.

Assessment. Pertussis manifests itself in three stages: catarrhal, paroxysmal, and convalescent. The **catarrhal stage** begins with upper respiratory symptoms such as coryza, sneezing, lacrimation, cough, and a low-grade fever. Children are irritable and listless. In some children, a mild cough is the only symptom during this stage. It lasts from 1 to 2 weeks (Scibano, 2000).

The paroxysmal stage lasts 4 to 6 weeks. During this time, the cough changes from a mild one to a paroxysmal one, involving five to ten short, rapid coughs, followed by a rapid inspiration, which causes the "whoop," or high-pitched crowing sound, of whooping cough. Children are in obvious distress while coughing. They may become cyanotic or red-faced, and their nose may drain thick, tenacious mucus. They often vomit after a paroxysm of coughing, and they are exhausted afterward from the effort. Attacks of coughing tend to be more severe at night.

During the convalescent stage, there is a gradual cessation of the coughing and vomiting. The cough may be present for some time, but as single, not paroxysmal, coughs. During the next year, if children develop an upper respiratory infection, they may again have a return of the paroxysmal coughing with vomiting.

Pertussis is diagnosed by its striking symptoms, although in children younger than age 6 months the "whoop" of the cough may be absent, making it more difficult to diagnose. The *B. pertussis* bacillus may be cultured from nasopharyngeal secretions during the catarrhal and paroxysmal stages. The white cell count, particularly the lymphocyte count, increases with whooping cough: it may be as high as 20,000 to 30,000/mm^3 at the end of the catarrhal stage (normal is 5,000 to 10,000/mm^3).

Therapeutic Management. Children with pertussis must be maintained on bedrest until the paroxysms of coughing subside. They need to be secluded from environmental factors, such as cigarette smoke, dust, and strenuous activity, that initiate coughing episodes. Nutrition may be a problem if the child is constantly coughing and vomiting. As a rule, frequent small meals are vomited less than larger meals. Infants with pertussis may be admitted to a health care facility for observation because they may have such tenacious secretions with coughing episodes that they need airway suction. Place an intercom in the infant's room so personnel can listen for paroxysms of coughing.

> **WHAT IF?** What if an adolescent with pertussis vomits after an episode of coughing? Should he try to eat again immediately, or do you think that he would be too nauseated to eat again?

A full 10-day course of erythromycin or penicillin may be prescribed. These drugs have the potential to shorten the period of communicability and may shorten the duration of symptoms. Droplet precautions are used until 5 days after the child starts effective therapy.

Complications of pertussis include pneumonia, atelectasis, or emphysema from plugged bronchioles. Seizures from asphyxia as a result of severe paroxysms of coughing may occur. Epistaxis, subconjunctival and subarachnoid bleeding from the force of coughing, may occur. If sufficient fluid intake cannot be maintained, alkalosis and dehydration from persistent vomiting can occur.

Prevention. Little passive immunity is transferred to the newborn, so children in their early months are particularly susceptible to this disease. This is why pertussis vaccine is one of the first immunizations scheduled. Infants who have not yet been immunized or are immunocompromised and are exposed may be given pertussis immune serum globulin to protect them from contracting the disease (Ogle & Anderson, 2001).

Anthrax

- Causative agent: *Bacillus anthracis,* a bacteria
- Incubation period: 1 to 7 days (inhalational), 1 to 12 days (cutaneous), 1 to 7 days (gastrointestinal)
- Mode of transmission: Originally contracted from contact with cow or sheep feces; not transmissible from person to person
- Immunity: Unstudied
- Active artificial immunity: A vaccine is available for people in high-risk occupations, such as veterinarians, but it is not recommended for children.
- Passive artificial immunity: Not available

Anthrax is an acute infectious disease that is contracted from exposure to the bacteria or its spores. Such bacteria live in the feces of infected cows or sheep. As the organism grows inside the human body, a toxin is produced that is the actual source of the symptoms. Children, like adults, may be affected by all three clinical forms: cutaneous, inhalational, or gastrointestinal (CDC, 2001).

Inhalational anthrax begins with a brief prodromal period of influenza-like symptoms, followed shortly by dyspnea, severe systemic shock, and marked evidence of mediastinal widening and pleural effusion on x-ray. The mortality for this form is over 90%.

Cutaneous anthrax is characterized by a skin lesion that begins as a papule, then passes through a vesicle stage to a painless depressed black eschar. Fever, malaise, and headache and regional lymphadenopathy may accompany the skin lesion. The mortality of cutaneous anthrax is as low as 1% with antibiotic therapy.

Gastrointestinal anthrax is contacted by eating undercooked meat infected with the organism. The child develops severe abdominal pain, fever, bloody diarrhea, and septicemia. Mortality is about 25%.

If a child is exposed to anthrax, prophylaxis with ciprofloxacin (Cipro) for those over 18 years and doxycycline for those younger should be started. Drug therapy is continued for 60 days because of the potential persistence of spores.

Tetanus (Lockjaw)

- Causative agent: *Clostridium tetani*
- Incubation period: 3 days to 3 weeks
- Period of communicability: None
- Mode of transmission: Direct or indirect contamination of a closed wound
- Immunity: Development of the disease gives lasting natural immunity.
- Active artificial immunity: Tetanus toxoid contained in DTaP vaccine
- Passive artificial immunity: Tetanus immune globulin

Tetanus, which is a highly fatal disease if untreated, is caused by an anaerobic, spore-forming bacillus. The bacillus, found in soil and the excretions of animals, enters the body through a wound. If the wound is deep, such as a puncture wound, where the distal end of the wound is shut off from an oxygen source, the tetanus bacilli begin to reproduce. The organism may also enter through a burn site, which crusts, creating an anaerobic environment. As the bacilli grow, they produce exotoxins that cause the disease symptoms by affecting the motor nuclei of the central nervous system (Callahan, 2000).

The entrance site of the bacillus does not appear infected (no pus or reddened area is present unless a secondary infection also exists). After the incubation period, the exotoxins have developed to such an extent, however, that they are capable of disrupting the nervous system.

Assessment. The first symptoms that are noticeable are stiffness of the neck and jaw (lockjaw). Within 24 to 48 hours, muscular rigidity of the trunk and extremities develops. The back becomes arched (opisthotonos), the abdominal muscles are stiff and boardlike, and the face assumes an unusual appearance, with wrinkling of the forehead and distortion of the corners of the mouth (a "sardonic grin" sign). Any stimulation, such as a sudden noise, a bright light, or a touch, causes painful, paroxysmal spasms. The sensorium is clear throughout the course of the disease, so the child is aware of the pain associated with muscle spasms. As these spasms begin to include laryngospasm, respiratory obstruction, and a collection of secretions in the respiratory tract, death by asphyxiation may occur.

Fever is an ominous sign accompanying tetanus. Children who survive the disease rarely have more than a low-grade fever.

Therapeutic Management. The child needs to be cared for in a quiet, stimulation-free room. If the wound has necrotic tissue, it may be debrided to ensure that no secondary infections arise. Enteral or total parenteral nutrition may be necessary to prevent aspiration from laryngeal spasm. Tetanus immune globulin (human) is administered to supply passive antitoxins to combat the extent of the disease involvement.

Parenteral penicillin G or erythromycin is administered to reduce the number of growing forms of the bacillus. Sedation and a muscle relaxant may be necessary to reduce the severity and pain of the muscle spasms. The child needs to be intubated, and mechanical ventilation is begun to maintain respiratory function after administration.

Prevention. Tetanus is a serious disease, but it can be prevented through active immunization and suitable booster immunization. Children routinely receive tetanus immunization as part of routine DTaP immunization and a booster dose at school age; thereafter they should receive a booster dose every 10 years. At the time of a wound, the wound site should be cleaned well with soap and water and a suitable antiseptic. If the wound is deep, such as a knife stab, a nail puncture, or a dog bite, it should not be sutured but should be left open to heal by secondary intention. This reduces the possibility of an anaerobic pocket forming in the wound. If the child received basic immunization against tetanus (five doses) and it has been fewer than 10 years since the last injection, no booster or antitoxin management is needed at the time of the wound.

If a child's immunization record cannot be obtained, or if it has been more than 10 years since the child received a booster injection or an initial injection for tetanus, the child will probably be treated with a booster injection and tetanus immune globulin. A booster injection provides tetanus antigen to the child. If the child received initial immunization for this disease, the booster will cause the body to "remember" how to make tetanus antibodies, and the body will begin to produce them rapidly. By the time the invading tetanus organisms from the wound have passed their long incubation period (3 days to 3 weeks), the child will have antibodies in the system prepared to eradicate the organisms. If the initial immunizations were incomplete or are unknown, in addition to tetanus antigen the child will also receive the passive antibodies included in tetanus immune globulin (Ogle & Anderson, 2001).

Lyme Disease

- Causative agent: *Borrelia burgdorferi,* a spirochete
- Incubation period: 3 to 30 days
- Period of communicability: Not communicable from one person to another
- Mode of transmission: Deer tick
- Active artificial immunity: Lyme disease vaccine

Lyme disease is caused by a spirochete, *Borrelia burgdorferi,* that is transmitted by a tick often carried on deer. The disease is the most frequently reported vector-borne infection in the United States, occurring most often in the summer and early fall. Almost immediately after the tick bite, an erythematous papule is noticeable at the site, which spreads over the next 3 to 30 days (the incubation period) to become a large, round ring with a raised swollen border (erythema chronicum migrans; Fig. 43-13). This is followed by systemic involvement that leads to cardiac, musculoskeletal, and neurologic symptoms. Cardiac involvement may be so severe that it includes heart block from atrioventricular conduction abnormalities. Neurologic symptoms commonly include stiff neck, headache, and cranial nerve palsy. Musculoskeletal symptoms occur in 50% of children and include painful swollen arthritic joints, particularly the knee.

Amoxicillin or penicillin V is administered at the time of the bite to young children. Doxycycline is given to those older than 8 years of age (Chalom, 2000). A vaccine

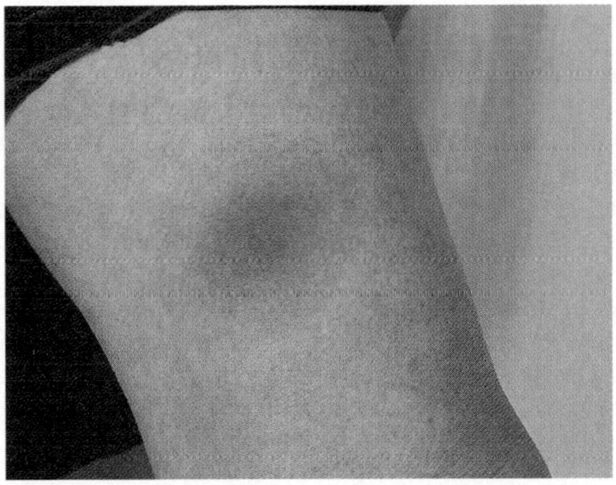

FIGURE 43.13 The rash of Lyme disease.

for the disease has been approved for use in adults who live or work in high-risk areas.

Parents should be cautioned to inspect the skin of children who have been playing in wooded areas for tick bites to help identify the disorder before debilitating symptoms occur. Other suggestions for avoiding Lyme disease are shown in Focus on Family Empowerment.

✔ CHECKPOINT QUESTIONS

13. What is the result of exotoxin production by diphtheria bacilli?
14. What is the major complication of pertussis?

OTHER INFECTIOUS PATHOGENS

Rickettsial Diseases

Rickettsiae are organisms that resemble viruses both in size and in their inability to reproduce except inside the cells of a host organism. They reproduce by fission, however, as bacteria do; like bacteria, they are complete organisms containing both RNA and DNA. They multiply inside ticks, lice, mites, or fleas (arthropods) without causing disease. They are transmitted to humans through the bite or feces of the infected arthropod. An exception is Q fever, which is spread by droplet infection. All rickettsial diseases include fever, and almost all include a rash caused by rickettsial multiplication in the endothelial cells of small blood vessels. Rickettsiae invasion triggers an immune response.

Rocky Mountain Spotted Fever

- Causative agent: *Rickettsia rickettsii*
- Incubation period: 3 to 12 days
- Period of communicability: Not communicable from one person to another
- Mode of transmission: Wood, dog, or rabbit tick
- Active artificial immunity: Rocky Mountain spotted fever vaccine

Rocky Mountain spotted fever is the most common rickettsial disease seen in the United States. It is most prevalent in the western United States and is transmitted by a tick. It is seen most often during the spring and early summer, when ticks are most commonly seen. A reddened area develops at the site of the tick bite. In 2 to 8 days, a typical rash, persistent headache, fever (as high as 104°F [40°C]), and mental confusion begin. The rash is distinctive, beginning with reddened macules, then changing to petechiae. It begins on the wrists and ankles, then spreads up the arms and legs onto the trunk. Unlike most rashes, it can cover the palms of the hands and soles of the feet (Fig. 43-14).

In untreated children, symptoms worsen to include central nervous system involvement (stiff neck and seizures) and cardiac and pulmonary symptoms such as heart failure and pneumonia. Nitrogen loss in the urine becomes extreme. An accompanying hyponatremia may also be present (Buckingham, 2002).

Therapy is with tetracycline for 7 to 10 days. Caution parents to administer the drug for the full course of therapy to ensure disease eradication and prevent the risk of complications. Rocky Mountain spotted fever was a serious childhood illness before antibiotic therapy was available,

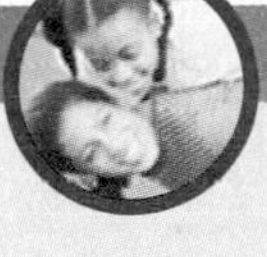

FOCUS ON FAMILY EMPOWERMENT

Tips For Avoiding Exposure to Lyme Disease

Q. My children love to play in the woods behind our house, but I'm so afraid that they'll get Lyme disease. What can I do to protect them?

A. Here are some suggestions for you and your children to help reduce the risk for exposure to Lyme disease:

- Wear protective clothing when hiking or playing in wooded areas: long sleeves, high necklines, long slacks. Tuck bottom of slacks into socks or boots.
- Wear light-colored clothing so any tick present on clothing can be readily observed.
- Inspect skin for ticks thoroughly after hiking or playing in wooded areas. Remove any present with tweezers.
- Report any area of inflammation that might be a tick bite to a health care provider for early diagnosis.
- Ask your primary care provider about the availability of Lyme disease vaccine. Currently, it is administered only to adults with high-risk occupations, but it is anticipated that the vaccine will soon be available for children living in high-risk areas.

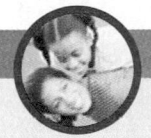

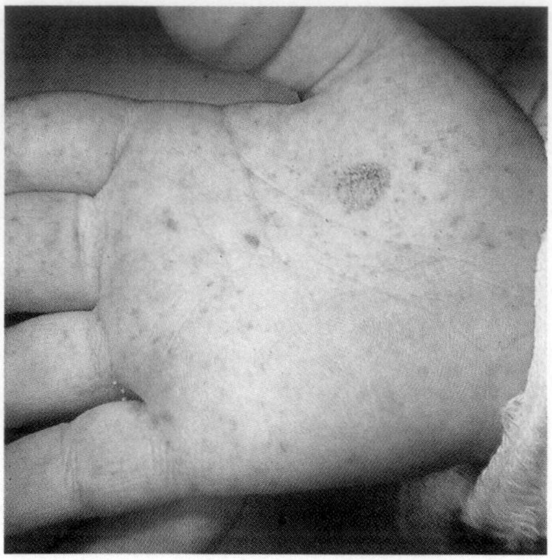

FIGURE 43.14 Typical rash of Rocky Mountain spotted fever.

and it still has the potential to be serious if the symptoms are not reported when they first occur (Woodward, 2000).

Murine Typhus

Murine typhus is seen almost exclusively in the southern United States. It is transmitted by mites and fleas that live on rats. It is almost identical in symptoms to Rocky Mountain spotted fever. It responds to tetracycline or a third-generation antibiotic such as ciprofloxacin (Cipro).

Chlamydial Infections

Chlamydiae are gram-negative nonmotile organisms similar to rickettsiae. Chlamydial pneumonia or vaginitis may occur (see Chaps. 40 and 47). Psittacosis is a chlamydial infection commonly found in children.

Psittacosis

Psittacosis, caused by *Chlamydia psittaci,* is a disease transmitted to children by birds, such as parakeets, lovebirds, parrots, chickens, turkeys, and pigeons. The bird has no apparent symptoms of illness. Children develop symptoms of an upper respiratory infection, possibly accompanied by a low-grade fever, a dry cough, weakness, and anorexia out of proportion to the fever. An enlarged spleen may also be present. Children may develop patchy bronchopneumonia. The course of the disease is as long as 3 to 4 weeks. Treatment is with erythromycin for young children and tetracycline for children over the age of 8 years (Tsarouhas, 2000b).

Parasitic Infections

Parasites are organisms that live and obtain their food supply from other organisms. Frequently seen parasites in children include head lice and scabies (Table 43-3). Parents are often embarrassed when they learn that their child has lice. Reassure them that this infestation can happen to any child (see Focus on Communication).

Helminthic Infections

Helminth (worm) refers to pathogenic or parasitic ones. They may be roundworms (nematodes), flukes (trematodes), or tapeworms (cestodes). Most helminths begin life when the eggs or larvae are eliminated in the feces or urine of humans. They are then transmitted to the oral cavity by contaminated foods or hands. Because children tend to be careless about washing their hands before eating or tend to suck their thumbs, they are prone to these infections.

Roundworms (Ascariasis)

The roundworm parasite lives in the intestinal tract. Eggs are excreted in the feces. Children typically ingest the eggs when they eat food with hands that are improperly

TABLE 43.3 Common Parasitic Infections

INFECTION	ORGANISM	SYMPTOMS	TREATMENT
Pediculosis capitis	Head lice	Small, white flecks on hair shaft (nits or eggs of lice) Extreme pruritus	Wash hair with shampoo such as lindane (Kwell). Comb nits from hair with fine-toothed comb. Wash bed sheets, recently worn clothes. Vacuum pillows, mattresses, or other items unable to be washed. Teach children not to exchange combs, hair barrettes, or other personal items.
Pediculosis	Pubic lice	Same as for head lice except on pubic hair	Same as head lice
Scabies	Female mite (*Acarus scabiei*)	Black burrow filled with mite feces ½ inch long, usually between fingers and toes, on palms, or in axilla or groin	Caution adolescent that groin infestations might be spread by physical intimacy. Wash area with lindane (Kwell) lotion or permethrin (Elimite).

FOCUS ON COMMUNICATION

Joshua is a 1-year-old boy you see in an ambulatory clinic. He has scratch marks on his neck and forehead. His hair shafts are covered by sandlike particles. He is diagnosed as having pediculosis capitis.

Less Effective Communication

Nurse: Hello, Mrs. Ireland. Did the doctor tell you what is wrong with Joshua?
Mrs. Ireland: No.
Nurse: I heard him tell you that Joshua has head lice. I have the prescription for you that you need for shampoo.
Mrs. Ireland: The doctor hasn't done any tests yet.
Nurse: There aren't any tests for head lice. Take the prescription to your drugstore and buy the shampoo.
Mrs. Ireland: What about the itchiness? Or these white marks?
Nurse: The shampoo will take care of it.
Mrs. Ireland: I'm not putting anything on his head for lice.
Nurse: Okay. I'll leave the prescription and you can think about it.

More Effective Communication

Nurse: Hello, Mrs. Ireland. Did the doctor tell you what is wrong with Joshua?
Mrs. Ireland: No.
Nurse: I thought that I heard him tell you that Joshua has head lice.
Mrs. Ireland: The doctor hasn't done any tests yet.
Nurse: Do you have any questions about what he said?
Mrs. Ireland: He said Joshua has head lice. But how could that be? We're not that poor.
Nurse: Let's talk about head lice, and how easy it is for anyone to get them.

The above scenario is an example of what can happen if people believe one of the stories that circulate related to communicable diseases. By allowing the mother to explain why she thinks the diagnosis could not be right rather than just proceeding with instructions, the nurse makes it possible for her to learn the correct information. This should increase compliance.

washed. Larvae, which hatch from the ingested eggs, penetrate the intestinal wall and enter the circulation. From there, they may migrate to any body tissue. Children have a loss of appetite and perhaps nausea and vomiting. Intestinal obstruction may occur from a mass of roundworms in the intestinal tract. Ascariasis can be prevented by the sanitary disposal of feces to prevent contamination of the soil. A single dose of an anthelmintic such as pyrantel pamoate (Antiminth) controls the infection (Weinberg & Levin, 2001).

Hookworms

Hookworm eggs, like roundworm eggs, are found in human feces. They enter children's bodies through the skin and then migrate to the intestinal tract, where they attach themselves onto the intestinal villi. They suck blood from the intestinal wall to sustain themselves. If a great number of hookworms are present, severe anemia may result. Treatment is with anthelmintics to destroy the worms. Children may also need therapy for the anemia.

Pinworms

Pinworms are small, white, threadlike worms that live in the cecum. At night, the female pinworm migrates down the intestinal tract and out the anus to deposit eggs in the anal and perianal region. The anal area itches, and the child awakens at night crying and scratching. Some of the eggs are then carried from the child's fingernails to the mouth. They hatch in the child's intestinal tract, and the cycle is repeated.

The worms are large enough that they can be seen if the child's buttocks are separated when he or she is sleeping. Pressing a piece of cellophane tape against the anus and then looking at it under a microscope will generally reveal pinworm eggs.

Treatment is with a single dose of mebendazole (Vermox) or pyrantel pamoate (Antiminth; Silver, 2000). Both drugs destroy pinworms. All family members are treated for pinworm infestation because the worms are easily transmitted from person to person. Underclothing, bedding, towels, and nightclothes should be washed before reuse. Teach children to avoid nailbiting and to wash their hands before food preparation or eating to avoid transfer of pinworm eggs to the gastrointestinal tract.

Protozoan Infections

Protozoa are unicellular organisms. They absorb fluid through the cell membrane and can move from place to place by pseudopod, flagella, or cilia action. They are most pathogenic in the gastrointestinal, genitourinary, and circulatory systems. Some protozoa reproduce by simple binary fission; other forms have complex life cycles. Protozoa have the ability to form cysts or surround themselves with a membrane; this makes them resistant to destruction.

Giardiasis

Giardia lamblia is a protozoan infection that is responsible for epidemic outbreaks of diarrhea, particularly in travelers to Europe and in day care centers in the United States.

Transmission occurs when the child ingests the cysts of the organism on unclean hands. In the intestine, the cysts develop into the mature form of the organism, causing symptoms such as diarrhea, weight loss, abdominal cramps, and nausea.

Diagnosis is made by history and recognition of the mature form of the organism in the stool or on duodenal aspiration. Therapy is with metronidazole (Flagyl) for 7 days (Gardner & Hill, 2001). Flagyl is contraindicated during early pregnancy.

Fungal Infections

Fungi are larger than bacteria; some are unicellular (yeasts), but generally they are multicellular (molds). Fungal infections are most often divided into groups according to the body tissue they infect. Deep mycoses invade internal organs. Transmission is by the inhalation of spores. Subcutaneous mycoses invade skin, subcutaneous tissue, and bone. Infections usually occur from introduction of the fungi into a wound. Superficial mycoses invade only the hair, skin, or nails.

Superficial Fungal Infections

Four superficial fungal infections are seen frequently in children: tinea cruris, pedis, capitis, and corporis.

Tinea Cruris. Tinea cruris (jock itch) occurs on the inner aspects of the thighs and scrotum. It is pruritic. Local application of clotrimazole (Lotrimin) liquid or powder destroys the infection (Morelli & Weston, 2001).

Tinea Pedis. Tinea pedis (athlete's foot) produces skin lesions between the toes and on the plantar surface of the foot. Pruritic, pinpoint vesicles and fissuring, especially between the toes, may occur. It is treated with liquid preparations of clotrimazole (Lotrimin; Morelli & Weston, 2001).

Tinea Capitis. Tinea capitis (ringworm) is a fungal infection that begins as an infection of a single hair follicle but spreads rapidly in a circular pattern to produce a lesion usually approximately 1 inch in diameter (Fig. 43-15). The hairs involved in the lesion generally break off. The circle becomes filled with dirty-appearing scales. Some strains of tinea capitis may be detected because they glow green under a Wood's light. Newer strains of the organism do not do this, so the test is losing its accuracy.

Treatment is with griseofulvin given orally. Adolescents should be warned not to use alcohol while taking this drug; this may cause tachycardia. Safety during pregnancy is not established. Children need to avoid strong sunlight during therapy because photosensitivity may occur.

Tinea capitis is not as contagious as was once assumed. Children need not be kept home from school, although they should be cautioned not to exchange towels or combs or other potential fomites. The course of the disease may be long; it may be 3 months before all lesions have faded (Truong & Friedlander, 2001).

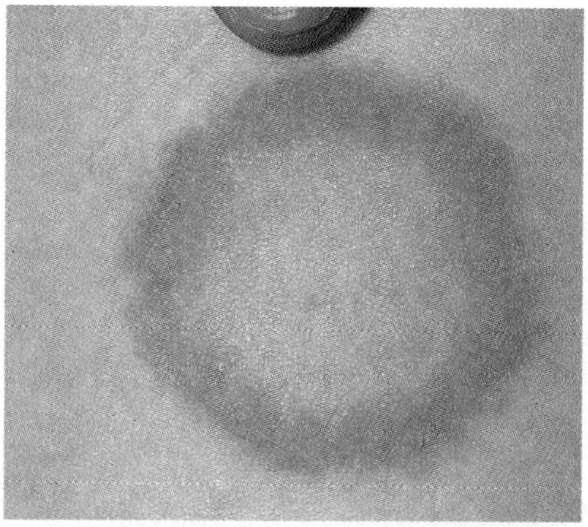

FIGURE 43.15 Ringworm. The fungus spreads rapidly, producing a circular, ringlike lesion.

Tinea Corporis. Tinea corporis is fungal infection of the epidermal layer of the skin. It presents as a scaly ring of inflammation with a clear area in the center. Treatment is with a topical antifungal agent such as clotrimazole (Lotrimin).

Candidiasis

Candida albicans is the fungus responsible for candidal (monilial) infections. Candidal organisms grow in the vagina of many adult women (candidal vaginitis). Newborns delivered vaginally may develop an infection of the mucous membrane of the mouth (thrush or oral candidal infection). Thrush is characterized by white plaques on an erythematous base on the buccal membrane and the surface of the tongue. It resembles a milk curd left from a recent milk feeding. Thrush plaques do not scrape away, however, whereas milk curds do. The mouth is painful, and the child does not eat well due to the inflammation and local pain. Adolescent girls may develop candidal vaginitis (Weinberg & Levin, 2001; see Chap. 47).

C. albicans also causes a severe, bright red, sharply circumscribed diaper-area rash (Fig. 43-16). Satellite lesions also may appear. The rash is marked by its intense color, and it does not improve with the usual diaper rash measures, such as Desitin, frequent changing of diapers, or exposure to air.

Nystatin is an effective antifungal drug. For oral thrush, it is generally administered by mouth approximately four times a day. It should be dropped into the mouth after feedings so it will remain in contact with the lesions rather than being washed away immediately by a feeding. For diaper rash, a nystatin ointment is prescribed.

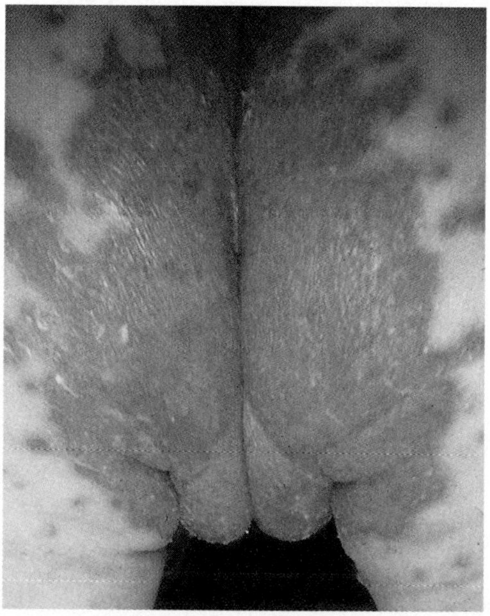

FIGURE 43.16 Monilial diaper rash. Note the intense red color of the rash.

Candidiasis can become a generalized infection, especially in a newborn. There is a tendency to think of thrush as a common, almost expected disease of infants. It needs treatment, however, to prevent it from becoming more serious or systemic (Weinberg & Levin, 2001).

✔ CHECKPOINT QUESTIONS

15. How are helminthic infections transmitted?
16. What organism is responsible for thrush?

KEY POINTS

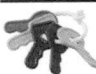

The incubation period of infectious disease is the time between the invasion of an organism and the onset of symptoms. The prodromal period is the time between the beginning of nonspecific symptoms and specific symptoms. Children are infectious during the prodromal period. Illness is the stage during which specific symptoms are evident. The convalescent period is the interval between the time symptoms begin to fade and the time the child returns to full wellness.

The chain of infection depends on the presence of a reservoir, a portal of exit, a means of transmission, a portal of entry, and a susceptible host. To reduce the spread of infection, use standard precautions. Transmission-based precautions—airborne, droplet, and contact—also may be necessary.

Common viral infections of childhood include exanthem subitum (roseola), rubella (German measles), measles (rubeola), chickenpox (varicella), herpes zoster, erythema infectiosum (fifth disease), pityriasis rosea, mumps (epidemic parotitis), infectious mononucleosis, and cat-scratch disease. Other important viral infections include poliomyelitis (now almost extinct), herpesvirus infections, verrucae (warts), and rabies.

Streptococcal diseases include scarlet fever and impetigo. Staphylococcal infections include furunculosis (boils), cellulitis, and scalded skin disease. Outbreaks of diphtheria, whooping cough (pertussis), and tetanus (lockjaw) still occur.

Important tick-borne diseases are Rocky Mountain spotted fever and Lyme disease. Parasitic infections are pediculosis capitis (head lice), pediculosis pubis, and scabies. Helminthic infections are roundworms, hookworms, and pinworms. Fungal infections are tinea capitis and tinea corporis (ringworm).

Teaching parents and children about infection control measures and the need for up-to-date immunizations is essential to reduce the risk of infectious disorders.

CRITICAL THINKING EXERCISES

1. Marty is the 10-year-old boy you met at the beginning of the chapter. He was diagnosed as having chickenpox (varicella) the morning after surgery for appendicitis. Is it likely that Marty contracted this infection while he was hospitalized, or is it more likely that the contact occurred before hospitalization? What is the typical pattern of chickenpox lesions? What would you recommend to his parents to help reduce the itchiness of the rash?
2. An adolescent is diagnosed with Lyme disease. She tells you, "I never eat limes. How did I get this disease?" How would you respond to her?
3. A newborn is found to have oral candidiasis (thrush). His mother asks you, "How did my newborn get this infection? Aren't they born sterile?" How would you respond to her?
4. Examine the National Health Goals related to infections in children. Most government-sponsored money for nursing research is allotted based on these goals. What would be a possible research topic to explore pertinent to these goals that would be fundable and would advance evidence-based practice?

REFERENCES

Bagarazzi, M. L., & Cohen, A. (2000). Scarlet fever. In M. W. Schwartz (Ed.). *The 5-minute pediatric consult* (pp. 728–729). Philadelphia: Lippincott Williams & Wilkins.

Bell, L. M. (2000a). Roseola infantum. In M. W. Schwartz (Ed.). *The 5-minute pediatric consult* (pp. 720–721). Philadelphia: Lippincott Williams & Wilkins.

Bell, L. M. (2000). Measles (rubeola, first disease). In M. W. Schwartz (Ed.). *The 5-minute pediatric consult* (pp. 520–521). Philadelphia: Lippincott Williams & Wilkins.

Buckingham, S. C. (2002). Rocky mountain spotted fever. *Pediatric Annuals, 31*(3), 163–169.

Burroughs, K. E. (2000b). Athletes resuming activity after infectious mononucleosis. *Archives of Family Medicine, 9*(10), 1122–1123.

Callahan, J. M. (2000). Tetanus. In M. W. Schwartz (Ed.). *The 5-minute pediatric consult* (pp. 802–803). Philadelphia: Lippincott Williams & Wilkins.

Centers for Disease Control. (2001). Investigation of anthrax associated with intentional exposure and interim public health guidelines. *MMWR, 50*(41), 889–893.

Centers for Disease Control. (2002). *Recommendations for isolation precautions in hospitals.* Washington, DC: CDC.

Chalom, E. C. (2000). Lyme disease. In M. W. Schwartz (Ed.). *The 5-minute pediatric consult* (pp. 510–511). Philadelphia: Lippincott Williams & Wilkins.

Chasens, E. R., & Umlauf, M. G. (2000). Post-polio syndrome. *American Journal of Nursing, 100*(12), 60–65.

Conrad, D. A. (2001). Treatment of cat-scratch disease. *Current Opinion in Pediatrics, 13*(1), 56–59.

Conway, D. H., & Bagarazzi, M. L. (2000). Staphylococcal scalded skin syndrome. In M. W. Schwartz (Ed.). *The 5-minute pediatric consult* (pp. 766–767). Philadelphia: Lippincott Williams & Wilkins.
Cordell, R. L. (2001). The risk of infectious diseases among child care providers. *Journal of the American Medical Women's Association, 56*(3), 109–112.
Department of Health and Human Services (2000). *Healthy people, 2010.* Washington, D.C.: DHHS.
Dibs, S. (2000). Rabies. In M. W. Schwartz (Ed.). *The 5-minute pediatric consult* (pp. 684–685). Philadelphia: Lippincott Williams & Wilkins.
Foster, J. A. (2000). Impetigo. In M. W. Schwartz (Ed.). *The 5-minute pediatric consult* (pp. 468–469). Philadelphia: Lippincott Williams & Wilkins.
Gardner, T. B., & Hill, D. R. (2001). Treatment of giardiasis. *Clinical Microbiology Reviews, 14*(1), 114–128.
Gould, J. M. (2000). Herpes simplex virus (HSV). In M. W. Schwartz (Ed.). *The 5-minute pediatric consult* (pp. 430–431). Philadelphia: Lippincott Williams & Wilkins.
Hanson, C. M. (2001). Fifth disease. *American Journal for Nurse Practitioners. 5*(8), 35–40.
Henderson, D. A. (2002). Countering the posteradication threat of smallpox and polio. *Clinical Infectious Diseases, 34*(1), 79–83.
Kim, H. J. (2000). Warts. In M. W. Schwartz (Ed.). *The 5-minute pediatric consult* (pp. 874–875). Philadelphia: Lippincott Williams & Wilkins.
Levin, M. J., & Weinberg, A. (2001). Infections due to herpesviruses. In W. W. Hay, A. R. Hayward, M. J. Levin, & J. M. Sondheimer (Eds.). *Current pediatric diagnosis and treatment* (15th ed.). New York: McGraw-Hill.
Morelli, J. G., & Weston, W. L. (2001). Common skin diseases in infants, children & adolescents. In W. W. Hay, A. R. Hayward, M. J. Levin, & J. M. Sondheimer (Eds.). *Current pediatric diagnosis and treatment* (15th ed.). New York: McGraw-Hill.
Nelson, J. S., & Stone, M. S. (2000). Update on selected viral exanthems. *Current Opinion in Pediatrics, 12*(4), 359–364.
Ogle, J. W., & Anderson, M. S. (2001). Bacterial and spirochetal infections. In W. W. Hay, A. R. Hayward, M. J. Levin, & J. M. Sondheimer (Eds.). *Current pediatric diagnosis and treatment* (15th ed.). New York: McGraw-Hill.
Papesch, M., & Watkins, R. (2001). Epstein-Barr virus infectious mononucleosis. *Clinical Otolaryngology & Allied Sciences, 26*(1), 3–8.
Ramos, M. M. et al. (2001). Infection with Sin Nombre hantavirus: Clinical presentation and outcome in children and adolescents. *Pediatrics, 108*(2), E27.
Sax, H., et al. (2001). Variation in nosocomial infection prevalence according to patient care setting. *Journal of Hospital Infection, 48*(1), 27–32.
Scribano, P. V. (2000). Pertussis In M. W. Schwartz (Ed.). *The 5-minute pediatric consult* (pp. 620–621). Philadelphia: Lippincott Williams & Wilkins.
Silver, D. L. (2000). Pinworms. In M. W. Schwartz (Ed.). *The 5-minute pediatric consult* (pp. 626–627). Philadelphia: Lippincott Williams & Wilkins.
Tangermann, R. H., et al. (2000). Eradication of poliomyelitis in countries affected by conflict. *Bulletin of the World Health Organization, 78*(3), 330–338.
Truong, A., & Friedlander, S. F. (2001). Superficial fungal infections in adolescence. *Adolescent Medicine, 12*(2), 213–227.
Tsarouhas, N. (2000a). Mumps/parotitis. In M. W. Schwartz (Ed.). *The 5-minute pediatric consult* (pp. 546–547). Philadelphia: Lippincott Williams & Wilkins.
Tsarouhas, N. (2000b). Psittacosis/Ornithosis (parrot fever). In M. W. Schwartz (Ed.). *The 5-minute pediatric consult* (pp. 666–667). Philadelphia: Lippincott Williams & Wilkins.
Watson, B. (2000). Varicella/Herpes zoster. In M. W. Schwartz (Ed.). *The 5-minute pediatric consult* (pp. 424–425). Philadelphia: Lippincott William & Wilkins.
Weinberg, A., & Levin, M. J. (2001). Infections: mycotic. In W. W. Hay, A. R. Hayward, M. J. Levin, & J. M. Sondheimer (Eds.). *Current pediatric diagnosis and treatment* (15th ed.). New York: McGraw-Hill.
Woodward, G. A. (2000). Rocky Mountain spotted fever. In M. W. Schwartz (Ed.). *The 5-minute pediatric consult* (pp. 718–719). Philadelphia: Lippincott Williams & Wilkins.

SUGGESTED READINGS

Berg, D., & Erickson, P. (2001). Fungal skin infections in children. *Postgraduate Medicine, 110*(1), 83–93.
Bielan, B. (1999). What's your assessment: Impetigo. *Dermatology Nursing, 11*(5), 354–355.
Gellin, B. G., Maibach, E. W., & Marcuse, E. K. (2000). Do parents understand immunization? *Pediatrics, 106*(5), 1097–1102.
Girouard, S., et al. (2001). Infection control programs at children's hospitals: A description of structures and processes. *American Journal of Infection Control, 29*(3), 145–151.
Healy, T. L. (2000). The impact of Lyme disease on school children. *Journal of School Nursing, 16*(2), 12–18.
Houston, S. (1999). Managing the outcome of infection: Nosocomial infection initiative. *Outcomes Management for Nursing Practice, 3*(2), 73–77.
Huskins, W. C. (2000). Transmission and control of infections in out-of-home child care. *Pediatric Infectious Disease Journal, 19*(10 Suppl), 106–110.
Kenny, H., & Lawson, E. (2000). The efficacy of cotton cover gowns in reducing infection in nursing neutropenic patients: An evidence-based study. *International Journal of Nursing Practice, 6*(3), 135–139.
Miller, L. C., & Hendrie, N. W. (2000). Health of children adopted from China. *Pediatrics, 105*(6), 76–78.
Orenstein, W. A., et al. (2000). Measles eradication: Is it in our future? *American Journal of Public Health, 90*(10), 1521–1525.
Ridgway, D. (2000). The logic of causation and the risk of paralytic poliomyelitis for an American child. *Epidemiology & Infection, 124*(1), 113–120.
Weber, L. G. & Bissell, M. G. (2002). Infectious diseases, confidentiality, and research ethics. *Clinical Leadership & Management Review, 16*(1), 35–36.

Nursing Care of the Child With a Hematologic Disorder

CHAPTER 44

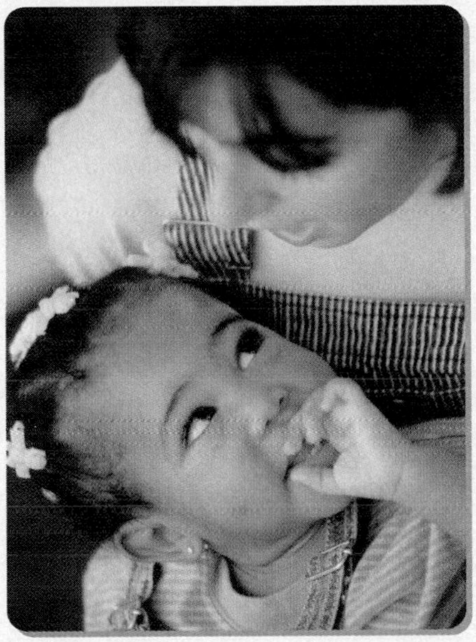

Key Terms

- agranulocytes
- allogeneic transplantation
- aplastic anemia
- autologous transplantation
- blood dyscrasias
- blood plasma
- direct bilirubin
- erythroblasts
- erythrocytes
- erythropoietin
- granulocytes
- Heinz bodies
- hemochromatosis
- hemoglobin
- hemolysis
- hemosiderosis
- hypodermoclysis
- leukocytes
- leukopenia
- megakaryocytes
- normoblasts
- pancytopenia
- petechiae
- plethora
- poikilocytic
- polycythemia
- priapism
- purpura
- reticulocytes
- sickle-cell crisis
- sickle-cell trait
- synergeneic transplantation
- thrombocytes
- thrombocytopenia

Objectives

After mastering the contents of this chapter, you should be able to:

1. Describe the major hematologic disorders of childhood.
2. Assess the child with a hematologic disorder.
3. Formulate nursing diagnoses for the child with a hematologic disorder such as sickle-cell anemia.
4. Identify outcomes for the child with a hematologic disorder.
5. Plan nursing care for the child with a hematologic disorder.
6. Implement nursing care related to the child with a hematologic disorder.
7. Evaluate outcomes for achievement and effectiveness of care for a child with a hematologic disorder.
8. Identify National Health Goals related to children with hematologic disorders that nurses could be instrumental in helping the nation to achieve.
9. Identify areas related to care of children with hematologic disorders that could benefit from additional nursing research or application of evidence-based practice.
10. Use critical thinking to analyze ways that nursing care for a child with a hematologic disorder could be more family-centered.
11. Integrate knowledge of hematologic disorders in children with nursing process to achieve quality maternal and child health nursing care.

Heather is a 2-year-old girl diagnosed with thalassemia major. She has a prominent mandible and wide-spaced upper teeth from the overgrowth of bone marrow centers. Her skin is bronze from the number of transfusions (64) she has received in her short lifetime. Joey is a 4-year-old boy seen at the same clinic. He is diagnosed as having thalassemia minor. He has no facial deformities or skin discoloration. "Why did this happen?" Heather's mother asks you. "How can two children with the same disease look so different?" What additional health teaching about thalassemia does Heather's mother need to help her better understand her daughter's disease?

Previous chapters described the growth and development of well children. This chapter adds information about the dramatic changes, both physical and psychosocial, that occur when children have a hematologic disorder. This is important information because it builds a base for care and health teaching.

After you've studied the chapter, answer the Critical Thinking Exercises at the end of the chapter and then access the on-line study activities (http://connection.lww.com) *to further sharpen your skills and test your knowledge.*

FOCUS ON NATIONAL HEALTH GOALS

A National Health Goal that addresses iron-deficiency anemia, the most common blood disorder in children, is:

- Reduce iron deficiency among young children aged 1 to 2 years to less than 5% and among women of child-bearing age to less than 7% from baselines of 9% and 11% (DHHS, 2000).

Nurses can be instrumental in helping the nation achieve this goal by educating parents about the importance of adding iron-rich cereal to infants' diets and women taking an iron supplement during pregnancy. Nursing research questions that could add important information for prevention include: what are ways of increasing compliance in pregnant women that would help ensure that all women take an iron supplement during pregnancy; and do infants maintain higher iron levels when cereal is eaten with milk or orange juice?

The blood and blood-forming tissues that make up the hematologic system play a vital role in body metabolism: transporting oxygen and nutrients to body cells, removing carbon dioxide from cells, and initiating blood coagulation when vessels are injured. As a result, any alteration in the substance or function of blood or its components can have immediate and life-threatening effects on the functioning of all body systems. For instance, an alteration in the process of coagulation can result in death from acute and uncontrollable blood loss. Inadequate red cell formation results in decreased oxygenation in tissues.

Hematologic disorders, often called **blood dyscrasias,** occur when components of the blood either increase or decrease in amount beyond normal ranges or are formed incorrectly. Most blood dyscrasias in children originate in the bone marrow, where blood cells are formed.

A common hematologic disorder in children is iron-deficiency anemia. The National Health Goals related to this disorder are shown in the Focus on National Health Goals box.

NURSING PROCESS OVERVIEW

For the Child With a Hematologic Disorder

Assessment

Many of the symptoms of hematologic disorders begin insidiously, with symptoms such as pallor, lethargy, and bruising (see Assessing the Child With a Hematologic Disorder). These seem to be such minor symptoms that parents may not bring their child to a health care facility for some time. They are surprised to learn that subtle symptoms such as these can signify the presence of a serious disease.

Many hematologic disorders are inherited. When one is diagnosed, parents may feel guilty or blame themselves or their partner for the child's disease. It is difficult for parents to support a child during an illness when they need intensive support themselves. Be certain both parents and children receive the support and comfort they need.

Asking at routine checkups about a child's dietary intake often reveals iron-deficiency anemia. Many babies with this problem have been drinking too much milk and not eating enough iron-containing foods. This makes them iron-deficient, but aside from paleness and irritability, they appear plump and "healthy." Their parents have not suspected that their baby's appearance masks a nutritional deficiency.

Nursing Diagnosis

Nursing diagnoses that might be used with children who have hematologic disorders may include:

- Deficient knowledge related to cause of illness
- Imbalanced nutrition, less than body requirements, related to parental lack of knowledge of need for iron-rich diet
- Anxiety related to frequent blood-sampling procedures
- Pain related to tissue ischemia
- Compromised family coping related to long-term care needs of child with chronic hematologic disorder

Outcome Identification and Planning

Be certain in helping parents plan outcomes that they are realistic. The number of blood-sampling procedures, for example, cannot be reduced, but the child can be helped, with distraction techniques, to deal with the pain and anxiety the procedures cause.

Children with hematologic disorders often are prescribed long-term medication such as a corticosteroid. When a child is very ill, parents are usually very conscientious about giving such medicine. When

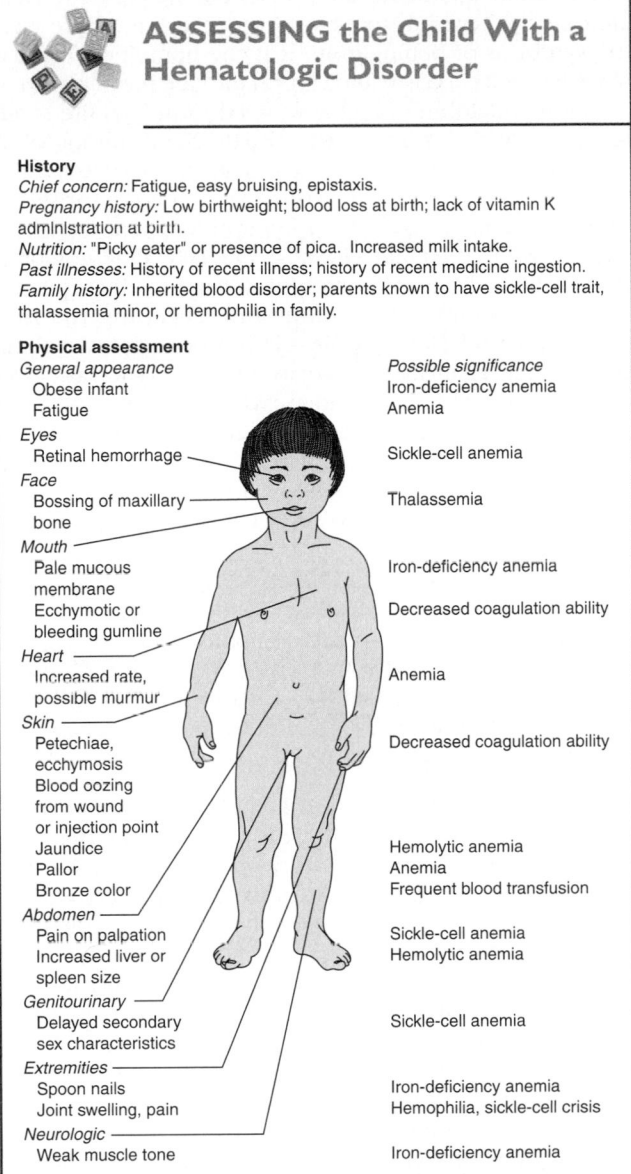

ASSESSING the Child With a Hematologic Disorder

History
Chief concern: Fatigue, easy bruising, epistaxis.
Pregnancy history: Low birthweight; blood loss at birth; lack of vitamin K administration at birth.
Nutrition: "Picky eater" or presence of pica. Increased milk intake.
Past illnesses: History of recent illness; history of recent medicine ingestion.
Family history: Inherited blood disorder; parents known to have sickle-cell trait, thalassemia minor, or hemophilia in family.

Physical assessment

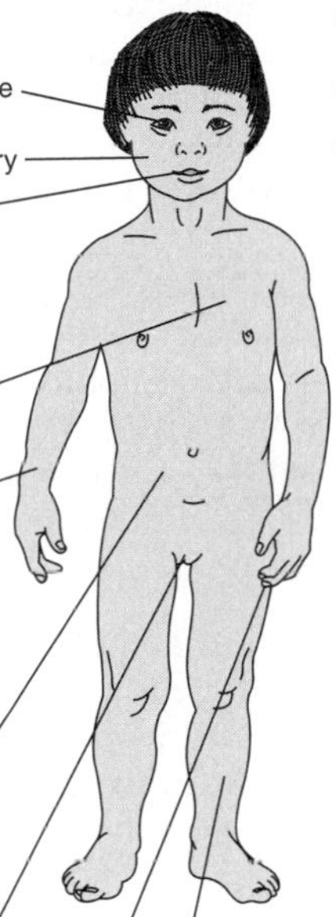

General appearance	*Possible significance*
Obese infant	Iron-deficiency anemia
Fatigue	Anemia
Eyes	
Retinal hemorrhage	Sickle-cell anemia
Face	
Bossing of maxillary bone	Thalassemia
Mouth	
Pale mucous membrane	Iron-deficiency anemia
Ecchymotic or bleeding gumline	Decreased coagulation ability
Heart	
Increased rate, possible murmur	Anemia
Skin	
Petechiae, ecchymosis	Decreased coagulation ability
Blood oozing from wound or injection point	
Jaundice	Hemolytic anemia
Pallor	Anemia
Bronze color	Frequent blood transfusion
Abdomen	
Pain on palpation	Sickle-cell anemia
Increased liver or spleen size	Hemolytic anemia
Genitourinary	
Delayed secondary sex characteristics	Sickle-cell anemia
Extremities	
Spoon nails	Iron-deficiency anemia
Joint swelling, pain	Hemophilia, sickle-cell crisis
Neurologic	
Weak muscle tone	Iron-deficiency anemia

a child has a disorder with few symptoms, however, it is easy for parents to forget to give the medication. In addition, the child may refuse to take the medication because it tastes bad or upsets the stomach. Planning includes helping the parents devise ways to disguise the taste or remember to give the medication over the long term.

Nutritional planning is another area that needs consideration. Parents of children with iron-deficiency anemia, for example, may need to modify meal plans not only for the child but also for the entire family. Iron-rich foods often are expensive. A parent on a limited budget may have difficulty, therefore, providing meals rich in iron. If the child is a "fussy eater," parents may need a great deal of support to insist that the child eat foods containing iron rather than giving the child what he or she wants. If the child will be restricted for long periods because the immune system is compromised as a part of the illness, planning must include ways to keep the child interested in activities to promote development. Investigate possible resources for parental and child support and education.

Implementation
Nursing interventions for children with hematologic disorders include helping with obtaining specimens for testing and assisting with blood or bone marrow transfusions. Remember that a finger stick for blood is often as painful as a venipuncture (and more painful afterward because the fingertip is irritated every time the child attempts to use it). Suggesting that blood be drawn by means of an intermittent device such as a heparin lock may reduce the number of times a child is subjected to venipuncture. Applying EMLA cream before finger sticks or venipunctures also helps to reduce pain and improve compliance with procedures. Even so, children may need some therapeutic playtime with a syringe and a doll to express their anger about constant invasion by needles.

Because of the chronicity of some of the hematologic disorders, parents and children often need the support of outside agencies. Some organizations helpful for referral are:

Aplastic Anemia Foundation of America (*www.aplastic.org*)
Sickle Cell Disease Association of America (*www.sicklecelldisease.org*)
American Society of Pediatric Hematology and Oncology (*www.aspho.org*)
National Hemophilia Foundation (*www.hemophilia.org*)

Outcome Evaluation
Evaluation focuses on achievement of short-term outcomes (e.g., the moderation of pain or elimination of anxiety in the child undergoing testing or treatment) and progress toward the achievement of long-term outcomes (e.g., improving the ability of the family to manage the stress of raising a child with a chronic illness or deal with frequently occurring health crises).

Examples suggesting achievement of outcomes may include:

- Parents state increased knowledge of cause of iron-deficiency anemia.
- Child states she feels better able to cope with blood-sampling procedures through the use of imagery.
- Parents describe realistic plans to ensure compliance with long-term medication administration.

STRUCTURE AND FUNCTION OF BLOOD

Blood Formation and Components

The formation of blood cells begins as early as week 2 of intrauterine life. The yolk sac is responsible for this early blood formation. By month 2 of intrauterine life, the liver and spleen begin forming blood components. At approximately month 4, the bone marrow becomes and remains the active center for the origination of blood cells. As in extrauterine life, the spleen serves as the organ for the destruction of blood cells once their normal lifetime has passed (Bondurant & Koury, 1999).

The total volume of blood in the body is roughly proportional to body weight: 85 mL/kg at birth, 75 mL/kg at age 6 months, and 70 mL/kg after the first year. The **blood plasma** (liquid portion containing proteins, hormones, enzymes, and electrolytes) is in equilibrium with the fluid of the interstitial tissue spaces. Although important in diseases causing vomiting and diarrhea (when it may become depleted, leading to dehydration), plasma is not a major site of hematologic disease. The formed elements—the **erythrocytes** (red blood cells), **leukocytes** (white blood cells), and **thrombocytes** (platelets)—are the portions most affected by hematologic disorders in children.

Erythrocytes (Red Blood Cells)

Erythrocytes (red blood cells [RBCs]) function chiefly to transport oxygen to and carry carbon dioxide from body cells. RBCs are formed under the stimulation of **erythropoietin,** a hormone produced by the kidneys. An increase in erythropoietin is stimulated whenever a child has tissue hypoxia. **Polycythemia,** or an overproduction of RBCs, is chronically present in children who experience prolonged systemic hypoxia. Children with kidney disease often have a low number of RBCs because erythropoietin secretion is inadequate in diseased kidneys.

RBCs form first as **erythroblasts** (large, nucleated cells), then mature through **normoblast** and **reticulocyte** stages to mature, nonnucleated erythrocytes. Approximately 1% of RBCs are in the reticulocyte stage at all times. An elevated reticulocyte count in children indicates rapid production of RBCs. This is seen in children with iron-deficiency anemia once iron therapy is begun and the body is again able to produce RBCs. The absence of a nucleus in the mature cell allows for increased space for oxygen transport, but it also limits the life of cells because metabolic processes are limited. At the end of their life span, erythrocytes are destroyed through phagocytosis by reticuloendothelial cells, found in the highest proportion in the spleen.

In infants, the long bones of the body are filled with red marrow actively producing RBCs. In early childhood, yellow marrow begins to replace this in long bones, so blood element production is then carried out mainly in the ribs, scapulae, vertebrae, and skull bones. The yellow marrow remaining in the extremities can be activated if necessary to produce additional blood products.

At birth, an infant has approximately 5 million RBCs per cubic millimeter of blood. This concentration diminishes rapidly in the first months, reaching a low of approximately 4.1 million per cubic millimeter at age 3 to 4 months. The number then slowly increases until adolescence, when adult values of approximately 4.9 million per cubic millimeter are reached.

Hemoglobin. The component of RBCs that allows them to carry out the transport of oxygen is **hemoglobin,** a complex protein. Hemoglobin comprises globin, a protein (like all protein) dependent on nitrogen metabolism for its formation, and heme, an iron-containing pigment. Deficiency of either iron stores or nitrogen will interfere with the synthesis of hemoglobin. It is the heme portion that combines with oxygen and carbon dioxide for transport.

The hemoglobin in erythrocytes during fetal life is different from that formed after birth. Fetal hemoglobin serves the fetus well because it can absorb oxygen at the low oxygen tension that exists in utero. It is comprised of two alpha and two gamma polypeptide chains. At birth, 40% to 70% of the child's hemoglobin is fetal hemoglobin (hemoglobin F). Fetal hemoglobin is gradually replaced by adult hemoglobin (hemoglobin A) during the first 6 months of life. Hemoglobin A is comprised of two alpha and two beta chains. For this reason, diseases such as sickle-cell anemia or the thalassemias, which are defects of the beta chains, do not become apparent clinically until this hemoglobin change has occurred (at approximately age 6 months). However, because beginning in early intrauterine life some hemoglobin A is present, they can be diagnosed prenatally.

The hemoglobin level of blood varies according to the number of RBCs present and the average amount of hemoglobin each cell contains. Hemoglobin levels are highest at birth (13.7 to 20.1 g/100 mL); they reach a low at approximately age 3 months (9.5 to 14.5 g/100 mL); and they gradually rise again until adult values are reached at puberty (11 to 16 g/100 mL).

Bilirubin. RBCs have a life span of approximately 120 days. After this time, they disintegrate and their protein component is preserved by specialized cells in the liver and spleen (reticuloendothelial cells) for further use. Iron is released for reuse by the bone marrow to construct new RBCs. As the heme portion is degraded, it is converted into protoporphyrin. Protoporphyrin is then further broken down into indirect bilirubin. Indirect bilirubin is fat-soluble and cannot be excreted by the kidneys in this state. It is therefore converted by the liver enzyme glucuronyl transferase into **direct bilirubin,** which is water-soluble and is combined and excreted in bile.

In the newborn, generally liver function is so immature that the conversion to direct bilirubin cannot be made. Therefore, bilirubin remains in the indirect form. When the level of indirect bilirubin in the blood rises to more than 7 mg/100 mL, it permeates outside the circulatory system, and the infant shows signs of yellowing from physiologic jaundice. If excessive **hemolysis** (destruction) of RBCs occurs, the child will also show signs of jaundice.

Leukocytes (White Blood Cells)

Leukocytes (white blood cells [WBCs]) are nucleated cells. They are few in number compared with RBCs, with approximately 1 WBC to every 500 RBCs. Their primary function is defense against antigen invasion. There are two main forms of WBCs: **granulocytes** (those with granules in the cell cytoplasm) and **agranulocytes** (those without granules in the cell cytoplasm). Granulocytes (often referred to as polymorphonuclear forms) are further differentiated as neutrophils, basophils, and eosinophils. The agranulocytic leukocytes are further differentiated as lymphocytes and monocytes.

The total WBC count in newborns is approximately 20,000 per cubic millimeter, a high level caused by the trauma of birth. In the newborn, granulocytes are the most common WBCs. By 14 to 30 days of life, the total WBC count falls to approximately 12,000 per cubic millimeter, and lymphocytes become the dominant type. By age 4 years, the WBC count reaches the adult level, and granulocytes are again the dominant type. Leukocytes are produced in response to need. The life span of leukocytes varies from approximately 6 hours to unknown intervals (Bondurant & Koury, 1999).

Thrombocytes (Platelets)

When blood is centrifuged in a test tube, plasma rises to the top as a clear yellow fluid; red cells sink to the bottom as a dark-red paste. Between these two layers a thin white strip (often termed a buffy coat) forms that comprises the WBCs and platelets. Thrombocytes are round, nonnucleated bodies formed by bone marrow. Their function is capillary hemostasis and primary coagulation. The normal range is 150,000 to 300,000 per cubic millimeter after the first year. Immature thrombocytes are termed **megakaryocytes.** If large numbers of these are present in serum, it indicates that rapid production of platelets is occurring.

Blood Coagulation

Effective blood coagulation depends on a complex series of events including a combination of blood and tissue factors released from the plasma (the intrinsic pathway) and from injured tissue (the extrinsic pathway). The plasma-released factors are factors VIII, IX, and XII. Factors released from injured tissues are a tissue factor (an incomplete thromboplastin or factor III), plus factors VII and X. Together, the pathways form factor V. The names for coagulation factors are given in Box 44-1.

BOX 44.1

BLOOD COAGULATION FACTORS

I: Fibrinogen
II: Prothrombin
III: Thromboplastin
IV: Calcium
V: Labile factor (platelet phospholipids)
VII: Stable factor
VIII: Antihemophilic factor
IX: Christmas factor; antihemophilic factor B; plasma thromboplastin component
X: Stuart factor
XI: Plasma thromboplastin antecedent (antihemophilic factor C)
XII: Hageman factor
XIII: Fibrin stabilizing factor

Numbers refer to the order in which factors were discovered, not to the order of action in coagulation.

When a vessel is injured, vasoconstriction occurs in the area proximal to the injury, narrowing the vessel lumen and reducing the amount of blood to the injured area. Platelets begin to adhere to the damaged vessel site and to one another, forming a platelet plug. This is the first stage of clotting (Fig. 44-1).

In the second stage, factors from either the intrinsic or the extrinsic system combine with platelet phospholipid to form complete thromboplastin.

In the third stage, thromboplastin converts prothrombin (factor II) to thrombin if ionized calcium is present. The production of prothrombin and factors VII, IX, and X depends on the presence of vitamin K. This stage will be incomplete if any of factors VIII through XII or calcium is deficient.

In the fourth stage, thrombin converts fibrinogen (factor I) to fibrin. Fibrin strands form a mesh, incorporating RBCs, WBCs, and platelets to form a permanent protective seal at the site of injury. Factor XIII (fibrin stabilizing factor) acts to make the fibrin clot insoluble and permanent.

To prevent too much coagulation, plasminogen may be converted to plasmin (a fibrinolysin) near the injury. Blood coagulation problems will result if any step or factor in the process is inadequate. Common tests for blood coagulation are described in Table 44-1.

✔ CHECKPOINT QUESTIONS

1. What hormone is responsible for stimulating the production of RBCs?
2. What are the two major forms of WBCs?
3. What term is used to denote immature platelets?

ASSESSMENT OF AND THERAPEUTIC TECHNIQUES FOR HEMATOLOGIC DISORDERS

Bone Marrow Aspiration and Biopsy

Bone marrow aspiration provides samples of bone marrow for determining the type and quantity of cells present. In children, the aspiration sites include the iliac crests or

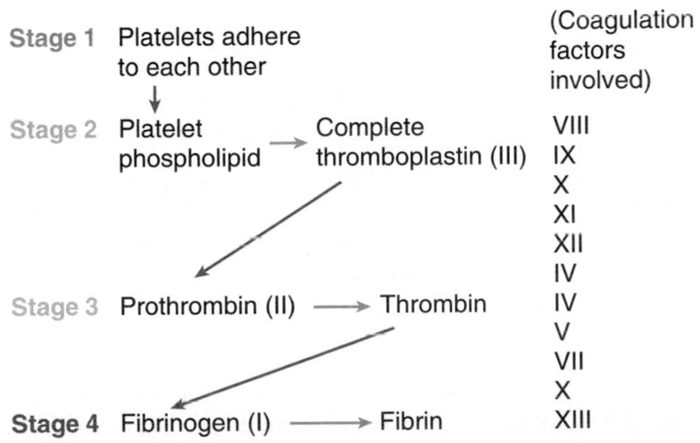

FIGURE 44.1 Steps in blood coagulation.

TABLE 44.1 Tests for Blood Coagulation

TEST	DEFINITION	NORMAL VALUE
Prothrombin time (PT)	Measures action of prothrombin after complete thromboplastin is added to the blood in a test tube; reveals deficiencies in prothrombin, factors V, VII, and X (International Normalized Ratio [INR]—a comparative rating of PT ratios that allows for more sensitive control)	11–13 sec (PT) 2.0–3.0 (INR)
Partial thromboplastin time (PTT)	Measures activity of thromboplastin after incomplete thromboplastin is added to blood in a test tube; reveals deficiencies in thromboplastin, factors VIII–XII	30–45 sec
Bleeding time	Measures the time required for bleeding at a stab wound on the earlobe to cease; reveals deficiencies in platelet formation and vasoconstrictive ability	3–10 min
Clot retraction	Measures platelet function; interval from placement of blood in a tube to the point clot shrinks and expels serum	Retraction at side of test tube in 1 h; complete in 24 h
Tourniquet	Measures capillary fragility and platelet function; response of tissue to application of tourniquet to forearm for 5–10 min	0–2 petechiae per 2-cm area
Prothrombin consumption time	Evaluates thromboplastin function; child's blood is allowed to clot and PT is then done on the serum; if clot formation used a great deal of prothrombin (as it should), serum prothrombin time will be low; increase denotes defects in thromboplastin function	Approximately 20 sec
Thromboplastin generation time	Tests basic ability to form thromboplastin; difficult test to do; ordered rarely to distinguish factor VIII from factor IX defects	12 sec or less
Plasma fibrinogen	Measures stage 4 clotting process; level of fibrinogen in blood	200–400 mg/100 mL plasma
Venous clotting time (Lee-White)	Measures factor defects in stages 2 and 4; time it takes venous blood to clot in a test tube	9–12 min

spines (rather than the sternum, which is commonly used in adults; Fig. 44-2) because these sites have larger marrow compartments during childhood. Also performing the test here is usually less frightening for children. In neonates, the anterior tibia can be used (Perkins, 1999).

The child lies prone on a treatment table. Use of a hard table is advantageous because pressure is needed to insert

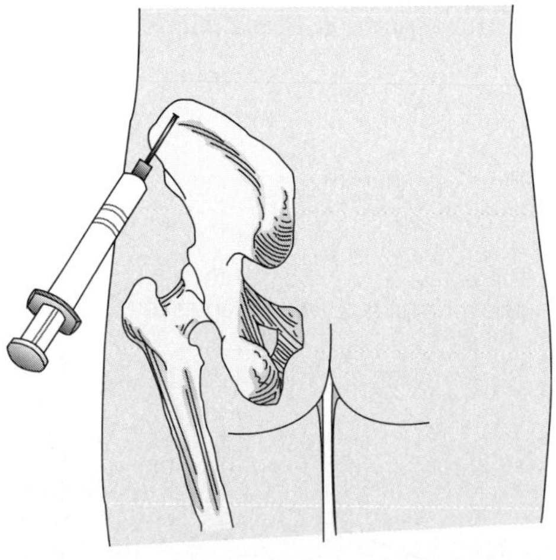

FIGURE 44.2 A common site used for bone marrow aspiration in children is the iliac crest. In neonates, the anterior tibia may be used.

the needle through the surface of the bone into the marrow compartment. Conscious sedation may be used to help reduce the child's fear of the procedure. Topical anesthesia helps reduce pain.

The area of the aspiration is cleaned with an antiseptic solution and draped. The overlying skin is infiltrated with a local anesthetic. After a few minutes, a large-bore needle with stylus is introduced through the overlying tissue into the bone. This involves considerable pressure. When the marrow cavity is reached, the stylus is removed, a syringe is attached to the needle, and bone marrow is aspirated (appears as thick blood in the syringe). The syringe is then removed, and marrow is expelled onto a slide and allowed to dry. After being sprayed with a preservative, it is taken to the laboratory for analysis. The aspiration needle is removed, and pressure is applied to the puncture site to prevent bleeding. After another few minutes, a pressure dressing is applied.

The child feels the pain of the local anesthetic injection and the hard pressure while the needle is inserted. Some report a sharp pain when the marrow is actually aspirated. If conscious sedation is used, monitor vital signs until the child is fully awake. Monitor pulse and blood pressure and observe the dressing every 15 minutes for the first hour after the procedure to be certain that no bleeding is occurring. Keep the child fairly quiet for the first hour by playing a quiet game or other activity. Allow young children an opportunity for therapeutic play with a doll and syringe to help them express their feelings about such a painful, invasive procedure. Instruct parents to take the child's temperature 12 and 24 hours after the procedure to detect infection.

Blood Transfusion

Transfusions of blood or its products are used in the treatment of many disorders, including the anemias and primary immunodeficiency disorders (see Chap. 42). A variety of forms are available, including whole blood, packed RBCs, washed RBCs (as much "foreign" matter is removed as possible to reduce the possibility of blood reaction), plasma, plasma factors, platelets, WBC transfusion, and albumin. No matter what the blood product, it is important to be certain that it has been carefully matched with the child's blood type. Blood must be infused with a solution as nearly isotonic as possible (normal saline). If blood is given with a hypertonic solution, fluid will be drawn out of the RBCs, causing them to shrink; if infused with a hypotonic solution, fluid will be drawn into the cells, and they will burst. In both instances, they will be worthless.

Packed RBCs are the most common form of transfusion because they help minimize the risk of fluid overload. The usual amount of blood transfused to children is 15 mL/kg body weight. The commonly accepted rate for transfusions in a child is 10 mL/kg/h unless the child has hypovolemic shock and volume equilibrium needs to be established. An infusion of packed RBCs at a proportion of 15 mL/kg can be expected to raise the hematocrit level 5 points. Platelets last only approximately 10 days, so transfusions must be repeated every 10 days. A transfusion of platelets will elevate the platelet count by approximately 10,000 (Schroeder, 1999).

Even if given slowly, a blood transfusion is always a strain on a child's circulation beyond that of a regular intravenous infusion, because the circulatory system must accommodate a thick, difficult-to-mobilize fluid.

Before any transfusion, ensure that a signed consent form is on the child's chart and that permission for blood transfusion is obtained to respect sociocultural or religious beliefs. Also obtain vital signs to establish a baseline. Monitor vital signs every 15 minutes during the first hour and approximately every half hour for the remainder of the transfusion. Give the infusion slowly for the first 15 minutes; then increase the rate if no reaction occurs. Common symptoms of blood transfusion reactions are shown in Table 44-2.

Provide an enjoyable activity for the child during a transfusion. Without this, the child can become bored and may attempt to increase the infusion rate.

Bone Marrow Transplantation

Bone marrow transplantation is the intravenous infusion of hematopoietic stem cells from bone marrow obtained by marrow aspiration or peripheral blood from a donor to reestablish marrow function in a child with defective or nonfunctioning bone marrow. Donors are compatible when their human leukocyte antigen (HLA) system matches that of the recipient. **Allogeneic transplantation** involves the transfer of stem cells from an immune-compatible (histocompatible) donor, usually a sibling, although a national registry allows compatible volunteer donors to be located. The term **synergeneic transplantation** is used when the donor and recipient are genetically identical (i.e., identical twins). In **autologous transplantation,** the child's own stem cells are used. The stem cells are aspirated from the bone marrow or obtained from circulating blood, treated to remove abnormal cells, and then reinfused. Umbilical cord blood is a third source of stem cells (Ende et al., 2001).

Hematologic stem cell transplantation has become a relatively common procedure for children with blood disorders such as acquired aplastic anemia, sickle-cell anemia, thalassemia, and leukemia and some forms of immune dysfunction. Stem cells can be recovered from circulating peripheral blood after the stimulation of stem cell production by a cytokine or stem cell colony-stimulating factor. Stem cell transplants are most successful when the recipient has not already received multiple blood transfusions that have sensitized him or her to blood products. Success also depends on the compatibility of donated stem cells to a child's blood. An identical twin is the ideal donor; a parent or sibling may be next best, although compatibility is not guaranteed. Siblings have a 25% chance of being compatible. Donors registered with regional or national bone marrow banks have provided closer matches in some instances (Nash, 1999).

All potential donors are typed for HLA compatibility. Parents who are found to be incompatible often feel guilty and frustrated that they could not do more for their child. If the most compatible person is a young sibling, health care personnel and parents alike may have some reservations about submitting a child to bone marrow aspiration. There is no guarantee that the graft will be accepted by the recipient, or that improvement will occur. However, with good tissue compatibility in the absence of infection, this can be effective in 80% to 90% of children.

To prevent a child from rejecting newly transplanted donor stem cells by the T lymphocytes, a drug such as cyclophosphamide (Cytoxan) is administered intravenously to the child to suppress marrow and T-lymphocyte production. This may cause nausea and vomiting. Total body irradiation to destroy the child's marrow also may be done. This is a difficult time for the child because total body irradiation causes extreme nausea, vomiting, and diarrhea.

WHAT IF? What if a child donates stem cells to a sibling but the transplant does not "take"? How would you explain to the donor child that he or she did not fail?

On the day of the procedure, the donor is admitted to the hospital for a 1-day stay and receives general or epidural anesthesia or conscious sedation as stem cells will be obtained by multiple bone marrow aspirations from the posterior iliac crests. The marrow is strained to remove fat and bone particles and any other unwanted cells. An anticoagulant is added to prevent clotting. It is then infused intravenously into the recipient's bloodstream. Because the infused solution is fairly thick, this infusion takes 60 to

TABLE 44.2 Common Blood Transfusion Reaction Symptoms

SYMPTOMS	CAUSE	TIME OF OCCURRENCE	NURSING INTERVENTIONS
Headache, chills, back pain, dyspnea, hypotension, hemoglobinuria (blood in urine)	Anaphylactic reaction to incompatible blood; agglutination of red blood cells occurs; kidney tubules may become blocked, resulting in kidney failure	Immediately after start of transfusion	Discontinue transfusion. Maintain normal saline infusion for accessible intravenous line. Administer oxygen as necessary. Anticipate physician order for diuretic to increase renal tubule flow and reduce tubule plugging and/or heparin to reduce intravascular coagulation.
Pruritus, urticaria (hives), wheezing	Allergy to protein components of transfusion	Within first hour after start of transfusion	Discontinue transfusion temporarily. Give oxygen as needed. Anticipate physician order for antihistamine to reduce symptoms.
Increased temperature	Possible contaminant in transfused blood	Approximately 1 hour after start of transfusion	Discontinue transfusion. Obtain blood culture to rule out bacterial invasion as ordered.
Increased pulse, dyspnea	Circulatory overload	During course of transfusion	Discontinue transfusion. Give oxygen as needed. Provide supportive care for pulmonary edema and congestive heart failure. Anticipate physician order for diuretic to increase excretion of fluid.
Muscle cramping, twitching of extremities, convulsion	Acid-citrate-dextrose anticoagulant in transfusion is combining with serum calcium and causing hypocalcemia	During course of transfusion	Discontinue transfusion. Anticipate physician order for calcium gluconate intravenously to restore calcium level.
Fever, jaundice, lethargy, tenderness over liver	Hepatitis from contaminated transfusion	Weeks or months after transfusion	Obtain transfusion history of any child with hepatitis symptoms. Refer for care of hepatitis.
Bronze-colored skin	Hemosiderosis or deposition of iron from transfusion in skin	After repeated transfusions	Support self-esteem with altered body image. Administer iron-chelating agent (deferoxamine) as ordered to help reduce level of accumulating iron.

90 minutes. Do not use a filter that is normally used for the infusion of blood products because this would filter out marrow tissue. Monitor the child's cardiac rate and rhythm during the infusion to detect circulatory overload or pulmonary emboli from unfiltered particles.

To obtain stem cells from peripheral blood, donors receive 5 days of a colony-stimulating factor to promote release of stem cells into the peripheral blood. Blood is then collected by the leukopheresis technique. Umbilical cord blood is drained from placentas immediately after birth.

Fever and chills are common reactions to a stem cell transplant infusion. Acetaminophen (Tylenol), diazepam (Valium), and diphenhydramine hydrochloride (Benadryl) may be prescribed to reduce this reaction.

After the infusion, take the child's temperature at 1 hour and then every 4 hours to detect infection that could occur because the child's WBCs are nonfunctioning from radiation. Reinforce strict handwashing, and limit the child's diet to cooked foods to reduce the presence of bacteria. The WBC count must be measured daily; bone marrow aspirations or venous blood samples are scheduled at regular intervals to assess the growth of the new marrow.

Almost immediately after the infusion, stem cells begin to migrate from the child's bloodstream into the marrow.

If engraftment occurs (the transplant is accepted), new RBCs can be detected in peripheral blood in approximately 3 weeks. WBCs and platelet cells may not return to normal for up to 1 year after the transplant.

NURSING DIAGNOSES AND RELATED INTERVENTIONS

Nursing Diagnosis: Anxiety related to lack of knowledge about procedure and expected outcome of transplant

Outcome Identification: Parents and child will demonstrate an understanding of the transplant procedure and possible uncertainty of outcome from therapy by 24 hours.

Outcome Evaluation: Parents state the reasons for the transplant; verbalize that they know the transplant may not work, depending on immunologic factors that are not totally known to science, but are agreeable to the procedure.

Stem cell transplantation is an emotional experience not only for the child but also for the parents and the marrow donor. Be certain that the child who receives the transplant and the donor understand that they are not responsible for the outcome of the transplant. Its success does not depend on their behavior or what kind of person they are but on immunologic factors over which they have no control. If a sibling was the donor, he or she may become jealous of the recipient child who is the center of attention. Be certain that donors know that the donor sites will feel tender afterward. General anesthesia or conscious sedation will leave them feeling exhausted for several days. Donors who have undergone bone marrow aspiration generally return to their primary care provider in 24 to 48 hours for evaluation to ensure that the aspiration sites are not infected (no local swelling, redness, intense pain, or fever).

Nursing Diagnosis: Risk for delayed growth and development related to extended restrictions and infection control precautions in hospital or at home

Outcome Identification: Child will demonstrate age-appropriate growth in motor skills and social, cognitive, and emotional behaviors during course of therapy.

Outcome Evaluation: Parents express satisfaction with child's ongoing development. Objective tests of developmental stage show child within age-appropriate ranges.

Children may be restricted from others to prevent them from contracting an infection. Be certain that children are not socially isolated as well. Visit the room frequently; provide sterilized play materials as appropriate. Most children grow tired of a restricted diet and may crave fresh fruits and vegetables that are usually not their favorite foods. Thick-skinned fruits such as bananas and oranges can be given soon after the procedure, but unwashed foods should be avoided (see Focus on Multidisciplinary Care).

FOCUS ON MULTIDISCIPLINARY CARE

Many health care professionals such as physicians, advanced-practice nurses, play therapists, laboratory technicians, phlebotomists, and social workers participate in the care of children with long-term hematologic disease, especially those who have received stem cell transplants. Measures to minimize the child's risk for infection are paramount. Be certain that all personnel understand that until these children's immune response returns to normal, they should not be offered foods such as unwashed fruit that could carry microorganisms, or toys or other equipment that has not been sterilized. Review specific infection control precautions as necessary. Be certain too that all personnel understand that if they have an infection such as herpes simplex or an upper respiratory infection, they should not care for the child.

Be certain that children are well prepared for all procedures. Allow them to make as many choices as they can about their care to help them preserve a sense of control over their life. Children who receive a transplant need periods of therapeutic play incorporated into their care so they can begin to express their anger and frustration at the number of intravenous therapies or follow-up bone marrow aspirations they require. Measures to help children cope with pain, such as imagery, can help a child to accept one more painful procedure. Encourage parents to spend time with their child during long periods of hospitalization for additional support.

If children are prepared adequately for these painful procedures and supported throughout, they should have no long-term consequences. Not all transplants are successful, however, and some children will die of the original disease that necessitated the transplant. Some children develop an infection despite all precautions and die in the weeks immediately after the transplant.

Provisions for completing schoolwork need to be made as soon as the child has a return of RBCs in the peripheral blood (approximately 3 weeks). On the day of discharge, parents may be surprised that the child's blood replacement is not complete and that they will need to continue infection control measures and restrictions at home. Help them locate a support group in the community if possible. Be certain that they feel free to call the transplant center after discharge if they have any problems. Once the danger of infection has passed and the restrictions can be discontinued, parents may still be reluctant to allow their child outside, fearing that the child may still be susceptible to infection. Frequent follow-up for the next year is necessary to ensure that the child is free of infection until WBCs have risen to normal levels. Follow-up should also address the parents' commitment to allowing their child to pursue age-appropriate activities and avoiding overprotecting him or her.

Graft-Versus-Host Disease

Graft-versus-host disease (GVHD) is a potentially lethal immunologic response of donor T cells against the tissue of the recipient. The symptoms range from mild to severe and include a rash and general malaise beginning 7 to 14 days after the transplant. Latent virus infections may become active. Severe symptoms include high fever and diarrhea and liver and spleen enlargement as cells are destroyed.

Because there is no known cure for GVHD, prevention is essential. Careful tissue typing; intravenous administration of methotrexate, a corticosteroid, or cyclosporine; and irradiation of blood products (which helps to inactivate mature T lymphocytes) before stem cell infusion all can help reduce the incidence of this complication. Drugs such as methotrexate and cyclosporine kill all rapidly growing cells, including WBCs and T lymphocytes, so administration of these drugs after transplantation cannot be continued because they would also slow the growth of the host's stem cells. Depletion of mature T lymphocytes from donor bone marrow before infusion into the child offers good results, as does the administration of corticosteroids or antithymocyte globulin (ATG).

Splenectomy

One of the purposes of the spleen is to remove damaged or aged blood cells. This poses a difficulty with diseases such as sickle-cell anemia and the thalassemias because the spleen recognizes the typical cells of these diseases as damaged and destroys them. This causes these children to have a continuous anemia, with hemoglobin as low as 5 to 9 g/mL. In some children, therefore, removal of the spleen (splenectomy) will not cure the basic defect of the blood cells but will limit the degree of anemia.

Splenectomy is considered major surgery. It formerly required an abdominal incision, but today it is usually performed by laparoscopy (Esposito et al., 2001).

A second function of the spleen is to strain the plasma for invading organisms so phagocytes and lymphocytes can destroy them. Children who have had their spleen removed appear to be very susceptible to the pneumococcal infections. After surgery, oral penicillin is given as a prophylactic antibiotic for a year or two. The child should receive pneumococcal and meningococcal vaccines as well as routine immunizations. Instruct parents about signs of infection (cough, fever, general malaise), and encourage them to report any such signs immediately.

> ✔ **CHECKPOINT QUESTIONS**
>
> 4. Where is the preferred site for bone marrow aspiration in a child?
> 5. All bone marrow donors are screened for what type of compatibility?

HEALTH PROMOTION AND RISK MANAGEMENT

Many hematologic disorders such as sickle-cell anemia and hemophilia are inherited disorders. Thus, health promotion and disease prevention begin with ensuring that families have access to genetic counseling so they can be aware of the incidence of the disorder in their family and, therefore, the potential for the disease to develop in their child.

The most frequently occurring anemia in children, iron-deficiency anemia, is preventable. This condition could be eradicated in infants if all bottle-fed infants were fed iron-fortified formula for the first year and when cereal is introduced, iron-fortified types are used. The disorder occurs again at a high incidence in adolescents because their diets tend to be low in meat and green vegetables, the chief dietary sources of iron. Adolescents who begin vegetarian diets become especially prone to developing the disorder. Counseling parents of young children to maintain well-child visits and urging adolescents to ingest iron-rich foods could have a major impact on decreasing the incidence of the disorder.

Aplastic anemia, or the inability to form blood elements, can be acquired if a child is exposed to a toxic drug or chemical. Educating parents about the importance of keeping poisons locked and out of the reach of children could help decrease the incidence of this disorder.

Because many of the disorders are inherited, nurses cannot play a role in prevention. However, nurses can be instrumental in making the therapy for these disorders much less painful and distressing than it was in the past. All hematologic disorders require obtaining blood specimens for diagnosis and continued testing for follow-up. Many therapies include blood product transfusion. The use of EMLA cream or topical lidocaine can greatly reduce the pain of venipuncture. Helping a child to use a distraction technique such as imagery can reduce any apprehension or fear associated with the procedures or treatments.

DISORDERS OF THE RED BLOOD CELLS

Most RBC disorders fall into the category of the anemias, or a reduction in the number or function of erythrocytes. Polycythemia, or an increase in the number of RBCs, can also occur and may be as dangerous to the child as a reduction in RBC production can be (see Focus on Cultural Competence).

Anemia occurs when the rate of RBC production falls below that of cell destruction, or when there is a loss of RBCs, causing their number, or the hemoglobin level, to fall below the normal value for a child's age. Anemias are classified according to the changes seen in RBC numbers or configuration, or according to the source of the problem. Although any reduction in the amount of circulating hemoglobin lessens the oxygen-carrying capacity, clinical symptoms of this are not apparent until the hemoglobin reaches 7 to 8 g/100 mL. Average values for hemoglobin and RBC number are shown in Appendix F.

FOCUS ON CULTURAL COMPETENCE

Blood dyscrasias do not occur at equal rates in all countries because many of them are inherited. Sickle-cell anemia occurs mainly in African Americans; thalassemia occurs in children from Mediterranean countries. Iron-deficiency anemia, an example of a noninherited disorder, tends to occur in children from lower socioeconomic areas of many countries because iron-rich foods often are expensive. Being aware of the differences in the incidence of blood dyscrasias can be helpful in planning care and providing health care services for an individual community.

Blood transfusions are often the therapy for blood disorders. Jehovah's Witnesses may refuse such transfusions on religious grounds.

Normochromic, Normocytic Anemias

Normochromic, normocytic anemias are marked by impaired production of erythrocytes by the bone marrow, or by abnormal or uncompensated loss of circulating RBCs, such as in acute hemorrhage. The remaining RBCs are normal in both color and size, but they are simply too few in number.

Acute Blood-Loss Anemia

Blood loss sufficient to cause anemia might occur from trauma such as an automobile accident with internal bleeding; from acute nephritis in which blood is being lost in the urine; or, in the newborn, from disorders such as placenta previa, premature separation of the placenta, maternal-fetal or twin-to-twin transfusion, or trauma to the cord or placenta, as might occur with cesarean birth.

Children are in shock from acute blood loss and appear pale. As the heart attempts to push the reduced amount of blood through the body more rapidly, tachycardia will occur. Loss of RBCs needed for oxygen transport causes body cells to register an oxygen deficit, and children experience tachypnea. Newborns may have gasping respirations, sternal retractions, and cyanosis. They will not respond to oxygen therapy because they lack RBCs to transport and use the oxygen. Such infants will be listless and inactive.

This type of acute blood-loss anemia generally is transitory because the sudden reduction in available oxygen stimulates a regeneration response in the bone marrow. The reticulocyte count becomes elevated, evidence that the bone marrow is trying to increase production of erythrocytes to meet the sudden shortage.

Treatment involves control of bleeding by addressing its underlying cause. The child or infant should be placed in a supine position to provide as much circulation as possible to brain cells. Keep the child warm with blankets; place an infant in an incubator. Blood transfusion may be necessary for an immediate increase in the number of erythrocytes. Until blood is available for transfusion, a blood expander such as plasma or intravenous fluid such as normal saline or Ringer's lactate may be given to expand the blood volume and improve blood pressure.

Anemia of Acute Infection

Acute infection or inflammation, especially in infants, may lead to increased destruction of erythrocytes and therefore to decreased erythrocyte levels. Common conditions include osteomyelitis, ulcerative colitis, and advanced renal disease. Impaired production of erythrocytes due to the infection may also contribute to the anemia. Management involves treatment of the underlying condition. When this is reversed, the blood values will return to normal.

Anemia of Renal Disease

Renal disease causes loss of function in kidney cells, with an accompanying decrease in erythropoietin production. This decreases the stimulation for RBC production in bone marrow and a resultant normocytic normochromic anemia. Administration of recombinant human erythropoietin can increase RBC production and correct the anemia, but not the renal disease.

Anemia of Neoplastic Disease

Malignant growths such as leukemia or lymphosarcoma (common neoplasms of childhood) result in normochromic, normocytic anemias because invasion of bone marrow by proliferating neoplastic cells impairs RBC production. There may be accompanying blood loss if platelet formation also has decreased. The treatment of such an anemia involves measures designed to achieve remission of the neoplastic process and transfusion to increase the erythrocyte count.

Aplastic Anemias

Aplastic anemias result from depression of hematopoietic activity in the bone marrow. The formation and development of WBCs, platelets, and RBCs are affected.

Congenital aplastic anemia (Fanconi's syndrome) is inherited as an autosomal recessive trait. The child is born with a number of congenital anomalies, such as skeletal and renal abnormalities, hypogenitalism, and short stature. Between 4 and 12 years of age, the child begins to manifest symptoms of **pancytopenia** (reduction of all blood cell components).

Acquired aplastic anemia is a decrease in bone marrow production that can occur if the child has excessive exposure to radiation, drugs, or chemicals known to cause bone marrow damage. Drugs that may contribute include chloramphenicol, sulfonamides, arsenic (contained in rat poison, sometimes eaten by children), hydantoin, benzene, or quinine. Exposure to insecticides also may cause such bone marrow dysfunction. Chemotherapeutic drugs temporarily reduce bone marrow production. A serious infection such as meningococcal pneumonia might cause autoimmunologic suppression of the bone marrow.

Assessment. As symptoms begin, the child appears pale, fatigues easily, and has anorexia. These symptoms reflect the lower RBC count (anemia) and tissue hypoxia. Because of reduced platelet formation (**thrombocytopenia**), the child bruises easily or has **petechiae** (pinpoint, macular, purplish-red spots caused by intradermal or submucous hemorrhage). The child may have excessive nosebleeds or gastrointestinal bleeding. As a result of a decrease in WBCs (**leukopenia**), the child may contract an increased number of infections and respond poorly to antibiotic therapy. Observe closely for signs of cardiac decompensation (e.g., tachycardia, tachypnea, shortness of breath, or cyanosis) from the long-term increased workload on the heart (see Assessing the Child With a Hematologic Disorder earlier in this chapter). Ask about any exposure to drugs or chemicals or recent infection.

Bone marrow samples will show a reduced number of hematopoietic forms; blood-forming spaces are infiltrated by fatty tissue (Derivan & Ferrante, 2001).

Therapeutic Management. The treatment for congenital and acquired aplastic anemia is bone marrow transplantation. If a donor cannot be located, the disease is managed by procedures to suppress T-lymphocyte-dependent autoimmune responses with antithymocyte globulin (ATG) and cyclosporine (Lane et al., 2001), testosterone to stimulate RBC growth, or transfusion of new blood elements. Any drug or chemical suspected of causing the bone marrow dysfunction must be discontinued at once. ATG, given intravenously, must be administered cautiously because of the high risk for anaphylaxis. Packed RBCs and platelet transfusions are generally necessary to maintain adequate blood elements. An RBC-stimulating factor (erythropoietin) may be helpful. Colony-stimulating factors may also improve bone marrow function. Some children show improvement with a course of an oral corticosteroid (prednisone).

For children who receive a stem cell transplant, chances of complete recovery are good. For others, the course is uncertain. A decreased platelet count may persist for years after other blood elements have returned to normal. Hence, bleeding, especially petechiae or purpura, may be a long-term problem. If the disease was caused by exposure to a drug or chemical, children must never be exposed to that substance again.

When discussing with parents the outcome of this disease, be conservatively optimistic. For some children, the outcome will be fatal. It may be easier for parents to deal with this problem if they face only one day or one blood test at a time rather than trying to predict the outcomes of all the blood tests to come. They need to feel that they can discuss their frustration and bitterness about continual abnormal results with health care personnel. Establishing good communication with these parents does much to reestablish their trust in everyone caring for their child.

NURSING DIAGNOSES AND RELATED INTERVENTIONS

Children with aplastic anemia are apt to be irritable because of their fatigue and recurring symptoms. Their parents may feel responsible for causing the illness if it originated from exposure to a chemical such as an insecticide. Many parents will have less confidence in health care personnel if the illness followed treatment with a drug such as chloramphenicol. They wonder how they can trust in a drug to cure the illness if they believe that one drug caused the illness. How can they trust that their child will not be harmed further?

Nursing Diagnosis: Risk for infection related to dramatic decrease in number of WBCs

Outcome Identification: Child will remain free of any signs and symptoms of infection during treatment period.

Outcome Evaluation: Child's temperature is below 100°F (38.0°C) axillary; symptoms such as cough, vomiting, or diarrhea are absent.

Exposure to other children must be limited as long as WBC production is inadequate to prevent infection. Remind parents of the signs and symptoms of infection and advise them to come for treatment promptly if the child shows any of these signs. In the absence of granulocytes, however, antibiotic therapy may be ineffective, and severe septicemia can result. WBCs (granulocytes) may be transfused for a severe infection.

Nursing Diagnosis: Risk for disturbed body image related to changed appearance occurring as medication side effect

Outcome Identification: Child will demonstrate adequate self-esteem during therapy.

Outcome Evaluation: Child states that he or she is a worthwhile person; does not appear to be excessively shy or reluctant to interact with peers.

Children who receive corticosteroids such as prednisone for a long period almost always experience some of the side effects, such as a cushingoid appearance, hirsutism, hypertension, and marked weight gain. Masculinizing effects, such as growth of facial and body hair, the development of acne, and deepening of the voice, may occur as the result of long-term therapy with testosterone. Both the child and the parents need to be prepared for these effects; they should know that the effects are related to the medication and that they will remain for an extended period but will fade when the medication is withdrawn.

Adolescents may have an especially difficult time accepting weight gain and increased acne. They need a chance to express their feelings about their changed appearance. Reinforce and emphasize positive attributes.

Nursing Diagnosis: Risk for injury related to ineffective blood clotting mechanisms secondary to inadequate platelet formation

Outcome Identification: Child will remain free of excessive bleeding episodes while condition is resolving.

Outcome Evaluation: Child exhibits absence of ecchymotic skin areas, gingival bleeding, or epistaxis; stools negative for occult blood.

Inadequate platelet formation interferes with blood coagulation, placing the child at risk for bleeding. Techniques for reducing bleeding due to inadequate platelet formation include the following:

- Limit the number of blood-drawing procedures; combine samples whenever possible; use a blood pressure cuff instead of a tourniquet to reduce the number of petechiae.
- Apply pressure to any puncture site for a full 5 minutes before applying a bandage.
- Minimize use of adhesive tape to the skin (pulling for removal may tear the skin and cause petechiae).
- Pad side and crib rails to prevent bruising.
- Protect intravenous sites to avoid numerous reinsertions.
- Administer medication orally or by intravenous infusion to minimize the number of injection sites.
- Assess diet for foods that the child can chew without irritation (e.g., avoid toast crusts).
- Urge the child to use a soft toothbrush.
- Check toys for sharp corners, which may cause scratches. Urge the child to be careful with paper, because paper cuts can bleed out of proportion to their size.
- Assess the need for routine blood pressure determinations. Tight cuffs could lead to petechiae.
- Distract the child from rough play; suggest stimulating but quiet activities to minimize risk of injury.
- Keep a record of blood drawn; do not draw extra amounts "just in case."

These measures require conscientious nursing care.

Hypoplastic Anemias

Hypoplastic anemias also result from depression of hematopoietic activity in bone marrow; they can be either congenital or acquired. Unlike aplastic anemias, in which WBCs, RBCs, and platelets are affected, in hypoplastic anemias only RBCs are affected.

Congenital hypoplastic anemia (Blackfan-Diamond syndrome) is a rare disorder revealed in the first 6 to 8 months of life. It affects both sexes and is apparently caused by an inherent defect in RBC formation (Lane et al., 2001). No changes in the leukocytes or platelets occur. An acquired form is caused by infection with parvovirus, the infectious agent of fifth disease.

The onset of hypoplastic anemia is insidious and must be differentiated from iron-deficiency anemia. The blood cells appear hypochromic and microcytic in iron-deficiency anemia; in hypoplastic anemia, they are normochromic and normocytic.

With acquired hypoplastic anemia, the reduction of RBCs is transient, so no therapy is necessary. Children with the congenital form show increased erythropoiesis with corticosteroid therapy. Long-term transfusions of packed RBCs are needed to raise erythrocyte levels. As a result of the necessary number of transfusions, **hemosiderosis** (deposition of iron in body tissue) occurs. Therefore, an iron chelation program such as subcutaneous infusion (**hypodermoclysis**) of deferoxamine (Desferal) is begun concurrently with transfusions. Deferoxamine binds with iron and aids its excretion from the body in urine; it is given 5 or 6 days a week over an 8-hour period. This is one of the few times that an infusion is given subcutaneously. Parents can do this at home after careful instruction, often when the child is asleep at night. The parent must assess that voiding is present and specific gravity is normal (1.003 to 1.030) before administration.

For a subcutaneous infusion, an area beside the scapula or on the thigh is cleaned with alcohol; a short 25-gauge needle is inserted at a low angle into only the subcutaneous tissue. The medication is then allowed to infuse slowly. Periodic slit-lamp eye examinations should be scheduled to check for cataract formation, a possible adverse effect of the drug.

Congenital hypoplastic anemia is a chronic condition. However, approximately one fourth of affected children undergo spontaneous permanent remission before age 13 years. If not, they are candidates for stem cell transplantation. Both the child and the parents need support from health care personnel to help them accept the many procedures and tests required.

Hypersplenism

Under normal conditions, blood is filtered rapidly through the spleen. If the spleen is enlarged and functioning abnormally, blood cells pass through more slowly, with more cells being destroyed in the process. The increased destruction of RBCs causes anemia and may lead to pancytopenia (deficiency of all cell elements of blood). Virtually any underlying splenic condition can cause this syndrome.

Therapeutic management consists of treating the underlying splenic disorder, including possible splenectomy. Although the spleen's role in the body's defense mechanisms against infection is not well documented, the organ appears to be relatively important in early infancy. Its function decreases as the child grows older and it may serve no function at all in adulthood. If the spleen is removed, there is no decrease in general immunity or in gamma globulin or antibody formation. With the removal of the spleen's filtering function, however, there seems to be an increased susceptibility to meningitis or pneumonia due to pneumococci (Esposito et al., 2001). For this reason, a splenectomy may be delayed until after age 2 years, when the risk of meningitis decreases. Such children should receive immunization against pneumococci and *H. influenzae* in addition to prophylactic penicillin for 2 years after the splenectomy.

> ✔ **CHECKPOINT QUESTIONS**
>
> 6. What blood cells are affected in aplastic anemia?
> 7. What problem indicates the need for iron chelation therapy?

Hypochromic Anemias

When hemoglobin synthesis is inadequate, the erythrocytes appear pale (hypochromia). Hypochromia is generally accompanied by a reduction in the diameter of cells (RBCs are also microcytic).

Iron-Deficiency Anemia

Although the incidence of iron-deficiency anemia is decreasing in the United States due to improved infant nutrition, it is still the most common anemia of infancy and childhood, occurring when the intake of dietary iron is inadequate (Sherry et al., 2001). This prevents proper hemoglobin formation. Most iron in the body is incorporated in hemoglobin, but an additional amount is stored in the bone marrow to be available for hemoglobin production. With iron-deficiency anemia, RBCs are both small in size (hypocytic) and pale (hypochromic) due to the stunted hemoglobin (Mahoney, 2000).

Children are at high risk for iron-deficiency anemia because they need more daily iron in proportion to their body weight to maintain an adequate iron level than do adults. A daily intake of 6 to 15 mg of iron is necessary. Iron-deficiency anemia occurs most often between ages 9 months and 3 years; its frequency rises again in adolescence, when iron requirements increase for girls who are menstruating (Shusterman, 2000).

Prevention. Iron-deficiency anemia can be prevented in formula-fed infants by giving them iron-fortified formula for the first year. If an infant is breast-fed, iron-fortified cereal should be introduced when solid foods are introduced in the first year. Fortunately, these cost no more than nonfortified foods. Occasionally, an infant becomes constipated while ingesting iron-rich formula, but this is the exception rather than the rule.

Causes in Infants. When an infant's diet lacks sufficient iron, he or she usually has enough in reserve to last for the first 6 months. After that, if the infant continues to be iron-deficient, he or she will have difficulty forming the RBCs needed. Infants of low birthweight have fewer iron stores than those born at term because the iron stores develop near the end of gestation. Because low-birthweight infants grow rapidly and their need for RBCs expands accordingly, they will develop an iron-deficiency anemia before 5 to 6 months. As a preventive measure, they are given an iron supplement beginning at about 2 months of age.

Women with iron deficiency during pregnancy tend to give birth to iron-deficient babies because of their lack of iron stores. Low hemoglobin levels from iron-deficiency anemia lead to diffusion of plasma proteins such as albumin and gamma globulin out of the bloodstream by osmosis. The loss of transferrin, a plasma protein responsible for binding iron to protein to facilitate its transportation to bone marrow after absorption from the gastrointestinal tract, further depletes this system of iron transport.

Infants born with structural defects of the gastrointestinal system, such as gastroesophageal reflux (chalasia—immature valve between the esophagus and stomach, resulting in regurgitation) or pyloric stenosis (narrowing between the stomach and duodenum, resulting in vomiting), are particularly prone to iron-deficiency anemia. Although their diet is adequate, they cannot make use of the iron because it is never adequately digested. Infants with chronic diarrhea are also prone to this form of anemia due to inadequate absorption. Some infants develop minimal gastrointestinal bleeding if fed cow's milk; this is why breastfeeding or commercial formula is recommended for the first year.

Causes in Older Children. In children older than 2 years, chronic blood loss is the most frequent cause of iron-deficiency anemia. This results from gastrointestinal tract lesions such as polyps, ulcerative colitis, Crohn's disease, protein-induced enteropathies, parasitic infestation, or frequent epistaxis.

Many adolescent girls are iron-deficient because their frequent attempts to diet and overconsumption of snack foods result in low iron intake. Without sufficient iron, their body cannot compensate for the iron lost with menstrual flow.

Assessment. Common symptoms of iron-deficiency anemia are shown in Assessing the Child With Iron-Deficiency Anemia. Children with iron-deficiency anemia appear pale. Because the pallor develops slowly, however, parents may not realize how extensive it is. They may describe their child as "fair-skinned" even though the child's pallor is so extreme that the skin is transparent. In dark-skinned infants, pale mucous membranes may be the most significant finding.

Infants may show poor muscle tone and reduced activity. They are generally irritable from fatigue. The heart may be enlarged, and there may be a soft systolic precordial murmur as the heart increases its action, attempting to supply blood cells better. The spleen may be slightly

ASSESSING the Child With Iron-Deficiency Anemia

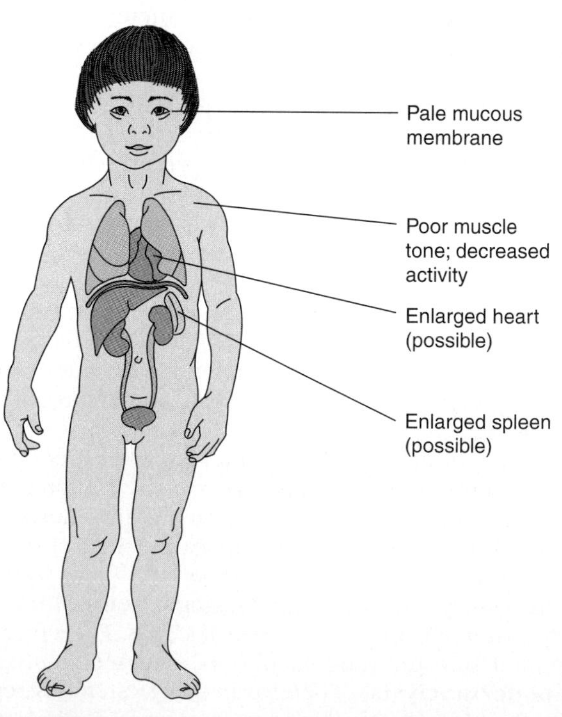

enlarged. Fingernails become typically spoon-shaped or depressed in contour.

A dietary history generally reveals an abnormally high milk intake. As a rule, infants should not ingest more than 32 oz of milk a day. Infants with iron-deficiency anemia may be drinking up to 50 oz a day. One quart of milk provides only approximately 0.5 mg of iron. In contrast, 1 tablespoon of iron-fortified baby cereal supplies 2.5 to 5.0 mg of iron.

With iron-deficiency anemia, laboratory studies reveal a decreased hemoglobin (a hemoglobin level less than 11 g/100 mL of blood) and hematocrit (below 33%). The RBCs are microcytic and hypochromic and possibly **poikilocytic** (irregular in shape). The mean corpuscular volume is low. The mean corpuscular hemoglobin may be reduced. Serum iron levels are normally 70 μg/100 mL; with iron-deficiency anemia the level is often as low as 30 μg/100 mL, with an increased iron-binding capacity (more than 350 μg/100 mL). The level of serum ferritin reflects the extent of iron stores and is less than 10 μg/100 mL (normal is 35 μg/mL). Without iron, heme precursors cannot be used, so free erythrocyte protoporphyrins increase to more than 10 μg/g from a normal of 1.9 μg/g.

Monoamine oxidase (MAO) is an enzyme important for central nervous system maturation. Iron is incorporated into MAO, so without iron this necessary enzyme is absent and CNS maturation may be affected.

Infants with iron-deficiency anemia tend to be more fearful, less active, and less persistent than other infants. School-age children with iron-deficiency anemia score lower on tests than their healthy counterparts, but there is little documentation that supplementing iron improves this (Logan et al., 2001). Iron-deficiency anemia is also associated with pica (the eating of inedible substances such as dirt and paper). Eating ice cubes is common in adolescents. Until the anemia is corrected, parents need to supervise the child's environment to keep inedible materials out of the child's reach.

Therapeutic Management. Therapy for iron-deficiency anemia focuses on the treatment of the underlying cause. Sources of gastrointestinal bleeding must be ruled out. The diet must be rich in iron and should contain extra vitamin C, which will enhance iron absorption. Infants who are bottle-fed should be given iron-fortified formula for a full year. Ferrous sulfate for 4 to 6 weeks is the drug of choice to improve RBC formation and replace iron stores (Lane et al., 2001; see Focus on Nursing Care Planning and Focus on Pharmacology).

NURSING DIAGNOSES AND RELATED INTERVENTIONS

Nursing Diagnosis: Imbalanced nutrition, less than body requirements, related to inadequate ingestion of iron

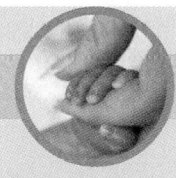

FOCUS ON *Nursing Care Planning*

A CHILD WITH IRON-DEFICIENCY ANEMIA

A 4-year-old boy is brought to the clinic by his mother after being diagnosed with iron-deficiency anemia at a routine health maintenance visit. He is scheduled to start oral iron therapy. His mother asks, "How could this have happened?"

Assessment: Thin, black boy whose weight is at approximately 25th percentile for age. Has a history of frequent nosebleeds. "Sometimes he has three or four in one day." Mucous membranes and conjunctivae pale. Mother reports child is a "picky eater but loves cheese and yogurt." Hemoglobin 10 g/100 mL; hematocrit 31%; serum iron level 50 ug/100 mL; serum ferritin 10 ug/100 mL. The physician orders ferrous sulfate elixir t.i.d. for 6 weeks. Mother is asking many questions about her son's condition and medication therapy. "I don't know how I'll get him to take this medication. I always have trouble giving him any kind of medicine."

Nursing Diagnosis: Deficient knowledge related to causes and treatment of iron-deficiency anemia

Outcome Identification: Parent and child will verbalize accurate information about the disorder and its treatment.

Outcome Evaluation: Parent identifies possible causes; demonstrates proper administration methods for iron elixir; identifies signs and symptoms of iron toxicity; identifies foods high in iron; states the need for medication compliance; describes measures to involve child in medication therapy. Child states reason for iron therapy; identifies appropriate high-iron food choices; states he takes the medication three times a day.

(continued)

Interventions	Rationale
1. Assess parent and child's current knowledge about iron-deficiency anemia.	1. Obtaining a baseline knowledge assessment provides a foundation on which to build future teaching strategies.
2. Explore with the child and mother possible contributing factors associated with iron-deficiency anemia.	2. A dietary intake of large amounts of milk products and chronic blood loss, such as from frequent epistaxis, are common contributing factors to the development of iron-deficiency anemia.
3. Question child about his food likes and dislikes.	3. Ascertaining the child's likes and dislikes provides a baseline for future suggestions for food choices that would be followed.
4. Instruct the mother in foods that are high in iron and measures to include iron-rich foods in diet. Refer for financial assistance for food purchases, if appropriate.	4. Foods high in iron provide an additional means for supplementing needed iron. These foods are typically more expensive than other foods; therefore, financial assistance may be necessary to ensure appropriate food purchases.
5. Allow the child to choose foods from a list of high-iron foods. Develop a simple contract with the child for including one high-iron food with each meal.	5. Contracting and providing the child with choices promote active participation in his care and a feeling of control, enhancing the chances for success.
6. Review the rationale for ferrous sulfate therapy.	6. Ferrous sulfate improves red blood cell formation and replaces iron stores.
7. Instruct the mother to administer the elixir 1 hour before or 2 hours after a meal, mixed with water or juice. Advise the mother to have the child drink the medication through a straw.	7. Mixing the elixir with water or juice helps to mask its taste. Using a straw prevents staining of the teeth.
8. Suggest administering the medication with a citrus juice.	8. Vitamin C enhances iron absorption.
9. Teach the parent about possible adverse effects such as gastrointestinal upset, constipation, and black tarry stools. Encourage the addition of high-fiber foods to the diet.	9. Knowledge of possible adverse effects is important for early detection and prompt intervention should any occur. Adding fiber to the diet helps to reduce the risk of constipation.
10. Instruct the mother to give the medication exactly as prescribed and not to increase the dosage or frequency unless directed to do so by the physician. Advise the parent to call the health care provider if the child experiences any nausea, vomiting, abdominal pain, or blood in emesis or stool (signs of iron toxicity).	10. Giving iron more frequently or in greater doses than ordered can lead to iron toxicity.
11. Encourage the child to brush his teeth thoroughly after each meal.	11. Thorough, regular brushing helps to prevent staining of the teeth.
12. Reinforce the need for compliance with therapy. Arrange for follow-up appointment and blood studies within 4 weeks.	12. Follow-up is essential for assessing compliance and evaluating the effectiveness of therapy and teaching.

Outcome Identification: Child will demonstrate an increase in oral intake of iron by 24 hours.

Outcome Evaluation: Parents report child's dietary intake includes iron-rich foods; parents administer ferrous sulfate as prescribed; serum iron levels increase to normal by 6 months.

When planning care for the infant with iron-deficiency anemia, minimize the child's activities to prevent fatigue, particularly at mealtime. A fatigued child will not be able to eat, let alone eat iron-rich foods.

Counsel parents on measures to improve their child's diet, such as adding iron-rich foods while decreasing milk intake to maintain the iron levels and prevent recurring anemia. If the child is not fond of meat, suggest that parents substitute cheese, eggs, green vegetables, or fortified cereal. Because iron-rich foods are often expensive, remind parents that these items are important and that they should not substitute less expensive, high-carbohydrate foods.

Before iron therapy is started, alert parents to possible side effects, such as stomach irritation. If oral iron is not tolerated or if there is a doubt that the

FOCUS ON PHARMACOLOGY

Ferrous Sulfate (Feosol)

Action: Ferrous sulfate is an iron salt that acts to supply iron for red cell production. It elevates the serum iron concentration and then is converted to hemoglobin or trapped in the reticuloendothelial cells for storage and eventual conversion to a usable form of iron.

Pregnancy risk category: A

Dosage: For severe iron-deficiency anemia: 4 to 6 mg/kg/day in three divided doses. For mild iron-deficiency anemia: 3 mg/kg/day in two divided doses.

Possible adverse effects: Gastrointestinal upset, anorexia, nausea, vomiting, constipation, dark stools, stained teeth (liquid preparations)

Nursing Implications

- Instruct parents to administer the drug on an empty stomach with water to enhance absorption. If this causes GI irritation, administer it after meals. Avoid giving it with milk, eggs, coffee, or tea.
- If the liquid preparation is ordered, advise parents to mix it with water or juice to mask the taste and prevent staining of teeth. Encourage the parents to have the child drink the medication through a straw to avoid staining of the teeth.
- Keep in mind that iron is absorbed best in the presence of vitamin C. Suggest parents give the iron with a citrus juice such as orange juice to help absorption. Some children may be prescribed vitamin C to take concurrently to increase absorption.
- Educate child and parents that iron may turn stools black.
- Encourage parents to include high-fiber foods in the child's diet to minimize the risk of constipation.
- Reinforce the need for thorough brushing of teeth to prevent staining.
- Remind parents about the need for follow-up blood studies to evaluate the effectiveness of the drug.

child will take it, an iron-dextran injection (Imferon) can be given intramuscularly. Imferon stains the skin and is extremely irritating unless it is given by deep z-track intramuscular injection.

Of all age groups, adolescents tend to do the least well with medicine compliance. Help them plan a daily time for taking their iron supplement with a medication reminder chart. At first, they may reject this as childish, but assure them that everyone needs these charts. Review with them the iron-rich foods they will need to eat daily. An iron supplement is effective only if taken with iron-rich foods.

After 7 days of iron therapy, a reticulocyte count is usually done. If elevated, this means that the child is receiving adequate iron and that the rapid proliferation of new erythrocytes is correcting the anemia. Iron medication must be taken for at least 4 to 6 weeks after the RBC count is normal to rebuild iron levels in the blood. In some children, maintenance therapy may continue for as long as 1 year.

Chronic Infection Anemia

Acute infection interferes with RBC production, producing a normochromic, normocytic anemia. When infections are chronic, anemia of a hypochromic, microcytic type occurs. This is probably caused by impaired iron metabolism as well as impaired RBC production.

The degree of anemia is rarely as severe as that occurring with iron deficiency. Administration of iron has little effect until the infection is controlled.

Macrocytic (Megaloblastic) Anemias

A macrocytic anemia is one in which RBCs are abnormally large. These cells are actually immature erythrocytes or megaloblasts (nucleated immature red cells). For this reason, these anemias are often referred to as megaloblastic anemias. Because these anemias are caused by nutritional deficiencies, they occur less frequently in the United States than in developing countries.

Anemia of Folic Acid Deficiency

A deficiency of folic acid combined with vitamin C deficiency produces an anemia in which erythrocytes are abnormally large. There is accompanying neutropenia and thrombocytopenia. Mean corpuscular volume and mean corpuscular hemoglobin are increased, whereas mean corpuscular hemoglobin concentration is normal. Bone marrow will contain megaloblasts, indicating inhibition of the production of erythrocytes at an early stage. Megaloblastic arrest, or inability of RBCs to mature past an early stage, may occur in the first year of life from the continued use of infant food containing too little folic acid or goat's milk, which tends to be deficient in folic acid. Treatment is daily oral administration of folic acid (Lane et al., 2001). Response to treatment is dramatic.

Pernicious Anemia (Vitamin B_{12} Deficiency)

Vitamin B_{12} is necessary for maturation of RBCs. Pernicious anemia results from deficiency or inability to use the vitamin. Vitamin B_{12}, found primarily in food of animal origin, including both cow's milk and breast milk, usually is readily available to infants. An adolescent may be deficient in vitamin B_{12} if he or she is on a long-term, poorly formulated vegetarian diet.

For absorption of vitamin B_{12} from the intestine, an intrinsic factor must be present in the gastric mucosa. Lack of the intrinsic factor is the most frequent cause of the disorder. Symptoms of intrinsic factor deficiency generally occur in the first 2 years of life (once the intrauterine stores of vitamin B_{12} have been exhausted). The child appears pale, anorexic, and irritable, with chronic diarrhea. The tongue appears smooth and beefy-red due to papillary atrophy. In children, neuropathologic findings such as ataxia, hyporeflexia, paresthesia, and a positive Babinski reflex are less noticeable than in adults.

Laboratory findings reveal low serum levels of vitamin B_{12}. The rate and efficiency of absorption of vitamin B_{12} can be tested by the ingestion of the radioactively tagged vitamin. The dose absorbed in the presence and absence of a dose of intrinsic factor can be measured (a Schilling test; Al-Khatti, 2001).

Pernicious anemia is treated with lifelong monthly intramuscular injections of vitamin B_{12}. Parents and the child need to understand that lifelong therapy is necessary.

✔ **CHECKPOINT QUESTIONS**

8. What is the drug of choice for treating iron-deficiency anemia?
9. What must be present for vitamin B_{12} absorption?

Hemolytic Anemias

Hemolytic anemias are those in which the number of erythrocytes decreases due to increased destruction of erythrocytes. This may be caused by fundamental abnormalities of erythrocyte structure or by extracellular destruction forces.

Congenital Spherocytosis

Congenital spherocytosis is a hemolytic anemia that is inherited as an autosomal dominant trait. It occurs most frequently in the white Northern European population (Lane et al., 2001). The cells are small and defective, apparently due to abnormalities of the protein of the cell membrane that make them unusually permeable to sodium. The life span of erythrocytes is diminished.

The disease may be noticed shortly after birth, although symptoms may appear at any age. The hemolysis of RBCs appears to occur in the spleen, apparently from excessive absorption of sodium into the cell. The abnormal cell swells and ruptures and thus is destroyed. Chronic jaundice and splenomegaly are present. The mean corpuscular hemoglobin concentration is increased because the cells are small. Gallstones may be present in the older school-age child and adolescent because of the continuous hemolysis, bilirubin release, and incorporation of bilirubin into gallstones.

Infections may precipitate a crisis involving bone marrow failure. During such a period, the anemia increases rapidly as the hemolysis continues. Blood transfusion will be necessary to maintain a sufficient number of circulating erythrocytes.

The diagnosis of the disease is based on family history, the obvious hemolysis, and the presence of the abnormal spherocytes. The medical treatment is generally splenectomy at approximately 5 to 6 years. This measure will increase the number of RBCs present but will not alter their abnormal structure.

Glucose-6-Phosphate Dehydrogenase (G6PD) Deficiency

The enzyme glucose-6-phosphate dehydrogenase (G6PD) is necessary for maintenance of RBC life. Lack of the enzyme results in premature destruction of RBCs if the cells are exposed to an oxidant, such as acetylsalicylic acid. Deficiency of the enzyme occurs most frequently in children of African-American, Asian, Sephardic Jewish, and Mediterranean descent. The disease is transmitted as a sex-linked recessive trait. Approximately 15% of African-American males have the disorder (Rheingold, 2000). Because the disease is sex-linked, males of high-risk groups should be screened in infancy.

G6PD occurs in two identifiable forms. Children with congenital nonspherocytic hemolytic anemia have hemolysis, jaundice, and splenomegaly and may have aplastic crises. Other children have a drug-induced form in which the blood patterns are normal until the child is exposed to fava beans or drugs such as antipyretics, sulfonamides, antimalarials, and naphthaquinolones (the most common drug in these groups is acetylsalicylic acid [aspirin]). Approximately 2 days after ingestion of such an oxidant drug, the child begins to show evidence of hemolysis.

A blood smear will show **Heinz bodies** (oddly shaped particles in RBCs). The degree of RBC destruction depends on the drug and the extent of exposure to it. The child may have accompanying fever and back pain. Occasionally a newborn is seen with marked hemolysis because the mother ingested an initiating drug during pregnancy.

Drug-induced hemolysis usually is self-limiting, and blood transfusions are rarely necessary. G6PD deficiency may be diagnosed by a rapid enzyme screening test or electrophoretic analysis of RBCs. Both parents and children must be told of the defect in the child's metabolism so they can avoid common drugs such as acetylsalicylic acid.

Sickle-Cell Anemia

Sickle-cell anemia is the presence of abnormally shaped (elongated) RBCs. It is an autosomal recessive inherited defect of the beta chain of hemoglobin; the amino acid valine takes the place of the normally appearing glutamic acid. The erythrocytes become characteristically elongated and crescent-shaped (sickled) when they are submitted to low oxygen tension (less than 60% to 70%), a low blood pH (acidosis), or increased blood viscosity, such as occurs with dehydration or hypoxia. When RBCs sickle, they do not move freely through vessels. Stasis and further sickling occur (a sickle-cell crisis). Blood flow halts and tissue distal to the blockage becomes ischemic, resulting in acute pain and cell destruction (Smith-Whitley, 2000).

Because fetal hemoglobin contains a gamma, not a beta, chain, the disease usually will not result in clinical symptoms until the child's hemoglobin changes from the fetal to the adult form at approximately 6 months. However, the disease can be diagnosed prenatally by chorionic villi sampling or from cord blood during amniocentesis. The abnormal form of hemoglobin in this disorder is designated hemoglobin S. A child with sickle-cell disease is said to have hemoglobin SS (homozygous involvement).

Sickle-cell disease occurs almost exclusively among African Americans. Both parents of the child with the disease will have both normal adult and hemoglobin S or be carriers (heterozygous) of the **sickle-cell trait** (have hemoglobin AS). In people with the trait, approximately 25% to 50% of hemoglobin produced is abnormal. They produce enough normal hemoglobin to compensate for the defect and therefore show no symptoms. Sickle-cell trait occurs in approximately 1 in 12 African Americans. A child with the disease (homozygous) produces no normal hemoglobin and so shows characteristic symptoms of sickle-cell anemia. Approximately 1 in 400 African Americans has the disease (Westerman et al., 2002). A very few children have combinations of hemoglobin S and hemoglobin C or E, leading to mild anemia.

Assessment. Hemoglobin electrophoresis is used to diagnose sickle-cell anemia. At approximately 6 months of age, children with sickle-cell disease begin to show initial signs of fever and anemia. Stasis of blood and infarction may occur in any body part, leading to local disease. Some infants have swelling of the hands and feet (a hand–foot syndrome). This is probably caused by aseptic infarction of the bones of the hands and feet. Children with sickle-cell anemia tend to have a slight build and characteristically long arms and legs. They may have a protruding abdomen because of an enlarged spleen and liver. In adolescence, the spleen size may be decreased from repeated infarction and atrophy. An atropic spleen leaves a child more susceptible to infection than normal because the spleen can no longer filter bacteria. Pneumococcal meningitis and salmonella-induced osteomyelitis are frequent illnesses. A chest syndrome with symptoms similar to pneumonia may occur. To prevent infection, many children are given prophylactic penicillin from about 6 months to 6 years of age. The liver may become enlarged from stasis of blood flow. Eventually, cirrhosis (fibrotic degeneration) will occur from infarcts and tissue scarring. The kidneys may have subsequent scarring also, and kidney function may be decreased. The sclerae are generally icteric (yellowed) from chronic destruction of the sickled cells; small retinal occlusions may lead to decreased vision. Regular eye examinations are necessary in children with sickle-cell disease to detect this. Cell clusters in the blood vessels of the penis may cause **priapism,** or persistent, painful erection (Gbadoe et al., 2001).

Sickle-Cell Crisis. **Sickle-cell crisis** is the term used to denote a sudden, severe onset of sickling. Symptoms of crisis occur from pooling of the many new sickled cells in vessels and consequent tissue hypoxia (a vaso-occlusive crisis). A sickle-cell crisis can occur when a child has an illness causing dehydration or a respiratory infection that results in lowered oxygen exchange and a lowered arterial oxygen level, or after extremely strenuous exercise (enough to lead to tissue hypoxia). Sometimes no obvious cause of a crisis can be found. Symptoms are sudden, severe, and painful (see Assessing the Child With Sickle-Cell Crisis). Aseptic necrosis of the head of the femur or humerus with increased joint pain may occur. Laboratory reports reveal a hemoglobin level of only 6 to 8 g/100 mL. A peripheral blood smear demonstrates sickled cells. The WBC count is often elevated to 12,000 to 20,000/mm^3. Bilirubin and reticulocyte levels are increased.

If a cerebrovascular accident occurs from a blocked artery, the central nervous system will be affected and the child may have coma, seizures, or even death. If there is renal involvement, hematuria or flank pain may result.

Less frequent forms of crisis may occur when there is splenic sequestration of RBCs or severe anemia due to pooling and increased destruction of sickled cells in the liver and spleen (a sequestration crisis). This leads to shock from hypovolemia. The spleen is enlarged and tender. An aplastic crisis is manifested by severe anemia due to a sudden decrease in RBC production. This form usually occurs with infection. A hyperhemolytic crisis can occur when there is increased destruction of RBCs. A megaloblastic crisis may occur if the child has folic acid or vitamin B deficiency (new RBCs cannot be fully formed due to lack of these ingredients).

ASSESSING the Child With Sickle-Cell Crisis

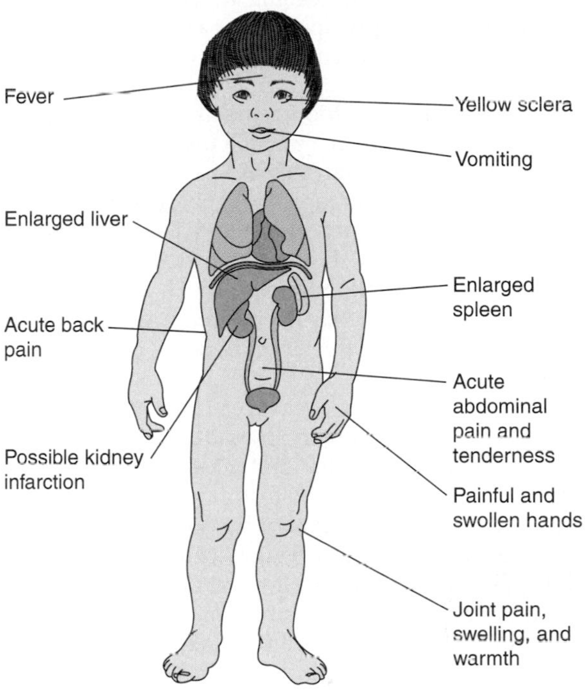

Acute Chest Syndrome. Acute chest syndrome has become the leading cause of death in patients with sickle-cell disease. Children exhibit hypoxia, decreased hemoglobin levels, and a persistent diffuse pneumonia so severe that ventilator care may be needed. Blood transfusion is used to increase the oxygen-carrying capacity of blood, and broad-spectrum antibiotics are given to resolve the pneumonia (Vichinsky et al., 2000).

Therapeutic Management. The child in sickle-cell crisis has three primary needs: pain relief and adequate hydration and oxygenation to prevent further sickling and halt the crisis (Jakubic & Thompson, 2001).

Acetaminophen (Tylenol) may be adequate pain relief for some children; for others, a narcotic analgesic such as intravenous morphine may be needed. Once the child is pain-free, he or she is able to relax, reducing the metabolic demand for oxygen and helping to end the sickling. Hydration is generally accomplished with intensive intravenous fluid replacement therapy. Tissue hypoxia leads to acidosis. The acidosis must be corrected by electrolyte replacement. Some kidney infarction may have occurred, so do not administer potassium intravenously until kidney function has been determined. Otherwise, excessive potassium levels may occur, possibly leading to cardiac arrhythmias. Infection may be the precipitator for a sickling crisis. If this occurs, blood and urine cultures, a chest x-ray, and a complete blood count will be taken and the infection will be treated by antibiotics. Blood transfusion (usually packed RBCs) may be necessary to maintain the hemoglobin above 12 g/dL (termed hypertransfusion).

Hydroxyurea, an antineoplastic agent that has the potential to increase the production of hemoglobin F (fetal hemoglobin), can be used in children with sickle-cell disease to increase their overall hemoglobin level. The drug, given orally, may cause anorexia. Therefore, monitor the child's nutrition intake during this drug therapy (Davies & Olujohungbe, 2001).

If none of the above measures appears to be effective, children may be given an exchange transfusion to remove most of the sickled cells and replace them with normal cells. Exchange transfusion (see Chap. 26) must be done with small amounts of blood at each exchange. Otherwise, the pressure changes can cause such irregularities in blood volume that heart failure results. Bone marrow stem cell transplantation is possible for the child who does not respond to usual therapies (Smith-Whitley, 2000).

NURSING DIAGNOSES AND RELATED INTERVENTIONS

Nursing Diagnosis: Ineffective tissue perfusion related to generalized infarcts due to sickling

Outcome Identification: Child will remain free of detrimental effects of sickle-cell crisis during crisis.

Outcome Evaluation: Child's respiratory rate is 16 to 20/min; cyanosis absent; arterial blood gases within acceptable parameters including PCO_2 = 40 mm Hg; PO_2 = 80 to 90 mm Hg; oxygen saturation of 95%; urine output greater than 1 mL/kg/h.

Oxygen may be administered by nasal cannula or mask if arterial blood gases reveal a low PO_2 level. Oxygen may not reach every distal body part effectively if blood flowing to the part is obstructed by the sickled cells. When hemoglobin S is below 40%, there is adequate blood flow to body cells. High concentrations of oxygen are not used because hypoxia is a stimulant to erythrocyte production—production badly needed to replace damaged cells. Monitor the flow rate carefully and use pulse oximetry to evaluate oxygen saturation levels for changes. Encourage bedrest to relieve the pain and reduce oxygen expenditure.

It is important to maintain accurate intake and output records, test urine for specific gravity, and hematuria to detect the extent or presence of kidney damage from infarcts.

Nursing Diagnosis: Ineffective health maintenance related to lack of knowledge regarding long-term needs of child with sickle-cell anemia

Outcome Identification: Family will demonstrate ability to carry out necessary measures to maintain child's health in the future.

Outcome Evaluation: Mother or father accurately describes disease process and identifies special precautions necessary to prevent sickle-cell crisis.

In many children, episodes of sickling grow less severe as the child reaches adolescence. These children may have a normal life expectancy but still experience the stresses of chronic illness. Other children experience such devastating episodes in early childhood that the disease is fatal at an early age. Parents need support to supervise children carefully day by day when they are aware that, due to the intense episodes, the child may die despite the precautions.

Between crises, care focuses on preventing recurring crises. Although the hemoglobin level of children may remain as low as 6 to 9 g/100 mL, children adjust well to this chronic state. Children who receive frequent blood transfusions should not be given supplementary iron or iron-fortified formula or vitamins or they may receive too much iron; high levels of excess iron are deposited in body tissues (hemosiderosis) to a point of destroying RBCs (**hemochromatosis**). Oral folic acid may be prescribed to help rebuild hemolyzed RBCs.

Children with sickle-cell anemia need to be followed at regular health care visits. They must receive childhood immunizations so they are not vulnerable to common childhood infections such as measles or pertussis. They may be prescribed oral penicillin as prophylaxis for the first 5 years. They are also candidates for meningococcal and pneumococcal vaccines to prevent infection. Puberty may be delayed, and both parents and children may need counseling to accept this. Once puberty changes do occur, they are adequate, just later than normal. Parents and children with sickle-cell disease also need support and positive reinforcement to enhance the child's self-esteem and to learn how to deal with problems that occur as a result of this chronic hematologic disorder (see Focus on Evidence-Based Practice).

Caution parents to bring their child to a health care facility at the first indication of infection. Some parents are reluctant to do this, afraid that they will be labeled overprotective. Assure them that health care personnel are knowledgeable about sickle-cell anemia, and they know that a child with even a minor infection could become very ill. Respiratory illness will lead to sickling for two reasons. the accompanying dehydration and the lowered oxygen tension from altered oxygen–carbon dioxide exchange.

Parents must make decisions regarding children's activity levels. Children should attend regular school and should be allowed to participate in all school activities except contact sports (such as football), which could result in rupture of an enlarged spleen. Long-

FOCUS ON EVIDENCE-BASED PRACTICE

What Are Common Problems That Occur From Care of the Child With a Chronic Illness?

To analyze what school problems occur when a child has a chronic illness such as a blood dyscrasia, researchers interviewed 21 parents and 24 school personnel. Results of the study revealed five prominent areas of concern: how parents should inform the school about the child's illness, what the process related to the child's re-entry into the school should be, how ongoing monitoring of the child's health status will be conducted, how school personnel will be taught about unexpected health problems, and what school personnel's expectations for the child should be.

In a second study, to investigate how parents feel about having a child with a chronic illness, 190 mothers were asked what positive things they could list about their experience. Eighty-eight percent of mothers in this study said they felt better about themselves because they were able to manage a child's chronic condition, 70% felt their families were stronger because of their child's condition, and 80% felt their family had benefited in some way from having a child with a chronic illness.

These are important studies for nurses because nurses are the health care providers frequently asked to solve difficulties that arise in the care of children with a chronic hematologic disorder. Knowing what school personnel believe are prime problems aids in building communication bridges with teachers and other school personnel for better problem-solving and overall continuity of the child's care. Knowing that having a child with a chronic illness can create positive feelings in the family is a key element in developing teaching plans to enhance the family's ability for problem-solving.

Chernoff, R. G., et al. (2001). Maternal reports of raising children with chronic illnesses: The prevalence of positive thinking. *Ambulatory Pediatrics, 1*(2), 104–107.

Kliebenstein, M. A., & Broome, M. E. (2000). School re-entry for the child with chronic illness: Parent and school personnel perceptions. *Pediatric Nursing, 26*(6), 579–584.

distance running is also inadvisable because it can lead to dehydration. Caution parents to give the child fluids frequently, especially on long hikes and at the beach. Caution them against taking the child on board an unpressurized aircraft in which the oxygen concentration may fall during flight. During the summer, parents need to be certain that they offer the child frequent drinks to prevent dehydration.

Some children who have had kidney infarcts and lessened ability to concentrate urine have chronic nocturnal enuresis (bedwetting) (see Focus on Family Empowerment).

WHAT IF? What if a parent tells you she restricts her child, who has sickle-cell anemia, from drinking any fluid after 4 PM to prevent bedwetting? Is this a good solution to bedwetting for this child? How would you counsel this parent?

Children with sickle-cell disease are at high risk if they need surgery. The hours of being on nothing-by-mouth status, as well as being unable to eat afterward, may lead to dehydration. Anesthesia may cause a transient hypoxia leading to sickling. Parents must be cautioned that even for such a simple operation as tooth extraction, they must alert health care personnel about their child's condition.

✔ CHECKPOINT QUESTIONS

10. What is the treatment of choice for congenital spherocytosis?
11. With sickle-cell anemia, do children need less or more fluid in the summer, and why?

Thalassemias

The thalassemias are anemias associated with abnormalities of the beta chain of adult hemoglobin (HgbA). Although these anemias occur most frequently in the Mediterranean population, they also occur in children of African and Asian heritage (Al-Awamy & Pearson, 2001).

Thalassemia Minor (Heterozygous Beta-Thalassemia)

Children with thalassemia minor, a mild form of this anemia, produce both defective beta hemoglobin and normal hemoglobin. Because there is some normal production, the RBC count will be normal, but the hemoglobin concentration will be decreased 2 to 3 g/100 mL below normal levels. The blood cells are moderately hypochromic and microcytic because of the poor hemoglobin formation.

Children may have no symptoms other than pallor. They require no treatment, and life expectancy is normal. They should not receive a routine iron supplement because their inability to incorporate it well into hemoglobin may cause them to accumulate too much iron. The condition represents the heterozygous form of the disorder or can be compared with children having the sickle-cell trait.

Thalassemia Major (Homozygous Beta-Thalassemia)

Thalassemia major is also called Cooley's anemia or Mediterranean anemia. Because thalassemia is a beta chain hemoglobin defect, symptoms do not become apparent until the child's fetal hemoglobin has largely been replaced by adult hemoglobin during the second half of the first year of life. Effects of thalassemia major on body systems are

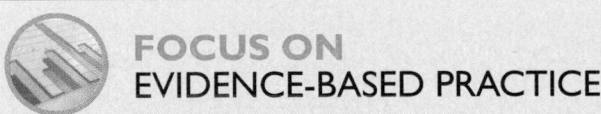

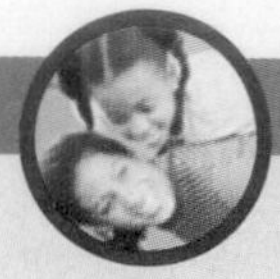

FOCUS ON FAMILY EMPOWERMENT
Safety Precautions for School

Q. Our son has sickle-cell disease. What can we do to help keep him safe, especially at school?

A. Use these guidelines to help ensure your son's safety at school:

- Be certain your child either takes fluid with him or buys adequate fluid for lunch. Children with sickle-cell anemia need to maintain a high fluid intake to prevent their blood from becoming thick.
- Provide additional fluid in the summer when dehydration is more apt to happen. Anticipate ways to provide fluid during long hikes or school trips; time spent on a hot beach may need to be limited.
- Learn about sources high in folic acid, such as vegetables and fruit, and be certain these are included in your son's diet every day.
- Encourage the boy to get adequate sleep at night as a general measure to prevent illness.
- With the exception of contact sports (to avoid damage to an enlarged spleen) and long-distance running (to prevent dehydration), encourage your son to participate in normal school activities.
- Know that bedwetting may occur as part of the illness. Encourage your son to take baths in the morning if this occurs so his clothes don't smell of urine.
- Maintain routine health care such as immunizations to prevent common childhood illnesses such as measles and mumps.
- Call your primary health care provider at the first sign of illness, such as an upper respiratory infection, so therapy can be begun immediately.

summarized in Table 44-3. Unable to produce normal beta hemoglobin, the child shows symptoms of anemia: pallor, irritability, and anorexia.

RBCs are hypochromic (pale) and microcytic (small). Fragmented poikilocytes and basophilic stippling (unevenness of hemoglobin concentration) are present. The hemoglobin level is less than 5 g/100 mL. The serum iron level is high because iron is not being incorporated into hemoglobin; iron saturation is 100%.

Assessment. To maintain a functional level of hemoglobin, the bone marrow hypertrophies in an attempt to produce more RBCs. This may cause bone pain; the ineffective attempt often leads to the formation of target cells or large macrocytes that are short-lived and nonfunctional. As bone marrow becomes hyperactive, this results in the characteristic change in the shape of the skull (parietal and frontal bossing) and protrusion of the upper teeth, with marked malocclusion. The base of the nose may be broad and flattened; the eyes may be slanted with an epicanthal fold, as in Down syndrome. An x-ray of bone shows marked osteoporotic (of lessened density) tissue, possibly resulting in fractures. The child may have hepatosplenomegaly due to excessive iron deposits and fibrotic scarring in the liver and the spleen's increased attempts to destroy defective RBCs. Abdominal pressure from the enlarged spleen may cause anorexia and vomiting. Epistaxis is common, as is diabetes mellitus due to pancreatic siderosis and cardiac dilatation with an accompanying murmur. Arrhythmias and heart failure are frequent causes of death.

TABLE 44.3 Effects of Thalassemia Major

BODY ORGAN OR SYSTEM	EFFECT OF ABNORMAL CELL PRODUCTION
Bone marrow	Overstimulation of bone marrow leads to increased facial-mandibular growth
Skin	Bronze-colored from hemosiderosis and jaundice
Spleen	Splenomegaly
Liver and gallbladder	Cirrhosis and cholelithiasis
Pancreas	Destruction of islet cells and diabetes mellitus
Heart	Failure from circulatory overload

Therapeutic Management. Digitalis, diuretics, and a low-sodium diet may be prescribed to prevent heart failure, which could result from the decompensation that accompanies anemia, and from myocardial fibrosis caused by invasion of iron (hemochromatosis). Transfusion of packed RBCs every 2 to 4 weeks (hypertransfusion therapy) will maintain hemoglobin between 10 and 12 g/100 mL. With this level of hemoglobin, erythropoiesis is suppressed and cosmetic facial alterations, osteoporosis, and cardiac dilatation are minimized. Hypertransfusion therapy also reduces the possibility that splenectomy will be necessary. Frequent blood transfusions, unfortunately, increase the risk of blood-borne disease, such as hepatitis B, and deposition of iron in body tissues (hemosiderosis). Children may receive an iron-chelating agent to remove this excessive store of iron, such as deferoxamine (given subcutaneously over 6 to 8 hours as they sleep at night; Shankar, 2000).

Splenectomy may become necessary to reduce discomfort and also to reduce the rate of RBC hemolysis and the number of necessary transfusions. Bone marrow stem cell transplantation can offer a cure. With treatment, the overall prognosis of thalassemia is improving but still grave. Most children with the disease die of cardiac failure during adolescence or as young adults.

NURSING DIAGNOSES AND RELATED INTERVENTIONS

Nursing Diagnosis: Risk for situational low self-esteem related to changed physical appearance

Outcome Identification: Child will demonstrate an adequate level of self-esteem during course of illness.

Outcome Evaluation: Child states he can accept altered appearance and interacts with peers.

Children with thalassemia major may have delayed growth and sexual maturation. They usually develop a marked change in facial appearance because of the overgrowth of marrow-producing centers of the facial bones. This can be demoralizing because these changes will be permanent. In addition, the child who receives frequent blood transfusions may develop such hemosiderosis that his or her skin appears bronze.

Children should be allowed as much activity as possible and should attend regular school, if possible, to maintain a nearly normal childhood. Discussions about other children's reactions to their changing facial appearance can be helpful.

Autoimmune Acquired Hemolytic Anemia

Occasionally, autoimmune antibodies (abnormal antibodies of the IgG class) attach themselves to RBCs, destroy them, and cause hemolysis. This may occur at any age, and its origin is generally idiopathic, although the disorder may be associated with malignancy, viral infections, or collagen diseases such as rheumatoid arthritis or systemic lupus erythematosus. A child may recently have had an upper respiratory infection, measles, or varicella virus infection (chickenpox). Such hemolysis may occur after the administration of drugs such as quinine, phenacetin, sulfonamides, or penicillin.

The exact cause is unknown but may involve a change in the RBCs themselves, making them antigenic, or a change in antibody production, making antibodies destructive to other substances.

Assessment. The onset is insidious. Children have a low-grade fever, anorexia, lethargy, pallor, and icterus from release of indirect bilirubin from the hemolyzed cells. Both urine and stools appear dark because the excess bilirubin is being excreted. In some children, the illness begins abruptly with high fever, hemoglobinuria, marked jaundice, and pallor. There may be an enlarged liver and spleen.

Laboratory findings reveal that the RBCs are extremely small and round (spherocytosis), resembling hereditary spherocytosis. The reticulocyte count is increased as the body attempts to form replacement RBCs. A direct Coombs' test result is positive, indicating the presence of antibodies attached to red cells. Hemoglobin levels may fall as low as 6 g/100 mL.

Therapeutic Management. In some children, the disease process runs a limited course and no treatment is necessary. In others, a single blood transfusion may correct the disturbance. For these children, it is difficult to cross-match blood for transfusion because the red cell antibody tends to clump or agglutinate all blood tested. If cross-matching is impossible, the child may be given type O Rh-negative blood. Observe the child carefully during any transfusion for signs of transfusion reaction.

If the anemia is persistent, corticosteroid therapy (oral prednisone) is generally effective, increasing the RBC count and hemoglobin concentration in a short period (Lane et al., 2001). If this is ineffective, splenectomy may be necessary. For some children, immunosuppressive agents (e.g., cyclophosphamide [Cytoxan] or azathioprine [Imuran]) are effective in reducing antibody formation.

Often it is difficult for parents to understand the process. How could a child's body turn on itself? What caused this? How long will it last? What will stop it from happening again? There are no answers to these questions. Provide the parents and child with support as they wait for this unexplainable process to run its course and for the child to be well again.

Polycythemia

Polycythemia is an increase in the number of RBCs that results as a compensatory response to insufficient oxygenation of the blood. With this disorder, erythropoiesis is increased to attempt to supply enough RBCs to supply oxygen to cells. Chronic pulmonary disease and congenital heart disease are the usual causes of polycythemia in childhood. Also, it may occur from twin transfusion at birth (one twin receives excess blood while a second twin is anemic).

Plethora (marked reddened appearance of the skin) occurs because of the increase in total RBC volume. The erythrocytes are usually macrocytic (large) and the hemoglobin content is high. This means that the mean corpuscular hemoglobin will be elevated; the mean corpuscular hemoglobin concentration, however, will be normal, indicating that, although many in number, each erythrocyte is normally saturated with hemoglobin. The RBC count may be as high as 7 million/mm^3. Hemoglobin levels may be as high as 23 g/100 mL.

Treatment of polycythemia involves treatment of the underlying cause. Because of the high blood viscosity from so many crowded blood cells, cerebrovascular accident or emboli may occur. The risk increases particularly if the child becomes dehydrated, such as with fever or during surgery. Exchange transfusion to reduce the RBC count may be necessary.

✔ CHECKPOINT QUESTIONS

12. What body appearance is associated with thalassemia major?
13. What laboratory test results would be seen with a child with autoimmune acquired hemolytic anemia?

DISORDERS OF THE WHITE BLOOD CELLS

Most disorders characterized by a decrease or increase in the number of WBCs or specific WBC components occur in response to another disease (often infection or an allergic reaction) in the body (Table 44-4). Laboratory values of WBCs, therefore, provide one of the first objective indicators of disease, often aiding in specific diagnosis.

DISORDERS OF BLOOD COAGULATION

Platelets are necessary for blood coagulation. Thus, platelet disorders limit the effectiveness of this process. A normal platelet level is 150,000/mm^3. Thrombocytopenia (decreased platelet count) may be defined as a platelet count of less than 40,000/mm^3. In one disorder, children are born with thrombocytopenia and also are missing the radius bone in the forearm (TAR [thrombocytopenia/absent radius] syndrome). Thrombocytopenia leads to purpura or blood seeping from vessels into the skin.

Purpuras

Purpura is a hemorrhagic rash or small hemorrhages occurring in the superficial layer of skin. Two main types of purpura occur in children: idiopathic thrombocytopenia purpura and Henoch-Schönlein syndrome.

Idiopathic Thrombocytopenic Purpura

Idiopathic thrombocytopenic purpura (ITP) is the result of a decrease in the number of circulating platelets in the presence of adequate megakaryocytes (precursors to platelets). The cause is unknown, but it probably results from an increased rate of platelet destruction due to an antiplatelet antibody that destroys platelets (making this an autoimmune illness) (Buchanan, 2001).

In most instances, ITP occurs approximately 2 weeks after a viral infection such as rubella, rubeola, varicella, or an upper respiratory tract infection. Congenital ITP may occur in the newborn of a woman who has had ITP during pregnancy. An antiplatelet factor apparently crosses the placenta and causes platelet destruction in the newborn. If it occurs in an infant whose mother did not have ITP, the disease appears to develop in the same way as Rh incompatibility or hemolytic disease of the newborn. However, in ITP, the platelets, not the RBCs, are sensitized (see Chap. 26).

Assessment. Manifestations often begin abruptly, first evidenced as miniature petechiae or as large areas of asymmetric ecchymosis most prominent over the legs, although they may occur anywhere on the body (Fig. 44-3). Epistaxis or bleeding into joints may be present.

Laboratory studies reveal marked thrombocytopenia. The platelet count may be as low as 20,000/mm^3. Bone marrow examination shows a normal number of megakaryocytes. A tourniquet test may be performed. For this, the child's blood pressure is taken. Then the cuff is reinflated on the child's arm to a point halfway between systolic and diastolic pressure and left inflated for 5 minutes.

TABLE 44.4 Disorders of White Blood Cells

DISORDER	DESCRIPTION	CAUSES/TREATMENT
Neutropenia	Reduced number of white blood cells	Transient phenomenon with nonpyrogenic infections such as viral disease Response to therapy with some drugs, such as 6-mercaptopurine or nitrogen mustard Possible side effect from drugs such as phenytoin sodium (Dilantin), chloramphenicol, or chlorpromazine Treatments: Possibly white blood cell transfusion; prophylactic antibiotics
Neutrophilia	Increased number of circulating white blood cells, primarily neutrophils (total number of cells increases and the proportion of mature neutrophils changes, with an increase in immature cells)	Usually in response to infection or inflammation (see Chap. 43) Treatment: antibiotic therapy to eliminate infectious organisms
Leukemia	Uncontrolled proliferation of white blood cells	Neoplastic disorder (see Chap. 53)
Eosinophilia	Increased number of eosinophils	Associated with many allergic disorders, such as atopic dermatitis, and with parasitic invasion (see Chaps. 42 and 43)
Lymphocytosis	Increased number of lymphocytes	Normally occurs in the preschool period, when there is a marked predominance of lymphocytes in relation to neutrophils Abnormally elevated in childhood illnesses such as pertussis, infectious mononucleosis, and lymphocytic leukemia Treatment: Therapy for the underlying condition

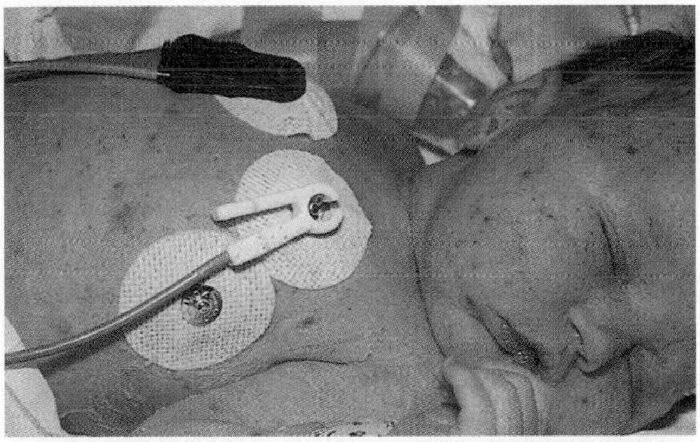

FIGURE 44.3 The infant with ITP. Notice the tiny petechiae and large ecchymotic areas.

In a child with normal coagulation ability, this extended pressure should result in fewer than two petechiae marks on an area of skin on the forearm 2 cm square. The child with decreased platelets will have more petechiae.

Therapeutic Management. Oral prednisone to reduce the immune response and intravenous immunoglobulin (IVIG) or, in Rh-positive children, anti-D immunoglobulin to supply anti-ITP antibodies are used to treat ITP (Bolton-Maggs, 2000). Platelet transfusion will temporarily increase the platelet count, but because the lifespan of platelets is relatively short, a platelet transfusion will have limited effect. Children with central nervous system bleeding may require more vigorous treatment, but even with these symptoms, a splenectomy is rarely necessary.

If the child experiences joint pain from bleeding, do not give salicylates or ibuprofen. These agents interfere with blood clotting by preventing the aggregation of platelets at wound sites.

In most children, ITP runs a limited, 1- to 3-month course. A few children develop chronic ITP. A course of immunosuppressive drugs may be attempted if the chronic state persists.

All children need to be vaccinated against the viral diseases of childhood so that diseases such as rubella, rubeola, and varicella are eradicated and can no longer lead to this defective coagulation process.

NURSING DIAGNOSES AND RELATED INTERVENTIONS

Nursing Diagnosis: Health-seeking behaviors related to injury-prevention measures

Outcome Identification: Parents will demonstrate measures to prevent injury that would result in bleeding during child's illness.

Outcome Evaluation: Parents state precautions they will take to reduce possibility of bleeding injury; repeat correct dose and timing of medication therapy; child's skin is free of ecchymotic areas; platelet count rises to within normal values.

The techniques for reducing bleeding described earlier in the chapter can be used to reduce the possibility of bleeding (e.g., padding the surfaces where the child plays) for the child with ITP. Parents cannot eliminate the possibility of a serious bleeding injury, however, until the platelet count returns to normal. The chief danger to the child from ITP, aside from the psychological stress of a perplexing illness, is intracranial hemorrhage. Although this is rare, be alert for signs such as persistent headache, nuchal rigidity, and lethargy.

Nursing Diagnosis: Risk for compromised family coping related to diagnosis of child's illness

Outcome Identification: Parents demonstrate ability to cope with life-threatening circumstances during course of illness.

Outcome Evaluation: Parents state that they understand the nature of their child's illness and have identified ways to carry out daily activities despite the illness.

Because the symptoms (e.g., easy bruising) of ITP mimic the beginning ones of leukemia, parents may be extremely frightened. Assure them that this bruising is not leukemia. If the ITP follows a long course (2 or 3 months), reassure them that this process will not later become leukemia. A child may have so many bruises that the parents are initially suspected of child abuse. They may become very defensive and angry at health care personnel. They need time to express their anger and regain confidence in the health care team.

It is also bewildering for parents to be told that no one knows exactly what is causing their child's disease. To be convinced that health care personnel can manage their child's care without knowing the exact cause, they need careful explanations of all procedures.

Henoch-Schönlein Syndrome

Henoch-Schönlein purpura (also called anaphylactoid purpura) is caused by increased vessel permeability. Although no definite allergic correlation can be identified, it is generally considered to be a hypersensitivity reaction to an invading allergen. It occurs most frequently in children between 2 and 8 years of age, and more frequently in boys than girls (Gusic, 2000). Usually, there is a history of a mild infection before the outbreak of symptoms. The syndrome presents (because of the purpura) as a possible platelet disorder until a differential diagnosis is made.

Assessment. The purpural rash occurs typically on the buttocks, posterior thighs, and extensor surface of the arms and legs (Fig. 44-4). The tips of the ears may be involved. The rash begins as a crop of urticarial lesions that change to pink maculopapules. These become hemorrhagic (bright red) and then fade, leaving brown macular spots that remain for several weeks. The child's joints are tender and swollen. The child may have gastrointestinal symptoms such as abdominal pain, vomiting, or blood in stools. Gross or microscopic hematuria may be present

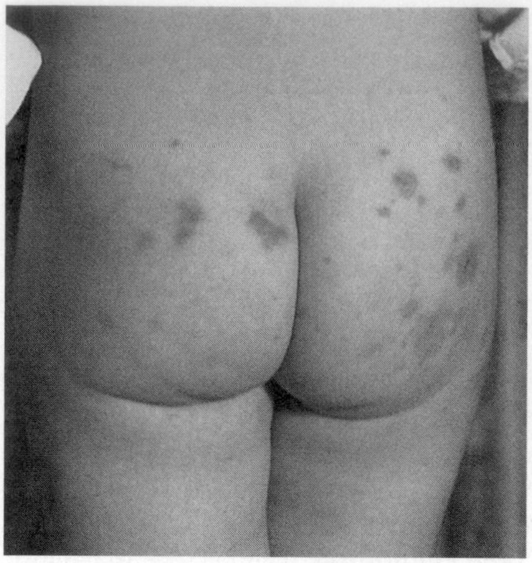

FIGURE 44.4 The distinctive purpural rash of Henoch-Schönlein syndrome appearing on the buttocks of a young child.

from kidney involvement. A biopsy shows granulocytes in the walls of small arterioles.

Laboratory studies show a normal platelet count. Sedimentation rate, WBC count, and eosinophil count are elevated.

Therapeutic Management. Treatment involves oral corticosteroid therapy (prednisone) and mild analgesics for a short period. Nose and throat cultures rule out continuing bacterial involvement. Urine should be assessed for protein and glucose to detect kidney involvement. Typically the disease runs a course of 4 to 6 weeks. A few children develop chronic nephritis as a complication (Gusic, 2000).

Disseminated Intravascular Coagulation

Disseminated intravascular coagulation (DIC) is an acquired disorder of blood clotting that results from excessive trauma or some similar underlying stimulus.

Normal blood clotting is a balance between the hemostatic (clotting) system and the fibrinolytic (dissolving) system of the bloodstream. After a blood vessel injury, local vasoconstriction rapidly prevents additional blood loss at the site. With the tear in the vessel wall, the underlying collagen is exposed. This causes platelets to swell and become adherent and irregular in shape. They release adenosine diphosphate, which attracts additional platelets and binds them together (platelet aggregation). This phenomenon results in a platelet plug to seal the vessel. The plug is strengthened by fibrin threads that form as a result of an intrinsic and extrinsic coagulation process into a firm, fixed structure. To prevent too much clotting from occurring, plasmin or fibrinolysin, a proteolytic enzyme formed from plasminogen, digests fibrin threads and causes lysis of the clot along with consumption of blood clotting factors. As plasmin, fibrinogen, and fibrin are lysed, fibrin degradation products are formed. These products prevent the laying down of further fibrin and platelet aggregation.

With DIC, an imbalance occurs between clotting activity and fibrinolysis. Extreme clotting due to endothelial damage begins at one point in the circulatory system, depleting the availability of clotting factors such as platelets and fibrin from the general circulation. A secondary initiation of fibrinolysis begins as well. A paradox exists: the person has both increased coagulation and a bleeding defect at the same time. Many of the complications of pregnancy (abruptio placentae or death of a fetus) initiate DIC, so this is a common complication seen accompanying bleeding during pregnancy (see Chap. 15). DIC can occur in children with acute infections.

Assessment. A child begins to have uncontrolled bleeding from puncture sites from injections or intravenous therapy. Ecchymoses and petechiae form on the skin. The toes and fingers may appear pale, cyanotic, or mottled and feel cold because small blood vessels are so filled with coagulated blood that circulation to the extremities is impaired. If coagulation is acute, neurologic or renal symptoms may occur from occlusion of vessels supplying the brain and kidneys. Observe all children with a serious illness carefully for signs of increased bleeding such as skin petechiae or oozing from blood-drawing sites.

With DIC, laboratory tests usually show the following:

- Thrombocytopenia (level depends on the rate at which bone marrow is able to replace platelets)
- Large-appearing platelets on blood smear, possibly fragmented (from passing through meshes of collecting fibrin)
- Prolonged prothrombin and partial thromboplastin times
- Markedly low serum fibrinogen levels (less than 100 mg/100 mL)
- Elevated fibrin split products

Therapeutic Management. To stop DIC, the underlying insult that began the phenomenon must be halted. Intravenous heparin administration helps to interfere with the marked coagulation. Although blood transfusion may be necessary to correct blood loss, it may be delayed until after heparin has been administered so that the new blood factors are not also consumed by the coagulation process. Fresh-frozen plasma, platelets, or fibrinogen may be administered.

With adequate therapy, the results of blood coagulation studies will return to normal. If renal or brain cells were damaged from occluded capillaries, permanent injury to these areas may result.

NURSING DIAGNOSES AND RELATED INTERVENTIONS

Nursing Diagnosis: Deficient knowledge about blood clotting disorder related to its paradoxical nature

Outcome Identification: Client or parents will demonstrate increased knowledge of the illness by 1 hour.

Outcome Evaluation: Client or parents accurately state nature of illness and proposed therapy; state signs and symptoms of disease; verbalize understanding of treatments.

Parents may be bewildered by the paradoxical problems of bleeding on the one hand and clotting on the other. If they understand the action of heparin—to discourage blood coagulation—their child's need and the medication seem directly contradictory. Be certain that both children and parents are given a full explanation. The child has an increased risk of hemorrhage because part of the coagulation system has used up coagulation factors; heparin is acting to stop this coagulation. This effort will help parents understand what is happening and foster trust and confidence in caregivers.

✔ CHECKPOINT QUESTIONS

14. What WBC disorder is commonly associated with allergies?
15. Why should ibuprofen be avoided for the child with ITP?
16. What is the drug of choice for treating DIC?

Hemophilias

Hemophilia is an inherited interference with blood coagulation. There are numerous hemophilia types, each involving deficiency of a different blood coagulation factor.

Hemophilia A (Factor VIII Deficiency)

The classic form of hemophilia is caused by deficiency of the coagulation component factor VIII, the antihemophilic factor, which is transmitted as a sex-linked recessive trait. In the United States, the incidence is approximately 1 in 10,000 white males. The female carrier may have slightly lowered but sufficient levels of the factor VIII component so that she does not manifest a bleeding disorder. Males with the disease also have varying levels of factor VIII, and their bleeding tendency varies accordingly, from mild to severe (Kelly, 2000).

Factor VIII is an intrinsic factor of coagulation, so the intrinsic system for manufacturing thromboplastin is incomplete. The child's coagulation ability is not absent because the extrinsic or tissue system remains intact. Thus, the child's blood will eventually coagulate after an injury.

Assessment. Hemophilia often is recognized first in the infant who bleeds excessively after circumcision. If the disease has not shown itself for several generations in a family, the parents may be unaware of its existence. For this reason, all infants need careful and thoughtful observation after circumcision.

Because infants do not receive many injuries, the child's bleeding tendency may not become apparent until he or she begins to walk. Suddenly the lower extremities (where the child bumps things) become heavily bruised. There is soft tissue bleeding and painful hemorrhage into the joints, which become swollen and warm. The child holds the injured joint stiffly. Repeated bleeding into a joint causes damage to the synovial membrane (hemarthrosis), possibly resulting in severe loss of joint mobility.

Severe bleeding may also occur into the gastrointestinal tract, peritoneal cavity, or central nervous system. Interestingly, nosebleeds are common but are not as severe as with the platelet deficiency syndromes. The child must be identified as having hemophilia before surgery is performed for any reason; otherwise, fatal bleeding could occur.

With hemophilia, the platelet count and prothrombin time are normal. The whole blood clotting time is markedly prolonged or normal, depending on the level of factor VIII present. A thromboplastin generation test is abnormal. PTT is the test that best reveals the low levels of factor VIII.

Therapeutic Management. With even minor abrasions, bleeding must be controlled by the administration of factor VIII. This may be supplied by fresh whole blood or by fresh or frozen plasma, but it is best supplied by a concentrate of factor VIII. One bag of concentrate per 5 kg body weight is usually sufficient. This provides protection for approximately 12 hours; another transfusion may be necessary after that time. Powdered forms of factor VIII that can be stored at home and reconstituted as needed are available. Prophylactic administration may best reduce bleeding episodes (Kelly, 2000). In some children, administration of desmopressin (DDAVP), which stimulates the release of factor VIII, may be helpful.

In a few children, antibodies (termed inhibitors) to factor VIII develop, rendering the factor ineffective. If this happens, epsilon-aminocaproic acid, a fibrinolytic enzyme that helps to stabilize clot formation and promote wound healing, can be self-administered every 6 hours if needed. Children with inhibitors to factor VIII can also be given a factor IX concentrate (Proplex or Konyne). This concentrate enters the coagulation cascade after factor VIII and halts bleeding (Yaish, 2001).

NURSING DIAGNOSES AND RELATED INTERVENTIONS

Nursing Diagnosis: Parental health-seeking behaviors related to strategies for protecting the child from injury

Outcome Identification: Parents will develop plan for preventing injury to the child; child will not experience major bleeding episodes during childhood.

Outcome Evaluation: Child's skin is free of ecchymotic areas; absence of frequent epistaxis; blood pressure within age-appropriate parameters; absence of swelling or warmth at joints.

Prevention of injury is the most important intervention with these children. Parents need information about how to prevent bleeding episodes and also how to respond when one occurs (see Focus on Communication). Help parents to set appropriate limits. An active infant may need to have his crib sides padded; all toys need to be inspected for sharp edges or parts.

Parents (and the child as soon as he is approximately 10 years old) can be taught to administer a

FOCUS ON COMMUNICATION

Murray Harrow is an 8-year-old boy with hemophilia you see in an emergency room. His right knee is covered by a large brush burn and is swollen, discolored, and warm to touch.

Less Effective Communication

Nurse: Hello, Mrs. Harrow. I need to take a history of Murray's accident.
Mrs. Harrow: He doesn't know how he hurt it.
Nurse: It looks like he fell. Were you running, Murray? Riding a bicycle? Skateboarding?
Mrs. Harrow: He's never ridden a bicycle. I don't allow it. Or skateboarding. He better not say that he was doing that!
Nurse: Murray, how do you think you hurt your knee?
Murray: I don't know.
Nurse: You must have hit it hard to cause so much damage to the surface skin. You didn't notice hitting it so hard?
Murray: No.
Nurse: Okay. Let's get your factor replacement started and get the swelling down.

More Effective Communication

Nurse: Hello, Mrs. Harrow. I need to take a history of Murray's accident.
Mrs. Harrow: He doesn't know how he hurt it.
Nurse: It looks like he fell. Were you running, Murray?
Mrs. Harrow: He better not say that was what he was doing. He knows better than that.
Nurse: What about riding a bicycle?
Mrs. Harrow: He's never ridden a bicycle. I don't allow it.
Nurse: How about skateboarding?
Mrs. Harrow: He better not say he was doing that!
Nurse: Mrs. Harrow, I need to get an accurate history of what happened. I'd like Murray to tell us how he thinks the accident happened. Then later on, we can talk about what are good rules for him to be following.

Children with bleeding disorders have to follow a great many rules to avoid bleeding episodes, such as not playing contact sports or skateboarding. Because these forbidden activities are appealing, children occasionally break the rules. In an emergency room, it is important that children and parents both recognize that the priority at the moment is obtaining an accurate history. Until they realize this, they may be so concerned with the broken rule that they are unable to move beyond that to secure adequate therapy.

replacement factor intravenously to prevent bleeding immediately after an injury. This action, combined with immobilization of the injured extremity and an ice pack applied locally, almost always eliminates the need for hospital admission. Pressure should be applied to a laceration to halt bleeding directly. Suturing of lacerations is avoided whenever possible, because the sutures make additional puncture sites that may bleed.

Nursing Diagnosis: Pain related to joint infiltration by blood

Outcome Identification: Child will experience a tolerable level of pain after injury.

Outcome Evaluation: Child states that pain is at a tolerable level.

The child with hemophiliac bleeding experiences discomfort because of the bleeding into joints and may be frightened because the parents are so frightened. Immobilization of the affected joint helps to decrease bleeding and also provides relief. Be certain that immobilized joints are in good alignment. As soon as the acute bleeding episode has halted (approximately 48 hours), perform passive range of motion as ordered to maintain function. Ibuprofen is not ordered as an analgesic because it may prolong bleeding. As soon as effective levels of factor VIII have been provided, the pain in the bleeding joint is generally relieved, despite the continued heat or swelling.

Nursing Diagnosis: Risk for interrupted family processes related to fears regarding child's prognosis and long-term nature of illness

Outcome Identification: Family members will demonstrate adequate coping behaviors by 1 month.

Outcome Evaluation: Family members voice their fear regarding illness; state that they can cope despite stress level; demonstrate positive coping responses.

Parents of children with hemophilia are frightened during a time of acute bleeding, not just because of what is currently happening but also because they may have seen other family members or even a previous child die of the disease. Be certain to give them a chance to talk about how the bleeding began (e.g., "I should have noticed that toy had a sharp edge," "He fell from his bike. I should have watched him more closely"). It is extremely important for parents to allow the child to lead a normal life—for example, with toys and bicycle riding. Remind them that it is impossible to prevent all injuries. Assist them with measures that offer them a sense of control over the situation. As the child reaches school age, he must learn to monitor his own activities.

Von Willebrand's Disease

Von Willebrand's disease, an inherited autosomal dominant disorder affecting both sexes, is often referred to as angiohemophilia. Along with a factor VIII defect, there is also an inability of the platelets to aggregate. In addition, the blood vessels cannot constrict and aid in coagulation. Bleeding time is prolonged, with most hemorrhages occurring from mucous membrane sites.

Epistaxis is a major problem, because children tend to rub or pick at their noses as a nervous mechanism. In girls, menstrual flow is unusually heavy and may cause embarrassment from stained clothing. Childbirth is obviously a risk for women with von Willebrand's disease. Bleeding is controlled with factor VIII replenishment as with hemophilia, or by administration of arginine desmopressin (DDAVP), a vasoconstricting agent (Montgomery & Kroner, 2001).

Christmas Disease (Hemophilia B, Factor IX Deficiency)

Christmas disease, caused by factor IX deficiency, is transmitted as a sex-linked recessive trait. Only approximately 15% of people with hemophilia have this form. Treatment is with a concentrate of factor IX, available for home administration (Lane et al., 2001).

Hemophilia C (Factor XI deficiency)

Hemophilia C or plasma thromboplastin antecedent deficiency, caused by factor XI deficiency, is transmitted as an autosomal recessive trait occurring in both sexes. The symptoms are generally mild compared with those in children with factor VIII or factor IX deficiencies. Bleeding episodes are treated with administration of desmopressin (DDAVP) or transfusion of fresh blood or plasma (Lane et al., 2001).

✔ CHECKPOINT QUESTIONS

17. What coagulation factor is deficient in hemophilia A?
18. What intervention is crucial for any child with hemophilia?

KEY POINTS

Bone marrow stem cell transplantation is the main therapy for several blood dyscrasias. Transplantation can be allogeneic (from a histocompatible donor) or autologous (using the child's own marrow). Splenectomy, another possible treatment, may increase a child's susceptibility to pneumococcal infections. Assess whether the child has received pneumococcal vaccine after a splenectomy.

Disorders of the red blood cells that commonly occur in children include acute blood-loss anemia and anemia of acute infection. Aplastic and hypoplastic anemias occur from depression of hematopoietic activity in bone marrow. These anemias can be congenital or acquired.

A major hypochromic anemia that develops in children is iron-deficiency anemia. Children invariably fatigue easily because they cannot oxygenate body cells well. Their care must include measures to keep them from tiring; oxygen administration may be necessary.

Macrocytic anemias occur from folic acid deficiency and pernicious anemia (vitamin B_{12} deficiency).

Hemolytic anemias include congenital spherocytosis, glucose-6-dehydrogenase deficiency, sickle-cell anemia, thalassemia, and autoimmune acquired hemolytic anemia. Sickle-cell anemia occurs most often in African-American children.

Disorders of white blood cells that occur include neutropenia (reduced number of white blood cells) and neutrophilia (increased number). Neutropenia makes children susceptible to infection.

Disorders of blood coagulation include the purpuras (idiopathic thrombocytopenic purpura and Henoch-Schönlein syndrome), disseminated intravascular coagulation (DIC), and the hemophilias.

Children with blood coagulation disorders must carefully guard against injury. This includes monitoring types of toys and activities. It may include padding a crib or side rails.

Disorders of the blood tend to be long-term illnesses. Education of the parents and child is important to promote adaptation to the condition and enhance compliance with long-term medication therapy.

CRITICAL THINKING EXERCISES

1. Heather is the 2-year-old girl with thalassemia major you met at the beginning of the chapter. Her mother asked you why Heather has developed a prominent mandible while another patient with thalassemia minor has no such facial changes. What additional health teaching does Heather's mother need to help her understand what is happening to her daughter? How would you explain why skin color changes have happened to her daughter?
2. A 12-year-old girl has been diagnosed with sickle-cell disease. You have noticed that every summer for the past 5 years, while she has been home from school on summer vacation, she has had an acute episode of her illness. What assessments would you want to make of her family before this summer? What precautions would you want to discuss with them?
3. A 5-year-old boy with hemophilia wants to join a preschool soccer program. How would you counsel his family regarding this?
4. Examine the National Health Goals related to hematologic disorders in children. Most government-sponsored money for nursing research is allotted based on these goals. What would be a possible research topic to explore pertinent to these goals that would be fundable and would advance evidence-based practice?

REFERENCES

Al-Awamy, B. H., & Pearson, H. A. (2001). Thalassemia. In A. Y. Elzoui, H. A. Harfi, & H. Nazer. (2001). *Textbook of clinical pediatrics* (pp. 887–891). Philadelphia: Lippincott Williams & Wilkins.

Al-Khatti, A. (2001). Anemias resulting from deficient or ineffective utilization of necessary elements. In A. Y. Elzoui, H. A. Harfi, & H. Nazer. (2001). *Textbook of clinical pediatrics* (pp. 863–867). Philadelphia: Lippincott Williams & Wilkins.

Bolton-Maggs, P. H. B. (2000). Idiopathic thrombocytopenic purpura. *Archives of Disease in Childhood, 83*(3), 220–222.

Bondurant, M. C., & Koury, M. J. (1999). Origin and development of blood cells. In G. R. Lee et al. (Eds.). *Wintrobe's clinical hematology.* Philadelphia: Lippincott Williams & Wilkins.

Buchanan, G. R. (2001). Idiopathic thrombocytopenic purpura in childhood. *Pediatric Annals, 30*(9), 527–533.

Chernoff, R. G. et al. (2001). Maternal reports of raising children with chronic illnesses. *Ambulatory Pediatrics, 1*(2), 104–107.

Davies, S., & Olujohungbe, A. (2001). Hydroxyurea for sickle cell disease. *The Cochrane Library* (Oxford) 2001, issue 3.

Department of Health and Human Services (2000). *Healthy people, 2010.* Washington, DC: DHHS.

Derivan, M., & Ferrante, C. (2001). Aplastic anemia. *Clinical Journal of Oncology Nursing, 5*(5), 227–229.

Ende, N., et al. (2001). Pooled umbilical cord blood as a possible universal donor for marrow reconstitution and use in nuclear accidents. *Life Sciences, 69*(13), 1531–1539.

Esposito, C., et al. (2001). Experience with laparoscopic splenectomy. *Journal of Pediatric Surgery, 36*(2), 309–311.

Gbadoe, A. D., et al. (2001). Management of sickle cell priapism with etilefrine. *Archives of Disease in Childhood, 85*(1), 52–53.

Gusic, B. R. (2000). Henoch-Schönlein purpura. In M. W. Schwartz (Ed.). *The 5-minute pediatric consult* (pp. 424–425). Philadelphia: Lippincott Williams & Wilkins.

Jakubik, L. D., & Thompson, M. (2000). Care of the child with sickle cell disease: Acute complications. *Pediatric Nursing, 26*(4), 373–381.

Kelly, K. M. (2000). Hemophilia. In M. W. Schwartz (Ed.). *The 5-minute pediatric consult* (pp. 420–421). Philadelphia: Lippincott Williams & Wilkins.

Kliebenstein, M. A. & Broome, M. E. (2000). School re-entry for the child with chronic illness. *Pediatric Nursing, 26*(6), 579–584.

Lane, P. A., Nuss, R., & Ambruso, D. R. (2001). Hematologic disorders. In W. W. Hay, A. R. Hayward, M. J. Levin, & J. M. Sondheimer (Eds.). *Current pediatric diagnosis and treatment* (15th ed.). New York: McGraw-Hill.

Levi, M. (2001). Pathogenesis and treatment of disseminated intravascular coagulation in the septic patient. *Journal of Critical Care, 16*(4), 167–177.

Logan, S. et al. (2001). Iron therapy for improving psychomotor development and cognitive function in children with iron deficiency anemia. *Cochrane Database System Review, (2),* CD001 444.

Mahoney, M. C. (2000). Putting prevention into practice: Screening for iron deficiency anemia among children and adolescents. *American Family Physician, 62*(3), 671–673.

Montgomery, R. R., & Kroner, P. A. (2001). Von Willebrand disease. A common pediatric disorder. *Pediatric Annals, 30*(9), 534–540.

Nash, R. A. (1999). Hematopoietic stem cell transplantation. In G. R. Lee et al. (Eds.). *Wintrobe's clinical hematology.* Philadelphia: Lippincott Williams & Wilkins.

Perkins, S. L. (1999). Examination of the blood and bone marrow In G. R. Lee et al. (Eds.). *Wintrobe's clinical hematology.* Philadelphia: Lippincott Williams & Wilkins.

Rheingold, J. R. (2000). Idiopathic thrombocytopenic purpura. In M. W. Schwartz (Ed.). *The 5-minute pediatric consult* (pp. 460–461). Philadelphia: Lippincott Williams & Wilkins.

Schroeder, M. L. (1999). Principles and practice of transfusion medicine. In G. R. Lee et al. (Eds.). *Wintrobe's clinical hematology.* Philadelphia: Lippincott Williams & Wilkins.

Shankar, S. M. (2000). Thalassemia. In M. W. Schwartz (Ed.). *The 5-minute pediatric consult* (pp. 806–807). Philadelphia: Lippincott Williams & Wilkins.

Sherry, B., Mei, Z., & Md, R. Y. (2001). Continuation of the decline in prevalence of anemia in low-income infants and children in five states. *Pediatrics, 107*(4), 677–682.

Shusterman, S. (2000). Iron deficiency anemia. In M. W. Schwartz (Ed.). *The 5-minute pediatric consult* (pp. 488–489). Philadelphia: Lippincott Williams & Wilkins.

Smith-Whitley, K. (2000). Sickle-cell disease. In M. W. Schwartz (Ed.). *The 5-minute pediatric consult* (pp. 756–757). Philadelphia: Lippincott Williams & Wilkins.

Vichinsky, E. P., et al. (2000). Causes and outcomes of the acute chest syndrome in sickle cell disease. *New England Journal of Medicine, 342*(25), 1855–1865.

Westerman, M. P. et al. (2002). Coagulation changes in individuals with sickle cell trait. *American Journal of Hematology, 69*(2). 89–94.

Yaish, H. M. (2001). Hemostasis and coagulation disorders. In A. Y. Elzoui, H. A. Harfi, & H. Nazer (2001). *Textbook of clinical pediatrics* (pp. 920–938). Philadelphia: Lippincott Williams & Wilkins.

SUGGESTED READINGS

Altemeier, W. A. (2001). Interpreting bruises in children. *Pediatric Annals, 30*(9), 517–520.

Brigden, M. L. (2001). Hematologic and oncologic emergencies. Doing the most good in the least time. *Postgraduate Medicine, 109*(3), 143–157.

Dix, H. M. (2001). New advances in the treatment of sickle cell disease: Focus on perioperative significance. *AANA Journal, 69*(4), 281–286.

Fung, E. B., et al. (2001). Energy expenditure and intake in children with sickle cell disease during acute illness. *Clinical Nutrition, 20*(2), 131–138.

Gould, D., Thomas, V., & Darlison, M. (2000). The role of the haemoglobinopathy nurse counselor. *Journal of Advanced Nursing, 31*(1), 157–164.

Graumlich, S. E., et al. (2001). Multidimensional assessment of pain in pediatric sickle cell disease. *Journal of Pediatric Psychology, 26*(4), 203–214.

Kulkarni, R. (2001). Bleeding in the newborn. *Pediatric Annals, 30*(9), 548–557.

Pederson, C., Parran, L., & Harbaugh, B. (2000). Children's perceptions of pain during 3 weeks of bone marrow transplant experience. *Journal of Pediatric Oncology Nursing, 17*(1), 22–32.

Sadowitz, P. D. et al. (2002). Hematologic emergencies in the pediatric emergency room. *Emergency Medicine Clinics of North America, 20*(1), 177–198.

Salsbury, D. C. (2001). Anemia of prematurity. *Neonatal Network: Journal of Neonatal Nursing, 20*(5), 13–20.

Warrier, I. (2001). Thrombotic disorders in infancy and childhood. *Pediatric Annals, 30*(9), 558–563.

CHAPTER 45

Nursing Care of the Child With a Gastrointestinal Disorder

Key Terms

- achalasia
- aganglionic megacolon
- appendicitis
- beriberi
- celiac disease
- Crohn's disease
- dehydration
- gastroesophageal reflux
- hepatitis
- hiatal hernia
- inguinal hernia
- insensible loss
- intussusception
- irritable bowel syndrome
- keratomalacia
- kwashiorkor
- liver transplantation
- McBurney's point
- Meckel's diverticulum
- necrotizing enterocolitis
- nutritional marasmus
- overhydration
- pellagra
- peptic ulcer
- pyloric stenosis
- rickets
- scurvy
- steatorrhea
- ulcerative colitis
- volvulus
- xerophthalmia

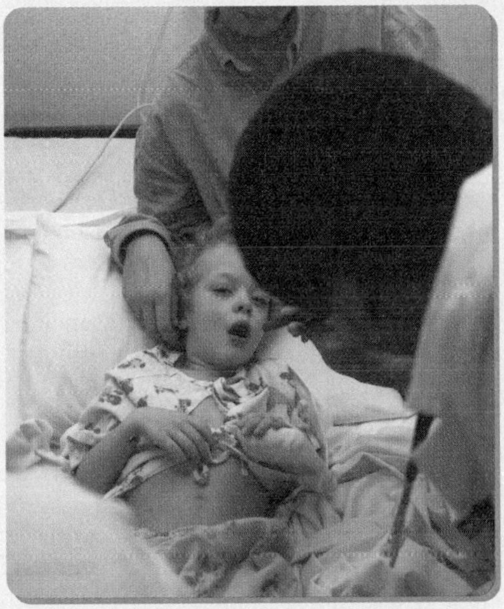

Objectives

After mastering the contents of this chapter, you should be able to:

1. Describe common gastrointestinal disorders seen in children.
2. Assess the child with a gastrointestinal disorder.
3. Formulate nursing diagnoses for the child with a gastrointestinal disorder.
4. Develop outcomes for the child with a gastrointestinal disorder.
5. Plan nursing care with specific goals for the child with a gastrointestinal disorder.
6. Implement nursing care for the child with a gastrointestinal disorder.
7. Evaluate outcomes for effectiveness and achievement of care.
8. Identify National Health Goals related to gastrointestinal disorders and children that nurses could be instrumental in helping the nation achieve.
9. Identify areas of care related to gastrointestinal disorders and children that could benefit from additional nursing research or application of evidence-based practice.
10. Analyze ways that nursing care of the child with a gastrointestinal disorder can be more family centered.
11. Integrate knowledge of gastrointestinal disorders with nursing process to achieve quality maternal and child health nursing care.

Barry is a 2-year-old boy diagnosed with celiac disease that you see at a birthday party. His abdomen is protuberant, yet his arms and legs seem thin and wasted. He refuses to eat a piece of birthday cake even though his mother sits beside him insisting on it. "See the problem I have with him?" she asks you. "He eats nothing. When he does, he gets diarrhea."

Does Barry's mother understand her son's disease? Is she choosing wise food selections for him?

Previous chapters described the growth and development of well children and the nursing care for children with disorders of other systems. This chapter adds information about the dramatic changes, both physical and psychosocial, that occur when children develop gastrointestinal disorders. This is important information because it builds a base for care and health teaching.

After you've studied the chapter, answer the Critical Thinking Exercises at the end of the chapter and then access the on-line study activities (http://connection.lww.com) *to further sharpen your skills and test your knowledge.*

The gastrointestinal (GI) system involves a long body tract with numerous organs. Because it is so long and diverse, a multitude of possible disorders can occur in it, including both congenital defects and acquired illnesses. (Developmental physical defects involving the GI system discovered at birth are discussed in Chapter 39.) Because the GI system is responsible for taking in and processing nutrients for all parts of the body, any problem can quickly affect other body systems and, if not adequately treated, can affect overall health, growth, and development.

Health education is extremely important for children with GI disorders and their families because many parents do not appreciate the seriousness of GI illness. Often, they are surprised to find that what they thought was a simple "stomach flu" has caused serious electrolyte imbalances and possibly a life-threatening state for their child. Some GI disorders require both parents and child to learn about new nutritional patterns. When the child is young, the parents need education concerning this topic as well as other care measures. As the child grows older, counseling to help the child maintain self-esteem and learn nutritional requirements becomes important.

Hepatitis in children has received much attention as a national health goal. Goals concerning this health concern are highlighted in the Focus on National Health Goals.

FOCUS ON NATIONAL HEALTH GOALS

Hepatitis is a gastrointestinal condition growing in incidence. For this reason, National Health Goals address this topic in a variety of ways. Goals addressing hepatitis include the following:

- Reduce chronic hepatitis B viral infections in infants and young children (perinatal infections) from a baseline of 1,682 cases per year to a target level of 400 cases per year.
- Reduce hepatitis B in adolescents 19 to 24 years of age from 24/100,000 population to 2.4/100,000 population.
- Reduce hepatitis C from a baseline of 2.4 new cases/100,000 population to 1 new case/100,000 population.
- Reduce hepatitis A from a baseline of 11.3/100,000 to 4.5/100,000 (DHHS, 2000).

Nurses can be instrumental in helping the nation achieve these goals by serving as consultants to day care providers to reduce the spread of stool contamination in these settings and actively administering hepatitis B vaccine to infants and adolescents to eradicate this form of the illness in another generation. Nursing research in a number of areas could be helpful: Does the brand of diapers used by children in day care influence the spread of infectious stool; how many infants are not being brought for follow-up care and thus do not receive all three immunizations against hepatitis B; and do the majority of parents appreciate the devastating outcome that can result from hepatitis?

NURSING PROCESS OVERVIEW

For the Child With a Gastrointestinal Disorder

Assessment

Children with GI disorders quickly become dehydrated, especially if vomiting or diarrhea is a symptom. They need to be assessed for signs of fluid loss, such as poor skin turgor, dry mucous membranes, or lack of tearing (see Assessing the Child With Altered GI Function). When talking to parents about a child's symptoms, ask exactly what they mean when they say "spitting up" or "a little vomiting." Also ask how many times a child has voided or how many diapers have been wet in the past 24 hours, and whether this is less than usual. Compare the child's current weight with past weight measurements, if available. Unless the child is an adolescent who has been actively dieting, there is never a normal reason for weight loss in children.

Ask parents to describe what they mean by diarrhea. Some parents mistakenly confuse normal newborn stools with diarrhea. As a rule, all children with diarrhea, especially small children, need to be seen by a health care provider because fluid and electrolyte changes occur rapidly in children because of the greater percentage of fluid held extracellularly rather than intracellularly.

For many children, a GI tract disorder is diagnosed largely by presenting symptoms such as those just described. In other instances, x-ray studies with a contrast medium (barium) or an endoscopic examination may be needed to confirm the presence of an anomaly. Ultrasound or magnetic resonance imaging (MRI) also may be helpful. Another important assessment area is laboratory testing for electrolyte balance through serum analysis, or fluid concentration through urinalysis.

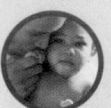

ASSESSING the Child With Altered GI Function

History

Chief concern: Vomiting, diarrhea, constipation, abdominal pain, abdominal distention, weight below normal standard, lethargy, paleness.

Past medical history: History of past vomiting or diarrhea or abdominal pain; hydramnios in pregnancy.

Family history: Relatives have a similar disorder; high stress level because of home or school environment.

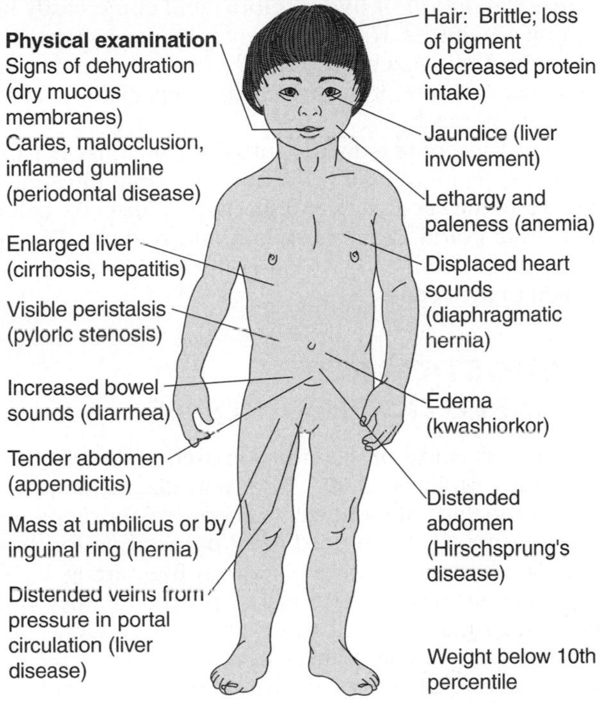

Nursing Diagnosis

Nursing diagnoses relevant to children with GI disorders invariably center on imbalanced nutrition, because most GI diseases alter the kind and amount of nutrients ingested or absorbed into the body in some way. However, GI disorders also take an emotional toll on the ill child and family. Feeding is one of the primary ways mothers bond with their newborns, and bonding can be seriously threatened when the infant develops a GI disorder, especially when hospitalization is required. The process of eating and the types of food eaten are also integral components of family life and culture, so any disruption caused by illness can place a strain on the entire family. Examples of nursing diagnoses may include:

- Impaired parenting related to interference with establishing parent–infant bond
- Interrupted family processes related to chronic illness in child
- Risk for deficient fluid volume related to chronic diarrhea
- Imbalanced nutrition, less than body requirements, related to malabsorption of necessary nutrients
- Situational low self-esteem related to feelings of being different resulting from special dietary restrictions

Outcome Identification and Planning

Planning care for the child with a GI disorder often includes nutritional planning with the child and parents. Be certain when helping to plan a new nutritional pattern that the person who actually prepares or supervises the child's diet is included. In many instances, some of the foods that the child eats may be prepared by a baby sitter, day care center staff, the child's other parent, or a grandparent. Many children eat breakfast and lunch at school cafeterias. It may be necessary to contact school staff to ask them to make meal exceptions for the child or to supervise a choice of foods (or to see that a child eats only the packaged lunch he or she brought to school, not extra items the child trades for with friends).

Some parents are unfamiliar with the basic food categories and the importance of providing food from a food pyramid in children's diets. They may have little understanding of which foods have high or low fiber content, or which foods are "bland" or "clear." Many parents have difficulty keeping children restricted to "nothing by mouth" (NPO) for tests or to rest the GI tract. They have been told that dehydration happens quickly in infants (which it does); they need support to follow the necessary restrictions when those restrictions are so opposed to basic parenting, which involves giving food.

If feedings will be given by nasogastric or gastrostomy tube, parents need enough practice time to be comfortable with the equipment and the technique before they are given the responsibility of doing it alone at home. If a child is going to gag or become distressed when a new tube is passed, parents need to have this happen where there are calm, supportive people nearby, not when they are by themselves at home.

Because GI disorders interfere with common body functions such as eating and elimination, long-term therapies such as gastrostomy feedings or colostomy care may be needed. These therapies are difficult for children and parents to accept without the support of concerned health care providers.

Implementation

Never underestimate the difficulty family members may experience adapting to alternative nutrition methods such as total parenteral nutrition or enteric feeding tubes, or caring for a child with a colostomy. Parents need a great deal of support to adapt their busy life to these alternative methods of care.

Insertion of a nasogastric tube, enteral and parenteral nutrition, and administration of an enema are discussed in Chapter 36. Be certain to give clear, simple explanations, and praise the parents and child after they demonstrate these procedures. Children can easily interpret enemas as punishment because of the extreme intrusiveness. Provide therapeutic play before and after these procedures to reduce children's anxiety.

Anticipate the need for additional support for the family and child with a chronic GI disorder. Agencies that might be helpful for referral are:

Celiac Disease Foundation (*www.celiac.org*)
Crohn's & Colitis Foundation of America (*www.ccfa.org*)
International Foundation for Functional Gastrointestinal Disorders (*www.iffgd.org*)
North American Society for Pediatric Gastroenterology, Hepatology and Nutrition (*www.naspgn.org*)

Outcome Evaluation

Recording children's height and weight is a primary method to evaluate nutritional outcomes. Even if a diet is limited in a special way, if it is adequate, children should gain weight and maintain growth.

Because children will ultimately be responsible for their own nutrition, evaluation should include making certain that children gradually learn more about their specific nutritional measures so they can become increasingly responsible for their own intake. Often, only when they are at this stage can their parents feel secure enough to let them stay overnight with a friend, visit a relative in a distant city, go to summer camp—activities that become important to children as they reach school age.

The saying "people are what they eat" has some relevance. Children who require special nutritional plans need to be evaluated for self-esteem at periodic health visits. Does the child think of himself or herself as inferior to or different from others because of food restrictions? What kind of positive experiences can be offered to such a child, or what can parents do to provide the child with experiences that would improve the child's self-esteem?

Some examples suggesting outcome achievement may include:

- Child lists examples of bland foods to select for lunch from school cafeteria menu.
- Parent states steps she will take to seek medical care if child has a second episode of severe diarrhea.
- Family members state they have adjusted to care of a child with celiac disease.

ANATOMY AND PHYSIOLOGY OF THE GASTROINTESTINAL SYSTEM

Embryonic development of the GI tract is discussed in Chapter 8. Digestion begins in the mouth, where food is broken down into small particles and mixed with saliva from the sublingual, submandibular, and parotid glands. Both gagging and swallowing reflexes are present even in newborns to prevent aspiration with swallowing. Digestion continues in the stomach and small intestine, the same as in adults.

The esophagus pierces the diaphragm to serve as a passageway to the stomach. (Fig. 45-1). Occasionally, an infant is born with a portion of the bowel or stomach protruding through the diaphragm's esophageal opening (hiatal or diaphragmatic hernia). At the junction of the esophagus and the stomach is the gastroesophageal (cardiac) sphincter. In some newborns, this sphincter is so lax that fluid regurgitates into the esophagus (gastroesophageal reflux or **chalasia**). At the distal end of the stomach is the pyloric *sphincter. In some infants, this valve is narrowed (stenosed), preventing food from flowing out of the stomach freely (pyloric stenosis). Originally, it was believed that the stomach was sterile because the action of hydrochlo*ric acid could easily kill invading organisms. However, since the discovery that a bacterium, Helicobacter pylori (*H pylori*) is the cause of peptic ulcer disease, it is obvious that organisms can survive in the stomach.

The small intestine is divided into three sections. (1) duodenum, (2) jejunum, and (3) ileum. The large intestine is divided into the cecum, ascending colon, transverse colon, descending colon, sigmoid colon, and rectum. The appendix, which frequently becomes diseased in children, is attached to the cecum.

DIAGNOSTIC AND THERAPEUTIC TECHNIQUES

A number of typical procedures are used in the diagnosis and therapy of GI disorders. Common diagnostic procedures used include fiberoptic endoscopy, colonoscopy, and barium enema. Children need good preparation for these procedures because they are potentially frightening. If children receive conscious sedation for a procedure, they need preparation for this as well as the actual procedure.

Therapy may include alternative methods of feeding such as enteral (nasogastric or gastrostomy tube feedings), total parenteral nutrition, and intravenous (IV) therapy to rest the GI tract. A colostomy or ileostomy may be created for the same reason. These tests and procedures, their meaning, impact on children, and nursing responsibilities for them are discussed in Chapters 36 and 37.

HEALTH PROMOTION AND RISK MANAGEMENT

Health promotion related to GI disorders focuses on a wide area because the causes of these disorders cover a wide and varied range. Some disorders, such as appendicitis, cannot be prevented because they occur for unpredictable causes. Some, such as celiac disease, involve genetic aspects that cannot be changed. Some, such as Crohn's disease and ulcerative colitis, are associated with an autoimmune response. Other conditions, such as vomiting and diarrhea, often caused by foods that were refrigerated improperly or spread through contaminated food from improper handwashing, can be prevented. Additionally, hepatitis can be prevented through good handwashing (hepatitis A) and immunization (hepatitis A and B). Vitamin and protein deficiency disorders can be prevented by educating parents about the food pyramid and how to select foods that fit each of the sections.

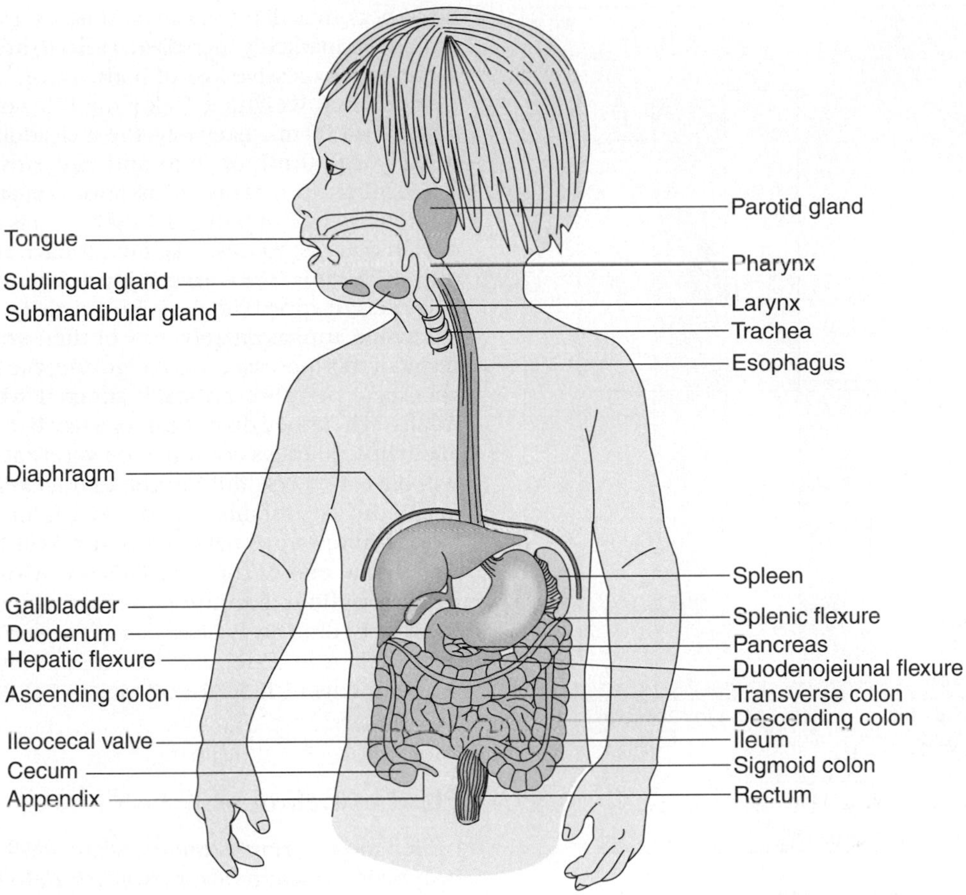

FIGURE 45.1 The gastrointestinal tract.

Because an interference in nutrition pervades many aspects of children's lives, families often need help with planning care. Help families plan the necessary adaptations to their lifestyle to prevent the disease from interfering with family functioning (e.g., will day care center personnel do gastrostomy feedings? Will a nursery school accept a child with a colostomy? Can a child select a gluten-free diet at the school cafeteria?). All families should be encouraged to eat at least one meal together so they can have time to share experiences and "touch base" with each other. For the family with a child who has a special feeding problem such as a gastrostomy feeding or total parenteral nutrition, this can be difficult. Urge such families to bring the child to the table for a social time even if the child cannot eat with the family. If watching family members eat while the child cannot is too difficult, urge the family to provide a "together" time in some other way so they do not miss out on this valuable family activity.

Some GI disorders in children such as aganglionic megacolon are diagnosed late because parents think the child's refusal to eat is just the sign of being a "picky eater" or a manifestation of 2-year-old autonomy. Educating parents about normal nutrition and how to distinguish things such as vomiting from illness from normal "spitting up" or severe diarrhea from a simple GI upset helps parents bring their children for care at the first possible time. Early intervention prevents the child from becoming dehydrated and seriously ill (Sondheimer, 2001a).

FLUID, ELECTROLYTE, AND ACID–BASE IMBALANCES

The GI system plays a major role in maintaining fluid, electrolyte, and acid–base balance. It is the main route by which substances are taken into the body and can be a major source of loss if vomiting or diarrhea occurs.

Fluid Balance

Retaining fluid is of greater importance in the body chemistry of infants than that of adults because fluid constitutes a greater fraction of the infant's total weight. In adults, body water accounts for approximately 60% of total weight. In infants, it accounts for as much as 75% to 80% of total weight; in children, it averages approximately 65% to 70%.

Fluid is distributed in three body compartments: (1) intracellular (within cells), 35% to 40% of body weight; (2) interstitial (surrounding cells and bloodstream), 20% of body weight; and (3) intravascular (blood plasma), 5% of body weight. The interstitial and the intravascular fluid together are often referred to as the *extracellular fluid (ECF)*, totaling 25% of body weight. In infants, the extracellular portion is much greater, totaling up to 45% of total body weight (Fig. 45-2). In young children, this amount is 30%; in adolescents, it is 25%.

Fluid is normally obtained by the body through oral ingestion of fluid and by the water formed in the metabolic

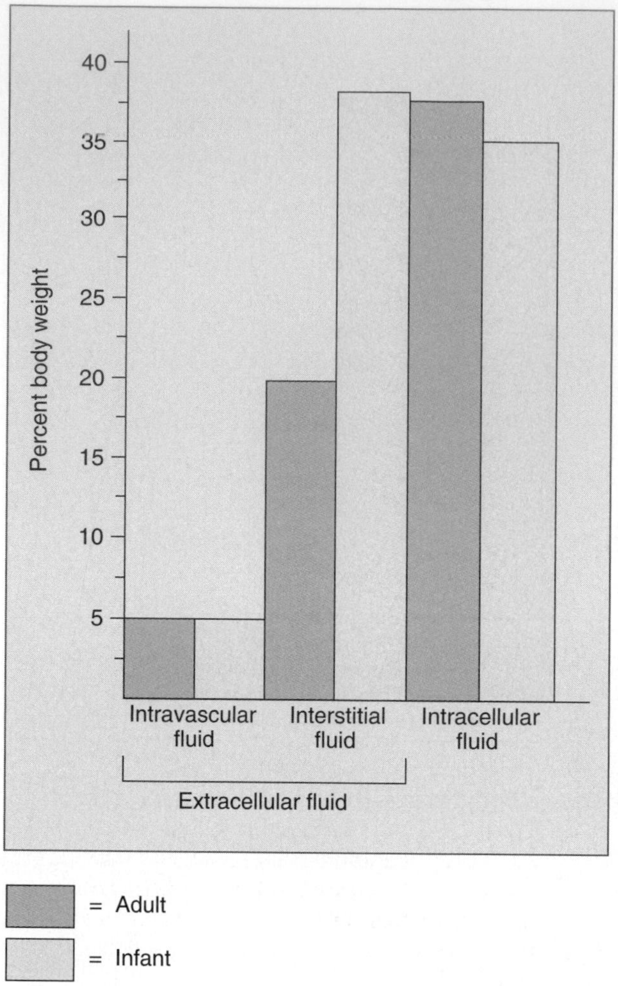

FIGURE 45.2 Distribution of fluid in body compartments.

breakdown of food. Primarily, fluid is lost from the body in urine and feces. Minor losses, **insensible losses,** occur from evaporation from skin and lungs and from saliva (of little importance except in children with tracheostomies or those requiring nasopharyngeal suction). Infants do not concentrate urine as well as adults because their kidneys are immature. As a result, they have a proportionally greater loss of water in their urine. In infants, the relatively greater surface area to body mass also causes a greater insensible loss. Fluid intake is altered when a child is nauseated and unable to ingest fluid or is vomiting and losing fluid ingested. When diarrhea occurs, or when a child becomes diaphoretic because of fever, the fluid output can be markedly increased. **Dehydration** occurs when there is an excessive loss of body water.

In an adult weighing 70 kg, the ECF volume is approximately 14,000 mL. Each day, the well adult ingests approximately 2,000 mL of fluid and excretes approximately 2,000 mL as urine. This means approximately 14% of his or her total ECF (2,000 mL of 14,000 mL) is exchanged each day. In contrast to this, 7-kg infants have an ECF volume of only 1,750 mL. They ingest approximately 700 mL daily and excrete approximately 700 mL daily. Therefore, they exchange approximately 40% of their volume daily. As a result of this increased exchange rate, the infant's fluid balance may be more critically affected when they are ill. Adults, when they do not eat for a day because of GI upset, and whose kidneys continue to excrete at the normal rate, will have 14% less fluid in the extracellular space by the end of the day. Infants who do not eat for a day (providing kidney function remains constant) will be 40% short of ECF by the end of the day. This is obviously a more critical loss of fluid than the same loss would be in an adult; thus, dehydration is always a more serious problem in infants than in older children and adults. Maintenance requirements of fluid for infants and children are shown in Table 45-1.

Fluid Imbalances

Under most circumstances, water and salt are lost in proportion to each other (*isotonic dehydration*). Occasionally, water is lost out of proportion to salt (i.e., water depletion or *hypertonic dehydration*). Occasionally, electrolytes are lost out of proportion to water (*hypotonic dehydration*). Each of these abnormal states produces specific symptoms.

Isotonic Dehydration

When the body loses more water than it absorbs (such as with diarrhea) or absorbs less fluid than it excretes (such as with nausea and vomiting), the first result will be a decrease in the volume of blood plasma. The body compensates for this fairly rapidly by shifting interstitial fluid into the blood vessels. The composition of fluid in these two spaces is similar, so the replacement by this fluid does not change plasma composition. However, this replacement phenomenon will only proceed until the interstitial fluid reserve is depleted—a danger point for the child because it is difficult for the body to replace interstitial fluid from the

TABLE 45.1 Maintenance Requirements of Fluid Based on Caloric Expenditure

BODY WEIGHT (KG)	CALORIC EXPENDITURE	DAILY FLUID REQUIREMENT
3–10	100 cal/kg/d	100 mL/kg
10–20	1000 cal + 50 cal/kg for each kg of body wt more than 10 kg	1000 mL + 50 mL/kg for each kg of body wt more than 10 kg
More than 20	1500 cal + 20 cal/kg for each kg of body wt more than 20 kg	1500 mL + 20 mL/kg for each kg of body wt more than 20 kg

intracellular fluid (the fluids in these two compartments have different electrolyte contents). If an infant continues to lose fluid after this point, the volume of the plasma will continue to fall rapidly, resulting in cardiovascular collapse. Typical signs and symptoms of isotonic dehydration are summarized in Table 45-2.

Hypertonic Dehydration

Water is apt to be lost in a greater proportion than electrolytes when fluid intake decreases in conjunction with a fluid loss increase, such as might occur in a child with nausea (preventing fluid intake) and fever (increased fluid loss through perspiration); profuse diarrhea, where there is a greater loss of fluid than salt; or renal disease associated with polyuria (i.e., diabetes insipidus or nephrosis with diuresis). Fluid loss is out of proportion to the loss of electrolytes, and, with such an increased loss of fluid, electrolytes concentrate in the blood. Fluid shifts from the interstitial and intracellular spaces to the bloodstream (from areas of less osmotic pressure to areas of greater pressure). Dehydration in the interstitial and intracellular compartments occurs. The red blood cell count and hematocrit will be elevated because the blood is more concentrated than normally. Electrolytes (i.e., sodium, chloride, and bicarbonate) will also likely be increased. Additional signs and symptoms of this are summarized in Table 45-2.

Hypotonic Dehydration

With hypotonic dehydration, there is a disproportionately high loss of electrolytes relative to fluid lost. The plasma concentration of sodium and chloride will be low. This could result from excessive GI loss by vomiting or from low intake of salt associated with extreme losses through therapeutic diuresis. It also occurs when there is extreme loss of electrolytes in diseases such as adrenocortical insufficiency or diabetic acidosis. When low levels of electrolytes occur, the osmotic pressure in extracellular spaces decreases. The kidneys begin to excrete more fluid to decrease ECF volume and bring the proportion of electrolytes and fluid back into line. This may lead to a secondary extracellular dehydration (see Table 45-2).

TABLE 45-2 Signs and Symptoms of Dehydration

	ISOTONIC	HYPOTONIC	HYPERTONIC
Thirst	Mild	Moderate	Extreme
Skin turgor	Poor	Very poor	Moderate
Skin consistency	Dry	Clammy	Moderate
Skin temperature	Cool	Cool	Warm
Urine output	Decreased	Decreased	Decreased
Activity	Irritable	Lethargic	Very lethargic
Serum sodium level	Normal	Reduced	Increased

Overhydration

Overhydration is as serious as dehydration. It generally occurs in children who are receiving IV fluid. The excess fluid in these instances is usually extracellular. The condition is serious because the ECF overload may result in cardiovascular overload and cardiac failure.

When large quantities of salt-poor fluid (hypotonic solutions) such as tap water are ingested or are given by enema, the body transfers water from the extracellular space into the intracellular space to restore the normal osmotic relationships. This transfer results in intracellular edema manifested by headache, nausea, vomiting, dimness and blurring of vision, cramps, muscle twitching, and seizures. A situation in which intracellular edema may occur is when tap water enemas are given in the presence of aganglionic disease of the intestine.

Acid–Base Imbalance

The GI system often is involved with two severe acid–base imbalances, metabolic acidosis and metabolic alkalosis. These may occur with severe vomiting or diarrhea.

When dealing with acid–base balance, a key component is pH. The abbreviation "pH" refers to two French words that mean the "power of hydrogen." pH denotes whether a solution is acid or alkaline, determined by the proportion of hydrogen (H^+) ions in relation to hydroxide (OH^-) ions—the two substances that disassociate when water is broken down into its basic components ($H_2O = H^+$ and OH^-). A solution is acid (pH below 7.0) if it contains proportionately more H^+ ions than OH^- ions. It is alkaline (pH above 7.0) if the proportion of OH^- ions exceeds that of H^+ ions.

Whether body serum is becoming acidotic is determined by analyzing a sample of arterial blood for blood gases. The pH of blood is normally slightly alkaline, ranging from 7.35 to 7.45. Pco_2 (the amount of dissolved carbon dioxide in arterial blood) is normally 35 to 45 mmHg. Bicarbonate (HCO_3) in arterial blood is normally 22 to 26 mEq/L (Ford, 2001).

Metabolic Acidosis

Metabolic acidosis may result from diarrhea. When diarrhea occurs, a great deal of sodium is lost with stool. This excessive loss of Na^+, in turn, causes the body to conserve H^+ ions in an attempt to keep the total number of positive and negative ions in serum balanced. As a result, a child becomes acidotic as the number of H^+ ions in the blood increases proportionately over the number of OH^- ions present. With metabolic acidosis, arterial blood gas analysis will reveal a decreased pH (under 7.35) and a low HCO_3 value (near or below 22 mEq/L). The lower the HCO_3 value is, presumably the larger the number of Na^+ ions that have been lost or the more extensive the diarrhea has been.

To correct this problem (a blood serum over 7.45 is incompatible with life), the body uses both its kidney and respiratory buffering systems. The respiratory buffering system attempts to correct the imbalance quickly. H^+ ions combine with HCO_3^- ion to form carbonic acid. This, in turn, is broken down into CO_2 and water, which is then eliminated by the lungs during expiration. This process works immediately, and, as it continues for a time, the bicarbonate level in the serum falls lower and lower as the body uses up its bicarbonate store.

In the kidneys, H^+ ions are excreted directly or combine with other substances, such as phosphate and ammonia to form a weak acid, which is excreted. Unfortunately, this process is slow, taking up to 24 h to complete.

The child breathes rapidly (hyperpnea) to "blow off" CO_2 to prevent it from combining with H_20 and reforming HCO_3. Urine becomes more acid as ammonia formation in the urine is increased.

Metabolic Alkalosis

With vomiting, a great deal of hydrochloric acid is lost. When Cl^- ions are lost this way, the body has to decrease the number of H^+ ions present so the number of positive and negative charges remains balanced. This causes the child to become alkalotic as the number of H^+ ions becomes proportionately lower than the number of OH^- ions present. To reduce the number of H^+ ions, the lungs conserve CO_2 and water by slowing respirations (hypopnea). The excessive CO_2 retained by this maneuver dissolves in the blood as carbonic acid and then is converted into excessive H^+ and HCO_3^-. With metabolic alkalosis, therefore, the serum HCO_3 invariably will be high. The higher the value is, presumably the larger the number of Cl^- ions that have been lost or the more extensive the vomiting has been.

The child will breathe slowly and shallowly; pH will be elevated (near or above 7.45), and HCO_3 level will be near or above 28 mEq/L.

When alkalosis occurs from vomiting, a secondary electrolyte problem often occurs. As the kidneys begin to help conserve H^+ ions, K^+ ions are exchanged for H^+ ions. That is, K^+ ions are excreted in order to retain H^+ ions. As a result of this loss of K^+ into the urine, low K^+ levels (hypokalemia) invariably accompany metabolic alkalosis.

✔ CHECKPOINT QUESTIONS

1. Which body fluid compartment accounts for a greater percentage of body weight in infants than in adults?
2. With isotonic dehydration, how does the body compensate initially?
3. What denotes whether a solution is acid or alkaline?
4. What secondary electrolyte problem often occurs when metabolic alkalosis results from vomiting?

COMMON GASTROINTESTINAL SYMPTOMS OF ILLNESS IN CHILDREN

Vomiting and diarrhea in children commonly occur as symptoms of disease of the GI tract as well as symptoms of disease in other body systems. Pneumonia or otitis media, for example, may present first with vomiting or diarrhea. The danger is that either can lead to a disturbance in hydration, electrolyte, or acid-base balance. In many infants, these secondary disturbances can be more threatening to the child than the primary disease (McCance & Huether, 2002).

Vomiting

Many children with vomiting are suffering from a mild gastroenteritis (infection) caused by a viral or bacterial organism. The adolescent who is pregnant may also experience vomiting. The condition is always potentially serious because a metabolic alkalosis may result.

Assessment

In describing symptoms of vomiting, be certain to differentiate between the various terms that are used (Table 45-3). It is important that vomiting be described correctly because different conditions are marked by different forms of vomiting, and a correct description of the child's actions can aid greatly in diagnosis (see Focus on Multidisciplinary Care).

Therapeutic Management

The treatment for vomiting is to withhold food from the stomach for a time. If there is nothing in the stomach, vomiting cannot occur. Most parents treat vomiting in the opposite way. Every time the child vomits, they attempt to feed the child again. The child vomits again and they feed again, and so on. This prolongs the vomiting and intensifies the potential for electrolyte imbalance.

NURSING DIAGNOSES AND RELATED INTERVENTIONS

Nursing Diagnosis: Risk for deficient fluid volume related to vomiting

Outcome Identification: Child will maintain an adequate fluid volume until vomiting ceases.

Outcome Evaluation: Skin returns quickly when turgor is assessed; specific gravity of urine is 1.003 to 1.030; urine output is more than 1 mL/kg/h; episodes of vomiting decrease in frequency and amount.

To decrease vomiting, withhold food and fluid for a time (nothing by mouth [NPO]), depending on the age of the child. On the average, 3 to 6 h are usually sufficient. In the older child, after this period of fasting, offer a few ice chips, then water in small amounts—approximately 1 tbsp every 15 min, four times; then 2 tbsp every ½ h, four times. Popsicles can be substituted for water. If this is retained, children can be given small sips of clear liquids, such as tea, ginger ale, or sports drinks, such as Gatorade. Children may become hungry and want whole glasses, but keeping the quantity to small sips prevents vomiting. If the child retains sips of clear liquids, he or she can be offered portions of broth, clear soup, and skim milk in addition to clear liquids. Dry crackers or toast will help hunger. By the second day, children can take a soft diet; by the third day, they should be back to their regular diet.

For the infant, introduce fluid after a fasting period of approximately 3 h in the same slow manner. 1 tbsp every 15 min for 2 h, then 1 oz every 2 h for the next

TABLE 45.3 Differentiation Between Regurgitation and Vomiting

CHARACTERISTIC	REGURGITATION	VOMITING
Timing	Occurs with feeding	Timing unrelated to feeding
Forcefulness	Runs out of mouth with *little force*	Forceful; often projected 1 ft away from the infant; *projectile vomiting*—projected as much as 4 ft (most often related to increased intracranial pressure in newborns; in infants age 4–6 wk, possibly due to pyloric stenosis)
Description	Smells barely sour; only slightly curdled	Extremely sour smelling, appearing curdled, yellow, green, clear or watery, or black; perhaps fresh blood or old blood staining from swallowed maternal blood (in newborns)
Distress	Nonpainful; child does not appear to be in distress and may even smile as if sensation is enjoyable	Possible crying just before vomiting as if abdominal pain is present, and after vomiting as if the force of action is frightening
Duration	Occurs once per feeding	Continuing until stomach is empty; followed by dry retching
Amount	1–2 tsp	Full stomach contents

12 to 18 h. Glucose water or a commercial electrolyte solution such as Pedialyte may be given as fluid during this time to help the infant maintain electrolyte balance. Infants progress, as do older children, gradually to clear liquids or breast milk, then a soft diet, then a regular diet. If vomiting is prolonged, infants need IV therapy to restore hydration (Sondheimer, 2001b).

Teach parents the importance of following these routines of gradually increasing fluid at intervals. Assure them that if children receive a small amount of fluid and do not vomit it they will ultimately receive more fluid than if they take a large amount but, because of a gastroenteritis, vomit that amount. Parents are capable of understanding that stomach secretions are lost along with vomitus each time, and the preservation of these stomach secretions is important to keep their child well. Antiemetics are rarely necessary for children. Always ask parents if they have used an herbal remedy to be certain that any medication prescribed will be safe (see Focus on Cultural Competence). Urge parents not to give these or over-the-counter preparations for vomiting to children, but to control vomiting by dietary management.

FOCUS ON MULTIDISCIPLINARY CARE

Children with gastrointestinal disorders often receive care from a number of different health care providers: nutritionist, gastroenterologist, primary care provider, and, to ensure that they are following their prescribed therapy at home, a community health nurse. In addition, unlicensed assistive personnel often contribute to care by feeding or assisting with preparing children's food in hospital settings. Be certain that all personnel involved with care understand how to differentiate between simple "spitting up," which is normal in infants, and vomiting so this important symptom is not overlooked. Additionally, if the personnel are involved in changing diapers, be certain they can distinguish between normally loose infant bowel movements and a diarrheal stool. Also, reinforce the need for personnel, when talking with parents, not to dismiss the importance of seeking help for either vomiting or diarrhea. Teach them as well as parents that there is no such thing as "simple" diarrhea in infants.

Diarrhea

Diarrhea caused by a virus is the major cause of infant gastroenteritis in developing countries (Sondheimer, 2001b). The most common viral pathogens that invade the GI tract include rotaviruses and adenoviruses. The most common

FOCUS ON CULTURAL COMPETENCE

Incidence of gastrointestinal illnesses is not the same in all communities. Vomiting and diarrhea, for example, tend to occur in communities where refrigeration is less than optimal because of food poisoning. Celiac disease occurs most frequently in children of Northern European ancestry. Because constipation, vomiting, and diarrhea are so common, every culture has home remedies for these: cascara for constipation; psyllium for diarrhea; ginger, peppermint, licorice, or chamomile tea for nausea or vomiting. To be certain that a child seen in a health care facility does not receive two forms of the same drug (one prescribed and one given in an herb form by a parent), always ask what home remedies have been given and document these on the child's plan of care.

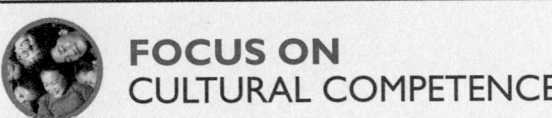

bacterial pathogens include *Campylobacter jejuni, Salmonella, Giardia lamblia,* and *Clostridium difficile.* Diarrhea in infants is always serious because infants have such a small extracellular fluid reserve that sudden losses of water exhaust the supply quickly. The loss of extracellular sodium leads to a decrease in plasma volume (additional water is excreted) and possible circulatory collapse. Renal failure results, with irreversible acidosis and death. Breastfeeding may actively prevent diarrhea by providing more antibodies and possibly an intestinal environment less friendly to invading organisms and so should be advocated. Diarrhea that is acute is usually associated with infection; that which is chronic is more likely related to a malabsorption or inflammatory cause.

✔ CHECKPOINT QUESTIONS

5. For approximately how long should a child be NPO if he is experiencing vomiting?
6. Does breastfeeding or formula feeding best prevent diarrhea?

Mild Diarrhea

Assessment. Normal and diarrheal stool characteristics are compared in Table 45-4. In mild diarrhea, fever of 101°F to 102°F (38.4°C to 39.0°C) may be present. Children usually are anorectic, irritable, and appear unwell. The episodes of diarrhea consist of 2 to 10 loose, watery bowel movements per day.

The mucous membrane of the infant's mouth with mild diarrhea will appear dry. Pulse will be rapid and out of proportion to the low-grade fever. Skin feels warm. Skin turgor is not yet decreased. Urine output is usually normal.

Therapeutic Management. At this stage, diarrhea is not yet serious, and children can be cared for at home. As with vomiting, treatment for diarrhea must involve resting the GI tract, but this is only necessary for a short time. At the end of approximately 1 h, parents can begin to offer an oral rehydration solution such as Pedialyte in small amounts on a regimen similar to that for vomiting. If infants are breastfed, breastfeeding should continue. Again, it may be difficult for parents to restrict fluid for a short time if they think they should overfeed children to make up for the fluid loss. Children also need measures to reduce the elevated temperature. Caution parents not to use over-the-counter drugs such as loperamide (Imodium) or kaolin and pectin (Kaopectate) to halt diarrhea. As a rule, these are too strong for young children (Armon et al., 2001). Also caution parents to wash their hands after changing diapers to prevent the spread of possible infection and to notify their health care provider if fever, pain, or diarrhea worsens.

Infants may develop a lactase deficiency after diarrhea. This leads to lactose intolerance. With lactose intolerance, the child is unable to take formula or breast milk or new diarrhea will begin. Such an infant will need to be introduced to a lactose-free formula initially before being returned to the usual formula or to breast milk.

TABLE 45.4 Differentiation Between Infant Normal Stool and Diarrheal Stool

CHARACTERISTIC	INFANT NORMAL STOOL	DIARRHEAL STOOL
Frequency	1–3 daily	Unlimited number
Color	Yellow	Green
Effort of expulsion	Some pushing effort	Effortless; may be explosive
pH	More than 7.0 (alkaline)	Less than 7.0 (acidic)
Odor	Odorless	Sweet or foul smelling
Occult blood	Negative	Positive; blood may be overt
Reducing substances	Negative	Positive

Severe Diarrhea

Assessment. Severe diarrhea may result from progressive mild diarrhea, or it may begin in a severe form. Infants with severe diarrhea are obviously ill. Rectal temperature is often as high as 103°F to 104°F (39.5°C to 40.0°C). Both pulse and respirations are weak and rapid. The skin is pale and cool. Infants may appear apprehensive, listless, and lethargic. They have obvious signs of dehydration such as a depressed fontanelle, sunken eyes, and poor skin turgor. The episodes of diarrhea usually consist of a bowel movement every few minutes. The stool is liquid green, perhaps mixed with mucus and blood, and it may be passed with explosive force. Urine output will be scanty and concentrated. Laboratory findings will show an elevated hematocrit, hemoglobin, and serum protein levels due to the dehydration. Electrolyte determinations will indicate a metabolic acidosis.

It is difficult to measure the amount of fluid the child has lost, but an estimate can be derived from the loss in body weight, if known. For example, if a child weighed 10.4 kg yesterday at a health maintenance visit and today weighs 8.9 kg, he or she has lost more than 10% of body weight. Mild dehydration occurs with a loss of 2.5% to 5% of body weight. In contrast, severe diarrhea quickly causes a 5% to 15% loss. Any infant who has lost 10% or more of body weight requires immediate treatment.

Therapeutic Management. Treatment focuses on regulating electrolyte and fluid balance by oral or IV rehydration therapy initiating rest for the GI tract, and discovering the organism responsible for the diarrhea.

All children with severe diarrhea should have a stool culture taken so definite antibiotic therapy can be prescribed. Stool cultures may be taken from the rectum or from stool in the diaper or a bedpan. Blood specimens need to be drawn for a hemoglobin level (an estimation of hydration as well as anemia); white blood cell and differential counts (to attempt to establish whether infection is present); and determinations of PCO_2, Cl^-, Na^+, K^+, and pH (to establish electrolyte needs). If the child cannot drink, an IV solution such as normal saline or 5% glucose in normal saline is started. The solution will provide replacement of fluid, sodium, and calories. Although infants usually have a potassium depletion, potassium cannot be given until it is established that they are not in renal failure. Giving potassium IV when the body has no outlet for excessive potassium can lead to excessively high potassium levels and heart block. *Before this initial fluid is changed to a potassium solution, therefore, be certain that the infant or child has voided—proof that the kidneys are functioning.*

Fluid must be given to replace the deficit that has occurred, for maintenance therapy, and to replace the continuing loss until the diarrhea improves. If infants have lost less than 5% of total body weight, their fluid deficit is approximately 50 mL/kg of body weight. If infants have lost 10% of body weight, they need approximately 100 mL/kg of body weight to replace their fluid deficit. If the weight loss suggests a 12% to 15% loss of body fluid, they require 125 mL/kg of body weight to replace the fluid lost. This fluid will be given rapidly in the first 3 to 6 h, then it will be slowed to a maintenance rate. Once infants void, a potassium additive may be ordered to restore serum potassium.

NURSING DIAGNOSES AND RELATED INTERVENTIONS

Nursing Diagnosis: Deficient fluid volume, related to loss of fluid through diarrhea

Outcome Identification: Child will maintain an adequate fluid balance until normal elimination pattern is restored.

Outcome Evaluation: Skin returns quickly when turgor is assessed; specific gravity of urine is 1.003 to 1.030; urine output is more than 1 mL/kg/h; bowel movements are formed and fewer than four per day. Stool tests negative for reducing substances and blood pH = more than 7.

Promote Hydration and Comfort. For a short time, infants are NPO to minimize the risk of vomiting, which, at this point, would compound the problem by adding to the dehydration. Wet infants' lips with a moisturizing jelly (Vaseline) if they appear to be dry. Give them a pacifier to suck if this seems to comfort them. (They want to suck because they are very thirsty, and, if they have intestinal cramping with the diarrhea, they interpret this as hunger.)

After a short time, infants may be allowed small sips of clear fluid, an oral rehydration solution, or breast milk. Gradually, the infant's oral intake is increased, changing to a soft then regular diet. Some children become lactose-intolerant after diarrhea and will need a lactose-free formula for rehydration (Semeao & Mulberg, 2000). If the child with severe diarrhea also has a fever, measures to reduce the fever will be necessary (see Chapter 36). Do not obtain rectal temperatures to assess fever, because stimulating the anal sphincter could initiate more diarrhea. Assess perianal skin for irritation from liquid stools and keep the skin clean and dry.

WHAT IF? What if a parent tells you that her doctor told her to "force fluids" for her child with diarrhea? She asks how much she should force the child to drink. How would you answer her?

Record Fluid Intake and Output. Much of the nursing care of children with diarrhea focuses on careful recording of fluid intake and output. Because children have dehydration when first seen, their IV therapy serves as their lifeline. Be sure to maintain proper functioning of the infusion and site. An arm board may be necessary to prevent catheter dislodgment or interference with the infusion. Instruct the child and parents about the need to refrain from touching or playing with any part of the IV setup. If the child is too young to understand, soft restraints applied to the affected and unaffected extremities may be necessary to prevent pulling, playing with, or poking at the tubing or site. If soft restraints are used, be sure to release them every hour and passively exercise the child's extremities. Give parents an explanation of why the IV infusion is important so they will understand the necessity of the soft restraints.

In children who are not toilet trained, apply a disposable urine collection bag to help separate urine from feces. This makes it obvious that the child is voiding, confirming adequate kidney function. Confirmation of adequate kidney function is necessary for IV K^+ replacement therapy, if ordered.

Separating urine from stools also helps to judge the appearance of stools or their water content better. For each stool passed, record its color, consistency, odor, size, and the presence of any blood or mucus. Weigh soiled diapers to reveal the number of grams of stool in the diaper (1 g = 1 mL fluid). Testing the stool for acidity and for reducing substances (sugars) indicates how quickly the stool is passing through the irritated tract. A stool positive for sugar indicates that little absorption has occurred because sugar is absorbed rapidly from ingested food. Acid stool (pH less than 7.0) shows the presence of unabsorbed sugar also (a process occurs similar to the process that causes acid to invade tooth enamel in the presence of glucose on teeth). Diarrheal stools are green from lack of time for bile to be modified in the intestine. As diarrhea improves and stool remains in the intestine for a longer period, the stool deepens in color, and the acid and sugar content fade. Testing stools for occult blood shows the extent of bowel irritation that is occurring from the acid stool. As the diarrhea improves and the irritation to the bowel lessens, occult blood disappears.

Nursing Diagnosis: Risk for impaired skin integrity related to presence of diarrheal stool on skin

Outcome Identification: Child's skin will remain intact during period of diarrhea.

Outcome Evaluation: Skin in diaper area is not erythematous or with ulcerations.

Because diarrheal stool is extremely irritating to the skin, change diapers immediately after infants pass any stool. Wash the skin of the diaper area well after each stool, and cover it with an ointment such as Vaseline or A and D to protect it from further irritation. If the child is older, caution him or her to wipe away stool thoroughly.

If infants already have skin excoriation from the number of stools they have had at home, an ointment such as Desitin may be helpful in soothing the irritated skin. Exposing infants' buttocks to air is generally helpful in healing irritation. Assure older children that loss of stool by diarrhea is not "shameful" or "babyish" but to be expected because he or she is ill.

Nursing Diagnosis: Anxiety related to traumatic experience

Outcome Identification: Child will not suffer long-term effects of experience.

Outcome Evaluation: Child interacts with parents in age-appropriate way; is able to be comforted after painful procedures.

All children with diarrhea are assumed to have an infectious form of gastroenteritis and, therefore, need contact precautions and standard precautions. Children usually are uncomfortable from the diarrhea, exhausted, and confused with these new body sensations. They need the security of someone to stay with them. When a child with severe diarrhea is admitted to the hospital, many emergency procedures must be performed, such as establishing the IV route, collecting specimens, and reducing temperature. During all of these procedures, try to remember how all of this must seem to the child in the bed. Be sure to take time during initial procedures to touch and soothe children and talk to them; once the initial admission procedures are done, sit by the bed and hold the child or gently stroke the child's head. Teach parents how to adhere to standard precautions and follow contact precautions if necessary. Encourage them to give any care possible. Children need this support to counteract the strange world into which they have suddenly been plunged.

Bacterial Infectious Diseases That Cause Diarrhea and Vomiting

Salmonella

- Causative agent: One of the *Salmonella* bacteria
- Incubation period: 6 to 72 h for intraluminal type; 7 to 14 days for extraluminal type
- Period of communicability: As long as organisms are being excreted (may be as long as 3 months)
- Mode of transmission: Ingestion of contaminated food

Salmonella is the most common type of food poisoning in the United States and a major cause of diarrhea in children. The diagnosis of the infection can be made from stool culture. Children develop diarrhea, abdominal pain, vomiting, high temperature, and headache. They are listless and drowsy. The diarrhea is severe and may contain blood and mucus. *Salmonella* infection may remain in the bowel as an intraluminal disease. When it does, it is treated, like severe diarrhea, with fluid and electrolyte replacement. It also may become systemic (extraluminal disease), and, in that instance, it is treated with the addition of an antibiotic such as ampicillin or a third-generation cephalosporin (Osterhoudt, 2000).

Complications such as meningitis, bronchitis, and osteomyelitis may occur. Although the source of *Salmonella* generally is infected food (contaminated chicken and eggs are common sources), it may be transmitted to children by infected turtles (Olsen et al., 2001; see Focus on Family Empowerment).

Shigellosis (Dysentery)

- Causative agent: Organisms of the genus *Shigella*
- Incubation period: 1 to 7 days
- Period of communicability: Approximately 1 to 4 weeks
- Mode of transmission: Contaminated food, water, or milk products

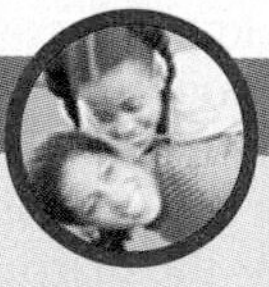

FOCUS ON FAMILY EMPOWERMENT

Preventing *Salmonella*-Caused Gastroenteritis

Q. Our daughter had severe diarrhea from food poisoning. The doctor said it was *Salmonella.* How can we make sure she doesn't get this again?

A. Anyone can get *Salmonella* food poisoning. However, it can be prevented by using the following measures:

- Wash your hands well before preparing any foods, but especially chicken and eggs.
- Remember that chicken may become contaminated with *Salmonella* at the factory where it was prepared. Wash your hands well after handling raw chicken to prevent the spread of infection to other foods being prepared.
- Clean cutting boards or food preparation surfaces with hot, soapy water and dry thoroughly after use to prevent them from becoming reservoirs of infection.
- Make a habit of preparing chicken last, after other foods are prepared.
- Cook eggs well (do not use raw eggs in milkshakes; cook soft-boiled or poached eggs at least 3 min).
- Refrigerate chicken and eggs after preparation.
- Wash hands well after playing with or feeding a pet turtle or changing the turtle's water.

Shigella organisms, like the *Salmonella* group, cause extremely severe diarrhea that contains blood and mucus. As the organism becomes more resistant, ampicillin or trimethoprim-sulfamethoxazole, typical drugs for therapy in the past, are being replaced by cephalosporins. The child needs intense fluid and electrolyte replacement. *Shigella* infection can be prevented by safe food handling and cautioning families to drink only from safe water sources.

Staphylococcal Food Poisoning

- Causative agent: Staphylococcal enterotoxin produced by some strains of *Staphylococcus aureus*
- Incubation period: 1 to 7 h
- Period of communicability: Carriers may contaminate food as long as they harbor the organism
- Mode of transmission: Ingestion of contaminated food

With staphylococcal food poisoning, the child has severe vomiting and diarrhea, abdominal cramping, excessive salivation, and nausea. Organisms are most often spread through creamed foods. It is often difficult to culture the causative organism from the contaminated food because, although the staphylococci may have been destroyed by inadequate cooking, the enterotoxin that actually causes the disorder will not have been destroyed. The child needs intensive supportive therapy with fluid and electrolyte replacement and administration of a drug effective against *Staphylococcus,* such as cefotaxime. Food poisoning from this source is prevented by proper food refrigeration.

✔ CHECKPOINT QUESTIONS

7. What acid-base imbalance is typical with severe diarrhea?
8. What causative organism would you suspect if a child develops diarrhea from eating raw eggs?

DISORDERS OF THE STOMACH AND DUODENUM

Gastroesophageal Reflux (Achalasia)

Gastroesophageal reflux (commonly called achalasia in infants) is a neuromuscular disturbance in which the gastroesophageal (cardiac) sphincter and the lower portion of the esophagus are lax and, therefore, allow easy regurgitation of gastric contents into the esophagus. It usually starts within 1 week after birth and may be associated with a hiatal hernia. Children with cerebral palsy or other neurologic involvement are at particular risk. The regurgitation occurs almost immediately after feeding or when the infant is laid down after a feeding. If the reflux is large, the infant does not retain sufficient calories and will fail to thrive. In addition, aspiration pneumonia or esophageal stricture from the constant reflux of hydrochloric acid into the esophagus may occur (Thilot & Rosenberg, 2001).

Assessment

The diagnosis is suggested by the history. Vomiting appears effortless and is nonprojectile, beginning much earlier in life than vomiting associated with pyloric stenosis. The child may be irritable and may experience periods of apnea. Inserting a probe or catheter through the nose into the distal esophagus, and determining the pH from secretions can show whether gastric secretions are entering the esophagus (if pH is less than 7.0, then acid is present). Fiberoptic endoscopy or esophagography (barium swallow) will show the lax sphincter and the reflux of stomach contents into the esophagus, especially if the infant's head is tilted down.

Therapeutic Management

The traditional treatment of GI reflux is to feed infants a formula thickened with rice cereal (1 tbsp of cereal per 1 oz of formula) while holding them in an upright position and then keeping them upright in an infant chair for 1 h after feeding so gravity can help prevent reflux. An H_2 receptor antagonist such as ranitidine (Zantac) or a proton pump inhibitor such as omeprazole (Prilosec) may be prescribed daily to reduce the possibility of the stomach acid contents irritating the esophagus.

Gastroesophageal reflux is usually a self-limiting condition. As the esophageal sphincter matures and the child begins to eat solid food and is maintained in a more upright position, the problem disappears. However, it is a problem that needs treatment. Otherwise, serious consequences can result from dehydration, alkalosis, or damage to the esophagus. If medical therapy is ineffective, laparoscopic or surgical procedure (tightening or suturing of the esophageal sphincter) may be performed (Patti et al., 2001). After this, the child returns with a nasogastric tube inserted and attached to intermittent low suction. It is usually irrigated with normal saline every 2 h to ensure its patency. Assess nasogastric tube drainage and any vomitus for coffee-colored drainage (although this is normal for the first 24 h) that would indicate bleeding from the surgical site. When infants are first fed after surgery, they may display symptoms of abdominal discomfort and distention because food can no longer reflux into the esophagus as readily as it could before surgery. As their stomach adjusts to this, symptoms fade. Before this happens, however, the distention may be so extreme that it leads to bradycardia and dyspnea. Be alert for the development of these important signs and symptoms.

NURSING DIAGNOSES AND RELATED INTERVENTIONS

Nursing Diagnosis: Risk for imbalanced nutrition, less than body requirements related to regurgitation of food with esophageal reflux

Outcome Identification: Infant will receive adequate nutrition during course of therapy.

Outcome Evaluation: Skin returns quickly when turgor is assessed; specific gravity of urine is 1.003 to 1.030; intake is 50 cal/lb/24 h.

Teach parents the importance of monitoring intake, output (urination), and weight. Also reinforce the need to keep the infant upright, such as in an infant car seat, after a feeding. Be certain parents understand how much cereal to mix with formula. Mothers who are breastfeeding may manually express breast milk and mix it with rice cereal for feedings. Encourage parents to feed the infant during the short time that the infant remains in the hospital after surgery to regain confidence as parents.

Pyloric Stenosis

The pyloric sphincter is the opening between the lower portion of the stomach and the beginning portion of the intestine, the duodenum. If hypertrophy or hyperplasia of the muscle surrounding the sphincter occurs, it is difficult for the stomach to empty, a condition called **pyloric stenosis** (Fig. 45-3). With this condition, at 4 to 6 weeks of age, children begin to vomit almost immediately after each feeding. The vomiting grows increasingly forceful until it is projectile, possibly projecting as much as 3 to 4 feet. Pyloric stenosis tends to occur most frequently in first-born white male infants. The incidence is high, approximately 1:150 in males and 1:750 in females. The exact cause is unknown, but multifactorial inheritance is the likely cause. It occurs less frequently in breastfed infants than in formula-fed infants. Infants fed on formula who will develop the condition typically begin having symptoms at approximately 4 weeks of age. Breastfed infants begin developing symptoms at approximately 6 weeks because the curd of breast milk is smaller than that of cow's milk, and it passes through a hypertrophied muscle more easily. An increased incidence is seen in infants who received a macrolide antibiotic such as erythromycin (Mahon et al., 2001).

Vomitus usually smells sour because it has reached the stomach and has been in contact with stomach enzymes. There is never bile in the vomiting of pyloric stenosis because the feeding does not reach the duodenum to become mixed with bile. The infant is usually hungry immediately after vomiting because he or she is not nauseated. Although it is difficult to assess whether nausea is present in infants, symptoms such as a disinterest in eating, excessive drooling, or chewing on the tongue may suggest this.

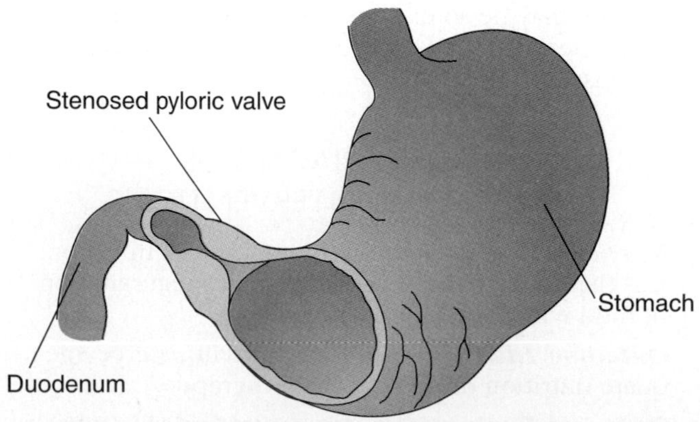

FIGURE 45.3 Pyloric stenosis. Fluid is unable to pass easily through the stenosed and hypertrophied pyloric valve.

Assessment

The diagnosis of pyloric stenosis is made primarily from the history. Whenever parents say that their baby is vomiting or spitting up, be certain to get a full description.

- What is the duration?
- What is the intensity?
- What is the frequency?
- What is the description of the vomitus?
- Is the infant ill in any other way?

Many infants have signs of dehydration from the vomiting at the time they are first seen. Lack of tears (many infants younger than age 6 weeks do not tear), dry mucous membrane of the mouth, sunken fontanelles, fever, decreased urine output, poor skin turgor, and loss of weight are common signs of dehydration. Alkalosis also may be present because of the excessive loss of Cl^- ions from stomach fluid, along with accompanying hypochloremia, hypokalemia, and starvation. Hypopnea (slowed respirations) occurs as the body attempts to compensate for the alkalosis. This will cause the HCO_3 content of plasma generally to be above 30 mEq/L (normal is 22 mEq/L to 28 mEq/L). Tetany may occur with alkalosis because the increased HCO_3^- ions may combine with Ca^{++} ions, trying to effect homeostasis and thereby lowering the level of ionized calcium. Low serum calcium leads to tetany.

A definitive diagnosis is made by watching the infant drink. Before the child drinks, attempt to palpate the right upper quadrant of the abdomen for a possible pyloric mass. If one is present, it feels round and firm, approximately the size of an olive. As the infant drinks, observe for gastric peristaltic waves passing from left to right across the abdomen. The olive-size lump becomes more prominent. The infant vomits with projectile emesis. If the diagnosis is still in doubt, the child may have an ultrasound, which will show the hypertrophied sphincter (Sondheimer, 2001b). Endoscopy also may be used for diagnosis by directly visualizing the hypertrophied sphincter.

Therapeutic Management

Treatment is surgical or laparoscopic correction (a pyloromyotomy) before electrolyte imbalance from the vomiting or hypoglycemia from the lack of food intake occurs. Before surgery, the electrolyte imbalance, dehydration, and starvation must be corrected by administration of IV fluid, usually isotonic saline or 5% glucose in saline because this contains an excess of Cl^- ions. Oral feedings are withheld to prevent further electrolyte depletion. An infant who is receiving only IV fluid generally needs a pacifier to meet nonnutritive sucking needs and be comfortable. If tetany is present, IV calcium also must be administered. The infant usually needs additional potassium, but, as a rule, this must not be administered until it is ascertained that the child's kidneys are functioning (i.e., the child is voiding). Otherwise, the potassium buildup could cause cardiac arrhythmias.

For surgical correction, the muscle of the pylorus is split down to the mucosa, allowing for a larger lumen. Although the procedure sounds simple, it is technically difficult to perform, and there is high risk for infection afterward because the abdominal incision is near the diaper area.

The prognosis for infants with pyloric stenosis is excellent if the condition is discovered before the electrolyte imbalance occurs.

NURSING DIAGNOSES AND RELATED INTERVENTIONS

Nursing Diagnosis: Risk for deficient fluid volume related to inability to retain food

Outcome Identification: Infant will remain well hydrated until condition is corrected.

Outcome Evaluation: Skin returns quickly when turgor is assessed; specific gravity of urine is 1.003 to 1.030; vomiting episodes have ceased; weight within acceptable age-appropriate parameters.

Preoperative Care. Preoperative management consists of fluid and electrolyte replacement based on laboratory determinations. A baseline weight is essential for establishing the extent of dehydration. Note carefully the frequency of urination, the specific gravity of the urine, and the number of stools passed to help assess dehydration and starvation. Parents may be impatient with preoperative management because it may take 24 h or more to restore a severe fluid imbalance. They need an explanation that infants cannot go to surgery with an electrolyte imbalance; these hours before surgery are as important to the welfare of their child as the operation itself.

Postoperative Care. Infants may return from surgery or laparoscopy with an IV line in place. The postoperative feeding regimen differs from one surgeon to another but usually is based on a regimen requiring frequent feedings of small amounts of fluid. Approximately 4 to 6 h after surgery, children are started on a small amount of an oral rehydrating solution by bottle. If no vomiting occurs, the amount is increased or half-strength formula or breastfeeding is begun. Finally, by 24 to 48 h, infants are taking their full formula diet or being fully breastfed. They are usually discharged from the hospital at the end of 48 h.

Postoperatively, it is important that infants be given no more than the amount of fluid ordered at a time so the surgical repair site is not overwhelmed. Infants need to ingest these small amounts because a small quantity of fluid passing through the sphincter in the immediate postoperative days helps to keep adhesions of the sphincter from forming. As the amount taken orally increases, the IV fluid will be decreased and then discontinued. Infants should be bubbled well after a feeding so there is no pressure from air in the stomach. Lay them on their side after feeding so if vomiting does occur, there is little chance of aspiration. Laying them on their right side possibly aids the flow of fluid through the pyloric valve by gravity. Continue to monitor daily weights to confirm that children are receiving adequate intake. Usually no vomiting occurs postoperatively. However, if it does occur, report it immediately. The feeding regimen may need to be adjusted accordingly, and the infant may require a longer hospital stay. Some infants have a short-term diarrhea (dumping syndrome) after surgery because of rapid functioning of the pyloric sphincter. However, this tends to resolve without additional therapy.

Nursing Diagnosis: Risk for infection at site of surgical incision related to danger of contamination from feces due to proximity of incision to diaper area

Outcome Identification: Infant's surgical incision will exhibit signs and symptoms of healing without infection.

Outcome Evaluation: Infant's temperature is below 98.6°F (37.0°C) axillary; incision is clean, dry, and intact without erythema or drainage.

The surgical incision for pyloric stenosis may be covered with collodion, a solution similar to clear nail polish, to help keep urine and feces from touching it. Keep diapers folded low to prevent the incision from being contaminated, and change diapers frequently. If the incision should be exposed to feces, wash the collodion well with soap and water.

Nursing Diagnosis: Risk for impaired parenting related to infant's feeding difficulty and illness

Outcome Identification: Parents will demonstrate positive bonding behaviors with the infant both preoperatively and postoperatively.

Outcome Evaluation: Parents hold and feed infant; express positive characteristics about infant.

Encourage the parents of a baby this young who may remain overnight in the hospital to room in so they can grow comfortable and confident in caring for their child again. When the child first began vomiting so forcefully, parents may have felt they were doing something wrong, possibly losing confidence in themselves as parents. Explain to them that the vomiting was caused by a physical problem and not by anything they did.

Hospitalization often occurs near the infant's second month, when the child would normally receive diphtheria-tetanus-pertussis, oral poliomyelitis, and *Haemophilus influenzae* immunization. Ask if this could be administered before discharge so the child's immunization status remains current. This also might serve to remind parents that getting back to normal means regular health care visits for vaccines and checkups.

✔ CHECKPOINT QUESTIONS

9. What is the best position for a child with GI reflux after being fed?
10. What type of vomiting is associated with pyloric stenosis?

Hiatal Hernia

Hiatal hernia is the intermittent protrusion of the stomach up through the esophageal opening in the diaphragm. When this occurs, the volume of the stomach is suddenly restricted, leading to periodic vomiting similar to that of gastroesophageal reflux. With a hiatal hernia, however, pain usually accompanies the vomiting. Shortness of breath may occur from compression of the lung space by the stomach (Sondheimer, 2001a).

Hiatal hernia is diagnosed by history and a sonogram or barium swallow. A baby can be kept in an upright position to help prevent the condition from recurring. Medication to reduce acid secretions may be helpful. If the condition has not corrected itself by the time the infant is 6 months old even with maintaining an upright position most of the day, laparoscopic surgery may be performed to reduce the ability of the stomach to protrude through the diaphragm.

Peptic Ulcer Disease

A **peptic ulcer** is a shallow excavation formed in the mucosal wall of the stomach, the pylorus, or the duodenum. In infants, ulcers tend to be gastric; in adolescents, usually duodenal. Such ulcers occur in a primary form caused by infection of *H. pylori* bacteria and a secondary form that follows severe stress such as burns or chronic ingestion of medications such as acetosalicylic acid or prednisone. A small ulceration of the gastric or duodenal lining will lead to symptoms of pain, blood in the stools, and vomiting (with blood). If left uncorrected, peptic ulcer disease can lead to bowel or stomach perforation with acute hemorrhage or pyloric obstruction. A chronic ulcer condition may lead to anemia from the constant, gradual blood loss.

Peptic ulcer disease occurs in only 1% to 2% of children. It occurs more frequently in males than in females. In addition to infection from *H. pylori,* associated factors in adolescents may include genetic tendency and use of alcohol, caffeine, and cigarettes (Sondheimer, 2001a).

Assessment

An ulcer occurring in a neonate usually presents with hematemesis (blood in vomitus) or melena (blood in the stool). Such ulcers are usually superficial and heal rapidly, although they can lead to rupture, with symptoms of respiratory distress, abdominal distention, vomiting, and, if extensive, cardiovascular collapse. If the ulcer occurs in the toddler, the first symptoms are usually anorexia or vomiting. Bleeding follows in several weeks. If the ulcer begins when children are of preschool or early school age, pain may be the presenting symptom. They may report pain as mild, severe, colicky, or continuous. It is often poorly localized, although it may be in the epigastric area as in adult clients. It may occur in the right lower quadrant and be confused with appendicitis.

In older, school-age children and adolescents, the symptoms are generally those of the adult: a gnawing or aching pain in the epigastric area before meals that is relieved by eating. Vomiting (due to spasm and edema of the pylorus) also may occur in a small number of children. On abdominal palpation, epigastric tenderness is noted.

Fiber-optic endoscopy, the most reliable diagnostic test to confirm the diagnosis of peptic ulcer disease, allows for visual inspection and cultures for *H. pylori* (Hassall, 2001). Because childhood ulcers are shallow, they may not show well on radiographs. In many children, little increase in gastric activity is demonstrable by gastric analysis. Children with this condition must have blood tests done periodically to be monitored for hypochromic, microcytic anemia (blood loss anemia).

Therapeutic Management

Children with peptic ulcer disease are treated with a combination of medications to reduce bacterium count and suppress gastric acidity. Adolescents are prescribed an antibiotic such as amoxicillin or clarithromycin (Biaxin) and a proton pump inhibitor such as omeprazole (Prilosec). Bismuth subsalicylate (Pepto-Bismol) is soothing and mildly antibiotic and so may be prescribed concurrently. Younger children are prescribed cimetidine (Tagamet) because safe levels of omeprazole have yet to be established. With current therapy, only a few children experience the potential complications of perforation, blood loss anemia, and intestinal obstruction, although a number of school-age children and adolescents will have recurring symptoms as they grow older.

NURSING DIAGNOSES AND RELATED INTERVENTIONS

Having peptic ulcer disease can be difficult for children because it is painful, and remembering to take medicine daily may be problematic for children.

Be certain that outcomes planned are realistic. It may not be possible to relieve symptoms of peptic ulcer immediately. Children can be helped immediately to understand why the pain occurs, however, and what they can do to help relieve it.

Nursing Diagnosis: Pain related to ulceration in intestinal tract

Outcome Identification: Child will report pain is at an acceptable level during course of illness.

Outcome Evaluation: Child exhibits verbal and nonverbal signs of decreased pain; the infant appears comfortable without excessive crying.

Encourage children to adhere to their prescribed medication therapy. Children with peptic ulcer disease should be able to eat a normal diet, avoiding heavily spiced food such as pizza or sausage if such food causes discomfort. Work with them to devise a schedule they can remember for taking their prescribed medications.

✔ CHECKPOINT QUESTIONS

11. What diagnostic test is the most reliable for diagnosing peptic ulcer disease?
12. For what three complications is the child with peptic ulcer disease at risk?

HEPATIC DISORDERS

Hepatic disorders include both acquired disorders, such as hepatitis or cirrhosis, and congenital disorders, such as obstruction or atresia of the biliary duct.

Liver Function

The liver lies immediately under the diaphragm on the right side. (In infants, 1 or 2 cm of liver is readily and normally palpable.) The organ is essential for the normal metabolism of carbohydrates, proteins, and fats. It plays a role in the maintenance of normal blood sugar level by changing glucose to glycogen and storing it until needed by body cells. It then reverses the process and changes glycogen back to glucose and releases it into the blood when cells need it.

The liver assists in the catabolism of fatty acids and protein and serves as a temporary storage space for both fat and protein. The liver, by the means of the enzyme glucuronosyltransferase, converts indirect (or unconjugated) bilirubin into direct (or conjugated) bilirubin so it can be excreted in bile and eliminated from the body. This is an important function in the newborn, and jaundice can result if the enzyme glucuronosyltransferase is low because of immaturity.

The liver manufactures bile, a secretion necessary for the digestion of fat; fibrinogen and prothrombin, substances essential for blood clotting; heparin, a substance necessary to keep blood from clotting in intact vessels; and blood proteins. It produces large amounts of body heat. It destroys red blood cells and detoxifies many harmful absorbed substances, such as drugs. Because the liver, a life-sustaining organ, performs all of these functions, any disorder involving the liver is always serious. A number of common liver function tests are used to diagnose the nature of liver pathology. These are summarized in Table 45-5.

Hepatitis

Hepatitis (inflammation and infection of the liver) is caused by the invasion of hepatitis A, B, C, D, and E viruses.

Hepatitis A

- Causative agent: A picornavirus; hepatitis A virus (HAV)
- Incubation period: 25 days on average
- Period of communicability: Highest during 2 weeks preceding onset of symptoms
- Mode of transmission: In children, ingestion of fecally contaminated water or shellfish; day care center spread from contaminated changing tables
- Immunity: Natural; one episode induces immunity for the specific type of virus
- Active artificial immunity: HAV vaccine (recommended for workers in day care centers)
- Passive artificial immunity: Immune globulin

Hepatitis B

- Causative agent: A hepadnavirus; hepatitis B virus (HBV)
- Incubation period: 120 days on average
- Period of communicability: Later part of incubation period and during the acute stage
- Mode of transmission: Transfusion of contaminated blood and plasma or semen; inoculation by a contaminated syringe or needle through IV drug use; may be spread to fetus if mother has infection in third trimester of pregnancy
- Immunity: Natural; one episode induces immunity for the specific type of virus

TABLE 45.5 Liver Function Tests

TEST	DESCRIPTION
Serum bilirubin	Indirect bilirubin found in large quantities in bloodstream indicates that the child is not converting it to direct bilirubin; hence, liver cell function may be impaired; the normal value of total bilirubin in serum is 1.5 mg per 100 mL; if large amounts of direct bilirubin are found in serum, it implies obstruction of the bile duct, preventing the excretion of the converted substance.
Stool and urine bilirubin	If bile pigments can be obtained from stool (excreted as urobilinogen in stool and urine), it is evidence that bile is being manufactured and excreted from the liver; without the presence of bile pigment, stool appears light in color (clay colored). Even trace amounts of bilirubin in urine are abnormal, possibly indicating liver dysfunction.
Alkaline phosphatase	Alkaline phosphatase is an enzyme produced by the liver and bone and excreted in the bile; with bile duct obstruction, increased levels of alkaline phosphatase will be in the blood.
Prothrombin time	This test is associated with blood coagulation. In chronic liver disease, the level of prothrombin produced by the liver may fall so severely that the prothrombin time is increased; there is little change in prothrombin time in mild or short-term liver disease.
Aspartate transaminase (AST; serum glutamic-oxaloacetic transaminase [SGOT])	AST (SGOT) is an enzyme found in the heart and liver; when there is acute cellular destruction in either organ, the enzyme is released into the bloodstream from the damaged cells; the blood levels are increased by 8 h after injury; the level reaches a peak in 24 or 36 h and then falls to normal in 4 to 6 days.
Alanine transaminase (ALT; serum glutamate pyruvate transaminase [SGPT])	ALT (SGPT) is an enzyme found mostly in the liver; it rises for the same reasons as AST (SGOT) but is not as sensitive an indicator of liver damage.
Lactic dehydrogenase (LDH)	LDH is another enzyme found in the heart and liver; it is a relatively insensitive indicator of liver destruction, however; infectious mononucleosis is the one disease in which increased levels of LDH seem to be seen frequently.
Serum albumin	Albumin, a serum protein, is chiefly synthesized in the liver; most acute or chronic liver disease will show decreased serum albumin.

- Active artificial immunity: Vaccine for the HBV virus (recommended for routine immunization series and health care providers)
- Passive artificial immunity: Specific hepatitis B immune serum globulin

Hepatitis C, D, and E

Although hepatitis A and B are the most frequent viruses to cause hepatitis, hepatitis C, D, and E viruses may also be involved. Hepatitis C (HCV) is a single-strand RNA virus. Transmission, as with HBV, is primarily by blood or blood products, IV drug use, or sexual contact. The virus produces mild symptoms of disease. There is, however, a high incidence of chronic infection with the virus (Sokol & Narkewicz, 2001).

Hepatitis D (HDV) or the delta form is similar to HBV in transmission, although it requires a coexisting HBV infection to be activated. Disease symptoms are mild, but there is a high incidence of fulminant hepatitis after the initial infection. The E form of hepatitis is enterically transmitted similarly to hepatitis A (fecally contaminated water). Disease symptoms from the E virus are usually mild, except in pregnant women, in whom they tend to be severe (Tung, 2000).

Chronic Hepatitis

Hepatitis becomes chronic when it persists for longer than 6 months (Tung, 2000). This is most often the result of hepatitis B, D, or C infection. Abnormal liver enzyme levels and a liver biopsy establish the diagnosis and can also predict the severity. With chronic hepatitis, fatty infiltration and bile duct damage are present. The disease may progress to cirrhosis and eventually liver failure. Therapy is supportive to compensate for decreased liver function.

Fulminant Hepatic Failure

Fulminant hepatic failure is present when acute, massive necrosis or sudden, severe impairment of liver function occurs leading to hepatic encephalopathy. Hepatic encephalopathy is the result of ammonia intoxication caused by the inability of the liver to detoxify the ammonia being constantly produced by the intestine in the process of digestion. Children show signs of mental aberrations such as confusion, drowsiness, or disorientation. Treatment is to reduce protein intake and administer lactulose to prevent absorption of ammonia in the colon or to administer nonabsorbable antibiotics such as neomycin to decrease the production of ammonia by the intestinal bacteria. Liver transplantation may be necessary. Unfortunately, many children may not be able to survive the long wait for a donor organ.

Assessment

Hepatitis is a generalized body infection with specific intense liver effects. Type A occurs in children of all ages and accounts for approximately 30% of infections. Hepatitis B tends to occur in adolescents after intimate contact or the use of contaminated syringes for drug injection, accounting for approximately 40% of hepatitis infections (Tung, 2000).

Clinically, it is impossible to differentiate the type of hepatitis from the signs that are present. All hepatitis viruses cause liver cell destruction, leading to increased serum aspartate transaminase (AST; serum glutamic-oxaloacetic transaminase [SGOT]) and alkaline phosphatase levels. Albumin synthesis decreases, and bile formation and excretion are impaired. The type of virus causing the disease can be determined by the recognition of a specific antibody against the virus (anti-HAV IgM; anti-HBV IgM, and so forth).

Children notice headache, fever, and anorexia. Symptoms with hepatitis A are generally mild. Jaundice occurs as liver function slows. This lasts for approximately a week, then symptoms fade with full recovery. Symptoms of hepatitis B are more marked. Children report generalized aching, right upper quadrant pain, and headache. They may have a low-grade fever. They feel ill; they are irritable and fretful from pruritus. After 3 to 7 days of such symptoms, the color of the urine becomes darker (brown) because of the excretion of bilirubin. In another 2 days, scleras become jaundiced; soon they have generalized jaundice. With the generalized jaundice, there is little excretion of bilirubin into the stool, so the stool color becomes white or gray. This icteric (jaundiced) phase lasts for a few days to 2 weeks. Some children have an anicteric form of infection, in which they develop the beginning symptoms but then never develop the jaundice. They are as infectious, however, as children with overt jaundice.

Laboratory studies will show elevations of AST (SGOT) and serum alanine transaminase (ALT; serum glutamate pyruvate transaminase [SGPT]). Measurement of bilirubin in the urine shows increased levels. Bile pigments in the stool are decreased. Serum bilirubin levels will be increased.

Therapeutic Management

Strict handwashing and infection control precautions are mandatory when caring for children with hepatitis. Feces must be disposed of carefully because the type A virus may be cultured from feces. Syringes and needles must be disposed of with caution because the type B virus can be transmitted by blood. Contacts should receive immune globulin (hepatitis A) or hepatitis B immune globulin (HBIG) as appropriate. All health care providers should receive prophylaxis against hepatitis by the hepatitis vaccine. Children should receive routine immunization against HBV (see Focus on Evidence-Based Practice). All women should be screened during pregnancy for hepatitis B surface antigen (HBsAg). Infants born of hepatitis-positive mothers receive both HBIG and active immunization at birth to prevent their contracting the disease. A hepatitis A vaccine is available for health care providers and may soon be included in routine immunization programs (Van Damme & Van der Wielen, 2001).

The treatment for hepatitis A is increased rest and maintenance of a good caloric intake. A low-fat diet, once recommended, is not required and, in any event, is difficult to enforce. Children are generally hungrier at breakfast than later in the day, so a good intake should be encouraged for breakfast. Children can be cared for at home. They should

FOCUS ON EVIDENCE-BASED PRACTICE

Do Adolescents Appreciate the Importance of Hepatitis B Vaccine to Reduce Their Risk of Contracting the Disease?

To answer this question, 943 adolescents received a standard education program about hepatitis B and the availability of a vaccine. They then completed a questionnaire asking about demographic factors, self-reported risk behaviors, and their attitude toward hepatitis B including their likelihood of acquiring the disease. Results from the questionnaire showed that the majority of adolescents did not think that they were at significant risk for contracting hepatitis B. Adolescents who had had sexual intercourse or already contracted a sexually transmitted disease were more likely to report that they were vulnerable to contracting the disease so hepatitis B immunization was important to their health.

This is an important study for nurses because nurses are often the health care providers who teach about the importance of immunization and, as school nurses, advocate that adolescents who did not receive immunization against hepatitis B early in life, receive it as teenagers. Knowing that adolescents do not readily classify hepatitis B as a sexually transmitted disease that they could contract should alert all health care providers that more education in this area may be necessary. Information from this study could be used to substantiate the need for additional educational programs for adolescents.

Schmidt, R. M., & Middleman, A. B. (2001). The importance of hepatitis B vaccination among adolescents. *Journal of Adolescent Health, 29*(3), 217–222.

not return to school or a day care center until 2 weeks after the onset of symptoms.

Lamivudine (Epivir), an antiviral agent, may be effective in reducing viral replication with hepatitis B. Interferon also may be prescribed. Of those with type B, 90% will also recover completely, but 10% will develop chronic hepatitis and become hepatitis carriers. Infants who contracted the disease at birth have an increased risk for liver carcinoma later in life (Tung, 2000).

NURSING DIAGNOSES AND RELATED INTERVENTIONS

Nursing Diagnosis: Pain related to pruritus of jaundice and liver inflammation

Outcome Identification: Child will not experience extreme discomfort during course of illness.

Outcome Evaluation: Child states level of itching is tolerable; no scratch marks on skin are present; reports right upper quadrant pain is minimal.

Jaundice commonly causes pruritus, and, for some children, this can result in extreme discomfort. Being certain that the child is not overheated and not perspiring reduces the itching. A cool bath is often comforting. Skin moisturizers such as Eucerin or an antihistamine may be prescribed. Teach the child distractive techniques such as putting pressure on a pruritic area or trying imagery to lessen the urge to scratch.

✔ CHECKPOINT QUESTIONS

13. Which hepatitis viruses are spread through fecally contaminated water?
14. When is hepatitis considered to be chronic?

Obstruction of the Bile Ducts

Obstruction of the bile ducts in children generally occurs from congenital atresia, stenosis, or absence of the duct. Although rare, it also can occur from a plugging of biliary secretions. When the bile duct is obstructed, bile, unable to enter the intestinal tract, accumulates in the liver. Bile pigments (direct bilirubin) enter the bloodstream and jaundice occurs, increasing in intensity daily.

Assessment

Although bile duct obstruction is a congenital disorder, the chief sign (jaundice) does not develop until approximately 2 weeks. This delay in development differentiates it clinically from physiologic jaundice, which occurs in almost all newborns on the third day of life, or the jaundice of Rh isoimmunization, which typically occurs during the first 24 h of life. Laboratory findings will also distinguish this type of jaundice from other types. Physiologic jaundice and Rh isoimmunization jaundice occur from a rise in indirect bilirubin, whereas the jaundice of bile duct obstruction is a result of a rise in direct bilirubin. Alkaline phosphatase levels will be elevated. AST (SGOT) level is normal in the early phase and later becomes abnormal, when prolonged obstruction and back pressure cause liver cell damage. In addition, because bile salts (necessary for fat absorption) are not reaching the intestine, absorption of fat and fat-soluble vitamins (i.e., vitamins A, D, E, and K) is poor. Calcium absorption, which depends on vitamin D absorption, also is poor. Infant's stools appear light in color from lack of bile pigments. The pressure on the liver from the obstruction becomes so acute with time that cell destruction or cirrhosis occurs. Ultimately, without liver transplantation, death of liver failure will result (Haber, 2000).

Therapeutic Management

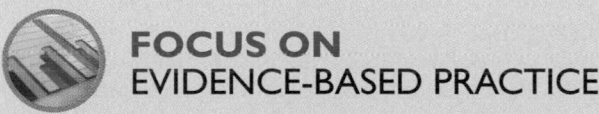

Before treatment is begun, appropriate blood work and a liver biopsy under a local anesthesia may be done to rule out hepatitis. Duodenal secretions may be collected by endoscopy to assess for bile. Radionuclide imaging, in which the infant is given an IV radioactive isotope that, when taken up by the liver would normally be seen flowing through the bile ducts, also may be performed. If a mucus plug in the duct is suspected, children may be given a course of magnesium sulfate (installed into the duodenum to relax the bile duct) or given dehydrocholic acid (Decholin) IV to stimulate the flow of bile. If atresia of the bile duct appears to be the problem, surgical correction is the treatment (a Kasai procedure). With this surgery, a loop of bowel is sutured next to the liver to create a fistula for bile flow between the liver and intestine. A double-barreled colostomy is then created (enterostomy). Bile flows out of the proximal loop into a collecting bag. It is periodically returned to the distal loop of intestine by injection. After 6 to 12 weeks, the colostomy is closed when a normal bile flow has been established. Unfortunately, surgical correction is impossible in all infants with atresia because the atresia tends to occur too far back in the liver to be in an operable area. Liver transplantation is needed for those children with extensive involvement (Sokol & Narkewicz, 2001).

NURSING DIAGNOSES AND RELATED INTERVENTIONS

Nursing Diagnosis: Risk for imbalanced nutrition, less than body requirements, related to inability to digest fat

Outcome Identification: Child will ingest adequate nutritional requirements until surgical correction is complete.

Outcome Evaluation: Infant's weight remains in same percentile on standardized growth curve; absence of vitamin deficiency (e.g., cracked lips or altered bone growth); dietary record reflects intakes of adequate nutrients.

Preoperative Care. Infants who are admitted for surgery for bile duct obstruction are placed on a low-fat, high-carbohydrate diet preoperatively. They are given water-soluble forms of vitamins A, D, and K to improve vitamin levels. If vitamin K level is too low, coagulation may be affected, increasing surgical risk. Vitamin K may be administered parenterally until the prothrombin levels rise to normal limits. Infants will also be well hydrated with parenteral fluids.

Postoperative Care. After surgery, infants return with a nasogastric tube in place attached to low intermittent suction. Observe carefully for abdominal distention because paralytic ileus is a frequent complication of this type of surgery. The nasogastric tube will be left in place until bowel peristalsis has returned. Gradually, children will be introduced to oral fluids and eventually to a normal diet. If the repair is successful, the child's stools change to a yellow and then brown (normal stool) color after surgery. Description of stools is, therefore, an important postoperative observation.

If bile flow is inadequate after surgery, infants will remain on a medium-fat, high-carbohydrate diet or receive total parenteral nutrition while they await transplantation surgery.

Cirrhosis

Cirrhosis is fibrotic scarring of the liver. Cirrhosis means "yellow" or the typical color of hepatic scar tissue. It occurs rarely in children, although it may be seen as a result of congenital biliary atresia or as a complication of chronic illnesses such as protracted hepatitis, sickle cell anemia, or cystic fibrosis.

When fibrotic infiltrates replace normal liver cells, liver function is impaired, resulting in a decreased ability to detoxify toxic substances, decreased protein synthesis, inability to produce prothrombin, decreased ability to produce bile, and, possibly, hypoglycemia. Children will have large, fatty stools resulting from the decrease in bile production; avitaminosis of fat-soluble vitamins; symptoms of hemorrhage from decreased clotting ability; and anemia.

Fibrotic infiltration interferes not only with the function of liver cells but also with the hepatic blood flow. This leads to portal hypertension from the back pressure of blood that cannot flow readily through the scarred organ (Fig. 45-4). Children will have compromised heart action, *ascites* (an exudate of fluid into the abdomen), possibly esophageal varices (back pressure causing them to dilate), and hypersplenism (Sokol & Narkewicz, 2001).

Once fibrotic infiltration begins, there is no way to reverse the changes. Nursing care focuses on promoting comfort, providing adequate nutrition by a high-carbohydrate, medium-chain-triglyceride diet, and preventing further involvement until liver transplantation can be scheduled. Cholestyramine (Questran) may be prescribed to stimulate bile flow and reduce reabsorption of bile into the circulation (this will minimize jaundice).

Esophageal Varices

Esophageal varices (distended veins) can be a frequent complication of liver disorders such as cirrhosis (Senyuz et al., 2001). They generally form at the distal end of the esophagus near the stomach secondary to back pressure on the veins due to increased blood pressure in the portal circulation. Bleeding of varices may occur if children cough vigorously or strain to pass stool. Gastric reflux into the distal esophagus may irritate and erode the fine covering of the distended vessels, causing rupture.

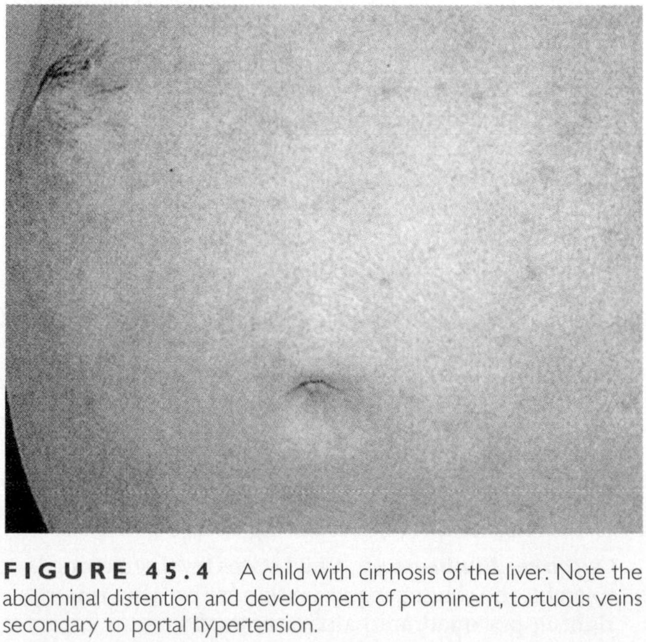

FIGURE 45.4 A child with cirrhosis of the liver. Note the abdominal distention and development of prominent, tortuous veins secondary to portal hypertension.

Rupture of esophageal varices is an emergency situation because children can lose a large quantity of blood quickly from the ruptured, engorged vessels. Vasopressin or nitroglycerin may be given IV to lessen hypertension and reduce the hemorrhage. Injection of a sclerosing agent into veins may be attempted. Iced saline nasogastric lavage may be instituted to promote vasoconstriction. A Sengstaken-Blakemore tube or Linton-Nachlas catheter may be passed into the stomach. After insertion, balloons on the sides of the catheter are inflated to apply pressure against the bleeding vessels. As with an external tourniquet, the compression in such a catheter must be reduced for 5 to 10 min every 6 to 8 h or tissue necrosis can result.

Children must be monitored for future bleeding episodes. Frequent vital sign measurements and testing of stool and any vomitus for the presence of blood will indicate new GI system bleeding.

Liver Transplantation

Liver transplantation is the surgical replacement of a malfunctioning liver by a donor liver. Donor livers are not readily available, so the waiting time for surgery may be months (see Focus on Communication). Finding an acceptable, child-sized liver may be especially difficult, so adult livers can be reduced in size for transplantation. Additionally, a lobe of a liver from a living donor can be used (Campbell et al., 2001). Often, a child is extremely ill with ascites, GI bleeding, extreme pruritus, hepatic encephalopathy, or renal dysfunction before the surgery can be accomplished. Nursing care after liver transplantation in a child is compounded because it involves taking care of a child who has had major surgery, and also one who normally would be categorized as too ill to undergo surgery. Despite the severity of illness and the length of surgery, children tend to recover quickly after liver transplantation. The survival rate is over 80% (Sokol & Narkewicz, 2001). Both children and parents must have thorough preoperative preparation so they understand the seriousness of the surgery and the possibility that the graft will be rejected. It helps to introduce the parents to others whose children have successfully undergone the procedure so they have support people available.

Preoperative Management

Preoperative management consists of keeping the child in the best physical condition possible so that, when a liver is available, transplantation can be performed. For many children, this includes dialysis and severe nutritional restrictions.

Surgical Procedure

Liver transplantation requires a wide subcostal incision. The vena cava is temporarily clamped during the removal of the natural liver to prevent bleeding, which means that all IV lines must be placed in the upper extremities (if placed in lower extremities, fluid could not return through the clamped venous circulation to the upper body). The total operation takes 10 to 14 h to complete.

FOCUS ON COMMUNICATION

Baxter Commons is a 2-year-old boy who was born with congenital obstruction of the bile duct. Unable to be surgically repaired, his condition has progressed to severe cirrhosis. Baxter's doctors spoke with his mother yesterday about the need for a liver transplantation. Today, you see Mrs. Commons filling out forms by Baxter's bedside.

Less-Effective Communication

Nurse: Mrs. Commons? Can I help you with anything?

Mrs. Commons: No. Baxter's going to have a transplantation. With him well again, I'll be free to start back to college. I'm filling out the forms.

Nurse: Will the transplantation really be that soon?

Mrs. Commons: As soon as tomorrow. Because Baxter won't be able to wait a long time.

Nurse: Do you think the doctors meant it could be that soon? But sometimes there's a long waiting period?

Mrs. Commons: No. Because Baxter can't wait long. If he has to, he'll die.

Nurse: It's lucky then that a liver is available.

More-Effective Communication

Nurse: Mrs. Commons? Can I help you with anything?

Mrs. Commons: No. Baxter's going to have a transplantation. With him well again, I'll be free to start back to college. I'm filling out the forms.

Nurse: Will the transplantation really be that soon?

Mrs. Commons: As soon as tomorrow. Because Baxter won't be able to wait a long time.

Nurse: Do you think the doctors meant it could be that soon? But sometimes there's a long waiting period?

Mrs. Commons: No. Because Baxter can't wait long. If he has to, he'll die.

Nurse: Let's review exactly what the doctor has told you.

People under stress often do not hear instructions well. When this happens, they may need them repeated several times before they truly comprehend what was said. An easy solution when you are aware that a parent has not heard potentially bad news is to ignore the loss of information, as in the first scenario above. A better solution is to explore with the parents what they did hear and help them receive more accurate information.

Postoperative Management

If a liver transplantation is rejected, it is most often rejected because of the function of T lymphocytes. Careful tissue matching (HLA matching) is necessary to reduce the possibility of stimulating T-cell rejection. To further reduce the action of T lymphocytes, children are administered a course of an immunosuppressive drug such as cyclosporine or tacrolimus (Prograf) before the transplantation.

Nursing care after liver transplantation surgery focuses on preventing complications that may arise from the surgery and continued immunosuppression. Children may need assisted ventilation for approximately 24 h postoperatively to prevent pulmonary complications such as atelectasis and pneumonia because the large abdominal incision makes coughing and deep breathing difficult. In addition, ascites has placed pressure against the diaphragm, interfering with lung expansion. Thus, preoperative pulmonary edema may be present. After discontinuation of mechanical ventilation and extubation, chest physiotherapy may be started to mobilize lung secretions.

Advocate for adequate pain control. Assess blood pressure, capillary refilling, peripheral pulses, and skin color frequently to ensure adequate cardiovascular function, important for good tissue perfusion of the transplanted liver. The child may have a central venous pressure line or an arterial line such as a Swan-Ganz catheter inserted to assess hemodynamic status. Assess neurologic status hourly using a modified Glasgow coma scale (see Chapter 52).

Usually, the child is positioned flat for the first 24 h to prevent cerebral air emboli, which may result from any air remaining in the transplanted liver. Typically, children have a nasogastric tube inserted during surgery attached to low intermittent suction postoperatively. Irrigate the tube according to agency policy to maintain patency. Assess the gastric pH by aspirating stomach contents every 4 h, and, based on this assessment, administer antacids or H_2 receptor antagonists such as cimetidine or mucosal protectants as prescribed to help prevent stress ulcer. If preoperative esophageal varices are present, assess nasogastric drainage carefully for frank or occult blood.

A T-tube inserted into the bile duct for drainage allows the amount of bile being produced by the new liver to be evaluated. Once bowel sounds become active, nasogastric suction and the T-tube are usually discontinued and liquids and then solid foods are introduced gradually. If vomiting occurs and is persistent, total parenteral nutrition may be used for 3 or 4 days to rest the intestinal tract before fluid is reintroduced.

Hypoglycemia is a danger postoperatively because glucose levels are regulated by the liver, and the transplanted organ may not function efficiently at first. Assess serum glucose levels hourly by fingerstick puncture. A 10% solution of dextrose may be necessary to prevent hypoglycemia.

Sodium, potassium, chloride, and calcium levels are evaluated approximately every 6 to 8 h to be certain that an electrolyte balance is maintained. Even if a low potassium level is detected, potassium is rarely added to IV solutions because of the risk of renal failure due to the stress of surgery. Plus, if the graft begins to necrose, the breakdown of cells will release potassium, elevating the level even more. Continuous cardiac monitoring is usually necessary to detect hyperkalemia (hyperkalemia causes elevation of T waves or ventricular fibrillation), hypokalemia (causes small T waves and the presence of a U wave), or other arrhythmias.

Many children develop hypertension within 72 h after surgery. This occurs because of alterations in the renin-angiotensin system due to the not yet fully functioning transplanted liver or as a side effect of cyclosporine, tacrolimus, and steroid therapy continued postoperatively to guard against transplant rejection. IV therapy with hypotensive agents such as hydralazine (Apresoline) and nitroprusside may be needed to reduce hypertension. Hypotension will occur if the transplanted liver becomes dysfunctional or there is bleeding caused by poor blood coagulation. The child also has an increased risk for bleeding because of the number of sites for anastomosis involved with the procedure. Observe and record abdominal girth, the incision line, and drainage from any catheters or tubes placed in the incision to allow peritoneal secretions to drain to help detect bleeding.

A warming blanket may be required postoperatively to maintain normal body temperature after the long exposure of surgery. Take axillary or tympanic, not rectal, temperatures, because many children with liver damage have rectal hemorrhoids that could rupture from the trauma of a thermometer insertion. Prevent the child from unnecessary exposure during procedures and care to help maintain normal body temperature.

NURSING DIAGNOSES AND RELATED INTERVENTIONS

Nursing Diagnosis: Risk for infection related to administration of immunosuppressive medication

Outcome Identification: Child will remain free of signs and symptoms of infection postoperatively.

Outcome Evaluation: Temperature remains within normal range; no presence of exudate or inflammation around abdominal incision.

Successful liver transplantation is possible because of the preoperative administration of an immunosuppressive agent, which effectively suppresses T lymphocytes, the lymphocytes responsible for rejecting transplanted organs. In addition, immunosuppressive agents are administered IV immediately postoperatively to prevent graft rejection. Because children are prone to infection while receiving immunosuppressive therapy, be sure to use strict aseptic techniques, standard precautions, and careful handwashing. Clean the skin around any abdominal drains every 4 h to prevent skin breakdown, thus preventing a portal of entry for microorganisms.

Serum transaminases (AST [SGOT] and ALT [SGPT]), alkaline phosphatase, serum bilirubin, and ammonia levels are assessed at least daily to detect rejection. However, children usually do not show signs of liver rejection until 5 to 7 days after surgery. In addition to changes in these laboratory values, with liver rejection the child also may develop fever and increasing abdominal girth. Also, the urine turns orange from increased urobilinogen excretion. If signs of rejection appear to be occurring, doses of cyclosporine, tacrolimus, and a corticosteroid such as methylprednisolone are increased to maximum levels.

Nursing Diagnosis: Interrupted family processes related to stress of surgery and uncertainty of transplantation outcome

Outcome Identification: Child and family will demonstrate adequate coping techniques postoperatively.

Outcome Evaluation: Child and family state that, although waiting is difficult, they are able to do so; identify ways they have changed their family life at home to accommodate child's illness and surgery.

Children and parents need continued support during the postoperative period while they wait to see if the graft will be rejected. They need continued contact with health care personnel through telephone calls and clinic visits.

After successful liver transplantation, a child should be able to function normally, attending school and enjoying age-appropriate activities. Be certain by hospital discharge that parents have a return appointment for evaluation and are aware of the symptoms of graft rejection, such as jaundice, lethargy, and fever.

✔ CHECKPOINT QUESTIONS

15. For the child with bile duct obstruction, absorption of what substances will be impaired?
16. The child with esophageal varices secondary to cirrhosis is at high risk for what complication?
17. Why is hypoglycemia a complication of liver transplantation?

INTESTINAL DISORDERS

Intussusception

Intussusception is the invagination of one portion of the intestine into another (Fig. 45-5). This generally occurs in the second half of the first year of a child's life (Mulberg, 2000).

In infants younger than 1 year, intussusception generally occurs for idiopathic reasons. In infants older than 1 year, a "lead point" on the intestine likely cues the invagination. Such a point might be a Meckel's diverticulum; a polyp; hypertrophy of *Peyer's patches* (lymphatic tissue of the bowel that increases in size with viral diseases); or bowel tumors. A number of children apparently developed intussusception from administration of a rotavirus vaccine before it was withdrawn from the market (Dennehy & Bresee, 2001). The point of the invagination is generally the juncture of the distal ileum and proximal colon.

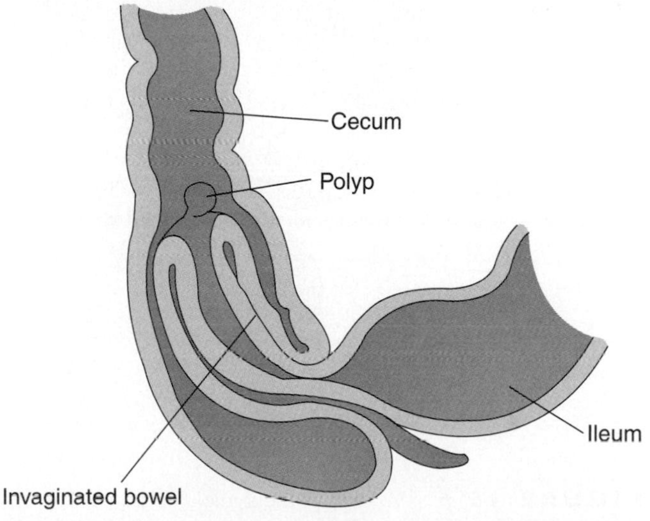

FIGURE 45.5 Intussusception. The distal ileal segment of bowel has invaginated into the cecum. A polyp serves as a lead point.

This condition is a surgical emergency. Reduction of the intussusception must be done promptly by either instillation of solution (or air) or surgery before necrosis of the invaginated portion of the bowel occurs.

Assessment

Children with this disorder suddenly draw up their legs and cry as if they are in severe pain and possibly vomit. After the peristaltic wave that caused the discomfort, they are symptom free. They play happily. In approximately 15 min, the same phenomenon of intense abdominal pain strikes again. Vomitus will begin to contain bile because the obstruction is invariably below the ampulla of Vater, the point in the intestine where bile empties into the duodenum. After approximately 12 h, children develop blood in stool, described as a "currant jelly" appearance. Their abdomen becomes distended as the bowel above the intussusception distends (D'Agostino, 2002).

If necrosis has occurred, children generally have an elevated temperature, peritoneal irritation (their abdomen will feel tender; they may "guard" it by tightening their abdominal muscles), an increased white blood cell count (WBC), and often a rapid pulse.

Diagnosis is suggested by the history. Any time a parent is describing a child who is crying, be certain to ask enough questions to recognize a possible history of intussusception.

- What is the duration of the pain? (It lasts a short time with intervals of no crying in between.)
- What is the intensity? (Severe.)
- What is the frequency? (Approximately every 15 to 20 min.)
- What is the description? (The child pulls up his or her legs with crying.)
- Is the child ill in any other way? (Yes. Vomits; refuses food; states his or her stomach feels "full.")

The presence of the intussusception is confirmed by sonogram.

Therapeutic Management

Intussusception requires surgery to straighten the invaginated portion, or reduction by instillation of a water-soluble solution, barium enema, or air (pneumatic insufflation). If there is no lead point, just the pressure of these nonsurgical techniques may successfully reduce the intussusception. After this type of reduction, children are observed for 24 h because a number of children will have a recurrence of the intussusception within 24 h. If this occurs, they are scheduled for an additional reduction or surgery (Mulberg, 2000).

NURSING DIAGNOSES AND RELATED INTERVENTIONS

Nursing Diagnosis: Pain related to abnormal abdominal peristalsis

Outcome Identification: Child will exhibit verbal and nonverbal indicators of pain at a tolerable level throughout illness.

Outcome Evaluation: Child is able to be comforted between spasms of pain, demonstrates interest in toys or social interactions.

Infants with intussusception have episodes of acute pain. They are bewildered by this type of pain because it is so different from any they have experienced before. Ordinarily, if they pinch a finger on a toy and it hurts, a parent picks them up, kisses their fingers, and the pain goes away. A parent picks them up now and the pain goes away, but it returns repeatedly. Infants need to be held and rocked and comforted in an attempt to relieve their frustration at this strange happening.

Nursing Diagnosis: Risk for deficient fluid volume related to bowel obstruction

Outcome Identification: Infant will exhibit signs of adequate fluid volume balance.

Outcome Evaluation: Infant's skin turgor is good; pulse is 90 to 100 beats/min. Amount of diarrhea and blood loss in stool is minimal. Episodes of vomiting decrease in frequency.

Infants are kept on NPO status before surgery or nonsurgical reduction. Because they have abdominal pain, they may find comfort in sucking a pacifier. Because they have been vomiting, IV fluid therapy may be started to reestablish their electrolyte balance and to supply adequate fluid to hydrate them.

If a nonsurgical reduction is accomplished, infants are kept NPO for a few hours and then introduced gradually to regular feedings. Infants who have surgery will return with a nasogastric tube attached to low intermittent suction and an IV infusion in place. The nasogastric tube will remain in place until the suture line is healing and peristaltic function has returned. Once bowel sounds are present, oral feedings will be started gradually.

Nursing Diagnosis: Risk for impaired parenting related to infant's illness

Outcome Identification: Parents will demonstrate positive bonding behavior with the infant during illness.

Outcome Evaluation: Parents hold and talk to infant; express positive characteristics about infant.

Parents need to hold infants after reduction or postoperatively to promote bonding and also to comfort the infant. Provide guidance and support as they hold the infant. When oral feeding is resumed, encourage the parents to participate with this aspect of care. It provides them with an opportunity to regain confidence in themselves as parents. Reassure them that this did not occur because of anything they did. Whenever a child's disorder begins with vomiting, many parents worry that the vomiting is somehow related to the child's method of feeding. Urge them to hold and be with the child as recovery proceeds to reassure themselves that the child is now all right again.

Volvulus

A **volvulus** is a twisting of the intestine (Fig. 45-6). The twist leads to obstruction of the passage of feces and compromise of the blood supply to the loop of intestine involved. This occurs most often because, in fetal life, a portion of the intestine first protrudes into the base of the umbilical cord at approximately age 6 weeks. At approximately age 10 weeks, it returns to the abdominal cavity. As the intestine returns to the abdominal cavity, it rotates to its permanent position. After the rotation, the mesentery

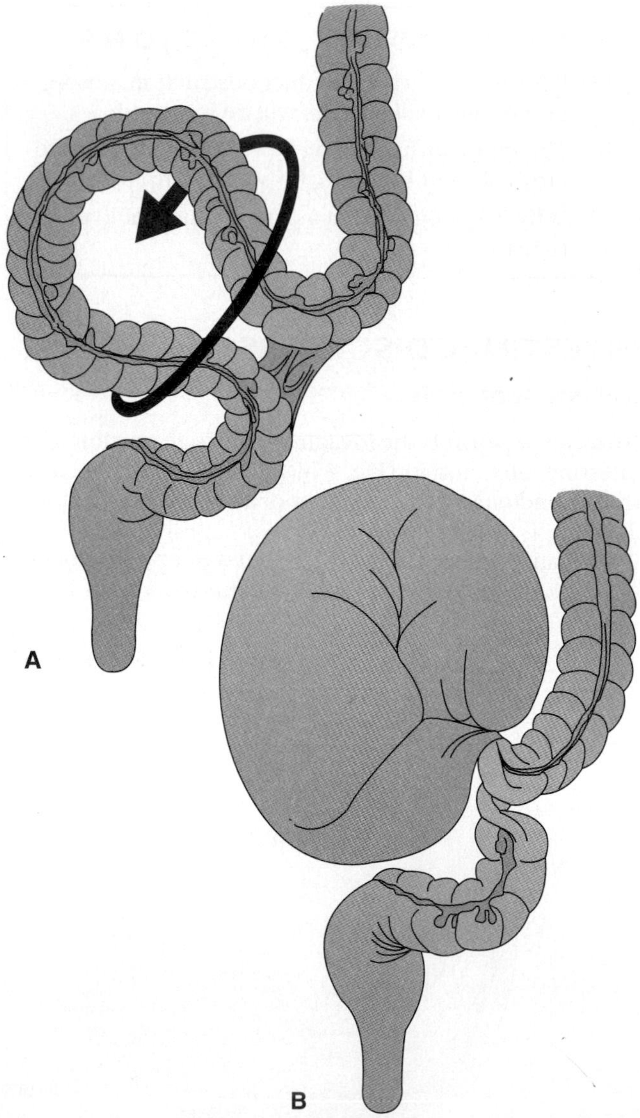

FIGURE 45.6 Volvulus of the sigmoid colon. (*A*) The unattached loop of bowel twists. (*B*) The bowel lumen is obstructed, leading to inability of stool to pass and compression of the blood supply to the looped bowel segment.

becomes fixed in this position. In an instance of volvulus, the action is incomplete, so that the mesentery does not attach to a normal position. The bowel is left free to move and twist (Sondheimer, 2001a).

Usually, the symptoms are those of intestinal obstruction and occur during the first 6 months of life. Symptoms may include intense crying and pain, pulling up the legs, abdominal distention, and vomiting. Diagnosis is made on the history and on abdominal examination, which reveals an abdominal mass. A sonogram or lower barium radiograph also will show the obstruction. Surgery is used to relieve the volvulus and reattach the bowel so it is no longer so free moving. This must be done promptly before necrosis of the intestine occurs from a lack of blood supply to the involved loop of bowel. Preoperative and postoperative care will be the same as for infants with intussusception.

✔ CHECKPOINT QUESTIONS

18. In what condition would you expect to see currant jelly–like stools?
19. At what age does volvulus usually occur?

Necrotizing Enterocolitis

Necrotizing enterocolitis (NEC) is a condition that develops in approximately 5% of all infants in intensive care nurseries. The bowel develops necrotic patches, interfering with digestion and possibly leading to a paralytic ileus. Perforation and peritonitis may follow.

The necrosis appears to result from ischemia or poor perfusion of blood vessels in sections of bowel. The ischemic process may occur when, owing to shock or hypoxia, there is vasoconstriction of blood vessels to nonessential organs such as the bowel. The entire bowel may be involved, or it may be a localized phenomenon. The incidence of NEC is highest in immature infants, those who have suffered anoxia or shock, and those fed by enteral feedings. Infants with infections may develop it as a further complication of their already stressed state (Loh et al., 2001).

Assessment

There is a lower incidence of the condition in infants who are fed breast milk than in those who are formula fed because intestinal organisms grow more profusely with cow's milk than breast milk (cow's milk lacks antibodies). A response to the foreign protein in cow's milk may be a mechanism that starts the necrotic process. Therefore, encouraging breastfeeding may help prevent the development of this disorder.

Signs of NEC usually appear in the first week of life. The abdomen becomes distended and tense. The infant does not empty the stomach by the next feeding time because of poor intestinal action, so, if stomach contents are aspirated before a feeding, a return of undigested milk of more than 2 mL will be obtained. Stool may be positive for occult blood. Periods of apnea may begin or increase in number if they were already present. Signs of blood loss due to intestinal bleeding, such as lowered blood pressure and inability to stabilize temperature, also may be present.

Abdominal x-ray films show a characteristic picture of air invading the intestinal wall; if perforation has occurred, there will be air in the abdominal cavity. Abdominal girth measurements made just above the umbilicus every 4 to 8 h show increases.

Therapeutic Management

As soon as the condition is recognized, feedings must be discontinued, and the infant is maintained on IV or total parenteral nutrition solutions to rest the GI tract. A course of an antibiotic may be given to limit secondary infection. Handle the abdomen gently to lessen the possibility of bowel perforation.

If bowel obstruction occurs, the infant may need a temporary colostomy performed to allow for bowel function. If the area of necrosis appears to be localized, surgery to remove that portion of the bowel may be successful. If a large portion of the bowel is removed, the infant may be prone to "short-bowel" syndrome or have a problem with digestion of nutrients in the future. If the bowel perforates, peritoneal drainage or a laparotomy will be necessary to help remove fecal secretions from the abdomen (Moss et al., 2001).

NEC is a grave insult to an infant already stressed by immaturity. The prognosis is guarded until it can be demonstrated that the infant can again take oral feedings without bowel complications.

Appendicitis

Appendicitis is inflammation of the appendix. This is the most common cause of abdominal surgery in children. It is seen most frequently in school-age children and adolescents, although it can occur in preschoolers and even in newborns (Sondheimer, 2001a). It occurs more commonly in some families than in others (Gauderer et al., 2001). The *appendix,* a blind-end pouch attached to the cecum, may become inflamed after an upper respiratory or other body infection, but the cause of appendicitis is generally obscure. In most instances, fecal material apparently enters the appendix, hardens, and obstructs the appendix lumen. Inflammation and edema develop, leading to compression of blood vessels and cellular malnutrition. Necrosis and pain result. If the condition is not discovered early enough, the necrotic area will rupture, and fecal material will spill into the abdomen, causing peritonitis—a potentially fatal condition.

Assessment

Most people assume that appendicitis begins with sharp pain, so they may dismiss their children's early symptoms for some time as simple gastroenteritis. Actually, pain is a late symptom in appendicitis. The history typically begins with anorexia for 12 to 24 h. Children do not eat and "just do not act like themselves." They may then report nausea and vomiting. The abdominal pain, when it does start, is at first diffuse. Gradually, it becomes localized to the right lower quadrant. The point of sharpest pain is often one third of the way between the anterior superior iliac crest and the umbilicus (**McBurney's point**). Keep in mind that, if the child's appendix is displaced from the usual position, the pain will not be at this typical point, so pain at any other point does not rule out appendicitis. Fever is a late symptom.

It is important in history taking to document the progress of the disease, for example:

- How was the child on Monday? (Not herself. She was not eating.)
- How was she Monday night? (Had generalized abdominal pain.)
- Tuesday morning? (Had sharp localized pain.)
- Now? (Has localized pain, vomiting, and fever.)

Until the pain becomes localized, appendicitis is difficult to distinguish from acute gastroenteritis. On abdominal examination, right lower quadrant tenderness may be elicited. Often, it is difficult to palpate children's abdomens because they guard their abdomen and make them stiff and hard by tensing their abdominal muscles. Although this interferes with abdominal examination, it is in itself an important sign that children have abdominal pain. To assist in a diagnosis of a painful abdomen, always palpate the anticipated tender area last.

Rebound tenderness is a phenomenon in which the child feels relatively mild pain when the area over his or her appendix is palpated, but, once the examiner's hand is withdrawn, the child experiences acute pain caused by the shifting of the abdominal contents. This is diagnostic for appendicitis, but it should be done with children only when absolutely necessary because it does cause acute pain. Caution children that the maneuver may cause pain. On auscultation, bowel sounds will be reduced. Only one or two are heard in the same length of time that 30 are normally heard. Absence of bowel sounds on auscultation suggests peritonitis or an appendix that has already ruptured.

Laboratory findings usually indicate leukocytosis (white blood cells [WBC] between 10,000 and 18,000/mm^3), which is actually low for the extent of the infection that may be present. Ketones in the urine are inordinately elevated as a symptom of starvation from poor intestinal absorption.

A CT scan reveals the swollen appendix (Gwynn, 2001). It can also be confirmed by sonogram. Pain in the right lower quadrant may occur as a manifestation of right lower lobe pneumonia. Therefore, children may have a chest radiograph taken to rule this out as the source of pain.

Therapeutic Management

Therapy for appendicitis is surgical removal of the appendix by laparoscopy before it ruptures. Achieving surgery before rupture occurs is easier in older children, who are more capable of relating the progression of symptoms. It is more difficult in young children, whose history is not as accurate, who do not have the words to describe their symptoms, or who will not relax their abdominal muscles enough to allow for manual examination. Also, the wall of the appendix is thinner and perforates more readily in young children.

NURSING DIAGNOSES AND RELATED INTERVENTIONS

Priorities for nursing care must be established quickly because this is an emergency situation, and the child must be prepared immediately for surgery (see Focus on Nursing Care Planning).

Nursing Diagnosis: Pain related to inflamed appendix

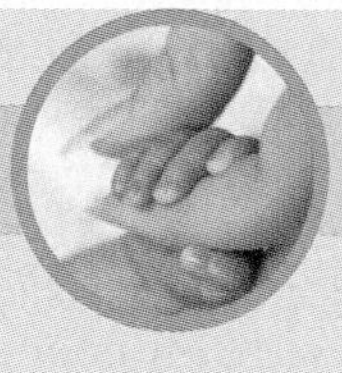

FOCUS ON *Nursing Care Planning*

A CHILD WITH APPENDICITIS

A 10-year-old male is brought to the emergency department by his parents because of nausea, vomiting, and abdominal pain since yesterday. "We thought it was just an upset stomach, but it isn't getting any better, and the pain is much worse now."

Assessment: Well-nourished, 10-year-old male without a history of major medical problems. Temperature 101.2°F; pulse 100; respirations 24. Mother reports that yesterday the child stated he was not feeling well. "He wasn't eating, and he had pains in his stomach. Last night, the pain got worse and he started vomiting." Pain now localized in right lower quadrant. Legs drawn up against abdomen. Bowel sounds sluggish. Rebound tenderness present. White blood cell count of 17,000/mm^3. Ultrasound confirms appendicitis. Child is scheduled for emergency appendectomy.

Nursing Diagnosis: Pain related to effects of appendicitis

Outcome Identification: Child will state pain is within tolerable limits until surgery.

Outcome Evaluation: Child demonstrates comfortable position; states pain is controlled with nonpharmacologic techniques.

(continued)

Interventions	Rationale
1. Assess the child's pain using a 10-point pain-assessment tool.	1. Assessment provides baseline information for planning. Using a pain-assessment tool provides an objective means for determining the extent and intensity of the child's pain.
2. Do not administer any analgesic. Give nothing by mouth (NPO).	2. Analgesics can mask the signs of possible rupture and subsequent peritonitis. NPO minimizes the risk for further vomiting and prevents abdominal distention, which could exacerbate the child's pain. NPO is also necessary preoperatively to reduce the risks of surgery and anesthesia.
3. Assist child with finding a position of comfort. Use pillows as appropriate.	3. Finding a position of comfort helps to minimize the sensation of pain. Pillows offer additional support to maintain the position of comfort.
4. Assist the child with using nonpharmacologic methods of pain control, such as imagery, distraction, and thought stopping.	4. Imagery, distraction, and thought stopping are gate control theory techniques useful in relieving pain.
5. Encourage the child to use these techniques at the onset of pain.	5. Using the techniques early on enhances their effectiveness in controlling pain.

Nursing Diagnosis: Risk for infection related to possible rupture of appendix

Outcome Identification: Child will remain free of any signs and symptoms of rupture until surgery.

Outcome Evaluation: Child's vital signs remain within age-acceptable parameters; states pain remains at current level or decreases; white blood cell count remains less than 20,000/mm^3. Abdomen does not become rigid.

Interventions	Rationale
1. Assess abdomen and extent of pain frequently for changes. Avoid palpating the abdomen unless absolutely necessary.	1. An increase in pain and boardlike abdomen are signs of peritonitis from a ruptured appendix.
2. Monitor vital signs every 15 to 30 min. Report any elevations in temperature or shallow respirations.	2. Elevated temperature indicates acute infection. Shallow respirations occur because deep breathing increases pressure on the abdomen, causing pain.
3. Obtain laboratory tests, including white blood cell count, as ordered.	3. A white blood cell count over 20,000/mm^3 suggests rupture.
4. Position the child comfortably with head of bed elevated in semi-Fowler's position.	4. Semi-Fowler's position keeps infected drainage localized to the lower abdominal cavity should the appendix rupture.
5. Administer intravenous (IV) fluid therapy as ordered. Anticipate the need for IV antibiotic therapy.	5. IV fluid therapy provides adequate hydration. IV antibiotics help to combat infection should rupture occur.
6. Avoid applying heat to the abdomen or using laxatives or enemas.	6. These measures could lead to rupture.

Nursing Diagnosis: Risk for deficient fluid volume related to vomiting, lack of oral intake, and NPO status

Outcome Identification: Child will maintain signs and symptoms of adequate hydration before surgery.

Outcome Evaluation: Child's skin turgor is good; weight, urine output, and urine specific gravity within acceptable parameters. Mucous membranes moist.

(continued)

Interventions	Rationale
1. Assess overall hydration status on admission, including skin turgor, mucous membranes, and weight.	1. Admission assessment provides a baseline for planning and evaluating changes. Weight is a reliable indicator of fluid balance.
2. Maintain NPO status as ordered. Institute IV fluid therapy with electrolytes as ordered.	2. NPO status is necessary to minimize the risks of surgery. IV fluid therapy with electrolytes helps to replace any lost through vomiting and lack of oral intake and also maintains adequate hydration in light of child being NPO.
3. Monitor intake and output as ordered, including IV fluid, urine, stool, and emesis.	3. Monitoring intake and output provides an objective estimate of overall fluid balance.

Nursing Diagnosis: Fear related to emergency nature of condition and surgery

Outcome Identification: Child and parents will demonstrate positive coping behaviors to deal with situation.

Outcome Evaluation: Child and parents verbalize concerns and fears; work with caregivers in measures preoperatively; participate in decision making and relaxation measures.

Interventions	Rationale
1. Allow child and parents to verbalize feelings and concerns. Assess for possible feelings related to "cause" of appendicitis.	1. Verbalization and assessment of feelings provide a safe outlet for emotions and help to dispel any misconceptions about the cause of appendicitis.
2. Approach the client in a calm, consistent, unhurried manner. Explain all actions and procedures. Attempt to minimize environmental stimuli.	2. Using a calm, consistent, unhurried approach with explanations helps to minimize the threat of the situation. Minimizing environmental stimuli can help reduce increasing fear and anxiety.
3. Include child and parents in treatment process and inform them about things ahead of time if possible.	3. Child and parent participation enhances their control over the situation and may help to instill hope and promote decision making.
4. Perform preoperative teaching about the child's condition, events before surgery, and what to expect after surgery. Allow time for the child and parents to ask questions.	4. Adequate preoperative teaching aids in preparing the child and parents for what is to come, helping to decrease the fears of the unknown. Time for questions helps clarify and individualize information and promotes feelings of control and trust.
5. Assist the child and parents with using relaxation techniques, such as muscle relaxation, breathing, and music.	5. Relaxation techniques help to decrease anxiety and fear, enhancing feelings of control.
6. Provide frequent updates about the child's progress.	6. Frequent updates about progress help to minimize fear about the unknown.

Outcome Identification: Child will not experience pain above a tolerable level throughout course of therapy.

Outcome Evaluation: Child voices that level of pain is tolerable.

In the period before surgery, analgesics must not be given because they obscure diagnostic signs such as tenderness and localizing pain. Cathartics and heat to the abdomen are also contraindicated because they may lead to rupture of the appendix. In adolescents, the abdomen will be shaved and washed with an antiseptic solution immediately before surgery. If assisting with the procedure, be gentle because the abdomen is tender, and compression could cause an appendix to rupture. Use lukewarm, not hot water, because heat can increase the possibility of appendix rupture by increasing edema in the appendix. Urge the child to find the best position of comfort and assure both parents and the child that emergency steps are in place and being carried out.

Nursing Diagnosis: Fear related to emergency nature of disorder and immediate surgery

Outcome Identification: Both parents and child will demonstrate positive coping behaviors during hospital stay.

Outcome Evaluation: Parents and child voice that they understand what interventions are necessary and cooperate as necessary.

Admission for appendicitis often occurs rapidly. A parent telephones the primary care provider, who recommends the child be seen in an emergency room. Surgery is scheduled as soon as it can be arranged. A mere 30 min may pass from the time of the first phone call until a child is wheeled to surgery. During this time, the parent and child both need to be told exactly what is happening ("I'm going to take some blood; I'm putting your name tag on your arm"); who the people are who are caring for them ("This is Dr. Brown, the anesthesiologist. I'm Ms. Henry, a registered nurse.") Parents do not think clearly in this type of emergency, and their reactions to situations may not be their usual ones. Explain that the procedures being done for their child (e.g., blood studies or a short wait while a surgery room is prepared) are necessary for safe surgery and that the danger of the appendix rupturing is not as acute a danger as they may have believed.

Remember that these children have had no preparation for hospitalization. The axiom "What they don't know won't hurt them" is not true. This can make appendicitis a harrowing experience for both parents and children. Praise them for those things they did well, such as recognizing their child was ill and bringing the child immediately for care.

WHAT IF? What if a parent tells you she "dropped everything" to rush her child to the emergency room because of appendicitis? What questions would you want to ask her to see if she has thought through the situation?

Nursing Diagnosis: Risk for deficient fluid volume related to NPO status

Outcome Identification: Child will exhibit signs of adequate hydration during treatment period.

Outcome Evaluation: Child's skin returns quickly when turgor is assessed; pulse and blood pressure are within normal age limits; weight maintained.

Preoperatively, obtain a urine sample for urinalysis and blood for a complete blood count. IV fluid therapy may be initiated to hydrate a child who has been vomiting a great deal.

Postoperatively, they will be maintained on IV fluids until they can take adequate oral feedings (approximately 24 h). With unruptured appendicitis, the postoperative course is uneventful; children are up a few hours after surgery and are discharged within a number of days. They generally return to school in another week.

Ruptured Appendix

If a child's appendix has already ruptured when the child is seen in the emergency department, the potential for peritonitis is great. When rupture occurs, children generally appear severely ill. WBC rises to more than 20,000/mm^3. Position them in a semi-Fowler's position so that infected drainage from the cecum drains downward into the pelvis rather than upward to the lungs. They need an IV fluid line inserted for hydration. Antibiotics will be begun preoperatively or at the point the ruptured appendix is confirmed.

During surgery, children will have drains placed beside the surgery incision so any infectious material in the abdomen can continue to drain. Warm soaks to these dressings may be ordered three or four times a day to encourage drainage. Examine the wound carefully at each dressing change. Be certain not to dislodge drains while removing soiled dressings; report immediately any drain that is expelled; the surgeon may want to replace it to ensure a patent drainage route. Often, drains are shortened with each dressing change to encourage initially deep areas, then areas closer to the skin to drain. IV fluid and antibiotic therapy are continued until full bowel function is restored.

Assess for signs of peritonitis. These may include a boardlike (rigid) abdomen, generally shallow respirations (because breathing deeply puts pressure on the abdomen and causes pain), and increased temperature. Although the postoperative course is slower (approximately 3 weeks) after a ruptured appendix, the prognosis is still good. A local abscess or intestinal adhesions may result. Adhesion formation, a long-term effect, could interfere with fertility in girls or cause bowel obstruction in both sexes later in life (Sondheimer, 2001a).

✔ CHECKPOINT QUESTIONS

20. When do signs of necrotizing enterocolitis generally begin?
21. When assessing the pain of a child with appendicitis, where, typically, is the point of sharpest pain?

Meckel's Diverticulum

In embryonic life, the intestine is attached to the umbilicus by the omphalomesenteric (vitelline) duct. This duct becomes a vestigial ligament as infants reach term. In 2% or 3% of all infants, a small pouch of this duct off the ileum, approximately 18 inches from the ileum–colon junction, remains: a **Meckel's diverticulum** (Sondheimer, 2001a). In this structure, there may be some misplaced gastric mucosa, which secretes gastric acids that flow into the intestine and irritate the bowel wall. Ulceration and bleeding may result. Infants will have painless, tarry (black) stools or grossly bloody stools. On occasion, the diverticulum may serve as the lead point causing an intussusception. In some instances, a fibrous band extending from the diverticulum pouch to the umbilicus acts as a constricting band, causing bowel obstruction. The history of the child suggests the diagnosis. Because the pouch is small, it does not fill and, therefore, may not be evident on x-ray or sonogram. Treatment is surgical exploration and removal of the vestigial structure.

Celiac Disease (Malabsorption Syndrome; Gluten-Induced Enteropathy)

The basic problem in **celiac disease** is a sensitivity or immunologic response to protein, particularly the gluten factor of protein found in grains—wheat, rye, oats, and barley. When children with celiac disease ingest gluten, changes occur in the intestinal mucosa or villi that prevent the absorption of foods across the intestinal villi into the bloodstream. Most noticeably, children develop an inability to absorb fat. As a result, they develop **steatorrhea** (bulky, foul-smelling, fatty stools); deficiency of fat-soluble vitamins A, D, K, and E (the vitamins are not absorbed because the fat is not absorbed); malnutrition; and a distended abdomen from the fat, bulky stools. Because vitamin D is one of the fat-soluble vitamins, rickets may occur. Hypoprothrombinemia may occur from loss of vitamin K. In addition, children may have hypochromic anemia (iron-deficiency anemia) and hypoalbuminemia from poor protein absorption.

Although gluten-induced enteropathy is a relatively rare condition, early recognition is essential for therapy and to provide early support and nutritional guidance for the parents. The illness occurs most frequently in children of a northern European background. It is apparently a dominantly inherited illness; children have different degrees of involvement. There is also an increased incidence in children with Down syndrome (Mackey et al, 2001).

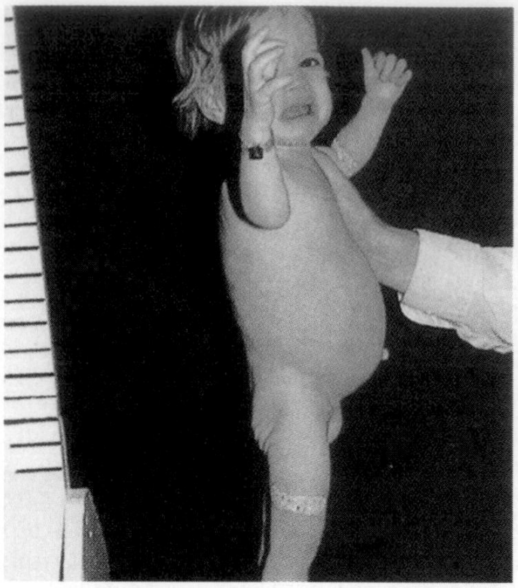

FIGURE 45.7 A child with celiac disease. Typically, the child's abdomen will be distended from the fat, bulky stools. Note the wasted appearance of the buttocks.

Assessment

Children with the syndrome tend to be anorectic and irritable. They gradually fall behind other children their age in height and weight. They appear skinny with spindly extremities and wasted buttocks. Their face, however, in contrast to children with true starvation, may be plump and well-appearing (Fig. 45-7).

Symptoms such as bulky stools, malnutrition, distended abdomen, and anemia become noticeable between 6 and 18 months of age. The diagnosis is based on history; clinical symptoms; serum analysis of antibodies against gluten (IgA antigliadin antibodies); and a biopsy of intestinal mucosa (done by endoscopy), which establishes the typical changes in intestinal villi. Children may have an oral glucose tolerance test, which will reveal poor absorption, and their stool may be collected to test for fat content, which will be increased.

In addition, response to gluten is observed by placing children on a gluten-free diet. In most instances, the response to this diet is dramatic. Children begin to gain weight, steatorrhea improves, and the irritability fades.

Therapeutic Management

Treatment is to continue children on a gluten-free diet for life because there is some suggestion that they are more prone to GI carcinoma later in life if they do not continue the diet into adulthood (Sondheimer, 2001a). In addition to this, children need to have water-soluble forms of vitamins A and D administered. Both iron and folate may be necessary as well to correct any anemia present.

NURSING DIAGNOSES AND RELATED INTERVENTIONS

Nursing Diagnosis: Imbalanced nutrition; less than body requirements, related to malabsorption of food

Outcome Identification: Child will receive adequate nutritional intake on gluten-free diet.

Outcome Evaluation: Child's weight is maintained on a percentile curve on a growth chart; skin turgor is good; steatorrhea is minimal; parents verbalize appropriate gluten-free food choices.

Parents need to record the consistency, appearance, size, and number of stools children pass. The disappearance of steatorrhea is a good indicator that children's ability to absorb nutrients is improving.

Parents need a great deal of nutritional counseling when children are first placed on a gluten-free diet so they can recognize foods that contain gluten (i.e., wheat, rye, oats, and barley products). Gluten is a part of wheat flour, gravy, soups, and sauces. Packaged and frozen foods usually contain gluten as fillers. Teach parents to be careful shoppers and read food labels carefully. Because children are anorectic when they are first introduced to the diet, getting them to eat it may be a problem. Remember that small servings are often eaten better by toddlers than larger servings are. Help parents create incentives to eat such as inviting dolls to "tea" or eating a picnic outside in nice weather.

As children reach school age, preparing a gluten-free diet grows more and more difficult, because favorite school-age foods (e.g., spaghetti, pizza, hot dogs, cake, and cookies) are not allowed. Selecting a diet in a school cafeteria may be impossible. Holidays pose special problems—birthday cake, turkey stuffing, and holiday cookies are prohibited. Until children are able to recognize which foods they can or cannot eat, parents often find it difficult to let them stay at friend's houses or go to summer camp—activities important to children's learning independence.

Celiac Crisis

When children with celiac disease develop any type of infection, a crisis of extreme symptoms may occur. Both vomiting and diarrhea become acute. Children can quickly experience electrolyte and fluid imbalances and need intensive therapy to replace them (see nursing care for children with vomiting and diarrhea earlier in chapter). Gradually, after such an episode, they are placed back on a gluten-free diet.

> ✔ **CHECKPOINT QUESTIONS**
>
> 22. What are the four most common symptoms in a child with celiac disease?
> 23. What substance must be restricted in a child with celiac disease?

DISORDERS OF THE LOWER BOWEL

Constipation

Constipation, or difficulty passing hardened stools, may occur in children of any age. Constipation is distressing to a child because passing hardened stool is painful and may cause anal fissures. The child then represses the next urge to defecate because of pain. The rectum gradually becomes distended and adjusts to the ever-present bulk of stool. The urge to defecate becomes less frequent. When the child does pass stool, it is larger and firmer than before and causes even more anal pain. This vicious cycle continues until the child becomes severely constipated. Children may have episodes of diarrhea or *encopresis* (involuntary release of stool) when their rectum can hold no more. They may have abdominal pain from forceful intestinal contractions.

Some children begin holding stool for psychological reasons. Once the process begins, however, the hardened stool, the anal fissures, and the pain on defecation soon occur, and what began for an emotional reason becomes a physical ailment. This is important to understand, because with these children, the therapy involves both counseling to correct the initial problem and treatment of the physical symptoms (Guerrero & Cavender, 1999).

Assessment

When taking a history of the condition, be certain to have parents describe what they mean by constipation. Some children have normal defecation habits of passing stool only every other day or every 3 days. As long as the stool is not hard and there is no discomfort associated with passing stool, this is not constipation. Examine the circumstances that may have led to constipation (diet low in fiber; little privacy in bathroom; family stress).

Children with constipation should be examined carefully to see if they have anal fissures. If these are present, sexual abuse must be ruled out. Constipation must be differentiated from aganglionic disease of the intestine. In constipation, on rectal examination, hard stool will be found in the rectum; in aganglionic disease of the intestine, no stool will normally be present.

Therapeutic Management

Treatment of chronic constipation is aimed at softening stool so it will pass painlessly. Children also need help to form bowel habits to evacuate their bowels frequently enough to prevent stool from becoming large and hardened before evacuation.

NURSING DIAGNOSES AND RELATED INTERVENTIONS

Nursing Diagnosis: Constipation related to pain from anal fissure and hardened stool

Outcome Identification: Child will achieve a normal elimination pattern by 2 weeks.

Outcome Evaluation: Child has a soft bowel movement without pain every other day.

For initial therapy, an enema may be administered to loosen hard stool. After this, a stool softener such as docusate sodium (Colace) is prescribed. Children need to ingest a high-fiber, high-fluid diet and be urged to evacuate their bowels at the same time every day to form a habit (Parker, 1999).

Inguinal Hernia

Inguinal hernia is a protrusion of a section of the bowel into the inguinal ring. It occurs usually in boys (9 : 1) because, as the testes descend from the abdominal cavity into the scrotum late in fetal life, a fold of parietal peritoneum also descends, forming a tube from the abdomen to the scrotum (Sondheimer, 2001a). In most infants, this tube closes completely. If it fails to close, intestinal descent into it (hernia) may occur at any time when there is an increase in intra-abdominal pressure. In girls, the round ligament extends from the uterus into the inguinal canal to its attachment on the abdominal wall. In girls, an inguinal hernia may occur because of a weakness of the muscle surrounding the round ligament.

Assessment

The hernia appears as a lump in the left or right groin. In some instances, the hernia is apparent only on crying (when abdominal pressure increases) and not when children are less active. Inguinal hernias are painless. Pain at the site implies that the bowel has become incarcerated in the sac, an emergency situation that requires immediate action to prevent bowel obstruction and ischemia.

The diagnosis is established on history and physical appearance. When taking a history of a well child, be certain to ask parents whether they have ever noticed any lumps in the child's groin area. The hernia may not be noticeable at the time of the visit, so, unless asked specifically, parents may not mention it. If present, the herniated intestine may be palpated in the inguinal ring on physical examination (Schier, 2000).

Therapeutic Management

Treatment of inguinal hernia is surgery. The bowel is returned to the abdominal cavity and retained there by sealing the inguinal ring. Pneumoperitoneum (instillation of carbon dioxide into the perineal cavity) during surgery may be performed to reveal the presence of an enlarged inguinal ring on the opposite side. If this is the case, both sides may be repaired, and the child will return from surgery with dressings on both groins.

Formerly, surgery for inguinal hernia was delayed until children were 3 or 4 years of age. Today, to prevent the complication of bowel strangulation—a surgical emergency—infants with inguinal hernia may have surgery before 1 year of age. If surgery is projected for children as a prophylactic measure, outcome setting may be difficult for parents as they weigh the value of surgical repair against the risk of anesthesia and surgery.

After surgery, keep the suture line dry and free of urine or feces to prevent infection. Most incisions in this area are closed by a tissue adhesive, which is waterproof and seals the incision from urine and feces. Even so, the infant will need frequent diaper changes and good diaper-area care. Assess circulation in the leg on the side of the surgical repair to be certain that edema of the groin is not compressing blood vessels and obstructing blood flow to the leg.

Hirschsprung's Disease (Aganglionic Megacolon)

Hirschsprung's disease, **aganglionic megacolon,** is absence of ganglionic innervation to the muscle of a section of the bowel. In most instances, this is the lower portion of the sigmoid colon just above the anus. The absence of nerve cells means there are no peristaltic waves at this section to further the passage of fecal material through that segment of intestine. This results in chronic constipation or ribbonlike stools (stools passing through such a small, narrow segment look like ribbons). The portion of the bowel proximal to the obstruction dilates, distending the abdomen (Fig. 45-8).

There is a familial incidence of aganglionic disease occurring at a greater incidence in siblings of a child with the disorder than in other children. It also occurs more often in males than in females. It is caused by an abnormal gene on chromosome 10. The incidence is approximately 1 in 5,000 live births (John-Kelly & Mulberg, 2000).

Assessment

Because newborn stools are normally soft, symptoms of aganglionic megacolon generally do not become apparent until 6 to 12 months of age. Occasionally, infants are born

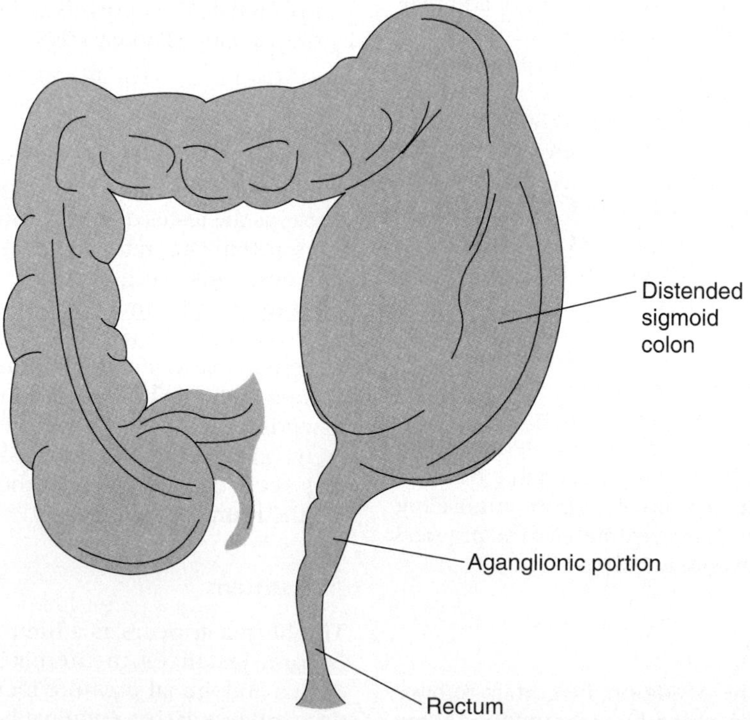

FIGURE 45.8 Aganglionic megacolon (Hirschsprung's disease). The distal portion of the bowel lacks nerve innervation. Because there is no peristalsis in this narrowed segment, the bowel proximal to it distends markedly.

with such an extensive section of bowel involved that even meconium cannot pass. The defect is suggested if infants fail to pass meconium by 24 h of age and have increasing abdominal distention.

By the time children are seen by a health care provider, they generally have a history of constipation or intermittent constipation and diarrhea. A careful history helps to document the illness:

- What is the duration of the constipation? (With this disease, it may be a problem from birth.)
- What do parents mean by constipation? (With this disease, children do not have a bowel movement more than once a week.)
- What is the consistency of the stool? (Ribbonlike or watery.)
- Is the child ill in any other way? (Children with aganglionic disease of the intestine tend to be thin and undernourished, sometimes deceptively so because their abdomen is large and distended.)

If a finger covered with a glove is inserted into the rectum of a child with true constipation, the examining finger will touch hard, caked stool. With aganglionic colon disease, the rectum is empty because fecal material cannot pass into the rectum through the obstructed portion. A barium enema is generally ordered to substantiate the diagnosis. The barium will outline on x-ray film the narrow, nerveless portion and the proximal distended portion of the bowel. Barium enema must be used cautiously because children cannot expel this afterward any more effectively than they can stool. The definitive diagnosis is by a biopsy of the affected segment to show the lack of innervation or by anorectal manometry, a technique to test the strength or innervation of the internal rectal sphincter by inserting a balloon catheter into the rectum and measuring the pressure exerted against it.

Therapeutic Management

Repair of aganglionic megacolon involves dissection and removal of the affected section with anastomosis of the intestine. Because this is a technically difficult surgery to perform in a small abdomen, the condition is generally treated in the newborn by two-stage surgery establishing a temporary colostomy followed by bowel repair at 12 to 18 months of age.

After the final surgery, children should have a functioning, normal bowel. In those few instances in which the anus is deprived of nerve endings, a permanent colostomy may be established.

NURSING DIAGNOSES AND RELATED INTERVENTIONS

Nursing Diagnosis: Constipation related to reduced bowel function

Outcome Identification: Child will accomplish adequate bowel elimination with some adaptation until normal bowel function can be established.

Outcome Evaluation: Child has a daily bowel movement through either a colostomy or by enema.

Before surgery, the child may be prescribed daily enemas to achieve bowel movements. The fluid used for enemas must be normal saline (0.9% NaCl) and not tap water. Tap water is hypotonic. If it is instilled into the bowel, it moves rapidly across the intestine into interstitial and intravascular fluid compartments to equalize osmotic pressure (by the laws of osmosis, fluid moves from an area of less to greater concentration). This has led to death of infants from cardiac congestion or cerebral edema (water intoxication). Teach parents how to prepare and administer saline enemas at home. Parents can buy a ready-made saline preparation at a pharmacy, or they can prepare their own by mixing 2 tsp of noniodized salt to 1 quart of water. Although adding salt to water does not seem important, be certain that the parents understand the rationale for doing so and can demonstrate the proper technique and the proportion of salt to water for the enema.

Caring for a child with a colostomy is discussed in Chapter 36. Children may have an antibiotic solution or saline prescribed to be infused into the distal bowel to reduce the possibility of infection.

Nursing Diagnosis: Imbalanced nutrition, less than body requirements, related to reduced bowel function

Outcome Identification: Child will receive adequate nutrition during course of illness.

Outcome Evaluation: Child ingests a low-residue diet; weight follows a percentile curve on a growth chart.

Preoperatively, older children may be in poor physical health from poor food intake over a long period at the time the condition is diagnosed. If this is so, they may be returned home on a minimal-residue diet, stool softeners, vitamin supplements, and perhaps daily enemas until their condition improves. Total parenteral nutrition is helpful to offer another source of nutrition. If a child is to be cared for at home, help the parents learn about a minimal-residue diet (i.e., one that is low in undigestible fiber, connective fiber, and residue.) Fried foods and highly seasoned foods are omitted to eliminate chemical irritants from the intestinal tract.

Help parents to make out a reminder sheet for the stool softener so it is given daily. When children are beginning a special diet, it may be advisable to have parents refrain from introducing new feeding methods, such as a cup or spoon, unless children are at that developmental point where they will quickly adapt to the new procedure and are, in fact, so anxious to feed themselves that they will actually eat better this way.

Postoperatively, after removal of the aganglionic portion and anastomosis of the colon at the time of the second step of the repair, infants will return with a nasogastric tube in place attached to low suction, an IV infusion, and probably an indwelling urinary (Foley) catheter. Observe the infant for abdominal distention. Assess bowel sounds and observe also for passage of flatus and stools. As soon as peristalsis has returned (approximately 24 h after surgery), the nasogastric tube may be removed and children may be offered small, frequent feedings of fluids, such as water or gelatin. They are then introduced gradually to full fluids, a soft diet, then a minimal-residue diet, and, finally, a normal diet for age.

Nursing Diagnosis: Risk for compromised family coping related to chronic illness in child

Outcome Identification: Parents will demonstrate adequate coping behavior during course of child's illness.

Outcome Evaluation: Parents state they are able to cope with the level of stress present from their child's condition.

Most parents feel tremendous relief after the second-stage surgery is complete. Caution parents that children may still remain "fussy" eaters for a few months because feeding problems that begin for physical reasons can continue for emotional or psychologic reasons. Help parents to diminish the importance of meals gradually; to schedule periods during the day when they give their full attention to the child, such as reading a story or putting a puzzle together; and to offer praise for pleasant, not difficult, behavior. These measures will help mealtime problems gradually diminish.

Inflammatory Bowel Disease: Ulcerative Colitis and Crohn's Disease

Two conditions are categorized as inflammatory bowel disease: ulcerative colitis and Crohn's disease. They both involve the development of ulceration of the mucosa or submucosa layers of the colon and rectum. They both occur most frequently in young adults and adolescents, although, more and more frequently, symptoms first appear during school age. Both diseases occur most frequently in males than in females and show familial tendencies (Baldassano, 2000).

The causes of these disorders are obscure, but they probably represent an alteration in immune system response or are autoimmune processes. There is an increased number of immunoglobulins IgA and IgG present on intestinal mucosa. IgE immunoglobulins and the eosinophil count also may possibly be elevated. Psychologic factors have not been supported as a primary contributory factor to inflammatory bowel disease, but psychological problems often occur secondary to the disease, possibly intensifying symptoms. Smoking and frequent use of antibiotics or aspirin are correlated with the occurrence of Crohn's disease (Baldassano, 2000).

Crohn's disease is an inflammation of segments of the intestine, affecting any part of the GI tract, but most commonly the terminal ileum. Involved segments are separated by normal bowel tissue. The wall of the colon becomes thickened, and the surface is inflamed, leading to a "cobblestone" appearance of mucosa. Usually, the areas of the bowel affected are higher in the intestine than that which occurs with ulcerative colitis. In **ulcerative colitis,** typically the colon and rectum are involved, with the distal colon and rectum most severely affected, and inflammation involves continuous segments (Hyams, 2000).

As inflammation becomes acute with these disorders, children develop abdominal pain from contractions of the irritated portions. These areas do not absorb nutrients or fluid well, so diarrhea and malnutrition develop. To reduce abdominal pain (which is most acute after eating when the bowel becomes active), children begin to omit meals. They may be malnourished and have a vitamin or iron deficiency at the time the condition is diagnosed.

A number of complications may occur during the course of these diseases. Hemorrhage from bowel perforation during the active disease is a possibility. If perforation occurs, it can lead to peritonitis or the formation of fistulas between bowel loops. Rectal fistula is present in as many as 20% of children. A relapse is apt to occur 6 to 12 months after therapy. With ulcerative colitis, there is an association between the disease and bowel carcinoma if the disease persists over 10 years (Bliss & Sawchuk, 2001).

Assessment

Children develop diarrhea and steatorrhea from the irritation and the unabsorbed fluid from both conditions. If inflamed portions ulcerate, there will be blood in the stool. Weight loss occurs; growth failure occurs in prepubertal children. A recurring fever may be present (Table 45-6).

Diagnosis is established by colonoscopy and barium enema. On colonoscopy, the shallow ulcerations along the bowel can be seen; the mucosa is friable (easily irritated) and bleeds easily from inflammation. A biopsy may be performed for definite diagnosis. Observe children carefully after a bowel biopsy to detect rectal bleeding from an internal bleeding point (take blood pressure and pulse, and assess stool for occult blood).

Therapeutic Management

The child's bowel heals best if it is allowed to rest for a time. Enteral or total parenteral nutrition is usually provided for nutrition during the resting period. The child can remain home during this period as long as parents have thorough education about the child's care (see Chap. 36).

TABLE 45.6 Comparison of Crohn's Disease and Ulcerative Colitis

COMPARISON FACTOR	CROHN'S DISEASE	ULCERATIVE COLITIS
Part of bowel affected	Ileum	Colon and rectum
Nature of lesions	Intermittent	Continuous
Diarrhea	Moderate	Severe and bloody
Anorexia	Severe	Mild
Weight loss	Severe	Mild
Growth retardation	Marked	Mild
Anal and perianal lesions	Common	Rare
Association with carcinoma	Rare	Common

When food is reintroduced after the resting period, a high-protein, high-carbohydrate, high-vitamin diet is prescribed to replace nutrients. Children may eat cautiously at first to avoid reintroducing diarrhea; assess intake and output. An anti-inflammatory drug, such as prednisone (a corticosteroid), sulfasalazine (Azulfidine; a sulfonamide and salicylic acid), or azathioprine (Imuran; an immunosuppressive agent) generally brings about a great improvement in symptoms (see Focus on Pharmacology). If medical therapy is ineffective, bowel resection to remove a portion of the bowel (colectomy) followed by an ileoanal pull-through may be necessary. In some children, such a large portion of the bowel may be removed that a colostomy or a continent ileostomy needs to be constructed (for continent ileostomy, an internal reservoir is created by a section of bowel and emptied by insertion of a catheter; Fig. 45-9). Bowel surgery is a serious step for a child. Because it reduces the possibility of the child's developing intestinal cancer in association with ulcerative colitis, it may be necessary in children whose disease is running a long-term, debilitating course that does not improve.

NURSING DIAGNOSES AND RELATED INTERVENTIONS

Nursing Diagnosis: Imbalanced nutrition related to poor absorption because of disease process

Outcome Identification: Child will receive adequate nutrients during course of illness.

FOCUS ON PHARMACOLOGY

Sulfasalazine (Azulfidine)

Action: Sulfasalazine is a combination anti-inflammatory agent and antibiotic used to reduce the inflammation of ulcerative colitis and Crohn's disease

Pregnancy risk category: C (D at term)

Dosage: Varied, based on severity of illness, 20 to 75 mg/kg/day. Initially, 40 to 60 mg/kg/24 h orally in four to six divided doses in children older than age 2 years. Maintenance therapy usually 20 to 30 mg/kg/day in four equally divided doses.

Possible adverse effects: Sensitivity to sunlight; dizziness; drowsiness, nausea, abdominal pains, crystalluria, and hematuria

Nursing Implications

- Warn the parents and child that the drug may turn urine orange-red and soft contact lenses yellow.
- Advise children to take with or just after meals to avoid GI irritation.
- Ensure adequate fluid intake to avoid crystallization of sulfa component in urine.
- Anticipate prescription for folic acid concurrently. Drug decreases folic acid absorption.
- Instruct the child and parents about the need for using sunscreens and protective clothing while outside.

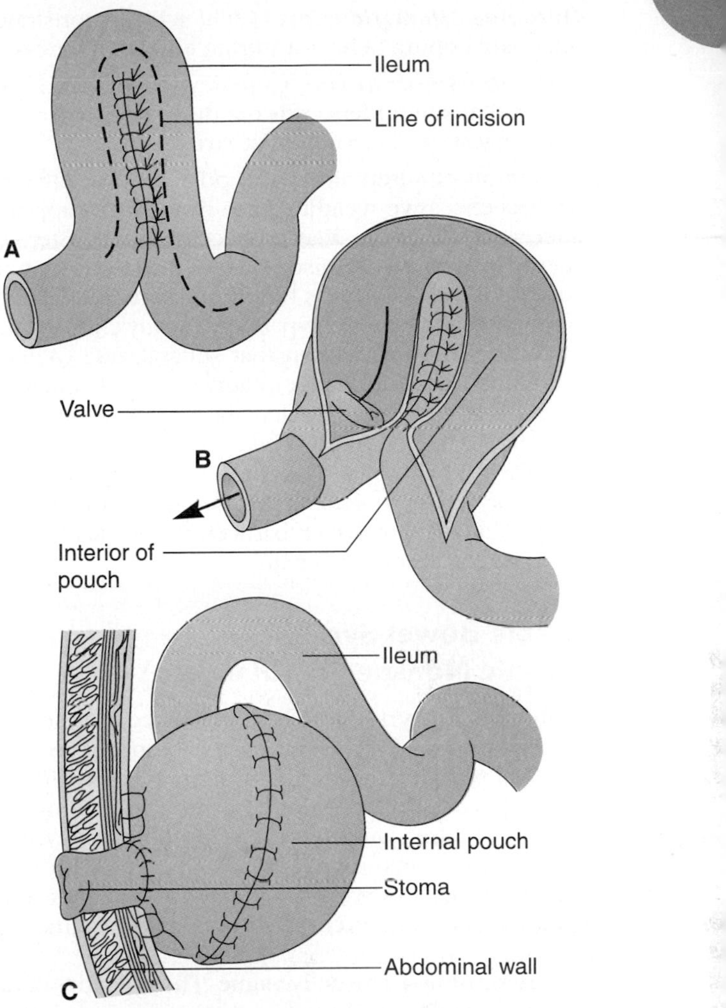

FIGURE 45.9 A continent ileostomy. (*A*) Segment of bowel is anastomosed. (*B*) Pouch for stool collection is formed. (*C*) Liquid stool is contained in pouch until drained by catheter.

Outcome Evaluation: Child's weight follows a percentile growth curve; urine specific gravity is 1.003 to 1.030. Child states that alternative feeding method is tolerable.

Nutrition must be a priority concern with both Crohn's disease and ulcerative colitis or malnutrition can occur from the combination of poor intestinal absorption and chronic diarrhea. Anorexia compounds the problem. Unless active steps are taken to replace nutrition, children with inflammatory bowel disease can be left both short in stature and light in weight. Protein, vitamin, fat, and mineral deficiencies all may occur.

When nutrition is supplied by enteral or total parenteral nutrition solutions, allowing the enteral infusion to flow during the night and removing the tube during the day can make feedings more tolerable. Remember that food provides social experiences as well as nutrition. Help parents provide opportunities for mealtime stimulation in other ways.

Nursing Diagnosis: Risk for ineffective coping related to chronic illness

Outcome Identification: Child will demonstrate adequate coping behavior during course of illness.

Outcome Evaluation: Child expresses feelings, voices that she understands the disease and therapy, and suggests ways to minimize stress.

Caution children about the possible side effects, such as excessive weight gain, a round facial appearance, and facial acne, that may occur if corticosteroid therapy, such as prednisone, is used so they are not surprised by this. Assess blood pressure, intake and output, weight, and sleep patterns for any child taking steroids. Caution children that sulfasalazine (Azulfidine) turns urine an orange-yellow so they do not mistake this color change as bleeding.

Provide time to listen so children have someone outside their family to talk to about their symptoms and family or stress problems. The disorder runs a chronic course and can involve embarrassing episodes of diarrhea or acute abdominal pain.

Irritable Bowel Syndrome (Chronic Nonspecific Diarrhea)

Irritable bowel syndrome is the presence of either intermittent episodes of loose and normal stools or recurrent abdominal pain. It appears slightly more often in girls than in boys. It is most often seen in infants 6 to 36 months of age. Most children outgrow the symptoms by 3 years of age. The cause is unknown, but it is associated with low fat intake (without fat slowing absorption, stool passes rapidly through the bowel). Excessive fluid intake also may play a role.

The symptoms are usually vague. The episodes of diarrhea may occur several times a week or as frequently as twice a day. There is seemingly no relationship to meals. Children are encouraged to eat a regular diet. Psyllium bulk agents will almost always reduce the frequency of symptoms.

Chronic Recurrent Abdominal Pain

A number of children develop episodes of recurring abdominal pain. Although such episodes can occur for reasons such as lactose intolerance or muscle strain from sports activities, in most instances, recurrent abdominal pain occurs for unknown reasons (Ashcraft, 2000). Children who experience this are commonly 6 or 7 years of age or in prepuberty (11 to 12 years of age). The pain is not accompanied by a change in bowel habits. There is no association with meals. Episodes of pain can last for only a few minutes or last for hours. The intensity of the pain is mild or "annoying" rather than severe. It is generally poorly localized, although children may point to the umbilicus as the primary site. On physical examination, there is no abdominal tenderness, distention, guarding, or muscle spasm.

Symptoms of stress such as sleep disturbances, fears, or eating problems may be present. A family history may indicate problems in the family such as marital discord, financial problems, or physical illness in parents or siblings.

Keep in mind that, although the cause of the pain cannot be identified, the pain is real. For some children, just having the opportunity to talk to an understanding person about the problem is all that is necessary to stop the attacks of pain. Other families need counseling regarding the underlying problem, such as allowing children to express their anger, reducing excessive demands on them, or giving them more attention through spending more time on activities with them. The family may need to be referred to a family service agency to secure more extensive counseling.

✔ CHECKPOINT QUESTIONS

24. What type of diet is usually ordered for the child with aganglionic megacolon?
25. What is the cause of inflammatory bowel disease?

DISORDERS CAUSED BY FOOD, VITAMIN, AND MINERAL DEFICIENCIES

There are many underfed and malnourished children in every part of the world. Although extreme diseases of food or vitamin deprivation are rare in the United States, they do exist. Such children need early identification so they can receive better nutrition before permanent damage occurs.

The average child does not develop a deficient intake of essential nutrients because, even if the child is occasionally a fussy eater, over 1 week, he or she does ingest foods containing the necessary nutrients. Always carefully assess any child who has an interference in nutrition such as a GI illness or the child placed on enteric feedings or total parenteral nutrition to see that nutrient deficiencies do not exist. Assess abused or neglected children closely for nutritional deficiencies because they may not have been given adequate food.

Kwashiorkor

Kwashiorkor is a disease caused by protein deficiency. It occurs most frequently in children ages 1 to 3 years because this age-group requires a high protein intake. It is a disease found almost exclusively in developing countries such as Africa, Asia, and Latin America, although it does occur in the United States (John-Kelly, 2000). It tends to occur after weaning, when children change from breast milk to a diet consisting mainly of carbohydrates. Growth failure is a major symptom. Because edema is also a symptom, however, children may not appear light in weight until the edema is relieved. There is a severe wasting of muscles, but, again, this is masked by the edema.

Edema results from hypoproteinemia, which causes a shift of body fluid from the intravascular compartments to the interstitial space, causing ascites (Fig. 45-10). This is the same phenomenon that causes extensive edema in children with nephrosis. The edema tends to be dependent, so it is first noted in children's lower extremities. Children are generally irritable and uninterested in their surroundings. They grow behind other children of the same age in motor development.

If children had a period of good protein intake, then poor protein intake, then good intake again, individual hair

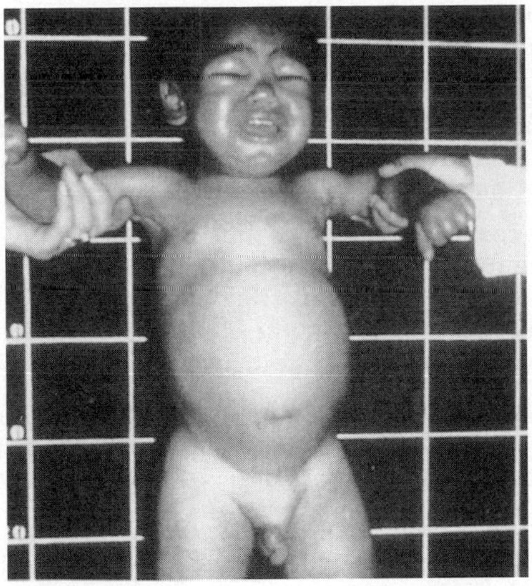

FIGURE 45.10 A child with kwashiorkor. Here the extensive generalized edema masks the severe muscle wasting. Notice the severe abdominal distention from ascites.

shafts develop a striped appearance of brown, then white, and so on—a zebra sign. Children also have diarrhea, iron-deficiency anemia, and hepatomegaly.

Without treatment, kwashiorkor is fatal. For therapy, a diet rich in protein is essential. Even so, there is evidence to suggest that protein malnutrition early in life, even if corrected later, may result in failure of children to reach their full potential of intellectual and psychological development (John-Kelly, 2000).

Nutritional Marasmus

Nutritional marasmus is a disease caused by deficiency of all food groups, basically a form of starvation. Although it is seen most commonly in developing countries where food supplies are short, it is seen in grossly neglected children or those with failure to thrive in the United States. These children are most commonly younger than 1 year of age. They have many of the same symptoms as children with kwashiorkor, including growth failure, muscle wasting, irritability, iron-deficiency anemia, and diarrhea. Whereas children with kwashiorkor are anorectic, children with nutritional marasmus are invariably hungry (starving) and will suck at any object offered them, such as a finger or their clothing. Treatment is to supply children with a diet rich in all nutrients (see Chap. 55).

Vitamin and Mineral Deficiencies

Both vitamin and mineral deficiencies occur at a low rate in children of the United States because so many foods are enriched (restoration of ingredients removed by processing) or fortified (additional vitamins and minerals not normally present added). Milk, for example, is fortified with vitamins D and A. Orange juice is fortified with calcium. White bread is enriched with B vitamins. Vitamin deficiency diseases are summarized in Table 45-7.

Iodine Deficiency

Because iodine is not supplemented in food except as iodized salt, a diet deficient in iodine may lead to hyperplasia of the thyroid gland (*goiter*) or hypothyroidism. In

TABLE 45.7 Vitamin Deficiency Disorders

VITAMIN	CAUSE OF DEFICIENCY	SIGNS AND SYMPTOMS
Vitamin A	Lack of yellow vegetables in diet	Tender tongue; cracks at corners of mouth Night blindness **Xerophthalmia** (dry and lusterless conjunctivae of the eye) **Keratomalacia** (necrosis of the cornea with perforation, loss of ocular fluid, and blindness)
Vitamin B_1	Most common in children who eat polished rice as dietary staple, because B_1 is contained in hull of rice.	**Beriberi** (tingling and numbness of extremities; heart palpitations; exhaustion) Diarrhea and vomiting Aphonia (cry without sound) Anesthesia of feet
Niacin	Commonly in children who eat corn as dietary staple, because corn is low in niacin.	**Pellagra** (dermatitis; resembles a sunburn) Diarrhea Mental confusion (dementia)
Vitamin C	Lack of fresh fruits in diet	**Scurvy** (muscle tenderness; petecchiae)
Vitamin D	Lack of sunlight	Poor muscle tone; delayed tooth formation. **Rickets** (poor bone formation) Craniotabes (softening of the skull) Swelling at joints, particularly of wrists and cartilage of ribs Bowed legs Tetany

the United States, areas where goiter is endemic are mainly the states bordering Canada, especially the Great Lakes area, and those states between the Rocky Mountains and the Appalachians (Dudek, 2001). When the thyroid gland does not have adequate iodine to make thyroxine, its chief hormone, the gland is overstimulated by the pituitary gland, ultimately leading to the hyperplasia. Goiter tends to occur most commonly in girls at puberty and during pregnancy. An enlarged thyroid gland may lead to difficulty breathing.

Supplemental iodine or synthetic thyroxine (Synthroid) is needed. Children must also be maintained on a diet adequate in iodine, found most abundantly in seafood (Dudek, 2001).

✔ CHECKPOINT QUESTIONS

26. What nutrient does the child with kwashiorkor lack?
27. Lack of vitamin D prevents adsorption of which mineral?

KEY POINTS

Children with GI disorders need to join the family for mealtime if possible. Even if they cannot eat the same foods as other family members, they benefit from the social interaction.

Some GI disorders lead to long-term therapies such as colostomy or gastrostomy feedings. Because these disorders interfere with common body functions such as eating and elimination, they are difficult for children to accept without the support of concerned health care providers.

Remember that children lose proportionately more fluid with vomiting and diarrhea than adults do. For this reason, they need rapid assessment and interventions to avoid dehydration.

Fluid, electrolyte, and acid–base imbalances tend to occur rapidly with vomiting and diarrhea. Vomiting leads to alkalosis. Diarrhea leads to acidosis.

GI disorders almost always interfere with nutrition to some degree. This is a greater problem in children than adults because children need to ingest adequate nutrients and fluid daily for growth as well as body maintenance.

Gastroesophageal reflux (achalasia) is a neuromuscular disturbance in which the cardiac sphincter is lax, allowing for easy regurgitation of gastric contents into the esophagus. It is treated by feeding a thickened formula and keeping the infant upright after feedings.

Pyloric stenosis is hypertrophy of the valve between the stomach and duodenum. It impedes the passage of feedings leading to vomiting.

Peptic ulcer disease may occur in young children. This is a shallow excavation formed in the mucosal wall of the stomach. It is treated, like adult ulcers, with antibiotics and agents to suppress gastric acidity.

Forms of hepatitis seen in children include hepatitis A and C (caused usually by eating contaminated shellfish) and hepatitis B, D, and E (caused by contaminated blood or placental spread).

Congenital obstruction of the bile ducts occurs from failure of the bile duct to recanalize in utero. This can lead to fibrotic scarring of the liver (cirrhosis). Most of these children need a liver transplantation to restore liver function.

Intussusception is the invagination of one portion of the intestine into another. Volvulus is twisting of intestine. Both may lead to bowel obstruction.

Necrotizing enterocolitis is the development of necrotic patches on the intestine. It occurs almost exclusively in immature infants.

Appendicitis is inflammation of the appendix. It is always an emergency situation and is the most common cause of abdominal surgery in children. Laparoscopy is done to remove the appendix before it ruptures.

Celiac disease (gluten-induced enteropathy) is a change in the ability of the intestinal villi to absorb. It is apparently a dominantly inherited illness.

A number of hernias such as inguinal and hiatal hernia can occur in children. These are surgically corrected when recognized.

Hirschsprung's disease (aganglionic megacolon) is absence of ganglionic innervation in a section of the lower bowel. The therapy is possibly a temporary colostomy followed by surgery in 6 to 12 months to remove the affected portion.

Inflammatory bowel disease can occur as either ulcerative colitis or Crohn's disease. Therapy is long-term. If medical therapy is unsuccessful, children may have portions of their bowel surgically removed to relieve these conditions.

Kwashiorkor (protein deficiency), nutritional marasmus (starvation), vitamins A and D (rickets), B_1 (beriberi), and C (scurvy) deficiencies or iodine deficiencies occur in children when they are not provided or cannot absorb adequate nutrients. Although associated with developing countries, they can occur in a child in any community.

CRITICAL THINKING EXERCISES

1. Barry is the 2-year-old boy you met at the beginning of the chapter. He was diagnosed as having celiac disease. When you met him, his mother was insisting that he eat a piece of birthday cake. What health education does his mother need to help her

choose a better diet for her son? What would have been a better food, probably available at a birthday party, that he could have eaten?

2. An 8-month-old girl is seen in a hospital emergency department with severe diarrhea. What emergency interventions does she need to prevent an electrolyte or fluid imbalance? What measures could you take to reduce her fear of the strange hospital environment?
3. A 12-year-old child with Crohn's disease is being cared for at home with total parenteral nutrition. How can you help him keep pace with his friends at school? How can you help him maintain a sense of high self-esteem in light of many hospitalizations and home care?
4. A 4-year-old girl is being transferred to a distant city to have a liver transplantation because of congenital biliary atresia. Her parents ask you what they can expect at the distant hospital. How would you prepare them for this?
5. Examine the National Health Goals related to GI disorders. Most government-sponsored money for nursing research is allotted based on these goals. What would be a possible research topic to explore pertinent to these goals that would be both fundable and would advance evidence-based practice?

REFERENCES

Armon, K., et al. (2001). An evidence and consensus based guideline for acute diarrhoea management. *Archives of Disease in Childhood, 85*(2), 132–141.

Ashcraft, K. W. (2000). Consultation with the specialist: Acute abdominal pain. *Pediatrics in Review, 21*(11), 363–367.

Baldassano, R. N. (2000). Crohn disease. In M. W. Schwartz (Ed.). *The 5-minute pediatric consult* (pp. 290–291). Philadelphia: Lippincott Williams & Wilkins.

Bliss, D. Z., & Sawchuk, L. (2001). Lower gastrointestinal problems. In S. M. Lewis et al. (Eds.). *Medical-surgical nursing* (pp. 1136–1190). St. Louis: Mosby.

Campbell, D. A., et al. (2001). Transplantation and immunology: Hepatic transplantation. In W. W. Hay, A. R. Hayward, M. J. Levin & J. M. Sondheimer (Eds.). *Current pediatric diagnosis and treatment* (15th ed.). New York: McGraw-Hill.

D'Agostino, J. (2002). Common abdominal emergencies in children. *Emergency Medicine Clinics of North America, 20*(1), 139–153.

Dennehy, P. H., & Bresee, J. S. (2001). Rotavirus vaccine and intussusception. *Infectious Disease Clinics of North America, 15*(1), 189–207.

Department of Health and Human Services. (2000). *Healthy people 2010.* Washington, DC: DHHS.

Dudek, S. G. (2001). *Nutrition. Essentials for nursing practice* (4th ed.). Philadelphia: Lippincott Williams & Wilkins.

Ford, D. M. (2001). Fluid, electrolyte & acid-base disorders & therapy. In W. W. Hay, A. R. Hayward, M. J. Levin & J. M. Sondheimer (Eds.). *Current pediatric diagnosis and treatment* (15th ed.). New York, NY: McGraw-Hill.

Gauderer, M. W., et al. (2001). Acute appendicitis in children: The importance of family history. *Journal of Pediatric Surgery, 36*(8), 1214–1217.

Guerrero, R. A., & Cavender, C. P. (1999). Constipation: Physical and psychological sequelae. *Pediatric Annals, 28*(5), 312–316.

Gwynn, L. K. (2001). The diagnosis of acute appendicitis: Clinical assessment versus computed tomography evaluation. *Journal of Emergency Medicine, 21*(2), 119–123.

Haber, B. (2000). Biliary atresia. In M. W. Schwartz (Ed.). *The 5-minute pediatric consult* (pp. 180–181). Philadelphia: Lippincott Williams & Wilkins.

Hassall, E. (2001). Guidelines for approaching suspected peptic ulcer disease or *Helicobacter pylori* infection: Where we are in pediatrics and how we got there. *Journal of Pediatric Gastroenterology and Nutrition, 32*(4), 405–406.

Hyams, J. S. (2000). Inflammatory bowel disease. *Pediatrics in Review, 21*(9), 291–295.

John-Kelly, H. A. (2000). Kwashiorkor. In M. W. Schwartz (Ed.). *The 5-minute pediatric consult* (pp. 496–497). Philadelphia: Lippincott Williams & Wilkins.

John-Kelly, H. A., & Mulberg, A. E. (2000). Hirschsprung disease. In M. W. Schwartz (Ed.). *The 5 minute pediatric consult* (pp. 434–435). Philadelphia: Lippincott Williams & Wilkins.

Loh, M., et al. (2001). Outcome of very premature infants with necrotising enterocolitis cared for in centers with or without on site surgical facilities. *Archives of Disease in Childhood, 85*(2), 114–118.

Mackey, J., et al. (2001). Frequency of celiac disease in individuals with Down syndrome in the United States. *Clinical Pediatrics, 40*(5), 249–252.

Mahon, B. E., et al. (2001). Maternal and infant use of erythromycin and other macrolide antibiotics as risk factors for infantile hypertrophic pyloric stenosis. *The Journal of Pediatrics, 139*(3), 380–384.

McCance, K. L., & Huether, S. E. (2002). *Pathophysiology* (4th ed.). St. Louis: Mosby.

Moss, R. L., et al. (2001). A meta-analysis of peritoneal drainage versus laparotomy for perforated necrotising enterocolitis. *Journal of Pediatric Surgery, 36*(8), 1210–1213.

Mulberg, A. E. (2000). Volvulus. In M. W. Schwartz (Ed.). *The 5-minute pediatric consult* (pp. 870–871). Philadelphia: Lippincott Williams & Wilkins.

Olsen, S. J., et al. (2001). The changing epidemiology of salmonella: Trends in serotypes isolated from humans in the United States. *Journal of Infectious Diseases, 183*(5), 753–761.

Osterhoudt, K. E. (2000). Salmonella infections. In M. W. Schwartz (Ed.). *The 5-minute pediatric consult* (pp. 722–723). Philadelphia: Lippincott Williams & Wilkins.

Parker, P. H. (1999). To do or not to do? That is the question. *Pediatric Annals, 28*(5), 283–291.

Patti, M. G., et al. (2001). Laparoscopic Heller myotomy and Dor fundoplication for esophageal achalasia in children. *Journal of Pediatric Surgery, 36*(8), 1248–1251.

Schier, F. (2000). Direct inguinal hernias in children: Laparoscopic aspects. *Pediatric Surgery International, 16*(8), 562–564.

Schmidt, R. M., & Middleman, A. B. (2001). The importance of hepatitis B vaccination among adolescents. *Journal of Adolescent Health, 29*(3), 217–222.

Semeao, E., & Mulberg, A. E. (2000). Acute diarrhea. In M. W. Schwartz (Ed.). *The 5-minute pediatric consult* (pp. 326–327). Philadelphia: Lippincott Williams & Wilkins.

Senyuz, O. F., et al. (2001). Sugiura procedure in portal hypertensive children. *Journal of Hepato-Biliary-Pancreatic Surgery, 8*(3), 245–249.

Sokol, R. J., & Narkewicz, M. R. (2001). Liver & pancreas. In W. W. Hay, A. R. Hayward, M. J. Levin & J. M.

Sondheimer (Eds.). *Current pediatric diagnosis and treatment* (15th ed.). New York: McGraw-Hill.

Sondheimer, J. (2001a). Gastrointestinal tract. In W. W. Hay, A. R. Hayward, M. J. Levin & J. M. Sondheimer (Eds.). *Current pediatric diagnosis and treatment* (15th ed.). New York: McGraw-Hill.

Sondheimer, J. M. (2001b). Vomiting in children. In W. W. Hay, A. R. Hayward, M. J. Levin & J. M. Sondheimer (Eds.). *Current pediatric diagnosis and treatment* (15th ed.). New York: McGraw-Hill.

Thilo, E. H., & Rosenberg, A. A. (2001). Gastrointestinal & abdominal surgical conditions in the newborn infant. In W. W. Hay, A. R. Hayward, M. J. Levin & J. M. Sondheimer (Eds.). *Current pediatric diagnosis and treatment* (15th ed.). New York: McGraw-Hill.

Tung, J. (2000). Viral hepatitis. In M. W. Schwartz (Ed.). *The 5-minute pediatric consult* (pp. 868–869). Philadelphia: Lippincott Williams & Wilkins.

Van Damme, P., & Van der Wielen, M. (2001). Combining hepatitis A and B vaccination in children and adolescents. *Vaccine, 19*(17–19), 2407–2412.

SUGGESTED READINGS

Arguedas, M. R., & Fallon, M. B. (2001). Prevention in liver disease. *American Journal of Medical Science, 321*(2), 145–151.

Balling, K., & McCubbin, M. (2001). Hospitalized children with chronic illness: Parental caregiving needs and valuing parental expertise. *Journal of Pediatric Nursing, 16*(2), 110–119.

Campo, J. V., et al. (2001). Adult outcomes of pediatric recurrent abdominal pain: Do they just grow out of it? *Pediatrics, 108*(1), E1–E5.

Caplan, M. S., & Jilling, T. (2001). New concepts in necrotising enterocolitis. *Current Opinion in Pediatrics, 13*(2), 111–115.

Carney, D. E. & Meguid, M. M. (2002). Current concepts in nutritional assessment. *Archives of Surgery, 137*(1), 42–45.

Cheng, W., et al. (2001). Hirschsprung's disease: A more generalized neuropathy? *Journal of Pediatric Surgery, 36*(2), 296–300.

Christensen, J., & Miftakhov, R. (2001). Hiatus hernia: A review of evidence for its origin in esophageal longitudinal muscle dysfunction. *American Journal of Medicine, 108*(54A), 3S–7S.

Davis, R. L., et al. (2001). Measles-mumps-rubella and other measles-containing vaccines do not increase the risk for inflammatory bowel disease. *Archives of Pediatrics & Adolescent Medicine, 155*(3), 354–359.

DeLucas, C., et al. (2000). Transpyloric enteral nutrition reduces the complication rate and cost in the critically ill child. *Journal of Pediatric Gastroenterology and Nutrition, 30*(2), 175–180.

Jonas, M. M. (2000). Viral hepatitis: From prevention to antivirals. *Clinics in Liver Disease, 4*(4), 849–877.

Jordan, P. H. (2001). Long term results of esophageal myotomy for achalasia. *Journal of the American College of Surgeons, 193*(2), 137–145.

Kolsteren, M. M., et al. (2001). Health-related quality of life in children with celiac disease. *Journal of Pediatrics, 138*(4), 593–595.

Lacy, B. E., & Rosemore, J. (2001). *Helicobacter pylori* ulcers and more: The beginning of an era. *Journal of Nutrition, 131*(10), 2789S–2793S.

Lee, A. C., Munro, F. D., & MacKinlay, G. A. (2001). An audit of post-pyloromyotomy feeding regimens. *European Journal of Pediatric Surgery, 11*(1), 12–14.

Lobritto, S. J. (2001). Endoscopic considerations in children. *Gastrointestinal Endoscopy Clinics of North America, 11*(1), 93–109.

Martucciello, G., et al. (2000). Pathogenesis of Hirschsprung's disease. *Journal of Pediatric Surgery, 35*(7), 1017–1025.

Pineiro-Carrero, V. M., et al. (2001). Etiology and treatment of achalasia in the pediatric age group. *Gastrointestinal Endoscopy Clinics of North America, 11*(2), 387–408.

Reid, J. R., et al. (2000). The barium enema in constipation: Comparison with rectal manometry and biopsy to exclude Hirschsprung's disease after the neonatal period. *Pediatric Radiology, 30*(10), 681–684.

Seid, M., et al. (2001). Correlates of vaccination for hepatitis B among adolescents: Results from a parent survey. *Archives of Pediatrics & Adolescent Medicine, 155*(8), 921–926.

Shulman, R. J. (2000). New developments in total parenteral nutrition for children. *Current Gastroenterology Reports, 2*(3), 253–258.

Tiao, M. M., et al. (2001). Sonographic features of small-bowel intussusception in pediatric patients. *Academic Emergency Medicine, 8*(4), 368–373.

46

CHAPTER

Nursing Care of the Child With a Renal or Urinary Tract Disorder

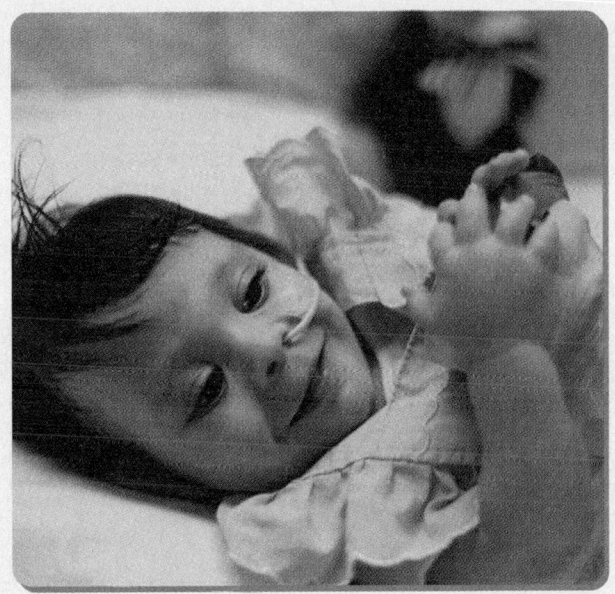

Key Terms

- acute transplant rejection
- Alport's syndrome
- azotemia
- Bowman's capsule
- dialysis
- enuresis
- epispadias
- exstrophy of the bladder
- glomerular filtration rate
- glomerulonephritis
- hydronephrosis
- hypospadias
- nephrosis
- patent urachus
- polycystic kidney
- postural proteinuria
- prune-belly syndrome
- vesicoureteral reflux

Objectives

After mastering the contents of this chapter, you should be able to:

1. Describe common renal and urinary disorders that occur in children.
2. Assess a child for a renal or urinary tract disorder.
3. Formulate nursing diagnoses related to renal or urinary disorders.
4. Establish outcomes related to the care of a child with a renal or urinary disorder.
5. Plan nursing care related to urinary or renal disorders.
6. Implement nursing care for the child with a renal or urinary disorder.
7. Evaluate outcomes for achievement and effectiveness of care.
8. Identify National Health Goals related to renal or urinary tract disorders and children that nurses can be instrumental in helping the nation achieve.
9. Identify areas related to care of the child with a renal or urinary disorder that would benefit from additional nursing research or application of evidence-based practice.
10. Analyze methods for making nursing care of the child with a renal or urinary disorder more family centered.
11. Integrate knowledge of renal and urinary tract disorders with the nursing process to achieve quality maternal and child health nursing care.

Carol is a 4-year-old girl admitted to the hospital with nephrotic syndrome. She has marked ascites and edema. "I kept asking everyone how she could be gaining so much weight, yet she doesn't eat anything," her parent tells you. "My aunt said this happened because Carol drank part of a beer I left on the coffee table. I didn't give her the beer, she just picked it up and drank it. Do you think that's what caused it? What if she needs a kidney transplant? Will I be allowed to give my kidney for that?"

How would you answer Carol's mother? What information does she need to better understand her child's condition?

Previous chapters described the growth and development of well children and the nursing care of children with disorders of other systems. This chapter adds information about the dramatic changes, both physical and psychosocial, that occur when children develop urinary tract or renal disorders. This is important information because it builds a base for care and health teaching.

After you've studied the chapter, answer the Critical Thinking Exercises at the end of the chapter and then access the on-line study activities (http://connection.lww.com) *to further sharpen your skills and test your knowledge.*

Normally, the urinary system maintains the proper balance of fluid (water) and electrolytes in the blood. When disease occurs, such as with structural abnormalities or kidney malfunction, a child may be left with excessive amounts of fluid in the body or with an imbalance of electrolytes and other substances essential to the body's functioning. Disorders involving the kidneys and urinary tract often are long term. Any urinary tract disorder can ultimately (if not originally) affect the kidneys, resulting in kidney dysfunction with potentially fatal consequences.

Unfortunately, because symptoms may be vague, or because the child or parents do not realize the seriousness of urinary disease or are embarrassed to discuss it, children may not be evaluated at the first sign of illness.

Health education to increase awareness of the symptoms of urinary tract and kidney disorders is an important area of family health teaching. National Health Goals related to renal or urinary tract disorders and children are shown in the Focus on National Health Goals box.

FOCUS ON NATIONAL HEALTH GOALS

Renal disease can lead to long-term illness so preventing it is important to improving the health of the nation. The following National Health Goals address this:

- Reduce the rate of new cases of end-stage renal disease from a baseline of 289/million population to a target rate of 217/million population.
- Increase the proportion of patients with treated chronic kidney failure who receive a transplant within 3 years of registration on waiting list from a baseline of 41/1,000 to 51/1,000 (DHHS, 2000).

Nurses can be instrumental in helping the nation achieve these goals by educating parents to give antibiotics conscientiously for streptococcal throat infections and being active advocates for organ transplant procedures.

Areas that would benefit from nursing research could include: determining parents' or children's ability to accurately self-assess for proteinuria after streptococcal infections, identifying the specific needs of children on ambulatory peritoneal dialysis, designing ways to make low-potassium diets more appealing to children with end-stage renal disease, or designing ways that organ donation can be presented to make it more appealing to potential donors.

NURSING PROCESS OVERVIEW

For Care of the Child With a Renal or Urinary Tract Disorder

Assessment

Because the symptoms of many urinary tract and renal disorders (e.g., mild abdominal pain, slowly growing edema, or low-grade fever) are subtle, parents may not bring their child for evaluation as early in the disease as they might if symptoms were more definite. School nurses can play an important role in recognizing the seriousness of minor symptoms and making proper referrals for care.

Common findings from a health history and physical examination are shown in Assessing the Child for Renal and Urinary Tract Dysfunction. The hallmark of kidney or bladder infection is pain. If children have had bladder surgery, they also may experience pain on urination or pain from bladder spasms. Be sure to assess the degree of pain, including its location and intensity, before administering an analgesic or antispasmodic. Urine specimens also provide very valuable assessment information. Techniques for obtaining urine samples (i.e., clean-catch, catheterization, 24-h collections, suprapubic aspiration, and urinalysis) are described in Chapter 36.

Nursing Diagnosis

Examples of nursing diagnoses for children with urinary tract or renal disorders may include the following:

- Pain related to effects of urinary tract infection
- Excess fluid volume related to decreased kidney function and fluid accumulation
- Fear related to outcome of kidney transplantation
- Imbalanced nutrition, less than body requirements, related to effects of dietary restrictions
- Social isolation related to immunosuppressant therapy
- Risk for injury related to body's inability to excrete waste products properly

Because the entire family becomes involved in long-term renal disease, other appropriate nursing diagnoses may include:

ASSESSING the Child for Renal and Urinary Tract Dysfunction

History

Chief concern: Child reports burning or cries on urination; blood or "dark" urine, frequency of urination; abdominal pain, flank pain, enuresis. Parents report increase in size of abdomen, periorbital edema, poor appetite, frequent thirst, weight gain, strong odor to urine; diaper rash in infants. A school-age child may be described as a behavior problem because he or she frequently asks to use the bathroom.
Family history: History of renal disease, such as polycystic kidney, enuresis; hypertension.
Pregnancy history: Exposure to nephrotoxic drugs (antibiotics) during pregnancy. Oligohydramnios at birth.
Past illness history: Child recently had a throat or skin infection.

Physical assessment

General appearance
Fatigue, paleness
Growth retardation
Low-grade temperature

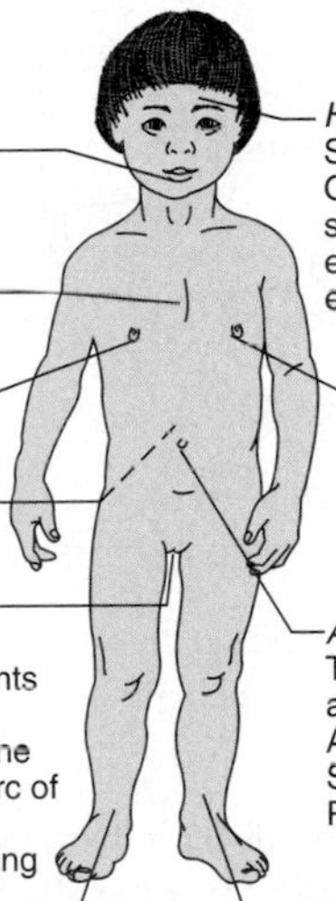

Mouth
Pale mucous membrane, caries

Cardiovascular
Hypertension

Respiratory
Rapid respirations

Back
Pain over kidney area

Genitals
Reddened urethra
Diaper area rash in infants
Round urethra in males
Constant dripping of urine
A stronger than usual arc of urine in males
Displaced urethra opening

Skin
Poor skin turgor
White crystals on skin
Edema

Head
Swelling around eyes
Odd facies; beaklike nose, small chin, prominent epicanthal folds, low-set ears

Chest
Gynecomastia

Abdomen
Tenderness over bladder area
Abdominal mass
Slack abdominal muscles
Protuberant abdomen

Extremities
Bowed legs

Neurologic
Confusion, muscle twitching

- Interrupted family processes related to the effects and stresses of the child's chronic illness
- Compromised family coping related to the chronicity of the child's illness

Outcome Identification and Planning

Be certain that outcomes established for care are relevant to the child's age and condition. Because renal disease may become chronic, outcomes need to be modified frequently to meet changing needs.

Planning for the child with a urinary tract or renal disorder often involves helping parents plan how to remember to give medicine. The child with nephrotic syndrome, for example, may take three or four different types of medicine every day at home. Be certain that parents understand the types of medicine they are being asked to administer and the expected action of each. School-age children need a schedule that allows them to take medicine before they leave home in the morning or after they return in the afternoon. Some schools allow medications to be given during school hours. In these cases, an order from the prescriber and the reason for the medication are required.

If a child has severe renal impairment, parents may be asked to make decisions regarding kidney removal and transplantation. Be sure to provide them with ample time for discussion. If a kidney donor is sought among relatives, the parents must help decide whether the person whose tissue matches the child's really wants to donate a kidney or is being pressured to do so. Helping parents to schedule times for hemodialysis or peritoneal dialysis or to supervise continuous ambulatory peritoneal dialysis (CAPD), to care for their other children, and to provide a life apart from their child requires nursing planning. Investigate possible community sources for additional family support.

Implementation

Parents may or may not understand the function of the urinary system because it is not a system that receives much discussion. For example, they may confuse the words ureter and urethra. You can play a major role as a resource person, explaining anatomy, and tests and procedures including the reason they are being done.

Many children with kidney disease take steroids and develop a typical cushingoid appearance. They may have edema or ascites, which makes them appear obese. The child may be teased or criticized by some classmates because of the "different" appearance. Contacting the school nurse or making the reason for the child's appearance known to the child's teacher may be necessary to help minimize this. Frequent contact and discussion with the child's siblings are important in helping them to understand the reason for so many tests and health care visits and why this one child in the family is receiving so much attention. It also aids in opening up the channels of communication with all members of the family.

Referrals to support organizations may be helpful. Organizations that can be of help may include the following:

National Kidney Foundation (*www.kidney.org*)
Kidney Dialysis Foundation (*www.kdf.org*)

If kidney damage is extensive and the child's kidneys fail or a transplant is rejected, nursing care needs to be refocused on assisting the family facing the possibility of the child's death. Nursing interventions can begin to prepare the child, parents, and family for this event (see Chap. 56).

Outcome Evaluation

Children with urinary or renal disease often need follow-up care after their acute illness. Because they are followed by a specialty renal group or clinic, parents may assume that routine health maintenance care is being given as well. Check to see that children are receiving their routine childhood immunizations (remember that children on steroid or other immunosuppressive therapy should not receive live virus immunizations) and that parents have their questions about day-to-day childrearing concerns answered.

Children returning to health care agencies for reevaluation usually need as much preparation for procedures as those having them for the first time. Memory blurs events and sometimes confuses children. For example, they may recall that a particular test involved an injection when it did not, worrying needlessly unless their memories are refreshed. Parents wait anxiously for the results of reevaluation studies. Work to ensure that they are given test results as soon as a comprehensive opinion of the child's progress is available. Be sure that all involved are aware of how anxious a particular parent is to hear the results of the reevaluation.

Examples suggesting achievement of outcomes might include the following:

- Child reports pain is controlled and decreasing in intensity after treatment.
- Family states they are able to cope with long-term illness in child.
- Child states the value of a low-sodium diet and lists the ingredients of a low-sodium meal.
- Child states she can accept the necessity of kidney transplantation.
- Child states the necessary precautions he must follow to reduce possibility of infection while on immunosuppressive therapy.
- Child remains free of any signs and symptoms of complications related to accumulated waste products.

ANATOMY AND PHYSIOLOGY OF THE KIDNEYS

Embryonic development of the urinary tract is discussed in Chapter 8. Figure 46-1 identifies the structures of the tract.

Kidneys are more susceptible to trauma in children than in adults, because they are located slightly lower in relation to the ribs than in adults. They also do not have as much perinephric fat to pad them.

Nephron

A *nephron,* the functioning unit of the kidney, is comprised of a glomerulus (a filtrating unit) and a complex set of tubules with accompanying blood supply (Fig. 46-2).

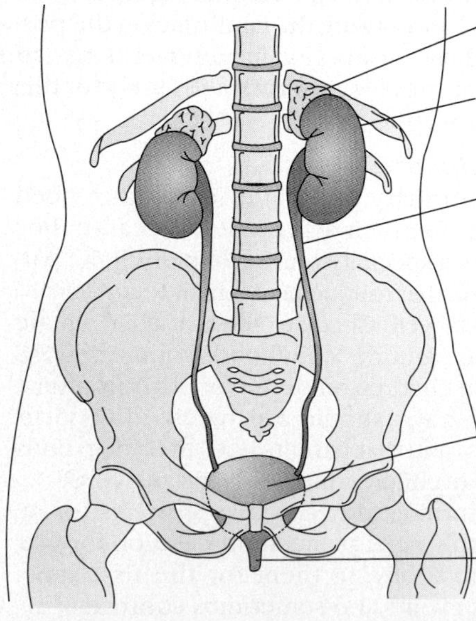

FIGURE 46.1 The urinary system.

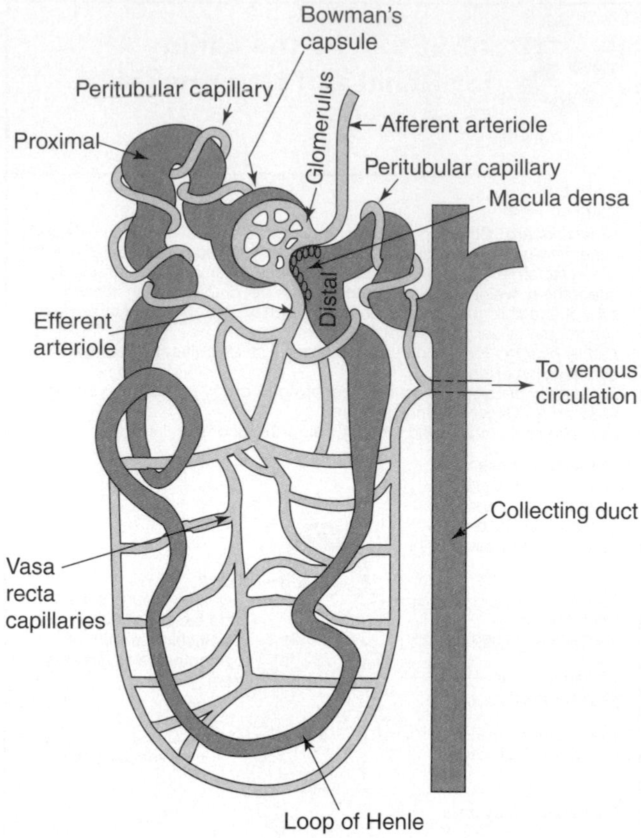

FIGURE 46.2 Basic structure of a nephron with its accompanying blood vessels.

Enclosed by a double-walled chamber, called a **Bowman's capsule,** the *glomerulus* is a capillary tuft supplied by a large afferent (ingoing) and a small efferent (outgoing) arteriole. It is invaginated within a tubule with a proximal and distal portion. In the glomerulus, water and solutes are filtered from the blood. This passage of water and solutes from the blood into the glomeruli is effective only as long as the blood pressure in glomerular arteries exceeds that in the tubule. The smaller efferent arteriole causes back pressure in the glomerular arterioles, increasing the existing pressure and allowing filtration to occur readily. If blood pressure in these arterioles should fall below the tubular pressure or the tubular pressure should rise above that of the arterioles, little or no filtration will occur. For this reason, renal function must be assessed carefully in children who are hemorrhaging or are in shock with lowered blood pressure for any reason.

The solution that filtered into the tubule passes through the proximal portion, the loop of Henle, and then the distal portion. Beginning with the loop of Henle, water and electrolytes diffuse back into blood capillaries, reducing the vol- ume of the filtrate by approximately 90%.

The glomerular filtrate enters the proximal tubule at a rate of approximately 120 mL/min. So much water is reabsorbed that the final end product (urine) left in the tubule is excreted at a rate of only approximately 1 mL/min. The proximal portion of the tubules reabsorbs most of the water, glucose, sodium chloride, phosphate (PO_4^-), sulfate (SO_4^-), and some bicarbonate (HCO_3^-) ions. This is a passive process, not particularly affected by body needs. The distal portion of the tubules responds selectively to body needs. If necessary, Na^+ and HCO_3^- ions and additional water are reabsorbed. The functions of nephron structures are summarized in Table 46-1.

Urine

The amount of urine excreted in a 24-h period depends on fluid intake, state of kidney health, and age. Approximate urine output from different age-groups is shown in Table 46-2. A significant decrease in urine production is termed *oliguria;* absence of urine production is *anuria.*

When renal disease occurs, and glomerular or tubular function becomes impaired, nonprotein nitrogenous substances such as creatinine, urea, ammonia, and purine bodies are retained in the blood rather than being excreted. Urea is formed from the breakdown of amino acids by the liver. Measuring the amount of urea in urine indirectly measures kidney and liver function (Ford, 2001).

Creatinine is a product released during muscle cell metabolism. The concentration in urine remains constant, regardless of the amount of protein in the diet or body processes. Its presence or amount, therefore, can be used when comparing urine specimens. When kidney function is impaired, not only are substances retained, but some constituents that normally are retained will be allowed to enter the urine. These include albumin, glucose, blood, bile pigments, and casts. Bile pigments appear in the urine when the child has elevated levels of indirect or direct bilirubin in the blood plasma (hemolysis of red blood cells and obstructed jaundice will cause this). Bile pigments stain urine a greenish yellow-brown color. Casts are formed when there is an abnormal condition that causes the kidney tubule to become lined with protein formed from red and white blood cells, epithelial cells, or fatty cells that hardens into the shape of the tubule. After urine washes the casts out, they can be detected by microscopic examination of urine. As protein only deposits in this way when fluid is slow moving, their presence suggests slow filtration. Normal constituents of urine are shown in Table 46-3.

> ✔ **CHECKPOINT QUESTIONS**
>
> 1. What is the major functioning unit of the kidney?
> 2. What substance in urine remains constant regardless of protein intake?

ASSESSMENT OF RENAL AND URINARY TRACT DYSFUNCTION

Laboratory/Diagnostic Tests

A variety of diagnostic tests may be performed, either in an ambulatory department or on an inpatient basis, to document renal or urinary tract disease (see Focus on Cultural Competence).

Urinalysis

One of the most revealing tests of kidney function is also one of the simplest: urinalysis. For best results, specimens collected should be fresh because urine that stands at room temperature for any length of time changes composition. Devices used to collect urine specimens and the method for obtaining urine specimens from diapers are described in Chapter 36. A chemical reagent strip can be used to detect glucose, protein, and occult blood and to measure pH (see Focus on Multidisciplinary Care). Specific gravity is best determined by use of a refractometer (requires only a single drop [see Chap. 36]).

Creatinine Clearance Rate

Glomerular filtration rate is the rate at which substances are filtered from the blood to the urine. It is measured by the amount of creatinine (the breakdown product of creatine from muscle contraction) excreted in 24 h as determined by a 24-h urine sample. This is known as a creatinine clearance test. A venous blood sample is taken during the 24-h period and compared with the urine findings. A normal creatinine clearance rate is 100 mL/min. A normal urine creatinine level is 0.7 to 1.5 mg/100 mL; serum creatinine rarely exceeds 1 mg/dL (Lum, 2001).

Radioisotope Scanning

The administration of radioisotopes (a technetium scan) also may be used to assess glomeruli filtration ability. Radioactively tagged substances are given intravenously (IV); the rate at which these substances can be observed flowing through the kidney and excreted in urine is then scanned. Parents and the child can be assured that the level of radioisotopes used in these studies is small, and urinating removes the substance from the body immediately afterward. Thus, parents do not need to feel that children remain

TABLE 46.1 Functions of the Nephron

SITE	ACTIVITY
Glomerulus	Secretion of water and all solutes except protein from blood
Proximal convoluted tubule	Reabsorption of 80% of glomerular filtrated water, all of glucose amino acids, vitamins, and proteins; most of sodium, chloride, and ascorbic acid; secretion of creatinine
Descending and ascending loop of Henle	Reabsorption of additional water; fluid becomes neutral in reaction; specific gravity 1.010; additional reabsorption of sodium and chloride
Distal convoluted tubule	Reabsorption of water, sodium, chloride, phosphate, and sulfate as needed; secretion of potassium, H^+ ions, and ammonia (secretion of NH_4^+ and H^+ ions conserves base because H^+ ions are substituted for sodium ions; sodium is reabsorbed as sodium bicarbonate)

TABLE 46.2 Child's Average Urine Output in 24 Hours

AGE	AMOUNT OF URINE (mL)
6 mo–2 yr	540–600
2–5 yr	500–780
5–8 yr	600–1,200
8–14 yr	1,000–1,500
Over 14 yr	1,500

radioactive. They should not be afraid to stay near them or, with infants, to hold them after such a study.

Urine Culture

The presence of urinary tract infection (UTI), the presence of bacteria in urine, is established by urine culture. Because bladder catheterization can introduce bacteria into the bladder and also is painful and intrusive, most urine specimens in children are obtained by a clean-catch procedure or sterile suprapubic aspiration (see Chap. 36).

TABLE 46.3 Normal Urinalysis Findings

ASSESSMENT	NORMAL FINDING	DESCRIPTION/IMPLICATIONS
Color	Pale yellow	Color is influenced by urine concentration and ingredients; if fresh blood is present, urine may be red; if old blood, it may be brown or black.
Appearance	Clear	Bacteria, excessive crystals, or cells cause cloudiness; if protein content is high, it foams like beer when it is poured.
pH	4.6–8.0	Urine becomes alkaline (pH more than 7) with urinary tract infection or severe alkalosis; urine left at room temperature becomes alkaline.
Specific gravity	1.003–1.030	Specific gravity is elevated in dehydration as kidneys try to conserve fluid, and decreased in overhydration as they try to rid the body of fluid.
Protein	0	Due to inflammation, protein molecules pass into urine; in adolescent girls, protein in urine may occur as a result of pregnancy; some children have *orthostatic proteinuria,* slight to mild proteinuria occurring only when they are standing.
Ketones	0	Ketones are released after breakdown of body protein, because of starvation.
Glucose	0	Glucose in urine occurs most frequently as a symptom of diabetes mellitus; in adolescent girls, glucosuria may occur with pregnancy.
Red blood cells	Less than 1 per high-power field Negative on dipstick	Blood may be present in urine as a result of such diseases as glomerulonephritis, urinary tract infection, or trauma; may also suggest systemic diseases such as leukemia or blood dyscrasias.
White blood cells	Less than 5 per high-power field	White blood cells are round, small configurations on a microscopic slide; they are present with bacteriuria.
Casts	0	Casts (protein configurations) are found most often in concentrated urine specimens; with cast formation, there is invariably proteinuria; casts comprise red blood cells, white blood cells, or desquamated renal epithelium; as an epithelial cast moves along the nephron, the cells begin to disintegrate, leaving a coarse granular cast; some disintegrate still further to become fine granular casts. The last stage of the process is a configuration in the shape of the tubule, termed a *waxy cast* (translucent and may be shiny and reflect light). The stage of the cast is important in indicating the flow of urine through the kidney. Hyaline casts are formations of protein appearing dull and reflecting light poorly; fatty casts are casts caused by the degeneration of tubular epithelial cells and are found in children with nephrosis. Red blood cells, white blood cells, and fatty casts are evidence of disease; other casts suggest urine stasis and probably proteinuria.
Crystals	Possibly present or not	Crystal formation is possibly indication of urine pH; uric acid, cystine, and calcium oxalate crystals are examples of crystals found in acid urine; phosphate crystals tend to be present in alkaline urine. Infection (particularly *Proteus* infection) is the most usual cause of alkaline urine. Sulfur crystals may be present if the child is receiving a sulfa drug (such as sulfamethoxazole [Gantanol]).

FOCUS ON CULTURAL COMPETENCE

The ease with which parents and children are able to discuss illnesses of the kidneys or urinary tract is culturally influenced. As a general rule, because elimination functions are typically regarded as private, this is not a body system that people discuss as comfortably as they do illnesses of other body systems. The more that modesty is stressed in a culture, the more difficult it may be for people to ask questions about kidney or urinary tract disorders. As a result, parents may wait to bring a child in to be evaluated. By being aware that this is a difficult area for parents to discuss, health care personnel can observe whether added health education is needed when caring for a child with one of these disorders.

A number of instant-read commercial kits for culturing urine are available for use in ambulatory settings.

Blood Studies

A blood urea nitrogen (BUN) test measures the level of urea in blood and, therefore, is a test of glomerular function, or how well the kidneys can clear this from the bloodstream. However, this level may not increase until approximately 50% of glomeruli are destroyed, because the remaining glomeruli are able to increase in size and function to accommodate urine production. A normal value is 5 to 20 mg/100 mL.

Sonography and Magnetic Resonance Imaging

A *sonogram* or *magnetic resonance imaging (MRI)* will detect differing sizes of kidneys or ureters and will differentiate between solid or cystic kidney masses. Parents can be assured that these techniques do not use x-rays, and so may be repeated at frequent intervals for follow-up without danger of radiation exposure to their child.

FOCUS ON MULTIDISCIPLINARY CARE

Many different disciplines can be involved in the care of a child with a urinary tract or renal disorder. A nutritionist may meet with the parents and child to plan a sodium-restricted or low-phosphorus diet. A nurse practitioner skilled in ambulatory peritoneal dialysis may talk to parents and the child about ways to incorporate this procedure into the family's lifestyle. Both physicians and nurses will be involved in helping the child and family maintain a long-term medication program. Unlicensed assistive personnel may be the individuals asked to collect and test urine specimens for substances such as glucose or protein. Be certain they understand how important these measurements are so that they perform them accurately. Recognizing protein present with such a test is often the first indication that a child has a serious renal disorder.

Computed Tomography

Computed tomography (CT) scans of the kidneys are used to show the size and density of kidney structures and adequacy of urine flow. Conscious sedation may be given before a CT scan because the child must lie still for an extended time during the procedure, and the size of a CT scanner and the fact that it surrounds the child may be frightening. Be sure to prepare the child for this. A contrast medium may be injected before the procedure to better outline urine flow. If this medium is iodine based, be certain to ask about allergy to iodine before the study. Because a support person is not allowed to remain in the room during the procedure, be certain to thoroughly prepare children so they can comfortably handle the procedure by themselves.

X-ray Studies

A plain flat-plate abdominal x-ray film can provide information about the size and contour of the kidneys. A small kidney shown this way is generally a hypoplastic or an underdeveloped organ. A large kidney may indicate hydronephrosis or a polycystic kidney. Such an x-ray may be referred to as a *KUB: kidney, ureters,* and *bladder*.

Intravenous Pyelogram. An *intravenous pyelogram (IVP)* is an x-ray study of the upper urinary tract. A radiopaque dye is injected into a peripheral vein, circulates through the bloodstream, and is almost immediately identified as a foreign substance by the kidney and filtered out into the urine by the glomeruli. X-ray films taken at frequent intervals show the outline of collecting systems in the kidney and of the ureters as the radiopaque dye passes through them.

In preparing children for an IVP, tell them that they will receive an injection. Say "medicine," not "dye" (or compare coloring kidneys to coloring with crayons or coloring Easter eggs) to help children not mistake "dye" for "die." Be sure children know that, after this injection, they must lie still in whatever position they are placed until all films are taken. This may be difficult for young children because x-ray tables are hard and cold and the x-ray camera overhead can be frightening. When explaining the test, compare x-ray machines to cameras to reduce possible fear. Warn children that they may experience flushing of the face, warmth, and a salty taste in their mouth after the injection of dye. Because the dye used is iodine based, ask the parents if the child has a known allergy to iodine. This is rarely known in children, because they may have had no previous studies of this kind.

Voiding Cystourethrogram. A *voiding cystourethrogram (VCUG)*, a study of the lower urinary tract, reveals the structure of the urethra and bladder and the presence of reflux into the ureters. For this test, after bladder catheterization, a radiopaque dye is injected into the bladder, and the catheter is then removed. The child is asked to void into a bedpan while serial x-ray films are taken. Although the catheterization is unpleasant, being asked to void while they are observed on the x-ray table is the most stressful part of the procedure for the majority of children because they have been taught that voiding is a private act. Children need to be told in advance that they will be asked to do this as a necessary part of the study. Caution children that a first voiding this way after catheterization may be painful. A few children have difficulty voiding a second time later in the day because they worry that the second voiding will also sting. Pouring warm water over the perineal area while sitting on the toilet or sitting in a bathtub of warm water and voiding into the water may help relieve pain. Most children, once they void this second time and realize that it is not painful, usually have no further difficulty.

A VCUG should not be done if the child has an active UTI because there is danger that the radiopaque material injected into the bladder could spread, carrying bacteria with it from the infection into the ureters and kidneys. Report any symptoms of UTI such as frequency, pain on voiding, or low back pain to the radiologic physician. A clean-catch urine specimen for culture may be ordered before the VCUG to rule out infection.

Cystoscopy

Cystoscopy, examination of the bladder and ureter openings by direct examination with a cystoscope introduced through the urethra, is done to evaluate for possible vesicoureteral reflux or urethral stenosis. Radiopaque dye may be introduced into the bladder at the time of cystoscopy so the bladder can be visualized on x-ray (cystography). Small catheters also can be threaded into the ureters for the introduction of dye to outline them (retrograde pyelography). Because the procedure is painful and requires the child to lie still for the procedure, it is usually done under conscious sedation. After the procedure, the first voiding may be painful. Once allowed, urge the child to drink plenty of fluids so he or she urinates frequently to flush out any possible pathogens introduced at the time of the procedure.

Renal Biopsy

Renal biopsy, which involves passing a thin biopsy needle into the kidney through the skin over the kidney, is used to diagnose the extent of renal disease and thereby predict disease outcome or progress or beginning rejection of a transplanted kidney. Renal biopsy may be done in the older child under only a local anesthetic. Conscious sedation may be necessary for the younger child who cannot cooperate easily. The kidney is located first by sonogram to accurately locate the place of the biopsy. The child lies prone with a sandbag under the abdomen for firmness. If the procedure is done under a local anesthetic, prepare children for the feel of a pinprick as the local anesthetic is injected; after this, they should not feel any further pain. What they may feel is pressure as the biopsy needle is inserted. Caution children that they need to lie still while the biopsy specimen is taken (if the child moved suddenly, the needle might puncture a renal artery or vein or tear vital glomeruli). Be certain children have support people to accompany them for this procedure so that they have someone to hold their hand or comfort them during the time they feel the pressure of the needle.

After the biopsy, press a sterile gauze square against the biopsy site for approximately 15 min to halt bleeding. Follow this with the application of a pressure dressing. Caution parents that a large dressing will be used and that the size of this dressing does not reflect the size of the specimen taken (the amount of tissue removed is no more than the lumen of the needle used or approximately the size of a pencil lead).

If the procedure was done on an ambulatory basis, children can be discharged 2 to 4 h after the procedure if vital signs are stable and they have voided. This first voiding after renal biopsy is invariably blood-tinged. Advise parents to keep children on restricted activity for 24 h or until no more hematuria is present. Instruct parents how to keep serial urine samples, comparing each specimen with the previous one, to detect whether hematuria is becoming more or less marked. When urine no longer appears bloody, teach them to test it for occult blood to confirm that bleeding has completely stopped.

Measure vital signs and observe the biopsy site every 15 min for at least the first hour. Do not lift the dressing to assess bleeding because doing so destroys the protective function of the pressure dressing. Encourage children to drink a considerable amount of fluid (a glass every hour while awake) during the first 24 h to keep urine flowing freely and prevent blood from clotting in the kidney tubules and blocking urine flow. Play games with a child, if necessary, to encourage a high fluid intake (the child must take a drink each time before his or her turn at a game; play "Simon Says" and have Simon frequently say, "Drink").

A hematocrit may be ordered 24 h after the procedure to provide additional proof that no bleeding is continuing.

✔ CHECKPOINT QUESTIONS

3. Which diagnostic test establishes that a UTI is present?
4. Why is voiding cystoscopy a difficult test for many children?

THERAPEUTIC MEASURES FOR THE MANAGEMENT OF RENAL DISEASE

When kidney function deteriorates, some method to replace kidney function must be instituted.

Peritoneal Dialysis

Dialysis is the separation and removal of solutes from body fluid by diffusion through a semipermeable membrane. *Peritoneal dialysis* uses the membrane of the peritoneal cavity to do this. The technique has the advantage over hemodialysis of not requiring elaborate equipment or expense. It has the disadvantage of requiring more time than hemodialysis.

Peritoneal dialysis may be used as a temporary measure for children who experience sudden renal failure caused by trauma or shock. It is used for fairly long periods with children with chronic renal disease both in the hospital or at home to allow them to live until a kidney transplantation can be arranged. It is usually begun when the serum creatinine level reaches 10 mg/100 mL. Other indications are congestive heart failure, BUN of more than 100 mg/100 mL, hyperkalemia (potassium of more than 6 mEq/L), and uremic encephalopathy (confusion or coma). *Continuous cycling peritoneal dialysis* allows the procedure to be done at home because less close monitoring of the procedure is necessary.

Method for Performing Peritoneal Dialysis

Before peritoneal dialysis begins, a child's weight and vital signs are obtained to provide baseline information. Ask the child to void to reduce bladder size so that the bladder occupies as little anterior space as possible. If a child cannot void, catheterization may be necessary. The child's abdomen is cleaned just below the umbilicus with an antiseptic solution and covered with a sterile drape; a local anesthetic is injected into the abdominal wall, and a large-bore needle is inserted into the peritoneal cavity. If ascites fluid is present, a quantity of this fluid is removed and then a warmed hypertonic glucose solution (approximately 50 to 100 mL/kg of body weight) or a commercial dialysis solution is infused by gravity flow into the peritoneal cavity. This distends the abdominal wall and allows insertion of a peritoneal catheter, which is sutured in place and covered with a sterile dressing (Fig. 46-3). This catheter will remain in place for the period of dialysis.

A prescribed amount of dialysis solution is then infused into the peritoneal cavity by gravity drainage. This takes approximately 10 min and is recorded as inflow time. Be certain that the infusion fluid is warmed to room temperature to prevent the child from becoming chilled; moreover, warming the solution to near body temperature appears to improve diffusion efficiency. It can be warmed in a basin of warm water or with the use of commercial warm packs at the child's bedside. Heparin is generally added at least to the first infusion to keep any blood from the abdominal puncture from plugging the tube.

Infused fluid is allowed to remain in the child's peritoneal cavity for 15 to 60 min (called the *equilibrium or dwell time*). Because the infused solution is hypertonic, fluid from extracellular spaces diffuses across the semipermeable peritoneal membrane to dilute the hypertonic solution. Urea and electrolytes diffuse with this fluid. After this designated equilibrium time, allow the fluid to drain from the peritoneal catheter into a collecting bottle (this takes approximately 10 min and is recorded as outflow time). More fluid generally drains from the peritoneal cavity than was infused, because excessive fluid has diffused across the peritoneum, reducing peritoneal or ascitic fluid. After a cycle of inflow, equilibrium, and outflow time, a new cycle is begun. Peritoneal dialysis may be conducted continuously for periods of 12 to 72 h, depending on the effectiveness of the procedure in restoring the serum creatinine and BUN levels to normal.

Monitor vital signs at least every hour while children are undergoing peritoneal dialysis. During each new infusion period and during the time the solution is in the abdomen, carefully observe for shortness of breath because the fluid exerts upward pressure on the diaphragm. Elevating the head of the bed helps to increase breathing space and ease respirations. If tachycardia or hypotension occurs, hypovolemia may be present. An increasing temperature (after 24 h) may indicate peritoneal infection, a serious complication. Frequent blood studies are necessary during periods of peritoneal dialysis to determine electrolyte concentrations. If electrolyte imbalances occur, electrolytes may be added to the infusion solution or administered IV.

The longer the peritoneal catheter remains in place, the greater the risk of peritoneal infection from the catheter insertion site (Verrina et al., 2000). Assess the insertion site daily for signs of infection, such as redness or drainage. Obtain temperature about every 4 h. Ask children to report any abdominal pain or diarrhea. Assess for abdominal guarding or tenderness once daily by palpating their abdomen. A rigid abdomen suggest peritonitis or infection. Follow the agency's policy for cleaning and covering the end of the peritoneal catheter (Fig. 46-4).

As for any procedure, children need to be well prepared for peritoneal dialysis. If the procedure is presented in a matter-of-fact way, children usually accept it with no more apprehension than IV therapy. Both procedures involve a needle penetration. Children can be assured that they will

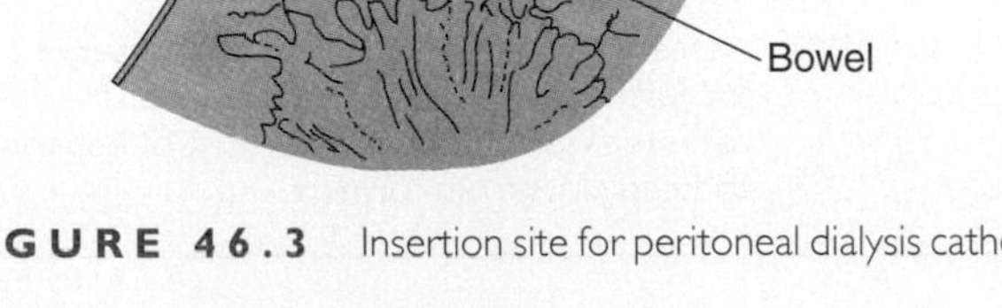

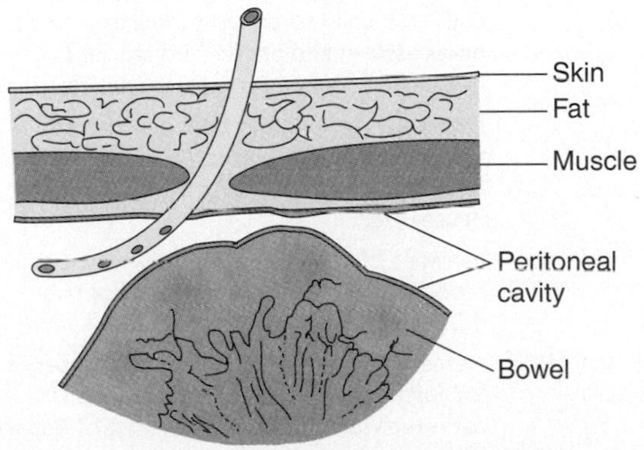

FIGURE 46.3 Insertion site for peritoneal dialysis catheter.

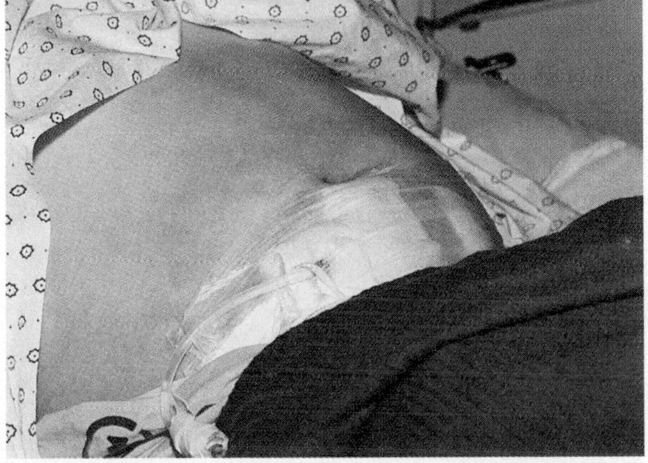

FIGURE 46.4 Peritoneal catheter inserted into a child's abdomen. A secure dressing surrounds the insertion site to prevent infection.

feel the initial prick of the needle that administers the local anesthetic and they will feel pressure after that as the peritoneal needle or catheter is inserted. It is intrusive, however, and frightening. Provide opportunities for therapeutic play (e.g., use a cloth doll, a dialysis tube, IV tubing, a doll's bed, or syringes and needles).

Once cycles of dialysis begin, children often grow bored lying in bed waiting for this procedure to be finished. They need planned interaction for these times—perhaps a toy or game that is allowed only during the procedure, so that it remains special. Children generally do not feel hungry while having peritoneal dialysis, because the bulk of peritoneal fluid causes pressure on the stomach and makes them feel uncomfortably full. They do well on a liquid diet or small frequent feedings during this time. So that children can feel that they have a sense of control over what is happening, let them help with the procedure by doing such things as recording the amount of solution infused and drained, and allowing them to select liquids they like for meals.

Peritoneal dialysis is a simple yet important concept. Help parents understand its importance so they can demonstrate a positive attitude toward it. The parents' acceptance of the procedure helps the child to accept it positively also.

Continuous Ambulatory Peritoneal Dialysis

Continuous ambulatory peritoneal dialysis (CAPD) allows a child to go to school or participate in other activities while receiving dialysis. With CAPD, a permanent dialysis catheter is inserted and sutured into place on the abdomen. Each day, the child or parent attaches a bag of dialysis fluid and tubing to this and infuses a prescribed dialysis solution by gravity drainage; the bag and tubing are then rolled into a compact square and carried with the child. The infused solution remains in the child for 4 to 6 h during the day (8 h at night); the dialysate bag is then lowered and the solution drains from the peritoneal cavity into it; the bag and fluid are then discarded and a new bag of dialysate solution is attached and raised and new solution is infused.

CAPD requires careful monitoring and attention by the child or family. The parent or child must keep accurate records of infusions. Children can participate in gym programs but should not participate in contact sports or swimming. Teach parents to think ahead for holidays or family trips so they don't run short of supplies at these times.

Because CAPD is continuous, electrolytes in the bloodstream are maintained at more constant levels than when intermittent dialysis is used. CAPD also allows greater freedom because children can return home and go back to school. There are disadvantages, however. Infection can occur because of the long-term placement of the catheter. Dehydration or hypernatremia may occur because of excess fluid removal. Because the tube remains in place at all times and the peritoneal solution constantly distends the abdomen, making the child appear obese and clothing difficult to fit, the child is frequently reminded of the illness and may have difficulty accepting this change in body image. Possible complications of CAPD are listed in Table 46-4.

Hemodialysis

Hemodialysis removes body wastes by using an external membrane as the diffusion surface. For hemodialysis, a catheter is inserted into an artery and blood is removed from the child and circulated through a dialysis coil. Urea

TABLE 46.4 Possible Complications of CAPD

ASSESSMENT	PROBLEM	INTERVENTIONS
Redness or pain or swelling at tubing insertion	Infection	Take culture at site; administer antibiotics as prescribed; continue site care as ordered; notify physician.
Abdominal pain, increased temperature, nausea and vomiting, cloudy return in drainage solution	Peritonitis	Notify physician; administer antibiotics as prescribed; auscultate for bowel sounds.
Cramps as fluid is infused	Irritation of peritoneal cavity	Infuse solutions more slowly; warm temperature of solution to body temperature.
Difficulty with infusion or drainage of fluid	Kinked or clotted tubing; malpositioned catheter	Assess tubing for kinking; change position of child; ask child to cough to increase abdominal pressure; add prescribed amount of heparin to dialysate bag (prevents clotting).
Weight increase; moist cough, shortness of breath	Fluid overload	Decrease sodium and fluid oral intake; assess blood pressure and weight; use 4.25% exchange solution until weight is again decreased.
Weight loss, hypotension, poor skin turgor, tachycardia	Fluid loss	Increase fluid and sodium intake; assess blood pressure and weight; do not use 4.25% solution.
Blood-tinged dialysis return	Ruptured blood vessel	Assess pulse and blood pressure; observe for further bleeding in drainage; flush catheter with prescribed amount of heparin to keep clots from forming.

and electrolytes in the blood diffuse into the surrounding fluid bath as the blood passes through the coil. After diffusion is complete, the blood is returned to the child's venous circulation (Fig. 46-5).

Hemodialysis can be done as a continuous process, but it is so effective that 3 h of hemodialysis accomplishes as much as 12 h of peritoneal dialysis. Children who have renal failure or whose kidneys have been removed can be maintained almost indefinitely by hemodialysis sessions two or three times a week or by continuous ultrafiltration or continuous arteriovenous hemofiltration (Gong et al., 2001). To establish a site for blood removal, children may have a double-lumen central catheter inserted into a central vein, such as the subclavian or internal jugular vein.

A permanent technique is subcutaneous anastomosis of a vein and artery creating an arteriovenous fistula (usually the brachial artery and brachiocephalic vein; Fig. 46-6*A*) or internal anastomosis of the artery and vein using a subcutaneous graft (Fig. 46-6*B*). The possibility of infection is reduced with this method, although, unfortunately, two venipunctures, one from a low point in the shunt to remove blood and one high in the shunt to return it, are necessary for dialysis (use lidocaine or EMLA cream first to reduce pain). The ability to feel a thrill (vibration) or hear a bruit over the fistula or graft site is proof that it is open.

The risks of hemodialysis include infection introduced with venipuncture (severe because the infection automatically is septicemia) and clotting of the access site, which can lead to emboli. During hemodialysis, children may begin to show signs of confusion, vomiting, visual blurring, or hallucinations from a *dialysis disequilibrium syndrome.* This occurs because the hemodialysis is removing urea from the blood at too rapid a rate—faster than urea can be shifted from the brain to the blood. This causes fluid to shift into the brain, resulting in cerebral edema. The procedure must be temporarily halted to allow equalization to return. Muscle cramping may occur from sodium depletion. A "first use" syndrome (i.e., dizziness or muscle cramping) may occur from a reaction to the fibers in the dialysis machine coil.

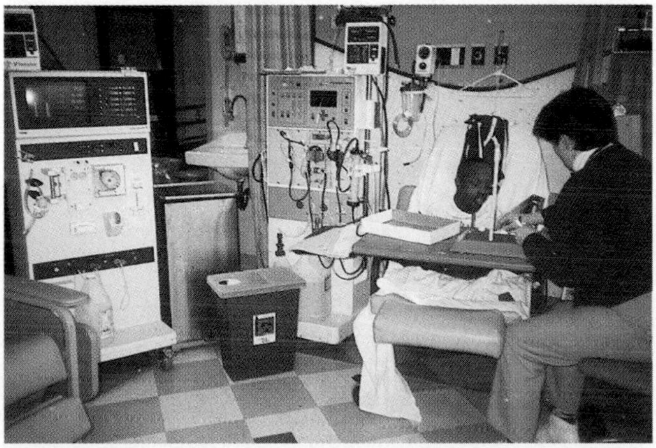

FIGURE 46.5 An adolescent receiving hemodialysis. A catheter from the child is connected to the hemodialysis equipment (in the background). Blood flows from the child through the catheter to the hemodialysis equipment for waste removal and is then returned to the child's venous circulation.

Children grow bored during hemodialysis as they do during peritoneal dialysis. They need entertainment provided for them so the procedure remains acceptable. Help parents provide stimulating activities such as a play board, a ball to throw, or rings to stack for the infant. Parents may envision the infant as so ill that lying still without an activity would be the best for him or her. Children need stimulation and play to avoid missing normal developmental milestones even during a long therapy such as dialysis.

When children's kidneys are removed and they must remain on a continuous program of hemodialysis, they may come to resent a machine as "owning" or "controlling" them. They become aware that they cannot exist apart from it. Planning special activities to do during hemodialysis time helps to give them a feeling of control (Haffner & Schurman, 2001).

HEALTH PROMOTION AND RISK MANAGEMENT

A number of important interventions can help prevent urinary and renal disease in children. First of these is the prevention of UTI in girls by educating them about perineal hygiene measures from the time they are first toilet-trained. Second is educating parents about the importance of giving the full course of antibiotic prescription for UTI to prevent reinfection. Also important is educating parents about the importance of giving the full course of antibiotic after a streptococcal infection to prevent acute glomerulonephritis.

Teach parents to recognize the normal appearance of urine (clear and yellow) so that they can recognize abnormalities, such as red, black, or cloudy urine. Also teach parents about the signs and symptoms of UTI, such as urgency, frequency, and pain. Additionally, remind them of the simple measures such as not allowing children to bathe with bubble bath as a means to prevent UTI.

WHAT IF? What if a parent telephones you and says her child is voiding black urine? Is there a possibility this is blood? What questions would you ask to elicit additional information? What recommendations would you make to the mother?

STRUCTURAL ABNORMALITIES OF THE URINARY TRACT

Patent Urachus

When a bladder first forms in utero, it is joined to the umbilicus by a narrow tube, the *urachus.* When this fails to close properly during embryologic development, a fistula is left between the bladder and umbilicus (**patent urachus**). This occurs more commonly in males than in females. Nurses are frequently the ones to discover this condition as they notice clear fluid draining from the base of the umbilical cord while changing newborn diapers. If the fluid is tested with Nitrazine paper for pH, its acid content will identify it as urine. A sonogram will confirm the patent connection is present.

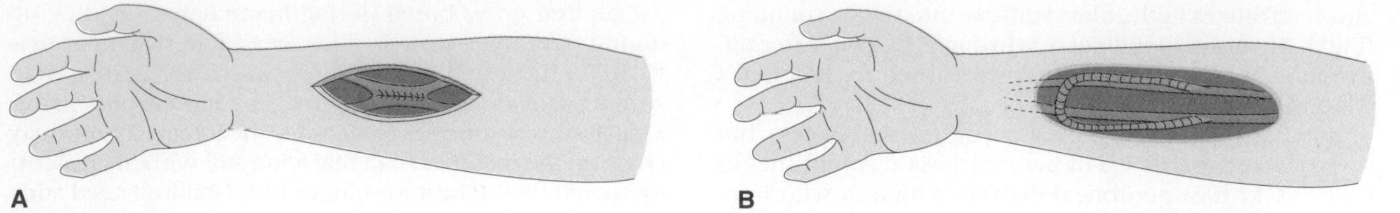

A B

FIGURE 46.6 (*A*) An internal arteriovenous fistula. (*B*) An internal arteriovenous graft.

A few patent urachus abnormalities heal spontaneously. Most require surgical correction to prevent pathogens from entering the fistula site and causing persistent bladder infection. This can be done in the immediate neonatal period using only a small subumbilical incision.

Exstrophy of the Bladder

Exstrophy of the bladder is a midline closure defect that occurs during the embryonic period of gestation (first 8 weeks). As a result, the bladder lies open and exposed on the abdomen. It occurs more frequently in males than females at a ratio of 2:1 (Master, 2000a).

Assessment

Exstrophy can be revealed by fetal sonogram. With the condition, there is no anterior wall of the bladder and no anterior skin covering on the lower anterior abdomen (Fig. 46-7*A*). The bladder appears bright red and continually drains urine from the open surface. In females, the urethra may also be abnormally formed. In males, the penis is often unformed or malformed. Pelvic bone defects, particularly nonclosure of the pubic arch, and urethral defects such as **epispadias**—opening of the urinary meatus on the dorsal or superior surface of the penis—may be present. The skin around the bladder quickly becomes excoriated because of constant exposure to acid urine. Untreated bladder exstrophy leads to kidney infection from ascending organisms. When children with this disorder begin to walk, they may demonstrate a "waddling" gait from the effect of the nonfused pubic arch.

Therapeutic Management

The treatment of bladder exstrophy begins with surgical closure of the bladder and, if necessary, the anterior abdominal wall with construction of a urethra (see Fig. 46-7*B*). Surgical repair may be limited if inadequate bladder tissue is present. For this reason, in some instances, the bladder is surgically removed, and a ureterocecal implantation (ureters directed into the small intestine) or a *continent urinary reservoir* (an artificial bladder) is constructed (Fig. 46-8; Master, 2000a).

To construct a continent urinary reservoir, a small segment of the intestine, usually the cecum, is separated from the intestinal tract. The intestinal tract is then anastomosed so that a normal gastrointestinal (GI) tract is maintained. The separated segment is attached to the internal abdominal wall using the appendix to create an artificial urethra. The ureters are anastomosed to this segment.

Urine drains from the kidneys into the ureters, and then into the collecting bowel segment. The parent or child catheterizes the abdominal urethra three or four times daily to empty urine. The procedure is theoretically simple, but it is technically difficult to accomplish. Parents need a good review of anatomy to aid their understanding of the procedure. As the child reaches school age and begins school activities, such as showering, that expose the condition to others, adjusting to a continent urinary reservoir can be difficult. Ensure that the child has a plan for follow-up care during the school years and in adolescence so the function of the reservoir and also the child's adjustment can continue to be assessed.

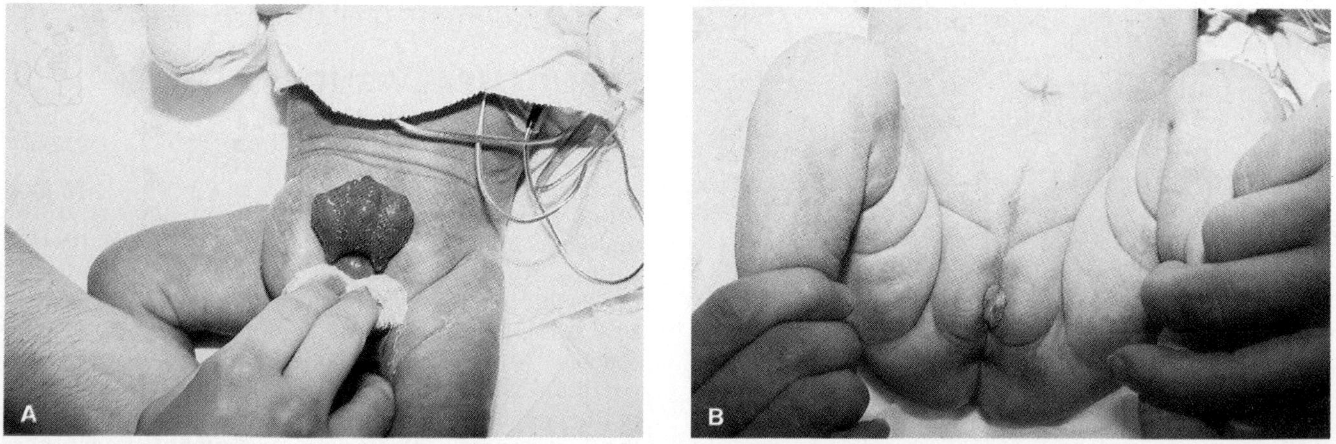

FIGURE 46.7 Bladder exstrophy. (*A*) Prior to surgical reconstruction. Note the bright-red color of the bladder. (*B*) Following surgical reconstruction.

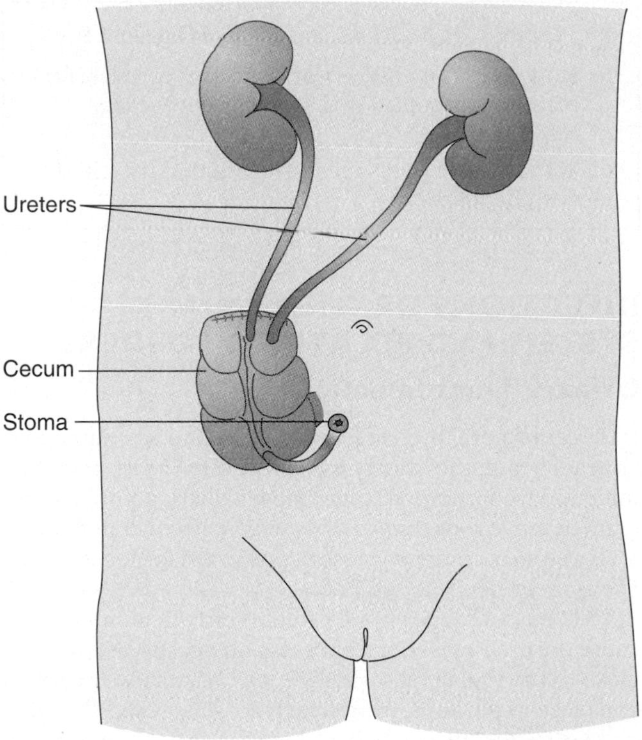

FIGURE 46.8 A continent urine reservoir. A portion of intestine is isolated; the attached ureters drain into it. The appendix creates an abdominal stoma for catheterization.

Preoperative Interventions. To minimize the possibility of infection in the bladder while the infant is waiting for surgery, keep the exposed bladder covered by a sterile plastic bowel bag. This prevents the bladder surface from adhering to bedclothes or diapers and the mucosal surface from being injured. To prevent the skin of the abdomen from excoriation due to the constant irritation of urine, protect it with a substance such as A & D Ointment, Karaya Gum, or Maalox. Consult a wound, ostomy, continence nurse for the best approach. To reduce pressure and prevent further separation of the symphysis, the orthopedic physician may ask that the infant's legs be flexed and brought together and wrapped in Ace bandages to hold them in that position. If this is done, do not separate the infant's legs to apply diapers. Just place them under the child instead. Be certain to change diapers promptly after defecation so feces are not brought forward to the open bladder. Position the infant on his or her back, the same as for all infants, so urine drains freely. Sponge bathe rather than tub bathe the infant to prevent water from entering the ureters and becoming a source of infection.

Parents often need support to view their child as normal in all other ways but the unusual bladder formation. In some instances, the bladder repair will not be made immediately, so parents will need instructions on how to care for the child at home while waiting for surgery.

Postoperative Interventions. Surgery may be completed either as a one-step or two-step procedure. In the first step, the bladder tissue is constructed; in the second, a urethra is created. After bladder construction, the surgical incision over the bladder area must be kept free of infection. Position the infant on his or her back or in an infant chair to prevent feces from coming forward and contaminating the incision line. A suprapubic or indwelling urethral catheter for urine drainage will be inserted to allow the newly constructed bladder to rest. Immediately after surgery, urine draining from the catheter may be blood-stained but should clear after the first few hours. Children may notice sharp painful bladder contractions for the first few days after surgery. Analgesics and antispasmodics may be needed to keep the child comfortable. To prevent the nonfused pubic bone from separating and putting stress on the suture line, at the time of surgery, the child may be fitted with an external fixation device after an osteotomy to hold the pubic bones in approximation until they fuse.

After the second-stage urethra repair, children can be expected to experience some stress incontinence (loss of urine on physical exertion) from the constructed urethra. Kegel exercises can be helpful in strengthening perineal muscles.

Hypospadias

Hypospadias is a urethral defect in which the urethral opening is not at the end of the penis but on the ventral (lower) aspect of the penis (Fig. 46-9*A*). The meatus may

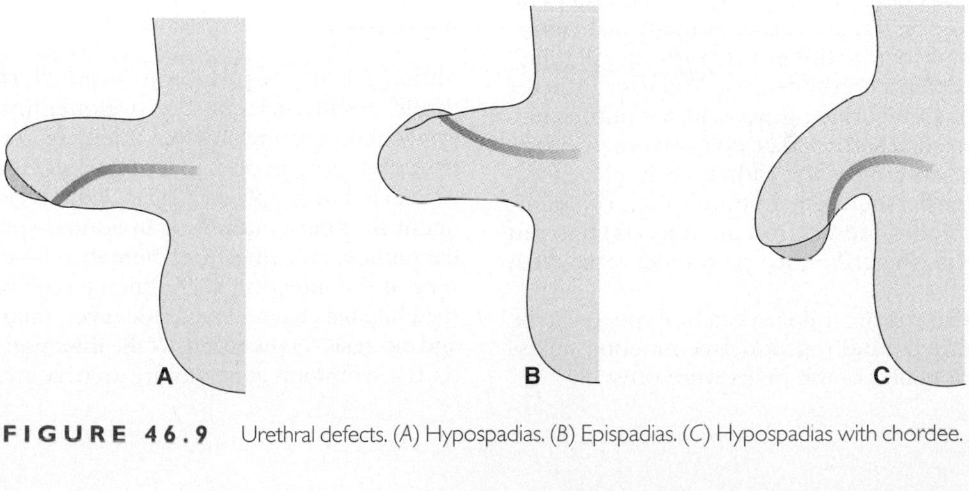

FIGURE 46.9 Urethral defects. (*A*) Hypospadias. (*B*) Epispadias. (*C*) Hypospadias with chordee.

be near the glans, midway back, or at the base of the penis. This anomaly is fairly common, occurring in approximately 1 in 300 male newborns. It tends to be familial or may occur from a multifactorial genetic focus. Epispadias is a similar defect in which the opening is on the dorsal surface of the penis (Fig. 46-9*B*); this is corrected the same way.

Assessment

Be certain to inspect all male newborns at birth for hypospadias or epispadias as part of the routine physical examination. The degree of hypospadias may be minimal (on the glans but inferior in site) or maximal (at the midshaft or at the penal-scrotal junction). Many newborns with hypospadias have an accompanying short *chordee*—a fibrous band that causes the penis to curve downward (often called a cobra-head appearance; Fig. 46-9*C*). Also inspect carefully for *cryptorchidism* (undescended testes), often found in conjunction with hypospadias.

If the penis defect is so extensive that sex determination is unclear, sex cell karyotyping (see Chap. 7) will be done. Hypospadias can be a difficult medical diagnosis for parents to accept because they may view it as a threat to the child's masculinity. This may cause them to have difficulty discussing this defect with relatives or health care personnel. Help parents work through these feelings by allowing them to talk about the disorder and by answering their questions honestly and openly.

Therapeutic Management

Children with hypospadias should not be circumcised because, at the time of the plastic surgical repair, the surgeon may wish to use a portion of the foreskin for the repair. In the newborn, a *meatotomy*—a surgical procedure in which the urethra is extended to a normal position—may initially be performed to establish better urinary function. When the child is older (age 12 to 18 months), adherent chordee may be released. If the repair will be extensive, all surgery may be delayed until the child is age 3 to 4 years. To encourage penis growth and make the procedure easier, the child may have testosterone cream applied to the penis or receive daily injections of testosterone. It is important that hypospadias be corrected before school age so the child looks and feels normal. If left uncorrected, in later years, a meatal opening at an inferior penile site may interfere with fertility, because it does not allow sperm to be deposited close to the female cervix as in normal coitus. Repair must be made before this time to prevent infertility.

After surgical repair, a urethral urinary drainage catheter will be inserted to allow urine output without putting tension against the urethral sutures. The child may notice painful bladder spasms as long as the catheter is in place (3 to 7 days). An analgesic such as acetaminophen (Tylenol) and an antispasmodic medication such as oxybutynin (Ditropan) may be prescribed for pain relief (Ellsworth et al., 1999).

After hypospadias repair, children can be expected to be normal in both urinary and reproductive function unless accompanying anomalies of the penis were present.

✔ CHECKPOINT QUESTIONS

5. How does the child empty urine after repair for bladder exstrophy with a continent urinary reservoir?
6. Where is the penis meatus located in the child with hypospadias?

INFECTIONS OF THE URINARY SYSTEM AND RELATED DISORDERS

Urinary Tract Infection (UTI)

UTI occurs more often in females than in males. Pathogens appear to enter the urinary tract most often as an ascending infection from the perineum. Most urinary pathogens are gram-negative rods; *Escherichia coli* is a frequent offender. UTIs also are a common cause of nosocomial infections (see Focus on Evidence-Based Practice).

UTIs tend to occur more often in girls than in boys because the urethra is shorter in girls and because it is located close to the vagina (allowing the spread of vulvovaginitis) and close to the anus, from which *E coli* spread. Changing diapers frequently can help reduce the risk for infection in infants. Girls should be taught early (when they are toilet trained) to wipe themselves from front to back after voiding and defecating to avoid contaminating the urethra. There is a suggested correlation between the use of products such as bubble bath, feminine hygiene sprays, and hot tubs and UTI in girls (Lum, 2001). Use of these should be discouraged. Infection also often occurs after sexual intercourse. Teach females to void after sexual intercourse. Measures to prevent UTI are summarized in Focus on Family Empowerment.

UTIs need vigorous treatment in childhood so they do not spread to involve the kidneys (pyelonephritis). Girls who have more than three UTIs or boys with their first UTI should be referred to a urologist for further evaluation to determine whether they may have a congenital anomaly such as urethral stenosis or bladder–ureter reflux that causes recurrent urinary stasis. The existence of a secondary problem is most apt to be true in boys with a UTI (Lum, 2001).

Assessment

Although it may be possible to locate a UTI precisely as urethritis, cystitis, ureteritis, or pyelonephritis, the signs and symptoms in young children often are not clear cut. When the exact location or extent of the infection is unknown, it is referred to simply as a UTI. The typical symptoms that occur in older children or in adults—pain on urination, frequency, burning, and hematuria—may not be present. If the infection is confined to the bladder (cystitis), the child may have a low-grade fever, mild abdominal pain, and enuresis (bedwetting). If the infection is a pyelonephritis, the symptoms generally are more acute, with high fever,

FOCUS ON EVIDENCE-BASED PRACTICE

Are Children at Risk for Developing a Urinary Tract Infection (UTI) While Hospitalized?

To look at the incidence of nosocomial or hospital-based UTI, researchers conducted a survey of hospitalized patients' charts for 7 years. Based on this chart review, they discovered that UTI was the fifth most commonly occurring nosocomial infection in all patients although the incidence did gradually decrease over the 7 years. Surprisingly, UTI occurred at a disproportionately high rate in newborns and infants: 20/1,000 patient days in infants 0 to 28 days of age and 40/1,000 patient days in infants 1 to 3 months of age compared to 15/1,000 patient days in children 2 to 12 years of age, and 10/1,000 patient days in adolescents 13 to 15 years of age. As expected, the most frequently found pathogen was *Escherichia coli* (28%). Although catheterization has always been considered a risk for urinary tract infection, only 50% of the participants in this study had had a urinary catheterization before the study.

Based on these findings, the researchers concluded that children in the very young age groups are at particular risk for contracting UTI during a hospital stay. Elevated temperature, crying on voiding, and general irritability would be signs for nurses to observe for to help detect such nosocomial infections.

This is an important study for nurses because it is a good example of the way that patient charts can be surveyed to discover incidence of disease. Because nurses give direct care to infants, they may be the first care providers to realize that the child is developing a UTI in addition to a primary illness.

Langley, J. M., Hanakowski, M., & Leblanc, J. C. (2001). Unique epidemiology of nosocomial urinary tract infection in children. *American Journal of Infection Control, 29*(2), 94–98.

abdominal or flank pain, vomiting, and malaise. Any child with a fever and no demonstrable causes on physical examination should be evaluated for UTI (Shaw, 2000).

Urine for culture can be collected by a clean-catch technique, suprapubic aspiration, or catheterization, so that bacteria from the vulva or foreskin do not contaminate the sample. Suprapubic aspiration is generally limited to infants because the sight of the syringe is so frightening to older children. Plus, the procedure can introduce infection. Catheterization, also frightening and a potential source of infection, is limited in children of all ages.

Urine obtained from suprapubic aspiration is generally sterile, so any growth from this source is significant. A clean-catch urine specimen is said to be positive for bacteriuria if the bacterial colony count is more than 100,000/mL. A count of less than 10,000/mL is considered a negative culture. Counts between 10,000 and 100,000/mL are repeated. Usually, the urine also is positive for proteinuria (because of the presence of bacteria). Microscopic examination may indicate the presence of red blood cells (hematuria) because of mucosal irritation. The presence of red or white blood cells and bacteria tends to make urine more alkaline. Thus, the pH will be elevated (more than 7).

Therapeutic Management

The medical treatment for UTI is the oral administration of an antibiotic specific to the causative organism that is cultured (Santen & Altieri, 2001).

In addition to the antibiotic, the child needs to drink a large quantity of fluid to "flush" the infection out of the urinary tract. Cranberry juice is often recommended as being highly effective in acidifying urine and making it more resistant to bacterial growth. In actual practice, there is little proof of its effectiveness, so offer any fluid the child drinks readily. If the child experiences moderate to severe pain on urination that interferes with his or her ability to void, suggest that the child sit in a bathtub of warm water and void into the water. A mild analgesic, such as acetaminophen (Tylenol), may help reduce pain enough to allow voiding.

With a first UTI, treatment with antibiotics must be continued for the full prescription or the infection will return (Jantunen et al., 2002). Create a reminder sheet for them to post in a readily visible location, such as on the refrigerator door, to help ensure compliance. A repeat clean-catch urine is usually obtained at 72 h to assess the effectiveness of the antibiotic treatment (see Focus on Nursing Care Planning).

After antibiotic therapy is stopped, at least three sterile urine specimens must be obtained to prove that bacteria are not still present. After recurrent UTIs, children may be prescribed a prophylactic antibiotic for 6 months. At periodic health checkups for the next few years, a child should void a clean-catch specimen for culture or microscopic analysis (Lum, 2001).

"Honeymoon" Cystitis

Honeymoon cystitis refers to lower UTI seen in young women shortly after they initiate a first sexual relationship. Such infections occur in connection with the local irritation and inflammation caused by initial sexual coitus. Cystitis of this nature is occurring more and more frequently in young adolescent girls as more girls of this age group begin to engage in sexual relations. Such UTIs respond quickly to antibiotic therapy. Voiding as soon as possible after coitus may help to flush pathogenic organisms from the urethra and prevent such infections from occurring. When cystitis is seen in adolescent girls, it should alert health care providers to the possibility that a girl may be sexually active. In addition to needing counseling about personal hygiene measures to prevent UTI, the girl may need information on sexually transmitted diseases, reproductive planning, and her responsibility for her maturing body.

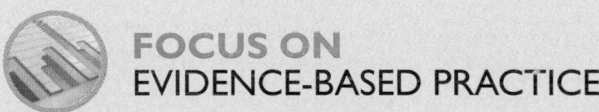

FOCUS ON FAMILY EMPOWERMENT
Preventing Urinary Tract Infection (UTI) in Females

Q. My 10-year-old daughter had a urinary tract infection. How can we prevent this from happening again?

A. Here are some important tips to help prevent UTI:

- Encourage your daughter to drink periodically during the day, especially in warm weather or during exercise, to keep urine flowing freely and prevent stasis of urine in ureters.
- Urge her to urinate at least every 4 h to prevent stasis of urine in bladder.
- Teach her not to bathe with bubble bath; this can cause vulvar and urethral irritation.
- Help your daughter learn to wipe from front to back after moving her bowels or urinating to prevent moving rectal contamination forward to urethra.
- Have your daughter wear cotton, not synthetic, underwear to decrease perineal irritation.
- Instruct your daughter to wash vulva daily to lower the bacterial count on the perineum.
- When your daughter begins menstruating, encourage her to change sanitary pads at least every 4 h to reduce the possible growth of bacteria near the urethra.
- If symptoms of UTI should occur (pain on urination, frequency, blood in urine), call your primary health care provider. If an antibiotic is prescribed, make sure that your daughter takes it for the full prescribed course so all bacteria are completely eradicated. Otherwise, after a short time, bacteria will proliferate, and the infection will recur.
- When your daughter becomes sexually active, teach her to urinate immediately after intercourse to remove any bacteria forced into the urethra by pressure.

Vesicoureteral Reflux

Normally, urine flows from the ureters into the bladder with almost no flow reentering the ureters from the bladder. This is because the ureters enter the bladder obliquely, and a bladder skin flap or "valve" obscures the end of the ureter, preventing backflow. **Vesicoureteral reflux** refers to retrograde flow of urine from the bladder into the ureters. This occurs because the valve that guards the entrance from the bladder to the ureter is defective, either from birth or because of scarring from repeated UTIs, bladder pressure that is stronger than usual, or ureters that are im-

FOCUS ON *Nursing Care Planning*
A CHILD WITH A URINARY TRACT INFECTION (UTI)

A 4-year-old female is brought to the clinic by her mother for evaluation. "She started wetting the bed just recently, and she's been running a low-grade fever."

Assessment: Well-nourished 4-year-old female. Height and weight appropriate for age. Mother denies any past history of medical problems. Toilet training completed at approximately 2½ years of age. Temperature 100.8°F. Other vital signs within age-appropriate parameters. Child states she has mild abdominal pain. Urinalysis and clean-catch urine specimen obtained; positive for bacteriuria and proteinuria. Urine pH of 7.5. A diagnosis of UTI is made, and child is prescribed antibiotic therapy. Mother asking many questions. "How could this have happened? She takes a bath every day. Recently, she's started using some bubble bath that she got for her birthday."

Nursing Diagnosis: Deficient knowledge related to causes and treatment of UTI

Outcome Identification: Parent will verbalize accurate information about UTI.

Outcome Evaluation: Parent states possible causes and contributing factors associated with UTI; identifies measures to prevent UTI; describes antibiotic therapy regimen.

(continued)

Interventions	Rationale
1. Assess the mother's understanding of UTI and its causes.	1. Obtaining a baseline knowledge assessment provides a foundation on which to build future teaching strategies.
2. Review the structure and function of the urinary tract and development of UTI. Clarify any misconceptions the mother might have.	2. Reviewing and clarifying aids in learning and strengthening understanding. UTIs are believed to be more common in girls because the urethra is located in close proximity to the vulva and is shorter in girls than boys.
3. Discuss with the mother possible contributing factors associated with UTI, such as using bubble bath and improper wiping after voiding and defecation.	3. Products such as bubble baths can irritate the vulva and urethra. Wiping from front to back minimizes the risk of urethral contamination after elimination.
4. Instruct the mother in measures to prevent UTI, including adequate fluids and frequent voiding, avoidance of irritating products, and use of cotton underwear.	4. Adequate fluids and frequent voiding help to prevent urinary stasis. Avoidance of products that are irritating reduces the risk of further irritation. Use of cotton underwear helps to reduce risk of perineal irritation from accumulated moisture.
5. Discuss antibiotic regimen prescribed and need for continuation for at least 10 days. Remind the mother that, although the child's signs and symptoms may decrease after 1 to 2 days, the full course of antibiotic must be given.	5. Antibiotic administration based on the results of a clean-catch urine specimen is the treatment of choice for UTI. A full course of therapy is required to eradicate the organism and prevent recurrence.
6. Assist mother with setting up a schedule for antibiotic administration.	6. A schedule individualized to the child helps to reinforce the importance of the medication and need for compliance.
7. Instruct the mother to encourage large quantities of fluid intake. Provide suggestions for fluid choices, offering fluids the child likes.	7. Fluid intake is important in preventing urinary stasis, helping to flush the organisms out of the urinary tract. Suggestions about possible fluid choices provide variety, helping to ensure compliance.
8. Reinforce all instructions with the child at her level of understanding.	8. Reinforcement based on the child's level helps her better understand the need for treatment and compliance with therapy.
9. Provide ample time for questions and concerns.	9. Providing time for questions and concerns helps clarify and individualize information and promotes a feeling of control and trust.
10. Demonstrate the procedure and provide the mother with written instructions for obtaining a clean-catch urine specimen for next scheduled visit. Include both the mother and child in the demonstration.	10. Demonstration aids in learning and helps to reduce the child's anxiety about the procedure, preparing her for what to expect. Written instructions provide an additional source of information to ensure appropriate specimen collection.
11. Schedule a follow-up visit in 2 weeks, including arrangements for a repeat clean-catch urine specimen.	11. Follow-up visit allows time for evaluation, feedback, and review of compliance. A repeat clean-catch urine specimen aids in assessing the effectiveness of antibiotic therapy and helps determine resolution of infection.

planted at abnormal sites or angles. This backflow of urine happens at micturition (voiding) when the bladder contracts (Fig. 46-10).

Reflux leads to bladder infection because urine is retained in ureters after voiding. Stasis of this urine leads to infection. It also appears that the capacity for normal bladder tissue to lyse bacteria becomes reduced due to the large residual urine volume that is always present. In addition, reflux is a potentially serious condition because it can lead to back pressure on the kidneys, possibly leading to nephron destruction and, subsequently, hydronephrosis or dilatation of the renal pelvis. One form of reflux is inherited as a polygenic disorder.

Assessment

A child with reflux is usually first seen by health care personnel because of a history of repeated UTI. A voiding cystourethrogram, CT scan, cystoscopy, or cystography with contrast material will show the ureteral reflux. Based on diagnostic studies, reflux is graded from I to V by degree of reflux, V being the most serious (Master, 2000b).

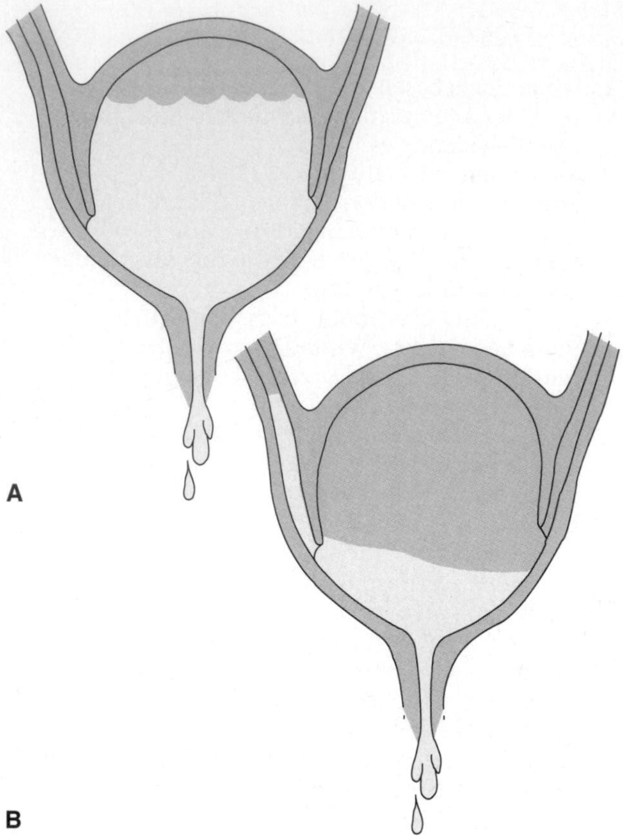

FIGURE 46.10 Vesicoureteral reflux. (*A*) Normal voiding pattern. (*B*) Reflux into ureters with voiding.

Therapeutic Management

The majority of grades of reflux resolve with maturity without a need for surgical intervention. Until this normal growth occurs, reflux must be rigorously treated to decrease the possibility of glomerular scarring from infection or back pressure. Teaching double voiding (having the child void, then in a few minutes attempt to void again) may help to empty the bladder and prevent recurrent infection from urinary stasis. Some children need to remain on prophylactic antibiotics to prevent bladder infection. Long-term maintenance with antibiotics may be as effective in reducing renal scarring as is surgical intervention in lower grades of reflux.

Reflux can be corrected by cystoscopy. Under general anesthesia or conscious sedation, a cystoscope is passed, and polytetrafluoroethylene (Teflon) paste is injected to stabilize the ureter valves. Laparoscopic surgery to correct the placement of ureters may be scheduled to reinsert the ureters at a more oblique angle, creating the normal valve effect.

After surgery, a suprapubic catheter remains in place to keep the bladder empty and prevent pressure against the surgical area. Two ureteral catheters (stents), threaded into the ureters to drain urine directly from the kidney pelvis, also exit at the suprapubic tube site. These are all attached as a closed drainage system to collecting bags. Sterile gauze dressings and antibiotic cream are placed around the tube insertion sites.

In preparing children for this type of surgery, be certain to prepare them for the number of tubes that will be inserted. Explain that, even with the tubes in place, the child will be allowed to walk and move about soon after the operation (and should do this). Be sure that the child and parents understand the importance of keeping the urine collection bags below the level of the child's bladder to prevent urine from flowing back into the bladder. Urge them not to raise the bags above the child's bladder level when helping the child out of bed.

Observe the catheter drainage tubes closely, every hour for the first 24 h and then at least every 4 h. Note the color and the amount of drainage (urine), and carefully measure and record it. Initially, drainage will be bloody, but should clear in 1 or 2 days. Assess drainage for clots (should not be over pinpoint in size). The stents should drain an equal amount, to ensure that kidney production is equal on both sides. Urine will drain primarily from the stents for approximately the first 3 days after surgery. Thereafter, drainage will flow around the stents and be mainly from the suprapubic tube.

Be sure that the ends of the catheters do not become contaminated, because then infection can spread to the surgical area or the kidneys. An antibiotic solution may be ordered placed in the drainage bags to limit the growth of bacteria in the collecting urine. Be certain any amount added is subtracted from the output amount. As soon as urine drainage from the stent catheters has decreased and blood has cleared, the stent catheters will be removed. To show that urine is clearing of blood, obtain serial urine specimens each time collecting bags are emptied and label with the time of removal. Comparing the color of these samples will show that urine is clearing of blood. School-age children can help with labeling the containers, which can help to improve their sense of accomplishment and control over the situation. Many children become frightened when they learn the stent catheters will be removed. Assure them that this will not be painful and can be done at an ambulatory visit without anesthetic.

Incisional pain and painful bladder spasms may occur for the first 3 days after surgery so antispasmodics may be prescribed to reduce bladder spasm. Also, not touching or not moving the suprapubic tube helps to reduce spasms because this limits bladder irritation. The suprapubic tube is removed between 4 and 7 days after surgery (again, a nearly painless procedure). There may be slight urine leakage from the puncture site of the tube for 1 or 2 days after removal of the tube. Keep a sterile dressing in place to absorb the leaking urine. Remind the child and parents to avoid tub baths until the suprapubic tube site has closed completely.

A small number of children continue to have bladder reflux after ureter reimplantation. All children need follow-up care (i.e., repeated urine cultures or perhaps an IVP or VCUG at a later date) to establish that surgery was effective in halting the reflux.

Hydronephrosis

Hydronephrosis is enlargement of the pelvis of the kidney with urine as a result of back pressure in the ureter. The back pressure is generally caused by obstruction, either of the ureter or of the point where the ureter joins the bladder, such as happens with vesicoureteral reflux. Although this may occur at any age, it occurs most often in the first 6 months of life. If it occurs during intrauterine life, it can be shown by fetal sonography.

Children with hydronephrosis are usually asymptomatic. They may have repeated UTIs from urinary stasis (difficult to detect in a child this age except as general irritability or crying on voiding). Elevated blood pressure caused by increasing tubular pressure (which activates the renin-angiotensin system) may be detected on a routine health assessment, although blood pressure is not taken routinely in a child of this age. With severe back pressure, the infant experiences flank or abdominal pain. Abdominal palpation may reveal an abdominal mass (the dilated kidney pelvis). An IVP will show the enlarged pelvis and the point of obstruction (Thilo & Rosenberg, 2001).

Hydronephrosis is a serious disorder because, if the pressure in the pelvis becomes too acute, back pressure on the kidney will interfere with tubular function or destroy the nephrons. The treatment is surgical correction of the obstruction before glomerular or tubular destruction occurs.

> ✔ **CHECKPOINT QUESTIONS**
>
> 7. What organism is the most common cause of UTI?
> 8. What is a common symptom usually reported by the child with vesicoureteral reflux?

DISORDERS AFFECTING NORMAL URINARY ELIMINATION

Enuresis

Enuresis is involuntary passage of urine past the age when a child should be expected to have attained bladder control. Because this is expected at age 2 to 3 years for daytime and age 4 years for nighttime, enuresis is said to occur at approximately 5 to 7 years. Enuresis may be nocturnal (occurs only at night), diurnal (occurs during the day), or both. It is primary if bladder training was never achieved; acquired or secondary if control was established but has now been lost.

Functional nocturnal enuresis (that with no known cause) occurs in approximately 8% to 12% of children age 8 years or younger. It is found more frequently in boys than girls. It also tends to be familial (if it is present in a child, one of the parents probably experienced it, too).

Assessment

Most enuresis is nocturnal; only rarely does daytime enuresis occur. Children who are older than age 5 years need an evaluation to determine whether there is an organic cause for the disorder. During the history, ask how parents have tried to correct the problem; identify whether it is primarily a problem for the child or the parents (treatment will be most effective if the child wants the situation corrected). Assess whether there are stresses in the family such as parents who expect more mature behavior of a child than he or she can handle, a new brother or sister, an uncomfortable school situation such as being assigned to a "shouting" teacher, or marital discord between the parents.

If a child wets only when he or she is engrossed in an interesting activity, he or she may simply need more frequent reminding to empty the bladder. If a child wets only on nights when he or she is exceptionally tired or troubled, a functional rather than an organic cause is suggested. If the child has symptoms other than bedwetting, such as abdominal pain, burning, or frequency, UTI is suggested. It is a common practice for many parents to get children out of bed every night and take them to the bathroom. At any point parents stop this practice, children may begin bedwetting because they have been conditioned to empty their bladder at that time of night.

Some children with enuresis have abnormal electroencephalographic patterns. Other children with the same abnormal patterns do not have enuresis, however, so this by itself is not a sufficiently specific finding to be helpful. In others, bedwetting seems to occur as children pass from a period of rapid eye movement sleep pattern to a type IV level, or it is primarily a sleep disorder. It may be associated with small bladder capacity (which would account for why the condition is familial).

Although usually not necessary to aid diagnosis, an IVP, VCUG, or sonogram may be done to rule out organic disease. A clean-catch urine specimen should be collected to rule out bacteriuria. Specific gravity is assessed to rule out a defect in urine concentration. Protein and glucose levels are evaluated to determine evidence of kidney disease.

Therapeutic Management

The treatment of enuresis may be complex because the cause is generally unknown. If stress factors have been identified, an attempt should be made to correct these. Some stress factors, such as birth of a new sibling, cannot be changed, but frank discussion with children regarding what causes the stress and attempts to help children cope better with their daytime activities may improve enuresis. Therapy will be most effective if the child wants the enuresis to end.

In many children, it helps to limit fluids after dinner. Urge parents to exercise common sense in this area. Remind them that a child may not be able to go every night without a drink from dinner until breakfast. Caution parents of children with sickle cell anemia not to restrict fluid this way. Increased sickling of cells occurs with dehydration.

Synthetic antidiuretic hormone (ADH; desmopressin [DDAVP]) administered intranasally or orally is the drug of choice to reduce urinary output (Caudle, 2000; see Focus on Pharmacology). Imipramine (Tofranil), an anticholinergic drug that inhibits urination given an hour before bedtime, is also effective. Unfortunately, this has side effects of insomnia, anxiety, and arrhythmias that limit its use.

Alarm bells that ring when children wet at night may be effective in some children. This type of system does not actually stop bedwetting. The alarm wakes the child, he or

FOCUS ON PHARMACOLOGY

Desmopressin acetate (DDAVP)

Action: A synthetic form of human antidiuretic hormone that promotes resorption of water in the renal tubule or decreases bladder filling; drug of choice for enuresis.

Pregnancy Risk Category: B

Dosage: In children 6 years of age and older, 20 µg (0.2 mL) intranasally at bedtime, possibly increasing the dose up to 40 µg if necessary or 0.2 mg at bedtime, titrated up to 0.6 mg to obtain the desired response.

Possible Adverse Effects: Transient headache, nausea, flushing, mild abdominal cramps, fluid retention

Nursing Implications

- Instruct parents and child that child should restrict fluid after dinner time in addition to taking medication.
- If given intranasally, advise parents to refrigerate the solution
- Teach parents and child the proper method for intranasal administration
- Caution child and parents that nasal administration is less effective if the child develops a cold with draining rhinitis.

she stops voiding, and then the child gets up and uses the bathroom. Over time, this type of conditioning may be effective, but once the urine alarm is removed, children may relapse to enuresis. Bladder-stretching exercises—drinking a large quantity of water and then refraining from voiding as long as possible—to increase the functional size of the bladder may be helpful in some children. A bladder that can hold 300 to 350 mL of fluid will generally be large enough to contain urine during a night's sleep.

Enuresis is not a minor problem for either parents or for the child. Parents find it difficult to include the child on vacation trips. They may resent the daily linen washing. Children may exclude themselves from activities such as slumber parties or camping trips with friends to avoid embarrassment. As a general measure, children who wet their beds need to take baths in the morning rather than at bedtime to minimize urine odor and also reduce the risk of possible ridicule from other children if they notice the odor.

Enuresis may occur in hospitalized children because of the stress of their new surroundings. Preschool children may experience it because they are uncomfortable using strange bathrooms or do not understand which bathroom is theirs to use. As a rule, place as little stress or importance on enuresis as possible during an illness and encourage parents to do the same.

Postural (Orthostatic) Proteinuria

A small number of children will spill albumin into the urine when they stand upright for an extended period (**postural proteinuria** [postural albuminuria]). The amount of spilling decreases when they rest in a supine position. Children with this condition have no apparent disease; the phenomenon is apparently attributable to the effect of gravity on glomerular function.

To determine postural proteinuria, urine is collected after the child has been recumbent during the night (a first-voided specimen) and then again after the child has been up and active for a number of hours. Make certain when collecting this urine specimen to record the child's activity accurately. If the child stood by the crib rail crying for a parent or was held in a nurse's lap for most of the night, the urine may show protein in the morning specimen because it is not truly a "resting specimen." Likewise, for the specimen to be collected after the child has been active, make certain that he or she is up and active, not lying in a supine position reading a book for most of the time. Play a game if necessary, such as follow the leader, so the child is active.

Postural proteinuria needs no therapy. However, be sure to document the condition because a certain percentage of these children develop some form of kidney disorder later in life.

✔ CHECKPOINT QUESTIONS

9. In which gender is enuresis more commonly seen?
10. What is orthostatic proteinuria?

DISORDERS OF ALTERED KIDNEY FUNCTION

Renal disorders occur because of faulty kidney formation or illness that causes glomeruli changes.

Kidney Agenesis

Agenesis means lack of growth (literally, lack of a beginning) or that no organ has formed in utero. Absence of kidneys in a newborn is suggested when the volume of amniotic fluid on sonogram or at birth is less than normal (oligohydramnios). This occurs because urine normally adds to the volume of amniotic fluid in utero. The infant with kidney agenesis often has Potter's syndrome or accompanying misshapen, low-set ears and hypoplastic (stiff, inflexible) lungs. He or she will void no urine. Bilateral absence of kidneys is obviously incompatible with life unless a renal transplantation can be accomplished. The associated condition of nonfunctioning lungs makes a successful transplantation highly unlikely.

Polycystic Kidney

Polycystic kidney means that large, fluid-filled cysts have formed in place of normal kidney tissue. The most frequent type of polycystic kidney seen in children is inherited as an autosomal recessive trait (Lum, 2001). With this, there is abnormal development of the collecting tubules. The kidneys are large and feel soft and spongy. If the disorder is bilateral, an infant will not pass urine. The mother will have had oligohydramnios during pregnancy. Children often have a typical appearance (i.e., *hypertelorism*—

wide-spaced eyes, epicanthal folds, flattened nose; or *micrognathia*—small jaw), findings described as a "Potter facies." Either *transillumination* or *sonography* will show the fluid-filled cysts. In many children, the liver is filled with identical cysts. This is most evident later in life when increased portal circulation occurs (blood cannot perfuse the cystic liver structures, either). Because this kidney disease is inherited, parents and children at adolescence need genetic counseling to fully inform them that future children may also have this problem.

If the condition is unilateral, urine production will be decreased (oliguria). Because kidneys are difficult to locate in newborns, a unilateral polycystic kidney may be missed until later in life, when, with increased kidney growth, an abdominal mass can be palpated. The cystic growth offers such resistance to blood circulation that systemic hypertension often results by school age.

The treatment for polycystic formation is surgical removal of a kidney if only one is cystic. If both kidneys are cystic, treatment is renal transplantation (difficult in the young child, because few infant kidneys are available for transplantation and because of the technical challenge of such small blood vessels).

Renal Hypoplasia

Hypoplasia means reduced growth. Hypoplastic kidneys contain fewer lobes than normal kidneys and are small and underdeveloped. The child with hypoplastic kidneys, in addition to having poor kidney function, may develop hypertension from stenosis of the renal arteries. If hypoplasia is bilateral, the child may need a kidney transplantation performed in later life to maintain kidney function.

Prune-Belly Syndrome

Prune-belly syndrome is severe urinary tract dilation that develops as early as intrauterine life from an unknown cause. Occurring mainly in boys, the severe dilation causes back pressure and destruction of kidneys. The infant is born with oligohydramnios and pulmonary dysplasia because of the lack of amniotic fluid in utero.

The condition is marked by the presence of three symptoms: deficiency of usual abdominal muscle tone, bilateral undescended testes, and the dilated faulty development of the bladder and upper urinary tract. The infant's abdomen appears wrinkled (like a prune) because of the poorly developed abdominal muscles (Fig. 46-11). Without surgical remodeling, the infant can develop repeated UTIs, leading to end-stage renal disease. Teach parents to protect their child's abdomen from trauma that could be caused by lap belts or baby walkers, because their child lacks abdominal support. A number of children need kidney transplantation because of destruction of glomeruli from back pressure (Leonard, 2000).

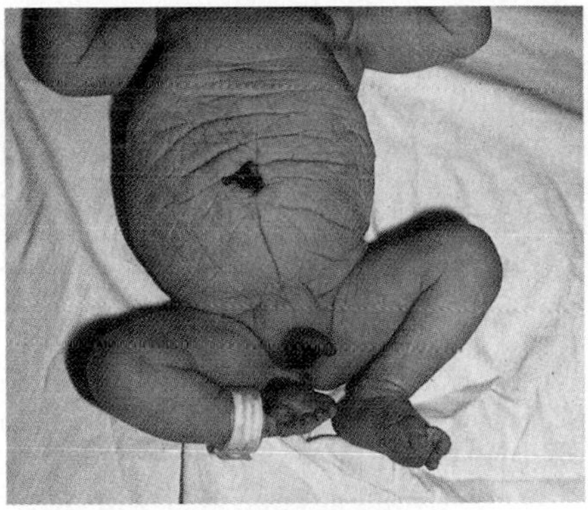

FIGURE 46.11 Prune belly syndrome.

Acute Poststreptococcal Glomerulonephritis

Glomerulonephritis, inflammation of the glomeruli of the kidney, may occur as a separate entity but usually occurs as an immune complex disease after infection with nephritogenic streptococcus (most commonly subtypes of group A beta-hemolytic streptococci). Tissue damage occurs from a complement fixation reaction in the glomeruli (*complement* is a cascade of proteins activated by antigen–antibody reactions and actually plugs or obstructs glomeruli). IgG antibodies against *Streptococcus* may be detected in the bloodstream of children with acute glomerulonephritis, proof that the illness follows a streptococcal infection (Kasahara et al., 2001).

Intravascular coagulation in minute renal vessels occurs. Ischemic damage leads to scarring and decreased glomerular formation. This results in a reduction in the glomerular filtration rate, leading to an accumulation of sodium and water in the bloodstream. Inflammation of the glomeruli increases permeability, allowing protein molecules to escape into the filtrate.

Assessment

Acute glomerulonephritis is most common in children between the ages of 5 and 10 years, the age group most susceptible to streptococcal infections. Boys appear to develop the disease more often than girls; it occurs more often during the winter and spring months, as do pharyngeal streptococcal infections (Meyers, 2000a). The child typically has a history of a recent respiratory infection (within 7 to 14 days) or impetigo (within 3 weeks). All children who have had a "strep" throat, tonsillitis, otitis media, or impetigo caused by streptococcal infection should have a urinalysis 2 weeks after the infection to evaluate for glomerulonephritis. Without frightening them unduly, tell parents that this is an extremely important follow-up test.

Acute glomerulonephritis is characterized by a sudden onset of hematuria and proteinuria. The protein content both of individual urine specimens and of total 24-h urine volume is measured. Testing a single specimen will show 1^+ to 4^+ protein; a 24-h urine specimen may contain as much as 1 g protein. Normally, urine contains none.

The hematuria associated with acute glomerulonephritis is usually so gross that the child's urine appears tea-colored, reddish-brown, or smoky. Urinary sediment will contain white blood cells, epithelial cells, and hyaline, granular, and red blood cell casts. After these initial urine changes, the child develops oliguria. Specific gravity of urine will be elevated. Hypertension from hypervolemia occurs. The child may have abdominal pain, a low-grade fever, edema, anorexia, vomiting, or headache. There may be cardiac involvement related to the difficulty in managing the excessive plasma fluid. Such children show signs of orthopnea, cardiac enlargement, enlarged liver, pulmonary edema, and a galloping heart rhythm. Electrocardiographic changes such as T-wave inversion and prolongation of the PR interval may be seen. Heart failure may occur from circulatory overload.

Blood analysis will indicate a lowered blood protein level (hypoalbuminemia) caused by the massive proteinuria. Low serum complement will be present, and, as the blood volume expands, a mild anemia also will occur. As in all inflammatory diseases, the erythrocyte sedimentation rate will increase. Because the glomeruli cannot filter properly, concentrations of urea, nonprotein nitrogen (BUN), and creatinine in blood will increase. The antistreptolysin O (anti-DNase B) titer or antibody formation against *Streptococcus* is generally elevated, indicating that a recent hemolytic streptococcal infection has occurred.

If blood pressure reaches 160/100 mm Hg as part of the acute process, encephalopathy may occur, with symptoms of headache, irritability, seizures, vomiting, coma or lethargy, and perhaps transitory paralysis. This extreme elevation in blood pressure is probably related to the expanded circulatory volume. The cerebral symptoms are caused by *cerebral ischemia* (vasoconstriction of cerebral vessels to reduce cranial pressure).

Therapeutic Management

The course of acute glomerulonephritis is 1 to 2 weeks. During this time, there is little therapy specific for the disorder. Antibiotics usually are ineffective because the disease is caused not by an active infection but by an antigen–antibody inflammatory response to a past infection. Diuretics are of little value because obstructed glomeruli bases cannot be made to function; a course of ethacrynic acid or furosemide (Lasix) may be tried. If heart failure occurs, specific measures such as placing the child in a semi-Fowler's position, digitalization, and oxygen administration may be necessary. If diastolic blood pressure rises to more than 90 mm Hg, antihypertensive therapy with a calcium channel blocker may be necessary. Phosphate binders, such as aluminum hydroxide to reduce phosphate absorption in the GI tract or a potassium-removing resin agent, such as sodium polystyrene sulfonate (Kayexalate), may be necessary in children who are severely affected.

Bedrest is unnecessary, although children should be encouraged to participate in quiet play activities. They can attend school and engage in normal activities after 1 or 2 weeks, but competitive activity is limited until kidney function has returned to normal to avoid overstressing the kidneys.

Diet is controversial. Although limiting protein intake reduces the amount of protein lost in urine, many children who are losing large quantities of protein need high-protein diets to supplement this loss. Salt restriction may be needed to reduce severe edema. Most children do well on a normal diet for their age, however, with normal salt and protein content. Weighing the child every day and calculating intake and output are important assessments in following the course of the disease. In most children, acute glomerulonephritis runs a limited, benign course. After most symptoms fade, proteinuria and impaired clearance of urea and creatinine may remain for as long as 2 months. Caution parents that the results of a urine protein test may remain abnormal for up to a year, so that, if their child has this test as a routine screening procedure at a health checkup, they should not worry that this finding means reinfection or the beginning of further disease (Kasahara et al., 2001). A small number of children will not completely recover from acute glomerulonephritis but will develop chronic nephritis. These children appear to suffer destruction from the initial inflammation that resulted in chronic renal insufficiency.

NURSING DIAGNOSES AND RELATED INTERVENTIONS

Nursing Diagnosis: Situational low self-esteem, related to feelings of responsibility for onset of serious illness

Outcome Identification: Child (parent) will verbalize positive aspects about self and interact appropriately with others in 1 month.

Outcome Evaluation: Child (parent) states feelings about becoming ill; discusses future plans and ways to maintain health; participates in care.

Glomerulonephritis is a frightening disease for both children and their parents. Children may be frightened by the initial hematuria. They may be upset at the appearance of periorbital edema, which makes their reflection in the mirror so strange to them. Children as young as early school age are aware that kidneys are necessary for life. This means they recognize the seriousness of kidney disease.

If children were prescribed penicillin for a pharyngitis 2 weeks before the development of the nephritis but refused to take it, they may believe that they caused this disease. The parents may feel guilty because they did not force the child to take the medicine. They worry that their child will develop chronic glomerulonephritis or die during the acute phase of this attack. These parents and children need to talk about their feelings openly. Provide frequent reports of subtle positive changes in a child's condition (e.g., "His blood pressure is staying down by itself now; he does not need medicine for that any more." "He weighs 2 pounds less today than 4 days ago; that generally means his kidneys are beginning to function more efficiently again").

Be certain that parents know the date and place of a return visit for follow-up care. Because this is a perplexing disease, be sure they have a telephone number to call if they have questions about their child's care or condition.

The most frequent type of acute glomerulonephritis can be avoided by the prevention or effective early treatment of group A beta-hemolytic streptococcal infections. Acute glomerulonephritis tends not to recur with subsequent streptococcal infections, so prophylactic penicillin to prevent further streptococcal infections is unnecessary.

Chronic Glomerulonephritis

Although chronic glomerulonephritis occasionally may follow acute glomerulonephritis or nephrotic syndrome, it also occurs as a primary disease (or after acute glomerulonephritis that was clinically so mild it was undiagnosed). The child is found to have proteinuria at a routine checkup. Further investigation may indicate hypertension and the presence of red cell or white cell casts and occult blood in urine. The specific gravity of the child's urine is below normal (below 1.003). Blood studies may indicate an increased BUN or creatinine level. A renal biopsy will show permanent destruction of glomeruli membranes.

Chronic glomerulonephritis may result in either diffuse or local nephron damage. The remaining functioning nephrons increase their glomerular filtration rate to compensate for those that are damaged. At some point in this chronic disease destruction process, however, compensatory mechanisms fail, and renal insufficiency or failure will result. **Alport's syndrome** is a progressive chronic glomerulonephritis inherited as an autosomal dominant disorder.

During the course of the illness, if the child has acute symptoms of edema, hematuria, hypertension, or oliguria, bedrest may be necessary. If children have only a chronic manifestation, such as proteinuria, and if they feel well, they can maintain normal activity, including attending school. Children should not engage in competitive activities such as contact sports, however, because of the risk for kidney injury.

Therapy is nonspecific and directed at symptom relief rather than the disease process itself, because the cause of the disease is unknown. Therapy with antihypertensive drugs such as hydralazine (Apresoline) or with diuretics to increase urine output such as ethacrynic acid (Edecrin) may be necessary. *Corticosteroid therapy* may reduce or halt the progress of the disorder by reducing inflammation. Children have difficulty accepting long-term corticosteroid therapy because of the side effects, in particular, a typical moon face and extra body hair (Cushing's syndrome). Talk with them about these body changes and assure them that these changes will be reversed when the drug is discontinued.

Children receiving corticosteroids are at an increased risk for infection because of immunosuppressive activity of these drugs. They need to be shielded from other children and health care personnel with infection. Parents need to learn to take their child's temperature and recognize and report the earliest signs of infection.

Generally, the prognosis for children with chronic glomerulonephritis is poor. Although the illness may run a long-term course, eventually it leads to renal insufficiency and renal failure. Children may be maintained for long periods by peritoneal dialysis or hemodialysis. Kidney transplantation is a possibility.

Because children as young as early school age are aware of the importance of kidney function to life, most children with chronic renal disease are aware of the likely outcome of their disease. Most children are adolescents or young adults before the disease runs its ultimate course. They indicate that they appreciate having health care personnel face this outcome with them honestly if kidney transplantation cannot be performed to prolong their life.

Nephrotic Syndrome (Nephrosis)

Nephrosis, altered glomeruli permeability due to fusion of the glomeruli membrane surfaces, causes abnormal loss of protein in urine. Immunologic mechanisms are involved in instigating the process. The cause may be hypersensitivity to an antigen–antibody reaction or an autoimmune process. A T-lymphocyte dysfunction may be responsible. The highest incidence is at 3 years of age, occurring more often in boys than in girls (Meyers, 2000b).

Nephrotic syndrome in children occurs in three forms: (1) congenital; (2) secondary, as a progression of glomerulonephritis or in connection with systemic diseases such as sickle cell anemia or systemic lupus erythematosus (SLE); or (3) idiopathic (primary). In children, the idiopathic form is seen most commonly.

Nephrosis can be further classified according to the amount of membrane destruction present. Minimal change nephrotic syndrome (MCNS) is the type most often seen in children. As the name implies, little scarring of glomeruli occurs. Children with this degree of scarring respond well to therapy. Other types are focal glomerulosclerosis (FGS) and membranoproliferative glomerulonephritis (MPGN). Both of these types involve scarring of glomeruli. These children will have a poor response to therapy. Fortunately, most children (80%) develop only MCNS (Meyers, 2000b).

The four characteristic symptoms of nephrotic syndrome include (1) proteinuria, (2) edema, (3) low serum albumin (hypoalbuminemia), and (4) hyperlipidemia (increased blood lipid level). Proteinuria occurs because increased glomeruli permeability leads to protein loss in the urine and, subsequently, hypoalbuminemia. With a low level of protein in the bloodstream, osmotic pressure causes fluid to shift from the bloodstream into interstitial tissue, causing edema. As the blood volume decreases, the kidneys begin to conserve sodium and water, adding to the potential for edema. The hyperlipidemia occurs because the liver increases production of lipoproteins to try to compensate for protein loss. Lipids are too large to be lost in urine and, thus, rise to high levels in the blood serum. Some children have such high cholesterol levels that, when blood is drawn and placed into a test tube, a circle of white fat forms on the top of it. Figure 46-12 illustrates the process that leads to the common symptoms.

Assessment

Symptoms usually begin insidiously. Children develop edema around the eyes (periorbital edema), most noticeable when they wake in the morning from a head-dependent position. Parents may notice that clothing no longer fits a child around the waist, because edematous fluid is beginning to collect in the abdominal cavity (ascites). It is easy to dismiss these first symptoms as those of an upper respiratory tract infection and the normal "paunchy" belly of a toddler or preschooler. As edema progresses, the child's skin becomes pale, stretched, and taut.

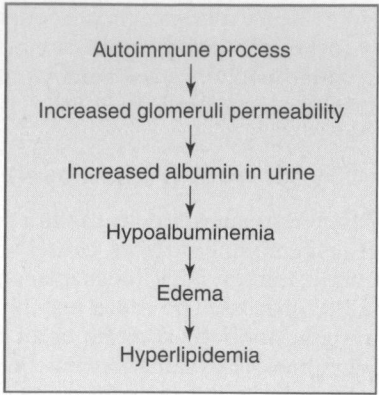

Autoimmune process
↓
Increased glomeruli permeability
↓
Increased albumin in urine
↓
Hypoalbuminemia
↓
Edema
↓
Hyperlipidemia

FIGURE 46.12 The process that results in the signs and symptoms of nephrotic syndrome.

In boys, scrotal edema becomes extremely marked. Ascites may become so extensive that the resultant pressure on the stomach leads to anorexia or vomiting. Children may have diarrhea caused by intestinal edema and poor absorption by the edematous membrane. Because of poor nutrition, growth may stop. The child may become malnourished but yet appear deceptively obese, because of the extensive edema (Fig. 46-13). When the ascites becomes even more extensive, children may have difficulty breathing as the abdominal fluid presses against the diaphragm, decreasing lung expansion. Parents report that children are irritable and fussy, probably from the feeling of abdominal fullness and generalized edema. An increased risk for clotting can occur from the decreased intravascular fluid volume.

Laboratory studies will reveal marked proteinuria. A single test will show a 1^+ to 4^+ protein; a 24-h total urine test will show up to 15 g protein when normally urine contains no protein. The protein loss with nephrotic syndrome is almost entirely albumin, differentiating it from the proteinuria of glomerulonephritis, in which protein loss tends to be nonspecific. Some children with nephrotic syndrome exhibit hematuria at the onset, but it is minimal in contrast to that seen with acute glomerulonephritis. The erythrocyte sedimentation rate (demonstrating the inflammation of the glomeruli membrane) is elevated. Features of acute glomerulonephritis and nephrotic syndrome are compared and contrasted in Table 46-5.

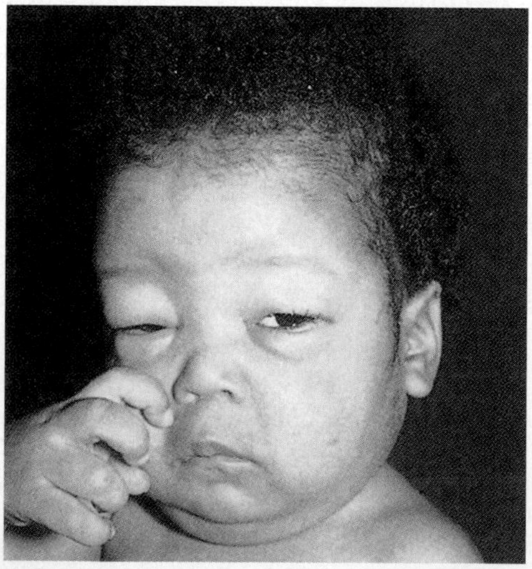

FIGURE 46.13 A 2-year-old with nephrotic syndrome. Note the extensive edema of the face and hand.

A renal biopsy may be done to determine whether there is scarring of the glomerular membrane.

Therapeutic Management

Therapy for the child with nephrotic syndrome is directed toward reducing the proteinuria and subsequently the edema with a course of corticosteroid therapy, such as oral prednisone, and keeping the child free of infection while the immune system is suppressed. An initial dose of prednisone is given until diuresis without protein loss is accomplished; dosage is then reduced for maintenance and continued for as long as 1 to 2 months.

Instruct parents to test the first urine specimen of the day for protein with a chemical reagent strip and keep an accurate chart showing the pattern of protein loss. Approximately once a week, they are usually asked to collect a 24-h urine specimen so total protein loss can be measured.

After the initial 4 weeks, prednisone is generally given every other day rather than every day. Prednisone has the potential to halt growth and to suppress adrenal gland secretion. However, growth is apparently not delayed when the drug is given on alternate days and there is less alteration of adrenal steroid production (Karch, 2001). Parents may need to be assured that alternate-day therapy is best to keep them from changing the schedule to every day or giving twice the calculated dose by adding extra tablets on alternate days. To help parents remember to give medication on alternate days, have them choose either even or odd calendar days as the day of administration. Help them design a reminder chart. Prednisone tastes bitter. Parents may welcome suggestions as to how to disguise the taste, such as by mixing it with applesauce.

Be certain both the parents and the child are aware that prednisone causes a cushingoid appearance (i.e, moon face, extra fat at the base of the neck, and increased body hair). Caution parents to plan ahead when getting refills of prescriptions, so that the prednisone therapy is not stopped abruptly because they ran out of medication. This abrupt stop can lead to adrenal insufficiency.

Diuretics are not commonly used to reduce the edema, because they tend to decrease blood volume, which is already decreased. This could lead to acute renal failure. Children who respond poorly to prednisone alone, however, may need diuretic therapy with a drug such as furosemide (Lasix). When children are taking furosemide for extended periods, there is always a danger that too much potassium will be excreted, causing hypokalemia. Children on long-term diuretic therapy need frequent blood studies to determine that electrolyte levels, especially the potassium level, are adequate. They may need supplemental potassium and should have foods high in potassium included in their diet. IV albumin may be administered to temporarily correct hypoalbuminemia. As the serum albumin level rises, fluid shifts from subcutaneous spaces into the bloodstream. Children are then administered a rapidly acting diuretic to remove the extra fluid. It is important that the diuretic be

TABLE 46.5 Comparison of Features of Acute Glomerulonephritis and Nephrotic Syndrome

FACTOR	ACUTE GLOMERULONEPHRITIS	NEPHROTIC SYNDROME
Cause	Immune reaction to group A beta-hemolytic streptococcal infection	Idiopathic; possibly a hypersensitivity reaction
Onset	Abrupt	Insidious
Hematuria	Profuse	Rare
Edema	Mild	Extreme
Hypertension	Marked	Mild
Hyperlipidemia	Rare or mild	Marked
Peak age frequency	5–10 yr	2–3 yr
Interventions	Limited activity; antihypertensives as needed; symptomatic therapy for congestive heart failure	Corticosteroid administration; cyclophosphamide administration; possibly a diuretic and potassium supplement
Diet	Normal for age	High-protein, low-sodium diet
Prevention	Prevention or thorough treatment of group A beta-hemolytic streptococcal infections	None known

administered after the albumin infusion or the child could develop a fluid overload and, subsequently, heart failure.

A course of cyclophosphamide (Cytoxan), because of its immunosuppressant action, may be effective in reducing symptoms or preventing further relapses of the disease in children who do not respond to corticosteroid therapy. It is important to ensure adequate fluid intake with cyclophosphamide to prevent bladder irritation and bleeding. Cyclophosphamide is also used in chemotherapy for malignancy (see Chap. 53). Be certain that parents are not misled into believing that their child has cancer because he or she is receiving a chemotherapeutic drug. Cyclosporine (Sandimmune) is another immunosuppressant that may be used.

The prognosis for children with nephrotic syndrome varies. Almost all children with MCNS respond initially to steroid therapy. Although they may have a relapse, they will then remain free of the disease. Those with FGS and MPGN types will have relapses at frequent or infrequent intervals over the next several years. Children who have frequent relapses have a relatively poor chance of ever being free of the disorder. Many develop renal failure later. Kidney transplantation may be necessary to sustain life.

NURSING DIAGNOSES AND RELATED INTERVENTIONS

Nursing Diagnosis: Imbalanced nutrition, less than body requirements, related to poor appetite, restricted diet, and protein loss

Outcome Identification: Child will demonstrate adequate intake of nutrients for growth needs throughout course of illness.

Outcome Evaluation: Child follows normal growth curve on standard assessment scale.

Because children with nephrosis have poor appetites, maintaining them on restricted diets is difficult. A good protein intake is necessary to offset protein loss. A good potassium intake through consumption of fruits and fruit juices, particularly bananas, is necessary to maintain sufficient serum potassium levels, especially if the child is receiving diuretics (Table 46-6). During acute phases of the disease, fluid or sodium may be temporarily restricted. If this is so, most children are happiest with many small glasses of fluid spaced throughout the day, rather than several large drinks. It helps to make a chart showing the amount of fluid the child is allowed each day. As fluid is given, color in a portion of the chart corresponding to the amount given. The child can tell from the uncolored portion how much more he or she is allowed that day. This is easier for toddlers and preschoolers (the age group usually affected by this disease) to understand rather than talking in terms of milliliters or even glassfuls.

Parents need to weigh children daily to detect fluid accumulation (use the same scale with the child in the same clothing at the same time of day) and to measure intake and output accurately. If the child is hospitalized, taking pulse rate and blood pressure every 4 h will detect hypovolemia from excessive fluid shifts to interstitial tissue.

TABLE 46.6 Foods High in Potassium

FOOD GROUP	EXAMPLES
Fruits	Bananas, peaches, prunes, raisins, oranges, and orange juice
Vegetables	Carrots, celery, lima beans, potatoes, collards, dandelion greens, spinach
Meat	Nuts, peanuts, red meat
Dairy products	Milk, whole or skim; low-sodium milk
Miscellaneous	Salt substitutes, chocolate and cocoa, bran

Nursing Diagnosis: Risk for impaired skin integrity related to edema

Outcome Identification: Child's skin will remain intact through course of illness.

Outcome Evaluation: Child's skin is intact, clean, and dry without erythema.

The edematous skin of children with nephrotic syndrome tends to break down easily, so they need frequent position changes while in bed. Check clothing to make certain that the elastic band at the waist of pajamas or other constricting parts is not tight. Soft gauze placed between skin surfaces, especially of boys' scrotums, tends to prevent skin irritation and breakdown. Edematous tissue does not heal well, so breaks in the skin easily become secondarily infected. The child who is not toilet-trained needs frequent diaper changes and thorough cleaning at each change to prevent skin breakdown in the diaper area.

Generally, children are more comfortable if they sleep with their head elevated in a semi-Fowler's position rather than the supine or prone position because this reduces periorbital edema. If children sleep in a head-flat position, edema can be so severe by morning that children's eyes are swollen completely shut; their tongue is also swollen, so they cannot speak. At home, parents can provide a semi-Fowler's position by placing extra pillows on children's beds or slipping a cardboard box under the head of the mattress to raise the end of the mattress.

Because medications are poorly absorbed from edematous skin areas, intramuscular (IM) injections should be kept to a minimum. Medication should be administered orally if possible.

WHAT IF? What if you needed to give an IM injection to a child with extensive dependent edema from nephrotic syndrome? Would it be best to give it in a thigh or deltoid muscle and why?

Nursing Diagnosis: Knowledge deficit related to chronic illness

Outcome Identification: Parents will demonstrate increased knowledge concerning nephrotic syndrome in 1 week.

Outcome Evaluation: Parents describe course and nature of nephrosis and their role in care of child at home.

Parents often need support to manage children at home. They need clear instructions about their responsibilities, including keeping the child free of infection, perhaps by limiting exposure to friends, and giving prednisone or oral diuretics and a potassium supplement. Review medication instructions with parents and have them repeat the instructions. Make certain they understand where and when they are to return for a follow-up visit and make certain they have a telephone number to call if they have questions or concerns about their child's care or health.

Henoch-Schönlein Syndrome Nephritis

Henoch-Schönlein purpura is discussed in Chapter 44. Approximately one quarter of the children who develop this type of purpura develop renal disease as a secondary complication. The renal involvement becomes apparent within a few days after the manifestations of purpuric symptoms. Children may show only urinary abnormalities such as proteinuria or may have a rapidly progressing glomerulonephritis. Most children recover completely. Only a few develop chronic symptoms. In those who do, long-term kidney disease can develop (Gusic, 2000).

✔ CHECKPOINT QUESTIONS

11. What is typically the first symptom of acute glomerulonephritis?
12. What are the four characteristic symptoms of nephrotic syndrome?

Systemic Lupus Erythematosus

SLE is an autoimmune disease in which autoantibodies and antigens cause deposits of complement on the kidney glomerulus (see Chap. 14). Because of this, a number of children with SLE develop symptoms of acute or chronic glomerulonephritis, the ultimate cause of death in many adults with SLE. Therapy with corticosteroids or cytotoxic agents may be effective. If kidney transplantation is required, the same damage rarely occurs in the transplanted kidney (Chalom, 2000).

Hemolytic-Uremic Syndrome

With hemolytic-uremic syndrome, the lining of glomerular arterioles become inflamed, swollen, and occluded with particles of platelets and fibrin. Red blood cells and platelets are damaged as they flow through the partially occluded blood vessels. As the damaged cells reach the spleen, they are destroyed by the spleen and removed from circulation. This leads to hemolytic anemia.

Ninety percent of children who develop this syndrome have recently experienced an *E. coli* GI infection. The most likely source of the *E. coli* is undercooked hamburger because *E. coli* is found in the intestine of beef cattle. It occurs more frequently in infants who have their initial *E. coli* infection treated with an antibiotic (Farquhar, 2000). The syndrome occurs during summer months in children 6 months to 4 years of age.

Assessment

Children usually develop only a transient diarrhea, although this can progress to severe fluid loss and bowel wall necrosis. Fever may be so elevated that the child experiences stupor and hallucinations. Oliguria accompanied by proteinuria, hematuria, and urinary casts in urine follows. Extensive edema may occur. The oliguria will lead to increased serum creatinine and BUN. Children appear pale from the anemia; easy bruising or petechiae may be present from *thrombocytopenia* (reduced platelet level). Laboratory studies will show fibrin-split products in the serum as the fibrin deposits in glomerular vessels are degraded. Thrombocytopenia is present because platelets are damaged by the irregular blood vessels. An increased reticulocyte count indicates that red blood cells are rapidly being replaced.

Therapeutic Management

The child needs supportive therapy to maintain kidney and heart function. The extreme oliguria can be treated with peritoneal dialysis; anemia can be corrected by careful transfusion of packed red cells. Peritoneal dialysis can be extremely frightening to parents and the child because it involves penetration of the child's abdomen. Be certain they understand that the actual dialysis procedure is not painful and they can hold the child during it.

Ensure that parents understand the importance of follow-up care and have an appointment for this. Help them begin to view the child as well again so they do not continue to shelter him or her unnecessarily but allow for normal growth and development. Despite the extent of the illness, most infants with hemolytic-uremic syndrome recover completely. A number of children, unfortunately, will continue to have chronic renal involvement (Farquhar, 2000).

Acute Renal Failure (ARF)

Renal failure occurs in either an acute or chronic form. The acute form most often occurs because of a sudden body insult, such as dehydration. The chronic form results from extensive kidney disease, such as hemolytic-uremic syndrome or glomerulonephritis (Lum, 2001).

Other causes of ARF include prolonged anesthesia, hemorrhage, shock, severe diarrhea, or sudden traumatic injury. ARF also can occur in a child who is placed on cardiopulmonary bypass while undergoing heart surgery, who receives common antibiotics (aminoglycosides, penicillin, cephalosporins, and sulfonamides), who swallows poisons such as arsenic (found in rat poison), or who is exposed to industrial wastes such as mercury. The active course of acute glomerulonephritis may result in renal failure. All of these conditions appear to lead to renal ischemia, which ultimately leads to ARF.

Assessment

One of the first symptoms noted with acute renal failure is *oliguria,* defined as a urine output of less than 1 mL/kg of the child's body weight/h. An indwelling urinary catheter may be inserted to rule out the possibility that urinary retention in the bladder rather than kidney dysfunction is causing the oliguria.

Azotemia (accumulation of nitrogen waste in the bloodstream) will occur because of the oliguria. *Uremia* (extra accumulation of nitrogen wastes in the blood with additional toxic symptoms such as cerebral irritation) also may occur. The BUN level rises progressively as renal insufficiency continues and the breakdown products of protein cannot be excreted. A level greater than 80 to 100 mg/100 mL is toxic and needs correction, usually by dialysis. Urine creatinine level is another measure that can be used as an indicator of function, because it is normally excreted at a uniform rate. A rate of less than 10 mg/100 mL indicates severe renal failure. As the kidneys become unable to dilute or concentrate urine, the specific gravity of urine often becomes "fixed" at 1.010.

Hyperkalemia (elevated potassium level) may occur if potassium cannot be excreted. Hyperkalemia is manifested by a weak, irregular pulse, abdominal cramps, lowered blood pressure, and muscle weakness. Acidosis will follow shortly with ARF from the inability of H^+ ions to be excreted. As total output decreases, phosphorus will rise in the bloodstream. A high serum phosphorus level leads to a low calcium serum level (recall that phosphorus and calcium have an inverse proportional relationship). Severe hypocalcemia can lead to muscle twitching and seizures (*tetany*); chronic hypocalcemia can lead to withdrawal of calcium from bones (*osteodystrophy*).

An IVP or radioactive uptake scan may be ordered to substantiate the lack of kidney function. Parents and children need support for this type of study, because the results may be disappointing and so different from what they hoped they would be.

Therapeutic Management

Because acute renal failure is a reaction to body stress caused by acute disease or insult, attempts to treat it focus on supporting the child's body systems while correcting the underlying condition. If the child is dehydrated (as with diarrhea or hemorrhage), IV fluid is needed to replace plasma volume. Be certain to administer such fluid slowly enough to avoid heart failure; extra fluid cannot be removed by the kidneys because the kidneys are not functioning. The fluid should not contain potassium until it is established that kidney function is adequate; buildup of potassium may otherwise cause heart block. Potassium levels greater than 6 mEq/L are corrected either by the IV administration of calcium gluconate (as the glucose moves into cells, it carries potassium with it), the oral administration of a cation exchange resin such as Kayexalate, or by dialysis. Administering sodium bicarbonate may cause a shift of potassium from the bloodstream into cells, temporarily reducing the circulating potassium level. Administration of a combination of IV glucose and insulin may be effective (insulin helps glucose move into cells).

A diuretic such as furosemide (Lasix) may be ordered in an attempt to increase urine production. Diet should be low in protein, potassium, and sodium and high in carbohydrate to supply enough calories for metabolism yet limit urea production and control serum potassium levels. Fluid intake may be limited to prevent heart failure from accumulating fluid that cannot be excreted. Weigh children daily (same scale, same clothing, same time of day) and maintain accurate intake and output recordings to evaluate fluid status. If children are so ill that they cannot eat, total parenteral nutrition may be used. Regulate amounts carefully to prevent fluid overload (see Chap. 36 for total parental nutrition administration techniques).

When recovery from acute renal failure begins, children generally have a degree of diuresis as the extra fluid accumulated by the body is cleared. The increase in urine must be noted, because children may need additional fluid intake at this point to prevent hypovolemia, which could lead once more to renal failure. Parents usually remain anxious for an extended period after an episode of ARF because they are afraid that the restoration of kidney function is only temporary. Give them reassurance that urine output is remaining at a normal level. This helps them to relax and interact effectively with their child.

Chronic Renal Failure

Chronic renal failure results from developmental abnormalities, when acute failure becomes long-term or when chronic kidney disease has caused extensive nephron destruction (Lum, 2001). The nephrons that are not destroyed by long-term disease appear to function normally. They simply are inadequate in number to sustain kidney function. Glomeruli are capable of adjusting so that they enable kidney function to continue normally until 50% of nephrons are destroyed. After this point, kidney function diminishes by degrees until the child develops end-stage kidney disease, where the kidneys are unable to maintain normal function.

Assessment

With loss of nephron function, kidneys are unable to concentrate urine. This results in polyuria, possibly manifested as enuresis. The few functioning nephrons present are unable to reabsorb enough sodium to maintain a functioning level of body fluid, so dehydration occurs. As additional nephrons are lost, oliguria and anuria occur. Inability to excrete H^+ ions leads to acidosis. Hypocalcemia and hyperphosphatemia occur from the kidney's inability to excrete phosphate. Osteodystrophy occurs as calcium is withdrawn from bones to compensate. Kidneys are responsible for synthesizing vitamin D to its active form. With poor kidney function, vitamin D cannot be used. Without this, calcium cannot be absorbed from the GI tract and deposited in bones. Bones become so calcium depleted that growth halts and the bones lose strength (renal rickets).

Erythropoietin, formed by the kidneys, stimulates red cell production. With decreased erythropoietin production, anemia develops. Pruritus may be present from skin irritation from excretion of nitrogenous wastes in sweat from high levels of BUN and serum creatinine. These changes are summarized in Figure 46-14.

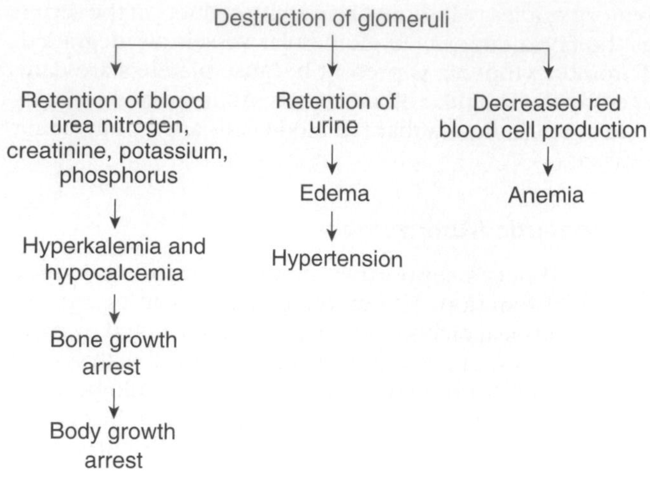

FIGURE 46.14 Pathology of chronic renal failure.

Therapeutic Management

Children with chronic renal failure are generally placed on a low-protein, low-phosphorus diet to prevent rapid urea and phosphate buildup. Children may take aluminum hydroxide gel with meals to bind phosphorus in the intestines and prevent absorption. Milk usually is not given because it is high in sodium, potassium, and phosphate—electrolytes children may have difficulty clearing. Meat is restricted and even beans are high enough in protein to be eliminated from the diet. This can be difficult for parents and children to understand because they are taught that meats are high in protein but vegetables are not. Letting children have some choice about foods they eat each day helps to promote compliance with this restricted diet. Whoever prepares meals needs good instructions on selecting low-protein foods. Low-electrolyte, low-protein formulas are commercially available for infants with renal failure.

Daily fluid intake may need to be restricted, although restriction should be as minimal as possible or it will present an area of tremendous conflict between the child and parents. Many children need sodium intake restricted, and others need a normal sodium intake (but no excessively salty foods such as luncheon meats, potato chips, or pretzels). Other children may actually need additional salt because, due to poor tubular reabsorption, they dump sodium in urine. Low-sodium formulas such as Lonalac are recommended for children with heart failure who need a low-sodium intake. Use them cautiously with children with renal insufficiency, because their high potassium content can lead to toxic potassium blood levels. Diuretics may be ordered to help children regulate sodium and fluid levels and prevent edema.

As renal failure becomes prolonged, the child may need supplemental calcium to prevent muscle cramping, rickets, tetany, or seizures. As hypertension becomes more and more acute from the accumulating blood volume, a daily antihypertensive drug may be ordered. A blood transfusion may be needed to correct anemia, but it must be given cautiously so volume overload does not occur. Recombinant human erythropoietin may be prescribed to stimulate red blood cell formation. Effective excretion of urea can be accomplished by dialysis or by replacing the nonfunctioning kidneys with kidney transplantation.

NURSING DIAGNOSES AND RELATED INTERVENTIONS

Nursing Diagnosis: Risk for interrupted family processes related to chronically ill family member

Outcome Identification: Family members will maintain functional system of mutual support for each other during course of child's illness.

Outcome Evaluation: Family members express feelings about illness to each other and to nurses; participate in care of ill member.

Children with renal failure grow poorly because of the alteration in calcium metabolism. Their height begins to fall below normal. It is easy for them to become depressed because of chronic fatigue and an unappetizing diet. If children are on corticosteroids or other immunosuppressive drugs because of glomerulonephritis, they may be angry or disheartened about their change in appearance.

Caring for a child with chronic renal disease is not only time consuming but financially and socially devastating for parents. Parents caring for such children at home need opportunities at periodic health assessments to voice their frustrations, fears, and anxieties. They need time to do those things important to them as individuals, whether taking a weekend trip or attending an evening show or program. Ask parents at clinic or follow-up visits, "Do you ever get out of the house or have the opportunity to do anything for yourself?" "What can we do for *you?*" Help of this kind ultimately improves children's care, because it improves the lives and mental attitudes of those around them.

✔ CHECKPOINT QUESTIONS

13. What is the first symptom typically seen in a child with acute renal failure?
14. What type of diet is usually ordered for a child with chronic renal failure?

KIDNEY TRANSPLANTATION

The ultimate possibility for prolonging the life of children with renal failure is kidney transplantation. With complete renal failure, children who have extensive hypertension may have their damaged kidneys removed and may be placed on hemodialysis or CAPD to await kidney transplantation. Kidney removal this way is an important step for parents and the child. Although parents realize that their child's kidneys are no longer functioning, this step removes all hope that a miracle might happen and make them function once more. Parents may ask whether it is possible to leave one of the child's kidneys, because only one kidney will be transplanted (this is not recommended because the hypertension would continue). Parents need a thorough explanation of why hypertension is destructive (i.e., it will lead to cerebral vascular accident or coronary artery disease). They must understand that renal biopsy shows that, short of a miracle, their child's kidneys will not function again, so that removal of them is not a loss but only recognition of a loss.

Preoperative Care

Kidney transplantation is most effective (the kidney is less likely to be rejected) if the kidney is taken from a living twin or sibling. Rejection occurs at a higher incidence if a kidney comes from a cadaver or recently deceased child. If a relative's tissue-compatible kidney is used, the success rate is as high as 90% (Merion & Magee, 2001). Most people consider that children should be of legal age to give consent to supply a kidney for transplantation, so few children have a sibling who is eligible to donate such a kidney. Tissue studies done to determine the best donor (matched for human leukocyte antigens) may show that the person in a family most willing to donate a kidney is not the best person in terms of tissue compatibility. This can cause bitterness and hopelessness in the family, compounding an already stressed family life. Many children anticipate that the characteristics of the donor will be transmitted to them by the kidney, and thus they are reluctant to accept the kidney of a family member with a character trait they do not like (perhaps a bad temper). They need to be assured that transplanted organs do not carry this type of problem with them. Adult-sized kidneys may be transplanted into children, although, if the child weighs less than 10 kg, this large a kidney may lead to hypertension, excessive diuresis, and abdominal complications because of the lack of space. Transplanted kidneys are placed in the abdomen, not the usual kidney space.

Tests that kidney donors can expect to have preoperatively include an HLA (human leukocyte antigen) typing, electrolyte blood analysis, complete blood count, bleeding time, urinalysis and urine culture, 24-h urine for protein, renal arteriogram, and IV pyelography. People who are unable to donate a kidney include those with multiple bilateral small renal arteries, bilateral renal disease, renal infection, advanced medical illness, severe obesity, or hypertension. Although kidney removal can be done by laparoscopy, donors must understand that removal of a kidney involves major surgery. They will have urine samples collected after surgery to assess that their remaining kidney is capable of maintaining full function and they are still in good health.

Before surgery, children who are to receive a transplantation may be dialyzed to clear their body of excessive potassium and fluid. If the donated kidney will be from a relative, there is adequate time for thorough preoperative preparation. If the donor kidney is from a cadaver, the announcement of surgery may be sudden and time for preoperative instruction and procedures may be limited.

Children who receive pretransplantation blood transfusions have an improved chance of transplant success. Most children receive at least five blood transfusions while awaiting surgery. The mechanisms by which this operates are unclear, but transfusion-induced production of antibodies or immune complexes mediates graft survival (Merion & Magee, 2001).

HLA (Human Leukocyte Antigen) Typing

The presence of antigens on erythrocytes has been documented for years. Antigens serve as the basis for blood transfusion typing and reactions. HLA is a group of antigens found on the surfaces of all cells with a nucleus, including blood components such as leukocytes and platelets. The name is derived from the fact that they were first identified on white blood cells. Such antigens are inherited from both parents and are specific for each individual. They denote tissue type or determine which tissue the immune system identifies as foreign tissue. They are carried on the short arm of chromosome 6 in each cell.

Such antigens also serve as the basis for paternity typing; they may cause reactions to blood product transfusions, bone marrow, and organ transplantation. When two people have like HLA antigens, they are said to be *histocompatible.* Identical twins have complete histocompatibility, family members have partial histocompatibility; any two people can have histocompatibility at least on one antigen site.

Children who are awaiting kidney transplantation are tissue typed, and this information is circulated to major medical centers. When a kidney is available for transplantation, the child's tissue type is compared with the donor kidney. For tissue typing, lymphocytes from both a donor and recipient are grown together in a culture medium and then examined for like characteristics.

Postoperative Care

After renal transplantation, children are cared for in an environment that is as sterile as possible. They are placed on immunosuppressive therapy (administration of cyclosporine, azathioprine [Imuran], and methylprednisolone [Solu-Medrol]) to reduce the possibility of kidney rejection. Antilymphocyte globulin and antithymocyte globulin may be administered to aid immunosuppression.

Children need supportive care postoperatively. Although some transplanted kidneys begin to function immediately, hemodialysis may be continued until the implanted kidney can fully function after the insult of transplantation. Be prepared to help the child and parents through the "honeymoon" period after the transplantation (see Focus on Communication).

Help children understand that acceptance or rejection of a kidney depends on a multitude of factors—the condition of renal veins and arteries, the transplanted kidney, or antigen–antibody formation—but none of these factors is related to whether the child is good or bad or deserves or does not deserve to have the transplantation work.

Children with end-stage renal disease usually fail to grow despite treatment. Although children's rate of growth is improved after kidney transplantation, they will probably never reach full height. Part of this growth retardation is related to the need for corticosteroid maintenance therapy.

Transplant Rejection

Acute transplant rejection, if it occurs, usually occurs within the first 3 months after transplantation. Children begin to develop fever, proteinuria, oliguria, weight gain, hypertension, and tenderness over the kidney. Serum creatinine and BUN levels will rise. Increasing the dose of immunosuppressants may be effective in relieving this type of rejection.

Rejection may also be *chronic,* in which the transplanted kidney gradually loses function after the first 6 months. Hypertension and anemia result. A biopsy will show vascular changes such as narrowing of arterial lumens and interstitial changes such as fibrosis and tubular atrophy. This type of rejection is difficult to halt, although it may be such a slow, steady process that it is 2 or 3 years before the kidney fails. If a kidney is rejected, it is removed, and a child is returned to a program of hemodialysis. Because one kidney was rejected does not mean that a second transplantation will be rejected also. Unfortunately, however, the number of kidneys available for transplantation is limited, so kidney rejection becomes an ominous sign for the child's long-term survival.

The incidence of malignant disease is six times more frequent in transplantation recipients than in the normal population, probably because of the long-term immunosuppression (Merion & Magee, 2001). The original disease for which the child had the transplantation may recur in the transplanted kidney. This is most apt to occur in glomerulonephritis. During adolescence, typically an age of poor

FOCUS ON COMMUNICATION

Shasha is a 9-year-old recipient of a kidney transplant whom you visit at home. Her mother tells you that Shasha has "changed completely" since the transplantation. She thinks this is as wonderful as the transplantation itself.

Less Effective Communication

Nurse: Mrs. Maronia? In what way has Shasha changed?

Mrs. Maronia: She used to whine all the time. And constantly ask for things. Now she entertains herself. It's like heaven.

Nurse: How does she behave with her brother?

Mrs. Maronia: Perfect. She never used to share with him. Yesterday, she gave him her magic markers. She even lets him watch his television programs instead of hers.

Nurse: That sounds wonderful. Let's review her medicine routine to be sure that's going well.

Mrs. Maronia: That's another thing she does perfectly. Never fusses a bit about anything she has to take.

More Effective Communication

Nurse: Mrs. Maronia? In what way has Shasha changed?

Mrs. Maronia: She used to whine all the time. And constantly ask for things. Now she entertains herself. It's like heaven.

Nurse: How does she behave with her brother?

Mrs. Maronia: Perfect. She never used to share with him. Yesterday, she gave him her magic markers. She even lets him watch his television programs instead of hers.

Nurse: Do you think she's acting a little too perfect?

Mrs. Maronia: Well, it does seem a bit strange for her.

Nurse: Do you think she could be worrying that if she misbehaves, her transplant might not take?

Mrs. Maronia: I never thought of that. I would feel better if she started to act like her old self.

What the mother above is describing is a "honeymoon" period that children may pass through after transplantation. Parents often need help seeing this for what it is so they can begin to reassure the child that behaving perfectly will not influence the transplantation and because they loved them as they were, they will continue to love them regardless.

medicine compliance, kidney recipients need to be followed closely to be certain they are taking their immunosuppressive therapy. Parents cannot help but overprotect the child; they worry that a rough-housing session with a sibling or playing a game such as baseball may injure the transplanted kidney. The child may be afraid to engage in any activity for the same reason.

✔ CHECKPOINT QUESTIONS

15. What are major problems of transplanting adult kidneys into children?
16. Where are transplanted kidneys placed?

KEY POINTS

Many urinary tract disorders such as polycystic kidneys, urethral obstruction, and bladder exstrophy are evident on fetal sonogram. Early identification allows therapy to begin immediately at birth.

Many urinary tract disorders such as polycystic kidneys or chronic renal failure are long-term conditions requiring years of therapy. Be certain that parents are well informed about the child's condition so they can continue to participate in planning the child's care.

Congenital structural abnormalities of the urinary tract include patent urachus, exstrophy of the bladder, hypospadias, and epispadias. Surgical correction is required for all of these.

UTI tends to occur more often in girls than boys. "Honeymoon cystitis" refers to a UTI occurring with first-time sexual intercourse.

Vesicoureteral reflex is the backflow of urine into ureters with voiding. It occurs because the valve that guards the entrance to the ureters is defective. Surgical correction may be necessary to prevent repeated UTI.

Renal dysfunction can occur for structural reasons such as kidney agenesis, polycystic kidney, and renal hypoplasia. Acute poststreptococcal glomerulonephritis is inflammation of the glomeruli after a streptococcal infection. It is characterized by an acute episode of hematuria and proteinuria.

Diminished kidney function leads to both fluid and electrolyte imbalances. Creative techniques are necessary to encourage children to continue to ingest a restricted-protein diet.

Nephrotic syndrome is an immunologic process that results in altered glomeruli permeability. Nursing diagnoses associated with this condition may include imbalanced nutrition, risk for impaired skin integrity, and deficient knowledge.

Renal failure can be acute or chronic. Peritoneal dialysis or hemodialysis may be used to remove body waste until kidney function can be restored.

Kidney transplantation may be a therapy option for some children with kidney disorders. This is extensive surgery and requires the child to remain on immunosuppressive therapy to counteract transplant rejection.

CRITICAL THINKING EXERCISES

1. Carol is the preschooler with nephrotic syndrome whom you met at the beginning of the chapter. Her parent asked you whether when Carol accidentally drank beer off the coffee table if this could have caused the kidney disease. What would you tell her is the cause of nephrosis? What discharge instructions can you anticipate you will need to review with Carol's mother?
2. A 12-year-old girl comes to a pediatric clinic with her third UTI this year. Her mother asks you whether there is anything she should be doing to help prevent these. How would you answer her?
3. A child with end-stage renal disease is awaiting kidney transplantation. He tells you he hopes he has been good enough to deserve being chosen for the next kidney available. What would you want to teach him about the transplantation selection process?
4. A 6-year-old girl is receiving continuous ambulatory peritoneal dialysis. She wants to go to her church camp this summer. Her parents ask you whether this would be a good experience for her. What factors would you want to know about the camp? About the child? About her procedure?
5. Examine the National Health Goals related to renal disorders. Most government-sponsored money for nursing research is allotted based on these goals. What would be a possible research topic to explore pertinent to these goals that would be both fundable and advance evidence-based practice?

REFERENCES

Caudle, S. S. (2000). Enuresis. In M. W. Schwartz (Ed.). *The 5-minute pediatric consult* (pp. 350–351). Philadelphia: Lippincott Williams & Wilkins.

Chalom, E. C. (2000). Lupus erythematosis. In M. W. Schwartz (Ed.). *The 5-minute pediatric consult* (pp. 508–509). Philadelphia: Lippincott Williams & Wilkins.

Department of Health & Human Services. (2000). *Healthy people 2010*. Washington, DC: DHHS.

Ellsworth, P., et al. (1999). Hypospadias repair in the 1990s. *AORN Journal, 69*(1), 148–161.

Farquhar, D. (2000). *E. coli*, antibiotics and hemolytic-uremic syndrome in children. *Canadian Medical Association Journal, 163*(4), 438–440.

Ford, D. M. (2001). Fluid, electrolyte & acid-base disorders & therapy. In W. W. Hay, A. R. Hayward, M. J. Levin & J. M. Sondheimer (Eds.). *Current pediatric diagnosis and treatment* (15th ed.). New York: McGraw-Hill.

Gong, W. K., et al. (2001). Eighteen years experience in pediatric acute dialysis: Analysis of predictors of outcome. *Pediatric Nephrology, 16*(3), 212-215.

Gusic, B. R. (2000). Henoch-Schönlein purpura. In M. W. Schwartz (Ed.). *The 5-minute pediatric consult* (pp. 424-425). Philadelphia: Lippincott Williams & Wilkins.

Haffner, J. C., & Schurman, S. J. (2001). The technology-dependent child. *Pediatric Clinics of North America, 48*(3), 751-764.

Jantunen, M. E. et al. (2002). Recurrent urinary tract infections in infancy: Relapses or reinfections? *Journal of Infectious Diseases, 185*(3), 375-379.

Karch, A. M. (2001). *Lippincott's nursing drug guide.* Philadelphia: Lippincott Williams & Wilkins.

Kasahara, T., et al. (2001). Prognosis of acute poststreptococcal glomerulonephritis (APSGN) is excellent in children, when adequately diagnosed. *Pediatrics International, 43*(4), 364-367.

Langley, J. M., Hanakowski, M., & Leblanc, J. C. (2001). Unique epidemiology of nosocomial urinary tract infection in children. *American Journal of Infection Control, 29*(2), 94-98.

Leonard, M. B. (2000). Prune-belly syndrome. In M. W. Schwartz (Ed.). *The 5-minute pediatric consult* (pp. 662- 663). Philadelphia: Lippincott Williams & Wilkins.

Lum, G. M. (2001). Kidney and urinary tract. In W. W. Hay, A. R. Hayward, M. J. Levin & J. M. Sondheimer (Eds.). *Current pediatric diagnosis and treatment* (15th ed.). New York: McGraw-Hill.

Master, C. L. (2000a). Exstrophy of the bladder. In M. W. Schwartz (Ed.). *The 5-minute pediatric consult* (pp. 364-365). Philadelphia: Lippincott Williams & Wilkins.

______. (2000b). Vesicoureteral reflux. In M. W. Schwartz (Ed.). *The 5-minute pediatric consult* (pp. 866-867). Philadelphia: Lippincott Williams & Wilkins.

Merion, R. M., & Magee, J. C. (2001). Transplantation and immunology: Renal transplantation. In W. W. Hay, A. R. Hayward, M. J. Levin & J. M. Sondheimer (Eds.). *Current pediatric diagnosis and treatment* (15th ed.). New York: McGraw-Hill.

Meyers, K. E. (2000a). Glomerulonephritis. In M. W. Schwartz (Ed.). *The 5-minute pediatric consult* (pp. 388-389). Philadelphia: Lippincott Williams & Wilkins.

______. (2000b). Nephrotic syndrome. In M. W. Schwartz (Ed.). *The 5-minute pediatric consult* (pp. 566-567). Philadelphia: Lippincott Williams & Wilkins.

Santen, S. A., & Altieri, M. G. (2001). Pediatric urinary tract infection. *Emergency Medicine Clinics of North America, 19*(3), 675-690.

Shaw, K. N. (2000). Urinary tract infection. In M. W. Schwartz (Ed.). *The 5-minute pediatric consult* (pp. 852-853). Philadelphia: Lippincott Williams & Wilkins.

Thilo, E. H., & Rosenberg, A. A. (2001). Renal disorders in the newborn infant. In W. W. Hay, A. R. Hayward, M. J. Levin & J. M. Sondheimer (Eds.). *Current pediatric diagnosis and treatment* (15th ed.). New York: McGraw-Hill.

Verrina, E., et al. (2000). Prevention of peritonitis in children on peritoneal dialysis. *Peritoneal Dialysis International, 20*(6), 625-630.

SUGGESTED READINGS

Balling, K., & McCubbin, M. (2001). Hospitalized children with chronic illness: Parental caregiving needs and valuing parental expertise. *Journal of Pediatric Nursing, 16*(2), 110-119.

Baskin, L. S. (2000). Hypospadias and urethral development. *Journal of Urology, 163*(3), 951-956.

Bensman, A. (2002). Should children with asymptomatic bacteriuria undergo imaging studies of the urinary tract? *Pediatric Nephrology, 17*(1), 76-77.

Freedman, A. L., Johnson, M. P., & Gonzalez, R. (2000). Fetal therapy for obstructive uropathy: Past, present, future. *Pediatric Nephrology, 14*(2), 167-176.

Hodson, E. M., et al. (2000). Corticosteroid therapy for nephrotic syndrome in children. *Cochrane Database of Systematic Reviews,* (4), CD001533.

Jennings, R. W. (2000). Prune belly syndrome. *Seminars in Pediatric Surgery, 9*(3), 115-120.

Jeong, H. J., et al. (2001). Glomerular growth under cyclosporine treatment in childhood nephrotic syndrome. *Clinical Nephrology, 55*(4), 289-296.

Kliebenstein, M. A., & Broome, M. E. (2000). School re-entry for the child with chronic illness: Parent and school personnel perceptions. *Pediatric Nursing, 26*(6), 579-584.

Weidner, I. S., et al. (1999). Risk factors for cryptorchidism and hypospadias. *Journal of Urology, 161*(5), 1606-1609.

Weir, M., & Brien, J. (2000). Adolescent urinary tract infections. *Adolescent Medicine, 11*(2), 293-313.

47

CHAPTER

Nursing Care of the Child With a Reproductive Disorder

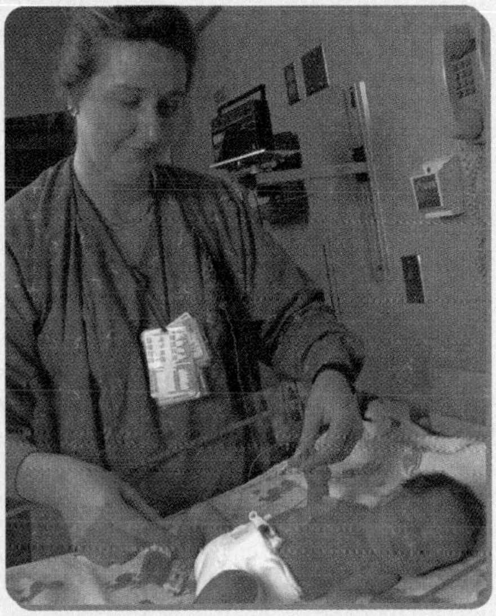

Key Terms

- amenorrhea
- anovulatory
- cryptorchidism
- dysmenorrhea
- endometriosis
- fibrocystic breast disease
- gynecomastia
- hermaphrodite
- hydrocele
- menorrhagia
- metrorrhagia
- mittelschmerz
- orchiectomy
- orchiopexy
- pelvic inflammatory disease
- premenstrual dysphoric disorder
- pseudo-hermaphrodite
- sexually transmitted disease (STD)
- toxic shock syndrome
- varicocele
- vulvovaginitis

Objectives

After mastering the contents of this chapter, you should be able to:

1. Describe common reproductive disorders in children.
2. Assess children with a reproductive disorder.
3. Formulate nursing diagnoses related to a child's reproductive illness.
4. Develop outcomes for children with a reproductive disorder.
5. Plan nursing care related to preventing reproductive disorders in children.
6. Implement nursing care for the child with a reproductive disorder.
7. Evaluate outcomes for achievement and effectiveness of care.
8. Identify National Health Goals related to reproductive disorders that nurses can help the nation achieve.
9. Identify areas related to the care of children with reproductive disorders that could benefit from additional nursing research or application of evidence-based practice.
10. Analyze ways to implement more family-centered nursing care for the child with a reproductive disorder.
11. Integrate knowledge of reproductive disorders in children with the nursing process to achieve quality maternal and child health nursing care.

Navi is a 15-year-old girl seen in a pediatric clinic. She has been diagnosed with gonorrhea because of a purulent vaginal discharge and burning on urination. When you ask her if she is sexually active, she says no; she thinks she contracted the infection from sharing a towel in a locker room after gym class. As she leaves the clinic, you hear her tell the receptionist, "I'm glad I got this early in life. Now I won't have to worry about getting it again." What kind of health education does Navi need?

Previous chapters described the growth and development of well children. This chapter adds information about the dramatic changes, both physical and psychosocial, that occur when children develop reproductive disorders. This is important information because it constitutes a basis for care and health teaching.

After you have studied the chapter, answer the Critical Thinking Exercises at the end of the chapter and then access the on-line study activities (http://connection.lww.com) *to further sharpen your skills and test your knowledge.*

Reproductive disorders in children range from mild infections to serious anatomic malformations that can interfere with fertility. All of these disorders, however, require prompt and careful treatment so that children can reach adulthood in reproductive health and with a positive sense of sexuality.

Parents are not always as comfortable inquiring about disorders of the reproductive tract as they are about other disorders. Unless they have clear, thorough explanations of the disease process and prescribed therapy, their reluctance to pursue the subject may leave them confused or misinformed. Even young children can sense that illness affecting genitalia or reproductive ability is viewed by some adults as different from other diseases. As they reach puberty, they need honest explanations about any effect such a condition will have on interpersonal relationships, sexual functioning, or childbearing. National Health Goals related to reproductive disorders in children are highlighted in the Focus on National Health Goals box.

FOCUS ON NATIONAL HEALTH GOALS

Because sexually transmitted diseases (STDs) not only cause short-term distress because of painful lesions but can also have long-term implications for fertility and future childbearing, a number of National Health Goals specifically address them. These are:

- Reduce the proportion of adolescents and young adults with *Chlamydia trachomatis* infections from baselines of 12% (females) and 15% (males) to a target of 3%.
- Reduce new cases of gonorrhea to an incidence of no more than 19 new cases/100,000 people from a baseline of 123/100,000.
- Reduce primary and secondary syphilis to an incidence of no more than 0.2 cases/100,000 people from a baseline of 3.2 per 100,000.
- Reduce genital herpes to an incidence of no more than 14% from a baseline of 17%.
- Reduce pelvic inflammatory disease to an incidence of no more than 5% of women aged 15 through 44 from a baseline of 8% (DHHS, 2000).

Nurses can be instrumental in helping the nation achieve these goals by educating adolescents about effective ways to prevent STDs and how to recognize the signs and symptoms of these illnesses. Areas that could benefit from additional nursing research and evidence-based practice in this area include: the most effective ways to teach adolescents about safer sex practices, the reasons adolescents continue to believe that they cannot contract infectious diseases, and strategies that would make it easier for parents to discuss this topic with adolescents.

NURSING PROCESS OVERVIEW

For Care of the Child With a Reproductive Disorder

Assessment

Assessment of reproductive health begins with the first physical examination at birth and continues at health assessments throughout childhood (see Assessing the Child for Reproductive Disorders). As with other parts of the health interview, questions regarding reproductive health and illness are generally addressed to the parents until the child is able to answer history questions reliably and independently. Once the girl has reached adolescence, a gynecologic history (Box 47-1) should be included in the health assessment. To preserve their privacy, adolescents of both genders may prefer not to be accompanied by a parent during a physical examination for reproductive dysfunction.

Some adolescents visit health care facilities on their own. They may be worried that they have contracted a sexually transmitted disease (STD; a disease spread by sexual relations) or that they have become pregnant, or they want to receive some form of contraception. Before they can admit their chief concern to health care providers, however, they may "test" the health care provider by eliciting a reaction to a minor problem. Be aware that an adolescent who consults a health care provider with a seemingly minor concern may only be misinterpreting symptoms and is truly worried that a minor symptom is serious. On the other hand, the adolescent actually may be seeking help for another problem. Asking the adolescent, "Is there anything else that worries you? Is there any other way we can help you today?" may help you elicit the adolescent's primary concern (see Focus on Communication).

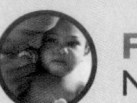

A pelvic examination is unnecessary for girls who have not yet reached adolescence, but, if vaginal walls need to be inspected (because of an inflamma-

ASSESSING the Child for a Reproductive Disorder

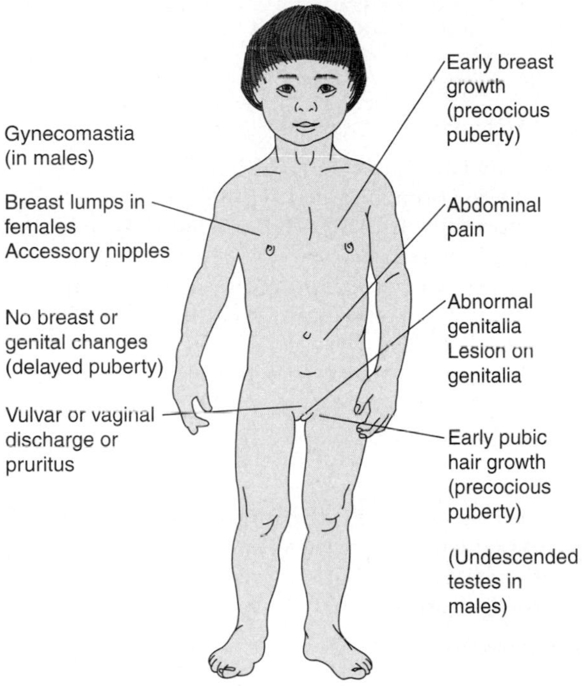

tion or infection), an otoscope and ear tip can be used. Cotton-tipped applicators moistened with sterile normal saline solution can be used to take culture specimens without causing discomfort. For the adolescent girl, the pelvic examination becomes an important part of health assessment. Because the first pelvic examination can be frightening and embarrassing, spend time with the girl before the procedure to teach her about what is being assessed. A three-dimensional model of internal organs and some representative instruments may be more useful when describing the examination than a verbal description of anatomy. Let her look at and handle a speculum. A small speculum should be used for examining young girls. For their comfort, warm the speculum first.

Remaining beside her as a support person helps to make the examination less embarrassing. To protect her self-esteem, be sure the girl meets the person who will examine her before she is placed in a lithotomy position (see Focus on Cultural Competence).

A young adolescent may be uncomfortable in a lithotomy position and can be examined in a dorsal recumbent one instead (see Chap. 10 for information on assisting with a pelvic examination). Allow the adolescent to choose whether she wants a parent to remain in the room with her.

Nursing Diagnosis

Selected nursing diagnoses used for children with reproductive disorders include the following:

- Pain related to vaginal infection
- Disturbed body image related to fibrocystic breast disease
- Anxiety related to absence or irregularity of menstrual periods in adolescent
- Fear related to surgery on genital organs

Outcome Identification and Planning

Assessment of the child's knowledge about the reproductive system and ways that illness can affect reproductive and sexual functioning forms the foundation for developing appropriate outcomes. Educating the child about reproductive health may be one of the first areas to plan. When establishing outcomes with adolescents, remember that it will be difficult to meet those that require an entire change in lifestyle. It may be more effective to plan for change one step at a time.

Implementation

Interventions for children with reproductive disorders should always include education about reproductive functioning and measures for maintaining reproductive and sexual health and preventing illness. Health education regarding the importance of testicular self-examination for adolescent males and breast self-examination for adolescent females should be stressed at all health care visits (see Chap. 33). Guidelines for teaching about menstrual health and safer sex are covered in Chapter 4. Organizations helpful for referral for adolescents include:

National Women's Health Network
(*www.womenshealthnetwork.org*)
National Adolescent Health Information Center
(*www.youth.ucsf.edu*)

Essential nursing interventions also include supporting parents and children through difficult decisions and frightening procedures and providing close observation and empathic counseling after surgery. For example, surgery for undescended testes is a procedure that can be traumatic for the child, especially if performed during a developmental stage in which he views such surgery as castrating. Being certain that the child receives good preparation for surgery and reassurance that he will not be mutilated is an essential nursing intervention.

Outcome Evaluation

The responses of children to reproductive dysfunction vary both with the severity of the illness and the specific age and fears of the child. It is safe to assume, however, that children who have experienced such an illness are at risk for a loss of self-esteem or confusion about their body image. Therefore, outcome evaluation must include long-term evaluation of the child's coping abilities and self-image. If the child contracts an STD, evaluation should also address the child's knowledge about avoiding STDs in the future

BOX 47.1

TAKING A GYNECOLOGIC HISTORY

When assessing an adolescent for a gynecologic health history be especially conscious of the patient's sense of modesty and need for privacy. To ensure privacy, conduct the interview without the parent or caregiver present.

Menstrual History

At what age did you begin menstruating?
How often do your menstrual periods occur and how long do they usually last?
What is the amount of menstrual flow? (Document by amount of pads or tampons used.)
Do you experience discomfort? (Document if first day, all days, and so forth, and action taken to relieve it.)
Do any sisters or your mother have discomfort or pain during their menstrual periods (dysmenorrhea) also (endometriosis is familial)?
Do you experience any symptoms of irritability, moodiness, headache, or diarrhea (premenstrual dysphoric disorder) 1 or 2 days before menses?
What were the dates of your last two menstrual periods, how long did they last (duration), and what was the flow like (type of flow)?

Reproductive Tract History

Have you had any vaginal discharge? (Document amount and whether pad is necessary or not—include duration, frequency, description, associated symptoms, actions taken.)
Is there vaginal itching (pruritus)?
Is there any vaginal odor?
Have you had reproductive tract surgery? Have you ever been pregnant? Have you ever had an abortion or miscarriage?

Sexual History

Have you had a sexually transmitted disease (STD; eg, herpes, gonorrhea, and syphilis)?
Are you currently sexually active? What is the gender of your partner?
Do you experience any discomfort during sexual activity (dyspareunia) or any spotting afterward (postcoital spotting)?
Do you have any concerns (worried about frequency, position, partner's satisfaction with coitus)?
Is orgasm experienced?

Contraception History

Do you use any type of birth control? If so, what contraceptive currently do you use? (Document length of time used, satisfaction, any problems.)
Have you used any other type in the past?

Breast Health

Have you ever noticed any abnormality such as a lump, discharge, or pain in your breasts?
Have you ever had breast surgery?
Have you breastfed a child?

and willingness to seek help should an infection recur. An STD in a young child should be investigated as the result of possible sexual abuse.

The following are examples suggesting achievement of outcomes:

- Child states discomfort from vaginal infection is tolerable after beginning medication.
- Child states she is able to view self as confident despite fibrocystic breast disease.
- Child states she is able to wait 6 months without worrying about not yet having a menstrual period.
- Child states he feels less fearful about impending surgery after talking with the health care provider.

DISORDERS CAUSED BY ALTERED REPRODUCTIVE DEVELOPMENT

Genetic sex or *biologic gender* (sex chromosome XX or XY) is determined at conception. However, development of the reproductive system, including external genitalia, occurs over two distinct periods. Reproductive organs and genitalia begin to differentiate in utero by the 8th week, with growth and refinement occurring over the next several months. This period constitutes the first phase of reproductive development. The second phase occurs with specific endocrine changes that are triggered during puberty; this is a period of maturation of primary and secondary sexual characteristics.

Ambiguous genitalia, which is a rare condition with different causes that occur during fetal development, and precocious puberty or delayed puberty, second phase disorders, are examples of altered reproductive development. (For a discussion of genetic disorders, see Chap. 7.)

Ambiguous Genitalia

Understanding how reproductive organs develop in utero is important to understand ambiguous genitalia. Although external sexual characteristics generally follow from the XX or XY chromosome, under certain circumstances it is possible for structures generally considered "male" or "female" to develop in either chromosomal gender. Usually, a diagnosis of ambiguous genitalia means that external sexual organs in the child did not follow the normal course of development, so that, at birth, the external sexual organs are so incompletely or abnormally formed that it is impossible to clearly determine the child's gender by simple observation. For instance, a male infant with *hypospadias* (urethral opening on the underside of the penis)

FOCUS ON COMMUNICATION

Terry is a 16-year-old boy you see at a pediatric clinic. He has mild upper respiratory symptoms.

Less Effective Communication

Nurse: Terry? Doctor Jensen doesn't believe you need anything for your cold. Just drink a little extra fluid and take it easy for a couple days.
Terry: Don't I need a prescription? Some penicillin or something?
Nurse: No. Colds are caused by viruses. Penicillin isn't necessary.
Terry: I want to be sure I get over this. I'd really like an antibiotic of some kind.
Nurse: One really isn't necessary.
Terry: I have a bad cough. I don't think I mentioned that.
Nurse: Doctor Jensen listened to your chest. You don't have anything serious there.
Terry: My stomach doesn't feel very good either. Can't I have something?
Nurse: Sorry. Goodbye now.

More Effective Communication

Nurse: Terry? Doctor Jensen doesn't believe you need anything for your cold. Just drink a little extra fluid and take it easy for a couple days.
Terry: Don't I need a prescription? Some penicillin or something?
Nurse: No. Colds are caused by viruses. Penicillin isn't necessary.
Terry: I want to be sure I get over this. I'd really like an antibiotic of some kind.
Nurse: One really isn't necessary.
Terry: I have a bad cough. I don't think I mentioned that.
Nurse: Doctor Jensen listened to your chest. You don't have anything serious there.
Terry: My stomach doesn't feel very good either. Can't I have something?
Nurse: It seems that you have a couple more symptoms that you didn't mention before? Is there anything else?
Terry: Well, I have this rash and . . . . . .
Nurse: And . . . . . go on . . . .
Terry: And I'm scared I might have a sex disease.

Adolescents can have difficulty discussing reproductive tract symptoms. If they have too much difficulty, they can try to obtain an antibiotic by describing respiratory or abdominal symptoms. Being alert that adolescents do this helps you to recognize a "growing" history of this type.

FOCUS ON CULTURAL COMPETENCE

Different cultures have different attitudes toward reproductive disorders. Adolescents in Middle Eastern countries, for example, are extremely modest, and so are extremely uncomfortable having pelvic examinations done for reproductive disorders. Girls from these countries may be more comfortable if the examiner is a woman.

and **cryptorchidism** (undescended testes) may appear more female than male on first inspection (see Chap. 46 for a discussion of hypospadias). Alternatively, a chromosomal female (XX) fetus may become "masculinized" with exposure to androgen in utero (the clitoris is so enlarged that it appears more like a penis, labia may be partially fused so it is difficult to tell them from a male perineum, or the urethra may be displaced so far forward that it is located on the clitoris). When this occurs, the newborn will appear to be a boy on initial inspection. Likewise, under certain conditions, a chromosomal male (XY) may become "feminized," with a lack of fusion of the labioscrotal folds and an incompletely formed penis.

The most common cause of in vitro virilization of females is *congenital adrenocortical syndrome.* The adrenal gland produces androgen instead of adequate cortisone, causing the clitoris to become the size of a typical newborn male's penis (see Chap. 48).

If testosterone was produced in utero but the mullerian duct (female) development was not suppressed, a child may be a **hermaphrodite** (having both ovaries and testes and either male or female external genitalia). Children with ambiguous genitalia are often termed **pseudohermaphrodites** because, as infants, they have some external features of both sexes, although only either ova-ries or testes (or neither) are present (Kappy, Steelman & Travers, 2001).

Assessment

If there is any question about the child's gender, karyotyping will help to establish whether the child is genetically male or female (see Chap. 7). This involves drawing a specimen of blood, allowing the white blood cells to reach a division stage, then examining them. *Laparoscopy* (introduction of a narrow laparoscope into the abdominal cavity through a half-inch incision under the umbilicus) or possibly exploratory surgery may be necessary to determine if ovaries or undescended testes are present. Intravenous (IV) pyelography or sonogram can be used to establish whether a male has a complete urinary tract.

Therapeutic Management

Once the child's true gender is determined, the extent of necessary reconstructive surgery is determined in consultation with the parents. This may involve correction of a hypospadias or cryptorchidism, removal of labial adhesions, or surgical removal of an enlarged clitoris. When removal of an enlarged clitoris is involved, the parents must consider what the absence of this organ will mean to the girl in terms of later sexual enjoyment. Parents may be well advised to delay this type of surgery until the girl can decide for herself whether she wants it done. Nonfunctioning ovaries or testes are generally removed to prevent malignancy later in life.

If an infant is chromosomally male but does not have an adequate penis, a decision to raise the child as a female might be made, although construction of an artificial penis is more likely.

NURSING DIAGNOSES AND RELATED INTERVENTIONS

When identifying outcomes, be aware that parents under stress may have difficulty making long-range plans. The birth of a child with a perplexing defect produces a particularly high level of stress, hampering parents' ability to think clearly and calmly about their situation.

Nursing Diagnosis: Anxiety related to ambiguous sex of child at birth

Outcome Identification: Parents will demonstrate confidence in health care team and increased knowledge about child's condition and necessary care.

Outcome Evaluation: Parents voice willingness to support treatment plan, including additional necessary tests, and state they are prepared to make decisions with guidance from health care team.

If the gender of the child is unclear, parents should be told this immediately. If told first that their child is a boy, only to be told 24 hours later that "he" is really a girl, parents can have difficulty accepting this drastic change. During this period when the baby's gender is yet to be determined, avoid calling the baby "it." Rather, say "the baby" or "your child." Explain how sexual organs form in utero and that every child has the potential to be externally female or male.

To promote bonding, help parents understand that their child is otherwise perfect (assuming this is true). As the child grows, additional counseling may be needed to help the child adjust to an abnormal appearance or function.

Precocious Puberty

The development of breast or pubic hair before age 8 years or menses before age 9 years is considered precocious sexual development. Often, such development is expressed as isolated breast or pubic hair growth but can proceed to complete spermatogenesis and menstrual function. Precocious puberty occurs more often in girls than in boys (Ferry & Satin-Smith, 2000).

This condition is caused by the early production of gonadotropins by the pituitary gland; gonadotropins stimulate the ovaries or testes to produce sex hormones. Such stimulation can occur because of a pituitary tumor, cyst, or traumatic injury to the third ventricle next to the pituitary gland. It also can occur because of estrogen-secreting cysts or tumors of the ovary or testosterone-secreting cysts of the testes. In rare instances, it occurs because of an estrogen- or testosterone-secreting adrenal tumor. In girls, ingestion of a mother's oral contraceptives can also initiate menarchelike changes.

In children affected by precocious puberty, a tumor must be ruled out. When no physical cause, such as a tumor, is detected, the phenomenon appears to occur only because the *gonadostat* of the hypothalamus (the trigger that begins the development of secondary sex characteristics) was turned on several years too early.

Assessment

With precocious puberty, children have increased breast development and accelerated skeletal maturation. Girls have menstrual bleeding with little pubic or axillary hair because of still low androgen secretion. Boys have obvious genital growth. The diagnosis of early puberty is confirmed by serum analysis for estrogen or androgen; these will be at adult levels.

Therapeutic Management

A synthetic analogue to gonadotropin-releasing hormone (GnRH) is available as leuprolide acetate (Lupron; see Focus on Pharmacology). Administration of this analogue desensitizes GnRH receptors, making stimulation of GnRH ineffective. The preparation is administered subcutaneously daily. When discontinued at age 12 or 13 years, puberty progresses normally.

NURSING DIAGNOSES AND RELATED INTERVENTIONS

Nursing Diagnosis: Disturbed body image related to precocious puberty

FOCUS ON PHARMACOLOGY

Leuprolide acetate (Lupron)

Action: Leuprolide is a hormonal agent, specifically an LH-RH agonist, that occupies pituitary gonadotropin-releasing hormone receptors preventing GnRH from functioning.

Pregnancy Risk Category: X

Dosage: Daily SQ or monthly intramuscular (IM) injection

Possible adverse effects: Nausea, vomiting, anorexia, hot flashes, headache, pain at injection site.

Nursing Implications

- Administer only with the syringes supplied with the drug
- Vary injection sites to decrease local irritation
- Monitor injection sites for bruising and rash
- Instruct parents in method for proper administration
- When monthly doses are prescribed, assist parents with preparing a realistic schedule for administration. Encourage the use of a calendar for accurate timing

Outcome Identification: Child will demonstrate adequate level of confidence in self and body in 3 months.

Outcome Evaluation: Child voices an understanding of what is happening and does not evidence excessive shyness or reluctance to interact with peers.

Children who develop precociously may have difficulty interacting with peers because they appear so different from other members of their group. Parents may worry about the children becoming sexually active, particularly about girls becoming pregnant.

Both parents and children need reassurance that, after reaching the age of normal puberty, the child will again be the same as other children; the fact that the child's sexual growth started early does not mean the genitals will be out of proportion to the rest of the body as an adult.

Parents must also understand that the child is fully fertile and able to inseminate or conceive when early puberty occurs. Oral contraceptives are not advisable for girls this young because the increased load of estrogen will hasten the closing of epiphyseal lines of long bones too early and possibly stunt their growth permanently.

Parents may need to be reminded that, although their child appears to be much older, the changes are only in sexual characteristics. Household tasks, responsibility, and expectations must be geared to the child's chronologic age, not to outward appearance.

Delayed Puberty

Secondary sex characteristics normally are present by age 14 in girls and age 15 in boys. Delayed puberty, as the name implies, is the failure of pubertal changes to occur at the usual age. The family history of many children reveals a family tendency for late maturation. If so, the child needs a thorough physical examination that will disclose whether some secondary sex characteristics are present or if endocrine stimulation is beginning.

If girls have not begun to menstruate by age 17 years and pathology has been ruled out, menstrual cycles can be started by administering estrogen. Many girls worry considerably about delayed menstruation, but, once reassured that development is merely delayed, they are usually willing to wait for menarche to occur on its own.

Similarly, boys who are distressed by their lack of development may receive testosterone supplements to stimulate hair and genital growth (Kappy, Steelman & Travers, 2001).

> ✔ **CHECKPOINT QUESTIONS**
>
> 1. Does precocious puberty occur more often in males or females?
> 2. Secondary sex characteristics usually are present by the time a girl is what age?

REPRODUCTIVE DISORDERS IN MALES

Common reproductive disorders in males include structural alterations in the penis or testes such as phimosis and cryptorchidism, inflammation such as balanoposthitis, and, in adolescents, testicular cancer.

Balanoposthitis

Balanoposthitis is inflammation of the glans and prepuce of the penis. It is generally caused by poor hygiene and may accompany a urethritis or a regional dermatitis.

Assessment

The prepuce and glans become red and swollen; a purulent discharge may be present. The boy may have difficulty voiding because of crusting at the meatal opening and because acidic urine touching the denuded surface of the glans causes pain.

Therapeutic Management

Medical treatment involves local application of heat; this can be carried out with warm wet soaks or warm baths (Master, 2000). A local antibiotic ointment may be prescribed. If *phimosis* (a tight foreskin) appears to be contributing to the condition, circumcision may be advocated after the inflammation subsides. This will prevent the condition from recurring.

Although balanoposthitis is painful, a boy may tolerate the discomfort for several days because he is too embarrassed to discuss the problem. He may think it was caused by masturbation (which can contribute to the irritation) or sexual activity, and is reluctant to seek help for fear of being criticized. He can be reassured that the problem is local and will have no long-range effect. Any discharge should be cultured to rule out an STD such as gonorrhea.

Phimosis

In the normal infant, the foreskin is tight at birth and may be even held by adhesions. Generally, it cannot be retracted. After a few months, the adhesions dissolve and the foreskin will become retractable. If not, the infant may have phimosis. With this, the foreskin remains so tight that it interferes with voiding. Balanoposthitis may develop because the foreskin cannot be retracted for cleaning. True phimosis is rare but can be corrected by circumcision (Master, 2000). The technique of circumcision is discussed in Chapter 23.

Cryptorchidism

Cryptorchidism is failure of one or both testes to descend from the abdominal cavity to the scrotum. The testes descend into the scrotal sac during months 7 to 9 of intrauterine life. They may descend any time up to 6 weeks after birth; they rarely descend after that time.

The cause of undescended testes is unclear. Fibrous bands at the inguinal ring or inadequate length of spermatic vessels may prevent descent. Testes apparently descend because of stimulation by testosterone; hence, it is possible that a lower than normal level of testosterone production prevents descent. About 17% of premature infants and 3% to 4% of term infants are born with undescended testes (Master, 2000).

Assessment

Early detection of undescended testes is important, because the warmth of the abdominal cavity may inhibit development of the testes, ultimately affecting spermatogenesis. After puberty, sperm production deteriorates rapidly in undescended testes, and the testes may undergo a malignant change. Anchoring the testes in the scrotal sac may not prevent malignancy but will allow the boy to perform preventive measures such as testicular self-examination.

It is more common for the right testis to remain undescended than the left one. In approximately 20% of all cases, both testes remain undescended. Some children may be diagnosed with undescended testes when, in fact, poor examining technique caused the testes to retract. If the child is supine or the examining room is chilly, the scrotal sac may appear to be empty. Excessive palpation or stroking the inner thigh may also stimulate the cremasteric reflex and cause retraction. In these instances, testes descend when the child is standing or after a warm bath.

An undescended testis may be at the inguinal ring (true undescended testis) or ectopic (still in the abdomen). Laparoscopy is effective in identifying undescended testes. Because testes arise from the same germ tissue as the kidneys, the kidney function of children with ectopic testes is usually evaluated. If undescended testes and other factors (e.g., ambiguous genitals) pose questions about the child's gender, a *karyotype* may be done to determine true gender.

Therapeutic Management

Sometimes, the testes descend spontaneously during the first year of life, so treatment is usually delayed until 6 to 12 months. Children may be given chorionic gonadotropin hormone to stimulate testicular descent, but this therapy is successful only in approximately 20% of cases. If necessary, surgery (**orchiopexy**) by laparoscopy by 1 year of age will correct the condition (Kappy, Steelman & Travers, 2001).

NURSING DIAGNOSES AND RELATED INTERVENTIONS

If an orchiopexy is scheduled, the focus is on parent and child teaching, preoperative preparation, and postoperative care.

Nursing Diagnosis: Deficient knowledge related to parents' and child's inexperience with surgical procedure and postoperative treatment plan

Outcome Identification: Parents and child (if old enough) will demonstrate increased level of knowledge about surgical procedure by time of admission.

Outcome Evaluation: Parents (and child) state what will be done during surgery.

Boys who are old enough to understand need good preparation for this type of surgery. Use an anatomically correct picture to point out the exact site at which surgery will be performed. Reassure the boy that his penis itself will not be cut. The child may not voice a fear of mutilation, but you can assume that it exists, especially in preschool children.

During surgery, internal sutures may be inserted to hold the testis in place. Although the child may be discharged from the hospital the same day, his activity will be limited until approximately the second day after surgery to ensure that the internal suture line remains intact.

Nursing Diagnosis: Disturbed body image related to change in physical appearance

Outcome Identification: Child will show evidence of an adequate level of self-acceptance during surgical experience.

Outcome Evaluation: Child (if verbal) states he views self as whole person and interacts with peers without excessive shyness or hesitancy.

Postoperative evaluation should reveal that the suture line is healing well and that both testes can be palpated in the scrotum. It should also address the boy's feelings about the surgery and the changes in his body. He may need an opportunity to express his fears about mutilation or castration by playing with puppets or dolls after surgery. Boys who have bilateral cryptorchidism are apt to be less fertile as adults (Lee & Coughlin, 2001). When boys reach puberty, teach them testicular self-examination to assess any early symptoms of malignancy, such as nodules or abnormal growth (see Chap. 33).

Hydrocele

When a testis descends into the scrotum in utero, it is preceded by a fold of tissue, the *processus vaginalis.* Occasionally, fluid collects in this fold. If this occurs, **hydrocele** (the fluid) can be revealed by prenatal sonogram. At birth, the collection of fluid makes the scrotum of the newborn appear enlarged. On *transillumination* (the shining of a light through the scrotal sac), the area is illuminated by the water and shines or glows. Sonogram also will reveal this fluid collection. If the hydrocele is uncomplicated, the fluid will gradually be reabsorbed into the body and no treatment is necessary. The child's parents can be assured that the hydrocele is only excess fluid and that the scrotal enlargement is not due to an abnormal testis, tumor, or hernia.

A hydrocele may form later in life due to *inguinal hernia* (abdominal contents extruding into the scrotum through the inguinal ring, with accompanying fluid). If this happens, the hernia must be repaired for the hydrocele to be reabsorbed (see Chap. 45). Injection of a drug to decrease fluid production (*sclerotherapy*) may also be effective.

Varicocele

A **varicocele** is abnormal dilation of the veins of the spermatic cord (Esposito et al., 2001; Fig. 47-1). Although asymptomatic, identifying a varicocele is important in adolescents because the increased heat and congestion in the testicles can lead to infertility. No treatment is necessary unless fertility becomes a concern, at which time the varicocele can be surgically removed. The patient may report some local tenderness and edema for a few days after surgery. Edema can be minimized by applying ice for the first few hours postoperatively.

Testicular Torsion

Testicular torsion (twisting of the spermatic cord) is a surgical emergency. Although it can be present in newborns, it occurs most frequently in early adolescence (Seng & Moissinac, 2000). Less than normal testicular support apparently allows the spermatic cord to twist. Testicular torsion usually results from a sports activity. The boy experiences severe scrotal pain and perhaps nausea and vomiting from the severity of the pain. The testis feels tender to palpation, and edema begins to develop. If the condition is not recognized promptly (within 4 h), irreversible change in the testis may occur from lack of circulation to the organ. Boys need to be educated about the phenomenon so that they report symptoms promptly. Laparoscopic surgery is necessary to reduce the torsion and reestablish circulation (Porpiglia et al., 2001).

Testicular Cancer

Testicular cancer is rare (only 1% of all malignancies). It usually occurs between ages 15 and 35 years, often in association with cryptorchidism. If discovered early, testicular cancer is one of the most curable cancers (Dearnaley, Huddart & Horwich, 2001).

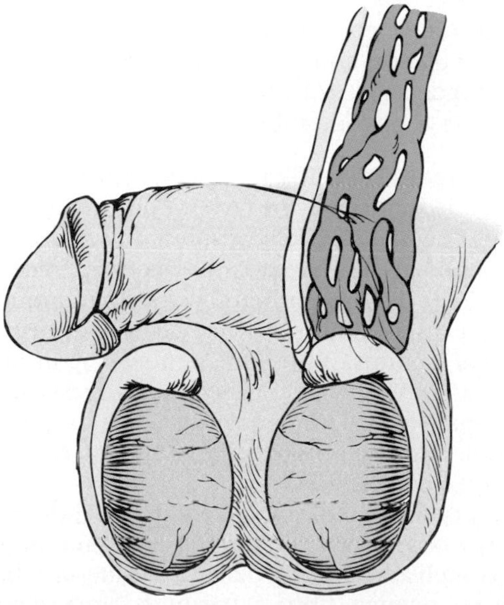

FIGURE 47.1 A varicocele. Identifying and correcting varicocele in adolescent males is important because the condition is associated with infertility.

Symptoms include painless testicular enlargement and a feeling of heaviness in the scrotum. The disease metastasizes rapidly, leading to abdominal and back pain due to retroperitoneal node extension, weight loss, and general weakness. **Gynecomastia** (enlargement of the breasts) may arise from human chorionic gonadotropins (HCG) produced by the tumor. HCG and alpha-fetoprotein, tumor markers, can be detected in blood serum.

Therapy for testicular malignancy is **orchiectomy** (removal of the testis) followed by radiation or chemotherapy. After surgical removal, a gel-filled prosthesis may be inserted to provide a symmetrically appearing scrotum. Infertility in the opposite testis results after radiation therapy. For some patients, "sperm banking," or preserving frozen sperm before the procedure, may be presented as an option for future family planning.

Teaching males to perform testicular self-examination for early cancer detection is as important as teaching females to perform breast self-examination (see Chap. 33).

✔ CHECKPOINT QUESTIONS

3. Why is it important that undescended testes be brought down into the scrotal sac before puberty?
4. What is the first symptom of testicular torsion?

REPRODUCTIVE DISORDERS IN FEMALES

The most frequent reproductive disorders in females involve vaginal or menstrual irregularities. Other disorders are caused by structural alterations of the reproductive organs, such as imperforate hymen, pelvic inflammatory disease (PID), or infections caused by STD.

Menstrual Disorders

Because menstruation is an ongoing process throughout half of a woman's life, it affects her self-image significantly. An irregularity such as a painful cycle can exert a major influence on daily activities. Therefore, it is a health concern requiring as much time and attention as that given to other concerns.

Menstrual disorders generally fall into two categories: (1) menstruation that is painful or uncomfortable and (2) infrequent or too-frequent cycles.

Mittelschmerz

Some women may experience abdominal pain during ovulation from the release of accompanying prostaglandins. It may also be caused by a drop or two of follicular fluid or blood spilling into the abdominal cavity. This pain, called **mittelschmerz,** may range from a few sharp cramps to several hours of discomfort. It is typically felt on one side of the abdomen (near an ovary) and may be accompanied by scant vaginal spotting (Kaplan & Love, 2001).

An advantage of mittelschmerz is that it clearly marks ovulation. If pain is felt in the right lower quadrant, it can be differentiated from appendicitis by the lack of associated symptoms (i.e., nausea, vomiting, fever, abdominal guarding, and rebound tenderness) as well as by its occurrence in the menstrual cycle. Usually mittelschmerz is of limited duration and intensity and, therefore, not a great source of discomfort.

Dysmenorrhea

Dysmenorrhea is painful menstruation. For generations, it was thought to be mainly psychological, needing no treatment other than reassurance that it was a normal phenomenon and something women should endure. Today, it is known that the pain is due to the release of prostaglandins in response to tissue destruction during the ischemic phase of the menstrual cycle (Davis & Westhoff, 2001). Prostaglandin release causes smooth muscle contraction in the uterus.

Dysmenorrhea can also be a symptom of an underlying illness such as PID, uterine myomas (tumors), or endometriosis (abnormal formation of endometrial tissue).

Assessment. Dysmenorrhea can be categorized as mild (no interference with normal activities), moderate (some interference with normal activities), and severe (interference with the majority of everyday activities). As many as 80% of adolescents have some discomfort with menstruation; in approximately 10%, the discomfort seriously interferes with daily living (Clark, 2000). Dysmenorrhea is *primary* if it occurs in the absence of organic disease; it is *secondary* if it occurs as a result of organic disease. There may be a "bloating" feeling and light cramping 24 h before menstrual flow. Pain is mainly noticed, however, when the flow begins. Colicky (sharp) pain is superimposed on a dull, nagging pain across the lower abdomen. Accompanying this is an "aching, pulling" sensation of the vulva and inner thighs. Some adolescents have mild diarrhea with the abdominal cramping. Mild breast tenderness, abdominal distention, nausea and vomiting, headache, and facial flushing may be present.

Therapeutic Management. Painful symptoms can generally be controlled by an analgesic such as acetylsalicylic acid (aspirin) or ibuprofen (Advil, Motrin). Acetylsalicylic acid works well as an analgesic for dysmenorrhea because it is a mild prostaglandin inhibitor. Although adolescents are generally advised not to take aspirin because of its link to Reye's syndrome, girls may take it safely at the beginning of a menstrual period as long as they do not have additional flulike symptoms. Ibuprofen is a stronger prostaglandin inhibitor and relieves more severe menstrual pain. Naproxen sodium (Aleve) is also effective. Low-dose oral contraceptives to prevent ovulation may also be effective if pregnancy is not desired. One disadvantage of this is the possible adverse effects of long-term estrogen administration (Davis & Westhoff, 2001).

During the first year or two of menstruation, dysmenorrhea rarely occurs, because early menstrual cycles are usually **anovulatory** (without ovulation). As ovulation begins, typical menstrual discomfort begins.

NURSING DIAGNOSES AND RELATED INTERVENTIONS

Nursing Diagnosis: Pain related to dysmenorrhea

Outcome Identification: Client will not experience pain above a tolerable level.

Outcome Evaluation: Client states that she has some control over pain through nonpharmacologic or pharmacologic methods.

Several nonpharmacologic solutions may help relieve dysmenorrhea. St. John's wort is an herb that can be used to promote general well-being. Decreasing sodium intake a few days before an expected menstrual flow by omitting salty foods, such as potato chips, pretzels, and ham and other luncheon meats, and by not adding salt to foods, may help reduce "bloated" feelings. Abdominal breathing (breathing in and out slowly, allowing the abdominal wall to rise with each inhalation) may also be helpful. Applying heat to the abdomen with a heating pad or taking a hot shower or tub bath may relax muscle tension and relieve pain. Caution young girls not to apply heat to their abdomen for abdominal pain unless they are actually menstruating; if the pain results from an inflamed appendix, heat can cause rupture of the appendix and life-threatening peritonitis. Resting may help to relieve vulvar pain; abdominal massage (effleurage or light massage) may feel soothing. Adolescents who remain sexually active during their menses may discover that orgasm helps relieve pelvic engorgement and, therefore, cramping.

Menorrhagia

Menorrhagia is an abnormally heavy menstrual flow usually defined as greater than 80 mL per menses (Kadir & Lee, 2001). It may occur in girls close to puberty and in women nearing menopause because of anovulatory cycles. Without ovulation and subsequent progesterone secretion, estrogen secretion continues and causes extreme proliferation of endometrium.

Assessment. It is difficult to determine when a menstrual flow is abnormally heavy, but one method is to ask the client how long it takes her to saturate a sanitary napkin or tampon. A sanitary napkin or tampon holds approximately 25 mL of fluid. Saturating a pad or tampon in less than 1 h means the flow is heavier than usual. There is often an unusual amount of flow in clients using intrauterine devices (IUD). With oral contraceptives, the flow is often light but may seem alarmingly heavy once the pills are discontinued. Usually, however, this is just a return of the adolescent's normal flow.

A heavy flow can indicate endometriosis (see discussion later in the chapter), a systemic disease (anemia), blood dyscrasia such as a clotting defect, or a uterine abnormality such as a myoma (fibroid) tumor. It can be a symptom of infection such as PID or an indication of early pregnancy loss that is coincidentally occurring at the time of an expected menstrual period.

Determining the cause of menorrhagia is important because it can lead to anemia from excessive iron loss, thus requiring iron supplements to achieve sufficient hemoglobin formation. The adolescent who is losing excessive blood because of anovulatory cycles may be prescribed progesterone during the luteal phase to prevent proliferative growth during this phase of the cycle; if the ability to conceive is unimportant, adolescents may be placed on a low-dose oral contraceptive or GnRH inhibitor to decrease the flow.

Metrorrhagia

Metrorrhagia is bleeding between menstrual periods. This is normal in some adolescents who have spotting at the time of ovulation ("mittelstaining"). It may also occur in clients on oral contraceptives (breakthrough bleeding) for the first 3 or 4 months. Additionally, vaginal irritation from infection may cause midcycle spotting. Spotting may also represent a temporarily low level of progesterone production and endometrial sloughing (dysfunctional uterine bleeding or a luteal phase defect), a condition that tends to occur near the end of the reproductive years.

If metrorrhagia occurs for more than one menstrual cycle and the client is not on oral contraceptives, she should be referred to her primary care provider for examination, because vaginal bleeding is also an early sign of uterine carcinoma or ovarian cysts.

Endometriosis

Endometriosis is the abnormal growth of extrauterine endometrial cells, often in the cul-de-sac of the peritoneal cavity, the uterine ligaments, and the ovaries. This abnormal tissue results from excessive endometrial production and a reflux of blood and tissue through the fallopian tubes during menstrual flow. As many as 25% of women in the United States have endometriosis; as many as 50% of adolescents seen for dysmenorrhea have endometriosis (Schenken, 2000). It tends to occur most often in white nulliparous women, but there is also a familial tendency. Daughters of women with endometriosis may develop symptoms of dysmenorrhea early in life and so may want to consider having children before overgrowth of the endometrium becomes so extensive that it interferes with conception.

The excessive production of endometrial tissue may be related to a deficient immunologic response. In many women, it appears to be related to excess estrogen production or a failed luteal menstrual phase. Many women with endometriosis do not ovulate or ovulate irregularly. Thus, it is discovered at a higher than usual rate in women undergoing infertility testing (Schenken, 2000). Estrogen secretion continues through the cycle rather than becoming secondary to progesterone late in the cycle, as happens with normal ovulation. This proliferation of tissue then forces the blood back into the fallopian tubes.

Endometriosis causes dysmenorrhea when the abnormal tissue responds to estrogen and progesterone stimulation by swelling and then sloughing its layers in the same manner as the uterine lining. This causes inflammation of surrounding tissue in the abdominal cavity and an even greater release of prostaglandins. Abnormal tissue in the pelvic cul-de-sac may cause *dyspareunia* (painful coitus) because it puts pressure on the posterior vagina. Infertility may result when the fallopian tubes become immobilized and blocked by tissue implants or adhesions, preventing peristaltic motion and ova transport (see Chap. 4).

Assessment. Pelvic examination may show that the uterus is displaced by tender, fixed, palpable nodules. Nodules in the cul-de-sac or on an ovary may be palpable as well. If the endometriosis is minimal, the woman will not experience related symptoms. If the condition is moderate or extensive, she may experience dysmenorrhea or dyspareunia.

Therapeutic Management. Treatment for endometriosis can be medical or surgical, depending on the extent of the disease. Estrogen–progesterone-based oral contraceptives may stimulate implant regression as the tissue sloughs under the influence of the progesterone. Danazol (Danocrine), a synthetic androgen, can be prescribed to help shrink the abnormal tissue. Administration of a GnRH agonist, such as leuprolide acetate (Lupron), can reduce hormone stimulation (see Focus on Pharmacology earlier in this chapter). Laparotomy and excision by laser surgery are the most effective measures, but, because it is a highly invasive procedure, a course of conservative medical treatment may be tried first (Chapron & Dubuisson, 2001).

Amenorrhea

Amenorrhea, or absence of a menstrual flow, strongly suggests pregnancy but is by no means definitive because it may also result from tension, anxiety, fatigue, chronic illness, extreme dieting, or strenuous exercise. Competitive swimmers, long distance runners (50 to 75 miles weekly), and ballet dancers notice that intensive training causes their periods to become scant and irregular. This appears to be associated with their low ratio of body fat to body muscle, which leads to excessive secretion of prolactin. An elevation in prolactin causes a decrease in GnRH from the hypothalamus, followed by a decline in follicle-stimulating hormone, follicular development, and estrogen secretion. Menstrual cycles generally return to normal within 3 months of discontinuing strenuous training and conditioning.

Adolescents who wish to maintain a normal cycle while training for a sports event may take bromocriptine (Parlodel), which can reduce high prolactin levels by acting on the hypothalamus and initiating menstruation each month. Many adolescents, however, view the absence of menstrual periods as a benefit during sports training. If a menstrual flow is delayed and pregnancy is suspected, bromocriptine should be discontinued, because it is potentially teratogenic.

Amenorrhea also occurs when females diet excessively, partially as a natural defense mechanism to limit ovulation and as a means of conserving body fluid. Women with *anorexia nervosa* or *bulimia* (eating disorders described in Chapter 54) often develop amenorrhea after approximately 3 months of excessive dieting or bingeing and dieting; as in athletes, this is due to an increase in prolactin. Amenorrhea as a sign of pregnancy is discussed in Chapter 9.

Premenstrual Dysphoric Disorder

Premenstrual dysphoric disorder (PDD) is a condition occurring in the luteal phase of the menstrual cycle and relieved by the onset of menses that has both behavioral and physiologic symptoms. Because of the variety of possible symptoms, as many as 30% of women experience some degree of PDD, a cluster of symptoms that include anxiety, fatigue, abdominal bloating, headache, appetite disturbance, irritability, and depression (Kaplan & Love, 2001). For some women, these symptoms are so extreme that they are incapacitating.

The cause of PDD is unproven but, contrary to previous beliefs, must be due to more than a drop in progesterone just before menses. A syndrome similar to PDD may occur in women after tubal ligation as a decrease in the blood supply to the ovary apparently results in decreased luteal function. In some women, a vitamin B–complex deficiency may lead to estrogen excess, causing an abnormal ratio of estrogen to progesterone; other related causes may be poor renal clearance leading to water retention or hypoglycemia leading to a surge of adrenalin and low calcium levels and interference with serotonin synthesis (Hammond & Riddick, 2000).

Symptoms of PDD vary from cycle to cycle and throughout life. Therapy is aimed at correcting specific symptoms.

Adolescents who think they have PDD should keep a diary of when symptoms occur. If they are aware of recurring patterns that indicate PDD, they will be better able to recognize the cause. They should be certain their diet is high in vitamins and calcium and low in salt. Agents that suppress ovarian function, such as oral contraceptives or the GnRH agonist leuprolide (Lupron), may be prescribed. If depression is a major symptom, an antidepressant such as buspirone (BuSpar) can be helpful. Paroxetine (Paxil) is a serotonin reuptake inhibitor that is specifically designed for PDD therapy in adults. Its safe use with children is not yet established (Bourin, Chue & Guillon, 2001).

Other Reproductive Disorders in Females

Imperforate Hymen

The *hymen* is a membranous ring of tissue partly obstructing the vaginal opening. An *imperforate hymen* totally occludes the vagina, preventing the escape of vaginal secretions and menstrual blood.

Before menarche, the child with an imperforate hymen generally has no symptoms. With onset of menstruation, the menstrual flow is obstructed. It builds up in the vagina, causing increased pressure in the vagina and uterus and eventual abdominal pain. Palpation of the abdomen will reveal a lower abdominal mass. On vaginal examination, an intact, bulging hymen is evident.

The treatment is surgical incision or removal of the hymenal tissue. The girl may have local pain after the incision, which can be relieved by a mild analgesic and warm baths.

Careful explanation of this condition will help the girl understand that this will not interfere with sexual relations or future childbearing. Because most girls of early menstrual age have scant knowledge of anatomy, pictures of the reproductive tract will help to explain that this is a local and minor problem.

Toxic Shock Syndrome

Toxic shock syndrome (TSS) is an infection usually caused by toxin-producing strains of *Staphylococcus aureus* organisms. Although organisms can enter the body by other means, they typically enter through vaginal walls damaged by the insertion of tampons at the time of a menstrual period.

Assessment. The symptoms of TSS appear in Box 47-2. Any female who develops fever with diarrhea and vomiting during a menstrual period should suspect TSS. Remember, however, a number of females have mild diarrhea as a normal accompaniment to dysmenorrhea.

Therapeutic Management. Women or adolescents with suspected TSS need a careful vaginal examination and removal of any tampon particles, as well as cervical and vaginal cultures for *S. aureus.* Iodine douches may reduce the number of organisms present vaginally. *S. aureus* is generally resistant to penicillin but not to penicillinase-resistant antibiotics (ie, cephalosporins, oxacillins, or clindamycins). IV fluid therapy to restore circulating fluid volume and increase blood pressure or vasopressors such as dopamine (Intropin) may be necessary to increase the

BOX 47.2

SYMPTOMS OF TOXIC SHOCK SYNDROME*

- Temperature more than 102°F (38.9°C)
- Vomiting and diarrhea
- A macular (sunburn-like) rash that desquamates on palms and soles 1 to 2 weeks after illness
- Severe hypotension (systolic pressure less than 90 mmHg)
- Shock, leading to poor organ perfusion
- Impaired renal function with elevated blood urea nitrogen or creatinine at least twice the upper limit of normal
- Severe muscle pain or creatine phosphokinase at least twice the upper limit of normal
- Hyperemia of mucous membrane
- Impaired liver function with increased total bilirubin and increased serum glutamic-oxaloacetic transaminase at twice the upper limit of normal
- Decreased platelet count
- Central nervous system symptoms of disorientation, confusion, severe headache

*Three symptoms must be present for diagnosis.

blood pressure. Diuretic therapy to shift fluid back to the intravascular circulation and to prevent renal and cardiac failure may be necessary. Recovery occurs in 7 to 10 days; fatigue and weakness may remain for months afterward.

The rate of TSS recurrence is 28% to 64%, generally within 2 months of the first attack. Recurrence probably happens because the organism is not completely eliminated from the body. Therefore, be certain that girls complete their entire antibiotic prescription. Girls who have TSS should avoid tampon use in the future (Eschenbach, 2000). Also be sure to educate females about menstrual hygiene (see Focus on Family Empowerment).

Vulvovaginitis

Vulvovaginitis, inflammation of the vulva or vagina, is accompanied by pain, odor, pruritus, and a vaginal discharge. Vaginal bleeding may be present. This condition may occur in a girl of any age but tends to be more frequent as girls reach puberty, and a change to adult pH and the presence of vaginal secretions make the vagina more receptive to infections. Focus on Family Empowerment discusses common measures to relieve discomfort.

Preschool and School-Age Children. Vaginal discharge may occur before menarche, but bleeding is rarely seen at this age. If bleeding is present, its cause must be determined. A cystitis can cause urethral bleeding; scratching from rectal pruritus will lead to rectal bleeding. The cause of true vaginal bleeding in this early age group is generally either irritation of an inserted foreign object in the vagina, infestation of pinworms, or *vaginitis* (inflammation or infection). Sexual abuse must also be investigated as a cause of any bleeding, tenderness, or infection (see Chap. 55). Precocious puberty must also be ruled out.

Treatment for pinworm is discussed in Chapter 43. If there is a foreign body in the vagina, it should be removed. Vaginal examination is necessary first to locate the object and then to confirm that it has been fully removed. This may be difficult for girls to accept, and vaginal manipulation and stretching can be painful. A small speculum helps reduce the pain. A local antibiotic ointment or warm bath may be ordered to reduce accompanying infection and inflammation afterward.

Sometimes, daily bubble baths can cause vulvar irritation. This can be quickly remedied by discontinuing the bubble baths; irritation from such a compound can lead not only to local discomfort but to urinary tract infection as well (Kaplan & Love, 2001).

A few preschool or school-age children develop a vaginitis from *Streptococcus* or from *Escherichia coli* introduced from the anus by improper perineal care after voiding or bowel movements. A tight hymen then traps the microorganisms in the vagina and leads to infection. The girl needs to be reminded to wipe from front to back after voiding or bowel movements.

Adolescents. As a girl enters puberty, she may notice a slight vaginal discharge due to increased vaginal secretions. She can be reassured that this is normal. To keep from developing vulvar irritation, girls should wear cotton underpants rather than nylon (so moisture is absorbed better) and dry the vulva thoroughly after bathing or swimming.

Some girls may develop vulvar irritation from personal hygiene sprays or douches. These products are unnecessary. Good hygiene can be achieved by daily washing and frequent changing of tampons or sanitary pads during menstruation. This will prevent chafing or stasis of menstrual blood and help prevent irritation and excessive odor.

FOCUS ON FAMILY EMPOWERMENT
Preventing Toxic Shock Syndrome

Q. I've heard so much about this disease called toxic shock syndrome. What is it and how can I make sure that I don't get it?

A. Although toxic shock syndrome can occur for other reasons, it most often occurs during a menstrual flow when tampons are used. The following are measures to help prevent the syndrome:

- Use only tampons made of natural materials such as cotton, not synthetics such as cellulose or polyester; avoid high-absorbency tampons.
- Change tampons at least every 4 h during use.
- Alternate the use of tampons with sanitary pads.
- Avoid handling the portion of the tampon that will be inserted vaginally.
- Do not use tampons near the end of a menstrual flow when excessive vaginal dryness can result from scant flow.
- Do not insert more than one tampon at a time to avoid abrasions and to keep the vaginal walls from becoming too dry.
- Avoid deodorant tampons, sanitary pads, and feminine hygiene sprays; these products can irritate the vulvar–vaginal lining.
- If fever, vomiting, or diarrhea occurs during a menstrual period, discontinue tampon use and immediately consult a healthcare provider because these are symptoms of TSS.
- Anyone who has had one episode of TSS is well advised not to use tampons again or at least not until two vaginal cultures for *Staphylococcus aureus,* the bacteria usually responsible for TSS, are negative.

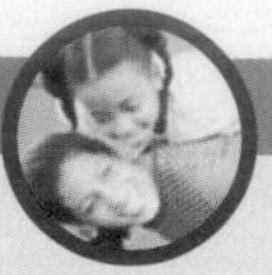

FOCUS ON FAMILY EMPOWERMENT
Tips for Relieving the Pain of Vulvitis

Q. The doctor says that I have vulvitis. The pain is awful. Is there anything I can do to relieve it?

A. Here are some tips that might help:

- Wash the area twice a day with mild, nonperfumed soap and water, and pat dry. This removes secretions and decreases irritation. Wash and dry from front to back to prevent spreading rectal contamination forward.
- Take sitz baths or apply warm, moist compresses three times a day to soothe the area and keep it free of irritating drainage.
- After drying the cleansed area, apply cornstarch for comfort and to absorb residual moisture.
- Avoid bubble baths and feminine hygiene sprays because the ingredients may cause additional local irritation or contribute to urinary tract infections.
- Take acetaminophen (Tylenol) every 4 h. Acetaminophen is an analgesic that relieves pain and reduces itching, a mild pain sensation.
- Avoid scratching, which may increase abrasions and introduce a secondary infection. Instead, apply a cold compress to relieve itching sensation.
- Wear cotton underwear, which allows air to circulate and moisture to evaporate, rather than nylon or silk, which prevents air circulation and retains moisture.
- Sleep without underwear.
- Use an anesthetic spray or hydrocortisone cream only as prescribed.
- Carefully follow the instructions from the health care provider about caring for a vaginal infection; only when the infection subsides will the vulvitis clear.

Pelvic Inflammatory Disease

Pelvic inflammatory disease (PID) is infection of the pelvic organs: the uterus, fallopian tubes, ovaries, and their supporting structures. The infection can extend to cause pelvic peritonitis. Although sexual transmission accounts for approximately 75% of all PID (gonorrheal and chlamydial organisms are frequently responsible), infections from other causes such as *E. coli* and *Streptococcus* are beginning to occur more frequently and may be as severe. Adolescents have the highest incidence of PID when compared with any other age group (Nyquist, Levin & Sigel, 2001).

PID begins with a cervical infection that spreads by surface invasion along the uterine endometrium and then out to the fallopian tubes and ovaries. It is most likely to occur at the end of a menstrual period, because menstrual blood provides an excellent growth medium for bacteria and there is loss of the normal barrier of cervical mucus during this time.

Assessment. As peritoneal tissue becomes inflamed and edematous, a purulent exudate forms. If the process is untreated, it enters a chronic phase and fibrotic scarring with stricture of the fallopian tubes will result. With acute PID, the adolescent notices severe pain in the lower abdomen. She may have an accompanying heavy purulent discharge. As the infection progresses, she will develop a fever. Leukocytosis and an elevated erythrocyte sedimentation rate will be present on laboratory testing. During a pelvic examination, any manipulation of the ᵣvix causes severe pain. It may be difficult to palpate ᵥvaries because of tenderness and abdominal guard- the PID enters a chronic phase, the abdominal ᵉns but dyspareunia and dysmenorrhea may be the ovaries are affected, intermenstrual spot- ʳr. Diagnosis can be aided by sonogram or

Therapeutic Management. Therapy involves administration of analgesia for comfort plus specific broad-spectrum antibiotics such as cefoxitin (Mefoxin), doxycycline (Vibramycin), or clindamycin (Cleocin). Limiting activity also helps relieve the pain. In some women, a pelvic abscess forms and must be drained through the cul-de-sac before healing will occur.

Women who have had one episode of PID have an increased chance of a second occurrence because the immune protection of the tubes and ovaries may be damaged. They should not have coitus with an infected partner, and they should avoid coitus during menstruation, when their protective mechanisms are lowest. Early childbearing may be recommended if they plan to have children, because extensive tubal scarring could impair fertility. It is important for adolescents to recognize the symptoms of PID and to seek early help for the best outcome.

✔ CHECKPOINT QUESTIONS

5. How does endometriosis lead to dysmenorrhea?
6. What condition must be ruled out in young girls with vulvovaginitis?

BREAST DISORDERS

Males have few breast disorders. Gynecomastia (enlarged breast tissue) may occur temporarily in preadolescent boys in response to a rising estrogen level. Particularly noticeable in obese males, this enlargement fades with a normal increase in testosterone production (Boom, 2000). It may also occur in teens as a result of steroid use in body-building sports. If this is the cause, counseling regarding drug use is crucial. Breast disorders that concern adolescent females include accessory nipples, lesions such as cysts, infection, and injury.

Accessory Nipples

As the name implies, *accessory nipples* are additional breast nipples. They occur along the mammary lines (Fig. 47-2). They are generally not as protuberant as true nipples; they also lack areolar pigmentation. Many girls are unaware that they have an accessory nipple, and think it is a large mole. Accessory nipples are present at birth; and parents should be told what they are so they can inform their daughters later, as some growth in accessory nipples may occur at puberty or during pregnancy in response to estrogen stimulation.

In a few instances, actual breast tissue is present beneath the accessory nipple. If so, it is subject to the same diseases as other breast tissue. If the accessory nipple or accessory breast tissue is cosmetically distressing to the adolescent, it can be removed by simple surgical excision.

WHAT IF? What if an adolescent girl has an accessory nipple with breast tissue underneath? How would you counsel her about breast self-examination?

Breast Hypertrophy

Breast hypertrophy is abnormal enlargement of breast tissue. In the average girl, breast development halts after puberty as soon as progesterone levels rise to mature strength. Progesterone levels remain low until menstruation cycles are fully established. If this process is a lengthy one, breast growth may last for several years.

Breast hypertrophy can lead to both physical and emotional stress. The girl may feel pain and fatigue in the back or shoulders from attempting to maintain good posture despite the weight of heavy breast tissue. She may feel self-conscious and try to minimize her breast size by slouching and develop poor posture or rounded shoulders.

Adolescent girls with large breasts may find it difficult to adapt to such a new appearance. They may be treated as provocative sex objects and believe they should live up to this image. This can make it difficult for them to find their own identity. They may hear comments such as "I wish I had your problem" rather than receiving support and understanding from parents, peers, and health care providers.

If breast hypertrophy interferes with the girl's physical and emotional well-being, surgical breast reduction is a possibility. Adolescents need to seriously consider the consequences of this procedure before undertaking it. If a large amount of glandular tissue is removed, breastfeeding may no longer be possible. The adolescent needs to be told realistically that changing her physical appearance will reduce physical discomfort, but changing her self-concept must come from within. An adolescent with large breasts must conscientiously perform breast self-examination, because it is easier for a cancerous lesion to escape detection in large amounts of breast tissue than in a smaller breast. Pregnancy and lactation may be particularly difficult times because breasts that are already large become even heavier with milk formation.

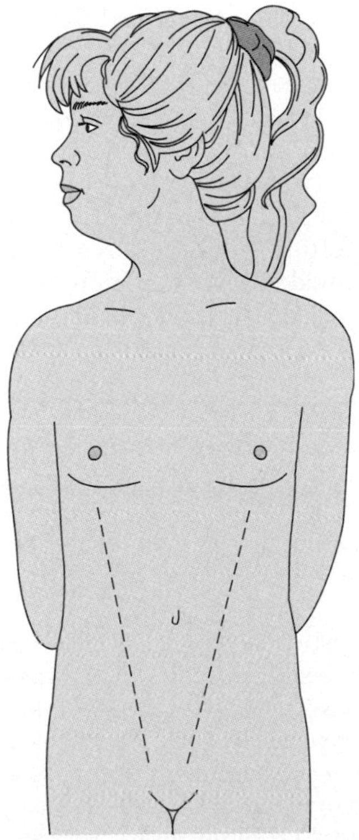

FIGURE 47.2 Nipple lines along which accessory nipples occur.

Breast Hypoplasia

Breast hypoplasia is less-than-average breast size. In most instances, this does not represent a decreased amount of glandular or functional breast tissue but a reduced amount of fatty tissue, which, as a rule, will not interfere with breastfeeding. If an adolescent feels that having small breasts interferes with self-esteem, she can have surgical augmentation to increase breast size.

For augmentation, an incision is made under the breast and a saline implant is inserted under the breast tissue next to the musculus pectoralis major. It is important for the adolescent to realize that her breast tissue is not being replaced by the implant; she still needs to do monthly breast self-examination. Because the original breast tissue is in front of the implant, she will be able to perform this without difficulty.

The client may notice decreased nipple sensation for approximately 1 year after the procedure. Breasts with implants in place may feel firmer than normal on palpation due to the formation of a fibrotic band or capsule around the implant.

Some women elect not to breastfeed with implants in place because a breast infection would necessitate removal of the implant. A traumatic blow to the breast, for example, from an automobile accident, requires examination by the augmentation surgeon to be certain that the implant did not rupture and cause the contents of the implant to leak into the breast tissue.

Breast Tenderness or Fullness

Many women notice a day or two of premenstrual breast fullness and tenderness each month. Some may find palpable granular or fine nodular lumps in their breasts during this time. This is a benign occurrence and part of the monthly change in hormone stimulation. For accurate assessment, breast self-examination should be done after, not before, a menstrual period. If a lump or tenderness persists, the woman should consult a health care provider for additional assessment and care, because the change might signal a lesion or other problem.

Fat Necrosis

If struck during a fall or other traumatic injury, breast tissue will be tender, painful, inflamed or reddened, and possibly bruised. A few days later, necrosis or disintegration may occur in the fatty layer. As the area heals, fibrotic scar tissue forms. This may leave a firm, palpable lump in the breast. It is not freely movable; it may cause skin or nipple retraction or dimpling on the skin surface. Unlike malignant breast growths, post-traumatic breast lumps tend to be well delineated.

It is generally recommended that such fibrotic areas be biopsied and then excised. The surgical procedure usually leaves little scarring, and the woman no longer needs to worry about the lump in her breast. Although, at one time, breast trauma was thought to be a precipitating factor of breast carcinoma, no direct correlation between the two has been established. The association may exist because a woman who examines her breasts after an injury may find an already existing carcinoma (Givens & Luszczak, 2002).

Fibrocystic Breast Disease

Fibrocystic breast disease is the most common benign breast condition in women of all ages. It can occur as early as puberty when estrogen rises to adult levels. More commonly, however, it affects women between the ages of 20 and 45 years. Round, fluid-filled cysts form in the connective breast tissue (Fig. 47-3). The woman is able to palpate freely movable, well-delineated breast lumps. Lumps may also be visible on the surface of the breasts (most often in the upper outer quadrant). The consistency of these lesions varies with the menstrual cycle, changing from firm and hard to soft and flexible, depending on the amount of serous fluid present. Oral contraceptives help reduce the incidence and size of cysts. The lesions tend to shrink or even disappear during pregnancy and lactation, and they totally disappear with menopause.

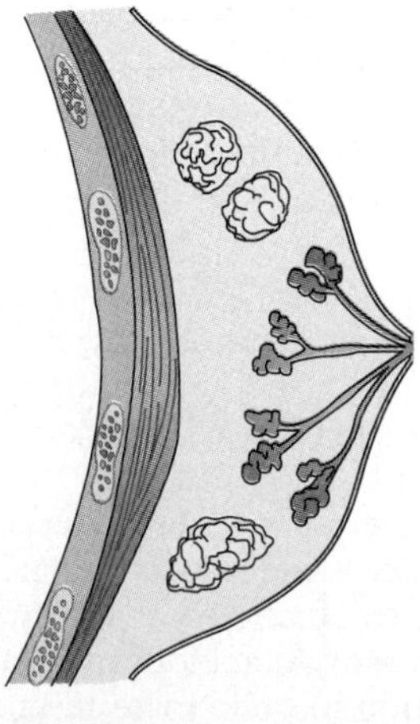

FIGURE 47.3 Round, fluid-filled cysts form in breast tissue in fibrocystic breast disease.

Fibrocystic breasts can be painful; the breasts may feel tender and "stretched," interfering with active sports and other strenuous activity. This discomfort can be relieved with a simple analgesic, such as acetaminophen (Tylenol), or warm compresses. The formation of fibrocystic lesions may be increased in some women with the use of methylxanthines found in caffeine, theophylline, and theobromine. Advise these women to avoid coffee, cola drinks, tea, chocolate, some toffee candy, and medications such as aspirin compound or Excedrin. Discontinuing smoking can also decrease the occurrence of fibrocystic lesions. Decreasing sodium and caffeine intake as well as short-term use of a mild diuretic can reduce the fluid retention just before menses (Fiorica, 2000).

If these measures do not decrease the fibrocystic symptoms, cysts may be aspirated under a local anesthetic by injection of a thin sterile needle attached to a small syringe. This procedure not only reduces the size of the cyst but also provides fluid for biopsy.

Oral contraceptives may be prescribed to reduce the symptoms. Danazol (Danocrine), a synthetic androgen, may help to reduce the symptoms of fibrocystic breast disease by suppressing estrogen formation in the ovaries.

In addition to being physically distressed, women with fibrocystic breasts may worry that each lump could be malignant. They can be reassured that the disease itself does not lead to breast carcinoma. Breast carcinoma can occur in a woman with fibrocystic breast condition, however, and may even metastasize before she seeks health consultation, having assumed that all her breast lesions are benign. As a result, she needs more consultation than the average woman. In addition to a yearly breast examination, she needs to perform monthly breast self-examinations, and have an annual breast sonogram, which involves no x-ray exposure and can efficiently locate fluid-filled cysts.

Fibroadenoma

Fibroadenomas are tumors consisting of both fibrotic and glandular components that occur in response to estrogen stimulation. The tumors may increase in size during adolescence and during pregnancy and lactation, or when a woman takes an estrogen source such as an oral contraceptive.

Unlike fibrocystic lesions, fibroadenomas are round and well delineated, feeling firmer and more rubbery than fluid-filled cysts. Occasionally, they calcify and feel extremely hard. They are typically painless, freely movable, and tend not to cause skin retraction. Like fibrocystic lesions, they do not become malignant.

Such tumors can be surgically excised so that the woman no longer has to worry about them. Because the incision is small, it leaves little scarring at the site.

✔ CHECKPOINT QUESTIONS

7. If an adolescent girl has breast augmentation, can she still breastfeed?
8. Why do adolescents with fibrocystic breasts need to continue to do breast self-examinations?

SEXUALLY TRANSMITTED DISEASES

Sexually transmitted diseases (STDs) are those diseases spread through sexual contact. They range in severity from easily treated infections, such as trichomoniasis, to human immunodeficiency virus (HIV) which, despite advances in therapy, is life threatening. If these diseases occur in young children, the possibility of sexual abuse must be considered (Ingram et al., 2001).

Abstinence or condom use provides the best protection against STDs. Condoms should always be used in addition to washing the genitals well with soap and water, voiding immediately after coitus, and choosing sexual partners who are at low risk for infection (avoiding persons who are IV drug users or those with multiple sexual partners). Educate adolescents about safer sex practices including the need for condom use (see Focus on Evidence-Based Practice). Also reinforce with them that little immunity develops from STDs, which means such diseases can be contracted repeatedly. STDs are becoming more difficult to treat because these organisms are becoming more and more resistant to antibiotics. The effects of STDs on pregnancy and the fetus are discussed in Chapter 14.

WHAT IF? What if an adolescent girl tells you that she feels safe from contracting an STD because she knows that she is up to date with her immunizations? How would you counsel her?

Candidiasis

The candidal organism is a fungus that thrives on glycogen. As many as 40% of adult females have asymptomatic candidal vaginal infections; this rate rises even higher during pregnancy when high estrogen levels lead to glycogen levels that produce a favorable environment for fungal growth. Because oral contraceptives produce a pseudopregnancy state, pill users also have frequent vaginal candidal infections. When a woman is being treated with an antibiotic (which destroys normal vaginal flora and lets fungal organisms grow more readily), she is particularly susceptible to this infection. Incidence is also strongly associated with diabetes mellitus because hyperglycemia provides a glucose-rich environment for candidal growth.

Assessment

Because of the scant mucus production in the premenses period, symptoms may be most acute at this time. The adolescent notices vulvar reddening, burning and itching, and even bleeding from hairline fissures. The vagina sometimes shows white "patches" on the walls. The patches are adherent and cannot be scraped away without bleeding. A thick, cream cheese–like discharge can usually be observed at the vaginal introitus. The adolescent may notice pain on coitus or tampon insertion (Nyquist, Levin

FOCUS ON EVIDENCE-BASED PRACTICE

We Tell Adolescents to Be Certain to Use Condoms. How and Where Do the Majority of Adolescents Obtain Them and How Much Does Peer Influence Determine Their Use?

To answer this question, researchers conducted a telephone survey in upstate New York of 259 adolescents, ages 14 to 19 years of age (Klein, 2000). Stores in the area were then investigated as to whether they sold condoms and how openly they displayed them. Results of the study revealed that the majority of adolescents who completed the survey reported that they obtained condoms from retail stores rather than free health care settings. All drug stores and 75% of supermarkets in the investigation area were found to sell condoms and display them openly. Ninety-two percent of small grocery stores also sold condoms, although they did not display them as openly. Those areas that had the higher STD rates had more stores that sold condoms than those with lower STD rates. Interestingly, no stores in the area displayed or provided safer sex information. The researchers suggest that a more open display of condoms in smaller stores could help improve condom use by adolescents.

In a second study (Dilorio et al., 2001), researchers interviewed 405 adolescents, ages 13 to 15 years, to discover if peer influence was important in their using condoms. Results of this study showed that, among sexually active adolescents, those who expressed confidence in putting on a condom, who were more able to refuse sex with a sexual partner, and who expressed more favorable outcome expectancies of using a condom were those most likely to use condoms.

These are important studies because they attempt to look at whether health information about safer sex and condom use is reaching adolescents. Nurses often are the primary people providing adolescents with this information. These studies provide some guidelines as to how important it is for adolescents to not only believe that condoms can protect them but for their friends to believe this as well. Information from these studies could be used as a foundation for developing community and school teaching programs for adolescents.

Klein, J., et al. (2001). Where do adolescents get their condoms? *Journal of Adolescent Health, 29*(3), 186–193; DiIorio, C., et al. (2001). Social cognitive correlates of sexual experience and condom use among 13- through 15-year-old adolescents. *Journal of Adolescent Health, 29*(3), 208–216.

& Sigel, 2001). Candidal infections may also be present at other body sites, such as the oral cavity or a moist area such as the umbilicus.

Candidal infections are diagnosed by removing a sample of discharge from the vaginal wall and placing it on a glass slide; three or four drops of a 20% potassium hydroxide (KOH) solution are then added, and the mixture is protected by a coverslip. Under a microscope, typical fungal hyphae indicate the presence of *Candida* organisms (Table 47-1).

Therapeutic Management

Therapy for candidal infections includes vaginal suppositories or cream applications of antifungal preparations such as miconazole (Monistat) or clotrimazole, once a day for 3 to 7 days. Oral fluconazole (Diflucan) can be administered as a one-time oral dose (see Focus on Pharmacology). Vaginal creams or suppositories generally are inserted at bedtime so the drug does not drain from the vagina immediately afterward. During the day, the girl may want to wear a sanitary pad to avoid staining from vaginal discharge. If the adolescent is sexually active, treatment of the male partner may be necessary to break a reinfection cycle. Treatment should not be interrupted until it is complete, even during a menstrual period. Because miconazole and clotrimazole are available without a prescription, the adolescent needs to be advised how to differentiate a candidal infection from other infections or to consult a health care provider for assistance and treatment (see Focus on Nursing Care Planning).

If a girl has frequent candidal infections, her urine should be tested for glucose to rule out diabetes mellitus. If she is using an oral contraceptive, she might be counseled to use another contraceptive method.

Trichomoniasis

Trichomonas vaginalis is a single-cell protozoan that is spread by coitus. Up to 25% of adult men and women have asymptomatic trichomoniasis. The incubation period is 4 to 20 days (Eschenbach, 2000).

With a trichomonal infection, females will notice vaginal irritation and a frothy white or grayish-green vaginal discharge. The frothiness of the discharge is an important typical finding. The upper vagina is reddened and may have pinpoint petechiae. Extreme vulvar itching is present. By contrast, males with the same infection rarely report any symptoms.

Assessment

The infection is diagnosed by microscopic examination of vaginal discharge combined with lactated Ringer's or normal saline solution. Trichomonads typically appear as rounded, mobile structures.

TABLE 47.1 Common Vulvovaginitis Infections

CAUSATIVE AGENT	SYMPTOMS	COMMON THERAPY
Candida	Vulvar reddening and pruritus; thick, white, cheeselike vaginal discharge	Nystatin or miconazole (Monistat) suppositories or fluconazole (Diflucan) orally; bathing with dilute sodium bicarbonate solution may relieve pruritus
Trichomonas	Thin, irritating, frothy, gray-green discharge; strong, putrid odor; itching	Metronidazole (Flagyl) orally; douching with weak vinegar solution to reduce pruritus
Herpesvirus type II	Painful pinpoint vesicles on an erythematous base with a watery vaginal discharge possible; voiding may be irritating and painful	Bathing with dilute sodium bicarbonate solution, applying lubricating jelly to lesions or an oral analgesic such as aspirin may be necessary for pain relief; topically applied acyclovir (Zovirax) helps heal lesions
Gardnerella	Edema and reddening of vulva, milky gray discharge, fishlike odor	Metronidazole (Flagyl) or clindamycin
Chlamydia trachomatis	Watery, gray-white vaginal discharge, vulvar itching	Tetracycline or doxycycline; erythromycin during pregnancy
Neisseria gonorrhoeae	Possibly symptomless; may have profuse yellow-green vaginal discharge	Ceftriaxone and doxycycline; oral amoxicillin
Enterobius vermicularis (pinworm)	Rectal pruritus, especially on rising in the morning	Oral administration of an anthelmintic, such as mebendazole (Vermox)
Treponema pallidum (syphilis)	Painless ulcer on vulva or vagina	Benzathine penicillin, administered intramuscularly
Streptococcus	Vaginitis, vulvar itching; edema and reddening of vulva	Antibiotic (e.g., amoxicillin)
Foreign body	Vaginal discharge; odor	Removal of foreign body during pelvic examination

FOCUS ON PHARMACOLOGY

Fluconazole (Diflucan)

Action: Antifungal agent that increases fungal cell wall permeability, thus exerting fungicidal or fungostatic action

Pregnancy Risk Category: C

Dosage: 150 mg orally as a single dose

Possible Adverse Effects: Nausea, vomiting; diarrhea, abdominal pain, headache.

Nursing Implications

- Instruct the adolescent that this drug is given as a one-time single dose.
- Teach the adolescent about safer sex measures and hygiene practices to help prevent reinfection after therapy.
- Urge the adolescent to watch for signs and symptoms of possible reinfection and report any to the primary care provider.

Therapeutic Management

Oral metronidazole (Flagyl) eradicates trichomonal infections. However, a pregnancy test should be performed before Flagyl is prescribed, because this drug may be teratogenic. Treatment with Flagyl and use of condoms by her sexual partner will help prevent recurrence of *Trichomonas* in both parties. Be aware that *Trichomonas* infections cause such inflammatory changes in the cervix or vagina that a Pap test taken during this time may be misinterpreted as showing abnormal tissue. Because the drug interacts with alcohol to cause acute nausea and vomiting, advise the adolescent not to drink alcoholic beverages during the course of treatment.

Bacterial Vaginosis

Bacterial vaginosis is the invasion of an organism such as *Gardnerella vaginalis.* This organism thrives in the vagina, a body area with a reduced oxygen level. Vaginal discharge is milk-white to gray and has a fishlike odor. Pruritus may be intense. Microscopic examination of the discharge in normal saline solution shows gram-negative rods adhering to vaginal epithelial cells, which are termed *clue cells* (Nyirjesy, 1999).

The treatment is oral metronidazole for 7 days; the woman's sexual partner should also be treated to prevent recurrence of the infection.

Chlamydia trachomatis Infection

Chlamydia trachomatis infections have become so common that they are the most common bacterial cause of STD in the United States (Nyquist, Levin & Sigel, 2001). Symptoms include a heavy grayish-white discharge and vulvar itching. The incubation period is 1 to 5 weeks. Diagnosis is made by culture of the organism. Therapy is oral doxycycline or tetracycline for 7 days. *Chlamydia* infection in a mother may cause eye infection or pneumonia in the newborn (see Chap. 14). During pregnancy, the infection is treated with erythromycin, because tetracycline is teratogenic. Because it has become so common, most public health departments require that any cases be reported.

Genital Warts (Human Papilloma Virus)

Genital warts are lesions caused by the human papilloma virus (HPV). They are rapidly growing structures on the

FOCUS ON *Nursing Care Planning*

AN ADOLESCENT WITH CANDIDIASIS

An 18-year-old female college freshman is seen at the student health center. She describes intense vaginal itching. "It started a couple of days after I started taking the antibiotic the dentist prescribed for my abscessed tooth."

Assessment: Well-proportioned female; sexual maturity stage 5. Menarche at age 12 years. Menses regular, every 29 days with moderate flow. Denies history of oral contraceptive use or other reproductive or health problems. Sexually active for approximately 1 year with same partner. "We always use a condom. You can never be too careful."

On examination, vulva reddened and excoriated. "It burns and itches terribly. It even hurts to sit. I've tried not scratching, but sometimes, I just can't help it." Thick, white, cheeselike discharge noted at vaginal introitus. White adherent patches noted on vaginal walls. Specimen of discharge examined and is positive for *Candida.* Fluconazole (Diflucan) prescribed as a one-time oral dose. She asks, "How did I get this? From my boyfriend? Does he need to be treated too?"

Nursing Diagnosis: Pain related to irritation, excoriation, and pruritus associated with candidal infection

Outcome Identification: Adolescent will verbalize relief within 24 hours.

Outcome Evaluation: Adolescent identifies appropriate measures to promote comfort; reports relief of pain after use of comfort measures.

(continued)

Interventions	Rationale
1. Instruct adolescent about the use of fluconazole.	1. Fluconazole is an antifungal agent effective in treating candidal infections, the source of the adolescent's discomfort.
2. Strongly urge that the adolescent refrain from scratching. Suggest use of cool compresses to perineal area.	2. Scratching exacerbates the irritation and may lead to further excoriation and possible secondary infection. Cool compresses help to minimize the itching sensation.
3. Instruct the adolescent to gently wash the perineal area at least two times per day with mild unscented soap and water and to pat rather than rub dry.	3. Frequent cleansing of the perineal area removes irritating drainage. Use of unscented mild soap prevents exposing the perineal area to additional irritants. Rubbing an area increases blood flow to the area, increasing the edema and inflammation, thus increasing the risk for further irritation and subsequent itching.
4. Recommend the use of sitz baths three to four times a day.	4. Sitz baths are soothing and help keep the area free of irritating discharge.
5. Encourage the adolescent to wear cotton underwear.	5. Cotton underwear permits air to circulate and moisture to evaporate, minimizing the risk for further irritation.
6. Recommend the use of an over-the-counter analgesic such as acetaminophen or ibuprofen.	6. Acetaminophen and ibuprofen are effective analgesics for mild pain.

Nursing Diagnosis: Deficient knowledge related to cause and treatment of candidal infection

Outcome Identification: Adolescent will verbalize accurate information about candidiasis.

Outcome Evaluation: Adolescent reports contributing factors associated with development of infection; reports boyfriend has an appointment within 48 hours for evaluation.

Interventions	Rationale
1. Explore what the adolescent knows about candidal infections. Explain the possible relationship between this infection and use of antibiotics for tooth abscess.	1. Exploration provides a baseline for building teaching strategies. Antibiotics destroy the normal vaginal flora, promoting the overgrowth of fungal organisms.
2. Encourage the adolescent to have her boyfriend come in for an evaluation. Urge her to avoid sexual activity until infection is resolved. If not possible, instruct her to have partner wear a condom.	2. Although sexual contact is not the only means of contracting the initial infection, a reinfection cycle can occur with sexual activity, thus necessitating treatment of the partner. Avoidance of sexual activity and use of a condom help to minimize the risk for reinfection.
3. Recommend that the adolescent notify her dentist for a possible change in antibiotic for the abscessed tooth.	3. Some antibiotics are more prone to promoting candidal growth than others. A switch to another antibiotic may be necessary to resolve the abscess and minimize the risk for a recurrent candidal infection.
4. Instruct the adolescent in signs and symptoms of recurrent candidal infection.	4. Knowledge of these signs and symptoms allows for early recognition and prompt treatment should the infection recur.

vulva, vagina, or cervix. Large growths may be excised by cautery or cryotherapy, because they can become cancerous. Small growths may be removed by applying podophyllin (see Chap. 14).

Herpes Genitalis

Genital herpes is caused by the *Herpesvirus hominis* type 2 (HSV-2). This is one of four similar herpes viruses: cytomegalovirus, Epstein-Barr, varicella-zoster, and herpes type 1 and type 2. Genital herpes occurs in epidemic proportions in the United States, and its incidence appears to be growing yearly (Sandhaus, 2001). Unlike most other STDs, there is no known cure. The disease involves a lifelong process, and, although it is not a precursor to cervical cancer, women with cervical cancer have more antibodies against herpes genitalis than others do (Eschenbach, 2001). The virus, spread by skin-to-skin contact, enters a break in the skin or mucous membrane. For the newborn, the virus can be systemic and even fatal (see Chap. 26).

Assessment

Herpes is diagnosed by a culture of the lesion secretion from its location on the vulva, vagina, cervix, or penis or by isolation of HSV antibodies in serum. The incubation period is 3 to 14 days. On first contact, extensive primary lesions originate as a group of pinpoint vesicles on an erythematous base. Within a few days, the vesicles ulcerate and become moist, draining, open lesions. The client may have accompanying flulike symptoms with an increased temperature; vaginal lesions may cause profuse discharge. Pain is intense on contact with clothing or acidic urine.

After the primary stage that lasts approximately 1 week, lesions heal but the virus lingers in a latent form, affecting the sensory nerve ganglia. The condition will flare up and become an active infection during illness, premenstrual dysphoric disorder, fever, overexposure to sunlight, or stress. A secondary response usually produces only local lesions rather than systemic symptoms.

Therapeutic Management

Acyclovir (Zovirax) controls the virus by interfering with deoxyribonucleic acid reproduction and decreasing symptoms. The drug is available as a topical ointment. If applying this to a client, protect yourself with a finger cot or glove so you do not contract the virus or absorb the drug. Sitz baths three times a day and applying a soothing substance such as cornstarch to reduce discomfort afterward may be helpful. An emollient (A & D Ointment) also reduces discomfort, but its moisture tends to prolong the active period of the lesions. Topical imiquimod (Aldara) may be prescribed for resistant lesions (Gilbert, Drehs & Weinberg, 2001).

Because of the possible association with cervical cancer, any female with genital herpes should have a yearly Pap test for the rest of her life. Condoms will help prevent the spread of herpes among sexual partners.

People with herpes may have difficulty establishing sexual relationships for fear of infecting a partner. Because herpes is communicated only by direct contact, infected people need to inform their partner when they have any active lesions and avoid sexual contact or use a condom to decrease the danger of spreading the virus.

Hepatitis B and C

Both hepatitis B and C can be spread by semen as well as blood and, therefore, are considered STDs. These are discussed in Chapter 45 with other forms of hepatitis. Because hepatitis B can be spread by sexual intercourse, adolescents need immunization against hepatitis B (Schmidt & Middleman, 2001).

Gonorrhea

Gonorrhea is transmitted by *Neisseria gonorrhoeae,* a gram-positive diplococcus that thrives on columnar transitional epithelium of the mucous membrane. Symptoms, which begin after a 2- to 7-day incubation period, in males include *urethritis* (pain on urination and frequency of urination) and a urethral discharge. Without treatment, the infection may spread to the testes, scarring the tubules and causing permanent sterility. Untreated, the infection is easily spread among sexual partners. It often occurs concurrently with chlamydial infection (Robinson & Ridgway, 2000)

Although symptoms of gonorrhea in females are not as visible, there may be a slight yellowish vaginal discharge. Bartholin's glands may become inflamed and painful. If left untreated, the infection may spread to pelvic organs, most notably the fallopian tubes (PID). Tubal scarring can result in permanent sterility. In both males and females, untreated gonorrhea can lead to arthritis or heart disease from systemic involvement (Stevens, 2000).

An infant may contract gonorrhea in the birth canal from its mother. This leads frequently to gonorrheal ophthalmia (discussed in Chap. 14).

Assessment

A urine culture for gonococcal bacillus, in addition to vaginal and urethral cultures, should be done on all children with vulvovaginitis or urethral discharge. In males, a first voiding may reveal gonococci if a midstream specimen is inconclusive.

Therapeutic Management

The treatment for gonorrhea is one intramuscular (IM) injection of ceftriaxone (Rocephin) plus oral doxycycline (Vibramycin) for 7 days (Centers for Disease Control [CDC], 2001). This treatment regimen is effective for both gonorrhea and chlamydia. Sexual partners should receive the same treatment.

Approximately 24 h after treatment, the gonorrhea is no longer infectious. Approximately 7 days after treatment, a client should return for a follow-up culture to verify that the disease has been completely eradicated (few people take this precaution). A sexually active client should be given a serologic test for syphilis along with the gonorrheal culture, although the dose of ceftriaxone and doxycycline is also effective treatment for syphilis. Most states require that gonorrhea be reported to the health department; adolescents are asked to name sexual contacts.

NURSING DIAGNOSES AND RELATED INTERVENTIONS

Nursing Diagnosis: Anxiety related to having contracted a reportable STD

Outcome Identification: Client will demonstrate reduced anxiety by end of health care visit.

Outcome Evaluation: Client voices confidence in ability to cope with this problem and demonstrates understanding of both illness and treatment regimen.

People who seek treatment for an STD need to believe they can trust health care personnel and reveal information without fear of criticism. Assure the client of absolute confidentiality in naming his or her sexual contacts. Without being told who put them at risk, these people can then be notified by a health department investigator that they have been exposed to a particular STD. This vital information will help prevent further spread of the disease.

Some people are reluctant to seek treatment for gonorrhea because they have heard stories that therapy involves 10 to 15 days of IM injections. Because they have no symptoms, some girls may avoid going for what they think will be extremely painful treatment. Alert them that treatment is simple. This is an insidious disease, and, even though no symptoms are apparent, it can have disastrous long-term effects if left untreated.

Syphilis

Syphilis is a systemic disease caused by the spirochete *Treponema pallidum.* It is transmitted by sexual contact with a person who has an active spirochete-containing lesion (Satcher, 2000). Like gonorrhea and chlamydia, it must be reported to public health departments.

After an incubation period of 10 to 90 days, a typical lesion appears, generally on the genitalia (penis or labia) or on the mouth, lips, or rectal area from oral–genital or genital–anal contact. The lesion (termed a *chancre*) is a deep ulcer and generally painless despite its size. Lymphadenopathy may be present but is unlikely to be noticed by the affected person. A lesion in the vagina may not be immediately evident. Without treatment, a chancre lasts approximately 6 weeks and then fades.

Approximately 2 to 4 weeks after the chancre disappears, a generalized, macular, copper-colored rash appears. Unlike many other rashes, it affects the soles and the palms. A serologic test for syphilis yields a positive result at this time. There may be secondary symptoms of generalized illness such as low-grade fever and adenopathy. With or without treatment, this stage of syphilis will also fade.

The next stage is a latency period that may last from only a few years to several decades. The only indication of the disease is the serologic test, which continues to yield a positive result.

The final stage of syphilis is a destructive neurologic disease that involves major body organs such as the heart and the nervous system. Typical symptoms are blindness; paralysis; severe, crippling neurologic deformities; mental confusion; slurred speech; and lack of coordination. This third stage must be identified before it becomes fatal.

Assessment

Syphilis is diagnosed by the recognition of the various symptoms of the three stages and by serologic serum tests, usually VDRL (Venereal Disease Research Laboratory), ART (automated reagin test), RPR (rapid plasma reagin test), or FTA-ABS (fluorescent treponemal antibody absorption test).

Therapeutic Management

The therapy effectively arrests the disease at whatever stage it has reached. Benzathine penicillin G given IM in two sites is effective therapy. For the adolescent sensitive to penicillin, either oral erythromycin or tetracycline can be given for 10 to 15 days. As with gonorrhea, sexual partners are treated in the same way as the person with the active infection.

Because syphilis can be treated so easily, one would think it would be easy to eradicate. In reality, however, because the primary chancre is painless, many people are either unaware of it or choose to ignore it, thereby transmitting the disease to unsuspecting partners. Adolescents, in particular, need accurate information about syphilis to become aware of the symptoms. They should believe they can report the disease to health care personnel and that they can name sexual contacts without fear of being criticized. If a woman develops syphilis during pregnancy, the disease can be spread to the fetus (DHHS, 2001).

Human Immunodeficiency Virus

HIV is carried by semen as well as other body fluids so is considered an STD. Invasion of the virus is discussed with other immune disorders in Chapter 42, and in relation to pregnancy in Chapter 14.

✔ CHECKPOINT QUESTIONS

9. What are the typical symptoms of a candidal vaginal infection?
10. Why is gonorrhea an especially serious STD?

KEY POINTS

Children who are born with a reproductive tract disorder frequently adjust well when young. They may need counseling at puberty or when they become aware of the impact of their disorder on their sexual functioning or their ability to reproduce.

The cause of ambiguous genitalia is unknown but may be related to the level of testosterone produced in utero. The true gender of children is established by a karyotype of chromosomes.

The development of breast or pubic hair before age 8 years or menses before age 9 years is considered precocious sexual development. Children may be treated with a synthetic analogue of gonadotropin-releasing hormone to reduce development. Without effective support, such children are at high risk for disturbed body image.

Delayed puberty is the failure to develop secondary sex characteristics by the age of 17 years. Girls may be administered estrogen to promote development; boys may be administered testosterone.

Balanoposthitis (inflammation of the glans and prepuce) and phimosis (constricted foreskin) occur in boys. Phimosis can be treated with circumcision.

Cryptorchidism is failure of one or both testes to descend during intrauterine life. The condition is surgically corrected to prevent infertility and detect testicular cancer later in life.

Testicular cancer is rare but tends to occur in young men. Boys need to be taught testicular self-examination for early detection.

Dysmenorrhea is a menstrual disorder that occurs frequently in adolescent girls. Therapy for this is a prostaglandin inhibitor such as ibuprofen.

Untreated endometriosis (the abnormal growth of extrauterine endometrial tissue) can lead to infertility later in life. Therapy is administration of a synthetic androgen or GnRH receptor inhibitor or surgery to reduce the size of the abnormal tissue.

Vulvovaginitis (inflammation of the vulva and vagina) and PID are infections that can occur in adolescents. Therapy to prevent fallopian tube scarring and infertility later in life is essential. Girls need to be taught, in addition, ways to avoid toxic shock syndrome.

Conditions such as fibrocystic breasts can occur in adolescents. Adolescent girls need to learn breast self-examination to detect and monitor abnormalities that could be signs of breast cancer.

STDs such as candidiasis, trichomoniasis, *Chlamydia trachomatis,* genital warts, herpes genitalis, gonorrhea, and syphilis are increasing in incidence in the adolescent population. An important health-teaching area with children is the need to follow safer sex practices.

When teaching about STDs, it is important to stress that they do not confer immunity and thus can be contracted more than once.

CRITICAL THINKING EXERCISES

1. Navi is the 15-year-old girl that you met at the beginning of the chapter who had been diagnosed as having gonorrhea. She said she was glad she had contracted the disease early in life because now she will never get it again. What health teaching does Navi need to be better informed about her disease?
2. You care for a 15-year-old girl who has no breast development and also has not menstruated yet. She asks you if it is time to worry. How would you counsel her?
3. A 12-year-old boy was born with undescended testes. He had surgery for this at age 2 years. He is concerned now that he is at high risk for testicular cancer. How would you counsel him?
4. Examine the National Health Goals related to reproductive disorders in children. Most government-sponsored money for nursing research is allotted based on these goals. What would be a possible research topic to explore pertinent to these goals that would be both fundable and advance evidence-based practice?

REFERENCES

Boom, J. A. (2000). Gynecomastia. In M. W. Schwartz (Ed.). *The 5-minute pediatric consult* (pp. 404–405). Philadelphia: Lippincott Williams & Wilkins.

Bourin, M., Chue, P., & Guillon, Y. (2001). Paroxetine: a review. *CNS Drug Reviews,* 7(1), 25–47.

Centers for Disease Control (2000). Gonorrhea. *MMWR, 49*(24), 538–542.

Chapron, C., & Dubuisson, J. B. (2001). Management of endometriosis. *Annals of the New York Academy of Sciences, 943*(9), 276–280.

Clark, L. R. (2000). Dysmenorrhea. In M. W. Schwartz (Ed.). *The 5-minute pediatric consult* (pp. 340–341). Philadelphia: Lippincott Williams & Wilkins.

Davis, A. R., & Westhoff, C. L. (2001). Primary dysmenorrhea in adolescent girls and treatment with oral contraceptives. *Journal of Pediatric & Adolescent Gynecology, 14*(1), 3–8.

Dearnaley, D., Huddart, R. A., & Horwich, A. (2001). Managing testicular cancer. *British Medical Journal, 322*(7302), 1583–1588.

Department of Health and Human Services. (2000). *Healthy people 2010.* Washington, DC: DHHS.

Department of Health and Human Services. (2001). Congenital syphilis—United States, 2000. *Morbidity & Mortality Weekly Report, 50*(27), 573–577.

Dilorio, C., et al. (2001). Social cognitive correlates of sexual experience and condom use among 13- through 15-year-old adolescents. *Journal of Adolescent Health, 29*(3), 208–216.

Eschenbach, D. A. (2000). Pelvic infections and sexually transmitted diseases. In J. R. Scott et al. (Eds.). *Danforth's obstetrics and gynecology* (8th ed., pp. 579–600). Philadelphia: Lippincott Williams & Wilkins.

Esposito, C., et al. (2001). Results and complications of laparoscopic surgery for pediatric varicocele. *Journal of Pediatric Surgery, 36*(5), 767–769.

Ferry, R. J., & Satin-Smith, M. (2000). Sexual precocity. In M. W. Schwartz (Ed.). *The 5-minute pediatric consult* (pp. 752–753). Philadelphia: Lippincott Williams & Wilkins.

Fiorica, J. V. (2000). The breast. In J. R. Scott et al. (Eds.). *Danforth's obstetrics and gynecology* (8th ed., pp. 631–648). Philadelphia: Lippincott Williams & Wilkins.

Gilbert, J., Drehs, M., & Weinberg, J. (2001). Topical imiquimod for acyclovir-unresponsive herpes simplex virus 2 infection. *Archives in Dermatology, 137*(8), 1015–1017.

Givens, M. L. & Luszczak, M. (2002). Breast disorders: A review for emergency physicians. *Journal of Emergency Medicine, 22*(1), 59–65.

Hammond, C. B., & Riddick, D. H. (2000). Menstruation and disorders of menstrual function. In J. R. Scott et al. (Eds.). *Danforth's obstetrics and gynecology* (8th ed., pp. 601–614). Philadelphia: Lippincott Williams & Wilkins.

Ingram, M., et al. (2001). Risk assessment for gonococcal and chlamydial infections in young children undergoing evaluation for sexual abuse. *Pediatrics, 107*(5), 73–78.

Kadir, R. A., & Lee, C. A. (2001). Menorrhagia in adolescents. *Pediatric Annals, 30*(9), 541–547.

Kaplan, D. W., & Love, K. A. (2001). Gynecologic disorders in adolescence. In W. W. Hay, A. R. Hayward, M. J. Levin, & J. M. Sondheimer (Eds.). *Current pediatric diagnosis and treatment* (15th ed.). New York: McGraw-Hill.

Kappy, M. S., Steelman, J. W., & Travers, S. H. (2001). The gonads. In W. W. Hay, A. R. Hayward, M. J. Levin, & J. M. Sondheimer (Eds.). *Current pediatric diagnosis and treatment* (15th ed.). New York: McGraw-Hill.

Klein, J., et al. (2001). Where do adolescents get their condoms? *Journal of Adolescent Health, 29*(3), 186–193.

Lee, P. A., & Coughlin, M. T. (2001). Fertility after bilateral cryptorchidism. *Hormone Research, 55*(1), 28–32.

Master, C. L. (2000). Cryptorchidism. In M. W. Schwartz (Ed.). *The 5-minute pediatric consult* (pp. 296–297). Philadelphia: Lippincott Williams & Wilkins.

Nyirjesy, P. (1999). Vaginitis in the adolescent patient. *Pediatric Clinics of North America, 46*(4), 733–745.

Nyquist, A. C., Levin, M. J., & Sigel, E. (2001). The spectrum of sexually transmitted infections. In W. W. Hay, A. R. Hayward, M. J. Levin, & J. M. Sondheimer (Eds.). *Current pediatric diagnosis and treatment* (15th ed.). New York: McGraw-Hill.

Porpiglia, F., et al. (2001). Laparoscopic diagnosis and management of acute intra-abdominal testicular torsion. *The Journal of Urology, 166*(2), 600–601.

Robinson, A. J., & Ridgway, G. L. (2000). Concurrent gonococcal and chlamydial infection: How best to treat. *Drugs, 59*(40), 801–813.

Sandhaus, S. (2001). Genital herpes in pregnant and non-pregnant women. *Nurse Practitioner, 26*(4), 15–22.

Satcher, D. (2000). National Syphilis Elimination Launch. *Sexually Transmitted Diseases, 27*(2), 66–67.

Schenken, R. S. (2000). Endometriosis. In J. R. Scott et al. (Eds.). *Danforth's obstetrics and gynecology* (8th ed., pp. 669–675). Philadelphia: Lippincott Williams & Wilkins.

Schmidt, R. M., & Middleman, A. B. (2001). The importance of hepatitis B vaccination among adolescents. *Journal of Adolescent Health, 29*(3), 217–222.

Seng, Y. J., & Moissinac, K. (2000). Trauma induced testicular torsion. A reminder for the unwary. *Journal of Accident & Emergency Medicine, 17*(5), 381–382.

Stevens, M. W. (2000). Gonococcal infections. In M. W. Schwartz (Ed.). *The 5-minute pediatric consult* (pp. 394–395). Philadelphia: Lippincott Williams & Wilkins.

SUGGESTED READINGS

Baines, P. A., & Allen, G. M. (2001). Pelvic pain and menstrual related illnesses. *Emergency Medicine Clinics of North America, 9*(3), 763–780.

Blythe, M. J., & Rosenthal, S. L. (2000). Female adolescent sexuality: Promoting healthy sexual development. *Obstetrics & Gynecology Clinics of North America, 27*(1), 125–141.

Carvajal, S. C. (1999). Psychosocial predictors of delay of first sexual intercourse by adolescents. *Health Psychology, 18*(5), 443–452.

Dwivedi, A. J. et al. (2002). Abdominal wall endometriomas. *Digestive Diseases & Sciences, 47*(2), 456–461.

Frank, D., & Williams, T. (1999). Attitudes about menstruation among fifth-, sixth-, and seventh-grade pre- and post-menarcheal girls. *Journal of School Nursing, 15*(4), 25–31.

Granot, M., et al. (2001). Pain perception in women with dysmenorrhea. *Obstetrics & Gynecology, 98*(3), 407–411.

Griffin, C. M. (1999). Reframing menarche education: A developmental perspective. *Advance for Nurse Practitioners, 7*(11), 53–57.

Hogan, D. P., Sun, R., & Cornwell, G. T. (2000). Sexual and fertility behaviors of American females aged 15–19 years. *American Journal of Public Health, 90*(9), 1421–1425.

Lammers, C., et al. (2000). Influences on adolescents' decision to postpone onset of sexual intercourse. *Journal of Adolescent Health, 26*(1), 42–48.

Long, F. W. (2000). Recognizing and treating premenstrual dysphoric disorder in the obstetric, gynecologic and primary care practices. *Journal of Clinical Psychiatry, 61*(12 Suppl), 9–16.

Marcozzi, D., & Suner, S. (2001). The nontraumatic, acute scrotum. *Emergency Medicine Clinics of North America, 19*(3), 547–568.

Santelli, J. S., et al. (2000). The association of sexual behaviors with socioeconomic status, family structure, and race/ethnicity among US adolescents. *American Journal of Public Health, 90*(10), 1582–1588.

Wolf, C. K., Maizels, M., & Furness, P. D. (2001). The undescended testicle. *Comprehensive Therapy, 27*(1), 11–17.

Nursing Care of the Child With an Endocrine or Metabolic Disorder

Key Terms

- carpal spasm
- exophthalmos
- glycosuria
- hormones
- hyperfunction
- hyperglycemia
- hypofunction
- hypoglycemia
- hypothalamus
- ketoacidosis
- latent tetany
- manifest tetany
- pedal spasm
- polydipsia
- polyuria
- sella turcica
- Somogyi phenomenon

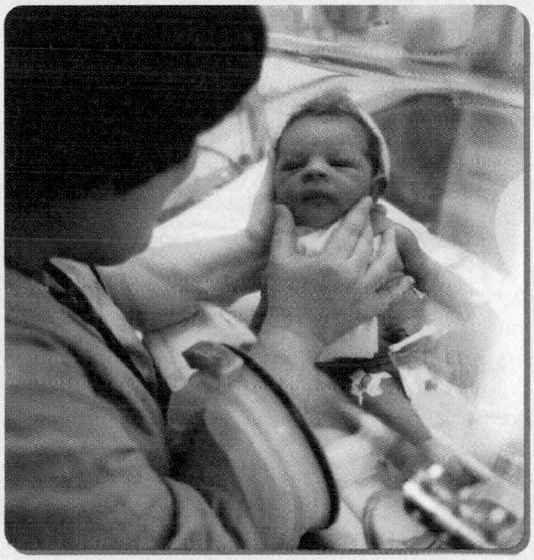

Objectives

After mastering the contents of this chapter, you should be able to:

1. Describe the structure and function of the different endocrine glands.
2. Assess a child with a disorder of endocrine function.
3. Formulate nursing diagnoses for a child with altered endocrine or metabolic function.
4. Develop appropriate outcomes for the child with endocrine or metabolic dysfunction.
5. Plan nursing care (e.g., health teaching) for the child with altered endocrine or metabolic function.
6. Implement nursing care (e.g., teaching insulin administration) for the child with an endocrine or metabolic disorder.
7. Evaluate outcomes to be certain that goals of nursing care were achieved.
8. Identify National Health Goals related to childhood endocrine or metabolic disorders that nurses could be instrumental in helping the nation achieve.
9. Identify areas related to care of children with endocrine or metabolic disorders that could benefit from additional nursing research or application of evidence-based practice.
10. Analyze ways that care of the child with altered endocrine or metabolic function can be family centered.
11. Synthesize knowledge of endocrine and metabolic dysfunctions and the nursing process to ensure quality maternal and child health nursing care.

Rob is a 16-year-old boy with type 1 diabetes whom you see in an ambulatory clinic. His diabetes was diagnosed when he was 7 years old. His records indicate that his disease control has been generally good over the years, but, in the last 6 months, he has "forgotten" to take his insulin at least once a week. When you ask him about this, he mentions that sports after school plus a weekend job, a new girlfriend, and a new car have occupied his time and interrupted what used to be a strict schedule of home-cooked meals and rigid bedtimes. Is Rob's history unusual for an adolescent? What health teaching do you think will most help him reestablish control?

Previous chapters described the growth and development of well children. This chapter adds information about the dramatic changes, both physical and psychosocial, that occur when children develop an endocrine or metabolic disorder. This is important information because it builds a base for care and health teaching.

After you've studied the chapter, answer the Critical Thinking Exercises at the end of the chapter and then access the on-line study activities (http://connection.lww.com) *to further sharpen your skills and test your knowledge.*

The endocrine system is composed of a small group of ductless glands that work together with the neurologic system to regulate and coordinate all body systems (**Fig. 48-1**). The glands produce chemicals called *hormones,* which are secreted into surrounding tissue and picked up by the bloodstream where they act individually and in concert to affect various organ systems. (The word *hormone* is from the Greek hormaein, which means "to set in motion.") Each gland of the endocrine system has specific functions that are necessary for regulating body processes; each hormone secreted acts on a specific target (or designated) organ.

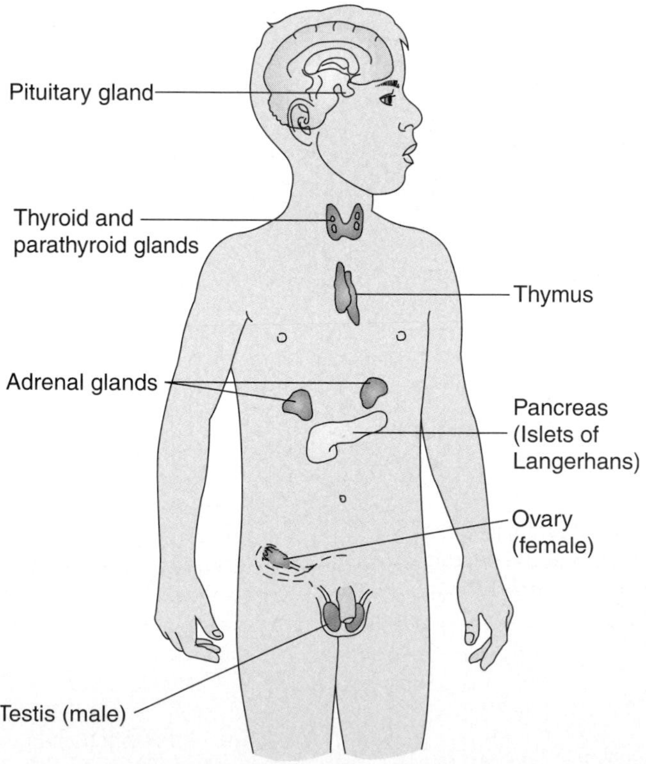

FIGURE 48.1 Location of the endocrine glands.

Dysfunction of the glands or action of the hormones results in a variety of disorders, most of which have long-term implications. Parents—and children as soon as they are old enough—need to understand these diseases to the best of their ability and to participate in their long-term plan of care. National Health Goals related to endocrine and metabolic disorders in children are presented in the Focus on National Health Goals box.

NURSING PROCESS OVERVIEW

For Care of the Child With an Endocrine or Metabolic Disorder

Assessment

Endocrine and metabolic disorders as a group commonly cause changes in normal growth or activity patterns. This is usually detected when height and weight are assessed and compared with standards for the child's age at a health visit (see Focus on Multidisciplinary Care). Obese children may have thyroid deficiencies. Short children may have pituitary difficulties. An acute loss in weight is often the first symptom of type 1 diabetes mellitus in children.

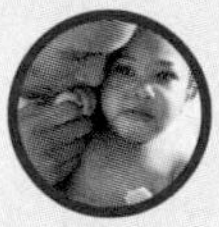

FOCUS ON NATIONAL HEALTH GOALS

Diabetes mellitus is a disorder with serious consequences in both children and pregnant women. A number of National Health Goals address reducing the incidence of this disease:

- Reduce diabetes-related deaths to no more than 7.8/1,000 people from a baseline of 8.8/1,000.
- Increase the proportion of persons with diabetes who receive formal diabetes education from a baseline of 45% to a target of 60%.
- Decrease the proportion of pregnant women with gestational diabetes (DHHS, 2000).

Nurses can be instrumental in helping the nation achieve these goals by educating women about the possible effects the illness can have on pregnancy and by educating children about ways to prevent the long-term effects of the illness. Nursing research could shed additional light on these goals by asking questions such as: How should women be taught that fetal anomalies from hyperglycemia occur very early in pregnancy so they must be certain to enter pregnancy in good glucose control? Long-term effects of diabetes are not noticeable in childhood, but how can children be educated to plan a healthy lifestyle to prevent these effects in adult life? At what age can children be expected to be responsible for glucose monitoring and insulin injection? What methods are best for encouraging children to be in charge of their own nutrition?

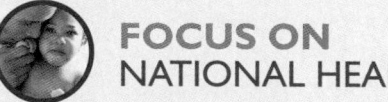

FOCUS ON MULTIDISCIPLINARY CARE

Children with endocrine or metabolic disorders interact with many different health care professionals such as endocrinologists, nurse practitioners, physicians, physical therapists, pharmacists, nutritionists, and nurses. The disorder is often identified first through routine height and weight measurements taken by nurses. Any changes need to be communicated clearly to other health care personnel involved with the child's care. In addition, the child's therapy regimen may be complex, requiring careful and consistent communication among team members.

Weighing babies at birth and at health visits is often done by unlicensed assistive personnel. Be certain that they understand the importance of these measurements in detecting disease so they obtain these measurements as accurately as possible. Help them learn to compare a new reading with the previous reading so they can identify a marked difference in height or weight (or a gradual trend) and can alert the primary care provider to a change in these measurements.

To obtain information on activity, take a day history by asking the parent or child to describe all the child's actions on a typical day. This type of information yields clues that are helpful in distinguishing between a normally "quiet" child and one experiencing inactivity and chronic fatigue resulting from decreased endocrine function. For example, the quiet child lies down after school and reads; the ill child lies down and sleeps. Taking a day history also helps to differentiate between a child who is merely active and one who is overly active because of hyperthyroidism. For example, the healthy child appears to "go constantly" but can sit through a favorite television program or a meal. The child with increased thyroid hormone production may be unable to sit quietly at all.

Also assess dietary and elimination habits. Extreme thirst or appetite may occur with an endocrine disorder such as diabetes insipidus or type 1 diabetes mellitus. Frequent voiding in children most often reflects a urinary tract infection, but it may be evidence of excessive urine excretion (polyuria), possibly from pituitary dysfunction or diabetes mellitus.

On physical examination, observe the child's general appearance, noting any excessive tiredness, scaling or dry skin, drooping eyelids, or protrusion of the eyeballs (**exophthalmos**), and poor muscle tone (see Assessing the Child With an Endocrine Disorder).

Nursing Diagnosis

Nursing diagnoses relevant to children with endocrine or metabolic disorders may include the following:

- Deficient fluid volume related to constant excessive loss of fluid through urination
- Risk for imbalanced nutrition, less than body requirements related to inability to use glucose because of diabetes mellitus
- Disturbed body image related to abnormal height
- Health-seeking behaviors related to self-administration of insulin
- Deficient knowledge related to treatment needs
- Fear related to illness outcome
- Anticipatory grieving related to presumed losses associated with diagnosis of long-term illness
- Interrupted family processes related to child's chronic illness

ASSESSING the Child With an Endocrine Disorder

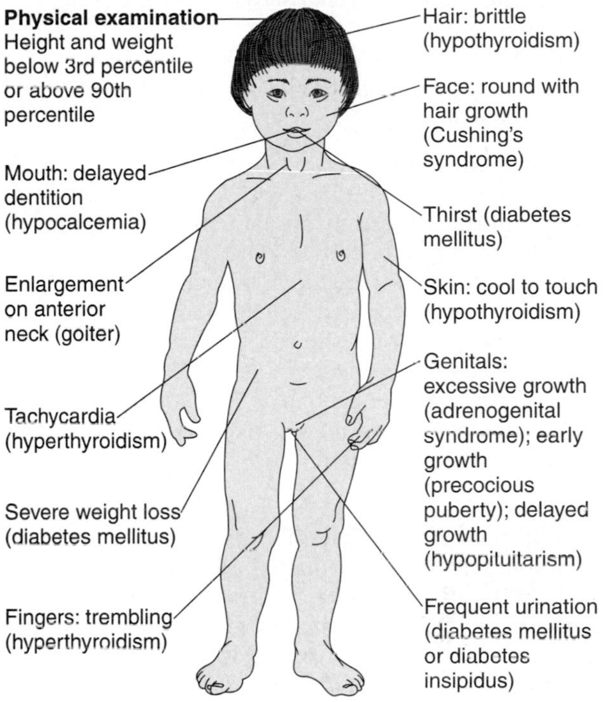

Outcome Identification and Planning

Although most endocrine and metabolic disorders have long-term implications, parents and children may find it easier to work with outcomes initially that are short-term—particularly if they are having difficulty accepting the diagnosis and the long-term nature of the disorder. Because symptoms usually are not acute, children may easily forget to take medications or the parents may forget to give the medications. Helping parents create reminder charts is an effective measure to increase therapeutic compliance.

Evaluate the school as well as the home situation for any child with a chronic illness. You may need to instruct teachers about the child's health problem (with the parents' permission) so they do not make excessive or inappropriate demands (e.g., insisting that the child with hyperthyroidism submit neat handwriting assignments when the child cannot do so).

Selected organizations for referral include the following:

American Diabetes Association (*www.diabetes.org*)
Congenital Adrenal Hyperplasia Support Group (*www.cah.org.uk*)
Little People of America (*www.lpaonline.org*)
National Tay-Sachs and Allied Diseases Association (*www.ntsad.org*)

Implementation

Interventions for children with endocrine or metabolic disorders must always be carried out with the long-term aspects of care in mind. Bribing children to take a medicine, for example, is never good practice. It has no place with children who must continue to take a medication for the rest of their lives (bribery quickly becomes ineffective). As children grow older and can better understand their disorder, explanations of why they must continue to take medication need to become more detailed.

Outcome Evaluation

Children with disorders of endocrine or metabolic function need to be evaluated periodically throughout childhood because growth and changing activity necessitate changes in medication dosages or schedules. These checkups provide good opportunities for health teaching to equip children to meet new situations that arise as they mature. Body appearance becomes increasingly important as children enter adolescence, for example, because being like, not unlike, their peers grows even more important. Because of this, seemingly well-adjusted school-age children develop extreme difficulty continuing to accept their illness. Compliance with a medication program may become erratic. Only by periodic reevaluation can these problems be identified so that health care plans can be modified and adapted to the child's needs, enabling the child and family to continue coping with a long-term illness.

The following are examples suggesting achievement of outcomes:

- Child demonstrates written record illustrating compliance with medication regimen.
- Parents list developmentally appropriate, not size appropriate, activities for their child with short stature.
- Child's blood pressure and pulse remain within normal limits for age; specific gravity of urine is between 1.003 and 1.030; skin turgor is good; child states thirst is not excessive.
- Parents demonstrate correct insulin injection technique and state they are comfortable administering an injection to their child.

THE PITUITARY GLAND

The work of the pituitary gland is directed by the **hypothalamus,** an organ located in the center of the brain that is the regulator of the autonomic nervous system. About 1 cm long, 1.0 to 1.5 cm wide, and 0.5 cm thick, the pituitary rests in the **sella turcica,** a depression of the sphenoid bone. It is covered by a tough membrane, which also joins the gland to the hypothalamus.

The pituitary gland has several distinct regions: the anterior lobe, or *adenohypophysis;* the posterior lobe, or *neurohypophysis;* and the intermediate lobe (*pars intermedia*), which lies between the anterior and posterior lobes. Each of these regions appears to have its own function and secretes specific hormones.

Pituitary Hormones

The regions of the pituitary gland store and release eight hormones; four of these—antidiuretic hormone (ADH), thyrotropin, corticotropin, and somatotropin—are prominently involved in childhood illnesses (Table 48-1).

PITUITARY GLAND DISORDERS

Illnesses caused by pituitary dysfunction result from tumor growth of the pituitary or hypothalamus, interference with circulation to the gland, trauma, inflammation, structural abnormalities, erratic or nonfunctional feedback mechanisms, and, possibly, autoimmune responses.

Growth Hormone Deficiency

When production of human growth hormone (GH; somatotropin) is deficient, children cannot grow to full size. As a result, they remain in proportion but well below the average on a standard growth chart. Deficient production of GH may result from a nonmalignant cystic tumor of embryonic origin that places pressure on the pituitary gland or from increased intracranial pressure from a cause such as a trauma. In most children with hypopituitarism, the cause of the defect is unknown (Ferry & Collett-Solberg, 2000a).

If a child with hypopituitarism is not treated, predicting exactly what height will be reached is difficult because height varies with each individual. Without treatment, however, most children will not reach a height over 3 or 4 ft.

Assessment

The child with deficient production of GH is generally normal in size and weight at birth. Within the first few years of life, however, the child begins to fall below the third percentile of height and weight on growth charts. The face appears infantile because the mandible is recessed and immature; the nose is usually small. The child's teeth may be crowded in a small jaw (and may erupt late). The child's voice may be high pitched, and the onset of pubic, facial, and axillary hair and genital growth is delayed. History, physical findings, and a decreased level of circulating GH contribute to the diagnosis.

Evaluate the family history for traits of short stature or to detect if the main problem is constitutional delay (familial late development). If at all possible, obtain estimates of the parents' height and siblings' height and weight during their periods of growth. Assess thoroughly the child's prenatal and birth history for suggestion of intrauterine growth retardation or severe head trauma at birth, which could

TABLE 48.1 Common Pituitary Hormones and Their Purposes

PITUITARY HORMONE	SOURCE AND TARGET ORGANS	ACTIONS AND EFFECTS
Antidiuretic hormone (ADH)	Secreted by the neurohypophysis *Target organ:* Kidney	• ADH helps regulate fluid volume and urine output. It decreases urinary output by increasing water reabsorption. This increases extracellular fluid volume, resulting in a vasopressor effect (increased blood pressure). When the plasma concentration increases or overall circulating vascular volume decreases, more ADH will be released. • If blood pools in the body periphery, decreasing core body volume, ADH will be released. • Postural changes (from a lying to a standing position) and exposure to high temperatures (blood shifts to peripheral structures to begin the cooling process) stimulate ADH release. • Trauma, pain, and anxiety increase ADH release. • When ADH levels fall, little or no water is reabsorbed, and urinary output increases. • Alcohol consumption inhibits ADH secretion; as a result, urine output increases.
Corticotropin (ACTH)	Secreted by the adenohypophysis *Target organ:* Kidney	• ACTH stimulates the adrenal gland to produce glucocorticoid and mineralocorticoid hormones. Increased production of adrenal gland secretions decreases ACTH production and vice versa. • If a child receives synthetic ACTH or a corticosteroid, natural ACTH production is temporarily depressed. If these synthetic hormones are given for a long time, then stopped abruptly, the decreased amount of natural ACTH may not be enough to stimulate adrenal gland activity. The child will experience symptoms of adrenal insufficiency. • When discontinuing ACTH and high doses of long-term corticosteroids, dosage must be reduced gradually to protect adrenal function. The medication should never be stopped abruptly.
Somatotropin (growth hormone; GH)	Secreted by the adenohypophysis *Target organ:* None; acts on all body cells	• GH increases bone and cartilage growth and increases gastrointestinal absorption of calcium. If GH production is inhibited, dwarfism will occur; if GH production is excessive, gigantism or overgrowth will occur. • GH decreases catabolism of protein in cells by freeing fatty acids for energy, which, in turn, frees glucose for glycogen storage (GH is both protein and glucose sparing). • GH production increases when hypoglycemia occurs and during sleep. • GH is released from the adenohypophysis based on a release factor from both the hypothalamus and the liver. • The amount of GH secretion is influenced by exercise, sleep, nutrition, and thyroid and adrenal function.
Thyrotropin (TSH)	Secreted by the adenohypophysis *Target organ:* Thyroid gland	• TSH stimulates the thyroid gland to produce thyroid hormones (thyroxine and triiodothyronine). • Too little TSH leads to atrophy and inactivity of the thyroid gland; too much TSH causes hypertrophy (increase in size) and hyperplasia (increase in the number of cells) of the gland. • A feedback message of increased thyroid secretion lowers TSH production; decreased thyroid production increases TSH production.

have injured the pituitary gland. Assess the health history for any chronic illness, such as heart, kidney, or intestinal disorders, that could contribute to the decreased level of growth. Take a 24-h nutrition history and ask carefully about urinary and bowel function. Parents often report that their child is a "picky eater," yet the 24-h history does not reveal a poor appetite that is extensive enough to halt growth. Be certain to assess not only the child's actual height but also his or her feelings about being short.

A pituitary tumor must be ruled out as the cause of decreased GH production. Sudden halted growth suggests a tumor; gradual failure suggests an idiopathic involvement. A history of vision loss, headache, increase in head circumference, nausea, and vomiting (signs of increased intracranial pressure) also suggests a pituitary tumor. The history of a child with GH deficiency typically reveals a well child except for the abnormal lack of growth.

A physical assessment, including a funduscopic examination and neurologic testing, is necessary to detect a lesion or tumor. Blood studies for hypothyroidism, hypoadrenalism, and hypoaldosteronism are performed, because these conditions also influence growth. The wrist is examined by x-ray to determine bone age. Epiphyseal closure of long bone is delayed with GH deficiency but is proportional to the height delay. A skull series, computed tomography (CT) scan, magnetic resonance imaging (MRI), or sonogram will be performed to detect possible enlargement of the sella turcica, which would suggest a pituitary tumor.

Normally, GH level rises after a period of sound sleep or a period of activity. If the level is low during these test periods, the hormone's response to artificial stimulation can be tested. If normal children are given a test dose of insulin, for example, they will become hypoglycemic. **Hypoglycemia** (low blood glucose level) stimulates the release of circulating GH. Intravenous (IV) infusion of arginine or oral administration of clonidine (Catapres) will have the same effect. In children with GH deficiency, an increase in the level of GH does not occur in these instances.

These studies obviously call for careful nursing attention so children do not become extremely hypoglycemic or refuse to cooperate with the number of blood samples and the IV line necessary for the study. If a child is not yet concerned about being short, these studies may not seem important; this makes it difficult to tolerate the pain associated with the procedures (although application of EMLA cream and use of an intermittent infusion device such as a heparin lock, so that blood sampling will involve as few venipunctures as possible, greatly reduces the discomfort).

Therapeutic Management

GH deficiency is treated by the administration of intramuscular (IM) recombinant human GH injection two or three times a week (Sandberg & MacGillivray, 2000; see Focus on Pharmacology). Because the time of the dose affects the hormone's effectiveness, GH is usually given at bedtime, the time of day that GH normally peaks. Fortunately, because these children have delayed epiphyseal closure, if treatment is started early, they will be able to reach a targeted height. Some may need luteinizing hormone-releasing hormone to delay epiphyseal closure. Some children may need supplements of gonadotropin or other pituitary hormones because these are deficient as well.

A slight increase in the incidence of leukemia in children treated with GH has been noted (Ferry & Collett-Solberg, 2000a). Parents need to be aware of, but not unduly frightened by this association because this may be due to other predisposing factors rather than just the administration of GH.

FOCUS ON PHARMACOLOGY

Somatropin (Nutropin, Humatrope)

Action: Somatropin is a recombinant human growth hormone used for the long-term treatment of children who have growth failure from inadequate production of pituitary hormone, renal failure, and Turner's syndrome; may be used to promote healing in severe burns

Pregnancy risk category: C

Dosage: Somatropin dosage is individualized. The drug is administered by injection.

Possible adverse effects: Injection site pain, glucose intolerance, hypothyroidism, bone problems (particularly the hip), blood abnormalities, rare intracranial hypertension in first 8 weeks of therapy

Nursing Implications

- Advise parents that wrist or hip x-rays are performed before therapy begins. Thereafter, parents should be alert for limping or knee or hip pain, which should be reported to their primary care provider. Slipped capital epiphysis is associated with growth hormone supplementation.
- Reinforce the need for periodic thyroid function tests and funduscopic examination (to detect rare intracranial hypertension).
- Tell parents that growth hormone may interact with glucocorticoid therapy (e.g., prednisone), causing a decrease in the effectiveness of the growth hormone. Urge parents to inform all health care practitioners that the child is receiving growth hormone.
- Keep in mind that administration of growth hormone is associated with a possible increased risk of leukemia.

NURSING DIAGNOSES AND RELATED INTERVENTIONS

Nursing Diagnosis: Situational low self-esteem related to short stature

Outcome Identification: Child will demonstrate adequate self-esteem by the end of the treatment period.

Outcome Evaluation: Child speaks positively about self; identifies friends and activities enjoyed with peers.

If a child has been consistently behind in growth since early life, parents may simply assume in early childhood that the child is going to be short as an adult. The parents become concerned only when the child reaches puberty and fails to develop secondary sex characteristics. When investigation reveals the child's true problem, parents may feel guilty that they did not become alarmed earlier. They may feel resentment toward health care personnel who did not alert them to the problem earlier. Encourage parents to discuss these feelings and provide support to help them accept their child in this new light as well as participate in making the new plan of care a success. You may need to remind parents to assign duties and responsibilities to children that match their chronologic age, not physical size, to promote their feelings of maturity and self-esteem. Children, too, may need some help in accepting themselves at the ultimate height they achieve, especially if this is only in the 5th percentile, not the 50th (see Focus on Communication).

Growth Hormone Excess

Overproduction of GH is generally caused by a tumor of the anterior pituitary (an adenoma). If an overproduction occurs before the epiphyseal lines of the long bones have closed, excessive growth results. Weight is excessive also, but it is proportional to height. The skull circumference generally exceeds normal, and the fontanelles may close late or not close at all. Such excessive growth generally becomes evident at puberty when prepubertal growth is great. *Acromegaly* (enlargement of the bones of the head and soft parts of the hands and feet) may accompany the early excessive growth in stature, although acromegaly becomes more pronounced after the epiphyseal lines of the long bones close and linear growth is no longer possible. Acromegaly may cause the tongue to be so enlarged and thickened that it protrudes from the mouth, giving the child a dull, apathetic appearance and difficulty in articulating words. Untreated, a child may reach a height of over 8 ft. X-rays or sonograms of the skull reveal enlargement of the sella turcica.

FOCUS ON COMMUNICATION

Peggy, a 10-year-old fifth grader, has been diagnosed with hypopituitarism. She is only three ft tall and has shown no secondary sex development as yet. The physician has prescribed injections of growth hormone three times weekly. While observing her and her mother, you notice that Peggy is wearing a dress more suitable for a first grader than a fifth grader.

Less Effective Communication

Nurse: Mrs. Stone, do you have any questions about Peggy's care?

Mrs. Stone: Not really. I think everyone is exaggerating the importance of being tall, though. Look how cute she is playing with that puzzle on that little table over there.

Nurse: She is cute, but is she happy with being so short?

Mrs. Stone: Well, her size has made her better at gymnastics than the taller girls—and tap dancing. She's won two contests—probably because she looks so much younger than she is.

Nurse: But how does she feel about her size? Have you talked to her about how she thinks she will feel about her size in the future when she's grown up?

Mrs. Stone: I can't imagine her grown up—not when she's so tiny and cute now.

Nurse: Well, you realize that the growth hormone injections that I will be teaching you to give will make her grow.

Mrs. Stone: Yes, but I hope she doesn't grow too much. I don't want to lose my baby.

Nurse: Let's go over the injection technique now so I'm sure you can give them effectively.

More Effective Communication

Nurse: Mrs. Stone, do you have any questions about Peggy's care?

Mrs. Stone: Not really. I think everyone is exaggerating the importance of being tall, though. Look how cute she is playing with that puzzle on that little table over there.

Nurse: Yes, she is a very cute girl. Is she happy with being so short?

Mrs. Stone: Well, her size has made her better at gymnastics than the taller girls—and tap dancing. She's won two contests—probably because she looks so much younger than she is.

Nurse: But how does she feel about her size? Have you talked to her about how she thinks she will feel about her size in the future when she's grown up?

Mrs. Stone: I can't imagine her grown up—not when she's so tiny and cute now.

Nurse: Well, you do understand that the growth hormone injections that your physician has prescribed will make her grow.

Mrs. Stone: Yes, but I hope she doesn't grow too much. I don't want to lose my baby.

Nurse: Let's talk a little bit about how Peggy's growing up makes both you and Peggy feel before we review the injection technique.

Children with hypopituitarism are often viewed as cute and petite by parents and treated as if they were the age of a child their size, not their chronologic age. When therapy to make them taller begins, some parents have difficulty accepting that growth may change not only the child's appearance, but also the parent–child relationship—that growing up means growing away toward independence. Exploring how the parents and the child feel about this may help them view the coming change as a positive and exciting new stage in their relationship. In such instances, a positive outlook on growth will help ensure adherence to and acceptance of therapy.

If the cause of the increased hormone production is a tumor, laser surgery to remove the tumor or cryosurgery (freezing of tissue) is the primary treatment. If no tumor is present, irradiation or radioactive implants of the pituitary may be successful in reducing the abnormal GH production. Other hormones may be affected when GH secretion is halted in this way, so it may be necessary for the child to receive supplemental thyroid extract, cortisol, and gonadotropin hormones in later life.

It is difficult for a child always to be bigger and taller than playmates, and the problem continues to be very real and distressing in adulthood. These children need to be identified during regular health screening to determine the cause of such excessive growth and to offer treatment.

Diabetes Insipidus

Diabetes insipidus is a disease in which there is decreased release of antidiuretic hormone (ADH) by the pituitary gland. This causes less reabsorption of fluid in the kidney tubules. Urine becomes extremely dilute, and a great deal of fluid is lost from the body. Diabetes insipidus may reflect an X-linked dominant trait, or it may be transmitted by an autosomal recessive gene. It may result from a lesion, tumor, or injury to the posterior pituitary; or it may have an unknown cause. In a rare type of diabetes insipidus, pituitary function is adequate, but the kidneys' nephrons are not sensitive to ADH (a kidney etiology).

Assessment

The child with diabetes insipidus experiences excessive thirst (**polydipsia**), relieved only by drinking water, not breast milk or formula, and excessive urination (**polyuria**). The specific gravity of the urine will be low (1.001 to 1.005); the normal values are more often 1.010 to 1.030. Urine output may reach 4 to 10 L in a 24-h period (the normal is 1 to 2 L), depending on age.

Signs and symptoms of diabetes insipidus usually present gradually. Parents may notice the polyuria first as bedwetting in the toilet-trained child. Weight loss from the large loss of fluid occurs. Untreated, the child will lose a sufficient quantity of water that dehydration and death may result (Ferry & Collett-Solberg, 2000b).

X-ray, CT scan, or ultrasound study of the skull reveals whether a lesion or tumor is present. A further test is the administration of vasopressin (Pitressin) to rule out kidney disease. After measuring a child's urine output to establish a baseline, vasopressin is then administered. The drug decreases the blood pressure, alerting the kidney to retain more fluid to maintain vascular pressure. If the fault of the dilute urine is with the pituitary, not the kidney, the child's urine output will decrease; if the fault is with the kidney, urine will remain dilute and excessive in amount.

Therapeutic Management

Surgery is the treatment of choice if a tumor is present. If the cause is idiopathic, the condition can be controlled by the administration of desmopressin (DDAVP), an arginine vasopressin. In an emergency, this can be given IV. For long-term use, it is given intranasally or orally. If desmopressin is given as an intranasal spray, children use the small tube supplied with the medication to deposit the prescribed dose well into the nose. Nasal irritation may result from intranasal administration; intranasal administration will not be effective if the child has an upper respiratory infection and swollen mucous membranes. Caution children that they will notice an increasing urine output just before the next dose is due (Karch, 2001).

NURSING DIAGNOSES AND RELATED INTERVENTIONS

Nursing Diagnosis: Risk for deficient fluid volume related to constant, excessive loss of fluid through urination

Outcome Identification: Child will maintain adequate fluid volume during the illness.

Outcome Evaluation: Child's blood pressure and pulse are within normal limits for age; specific gravity of urine is between 1.003 and 1.030; skin turgor is good; child states thirst is not excessive.

Teach About Long-Term Therapy. If an IM medication is prescribed, the child and at least one parent must learn the injection technique to ensure compliance. Be sure to explain the difference between diabetes insipidus and diabetes mellitus, the disorder most people think of when they hear the word diabetes, so that the family is not confused about differences in therapy. Help the parents and child establish a routine to ensure that the child receives adequate fluid to discourage a feeling of thirst and has access to bathroom facilities possibly more frequently than others.

Encourage Communication. Caution parents that, when seeking any type of health care, they should always notify health care providers that the child has diabetes insipidus. For example, surgery poses particular dangers because of the fluid restrictions that accompany most procedures. Encourage children to wear a MedicAlert tag identifying them as having diabetes insipidus. With the child's and parents' permission, inform school personnel that the child may need to use the bathroom frequently; help the child and family plan frequent bathroom stops and adequate fluid intake on long trips or activity-filled days.

✔ CHECKPOINT QUESTIONS

1. Why must children be monitored closely after insulin or arginine testing for GH deficiency?
2. What special arrangement might need to be made at school for a child with diabetes insipidus?

THE THYROID GLAND

The thyroid gland is responsible for controlling the rate of metabolism in the body through production of the hormones thyroxine (T_4) and triiodothyronine (T_3) by its follicular cells.

A third hormone, thyrocalcitonin, is produced by the interstitial cells of the gland. Thyrocalcitonin is released if a high serum calcium level occurs. This hormone inhibits bone resorption, thereby slowing the rate of release of calcium from bone to plasma and a resulting lowered serum calcium level. It reflects the reverse action of parathyroid hormone, which elevates serum calcium levels.

Assessment of Thyroid Function

Radioimmunoassay of T_4 and T_3 is a specific blood study to determine how much protein-bound iodine (PBI) is present. If a child has recently taken large amounts of cough medicine containing iodide or had an iodine-based, contrast-media study, such as urography or bronchography, the PBI level may be abnormally elevated. The small amount of iodine ingested from iodized salt does not affect PBI levels.

Children who have low circulating albumin levels can have abnormally low PBI levels, because iodine is carried bound to protein. Phenytoin (Dilantin), a common anticonvulsant medication prescribed for children with recurrent seizures, may displace thyroxine from binding globulin and further contribute to these low PBI levels.

Another test of thyroid function is a radioactive iodine uptake test. The child is given an oral dose of a solution containing radioactive iodine (^{123}I). The thyroid gland "traps" this iodine, and 24 h later, after the maximum amount has been trapped, the amount of radioactive iodine present can be determined. It is important in this type of test that the child swallow all the solution. In infants, this is generally given as a gavage feeding so accuracy of the dose can be ensured.

An uptake of less than 10% of the test dose suggests hypothyroidism. If the child vomits after ingesting the substance, this event should be recorded and called to the attention of the laboratory; it will obviously result in a lower uptake value, because only a part of the actual dose was available for uptake. Be certain the child does not receive iodine or thyroid extract in any other form during the test time; it will compete with the uptake of the radioactive iodine and, again, the value will be falsely low.

THYROID GLAND DISORDERS

Congenital Hypothyroidism

Thyroid hypofunction causes reduced production of both T_4 and T_3. Congenital *hypofunction* usually occurs as a result of an absent or nonfunctioning thyroid gland. The condition may not be noticeable initially, because the mother's thyroid hormones maintain adequate levels in the fetus during pregnancy. The symptoms of congenital hypothyroidism become apparent, however, during the first 3 months of life in a formula-fed infant and at about 6 months in a breastfed infant. The disorder occurs in 1 in 4,000 live births and about twice as often in girls as in boys (Grimberg & Satin-Smith, 2000). Because congenital hypothyroidism causes progressive physical and cognitive challenges, early diagnosis is crucial. In most states, a screening test for hypothyroidism is mandatory at birth (using the same few drops of blood obtained for a Guthrie or phenylketonuria [PKU] test).

Assessment

Parents may report that their child sleeps excessively. The tongue becomes enlarged, causing respiratory difficulty, noisy respirations, or obstruction. The child may suck poorly because of sluggishness or choking. The skin of the extremities usually feels cold, and the overall body temperature may be subnormal because of slowed metabolism. A slow metabolic rate is also revealed by slow pulse and respiratory rates. Prolonged jaundice, due to the immature liver's inability to conjugate bilirubin, may be present. Anemia may increase the child's lethargy and fatigue.

The child's neck becomes short and thick. The facial expression becomes dull, as the result of being cognitively challenged, and open-mouthed because of the child's attempts to breathe around the enlarged tongue. The extremities appear short and fat, with hypotonic muscles, giving the infant a floppy, rag-doll appearance. Deep tendon reflexes are slower than normal. Generalized obesity usually occurs. Hair is brittle and dry. Dentition is delayed, or teeth may be defective when they do erupt.

The hypotonia affects the intestinal tract as well, so the infant develops chronic constipation; the abdomen enlarges because of intestinal distention and poor muscle tone (Fig. 48-2). Many infants have an umbilical hernia. Overall, the skin is dry and perhaps scaly, and the child does not perspire. Infants will have low radioactive iodine uptake levels, low serum T_4 and T_3 levels, and elevated thyroid-stimulating factor. Blood lipids will be increased. X-ray may reveal delayed bone growth.

Therapeutic Management

The treatment for hypothyroidism is oral administration of synthetic thyroid hormone, sodium levothyroxine. A small dose is given at first, and then the dose is gradually increased to therapeutic levels. The child will need to continue taking medication indefinitely to supplement that which the thyroid does not make. Supplemental vitamin D may also be given to prevent the development of rickets when, with the administration of thyroid hormone, rapid bone growth begins.

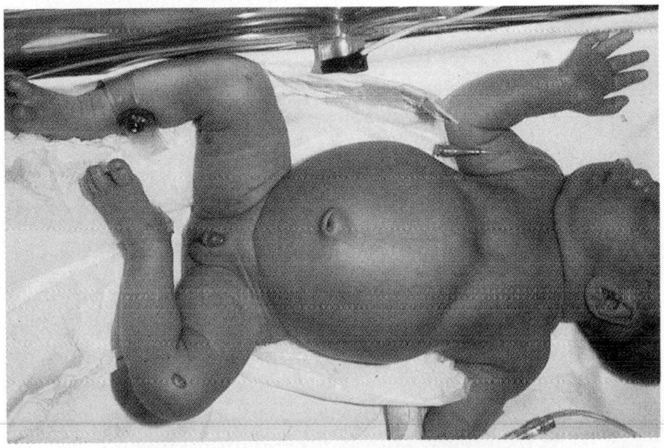

FIGURE 48.2 An infant with congenital hypothyroidism Notice the short, thick neck and enlarged abdomen.

Further cognitive challenges can be prevented as soon as therapy is started, but any degree of impairment already present cannot be reversed.

Helping parents administer medication over a long period of time is a major nursing role. Be certain that parents know the rules for long-term medication administration with children, particularly the rule about not putting medicine in a large amount of food (thyroxine tablets must be crushed and added to food or a small amount of formula or breast milk; see Focus on Family Empowerment). Periodic monitoring of T_4 and T_3 will help to ensure an appropriate medication dosage. If the dose of thyroid hormone is not adequate, the T_4 level will remain low, and there will be few signs of clinical improvement. If the dose is too high, the T_4 level will rise, and the child will show signs of hyperthyroidism: irritability, fever, rapid pulse, and perhaps vomiting, diarrhea, and weight loss.

Acquired Hypothyroidism (Hashimoto's Disease)

Hashimoto's disease is the most common form of acquired hypothyroidism in childhood; the age of onset is often 10 to 11 years, and there may be a family history of thyroid disease. It occurs more often in girls than in boys. The decrease in thyroid secretion is caused by the development of an autoimmune phenomenon that interferes with thyroid production. Excretion of thyroid-stimulating hormone (TSH) from the pituitary increases when thyroid hormone production decreases in an attempt to cause the thyroid to be more effective.

Assessment

In response to TSH, hypertrophy of the thyroid (goiter) occurs, and body growth is impaired by lack of thyroxine. In infants, congenital goiter can lead to airway obstruction; in children, the condition leads to obesity, lethargy, and delayed sexual development.

Antithyroid antibodies will be present in serum if the illness was caused by an autoimmune process. The thyroid not only enlarges but may become nodular in response to the oversecretion of TSH. Although in childhood, a nodular thyroid is usually benign, an investigation into the possibility of thyroid malignancy must be considered. For diagnosis, children are administered radioactive iodine. If the nodes are benign, there is generally a rapid uptake of radioactive iodine ("hot nodes"). If there is no uptake ("cold nodes"), carcinoma is a much more likely diagnosis (rare at this age).

Therapeutic Management

Treatment for acquired hypothyroidism is the administration of synthetic thyroid hormone (sodium levothyroxine), the same as for congenital hypothyroidism. With adequate dosage, the obesity will diminish and growth will begin again. It is important that the disease be recognized as early as possible so there is time to stimulate growth before the epiphyseal lines close at puberty.

If acquired hypothyroidism exists in a woman during pregnancy, her infant can be born cognitively challenged. Therefore, it is important that girls with this syndrome be identified before they reach childbearing age (Klein et al., 2001).

Hyperthyroidism (Graves' Disease)

Hyperthyroidism is oversecretion of thyroid hormones by the thyroid gland. In children, it usually occurs at the time of puberty or during adolescence and is more common in girls than in boys (Grimberg & Satin-Smith, 2000). Overactivity of the thyroid gland can occur from the gland being overstimulated by TSH of the pituitary gland due to a pitu-

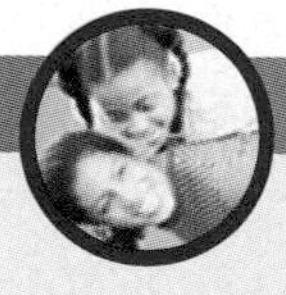

FOCUS ON FAMILY EMPOWERMENT
Guidelines for Successful Long-Term Medicine Administration

Q. What can we do to make sure that our son will continue to take the prescribed medication for the remainder of his life?

A. Here are some helpful tips to increase the success of long-term medication therapy:

1. Teach children about the type and purpose of medicine they will be taking. Knowing the purpose of something maintains interest and cooperation.
2. If mixing a medication with food or fluid, use only a small amount to avoid opposition from the child and ensure that the child takes the necessary dose.
3. Always be certain to anticipate obtaining prescriptions so a ready supply is on hand before vacations, summer camp, holidays.
4. Avoid bribing children to get them to take their medicine. After a time, a bribe becomes too difficult to maintain.
5. Begin involving your child early in administering his own medication. The earlier you can involve children in administering their own medication, the sooner they can achieve an independent lifestyle.
6. Be aware of the lifespan of the medicine being administered so outdated medication is not used.
7. Do not store medicine carelessly. Consider all medicine a potential poison and keep it out of the reach of small children.
8. Use a dose-reminder system such as a chart on the refrigerator, bathroom door, or school locker.
9. Plan times for medication administration that allow for a normal lifestyle (e.g., not getting up at 2 AM, or having to interrupt a school class for an injection).

itary tumor. More frequently, hyperthyroidism in children is caused by an autoimmune reaction that results in production of immunoglobulin G (IgG), which stimulates the thyroid gland to overproduce thyroxine. An exophthalmos-producing pituitary substance causes the prominent-appearing eyes that accompany hyperthyroidism in some children.

Assessment

Graves' disease often follows a viral illness or a period of stress. Some children may have a genetic predisposition to development of the disorder. With overproduction of T_3 and T_4, children gradually experience nervousness, loss of muscle strength, and easy fatigue. Their basal metabolic rate is high; blood pressure and pulse are increased. They perspire freely. They are always hungry, and, although they eat constantly, they do not gain weight and may even lose weight because of the increased basal metabolic rate. On x-ray, bone age will appear advanced beyond the chronologic age of the child. Unless the condition is treated, the child will not be able to reach normal adult height, because epiphyseal lines of long bones will close before normal height is attained.

The thyroid gland, which is usually not prominent in children, appears as a swelling on the anterior neck (goiter). This enlargement can be confirmed by ultrasound. When the child protrudes the tongue or extends the hands, fine tremors are noticeable. In a few children, the eye globes will be prominent (exophthalmos), giving the child a wide-eyed, staring appearance. Laboratory tests will show elevated T_4 and T_3 levels and an increased radioactive iodine uptake. TSH level will be low or absent because the thyroid is being stimulated by antibodies, not by the pituitary gland.

Therapeutic Management

Therapy consists first of a course of a beta-adrenergic blocking agent, such as propranolol, to decrease the antibody response. After this, the child is placed on an antithyroid drug, such as propylthiouracil (PTU) or methimazole (Tapazole), to suppress the formation of thyroxine (Kraiem & Newfield, 2001). While the child is taking these drugs, monitor the white blood cell count for leukopenia (decreased white blood cell level) and thrombocytopenia (decreased platelet count), side effects of the drugs. If either of these results, expect to discontinue the drug until the white blood cell or platelet count returns to normal so the child does not develop an infection or experience spontaneous bleeding.

Because the thyroid stores considerable thyroid hormone that must be used up first, it will take about 2 weeks for these drugs to have an effect. The child will generally have to take the drug for 2 to 3 years before the condition "burns itself out." The exophthalmos may not recede but will not become worse from the time therapy is instituted.

If the child has a toxic reaction to medical management (severe lowered white blood cell or platelet count) or is noncompliant about taking the medicine, radioiodine ablative therapy with ^{131}I to reduce the size of the thyroid gland can be accomplished (Allahabadia et al., 2001). Surgical removal of part or almost all of the thyroid gland, which may be necessary in a young adult, also can be completed safely. After both radioiodine ablative therapy and thyroidectomy, supplemental thyroid hormone therapy may be needed indefinitely because the gland is no longer able to produce an adequate amount.

NURSING DIAGNOSES AND RELATED INTERVENTIONS

Nursing Diagnosis: Situational low self-esteem related to lack of coordination and presence of prominent goiter

Outcome Identification: Child will demonstrate adequate self-esteem by the end of the treatment period.

Outcome Evaluation: Child states positive traits about self and identifies friends and activities enjoyed.

Hyperthyroidism begins gradually and may become fairly involved before it is detected. Suspect children at puberty of having hyperthyroidism if they are losing weight or having behavior problems in school because of hand tremors and tongue tremors that make it hard for them to write or speak. Behavior problems may also arise because of the nervousness and inability to sit still during class.

Offer parents support to supervise medication administration so they can be certain that the child takes the medicine every day. Caution children not to stop taking the medicine abruptly or a thyroxine crisis (sudden onset of extreme symptoms of hyperthyroidism) can occur. Parents may ask if their child can have surgery as a cure so that long-term administration of medicine will not be required. Help them understand that surgery may not dispel the need for medication; if a large portion of the thyroid gland is removed, it may be necessary to give medicine indefinitely to make up for the missing gland. In any event, it is preferable to try a course of medical management before resorting to surgery.

Because the onset of hyperthyroidism is gradual, children may be aware of their difficulties in school before their parents are. Exophthalmos may lead to an appearance about which other children tease them. After therapy, encourage children to return to activities that require fine coordination or social interaction and to think of themselves as well again.

✔ CHECKPOINT QUESTIONS

3. What is the chief (most serious) effect of congenital hypothyroidism?
4. Why are children who develop hyperthyroidism at puberty often seen as behavior problems in school?

THE ADRENAL GLAND

The two adrenal glands are located retroperitoneally just above each kidney. (Because of their location, they are also referred to as suprarenal glands.) The adrenal glands are made up of two distinct parts, which differ not only in tissue origin, but also in function. The *adrenal medulla* is a small core surrounded by the *adrenal cortex*. Although each of these parts has different functions and releases different hormones, together they protect the body against acute and chronic forms of stress.

Adrenal Hormones

The adrenal cortex produces cortisol (a glucocorticoid), androgen, and aldosterone (a mineralocorticoid)—three hormones that can cause childhood illness. Norepinephrine and epinephrine, hormones important for maintaining blood pressure, are produced by the adrenal medulla.

Cortisol

Cortisol, a glucocorticoid that is necessary for glucose and protein metabolism, is released by the adrenal cortex in response to adrenocorticotropic hormone (ACTH) stimulation from the pituitary gland. ACTH is strongly influenced by biorhythm or circadian rhythms. In the hours just before and after a person awakens, ACTH reaches its highest peak. The level decreases again gradually throughout the day and night. The level of ACTH secretion also increases during periods of emotional stress, leading to increased production of cortisol. Severe trauma, major surgery, hypotension, extreme cold, and acute or chronic illness also increase production of cortisol.

Cortisol is necessary during a time of stress to provide the body with readily available glucose and protein for emergency processes. It elevates serum glucose by increasing the amount of glucose formed by the liver (gluconeogenesis), decreasing use of glucose by tissue, and releasing free fatty acids from tissue stores into the plasma, to make these available for energy. To increase available protein, protein synthesis in cells is halted, which frees up amino acids for liver production of protein.

Cortisol is also important in decreasing an inflammatory response. In the bloodstream, it causes a reduced number of eosinophils and lymphocytes whereas red blood cell and platelet production are increased. A drawback of this response is that the decreased number of lymphocytes may allow infection to occur.

Aldosterone

Aldosterone is secreted in response to the renin-angiotensin system, serum potassium, and sodium levels. Renin is released from kidney nephrons in response to a lowered blood pressure; shortly thereafter, it is converted to angiotensin II. In the presence of angiotensin II, aldosterone is released from the adrenal cortex. This causes retention of sodium and water and elevates blood pressure. When angiotensin is decreased, the production of aldosterone stops. When serum potassium levels rise, aldosterone secretion increases. Lowered levels of potassium decrease aldosterone secretion. Sodium influences aldosterone by a reverse process (when sodium levels are low, aldosterone secretion increases; an increased sodium concentration inhibits aldosterone secretion).

The end result of aldosterone secretion is always sodium retention by the body. As sodium is retained, fluid is also retained. Aldosterone plays a direct role in stabilizing blood volume and pressure because of its role in maintaining sodium balance. Infants born with an inability to produce aldosterone will quickly become dehydrated, and their lives can be in immediate danger.

Androgen

Androgen is the hormone responsible for muscular development, increase in linear size, growth of body hair, and the increase in sebaceous gland secretions that cause typical acne at puberty (see Chapters 32 and 47).

ADRENAL GLAND DISORDERS

Disorders of the adrenal gland include those related to **hypofunction,** which can lead to acute or chronic insufficiency, and those related to **hyperfunction,** which most often leads to overproduction of androgen or cortisol.

Acute Adrenocortical Insufficiency

Insufficiency (hypofunction) of the adrenal gland may be either acute or chronic. In many adrenal syndromes, only one hormone is involved, and the symptoms are directly related only to that hormone. In acute adrenocortical insufficiency, the entire cortical adrenal gland function suddenly becomes insufficient. Generally, this occurs in association with severe overwhelming infections usually involving hemorrhagic destruction of the adrenal glands. It is seen most commonly in meningococcemia. It also can occur when corticosteroid therapy, which has been maintained at high levels for long periods, is abruptly stopped.

Assessment

The symptoms of acute adrenocortical insufficiency are acute and sudden. The blood pressure drops to extremely low levels; the child appears ashen gray and may be pulseless. Temperature becomes elevated; dehydration and hypoglycemia are marked. Sodium and chloride blood levels will be very low, but serum potassium will be elevated, because there is usually an inverse relationship between sodium and potassium values. The child is prostrate, and seizures may occur. Without treatment, death may occur abruptly (Kappy, Steelman & Travers, 2001).

Therapeutic Management

Treatment involves the immediate replacement of cortisol (IV hydrocortisone sodium succinate [Solu-Cortef]); deoxycorticosterone acetate (DOCA), the synthetic equivalent of aldosterone; and IV 5% glucose in normal saline solution to restore blood pressure, sodium, and blood glucose levels. A vasopressor may be necessary to elevate the blood pressure further.

Acute adrenal cortical insufficiency is a medical emergency. Although seen less often than in the past because of antibiotics that quickly halt the course of infectious disease, it is not an obsolete entity. Now that more conditions are being treated with corticosteroids, the chances that acute adrenal cortical insufficiency will occur from sudden withdrawal of high-dose steroids is actually increasing.

Congenital Adrenogenital Hyperplasia

Congenital adrenogenital hyperplasia is a syndrome inherited as an autosomal recessive trait. The primary defect is an inability by the adrenal glands to synthesize cortisol from its precursors. Because the adrenal gland is unable to produce cortisol, the amount of ACTH increases, stimulating the adrenal glands to improve function. Although the adrenals enlarge (hyperplasia), they still cannot produce cortisol, but they overproduce androgen.

Assessment

The excessive androgen production masculinizes the female fetus or increases the size of genital organs in a male fetus. Because this process begins as early as fetal life, the female infant is born with a clitoris so enlarged it appears more like a penis (Fig. 48-3). Internal female organs are generally normal, although a sinus between the urethra and vagina may be present (see discussion of ambiguous genitalia in Chapter 47). Because labia are typically fused as well, the girl resembles a boy with undescended testes and hypospadias. If the condition is not recognized at birth and the child remains untreated, pubic and axillary hair and acne will appear precociously and a deep masculine voice will develop. The bone age is usually advanced, so the epiphyseal line of the long bones closes early. This closure will prevent the child from reaching adult height unless treatment is initiated. At puberty, there will be no breast development or menstruation.

The male child may appear normal at birth, but by 6 months of age signs of sexual precocity appear. By 3 or 4 years of age, boys will have pubic hair and enlargement of the penis, scrotum, and prostate. They may have acne and a deep, mature voice. The testes do not enlarge, however, and, although they are normal in size, they appear small in relation to the size of the penis. Spermatogenesis does not occur, so the child is infertile.

Children with congenital adrenogenital hyperplasia will have increased levels of androgen, an important point for diagnosis. By determining the amount of other adrenal hormones, the exact level of the metabolic defect in the production of cortisol can be measured (Merke et al., 2000).

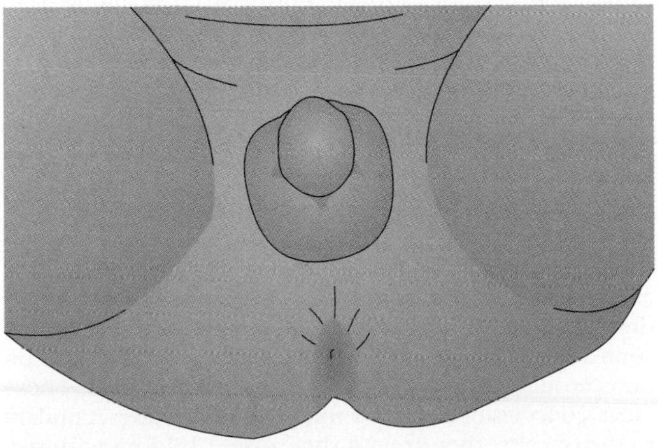

FIGURE 48.3 A female infant with congenital adrenogenital hyperplasia. Note the fused labia and abnormally enlarged clitoris.

Therapeutic Management

Both male and female infants are placed on a corticosteroid agent, such as oral hydrocortisone, to replace what they cannot produce naturally. When corticosteroids are given to the child in this way, stimulation by ACTH will decrease, the production of androgen will return to normal limits, and no further masculinization will occur. Corticosteroid therapy needs to continue indefinitely. The child will need periodic analysis of serum cortisol levels and growth measurements to estimate the effectiveness of the therapy.

It is possible to identify the fetus with congenital adrenogenital hyperplasia as early as at 6 to 8 weeks of pregnancy by means of chorionic villi sampling and at 15 weeks by amniocentesis (see Chapter 7). Treating the mother with dexamethasone (a corticosteroid), which will cross the placenta to the fetus, can prevent masculinization in the fetus for the remainder of pregnancy.

NURSING DIAGNOSES AND RELATED INTERVENTIONS

Nursing Diagnosis: Situational low self-esteem related to genital formation at variance with true gender

Outcome Identification: Child will demonstrate adequate self-esteem throughout life.

Outcome Evaluation: Child identifies positive traits about self and describes activities enjoyed with peers; expresses satisfaction with gender identity.

When children with congenital adrenogenital hyperplasia are not closely scrutinized at birth, they can be wrongly identified as boys when chromosomally they are actually girls. Therefore, all newborns require an extensive physical examination at birth. It is sometimes recommended that a girl's enlarged clitoris be reduced by plastic surgery early in life. This treatment is controversial, however, because clitoral reduction can also result in reduced clitoral sensation. Fortunately, with finer surgical techniques, this problem is now minimal.

Parents of females with congenital adrenogenital hyperplasia may need a great deal of support during the first few days of their child's life if they feel that their child is imperfect in an embarrassing, hard-to-explain way. When they are told the results of the chromosome analysis, parents may react with grief for the loss of the son they thought was born to them. Parents need support from health care personnel who recognize that the child is simply lacking a completely formed hormone but is complete in every other way.

Nursing Diagnosis: Health-seeking behaviors related to lack of knowledge about long-term treatment needed to sustain adequate growth and development

Outcome Identification: Parents will understand the importance of giving prescribed medication through the child's growing years.

Outcome Evaluation: Parents state plans for incorporating medication administration into daily routine and other occasions (e.g., trips away from home).

Parents, and children as they grow older, need to understand the importance of continuing to take the oral medication prescribed. When this condition is first diagnosed, it is easy for parents to remember to give the drug. As the years pass, however, it becomes more difficult to remember medication administration because the child has no acute symptoms. Cortisol is necessary for glucose and protein metabolism. The body needs adequate levels to allow it to react to physical and emotional stress. When plans are made for summer camp or vacation away from home, special arrangements for regular medicine administration must be made. Children may need to have a routine dose increased when they are undergoing periods of stress, such as surgery or infection. They may need support throughout life if their body image is distorted from body changes at birth.

Salt-Losing Form of Congenital Adrenogenital Hyperplasia

When there is a complete blockage of cortisol formation, aldosterone production will also be deficient. Without adequate aldosterone, salt is not retained by the body, so fluid is not retained. Almost immediately after birth, infants begin to have vomiting, diarrhea, anorexia, loss of weight, and extreme dehydration. If these symptoms are untreated, the extreme loss of salt and fluid can lead to collapse and death as early as 48 to 72 h after birth.

About one third of children with congenital adrenogenital hyperplasia are affected by this complete deficiency. Because boys with this syndrome appear normal at birth, the symptoms may be incorrectly diagnosed as pyloric stenosis, intestinal obstruction, or failure to thrive. In girls, because of the ambiguous genitalia, the correct diagnosis can be made more easily.

Assessment

The salt-losing form of congenital adrenogenital hyperplasia must be detected in infants before they reach an irreversible point of salt depletion. Weighing a newborn at birth and again at 24 h aids in detecting this condition. Weighing infants at each well-child health checkup is also important. In boys, the inability to gain back their birth weight may be the first sign of the syndrome.

Therapeutic Management

Children with the salt-losing form of congenital adrenogenital hyperplasia need to take supplements of hydrocortisone in conjunction with a high amount of salt and DOCA, a synthetic aldosterone, to maintain a balance of fluid and electrolytes. A long-acting form of DOCA can be given once a month IM. Capsules of DOCA can be implanted subcutaneously (SC) as another form of long-acting therapy. As the child grows older, fludrocortisone (Florinef), a mineralocorticoid, may be given orally to aid salt retention.

NURSING DIAGNOSES AND RELATED INTERVENTIONS

Nursing Diagnosis: Risk for deficient fluid volume related to loss of body fluid

Outcome Identification: Child will remain well hydrated throughout childhood.

Outcome Evaluation: Child's skin turgor remains good; specific gravity of urine is between 1.003 and 1.030.

Teach parents about the body's critical need to balance aldosterone, salt, and water so that they understand the drastic consequences if their child skips taking a dose of medication. Help them set up a schedule as necessary for measuring the child's weight, giving medication, or measuring urine output. Help them to understand that, although salt seems to be an "extra" in their own diet, it is as vital to their child's intake as digitalis is in heart disease or insulin is in diabetes.

Cushing Syndrome

Cushing's syndrome is caused by the overproduction of the adrenal hormone, cortisol; this usually results from increased ACTH production by a pituitary tumor. It may occur from a malignant or benign tumor of the adrenal cortex. The peak age of occurrence is 6 or 7 years, but the syndrome can occur as early as infancy (Katz, 2000). Overproduction of cortisol results in increased glucose production; this causes fat to accumulate on the cheeks, chin, and trunk causing a moon-faced, stocky appearance. Cortisol is catabolic so protein wasting occurs. This leads to muscle wasting, making the extremities appear thin. Loss of protein matrix in bones causes osteoporosis (loss of calcium in bones). Cortisol also suppresses the immune system, so humoral immunity is decreased, leaving children susceptible to infection. Additionally, it causes vasoconstriction so extreme hypertension may occur.

Hyperpigmentation occurs from melanin-stimulation properties of ACTH. This causes the child's face to be unusually red, especially the cheeks. Signs of abnormal masculinization or feminization may occur from overproduction of androgen or estrogen. Purple striae resulting from collagen deficit appear on the child's hips, abdomen, and thighs, similar to those seen in pregnancy (Fig. 48-4).

Polyuria develops as the body tries to excrete increased glucose levels. Growth ceases, and, if the condition is not reversed before epiphyseal lines close, short stature will result.

Children who receive high doses of synthetic corticosteroids, such as prednisone, over a long time may develop the same symptoms as in Cushing syndrome. Such children are said to have a *cushingoid appearance.* Cushing syndrome is often suspected as the cause of obesity in children; some obese children do have elevated levels of plasma corticosteroids, a fact that complicates the diagnosis. These elevated levels of corticosteroids, however, are secondary to the obesity; they are not the cause. Children with natural obesity are generally tall; those with Cushing syndrome are short.

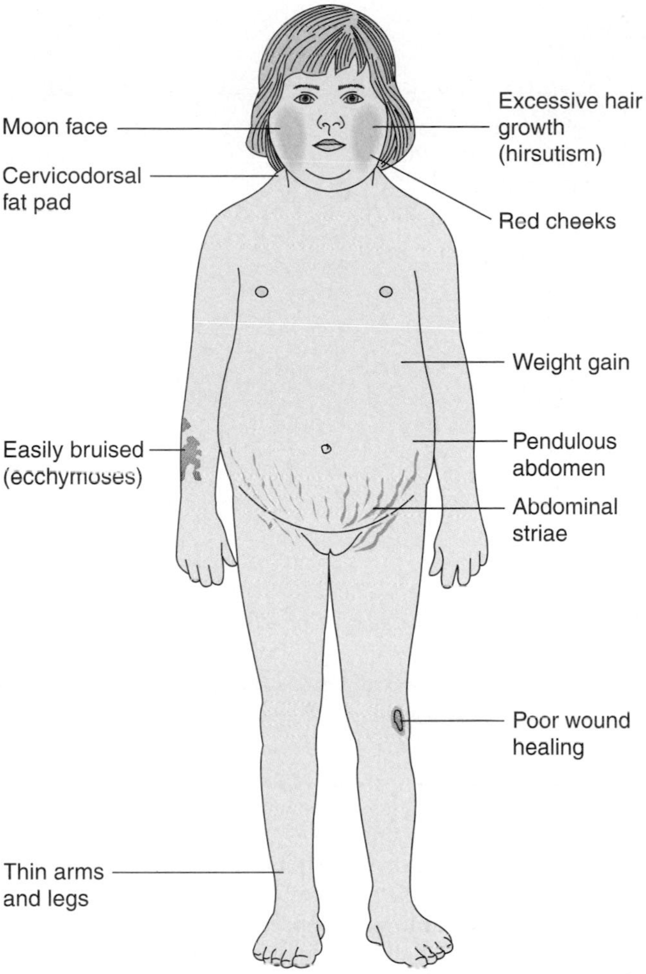

FIGURE 48.4 Signs and symptoms of Cushing syndrome.

Assessment

Children with Cushing syndrome have elevated plasma cortisol and increased urinary free-cortisol levels. A dexamethasone suppression test confirms the diagnosis. If a normal child is given a test dose of dexamethasone (a glucocorticoid), the plasma level of adrenal cortisol will fall. It will not fall in children with adrenal cortical tumors because the tumor continues to stimulate the adrenal glands to oversecretion. If cosyntropin (Cortrosyn), a synthetic corticotropin, or ACTH is administered, plasma cortisol levels will normally rise. With an adrenal tumor, the gland is already functioning at full capacity so no cortisol elevation occurs. A CT scan or ultrasound will reveal the enlarged adrenal or pituitary gland, confirming the diagnosis.

Therapeutic Management

Treatment of Cushing syndrome is surgical removal of the causative tumor. The prognosis will depend on whether the tumor is benign or malignant; carcinoma of this type tends to metastasize rapidly. If a major part of the adrenal gland is surgically removed, the child will need replacement cortisol therapy indefinitely.

If a major portion of the pituitary gland is removed, replacement of all pituitary hormones may be necessary. After adrenal surgery, observe the child carefully for signs of shock because, without epinephrine from the adrenal gland, the body's ability to maintain blood pressure is severely compromised. Severe hypotension can result.

> ✔ **CHECKPOINT QUESTIONS**
>
> 5. What is the appearance at birth of girls who have congenital adrenogenital hyperplasia?
> 6. What is the effect on a child when sufficient aldosterone cannot be produced?

THE PANCREAS

The pancreas is a unique organ in that it has both endocrine (ductless) and exocrine (with duct) types of tissue. The *islets of Langerhans* form the endocrine portion; these cells are scattered throughout the exocrine cells like small islets, hence their name. The islet cells compose only about 1% of the total weight of the pancreas. Alpha islet cells secrete glucagon; beta islet cells secrete insulin.

Insulin is essential for carbohydrate metabolism and is important to the metabolism of fats and protein. It is formed by two amino acid chains from a precursor, *proinsulin,* at a rate of 35 to 50 U/day in adults and proportionately less in children. The actual amount of insulin produced is regulated by serum glucose levels. When serum glucose that passes through the pancreas exceeds 100 mg/dL, beta cells immediately increase insulin production. When blood serum levels are lowered, production decreases. Both the ability to secrete additional insulin and the action to decrease production are immediate responses.

Also important in the secretion of insulin is the presence of gastrointestinal (GI) hormones, such as gastrin, that rise when the stomach is full, because these also stimulate the pancreas to produce the necessary insulin. Other hormones that stimulate insulin production include glucagon, cortisol, GH, progesterone, and estrogen. In contrast, increasing levels of epinephrine or norepinephrine inhibit the secretion of insulin.

The principal childhood disorders associated with pancreatic dysfunction are type 1 diabetes mellitus and cystic fibrosis. Because the nursing care for children with cystic fibrosis includes many respiratory care procedures, it is discussed in Chapter 40.

Type 1 Diabetes Mellitus

Diabetes is a disorder involving an absolute or relative deficiency of insulin. There are two main types of diabetes, as shown in Table 48-2. Type 1 diabetes (formerly referred to as juvenile diabetes or insulin-dependent diabetes) most commonly occurs in childhood. The disease affects as many as 1 in 1,500 children under the age of 5 years and increases to 1 in 350 by age 16 (Weinzimer, 2000). It results from immunologic damage to insulin-producing cells in susceptible individuals. Environmental effects are necessary to create the immunologic response (Chase & Eisenbarth, 2001).

TABLE 48.2 Comparison of Type I and Type 2 Diabetes

ASSESSMENT	TYPE I	TYPE 2
Age of onset	5–7 years or at puberty	40–65 years (may occur in adolescents as maturity onset diabetes of youth [MODY])
Type of onset	Abrupt	Gradual
Weight changes	Marked weight loss often initial sign	Associated with obesity
Other symptoms	Polydipsia	Polydipsia
	Polyuria (often begins as bedwetting)	Polyuria
	Fatigue (marks fall in school)	Fatigue
	Blurred vision (marks fall in school)	Blurred vision
	Glycosuria	Glycosuria
	Polyphagia	
	Pruritus	Pruritus
	Mood changes (may cause behavior problems in school)	Mood changes
Therapy	Hypoglycemia agents never effective; insulin required	Diet, oral hypoglycemic agents, or insulin
	Diet recommended as 55% carbohydrates, 15% protein, and 30% fat; no dietary foods used	Nutrition concentrating on no excess weight gain and balanced intake of carbohydrates, protein, and fat
	Common-sense foot care for growing children	Meticulous skin and foot care necessary
Period of remission	Period of remission for 1–12 months ("honeymoon period") generally after initial diagnosis	Not demonstrable

Children with this type of diabetes must take insulin to replace what their pancreas can no longer produce. This is a separate disease from type 2 diabetes (formerly known as non–insulin-dependent diabetes) characterized by diminished insulin secretion. Usually individuals with type 2 diabetes do not need daily insulin, because their disease can be managed with diet alone or diet and oral hypoglycemic agents. Once thought to occur only in older people, type 2 diabetes is also seen in overweight adolescents (maturity onset diabetes of youth [MODY]) (Guazzarotti et al., 2001).

Etiology

Why autoimmune destruction of islet cells occurs in some children and not in others is unknown, but children with this disorder have a high frequency of specific human leukocyte antigens (HLA), particularly HLA-DR3 and HLA-DR4, located on chromosome 6 (Chase & Eisenbarth, 2001).

Although specific HLA antigens predispose a child to developing diabetes, they do not always result in the actual disease. An environmental factor, such as a viral infection, must trigger active pancreatic dysfunction through an autoimmune process. Symptoms of the disease generally do not manifest themselves until preschool or school age. The incidence is equal among girls and boys (Weinzimer, 2000).

If one child in a family has diabetes, the chance of a sibling also developing the illness is higher than normal, because siblings also tend to have one of the specific HLA antigens that lead to the development of the disease. Because no prevention measures are available to stop diabetes from developing, children are not routinely tissue-typed for the disorder, although this may be done experimentally. Administration of immune suppressors to stop destruction of insulin-secreting cells is a possibility, although the long-term effects of immune suppression, such as development of opportunistic infections, limit the use of these drugs (Chase & Eisenbarth, 2001).

Progress of Disease

Insulin can be thought of as a compound that opens the doors to body cells, allowing them to admit the glucose needed to function. It does not play a major role in glucose transport into the brain, erythrocytes, leukocytes, intestinal mucosa, or kidney epithelium. These cells can survive insulin deficiency but not glucose deficiency.

When glucose is unable to enter body cells because of lack of insulin, it builds up in the bloodstream (**hyperglycemia**), the underlying defect that leads to other metabolic consequences. When the kidneys detect hyperglycemia (above the renal threshold of about 160 mg/dL), the kidneys attempt to lower it to normal levels by excreting excess glucose into the urine causing **glycosuria.** While attempting to excrete this excess glucose, the body also excretes a large amount of fluid as well (polyuria). Excess fluid loss triggers the thirst response (polydipsia).

Because the body cells are unable to use glucose but still need a source of energy, the body begins to break down protein and fat for cell utilization. When large amounts of fat are metabolized this way, weight loss occurs and ketone bodies, the acid end-product of fat breakdown, begin to accumulate in the bloodstream and spill into the urine. Because the blood bicarbonate cannot effectively continue to buffer this high of an acid level, the pH of the blood becomes acidic, resulting in severe acidosis. The breakdown of fat also leads to increased serum cholesterol levels. Potassium and phosphate, attempting to serve as buffers, pass from body cells into the bloodstream. As they are evacuated, the body loses these important electrolytes.

Untreated diabetic children, therefore, lose weight, are acidotic due to the buildup of ketone bodies in their blood, are dehydrated because of the loss of water, and experience an electrolyte imbalance because of the loss of electrolytes in urine. Because large amounts of protein and fat are being used for energy instead of glucose, these children will remain short in stature and underweight because they lack the necessary components for growth.

Assessment

Although children may be prediabetic for some time, the onset of symptoms in childhood is generally abrupt (McCance & Huether, 2002). The first symptoms likely to be reported are increased thirst (polydipsia) and increased urination (polyuria). Increased urination may begin as bedwetting (enuresis) in the previously toilet-trained child. Children may have constipation because of the dehydration.

Laboratory Studies. In some children, diabetes is detected at a routine health screening. For others, although the disease has been progressing internally for some time, outward symptoms have such an abrupt onset that children will be in coma from acidosis and hyperglycemia by the time it is detected. Laboratory studies usually show a random plasma glucose level (above 200 mg/dL; normal is 70 to 110 mg/dL fasting and 90 to 180 mg/dL not fasting) and significant glycosuria (Table 48-3).

Two diagnostic tests, fasting blood glucose and random blood glucose are used to diagnose diabetes. A diagnosis of diabetes is confirmed based on finding one of the following three criteria on two separate occasions:

- Symptoms of diabetes with a random blood glucose level over 200 mg/dL
- Fasting blood glucose level greater than 126 mg/dL
- Two-hour plasma glucose level greater than 200 mg/dL during an oral glucose tolerance test (GTT)

Typically, a GTT, which involves oral ingestion or IV administration of a concentrated glucose solution followed by blood glucose levels drawn at fasting, then 1 h, and 2 h, is rarely performed with children. This test is difficult for children to undergo, because it requires them to fast and submit to painful, intrusive procedures (routinely applying EMLA cream to fingerstick or venipuncture sites and using intermittent infusion devices greatly reduces this problem). Do not take blood for glucose analysis from functioning IV tubing because the glucose in the IV solution will cause the serum reading to be abnormally high.

TABLE 48.3 Acceptable Blood Glucose Ranges for Young Children

TIMING	VALUE
Before a meal	70–110 mg/dL
1 h after a meal	90–180 mg/dL
2 h after a meal	80–150 mg/dL
Between 2 and 4 AM	70–120 mg/dL

Other Diagnostic Tests. If diabetes is detected, the diagnostic workup also usually includes analysis of blood samples for pH, PCO_2, sodium, and potassium levels; a white blood cell count; and glycosylated hemoglobin evaluation. Normally, red blood cells carry only a trace of glucose incorporated into the hemoglobin. If the serum glucose is excessive, however, it attaches itself to hemoglobin molecules, causing glycosylated hemoglobin. The higher the serum glucose level, the higher the hemoglobin A_{1c} becomes. In nondiabetic children, the usual hemoglobin A_{1c} value is 1.8 to 4.0. A value above 6.0 reflects an excessive level of serum glucose. Measuring glycosylated hemoglobin provides information about what the child's glucose levels have been during the preceding 3 to 4 months, because red blood cells have a lifespan of less than 120 days.

If the potassium level of the blood is low, children may need an electrocardiogram to observe for T-wave abnormalities, the mark of potassium deficiency. The white blood cell count of a child with diabetes may be elevated, even though no infection is present, apparently as a response to the ketoacidosis. The presence of infection must always be suspected, however, because it is often a precipitant to a diabetic crisis. For this reason, nose and throat cultures may be obtained as well.

Therapeutic Management

Therapy for children with type 1 diabetes involves five measures: insulin administration; regulation of nutrition and exercise; stress management; and blood glucose and urine ketone monitoring. Children with newly suspected diabetes mellitus may be admitted to the hospital for a few days for diagnosis, regulation of insulin dosage, and education. This may not be necessary if the child's symptoms are minimal. Teaching parents and the child intensive management (frequent insulin injections and adherence to nutritional guidelines with regulation of exercise) produces immediate well-being and reduces the incidence of long-term complications. Allow parents and children time to adjust to an illness such as diabetes that will require constant vigilance in the months and years to follow.

Initial Regulation of Insulin. When children are first diagnosed with diabetes, they are generally hyperglycemic and perhaps ketoacidotic. To correct the metabolic imbalance, they are given insulin. This is usually administered IV at a dose of 0.1 U/kg to 0.2 U/kg of body weight per hour, depending on the severity of the symptoms. This initial IV infusion of insulin is followed by further dose reductions once the blood glucose level is below 200 mg/dL. The dosage will depend on the change in the acidosis and the degree of glycosemia and ketonuria. Some controversy exists surrounding the belief that insulin binds to the plastic IV tubing. Therefore, check your institution's policy and be prepared to change the IV tubing as required. Insulin may be given intranasally, but the inconsistency of absorption does not make this a preferred route (Karch, 2001). Ideally, within 12 h, the acidosis is considerably less than when the child was admitted to the hospital, and the serum glucose level is close to the normal range. The insulin given for emergency replacement is always regular (short-acting) insulin (Humulin-R), because this is the form that takes effect most quickly when administered IV in normal saline. Lispro (Humalog), which is also rapid acting, is another possibility.

It may seem that, in the diabetic child in a state of acidosis, the administration of glucose would not be warranted. Because children are being administered insulin, however, body cells soon become ready to use glucose, so incorporate and use available glucose quickly. If more is not provided, cells are forced to continue to break down fats and protein, and the acidosis can increase, not decrease. Glucose may be added to the infusion if necessary to meet this need.

After 24 h, as the child begins to improve, oral feedings may replace the IV route. Further management of the child in the days after this first crucial 24-h period will be based on the serum glucose determinations. Children may remain on regular insulin alone (given three or four times a day) for the first 1 or 2 days. Typically, intermediate-acting insulin is started as soon as oral fluids are taken, usually on the second day of therapy.

Insulin Administration. Before insulin was discovered in 1920, few children with diabetes lived to adulthood. Even after its discovery, not all children responded well to insulin administration, because early forms were manufactured from a pork or beef base that caused development of antibodies against insulin, making the therapy less effective than predicted. Today, insulin is manufactured by a recombinant DNA technique to simulate human insulin (Humulin, Novolin), largely eliminating the problem of antibody reaction. Types of insulin vary as to their time of onset, peak action, and duration of action. These differences are shown in Table 48-4. Regular insulin is usually referred to as a short-acting insulin; Humulin-L and Humulin-N are examples of intermediate-acting insulins; Humulin-U is long acting. Children are regulated on a variety of insulin programs, but most receive a dose of 0.4 to 0. 7 U/kg daily in two divided doses (one before breakfast and one before dinner); adolescents may need as much as 1.2 U/kg daily. The most common mixture of insulin used with children is a combination of an intermediate-acting insulin and a regular insulin; this is usually mixed at a ratio of ⅔ U of the intermediate-acting insulin to ⅓ U regular insulin and given in the same syringe, although this prescription will vary for individual children. The morning dose is two thirds of the total daily dose; the evening dose is the remaining one third. The peak effects of the short-acting insulins are at 3 to 4 h (see Table 48-4). This means that the child who takes insulin before breakfast will notice a peak effect between 10 am and 12 noon; that is the time of day when hypoglycemia (a reaction to an excessive insulin level) is most likely to occur. The peak effect period of the intermediate-acting insulins is 8 to 14 h, or late afternoon, just before dinner. That makes this another prime time for hypoglycemia.

TABLE 48.4 Common Types of Insulin

PREPARATION	ONSET (H)	PEAK EFFECT (H)	DURATION OF EFFECT (H)
Human Insulin			
Lispro (Humalog)	Immediate	½–1	3–4
Regular (Humulin-R)	0.5–1.0	2–4	5–7
Lantus	1	5	24
Humulin-N	1–2	4–12	24+
Humulin-L	1–3	6–14	24+
Humulin-U	6	16–18	36+

Skidmore-Roth, L. (2002). *Mosby's nursing drug reference.* St. Louis: Mosby.

Some children require a program of insulin therapy that includes three injections daily (a short-acting and intermediate-acting insulin before breakfast, a short-acting insulin before supper, and a bedtime injection of an intermediate-acting insulin). Still others may receive an injection of regular or Humalog insulin before each meal, followed by a bedtime injection of intermediate-acting insulin (a total of four injections daily). Although a regimen with the fewest injections daily at first seems advantageous, multiple injections allow for greater variation in activity and meal consumption.

In the past, fixed doses of insulin were prescribed, and parents were advised not to vary the dose. Today, parents are educated to be able to vary the dose based on an insulin algorithm or protocol determined by the child's level of activity, the size of meals consumed, and the time of the injection (referred to as "thinking scales"). The time between the insulin injection and a meal is known as "lag time." If a child's premeal blood glucose level is above a target range, parents learn that increasing the lag time will help prevent hyperglycemia. If the blood glucose is low at a premeal test, decreasing the lag time could help prevent hypoglycemia. If it is anticipated that the child will eat an unusually large meal (e.g., a birthday dinner), parents can increase the size of the premeal regular insulin injection. If the child will participate in a strenuous sport in the afternoon, the regular insulin injection can be decreased. Lantus is a new long-acting insulin that lasts 24 h. A disadvantage of this insulin is its pH, which is so low it cannot be mixed in a syringe with other insulins. Children can be regulated on it plus three doses of Humalog before meals (Chase & Eisenbarth, 2001).

Injection Technique. When insulins are mixed in one syringe, the regular or short-acting insulin should be drawn into the syringe first. Then, if mixing accidentally occurs in the bottle, the time of effectiveness of the short-acting insulin (which needs to be kept short-acting for emergency treatment) will not be lengthened by the addition of the intermediate-acting insulin.

Insulin is always injected SC except in emergencies, when half the required dose may be given IV. Children should be encouraged to rotate sites in a pattern based on their planned activity. Absorption is increased if the muscles at the injection site are exercised after the injection, so it is best to choose sites that will not be exercised soon after the injection. Subcutaneous tissue injection sites include those of the upper outer arms and the outer aspects of the thighs (Fig. 48-5). The abdominal subcutaneous tissue injection sites may be the preferred site for injection because many children have a greater amount of subcutaneous tissue there. However, most children dislike this site. If a child will be jogging after an injection, the thigh should probably not be used for injection. Similarly, if the child will be playing tennis, the injection should probably not be given in the dominant arm.

Work out a plan of rotation for each child so that everyone who will be working with the child and injections knows what injection site should be used next. In the hospital, record the injection site in the child's chart or nursing plan of care so each nurse can check it before an injection and not repeat an injection site. If the same injection site is used repeatedly, a great deal of subcutaneous atrophy (lipodystrophy) occurs at the site, causing deep, obvious pockmarks. However, this is less of a problem now that synthetic human insulin is available.

Children quickly learn that, if they continuously give injections in the same site, scar tissue (lipohypertrophy) forms there, and no pain will be felt on injection. This is a dangerous practice, however, because insulin no longer absorbs well from this site; the child will have to increase the dose beyond what he or she actually needs for glucose metabolism, because a portion of each dose is "locked" in the tissue. Should the child then inject this larger dose of insulin into a new site, there is a potential for overdose (which would cause hypoglycemia).

Insulin should be given at room temperature. This diminishes subcutaneous atrophy and ensures its peak effectiveness. Parents may keep additional bottles in the refrigerator to increase the insulin's shelf life.

When a short needle (less than 0.4 inch) is used, children can administer insulin without bunching skin at the site and give the injection to themselves at a 90-degree angle, a technique more closely resembling that of IM than SC injection. With this technique, because the needle is so short, the insulin is deposited in the subcutaneous tissue. This technique is easier for children to learn because it takes less coordination to administer an injection at a 90-degree angle than at a 45-degree subcutaneous angle (Fig. 48-6). Automatic injection devices, such as pens and jet injectors, are easy for children to use, promote early independence, and can be given with the 90-degree technique (Fig. 48-7).

Insulin Pumps. An insulin pump is an automatic device approximately the size of a transistor radio. It delivers insulin at a constant rate, thus better regulating serum glucose levels than periodic injections. It has the potential to decrease future complications (Lenhard & Reeves, 2001). To use a pump, a syringe of regular insulin is placed in the pump chamber; a thin polyethylene tubing leads to the child's abdomen where it is implanted into the subcutaneous tissue by a small-gauge needle. Throughout the day, the pump edges the syringe barrel forward, infusing insulin at a continuous rate into the subcutaneous tissue. Before a snack or meal, the parent or child presses a button on the pump and forces a bolus of insulin forward to

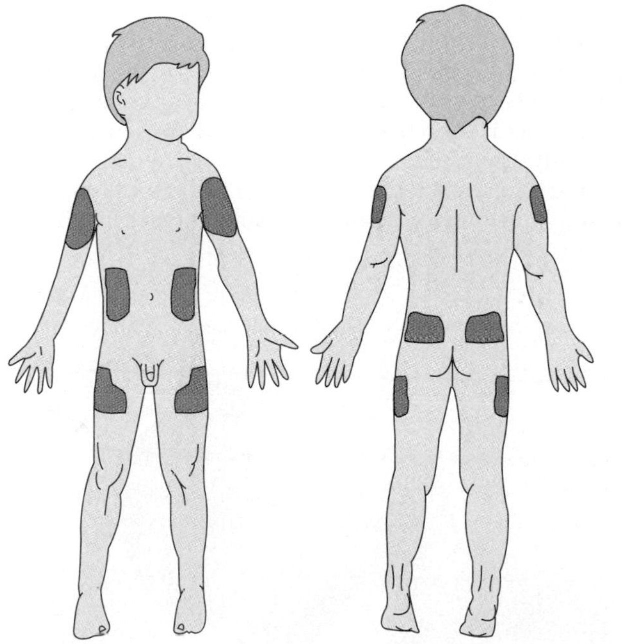

FIGURE 48.5 According to the American Diabetes Association, insulin injection sites in children and adults are the upper outer portions of the arms; the thighs—4 inches below the hip and 4 inches above the knee (adjusted proportionally for children); and the abdominal area just above and just below the waist. The navel and a circular area just around it are excluded as injection sites. In some children the abdominal area may not be an appropriate injection site.

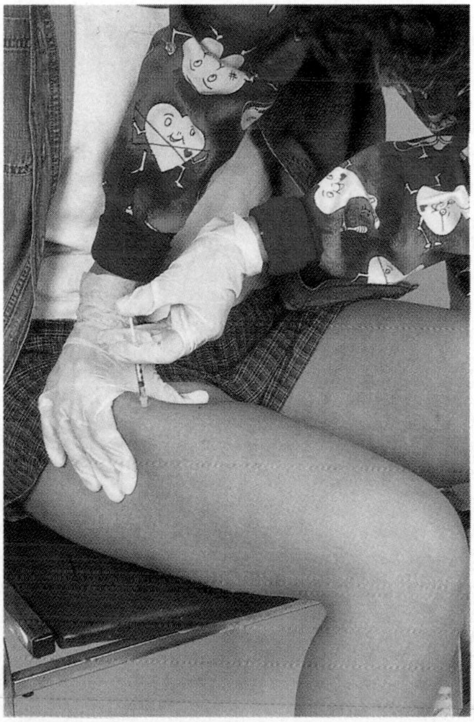

FIGURE 48.6 Insulin is usually injected at a 90-degree angle with a short needle. This angle places the insulin in the subcutaneous space.

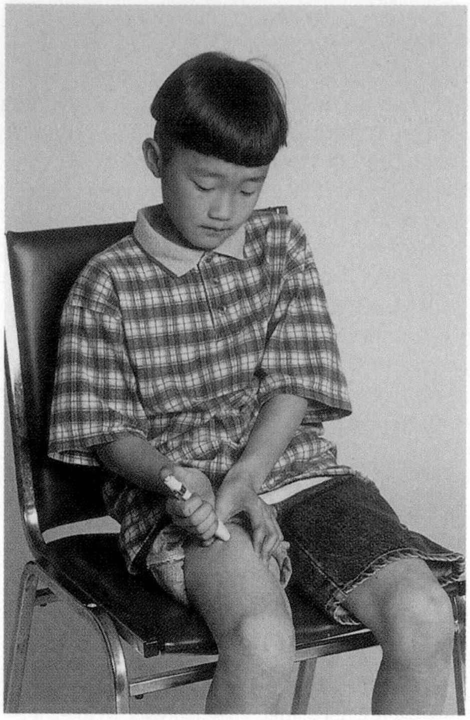

FIGURE 48.7 Injection of insulin by an automatic device.

increase the insulin injected for managing these times of high carbohydrate intake. Children need to inspect the site of the pump insertion to make sure that the site is not inflamed; the site is cleaned and changed every 48 to 72 h to ensure that absorption is still optimal.

Restrictions with pump therapy include keeping it dry; a child must remove the pump (not the syringe and tubing) while showering unless it is a brand that is waterproof or is equipped with a waterproof pouch so it can be taken into the shower or swimming pool. A disadvantage of pump therapy is that the pump is always present. Children usually prefer to wear clothing that hides the pump's outline (it can be held against the abdomen by an over-the-shoulder sling or hung from a belt around the waist). To assess the pump's delivery of insulin, the child must do blood glucose determinations about four times a day. When pump therapy first begins, a parent must wake at 2 am and test the child's blood glucose level because this is such a vulnerable time for hypoglycemia (the pump is delivering insulin, but the child has not eaten since bedtime).

Inhalation Insulin. In the future, insulin may be administered by way of inhalation because it is absorbed well across mucous membranes. This will release the child from the chore of daily injections. However, if the child develops a cold or allergies that cause edema of the nasal membrane, drug absorption is reduced. Absorption also can be influenced by whether the insulin is inhaled while the child is upright or lying down at the time of administration.

Nutrition. Children with type 1 diabetes need to consume a diet appropriate for their age in the proportion of 55% carbohydrate, 15% protein, and 30% fat. The meal pattern should be three spaced meals with a snack in the midmorning, midafternoon, and evening (Weinzimer, 2000).

Urine Testing. Urine testing has the disadvantage of not being as accurate as blood serum testing and is now used only to test for ketonuria when the child's blood glucose level is above 200 mg/dL. A dipstick technique may be used. Acetone appearing in the urine is a sign that fat is being used for energy, which occurs with infection or when not enough food has been ingested.

Self Blood Glucose Monitoring (SBGM). Children as young as early school age can learn the techniques of finger puncture (fingerstick) and reading a computerized monitor. Using a spring-loaded puncture device to obtain the blood sample helps minimize pain, and an automatic readout monitor, such as a Glucometer, simplifies the procedure and gives a more accurate reading than matching the shade of blood on a test strip to the colors on the test strip container (Fig. 48-8). Some meters measure whole blood value, not the serum glucose level. This means that the result will be about 15% higher than a serum determination (ie, a blood determination of 115 mg/dL equals 100 mg/dL of serum). However, some newer meters automatically convert the whole blood level value to a plasma level value. Be sure that parents and children understand the type of monitor they are using.

The "Honeymoon" Period. After the child's diagnosis has been confirmed and the blood glucose level has been initially regulated by insulin, a honeymoon period may follow when only a minimal amount of insulin, or none at all, is needed for glucose regulation. Apparently, this occurs because the exogenous insulin stimulates the islet cells to produce natural insulin, as if they are being reminded of their true function. Unfortunately, after a month or even up to a year, the islet cells begin to fail once again and diabetic symptoms recur. This can be upsetting to parents if they began to believe that their child was wrongly diagnosed or that a cure had taken place. Caution both the parents and child that symptoms will inevitably recur. Sometimes, the child is maintained on a minimum

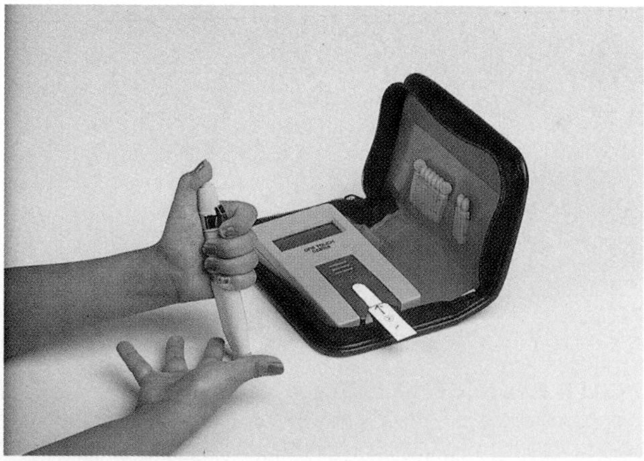

FIGURE 48.8 A child uses an automatic lancet for blood sampling (*left*). Blood glucose level will be determined by the glucometer (*right*).

amount of insulin during this period to prevent unrealistic expectations of a cure. This practice may also help to reduce islet cell destruction.

Stress Adjustment. Whenever children with diabetes undergo a stressful situation, either emotionally or physically, they may need increased insulin to maintain glucose homeostasis. When seen at health care facilities for periodic checkups, ask them about whether they are having any difficulty with blood testing or insulin injection and how things are at home and at school.

Try to interview children separately from their parents so they can feel free to talk about anything that may be happening or going wrong. There must be cooperation between primary health care personnel and school health care personnel so conflicts about the children's regimen do not cause problems or tensions while at school. Parents may have to meet with schoolteachers to help them view the child as well, not ill, so they will allow participation in all activities, including sports. Sometimes, children are embarrassed to have to do blood glucose testing in school, especially in the public lavatory. It may be easier for them if they can go to the nurse's office for privacy when testing (see Focus on Cultural Competence).

WHAT IF? What if your patient is a diabetic 13-year-old boy who wants to play soccer and baseball on his school teams? His parents tell you that both teams are coached by the same teacher, who thinks that diabetic children should be excluded from sports. The parents prefer not to dispute the coach's decision. What information can you give the parents and the patient about diabetes and diabetes control that they can share with the coach? How can you present this information to benefit the patient and/or help change the coach's mind?

FOCUS ON CULTURAL COMPETENCE

How people view endocrine disorders can be culturally influenced. Because many of these disorders are inherited, they tend to cluster in various populations so that either there is a high incidence of the condition in family or friends or else people know nothing about the condition. In the past, because many endocrine disorders led to changes in body appearance, particularly overgrowth or undergrowth, and because the reason for these changes was poorly understood, children with these disorders found themselves poorly accepted by peers. Being aware of the way that these diseases used to be viewed aids in understanding a parent's anxiety at diagnosis of these disorders and helps with nursing care planning to include reassurance and modern concepts of therapy in education. Also, be sure to ask parents if they are using alternative therapies because many advertised herbs suggest that they increase growth.

Complications. When temperature rises and infection occurs, counter-regulatory hormones increase, causing insulin resistance and increasing the need for more insulin. Teach parents to notify their primary health care provider when their child appears to be ill (particularly if the child is nauseated or vomiting) for careful observation and a change in insulin dosage if necessary. If a child with diabetes is scheduled for surgery, careful regulation on the day of surgery and in the immediate postoperative period is essential, especially if oral fluids will be restricted.

Many long-term body changes occur because of long-term hyperglycemia but may not be a part of childhood management because their onset does not begin until late adolescence or adulthood. These changes may include arteriosclerosis (hardening of artery walls), which can lead to general poor circulation and kidney disease, and thickening of retinal capillaries and cataract formation, which ultimately can result in blindness. Some children may notice blurred vision when their disease is not in control, but this should not be confused with the final retinopathy that may result with older age. It is a temporary change in depth of the eye globe related to hyperglycemia. Because women with diabetes eventually develop some degree of arteriosclerosis in adulthood, women are encouraged not to delay childbearing past age 35. Current research supports the use of low-dose progestin and estrogen combination oral contraceptives (high doses of estrogen can elevate blood glucose). Alternative measures of birth control, such as the diaphragm or vaginal foam along with condoms for their sexual partner, also should be discussed. Care of the woman with diabetes mellitus during pregnancy is discussed in Chapter 14.

Pancreas Transplant. For children who develop severe kidney disease or retinopathy, pancreas transplantation may be considered. Unlike other organ transplantation, the original pancreas is not removed entirely. The portion that supplies digestive enzymes is still functioning and is left in place. During surgery, the new pancreas is grafted to the iliac artery and vein to allow insulin from the new organ to enter the systemic circulation. For this reason, pancreatic replacement is more accurately called grafting. The digestive enzymes of the new pancreas can be diverted into the intestine or bladder, or the pancreatic ducts can be sclerosed so the digestive enzymes do not leave the transplanted organ. Grafts may be taken from cadavers or from live donors, who can lose up to 45% of their pancreas and still maintain a functioning organ for themselves.

To reduce their immune response and protect against graft rejection, drugs such as antilymphocyte globulin, cyclosporine, prednisone, or azathioprine (Imuran) are administered after surgery. If rejection does start to occur, they are then given monoclonal T-cell antibodies (OKT3).

Pancreatic transplantation is a last-resort solution for children, because the outcome is guarded (about 50% of transplanted organs will be rejected) and the outcome—continuous immune-suppressive medication for life—may not be regarded as a major improvement over the original illness, for which they would take continuous daily insulin for life.

NURSING DIAGNOSES AND RELATED INTERVENTIONS

Nursing Diagnosis: Health-seeking behaviors related to self-administration of insulin, balanced exercise, and hygiene

Outcome Identification: Child will demonstrate ability to self-administer insulin and identify an exercise and hygiene program within 3 days.

Outcome Evaluation: Child demonstrates insulin injection technique to nurse, describes steps correctly, and discusses plans for an exercise and hygiene program.

Self-Administration of Insulin. From about 8 years of age, children can be taught to administer their own insulin (Fig. 48-9). Many children younger than this do not have the dexterity to handle a syringe or an understanding of the importance of sterile technique and proper dosage. They may not always give it if they are tired or busy.

Do not underestimate how difficult it is for children to learn to give injections to themselves. After giving injections for some time, it seems as if it is a two-step process: (1) draw up the medication, and (2) give it. In actuality, more than 25 steps are involved.

When children have to mix insulins, the number of steps increases. Besides lacking dexterity and adult-level fine motor skills, children have to face *injecting themselves.* There is no such thing as getting used to injections. Children grow used to the *idea* of self-injection, not to the injections themselves.

Even if children are taught to give their own insulin from the beginning, at least one adult in the family should be taught to give it as well. There will be days when children refuse to administer their own insulin or are not feeling well and need to have or appreciate having someone do it for them. Parents may have a hard time giving their child a painful injection; teaching them to view it as a helping action will help alleviate their distress.

Exercise. Exercise is an important component of care, because it uses carbohydrates and helps reduce hyperglycemia. No type of exercise is restricted for children with diabetes (see Focus on Nursing Care Planning).

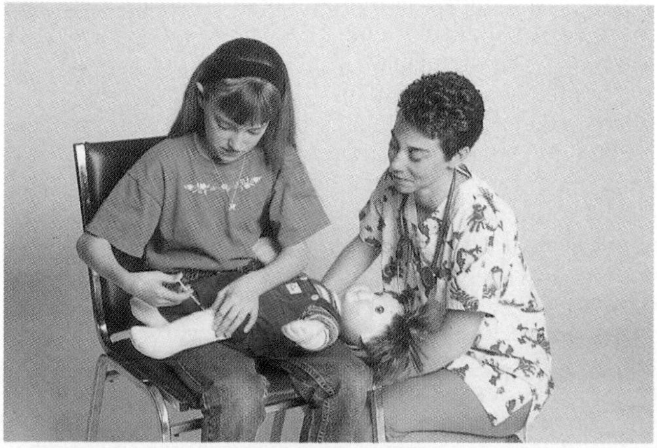

FIGURE 48.9 A school-age child is taught insulin administration using a teaching doll for practice.

A problem that arises with vigorous exercise, however, is the development of hypoglycemia because of the increased absorption of insulin from the injection site and utilization of glucose by active body cells. One way to minimize this effect is to choose an injection site least likely to be exercised. Another method is to eat additional carbohydrate or decrease the regular insulin injection according to an established protocol (algorithm) before exercise (ADA, 2002). Keep in mind that hypoglycemia may be delayed for up to 18 h after exercise.

Teach children to design a consistent daily exercise program. Once a daily program (eg, briskly walking the dog or 10 min of aerobics every day before school) is established, children need to continue this type of exercise every day (on weekends, too) or they may become hyperglycemic on those days.

Hygiene. Skin care, particularly foot care, is extremely important for adults with diabetes, because arteriosclerosis causes loss of circulation to the feet, and decreased circulation leads to poor healing ability. This is not as important a concern with children, but teach them to cut their toenails straight across to prevent ingrown toenails (as should all children) and to tend to cuts and scrapes promptly so healing can begin right away. Properly fitting shoes are essential. Girls may need to be reminded of good perineal care to prevent vaginal infection.

Nursing Diagnosis: Parental anxiety related to newly diagnosed diabetes mellitus in a child

Outcome Identification: Parents will demonstrate a full understanding of the disease process and their role in their child's care. They will state their ability to deal with new responsibilities within 1 month.

Outcome Evaluation: Parents accurately describe child's illness and treatment and ways the disease will affect their lifestyle. They state a specific plan for daily routine child care and identify potential problems in the schedule and ways these can be handled.

Parents with a child newly diagnosed with diabetes mellitus have a great deal of new responsibility. Ensure that they have the telephone number of the health care facility, liaison, or home care person to call for the first days of home management. During these days, most parents appreciate having someone to consult before they give insulin, for reassurance that they are giving the correct dose.

Encourage Expression of Feelings. Although parents may be aware of the disease occurring in other family members, they may be surprised that it has occurred in their child. Both parents and the child need time to describe their perceptions of diabetes. If there are other family members with the illness, children may have heard many false stories about the disorder. These misconceptions need to be corrected before they can begin to accept the diagnosis and view themselves as basically well except for faulty insulin release.

Teach About Disease and Principles of Care. Teaching is one of the main interventions necessary for children

FOCUS ON *Nursing Care Planning*

A CHILD WITH TYPE I DIABETES MELLITUS

An 8-year-old female is brought to the primary health care provider's office by her parents for a follow-up appointment after being diagnosed with type 1 diabetes mellitus. "She wants to play on the soccer team, which starts practice in a few weeks. How can we make sure that she'll be okay?"

Assessment: 8-year-old female. Height and weight appropriate for age. Diagnosed with type I diabetes approximately 5 months ago. Currently receiving short-acting and intermediate-acting insulin every morning before breakfast and intermediate-acting insulin before dinner. Child self-injects with automatic injection device with some parental supervision. Child performs fingerstick blood glucose levels four times a day. Blood glucose levels range between 105 and 115 mg/dL. Dietary history reveals three meals per day with midmorning, afternoon, and bedtime snack. Denies any signs and symptoms of hypoglycemia. Parents report child is active, playing outside and occasionally riding her bicycle. Voicing concerns about her increased activity level on diabetic control. Soccer practice scheduled for three times per week after school.

Nursing Diagnosis: Health-seeking behaviors related to participation in active sports program and effects on glucose control

Outcome Identification: Child and parents will verbalize measures to maintain blood glucose control.

Outcome Evaluation: Child and parents describe the effects of exercise on glucose control; identify signs and symptoms of hypoglycemia; state measures to prevent hypoglycemia and other possible complications.

Interventions	Rationale
1. Explore with the child and parents their understanding about the interrelationship of nutrition, exercise, and diabetes. Review with them the current routine for insulin administration, blood glucose monitoring, and snacks.	1. Exploration and review provide baseline information for identifying teaching needs and developing possible strategies.
2. Discuss the possibility of an insulin protocol for regulating blood glucose with the primary health care provider. Instruct the parents and child in this protocol if ordered.	2. Insulin needs are determined by activity level, diet, and timing of injection. A protocol helps to maintain blood glucose control based on the child's needs.
3. Advise the parents to pack a carbohydrate snack for the child to consume before practice. Encourage the child to ingest the snack before practice.	3. Exercise uses carbohydrates for energy. Intake of carbohydrates before exercise reduces the risk for hypoglycemia.
4. If insulin is prescribed to be administered before practice, instruct the child to use the upper extremity sites for injection and to avoid injecting the insulin into lower extremity sites.	4. Injection of insulin into a site that is to be exercised after the injection increases absorption of insulin from that site, increasing the risk for hypoglycemia.
5. Review the signs and symptoms of hypoglycemia with the child and parents. Instruct the child to check blood glucose level if she experiences any symptoms and to always carry an additional source of carbohydrate in case any signs or symptoms occur.	5. Knowledge of possible problems allows for early detection and prompt intervention should they occur. Testing blood glucose levels confirms hypoglycemia. Having a readily available source of carbohydrate helps raise blood glucose levels quickly should hypoglycemia occur.
6. Encourage the parents to discuss the child's needs and possible emergency measures necessary with the soccer coach. Suggest parents give the coach a written handout of signs and symptoms of hypo- and hyperglycemia and treatment measures.	6. Communication with the coach helps to alert him to the child's condition and inform him of any emergency measures that may be necessary. It also provides supervision for the child, which may help to alleviate some parental concerns.

(continued)

Interventions	Rationale
7. Encourage the use of protective equipment such as shin guards. Instruct the parents and child in measures to reduce complications, such as wearing properly fitting shoes and cleaning any cuts or scrapes promptly.	7. Protective equipment is necessary for any child to prevent injury. Diabetes can result in decreased circulation to the feet and slowed healing, increasing the possibility for infection, which can ultimately affect glucose control.
8. Advise the child to keep a written diary of insulin administration, blood glucose level results, dietary intake (including any snacks), and any symptoms of hypoglycemia and measures used.	8. A written diary provides objective evidence for evaluation of the regimen, indicating the need for possible changes or adjustments.
9. Arrange for a follow-up appointment for 1 week after the start of soccer practice. Give the parents the health care provider's office number and encourage them to call with any questions or concerns.	9. Follow-up visit provides a means for evaluating the effectiveness of the regimen and child's adaptation to activity, allowing opportunities for feedback, review of compliance, and further teaching. Availability of a contact person and telephone number provides additional support for the parents.

newly diagnosed with diabetes. Review general principles of care, including the fact that insulin injections, supervised intake of food, and exercise will decrease the blood glucose level, and increased intake of food will increase it. Infection and emotional upset also increase insulin requirements. If this process is not explained, parents may attempt to keep the child relatively quiet, unaware of the fact that exercise is actually healthful.

Teach that hypoglycemia is an extremely serious condition and must be prevented, if possible. Otherwise, parents may view continuous low blood glucose levels as a positive sign rather than as a potentially threatening condition that deprives body cells of glucose. If early signs are not recognized and treated, they can lead to coma and seizures. Severe glucose depletion can lead to permanent brain damage with mental and motor impairment, because brain cells need glucose for metabolism.

Be certain that parents have opportunities to practice supervised insulin injection and blood glucose testing so they become familiar with these procedures and any accompanying problems. Help them make a fair appraisal of how much care a child will be able to undertake for himself or herself. In the beginning, it is often better to limit the child's share of care to one blood glucose testing session and one self-administered insulin injection per day. This helps parents to avoid expecting too much from their child, possibly growing frustrated when the child does not meet their expectations. It makes successful management of their child's diabetes a rewarding experience rather than a chore.

Teach parents about the type of insulin that their child will use. However, avoid giving too much confusing detail about all the different types. If the insulin is changed at a later date, the new form can be described in greater depth at that time. Also, urge the parents or the child to begin keeping a log of blood glucose test results in a permanent notebook so these numbers can be evaluated for any unusual patterns at periodic checkups.

Establish Mode of Supervision and Support. Children with diabetes need frequent health supervision visits, approximately every 3 months. Those who appear to accept their diagnosis initially may have difficulty later when their true feelings about their disorder surface. Adolescents who are rebelling against a multitude of things may choose to rebel against blood glucose testing and insulin administration. Assess that children with diabetes have supportive friends to help them through "bad days." Sometimes what is needed most from health care personnel is understanding and appreciation of the difficulties encountered by children living with diabetes.

Serving as an active support person to parents is also necessary. Often, parents are so concerned with learning the techniques of insulin administration and blood glucose testing that they are not aware of other problems of everyday living that will arise later. Make sure that the parents can identify support people and others to contact if they have problems or questions.

Nursing Diagnosis: Risk for imbalanced nutrition, less than body requirements related to decreased insulin level

Outcome Identification: Child will demonstrate ability to plan nutrition to achieve normal serum glucose values within 1 month.

Outcome Evaluation: Child's growth follows percentile curve on standard growth chart; serum glucose is between 70 and 110 mg/dL fasting; child states that nutrition and exercise program are being followed.

Plan Nutrition Program. At one time, children with diabetes were placed on rigidly specified diets in which each food item had to be weighed. Then followed a period when children were allowed free diets, and any resulting glycosuria was managed by increasing insulin doses. Today, it is generally accepted that conscientious diet modification is necessary, because chronic hyperglycemia can lead to vascular disease in later years. The American Diabetes Association no longer recommends a food exchange list. Rather they recommend that children follow a nutrition pattern consistent with their lifestyle and cultural preferences. General guidelines for good nutrition are shown in Focus on Family Empowerment.

FOCUS ON FAMILY EMPOWERMENT

Nutritional Guidelines

Q. How can we make sure that our child who has diabetes gets adequate nutrition?

A. Here are some nutritional guidelines to help you:

- Plan well-balanced and appealing meals. Caloric content should be appropriate for your child's age group.
- Provide three meals throughout the day plus snacks. Total daily caloric intake is divided to provide 20% as breakfast, 20% as lunch, 30% as dinner, and 10% as morning, afternoon, and evening snacks. Distribution of calories should be 55% carbohydrate, 30% fat, and 15% protein.
- Do not use dietetic food. This is expensive and not necessary.
- Urge your child not to omit meals. This calls for creative planning so the child likes the foods served and eats readily.
- Maintain a positive outlook by stressing the foods your child is allowed to eat, not those to be avoided.
- Steer clear of concentrated carbohydrate sources, such as candy bars; be sure to include adequate fiber, such as broccoli, because this helps prevent hyperglycemia.
- Keep complex carbohydrates available to be eaten before exercise, such as swimming or a softball game, to provide sustained carbohydrate energy sources.
- Teach children about meal planning so they can wisely select what to eat at school or at a friend's home. This will promote independent self-care.

Teach Hypoglycemic Management. Symptoms of hypoglycemia occur when the blood glucose level falls to about 60 mg/dL. At this point, there will be no glycosuria. Parents and children, as soon as they are old enough to understand, must be aware of the reasons for hypoglycemia and what measures they must take to counteract it if it occurs.

Hypoglycemia can result from the administration of too much insulin, excessive exercise (because exercise uses up glucose), or failure to eat enough food. Typically, beginning symptoms include nervousness, weakness, dizziness, sweating, or tremors. In many children, the first signs of hypoglycemia are behavior problems: temper tantrums, stubbornness, silliness, irritability, or simply "not acting like himself." A few children become insensitive to the symptoms of hypoglycemia (termed *hypoglycemia unawareness*) and are then unable to recognize that it is occurring. Such children need more blood glucose determinations built into their routine than others.

When the signs of hypoglycemia are recognized, the child needs an immediate source of carbohydrate. Fifteen grams of a fast-acting carbohydrate are recommended, such as a half glass of orange juice or regular soda. It is easy for children always to carry glucose tablets or hard candy such as Lifesavers with them and have them available for these times (see Focus on Evidence-Based Practice). If there is no improvement in symptoms and the blood glucose level has not risen by 15 mg/dL after 15 min, more carbohydrate, such as juice, should be given.

For children who are comatose when they are first discovered or too upset or uncooperative to take oral sugar, parents can inject a specified dose of glucagon hydrochloride. This converts the glycogen that is stored in the liver to glucose. Generally, enough glycogen is converted after the drug injection to bring the child out of coma so that an oral form of glucose can then be given. The drug is not effective if the child's supply of glycogen is depleted.

If parents cannot give their child an injection and oral sugar cannot be given, honey, corn syrup, cake icing gel, or glucose can be rubbed onto the gums or inside the cheek (of course, parents should be taught how to prevent aspiration). As soon as children are out of coma or are cooperative, they must take a source of complex carbohydrate to prevent further hypoglycemia. Their primary health care provider needs to be notified of the incident so its cause can be determined and steps taken to prevent it from occurring again.

Urge parents to anticipate occasions when hypoglycemia is likely to occur and to take preventive measures. Hypoglycemia is most likely to occur at the peak effective time of the insulins being given (ie, just before lunch or just before dinner). This means that many children who are attending school need to be scheduled for the first lunch period, not the second, or need a snack before lunch. Encourage the child and parents to discuss lunch times with the physician and dietitian so appropriate meal planning is coordinated with the child's insulin schedule. Follow-up at 6-month intervals is advised to make adjustments for changes in growth and school schedules. Children also should eat dinner at a regular time or have a snack to tide them over until dinner. Additionally, children need a snack before bedtime to prevent hypoglycemia from developing during the night.

If children are going to engage in an active sport, such as swimming, tennis, or basketball, they should take a source of sugar before participation. This precaution is extremely important before swimming, because a child who suddenly becomes weak in the middle of a pool may be unable to reach the side safely. Although eating before swimming is something that children typically are taught not to do, the child with diabetes must be taught to break this rule (sensibly, of course; before swimming, the child eats a complex carbohydrate, such as crackers, not a full meal). Day and residential camps are available to help the child learn more

FOCUS ON EVIDENCE-BASED PRACTICE

Do Children With Diabetes Conscientiously Carry a Source of Sugar With Them?

Children with diabetes should carry with them an easily dissolved sugar in the event they experience hypoglycemia while at school or during some other activity. To determine whether young diabetics follow this rule, 263 children (a total of 112 boys and 151 girls) either from Kansas in the United States or from Silesia, Poland, were sent a questionnaire asking various questions about their disease management. The mean age of the children was 12, and the mean duration of their illness was 4.77 years. Results of the study revealed that 79% of children said they carried some food daily but only 59% carried a soluble sugar. Only 53% of children said they never forgot insulin injections. Children with diabetes of a longer duration were more apt to forget these. Older girls with longer duration of disease demonstrated worse metabolic control and checked for serum glucose less frequently as well as forgot insulin injections more frequently. The researchers concluded that children, as a group, need additional education about what are the best foods to carry to treat hypoglycemia and how to better remember insulin injections.

This is an important study for nurses because it documents what a worldwide problem diabetes can be among young people. In addition, it illustrates, when there are so many instructions that need to be given to children with this disorder, how easy it is for them to misunderstand (in this instance, the difference between "a readily dissolved sugar" and carrying just any food). The information from this study is appropriate for use as a foundation when designing initial teaching plans for children with diabetes. It can also be used as a guide for developing supplemental teaching plans as children grow older.

Jarosz-Chobot, P., Guthrie, D. W., Otto-Buczkowski, E., & Koehler, B. (2000). Self-care in young diabetics in practice. *Medical Science Monitor, 6*(1), 129–132.

about diabetes and common measures others use to prevent hypoglycemia.

Occasionally, insulin overuse and persistent hypoglycemia cause a rebound hyperglycemic response referred to as the **Somogyi phenomenon.** This phenomenon is suspected when children have nighttime (2 or 3 am) hypoglycemia followed by high early-morning hyperglycemia. These children need to be referred to their health care provider because they actually need less insulin rather than more to correct the problem.

Teach Signs of Ketoacidosis. It is often difficult to distinguish between hypoglycemia (occurring from too much insulin) and hyperglycemia (occurring from too little insulin for the level of glucose present in the bloodstream). Hyperglycemia leads to **ketoacidosis** with symptoms of vomiting and abdominal pain and the same kind of behavior changes exhibited with hypoglycemia.

When a parent does not know the cause of the upset, children should be offered a carbohydrate as if the problem were hypoglycemia. The added carbohydrate will do no harm if the problem is already hyperglycemia, whereas giving insulin is harmful if the cause is hypoglycemia. The child's inability to void suggests that the problem is hypoglycemia. With hyperglycemia, urine output is copious—one of the primary signs of diabetes. The real key to differentiating ketoacidosis from hypoglycemia is blood glucose levels. Assessing a blood glucose level by fingerstick solves the problem of whether symptoms relate to hypoglycemia or hyperglycemia.

When ketoacidosis is severe, children's respirations become deep and rapid (Kussmaul breathing) in an attempt to "blow off" carbon dioxide and lessen the acidotic state. Breath smells sweet because of the presence of ketone bodies, and the pulse rate may be rapid. Children may have signs of dehydration: dry mucous membranes and skin, sunken eyeballs, and no tears. This may be the picture when children with diabetes are first diagnosed. It is often seen in children with diabetes who develop gastroenteritis and hence eat poorly for a number of meals. Because the child is not eating well, parents may omit giving insulin. In actuality, because of an increased metabolic rate due to fever, children may need more insulin and glucose than usual during these times.

A comparison of hypoglycemia and hyperglycemia appears in Table 48-5.

✔ CHECKPOINT QUESTIONS

7. Which type of diabetes mellitus is seen most often in children?
8. What is meant by the "honeymoon period" in type 1 diabetes?
9. What is the usual peak time for regular insulin when given SC?
10. What are the typical symptoms of hypoglycemia?

THE PARATHYROID GLANDS

The parathyroid glands, four of them located posterior and adjacent to the thyroid gland, function to regulate serum levels of calcium in the body and control the rate of bone metabolism by the secretion of parathyroid hormone. This hormone is not under the control of the pituitary gland but is controlled by a negative feedback of the circulating serum levels of calcium. If blood calcium levels fall, parathyroid hormone secretion increases; if blood calcium levels increase, hormone production decreases. Vitamin D is necessary for calcium absorption from the GI tract into the bloodstream, so it also influences parathyroid hormone secretion. Calcitonin (thyrocalcitonin) secreted by the thyroid gland opposes the action of parathyroid hormone and, therefore, decreases blood calcium levels.

TABLE 48.5 Comparison of Hypoglycemia and Hyperglycemia

COMPARISON FACTOR	HYPOGLYCEMIA	HYPERGLYCEMIA
Cause	Excessive insulin injection	Inadequate insulin injection
	Excessive exercise	Excessive food intake
	Limited food intake	Stress from infection, surgery, etc.
Symptoms	Hunger	Glycosuria and ketonuria
	Lethargy	Polyuria, polydipsia
	Sensorium changes	Kussmaul respirations
	Pallor	Flushing
	Sweating	
	Seizures	Sweet (acetone) breath
	Coma	Decreased CO_2 combining power
		Dehydration
		Lowered sodium, potassium, bicarbonate, chloride, and phosphate levels
		Vomiting, abdominal pain
		Coma
Danger	Brain cells need glucose for function and survival	Fatty acids are used and acidosis develops
Major nursing interventions	Administration of source of glucose by oral or IV route	Reestablishment of electrolyte balance and hydration
	Education to prevent recurrences	Education to prevent recurrences

Hypocalcemia

Hypocalcemia is a lowered blood calcium level. It occurs to some extent in all newborns before they begin eating well (Thilo & Rosenberg, 2001). Phosphorus and calcium levels are maintained in an inverse proportion to each other in the bloodstream (i.e., if phosphorus levels rise, calcium levels decrease; if calcium levels rise, phosphorus levels decrease). Hypocalcemia, therefore, may be caused by changes in either calcium or phosphorus metabolism.

Assessment

Hypocalcemia tends to occur in infants who experienced birth anoxia (phosphorus is released with anoxia), immature infants (the parathyroid gland is immature), and infants of diabetic mothers (it tends to accompany the hypoglycemia that occurs in these infants shortly after birth). It may be caused by the imbalance between phosphorus and calcium in milk (such an imbalance does not exist in breast milk and is modified in commercial formulas).

Latent Tetany. The chief sign of hypocalcemia is neuromuscular irritability, often referred to as **latent tetany.** This occurs if the blood calcium level is less than 7.5 mg/dL. Newborns with latent tetany are jittery when they are handled, or they cry for extended periods.

Four ways can be used to produce the clinical manifestations of tetany for diagnosis of hypocalcemia; these are shown in Table 48-6. These are all useful tests to determine or suggest whether newborn jitteriness is from hypocalcemia, a central nervous system problem, or some other cause.

If tetany is caused by infant formula, it occurs at about day 7 of life. A community health nurse making a follow-up visit after a home birth might be the one to recognize the problem initially.

Manifest Tetany. If the blood calcium level falls well below 7 mg/dL, **manifest tetany** may result, commonly manifested by muscular twitching and carpopedal spasms.

TABLE 48.6 Detection of Hypocalcemia

SIGN	DESCRIPTION
Chvostek's	When skin anterior to external ear (just over sixth cranial nerve) is tapped, facial muscles surrounding eye, nose, and mouth contract unilaterally.
Trousseau's	When upper arm is constricted by tourniquet for 2–3 min and area becomes blanched, carpal spasm is elicited (hand abducts, wrist flexes, thumb is positioned across cupped palm).
Peroneal	When fibular side of leg over peroneal nerve is tapped, foot abducts and dorsiflexes.
Erb's	This test is dramatic to see demonstrated, although it requires a mild galvanic current so is not used routinely. A person with tetany has greater muscular irritability than a person with a normal calcium level; therefore, when a mild current is applied over the peroneal nerve just below the head of the fibula, the foot on that side will abduct and dorsiflex.

A **carpal spasm** (hand spasm) involves abduction of the hand and flexion of the wrist with the thumb positioned across the palm. In **pedal (foot) spasm,** the foot is extended, the toes flex, and the sole of the foot cups. Generalized seizures may occur. There may be spasm of the larynx. Because of this spasm, the infant emits a high-pitched, crowing sound on inspiration because of the constricted airway. If the spasm is prolonged, respirations may cease.

Therapeutic Management

Treatment is aimed at increasing the calcium level in the blood above the point that leads to latent tetany. Calcium may be administered orally as 10% calcium chloride if the infant can and will suck. It can be given IV as a 10% solution of calcium gluconate if the tetany has progressed to a point at which the child does not have enough muscular coordination to take oral fluid safely. Calcium gluconate should not be given IM or SC because necrosis may occur at the injection site. Newborns who are having generalized seizures may require anticonvulsant therapy in addition to the calcium gluconate to halt the seizures. Emergency equipment for intubation to relieve laryngospasm should be available.

After immediate therapy to increase the low blood calcium levels, infants will be placed on oral calcium therapy until their calcium level stabilizes above 7.5 mg/dL. Because vitamin D is necessary for the absorption of calcium and phosphorus from the GI tract, the infant also may be given a vitamin D supplement.

METABOLIC DISORDERS

Earlier in this chapter, overproduction or underproduction of certain hormones and ways these can seriously hinder body metabolism, creating such problems as hypothyroidism, congenital adrenogenital hyperplasia, and type 1 diabetes mellitus, were discussed. There are many causes for hormonal deficiency or excess, most of which are related to the endocrine glands and the highly complex system of feedback and communication between these glands and the hypothalamus. The neuroendocrine regulation of hormonal balance is so sensitive that it is affected by the body's internal and external environments (i.e., injury, stress, and emotional changes).

In addition to endocrine disorders, a group of hereditary biochemical disorders also affect metabolism. These are caused largely by some specific defect in the body biochemistry that disrupts one step of the metabolic process. The term *inborn errors of metabolism* is used to refer to these disorders. Most of them are caused by a lack of or deficiency in a particular enzyme, which seriously impairs the ability of the body to metabolize properly the components of food for energy.

Inborn errors of metabolism affect amino acid and protein, carbohydrate, and lipid metabolism. Many of these disorders are evident at or soon after birth and can cause severe symptoms rapidly. Early detection and treatment are essential to the prevention of irreversible cognitive challenge and early death.

Phenylketonuria (PKU)

Phenylketonuria is a disease of metabolism inherited as an autosomal recessive trait. Absence of the liver enzyme phenylalanine hydroxylase prevents conversion of phenylalanine, an essential amino acid, into tyrosine (a precursor of epinephrine, thyroxine, and melanin). As a result, excessive phenylalanine builds up in the bloodstream and tissues, causing permanent damage to brain tissue leading to children who become severely cognitively challenged.

The metabolite phenylpyruvic acid (a breakdown product of phenylalanine) spills into the urine to give the disorder its name. It causes urine to have a typical musty or "mousy" odor that is so strong it often pervades not only the urine but the entire child.

Tyrosine is necessary for building body pigment and is incorporated into thyroxine. Without it, body pigment fades and the child becomes very fair skinned, light blonde haired, and blue eyed. The child fails to meet average growth standards because of the lack of thyroxine production. Many children develop an accompanying seizure disorder. The skin is prone to eczema (atopic dermatitis). There is such a strong association between these two disorders that all infants with atopic dermatitis need to be rescreened for PKU.

Phenylketonuria is found in 1 in 10,000 births in the United States. It occurs rarely in people of African or Jewish ancestry (Greene, Thomas & Goodman, 2001). Untreated, the child with PKU will have an IQ that is generally below 20. In addition, about one third of affected children have recurrent seizures, and about half have muscular hypertonicity and spasticity. PKU cannot be detected by amniocentesis or percutaneous umbilical cord blood sampling as a routine screening measure, because the phenylalanine level does not rise in utero while the infant is still under the control of the mother's enzyme system. Recombinant DNA techniques can be used for carrier detection and prenatal diagnosis.

Assessment

Early identification of the disorder is essential to prevent the child from becoming severely cognitively challenged. Infants are screened at birth after receiving 2 full days of feedings (at least 120 mL of formula at a concentration of 20 calories per ounce, or the equivalent amount obtained by breastfeeding). The screening is done by pricking the infant's heel with a blood lancet, and letting a few drops of blood fall onto a specially prepared filter paper. The filter paper is then analyzed by a bacterial inhibition process for the amount of phenylalanine contained in the infant's blood (the Guthrie test). If an infant is born at home or discharged from a hospital or birthing center before the second day of life, the parents will need to have the test performed on the second or third day after birth. If the infant is being breastfed and there is a question as to whether only colostrum has been received, a repeated Guthrie test should be performed by the second week of life during a health care visit.

Some infants demonstrate a benign, transitory elevated level of phenylalanine shortly after birth, apparently due to immature processing of amino acids. This benign, transitory form needs to be differentiated from the actual disease so parents are not frightened unnecessarily and the child is not unnecessarily placed on a restricted diet.

Therapeutic Management

Infants in whom this disease is detected in the first few days of life can be placed on an extremely low phenylalanine formula, such as Lofenalac. Beginning the diet early helps to prevent the child from becoming cognitively challenged. A dietitian may recommend that a small amount of milk be added to the infant's diet every day so the child does receive some phenylalanine (this essential amino acid is necessary for growth and repair of body cells). As a result, a mother who wants to breastfeed may be able to do this on a limited basis.

Parents of children with PKU need a realistic prognosis of their child's potential. If the disorder was detected in the first few days of life and the child's diet is well controlled to avoid any abnormal high level of phenylalanine, the child's IQ will not be adversely affected. On the other hand, if the disorder was not detected until some brain involvement or other symptoms were noticeable, such symptoms cannot be reversed.

Providing nutrition for a child with PKU is a difficult task. There is no natural protein with both a low phenylalanine concentration and a normal concentration of other essential amino acids. A diet of just protein restriction, therefore, would result in restriction of all essential amino acids—a diet that is incompatible with life. Specially manufactured formulas such as Lofenalac are synthetic compounds that have a low phenylalanine concentration but contain enough other essential nutrients that, with the exception of some additional milk, they are the only food required in early infancy. Amino acid formulas have a rather disagreeable taste. When infants are placed on these in the first few days of life, however, they do not seem to react to the flavor and will drink such formulas readily into adulthood. These formulas may cause stools to be loose. As children grow older and have solid foods added to their meals, these foods also must be low in phenylalanine so that the phenylalanine level of the child's blood stays below 8 mg/dL. Foods highest in phenylalanine are those that are rich in protein, such as meats, eggs, and milk. Foods low in phenylalanine include orange juice, bananas, potatoes, lettuce, spinach, and peas. A formula such as Lofenalac can be used to make treat foods, such as ice cream, milk shakes, birthday cakes, and puddings (foods that would otherwise be forbidden because they are made with milk). Children need their blood and urine monitored frequently for phenylalanine levels. Hemoglobin levels should also be closely monitored to ensure that the child is not becoming anemic because iron is found primarily in protein-rich foods, which are to be avoided.

At health visits, offer parents an opportunity to express their feelings about the difficulty of maintaining a young child on such a restricted diet. In addition, assess the child's ability to cope with the illness. Adolescents appreciate the chance to meet other teenagers who have this condition and find out how they are solving nutritional problems (Singh et al., 2000).

When to discontinue the diet is controversial because of reports of progressive neurologic deterioration in children no longer following a restricted diet. Generally, current advice is for children to follow the diet indefinitely (Greene, Thomas & Goodman, 2001). A woman who has PKU must anticipate when she wants to have children as an adult and, if not following her diet conscientiously, return to a low-phenylalanine diet for about 3 months before conception and remain on the diet during pregnancy. If not, the fetus will be exposed to high levels of phenylalanine during pregnancy and will be born cognitively challenged. (see Chapter 12).

WHAT IF? What if you are helping at a preschool and notice the teacher urging a little boy with PKU to drink his milk? When you suggest that milk might not be good for him, the teacher says, "Of course it is. Milk is nature's perfect food." How would you respond? What would you do?

Maple Syrup Urine Disease

Maple syrup urine disease is a rare disorder, inherited as an autosomal recessive trait, in which there is a defect in amino acid metabolism of leucine, isoleucine, and valine that leads to cerebral degeneration similar to that of PKU.

Assessment

Infants appear well at birth but quickly begin to show signs of feeding difficulty, loss of the Moro's reflex, and irregular respirations. The symptoms progress rapidly to *opisthotonos,* generalized muscular rigidity, and seizures. Untreated, the child may die of the disease as early as 2 to 4 weeks of age.

Although the disorder is rare, it is mentioned because it is relatively easy to detect: by the first or second day of life, the urine of the child develops the characteristic odor of maple syrup, hence the name of the disease. The odor is due to the presence of ketoacids, the same phenomenon that makes the breath of diabetic children in severe acidosis smell sweet. Because nurses are most likely to detect the characteristic urine odor in the first few days of life, it is a disorder that nurses caring for newborns should be aware of so they do not discount the pleasant urine odor as an innocent finding. Prenatal detection is possible by analyzing cells obtained by amniocentesis.

Therapeutic Management

If maple syrup urine disease is diagnosed in the first day or two of life and the child is placed on a well-controlled diet high in thiamine and low in the amino acids leucine, isoleucine, and valine, the cerebral degeneration can be prevented, just as it can be prevented in PKU (Robinson & Drumm, 2001). Such a diet is extremely difficult to maintain, however, because of its low protein content. Parents need intensive nutritional counseling. Hemodialysis or peritoneal dialysis can be used to temporarily reduce abnormal serum levels at birth or during a childhood infection when catabolism of cells releases increased amino acid into the bloodstream.

Galactosemia

Galactosemia is a disorder of carbohydrate metabolism characterized by abnormal amounts of galactose in the blood (*galactosemia*) and in the urine (*galactosuria*). It occurs in about 1 in 40,000 births, most often as an inborn error of metabolism, transmitted as an autosomal recessive trait, in which the child is deficient in the liver enzyme galactose 1-phosphate uridyltransferase (Greene, Thomas & Goodman, 2001).

Lactose (the sugar found in milk) normally is broken down into galactose and glucose; galactose is then further broken down into additional glucose. Without the galactose 1-phosphate uridyltransferase enzyme, this second step, the conversion of galactose into glucose, cannot take place, and galactose builds up in the bloodstream and spills into the urine. When it reaches toxic levels, it destroys body cells.

Assessment

Symptoms appear when the child begins formula feeding or breastfeeding and include lethargy, hypotonia, and perhaps diarrhea and vomiting. Next, the liver enlarges as cirrhosis develops. Jaundice is often present and persistent; bilateral cataracts develop. The symptoms begin abruptly and worsen rapidly. Untreated, the child may die by 3 days of age. Untreated children who do survive beyond this time may be cognitively challenged or have bilateral cataracts. Because early detection is the key to preventing brain damage, nursing assessment is particularly important in this disorder.

Diagnosis is made by measuring the level of the affected enzyme in the red blood cells. A screening test (the Beutler test) can be used to analyze cord blood when the child is known to be at risk for the disorder.

Therapeutic Management

The treatment of galactosemia consists of placing the infant on a diet that is free of galactose or on a formula made with milk substitutes like casein hydrolysates (eg, Nutramigen). Once the child is regulated on this diet, symptoms of the disease do not progress; however, any neurologic or cataract damage already present will persist. The duration of the restricted diet is controversial, but probably it should be followed for life (Greene, Thomas & Goodman, 2001).

Glycogen Storage Disease

Glycogen storage disease is actually a group of genetically transmitted disorders involving altered production and use of glycogen in the body. All but 1 of the 13 types described are inherited as autosomal recessive traits; the remaining 1 is a sex-linked disorder.

Glycogen is normally stored in the liver as a reserve supply of glucose. When the body needs glucose for energy, this glycogen is transformed back to glucose. In children with glycogen storage disease, glycogen is deposited normally, but an enzyme deficiency prevents retransformation of the glycogen back to glucose. As a result, children's livers rapidly increase in size from the stored glycogen. Children with this disorder are susceptible to periods of hypoglycemia because their only source of ready glucose is oral intake (Greene, Thomas & Goodman, 2001).

In one form of this disorder (type II or Pompe's disease), children deposit large stores of glycogen not only in the liver, but in the muscle and heart as well. The muscles begin to feel hard to palpation from the deposits of glycogen. The heart will be enlarged, and many children have an arrhythmia. Children with this form will usually die of heart failure before they reach adulthood.

Assessment

A common sign of glycogen storage disease is liver enlargement because the liver must store such a large supply of glycogen (Pozzato et al., 2001). Consequently, the abdomen protrudes. Over a long period of time, the child's growth is stunted because there is not enough glucose for any function but immediate energy. If hypoglycemic episodes have been severe, brain damage may result. Many children have a tendency toward epistaxis or hemorrhage and are at risk when having surgery performed because of impaired clotting ability due to decreased platelet adhesiveness.

Therapeutic Management

Children with glycogen storage disease need to be maintained on a high-carbohydrate diet with snacks between meals to prevent hypoglycemia. In addition, a continuous glucose nasogastric or gastrostomy feeding during the night may be necessary to prevent hypoglycemia while sleeping. Therapy with diazoxide (Proglycem), an antihypoglycemic drug that inhibits insulin release, may help regulate the glucose level to give additional growth. Liver transplantation may be a possibility but will not cure the enzyme deficiency.

Tay-Sachs Disease

Tay-Sachs disease is an autosomal recessively inherited disease in which the infant lacks hexosaminidase A, an enzyme necessary for lipid metabolism. Without this enzyme, lipid deposits accumulate on nerve cells, leading to cognitive challenge when deposits are on brain cells and blindness when deposits are on optic nerve cells (Moe & Seay, 2001).

Tay-Sachs disease is found primarily in the Ashkenazi Jewish population (Eastern European Jewish ancestry). Children generally appear normal in the first few months of life except for an extreme Moro's reflex and mild hypotonia. At about 6 months of age, they begin to lose head control and are unable to sit up or roll over without support. On ophthalmoscopic examination, a cherry-red macula is noticeable (caused by lipid deposits). By 1 year of age, children have developed symptoms of spasticity and are unable to perform even simple motor tasks. By 2 years of age, generalized seizures and blindness have occurred. Most children die of cachexia (malnutrition) and pneumonia by 3 to 5 years of age.

Unfortunately, there is no cure for Tay-Sachs disease. The disorder may be detected in utero by amniocentesis. Carriers for the disease trait may be identified by hexosaminidase A assay.

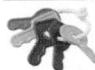

✔ CHECKPOINT QUESTIONS

11. What is the chief symptom of latent tetany?
12. Why are children with glycogen storage disease prone to hypoglycemia?

KEY POINTS

Endocrine disorders are almost all long-term disorders. Helping parents and children remember to take medicine on a long-term basis is an important nursing responsibility.

Children with endocrine disorders often develop height or weight discrepancies. The nurse should help children continue to feel high self-esteem by concentrating on the things they are able to do despite a growth lag.

Growth hormone (GH) deficiency, a pituitary disorder, results in children who are short in stature. Therapy for children is the injection of synthetic GH. Children can experience situational low self-esteem if they do not receive adequate emotional support from significant others.

Other pituitary disorders include GH excess and diabetes insipidus. As the name implies, with GH excess, there is overproduction of GH. With diabetes insipidus, there is decreased release of antidiuretic hormone (ADH). Urine becomes dilute, and large amounts are excreted. Therapy is administration of desmopressin (DDAVP), an arginine vasopressin. Children with this are at high risk for fluid volume deficit.

Congenital hypothyroidism occurs as a result of an absent or nonfunctioning thyroid gland. The condition is discovered by a blood test at birth. The therapy is oral administration of synthetic thyroid hormone.

Acquired hypothyroidism (Hashimoto's disease) is an autoimmune phenomenon that interferes with thyroid gland function. Therapy is administration of synthetic thyroid hormone.

Acute adrenocortical insufficiency can occur in children from causes such as an overwhelming infection in which there is hemorrhagic destruction of the adrenal gland. A more common disease in children is congenital adrenogenital hyperplasia. Girls are born masculinized; either sex may be unable to retain sodium, which results in rapid fluid loss. Therapy is administration of corticosteroid.

Cushing's syndrome is overproduction of cortisol by the adrenal gland. This usually results from a tumor in the gland. Children appear abnormally obese. Therapy is surgical removal of the tumor.

The most frequently occurring pancreatic disorder is type 1 diabetes mellitus. This may be an autoimmune process in which there has been destruction of insulin-producing islet cells. Therapy is a combination of administration of insulin, diet, and exercise.

Hypocalcemia, a parathyroid gland disorder, results in a lowered blood calcium level. In children, tetany develops. Therapy is the administration of calcium.

Various disorders of metabolism that interfere with carbohydrate, amino acid, or fat metabolism occur in children. Representative of these are PKU, galactosemia, and Tay-Sachs disease.

CRITICAL THINKING EXERCISES

1. Rob is the 16-year-old boy diagnosed as having type 1 diabetes you met at the beginning of the chapter. In the last 6 months, he has "forgotten" to take his insulin at least once a week. Is Rob's history unusual for an adolescent? What health teaching do you think will most help him reestablish control?
2. A 12-year-old girl with GH deficiency is only 3 ft tall at present and has been told she probably will not grow taller than 4 ft, 6 in. Her parents tell you they find her "cute," so they do not want her to receive GH. How would you approach this family? How much should the child be able to contribute to this decision?
3. A newborn is diagnosed as having salt-losing form of congenital adrenogenital hyperplasia. What would be the most important measure to teach her parents before she is discharged from the hospital? How may having a child with this disorder change this family's life?
4. Examine the National Health Goals related to endocrine or metabolic disorders. Most government-sponsored money for nursing research is allotted based on these goals. What would be a possible research topic to explore pertinent to these goals that would both be fundable and advance evidence-based practice?

REFERENCES

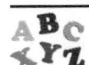

Allahabadia, A., et al. (2001). Radioiodine treatment of hyperthyroidism-prognostic factors for outcome. *Journal of Clinical Endocrinology & Metabolism, 86*(8), 3611–3617.

American Diabetes Association. (2002). Evidence-based nutrition principles and recommendations for the treatment and prevention of diabetes. *Diabetes Care, 25*(1), 550–560.

Chase, H. P., & Eisenbarth, G. S. (2001). Diabetes mellitus. In W. W. Hay (Ed.). *Current pediatric diagnosis & treatment* (15th ed.). New York: McGraw-Hill.

Department of Health and Human Services. (2000). *Healthy people 2010.* Washington, DC: DHHS.
Ferry, R. J., & Collett-Solberg, P. F. (2000a). Growth hormone deficiency. In M. W. Schwartz (Ed.). *The 5 minute pediatric consult* (pp. 400–401). Philadelphia: Lippincott Williams & Wilkins.
Ferry, R. J., & Collett-Solberg, P. F. (2000b). Diabetes insipidus. In M. W. Schwartz (Ed.). *The 5 minute pediatric consult* (pp. 316–317). Philadelphia: Lippincott Williams & Wilkins.
Greene, C. L., Thomas, J. A., & Good, S. I. (2001). Inward errors of metabolism. In W. W. Hay (Ed.). *Current pediatric diagnosis & treatment* (15th ed.). New York: McGraw-Hill.
Grimberg, A., & Satin-Smith, M. (2000). Congenital hypothyroidism. In M. W. Schwartz (Ed.). *The 5 minute pediatric consult* (pp. 274–275). Philadelphia: Lippincott Williams & Wilkins.
Guazzarotti, L., et al. (2001). Diagnosis of MODY in the offspring of parents with insulin-dependent and non-insulin-dependent diabetes mellitus. *Journal of Pediatric Endocrinology, 14*(51), 61–67.
Jarosz-Chobot, P., Guthrie, D. W., Otto-Buczkowski, E., & Koehler, B. (2000). Self-care in young diabetics in practice. *Medical Science Monitor, 6*(1), 129–132.
Kappy, M. S., Steelman, J. W., & Travers, S. H. (2001). Endocrine disorders. In W. W. Hay (Ed.). *Current pediatric diagnosis & treatment* (15th ed.). New York: McGraw-Hill.
Karch, A. M. (2001). *Lippincott's nursing drug guide.* Philadelphia: Lippincott Williams &Wilkins.
Katz, L. (2000). Cushing syndrome. In M. W. Schwartz (Ed.). *The 5 minute pediatric consult* (pp. 300–301). Philadelphia: Lippincott Williams & Wilkins.
Klein, R. Z., et al. (2001). Relation of severity of maternal hypothyroidism to cognitive development of offspring. *Journal of Medical Screening, 8*(1), 18–20.
Kraiem, Z., & Newfield, R. S. (2001). Graves' disease in childhood. *Journal of Pediatric Endocrinology, 14*(3), 229–234.
Lenhard, M. J., & Reeves, G. D. (2001). Continuous subcutaneous insulin infusion: A comprehensive review of insulin pump therapy. *Archives of Internal Medicine, 161*(19), 2293–3000.
McCance, K. L. & Huether, S. E. (2002). *Pathophysiology*. St. Louis: Mosby.
Merke, D. P., et al. (2000). Adrenomedullary dysplasia and hypofunction in patients with classic 21-hydroxylase deficiency. *New England Journal of Medicine, 343*(19), 136–138.
Moe, P. G., & Seay, A. R. (2001). Neurologic and muscular disorders. In W. W. Hay (Ed.). *Current pediatric diagnosis & treatment* (15th ed.). New York: McGraw-Hill.
Pozzato, C. et al. (2001). Sonographic findings in type I glycogen storage disease. *Journal of Clinical Ultrasound, 29*(8), 456–461.
Robinson, D., & Drumm, L. (2001). Maple syrup disease: A standard of nursing care. *Pediatric Nursing, 27*(3), 255–258.
Sandberg, D. E., & MacGillivray, M. H. (2000). Growth hormone therapy in childhood-onset growth hormone deficiency: Adult anthropometric and psychological outcomes. *Endocrine Journal—UK, 12*(2), 173–182.
Singh, R. H., et al. (2000). Impact of a camp experience on phenylalanine levels, knowledge, attitudes, and health beliefs relevant to nutrition management of phenylketonuria in adolescent girls. *Journal of the American Dietetic Association, 100*(7), 797–803.
Skidmore-Roth, L. (2002). *Mosby's nursing drug reference.* St. Louis: Mosby.
Thilo, E. H., & Rosenberg, A. A. (2001). Metabolic disorders in the newborn infant. In W. W. Hay (Ed.). *Current pediatric diagnosis & treatment* (15th ed.). New York: McGraw-Hill.
Weinzimer, S. A. (2000). Diabetic mellitus. In M. W. Schwartz (Ed.). *The 5-minute pediatric consult* (pp. 320–321). Philadelphia: Lippincott Williams & Wilkins.

SUGGESTED READINGS

American Academy of Pediatrics. (2000). School health assessments. *Pediatrics, 105*(4), 875–877.
American Association of Diabetes Educators. (2000). Management of children with diabetes in the school setting. *Diabetes Educator, 26*(1), 32–35.
Andrews, M. (2000). A parent's view of short stature. *Pediatric Annals, 29*(9), 582–584.
Anhalt, H., & Chin, D. (2000). Endocrine treatments for short stature. *Pediatric Annals, 29*(9), 576–581.
Drake, W. M., et al. (2001). Optimizing GH therapy in adults and children. *Endocrine Reviews, 22*(4), 425–450.
Hopwood, N. J. (2000). The dilemma of the short child without a clear diagnosis. *Pediatric Annals, 29*(9), 542–548.
Hoyme, H. E. (2000). A clinical genetics and dysmorphology approach to growth deficiency. *Pediatric Annals, 29*(9), 549–557.
Jaruratanasirkul, S., et al. (2001). The clinical course of Hashimoto's thyroiditis in children and adolescents. *Journal of Pediatric Endocrinology, 14*(2), 177–184.
Lindholm, J., et al. (2001). Incidence and late prognosis of Cushing's syndrome: A population-based study. *Journal of Clinical Endocrinology & Metabolism, 86*(1), 117–123.
MacGillivray, M. H. (2000). The basics for the diagnosis and management of short stature. *Pediatric Annals, 29*(9), 570–575.
Prinz, R. A. et al. (2002). Difficult problems in thyroid surgery. *Current Problems in Surgery, 39*(1), 5–9.
Savage, M. O., et al. (2001). Cushing's disease in childhood: Presentation, investigation, treatment and long-term outcome. *Hormone Research, 55*(51), 24–30.

CHAPTER 49

Nursing Care of the Child With a Neurologic Disorder

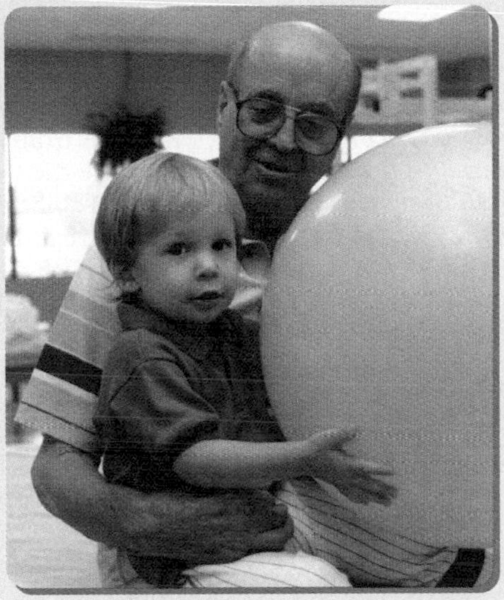

Key Terms

- astereognosis
- automatisms
- autonomic dysreflexia
- central nervous system (CNS)
- cerebrospinal fluid (CSF)
- choreoathetosis
- choreoid
- decerebrate posturing
- decorticate posturing
- diplegia
- dyskinetic
- graphesthesia
- hemiplegia
- infantile spasms
- kinesthesia
- neuron
- paraplegia
- peripheral nervous system (PNS)
- pulse pressure
- quadriplegia
- status epilepticus
- stereognosis

Objectives

After mastering the contents of this chapter, you should be able to:

1. Describe common neurologic disorders in children.
2. Assess a child with a neurologic disorder.
3. Formulate nursing diagnoses for the child with a neurologic disorder.
4. Establish appropriate outcomes for the child with a neurologic disorder.
5. Plan nursing care for the child with a neurologic disorder.
6. Implement nursing care, such as monitoring medicine compliance, for the child with a neurologic disorder.
7. Evaluate outcomes for achievement and effectiveness of care.
8. Identify National Health Goals related to neurologic disorders and children that nurses could be instrumental in helping the nation achieve.
9. Identify areas related to care of children with neurologic disorders that could benefit from additional nursing research or application of evidence-based practice.
10. Analyze ways that care of the child with a neurologic disorder can be optimally family centered.
11. Integrate knowledge of neurologic disorders and the nursing process to achieve quality maternal and child health nursing care.

Tasha is a 2-year-old girl who has just been diagnosed with cerebral palsy. Her parents are visibly upset by this information. Her father says, "My poor little girl, what's going to happen to her? What are we going to do?" Her mother asks, "How can we take care of her? How will she ever be independent?"

The discovery of a neurologic disorder in a child can be devastating to the parents. Helping the family deal with the possible long-term and permanent effects of the disorder is essential. Nurses play a key role in providing support and education to the parents and child to promote the child's optimal level of functioning.

Previous chapters described the normal growth and development in children and the nursing care of the child with a disorder of other systems. This chapter adds information about the dramatic changes, both physical and psychosocial, that occur when a child develops a neurologic disorder. This is important information because it builds a base for care and health teaching for children with these disorders.

After you've studied the chapter, answer the Critical Thinking Exercises at the end of the chapter and then access the on-line study activities (http://connection.lww.com) *to further sharpen your skills and test your knowledge.*

Neurologic disorders encompass a wide array of problems resulting from congenital disorders, acquired dysfunction, infection, or trauma. Many of these disorders can cause severe illness. Even if the problems are considered minor, they can result in life-threatening complications. In addition, because neural tissue does not have the regenerative power of other body tissue, any nervous system degeneration is permanent. Whenever possible, prevention must be the highest priority for keeping the nervous system healthy. When degeneration has already occurred, nursing care often focuses on helping the child and family develop strategies for dealing with the associated loss in mental or physical functioning, in making the child comfortable, and in providing an environment conducive to the child's growth and self-esteem. Two major causes of neurologic dysfunction in children have been addressed by the National Health Goals. These are shown in the Focus on National Health Goals box.

FOCUS ON NATIONAL HEALTH GOALS

Bacterial meningitis and head injuries are major causes of neurologic damage and subsequent disability in children. Three National Health Goals address children with disabilities:

- Reduce the proportion of children and adolescents with disabilities who report being sad, unhappy, or depressed from a baseline of 31% to a target level of 17%.
- Reduce the number of people 21 years of age and younger with disabilities in congregate care facilities from a baseline of 24,300 to 0.
- Increase the proportion of children and youth with disabilities who spend at least 80% of their time in regular education programs from 45% to 60% (DHHS, 2000).

Nurses can be instrumental in helping the nation achieve these goals through prevention of neurologic injury by educating children and parents about the use of helmets for bicycle and motorcycle safety, by administering and teaching paramedical personnel to administer safe care at accident scenes so children's heads and necks are protected, and by decreasing the possible spread of bacterial meningitis by using good handwashing and infection control precautions in hospitals.

Topics of nursing research that might help in the prevention of neurologic injury or disease and subsequent disability include: What kind of programs can school nurses initiate that would effectively teach bicycle safety? Could serious outcomes of bacterial meningitis be reduced if parents were educated about the symptoms of meningitis and thus were able to bring children with such symptoms to health care facilities earlier?

NURSING PROCESS OVERVIEW

For Care of the Child With a Neurologic System Disorder

Assessment

Neurologic disorders often present with vague symptoms of something being wrong. Parents may indicate that their child "seems to be walking strangely" or is "just not herself." A thorough history and neurologic examination provide the best source of information regarding the cause of the child's problem. Possible findings are highlighted in Assessing the Child for Signs and Symptoms of a Neurologic Disorder.

The neurologic examination covers six areas of neurologic functioning, including mental or cognitive processes as well as motor and sensory functioning. When more information is needed, numerous diagnostic laboratory tests may be ordered. The parents and child will need considerable support throughout the assessment process. Although the neurologic examination may be made "fun" for a child, other procedures such as a computed tomography (CT) scan or lumbar puncture can be frightening. Additionally, the anxiety of not knowing what is wrong and fearing the worst can make the waiting period for test results especially difficult for the child's parents.

Nursing Diagnosis

Nursing diagnoses for children with neurologic disorders vary according to the child's needs. Initially, the child may need emergency care and constant observation, and the parents may need to discuss their fears about their child's illness. If the child undergoes surgery, nursing diagnoses should address immediate preoperative and postoperative care and long-term

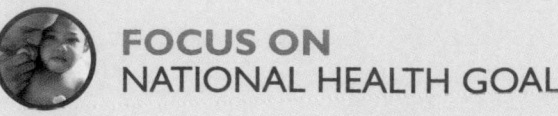

ASSESSING the Child for Signs and Symptoms of a Neurologic Disorder

History

Chief concern: Seizure, loss of consciousness, delay in developmental tasks, headache, clumsiness at motor tasks.
Past medical history: Infection during pregnancy; difficult birth; difficulty with initiating respirations at birth; head injury from fall or accident.
Family medical history: History of seizures or headache in other family members.

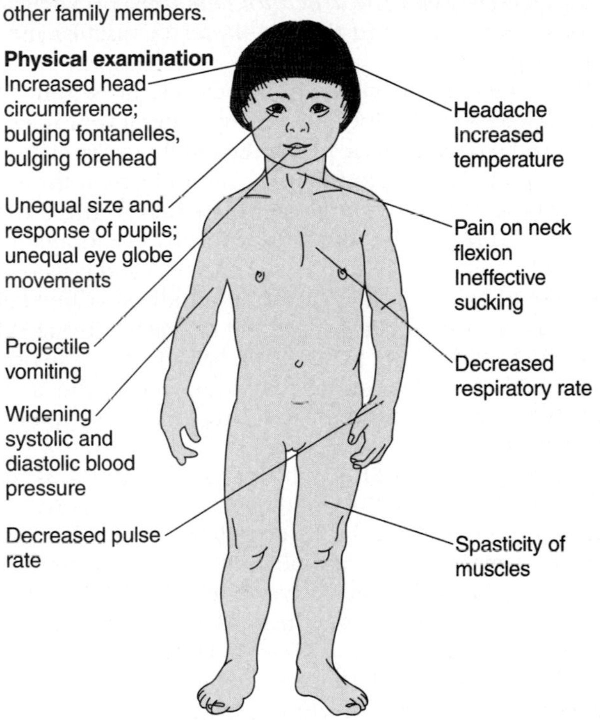

care such as rehabilitation and home care, taking into account the child's specific limitations and health care needs. Two nursing diagnoses should be kept in mind throughout these treatment phases:

- Risk for disuse syndrome related to neurologic deficit affecting one area of functioning
- Interrupted family processes related to stress associated with the long-term effects of the neurologic dysfunction

Other nursing diagnoses are described along with specific disorders in this chapter.

Outcome Identification and Planning

Be realistic when establishing outcomes. Children who have permanent limitations may not be able to achieve in some areas. When neurologic disorders are first diagnosed, parents may be able to focus only on the short term, such as the child will survive meningitis; the child has stopped convulsing. Later, they may need help to look at the long-term picture: Will they need assistance to care for the child at home? What type of education can be obtained? What type of exercise program will be required?

Before a diagnosis is confirmed, parents may attribute their child's functional deficits to immaturity (she is not walking yet because she is simply too young). They insist that, with age, her ability to function will improve. They are unable to make plans because they have not accepted their child's neurologic deficits. Until this occurs, they will not be ready for specific planning. When parents begin to adjust to the new reality, they will need support and help in solving problems. Anticipate the need for assistance from outside organizations.

Implementation

Nursing interventions for the child with a neurologic problem must address both short- and long-term needs. For instance, while feeding an infant with increased intracranial pressure (ICP), demonstrate a caring attitude by showing her parents how to handle her gently. For parents of a child with seizures, explain that turning him gently to his side will prevent him from choking. This will help them feel less anxious about future seizures. The child, too, will feel more in control of his illness if he believes that both he and his parents will be able to handle any acute symptoms. Providing nursing care that meets everyone's needs takes a great deal of sensitivity and planning (see Focus on Multidisciplinary Care).

Long-term care needs can be a source of stress, physically, emotionally, socially, and financially. Numerous organizations are available for assistance and support. Some organizations concerned with children with neurologic disorders include the following:

Epilepsy Foundation of America (*www.efa.org*)
National Information Center for Children and Youth with Disabilities (*www.nichcy.org*)

FOCUS ON MULTIDISCIPLINARY CARE

A large number of health care providers are often necessary to give comprehensive care to a child with a neurologic disorder: a neurologist; a primary care provider; physical therapists; technicians to complete electroencephalograms (EEG), laboratory tests, or CT scans; nurses skilled in neurosurgical care; and the school nurse who monitors long-term follow-up. Unlicensed assistive personnel may be assigned to accompany children to hospital departments for diagnostic tests such as EEG and CT scan because these tests are time consuming.

Any of these people may be present when a child with a neurologic disorder has a seizure. Reinforce the need to remain calm in the light of this very sudden change in behavior. Modeling calm behavior helps keep the child safe and also helps the parents and the child to accept a diagnosis of recurrent seizures.

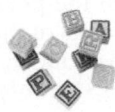

National Fibromatosis Foundation (*www.nf.org*)
National Spinal Cord Injury Association (*www.spinalcord.org*)
United Cerebral Palsy Association (*www.ucp.org*)

Outcome Evaluation

Evaluation of the child with a neurologic disorder should address not only the child's progress in regaining physical function but also his or her level of self-esteem. Further planning to increase the child's self-esteem is necessary if the disorder is long-term. Some examples indicating achievement of possible outcomes may include:

- Child is aware of potential for injury related to recurrent seizures.
- Family members state they are able to maintain family cohesiveness yet maintain contact with hospitalized child.
- Child practices exercises daily to reduce possibility of contracture from disuse syndrome.

ANATOMY AND PHYSIOLOGY OF THE NERVOUS SYSTEM

Nerve cells (**neurons**) are unique among body cells in that, instead of being compact, they consist of a cell nucleus and extensions: one axon and several dendrites. The *dendrite* transmits impulses to the cell nucleus; the *axon* transmits impulses from the cell nucleus to body organs. These cells vary in size, ranging from a few inches to several feet long, reaching from distant body sites such as the feet, through the spinal cord, and to the brain. Although their great length is vital to motor and sensory function, it also makes nerve cells more susceptible to injury than other body cells are.

The nervous system continues to mature through the first 12 years of life. It actually consists of two separate systems: the **central nervous system (CNS)** and the **peripheral nervous system (PNS).** The PNS consists of the cranial nerves, the spinal nerves, and the somatic and visceral divisions. The visceral division includes the autonomic system.

The CNS consists of the brain, the spinal cord, and the surrounding membranes or meninges that protect the delicate tissues from normal trauma. These tissues are also protected by the skull, the vertebral column, and the **cerebrospinal fluid (CSF),** the fluid in the subarachnoid space, which serves as a cushion.

The brain is covered by three membranes: the *dura mater* (a fibrous, connective tissue structure containing many blood vessels), the *arachnoid membrane* (a delicate serous membrane), and the *pia mater* (a vascular membrane; Fig. 49-1).

Four fluid-filled cavities, or ventricles, lie within the brain (Fig. 49-2). CSF forms in the two lateral ventricles in the choroid plexus of the pia mater and flows through the foramens of Monro into the third ventricle, then through a narrow canal (the aqueduct of Sylvius) to the fourth ventricle. It leaves the fourth ventricle by the foramen of Magendie and the two foramens of Lushka and flows into the cisterna magna, a collection pool at the base of the skull. From the cisterna magna, the fluid circulates to the subarachnoid space of the spinal cord, bathing both the brain and spinal cord. The fluid is then absorbed by the arachnoid membrane. The time span for replacement is approximately 6 h.

The properties of CSF are shown in Table 49-1. It is basically a colorless, alkaline fluid with a specific gravity of approximately 1.004 to 1.008, containing traces of protein, glucose, lymphocytes, and body salts. The fluid circulates downward to the second sacral vertebral level (S2). In infants, the spinal cord ends at the third lumbar vertebra (L3); in adolescents and adults, at L1 or L2. Thus, a space near the cord base contains CSF that can be tapped safely (lumbar puncture) without fear of causing spinal cord damage.

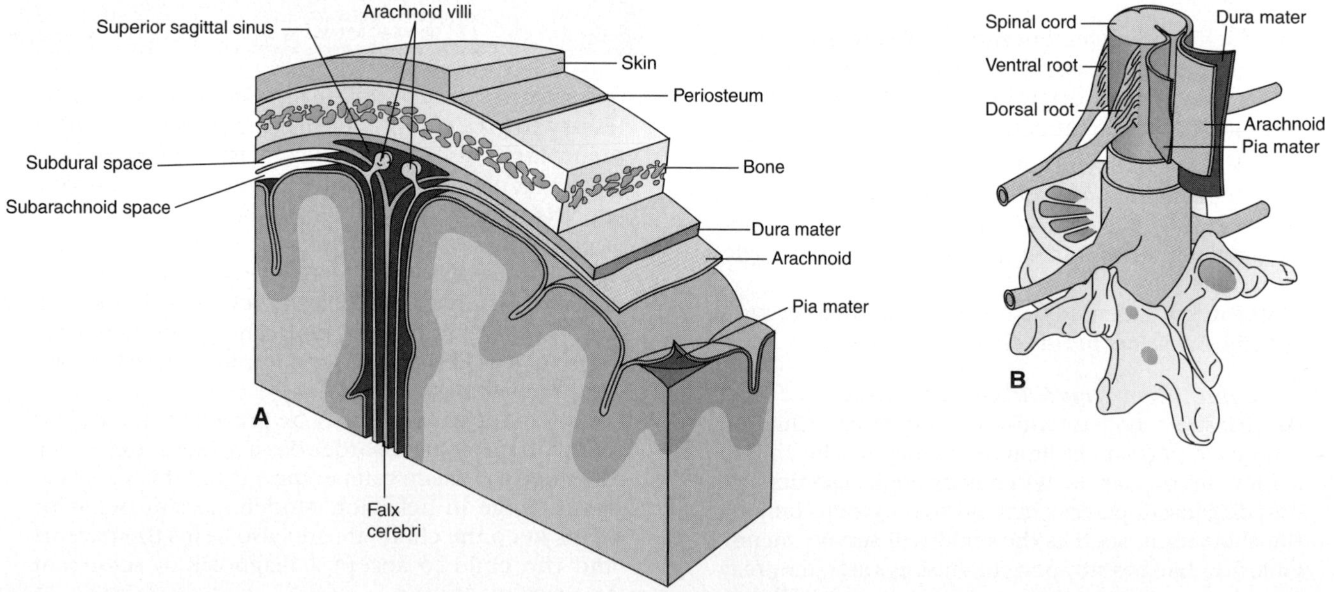

FIGURE 49.1 Meninges of the (*A*) brain and (*B*) spinal cord.

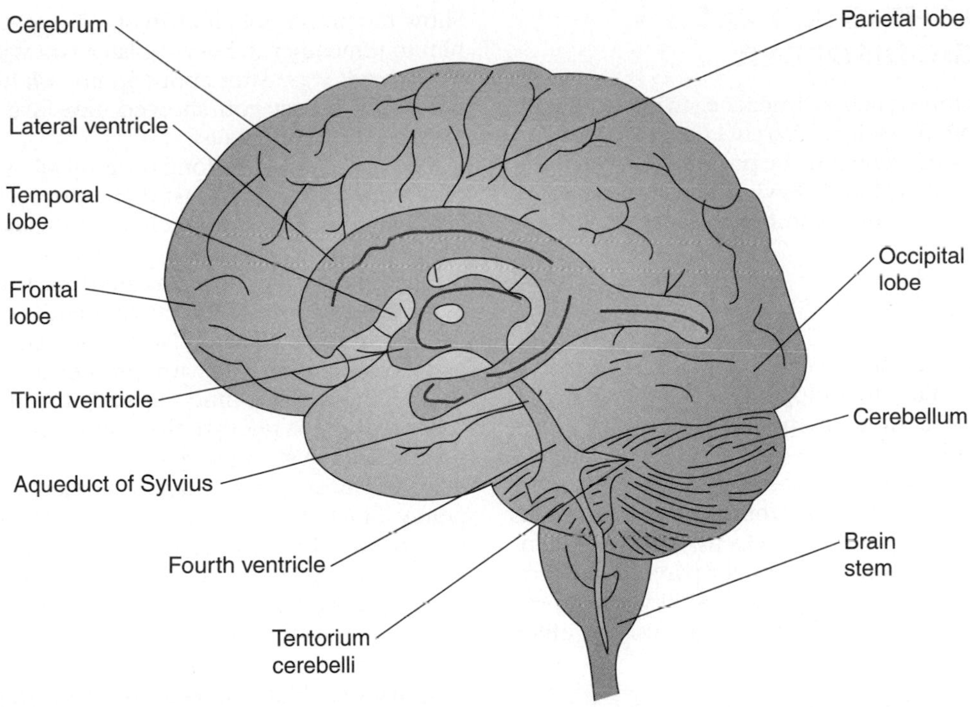

FIGURE 49.2 Ventricles of the brain. Cerebrospinal fluid flows from the lateral ventricles into the third ventricle, then through the narrow aqueduct of Sylvius to the fourth ventricle.

TABLE 49.1 Normal Properties of Cerebrospinal Fluid

PARAMETER	NORMAL FINDING	POSSIBLE SIGNIFICANCE
Opening pressure	60–160 cm H_2O	Lowered pressure generally indicates that there is subarachnoid obstruction in the spinal column above the puncture site.
		Elevated pressure suggests intracranial compression, hemorrhage, or infection.
		Pressure will increase if a child coughs or pressure is applied to the external jugular vein (Valsalva maneuver).
Appearance	Clear and colorless	If cloudy, possible infection and an increased number of white blood cells.
		If reddened, probably red blood cells.
Cell count	0–8 mm^3	Granulocytes are suggestive of CSF infection.
		Lymphocytes suggest meningeal irritation and inflammation.
		A few of both red and white blood cells are present in the newborn from the trauma of birth.
Protein	15–45 mg/100 mL	Elevated count (over 45/100 mL) occurs if red blood cells are present.
		If both protein content and red blood cell count are elevated, meningitis or subarachnoid hemorrhage is suggested.
		If protein content alone is elevated, it is more suggestive of a degenerative process such as multiple sclerosis.
Glucose	60%–80% of serum glucose level	Decreased glucose level suggests that a glycolytic process is occurring.
		Bacterial meningitis causes a marked decrease in CSF glucose; invasion of fungi, yeast, tuberculosis, or protozoans into the CSF will result in some decrease in glucose level.
		Viral infections do not cause a decrease in CSF glucose level and may occasionally cause a slight increase.
Albumin/globulin (A/G)	8:1	Increase suggestive of infection or A/G ratio neurologic disorder.

ASSESSING THE CHILD WITH A NEUROLOGIC DISORDER

Neurologic symptoms, such as headache, an unsteady gait, or lethargy, are often insidious. Parents need support during diagnostic procedures while the possible cause of these symptoms is being explored. Review the tests and any results with parents so they can better understand their child's disease.

Health History

The child's history may be the first clue in assessing a neurologic disorder. Many neurologic problems may result from fetal injury. The mother's pregnancy history, therefore, is important to obtain.

At primary care visits, ask parents about their child's developmental milestones and ability to perform age-appropriate tasks successfully. The Denver Developmental Screening Test can indicate whether a parent's concern about a preschool child is well founded. Ability to perform well in school is important documentation for the older child.

Neurologic Examination

A complete neurologic examination takes at least 20 min. It requires patience and skill to keep the child's attention while observing for possible indications of neurologic disease. For a full examination, six areas are assessed: cerebral, cranial nerve, cerebellar, motor, sensory, and reflex function.

Cerebral Function

Both general and specific cerebral functions are evaluated. General cerebral function is indicated by level of consciousness, orientation, intelligence, performance, mood, and general behavior.

Evaluate the child's level of consciousness through conversation. Note any drowsiness or lethargy and whether the child is oriented to his surroundings. Allow the child to answer questions without prompting, and listen carefully that the answer is appropriate to the question.

Orientation refers to whether a child is aware of who he is, where he is, and what day it is (person, place, and time). Be careful to take into account the child's age and development; children younger than 4 years of age may not know both their first and last names. Children may be of school age before they know their address. Children younger than 7 or 8 years of age may have difficulty with the days of the week, confusing "yesterday" with "today" or "tomorrow." Generally, you will be able to sense whether they are in touch with their surroundings and have a clear sense of self.

Intellectual performance can be determined by the child's score on a standard intelligence test. Estimates of intellectual function can be made by asking the child questions on several topics. *Immediate recall* is the ability to retain a concept for a short time. Ask the child to repeat numbers after you. The child who is 4 years old can usually repeat three digits. The child older than 6 years can repeat five digits. *Recent memory* covers a slightly longer period. Show the preschool child an object such as a key and ask him to remember it, because later you will ask him to tell you what it was. After about 5 min, ask him if he remembers what object you showed him. Ask the older child what he ate for breakfast.

Remote memory is long-term recall. Ask preschoolers what they ate for breakfast that morning (to them, it was a long time ago); ask older children the name of their first-grade teacher.

Specific cerebral function can be measured by assessing language, sensory interpretation, and motor integration. When assessing language, listen to the child's ability to articulate. Remember that many preschoolers substitute "w" for "r," saying "west time" instead of "rest time."

Stereognosis refers to the ability to recognize an object by touch and tests sensory interpretation. Ask the child to close her eyes; place a familiar object, such as a key, a penny, or a bottle cap, in her hand and ask her to identify it. This is something even preschoolers are able to do.

Graphesthesia is the ability to recognize a shape that has been traced on the skin. Ask a preschooler to close his eyes, then trace first a circle, then a square, on the back of his hand; ask him if the shapes are the same or different. Be sure that the child understands the concept of "different" by first showing him objects such as two keys and a bottle cap and document that he is able to identify the keys as being the same and the bottle cap as being different. For the older child, trace a number (8, 3, 0, and 1 work well) and ask the child to identify each one.

Kinesthesia is the ability to distinguish movement. Have the child close her eyes and extend her hands in front of her. Raise one of her fingers and ask her if it is up or down. Hold the finger by its sides so that your other fingers do not brush against the child's palm or the back of her hand (this will reveal the finger position). Repeat the same movement with a toe on each foot. For preschoolers, first determine whether the child understands the concept of up and down.

Measure motor integration by asking the child to perform a complex motor skill, such as folding a piece of paper and putting it into an envelope. A child of 4 years and older should be able to do this neatly.

Children do best when these tests are presented as a game. Be certain to convey that there are no right or wrong answers. A child who believes that he has failed these tests may not respond well to further testing.

Cranial Nerve Function

Testing for cranial nerve function consists of assessing each pair of cranial nerves separately. This is described in Table 49-2.

Cerebellar Function

Tests for cerebellar function are tests for normal balance and coordination. Observe the child walking. Does he do so naturally and freely? (Most children walk self-consciously when being observed.) Ask the child to stand on one foot. A child as young as 4 years should be able to do this for as long as 5 seconds. Ask him to attempt a tandem walk (walk a straight line, one foot directly in front of the other, heel

TABLE 49.2 Cranial Nerve Function

CRANIAL NERVE	FUNCTION	ASSESSMENT
I (olfactory)	Sense of smell	Assess child's ability to recognize common odors (eg, peanut butter or an orange) while eyes are closed.
II (optic)	Vision	Assess vision fields and visual acuity, and examine retinas.
III (oculomotor)	Motor control and sensation for eye muscles and upper eyelid elevation	Assess ability to move eyes to follow an object in all directions. Note nystagmus (jerking motion). Assess pupillary size, equality, and reaction to light. Cranial nerves II, IV, and VI tested together.
IV (trochlear)	Movement of major eye globe muscles	As above.
V (trigeminal)	Mastication muscles and some facial sensations	Assess ability to discern light touch to test sensory component; assess symmetry and strength of bite to test motor component.
VI (abducens)	Movement and muscle sense of eye globe	As with nerves III and IV.
VII (facial)	Impulses for hyoid and facial muscles, salivation, and taste	Assess motor strength by asking child to close eyes while you attempt to open them. Note symmetry of facial expression (such as smile) and movement (such as wrinkling forehead). Assess taste by asking child to identify salt or sugar.
VIII (acoustic)	Equilibration and hearing	Assess hearing by the response to a whispered word or a Weber or Rinne test. Equilibrium is not tested routinely.
IX (glossopharyngeal)	Motor impulses to heart and other organs; sensation from pharynx, thorax, and abdominal organs	Assess gag reflex by pressing on rear of tongue with tongue blade. Note midline uvula (tested together with 10th cranial nerve).
X (vagus)	Swallowing and gag reflexes	Assess ability to swallow; elicit gag reflex by pressing a tongue blade on posterior tongue.
XI (accessory)	Impulses to striated muscles of pharynx and shoulders	Ask child to turn head to the side; try to turn it to center. Ask the child to elevate shoulders while you press down on them.
XII (hypoglossal)	Motor impulses to tongue and skeletal muscles; sensation from skin and viscera	Ask child to protrude tongue. Assess for tremors. Ask child to press on side of cheek with tongue; assess tongue strength.

touching toe; Fig. 49-3*A*). A child older than 4 years should be able to do this for about four consecutive steps. Ask the child to touch his nose with his finger, then reach and touch your finger with the same hand (held about 1½ feet in front of him; Figure 49-3*B*). Tell him to repeat this action; move your finger to a new position each time. The average child rarely reaches past your finger or stops before touching it.

Ask the child to pat one knee with the palm of her hand, then quickly turn the hand over and pat the knee with the back of her hand; repeat over and over. Children should be able to do this rapid, coordinated motion without much difficulty. Ask her to do this one hand at a time. Preschoolers will mirror the movement of the actively moving hand by moving the inactive hand as well. Older children should not demonstrate this (or should show only a small amount of movement).

Ask the child to touch each finger on one hand with the thumb of that hand in rapid succession. Ask him to run the heel of one foot down the front of his other leg while he is lying supine (he should be able to do this without "running off" the leg). While he is still lying on the examining table, ask him to close his eyes and to draw a circle or figure 8 in the air with his foot.

Tests of cerebellar function are all fun for children to do, as long as they know that there are no passes or failures. Show approval for effort even if they are having difficulty with the task, so they have confidence to try another one.

Motor Function

Muscle size, strength, and tone are part of motor function assessment. Compare the size of the extremities on each side. If in doubt about symmetry, measure the circumference of the calves or thighs or upper and lower arms for comparison. Palpate muscles for tone. Move the extremities through passive range of motion; evaluate for symmetry, spasticity, and flaccidity bilaterally. Ask the child to extend her arms in front of her and resist your action as you push down or up on her hands, or push them out to the side. Do the same with the lower extremities.

Sensory Function

If children's sensory systems are intact, they should be able to distinguish light touch, pain, vibration, hot, and cold. Have a child close his eyes and then ask him to point to the

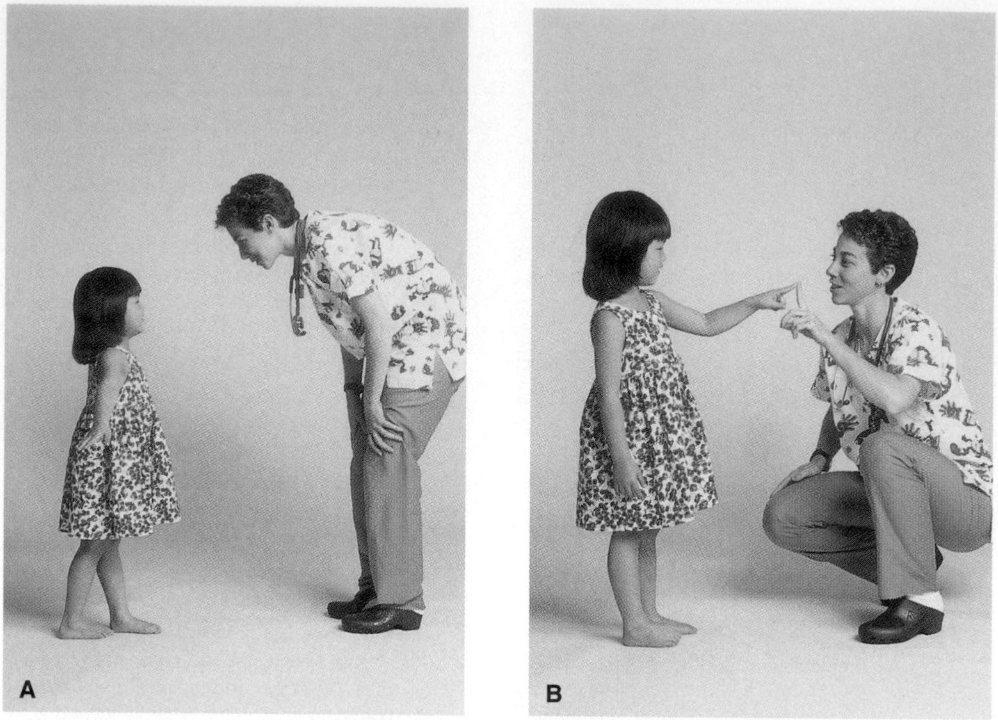

FIGURE 49.3 Cerebellar function tests. (*A*) A child attempting a tandem walk. (*B*) Nose-to-finger test.

spot where you touch him with an object. Light touch is tested by using a wisp of cotton, deep pressure by pressure of your finger, pain by a safety pin, temperature by test tubes filled with hot or cold water. Vibration is tested by touching the child's bony prominences (iliac crest, elbows, knees) with a vibrating tuning fork. Warn the child that on pin testing, he will feel a momentary prick. Otherwise, he may be unwilling to close his eyes again for further testing.

Reflex Testing

Deep tendon reflex testing, which is part of a primary physical assessment (see Chapter 33), is also a basic part of a neurologic assessment. In newborns, reflex testing is especially important, because the infant cannot perform tasks on command to demonstrate the range of neurologic function (see Chapter 23).

Diagnostic Testing

A variety of diagnostic tests may be ordered to provide more information should any abnormalities be detected in the health history, physical examination, or neurologic examination. Many of these tests are invasive, and it is best to try to schedule the least invasive procedures first, before the painful or more frightening procedures are done, to help promote the child's cooperation. Ensuring that the child and the child's family are well prepared for these procedures is an important nursing responsibility. When explaining tests, take into account not only the child's chronologic age but also the child's level of cognitive functioning. Otherwise, explanations may not be well understood. Be sure also to provide an explanation that includes a description of all of the sensory experiences the child might undergo, that is, not only what will be done but also how the child might feel, or what he or she might see or hear or even smell or taste (if appropriate).

Lumbar Puncture

Lumbar puncture involves the introduction of a needle into the subarachnoid space (under the arachnoid membrane) at the level of L4 or L5 to withdraw CSF for analysis. The procedure is used most frequently to diagnose hemorrhage or infection in the CNS or to diagnose an obstruction of CSF flow. Lumbar puncture is contraindicated if the skin over the needle insertion site is infected (to avoid introducing pathogens into the CSF) or if there is a suspected elevation of CSF pressure. In the latter instance, if fluid is removed, the increased pressure in the intracranial space could cause the brain stem to be drawn down into the spinal cord space, compressing the medulla and compromising the action of the cardiac and respiratory centers. EMLA or lidocaine can be applied to the puncture site 1 h before the procedure to reduce pain. Alternatively, the child may receive conscious sedation (see Chapter 38).

For the procedure, the newborn is seated upright with the head bent forward (Fig. 49-4*A*). The older infant or child is placed on one side on the examining table. The head is flexed forward, the knees are flexed on his abdomen, and the back is arched as much as possible. This position opens the space between the lumbar vertebrae, facilitating needle insertion (Fig. 49-4*B*). Children younger than school age need to be held in this position, because they may be so frightened by someone working on their back unseen that they are unable to hold this arched posi-

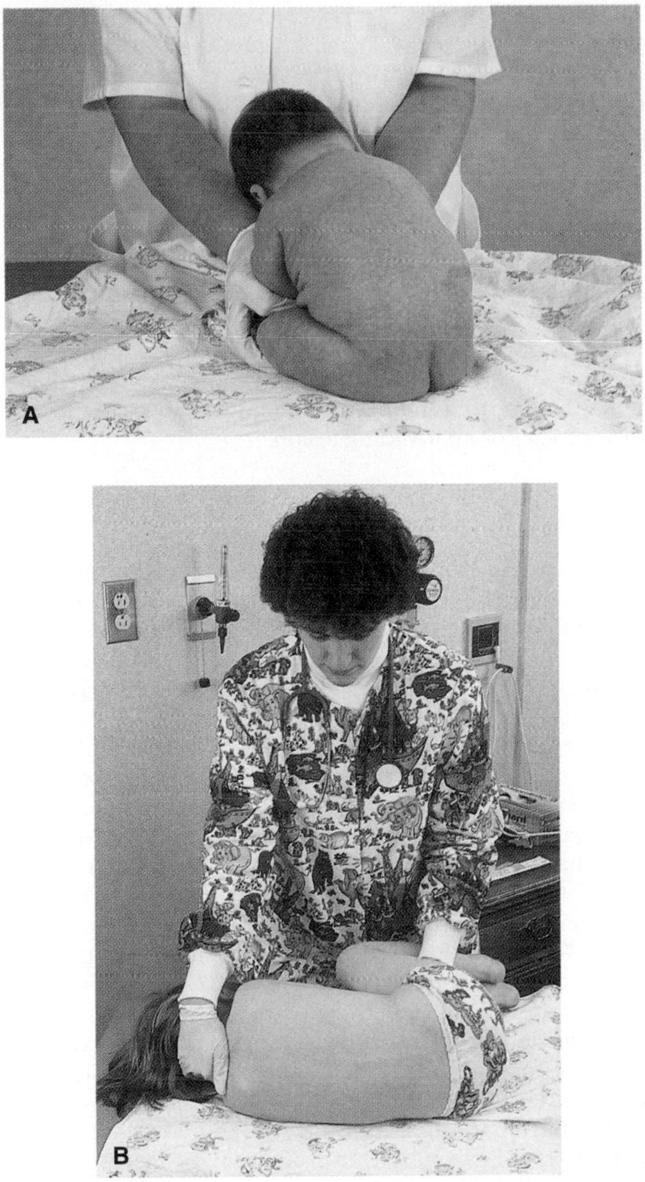

FIGURE 49.4 (A) Positioning an infant for a lumbar puncture. (B) Positioning a young child for a lumbar puncture.

tion; they may try to turn over or turn their head to see what is happening. It helps a school-age child or adolescent if you stand by the table facing him and gently rest your hand on the back of his head, keeping it bent forward. This helps to maintain good position without the impression of restraining him.

Children need good preparation for a lumbar puncture, because they cannot see what is happening. Be certain that they know that the health care provider performing the procedure will wash their back with a solution that feels cold and inject a local anesthetic that might sting like a mosquito bite (if an analgesic cream was not applied before the procedure). Caution children that they probably will feel pressure but not pain as the lumbar puncture needle is inserted. Remind them to remain absolutely still throughout the procedure. You might describe the position as "rolling into a ball" or "folding up like an astronaut in a small spaceship." Occasionally during a lumbar puncture, the needle will press against a dorsal nerve root and the child will experience a shooting pain down one leg. If this happens, reassure the child that this feeling passes quickly and does not indicate an injury.

When the insertion stylette is removed and CSF drips from the end of the needle, the procedure has been successful. An initial pressure reading is made, which varies with the child's age. To confirm that the subarachnoid space in the cord is patent with that in the skull, the examiner may ask a child who is older than 3 years to cough, or ask you to press on the child's external jugular during the procedure. Either of these measures will cause an increase of CSF pressure if fluid can flow freely through the subarachnoid space. Typically, three tubes of CSF, containing 2 to 3 mL each, are collected, a closing pressure reading is taken, and the needle is withdrawn. Samples are usually sent for culture, sensitivity, glucose, and presence of red blood cells. Determining if there is an alteration in the albumin–globulin ratio in the CSF and gamma globulin levels also may be evaluated. An increased level of gamma globulin is suggestive of multiple sclerosis or meningitis. The first sample obtained may contain blood or skin pathogens from the puncture, so it should not be the sample sent for determination of red blood cell content or culture. Throughout the procedure, sterile technique must be strictly observed to ensure that an uncontaminated sample of fluid is sent for culture and also to prevent introducing pathogens into the CSF.

Lumbar puncture involves at least momentary pain, so children need to be comforted afterward. Although rare because of the small needle used for insertion, a child may develop a headache after a lumbar puncture as a result of the reduction in CSF volume or invasion of a small air pocket during the puncture. Asking the child to lie flat for about 30 min and drink a glass of fluid can help prevent cerebral irritation caused by air rising in the subarachnoid space and can increase the amount of CSF in the body. Some children may have a headache despite these precautions and may need an analgesic for pain relief. Although post–lumbar puncture headache is seen less frequently in young children than in adults, assessing for it is important to reduce the risk of pain for the child.

If a child had minimally increased CSF pressure at the time of the puncture, closely observe the child after the procedure to prevent respiratory and cardiac difficulty from medulla pressure. An increase in blood pressure or a decrease in pulse and respiration is an important sign of increased intracranial compression. Other important signs include a change in consciousness, pupillary changes, or decrease in motor ability.

Ventricular Tap

In infants, CSF may be obtained by a subdural tap into the ventricle through the coronal suture or anterior fontanelle. A small space on the scalp over the insertion site must be shaved or the hair clipped and the area prepared with an antiseptic. The infant's head must be held firmly while in a supine position to prevent movement during the procedure, which could cause the needle to strike and lacerate meningeal tissue.

Fluid must be removed from this site slowly, rather than suddenly, to prevent a sudden shift in pressure that could cause intracranial hemorrhage. After the procedure, a pressure dressing is applied to the site, and the infant is placed in a semi-Fowler's position to prevent prolonged drainage from the puncture site. After the procedure, comfort the infant or allow the parents to do this to both reduce the stress of a painful procedure and prevent him from crying excessively, an action that could increase ICP.

X-ray Techniques

A flat-plate skull x-ray film may be used to obtain information about increased ICP or skull defects such as fracture or craniosynostosis (premature knitting of cranial sutures). Increased ICP is suggested when skull sutures are separated. When the process is chronic, other subtle changes such as a flattening of the sella turcica or an increase in the convolutions of the inner table of the skull may be present.

Cerebral Angiography. Cerebral angiography is an x-ray study of cerebral blood vessels involving the injection of a contrast material into an extracranial artery. Serial radiographs are taken as the dye flows through the blood vessels of the cerebrum. The injection site chosen is often a femoral artery, although a carotid artery may be used. The study will show any vessel defects or space-occupying lesions that are occluding blood vessels.

Myelography. Myelography is an x-ray study of the spinal cord involving the introduction of a contrast material into the CSF by lumbar puncture. It is used to show the presence of space-occupying lesions of the spinal cord. After the procedure, keep the head of the child's bed elevated to prevent contrast medium from reaching the meninges surrounding the brain.

Computed Tomography. CT involves the use of radiographic images to reveal densities at different levels or layers of brain tissue. It is helpful in confirming the presence of a brain tumor or other encroaching lesions. The study is discussed in further detail in Chapter 36. Single-photon-emission computed tomography (SPECT) is a similar procedure used mainly for blood flow evaluation.

Magnetic Resonance Imaging

Magnetic resonance imaging (MRI) uses magnetic fields to show differences in tissue composition, revealing normal versus abnormal brain tissue very effectively. This is discussed in greater detail in Chapter 36.

Nuclear Medicine Studies

Brain Scan. For a brain scan, a radioactive material is injected intravenously (IV), and, after a fixed time during which the injected material is deposited in cerebral tissue, radioactivity levels over the skull are measured. If the blood–brain barrier is not functioning, the radioactive material will accumulate in specific areas, suggesting possible tumor, subdural hematoma, abscess, or encephalitis.

Positron Emission Tomography. The diagnostic technique of positron emission tomography (PET) involves imaging after injection of positron-emitting radiopharmaceuticals into the brain. These radioactive substances accumulate at diseased areas of the brain or spinal cord. It is extremely accurate in identifying seizure foci.

Echoencephalography

Echoencephalography involves the projection of ultrasound (high-frequency sound waves above the audible range) toward the child's head or spinal cord (a sonogram). Sonography may be used to outline the ventricles of the brain. Because this technique of scanning is noninvasive, produces no discomfort, and has no known complications, it may be repeated frequently to follow changes in the size of ventricles or an invading lesion.

Electroencephalography

The electroencephalogram (EEG) reflects the electrical patterns of the brain. It summarizes the physical and chemical interaction within the brain at the time of the test. Normally, a tracing indicates four types of waves: delta (1 to 3 waves/s), theta (4 to 7 waves/s), alpha (8 to 12 waves/s), and beta (13 to 20 waves/s).

To reduce extraneous movements of the eyes, head, or muscles that will affect the tracing, children must be cooperative and quiet during the procedure. Therefore, good preparation and encouragement are crucial. Caution children that the room will probably be darkened to help them rest. Compare the electrode wires attached to their scalp with adhesive paste to those attached to astronauts in space. Reassure them that these electrodes are not painful. Be careful not to use the word *electrical.* Children as young as 3 years know that electrical wires are ordinarily dangerous and can hurt them. They cannot relax if they are worried that they may be shocked or even electrocuted by the procedure.

If children are unable to lie still and cooperate even after careful explanation, they may need conscious sedation (Olson et al., 2001). Unfortunately, sedation alters the electrical pattern of the cortex and should be avoided if possible. For example, chloral hydrate, a frequently used sedative for this procedure may increase the fast activity of brain waves; chlorpromazine (Thorazine) may increase slow activity. Because phenobarbital and phenytoin sodium (diphenylhydantoin; Dilantin) also cause an increase in fast activity, be sure to inform the person interpreting the recording what medication the child is receiving. Although usually unnecessary, be sure parents know if anticonvulsant medication should be withheld on the morning of an EEG to reduce the effect of medications on tracings.

Although EEGs can show important information about brain activity, they are not helpful in all circumstances. For example, approximately 15% of children who are absolutely normal clinically demonstrate some abnormality on an EEG. Most brain tumors in pediatric patients are in the posterior fossa. The activity of this region does not show up well on an EEG. An EEG may appear normal even when there is a brain tumor, unless the tumor is pressing on more distal brain portions. On inspecting the symmetry of hemispheres, local lesions may be suggested. Where there is a lesion, there will be slower waves, a higher voltage pattern, and an overall more irregular pattern. A subdural lesion (perhaps from a hematoma) can interfere with the transmission of the electrical impulses, and the voltage pattern will be lower.

An EEG is most beneficial in diagnosing absence seizures. The typical pattern with this disorder is discussed later in the chapter.

Visual stimulation, such as having children look at a whirling disk, may be used in connection with EEG, because various types of electrical discharges increase with rapid eye movements. In a child who is sensitive to this type of stimulation, the testing may produce a seizure. If this occurs, the child may be very disturbed and disoriented after the procedure. Describe what has happened, letting him know that things are all right to help him relax.

After an EEG, children will be sleepy if they have been sedated. Allow them to sleep as long as needed.

✔ CHECKPOINT QUESTIONS

1. How would you assess for graphesthesia?
2. What cranial nerve is assessed when you ask a child to raise his shoulders as you push against them?

HEALTH PROMOTION AND RISK MANAGEMENT

Health promotion for nervous system health begins prenatally with measures to ensure optimal fetal growth and development and prevention of problems associated with anoxia. It continues throughout childhood with routine health maintenance visits, screening for possible neurologic or developmental problems, and ensuring immunizations to prevent sequelae of typical childhood infections such as measles or chickenpox. Nurses play a key role in providing education to parents about the importance of obtaining immunizations and completing medication therapy to ensure complete resolution of an infection.

Parents also need anticipatory guidance about safety measures to prevent injury, specifically, head and spinal cord injury. Reinforce the need for seat belts and child restraints while riding in automobiles, and use of protective gear, such as helmets, for bicycle and motorcycle riding.

For the child with seizures, parents need instructions to prevent injury during a seizure (see discussion later in the chapter) and to administer anticonvulsants conscientiously. Guidelines for safe administration of anticonvulsants include the following:

- Caution children to be careful around motor vehicles and electrical equipment because many anticonvulsants cause drowsiness.
- Advise the child and parents to observe for easy bruising because several anticonvulsants may suppress bone marrow function.
- Caution the adolescent to avoid alcohol while taking anticonvulsants because alcohol can potentiate the CNS effects of some anticonvulsants.
- Use caution when administering anticonvulsants to children with liver disease, because many of these drugs are metabolized by the liver.
- Caution the child and parents not to discontinue anticonvulsant therapy abruptly, because this may lead to uncontrolled seizures.
- Remind parents about the need for follow-up blood tests to evaluate the drug level. Maintaining a therapeutic blood level enhances the drug's effectiveness and minimizes the risk for toxicity.

For the child with a long-term neurologic disorder, rehabilitation and early intervention play a major role in reducing the risk of complications and in promoting the child's and family's optimal level of functioning.

INCREASED INTRACRANIAL PRESSURE

Increased ICP is not a single disorder but a sign that may occur with many neurologic disorders. When caring for a child with a potential neurologic disorder, it is important to observe him or her closely for this sign.

Increased ICP may occur with an increase in the CSF volume, blood entering the CSF, cerebral edema, or space-occupying lesions such as tumors. Examples that lead to increased ICP may include:

- Birth trauma or hydrocephalus
- Head trauma from an accident
- Infection
- Brain tumor
- Guillain-Barré syndrome

The rate at which symptoms develop depends on the cause and the ability of the child's skull to expand to accommodate the increased pressure. Children with open fontanelles can withstand more pressure without brain damage than older children, whose suture lines and fontanelles have already closed.

Assessment

Assessment of neurologic function may involve only a few quick procedures, such as obtaining vital signs, evaluating pupil response, determining level of consciousness and motor and sensory function, or more elaborate electronic monitoring. Signs and symptoms of ICP are shown in Table 49-3.

With increased ICP, symptoms are often subtle at first. The child may report a headache, irritability or restlessness. Infants with a headache become increasingly fussy or difficult to comfort. Changes in vital signs may be important indicators of ICP. Growing pressure on the brain stem, which controls respiration and cardiac activity, causes pulse and respirations to slow. Compression of cranial vessels leads to a compensatory increase in blood pressure (or **pulse pressure,** the gap between systolic and diastolic blood pressure). Pressure on the hypothalamus, the temperature-regulating center of the body, causes an increase in temperature. These changes may occur gradually, so a single measurement may not show the extent of the change. Always compare the new information against all recordings taken in the last 24 h.

TABLE 49.3 Signs and Symptoms of Increased Intracranial Pressure

SIGN OR SYMPTOM	INDICATION OF INCREASED ICP
Increased head circumference	An increase >2 cm/month in first 3 months of life, >1 cm/month in the second 3 months, and >0.5 cm/month for the next 6 months
Fontanelle changes	Anterior fontanelle tense and bulging; closing late
Vomiting	Occurring in the absence of nausea, on awakening in morning or after nap. Possibly projectile
Eye changes	Diplopia (double vision) from pressure on abducens nerves; white of sclera evident over pupil (setting sun sign); limited visual fields, papilledema
Vital sign changes	Elevated temperature and blood pressure; decreased pulse and respiration rates
Pain	Headache, often present on awakening and standing.
	Increasing with straining at stool (Valsalva maneuver) or holding breath
Mentation	Irritability, altered consciousness such as sleepiness

Ocular changes may indicate that pressure is increasing posterior to the eye globe. One obvious abnormality may be a dilated pupil suggesting third cranial nerve compression. Test pupil reactivity by shining a light into each eye. To elicit the most dramatic and sudden response, bring the light to the child's eye from the side or down from the forehead, to make it appear suddenly rather than gradually. Repeat this with the other eye. Each pupil should constrict, and the constriction should be equal bilaterally.

Consensual constriction should also be noted. As you shine the light on the right pupil, the left pupil also should constrict. The same is true when testing the left eye (the right pupil should constrict).

If the child is alert and able to cooperate, have him follow the light through the six cardinal positions of gaze and test convergence (ability to follow the light as it approaches closer and closer to the nose). Note any tendency toward strabismus, nystagmus (constant eye movement), "sunset eyes" (white sclera showing over the top of the cornea), or inability to follow the light into any quadrant. Be specific about what you document. "Inability to follow light" is not nearly as informative as "inability to follow light into left superior field. Vertical nystagmus noted as child follows light into other fields."

While lying supine, normally, a child will turn his eyes to the left if you turn his head gently but rapidly to the right, and vice versa (doll's eye reflex). If a child has increased ICP, this phenomenon will be absent. (This is useful in assessing a comatose child who is unable to cooperate by following a light.) An older child may be able to report symptoms such as diplopia. On funduscopic examination, papilledema may be detected (Moe & Seay, 2001).

Assess the child's level of consciousness. If the child is alert but unable to comprehend surroundings, time, or place, this may be the first indication of increased ICP. As pressure increases, this may be followed by a pseudoawake state, in which the child is awake but unable to follow light or noise. Finally, the child may be comatose, unable to be roused by any stimuli. Levels of coma are rated by a Glasgow coma scale. This is discussed in Chapter 52 in connection with assessment for head injury.

Children, like adults, generally become disoriented about time first, then place, then self. It is useful, therefore, to assess that the child is alert enough to answer these questions. Explain that you will be asking these seemingly simple questions periodically to make sure the child can answer them accurately each time. Otherwise, the child may quickly become annoyed with your questions and may refuse to answer them or make up silly answers instead. Or she may pretend to be asleep to avoid being asked.

Be aware that many children, even when healthy, are groggy when they first wake up and, until fully awake, may not be able to say who or where they are. This happens especially when the child is awakened from a dream. Make sure the child is fully awake before attempting to determine his or her level of consciousness.

Be certain that you ask questions appropriate to a child's age. Preschoolers do not usually know the day of the week or concepts such as *morning* or *night*. They do not necessarily know their whole name. With children of this age, it is often more helpful to identify an area of knowledge, for example, colors, with which they are familiar. Every half hour or hour, show them a colored block and ask them its color. Even if they give the wrong answer, it does not matter. Your concern is that they understood your request, not that they actually recognize colors. Also remind parents that you are asking these questions to assess their child's level of consciousness, not to quiz for right answers or to be intrusive. Remind them not to answer for the child.

A good way to test an infant's level of consciousness is to see whether he or she will respond to sounds such as a music box or voices or will reach for an attractive object.

Evaluate motor ability by asking a child to perform some simple motor task such as squeezing your hands. Have her push against your hand with both feet. Have her perform rapid, alternating hand movements, such as turning her hand over and back several times. Evaluate cranial nerves grossly by having her make a face, close her eyes tightly, and show you her teeth. With all these assessments, be sure to evaluate whether the responses are equal and symmetric bilaterally.

Test deep tendon reflexes because these decrease in intensity with decreased level of consciousness. Carefully observe the child's resting posture. When motor control grows weaker because of loss of cell function, characteristic posturing (primitive reflexes) occurs. Cerebral loss is shown mainly by **decorticate posturing.** A child's arms are adducted and flexed on the chest with wrists flexed, hands fisted. The lower extremities are extended and internally rotated, and the feet are plantar flexed (Fig. 49-5*A*). **Decerebrate posturing,** which occurs when the midbrain is not functional, is characterized by rigid extension and adduction of arms and pronation of the wrists with the fingers flexed. The legs are extended, and the feet are plantar flexed (Fig. 49-5*B*).

Observe the child carefully for any seizure activity. However, keep in mind that this is a late sign of increased ICP.

Intracranial Pressure Monitoring

ICP can be measured by several methods:

- An intraventricular catheter inserted through the anterior fontanelle
- A subarachnoid screw or bolt inserted through a burr hole in the skull
- A fiber-optic sensor implanted into the epidural space (or anterior fontanelle in an infant)
- A disposable fiber-optic transducer–tipped catheter inserted through a subarachnoid bolt into the white matter of the brain (Fig. 49-6).

The most accurate of these is the intraventricular catheter (Fig. 49-6*C*). It is threaded into the lateral ventricle, filled with normal saline, and then connected to an external pressure monitor. As pressure in the ventricle changes, it is registered through the filled catheter on an oscilloscope screen and a written printout. This method is also advantageous because it allows for CSF drainage and administration of medication through the catheter (Carpenter et al., 2001).

ICP normally ranges from 1 to 10 mm Hg. A level over 15 mmHg is considered abnormal. As blood pressure rises and falls with the influx of blood through vessels, so does ICP. On a monitor, it appears as A waves (plateau waves) or transient paroxysmal elevations that last for 5 to 20 min with an amplitude of 50 to 100 mm Hg. If brain ischemia is present, these waves increase before other signs, such as a change in blood pressure or pulse rate, become apparent. B waves are short-duration waves ($\frac{1}{2}$ to 2 min) with low amplitude (up to 50 mm Hg). C waves are small, rhythmic waves at a frequency of approximately 6 waves/min. They are related to deviations in the arterial blood pressure (Fig. 49-7). Because A waves appear to reflect brain ischemia, they can be used to signal when the child needs more oxygen.

ICP monitoring also can be used to estimate cerebral perfusion pressure (CPP) or cerebral blood flow (Box 49-1). Normal cerebral perfusion pressure is at least 50 mmHg. Cerebral circulation ceases if ICP ever exceeds arterial pressure, because this obstructs blood flow through the cerebral vessels (McCance & Huether, 2002).

Parents may have difficulty accepting procedures such as the insertion of intraventricular catheters or screws. Explaining the brain's anatomy will help them see that the catheter or screw does not puncture or tear brain tissue. Also be sure to explain that this type of monitoring is advantageous, allowing for early detection should problems arise, thus helping to reduce the risk of further injury or complications.

Therapeutic Management

When ICP increases, the cause of the problem must be identified and removed as quickly as possible to prevent brain injury. In addition to local injury, severe pressure ele-

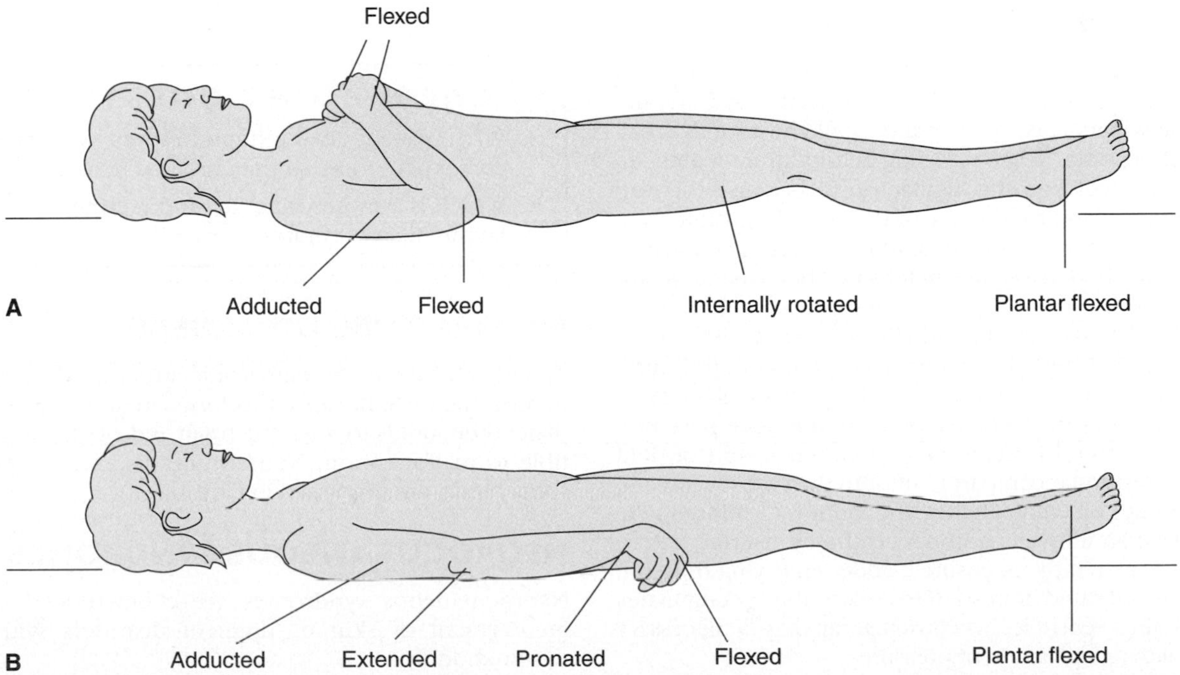

FIGURE 49.5 (*A*) Decorticate posturing. (*B*) Decerebrate posturing.

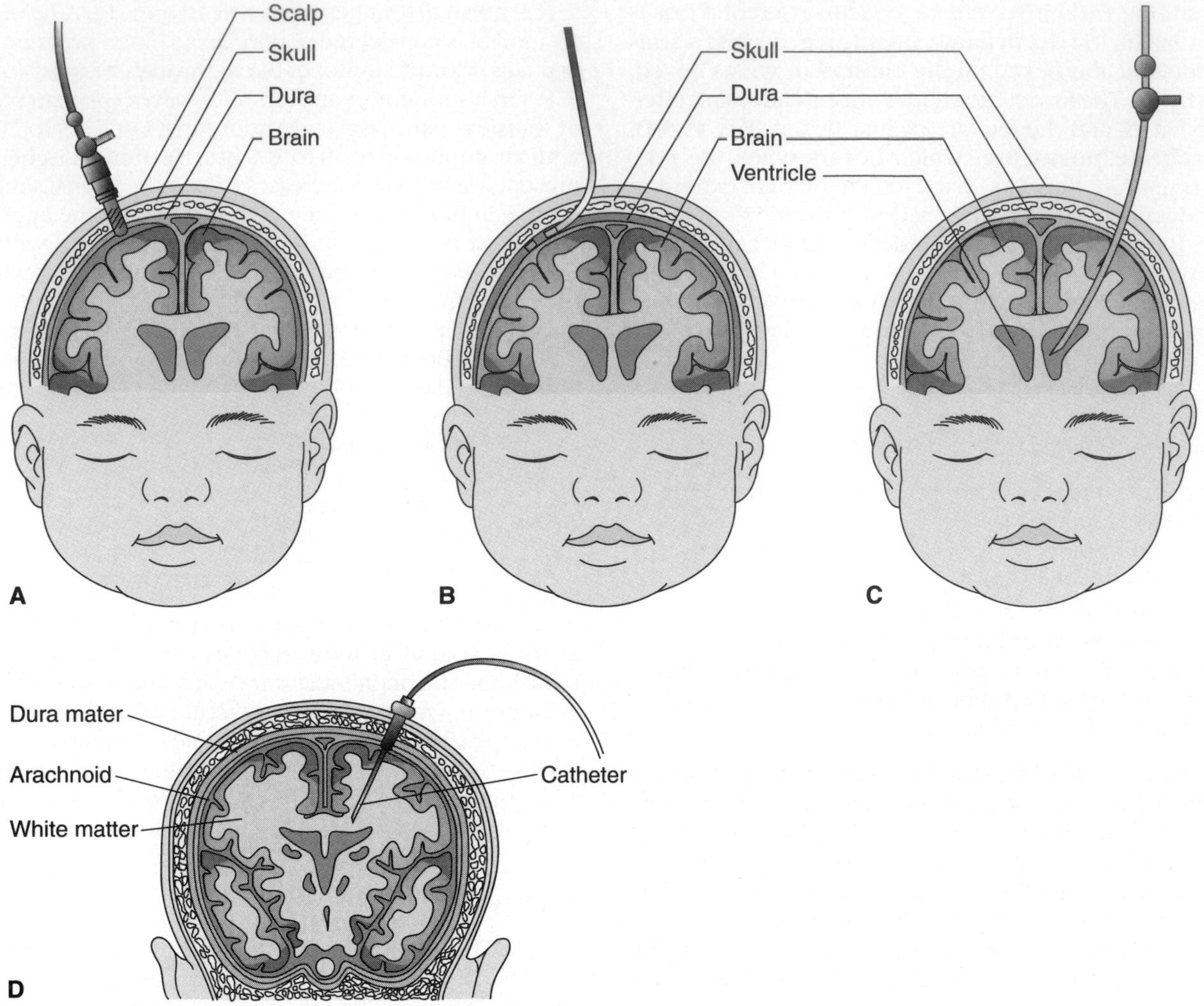

FIGURE 49.6 Devices used to monitor intracranial pressure. (*A*) Subarachnoid screw. (*B*) Epidural sensor. (*C*) Intraventricular catheter. (*D*) Intraparenchymal monitoring.

vation will compress the brain stem and lead to cardiac and respiratory failure. Actions such as coughing, vomiting, and sneezing will increase the ICP and should be kept to a minimum, if possible. When bubbling infants after feeding, do not put pressure on the jugular veins, because this can increase ICP. Monitor the rate of IV fluid administration in such children because overhydration also can increase ICP. Placing the child in a semi-Fowler's position (use an infant seat for babies) can reduce cerebral pressure. A corticosteroid such as dexamethasone (Decadron) may effectively reduce cerebral edema and its accompanying pressure. An osmotic diuretic, such as mannitol, may be given IV to remove fluid from interstitial tissue and reduce pressure. Because mannitol is hypertonic, it causes a shift of fluid from extravascular compartments into the vascular stream, where it can be eliminated by the kidneys. Children generally have an indwelling urinary catheter inserted before starting this therapy, to ensure bladder emptying from the drug-induced rapid diuresis. If excessive fluid accumulates in the brain's ventricles, a ventricular tap may be necessary for immediate reduction of pressure.

✔ CHECKPOINT QUESTIONS

3. When testing deep tendon reflexes, what would you expect to see if the child has increased ICP?
4. Which ICP-monitoring method is considered to be the most accurate?

NEURAL TUBE DISORDERS

The neural tube is the embryonic structure that matures to form the CNS. Because this forms in utero first as a flat plate, then molds to form the brain and cord, it is susceptible to malformation. Neural tube disorders, including spina bifida, are discussed in Chapter 39.

NEUROCUTANEOUS SYNDROMES

Neurocutaneous syndromes are characterized by the involvement of skin or pigment disorders with CNS dysfunction.

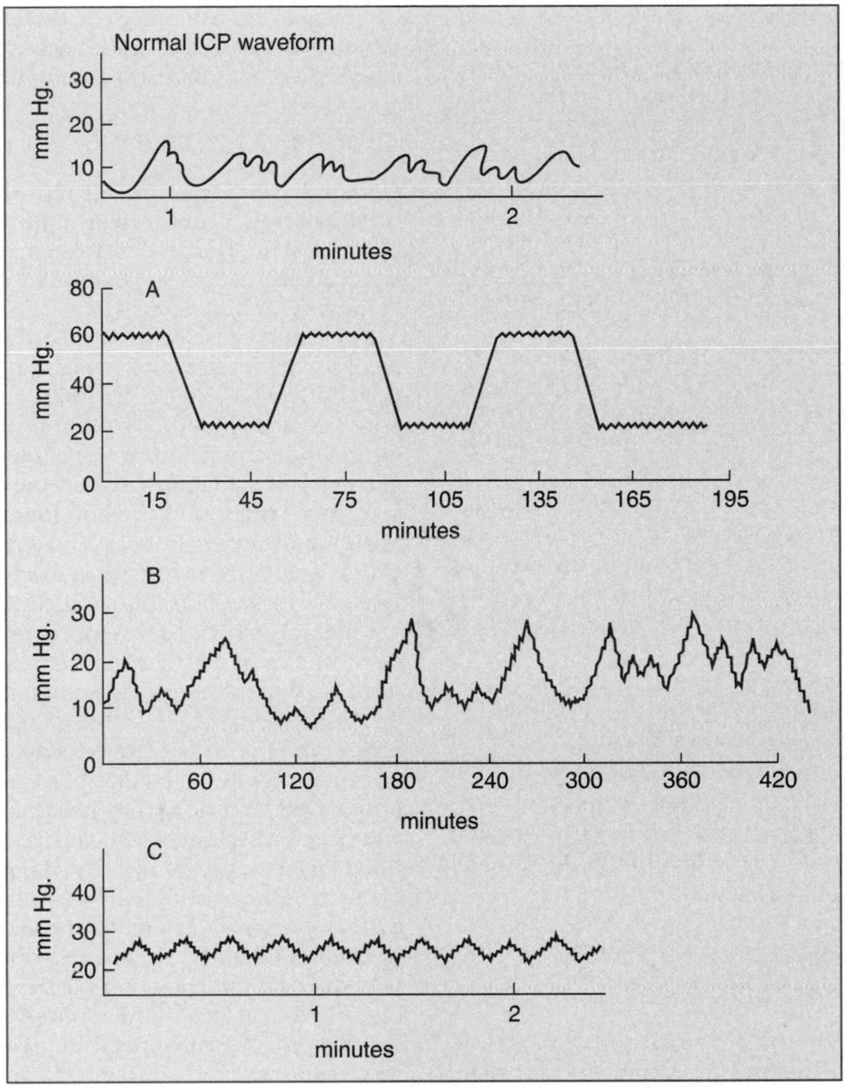

FIGURE 49.7 Normal ICP waveform and generalized shapes of the three types of intracranial pressure waves: A waves or plateau waves, B waves, and C waves.

BOX 49.1

CALCULATING CEREBRAL PERFUSION PRESSURE

Cerebral perfusion pressure (CPP) is calculated by subtracting the mean intracranial pressure (ICP) from the mean arterial pressure (MAP):

MAP – ICP = CPP

Mean arterial pressure is determined by subtracting the diastolic blood pressure (DBP) reading from the systolic blood pressure (SBP) reading, dividing this by 3, then adding that sum to 80:

MAP = SBP – DBP/3 + 80

Follow this example: A child has a blood pressure of 100/70 and an intracranial pressure of 10 mmHg. Using the formulas above, first calculate the MAP:

100 mmHg – 70 mmHg/3 + 80 = 90 mmHg

Next calculate the CPP:

90 mmHg – 10 mmHg = 80 mmHg

Therefore, a child with a blood pressure of 100/70 and an intracranial pressure of 10 would have a cerebral perfusion pressure of 80 mmHg.

Sturge-Weber Syndrome

Sturge-Weber syndrome (encephalofacial angiomatosis) involves a congenital port-wine birth mark on the skin of the upper part of the face that extends inward to the meninges and choroid. The skin manifestation follows the distribution of the first division of the fifth cranial nerve (trigeminal nerve). Because the defect is generally unilateral, the port-wine stain ends abruptly at the midline. In many children, only the ophthalmic branch of the nerve is involved, so the lesion is confined to the upper aspect of the face.

Because of involvement of the meningeal blood vessels, blood flow is sluggish, and anoxia may develop in some portions of the cerebral cortex. The child may have symptoms of hemiparesis (numbness) on the side opposite the lesion from destruction of motor neurons. The child may experience intractable seizures, be cognitively challenged, and develop blindness from glaucoma. A CT scan or MRI of the skull will generally show calcification in the involved cerebral cortex. Such calcification follows a diagnostic "railroad track" or double-groove pattern. An EEG shows areas of decreased voltage.

When the syndrome is first diagnosed, parents may hope that the defect does not extend beyond the skin lesion. They may ask to have the skin lesion surgically removed in the belief that this will correct their child's condition completely. Ensure that parents understand the need for long-term follow-up, particularly if the child has accompanying seizures that require long-term anticonvulsant therapy (Moe & Seay, 2001).

Neurofibromatosis (von Recklinghausen's Disease)

Neurofibromatosis is the unexplained development of subcutaneous tumors. The disorder can occur as a mutation or can be inherited as an autosomal dominant trait carried on the long arm of chromosome 17 and may be diagnosed prenatally. It occurs in approximately 1 in 4,000 live births (Moe & Seay, 2001). The famous "Elephant Man" is thought to have had an extreme case of multiple neurofibromatosis involving skeletal changes as well. As an infant, the child with neurofibromatosis has irregular but excessive skin pigmentation. Later in childhood, pigmented nevi or "café-au-lait" (coffee with cream) spots appear that tend to follow the paths of cutaneous nerves. The presence of more than six spots larger than 1 cm in diameter is suggestive of the disorder. By puberty, multiple soft cutaneous tumors begin to form in the child's skin along nerve pathways. Subcutaneous tumors develop by young adulthood. The acoustic nerve (eighth cranial nerve), is frequently involved, leading to hearing loss. Involvement of the optic nerve will cause vision loss. Approximately 15% of children with the disorder develop neurologic complications such as seizures. Approximately 8% become cognitively challenged from cerebral deterioration. Symptoms and growth of tumors increase at puberty and during pregnancy (Moe & Seay, 2001).

Little therapy is available to halt the tumor growth. Mast cell blockers have some effect. If lesions are causing acoustic or optic degeneration, surgical removal of the tumors may be attempted. Be certain that the parents and child have a source of emotional support through the disease's slow but invariably fatal course.

CEREBRAL PALSY

Cerebral palsy (CP) is a group of nonprogressive disorders of upper motor neuron impairment that result in motor dysfunction. A child also may have speech or ocular difficulty, seizures, cognitive challenges, or hyperactivity (Gormley, 2001).

The exact cause of CP is unknown, but the disorder is associated with low birth weight, prebirth, or birth injury (Decoufle et al., 2001). It apparently occurs when brain anoxia leads to cell destruction of the motor tracts. If intrauterine anoxia occurs for some reason (such as faulty placental implantation, placenta previa, or abruptio placentae), this type of brain cell dysfunction may result. Nutritional deficiencies, drugs, or maternal infections (such as cytomegalovirus or toxoplasmosis) as well as direct birth injury may also contribute to the cause.

Cerebral palsy occurs in approximately 2 in 1,000 births, occurring most frequently in very-low-birth-weight infants or those who are small for gestational age. It is increasing in incidence because of the number of very-low-birth-weight infants who survive today. Cerebral palsy occurs more frequently in infants born from occipitoposterior rather than anterior birth positions. In these instances, anoxia and resulting brain damage may occur with birth. In all instances, however, the damage may already have occurred. This may be why the infant is born abnormally early or presents in an unusual position. Head injury, such as from child abuse or shaken baby syndrome or severe dehydration in the newborn, with resulting venous thrombosis, also may lead to these symptoms.

In the past, kernicterus from neonatal hyperbilirubinemia was considered a cause of the athetoid type of cerebral palsy (slow writhing, involuntary movements). This is rarely seen today because of improved management of hyperbilirubinemia. Infections such as meningitis or encephalitis in the newborn also may result in cerebral palsy.

Types of Cerebral Palsy

Cerebral palsy has been classified in various ways. Traditionally, it is divided into two main categories based on the type of neuromuscular involvement: pyramidal or spastic (approximately 40% of affected children) and extrapyramidal, which is further subdivided into ataxic (approximately 10%), dyskinetic or athetoid (approximately 30%), and mixed (10%; Pelligrino, 2000).

Spastic Type

Spasticity is excessive tone in the voluntary muscles (loss of upper motor neurons). The child with spastic CP has hypertonic muscles, abnormal clonus, exaggeration of deep tendon reflexes, abnormal reflexes such as a positive Babinski reflex, and continuation of neonatal reflexes, such as the tonic neck reflex, past the age at which these usually disappear. When infants with CP are held in a ventral suspension position, they arch their backs and extend their arms and legs abnormally. They fail to demonstrate a parachute reflex if lowered suddenly, failing to hold out their arms as if to break their fall. Children tend to assume a "scissors gait" because tight adductor thigh muscles cause their legs to cross when held upright. This involvement may be so severe that it leads to a subluxated hip. Tightening of the heel cord usually is so severe that children walk on their toes, unable to stretch their heel to touch the ground.

Spastic involvement may affect both extremities on one side (**hemiplegia**), all four extremities (**quadriplegia**), or primarily the lower extremities (**diplegia** or **paraplegia**). When a child has hemiplegia, the arm is usually more involved than the leg. This may be demonstrated by asking the child to extend his arms and pronate them. When the child is asked to supinate the arm, the child's elbow flexes on the involved side. The involved arm may be shorter with a smaller muscle circumference than the other arm. Most children with hemiplegia have difficulty identifying objects placed in their involved hand when their eyes are closed (**astereognosis**).

In older children, leg involvement may be detected most easily by examining the child's shoes. One heel will be much more worn than the other because the child does not put the heel all the way down on the involved side. On physical examination, it may be difficult to abduct the involved hip fully, extend the knee, or dorsiflex the foot (Fig. 49-8).

A child with quadriplegia invariably has impaired speech (pseudobulbar palsy) but may or may not be cognitively challenged. Swallowing saliva may be so difficult that the child drools continually and has difficulty swallowing food as well. The upper extremity involvement may be limited to an abnormal, awkward hand movement. If there is no involvement of the arms at all, this is a true spastic paraplegia, and a spinal cord anomaly rather than cerebral anomaly is suggested.

Dyskinetic or Athetoid Type

This type of CP involves abnormal involuntary movement. *Athetoid* means "wormlike." Early in life, the child is limp and flaccid. Later, in place of voluntary movement, he or she makes slow, writhing motions. This may involve all four extremities, plus the face, neck, and tongue. Because of poor tongue and swallowing movements, the child drools and speech is difficult to understand. With emotional stress, the involuntary movements may become irregular and jerking (**choreoid**) with disordered muscle tone (**dyskinetic**).

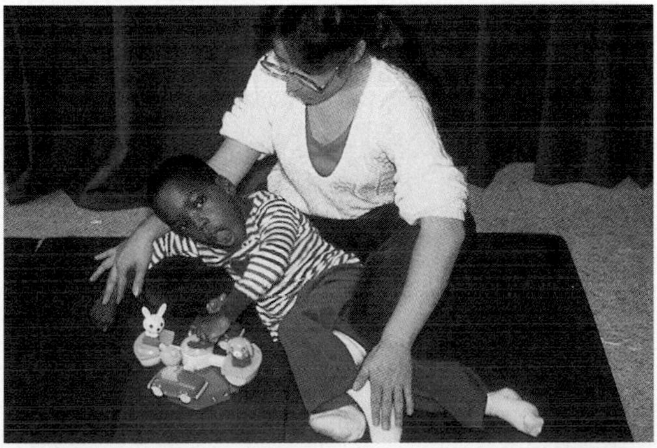

FIGURE 49.8 A physical therapist working with a child with cerebral palsy to maximize mobility.

Ataxic Type

Children with ataxic involvement have an awkward, wide-based gait. On neurologic examination, they are unable to perform the finger-to-nose test or perform rapid, repetitive movements (tests of cerebellar function) or fine coordinated motions.

Mixed Type

Some children show symptoms of both spasticity and athetoid movements. Ataxic and athetoid movements also may be present together. This combination results in a severe degree of physical impairment.

Assessment of Cerebral Palsy

The diagnosis of CP is based on history and physical assessment. On history, an episode of possible anoxia during prenatal life or at birth should be documented. Determining the extent of involvement in an infant can be difficult because a neurologic assessment in infants is difficult. The full extent of the disorder may be recognizable only when children are older and attempt more complex motor skills such as walking. All infants need careful neurologic assessment during the first year of life, however, so that small signs of impairment can be tracked and also so that the child can be followed closely for further testing and assessment. Important physical findings that suggest cerebral palsy are shown in Table 49-4.

Children with all forms of CP may have sensory alterations such as strabismus, refractive disorders, visual perception problems, visual field defects, and speech disorders such as abnormal rhythm or articulation. They also may show an attention deficit disorder. Deafness caused by kernicterus occurs in connection with athetoid cerebral palsy.

Twenty-five percent to 75% of children with symptoms of cerebral palsy are cognitively challenged. As many as 50% of children with cerebral palsy have recurrent seizures (Moe & Seay, 2001).

A skull x-ray or sonogram may show cerebral asymmetry. However, generally, the skull shape is normal. A CT or MRI scan usually is negative. The EEG may be abnormal, but the pattern is highly variable. The abnormality may be asymmetry or a spike seizure discharge. An abnormality is noteworthy but not diagnostic in itself.

NURSING DIAGNOSES AND RELATED INTERVENTIONS

Parents who are reacting to the revelation that their child has multiple physical disabilities often find it difficult to make long-range plans. Therefore, focus out-

TABLE 49.4 Physical Findings That Suggest Cerebral Palsy

FINDING	DESCRIPTION
Delayed motor development	Children with this disorder generally do not meet motor developmental milestones such as sitting, walking, saying sentences, or changing objects from hand to hand when they should, especially if there is associated cognitive impairment.
Abnormal head circumference	The child's head circumference may be smaller than normal for age, because the head grows as the brain grows. If the brain cortex is severely involved, it grows more slowly than normal.
Abnormal postures	When infants lie on their back, they usually flex their legs; infants with cerebral palsy straighten or "scissor" them; they often hold feet plantar flexed (toes down). Scissoring is also evident when the infant is held upright and you try to make him or her bear weight. In a prone position, an infant tends to raise the head higher than normal because of arching of the back. The child may flex arms and legs abnormally under trunk.
Abnormal reflexes	Newborn reflexes tend to be persistent or last long past the point they should fade: tonic neck reflex or grasp reflex beyond 5 months, Moro beyond 6 months. Hyperreflexia (extreme reflexes) is also present. Ankle clonus (persistent movement of the ankle after you have repeatedly flexed it) often occurs.
Abnormal muscle performance and tone	These infants often show abnormal use of muscle groups. They often tend to move about not by crawling on their abdomen but by scooting on their back. When they begin walking, they walk by placing their toes down first. Tight adductus muscles at the hip (which also causes scissoring) tend to pull the femoral head out of the acetabulum so that subluxation of the hip occurs not because of faulty bone formation but because of muscle spasticity.

comes on short-term concerns to assist with family functioning.

Nursing Diagnosis: Deficient knowledge related to understanding of complex disease condition

Outcome Identification: Parents will verbalize accurate information about the cause and prognosis of CP by next visit.

Outcome Evaluation: Parents state they understand that cause of disease is unknown and that disease is not progressive.

Help parents to understand that CP is a nonprogressive disease. The brain damage that occurred during pregnancy or at birth will not recur, but the child's condition may seem to grow more apparent with age. Motor deficits of the upper extremities, for example, may not be strikingly evident until the child attempts fine motor tasks in school. Without follow-up care, contractures from spasticity may result, further reducing existing motor function.

Caution parents also that CP is a single name for a wide variety and extent of diseases. Although another child may have such severe CP that he has no useful function in his extremities, their own child may not be affected to the same extent. Conversely, although they know someone with CP who is able to hold a full-time job, their child may not necessarily be able to do as well some day. Each child's potential must be evaluated individually.

Nursing Diagnosis: Risk for disuse syndrome related to spasticity of muscle groups

Outcome Identification: Child will achieve maximum mobility possible during childhood.

Outcome Evaluation: Child walks with a minimum of support or equipment; skin and tissue remain intact.

Children with CP need promotion of any function that is not already impaired to prevent further loss of function. Major areas to be addressed include self-care, communication, ambulation, education, safety, nutrition, parental support, and establishment of self-esteem.

Learning to be ambulatory is an important part of self-care because it helps determine how independent the child can become. This is difficult for the child to achieve because of lack of muscle group coordination. Surgery to lengthen heel tendons may be needed. Assisted ambulation devices such as wheeled walkers may be necessary (Fig. 49-9). Medication to reduce spasticity has little effect, although baclofen (Lioresal) may be prescribed for some children to improve motor function. Cerebellar pacemakers may reduce spasticity in some children. Administration of botulism toxin (Botox) has shown success in relieving spasticity and aiding in walking (O'Donnell, 2001).

Preventing contractures is important to maintain motor function. Formerly, children were fitted with extensive braces. The weight of these braces, however, often impeded muscle movement and actually prevented children from learning to walk. Partial leg braces, however, may be used to encourage children to bring their heels down and keep heel cords from tightening. If leg braces are prescribed, parents may need some encouragement and support to insist that their children wear them. Remind parents that partial leg braces for stretching the heel cords should be worn for long periods during the day to be effective.

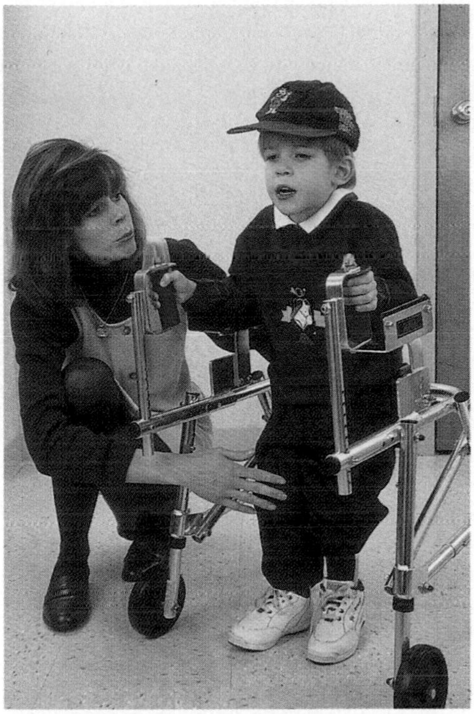

FIGURE 49.9 Wheeled walkers give a child added stability for walking and keep heel cords from shortening.

Just putting them on when the child is going outside is not enough.

Passive and active muscle exercises also are important to prevent contractures. Teach parents passive exercises and games to play with the child that encourage active exercise. At health care visits, remind parents that these exercises are an important part of their child's therapy and must be done consistently each day.

Nursing Diagnosis: Risk for self-care deficit related to impaired mobility

Outcome Identification: Child will achieve independent self-care by puberty.

Outcome Evaluation: Child feeds and dresses self; manages elimination independently.

Children need to learn self-care measures such as dressing, toothbrushing, bathing, and toileting so they can gain self-esteem from accomplishing these tasks and achieve optimal independence. Modifications such as straps attached to their toothbrush or feeding utensils may be necessary so they can hold these more securely. Advise parents to always supervise children during bathing. Children's lack of coordination could cause them to slip underwater and drown. However, encourage the parents to allow children to scrub themselves and wash their hair. Toileting is often difficult because they do not have the muscle group coordination to achieve successful bowel evacuation. A high-roughage diet will help prevent constipation and aid bowel evacuation. Voiding may be equally difficult because the child may lack sufficient voluntary muscle control.

The parents need considerable support and guidance. Helping the child with self-care activities often requires patience to allow the child to accomplish the task. Doing so, however, helps to instill confidence and self-esteem in the child.

Nursing Diagnosis: Risk for delayed growth and development related to activity restriction secondary to cerebral palsy

Outcome Identification: Child will demonstrate age-appropriate developmental milestones within the limits of his disease.

Outcome Evaluation: Child receives environmental stimulation; expresses interest in people and activities around him; attends school setting that is as free of restrictions as possible.

Children with CP may be unable to pursue stimulating activities and surroundings. Therefore, these things must be brought to them. Some children may need more stimulating activities than others because they have difficulty concentrating on one activity for any length of time. An activity should be neither too difficult nor too easy for the child. Choose toys and activities appropriate to the child's intellectual, developmental, and motor levels, not chronologic age.

A preschool program is important for providing exposure to the outside world. If at all possible, school-age children with cerebral palsy should be mainstreamed so they can be among other children. Under federal law, children who are physically or cognitively challenged must be provided an education in the least restrictive setting possible. If they are both cognitively and physically challenged, the combined mental and motor deficits may severely limit their abilities, making school placement difficult. You may need to advocate that a child be placed in a school setting that is consistent with his or her intellectual abilities.

Nursing Diagnosis: Risk for imbalanced nutrition, less than body requirements, related to difficulty sucking in infancy and in feeding self as older child

Outcome Identification: Child will demonstrate intake of adequate nutrients throughout childhood.

Outcome Evaluation: Child's weight will remain within 5th to 95th percentile on height–weight chart; skin turgor remains good; specific gravity of urine is 1.003 to 1.030.

Providing adequate nutrition to children with CP is often difficult. As infants, they often suck poorly because uncoordinated movements of the tongue, lips, and jaw and tongue thrusting cause them to push food out of their mouth (a retained primitive reflex). Their lip and tongue control may be poor, with weak or uncoordinated jaw muscles. Older children may have difficulty holding and controlling a spoon to bring food to their mouth. Spasticity causes children to hyperextend the head when leaning forward to take a bite, so they never feel comfortable while eating. Parents may need guidance in finding a feeding pattern that works for their child. Manually controlling the jaw may help control the head, correct neck and trunk hyperextension, and stabilize the jaw and assist with feeding. If children cannot chew or swallow well, a liquid or soft diet may be necessary. Other children can handle solids and finger foods but may take longer to eat than the average child. They may need protection for their clothing and the floor. It may take longer for them to eat than the rest of the family, so people will need to wait patiently for them to finish.

A hyperactive gag reflex may cause children to vomit after feeding. Be certain that infants are positioned on their side or upright after feeding to prevent aspiration.

Nursing Diagnosis: Impaired verbal communication related to neurologic impairment

Outcome Identification: Child will achieve satisfactory communication with caregivers and significant others by school age.

Outcome Evaluation: Child can verbally make needs known to strangers and family members.

Most children with CP benefit from speech therapy, which helps them learn to speak slowly and coordinate their lips and tongue to form speech sounds. Be patient with children, and allow them to form words deliberately. If they try to hurry to please you, their speech will be much less clear, and communication will be impaired. For the child who cannot speak clearly, provide an alternative form of communication, such as flash cards or a picture board. Touch-screen computer programs are often used in school settings to aid communication.

Long-Term Care

Because CP is not always diagnosed early in infancy, parents may not learn that their child has a chronic disease until nearly 2 to 4 years later. Help them to encourage children with CP to reach their fullest potential within the limits of their disorder. Evaluations at health care visits should note not only whether the child is achieving this goal but also whether he and his family members find satisfaction and acceptance in his achievements. Listen to parents during health care visits and encourage them to discuss the difficulties of daily living, such as feeding problems. They may grieve because their child is not able to accomplish all of the major things they had wished for during pregnancy, and they may feel defeated by the day-to-day strain of caring for the child's multiple special needs. Care of the child with a chronic illness is discussed further in Chapter 56.

✔ CHECKPOINT QUESTIONS

5. What are the four types of cerebral palsy?
6. What measures to prevent contractures should you teach the parents of a child with cerebral palsy?

INFECTION

Nervous system tissue is as susceptible to infection as all other body tissue. Common major infections include meningitis, encephalitis, Guillain-Barré syndrome, Reye's syndrome, and botulism.

Bacterial Meningitis

Meningitis is an infection of the cerebral meninges, occurring most often in children under 24 months of age. Although the disease may occur in any month, its peak incidence appears to be in the winter. In the United States, it is caused most frequently by *Neisseria meningitidis, Streptococcus pneumoniae,* or group B *Streptococcus.* In children under 2 months of age, group B *Streptococcus* and *Escherichia coli* are common causes of meningitis (Bell, 2000). In children with myelomeningocele who develop meningitis, *Pseudomonas* infection is common. Children who have had a splenectomy are particularly susceptible to pneumococcal meningitis unless they have received a pneumococcal vaccine. *Hemophilus influenzae,* once a major cause, is now rarely seen because of routine immunization against this organism.

Pathologic organisms generally are spread to the meninges from upper respiratory tract infections, by lymphatic drainage possibly through the mastoid or sinuses, or by direct introduction by a lumbar puncture or skull fracture. Once organisms enter the meningeal space, they multiply rapidly and spread throughout the CSF. Organisms invade brain tissue through meningeal folds that extend down into the brain itself. The inflammatory response that occurs may lead to a thick, fibrinous exudate that blocks CSF flow. Brain abscess or invasion of the infection into cranial nerves may result in blindness, deafness, or facial paralysis. Pus that accumulates in the narrow aqueduct of Sylvius may cause obstruction leading to hydrocephalus. Brain tissue edema can put pressure on the hypopituitary gland, causing increased production of antidiuretic hormone (syndrome of inappropriate antidiuretic hormone [SIADH]). This causes increased edema because the body cannot excrete adequate urine (Ferry & Collett-Solberg, 2000).

Assessment

The symptoms of meningitis may occur insidiously or suddenly. Children generally have 2 or 3 days of upper respiratory tract infection. They become increasingly irritable because of headaches. They may have seizures. In some children, seizures or shock is the first noticeable sign of illness. As the disease progresses, signs of meningeal irritability occur, as evidenced by a positive Brudzinski's and Kernig's signs (Fig. 49-10). Their back may become arched and their neck hyperextended (opisthotonos). Cranial nerve paralysis, most typically of the third and sixth nerves, may occur, so that children are not able to follow a light through full visual fields. If open, the fontanelles are bulging and tense; if they are closed, children may develop papilledema. If the meningitis is caused by *H. influenzae,* children may develop septic arthritis. If it is caused

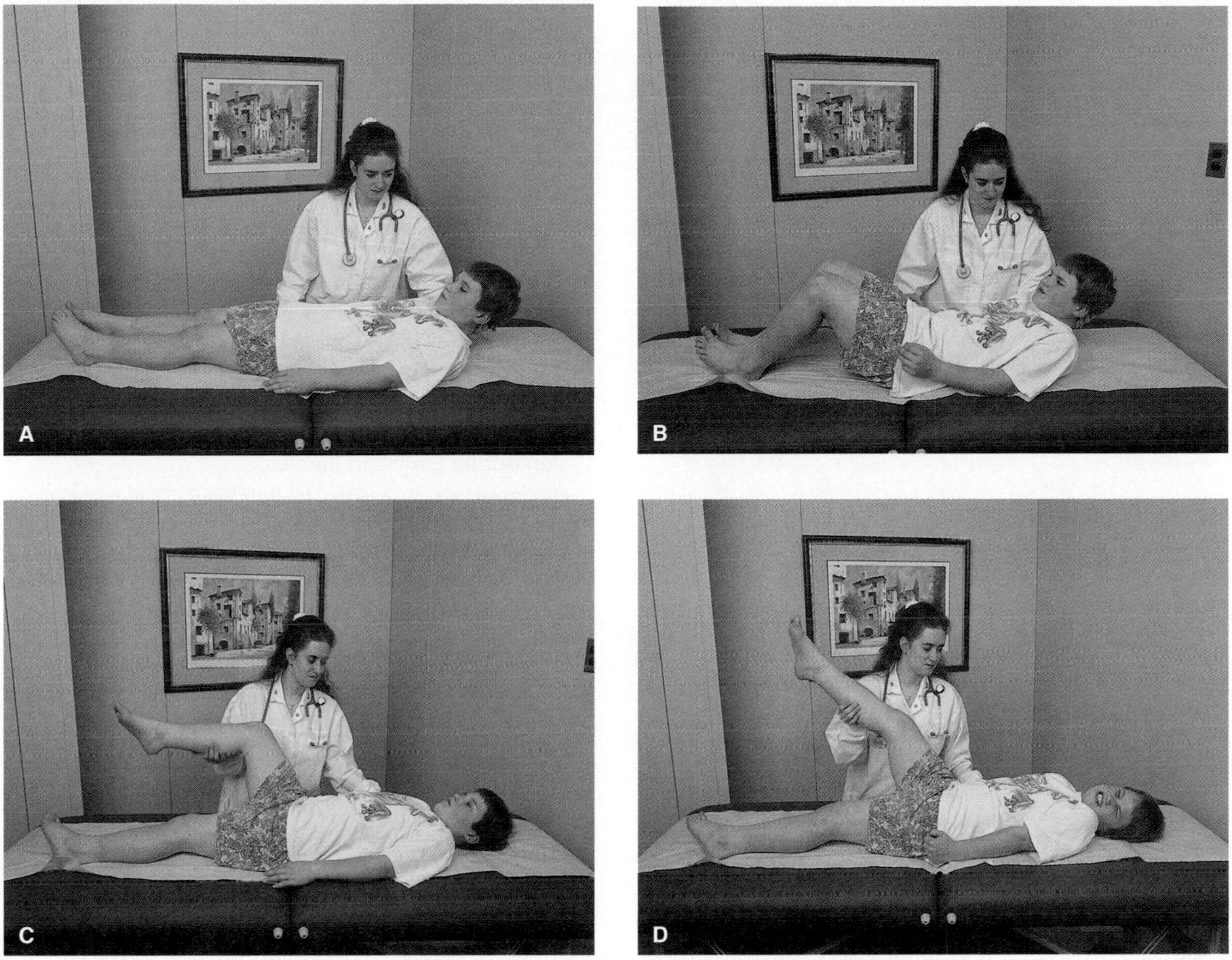

FIGURE 49.10 (*A*) Brudzinski's sign. The nurse flexes the child's neck forward. (*B*) Positive response. Bilateral hip, knee, and ankle flexion indicates meningeal irritation. (*C*) Kernig's sign. The nurse flexes the child's hip and knee, forming a 90-degree angle. (*D*) Positive response. As the leg is extended, pain, resistance, and spasm are noted, indicating meningeal irritation.

by *N meningitidis,* a papular or purple petechial skin rash may develop (Friday, 2000).

In the newborn, the symptoms are often vague, for example, poor sucking, weak cry, and lethargy. After this generalized beginning, sudden cardiovascular shock, seizures, or apnea may occur. Because the infant has open fontanelles, nuchal rigidity appears late and is not as useful a sign for diagnosis as in the older child.

Meningitis is diagnosed by history and analysis of CSF obtained by lumbar puncture. A child with a febrile seizure should be assumed to have meningitis until CSF findings prove otherwise. CSF results indicative of meningitis include an increase in white blood cell and protein levels and a lowered glucose level (bacteria have fed on the glucose). In a healthy child, the glucose level in the CSF is 60% of that of the serum glucose. Because meningitis often spreads and causes septicemia, a blood culture also is done. A fulminating (overwhelming) meningitis often leads to leukopenia. If children have had close association with someone with tuberculosis, a tuberculin skin test to rule out tuberculosis meningitis should be done. A CT scan, MRI, or ultrasound may be ordered to examine for abscesses. Typically, ICP is often severely elevated.

Therapeutic Management

Antibiotic therapy as indicated by sensitivity studies is the primary treatment measure. Usually given IV for rapid effect, intrathecal injections (directly into the CSF) may be necessary to reduce the infection, because the blood–brain barrier may prevent an antibiotic from passing freely into the CSF. If the organism is identified as *H influenzae,* ampicillin generally is the drug of choice. In other instances, a third-generation cephalosporin, such as cefotaxime (Claforan) or ceftriaxone (Rocephin) may be used for 8 to 10 days. In some children, it will take a month before the CSF cell count returns to normal. A corticosteroid such as dexamethasone or the osmotic diuretic, mannitol, may be administered to reduce ICP and help prevent hearing loss.

In addition to standard precautions, children with meningitis are placed on respiratory precautions for 24 h after the start of antibiotic therapy to prevent infection transmission (Meyers, 2000). Antibiotics also may be prescribed prophylactically for the immediate family members of the ill child or others who were in close contact with the child.

Meningitis is always a serious disorder because it can run a rapid, fulminating, possibly fatal course, although, if symptoms are recognized early enough and if treatment is effective, the child will recover with no sequelae. Neurologic sequelae, such as learning problems, seizures, hearing and cognitive challenges, and inability to concentrate urine, must be assessed after the infection.

NURSING DIAGNOSES AND RELATED INTERVENTIONS

When a child has meningitis, the parents may feel responsible for the illness. They knew the child had a cold, and they wonder whether they could have prevented meningitis if only they had taken him to a physician as soon as the cold symptoms started. Assure them that the symptoms of meningitis occur insidiously and that no one could have predicted the full extent of the disease from the first signs.

Encourage parents to care for the child during the illness, both to help make the child more comfortable and to help them manage their own anxiety. Teach them good infection control techniques so they can perform these tasks safely.

Nursing Diagnosis: Pain related to meningeal irritation

Outcome Identification: Child will experience a tolerable degree of pain during the course of illness.

Outcome Evaluation: Child states that pain is tolerable; shows no facial grimacing or other signs of discomfort.

For a child with meningitis, dealing with hospitalization and the numerous invasive treatments and procedures is usually difficult. If the child had a lumbar puncture on admission, an initial impression may become one of people restraining him for a painful procedure. Continuous IV infusions contribute to this impression. Remember that the child feels pain when the head is flexed forward and will usually be more comfortable without a pillow. Be careful not to flex the child's neck when turning or positioning him.

On admission, a child may be extremely irritable. Although he would benefit from puppet play or drawing that would help him express how he feels about so many intrusive procedures, frequently he is too uncomfortable to play, appearing as though nothing seems to comfort him. This is the result of the disease process, and he cannot help feeling this way. Be aware of this so as not to interpret the child's withdrawal as unfriendliness and feel hurt when advances are rebuffed. Parents also need to understand that the child's behavior is because of the disease and not anything that they did or are doing. The child needs a good explanation of everything that is happening. He needs extra attention from health care personnel consistently, not just when they perform painful procedures. As the child recovers, irritability lessens and the child usually will show more interest in communicating his feelings. Promote rest for the child by keeping stimulation in the room to a minimum.

Nursing Diagnosis: Risk for ineffective tissue perfusion (cerebral), related to increased ICP

Outcome Identification: Child will remain free of signs and symptoms of altered cerebral tissue perfusion during course of illness.

Outcome Evaluation: Child's vital signs return to normal; child is alert and oriented; motor, cognitive, and sensory function are within acceptable parameters for the child's age; specific gravity of urine is 1.003 to 1.030.

Observe the child carefully for signs of increased ICP. Carefully monitor the rate of all IV infusions to prevent overhydration. Measure urine specific gravity to detect oversecretion or undersecretion of antidiuretic hormone from pituitary pressure. Measure the child's head circumference, and weigh him or her daily.

Monitor hearing acuity (reduced if there is compression of the eighth cranial nerve) by asking the child a question or observing whether the infant listens to a music box or your voice.

Group B, Beta-Hemolytic Streptococcal Meningitis

A major cause of meningitis in newborns is the group B, beta-hemolytic streptococcal organism. The organism is contracted either in utero or from secretions in the birth canal at delivery. It can spread to other newborns if good handwashing technique is not used.

Group-B beta-hemolytic streptococci colonization may result in early-onset or late-onset illness. With the early-onset form, symptoms of pneumonia become apparent in the first few hours of life.

The late-onset type often leads to meningitis instead of pneumonia. At approximately the age of 2 weeks, the infant may gradually become lethargic, developing a fever and upper respiratory symptoms. The fontanelles will bulge from increased ICP. Mortality from group B streptococcal infections is approximately 25%; surviving infants may develop neurologic consequences such as hydrocephalus (Thilo & Rosenberg, 2001). Treatment is with antibiotics, such as ampicillin and cephalosporins, effective against group B, beta-hemolytic streptococcal infections.

It can be difficult for parents to understand how their infant suddenly became so ill. They may need considerable support in caring for the infant who is left neurologically challenged.

✔ **CHECKPOINT QUESTIONS**

7. What important sign would you use to evaluate for meningeal irritation in the child with meningitis?
8. For how long should the child with bacterial meningitis be placed on respiratory precautions?

Encephalitis

Encephalitis is an inflammation of brain tissue and, possibly, the meninges as well (Bergqvist, 2000). It can arise from protozoan, bacterial, fungal, or viral invasion. Enteroviruses are the most frequent cause, followed by arboviruses (togavirus). A number of encephalitis viruses, such as St. Louis encephalitis and eastern equine encephalitis, are borne by mosquitoes and are seen most during the summer months. In endemic areas, mosquito repellents are strongly suggested. Encephalitis also can result from direct invasion of the CSF during lumbar puncture. It may occur as a complication of common childhood diseases, such as measles, mumps, or chickenpox. Therefore, it is crucial that children receive immunization against these childhood diseases.

Assessment

Symptoms of encephalitis may begin gradually or suddenly. These include headache, high temperature, and signs of meningeal irritation, such as nuchal rigidity (positive Brudzinski's sign and Kernig's sign). Symptoms of ataxia, muscle weakness or paralysis, diplopia, confusion, or irritability also may occur. The child becomes increasingly lethargic and eventually comatose.

The diagnosis is made by the history and physical assessment. CSF evaluation generally reveals an elevated leukocyte count and elevated protein and glucose levels. An EEG shows widespread cerebral involvement. A brain biopsy, usually from the temporal lobe, may be done to identify the possible virus.

Therapeutic Management

Treatment for the child with encephalitis is primarily supportive. An antipyretic is given to control fever. Take and record vital signs frequently, because brain stem involvement may affect cardiac or respiratory rates. Mechanical ventilation may be required to maintain the child's respirations during the acute phase. An antiviral agent, such as acyclovir (Zovirax) will be prescribed. Anticonvulsants, such as carbamazepine (Tegretol), phenobarbital, or phenytoin (Dilantin), may be prescribed for seizures. A steroid such as dexamethasone or an osmotic diuretic such as mannitol may be prescribed to decrease brain edema and ICP.

Encephalitis is always a serious diagnosis because, although the child may recover from the initial attack, there may be residual neurologic damage, such as seizures or learning disabilities. Parents may find it hard to believe that their child is seriously ill because she only seemed tired and had a slight headache. They will find it even harder to accept a diagnosis of permanent impairment such as a learning disability. Follow-up care after the hospitalization is important for the child's rehabilitation and to help parents deal with their grief, shock, and anger. Although complete recovery is possible, parents may find themselves with a child whose health and abilities have been permanently changed.

Reye's Syndrome

Reye's syndrome is acute encephalitis with accompanying fatty infiltration of the liver, heart, lungs, pancreas, and skeletal muscle. It occurs in children from 1 to 18 years of age regardless of gender (Mulberg, 2000).

The cause is unknown, but it generally occurs after a viral infection such as varicella (chickenpox) or influenza if the child is treated with a salicylate such as acetylsalicylic acid (aspirin) during the viral infection. Anticipatory guidance to parents and children about avoiding the use of aspirin during viral infections has led to almost total prevention of the syndrome.

Assessment

After seeming to recover from an initial viral illness, children become ill again 1 to 3 weeks later, with lethargy, vomiting, agitation, anorexia, confusion, and combativeness. Symptoms in adolescents may be so extreme that they mimic those of drug intoxication and may be mistaken for it. As fatty droplets invade the liver, enzyme abnormalities, hypothrombinemia, hypoglycemia, and elevated blood ammonia levels occur. Although CSF findings remain normal, cerebral symptoms progress from confusion to stupor to deep coma, with seizures and respiratory arrest resulting from pressure on the brain stem.

Laboratory diagnosis of Reye's syndrome is confirmed by elevated liver enzyme levels (ALT [SGPT] and AST [SGOT]), elevated serum ammonia, normal direct bilirubin, delayed prothrombin time and partial thromboplastin time, decreased blood glucose, elevated blood urea nitrogen, elevated serum amylase, elevated short-chain fatty acids, and an elevated white blood count. A lumbar puncture is usually done to rule out other infection. CSF findings are normal, except for slightly elevated opening pressure. A skull CT scan or sonogram will be normal at first. Later, this will show cerebral edema and decreased ventricle size. A liver biopsy will show fatty infiltration, establishing a definitive diagnosis.

Therapeutic Management

If left untreated, Reye's syndrome is rapidly fatal. If diagnosed early and promptly treated, the child usually recovers quickly and generally without any residual neurologic effects.

Reye's syndrome is not infectious. It is categorized by stages of involvement from 1 to 5, depending on the amount of the child's lethargy or presence of coma. In stages 1 and 2, the child responds to stimuli but may exhibit lethargy or delirium and possibly combativeness. With stages 3 through 5, the child is unresponsive to stimuli with a progressively deepening coma. Frequent neurologic assessments are necessary to evaluate the child's status and possible progression to a more serious stage of involvement. Therapy is directed toward supporting respiratory function, controlling hypoglycemia, and reducing brain edema.

Guillain-Barré Syndrome

Guillain-Barré (inflammatory polyradiculoneuropathy) is a perplexing syndrome involving both motor and sensory portions of peripheral nerves. It affects both sexes and occurs most often in school-age children to adolescents (Teener, 2000).

The cause of the condition is unknown, but it is suspected that the reaction is immune mediated, following upper respiratory and gastrointestinal illnesses and immunization. Inflammation of the nerve fibers apparently causes temporary demyelinization of the nerve sheaths.

Assessment

Children experience peripheral neuritis several days after the primary infection. Tendon reflexes are decreased or absent. Muscle paralysis and paresthesia (loss of sensation) begin first in the legs and then spread to involve the arms and trunk and head. The symmetric nature of the disorder helps to differentiate it from other types of paraplegia. Cranial nerve involvement leads to facial weakness and difficulty in swallowing. As the respiratory muscles become involved, spontaneous respirations are no longer possible. This can lead to respiratory involvement severe enough to warrant mechanical ventilation (Moe & Seay, 2001).

A significant laboratory finding is an elevated CSF protein level. An EEG may show denervation and decreased nerve conduction velocity.

Therapeutic Management

Treatment of Guillain-Barré syndrome is supportive until the process runs its course (paralysis peaks at 3 weeks, followed by gradual recovery). A course of prednisone to halt the autoimmune response may be tried, but its use is controversial. Plasmapheresis or transfusion of immune serum globulin may shorten the course of the illness (Moe & Seay, 2001).

Care of the child with Guillain-Barré includes preventing all of the effects of extreme immobility while guarding respiratory function. The child's cardiac and respiratory function must be closely monitored. An indwelling urinary catheter is usually inserted to monitor urine output. Enteral or total parenteral nutrition may be used to maintain protein and carbohydrate needs. If the child has discomfort from neuritis, adequate analgesia needs to be administered.

To prevent muscle contractures and effects of immobility, the child should have passive range-of-motion exercises every 4 h. Turning and repositioning the child every 2 h also is important to protect skin integrity. Providing adequate stimulation for the long weeks when the child is unable to perform any care for himself or herself is also important. Most children recover completely, without any residual effects of the syndrome, although they may continue to have minor problems such as residual weakness.

Botulism

Botulism occurs when spores of *Clostridium botulinum* colonize and produce toxins in the immature intestine. The source of the spores is generally unknown, but honey and corn syrup are frequent contaminants so should be avoided in infants. The disease is not infectious and generally occurs in infants younger than 6 months of age (Callahan, 2000).

With infant botulism, symptoms occur within a few hours of ingestion of contaminated food. Almost immediately, there is generalized weakness, hypotonia, listlessness, a weak cry, and a diminished gag reflex. This is followed by a flaccid paralysis of the bulbar muscles that leads to diminished respiratory function. The organism can be cultured from stools or serum. Electromyography may be helpful to support the diagnosis.

Treatment is supportive care. The antitoxin for botulism is rarely given to infants because it is made from a horse serum base and can cause a hypersensitivity reaction and it is generally not necessary for full recovery. Infant botulism may account for some fatalities credited to sudden infant death syndrome.

✔ CHECKPOINT QUESTIONS

9. What is the most frequent cause of encephalitis?
10. What factors are associated with the development of Reye's syndrome?
11. What is a frequent source of botulism spores, so should not be given to infants?

PAROXYSMAL DISORDERS

A paroxysmal disorder is one that occurs suddenly and recurrently. Seizures, headaches, and breath-holding spells are the most frequent types seen in childhood.

Recurrent Seizures

A *seizure* is an involuntary contraction of muscle caused by abnormal electrical brain discharges. Approximately 2% to 3% of children will have at least one seizure by the time they reach adulthood (Moe & Seay, 2001). These episodes are always frightening to parents and other children. Although seizures may be idiopathic (without cause), they also can be attributed to infection, trauma, or tumor growth. Familiar or polygenic inheritance may be responsible. Fifty percent of seizures are unexplainable. They are not so much a disease as symptoms of an underlying disorder and should be investigated carefully (see Focus on Cultural Competence).

The term *epilepsy* comes from a Greek word meaning "to take hold of" and refers to a person with chronic seizures. The preferred term now is *recurrent seizures* because epilepsy carries the stigma of cognitive challenge, behavioral disorders, institutionalization, or just unexplainable strangeness.

The types and causes of seizures vary according to the child's age. They have been classified into two major categories: partial seizures and generalized seizures (Box 49-2).

FOCUS ON CULTURAL COMPETENCE

The degree of understanding about the cause of disorders such as recurrent seizures varies in different cultures. Because the cause of recurrent seizures is often unknown (idiopathic), it has in the past been attributed to an invasion by evil spirits. Many people today still fear that recurrent seizures will lead to cognitive impairment. Adults with recurrent seizures may be refused jobs because they are viewed as undependable. Being aware of these common misconceptions can help you appreciate parents' anxiety about the diagnosis of recurrent seizures. It can accentuate the need for parent education and careful planning to maintain self-esteem in the child.

With partial seizures, only one area of the brain is involved; with generalized seizures, the disturbance involves the entire brain, and loss of consciousness usually occurs. It is important that seizures be differentiated by their degree of severity so that appropriate management and drug therapy can be instituted.

Seizures in the Newborn Period

Seizure activity in the newborn period may be difficult to recognize because it may consist only of twitching of the head, arms, or eyes; slight cyanosis; and perhaps respiratory difficulty or apnea. Afterward, the infant may appear limp and flaccid. Whereas older children often have seizures of unknown cause, 75% of seizures in neonates have a known cause. Some possible causes include:

- Trauma and anoxia (head trauma involved with the birth process, tight maternal cervix, poor use of forceps, or placenta previa)
- Metabolic disorders (hypoglycemia [glucose level below 40 mg/100 mL in the full-term infant; 20 mg/100 mL in the preterm infant]; infants of diabetic mothers; hypocalcemia; and lack of pyridoxine [vitamin B_6])
- Neonatal infection (CNS infection or prolonged rupture of membranes before delivery)
- Kernicterus

Because of the nervous system's immaturity, EEGs in the newborn may be normal, despite extensive disease. Therefore, a noticeably abnormal EEG generally means a poor prognosis, indicating that the involvement this early in life must be severe. Because nearly 20% of all newborns have abnormal CSF values as compared with adult standards, lumbar puncture also is not conclusive. Protein is increased, and there may be a few red blood cells from rupture of subarachnoid capillaries from the pressure of birth.

A high dosage of anticonvulsant medication may be needed to control seizures in newborns because they metabolize drugs more rapidly than older infants. In adults, for example, phenobarbital may be administered in the range of 1.5 mg/kg body weight/day. In newborns, the dose might be as high as 3 to 10 mg/kg/day.

BOX 49.2

CLASSIFICATION OF SEIZURES

Partial (Focal) Seizures

- Simple partial seizures (no altered level of consciousness)
  Simple partial seizures with motor signs (includes aversive, rolandic, and jacksonian march)
  Simple partial seizures with sensory signs
- Complex partial (psychomotor) seizures (some impairment or alteration in level of consciousness)

Generalized Seizures

- Tonic-clonic seizures (formerly grand mal)
  Tonic
  Clonic
- Absence seizures (formerly petit mal)
- Atonic seizures (formerly "drop attacks")
- Myoclonic seizures
- Infantile spasms

Seizures in the Infant and Toddler Periods

Seizures commonly seen in this age group are **infantile spasms,** a form of generalized seizures—"salaam" and "jackknife"—or infantile myoclonic seizures, characterized by very rapid movements of the trunk with sudden strong contractions of most of the body including flexion and adduction of the limbs. The infant suddenly slumps forward from a sitting position or falls from a standing position. These episodes may occur singly or in clusters as frequently as 100 times a day. They are most common in the first 6 months of life (Brooks-Kayal, 2000).

The cause is unknown, but the spasms apparently result from a failure of normal organized electrical activity in the brain. Sometimes, the seizures accompany a preexisting form of neurologic damage. In approximately 50% of those affected, there is an identifiable cause such as trauma or a metabolic disease such as phenylketonuria. In the other 50%, there may be no identifiable cause. They may follow invasion by viruses such as herpes or cytomegalovirus. Approximately 90% of these infants are developmentally delayed (Brooks-Kayal, 2000).

In infants whose development was previously normal, intellectual development appears to halt and even regress after seizures start. Most children with infantile spasms show high-amplitude slow waves and spikes, a chaotic discharge called *hypsarrhythmia,* on an EEG tracing.

The response to treatment with anticonvulsant therapy is poor. Parenteral adrenocorticotropic hormone (ACTH) and pyridoxine (vitamin B_6) therapy is commonly used. High-dose valproic acid or a newer anticonvulsant agent such as topiramate (Topamax) may be used in children who do not respond to usual therapy. The infantile seizure phenomenon seems to "burn itself out" by 2 years of age.

The associated cognitive or developmental delay remains, however, so children need follow-up planning and care.

Seizures From Poisoning or Drugs. The possibility of poisoning must be considered in all children who have a first seizure. Although poisoning is most likely in the age group between 6 months and 3 years, it must be considered again in adolescence when drugs may be intentionally self-administered. Seizures also can be a late symptom of encephalopathy caused by lead poisoning (see Chapter 52).

Seizures in Children Older Than 3 Years of Age

Febrile Seizures. Seizures associated with high fever (102°F to 104°F [38.9°C to 40.0°C]) are the most common in preschool children, or between 5 months and 5 years of age, although seizures may occur as early as 3 months and as late as 7 years. The seizure shows an active tonic-clonic pattern, which lasts 15 to 20 seconds. The EEG tracing usually is normal. There usually is a history of other family members having had similar seizures. Febrile seizures may occur after immunization because of the fever that may accompany these (Barlow et al., 2001).

It is unclear whether this type of seizure is initiated by a consistently high fever or a sudden spike of temperature. The seizure subsides quickly once the fever is lowered.

Prevention of Febrile Seizures. Because these seizures arise with high fever, they are largely preventable. If acetaminophen is given to keep a developing fever below 101°F (38.4°C), seizures rarely occur. They happen most often when children develop a fever at night, when the parent is not aware of it, when the temperature is already high, or when a parent is reluctant to give acetaminophen in large enough doses to be therapeutic. Although this type of seizure can be prevented by phenobarbital, prophylactic use during an upper respiratory infection is not recommended (Baumann & Duffner, 2000). Phenobarbital takes 2 or 3 days to reach therapeutic blood levels. By this time, seizures would already have occurred. In addition, phenobarbital is associated with sleepiness, thus possibly reducing cognitive function in children.

Instruct parents that every child who has a febrile seizure must be seen by a health care provider. A good rule of thumb is to assume that the child in this situation has meningitis until it is ruled out by a complete neurologic workup (Reuter & Brownstein, 2002).

Therapeutic Management. Teach parents that, after the seizure subsides, they should sponge the child with tepid water to reduce the fever quickly. Advise them not to put the child in the bathtub, however, because it would be easy for the child to slip underwater should a second seizure occur. Applying alcohol or cold water is also not advisable. Extreme cooling causes shock to an immature nervous system, and alcohol can be absorbed by the skin or the fumes inhaled in toxic amounts, compounding the child's problems. Parents should not attempt to give oral medications such as acetaminophen, because the child will be in a drowsy, or *postictal,* state after the seizure and might aspirate the medicine. If attempts to reduce the child's temperature by sponging are unsuccessful, advise parents to put a cool washcloth on the child's forehead, axillary, and groin areas and transport the child, lightly clothed, to a health care facility for immediate evaluation.

Additional treatment will depend on the underlying cause of the fever. A lumbar puncture will be performed to rule out meningitis. Antipyretic drugs to reduce the fever below seizure levels will be administered. Appropriate antibiotic therapy will be started, depending on the type of infection.

Many parents need to be assured that febrile seizures do not lead to brain damage and that the child is almost always completely well afterward.

Complex Partial (Psychomotor) Seizures. More than half of children who develop recurrent seizures during school age have an idiopathic type—the cause of the seizures cannot be discovered. Fortunately, even without a clearly understood cause, medication controls these idiopathic seizures in almost all affected children. Other seizures in this age group occur because of organic causes. They generally result from focal or diffuse brain injury that has left residual damage. The injury may have been the result of laceration of brain tissue in a car accident or fall, hemorrhage due to blood dyscrasia, infection (meningitis or encephalitis), anoxia, or toxic conditions such as lead poisoning. The possibility that a growing brain tumor is causing brain irritation also must be considered.

Complex partial (psychomotor) seizures vary greatly in extent and symptoms and tend to be the most difficult to control. The child may have a slight aura, but it is rarely as definite as that seen with tonic-clonic seizures. A CT or MRI scan and EEG invariably are all normal.

This type of seizure may begin with a sudden change in posture, such as an arm dropping suddenly to the side. Other motor, sensory, and behavior signs may include **automatisms** (complex purposeless movements, such as lip smacking, or fumbling hand movements). The child then slumps to the ground, unconscious. Circumoral pallor may develop due to a halt in respirations. The child usually regains consciousness in less than 5 min. He or she may feel slightly drowsy afterward but does not have an actual postictal stage as in tonic-clonic seizures.

Common drugs used include carbamazepine (Tegretol), valproic acid (Depakene), phenytoin (Dilantin), and phenobarbital (see Focus on Pharmacology displays). Carbamazepine can lead to neutropenia, so white blood cell counts need to be monitored during therapy. If these drugs are not effective, surgery to remove the epileptogenic focus may be attempted (Dlugos, 2001).

Partial (Focal) Seizures. Partial seizures originate from a specific brain area. A typical partial seizure with motor signs begins in the fingers and spreads to the wrist, arm, and face in a clonic contraction. If the movement remains localized, there will be no loss of consciousness. When the spread is extensive, the seizure may become generalized and then is impossible to differentiate from a tonic-clonic seizure. Thus, it is important to observe children carefully as a seizure begins. A partial seizure with sensory signs may include numbness, tingling, paresthesia, or pain originating in one area and spreading to other parts of

FOCUS ON PHARMACOLOGY

Phenytoin (Dilantin)

Action: Phenytoin is an anticonvulsant that stabilizes neuronal membranes, prevents hyperexcitability caused by excessive stimulation, and limits the spread of seizure activity without causing general central nervous system depression

Pregnancy risk category: D

Dosage: Initially, 5 mg/kg/day in two to three equally divided doses up to a maximum of 300 mg/day with a maintenance dose of 4 to 8 mg/day.

Possible adverse effects: Nystagmus, ataxia, slurred speech, confusion, fatigue, irritability, nausea, gingival hyperplasia, liver damage, and blood dyscrasias

Nursing Implications

- Administer the drug with food to minimize gastrointestinal upset and enhance absorption. Instruct parents to do the same.
- Advise parents to have the prescription filled each time with the same brand of drug, because differences in bioavailability have been reported.
- Obtain serum drug levels as ordered to monitor for drug's effectiveness and prevent possible toxicity. Keep in mind that the therapeutic range is 10 to 20 μg/mL.
- Monitor liver function studies and blood counts periodically.
- Inform parents about the need for follow-up laboratory tests.
- Instruct the child and parents about oral hygiene measures to prevent gum problems. Encourage frequent dental checkups.
- Suggest that the parents obtain a medical alert bracelet and have the child wear it in case of an emergency.
- Warn parents not to discontinue the drug abruptly or change the dose unless ordered by the health care provider.
- Instruct parents to notify the health care provider if the child develops nystagmus, ataxia, or diminished mental capacity. These are signs of possible toxicity.

FOCUS ON PHARMACOLOGY

Carbamazepine (Tegretol)

Action: Carbamazepine is an anticonvulsant whose exact mechanism of action is unknown. It is believed to inhibit polysynaptic responses and block post-tetanic potentiation.

Pregnancy risk category: C

Dosage: Initially in children 6 to 12 years of age, 100 mg orally bid on the first day, increased gradually in 100-mg increments at 6- to 8-h intervals until best response is achieved, or 10 to 30 mg/kg/day in divided doses tid or qid. Not to exceed 1,000 mg/day.

Possible adverse effects: Dizziness, drowsiness, behavioral changes, nausea, vomiting, gastrointestinal upset, abnormal liver function tests, bone marrow depression, rash, photosensitivity

Nursing Implications

- Administer the drug with food to minimize gastrointestinal upset. Instruct parents to do the same.
- Obtain serum drug levels as ordered to monitor for drug's effectiveness and prevent possible toxicity. Keep in mind that the therapeutic range is 4 to 12 μg/mL.
- Monitor liver function studies and blood counts periodically.
- Inform parents about the need for follow-up laboratory tests.
- Suggest that the parents obtain a medical alert bracelet and have the child wear it in case of an emergency.
- Instruct parents and child about avoiding alcohol and sleep-inducing or over-the-counter drugs, which could cause dangerous synergistic effects.
- Warn parents not to discontinue the drug abruptly or change the dose unless ordered by the health care provider.
- Instruct parents to notify the health care provider if the child develops bruising, bleeding, or signs of infection. These are signs of possible bone marrow depression.

the body. These types of seizures may be caused by something as specific as a rapidly growing brain tumor. Documenting the spread can help localize the spot where the seizure first began.

Absence Seizures. Absence seizures, formerly known as *petit mal,* are classified as generalized seizures. They usually consist of a staring spell that lasts for a few seconds. A child might be reciting in class when he pauses and stares for 1 to 5 seconds before continuing the recitation; he is unaware that time has passed. Rhythmic blinking and twitching of the mouth or an extremity may accompany the staring. Absence seizures can occur up to 100 times per day. An EEG usually shows a typical 3 wave/s spike and slow-wave discharge. Such seizures tend to occur more frequently in girls than boys. The usual age of occurrence is 6 to 7 years (Moe & Seay, 2001).

Children with absence episodes may be accused of daydreaming in school and may be referred to the school nurse for behavior problems. These children generally have normal intelligence, although, if they have frequent episodes, they may be doing poorly in school because they are missing instructional content.

Absence seizures can usually be demonstrated in children by asking them to hyperventilate and count out loud. If they are susceptible to such seizures, they will breathe in and out deeply, possibly 10 times, stop and stare for 3 sec-

FOCUS ON PHARMACOLOGY

Phenobarbital

Action: Phenobarbital is a central nervous system (CNS) depressant that acts as an anticonvulsant.

Pregnancy risk category: D

Dosage: 3 to 6 mg/kg/day orally or 4 to 6 mg/kg/day parenterally for 7 to 10 days until achievement of a blood level of 10 to 15 μg/mL, or 10 to 15 mg/kg/day IV or IM. In status epilepticus, 15 to 20 mg/kg IV administered over 10 to 15 min.

Possible adverse effects: Somnolence, sedation, confusion, ataxia, lethargy, hangover, paradoxical excitement, nausea, vomiting, constipation, diarrhea, epigastric pain, bradycardia, hypotension, syncope, hypoventilation, respiratory depression, pain or tissue necrosis at the injection site.

Nursing Implications

- When giving phenobarbital parenterally, administer IV doses slowly directly into tubing or running infusion. Inject a partial dose and assess response before continuing. If giving phenobarbital IM, administer deeply into a large muscle.
- Monitor IV site carefully for signs of irritation or extravasation.
- Assess vital signs closely—especially pulse, blood pressure, and respiratory rate—during IV administration.
- Administer the oral form of the drug with food to minimize gastrointestinal upset. Instruct parents to do the same.
- Warn the parents and child that the drug will make the child drowsy. Advise the child to change positions slowly and sit at the edge of the bed for a few minutes before arising. Assist parents with safety measures to protect the child from injury.
- Monitor laboratory tests for liver and renal function and blood counts if the child is on long-term therapy.
- Inform parents about the possible need for follow-up laboratory tests.
- Suggest that the parents obtain a medical alert bracelet and have the child wear it in case of an emergency.
- Instruct parents and child about avoiding alcohol and sleep-inducing or over-the-counter drugs, which could cause increased CNS depression.
- Warn parents not to discontinue the drug abruptly or change the dose unless ordered by the health care provider.
- Instruct parents to notify the health care provider if the child develops severe dizziness, weakness, or drowsiness that persists.

onds, then continue to hyperventilate and count, unaware that they paused.

No first aid measures are necessary for absence seizures. Down playing the importance of these episodes will help children maintain a positive self-image.

Absence seizures can be controlled by ethosuximide (Zarontin) or by valproic acid. If seizures are fully controlled by medication, children can participate in normal school activities and ride a bicycle. If seizures cannot be controlled fully, parents need to anticipate potentially hazardous situations during the child's day, such as crossing a busy street on the way to school or learning to drive. This is crucial for adolescents who are eager to get a driver's license. The tendency for developing seizures should be evaluated carefully, for the child's own safety as well as others.

Approximately one third to one half of all children with absence seizures "outgrow them" by adulthood. This does not mean that treatment is not necessary during childhood. Absence seizures usually occur independently of tonic-clonic seizures, although it is possible for children to manifest both types. Some children's seizure pattern changes from absence involvement to tonic-clonic involvement as they approach adulthood.

Tonic-Clonic Seizures. Typical tonic-clonic seizures (formerly termed *grand mal seizures*) are generalized seizures, consisting of four stages. There may be a *prodromal* period of hours or days; an *aura,* or warning, immediately before the seizure; the tonic-clonic stage; and, finally, a postictal stage. Not all four stages occur with every seizure.

The prodromal period may consist of drowsiness, dizziness, malaise, lack of coordination, or tension. Parents may observe simply that the child is "not himself." As the child reaches school age, he may be able to predict from these vague preliminary feelings when he is going to have a seizure.

The aura, or second phase, may reflect the portion of the brain in which the seizure originates. Smelling unpleasant odors (often reported as feces) denotes activity in the medial portion of the temporal lobe. Seeing flashing lights suggests the occipital area; repeated hallucinations arise from the temporal lobe; numbness of an extremity relates to the opposite parietal lobe; and a "Cheshire cat grin" relates to the frontal lobe. Young children, unable to describe or understand an aura, may scream in fright or run to their parent with its onset. Note exactly what symptoms the child experiences during this time, because this may help to localize the involved brain portion.

The third phase is the tonic stage. All muscles of the body contract, and the child falls to the ground. Extremities stiffen; the face distorts. Although this phase lasts only about 20 seconds, the respiratory muscles are contracted, and the child may experience hypoxia and turn cyanotic. Contraction of the throat prevents swallowing, so saliva collects in the mouth. The child may bite the tongue when the jaws contract. As the chest muscles contract initially, air is pushed through the glottis, producing a guttural cry.

The seizure then enters a clonic stage, in which muscles of the body rapidly contract and relax, producing quick, jerky motions. The child may blow bubbles or foamy saliva and, if he bit his tongue when his jaw spasmed shut, he may have blood in his mouth. He may be incontinent of stool and urine. This phase usually lasts about 20 to 30 seconds.

After the tonic-clonic period, the child falls into a sound sleep, called the *postictal period*. He will sleep soundly for 1 to 4 h and will rouse only to painful stimuli during this time. When he awakens, he often experiences a severe headache. He has no memory of the seizure.

Seizures may occur only at night. The child wakes in the morning with a bitten tongue, blood on the pillow, or a bed wet with urine. In the child with persistent bed-wetting, the possibility of nocturnal seizures must be considered.

Although not always true, children with this type of seizure generally have an abnormal EEG pattern. Other family members may have similarly abnormal EEG patterns without any symptoms.

Therapy usually includes the daily administration of anticonvulsants such as valproic acid (Depakene) and carbamazepine (Tegretol). Phenobarbital has the advantage of being an inexpensive anticonvulsant (see Focus on Pharmacology). However, drowsiness and sleepiness may interfere with the child's ability to perform in school. Phenobarbital dosages should be tapered, never stopped suddenly, because the body becomes dependent on it. Rapid withdrawal may precipitate a seizure.

Children with tonic-clonic seizures also may be given phenytoin sodium (Dilantin) for control. One nontoxic side effect of phenytoin is painless hypertrophy of the gums. Unless the gum hypertrophy is extensive, however, it is not sufficient reason to discontinue the drug. Medications are usually continued until the child has been seizure free for 2 to 3 years.

Some children may be placed on a ketogenic diet. This diet is high in fat and low in protein and carbohydrate. It causes the child to have a high level of ketones, which is believed to decrease myoclonic or tonic-clonic seizure activity. Because a ketogenic diet is monotonous for children and difficult for parents to prepare, however, it is hard to maintain for very long (Moe & Seay, 2001).

WHAT IF? A child with a history of seizures controlled with phenobarbital is brought to the clinic. His mother states that he's been very sleepy, especially in school. To correct this, she reported that she cut his phenobarbital dosage in half. How would you respond to this parent?

Status Epilepticus. **Status epilepticus** refers to a seizure that lasts continuously for more than 30 min or a series of seizures from which the child does not return to his or her previous level of consciousness (Altemeier, 1999). This is an emergency situation requiring immediate treatment. Otherwise, permanent brain injury, exhaustion, respiratory failure, and death may occur. Oxygen may be necessary to relieve cyanosis. An IV benzodiazepine, such as diazepam (Valium) or lorazepam (Ativan) halts seizures dramatically. This may be followed by IV phenobarbital or phenytoin (Dilantin). Diazepam must be administered with extreme caution because the drug is incompatible with many other drugs, and any accidental infiltration into subcutaneous tissue causes extensive tissue sloughing. Parents may administer diazepam by enema at home. Lorazepam (Ativan) is a long-acting benzodiazepine, thus providing a longer duration of action and also less respiratory depression in children older than 2 years of age.

✔ CHECKPOINT QUESTIONS

12. A parent describes the child's seizure as starting with a twitch in the fingers and progressing to the arm and face. What type of seizure is the parent describing?
13. How can you assess for the occurrence of absence seizures in a child?

Assessment of the Child With Seizures

A thorough pregnancy history must be obtained on children with seizures. Events immediately before the seizure as well as an accurate description of the seizure itself also should be recorded. Investigate the child's overall behavior in the last few weeks. Is the child an A student who has been getting Ds lately? Has the parent noticed bed-wetting? These might be possible signs of absence or nocturnal seizures.

A complete physical and neurologic examination and blood studies are necessary to rule out metabolic or infectious processes. Prepare the child for a lumbar puncture to rule out meningitis or bleeding in the CSF. A CT scan, MRI, skull x-ray film, or EEG may be done if indicated. During the EEG, the child may be stimulated with rhythm patterns or flashing lights or may be asked to hyperventilate to see whether a seizure can be provoked.

NURSING DIAGNOSES AND RELATED INTERVENTIONS

Nursing Diagnosis: Risk for injury related to tonic-clonic seizure

Outcome Identification: Child will remain free of injury during seizure.

Outcome Evaluation: Child exhibits no signs of aspiration or traumatic injury.

Protecting the child from hurting himself during a tonic-clonic seizure is crucial (see Focus on Family Empowerment). Restraining the child's thrashing extremities is not advisable, because it is difficult for the adult and could result in injury to either person because of the amount of force needed to keep the child still. In early school-aged children, it is particularly important to avoid inserting a tongue blade between the teeth because these children often have loose anterior teeth that are on the verge of falling out.

Remaining calm is also important; be aware that people are frightened by the sight of a child having a seizure because the action is so forceful and violent. It is reassuring for them to see someone calm and in control of the situation and that there is no reason to be afraid. If the child passes rapidly from one seizure into another (status epilepticus), be prepared to provide supplemental oxygen and administer anticonvulsant therapy to counteract this as needed.

FOCUS ON FAMILY EMPOWERMENT
Safety During Seizures

Q. What can we do to make sure that our son doesn't get hurt when he is having a seizure?

A. When your son has a seizure, here are some tips to help keep him safe:

- Remain calm.
- Move away furniture or any sharp object.
- Turn your child gently on his side or abdomen with his head turned to the side to prevent aspiration of unswallowed mouth secretions.
- Don't restrain him other than to keep his head turned to the side so that mouth secretions continue to drain. Restraining the child could result in injury because of the amount of force necessary.
- Do not attempt to place a stick or padded tongue blade between the child's teeth. Trying to force a tongue blade into the mouth this way could break the tongue blade or loosen teeth.
- Try to keep onlookers from crowding the area. A convulsing child is an abnormal sight and always attracts a crowd. Ask people who are only interested spectators to move away.
- Be aware that a child having this type of seizure may have some slight cyanosis during the tonic and clonic stages, but these stages are so short that administering oxygen is not needed.
- After any seizure, telephone your primary care provider and notify him or her of the seizure so arrangements for any necessary follow-up care can be made.
- If your child should pass rapidly from one seizure into another (status epilepticus), he may need supplemental oxygen and you may need to administer diazepam. If this happens, telephone your emergency medical service number.

Nursing Diagnosis: Interrupted family processes related to diagnosis of long-term illness in child

Outcome Identification: Family will maintain functional system of support for each member throughout the course of the illness.

Outcome Evaluation: Child, parents, and other family members express fears and questions about disease to health care team; parents discuss ways to accommodate illness (eg, medication schedules, school, sports activities, plans for vacation, and discipline) in their daily life.

As soon as the diagnosis of a seizure disorder is made, parents and children need to be told that it is likely to signify a long-term disease. Although the seizures can be controlled with medication, the disease is not cured. If children neglect their medication, seizures are apt to recur (see Focus on Nursing Care Planning). Most children are given tablets rather than liquid medication, because the latter tends to settle at the bottom of the bottle, resulting in overdiluted or overconcentrated doses that might allow seizures to break through. Parents need instruction on planning to ensure an adequate supply of medications, especially for a trip away from home or for summer camp. Abrupt discontinuation of seizure medications (particularly phenobarbital) may result in severe seizures.

The child will need to be monitored frequently during childhood to be certain that a medication dosage is adequate. He or she will need periodic blood sampling to ascertain whether therapeutic blood levels of the medication are being maintained.

Provide parents with as much information as possible about the cause of their child's seizures. This will help them feel that they are dealing with a known disease, not an unexplainable and unpredictable illness. If the cause of the seizures is unknown, parents can be reassured that the treatment is known. Many new anticonvulsant medications are available today and being introduced into therapy. These include topiramate (Topamax), lamotrigine (Lamictal) and tiagabine (Gabitril). This means that the child can be expected to respond to anticonvulsant medication as well as the child whose seizures have a known cause such as recent trauma (Wallace, 2001).

Although it may be difficult, parents need to treat children with seizures as a normal member of the family. Alert them that scolding children, asking them to do household chores, or insisting that they do their homework will not cause seizures. A few children with absence seizures can initiate them by hyperventilating and may try to manipulate those around them by doing this to gain sympathy. The few children who use this extreme form of manipulation may need to be referred for counseling.

Assure parents that occasional seizures in children are not harmful. Unless status epilepticus occurs and the child becomes anoxic, the chance that their child will be injured during a seizure is remote. Knowledge of this helps them not to worry about the child becoming cognitively challenged or heed other misconceptions about seizures. Although some children who have seizures are cognitively challenged, this and the seizures were caused by the same event; the seizures did not cause the impairment. At every health care visit, be certain that parents have time to ask questions about their child's care and to express any concerns they have. There are so many "scare stories" about seizures that every parent is likely to believe

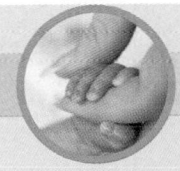

FOCUS ON *Nursing Care Planning*

A CHILD WITH RECURRENT SEIZURES

A 12-year-old male is admitted to the acute care facility after a tonic-clonic seizure. His mother states, "He hasn't had a seizure in over a year."

Assessment: Well-proportioned male sleeping soundly on left side since admission. Seizure episode occurred approximately 1 h ago. Vital signs within age-appropriate parameters. Reacts to painful stimuli only. Deep tendon reflexes depressed. "He was watching television this morning and then told me the light was hurting his eyes and that everything was turning orange. Suddenly, he just fell to the floor and started shaking. His face became distorted, and he started foaming from his mouth. Some had little specks of blood in it. I called 911, and they brought him here." Diagnosed with seizures 3 years ago. Currently taking phenobarbital and phenytoin (Dilantin) four times a day. "Since my husband and I divorced 6 months ago, he's been taking charge of his own medicines because I went back to work full time. He's told me he hates to take them because he feels like they slow him down. Now I'm not sure if he really has been taking them like he should." Child leaves for school when mother leaves for work at 7 AM and takes the late bus home from school after baseball practice, getting home around 6 PM. Mother noticed some small blood spots on the child's pillow twice in the last week. "Maybe he had a seizure during the night?" Child is in seventh grade and is a B student. Plays on the middle school baseball team. Has a 7-year-old sister. Mother states, "They get along fairly well, except for their occasional fights." Lumbar puncture performed; pressures within normal limits; specimens sent for cell count, glucose, and culture. Serum drug levels obtained: phenobarbital level 7 μg/mL; phenytoin level 6 μg/mL.

Nursing Diagnosis: Risk for injury related to diminished level of consciousness resulting from seizure episode

Outcome Identification: Child will remain free of injury now and during future seizures.

Outcome Evaluation: Child and parent state safety measures to prevent injury. Child exhibits no signs of aspiration or traumatic injury.

Interventions	Rationale
1. Maintain a patent airway with the child lying on his side until alert and responsive. Provide privacy and institute seizure precautions.	1. Side-lying position reduces the risk for aspiration. Privacy minimizes possible embarrassment for the child. Seizure precautions minimize the risk of injury when the child's level of consciousness is diminished and also if another seizure should occur.
2. Monitor vital signs and neurologic status every 15 min until the child is fully awake.	2. Frequent monitoring provides information about the extent of involvement and resolution of the seizure.
3. Observe for signs and symptoms of respiratory distress. Administer oxygen as ordered, and monitor oxygen saturation levels with pulse oximetry.	3. Respiratory distress may indicate aspiration. Oxygen administration aids in preventing hypoxemia. Oxygen saturation levels provide objective evidence of tissue perfusion.
4. Provide a calm, restful environment. Minimize the child's exposure to external stimuli. Administer anticonvulsants as ordered.	4. After a tonic-clonic seizure, a calm, restful environment is necessary to allow the child to sleep. The child's drug levels are subtherapeutic. Administering anticonvulsants reduces the risk for further seizure activity by increasing serum drug levels.

(continued)

Interventions	Rationale
5. As the child begins to awaken, orient him. Do not give anything by mouth until the child is fully awake, alert, and oriented and the gag reflex is intact.	5. Children experiencing tonic-clonic seizures have no memory of the event. Orienting the child decreases confusion. Giving fluids too early increases the risk for aspiration.
6. Instruct the mother (and the child when alert and oriented) in safety measures to use during future seizures.	6. Anticipatory guidance about safety measures minimizes the risk of injury in the future.
7. Advise the mother and child to report any unusual sensations such as flashing lights or strange smells.	7. The ability to identify an "aura," if present, helps to alert those nearby that a seizure may be imminent, prompting them to initiate safety measures.
8. Caution parent not to restrain the child during a seizure.	8. The force needed to restrain a person experiencing a tonic-clonic seizure may result in further injury to the child or the person attempting to restrain him.

Nursing Diagnosis: Ineffective therapeutic regimen management related to age, lack of knowledge, effects of medication, and inadequate supervision

Outcome Identification: Child will demonstrate responsibility for self-medication.

Outcome Evaluation: Child states accurate information about the drugs prescribed; reports adherence to medication schedule. Serum drug levels of anticonvulsants at therapeutic levels.

Interventions	Rationale
1. Administer anticonvulsant medications as ordered while hospitalized.	1. Administration during hospitalization helps to raise serum drug levels before discharge.
2. Explore with the child possible reasons for problems with the medications. Work with the child to develop ways to overcome these problems. Anticipate the need for a change in medication if the adverse effects of the drug are interfering with the child's adhering to therapy.	2. Exploration provides clues to the child's behavior and provides a base from which to develop appropriate actions. A change in medication with fewer adverse effects for the child may help to improve compliance while still maintaining seizure control.
3. Review the seizure medications ordered with the child and parent, including any new medications, changes in dosages or frequency, and follow-up laboratory testing.	3. Providing accurate information about the regimen helps the child and parent understand the importance of drug therapy in controlling the seizures.
4. Caution the child and parent to measure the dosage accurately and to administer the medication on time.	4. Accurate dosages and scheduling aid in maintaining therapeutic serum drug levels.
5. Work with the child to develop a medication schedule that fits his usual daily routine. Contact the child's school nurse, as appropriate, to assist with medication administration during school hours. Help the child make out a written reminder chart for medication administration.	5. Proper scheduling of medications, including during school hours, is necessary to maintain therapeutic drug levels. A written reminder chart promotes active participation and helps to promote compliance.
6. Remind the mother to check the reminder chart daily and offer positive reinforcement for adherence.	6. A 12-year-old child, although feeling the need for independence and increased responsibility, still requires some supervision. Positive reinforcement aids in promoting compliance and also in fostering a sense of self-esteem and accomplishment.
7. Arrange for a home care referral as needed.	7. Home care follow-up provides opportunities for additional support, assessment, education, and evaluation of compliance.

(continued)

Nursing Diagnosis: Deficient knowledge related to recurrent seizures

Outcome Identification: Child and parent will verbalize accurate information about seizures.

Outcome Evaluation: Child and parent state causes and possible contributing factors associated with seizures; identify measures to control seizures; demonstrate knowledge of prognosis and future planning needs.

Interventions	Rationale
1. Review what each knows about seizures so they do not view this as an uncontrollable disorder.	1. Review of what they already know provides a baseline for teaching and prevents repetition. Increased knowledge can help to improve compliance.
2. Caution them that seizure activity may increase with adolescence.	2. Glandular changes or growth spurts requiring increased medication dosages can occur with puberty. Awareness of this can help the child and parent plan for future growth and development needs.
3. Inform the child and parent about precipitating factors such as alcohol, fatigue, and excessive stress. Encourage the child to continue to participate in activities.	3. Knowledge of precipitating factors helps the child and parent avoid them, enhancing their feelings of control over the situation. Physical activity has been shown to reduce the frequency of seizures.
4. Assist the child and parent with planning for future events, such as obtaining a driver's license.	4. Obtaining a driver's license is usually highly valued by adolescents. Most states require a specific amount of time for the person to be seizure free. This information may provide the child with motivation for improved compliance.
5. Reinforce instructions about safety measures during a seizure.	5. A thorough understanding of safety measures minimizes the risk for injury should the child experience a seizure.
6. Encourage the child and parent to obtain a medical alert bracelet or tag and strongly encourage the child to wear it.	6. Alert bracelets or tags help to ensure safety for the child should a seizure occur if he is away from home.

some of these stories unless counseled otherwise (see Focus on Communication).

As a rule, children with seizures should attend regular school and participate in physical education classes and active sports (possible exceptions include scuba or sky diving or rock climbing). Many teachers are concerned about the responsibility of having a child with seizures assigned to their classes. Help them learn about the success of modern seizure control. State regulations differ, but most states allow teenagers to apply for a driver's license after they have been seizure free for 1 year (Moe & Seay, 2001).

In many children, seizures increase at puberty. This may be the result of glandular changes or of sudden growth and the need for an increased medicine dosage. It may result in part from adolescent rebellion against following prescribed medication routines. Respect the adolescent's feelings and need for independence, but assist the adolescent with channeling feelings to a more positive area.

All anticonvulsant medications are potentially teratogenic to a fetus. Be certain that adolescent girls are made aware of this so they can choose to delay childbearing until later in life, when their medication can be reduced or even discontinued.

Breath Holding

Breath holding is a phenomenon that occurs in young children when they are stressed or angry. The child breathes in and, because he is upset, does not breathe out again or else breathes out and then does not inhale again (Blum, 2000). As brain cells become anoxic, the child becomes cyanotic and slumps to the floor, momentarily unconscious. With loss of consciousness, the child begins breathing again. The child's color returns to normal, and he awakens. Breath holding is frightening but represents the immaturity of the child's neurologic control. This differs from a temper tantrum in which a child deliberately attempts to hold his breath and pass out (see Chapter 29). The child needs no therapy except reassurance that he is all right.

Headache

Headache in children younger than school age is rare, although children may report "headache" in imitation of their parents. Preschoolers may have headache with a

FOCUS ON COMMUNICATION

Melissa is a 5-year-old girl with a history of tonic-clonic seizures, which have been controlled with anticonvulsant therapy. Her father brought her into the clinic for evaluation after a seizure over the weekend.

Less Effective Communication

Nurse: Mr. Jarman, can you tell me what happened?
Mr. Jarman: She just started shaking all over. It was really frightening.
Nurse: Did she voice any symptoms before the seizure?
Mr. Jarman: No, she just started shaking.
Nurse: Is she taking her medicines?
Mr. Jarman: Yes, I make sure she does. I don't want her to become retarded from the seizures.
Nurse: Let's get a blood test to check her drug level and then I'll examine her.

More Effective Communication

Nurse: Mr. Jarman, can you tell me what happened?
Mr. Jarman: She just started shaking all over. It was really frightening.
Nurse: Did she voice any symptoms before the seizure?
Mr. Jarman: No, she just started shaking.
Nurse: Is she taking her medicines?
Mr. Jarman: Yes, I make sure she does. I don't want her to become retarded from the seizures.
Nurse: Retarded from the seizures?
Mr. Jarman: Yes. Our neighbor's son has seizures and he's severely retarded.
Nurse: Mr. Jarman, let's talk about this a little more. What do you know about seizures?

In the first scenario, the nurse fails to identify a misconception verbalized by the father, being more intent on evaluating what may have precipitated Melissa's seizure. In the second scenario, the nurse identifies the concern and attempts to clarify it, providing an opportunity for teaching.

fever because of increased ICP caused by increased cerebral blood flow. As the child reaches school age, headaches may occur as a result of conditions as simple as eyestrain and sinusitis or as serious as a brain tumor. Headache pain results from meningeal or vascular irritation. The brain is insensitive to pain, so a cerebral tumor may be present for a long time before meningeal irritation occurs and pain symptoms are apparent. With a brain tumor, pain becomes evident on changing body position, so a young child who reports headache after getting up should be carefully evaluated. Pain from a brain tumor is also generally occipital, so asking the child to indicate where it hurts will help determine whether a tumor could be the cause.

Tension or Stress Headache

When children are studying intently or taking a test, contraction of their neck muscles from tension may cause temporary ischemia. This is experienced as a dull, steady pain in the head. Children with these symptoms should have their vision tested, because poor eyesight may be causing them to hunch over their books. Tension or stress is relieved by simple analgesics, such as acetaminophen, or by sleep or application of a cool compress.

Sinus Headache

Sinus headache usually accompanies sinusitis and is associated with inflammation and possible obstruction of the sinuses. Sinusitis is discussed in Chapter 40.

Migraine Headache

Migraine headache refers to a specific type of headache that may or may not begin with an aura of visual disturbance such as diplopia or a zigzag pattern across the visual field. The pain that follows is generally unilateral and extremely intense with throbbing that is moderate to severe. The headache is aggravated by routine physical activity and may be compounded by nausea and vomiting and intolerance to bright lights and noise (Lewis, 2001).

The cause of migraine headache in any age group is not well understood. It probably results from abnormal constriction of intracranial arteries, temporarily reducing cerebral blood supply. This is followed by compensating overdistention of cranial blood vessels. The aura accompanying such headaches is the result of the temporary ischemia, whereas the headache is the result of the overdistention. Some children who have migraine headaches have an abnormal EEG.

Most children with migraine headache have a positive family history. This syndrome may be inherited as a dominant trait.

Assessment. To help assess the cause of a headache, obtain a thorough history, including

- When the headache generally occurs
- The events preceding it (to detect an aura)
- Its duration, frequency, intensity, description, and associated symptoms
- Any actions taken to treat the headache

The child needs a thorough physical examination, including funduscopic examination, to rule out papilledema. Blood pressure must be measured to rule out hypertension. If an aura is documented, an EEG will be ordered.

Therapeutic Management. A drug commonly prescribed for migraine headache in children is ergotamine tartrate (Cafergot), which constricts cerebral arteries. Sumatriptan, a serotonin agonist approved for adults, has even greater potential for relief (Molloy, 2000). Beta blockers or calcium channel blockers that result in vasodilation may be prescribed prophylactically. At the time of the headache, sleep or lying down may be necessary to relieve the pain and vomiting. Frequent headaches interfere with a child's ability to achieve in school. Children need to be reassured that migraine headaches are benign, although painful and incapacitating, and not signs of a developing brain tumor. Follow-up visits are necessary to confirm that there is no progressive disease.

If other family members have migraine headaches, counsel them on how their reactions to their headaches influence their child's reaction to his or her own headaches. If the mother goes to bed for the day when she has a migraine headache, she cannot expect her child to go to school when he has one.

> **✔ CHECKPOINT QUESTIONS**
>
> 14. What are two reasons for an increase in seizure activity at puberty?
> 15. How does breath holding differ from a temper tantrum?

ATAXIC DISORDERS

Ataxia is the failure of muscular coordination, or irregularity of muscle action. Ataxic disorders are often manifested by an awkward gait or lack of coordination. Causes of ataxias differ, but degeneration of cerebellar or vestibular function is always involved.

Ataxia-Telangiectasia

Ataxia-telangiectasia, transmitted as an autosomal recessive trait attributable to a defect of chromosome 11, is a primary immunodeficiency disorder that results in progressive cerebellar degeneration. This is a multisystem disease with neurologic and immunologic aspects. In addition, endocrine abnormalities may occur, and there is an increased risk of cancer, particularly brain tumor. Telangiectasia (red vascular markings) appear on the conjunctiva and skin at the flexor creases (Moe & Seay, 2001).

Both immunologic and neurologic symptoms of this disorder vary in severity and onset. Serum IgA and IgE levels may be low, and there is often evidence of reduced T-cell function. Children generally develop frequent infections (primarily sinopulmonary) because of the immunologic deficits. Tonsillar tissue in the pharynx is scant.

Neurologic symptoms from the degeneration process can usually be detected in early infancy when developmental milestones are not met. Children develop an awkward gait when they begin to walk. **Choreoathetosis** (rapid, purposeless movements), nystagmus, an intention tremor, or scoliosis may develop. They may be unable to move their eyes on demand or follow through visual fields. Eye changes (conjunctival telangiectasia) develop by 5 years of age. There is no effective treatment. Children with this disorder often die in late adolescence of infection, respiratory failure, or a malignant brain tumor.

Friedreich's Ataxia

Friedreich's ataxia involves a variety of degenerative symptoms, carried on the short arm of chromosome 9 as an autosomal recessive trait. Symptoms, such as progressive cerebellar and spinal cord dysfunction, occur in late adolescence. Teenagers develop a progressive gait disturbance or a lack of coordinated arm movements. They also develop a high-arched foot (pes cavus), hammer toes, and scoliosis. The combined symptoms of a positive Babinski reflex, absence of deep tendon reflexes in the ankle, and ataxia are strongly diagnostic. Neurologic examination shows difficulty in recognizing foot position (whether the foot is moved up or down). Death occurs in young adulthood from myocardial failure attributable to cardiac muscle fiber degeneration.

SPINAL CORD INJURY

Because of the resilience of their vertebrae, children have fewer spinal cord injuries than adults. Because more adolescents are commonly involved in accidents, however, particularly motorcycle accidents, spinal cord injuries in this age group are increasing. Another major cause of spinal cord injury is diving into too-shallow water (see Focus on Evidence-Based Practice). Any patient with multiple traumatic injuries should be assessed for spinal cord damage. Spinal cord injury without radiographic abnormality (SCIWRA syndrome) may occur. Stabilizing the neck is the best protection against further injury when this happens (Brown, Brunn & Garcia, 2001).

Recovery Phases

Spinal injuries result when the cord becomes compressed or severed by the vertebrae; further cord damage can be caused by hemorrhage, edema, or inflammation at the injury site as the blood supply becomes impeded. Table 49-5 summarizes functional ability after spinal cord injury. The first questions asked by the parents or the child after the injury are: How much damage is there? Will our child be able to walk again? Predictions of useful body function can-

> **FOCUS ON EVIDENCE-BASED PRACTICE**
>
> *What Sports Cause the Most Spinal Cord Injuries in Children?*
>
> To examine what sports cause sport-related spinal cord injuries that resulted in paraplegia or quadriplegia, researchers reviewed the charts of 1,016 children who had experienced a traumatic spinal cord injury. Results showed that, of this large sample, 15% of injuries were caused by sport or diving accidents. The sport accidents included 16 from downhill skiing, 9 from horseback riding, 7 from air sports such as paragliding, 6 from gymnastics, 5 from trampolining, and 26 from other active sports.
>
> This is an important study for nurses because they are the health care providers who are frequently most active in teaching about accident prevention. Mention that, although participating in sports is a healthy activity, it also carries some risk. This is important information to include in any teaching plan for parents and children.
>
> Schmitt, H., & Gerner, H. J. (2001). Paralysis from sport and diving accidents. *Clinical Journal of Sport Medicine, 11*(1), 17–22.

TABLE 49.5 Functional Ability After Spinal Cord Injury

INJURY SITE	HIGHEST KEY FUNCTIONS STILL PRESENT	EFFECTS AND POSSIBLE INTERVENTIONS
C1–3	Head and neck muscles intact	Respiratory paralysis from loss of phrenic nerve innervation; will need ventilatory assistance No voluntary motion below chin; possibly able to learn to use mouth to control pen for writing and mouthstick to reach objects
C4	Diaphragm intact	Loss of motor function of upper and lower extremities and trunk; able to learn to use abdominal muscles to breathe independently
C5	Shoulder control; biceps, deltoid function	Able to feed self and operate wheelchair if fitted with self-care aids
C6	Forearm pronation; wrist extension	Use of upper extremities for self-care. Can transfer to wheelchair and so have increased independence
C7	Triceps function	Able to transfer to wheelchair readily; increasing independence
C8	Thumb and finger function	Able to do fine motor tasks; increases self-care ability
T1–7	Intercostal muscle (able to breathe with chest, not abdominal, muscles)	Full use of upper extremities but is still dependent on wheelchair Possibly able to drive car with hand controls Possibly able to have high leg braces fitted for standing
T10–12	Abdominal muscles	Use of long leg braces and four-point crutch to ambulate
L2–4	Hip flexion Leg extension	Use of long or short leg braces to ambulate
L5–S1	Gluteus maximus muscle function	Walking without aids
S4	Bladder and anal sphincter control	Controlling of bladder and bowel function Penile erection and ejaculation

not be made at the time of the accident, however. Three phases of recovery must first take place.

First Recovery Phase

Immediately after the injury, the child experiences spinal shock syndrome or loss of autonomic nervous system function (anterior nerve fibers traveling through the anterior horn of the spinal canal). This leads to loss of motor function, sensation, and reflex activity, and flaccid paralysis in body areas below the level of the injury. If a cervical injury is present, this will mean loss of respiratory function attributable to flaccidity of the diaphragm. In high thoracic lesions, use of accessory muscles of the chest is lost, so the child has difficulty maintaining effective respirations. The child has no ability to sweat or shiver to change body temperature below the level of the lesion because of loss of autonomic nerve control; hypothermia or hyperthermia becomes a threat. Blood vessels below the level of the injury are no longer able to constrict, so blood tends to pool in the lower body, leading to hypotension, especially if the upper body is elevated. Loss of bladder control will occur (when flaccid, the bladder overdistends and continually empties). The bowel becomes equally distended, and bowel sounds are absent. This phase of spinal cord injury lasts from 1 to 6 weeks. As a rule, the shorter the phase of spinal shock, the better the final outcome.

Administration of a corticosteroid helps to reduce edema and hopefully protect function of the spinal cord during this phase. A vasopressor agent such as dopamine may be prescribed to maintain blood pressure and perfusion to the cord.

Second Recovery Phase

During the second phase of recovery, the flaccid paralysis of the shock phase is replaced by spastic paralysis. Normally, motor impulses begin in the brain cortex; are transmitted to the medulla, where they cross to the opposite side of the cord; and then travel down the descending motor tracts of the spinal cord. They synapse in the anterior horn of the spinal cord and travel by way of the spinal and peripheral nerves to the designated muscle group, which they set in motion. The nerve pathways of the brain and the descending tracts are termed *upper motor neurons.* Those in the anterior horn cells and the spinal and peripheral nerves are termed *lower motor neurons.* Whether a motor neuron has upper or lower function, therefore, does not depend as much on its height in the spinal tract as on its position in relation to an anterior horn (between the brain and the anterior horn, it is an upper motor neuron; between the anterior horn and the point of innervation, it is a lower motor neuron; Fig. 49-11).

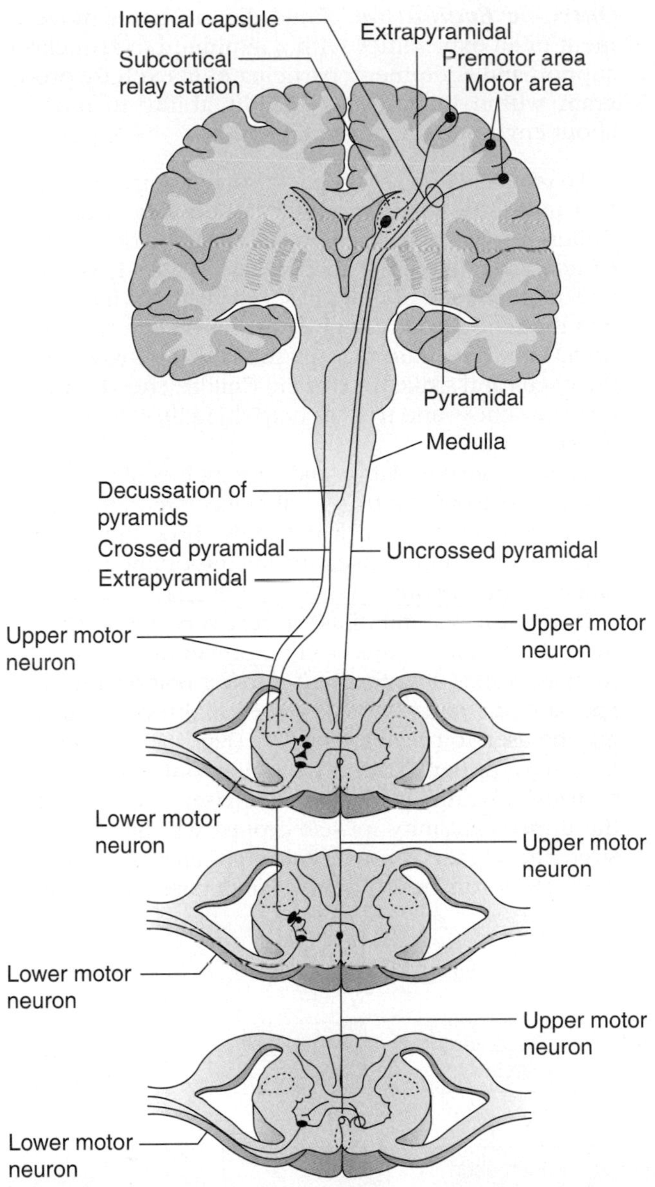

FIGURE 49.11 Diagram of motor pathways between the cerebral cortex, one of the subcortical relay stations, and lower motor neurons in the spinal cord. Decussation (crossing of fibers) means that each side of the brain controls skeletal muscles on the opposite side of the body.

Spasticity in the second phase is due to the loss of upper level control or transmission of meaningful innervation to the lower muscles. Lacking upper motor neuron function because of a severed cord, lower motor neurons, or reflex arcs causes the muscles to contract and remain that way. Parents and children are quick to interpret the sudden spastic movement of a lower extremity as meaningful activity. This is particularly easy to believe with an infant, who cannot tell you that he has no control over his leg movement. Differences between upper and lower neuron damage are listed in Table 49-6. If the injury is very low in the spinal tract, affecting mostly lower motor neurons, muscles will remain flaccid, because lower motor neurons cannot send impulses for contraction.

During this phase, if the child's bladder is allowed to fill, the resultant sensory stimulation relayed to the damaged cord will initiate a powerful sympathetic reflex reaction (**autonomic dysreflexia**), and the child will show signs of hypertension, tachycardia, flushed face, and severe occipital headache. This is an emergency situation, and, if the severe hypertension is not relieved, cerebral vascular accident can result (Patel et al., 2001).

Third Recovery Phase

The third phase of recovery from spinal cord injury is the final outcome, or permanent limitation of motor and sensory function. If the compression of the spinal cord is caused by edema that is then relieved, no permanent motor and sensory disability will occur.

Assessment of Spinal Cord Injury

Spinal cord injury should be suspected whenever a child has sustained a forceful trauma of any kind. The signs of spinal cord injury vary according to the level of the injury. The cervical and thoracolumbar areas of the spine are the ones most likely to sustain injury.

Do not move a child with suspected spinal cord injury until the back and head can be supported in a straight line to prevent further injury to the spinal column from twisting or bending. In the emergency department, do not attempt to move the child from the stretcher to an examining table until spinal x-ray films are done. This will reduce any unnecessary movement. When moving the child onto the x-ray table, log-roll him gently so additional injury does

TABLE 49.6 Characteristics of Upper and Lower Motor Nerve Lesions After Spinal Shock Phase

FINDING	UPPER MOTOR LESION	LOWER MOTOR LESION
Spasticity	Present	Absent (flaccidity present)
Clonus	Present, increased	Absent
Tendon reflexes	Increased	Absent
Babinski reflexes	Present	Absent
Reflexes below level of lesion	Present	Absent
Reflex at level of lesion	Absent	Absent
Atrophy of muscles	Absent or present only to slight degree	Present (muscle fasciculations may be present)

not result. If resuscitation is necessary, maintain the head in a neutral position; do not hyperextend it. To keep the neck immobilized, do not remove a child's football or motorcycle helmet or neck brace.

The child will need a thorough neurologic assessment to determine the level of injury. Help maintain spinal immobilization during procedures.

> **WHAT IF?** You are caring for the child with a spinal cord injury and he suddenly develops hypertension, tachycardia, diaphoresis, and headache. What would you initially assess for? How would you intervene?

NURSING DIAGNOSES AND RELATED INTERVENTIONS

During the first phase of recovery, the child's major problems are those resulting from almost complete immobility: pressure ulcers on bony prominences; loss of appetite and subsequent poor nutrition from depression or being in the supine position; urinary calculi from excessive calcium loss; atrophy of flaccid muscle groups; and urinary retention and bladder infection. These effects of immobility are shown in Figure 49-12.

Nursing Diagnosis: Impaired physical mobility related to effects of spinal cord injury

Outcome Identification: Child will achieve the optimal level of mobility possible after injury.

Outcome Evaluation: Child demonstrates movement of all extremities with a minimum of artificial support and equipment; participates in exercise program within limitations; exhibits ability to move about environment within limitations.

To relieve edema at the injury site and prevent further injury, IV corticosteroids will be administered. Children may be placed in cervical traction with Crutchfield tongs and a traction belt (Fig. 49-13) or by halo traction (see Chapter 51). Having tongs inserted into the skull is a very frightening procedure for children. They are afraid that the tongs will burrow into their skull and strike their brain. Children need someone they know and trust to help them lie still during the procedure.

To promote circulation and prevent loss of calcium that results from inactivity, full range-of-motion exercises must be done approximately three times per day. These are time consuming but important in maintaining joint function.

During the second phase of recovery, when spasticity of muscle groups occurs, preventing contractures becomes an important nursing responsibility. Specialized splints, boots, or even hightop sneakers may be used to prevent footdrop (Fig. 49-14). If children have upper extremity mobility but will be left with lower extremity paralysis, exercises to strengthen the upper extremity muscle groups will be started. Strengthening the arms will help children be able to lift themselves from bed to wheelchair or raise themselves

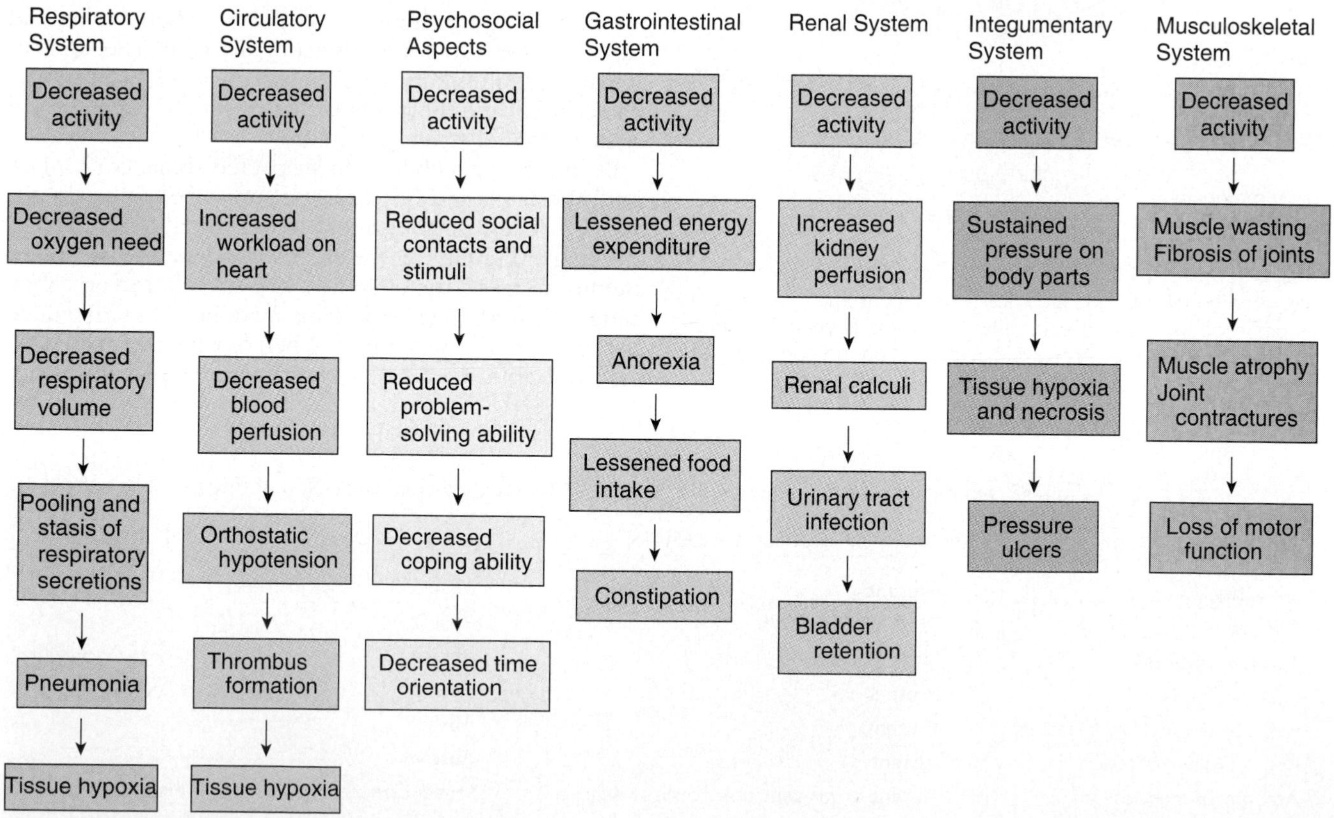

FIGURE 49.12 Effects of immobilization.

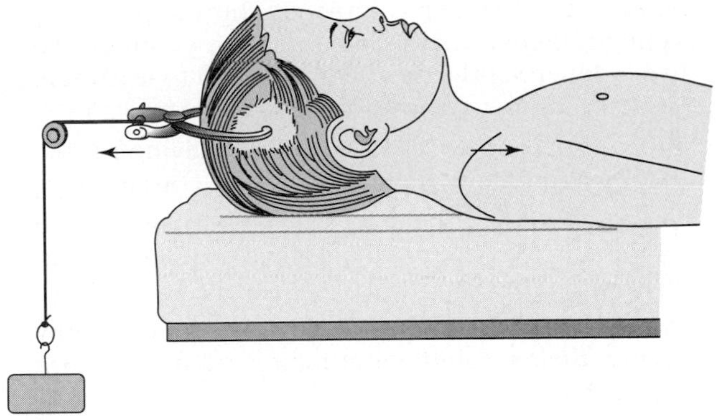

FIGURE 49.13 Crutchfield tongs used to create spinal traction.

with a trapeze over the bed when changing positions. Holding legs and arms at the joints while moving them helps reduce the spasms.

One major problem of ambulation after spinal cord injury is helping a child's body readjust to a vertical position after being maintained in the supine position for so long. When the child is raised, blood tends to pool in dilated blood vessels below the level of the lesion. This pooling of blood results in pseudohypovolemia and hypotension, and the child may faint. Gradually increasing the angle of the bed will help the child become acclimated to the upright position without experiencing vascular pooling.

Nursing Diagnosis: Self-care deficit related to spinal cord injury

Outcome Identification: Child will demonstrate ability to perform as many activities of daily living as possible within his level of functioning.

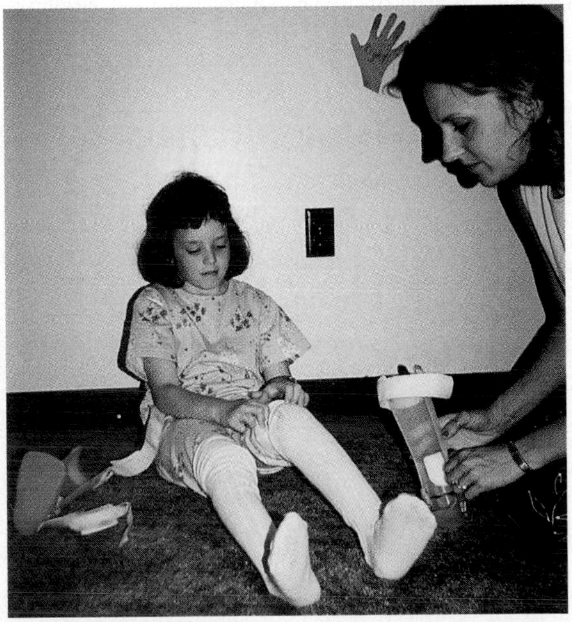

FIGURE 49.14 Specialized splints are used for a child with a low spinal cord injury to prevent contractures and foot drop. Here the physical therapist prepares to apply the splint to the child's leg.

Outcome Evaluation: Child states intention of taking over self-care; practices using equipment for eating, bathing, and toileting; participates in one new aspect of self-care each week.

As soon as possible, children should be introduced to self-help methods for activities of daily living. Most parents need to be encouraged to allow the child to become as self-sufficient as possible and not to take over complete care. The child may well outlive them and will some day need to be able to function as independently as possible.

With autonomic nervous system dysfunction, the child will be unable to sweat and will become hyperthermic if covered too warmly; if not covered warmly enough, the capillaries will dilate, and he or she will lose considerable heat into the environment. If the room temperature cools at night, be careful to dress the child appropriately for sleeping.

Specific measures for bowel evacuation may be necessary, depending on the level of the injury. A bowel program incorporating the use of stool softeners, suppositories, and bowel retraining may be required. The child and parents need support and instructions in accomplishing this task and gaining independence.

For some children and parents, the first day of using a wheelchair is exciting (proof they can be partially ambulatory). For others, it is the day they must face the reality that they cannot undo the results of the accident and are faced with a lifelong disability. For some parents who have nearly overcome their grief and almost accepted their child's disability, the day they are introduced to a symbol of disability such as a wheelchair or long-leg braces may bring new grieving and a sense of loss.

When the child reaches sexual maturity, limitations in this area may become apparent. If a male has had an upper motor neuron injury, he will not be able to achieve spontaneous erection or ejaculation. With manual stimulation of the penis, however (stimulation of lower motor neuron function), he may be able to achieve an erection and engage in coitus. Ejaculation and fertility remain limited. At the time of injury, lack of lower extremity motor control may seem the greatest loss. In adolescence, loss of normal sexual function may become even more disturbing. With most spinal cord injuries, a female is not able to experience orgasm but is able to conceive and bear children.

The limitations caused by a spinal cord injury will become especially evident to the child (and the parents) when choosing a vocation and selecting an appropriate school program (children cannot be denied normal schooling by federal law in the United States, even with a severe physical disability).

Counseling and rehabilitation are crucial aspects to achieve an optimal level of functioning and independence.

Nursing Diagnosis: Risk for impaired gas exchange related to spinal cord injury

Outcome Identification: Child will achieve optimum respiratory function possible.

Outcome Evaluation: Respiratory rate is within acceptable parameters; lungs clear; airway patent.

If the cervical level of the cord is involved, the child will need ventilatory assistance. He may be intubated at first, but orotracheal or nasotracheal intubation is only a temporary measure to maintain a patent airway. A tracheostomy may be done for long-term airway management and to prevent sloughing of pharyngeal tissue from the pressure of the intubation tube. If this is required, the parents will need instruction about caring for the tracheostomy and working with a mechanical ventilator. A phrenic nerve pacemaker may be used to stimulate the diaphragm to contract and initiate respirations. If the child has a thoracic level injury, rare because the rib cage gives extra strength to thoracic vertebrae, the child will be able to breathe on her own but will have reduced vital capacity. Periodic positive-pressure breathing treatments may be necessary to encourage increased lung filling. Be careful when positioning the child to prevent compromising chest movement with equipment or other restricting objects. Other respiratory care measures, such as suctioning and chest physiotherapy, are also important.

Nursing Diagnosis: Risk for impaired skin integrity related to immobility

Outcome Identification: Child's skin will remain intact.

Outcome Evaluation: Child's skin remains clean, dry, and intact without signs of erythema or ulceration.

To prevent skin breakdown, the child should be turned about every 2 h (always be sure to log-roll or maintain immobilization with a striker frame or continuously moving, automatically controlled bed). The use of an alternating-pressure mattress may be helpful. With loss of sensation in body parts, the child is unable to report skin irritation from a wrinkled sheet or wet clothing. If incontinent, the bedding must be changed immediately to prevent skin breakdown. Once children begin to be ambulatory, their legs and buttocks should be checked regularly to prevent pressure ulcers from developing from sitting in a wheelchair or using leg braces.

Nursing Diagnosis: Risk for impaired urinary elimination related to spinal cord injury

Outcome Identification: Child will demonstrate ability to eliminate urine within limits of injury.

Outcome Evaluation: Child's urine output is adequate for intake; child identifies measures to assist with voiding; child demonstrates procedure for self-catheterization.

To prevent urinary retention during the first phase of recovery, a Foley catheter will be inserted, or the bladder can be emptied by periodic suprapubic aspiration, or intermittent catheterization. Second-stage spasticity causes periodic reflex emptying. This rarely empties the bladder completely, however, so the same problems of stasis and infection continue. To live independently, the child will need to learn self-catheterization to empty the bladder.

Nursing Diagnosis: Anticipatory grieving related to loss of function secondary to spinal cord injury

Outcome Identification: Child and parents will express their grief regarding spinal cord injury during recovery period.

Outcome Evaluation: Child and parents openly discuss their feelings about injury and its effect on their lives.

The second recovery phase is the time for parents and children to begin thinking about what this degree of disability will mean to them and to face its full extent. Children and parents typically react to the initial diagnosis with grief. They may still be in denial or shock when the second phase begins. With no sudden miracle cure in sight, they may begin to move through stages of anger, bargaining, depression, and then acceptance (the accident happened; we must go on from this point). They need assistance and support to work through these feelings. Both the parents and the child may need counseling to reach acceptance. Incorporation of a rehabilitation program can help in maximizing the child's potential despite the limitations imposed by the injury (Fig. 49-15).

✔ CHECKPOINT QUESTIONS

16. During which recovery phase would you expect to observe loss of autonomic nervous system function?
17. Why does spastic paralysis occur in a child with spinal cord injury?
18. Which area of the spinal cord is most likely to sustain an injury in a child?

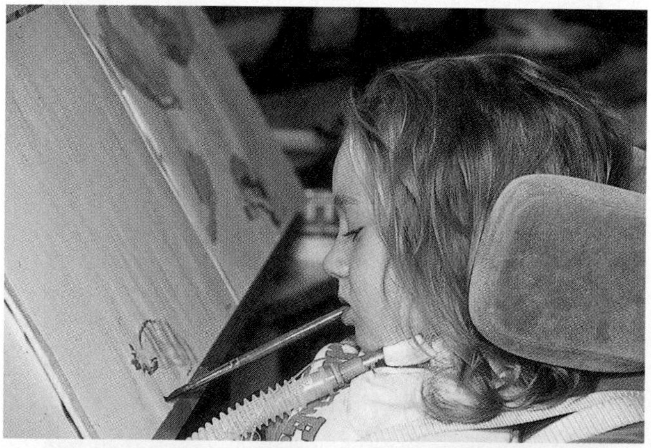

FIGURE 49.15 A 6-year-old girl with a cervical spine injury adapts to her disability by using her mouth to hold a paintbrush and participate in age-appropriate activities.

KEY POINTS

Nerve cells are unique in that they do not regenerate if damaged. This makes neurologic disease a long-term type of illness. Parents and children alike need support from health care providers to cope with problems that continue to occur over a long period.

Increased ICP arises from an increase in the CSF volume or from blood accumulation, cerebral edema, or space-occupying lesions. Neurologic changes, such as increased temperature and blood pressure and decreased pulse and respirations that occur with this, are subtle. Always compare assessments with previous levels to detect that a consistent, although minor, change is occurring.

Cerebral palsy is a nonprogressive disorder of upper motor neurons. The exact cause is generally unknown, but the condition is associated with anoxia before, during, or shortly after birth. Four major types are identified: spastic (there is excessive tone in the voluntary muscles), dyskinetic or athetoid (abnormal involuntary movement), atonic (decreased muscle tone), and mixed (symptoms of both spasticity and athetoid movements are present).

Meningitis is infection of the cerebral meninges. It is caused most frequently by bacterial invasion. Children need follow-up afterward to monitor for hearing acuity and impaired secretion of antidiuretic hormone.

Encephalitis is inflammation of brain tissue. This is always a serious diagnosis, because the child may be left with residual neurologic damage such as seizures or learning disabilities.

Reye's syndrome is acute encephalitis with accompanying fatty infiltration of the liver, heart, and lungs associated with the use of aspirin in children with a viral infection. Its incidence is declining.

Guillain-Barré syndrome is inflammation of motor and sensory nerves. The reaction may be immune mediated, after an upper respiratory illness. Temporary demyelinization of the nerve sheaths occurs with loss of function.

Botulism occurs when spores of *Clostridium botulinum* produce toxins in the intestine. Because honey and corn syrup may be sources of the organism, they should not be given to infants.

Recurrent seizures are involuntary contractions of muscle caused by abnormal electrical brain discharges. Common types seen in children include febrile seizures, infantile spasms, partial (focal), absence, and tonic-clonic. Therapy is administration of anticonvulsant drugs.

Spinal cord injury is occurring at increased rates in children from sports and motor vehicle accidents. Children pass through a first, second, and third recovery phase after the injury.

CRITICAL THINKING EXERCISES

1. Tasha is the 2-year-old girl newly diagnosed with cerebral palsy you met at the beginning of the chapter. Her parents are concerned about long-term problems. Would you encourage them to concentrate on these or on more short-term concerns?
2. A 2-year-old girl diagnosed with bacterial meningitis has severe neck pain when she is moved. Her mother asks you not to worry so much about measuring intake and output so her daughter can rest. How would you answer her mother? Suppose you call the child's name and she does not answer you? Why is this a particular cause of concern with a child with meningitis?
3. A high school senior who is your neighbor tells you that he thinks he has the flu and that he took some aspirin for it. When you tell him it is not wise for children to take aspirin for flulike symptoms, he tells you that advice is "just for babies." How would you respond and how would you pursue the matter with him?
4. A spinal cord injury can cause severe disability in adolescents. If you were designing a program to teach measures to prevent spinal cord injury, what topics would you include in your presentation?
5. Examine the National Health Goals related to neurologic disorders. Most government-sponsored money for nursing research is allotted based on these goals. What would be a possible research topic to explore pertinent to these goals that would be fundable and also would advance evidence-based practice?

REFERENCES

Altemeier, W. A. (1999). A pediatrician's view: Status epilepticus. *Pediatric Annals, 28*(4), 206–217.

Barlow, W. E., et al. (2001). The risk of seizures after receipt of whole-cell pertussis or measles, mumps and rubella vaccine. *New England Journal of Medicine, 345*(9), 656–661.

Baumann, R. J., & Duffner, P. K. (2000). Treatment of children with simple febrile seizures: The AAP practice parameter. *Pediatric Neurology, 23*(1), 11–17.

Bell, L. M. (2000). Meningitis. In M. W. Schwartz (Ed.). *The 5 minute pediatric consult* (pp. 526–527). Philadelphia: Lippincott Williams & Wilkins.

Bergqvist, A. G. (2000). Encephalitis. In M. W. Schwartz (Ed.). *The 5 minute pediatric consult* (pp. 344–345). Philadelphia: Lippincott Williams & Wilkins.

Blum, N. J. (2000). Breath-holding spells. In M. W. Schwartz (Ed.). *The 5 minute pediatric consult* (pp. 206–207). Philadelphia: Lippincott Williams & Wilkins.

Brooks-Kayal, A. R. (2000). Infantile spasms. In M. W. Schwartz (Ed.). *The 5 minute pediatric consult* (pp. 474–475). Philadelphia: Lippincott Williams & Wilkins.

Brown, R. L., Brunn, M. A., & Garcia, V. F. (2001). Cervical spine injuries in children. *Journal of Pediatric Surgery, 36*(8), 1107–1114.

Callahan, J. M. (2000). Botulism. In M. W. Schwartz (Ed.). *The 5 minute pediatric consult* (pp. 190–191). Philadelphia: Lippincott Williams & Wilkins.

Carpenter, T. C., et al. (2001). Critical care. In W. W. Hay, A. R. Hayward, M. J. Levin & J. M. Sondheimer (Eds.). *Current pediatric diagnosis & treatment* (15th ed.). New York: McGraw-Hill.

Decoufle, P., et al. (2001). Increased risk for developmental disabilities in children who have major birth defects. *Pediatrics, 108*(3), 728–734.

Department of Health and Human Services. (2000). *Healthy people 2010.* Washington, DC: DHHS.

Dlugos, J. (2001). The early identification of candidates for epilepsy surgery. *Archives of Neurology, 58,* 1543–1546.

Ferry, R. J., & Collett-Solberg, P. R. (2000). Inappropriate antidiuretic hormone secretion. In M. W. Schwartz (Ed.). *The 5-minute pediatric consult* (pp. 470–471). Philadelphia: Lippincott Williams & Wilkins.

Friday, J. H. (2000). Meningococcemia. In M. W. Schwartz (Ed.). *The 5-minute pediatric consult* (pp. 528–529). Philadelphia: Lippincott Williams & Wilkins.

Gormley, M. E. (2001). Treatment of neuromuscular and musculoskeletal problems in cerebral palsy. *Pediatric Rehabilitation, 4*(1), 5–16.

Lewis, D. W. (2001). Headache in the pediatric emergency department. *Seminars in Pediatric Neurology, 8*(1), 46–51.

McCance, K. L., & Huether, S. E. (2002). *Pathophysiology* (4th ed.). St. Louis: Mosby.

Meyers, F. (2000). Meningitis: The fears, the facts. *RN, 63*(11), 52–57.

Moe, P. G., & Seay, A. R. (2001). Disorders affecting the nervous system in infants and children. In W. W. Hay, A. R. Hayward, M. J. Levin & J. M. Sondheimer (Eds.). *Current pediatric diagnosis & treatment* (15th ed). New York: McGraw-Hill.

Molloy, P. T. (2000). Headache. In M. W. Schwartz (Ed.). *The 5-minute pediatric consult* (pp. 410–411). Philadelphia: Lippincott Williams & Wilkins.

Mulberg, A. E. (2000). Reye syndrome. In M. W. Schwartz (Ed.). *The 5-minute pediatric consult* (pp. 704–705). Philadelphia: Lippincott Williams & Wilkins.

O'Donnell, M. E. (2001). Randomized double-blind placebo controlled trial of the effect of botulinum toxin on walking in cerebral palsy. *Journal of Pediatrics, 139*(1), 163–165.

Olson, D. M., et al. (2001). Sedation of children for electroencephalograms. *Pediatrics, 108*(1), 163–165.

Patel, J. C., et al. (2001). Pediatric cervical spine injuries: Defining the disease. *Journal of Pediatric Surgery, 36,* 373–376.

Pelligrino, L. (2000). Cerebral palsy. In M. W. Schwartz (Ed.). *The 5-minute pediatric consult* (pp. 236–237). Philadelphia: Lippincott Williams & Wilkins.

Reuter, D., & Brownstein, D. (2002). Common emergent pediatric neurologic problems. *Emergency Medicine Clinics of North America, 20*(1), 155–176.

Schmitt, H., & Gerner, H. J. (2001). Paralysis from sport and diving accidents. *Clinical Journal of Sport Medicine, 11*(1), 17–22.

Teener, J. W. (2000). Guillain-Barré syndrome. In M. W. Schwartz (Ed.). *The 5-minute pediatric consult* (pp. 42–43). Philadelphia: Lippincott Williams & Wilkins.

Thilo, E. H., & Rosenberg, A. A. (2001). Neurological problems in the newborn infant. In W. W. Hay, et al. (Eds.). *Current pediatric diagnosis & treatment* (15th ed.). New York: McGraw-Hill.

Wallace, S. J. (2001). Newer antiepileptic drugs: Advantages and disadvantages. *Brain & Development, 23*(5), 277–283.

SUGGESTED READINGS

Bebin, M. (1999). The acute management of seizures. *Pediatric Annals, 28*(4), 225–230.

Bottos, M., et al. (2001). Functional status of adults with cerebral palsy and implications for treatment of children. *Developmental Medicine & Child Neurology, 43*(8), 516–528.

Brown, F. D., Brown, J., & Beattie, T. F. (2000). Why do children vomit after minor head injury? *Journal of Accident & Emergency Medicine, 17*(4), 268–271.

Geddes, J. F., et al. (2001). Neuropathology of inflicted head injury in children. *Brain, 124*(7), 1290–1298.

Huff, J. S., et al. (2001). Emergency department management of patients with seizures. *Academic Emergency Medicine, 8*(6), 622–628.

Jolly, K., & Stewart, G. (2001). Epidemiology and diagnosis of meningitis. *Communicable Disease & Public Health, 4*(2), 124–129.

Lai, A. M., et al. (2000). The young athlete with physical challenges. *Clinics in Sports Medicine, 19*(4), 793–819.

Mannix, L. K. (2001). Epidemiology and impact of primary headache disorders. *Medical Clinics of North America, 85*(4), 887–895.

McAbee, G. N., & Wark, J. E. (2000). A practical approach to uncomplicated seizures in children. *American Family Physician, 62*(5), 1109–1116.

Merenda, L. A. (2001). The pediatric patient with spinal cord injury: Not a small adult. *SCI Nursing, 18*(1), 43–44.

Motion, S., et al. (2002). Early feeding problems in children with cerebral palsy. *Developmental Medicine & Child Neurology, 44*(1), 40–43.

Murdoch-Eaton, D., Darowski, M., & Livingston, J. (2001). Cerebral function monitoring in paediatric intensive care: Useful features for predicting outcome. *Developmental Medicine & Child Neurology, 43*(2), 91–96.

Rothner, A. D., et al. (2001). Chronic nonprogressive headaches in children and adolescents. *Seminars in Pediatric Neurology, 8*(1), 34–39.

50

CHAPTER

Nursing Care of the Child With a Disorder of the Eyes or Ears

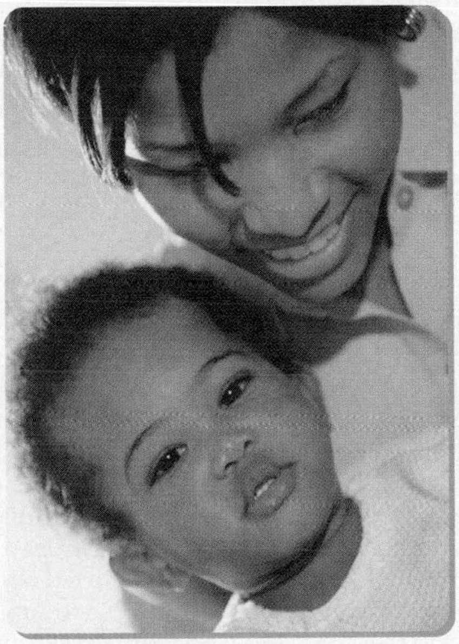

Key Terms

- **accommodation**
- **amblyopia**
- **astigmatism**
- **diplopia**
- **enucleation**
- **fovea centralis**
- **goniotomy**
- **hyperopia**
- **light refraction**
- **myopia**
- **nystagmus**
- **orthoptics**
- **photophobia**
- **ptosis**
- **stereopsis**
- **strabismus**
- **tympanocentesis**

Objectives

After mastering the contents of this chapter, you should be able to:

1. Describe the structure and function of the eyes and ears and disorders of these organs that affect children.
2. Assess the child who has a disorder of vision or hearing.
3. Formulate nursing diagnoses related to the child with a disorder of vision or hearing.
4. Establish appropriate outcomes for the child with a disorder of vision or hearing.
5. Plan nursing interventions for the child with a disorder of vision or hearing.
6. Implement nursing care to meet the specific needs of the child who has a disorder of the eyes or ears.
7. Evaluate outcomes for achievement and effectiveness of care.
8. Identify National Health Goals related to vision and hearing disorders of children that nurses could be instrumental in helping the nation achieve.
9. Identify areas related to care of children with vision or hearing disorders that could benefit from additional nursing research or application of evidence-based practice.
10. Use critical thinking to analyze ways that nursing care of children with a dysfunction of vision or hearing could be more family centered.
11. Integrate knowledge of childhood disorders of the eyes or ears with the nursing process to achieve quality maternal and child health nursing care.

Carla Vander, a 4-year-old child, is brought to the clinic for evaluation. Her mother states, "I think she has another ear infection. She's had a fever for 2 days and says that her ear hurts. This is just like what happened 2 weeks ago when she had an ear infection. Why does this keep happening?" How would you answer Ms. Vander? What information does she need to know about ear infections?

Previous chapters discussed the growth and development of well children. This chapter adds information about the changes, physical and psychosocial, that occur when a child develops a disorder of the eyes (vision) or ears (hearing). This is important information because it builds a base for care and health teaching.

After you've studied this chapter, answer the Critical Thinking Exercises at the end of the chapter and then access the on-line study activities (http://connection.lww.com) *to further sharpen your skills and test your knowledge.*

Any interference with vision or hearing always poses a threat to normal growth and development, because so much of what and how a child learns about the world is achieved through these sensory organs. Infants first learn how to interact with others by watching their parents' faces. They learn to speak by listening to words spoken to them. They continue to depend on sensory input for stimulation throughout life.

Eye and ear disorders may be transitory. However, they always have the potential for becoming long-term illnesses if they permanently affect vision and hearing. This is an area in which health promotion, illness prevention, and health rehabilitation are important aspects of nursing care. Because of the importance of vision and hearing, National Health Goals have been established in relation to them (see the Focus on National Health Goals box).

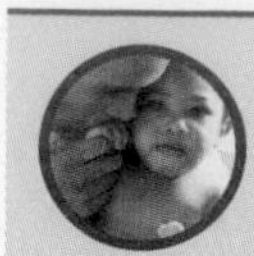

FOCUS ON NATIONAL HEALTH GOALS

Adequate vision and hearing ability are necessary for normal growth and development. Four National Health Goals address these areas.

- Reduce otitis media in children and adolescents from 344 health care visits yearly per 1000 children to 294 visits yearly.
- Reduce blindness and vision impairment in children and adolescents aged 17 years and under from a baseline of 24/1,000 to 20/1,000 children.
- Reduce noise-induced hearing loss in children and adolescents aged 17 years and under.
- Increase the proportion of preschool children who receive vision screening (DHHS, 2000).

Nurses can be instrumental in helping the nation achieve these goals by screening for vision and hearing at all well-child assessments, paying particular attention to those children who were low birth weight or cared for in neonatal intensive care units or excessively exposed to loud noises such as music. Nursing research questions that might yield helpful information include: Can infants who are prone to hearing and vision disorders be better identified before discharge from a neonatal intensive care unit? What are effective techniques for teaching adolescents to avoid excessive sound levels, such as those associated with loud music? What are effective ways to teach school-age children to avoid eye injury?

NURSING PROCESS OVERVIEW

For Care of the Child With a Vision or Hearing Disorder

Assessment

All newborns should be assessed for their ability to focus on or see an examiner's face and to follow an object from the periphery to midline. Observe the infant closely to ensure that the newborn's interest is evoked by sight, not sound. Newborn vision can be further tested by optokinetic nystagmus testing (the infant is shown alternating black and white stripes), visual-evoked potential testing (similar but checkerboard-appearing pictures are shown), and forced-choice preferential looking testing (the infant is shown a pattern and a plain picture; the seeing child focuses on the pattern).

Assessing newborn infants for hearing loss is an equally important part of newborn care. Newborns should quiet to the sound of a soothing voice. (For this, you need to stay out of sight so you are certain the infant is not quieting to your face.) Many hospitals routinely test newborn hearing before the newborn is discharged from the facility.

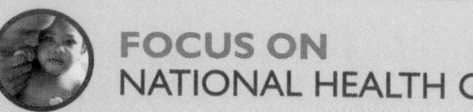

Throughout childhood, children should be assessed for vision problems and hearing loss by their history. (Is a parent or teacher concerned about vision? Does a parent worry that a child may not be hearing well? Is a child having any difficulty in school?) Vision should also be assessed by inspection: Do the child's eyes follow a moving light into all six fields of vision? Is a red reflex present? Do the child's eyes appear to be in straight alignment? Both vision and hearing acuity should be checked periodically. Children also should be assessed for their ability to speak clearly and age-appropriately, because language development is influenced by hearing. Detailed vision and hearing assessment is discussed in Chapter 33 with other aspects of physical assessment (see Assessing the Child for Signs and Symptoms of Vision or Hearing Disorders).

Nursing Diagnosis

Health promotion in regard to safety measures for eye and ear health is a major responsibility of the nurse. Related nursing diagnoses include the following:

- Health-seeking behaviors related to prevention of trauma to eyes or ears

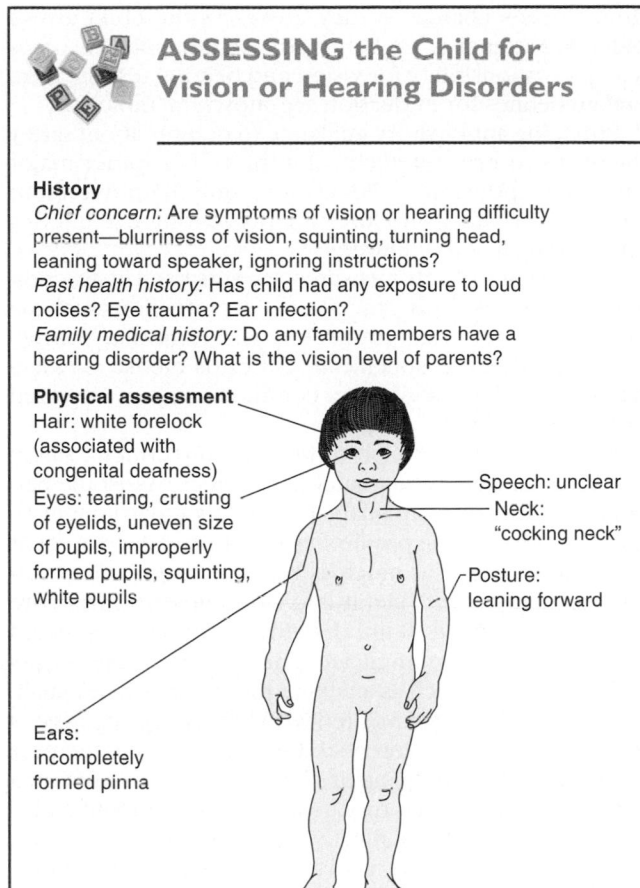

ASSESSING the Child for Vision or Hearing Disorders

History

Chief concern: Are symptoms of vision or hearing difficulty present—blurriness of vision, squinting, turning head, leaning toward speaker, ignoring instructions?

Past health history: Has child had any exposure to loud noises? Eye trauma? Ear infection?

Family medical history: Do any family members have a hearing disorder? What is the vision level of parents?

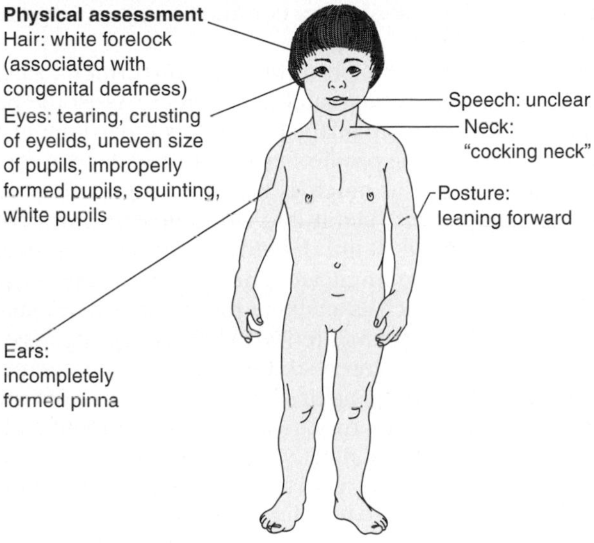

- Deficient knowledge related to importance of early diagnosis and treatment of ear infection

Nursing diagnoses for the child with vision or hearing impairment should focus on the child and parents' responses to loss of sight or hearing, not on the deficit itself (Carpenito, 2001). Such nursing diagnoses might include:

- Self-care deficit related to impaired visual acuity
- Risk for injury related to hearing loss
- Risk for situational low self-esteem related to long-term vision deficit
- Impaired verbal communication related to congenital hearing deficit
- Social isolation related to effects of hearing loss
- Dysfunctional grieving related to child's loss of sight
- Readiness for enhanced family coping related to child's traumatic injury and subsequent loss of vision in one eye

Outcome Identification and Planning

Be certain that outcomes established are realistic and address areas in which you can have some impact. By listening attentively to parents' concerns and providing useful anticipatory guidance, you can help to increase the child's ability to function effectively. Because many eye and ear disorders cause pain, helping parents reduce pain is a major nursing responsibility. Outcomes should always address preventive aspects of care in all areas of daily living.

When parents learn that a child has a vision or hearing impairment, they generally need help in planning for schooling and activities such as toilet training and self-care. You need to discuss with these parents the importance of talking to and touching their infant; of teaching her how to communicate and learn about the world around her through touch as well as through her other functioning senses.

Children with sensory impairment benefit from very early preschool education programs. They are exposed to interesting and stimulating tasks when their sense of initiative is strongest, allowing them to accomplish learning tasks despite their disability. It may be difficult for parents to relinquish their children to such programs during the day, especially at such an early age. It takes careful planning to enable parents to accept this separation.

Parents of children with hearing impairments may need to be encouraged to talk to their children, even in infancy. Although the infant may not be able to hear what the parents are saying, observing facial expressions and spontaneous body movements that accompany verbal speech will help him or her learn important aspects of communication. For example, although the older child may not be able to hear her mother say, "I'm so proud of you," the child can see the positive reaction displayed on the mother's face.

Implementation

Nursing interventions for the child with a disorder of the eyes or ears range from providing anticipatory guidance and teaching children and parents measures to promote eye and ear health to preparing a child for surgery. Nursing interventions also include helping a child and parents adjust to aids that will improve hearing, speech, or sight. Referrals to organizations that can provide information and support to parents of children with vision or hearing impairment can be particularly useful, especially when the impairment will be long term. Some of the organizations concerned with sensory impairment include the following:

Alexander Graham Bell Association for the Deaf and Hard of Hearing (*www.agbell.org*)
American Foundation for the Blind (*www.afb.org*)
American Speech-Language-Hearing Association (*www.asha.org*)
National Association for Visually Handicapped (*www.navh.org*)
National Federation of the Blind Deaf-Blind Division (*www.nfb-db.org*)
Recording for the Blind & Dyslexic (*www.rfbd.org*)
National Association of the Deaf (*www.nad.org*)

Outcome Evaluation

As stated before, a disorder of the eyes or ears can range from an acute, one-time illness to a chronic and developmentally debilitating condition if steps are not taken to treat the initial problem quickly and completely. Even the most rigorous preventive care and attention, however, cannot avert the occurrence of some serious disorders affecting vision and hearing. Nursing care must then focus on helping the child and parents adjust to this condition, ensuring that the child receives the stimulation needed to grow and develop on a normal continuum.

Continuous follow-up is essential, too. Self-esteem is an important factor to be evaluated. Does the child see herself as well or ill; as a person able to do things or as helpless? Plans to promote self-esteem may have to be devised. Some parents may require help with their own feelings of worth. (Feeling inferior to other parents is common in parents of children with disabilities.) They may need help in letting go as children begin school. The growth of parents in allowing their child to be independent is just as important to evaluate as the child's own progress toward independence.

The following are examples of achievement of outcomes:

- Parent voices importance of giving full 10-day supply of antibiotic to child for otitis media therapy.
- Parents state concrete plans for enrolling child in preschool program.
- Child wears corrective lenses for major portion of each day.
- Child demonstrates method to communicate effectively with health care providers.

HEALTH PROMOTION AND RISK MANAGEMENT

All children should be screened routinely for vision and hearing problems. A history and physical examination performed at each health maintenance visit can provide important clues to possible problems and need for further evaluation. Pay special attention to any questions or concerns voiced by the parents at these visits because children's needs change as they grow. As the child grows older and attends school, often the school nurse assumes a major responsibility for vision and hearing testing. General guidelines for evaluation are shown in Table 50-1.

Providing anticipatory guidance to parents about safety measures to prevent accidental injury is another major nursing responsibility. Focus on Family Empowerment summarizes safety measures for preventing eye injuries and hearing loss in children.

In addition to safety measures, parents need instruction about measures to prevent eye and ear infections so these do not lead to long-term problems. Promoting compliance with therapy, specifically for otitis media, is essential because this disorder is a common cause of impaired hearing in children.

If the child has a vision or hearing impairment, safety measures take on even greater importance. Assist the parents with measures to adapt the child's environment to meet his needs while promoting growth and development and independence as much as possible. Supplement verbal explanations with tactile and visual aids as appropriate and allow the child to use drawings, writing, or gestures to respond and communicate. Encourage the use of specialized devices, such as a talking picture board or e-mail, if the child is hearing impaired with limited speech. Assess whether parents are interested in investigating cochlear implants for a hearing-impaired child. Provide ample time for interaction and incorporate the use of therapeutic play (see Focus on Multidisciplinary Care). Children with vision or hearing impairments need to attend regular classrooms in school, if possible, so they have contact with seeing and hearing children to promote normal growth and development (Brambring, 2001). School nurses or preschool nurse consultants need to advocate for such placements.

VISION

Vision occurs because light rays reflect from an object through the corneas, aqueous humors, lenses, and vitreous

TABLE 50.1 Health Promotion Guidelines

AGE	VISION ASSESSMENT PARAMETERS	HEARING ASSESSMENT PARAMETERS
Infant	Ability to follow objects Corneal reflex Ability to turn to light stimuli	Startle reflex (at birth) Ability to track sounds (3–6 months) Ability to recognize sounds (6–8 months) Ability to locate sounds (8–12 months)
Toddler	Corneal light reflex Cover test Smooth ocular movements Hand–eye coordination	Ability to react to soft sounds (whispers) Ability to track source of sounds Ability to form a noun–verb sentence by 2 years Ability to follow simple directions Awareness of pitch and tone
Preschooler	Corneal light reflex Cover test Snellen E chart (or modification)	Pure tone audiometry (starting at age 4 years) Understandable language with increasing vocabulary
School age	Visual acuity testing every 1–2 years	Pure tone audiometry at ages 6, 8, and 11 years
Adolescent	Visual acuity testing every 1–2 years	Pure tone audiometry at ages 14 and 18 years

FOCUS ON FAMILY EMPOWERMENT
Protecting Vision and Hearing

Q. What can we do to protect our children from having problems with their eyes and ears?

A. Here are some helpful tips to protect your children's vision and hearing:

To protect vision:

- Place infants and small children in a car seat (older children, a seat belt) when in a car to prevent hitting the dashboard or front seat in an accident.
- Don't allow infants to hold sharp objects. If an infant is holding such an object in his hand, there is the danger that the object could strike his eye as he brings his fist to his mouth to suck his thumb.
- Don't allow toddlers to carry sharp objects such as lollipop sticks in their hands while walking. They fall readily because of their unsteady gait.
- Don't allow older children to run with sharp objects in their hands, because they can fall while running and puncture an eye.
- Caution older children to use eye-protection measures, such as goggles, when working with projects such as soldering metal in school.
- Encourage the use of face masks for hockey players.
- Teach children not to place any medication in their eyes not prescribed by a health care provider; don't use outdated eye medication, because it may become contaminated with bacteria or change in composition with time.
- Caution children that chemicals can cause burns to the eye; alert them to the emergency shower installations in science rooms to use to wash away any spilled chemical from their eye. Chemical burns may be worse in children with contact lenses in place, because chemicals may flow under the lens and remain longer in contact with the cornea.
- Teach children not to wear contact lenses for longer intervals than recommended by the manufacturer to prevent drying and lack of oxygen to the cornea.

To prevent hearing loss:

- Teach children to avoid chronic exposure to loud noises, such as can occur with radios and using earphones.
- Secure prompt treatment for symptoms of otitis media (fever and ear pain) and administer any antibiotic prescribed for the full prescribed course to prevent damage to the middle ear from infection.
- Be certain children's immunizations are up to date, because illnesses such as parotitis (mumps) or bacterial meningitis can lead to hearing loss.

humors to the retinas (Fig. 50-1). If any of these structures have defects, light rays may not be able to reach the retinas or focus correctly there, resulting in a vision disturbance. The retinas are studded with rods (instrumental for night vision and movement in the visual field) and cones (regis-

FOCUS ON MULTIDISCIPLINARY CARE

A number of different health care professionals in addition to the child's primary care provider can be involved with a child who is experiencing a vision or hearing impairment. Be certain that everyone participating in the child's care knows to speak to visually impaired children before they touch them and to allow hearing-impaired children to see them before they touch them. Be certain, also, that they think through safety precautions for such children. Children with hearing impairments can easily miss instructions such as "Don't touch that" or "That is hot." Visually impaired children explore their environment by feeling. This means they can be injured by a sharp instrument left at the bedside. If an interpreter such as a sign language specialist is involved, you may need to assist other health care providers who are inexperienced with working with this type of interpreter about how to perform this task effectively and without ignoring the child while speaking with the interpreter.

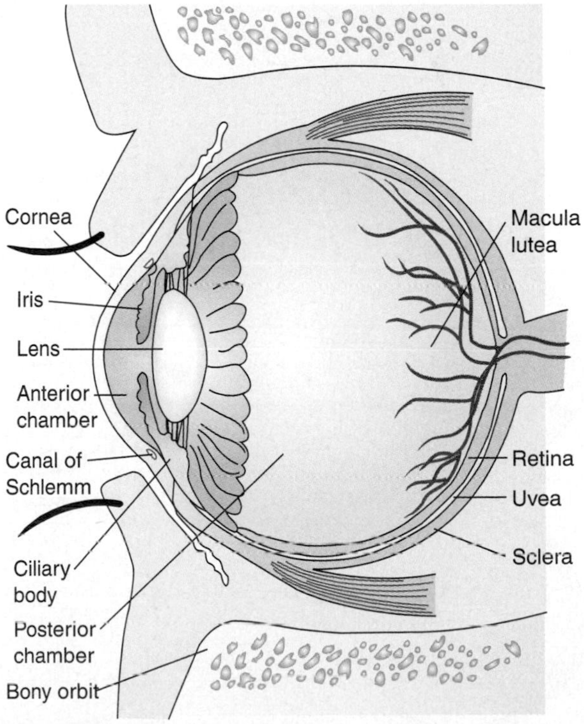

FIGURE 50.1 Anatomy of the eye.

ter daylight and color vision). Rods and cones join in a major network to register at the optic nerve. The **fovea centralis** (the center of the macula) is an area of closely packed cones on the retinas where color is best perceived.

Each eye globe must develop good central and peripheral vision. However, in addition, *fusion* must occur—that is, both eyes must interpret a visual image as one image, fusing visual perception into a single image. This is called *single binocular vision.* Infants with poor eye alignment cannot establish single binocular vision but have **diplopia,** or double vision.

Stereopsis

Stereopsis is depth perception, or the ability to locate an object in space relative to other objects. The right eye sees more of the right side of an object whereas the left sees more of the left side. This makes the object appear to be three-dimensional. Children with vision loss in one eye do not develop stereopsis and, consequently, reach farther than or closer to an object to grasp it. They have difficulty learning to ride a bicycle and have great difficulty driving a car safely. Children without stereopsis do not realize that their sight is different from that of other people. The *Stereo-Fly* or random dot test, simple tests for depth perception, is a specially constructed picture of a large fly or colored dots. When asked to touch the fly's wings or colored dots, a child with good depth perception touches them accurately. A child with poor depth perception touches a spot 2 or 3 inches above the pattern (Eisenbaum & Ornitz, 2001).

Accommodation

Accommodation is the adjustment of the eye to focus on a close image. To focus on a close object, the ciliary bodies of the eye contract, changing the curvature of the lens. The action of the ciliary body allows accommodation but also causes the eye to converge (look medially) and the pupil to constrict. To test accommodation, ask a child to follow a penlight as it moves in toward the nose. Children should be able to do this by 6 months of age and older. Actually, convergence is demonstrated with this test, but convergence does not occur without accommodation. So this test indirectly measures accommodation. Children who cannot accommodate have double vision (diplopia) or are unable to focus on objects near their eyes.

DISORDERS THAT INTERFERE WITH VISION

Eye disease in children is always potentially serious. If permanent vision impairment occurs, a child's functioning at many everyday tasks can be severely compromised.

Refractive Errors

The largest category of vision defects in children is refractive errors (Shields, 2000). **Light refraction** refers to the manner in which light is bent as it passes through the lens. Normally, this bending causes a ray of light to fall directly on the retina (Fig. 50-2*A*). Because the depth of

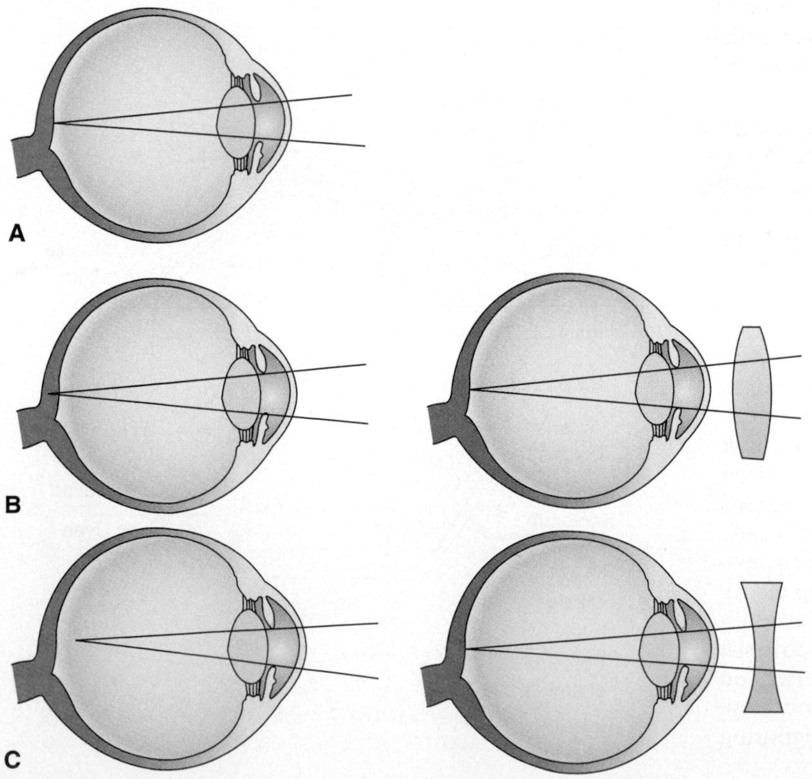

FIGURE 50.2 Corrective lenses for refractive errors of vision. (*A*) Normal vision. (*B*) Convex lens for hyperopia (farsightedness). (*C*) Concave lens for myopia (nearsightedness).

the eye globe in infants and children increases with age, the light rays do not always focus onto the retina accurately, but at a point behind the retina. This results in **hyperopia** (farsightedness) in which vision is blurry at a close range and clear at a far range. The normal hyperopia of a preschooler needs no correction. It is important that you keep this in mind when performing vision screening with children this age. At about 5 years of age, as a result of developmental changes, hyperopia begins to diminish. In some children, however, eyesight does not change in the early school years, and so they remain hyperopic. Focusing on close objects requires such strong accommodation that these children often have headaches or dizziness after completing schoolwork. A finding of hyperopia in a school-age child is cause for referral so that the child may get a prescription for glasses with a convex lens.

Approximately 10% of school-age children have eye changes that result in **myopia** (nearsightedness), meaning that the light rays focus at a point in front of the retina (Eisenbaum & Ornitz, 2001). These children are able to read a book or a computer screen immediately in front of them but are unable to read the blackboard clearly in a classroom. They have difficulty reading signs across the street or playing baseball. Once myopia begins, it often progresses into the teen years, when it plateaus. Children with myopia need corrective (concave) lenses to enable them to see at a distance.

Myopia tends to be familial. If both parents are myopic, children should be screened yearly during the early school years. Any child who reports difficulty seeing or who shows mannerisms suggestive of refraction errors—rubbing eyes, tearing, red-rimmed eyes, blinking, squinting, or pressing on their eyes—should be screened for visual difficulty. Children with myopia try to focus on objects by squinting and rubbing their eyes, which changes the shape of their eye globe.

In the past, the only correction for refractive errors of vision was by eyeglasses or contact lenses (Fig. 50-2*B,C*). Today, adolescents may have laser surgery (LASIK) to permanently change the depth of the eye globe and correct refractive vision errors.

If parents are going to purchase eyeglasses, advise them to choose frames fitted with plastic or safety glass (shatterproof) lenses so that, if the lenses accidentally break, the child's eye is not injured. It is possible for contact lenses to be fitted for even young infants. Children as young as 5 years of age are capable of putting them in and taking them out if taught properly. Contact lenses are a big responsibility requiring conscientious cleaning to prevent eye irritation or infections. Until children are about 12 years of age or older, they generally cannot be relied on to take care of contact lenses independently.

Although wearing glasses is more acceptable today, children still may encounter name calling. Encourage them to give glasses a fair try. In most instances, glasses usually improve vision to such an extent after trying them that children will continue to wear them. However, throughout their development, they may need continued encouragement to keep wearing the glasses.

Laser in Situ Keratomileusis (LASIK)

Laser in situ keratomileusis (LASIK) is laser surgery for correction of myopia. It involves an incision under the cornea to change the contour of the eye globe so light rays fall more accurately on the retina. Because having the procedure carried out before the child's eye globe has reached its adult size would require that surgery be repeated with maturity, the youngest age at which LASIK therapy should be accomplished is controversial. As the technique improves, it will become a major method of correcting refractive vision errors in children (Sugar et al., 2002).

Astigmatism

Astigmatism is congenital or acquired unevenness of the curvature of the cornea (Gwiazda et al., 2000). All light rays coming to the retina are not refracted in the same way, resulting in an uneven quality of vision. When children with astigmatism look at the letter T, for example, they see the crossbar but not the letter stem. If they focus on the stem, they cannot see the crossbar. On any given page of print, therefore, they may see only half the letters. Because of this, they will have difficulty reading or following written instruction. They report headache and vertigo after doing close work. Their vision may appear deceptively normal by vision screening because, by tilting their head, they may be able to see all numbers on a chart enough to pass a vision screening test. They need to be referred to an ophthalmologist, however, on the basis of their other difficulties: vertigo, headaches, and difficulty with reading. Corrective lenses for close work relieve the symptoms and restore functional vision. Contact lenses may be even more helpful because they actually smooth out the curvature of the cornea.

Nystagmus

Nystagmus is rapid, irregular eye movement. It is not a disease in itself but rather a symptom of an underlying disease condition. Ocular nystagmus is seen in children with vision-impairing lesions, such as congenital cataracts. It also occurs as a neurologic sign when there is a lesion of the cerebellum or brain stem. Children with nystagmus must be referred to a physician so the underlying cause of the symptom can be determined.

Amblyopia

Amblyopia is "lazy eye," or subnormal vision in one eye, or children are using only one eye for vision while "resting" the other eye. If this process continues too long, children fail to develop central vision (or the central vision that had developed fades) and they become functionally blind in one eye (Hertle, 2000a). This can occur if children have a refractive error in one eye that is significantly different from that of the other eye. Because one eye focuses more readily than the other, children come to depend on only the easily focused eye (Simon & Kaw, 2001).

Amblyopia can also develop from **strabismus** (crossed eyes). With strabismus, one eye looks straight ahead while the other "wanders." Children whose one eye wanders will constantly be looking at two separate images rather than one fused image. To make sense out of what they see, they suppress one visual image, leading to suppression of central vision in that eye, or amblyopia. The same phenomenon occurs if the vision in one eye is obscured by a lid that does not open fully (**ptosis**).

Assessment

All preschool children should be screened for amblyopia by vision testing with a preschool E chart at routine health visits (Eibschitz-Tsimhoni et al., 2000; see Chapter 33). The child with amblyopia will have 20/50 vision (normal for preschool age) in one eye. The other eye will show lessened vision (perhaps 20/100).

Therapeutic Management

Amblyopia is correctable if treated during the preschool period. After 6 years of age, the prognosis for correction is considerably diminished. After 10 years of age, little improvement in vision can be achieved (Hertle, 2000a). For treatment, the good eye is covered by a patch held firmly in place. This forces a child to use the poor eye to develop vision in that eye. Generally, the child has some difficulty initially adjusting to the patch, and, being unable to see well from the unpatched eye, possibly develops headaches and dizziness. Only constant attempts to see with the poor eye, however, can improve binocular vision. The patch is removed for 1 h/day to prevent amblyopia from developing in the nonamblyopic eye. Administration of levodopa in addition to occlusion therapy may also be prescribed (Mohan et al., 2001). Atropine, to produce pupil dilation, may be another solution (PEDIG, 2002).

NURSING DIAGNOSES AND RELATED INTERVENTIONS

Nursing Diagnosis: Deficient knowledge deficit related to need for consistent wearing of patch

Outcome Identification: By 1 week, parents and child will demonstrate understanding of the importance of early and constant wearing of patch to achieve correction of amblyopia.

Outcome Evaluation: Parents state that the reason for child to wear a patch over the functioning eye is to improve vision in the poorly functioning eye. Child wears patch over functioning eye for all but 1 h/day.

Parents need support to be firm with their child about keeping the patch in place. A child may beg to remove the patch for special occasions, such as a birthday party or a family wedding, or just for an hour, because she or he finds the patch embarrassing and uncomfortable. Soon, however, the "special occasions" become so frequent that children are wearing the patch only half the time. Remind parents how important compliance with occlusion therapy is so that their child will achieve good vision (see Focus on Evidence-Based Practice). If amblyopic eyes are not corrected by 6 years of age, the time for correction runs out. If amblyopia occurs secondary to another defect (strabismus, ptosis, or refraction error), this primary problem will need to be corrected also. Otherwise, the amblyopia will recur after the patching is completed.

Color Vision Deficit (Color Blindness)

Color blindness is the inability to perceive color correctly. It occurs because one of the sets of cones of the retina that perceive red, green, or blue is absent. It is inherited as a sex-linked disorder and occurs in about 8% of boys. There is a high incidence of color vision deficit in children with hemophilia, congenital nystagmus, and glucose-6-phosphate dehydrogenase deficiency. It may be associated with exposure to occupational solvents during pregnancy (Till et al., 2001).

The vision problem may involve the inability to see red and green or blue and yellow. A small proportion of children are unable to see all colors. Color plates or discs may be used to detect color deficit in children as young as preschool age. Children with normal vision see numbers or patterns on these plates, whereas children with a color

FOCUS ON EVIDENCE-BASED PRACTICE

How Well Do Parents Enforce Occlusion Therapy for Amblyopia?

To answer this question, 60 parents of children ranging in age from 2 to 7 years whose child had been prescribed at least an hour of occlusion therapy daily were asked to keep a diary and answer a questionnaire about the procedure. Results of the study showed that 57 parents or 95% of the participants admitted to not always encouraging their child to keep the eye patch in place. Parental knowledge was especially poor in areas of knowing what is the critical period involved in patching (23%). The researchers concluded that increased parental awareness of the rationale and urgency of the treatment with better reinforcement of details of the regimen would help to increase compliance with occlusion therapy.

This is an important study for nurses because nurses are often the health care professionals who give instructions regarding eye therapies. As school nurses, they are in optimal positions to monitor and reinforce compliance. Knowledge of this study provides the rationale for thorough explanations for parents about occlusion therapy and need for compliance.

Newsham, D. (2000). Parental non-concordance with occlusion therapy. *British Journal of Ophthalmology, 84*(9), 957-962.

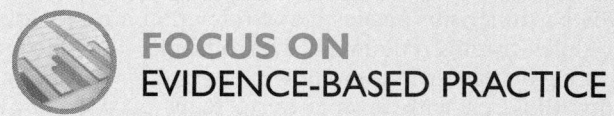

vision deficit see only a jumble of dots or unclear images (Shute & Westall, 2000).

There is no therapy for color blindness, but the condition should be detected early so children are not asked to complete color identification assignments in school and so they can be educated about traffic signals and other color-dependent signs necessary for safety.

Some children associate color blindness with total "blindness" and fear that they will eventually lose their eyesight. Reassure them that, although color blindness means that they have a loss of color discrimination, this loss will be limited to that one area.

✔ **CHECKPOINT QUESTIONS**

1. What type of corrective lens is used to correct myopia?
2. What is nystagmus and why do children with nystagmus need a referral for an ophthalmologist?

STRUCTURAL PROBLEMS OF THE EYE

Coloboma

A *coloboma* is a congenital incomplete closure of the facial cleft. The incomplete closure may involve only the lower eyelid (there is a notch in the lid); it may involve the iris, which will appear as a keyhole, not a circle (Fig. 50-3). It may involve the ciliary body, the lens, the choroid, the retina, and the optic nerve. Children with any degree of coloboma should be referred to an ophthalmologist for further investigation to determine the extent of the condition. Children with retina and optic nerve coloboma will have some vision impairment in the affected eye.

Hypertelorism

Hypertelorism is a congenital condition involving abnormally wide-spaced eyes. Children with wide epicanthal folds by the inner canthus may appear to have wide-spaced eyes, but, when the distance between the pupils is measured and compared with standards for that age, the true condition is revealed. Detecting true hypertelorism in children is important because this condition is associated with chromosomal abnormalities, most notably Waardenburg's syndrome, which also involves congenital hearing impairment. These children also have a white forelock of hair, different-colored irises, and eyebrows that tend to grow together in the center line. These signs may not be noticeable in newborns. Thus, the wide-spaced eyes, because of a broad-bridged nose, then, is the chief clue in the newborn that the child can hear no sound and will need close follow-up to determine whether cochlear implants or hearing aids can provide ability to hear (Read, 2000).

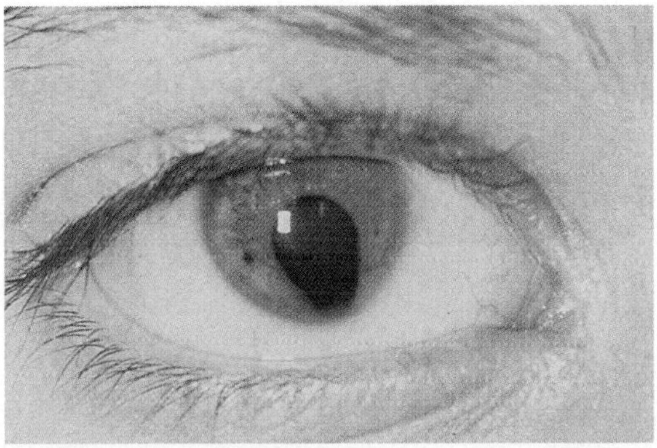

FIGURE 50.3 Coloboma involving the iris showing a "keyhole" appearance.

Ptosis

Ptosis is the inability to raise the upper eyelid normally. Thus, the eyelid always remains slightly closed. The condition may be congenital (frequently hereditary and bilateral) or acquired (generally unilateral). It may be a result of injury to the third cranial nerve (neurogenic) or to the lid or levator muscle. With injury to the third cranial nerve, there is generally paralysis of one or more of the other muscles supplied by the third cranial nerve. In addition, children may exhibit the following:

- Dilated pupil
- Inability to rotate the eye globe upward, medially, or downward
- Weakness of accommodation (looking at near objects)

Myasthenia gravis, which produces generalized muscle weakness, must always be ruled out as the cause of bilateral ptosis.

Children with ptosis tend to wrinkle their forehead and raise their eyebrows more than usual in an attempt to lift the eyelid further. Also, they may cock their heads back to see under the lowered lid.

After careful investigation of the cause has been completed, ptosis is corrected surgically. The correction is usually important to the child from a cosmetic standpoint. More importantly, however, if the lid obstructs vision, early surgery is necessary to prevent the development of amblyopia (from lack of use of the eye). Be sure that parents understand the importance of surgical correction. Otherwise, they may insist on delaying a corrective procedure "until the child is older." When the child is older, although the ptosis can be corrected, the amblyopia cannot be corrected.

Strabismus

Strabismus is unequally aligned eyes (cross-eyes). Approximately 1% to 2% of children have some degree of strabismus. The condition occurs without regard for gender, social status, or geographic area. Approximately 30% of children with strabismus have a history of someone else in the family having a similar strabismus. When there is a family history of strabismus, children need to be observed and examined yearly for this problem (Hertle, 2000b).

The movement of each eye globe is controlled by extraocular muscles. These can be compared in movement to the handling of reins of a horse (Fig. 50-4).

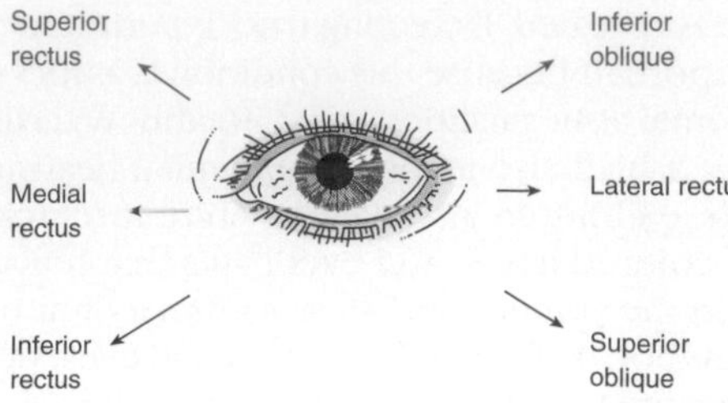

Eye muscle	Action	Innervation
Superior rectus	Turns eye up and medially	Oculomotor (third cranial) nerve
Medial rectus	Turns eye inward	Oculomotor (third cranial) nerve
Inferior rectus	Turns eye down and medially	Oculomotor (third cranial) nerve
Lateral rectus	Turns eye out	Abducens (sixth cranial) nerve
Superior oblique	Turns eye down and laterally	Trochlear (fourth cranial) nerve
Inferior oblique	Turns eye up and laterally	Oculomotor (third cranial) nerve

FIGURE 50.4 Extraocular eye muscles.

Normally, with good eye alignment, the resting position of the eyes is straight, largely the result of neuromuscular influences that the child cannot control. In strabismus, the resting position of one eye may be *divergent* (turned out) or *convergent* (turned in). One pupil may be higher than the other (vertical strabismus). The strabismus may be monocular, in which the same eye deviates constantly. Or it may be an alternating strabismus, in which one eye deviates first, then the other.

Both the resting position of eyes and the amount of turning necessary to read small print depend on the eyes' ability to fuse and see only one image. In infancy, this ability is minimal but becomes stronger with practice. In adulthood, it is automatic. If children do not learn to fuse vision effectively early in life, they are never able to achieve it later on or to maintain good eye position.

It takes muscular effort to look medially (turn an eye in toward the nose). When children read small print, they turn both eyes medially, or *converge,* to focus at the short distance. If they are farsighted in one eye, they have to turn the affected eye in more than the other, causing strabismus. If they have one eye that is nearsighted, they will not need to turn that eye in as far as the other one. This results in divergence of that eye. Although these children have good eye alignment at rest, they "cross their eyes" when attempting to focus at a reading distance.

Assessment

Infants' eyes may cross occasionally until 6 weeks of age. If infants demonstrate strabismus past this age, they should be referred for diagnosis and treatment. Infants who demonstrate a constant strabismus before 6 weeks of age need referral right away.

Definite deviations will be obvious (Fig. 50-5). These can be *exotropia* (eye turning out), *esotropia* (eye turning in), or *hypertropia* (eye turning up). If the deviation is not so obvious but only occurs when the child is fatigued or ill and, therefore, less able to maintain fixation, the terms used are *exophoria, esophoria,* and *hyperphoria.* If the parents report that the deviation only occurs when the child is tired or sick, attempt to assess it at this time because the deviation will be most striking.

Some children have a latent strabismus, but, because they are able to maintain fusion, the strabismus is not overt. They maintain this fusion at the expense of eyestrain, however. They may experience headaches; tired, irritated eyes; and perhaps even nausea and vomiting.

Children who have flat, broad-bridged noses, a narrow interpupillary distance, and an epicanthal fold or oval-shaped palpebral fissures may appear to have strabismus when they truly do not (pseudostrabismus). When you observe these children, you see less white sclera in the inner margin of the eye than normally, and so the eye appears to be turned in (*pseudoesotropia*).

A cover test will reveal the true condition. If pseudostrabismus is present, the covered eye will not move after being uncovered. It only appears to be turned medially because of the obscured sclera at the inner canthus. Hirshberg's test is another method of detecting strabismus (see Chapter 33).

Once strabismus is detected, it is important to attempt to discern whether it is concomitant (measures the same in all directions of gaze) or nonconcomitant (greater in one direction than another; often called *paralytic strabismus*).

Concomitant (nonparalytic) strabismus is the most usual type found in children. All the muscles of the eye are capable of function, but they are not functioning together. This deviation is equally apparent in all directions of gaze.

Paralytic strabismus is caused by paralysis of a muscle or nerve, perhaps from an injury, such as a birth injury, or invading lesion. The eyes appear straight except when they are moved in the direction of the paralyzed muscle. Then double vision occurs, and the crossed eye is evident. Such children often close one eye or tilt their head to decrease the double vision. They may tilt their head so much they appear to have a torticollis, or "wry neck"—

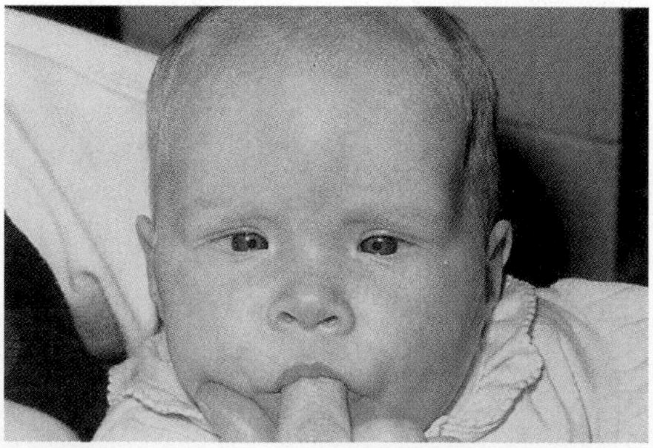

FIGURE 50.5 Strabismus (esotropia) in an infant.

an orthopedic rather than an eye problem. They are often fussy or clumsy because of the diplopia. They cannot see well and may be too young to describe what is happening to them through any means other than fussiness.

Therapeutic Management

The therapy for strabismus depends on the cause of the problem. If the fusion mechanism is weak, eye exercises (**orthoptics**) may be necessary. If eyes are diverging with convergence because of farsightedness or nearsightedness, the child needs glasses to correct the basic visual defect. If the misalignment is caused by unequal muscle strength, eye-muscle surgery is generally necessary to correct it, although injection of botulinum toxin into the eye muscle may be done first as temporary therapy (Han et al., 2001). This paralyzes the muscle, temporarily aligning vision.

Nursing care for the child having eye surgery is discussed later in the chapter. After strabismus surgery, eye patches are not required. Postoperatively, antibiotic ointment is applied to the eye for 2 to 3 days. After eye muscle surgery, the child may experience some pain on eye movement for the first day.

Follow-up visits after surgery are necessary to determine the success of the surgery. Retest children who have had this surgery periodically at health maintenance visits to be certain that their vision remains equal and eye alignment remains straight.

Because strabismus causes the eyes to be viewing two different fields of vision, diplopia, or double vision, occurs. To prevent this, the child suppresses the vision in one eye or only looks with one eye (amblyopia). Even if diplopia is not present, the lack of fusion leads to the same consequence. For this reason, eye correction for strabismus must be done early in life, before 6 years of age. It is true that some children whose eyes are crossing because of an accommodation problem caused by hyperopia in one eye will outgrow the condition as the normal hyperopia of the preschooler lessens. This is not always true. Even if the child's eyes appear to be straighter later, an amblyopia may be present that could have been prevented by earlier treatment (Hertle, 2000b).

> ✔ **CHECKPOINT QUESTIONS**
>
> 3. What conditions may result in ptosis?
> 4. What are two common tests for strabismus?

INFECTION OR INFLAMMATION OF THE EYE

In children, many different types of eye infection or inflammatory conditions can occur (Table 50-2). Regardless of the condition, parents need specific instructions about instilling eye drops or applying ointment, preventing the transmission of infection, applying compresses, and completing systemic antibiotic therapy (Thilo & Rosenberg, 2001). Having eye medication applied can be frightening for older children because they worry that the health care provider's or parent's hand might slip and cut their eye. If they have pain, they may be especially reluctant to let anyone touch the eye.

TRAUMATIC INJURY TO THE EYE

The primary cause of vision impairment in children today is from ocular trauma, such as dirt or sand, baseballs, pieces of broken plastic toys, or flying glass in car accidents that strike and even enter the eye globe. Fights with other children, cigarette burns, and fingernail scratches are also causes. Fireworks and sports injuries are growing in number (Barr et al., 2000).

Assessment

Children who have eye injuries are generally in acute pain immediately after the accident. Their eyes tear and are sensitive to light, and they blink rapidly. Vision may be blurred or lost in the affected eye. Because of the pain and the fear of not being able to see clearly, most children are very reluctant to let anyone touch their injured eye for examination. A few drops of a topical anesthetic instilled into the eye may be necessary to relieve the pain and allow their eye to be opened for examination. Even after the anesthetic is applied, the child needs a thorough explanation of what is happening and that an examiner is "just looking" (provided this is the case). Even after anesthetic application, children may not be able to open their eye readily for inspection, because the acute pain of the injury can cause the eyelid to close by reflex spasm. Eyelid edema also may form quickly, interfering with the eye's ability to open. Do not confuse these physical problems with a child's unwillingness to open an eye.

To visualize the inner surface of the lower lid and bottom half of the eye globe, press firmly on the lower lid with your fingertip until it turns out. The inner surface of the upper lid and the upper portion of the eye globe can best be visualized if the upper eyelid is everted. Ask the child to look downward. Grasp the eyelash and gently stretch the upper eyelid downward. Place the stick of a cotton-tipped applicator horizontally against the center of the upper lid. While still grasping the eyelash, pull the eyelid upward and over the applicator until it is everted (Fig. 50-6). Gently press the everted eyelid against the eyebrow to maintain the everted position. Be careful not to exert pressure on the eye globe during the procedure in case a penetrating injury from a foreign body is present. Pressure would further embed the object in the eye globe.

A foreign body, such as a speck of dirt or a fragment of glass, often clings to the inside of the upper lid and can be readily removed by being touched with a moistened, sterile, cotton-tipped applicator when the lid is everted. Keep an eyelid everted no longer than is necessary because the eye globe tends to become dry when it is exposed. Magnetic resonance imaging (MRI) is an excellent method for documenting internal eye damage after an injury (Adler et al., 2001).

TABLE 50.2 Infectious and Inflammatory Eye Disorders

DISORDER	DESCRIPTION/CAUSE	SIGNS AND SYMPTOMS	TREATMENT
Stye	Infection of a ciliary gland (a modified sweat gland) that enters into the hair follicle at the lid margin; most commonly caused by *Staphylococcus*	Pain and redness at a localized point on the lid margin Possible edema of the lid out of proportion to the severity of the disease Preauricular lymph node swelling and tenderness	Hot, moist compresses for 15–20 min four times a day Antibiotic ointment application after the compresses (possible); incision and drainage (when the stye points [develops a head]) Nose and throat cultures for *Staphylococcus* Follow-up evaluation for repeated episodes to rule out other debilitating diseases such as diabetes mellitus or anemia Visual acuity assessment (although styes are not associated with refraction error, they occur when children rub their eyes excessively because of this)
Chalazion	Low-grade granulation tissue tumor of the *meibomian,* or tarsal, gland on the eyelid; cause unknown, but may be a result of a low-grade infection produced by retained secretion in the gland	Small, slow-growing, hard but painless nodule on the lid Skin freely movable over it; absence of inflammation or edema	None; may resolve itself spontaneously, evacuating itself onto the conjunctival surface of the lid Incision and drainage if no spontaneous remission, followed by antibiotic ointment application to prevent secondary gland infection after incision and drainage If ptosis is present in child under age 8, surgical removal performed to prevent possible subsequent amblyopia
Blepharitis marginalis	Inflammation of the eyelid margin; generally a local infection caused by *Staphylococcus;* possibly an extension of seborrheic dermatitis (cradle cap)	Eyelid margin reddened, possibly covered by hard, dirty-yellow crusts that stick tenaciously to the lid margin and lashes Styes possibly present secondary to the presence of *Staphylococcus*	Application of an antibiotic ointment six to eight times a day to the lower conjunctival rim Removal of crusts with a moistened cotton applicator after the lid margins have been covered by wet compresses for 10–15 min If condition persists, systemic antibiotic therapy to reduce the presence of *Staphylococcus* on the skin surface
Conjunctivitis	Inflammation of the conjunctiva; causes are numerous, including bacterial (most serious—ophthalmia neonatorum [exposure to gonococcus bacillus]; see Chapter 26), viral, and fungal	Eyes watery with reddened conjunctiva and sensitivity to light Sticking of eyelids with pustular drainage	Application of an antibiotic ointment Follow-up visit mandatory to be certain infection clears
Inclusion blennorrhea	*Chlamydia* organism	Acute inflammation usually occurring on the 5th to 14th day after birth Conjunctiva reddened with tearing Eye discharge	Systemic antibiotic such as erythromycin
Acute catarrhal conjunctivitis	Commonly called "pinkeye," usually caused by a virus or irritation from a foreign body; most frequently caused by *Hemophilus influenzae* and *Streptococcus pneumoniae*	Conjunctiva fiery red with tearing Mucopurulent or purulent discharge	Antibiotic ointment or drops three to four times a day for 7 days (redness usually disappears within 48 h) Avoidance of rubbing and transmission of infection to unaffected eye Cool moist compresses to affected eye

(continued)

TABLE 50.2 Infectious and Inflammatory Eye Disorders *(Continued)*

DISORDER	DESCRIPTION/CAUSE	SIGNS AND SYMPTOMS	TREATMENT
Herpetic conjunctivitis	Herpes simplex viral infection (may occur along with development of facial herpes lesion)	Series of pinpoint vesicles on the conjunctiva On fluorescein stain, vesicles stain bright green and are readily evident	Referral to ophthalmologist (can spread easily and become a corneal infection with resultant opacity and permanent scarring) Antibiotics ineffective; steroids avoided Idoxuridine (Herplex) specific for herpes virus, possibly effective in limiting corneal involvement
Allergic conjunctivitis	Hypersensitivity to specific allergen; usually seasonal	Eyelid edema and conjunctiva Profuse tearing and severe itching	Treatment of underlying allergy Cool, moist compresses
Keratitis	Inflammation and infection of the superficial layers of the cornea; may accompany or be a complication of conjunctivitis. May result when a foreign body strikes the cornea, with the invading organism fungal, bacterial, or viral	Acute pain, tearing, photophobia (intolerance to light), and redness	Referral to ophthalmologist for therapy (infection could lead to corneal scarring, resulting in vision impairment [light rays unable to enter the eye normally])
Periorbital cellulitis	Cellulitis (infection of subcutaneous tissue) most often due to extension of a superficial infection after an open break in the skin, such as mosquito bite or scratch by the eye	Swelling around and in the eye with possible damage to eye globe or optic nerve	IV antibiotic therapy
Dacryostenosis	Blockage of the nasolacrimal duct; primarily in newborns due to a membrane obscuring distal end of duct or plugging by epithelial debris	Painless lump in the inner canthus Tearing Usually unilateral	Gentle pressure to inner aspect of each eye at each feeding in attempt to "milk" secretions down into duct Ophthalmologic probing of gland duct if condition not corrected spontaneously after age of 6 months
Dacryocystitis	Inflammation of nasolacrimal duct; possibly secondary to dacryostenosis (from fluid stasis) or from nasal mucosal swelling and infected mucus being forced back into duct	Acute pain in inner canthus (from presence of infected sac); complaints of pain in back of eye or possibly eye itself	Local and systemic antibiotics Possible probing of duct to free obstruction and allow for free drainage Antihistamines for children with chronic allergies or sinusitis

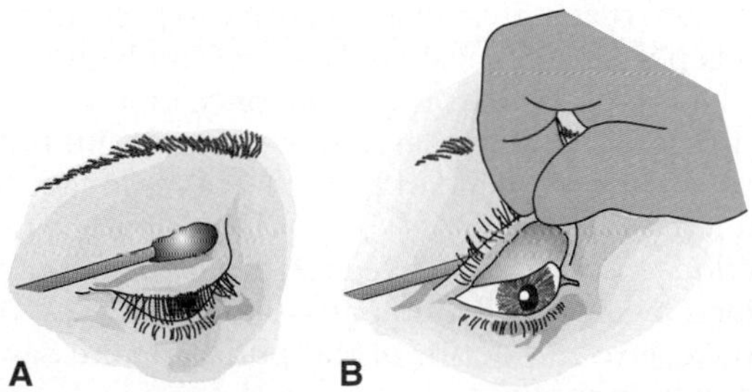

FIGURE 50.6 Technique for everting the upper eyelid for examination and foreign body removal. (*A*) Place a cotton applicator across the upper eyelid. (*B*) Pull the eyelid outward and upward over the applicator.

NURSING DIAGNOSES AND RELATED INTERVENTIONS

Nursing Diagnosis: Parental role conflict related to feelings of guilt about accident affecting child's vision

Outcome Identification: Parents will demonstrate confidence in their ability to care for child and verbalize feelings of guilt about the accident by 1 h.

Outcome Evaluation: Parents accurately state child's treatment plan and expected outcome; child and parents talk openly about accident and ways to prevent future ones; parents participate actively in child's care and in decision making with health care providers regarding follow-up and long-term care.

Eye injuries are almost always serious in children because of the pain and the potential threat to vision. Both parents and children are apt to feel guilty about the accident. Parents may have difficulty handling this emergency because they feel angry at their children and even more angry at themselves for not supervising them or teaching them better about eye safety. Children remember being told many times to be careful of their eyes. Children may need help in understanding that, although this accident might have been prevented, accidents do happen. Doing so helps them to maintain a sense of self-esteem. Parents also may need counseling to understand that accidents can happen even under the most watchful care; this will help them reestablish their feelings of worth as parents (see Focus on Communication).

After eye trauma, the degree of vision in the child's affected eye, as well as the status of the parent–child relationship, needs to be evaluated. Guilt over the accident, whether parental or child, can interfere with the parent–child relationship. After an eye injury, most children do not need future warnings about protecting their eyes.

WHAT IF? What if you are working as a school nurse and learn that many children in your school buy fireworks to celebrate holidays? How would you go about providing safety teaching for them?

FOCUS ON COMMUNICATION

Jon Crisp, an 8-year-old boy, is brought to the emergency department by his mother after being hit by a baseball on the right side of his face at his right eye.

Less Effective Communication

Nurse: Mrs. Crisp, how did the injury occur?
Mrs. Crisp: He was playing catch with his older brother in the backyard.
Nurse: Was he hurt anywhere else?
Mrs. Crisp: No, but I didn't see exactly what happened. I should have been watching him more closely.
Nurse: Does he have pain?
Mrs. Crisp: Just a little, but I didn't see what happened. I shouldn't have left him out there with his brother. He's too young to play baseball.
Nurse: Okay, wait here. The doctor will be in shortly to examine Jon.

More Effective Communication

Nurse: Mrs. Crisp, how did the injury occur?
Mrs. Crisp: He was playing catch with his older brother in the backyard.
Nurse: Was he hurt anywhere else?
Mrs. Crisp: No, but I didn't see exactly what happened. I should have been watching him more closely.
Nurse: Watching him more closely?
Mrs. Crisp: Yes, I was inside checking on them through the kitchen window. I should have been outside supervising them.
Nurse: It sounds like you're blaming yourself.
Mrs. Crisp: It's my fault.
Nurse: Your fault?
Mrs. Crisp: Yes, I should have been out there instead of inside making dinner. He's too young to be playing baseball.
Nurse: You believe he's too young? Let's talk a little more about this.

In the first scenario, the nurse focuses on assessing the events surrounding the injury. Although this is important information, the nurse fails to identify the mother's feelings. In the second scenario, the nurse actively listens to the mother to elicit more information about her feelings.

Foreign Bodies

Foreign bodies such as sand or dirt that are loose on the conjunctiva can be removed by irrigation with a sterile normal saline solution or by gentle wiping with a well-moistened, sterile, cotton-tipped applicator after the eyelid is everted. After the removal, if the conjunctiva is touched with a strip of filter paper impregnated with fluorescein stain, any corneal ulceration or abrasion from the foreign body will stain green and be readily apparent. If the foreign body is easily removed and no corneal ulceration or injury is present, no further treatment is necessary. Children will blink a few times after their upper lid is returned to place, but, in a matter of minutes, they will report feeling "fine" again. If the fluorescein stain shows any corneal ulceration, refer the child to an ophthalmologist for follow-up care.

If a foreign body adheres to the cornea, it needs to be removed by an ophthalmologist. If the foreign body is metallic, and it has been in contact with the cornea for a period of hours, a rust ring forms around the particle. This rust ring must be removed as well as the original particle or it will continue to act as a foreign body. After corneal injury, corneal tissue will regenerate. To allow for this, the eye is washed with an antibiotic solution and then closed and patched. The patch must be secure enough to keep the eyelid closed yet not put undue pressure on the eye. Caution children that it must be left in place to prevent the delicate regenerating corneal epithelium from being rubbed off until it is well healed and secure once more.

If a foreign object is a large one such as a BB bullet, a lollipop stick, or a piece of broken glass, the fact that it has punctured the eye globe is usually apparent on first inspection. In these instances, children also need to be examined by an ophthalmologist. Surgery may be necessary to explore the depth of the puncture and save the child's sight in that eye.

An extremely serious complication called *sympathetic iritis,* or inflammation of the opposite eye, may result if the ciliary body was involved in a penetrating injury. As a result, blindness in the noninjured eye may occur. This complication can be prevented by administration of corticosteroid and antibiotics to reduce inflammation. If this is unsuccessful, removal (**enucleation**) of the injured eye may be necessary. If the vision in the injured eye appears to be destroyed, a decision for removal is not difficult for parents to make. If the vision is not totally destroyed, however, deciding to remove the injured eye is extremely difficult for parents. Fortunately, immediate treatment with corticosteroids and antibiotics has significantly reduced the incidence of this complication.

Contusion Injuries

Many eye injuries happen not from a sharp object striking the eye but from blunt trauma such as a baseball, a fist, a soccer ball, or an automobile dashboard striking the eye. With this type of injury, the eyelid and the surrounding tissue, including the intraorbital tissue, may hemorrhage and become edematous.

The simplest form of contusion injury is a "black eye." After this occurs, inspect the eye globe (including a funduscopic examination) and assess vision in the eye. If a vision chart is not available, vision can be assessed by having children tell you how many fingers they can count at a distance of about 6 feet (assuming they are old enough to count accurately) or by having them read a printed page at reading distance (assuming they are old enough to read). Ask children if they are having any difficulty seeing. Evaluate extraocular eye movement for adequate function. Children should be able to look up and down, left and right, upward obliquely, and downward obliquely—the six cardinal positions of gaze.

If there is no apparent eye injury, ocular movement is good, and vision is normal (for them), the only treatment necessary is an ice pack applied to the eye to minimize swelling (20 min on, 20 min off, and repeat). Reabsorption of hemorrhage in the tissue surrounding the eye will take place over the next 1 to 3 weeks. Often, tissue hemorrhage extends across the nose and surrounds the other eye the day after the injury. Assure both parents and child that this is not a worsening of the condition but mainly evidence of the severity of the initial blow.

Limited eye movement or reports of diplopia (double vision) are strong evidence that a "blow out" fracture of the floor of the orbit (the maxillary bone) has occurred. This fracture line is trapping intraorbital tissue and preventing the eye globe from moving freely. Refer these children to an ophthalmologist. Surgery is needed to free the entrapped tissue, prevent interference with vascular flow, and restore normal eye movement (Hatton et al., 2001).

After a blunt contusion to the eye globe, a number of serious findings in addition to limited motion may be present. These include disturbances of the pupil, such as a dilated, fixed, or cloudy pupil; cloudy lens or cornea; loss of vision in the eye; and visible blood in the anterior chamber (hyphema). These may indicate dislocation of the lens or retinal detachment requiring evaluation by an ophthalmologist.

Eyelid Injuries

Eyelid injuries may accompany eye globe injuries or may be the only finding present after a foreign body has struck the eye. Although such injuries appear to be trivial, do not dismiss them lightly. Refer the child to an ophthalmologist for care. A deep laceration of the eyelid can cause a permanent ptosis. A laceration to the inner canthal area may disrupt the lacrimal drainage system (dacryostenosis).

✔ **CHECKPOINT QUESTIONS**

5. How should you remove a speck of dirt clinging to the inside of the child's upper eyelid?
6. What are important assessments after a contusion injury to the eye?

INNER EYE CONDITIONS

Congenital Glaucoma

Glaucoma is increased intraocular pressure (IOP) in the eye globe because of inadequate or blocked drainage of aqueous humor. Aqueous humor, produced by the ciliary body, flows from the posterior chamber through the pupil to the anterior chamber and is excreted through the canal of Schlemm at the lateral angle into the venous circulation (Fig. 50-7). When glaucoma is congenital, a developmental anomaly in the angle of the anterior chamber prevents proper drainage at the canal. Later in life, glaucoma occurs when the canal becomes blocked. The increased fluid content causes the globe of the eye to increase in size. After the eye globe has increased in size

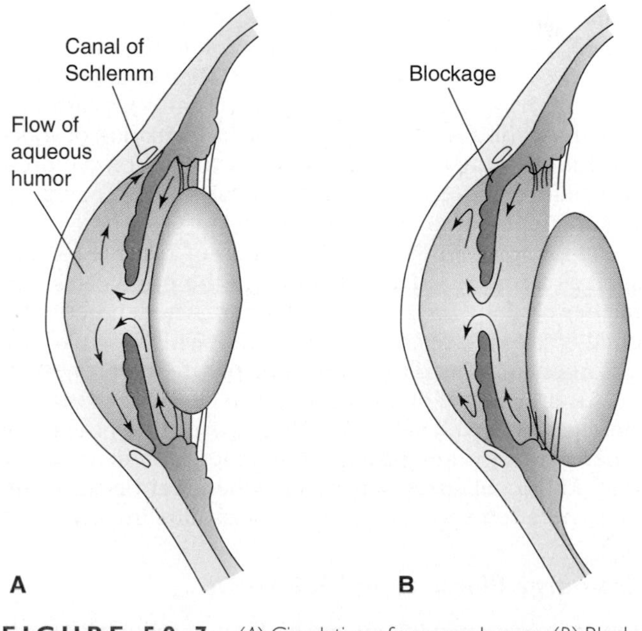

FIGURE 50.7 (*A*) Circulation of aqueous humor. (*B*) Blockage of canal of Schlemm in congenital glaucoma.

to the extent that it can, the pressure in the eye globe continues to rise, compressing and ultimately destroying the optic nerve. Glaucoma (meaning "gray") gets its name from the color of the retina or red reflex (gray to green) in the eye after the sight has been lost. The condition occurs as often as 1 in 10,000 live births (Quinn, 2000).

Assessment

Although congenital glaucoma is a rare disease, all infants must be assessed for it because the disease accounts for vision impairment in 5% to 13% of children in schools for the visually impaired. In most infants, the condition is bilateral and caused by a recessive gene inheritance pattern. In the majority of children with this condition, symptoms are noticeable shortly after birth; in almost all children, glaucoma is apparent at 1 year of age. It occurs more often in females than in males (Quinn, 2000).

The cornea, which appears enlarged, may be edematous and hazy. In addition, the newborn may have tearing, pain, and **photophobia** (sensitivity to light), all difficult to identify in a newborn. The eye globe may feel tense to finger palpation.

Eye pressure is measured by means of a *tonometer,* a pressure-sensitive device that is placed against the anterior eye globe or measures eye pressure by a beam of light directed toward the eye. Tension above the normal range of 12 to 20 mmHg is suggestive of glaucoma. If local anesthesia is needed for tonometry, caution parents to avoid allowing children to rub their eyes after the procedure (an infant's arms may need to be gently restrained to prevent eye rubbing for about 4 h after such an examination). Otherwise, corneal abrasions may occur because of the cornea's lack of sensitivity.

Therapeutic Management

Immediate surgery—a **goniotomy,** or trabeculotomy, in which a new opening to the canal of Schlemm is constructed—is scheduled for the infant (Eisenbaum & Ornitz, 2001). A drug such as acetazolamide (Diamox), a carbonic anhydrase inhibitor that suppresses the formation of aqueous humor, may be used temporarily to reduce eye pressure before the surgery can be scheduled. Newer surgical techniques include laser therapy (Quinn, 2000).

Before surgery, the infant should not receive a drug, such as atropine sulfate, that dilates the pupil. This will further occlude the canal of Schlemm. After surgery, the child is asked to restrict rough play activities for 1 week.

Surgery may need to be repeated before the new opening for drainage of fluid is adequate to keep eye globe tension at a normal level. Inform parents of this possibility when surgery is first proposed, so that they will not think that additional surgery is being scheduled because the first operation was inadequate or was done incorrectly.

Discharge Planning and Follow-Up

Eye examination in infants and children at regular intervals is important so that congenital glaucoma can be recognized before damage to the optic nerve occurs. Glaucoma may occur after eye trauma if there is scarring at the canal of Schlemm. Children who have eye injuries are usually asked to return for a follow-up appointment in a month for eye pressure assessment. Stress the importance of this visit without alarming parents or child about the possible complication.

Cataract

A *cataract* is a marked opacity of the lens. This may be present at birth or may become apparent in early childhood. A few cases may occur from steroid use or radiation exposure. It can occur as a result of trauma to the eye if the lens is injured. Some are familial as a dominantly inherited condition (Schaffer, 2000). When the opacity is on the anterior surface of the lens, the cause is thought to be birth injury or possibly contact between the lens and the cornea during intrauterine life. When the opacity is located at the edge of the lens, it may be the result of nutritional deficiency during intrauterine life, such as rickets or hypocalcemia. Infants who contract rubella prenatally may develop opacity throughout the lens.

Assessment

When you inspect the pupil of a child with a cataract, the pupil opening appears to be white (leukocoria). The red reflex elicited by shining a light into the pupil appears white. Older children report blurred vision from cataract formation. In the infant, this can be detected by a lack of response to a smile or inability to reach and grasp a nearby object. The infant will also demonstrate nystagmus, being unable to focus the eye on objects. A few other conditions such as retinoblastoma, retinopathy of prematurity, or an abscess of the posterior chamber simulate this appearance. In congenital glaucoma, the lens may be opaque from edema. This can be differentiated from simple cataract by the accompanying enlargement of the eye and pupil opening.

Therapeutic Management

Treatment of childhood cataract is surgical removal of the cloudy lens, followed by insertion of an internal intraocular lens. If the total lens is involved, this may be done as early as 3 months of age. If this is not done before 6 months of age, amblyopia may result (Schaffer, 2000).

With modern surgical techniques, the incision is so small that eye patching is not necessary. Infants may be given a sedative to help them rest for 24 h. Introduce fluids cautiously after eye surgery so nausea and vomiting do not occur. Vomiting increases IOP, which could injure the suture line. Encourage parents to stay with the infant, helping with care so the infant does not cry after surgery, because this also increases eye pressure. Infants can be expected to have some discomfort but, generally, should not have acute eye pain after surgery. If they are unusually restless, fussy, or crying and seem to be in pain, notify the physician immediately. Although this could be caused by an unrelated reason, this may be a sign of increased IOP from hemorrhage or from occlusion of the canal of Schlemm, causing a developing glaucoma.

As a rule, children will be given a mydriatic (to dilate the pupil) and steroids to prevent postoperative development of pupillary adhesions. If the eye that had the cataract is now amblyopic, patching of the normal eye as with usual amblyopia correction may be necessary to restore vision.

Parents of children with congenital cataracts need support to carry out the procedures necessary and to give the long-term medication and corrective measures needed. Outcome evaluation should include the child's current vision status and also how the child views himself or herself in light of this early life problem.

✔ CHECKPOINT QUESTIONS

7. What are signs and symptoms of congenital glaucoma?
8. After cataract surgery, why should vomiting be prevented if at all possible?

THE CHILD UNDERGOING EYE SURGERY

Surgery to treat cataracts or glaucoma in childhood is generally performed on infants. Thus, preparation for this surgery primarily consists of helping the baby to adjust to the strange environment and encouraging parents or a primary care person to spend as much time with the baby as possible. This is particularly important if eyes will be patched after surgery. Surgery for strabismus is often done during the preschool period. The operation can be explained to the preschooler through the use of puppets or dolls. As with all surgical procedures, talk about the child's affected parts, in this case, the eyes, being "fixed" or "made better," never "cut." Even a very young child knows how important his or her eyes are and will agree to having them made better, but not cut.

NURSING DIAGNOSES AND RELATED INTERVENTIONS

Nursing Diagnosis: Anxiety related to lack of knowledge about eye surgery and postoperative experience

Outcome Identification: Child will demonstrate confidence in and cooperate with health care providers postoperatively.

Outcome Evaluation: Child asks questions and expresses fears about surgery; child states plans for postoperative period and practices putting on eye patches, if appropriate.

Most eye surgery is completed as ambulatory surgery. A major nursing role is preparing the parents to support the child through the procedure.

If the child's eyes are going to be patched after surgery, it is helpful to allow the child to become accustomed to the feeling of the patches beforehand. Even when only one eye is going to be operated on, it is not unusual for both eyes of children to be patched because eyes move conjugately. When the right eye looks to the right, so does the left eye. The repaired eye, therefore, will only stay immobile under a bandage if both eyes are patched.

Parents could show the child a doll with eye patches, and let the child practice wearing them. They could play a game such as "pin the tail on the donkey" or "blindman's bluff" to adjust to the sensation of the eyes being covered. Another helpful game is to have the child pull out familiar objects from a paper bag—a key, an orange, a spoon, and a penny—and, with eyes covered, try to guess what they are.

When you meet the child before surgery, be certain to speak with the child so he or she will be able to recognize your voice afterward. Practice having the child identify their parents' voice by covering the eyes and then guessing whether you or the parent is speaking.

Postoperatively, check that the young child's favorite toy is within reach if his or her eyes are patched. If children will require arm restraints to prevent them from pressing on their eyes or removing the patches, urge parents to introduce these preoperatively as well. Children who awaken from conscious sedation and find their arms tied down can be extremely frightened or believe they are being punished.

THE HOSPITALIZED CHILD WITH A VISION IMPAIRMENT

Like other children, those with vision impairment experience disorders such as appendicitis or pneumonia that may require hospitalization. Severe vision impairment or blindness can cause increased difficulty adjusting to a hospital environment. The World Health Organization defines severe vision impairment as testing 20/60 to 20/200 in the better eye on a standard eye examination. Blindness is defined as vision less than 20/200 or peripheral vision less than 10 degrees (Bodaghi et al., 2001).

NURSING DIAGNOSES AND RELATED INTERVENTIONS

Nursing Diagnosis: Powerlessness related to difficulty adjusting to strange environment, secondary to vision impairment

Outcome Identification: Child will state that she feels secure during hospitalization.

Outcome Evaluation: Child identifies specific fears and concerns; is able to make age-appropriate decisions regarding self-care.

Vision impairment can range from very mild to total blindness. Assess children carefully for the degree of their vision impairment to better gauge their abilities, helping them neither too much nor not enough. Children who are blind need to feel secure in a strange hospital environment. Be sure to thoroughly orient them to the experience and their surroundings. Remember that they may think that a parent has left them when the parent has only moved a few feet away. Also, keep in mind that severe vision impairment can lead to chronic depression as a child grows older and realizes more and more the many ways that lack of vision affects life (Koenes & Karshmer, 2000).

Before you approach a child who is blind, speak first to avoid startling her. The child who is blind is very aware of another person's presence in the room and may be frightened if you slip in quietly to straighten another child's bed or pick up some equipment without speaking to her.

Remember that the sounds of a hospital are strange sounds to any child. The whirring noise of a floor-polishing machine or another child's oxygen administration, the hissing of a ventilator, and the clanking of waste baskets being emptied can be frightening sounds if you do not know what they are. Stand by the child's bed and explain the sounds you both hear. Sound is a major way in which visually impaired children experience their environment.

Children who are blind need to learn self-care like other children; they can be taught to bathe themselves, brush their teeth, brush their hair, and put on their clothes like other children their age. Toilet training may come later, because they cannot see the excretions that parents are asking them to dispose of in a special place. They must be able to understand cognitively what is expected of them.

Blind children often want to be told what is on their food tray when it is first presented to them. Name the foods so they can identify tastes with names. Do not hesitate to use food colors: "Those are green beans; this is an orange; those are red beets." These words are names as well as colors. Visually impaired preschoolers enjoy the same finger foods as sighted children. Children with severe vision impairments have difficulty getting food from spoons or forks to their mouths neatly. They should not be fed just because it is neater and faster, however; eating is important self-care for the blind child to learn to be independent as an adult.

Be certain to offer frequent descriptions of what is happening or planned for them. They cannot see their surgical dressing, for example, so urge them to feel it. They cannot see the intravenous infusion, but they could feel the tubing and the arm board that is holding their arm in place.

Parents of a severely visually impaired child usually plan to room in with their child during a hospitalization experience. Demonstrate competence and consistency when caring for their child by using good techniques and by relating to him or her warmly. Ask the parents about the child's routines at mealtime and bedtime, his or her favorite toy, what word is used for voiding, and so on, and pass the information on to the entire nursing staff. Only when parents have confidence in you and the other staff members will they be able to leave their child to meet their own needs.

✔ CHECKPOINT QUESTIONS

9. What criteria are used to identify that a child is legally blind?
10. For the child who is visually impaired, what sense is most used to experience the environment?

STRUCTURE AND FUNCTION OF THE EARS

Ear anatomy is shown in Figure 50-8. Most ear disease in children involves the external and middle portions.

Physiology of Hearing Loss

Hearing loss is termed a *conduction loss* if there is interference with sound reaching the inner ear (difficulty with the external canal, the tympanic membrane, or the ossicles). It is termed *nerve* or *sensorineural loss* if the inner ear or the eighth cranial nerve is affected. Conduction loss can occur if the external canal is obstructed with cerumen (wax) or a foreign object, the tympanic membrane is damaged or immobile, or the middle ear is filled with fluid, as occurs in *serous otitis media.* Sensorineural loss occurs from disease that affects the transmission of sound sensation to the cerebral cortex or a pathologic condition of the cochlea. In children, this condition is usually congenital, although it can occur from drug therapy or infection from an illness such as meningitis. It also can occur from exposure to loud sound.

Hearing Impairment

Hearing impairment occurs in many different degrees and can be rated by levels of severity. Usual classifications are shown in Table 50-3. Approximately 1 in 1,000 children in

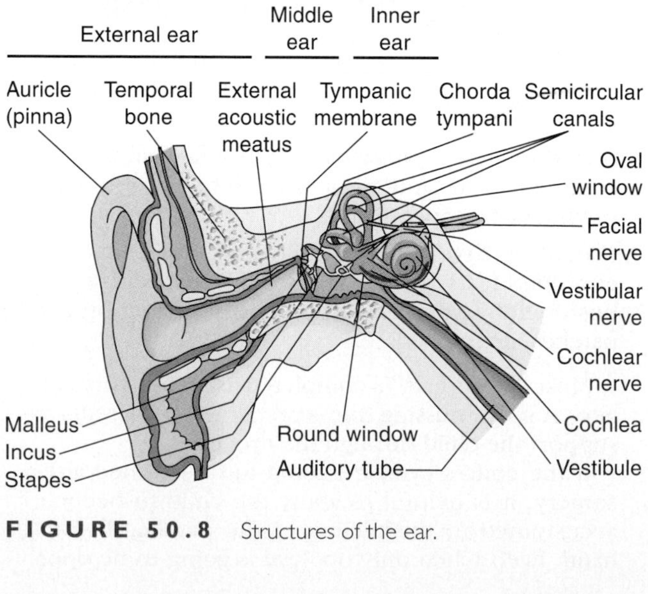

FIGURE 50.8 Structures of the ear.

TABLE 50.3 Levels of Hearing Impairment

dB LEVEL	HEARING LEVEL PRESENT
Slight (<30)	Unable to hear whispered words or faint speech
	No speech impairment present
	May not be aware of hearing difficulty
	Achieves well in school and home by compensating (eg, leaning forward, speaking loudly)
Mild (30–50)	Beginning speech impairment may be present
	Difficulty hearing if not facing speaker; some difficulty with normal conversation
Moderate (55–70)	Speech impairment present; may require speech therapy
	Difficulty with normal conversation
Severe (70–90)	Difficulty with any but nearby loud voice
	Hears vowels more easily than consonants
	Requires speech therapy for clear speech
	May still hear loud sounds, such as jets or train whistles
Profound (>90)	Hears almost no sound

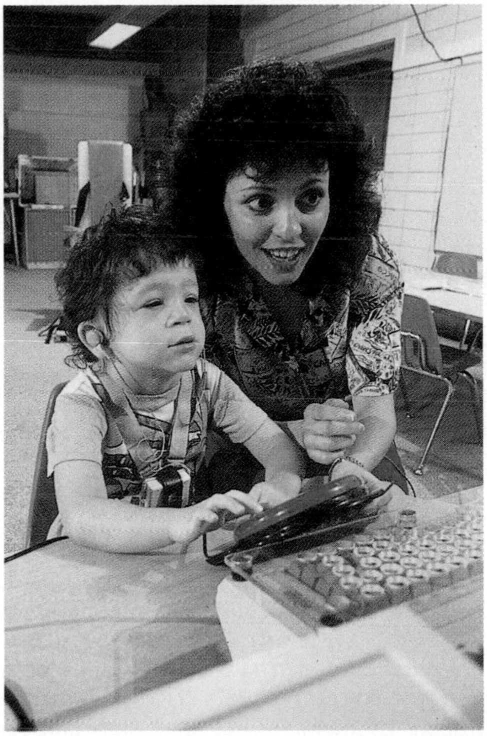

FIGURE 50.9 A hearing-challenged young girl learning to use the computer with the aid of a speech therapist.

the United States are profoundly hearing impaired; 25 of 1,000 children have a moderate to severe hearing impairment. Congenital sensorineural hearing loss occurs in 2 to 3 of 1,000 live births (Berman, Johnson, Chan & Kelley, 2001). Prenatal rubella infection accounts for another large percentage. Treacher Collins syndrome, otosclerosis, osteogenesis imperfecta, and Waardenburg's syndrome, all diseases transmitted by autosomal dominant inheritance, are examples of diseases causing congenital deafness. Causes of slight hearing impairment include serous otitis media, trauma, or untreated acute otitis media with rupture of the tympanic membrane.

Children with congenital hearing impairment should be enrolled in special programs for hearing-challenged children as soon as the hearing loss is discovered. This early exposure is necessary to learn effective speech (Fig. 50-9). For children who have conductive losses, an improvement in hearing can generally be achieved by use of a hearing aid (which intensifies the level of sound waves). Children who have inner ear or nerve deafness cannot expect this kind of improvement. Parents of children with neural deafness need an explanation of the difference so they do not continue to search for a "cure" for their child or spend a great deal of money for hearing aids, hoping a different brand or model will help their child. Acupuncture, often recommended to parents by friends as therapy for nerve deafness, has no documented effect.

Cochlear implants are available to replace a nonfunctioning inner ear with nerve damage (Balkany et al., 2001). After implantation, hearing is often reported as "muffled" but adequate. Hearing-challenged adults may be reluctant to consent to a cochlear implant in their child, feeling that to move from hearing-impaired to non–hearing-challenged status would remove the child from their culture. Children who spoke with an impediment before an implantation usually need speech therapy afterward to improve their speech pattern.

Because the diseases that lead to inherited hearing challenge tend to be autosomal dominant, there is a strong chance that they will occur in future siblings of the hearing-challenged child. Genetic counseling can aid in increasing parental awareness.

Hearing Aids

Hearing aids pick up sound through a microphone, convert sound waves into electrical impulses, and amplify them across the tympanic membrane. They are powered by batteries that must be changed periodically.

Hearing aids are designed to be as inconspicuous as possible so children will not feel self-conscious wearing them. The receiver of the hearing aid may be incorporated into eyeglasses, molded into a plastic form that fits behind or in the ear, or housed in a small box resembling a small transistor radio that children wear on a cord around their neck or carry in a blouse or shirt pocket. Teach children to remove hearing aids before washing their hair, showering, or swimming. Hearing aids should be turned off when removed to preserve the life of the batteries.

Children with a hearing impairment may grow self-conscious about wearing a hearing aid during school years. Encourage such children to view themselves as whole persons despite their need for such devices, rather than as someone with something to hide (Fig. 50-10).

WHAT IF? What if you discover than an adolescent is failing a history course because he refuses to wear his hearing aid, which makes him self-conscious? As a school nurse, what would you recommend?

Speech Therapy

If children who are hearing-challenged are to interact as fully as possible with the world around them, they need an intensive program of speech therapy. Some therapists believe that learning sign language early is helpful because it allows children to express their needs early. Others believe that, by learning sign language, children decrease their need to learn to articulate speech sounds or to lip read and, for this reason, learning sign language should not be encouraged. It is true that, for real independence and to perform in regular school classes, children need to communicate by means other than sign language. For children with a profound impairment, however, learning speech sounds may be a long-term process, making sign language necessary for contact with the world around them until they learn to speak.

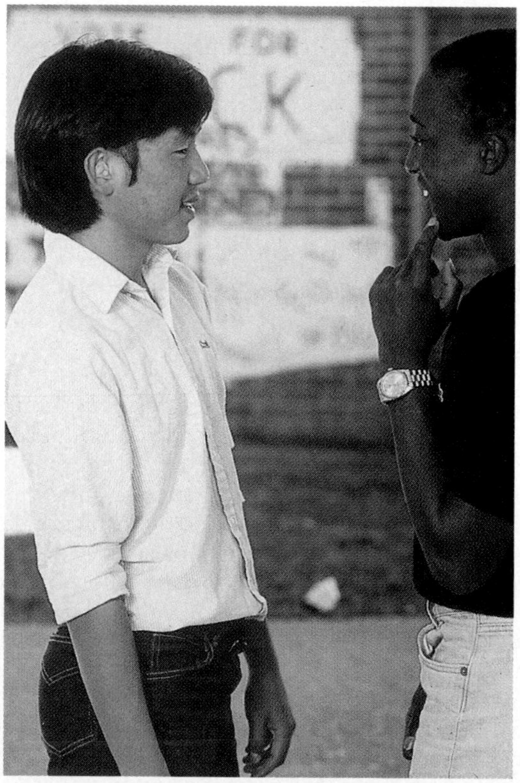

FIGURE 50.10 Maintaining peer relationships is important for an adolescent. Here, a hearing-challenged teen communicates with a friend.

DISORDERS OF THE EAR

Ear disorders are always serious in children because hearing is such an important function for the growing child. Some parents need to be cautioned that there is no such thing as "only an earache." "Only an earache" today may mean "only a hearing impairment" when the child reaches maturity. Assessment of hearing is discussed in Chapter 33.

External Otitis

External otitis is inflammation of the external ear canal. Although external ear inflammation rarely threatens hearing or causes permanent damage, it does cause discomfort in the form of itching and sometimes extreme pain.

Assessment

The history of children with external otitis generally indicates that they have recently been swimming, which is why this condition is popularly called *swimmer's ear.* It also can occur if a young child pushes a foreign object, such as a peanut, into the ear canal. Unlike middle ear infection (otitis media), there is no history of a recent respiratory infection. Children first notice itching of the canal, then pain. When you touch the external ear, the pain becomes acute. The moisture in the canal left from swimming has caused inflammation; a secondary infection may occur in the closed space. *Pseudomonas* and *Candida* are frequent agents involved in infection. Otoscopic examination may indicate only a sharply localized, tender swelling of a furuncle, or the entire canal may be swollen shut and tender to the touch. If a fungal infection is present, the entire canal may appear brown or black. If the inflammation is from a foreign body such as a peanut or the tip of a cotton applicator being present, white or gray debris may surround the object; the skin under the object is moist, red, and eroded.

In external otitis, the tympanic membrane must be visualized to ensure that there is no extension of the external otitis into the middle ear (Biggs, 2000a). In some instances, the eardrum is so inflamed from the external infectious process that it is difficult to tell whether the middle ear is free of disease. Before the tympanic membrane can be visualized, it is often necessary to remove superficial debris from the canal. A Weber test (discussed in Chapter 33) should show that hearing is equal. A tuning fork vibration that sounds louder in the affected ear suggests that otitis media (middle ear infection) is present.

Removal of debris from an infected external canal requires patience and skill. Foreign material should not be irrigated until it is shown that the tympanic membrane is intact. Otherwise, infected material could be washed through a rupture into the middle ear. Material should be removed by an ear curette using extremely gentle pressure. Children must be securely restrained for the procedure to prevent them from suddenly turning their head, causing the curette to puncture their tympanic membrane. If the debris is hard and difficult to remove, it can be softened and loosened by touching it with a hydrogen peroxide-soaked, soft, cotton applicator, or 2% acetic acid can be instilled into the canal and allowed to stand for a few minutes.

Therapeutic Management

The treatment of an external otitis differs according to the organism causing the infection. If the canal is so swollen shut that ear drops will not be able to flow back into the canal, a cotton wick moistened with Burow's solution may be threaded into the canal. The cotton extending out into the auricle is kept moistened by rewetting it for 24 h with Burow's solution. This generally reduces the swelling of the canal to a point that further treatment can be initiated.

The parents are then instructed to use ear drops containing hydrocortisone and an antibiotic or an antifungal mixture. Hydrocortisone reduces inflammation; the antibiotic or antifungal preparation will reduce the infection. Some ear drops have an additional alcohol base, which serves to dry the external canal further. If ear pain is present, an analgesic, such as acetaminophen or ibuprofen, may be necessary to control discomfort. Children must keep the ear canal dry, avoiding swimming or hair washing during this time. If children shower, they should first insert ear plugs into the external meatus to keep the moisture out.

NURSING DIAGNOSES AND RELATED INTERVENTIONS

Nursing Diagnosis: Deficient knowledge related to technique for ear drop instillation and preventive care measures

Outcome Identification: Parents will demonstrate effective ear drop administration technique by 1 h.

Outcome Evaluation: Parents demonstrate proper instillation of ear drops; state the importance of continuing prescribed treatment to completion.

Putting in ear drops can be a challenging task. Show parents how this is done (see Chapter 37) before they leave the health care facility. Encourage them to give the medication for the full time prescribed. Otherwise, because ear drops are difficult to give, they may give them only until the pain subsides (24 to 48 h). A week later, the infection may recur. Caution parents not to put anything but the ear drops into their child's ear.

Follow-Up

Evaluation after external otitis should include not only whether the inflammation and pain have decreased but also whether children and parents are aware of how to prevent the condition in the future. This includes knowing not to put any object into the ear canal and use of ear plugs during swimming. Instillation of a dilute alcohol or acetic acid solution by dropper after swimming is a prophylactic measure that helps keep the ear canal dry (Biggs, 2000a). This is often recommended for children who swim competitively or spend a great deal of time in water.

Impacted Cerumen

Cerumen (ear wax) serves the important function of cleansing the external ear canal as it gradually moves outward, bringing with it shed epithelial cells and any foreign objects. Parents are often concerned that ear wax will lead to loss of hearing (or view it as dirty) and will ask to have it removed. Wax accumulation rarely is enough to interfere with hearing. Cerumen serves a protective function and should not be removed routinely. Caution parents not to clean ears with cotton-tipped applicators as a regular practice because they may scratch the ear canal, causing an invasion site for a secondary infection. This practice may also push accumulated cerumen farther into the ear canal, causing a true plugging of wax.

Commercial softeners are available if cerumen accumulates to such an extent that hearing is affected. Some physicians advise a dilute solution of hydrogen peroxide to dissolve cerumen. This may be done once in a while but, again, should not be done regularly because this will keep the ear canal constantly moist, an environment that leads to external otitis. For most children, the basic rule of thumb—never put anything smaller than an elbow in a child's ear—is the best rule.

Acute Otitis Media

Inflammation of the middle ear (otitis media) is the most prevalent disease of childhood after respiratory tract infections. It occurs most often in the child 6 to 36 months of age and again at 4 to 6 years. It is seen most frequently in males, Alaskan and Native American, and children with cleft palate. There is a higher incidence of otitis media in formula-fed infants than those who are breast-fed because of the more slanted position that formula-fed infants are held in while feeding. This allows milk to enter the eustachian tube. The incidence of otitis media is highest in the winter and spring and higher in homes in which a parent smokes cigarettes (Berman et al., 2001). It is also associated with constant pacifier use (Post & Goessier, 2001).

Otitis media is an extremely serious disease of childhood because, if it is not treated, permanent damage can occur to middle ear structures, leading to hearing impairment.

Assessment

Acute otitis media generally follows a respiratory infection. Children have a "cold," rhinitis, and perhaps a low-grade fever for a number of days. Suddenly, they have a fever of about 102°F (38°C) and a sharp, constant pain in one or both ears. Older children can verbalize reports of pain. The infant becomes extremely irritable and frequently pulls or tugs at the affected ear in an attempt to gain relief from pain. The external canal is generally free of wax because the warmth of the inflammation and fever melts the wax and moves it more readily out of the canal. In contrast to an external ear canal infection, the discomfort does not increase on manipulation of the auricle. The mastoid process behind the ear should not be tender to touch. If it is, the infection probably has spread out of the middle ear into the mastoid cells, a very serious complication.

The appearance of a normal eardrum shows the outline of the malleus (see Chapter 33). With infection, the tympanic membrane appears inflamed on otoscopic examination. It may be seen bulging into the external canal. The light reflex of the otoscope will not be as definite as usual because of the convex shape of the eardrum. The landmarks of the tympanic membrane, the malleus and incus, will not be present or can only be poorly visualized. There will be decreased mobility on a pneumatic examination. A **tympanocentesis** (withdrawal of fluid from the middle ear through the tympanic membrane) may be performed by a physician to obtain fluid for culture at the time of assessment.

Therapeutic Management

Most middle ear infections are caused by *Streptococcus pneumoniae, Haemophilus influenzae* (especially in children younger than 5 years), or group A beta hemolytic streptococci (Biggs, 2001b). Many otitis media infections resolve spontaneously without therapy (Takata et al., 2001), but, to avoid the possibility of complications, most children with otitis media are treated with antibiotics such as ampicillin or amoxicillin (antibiotics that eliminate *H influenzae* organisms). With more and more organisms becoming resistant, erythromycin and a sulfonamide may be added to the therapy. Chronic otitis media may be caused by *Staphylococcus,* which would require treatment with an antibiotic, such as a cephalosporin that is effective against *Staphylococcus.*

Caution parents to give the prescribed antibiotic for the full length of treatment, usually 10 to 14 days. Otherwise, parents may give it only until the pain is gone (24 to 48 h), and the child will return in about 2 weeks with recurrent otitis media. It is actually still the first infection, which was not properly eradicated. Also, because the cause of the infection may be *Streptococcus,* children are susceptible to the complications of streptococcal infection such as rheumatic fever or glomerulonephritis unless properly treated.

During the course of otitis media, most children have a conductive hearing loss, which may last for up to 6 months after an acute infection. Caution parents about this so they will not think the infection is growing worse if they first notice the impairment after they arrive home from the health care facility. They also need to know about the hearing loss so that, if children are routinely screened for hearing in school during the next 6 months, they can account for the loss. If children still have a conductive hearing loss after 6 months (or have other symptoms), they should be examined again to see whether a new infection or serous otitis media is present (see Focus on Nursing Care Planning).

Children need an analgesic and antipyretic such as acetaminophen (Tylenol). Some health care providers may prescribe decongestant nose drops to open the eustachian tubes and allow air to be admitted to the middle ear. Although not proven, this may be helpful in preventing the infection from becoming a serous or long-term otitis media. Nasal decongestant drops usually are only given for 3 days. If given longer, a rebound effect may occur, causing edema and a subsequent increase in mucous membrane size.

Otitis Media With Effusion

Otitis media with effusion is a result of chronic otitis media. Normally, the middle ear is an air-filled cavity, air being supplied to it by the eustachian tube. The tube opens with swallowing, yawning, or chewing. If the source of air to the middle ear is shut off, the epithelial cells of the middle ear change in function, becoming secretory cells. The middle ear fills with these secretions. Over time, the fluid becomes so thick and tenacious that it is described as "gluelike." Some children notice a feeling of fullness or the sound of popping or ringing in their ears. There may be a drop in hearing of 20 to 40 dB because of the fluid content. Because the loss is gradual, parents and children may not be aware of it until it is noticed on a routine hearing screening. Involvement is generally bilateral. It occurs most frequently in children 3 to 10 years of age (MOMSC, 2001).

Assessment

The child experiences muffled hearing and a feeling of pressure in the ear. Examination of the ears may show a level of fluid behind the tympanic membrane. This is visible, however, only if there is also a quantity of air in the middle ear as well, to contrast with the fluid line. As the collected fluid becomes thick, it tends to retract the eardrum. This makes the malleus more prominent and perhaps displaced to a horizontal angle as the membrane is retracted around it; the light reflex from the otoscope light becomes distorted. If a pneumatic otoscope is used, when air is gently introduced against the eardrum, there is no movement of the tympanic membrane (as there would be normally).

Therapeutic Management

Therapy for otitis media with effusion may be long-term. If the condition appears to be intensified by inflammation from an allergy, measures to control the allergy must be instituted: avoidance of the allergen, hyposensitization, or pharmacologic alteration of the allergic response. Treatment of children with allergies is discussed in Chapter 42.

Definitive medical treatment is aimed at supplying air to the middle ear. For mild involvement, the daily administration of an antihistamine or a nasal decongestant to shrink the mucous membrane of the eustachian tube may be enough to achieve this. In a few children, the eustachian tube is blocked by enlarged adenoids, and their removal is indicated. This is not often needed, however. Fluid from the middle ear can be removed by tympanocentesis (needle inserted through the tympanic membrane). Fluid usually returns, however, unless some intervention to introduce air to the middle ear (tubal myringotomy) is undertaken.

Tubal Myringotomy. A source of air can be supplied to the middle ear by the insertion of small plastic (Teflon) tubes through the tympanic membrane (a tympanostomy). The insertion of such tubes is done after a myringotomy at a point in the tympanic membrane that is not instrumental for hearing, so as not to interfere with this (Fig. 50-11). Myringotomy tubes can be placed in one or both ears as an ambulatory procedure after the local injection of lidocaine (Xylocaine). Tubes tend to be extruded after 6 to 12 months. For many children, this period is enough to halt the secretory process of the middle ear. In others, tubes must be reinserted to continue the aeration.

FOCUS ON *Nursing Care Planning*

A CHILD WITH OTITIS MEDIA

A 10-month-old boy is seen at the ambulatory clinic for a fever. His mother states, "I think he has another ear infection."

Assessment: 10-month-old male with a history of two previous ear infections in the past 8 months. Mother reports that the child was well until 3 days ago when he started with a "cold." Child had a clear, watery nasal discharge and slight cough. Last evening, the child developed a fever of 102.2°F (39.0°C). Temperature now 100.8°F (38.2°C). "He was really irritable and fussy all day yesterday, and he barely drank his night time bottle. He was up crying most of the night, even screaming out a few times. I noticed him pulling on his right ear."

Child sitting in mother's lap, restless, irritable, and crying continuously. Observed tugging vigorously on right ear. Thick, purulent, white nasal drainage noted from both nostrils. On examination, right tympanic membrane erythematous and bulging, with poor mobility on pneumoscopy. Left ear examination unremarkable. Child is diagnosed with otitis media of the right ear. "I can't believe he has another ear infection. I'm so frustrated. It seems like everything we do is useless."

Nursing Diagnosis: Pain related to inflammation and erythema secondary to ear infection

Outcome Identification: Child will exhibit behaviors indicative of pain relief within 24 h.

Outcome Evaluation: Child no longer tugging at right ear; crying has diminished in frequency and intensity. Mother reports child is able to nap for short periods and sleeps most of night.

Interventions	Rationale
1. Explore measures used by mother to console and comfort the child.	1. Exploration of currently used measures provides a baseline from which to develop future teaching strategies.
2. Suggest alternative measures for comfort, such as gentle rocking and close cuddling. Caution the mother to position the child on the unaffected ear.	2. Gentle rocking and close cuddling aid in providing a sense of a secure, warm environment. Positioning on the unaffected side prevents pressure on and subsequent pain in the affected ear.
3. Instruct the mother to administer acetaminophen every 4 h or ibuprofen every 8 h.	3. Acetaminophen and ibuprofen are effective analgesics and antipyretics for this degree of pain.
4. Institute antibiotic therapy as ordered. Strongly reinforce need for completion of a full course of therapy.	4. Antibiotics treat the infection and decrease inflammation. As the inflammation decreases, so does the pain. A full course of therapy is necessary to ensure complete eradication of the infection and prevention of possible sequelae.
5. Suggest use of saline nose drops or nasal spray.	5. Saline nose drops or nasal spray helps to relieve nasal inflammation and subsequent pressure on the eustachian tube.
6. Encourage the mother to offer liquids and soft finger foods.	6. Movement of the eustachian tube, such as with chewing, may increase pain.
7. Instruct the mother to contact the clinic or the health care provider if there is no improvement within 24 to 48 h or if the child exhibits increased pain or a sudden relief of pain.	7. Lack of improvement within 24 to 48 h indicates the need for further evaluation. Increased pain may indicate excessive fluid accumulation, which could lead to tympanic rupture, evidenced by a sudden relief of pain.

(continued)

Nursing Diagnosis: Powerlessness related to repeated episodes of otitis media

Outcome Identification: Parent will demonstrate behaviors to control the situation.

Outcome Evaluation: Parent identifies factors within her control; demonstrates positive behaviors to manage situation; participates in decisions when possible.

Interventions	Rationale
1. Assess mother for possible contributing factors related to feelings of loss of control.	1. Assessment of factors provides a baseline for developing future strategies.
2. Slowly and clearly explain the events and changes occurring with this and previous episodes of otitis media. Inform the mother of things that can and cannot be controlled.	2. Explanation provides the mother with an understanding of what is happening and why. Information about things that can be controlled provides a means for focused participation.
3. Educate the mother about the common characteristics of otitis media.	3. Education promotes better understanding of the problem, alleviating some of the stress and anxiety associated with it.
4. Reassure the mother that she did nothing to cause the repeated episode and that the infection will resolve with proper treatment.	4. Parents may feel guilty if they are unable to soothe their child. Reassurance that the problem is not her fault can aid in objective problem solving, help to minimize anxiety, and increase motivation and hope.
5. Emphasize positive aspects of situation and what can be controlled.	5. Positive emphasis on controllable aspects helps to shift the focus of fears, enhancing feelings of control. Feelings of lack of control can diminish attention to and retention of information.
6. Praise the mother for her ability to recognize the signs and symptoms and seek treatment.	6. Praise enhances the mother's self-esteem, helping to promote feelings of control.
7. Provide emotional support throughout diagnosis and treatment.	7. Emotional support assists in reinforcing positive behaviors, enhancing self-esteem.

With myringotomy tubes in place, water should not be allowed to enter the child's ears. Most physicians prefer children to bathe rather than shower, but using ear plugs in their ears while showering may be allowed. Hair washing should be done with ear plugs in place. Similarly, swimming is either contraindicated or allowed only with ear plugs in place.

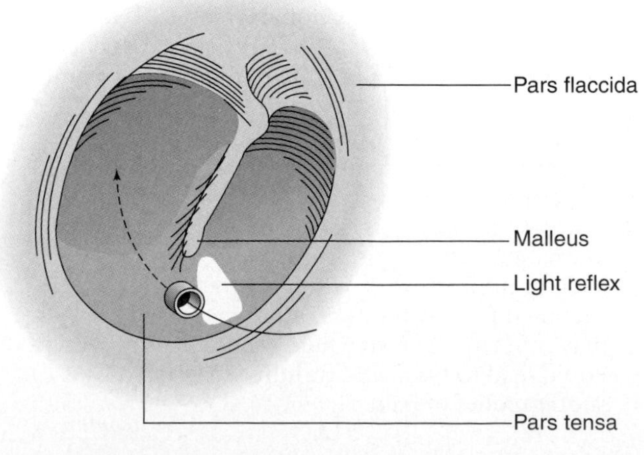

FIGURE 50.11 A myringotomy tube provides air to the middle ear to prevent otitis media with effusion.

Otitis media with effusion runs a long-term course in many children. Teach parents to continue giving medications as prescribed. They often need a great deal of support to accept the insertion of myringotomy tubes. They are afraid that cutting the eardrum will do more harm than if they just leave the situation alone. Because the course of the process is long, the hearing impairment associated with it may also be long term. Urge parents to notify the school nurse of the problem. Children may need to be changed to a front seat in a classroom so they do not miss important class content or discussion. They need support through this puzzling and annoying condition.

Cholesteatoma

Cholesteatoma is a lesion of the pars flaccida or upper portion of the tympanic membrane. A retraction cyst forms, and there is necrosis of the pars flaccida with foul-smelling drainage from the ear. If the retraction cyst is not discovered and surgically removed at this point, it grows gradually deeper and deeper until it eventually invades the mastoid cells. It can progress to mastoiditis, meningitis, and possibly facial nerve paralysis if it is not surgically removed.

Any child with foul-smelling drainage from the ear should be referred to a primary care provider for further investigation to rule out this problem. If you are inspecting children's tympanic membranes during health maintenance visits, be certain to inspect the pars flaccida and pars tensa to detect cholesteatoma (Hasebe et al., 2001).

THE HOSPITALIZED CHILD WITH A HEARING IMPAIRMENT

Children who have a hearing loss greater than 49 dB have a hearing impairment sufficient enough to interfere with hearing normal conversation and developing language. Like visually challenged children, they may be hospitalized for other health problems as well.

It can be difficult for parents to prepare children who cannot hear for hospitalization. Words such as *surgery, tonsils, hurts, operating room,* and *recovery room* are new to them. Showing a child a book with good pictures demonstrating what is going to happen is helpful. Allowing them time to play with dolls or puppets can help them understand hospital routine. Because children who are hearing challenged may not be as well prepared for hospitalization as children without a hearing impairment, make an extra effort on admission to ensure that they receive such instruction.

Always allow hearing-challenged children to see you before you touch them. They will not find this nearly as intrusive as being touched without warning. If children are sleeping when you approach them, use a light touch to waken them gently. Some children turn off their hearing aid or remove it while they sleep. You may need to turn it on before you call them to wake them, or they may need to replace the hearing aid as soon as they awaken. Children as young as 2 years of age are effective lip readers as long as you are facing them. Position yourself at eye level to the child so he can view your face. In a group, help a child follow conversation by directing him to who is speaking. Assign consistent staff members to decrease the number of persons with whom a child must attempt to communicate. Have a staff person accompany the child and stay with him or her in all departments to help with communication.

Do not underestimate the intelligence level of hearing-challenged children. Because they do not speak clearly, others may assume that hearing-challenged children are cognitively challenged. As a result, they may not be given information that the average hearing child receives, such as explanations of how things work. On a hospital unit, hearing-challenged children, locked in a silent world, are unable to express how they feel about procedures. They need help from health care personnel who understand this and take more than the usual amount of time to offer them explanations and support.

Ask parents of children who are hearing challenged to draw pictures or demonstrate the sign language symbols children use for important words such as *pain, drink,* and *bathroom.* Encourage children to use or draw pictures of what they want if they are still too young to write words and you cannot understand what they are saying.

Hearing-challenged children have the right to be provided with an interpreter during care. Advocate for this, especially if parents will not be present during care.

✔ CHECKPOINT QUESTIONS

11. How does acute otitis media differ from otitis media with effusion?
12. Why should you assess for cholesteatoma?
13. When approaching a hearing-challenged child, what should you do first before touching them?

KEY POINTS

Teaching preventive measures to avoid eye and hearing injuries (using proper eye protection during sports or play and wearing goggles or ear protection as appropriate) and screening children for sensory impairments are important nursing roles.

Refractive errors of vision such as myopia and hyperopia are the most common eye disorders in children. Amblyopia (lazy eye) is subnormal vision in one eye. Children with these disorders need correction at the time the disorder is recognized to prevent further vision distortion.

Coloboma is congenital incomplete closure of the pupil or lower eyelid. Ptosis is the inability to open the upper eyelid normally. Ptosis needs correction to avoid development of amblyopia. Strabismus is unequally aligned eyes. Like ptosis, it may lead to amblyopia if not corrected.

Infections of the lids such as styes or chalazions can occur in children. Conjunctivitis (inflammation of the conjunctiva) often presents with acute symptoms. An antibiotic is necessary for therapy.

Eye injuries such as penetration by a foreign body need follow-up after treatment to be certain that vision remains adequate.

Children who are either vision or hearing challenged need special preparation and orientation for a hospital or ambulatory health visit so they can fully understand what is going to happen during the visit.

Help children who are vision challenged work through new experiences by letting them feel equipment as much as possible. Guide their hands through the steps of a new procedure you are teaching them.

Otitis media (middle ear infection) is a common childhood illness. Children need therapy with antibiotics to correct this. With otitis media with effusion, some children have myringotomy tubes inserted to relieve pressure and supply air access to the middle ear.

Use photographs, drawings, or demonstration with hearing-challenged children to help them learn new skills. Contact a signing interpreter as appropriate to be certain that children understand instructions.

CRITICAL THINKING EXERCISES

1. Carla is the 4-year-old girl with an ear infection you met at the beginning of the chapter. What information would be important to ascertain from her mother about Carla's previous ear infection? How would you counsel this parent about preventing future episodes?
2. A 4-year-old boy is going to have eye surgery. What special steps do you want to take to prepare him for this surgery? Is he old enough to appreciate the importance of seeing? Please support your response.
3. A 14-year-old boy who is profoundly hearing challenged from developing meningitis as a preschooler uses sign language to communicate. How could you communicate effectively with him while he's hospitalized? What are his rights as a patient in regard to having an interpreter provided for him?
4. You are going to teach a first-grade class on ways to prevent eye and hearing injuries. What would you include in your class? How would your teaching plan be different if the class was for 16-year-old students?
5. Examine the National Health Goals related to sensory disorders. Most government-sponsored money for nursing research is allotted based on these goals. What would be a possible research topic to explore pertinent to these goals that would be fundable and also would advance evidence-based practice?

REFERENCES

Adler, I. N., et al. (2001). Ophthalmologic disease in children. *Magnetic Resonance Imaging Clinics of North America, 9*(1), 191-206.

Balkany, T. J., et al. (2001). Cochlear implants in children. *Otolaryngologic Clinics of North America, 34*(2), 455-467.

Barr, A., et al. (2000). Ocular sports injuries: The current picture. *British Journal of Sports Medicine, 34*(6), 456-458.

Berman, S., Johnson, C., Chan, K., & Kelley, P. (2001). Ear, nose & throat. In W. W. Hay, A. R. Hayward, M. J. Levin, & J. M. Sondheimer (Eds.). *Current pediatric diagnosis & treatment* (15th ed.). New York: McGraw-Hill.

Biggs, L. M. (2000a). Otitis externa. In M. W. Schwartz, M. W. (Ed.) *The 5-minute pediatric consult* (pp. 588-589). Philadelphia: Lippincott Williams & Wilkins.

Biggs, L. M. (2000b). Otitis media. In M. W. Schwartz, M. W. (Ed.) *The 5-minute pediatric consult* (pp. 590-591). Philadelphia: Lippincott Williams & Wilkins.

Bodaghi, B., et al. (2001). Chronic severe uveitis: Etiology and visual outcome in 927 patients from a single center. *Medicine, 80*(4), 263-270.

Brambring, M. (2001). Integration of children with visual impairment in regular preschools. *Child, Health & Development, 27*(5), 425-438.

Carpenito, L. J. (2001). *Handbook of nursing diagnosis* (9th ed.). Philadelphia: Lippincott Williams & Wilkins.

Department of Health and Human Services. (2000). *Healthy people 2010.* Washington, DC: DHHS.

Eibschitz-Tsimhoni, M., et al. (2000). Early screening for amblyogenic risk factors lowers the prevalence and severity of amblyopia. *Journal of the American Association for Pediatric Ophthalmology & Strabismus, 4*(4), 194-199.

Eisenbaum, A. M., & Ornitz, D. B. (2001). The eye. In W. W. Hay, A. R. Hayward, M. J. Levin, J. M. Sondheimer (Eds.). *Current pediatric diagnosis & treatment* (15th ed.). New York: McGraw-Hill.

Gwiazda, J., et al. (2000). Astigmatism and the development of myopia in children. *Vision Research, 40*(8), 1019-1026.

Han, S. H., et al. (2001). Effect of botulinum toxin A chemodenervation in sensory strabismus. *Journal of Pediatric Ophthalmology & Strabismus, 38*(2), 68-71.

Hasebe, S., et al. (2001). Mastoid condition and clinical course of cholesteatoma. *Journal of Oto-Rhino-Laryngology & Its Related Specialties, 63*(3), 160-164.

Hatton, M. P., et al. (2001). Orbital fractures in children. *Ophthalmic Plastic & Reconstructive Surgery, 17*(3), 174-179.

Hertle, R. W. (2000a). Amblyopbia. In M. W. Schwartz, M. W. (Ed.) *The 5-minute pediatric consult* (pp. 112-113). Philadelphia: Lippincott Williams & Wilkins.

Hertle, R. W. (2000b). Strabismus. In M. W. Schwartz, M. W. (Ed.) *The 5-minute pediatric consult* (pp. 774-775). Philadelphia: Lippincott Williams & Wilkins.

Koenes, S. G., & Karshmer, J. F. (2000). Depression: A comparison study between blind and sighted adolescents. *Issues in Mental Health Nursing, 21*(3), 269-279.

Mohan, K., et al. (2001). Visual acuities after levodopa administration in amblyopia. *Journal of Pediatric Ophthalmology & Strabismus, 38*(2), 62-67.

Multi-centre Otitis Media Study Group. (2001). Risk factors for persistence of bilateral otitis media with effusion. *Clinical Otolaryngology & Allied Sciences, 26*(2), 147-156.

Newsham, D. (2000). Parental non-concordance with occlusion therapy. *British Journal of Ophthalmology, 84*(9), 957-962.

Pediatric Eye Disease Investigator Group. (2002). A randomized trial of atropine vs. patching for treatment of moderate amblyopia in children. *Archives of Ophthalmology, 120*(3), 268-278.

Post, J. C. & Goessier, M. C. (2001). Is pacifier use a risk factor for otitis media? *Lancet, 357*(9259), 823-824.

Quinn, G. E. (2000). Glaucoma-congenital. In M. W. Schwartz, M. W. (Ed.) *The 5-minute pediatric consult* (pp. 386-387). Philadelphia: Lippincott Williams & Wilkins.

Read, A. P. (2000). Waardenburg syndrome. *Advances in Oto-Rhino-Laryngology, 56*(1), 32-38.

Schaffer, D. B. (2000). Cataracts. In M. W. Schwartz, M. W. (Ed.) *The 5-minute pediatric consult* (pp. 224-225). Philadelphia: Lippincott Williams & Wilkins.

Shields, S. R. (2000). Managing eye disease in primary care. *Postgraduate Medicine, 108*(5), 69-78.

Shute, R. H., & Westall, C. A. (2000). Use of the Mollon-Reffin minimalist color vision test with young children. *Journal of AAPOS: American Association for Pediatric Ophthalmology & Strabismus, 4*(6), 366-372.

Simon, J. W., & Kaw, P. (2001). Commonly missed diagnoses in the childhood eye examination. *American Family Physician, 64*(4), 623-628.

Sugar, A., et al. (2002). Laser in situ keratomileusis for myopia and astigmatism. *Ophthalmology, 109*(1), 175-187.

Takata, G. S. et al. (2001). Evidence assessment of management of acute otitis media. *Pediatrics, 108*(2), 239–247.
Talbot, A. W., & Russell-Eggitt, I. (2000). Pharmaceutical management of the childhood glaucomas. *Expert Opinion on Pharmacotherapy, 1*(4), 697–711.
Thilo, E. H. & Rosenberg, A. A. (2001). Infections in the newborn infant. In W. W. Hay, A. R. Hayward, M. J. Levin, & J. M. Sondheimer (Eds.). *Current pediatric diagnosis & treatment* (15th ed.). New York: McGraw-Hill.
Till, C., et al. (2001). Effects of maternal occupational exposure to organic solvents on offspring visual functioning. *Teratology, 64*(3), 134–141.
Wetmore, R. F. (2000). Complications of otitis media. *Pediatric Annals 29*(10), 637–647.

SUGGESTED READINGS

Danis, R. P., Hu, K., & Bell, M. (2000). Acceptability of baseball face guards and reduction of oculofacial injury in receptive youth league players. *Injury Prevention, 6*(3), 232–234.
Davis, N. M., et al. (2001). Auditory function at 14 years of age of very-low-birthweight children. *Developmental Medicine & Child Neurology, 43*(3), 191–196.
Gabriel, K. O. S., & Getch, Y. Q. (2001). Parental training and involvement in sexuality education for students who are deaf. *American Annals of the Deaf, 146*(3), 287–293.
Ghaffar, F. A., et al. (2001). Acute mastoiditis in children: A seventeen-year experience in Dallas, Texas. *Pediatric Infectious Disease Journal, 20*(4), 376–380.
Giannoni, C. (2000). Swimming with tympanostomy tubes. *Archives of Otolaryngology, 126*(12), 1507–1508.
Hargrave, S., Weakley, D., & Wilson, C. (2000). Complications of ocular paintball injuries in children. *Journal of Ophthalmic Nursing & Technology, 19*(5), 234–239.
Hoberman, A., & Paradise, J. L. (2000). Acute otitis media: Diagnosis and management in the year 2000. *Pediatric Annals, 29*(10), 609–622.
Katelaris, C. H., et al. (2000). A springtime Olympics demands special consideration for allergic athletes. *Journal of Allergy & Clinical Immunology, 106*(2), 260–266.
Kemper, A. R., et al. (1999). A systematic review of vision screening tests for the detection of amblyopia. *Pediatrics, 104*(5.2), 1220–1222.
Lai, J. C., et al. (2001). Traumatic hyphema in children: Risk factors from complications. *Archives of Ophthalmology, 119*(1), 64–70.
Luntz, M., et al. (2001). Cochlear implantation in healthy and otitis-prone children: A prospective study. *Laryngoscope, 111*(9), 1614–1618.
McCracken, G. H. (2002). Diagnosis and management of acute otitis media in the urgent care setting. *Annals of Emergency Medicine, 39*(4), 413–421.
Mills, M. D. (1999). What is amblyopia and how is it treated? *American Family Physician, 60*(3), 918.
Moores, D. F. (2001). Testing . . . 3, 2, 1. *American Annals of the Deaf, 146*(3), 243–244.
Pandey, S. K., et al. (2001). Pediatric cataract surgery and intraocular lens implantation. *International Ophthalmology Clinics, 41*(2), 175–196.
Raivio, V. E., et al. (2001). Transcleral contact krypton laser cyclophotocoagulation for treatment of glaucoma in children and young adults. *Ophthalmology, 108*(10), 1801–1807.
Roddey, O. F., & Hoover, H. A. (2000). Otitis media with effusion in children. *Pediatric Annals, 29*(10), 623–629.
Woolfe, T., & Smith, P. K. (2001). The self-esteem and cohesion to family members of deaf children in relation to the hearing status of their parents and siblings. *Deafness & Education International, 3*(2), 80–96.

CHAPTER 51

Nursing Care of the Child With a Musculoskeletal Disorder

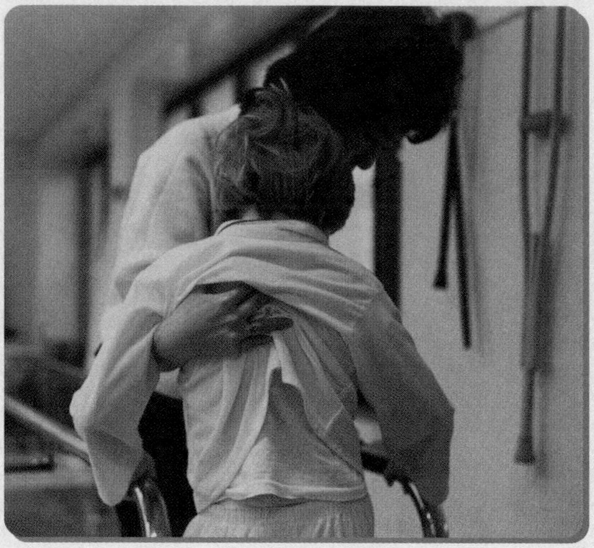

Key Terms

- apposition
- arthroscopy
- cartilage
- diaphysis
- distraction
- epiphyseal plate
- epiphysis
- fracture
- malleoli
- metaphysis
- myopathy
- periosteum
- remodeling
- resorption
- sequestrum
- traction

Objectives

After mastering the contents of this chapter, you should be able to:

1. Describe common musculoskeletal disorders in children.
2. Assess the child with a musculoskeletal disorder.
3. Formulate nursing diagnoses related to the child with a musculoskeletal disorder.
4. Establish appropriate outcomes for the child with a musculoskeletal disorder.
5. Plan nursing care, such as age-appropriate diversional activities, for the child with a musculoskeletal disorder.
6. Implement nursing care for the child with a musculoskeletal disorder.
7. Evaluate outcomes for achievement and effectiveness of care.
8. Identify National Health Goals related to musculoskeletal disorders and children that nurses can be instrumental in helping the nation to achieve.
9. Identify areas related to care of the child with a musculoskeletal disorder that could benefit from additional nursing research or application of evidence-based practice.
10. Use critical thinking to analyze ways that care of the child with a musculoskeletal disorder can be more family centered.
11. Integrate knowledge of musculoskeletal disorders with nursing process to achieve quality maternal and child health nursing care.

Jeffrey, 10 years old, is brought to the clinic because of pain in his left lower leg. He is irritable, has a fever, and his left lower leg is warm to the touch and edematous. His mother tells you that he had a skin abscess in that area about 2 weeks ago. After further evaluation, Jeffrey is diagnosed with osteomyelitis. His mother asks, "How could he get an infection in his bone? It was his skin that was the problem. I thought he was just having growing pains." What does Jeffrey's mother need to know? How would you explain what has happened?

Previous chapters described the growth and development of well children and the nursing care of children with a disorder of other body systems. This chapter adds information about the dramatic changes, both physical and psychosocial, that occur when a child develops a musculoskeletal disorder. This is important information because it builds a base for care and health teaching.

After you've studied the chapter, answer the Critical Thinking Exercises at the end of the chapter and then access the on-line study activities (http://connection.lww.com) *to further sharpen your skills and test your knowledge.*

The skeletal system, composed of more than 200 bones connected by the joints and tendons, provides a structural casing or protective armor for the internal organs of the body. Skeletal muscles, attached to the bones by connective tissue, tendons, and ligaments, allow for voluntary movement—including gross motor activity, such as running, and fine motor activity, such as writing. Together, the skeletal and muscular systems support the body and make coordinated movement possible.

Because their bones and muscles are still growing, children suffer from disorders of the musculoskeletal system more frequently than adults do. Fortunately, with fractures, because bones are still growing, healing occurs much more quickly for the child than for the adult. If a growth plate is injured (which results in halting of bone growth), however, an injury that might be simple in an adult becomes serious in a child. Because many musculoskeletal system disorders lead to problems with locomotion and thus possibly limit activity, they can threaten a child's ability to develop optimally in other ways. Some problems of locomotion may be slight and self-limiting, whereas others can be extensive and incapacitating. In either instance, because children gain much of their knowledge by interacting with people and exploring the environment around them, a problem of locomotion can be a serious impairment during childhood. Nurses play a key role in teaching parents ways to expose their children to the same sorts of stimuli that might be experienced if the child were able to move around independently.

Maintenance of musculoskeletal function is addressed by the National Health Goals. These are shown in the Focus on National Health Goals box.

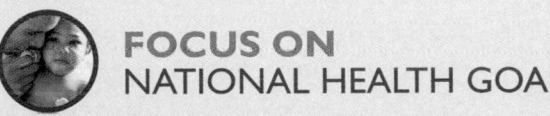

FOCUS ON NATIONAL HEALTH GOALS

To maintain a healthy musculoskeletal system, proper exercise is necessary. Several National Health Goals address this issue:

- Increase the proportion of the nation's public and private schools that require daily physical education for all students from 17% to 25%.
- Increase to at least 30% from a baseline of 27% the proportion of adolescents who participate in moderate physical activity for at least 30 min on 5 of 7 days.
- Increase the proportion of adolescents who view television 2 or fewer hours on a school day from 57% to 75%.
- Increase the proportion of trips made by walking in children and adolescents from 31% to 50% (DHHS, 2000).

Nurses can be instrumental in helping the nation achieve these goals by educating children about the importance of physical activity, serving as consultants for school systems in designing physical education programs, and being certain to ask children about their usual activity level at health maintenance visits. Nursing research that would be helpful in adding to nursing knowledge includes whether children sustain interest longer in group or single-person exercise programs; whether adolescents are accurate in reporting the time and intensity of exercise in which they engage; and whether designing exercise programs for well children and those with chronic illness can be a nursing role.

NURSING PROCESS OVERVIEW

For Care of the Child With a Musculoskeletal Disorder

Assessment

Unlike many other diseases in children, disorders of the skeletal system usually present with specific, localized symptoms. Parents usually bring children to health care facilities early in the course of such illnesses. On the other hand, disorders of the muscles or joints (such as juvenile rheumatoid arthritis [JA]) may present insidiously, and, when the disorder is diagnosed, parents may feel guilty for not having sought health care earlier.

One condition whose seriousness parents may underestimate is a childhood limp. A limp is never normal, however, and may be the first manifestation of a serious hip or knee problem. When weighing or measuring a child, there is ample opportunity to assess gait (whether the child walks naturally or stiffly, tiptoes, or walks on the whole foot; whether

ASSESSING the Child for Possible Signs and Symptoms of a Musculoskeletal Disorder

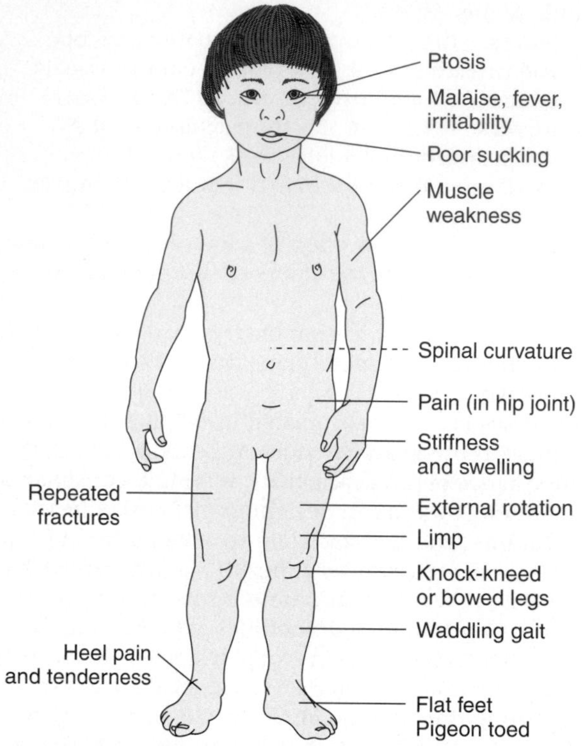

the feet are in good alignment; whether the back is held straight). Such assessments, for example, may detect that a child brought to a health care center because of an upper respiratory condition, has another, perhaps more important, musculoskeletal problem requiring evaluation (see Assessing the Child for Possible Signs and Symptoms of a Musculoskeletal Disorder). Because scoliosis is a common spinal deformity requiring early detection, school nurses have direct responsibility for instituting scoliosis screening programs in their schools.

In addition, because skeletal injuries may be a sign of abuse, careful history taking is necessary to rule this out.

Nursing Diagnosis

The nursing diagnoses most frequently identified for children with musculoskeletal disorders include those that deal with pain, lack of mobility, and, because of immobilization, a need for diversional activities. Children, especially adolescents, requiring a walker or other equipment to aid in skeletal support or locomotion may encounter problems with self-concept. Some common nursing diagnoses may include the following:

- Pain related to chronic inflammation of joints
- Impaired physical mobility related to cast on leg
- Deficient diversional activity related to need for imposed activity restriction for 4 weeks
- Situational low self-esteem related to continuous use of body brace

Outcome Identification and Planning

Many musculoskeletal problems in children require long-term care. Despite current therapies, some disorders may leave the child with a permanent disability. Before children are discharged from an ambulatory or inpatient setting, help parents plan how they will care for the child at home. At first, a cast on an arm seems exciting to a school-age child: It is something to show off, an injury to describe, an excuse not to write in school. After a few days, the cast may become more frustrating than enjoyable. Take the time to review what wearing the cast will mean to the child in everyday situations. For example, the cast may not fit through shirts with tight cuffs. In this instance, dressing for school might be a problem. Planning transportation, for example, if the child has a large cast and will not be able to fit in a car seat, may be a problem. If the child will have to stay home from school, plans for tutoring need to be made. If both parents work, child care may be necessary.

Depending on the child's and family's circumstances, the answers to these problems differ. However, taking the time to sit down with the parents and asking them if these concerns will be problems initiates problem solving. Doing so helps parents plan and prepare solutions with a concerned person rather than by themselves at home. In some instances, additional support from organizations and associations may be needed. Investigate possible referral sources.

Implementation

Many nursing interventions for children with musculoskeletal disorders involve care of a child in a cast or in traction or teaching about common concerns, such as posture or children's shoes. Parents and children who are kept well informed in these matters are much more likely to be able to cope with changing circumstances. Referrals to appropriate organizations may be helpful. Organizations that can be used for referral include the following:

Arthritis Foundation (*www.arthritis.org*)
Muscular Dystrophy Association of America, Inc. (*www.mdausa.org*)
National Institutes of Health Osteoporosis and Related Bone Diseases—National Resource Center (*www.osteo.org*)
Osteogenesis Imperfecta Foundation, Inc. (*www.oif.org*)

Outcome Evaluation

Children with musculoskeletal disorders invariably need follow-up care after discharge from an ambulatory visit or inpatient care, because bone healing is a slow process. Parents may ask to have x-rays taken frequently to evaluate healing progress. They may need to be reminded that x-rays are never taken on children unless there is a documented need for them (excessive radiation at epiphyseal plates can lead to uneven growth and also have been associated with the development of leukemia in children; Shankar, 2000).

Both parents and children may need support at reevaluation visits when learning that a cast or brace must stay on longer or that they must continue exercises. Praise for their management thus far is an effective intervention for helping parents realize that they can cope with the situation in the future.

During reevaluation visits, spend time assessing the child's body image and self-esteem. Does the child view himself or herself as a well person with, for example, a right leg shorter than the left leg, or as a deformed person who is inferior to others? Success of treatment is incomplete if a child's self-concept is impacted.

Some examples indicating achievement of outcomes may include the following:

- Child states he feels no pain or numbness in extremity after application of a cast.
- Child demonstrates allowable weight-bearing activities with casted lower extremity.
- Parents accurately state child's care needs to be met both in and out of the hospital.
- Child states positive aspects of self, participates in activities, establishes friendships with peers.

THE MUSCULOSKELETAL SYSTEM

Bones and Bone Growth

Bones are generally classified by their shape as long, short, flat, or irregular. Long bones are the bones of the extremities, including the fingers and toes, in which most childhood bone disorders are found. The short bones are those found in the ankle and wrist. Flat bones are found in the skull, ribs, scapula, and clavicle. Irregular bones are found in the vertebrae, the pelvis, and the facial bones of the skull.

Long bones are composed of a long central shaft (the **diaphysis**), a rounded end portion (the **epiphysis**), and a thin area between them (the **metaphysis**) (Fig. 51-1). Increase in the length of long bones occurs at the cartilage segment (the **epiphyseal plate**). As **cartilage** (connective tissue) cells grow away from the shaft, they are replaced by bone, thereby increasing bone length. Injury to this area in a growing child is always potentially serious, because it may halt growth, stimulate abnormal growth, or cause irregular or erratic growth. The central shafts of long bones are covered by an outer sensitive layer of **periosteum.** Bone width increases by growth at the inner surface of the periosteum. Injury to the periosteum, such as may occur with osteomyelitis, can also threaten bone growth.

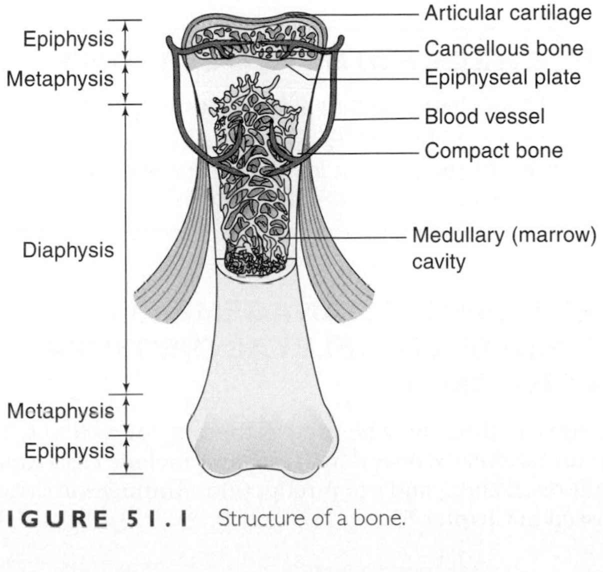

FIGURE 51.1 Structure of a bone.

Although it is easy to think of bones as rigid, solid structures, they are, in fact, living tissue, for which nutrients must be supplied for growth. Calcium, one of the main components of bone, is an important element for bone formation, **remodeling** (new bone tissue replacing old bone tissue), and **resorption** (bone breakdown). These processes are influenced by parathyroid hormone, calcitonin, vitamin D, other minerals, nutrients, and enzymes. "Bone age" can be determined by an x-ray of the wrists that shows the ossification level of bones. The inner core of long bones is filled with yellow and red marrow, and is responsible for platelet, red blood cell, white blood cell, and adipose cell formation. Red marrow is primarily involved with blood component production, whereas yellow marrow is chiefly involved with adipose cell formation. The blood supply to bones is abundant so that the marrow can actively supply enough blood components for the body. As with other tissues, if the blood supply is cut off, bone cells die.

The bones of children tend to be more resilient than the bones of adults. This means that accidents that might result in severe breaks to adult bones are apt to result in lesser breaks or only torsional twists in children. Bones tend to heal more quickly in children than in adults; therefore, children usually are incapacitated for a shorter time after an injury.

Muscle

The skeletal muscular system is composed of one type of muscle, called striated muscle, which is the predominant muscle in the body (differentiated from smooth muscle, which is responsible for, among other things, gastrointestinal peristalsis). Activation of skeletal muscle occurs with innervation from a motor nerve and is under voluntary control. **Myopathy,** or disease of the muscular system, can be inherited (as in muscular dystrophy) or acquired (as in myasthenia gravis).

ASSESSMENT OF MUSCULOSKELETAL FUNCTION

In addition to the history and physical examination, diagnostic tests frequently are necessary to detect musculoskeletal dysfunction in children. These may include x-rays and bone scans, bone and muscle biopsies, electromyography, and arthroscopy. Ultrasound and magnetic resonance imaging (MRI) studies may reveal soft-tissue disease.

X-ray

Because bones are opaque, they outline well on x-ray. Bone x-rays provide information about a specific bone, groups of bones, or a joint. They can also provide information about soft-tissue structure, swelling, or calcification. However, other tests are indicated to confirm problems with cartilage, tendons, and ligaments.

Bone Scan

A bone scan is a study of the uptake of intravenously (IV) injected radioactive substances by the bone. The distribution and concentration of the substance are evaluated to determine the problem. For example, areas of increased metabolic activity will cause the substance to concentrate in that area. A bone scan provides information of very early bone disease and healing, often before it is visible in x-rays.

Electromyography

Electromyography studies the electrical activity of skeletal muscle and nerve conduction. It can determine the location and cause of several disorders, such as myasthenia gravis and muscular dystrophy and lower motor neuron and peripheral nerve disorders.

For the test, needle electrodes are inserted into muscle masses; the electrical activity of the muscle at rest and in motion is detected by audioamplification and recorded on an oscilloscope. Normally, resting muscle is quiet. If defects, such as fasciculations, are present, abnormal noises or oscilloscope spikes will be observed.

Although the needle electrodes are small, the test may be frightening for children because they are pricked by needles. They need support from someone they know during the procedure. Before and after the procedure, provide opportunities for therapeutic play so they can express their anxiety and feelings.

Muscle or Bone Biopsy

A muscle or bone biopsy involves removal of a tissue sample for examination of its microscopic structure. It can provide evidence about infection, malignant bone growth, inflammation, or atrophy of the area. Either type may be done during surgery or as an ambulatory procedure.

Muscle biopsy is generally done using conscious sedation or a local anesthetic. Caution children that, if local anesthesia is not used, they will feel the initial prick of an anesthetizing needle; as the actual biopsy needle enters the muscle mass, they will feel an additional momentary pain. They can be assured that the amount of tissue taken from them is no larger than the inner bore of the biopsy needle, comparable to the size of the lead in a pencil.

Arthroscopy

Arthroscopy involves direct visualization of a joint with a fiberoptic instrument. It is usually done under local anesthesia in an ambulatory care setting. Arthroscopy allows a joint, most commonly the knee, but also the hip, shoulder, elbow, or wrist, to be examined without a large incision. It is most commonly used to diagnose athletic injuries and to differentiate between acute and chronic joint disorders.

HEALTH PROMOTION AND RISK MANAGEMENT

Health promotion focuses on thorough assessment at all health maintenance visits. The child's ability to achieve developmental milestones, specifically gross and fine motor abilities, provides important information about his or her musculoskeletal function. In addition, the ability to get around directly influences a child's exploration of the environment and exposure to stimuli. If this is impaired, it also can interfere with his or her growth and development. Screening, such as for scoliosis in the prepubescent child and adolescent, is also an important health promotion measure.

Safety is paramount for any child to prevent injury. Anticipatory guidance for parents is essential to minimize the risk of injury, specifically to the extremities, in all aspects of every day life. As the child grows and becomes active in sports, parental and child education about the importance of face masks for hockey, batting helmets for baseball, and mouth guards for football, takes on an even greater role.

Nutrition education is important to ensure adequate calcium intake necessary for bone growth and healing. However, if the child requires bedrest, calcium intake should be moderated to reduce the risk of renal calculi formation resulting from immobilization. The teenage years are an important time for males and females to build calcium stores to protect against osteoporosis later in life (Weaver, 2000).

If the child experiences a musculoskeletal disorder, education helps to prevent complications, maximize the child's ability to function, and minimize the risk of residual impaired physical mobility. Parents and children need instruction about all aspects of treatment and follow-up, for example, caring for the child requiring a cast, traction, body brace, or drug therapy, such as antibiotics for osteomyelitis or nonsteroidal anti-inflammatory drugs (NSAIDs) for JA. Teaching provides a basis for enhancing compliance, maximizing the effectiveness of treatment, and minimizing the possible long-term risk for problems.

> ✔ **CHECKPOINT QUESTIONS**
>
> 1. At what part of the long bone does an increase in bone length occur?
> 2. What diagnostic test involves inserting needle electrodes into the child's muscles?

THERAPEUTIC MANAGEMENT OF MUSCULOSKELETAL DISORDERS IN CHILDREN

Various methods may be used as therapy for a child with a musculoskeletal disorder. These may include casts, traction, distraction, and open reduction. Amputation is discussed in Chapter 53.

Casting

Casts may be used to treat a variety of musculoskeletal system disorders—from simple fractures in the extremities to correction of congenital structural bone disorders (see Chapter 39 for a discussion of the latter).

Cast Application

Casts are created from either plaster of Paris or synthetic material, such as fiberglass. Fiberglass is an attractive material to use for children's casts because it is light, comes in colors, and is water resistant. A special waterproof liner can be used, allowing the cast to be immersed in water. Unfortunately, it is more expensive and may not be practical for casts that need frequent changing, such as those used to correct talipes disorders.

Children need an explanation of what to expect with casting. To maintain alignment of body parts, a physician gently exerts a pull on the body part (manual traction) being casted during cast application. If a large body cast is being applied, children may be positioned on a special cast table with traction apparatus at the chin and pelvis. These tables are stark, steel tables and may resemble torture racks children have seen in horror movies. Allow someone to accompany them to the cast room to hold their hand or talk to them during the application. Most children (and adults) are unaware that casts are formed from strips or rolls of material impregnated with the casting material. The normal curiosity of children as they watch a cast grow and mold to their body part makes casting a pleasant procedure. Some children look forward to having a cast applied. It may be a badge of courage or a conversation piece.

Before the cast is applied, a tube of stockinette is stretched over the area, and a soft cotton sheet is placed over bony prominences. This stockinette is pulled up and over the raw edges of the cast as it is applied to form a smooth, padded surface (Fig. 51-2). If a plaster cast is to be applied, caution children that, at first, the wet strips of plaster of Paris feel cool. Almost immediately, the strips begin to generate heat as evaporation begins, and body parts feel warm. If the cast is a full-body cast, children may become uncomfortably warm with perspiration possibly running from their forehead. Assure them that this feeling of warmth is transient and is never enough to cause a burn.

A plaster cast takes from 10 to 72 h to dry depending on its size. Fiberglass casts usually dry within 5 to 30 min.

A window may be placed in a cast if an infection is suspected. It also may be used with an open fracture to permit observation and care of the wound site. If the child has a body or hip spica cast, windowing may prevent uncomfortable abdominal distention.

NURSING DIAGNOSES AND RELATED INTERVENTIONS

Nursing Diagnosis: Risk for ineffective peripheral tissue perfusion related to pressure from cast

Outcome Identification: Child will exhibit signs and symptoms of adequate tissue perfusion during the time the cast is in place.

Outcome Evaluation: Child states she feels no pain or numbness in extremity; distal nail bed blanches and refills in less than 5 s; pedal pulses are palpable.

If an extremity has been casted, keep it elevated to prevent edema in the part. Check circulation frequently, such as every 15 min during the first hour, hourly for the first 24 h, and then every 4 h thereafter. Assess for color, warmth, presence of pedal pulses, and sensations of numbness or tingling. Signs of impaired neurovascular function include pallor (including blueness or coldness of a distal part), pulselessness, pain in the casted part, or paresthesia, such as numbness or tingling in the part as if it were "asleep," and paralysis. Keep in mind that children younger than 6 or 7 years have difficulty describing paresthesia; however, they may whine or cry with the discomfort of the sensation. Edema that does not improve with elevation is also an important sign. Any of these symptoms requires immediate attention, because neurovascular impairment can lead to nerve ischemia and destruction, possibly causing permanent paralysis of an extremity.

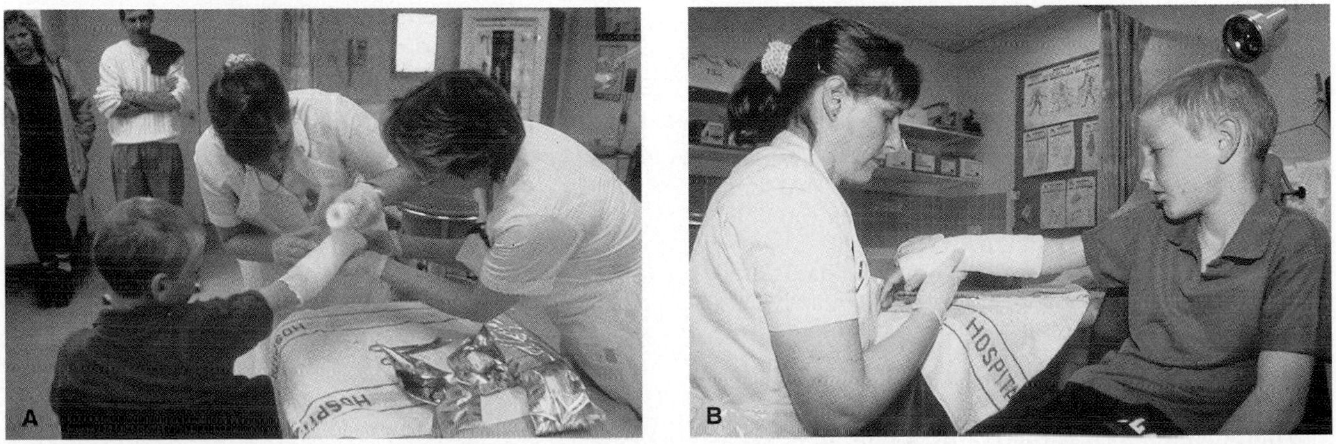

FIGURE 51.2 Cast application. (*A*) A fiberglass cast is applied to a young boy's arm over a stockinette already in place. (*B*) While applying the finishing touches to the young boy's cast, a nurse assesses the extremity.

Nursing Diagnosis: Risk for impaired tissue integrity related to pressure from cast

Outcome Identification: Child's skin will remain intact during time cast is in place.

Outcome Evaluation: Child reports no pain under cast; cast remains dry and free of stains; skin surrounding cast edges is clean, dry, and free of erythema or irritation.

If a cast surrounds the genital area of a non–toilet-trained child, cover the edges of the cast surrounding the genital area with plastic or waterproof material. Keeping urine from flowing under the edges of a cast can be a problem with full body or high leg casts. Keeping children in a semi-Fowler's position by using pillows or raising the head of the bed helps to direct urine and feces downward and can help prevent this. Because a cast is heavy, an infant tends to slip down a great deal, so he or she needs frequent repositioning to remain in the raised position.

Make certain that when children are being fed or are feeding themselves, they have a bib or a cover over the top edge of a cast so crumbs and fluid are not spilled inside. Toys should be chosen carefully for the same reason. A piece of food inside a cast will mold and macerate the skin; a small part of a toy dropped inside a cast can cause irritation and a pressure ulcer. If a child spills food on a cast or the cast becomes soiled, it can be cleaned with a damp cloth.

Nursing Diagnosis: Parental health-seeking behaviors related to care of child with cast at home

Outcome Identification: Parents will demonstrate ability to care for child after cast application.

Outcome Evaluation: Parents state plans for adapting home environment and lifestyle to accommodate child with cast; parents demonstrate measures to check neurovascular status.

If the child has an upper extremity cast, be sure parents understand how to position the extremity properly, such as with a sling. If the cast is on a lower extremity, instruct the child and parents in the amount of weight bearing allowed to the affected extremity and in the use of crutches, if prescribed. Caution parents that fiberglass casts, because they are porous, should not be autographed.

Handling a child in a large cast is a major task for parents. For many, it may seem so overwhelming that they do not see how they will be able to care for the child at home. Assure them that the child is quite comfortable in the cast, despite its awkward, constricting appearance. Role model moving the child and positioning him or her to give them direction. Be sure to caution them that, if an abduction bar is used with a cast, it must never be used as a handle for lifting the cast. Such use can break the bar from the cast or weaken its support.

A body cast is heavy, so caution parents to use good body mechanics (lift with the thighs, not the back) when turning or positioning the child. If a cast is bulky, parents often appreciate suggestions on ways to help move the child from room to room, such as using a toy wagon with a flat board on top or using a skateboard for the child to propel himself forward. It is important to point out that all children thrive on being touched. Children in a large body cast need their head and arms stroked (or any areas of the body that are not covered by a cast). Demonstrate how even a child in a large hip spica cast can be held, cuddled, and supported for feeding. Otherwise, parents may neglect this aspect of care.

Many children report a sensation of itching inside a cast at about the end of the first week. If the area is immediately under the edge of the cast, the itching is probably the result of dry skin caused by the drying effect of the cast. Reaching a hand under the edge of the cast and massaging the area generally relieves the itching. Applying hand lotion may relieve the dryness. If the area is unreachable, blowing cool air through the cast with a fan, a hair dryer set on cool air, or a vacuum cleaner attachment may relieve the uncomfortable feeling. Caution the child and parents not to use implements such as a coat hanger or knitting needle to scratch the area. These can injure the skin, causing infection under a cast (see Focus on Family Empowerment).

Transporting the child in the car, particularly fitting a bulky cast into an infant car seat, can be a major problem. Before a child is discharged, give parents a telephone number to call if they have any questions about their child's care or condition.

Cast Removal

Most casts remain in place for 4 to 8 weeks and are then removed, using an electric cast cutter with a rapidly vibrating, circular disk (Fig. 51-3). The disk makes a very loud noise as it cuts through the cast material and also generates heat. To the child, the disk appears capable of cutting through not only the plaster but an arm or leg as well. The person removing the cast generally demonstrates that the disk does not cut skin by touching a thumb to the edge of it. Not all children are totally convinced by the demonstration, however, and may require additional support while the disk moves from one end of a cast to the other, such as saying, "It's all right to cry; I know this looks scary" or by holding your hands over the child's ears to lessen the noise.

The skin of the child's extremity looks macerated and dirty after the cast is removed; a good bath usually washes away most of this. If an arm has been casted in flexion, the elbow may feel stiff and even sore as the child is asked to extend it for the first time. Children often use extremities with caution after a cast has been removed. Therefore, advise parents to allow the child to begin using the extremity again at his or her own pace. As children naturally play and reach for objects, they gradually forget to favor the arm or leg, and full function then returns. Once healing has taken place, the extremity is as strong as it was before the fracture. The child does not need to continue to favor the extremity to protect it from a second fracture.

Crutches

Crutches are prescribed for children for one of three reasons: to keep weight off one or both legs, to support weakened legs, or to maintain balance. Usually, a physical

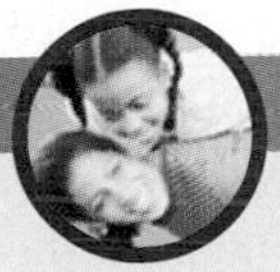

FOCUS ON FAMILY EMPOWERMENT
Cast Care at Home

Q. What should we do now that our child has a fiberglass cast on her arm?

A. Here are some helpful tips to care for your child's cast at home:

- Keep the casted body part elevated on a pillow for the first day to decrease swelling.
- Observe the hands and fingers (the body part distal to the cast) for swelling or blueness, and ask your child to move the part about every 4 h for the first 24 h. If he is unable to move the part or if swelling, blueness, or pain is present, telephone your health care provider (this could mean the cast is pressing on a nerve or constricting a blood vessel).
- Monitor strenuous activities, such as roughhousing, while the cast is in place; urge usual activities so your child remains active.
- Ask your child to think through how wearing a cast will change his day, such as making it difficult to eat in a cafeteria at school or carry books to classes, and brainstorm how to solve these problems.
- Be certain your child knows not to put anything inside the cast. If itching occurs inside the cast, blowing some cool air into it from a hair dryer can be comforting.
- Be sure that your child keeps the cast dry (cover with a plastic bag to shower); no swimming is allowed. Remind children that autographs are not allowed because fiberglass is a porous material.
- Be certain to keep your return appointment for follow-up care. Because children grow so rapidly, they can outgrow a cast rapidly. This could put pressure on nerves and lead to permanent disability.

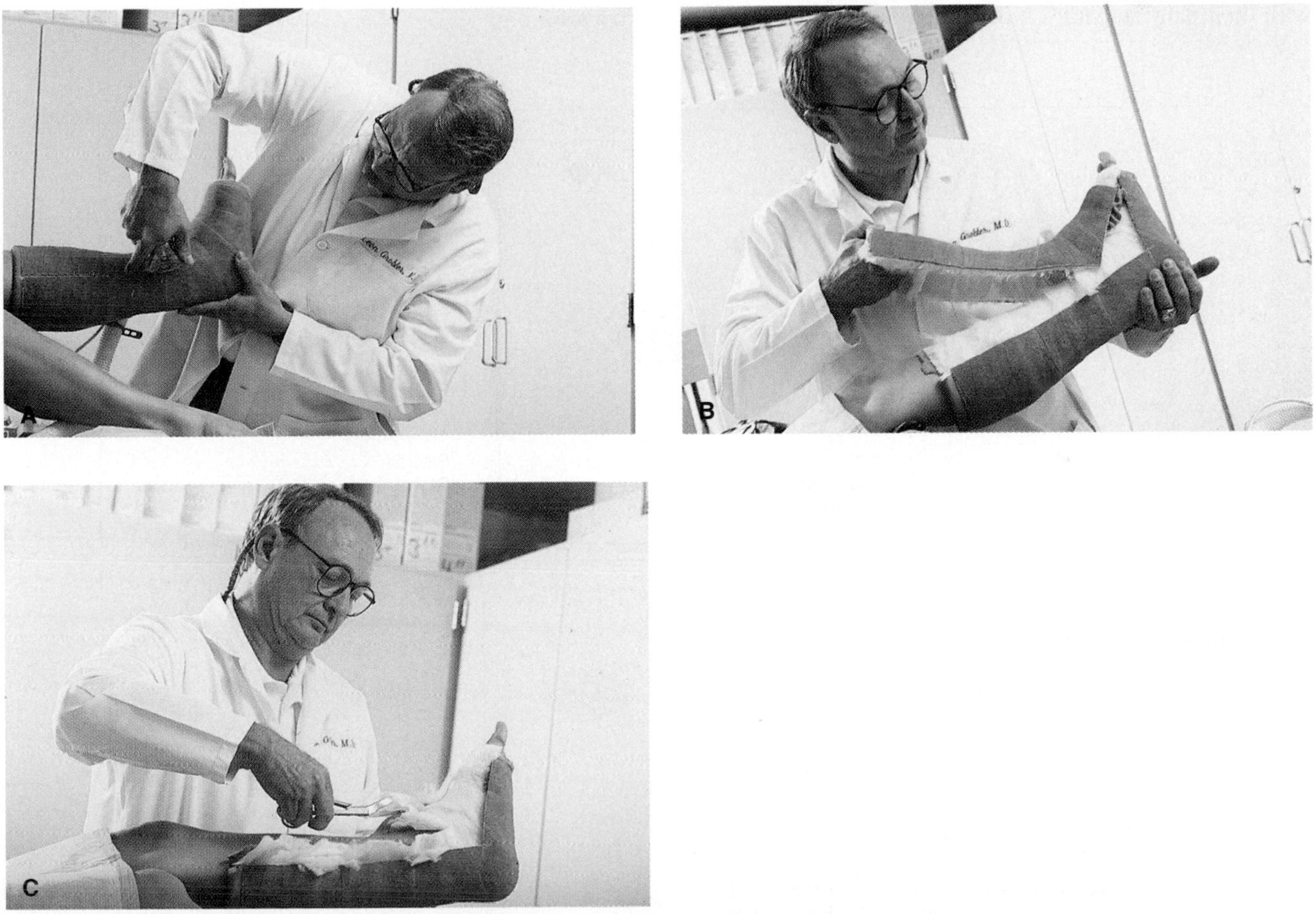

FIGURE 51.3 Cast removal. (*A*) A cast cutter is used to begin the removal of a fiberglass cast on an adolescent's leg. (*B*) The fiberglass cast is lifted off the leg. (*C*) Underlying stockinette and padding are removed.

therapist measures crutch length and gives beginning instruction in crutch walking. Be familiar with measuring and supervising crutch walking to offer emotional support to children as they learn and to assess progress at follow-up visits.

Fit and Adjustment

If crutches are properly fitted, there should be a space of 1 to 1½ inches between the axilla crutch pad and the child's axilla. When the child stands upright and places his hands on the handrests of the crutches, the elbows should flex about 20 degrees. This degree of flexion ensures that, when the child bears weight on the crutch, the body weight will be borne by the arm, not the axilla. Pressure of a crutch against the axilla could lead to compression and damage of the brachial nerve plexus crossing the axilla, resulting in permanent nerve palsy. Teach children not to rest with the crutch pad pressing on the axilla but always to support their weight at the hand grip.

Always assess the tips of crutches to see that the rubber tip is intact and not worn through. The tip prevents the crutch from slipping when it is in place. Be certain that the child is walking with the crutches placed about 6 inches to the side of foot. This distance furnishes a wide, balanced base for support.

Explore with children any problems crutches may cause with their daily activities. If they carry books to school, for example, they may prefer to wear a backpack until they are free of crutches so they can leave their hands free for the handrests. Caution parents to clear articles, such as throw rugs and small footstools, out of the paths at home. If there are small children at home, the parents will need to keep the traffic areas free of toys to prevent an accident.

Crutch Walking

Two main crutch-walking patterns are used (Fig. 51-4). A two-point gait is used when a child needs support for weakened muscles or balance but may bear weight on both lower extremities. The child places the right crutch and left foot forward, then left crutch and right foot forward, and so on. Using the crutch opposite a foot provides a wider base of support than using the crutch next to the foot. Caution children to take small steps until they feel confident.

A three-point swing-through gait is used when no weight bearing is allowed on one foot. For this, the crutches are both brought forward. The weight of the body is shifted forward as both legs are swung through the crutches. The child bears weight on the unaffected (good) leg and moves the crutches forward again. It takes strong arm support to bear full weight on crutches this way. Be certain the child is bearing weight on the hands and not the axillae when swinging through. Some children use a swing-through gait rather recklessly and need to be advised to slow their pace to a safer one.

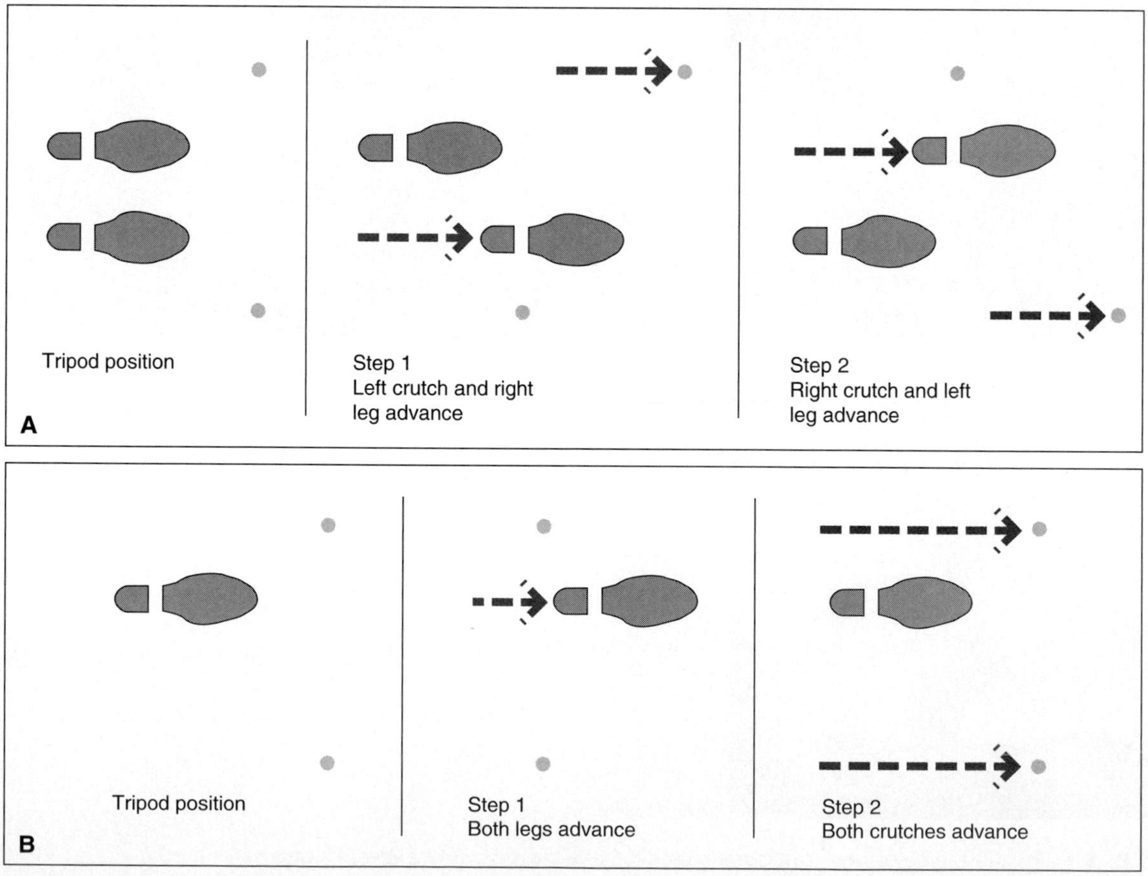

FIGURE 51.4 Crutch-walking patterns. (*A*) Two-point gait. (*B*) Swing-through gait.

To walk downstairs using a swing-through gait, children place the crutches on the lower step, then swing the unaffected (good) foot forward and down to that step. To go upstairs, they place their unaffected (good) foot on the elevated step, then raise the crutches onto the step and lift themselves up. To help children remember this pattern, a saying—"angels" (the good foot) go up; "devils" (the bad foot with the crutches) go down—is traditionally used.

A third type of crutch walking, the four-point gait, may be used. However, this method requires the ability to move both legs separately and bear weight on each leg.

Traction

Traction, used to reduce dislocations and immobilize fractures, involves pulling on a body part in one direction against a counterpull exerted in the opposite direction. Although still necessary for some conditions, its use is declining. In straight (running) traction, a child's body weight serves as the counterpull. In suspended or balanced traction, the body part is suspended by a sling, and the counterpull and primary pull are accomplished by pulleys and weights. Skin traction (in which skin provides the counterpull) or skeletal traction (in which bone provides the counterpull) may be used. Skin traction is used when only minimal traction is necessary; the child's skin must be in good condition for this procedure. Skeletal traction is used when a longer period of traction or greater strength of traction pull is needed. Types of traction are illustrated in Figure 51-5. Use of traction in the home allows the child to interact with family members and should be encouraged.

Skin Traction

Bryant's traction, used for fractured femurs in younger children (younger than 2 years), is an example of skin traction (Fig. 51-6). It also may be used in preparation

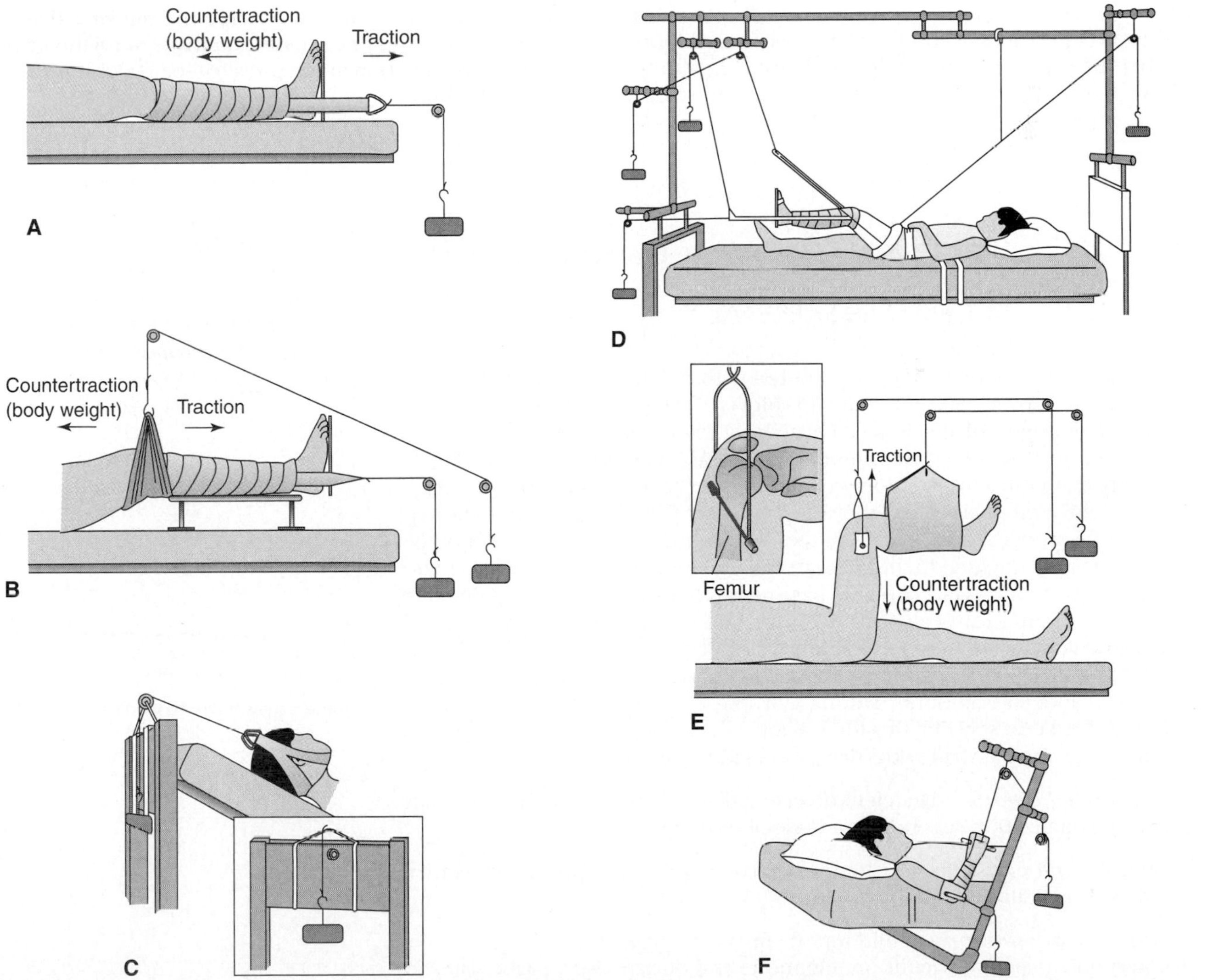

FIGURE 51.5 Types of skin traction: (*A*) Buck's extension, (*B*) Russell, (*C*) Cervical skin traction. Types of skeletal traction: (*D*) Balanced suspension, (*E*) 90-degree, (*F*) Dunlop's traction with pin insertion.

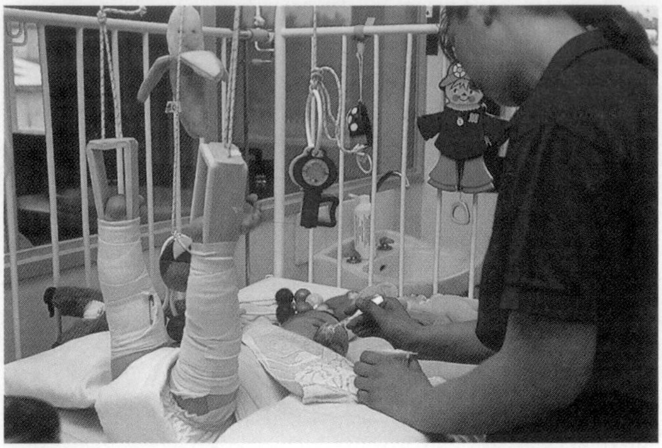

FIGURE 51.6 An infant in Bryant's traction. Here, the father feeds the infant while the infant is maintained in traction.

for surgical repair of congenital developmental defects, such as developmental hip dysplasia (see Chapter 39). This type of traction is being used less frequently because the elevation of the extremities causes blood to pool at the hips. This and the possible tourniquet effect of the traction strips, bandages, and traction itself increase the risk for possible vasospasm and avascular hip necrosis.

Buck's extension is an example of skin traction used for immobilizing lower extremity fractures in older children. Dunlop's traction is used to immobilize the upper extremity. This can be skin traction or skeletal traction if a wire or pin is used to immobilize. Cervical skin traction may be used to decrease muscle spasms in the back. This type of traction uses a halter-type device attached to weights. With this type of traction, the head of the bed is elevated to provide some countertraction.

Skeletal Traction

Skeletal traction involves the use of a pin, such as a Steinmann pin, or wire, such as a Kirschner wire, passed through the skin into the end of a long bone. The pin or wire can be inserted in an emergency department under local anesthesia if the child can hold absolutely still, but usually it is done under general anesthesia in the operating room. With skeletal traction, ropes strung over pulleys and attached to weights exert a pull on the extremity at the pin site. Cotton gauze squares usually are placed around the ends of the pin on the outside. Be sure to observe the pin sites daily for drainage. Odorous or excessive drainage or erythema may be a sign of infection at the pin site (see Focus on Nursing Care Planning).

FOCUS ON *Nursing Care Planning*

A CHILD IN SKELETAL TRACTION

A 10-year-old male with a fracture of the left femur was placed in skeletal traction 2 days ago. He is scheduled to remain hospitalized for the next week.

Assessment: 10-year-old male admitted with fracture of left femur after being struck by a car while riding his bicycle. Placed in balanced suspension traction with pin placed in distal portion of femur. Skin around pin insertion site slightly reddened. Small amount of serosanguinous drainage observed oozing from pin site. Traction weights attached and hanging freely. Left lower extremity pale, pink, and warm with pedal pulses present. Capillary refill of 3 seconds. Able to wiggle toes on command. States he does not feel numbness or tingling. Right lower extremity findings within normal limits. Vital signs within age-acceptable parameters. States he has some pain, rating it a 4 on a numerical scale of 1 to 10 (no pain to severe pain). Relieved with codeine and acetaminophen as ordered. Abdomen soft, nontender; bowel sounds active but slow. Bowel movement 2 days ago. Voiding clear yellow urine in adequate amounts. During morning assessment, child states, "I'm so bored. I have to stay like this for a whole week? I'll go stir crazy." Child enjoys playing baseball with friends and video games.

Nursing Diagnosis: Deficient diversional activity related to immobilization and hospitalization secondary to skeletal traction

Outcome Identification: Child will participate in age-appropriate activities during hospitalization.

Outcome Evaluation: Child reports fewer feelings of boredom; communicates with friends on telephone and during visits; participates in activities offered.

(continued)

Interventions	Rationale
1. Discuss typical interests, hobbies, and activities that the child likes and dislikes.	1. Ascertaining likes and dislikes provides a foundation on which to build future suggestions.
2. Work with the child to plan nursing care that allows time for rest and activities. Involve the child in care as appropriate.	2. Active participation lessens the feelings of boredom and passivity, enhancing the feelings of control, autonomy, and individualism.
3. Provide age-appropriate play items, such as video games, arts and craft supplies, and music, within easy access to the child. Use therapeutic play.	3. Play enhances a child's mental, emotional, and social well-being. Therapeutic play aids in ventilating feelings and anxiety.
4. Encourage the parents to bring in favorite items from home. Provide time for the child and parents to verbalize their feelings.	4. Items with personal meaning help to foster a sense of familiarity, promoting interest and stimulation. Verbalizing feelings aids in reducing frustration and anxiety.
5. Move the child to a room with another child of the same age, sex, and physical capabilities. Change the position of the child's bed in the room and transport the child in bed out of the room periodically.	5. Interaction between children with similar characteristics promotes socialization, fostering growth and development. Changing the bed's position or transporting the child in bed out of the room alters sensory stimuli and prevents monotony.
6. Encourage the child to telephone friends as appropriate. Urge the parents to have the child's friends visit.	6. Contact with peers is essential to maintain relationships and promote growth and development.

Nursing Diagnosis: Risk for peripheral neurovascular dysfunction related to the effects of the fracture and use of skeletal traction

Outcome Identification: Child will remain free of signs and symptoms of neurovascular compromise.

Outcome Evaluation: Child's extremities pink, warm, dry, with palpable pedal pulses and capillary refill of 3 s or less bilaterally. Child denies any numbness or tingling in extremity.

Interventions	Rationale
1. Assess neurovascular status of left lower extremity, including temperature, color, pedal pulse, edema, and capillary refill at least every 4 h or more often as indicated. Compare findings with unaffected extremity.	1. Changes in neurovascular function often begin with minor changes. Frequent assessment allows for early detection and prompt intervention should any problems occur. Comparing the affected with the unaffected extremity provides a basis for evaluation.
2. Monitor the child's ability to move his toes and detect sensation in the left lower extremity.	2. Ability to move toes and detect sensations indicate intact motor and sensory function.
3. Maintain traction with left leg in proper alignment.	3. Proper positioning with intact traction promotes adequate bone healing and circulation.
4. Instruct the child to report any numbness, tingling, increased pain, or feelings of coldness.	4. Symptoms such as these indicate decreased blood supply to nerve or muscle tissue.

Nursing Diagnosis: Risk for infection related to open wound at pin insertion site

Outcome Identification: Child will remain free of signs and symptoms of infection.

Outcome Evaluation: Pin site is clean and dry without purulent drainage. Temperature is within age-appropriate parameters.

(continued)

Interventions	Rationale
1. Assess vital signs, especially temperature, every 4 h or more often as indicated.	1. Vital signs, especially temperature, are reliable indicators of infection.
2. Inspect pin insertion site at least every 8 h for signs of redness, swelling, irritation, or drainage. Obtain culture of pin site as ordered.	2. The skin provides the first line of defense against infection; insertion of pin disrupts this defense, providing an entrance for microorganisms. Frequent monitoring of the pin insertion site allows for early detection of problems and prompt intervention should any signs be noted.
3. Perform pin site care according to the institution's policy. Adhere to standard precautions and use aseptic technique.	3. Pin site care helps keep the area clean, minimizing the risk for infection. Standard precautions and aseptic technique minimize the risk for infection transmission.
4. Provide a well-balanced diet with adequate protein and calories. Limit calcium intake as ordered.	4. Adequate nutrition is essential for overall body function. Calories and protein are needed for tissue repair. Calcium intake is necessary for bone healing. Too much calcium, however, increases the risk for renal calculi development from immobility.
5. Anticipate antibiotic administration based on culture reports.	5. Antibiotic therapy specific to the organism involved is necessary to treat the infection, should one occur.

Nursing Diagnosis: Risk for disuse syndrome related to prolonged bedrest and immobilization secondary to skeletal traction

Outcome Identification: Child remains free of any signs and symptoms of complications of immobility.

Outcome Evaluation: Child's skin integrity remains intact; lungs clear to auscultation. Child voids in adequate amounts; has a bowel movement at least every other day; maintains range of motion of unaffected extremities; exhibits signs of adequate peripheral blood flow.

Interventions	Rationale
1. Assess skin surfaces at least every 8 h for signs of redness, irritation, or pressure. Provide frequent skin care measures, padding bony prominences and using pressure-reducing devices as appropriate. Encourage frequent position changes within the limits of traction, and urge child to use over-bed trapeze bar to shift body weight.	1. Frequent position changes, skin care measures, and pressure-reducing devices reduce the risk for skin breakdown. Use of the over-bed trapeze allows the child to participate in care and activities.
2. Assess respiratory status at least every 4 h; auscultate lungs for abnormal breath sounds. Encourage coughing, deep breathing, and use of incentive spirometer at least every 2 h.	2. Immobilization leads to stasis of respiratory secretions, decreased chest expansion, and shallow respirations. Adventitious breath sounds are abnormal, indicating compromised respiratory function. Coughing, deep breathing, and incentive spirometry help to clear the airway, expand the lungs, and mobilize secretions for expectoration.
3. Assess urine elimination. Monitor intake and output. Encourage fluid intake of at least 2 L per day with limited calcium intake.	3. Immobilization leads to urinary stasis and increases the risk for urinary calculi (from bone demineralization). Increased fluid intake helps to promote urine excretion. Limiting calcium intake reduces the risk for renal calculi.

(continued)

Interventions	Rationale
4. Assess bowel sounds and elimination patterns. Institute a diet high in fiber and ensure adequate fluid intake. Allow child to use fracture pan in bed for elimination. Anticipate the need for a bowel program if no bowel movement in 3 days.	4. Immobilization leads to decreased peristalsis. High-fiber foods and adequate fluid intake promote peristalsis and enhance bowel elimination. A fracture pan may be helpful in allowing the child to assume the normal anatomic position for defecating without interfering with the traction. Additional assistance such as with a bowel program may be necessary for effective bowel elimination.
5. Have the child perform active range-of-motion exercises to unaffected extremities as appropriate. Encourage use of isometric exercises to the affected leg.	5. Exercise helps to maintain muscle strength and tone and prevent contractures.
6. Anticipate the need for antiembolism stockings or intermittent compression devices for the unaffected leg.	6. Immobility results in venous stasis. Antiembolism stockings or intermittent compression devices promote venous return.
7. Monitor vital signs and laboratory test results, such as serum calcium levels, coagulation studies, and white blood cell counts.	7. Vital signs are important indicators of overall body function. Immobility results in bone demineralization, which may lead to hypercalcemia. Increased serum calcium levels increase blood coagulability, which, when coupled with venous stasis, increases the child's risk for thrombosis. White blood cell count provides information about the possibility of infection.
8. Allow the child to participate in planning and to do as much as possible in all aspects of care. Vary the routine and physical environment whenever possible.	8. Participation in care activities promotes feelings of control and self-esteem. Varying the routine and environment reduces monotony of the situation and provides stimulation.

Traction-Related Care

Children in traction need to be assessed carefully for neurovascular impairment, as do children in casts. The extremity in traction should be checked every 15 min during the first hour, hourly for 24 h, and every 4 h thereafter for signs of pallor (or blueness), lack of warmth (coldness), tingling, absent peripheral pulse, edema, or pain. Traction can lead to hypertension because the head typically is positioned lower than the lower extremities. Assess once a day for this.

Be careful when changing the child's bed linens or carrying out nursing functions that you do not move the weights or interfere with the traction. Provide good skin care on the child's back, elbows, and heels, which may become irritated. A trapeze bar suspended over the bed provides a great deal of mobility and assists children in using a bedpan and positioning themselves in bed.

Being in traction is not as dramatic for children as being placed in a cast. There is an unspoken feeling from other children that "if what you have is really serious, you'd have a cast." Explain to children why this type of treatment is best for them. Keep them informed of x-ray reports, for example, "The fracture is being held in just the right position; the bone is beginning to re-form." Although they cannot see progress, they can be assured that it is happening.

Children need to maintain contact with their school friends through cards, letters, or tape-recorded messages. If hospitalized, their bed should be located so they can see unit activities. Whether at home or in the hospital, allow frequent visitors of their own age to help maintain peer relationships.

Children in traction are generally not "ill" children. They feel well except for the leg or arm being held in correct position. Therefore, they have the energy and need the stimulation of well children. Keeping them occupied and exposed to activities appropriate to their age group is a major part of nursing care (Fig. 51-7).

Distraction

Distraction involves the use of an external device to separate opposing bones, thus encouraging new bone growth. It can be used to lengthen the bone when one limb is shorter than the other. It also can be used to immobilize fractures or correct defects when the bone is rotated or angled.

A device such as the Ilizarov external fixator is used to achieve distraction (Fig. 51-8). It consists of wires that are inserted through the bone. The wires are attached to either full or half rings, which are secured to telescoping rods. If used for bone lengthening, each day the rods are adjusted approximately 1 mm to stimulate bone growth until the desired length is achieved. The device remains in place until consolidation is complete and there is no pain, limp, or edema. At this time, the bone is healed and can bear weight.

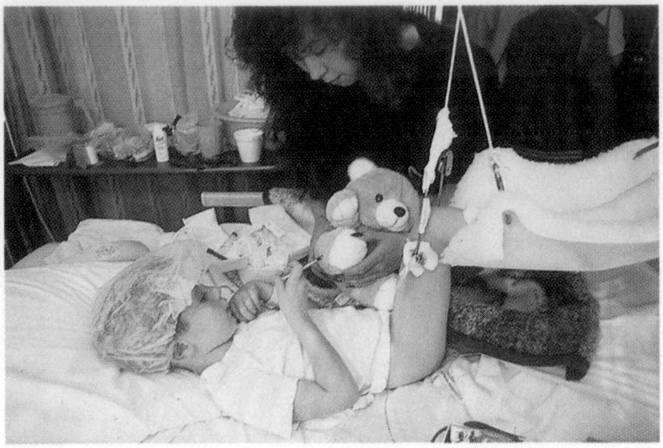

FIGURE 51.7 A child in skeletal traction engages in play.

The child and parents need thorough preparation for the surgery and application of the device. Because the device is external, large, and awkward, they need to be prepared for its appearance and the reactions of others to it. Provide suggestions for ways to minimize the device's appearance, such as wide-legged pants with adjustable closures. Parents also need instructions about adjusting the telescoping rods, if ordered; providing care to the wire insertion sites; assessing for signs and symptoms of infection; and instituting activity restrictions. Follow-up care is essential to ensure the optimal outcome for the child.

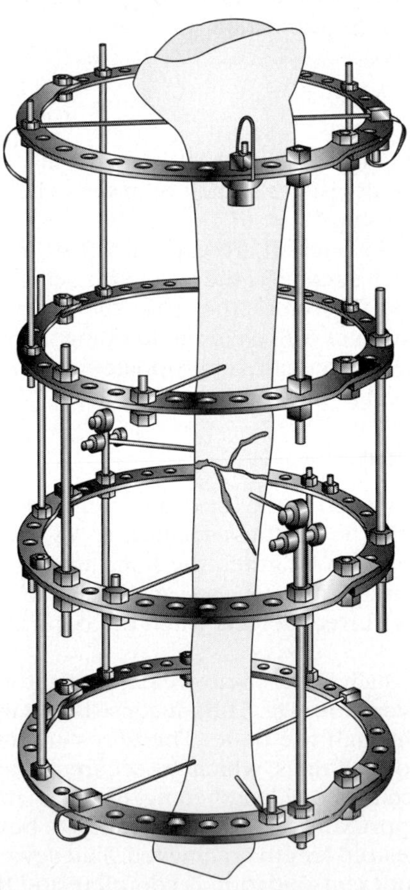

FIGURE 51.8 Ilizarov device in place to treat comminuted fracture.

Open Reduction

Open reduction is a surgical technique used to align and repair bone. If there is a spinal fracture or both bones of a forearm or lower leg are fractured, open reduction may be necessary to stabilize the bones. Internal fixation, such as the use of rods or screws, is rarely used with children except in those with scoliosis.

Once an open reduction is completed, the area is generally casted to provide support. Invariably, serosanguineous fluid oozes from an open-reduction site. Any stain on the cast that suggests oozing from a surgical incision should be outlined with a ballpoint pen so that an increase in the size of the mark can be noted. Do not use a magic marker for this, because the fluid tends to penetrate through the cast. Noting the time you make the pen mark on the cast allows you to tell how rapidly the spot is increasing in size. Children with an open-reduction incision are prone to incision infection as is any child after a surgical incision. Be aware of systemic symptoms (increased pulse, increased temperature, lethargy) and local signs (edema, pain, tingling, blueness or coolness of the distal extremity) of infection.

✔ CHECKPOINT QUESTIONS

3. Why might a window be used with a cast?
4. When using crutches, where should the child bear the weight?

DISORDERS OF BONE DEVELOPMENT

Flat Feet (Pes Planus)

The term *flat feet* refers to relaxation of the longitudinal arch of the foot. Many parents worry that their children have this problem. Only rarely, however, does this occur. Parents become concerned because, normally, a newborn's foot is flatter and proportionately wider than an adult's. A transverse arch rarely is visible. A longitudinal arch may not be present until a child has been walking for months. Parents notice that when their child walks in the sand or makes wet tracks on the bathroom floor, he or she makes an impression of a "flat foot."

Evaluate children's feet for this by having them stand on tiptoe. In this position, a longitudinal arch should be visible. If they can stand on their heels with the soles of the feet off the ground, the feet probably are normal. Examine the ankle joint to be certain a full range of motion is present to demonstrate that the Achilles' tendon is not shortened. Tarsal and metatarsal joints should normally show a full range of motion.

Some children experience foot pain at the end of the day. This probably occurs not from lack of a longitudinal arch, but from poor arch development. The arch can be strengthened and the pain usually can be eliminated if the child walks on tiptoe for 5 to 10 min daily or practices picking up marbles with the toes. For an older child, standing pigeon toed (toes pointed in) and throwing the weight forward onto the lateral aspect of the feet tends to strengthen arches.

Teach parents that children do not need a hightop or rigid shoe for foot development. If the child notices leg pain from poor arch support, a sports shoe is usually adequate to correct this (Eilert, 2001).

Bowlegs (Genu Varum)

Genu varum is the lateral bowing of the tibia. If present, the **malleoli** (rounded prominence on either side of the ankles) are touching and the medial surface of the knees is over 2 in (5 cm) apart (Fig. 51-9*A*). Children may develop this condition as part of normal development, but it is seen most commonly in 2-year-old children. Record the extent of the bowing at health maintenance visits by approximating the medial malleoli of the ankles and measuring the distance between the patellas (knees) for changes.

Genu varum gradually corrects itself by about 2 years of age and at the latest by school age. If the problem is unilateral, becoming rapidly worse or persists beyond this time, children need referral to an orthopedist for further evaluation (Do, 2000).

Blount's Disease (Tibia Vara)

Blount's disease is retardation of growth of the epiphyseal line on the medial side of the proximal tibia (inside of the knee), resulting in bowed legs. Unlike the normal developmental aspect of genu varum, however, Blount's disease is a serious disturbance in bone growth that requires treatment.

Because it is not possible to rule out Blount's disease by appearance alone, almost all children with bowed legs have an initial x-ray. With Blount's disease, the medial aspect of the proximal tibia will show a sharp, beaklike appearance on x-ray (Eilert, 2001).

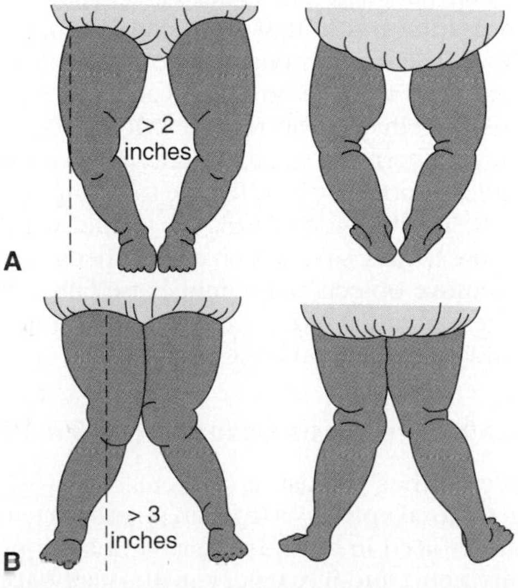

FIGURE 51.9 (*A*) Genu varum. (*B*) Genu valgum.

Bracing or osteotomy may be necessary to correct this deformity or prevent it from becoming more severe. Explain to the parents why their child requires treatment or surgery when another child on the block with a similar appearance (developmental genu varum) is expected to outgrow the problem.

Knock Knees (Genu Valgum)

Genu valgum or knock knee, appears as the opposite of genu varum. The medial surfaces of the knees touch, and the medial surfaces of the ankle malleoli are separated by more than 3 in (7.5 cm) (see Fig. 51-9*B*).

This is seen most commonly in children 3 to 4 years old. No treatment is necessary for genu valgum. The problem tends to correct itself as the child grows. By school age, few children continue to have the problem. Those children who do, or those in whom the abnormality is unilateral or becoming more pronounced, need a referral to an orthopedist for further evaluation. The severity of the deformity can be measured at regular health maintenance visits by approximating the medial aspects of the knees and measuring the distance between the medial malleoli of the ankles.

Toeing-In

Toeing-in (pigeon toe) in children may occur as a result of foot, tibial, femoral, or hip displacement. Assess for this when a parent describes a child as "always falling over her feet" or "awkward."

Metatarsus adductus is turning in of the forefoot. The heel is in good alignment; only the forefoot is turned in. This may develop or become more pronounced in infants who sleep prone with feet adducted or older children who watch television by kneeling, resting on their feet, and turning their feet in. If the child stood on a copying machine and made a print, the turning in of the foot would be well demonstrated.

Most instances of metatarsus adductus resolve without therapy. Those that persist beyond 1 year can be corrected by passive stretching exercises.

A few infants with extremely rigid, incorrect foot posture may require casts or splints for correction. Early detection is important. Treatment for metatarsus adductus is most effective if it is begun before an infant walks. With early treatment, the prognosis is excellent.

Inward tibial torsion also may be evidenced as toeing-in. This condition is diagnosed when a line drawn from the anterior superior iliac crest through the center of the patella intersects the fourth or fifth toe (or a position even more lateral; Fig. 51-10). Ordinarily, such a line should intersect the second toe.

Tibial torsion, a normal developmental finding, usually improves as the tibia grows and needs no treatment. Parents will need a good explanation of why no treatment is necessary. Reassure them at periodic health maintenance visits that patience and time will correct tibial torsion.

Inward femoral torsion can be detected if you have a child lie supine and attempt to rotate his or her leg internally and then externally at the hip. Normally, internal rotation is about 30 degrees, and outward rotation is

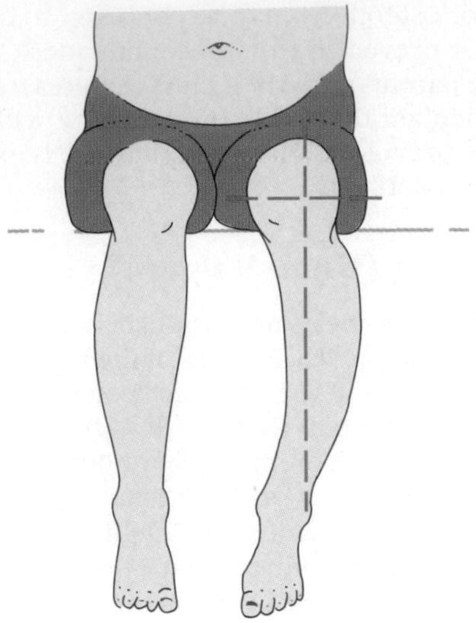

FIGURE 51.10 Toeing-in caused by inward tibial torsion. In good alignment, a line drawn from the anterosuperior iliac crest through the patella should intersect the second toe.

about 90 degrees. With inward femoral torsion, the degree of internal rotation is closer to 90 degrees. In some children, the femur rotates so far that the patellar bones face each other. As with tibial torsion, no treatment is necessary (Eilert, 2001). Inward femoral rotation will not correct itself, but a compensating tibial torsion will develop and make feet appear straight.

A fourth cause of toeing-in may be improper hip placement or developmental hip dysplasia, a problem that is very serious and needs early therapy for correction (see Chapter 39).

Limps

Observation of a child's gait is part of the health assessment at any health maintenance visit. Gait is a variable characteristic; however, limping is never normal. Although it may reflect a simple problem (a recently stubbed toe), it may also reflect serious bone or muscle involvement, such as with osteomyelitis or cerebral palsy.

History is important in determining the cause of the limp. When children have pain in the lower extremities, they protect their extremities by limping—stepping gingerly and quickly on an affected leg. Although children may seem to be favoring an ankle or a knee, ask them specifically what hurts. They may be favoring a hip. Because a hip hurts, they may be walking gingerly on the leg and causing pain in a knee.

The lower extremities need careful, thoughtful examination, including inspection, measurement of leg length, range of motion, palpation, and a neurologic examination. X-ray or bone scan may be necessary to rule out a pathologic process (Barkin, Barkin & Barkin, 2000).

Growing Pains

Listen to parents carefully when they state that their child has "growing pains." What they are reporting may be symptoms indicative of rheumatic fever or JA rather than a simple, transient phenomenon. Growing pains occur most frequently in the muscle of the calf, never in a joint. Children wake at night because of the pain. Such cramping generally is associated with a day of vigorous activity or wearing new shoes with a heel of a different height than before. Children with genu varum (bowlegs) tend to have more of such pain than other children do. Growing pains should be evaluated seriously at health maintenance visits to detect possible symptoms of disease.

WHAT IF? The parents of a child report that their child has been waking up at night because of pain in the calf. How would you evaluate this child further?

Osteogenesis Imperfecta

Osteogenesis imperfecta is a connective tissue disorder that, because of fragile bone formation, leads to recurring (pathologic) fractures (Dormans, 2000a). It occurs in two main forms: a severe autosomal dominant form that is recognized at birth (osteogenesis imperfecta type 1) and an autosomal recessive form that occurs later in life (osteogenesis imperfecta type 3).

Children with type 1 are born with countless fractures already present from the force of birth. They develop many more fractures during childhood. X-ray reveals a particular ribbonlike or mosaic pattern in bones, which aids in diagnosis. There is an unusual blueness of the sclera because of poor connective tissue formation. Children with the type 3 form may have associated deafness and dental deformities.

In both instances, the major clinical manifestation is a tendency to fracture easily due to poor collagen formation. In some children, their bones are so fragile, fracture results not only from trauma, such as a fall, but from simple walking.

As the child grows older, the multiple breaks tend to cause limb and spinal column deformities, interfering with alignment or growth. A number of therapies such as growth hormone to stimulate growth, calcitonin to aid bone healing, and bisphosphonates to increase bone mass may be prescribed, although no therapy is curative (Dormans, 2000a). Parents need to protect children from trauma; fractures need to be aligned and casted; and children need to be educated about a lifestyle that is productive yet minimizes the risk of trauma. Lightweight leg braces or intermedullary rods may be effective to strengthen bones.

Always be careful when caring for a child with this disorder. Be sure to raise side rails on cribs or beds. Keep floors dry, and remove objects that could cause falls. Always lift children gently and avoid lifting them by a single arm or leg to avoid placing strain on a bone.

Legg-Calvé-Perthes Disease (Coxa Plana)

Legg-Calvé-Perthes disease is avascular necrosis of the proximal femoral epiphysis from an unknown cause. This occurs more often in boys than girls and has a peak incidence between 4 and 8 years of age. It usually occurs unilaterally but may occur bilaterally (Dormans, 2000b).

The child notices pain in the hip joint accompanied by spasm and limited motion. X-ray studies are used to distinguish between Legg-Calvé-Perthes disease and simple synovitis (inflammation of the hip joint), which begins with the same symptoms. X-ray changes may not be apparent when a child is first seen but appear after about 3 weeks. For this reason, most children seen for synovitis of the hip joint are asked to return in 3 weeks for a repeat x-ray.

Children with Legg-Calvé-Perthes disease pass through four stages. First is the synovitis stage, or period of painful inflammation. Following this is a necrotic stage, during which bone in the femur head becomes smaller and shows increased density on x-ray. This stage lasts 6 to 12 months. A third stage is a fragmentation stage. Resorption of dead bone occurs over a 1- to 2-year period. The fourth stage, a reconstruction stage, marks final healing with deposition of new bone occurring.

Treatment for Legg-Calvé-Perthes disease focuses on pain reduction with nonsteroidal antiinflammatory drugs (NSAIDs) and on keeping the head of the femur within the acetabulum to act as a mold to preserve the shape of the femoral head and maintain range of motion.

Initially, rest is used to reduce inflammation and restore motion. To keep the head of the femur correctly positioned within the acetabulum, "containment" devices, such as abduction braces, casts, or leather harness slings, or weight-bearing devices, such as abduction ambulation braces or casts (after bedrest and traction), may be used.

A reconstructive surgery technique (an osteotomy to center the femur head in the acetabulum followed by cast application) also may be used. This technique returns the child to normal activity within 3 to 4 months.

Parents and children need thorough education about treatment and care because a majority of it occurs on an ambulatory basis. Be sure parents understand the need for a containment device. Without the apparatus, the femur head tends to remold in a mushroom shape, thereafter making the hip unstable. Because this shape does not conform well to the acetabulum, degenerative changes may occur later in life, leading to chronic pain, reduced mobility of the hip joint, and possible permanent disability.

It may be difficult for children to accept the extended treatment period involved with this disorder. Be certain that parents and children understand the long-term consequences. In addition, the parents may need assistance with devising appropriate activities for the child during treatment because of the device and limited weight bearing allowed.

Osgood-Schlatter Disease

Osgood-Schlatter disease is thickening and enlargement of the tibial tuberosity resulting from microtrauma. Children notice pain and swelling over the tibia tubercle. The pain is aggravated by running and squatting. This tends to occur in early adolescence or preadolescence in children who are athletic, probably because of rapid growth at these times.

Therapy depends on the extent of the bone changes. Limiting strenuous physical exercise may be all that is necessary. Occasionally, immobilization of a leg in a walking cast or immobilizer for about 6 weeks may be required.

Slipped Capital Femoral Epiphysis

Slipped epiphysis (coxa vera) is, as the name implies, a slipping of the femur head in relation to the neck of the femur at the epiphyseal line. The proximal femoral head displaces posteriorly and inferiorly. The cartilage covering the femur head may be destroyed by necrosis, resulting in permanent loss of motion of the femoral head. An avascular necrosis similar to Legg-Calvé-Perthes disease may occur. With both complications, surgical reconstruction of the hip joint will be necessary.

This disorder occurs most frequently in preadolescence. It is twice as frequent in African Americans as other races and twice as frequent in boys as in girls. It is more common in obese or rapidly growing children. This suggests that it occurs due to the influence of growth hormone and excessive weight bearing in the preadolescent child (von Scheven, 2000).

The onset of symptoms is gradual. On inspection, children often will be observed limping and holding their leg externally rotated to relieve stress and pain in the hip joint. They may report pain first in their knee, because favoring the hip joint puts abnormal stress on the knee. On physical examination, internal rotation of the hip is difficult and painful. X-ray will reveal the slipped epiphysis at the femoral head.

Early detection is important because correction is easiest if it is attempted before the condition has progressed to epiphyseal destruction. Surgery with pinning or external fixation, such as with skeletal traction, is used to stabilize the femur head. After surgery, the child may have activity restrictions or be confined to bed. Because it is most common in preadolescence, these children need continued support. Help them to understand the potential seriousness of the condition. Although they may not like being restricted or confined in this way, supportive communication and education can help them accept this as necessary to maintain good healing and function of the hip joint. Encourage frequent visits and telephone calls with friends to provide optimal growth and development.

Although this condition usually is unilateral, a number of affected children later develop the same condition in the opposite hip. All children with a slipped epiphysis, therefore, need follow-up care, with careful attention to the condition of the opposite hip.

✔ CHECKPOINT QUESTIONS

5. Are bowed legs common in 15-month-old children?
6. Should you prepare a child with Legg-Calvé-Perthes disease for a short or long period of therapy?

INFECTIOUS AND INFLAMMATORY DISORDERS OF THE BONES AND JOINTS

Osteomyelitis

Osteomyelitis is infection of the bone. It is most often caused by *Staphylococcus aureus* in older children and *Streptococcus pyogenes* in younger children. Children with sickle cell anemia have a special susceptibility to *Salmonella* invasion in long bones. The organism is carried to the bone site by septicemia (blood infection). It may follow extensive impetigo, burns, or something as simple as a furuncle (skin abscess). Osteomyelitis also may occur directly from outside invasion from a penetrating wound, open fracture, or contamination during surgery (Carek, Dickerson & Sack, 2001).

Osteomyelitis begins typically as a metaphysis infection because the blood supply is sluggish in that portion of the bone. An abscess forms, spreading along the shaft of the bone under the periosteum, possibly extending to and penetrating the bone marrow. Sinuses may form between the marrow and the periosteum or between the infected bone and the skin above. If the epiphyseal plate is infected, altered bone growth may result.

Assessment

Osteomyelitis generally begins with acute symptoms. Children show systemic malaise, fever, and irritability. They may have sharp pain at the bone metaphysis. By the second day, the area of skin over the infected bone will feel warm to the touch; edema will be present. Edema reduces the blood supply to vast expanses of bone, causing death of bone tissue. This dead bone tissue, which appears dense on x-ray, is called **sequestrum.**

Blood studies will reveal an increased white blood cell count, C-reactive protein, and sedimentation rate, and the blood culture generally is positive. X-ray may not reveal bone changes (formation of sequestrum) until 5 to 10 days after the beginning of the infection. Computed tomography may demonstrate early stage bone changes. Some children with osteomyelitis are not seen at health care facilities as soon as they should be, because parents account for the pain as "growing pain." Children with systemic symptoms, such as fever, malaise, and joint pain, must be evaluated carefully so developing osteomyelitis, if present, can be detected early.

Therapeutic Management

Medical therapy involves limitation of weight bearing on the affected part, bedrest, immobilization, and administration of an IV antibiotic such as oxacillin (Bactocil) as indicated by the blood culture. This therapy is usually initiated in the hospital and then continued at home for as long as 2 weeks, often using an intermittent infusion device or peripherally inserted central catheter. After this, the child will be prescribed an oral antibiotic for 3 to 4 more weeks.

If pus forms under the periosteum, it may be aspirated using a technique similar to bone marrow aspiration. After the procedure, a tube may be inserted into the area for instillation of an antibiotic solution. A drainage tube may be inserted and attached to suction to evacuate the subperiosteum area.

NURSING DIAGNOSES AND RELATED INTERVENTIONS

Nursing Diagnosis: Parental health-seeking behaviors related to care of the child with osteomyelitis

Outcome Identification: Parents will understand child's care needs within 24 h.

Outcome Evaluation: Parents accurately identify child's care needs to be met in the hospital and at home; parents demonstrate procedure for IV antibiotic administration.

When planning for the child with osteomyelitis, be certain that the long-term immobilization necessary for care will be considered. Parents may need to make major changes in their lifestyle for the child remaining in a hospital or to give care at home for an extended length of time.

Parents have many questions when osteomyelitis is diagnosed because the defect does not show on x-ray initially. They may be startled to hear their physician talking about the need for 6 weeks of antibiotic therapy. They may be suspicious, anxious, and afraid that hospitalization and administration of IV antibiotics are really unnecessary. At the point that the x-ray reveals the process, often they will become more supportive and understanding of the care given to their child.

Handle the extremity gently when giving care because the child has pain. Demonstrate to the parents how to do this. Provide instructions to the parents about good food sources of calcium and protein for bone healing. Keep in mind that young children are active, even if they are on bedrest. If the child had surgery and drainage tubes in place, institute infection-control precautions because the drain evacuates infected material.

When the child is discharged from the hospital, be sure to instruct the parents about the importance of follow-up antibiotic care at home even though the child's symptoms may have completely disappeared (Gomez et al., 2001). Review with them measures to care for the IV site and techniques for antibiotic administration. Also review the signs and symptoms of reinfection, measures for wound care and infection control, and possible adverse effects of antibiotic treatment. A referral for home care follow-up is important to ensure continued support and education.

If osteomyelitis is not entirely eradicated with the initial treatment, it will return and result in a chronic infectious process with open, draining sinuses and bone deformity in years to come. Growth plates can be destroyed, leading to shortening of an extremity (Chalom, 2000b).

Synovitis

Synovitis, an acute, nonpurulent inflammation of the synovial membrane of a joint, occurs most commonly in the hip joint in children. The peak age of incidence is between 2 and 10 years (Keenan, 2000). Children notice pain in their groin, the lower portion of the thigh or knee, or the buttocks. Pain is intense and most noticeable in the morning when they first awaken. Children may wake at night or in the morning, crying from the pain of turning over. Pain again becomes worse later in the day when children become tired.

Aside from the localized pain, children feel well except that they generally hold the joint flexed in a position of comfort. On physical examination, range-of-motion exercises will cause pain. An x-ray may reveal capsular swelling at the involved joint.

The treatment of synovitis is prescription of NSAID such as ibuprofen (Motrin) and limited activity until muscle spasm from pain has passed. In most children, 3 days of rest will reduce the synovitis. However, some children may need 10 to 14 days. A short course of oral corticosteroids may be necessary.

Synovitis must be differentiated from septic arthritis restricted to one joint. With septic arthritis, the child tends to be systemically ill, and blood studies will reveal an increased white blood cell count.

It is important that children and parents understand that synovitis is a simple inflammation process that will heal without sequelae. Rest is important for this recovery, however, and must be enforced.

Apophysitis

Adolescents who are growing rapidly are prone to apophysitis, or inflammation of the epiphysis of a heel bone. The heel feels tender, and pain on walking may be acute.

Pain generally can be relieved by adding a lift to the heel of the adolescent's shoe, reducing the tension on the heel cord. When pain has subsided, adolescents need to practice exercises to stretch the heel cord. This can be accomplished by having an adolescent stand on a slanting board, which elevates the foot and toes above the level of the heel, for 20 min about three times a day.

Apophysitis is an annoying condition, particularly for adolescents who feel a need to excel in sports to win peer approval. They need assurance that, although this annoying pain may persist for months, it is not a serious disorder. It helps to put the slant board by the telephone or somewhere where they will be reminded of it daily. Many adolescents believe that they are too busy and do not have the time for such an exercise three times a day unless they can combine it with another activity, such as talking on the telephone or watching television.

> ✔ **CHECKPOINT QUESTIONS**
>
> 7. What organism typically causes osteomyelitis in the older child?
> 8. Where does synovitis most commonly occur?

DISORDERS OF SKELETAL STRUCTURE

Scoliosis: Functional (Postural)

Scoliosis is a lateral (sideways) curvature of the spine. It may involve all or only a portion of the spinal column. It may be functional (a curve caused by a secondary problem) or structural (a primary deformity; Eilert, 2001).

Functional scoliosis occurs as a compensatory mechanism in children who have unequal leg lengths and sometimes in children with ocular refractive errors that cause them constantly to tilt their head sideways. The pelvic tilt caused by unequal leg length or the neck tilt results in a spinal deviation (necessary for the child to stand upright). The curve that occurs in functional scoliosis tends to be a C-shaped curve, in contrast to that in structural scoliosis, which tends to be S-shaped (composed of two separate curves). There is little change in the shape of vertebrae on x-ray with functional curves.

To rectify functional scoliosis, the difficulty causing the spinal curvature must be corrected. A lift inserted in one shoe will correct unequal leg length (leg length is measured from the anterior iliac spine to the bottom of the medial malleolus). Correcting ocular refractive errors will improve problems caused by head tilt. In addition, children must be reminded to maintain good posture during everyday activities. Walking with a book on the head for 10 min, three times a day, or hanging by the hands from a door frame (chinning themselves) stretches the back and is often helpful. Sit-ups and push-ups are good exercises. Swimming also is good exercise, because the reaching involved stretches the spine.

Parents and children need to be assured that functional scoliosis is a disorder that can be corrected. Children need to be aware of this to prevent problems with self-esteem and body image. Reinforce the need for good posture and exercise with the child and parents. Caution parents about nagging children of this age to do exercises or maintain good posture. Puberty is an age of rebellion and exertion of independence. Children may choose to ignore the parents' requests. Be open with them, helping them to understand the need for treatment. Let them know that you understand that children of their age believe they do not have to do everything their parents want them to do. Help them to find alternative, more positive ways to exert their independence.

Scoliosis: Structural

Structural scoliosis is idiopathic, permanent curvature of the spine accompanied by damage to the vertebrae. The spine assumes a primary lateral curvature. To allow children to hold their head level, a compensatory second curve develops, giving the spine an S-shaped appearance (Fig. 51-11). The primary curve is often a right thoracic convexity. As the original curve becomes severe, rotation and angulation of vertebrae occur. The thoracic rib cage will rotate to become very protuberant on the convex curve. Vertebral growth may halt because of extreme pressure changes (Killian, Mayberry & Wilkinson, 1999).

A family history of curvature of the spine is found in up to 30% of children with scoliosis, although no specific inheritance pattern has been documented. It is five times more common in girls than boys with a peak incidence age of 8 to 15 years. As long as children are growing, the spinal curves will become more severe. This is why the symptoms become most marked at prepuberty, a time of rapid growth (Killian et al., 1999).

Assessment

All children older than 10 years should be assessed for scoliosis at all health assessment visits.

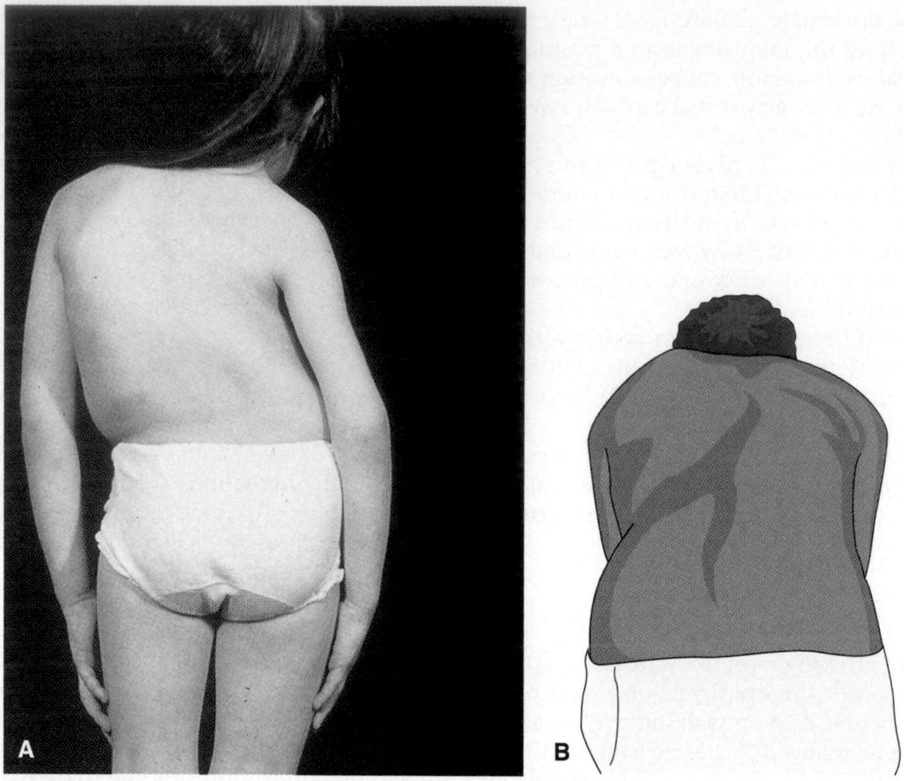

FIGURE 51.11 Assessing scoliosis. (*A*) Child with scoliosis (standing). (*B*) Child with scoliosis (bending over).

Often, the condition develops insidiously and may be very prominent before it is noticed, because of the preadolescent's and adolescent's need for privacy and the lack of pain. A parent might notice when doing laundry that the daughter's bra straps are adjusted to unequal lengths. The girl may find it difficult to buy jeans that fit correctly because of uneven iliac crests, or she may notice that her skirts or dresses hang unevenly. If the child bends forward, the curve becomes noticeable (see Nursing Procedure 33-2).

A scoliometer is a commercial device that can be used to document the extent of the spinal curve. With this device (a type of protractor), a reading over 7 degrees equals a 20-degree scoliotic curve detected by x-ray (Killian et al., 1999).

X-rays and photographs help to estimate the extent of the deformity and serve as a baseline description. Children's bone age is established by x-ray of the wrists or iliac bones. If children have a vertebral rotation causing rib imbalance, pulmonary function studies and a chest x-ray may be done to provide further baseline information. If bone growth is complete or nearly complete, little more deformity will result, so no correction may be necessary. On the other hand, if children have 1 to 2 years of bone growth remaining, some correction most likely will be undertaken.

Therapeutic Management

If the spinal curve is less than 20 degrees, no therapy is usually required except for close observation until the child reaches about 18 years of age (Eilert, 2001).

If the curve is greater than 20 degrees, treatment may be a conservative, nonsurgical approach using a body brace or traction, surgery, or a combination of both. Curves greater than 40 degrees require surgery with spinal fusion. Regardless of the type of treatment chosen, the child must be prepared for it to be long term. The goal of both surgery and mechanical bracing is to maintain spinal stability and prevent further progression of the deformity until bone growth is complete.

During prepuberty and adolescence, children are very concerned about body image and are very impatient with scoliosis correction, often wanting their problem corrected immediately. They need a great deal of support at health care visits to help them cope with the time needed for correction.

Bracing. If the spinal curve is greater than 20 degrees but less than 40 degrees and the child is still skeletally immature, bracing may be used. The Milwaukee brace was the first type used for this purpose. Although today's braces look much different, they may still be referred to by this name. Where originally braces extended to the neck, today, they are underarm thoracolumbar supports that are worn under clothing (Fig. 51-12). The brace is worn for 23 out of the 24 h of the day but can be removed so the child can participate in a school athletic program. At night, children may wear a Charleston Bending Brace that confines the spine to an overcorrected position.

Children and parents need thorough instructions on how to apply these braces. Frequent follow-up health care visits are necessary to check the fit of the device, making sure that

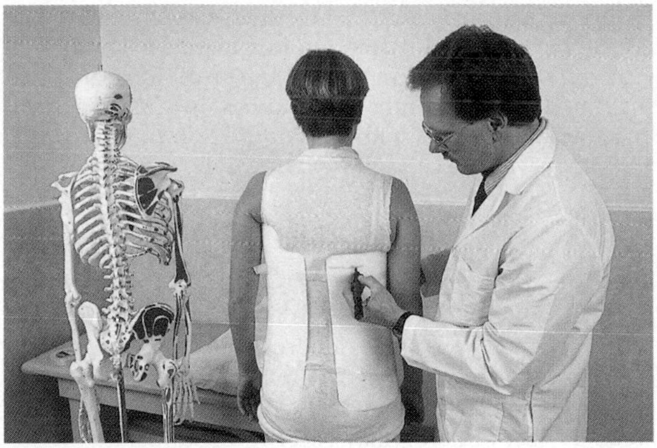

FIGURE 51.12 A teenage girl is fitted with a thoracic-lumbar-sacral orthotic device for treatment of scoliosis.

it fits snugly without rubbing on bony prominences, such as the iliac crests. Caution children and parents to notify the health care provider if rubbing occurs. Also caution them not to loosen straps to decrease the discomfort. This makes the brace fit loosely, and it will not exert adequate compression and traction this way.

During the first couple of weeks of wearing a brace, children may notice slight muscle aches resulting from the new alignment. If neck and pelvic traction were applied beforehand, this aching may be minimized. A mild analgesic such as acetaminophen (Tylenol) will decrease the discomfort in most children. Rest also provides considerable relief. Caution children not to remove the brace during this time because taking it off will compound the problem of discomfort by prolonging the period of adjustment.

Braces should be worn over a tee shirt to prevent the plastic pads from touching skin surfaces and causing skin excoriation. Children should remove the brace to bathe or shower.

NURSING DIAGNOSES AND RELATED INTERVENTIONS

Nursing Diagnosis: Situational low self-esteem related to obviousness of the brace used for scoliosis correction

Outcome Identification: Child will demonstrate positive self-concept by 1 week.

Outcome Evaluation: Child states positive aspects of self; participates in activities; establishes friendships with peers.

It may be easier for children to accept bracing today than it once was because the braces are more compact and because teenage clothing tends to be more casual and looser. Although choosing clothes is easier than it once was, it may still be a major problem for some children. They need time at health care visits to voice concerns about their appearance. Encourage children to voice what it feels like to have to wear a brace of this size constantly. Help them to concentrate on things they can do, such as having a friend over or going to the movies, rather than those they cannot do because of the brace (see Focus on Communication).

Encourage children in scoliosis braces to remain as socially active as possible. They may comment at first that they feel awkward or "so much taller" that they are afraid they will fall. The only way to get comfortable with this feeling is to walk and get used to the new sensation of actually being a little taller. Braces may be awkward at school if chairs are attached to desks. Advocate for the child with the school nurse for seating arrangements that are comfortable.

Friends typically ask questions about what happened to a child. The sooner children expose them-

FOCUS ON COMMUNICATION

Stacey is a 13-year-old girl who was diagnosed with structural scoliosis after a routine screening at school. She is being fitted with a scoliosis brace.

Less Effective Communication

Stacey: Look at this thing; it's so ugly!
Nurse: It is awkward, but it's not too bad.
Stacey: You don't have to wear it. All my friends are going to laugh at me now!
Nurse: You need to wear this brace to help correct your spine.
Stacey: I know, but . . . I'm going to look like such a freak!
Nurse: You need to wear it. Otherwise, your spine will be deformed.
Stacey: I know. I know.

More Effective Communication

Stacey: Look at this thing; it's so ugly!
Nurse: It is awkward, but it's not too bad.
Stacey: You don't have to wear it. All my friends are going to laugh at me now!
Nurse: You need to wear this brace to help correct your spine.
Stacey: I know, but . . . I'm going to look like such a freak!
Nurse: You'll feel like a freak?
Stacey: Yeah, how can I go to school? What can I wear?
Nurse: There are ways to try and make this brace look less obvious.
Stacey: Really? How?
Nurse: Let's talk about this. Now, what do you usually like to wear to school?

In the first scenario, the nurse focuses on stressing the need for wearing the brace but fails to identify and acknowledge the adolescent's concerns about how she will look. In the second scenario, the nurse picks up on the adolescent's clues about body image and self-esteem and works with her to develop possible strategies to enhance these areas and promote compliance with wearing the brace.

selves wearing a brace to friends and family, the sooner these questions will cease. A brace may need adjustment about every 3 months to accomplish more alignment. Children may need more frequent visits than this, however, to be able to express the problems they are having with social and school adjustment. However, do not underestimate an adolescent's ability to adjust to new situations. Children can see by looking in a mirror that their spine is curved, and they want this corrected. Often, they will endure discomfort if they have hope that they will emerge at the end of the correction period without an obvious physical deformity (see Focus on Cultural Competence).

In some instances, parents must be firm about insisting that the child wear the brace continuously to experience the maximum benefits. If bracing does not work, children must have spinal alignment and fusion surgery. Be certain that children do not think spinal surgery is a simple, quick procedure, similar to an appendectomy, and, therefore, preferable to bracing. If children think this, they may avoid wearing the brace, hoping that surgery will then be prescribed. However, do not depict surgery as horrible. In some children, the scoliosis continues to worsen despite good bracing, and surgery will be necessary.

A scoliosis brace typically is worn until the child's spinal growth stops (about $14\frac{1}{2}$ years in girls, $16\frac{1}{2}$ years in boys), as demonstrated by spinal x-ray. Bracing is not discontinued abruptly, however. When this point is reached, children are weaned from it gradually because some demineralization of vertebrae may have occurred during the long period of bracing. Gradual resumption of activity allows remineralization and continued spinal support. They may continue to wear the brace at night for a prolonged period (6 months).

Halo Traction. Halo traction is the use of opposing forces to straighten and reduce spinal curves that are severe when first diagnosed or progress despite bracing (Sink et al., 2001). Halo traction is achieved using a ring of metal (a halo) held in place with about four stainless steel pins inserted into the skull bones. Countertraction is applied by pins inserted into the distal femurs or iliac crests (Fig. 51-13). A halo traction apparatus is bulky and looks frightening. Children have some real fear that, when the pins are inserted into their skull (done under general anesthesia), the pins will slip and penetrate their brain. They may worry that the apparatus will be so heavy that it will strain or break their neck.

Halo traction is generally used when children have respiratory involvement, cervical instability, a high thoracic deformity, or decreased vital capacity from severe spinal curvature and rotation. Children need to see photographs of the apparatus or talk to children who have the apparatus in place before having it applied. They need time to express their feelings about being placed in such a cumbersome device. Children may react to the apparatus physically, such as with nausea or diarrhea, or emotionally, such as with chronic sadness until they see that they can adjust to it. Orientation must be as thorough for the parents as it is for the child. Parents may show symptoms similar to those of the child for the first few days after the application of such traction. Generally, during the first week, they may feel unsure about how to care for the child. Therefore, they need support to parent during this time.

Careful explanations about the child's care before it is given will help reduce anxiety. Stressing positive aspects, such as what the child can do, and explaining that the traction will help the spinal curvature may encourage children to accept such extreme traction

For the first 24 h after applying the apparatus, children generally experience a nagging level of pain at the pin insertion sites. A generalized headache may occur, requiring analgesia. Accepting halo traction is difficult, even without this pain. Offer adequate analgesia for comfort.

Children in halo traction need frequent hair care to keep the pin sites clean. Crusting around the pin sites can be reduced by cleaning the pin insertion sites daily with half-strength hydrogen peroxide or another appropriate solution. Encourage children to be as self-sufficient as possible. Be certain that parents or children have a telephone number they can call for help or if they have questions once the child returns home.

FOCUS ON CULTURAL COMPETENCE

The way that parents or a child reacts to the diagnosis of a musculoskeletal disorder can be culturally influenced. In a culture in which beauty and looking similar to others are important values, being asked to wear a corrective brace would be very difficult to accept. Because an adolescent culture is often one that respects athletics, beauty, and conformity, adolescence may be a very difficult time for a child to maintain body image and self-esteem when a musculoskeletal disorder is present and requires the use of an obvious corrective device.

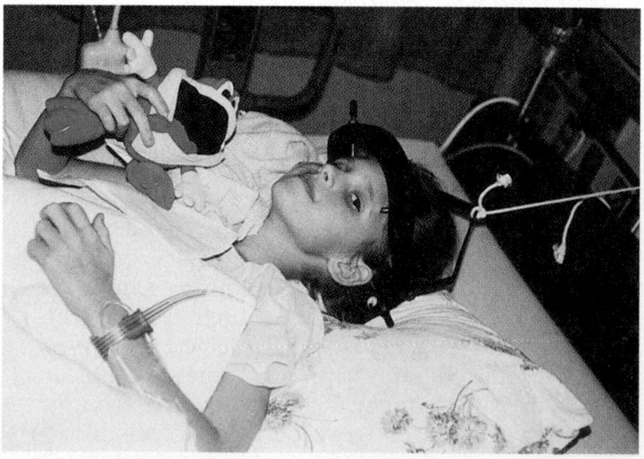

FIGURE 51.13 A 9-year-old girl in halo traction.

When optimal spinal correction has been achieved, halo traction equipment is removed easily. The pin sites in the skull heal within a week without obvious scarring.

Surgical Intervention: Spinal Instrumentation. Surgical correction is generally necessary when the degree of curvature is greater than 40 degrees. Instruments, such as rods, screws, and wires, are placed next to the spinal column to provide firm reduction of the curvature; the spine is then fused in the corrected position. Bone from the iliac crests may be used to strengthen the fusion procedure.

Preoperative Nursing Care. Before spinal instrumentation, extensive x-rays will be taken to plan the exact location of the rods. Introduce children to the postoperative deep-breathing exercises and incentive spirometry they will need to perform. Deep-breathing exercises are particularly important in children whose scoliosis has caused chronically reduced lung capacity.

Ensure that children have a good explanation of what they can expect after surgery. This surgery involves bone destruction and major muscle and tendon shifts, so they can expect to have pain. It is a major operation, so they can expect to feel tired and "not themselves" for a number of days. Teaching young adolescents about these events helps them adjust to the postoperative period, and they appreciate being treated like adults. Be aware, however, that early adolescents are not adults, and, although they seem eager to breathe deeply and cooperate with routines before surgery, these requests may be overwhelming for them postoperatively, and their behavior may not be nearly as adult as they anticipate. Epidural anesthesia offers a great deal of pain relief. Allowing children to use an IV or epidural patient-controlled analgesia system offers both pain relief and a feeling of control (Lamontagne et al., 2001).

The type of rods used depends on the degree of spinal curvature and the age of the child. Harrington rods were the first such rods manufactured, so the surgery is frequently referred to as Harrington rod placement, although newer types of rods are now more commonly used. Luque rods and Wisconsin segmental spinal instrumentation use a segmental approach. Cotrel-Dubousset rods also are commonly used. These are attached to the vertebrae using hooks or screws (Fig. 51-14*A*).

Postoperative Care. After surgery, the child's bed must not be gatched because, once rods are in place and the spinal fusion has been done, the back must not be bent. Tape the gatch of the bed in place or unplug electric controls so the bed cannot be raised by accident by a parent or by uninformed auxiliary personnel (see Focus on Multidisciplinary Care). A nasogastric tube generally is inserted before surgery to prevent abdominal distention; major surgery may cause paralytic ileus and lack of bowel tone.

Depending on the type of rods inserted, when the child returns from surgery, he or she may need to lie flat and be log-rolled (always by two people) to a side-lying position every 2 h to enhance respiratory status (see Fig. 51-14*B*). Perform neurovascular assessment of lower-extremity function every hour for the first 24 h. Assess the lower extremities for warmth. Ask the child if he or she can feel you touch a foot. Also, ask the child to wiggle his or her toes. Neurologic dysfunction may result from bleeding or compression caused by a bone particle dislodged during the spinal fusion. Assess and record vital signs carefully. Circulatory pressure changes resulting from realignment of the chest cage and reduced rotation of the spine may result in circulatory impairment. There is usually extensive blood loss during spinal fusion surgery. A drainage system, such as a Hemovac, may be inserted next to the incision to evacuate any accumulating drainage. The procedure itself or the blood loss may cause shock and hypotension.

The child will have nothing by mouth until bowel sounds return (usually 12 to 24 h). An indwelling urinary catheter is generally in place for 24 h because voiding may be difficult due to the horizontal position that must

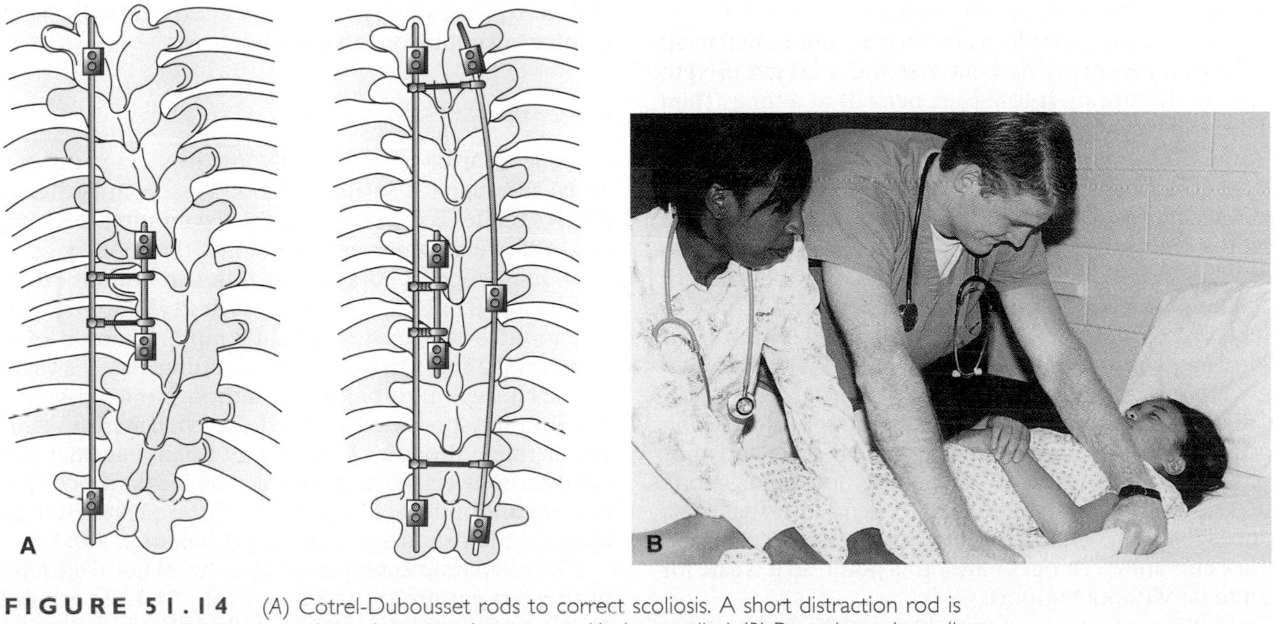

FIGURE 51.14 (*A*) Cotrel-Dubousset rods to correct scoliosis. A short distraction rod is linked to a longer one to correct the major curve. A convex rod is then applied. (*B*) Preparing to log roll. Two nurses use a drawsheet to roll the child in one coordinated movement to the side-lying position.

FOCUS ON MULTIDISCIPLINARY CARE

A number of health care personnel can be involved in a child's care when the child has a musculoskeletal disorder, including physical therapists, occupational therapists, orthopedists, x-ray technicians, and advanced practice rehabilitation nurses. After orthopedic surgery, health care professionals that form pain management teams also may be involved in care.

Unlicensed assistive personnel are often assigned to help with the application or removal of casts in emergency departments. Be certain they understand that cast application must be followed by instructions on cast care and ways the child can take active measures to accommodate the cast to his or her lifestyle.

Most children with orthopedic disorders do not feel so ill that they do not want to play. Therefore, they need activities provided for them to occupy their time. Urge all health care professionals to assess that the play activities children are choosing are not activities that could interfere with healing (eg, an activity that requires weight bearing when weight bearing is restricted).

---

be maintained and the edema at the lower spinal cord innervation points.

Although the parents have been prepared for the fact that spinal fusion is major surgery, they may be shocked by the child's appearance after surgery. This can cause them to be afraid to touch the child to provide comfort at a time when he or she would probably enjoy being touched because of feeling so ill and frightened.

As soon as bowel sounds are present, the child can take fluids and then solids. If the child needs to remain flat, there can be rapid release of calcium from bones. Calcium intake should, therefore, be moderate at first rather than extensive to prevent renal calculi.

After 2 to 4 days, children are allowed out of bed to sit up. They may feel very dizzy at first and must get used to sitting by attempting it for short periods at a time. Then activity is increased to a normal level with few restrictions.

Because removing rods is as extensive a procedure as inserting them, instrumentation rods are left in place permanently unless they cause irritation later. The average child becomes unaware that the rods are in place. However, they must always be conscious of good posture (not slumping in chairs; stooping, not bending, to pick up objects from the floor). Extremely active gymnastics or trampoline work is contraindicated. The rods do not interfere with other sports.

Children may be afraid to move freely after spinal fusion because, if they have had a brace applied beforehand, they have been in some type of restraining device for a long time. They may need to be reassured frequently that, with the spinal fusion, their problem finally is corrected. No further curvature can occur after this point, so it is safe for them to be without support.

Correction of scoliosis may have taken years. After surgery, children need an opportunity to talk at health care assessments about how they feel to be free of this problem. If the correction was not as complete as the child wished (children with severe scoliosis cannot expect 100% correction), they need time to talk about their disappointment and to adjust to their new appearance. They may believe their disorder has caused them to miss adolescence or "the best time of their lives." Emphasize positive experiences and point out positive attributes to help the adolescent gain self-esteem.

Osteoporosis

Osteoporosis is the loss of bone mass that leaves bones brittle and easily fractured. Stress on the weakened spinal vertebrae often result in a severe kyphosis. It tends to occur most often in postmenopausal white women as their estrogen levels decrease with aging (Marcus, 2001). Although osteoporosis is not apt to occur in adolescents, adolescence is the time when sufficient bone density is massed (Leonard & Zemel, 2002). Osteoporosis can be prevented by a program of weight-bearing physical exercise, a dietary calcium intake of 1,200 mg/day, and an adequate vitamin D intake (Weaver, 2000).

✔ CHECKPOINT QUESTIONS

9. What are the two types of scoliosis?
10. Does bracing for scoliosis always prevent the need for spinal surgery?

DISORDERS OF THE JOINTS AND TENDONS: COLLAGEN-VASCULAR DISEASE

Collagen is composed of bundles of protein-rich fibers and forms the connective tissue of the tendons, ligaments, and bones. Because this tissue is found throughout the body, collagen diseases are systemic. They also tend to be painful, involve inflammation, and are long term.

Juvenile Arthritis

Juvenile arthritis (JA) primarily involves the joints of the body, although it also affects blood vessels and other connective tissue. To be classified as JA, symptoms must begin before 16 years of age and last longer than 3 months. The peak incidence occurs at two times in childhood: 1 to 3 years and 8 to 12 years. It can occur in children as young as 6 months of age and is slightly more common in girls than boys. Acute changes rarely continue past 19 years.

The cause of JA is unknown, although it is probably an autoimmune process in which the child has developed circulating antibodies (immunoglobulins) against his or her own body cells. This is revealed by the presence of antinuclear antibodies (ANA). A genetic predisposition may increase the risk in some people (Chalom, 2000a).

Three separate subtypes of JA exist. Major distinctions of these types are outlined in Table 51-1. Types differ mainly by the type of joint affected and the severity of systemic effects.

TABLE 51.1 Comparing Different Types of Juvenile Arthritis

CHARACTERISTIC	POLYARTICULAR	PAUCIARTICULAR	SYSTEMIC ONSET
Number of joints involved	Five or more	Four or less	Any number
Joints affected	Usually small joints of fingers and hands	Usually large joints, such as knees, ankle, or elbow	Any joint
	Also possibly weight-bearing joints		
	Often same joint on both sides of body	Usually particular joint on one side of body	
Gender affected	More girls than boys	More girls than boys (most common type)	Boys and girls equally
Body temperature	Low-grade fever	Low-grade fever	High spiking fever lasting for weeks or months
Other symptoms	Stiffness and minimal joint swelling, leading to limited motion	Iridocyclitis (eye inflammation)	Macular rash on chest, thighs
	Rheumatoid nodules or bumps on elbow or other body area receiving pressure from chairs, shoes, or other object	Painless joint swelling with little redness (+)ANA titer (possible)	Inflammation of heart and lungs Anemia
	(+)Rheumatoid factor (in approximately 20% of cases)	(+)HLA antigen (possible in boys)	Enlarged lymph nodes, liver, and spleen
	(+)ANA titer (possible)		Rarely + rheumatoid factor and ANA titer
	Elevated white blood cell count, complement, and sedimentation rate		Elevated white blood cell count

Assessment

Children with systemic JA may be brought to a health care provider because of their persistent fever and rash. These may be manifested before joint involvement is present. When arthritis is diagnosed, parents may be surprised, believing that arthritis is a disease of older adults only. Regardless of the type of JA, assess children for signs and symptoms of the disease (Fig. 51-15) and for the effect their disease is having on self-care. (Do they need help eating, dressing, ambulating, or toileting?) An activity such as sitting on the toilet may be uncomfortable if hip and knee joints are painful. An elevated toilet seat may be helpful because it reduces bending. Children may be unable to dress themselves independently because they cannot manage buttons or zippers with painful finger joints. Modifying these activities by using hoop and loop or Velcro strips not only helps children feel good about themselves, but increases their overall level of activity.

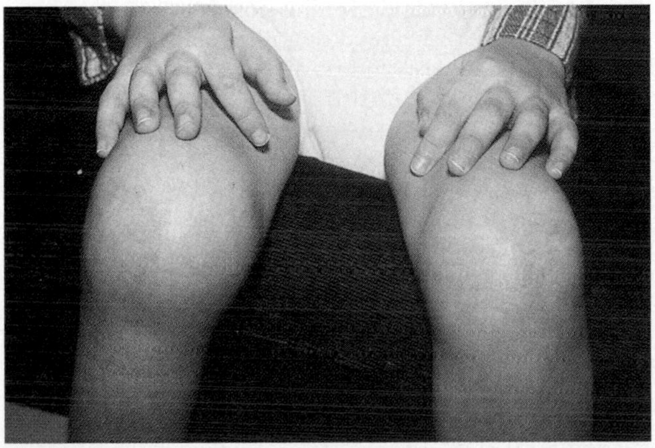

FIGURE 51.15 The knees of a child with juvenile arthritis. Note the degree of joint enlargement and swelling.

Also assess the child's and parents' understanding of the illness and planned therapy. Children and parents typically bear the major responsibility for carrying out therapy at home.

Children with pauciarticular arthritis need screening with a slit lamp examination every 6 months for uveitis (inflammation of the iris, ciliary body, and choroid membrane of the eye), because severe uveitis can lead to blindness (Hollister, 2001).

Therapeutic Management

Because JA is a long-term illness, therapy includes a balanced program of exercise, rest, and medication administration to relieve pain, restore function, and maintain joint mobility.

Exercise. To preserve muscle and joint function, children need a set program of daily range-of-motion exercises to strengthen muscles and put joints through their full range of motion. It is best if these exercises can be incorporated into a dance routine or a game, such as "Simon Says." This not only makes exercises enjoyable, but it also can make the exercise a family participation time to be anticipated rather than a dull routine that must be followed. Swimming and tricycle or bicycle riding are excellent activities because these provide smooth joint action. Also encourage children to do as much self-care as they can because the natural motions of activities such as dressing and brushing teeth exercise joints. In contrast, to reduce joint destruction, activities that place excessive strain on joints, such as running, jumping, prolonged walking, and kicking, should be avoided. School-age children can cooperate to avoid these activities. Parents of preschool children need to create interesting alternative activities so the child avoids these motions.

Children should attend school, if possible, because active children tend to show fewer contractures and less decalcification of bones than do inactive children. Children with JA fatigue easily, however, so may need a shortened school day. If a school day is to be shortened, it is often better if the starting time is moved to midmorning. This allows the child time for a warm bath in the morning before school, an activity that reduces the pain and increases movement of involved joints.

Heat Application. Heat reduces pain and inflammation in joints and increases comfort and motion. Heat can be applied by the use of warm water soaks for 20 to 30 min. Paraffin soaks can be useful for wrist and finger inflammation.

Splinting. Splinting once used extensively to immobilize inflamed joints in good body alignment are rarely prescribed today because NSAIDs are effective and efficient in reducing joint inflammation.

Nutrition. Children with JA, as with almost all chronic diseases, may eat poorly because of joint pain and fatigue. Some children experience mild gastric irritation from NSAID therapy. Help parents plan mealtimes for "best times" of the day to overcome these problems.

Medication. NSAIDs are the drugs of choice for children with JA. Those approved for use in children 12 years and older include tolmetin (Tolectin), naproxen (Naprosyn), and ibuprofen (Motrin). If these agents cause gastric upset, celecoxib (Celebrex) or rofecoxib (Vioxx) may be prescribed because these agents cause less stomach irritation (Hollister, 2001).

NSAIDs are taken one to four times a day. They not only control pain and inflammation, thereby reducing joint swelling, joint discomfort, and morning stiffness, but they may contribute to improvement in malaise and irritability. NSAIDs must be taken for at least 6 to 8 weeks to ensure effectiveness.

Educate parents that NSAIDs may cause gastrointestinal upset and bleeding. Therefore, advise parents always to give the medication with food. Most parents think of NSAIDs as a drug to give children only when they have pain. Teach that they should continue to give the drug even if the child has no noticeable pain at the time of administration. Its anti-inflammatory action is important in preventing pain.

Slow-acting anti-rheumatic drugs (SAARDs), also called disease-modifying antirheumatic drugs (DMARDS), are used when NSAIDs have been ineffective. In contrast to the immediate pain relief or anti-inflammatory effect, these drugs modify the natural progress of the disease over weeks to months. Examples include gold salts, penicillamine, and hydroxychloroquinine.

Cytotoxic drugs, such as cyclophosphamide, azathioprine, chlorambucil, and methotrexate, may be used in children who have severely debilitating disease that has not responded to NSAIDs or SAARDs. Steroids, such as prednisone, may be added to the drug therapy if the disease is severe or is an incapacitating systemic disease that has not responded to other anti-inflammatory agents. Although they are the most potent anti-inflammatory drugs, they are avoided if at all possible because of the numerous adverse effects. When they are prescribed, usually the lowest possible dose given for the shortest time is the rule.

WHAT IF? A child with juvenile arthritis states, "It seems like I've had this disease forever. Will it ever go away, or will I be a cripple the rest of my life?" How would you respond?

NURSING DIAGNOSES AND RELATED INTERVENTIONS

Nursing Diagnosis: Deficient knowledge related to care necessary to control disease symptoms

Outcome Identification: Parents and child will demonstrate increased knowledge of care regimen within 1 week.

Outcome Evaluation: Parents and child follow instructions regarding exercise and medication.

Help parents and children to understand the necessity for them to take an active role in therapy. Help them plan exercise and medication programs around school and other activities. Children with JA commonly experience irritability and fatigue, which may interfere with the plans. Assist them with planning a schedule that allows for a balance of rest periods with exercise to maximize the possibility of success.

Children with JA need ongoing follow-up care to evaluate the disease and how they view themselves. Assist them with measures that allow them to view themselves as well again after such a long period of pain and illness. The few children who are left with joint contractures may require soft-tissue surgery, such as contracture release, tendon reconstruction, and synovectomy, or orthopedic surgery, such as equalization of leg length and orthoplasty, at a later date. Surgery may be delayed until growth is complete so further growth will not influence the outcome.

About half of children with JA will recover without chronic joint involvement. The others will continue to have the disease into adulthood (Chalom, 2000a). Until the disease does reach remission, children need a great deal of support to perform exercises and take daily medication as prescribed.

✔ CHECKPOINT QUESTIONS

11. What are the drugs of choice for treating JA?
12. What is a common nonpharmacologic method to reduce pain with JA?

DISORDERS OF THE SKELETAL MUSCLES

Myasthenia Gravis

For nerve conduction to cause muscles to contract effectively, a neurotransmitter, acetylcholine, must be released at synaptic junctions. Myasthenia gravis is an interference in this process, leading to symptoms of progressive muscle weakness. The fault may be the impaired synthesis or storage of acetylcholine, insufficient acetylcholine release, blockage of acetylcholine factor present at motor end plates, or opposition of acetylcholine by an antiacetylcholine factor. The defect is probably a motor end plate insufficiency (a decreased number of acetylcholine receptors present). This probably occurs from an autoimmune process (autoantibodies may block receptor sites for acetylcholine; Porter, 2000). It occurs in three forms in childhood: neonatal transient myasthenia, congenital myasthenia, and juvenile myasthenia.

Assessment

With neonatal transient myasthenia, the mother has myasthenia gravis and the infant demonstrates transient disease symptoms at birth due to the transfer of antibodies from the mother. The newborn is "floppy," sucks poorly, and has weak respiratory effort. Ptosis (drooping eyelids) may be present. The symptoms disappear within 2 to 4 weeks, but, if not recognized when they occur, they could prove fatal because of respiratory muscle dysfunction.

Congenital myasthenia appears to be an inherited disorder that results in faulty acetylcholine transmission. Juvenile myasthenia gravis is an autoimmune process; it occurs most typically at 10 to 13 years of age and in more girls than in boys. Most children with this form have thymus hypertrophy that helps document the autoimmune process (Porter, 2000).

With all forms, children gradually begin to develop double vision (diplopia). Ptosis is present because of weakness of the extraocular muscles. Symptoms grow more intense as facial, neck, jaw, swallowing, and intercostal muscles become affected. Fatigue is extreme, becoming more noticeable as the day progresses. Symptoms increase with emotional stress, fatigue, menstruation, respiratory infections, and alcohol intake. In the most severe form, all muscles, including those of respiration, become unable to contract.

Obtaining an accurate history, especially documenting if children can perform repetitive movements, is important. To do this, ask a child to look upward and hold that position; with myasthenia gravis, the child will gradually demonstrate ptosis. Most children have myography performed to document the poor muscle function. Chest x-ray and computed tomography will demonstrate an enlarged thymus gland. Administration of edrophonium (Tensilon), which prolongs the action of acetylcholine and, therefore, increases muscle strength, renews exhausted muscles in a few minutes. If this occurs, the diagnosis is positive for myasthenia gravis.

Therapeutic Management

Myasthenia gravis is treated by the administration of neostigmine (Prostigmin) or pyridostigmine bromide (Mestinon), acetylcholinesterase inhibitors that prolong the action of acetylcholine (see Focus on Pharmacology). The dose of these agents must be individually determined. If toxicity occurs, it is similar to the symptoms of the origi-

FOCUS ON PHARMACOLOGY

Neostigmine (Prostigmin)

Action: Neostigmine is an antimyasthenic agent that increases the concentration of acetylcholine, prolonging and exaggerating its effects and facilitating neuromuscular transmission.

Pregnancy risk category: C

Dosage: Orally, 2 mg/kg daily in divided doses every 3 to 4 h or 0.01 to 0.04 mg/kg per dose intramuscularly, intravenously, or subcutaneously every 2 to 3 h as needed

Possible adverse effects: Salivation, dysphagia, nausea, vomiting, increased peristalsis, abdominal cramps, cardiac arrhythmias, increased respiratory secretions, urinary frequency, pupil constriction, and diaphoresis

Nursing Implications

- If ordered intravenously, administer the drug slowly directly into a vein or into the tubing's injection port of an intravenous infusion.
- Assess the child for increased muscle weakness, indicating possible cholinergic crisis. Keep atropine sulfate readily available as the antidote.
- If given orally, administer the drug with food or milk to minimize gastrointestinal upset. Instruct parents to administer the drug exactly as prescribed.
- Anticipate administering larger portions of the divided doses approximately one half hour before times of greater fatigue.
- Review possible adverse effects with parents and child. Advise parents to watch for signs of excessive salivation, emesis, or frequent urination and to notify the health care provider if any occur.
- Encourage parents to control the child's environmental temperature as much as possible to prevent diaphoresis from too hot or too humid an environment.
- Inform parents that an increase in muscle weakness may be related to drug overdose or exacerbation of the disease. Urge them to report any signs of increased weakness to the health care provider.

nal disease. Atropine, an anticholinergic agent and the antidote for an overdose of anticholinesterase drugs, should be available when the dosage is first being determined. In other children, prednisone may be added to their medication regimen to decrease the amount of anticholinesterase medication required. In some children, plasmapheresis to remove immune complexes from the bloodstream is effective in reducing symptoms. Excision of the thymus gland may also reduce symptoms, although removing the thymus gland may leave the child open to additional autoimmune disorders.

Teach parents and children that symptoms become worse under stress so parents will need to prepare children well for new experiences (menstruation, high school, a parental divorce, surgery) to minimize stress. Help children plan their day to include rest periods, possibly advocating for a special school schedule if necessary. If chewing and swallowing are difficult, ensure a rest period before meals. Children may need to eat a soft diet and learn to eat slowly and cautiously to avoid choking and aspiration. Scheduling medication administration for about an hour before mealtime is often helpful. If symptoms of muscle weakness suddenly become very severe, children should be seen at a health care facility, because paralysis of intercostal muscles may lead to respiratory arrest.

Dermatomyositis

Dermatomyositis occurs from degeneration of skeletal muscle fibers. The cause of the disorder is unknown. However, an autoimmune basis is suspected. It is more common in girls, occurring between the ages of 5 and 14 years (Hollister, 2001).

Symptoms generally begin insidiously with muscle weakness that prevents children from performing tasks that they could manage previously, such as competing in gym classes, lifting objects, or climbing onto a high stool. Muscle pain is infrequent. Skin symptoms are present (swollen upper eyelids, a confluent rash on the cheeks that increases to become telangiectatic and scaling). Subcutaneous calcifications may appear, making the skin feel unusually firm. Muscle breakdown leads to creatinine appearing in the urine. A muscle biopsy will reveal lack of electrical activity in muscle fibers.

High-dose corticosteroids or methotrexate is prescribed to improve muscle strength. Immune globulins may also be helpful. Children who survive beyond the first year after diagnosis have a good prognosis for prolonged remissions.

Muscular Dystrophies

Muscular dystrophies are a group of inherited disorders that lead to progressive degeneration of skeletal muscles, apparently from lack of a protein (merosin) necessary for muscle contraction.

Types

Muscular dystrophies are classified into three types: congenital myotonic dystrophy, facioscapulohumeral muscular dystrophy, and pseudohypertrophic muscular dystrophy (Duchenne's disease).

Congenital Myotonic Dystrophy. Congenital myotonic dystrophy is inherited as an autosomal dominant trait. As the disease process begins in utero, the newborn may already have severe myotonia (muscle weakness). Muscle degeneration continues until adequate respiratory muscle movement becomes difficult. Diagnosis is by serum enzyme analysis and muscle biopsy. Most of these infants die before they are 1 year old because they cannot sustain respiratory function.

Facioscapulohumeral Muscular Dystrophy. Facioscapulohumeral muscular dystrophy is inherited as a dominant trait, carried on the number 4 chromosome. Symptoms begin after the child is 10 years old. The predominant symptom is facial weakness. The child is unable to wrinkle his or her forehead and cannot whistle. Serum enzyme analysis and muscle biopsy are used in diagnosis. The symptoms generally progress so slowly that a normal lifespan is possible.

Pseudohypertrophic Muscular Dystrophy (Duchenne's Disease). Duchenne's disease, the most common form of muscular dystrophy, is inherited as a sex-linked recessive trait. Therefore, it occurs only in boys. Symptoms are usually apparent by 3 years of age.

Assessment

Children with Duchenne muscular dystrophy generally have a history of meeting motor milestones, such as sitting, walking, and standing, but they reach these milestones later than the average infant does. By about 3 years of age, symptoms become acute and obvious as they develop a waddling gait and have difficulty climbing stairs. They can rise from the floor only by rolling onto their stomachs, then pushing themselves to their knees. To stand, they press their hands against their ankles, knees, and thighs (they "walk up their front"); this is Gower's sign. They may walk on their toes, which leads to the development of a short heel cord. Speech and swallowing become difficult. It can be difficult to lift the young child with this condition by placing your hands under the axillae. The child seems to slip through your hands because of the lax shoulder muscles. In contrast, calf muscles are hypertrophied (measure larger than normal) because the muscles become so degenerated that they are replaced by fat and connective tissue (Thorarenson, 2000).

As the disease progresses, the muscle weakness becomes more pronounced. Scoliosis of the spine and fractures of long bones may occur from abnormal muscle tension and lack of muscle support. By junior high school age, most boys become wheelchair dependent. Tachycardia occurs as heart muscle weakens and enlarges. Pneumonia develops easily as the child's cough reflex becomes weak and ineffective. Death from heart failure may occur at about 20 years (Thorarenson, 2000).

The diagnosis is based on the history and physical findings, muscle biopsy showing fibrous degeneration and fatty deposits, electromyography showing a decrease in amplitude and duration of motor unit potentials, and an elevated level of serum creatine phosphokinase.

Therapeutic Management

Encourage boys with muscular dystrophy to remain ambulatory for as long as possible. Help the child and family plan a program of active and passive daily range-of-motion exercises. Splinting and bracing may be necessary to maintain lower extremity stability and avoid contractures. If children become overweight, remaining ambulatory becomes more difficult for them. Therefore, encourage a low-calorie, high-protein diet to avoid this. In addition, to prevent constipation, encourage a high-fiber and high-fluid diet. Advocate for a stool softener if necessary.

Because the disease is progressive, assist the child and family with achieving the optimal level of activity within the child's limitations. Provide support and education to assist them with coping. Help children and parents locate a parent support group. Organizations such as the Muscular Dystrophy Association (*www.mdausa.org*) can be helpful in supplying information about the disease and support through the long period of illness.

✔ CHECKPOINT QUESTIONS

13. What is the underlying pathophysiologic problem associated with myasthenia gravis?
14. What is the most common form of muscular dystrophy?

INJURIES OF THE EXTREMITIES

Finger Injuries

It is not uncommon for a child to sustain a finger injury from a slammed car door. This injury, which causes a crushing blow to the tip of the finger, is excruciatingly painful. The fingernail may be lacerated and detached. As blood accumulates under an attached fingernail, pain continues to increase. An incision under the distal end of the nail or a stab wound through the attached nail helps to relieve pain. Fingernails often are lost after these injuries, but they grow back readily with little scarring. Reassure parents that, although fingernails may be lost, the cosmetic effect will invariably not be a problem.

Parents may feel embarrassed and guilty when they bring in a child for this type of injury. The accident usually occurred because they closed a door without looking for the child's finger. They appreciate how much this hurts and are angry with themselves for being so careless. Reassure parents that this is a common childhood injury.

The fingertip will be x-rayed to make certain that the tip of the distal phalanx is not broken. The rule, "If the child can bend it, it's not broken," does not apply to this injury, because the fracture is often distal to the last phalangeal joint. Any open wound is cleaned well. If the distal phalanx is fractured, a splint should be applied to the finger. A follow-up visit is necessary to ensure that healing has occurred.

Bicycle-Spoke Injuries

Children who ride in child bicycle seats or over the back wheel of a bicycle can catch a foot or ankle between the spoke and the frame of the bicycle, resulting in a crushing, lacerating injury that quickly becomes edematous. Children can also injure their fingers in bicycle spokes. An x-ray is needed to rule out a fracture.

The wound, which usually is contaminated with spoke grease, needs cleaning with an antiseptic. It may be necessary to soak the area first with a solution of lidocaine, a local anesthetic, because of the amount of pain present. Sutures and a splint may be necessary. If it is a foot injury, the child may need to limit weight bearing by using crutches.

Soft-tissue injuries are painful. Edema and ecchymosis are extensive. Elevating the body part on pillows helps to reduce pain and edema. Such a major tissue injury may take up to 6 weeks to heal. Advise parents of this at the time of the injury. Otherwise, they may worry that the child's injury is not healing.

Fractures

A **fracture** is a break in the continuity or structure of bone. Because children experience falls during their growth years, fractures of long bones are common childhood injuries. Many fractures in early childhood are the greenstick variety (one side of a bone is broken; the other is only bent) because of the high resilience of immature bone. These fractures cause minimal pain, swelling, or deformity, the usual hallmarks of fracture. The various types of fractures are described in Table 51-2. Fractures in children tend to be different than in adults because of the following:

- Bone in childhood is fairly porous (allowing bone to bend rather than break).
- The periosteum is thick (causes greenstick fractures).
- Epiphyseal lines may cushion a blow so bone does not break.
- Healing is rapid as a result of overall increased bone growth.

Many fractures in children occur at the epiphyseal line. These are always serious fractures because bone growth occurs at this point. Damage to the area may lead to complications of bone growth (undergrowth, overgrowth, or uneven growth, resulting in angulation). If a child is involved in an accident that causes severe trauma, such as an automobile accident, compound (open) fractures may result. These are always serious injuries because the severed bone may lacerate nerves or blood vessels. The open wound may become infected, and correction will most likely involve a surgery with the risks of anesthesia.

If a fall is from a high distance or caused by a violent force, such as a speeding automobile, breaks may be complex or the formation may be compounded (the bone pierces the skin) or comminuted (the parts of the bone are fragmented).

Fractures heal relatively slowly compared with other body injuries. Immediately after a fracture, a hematoma forms at the site of the break; over the next several days, this is infiltrated by capillaries to lay down granulation tissue.

TABLE 51.2 Common Fractures in Children

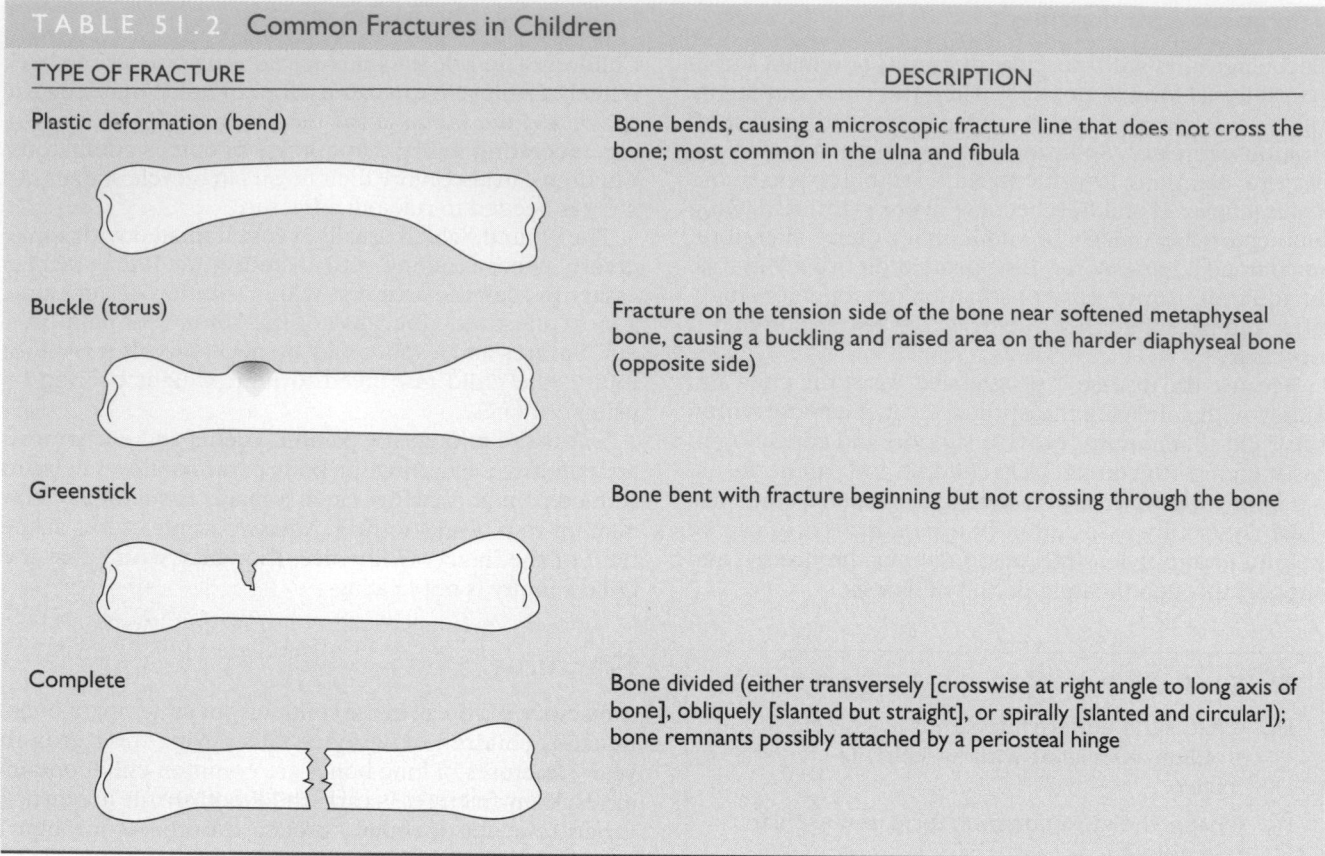

TYPE OF FRACTURE	DESCRIPTION
Plastic deformation (bend) 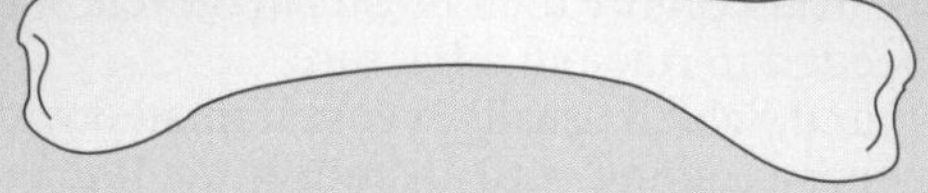	Bone bends, causing a microscopic fracture line that does not cross the bone; most common in the ulna and fibula
Buckle (torus) 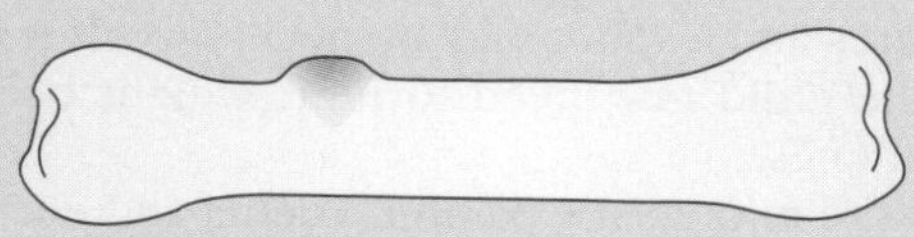	Fracture on the tension side of the bone near softened metaphyseal bone, causing a buckling and raised area on the harder diaphyseal bone (opposite side)
Greenstick 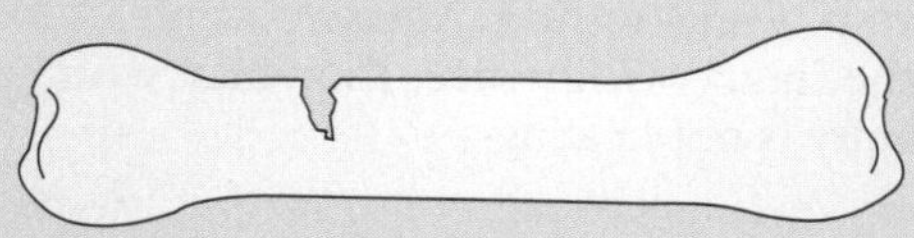	Bone bent with fracture beginning but not crossing through the bone
Complete 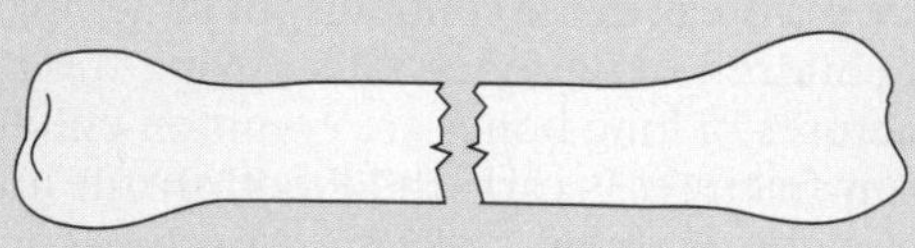	Bone divided (either transversely [crosswise at right angle to long axis of bone], obliquely [slanted but straight], or spirally [slanted and circular]); bone remnants possibly attached by a periosteal hinge

Over the next several weeks, osteoblasts invade the new tissue, and calcium is deposited (termed *callus*) to form new bone. When callus formation is extensive (enough for movement at the fracture site to be impossible), clinical healing or clinical union has occurred. Complete healing does not occur until all the temporary callus formation has been replaced by mature bone cells and the bone has once more regained its normal shape and contour.

A number of complications may occur after traumatic fractures. One is fat embolus or the release of fat from the broken bone into the bloodstream. This can travel to the brain and cause symptoms of confusion or hallucinations. It also could become a pulmonary embolus, producing dyspnea, tachycardia, and cyanosis. A second problem is compartment syndrome. This occurs when excessive swelling around the injury site causes increased pressure. The child notices severe pain that is aggravated by passive stretching. Color and warmth of the extremity may remain normal. Any constricting devices such as a cast need to be removed to reduce the pressure in the compartment. A long-term complication of fracture may be interference with growth if the growth plate was involved. Some children need bone lengthening or shortening procedures later in life.

Assessment

When children are seen in an emergency department for multiple trauma, the extremities should be observed closely for signs of fracture (deformity, edema, pain). If a fracture is suspected, splint the extremity to avoid further trauma. Splinting also reduces pain, because it prevents further movement of the bone. If the extremity is so seriously deformed by the break that it will not conform to the contour of a splint, do not attempt to move it into a splint position. Immobilize the extremity (eg, by placing sandbags on the sides of the arm or leg), and leave it in that position. Apply splints so they reach a joint above and a joint below the suspected fracture site. For example, for a fracture of the forearm, the splint should reach above the elbow and below the wrist. Immobilizing the joint below and above the injury prevents movement and muscle tension and, thus, further dislocation of the fracture. Take a thorough history of the accident. Some fractures in childhood occur from child abuse. This must be ruled out with all accidents.

Therapeutic Management

All children with a suspected fracture will need an x-ray to confirm the diagnosis and to determine the alignment and apposition of the fractured segments of bone. **Apposition** (the amount of end-to-end contact of the bone fragments) is not as important in children as in adults. Bayonet or side-to-side apposition may be established or left in children up to 10 to 12 years old, because, as the child grows and remodeling occurs, the bone will develop with normal contour and length. Side-to-side apposition results in a rapid, strong union and actually is the preferred position in some fractures.

If skin has been broken, children may need tetanus immunization. A hematocrit determination to estimate blood loss and cross-matching for replacement therapy may be necessary. An IV line is generally established to provide a route for fluid or blood replacement or for administration of an IV antibiotic to reduce the possibility of infection through the open wound.

All children with fractures are in some pain. Generally, they are frightened not only from the pain, the appearance of the fracture, and their inability to use the extremity, but also from the frightening situation that led to the fracture (a fall, an automobile accident). Spend time comforting and helping children to realize that they are now safe and will not be injured further. If they can relax enough to lie still and not move the fractured extremity, pain will decrease. When children have a compound fracture, they are as frightened at the sight of blood as they are of the deformity and pain. However, assure children and parents that, unless the bone has been crushed, the bone fragments can be brought back into line. After this, the bone will heal with the same strength as before.

Forearm Fractures

Because a child often falls on an outstretched arm, fractures of the forearm are common. In children, most fractures of the forearm involve the distal third; a smaller number of such accidents occur in the middle or proximal third. The injury may involve a fracture of the radius, a fracture of both the radius and ulna, or a displacement of the epiphyseal plate of the radius. In young children, the injury usually is a greenstick fracture. Sometimes greenstick fractures are broken completely before casting to prevent the bone's resuming its "bent" position within the cast. Refer to this as "straightening" the bone, rather than "breaking" the bone. If a greenstick fracture is slight so that the degree of angulation is not great, it may not be reduced or brought into a straight line. As callus is formed and the bone remodels itself, it will naturally straighten into good alignment.

If the fracture is complete and overriding is excessive, traction to the fingers may be used as a part of the cast. This "banjo" traction is cumbersome and limits the child's use of that hand. With almost all casts, the hand is covered up to the first phalangeal knuckle to prevent the child from moving the hand excessively and damaging the edge of the cast, which will loosen it and put the arm into poor alignment.

Volkmann's Ischemic Contracture

When an arm is flexed and put into a cast, the radial artery and nerve may be compressed at the elbow, causing nerve injury or severe impairment of circulation. If the fracture is in the proximal third of the radius, parents need to assess for signs of circulatory or nerve impairment for 24 h to ensure that the nerve injury or circulatory impairment does not develop.

If symptoms of compression are present but not detected within 6 h, Volkmann's contracture and possible permanent damage to the arm will result. The arm is left permanently flexed at the elbow. The wrist is hyperextended, and the fingers assume a flexed, clawlike, useless position. If a child is going to be discharged after application of a cast, inform parents about the symptoms of compression so that its development can be detected. If a child is admitted to the hospital for 24 h, the radial pulse (if palpable at the edge of the cast) should be taken hourly along with checks for coldness, blanching, and color for the first 8 h. In some instances, the cast will be applied incompletely for 24 h, the elbow portion just being splinted and wrapped with elastic bandages. After 24 h, when edema has subsided and the chance of compression is less, the rest of the arm is casted.

Elbow Fractures

If a child falls and stops the fall with a hand, the elbow may hyperextend, transmitting the force of the blow to the distal humerus and causing a supracondylar fracture of the humerus. The fracture of the humerus is reduced and stabilized with an arm cast, a splint, or traction, depending on the position of the fracture. Although the fracture may be minor, the child needs to be assessed for signs of Volkmann's contracture. Elevating the cast on pillows or suspending the hand by a strip of gauze or traction apparatus reduces edema.

Epiphyseal Separations of the Radius

When children break a fall with an outstretched arm, they may cause a separation of the epiphysis of the distal radius. When this occurs, the wrist must be casted to restabilize the epiphysis. Although epiphyseal injuries are always serious because injury to an epiphysis may cause growth disturbances, distal radial injury rarely causes serious sequelae in children. Advise parents that it is important to keep appointments for follow-up visits, however, so growth disturbances can be detected early and correction started. Stapling the epiphysis may be done to arrest abnormal growth if it occurs. Stimulation of the epiphyseal line may increase growth if growth retardation occurs.

Clavicle Fractures

When young children fall and catch themselves with an outstretched arm, the force of the blow may be transmitted to the clavicle, causing fracture of the clavicle rather than of the arm. Clavicles also may be fractured during birth.

Swelling is often present at the site of the break. The child refuses to use the arm, with the arm hanging at the side. Crepitus can be felt over the clavicle (Manko, 1999). In the newborn, Moro's reflex is demonstrated only on the unaffected side and the affected arm is immobilized against the chest. After x-ray diagnosis, an older child is placed in a commercially manufactured or figure-eight splint of stockinette placed over the shoulders and under the axilla, keeping the arm adducted and flexed across the chest. This is left in place for about 3 weeks. The child should keep it dry—no swimming or showering during this time. The parent often needs to tighten it every morning to keep it firmly in place. These stockinette wraps tend to get soiled in 3 weeks. Parents are usually apologetic about the appearance of the stockinette when they return for a repeat x-ray after 3 weeks; they are worried that the soiled appearance of the splint reflects the quality of their housekeeping or child care. Assure them that the soiled splint proves that they followed instructions well and left the splint in place for 3 weeks.

Parents may need reassurance that this splint is adequate therapy. They may ask, "The bone is broken, after all—why is my child not being placed in a cast?" Acknowledge their concern with a statement such as, "Most people think that when there is a broken bone, a cast is needed, but this is an exception." Doing so allows parents to voice their concern and receive further assurance.

Fracture of the Femur

Children who are involved in automobile accidents or who fall from considerable heights and land on their feet may suffer a fractured femur. Child abuse should be considered in an infant who sustains a fractured femur because there are few normal instances when this could occur in an infant.

Even if these fractures are closed so the skin is not broken, blood loss may be extensive because of the size of the bone broken. As the child lies on the examining table in the emergency department, the child holds the leg externally rotated; the thigh may appear abnormally short or deformed. Often, the child is in a great deal of pain, possibly with signs of shock from pain and blood loss. Children are always frightened from the force of the accident that caused such a severe injury.

Fractured femurs usually cannot be casted immediately because strong tendon spasm causes poor alignment and overriding of the femur segments. Therefore, alignment must be initiated first by traction.

For a child younger than 2 years old, Bryant's traction is used (see Figure 51-6). For the older child with a fractured femur, skeletal traction with a pin through the distal femur is used. When muscle spasm has been reduced enough to allow close approximation of the bone edges and callus formation is good (7 to 14 days), the child is removed from traction and placed in a hip spica cast. A young child will remain in a cast for an additional 3 to 4 weeks. In older children, healing of a fractured femur requires an extended time. In a child who is 12 years old, firm union of the bone fragments will take about 12 weeks. Help the child and family identify ways for the child to continue school work and contact with friends if he or she is unable to attend school because of the large cast during this time.

Dislocation of the Radial Head

If a small child is lifted by one hand, as happens when a parent pulls on one arm to lift the child over a curb or up a step, the head of the radius may escape the ligament surrounding it and become dislocated (nursemaid's elbow). The child holds the arm flexed at the elbow with the forearm pronated. The child winces with pain when the radial head is palpated.

A simple dislocation of the radial head can be reduced by a physician, using gentle pressure on the radial head while the arm is flexed and supinated. Relief of pain is immediate, and the child begins to use the arm again.

Assure parents that this is a common injury in small children. Parents feel guilty because they caused this dislocation. They rarely need to be cautioned that lifting a child in this manner is not wise. Be aware, however, that a dislocation of the radial head can occur from extremely rough handling as is seen in child abuse. Investigate the circumstances of the injury very closely.

Athletic Injuries

Although participating in athletics promotes growth and development, participation can lead to injury (see Focus on Evidence-Based Practice).

Knee Injuries

Participation in sports, such as football, skiing, soccer, or track, can cause knee injuries in children. These injuries generally involve the ligaments (the medial, lateral, posterior, or cruciate ligaments [figure-eight ligaments that stabilize the knee]) surrounding the knee. After the injury, the child has severe pain in the knee with localized edema. An x-ray will be taken to rule out fracture.

FOCUS ON EVIDENCE-BASED PRACTICE

Is Trampoline Exercise a Safe Activity for Children? Trampolines cause over 80,000 injuries (mainly fractures) in US children yearly. Thus the American Academy of Pediatrics has recommended that they should only be used in supervised training programs, never in the home, in routine physical education classes or at outdoor playgrounds (American Academy of Pediatrics [AAP], 1999).

To determine what type of injuries that playing on trampolines causes, researchers reviewed medical records of all trampoline injuries admitted to their hospital over a 7-year period (727 patients total). The results showed that patients were 53% female with a median age of 7 years. Privately owned trampolines accounted for 99% of injuries. Forty-five percent of patients had fracture injuries; spinal injuries occurred in 12%. The researchers concluded that the AAP recommendations on restricting trampoline use are justified.

This is an important study for nurses because nurses play a key role in educating parents and children about injury prevention. Nurses could integrate the findings from this study into a teaching program that addresses the types of activities that are the least likely and most likely to cause injury.

American Academy of Pediatrics Committee on Injury and Poison Prevention and Committee on Sports Medicine and Fitness. (1999). Trampolines at home, school, and recreational centers. *Pediatrics, 103*(5.1), 1053–1056; and Furnival, R. A., Street, K. A., & Schunk, J. E. (1999). Too many pediatric trampoline injuries. *Pediatrics, 103*(5), 257.

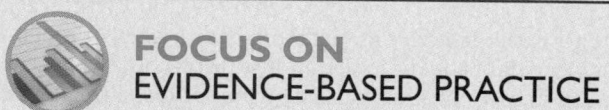

If the injury is mild (only a few torn fibers), bedrest with ice applied to the knee is often the only therapy needed. Local infiltration of an anesthetic may be necessary to minimize pain. After 24 h, heat is applied to the leg to hasten healing.

If the injury is more severe, the knee joint may fill with fluid. The child will need bedrest and ice applied to the joint. The abnormal synovial fluid will be aspirated, and a compression dressing will be applied to discourage accumulation of further fluid. After 24 h, heat treatments will be started to hasten healing.

If the injury is severe, a cast may be applied for complete immobilization. It takes as long for a severe ligament injury to heal as it does for a bone fracture, so the cast will remain in place for about 8 weeks. Arthroscopy may be done to visualize and surgically repair the knee ligaments. Arthroscopic surgery makes repair of ligaments or cartilage a minor procedure and limits the necessity for immobilization and a cast.

A severe twisting motion to the knee may cause a dislocation of the kneecap (it moves to the posterior surface of the knee). The knee appears deformed, and the child is in acute pain. Immediate treatment for a dislocated kneecap is to slide it again to the front of the knee. After this, the child will usually have to use a leg immobilizer for 1 week. If the problem is chronic or occurs frequently, surgery to strengthen the ligaments may be necessary. Quadriceps exercises (straight leg raising) are important to prevent the dislocation from occurring again (Johanson & Pellicci, 2000).

Throwing Injuries

Throwing places repeated stress on the upper extremity, particularly the elbow joint. The injury tends to occur during the forward motion of the arm or the follow-through. Children are unable to extend their elbow completely because of minute tears and fibrous contractures in the muscle. They notice pain and tenderness and loss of complete elbow extension for 24 to 48 h after the injury. Resting the arm and applying ice packs for 15 to 20 min three times a day relieves the pain. An anti-inflammatory agent may be helpful. A limited number of cortisone injections into the elbow musculature may be helpful. Exercises to strengthen flexor muscles help to prevent this type of injury.

"Little Leaguer's elbow" is epiphysitis of the medial epicondylar epiphysis (Williams & Wickiewicz, 2000). Throwing curve balls and breaking pitches increases the stress in this area because of the forceful flexion and pronation required. An x-ray of the elbow may reveal increased growth, separation, and fragmentation of the medial epicondylar epiphysis.

Children generally need extra protection against injury until the epiphyseal growth centers at the elbow have fused at 14 to 17 years of age. Children who participate in Little League sports need time for proper warm-up. They should be encouraged to refrain from throwing curve balls or breaking pitches and should be limited to pitching about six innings per week with a 3-day rest between games. Treatment for Little Leaguer's elbow is rest and immobilization until pain, tenderness, and limitation of movement have passed. If the injury is not treated adequately, permanent damage to the epiphyseal line and elbow deformity can occur.

Strains and Sprains

A strain is a muscle-tendon injury. A sprain is a ligament injury. Strained or sprained ankles are common but difficult childhood injuries. The joint is painful and swollen. They are typical injuries that occur with inline skating or snow- or skateboarding. When the x-ray reveals no fracture, the child may feel as though someone has said that the injury is not serious but "just a sprain." He or she finds the extent of the swelling and pain baffling. Some children may be accused by parents of "putting on" pain, because the injury is "only a sprain."

Help the child and parents to understand that strains and sprains are truly painful. Because a cast is not used and an ankle is not immobilized completely, strains and sprains are often more painful than fractures, which are casted.

If the injury is recent, an ice pack should be applied for approximately 20 min at a time to reduce edema at the site. An elastic bandage may be applied for firm support. The child may be given crutches to limit weight bearing for the next 3 or 4 days. Make certain that the parents of the child understand how the elastic bandage is applied so that it can be rewrapped if it loosens and that the child is using the crutches properly before being discharged from the emergency department.

✔ CHECKPOINT QUESTIONS

15. What is a "greenstick" fracture?
16. Why is casting an elbow a potentially dangerous type of cast application?

KEY POINTS

- Bone and muscle disorders tend to be long-term disorders. Help children and their families to think about how the disorder will affect tasks of daily living to help the child better adjust to interventions such as a cast or brace. Help children plan self-diversional activities as necessary so they continue to grow developmentally while confined to a cast or traction.
- As a rule, if a bone is broken, children need additional calcium in their diet to aid bone healing. If they are on strict bedrest, however, this should only be a moderate addition to their diet to prevent renal calculi from forming.
- Many children have casts applied to allow broken bones to heal. If broken bones are not easily aligned, children are placed in traction.
- Developmental disorders that occur in children include flat feet (pronation), genu varum

(bowlegs), and genu valgum (knock knees). The majority of these disorders are corrected naturally by normal growth.

Slipped epiphysis is slipping of the femur head in relation to the neck of the femur at the epiphyseal line. It occurs most frequently in obese or rapidly growing boys.

Osteomyelitis is infection of the bone. It can result in extensive destruction of the bone. Antibiotic therapy is necessary to combat the infection.

Scoliosis is a lateral curvature of the spine. It is treated by bracing or surgery.

Juvenile arthritis occurs in a number of different forms: polyarticular, pauciarticular, and systemic onset. Therapy is exercise, heat application, and administration of medications, such as NSAIDs, or methotrexate.

Myasthenia gravis can occur in three types: neonatal transient, congenital myasthenia, and juvenile myasthenia. Anticholinesterase drugs, such as neostigmine (Prostigmin), that prolong acetylcholine action are used.

Muscular dystrophies are a group of disorders that lead to progressive degeneration of skeletal muscles. Different types that can occur include congenital myotonic, facioscapulohumeral, and pseudohypertrophic. Children and parents need long-term support throughout this long-term illness.

A fracture or bruise of soft tissue could result from any trauma, including child abuse. Be certain to secure a detailed history of an injury to be certain that the history is consistent with the degree of injury.

Volkmann's ischemic contracture is a complication that occurs when an arm is casted in a bent position and a radial artery and nerve are compressed at the elbow. Frequent assessments of finger color and warmth are safeguards to prevent this from occurring.

CRITICAL THINKING EXERCISES

1. Jeffrey is the 10-year-old boy with osteomyelitis that you met at the beginning of the chapter. How would you explain what has happened to Jeffrey's mother? Develop a teaching plan to address this issue.
2. A 14-year-old girl is required to wear a brace 23 h a day for treatment of scoliosis. During the last month, she turned down an invitation to the high school prom and has dropped out of the high school band and the one after-school club to which she belonged. She tells you she is dropping activities to have more "time to study." Would you be concerned about her? What areas would you need to assess, and how would you intervene?
3. Your patient is a 3-year-old boy with JA. You notice when he returns for a follow-up visit to the arthritis clinic that the inflammation in his joints is worse than at his last visit. He has a great deal of pain. His mother tells you she has been giving him acetaminophen instead of his prescribed NSAID because she read that NSAIDs cause stomach irritation. Was she wise to substitute another medication this way? How would you suggest that she proceed at this point?
4. A parent has three athletically inclined boys in grade school. She is concerned with guiding them into sports that will be safe for them during their growing years. What suggestions and directions would you give her?
5. Examine the National Health Goals related to musculoskeletal disorders in children. Most government-sponsored money for nursing research is allotted based on these goals. What would be a possible research topic to explore pertinent to these goals that would be fundable and would also advance evidence-based practice?

REFERENCES

American Academy of Pediatrics Committee on Injury and Poison Prevention and Committee on Sports Medicine and Fitness. (1999). Trampolines at home, school, and recreational centers. *Pediatrics, 103*(5.1), 1053–1056.

Barkin, R. M., Barkin, S. Z., & Barkin, A. Z. (2000). The limping child. *Journal of Emergency Medicine, 18*(3), 331–339.

Carek, P. J., Dickerson, L. M., & Sack, J. L. (2001). Diagnosis and management of osteomyelitis. *American Family Physician, 63*(12), 2413–2420.

Chalom, E. C. (2000a). Arthritis—juvenile rheumatoid. In M. W. Schwartz (Ed.). *The 5-minute pediatric consult* (pp. 138–139). Philadelphia: Lippincott Williams & Wilkins.

Chalom, E. C. (2000b). Osteomyelitis. In M. W. Schwartz (Ed.). *The 5-minute pediatric consult* (pp. 584–585). Philadelphia: Lippincott Williams & Wilkins.

Department of Health and Human Services. (2000). *Healthy people 2010.* Washington, DC: DHHS.

Do, T. T. (2001). Clinical and radiographic evaluation of bowlegs. *Current Opinion in Pediatrics, 13*(1), 42–46.

Dormans, J. P. (2000a). Osteogenesis imperfecta. In M. W. Schwartz (Ed.). *The 5-minute pediatric consult* (pp. 582–583). Philadelphia: Lippincott Williams & Wilkins.

Dormans, J. P. (2000b). Perthe disease. In M. W. Schwartz (Ed.). *The 5-minute pediatric consult* (pp. 618–619). Philadelphia: Lippincott Williams & Wilkins.

Eilert, R. E. (2001). Growth disturbances of the musculoskeletal system. In W. W. Hay, A. R. Hayward, M. J. Levin & J. M. Sondheimer (Eds.). *Current pediatric diagnosis & treatment* (15th ed.). New York: McGraw-Hill.

Furnival, R. A., Street, K. A., & Schunk, J. E. (1999). Too many pediatric trampoline injuries. *Pediatrics, 103*(5), 257.

Gomez, M., et al. (2001). Complications of outpatient parenteral antibiotic therapy in childhood. *Pediatric Infectious Disease Journal, 20,* 541-543.

Hollister, J. R. (2001). Juvenile rheumatoid arthritis. In W. W. Hay, A. R. Hayward, M. J. Levin & J. M. Sondheimer (Eds.). *Current pediatric diagnosis & treatment* (15th ed.). New York: McGraw-Hill.

Johanson, N. A., & Pellicci, P. (2000). Knee pain. In S. A. Paget, A. Gibofsky & J. F. Beary (Eds.). *Manual of rheumatology & outpatient orthopedic disorders.* Philadelphia: Lippincott Williams & Wilkins.

Keenan, G. F. (2000). Synovitis. In M. W. Schwartz (Ed.). *The 5-minute pediatric consult* (pp. 792-793). Philadelphia: Lippincott Williams & Wilkins.

Killian, J. T., Mayberry, S., & Wilkinson, L. (1999). Current concepts in adolescent idiopathic scoliosis. *Pediatric Annals, 28*(12), 755-761.

Lamontagne, L. L., Hepworth, J. T., & Salisbury, M. H. (2001). Anxiety and postoperative pain in children who undergo major orthopedic surgery. *Applied Nursing Research, 14,* 119-124.

Leonard, M. B., & Zemel, B. S. (2002). Current concepts in pediatric bone disease. *Pediatric Clinics of North America 49*(1), 143-173.

Manko, J. (1999). Clavicle fracture. In P. Rosen et al. (Eds.). *The 5-minute emergency medicine consult.* Philadelphia: Lippincott Williams & Wilkins.

Marcus, R. (2001). Role of exercise in preventing and treating osteoporosis. *Rheumatic Diseases Clinics of North America, 27*(1), 131-141.

Porter, B. (2000). Myasthenia gravis. In M. W. Schwartz (Ed.). *The 5-minute pediatric consult* (pp. 552-553). Philadelphia: Lippincott Williams & Wilkins.

Shankar, S. M. (2000). Acute lymphoblastic leukemia. In M. W. Schwartz (Ed.). *The 5-minute pediatric consult* (pp. 100-101). Philadelphia: Lippincott Williams & Wilkins.

Sink, E. L., et al. (2001). Efficacy of perioperative halo-gravity traction in the treatment of severe scoliosis in children. *Journal of Pediatric Orthopedics, 21*(4), 519-524.

Thorarenson, O. (2000). Muscular dystrophies. In M. W. Schwartz (Ed.). *The 5-minute pediatric consult* (pp. 550-551). Philadelphia: Lippincott Williams & Wilkins.

Von Scheven, E. (2000). Dermatomyositis/polymyositis. In M. W. Schwartz (Ed.). *The 5-minute pediatric consult* (pp. 310-311). Philadelphia: Lippincott Williams & Wilkins.

Weaver, C. M. (2000). The growing years and prevention of osteoporosis in later life. *Proceedings of the Nutrition Society, 59*(2), 303-306.

Williams, R., & Wickiewicz, T. L. (2000). Sports injuries. In S. A. Paget, A. Gibofsky & J. F. Beary (Eds.). *Manual of rheumatology & outpatient orthopedic disorders.* Philadelphia: Lippincott Williams & Wilkins.

SUGGESTED READINGS

Adkins, S. B., & Figler, R. A. (2000). Hip pain in athletes. *American Family Physician, 61*(7), 2109-2118.

D'Amato, C. R., Griggs, S., & McCoy, B. (2001). Nighttime bracing with the Providence brace in adolescent girls with idiopathic scoliosis. *Spine, 26*(18), 2006-2012.

Do, T. T. (2002). Orthopedic management of the muscular dystrophies. *Current Opinion in Pediatrics, 14*(1), 50-53.

Gerloni, V., et al. (2001). Efficacy and safety of cyclosporin A in the treatment of juvenile chronic (idiopathic) arthritis. *Rheumatology, 40*(8), 907-913.

Hamilton, J., & Capell, H. (2001). The treatment of juvenile arthritis. *Expert Opinion on Pharmacotherapy, 2*(5.1), 1085-1092.

Karol, L. A. (2001). Effectiveness of bracing in male patients with idiopathic scoliosis. *Spine, 26*(18), 2001-2005.

Kothari, N. A., Pelchovitz, D. J., & Meyer, J. S. (2001). Imaging of musculoskeletal infections. *Radiologic Clinics of North America, 39*(4), 653-671.

Mason, D. E. (1999). Back pain in children. *Pediatric Annals, 28,* 727-739.

Roy, D. R. (1999). Current concepts in Legg-Calvé-Perthes Disease. *Pediatric Annals, 28*(12), 748-754.

Sherry, D. D. (2000). An overview of amplified musculoskeletal pain syndromes. *Journal of Rheumatology, 27*(58S), 44-48.

Thastum, M., Zachariae, R., & Herlin, T. (2001). Pain experience and pain coping strategies in children with juvenile idiopathic arthritis. *Journal of Rheumatology, 28*(5), 1091-1098.

Vitale, M. G., et al. (2001). Capturing quality of life in pediatric orthopaedics: Two recent measures compared. *Journal of Pediatric Orthopedics, 21*(5), 629-635.

52

CHAPTER

Nursing Care of the Child With a Traumatic Injury

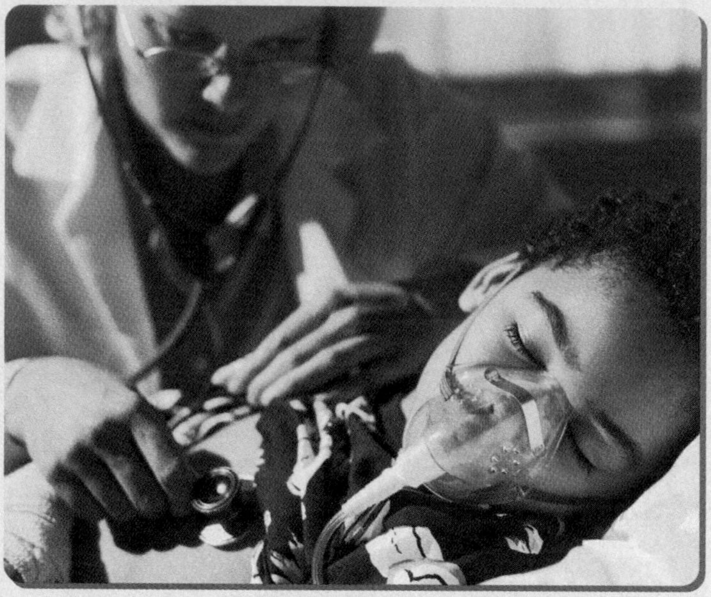

Key Terms

- allografting
- autografting
- contrecoup injury
- débridement
- drowning
- escharotomy
- heterografts
- homografting
- near drowning
- otorrhea
- plumbism
- rhinorrhea
- stupor

Objectives

After mastering the contents of this chapter, you should be able to:

1. Describe the causes and consequences of common accidents and injuries in childhood and measures to prevent them.
2. Assess a child traumatically injured from an accident.
3. Formulate nursing diagnoses related to the traumatically injured child.
4. Establish appropriate outcomes for the traumatically injured child.
5. Plan nursing care related to the traumatically injured child.
6. Implement nursing care for the child with a traumatic injury.
7. Evaluate outcomes for achievement and effectiveness of care.
8. Identify National Health Goals related to children who have experienced trauma that nurses can be instrumental in helping the nation to achieve.
9. Identify areas related to care of children with traumatic injuries that could benefit from additional nursing research or application of evidence-based practice.
10. Use critical thinking to analyze ways that accidents and traumatic injuries can be prevented in childhood.
11. Integrate knowledge of traumatic injuries in childhood with nursing process to achieve quality maternal and child health care.

Jason, a 4-year-old boy, is seen in the emergency room after an automobile accident. He is lethargic and stuporous, although the only visible signs of trauma are a reddened and edematous area on the middle of his forehead. Vital signs reveal the following: temperature, 99.4°F (37.5°C); respirations, 18; pulse, 62; and blood pressure, 110/62. His left pupil is more dilated than his right; it reacts sluggishly to light. His Glasgow Coma score is 8. His mother tells you, "I'm sure he's not injured badly. He was wearing his seat belt." You are the triage nurse. Would you rate Jason as a child to be seen immediately, or could he be given second priority?

Previous chapters described the growth and development of well children and care of children with disorders of specific body systems. This chapter adds information about the characteristic changes, both physical and psychosocial, that occur when children experience a traumatic injury. This is important information because it provides a base for care and health teaching.

After you've studied the chapter, answer the Critical Thinking Exercises at the end of the chapter and then access the on-line study activities (http://connection.lww.com) *to further sharpen your skills and test your knowledge.*

Accidents, such as those involving motor vehicles, falls, burns, and water immersions, cause more deaths in the 1- to 4-year age group than the next six most prevalent diseases combined. In the 15- to 24-year age group, they cause more deaths than all other combined causes (Battan & Dart, 2001). Thus, if accidents could be prevented, a major cause of childhood morbidity and mortality would be eliminated. However, total accident elimination may not be possible. Children commonly believe that accidents will not happen to them and, as a result, fail to take sensible precautions against them. Some parents may predispose their children to accidents by overestimating their development and giving them responsibility beyond their capabilities.

Family stress plays a large role in childhood poisoning accidents because these types of accidents tend to occur when parents are preoccupied. Many accidental poisoning ingestions occur on the same day that the medicine was purchased, implying that the stress of family illness plays a major role (Ozanne-Smith et al., 2001). Eliminating accidents in children, therefore, is not a simple procedure, because it involves reducing family stress as well. National Health Goals related to children and trauma are shown in the Focus on National Health Goals box.

The frequency of different types of accidents varies according to age group (Table 52-1). Because the anatomy and physiology of children are different from those of adults, they are not only involved in different types of accidents than adults, but they are affected by accidents differently.

FOCUS ON NATIONAL HEALTH GOALS

Because injury prevention could have immediate and long-term effects on the nation's health, a number of National Health Goals are concerned with accidents, traumatic injuries, and children:

- Reduce drownings from 1.6/100,000 to 0.9/100,000.
- Reduce firearm-related deaths from a baseline of 11.3/100,000 to 4.1/100,000 population.
- Reduce nonfatal poisonings from 348/100,000 to 292/100,000.
- Reduce deaths caused by suffocation from 4/100,000 to 3/100,000.
- Reduce deaths caused by unintentional injury from 36/100,000 to 17.5/100,000.
- Reduce deaths caused by motor vehicle crashes from 15.6/100,000 to 9.2/100,000.
- Increase the use of child safety restraints from 92% to 100%.
- Increase the use of helmets by bicyclists.
- Reduce residential fire deaths from 1.2/100,000 to 0.2/100,000 (DHHS, 2000).

Nurses can be instrumental in helping the nation achieve these goals by being primary care providers who provide counseling on safety precautions to parents and children. Additional nursing research would be helpful in areas such as the following: what are effective ways to communicate safety information to parents at well-child visits when time is at a premium; in what ways should safety teaching given after an accident to prevent a further accident be different from that given as primary prevention; and is there an association between children setting fires and their exposure to fire experiences with fireplaces or candles?

NURSING PROCESS OVERVIEW

For Care of the Child With a Traumatic Injury

Assessment

When children are seen at health care facilities because of traumatic injuries, neither they nor their parents may be functioning at their optimal level because of the stress of the situation. They may be apprehensive and frightened not only about what *has* happened, but also about what could have happened. Children often feel guilty and fear that they will be

TABLE 52.1 Most Frequent Accidents in Children by Age Group

AGE (y)	TYPE OF ACCIDENT
0–1	Falls, inhalation of foreign objects, poisoning, burns, drowning
2–4	Falls, drowning, motor vehicles, poisoning, burns
5–9	Motor vehicles, bicycle accidents, drowning, burns, firearms
10–14	Motor vehicles, drowning, burns, firearms, falls, bicycle accidents
15–18	Motor vehicles, drowning, firearms

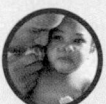

scolded or punished. Their parents may feel equally guilty; for example, they may feel that if they were really "good" parents, they would have been watching more closely. They may feel defensive because they are worried about being criticized. People under stress do not hear well and may not perceive the information given to them correctly. Information they receive in the emergency department may be grossly misinterpreted or not heard at all.

Children are likely to be in pain. They are frightened not just from the pain of the injury, but also from the circumstance of the injury. Children count on their parents to keep them safe, yet they have been hurt. The trust is broken momentarily. How can they be safe here if their parents no longer are protecting them?

Because the emergency department nurse is often the first person who sees a child after an injury, be ready to make a preliminary assessment of the extent of the child's injuries before a physician arrives. Remember that children may be seriously hurt but will not cry because they are in shock. They may be hemorrhaging, but, if they are bleeding internally, blood may not be visibly evident. Accidents become fatal when lung, heart, or brain function becomes inadequate. These three body systems, therefore, must be evaluated first. Table 52-2 lists signs and symptoms to assess when determining the respiratory, cardiovascular, and neurologic status of an injured child.

TABLE 52.2 Important Assessment on Initial Examination of an Injured Child

BODY SYSTEM	ASSESSMENT
Respiratory system	Quality of respirations
	Rate of respirations
	Sound of obstruction (wheezing, stridor, retractions, coughing?)
	Color (cyanotic?)
	Oxygen hunger (restlessness, inability to lie flat?)
Cardiovascular system	Color (pallor from hemorrhage or cardiovascular collapse?)
	Gross bleeding
	Pulse rate (increases with hemorrhage)
	Blood pressure (decreases with hemorrhage)
	Feeling of apprehension from altered vascular pressure
Nervous system	Level of consciousness (child answers questions coherently?; infant attunes to parent's voice?)
	Pupils (equal and reacting to light?)
	Bumps or bruises on head or spinal column
	Loss of motion or sensory function in a body part

While conducting a preliminary assessment of a child's major body systems, take a brief history of the accident. What happened? How long ago did it happen? What have the parents done? If the child fell, how far did he or she fall? On what body part did the child land? (A head injury is more likely to be serious than an ankle injury, although a child may be in more pain and have more obvious symptoms with the lesser injury.) Ask parents what they think are a child's major injuries. Children may report one body part hurts at first, but then a small cut elsewhere begins to bleed, and they focus on the minor bleeding as their major injury. If parents say, "At first, he acted as if his stomach hurt," this may be the first suggestion that he has a serious abdominal injury such as splenic rupture.

Evaluating children in an emergency department is difficult, because they are so frightened that they cannot stop crying to report which body parts are painful or to indicate which parts should be assessed first. Spend a few minutes attempting to calm children and get them past this initial fright unless symptoms of major body system disturbances require that you direct your immediate efforts elsewhere. Parents need frequent explanations of care given or planned because, as long as they are worried and tense, children cannot be calmed easily.

A proportion of traumatic injuries in children result from child abuse. Ask yourself if this could be a possibility (see Chapter 55).

Nursing Diagnosis

The nursing diagnosis used most frequently with injured children is Pain. Depending on the particular injury, a number of other nursing diagnoses are relevant, as are those that relate to the suffering that parents experience when their child is injured. Examples of possible nursing diagnoses include the following:

- Ineffective airway clearance related to burned esophageal tissue
- Impaired physical mobility related to severe burn injury
- Disturbed body image related to change in physical appearance with thermal burns
- Parental fear related to outcome after head injury in child
- Interrupted family processes related to child's accident
- Anxiety related to apprehension and lack of knowledge regarding medical treatment of child

Outcome Identification and Planning

Parents in an emergency department are rarely ready for long-term planning. They have great difficulty in coming up with answers even to the most straightforward questions. Therefore, long-term planning may have to be delayed until the immediate concern of the injury has passed.

On discharge from the emergency department, parents need printed instructions about the child's care at home and the name and number of the person to call if they have questions about care or progress. They also need an appointment (or the number to call for a return appointment) for follow-up care. If the child is admitted to the hospital from the emergency department, it is helpful if the nurse who cared for the child in the emergency department can accompany him or her to the hospital unit. The first people who care for a child after an injury become very important to the child and parents because that person was the first one to recognize their stress. Parents have difficulty letting them go and accepting new caregivers. A transition period, a "passing on of care," helps a parent to accept the child's new caregivers as being as dependable and trustworthy as the emergency department staff.

Implementation

The extent of a child's injury depends on the injuring agent, the part of the body that was injured, and often the immediate care, including both physical and psychological management that the child received.

The diameter of the airway in children is smaller than in adults, so an injury to this body area almost always results in a greater danger of airway closure than in adults. This could happen from the child inhaling a substance, such as water, that directly obstructs the airway or from inhaling toxic fumes that cause inflammation along the lining of the airway, resulting in obstruction. A blow to the neck can result in edema of surrounding tissues, causing the airway to close.

Most injuries involve some blood loss. Fortunately, a child's circulatory system is capable of rapid compensation for blood loss by vasoconstriction. Because the total volume of blood in a child is reduced, however, blood loss in children is always potentially serious.

Often, in the emergency department, large portions of the child's body must be exposed to view so that care can be given easily. This means that rapid cooling can occur. Because of the large body surface area of children in relation to weight, always be conscious of body temperature and take active measures to decrease cooling by keeping the child covered as much as possible during examination times.

Standard precautions are maintained in emergency situations, the same as at any other time. Parental consent must be obtained for treatment procedures even in an emergency, except for life-saving actions, such as cardiopulmonary resuscitation procedures. In these instances, action can and should be taken to save the child's life with or without parental permission (it is assumed that parents would consent to life-saving procedures). Delaying emergency procedures until parents can be located may result in permanent disability or death.

A key component of nursing intervention in an emergency department is to help parents understand why an injury happened and plan ways to make their immediate or community environment safe for children. An organization that might be appropriate for referral is the American Association of Poison Control Centers (*www.aapcc.org*).

Outcome Evaluation

After an injury, children need follow-up care to be certain that the immediate interventions were adequate and that healing is taking place. Evaluation visits are also the time to determine if the child's environment has been changed and is safer now than at the time of the accident (if applicable). At that time, parents may have been too anxious to hear health supervision information. Now, with the accident behind them, they are ready for such information and prepared to make changes.

When an injury could not have been anticipated, parents appreciate hearing one more time that such an accident could not have been avoided and that they are good parents. This helps them maintain adequate self-esteem to continue to function well as parents.

Examples of suggesting outcome achievement may include:

- Child swallows fluids without distress after esophageal burns.
- Child states pain is at tolerable level within half hour.
- Child demonstrates full range of motion in hand after thermal injury.

HEALTH PROMOTION AND RISK MANAGEMENT

In every care setting, nurses have the unique opportunity among health care professionals to provide child and family teaching concerning the prevention of accidents. Even in the acute care setting when an accident has already occurred, nurses can provide invaluable instruction to families about safeguarding their children against future accidents. In the community setting, nurses have a greater opportunity for assessment of the unique threats present in particular environments (eg, lead-based paint in older homes, the presence of kerosene heaters in a home, the risk of drowning in a home that has a swimming pool, the danger for children in pickup trucks [Winston et al., 2002]). Nurses, therefore, need to be knowledgeable about the interventions to be used and the measures to prevent injury.

Poisoning is an important cause of serious injuries in children younger than 6 years. Over 1 million episodes occur per year (Shannon, 2000). Common household agents are often the cause. Since the Poison Prevention Packaging Act of 1970, potentially hazardous products must be sold in child-resistant containers. Passage of this Act initiated a decrease in the incidence of childhood poisonings.

The home environment may still contain products that may be hazardous and poisonous to children if handled improperly. Plants, cosmetics, and cleaning products may be considerably dangerous to children if ingested or absorbed through the skin. Parents must be made aware of these dangers and taught strategies for maintaining a safe home environment, including learning basic first aid.

Measures for a safe home environment include actions such as installing child-resistant locks on low cabinets where household products are stored and moving plants to a higher surface or removing them from the home until the child is older, keeping matches in safe places and teaching street safety. In addition, parents should anticipate that, even in the safest environment, a child can be injured. Along with knowledge of basic first aid, the phone number of the local poison control center should be posted by the phone. Parents should also have an emergency first aid kit and syrup of ipecac on hand (see Focus on Pharmacology: Syrup of Ipecac later in this chapter) as recommended by the Poison Control Center.

✔ CHECKPOINT QUESTIONS

1. What types of accidents are the most common in children between the ages of 5 and 9 years?
2. What legislation has contributed to a decrease in the number of childhood poisonings?

HEAD TRAUMA

Children receive head injuries when they are involved in multiple trauma accidents, such as automobile accidents. Falls from swing sets, porches, and bunk beds also cause many head injuries. Other children are injured by being struck on the head by an object, such as a baseball, rock, or hockey puck, or they fall from a bicycle (Matthews & Wilson, 2001).

Head injuries are serious not only because they cause an immediate life threat to the child, but also because a number of complications may follow. With a depressed skull fracture, for example, recurrent seizures can occur (Chiaretti et al., 2000). Many of these children show focal abnormalities on an electroencephalogram (EEG) from scar tissue formation. A number of children with seizure involvement will have a normal EEG, however, so, by itself, EEG is of limited value in predicting post-traumatic seizures.

Some children experience memory deficits or minor personality changes after head injury. Symptoms such as headache, irritability, and postural vertigo (sensation of faintness or an inability to maintain normal balance—also known as post-trauma syndrome) also may occur. Behavioral manifestations may include aggressiveness or poor school performance. It often is difficult to determine whether these symptoms are organic or the result of being treated differently than usual by anxious parents.

Immediate Assessment

All children with head trauma require a neurologic assessment as soon as they are seen and again at frequent intervals to detect signs and symptoms of increased intracranial pressure (ICP). Increasing pressure puts stress on the respiratory, cardiac, and temperature centers, causing dysfunction in these areas. With increased pressure, the pupils become slow or unable to react immediately. Level of consciousness and motor ability decrease, pulse and respiratory rates decrease, and temperature and pulse pressure increase.

Assess vital signs to detect these changes and observe children's pupils to be certain that they are equal and react to light. Assess children's level of consciousness and motor function. Stabilize the neck with a brace until cervical trauma has been ruled out.

Immediate Management

After a head injury, brain edema is likely because fluid rushes into the inflamed and bruised area. Both central venous and central arterial lines may be inserted. ICP monitoring may be initiated (see Chapter 49). A computed tomography (CT) scan or magnetic resonance imaging (MRI) will be ordered to determine areas of edema or bleeding. An attempt may be made to decrease brain edema by intravenous (IV) administration of a hypertonic solution, such as mannitol. This will increase intravascular pressure and shift edema fluid back into the blood vessels. Steroids such as dexamethasone may be added to decrease inflammation and edema. Keeping the head elevated is also effective in reducing ICP.

NURSING DIAGNOSES AND RELATED INTERVENTIONS

Nursing Diagnosis: Risk for excess fluid volume related to administration of hypertonic solution

Outcome Identification: Child will remain free of effects of increased fluid load during the course of treatment.

Outcome Evaluation: The child's respiratory rate remains between 16 to 24 per minute; specific gravity of urine is between 1.003 and 1.030; pulse remains between 60 to 100 beats per minute; blood pressure remains consistent for age group; lungs are clear to auscultation.

When hypertonic solutions are being infused into children, assess vital signs frequently to be certain that the fluid load being pulled into the intravascular system does not overtax it. This fluid must be excreted by the kidneys to keep the vascular system from becoming overloaded. Keep accurate intake and output records, and test the specific gravity of urine to detect the development of pituitary compression and resultant overproduction or underproduction of antidiuretic hormone from the posterior pituitary.

Nursing Diagnosis: Risk for delayed growth and development related to late sequelae of head injury

Outcome Identification: Child will maintain normal function after head trauma.

Outcome Evaluation: Child shows no evidence of any alteration in thought processes, seizure activity, or memory at follow-up visits. Cognitive and physical development are appropriate for age.

Helping care for the child with a head injury may be difficult for parents because they are so worried. Offer information on the child's progress as it is available to you. Urge parents to help care for the child to increase their sense of control.

During the acute phase of illness, ensure that parents are informed about the dangers of trauma. If they ask about the possibility that personality changes or seizures will develop later in life, their questions should be answered truthfully. At the same time, don't give unnecessary warnings about observing the child carefully in the months to come. Head injuries by themselves are worrisome enough to parents and children without adding to their burden.

Skull Fracture

A skull fracture is a crack in the bone of the skull. Recognizing skull fractures in children is important because associated cerebral injury often occurs under the fracture. Many skull fractures are simple linear types, most often involving the parietal bones. In some children, the skull does not fracture, but the suture lines separate. This occurs more commonly in the lambdoid suture line; a coronal suture separation is rare and, if present, indicates severe trauma (Fig. 52-1).

Assessment

If the base of the skull is fractured, children generally exhibit orbital or postauricular ecchymosis. They may have **rhinorrhea** or **otorrhea** (clear fluid draining from the nose or ear). This is escaping cerebrospinal fluid (CSF)—a serious finding, because it means the child's central nervous system is open to infection. Nasal discharge may be tested with a glucose reagent strip if there is doubt about the source of the drainage. CSF will be positive for glucose, whereas the clear, watery drainage from the upper respiratory tract infection will not.

Skull fractures are confirmed by skull x-ray. Take a careful history of the accident so the strength of the blow to the head can be judged. Shock with hypotension rarely occurs with an isolated head injury. If children are in shock, bleeding points other than the head injury should be investigated.

If a skull fracture is linear with no underlying pathology, no treatment except observation and prescription of an analgesic is necessary. In about 3 weeks, children need a repeat x-ray to confirm that healing has taken place. Parents can be assured that a second x-ray this soon is not harmful but necessary.

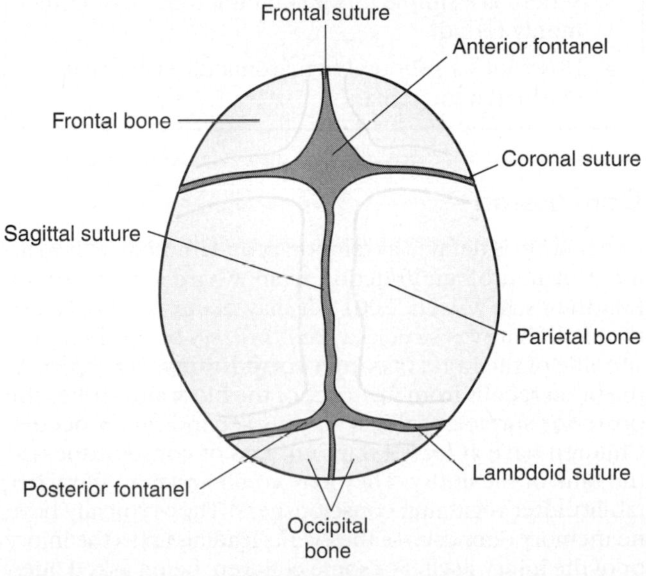

FIGURE 52.1 Location of sutures.

If a fracture is depressed (a bone fragment is pressing inward) or compounded (bone is broken into pieces), surgery will be necessary to remove or repair broken fragments. Cranial surgery is discussed in Chapter 49.

Therapeutic Management

If CSF is draining from the nose, children will be admitted for observation. Keep them in a semi-Fowler's position so fluid drains out, not inward, to reduce the possibility of introducing infection. Make certain that they do not attempt to hold their nose or pack their nostrils with something to halt the drainage. Because coughing and sneezing may allow air to enter the meningeal space, coughing may be suppressed by medication. If the drainage is excoriating to the upper lip, coat the space with petrolatum. Children may be placed on a prophylactic antibiotic to reduce the risk for meningitis. If the drainage does not stop within a few days, surgery will be necessary to repair the fracture and reduce the danger of meningitis. Air that enters intracranial spaces generally is absorbed rapidly. If x-rays at 72 h still show air in the cerebral spaces, it implies that a skull defect remains. Surgery may be indicated to close the defect.

Potential Complications

A long-term complication of even a linear fracture may be a *leptomeningeal cyst.* This results from projection of the arachnoid membrane into the fracture site. With the interfering tissue, bone cannot heal and actually erodes so that the fracture site becomes progressively larger, not smaller. This will be evident on a follow-up x-ray. It may be suspected if a child develops focal seizures or symptoms of increased ICP. The defect may be palpated on the skull as an underlying indentation. Surgical resection will be necessary to remove the cyst.

Subdural Hematoma

Subdural hematoma is venous bleeding into the space between the dura and arachnoid membrane (Fig. 52-2A). It occurs when head trauma lacerates minute veins in this area. The collection of blood generally is bilateral.

Subdural hematomas tend to occur in infants more than in older children. Symptoms may occur within 3 days of trauma or as late as 20 days. Infants generally have symptoms of increased ICP. Seizures, vomiting, hyperirritability, and enlargement of the head may occur. Anemia from the substantial blood loss is a prominent sign. Angiocardiography or sonogram will reveal the extent of the hematoma (Hilton, 2001).

In infants, accumulated subdural blood may be removed by a subdural puncture through the lateral aspect of a patent anterior fontanelle. The procedure is similar to a lumbar puncture. Infants receive conscious sedation or must be held extremely still during the procedure so they do not move and cause the aspiration needle to be inserted incorrectly. Without conscious sedation, half of the success of subdural puncture depends on the ability of the person to hold the child still.

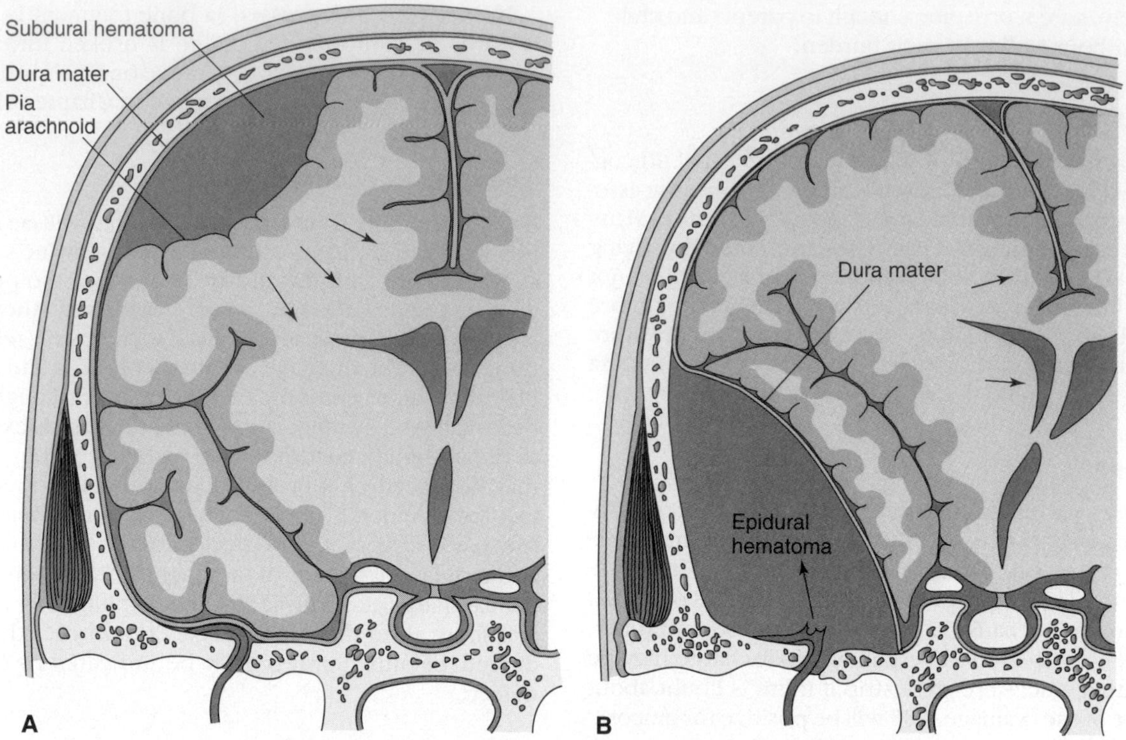

FIGURE 52.2 (*A*) Subdural hematoma. The dark area in the upper left area of the drawing is the hematoma. Note the shift of structures. (*B*) Epidural hematoma. The dark area in the lower left area of the drawing is the hematoma. Note the broken blood vessel and the shift of midline structures.

Subdural punctures may need to be repeated daily to empty the subdural space. When the space is empty, it will be occluded by expanding brain tissue. If the space has not been occluded after 2 weeks of daily punctures, active bleeding is still present, and surgery generally is necessary to reduce the space and halt bleeding.

In older children, surgery generally is necessary because the anterior fontanelle is closed, and the space cannot be reached by puncture.

Epidural Hematoma

Epidural hematoma is bleeding into the space between the dura and the skull (Figure 52-2*B*). This happens when head trauma is severe. Subdural hemorrhage is generally venous bleeding, but epidural hemorrhage is usually a result of rupture of the middle meningeal artery and is, therefore, arterial bleeding. It usually is intense and causes rapid brain compression.

At the time of the injury, usually children are momentarily unconscious. They then regain consciousness and, to the untrained eye, appear to be well for minutes or hours. Then signs of cortical compression—vomiting, loss of consciousness, headache, seizures, or hemiparesis (paralysis on one side)—are observed. On physical examination, unequal dilatation or constriction of the pupils may be present. Decorticate posturing (see Chapter 49) may be seen, indicating extreme pressure on upper cortical centers. If the pressure is allowed to continue unchecked, cortical compression may be so great that brain stem, respiratory, or cardiovascular function is impaired.

As a rule, the closer to the time of the injury that symptoms of compression occur, the more extreme the amount of blood loss. The treatment is surgical removal of the accumulated blood and cauterization or ligation of the torn artery. The earlier the process is recognized and treated, the lesser the chance of residual damage from extreme pressure or anoxia to the involved portion of the brain.

✔ CHECKPOINT QUESTIONS

3. Where is a simple linear skull fracture most commonly found?
4. How does a subdural hematoma differ from an epidural hematoma?

Concussion

Concussion is defined as temporary and immediate impairment of neurologic function from a hard, jarring shock (Matthews & Wilson, 2001). It may occur on the side of the skull that was struck (a *coup injury*) or on the opposite side of the brain (a **contrecoup injury;** Fig. 52-3). As the brain recoils from the force of the blow and strikes the posterior surface of the skull, this second injury occurs. Children have at least a transient loss of consciousness at the time of the injury. They may vomit and may show irritability after regaining consciousness. They typically have no memory (amnesia) of the events leading up to the injury or of the injury itself. For some children, being asked questions about the accident is extremely upsetting because

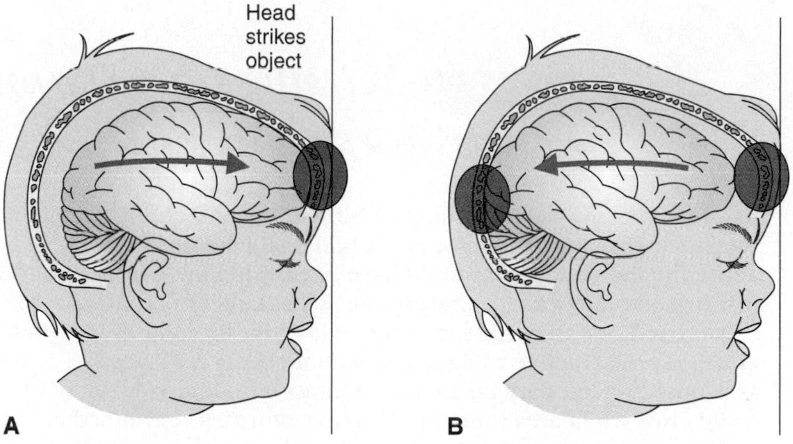
Head
strikes
object
A
B
COUP INJURY
Anterior of brain strikes
skull and is injured
CONTRECOUP INJURY
Brain recoils and strikes
posterior skull, so is
injured twice

FIGURE 52.3 Etiology of (*A*) coup and (*B*) contrecoup injuries.

they do not remember anything that happened and feel a frightening loss of control. The child requires a skull x-ray to rule out skull fracture and observation for 24 h to rule out severe brain trauma, edema, or laceration. The child usually can be observed at home by the parents, who are instructed to rouse him or her every 1 to 2 h while awake to check the level of consciousness. Parents usually are instructed not to keep waking children during the night because multiple wakings are disorienting and can be confused with unconsciousness. Parents should wake the child at least once during the night, however, and assess that the pulse rate is more than 60 beats per minute.

To be certain that children are alert, parents can ask them to name a familiar object, such as a favorite toy, or to name the color of some object shown to them. Telling parents their name or where they live is equally revealing.

Give parents the telephone number to call if they have any questions about their child's care. Advise them to call if their child's behavior changes in any way that makes them suspicious. Many parents will need to set an alarm clock to wake themselves during the night to assess their child's status. There is an old belief that, if children fall asleep after a head injury, they will die in their sleep; thus, some parents may keep shaking children awake or make them walk continuously. Be certain they understand that it is all right for children to sleep, but they must wake them at least once to assess their status (see Focus on Nursing Care Planning).

WHAT IF? In the emergency room, parents state that their 5-year-old daughter has been vomiting, is lethargic, and seems "clumsy." What is the priority intervention? What questions would you want to ask to learn more about the child? What might the medical diagnosis reveal?

Contusion

A brain contusion occurs when there is tearing or laceration of brain tissue (Fig. 52-4). The symptoms are the same as those for concussion except that they are more severe. In addition, there are specific symptoms related to the lacerated brain area (focal seizure, eye deviation, loss of speech). Surgery may be necessary to halt bleeding. The child's prognosis depends on the extent of the injury and effectiveness of therapy.

Coma

Coma (unconsciousness from which children cannot be roused) or **stupor** (grogginess from which children can be roused) may be present in children after severe head trauma. Coma and stupor are both symptoms of underlying disorders; a history of the injury must be obtained so treatment can be directed specifically toward the cause.

Obtain a history to determine the circumstances immediately before the time the child became comatose. Assess children in coma carefully and completely so the cause of the decreased consciousness can quickly be determined.

Assessment

Undress children completely so all body parts can be inspected. Although head injury is most likely to be the underlying cause of coma or seizure, metabolic disturbances, such as diabetes mellitus, dehydration, severe hemorrhage, or drug ingestion, also must be considered as possible causes. Count respirations and pulse and measure blood pressure to establish baseline values because changes in these often provide good clues. A child with increased ICP will show decreased pulse and respiratory rates, and increased blood pressure. Diabetes leads to increased respirations. Hemorrhage leads to an increased pulse rate and a decreased blood pressure. Drug ingestion may lead to increased or decreased measurements, depending on the drug ingested.

If bulbar (brain stem) compression is present, children cannot swallow effectively or safely. If this is suspected, turn them on the side to prevent aspiration. Observe the eyes for signs of increased ICP. If both pupils are dilated, irreversible brain stem damage is suggested, although such a finding may be present with poisoning from an atropine-

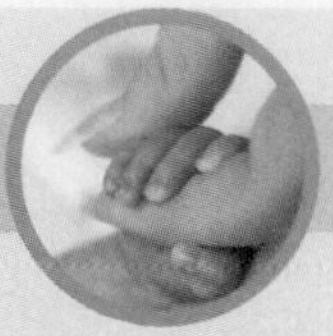

FOCUS ON *Nursing Care Planning*

A CHILD WITH A CONCUSSION

A $3\frac{1}{2}$-year-old child clutching her teddy bear is brought to the emergency department by her parents. Her parents state that she was playing on the swings in the backyard, when she fell off, hitting her head on the metal support. "She was out for a minute or two."

Assessment: $3\frac{1}{2}$-year-old female visibly upset and crying. Height and weight at 75th percentile for age. Child unable to report or recall anything about the incident. "We should have been watching her more closely. We just turned our backs for one minute. What kind of parents are we?"

Alert and oriented. Able to name teddy bear brought in with her. Pupils equal, round, reactive to light and accommodation bilaterally. 1.5-cm raised area noted on left parietal area. Skin intact without evidence of bleeding. Child cries when area touched. Negative otorrhea or rhinorrhea. Small 2-cm abrasion noted on right knee; 3-cm abrasion noted on right hand. No other injuries noted. Able to move all extremities through range of motion.

Vital signs: Temperature: 98.2°F (36.8°C); pulse: 128; respirations: 32; blood pressure: 110/70. A diagnosis of concussion is made, and child is to be discharged home to parents.

Nursing Diagnosis: Risk for injury related to effects of concussion

Outcome Identification: Child will remain free of signs and symptoms of injury after concussion.

Outcome Evaluation: Child remains alert and oriented; easily arousable. Pupils equal, round, react to light and accommodation; vital signs within age-acceptable parameters; exhibits no signs or symptoms of neurologic dysfunction.

Interventions	Rationale
1. Assess the child's vital signs, level of consciousness, and neurologic function initially, and then every $\frac{1}{2}$ h or according to institution's policy until discharge.	1. Assessment provides a baseline for evaluation. Changes in vital signs, level of consciousness, or neurologic function indicate a worsening of the child's condition and possibly increasing intracranial pressure.
2. Orient the child to her surroundings and explain what has happened. Offer explanations about any treatments or procedures that are to come.	2. Children often have no memory of events leading up to or at the time of the injury. Orientation and explanation help to minimize the child's fear of the unknown and of her situation.
3. Obtain a skull x-ray and other diagnostic tests as ordered, such as CT scan or MRI.	3. Skull x-ray rules out a possible skull fracture secondary to the trauma. CT scan or MRI helps determine any areas of bleeding or edema if present.
4. Institute measures to calm the child. Speak slowly and softly and minimize distractions. Encourage the parents to hold and stroke the child.	4. Crying increases intracranial pressure. Involving the parents provides them with a concrete activity, helping to provide some sense of control over the situation.
5. Instruct the parents to observe the child for the next 24 h for changes. Advise them to rouse the child approximately every 2 h during daytime hours and at least once during the night, asking the child to name a familiar object, color, or something she's been shown or to state her name or where she is.	5. Observation is necessary to rule out the possibility of severe brain trauma, edema, or laceration. Waking the child every 2 h provides time for assessing the child's level of consciousness.
6. Caution parents not to awaken the child too frequently.	6. Multiple frequent waking can be disorienting to the child and be confused with altered levels of consciousness.

(continued)

Interventions	Rationale
7. Review the signs and symptoms of increased intracranial pressure or decreased neurologic function with the parents. Give them a telephone number to call if they have any questions or notice any behavior changes that are suspicious.	7. Understanding of what to look for allows the parents to be comfortable with caring for the child at home. Availability of contact, if necessary, provides the parents with a sense of reassurance and support.
8. Recommend that the parents call their primary health care provider for an appointment once they are at home.	8. Appointment with the child's health care provider allows for additional follow-up.

Nursing Diagnosis: Situational low self-esteem related to feelings of guilt about the child's accident

Outcome Identification: Parents will express positive feelings about themselves as parents.

Outcome Evaluation: Parents state the impact of the child's accident on their view of themselves as parents; identify steps taken after child's fall, participate actively in child's care, and report some degree of control over the situation.

Interventions	Rationale
1. Attempt to identify the meaning and effect of the child's accident on the parents.	1. Identification of the meaning and effect of the child's accident assists in determining the degree of impact of the situation on the parents.
2. Encourage the parents to express their feelings about themselves as parents and their role in the child's accident.	2. Sharing of feelings permits a safe outlet for emotions and also aids in highlighting the parents' awareness of the possible impact on their self-esteem.
3. Review and reinforce positive actions as parents. Point out positive behaviors related to maintaining the child's safety and prompt action when the accident happened.	3. Positive actions and behaviors provide a foundation for rebuilding self-esteem.
4. Clarify any misconceptions that the parents may have. Reinforce with them that, even with the most constant supervision, it is not always possible to prevent all accidents.	4. Understanding that accidents can happen even with the best of supervision helps to alleviate possible feelings of guilt and anxiety.
5. Assist the parents with participating in the child's care during hospitalization and after discharge. Reinforce previous instructions about observing the child.	5. Ability to perform one's role promotes self-esteem; active participation enhances feelings of control.
6. Reinforce with the parents about calling the institution with any questions.	6. Awareness of additional support helps to reduce feelings of anxiety.

like drug. Pinpoint pupils suggest barbiturate or opiate intoxication. One pupil dilated more than the other suggests third cranial nerve damage. The eye may be deviated downward and laterally as well. This also may be caused by a tentorial tear (the membrane between the cerebellum and cerebrum) and herniation of the temporal lobe into the torn membrane. This situation requires immediate surgery to correct temporal compression.

The retina of the eye should be examined for papilledema, which will be present if increased pressure is longstanding (more than 24 to 48 h). Lack of a doll's eye reflex suggests that compression of the oculomotor nerves (third, fourth, or sixth) or the brain stem is involved. Observe for posturing, such as decerebrate posturing, which suggests cerebral compression and dysfunction.

Coma is usually graded according to a standard scale so changes can be evaluated accurately. Figure 52-5 shows the Glasgow Coma Scale, a commonly used evaluation system. Because this system was devised to be an adult assessment scale, it must be modified for use with children; such a modification is shown in Box 52-1.

A score of 3 to 8 suggests severe trauma (less than 5 carries a very severe prognosis); a score of 9 to 12, moderate trauma; and 13 to 15, slight trauma. Many laboratory

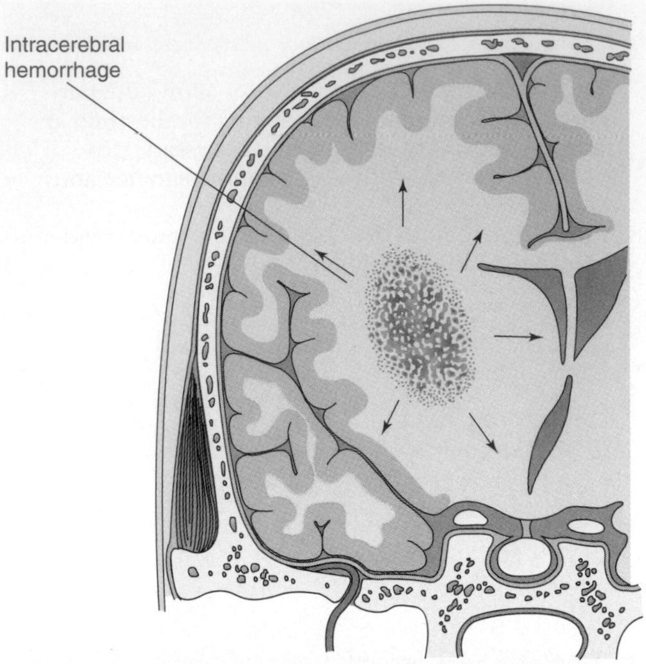

FIGURE 52.4 Intracerebral hemorrhage. The central large dark area represents the hemorrhage. Note the midline shift.

studies are helpful in determining the cause of coma. Blood glucose, blood electrolytes, blood urea nitrogen (BUN), liver function tests, blood gas studies, lumbar puncture, and toxicology tests may be ordered to rule out possible causes, such as bacterial meningitis or hemorrhage.

Therapeutic Management

If children are unconscious for more than a transient period, they generally are admitted to an observation unit for further assessment. As a general rule, place children who are comatose on their side to reduce the risk of aspiration. Oral suctioning to remove mucus from their mouths and pharynx may be necessary. If children have acute signs of respiratory difficulty, endotracheal intubation or tracheostomy may be necessary to ensure respiratory function.

An IV route is established so that when specific measures are determined (blood replacement, electrolyte replacement, fluid replacement), a route for immediate administration will be available. Blood will be drawn for a complete blood count, electrolyte determination, toxicology tests, and cross-matching. If the cause of the coma is unknown, a lumbar puncture and EEG may be done. Skull x-rays, CT scan, or MRI may be done.

Lumbar puncture has little value at first in predicting the severity of a head injury, because any degree of cerebral contusion generally leads to increased CSF pressure. Lumbar punctures are contraindicated if increased ICP is present. Otherwise, brain stem compression can result. Obtain children's vital signs and assess neurologic status, such as state of consciousness and the ability of pupils to react to light, every 15 to 20 min or as ordered. Accurately and carefully record this information so a picture of gradual change will become apparent.

A child's prognosis after coma depends on the initial cause of the coma. If the increased ICP can be relieved before any permanent brain damage results, the effects of the coma will be transient. Prognosis is always guarded,

Glasgow Coma Scale			A.M.		P.M.						A.M.				
Assessment	Reaction	Score	8	10	12	2	4	6	8	10	12	2	4	6	8
Eye Opening	Spontaneously	4	X						X	X	X	X	X		
Response	To speech	3		X				X							
	To pain	2			X	X	X								
	No response	1													
Motor Response	Obeys verbal command	6	X						X	X	X	X	X		
	Localizes pain	5		X	X										
	Flexion withdrawal	4				X		X							
	Flexion	3					X								
	Extension	2													
	No response	1													
Verbal Response	Oriented x3	5	X						X	X	X	X	X		
	Conversation confused	4		X				X							
	Inappropriate speech	3			X										
	Incomprehensible sounds	2				X	X								
	No response	1													

FIGURE 52.5 Glasgow Coma Scale scoring for a child. A score of 3 to 8 denotes severe trauma; 9 to 12, moderate trauma; 13 to 15, slight trauma. Notice the gradual improvement from coma in this example.

BOX 52.1

SCORING FOR GLASGOW COMA SCALE

Eye Opening

4. Child opens his or her eyes spontaneously when you approach.
3. Child opens his or her eyes in response to speech (spoken or shouted).
2. Child opens his or her eyes only in response to painful stimuli, such as pressure on a nail bed.
1. Child does not open his or her eyes in response to painful stimuli.

Motor Response

6. Child can obey a simple command such as "hand me a toy" (infant smiles or attunes).
5. Child moves an extremity to locate a painful stimuli applied to the head or trunk and attempts to remove the source.
4. Child attempts to withdraw from the source of pain.
3. Child flexes his or her arms at the elbows and wrists in response to painful stimuli to the nail beds (decorticate rigidity).
2. Child extends his or her arms (straightens the elbows) in response to painful stimuli (cerebrate rigidity).
1. Child has no motor response to pain on any extremity.

Verbal Response

5. Child is oriented to time, place, and person (child over age 4 years knows name, date, and where he or she is; infant appears to recognize parent).
4. Child is able to converse, although not oriented to time, place, or person (does not know who or where he or she is; infant says words but does not appear to differentiate parents from others).
3. Child speaks only in words or phrases that make little or no sense ("I want frazzle no"; infant's vocabulary is less than it is normally).
2. Child responds with incomprehensible sounds, such as groans.
1. Child does not respond verbally at all.

Modified from Teasdale, G., & Bennett, B. (1974). Assessment of coma and impaired consciousness: A practical scale. *Lancet, 2*(7872), 81–84.

however, because coma reflects a major health problem to children.

NURSING DIAGNOSES AND RELATED INTERVENTIONS

Care of the child in coma is directed toward maintaining body function in an optimum state until the child reawakens.

Nursing Diagnosis: Risk for ineffective airway clearance related to brain stem pressure

Outcome Identification: Child's airway will remain unobstructed during course of illness.

Outcome Evaluation: Child's respiratory rate remains between 16 and 20 breaths per minute; there are no retractions or signs of obstruction.

Some children who are comatose will require endotracheal intubation or tracheostomy to ensure an open airway. Some will be placed on mechanical ventilation. Oxygen may be prescribed if arterial blood gases reveal poor oxygenation of body cells (Po_2 below 80 mmHg). Endotracheal tubes are replaced with a tracheostomy after 3 or 4 days to prevent necrosis of the pharynx from pressure of the tube.

Nursing Diagnosis: Risk for impaired skin integrity related to lack of mobility

Outcome Identification: Skin will remain intact during the period of coma.

Outcome Evaluation: Child exhibits no areas of broken or irritated skin.

Bathe children who are comatose daily to stimulate skin circulation. Include the hair as part of the bath about every 3 days. Change their position at least every 2 h to prevent pressure ulcer formation and development of hydrostatic pneumonia from pooled secretions. When turning, assess skin for reddened points. Keep linen dry and free from wrinkles. Perform thorough passive range-of-motion exercises to maintain muscle tone and prevent contractures. Using sheepskin, an egg carton, or an alternating pressure or water mattress also can be important in decreasing pressure to the skin.

Nursing Diagnosis: Risk for imbalanced nutrition, less than body requirements related to inability to take in oral food or fluid

Outcome Identification: Child will remain well nourished during period of coma.

Outcome Evaluation: Child's skin turgor is normal; weight remains within acceptable percentile; hourly urine output remains over 1 mL/kg/h.

Children who are unconscious cannot be fed orally or they might aspirate. Therefore, nutrition must be maintained by nasogastric (NG) or gastrostomy tube feedings, IV fluid, or total parenteral nutrition. IV fluid is only a short-term answer because adequate protein and fat cannot be supplied solely by this route. NG or gastrostomy feedings can supply total nutrient needs. Always aspirate the tube for stomach contents before giving a feeding to check tube placement and assess gastric residual amounts. Always return any amount of stomach residue aspirated because if this is discarded each time, the child will lose a large amount of stomach acid, possibly leading to alkalosis. Check whether the amount of the feeding should be reduced by the amount of fluid remaining in the stomach before feeding the full amount of prescribed formula.

Give mouth care at least twice daily with clear water and a padded tongue blade. Coat lips with petrolatum to prevent drying and cracking. If the child's eyes tend to dry, close them to prevent corneal ulceration. Artificial tears (methylcellulose) may be prescribed to keep eyes from drying.

✔ CHECKPOINT QUESTIONS

5. What is the most common underlying cause of a coma in a child?
6. A child has a Glasgow Coma score of 10. What does this score indicate?

ABDOMINAL TRAUMA

When children are brought to a health care facility after suffering a multiple-injury trauma, several medical specialists may be required: a neurosurgeon for consultation about a head injury; an orthopedic physician for consultation about a fractured extremity; and a thoracic surgeon to intubate or investigate lung trauma. The nurse may serve the important function as the person who is best able to observe a total child and recognize subtle signs such as abdominal trauma.

Assessment

Abdominal trauma can result from any object striking the abdomen, such as a baseball bat or a seat belt drawing tight after a motor vehicle crash (Jordan, 2001). Assess vital signs frequently until they are stable. Hypotension (under 80 mmHg systolic pressure in older children; under 60 mmHg in infants) generally suggests hemorrhage, which may be hidden abdominal bleeding. In addition, children may have increasing pallor and rapid respirations. If internal bleeding is present, blood pressure will show little improvement when IV fluid is administered.

When abdominal trauma is suspected, an NG tube is passed and stomach contents are aspirated to be checked visually for blood and to test for occult blood. Attach the tube to low intermittent suction if the presence of blood is established. An indwelling urinary (Foley) catheter is also inserted to evaluate urine for blood and urine output. Evidence of blood in the urine or decreased output may indicate accompanying kidney or bladder trauma. If the urine contains blood, an emergency IV pyelogram may be ordered. Be aware that having NG tubes or catheters passed is always frightening for children (unsure of their anatomy, they have no clear idea where the tubes are going). After an accident, when they are already frightened, they need a great deal of support to accept these procedures (see Focus on Communication).

An abdominal x-ray or sonogram may be ordered to rule out a fractured pelvis, a condition that could contribute to blood loss. Air under the diaphragm on the x-ray suggests gastric or intestinal rupture with the escape of air from these organs into the peritoneal cavity. Free fluid in the abdomen, shown on x-ray when children are turned on their side, suggests leakage of bowel fluid or splenic rupture and pooling of blood. If the x-ray does not suggest the source of the fluid, an abdominal paracentesis may be done. This procedure is very frightening to children not only because it is intrusive, but also because children's abdomens are likely to be tender. Parents may be so frightened by the sight of the procedure that they are unable to remain with a child while this is done. A nurse, therefore, needs to be present to offer support (Fig. 52-6).

For a paracentesis, children are placed in a sitting or side-lying position; their abdomen is cleaned with an antiseptic and covered with a sterile drape. Caution children

FOCUS ON COMMUNICATION

Danny, a 6-year-old boy with multiple trauma, comes into the emergency room with his father. He is being assessed for abdominal injuries.

Less Effective Communication

Mr. Varton: Why are you looking at his belly? He didn't hurt that.

Nurse: We need to investigate his entire body just to make sure that there aren't any problems. He's had major trauma. He needs to have a central intravenous line and indwelling urinary catheter inserted and a CT scan to rule out any problems.

Mr. Varton: Are you sure? I don't want to put him through any more. He's already in so much pain, and he's so upset. I'm just not sure about all this stuff. What if something else goes wrong?

Nurse: If you don't consent to these tests and treatments, we cannot take care of your child.

Mr. Varton: He needs help. Do what you have to. But I'm still not sure.

More Effective Communication

Mr. Varton: Why are you looking at his belly? He didn't hurt that.

Nurse: We need to investigate his entire body just to make sure that there aren't any problems. He's had major trauma. He needs to have a central intravenous line and indwelling urinary catheter inserted and a CT scan to rule out any problems.

Mr. Varton: Are you sure? I don't want to put him through any more.

Nurse: If you consent to these tests, we will be better able to care for your child.

Mr. Varton: He's already in so much pain and he's so upset. I'm just not sure about all this stuff. What if something else goes wrong?

Nurse: This must be very difficult for you to see your child in such pain. Can you tell me how you're feeling or what you're afraid of?

Mr. Varton: I'm really not sure. I'm just so scared that he might die.

Nurse: That's understandable. Let me explain a little more about what we're doing and why these things are necessary. Maybe I can help to calm some of those fears.

In the first scenario, the nurse focuses on obtaining the parent's consent but fails to recognize the fear and apprehension in the parent. In the second scenario, the nurse recognizes and attends to the fears of the parent, helping to establish a sense of support and trust.

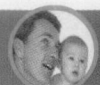

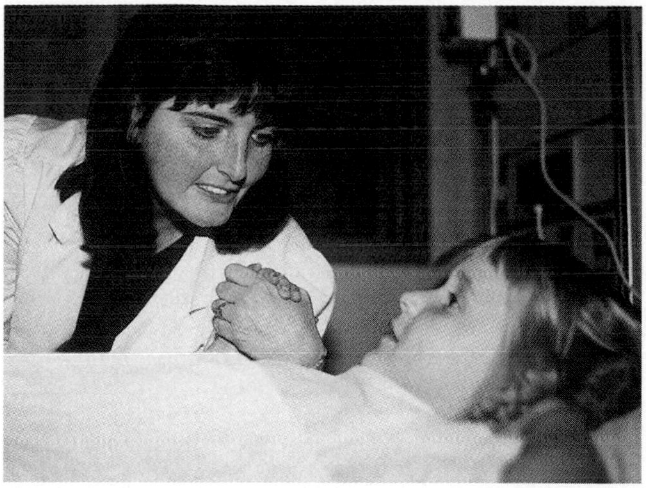

FIGURE 52.6 Prior to a paracentesis, a nurse provides support to the child to help alleviate her fears.

that they will feel a pinprick as a local anesthetic is inserted into their abdominal wall and feel pressure as the paracentesis needle is inserted. Appreciate children's concern. It is almost impossible for them to lie or sit still while the procedure is being done. Comments such as "Don't cry; be a good boy" are not therapeutic. "It's all right to cry; I know this is scary" is much more comforting and achieves better results, because it lets children know that you understand what you are asking of them.

Parents often find it difficult to appreciate the seriousness of abdominal trauma, because the signs are not as dramatic or obvious as those of fractured extremities or lacerations. Some parents may not bring a child to an emergency department immediately after abdominal trauma, because they are unaware that serious injury can result to this part of the body. Without frightening them, explain that an injury need not be obvious at first glance to be serious and need care. They may ask why an x-ray is necessary. When children are asked to turn on the x-ray table so that an abdominal fluid level can be revealed, they may perceive this as unnecessary manipulation of an injured child.

NURSING DIAGNOSES AND RELATED INTERVENTIONS

Nursing Diagnosis: Pain related to abdominal injury

Outcome Identification: Child will experience a tolerable level of pain during period of recovery.

Outcome Evaluation: Child states that level of pain is tolerable; child does not grimace when body parts are touched.

Routinely, analgesics are not administered to most children after abdominal trauma so that pain is not masked and that the location of the pain can help identify which organs may be injured. If parents did not recognize that the child was injured, guilt and fear may compound the problem. Goal setting is usually concerned with the immediate diagnostic procedures or surgery that is anticipated. Interventions differ according to the specific injury present.

Splenic Rupture

In children, the spleen is the most frequently injured organ in abdominal trauma because the organ is usually palpable under the lower left ribs. It is an organ frequently injured from inappropriately applied seat belts in automobiles and from handlebar injuries in bicycle accidents (Jordan, 2001). Children with splenic injury will have tenderness in the left upper quadrant, especially on deep inspiration, when the diaphragm moves down and touches the spleen. They may hold their left shoulder elevated to keep the diaphragm raised on the left side to keep this from happening. Occasionally, children will notice radiated left shoulder pain when they lie in a supine position (Kehr's sign). An abdominal x-ray will show little about the spleen itself but perhaps will reveal a broken rib over the spleen, suggesting the extent of the trauma to that area. Fluid in the abdomen will suggest bleeding from some source. Obtaining blood on abdominal paracentesis strongly suggests splenic rupture.

An IV line is started immediately for fluid replacement, and an IV pyelogram will be done to rule out damage to the left kidney, which, because of its location in that area, may also have suffered trauma. A complete blood count is done to estimate the extent of the blood loss. Blood is typed and cross-matched so blood for replacement can then be readied if necessary. Children will be admitted to an observation unit if the blood loss from rupture appears mild. If bleeding is severe, immediate surgery such as a partial or total splenectomy may be necessary to halt bleeding and save their life.

After a splenectomy, children are very susceptible to infection, particularly pneumococcal infections. Therefore, a large percentage of children are managed expectantly to see if the bleeding will halt without spleen removal (Leone & Hammond, 2001).

Liver Rupture

Children with liver rupture or laceration usually have severe abdominal pain, most marked on inspiration when the diaphragm descends and touches the liver. They show symptoms of blood loss, including tachycardia, hypotension, anxiety, and pallor. Their hematocrit will be low or falling. Such children need to be prepared for immediate surgery, because the liver is a highly vascular organ, and blood loss from it is acute and possibly life threatening.

Occasionally, a communication between an artery and a bile duct occurs at the time of trauma. With this, symptoms are not immediate, but gastrointestinal (GI) bleeding, such as hematemesis, or melena may occur in a few days. The child may have colicky upper abdominal pain that may be relieved by emesis. Liver studies, such as a liver arteriogram, will be necessary to reveal the extent of the problem.

After both liver and spleen surgery, children need careful observation for return of bowel function, assessment for the possibility that peritonitis may develop, and careful reintroduction of oral nutrition.

DENTAL TRAUMA

Injuries to teeth occur most often from falls in which children strike their upper front incisors and from blows to the face by objects such as baseball bats or hockey sticks. They are always potentially serious because they can lead to aspiration of the injured teeth or malalignment of future teeth. When a tooth is knocked out, parents should rinse the tooth in water and replace it in the child's mouth or drop the tooth in a salt solution or milk and bring it to the emergency department with them (McTigue, 2000). If permanent teeth that have been knocked out recently are washed with saline in the emergency department and replaced, there is a good chance that they will reimplant successfully. Some dentists advocate immersing the tooth in an antiseptic and then an antibiotic solution before replacing it. If a tooth is replaced, it generally is wired into place to hold it in good alignment. Children receive a course of oral antibiotics, such as penicillin, to prevent infection. They must eat only soft food until the tooth has firmly adhered, approximately 2 weeks.

If a blow to a child's teeth was extensive, an x-ray may be taken to rule out a mandibular or maxillary fracture. If a portion of a tooth cannot be located, the possibility of aspiration must be considered and confirmed or ruled out by a chest x-ray. In young children, often a tooth is not knocked out but is pushed back up into the gum. These teeth gradually regrow, and, although they may darken in color, they usually are healthy. If the affected tooth is a deciduous tooth, the permanent tooth is rarely injured even though it is already formed in the gum. At the appropriate time, the permanent tooth will erupt normally.

✔ CHECKPOINT QUESTIONS

7. What does air under the diaphragm on abdominal x-ray suggest?
8. Which organ is most frequently injured in the child with abdominal trauma?

NEAR DROWNING

Drowning is defined as death due to suffocation from submersion in liquid. Inhaled water fills and, therefore, blocks the exchange of oxygen in the alveoli. More than 3,500 children die from drowning annually. It is the second most common cause of death by unintentional injury among children (Battan & Dart, 2001). The term **near drowning** is used to describe the child with a submersion injury who requires emergency treatment and who survives the first 24 h after injury (Shaw, 2000).

Most infant drownings occur in bathtubs; 1- to 4-year-old children most frequently drown in artificial pools; older children most frequently drown in bodies of fresh water (Brenner et al., 2001). The majority of drowning accidents that take place outside the home occur in the summer months, when more children are swimming and boating. Particularly at risk are male adolescents because they may take dares to swim farther than their ability allows or swim under the influence of alcohol, which impairs their decision-making ability and their physical coordination.

Pathophysiology of Drowning

When children's heads are submerged, and they first inhale water, they cough violently from the irritation of the water in their nose and throat. If they cannot get their head out of water at this point, water will enter the larynx. This causes the larynx to spasm, preventing any further water but also air from entering the trachea, so asphyxia results. If children are ventilated at this point, treatment generally is very effective because there is little water in the lungs. The condition more closely simulates asphyxia that occurs with croup or when a foreign body, such as a nut, lodges in the larynx and stops air flow.

If treatment is not given at this point, the larynx relaxes from the asphyxia and water enters the lungs. Children can no longer exchange oxygen, because the alveoli fill with water. Hypoxia deepens, and cardiac arrest occurs.

Additional changes that occur when water enters the lungs depend on whether the water is fresh or salt. Salt water is hypertonic, causing fluid to osmose from the bloodstream and enter the alveoli, increasing the amount of fluid in the lung tissue. Tachycardia and decreased blood pressure from hypovolemia will result. Blood viscosity will increase (increased hematocrit level). The presence of pulmonary edema will cause increased hypoxia.

Fresh water is hypotonic, so fluid in the lungs shifts into the bloodstream due to changes in osmotic pressure. This may lead to hemolysis of red blood cells, a dilution of plasma, and possible hypervolemia with tachycardia and increased blood pressure. If the release of potassium from destroyed red blood cells is great enough with freshwater drowning, cardiac arrhythmias may occur. In both instances, loss of surfactant from the lung alveoli, caused by introduction of water, can lead to alveolar collapse.

Hyperventilating before swimming should be discouraged. When children blow off carbon dioxide this way, during an extended period of underwater swimming, carbon dioxide levels rise, but not adequately to cause them to experience distress. This results in decreased oxygen levels with drowsiness and listlessness (children drown without struggling or realizing their danger).

Very young children display a mammalian diving reflex when they plunge under cold water. Immediately, a lifesaving bradycardia and shunting of blood away from the periphery of their body to their brain and heart occur. This is triggered when water is 70°F (21°C) or less and their face is submerged first. This explains why very young children can survive better than other children after being submerged in water that is very cold (32°F to 60°F; 0°C to 15°C; Gheen, 2001).

Emergency Management

When children are pulled from the water after near drowning, mouth-to-mouth resuscitation should be started at once. If cardiac arrest has occurred from hypoxia, simultaneous measures to initiate cardiac action must be taken. The techniques of cardiopulmonary resuscitation for infants and children are discussed in Chapter 41.

Assuming that cardiopulmonary resuscitation is effective, children need follow-up care at a health care facility, because they are certain to be acidotic from accumulated carbon dioxide and hypoxia (from lack of oxygen because of the water in the alveoli) and are at risk for respiratory infection from contaminants in the water.

Follow-up care aims to increase children's oxygen and carbon dioxide exchange capacity, using the lung areas that are not filled with water. Typically, children are intubated with a cuffed intratracheal tube; mechanical ventilation with positive end-expiratory pressure may be necessary to force air into the alveoli. Because children swallow water, vomiting usually occurs as the child is revived. The cuff of the intratracheal tube prevents vomitus from being aspirated. Children are given 100% oxygen so that as much space as possible in the available lung alveoli can be used. An NG tube is inserted to decompress the stomach, prevent vomiting, and free up breathing space. Generally, albuterol is administered by aerosol to prevent bronchospasm and, again, to allow children to make maximum use of the oxygen administered. If a child aspirated salt water, plasma may be administered to replace protein being lost into the lungs and prevent hypovolemia.

If the child's body temperature is very low, gradual warming (not using a warming blanket) is advised so metabolism need does not rise sharply before alveolar space is ready to accommodate this. Extracorporeal membrane oxygenation may be used.

Unfortunately, neurologic damage occurs in as many as 21% of near-drowning incidents. If the child is awake or only lethargic at the scene of the accident and immediately afterward in the hospital, the prognosis is greatly improved over that of the child who is comatose (Battan & Dart, 2001).

NURSING DIAGNOSES AND RELATED INTERVENTIONS

Nursing Diagnosis: Risk for infection related to foreign substance in respiratory tract

Outcome Identification: Child will remain free of signs and symptoms of infection after near drowning.

Outcome Evaluation: Child's temperature remains within age-acceptable parameters orally; crackles are absent on lung auscultation; respiratory rate is within age-acceptable parameters.

Children may be placed on a prophylactic antibiotic therapy to prevent pneumonia and additional airway interference. Assess vital signs and auscultate lung sounds for adventitious sounds, such as crackles or fine rhonchi. Turning the child every 2 h if on bedrest and encouraging deep breathing and incentive spirometry every hour help to aerate the lungs fully and prevent the accumulation of fluid, which promotes infection.

Nursing Diagnosis: Fear related to near-drowning experience

Outcome Identification: Child will demonstrate that she can manage this degree of fear.

Outcome Evaluation: Child discusses fears; child states that he or she understands that, although frightening, the experience is over, and she is now safe.

Children may be admitted to an observation unit for monitoring of blood gases until water from the alveoli is absorbed and they once again can ventilate effectively on their own. Children may wake at night from a nightmare that they are drowning. They need parents to reassure them that they are now safe and definitely out of the water. Near drowning is a thoroughly frightening experience. Encourage children to verbalize this fright. They will need support from parents before they engage in an activity such as swimming again after such a frightening experience.

✔ CHECKPOINT QUESTIONS

9. What do very young children display when they plunge into cold water?
10. What is the rationale for prophylactic antibiotic therapy after a near-drowning episode?

POISONING

Poisoning occurs most commonly in children between the ages of 2 and 3 years and in all socioeconomic groups. Common agents in childhood poisoning include soaps, cosmetics, detergents or cleaners, and plants. Poisoning can occur from over-the-counter drugs, such as vitamins, iron compounds, aspirin, or acetaminophen, or prescription drugs, such as antidepressants. Poisoning is entirely preventable. Parents need education about the high risk for poisoning and strategies for maintaining a home environment that is safe for children of all ages. Be aware that when poisoning occurs in an older child, it may be a suicide attempt (Gauvin, Bailey & Bratton, 2001).

NURSING DIAGNOSES AND RELATED INTERVENTIONS

Nursing Diagnosis: Risk for injury related to maturational age of child and presence of poisons

Outcome Identification: Child will not ingest a poison during childhood.

Outcome Evaluation: Parents identify poisonous and toxic items in the home and describe how they are stored safely; parents state local poison control center number; parents describe measures to seek help immediately if poisoning occurs.

Emergency Management of Poisoning at Home

Teach parents that, if they discover that a child has swallowed a poison, they should immediately call the emergency poison control center number in their community. Information they need to provide includes the following:

- Child's name, telephone number, address, weight, and age and what the child swallowed
- How long ago the poisoning occurred
- The route of poisoning (oral, inhaled, sprayed on skin)

- How much of the poison the child took (This may be difficult for parents to judge if they do not know how much was in the bottle. If they just answer, "a whole bottle," ask them to read from the bottle how much that is.)
- If the poison was in pill form, whether there are pills scattered under a chair or if they are all missing and presumed swallowed
- What was swallowed; if the name of a medicine is not known, what it was prescribed for and a description of it (color, size, shape of pills)
- The child's present condition (sleepy, hyperactive, comatose)

If one child has swallowed a poison, parents should investigate whether other children have also poisoned themselves. A preschooler often gives a younger sibling some of the "candy" he or she has been eating. Ask if parents have transportation to the health care facility or if they need an ambulance.

Although syrup of ipecac is rarely used in emergency departments today, the American Academy of Pediatrics recommends that parents keep a bottle of syrup of ipecac (an emetic) with their emergency first aid supplies (see Focus on Pharmacology: Syrup of Ipecac) for use in home poisoning emergencies. Before they administer this emetic, however, they should call a poison control center to make certain that vomiting is desirable (Shannon, 2000). Unless the poison was a caustic, corrosive, or a hydrocarbon, vomiting is an effective way to remove the poison from the body. In 90% of children, vomiting will occur within 20 min of being given ipecac. If vomiting does not occur in 20 to 30 min, another dose of ipecac can be given. Parents may be asked to bring any vomited material with them to the health care facility so it can be analyzed for content.

FOCUS ON PHARMACOLOGY

Syrup of Ipecac

Action: Syrup of ipecac is an emetic agent used in the treatment of drug overdose and poisoning. Commonly recommended for parents to administer at home after childhood poisoning, it produces vomiting by locally irritating the gastrointestinal mucosa and stimulating the brain's chemotrigger receptor zone for vomiting.

Pregnancy risk category: C

Dosage: For children <1 year: 5 to 10 mL orally followed by 1 glass (200 mL) of water or clear fluid. For children >1 year: 15 mL orally followed by 2 to 3 glasses of water or clear fluid. Dosage may be repeated if vomiting does not occur within 20 min.

Possible adverse effects: Mild CNS depression, nausea, diarrhea.

Nursing Implications

- Keep in mind that, in the emergency department, activated charcoal will be administered if vomiting of ipecac does not occur or if ipecac overdose occurs.
- If the child doesn't vomit within 30 min of the dose, prepare to repeat the dose.
- Know that ipecac is administered to a conscious child only. Do not give ipecac after activated charcoal is given; charcoal will inactivate the ipecac.
- Instruct parents to keep this drug readily available in the home in case of accidental poisoning. Advise them to call the local poison control center for instructions before administering it.
- If vomiting is indicated for poisoning, tell parents to administer the drug as soon as possible after poisoning.
- Teach parents about the possible sources of poisons in the home and how to minimize the risk of poisoning.

Emergency Management of Poisoning at the Health Care Facility

In the emergency department, the best method to deactivate a poison is the administration of activated charcoal, either orally or by way of NG tube.

Activated charcoal is supplied as a fine black powder that is mixed with water for administration. A sweet syrup may be added to the mixture to make it more palatable. As the charcoal is excreted through the bowel over the next 3 days, stools will appear black (see Focus on Pharmacology: Activated Charcoal).

Always follow emergency measures with an education program for the family to prevent poisoning from happening again. Specific measures for each age group are discussed in previous chapters with problems and concerns of the age group.

Acetaminophen Poisoning

Acetaminophen (Tylenol) is the most frequent drug causing childhood poisoning today because parents use acetaminophen to treat childhood fevers (Shannon, 2000). Told that acetaminophen is safer than aspirin, parents may not be as careful about putting this substance away as they were with aspirin. If their child swallows acetaminophen, they may delay bringing him or her for help, thinking it is a harmless drug.

Acetaminophen in large doses, however, is not an innocent drug. It can cause extreme liver destruction. Immediately after ingestion, the child will experience anorexia, nausea, and vomiting. Soon, serum aspartate transaminase (AST [SGOT]) and serum alanine transaminase (ALT [SGPT]) liver enzymes become elevated. The liver may be tender as liver toxicity occurs.

Parents should call their local poison control center and may be advised to administer syrup of ipecac to induce vomiting. In the emergency department, activated charcoal or acetylcysteine, the specific antidote for acetaminophen poisoning, will be administered. Acetylcysteine prevents hepatotoxicity by binding with the breakdown product of acetaminophen so it will not bind to liver cells. Unfortunately, acetylcysteine has an offensive odor and taste. Administer it in a carbonated beverage to help the child swallow it. In small children, it is administered directly

FOCUS ON PHARMACOLOGY

Activated Charcoal

Action: Activated charcoal, an antidote for poisoning, absorbs toxic substances that have been swallowed to prevent them from being absorbed from the stomach

Pregnancy Risk Category: C

Dosage: Provided as a powder that must be mixed with water and administered orally or by way of nasogastric (NG) tube.

Possible Adverse Effects: Vomiting, diarrhea, black stools.

Nursing Implications

- Administer orally to conscious victims only.
- Give the drug as soon as possible after poisoning.
- Store the drug in a closed container because it absorbs gases from the air and is inactivated.
- Know that the solution feels gritty and tastes disagreeable so young children have difficulty swallowing the drug. May need to be administered by NG tube.
- Caution child or parent that stools will be black for several days after administration.

into an NG tube to avoid this difficulty. If the child is admitted to an observation unit, continue to observe for jaundice and tenderness over the liver; assess ALT and AST levels as ordered.

NURSING DIAGNOSES AND RELATED INTERVENTIONS

Nursing Diagnosis: Situational low self-esteem related to child's poisoning

Outcome Identification: Parents demonstrate confidence in their ability to provide safe care for the child (and other family members) within 24 h.

Outcome Evaluation: Parents state guidelines for continued assessment of child at home; parents state ways they can improve "childproofing."

After the child is stabilized, take some time to talk to parents about how they feel about this event. Remember that poisoning tends to happen in homes where there is stress. If stress was already present, how has this poisoning added to it?

Before children are discharged from a health care facility, be certain parents are comfortable with any further assessment measures they will need to continue at home, such as temperature taking and urging a high fluid intake. Talk to the parents about childproofing their home.

Caustic Poisoning

Ingestion of a strong alkali, such as lye, often contained in toilet bowl cleaners or hair care products, may cause burns and tissue necrosis in the mouth, esophagus, and stomach.

Assessment

After a caustic ingestion, the child has immediate pain in the mouth and throat and drools saliva from oral edema and an inability to swallow. The mouth turns white immediately from the burn. Later, the mouth turns brown as edema and ulceration occur. There may be such marked edema of the lips and mouth that it is difficult to examine them. The child may immediately vomit blood, mucus, and necrotic tissue. The loss of blood from the denuded, burned surface may lead to systemic signs of tachycardia, tachypnea, pallor, and hypotension.

A chest x-ray may be ordered to determine if pulmonary involvement has occurred from any aspirated poison or an esophageal perforation has allowed poison to seep into the mediastinum. An esophagoscopy under conscious sedation may be done to assess the esophagus, although this test may be omitted because there is a possibility an esophagoscope might perforate the burned esophagus. After 2 weeks, a barium swallow may be ordered to reveal the final extent of the esophageal burns.

Therapeutic Management

Parents should always call a poison control center to ask for advice on how to proceed. With caustic poisoning, vomiting should not be induced, because the corrosive substance will burn as it comes up just as it did going down. Parents will be advised to immediately take the child to a health care facility for treatment.

There is a high possibility that pharyngeal edema will be severe enough to obstruct a child's airway by even 20 min after the burn. Intubation may be necessary to provide a patent airway.

To detect respiratory interference, assess vital signs closely, especially respiratory rate. In infants, increasing restlessness is an important accompanying sign. Assess children for the degree of pain involved. A strong analgesic, such as morphine, may need to be ordered and administered to achieve pain relief.

NURSING DIAGNOSES AND RELATED INTERVENTIONS

Nursing Diagnosis: Risk for ineffective airway clearance related to burns of esophagus and mouth

Outcome Identification: Child will maintain adequate respiratory function.

Outcome Evaluation: Child's respiration rate will remain within 16 to 20 breaths per minute.

Starting therapy immediately with a steroid such as dexamethasone (Decadron) and continuing it for about 4 weeks may be prescribed to reduce the chance of permanent esophageal scarring. In addition, children may be placed on a prophylactic antibiotic to reduce the possibility of infection and additional inflammation in the denuded mouth and esophageal area.

Children who respond well to steroid therapy usually will recover with no important sequelae. Children who do not receive steroid therapy for some reason may be left with scarring of the esophagus, resulting in complete obstruction. To correct complete obstruction, repeated surgical procedures are necessary. Sometimes transplantation of intestinal tissue or a synthetic graft is required to replace stenosed esophageal tissue.

Nursing Diagnosis: Risk for imbalanced nutrition, less than body requirements related to esophageal stricture from burn scarring

Outcome Identification: Child will ingest an adequate intake for age after ingestion.

Outcome Evaluation: Child's diet meets recommended daily allowance requirements for age.

Oral intake commonly will be a problem for the first week because of soreness in the child's mouth. Observe children carefully the first time they drink to observe for signs, such as coughing, choking, or cyanosis, indicative of esophageal perforation. IV fluid may be needed as a supplement. If a child is totally unable to swallow, gastrostomy feedings or total parenteral nutrition may be necessary. When children are able to take food, they should begin with a liquid diet. Liquid passing through the burned and scarring esophagus tends to maintain esophageal patency, so it is therapeutic for the burn and nutritious for the child.

Hydrocarbon Ingestion

Hydrocarbons are substances contained in products such as kerosene and furniture polish. Because these substances are volatile, fumes rise from them, and their major effect is respiratory irritation (see Chapter 40).

✔ CHECKPOINT QUESTIONS

11. What is the specific antidote for acetaminophen poisoning?
12. When is vomiting contraindicated with poisoning in a child?

Iron Poisoning

Iron is frequently swallowed by small children because it is an ingredient in vitamin preparations, particularly pregnancy vitamins. When it is ingested, it is corrosive to the gastric mucosa, so leads to the signs and symptoms of that. The immediate effects include nausea and vomiting, diarrhea, and abdominal pain. After 6 h, these symptoms fade, and the child's condition appears to improve. By this time, however, hemorrhagic necrosis of the lining of the GI tract has occurred. By 12 h, melena (blood in stool) and hematemesis (blood in emesis) will be present. Lethargy and coma, cyanosis, and vasomotor collapse may occur. Coagulation defects may occur; hepatic injury also can result. Shock from an increase in peripheral vascular resistance and decreased cardiac output can occur. Long-term effects can be gastric scarring from fibrotic tissue formation (Fine, 2000).

Assessment

It is difficult to estimate the amount of iron a child has swallowed, because parents can only guess at the number of pills in the bottle. In addition, the amount of elemental iron in compounds varies. Serum iron level should be measured to establish a baseline.

Therapeutic Management

Parents should contact their poison control center, which may advise them to administer syrup of ipecac to remove any iron not yet absorbed. A cathartic may be given to help a child pass enteric-coated iron pills. Activated charcoal has no effect.

A child who has ingested a potentially toxic dose is given a chelating agent, such as IV or intramuscular (IM) deferoxamine. Chelating agents combine with metal and allow metal to be excreted from the body. Deferoxamine causes urine to turn orange as iron is excreted.

An exchange transfusion is another way that excess iron can be removed from the body (Batton & Dart, 2001). An upper GI series and liver studies may be ordered 1 week after ingestion to screen for long-term effects. The hope is that the iron load was removed from the stomach in time so that not all of it was absorbed.

Assist with emergency measures, such as gastric lavage, and administer chelating agents as ordered. Parents may be asked to test any stool passed for the next 3 days for occult blood to assess for stomach irritation and subsequent GI bleeding. Be certain that parents understand how to do this accurately.

NURSING DIAGNOSES AND RELATED INTERVENTIONS

Nursing Diagnosis: Deficient parental knowledge related to the danger of iron as a poison

Outcome Identification: Parents will acknowledge that iron is a dangerous substance to children in toxic dosages after the ingestion.

Outcome Evaluation: Parents state ways they have safeguarded their child from future iron exposure.

Iron poisoning occurs frequently because parents do not think of iron pills or vitamins containing iron as real medicine. Additionally, because many children's vitamins are manufactured as familiar television or cartoon characters, children often think of vitamins as candy.

When you instruct parents to use an iron supplement for themselves or their children, stress that overdoses can be fatal to small children. Teach them to think of iron as they would any other medicine and keep it out of the reach of small children.

WHAT IF? A 3-year-old girl is seen in the emergency room after ingesting prenatal vitamins. For what clinical manifestations of systemic toxicity would you observe?

Lead Poisoning

Lead in the body interferes with red blood cell function by blocking the incorporation of iron into the protoporphyrin compound that makes up the heme portion of hemoglobin in red blood cells (Godwin, 2001). This leads to a hypochromic, microcytic anemia. Kidney destruction may occur, causing excess excretion of amino acids, glucose, and phosphates in the urine. The most serious effects include lead encephalitis or inflammation of brain cells from the toxic lead content. Lead poisoning (**plumbism**), like all forms of poisoning in children, tends to occur most often in the toddler and preschool child (see Chapter 29 for measures to prevent lead poisoning).

Assessment

The usual source of ingested lead is from paint chips or paint dust, home-glazed pottery or fumes from burning batteries (Battan & Dart, 2001). Paint tastes sweet, and a child will repeatedly pick chips up off the floor or off the walls. If a crib rail is painted with lead paint, a child will ingest it as he or she teethes on the rail. Chewing on windowsills is also common. In fishing communities, swallowing lead sinkers can be a common source. Restoring an older home saturates the air with lead dust. In such homes, lead plumbing also may contaminate the drinking water.

The most widely used method of screening for lead levels is the blood lead determination (serum ferritin). Unfortunately, this test requires using atomic absorption spectrophotometry, which is a costly procedure. Free erythrocyte protoporphyrin tests are a simple screening procedure, involving only a finger stick. Because protoporphyrin is blocked from entering heme by lead, it will be elevated in lead poisoning.

Many children with fairly high blood lead levels are asymptomatic. Others show insidious symptoms of anorexia and abdominal pain from the presence of lead in the stomach. One of the major effects of excessive lead levels is encephalopathy. The child usually has beginning symptoms of lethargy, impulsiveness, and learning difficulties. As the child's blood level of lead increases, severe encephalopathy with seizures and permanent neurologic damage will result.

Basophilic stippling (an odd striation of basophils) may be apparent on a blood smear. An x-ray of the abdomen may reveal paint chips in the intestinal tract (Fig. 52-7*A*). "Lead lines" (areas of increased density) may be present near the epiphyseal line of long bones (see Figure 52-7*B*). The thickness of the line shows the length of time lead ingestion has been occurring. Damage to the kidney nephrons from the presence of lead leads to proteinuria, ketonuria, and glycosuria. CSF may have an increased protein level. Lead poisoning is usually said to be present when the child has two successive blood lead levels greater than 10 μg/dL. A classification of levels of lead poisoning is shown in Table 52-3.

Therapeutic Management

A child with a blood lead level between 10 and 14 μg/dL needs to be rescreened to confirm the level. If the lead level is 15 or above, the child needs active interventions to prevent further lead exposure. These interventions may include removing the child from the environment containing the lead source or removing the source of lead from the child's environment. Removing the lead source may be difficult. If the family lives in a rented apartment, the landlord may be legally obligated to remove the lead. Simple repainting or wallpapering does not remove a source of peeling paint adequately. After some months, the new paint will begin to peel because of the defective paint underneath. The walls must be covered by paneling or masonite. All children with lead levels over 20 μg/100 mL require treatment with an oral chelating agent such as succimer (see Focus on Pharmacology: Succimer [Chemet]).

Children with blood lead levels of greater than 45 μg/100 mL may be admitted to the hospital for chelating therapy with agents such as dimercaprol (BAL) or edetate calcium disodium (CaEDTA), administered IM (Campbell, 2000).

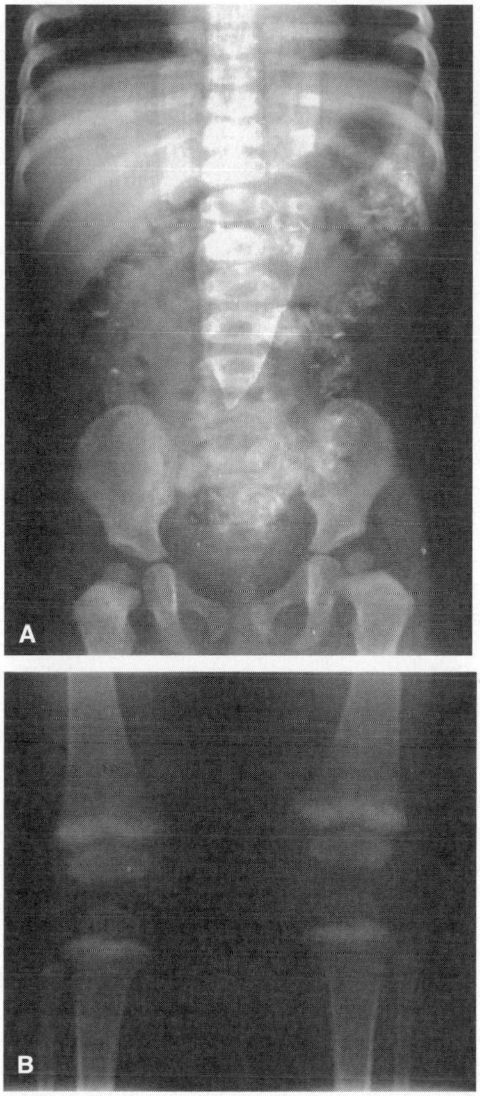

FIGURE 52.7 (*A*) Ingested paint chips (white crescents) in the intestinal tract. (*B*) A radiograph of the long bones of a child with chronic lead ingestion showing the characteristic "lead line" or white marking at the epiphyseal line.

TABLE 52.3 Classification of Lead Poisoning Risk

CLASS	LEAD BLOOD LEVEL CONCENTRATION (μg/dL)	RECOMMENDED ACTION
Class I (low risk)	Under 9	Retest at 24 months for children 6 to 35 months of age who are considered low risk; retest every 6 months for those 6 to 35 months of age who are considered high risk
Class IIa (rescreen)	10–14	Retest yearly; continue retesting yearly for children over 36 months of age until the age of 6 years
Class IIb (moderate risk)	15–19	Retest every 3 to 4 months for children 6 to 35 months of age
Class III (high risk)	20–44	Retest every 3 to 4 months; begin home abatement program
Class IV (urgent risk)	45–69	Initiate medical therapy and environmental remediation
Class V (urgent risk)	Greater than 70	Immediately treat with a chelating agent.

Centers for Disease Control and Prevention. (2001). *Preventing lead poisoning in young children.* Washington, DC: US Department of Health and Human Services, Public Health Service.

Chelating agents remove the lead from soft tissue and bone (although not from red blood cells) allowing it to be eliminated in the urine. Injections of EDTA, which must be given IM into a large muscle mass, are painful and may be combined with 0.5 mL of procaine. EDTA also removes calcium from the body; therefore, serum calcium must be measured periodically to determine whether it is at a safe level. Measure intake and output to ensure that kidney function is adequate to handle the lead being excreted. BUN, serum creatinine, and protein in urine may also be assessed. If kidney function is not adequate, EDTA may lead to nephrotoxicity or kidney damage.

BAL has the advantage of removing lead from red blood cells, but, because of severe toxicity, it is only used with children who have severe forms of lead intoxication. Penicillamine (Cuprimine) is another drug used for lead poisoning. It is given orally after BAL or EDTA. Weekly complete blood counts and renal and liver function tests accompany the administration of penicillamine. It may be given for as long as 3 to 6 months.

FOCUS ON PHARMACOLOGY

Succimer (Chemet)

Action: Agent forms water-soluble chelates with lead leading to increased urinary excretion of lead.

Pregnancy Risk Category: C

Dosage: Orally, starting with 10 mg/kg or 350 mg/m^2 every 8 h orally for 5 days then reducing dosage to 10 mg/kg or 350 mg/m^2 every 12 h for 2 weeks. The drug is taken for a total of 19 days.

Adverse Effects: Nausea; vomiting; loss of appetite; back, stomach, flank, head, or rib pain; chills; flulike symptoms.

Nursing Implications

- Obtain serum lead levels before beginning therapy and again at the close of therapy.
- Instruct parents and child about the need to take the full 19-day course for optimal effectiveness.
- If the child has difficulty swallowing capsules, encourage parents to open capsules and mix capsule contents with a small amount of soft food or administer capsule contents on a spoon followed by a fruit drink.
- Urge the child to drink increased amount of fluid to provide enough urine for removing the chelated lead from the body.
- Ensure that a lead abatement program is instituted concurrently to reduce the amount of lead to which the child is exposed.

NURSING DIAGNOSES AND RELATED INTERVENTIONS

Planning can be difficult because parents are upset at learning their child has been exposed to lead. They may experience a loss of self-esteem and sense of powerlessness when realizing that their financial circumstances or lifestyle has hurt their child.

Nursing Diagnosis: Deficient knowledge related to the dangers of lead ingestion

Outcome Identification: Parents will acknowledge the danger of lead ingestion to their child and potential sources of lead in their environment.

Outcome Evaluation: Parents state ways they have safeguarded their child against further lead ingestion; parents identify measures to reduce lead in the environment.

Parental education about the risk of lead poisoning is crucial. Teach parents to keep toddlers away from windowsills and other common sources of lead paint. Placing the television or an overstuffed chair against the windowsill may be effective as a temporary measure. As a rule, children's cribs should be placed about 3 ft away from walls in older homes to reduce the risk of children picking at loose wallpaper when they first wake in the morning or before they fall asleep at night (plaster, which contains lead, clings to the wallpaper).

All children with elevated lead levels need careful follow-up care to determine the seriousness of their condition and to ensure that they are kept from a lead source. Because children who recover from symptomatic lead poisoning have a high incidence of permanent neurologic damage, all children with elevated blood lead levels need appropriate follow-up care to evaluate development and intelligence (CDC, 2001).

Insecticide Poisoning

Insecticide poisoning can occur by accidental ingestion or through skin or respiratory tract contact when children play in an area that has recently been sprayed with one. Long-term exposure may result from exposure to a parent's clothing if he or she comes home covered with insecticide spray. Once thought to be only a rural problem, the increase in the use of lawn sprays by commercial companies now makes this a suburban problem as well (Battan & Dart, 2001).

Many insecticides have an organophosphate base that leads to an accumulation of acetylcholine at neuromuscular junctions. Within a few minutes to 2 h of exposure, children develop nausea and vomiting, diarrhea, excessive salivation, weakness of respiratory muscles, confusion, depressed reflexes, and possibly seizures.

In the emergency department, activated charcoal may be administered if the insecticide was swallowed. If clothing is contaminated, remove it and wash the child's skin and hair. To prevent coming in contact with the insecticide, wear gloves while bathing the child.

IV atropine and a cholinesterase reactivator, pralidoxime (Protopam chloride) are effective antidotes to reverse symptoms.

Plant Poisoning

Plant poisoning (ingestion of a growing plant) occurs because parents commonly do not think of plants as being poisonous. Common plants to which children may be exposed and the effects when they are ingested are shown in Focus on Family Empowerment.

Recreational Drug Poisoning

Adolescents and even grade-school children are brought to health care facilities by parents or friends because of a drug overdose or a "bad trip" caused by an unusual reaction or the effect of an unfortunate combination of drugs. Typical drugs involved include codeine and antidepressant drugs (Shannon, 2000).

Children are often extremely disoriented after this form of ingestion. They may be having hallucinations. Obtaining a history may be difficult because children may have no idea what they took except that it was a red or a yellow capsule. They may know but may be reluctant to name a drug if it was obtained illegally.

Assessment

Although the child may not appear to hear well or may not seem coherent, try to elicit a history from him or her. Avoid shouting or aggravating, with the knowledge that children who are having a paranoid reaction will be unable to cope rationally with this approach. If friends accompany an ill child, point out that your role is not that of a law enforcer. Your role is to help the child, and you cannot do that effectively unless the drug is identified. Approaching a child's friends this way is more likely to result in their naming the drug. If a child is brought in by parents who have no idea what drug could possibly have been taken, ask them to have someone at home check the child's bedroom for drugs (provided the child became ill while at home).

Try to determine whether the ingestion was an accident (a child was unaware that two drugs would react this way or took a wrong dose) or whether a child was actually attempting suicide. In the first instance, children will need counseling about drug use or about which drugs do not mix. If the incident was an attempted suicide, children will need observation and counseling toward more effective coping mechanisms in self-care. All poisonings or drug ingestions in children older than 7 years of age should be considered potential suicides until established otherwise.

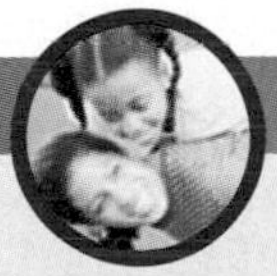

FOCUS ON FAMILY EMPOWERMENT
Identifying Poisonous Plants

Q. We never realized that plants could be poisonous to our children. Which ones should we be aware of?

A. A number of common plants can lead to poisoning in children. Here are some and the symptoms they produce:

English ivy: Nausea, vomiting, excess salivation, diarrhea, abdominal pain
Holly (berries): Vomiting, diarrhea, abdominal pain
Hydrangea: Nausea, vomiting, muscular weakness, seizures, dyspnea
Lily of the valley: Vomiting, abdominal pain, diarrhea, cardiac disturbances
Mistletoe: Vomiting, diarrhea, bradycardia
Morning glory (seeds): Nausea, diarrhea, hallucinations
Philodendron: Swelling of the tongue, lips, irritation of mouth
Poinsettia: Nausea, vomiting
Rhubarb (leaves): Irritant action on gastrointestinal tract
Rhododendron: Nausea, vomiting, abdominal pain, seizures, limb paralysis

Expect to obtain blood specimens for electrolyte levels and a toxicology screen. If a child is vomiting, save any vomitus for analysis.

Therapeutic Management

Children need supportive measures for their specific symptoms, including oxygen administration; electrolyte replacement (particularly if there is accompanying nausea and vomiting); and perhaps IV fluid administration in an attempt to dilute the drug.

Children who have swallowed a recreational drug need immediate treatment followed by empathic investigation into the events leading to the poisoning. This potentially lethal ingestion may act as a turning point in the child's life, possibly alerting the child and family to a drug problem and the need for help. Factors such as reduction of fear and anxiety, increased coping mechanisms, knowledge of the effects of drug use, and availability of referral sources for a drug problem are important areas to address (see Chapter 32 for more information related to adolescents and drug use).

✔ CHECKPOINT QUESTIONS

13. What type of agent is used for treating lead toxicity?
14. How might a child be poisoned by insecticides?

FOREIGN BODY OBSTRUCTION

Foreign bodies can become lodged in the throat or other body openings, causing stasis of secretions and infection. Direct obstruction or laceration of the mucous membrane may also result, leading to serious consequences.

Whether a foreign substance is inhaled or embedded elsewhere, nursing interventions will focus first on comforting the child and aiding in the substance's removal and then on teaching the child and parents ways to avoid such occurrences in the future.

Foreign Bodies in the Ear

Any child with a history of draining exudate from the ear canal needs an otoscopic examination to establish the reason for the drainage. In toddlers and preschoolers, the drainage often is the result of a foreign body in the ear canal. The object might be a small piece of a toy, a piece of paper, a small battery, or food, such as a peanut.

Removing foreign bodies from the ear is difficult because children are afraid that the instrument used will hurt them, so they have difficulty lying still for the procedure. If there is reason to think that the tympanic membrane is intact, irrigating the object from the ear canal with a syringe and normal saline may be possible. This should not be done if the object is a substance, such as a peanut, that will swell when wet. If it is possible that the tympanic membrane is ruptured, the ear canal must not be irrigated or fluid will be forced into the middle ear, possibly introducing infection (otitis media).

Often, it is better to wait for an otolaryngologist to care for the child, because trauma to the ear canal in an attempt to remove a foreign body will increase the edema and make removal even more difficult.

Foreign Bodies in the Nose

Foreign objects stuffed into the nose eventually cause inflammation and purulent discharge from the nares. The odor accompanying such impaction is often the first sign noticed by a parent. Objects pushed into the nose generally can be removed with forceps. A local antibiotic might be necessary after removal if ulceration resulted from the local irritation (Kalan & Tariq, 2000).

Foreign Bodies in the Esophagus

Children tend not to chew food well and to swallow portions that are too big to pass safely through the esophagus. Pieces of candy, such as Lifesavers, are common objects caught in the esophagus in young children; coins are swallowed by adolescents (Soprano & Mandl, 2001). Orthodontic appliances may become dislodged and also swallowed (Dibiase et al., 2000). Intense pain at the site where the object is lodged will result. If it is an object that will dissolve, such as a Lifesaver or a piece of digestible meat, offer the child fluid to drink to help flush the object into the stomach. Even after the object dissolves or passes into the stomach, children will feel transient pain at the original site of the obstruction.

An object that is a part of a toy or a chicken bone (other objects frequently swallowed) that will not dissolve and should not be passed is removed by esophagoscopy. Small coins, such as pennies and dimes, generally pass by themselves without difficulty.

Parents (or children themselves if adolescents) should observe stools over the next several days to determine when the coin passes through the GI tract (this takes about 48 h). Without frightening them, caution parents to observe for signs of bowel perforation or obstruction, such as vomiting or abdominal pain, until an object has passed. If there is any doubt, an x-ray taken 3 days to a week after ingestion will establish whether the object has been evacuated from the body.

WHAT IF? What if you received a call from your neighbor stating that her 2-year-old son swallowed a penny? What interventions would you expect to be necessary? What signs and symptoms would suggest obstruction?

Subcutaneous Objects

Children receive many wood splinters in hands and feet. These usually are removed easily by a probing needle and tweezers after cleaning with an antiseptic solution. If the penetrating object is metal, such as a sewing needle or nail, its presence can be detected by x-ray. If the object is one that would have been in contact with soil, such as a rusty nail, the child may need tetanus prophylaxis after extraction of the object.

TRAUMA RELATED TO ENVIRONMENTAL EXPOSURE

Frostbite

Frostbite is tissue injury caused by freezing cold. Cells at the site actually die. Cold exposure leads to peripheral vasoconstriction, so oxygen supply is cut off to surrounding cells. In children, the body parts involved usually are the fingers or toes (Hassi & Makinen, 2000).

Assessment

The affected part appears white or erythematous with edema and feels numb. Degrees of frostbite are summarized in Table 52-4. Explore the cause of frostbite by careful history taking. It occurs most frequently in children who are skiing or snowmobiling for long periods. If parents fail to provide adequate clothing because they underestimated the degree of cold outside, the possibility of neglect or child abuse must be ruled out as a cause. Frostbite also can occur from sucking on popsicles and inhalant abuse.

Therapeutic Management

Always warm frostbitten areas gradually. Sudden warming will increase the metabolic rate of cells. Without adequate blood flow to the area because of still-present vasoconstriction, additional damage will occur. Administration of a vasodilator and use of hyperbaric oxygen also may help (Salerno, 2000).

NURSING DIAGNOSES AND RELATED INTERVENTIONS

Nursing Diagnosis: Pain related to frostbite damage to cells

Outcome Identification: Child will experience a minimum amount of pain after injury.

Outcome Evaluation: Child states that pain is controlled at a tolerable level.

As soon as warming begins, the area becomes extremely painful from cells that are injured, but not destroyed, registering their anoxic state. Children need an analgesic for pain such as IV morphine. Morphine administered epidurally can be used for pain relief in lower body areas.

During the next few days after severe frostbite, necrosis of destroyed tissue will occur, and affected tissue will slough away. Apply a dressing as necessary to avoid secondary bacterial contamination of a necrotic injury site. Assess body temperature conscientiously to detect early symptoms of infection.

TABLE 52.4 Degrees of Frostbite

DEGREE	DESCRIPTION
First	Mild freezing of epidermis; appears erythematous with edema
Second	Partial- or full-thickness injury; appears erythematous with blisters and pain occurring after rewarming
Third	Full-thickness injury (epidermis, dermis, and subcutaneous tissue); appears white
Fourth	Complete necrosis with gangrene and possible ultimate loss of body part

✔ CHECKPOINT QUESTIONS

15. If a child swallowed a chicken bone, how would the child be treated?
16. What results if a frostbitten area is warmed too quickly?

BITES

Mammalian Bites

Dog bites account for approximately 90% of all bites inflicted on humans, and children and adolescents are involved in one third to one half of reported incidents. The dog is usually one owned by the child's family. Cat bites, wild animal bites, and human bites also constitute a threat, although less common to children. All of these bites can cause abrasions, puncture wounds, lacerations, and crushing injuries related to the size of the animal and location of the bite (Presutti, 2001). The biggest concerns associated with animal bites are the possibility of long-term scarring and disfigurement and the possibility of infection, especially rabies, from the presence of microorganisms in the animal's mouth. This latter subject is discussed in Chapter 43.

Snakebite

Snakebites tend to occur during the warm months of the year, from April to October. Most fatal snakebites (envenomation) in the United States are copperhead (found in Eastern and Southern states) and rattlesnake bites (found in almost every state). A few bites occur from cottonmouth moccasins or coral snakes (both found in Southeastern states). The effect of rattlesnake, copperhead, and cottonmouth bites (all pit viper types of snakes) is a failure of the blood coagulation system (Battan & Dart, 2001). Coral snakes are known for the small coral, yellow, and black rings encircling their body. Fortunately, they are shy and seldom bite. However, the venom injected through the bite of these snakes leads to neuromuscular paralysis.

Assessment

Reaction to a pit viper bite is almost immediate. A white wheal forms at the site, showing the puncture marks, accompanied by excruciating pain at the site. Purplish erythema and edema begin to extend rapidly from the site.

By the time children are seen at a health care facility, sanguineous fluid may ooze from the bite. Systemic symptoms, such as dizziness, vomiting, perspiration, and weakness, may be present. Because snake venom interferes with blood coagulation, children may have hematemesis or bleeding from the nose, intestines, or bladder from subcutaneous or internal hemorrhage. The pupils may be dilated, showing the potent effect on cerebral centers. If children are not treated, seizures, coma, and death may result.

Emergency Management at the Scene

At the scene of a snakebite, apply a cold compress to the bite in the hope of slowing the spread of the venom and to reduce edema formation. Urge the child to lie quietly to slow circulation. Keep the bitten extremity dependent, again to slow venous circulation. Commercial snakebite kits have rubber suction cups in them for suctioning out venom. These should be used, if available, at the site where the bite occurred. Excising the bite with a knife and sucking out the venom orally (often shown in old western movies) is of questionable value and contradicts rules of standard precautions. If the person administering the treatment has open mouth lesions, such as carious teeth, the procedure may be dangerous to that person (venom is not dangerous when swallowed, only when absorbed through open lesions). Excising the bite also may lead to secondary infection and, if done too vigorously, may injure tendon or muscle. No time should be wasted before the child is taken to a health care facility for treatment.

Emergency Management at the Health Facility

In the emergency facility, ask the child or a person who was with him or her to describe the snake. In areas where snakebites are frequent, keep available photographs of the venomous snakes commonly found. Even a preschooler may be able to identify the snake by pointing to a photograph. Specific antivenin will be administered. Because rattlesnakes, copperheads, and cottonmouth moccasins are all one type of snake (pit vipers), one form of antivenin acts against all of these bites. Specific antivenin is prepared for coral snake or cobra bites and is kept at most zoos. If the child receives antivenin promptly after a bite, the prognosis for full recovery is good. Tetanus prophylaxis is instituted if the child's immunization status is unknown or if it has been more than 10 years since a tetanus immunization was given.

Antivenin may contain a horse-serum base. Therefore, before the serum is injected IM or IV, a skin test may need to be performed first to prevent a possible anaphylactic reaction to the horse serum. If the serum is given IM, do not inject it into an edematous body part because poor medication absorption occurs. Giving antivenin in the limb opposite the bitten limb will be just as effective as administering it into the bitten limb.

NURSING DIAGNOSES AND RELATED INTERVENTIONS

Nursing Diagnosis: Fear related to seriousness of child's condition

Outcome Identification: Parents and child will demonstrate ability to keep fear within manageable limits.

Outcome Evaluation: Parents and child voice that they are able to cope with the degree of fear present.

Children with snakebites are extremely frightened. Their parents who have seen old western movies showing the agony of snakebite also are thoroughly frightened. Children need a great deal of support from health care personnel because parents may be too frightened to offer the support.

As a final care measure, teach children safety rules for avoiding snakebites:

- Look for snakes before stepping into underbrush.
- Do not lift up rocks without looking at what could be under them.
- Listen for the telltale sound of a rattlesnake.
- Be aware that snakes sun on rocks.
- Know the markings of poisonous snakes.

BURN TRAUMA

A burn is injury to body tissue caused by excessive heat (heat greater than 104°F [40°C]). They commonly occur in children of all ages after infancy. They are the second cause of accidental injury in children 1 to 4 years of age and the third cause in children 5 to 14 years (NCHS, 2001). Toddlers are often burned by pulling pans of scalding water off the stove and onto themselves or by biting into electrical cords. Older children are more apt to suffer burns from flames when they move too close to a campfire, heater, or fireplace; touch a hot curling iron; or if they play with matches or lighted candles (see Focus on Evidence-Based Practice). Some burns (particularly scalding) can be caused by child abuse (Sirotnak & Krugman, 2001). Any thermal burn tends to be more serious in children than in adults because the same size burn covers a larger surface of a child's body. As many as 50% of burns could be prevented with improved parent and child education.

Assessment

When children are brought to a health care facility with a thermal injury, the first questions must be, "Where is the burn and what is its extent and depth?" Burns are classified according to the criteria of the American Burn Association as major, moderate, or minor burns (McCance & Huether, 2002). These classifications are shown in Table 52-5. Along with the size and depth, be certain to assess and document the location of the burn. Face and throat burns are particularly hazardous because there may be unseen burns in the respiratory tract. Resulting edema could lead to respiratory tract obstruction. Hand burns are also hazardous because, if the fingers and thumb are not positioned properly during healing, adhesions will inhibit full range of motion in the future. Burns of the feet and genitalia are high risk for secondary infection. Genital burns are also hazardous because edema of the urinary meatus may prevent a child from voiding.

With adults, a "rule of nine" is a quick method of estimating the extent of a burn. Each upper extremity represents 9% of body surface; each lower extremity represents two 9s, or 18%, and the head and neck represent 9%. Because the body proportions of children are different from those of adults, this rule does not always apply and is mis-

FOCUS ON EVIDENCE-BASED PRACTICE

Do Curling Irons Cause Frequent Burn Injuries in Children?

To describe how many curling iron injuries are occurring, researchers surveyed data reported to the National Electronic Injury Surveillance System about children admitted to emergency rooms with curling iron injuries. Their results showed that there were 80,000 curling iron injuries over a 5-year period. Seventy percent of these injuries were to females. The average age for injury was 8 years. The most commonly seen injury was a thermal burn. In children under 4 years of age, the majority of burns occurred by grabbing or touching a hot iron, whereas in those older than that, burns occurred by contact with the appliance while it was in use. Surprisingly, 69% of burns were to the cornea.

This is an important study for nurses because, as a primary health care provider responsible for teaching safety to children and their families, nurses need to include this topic in safety education programs. Knowing that curling irons are a potential source of pediatric burns alerts nurses to include specific precautions for increased supervision when this electrical appliance is used.

Qazi, K., Gerson, L. W., Christopher, N. C., Kessler, E., & Ida, N. (2001). Curling iron–related injuries presenting to U.S. emergency departments. *Academic Emergency Medicine, 8*(1), 395–397.

leading in the very young child. Data for determining the extent of burns in children are shown in Figure 52-8. Computer analysis is now available (Neuwalder et al., 2002).

Depth of Burn

Assessing the depth of burns can be difficult on initial inspection. Descriptions of tissue at different burn depths appear in Table 52-6 and are illustrated in Figure 52-9.

TABLE 52.5 Classification of Burns

CLASSIFICATION	DESCRIPTION
Minor	First-degree burn or second-degree burn less than 10% of body surface or third-degree burn less than 2% of body surface; no area of the face, feet, hands, or genitalia burned
Moderate	Second-degree burn between 10% and 20% or on the face, hands, feet, or genitalia or third-degree burn less than 10% body surface or if smoke inhalation has occurred
Severe	Second-degree burn more than 20% body surface or third-degree burn more than 10% body surface

Partial-thickness burns include first- and second-degree burns. A first-degree burn involves only the superficial epidermis. The area appears erythematous. It is painful to touch and blanches on pressure (Fig. 52-10*A*). Scalds and sunburn are examples of first-degree burns. Such burns heal by simple regeneration and take only 1 to 10 days to heal.

A second-degree burn involves the entire epidermis. Sweat glands and hair follicles are left intact. The area appears very erythematous, blistered, and moist from exudate. It is extremely painful. Scalds can cause second-degree burns (see Figure 52-10*B*). Such burns heal by regeneration of tissue but take 2 to 6 weeks to heal.

A third-degree burn is a full-thickness burn involving both skin layers, epidermis and dermis. It may also involve adipose tissue, fascia, muscle, and bone. The burn area appears either white or black (Fig. 52-11). Because the nerves, sweat glands, and hair follicles have been burned, third-degree burns are not painful. Flames are a common cause of third-degree burns. Such burns cannot heal by regeneration because underlying layers of skin are destroyed. Skin grafting is usually necessary, and healing will take months. Scar tissue will cover the final healed site.

When estimating the depth of a burn, use the appearance of the burn and the sensitivity of the area to pain as criteria. Many burns are compound, involving first-, second-, and third-degree burns. There may be a central white area that is insensitive to pain (third degree), surrounded by an area of erythematous blisters (second degree), surrounded by another area that is erythematous only (first degree).

Undress children with burns completely so the entire body can be inspected. A first-degree burn is painful, whereas a third-degree burn is not. Therefore, a child may be crying from a superficial burn that is obvious on the arm, although the condition needing the most immediate attention is a third-degree burn on the chest, which is covered by a jacket.

Be certain to ask what caused the burn, because different materials cause different degrees of burn. Hot water, for example, causes scalding, a generally lesser degree of burn than a burn caused by flaming clothing. Ask where the fire happened. Fires in closed spaces are apt to cause more respiratory involvement than fires in open areas.

Ask if the child has any secondary health problem. In the anxiety over the present burn, parents may forget to report important facts (eg, that the child has diabetes or is allergic to a common drug). After a fire, parents may pick up the burned child and bring him or her to a health care facility, leaving other children unprotected at home. Ask about other children and where they are. Parents may have burned hands from putting out the fire on the child's clothes and need equal care, but in their anxiety about the child's condition, they do not mention this. Ask who put out the fire. Were any other family members or animals hurt? Does anyone else need care?

✔ CHECKPOINT QUESTIONS

17. What layer(s) of skin is (are) involved with a second-degree burn?
18. Why isn't a "rule of 9" applicable to burned children?

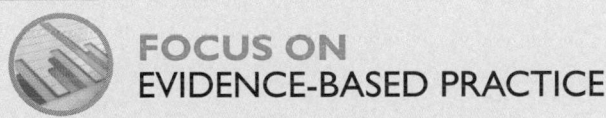

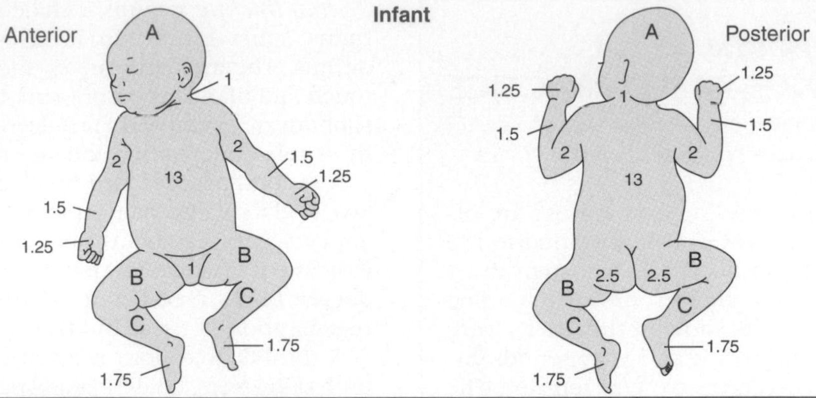

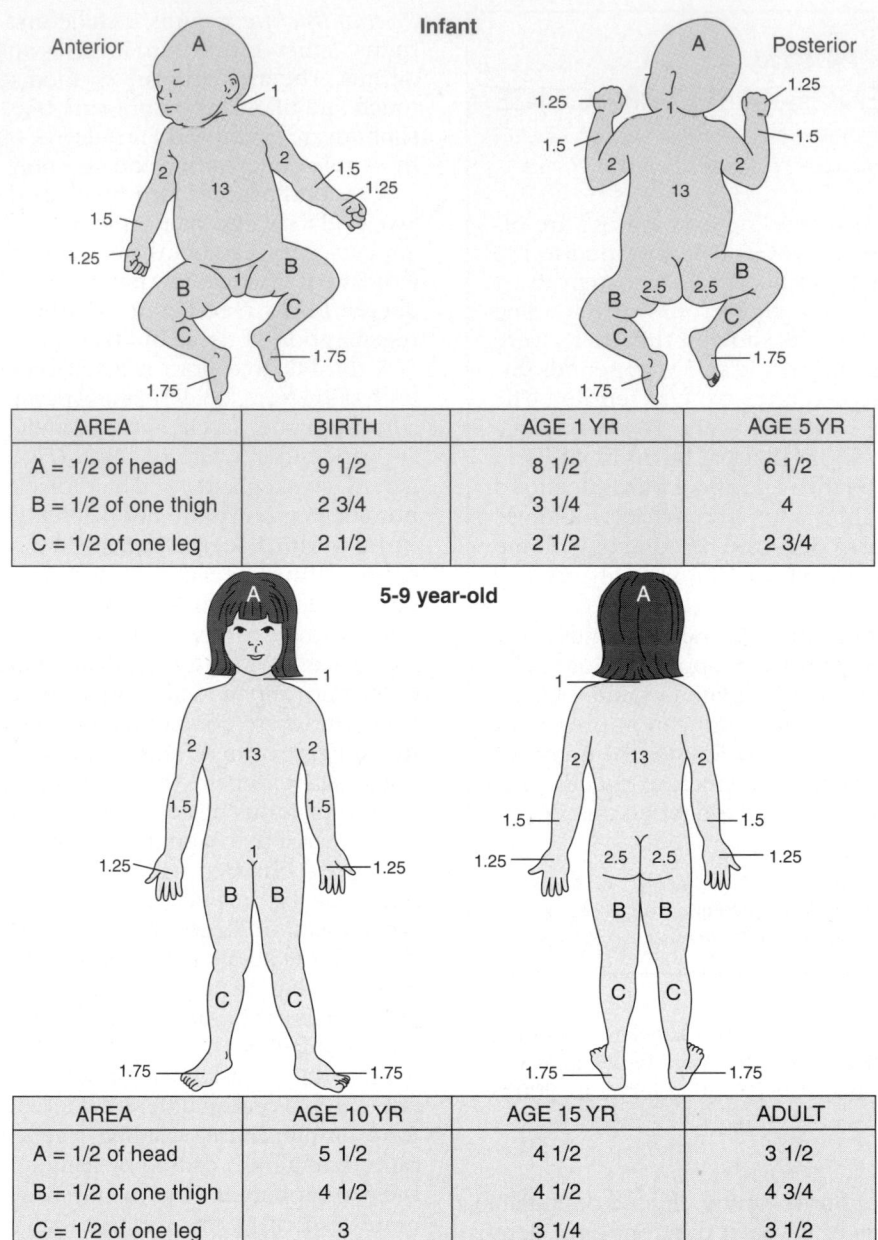

AREA	BIRTH	AGE 1 YR	AGE 5 YR
A = 1/2 of head	9 1/2	8 1/2	6 1/2
B = 1/2 of one thigh	2 3/4	3 1/4	4
C = 1/2 of one leg	2 1/2	2 1/2	2 3/4

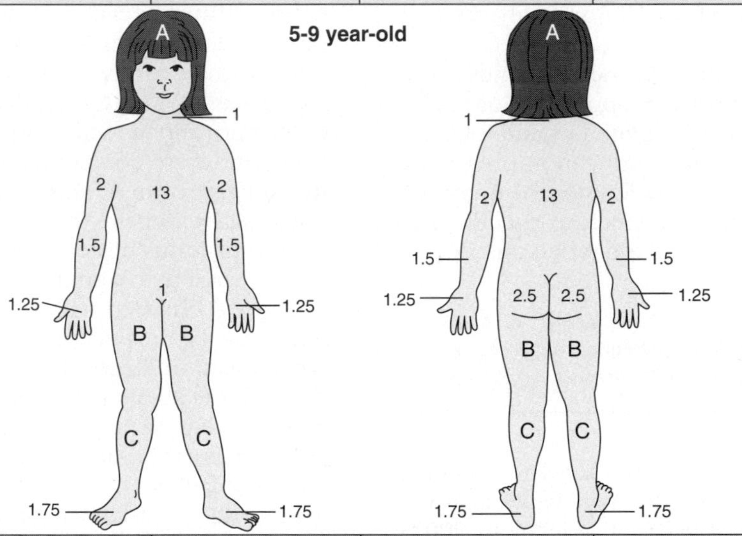

AREA	AGE 10 YR	AGE 15 YR	ADULT
A = 1/2 of head	5 1/2	4 1/2	3 1/2
B = 1/2 of one thigh	4 1/2	4 1/2	4 3/4
C = 1/2 of one leg	3	3 1/4	3 1/2

FIGURE 52.8 Determination of extent of burns in children.

Emergency Management

Minor Burns

Although minor burns (typically first-degree partial-thickness burns), are the simplest type of burn, they involve pain and death of skin cells, so they must be treated seriously. Applying an analgesic-antibiotic ointment and a gauze bandage to prevent infection is all that is usually required. The child should have a follow-up visit in 2 days to have the area inspected for a secondary infection and

TABLE 52.6 Characteristics of Burns

SEVERITY	DEPTH OF TISSUE INVOLVED	APPEARANCE	EXAMPLE
First degree (partial thickness)	Epidermis	Erythematous, dry, painful	Sunburn
Second degree (partial thickness)	Epidermis Portion of dermis	Blistered, erythematous to white	Scalds
Third degree (full thickness)	Entire skin, including nerves and blood vessels in skin	Leathery; black or white; not sensitive to pain (nerve endings destroyed)	Flame

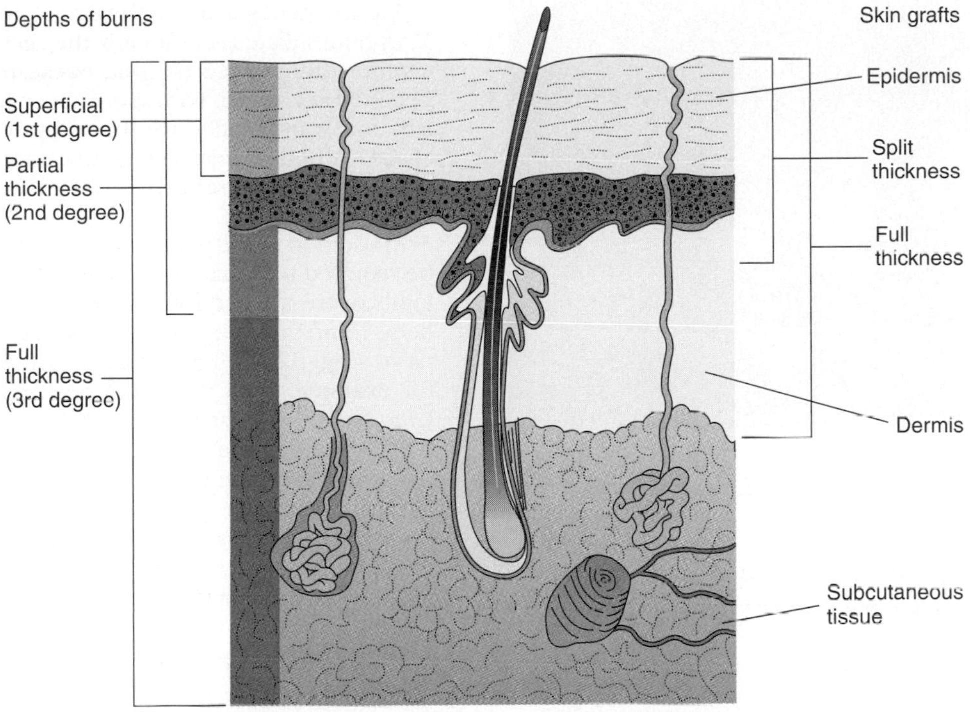

FIGURE 52.9 Depths of burns.

to have the dressing changed. Caution parents to keep the dressing dry (no swimming or getting the area wet while bathing for 1 week). A first-degree burn heals in about that time.

Moderate Burns

Moderate or second-degree burns may have blisters. Do not rupture these if present because doing so invites infection. Broken blisters may be débrided (cut away) to remove possible necrotic tissue. The burn will be covered with a topical antibiotic such as silver sulfadiazine and a bulky dressing to prevent the denuded skin from damage. The child usually is asked to return in 24 h to assess that pain control is adequate and there are no signs and symptoms of infection.

Severe Burns

The child with a severe burn is critically injured and needs swift, sure care including fluid therapy, systemic antibiotic therapy, pain management, and physical therapy to survive the injury without a disability caused by scarring, infection, or contracture.

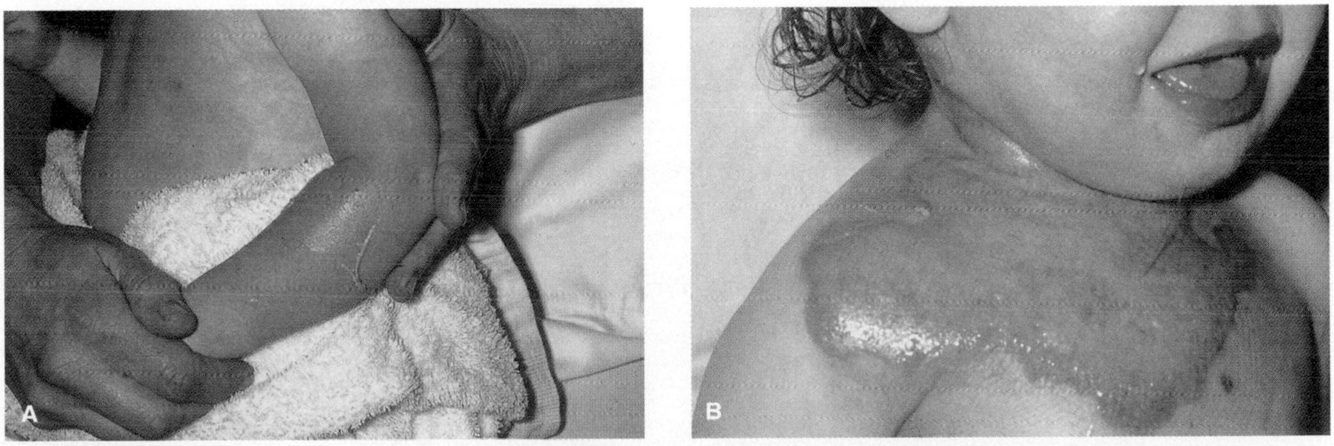

FIGURE 52.10 Partial-thickness burns. (*A*) An infant with a first-degree burn on the arm and chest caused by scalding with hot water. (*B*) A toddler with a second-degree burn caused by scalding. The area appears severely reddened and moist with some blistering.

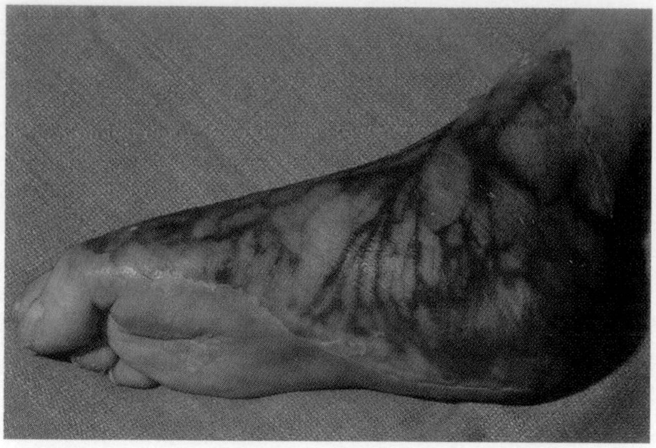

FIGURE 52.11 Full-thickness (third-degree) burn of the foot. Both layers of skin are involved with this type of burn.

NURSING DIAGNOSES AND RELATED INTERVENTIONS

Nursing Diagnosis: Pain related to trauma to body cells

Outcome Identification: Child will experience the minimum amount of pain possible (be certain that goal established is realistic; you cannot eliminate *all* pain).

Outcome Evaluation: Child states that pain is at a tolerable level.

Children who experience smoke inhalation may be unconscious from brain anoxia immediately after a burn. Most children, however, are awake and very aware of the pain and treatments involved. Therefore, a priority need is immediate pain relief. After the first week following a major burn, some children develop symptoms of delirium, seizures, and coma that result from toxic breakdown of damaged cells and sensory deprivation, isolation, and lack of sleep. Nursing care aimed at reducing unnecessary stimuli helps to prevent these late symptoms from occurring.

A child needs a potent analgesic to relieve pain. Morphine sulfate is commonly the agent of choice. It can be administered IM, but, because circulation is impaired in children with shock, IV or epidural administration is most effective. Use of patient-controlled analgesia before performing any burn care such as débridement is also effective. Be sure to assess for adequacy of pain relief.

In addition to the pain from the burn, children may be required to remain in awkward positions to keep joints overextended for most of every day. Doing so helps to prevent formation of contractures from scar tissue (Fig. 52-12). If their anterior throat is burned, for example, their head will be hyperextended to keep scar tissue that forms on the anterior neck from pulling their chin down against their chest in a contracture. It is difficult for children to watch television in this position or even to view activities on the unit. If they have burns at extremity joints, they may have splints applied over burn dressings to maintain joints in extension. Again, this makes activities very difficult for them and adds to their stress if they do not have adequate pain relief.

Nursing Diagnosis: Deficient fluid volume related to fluid shifts with severe thermal burn

Outcome Identification: Child will maintain normal balance of fluid and electrolytes during period of therapy.

Outcome Evaluation: Skin turgor remains good; hourly urine output is greater than 1 mL/kg, with specific gravity between 1.003 and 1.030; vital signs are within acceptable parameters.

Immediately after a severe burn, the child's circulatory system becomes hypovolemic, due to a loss of plasma that oozes from the burn site and fluid that sequesters in edematous tissue surrounding the site. This outpouring of plasma is caused by an increased

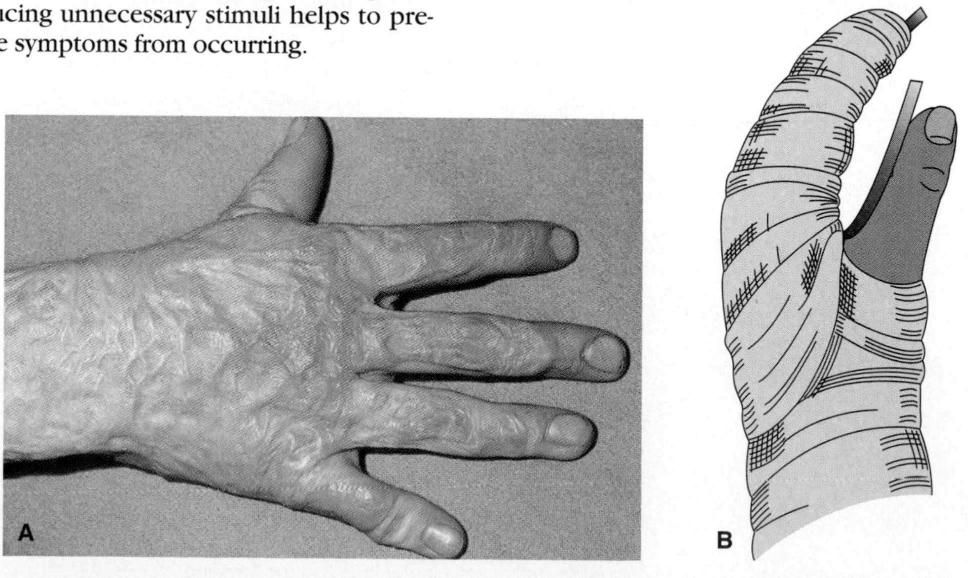

FIGURE 52.12 (*A*) An adolescent's hand scarred from third-degree burns. Note the proper extension and alignment of the hand and fingers, which were maintained by the use of splints (*B*) during healing.

permeability of capillaries (or damage to capillaries). It is most marked during the first 6 h after a burn. It continues to some extent for the first 24 h.

A primary response of the myocardium to the shock of thermal injury and the hypovolemia can lead to a marked reduction in cardiac output and decreased blood pressure. Therefore, even with relatively minor burns, vital signs must be monitored closely to allow early detection of this event. The child may be severely anemic because of injury to red blood cells by heat and loss of blood at the wound site, and he or she may have severe electrolyte abnormalities as a result of fluid shifts (Table 52-7). The large amount of sodium lost with the edematous burn fluid and the release of potassium from damaged cells can lead to an immediate hyponatremia and hyperkalemia.

Lactated Ringer's solution is the commercially available solution most compatible with extracellular fluid. It is one of the first fluids usually begun for fluid replacement, although normal saline may be used. The child may also need plasma replacement and additional fluid, such as 5% dextrose in water. Do not administer potassium immediately after a burn because kidney function must be evaluated first. IV fluid is generally administered by the most convenient venous access so that morphine sulfate can be administered to relieve pain. A more stable fluid line may then be inserted. The amount of fluid necessary is calculated carefully, based on predicted insensible fluid loss and loss due to the burn. A common formula (the Parkland formula) used to calculate fluid needed is: 4 mL/kg for percentage of body surface area burned for the first 24 h (Battan & Dart, 2001).

This fluid is administered rapidly for the first 8 h (half of the 24-h load), then more slowly for the next 16 h (the second half). It is important that it is continued beyond the time of increased capillary permeability (at least the first 24 h). The administration site, therefore, must be protected to prevent infiltration. A central venous pressure or pulmonary artery catheter may be inserted to determine hemodynamic and fluid volume status and evaluate that the child is receiving adequate fluid.

About 48 h after the burn, as inflammation decreases, the extracellular fluid at the burn site begins to be reabsorbed into the bloodstream. Edema begins to subside; the child will have diuresis and lose weight. The heart rate will increase because of temporary hypervolemia. The hematocrit level will be low because red blood cells will be diluted. The child will need frequent evaluation of electrolyte levels to determine fluid balance during this period. Potassium supplements may be necessary to maintain normal heart function because, although potassium was released into serum from destroyed cells, it is rapidly excreted by the kidneys. If the child needs continued electrolyte replacement at this time, carefully monitor the rate of flow so the blood volume does not exceed the child's tolerance. If many red blood cells were destroyed at the burn site, the child may need packed red blood cells to maintain an adequate hemoglobin level.

Nursing Diagnosis: Risk for ineffective tissue perfusion related to cardiovascular adjustments after thermal injury

Outcome Identification: Child's cardiovascular system will satisfactorily adjust to fluid shifts during therapy.

Outcome Evaluation: Child's vital signs stay within normal limits; hourly urine output remains greater than 1 mL/kg.

Take height, weight, and vital signs on admission, and continue to take vital signs every 15 min until they are stable. Once stabilized, record pulse, blood pressure, and central venous pressure hourly until the child passes the immediate danger of shock (at least 24 h). Another important period occurs 48 h after the injury when fluid is returning to the bloodstream. Remember that gradual but persistent changes in blood pressure may be as informative as sudden changes.

A complete blood count, blood typing and crossmatching, electrolyte and BUN determinations, and blood gas studies to ascertain blood levels of oxygen and carbon dioxide are also important.

Nursing Diagnosis: Risk for ineffective breathing patterns related to respiratory edema from thermal injury

Outcome Identification: Child will maintain respiratory function during course of illness.

Outcome Evaluation: Child's respiratory rate remains within 16 to 20 breaths per minute; lung auscultation reveals no rales.

If the child inhaled smoke from a fire, the injury from the smoke inhalation can be more serious than the skin surface burns. Smoke coming from a fire is at the temperature of the fire. Inhaling smoke, therefore, is the same as exposing the upper respiratory tract to open flame. In addition, toxic substances and soot given off from fire may cause even more irritation to the respiratory tract. If carbon monoxide is inhaled

TABLE 52.7 Fluid Shifts After Thermal Injury

FLUID SHIFTS IN FIRST 24 HOURS	REMOBILIZATION OF FLUID AFTER 48 HOURS
Burn	Edematous tissue surrounding burn area
↓	↓
Increased capillary permeability	Intravascular compartment
↓	↓
Hypoproteinemia	
Hyponatremia	Hypervolemia
Hyperkalemia	Hypernatremia
Hypovolemia	Hypokalemia

with the smoke, this enters red blood cells in place of oxygen, shutting off oxygen supply to body cells. If this is extensive, it can lead to loss of consciousness from cerebral anoxia. If the trachea is burned, edema fluid will pass into the injured bronchioles and trachea, causing pulmonary edema or obstruction limiting air inflow. This can lead to dyspnea and stridor. About a week after the smoke inhalation, the child is at risk for the development of pneumonia because of denuded tracheal and bronchial tract areas. That inhalation of smoke or flame from a fire can be more serious than the skin burns the child suffers may be difficult for parents to understand. They are relieved if they learn that the child has suffered only smoke inhalation. They may need an explanation of the physiologic consequences that can result from pulmonary injury.

To help rule out smoke inhalation, obtain a history to assess if the fire occurred in a closed space, such as a garage. Assess for burns of the face, neck, or chest, which means fire was near the nose and respiratory tract. Assess the quality of the child's voice (will be hoarse if the throat is irritated from smoke). Carefully, monitor the respiratory rate of all burned children because the respiratory rate increases with respiratory obstruction. The child also may become restless and thrash because of lack of oxygen. Measurement of blood gases will demonstrate the degree of hypoxia present from carbon monoxide intoxication. Administering 100% oxygen is the best therapy for displacing carbon monoxide and providing adequate oxygenation to body cells. The child may need endotracheal intubation or tracheostomy with assisted ventilation to ensure adequate oxygenation. Intubation is best because tracheostomies can lead to infection and this child is at a much higher risk for pneumonia than the average child.

Symptoms of smoke inhalation may not occur immediately but only 8 to 24 h after the burn. A chest x-ray taken at this time will reveal collecting edematous fluid and decreased aeration. Continue to assess the child's temperature every 4 h for the first week after the injury to detect that lung infection is not developing. Bronchodilators and antibiotics may be prescribed. High-frequency ventilation may be helpful to keep alveoli functioning. Some children need extracorporeal membrane oxygenation (ECMO) support because smoke inhalation has compromised their lung function to such a great extent.

Nursing Diagnosis: Risk for impaired urinary elimination related to thermal trauma

Outcome Identification: Child will not experience decreased urine output during course of illness.

Outcome Evaluation: Child's urine output will be greater than 1 mL/kg of body weight/h.

Because the child's blood volume decreases immediately after a burn, renal function is threatened by kidney ischemia just when renal function is needed to rid the body of breakdown products from burned cells. If the child is burned over 10% of his or her body surface, urinary output may decrease immediately. Blood volume must be maintained by IV fluid administration to establish good urinary output once more. Urine output should be 1 mL/kg of body weight/h. The specific gravity of urine also should be monitored to determine whether the kidneys can concentrate urine to conserve body fluid (failing kidneys lose this ability rapidly). In the days after the burn, because products of necrotic tissue and toxic substances must be evacuated by the kidney and antidiuretic hormone and aldosterone levels increase in response to low blood pressure, kidney function may fail again. If free hemoglobin from destroyed red blood cells plugs kidney tubules (acute tubular necrosis), urine color will be red to black from the hemoglobin present.

An indwelling urinary (Foley) catheter should be inserted in the emergency department, and an immediate urine specimen should be obtained for analysis. A diuretic, such as mannitol, may be administered to flush hemoglobin from the kidneys. If effective, urine returns to its usual straw color. Throughout the child's hospital stay, observing urinary output is a major nursing responsibility. An hourly urine output less than 1 mL/kg suggests renal insufficiency.

Nursing Diagnosis: Risk for imbalanced nutrition, less than body requirements, related to thermal trauma

Outcome Identification: Child will ingest adequate nutrients for increased metabolic needs during therapy.

Outcome Evaluation: Child's weight remains within normal age-appropriate growth percentiles; skin turgor remains normal; urine specific gravity remains between 1.003 and 1.030.

After burns, the metabolic rate increases in children as the body begins to pool its resources to adjust to the insult. If the child does not receive enough calories in IV fluid, he or she will begin to break down protein. This is particularly dangerous because the child needs protein now for burn healing. Additionally, breaking down protein can lead to acidosis.

After a severe burn, some children are nauseated from the systemic shock. An NG tube may be inserted and attached to low, intermittent suction as prophylactic therapy to prevent aspiration of vomitus. The tube must remain in place until bowel sounds are detected. This usually occurs within 24 h but may take as long as 72 h in severely burned children. The suction from the NG tube may be blood-tinged (coffee-ground fluid) due to bleeding caused by stomach vessel congestion. Closely observe this drainage for a change to fresh bleeding, which can be caused by a stress ulcer (Curling's ulcer). This type of ulcer can be prevented by administering a histamine-2 receptor antagonist, such as cimetidine (Tagamet) or a proton pump inhibitor such as omeprazole (Prilosec) in an attempt to reduce gastric acidity and ulcer formation.

If a bleeding ulcer occurs, gastric lavage with iced saline may be necessary. Blood for transfusion should be readily available, because the blood loss from a GI ulcer can be rapid and severe.

When children have burns over more than 30% of the body surface, paralytic ileus may occur. Symptoms of intestinal obstruction, such as vomiting, abdominal distention, and colicky pain, will appear within hours of the burn.

Children with severe burns usually are allowed nothing by mouth for 24 h because of the danger of vomiting or paralytic ileus. After this, most children are able to eat, so oral feedings are begun as soon as possible. To supply adequate calories for increased metabolic needs and spare protein for repairing cells, the diet is high in calories and protein (1,800 cal/m^2/24 h plus 22 cal/m^2 of burned area per 24 h). Children may also need vitamin (particularly B and C) and iron supplements. High-protein drinks may be necessary between meals to ensure an adequate protein intake (Dudek, 2001).

Because adequate nutrition is important, it may be necessary to supplement the child's diet with IV or parenteral nutrition solutions or NG tube feeding. As additional methods of stimulating interest in eating, encourage school-age children to help add intake and output columns, help the dietitian add a calorie-count list, or keep track of their own daily weight (taken at the same time each day in the same clothing). It may be helpful to make contracts with older children for a good nutritional intake.

Nursing Diagnosis: Risk for injury related to effects of burn, denuded skin surfaces, and lowered resistance to infection with thermal injury

Outcome Identification: Child will not develop an infection during time of denuded tissue.

Outcome Evaluation: Child's temperature remains at 98.6°F (37°C); skin areas surrounding burned areas show no signs of erythema or warmth.

There appears to be some defect in the ability of neutrophils to phagocytize bacteria after thermal injury. The formation of immunoglobulin G antibodies also apparently fails. For these reasons, the child has reduced protection against infection. *Staphylococcus aureus* and group A beta-hemolytic streptococci are the gram-positive organisms and *Pseudomonas aeruginosa* is the gram-negative organism that commonly invade burn tissue. Children are usually prescribed parenteral penicillin to prevent group A beta-hemolytic streptococcal infection and tetanus toxoid to prevent tetanus. In addition to bacteria, fungi also may invade burns. *Candida* species are the most frequently seen (Das & Kim, 2000).

Bacteria and fungi can penetrate the burn eschar readily, so this tissue offers little protection from infection. Fortunately, granulation tissue, which forms under the eschar 3 to 4 weeks after the burn, is resistant to microbial invasion.

Nose, throat, and wound cultures may be done immediately and daily to detect offending organisms. Until granulation tissue forms, the child has lost the integumentary defense against infection. Therefore, prophylactic treatment is important to prevent infection. Systemic antibiotics are not very effective in controlling burn-wound infection, probably because the burned and constricted capillaries around the burn site cannot carry the antibiotic to the area. Thus, any equipment used with the child must be sterile to avoid introducing infection. Children are placed on a sterile sheet on the examining table. Personnel caring for the severely burned child should wear caps, masks, gowns, and gloves, even for emergency care.

Although their burns may be covered by gauze dressings, children usually are cared for in private rooms. Helping children maintain their self-esteem and keeping them from withdrawing from social contacts are commonly difficult when infection control precautions are required.

Therapy for Burns

Second- and third-degree burns may receive open treatment, leaving the burned area exposed to the air, or a closed method, covering the burned area with an antibacterial cream and many layers of gauze. These two methods are compared in Table 52-8. A synthetic skin covering (Biobrane) or artificial skin (Integra) can be used to help decrease infection and protect granulation tissue. As a rule, burn dressings are applied loosely in the first 24 h to prevent interfering with circulation as edema forms. Be certain not to allow two burned body surfaces, such as the sides of fingers or the back of the ears and the scalp, to touch because, as healing takes place, a webbing forms between these surfaces. Do not use adhesive tape to anchor dressings to the skin. It is painful to remove and can leave excoriated areas providing additional entry for infection. Netting is useful to hold dressings in place because it expands easily and needs no additional tape.

Topical Therapy

Silver sulfadiazine (Silvadene) is the drug of choice for burn therapy to limit infection at the burn site for children. It is applied as a paste to the burn, and the area is

TABLE 52.8 Comparing Open and Closed Burn Therapy

METHOD	DESCRIPTION	ADVANTAGES	DISADVANTAGES
Open	Burn is exposed to air; used for superficial burns or body parts that are prone to infection, such as perineum	Allows frequent inspection of site; allows child to follow healing process	Requires strict isolation to prevent infection; area may scrape and bleed easily and impede healing
Closed	Burn is covered with nonadherent gauze; used for moderate and severe burns	Provides better protection from injury; is easier to turn and position child; allows child more freedom to play	Requires dressing changes that are painful; possibility of infection may increase because of dark, moist environment

covered with a few layers of mesh gauze. Silver sulfadiazine is an effective agent against both gram-negative and gram-positive organisms and even secondary infectious agents, such as *Candida.* It is soothing when applied and tends to keep the burn eschar soft, making débridement easier. It does not penetrate the eschar well, which is its one drawback.

Antiseptic solutions, such as povidone-iodine (Betadine), may be used to inhibit bacterial and fungal growth. Unfortunately, iodine stings as it is applied and stains skin and clothing brown. Dressings must be kept continually wet to keep them from clinging to and disrupting the healing tissue.

If *Pseudomonas* is detected in cultures, nitrofurazone (Furacin) cream may be applied. If a topical cream is not effective against invading organisms in the deeper tissue under the eschar, daily injections of specific antibiotics to the deeper layers of the burned area may be necessary.

If a burned area cannot be readily dressed, such as the female genitalia, it can be left exposed. The danger of this method is the potential invasion of pathogens.

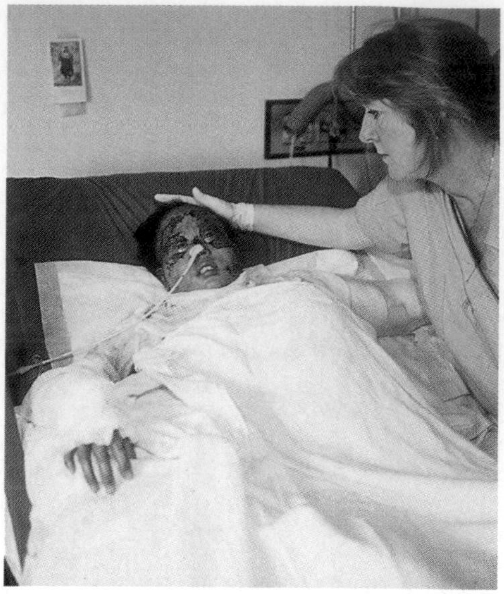

FIGURE 52.13 A nurse provides comfort and support to a child before débridement.

Escharotomy

An eschar is the tough, leathery scab that forms over moderately or severely burned areas. Fluid accumulates rapidly under eschars, putting pressure on underlying blood vessels and nerves. If an extremity or the trunk has been burned so both anterior and posterior surfaces have eschar formation, a tight band may form around the extremity or trunk, cutting off circulation to the distal body portions. Distal parts feel cool to the touch and appear pale. The child notices tingling or numbness. Pulses are difficult to palpate, and capillary refill is slow (more than 5 s). To alleviate this problem, an **escharotomy** (cut into the eschar) is performed. Some bleeding after escharotomy will occur. Packing the wound and applying pressure usually relieves this.

Débridement

Débridement is the removal of necrotic tissue from a burned area. Débridement reduces the possibility of infection because it reduces the tissue present for microorganisms to thrive. Children usually have 20 min of hydrotherapy before débridement to soften and loosen eschar, which then can be gently removed with forceps and scissors. Débridement is painful, and some bleeding occurs with it. Premedicate the child with a prescribed analgesic, and help the child use a distraction technique during the procedure to reduce the level of pain. Transcutaneous electrical nerve stimulation (TENS) therapy or patient-controlled analgesia may be helpful. Praise any degree of cooperation. Plan an enjoyable activity afterward to aid in pain relief and also to help reestablish some sense of control over the situation.

Children need to have a "helping" person with them, to hold their hand, to stroke their head, and to offer some verbal comfort during débridement: "It's all right to cry; we know that hurts. We don't like to do this, but it's one of the things that makes burns heal" (Fig. 52-13). Nursing personnel need a great deal of talk time to voice their feelings about assisting with or doing débridement procedures. Be careful in serving as the "helping" person that you do not project yourself as the healer and the comforter and a fellow nurse as the hurter, or "bad guy." It helps if people alternate this chore so that, on alternate days, each serves as the protector and the comforter.

If eschar tissue is débrided in this manner day after day, granulation tissue forms underneath. When a full bed of granulation tissue is present (about 2 weeks after the injury), the area is ready for skin grafting. In some burn centers, this waiting period is avoided by immediate surgical excision of eschar and placement of skin grafts. Another trend in débridement is the use of collagenase (Santyl), an enzyme that can dissolve devitalized tissue.

Grafting

Homografting (also called **allografting**) is the placement of skin (sterilized and frozen) from cadavers or a donor on the cleaned burn site. These grafts do not grow but provide a protective covering for the area. In small children, **heterografts** (also called *xenografts*) from other sources, such as porcine (pig) skin, may be used. **Autografting** is a process in which a layer of skin of both epidermis and a part of the dermis (called a *split-thickness graft*) is removed from a distal, unburned portion of the child's body and placed at the prepared burn site, where it will grow and replace the burned skin. Cultured epithelium is derived from a full-thickness skin biopsy. This can be grown into a coherent sheet or supply an unlimited source for autografts. Larger areas may require mesh grafts (a strip of partial-thickness skin that is slit at intervals so that it can be stretched to cover a larger area; Fig. 52-14). The advantage of grafting is that it reduces fluid and electrolyte loss, pain, and the chance of infection.

After the grafting procedure, the area is covered by a bulky dressing. So that the growth of the newly adhering cells will not be disrupted, this should not be removed or

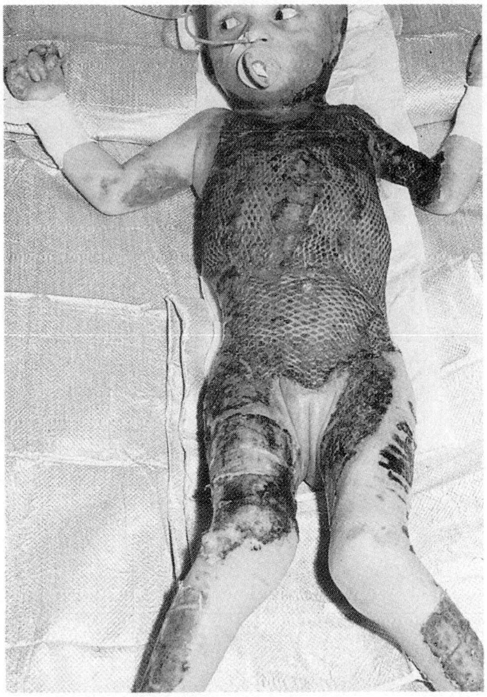

FIGURE 52.14 Mesh grafting is necessary to cover large areas of the body such as in this young child with third-degree burns.

changed. The donor site on the child's body (often the anterior thigh or buttocks) is also covered by a gauze dressing. Both donor and graft dressings should be observed for fluid drainage and odor. Observe the child to see if he or she has pain at either site, which might indicate infection. Monitor the child's temperature every 4 h. A rise in systemic temperature may be the first indication that there is infection at the graft or donor site. Autograft sites can be reused every 7 to 10 days, so any one site can provide a great deal of skin for grafting.

NURSING DIAGNOSES AND RELATED INTERVENTIONS

Nursing Diagnosis: Social isolation related to infection control precautions necessary to control spread of microorganisms

Outcome Identification: Child will demonstrate that he is able to cope with degree of restriction necessary during course of illness.

Outcome Evaluation: Child states that he understands the reason for infection control precautions; child accepts it as a necessary part of therapy.

Infection control measures involved in the care of children with major burns is more than just placing the child in a private room. Aseptic technique and appropriate barriers are necessary to reduce the risk of exposing the child to infection. Health care facilities differ in their policies for preventing infection for the child with a burn. Check your agency's policy. In some agencies, all the people who come into the room wear gowns, masks, caps, and sterile gloves. The child is doubly isolated: by distance and by strangers who never touch him or her directly.

It is easy for children with burns (who were told measures not to play with matches or go too close to the fireplace) to interpret these measures as punishment. Make every effort to make their environment as warm and comforting as possible, despite the infection control procedures. Place children's beds so they can see as much unit activity as possible. Decorate walls in front of them with cards they receive or with a changing gallery of pictures drawn by staff members of things in which the children appear interested.

Provide time for children to discuss their feelings about being kept in a room by themselves. A question such as, "It's hard to understand a lot of things about a hospital; do you understand why your bed is in this special room?" gives children a chance to express their feelings.

Show parents how to put on gowns, gloves, and masks (depending on agency policy), so they can participate in the child's care as much as possible. Parents often do not ask to do these things spontaneously when their children are severely burned. They are in a state of grief, so they do not react in a normal manner. They may believe the bulky dressings make it impossible for them to hold the child. Actually, the closed bulky dressings on the wound make it *possible* for the child to be held. If it is not possible for children to be held, help parents to see that stroking a child's face or touching a hand (even with gloves in place) gives the child a feeling of still being loved.

Nursing Diagnosis: Interrupted family processes related to the effects of severe burns in family member

Outcome Identification: The family will remain intact and functional during the period of rehabilitation.

Outcome Evaluation: Family members voice that they are able to cope effectively with the degree of stress to which they are subjected; family demonstrates positive coping mechanisms.

Children with severe burns always have a difficult hospitalization because of the pain, restrictions, and (at some point) awareness of the disfigurement that accompanies major burns.

Some parents grieve so deeply over the child's condition or are so concerned with other upsetting factors in their lives (many burns happen because of situational crises in the family) that their interaction with the child seems to falter or proves very difficult for them. They may avoid visiting because the sound of the child's crying when they leave is more than they can endure. At the same time, they may have lost their home and possessions to fire. They may need help in establishing priorities. It may be important that they wait at home one morning for an insurance inspector to make an estimate on damage caused by the fire to their house or furniture. Other tasks, such as shopping or housecleaning, could possibly be done by relatives or neighbors, leaving them time to visit the child.

Nursing Diagnosis: Deficient diversional activity related to restricted mobility after severe burn

Outcome Identification: Child remains interested in age-appropriate activities during rehabilitation.

Outcome Evaluation: Child expresses interest in obtaining school homework; child communicates with friends and relatives by way of telephone, letters, or e-mail.

Remember that, although children's chest, abdomen, and hands may be burned, they do not stop thinking. They need stimulation in their environment. A television set is good for passing time but should not be the child's main communication with the outside world. Listening to favorite tapes, having stories read to them, talking about what is going on at home or what they normally do at school, and doing schoolwork are important, too.

Toys and play material are important. Make certain to visit the child just to talk to him or her or come to play a game at times other than procedure or treatment times. The child may be hospitalized for a long time. He or she needs to view the nursing staff as friends and caregivers. Frequent visits convey that he or she is not alone and that others are aware of important needs.

Nursing Diagnosis: Disturbed body image related to changes in physical appearance with thermal injury

Outcome Identification: Child will maintain self-esteem during rehabilitation period.

Outcome Evaluation: Child expresses fears about physical appearance; demonstrates desire to resume age-appropriate activities.

Children with burns are often forced to become extremely dependent on the nursing staff due to the position in which they must lie and because of bulky dressings that cover their arms or hands and prevent them from feeding themselves. They respond to this forced dependence at first with gratitude. They are hurt, and someone is taking care of them. After a period, however, the response may become less healthy. The young school-age child or preschooler may revert to bedwetting or baby talk. Older children respond by becoming openly aggressive to counteract their feelings of helplessness. They attempt to reestablish independence in the ways that they can, often by refusing to eat or to lie in a position that is best for them. Although good nutrition is vitally important for rapid healing, it may suffer because of children's need to assert their independence. Make certain to allow independent decision making whenever possible. Children must take their 10 o'clock medicine, but they can choose the fluid they want to swallow after it. They must be fed meals because of the bulky dressings over their hands, but they can decide which food they will be fed first. They must have their dressings changed, but they can choose the story you will read them afterward.

Be careful not to give choices when there really are none to give. Inappropriate questions include, "Can I change your dressing now?" "Do you want dinner now?" "Will you swallow this pill?"

Immediately after a severe burn, children (if they are old enough to understand), parents, and probably the hospital staff are most concerned with whether they will live. When body systems have stabilized and it seems appropriate to assure parents that the child will live, thoughts turn to the child's cosmetic appearance. At first, it is easy for children and parents to ignore this problem because the burned areas are covered by dressings. Even when the dressings are removed for débridement or whirlpool, it is easy for children to assume that the appearance of the burned area is only temporary and the area will eventually heal and have a good appearance. They have probably never seen anyone with a scar from a second- or third-degree burn and have no reason to worry about it (Fig. 52-15).

When children see others on the unit with burn scars, they begin to realize what healing will look like. Depending on the extent and the site of the burn, parents and children will have varying degrees of difficulty accepting this. They may lose confidence in the health care personnel.

Parents and children need time to talk about their feelings. A girl may be extremely concerned if her chest is burned because she is worried that breast tissue will not develop (a very real concern, depending on the extent of the burn). Her parents may be most concerned because they can see that, although a blouse can cover her chest, her right hand will not have full function. Do not assume that your biggest concern is the same as the child's and parents' biggest concern. A father who dreamed his son would be a great track star may be most concerned about a leg scar; the child may be most concerned about a facial burn.

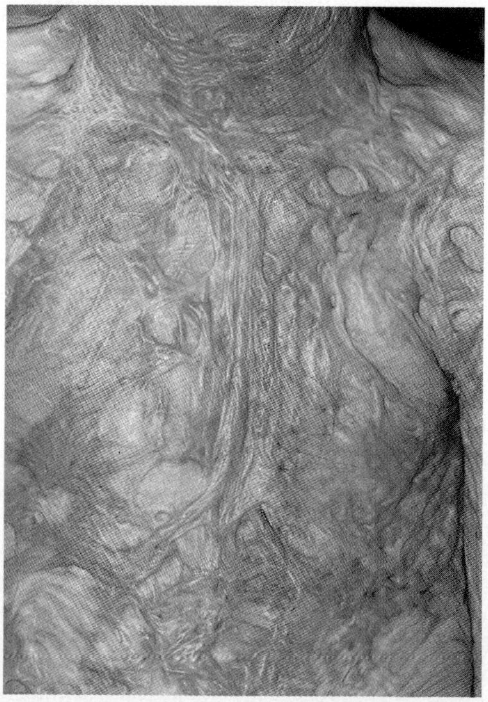

FIGURE 52.15 Extensive scarring on the chest of a 9-year-old boy with third-degree burns. The child and his family will need much support to help them deal with his appearance.

Children watch you as you care for them to see if you find them unattractive. As dressings are removed, children may expose parts of their body seemingly inappropriately, to see if you are shocked or revolted by them. It is easy to think that you will not react this way, but, for everyone, the first sight of a severe burn is a shock and it is difficult not to react accordingly. Imagining how the child feels, realizing that this mutilated skin is his or hers, helps health care providers maintain a professional attitude (see Focus on Multidisciplinary Care).

Returning to school may be difficult for children who have been hospitalized or receiving home care for a long time. Their old friends have new friends, so they may feel cut out of school activities. They look different if they have burn scars. The appearance of scar formation can be improved by the application of pressure dressings that the child wears 24 h a day. If the child has facial burns, facing friends with a compression bandage in place may be difficult. They need a great deal of support from health care personnel to be able to endure this. Some children may need referral for formal counseling. Some parents may need formal counseling also to help them accept the child's changed appearance.

Electrical Burns of the Mouth

If children put the prongs of a plugged-in extension cord into their mouth or chew on an electric cord, their mouth will be burned severely (Battan & Dart, 2001). Electrical current from the plug is conducted for a distance through the skin and underlying tissue so a tissue area much larger than where the prongs or cord actually touched is involved.

Tissue will be destroyed at the entry site, leaving an angry-looking ulcer. If blood vessels were burned, active bleeding will be present. The immediate treatment for electrical burns is to unplug the electric cord and control bleeding. Pressure applied to the site with gauze will usually control this. Most children are admitted to a hospital for at least 24 h in an observation unit after electrical burns of the mouth because edema in the mouth may lead to airway obstruction.

Clean the wound about four times a day with an antiseptic solution, such as half-strength hydrogen peroxide, to reduce the possibility of infection (a real danger in this area because bacteria are always present in the mouth).

Eating will be a problem for children because their mouth is so sore. They may be able to drink fluids from a cup best. Bland fluids, such as artificial fruit drinks, flat ginger ale, or milk products, are best.

Electrical burns of the mouth turn black as local tissue necrosis begins. They will heal with white, fibrous scar tissue, possibly causing a deformity of the lip and cheeks with healing. This can be minimized by the use of a mouth appliance, which helps maintain lip contour. Some children may have difficulty with speech sounds because of resulting lip scarring. They need follow-up care by a plastic surgeon to restore their lip contour and function again. Obviously, you need to review with parents the importance of not leaving "live" electrical cords where young children can reach them.

FOCUS ON MULTIDISCIPLINARY CARE

Children who experience major trauma, such as with severe burns, have many health care providers involved in their care: respiratory therapists, occupational and physical therapists, nutritionists, play therapists, physicians, intensive care nurses, and, possibly, social workers. For care to be effective, a great degree of coordination between professional disciplines is needed. Help everyone involved to remember that it takes a long time after an injury for the accompanying fear to be alleviated.

It is often a first reaction in people on seeing a child who has been injured to try and establish blame for the injury and then lecture on safety. Help personnel to react first to the child's needs (comfort, pain relief, airway) and secondarily to discovering the cause of the injury. This helps ensure that the child's needs are met and encourages parent cooperation, necessary for obtaining a factual history and planning for long-term care.

Be certain also that everyone understands that how burn tissue first looks is not how it will look eventually. This helps them to support the child through the many therapies necessary.

✔ CHECKPOINT QUESTIONS

19. What does debridement mean?
20. Where is skin taken from for autografting?

KEY POINTS

Children need total body assessment after a traumatic injury, because they may be unable to describe other injuries besides a primary one they may have suffered. Be aware that some trauma in children occurs from child abuse. Screen for this by history and physical examination. Use aseptic technique when caring for trauma victims so the child does not develop an additional unnecessary infection.

Head injuries are always potentially serious in children. Skull fractures, subdural hematomas, epidural hematomas, concussions, and contusions can occur. Coma (unconsciousness from which children cannot be roused) may be present in children after severe head trauma.

Abdominal trauma resulting in splenic or liver rupture may occur in connection with multiple trauma.

Near drowning can occur from salt or fresh water. The physiologic basis for complications after drowning differs depending on the type of water.

Common substances children swallow that result in poisoning include acetaminophen (Tylenol), caustic substances, and hydrocarbons. Teach parents to keep the number of the local poison control center next to their telephone and always to call first before administering an antidote for poisoning.

Lead poisoning most frequently occurs from the ingestion of lead chips from older housing. Preventing this is a major nursing responsibility.

Burns are classified as mild, moderate, and severe and can be divided into three types—first, second, and third degree—depending on the depth of the burn. Burns produce systemic body reactions and require long-term nursing care.

CRITICAL THINKING EXERCISES

1. Jason is the 4-year-old boy you met at the beginning of the chapter. He is admitted to the hospital confused and lethargic. What are the immediate nursing considerations? Why is frequent neurologic assessment necessary? What are the signs of deterioration and improvement of this child's status?
2. A 3-year-old child is seen in the emergency room for acetaminophen poisoning. Her father tells you they normally lock all medicine away carefully. His wife left acetaminophen on the counter because she was suffering from a headache. Would you want to discuss the necessity of poisoning prevention with these parents, or should they have learned from this experience that their actions were not safe?
3. A 10-year-old girl has third-degree burns on her legs from lighting a fire to burn leaves. She will probably have a lengthy hospitalization and may need skin grafts to improve healing. What precautions does this child need to prevent infection until healing is complete? What areas of care would you plan to address during the hospitalization?
4. Examine the National Health Goals related to trauma and children. Most government-sponsored money for nursing research is allotted based on these goals. What would be a possible research topic to explore pertinent to these goals that would be fundable and would also advance evidence-based practice?

REFERENCES

Battan, F. K., & Dart, R. C. (2001). Emergencies & injuries. In W. W. Hay, A. R. Hayward, M. J. Levin & J. M. Sondheimer (Eds.). *Current pediatric diagnosis & treatment* (15th ed.). New York: McGraw-Hill.

Brenner, R. A. et al. (2001). Where children drown. *Pediatrics, 108*(1), 85–89.

Campbell, C. (2000). Lead poisoning. In M. W. Schwartz (Ed.). *The 5-minute pediatric consult* (pp. 502–503). Philadelphia: Lippincott Williams & Wilkins.

Centers for Disease Control and Prevention. (2001). *Preventing lead poisoning in young children.* Washington, DC: Author.

Chiaretti, A., et al. (2000). Early post-traumatic seizures in children with head injury. *Child's Nervous System, 16*(12), 862–866.

Das, A., & Kim, K. S. (2000). Infections in burn injury. *The Pediatric Infectious Disease Journal, 19*(8), 737–738.

Department of Health and Human Services. (2000). *Healthy people 2010.* Washington, DC: DHHS.

Dibiase, A. T., et al. (2000). Hazards of orthodontic appliances and the oropharynx. *Journal of Orthodontics, 27*(4), 295–302.

Dudek, S. G. (2001). *Nutrition handbook for nursing practice* (4th ed.). Philadelphia: Lippincott Williams & Wilkins.

Fine, J. S. (2000). Iron poisoning. *Current Problems in Pediatrics, 30*(3), 71–90.

Gauvin, F., Bailey, B., & Bratton, S. L. (2001). Hospitalizations for pediatric intoxication in Washington State. *Archives of Pediatrics & Adolescent Medicine, 155*(10), 1105–1110.

Gheen, K. M. (2001). Near-drowning and cold water submersion. *Seminars in Pediatric Surgery, 10*(1), 26–27.

Godwin, H. A. (2001). The biological chemistry of lead. *Current Opinion in Chemical Biology, 5*(2), 223–227.

Hassi, J., & Makinen, T. M. (2000). Frostbite: Occurrence, risk factors and consequences. *International Journal of Circumpolar Health, 59*(2), 92–98.

Hilton, G. (2001). Assessment of subdural vs epidural hematoma. *American Journal of Nursing, 101*(9), 51–52.

Jordan, B. (2001). Lap belt complex: Recognition and assessment of seatbelt injuries in pediatric trauma patients. *Journal of Emergency Medical Services, 26*(5), 36–43.

Kalan, A., & Tariq, M. (2000). Foreign bodies in the nasal cavities. *Postgraduate Medical Journal, 76*(898), 484–487.

Leone, R. J. & Hammond, J. S. (2001). Nonoperative management of pediatric blunt hepatic trauma. *American Surgeon, 67*(2), 138–142.

Matthews, D. J., & Wilson, P. E. (2001). Common sports medicine issues and injuries. In W. W. Hay, A. R. Hayward, M. J. Levin & J. M. Sondheimer (Eds.). *Current pediatric diagnosis & treatment* (15th ed). New York: McGraw-Hill.

McCance, K. L. & Huether, S. E. (2002). *Pathophysiology* (4th ed.). St. Louis: Mosby.

McTigue, D. J. (2000). Diagnosis and management of dental injuries in children. *Pediatric Clinics of North America, 47*(5), 1067–1084.

National Centers for Health Statistics. (2001). *Child safety.* Washington, DC: Author.

Neuwalder, J. M. et al. (2002). A review of computer-aided body surface area determination. *Journal of Burn Care & Rehabilitation, 23*(1), 55–59.

Ozanne-Smith, J., et al. (2001). Childhood poisoning: Access and prevention. *Journal of Paediatrics & Child Heath, 37*(3), 262–265.

Presutti, R. J. (2001). Prevention and treatment of dog bites. *American Family Physician, 63*(8), 1567–1572.

Qazi, K., Gerson, L. W., Christopher, N. C., Kessler, E., & Ida, N. (2001). Curling iron-related injuries presenting to U.S. emergency departments. *Academic Emergency Medicine, 8*(4), 395–397.

Salerno, D. (2000). Frostbite. In M.W. Schwartz (Ed.). *The 5-minute pediatric consult* (pp. 372-373). Philadelphia: Lippincott Williams & Wilkins,

Shannon, M. (2000). Primary care: Ingestion of toxic substances by children. *The New England Journal of Medicine, 342*(3), 186-191.

Shaw, K. N. (2000). Near-drowning. In M. W. Schwartz (Ed.). *The 5-minute pediatric consult* (pp. 556-557). Philadelphia: Lippincott Williams & Wilkins.

Sirotnak, A. P. & Krugman, R. D. (2001). Child abuse and neglect. In W. W. Hay, A. R. Hayward, M. J. Levin, & J. M. Sondheimer (Eds.). *Current pediatric diagnosis and treatment* (15th ed.). New York: McGraw-Hill.

Soprano, J. V., & Mandl, K. D. (2001). Four strategies for the management of esophageal coins in children. *Pediatrics, 105*(1), 5-8.

Winston, F. K., et al. (2002). Risk of injury to child passengers in compact extended-cab pickup trucks. *JAMA 287*(9), 1147-1152.

ABC XYZ SUGGESTED READINGS

Agran, P. F., et al. (2001). Rates of pediatric and adolescent injuries by year of age. *Pediatrics, 108*(3), 45-48.

Barret, J. P., et al. (2000). Effects of tracheostomies on infection and airway complications in pediatric burn patients. *Burns, 26*(2), 190-193.

Beierle, E. A. (2000). Free fluid on abdominal computed tomography scan after blunt trauma does not mandate exploratory laparotomy in children. *Journal of Pediatric Surgery, 35*(6), 990-992.

Bernardo, L. M. (2002). Emergency nurses' role in pediatric injury and prevention. *Nursing Clinics of North America 37*(1), 135-143.

Berning, E. L., & Anderson, M. R. (2001). Respiratory support of the head-injured child. *Respiratory Care Clinics of North America,* 7(1), 39-57.

Broughan, T. A., & Soloway, R. D. (2000). Acetaminophen hepatotoxicity. *Digestive Diseases & Sciences, 45*(8), 1553-1558.

Burd, R. S., et al. (2001). Nutritional support of the pediatric trauma patient: A practical approach. *Respiratory Care Clinics of North America,* 7(1), 79-96.

Calkins, C. M., et al. (2001). Life-threatening dog attacks: A devastating combination of penetrating and blunt injuries. *Journal of Pediatric Surgery, 36*(8), 1115-1117.

Chisolm, J. J. (2001). The road to primary prevention of lead toxicity in children. *Pediatrics, 107*(3), 581-583.

Cohen, S. (2001). Lead poisoning: A summary of treatment and prevention. *Pediatric Nursing, 27*(2), 125-130.

Dise-Lewis, J. E. (2001). A developmental perspective on psychological principles of burn care. *Journal of Burn Care & Rehabilitation, 22*(3), 255-260.

Finnoff, J. T., et al. (2001). Barriers to bicycle helmet use. *Pediatrics, 108*(1), 4-7.

Giesbrecht, G. G. (2000). Cold stress, near downing and accidental hypothermia. *Aviation Space & Environmental Medicine, 71*(7), 733-752.

Kelly, K. D., et al. (2001). Sport and recreation-related head injuries treated in the emergency department. *Clinical Journal of Sport Medicine, 11*(2), 77-81.

Kurtzman, T. L., Otsuka, K. N., & Wahl, R. A. (2001). Inhalant abuse by adolescents. *Journal of Adolescent Health, 28*(3), 170-180.

Merk, T. (2001). Beyond the burns. Managing the pain and consequences of pediatric burns. *Journal of Emergency Medical Services, 26*(9), 66-77.

O'Neill, J. A. (2000) Advances in the management of pediatric trauma. *American Journal of Surgery, 180*(5), 365-369.

Powers, K. S. (2000). Diagnosis and management of common toxic ingestions and inhalations. *Pediatric Annals, 29*(6), 330-342.

Quang, L. S., & Woolf, A. D. (2000). Past, present, and future role of ipecac syrup. *Current Opinion in Pediatrics, 12*(2), 153-162.

Sheridan, R. L. (2001). Comprehensive treatment of burns. *Current Problems in Surgery, 38*(9), 657-756.

Smith, M. L. (2000). Pediatric burns: Management of thermal, electrical, and chemical burns and burn-like dermatologic conditions. *Pediatric Annals, 29*(6), 367-378.

Stallion, A. (2001). Initial assessment and management of the pediatric trauma patient. *Respiratory Care Clinics of North America,* 7(1), 1-11.

Stanken, B. A. (2000). Promoting helmet use among children. *Journal of Community Health Nursing, 17*(20), 85-92.

Zuckerman, G. B., & Conway, E. E. (2000). Drowning and near drowning: A pediatric epidemic. *Pediatric Annals, 29*(6), 360-366.

Nursing Care of the Child With Cancer

CHAPTER 53

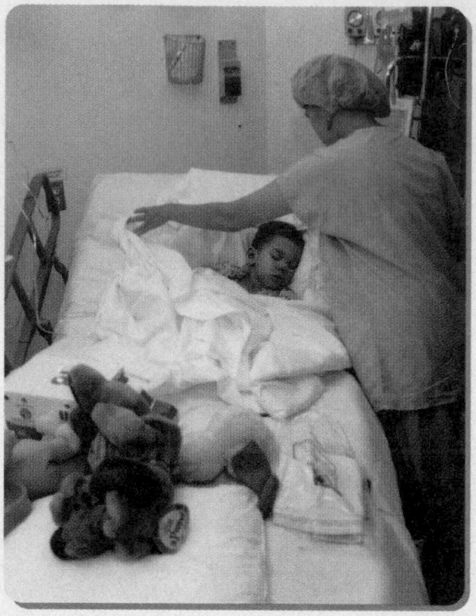

Key Terms

- biopsy
- chemotherapeutic agent
- Ewing's sarcoma
- leukemia
- lymphoma
- metastasis
- neoplasm
- neuroblastoma
- oncogenic virus
- osteogenic sarcoma
- rhabdomyosarcoma
- sarcoma
- tumor staging

Objectives

After mastering the contents of this chapter, you should be able to:

1. Define terms related to tumor growth, such as neoplasm, benign, malignant, sarcoma, and carcinoma.
2. Describe normal cellular growth and theories that explain how cells alter to become cancerous in children.
3. Assess the child with a cancerous process, such as a rhabdomyosarcoma, neuroblastoma, Wilms' tumor, and leukemia.
4. Formulate nursing diagnoses related to the child with cancer.
5. Establish appropriate outcomes for the child with cancer.
6. Plan nursing care specific to the child with cancer.
7. Implement nursing care for the child receiving cancer therapy.
8. Evaluate outcomes for the child with cancer.
9. Identify National Health Goals related to the care of the child with cancer that nurses can be instrumental in helping the nation to achieve.
10. Identify areas related to care of children with cancer that could benefit from additional nursing research or application of evidence-based practice.
11. Use critical thinking to propose ways that nursing care for the child with cancer can be more family centered.
12. Integrate knowledge of abnormal cell growth in children with the nursing process to achieve quality maternal and child health nursing care.

Geri is a 6-year-old boy you meet at a health maintenance organization clinic. He is there for a well-child checkup. His mother tells you that Geri wakes up every morning with a headache and then vomits. Immediately after that, he is fine. The problem began just after he started a new school in the fall, so she is certain it is related to this. His teacher has suggested that Geri needs an eye examination because he cocks his head to see the chalkboard. You notice that he has lost weight. "What do I do for school phobia?" his mother asks you.

Is his mother describing school phobia? What additional questions would you want to ask her to help discover if this is something more serious?

Previous chapters described the growth and development of well children and disorders associated with specific body systems. This chapter adds information about the dramatic changes, both physical and psychosocial, that occur when children develop cancer, a phenomenon that can present in any body system. This is important information because it forms a base for care and health teaching.

After you've studied the chapter, answer the Critical Thinking Exercises at the end of the chapter and then access the on-line study activities (http://connection.lww.com) *to further sharpen your skills and test your knowledge.*

The terms *malignant* and *cancerous* describe cells growing and proliferating in a disorderly, chaotic fashion. In adults, cancer usually occurs in the form of a solid tumor. In children, the most frequent type of cancer is that of an immature blood cell overgrowth, or leukemia (Albano et al., 2001).

Many parents assume that a diagnosis of cancer means that the child's life will be very limited. Because of the tremendous advances in cancer research and treatment over the last 20 years, however, the prognosis for children and the chances for a cure improve daily. To help parents and children adjust to this illness, however, nursing support is necessary from the time of diagnosis throughout the long-term therapy required. National Health Goals related to cancer and children are shown in the Focus on National Health Goals box.

FOCUS ON NATIONAL HEALTH GOALS

A number of National Health Goals concern cancer prevention and children:

- Reduce the overall cancer death rate from a baseline of 202/100,000 of the population to 159/100,000.
- Reduce the rate of melanoma cancer deaths from a baseline of 2.8/100,000 of the population to a target level of 2.5/100,000.
- Increase the proportion of adolescents in grades 9 through 12 who follow protective measures that may reduce the risk of skin cancer (DHHS, 2000).

Nurses can be instrumental in helping the nation achieve these goals by careful history taking at health assessments to reveal the symptoms of cancer, because these are often subtle in children, and by active teaching to stimulate self-screening measures, such as breast and testicular examination and measures to avoid excessive sun exposure.

Areas that could benefit from additional nursing research are effective ways to teach young clients about the dangers of tanning booths or excessive sun exposure; reasons adolescents give for avoiding self-examination; and reasons parents give for delaying health care consultation after discovering an abnormal growth, unexplainable bruising, or weight loss.

NURSING PROCESS OVERVIEW

For the Child With Cancer

Assessment

The symptoms of cancer in children are often insidious and difficult to define. Headaches or pain at a particular body site can often be explained away by other factors such as sports injuries or fatigue. Weight loss, however, a common symptom of cancer, is never normal in healthy children. Therefore, at every health care visit, plot and analyze a child's height and weight to document evidence of this important finding. Be sure to refer children with swelling or pain of major joints to their primary health care provider for further assessment so that bone tumors will not go undetected. See Assessing the Child for Signs of Cancer.

Nursing Diagnosis

Selected nursing diagnoses established for the child with cancer address specific symptoms caused by the cancer, side effects of the cancer therapy, or coping abilities of the child and family.

- Pain related to neoplastic process in bone
- Imbalanced nutrition, less than body requirements, related to stomatitis from radiation therapy
- Risk for infection related to immunosuppressive effects of chemotherapy
- Disturbed body image related to loss of hair following radiation treatment
- Compromised family coping, related to long-term chemotherapy program

Outcome Identification and Planning

When a neoplasm is first diagnosed in their child, parents may be able to deal only with short-term outcomes and plans. They may concentrate on learning about the effect or toxic properties of a particular chemotherapeutic drug given their child, or they may ask how long the child's surgical incision will be. Dealing with such specifics helps them to control their anxiety because it prevents them from dealing with the overall picture or prognosis—that their child has a potentially lethal condition.

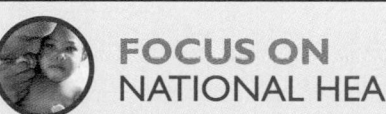

The family of the child with cancer needs support beginning with the diagnosis. When planning, sit down with parents and discuss the treatment proto-

ASSESSING the Child For Signs of Cancer

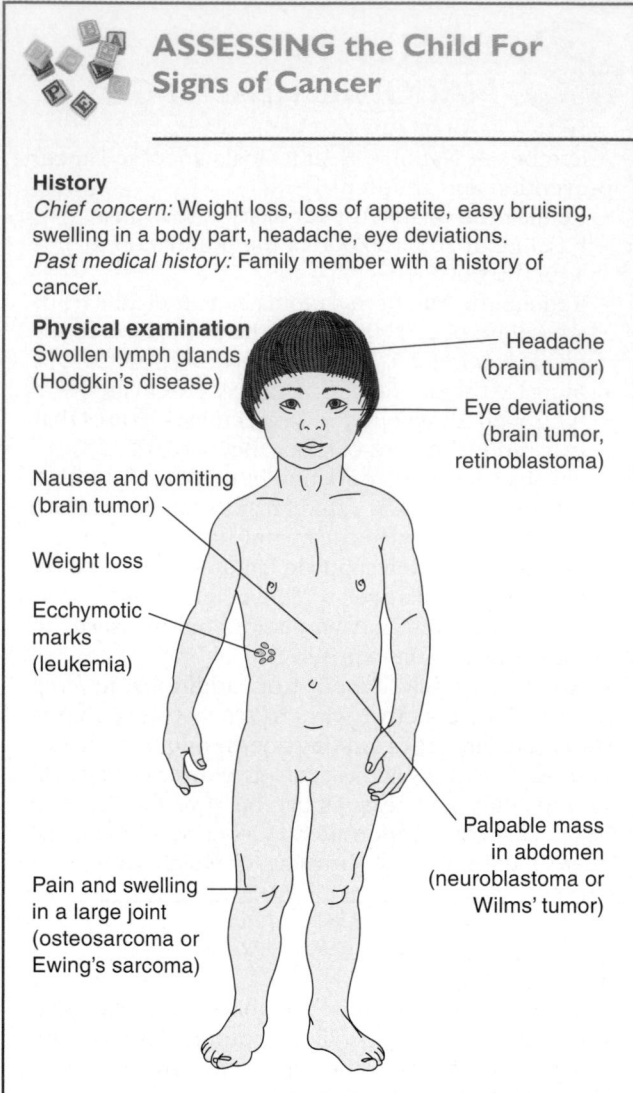

History

Chief concern: Weight loss, loss of appetite, easy bruising, swelling in a body part, headache, eye deviations.

Past medical history: Family member with a history of cancer.

Physical examination

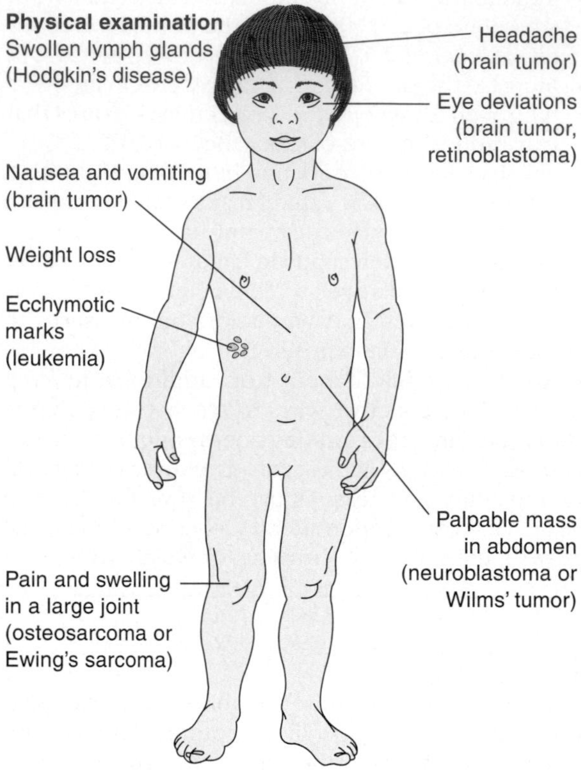

col. Explain measures they will need to take to make their child more comfortable during therapy (eg, not forcing food if the child is nauseated, playing games or reading stories while intravenous [IV] chemotherapy agent is administered).

Parents are usually eager for results of diagnostic tests. They may need support while waiting until all the findings have been assembled for an accurate assessment of staging and prognosis. Establishing a primary relationship with both the child and parents is important so that, no matter how many hospitalizations are necessary, they know a support person is waiting to help them through this long-term illness. Long-term therapy can be expensive, so consider the family's financial capabilities, helping them make any necessary financial arrangements for care. The siblings of the child with cancer should be included in planning care not only because the illness is serious, but also because the treatment may last for an extended period, further stressing the family.

Parents will hear of many questionable cancer cures from newspapers or friends during the course of their child's illness. Help them to voice their hope and concerns for these cures as they hear them. Open discussion helps parents keep such cures in perspective without putting any more emphasis on them than they warrant. If these questionable cures cannot be discussed with health care personnel, they appear to grow in importance, and parents may turn to them in preference to established therapy.

Parents can be expected to experience grief if they learn their child's prognosis is poor. They move slowly through stages of denial, anger, bargaining, depression, and acceptance. When planning with parents, be certain to take into account their current stage of grief (see Chapter 56).

Implementation

Nursing interventions for the child with cancer include supporting the child and parents from the time of diagnosis through procedures such as surgery, radiation therapy, chemotherapy, and continued health supervision. This is a stressful and long-term process because chemotherapy may be continued for 2 to 3 years after diagnosis. Increasingly, cancer treatment is offered on an ambulatory basis to keep hospitalization to a minimum, so many interventions include teaching the parents to give care or monitor for recurring signs.

Keep in mind that the stress of long-term treatment may put the child and family at risk for developmental or family coping problems. You can be a positive force in encouraging healthy adaptation to the demands of the child's illness and in reassessing the situation periodically during therapy to be certain the child is receiving appropriate stimulation for developmental growth. Providing comfort and alleviating pain are often primary concerns in oncology nursing. Measures for pain relief are discussed in Chapter 38.

Organizations that may be helpful in supplying information to parents include the following:

American Cancer Society (*www.cancer.org*)
National Cancer Institute (*www.cancer.gov*)
Children's Oncology Group
(*www.childrensoncologygroup.org*)
Candlelighters Childhood Cancer Foundation
(*www.candlelighters.org*)
The Leukemia & Lymphoma Society
(*www.leukemia-lymphoma.org*)

Outcome Evaluation

Because cancer therapy includes long-term care, children must be evaluated periodically to be certain that outcomes are being met and are still current. Some examples indicating outcome achievement may include:

- Child keeps all appointments for chemotherapy treatments.
- Child maintains passing grades in school despite interruptions for therapy.
- Parents voice that they can keep anxiety at an acceptable level between clinic appointments.

Children with cancer need the same well-child maintenance care that all children do, with one exception. While they are on chemotherapy, which causes a decreased immune response, they should not receive live-virus vaccines.

Returning for health care follow-up visits causes anxiety. The child seems well, but parents may be apprehensive while the health care practitioner palpates the child's abdomen or blood specimens are obtained. Some parents may find the strain of returning for follow-up visits too great and may miss appointments (not to know seems better than to be told bad news). Such parents need help in understanding that initial remissions can be maintained, second remissions can be achieved, so maintenance therapy must be continued. Because children with a tumor such as retinoblastoma or those who receive chemotherapy or radiation are more prone to developing a second cancer later in life than others, follow-up is an essential detection measure (Abramson et al., 2001).

Parents of the child with cancer may seek health maintenance care or evaluation for their other children more often than other parents would. This is because they are worried that what seems just a minor symptom is actually a sign of cancer in that child also. They need greater amounts of assurance that their other children are well than the average parent does.

Most children with cancer, even if no cure is possible, will be cared for at home, rather than being hospitalized. Their parents may need extensive preparation for home care (see Chapter 35). Help them to maintain close contact with health care personnel to prevent feeling abandoned. When the child dies, the parents may feel a need to return to their primary caregiver for support. This provides an opportunity to evaluate their adjustment to the child's death and offer support if needed. Being with a child who dies at home appears to make death a more understandable phenomenon for siblings and, in many instances, can be advocated (see Focus on Evidence-Based Practice). Care in a separate hospice setting is another option for the child in whom a remission cannot be achieved (see Chapter 56).

FOCUS ON EVIDENCE-BASED PRACTICE

Do Parents Adjust Best to the Death of a Child With Cancer If It Occurs During an Active Phase of Treatment or During Terminal Care?

To answer this question, the parents of 60 children who died while in terminal care and 26 children who died during a phase of active anticancer therapy were interviewed after the child's death. Parents in both groups reported physical and/or mental problems with similar frequency (39% and 34%); both groups of parents reported that their recovery time was similar (14 and 16 months); and their ability to return to work was also similar (over 70% returned to work by 1 month). In both groups, the mothers required a longer recovery time and returned to work later. The effect of the death on siblings showed significant differences with 18% of the terminal care group having problems such as fear, behavioral problems, problems with friends, and school-related issues compared with 32% in the active therapy group. The researchers concluded that when a child dies, there are few differences whether the death occurred during active therapy or after this has been discontinued. The loss of a child is a major event in either situation.

Although this study was conducted in Europe (Helsinki, Finland), it deals with such a universal concept (reaction to death of a child) that it has implications for nurses worldwide. Based on this study, it would be important to assess the siblings of a child who died at future well-child visits to see that they have resolved their reaction to the child's death, particularly if the death occurred during active treatment when there seemed to be hope that the child would live.

Sirki, K., Saarinen-Pihkala, U. M., & Hovi. L. (2000). Coping of parents and siblings with the death of a child with cancer: Death after terminal care compared with death during active anti-cancer therapy. *Acta Paediatrica, 89*(6), 717-721.

NEOPLASIA

All body tissue undergoes growth necessary to develop into that specific type of tissue. Normally, the body is able to maintain the proliferation necessary to replace old cells that die while also sustaining physical growth needs. Cancerous, or malignant, tissue, however, is unable to maintain this balance and begins to proliferate in disorderly, chaotic ways.

The word **neoplasm** means new growth; it usually refers to a new *abnormal* growth that does not respond to normal growth-control mechanisms. Whether this process is one that produces a solid tumor or one that involves blood-forming elements, growth begins insidiously. The process may have been ongoing for some time before parents or a child realize it is present. Even after parents or children are aware that a change exists, some time may pass before they realize that the changes are serious enough to require health care, particularly if the changes are not well defined.

Although cancer in children is rare, it still remains the leading cause of death due to disease in children under the age of 15 years. Approximately 8,000 new cases of cancer occur in children in the United States each year; approximately 1,700 deaths occur annually from this cause. Fortunately, the overall survival rate for children with cancer today has improved dramatically (National Cancer Institute, 2000). Knowing the processes involved in cell growth—both normal and abnormal—is essential to help parents understand what is happening to their child and why specific treatment measures are necessary at various stages of cell growth.

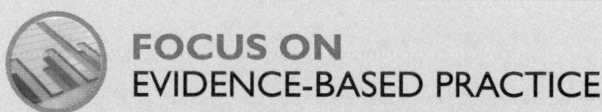

Cell Growth

The normal cell cycle consists of two main divisions: an interphase (resting phase) and a mitosis (dividing) phase. The interphase has four periods: G0, G1, S, and G2. Activity during these periods is summarized in Table 53-1. The time span of a cell's life cycle varies: a bone cell cycle is short—about 10 h; a nerve cell cycle is long—the lifetime of the person. The rate of cycles is slowed or increased by outside stimuli, such as hypoxia, genetic and immunologic factors, and physical and chemical agents. Normally, both resting and active cells are always present.

Body cells apparently have the ability to recognize their own type, possibly by recognizing surface enzymes or glucose particles on cell membranes. Normally, cells of like types do not migrate away from each other because they recognize and adhere to each other to form a solid mass. In neoplastic cells, the ability to keep together is defective (they are autonomous). This may be related to decreased calcium in the cell membrane or an increased negative charge that repels other cells rather than bonds them together.

Like cells appear to be able to recognize when they are being crowded for the space they must occupy and apparently communicate with one another to halt growth at the point they touch or become crowded. Neoplastic cells do not respond to this communication or cannot receive it, so, despite how crowded they are, they continue to grow. By the time a tumor mass is detected by palpation, it has probably doubled from its original aberrant cell about 30 times. In many instances, it may be necessary to kill as many as a billion cells to destroy the entire mass (McCance & Huether, 2002).

TABLE 53.1 Phases of the Cell Cycle

PHASE	ACTIVITY
G	Gap, or the phase between mitosis and synthesis.
G0	Cell at rest. Cells remain in this state until some stimulant, such as death of surrounding cells, triggers the cell to enter an active phase; it is difficult to destroy cells in this resting state.
G1	Period until DNA stabilization is complete; it remains difficult to destroy cells in this phase.
S (synthesis)	Period (6–8 h) during which DNA and chromosomes are duplicated or a cell readies itself for division into two daughter cells.
G2	Cell doubling in size as preparation for dividing into two daughter cells; if protein synthesis can be stopped at this point so that the cell cannot reach a "critical mass," mitosis (cell division) cannot take place.
M (mitosis)	Period of cell division into two like daughter cells.

Neoplastic Growth

Neoplasms can be either *benign* (growth is limited) or *malignant* (cancerous). Even when a tumor is benign, however, it may not be completely harmless. It can cause damage by pressing on adjacent tissue (eg, brain tumors in children are often benign, but they can cause extensive respiratory center depression from increasing pressure).

Causes of Neoplastic Growth

The exact origin of neoplastic growth is unknown, and any growth may actually involve more than one cause. In adults, tumors may grow because normal cell growth has been altered by environmental irritation, such as chronic exposure to chemical irritants or cigarette smoke. Tumors of the skin, bladder, lung, and intestines involve organs exposed to such outside influences and irritation. In children, tumors most frequently occur in organs unexposed to the environment (eg, leukemia of the bloodstream, Wilms' tumor of the kidney, brain tumors, and neuroblastoma in the abdomen). Because many tumors occur in children younger than 5 years, exposure to environmental carcinogens is limited, so this cause of tumors is probably not a great influence in childhood cancer. Two substances that lead to lung cancer and to which children may be exposed are secondary smoke and asbestos. Asbestos is a particular problem if the child's school or home is insulated with this material or a parent works in asbestos removal and brings home particles on clothing.

A child who has survived one cancer appears to be at higher than normal risk for the development of a second cancer. Radiation exposure used to treat the first malignancy may be responsible for this. In addition, there may be a predisposition to cancer in some families (Albano et al., 2001).

Another common theory of why neoplasms grow is the cell mutation theory. This suggests that carcinogenic agents and hereditary susceptibility combine to alter the nature of cells, leading to abnormal growth. A first stage of initiation may mark the cells for abnormal growth. A second stage of promotion actually begins the abnormal growth. Carcinogens can be living (viral), physical (radiation), or chemical. Radiation during intrauterine life is a documented cause of leukemia. Radiation of the thyroid in infancy may cause thyroid cancer later in life. Use of androgenic steroids may lead to hepatocellular cancer.

This theory explains why the growth of neoplastic cells is irreversible (the cells cannot return to a normal state because they are intrinsically changed) and why neoplasms occur in some people but not in others (both an intrinsic and extrinsic factor or an inherited tendency and an environmental insult must be present). It is difficult to document this process because it stipulates that two separate steps are necessary for a cell to become cancerous. If there is a lengthy time span between these steps, the cause-and-effect relationship is difficult to trace (McCance & Huether, 2002).

Yet another theory is that oncogenic (cancer-causing) viruses are responsible for tumor growth. According to the viral theory, **oncogenic viruses** have the ability to change the structure of DNA or RNA in cells. C-type RNA viruses may be implicated in leukemia. Epstein-Barr virus, a DNA virus, may be associated with Burkitt's lymphoma. This theory is supported by the fact that an immunodeficient state increases the risk for developing a neoplastic growth. With this state, both viral surveillance and removal of abnormal cells are lost; therefore, virus invasion and abnormal cell growth begin. Still another theory is that tumor suppressor cells exist in some individuals and not in others. Retinoblastoma is an example of a cancer that may occur when such cells are not present.

HEALTH PROMOTION AND RISK MANAGEMENT

Because childhood cancers do not seem to arise from environmental contaminants as much as adult cancers do, methods to reduce the risk are not as well defined. Urging parents to reduce children's exposure to secondary cigarette smoke and urging adolescents not to begin smoking can help reduce the incidence of lung cancer when they reach adulthood. Applying sunscreen and reducing the overall time of sun exposure for children can help reduce the development of skin cancer in later life. It is documented that children who receive chemotherapy or radiation for one cancer have a higher incidence of developing another cancer later in life. Therefore, urging these children to continue health appointments so additional tumor development can be discovered is another important preventive measure.

ASSESSING CHILDREN WITH CANCER

The incidence of various types of childhood cancers is shown in Figure 53-1. Because these cancers involve different body systems, signs and symptoms can vary greatly.

History

Many cancers in children have been developing for some time before the child is brought for care because the symptoms (bruising, nosebleeds, pain in a knee, constipation) are not perceived as important to parents. Thorough history taking at health care visits can help reveal these symptoms so the child can be further evaluated and the cancer discovered early in its growth. For example, symptoms of obstruction (such as constipation) or pressure (such as headache) may be revealed first by this method. As malignant tumors grow, they tend to cause systemic effects in the child. Cachexia (loss of weight, anorexia) occurs if the tumor is growing so rapidly that it takes nutrients from normal cells. Excessive hormone production (overproduction of antidiuretic, thyroid, or adrenocorticotropic hormone) may occur because of tumor growth in that specific body area leading to systemic symptoms. Although the warning signs of cancer listed by the American Cancer Society (Box 53-1) apply primarily to cancer in adults, they should also be kept in mind as general guidelines when assessing children (see Focus on Cultural Competence).

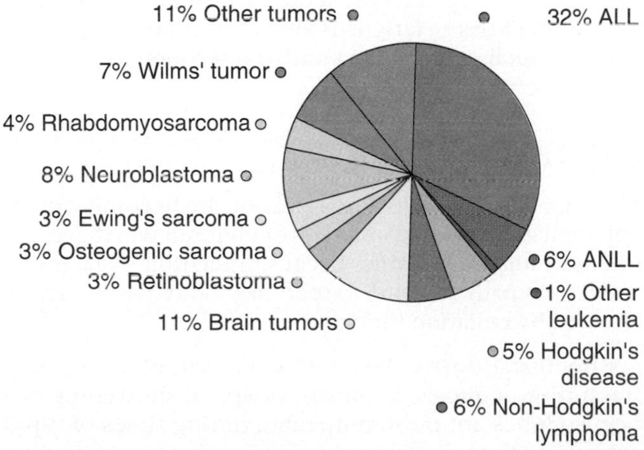

FIGURE 53.1 Approximate incidence of common childhood cancers (NCI, 2001).

Physical and Laboratory Examination

Any suspicion of a malignancy requires a thorough physical examination. Assessing height and weight of children is an important component. To confirm a diagnosis, a number of diagnostic procedures may be used, including x-ray, sonography, magnetic resonance imaging (MRI), blood analysis, and biopsy.

Biopsy

A **biopsy** is the surgical removal of tissue cells for laboratory analysis. Most children with a possible diagnosis of cancer will have a biopsy performed to confirm their ini-

BOX 53.1

WARNING SYMPTOMS AND SIGNS OF CANCER

General Symptoms

1. Unexplained weight loss
2. Fever
3. Fatigue
4. Pain
5. Skin changes (itching, darkening, reddening, hairiness)

General Signs

1. A change in bowel or bladder habits
2. A nonhealing sore
3. Unusual bleeding or discharge
4. A thickening or lump in the breast or other body part
5. Indigestion or difficulty swallowing
6. An obvious change in a wart or mole
7. A nagging cough or persistent hoarseness

The American Cancer Society. (1998). *Seven signs of cancer.* Atlanta: Author.

FOCUS ON CULTURAL COMPETENCE

People in different cultures have differing beliefs as to what causes cancer, ranging from evil spirits or evil past lives to totally environmental causes or unpredictable cell growth. Talking with parents and the child, if old enough, about what they think is the cause of cancer can add understanding to parents' actions; it can make explanations of therapy more meaningful to parents, because explanations can be geared to fit within their beliefs.

Additionally, many parents may ask if complementary therapies such as herbal medications or special diets will help cure their child. Provide time for discussion of these therapies because they offer parents a sense of control in an otherwise possibly bewildering environment of medical treatments.

tial diagnosis. Although biopsies are classified as minor surgery and usually done on an ambulatory basis, do not treat them lightly. They carry a definite surgical risk if conscious sedation or general anesthesia is used. Moreover, they are an anxiety-producing procedure for the parents and the child. Up to this point, parents can convince themselves that the child has something innocent. A biopsy clouds this hope because the word biopsy implies that cancer is at least a possibility. For this reason, parents and children need thorough preparation for the biopsy procedure and the care the child will need after the procedure. Anxious parents do not "hear" well and may need to have postoperative instructions repeated. Bone marrow aspiration is a frequent type of biopsy used with children. Although this can be done with only local anesthesia, it is equally frightening (see Chapter 44).

Staging

Tumor staging is a procedure by which a malignant tumor's extent and progress are documented. Knowing the stage of the tumor helps the health care team design an effective treatment program, establish an accurate prognosis, and evaluate the progress or regression of the disease. In general staging, stage I refers to a tumor that can be completely removed surgically. Stage II refers to a tumor that cannot be completely removed surgically. Stages III and IV designate tumors that have extended beyond the original site or have spread systemically (**metastasis**). There are various staging systems, but one of the most common is known as the TNM system, which describes the tumor's size (T), its presence in the lymph nodes (N), and its metastasis (M) or spread to other organs, if any. A TNM system is most applicable to carcinomas (tumors of the epithelial tissue). Because most childhood tumors are sarcomas (tumors derived from connective tissue), the system is not as useful for childhood cancers as it is for adult cancers.

✔ CHECKPOINT QUESTIONS

1. What does it mean when a tumor has metastasized?
2. What does stage II disease imply?

OVERVIEW OF CANCER TREATMENT MEASURES USED WITH CHILDREN

The treatment of a child with cancer focuses on devising ways to kill the growth of the abnormal cells while protecting normal surrounding cells. This is done by a combination of surgery, radiation, chemotherapy, bone marrow transplant, immunotherapy (biologic response modifiers), and general health measures. Bone marrow transplant is discussed in Chapter 44 with common blood disorders.

Radiation Therapy

Radiation therapy changes the DNA component of a cell nucleus to a point where the cell cannot replicate DNA material, thereby inhibiting further cell division and growth. Radiation is not effective on cells that have a low oxygen content (a proportion of cells in every tumor mass), nor is it effective at the time of cell division (mitosis). Therefore, radiation schedules are designed so that therapy occurs over 1 to 6 weeks. In this way, cells that are not in a susceptible stage on one day will be in a susceptible stage on another. Tumors that require such a massive dose of radiation that normal tissue through which the radiation must pass to penetrate the tumor would be destroyed in the process are said to be radioresistant.

Immediate Side Effects

Radiation has both systemic and localized effects. Radiation sickness (anorexia, nausea, vomiting) is the most frequently encountered systemic effect. This occurs if the gastrointestinal (GI) tract is radiated. It also can occur to a lesser degree from the release of toxic substances from destroyed tumor cells. The child may need to receive an antiemetic before each procedure to counter nausea and vomiting. Extreme fatigue is also very common. Skin reactions, such as erythema and tenderness, are typical local effects.

Long-Term Side Effects

The long-term side effects of radiation are becoming more apparent as increasing numbers of children who have had intense radiation survive. Because radiation damages all cells in its path to some extent, any body tissue can be affected by radiation therapy.

Effects on Bone. Asymmetric growth of bones, easy fracturing, scoliosis, kyphosis, or spinal shortening can occur. Bones are most vulnerable during times of rapid growth, such as the first year of life or during a prepubertal growth spurt. Scoliosis and kyphosis can be avoided if an entire vertebra is radiated rather than one side or the other; this means that a larger area of bone may be radiated than formerly so that both sides of the vertebra are in the radiation path.

Effects on Hormones. Radiation to the head and neck can result in long-term thyroid, hypothalamic, and pituitary gland dysfunction. This may result in growth hormone deficiency or hypothalamic-pituitary stimulation to the thyroid gland. Children's growth and thyroid function should be evaluated every 6 months for the next 3 years to detect these changes. Both hypothyroidism and hypopituitary growth failure can be treated with hormone replacement in coming years. Radiation to ovaries or testes can result in infertility. In girls, normal estrogen production may lag or fail, preventing the development of secondary sexual changes. In boys, testosterone production rarely fails. However, pretreatment sperm banking may be advocated for a boy past puberty before he undergoes radiation to the testes.

Effects on the Nervous System. Long-term effects of radiation to the nervous system are demyelination and necrosis of the white matter of the brain. This can result in symptoms of lethargy, sleepiness, and seizures. Effects on the gray matter can result in learning disabilities. There may be abnormal electroencephalograph tracings; the child may have low-intensity headaches, cataracts, salivary gland damage, and a chronic change in or loss of taste.

Effects on the Organs of the Chest and Abdomen. Radiation to the lungs may result in a chronic pneumonitis and pulmonary fibrosis or thickening. Heart effects may be pericardial thickening and reduced heart expandability. Radiation to the GI system can result in chronic malabsorption from changes in intestinal villi. Hepatic fibrosis can result in reduced liver function. Radiation to the kidney and bladder can result in nephritis and chronic cystitis.

The possibility of these long-term effects of radiation should be explained to parents when radiation is initially discussed as a part of obtaining informed consent. At the early stage of diagnosis, however, parents rarely are concerned with these long-term effects. Their thoughts are understandably filled with such short-term outcomes as the achievement of a remission or destruction of the tumor.

NURSING DIAGNOSES AND RELATED INTERVENTIONS

Nursing Diagnosis: Parental and child anxiety related to radiation procedure

Outcome Identification: Parents will demonstrate reduced anxiety about radiation by time of therapy.

Outcome Evaluation: Parents voice that they understand necessity of therapy and can help support child during therapy.

Before Treatment. The points where radiation therapy will be directed are marked on the child's skin, usually in indelible ink. As a rule, no cream or lotion should be applied to radiation areas until the treatment series is complete. If creams contain any metal, these could distort or interfere with the entrance of radiation. If the head will be irradiated, a dental consult may be suggested. This is because radiation therapy can slow healing if a tooth extraction is necessary.

During Treatment. Most children have had prior x-rays taken at the point that radiation therapy is begun and so are not frightened by the procedure. However, because the procedure requires them to lie still for a period of time possibly on an uncomfortable table, in a room away from personnel or their parents, they may experience extreme fear. Assure parents and the child that during the treatment, just as there is no sensation from x-ray exposure, the child will experience no sensation from radiation exposure. Infants are usually prescribed a sedative or conscious sedation before therapy to ensure that they lie still during the procedure. To make this approach effective, keep the child fairly active early in the day and introduce calming activities after the sedative is administered. The child will be sleepy and may fall asleep during radiation. An older child may want to plan an activity to think about during radiation, such as selecting 10 people to take on a camping trip (and why) or choosing 10 places to visit next year and so forth, mental activities that require no movement.

After Treatment. If the head area is involved in therapy, alopecia (hair loss) may result. Moreover, radiation to the head may reduce salivary gland function, leading to a constantly dry mouth. Tooth growth may be halted due to root atrophy. Radiation to bone marrow may depress white blood cell and platelet production. Children undergoing radiation therapy need their leukocyte and platelet counts monitored periodically for changes. Teaching points for parents to maintain skin integrity are summarized in Focus on Family Empowerment.

Chemotherapy

A **chemotherapeutic agent** is one that is capable of destroying malignant cells. In most instances, several chemotherapeutic agents are used to cause multiple damage to cells and thereby increase the chances that cells will no longer be able to reproduce. Like radiation, chemotherapy is scheduled over a period of time so that all cells can eventually be destroyed (cells undergoing meiosis and, therefore, not susceptible to the chemotherapeutic agent on one day will be susceptible on the next).

Types of Chemotherapeutic Agents

Several categories of chemotherapeutic agents are available. Typically, all agents that need mixing are prepared under a specialized hood in the pharmacy to prevent airborne drug residue. When administering such agents, wear gloves and wash your hands well afterward to prevent skin exposure and absorption of the drug.

Alkylating Agents. Alkylating agents interfere with DNA synthesis. They are cell cycle specific (ie, they are most effective against cells in the G1 and S phases of growth). Alkylating agents commonly used with children are cyclophosphamide (Cytoxan) and chlorambucil (Leukeran).

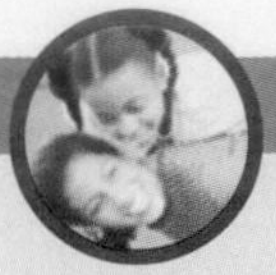

FOCUS ON FAMILY EMPOWERMENT

Caring for the Child Receiving Radiation Therapy

Q. What sorts of things do we need to do for our child who will be receiving radiation therapy?

A. In addition to preventing infection, you need to take some special actions to meet your child's needs. Here are some tips designed to promote therapeutic benefits and minimize adverse effects:

Skin Care

- Expose irradiated area to air but not direct heat or sunlight.
- Avoid lengthy soaks in bath water or swimming pools.
- Use mild shampoo on hair and rinse gently with water. Air dry or pat excess moisture gently. Avoid rough towels and hair dryers.
- Encourage loose clothing, particularly at waist, wrists, and neckline.
- Supply soft toothbrush to protect gums and oral mucous membranes. Keep dry mouth moist by offering frequent sips of water—particularly if radiation decreases salivary gland secretions.
- Because some skin preparations are drying and because some interfere with radiation, do not apply creams or lotions unless prescribed.

Nutrition

- To promote retention of nutrients, administer antiemetics as prescribed.
- Encourage high-calorie meals when child is least likely to be nauseated. Praise the child's efforts to eat. Strive for peaceful and pleasant meal and snack times.
- Provide foods identified by child as special favorites. Serve easy-to-swallow foods at tolerable temperatures.

Hydration

- Reduce fresh fruit and vegetables rich in cellulose, and eliminate apple juice from child's diet because these may contribute to diarrhea and subsequent fluid loss.
- If diarrhea occurs, administer antidiarrheal medication as prescribed.

Activity

- Provide adequate rest periods. Schedule activities to avoid waking child frequently at night.
- Structure the child's activities to be stimulating but not physically tiring.
- Recommend mild activity that does not stress bones that may be weakened by radiation and, therefore, easily fractured.

Instruction and Distraction

- Prepare the child for the effects of radiation therapy, particularly hair loss. Some comfort measures may include wearing a wig or special cap; introducing play things, such as dolls without hair; and stressing that people like people for themselves, not their appearance.
- Schedule a tour of the radiation department. As possible, let the child play act and become familiar with the equipment. Provide ample time to answer questions.
- Encourage active games before the procedure and quiet games afterward.
- Help the child devise "mind games" to play during the procedure (eg, listing 10 friends to take camping, 10 activities to do, or 10 favorite games to play).

Antimetabolites. Antimetabolites are drugs that so closely resemble natural products that a cell incorporates them into its structure. However, they are not the natural product. Thus, the cell cannot function or replicate with them in its structure and will die. They act only in the S (synthesis) phase of the cell cycle. Methotrexate (Folex PFS), a folic acid antagonist, is an example.

Plant Alkaloids. Plant alkaloids interfere with cell mitosis (M phase). Two commonly used plant alkaloids are vincristine (Oncovin) and vinblastine (Velban).

Antibiotics. A number of antibiotics are effective in destroying malignant cells by impairing DNA synthesis. These are not cell cycle specific, which means the agents can be effective at any cell phase (resting or dividing). Dactinomycin (Cosmegan) and doxorubicin (Adriamycin) are examples.

Nitrosoureas. Nitrosoureas disrupt protein synthesis, thereby interfering with DNA synthesis. Because these drugs cross the blood–brain barrier, they are effective as chemotherapy agents in brain tumor therapy. A common example is carmustine (BCNU).

Enzymes. Body cells need a ready supply of L-asparagine (an essential amino acid) to grow. L-Asparaginase (Elspar), a chemotherapeutic agent, is an enzyme that converts L-asparagine into L-aspartic acid, thereby making L-asparagine unavailable for leukemia cell growth.

Steroids. A corticosteroid, most frequently prednisone, binds to DNA to inhibit mitosis and probably RNA synthesis in cells. When added to therapy, the formation of new cells is prevented.

Immunotherapy. Immunotherapy is the stimulation of the body's immune system to attempt destruction of foreign or malignant cells. The administration of bacille Calmette-Guérin vaccine (the vaccine for tuberculosis) is an example of this type of therapy. The tuberculin antigen stimulates the immune system to identify and destroy an antigen in hopes that the system "recognizes" that foreign tumor cells are also present and acts against them as well. Interferon is an antiviral agent that prevents growth of viruses; stimulation of interferon or interferon therapy may be used to attempt to halt malignant cell growth.

Neuroblastoma is an example of a childhood cancer that appears to respond to antibody-based therapy (Cheung, 2000).

Immune therapy will be limited if the immune system has been so altered by the malignant process that it cannot respond when stimulated. It is also possible that the immune response to malignant cells is so different from the response to invading microorganisms that specific types of immunotherapy are necessary to stimulate it.

Chemotherapy Protocols

Chemotherapy is scheduled for children at set times and days and by different predetermined routes. At first, children may remain in the hospital for a few days of treatment; later, they may report on a specific day for therapy, or parents administer the designated therapy at home. Parents must learn about the child's treatment protocol so they know which drug the child will be receiving each day and on which day which drug must be administered. Knowing the protocol and specific drug therapy helps parents begin to prepare the child for it, such as increasing fiber in the child's diet for a few days before the beginning of a constipation-causing drug like vincristine. An example of such a protocol is shown in Table 53-2. Chemotherapy for acute lymphocytic leukemia (ALL; the most common cancer in children) is given first in a remission phase, next in a sanctuary or prophylactic phase, then a delayed intensification phase, and, finally, in a maintenance phase (up to 3 years; Shankar, 2000a).

While children are receiving chemotherapy, parents should not give them aspirin. In addition to increasing the child's susceptibility to Reye's syndrome, aspirin may interfere with blood coagulation, a problem already present due to lowered thrombocyte levels. Instead, they should use acetaminophen (Tylenol) or ibuprofen (Motrin) to relieve a headache or to reduce fever. A parent who wants to give the child vitamins should be certain that the vitamin preparation will not interfere with a chemotherapeutic agent. For example, administration of a vitamin that contains folic acid could interfere with the effectiveness of methotrexate, a folic acid antagonist.

Live virus vaccines should not be given. The child's immune mechanism is so deficient that these vaccines could cause widespread viral disease. The child is particularly susceptible to infections and should be kept away from people with known infections. Zoster immune globulin will be needed if the child has not been immunized against varicella and is exposed to chickenpox during chemotherapy.

Side Effects and Toxic Reactions

All chemotherapeutic agents have side effects and toxic effects. Table 53-3 lists commonly used chemotherapeutic agents, the specific side effects, and potential toxic effects for each agent. Malnutrition, nausea and vomiting, hair loss, stomatitis, constipation, diarrhea, cushingoid effects, and susceptibility to infection are side effects common to almost all of these agents. Nursing diagnoses and related interventions associated with these side effects are described below.

If an IV infusion of a chemotherapeutic agent that is a vesicant infiltrates into the subcutaneous tissue, there is apt to be extensive tissue sloughing and damage. Monitor IV infusions of chemotherapeutic vesicants carefully to prevent extravasation. Discontinue the infusion if it occurs. Then, apply an ice pack to the site to cause vasoconstriction and prevent further spread of the toxic solution. Hyaluronidase is an example of a drug that may be injected into the site to speed absorption. After this, application of warm compresses hastens absorption and clearance of the solution from subcutaneous tissue.

NURSING DIAGNOSES AND RELATED INTERVENTIONS

Nursing Diagnosis: Imbalanced nutrition, less than body requirements, related to nausea, vomiting, or anorexia resulting from chemotherapy

Outcome Identification: Child will take in adequate nutrients for needs during therapy period.

Outcome Evaluation: Child is able to eat frequent, small meals; calorie intake is adequate for age and size.

It is easy for the child with cancer to become malnourished. The fast-growing malignant cells take more than their share of nutrients from normal cells. Nausea and vomiting from chemotherapy make it difficult to

TABLE 53.2 Sample Protocol for Treating Acute Lymphocytic Leukemia

	REMISSION PHASE						SANCTUARY (OR CONSOLIDATION) PHASE							
Day	1	8	15	22	29	36	43	50	57	64	71	78	85	92
Week	1	2	3	4	5	6	7	8	9	10	11	12	13	14
	V	V	V	V	L	L	M		M		V	M		
							M′+			M′+				
	P	P	P	P	P	P								

V = vincristine; P = prednisone; M = intrathecal methotrexate; L = L-asparaginase; M′ = methotrexate IV;
+ = leucovorin.

TABLE 53.3 Commonly Used Chemotherapeutic Agents

DRUG	CLASSIFICATION	SIDE EFFECTS AND TOXIC EFFECTS	SPECIAL CONSIDERATIONS
Asparaginase (Elspar)	Enzyme; deprives leukemic cells of asparagine, leading to cell death	Anorexia, weight loss, nausea, vomiting, hepatotoxicity, central nervous system toxicity, anaphylactic reaction	Staying with child for first hour of infusion is important; take vital signs q15 min for first hour to detect anaphylactic reaction.
Carmustine (BCNU; BiCNU)	Nitrosourea compound; crosses blood–brain barrier	Nausea, vomiting, bone marrow depression (after 3–4 wk), hepatotoxicity	Child may notice burning sensation along vein during administration due to alcohol diluent.
Chlorambucil (Leukeran)	Nitrogen mustard derivative	Bone marrow depression	Monitoring of white blood cell count is necessary.
Cisplatin (Platinol)	Alkylating agent; reacts with and injures cell nucleus	Bone marrow depression, nephrotoxicity (renal dysfunction), nausea, vomiting, loss of taste, tinnitus, high-frequency hearing loss	Infusion bottle must be covered with aluminum foil to keep out light, or decomposition will result.
Cyclophosphamide (Cytoxan)	Alkylating agent (nitrogen mustard derivative)	Bone marrow depression, anorexia, nausea, vomiting, stomatitis, alopecia, cystitis, (hemorrhagic) hepatotoxicity	Fluid intake is encouraged; maintain IV line to limit bladder irritation; test urine for blood and specific gravity.
Cytosine arabinoside (Ara-C)	Antimetabolite (pyrimidine analogue)	Nausea, vomiting, bone marrow depression, stomatitis, alopecia, photosensitivity	Child may need to wear sunglasses in bright light.
Dacarbazine (DTIC)	Alkylating agent	Bone marrow depression	Extravasation causes severe tissue damage.
Dactinomycin (Cosmegan)	Antibiotic; inhibits DNA synthesis	Nausea, vomiting, bone marrow depression, stomatitis	Tissue inflammation occurs if it extravasates into tissue.
Daunorubicin (DaunoXome)	Antibiotic; vesicant	Alopecia, bone marrow depression	Extravasation causes severe tissue damage.
Etoposide (Toposar)	Mitotic inhibitor; inhibits DNA synthesis	Fatigue, alopecia, nausea and vomiting	Slow IV administration is necessary to avoid irritation.
Doxorubicin (Adriamycin)	Antibiotic; inhibits DNA synthesis; vesicant	Nausea, vomiting, bone marrow depression, alopecia, stomatitis, possible heart toxicity	Urine may turn red; take pulse for full minute to detect arrhythmia; tissue necrosis occurs if extravasated.
Ifosfamide (Ifex)	Alkylating agent; interferes with DNA synthesis	Leukopenia, alopecia, hemorrhagic cystitis	Maintaining hydration is important to prevent cystitis.

Lomustine (CCNU; CeeNu)	Alkylating agent (nitrosourea compound)	Nausea, vomiting in 6 h, bone marrow depression (after 3–4 wk)	Administration on an empty stomach enhances absorption.
Mercaptopurine (Purinethol)	Antimetabolite (purine analogue)	Bone marrow depression, nausea, vomiting, stomatitis, hepatotoxicity	Allopurinol delays the degradation of mercaptopurine and thus increases toxicity; question order if both are to be administered.
Methotrexate (MTX)	Antimetabolite	Stomatitis, bone marrow depression, nausea, vomiting, alopecia, hepatotoxicity, nephrotoxicity at high dosage	Decreased effect occurs if administered with salicylates; often followed by leucovorin to decrease toxicity to normal cells.
Prednisone	Corticosteroid; suppresses lymphocyte production	Weight gain, cushingoid facies, depressed systemic response to infection	Child needs support to accept changed appearance.
Procarbazine (Matulane)	Antineoplastic; interferes with DNA and RNA synthesis	Nausea, vomiting, bone marrow depression	Drug may cause blurriness of vision; avoid foods with high tyramine content.
Thioguanine	Antimetabolite	Bone marrow suppression	Monitoring of hepatic function tests is necessary.
Vincristine (Oncovin)	Plant alkaloid; vesicant	Constipation, alopecia, joint and muscle pain, muscle weakness	Paresthesia of fingers and toes, footdrop may occur; may need stool softener; tissue necrosis occurs if infiltrated.
Additional Agents			
Allopurinol (Allopurinol, Lopurin, Zyloprim)	Antigout agent; prevents uric acid formation from destroyed cells	Nausea, vomiting	
Bacillus Calmette-Guérin (BCG) vaccine*	Vaccine; stimulates immune system	Local inflammation	
Leucovorin (Wellcovorin)	Folic acid derivative; neutralizes the toxicity of methotrexate		
Interferon	Antiviral agent	Fever	
Filgrastim (Neupogen)	Granulocyte colony-stimulating factor	Nausea, vomiting	Leukocyte count increases.

*Otherwise used to vaccinate against tuberculosis.

maintain an adequate oral intake. If stomatitis occurs as a result of chemotherapy, eating becomes difficult due to mouth pain. Stomach and intestinal ulcers can interfere with absorption. Changes in fatty acid metabolism may alter the responsiveness of body cells to insulin metabolism. Unable to use glucose effectively, cells cannot function at an optimum level. This may account for the sense of fatigue that children with cancer frequently report (Davies et al., 2002). Anorexia may occur from a factor produced by the tumor that acts directly on the center for hunger in the hypothalamus, reducing appetite and altering taste perception. Cyclophosphamide, a commonly used chemotherapeutic agent, is associated with taste changes. Many children report that foods taste bitter; they do not describe foods as sweet until they are very sweet. Because of these taste changes, foods the child used to enjoy are no longer enjoyable. Unwilling to try new foods, the child's oral intake decreases.

To counteract these taste changes, you may need to suggest different foods or methods of food preparation or include a dietitian as a major health team member. Chicken, for example, often tastes less bitter than beef or pork. Sprinkling brown sugar on cereal gives a different sweet taste than plain sugar. Many children believe that sugar is bad for them so are reluctant to use a lot of it to make foods taste good. Assure them that eating is the most important thing to think about now. Carefully cleaning teeth after eating will preserve teeth even if a great deal of sugar is eaten. However, do not recommend honey as a sweetener. Botulism organisms may grow in honey, placing the immunosuppressed child at risk for infection.

Parents need to take specific actions to make mealtime a pleasant time. Urge them to allow the child to make choices whenever possible. Consultation with a nutritionist can help improve food selection. (Fig. 53-2).

A small meal that can be finished is more satisfying than a large meal half finished. Urge parents to make snack foods nutritious (eg, a malted milkshake rather than a cola beverage). Also suggest planning larger meals to be eaten early in the day before chemotherapy begins and when the child is less likely to be nauseated.

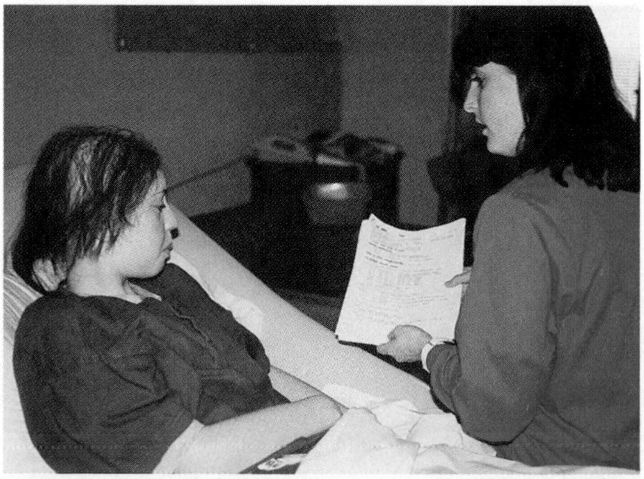

FIGURE 53.2 Children receiving radiation or chemotherapy often have reduced appetites. Here a nurse discusses nutrition and food choices with a 15-year-old with leukemia.

Nursing Diagnosis: Risk for deficient fluid volume related to nausea and vomiting resulting from chemotherapy

Outcome Identification: Child will remain adequately hydrated during therapy.

Outcome Evaluation: Skin turgor remains good; mucous membranes are moist; vomiting does not occur more than once a day.

Nausea and vomiting are common side effects of chemotherapy because the cells lining the stomach are fast growing, thereby being the first cells to incorporate the drug. Nausea and vomiting can often be prevented by administering an antiemetic, such as hydroxyzine (Atarax) or ondansetron (Zofran), before chemotherapy and at 4- to 8-h intervals during the course of therapy. These drugs effectively prevent nausea and vomiting in children but will not necessarily relieve it once it is present. It is necessary, therefore, to begin these medications prophylactically or before chemotherapy begins. For more information, see Focus on Pharmacology.

Do not encourage children to eat if they are nauseated. Encourage them to take clear fluids, however, because this helps prevent uric acid buildup in the kidneys from the malignant cells being destroyed. If

FOCUS ON PHARMACOLOGY

Ondansetron hydrochloride (Zofran)

Action: An antiemetic that blocks central and peripheral receptor sites to prevent chemotherapy-induced nausea and vomiting in adults and children older than 3 years

Dosage: 4 mg orally tid administered 30 min before beginning chemotherapy, with subsequent doses at 4 h and 8 h, continuing every 8 h for 1 to 2 days after chemotherapy treatment or three doses of 0.15 mg/kg IV with first dose being given over 15 min beginning 20 min before chemotherapy with subsequent doses at 4 h and 8 h.

Possible adverse effects: Dizziness, headache, pruritis, myalgia, pain at injection site

Nursing Implications

- Be aware of timing of chemotherapeutic treatment to ensure that first dose is given 20 to 30 min before beginning chemotherapy.
- Instruct parents to continue oral form for 1 to 2 days after completion of chemotherapy to maximize effects.
- Advise parents to administer the oral drug every 8 h around the clock for maximum results.

children are vomiting or cannot take even clear fluid, IV hydration therapy may be necessary. With a drug such as cyclophosphamide, known to cause cystitis when fluid intake is reduced, an IV line for adequate fluid intake is prescribed.

WHAT IF? What if a parent tells you that she does not want her child to have an antiemetic drug before chemotherapy because she sees the nausea and vomiting as proof that the chemotherapy is working? Would you give the drug?

Nursing Diagnosis: Risk for disturbed body image related to changes in physical appearance caused by chemotherapy

Outcome Identification: Child will accept side effects affecting appearance as temporary, inevitable components of treatment within 1 week.

Outcome Evaluation: Child discusses feelings about appearance changes with nurse and parents; states that, although she does not like them, they do not alter her in any other way.

Alopecia. *Alopecia,* or hair loss, is a side effect that occurs with almost all chemotherapeutic drugs because hair cells are fast-growing and easily killed when they incorporate the drug. Even when forewarned that such a consequence is likely, most children and parents are surprised at the suddenness of the hair loss (entire curls may fall out at a time; the child can be totally bald in 2 to 3 days). Even so, hair loss is often a greater problem for the parents than the child. Coping mechanisms may be enhanced by wearing a wig or a scarf, playing and identifying with a doll without hair, and being reminded that those who love the child love the whole person not just the packaging (Fig. 53-3).

Cushingoid Appearance. Children receiving long-term corticosteroid (prednisone) therapy will develop a typical "moon face," red cheeks, and increased body hair.

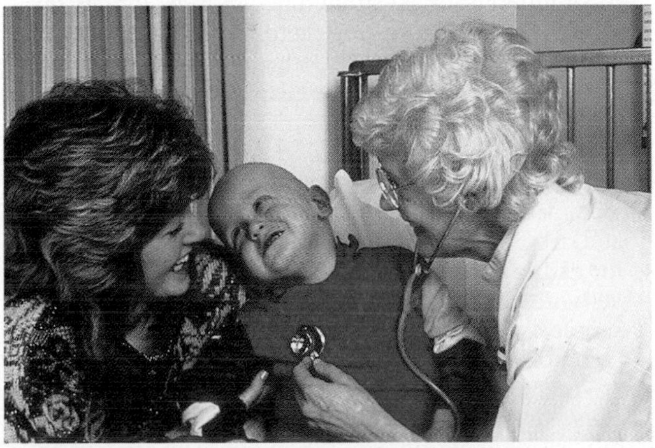

FIGURE 53.3 A child with alopecia. It helps the child to know that hair loss does not prevent meaningful interactions with people.

Like the loss of body hair, a cushingoid appearance may be devastating to children, the final insult in light of all the other things happening to them. Provide support and reassurance that this appearance is only temporary and will return to normal when they are no longer on therapy.

Nursing Diagnosis: Impaired oral mucous membrane related to effects of chemotherapy

Outcome Identification: Child will remain free of severe discomfort from stomatitis during course of chemotherapy.

Outcome Evaluation: Child states that mouth discomfort is at tolerable level; no signs of ulceration are present.

Stomatitis, or ulcers of the gumline and mucous membranes of the mouth, often occurs with antimetabolic drugs. The child may need a soft or light diet. Brushing the teeth with a soft swab rather than a brush or having the child just rinse the mouth with half-strength hydrogen peroxide and water is helpful. Viscous lidocaine (Xylocaine) may be prescribed to be swabbed on individual lesions for comfort. Lidocaine can cause paralysis of the gag reflex if it is swallowed, so it must be swabbed on individual lesions, *not* used for rinsing out the mouth as it is in adults. (Children younger than 8 years are most likely to rinse and swallow.) Measures to reduce stomatitis are summarized in the Focus on Family Empowerment.

Because mucous membrane ulcers may occur throughout the GI tract, avoid taking rectal temperatures for children on antimetabolic therapy to prevent aggravation or perforation of rectal ulcers.

Nursing Diagnosis: Risk for constipation related to effects of chemotherapeutic agents

Outcome Identification: Child will remain free of constipation during course of treatment.

Outcome Evaluation: Child maintains usual pattern of bowel elimination; child reports (and parent confirms) no existence of hard stools.

Some chemotherapeutic agents, particularly vincristine, cause constipation. Anticipate the use of a stool softener, such as docusate sodium (Colace), to prevent hard stools from exacerbating rectal ulcers. Record the frequency of bowel movements so constipation is recognized early in its course. Additional measures for dealing with constipation include increasing the intake of fluids and dietary roughage.

Nursing Diagnosis: Risk for diarrhea related to effects of chemotherapeutic agents

Outcome Identification: Child will remain free of episodes of diarrhea during course of treatment.

Outcome Evaluation: Child maintains usual pattern of bowel elimination; child reports (and parent confirms) no existence of watery stools.

Diarrhea may occur from effects of chemotherapeutic agents on the absorptive surfaces of the intestine. Keep careful records of the number and consistency of bowel movements in children receiving chemotherapy. If diarrhea is present, IV fluid will

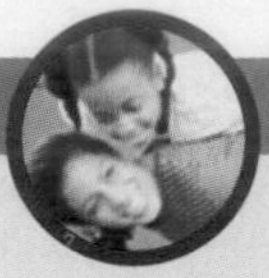

FOCUS ON FAMILY EMPOWERMENT
Tips for Relieving the Discomfort of Stomatitis

Q. Our son has developed ulcers in his mouth from the chemotherapy. What can we do to help him feel more comfortable?

A. Here are some tips for relieving the discomfort:

- Make oral hygiene fun. Use a soft toothbrush to keep the number of germs in the mouth to a minimum and hopefully prevent infection. Another way to promote oral hygiene is to make up a game about mouth care that the whole family can play.
- Serve soft foods like mashed potatoes and pudding, rather than hard ones, such as toast crusts or crunchy cereal, to avoid further abrasions to tender gumlines.
- Encourage your child to rinse his mouth with lukewarm water three times a day (half-strength hydrogen peroxide may be prescribed) both for comfort and to encourage healing.
- Provide nonacidic foods, such as gelatin instead of orange juice, which can sting if sores are present.
- Encourage your child to drink as much fluid as possible because this helps to keep lips from cracking.
- Keep lips well lubricated with petroleum jelly or a commercial product. This also prevents cracking.

usually be administered to supplement fluid loss; an antidiarrheal agent may be prescribed for older children. Be certain to change diapers frequently in infants to prevent excoriation of the skin from the acid stool content. Diarrhea is frightening for children because of the loss of control they experience. Offer support and comfort for this annoying side effect of their primary therapy.

Nursing Diagnosis: Risk for deficient diversional activity related to neuropathy resulting from chemotherapy

Outcome Identification: Child will maintain usual activity level during therapy.

Outcome Evaluation: Child identifies activities in which he can participate that do not require fine motor skills while neuropathy is present.

Almost all children receiving chemotherapy experience fatigue and, thus, are unable to participate in their usual activities. If they develop neutropenia, they may require temporary seclusion from other children to prevent exposure to and subsequent development of infection. Help children who are restricted in these ways to find an activity they enjoy, such as drawing, coloring, or playing hand-held video games so they can remain active.

Vincristine therapy will result in specific neurologic symptoms, such as weakness, tingling, and numbing of the extremities, and sometimes an inability to walk. These symptoms subside when the medication is discontinued. Children may be unable to hold a pen or pencil or maneuver small parts of toys because their fingers are so affected. Think of games they can accomplish until the numbness in the hands fades. Children on bedrest may develop foot drop with vincristine. In some children, physical therapy may be needed along with special braces or boots to prevent foot drop.

Nursing Diagnosis: Risk for infection related to therapy-induced depression of immune system

Outcome Identification: Child will remain free of an infection during treatment period.

Outcome Evaluation: Child's temperature remains below 98.6°F (37.0°C); no areas of erythema or other signs and symptoms of infection are present.

Children with cancer are very susceptible to infection not only because their immune system is depressed by chemotherapy, but also because they develop a degree of malnutrition that decreases the effectiveness of macrophage and phagocytosis functions, and possibly the production of interferon, which is important for destroying viral invaders. A malignant process in the body decreases the body's overall ability to recognize foreign invaders and respond with the usual efficient rejection process. Frequent insertion of IV devices, the development of dry and cracking mucous membranes, and ulcer formation throughout the GI tract provide ready sites for the entrance of microorganisms.

When infection occurs, it may be difficult to recognize because common findings such as local erythema, swelling, systemic fever, and swollen lymph glands may not be present or may be reduced in contrast to the degree of infection present.

Although not well studied in children, administration of colony-stimulating factors, such as filgrastim (Neupogen) can help the body quickly begin replacing damaged white blood cells (Karch, 2001). Even with this, bacterial infections are common. Gram-negative bacteria, such as *Escherichia coli, Pseudomonas aeruginosa,* and *Klebsiella pneumoniae,* and gram-positive bacteria, such as *Staphylococcus aureus* and streptococci, are common organisms responsible for causing infections. Viral infections, such as varicella (chickenpox), varicella zoster (shingles), herpes simplex, viral hepatitis, and cytomegalovirus, also are common invaders.

Treating bacterial infections with antibiotics may cause overgrowth of fungal infections such as candidiasis or aspergillosis. When children are treated with immunosuppressive drugs, protozoal infections, such as *Pneumocystis carinii* pneumonia (normally a very rare pneumonia), may occur.

When infection is discovered in children with cancer, the causative agent is identified by culture. Specific antibiotics are then prescribed. The most important nursing role in caring for children with cancer is to prevent infection. The Focus on Family Empowerment identifies interventions to reduce the possibility of infection in the child with neutropenia (lowered white blood cell count).

Bone Marrow Transplantation

Transplanting bone marrow that was previously harvested from a child with cancer or transplanting marrow from a well person to a child with cancer has become a frequently used treatment for children. This can allow higher doses of chemotherapy and radiation to be used because, in the event of severe bone marrow depression, the child can have healthy marrow restored. Immune cells in the transplanted marrow may actually help to kill remaining cancer cells in the child's circulation.

If the child's own marrow is used, this is *autologous* transfusion. Bone marrow may be donated by someone who is histocompatible (immune compatible) with the child. This is an *allogeneic* transplant. A *syngeneic* transplant is one between twins.

Before transplant, the child receives a chemotherapy agent, such as cyclophosphamide, and total-body irradiation to kill as many marrow cells as possible, suppress the child's immune response to the transplanted tissue, and create space in the bone marrow to allow the newly transplanted cells a place to grow.

Bone marrow is aspirated from the child and treated to reduce the number of abnormal cells present (called purging), or stem cells are removed from the circulating blood of a designated donor or donated placenta. Bone marrow or stem cells are then processed and transfused into the child intravenously. The new marrow migrates to the bone marrow in about 3 weeks. Until this time, the child is at extreme risk for infection. Everyone coming in contact with the child must wash their hands well, and

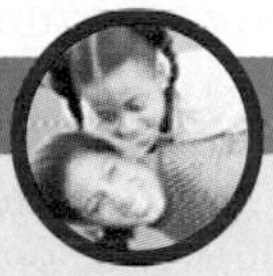

FOCUS ON FAMILY EMPOWERMENT
Preventing Infection in the Child With Neutropenia

Q. What special things should I do to help prevent my child from developing an infection until her white blood count returns to normal?

A. Here are some suggestions to help prevent infections:

- Arrange for your child to sleep in a single bed and room, if possible, to avoid close contact with other family members who may be developing upper respiratory infections.
- Limit the child's exposure to large crowds such at movie theaters.
- Screen and prohibit visitors who have signs of infection (eg, runny nose, oral herpes, rashes); who have been exposed to a communicable disease, such as chickenpox; or who have recently been vaccinated.
- Wash your hands frequently before child care and after handling potentially contaminated containers (eg, tissues, diapers, other containers of body secretions or fluids).
- Urge the child to wash hands well after using a bathroom and before eating.
- Keep child's immediate surroundings free of plants, flowers, and goldfish, all of which could harbor mold spores.
- Be sure the child has a daily bath or shower. Clean mouth with soft toothbrush to reduce opportunity for bacteria, always present in the mouth, to invade.
- Inspect mouth daily for breaks in the tissue, bleeding, or white patches, suggesting oral thrush (*Monilia*) infection. Apply a moisturizing and protective barrier, such as KY Jelly, to the lips to help prevent them from cracking.
- Take temperature and pulse and respiratory rates daily. Avoid taking rectal temperatures to protect against injuring rectal tissue.
- Inspect all skin surfaces daily for scratches that could become entrances for infection. Include IV or IM injection sites, venous access device insertion sites and the diaper area.
- Administer stool softeners, if prescribed, to promote soft stools and bowel movements to avoid rectal tears.
- Provide high-calorie, high-protein foods and food supplements to help rebuild white blood cells. Don't serve the child fresh fruit and vegetables because they have more potential to harbor infectious organisms than cooked foods.
- Assess for respiratory infection by listening for cough and throat clearing; inspect throat for redness and nasal passage for discharge. Keep child active and moving, (eg, playing games, such as "Simon Says," that encourage deep breathing).
- Assess for possible genitourinary infections. Note the color, clarity, frequency, and concentration of urine. If necessary, obtain a urine specimen using clean-catch method for testing. Promote increased fluid intake to keep urine flowing. Advise girls to wipe from front to back after voiding or defecating to avoid bringing organisms forward to the urethra. If a girl is menstruating, sanitary napkins do not have the potential to harbor as many germs as tampons; urge her to change pads frequently (every 4 h).
- Question the administration of any vaccine made with a live virus until the child's white blood count returns to normal.

specific infection control precautions must be maintained. Transfusion of blood products may be necessary to maintain functional blood components until the transplanted marrow begins to function (see Focus on Multidisciplinary Care).

Not all medical centers perform bone marrow transplants, so a family may have to travel a distance for the therapy. Complications of bone marrow transplant are discussed in Chapter 44, because this technique also is used with children with blood dyscrasias. Previously used only with children with leukemia, it is now being used in children with other cancers, such as neuroblastoma and Hodgkin's disease (Nash, 1999).

Pain Assessment

Because growing tumors displace cells, causing anoxia to those cells, pain is a common symptom experienced by children with cancer. Methods to assess pain and interventions to help children deal with pain are discussed in Chapter 38.

✔ CHECKPOINT QUESTIONS

3. Why does chemotherapy cause nausea and vomiting?
4. What are two common side effects of vincristine?

FOCUS ON MULTIDISCIPLINARY CARE

Children with cancer encounter a great many health care professionals because their care is complex and requires multidisciplinary interventions. Physicians, surgeons, imaging technicians, nutritionists, oncology nurses, physical and occupational therapists, and home care nurses are examples of the health care professionals that they may contact. Be certain that all health care professionals who may be assigned to care for children are made aware of major strides made in children's cancer therapy so that everyone can appreciate that most children with cancer (especially leukemia) have a favorable prognosis. This allows them to give care in a positive manner and helps keep the parents and children equally invested in care. Communication among all members of the health care team is essential.

Also be certain that all caregivers understand that children who are receiving chemotherapy or who have had bone marrow transplants are highly susceptible to infection. This helps them take responsibility for not spreading infection (washing hands well, not caring for an immunosuppressed child if they have an upper respiratory or herpes simplex infection, and the like).

THE LEUKEMIAS

Acute Lymphocytic Leukemia

Leukemia is the distorted and uncontrolled proliferation of white blood cells (leukocytes). It is the most frequently occurring type of cancer in children (Shankar, 2000a). The most frequent type of leukemia in children, acute lymphocytic leukemia (ALL) accounts for 75% of leukemias (Shankar, 2000a). The malignant cell involved is the lymphoblast, an immature lymphocyte. With the rapid proliferation of lymphocytes, the production of red blood cells and platelets falls, and invasion of body organs by the rapidly increasing white blood cell elements begins. Because the abnormally proliferating cells are so immature, they may be identifiable only at the immature, or "blast" or "stem," cell stage.

The highest incidence of ALL is in children between 2 and 6 years of age. The prognosis in children younger than 1 year or older than 10 years at the time of first occurrence is not as good as in those between 2 and 10 years of age. The prognosis in children who have more than 50,000 white blood cells per millimeter or who have more than 10% L2 cells (see classification of cells below) in bone marrow at the time of diagnosis is not as good as in those with a lower white blood cell count and fewer L2 cells at first diagnosis. The incidence of ALL is slightly higher in boys than girls, and the disease is seen more often in white children than in children of other races (Shankar, 2000a).

Although it can be shown that leukemia in mice and cats is of viral origin, the cause of leukemia in children is unknown. Radiation, exposure to chemicals, or genetic factors may have some influence on the occurrence. Children with Down syndrome or Fanconi's syndrome are more likely to develop leukemia than are other children (Hasle et al., 2000). It occurs more often in identical twins than in children who are only siblings. Bone irradiation may be implicated, so children should be submitted to as few x-rays as possible, including x-rays while in utero. An association between magnetic fields or power lines and leukemia is now disputed (Greenland et al., 2000).

Assessment

With ALL, bone marrow overproduces lymphocytes and so is unable to continue normal production of other blood components. Therefore, the first symptoms of ALL in children usually are pallor, low-grade fever, and lethargy (symptoms of anemia caused by decreased red blood cell production). A child may have petechiae and bleeding from oral mucous membranes and may bruise easily because of a low thrombocyte count. As the spleen and liver begin to enlarge from infiltration of abnormal cells, abdominal pain, vomiting, and anorexia will occur. As abnormal lymphocytes invade the bone periosteum, the child experiences bone and joint pain. Central nervous system (CNS) invasion leads to symptoms such as headache or unsteady gait.

Physical assessment will reveal painless generalized lymphadenopathy, especially of the submaxillary or cervical nodes. Laboratory studies will reveal a variable leukocyte count. In some children, the leukocyte count is normal or even slightly decreased but includes blast (very immature) cells; in other children, there is a marked leukocytosis of the blast cells. The platelet count and hematocrit will be low, but the red blood cells present will be normocytic and normochromic (of normal size and color).

A bone marrow aspiration is done to identify the type of white blood cell involved or document the type of leukemia. If there are more than 25% blast cells present, a leukemia diagnosis is established. In children, bone marrow is aspirated at the iliac crest rather than the sternum, both because this is less frightening and because it yields more marrow. X-rays of the long bones may reveal lesions caused by the invasion of abnormal cells. A lumbar puncture may show evidence of blast cells in the cerebrospinal fluid (CSF).

Therapeutic Management

Up to 95% of children will have a first remission. If a child experiences a relapse, the chances of long-term survival are reduced to approximately 70%. Although remission can be reinduced, the length of each subsequent remission tends to be shorter and less effective (Shankar, 2000a).

Disease Classification and Prognosis. Leukemia is classified to define subgroups of cells and to predict the usual response to treatment. Blasts with B-lymphocyte cell characteristics can be recognized by the presence of immunoglobulin and antigen–antibody receptors on their surfaces. B-lymphocyte cell types account for 85% of ALL. A specific antigen found on cell surfaces has been named CALLA. So cells are labeled as CALLA positive or CALLA negative. About 15% to 20% of children have T-lymphocyte cell involvement. T-lymphocytes are also categorized as CALLA positive or negative.

Cure as Goal. The goal of therapy for leukemia is complete cure, based on the use of chemotherapeutic agents. A chemotherapy program is aimed at, first, achieving a complete remission or absence of leukemia cells (induction phase); second, preventing leukemia cells from invading or growing in the CNS (sanctuary or consolidation phase); third, administering delayed intensive therapy; and fourth, maintaining the original remission (maintenance phase).

Chemotherapy in children is often administered by means of central venous catheter or port because administration into a major vessel helps prevent irritation to the vessel walls. These access devices have the secondary advantage of being able to be clamped or "trapped" so the child can be ambulatory between treatments.

Drugs frequently used to initiate a remission include vincristine, prednisone, and L-asparaginase, doxorubicin, and methotrexate. These are given over about a 1-month period. Because so many cells are destroyed by chemotherapy, a high level of uric acid is excreted during chemotherapy. This can lead to plugging of kidney glomeruli and loss of kidney function. To prevent this, a drug such as allopurinol to reduce formation of uric acid is often administered with chemotherapy. Keeping a child well hydrated also helps maintain safe uric acid excretion.

Because many chemotherapy drugs do not cross the blood–brain barrier in effective concentrations, leukemic cells in the CNS continue to flourish even with remission chemotherapy. A combination of intrathecal drug administration (injection of drugs into the CSF by lumbar puncture), such as methotrexate accompanied by oral administration of 6-mercaptopurine, is next instituted to eradicate this source of leukemic cells (called a *consolidation* or *sanctuary phase* because no "sanctuary" is given to malignant cells). Cranial radiation, once used extensively for this purpose, is less used today than previously because, over the long-term, minimal learning disorders may result.

The third phase of therapy intensifies the assault against leukemic cells using chemotherapeutic agents such as vincristine, prednisone, L-asparaginase, doxorubicin, cyclophosphamide, cytosine, arabinoside (ARA-C), or 6-thioguanine.

Maintenance and Monitoring. Maintenance chemotherapy aims to eliminate completely any remaining leukemic cells so the child's immune system can complete the eradication. Standard maintenance therapy includes a combination of daily 6-mercaptopurine, weekly methotrexate, and sporadic vincristine and prednisone, and intrathecal methotrexate. This is continued for 2 to 3 years. A drug such as leucovorin is usually given after systemic methotrexate to neutralize its action and protect normal cells from the effect of the drug. During the maintenance phase, the child's blood values must be monitored at least monthly. If there is serious bone marrow depression, medication levels may be reduced or a transfusion may be necessary.

If a bone marrow study during the maintenance phase shows that leukemic cells are again evident, a new induction phase will be initiated, followed by a new sanctuary, intensification, and maintenance phase. Children who are free of disease for 4 years are considered cured, and their maintenance therapy can then be stopped. Bone marrow transplantation or immunotherapy may be used with children who do not respond well to standard therapy. Newer drugs are constantly being researched to use for relapse therapy. Help parents evaluate the use of nonapproved drugs and the safety of using them with chemotherapeutic agents (see Focus on Communication).

Complications

Throughout therapy, the health care team and family need to be alert for complications of therapy. Among these problems are CNS, renal, and reproductive system disorders.

Central Nervous System Involvement. If CNS involvement occurs, it can be severe and intense. Blindness, hydrocephalus, and recurrent seizures are possible. The meninges and the sixth and seventh cranial nerves are the structures most often affected. With meningeal involvement, the child will develop nuchal rigidity, headache, irritability, and perhaps vomiting and papilledema. A lumbar puncture will reveal the presence of blast cells in the CSF. If these are discovered, children are treated with intrathecal injections of methotrexate. Always check that children are not prescribed oral or IV methotrexate at the same time, because some of the dose of intrathecal methotrexate is absorbed systemically, which could lead to a toxic reaction. Inserting Silicon tubing into a cerebral ventricle and threading it under the scalp (an Ommaya reservoir) provides easy access to the CSF for sampling or injection without the need for lumbar punctures (Fig. 53-4).

FOCUS ON COMMUNICATION

Len, a 10-year-old boy, was diagnosed with leukemia 3 months ago. His mother brings him into the emergency room because of a severe nose bleed. While you are putting pressure on his nose, you notice that both of Len's arms are covered with fresh ecchymotic bruises.

Less Effective Communication

Nurse: Is Len still having chemotherapy, Mrs. Miller?
Mrs. Miller: No. He's in remission.
Nurse: Is he taking anything that would lower his platelet count or clotting factors?
Mrs. Miller: All he takes is asparagus powder we get from Mexico.
Nurse: Why are you getting that from Mexico and not the clinic here?
Mrs. Miller: It's a new treatment and not legal here.
Nurse: If he's cured, why do you think he has so many new black and blue marks?
Mrs. Miller: I'm sure they're nothing.
Nurse: Well, let's focus right now on getting this bleeding stopped.

More Effective Communication

Nurse: Is Len still having chemotherapy, Mrs. Miller?
Mrs. Miller: No. He's in remission.
Nurse: Is he taking anything that would lower his platelet count or clotting factors?
Mrs. Miller: All he takes is asparagus powder we get from Mexico.
Nurse: You are getting the powder from Mexico and not from the clinic here?
Mrs. Miller: It's a new treatment and not legal here.
Nurse: Are you worried that he still has so many new black and blue marks?
Mrs. Miller: No, asparagus powder is a kind of chemotherapy.
Nurse: Well, let's get this nose bleed stopped. Then we can take a minute to talk about what they might mean and decide what to do about them.

Of all the diseases known, there is no other disease with as many "false cures" as cancer. It is important when talking with parents to see if they are using any of these unproven methods. Some of them do no harm, so parents can continue to give them along with proven therapies. Others, however, actually interfere with the action of a chemotherapy drug and are contraindicated. In the above scenario, the parent has chosen an unproven regimen. Ignoring that this choice may be an unhelpful one and denying a potential recurrence of cancer or other problem will not be therapeutic in the long term.

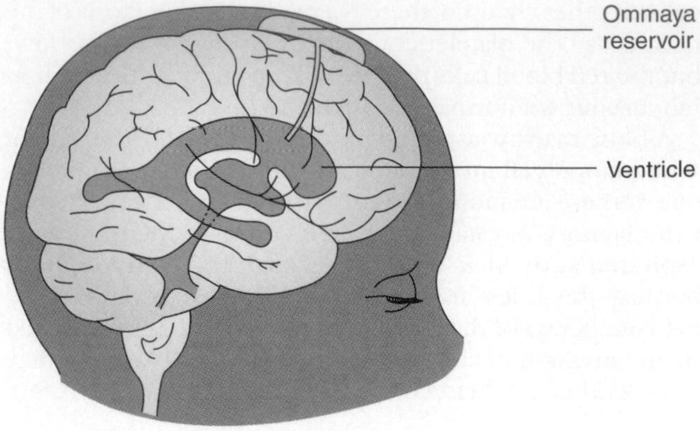

FIGURE 53.4 An Ommaya reservoir. Medication injected into the reservoir flows down to the ventricle and enters the cerebrospinal fluid.

Renal Involvement. Kidney involvement, resulting from invasion of leukemia cells, is a second serious complication. The kidneys may enlarge, and their function will be impaired. If uric acid levels rise as a result of the breakdown of leukemic cells during chemotherapy, plugging of renal tubules with uric acid crystals and kidney failure may result. Renal involvement may limit the use of chemotherapeutic agents, because they cannot be excreted effectively due to the kidney damage.

Testicular Invasion. In boys, leukemic cells tend to invade the testes. Unless this problem is specifically addressed, these cells will not be destroyed by chemotherapy. As a result, once chemotherapy is halted, the leukemic cells may grow and proliferate again. In most boys, therefore, the testes will be radiated to destroy this sanctuary site for cells. This will, unfortunately, lead to sterilization later in life. If a boy is past puberty and is forming sperm, sperm banking might be suggested before chemotherapy and radiation to preserve sperm for reproduction later in life.

NURSING DIAGNOSES AND RELATED INTERVENTIONS

Nursing Diagnosis: Risk for infection related to nonfunctioning white blood cells and immunosuppressive effects of therapy

Outcome Identification: Child will remain free of an infection during course of therapy.

Outcome Evaluation: Child's temperature will remain below 98.6°F (37.0°C); no areas of erythema or drainage are present on skin.

Because the number of functioning white blood cells is reduced and the drugs used for treatment are immunosuppressive, children with leukemia are at an extremely high risk for infection during chemotherapy. Most deaths in children result from infections, such as septicemia, pneumonia, or meningitis. *Pseudomonas* is commonly an invading organism.

While children are receiving care at home, parents must learn to observe them carefully and promptly report any indication of infection, such as low-grade fever or behavior that does not seem typical of the child. The sooner the symptoms are reported, the sooner anti-infective therapy can begin.

To increase the functioning leukocyte count, leukocytes may be transfused. Symptoms of fever and chills from leukocyte transfusion tend to be more common than with red blood cell transfusion. This is not a true transfusion reaction and generally not a reason to stop the transfusion.

Children may be placed on prophylactic antibiotics to reduce the possibility of infection. Parents may be advised to limit visitors, especially anyone with an infection, until the child's functioning white blood count improves.

Nursing Diagnosis: Risk for deficient fluid volume related to increased chance of hemorrhage from poor platelet production

Outcome Identification: Child will maintain an adequate fluid volume during course of therapy.

Outcome Evaluation: No evidence of hemorrhage is present (no epistaxis, hematuria, hematemesis); pulse rate and blood pressure remain normal for age group.

Because the platelet count is low due to poor platelet production and the effect of chemotherapy, children with leukemia also are extremely prone to massive hemorrhage. Epistaxis (nosebleed) is the most common kind of bleeding; GI, renal, or CNS bleeding also may occur.

Digital pressure is usually effective to stop epistaxis. The application of Gelfoam soaked in topical thrombin may be necessary. In some children, postnasal packing is necessary. Children may need a transfusion to replace the lost blood volume. Platelet-rich plasma or a concentrated preparation of platelets will be ordered to improve the platelet count. Unfortunately, the lifespan of transfused platelets is short (1 to 3 days), so frequent platelet transfusion may be necessary. After an intramuscular (IM) injection or the removal of an IV needle, apply firm pressure to the injection site to prevent bleeding.

Because children with leukemia have blood samples drawn frequently, receive transfusions, and have chemotherapeutic drugs given IV, they need the opportunity for therapeutic play with needles and syringes or IV tubing so they can work through some feelings about these intrusive, hurtful procedures. Advocate for intermittent infusion devices such as heparin locks or multilumen central venous catheters that minimize the need for repeated venipunctures.

Nursing Diagnosis: Pain related to invasion of leukocytes

Outcome Identification: Child will experience a tolerable degree of pain during course of illness.

Outcome Evaluation: Child states that pain is tolerable (if infant, not crying).

Children with acute leukemia experience pain because of the vast number of white blood cells that invade the periosteum of the bones. Assess pain using a standard scale for accuracy. Handle legs and arms gently to minimize pain. Using an alternating mattress device underneath body joints helps to reduce skin irritation caused by always resting in the same position.

Nursing Diagnosis: Ineffective health maintenance related to long-term therapy for leukemia

Outcome Identification: Child and parents demonstrate understanding of long-term health maintenance needs by hospital discharge.

Outcome Evaluation: Parents and child state importance of regular health maintenance visits; child continues chemotherapy regimen at home and keeps all ambulatory appointments.

During the maintenance phase of therapy, children are allowed normal activity and should attend regular school. Encourage parents to continue to report promptly any sign of infection so antibiotic therapy can be started early. Because chickenpox can be fatal to a child who is immunosuppressed, have parents ask the child's school to notify them if any other child in the school develops chickenpox so appropriate immune protection can be given. If the child did not receive immunization against varicella (chickenpox), they will need varicella immune globulin administered.

Evaluation of children at follow-up visits should include not only the state of their blood, but also whether they are making forward-thinking plans or think of themselves as well children again.

Parents may continue to need a great deal of support during the maintenance phase of therapy. They live from day to day, hoping that the remission will not end; they need a great deal of support if a relapse does occur. Parents who are told that their child has a heart defect that is not correctable know from the beginning that their child will die. In contrast, parents of the child with leukemia constantly hope that a remission is permanent, that their child will be one who is cured. In a sense, the child dies many times—at diagnosis and again if a relapse occurs. If death does occur, the reality of what has happened may be extremely difficult for the parents to accept. They may return to the hospital for visits weeks or months after the child's death in an effort to accept reality and work through their grief. Focus on Nursing Care Planning summarizes care for the child with leukemia.

Acute Myeloid Leukemia

Acute myeloid leukemia (AML) involves the overproliferation of granulocytes. It accounts for about 20% of all childhood leukemia (Shankar, 2000b). The frequency of the disorder increases in late adolescence. In its chronic form, it is the most common type of leukemia in adulthood.

With AML, granulocytes grow so rapidly that they often are forced out into the bloodstream still in the blast stage. As with ALL, the overproliferation of granulocytes limits the production of red blood cells and platelets.

Assessment

Children with AML have the same symptoms as those with ALL. Because they do not have mature granulocytes, they are susceptible to infection and may have noticed many recent upper respiratory infections at the time of diagnosis.

FOCUS ON *Nursing Care Planning*

A CHILD WITH LEUKEMIA RECEIVING MAINTENANCE CHEMOTHERAPY

A 6-year-old male with ALL is brought to the outpatient clinic for administration of maintenance chemotherapy. His father states, "He's been having trouble eating lately. He hates the way he looks."

Assessment: 6-year-old male diagnosed with ALL approximately 10 weeks ago. Completed induction phase of chemotherapy with some reports of nausea and vomiting; controlled with antiemetics. Weight maintained within 1 to 2 lb of baseline weight.

Child appears pale. Weight decreased 5 lb in last 2 weeks. "He's been having trouble keeping food down." Skin turgor sluggish. Oral mucous membranes red and irritated. Two ulcers noted on inner aspect of left cheek at gum line. "It hurts to eat."

Child's scalp is totally bald. Child states, "I'm so ugly. I look like an old man." Laboratory test results decreased from previous levels but within acceptable parameters.

Nursing Diagnosis: Imbalanced nutrition, less than body requirements, related to inadequate intake, secondary irritation and pain of mucosal ulceration and increased vomiting

Outcome Identification: Child will demonstrate an adequate intake of nutrients to return to baseline weight.

Outcome Evaluation: Child exhibits a 1- to 2-lb weight gain by next visit; states oral ulcers are healing and no further ulcers have developed; reports food intake is increasing with decreasing episodes of vomiting. Child and father verbalize measures to control vomiting and relieve ulceration.

Interventions	Rationale
1. Administer ordered antiemetic approximately 30 min before initiating chemotherapy and at prescribed intervals during therapy. Instruct parent to continue antiemetic therapy at home as ordered.	1. Antiemetics administered before chemotherapy help to prevent nausea and vomiting from developing. Continued therapy helps to control any nausea or vomiting that does develop.
2. If the child experiences nausea, encourage him to take clear fluids until feeling has passed.	2. Taking clear fluids helps to minimize irritation of the gastrointestinal tract and decreases the risk for vomiting.
3. When the child is comfortable, question him about his food likes and dislikes. Obtain a dietary recall from the child and his father.	3. Ascertaining likes and dislikes provides a baseline for future suggestions for food choices that would be followed. A dietary recall provides information about the child's current intake and aids in planning appropriate suggestions for nutritional intake.
4. Encourage the parent to offer food early in the day before chemotherapy. Suggest frequent high-calorie snacks, such as fortified breakfast foods, milk shakes, and high-energy snack bars. Enlist the aid of the dietitian.	4. Eating before chemotherapy enhances nutrition because the child is less likely to be nauseated at this time. Frequent high-calorie snacks provide additional calories needed without the additional expenditure of energy to eat a large meal. Assistance from the dietitian ensures nutritionally sound food choices.
5. Allow child to select items from a list of appropriate foods. Develop a simple contract with the child for including appropriate food choices. Praise the child for choices and eating behavior.	5. Contracting and providing the child with choices promotes active participation and feelings of control, thus enhancing the chances for success. Praising offers positive reinforcement.

(continued)

Interventions	Rationale
6. Encourage the child to eat small, frequent meals and to eat when hungry, even if it is not mealtime.	6. Small, frequent meals decrease the amount of energy expended for eating and also minimize the risk for abdominal distention, which may exacerbate the child's nausea and vomiting.
7. Instruct the parent and child in ways to enhance the taste, protein, and caloric content of food, such as adding brown sugar, eggs, or wheat germ.	7. Chemotherapy can alter the taste of foods. Increased calorie and protein intake is necessary to meet the child's increased metabolic needs.
8. Advise parent to offer nonacidic and soft, bland, moist foods, such as mashed potatoes, puddings, milk shakes, and cooked cereals rather than foods such as toast, cold cereal, and orange juice. Assist the parent with ways to make mealtime pleasant.	8. Soft, bland, moist, and nonacidic foods minimize irritation to the child's already ulcerated mucosa. Making mealtime pleasant may help to stimulate the child's appetite.
9. Instruct child and parent in oral care and advise using a soft toothbrush or swabs to cleanse teeth. Encourage the frequent use of warm water rinses and saline mouthwashes. Teach the parent about topical anesthetic application to the ulcers as appropriate.	9. Good oral care is essential to prevent further ulceration. It also helps to soothe the already ulcerated tissue. Topical anesthetics may help decrease the discomfort of the ulcers.
10. Encourage the child to drink as much fluid as possible.	10. Adequate fluid intake helps to keep mucous membranes moist and minimizes the risk of possible dehydration.
11. Reinforce with the parent the need to monitor the child's intake and output and to weigh the child twice a week at the same time each day, with the same scale, and with the child wearing similar clothing.	11. Intake and output and weight are valuable indicators of fluid balance and nutritional status if done consistently in the same manner each time. Because weight fluctuates from day to day, weighing the child twice a week rather than daily helps to deemphasize the problems, minimizing the risk for frustration.
12. Instruct the parent to keep a written record of the child's intake, weight, episodes of nausea and vomiting, and relief measures. Encourage the parent to involve the child with record keeping.	12. A written record provides objective evidence for evaluating the effectiveness of the plan and allows for feedback and further teaching. Involving the child in a concrete activity promotes active participation, helping to enhance feelings of self-esteem and control.
13. Urge the parent to contact the clinic if the child develops further ulcerations or experiences continued weight loss or an increase in nausea and vomiting.	13. Continued nausea and vomiting, weight loss, or development of more ulcers requires further evaluation and follow-up to minimize the risk of additional problems for the child.

Nursing Diagnosis: Disturbed body image related to hair loss secondary to the effects of chemotherapy

Outcome Identification: Child will verbalize positive feelings about himself.

Outcome Evaluation: Child states impact of hair loss on appearance and feelings; verbalizes measures to cope with hair loss; reports continued participation in age-appropriate activities.

Interventions	Rationale
1. Assess the child's understanding of hair loss and its cause. Review the structure and function of the hair and development of hair loss.	1. Obtaining a baseline knowledge assessment provides a foundation on which to build future teaching strategies. Reviewing and clarifying aid in learning and strengthen understanding.
2. Attempt to identify the meaning of his appearance and hair loss.	2. Identifying the meaning assists in determining the degree of its possible impact on the child.

(continued)

Interventions	Rationale
3. Encourage the child to express feelings and thoughts about self, appearance, and hair loss. Incorporate the use of therapeutic play.	3. Sharing of feelings and concerns permits a safe outlet for emotions and also aids in highlighting the child's awareness of possible impact on body image. Therapeutic play allows the child to express his feelings.
4. Reinforce with the child that hair is lost by breaking off at the skin surface. Remind child that the hair will grow back because the root is not damaged.	4. Reinforcement aids in clarifying any misconceptions, helping the child to understand that hair loss is temporary.
5. Assist the child with suggestions, such as the use of colorful caps, to minimize the appearance of the hair loss.	5. Minimizing the appearance of the hair loss may help the child cope better with the event and possibly enhance feelings of self-esteem and normalcy.
6. Include a few of the child's close friends as appropriate in discussion and suggestions.	6. Including the child's friends in these measures helps to decrease the child's feelings of being different and alone.

Therapeutic Management

The diagnosis is established by bone marrow aspiration and biopsy. Cells are typed (M1 to M6) to establish prognosis. After diagnosis, chemotherapy to effect remission will begin. Doxorubicin and cytosine arabinoside (ARA-C) are two drugs commonly used for therapy. It may take 1 to 2 months to reach a full remission.

During the maintenance phase, additional chemotherapeutic agents in common use are cyclophosphamide, and 6-thioguanine. Maintenance therapy is continued for 6 to 9 months (Shankar, 2000b).

Remission is more difficult to achieve in children with AML than in those with ALL; if one is achieved, it may be brief. Bone marrow transplantation may be attempted after the initial remission to ensure new growth of normal granulocytes.

✔ CHECKPOINT QUESTIONS

5. What are the first signs commonly seen in the child with ALL?
6. If a child has CNS involvement with leukemia, how will methotrexate be administered?

THE LYMPHOMAS

Lymphomas are malignancies of the lymph or reticuloendothelial system; they account for about 15% of all malignancies and are categorized as Hodgkin's or non-Hodgkin's lymphomas. Although Hodgkin's disease is better known, non-Hodgkin's lymphomas are more common worldwide in children (about 60% non-Hodgkin's to 40% Hodgkin's). They both occur more frequently in males than in females (Jordan, 2001).

Hodgkin's Disease

With Hodgkin's disease, lymphocytes proliferate, and special *Reed-Sternberg cells* (large, multinucleated cells that are probably nonfunctioning monocyte-macrophage cells) are found. Although Hodgkin's cells are capable of DNA synthesis and mitotic division, they are abnormal because they lack both B- and T-lymphocyte surface markers and cannot produce immunoglobulins.

As with all neoplastic diseases, the etiology of Hodgkin's disease is unknown. It is rarely seen in children younger than 7 years. The incidence increases greatly during adolescence and young adulthood. Metastasis is through lymphatic channels. Late in the disease, spread to lung, liver, and bone marrow occurs.

Assessment

Symptoms of Hodgkin's disease usually begin with only one painless, enlarged, rubbery-feeling lymph node, usually a cervical node. Other nodes then become involved, along with the liver, spleen, bone marrow, and, eventually, the CNS. The child usually has accompanying symptoms of anorexia, malaise, night sweats, and loss of weight. Fever may be present. The sedimentation rate will be elevated; anemia is usually present from reduced red blood cell survival.

Hodgkin's disease is confirmed by biopsy of the lymph nodes. Further studies (bone marrow, liver function, chest and abdominal computed tomography [CT] scan, lymphangiogram, and abdominal biopsy) are done to classify the clinical stage of the disorder. Chest x-ray reveals enlarged mediastinal nodes; the abdominal CT will reveal enlarged lymph nodes of the abdomen.

A lymphangiogram, performed by injecting dye into the hand or foot, allows visualization of the lymphatic system. A catheter is inserted into a lymph vessel, and radiopaque dye is added as in angiography. Lymphatic channels can be visualized on x-ray films. The lymph system does not eradicate opaque dye readily; in some children, lymph chains will still be outlined on x-ray films for up to 1 year. The original dye injected into the skin to visualize the lymph vessels stains the skin a bluish green. This dye will remain as a skin stain for about 1 year. Nodes opacified from lymphangiogram dye can be used as markers of disease progress on plain, flat-plate x-ray films for 6 to 12 months.

Therapeutic Management

Four subcategories of Hodgkin's disease can be documented: lymphocyte predominant, nodular sclerosing, mixed cellularity, and lymphocyte depletion. The most frequently occurring types in children are nodular sclerosing and lymphocyte predominant (Jordan, 2001).

The disease is staged according to regional involvement (Table 53-4). Such staging may be determined by a CT scan followed by multiple lymph node and bone marrow biopsies.

Treatment depends on the clinical stage of the disease at the time of diagnosis. Once treated mainly with radiation therapy, children today in all stages receive chemotherapy. Common agents include mechlorethamine (nitrogen mustard), vincristine (Oncovin), procarbazine, and prednisone, a protocol commonly called MOPP therapy. Other drugs used include cyclophosphamide and cytarabine (Jordan, 2001). Current therapy results in a 90% 5-year survival for children with stage I or stage II disease, and 60% to 90% for more advanced disease. If a relapse occurs, additional chemotherapy, radiation, or bone marrow transplantation will be scheduled.

Children need conscientious follow-up for symptoms of Hodgkin's disease relapse during adult life. A relapse is often retreatable, using a chemotherapy course different from that used initially.

NURSING DIAGNOSES AND RELATED INTERVENTIONS

The nursing diagnoses most often used with Hodgkin's disease address the child's impaired immune defenses and risk for infection, fear and feelings about the diagnosis, or changed body image (particularly in the adolescent). Both the parents and the child need opportunities to express their feelings about seriousness of this disease.

Nursing Diagnosis: Risk for powerlessness related to constant possibility of disease recurrence

Outcome Identification: Child will maintain positive attitude about self and ability of health care team to manage illness should a relapse occur.

Outcome Evaluation: Child states that he feels healthy during remission, participates in school and extracurricular activities, and voices confidence in health care team to treat symptoms if they recur.

The course of treatment for Hodgkin's disease is long. Some adolescents, in whom the disease is most prevalent, live from day to day wondering if symptoms will recur.

Encourage adolescents to attend regular school during periods of remission so they can lead as normal a life as possible. Keep them informed about the disease and their progress. Some adolescents want to know exactly what stage they are in; others prefer not to be told so they can continue to believe that a cure will be possible. Both adolescents and their parents need continued support from health care personnel during the long course of therapy.

TABLE 53.4 Stages of Hodgkin's Disease

STAGE	EXTENT OF DISEASE
I	Disease affects single lymph node or single extralymphatic organ or site.
II	Disease affects two or more lymph node regions on the same side of the diaphragm, or there is localized involvement of an extralymphatic organ or site.
III	Disease affects lymph node regions on both sides of the diaphragm, or there is localized involvement of an extralymphatic organ or site.
IV	There is diffuse or disseminated involvement of extralymphatic organs with or without associated lymph node involvement.

Non-Hodgkin's Lymphoma

Non-Hodgkin's lymphomas are malignant disorders of the lymphocytes. They involve stem cells and lymphocytes in varying degrees of differentiation. In the pediatric population, diffuse lymphoblastic, undifferentiated, and large-cell lymphomas are commonly seen. Unlike Hodgkin's disease, spread is through the bloodstream rather than directly by lymph flow. Thus, the course of the disease is unpredictable. Metastatic spread to the CNS tends to occur early in the disease. The most common age of occurrence is 5 to 15 years (Jordan, 2001).

The cause of non-Hodgkin's lymphomas may be an oncogenic virus because they occur with increased frequency in children with agammaglobulinemia and acquired immunodeficiency syndrome (AIDS) or those who are receiving long-term immunosuppressive therapy, such as would be given after organ transplantation. Such immunosuppressed states may reduce the body's ability to recognize and destroy oncogenic viruses or malignant cells.

Assessment

Non-Hodgkin's lymphomas of the lymphoblastic type involve the lymph glands of the neck and chest most commonly, although axillary, abdominal, or inguinal nodes may be the first involved. If mediastinal lymph glands are swollen, the child may first notice a cough or chest "tightness." If mediastinal nodes press on the veins returning blood from the head, edema of the face may result. Diffuse, undifferentiated types present most commonly with an abdominal mass. The child notices abdominal pain; he or she may have diarrhea or constipation, and a mass may be palpable on examination.

To establish the diagnosis, biopsy of the affected lymph nodes and bone marrow is performed. It is often difficult to distinguish between undifferentiated lymphoma cells and acute lymphoblastic leukemia. This can be established by bone marrow analysis (if a bone marrow biopsy shows more than 25% blasts, the diagnosis is acute leukemia). Areas of metastases are identified by chest x-ray; lymphangiogram; gallium, liver-spleen, and CT scans; and bone marrow aspiration.

Therapeutic Management

Non-Hodgkin's lymphomas are treated with systemic chemotherapy, similar to that used for acute lymphocytic leukemia. The initial phase of therapy is an induction phase (a time during which the child is put into remission, or no tumor can be detected by clinical means), followed by a maintenance phase up to 2 years long. Common drugs used are cyclophosphamide, vincristine, methotrexate, and prednisone (COMP therapy) and a multiple-agent program that includes cytosine arabinoside, cyclophosphamide, daunorubicin, vincristine, prednisone, L-asparaginase, thioguanine, and methotrexate. Intrathecal chemotherapy may be included in the therapy because of the tendency for non-Hodgkin's lymphoma metastasis to the CNS (Kramer, 2000b). Because the breakdown of cells is so rapid with chemotherapy, assess for hyperkalemia and hyperphosphatemia. Anticipate that allopurinol will be added to the therapy to prevent uric acid accumulation in the kidney. A granulocyte colony-stimulating factor may be given to prevent neutropenia.

Autologous bone marrow transfusion (bone marrow removed at diagnosis before the disease has spread to the marrow and then replaced at a point that blood components are destroyed by chemotherapy) allows more aggressive chemotherapy to be used than formerly.

Between 80% and 90% of children with non-Hodgkin's lymphoma with minimal symptoms will achieve remission.

Burkitt's Lymphoma

Burkitt's lymphoma (a non-Hodgkin's lymphoma) is a specifically named but rare form of cancer in the United States; it is generally seen in Africa. When this lymphoma does occur, however, it tends to affect children. Children 2 to 14 years old have the highest incidence; the peak age of incidence is 7 years (Jordan, 2001).

An association between Burkitt's lymphoma and Epstein-Barr virus, which causes infectious mononucleosis, exists. That is not to say that the virus causes the lymphoma, only that the virus is present at the same time as Burkitt's lymphoma.

The first indication of disease is an enlarged lymph node of the neck or abdomen. It is usually painless unless it blocks some body system.

A Burkitt's lymphoma is a rapidly growing tumor; the cell mass may double in size in 24 h. Surgery is used to remove the primary tumor. This is followed by chemotherapy; cyclophosphamide, methotrexate, doxorubicin, vincristine, and prednisone are commonly used agents. To prevent CNS involvement, intrathecal methotrexate may be given.

Because Burkitt's lymphomas are such rapidly growing tumors, they respond dramatically to chemotherapy (the cells are almost always in a susceptible state). As with other lymphomas, tissue breakdown may be so voluminous that the uric acid level of the urine may cause renal tubule plugging unless the child is kept well hydrated and a drug such as allopurinol is administered concurrently.

✔ CHECKPOINT QUESTIONS

7. At what age is Hodgkin's disease most likely to develop in a child?
8. What is usually the first sign of Hodgkin's disease?

NEOPLASMS OF THE BRAIN

Brain tumor is the second most common form of cancer in children and the most common solid tumor form (Albano et al., 2001). Tumors tend to occur between 1 and 10 years of age, with 5 years being the peak age of incidence. In children, brain tumors tend to occur at the midline in the brain stem or cerebellum located beneath the tentorial membrane; in contrast, they usually are lateral and above the tentorial membrane in adults. This makes them particularly difficult to remove in children without damaging normal brain tissue (Albano et al., 2001).

Types of Brain Tumors

Common sites for brain tumors in children are shown in Figure 53-5. The most common brain tumors include cerebellar astrocytomas, medulloblastomas, and brain stem tumors.

Astrocytomas are slow-growing, cystic tumors that arise from the glial or support tissue of neural cells. They account for about one fourth of all brain tumors in children. The peak age of incidence is 5 to 8 years.

Medulloblastomas are fast-growing tumors found most commonly in the cerebellum. The peak age of incidence is 5 to 10 years. Usually found at the midline, they cause fourth-ventricle compression and disturbances with the flow of CSF.

Brain stem tumors arise from the support tissue of the neural cells. They often cause paralysis of the fifth, sixth,

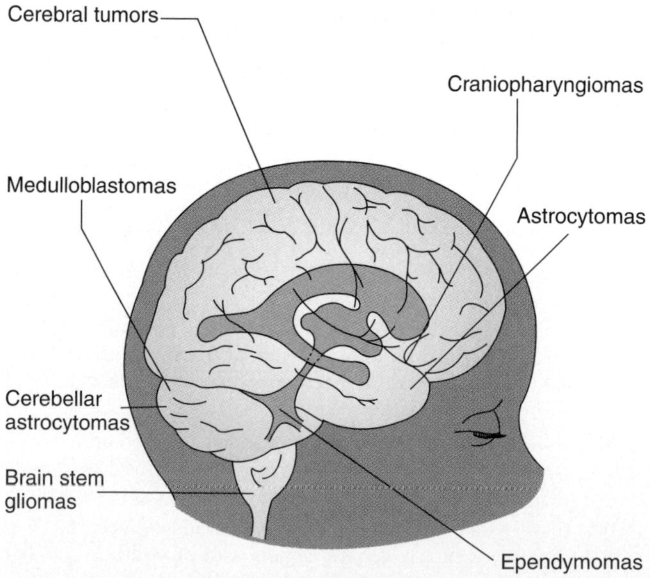

FIGURE 53.5 Common sites for brain tumors in children.

seventh, ninth, and tenth cranial nerves. They may produce symptoms of ataxia, nystagmus and changes in respiratory and pulse findings from pressure on these centers.

Assessment

Children with brain tumor develop symptoms of increased intracranial pressure: headache, vision changes, vomiting, an enlarging head circumference, or papilledema. Lethargy, projectile vomiting, and coma are late signs.

The headache associated with brain tumor usually occurs on arising in the morning. It may be intermittent because of pressure changes related to position and the ability of the cranium to expand to some degree and temporarily relieve the associated pressure. It becomes intense on straining, such as occurs with coughing or bowel movements. A parent may report these symptoms in the young child as an increasingly irritable child who is constipated because of reluctance to strain to pass stool. With some tumors, the pain is occipital. This is an important finding because this is an unusual location for a headache from any other cause.

Vomiting, like headache, more commonly occurs on arising. Unlike the child who vomits because of GI distress, the child with a brain tumor is not usually nauseated and will eat immediately afterward. The vomiting pattern occurs morning after morning. It will eventually become projectile after a long time, but projectile vomiting does not present as an initial symptom. Vomiting in this pattern may be discounted by parents as school phobia (reluctance to attend school) because the children are able to eat again immediately and seem to recover about a half hour after they are out of bed (at the same time the school bus leaves).

Diplopia due to sixth cranial nerve involvement or strabismus due to suppression of vision in one eye is usually noted. Children with strabismus may tend to tilt their head to the side or partially close one eye when viewing objects to compensate for the suppression and strabismus. The child may develop a torticollis (wry neck) or ptosis (lag of the eyelid). Papilledema (swelling of the optic nerve) may be evident on funduscopic examination.

Apart from these generalized symptoms of increased intracranial pressure, a growing tumor will produce specific localized signs, such as nystagmus (constant horizontal movement of the eye), cranial nerve paralysis, or visual field defects. Tumors of the cerebellum tend to cause a definite head tilt due to vision suppression. As the tumor growth continues, symptoms of ataxia, personality change (emotional lability, irritability), and seizures may occur.

Four to 6 months may pass from the time of initial symptoms until symptoms become localized enough to arouse suspicion of a brain tumor. When this suspicion arises, the child needs a thorough neurologic examination; skull films, a bone scan, sonogram or MRI, cerebral angiography, or a CT scan will be done as needed. Myelography may be done to identify tumors that have spread into the spinal column. Lumbar puncture must be done cautiously or the release of CSF may cause the brain stem (under pressure from the tumor) to herniate into the spinal cord and interfere with respiratory and cardiac function.

Therapeutic Management

Therapy for brain tumors includes a combination of surgery, radiotherapy, and chemotherapy, depending on the location and extent of the tumor. Because they are located so deeply, most tumors cannot be completely removed in children; this makes radiotherapy and chemotherapy measures increasingly important. Radiation therapy may be intense because, if tumor tissue is not rapidly proliferating, cells are not easily destroyed. Chemotherapy is limited because many chemotherapeutic agents do not cross the blood–brain barrier. Lomustine (CCNU) and vincristine are two drugs that do cross the barrier and so are used. Administration of the drug directly into the ventricular system by a reservoir (Ommaya) may increase drug effectiveness.

The diagnosis of brain tumor at any age is always a serious one. Closely observe the child who is admitted to the hospital for a possible diagnosis of brain tumor so that signs of increased intracranial pressure or new localizing signs are detected as they occur. Record pulse rate, blood pressure, and respiratory rate with extreme accuracy so subtle changes become apparent. Note and document episodes of irritability, drowsiness, speech difficulty, and eye involvement. Statements such as, "Child says he sees two forks when I show him one" or "Child is unable to see objects held in her left field of vision" are much more meaningful to a neurosurgeon than "Child has difficulty seeing." Completely describe any seizure activity observed, particularly the beginning movements of the seizure, because these may help to localize the point of maximum brain pressure. Side rails should be in place for protection if a seizure occurs when a child is in bed.

Preoperative Care

Before brain surgery, the child may receive a stool softener to prevent straining with bowel movements. Usually no preoperative enema is given, because expelling an enema will increase intracranial pressure.

Dexamethasone (Decadron) may be prescribed to reduce edema. An anticonvulsant such as phenytoin (Dilantin) will be ordered if the child is experiencing seizures or if surgery is apt to induce seizures (Albano et al., 2001). Also before surgery, a portion of the child's head is shaved. Prepare the child for this in a positive way by emphasizing that hair grows back very rapidly (Fig. 53-6).

If the child will go to an intensive care unit (ICU) for the first few days after surgery, a preoperative visit to meet the ICU staff should be made.

Postoperative Care

If laser surgery techniques were used for surgery, a postoperative course is simplified and shortened. Position the child as the surgeon prescribes. The position depends on the location of the tumor and the extent of surgery, but, generally, the child is positioned on the side opposite the incision. Keep the bed flat or only slightly elevated. Do not lower the head of the bed because this would increase intracranial pressure from accumulation of increased blood in the area. Note carefully how much movement of

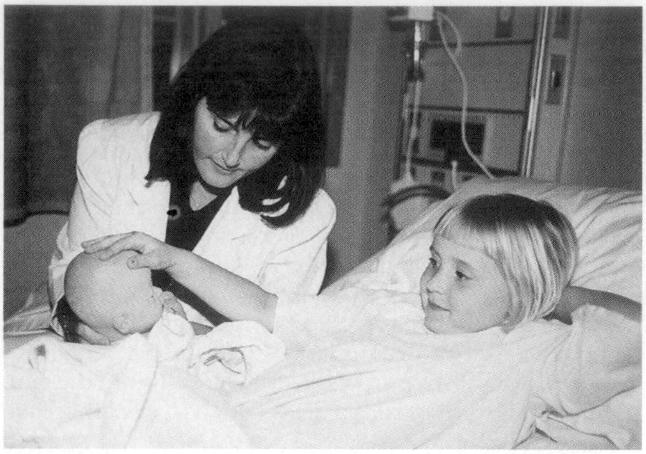

FIGURE 53.6 A nurse uses a doll to help prepare a child for shaving her head for brain surgery.

the child's neck is allowed. If surgery was in the low occipital area, the surgeon may want the child to be moved as though the head and neck were a single body part. A neck brace or cast can be applied to stabilize the head and neck and prevent movement.

You can expect the child to be comatose or extremely lethargic for a number of days after surgery due to brain irritation and edema. In addition, the child may require mechanical ventilation because of pressure on the respiratory center. Unless they are being ventilated, comatose children need to be positioned on their side so oral secretions drain from the mouth to prevent aspiration. Many children have such extreme facial edema that they cannot close their eyelids completely or their nasal breathing space is impaired. Saline eye drops or eye dressings (with the eyes carefully closed under the dressings) may be ordered to keep the cornea from drying and ulcerating. Cool compresses over the eyes may help to reduce edema. Carefully assess the pulse and respiratory rates, pupillary size and ability to react to light, muscle strength (by asking the child to squeeze your hands), and level of consciousness (by asking the child his or her name or giving a simple instruction to follow).

Obtain vital signs frequently, about every 15 min, until they are stable and there is no apparent increase in intracranial pressure. The child's temperature may be either elevated or decreased immediately postoperatively because of the effect of the edema on the hypothalamus. Measures to reduce hyperthermia (sponging, antipyretics given by gavage or rectal administration because of lethargy or coma, or a hypothermia blanket) may be necessary to reduce the elevated temperature to below 101°F (38.4°C).

Regulate the rate of IV fluid infusion carefully. An increase in the infusion rate will increase intracranial pressure. Children may receive solutions of mannitol or hypertonic dextrose to aid in evacuating the cerebral hemispheres of edematous fluid. As children regain consciousness, small amounts of oral fluid may be started. Make certain, when introducing fluid, that children are free of nausea from the anesthetic; vomiting increases intracranial pressure.

Observe head dressings carefully for serosanguineous drainage. A wet dressing is no longer a sterile dressing, because pathologic organisms may filter through its folds to reach the meninges and cause meningitis. Place a sterile towel under a wet dressing or reinforce the dressing with sterile compresses. Report signs of drainage, and estimate the extent of the seepage so you can tell later whether seepage has increased.

Children regaining consciousness after brain surgery generally are confused as to time and place; they may have difficulty performing simple tasks that they could do easily before. As the cerebral edema subsides and children begin to regain consciousness, they may need to be restrained to stop them from touching their head dressing or IV line. Use as few restraints as possible because, if they fight restraints, intracranial pressure will increase. Help the child gradually regain independence in self-care.

After the child is discharged from the hospital, parents should allow the child as near-normal activity as possible. Some children may need a football helmet to protect their head if a section of skull was removed or is not yet firmly closed. When the bulky head dressing is removed, the child may become aware of baldness for the first time. Some children need support to return to school because they are aware that other children will treat them differently now, having heard from their parents that they are dying or "had to have their head fixed." Urge parents to make the school administration aware of what has happened to the child; the school nurse should be encouraged to take an active role in helping the child readjust to school after a considerably long absence.

Late effects may occur in children who survive a malignant brain tumor. Long-term neurologic and pituitary dysfunction (especially lack of growth hormone) and cognitive challenge are not unusual in survivors of pediatric brain tumor, especially if they were treated with high doses of cranial radiation at a very young age.

NURSING DIAGNOSES AND RELATED INTERVENTIONS

Nursing Diagnosis: Fear related to diagnosis of brain tumor

Outcome Identification: Parents and child will demonstrate ability to cope with the level of fear present by 1 week.

Outcome Evaluation: Parents and child continue to maintain function as a family, visit in hospital, and plan appropriately for discharge and continued care.

Parents of children with brain tumors generally are not prepared for the severity of their child's diagnosis. They bring the child to a health care facility because of insidious symptoms—vomiting, headache, strabismus. They may think that the child has a mild GI upset or needs eyeglasses. They are shocked to learn that such benign symptoms are signs of a condition that may be fatal. This can cause such distress at the time of the initial diagnosis that they cannot think of questions to ask. In the hours or days after the diagnosis, they often have a great need to talk to people familiar with the care of children with brain tumors and to ask questions of the neurosurgeon.

Most parents want to hear a definite statement about prognosis—for example, "All the tumor can be removed; your child will be as good as new" or "Your child's chances are one in four of surviving surgery (or of having permanent effects)." Because the type of tumor, its exact location, and its extent are not fully known until the surgery, these predictions cannot be made with more than an informed guess. Assure parents that it is normal in these instances for a surgeon not to give more definitive information. Otherwise, they may interpret a surgeon's unwillingness to give them definite figures as incompetence or lack of interest. Help assure parents that earlier diagnosis would not have made a difference in the outcome. This makes it possible for them to live with themselves afterward and not be overwhelmed by the guilt that would come if they thought they could have prevented a bad outcome by recognizing symptoms earlier. Symptoms of brain tumor *are* insidious when they first begin, and the average parent cannot be expected to recognize them as important.

Help parents understand that, because of the importance of brain tissue, brain surgery is never minor surgery. Inform them how their child will appear after surgery: Their child will have a large, bulky head dressing; be drowsy or unresponsive; and have possible facial edema. Still, even parents who are well prepared are likely to be shocked at the actual sight of their child. Before you take them to the child's room after surgery, review with them once more that the child has a bulky dressing and is unconscious.

Some parents may not "hear" the full extent of their child's diagnosis before surgery. They cannot believe that the surgeon will not be able to remove the entire tumor and cure their child. After surgery, when they are told that the entire tumor could not be removed, a very genuine grief reaction occurs. As a result, they may be unable to sit and hold the child's hand, read to the child, and talk to him or her, because their minds have already jumped ahead to the time when the child might die. The child may have difficulty relating to them because they are no longer acting like the parents he or she knew before surgery (more like two strangers). Parents need a great deal of support from the time a child is first seen until the surgery, through discharge and readmissions, to the last hospital admission, when the child finally dies.

Children as young as 5 years old are aware that the head and the brain are important parts of the body. They are very aware of the feeling tone they detect in the words of parents and health care personnel. Because they undergo a number of diagnostic studies, followed by surgery and prolonged therapy, provide children with opportunities to express their feelings about intrusive procedures through play with puppets or hospital equipment. Remember that, when a patient becomes unconscious, hearing is often the last sense lost. Although children do not appear to respond after surgery, they may be able to hear what is said.

✔ CHECKPOINT QUESTIONS

9. Why may parents dismiss the vomiting that occurs with increased cranial pressure from tumors as unimportant?
10. Why may children be prescribed a stool softener before surgery for a brain tumor?

BONE TUMORS

Tumors derived from connective tissue, such as bone and cartilage, muscle, blood vessels, or lymphoid tissue, are called **sarcomas.** They are the second most frequently occurring neoplasms in adolescents (only lymphomas occur more frequently; Albano et al., 2001). Bone tumor may arise during adolescence because rapid bone growth is occurring at this time. Because girls have a puberty growth spurt earlier than boys, bone tumors tend to occur slightly earlier in girls than boys (13 compared with 14 or 15 years of age). The two most frequently occurring types are osteogenic sarcoma and Ewing's sarcoma (Fig. 53-7).

Osteogenic Sarcoma

An **osteogenic sarcoma** is a malignant tumor of long bone involving rapidly growing bone tissue (mesenchymal-matrix forming cells). It tends to occur more commonly in boys than girls. The most common sites of occurrence are the distal femur (40% to 50%), proximal tibia (20%), and

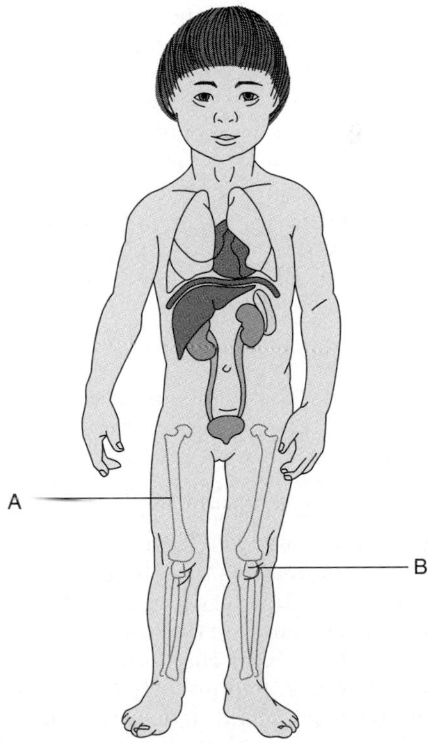

FIGURE 53.7 (*A*) The diaphysis (midshaft) is one of the most frequent sites of Ewing's sarcoma. (*B*) The epiphysis of a bone is a common site of osteogenic sarcoma.

proximal humerus (10% to 15%). Osteogenic sarcoma can occur in children who have had radiation for other malignancies as a later life effect. Children with retinoblastoma have a higher incidence than normal of osteosarcoma, as if a hereditary influence may be present.

Metastasis occurs early because of the high vascularity present in bones. Metastasis to the lungs is the most common site; as many as 25% of adolescents have lung metastasis already at the time of initial diagnosis. When this is present, the adolescent usually has a chronic cough, dyspnea, chest pain, and leg pain (if the tumor originates in the leg). Other common sites of metastasis are brain and other bone tissue.

Assessment

Children with osteogenic sarcoma are often taller than average, indicating rapid bone growth. They notice pain and swelling at the tumor site. Often, they report a history of recent trauma to the site (they fell playing basketball and bumped their knee) and attribute pain in the knee to this injury for some time. All adolescents with extremity pain and swelling, particularly near the knee, require evaluation because of the possibility that a malignant process may be at work. It is important that both adolescents and their parents understand that trauma did not cause the process; it merely called attention to the leg or arm where a malignant process was at work. This prevents adolescents from thinking they caused the tumor.

The area may be inflamed and feel warm, because tumors are highly vascular and, therefore, call increased blood into the area. As the tumor invades and weakens bone tissue, a pathologic fracture of the bone can occur.

For diagnosis, a biopsy is done of the area under suspicion. Because bone cells produce alkaline phosphatase, rapidly growing bone cells will raise the serum level of this markedly, so serum analysis for alkaline phosphatase will be obtained. To determine metastasis, a complete blood count, urinalysis, chest x-ray, chest CT scan, and bone scans will be done. Caution children not to bear weight on an affected appendage while waiting for tests or surgery. The bone may be so weakened by the growing tumor that weight bearing may cause a fracture at the tumor site.

Therapeutic Management

If the tumor is in the leg and the tumor is small at the time of diagnosis and if the child has reached adult height, the single bone involved may be surgically removed and replaced with an internally placed bone or metal prosthesis. This will preserve the child's leg. If the tumor is extensive at the time of diagnosis, the leg may be amputated at the joint above the tumor (this usually involves a total hip amputation). If the cancer has spread to the lung, metastases can usually be removed by thoracotomy.

An adolescent may have chemotherapy to shrink the tumor before surgery. Parents may be very concerned with the surgery delay and need an explanation that, with bone tumor, this is an accepted and helpful intervention before surgery. Common treatment drugs include methotrexate, cisplatin, doxorubicin, and ifosfamide (Albano et al., 2001).

Only a few years ago, a diagnosis of osteogenic sarcoma was ominous; only a few children survived into adulthood. Today, 60% to 65% of adolescents in whom the diagnosis is made early and who are treated rigorously can be cured.

NURSING DIAGNOSES AND RELATED INTERVENTIONS

Diagnosis of malignant bone tumor is a shock to both parents and children. The symptoms begin so insidiously that the diagnosis seems unreal. Parents can be assured that any delay in seeking treatment would not have had a marked effect on the chances for a cure. Neither the adolescent nor the parents could have been expected to seek medical attention any earlier. This is important preparation because guilt-ridden parents cannot function effectively to help a child through this extensive an illness.

Be certain that outcomes established are realistic. It is not realistic, for example, for adolescents to accept with understanding leg surgery that could compromise an athletic career. The highest you might be able to achieve is that they realize surgery is necessary to save their life.

Nursing Diagnosis: Risk for injury related to surgery and bone prosthesis

Outcome Identification: Adolescent will maintain good neurologic and circulatory function after surgery.

Outcome Evaluation: Extremity distal to surgical incision remains warm to touch; capillary filling is under 5 s; adolescent reports no tingling or numbness in distal extremity.

The major danger associated with surgery for excising osteosarcoma and placing a bone prosthesis (limb salvage surgery) is that the swelling that occurs during surgery or immediately afterward can disrupt neurologic or circulatory function. Therefore, position and handle the leg carefully to prevent further disruption. Assess frequently for signs that the neurologic and circulatory systems are intact distal to the surgery (toes are warm and pink; capillary filling is under 5 s; the client reports no numbness or tingling).

Adolescents who had pain in the leg before surgery may continue to feel this pain even though the involved bone has been removed. This is known as phantom pain, and it occurs because nerve tracts continue to report pain for a period after the pain has been relieved. Although you might think that phantom limb pain could be simply explained away, this is not true. The pain is very real. The adolescent may need an analgesic to control it.

Ewing's Sarcoma

Ewing's sarcoma is a malignant tumor occurring most often in the bone marrow of the diaphyseal area (midshaft) of long bones. It spreads longitudinally through the bone (see Figure 53-7). Ewing's sarcoma occurs primarily in young adolescents and older school-age children; it is slightly more common in boys than girls. It almost never occurs in African Americans. Metastasis is usually present at the time of diagnosis; the lungs and bones are the most common sites for this. Eventually, CNS and lymph node sites become involved (Widhe & Widhe, 2000).

Assessment

Most children have had pain at the site of the tumor for some time before seeing a physician. At first, the pain is intermittent, and the child attributes it to an injury (a friend punched her leg; she bumped it against a footstool). Finally, the pain becomes constant and so severe that the child cannot sleep at night. Because of this delay, at the time of the diagnosis, multiple areas of involvement are often found.

X-ray will reveal an unusual "onion skin" reaction (fine lines disclosed on the x-ray film) surrounding the invading tumor cells. A bone scan, bone marrow aspiration and biopsy, CT scan of the lungs, and IV pyelogram will probably be done to determine metastasis to the lung, bone, kidney, or lymph nodes. A biopsy of the tumor site will be done for a definite diagnosis. During tests, urge the child to avoid bearing weight on the affected extremity because this may cause a pathologic fracture at the site.

Therapeutic Management

With Ewing's sarcoma, therapy will be a combination of surgery to remove the primary tumor, radiation, and chemotherapy. Drugs often used are vincristine, dactinomycin, cyclophosphamide, doxorubicin, etoposide, and ifosfamide. Radiation to the entire involved bone may be scheduled.

About 50% of children achieve a 5-year survival rate; older children have a better survival rate than younger children (Albano et al., 2001). Caution adolescents to continue to be careful about stress on a leg that has received extensive radiation (no football, no weight lifting with pressure on that leg) because it may not be as strong as normal afterward.

✔ CHECKPOINT QUESTIONS

11. What is usually the first symptom of osteosarcoma?
12. What is a precaution to review with children waiting for surgery for Ewing's sarcoma?

OTHER CHILDHOOD NEOPLASMS

Neuroblastoma

Neuroblastomas are tumors that arise from the cells of the sympathetic nervous system; cells are highly undifferentiated and invasive, occurring most frequently in the abdomen near the adrenal gland or spinal ganglia. They are the most common abdominal tumor in childhood (Stern & Smith-Whitley, 2000). Neuroblastoma occurs primarily in infants and preschool children; it is slightly more common in boys than girls. They may occur so early in life that they are detected by fetal sonogram or at birth (Askin, 2000). There may be an association between the development of neuroblastomas and fetal alcohol syndrome or cigarette or marijuana smoking by parents. Common sites of metastasis include the bone marrow, liver, and subcutaneous tissue (De Roos et al., 2001).

Assessment

The growing tumor is most often discovered on abdominal palpation as an abdominal mass. The general symptoms of weight loss and anorexia may be present. Pressure on the adrenal gland from the tumor may cause excessive sweating, flushed face, and hypertension. Abdominal pain and constipation may be present. Compression on the spinal nerves or invasion into the intervertebral foramina may cause loss of motor function in lower extremities.

If the primary lesion is in the upper chest, children will report dyspnea; swallowing may be difficult, and neck and facial edema may occur from compression on the vena cava. If liver metastasis is present, children may have jaundice. If metastasis to the skin has occurred, blue or purplish nodules (prominent raised areas) on arms or legs may be seen.

The extent of the tumor and any metastases present are identified by an IV pyelogram (a mass growing on the adrenal gland just above the kidney will demonstrate kidney compression); an arteriogram (neuroblastomas are vascular tumors and incorporate veins and arteries into their structure as they grow); a sonogram, CT or MRI scan of the chest, abdomen, and pelvis; gallium bone scan; and bone marrow aspiration and biopsy. If an adrenal tumor is present, it will stimulate production of adrenal gland hormones or catecholamines. A urine sample will be tested for the presence of catecholamines or vanillylmandelic acid and homovanillic acid (the breakdown products of catecholamines). If children have a high level of serum ferritin, they have a poorer prognosis than those with low levels.

A biopsy of the tumor site will be planned so the tumor can be definitely identified and staged (Table 53-5).

Therapeutic Management

If the tumor is localized (stage I), therapy will consist of surgical removal of the primary tumor. If the tumor is stage II to IV, surgery will be followed by chemotherapy using agents such as doxorubicin, cyclophosphamide, etoposide, vincristine, ifosfamide, cisplatin, and carboplatin. A "second look" surgical procedure may be sched-

TABLE 53.5 Staging Neuroblastoma

STAGE	EXTENT OF DISEASE
I	Tumor is well encapsulated and completely removed by surgery.
II	Tumor cannot be completely removed by surgery or disease extends to lymph nodes.
III	Tumor extends beyond the midline; regional lymph nodes may be involved bilaterally.
IV	Distant metastases; bone, eyes, or liver is involved.

uled within several months to determine the effectiveness of therapy and to attempt the possible removal of further tumor. If aggressive chemotherapy is not effective, a bone marrow transplant to restore functioning bone marrow may be scheduled. Administration of cis-retinoic acid, a growth-inhibiting agent, improves eradication of residual disease. Immunotherapy is another possibility to eliminate residual disease after chemotherapy (Albano et al., 2001).

Stage IV disease is a unique form because it has a high rate of spontaneous regression (about 80%). This occurs because the tumor either spontaneously degenerates or undergoes differentiation to normal tissue (Grosfeld, 2000).

Overall, children with neuroblastoma have a 5-year survival rate of 70% to 90%. Although most children have a positive initial response to therapy, recurrence is common within the first year. The prognosis in children younger than 1 year of age is better than that in children older than 1 year of age (Stern & Smith-Whitley, 2000).

Rhabdomyosarcoma

A **rhabdomyosarcoma** is a tumor of striated muscle. It arises from the embryonic mesenchyme tissue that forms muscle, connective, and vascular tissue (Herz et al., 2000). The peak age of incidence of these tumors is 2 to 6 years; a second peak occurrence is during puberty. Common sites of occurrence include the eye orbit, paranasal sinuses, uterus, prostate, bladder, retroperitoneum, arms, or legs (Kelly, 2000). CNS invasion occurs from direct tumor extension. This results in cranial nerve palsy, nuchal rigidity, bradycardia, or bradypnea (due to brain stem compromise). Distant metastasis most commonly occurs in lungs, bone, or the bone marrow.

Assessment

The symptoms relate to the site of the tumor (Table 53-6). A biopsy specimen of the tumor is taken and examined for tissue identification. Metastasis is ruled out by bone scan, chest x-ray, CT scan, MRI, and bone marrow aspiration.

Therapeutic Management

The primary treatment is surgical removal of the tumor, followed by chemotherapy with agents such as vincristine, dactinomycin, cyclophosphamide, doxorubicin, etoposide, and ifosfamide. The child receives chemotherapy every 3 or 4 weeks for 18 to 24 months. If CNS extension has occurred, intrathecal chemotherapy may be included in the regimen.

A child's prognosis depends on the size of the tumor and whether metastasis was present at the time of initial diagnosis. If all the tumor can be removed and no lymph node metastasis has occurred, the chances are as high as 80% that the tumor will not recur. If some of the tumor has to be left because of its size or location, the chance of recurrence rises to about 50%. If metastasis to the lungs or bone was present at the time of the initial diagnosis, the prognosis drops still further (about 20% of children with this have long-term survival). In children who do survive, long-term complications, such as cardiomyopathy and infertility may occur from the side effects of chemotherapy.

TABLE 53.6 Common Sites and Associated Symptoms of Rhabdomyosarcoma

SITE OF TUMOR	SYMPTOMS
Orbit	Proptosis (extruding eye); visible and palpable conjunctival or eyelid mass
Neck	Hoarseness, dysphagia; visible and palpable mass in neck
Nasopharynx	Airway obstruction, epistaxis, dysphagia, visible mass in nasal or nasopharyngeal passages
Paranasal sinuses	Swelling, pain, nasal discharge, epistaxis
Middle ear	Pain, chronic otitis media, hearing loss, facial nerve palsy, mass protruding into external ear canal
Bladder and prostate	Dysuria, urinary retention, hematuria, constipation, palpable lower abdominal mass
Vagina	Mass protruding from uterus or cervix into vagina, abnormal vaginal bleeding
Trunk, extremities	Visible and palpable soft-tissue mass
Testicles	Visible and palpable soft-tissue mass

Wilms' Tumor

Wilms' tumor (nephroblastoma) is a malignant tumor that rises from the metanephric mesoderm cells of the upper pole of the kidney (Grosfeld, 2000). It accounts for 20% of solid tumors in childhood; there is no increased incidence for sex or race. It occurs in association with congenital anomalies, such as aniridia (lack of color in the iris), cryptorchidism, hypospadias, pseudohermaphroditism, cystic kidneys, hemangioma, and talipes disorders. Some children with the disorder have a deletion at chromosome 11 (Grosfeld, 2000). Metastatic spread is most often to the lungs, regional lymph nodes, liver, bone, and, eventually, brain by the bloodstream.

Assessment

A Wilms' tumor is usually discovered early in life (6 months to 5 years; peak at 3 to 4 years), although it apparently arises from an embryonic structure present in the child before birth (Albano et al., 2001). Wilms' tumors distort the kidney anteriorly so that the tumor is felt as a firm, nontender, abdominal mass. Parents sometimes are aware that their infant has a mass in the abdomen but bring him or her to a physician thinking that it is hard stool from chronic constipation. Fathers often discover the tumor when they toss a baby in the air, catch him or her by the abdomen, and feel the abdominal mass. Parents often report that the mass seemed to appear overnight. This actually can happen because tumors can hemorrhage into themselves, doubling their size in a matter of hours. Wilms' tumor may present with hematuria and a low-grade fever. Although hypertension may also occur from excessive renin production, blood pressure is not taken routinely in children of this age, so the tumor is rarely discovered by this method. The child may be anemic from lack of erythropoietin formation by the diseased kidney.

A CT scan or sonogram will reveal the primary tumor and any points of metastasis. Kidney function studies, such as glomerular filtration rate or blood urea nitrogen, will be done to assess function of the kidneys before surgery. Little time, however, can be allotted for preoperative testing, because these tumors metastasize rapidly as a result of the large blood supply to the kidneys and adrenal glands.

It is important that the child's abdomen not be palpated any more than is necessary for diagnosis, because handling appears to aid metastasis. Place a sign reading "No abdominal palpation" over the child's crib to prevent this.

Therapeutic Management

Wilms' tumors are staged according to the criteria of the National Wilms' Tumor Study Group (Table 53-7) to predict therapy and prognosis. The tumor will be removed by nephrectomy (excision of the affected kidney). This is generally followed immediately by radiation therapy (omitted in stage I tumors) and chemotherapy with dactinomycin, doxorubicin, or vincristine. The chemotherapy may be given at varying intervals for as long as 15 months. A second surgical procedure may be scheduled after 2 or 3 months to remove any remaining tumor.

If tumor involvement is bilateral, the operative decisions obviously become more complex. If tumors are small, both can be removed, leaving functioning kidney cells intact. Only the kidney with the larger tumor may be removed. Tumors may be treated with both radiation and chemotherapy.

Complications can occur from Wilms' tumor therapy. Both small bowel obstruction from fibrotic scarring and hepatic damage from radiation to the lesion can occur. Nephritis in the kidney also is a possibility. In girls, radiation to ovaries may result in sterility. Radiation to lungs may result in interstitial pneumonia; spine radiation can result in scoliosis.

TABLE 53.7 Staging Wilms' Tumor

STAGE	DESCRIPTION
I	Tumor confined to the kidney and completely removed surgically
II	Tumor extending beyond the kidney but completely removed surgically
III	Regional spread of disease beyond the kidney with residual abdominal disease postoperatively
IV	Metastases to lung, liver, bone, distant lymph nodes, or other distant sites
V	Bilateral disease

Therapy for Wilms' tumor is so effective that about 90% of children who had no metastatic spread survive for at least 5 years (Grosfeld, 2000).

WHAT IF? What if a father tells you that he discovered a Wilms' tumor in his son when he tossed him in the air and caught him, but his mother tells you that she thinks the father caused the tumor by his rough-housing? What would you want to discuss with the parents?

Retinoblastoma

Retinoblastoma is a malignant tumor of the retina of the eye (Askin, 2000). A rare tumor, it accounts for only 1% to 3% of childhood malignancies. A small number (about 10%) develop because of an inherited autosomal dominant pattern. An alteration of chromosome 13 is present. Parents who have one child with retinoblastoma have about a 4% chance of having a second child with a similar tumor. If two or more children have the tumor, the parents are probably carriers, and it can be predicted that up to 50% of their children will be affected. Because of the dominant pattern of inheritance, a person who survives retinoblastoma has a 90% chance of having a child with a tumor. Parents who may be carriers, or the parent who has survived the disease, need genetic counseling so they are aware of the risk to their children. Because the 5-year survival rate for children with retinoblastoma is good (at least 90%), this will become a very important counseling role in the future.

Retinoblastoma occurs most often, however, as spontaneous development, not the inherited type. Children with the inherited type tend to develop bilateral disease; those with the spontaneous type may or may not have the tumor in both eyes.

Assessment

Retinoblastoma occurs early in life, from about 6 weeks of age through the preschool period. It occurs equally in boys and girls, and there is no preference for either the right or left eye. One tumor or many individual tumors may be present. They are located on the retina or in the vitreous fluid or extend backward into the choroid, the optic nerve, and the subarachnoid space.

On examination, the child's pupil appears white (the red reflex is absent) or is described as a typical "cat's eye." The child will develop strabismus as the eye becomes nonfunctional. This tumor metastasizes readily along the course of the optic nerve to the subarachnoid space and brain; it quickly involves the second eye. Metastasis to distant body sites, such as the bone marrow and liver, occurs because of the rich blood supply to the brain.

Children with a family history should be examined at least three times yearly until they reach 5 years of age. When a tumor is suspected, an examination under general anesthesia or conscious sedation is scheduled because children this age do not comply well with eye examinations. CT scanning and sonography may be ordered to detect intraocular calcification or the presence of tumor. The possibility of distant metastasis is evaluated by lumbar puncture, liver and skeletal survey, and bone-marrow biopsy.

Therapeutic Management

Retinoblastomas are serious tumors because they involve the retina of the eye. If the tumor is very small at the time of diagnosis, it may be treated with cryosurgery (freezing the tumor to destroy local cells). This will preserve partial vision in the eye. Photocoagulation by way of laser surgery to destroy the blood vessels supplying the tumor may be used. Localized radioactive applicators or plaques sutured to the sclera over the tumor may be used. Such plaques remain in place for 4 to 7 days (Hogarty, 2000). The child may receive radiation treatment and chemotherapy (nitrogen mustard, vincristine, and cyclophosphamide are common drugs used) as well if the tumor has metastasized.

If the tumor is large when first discovered, enucleation of the eye may be necessary. After enucleation, the child has a large pressure dressing applied to the empty socket. Observe for bleeding on the dressing and assess vital signs frequently. To keep young children from tugging at the dressing and removing it, they may need to be restrained if a parent cannot be with them constantly. After about 48 h, the pressure dressing is removed (usually by the surgeon), and a small eye patch is applied. Irrigation of the empty socket with normal saline solution or application of an antibiotic ointment may be prescribed with future dressing changes.

An eye prosthesis is fitted about 3 weeks after surgery. Prostheses in children do not need to be removed and cleaned daily, and, in children this young, leaving the prosthesis in place prevents the child from playing with it (an interesting, colorful, round ball).

As discussed earlier, the long-term survival rate for children with retinoblastoma is as high as 90% (Hogarty, 2000). Evaluation of the child after retinoblastoma must include not only whether metastasis can be detected, but whether the child is adjusting to the loss of sight in one or both eyes. Children who do not have binocular vision this early in life generally do not have difficulty adjusting to this. They notice it most at school age when they are unable to compete in sports that require three-dimensional sight, such as baseball. They may be restricted from obtaining a driver's license. If radiation was used for therapy, cataracts may develop several years later. Any radiation therapy has the risk of leading to the development of leukemia later in life. The high incidence of osteogenic and soft-tissue sarcomas that occur may not be related to therapy as much as to a tendency for tumor growth (Albano et al., 2001).

NURSING DIAGNOSES AND RELATED INTERVENTIONS

Nursing Diagnosis: Decisional conflict related to approval of eye removal to save child's life

Outcome Identification: Parents and child will feel comfortable about decision regarding surgery postoperatively.

Outcome Evaluation: Parents and child state that they can accept removal of eye to save child's life.

With the diagnosis of retinoblastoma, parents may be asked to make a most difficult decision. To save their child's life, they must agree to the removal of an eye. Even after this procedure, the second eye may become involved or distant metastasis may occur.

Parents need support in the decision they make. If there is metastasis at a later date, they may feel guilty that they agreed to enucleation, thinking they have put the child through the surgery for nothing. They may feel guilty that they did not notice that the child's eye was abnormal before metastasis occurred. They may have noticed that the eye was abnormal but thought nothing more than that the child needed glasses and delayed seeking health care. Be certain that parents understand fully what surgery will entail (ie, loss of the eye). Provide time for discussion to help them work through this very emotional time in their life.

Skin Cancer

Skin cancer consists of three types: basal cell carcinoma (a surface epithelial growth that presents as a small ulcer that does not heal), squamous cell carcinoma (a tumor of the epidermis that presents as a white scaly lesion) and malignant melanoma (a tumor formed originating in melanocytes or nevi) that presents as a mole that changes in appearance. All three types of skin cancer are increasing in incidence and, although the symptoms do not usually appear until adulthood, the chief cause of it (excessive sun exposure) begins in childhood (McCance & Huether, 2001). Nurses can play major roles, therefore, in helping reduce the incidence of skin cancer by teaching parents and adolescents to better protect against excessive sun exposure including the following.

- Applying a sunscreen or wearing protective clothing if a child will be out in the sun for longer than 20 min
- Using tanning beds or ultraviolet light with the same precautions as sunlight
- Avoiding sunburn because there is a direct association between two or more episodes of sunburn in adolescence and the development of malignant melanoma in young adulthood

> **✔ CHECKPOINT QUESTIONS**
>
> 13. What must be avoided as much as possible for the child awaiting surgery for Wilms' tumor?
> 14. What is a common finding in the child with retinoblastoma?

KEY POINTS

After a diagnosis of cancer, parents and children need help to change their thinking from an older concept of cancer as being an always painful, fatal disease to a newer concept of it as a condition for which there is therapy and hope.

Because the therapy for cancer involves so many health care visits and so much parental concern, the siblings of children with cancer may begin to feel left out of family activities. Remind parents to incorporate the entire family in activities when possible to help them grow as a family during the course of therapy.

Radiation is an important treatment modality in cancer therapy. Immediate side effects include anorexia, nausea, vomiting, and hair loss if radiation is to the head. Long-term effects may include growth retardation or learning disabilities.

A chemotherapeutic agent is one capable of destroying malignant cells. Common side effects are the same as those for radiation therapy. Help children to use time during chemotherapy in constructive ways, such as playing a game, to keep them mentally stimulated yet quiet.

Be aware of the need to use gloves and mix preparations under a hood when preparing chemotherapy drugs to protect yourself from adverse effects of the medication.

Leukemia is the distorted and uncontrolled proliferation of white blood cells and is the most frequently occurring type of cancer in children. About 90% of children with an initially good prognosis now have long-term survival.

Hodgkin's disease and non-Hodgkin's lymphomas are malignancies of the lymphatic system. Hodgkin's disease occurs most often in adolescents; the initial symptom is often one painless, enlarged lymph node. Therapy is radiation and chemotherapy.

Brain tumors are the most common solid tumors to occur in childhood. Beginning symptoms are usually those of increased intracranial pressure. Therapy may include a combination of surgery followed by radiation and chemotherapy.

Bone tumors occur in two main forms: osteogenic sarcoma and Ewing's sarcoma. These tumors tend to be fast growing because of the ready blood supply to bone. Therapy is surgery followed by radiation and chemotherapy.

Neuroblastomas are tumors that arise from the cells of the sympathetic nervous system. They are the most common abdominal tumor in childhood. Therapy is surgery and chemotherapy.

Rhabdomyosarcomas are tumors of striated muscle. The peak age of incidence is 2 to 6 years. Therapy is surgery and chemotherapy.

Wilms' tumor (nephroblastoma) is a malignancy that arises from the metanephric mesoderm cells of the kidney. It is usually discovered early in life. Therapy is surgery followed by radiation and chemotherapy.

Retinoblastoma is a malignant tumor of the retina of the eye. It may be inherited as an autosomal dominant pattern. Therapy involves surgery, radiation, chemotherapy, and possibly enucleation if the tumor is large.

Skin cancer is a type of malignancy that begins in childhood. Cautioning children about sensible sun exposure can be an important health promotion role for nurses.

CRITICAL THINKING EXERCISES

1. Geri is the 6-year-old boy you met at the beginning of the chapter. His mother told you that he wakes up every morning with a headache and then vomits. She says this began just after school started, so she is certain it is related to school. The school nurse has suggested that Geri have an eye examination. What are some additional questions you would want to ask to see if you should pursue this problem further?
2. A 2-year-old child is going to be receiving chemotherapy after surgery for a neuroblastoma. How would you prepare the child for this? What activities would you propose to keep the child occupied while an IV solution is infusing?
3. An adolescent has been diagnosed as having Hodgkin's disease. How would you explain this disease to him? He is active in a school sports program and works part-time in a supermarket. How will you answer if he asks if these activities should be stopped?
4. Examine the National Health Goals related to cancer and children. Most government-sponsored money for nursing research is allotted based on these goals. What would be a possible research topic to explore pertinent to these goals that would be both fundable and that would advance evidence-based practice?

REFERENCES

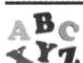

Abramson, D. H., et al. (2001). Third (fourth and fifth) monocular tumors in survivors of retinoblastoma. *Ophthalmology, 108*(10), 1868–1876.

Albano, E. A., et al. (2001). Neoplastic disease. In W. W. Hay, A. R. Hayward, M. J. Levin & J. M. Sondheimer (Eds.). *Current pediatric diagnosis & treatment* (15th ed.). New York: McGraw-Hill.

Askin, D. F. (2000). Neonatal cancer: a clinical perspective. *JOGNN: Journal of Obstetric, Gynecologic & Neonatal Nursing, 29*(4), 423–431.

Cheung, N. K. (2000). Monoclonal antibody-based therapy for neuroblastoma. *Current Oncology Reports, 2*(6), 547–553.

Davies, B. et al. (2002). A typology of fatigue in children with cancer. *Journal of Pediatric Oncology Nursing, 19*(1), 12–21.

Department of Health and Human Services. (2000). *Healthy people 2010.* Washington, DC: DHHS.

De Roos, A. J., et al. (2001). Parental occupational exposures to chemicals and incidence of neuroblastoma in offspring. *American Journal of Epidemiology, 154*(2), 106–114.

Greenland, S. et al. (2000). A pooled analysis of magnetic fields, wire codes, and childhood leukemia. *Epidemiology, 11*(6), 624-634.

Grosfeld, J. L. (2000). Risk-based management of solid tumors in children. *The American Journal of Surgery, 180*(5), 322-327.

Hasle, H., et al. (2000). Risks of leukaemia and solid tumours in individuals with Down's syndrome. *Lancet, 355*(9199), 165-169.

Herz, D., et al. (2000). Pediatric genitourinary tumors. *Current Opinion in Oncology, 12*(3), 273-281.

Hogarty, M. D. (2000). Retinoblastoma. In M. W. Schwartz (Ed.). *The 5-minute pediatric consult* (pp. 700-701). Philadelphia: Lippincott Williams & Wilkins.

Jordan, M. B. (2001). Lymphomas and lymphoproliferative disorders. In W. W. Hay, A. R. Hayward, M. J. Levin & J. M. Sondheimer (Eds.). *Current pediatric diagnosis & treatment* (15th ed.). New York: McGraw-Hill.

Karch, A. (2001). *Lippincott's nursing drug guide.* Philadelphia: Lippincott Williams and Wilkins.

Kelly, K. M. (2000). Rhabdomyosarcoma. In M. W. Schwartz (Ed.). *The 5-minute pediatric consult* (pp. 708-709). Philadelphia: Lippincott Williams & Wilkins.

Kramer, D. L. (2000a). Hodgkin lymphoma. In M. W. Schwartz (Ed.). *The 5-minute pediatric consult* (pp. 440-441). Philadelphia: Lippincott Williams & Wilkins.

Kramer, D. L. (2000b). Non-Hodgkin lymphoma. In M. W. Schwartz (Ed.). *The 5-minute pediatric consult* (pp. 576-577). Philadelphia: Lippincott Williams & Wilkins.

McCance, K. L. & Huether, S. E. (2002). *Pathophysiology.* St. Louis: Mosby.

Nash, R. A. (1999). Hematopoietic stem cell transplantation. In Lee, G. R., et al. (Eds.). *Wintrobe's clinical hematology.* Philadelphia: Lippincott Williams & Wilkins.

National Cancer Institute. (2001). *Young people with cancer.* Washington, D.C.: Author.

Shankar, S. M. (2000a). Acute lymphoblastic leukemia. In M. W. Schwartz (Ed.). *The 5-minute pediatric consult* (pp. 100-101). Philadelphia: Lippincott Williams & Wilkins.

Shankar, S. M. (2000b). Acute myeloid leukemia. In M. W. Schwartz (Ed.). *The 5-minute pediatric consult* (pp. 102-103). Philadelphia: Lippincott Williams & Wilkins.

Sirki, K., Saarinen-Pihkala, U. M., & Hovi, L. (2000). Coping of parents and siblings with the death of a child with cancer: Death after terminal care compared with death during active anti-cancer therapy. *Acta Paediatrica, 89*(6), 717-721.

Stern, J. W., & Smith-Whitley, K. (2000). Neuroblastoma. In M. W. Schwartz (Ed.). *The 5-minute pediatric consult* (pp. 570-571). Philadelphia: Lippincott Williams & Wilkins.

Widhe, B., & Widhe, T. (2000). Initial symptoms and clinical features in osteosarcoma and Ewing sarcoma. *JBJA: The Journal of Bone and Joint Surgery, 82-A*(5), 667-674.

SUGGESTED READINGS

Barr, R. D., et al. (2000). Health-related quality of life in survivors of Wilms' tumor and advanced neuroblastoma: A cross-sectional study. *Journal of Clinical Oncology, 18*(18), 3280-3287.

Biggar, R. J., Frisch, M., & Goedert, J. J. (2000). Risk of cancer in children with AIDS. *Journal of the American Medical Association, 284*(2), 205-209.

DeBaun, M. R., & Gurney, J. G. (2000). Environmental exposure and cancer in children. *Pediatric Clinics of North America, 48,* 1215-1221.

Grimer, R. J., et al. (2001). Early symptoms and diagnosis of bone tumors. *JBJS: The Journal of Bone and Joint Surgery, 83-A*(7), 1107-1108.

Han, H., & Belcher, A. E. (2001). Computer-mediated support group use among parents of children with cancer. *Computers in Nursing, 19*(1), 27-33.

Johnson, K., et al. (2001). Sun protection practices for children: Knowledge, attitudes, and parent behaviors. *Archives of Pediatrics & Adolescent Medicine, 155*(8), 891-896.

Lam, K. (2001). Characteristics of malignant tumors in young people. *Cancer Detection & Prevention, 25*(3), 223-230.

MacDonald, D. J., & Lessick, M. (2000). Hereditary cancers in children and ethical and psychosocial implications. *Journal of Pediatric Nursing, 15*(4), 217-225.

Mackey, H. T., & Klemm, P. (2000). Leukemia: Aggressive therapies predispose patients to a host of side effects. *American Journal of Nursing, 100*(1 Suppl), 27-31.

Silverberg, N. B. (2001). Update on malignant melanoma in children. *Cutis, 67*(5), 393-396.

Sparber, A., & Wootton, J. C. (2001). Surveys of complementary and alternative medicine: Use of alternative and complementary cancer therapies. *Journal of Alternative & Complementary Medicine, 7*(3), 281-287.

Tomlinson, D. (2001). The treatment of retinoblastoma: A case study. *Journal of Pediatric Oncology Nursing, 18*(2), 50-54.

Urquhart, A., & Berg, R. (2001). Hodgkin's and non-Hodgkin's lymphoma of the head and neck. *Laryngoscope, 111*(9), 1565-1569.

West, D. C. (2000). Ewing sarcoma family of tumors. *Current Opinion in Oncology, 12*(4), 323-329.

Wolfe, J., et al. (2000). Symptoms and suffering at the end of life in children with cancer. *New England Journal of Medicine, 342*(5), 326-333.

Yeh, C. H. (2002). Health-related quality of life in pediatric patients with cancer. *Cancer Nursing, 25*(1), 74-80.

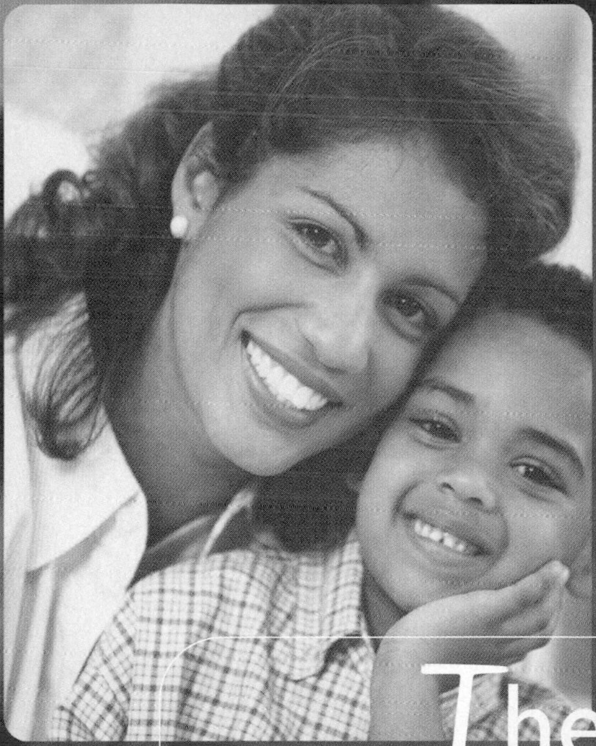

The Nursing Role in Restoring and Maintaining the Health of Children and Families With Mental Health Disorders

UNIT IX

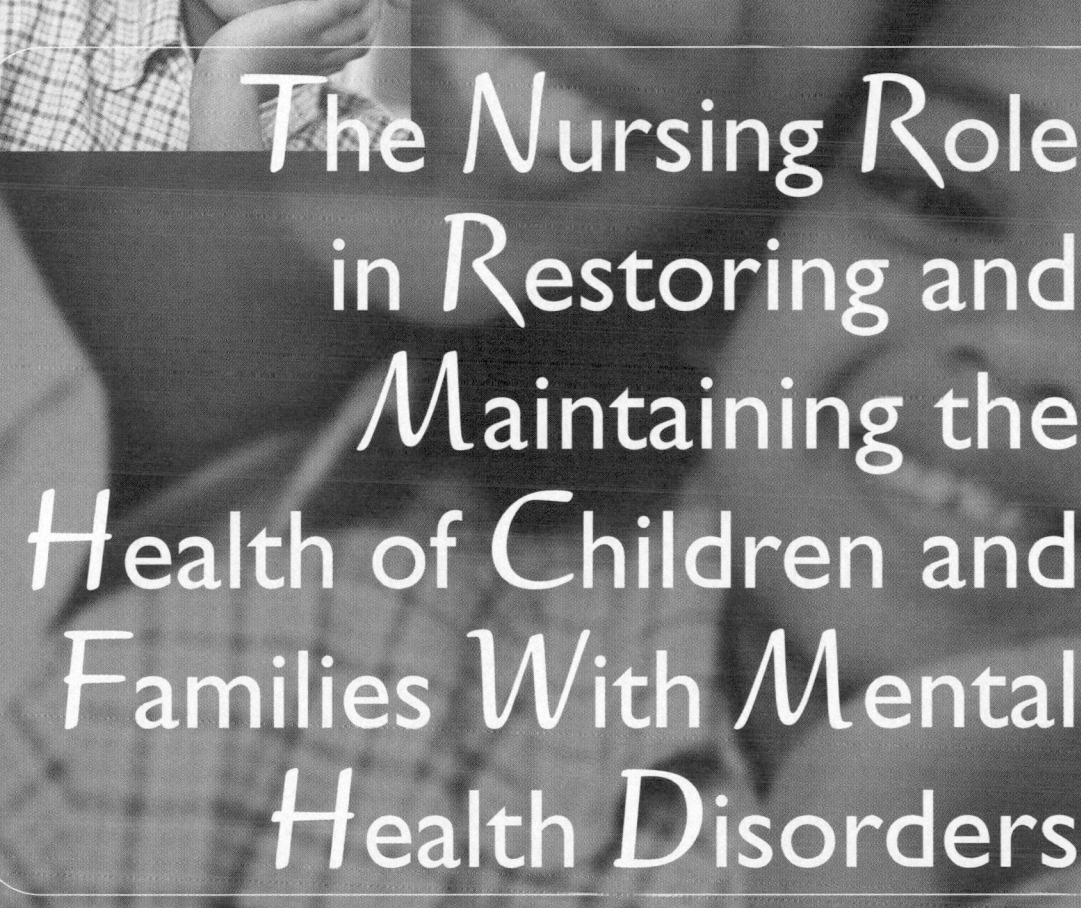

CHAPTER 54

Nursing Care of the Child With a Cognitive or Mental Health Disorder

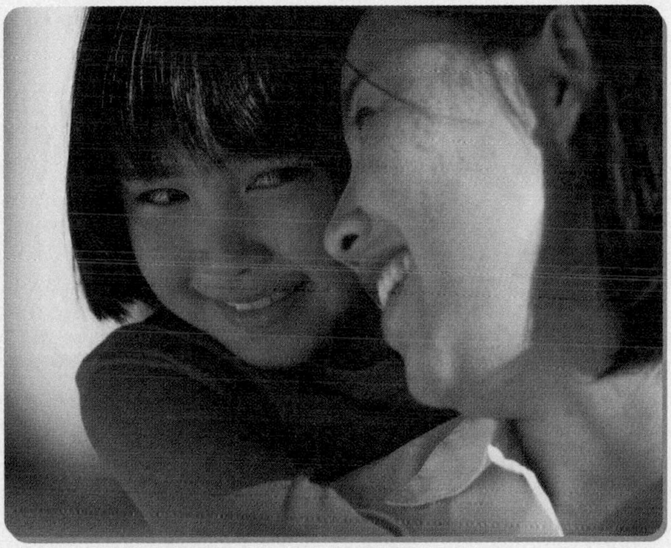

Key Terms

- anhedonia
- binge eating
- catatonia
- choreiform movements
- complex vocal tics
- coprolalia
- dyslexia
- echolalia
- flat affect
- graphesthesia
- hyperactivity
- labile mood
- motor tics
- palilalia
- purging
- stereognosis
- vocal tics

Objectives

After mastering the contents of this chapter, you should be able to:

1. Describe common cognitive and mental health disorders in children.
2. Assess a child for a cognitive or mental health disorder.
3. Formulate nursing diagnoses related to the cognitive or mental health disorders of childhood.
4. Establish appropriate outcomes for the child with a cognitive or mental health disorder.
5. Plan nursing care for the child with a cognitive or mental health disorder.
6. Implement nursing care for the child with a cognitive or mental health disorder.
7. Evaluate outcomes for achievement and effectiveness of care.
8. Identify National Health Goals related to cognitive or mental health disorders that nurses can be instrumental in helping the nation to achieve.
9. Identify areas related to cognitive or mental health that could benefit from additional nursing research or application of evidence-based practice.
10. Analyze ways that care of the child with a cognitive or mental health disorder can be more family centered.
11. Integrate knowledge of childhood cognitive and mental health disorders and nursing process to achieve quality maternal and child health nursing care.

Todd, a second grader, is brought to the clinic by his parents. He was diagnosed with attention-deficit hyperactivity disorder (ADHD) approximately 6 months ago. During the visit, Todd is observed coloring; running to the window; running over to the door, opening and closing it; and then throwing pamphlets out of the information rack. His mother tells you that she is at her "wits' end" because Todd's attention span is so short and his behavior so disruptive. His father tells you he's proud that his son is "all boy." How can you help this family?

Previous chapters described the growth and development of well children and care of the child with physiologic disorders. This chapter adds information about the dramatic changes that occur when children demonstrate a cognitive or mental health disorder. This is important information because it builds a base for care and health teaching.

After you have studied the chapter, answer the Critical Thinking Exercises at the end of the chapter and then access the on-line study activities (http://www.connection.lww.com) *to further sharpen your skills and test your knowledge.*

A child who is mentally healthy has successfully mastered the tasks of each developmental phase, developed the ability to trust adults, and possesses a positive self-concept and sense of contentment within his or her own limits. In addition, there is a good emotional relationship between the parents and the child and a sense of safety and security in the home environment. Promoting healthy family functioning during health care visits, providing anticipatory guidance for parents about developmental milestones and needs, and listening carefully to clients—the children *and* the parents—are all important in fostering both the physical and mental health of children.

Mental health also implies that a child is able to use adaptive coping mechanisms appropriately to meet the normal stressors of life. Often, these stressors provide the growth-producing challenges in life or help a child achieve the tasks of each developmental phase, for instance, establishing a sense of trust or independence. This is one of the reasons why providing age-appropriate stimulation is an essential nursing responsibility. Some stressors in life, however, go beyond what is considered "the norm." Acute illness and hospitalization are examples of increased stress. Chronic illness may provide an even greater stress, as the acute phase fades into recognition of long-term disability or an ultimately fatal prognosis. Nurses must be able to recognize the effects of illness and hospitalization on children and their families and also be able to provide interventions to prevent maladaptive coping mechanisms. Being aware of the potential emotional responses a child might have to a particular illness and implications for family functioning is essential to this ability (Fergusson & Woodward, 2002).

Children can develop the same mental health disorders that affect the adult population, such as depression or schizophrenia. In addition, a number of disorders (e.g., pervasive developmental disorders such as autistic disorder) appear to begin in childhood. Some problems, such as separation anxiety, may consist of behavior that is considered normal at one stage of development (infancy) but pathologic at another (adolescence). Current research attributes some of these disorders to genetic vulnerability, others to disruption in family life, temperament, or inadequate parent–child bonding and attachment difficulties. Children with mental illness, whatever the cause, must be evaluated and treated by specialists in the mental health field as early in their disease process as possible. It is often the child health nurse who is first aware of such problems and thus may be instrumental, through appropriate referrals, in helping the child and family adjust to the disorder.

Cognitive and mental health disorders addressed by the National Health Goals are shown in Focus on National Health Goals.

NURSING PROCESS OVERVIEW

For Care of the Child With Cognitive or Mental Illness

Assessment

Both a child's personality and mental growth potential are influenced by a number of factors, including genetic makeup, cultural background, family environment, and community resources. All of these need to be taken into account when assessing either a child's cognitive or mental health. Assess children for emotional as well as physical problems at regular health maintenance visits. When an emotional problem has been identified or is suspected, obtain a detailed history of the presenting problem, pre-

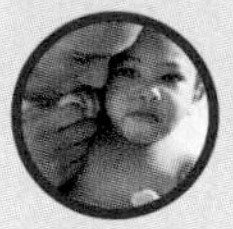

FOCUS ON NATIONAL HEALTH GOALS

Cognitive and mental health disorders in children produce major costs to a nation, as well as to individual families, because they have the potential to reduce the earning power and contributions of future citizens. Two National Health Goals directly address this:

- Increase the proportion of children with mental health problems who receive treatment.
- Reduce the proportion of children and adolescents with disabilities who are reported to be sad, unhappy, or depressed from a baseline of 31% to a target level of 17% (DHHS, 2000).

Nurses can be instrumental in helping the nation achieve these goals by educating parents to seek prenatal care so low birth weight and the threat of physical challenges can be reduced, educating about ways to reduce stress in families, and identifying children in school and health care agency settings who demonstrate a high level of stress or other symptoms of mental illness. Additional nursing research questions for this area include: What are the questions on a health history that would best reveal mental stress? Can nurses successfully identify adolescents who are at high risk for eating disorders? What support measures are most helpful to families of a child with mental illness or who is cognitively challenged.

sumed reason for its appearance, relevant past history, the child's school and social history, child's developmental history, family history, and current pattern of family functioning.

Table 54-1 lists some helpful observational and interview data for assessing these areas.

Nursing Diagnosis

Nursing diagnoses established for ill children often address mental health or the response of children and their families to their condition or treatment. Examples of these include:

- Anxiety related to surgical experience
- Deficient diversional activity related to lack of appropriate play materials for hospitalized child
- Fear related to potential loss of independence secondary to traumatic injury
- Situational low self-esteem related to disfiguring scars following accident
- Impaired social interactions related to hearing deficit
- Powerlessness related to loss of independence and control in hospital environment
- Decisional conflict related to lack of relevant information
- Hopelessness related to prolonged caretaking responsibilities for chronically ill child
- Compromised family coping related to overwhelming number of stressors placed on family at one time

Additional nursing diagnoses are appropriate when a problem of cognitive or mental health is present. Examples of these may include:

- Risk for self-directed violence related to impulsivity
- Impaired social interaction related to short attention span and distractibility
- Interrupted family processes related to inability of child to follow instructions
- Disturbed thought processes related to the effects of schizophrenia
- Impaired verbal communication related to depression and withdrawn behavior
- Ineffective health maintenance related to inattention to food or hygiene needs
- Situational low self-esteem related to lack of successful coping strategies
- Disturbed sleep pattern disturbance related to hallucinations
- Social isolation related to low self-esteem
- Compromised family coping, related to chronic mental health problems in child

Outcome Identification and Planning

Although the diagnosis of a mental health disorder or a referral to a child guidance or psychiatric clinic does not carry the stigma it once did, many parents still believe that such a referral is a mark of inadequacy or a sign of failure for themselves as parents. Help parents to see that this type of referral is no different from one to a cardiologist or orthopedist for a purely physical reason.

Parents can be assured that everyone recognizes the many pressures and stresses on children today that cannot be controlled or guarded against completely. Many parents find it reassuring to be told that their contact with a child guidance clinic, psychologist, or psychiatrist will be kept confidential. They also feel reassured by knowing that the health care personnel making the referral will continue to offer episodic or health maintenance care—that they are

TABLE 54.1 Guidelines for the Mental Health Interview of the Child

Observational Data	
General appearance	Height, weight, grooming and hygiene, nutrition, physical health, distinguishing features (deformities, tics), maturity level
Motor behaviors	Fine and gross, balance, bizarre motor activity
Speech and language	Receptive, expressive, content, tone, and articulation
Affect	Range of emotion, predominant emotion (depressed, angry, anxious, happy, irritable, labile), emotional reactions to process and/or content of interview (appropriate, inappropriate)
Thought process	Estimated intellectual level via language and knowledge base (organization and thought content), orientation (to person, place, time), perceptual distortions (hallucinations, illusions, tangentiality, obsessions, delusions), attention span, learning disabilities
Ability to relate to evaluator	Eye contact, attitude toward interviewer (negative, positive, shy, suspicious, withdrawn, friendly, self-centered)
Behaviors displayed during interview	Impulsivity, aggression, inhibition, distractibility, low frustration tolerance, ability to have fun, sense of humor, creativity
Interview Data	
Interpersonal relationships	Attitudes toward and perceptions of family, siblings, peers, transitional objects (inanimate objects used to allay anxiety), pets; social skills with peers, best friend; relationships with family, siblings, and peers; conflicts; behavior problems; adjustment to changes in routine or new situations
Self-concept and image	Self-appraisal (does child like self?), comparison of self with others (siblings, peers), what does child like most about self? what would he or she like to change about self? sense of pride in accomplishments, sex role, and gender identity
Conscience	Sense of right and wrong, acceptance of guilt, ability to accept limits in the evaluation, judgment

not being "transferred out" but asked to seek additional help only in this one area.

Implementation

Often what parents and children need most when a cognitive or mental health disorder is present is an empathic but uninvolved person to listen to their story objectively and to provide support for them as they try to resolve and manage the situation to a satisfactory conclusion. Recognizing when you are the person best able to serve this function requires professional judgment. Serving in this capacity can be important and can provide a source of personal satisfaction.

Additionally, outside organizations may be a source of support and education for the family. Organizations that might be helpful for referral include the following:

Anorexia Nervosa and Related Eating Disorders, Inc. (*www.anred.com*)
Autism Society of America (*www.autism-society.org*)
Tourette Syndrome Association, Inc. (*www.tsa-usa.org*)
National Association for Down Syndrome (*www.nads.org*)
National Mental Health Association (*www.nmha.org*)

Outcome Evaluation

Children who have a cognitive or mental health disorder need ongoing evaluation by health care personnel at health care visits because these disorders are long term. In addition, it is important to determine if any circumstances that led to a temporary problem have truly been corrected or, because the problem was only superficially changed, it is apt to resurface. On the whole, if the circumstances surrounding the child remain the same, the child's problem may return or be manifested later in another way.

Examples suggesting achievement of outcomes may include:

- Child does not injure himself during the coming month.
- Parents state they are able to cope with child's disruptive behavior since prescription of antipsychotic drug.
- Child ingests a minimum of 500 calories daily with no binge eating.
- Parents voice that they accept that their child is cognitively challenged.

HEALTH PROMOTION AND RISK MANAGEMENT

Nurses play a key role in assessing and promoting the mental and cognitive health of children and their families. A working knowledge of the typical growth and development of a child provides the basis for assessment. The knowledge also helps in developing appropriate educational strategies for parents so they can better identify problems early on. Like adults, children and adolescents are exposed to stress; however, they cope with these stresses differently. Nurses can help parents better understand how children respond to and cope with stress, also aiding in early identification should problems arise. Acting as educator, facilitator, and advocate, nurses can assist children and families to identify their needs and implement measures to meet them (see Focus on Multidisciplinary Care).

Various risk factors have been associated with an increased risk for mental health disorders in children. These include:

- Trauma or neglect
- Difficult temperament
- Attachment problems
- Experience of major losses
- Negative sibling relationships
- Medical problems and illnesses
- Exposure to high-risk activities, such as drug abuse
- Poverty and homelessness
- Parental substance abuse

A thorough assessment of the child and family can provide clues to the existence of possible risk factors and initiation of strategies to reduce their impact.

If a child develops a cognitive or mental health disorder, nurses act as advocates for referrals to support services and early intervention programs, thus helping to minimize the overall effects of the disorder on the child and family.

CLASSIFICATION OF MENTAL HEALTH DISORDERS

For many years, psychopathology in children was not classified according to a standard system; as a result, conditions were not clearly defined or described. Today, after several revisions, the American Psychiatric Association's (APA) *Diagnostic and Statistical Manual of Mental Disorders—Text Revised* (DSM-IV-TR; 2000) provides a standardized classification system that can be used by all members of the mental health care team. Major categories of disorders that have been devised are shown in Table 54-2.

FOCUS ON MULTIDISCIPLINARY CARE

A number of health care providers become involved in the care of children with cognitive or mental health disorders. These may include but are not limited to psychiatrists, psychologists, counselors, or psychiatric nurse practitioners. A key nursing responsibility is to ensure that, although children are seeing many specialists for health care, the children also receive routine health maintenance follow-up including well-child assessments and immunizations. Communication among all team members is crucial.

When a child is hospitalized, unlicensed assistive personnel often play a key role in providing day-to-day care. Encourage them to report any child who appears to be having more than the usual difficulty accepting an illness or undergoing a procedure so the child can receive necessary support to help modify his or her stress level.

TABLE 54.2 Disorders Usually First Diagnosed in Infancy, Childhood, or Adolescence

Developmental Disorders

Mental Retardation
- Mild Mental Retardation
- Moderate Mental Retardation
- Severe Mental Retardation
- Profound Mental Retardation
- Mental Retardation, Severity Unspecified

Learning Disorders
- Reading Disorder
- Mathematics Disorder
- Disorder of Written Expression
- Learning Disorder, Not Otherwise Specified

Motor Skills Disorders
- Developmental Coordination Disorder

Communication Disorders
- Expressive Language Disorder
- Mixed Receptive-Expressive Language Disorder
- Phonologic Disorder
- Stuttering
- Communication Disorder Not Otherwise Specified

Pervasive Developmental Disorders
- Autistic Disorder
- Rett's Disorder
- Childhood Disintegrative Disorder
- Asperger's Disorder
- Pervasive Developmental Disorder Not Otherwise Specified

Attention-Deficit and Disruptive Behaviors Disorders

Attention Deficit/Hyperactivity Disorder
- Combined Type
- Predominantly Inattentive Type
- Predominantly Hyperactive-Impulsive Type
- Attention-Deficit/Hyperactivity Disorder Not Otherwise Specified

Conduct Disorder

Oppositional Defiant Disorder

Disruptive Behavior Disorder Not Otherwise Specified

Feeding and Eating Disorders of Infancy or Early Childhood

Pica

Rumination Disorder

Feeding and Eating Disorders of Infancy or Early Childhood Not Otherwise Specified

Tic Disorders

Tourette's Disorder

Chronic Motor or Vocal Tic Disorder

Transient Tic Disorder

Tic Disorder Not Otherwise Specified

Elimination Disorders

Encopresis
- With Constipation and Overflow Incontinence
- Without Constipation and Overflow Incontinence

Enuresis (Not Due to a General Medical Condition)

Other Disorders of Infancy, Childhood, and Adolescence

Separation Anxiety Disorder

Selective Mutism

Reactive Attachment Disorder of Infancy or Early Childhood

Stereotypic Movement Disorder

Disorder of Infancy, Childhood, and Adolescence Not Otherwise Specified

American Psychiatric Association. (2000). *Diagnostic and statistical manual of mental disorders, text revised (DSM IV-TR)* (5th ed.). Washington, DC: American Psychiatric Association.

DEVELOPMENTAL DISORDERS

Developmental disorders, although not related by etiology, typically share a common feature in that there is a delay in one or more areas of development. These areas include attention, cognition, language, affect, and social and moral behavior. Because these behaviors are interrelated, a delay in one area may interfere with development in another area. Developmental disorders include mental retardation; pervasive developmental disorders; and specific developmental disorders such as learning disorders (reading, mathematics, disorders of written expression, and learning disorders not otherwise specified), motor skills disorders (developmental coordination disorder), and communication disorders (expressive language disorder, mixed receptive-expressive disorder, phonologic disorder, and stuttering). Mental retardation and pervasive developmental disorders are discussed in more detail below.

Mental Retardation

The DSM-IV-TR defines mental retardation on the basis of two criteria: significantly subaverage general intellectual functioning—an intelligence quotient (IQ) of 70 or below with an onset before 18 years of age—and concurrent deficits in adaptive functioning (APA, 2000). For infants, because available intelligence tests do not yield numerical values, a clinical judgment of significant subaverage intellectual function must be made.

Approximately 2% of children in the United States are cognitively challenged. This is not the result of a single cause, but conditions such as genetic abnormalities (e.g., fragile X syndrome and Down syndrome [trisomy 21]) and metabolic disorders (e.g., phenylketonuria). In addition, an interplay of several genes with environmental factors (polyfactorial causes) has been identified as a possible cause in some children (Box 54-1).

BOX 54.1

COMMON CAUSES OF COGNITIVE CHALLENGE

- Chromosomal abnormalities such as Down syndrome and fragile X syndrome
- Infection in utero, such as rubella or cytomegalic inclusion disease
- Anoxia at birth such as from umbilical cord compression
- Fetal alcohol syndrome
- Inherited metabolic disorders such as phenylketonuria
- Head trauma
- Lead poisoning
- Hypothyroidism
- Brain malformations such as anencephaly
- Very low birth weight
- Infection such as measles encephalitis

Children who are cognitively challenged are seen in health care settings for diagnosis, and they come to health settings throughout their lives for the same reasons as other children—for well-child care at ambulatory health maintenance visits; for treatment of lacerations or poisoning in emergency departments; or for treatment of illnesses such as pneumonia or appendicitis in in-service units. For these reasons, child health nurses need to be skilled in meeting the needs of cognitively challenged children.

Classification

It is unfair to categorize children only according to the results of intelligence tests, because children do not always perform well in testing situations. Commonly, cognitive challenge (mental retardation) is classified as mild, moderate, severe, or profound according to IQ. The level of 70 was chosen as the upper limit of cognitive challenge because most children with IQs below this are so limited in their functioning that they require special services, protection, and schooling. IQ tests are considered to have an error of measurement of about 5 points. Therefore, many children with an IQ of 75 are included in special schooling programs.

Mild Mental Retardation. About 85% of children who are cognitively challenged fall into this category (APA, 2000). In this group, a child's IQ is between 70 and 50. The category is equivalent to the educational category "educable." During early years, these children learn social and communication skills and are often not distinguishable from average children. They are able to learn academic skills up to about the sixth-grade level. As adults, they can usually achieve social and vocational skills adequate for minimum self-support. They can live independently but need guidance and assistance when faced with new situations or unusual stress.

Moderate Mental Retardation. Children in this category have an IQ between 55 and 35. About 10% of cognitively challenged children fall into this category (APA, 2000). During preschool years, these children learn to talk and communicate, but they have only poor awareness of social conventions. They can learn some vocational skills during adolescence or young adulthood and to take care of themselves with moderate supervision. They are unlikely to progress beyond the second-grade level in academic subjects. As adults, they may be able to contribute to their own support by performing unskilled or semiskilled work under close supervision in a sheltered workshop setting. They may learn to travel alone to familiar places. They need supervision and guidance when in stressful settings.

Severe Mental Retardation. Children in this group have an IQ between 40 and 20. About 4% of cognitively challenged children fall into this category (APA, 2000). During the preschool period, these children develop only minimal speech and little or no communicative speech. They usually have accompanying poor motor development. During school years, they may learn to talk and can be trained in basic hygiene and dressing skills. As adults, they may be able to perform simple work tasks under close supervision but, as a group, do not profit from vocational training. They need constant supervision for safety.

Profound Mental Retardation. The IQ of children in this group is below 20. Less than 1% of cognitively challenged children fall into this group (APA, 2000). During the preschool period, these children show only minimal capacity for sensorimotor functioning. They need a highly structured environment and a constant level of help and supervision. Some children respond to training in minimal self-care, such as toothbrushing, but only very limited self-care is possible.

Assessment

Assessment as to whether children are cognitively challenged is done by history taking and IQ testing. Early assessment is key and should be done as soon as parents become aware that their child is experiencing problems with development. Doing so helps to prevent them from developing unrealistic expectations of the child or punishing a child for doing things that he or she doesn't understand not to do. Assessment also allows parents to look at the things the child can do and to see where they can be of most help.

Intelligence is routinely measured with standardized tests, such as the Stanford-Binet test. Adaptive behavioral functioning, which may vary in different environments, is judged according to several methods, including standardized instruments for assessing social maturity and adaptive skills. A composite picture of life functioning is drawn from multiple sources.

Parents may react to the diagnosis of their child being cognitively challenged in the same way as parents who have been told that their child has a chronic or fatal illness—with a grief reaction. This may be manifested as disbelief, anger, or extreme sorrow. The grief may become chronic, always present, always waiting to strike a parent especially hard at times when the child would have reached milestones in his or her life, such as the first day of school or high school graduation. Work with the family in developing plans that are realistic. A child cannot achieve more than an individual disability will allow, but you can help parents better accept the outcome (see Focus on Cultural Competence).

✔ CHECKPOINT QUESTIONS

1. What are the four major categories of mental retardation (cognitive challenge)?
2. What level of development would you expect to see in a child who is cognitively challenged with an IQ of 45?

Therapeutic Management

To aid in planning, parents need a realistic prognosis for a child. This may be difficult to offer in early life, because infant intelligence tests are not accurate and more sophisticated tests are difficult to administer until the preschool years. Prediction based on these early tests involves some subjective input so a child's potential may be over- or underrated by them. Once parents have a realistic expectation based on the best judgment possible, however, they are ready, with guidance, to help children achieve their full potential.

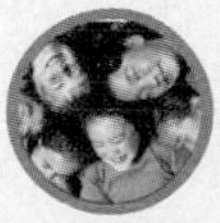

FOCUS ON CULTURAL COMPETENCE

Cognitive and mental health disorders have always been perplexing to people, and so there is a history of poor acceptance of children with such disorders. In ancient civilizations, physicians bored holes in children's heads to let out what they perceived to be evil spirits; modern television programs or movies still show distorted perceptions of behaviors associated with people who are cognitively challenged or have a mental illness. These misperceptions make it difficult for parents or siblings to accept these diagnoses. Taking time to talk with them about modern management of these disorders and the ways that children who are cognitively challenged can be integrated into a family can be a major intervention in helping families adjust to and grow with these disorders.

NURSING DIAGNOSES AND RELATED INTERVENTIONS

Nursing Diagnosis: Health-seeking behaviors related to increasing knowledge of care needs of the cognitively challenged child

Outcome Identification: Parents will demonstrate understanding of the needs of their child and care options before making any decisions.

Outcome Evaluation: Parents identify their particular options; identify child's care needs; demonstrate measures to care for child.

Parents of children who are cognitively challenged have a number of important decisions to make concerning care of their child.

Institutional Care Versus Home Care. At one time, if a child was born with a syndrome such as Down syndrome, parents were advised to place the child in an institution immediately. Today, very few institutions of this type are available. Parents are encouraged to keep children at home and maintain a home and school environment for them as near normal as possible. This plan has definite advantages for children who are mildly or moderately delayed. The give-and-take of a home environment improves their ability to relate to other people. Because a small group of people cares for them, stimulation and their desire to achieve are increased.

When children are severely delayed, keeping them at home becomes a more difficult task. If both parents work to earn an adequate family income, the responsibility for constant supervision of the child is on babysitters or older children in the family. Obtaining babysitters may be difficult, further compounding the problem. Day care and/or schooling outside the home may make home care more feasible.

Parents shoulder a great deal of responsibility to provide constant watchful care, especially for the child with problems affecting judgment. This responsibility increases as both the child and the parents grow older. The parents' freedom to go on vacation or have an adult life apart from the child is restricted. They may spend so much time with the child that other children in the family feel left out, unloved, or burdensome.

If parents are unable to care for a child at home, a suitable foster home placement may be possible to offer the child the advantage of a family setting. Halfway houses or group homes (6 to 12 children living in a home with assigned counselors) provide a care setting with a home atmosphere and community experiences.

Before giving advice to any family about where a child should be raised, consider the individual circumstances of the family. Every family has its own coping mechanisms, and individual parents may be at different stages of coping, especially in the first year after the birth of a child with a severe disability. Be certain to consider the feelings of each family member and how adequately they are coping.

Health Maintenance Needs. Children who are cognitively challenged need the same health maintenance supervision as other children. At health care visits, parents may need reinforcement and review of precautions against accidents. Remind them to treat children according to their intellectual age, not their chronologic age. All 2-year-old children would turn on the burners of the stove to see the flame if they could reach them. Most do not, however, because they cannot reach them. The mother of a 6-year-old child who thinks as a 2-year-old child must be exceedingly careful; her child can reach the same dangerous areas as any 6-year-old child but, unfortunately, may explore and touch them with a 2-year-old child's judgment.

Illness. It may be more difficult to detect illness in a child who is cognitively challenged because he or she may not be able to describe the problem. For example, children experiencing pain may respond to it by generalized crying, as infants do. Parents must observe them closely for symptoms such as tugging at an ear, refusing to swallow food, rapid breathing, or limping, because these will help to localize discomfort. When they call health care personnel, parents may be apologetic about their lack of ability to judge the child. Help parents to become advocates for their child. They know their child better than anyone else. The parents may not know exactly what is wrong, but they do know that something is wrong. Reassure parents that they have done the correct thing by calling to check out the problem.

When children with cognitive impairment are seen in an emergency department or an ambulatory setting for care, they need simple explanations of what will happen. The average 6-year-old child sees you with a thermometer in your hand and thinks, "She's going to take my temperature." Your explanation that you are going to do that only confirms what the child has already guessed. A child who is cognitively challenged may be unable to make this association between the thermometer and what you are going to do. Your explanation, therefore, is the first introduction to the event. Make certain that it is adequate.

When children are admitted to the hospital, nursing care must meet the needs of their intellectual age, not their chronologic one. For example, whether safety precautions such as side rails or possibly restraints will be necessary must be judged according to intellectual age. The explanations and preparation for procedures also must be geared to intellectual age (see Focus on Nursing Care Planning).

When cognitively challenged children are discharged from a hospital, parents need careful explanations of signs and symptoms to look for to ensure continued good health in the child. Remember that such signs may be more difficult to elicit, depending on the degree of the child's cognitive delay. Be sure parents have a telephone number they can call to seek further information or advice if they are unsure of their own observations in the period immediately after discharge.

Education. Most children who are cognitively challenged do well in preschool programs, possibly giving them a head start in learning to socialize with peers and to develop fine and gross motor coordination.

The school chosen for the child depends on the degree of intellectual delay and on the school situations available in the community. Children should be included in regular classes as much as possible (Fig. 54-1). This offers children a great deal of stimulation and helps them reach their best potential. It also helps them learn to work and socialize with people, something they will need to do for the rest of their lives. Advocating for school placement of a child in an inclusive program may be necessary. By federal law, children have the right to be educated in the least restrictive environment possible. Children who are cognitively challenged need an individualized education plan (IEP) developed based on the child's individual learning style and projected capabilities. In addition, they need safety instructions such as how to locate the correct bus for the trip home from school. If they walk to school, they need appropriate supervision to ensure safety when crossing streets.

Nursing Diagnosis: Delayed growth and development related to cognitive impairment

Outcome Identification: Child will reach and maintain optimum level of functioning possible.

Outcome Evaluation: Child is able to perform self-care within limits of disorder; exhibits feelings of satisfaction with accomplishments.

Self-Care Activities. Children who are cognitively challenged need to learn the maximum amount of self-care possible. Doing so provides them with a sense of control and accomplishment. Carefully assess whether children need special aids to achieve such skills as brushing teeth, combing hair, taking a bath, and eating. Even after children learn how to perform these skills, they may need con-

FOCUS ON *Nursing Care Planning*

A COGNITIVELY CHALLENGED ADOLESCENT WHO IS HOSPITALIZED

A 14-year-old female with moderate cognitive impairment is admitted to the hospital for knee surgery. After surgery, the child will be placed in a long leg cast and will remain hospitalized for approximately 4 days.

Assessment: 14-year-old, slightly overweight adolescent whose mother reports has an IQ of approximately 50. Sexual maturity rating: 3. Developmental age estimated at approximately 3 years. Child observed holding favorite doll tightly. Mother states, "She talks to the doll about what she wants to do." Some difficulty interacting and talking with others. "My daughter often repeats herself, asking 'What's your name?' 'What do you like to do?'" Able to feed self and use bathroom independently. Able to wash and dress self with supervision. Mother says, "She gets upset and cries easily if her routine changes." Attends mainstreamed classes at a local school. Mother planning to stay with child around the clock throughout the hospital stay.

Nursing Diagnosis: Self-care deficit (bathing/hygiene, dressing, toileting) related to application of cast and effects of hospitalization on daily routine

Outcome Identification: Child will maintain level of self-care achieved before hospitalization.

Outcome Evaluation: Child continues to feed self independently; verbalizes need to use bathroom and assists with toileting activities; participates in bathing and dressing activities with supervision.

Interventions	Rationale
1. Assess the child's daily routine at home.	1. Obtaining information about the usual routine helps in providing suggestions for modifying the hospital routine.
2. Modify care activities as much as possible to simulate the child's daily routine.	2. Maintaining as nearly normal a routine as possible minimizes the amount of stress to which the child is exposed and helps her adjust to hospitalization.
3. With each activity or procedure, offer simple, single explanations and instructions. Include the child's doll in these explanations.	3. Simple, single instructions are necessary to help the child understand what is happening. A child with cognitive impairment may be unable to associate a particular action with its meaning. Including the child's doll is therapeutic and may help to increase the child's understanding.
4. Encourage the mother to bring in personal care items from home, such as pajamas, toothbrush, and hair brush or comb.	4. Using the child's own personal care items helps to promote a more familiar, routine environment for self-care.
5. Break down each aspect of self-care into simple steps. Allow the child ample time to complete each step. Praise the child for accomplishments and provide help as necessary.	5. Breaking down a task into steps prevents overwhelming the child. Allowing ample time for task completion and praising for accomplishments helps to promote independence and foster self-confidence. Providing help as needed assists in minimizing the possible feelings of frustration, stress, and, ultimately, failure.
6. Instruct the child to use the call bell when she needs to use the bathroom. Arrange for a bedside commode, if appropriate, and assist as necessary, such as with transferring on and off the commode.	6. Because of cast placement, the child needs assistance with toileting. A bedside commode, similar in appearance to a toilet, may be less frightening for the child to use than a bedpan.

(continued)

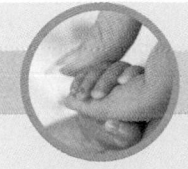

Nursing Diagnosis: Risk for injury related to impaired cognitive function and immobilization from cast application

Outcome Identification: Child will remain free of injury during hospitalization.

Outcome Evaluation: Child and mother use call bell when assistance is necessary. Child exhibits no signs or symptoms of injury. Mother informs staff when she is leaving the child's room.

Interventions	Rationale
1. Institute developmentally appropriate safety measures, such as raised side rails, for the child.	1. Although the child is chronologically an adolescent, she is developmentally a 3-year-old girl.
2. Instruct the child and mother in the use of the call bell, and keep the call bell within easy reach of both.	2. A call bell provides a ready access for help should it be needed.
3. Make frequent visits to the child's room and check on the child.	3. Frequent visits provide support and help to ensure safety.
4. Advise the child's mother to inform the staff about any plans to leave the child's room.	4. Knowledge that the child is alone allows for staff supervision to minimize the risk for injury.
5. Assess the neurovascular status of the affected extremity at least every 4 h.	5. A cast can interfere with circulatory and neurologic functioning of the affected leg, placing the child at risk for injury.
6. Institute measures to prevent complications related to immobility.	6. Immobility can adversely affect any body system. Preventive measures reduce the risk of their occurrence.

Nursing Diagnosis: Diversional activity deficit related to changes in routine and separation from school and family secondary to hospitalization.

Outcome Identification: Child will participate in developmentally age-appropriate activities while hospitalized.

Outcome Evaluation: Child participates in activities and demonstrates interest in staff and other children.

Interventions	Rationale
1. Explore with the mother and child the types of activities and interests that the child likes and dislikes.	1. Ascertaining likes and dislikes provides a basis for planning future activities.
2. Work with the mother and child to plan nursing care that allows time for rest and activities. Have the child participate in care based on the child's developmental level.	2. Active participation according to the child's developmental level minimizes feelings of boredom and enhances feelings of control and self-confidence. Expectations above the child's level promote failure.
3. Encourage the mother to bring in some of the child's favorite toys from home.	3. Items that are familiar provide stimulation and promote feelings of comfort and interest.
4. Contact the play therapist for assistance.	4. The play therapist can provide suggestions and support for developmentally appropriate activities.
5. Place the child in a room with another child who is school aged.	5. A school-aged child is younger chronologically but older developmentally. Such a roommate can provide social stimulation and act as a role model.
6. Include the child in play room activities and transport the child to the play room when possible.	6. Including the child in play room activities provides stimulation and offers opportunities for social interaction.
7. Encourage the mother to have family members and friends visit often.	7. Contact with family members and friends is essential to maintain relationships and foster growth and development, providing familiarity and additional support for the child and mother.

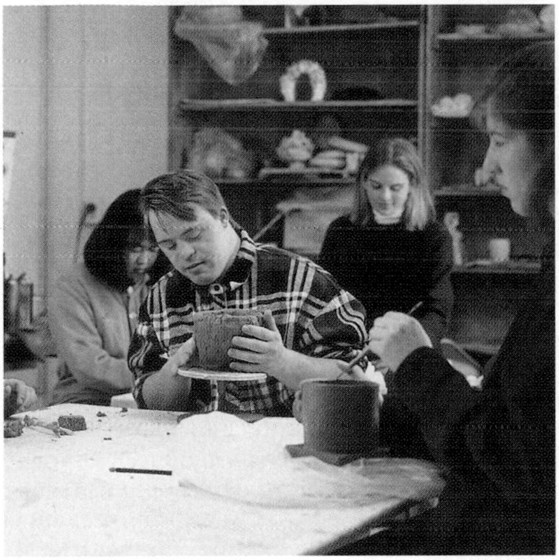

FIGURE 54.1 A teenage boy with Down syndrome participates in a high school art class.

tinued reminders to do them because they are unaware of the reason for or importance of the skill. If you do these skills for children, such as during a period of hospitalization, they can forget how to perform them and will need to be retaught after they return home (see Focus on Family Empowerment).

Play. Children with intellectual delays enjoy play like any child. Guide parents to choose toys that are appropriate for their child's developmental, not chronologic, age. Toys that cover a wide age range, such as music boxes or tape players, are good choices. Because children who are cognitively challenged may be older and stronger than the age stated for that toy, toys that are developmentally correct still may not be appropriate because they break too easily to be safe.

Social Relationships. The ability to communicate may be delayed in children who are cognitively challenged because the ability to develop language is often delayed. Speech therapy may be necessary to help them articulate correct sounds. Talking picture boards (boards with pictures on them, available commercially or made by parents) to which children can point if they want something can help speed communication.

Teaching early social behavior, such as saying "thank you" and "excuse me," shaking hands, and taking turns, is important to help children relate to other children and adults. Cognitively challenged children imitate this type of behavior the same as other children do. Providing good role models is an effective way of teaching social behavior.

Encourage parents to enroll children in preschool programs to help them learn to be comfortable with other children at the earliest time possible. Many programs enroll children as early as 1 year of age to begin education. As a school-age child, participating in organized groups such as Girl Scouts or Special Olympics is an important way to learn to interact with others and feel successful.

Preparation for Adulthood. As children who are cognitively challenged reach adolescence, they benefit from orientation to sexual responsibility, the same as all children. Girls can understand a simple explanation of menstruation and necessary menstrual hygiene. Both boys and girls need explanations of how pregnancy occurs and the measures they need to take to prevent this. Help them understand socially acceptable sexual activities.

If a girl is going to use a contraceptive and lives with a responsible adult, she can be given an oral contraceptive daily by that adult. Other longer-acting contraceptives, such as Depo-Provera and Norplant, which do not require daily administration, also are available. Sterilization is not

FOCUS ON FAMILY EMPOWERMENT
Teaching Guidelines for the Cognitively Challenged Child

Q. How can we help make sure that our cognitively challenged child can learn as much as he is able?

A. Here are some guidelines for teaching:

- Teach one step at a time. Short-term memory is often possible, whereas long-term memory is not. This means a child can only learn one step of a skill at a time (remembering three consecutive steps is long-term memory).
- Introduce motivators for learning, such as generous praise. Learning is not rewarding all by itself when intelligence is impaired.
- Reduce the number of extra stimuli present. With too many stimuli present, a child cannot focus attention on the task to learn (or realize that the task is more important than surrounding stimuli).
- Demonstrate the skill to be learned. Seeing a skill performed is generally better than just hearing it explained.
- Keep things simple. Cognitively impaired children may have difficulty with learning principles or abstractions. They may be able to learn to wash their hands, for example, but not why they should wash them (other than that it pleases you).
- Give praise accordingly. Remember that accomplishing even the most simple skill may be very difficult. Learning to tie shoes may take the same effort as another child spends learning mathematics. Learning to cross streets safely may be equivalent to earning a high school diploma.

usually recommended because it is difficult for a cognitively challenged adolescent to understand fully the implications of this (so consent is not fully informed). If pregnancy should occur, an adolescent who is cognitively challenged can be counseled but not forced to have an abortion. If the adolescent decides to continue the pregnancy, assist her through the pregnancy.

WHAT IF? A 15-year-old female who is mildly cognitively challenged comes to the clinic for a routine checkup with her mother. During your conversation, the girl asks you if she should have a baby. How would you respond?

Pervasive Developmental Disorders: Autistic Disorder

As a category, pervasive developmental disorders are characterized by impairment in social and communication skills and the display of stereotypical behaviors (APA, 2000). Autistic disorder is marked by severe deficits in language, perceptual, and motor development; defective reality testing; and an inability to function in social settings. These problems are evident before the age of 3 years. There often is a lack of responsiveness to other people, gross impairment in communication skills, and bizarre responses to various aspects of the environment, all developing within the first 30 months of age. It is a rare condition, occurring in only 2 to 10 children out of 10,000, although it may be increasing in incidence. A former concern that immunization may precede or cause the disorder has now been ruled out as a cause. It occurs more often in boys than in girls. As many as 50% of children with the disorder are also cognitively challenged (APA, 2000).

Assessment

Common symptoms of autistic disorder are summarized in Box 54-2. Because of the lack of responsiveness to people that is part of the syndrome, normal attachment behavior does not develop. Although often not diagnosed until the child is 2 to 3 years of age, parents report that they were worried much earlier because their infant failed to cuddle or make eye contact or exhibit facial responsiveness. Infants may not reach to be picked up. They are unable to play cooperatively or make friendships. Parents may first bring a child to a health care facility thinking he or she is deaf because of this inability to establish normal relationships.

The impairment in communication is shown in both verbal and nonverbal skills. Language may be totally absent. If a child does speak, grammatical structure may be impaired, such as the use of "you" when "I" is intended. There is inability to name objects (nominal aphasia) and abnormal speech melody, such as questionlike rises at the end of statements. **Echolalia** (repetitive words or phrases spoken by others) and concrete interpretation also may be present.

Bizarre responses to the environment include intense reactions to minor changes in the environment (screaming if a toy box is moved across the room) and attachment to odd objects (always carrying a string or a shoe). Repetitive hand movements, rocking, and rhythmic body movements are often observed. Children are intensely preoccupied by objects that move, such as a fan, the swirling water in the toilet bowl, or a spinning top. Music often holds a special interest for them. Hitting, head banging, and biting also may be present.

Children with autistic disorder have a **labile mood** (e.g., crying occurs suddenly followed immediately by giggling or laughing). They may react with overresponsiveness to sensory stimuli, such as light or sound, but then be unaware of a major event in the room, such as the sounding of a fire alarm.

In contrast to these mannerisms, long-term memory may be excellent. Autistic children may be able to recall dates and spoken words from conversations that took place years before. This excellent memory previously led to the belief that most of these children have normal intelligence. Actually, the majority of children with autistic disorder have an IQ below 70 (APA, 2000). Intelligence testing is difficult, however, because children with autistic disorder do not respond well to test situations and they score poorly on verbal parts of these tests. Tasks requiring manipulative or visual skills or immediate memory may be performed at above-normal levels.

BOX 54.2

COMMON SYMPTOMS IN THE CHILD WITH AUTISTIC DISORDER

Failure to develop social relations
Stereotyped behaviors such as hand gestures
Extreme resistance to change in routine
Abnormal responses to sensory stimuli
Decreased sensitivity to pain
Inappropriate or decreased emotional expressions
Specific, limited intellectual problem solving
Stereotyped or repetitive use of language
Impaired ability to initiate or sustain a conversation

Therapeutic Management

Autistic disorder is a perplexing condition. Parents need a great deal of support so that they do not reject the child because he or she seems to be rejecting them. Behavior modification therapy may be effective in controlling some of the bizarre mannerisms that accompany autism, but, because the basic cause of the disorder is not known, therapy will not always succeed.

As children mature, they develop greater awareness of and attachment to parents and other familiar adults. A day care program can help to promote social awareness. Some children may eventually reach a point where they can become passively involved in loosely structured play groups. Some children may be able to lead independent lives, although social ineptness and awkwardness may remain, especially if accompanied by cognitive challenges (Bechtold, 2001).

✔ **CHECKPOINT QUESTIONS**

3. What areas are important to address for the child who is cognitively challenged to reach his optimal level of functioning?
4. What assessment findings would you expect with a child with an autistic disorder?

Specific Developmental Disorders

Specific developmental disorders may be characterized by the more narrowed area of development involved with the delay. Typically, these include learning disorders, communication disorders, and motor skills disorders.

Learning disorders occur in approximately 5% of the children in the United States. Although the degree may vary, these disorders involve a discrepancy between actual achievement and what is expected based on the child's age and intelligence. Learning disorders may involve reading, such as **dyslexia** (reading reversal), mathematics, or writing. Children may develop accompanying low self-esteem and deficits in social skills (APA, 2000). Children need individualized educational plans to help them achieve at the highest level possible.

Communication disorders involve speech (motor aspect) or language (formulation and comprehension of verbal communication) problems. Categories include expressive disorder, mixed receptive-expressive disorder, phonologic disorder, and stuttering. Like learning disorders, these conditions can lead to a lack of self-esteem unless the child receives support and encouragement from parents, teachers, and health care providers. Fortunately, speech therapy can effectively improve these disorders and allow children to achieve sufficiently to become successful adults.

ATTENTION-DEFICIT AND DISRUPTIVE BEHAVIOR DISORDERS

Attention-deficit disorder and the disruptive behavior disorders, which include two subgroups: oppositional defiant disorder and conduct disorder (Steiner, 2000), may begin with behavior problems that are not so different from what most families experience. Thus, parents may be unaware of the need for intervention initially. By the time they seek help, they may already be extremely distressed about the seeming unmanageability of their child.

These disorders need to be diagnosed as early as possible, before the child's behavior leads to a deteriorating level of self-esteem and compromised social skills and social and legal complications in family functioning. The home environment may be the most important factor in determining whether the disorder turns into a more complicated psychopathologic process or whether it can be channeled into purposeful, productive activity.

Attention-Deficit Hyperactivity Disorder

Attention-deficit hyperactivity disorder (ADHD) is a persistent pattern of inattention and/or hyperactivity-impulsiveness revealed before the age of 7 years (APA, 2000). It is estimated to occur in about 3% to 7% of school-age children in the United States. Boys are affected more frequently than girls. Although the cause is unknown, it occurs more frequently among some families than in the general population, indicating a possible genetic etiologic component. ADHD has also been associated with child neglect, lead poisoning, and drug exposure in utero (APA, 2000). Both drug and behavior modification treatment methods have been used with success, which may support the theory of varying causes.

The disorder is characterized by three major behaviors: inattention, impulsiveness, and hyperactivity (Valente, 2001). In children, inattention makes them unable to complete tasks effectively. They become easily distracted and often may not seem to listen. Impulsiveness causes them to act before they think and have difficulty with such tasks as awaiting turns in games. With hyperactivity, children may shift excessively from one activity to another, exhibiting excessive or exaggerated muscular activity, such as excessive climbing onto objects, constant fidgeting, and aimless or haphazard running.

Assessment

The disorder is diagnosable by 36 months of age, although parents may excuse the behavior as "active" or "always on the go" until school age, when it is apparent that the child cannot sit still in school or concentrate on problem solving for longer periods. When the disorder is first suspected, a thorough initial history to reveal the extent of the problem should be recorded. The history is important because some children have enough control in a one-to-one situation that their extremes of behavior are not apparent in an ambulatory health care setting.

The pregnancy and birth history, the child's ability to meet developmental milestones, and a typical day for the child should be reviewed carefully. The term **hyperactivity,** or excess movement, is commonly carelessly used by parents to describe any active child. Have the parent give an exact description of what the child is unable to do, such as sitting still long enough to finish a full meal or running to the window 10 times in 15 min, to document that hyperactivity truly exists.

Assess for activity that is not only excessive but also disorganized. For example, in school, children with ADHD may run from the back of the room to the front of the room, to the window, to the teacher's desk, to their own desk throughout class. They perform repetitive activities such as pencil tapping, arm swinging, and finger tapping. At home, they may leave a project they are working on or a television program they are watching intently only to run to the window or open the refrigerator door, unaware of why they are running. This is driven or compulsive behavior.

Variability is another important symptom. Everyone has days when they perform at their peak and days when their performance is less than optimum. Children with ADHD may have behavior so variable that they have good and bad *moments.* This type of variability causes them to lose track of systems and methods, not just answers, so school performance may falter. When asked to add, for example, a child might add 4 and 3 correctly, but then lose track of the system and add 2 and 3 as 23 or 32.

A high level of impulsiveness can cause children to make statements without thinking, to touch objects they have just been told not to touch, or to speak or act before they have time to think about what they want to say or do. When angered, they may shout, strike out, or bite before they can be offered an explanation. They may be unable to wait in line for a drink of water—their impulsiveness tells them that they must have their drink immediately.

Usually, average children can filter out stimuli that are not important to them at that moment. Children with ADHD seem to have an "all-or-none" reaction to stimuli. They may block out all incoming stimuli and, as a result, do not hear their parents or a teacher calling them. They may be disciplined at school for something such as not answering a fire drill (unaware that a bell was ringing and that children around them were moving toward the exit). At other times, they may be unable to suppress any incoming stimuli. They mean to concentrate on a desk assignment in school, but, outside the window, they hear a bird singing; next to them, they smell a girl's perfume; they feel their watch on their wrist—so they cannot concentrate on the problem at hand. This may be reported by parents or teachers as an exceedingly short attention span.

Children with ADHD may also have difficulty with concepts such as *right* and *left, before* and *after, in front of, in back of, yesterday,* and *tomorrow,* because these concepts call for sequencing. If children cannot tell the difference between left and right, they can have difficulty forming common letters such as *b* and *d,* which vary only in the direction of the bottom loop. They can have difficulty with common tasks such as washing their hands, because they never know which way to turn a faucet. Turning door knobs and keys, tying shoe laces, and screwing on bottle caps are all complex tasks for a child who has difficulty with sequencing. They may show awkward motor movements and cannot work all muscles gracefully in proper sequence. These children may reach beyond an object, possibly spilling a glass of milk at the table at every meal.

Long after the average child is speaking in fluent sentences, children with ADHD may have difficulty using conjunctions or prepositions correctly (sequencing of words). They may have difficulty learning to read. To read words of more than one syllable, they must sound the first syllable, then retain that sound in their mind while they sound the second. If they have difficulty retaining the first syllable long enough to connect it with the second, they cannot construct the word. Similarly, they can have difficulty with arithmetic, because they may be unable to retain the sum of two numbers long enough to add the sum of a third. Spelling may be equally difficult. Not only are they unable to sequence the letters in a word correctly, but they also cannot retain memory rules such as "i before e" to help them.

Children with ADHD do not have a deficit in intelligence, although they may seem to because of their impulsive behavior. They may be unaware that their behavior is upsetting to family, friends, and teachers and, thus, are not anxious about their inability to conform to society's rules.

On physical assessment, these children often show many "soft" neurologic signs, such as inability to use a pencil or scissors well. A thorough neurologic examination often is difficult because their attention span is so short. On such an examination, they often have difficulty performing tests such as a finger-to-nose test or rapid hand movements, such as touching one finger after another with their thumb. They tend to show "mirroring" with this movement (the second hand imitates what the first hand attempts to do). Cerebellar difficulty may be evidenced further by inability to perform a tandem walk or a heel-to-shin test. They may be able to identify one touch but not two simultaneous touches on their body. They may not show the normal responses of **graphesthesia** (ability to recognize a shape that has been traced on the skin) or **stereognosis** (ability to recognize an object by touch). When asked to stand with arms outstretched, **choreiform movements** (aimless movements) and rising of the fingers are often present. More definite neurologic signs, such as a unilateral Babinski reflex or strabismus, may also be present. Testing children through the use of games may be necessary so their attention is maintained long enough to complete the assessment.

IQ testing is used to document the child's intelligence. The Wechsler Intelligence Scale for Children (WISC), the test most often chosen, consists of two portions: a verbal scale and a performance scale. The child is given three final scores: verbal IQ, performance IQ, and combination or full-scale IQ. The child with perceptual and motor deficits tends to do poorly on the performance scale but average or better on the verbal scale. Children with language difficulty typically do poorly on the verbal scale but average or above on the performance scale. Children with ADHD show a "scatter" pattern on both performance and verbal portions, doing well on some portions and poorly on others.

Children who have difficulty filtering out stimuli do poorly on group-administered intelligence tests because they are too distracted by those around them. These children, therefore, should take IQ tests individually. Neurologic examinations also should be performed in rooms free of distractions such as attractive toys.

Children with ADHD are often referred to a health care facility because they have had difficulty achieving in school. Parents may have been assured on previous occasions that, although their child had difficulty settling down to tasks, this was because he was "all boy" or "every child is different." They may need time to accept that their child has a condition that interferes with learning. Active listening is essential. This is a difficult situation that may have persisted for a long time. The parents may be unaware themselves of the strain this has produced until they start to describe it.

✔ CHECKPOINT QUESTIONS

5. What are the three major characteristics of ADHD?
6. What is the underlying problem associated with difficulty of concepts such as *before* and *after?*

Therapeutic Management

A variety of treatment methods are used, often in combination, in the management of ADHD.

Environment. Construction of a stable learning environment is crucial for children with ADHD. This may include special instruction, free from the distractions of an entire class. Parents may have difficulty accepting the fact that their child needs special schooling (the intelligence test, after all, said that he or she was above average). They may need help in seeing that the condition interferes with intellectual functioning and that a special program must be constructed for the child to succeed.

Parents having difficulty at home with discipline and management often appreciate support and advice. Encourage them to be fair but firm and set consistent limits. Although every child has a right to an opinion, many decisions that the average child enjoys making for himself or herself must be made for this child. "Do you want to wear your red or your blue shirt today?" is less effective than "Here is your blue shirt to wear today."

Children who are easily distracted have difficulty completing chores or picking up their toys. They can be assigned age-appropriate chores with the understanding that a parent must give many reminders to them to get the job completed. Teach parents to give instructions slowly and make certain that they have the child's attention before beginning instructions. Breaking down a chore into several steps may help (get the toy box is one step; pick up toys is a second). This helps to avoid confrontation that may arise later if children do not hear or do not process what is said to them.

All children like to participate in dinner conversation or discussions about their day. Children with ADHD often have difficulty telling a story or repeating a joke told to them (a sequencing problem). Suggest parents help them by asking questions such as "Why?" "Where?" or "Who?" to reach the point of the story. Also encourage parents that, when they correct behavior, their anger is about something the child has deliberately done wrong, not about some incident that happened because of the child's inability to sequence, filter, or integrate concepts. Punishment should follow an offense quickly because a child quickly forgets what he or she did. As with all children, parents should make sure the child understands that the parent is angry at the behavior, not the child. Children with ADHD commonly develop poor self-esteem because, although they are intelligent, they cannot succeed. Help parents to build, not hinder, the development of self-esteem at every stage possible.

Medication. A number of medications are helpful in controlling the excessive activity of the child with ADHD and lengthening the attention span or decreasing the distractibility so he or she can function in a normal classroom.

Methylphenidate hydrochloride (Ritalin, Concerta [extended-release form]) has been prescribed for this disorder (see Focus on Pharmacology). It works by stimulating dopamine receptors to achieve a more regular nerve transmission. Insomnia and anorexia are side effects. The insomnia may be relieved by administering the drug early in the day. The extended-release form is advantageous in that it only needs to be administered once a day. Children receiving the drug for extended periods of time need careful height and weight assessment to evaluate that long-term anorexia is not causing weight loss (Goldson & Hagerman, 2001).

FOCUS ON PHARMACOLOGY

Methylphenidate Hydrochloride (Ritalin, Concerta)

Action: Methylphenidate is a central nervous system stimulant that acts paradoxically in children with ADHD, possibly by stimulating dopamine receptors to calm rather than simulate activity.

Pregnancy risk category: C

Dosage: Initially, 5 mg orally before breakfast and lunch, gradually increasing the dosage in 5- to 10-mg increments weekly, not to exceed 60 mg/day. The extended-release form (Concerta) is administered once daily; dosage is determined by weight and symptoms.

Possible adverse reactions: Nervousness, insomnia, anorexia, pulse rate changes, hyper- or hypotension, tachycardia, leukopenia, anemia, and growth suppression.

Nursing Implications

- Administer the drug exactly as prescribed and instruct parents in same. Be sure that parents know which form of the drug they are to give. Reinforce the use of once-daily administration of extended-release form; instruct parents to have child swallow extended-release tablets whole and to refrain from chewing or crushing them.
- Instruct the parents to administer the drug before 6 PM to prevent interference with sleep.
- Advise the parents and child to avoid over-the-counter drugs, such as cold remedies and cough syrups that contain alcohol.
- Obtain baseline vital signs and monitor on follow-up visits for changes.
- Arrange for follow-up laboratory tests, including complete blood count for children on long-term therapy.
- Stress the need for adequate nutrition in light of possible anorexia. Monitor child's weight closely for changes.
- Assess child's growth on subsequent visits for possible growth suppression.
- Keep in mind that the safety of using Concerta for children under the age of 6 years has not been established.

Family Support. Parents of a child with ADHD often need frequent health care visits while their child is growing up. A responsive, listening ear is crucial to their ability to handle the challenge of raising a child with these symptoms. Any parent can grow short-tempered and irritable at times with a child who does not seem to hear them or follow what they say. They may need reminders at intervals that their child does not act this way on purpose. Help them to understand that, because of a very complex and as yet ill-understood syndrome, the behavior is the best their child can achieve.

Although hyperactivity fades, some children with ADHD continue to experience problems with impulsivity and inattention into adulthood. They achieve best if they can find careers that allow them to cope with these behaviors.

Oppositional Defiant Disorders

Oppositional defiant disorders consist of hostile, negativistic, or defiant behavior that results in disturbed functioning in academic and social domains and lasts for over 6 months (Steiner, 2000). Children typically have difficulty controlling their temper; their anger is often directed at an authority figure.

The disorder develops most frequently in late preschool or early school age. The cause may be a combination of temperament, inheritance, and adverse social factors. Therapy must be individually designed to meet the needs of individual children and includes such techniques as family therapy and anger management.

Conduct Disorders

Conduct disorders are persistent antisocial acts involving violations of personal rights or societal rules, such as disobedience, stealing, fighting, destruction of property, fire setting, and early sexual behavior (APA, 2000). Symptoms can be clustered as aggression to people and animals, destruction of property, deceitfulness and theft, and serious violations of rules. Many teenage runaways may fall into this category. Conduct disorders are the most frequently diagnosed psychiatric disorder in childhood (Steiner, 2000).

Children seem to develop an increasing loss of self-regulation or an inability to know when to stop an action.

Conduct disorders are seen more frequently in males than in females, particularly when property or violent crimes are involved; however, the prevalence of conduct disorders in girls is increasing, possibly reducing the male predominance over time. A number of etiologic factors have been described for this disorder, including genetic predisposition, neurologic deficit correlates, and sociologic factors related to poverty and cultural disadvantage. In addition, the home environment is frequently characterized by rejection, frustration, and harsh and inconsistent discipline. Parents may have marital conflicts or substance abuse problems, or children may have had a series of inconsistent caretaking by stepparents or foster parents.

Therapy for children with conduct disorders focuses on modifying the home environment and training in social and problem-solving skills. Social skills training teaches the child to recognize how his or her behavior affects others. Problem-solving skills training teaches the child to generate alternative solutions to situations, sharpen thinking about the consequences of choices, and evaluate his or her response. Parental training is also important but can be difficult until parents realize this is family problem. Removing the child from the home to a structured day care environment may be necessary. Unfortunately, the child may interpret this as more rejection, further compounding the problem. Any new environment that is created must be consistent and loving, not institutional, to be effective.

Numerous medications such as carbamazepine (Tegretol), propranolol (Inderal), and lithium carbonate may reduce the aggressive behavior. Long-term therapy with an agent such as buspirone (BuSpar) may be effective in helping control temper or explosive outbursts (Steiner, 2000).

✔ CHECKPOINT QUESTIONS

7. What medication is most frequently used to treat ADHD?
8. What methods are used as therapy for conduct disorders?

ANXIETY DISORDERS OF CHILDHOOD OR ADOLESCENCE

Because anxiety is considered a normal part of certain phases of development (e.g., stranger anxiety of the 6- to 8-month-old child, separation anxiety in the toddler, fear of mutilation and the dark in the preschooler, and performance anxiety or school avoidance of the school-age child or adolescent), genuine anxiety disorders in children may often be overlooked. When left untreated, children may cope with fear by becoming overdependent on others for support or by turning away from the problem and withdrawing into themselves (see Focus on Evidence-Based Practice). This can leave a child socially immature and unable to achieve in school. The DSM-IV-TR identifies separation anxiety disorder and anxiety-based school refusal as anxiety disorders in children (APA, 2000). School refusal is discussed with other concerns of the school-age child (see Chap. 31).

Separation Anxiety

Separation anxiety, a normal phase of development in the toddler (see Chapter 29), is considered a disorder when an older child shows excessive anxiety about separation or the possibility of separation from those to whom the child is attached. Children may worry when apart from parents that they will have an accident or become ill. They may have difficulty falling asleep at night or insist on sleeping with parents or just outside their parents' bedroom door. They may experience acute distress, frequent nightmares about separation, and reluctance and refusal to separate. Repeated reports of physical symptoms when separated or when separation is anticipated are also possible. Such a degree of anxiety can be incapacitating to children; it may prevent them from visiting at friends' houses, enjoying a camp experience, or actively participating in school.

Separation anxiety tends to run in families and occurs slightly more frequently in girls than in boys. Unresolved internal conflicts, uncertainty about one's caregiver, and parent-induced anxious attachment are psychodynamic factors attributed to this disorder. Temperament is also considered a contributing factor (Bechtold, 2001).

Treatment for separation anxiety includes individual counseling sessions combined with antidepressant med-

FOCUS ON EVIDENCE-BASED PRACTICE

Can Trauma Cause Post-traumatic Stress in Children?

Post-traumatic stress disorder (PTSD) is a syndrome that was formerly thought to apply only to adults, mainly those who had survived a particularly violent event such as war. Today, it is recognized as a syndrome that can apply to children as well. To discover if accidental injuries in children could lead to the syndrome, 48 children, aged 7 to 17 years, who had accidental injuries severe enough to warrant hospital admission, were assessed during hospitalization for measures such as any prior traumatization, prior psychopathology, the injury severity, the level of their parent's and own distress. At an ambulatory follow-up visit at least 1 month later, children were interviewed as to whether PTSD symptomatology was present. Parents were given a questionnaire. Results of the study showed that 12.5% of children demonstrated the full syndrome of PTSD at the follow-up visit and an additional 16.7% had partial symptoms (29.2% or a fourth of the children total). Those who had evidence of the syndrome were more apt to have had factors such as prior psychopathology and higher parental and child distress. The researchers concluded that the level of parents' and child's acute distress at the time of the injury may be useful predictors as to which children will need further counseling to help prevent PTSD.

This is an important study for nurses because nurses are often the health care professional on an emergency care service who has the most contact with the parents during the time the child is being treated so is in the best position to evaluate the level of parental distress. As nurses care for the child during the period of hospitalization, they are in excellent positions to evaluate the level of distress the child experienced by the injury. Documenting this distress could help to identify which children are most apt to have long-term psychological effects from the injury, thereby facilitating early intervention.

Daviss, W. B., et al. (2000). Predicting posttraumatic stress after hospitalization for pediatric injury. *Journal of the American Academy of Child & Adolescent Psychiatry, 39*(5), 576–583.

ication. In addition, family therapy may be helpful in allowing the family to gain greater insight into the dynamics of the problem and the child to gain more confidence in his or her ability to function independently.

EATING DISORDERS

Eating disorders in young children consist of pica, rumination, and feeding disorders. In older children, eating disorders include anorexia nervosa and bulimia (APA, 2000).

Pica

Children who persistently eat nonfood substances such as dirt, clay, paint chips, crayons, yarn, or paper are said to have pica. *Pica* is the Latin word for magpie (a bird that is an indiscriminate eater). The primary danger lies in the possibility of accidental poisoning. Other complications include constipation, gastrointestinal malabsorption, fecal impaction, and intestinal obstruction. The disorder is seen predominantly between the ages of 2 and 6 years, although it may be present into adolescence. Often, it is not diagnosed until the child presents with a pica-induced complication, such as lead poisoning (see Chapter 52).

The incidence of pica increases in children who are cognitively challenged, possibly because of their inability to distinguish edible from inedible substances as early as other children are. It is highly associated with iron deficiency anemia; it occurs at a high incidence in pregnant teenage girls (who also may be iron deficient). With these children, correcting the anemia also corrects the pica. An individualized therapy plan needs to be devised to meet the child's needs until the phenomenon fades. Keeping the child safe from ingesting inedible substances is a major responsibility until then (Chatoor, 2000).

Rumination Disorder of Infancy

The term *rumination* comes from the Latin word for "chewing the cud" (as cattle do). It is the act of regurgitating and then reswallowing previously ingested food. It is a rare disorder that generally affects infants between the ages of 3 to 12 months. It is seen most often in children who are cognitively challenged and appears to be pleasurable (Chatoor, 2000). Both organic and environmental theories have been explored to explain the disorder. In some children, an accompanying gastroesophageal reflux disorder has been implicated. It has also been postulated that rumination is a form of self-stimulation by the infant, similar to actions such as head banging and body rocking. It may be related to an understimulating environment, but attempts to implicate the role of the primary caregiver in contributing to the disorder have failed.

A parent may report that a child is constantly "spitting up" or vomiting or the child's breath smells sour. Children can lose a great deal of fluid and electrolytes through this process if they do not reswallow the regurgitated fluid and may show signs of failure to thrive. (Failure to thrive as a distinct problem is discussed in Chapter 55.) Distracting infants by holding, rocking, and talking to them tends to decrease rumination. Thickening formula with cereal occasionally is effective because this is more difficult to regurgitate. Attachment between the child and parent may be at risk because of the anxiety the parents suffer from their infant's constant regurgitation of food and lack of growth. Parents may need support, reassurance, and education to help them maintain or reestablish this bond.

Feeding Disorder

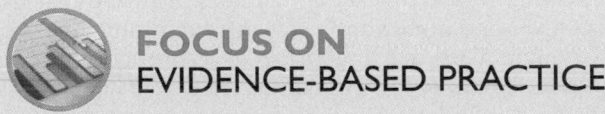

A feeding disorder is the persistent failure to eat adequately resulting in significant failure to gain weight or actual weight loss when no medical reason or lack of food is present. The disorder begins in infancy and is usually seen in children under 6 years of age. Meal time becomes a battlefield as parents insist on the child eating and the child persistently refuses food or exhibits extremely faddish or bizarre food preferences. As many as 35% of children may demonstrate some degree of the disorder (Steiner, 2000).

Therapy is a combination of counseling for the parents to help them appreciate that food refusal used this way can be a potent controlling measure and therapy for the child to learn to recognize hunger as a stimulant to eating rather than using food refusal as a controlling or attention mechanism (Steiner, 2000).

✔ CHECKPOINT QUESTIONS

9. Is separation anxiety seen more frequently in boys or girls?
10. What type of anemia is strongly associated with pica?

Anorexia Nervosa

Anorexia nervosa is a disorder characterized by refusal to maintain a minimally normal body weight because of a disturbance in perception of the size or appearance of the body (APA, 2000). Characteristics include:

- Body mass index (BMI) under 17.5 or less than 85% expected weight
- Intense fear of gaining weight or becoming fat even though underweight
- Severely distorted body image
- Refusal to acknowledge seriousness of weight loss
- Amenorrhea (in girls)

Anorexia nervosa occurs most often in girls (90%), usually at puberty or during adolescence, between 13 and 20 years of age. It is more common among sisters and daughters of mothers who also had the disorder. It may be preceded by a traumatic event such as a rape (APA, 2000).

The disorder may be manifested as severe weight restriction controlled by limiting food intake or with excessive exercise or by **binge eating/purging**—episodes of uncontrollable intake of large amounts of food over a specified period of time (binge eating) following by self-induced vomiting or the use of laxatives, enemas, or diuretics (purging)

Girls who develop this disorder tend to have a poor self-image (they cannot live up to their own expectations). Excessive dieting gives them a sense of control over their own body.

Lack of nutrition becomes so extreme that it causes delayed psychosexual development. With a lean, nearly starved appearance, girls do not appear as sexually developed or as old as they are. They may have significant symptoms of dehydration and acidosis from starvation.

Assessment

Because of an intense fear of becoming obese, children with anorexia come to perceive food as revolting and nauseating, and refuse to eat or else vomit food immediately after eating. Refusal to eat may be accompanied by the use of laxatives or diuretics and extensive exercising to further lose weight. Girls may ingest ipecac to induce vomiting. These measures lead eventually to excessive weight loss, acidosis, dependent edema, hypotension, hypothermia, bradycardia, and lanugo formation (fine, neonatal-like hair). Compulsive mannerisms such as handwashing may develop. If the process is allowed to continue without therapy, it can lead to starvation and death. The use of ipecac can be exceptionally damaging and possibly cardiotoxic.

Therapeutic Management

By the time most children are seen at health care facilities, they are often already extremely underweight, pale, and lethargic. Amenorrhea is commonly often present. Often, the child's parents have tried various methods of getting the child to eat, such as threatening, coaxing, and punishing; as a result, parent–child relationships may be strained. Parents may feel guilty for insisting their child lose weight if the girl was once overweight.

Planning and outcome identification need to be realistic. A girl who grows nauseated just looking at food cannot quickly begin to ingest a large amount of it. When caring for children with anorexia nervosa, remember that, although the condition began as a psychosocial problem, by the time a girl is seen for care, starvation and its effects are a second important component. For therapy, typically, oral foods are withheld and total parenteral nutrition is initiated to supply needed fat, protein, and calories. Children generally accept total parenteral nutrition well because they view it as medicine, not as food. Enteral feedings may also be accepted and used to restore weight.

In addition, establishing trust and effective communication are crucial to help the child resolve any interpersonal issues that are present (see Focus on Communication). Other therapeutic interventions include:

- Medications such as antidepressants
- Identification of emotional triggers
- Self-monitoring (awareness training)
- Education about normal nutritional needs

Gradual weight gain is recommended because rapid gain of weight may cause the child to begin dieting to reduce this weight gain. Weighing once a week is better than every day to reduce a concentration on weight. Box 54-3 describes common strategies for assisting family and friends to help the child with anorexia.

Children who have had anorexia nervosa need continued follow-up after weight is regained to be certain that they do not revert to their former dieting pattern (Fig. 54-2). Counseling may need to be continued for 2 to 3 years to be certain that self-image is maintained. With adequate counseling, most girls will achieve full recovery with adulthood.

WHAT IF? During a routine health maintenance visit, you notice that a teenage girl has lost 20 lb in the last 6 months. Her mother states, "She's the perfect daughter, always getting straight A's in school." How would you respond?

FOCUS ON COMMUNICATION

Brenda is a 15-year-old female who is diagnosed with anorexia nervosa. She is 5 feet, 8 inches tall and weighs 95 lb.

Less Effective Communication

Nurse: Let's talk about your weight, Brenda.
Brenda: I'm fat. Look at this belly of mine.
Nurse: You need to eat at least three good meals a day.
Brenda: I do. I eat a lot.
Nurse: You should have a healthy breakfast. After all, it is the most important meal of the day.
Brenda: I eat huge breakfasts. I'm just so active, I don't gain weight.

More Effective Communication

Nurse: Let's talk about your weight, Brenda.
Brenda: I'm fat. Look at me.
Nurse: You feel fat?
Brenda: Yes, just look at me.
Nurse: Tell me what you eat for a typical breakfast.
Brenda: A lot. I pig out for breakfast.
Nurse: Pig out? What did you eat this morning?
Brenda: A quarter piece of toast.
Nurse: Anything else? Tell me more about what it is that you eat.

In the first scenario the nurse is intent on getting the client to eat. In the second scenario. The nurse is attempting to obtain more information about the client, her image of herself, and her diet.

BOX 54.3

WHAT FAMILY MEMBERS AND FRIENDS CAN DO TO HELP THOSE WITH EATING DISORDERS

- Tell the person you are concerned, that you care and would like to help. Suggest that the person seek professional help.
- If the person refuses to seek help, encourage reaching out to an adult such as a teacher, school nurse, or counselor.
- Do not discuss weight, the number of calories being consumed, or particular eating habits. Try to talk about things other than food, weight, counting calories, or exercise.
- Avoid making comments about the person's appearance. Concern about weight loss may be interpreted as a compliment; comments about weight gain may be interpreted as criticism.
- Offer support but keep in mind that, ultimately, the responsibility and decision for accepting help and to change are with the person.
- Read and educate yourself about these disorders.

White, J. H., and Marshall, L. (2002). Eating disorders. In M. Boyd & M. Nihart. ***Psychiatric nursing: Contemporary practice.*** (2nd ed.). Philadelphia: Lippincott Williams and Wilkins.

Bulimia Nervosa

Bulimia refers to recurrent and episodic binge eating and purging, accompanied by an awareness that the eating pattern is abnormal but not being able to stop (APA, 2000). A period of depression or guilt usually follows the period of bingeing. Like anorexia nervosa, bulimia typically is seen in adolescence or early adult life and predominantly in girls. The disorder may last for months or years. Periods of normal eating may be interspersed, or the girl may constantly move from bingeing to fasting. Food consumed during a binge often has a high-caloric content and a texture that facilitates rapid eating. It may be eaten secretly, such as late at night or in the privacy of a bedroom. After ingestion of this food, the girl notices abdominal pain; she vomits to decrease the physical pain of abdominal distention and to improve self-concept (she feels more in control).

Children with bulimia may abuse purgatives, laxatives, and diuretics to aid in weight control. The combination of frequent vomiting and the use of these drugs can result in serious physical complications, notably electrolyte abnormalities, which can ultimately lead to changes as severe as cardiac arrest. People with bulimia may also have severe erosion of their teeth because of the constant exposure to acidic gastrointestinal juices from vomiting. Esophageal tears may also result.

Like adolescents with anorexia nervosa, these children exhibit great concern about their weight and overall body image and appearance. In contrast with anorexia, most children with bulimia are only slightly underweight or are of average weight and so may be discounted as merely slim unless a thorough history is obtained. As with anorexia nervosa, counseling is aimed at increasing the child's self-esteem and sense of control (APA, 2000).

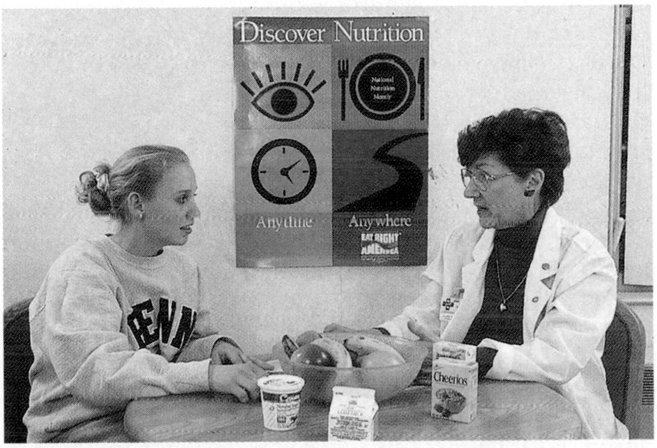

FIGURE 54.2 This anorexic teen, who is in the later stages of treatment, continues to meet with the counselor to discuss her food choices, exercise program, and overall well-being.

✔ **CHECKPOINT QUESTIONS**

11. Does anorexia nervosa also occur in boys?
12. How does bulimia differ from anorexia nervosa?

TIC DISORDERS

Tic disorders are abnormalities of semi-involuntary movement thought to result from dysfunction in the basal ganglia. *Tics* are rapid, repetitive muscle movements, such as rapid eye blinking or facial twitching. They generally become more pronounced during periods of stress and usually diminish in sleep. **Motor tics** include eye blinking, neck jerking, and facial grimacing. Simple **vocal tics** include coughing, throat clearing, snorting, and barking. Complex motor tics include facial gestures, grooming behaviors, jumping, touching, and smelling objects (McCracken, 2000).

Children are most prone to these disorders between the ages of 9 and 13. They occur more frequently in boys than in girls and in children who demonstrate obsessive—compulsive behavior. Some cases tend to be familial, possibly due to dopamine receptor inhibition. Tic disorders are subclassified into Tourette's syndrome, chronic motor or vocal tic disorder, and transient tic disorder. They occur so frequently that as many as 15% of children experience some form of transient tic disorder (McCracken, 2000). Because transient tics are associated with areas of high stress, treatment generally focuses on reducing areas of stress in a child's life. Pointing out the mannerism to the child is not usually helpful and may intensify the manifestation if it increases stress. Behavior modification may be successful in curing a particular tic. If the stress is not removed, however, a child may substitute another compulsive mechanism for the original tic.

Tourette's Syndrome

Tourette's syndrome is an inherited disorder in which the child suffers from a syndrome of motor and phonic vocal tics. **Complex vocal tics** include the repeated use of words or phrases out of context—specifically, **coprolalia** (use of socially unacceptable words, usually obscenities), **palilalia** (repeating one's own words), and echolalia. Some children with this syndrome have nonspecific electroencephalographic abnormalities and soft neurologic signs. Typically, the age of onset is around 7 years, with motor tics generally occurring before vocal tics. Although most children can suppress tics for short periods of time, the syndrome lasts a lifetime. It occurs three times more frequently in boys than in girls. Often, there is some other form of tic in other family members. Children with Tourette's syndrome can develop low self-esteem because of their uncontrollable actions before the syndrome is fully diagnosed. Fortunately, this syndrome responds to administration of neuroleptic agents such as haloperidol (Haldol) or pimozide (Orap).

ELIMINATION DISORDERS

Elimination disorders encompass functional enuresis (involuntary loss of urine) and encopresis (involuntary loss of feces). Developmental enuresis is discussed in Chapter 30 with the development of the preschooler.

Encopresis

Loss of feces is *encopresis* when there is repeated passage of feces at least once a month in places not culturally appropriate for that purpose. It is considered primary if a child was never fully toilet trained and secondary if the problem begins after effective training. Encopresis is considered to exist only after medical causes such as lactase deficiency, thyroid disease, hypercalcemia, Hirschsprung's disease, and infectious diarrhea have been ruled out. It is more common in boys than girls (Mikkelsen, 2000).

Isolated occurrences of encopresis may happen when a sibling is born (as part of an overall regression reaction) or when a child is visiting a strange house or new school and is too shy to ask for the bathroom. It can occur in school because a teacher may not allow children to use a bathroom when they wish or because some school bathrooms may be occupied.

In a few instances, encopresis occurs because of extreme constipation. Hard bowel movements cause anal fissures. Because it hurts to move the bowels, children avoid bowel movements, leading to chronically distended rectums. They are then no longer able to sense when they need to defecate, so involuntary or overflow defecation occurs. Encopresis is a distressing condition for children because other children in school can detect the odor of a bowel movement on their clothing.

Assessment

To document encopresis, take a careful history of the condition, including usual bowel evacuation habits, the number of bowel accidents, and the times they occur. Investigate any recent changes or stress factors on the child. A physical examination that includes a rectal examination should be done to establish whether there is proper anal sphincter control.

Therapeutic Management

Therapy is based on the apparent cause. Arranging to have children attempt to evacuate their bowels about two times daily (in the morning and after dinner) may create "habit" periods for them. Allowing children adequate time to sit on the toilet or encouraging them to take the time to do so may be helpful. If children evacuate their bowels before they leave for school in the morning, they are less likely to experience encopresis and embarrassment in school. The administration of 1 to 6 tablespoons of mineral oil daily for 2 or 3 months will often soften stools so that bowel movements are not painful. Children on long-term mineral oil therapy generally are given water-soluble forms of vitamins A, D, and K, because these vitamins tend to be removed from the gastrointestinal tract with the mineral oil. Imipramine (Tofranil), a tricyclic antidepressant, may be helpful in reducing encopresis, the same as it is effective for enuresis.

Emphasize to parents that children should not be punished for encopresis. Encourage them to pay as little attention as possible to bowel accidents and give praise for days when encopresis does not occur. Box 54-4 highlights an appropriate outcome and intervention using the terminology identified by the Nursing Outcomes Classification (NOC) and Nursing Interventions Classification (NIC).

BOX 54.4

NURSING OUTCOMES AND NURSING INTERVENTIONS CLASSIFICATION: ENCOPRESIS

NOC: Bowel Elimination

Bowel elimination is defined as the ability of the gastrointestinal tract to form and evacuate stool effectively (Johnson, Maas, & Moorhead, 2000). Some specific indicators suggesting achievement of this outcome include the following:

- Elimination patterns within expected range
- Stool color, odor, and fat within normal range with amount appropriate for diet
- Stool soft and firm
- Absence of bloating, painful cramping, discomfort with stool passage, constipation, diarrhea, and blood or mucus in stool
- Uncompromised sphincter control and muscle tone
- Ingestion of adequate fluids and fiber
- Uncompromised control of bowel movements

NIC: Bowel Incontinence Care, Encopresis

Bowel incontinence care, encopresis is defined as the promotion of bowel continence in children (McCloskey & Bulechek, 2000). Some important activities involved when implementing this intervention include:

- Obtaining information about child's toilet training history, duration of encopresis and measures tried to control the problem
- Attempting to determine the cause of incontinence as appropriate
- Recommending dietary changes or behavioral therapy as indicated
- Conducting family psychosocial assessment
- Using play therapy to assist child in working through feelings
- Investigating family communication patterns, strengths, and coping abilities
- Encouraging parents to foster security and demonstrate love and acceptance at home
- Discussing the psychosocial dynamics of encopresis with the family
- Referring for family therapy as appropriate

Enuresis

Enuresis is defined as repeated involuntary or intentional urination during the day or at night after children have attained or are at an age at which they should have attained control over bladder function, when no organic cause for the problem can be found (APA, 2000). Although stress may be a factor in occurrences of enuresis, its primary cause is unknown. Most children outgrow the problem by adolescence. Like encopresis, the most serious result of enuresis is related to the child's feelings of failure with each occurrence and associated rejection by peers, parents, or other caregivers. All this contributes to a lowered sense of self-esteem. The problem and associated nursing diagnoses are described in more detail in Chapter 46.

OTHER PSYCHIATRIC DISORDERS AFFECTING CHILDREN

Childhood Depression

Children and adolescents both have depressive episodes similar to those experienced by adults. The incidence ranges from 1% to 3% before puberty to 3% to 6% in adolescents (Bech, 2001). Depression is becoming an increasing concern in our society because the escalating suicide rate among children and adolescents has become a major societal problem. A child is considered to be depressed when symptoms such as loss of interest or pleasure, significant weight loss or gain, depressed mood, insomnia, psychomotor agitation, feelings of worthlessness or excessive or inappropriate guilt, diminished concentration, recurrent thoughts of death, and suicidal ideation exist for 2 weeks or more (APA, 2000). Because these symptoms are easily missed, a history should be taken from the child as well as from the parents. Depression can be differentiated from "normal" sadness when children report they cannot remember the last time they felt happy or had a good time (**anhedonia;** Fig. 54-3). Children who are depressed need treatment to prevent their depression from worsening. Counseling to discuss problems is necessary. Many children require antidepressant therapy, such as a selective serotonin reuptake inhibitor, to relieve the symptoms. In addition to the pharmacologic approach, family or individual counseling may be necessary to help the child regain self-esteem and the family to understand the level of depression that has occurred (Pataki, 2001). Attempted suicide as a result of depression is discussed in Chapter 32 with concerns of the adolescent.

Childhood Schizophrenia

Schizophrenia is actually a group of disorders of thought processes characterized by the gradual disintegration of mental functioning occurring in about 2 out of every 10,000 children (APA, 2000). It is a devastating mental illness that usually strikes in adolescence or young adulthood. Symptoms during childhood are usually undifferentiated or ill defined (Lambert, 2001).

Over the years, there has been a great deal of debate about the cause of schizophrenia. For a long time, it was hypothesized that schizophrenia resulted solely from an

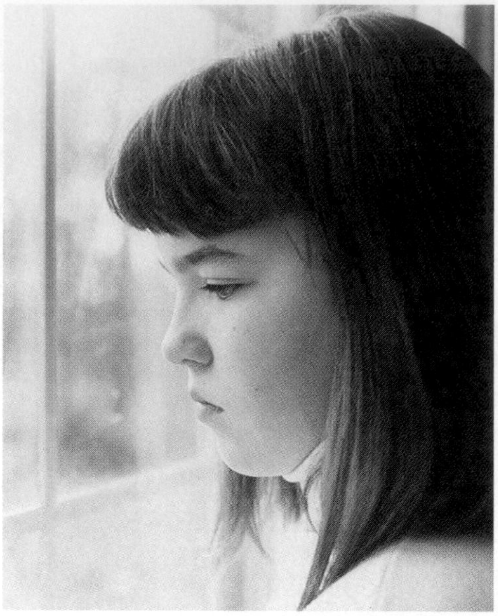

FIGURE 54.3 Symptoms of depression are easily missed in school-aged children unless history taking is thorough.

impaired parent–child relationship. Current research, however, indicates that there is as much a genetic as an environmental basis for this disorder. Magnetic resonance imaging has shown that cerebral involvement such as enlarged ventricles or decreased blood to the frontal lobe may be present (APA, 2000). Neurochemical mediators may influence or prolong the disorder.

Children with schizophrenia experience hallucinations (hear or see people or objects that other people cannot). They display rambling or illogical speech patterns. They may not be responsive (have a **flat affect**), or they may withdraw so completely that they are stuporous (**catatonia**). Although schizophrenic manifestations may occur suddenly after a major stress in a child's life (such as rejection by a boyfriend or girlfriend), subtle signs of mental illness have usually been present for some time.

A diagnosis of a psychotic disorder of this extent is a shock to parents. Fortunately, therapy with modern antipsychotic drugs is effective in reducing children's hallucinations and bizarre thinking. Parents need help to support a child during a long period of therapy. Many children who are diagnosed as having schizophrenia in childhood will continue to have mental illness as adults. Continuing support and long-term follow-up are essential (Bech, 2001).

✔ CHECKPOINT QUESTIONS

13. Is rumination usually a problem of infants or preschoolers?
14. What are symptoms of Tourette's syndrome?

KEY POINTS

Both cognitive and mental health disorders pose long-term care concerns for children and their families.

For children who are cognitively challenged, a stigma still may be present in many communities, although less so than previously. Parents may have a more difficult time accepting this diagnosis in their child than they would a physical illness. Help parents to gain the insight that cognitive challenges occur in a proportion of infants in every population and having a child with this merely reflects a chance occurrence.

Most children who are cognitively challenged benefit from early schooling. Urge parents to enroll children in early education and intervention programs.

Mental health disorders often begin subtly in children, often first manifested as a behavior problem in school. Assess thoroughly any child referred for disruptive behavior in class for the possibility that he or she has a serious mental health problem.

Autistic disorder is a pervasive developmental disorder that has a syndrome of behaviors, including fascination with movement, impairment of communication skills, and insensitivity to pain.

Attention-deficit and disruptive behavior disorders, such as oppositional defiant and conduct disorders may occur in childhood. Children with ADHD may be treated with methylphenidate hydrochloride (Ritalin, Concerta) to reduce the hyperactivity and allow them to achieve better in school and interact better at home.

Eating disorders seen in childhood include pica, rumination, anorexia nervosa, and bulimia. All of these disorders can lead to loss of weight and electrolyte imbalances if left unrecognized and untreated.

Tic disorders (e.g., Tourette's syndrome) are abnormalities of semi-involuntary movement thought to result from dysfunction of the basal ganglia or distorted dopamine reception.

Encopresis is the repeated passage of feces in places not culturally appropriate for that purpose. Therapy is both physiologic and psychological.

Children who are depressed are at high risk for committing suicide. They need thorough assessment and close observation to be certain this does not happen. Schizophrenia may occur in childhood. This usually presents as disorganized behavior. Long-term therapy is necessary.

CRITICAL THINKING EXERCISES

1. Todd is the second grader diagnosed with ADHD you met at the beginning of the chapter. His mother feels "at her wits' end" because his attention span is so short and his behavior so disruptive. His father is proud of his behavior. What suggestions could you make to his parents to help them adjust better to a child with ADHD?

2. A 3-year-old child who is cognitively challenged is critically ill with pneumonia. It is difficult to believe that her mother did not recognize how ill the child was becoming and bring her sooner for care. What reasons might explain a parent reacting this way?
3. You weigh a 12-year-old girl and discover that her body mass index is 16. You also notice that her school lunch consists of dry toast only. Would you be concerned? What questions would you want to ask to help discover why her weight is so low?
4. The parents of an adolescent tell you that he seems increasingly depressed, so much so that he sleeps almost all day on weekends. Does this adolescent need a referral, or is he simply demonstrating usual adolescent behavior? What questions would you want to ask to be able to tell?
5. Examine the National Health Goals related to cognitive and mental health disorders in children. Most government-sponsored money for nursing research is allotted based on these goals. What would be a possible research topic to explore pertinent to these goals that would be both fundable and would advance evidence-based practice?

REFERENCES

American Psychiatric Association. (2000). *Diagnostic and statistical manual of mental disorders, text revised (DSM IV-TR)* (5th ed.). Washington, DC: American Psychiatric Association.

Bechtold, D. W. (2001). Psychiatric disorders. In W. W. Hay, A. R. Hayward, M. J. Levin & J. M. Sondheimer (Eds.). *Current pediatric diagnosis & treatment* (15th ed.). New York: McGraw-Hill.

Chatoor, I. (2000). Feeding and eating disorders of infancy and early childhood. In H. I. Kaplan (Ed.). *Comprehensive textbook of psychiatry.* Philadelphia: Lippincott Williams & Wilkins.

Daviss, W. B., et al. (2000). Predicting posttraumatic stress after hospitalization for pediatric injury. *Journal of the American Academy of Child & Adolescent Psychiatry, 39*(5), 576–583.

Department of Health and Human Services. (2000). *Healthy people 2010.* Washington, DC: DHHS.

Fergusson, D. M. & Woodward, L. J. (2002). Mental health, educational, and social role outcomes of adolescents with depression. *Archives of General Psychiatry, 59*(3), 225–231.

Goldson, E., & Hagerman, R. J. (2001). Developmental disorders. In W. W. Hay, A. R. Hayward, A. R., M. J. Levin & J. M. Sondheimer (Eds.). *Current pediatric diagnosis & treatment* (15th ed.), New York: McGraw-Hill.

Johnson, M., Maas, M., & Moorhead, S. (2000). *Nursing outcomes classification* (2nd ed.). St. Louis: Mosby, Inc.

Lambert, L. T. (2001). Identification and management of schizophrenia in childhood. *Journal of Child & Adolescent Psychiatric Nursing, 14*(2), 73–80.

McCloskey, J., & Bulechek, G. (2000). *Nursing interventions classification* (3rd ed.). St. Louis: Mosby.

McCracken, J. T. (2000). Tic disorders. In H. I. Kaplan (Ed.). *Comprehensive textbook of psychiatry.* Philadelphia: Lippincott Williams & Wilkins.

Mikkelsen, E. J. (2000). Elimination disorders. In H. I. Kaplan (Ed.). *Comprehensive textbook of psychiatry.* Philadelphia: Lippincott Williams & Wilkins.

Pataki, C. S. (2000). Mood disorders and suicide in children and adolescents. In H. I. Kaplan (Ed.). *Comprehensive textbook of psychiatry.* Philadelphia: Lippincott Williams & Wilkins.

Steiner, H. (2000). Disruptive behavior disorders. In H. I. Kaplan (Ed.). *Comprehensive textbook of psychiatry.* Philadelphia: Lippincott Williams & Wilkins.

Valente, S. M. (2001). Treating attention deficit hyperactivity disorder. *Nurse Practitioner, 26*(9), 14–23.

White, J. H., & Marshall, L. (2002). Eating disorders. In M. Boyd & M. Nihart (Eds.). *Psychiatric nursing: Contemporary practice* (2nd ed.). Philadelphia: Lippincott Williams & Wilkins.

SUGGESTED READINGS

Armenteros, J. L. & Mikhail, A. G. (2002). Do we need placebos to evaluate new drugs in children with schizophrenia? *Psychopharmacology, 159*(2), 117–124.

Brugman, E., et al. (2001). Identification and management of psychosocial problems by preventive child health care. *Archives of Pediatrics & Adolescent Medicine, 155*(4), 462–469.

Falsafi, N. (2001). Pediatric psychiatric emergencies. *Journal of Child & Adolescent Psychiatric Nursing, 14*(2), 81–88.

Harrower, J. K., & Dunlap, G. (2001). Including children with autism in general education classrooms. *Behavior Modification, 25*(5), 762–784.

Hawkins-Walsh, E. (2001). Turning primary care providers' attention to child behavior: A review of the literature. *Journal of Pediatric Health Care, 15*(3), 115–122.

Hollis, C. (2001). Adult outcomes of child and adolescent onset schizophrenia: Diagnostic stability and predictive validity. *American Journal of Psychiatry, 157*(10), 1652–1659.

Kaplan, S., et al. (2001). Consumer satisfaction at a child and adolescent state psychiatric hospital. *Psychiatric Services, 52*(2), 202–206.

Leon, S. C., et al. (2000). Variations in the clinical presentations of children and adolescents at eight psychiatric hospitals. *Psychiatric Services, 51*(6), 786–790.

Pritchard, C., & Mason, T. (2000). Breaking the cycle of disadvantage: Young people, social exclusion and mental health. *Mental Health Care & Learning Disabilities, 4*(1), 14–17.

Tierney, J. A. (2000). Post-traumatic stress disorder in children: Controversies and unresolved issues. *Journal of Child & Adolescent Psychiatric Nursing, 13*(4), 147–158.

55

CHAPTER

Nursing Care of the Family in Crisis: Abuse and Violence in the Family

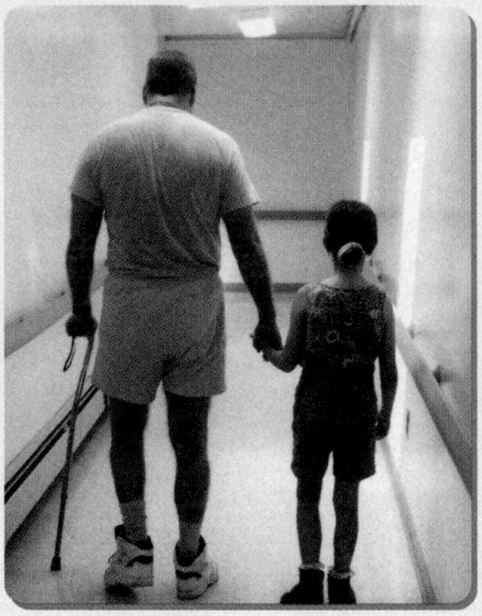

Key Terms

- abuse
- disorganization phase
- failure to thrive
- incest
- intimate partner abuse
- learned helplessness
- mandatory reporters
- molestation
- Munchausen syndrome by proxy
- pedophile
- permissive reporters
- rape trauma syndrome
- reorganization phase
- shaken baby syndrome
- silent rape syndrome

Objectives

After mastering the contents of this chapter, you should be able to:

1. Discuss the types of abuse seen in families and the theories explaining their occurrence.
2. Assess a family that is physically or emotionally abused.
3. Formulate nursing diagnoses related to the abused family.
4. Develop appropriate outcomes for an abused family.
5. Plan nursing care for the abused family, such as ways to role-model better parenting.
6. Implement nursing care for the family in which abuse occurred.
7. Evaluate outcomes for effectiveness and achievement of care.
8. Identify National Health Goals related to the abused family that nurses can be instrumental in helping the nation achieve.
9. Identify areas related to care of the abused family that could benefit from additional nursing research or application of evidence-based practice.
10. Analyze ways that nurses can be instrumental in preventing family abuse.
11. Integrate knowledge of family abuse with nursing process to achieve quality maternal and child health nursing care.

Marie is a 3-year-old you see in an emergency room. Her mother tells you that Marie fell off a swing in the back yard. Marie has a broken forearm, a broken rib, and multiple bruises on her chest and back. You notice in her chart that Marie was seen in the same emergency room a month ago for a burn on the palm of her hand. When you mention to her mother that Marie's injuries seem extreme for a simple fall, her mother says, "Marie isn't very pretty. I guess she's also clumsy." You suspect Marie may be a victim of child abuse. What questions would you want to ask to help determine if this is so?

Previous chapters described the normal growth and development of children and care of the child with disorders of specific body systems. This chapter adds information about the effect on children when abuse occurs in a family. This is important information because it builds a base for prevention of further abuse.

After you've studied the chapter, answer the Critical Thinking Exercises at the end of the chapter and then access the on-line study activities (www.connection.lww.com) *to further sharpen your skills and test your knowledge.*

Child abuse occurs at an incidence of 250,000 per year in the United States. It accounts for 2,000 deaths per year (Christian, 2000a). Abuse is associated with stress and has been linked to the inability of the family to handle external and internal stressors. Accordingly, abuse in the family is rarely an isolated event but rather an indication of how much the family needs care overall.

Abuse, defined as the "willful injury by one person of another" by the researchers who first identified the phenomenon (Helfer & Kempe, 1987), takes many forms: child abuse, which can be physical or emotional and includes neglect and sexual abuse; intimate partner abuse; and maltreatment of the elderly. Maternity, child health, and family nurses need to be especially observant for signs of possible family abuse and prepared to handle this highly emotional and complex problem objectively. The victim's safety is paramount, but ensuring this safety must be done with sensitivity to the importance of maintaining and improving overall family functioning.

Abuse has long-term consequences because as many as 30% of children from abusive families may become abusive parents themselves (Christian, 2000a). It may lead to a post-traumatic stress disorder (Beers & DeBellis, 2002). National Health Goals related to child abuse are shown in the Focus on National Health Goals box.

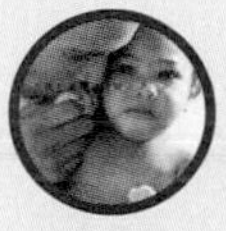

FOCUS ON NATIONAL HEALTH GOALS

Abuse of children is a national health disgrace and, thus, a national health concern. One National Health Goal specifically addresses this issue:

- Reduce maltreatment of children from a baseline of 12.9/1,000 under age 18 years to a target level of 10.3/1,000 children (DHHS, 2000).

Nurses can be instrumental in helping the nation achieve these goals by educating parents about how to parent more effectively and by identifying children in school or health care agency settings who have been abused or neglected. Additional nursing research would be helpful for the following questions: Can potentially abusing parents be identified on postpartum units and helped to avoid this? What counseling is necessary for adolescents who have been abused to help them be successful parents? What are the most helpful nursing interventions to use with parents when a child who has been abused is admitted to the hospital?

NURSING PROCESS OVERVIEW

For Care of the Family in Crisis

Assessment

Commonly, nurses are the first individuals to identify symptoms of possible family abuse because they are often the first to see a child undressed at a health care visit and recognize significant bruising; they are often the person in whom a pregnant woman or child confides about the problem (see Assessing the Child for Signs of Abuse). When abuse in any form is suspected, it is essential to get as full a picture as possible. When child abuse is suspected, talk with the parents first, without the child, and then interview the child to help to uncover any inconsistencies in the parents' explanations.

Nursing Diagnosis

Nursing diagnoses associated with abuse should address both the physical and emotional results of abuse and may include:

- Pain related to burn on hand
- Risk for injury related to previous abuse
- Risk for other directed violence related to admitted poor self-control
- Impaired parenting related to high level of stress
- Compromised family coping as manifested by child abuse related to alcohol use by father
- Disturbed self-esteem related to rape

Outcome Identification and Planning

Planning must center first on ensuring the safety of the abused family member and minimizing the effects of trauma. Long-term planning includes helping an abused family member find safe refuge and re-establishing self-esteem through a self-help or advocacy program. Teaching empowerment, or the ability to take charge of one's life, is particularly important for older children and women in abusing families. In addition, the abuser needs a program of therapy to help prevent future abuse.

Implementation

The most important intervention related to family abuse is prevention. Nurses can do much in all settings through serving as a role model or providing education to promote healthy patterns of child-rearing and optimal ways of handling family stress. They can

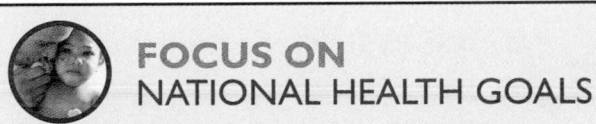

ASSESSING the Child for Signs of Abuse

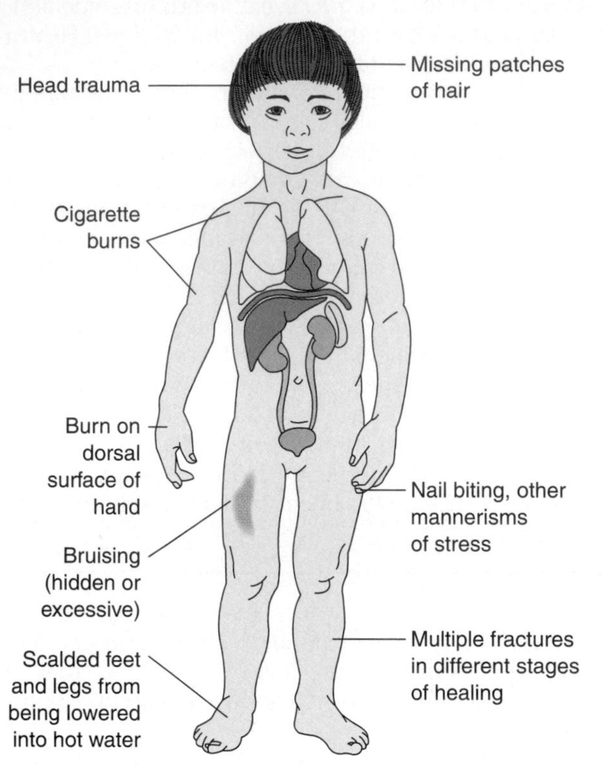

be particularly observant for families who seem to be at risk for abusive behavior. When instances of abuse are uncovered, further education is an intervention that can help parents who are ignorant about their children's needs and child behavior. Lecturing is not a useful intervention, but supportive education can be extremely valuable.

The following organizations are helpful for referral:

Parents Anonymous (*www.parentsanonymous.org*)
Child Abuse Prevention Network (*www.child-abuse.com*)
National Coalition Against Domestic Violence (*www.webmerchants.com/NCAD*)
Victims of Child Abuse Laws (VOCAL) (*www.vix.com*)
Women Organized Against Rape (WOAR) (*www.WOAR.org*)

Outcome Evaluation

Nurses are mandated by law to report child abuse; identifying and reporting this problem are therefore important nursing actions. Outcomes should focus on specific measures of improved interaction:

- Parent holds baby appropriately and maintains good eye contact.
- Parent admits to losing control with children at home and voices desire to undergo counseling for problem.
- Parent states she has the Crisis Center telephone number by the telephone and will call for help if she feels under threat by partner.
- Adolescent states she can still think of herself with high self-esteem in spite of rape by stepbrother.
- Parent attends monthly meetings of Parents Anonymous.

CHILD ABUSE

Because parenting is not an easy task and good parenting is not an automatic or truly instinctive ability, children in every community are injured because of abuse. Abuse may be physical (the child is beaten or burned) or it may be neglect (the child is not fed, clothed, supervised properly, or offered medical care or educational opportunities). Abuse may also be psychological or emotional. In some cases, women who threatened the health of their fetus by drug abuse have been viewed by the courts as child abusers (DeVille & Kopelman, 1999).

Abuse not only places a child at immediate risk but can also lead to long-term effects. For example, physically abused children are found to be more angry, noncompliant, and hyperactive than others; they may demonstrate poor self-control and low self-esteem. Children whose parents do not interact with them (emotional abuse) are apt to be more withdrawn and have a flatter affect than others. Because the abusive family is a disrupted one, children often have undiagnosed medical problems, such as anemia, otitis media, lead poisoning, and sexually transmitted diseases. Children who suffer sexual abuse can have long-term effects of depression, guilt, and difficulty enjoying sexual relations (Ruscio, 2001).

In addition, when children reach adulthood and begin parenting, they tend to rear their children in basically the same way as they were reared. Parents who themselves received little love or were abused as children may never form a basic sense of trust and so grow into nonloving and abusing parents unless there is effective intervention.

Theories of Child Abuse

The most commonly accepted theory as to why child abuse occurs is that a special triad of circumstances is present (Helfer & Kempe, 1987):

- A parent has the potential to abuse a child.
- A child is seen as "different" in some way by the parent.
- A special event or circumstance brings about the abuse.

Parents Who Abuse

Parents who abuse seem, on the surface, little different from others. Only a small fraction of them (probably less than 10%) have a history of mental illness. Many of these parents, however, were abused as children. Such parents may have less self-control than other parents. They may be unfamiliar with the normal growth and development of children and so have unrealistic expectations of a child. These parents may be socially isolated, with no support people readily available. The isolation may be by distance (a parent separated from other people in a farmhouse miles from neighbors), or it may be the type that exists in communities of apartment houses where neighbors do not routinely speak to one another. Abuse is strongly associated with excessive parental use of alcohol, a substance that removes inhibitions and self-control (Christian, 2000a).

Children Who Are Abused

Abused children are viewed as somehow "different" by parents. They may be more or less intelligent than other children in the family; they may have been unplanned. They may have a birth defect; they may have an attention span deficit. Because the child is perceived as somehow different, a good parent–child relationship does not develop. A category of children who are at high risk are those who are born prematurely or who have an illness at birth, because they are kept from parents or separated from them by special nurseries or equipment for the first weeks of life, which is when normal bonding occurs (Strathearn et al., 2001; AAP, 2001).

Special Circumstance: Stress

A third factor in child abuse is stress, which may be a response to an event that would not necessarily be stressful to an average parent. It might be something as common as a blocked toilet, an illness in the family, a lost job, a landlord asking for the rent, or a rainstorm that canceled a planned activity. Child abuse crosses all socioeconomic levels because stress occurs at all levels. Stress generally has a greater impact when people do not have strong support people around them. Families whose internal support system is faulty or who have not formed outside support systems are apt to have a higher incidence of abuse.

During a health crisis, parents unable to deal with stress may not show the usual degree of compassion for the child's pain or offer to comfort him or her. They may appear more concerned with how the injury affects them than how it affects the child: "Don't cry. You'll make me look like a bad parent," not "It's okay to cry. I know that it hurts."

To prevent abuse, a child may assume a role reversal with the parent or become the comforting, solacing person. These children recognize very early in life that when a parent is upset, they will be hurt. They learn to comfort the parent and reduce the parent's stress and anxiety, thereby avoiding the hurt. It is important to assess who is comforting whom during a child health crisis.

WHAT IF? What if you see a 4-year-old with severe burns in an emergency room who keeps telling her mother that everything is all right and that it wasn't the mother's fault, even though the mother reported that she spilled scalding coffee on the child? Is this a typical sign of abuse?

Reporting Suspected Child Abuse

State laws generally identify two types of responsibility in reporting child abuse: **mandatory reporters** and **permissive reporters.** Nurses are included in the mandatory category in most states; this means they *must* report suspected child abuse when they identify it. Failure to do so could result in a fine or possible loss of nursing licensure. The fact that the information was given in a confidential interview does not free the nurse from this responsibility.

All health care institutions and agencies have protocols on how the reporting of child abuse should be handled. It is important to learn the protocol required by your particular agency, community, and state. After an official report of child abuse has been made to a child protection agency, a health care agency has the right, in most instances, to hold the child for 72 hours for protection to give an appointed caseworker time to investigate if abuse has occurred. Following the 72 hours, a court proceeding will determine whether a child should be returned to the parents' care or kept in a safer location. Because child abuse is a crime, the health care record of the child can be subpoenaed and displayed in court. Be certain when charting information related to child abuse that you make specific and factual notes (observations, not interpretations), such as "parent spoke loudly and slurred his words" rather than "parent was intoxicated." Record conversations with parents using exact quotes when possible. Photographs of physical abuse enhance the strength of the testimony of abuse, so these are usually ordered.

A second provision in most state laws is protection from having a lawsuit brought against a health care provider for reporting suspected abuse that is then proved false. In other words, it is better to err on the side of reporting suspected abuse rather than not reporting it, from both a child safety and a legal perspective. When abuse is officially reported, parents should be told that child abuse is suspected, because open lines of communication with parents are important to protect the child and to arrange counseling for the parents.

✔ CHECKPOINT QUESTIONS

1. Are most parents who are child abusers mentally ill?
2. What is the triad that makes abuse possible?

Physical Abuse

Physical abuse is the action of a caregiver that causes injury to a child. It is commonly revealed by burns or head and hand injuries (see Focus on Nursing Care Planning).

Assessment

Interview. Always ask parents to account for any injury to a child's body. Remember, however, that most childhood injuries are from accidents caused by the child's inability to distinguish safe situations from dangerous ones, or because parents overestimate their child's ability to do such things as lighting a fire to burn trash or using a saw in a wood project. Most toddlers have a number of ecchymotic spots on their legs from bumping into tables or chairs. Some childhood diseases, such as leukemia or purpura, begin with easy bruising. Children with osteogenesis

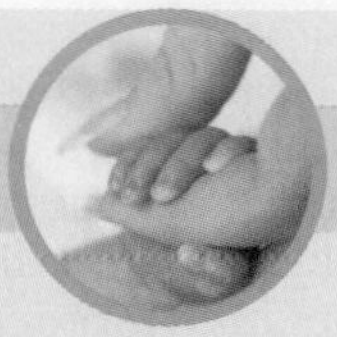

FOCUS ON *Nursing Care Planning*

A CHILD WHO HAS BEEN ABUSED

A 3-year-old boy is brought into the emergency department by his mother. "He got into the bathtub and burned himself because our water is so hot."

Assessment: 3-year-old boy dressed in wool coat and cap carried in by mother. Outside temperature 80°F. Mother's boyfriend present and protesting the removal of the child's clothing for examination: "It's too cold in here for that." Odor of alcohol noted on boyfriend's breath. On examination, superficial burns noted on lower extremities up to midcalf. Partial-thickness burns noted on plantar aspects of both feet. Area moist with some blistering apparent. Further examination reveals four ½-inch-diameter circular lesions on right arm; large 4-cm ecchymotic area on both buttocks and anterior left thigh. Sharp, pointed, triangular blistering and inflamed area noted on back of left hand. Mother states circular lesions are "mosquito bites"; mark on hand is a "birthmark." Child remained passive while being examined but drew back when mother's boyfriend approached. Mother divorced. Boyfriend lives with mother and child in one-bedroom apartment. Mother works as a waitress in a local restaurant from approximately 4 PM to midnight four nights a week. The physician approaches the mother and suggests that the child may have been beaten and burned. She states, "What can I do? My boyfriend is nice enough to watch him while I work."

Nursing Diagnosis: Fear related to repeated episodes of abuse and its effects

Outcome Identification: Child will demonstrate signs of increased comfort.

Outcome Evaluation: Child expresses fears verbally and through play; interacts with caregivers appropriately; demonstrates positive age-appropriate coping behaviors.

Interventions	Rationale
1. Approach the child in a calm manner and provide consistent caregivers for the child.	1. Approaching the child calmly and providing consistent caregivers help to foster a trusting relationship and minimize the child's exposure to stress.
2. Demonstrate acceptance of the child. Offer praise for positive behaviors.	2. All children need acceptance. Praise for positive behaviors helps to reinforce the behaviors and promote the child's self-esteem.
3. Explain all procedures and treatments in language the child can understand.	3. Explanations in the child's terms help to alleviate additional stress and anxiety associated with the experience.
4. Encourage the child to talk about what happened and incorporate the use of therapeutic play.	4. Talking and therapeutic play help the child express his feelings.
5. Reassure the child that he was not the cause of the abuse.	5. Because of their egocentric thinking, children often assume that they are responsible for maltreatment.
6. Make appropriate child abuse referral to keep child separate from abusing adult.	6. This is both a legal and child protective action.

Nursing Diagnosis: Disabled family coping related to situational stressors

Outcome Identification: The mother will demonstrate a beginning ability to arrange a caring family environment for child.

Outcome Evaluation: Mother identifies contributing factors to abusive situations; verbalizes existence of problem and need for assistance; uses community resources; demonstrates nurturing behaviors toward the child.

(continued)

Interventions	Rationale
1. Institute safety precautions for the child as appropriate. Anticipate the need for removing the boyfriend and/or child from the home environment.	1. Safety is essential for preventing further trauma. Removal is necessary to prevent probable future injury.
2. Approach the mother in an accepting, nonjudgmental, concerned manner. Inform her about notifying the appropriate agency about the abuse as required by law.	2. An accepting, nonjudgmental, concerned atmosphere helps to foster a sense of trust necessary for future interventions and action. Nurses are mandated by law to report child abuse.
3. Assess the situation for evidence of possible contributing factors, and assist mother in discussing events that preceded the incident. Stress her responsibility for making her home safe for her child.	3. Child abuse reflects a family in crisis and in need of help. Discussing difficulties and events in a controlled environment provides a safe outlet for emotions and also helps to increase awareness of the problem.
4. Explore her expectations of the child, listening for any complaints about him. Observe her responses and attitudes toward the child.	4. Exploration and observation provide clues to understanding possible influences on the mother's behavior.
5. Assist mother to view herself as responsible for her own and her child's safety.	5. Accepting responsibility is the first step in initiating change.
6. Review the typical growth and development of a child. Point out positive parenting behaviors, such as bringing the child in for care.	6. Review of normal growth and development helps to provide information and clarify any misconceptions that may have contributed to the abusive situation. Reinforcing positive parenting behaviors promotes feelings of accomplishment and self-esteem.
7. Take time to talk with the mother away from the child, focusing total attention on her.	7. Taking time away from the child to talk allows the mother to be the focus of attention, helping to meet her needs.
8. Explore with the mother how she responds to frustration. Caution her not to discipline the child when angry.	8. Exploration may help identify the responses that contribute to abuse. Disciplining when angry increases the risk for violence.
9. Role-model appropriate parental behavior. Involve the mother in the child's care as appropriate. Supervise her care as necessary.	9. Role-modeling provides the mother with objective examples of behaviors to follow, helping to promote more effective parenting skills. Involvement in care promotes active participation and opportunities for teaching and practicing these skills.
10. Offer praise and reinforcement for sound decision-making on childrearing practices that she demonstrates.	10. Praise and reinforcement for positive behaviors enhance self-esteem.
11. Empathize with the mother about the difficulties associated with single-parent families. Refrain from blaming.	11. Empathy aids in fostering acceptance and trust. Blaming serves only to further deflate the mother's self-esteem.
12. Emphasize alternative age-appropriate methods for discipline.	12. Alternative methods for discipline reduce the risk for violent behavior, enhancing family functioning and promoting the self-esteem of all family members.
13. Arrange for referrals to appropriate community resources such as hotlines, crisis centers, and parent groups to assist the mother. Refer to social services.	13. Community resources provide additional support and help reduce possible stress. Social services can assist the mother with measures to reduce situational stressors, such as finances and childcare.
14. Encourage the boyfriend to seek counseling for abusive behavior.	14. A demonstrated change in behavior is necessary before the boyfriend should return to the family unit.

imperfecta have frequent broken bones as a natural consequence of their disease. Because of inadequate fact-finding in these instances, false reports do occur. This can lead to severe stress on a family that has been falsely accused and can interfere with the relationship between the parents of an ill child and the health care personnel who will then give care to the child (see Focus on Cultural Competence).

When a child has been physically abused, the injury is usually out of proportion to the history of the injury given by the parent (Fig. 55-1). The parent may report, for exam-

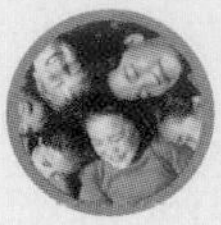

FOCUS ON CULTURAL COMPETENCE

Some health practices can be confused with child abuse. Coin-rolling, for example, a type of massage to draw illness out of the body used by the Vietnamese, leaves bruises on the back similar to those that would appear on a child who has been struck. Coin-rolling involves heating a coin and then vigorously rubbing it over the body, leaving red welts. Being aware of a practice such as coin-rolling aids understanding of the meaning of illness to parents and prevents false reports of child abuse.

ple, that the child was playing underneath the coffee table when he reared up quickly and hit his head, sustaining a large hematoma and temporary loss of consciousness, or that an infant "rolled off the couch" and now has two broken arms. In other instances, the parents may give conflicting stories (for example, the mother says that the child fell; the father says that the child broke his arm throwing a baseball) or can give no reason for the injury ("He woke up from his nap and couldn't move his arm; I don't know what could be wrong").

When questioned about the injury, abused children often repeat the parent's story; this loyalty to parents seems misplaced, but they may fear further beatings or simply believe that living with such parents is better than not having anyone. Ask about behavior problems in school, because the constant stress under which these children live can result in this type of manifestation.

It is often difficult to remain emotionally uninvolved and not grow angry when talking to the parents of an abused child. Emotional involvement is not constructive, however; it rarely helps the parents to change, and it may cause them to avoid seeking health care in the future, leaving the child totally unprotected.

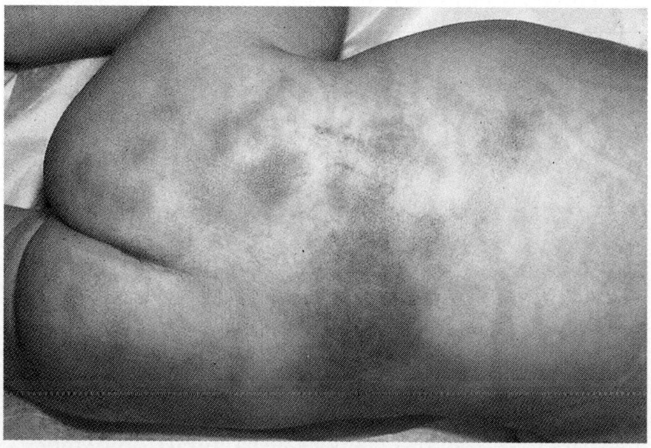

FIGURE 55.1 Large bruises on a child's body. With this type of injury, carefully assessing the history of the accident would be essential.

Always assume that the parents have done the best they could under the circumstances in which they found themselves. The fact that they have brought the child for care may mean they are seeking help; this may be their way of saying, "Help me; I don't want this to happen again." Child abuse is rarely an isolated phenomenon. Often the parent is also a victim and needs as much help and protection as the child.

Physical Examination. When children are examined at both well or ill child visits, be certain they are fully undressed (including removing all bandages and Band-Aids) so that their entire body can be observed. Plot height and weight on a standard growth chart. Delays in growth may suggest neglect.

A number of injuries in children clearly signal child abuse. Children who are beaten with electrical cords, belts, or clotheslines have peculiar circular and linear lesions (Fig. 55-2). Children beaten with a belt buckle have additional curved lacerations from the imprint of the buckle; few other weapons produce such contusions. Abrasions or ecchymotic areas on the wrists or ankles may be present if the child was tied to a bed or against a wall. Most parents protect their children's hands carefully; children who are abused have a higher incidence of hand injury than others.

Burns or scalds are frequent injuries in abused children. The peak age at which children accidentally burn themselves is 2 years; that of burns related to abuse is closer to 3 years. When children burn their hand by accident, they usually burn the palm; burns from abuse are often on the dorsal surface. Scalding with hot water may be seen. A child placed in a tub of hot water, buttocks first, often has no burn in the center of his buttocks because they touched the tub; a ring of burns causing a "hole in the doughnut" effect appears around this. Young children do accidentally step into bathtubs containing water that is hot enough to burn. When this happens, however, the child usually falls forward and so also has burns on the hands and splash marks on the chest or face. When a child is lowered into scalding water as punishment, only the feet and the skin up to the knees are scalded.

Cigarette burns are another common finding on the bodies of physically abused children. A fresh cigarette burn causes a blister that resembles the scab of impetigo or pediculosis; differentiation at this stage is often difficult. Impetigo lesions, however, heal without scarring. Cigarette burns and pediculosis heal with a definite circular scar.

Human bites or chunks of hair pulled off the scalp may be present. Head injury is common.

Broken bones are another frequent finding. Children who are preschool age and younger generally do not fall far enough in normal accidents to break bones; a broken bone at this age suggests the child was thrown or struck so hard that the bone broke. Common findings include multiple fractures in different stages of healing, a single fracture with multiple bruises, rib or occipital fractures, and metaphyseal-epiphyseal injuries. Bones are not always broken if a child is shaken roughly, but the periosteum is torn, so the x-ray reveals a strange haziness along both sides of the bone shaft. Tibial torsion (twisting) is often seen (Fig. 55-3). Deliberate poisoning is yet another form of child abuse;

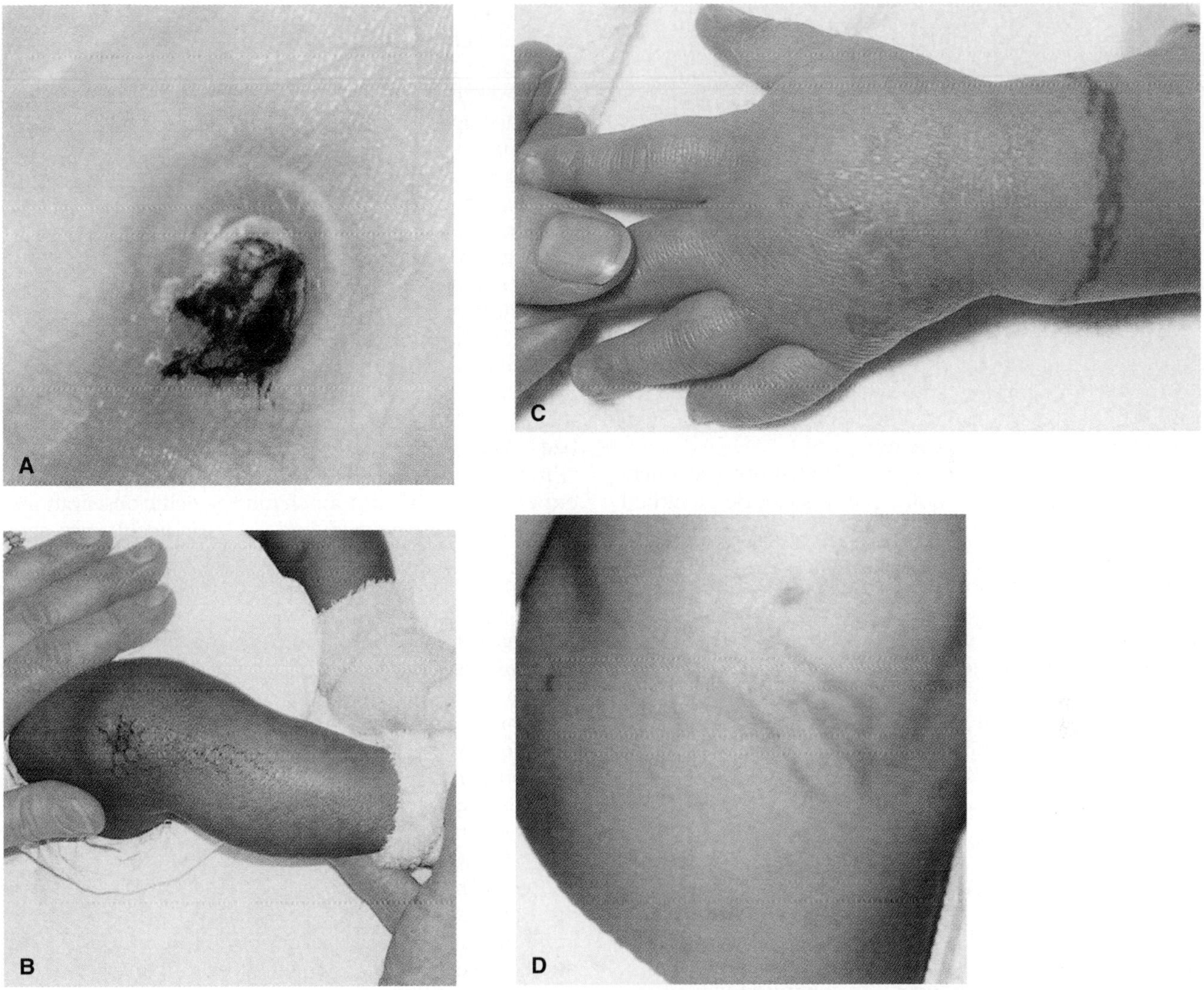

FIGURE 55.2 (*A*) Cigarette burn on child's foot. (*B*) Branding injury showing imprint of radiator cover. (*C*) Rope burn with edema and skin breakdown from being tied to crib rails. (*D*) Imprint marks from beating with a looped electrical cord.

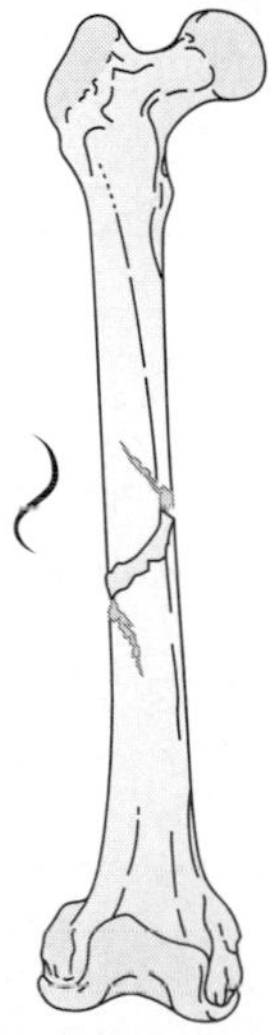

FIGURE 55.3 A spiral fracture around the bone is caused by a wrenching force and is frequently associated with child abuse.

this usually occurs in a child younger than 2.5 years. Bruises on a child who is too young to walk also are highly suspicious (Labbe & Caouette, 2001).

Listen to children while they are being examined. If they did not hear the parent's explanation of the accident, they may say something that is inconsistent with the parent's explanation. They may cry little in response to a painful procedure, such as an injection, because they are not used to receiving comfort for pain. They may draw back from an examiner more than the average child would because they are afraid of adults. These are very subjective observations, however, because children react in different ways to the fear produced by a recent injury.

NURSING DIAGNOSES AND RELATED INTERVENTIONS

Nursing Diagnosis: Risk for injury related to documented abuse by parent

Outcome Identification: Child will not experience further abuse for lifetime.

Outcome Evaluation: Child has no further physical injuries identifiable as being inflicted by abusing parent.

Prevent Further Abuse. When child abuse is discovered, it would be ideal if the abuser's behavior could be changed and the family kept intact. In reality, once child abuse has been discovered, the child must usually be removed from the home so that no more abuse occurs. Even so, it is impossible to reverse the damage that has been done to the child's sense of trust and self-esteem. The goal of health providers with child abuse, therefore, must be prevention (Box 55-1). Because many child abusers were abused themselves, stopping child abuse in any one generation helps prevent it in the next.

Identifying parents who are potential abusers is a necessary step in prevention. Some parents can be identified as potential abusers during pregnancy. Listen carefully to the way pregnant women or their partners talk about the child they are expecting. The parent who is overly concerned about the physical appearance or sex of the child ("This had better be a girl" or "He'd better not have his father's nose") may have difficulty accepting a child who does not meet these expectations. Listen for a parent who is concerned about "not letting children get the upper hand" or who says a child "had better be good." This parent may be conveying worry about how he or she will act when the child is "bad."

A parent may also be identified as a potential child abuser during the early postpartum period. Not all parents immediately bond or react warmly to their newborns. They may tentatively touch or pick up their infant. Be aware of parents who do not touch their infant within 24 hours or those who make disparaging remarks about the child's appearance. Risk factors during pregnancy and the early postpartum period are shown in Box 55-2.

Parents may also be identified as potential abusers during health maintenance visits for the infant (Gaffney et al., 2002). By the time a baby is brought to a health care agency for an initial health maintenance visit, a good parent–child interaction should have begun. Listen for parents who say the baby is "nothing but trouble," "cries all the time," or "is bad." Ask new parents how it feels to be a new parent. "I'm enjoying it" is a different answer from "not what I expected" or "it's not much fun." Specific observations to make during postpartum and pediatric health care check-ups are summarized in Box 55-3.

Helping parents to seek assistance from support people is another necessary step in prevention. Home visits and organizations for parents who abuse, such as Parents Anonymous, can be highly effective in encouraging parents to reach out for help in time of crisis. Interventions that appear promising are home visits, family counseling, and therapy.

Another nursing responsibility aimed at preventing child abuse is helping young parents learn about normal growth and development of children and how to be better parents (Fig. 55-4). Courses in high school that describe sound parenting and review normal growth and development of children and the responsibilities involved in parenting are important measures in preventing child abuse. Classes conducted in high-risk prenatal settings might also have an impact.

Provide Consistent Care and Support for the Abused Child. A major nursing role in caring for an abused child is supplying a consistent, caring adult presence for the abused child or furnishing a relationship that the child has never enjoyed.

Use a primary or case management type of nursing care assignment with abused children to offer them consistency

BOX 55.1

MEASURES TO PREVENT CHILD ABUSE

1. Advocate for high school courses on parenting and growth and development of children.
2. Help children learn problem-solving techniques so they are not overwhelmed by mounting problems as adults.
3. Foster high self-esteem in children so they are not dependent on others but are assertive (they will not become a passive observer to abuse).
4. Help parents with responsible reproductive planning so children are desired.
5. Help parents locate support people in their community, such as Parents of Retarded Citizens or church or social contacts.
6. Teach children to verbalize their problems and to seek help for problems so they do not mount to overwhelming proportions.
7. Role-model caring behaviors with children for parents.
8. Identify children who may be viewed as special in some way by parents (those separated at birth, premature, physically challenged).
9. Identify parents who were abused as children, and offer specific help to them to break the chain of child abuse.
10. Suggest that potential abusers join Parents Anonymous as an effective support group.

BOX 55.2

CHARACTERISTICS OF WOMEN AT HIGH RISK FOR CHILD ABUSE OR NEGLECT

1. Frequent changes of address in the year before child's birth
2. Past or present psychiatric treatment
3. Emotional problems
4. Lack of intellectual ability
5. Unrealistic expectations of the new baby
6. Changed decision about adoption
7. Abuse or neglect of a previous child
8. History of parental violence or neglect in childhood

BOX 55.3

QUESTIONS TO ASK TO DETECT CHILD ABUSE

1. Does the mother have fun with the baby?
2. Does the mother establish eye contact (direct *en face* position) with the baby?
3. How does the mother talk to the baby? Is everything she expresses a demand?
4. Are most of her verbalizations about the child negative?
5. Does she remain disappointed about the child's sex?
6. What is the child's name? Where did the name come from? When was the child named?
7. Are the mother's expectations for the child's development far beyond the child's capabilities?
8. Is the mother very bothered by the baby's crying?
9. Does the mother see the baby as too demanding during feedings? Does she ignore the baby's demands to be fed?
10. What is the mother's reaction to the task of changing diapers? Is she repulsed by the messiness?
11. When the baby cries, does she or can she comfort him or her?
12. Are the parents receiving adequate support?
13. Are there sibling rivalry problems?
14. Is the husband jealous of the baby's drain on the mother's time and affection?
15. When the mother brings the child to the physician's office, does she become involved and take control over the baby's needs and what is going to happen (during the examination and while in the waiting room)? Or does she relinquish control to the physician or nurse (e.g., undressing the child, holding him or her, allowing the child to express fears)?
16. Can attention be focused on the child in the mother's presence? Can the mother see something positive for her in that?
17. Does the mother report nonexistent symptoms in the baby? Does she describe to you a child that you do not see at all? Does she call with strange stories, such as the child has stopped breathing, changed color, or is doing something "on purpose" to aggravate the parent?
18. Does the mother make emergency calls to health care providers for very small things?

and the security of a one-to-one relationship. Many abused children are not used to playing for their own enjoyment but only to the point that a parent wants to play a game; this means that they may watch you carefully for signs that you approve of their behavior. They may not be used to activities such as rocking or talking. Be careful when asking questions not to imply that any one answer is the correct one, or they will supply what they think you want to hear rather than the truth. (A question such as, "That feels better, doesn't it?" will be followed by an instant "yes" even though the child feels no improvement in symptoms.)

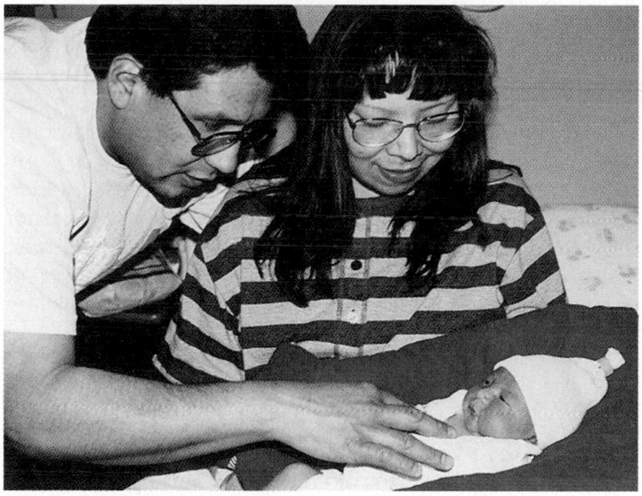

FIGURE 55.4 Teaching that all children have unique characteristics helps to prevent child abuse. Here, new parents explore the already noticeable unique aspects of their newborn.

Evaluate and Promote Family Health. Nurses can be instrumental in helping evaluate whether a child would be safe in the parents' care in the future. When parents who are suspected child abusers visit the health care facility, be certain they are given the same welcome and orientation to the facility and procedures as other parents are. When caring for such a child, point out positive characteristics about the child or growth and development markers he or she has reached and realistic expectations of the age, because lack of knowledge of normal growth and development may have contributed to the abuse.

For many parents, the response to a charge of child abuse is anger. For others, it is relief; now an unwanted child will be taken away from them. In some families, one of the parents is the abuser; the other is a victim also. The diagnosis of abuse may force the passive partner to make some important decisions about whether he or she wants to continue a marriage or a relationship with the abusive partner. These are not easy decisions to make; if decision-making of any kind were easy for this parent, the circumstances probably would never have reached the point where child abuse occurred.

Praise abusing parents for the things they do well; take time to talk to them away from the child so that your total attention is focused on them. Be certain they are referred for counseling.

Sometimes a child is removed temporarily from a home following child abuse, then returned to the home later when the stress that led to the abuse has been removed. Such children need careful follow-up, as parents may revert to an abuse pattern if stress should occur again.

If a child was injured seriously enough to be hospitalized so he or she has to be removed permanently from a parent's care, the foster family should visit before discharge from the hospital to make the change less frightening for the child. Children being removed from their parents in this way can feel an acute sense of loss and may grieve for the nonabusing parent or siblings very much. An abused child may also grieve for the abusing parent, especially if the child is convinced that he or she was responsible for the abuse and that the parent really was not to blame.

Outcome evaluation for abused children must include not only whether they are physically safe, but also whether they are developing self-esteem so that they can become adults who do not need role reversal with their children. It should include whether the abuser received counseling and changed his or her behavior.

Shaken Baby Syndrome

Shaken baby syndrome is repetitive, violent shaking of a small infant by the arms or shoulders, causing a whiplash injury to the neck, edema to the brain stem, and distinct retinal hemorrhages. In extreme instances, the infant may suffer brain hemorrhage and die (AAP, 2001). This is a particularly insidious form of child abuse because the damage inflicted on the infant is not readily apparent. Increased use of computed tomography scans and magnetic resonance imaging helps to detect these internal symptoms. Parents have used covert camcorders ("Nanny cams") to detect that a caregiver shook a baby this way.

Ritual Abuse

Ritual abuse is cult-based or religiously, spiritually, or satanically motivated. It can involve physical, sexual, or psychological abuse with bizarre or ceremonial activities. With this type of abuse, multiple perpetrators may abuse multiple victims over an extended period of time (Bernet, 2000).

✔ CHECKPOINT QUESTIONS

3. What national organizations are dedicated to helping potential abusers to avoid child abuse?
4. What is shaken baby syndrome?

Physical Neglect

Physical neglect is a more subtle form of abuse than physical abuse but can be just as damaging to a child's welfare. A neglected child might appear unwashed, thin, and malnourished or be dressed inappropriately, such as without mittens, a coat, or shoes in cold weather. In some families, no one has a warm coat to wear or receives enough food because there is no money for these things; that is different from the family in which parents do have these things, but the children or this particular child does not. This type of abuse may be overlooked because if you never see the other members of the family, it is easy to believe that all are dressed poorly.

Failing to bring a child for immunizations and failing to seek early medical care for an infection are other signs of neglect. Not requiring a child to attend school, deliberately keeping a child out of school without setting up a home school program, or allowing a child to go unsupervised after school may also be interpreted as neglect.

Neglect may be willful, or it may occur if parents simply do not realize the normal needs of a child. Such parents need guidance from health care personnel to understand their child's needs.

Psychological Abuse

Psychological abuse includes constant belittling or threatening, rejecting, isolating, or exploiting the child. Psychological neglect is the absence of positive parenting. Children who are psychologically abused are likely to have difficulty becoming emotionally confident adults. This type of abuse is the most difficult form of abuse to detect because it may occur only in the home, and its effects, although severe, may be subtle. However, it can be every bit as damaging to the child's ability to achieve as physical abuse is.

The parent who uses only negative terms to describe a child may be psychologically abusing a child. Be sure to include enough growth and development questions during a health assessment to reveal this, and observe parent–child interaction to determine whether this interaction is positive and healthy or negative and potentially unhealthy.

Munchausen Syndrome by Proxy

Munchausen syndrome by proxy refers to a parent who repeatedly brings a child to a health care facility and reports symptoms of illness when, in fact, the child is well. For example, a parent might report symptoms such as seizures, excessive sleepiness, or abdominal pain. The reporting of these symptoms causes the child to undergo needless diagnostic procedures or therapeutic regimens. The parent may deliberately inflict injury on the child (e.g., giving a laxative to induce diarrhea or slowly poisoning the child with a prescription drug). Two classic findings of the syndrome are always present: first, the symptoms are not easily detected by physical examination, only by history; second, the symptoms are present only when the abuser is providing care and disappear when care is provided by another person. The parent usually has some degree of medical or childcare knowledge; this knowledge may have been attained through formal education, reading, or Internet browsing. The parent tends to stay with the child constantly, offering to give the majority of care. This can be very deceptive because wanting to stay and give care is also the hallmark of a very conscientious and caring parent. To diagnose this disorder, covert video surveillance may be necessary (Hall et al., 2000). Because this syndrome reveals distorted perceptions on the part of the parent, it is almost always necessary to remove the child from the home to protect him or her (Hausman, 2000).

Failure to Thrive (Reactive Attachment Disorder)

Failure to thrive is a unique syndrome in which an infant falls below the fifth percentile for weight and height on a standard growth chart or is falling in percentiles on a growth chart. This condition can be divided into two categories: syndromes with organic causes, such as cardiac disease; and syndromes with nonorganic causes that occur because of a disturbance in the parent–child relationship, resulting in maternal role insufficiency. Sometimes both physical and emotional factors play a role in failure to thrive (Christian, 2000b).

The nonorganic type can be considered a form of child neglect, although this represents a very complex interplay between parent and child. In many instances, the parent feels little emotional attachment to the child and may have a history of frequent moves and little family support. The parent may not be offering enough food (the parent may not be aware of the hunger cues the infant is offering, or the parent does not have enough concern for a child to offer food regularly). Some infants are offered sufficient food, but the emotional deprivation they sense makes them so lethargic that they do not eat enough. A child may contribute to the poor parenting interaction by being an irritable, fussy, colicky, or "difficult" child. In some instances, the child may have neurologic dysfunction from a birth injury and may not respond as a normal child would. The mother may have interpreted this lethargic behavior as lack of response to her and so did not carry out her half of the interaction adequately. Failure to thrive must be taken seriously because it can lead to cognitive impairment in the child and even death if allowed to continue.

Assessment

Weigh all children at routine health assessments, and plot and compare their weight with standard growth curves so that children who are failing to thrive can be identified. Because of little parent–child interaction, accompanying motor and social developmental delays also may be present.

Take a detailed pregnancy history because in many instances a breakdown in the development of parenting began in the prenatal period. A pregnancy that was unplanned or not accepted; a boyfriend or husband who left during the pregnancy; the death of a close friend or parent; an economic catastrophe, such as loss of a job; or a long-distance move during pregnancy are all situations that can cause inadequate parenting after the child is born.

On physical examination, these infants generally demonstrate some typical characteristics, including the following:

- Lethargy with poor muscle tone, a loss of subcutaneous fat, or skin breakdown (Fig. 55-5)
- Inability to resist the examiner's manipulation the way the average infant does
- Rocking on all fours excessively, as if seeking stimulation, if emotionally deprived
- Possibly a greater reluctance to reach for toys or initiate human contact than the average infant
- Staring hungrily at people who approach them as if they are starved for human contact. Some health care personnel have an uneasy feeling when caring for these infants because this eye contact is so intense.
- Little cuddling or conforming to being held by the second month of life
- Achievement of developmental milestones in the prone position (e.g., lifting the head and chest and following an object with the eyes) by the third or fourth month, but delays in other behaviors that should appear in later months (e.g., sitting erect, pulling to a standing position, crawling, and walking)

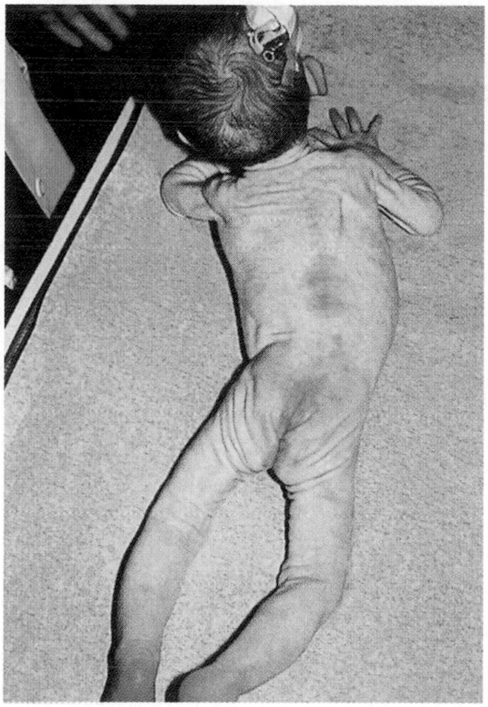

FIGURE 55.5 The child with failure to thrive experiences a loss of subcutaneous fat, muscle wasting, and skin breakdown.

- Markedly delayed or absent speech because of the lack of interaction
- Diminished or nonexistent crying

With advanced failure to thrive, the child's physical condition may be extremely poor; he or she may be nearing acidosis from starvation. If an upper respiratory infection develops, the child's resistance to infection may be so low that it could result in pneumonia.

Therapeutic Management

With rare exceptions, children with failure to thrive need to be removed from the parents' care for evaluation and therapy. If admitted to a hospital, studies other than routine admission blood work and urinalysis are usually delayed to avoid submitting these understimulated children to needless pain.

Severe failure to thrive in the early months must be treated rigorously, or it may lead to permanent neurologic damage or leave a child cognitively challenged because of protein deficits and interference with brain metabolism. Infants are placed on a diet appropriate for their ideal weight (the weight they would have been normally for their age). Gaining weight rapidly on this diet is diagnostic that their presenting illness was nonorganic failure to thrive (Christian, 2000b).

NURSING DIAGNOSES AND RELATED INTERVENTIONS

A nursing diagnosis commonly used with children who fail to thrive is "Imbalanced nutrition, less than body requirements, related to lack of desire to eat or parental neglect regarding nutritional needs." In addition, "Impaired parenting related to disturbance in parent–child bonding" is often appropriate. Be certain that the plan of care designed for the family is realistic. Parents cannot be made to form a bond with their children instantly, particularly if this lack of bonding has gone on for some time. On the other hand, one should never give up hope that this will happen. With the proper support and guidance over time, and when obstacles to bonding are removed, a healthy child–parent relationship could still develop.

Nursing Diagnosis: Imbalanced nutrition, less than body requirements, related to inadequate intake secondary to emotional deprivation

Outcome Identification: Child will take in adequate nutrients for growth by 24 hours.

Outcome Evaluation: Child shows interest in bottle feedings; child is able to establish a regular eating pattern; child begins to gain weight.

Ensure Adequate Nutrition. Keep a careful record of intake and output so that the number of calories being consumed every day can be evaluated. Assess stools for pH and reducing substances (glucose) to be certain the child is absorbing nutrients. If a stool tests positive for glucose or has an acid pH (less than 5.5), it suggests that not even carbohydrates, the easiest food to absorb, are being absorbed.

Evaluate how well the infant sucks or is able to take food from a spoon and swallow. Record any symptoms, such as pulling up the legs or crying after eating, that would suggest gastrointestinal discomfort.

Nurture the Child. Because children with failure to thrive are suffering from emotional deprivation, they need effective "parenting" from the nurses who care for them. This does not mean that everyone who passes the crib should stop and play with them for a few minutes; it means that a member of the nursing team should be chosen to be the child's "parent" during the hospital stay (a primary nursing or case management pattern of assignment). It is important that this person is able to spend time rocking the child, giving a leisurely bath, talking to the child, exposing the child to toys, and "parenting" the child rather than just giving routine care. Be certain that the person chosen for this role understands that interaction with the child must be active. Passive rocking without talking to the child or paying attention to him or her, for instance, may be no different than the parents' care (see Focus on Multidisciplinary Care).

Support and Encourage the Parents. Encourage the parents of children with failure to thrive to visit as much as possible while the child is hospitalized or in foster care; without encouragement, these parents may visit little or not at all. When they do visit, encourage them to feed the child if they want and interact with him or her as they choose. The parents cannot change their feelings about the child overnight. Telling them that they ought to pick up the baby more or hold him or her more while feeding is ineffective and may only increase the parents' feelings of inadequacy. Giving some suggestions about how the baby tries to communicate with them might be more effective: "Do you know what I think he's trying to say when he stops sucking like that? I think he's saying he's ready to be burped." Pointing out the infant's ability to respond to the parent may be helpful: "Look how he turns his head at the sound of your voice. He recognizes you."

FOCUS ON MULTIDISCIPLINARY CARE

Identifying and reporting abuse is a team effort that involves the coordination of a variety of health care providers, such as pediatricians, advanced practice nurses, counselors, and social workers, and legal authorities, such as judges and lawyers. Therefore, clear communication is essential. Be certain when caring for these children that all personnel understand the importance of interacting with the children to provide a nurturing environment.

Occasionally, a parent is so distraught by such factors as the illness or death of an older child or relative that he or she is simply unaware of how much energy is being drained by these events. These parents quickly can become good parents to a deprived child as soon as they realize what has been happening. More often, however, the disturbance in a parent–child interaction began long before or is so great that a parenting bond cannot be established at this point. If the infant is discharged from the hospital with the parents, the parents will need effective follow-up in the months to come to see that they maintain parenting at an acceptable level. There is a very thin line between the child who fails to thrive and one who is abused. Some of these children need to be placed in foster homes for their own safety and to ensure that they receive adequate care.

Ensure Evaluation and Follow-Up. Failure to thrive is easy to correct from a physiologic standpoint. When given proper food in a caring environment, the infant usually gains weight rapidly. Adequate follow-up to ensure that the emotional and physical needs continue to be met is a much larger issue, so big that the answer lies not in treatment but in prevention. Parents who may be at risk for poor parenting need to be identified during pregnancy so they can receive counseling and close follow-up in the postnatal period. At health maintenance visits, secure careful, thoughtful pregnancy histories to elicit information about the psychosocial events that could lead to parenting breakdown. Some parents may need respite care for their children when they are overwhelmed by the task of parenting. They may need extended counseling to prevent parenting breakdown. Nurses can be instrumental in all phases of this care.

✔ CHECKPOINT QUESTIONS

5. What behaviors can be classified as psychologically abusive?
6. What are two classic findings of Munchausen syndrome by proxy?
7. How is failure to thrive defined?

SEXUAL ABUSE

Sexual abuse may be broadly defined as any sexual contact between a child and an adult. Adolescents and older children may also be perpetrators. Sexual abuse involves the coercion of dependent, developmentally immature children and adolescents in sexual activities that they do not fully comprehend, to which they are unable to give informed consent, or that violate the social taboos of family roles. Adolescents have a higher rate of rape or sexual abuse than any other age group (5/1,000), and the abuse is often preceded by alcohol ingestion (Kaplan et al., 2001).

Sexual abuse is physically and emotionally destructive; it leaves children unable to trust others, and they have a sense of ambivalence toward intimacy and an overall sense of worthlessness. Children should be taught at an early age that their bodies are their own and to report anyone who tries to touch them in a way they do not like (Fig. 55-6).

Megan's Law is a federal law that requires law enforcement authorities to report when a sexual abuser moves into a neighborhood. Parents need to be aware of this law and insist that it be enforced. If they are aware that a former sexual abuser lives near them, they need to take appropriate precautions to protect their children's safety (Cole, 2000).

Molestation

Molestation is a vague term that includes "indecent liberties" such as oral–genital contact, genital fondling and viewing, or masturbation.

A **pedophile** is an adult who seeks out children for sexual gratification. In contrast to a rapist, whose crime is violent, the pedophile may be very gentle and limit the involvement to molestation. Such a person is usually a man who suffered sexual abuse as a child and repeatedly selects children who are of the same age at which his abuse occurred. The relationship may involve people with either homosexual or heterosexual orientations. Many pedophiles take photos or videotapes of their activities with children to use for sexual gratification at a later date (Shanahan & Donato, 2001).

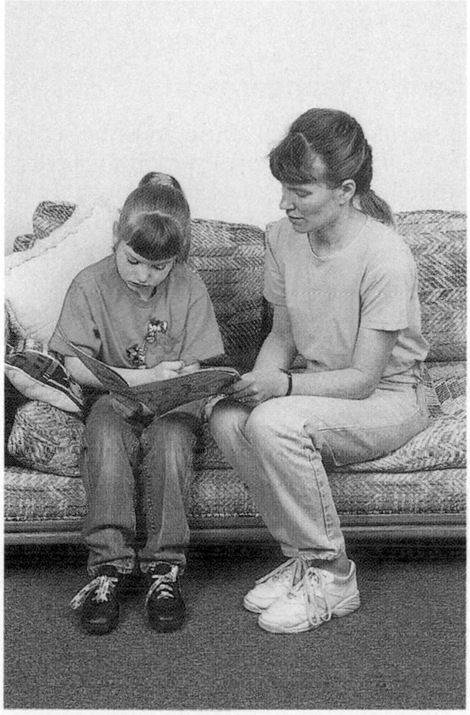

FIGURE 55.6 Teach children that their bodies are their own and that they have to give permission before anyone can touch them.

Rehabilitation of pedophiles is difficult because they are fixated emotionally at a childhood level (seeing themselves as children, they do not perceive relationships with children as wrong). Listen carefully to children who report that someone enjoys photographing them; ask children to describe what they mean by someone "touching" or "feeling" them to detect this type of abuse.

Incest

Incest is sexual activity between family members. It often involves an older man and a young girl, although it may involve an older woman and younger boy, brother or sister, or same-sex partners. It may involve foster, adopted, and stepchildren. Incest is a deviation from the norm and is so strongly viewed as such by most people that incest taboos are common to most cultures (Rudd & Herzberger, 1999).

Incest results in a destructive relationship because it causes a great deal of guilt and loss of self-esteem in both the abusing and the abused person. The abuser is aware that this act is not culturally approved but still is unable to end the relationship; the victim recognizes this act as wrong but is unable to resist the advances. Other members of the family are likely to suspect that something is wrong; this leads to guilt and feelings of worthlessness on their part for not being able to protect the victim.

Pornography and Prostitution

Child pornography involves photographing or describing sexual acts by any media involving children, or distributing such material in person or by mail or fax or over the Internet. Child prostitution involves arranging or participating in sexual acts with children. Both of these phenomena are demeaning to children. Child prostitution carries the additional risks of sexually transmitted disease and violence, the same as adult prostitution.

Assessment

Signs of sexual abuse are shown in the Focus on Family Empowerment. Symptoms of sexual abuse may be revealed on the health history (e.g., a young girl worrying that she is pregnant); it may be revealed by a child's abnormal anxiety about a parent returning home from a hospital stay or anxiety about being left with a particular individual in the family (see Focus on Communication). Young children who are the victims of this type of relationship often have been threatened or bribed to keep it a secret; they have extremely low self-esteem and may think that they are so bad that they deserve to be treated this way.

Allowing young children to play with anatomically correct dolls is a common way of determining whether

FOCUS ON FAMILY EMPOWERMENT
Identifying Signs of Sexual Abuse

Q. We just found out that our daughter's friend was sexually abused by her babysitter. Is there anything that would alert us to suspect if our daughter was also being sexually abused?

A. Here are some general indications that a child is being sexually abused:

- Verbal reports of sexual activity with an adult
- An awareness of sex and sexual vocabulary beyond age expectations
- Participation in sexual expression with dolls
- Pregnancy in a girl under age 15
- Perineal, vaginal, or anal inflammation
- Vaginal tears or anal fissures
- Presence of a sexually transmitted disease
- Symptoms of increased anxiety, such as sleep disturbance, development of tics, nail biting, or stuttering
- Change in school performance, school phobia, or truancy
- Fear of being left alone with a certain adult
- Vague abdominal pain or acting-out behavior

FOCUS ON COMMUNICATION

Cecily is a 4-year-old who is seen at a pediatric clinic for vulvovaginitis. You notice that on history taking, she uses a number of four-letter words to describe where it hurts.

Less Effective Communication

Nurse: Mrs. Holly, Cecily seems to know some words that are unusual for a 4-year-old.

Mrs. Holly: She gets that from watching cartoons on TV.

Nurse: Cartoon characters don't usually use the words Cecily uses.

Mrs. Holly: We're proud she's advanced for her age.

Nurse: Okay. I just want you to know I think her vocabulary is advanced. Here is the medicine to apply to her bottom.

More Effective Communication

Nurse: Mrs. Holly, Cecily seems to know some words that are unusual for a 4-year-old.

Mrs. Holly: She gets that from watching cartoons on TV.

Nurse: Cartoon characters don't usually use the words Cecily uses.

Mrs. Holly: We're proud she's advanced for her age.

Nurse: Using words with sexual connotations doesn't necessarily mean her vocabulary is advanced. It means she most likely keeps company with an adult who talks to her that way.

Mrs. Holly: That's probably her uncle. He babysits for us once a week.

Nurse: Does Cecily mind staying with him?

Mrs. Holly: A free babysitter doesn't happen every day.

Nurse: Let's talk some more about Cecily's vocabulary, especially in light of her infection.

It is often very difficult for families to face the fact that a family member could be guilty of child sexual abuse. In these instances, it is necessary to pursue the subject, rather than let yourself be distracted, to help a parent examine what could be happening.

sexual abuse is occurring. However, use of such dolls is controversial because there is a concern that without a common protocol for their use, the child's actions could be overinterpreted. For example, the average reaction of a preschooler or young school-age child who has not been abused is to undress the dolls, giggle for a moment or two about how they look, and then redress or put them aside. The child who is involved in an incestuous relationship is more apt to make the dolls perform a sexual act, such as placing the male doll's penis into the female doll's mouth. Asking the child to draw a picture of what happened may also be an effective way of revealing abuse.

WHAT IF? What if a stepbrother rapes his younger sibling? Because they are not blood relatives, would this be considered incest?

Therapeutic Management

Sexual abuse, like physical abuse, must be reported. The perpetrator will then be interviewed by the police because this is a criminal offense. It is important that this information be collected in such a way that the adult's rights are respected and the testimony is therefore admissible in court.

Both the adult and child involved in a sexual abuse relationship need psychological counseling—the child to improve self-esteem and the adult to channel sexual expression to less destructive outlets. To improve the child's self-esteem, the adult in the relationship needs to admit the fault is all his or hers. Follow-up care is best done by one of the people who sees the child initially so that he or she does not have to recount the incident to strangers again and again. Treatment for sexually transmitted diseases or protection against pregnancy should be provided if needed.

Parents may need as much counseling as the child so that they can help the child to work through his or her feelings about this situation. In many instances, the offender is a family member, such as an uncle, stepfather, or older brother. Often the relationship has been occurring for some time before it is reported. The parents may feel guilty that they allowed the family member to have access to the child or did not listen to the child's protestations that he or she did not like to be alone with this family member. If incest involves a parent, it may be extremely difficult for the parents to continue to relate to each other effectively enough to help the child. Encourage parents to teach children some simple rules to help them avoid sexual abuse (see Box 31-1 in Chap. 31).

RAPE

Rape is sexual activity that occurs under actual or threatened force. Forcible rape is defined by law in most states as intercourse or penetration of a body orifice by a penis or other object. Statutory rape is sexual activity with a person under the age of consent (in most states, younger than 18 years) and is considered to have occurred in spite of the apparent willingness of the underage person. Sexual assault is used to refer to other forced sexual acts, such as oral-genital or anal-genital acts (Kaplan et al., 2001).

Rape includes "date rape," a situation in which an individual forces a date or casual friend into having coitus despite a voiced unwillingness. The increasing misuse of flunitrazepam (Rohypnol), a drug easily dissolved in a drink, has led to an increase in the incidence of date rape (see Chap. 32). It may be very difficult for the victim of date rape to find a sympathetic ear because her companion insists he meant no harm; he simply didn't believe her. If the victim was given flunitrazepam, little or no memory of the event is present.

Both rape and sexual assault represent deviant behavior; they are crimes of violence, not acts of passion. They lack privacy and mutual consent, which are elements of "normal" sexual behavior, and so are degrading and dehumanizing, leaving the victim feeling completely helpless. Adolescent girls and boys should be informed about ways to prevent rape (including date rape) (see Box 32-3 in Chap. 32).

It is difficult to determine the actual incidence of rape; it may seem to be more prevalent because more people are reporting it. Many adolescents want to avoid the secondary, but no less severe, trauma associated with reporting rape and thus do not report it. This leaves them without the immediate treatment and follow-up care so important to a complete recovery.

Although victims can be any age and either male or female, the average rape victim is an adolescent girl. Up to 75% of girls know their attacker: the rapist may be a relative or family friend, and rapists frequently commit the act in the neighborhood where they live (Kaplan et al., 2001). Based on arrest data, the average rapist is a young adult man with a background of aggressive behavior. His motivation generally relates to expressions of power or anger; sexual satisfaction does not appear to be a dominant motive. An excessive amount of alcohol intake often precedes rape. Rape tends to be a repetitive, planned activity rather than an isolated event (Lim et al., 2001).

Assessment

Many rape victims demonstrate immediate physical and emotional symptoms that can last for weeks. The symptoms constitute what has been termed **rape trauma syndrome,** a form of post-traumatic stress syndrome, and generally occur in two stages: disorganization and reorganization. In the immediate **disorganization phase,** victims feel a combination of humiliation, shame and guilt, embarrassment, anger, and vengefulness. They feel that their lives have been completely disrupted by the crisis and that they were unable to protect themselves from the assault. They may tremble from fear and may be in great pain from perineal lacerations. They are apt to start visibly at the sound of anyone approaching or touching them. They need gentle, sympathetic support people with them in the days following the event to allow them to feel safe. They may have nightmares of the attack occurring again. This immediate stage of disruption and disorganization generally lasts about 3 days.

The second stage of rape trauma syndrome, termed the **reorganization phase,** may last for months or years. Many rape victims continue to report recurring nightmares, perhaps sexual dysfunction, and continuing inability to relate to men or face new and surprising situations. They may continue to have a great deal of difficulty discussing the rape. Many rape victims, trying to outlive this personal offense, change their residence at great sacrifice to finances and lifestyle. If not offered constructive counsel, victims may still feel guilt or shame when thinking about the rape as long as 20 to 30 years later.

When victims do not report rape and thus receive no counseling, symptoms indicative of **silent rape syndrome** can result. When the subject of rape is mentioned, people with silent rape syndrome may grow increasingly emotionally disturbed; it may be evident in their history that they altered their behavior toward men at a certain point in life and perhaps began to resist actions such as going outside or being alone in a house after that time. This can be devastating to their ability to maintain employment or remain independent. They need counseling as much as the person who reported a rape.

Emergency Care

Although most large city police forces have special officers assigned to investigate rape charges, victims can be confused and further traumatized by police officers who imply that they provoked the attack or could have at least done more to resist or prevent it. This increases the victim's feeling of shame and degradation. It may be especially harmful to adolescents because people they have been taught to respect have no concept of the degree of fright they have experienced or the strength of their attackers. Health care providers generally are the second group of people victims see following an attack, and they need to be extremely cautious that they do not show this type of callous behavior.

Most health care agencies where many rape victims are seen have a rape trauma team with specially educated counselors to talk to victims immediately following the rape and to offer long-term counseling as needed. Nurses serve as important members of such teams and may provide primary care after a rape. Any nurse should be able to offer emergency support, however, because it might be a long time before a specifically designated staff member arrives, and such services are not available in every community (McConkey et al., 2001).

Because rape is a crime, the hospital chart of a rape victim is often displayed as part of a court procedure. For the victim to bring charges against the attacker, information concerning the victim's appearance and history need to be detailed in the hospital chart. Therefore, statements in a chart must be accurate and unbiased. When recording a history, quote the victim's exact words whenever possible. Describe the victim's physical appearance carefully, including the presence and location of injuries, such as bruises, lacerations, teeth marks, or abrasions, and the condition of clothing. Ask if the victim bathed or washed before coming for care, because this can obscure evidence and obliterate the presence of sperm or DNA material. Ask if the woman was menstruating or using a tampon. The force of penis penetration with rape can cause a tampon to tear through the posterior vaginal wall into the abdominal cavity, causing an extreme loss of blood internally. Photographs should be taken as necessary to document the extent of injuries. Any clothing that is ripped or stained should be considered as evidence of violent assault and secured according to hospital policy.

Following this preliminary observation, a gynecologic or anal examination will be done to evaluate the physical condition of the victim and to document that rape occurred. This is done by recording the existence of any vaginal or perineal lacerations and aspirating sperm or acid phosphate from the vagina or rectum. Acid phosphate, a component of prostatic fluid, is a substance that is not normally present in vaginal or rectal secretions but is present in semen. The presence of acid phosphate is extremely important if the attacker is infertile or sterile, because sperm may not be present. Its presence is the best evidence that rape occurred. Vaginal and anal cultures are taken for gonorrhea and a Pap test is also performed. Blood is drawn for a pregnancy test and a VDRL for syphilis. Prophylactic administration of antibiotics against gonorrhea and syphilis is given. If the woman is not menstruating, she may be given oral contraceptives to avoid pregnancy. Victims may have a baseline blood sample drawn for human immunodeficiency virus (HIV) status.

Be certain during emergency care to provide privacy. Many people may want to ask the victim questions, including police officers or detectives, the victim's family, a rape trauma team, and the examining physician or nurse practitioner. Describing the experience is good, but lack of privacy during a perineal examination demonstrates little concern for the victim's self-esteem. Many female victims are uncomfortable with a male physician examining them after rape because they are temporarily fearful of men. Having a female nurse remain with the victim during this time may be helpful. A male nurse can be equally supportive because it is not the male–female contrast that a victim is seeking as much as an aggression versus caring contrast. Table 55-1 summarizes common tests and procedures for emergency care of rape victims.

Legal Considerations

Nurses working in emergency departments may be asked to testify in court about the victim's appearance after the assault, although the documentation in the chart is generally all that is necessary. Many victims, especially adolescents, do not press charges against their assailants because they were too frightened or unable at the time to observe the assailant's appearance and therefore cannot identify him later. They may fear that by naming him in court, he will return and kill them. Whether victims follow through with a legal action or not is their choice,

TABLE 55.1 Common Specimen Procedures Following Rape*

PROCEDURE	PURPOSE
Oral washing	Client rinses mouth with 5 mL sterile water, which is then collected in test tube. Analyzed for blood group antigens or sperm of attacker.
Fingernail scraping	Scraping under all of client's fingernails is done, and scrapings are placed in envelope. Analyzed for blood, skin, and clothing fibers of attacker.
Blood VDRL, HIV, and HbsAg	Blood is drawn for antibody titer for syphilis, HIV, and hepatitis B.
Blood typing	Blood is drawn for typing to differentiate it from attacker's type.
Pregnancy test	Either blood or urine specimen is collected; complete vaginal exam before woman voids.
Hair samples	Both scalp and pubic hairs of client (about 10) are removed for comparison with attacker's and placed in envelope.
Vaginal smear for sperm and DNA	Vagina is swabbed with dry applicator and smeared onto slide. Allow to dry. Sperm and DNA analysis performed.
Gonococcus smear	Cervix, vagina, rectum are cultured (also throat is cultured if oral coitus was attempted).
Vaginal washing	5 mL of sterile saline is placed in vagina and aspirated. Analyzed to detect sperm and acid phosphate.
Skin washings	Any dried stain of blood or semen on skin or clothing is touched with a moistened cotton swab, which is then dropped into test tube. Analyzed for attacker's blood and semen.
Clothing	Any clothing stained or torn is placed into a paper bag. Evidence of violent attack.

* Label all specimens carefully as to where they were obtained for medical therapy and legal evidence.

but the incidence of rape might be reduced if rapists were aware that they are not apt to escape without a penalty for their crime. Taking the rapist to court may be the opportunity and appropriate time for victims to "fight back" and therefore not be as helpless as they were during the attack.

NURSING DIAGNOSES AND RELATED INTERVENTIONS

Nursing Diagnosis: Rape trauma syndrome related to recent rape

Outcome Identification: Victim will demonstrate adequate coping behavior and eventually return to precrisis level of functioning.

Outcome Evaluation: Victim is able to discuss what happened and voice intense feelings about the crime; victim states ability to go forward with life.

One of the major needs of any victim following a violent act is to talk about what happened. A person who can describe an incident begins to "put a fence around" or contain the event. This process brings the event down from "something terrible has happened," a situation that leaves a person with a continuing high anxiety level, to "this specific thing has happened," a situation that allows the traumatic event to be examined and handled. Something that is concrete and describable is rarely as frightening as "something out there."

Ask the victim to describe the incident to you with an introduction such as, "Most people find it helps to talk about what happened to them." Table 55-2 lists areas to explore with victims to help them reduce the incident to a size they can begin to handle.

Victims should be given the number of a counseling service to telephone before they leave the emergency department. Because genital bruising may not be apparent until 24 hours after the rape, they may be asked to return for a re-examination the next day so this can be documented. Syphilis will not be apparent for up to 6 weeks in serum, so they should return for a repeat VDRL at that time. They may be advised to return in 6 weeks for HIV testing also. Be certain that victims have a support person to accompany them home. Be sure they know that if their distress becomes acute, they can return as needed to the health care facility for additional care or counseling. Inform them about any local support groups that provide follow-up counseling for victims of rape. One such organization, Women Organized Against Rape, is active in many communities.

Nursing Diagnosis: Disabling family coping related to recent rape of family member

Outcome Identification: Victim's partner and family will develop adequate coping mechanisms to be able to support victim.

Outcome Evaluation: Partner or other family members express their feelings about the rape to health care provider; they state confidence in their ability to support rape victim.

In many instances, the victim's usual sexual partner has difficulty being a support person to her after a rape because he has as much difficulty dealing with it as she does. Not infrequently, a relationship that was meaningful before the rape deteriorates because the partner now sees the victim as "soiled" or mistakenly believes she was somehow responsible for the trauma or actually enjoyed the experience. In

TABLE 55.2 Areas to Explore in Rape Counseling

AREA	CONSIDERATIONS
The event	Where did the attack occur? What was happening at the time? This information is important for the victim to discuss and work through; otherwise, any time she is in similar circumstances again, she may have uncontrollable fears related to the attack. Walking home from school or waiting for an elevator in a public building are everyday actions that she will do often during her life. If she was raped in these circumstances, she can be assured that she was acting sensibly and that the rape was not her fault.
The assailant	Allowing the victim to review the description of the rapist may help her to realize that she may react in negative ways in the future to a man with the same build or description. The man may have approached her with a simple gesture, such as a hand on her shoulder. Others will perform this gesture again. She must work through her revulsion to handle it when it occurs in friendly circumstances.
The conversation	Describing the conversation with the rapist helps the victim to convince herself that she did not provoke the attack.
Details of the assault	Describing the actual assault is extremely difficult for most victims, but doing so allows them to work through it. Until they can describe the attack or the sexual act to which they had to submit, they may have difficulty in performing these same acts with persons of their choice.
Resistance to the assault	Many victims do not struggle during an assault because they realize that it could result in further harm to them. If someone asks them what they did to try to fight off the assailant, they may feel again that they provoked or agreed to the attack. Reassure them that no action was probably the best action and the reason they are still alive. To improve self-esteem, counsel victims that rape is a violent crime and that usually the strength of an attacker is far too great for any woman to resist effectively.

other instances, the partner may become so overprotective (not allowing the victim to go out alone; checking on her constantly) that she is not free to maintain her identity. The man may be so filled with vengefulness and anger that he cannot relate to her without his anger surfacing toward her as well as toward the attacker. Parents of a young adolescent may feel the same way. Counseling for the victim's partner or family may help them to be truly supportive (Box 55-4).

✔ CHECKPOINT QUESTIONS

8. What is a pedophile?
9. Is rape a crime of passion or violence?

INTIMATE PARTNER ABUSE

Intimate partner abuse is abuse by a family member against other individuals living in a household (i.e., spouses, children, parents, or grandparents). The fact that spouse abuse and child abuse may both exist in a family strengthens the importance of providing family-centered nursing care so that both these situations can be identified and halted (Lemmey et al., 2001). Methods of assessing and caring for pregnant victims of intimate partner abuse are discussed in Chapter 14.

Intimate partner abuse can be destructive to children because they learn that violence is an acceptable method of managing aggression. This perpetuates it in the next generation.

Children exposed to intimate partner abuse may demonstrate conduct problems, noncompliance, and aggression.

BOX 55.4

GOALS OF CRISIS INTERVENTION FOR FAMILIES OF RAPE VICTIMS

Help the family to express openly their immediate feelings in response to a rape as a shared life crisis.

Help the family to be supportive of and reassuring to the victim.

Help the family work through immediate practical matters and initiate problem-solving techniques.

Help the family develop cognitive understanding of what the rape experience actually means to the victim and to the family.

Explain the possibility of future psychological and somatic symptoms that characterize a rape trauma syndrome and what the family can do to minimize these symptoms.

Activate qualities characteristic of healthy family functioning during the impact and resolution phases of the shared crisis.

Educate the family about rape as a *violent crime,* not a sexually motivated act, and eliminate focus on the victim's guilt or responsibility.

Eliminate the family's sense of guilt for not protecting the victim by assuring them that they could not have anticipated or prevented the rape.

Discourage violent, destructive, or irrational retribution toward the rapist (under the guise of being on the victim's behalf) by encouraging sharing of feelings of helplessness, sadness, hurt, and anger.

Encourage discussion of the sexual relationship between partners; suggest that the man let the victim know (a) that his feelings have not changed (when this is true) and that he still sexually desires her, (b) that he will wait for her to approach him, and (c) that sex therapy is available if they have difficulties that persist and want assistance in reestablishing normal sexual relations.

Explain the possibility of sexually transmitted disease and pregnancy that may result from a rape, the preventive care necessary for the victim and spouse or boyfriend, and the follow-up care indicated.

Explain that early crisis intervention often prevents long-term problems in resolving the crisis, and that to seek counseling at this time does not imply inadequacy (specify that crisis intervention usually lasts for 3–6 hours during the first few weeks after the rape).

Refer the family for direct counseling when members' shared responses to the crisis interfere with their ability to cope adaptively.

Provide factual data, resource lists for counseling, and follow-up care *in writing* (because highly stressed persons do not hear or recall information verbally communicated).

Let families know that some decisions, such as whether to prosecute the rapist or move to a safer residence, can be postponed while more immediate needs, such as medical care, are taken care of. (This action helps the family set priorities and organize decisions about what has to be done now and gain emotional distance from the urgency and confusion felt during a crisis state to permit sound decision-making later.)

Identify how the family has handled crises in the past, and encourage members to use adaptive coping mechanisms for this crisis.

Encourage contact with persons identified as supportive to the family, and offer to contact such persons.

Assign a primary nurse to spend time talking with the family in the emergency department waiting room while the victim receives medical care.

Allow time for thoughts and feelings in the decision-making process.

Use empathetic listening to convey understanding of the family's feelings and concerns.

Ask if you can check back with the family the next day to see how they are getting along and answer any questions they may have.

They may develop low levels of empathy, or display distress behaviors such as clinging, crying, abdominal pain, or sleeping disorders. They may regress in language or social developmental milestones. Effects may be long term if the abuse causes teenage girls to shy away from relationships with boys, afraid that they will be exposed to abuse in the same way as their mother, or they may develop a lack of respect for the abused parent because they blame that person for the abuse (Lemmey et al., 2001).

Like child abuse, intimate partner abuse affects all ethnic and social groups. If it appears to be more prevalent in the lower socioeconomic classes, it is because families at this level are more visible to service organizations and law enforcement officials. When it occurs in middle-class or upper-class houses, wives are often too embarrassed to let people know and keep the violence hidden longer.

TABLE 55.3 Levels of Intimate Partner Abuse

LEVEL	DESCRIPTION
I	Abuse is occasional; consists of slapping, punching, kicking, verbal abuse. Contusions occur.
II	Abuse is becoming more frequent; beatings are sustained and cause fractures, such as a broken jaw or rib fracture.
III	Abuse is even more frequent, perhaps daily. A weapon, such as a gun, baseball bat, or broom handle, may be used. Permanent disability or death from injuries, such as intracranial hemorrhage or concussion, may occur.

Theories About Intimate Partner Abuse

Violent family situations can be divided into two groups: those in which violence preceded the relationship or children and those in which the violence developed after the relationship was established or children were born.

In the first situation, which is more common, violence is usually brought into the family by a man with a history of violence (although the woman may be the offender). His violence-prone characteristics usually erupt early in the courtship and grow progressively worse. He uses violence to handle even small conflicts and provokes a pervasive feeling of powerlessness in the people around him. Such men usually have a history of early and prolonged exposure to family violence as children; alcohol is frequently associated with the expression of violence.

Intimate partner abuse often follows a cycle of violence that includes three phases: tension-building, acute violence, and a "honeymoon" or tranquil, loving phase. During the first phase, the abuser displays actions such as anger, arguing, and blaming the victim for external problems or for provoking the abuse. The acute violence phase is triggered by an internal response in the abuser or an external crisis. It can result in extreme physical harm to the victim. The tranquil, loving phase, characterized by kind and contrite behavior, follows this, lulling the victim into forgiveness and a wish to continue the relationship. Without intervention, however, this phase ends at some point, and the cycle of violence repeats.

Partners react to the situation in three phases (Table 55-3). During the impact phase (stage I), a light level of abuse, the woman uses denial as a defense mechanism. If she does not end the relationship at this point, the abuse grows more frequent and more violent; by not stopping it, the woman is indirectly giving the offender permission to continue. During this second stage, she can no longer deny that the violence is occurring. At the same time, she cannot stop it because she does not provoke the violence; she is only a convenient recipient of poorly controlled violent behavior. She is forced to use coping mechanisms such as becoming very obedient and cooperative and doing everything her abuser asks in a desperate effort to reduce the violence. This phase is termed psychological infantilism or **learned helplessness.** The level of abuse can continue until the woman is being almost constantly physically abused (stage III). A fetus is in danger if abuse of a pregnant woman occurs at this stage. During this stage, the woman is forced to become isolated; she sinks into hopelessness and depression. She has difficulty seeking help because she is unable to believe that outside people might want to help her (Berlinger, 2001).

In the second type of violent family, violence occurs as a last resort when all other attempts at communication have failed. The behavior of one partner threatens the psychological defenses of the other, and each projects his or her feelings and shortcomings onto the other. Such a situation, however, is not typical of intimate partner abuse: in most instances, one partner brought violence into the family.

Assessment

When any type of abuse against an individual family member is identified, it is important to investigate further for evidence of abuse against other family members. Asking about the possibility of abuse should be a priority with any woman seen for trauma. As many as 20% to 25% of women seen in emergency departments for trauma received their wounds from abuse. Common injuries suffered by abused women include burns, lacerations, bruises, and head injury. Asking all women at physical examinations to account for any bruise they have helps detect this. Asking them if they are ever concerned about their safety or well-being helps detect emotional abuse. In addition, screening for intimate partner abuse is important when parents bring children for health care visits (see Focus on Evidence-Based Practice).

Therapeutic Management

It may be difficult to understand how adults can tolerate abuse against themselves or their children. It is important, however, not to blame the victims. Hopelessness and powerlessness are consequences of continual abuse. Battered and emotionally abused individuals are often immobilized by a sense of guilt: they believe that if they were better people, their partners would not resort to beatings or verbal badgering. Because victims may have no access to money and no skills to earn any, they need a great deal of support to be able to leave their partners. Even if they have a skill

FOCUS ON EVIDENCE-BASED PRACTICE

What Are Barriers to Screening for Intimate Partner Violence at Pediatric Health Care Visits?

The American Academy of Pediatrics has recommended that health care providers should screen for intimate partner abuse in pediatric care settings because as many as 40% of women will report this if asked. To discover what problems make such screening difficult, questionnaires were mailed to 310 physicians with pediatric practices in Ohio. Results of the survey showed that physicians estimated the incidence of intimate partner abuse to be less than 5% in their practices, so only 8.5% of practitioners routinely screened for this. Barriers to screening they identified were lack of education about screening techniques (61%), office protocol (60%), time (59%), and support staff (55%). Family physicians were more likely to have had training in screening than pediatricians and to carry this out in their practice.

This is an important study for nurses because it reveals an important role that nurses could undertake in health care office practices: that of screening for intimate partner abuse.

Erickson, M. J., Hill, T. D., & Siegel, R. M. (2001). Barriers to domestic violence screening in the pediatric setting. *Pediatrics, 108*(1), 98–102.

and have supported themselves in the past, their self-esteem may be so low that they no longer believe they can put the skill to use. As the abuse becomes more violent, they may be afraid that their abusers will follow and kill them and their children if they leave. Other extended family members may be unwilling to shelter the victims for fear of being included in the violence. An important role for nurses is helping an abused family find a shelter where they can feel safe. Treatment for abusers needs to be scheduled, but safety is the first priority.

✔ CHECKPOINT QUESTIONS

10. What is a prime reason that women who experience intimate partner abuse do not seek help early in an abusive relationship?
11. What should be the first priority for nurses when intimate partner abuse is suspected?

KEY POINTS

A high suspicion for child abuse should be present when burns, head injury, or rib fractures are present or when the history of the accident seems out of context for the injury.

Child abuse may exist in many forms. It may be physical, emotional, or sexual and may encompass neglect and abuse.

Shaken baby syndrome involves repetitive, violent shaking of a small infant by the arms or shoulders, causing a whiplash injury to the neck, edema to the brain stem, and distinct retinal hemorrhages.

A triad of a "special parent, special child, special situation" is characteristic of the family in which child abuse occurs.

Failure to thrive is a syndrome in which an infant falls below the fifth percentile for weight and height on a standard growth chart. It is associated with a disturbance in the parent–child relationship.

Children who comfort parents in emergency settings may just be sensitive children, or they may be demonstrating role reversal, a behavior characteristic of abused children.

In families in which a child is abused, a parent may also be a victim of abuse. Ask enough questions at health care visits to be certain that this problem does not exist as well.

Child abuse is reportable by law. Nurses can initiate reporting as an independent action or through their health agency's referral network.

Methods to prevent abuse in which nurses can actively participate include teaching about the expected growth and development of children, educating teenage parents for parenting roles, and teaching empowerment, or a sense that children and adults have control of their own lives.

Sexual abuse of children can be prevented by teaching children to recognize abnormal advances and to know it is right to speak out about wrongs against them.

Abuse is a family, not an individual, problem. Therapy must include all family members to be effective.

Rape is a crime of violence, not of sexual intent. Rape victims need both short-term and long-term counseling.

CRITICAL THINKING EXERCISES

1. Marie is the 3-year-old you met at the beginning of the chapter. Although her mother told you that Marie fell from a swing, Marie has a broken forearm, a broken rib, and multiple bruises on her chest and back. Her mother tells you, "Marie isn't pretty. I guess she's also clumsy." What questions would you want to ask to determine if Marie has been abused?
2. You weigh a baby at a well child conference and discover that the infant's weight is below the sec-

ond percentile on a standardized growth chart. What questions would you want to ask the mother to see if you can account for this? What particular areas would you want to assess on a physical examination?

3. A 4-year-old girl is seen in an ambulatory clinic for a purulent vulvovaginitis. A culture reveals this is from gonorrhea. What questions would you want to ask the child to determine how she contracted this? Suppose her parents are influential people in your community. Would this influence what questions you ask?
4. Examine the National Health Goals related to child or intimate partner abuse. Most government-sponsored money for nursing research is allotted based on these goals. What would be a possible research topic to explore pertinent to the goals that would be fundable and would advance evidence-based practice?

REFERENCES

American Academy of Pediatrics: Committee on Child Abuse and Neglect. (2001). Shaken baby syndrome: Rotational cranial injuries: technical report. *Pediatrics, 108*(1), 206–210.

American Academy of Pediatrics: Committee on Child Abuse and Neglect and Committee on Children with Disabilities. (2001). Assessment of maltreatment of children with disabilities. *Pediatrics, 108*(2), 508–512.

Beers, S. R., & DeBellis, M.D. (2002). Neuropsychological function in children with maltreatment-related post-traumatic stress disorder. *American Journal of Psychiatry, 159*(3), 483–486.

Bernet, W. (2000). Child maltreatment. In H. I. Kaplan. *Comprehensive textbook of psychiatry.* Philadelphia: Lippincott Williams & Wilkins.

Christian, C. W. (2000a). Child physical abuse. In M. W. Schwartz (Ed.). *The 5-minute pediatric consult* (pp. 244–245). Philadelphia: Lippincott Williams & Wilkins.

Christian, C. W. (2000b). Failure to thrive. In M. W. Schwartz (Ed.). *The 5-minute pediatric consult* (pp. 36–37). Philadelphia: Lippincott Williams & Wilkins.

Cole, S. A. (2000). From the sexual psychopath statute to Megan's law. *Journal of the History of Medicine & Allied Sciences, 55*(3), 292–314.

Department of Health and Human Services (2000). *Healthy people 2010.* Washington, D.C.: DHHS.

DeVille, K. A., & Kopelman, L. M. (1999). Fetal protection in Wisconsin's revised child abuse law. *Journal of Law, Medicine, & Ethics, 27*(4), 332–346.

Erickson, M. J., et al. (2001). Barriers to domestic violence screening in the pediatric setting. *Pediatrics, 108*(1), 98–102.

Gaffney, K. F., et al. (2002). Early clinical assessment for harsh child discipline strategies. *MCN: American Journal of Maternal Child Nursing, 27*(1), 34–40.

Hall, D. E., et al. (2000). Evaluation of covert video surveillance in the diagnosis of Munchausen syndrome by proxy: Lessons from 41 cases. *Pediatrics, 105*(6), 1305–1312.

Hausman, C. L. (2000). Munchausen syndrome by proxy. In M. W. Schwartz (Ed.). *The 5-minute pediatric consult* (pp. 548–549). Philadelphia: Lippincott Williams & Wilkins.

Helfer, R. E., & Kempe, R. S. (1987). *The battered child.* Chicago: University of Chicago Press.

Kaplan, D. W., et al. (2001). Care of the adolescent sexual assault victim. *Pediatrics, 107*(6), 1476–1479.

Labbe, J., & Caouette, G. (2001). Recent skin injuries in normal children. *Pediatrics, 108*(2), 271–276.

Lemmey, D., et al. (2001) Intimate partner violence: Mothers' perspectives of effects on their children. *MCN: The American Journal of Maternal/Child Nursing, 26*(2), 98–103.

Lim, L. E., Gwee, K. P., & Woo, M. (2001). Men who commit statutory rape: How are they different from other rapists? *Medicine, Science & the Law, 41*(2), 147–154.

McConkey, T., Sole, M., & Holcomb, L. (2001) Assessing the sexual assault survivor. *The Nurse Practitioner, 26*(7), 28–33.

Rudd, J. M., & Herzberger, S. D. (1999). Brother-sister incest; father-daughter incest: A comparison of characteristics and consequences. *Child Abuse & Neglect, 23*(9), 915–928.

Ruscio, A. M. (2001). Predicting the child-rearing practices of mothers sexually abused in childhood. *Child Abuse & Neglect, 25*(3), 369–387.

Shanahan, M., & Donato, R. (2001). Counting the cost: Estimating the economic benefit of pedophile treatment programs. *Child Abuse & Neglect, 25*(4), 541–555.

Strathearn, L., et al. (2001). Childhood neglect and cognitive development in extremely low-birth-weight infants: A prospective study. *Pediatrics, 108*(1), 142–151.

SUGGESTED READINGS

Berlinger, J. (2001). Domestic violence: How can you make a difference. *Nursing 2001, 31*(8), 1958–1962.

Careaga, M. G., & Kerner, J. A. (2000). A gastroenterologist's approach to failure to thrive. *Pediatric Annals, 29*(9), 558–569.

Crouch, J. L., & Behl, L. E. (2001). Relationships among parental beliefs in corporal punishment, reported stress, and physical child abuse potential. *Child Abuse & Neglect, 25*(3), 413–419.

Haggerty, L. A., et al. (2001). Pregnant women's perceptions of abuse. *JOGNN: Journal of Obstetric, Gynecologic & Neonatal Nursing, 30*(3), 283–290.

Hayward, K. S., & Pehrsson, D. E. (2000). Interdisciplinary action supporting sexual assault prevention efforts in rural elementary schools. *Journal of Community Health Nursing, 17*(3), 141–150.

Halpern, C. T., et al. (2001) Partner violence among adolescents in opposite-sex romantic relationships. *American Journal of Public Health, 91*(10), 1679–1685.

Hughes, L. M., & Corbo-Richert, B. (1999). Munchausen syndrome by proxy: Literature review and implications for critical care nurses. *Critical Care Nurse, 19*(3), 1–78.

Kolko, D. J., et al. (2002). Children's perceptions of their abusive experience: Measurement and preliminary findings. *Child Maltreatment, 7*(1), 42–55.

Murry, S., Baker, A., & Lewin, L. (2001). Screening families with young children for child maltreatment potential. *Pediatric Nursing, 26*(1), 47–54.

Parkinson, G. W., Adams, R. C., & Emerling, F. G. (2001). Maternal domestic violence screening in an office-based pediatric practice. *Pediatrics, 108*(3), 43–46.

Robinson, J. R., Drotar, D., & Boutry, M. (2001). Problem-solving abilities among mothers of infants with failure to thrive. *Journal of Pediatric Psychology, 26*(1), 21–32.

56

CHAPTER

Nursing Care of the Family Coping With Long-Term or Terminal Illness

Key Terms

- anticipatory grief
- death
- grief process
- vulnerable children

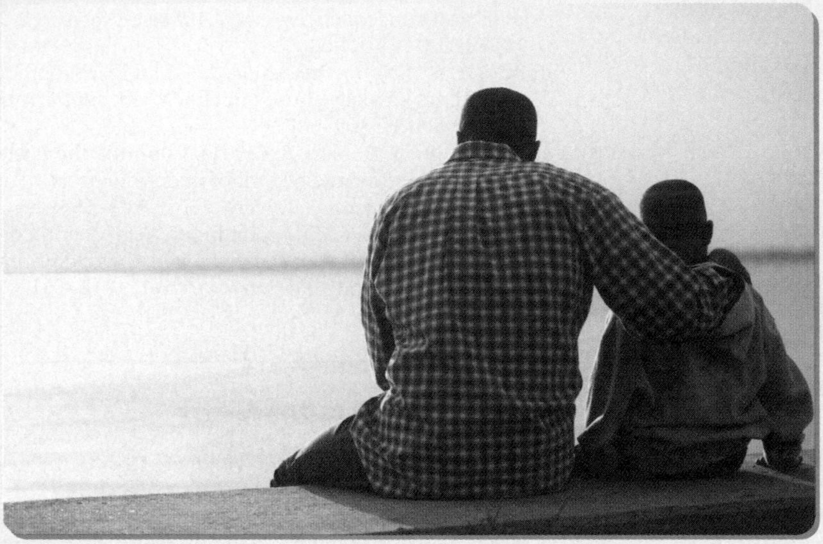

Objectives

After mastering the contents of this chapter, you should be able to:

1. Describe common concerns of parents of children with a long-term or terminal illness.
2. Assess adjustment of the child and family with a long-term or terminal illness.
3. Formulate nursing diagnoses for the child with a long-term or terminal illness.
4. Identify outcomes for the child with a long-term or terminal illness.
5. Plan nursing care for the child with a long-term or terminal illness.
6. Implement nursing care for the child with a long-term or terminal illness.
7. Evaluate outcomes for effectiveness and achievement for families whose child has a long-term or terminal illness.
8. Identify National Health Goals related to children with long-term or terminal illnesses that nurses could be instrumental in helping the nation achieve.
9. Identify areas related to the care of the child with a long-term or terminal illness that could benefit from additional nursing research or application of evidence-based practice.
10. Use critical thinking to analyze ways that nursing care of the child with a long-term or terminal illness can be more family-centered.
11. Integrate knowledge of long-term and terminal illness in children with nursing process to achieve quality maternal and child health nursing care.

Charlie is a 3-year-old who has had a relapse after 18 months of chemotherapy for leukemia. You meet him in an emergency room because he has developed a severe cough and high fever. He is diagnosed as having pneumonia. "He's been so sick for so long," his mother tells you. "And he's been through so much. How could he develop something else?" A fellow nurse asks you, "How could his parents let him get so sick before they brought him in? How could they not have known he was seriously sick?" What could be a reason his parents did not bring him for care sooner? What would you want to talk to them about?

Previous chapters described the growth and development of well children and the care of children with specific disorders. This chapter adds information about the care of chronically and terminally ill children. This is important information because it builds a base for care and health teaching and support for the parents and child.

After you've studied the chapter, answer the Critical Thinking Exercises at the end of the chapter and then access the on-line study activities (http://connection.lww.com) *to further sharpen your skills and test your knowledge.*

When children have acute illnesses, parents and the children may be frightened by the sudden onset and severity of symptoms. Because human beings have a great capacity for coping with stress, however, they can usually adjust to the strain of disrupted daily routines, hospital visits, and home care as long as they are given adequate support.

When a child's illness becomes long term or is one that can be projected to have a terminal outcome, a family's capacity to cope can become stretched beyond its limits. Support is essential for the family if it is to survive under this level of pressure and stress.

People cope with situations depending on their perception of the event, the type and kind of support they receive from people around them, and the ways that they have found successful in coping with stressful situations in the past. When working with parents of children with a long-term or terminal illness, discovering how the parents perceive the problem, what resources they have available, and how they plan to use these resources are crucial in planning nursing care.

Whether the medical diagnosis involves a permanent disability or impending death, a parent's first response will be grief. The parent has either lost the "perfect" child imagined during pregnancy or the well child he or she had up to the time of diagnosis. Depending on their age and maturity, children may also respond with a grief response. National Health Goals related to the care of the child with a long-term or terminal illness are shown in the Focus on National Health Goals box.

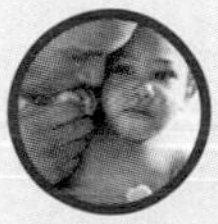

FOCUS ON NATIONAL HEALTH GOALS

Long-term illness or early death in children is a major cost to the nation and individual families because it has the potential to reduce the earning power and contribution of future citizens. A number of National Health Goals address this:

- Reduce the proportion of children and adolescents with disabilities who are reported to be sad, unhappy, or depressed from 31% to 17%.
- Increase the proportion of children and youth with disabilities who spend at least 80% of their time in regular education programs from 45% to 60%.
- Reduce infant deaths from a baseline of 7.2/100,000 to a target rate of 4.5/100,000.
- Reduce the death rate for children 1 to 4 years of age to no more than 18.6/100,000 children from a baseline of 34.6/100,000 and for children aged 5 to 9 years to 12.3/100,000 from a baseline of 17.7/100,000.
- Reduce the death rate for children 10 to 14 years of age to no more than 16.8/100,000 from a baseline of 22/100,000 and the death rate for adolescents 15 to 19 years of age from 70.6/100,000 to 39.8/100,000 (DHHS, 2000).

Nurses can be instrumental in helping the nation achieve these goals by educating women to seek care for themselves during pregnancy so congenital anomalies, a common cause of infant morbidity and mortality, are reduced and to seek immunizations for their children so diseases that can lead to long-term illness, such as rubeola and meningitis, can be prevented. Nursing research on the following areas would further these goals: What are special techniques for preparing children who are physically challenged to be more independent? How can children who use a wheelchair maintain a high sense of self-esteem? What specific measures are most helpful to parents when they learn their child has a terminal illness?

NURSING PROCESS OVERVIEW

For Care of the Family Coping With a Long-Term or Terminal Illness

Assessment

Because a family's coping abilities are best assessed gradually, over a period of many contacts, nurses' assessments of the degree of coping are often the most thorough and meaningful of all health care providers.

Observing children at home, where they are most comfortable, or at school in a familiar atmosphere often reveals a great deal more about their coping potential than does a formal test situation. Often a toy offered by a parent, sister, or brother will be grasped and manipulated by a child with a chronic disability; the same toy offered by a stranger will not be accepted. Children with a long-term illness, on the whole, have probably been through many tests and procedures in the diagnosis of their disorder; they may have reason to think of health care providers as hurting people, not people for whom they wish to achieve. It may be possible to change their perception by maintaining a reassuring, gentle manner during assessment and subsequent care procedures.

Nursing Diagnosis

Long-term illness takes many forms. A condition that requires daily attention, such as diabetes (insulin injections), but that is stabilized may not be as stressful to parents as an illness, such as muscular dystrophy, that slowly progresses in severity. In the former, although the child and family must adjust their lifestyle to incorporate the child's daily needs, they feel they have some control over the course of the illness and the child's overall health. In the latter, the child and family can feel powerless, lacking any ability to alter the course of the disease; they must simply wait for the next acute crisis to develop. Nursing diagnoses for children with long-term or terminal illnesses should address both the child and the family as a whole. Some examples of nursing diagnoses when a long-term illness is present are as follows:

- Interrupted family processes related to recent diagnosis of long-term or chronic illness in older child
- Compromised family coping related to child's disability
- Disabling family coping related to parents' inability to accept child's long-term illness
- Anticipatory grieving related to chronicity of the child's illness
- Risk for delayed growth and development related to lack of age-appropriate stimulation because of disability

New issues develop when the child's disorder is considered terminal. The family must learn to accept not only the child's illness, but also its eventual outcome. Some examples of nursing diagnoses when a terminal illness is present follow:

- Hopelessness related to steady progression of child's disease
- Anticipatory grieving related to child's terminal illness
- Powerlessness related to inability to prolong child's life
- Decisional conflict related to treatment options and choice of setting for child's final care

Outcome Identification and Planning

Be certain when planning care that the outcomes established are realistic. You probably cannot alter the course of a child's illness, but you can help parents cope with the illness or impending death and aftermath.

Parents who have not yet accepted the seriousness of their child's illness may make plans for a child that the child cannot possibly accomplish. These parents are holding on to the hope that their child will eventually be cured or restored to full health. Sometimes this level of denial is essential to the parents' ability to cope with the child's daily needs and the needs of the rest of the family. They may feel they must shield the child or other family members from the truth. Focusing on hopeful but realistic outcomes, such as the desire that the child will go through the day without experiencing pain or that the child will learn how to move about independently in a wheelchair, are helpful in moving a family forward toward final, realistic acceptance of a child's illness.

Implementation

When children have a long-term or terminal illness, parents may begin to overprotect them so much that they neglect to encourage their growth. They may forget to provide play materials or other stimulation appropriate for their age. Helping parents to look at their child's capabilities and arranging appropriate activities for him or her facilitate parents' acceptance of the diagnosis and the road ahead. Suggestions for helping children achieve developmental milestones are discussed with each age group in previous chapters.

Helping parents to learn better coping strategies and teaching them ways to remember to give medication for a number of years, ways to maintain quality care without becoming exhausted, and the importance of maintaining a lifestyle of their own are other important measures.

The following organizations are helpful for referral:

- Candlelighters Childhood Cancer Foundation (*www.candlelighters.org*)
- The Compassionate Friends (*www.compassionatefriends.org*)
- National Association of School Psychologists (*www.nasponline.org*)
- Centers for Loss in Multiple Births (CLIMB) (*www.climb-support.org*)

Outcome Evaluation

Children with long-term or terminal illness need periodic follow-up care because plans made when children are newborns may no longer be suitable as soon as the child becomes a toddler. Plans made in the early school years may need to be modified by the time the child is 12 years old, and they must change again with adolescence. In addition to follow-up of their specific therapy by a specialty clinic, children also need routine health maintenance care. Otherwise, children are well protected from the complications of a special illness but unprotected from common childhood illnesses that could be even more devastating.

Evaluation of whether outcomes for the family of a child who died were met helps to strengthen your planning with the next dying child you care for, improve your self-esteem, and build confidence in your ability to care for dying children. Evaluation will reveal discrepancies between the wish and the reality of care, identifying areas you need to strengthen to grow as a health care provider. Some examples suggesting achievement of outcomes may include:

- Parents state realistic plans for their child regarding school placement.
- Parents state they have been able to deal with their grief over child's diagnosis to maintain normal family functioning.

- Parents state they are able to cope with present stressors.
- Child states he or she is aware illness is chronic (long-term) but thinks of herself as a person able to accomplish many things in life.

THE CHILD WITH A LONG-TERM ILLNESS

Because families have different resources and everyone reacts to situations differently, each child with a long-term illness and his or her family need to be assessed for their potential to cope with the illness and provide necessary care. Through such assessment, appropriate interventions to help the family adapt can be started early in the course of the illness.

The Parents' Adjustment

Children have difficulty adjusting to events without good role-modeling from their parents. Thus, assessment begins with a look at how well the parents are responding to the diagnosis of a long-term illness.

Grief Response

Parents can be expected to experience a **grief process** or regulated steps in grieving when they are told their child will be physically or cognitively challenged or is terminally ill. The most commonly accepted steps or stages of grief are those outlined by Kübler-Ross (1969). Table 56-1 summarizes these stages. Most parents with a child who is physically or cognitively challenged never arrive at the final stage of acceptance; for parents with a terminally ill child, this may come only with the child's death.

During the first stage of grief (shock or denial), parents are unable to plan past immediate or short-term actions (learning to change a dressing or which pills to give each day). Trying to establish long-term outcomes at this point (what type of school the child will attend, the vocations that are open to him or her) is rarely productive because this all must be done again when parents are truly ready to look this far ahead. During the second stage, anger, parents may be unwilling to learn (the whole thing is so unfair; planning is asking too much of them; how can they trust you? If you were really helpful, you would cure their child). This becomes a time of waiting also, so be sure to refrain from giving any advice. During the bargaining stage of grief, parents are still not ready for planning. If their bargain is fulfilled (let their child be able to walk, and they will spend the rest of their life doing good), they see the plans they make now (such as purchasing a wheelchair) would have to be modified later.

During the next stage of grief, depression, parents are ready to make plans but need a great deal of help in planning because they feel so fatigued. Be careful in working with people who are depressed that you do not totally plan *for* them rather than *with* them. Many parents of children who are physically or cognitively challenged have low self-esteem (they believe if they were really good people, they would have had a normal child). This makes them feel that your suggestions must be better than any they could make. After they return home, however, they are the people who must live with these plans and so should participate in making them. Young adults who are physically or cognitively challenged show an above-average incidence of depression, probably from the chronic stress of the disability on their life, part of which occurs from poor planning (Bechtold et al., 2001).

Some parents need guidance in making plans to avoid becoming so self-sacrificing that the needs and wishes of the spouse and other children are ignored. For example, the parents spend every waking moment with the ill child. Being a martyr is a way of easing guilt, a part of grief bargaining, a way of proving that they are equal to others—perhaps even the best parents in the entire world. These parents need time to talk about possible reasons why they feel they must push themselves in this manner. Perhaps they can find a middle-of-the-road approach to a child's care that allows time for all family members. Helping them plan a respite from the care of a sick child, such as an evening out while a babysitter cares for the child, is a part of this.

TABLE 56.1 Stages of Grief

STAGE	PARENTS' REACTION	DESCRIPTION
1	Denial	Parents have difficulty realizing what has occurred. They ask, "How could this have happened?"
2	Anger	Parents react to the injustice of being singled out this way. They say, "It isn't fair this is happening."
3	Bargaining	Parents attempt to work out a "deal" to buy their way out of the situation. They say, "If my child gets well, I'll devote the rest of my life to doing good."
4	Depression	Parents begin to face what is happening. They feel sad and unprotected.
5	Acceptance	Acceptance is being able to say, "Yes, this is happening, and it is all right that it is happening." With a child with long-term illness, parents may never reach this stage but will always remain in the chronic sorrow of the depression stage.

(Modified from Kübler-Ross, E. [1969]. *On death and dying.* New York: Macmillan; with permission.)

WHAT IF? What if you arrange for a parent to spend an afternoon shopping so she can have some respite time away from an ill child, and she spends the time cleaning her kitchen cupboards instead? How would you respond? Would you consider this a good use of respite time?

By the time a child who is physically or cognitively challenged is of school age, parents should begin to make some concrete plans as to who will care for the child when they die. This is very difficult for parents; it asks them to contemplate their own mortality (something that people rarely want to do) and the vulnerability of their children when it occurs. They might consult with family members about guardianship and with a lawyer to help them write a will that will provide future caretaking and economic support for the child.

Factors Influencing Parental Adjustment

Certain circumstances appear to increase parents' difficulty in adjusting to a disabling or long-term illness in their child. These include the degree and timing of the illness, the experience of the parents, and the availability of support people.

Degree of Illness. The seriousness of an illness obviously affects the ability of parents to adjust. A child who needs total care will require a much more radical readjustment of the parents' lives than will a child who needs additional speech therapy for only an hour a day. In most instances, the parents' perception of the child's illness is as important as the child's condition (Fig. 56-1). A parent who envisioned a son as someday being an Olympic runner, for example, may perceive a son with developmental hip dysplasia as having a serious physical challenge. A parent whose mental image of the child is that of a lawyer doing mainly desk work may not view the hip problem as a serious illness.

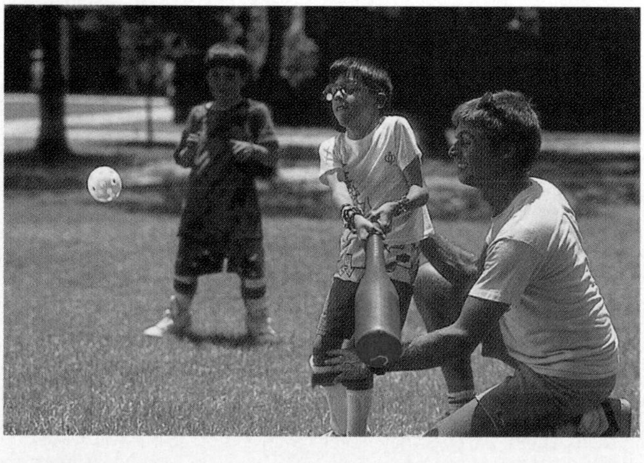

FIGURE 56.1 A parent's perception of a child's disability is important to how well the family adjusts. Often it is easier to accept a disability that allows for greater functioning in everyday activities.

Many parents are not aware of the mental image that they carry of their child, an image that began to form the moment the woman realized she was pregnant. Hidden desires are often revealed if you ask parents, "If things could have been different, what kind of person would you have liked your child to be?" A parent who answers, "a kind person" can still have that wish fulfilled, no matter what the degree of illness. A parent who says, "I always assumed my child would take over my business some day" may have some major mental readjustments to make.

Whether an illness is noticeable (spastic cerebral palsy) or not noticeable (controlled seizures) also can make a difference in how parents adjust to the illness. A mother who takes her child with cerebral palsy shopping (a child who walks unsteadily and knocks over a display) may hear other shoppers say, "Wouldn't you think a mother would watch her child more carefully?" On days that her child uses a wheelchair, however, shoppers' comments are more apt to be, "Poor little thing. Isn't it wonderful that his mother brings him shopping with her?" She is happy to have a signal (the wheelchair) that announces her child is different and cannot be held to standards for other children. Other parents might be more grateful that a child's illness is not a visible one: it makes the illness seem lesser in extent, and thus easier for them to accept.

Onset of the Illness. Whether a condition is apparent at birth (e.g., a myelomeningocele) or occurs at a later time (the child is struck by a car at school age) may make a difference in the parents' ability to adjust. For most parents, never having had a well child makes the child's illness easier to accept (Balling & McCubbin, 2001).

Effect of Parental Experience. First-time parents may have more difficulty caring for a child with a long-term illness than older, more experienced parents do because all phases of parenting are more difficult for them. They might have difficulty evaluating how much activity a child needs or what toys are appropriate, for example. On the other hand, first-time parents, because they have no preconceived opinions, may be more flexible than other parents. A young parent who has just this one child may have more time to spend in a daily exercise program than does a parent with five children.

Availability of Support People. The family that has few close friends and lives some distance from relatives is apt to have more difficulty adjusting to illness in a child than will the family that has close support people. People who have secondary support systems in the community, such as an organization for parents of children who are physically or cognitively challenged or a local church or synagogue, usually do better than parents without these resources. People who are able to use health care resources effectively adjust more easily than those who cannot do so. The ability to use health care resources depends on a number of factors, including:

- Transportation (it is difficult to take a child in a 50-lb cast on a bus)
- Language barriers (it is frustrating to go for care and be unable to make your needs known)

- Finances and insurance coverage (it is frustrating to be told you need to see a specialist when you have no money or your health coverage does not pay for one)
- Past experience with health care providers (if the best advice that has been given to the parents up to this point has been, "Take your baby home and treat him as near normally as possible," the parents may not see health care providers as a source of useful information or help)

Life Events. A child's illness generally appears to be more acute at times the child would normally reach developmental milestones: at 12 months, when the baby should be taking his or her first step and is not; 6 years, when the child should begin school; first communion or bar mitzvah; time for a driver's license; or voting age. When the child does not reach these milestones, parents are reminded of the illness in a particularly painful way.

Factors that indicate that a family will probably be able to adjust to caring for a child with a long-term illness are summarized in Table 56-2.

The Child's Adjustment

The child's reaction to being physically or cognitively challenged or having a long-term illness is strongly influenced by the family's reaction to the illness (Knafl & Zoeller, 2000). Family reactions may range from overprotectiveness to rejection and from denial to acceptance. The child's adjustment may also be influenced by peers and other support people, such as school personnel or health care providers. Social exclusion, discrimination, and physical barriers make it difficult for the child to adjust to a physical challenge or long-term illness. On the other hand, inclusion in school and social activities, acceptance by peers and support people, and the ability to function as normally as possible help the child adjust.

The child's ability to cope is further influenced by his or her personal attitude and temperament, self-concept, age and development, understanding of the condition, and degree of the disorder. As the child grows and life situations change, the child's ability to cope may improve or worsen. For example, an adolescent who is physically challenged may become more optimistic about her condition because she is successfully working at her first job; another adolescent may become angered by his deteriorating condition because he is suddenly confined to a wheelchair.

Nursing interventions to help the child better adjust include encouraging optimal growth and development (see Chapters 28 to 32), promoting self-care activities, enhancing self-esteem, preventing social isolation, providing health teaching, and aiding the child and family in accepting the child's condition.

Siblings' Adjustment

Siblings' reactions to a child with a long-term or terminal illness may be influenced by a number of factors; however, their reactions are most profoundly affected by the reactions and perceptions of the parents. Without counseling, they may react with jealousy, anger, hostility, resentment, competition, guilt, or withdrawal. They may feel that they take second place to the child who needs more care. These reactions are common when parents focus most of their attention on the ill child, allow the health problem and treatment to disrupt family life significantly, or grant the ill child special privileges and minimal discipline.

With counseling and support, siblings can develop acceptance, care, concern, and cooperation. Such reactions are common when parents make it a point to set aside time each day for special activities with the well siblings (playing a table game or walking in the park with them; teaching a child to swim), carefully explain the condition and the necessity for special care, include the siblings in the care of the ill child, provide the siblings with respite from care if needed, and establish realistic rules for all family members.

At any one time, the siblings may experience a mixture of these feelings. For example, if a boy's parents must take his sister for chemotherapy during his swim meet, the boy may feel both resentment that his parents missed the meet and sadness that his sister could not compete in that meet or any others as well.

TABLE 56.2 Factors Easing Parental Adjustment to a Child's Long-Term Illness

FACTOR	RATIONALE
Available support people	Caring for a child is a series of crises during which support people become very important.
A strong marital bond between the parents	A marriage partner can serve as the strongest support person.
A good relationship between the child's parents and their parents	The parents (because they had good care) have a firm sense of trust and the ability to give care to another.
The child is other than the first-born	The parents have had practice parenting.
The family lives close to shopping, schools, and transportation	The family is not isolated.
The family has a strong religious faith	Secondary support systems are important in times of stress.
The parents are told of the child's disability as soon as possible	A handicap is easier to accept if the parents never thought of the child as totally well.

The Nurse and the Ill Child

Caring for children with long-term illnesses can be a stressful role for nurses (Ford & Turner, 2001). To help parents and children with a long-term illness, learn specific aspects of the child's condition and the possible complications that could occur. Over a period of years, parents become experts on the care of a child with a particular condition (see Focus on Communication). This can make them grow impatient with health care providers who appear to be unaware of things that they know well. When young children are seen at an ambulatory care setting or admitted to a hospital for care, review with parents their typical way of carrying out a procedure so that you can continue to care for their child in the same way. As the child grows older, do this same review with the child. On the other hand, be available to show a parent or the child an easier way to do something if it seems appropriate. Frankly admitting to parents, "You're more familiar with Jennifer's care than I am; you'll have to teach me some things" is a refreshing approach; it not only allows parents to feel confidence in you (you are honest), but it also increases their self-esteem (they are knowledgeable people).

FOCUS ON COMMUNICATION

Samuel Circuso is a 1-year-old who was born with a number of congenital anomalies. He is admitted to the hospital for a second-stage revision of a colostomy. Although his abdominal skin was free of erythema on admission, 4 hours later you notice it is reddened, and Samuel cries when you touch the irritated skin.

Less Effective Communication

Nurse: Look at Samuel's skin. It looks really red and sore.
Mrs. Circuso: I think that's from the adhesive tape.
Nurse: Oh, I don't think so. I tape this way all the time.
Mrs. Circuso: I never use it, even on myself.
Nurse: Well, it usually works really well. I'll ask the doctor what she recommends.

More Effective Communication

Nurse: Look at Samuel's skin. It looks so red and sore.
Mrs. Circuso: I think that's from the adhesive tape.
Nurse: Oh, has Samuel had this type of reaction before?
Mrs. Circuso: Yes, that is why I never use it, even on myself. It always causes such a reaction.
Nurse: Of course, that makes perfect sense. I should have asked you earlier what you thought was causing the problem.

It is easy to believe that a fellow nurse who has spent a great deal of time caring for a child has become an expert in the child's care. It is often more difficult to remember that a parent can easily become this type of expert too. Asking parents for their input not only can simplify care, but also adds to the parents' feeling of self-esteem, improving their parenting.

Also be familiar with the community resources available for children with long-term illnesses. Advising parents to see a dentist who specializes in caring for children with cerebral palsy when there is no one of that description less than 200 miles away, for example, is not only unhelpful but is also actually destructive. It raises expectations in parents that cannot be met—accentuating, not solving, a problem.

Sometimes parents of children with long-term illnesses do not comply well with instructions or do not keep health care appointments consistently. This failure to comply usually is related to their adjustment to the illness. As long as denial, anger, bargaining, or depression is functioning (and there is rarely a parent who has successfully moved completely through these stages of grief to acceptance), coming for health care or evaluation is a major demand on parents. Each visit is more a reminder of the child's illness than a time of reassuring health assessment.

Developmental Tasks

Children with long-term illnesses often do not meet developmental milestones on schedule; achieving developmental tasks can be very difficult. When you are helping parents teach a child who is physically or cognitively challenged a developmental task, such as toilet training or using a spoon, help them to break the task down into its component parts (e.g., reach for the spoon; grasp it; move it toward you; push it under the chosen food; lift it toward the mouth). This allows parents to appreciate that they are asking the child to do a task that, although it looks easy, actually encompasses 20 or more coordinated motions. Helping them learn this technique allows them to be patient in teaching all tasks in future years.

Caring for a child with a long-term illness is never easy for parents. Support from interested health care personnel at all stages of the process is of great importance to their acceptance of their child's illness and their ability to give care (Lindeke et al., 2001). Ways to help children who are physically challenged achieve developmental tasks are discussed in Chapters 28 to 32. These include exposing them to normal events during a hospital stay or an ambulatory health care visit (Fig. 56-2).

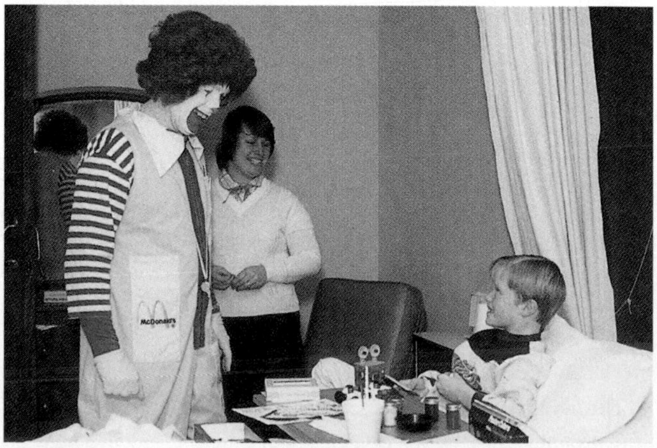

FIGURE 56.2 Ronald McDonald, a familiar face to many children, visits a young boy with a long-term illness. This helps him keep active and in touch with usual events during hospitalization.

Education

Children with a long-term illness often need special education programs or at least separate hours of individualized instruction to achieve in school. Most of these children benefit from preschool programs; these programs offer them a head start on school adjustment and learning. Children with a long-term illness tend to miss school more often than do their healthier classmates because of health care visits, and exacerbations of the illness can easily cause them to fall behind in school unless individualized plans to keep them with their school group are made. By federal law (Public Law 99-457, Education of the Handicapped Amendment), a school system must provide educational opportunities in the least structured setting possible for physically and cognitively challenged children, beginning with preschool. You may have to be a strong child advocate to see that the best educational program available is being provided for an individual child.

Home Care

Most children with a long-term illness receive care at home today; planning for this care is discussed in Chapter 35. Important aspects to consider include the best school setting, ways to involve the family in community activities, ways to include the child in a play group (children as young as preschool age may not choose an ill child as a playmate), ability to allow the child to stay alone for part of each day, and future plans, such as preparing a child for puberty or college.

Many parents today seek complementary or alternative therapies for children with long-term illnesses. Ask what therapies and medications they are using to document the full extent of treatment that the child is receiving (Sandler, 2001).

✔ CHECKPOINT QUESTIONS

1. What are the stages of a grief reaction as identified by Kübler-Ross?
2. Should you encourage a child with a long-term illness to attend a regular or special classroom?
3. How can parents help siblings better accept a child with a long-term illness?

THE CHILD WHO IS TERMINALLY ILL

Caring for a child who is terminally ill can be one of the hardest tasks in nursing. Most people are raised to accept the fact that elderly people die, but they have also lived a long life. Most people can accept the death of middle-aged people with the same philosophy—they experienced at least a portion of their life. It is often more difficult to accept the death of children because they have had so little opportunity to live. This can make it so difficult to work though your own feelings about a child's dying that you have difficulty caring for the child or supporting the parents (see Focus on Evidence-Based Practice).

FOCUS ON EVIDENCE-BASED PRACTICE

How Stressful for Nurses Is Caring for Children Who Are Dying?

A number of researchers have examined this problem because it is such an important one for the well-being of nurses involved in the care of children with a chronic or terminal illness.

To answer the question, Costello and Trinder-Brook (2001) used questionnaires, focus groups, and individual interviews to determine how 44 nurses who had cared for children dying in the hospital had been affected by the experience. Nurses reported that they experienced a sense of guilt and failure following the death of a child despite having no rational explanation to justify the feelings. They saw their role as needing to give support not only to the child but also to the child's parents to help them prepare for the death of the child. They also reported that although they gave this form of support to parents, there were few sources of support at the same level available to them when the child died.

Barnes (2001) conducted a literature review to determine the causes and effects of staff stress in a children's hospice. Results of this study revealed that the main causes of stress were related to conflicts within the staff group. Poor relationships with the child's family as well as the inability to relieve distressing symptoms in the child were also reported as common sources of stress. Methods that nurses used to relieve stress were teamwork, good communication, and the homelike atmosphere provided by the hospice setting. Staff support groups may or may not be beneficial, depending on their quality. The researcher concluded that nurses must be encouraged to take some responsibility for preventing and relieving stress themselves.

These are important studies for nurses because they help identify some of the reasons for stress that occur when caring for dying children. Both point out the importance of nurses taking active steps to reduce their own stress caused by this type of care.

Barnes, K. (2001). Staff stress in the children's hospice: Causes, effects and coping strategies. *International Journal of Palliative Nursing, 7* (5), 248–254; Costello, J., & Trinder-Brook, A. (2000). Children's nurses' experiences of caring for dying children in hospital. *Paediatric Nursing, 12* (6), 28–31.

Parental Grief Responses

Each family reacts in a unique way to the diagnosis of terminal illness in a child; the reaction is strongly influenced by culture (Ross, 2001). Being aware of the usual grief response that occurs in anticipation of a child's death helps in recognizing a response as grief and supporting a family through this very difficult period (Zeitlin, 2001).

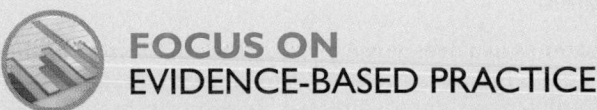

Denial

A parent's usual response to a diagnosis of a terminal illness in a child is denial, the first stage of grief (see Table 56-1). Although people are aware that children die, most proceed through life thinking, "it won't happen to my child." When it does, they respond with disbelief or denial. The likelihood of this response is enhanced by the fact that many terminal illnesses, such as brain tumor or leukemia, begin insidiously ("How can a few black-and-blue marks on her arms be the symptoms of a potentially terminal disease?").

How the parents handle this initial disbelief has a great deal to do with their relationship with health care personnel. If they have trusted health care personnel up to this point, they may be able to accept a diagnosis without questioning any further. If they do not have this relationship, they may feel the need to obtain a second opinion. This often involves considerable expense, but for many parents it is a necessary step in moving past this first reaction. Parents who feel a need for a third, fourth, or fifth opinion may be having an unusually difficult time resolving a "surely not me" response. They need a factual explanation of why it is certain their child has this disease, such as a copy of the blood report or the pathologist's biopsy report. They need time to talk about how they feel. Only when people can grasp that the illness is definitely present can they begin to accept that the disease will ultimately prove fatal.

During the stage of denial, parents' actions may be inappropriate to the child's condition. They may talk of an "upset stomach from the flu" when the child is vomiting blood or "his cold" when the child has cystic fibrosis. It is easy to view such denial as a step that should be hurried (parents cannot begin to deal with the problem as long as they deny that there is a problem). This is true, but neither can they deal with a problem when it hurts as much as this does. Denial is a temporary pain-relief measure that is a necessary step on the way to acceptance.

Anger

Parents can be expected to enter a stage of anger soon—a change from "Surely not me" to "It's not right that this is happening to me." When parents are angry about a diagnosis, they may be unable to direct their anger appropriately. They may find themselves angry with the child (scolding him or her for crying during a painful procedure). One parent may be angry with the other parent (criticizing him or her for reckless driving or for eating a fattening food for lunch). They may be angry with you (for not answering the child's call light immediately). They may be angry with the medical, x-ray, laboratory, and dietary staff or with the entire health care system. It can be difficult to react to this kind of angry attack because it seems unjustified (after all, you came as soon as you could). Be certain that your first reaction is not to be angry in return. This could result in your avoiding the child's room for the rest of the day to resist undergoing that kind of unfair criticism again, and therefore not meeting the child's basic need to have support people around him or her.

A more therapeutic reaction is to accept this angry response as the stage of grief that it is and respond accordingly: "I'm sorry it seemed to take me so long to answer your call bell, but you seem angry about more than just the light. Would it help to talk about it?"

Parents may "shop" for another health care provider during the stage of anger, although their reaction will depend to a great extent on their experience with death in the past and the meaning this child has to them. Because grandparents live longer today, for some parents fatal illness in a child is their first contact with death. Another influential factor is that different children mean different things to parents. A child born to them at a happy time in life can represent all that is good and happy in their life, so loss of this child could also mean loss of all the joy the child represents.

When you ask grieving parents to talk, therefore, they may talk not about the child, but about how they felt when a parent died, how hard their job is for them, or how they feel their marriage is failing. This is part of grief: gathering resources, reworking stress from the past, and arming themselves to face stress in the near future. Parents often receive support from other parents on the hospital unit whose children also are terminally ill. They are helped by seeing parents of other children adjusting to approaching death—or if not adjusting, at least functioning in what passes for a normal manner.

Bargaining

Although not everyone progresses through a grief response in a linear fashion, instead going back and forth between stages, bargaining is often the next stage to occur. Bargaining is an intermediate step in grief, a time when parents try to correct what is happening by making a bargain to be better people (a change from "This isn't right" to "I can make it right"). They vow to be better people or to function in a different way in exchange for their child's life. When parents realize that bargaining is ineffective, they are at a very low point: they have been let down not only by health care providers, but also by the superior power with whom they tried to bargain. They may need more support when bargaining fails than at any other point.

Depression

When parents have passed through stages of denial, anger, and bargaining, a further step occurs: developing awareness of the true meaning of what is happening, with accompanying depression. This is a change from "I can make it not happen" to "It is happening." Behavior such as crying is the most common sign that this stage has been reached. Parents may ask more questions about care, procedures, or medications than before. Be careful that you do not interpret this questioning as criticism. Parents are asking why a child must have continuous dialysis not to criticize care, but because this is the first time they are fully aware of its serious implication.

Parents may work through the expected loss of a child by talking about their plans for the child, the kind of child he or she was, or how the child was doing in school. They may suddenly shower him or her with expensive gifts or trips. They may have a great deal of difficulty leaving the child after visiting hours. On the surface, this reaction appears to be a step backward (they were accepting the diagnosis so well; now they seem demanding and overwhelmed by it). Actually, this is the first time they have actually begun to appreciate the diagnosis and what it means.

At about this stage, parents need to think about preparing other children in the family for the death of the ill child. If the ill child is hospitalized and siblings are not allowed to visit, they may interpret this as meaning that death is such a horrible sight that they are not allowed to be exposed to it, rather than that visiting is against the hospital rules. You may need to advocate for sibling visitation to overcome this concern.

Some siblings feel responsible for the death of the ill child. They may have wished the child dead, for example, so that they could have a room all by themselves or so they could have the child's bicycle. They were told not to wrestle with the ill sibling, and they did anyway. These children need assurance that wishing for something does not make it come true, and that the sibling's death is uncontrollable: it will happen no matter what they or their parents did or will do.

Acceptance

The acceptance stage of the grief process is resolution that the child will die (a change from "This is happening" to "It's all right that this is happening"). Few parents reach this stage by the time of the child's death; grief work will need to continue for years past the time of the death until this stage is reached.

Parental Coping Responses

Throughout the stages of grieving, parents will be developing important coping mechanisms to see them through this crisis. They may have already learned to cope positively with their child's illness and treatment measures, but the determination that the illness is terminal requires additional adjustments. Promoting the development of positive coping strategies while being sensitive to the unique needs of each family member is an important nursing responsibility. It may be difficult to determine when a coping strategy is truly helpful or when it has become maladaptive. For instance, seeking information, such as surfing the Internet and asking to have medical library access, is generally a very useful strategy for parents with ill children: knowing what to expect reduces anxiety. Some parents, however, continue these seeking procedures past the point at which information is helpful to them. They may believe that if they look hard enough, they'll discover a way to cure their child (prolonged denial), or they may "overintellectualize" their child's illness and impending death to block feelings of sadness.

Problem-solving is always an effective coping strategy as long as the parents are realistic about which problems they can solve. Seeking the support of others, including health care providers and families with similar needs, is another positive strategy to encourage; the nurse can provide the names of support groups or individual families (with their permission) who have gone through similar experiences. Nurses may also need to help parents who are not comfortable accepting the help of others learn how to do so or simply learn how to feel comfortable expressing their feelings to others.

Assuring parents that their child will be kept comfortable and will not die in pain can be extremely comforting. Parents may also be able to cope by searching for the meaning of their child's impending death in philosophical, spiritual, or religious terms. For these parents, body organ donation may be a meaningful way to give themselves some solace that their child will in some way continue to live and contribute to others.

Anticipatory Grief

If a child dies suddenly, such as in a car crash, the parents' grief response begins only with the actual death. Most parents, however, have some warning that death is expected, so they begin a preparatory or **anticipatory grief** phase in which they gradually incorporate the reality of their child's fate into their thoughts. Such anticipatory mourning prepares parents for their child's death and spares them the abrupt, devastating, intolerable grief reaction that comes to parents whose child dies suddenly from trauma, such as a car accident, or from sudden infant death syndrome (see Focus on Nursing Care Planning).

Although anticipatory grief does not shield the parents from experiencing renewed grief once their child has died, it can be a very useful process for them. A danger of anticipatory grief is that a parent may reach the acceptance stage of the grief process too far in advance of the child's death. If this happens, parents may accept the child's death so thoroughly that they begin to treat the child as if he or she had already died. They stop visiting. When they do visit, they may spend most of their time visiting other children on the unit or sitting in the waiting room talking to other parents. When once they spent time comforting their child, now they may fail to rock or touch the child as much. They may clean out the child's room and throw out or give away toys. Gradually they are drawing back from emotional attachment to shield themselves from the abrupt, stabbing pain that death will bring.

Children need a great deal of support if this happens, just as they did during the initial denial stage. Parents cannot help that the grief process did not time itself to coincide exactly with the child's death. They need understanding and not criticism for this reaction.

For some parents, when the child actually dies, the event may be anticlimactic. They have anticipated death so long that when it does occur, they cannot believe that it has actually happened. They may be so used to thinking constantly about their child's needs and having their child dependent on them that they do not know what to do. Some parents are reluctant to leave the hospital this final time. Leaving with the child's possessions is the step that will make the death real.

The Vulnerable or Fragile Child Syndrome

When anticipatory grief proceeds so effectively that parents begin to think of a youngster as already dead and then the child does not die, parents may find that their

FOCUS ON *Nursing Care Planning*

A FAMILY OF A CHILD WHO IS DYING

An 8-year-old girl diagnosed with an inoperable brain tumor is receiving hospice care at home.

Assessment: 8-year-old girl with history of brain tumor treated with radiation therapy and chemotherapy without results. Child considered terminal. Parents requesting no further treatment. "She's been through so much already. We wanted her to die at home with her family around her."

Child cachexic. Physiologic parameters deteriorating. Skin cool, damp, and mottled. Pulse rate 62 and weak; respirations 8. Rattling sounds noted from chest. Responsive only to deep pain stimuli. Parents and siblings (10-year-old brother and 6-year-old sister) at bedside.

Nursing Diagnosis: Anticipatory grieving related to impending death of child

Outcome Identification: Family members will demonstrate ability to cope with child's death.

Outcome Evaluation: Family members express feelings about anticipated death; demonstrate positive coping mechanisms.

Interventions	Rationale
1. Stay with the family and sit with them quietly if they prefer not to talk; allow them to cry. Arrange for visit by clergy if desired.	1. Staying with the family demonstrates caring and concern for their well-being and wishes and offers support. A visit by clergy provides the family with spiritual support.
2. Inform the family about what to expect. Explore their expectations and clarify any misconceptions.	2. Providing information helps to ease the family's fears and anxiety about the unknown.
3. Provide for the child's comfort, including positioning, turning, changing linens, applying lotion to her skin, moistening her lips, and alleviating any pain. Allow family members to provide care as desired without forcing them.	3. Providing comfort to the child is comforting to the family. Allowing family participation in care provides them with some sense of control over the situation, decreasing their feelings of powerlessness.
4. Allow family members to express their feelings. Listen to them and support their reactions, acknowledging their grief.	4. Expression of feelings provides a safe outlet for emotions. Listening, supporting, and acknowledging their grief helps to validate the family's feelings and promote trust.
5. Assist siblings with understanding the events and explore their perceptions. Allow them opportunities to express their feelings verbally and through stories, writing, or drawing pictures.	5. Siblings of dying children often experience a wide range of feelings, such as guilt, anger, jealousy, and fear. Children may have difficulty expressing their feelings verbally. Stories and pictures are effective methods for expression.
6. Provide the family with opportunities to review special memories or experiences with the child.	6. Reviewing memories and special experiences provides a positive method for coping with grief.
7. Assist family with making arrangements for what to do when the child dies and afterward (if not already accomplished).	7. Assistance with planning provides support and aids in grieving, allowing time to be spent with the child rather than on arrangements.
8. Maintain frequent contact with the family through phone calls and visits. Make sure that the family has the telephone number to call with any questions, problems, or concerns.	8. Frequent contact with the family provides them with emotional and physical support.
9. If not already accomplished, initiate referral to community organizations as appropriate.	9. Community organizations provide ongoing support.

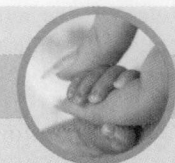

grief reaction was so complete that they are unable to reverse it; they cannot view the child as they did before. They begin to treat him or her in a cold and unfeeling way, as if the child were not really there but actually did die. Such children are termed **vulnerable** or fragile **children.** They may develop behavior problems as they grow older (acting-out behavior, such as temper tantrums, stealing in school, shoplifting as adolescents) as if to say, "Notice me! I'm not dead!" They require skilled counseling so that they can feel secure and learn to react effectively with others (O'Connor & Szekely, 2001).

✔ **CHECKPOINT QUESTIONS**

4. What stage of grief is apt to be most difficult for parents?
5. What is the purpose of anticipatory grief?

Children's Reactions to Impending Death

Children's reactions to death are strongly influenced by their previous experiences, the family's attitudes, and their developmental level (Christ, 2000). If children have little or no exposure to death, it can be a strange and frightening phenomenon. This is often the case when children are reared without pets or older relatives, forbidden to visit a dying relative, excluded from the rites of death, or discouraged from discussing the death of a loved one. To help ease the fear of death, encourage parents to maintain an open attitude, even if it is painful or uncomfortable. Children's reactions to death are also influenced by their stage of development and cognitive ability. Children's ability to understand death and the steps families can take to help their children cope with death are shown in the Focus on Family Empowerment.

Infants and Toddlers

Infants and toddlers are certainly too young to appreciate that their own death is about to occur. If the person who cared for them dies, they experience deep loss and a void in their life. If such a loss interferes with the development of a sense of trust, its implications for the child's ability to achieve warm, close relationships could last a lifetime.

Preschoolers

Preschoolers usually learn about the concept of death when a pet dies or they discover a dead bird or mouse. They envision death as temporary, however, and appear to have little of adults' fear of it. This casualness toward death is sometimes interpreted as callousness (the first response of a child who is told that his brother has just been killed in an automobile accident is to ask if he can have his brother's radio). This happens because he thinks of his brother as being gone for only a short time, making this a chance to take advantage of his property. This concept is strengthened by children's cartoons, in which characters frequently are killed and then immediately revive and go on with the story.

Because preschoolers fear separation greatly, they are stunned by the death of a parent. If children grasp the

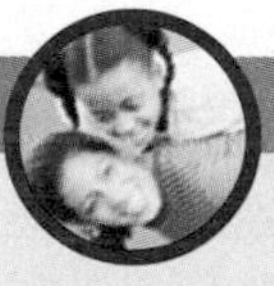

FOCUS ON FAMILY EMPOWERMENT

Guidelines to Help Children Cope With Death

Q. How can we help our children cope with death?

A. Here are some helpful guidelines for each age level:

- Infants have no understanding of their impending death. Important points for caring for an infant who is dying are to keep him or her comfortable and secure and to remain nearby to prevent loneliness and insecurity.
- Toddlers, likewise, do not understand death. Even though a close relative or friend may have died, they are unable to relate this to what is about to happen to them. Toddlers like routine, so allowing them opportunities to make choices and providing consistent care are the most important measures for them.
- Preschool children probably envision death as a long sleep. This makes them much more afraid of separation than of the thought of dying. Urge parents or family members to spend time with them.
- Early school-age children understand death as separation but tend to view the separation as temporary. Over 9 years of age, children are able to realize that death is final. They still, however, are not as fearful of death as they are sad at the thought of being away from their parents and frightened as to how they will manage without their parents. Answer questions about death honestly (no one knows what it is really like but because it happens to everyone, it must not be anything to be fearful of). It is important to praise children for accomplishments to help them maintain their self-esteem so they can face this coming change.
- Adolescents have adult concerns and understanding of death. They may ask if it will be painful; they may feel angry about all that they will miss in life by dying. They may be concerned that they will need to answer for past ill deeds after death. Providing time and opportunities for them to ask and talk about death is important to help them work through the coming change. Allowing them to continue their usual activities as much as possible helps them maintain self-esteem.

concept that they are dying, their major worry might be that they will be alone and separated. These children may need someone to stay with them constantly to assure them that they are not alone.

School-Age Children

School-age children begin to have additional experience with death, so their knowledge of it as a final measure increases. They may think of it, however, as something that happens only to adults. Children's books tend to deal only shallowly with the subject, although many books that deal specifically with death are available to children (Box 56-1). As children near 8 or 9 years, they begin to appreciate that death is permanent. It is the same feeling they experienced when their parents left them at camp or went away for a weekend, but this time the separation will be permanent.

Most children of school age are aware of what is happening to them when their disorder has a fatal prognosis. They may learn from other children on the unit ("Are you the kid who's dying?"), from their parents' strange responses to questions, or from overhearing snatches of conversation about reports or physical findings. Children, however, are accustomed to meeting new situations—starting school, visiting a museum for the first time, boarding an airplane for the first time—and they cope with these experiences very well, as long as they know that someone they care about will be there to support them. Dying can be viewed in this same light as another new experience for them. They are able to cope with it well if they know that there will be someone with them. If the parents become unable to relate to a child this age because of their grief, the nurse may need to fill the gap (Fig. 56-3).

Many children associate death with sleep (perhaps that was the explanation they were given for a grandparent's death), so they may be afraid to fall asleep without someone near them. They may need to have you sit with them while they fall asleep. The child may need the light left on because he or she may associate death with darkness, not with naptime. Often the child who is dying is moved to the end of the hallway, away from the nurses' station. This frees the room for a child who needs frequent procedures (a justifiable move in terms of efficiency). Unfortunately, it may further isolate a child who needs support and the child's parents, who also need your support and your presence nearby. Advocate as necessary for continued interaction with a child who is dying.

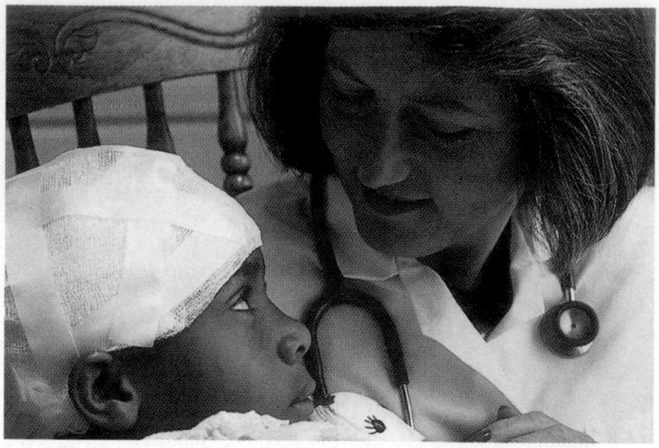

FIGURE 56.3 A one-to-one nursing relationship helps children with long-term illnesses not to feel deserted.

BOX 56.1

BOOKS ABOUT DEATH FOR CHILDREN

Breebaart, J., & Breebaart, P. (1993). *When I die, will I get better?* New York: P. Bedrick Books.
Brown, L. K. (1996). *When dinosaurs die: A guide to understanding death.* Boston: Little, Brown.
Davis, C. (1997). *For every dog an angel.* Portland, OR: Lighthearted Press.
Isherwood, S., & Isherwood, K. (1999). *Remembering Grandad.* London: Oxford Press.
Liss-Levenson, N. (1995). *When a grandparent dies: A kid's own remembering.* Woodstock, VT: Jewish Lights.
Mundy, M., & Alley, R. W. (1998). *Sad isn't bad: A good grief guidebook for kids dealing with a loss.* Meinard, IN: Abbey Press.
Tott-Rizzuti, K. (1992). *Mommy, what does dying mean?* Pittsburgh: Dorrance.
Weitzman, E. (1996). *Let's talk about when a parent dies.* New York: Rosen Group.

Adolescents

Although adolescents have an adult concept of death, they also may feel immune to death. Risky activities such as driving at high speeds reflect this judgment. They may deny symptoms for longer than usual because they believe it is impossible that anything serious could be happening to them. They appreciate time provided for discussion of how they view death and the ways they contributed to their family even though they are dying young. Continuing to participate in their typical activities helps them maintain a sense of control.

Environment for Death

The environment in which children die can influence their acceptance and their family's acceptance of death.

The Hospital

A few children who need a great deal of physical care (have a new tracheotomy, need lung ventilation) may remain in a hospital for care because their family does not have the skill, energy, or money to care for them at home. In a hospital setting, be certain that visiting hours are extended to parents and other family members so that a child is not left alone when he or she needs people around the most. Be certain the child has opportunities to maintain contact with peers.

The Home

Most children today are not kept in the hospital past the time it is determined that therapy is no longer effective. Many families prefer that a child die at home surrounded by family and familiar possessions rather than in a hospital. Time spent talking about arrangements—such as whom they should contact if the child suddenly becomes more ill than usual, how they will manage periodic checkups, or how they will purchase medicine or supplies—is important preparation for home care. Assess how the family will schedule its time to have some leisure periods free so they can balance the care of the ill child in their lives.

Home care can be an extremely satisfying experience both for the child who is dying and for the family, as long as safeguards exist for protecting the caregivers' health and for providing good care for the child. This is discussed further in Chapter 35.

The Hospice

In 1967, St. Christopher's Hospice in London opened as a facility for people who wanted to die in a homelike setting while still receiving skilled professional health care. Most large communities today have similar hospice settings, although places specifically for children are still not available in many communities. In a hospice, friends and family are allowed unlimited visiting; younger children and pets can visit. Children are invited to bring possessions that are important to them. They are urged to choose the degree of pain relief they want. Strong analgesia is often used to make a child pain-free (a criticism of hospice care is that this level of analgesia slows respiratory rates and actually hurries death).

A basic philosophy of hospice care is that death is an extension or part of life, not a separate entity; thus, it can be accepted not with separate or awkward rituals but with the same warm concern as other situations in everyday life. For many children, hospice care will be furnished as part of home care so that they are not separated from their families.

Preparation for a Nursing Role With Dying Children and Their Families

Caring for dying clients can be an emotionally draining experience for health care providers (see Focus on Evidence-Based Practice earlier in this chapter). Although it is best that nursing assignments be consistent so a child has meaningful support, for everyone there is a point at which he or she may need a respite from caring for a certain child or help in offering support for the parents. This is not admitting weakness but recognizing humanness and a sense of compassion that interferes with client need.

Self-Awareness

Before you can offer support to children in any circumstance, you need to be aware of your own reactions and feelings. Thus, to offer support to a child who is dying, examine how you feel about caring for someone who is dying.

Fear. Fear is a natural response to death because the phenomenon is new and strange. To overcome this fear, put it into perspective. In nursing, you care for many people who have illnesses and experiences you will never have; thus, caring for people with experiences beyond your own is not really strange but almost routine in nursing.

People who have never seen someone die are often afraid that the moment of death will be terrifying to watch. Death usually occurs gently, however, with body functioning gradually lessening until it stops in a pain-free, quiet manner. People who have been declared dead and were then resuscitated by heroic measures report that death was not frightening but involved a feeling of exceptional calm and comfort; a number of people have said afterward that they wished they had been allowed to die rather than be called back to their body because death seemed so appealing (Nelson, 2000).

Failure. Some health care professionals find themselves drawing back from caring for dying children because death symbolizes failure to them. This can make children feel as if they have failed—they have not been able to keep their body from dying despite everyone's best efforts.

Remind yourself that death is the ultimate outcome for everyone. At the point that death becomes unpreventable, the only failure that can exist is the failure of health care professionals to help a child achieve death with dignity and consideration and free of guilt that he or she has failed caregivers (Kelly, 2002).

Grief

Nursing care is so intense that the relationship formed may be closer than you realize until the child is diagnosed as having a terminal illness or dies; only then do you feel the depth of the relationship. Because nurses and staff can develop such close bonds with terminally ill children, they may experience profound grief when the children die or no longer require their care (see Focus on Multidisciplinary Care). The grief that accompanies caring for dying children can be broken down into the same stages of grief experienced by the children themselves when they learn that they are dying.

Denial. There is a danger that a nurse who is in a stage of denial may care for children without mentioning that they have more than a simple illness. This includes omitting the use of such common expressions as, "How are you this morning?" to avoid having to hear the answer. Denial may be so extensive that you avoid going into a child's room unless you have an important procedure to do. This is confusing and lonely for children, because they miss the normal exchange of conversation and contact.

Nurses sometimes change professions following the loss of a child to whom they felt close because they are unwilling to submit themselves to that level of hurt again.

Anger. Anger may be intense when a young child dies because the death seems so unfair. Nurses who are angry have difficulty offering effective care: they may perceive themselves as giving thorough, comforting care but are actually inflicting pain with sharp, abrupt movements. Anger clouds a nurse's judgment, such as which anal-

FOCUS ON MULTIDISCIPLINARY CARE

One of the most difficult aspects of caring for children with long-term illnesses or terminal care is letting go of them when their condition improves so they are no longer ill or when their condition worsens and they die. Be certain that all health care personnel involved with a child's care know not to continue a relationship past health agency discharge unless they are specifically asked by the family to do so. Unless they let go this way, the family cannot experience a sense of competency in the care of their now-well child. Help personnel to let go of a child who dies through a period of grieving and acceptance. Health care providers can have a difficult time establishing relationships with new children if they are still grieving for a former one. Holding debriefing sessions or support sessions for staff can be invaluable ways to help health care providers better care for children with terminal illnesses.

---

gesic would be best to administer. Dying children cannot approach angry caregivers or ask questions; they are left alone and perhaps feel guilty that they have caused this anger. Anger is always destructive.

WHAT IF? What if, while caring for a terminally ill child for an extended time, you notice yourself making poor judgments in your personal life (not following through on projects, spontaneous buying)? Could this be an expression of anger?

Bargaining. Caregivers begin to bargain for life just as children do. A statement such as, "If Tommy just makes it through the weekend while I'm off, I'll spend all my extra time with him next week" is a bargaining statement. Statements of this kind are easy to overlook in your coworkers or yourself. Listening for them helps you to evaluate when a fellow worker is having difficulty caring for a particular patient and perhaps needs to change assignments. Hearing yourself say them should alert you that you are more involved with a child than you perhaps realize. You need to talk to someone about your feelings or ask for help. Remember that when bargaining fails, people reach their lowest point in grief. Recognizing bargaining statements in yourself helps you to be prepared for the depression that will follow.

Depression. Nurses who enter this phase may be ineffective caregivers, because depressed people are poor problem-solvers (everything becomes a crisis). Nurses may make unwise decisions in their personal lives (e.g., drop out of a night school course, file for divorce) because they cannot solve problems effectively.

Depression is doubly destructive because when you are depressed, your reasoning processes are so slowed that you lose the ability to recognize that depression is the problem. When caring for a child who is expected to die, monitor your usual behavior to see if you are following your usual pattern. If irregularities occur (sleeping a great deal, not sleeping, loss of appetite), assess whether depression has overwhelmed you. When depressed, try to make no major decisions for at least a week to give your perspective time to change, or you may find later that you have made an unwise, irreversible decision.

Acceptance. The average person can reach a stage of acceptance in grief because he or she is subjected to few true losses in a lifetime. As a nurse on a unit where many terminally ill children come for care, you may find yourself facing loss or death repeatedly. Therefore, a stage of acceptance may never be reached. A caregiver who cannot reach a stage of acceptance is left in a stage of depression and cannot function.

To achieve a stage of acceptance, you may need to modify what it is you are accepting. You cannot accept the unfairness of death in children, but you can accept your ability to offer care that gives death dignity and compassion. Do not compensate for being unable to feel good by not feeling. This is a dangerous attitude because it also blocks your ability to feel happiness, love, and trust. You may need to ask for a temporary change of assignment to re-establish your perspective. You may need to concentrate on self-esteem therapy for yourself (doing something special for yourself, such as taking an evening to do nothing but meet your own needs).

Caring for the Dying Child

A child may live for days, weeks, or even months in a "dying phase." Attentive physical and emotional care is essential to the child's maintaining a sense of security and positive self-esteem during this time. It is also essential to the grieving process for both the child and the child's family. Frequent and substantive communication is a major part of providing this care. Children, like their parents, need the opportunity to talk about their fears and feelings about death. Practicing good communication skills when providing any care (e.g., when administering pain medication, starting intravenous lines, or providing basic comfort measures, such as a bath) will help to establish a trusting relationship with a child, making the child feel more comfortable about sharing feelings with you (Fig. 56-4). Box 56-2 provides some specific guidelines about communicating with the child who is dying.

The Child's Family

For many children, terminal illness involves a series of hospital admissions interspersed with ambulatory care or home visits. Parents need time during these visits to talk about the problems they are having, not only with physical care (Should the child attend regular school? Could he come on vacation? How many times a day are they supposed to give the immunosuppressant?) but also about how it feels to live with a child who is dying (Are they having any difficulty answering the child's or siblings' questions?). Although many parents are reluctant to tell a child that he or she is dying, this is probably the soundest

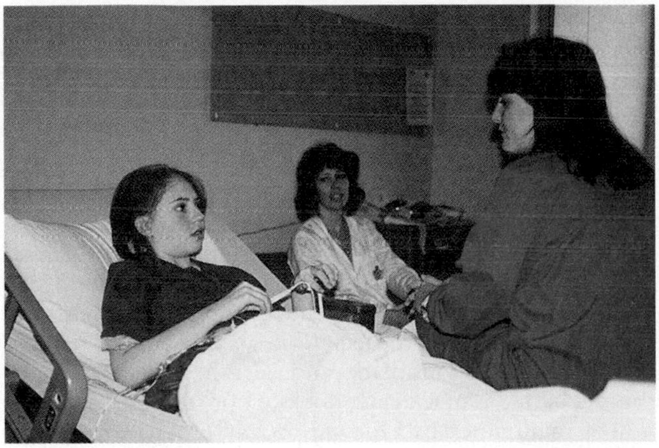

FIGURE 56.4 Good communication skills help build a trusting relationship, allowing the child to share feelings about being terminally ill.

course once the child can see that his or her condition is deteriorating. There is often less anxiety in knowing what is happening than in hearing people whispering or spelling out words around you.

If a child experiences an exacerbation of the disease, parents may again begin an anticipatory grief reaction: anger, bargaining, depression, acceptance. The process will be cut short by improvement, only to begin again at the next exacerbation. Parents of a child being admitted to the hospital for the 12th time for leukemia, therefore, may be in the same stage of grief as the parents of a child with newly diagnosed leukemia.

During health supervision visits, ask parents how other children in the family are managing. The parents may need to be reminded that although the dying child does need a lot of their time, other children find this illness in a sibling even more baffling than do the parents. When the ill child dies, siblings need active support to help them grieve.

The Onset of Death

As death nears in children, physiologic changes, such as slowed metabolism, decreased cell oxygenation, and cell dysfunction, begin to occur.

Stroke volume of the heart decreases, so the power to circulate blood is reduced. The child's skin feels cool and appears mottled or cyanotic because blood can no longer be pushed to distal sites. Just before death, blood will begin to pool in the dependent body parts, making them appear purple. As circulation fails, absorption of a drug from a muscle becomes virtually impossible; an emergency drug would need to be administered intravenously to have an effect.

As peripheral circulation fails, less heat is lost from the body, and the temperature rises. The child's body may compensate for this by increased perspiration to increase heat loss through evaporation. This makes the child's skin feel cool and damp. You may need to change linens frequently because of the increased moisture on the skin. Because perfusion of distal body parts is impaired, turn children slowly to allow their circulatory system to accommodate to the change in position.

BOX 56.2

APPROACHES TO COMMUNICATING WITH DYING CHILDREN

1. Continue active conversation. Children who are dying need stimulation in as near normal a way as possible.
2. Use moments of silence therapeutically. Such moments occur normally just as speech occurs normally. Do not feel you have to chatter to fill quiet intervals.
3. Use the words *death* and *dying* as appropriate in conversation. Trying to avoid a word makes interchanges awkward. Statements such as, "These flowers are dying," "That's a dead-end job," or "I'm dying to try that" may make it acceptable for the child you are caring for to voice for the first time what is happening to him or her—"I'm dying, too; let me tell you about dead-ending."
4. Preserve dying children's defenses. If they are using denial or bargaining, do not try to push them to the next step of grieving by confrontation. Children will move on to the next step when they are psychologically ready.
5. Remember that many children assume that they will die at night. Therefore, night is "owned" by the dying. A child may talk more freely at night about fears or an unfulfilled life ambition than during the day. Children may also be more frightened at night and enjoy having someone sit beside them until they fall asleep.
6. Be supportive, not trite. A statement such as "All of us are dying" is true but not helpful. A supportive statement such as, "This must be hard for you" is better.
7. Be aware that not all people's beliefs are the same as yours. A statement such as, "God works in mysterious ways" may explain death for you but can be little comfort to a family who does not envision that as true. A statement such as, "I believe God made some children die early to teach us to appreciate life" may evoke an angry response such as, "Who could believe in a God like that?" rather than be comforting.

Slowed respiration leads to increased secretions in the lungs and the appearance of crackles (rales—sound of air being pulled through fluid in the alveoli). To compensate for a few minutes of very slow respirations, a child may take a number of quick or extremely deep inhalations periodically. Be certain the child's chest is not compressed so he or she has optimal lung expansion to do this.

A decrease in muscular function leads to severe weakness and fatigue. More and more, a child maintains the exact position in which he or she was placed. As the throat muscles become lax, the possibility of aspiration increases. Assess children carefully for an intact gag reflex before offering oral fluid. If the gag or swallowing reflex is impaired, position children on their side to allow saliva to drain from the mouth and prevent aspiration. An often-noticed phenomenon is constant hand movement—picking at bedclothes, for example—that probably represents the loss of upper centers of voluntary muscular control. Neurologically, deep reflexes, such as the Achilles, begin to fade.

As children near death, they begin to demonstrate a lessened level of consciousness, although they may remain perfectly alert until seconds before death. Vision apparently blurs because children tend to turn toward a light. Touch seems to remain intact because children often quiet to a gentle stroking of the arm or shoulder; they grasp your hand meaningfully as if touch is appreciated and felt. Hearing remains intact; remind family members and, on occasion, other health care personnel of this. Continue to explain procedures to unconscious children as if they were conscious because they undoubtedly do hear you. Never make any comment in their presence that you would not make if they were alert. Continue to use the same gentle touch and nonverbal communication motions, such as holding a hand or brushing hair from the forehead, as if children were fully conscious. They may be fully aware of your actions even though they can give no indication of it.

Digestion slows as total body metabolism slows. Constipation due to poor bowel tone and decreased peristaltic action will occur. The abdomen may become distended from intestinal flatus. Dehydration with dry mucous membranes and conjunctivae will occur unless intravenous fluid replacement is initiated. Mouth dryness will lead to cracking and secondary infection and pain; prevent this by frequent cleaning of the mucous membrane with clear water and applying Vaseline to the lips. If the conjunctivae appear dry, ask a physician to prescribe moistening eye drops; keep any crusting at the eyelids washed away so that optimal vision is possible.

Keep skin surfaces from rubbing against one another by using supportive pillows and good positioning. Keep skin free of urine or feces from incontinence; this prevents the development of painful ulcers (normally not a major concern in children, but a concern here because of the lessened peripheral blood perfusion). Assess for pain (thrashing or moaning), and provide relief with appropriate comfort measures.

Documentation of Death

Defining when death occurs is controversial and involves both legal and ethical issues. Signs of death in a child not on ventilatory or mechanical assistance are the same as in adults and include the following:

- Absence of respirations
- No audible heart sounds by stethoscope
- No pulse by palpation
- No apparent blood pressure
- Absence of body movement or reflexes
- Dilated, fixed pupils

Death is officially determined by unreceptivity and unresponsivity; no spontaneous muscular movement or breath; no reflex response; and a flat electroencephalogram—again, the same as in adults. Emergency medical technicians make a preliminary assessment in the home or hospice setting, and then death is confirmed by the physician.

Organ Donation

Parents may be asked by their physician or a specifically designated transplant team before a child's death to grant permission for body organs to be transplanted following death. This is particularly important for liver and kidney transplants because it is difficult to transplant adult-size organs into children. If parents decide to allow organ donation, mark this information on the child's plan of care in a conspicuous place, and alert the physician about the decision. When death does occur, the child's body will be maintained by a life-support system to ensure that the organ remains perfused until it can be removed (Day, 2001). The donation of body organs may help parents accept their child's death more easily, because they can feel their child has helped another person live. Thus, after an adequate explanation of the process, the family may readily accept it (Verble & Worth, 2000). On the other hand, if parents are reluctant to agree to organ donation, you may need to advocate for them.

Aftercare

Before beginning any aftercare with a child following death in a health care facility or at home, check with family members to see if they want to spend a few minutes with the child or if there are any religious rites they want to complete before the body is transported to the morgue. Some parents need this time to comprehend that death has really occurred. Some people have special prayers they want to say; others want to say a final, private goodbye. In the hospital, check that the child's bed and room look neat and clean before you ask family if they would like to spend some time in the room, particularly if a final resuscitation attempt resulted in blood-soaked sponges or scattered equipment.

Remain in the room with the family in case they need your support, but be unobtrusive. Some parents fear touching a child's body after death, but touch is a strong and intimate communication technique that a family member may appreciate being shown how to use. Role-model touching by holding the child's hand or brushing hair away from the forehead as if the child were still alive. Some parents may seem unable to leave the room or to let go of the child's hand. You may need gradually to separate their hands, saying something such as, "I'll always remember Molly the way she was when I first met her—so full of life and always laughing. I'm sure that's how you'll always remember her, too." This helps parents begin to accept the fact that, in more than a physical sense, it is time to let go.

As a rule, crying is helpful for parents. You may need to tell them that it is all right to cry. On the other hand, do not interpret a lack of tears as a lack of feeling, because crying is not everyone's response to death. It is not unprofessional for nurses to cry when a child dies. A parent's warmest memory of a hospital experience may be that a nurse cried as she said goodbye to his or her child—the implication being that the child made an impact on people other than family.

FOCUS ON CULTURAL COMPETENCE

The way that death is viewed and the manner in which people express grief differ greatly across cultures. Some people are very expressive with grief; some are very restrained. The manner in which a child's body is handled after death also differs. Muslims, for example, forbid organ donations or transplants. Autopsies are not usually approved because it is important that children be buried quickly after death. Cremation is not permitted. Being aware that grief is expressed differently by different cultures allows for better understanding of parents' concerns and reactions during a child's terminal illness and when death occurs.

Autopsy Permission

If a child's death is a result of homicide, suicide, death within 24 hours after a hospital admission, suspected harmful (foul play) death, or death in an institution or home where the child was not under a physician's care, an autopsy is required by law; parents have no input as to whether one is done. In other instances, it would be helpful to medical programs or research if an autopsy could be done, but parents must give permission for this. Parents may refuse to allow an autopsy for a child, believing that this would protect the child from any more hurt or out of religious convictions (see Focus on Cultural Competence). Autopsies advance medical science, so they should be done if at all possible; on the other hand, parents have every right to refuse permission without being made to feel guilty for their actions. You may need to advocate for them.

✔ CHECKPOINT QUESTIONS

6. With dying, what is the last sense lost?
7. Why are donations of livers and kidneys from children so important?

KEY POINTS

Children with long-term illnesses need continual reassessment because, like all children, their needs change as they grow older. Larger doses of medicine will become necessary; things such as additional muscle-strengthening exercises may be necessary.

Factors that make it easier for parents to accept a long-term illness in a child include having support people present and being told about the child's condition as early as possible.

Long-term illness in a child is often most difficult for parents to accept at the times that the child would be achieving specific milestones of development. Extra support for both the parents and child may be necessary at these times.

Help children to do as much care for themselves as possible within the limits of the illness. This empowers them to be as independent as possible.

Children are about 9 years old before they are able to understand the meaning of death and that it is permanent. The child and parents can be expected to move through the stages of grief (denial, anger, bargaining, depression, and acceptance).

Children and parents are apt to need help to face a terminal diagnosis in the child. Urge parents and the child to ask for help to see them through this very difficult time in their lives.

CRITICAL THINKING EXERCISES

1. Charlie is the 3-year-old with leukemia you met at the beginning of the chapter. His parents tell you Charlie's disease has put them through a great deal of strain. What might you anticipate as a reason that Charlie was so ill with pneumonia before they brought him for care?
2. The parents of a newborn with a myelomeningocele are both 40 years old and live on a farm; finances are tight, and they have no health insurance. Two grown children have expressed resentment at their parents for spending so much time and money on a disabled child. How would you help this family? Do they have risk factors that might make adjusting to a disabled child more difficult than usual?
3. A 10-year-old in your care has an inoperable brain tumor. His parents have been told that he has only 6 months to live. You notice the parents in the waiting room of the hospital comforting a set of parents whose child was just hit by a car and killed instantly; you hear them say that losing a child suddenly is better than what they are experiencing. Why do you think the parents feel this way? What stage of grief could they be experiencing? How could you help them with their feelings?
4. An adolescent with leukemia wants to donate his corneas for transplant if he should die. His parents think this is totally wrong and say they will not allow it to happen. How would you counsel this family?
5. Examine the National Health Goals related to chronic or terminal illness and children. Most government-sponsored money for nursing research is allotted based on these goals. What would be a possible research topic to explore pertinent to these goals that would be fundable and would advance evidence-based practice?

REFERENCES

Balling, K., & McCubbin, M. (2001). Hospitalized children with chronic illness: Parental caregiving needs and valuing parental expertise. *Journal of Pediatric Nursing: Nursing Care of Children & Families, 16*(2), 110–119.

Barnes, K. (2001). Staff stress in the children's hospice. *International Journal of Palliative Nursing, 7*(5), 248–254.

Bechtold, D. W. (2001). Psychiatric disorders. In W. W. Hay, A. R. Hayward, M. J. Levin, & J. M. Sondheimer (eds.). *Current pediatric diagnosis and treatment* (15th ed.). New York: McGraw-Hill.

Christ, G. H. (2000). Impact of development on children's mourning. *Cancer Practice: a Multidisciplinary Journal of Cancer Care, 8*(92), 72–81.

Costello, J., & Trinder-Brook, A. (2000). Children's nurses' experiences of caring for dying children in hospital. *Pediatric Nursing, 12*(6), 28–31.

Day, L. (2001). How nurses shift from care of a brain-injured patient to maintenance of a brain-dead organ donor. *American Journal of Critical Care, 10*(5), 306–312.

Department of Health and Human Services. (2000). *Healthy people 2010.* Washington, D.C.: DHHS.

Ford, K., & Turner, D. (2001). Stories seldom told: Paediatric nurses' experiences of caring for hospitalized children with special needs and their families. *Journal of Advanced Nursing, 33*(3), 288–295.

Kelly, B. (2002). Dealing with employee grief. *Health Data Management, 10*(1), 110–112.

Knafl, K., & Zoeller, L. (2000). Childhood chronic illness: A comparison of mothers' and fathers' experiences. *Journal of Family Nursing, 6*(3), 287–302.

Kübler-Ross, E. (1969). *On death and dying.* New York: Macmillan.

Lindeke, L. L., et al. (2001). PNP roles and interventions with children with special needs and their families. *Journal of Pediatric Health Care, 15*(3), 138–143.

Nelson, H. R. (2000). The near death experience: Observations and reflections from a retired chaplain. *Journal of Pastoral Care, 54*(2), 159–166.

O'Connor, M. E., & Szekely, L. J. (2001). Frequent breast-feeding and food refusal associated with failure to thrive: A manifestation of the vulnerable child syndrome. *Clinical Pediatrics, 40*(1), 27–33.

Ross, H. M. (2001). Islamic tradition at the end of life. *MedSurg Nursing, 10*(2), 83–88.

Sandler, A. D. (2001). Counseling families who chose complementary and alternative medicine for their child with chronic illness or disability. *Pediatrics, 107*(3), 598–601.

Verble, M., & Worth, J. (2000). Overcoming families' fears and concerns in the donation discussion. *Progress in Transplantation, 10*(3), 155–160.

Zeitlin, S. V. (2001). Grief and bereavement. *Primary Care, 28*(2), 415–425.

SUGGESTED READINGS

Brown, K., & Bocock, J. (2002). Update in pediatric resuscitation. *Emergency Medicine Clinics of North America, 20*(1), 1–26.

Chernoff, R. G., et al. (2001). Maternal reports of raising children with chronic illnesses: The prevalence of positive thinking. *Ambulatory Pediatrics, 1*(2), 104–107.

Eiser, C., & Morse, R. (2001). A review of measures of quality of life for children with chronic illness. *Archives of Disease in Childhood, 84*(3), 205–211.

Fearnow-Kenney, M., & Kliewer, W. (2000). Threat appraisal and adjustment among children with cancer. *Journal of Psychosocial Oncology, 18*(3), 1–17.

Neufeld, S. M., Query, B., & Drummond, J. E. (2001). Respite care users who have children with chronic conditions: Are they getting a break? *Journal of Pediatric Nursing; Nursing Care of Children & Families, 16*(4), 234–244.

Oliver, R. C., et al. (2001). Beneficial effects of a hospital bereavement intervention program after traumatic childhood death. *Journal of Trauma-Injury Infection & Critical Care, 50*(3), 440–446.

Perry, D. F., & Ireys, H. T. (2001). Maternal perceptions of pediatric providers for children with chronic illness. *Maternal & Child Health Journal, 5*(1), 15–20.

Plant, W. A., Lobato, D., & Engel, R. (2001). Review of group interventions for pediatric chronic conditions. *Journal of Pediatric Psychology, 26*(7), 435–453.

Sartain, S. A., Clarke, C. L., & Heyman, R. (2000). Hearing the voices of children with chronic illness. *Journal of Advanced Nursing, 32*(2), 135–142.

Thies, K. M., & McAllister, J. W. (2001). The health and education leadership project: A school initiative for children and adolescents with chronic health conditions. *Journal of School Health, 71*(5), 167–172.

Wray, J., et al. (2001). Returning to school after heart or heart-lung transplantation: How well do children adjust? *Transplantation, 72*(1), 100–106.

Rights of Pregnant Women and Children

APPENDIX A

THE PREGNANT PATIENT'S BILL OF RIGHTS*

The Pregnant Patient has the right to participate in decisions involving her well-being and that of her unborn child, unless there is a clear-cut medical emergency that prevents her participation. In addition to the rights set forth in the American Hospital Association's "Patient's Bill of Rights," the Pregnant Patient, because she represents TWO patients rather than one, should be recognized as having the additional rights listed below.

1. *The Pregnant Patient has the right,* prior to the administration of any drug or procedure, to be informed by the health professional caring for her of any potential direct or indirect effects, risks or hazards to herself or her unborn or newborn infant which may result from the use of a drug or procedure prescribed for or administered to her during pregnancy, labor, birth or lactation.
2. *The Pregnant Patient has the right,* prior to the proposed therapy, to be informed, not only of the benefits, risks and hazards of the proposed therapy but also of known alternative therapy, such as available childbirth education classes which could help to prepare the Pregnant Patient physically and mentally to cope with the discomfort or stress of pregnancy and the experience of childbirth, thereby reducing or eliminating her need for drugs and obstetric intervention. She should be offered such information early in her pregnancy in order that she may make a reasoned decision.
3. *The Pregnant Patient has the right,* prior to the administration of any drug, to be informed by the health professional who is prescribing or administering the drug to her that any drug which she receives during pregnancy, labor and birth, no matter how or when the drug is taken or administered, may adversely affect her unborn baby, directly or indirectly, and that there is no drug or chemical which has been proven safe for the unborn child.
4. *The Pregnant Patient has the right,* if cesarean birth is anticipated, to be informed prior to the administration of any drug, and preferably prior to her hospitalization, that minimizing her and, in turn, her baby's intake of nonessential preoperative medicine will benefit her baby.
5. *The Pregnant Patient has the right,* prior to the administration of a drug or procedure, to be informed of the areas of uncertainty if there is *no* properly controlled follow-up research which has established the safety of the drug or procedure with regard to its direct and/or indirect effects on the physiological, mental and neurological development of the child exposed, via the mother, to the drug or procedure during pregnancy, labor, birth or lactation (this would apply to virtually all drugs and the vast majority of obstetric procedures).
6. *The Pregnant Patient has the right,* prior to the administration of any drug, to be informed on the brand name and generic name of the drug in order that she may advise the health professional of any past adverse reaction to the drug.
7. *The Pregnant Patient has the right* to determine for herself, without pressure from her attendant, whether she will accept the risks inherent in the proposed therapy or refuse a drug or procedure.
8. *The Pregnant Patient has the right* to know the name and qualifications of the individual administering a medication or procedure to her during labor or birth.
9. *The Pregnant Patient has the right* to be informed, prior to the administration of any procedure, whether that procedure is being administered to her for her or her baby's benefit (medically indicated) or as an elective procedure (for convenience, teaching purposes or research).
10. *The Pregnant Patient has the right* to be accompanied during the stress of labor and birth by someone she cares for, and to whom she looks for emotional comfort and encouragement.
11. *The Pregnant Patient has the right* after appropriate medical consultation to choose a position for labor and for birth which is least stressful to her baby and to herself.
12. *The Obstetric Patient has the right* to have her baby cared for at her bedside if her baby is normal, and to feed her baby according to her baby's needs rather than according to the hospital regimen.
13. *The Obstetric Patient has the right* to be informed in writing of the name of the person who actually delivered her baby and the professional qualifications of that person. This information should also be on the birth certificate.

*From Haire, D. B. (1975). The pregnant patient's bill of rights. *Journal of Nurse Midwifery, 20,* 29; from Committee on Patient's Rights, Box 1900, New York, NY 10001.

14. *The Obstetric Patient has the right* to be informed if there is any known or indicated aspect of her or her baby's care or condition which may cause her or her baby later difficulty or problems.
15. *The Obstetric Patient has the right* to have her and her baby's hospital medical records complete, accurate and legible and to have their records, including Nurses' Notes, retained by the hospital until the child reaches at least the age of majority, or to have the records offered to her before they are destroyed.
16. *The Obstetric Patient,* both during and after her hospital stay, *has the right* to have access to her complete hospital medical records, including Nurses' Notes, and to receive a copy upon payment of a reasonable fee and without incurring the expense of retaining an attorney.

It is the obstetric patient and her baby, not the health professional, who must sustain any trauma or injury resulting from the use of a drug or obstetric procedure. The observation of the rights listed above will not only permit the obstetric patient to participate in the decisions involving her and her baby's health care, but will help to protect the health professional and the hospital against litigation arising from resentment or misunderstanding on the part of the mother.

UNITED NATIONS DECLARATION OF THE RIGHTS OF THE CHILD†

Preamble

Whereas the peoples of the United Nations have in the Charter, reaffirmed their faith in fundamental human rights, and in the dignity and worth of the human person, and have determined to promote social progress and better standards of life in larger freedom,

Whereas the United Nations has, in the Universal Declaration of Human Rights, proclaimed that everyone is entitled to all the rights and freedoms set forth therein, without distinction of any kind, such as race, color, sex, language, religion, political or other opinion, national or social origin, property, birth or other status,

Whereas the child by reason of his physical and mental immaturity, needs special safeguards and care, including appropriate legal protection, before as well as after birth,

Whereas the need for such special safeguards has been stated in the Geneva Declaration of the Rights of the Child of 1924, and recognized in the universal Declaration of Human Rights and in the statutes of specialized agencies and international organizations concerned with the welfare of children,

Whereas mankind owes to the child the best it has to give.

Now therefore the general assembly proclaims

This Declaration of the Rights of the Child to the end that he may have a happy childhood and enjoy for his own good and for the good of society and rights and freedoms herein set forth, and calls upon parents, upon men and women as individuals and upon voluntary organizations, local authorities and national governments to recognize these rights and strive for their observance by legislative and other measures progressively taken in accordance with the following principles:

Principle 1

The child shall enjoy all the rights set forth in this Declaration. All children, without any exception whatsoever, shall be entitled to these rights, without distinction or discrimination on account of race, color, sex, language, religion, political or other opinion, national or social origin, property, birth or other status, whether of himself or of his family.

Principle 2

The child shall enjoy special protection, and shall be given opportunities and facilities, by law and by other means, to enable him to develop physically, mentally, morally, spiritually and socially in a healthy and normal manner and in conditions of freedom and dignity. In the enactment of laws for this purpose the best interests of the child shall be the paramount consideration.

Principle 3

The child shall be entitled from his birth to a name and a nationality.

Principle 4

The child shall enjoy the benefits of social security. He shall be entitled to grow and develop in health; to this end special care and protection shall be provided both to him and to his mother, including adequate prenatal care. The child shall have the right to adequate nutrition, housing, recreation and medical services.

Principle 5

The child who is physically, mentally or socially handicapped shall be given the special treatment, education and care required by his particular condition.

Principle 6

The child, for the full and harmonious development of his personality, needs love and understanding. He shall, wherever possible, grow up in the care and under the responsibility of his parents, and in any case in an atmosphere of affection and of moral and maternal security; a child of tender years shall not, save in exceptional circumstances, be separated from his mother. Society and the public authorities shall have the duty to extend particular care to children without a family and to those without adequate means of support. Payment of state and other assistance toward the maintenance of children of large families is desirable.

†United Nations. (1959). *Declaration of the rights of the child.* Geneva: The United Nations.

Principle 7

The child is entitled to receive education, which shall be free and compulsory, at least in the elementary stages. He shall be given an education which will promote his general culture, and enable him on a basis of equal opportunity to develop his abilities, his individual judgment and his sense of moral and social responsibility, and to become a useful member of society.

The best interests of the child shall be the guiding principle of those responsible for his education and guidance; that responsibility lies in the first place with his parents.

The child shall have full opportunity for play and recreation, which shall be directed to the same purposes as education; society and the public authorities shall endeavor to promote the employment of his right.

Principle 8

The child shall in all circumstances be among the first to receive protection and relief.

Principle 9

The child shall be protected against all forms of neglect, cruelty and exploitation. He shall not be the subject of traffic, in any form.

The child shall not be admitted to employment before an appropriate minimum age; he shall in no case be caused or permitted to engage in any occupation or employment which would prejudice his health or education, or interfere with his physical, mental or moral development.

Principle 10

The child shall be protected from practices which may foster racial, religious and any other form of discrimination. He shall be brought up in a spirit of understanding, tolerance, friendship among peoples, peace and universal brotherhood and in full consciousness that his energy and talents should be devoted to the service of his fellow men.

APPENDIX B

Composition and Ingredients of Infant Formulas

FORMULA	CALORIES (Per oz)	CALORIES (Per mL)	PROTEIN	FAT	CARBOHYDRATE	COMMENTS
Cow's milk	20	.67	80% casein, 20% whey	Butterfat	Lactose	
Enfamil 20†	20	.67	40% casein, 60% whey	45% soy, 55% coconut oils	Lactose	
Enfamil premature	20	.67	40% casein, 60% whey	40% MCT oil, soy and coconut oil	Corn syrup solids, lactose	Premature infants
Human milk	21	.70	40% casein, 60% whey	Human milk, fat	Lactose	
Isomil	20	.67	Soy protein	Coconut and soy oils	Corn syrup solids and sucrose	For cow's milk protein or lactose intolerance
Isomil SF	20	.67	Soy protein	Coconut and soy oils	Corn syrup solids	For cow's milk protein, lactose, or sucrose intolerance
Lofenalac	20	.67	Processed casein hydrolysate to remove most of the phenylalanine	Corn oil	Corn syrup solids and modified tapioca starch	For phenyl-ketonuria (PKU), low in phenylalanine
MJ 3232A‡	20	.67	Casein hydrolysate	MCT oil	Tapioca starch, mono- and disaccharide free	Management of disaccharidase deficiencies
Nursoy	20	.67	Soy protein	Coconut, safflower, and soy-bean oils	Sucrose	For cow's milk protein or lactose intolerance
Nutramigen	20	.67	Casein hydrolysate	Corn oil	Corn syrup solids, modified corn starch	Use for sensitivity to intact milk protein, or for lactose intolerance
Portagen	20	.67	Sodium caseinate	88% MCT oil, 12% corn oil	Corn syrup sucrose	Use in fat mal-absorption states, lactose intolerance (liver disease)
Pregestimil	20	.67	Casein hydrolysate with added L-cystine, L-tyrosine, L-tryptophan	60% corn oil, 40% MCT oil	Corn syrup solids, modified tapioca starch	Suitable for many malabsorption syndromes
Prosobee	20	.67	Soy protein isolate and methonine	Soy oil, coconut oil	100% corn syrup solids (glucose polymers)	Use for lactose and cow's milk protein intolerance; sucrose intolerance; galactosemia

(continued)

(*Continued*)

FORMULA	CALORIES (Per oz)	CALORIES (Per mL)	PROTEIN	FAT	CARBOHYDRATE	COMMENTS
RCF			Soy protein isolate	Coconut and soy oils	None	Contains no carbohydrates
Similac 20[†]	20[§]	.67	Nonfat cow's milk	Coconut and soy oils	Lactose	
Similac 24LLBW	24	.80	Nonfat cow's milk	MCT oil, coconut and soy oils	Lactose and corn syrup solids	Dilute initial feedings. For premature infants with fluid intolerance
Similac PM 60/40	20	.67	Casein and whey (60/40 ratio whey/ casein)	Coconut and soy oil	Lactose	(Ca:P=2:1) For infants predisposed to hypocalcemia; low salt content
Similac special care	20	.67	60% whey, 40% casein	MCT oil soy oil coconut oil	50% lactose 50% corn syrup solids	Premature infants Ca:P-2:1
Similac whey plus iron	20	.67	60% whey, 40% casein	Coconut, and soy oils	Lactose	
SMA 20	20	.67	Nonfat cow's milk, demineralized whey	Coconut safflower and soybean oils	Lactose	Low salt content
SMA Preemie	24	.80	60% whey, 40% casein	MCT oil coconut and soy oils	Lactose and glucose polymers	Premature infants

* Percentage of calories supplied
† Also comes with iron (12 mg/L)
‡ Mixed as 81 g diet powder plus 59 g added carbohydrate per quart
§ Varies with amount carbohydrate added
| Sibery, G. K. & Iannone, R. (2000). *The Harriet Lane handbook.* (15th ed.). St Louis: Mosby.
Values listed were provided by manufacturers except where indicated otherwise.)
(Oski, F. A., et al. [1999]. *Principles and practice of pediatrics* [3rd ed.]. Philadelphia: Lippincott Williams & Wilkins.)

Drug Effects in Lactation

APPENDIX C

Adrenergics	Parenteral *epinephrine* (Adrenalin) is excreted in breast milk; the status of other adrenergic bronchodilators is not known. *Albuterol* (Proventil, Ventolin) had tumorigenic effects in animals; if considered necessary, breast-feeding should be discontinued. Oral drugs used as nasal decongestants (e.g., *pseudoephedrine* [Sudafed], others) are contraindicated in nursing mothers because of higher than usual risks to infants from sympathomimetic drugs.
Analgesics	*Acetaminophen* (Tylenol) is excreted in breast milk in low concentrations. No adverse effects have been reported, and it is probably the analgesic-antipyretic drug of choice for nursing mothers. Salicylates (e.g., *aspirin*) are excreted in breast milk in small amounts. Adverse effects on nursing infants have not been reported but are a potential risk. Narcotic analgesics such as *meperidine* (Demerol) are excreted in breast milk, but amounts may not be enough to cause adverse effects in the nursing infant. Some authorities recommend waiting 4 to 6 h after a dose before nursing. *Alfentanil* (Alfenta) should probably not be given. Significant amounts were found in breast milk 4 h after a dose.
Angiotensin-Converting Enzyme (ACE) Inhibitors	*Captopril* (Capoten) is excreted in breast milk, but effects on the infant are unknown. It is not known whether *enalapril* (Vasotec) or *lisinopril* (Prinivil, Zestril) is excreted in breast milk. In general, nursing is not recommended while taking these drugs.
Antianginal Agents (Nitrates)	Safety for use in the nursing mother has not been established.
Antianxiety and Sedative-Hypnotic Agents (Benzodiazepines)	*Diazepam* (Valium) and other benzodiazepines should generally be avoided. They are excreted in breast milk and may cause lethargy and weight loss in the infant. The drugs and their metabolites may accumulate to toxic levels in neonates because of slow drug metabolism.
Antiarrhythmics	When these agents are required for a nursing mother, breast-feeding should generally be discontinued. *Quinidine* (Quinaglute), *disopyramide* (Norpace), and *mexiletine* (Mexitil) are excreted in breast milk; it is unknown whether *procainamide* (Pronestyl, Procan), *lidocaine* (Xylocaine), and *flecainide* (Tambocor) are excreted. There is a potential for serious adverse effects on infants.
Antibiotics	*Penicillins* are excreted in breast milk in low concentrations and may cause diarrhea, candidiasis, or allergic responses in nursing infants. *Cephalosporins* are excreted in small amounts and may alter bowel flora, cause pharmacologic effects, and interfere with interpretation of culture reports with fever or infection. *Aztreonam* (Azactam) is excreted in small amounts; discontinuing breast-feeding temporarily is probably indicated. It is unknown whether *imipenem/cilastatin* (Primaxin) is excreted. The aminoglycosides *netilmicin* (Netromycin) and *streptomycin* are excreted in small amounts. Because these drugs are nephrotoxic and ototoxic, the immature kidney function of neonates and infants should be considered. *Tetracyclines* are excreted in breast milk and should be avoided. *Sulfonamides* are excreted and generally contraindicated. They may cause kernicterus in the neonate and diarrhea and skin rash in the nursing infant. *Erythromycin* is excreted and may become concentrated in breast milk. No adverse effects on nursing infants have been reported. However, the potential exists for alteration in bowel flora, pharmacologic effects, and interference with fever workup. *Nitrofurantoin* (Macrodantin) is excreted in very small amounts. However, safety for use in nursing mothers has not been established, and infants with glucose-6-phosphate deyhydrogenase (G-6-PD) deficiency may be adversely affected. *Clindamycin* (Cleocin) is excreted. Breast-feeding is probably best discontinued if the drug is necessary, to avoid potential problems in the infant. *Cinoxacin* (Cinobac) and *norfloxacin* (Noroxin) are probably excreted, and there is a potential for severe adverse effects in nursing infants. Depending on the mother's need for the drug, either the drug or breast-feeding should be discontinued. *Isoniazid* (INH) and *rifampin* (Rifadin) are excreted in breast milk, and nursing infants should be observed for adverse drug effects. *Trimethoprim* (Proloprim, Bactrim) is excreted and may interfere with folic acid metabolism in the infant.
Anticholinergics	*Atropine* and others are excreted and may cause infant toxicity or decreased breast milk production. Safety for use is not established.
Anticoagulants	*Heparin* is not excreted in breast milk; *warfarin* (Coumadin) is excreted, but some evidence suggests no harm to the nursing infant. More data are needed, and heparin is preferred if anticoagulant therapy is required.

(*continued*)

(Continued)	
Anticonvulsants	*Phenytoin* (Dilantin) and other hydantoins are excreted and may cause serious adverse effects in nursing infants. The drug or breast-feeding should be discontinued. *Phenobarbital* is excreted in small amounts and may cause drowsiness in the infant.
Antidepressants	Tricyclic antidepressants such as *amitriptyline* (Elavil) and others are excreted in small amounts; effects on nursing infants are not known. Other antidepressants have not been established as safe for use.
Antidiabetic Drugs	*Insulin* does not enter breast milk and is not known to affect the nursing infant. However, insulin requirements of the mother may be decreased while breast-feeding. Oral agents *chlorpropamide* (Diabinese) and *tolbutamide* (Orinase) are excreted in breast milk; the status of other sulfonylureas is unknown. There is a potential for hypoglycemia in nursing infants.
Antidiarrheals	*Diphenoxylate* (Lomotil) and *loperamide* (Imodium) should be used cautiously during lactation; effects on the nursing infant are unknown.
Antiemetics	Although information is limited, most of the drugs (e.g., phenothiazines such as *promethazine* [Phenergan] and antihistamines such as *dimenhydrinate* [Dramamine]) are apparently excreted in breast milk and may cause drowsiness and possibly other effects in nursing infants. Antihistamines used for antiemetic effects also may inhibit lactation. *Metoclopramide* (Reglan) is excreted and concentrated in breast milk; it should be used cautiously, if at all.
Antihistamines	$Histamine_1$ receptor antagonists such as *diphenhydramine* (Benadryl) may inhibit lactation by their drying effects and may cause drowsiness in nursing infants. For most of the commonly used drugs, including over-the-counter allergy and cold remedies, little information is available about excretion in breast milk or effects on nursing infants. $Histamine_2$ receptor antagonists such as *cimetidine* (Tagamet) and *ranitidine* (Zantac) are excreted in breast milk. *Famotidine* (Pepcid) was excreted in animals, but it is not known whether it is excreted in human breast milk. It is generally recommended that either the drug or nursing be discontinued.
Antihypertensives	Beta-adrenergic blocking agents should generally be avoided by nursing mothers. *Propranolol* (Inderal) and *metoprolol* (Lopressor) are excreted in low concentrations; *acebutolol* (Sectral) and its major metabolite are excreted; it is unknown whether *nadolol* (Corgard) and *timolol* (Blocadren) are excreted. *Methyldopa* (Aldomet) is excreted; effects on nursing infants are unknown. It is unknown whether *hydralazine* (Apresoline) is excreted; safety for use is not established. *Captopril* (Capoten), *clonidine* (Catapres), *guanabenz* (Wytensin), and *guanfacine* (Tenex) are not generally recommended because information about effects on nursing infants is limited. Calcium channel blocking drugs should not be given to nursing mothers. *Verapamil* (Calan) and *diltiazem* (Cardizem) are excreted in breast milk.
Antimanic Agent	*Lithium* is excreted in breast milk and reaches about 40% of the mother's serum level. Infant serum and milk levels are about equal. If the drug is required, nursing should be discontinued.
Antipsychotic Drugs	Little information is available considering the extensive use of these drugs. *Chlorpromazine* (Thorazine) and *haloperidol* (Haldol) have been detected in breast milk in small amounts. Safety has not been established.
Antithyroid Drugs	Nursing is contraindicated for clients on the antithyroid drugs *propylthiouracil* and *methimazole* (Tapazole).
Beta-Adrenergic Blocking Agents	See **Antihypertensives**.
Bronchodilators (Xanthine)	*Theophylline* (Theo-Dur) enters breast milk readily; use in caution.
Calcium Channel Blocking Agents	See **Antihypertensives**.
Corticosteroids	*Prednisone* (Deltasone), *dexamethasone* (Decadron), and others appear in breast milk and could suppress growth, interfere with endogenous corticosteroid production, or cause other adverse effects in nursing infants. Advise mothers taking pharmacologic doses not to breast-feed.
Digitalis	*Digoxin* (Lanoxin) is excreted. However, infants receive very small amounts, and no adverse effects have been reported.
Diuretics	If diuretic drug therapy is required, nursing mothers should discontinue breast-feeding. Thiazide diuretics such as *hydrochlorothiazide* (HydroDIURIL) and the loop diuretic *furosemide* (Lasix) are excreted in breast milk. It is unknown whether *bumetanide* (Bumex) and ethacrynic acid (Edecrin) are excreted. Little information is available about potassium-sparing diuretics, such as *amiloride* (Midamor), *triamterene* (Dyrenium, Dyazide, Maxide), and *spironolactone* (Aldactone). They are not recommended for use.
Laxatives	*Cascara sagrada* is excreted in breast milk and may cause diarrhea in the nursing infant. It is not known whether *docusate* (Colace) is excreted.
Nonsteroidal Anti-inflammatory Drugs	Most of the drugs, such as *ibuprofen* (Motrin, Advil), are excreted in breast milk, and nursing is not recommended. However, occasional use of therapeutic doses is probably acceptable.
Thyroid Hormones	Small amounts are excreted in breast milk. The drugs are not associated with adverse effects on nursing infants but should be used with caution in nursing mothers.

(From Abrams, A. C. [1998]. *Clinical drug therapy* [5th ed.]. Philadelphia: Lippincott.)

APPENDIX D

Temperature and Weight Conversion Charts

Conversion of Pounds to Kilograms

POUNDS	0	1	2	3	4	5	6	7	8	9
0	—	0.45	0.90	1.36	1.81	2.26	2.72	3.17	3.62	4.08
10	4.53	4.98	5.44	5.89	6.35	6.80	7.25	7.71	8.16	8.61
20	9.07	9.52	9.97	10.43	10.88	11.34	11.79	12.24	12.70	13.15
30	13.60	14.06	14.51	14.96	15.42	15.87	16.32	16.78	17.23	17.69
40	18.14	18.59	19.05	19.50	19.95	20.41	20.86	21.31	21.77	22.22
50	22.68	23.13	23.58	24.04	24.49	24.94	25.40	25.85	26.30	26.76
60	27.21	27.66	28.12	28.57	29.03	29.48	29.93	30.39	30.84	31.29
70	31.75	32.20	32.65	33.11	33.56	34.02	34.47	34.92	35.38	35.83
80	36.28	36.74	37.19	37.64	38.10	38.55	39.00	39.46	39.91	40.37
90	40.82	41.27	41.73	42.18	42.63	43.09	43.54	43.99	44.45	44.90
100	45.36	45.81	46.26	46.72	47.17	47.62	48.08	48.53	48.98	49.44
110	49.89	50.34	50.80	51.25	51.71	52.16	52.61	53.07	53.52	53.97
120	54.43	54.88	55.33	55.79	56.24	56.70	57.15	57.60	58.06	58.51
130	58.96	59.42	59.87	60.32	60.78	61.23	61.68	62.14	62.59	63.05
140	63.50	63.95	64.41	64.86	65.31	65.77	66.22	66.67	67.13	67.58
150	68.04	68.49	68.94	69.40	69.85	70.30	70.76	71.21	71.66	72.12
160	72.57	73.02	73.48	73.93	74.39	74.84	75.29	75.75	76.20	76.65
170	77.11	77.56	78.01	78.47	78.92	79.38	79.83	80.28	80.74	81.19
180	81.64	82.10	82.55	83.00	83.46	83.91	84.36	84.82	85.27	85.73
190	86.18	86.68	87.09	87.54	87.99	88.45	88.90	89.35	89.81	90.26
200	90.72	91.17	91.62	92.08	92.53	92.98	93.44	93.89	94.34	94.80

Conversion of Pounds and Ounces to Grams for Newborn Weights

	OUNCES															
POUNDS	*0*	*1*	*2*	*3*	*4*	*5*	*6*	*7*	*8*	*9*	*10*	*11*	*12*	*13*	*14*	*15*
0	—	28	57	85	113	142	170	198	227	255	283	312	430	369	397	425
1	454	482	510	539	567	595	624	652	680	709	737	765	794	822	850	879
2	907	936	964	992	1021	1049	1077	1106	1134	1162	1191	1219	1247	1276	1304	1332
3	1361	1389	1417	1446	1474	1503	1531	1559	1588	1616	1644	1673	1701	1729	1758	1786
4	1814	1843	1871	1899	1928	1956	1984	2013	2041	2070	2098	2126	2155	2183	2211	2240
5	2268	2296	2325	2353	2381	2410	2438	2466	2495	2523	2551	2580	2608	2637	2665	2693
6	2722	2750	2778	2807	2835	2863	2892	2920	2948	2977	3005	3033	3062	3090	3118	3147
7	3175	3203	3232	3260	3289	3317	3345	3374	3402	3430	3459	3487	3515	3544	3572	3600
8	3629	3657	3685	3714	3742	3770	3799	3827	3856	3884	3912	3941	3969	3997	4026	4054
9	4082	4111	4139	4167	4196	4224	4252	4281	4309	4337	4366	4394	4423	4451	4479	4508
10	4536	4564	4593	4621	4649	4678	4706	4734	4763	4791	4819	4848	4876	4904	4933	4961
11	4990	5018	5046	5075	5103	5131	5160	5188	5216	5245	5273	5301	5330	5358	5386	5415
12	5443	5471	5500	5528	5557	5585	5613	5642	5670	5698	5727	5755	5783	5812	5840	5868
13	5897	5925	5953	5982	6010	6038	6067	6095	6123	6152	6180	6209	6237	6265	6294	6322
14	6350	6379	6407	6435	6464	6492	6520	6549	6577	6605	6634	6662	6690	6719	6747	6776
15	6804	6832	6860	6889	6917	6945	6973	7002	7030	7059	7087	7115	7144	7172	7201	7228

Conversion of Fahrenheit to Celsius

CELSIUS	FAHRENHEIT	CELSIUS	FAHRENHEIT	CELSIUS	FAHRENHEIT
34.0	93.2	37.0	98.6	40.0	104.0
34.2	93.6	37.2	99.0	40.2	104.4
34.4	93.9	37.4	99.3	40.4	104.7
34.6	94.3	37.6	99.7	40.6	105.2
34.8	94.6	37.8	100.0	40.8	105.4
35.0	95.0	38.0	100.4	41.0	105.9
35.2	95.4	38.2	100.8	41.2	106.1
35.4	95.7	38.4	101.1	41.4	106.5
35.6	96.1	38.6	101.5	41.6	106.8
35.8	96.4	38.8	101.8	41.8	107.2
36.0	96.8	39.0	102.2	42.0	107.6
36.2	97.2	39.2	102.6	42.2	108.0
36.4	97.5	39.4	102.9	42.4	108.3
36.6	97.9	39.6	103.3	42.6	108.7
36.8	98.2	39.8	103.6	42.8	109.0

$(°C) \times (9/5) + 32 = °F$
$(°F - 32) \times (5/9) = °C$

Growth Charts

APPENDIX E

Birth to 36 months: Boys
Length-for-age and Weight-for-age percentiles

NAME ____________________
RECORD # ____________

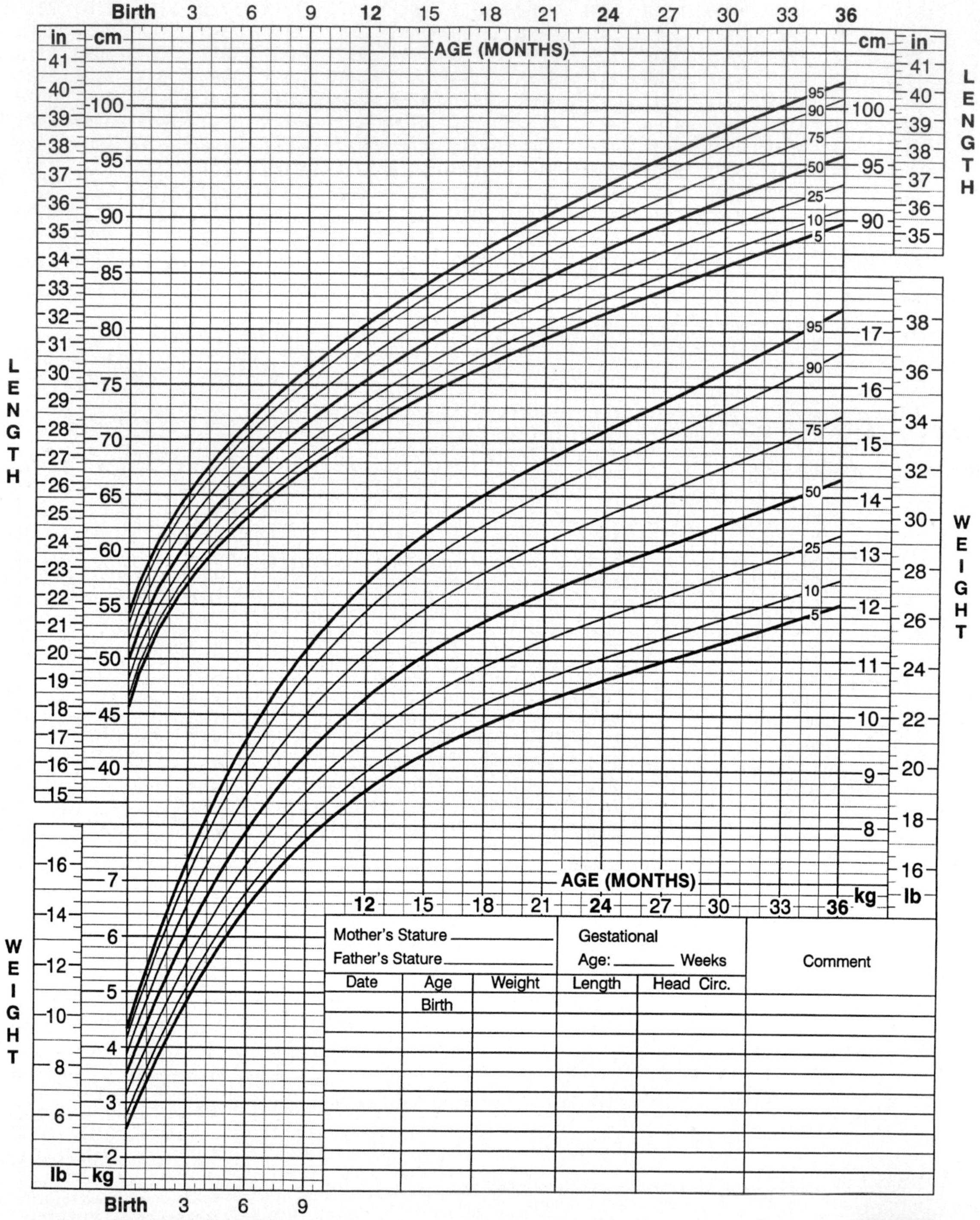

Published May 30, 2000 (modified 4/20/01).
SOURCE: Developed by the National Center for Health Statistics in collaboration with the National Center for Chronic Disease Prevention and Health Promotion (2000).
http://www.cdc.gov/growthcharts

CDC
SAFER · HEALTHIER · PEOPLE™

Birth to 36 months: Boys
Head circumference-for-age and Weight-for-length percentiles

NAME ______________________

RECORD # ______________________

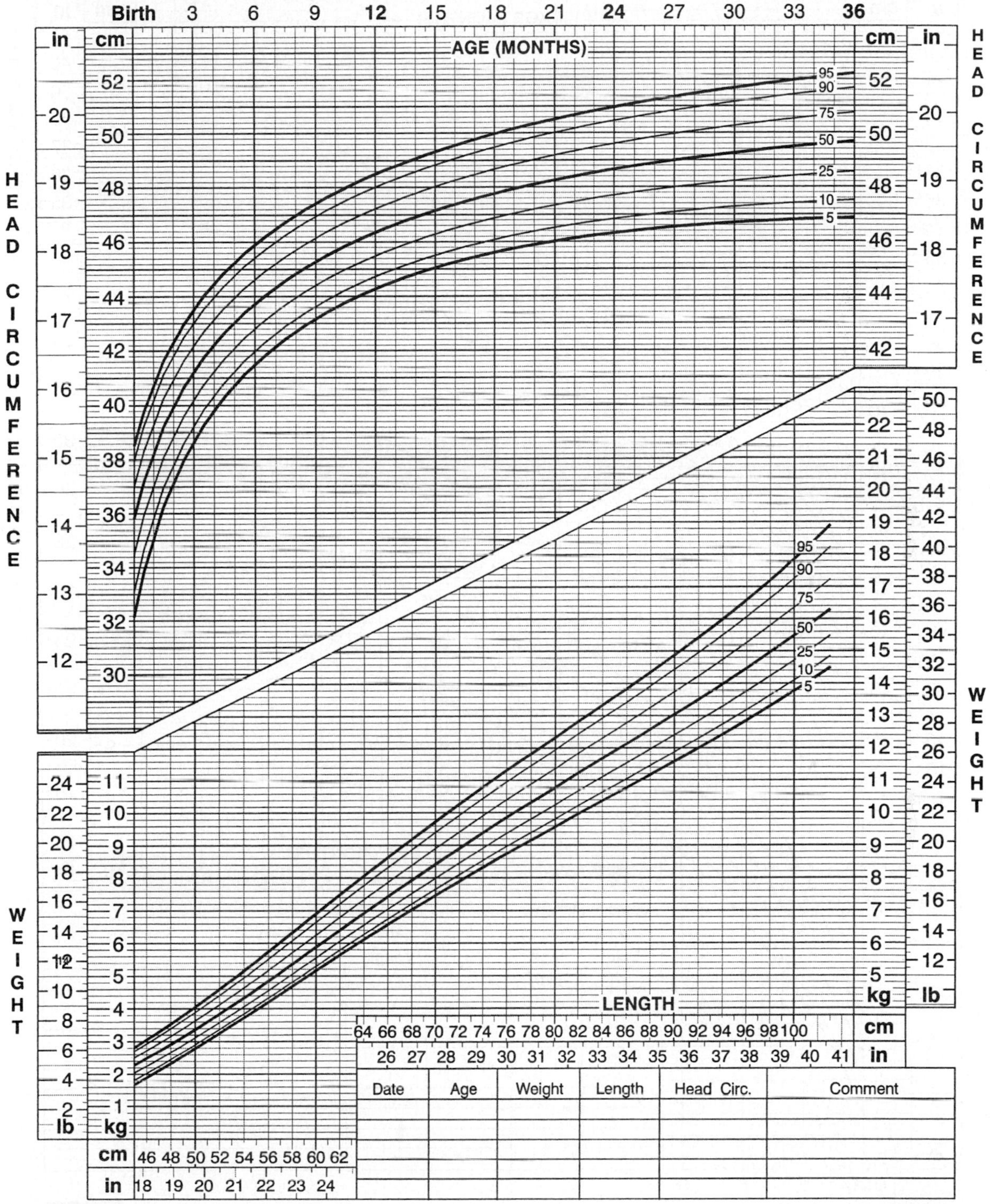

Published May 30, 2000 (modified 10/16/00).

SOURCE: Developed by the National Center for Health Statistics in collaboration with the National Center for Chronic Disease Prevention and Health Promotion (2000).

http://www.cdc.gov/growthcharts

CDC

SAFER · HEALTHIER · PEOPLE™

Birth to 36 months: Girls
Length-for-age and Weight-for-age percentiles

NAME ______________________

RECORD # ______________

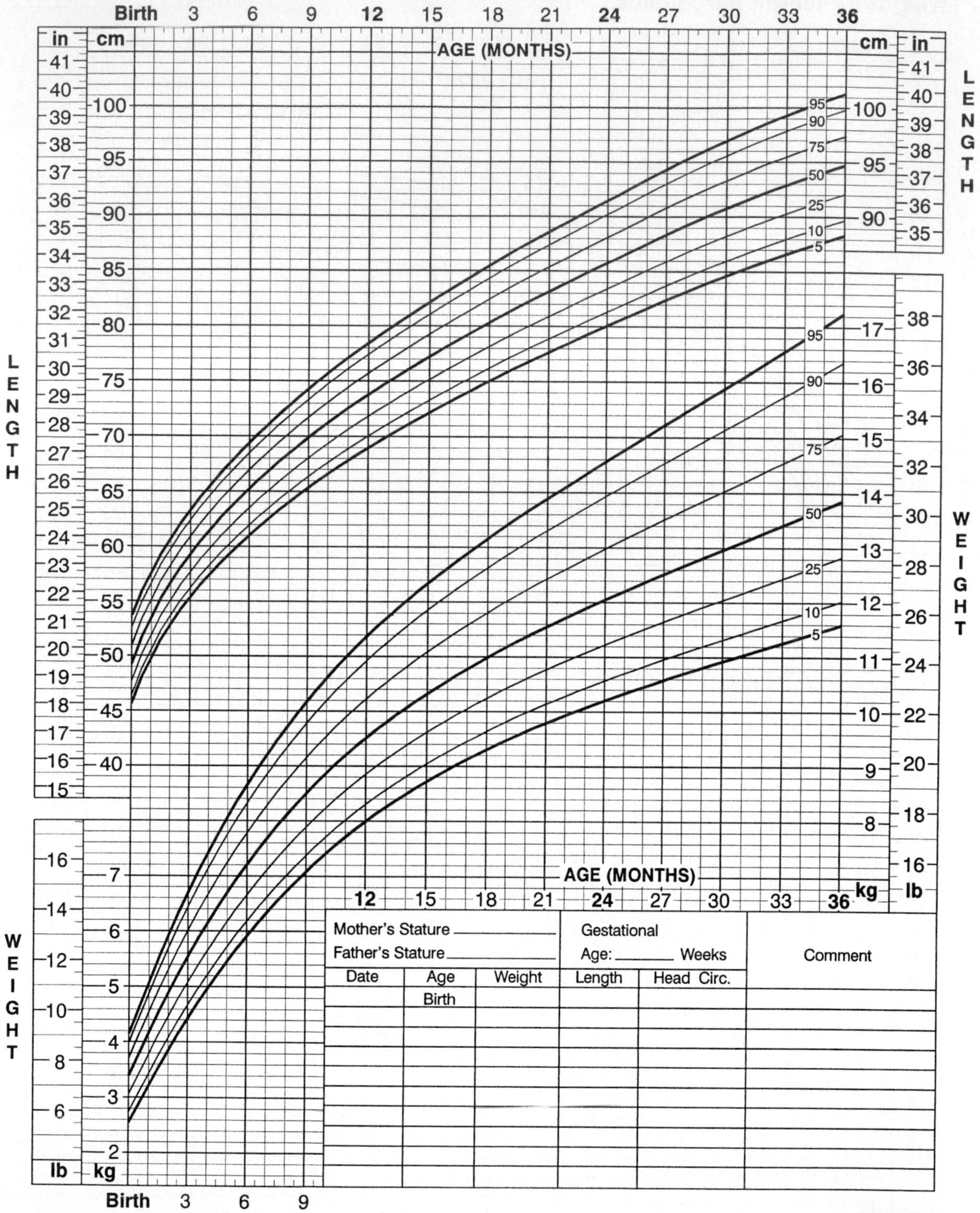

Published May 30, 2000 (modified 4/20/01).
SOURCE: Developed by the National Center for Health Statistics in collaboration with the National Center for Chronic Disease Prevention and Health Promotion (2000).
http://www.cdc.gov/growthcharts

CDC
SAFER · HEALTHIER · PEOPLE™

Birth to 36 months: Girls
Head circumference-for-age and Weight-for-length percentiles

NAME ____________________

RECORD # ____________

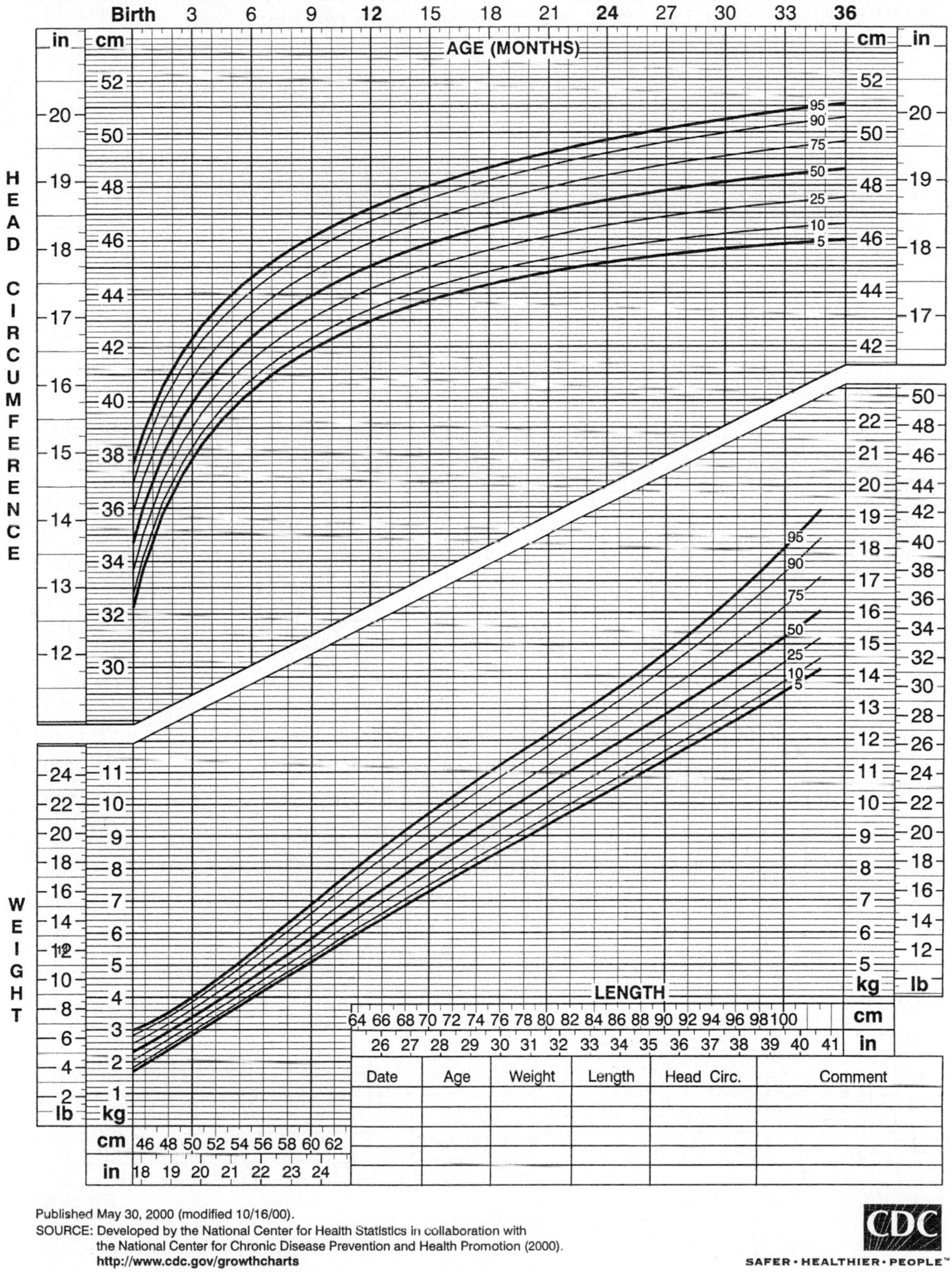

Date	Age	Weight	Length	Head Circ.	Comment

Published May 30, 2000 (modified 10/16/00).
SOURCE: Developed by the National Center for Health Statistics in collaboration with the National Center for Chronic Disease Prevention and Health Promotion (2000).
http://www.cdc.gov/growthcharts

SAFER · HEALTHIER · PEOPLE™

2 to 20 years: Boys
Stature-for-age and Weight-for-age percentiles

NAME ______________________

RECORD # ______________________

Mother's Stature ____________ Father's Stature ____________

Date	Age	Weight	Stature	BMI*

***To Calculate BMI**: Weight (kg) ÷ Stature (cm) ÷ Stature (cm) x 10,000
or Weight (lb) ÷ Stature (in) ÷ Stature (in) x 703

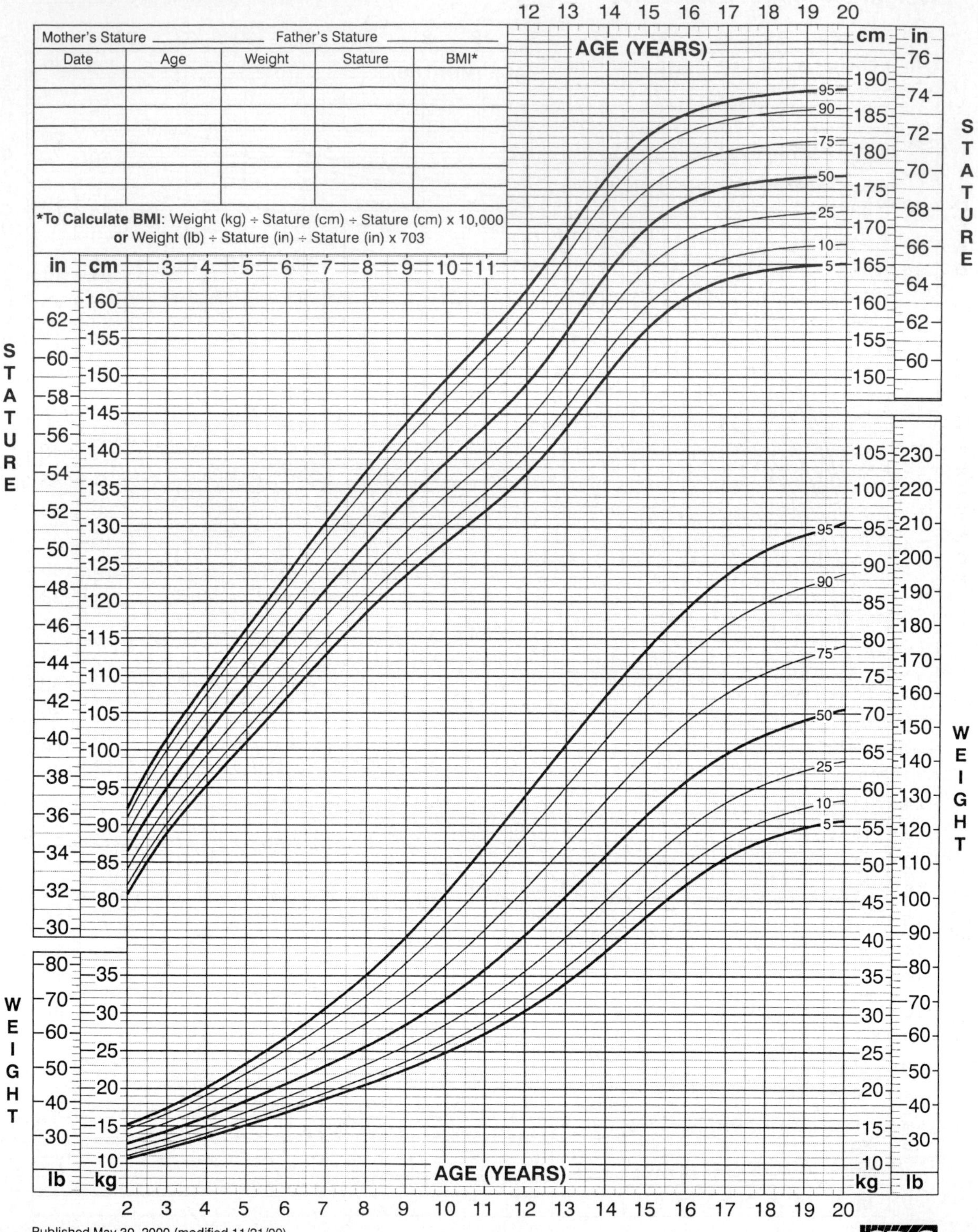

Published May 30, 2000 (modified 11/21/00).
SOURCE: Developed by the National Center for Health Statistics in collaboration with the National Center for Chronic Disease Prevention and Health Promotion (2000).
http://www.cdc.gov/growthcharts

CDC SAFER • HEALTHIER • PEOPLE

2 to 20 years: Boys
Body mass index-for-age percentiles

NAME ____________________

RECORD # ____________

Date	Age	Weight	Stature	BMI*	Comments

***To Calculate BMI:** Weight (kg) ÷ Stature (cm) ÷ Stature (cm) x 10,000
or Weight (lb) ÷ Stature (in) ÷ Stature (in) x 703

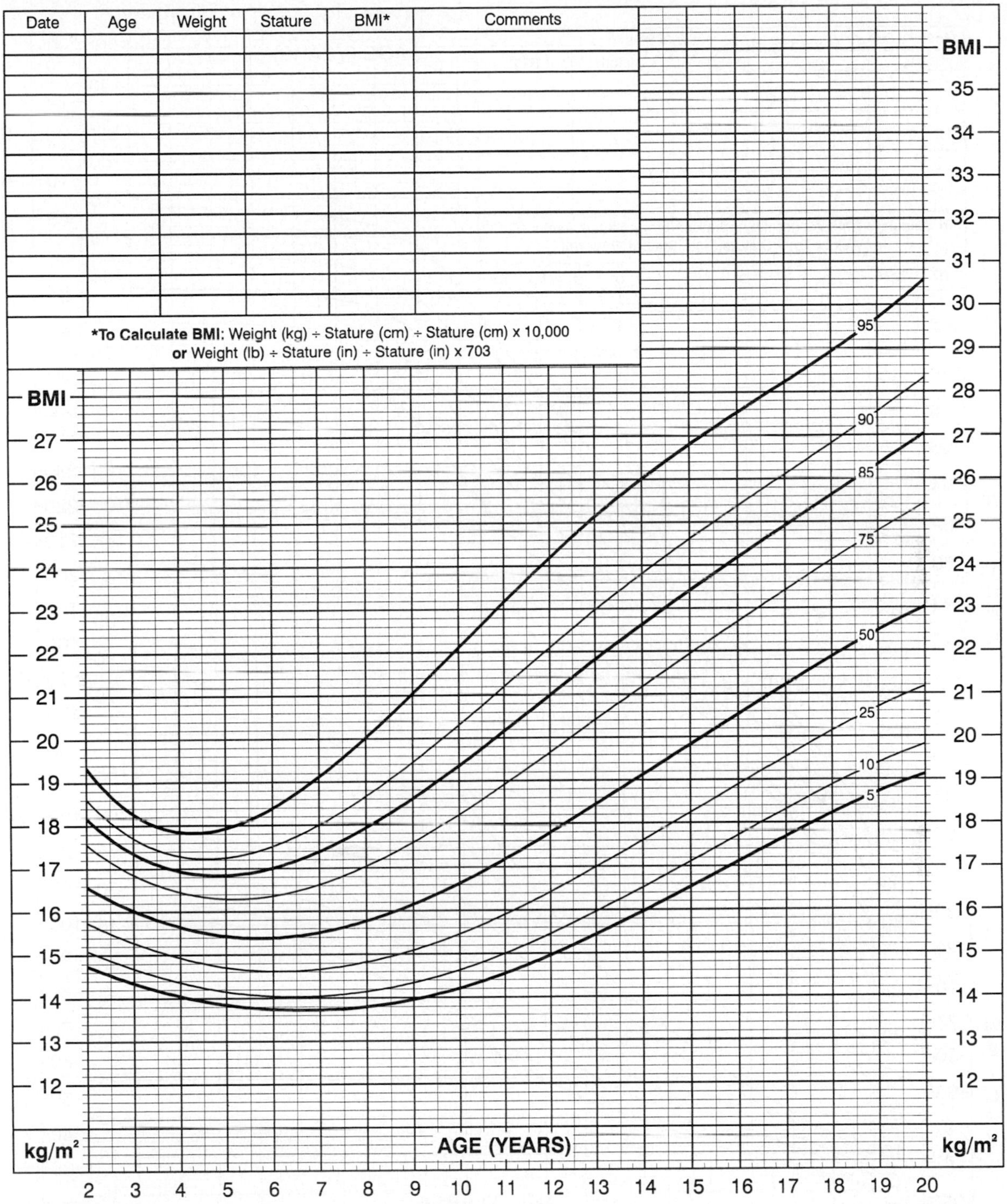

SOURCE: Developed by the National Center for Health Statistics in collaboration with the National Center for Chronic Disease Prevention and Health Promotion (2000).
http://www.cdc.gov/growthcharts

CDC

2 to 20 years: Girls
Stature-for-age and Weight-for-age percentiles

NAME ____________________

RECORD # ____________

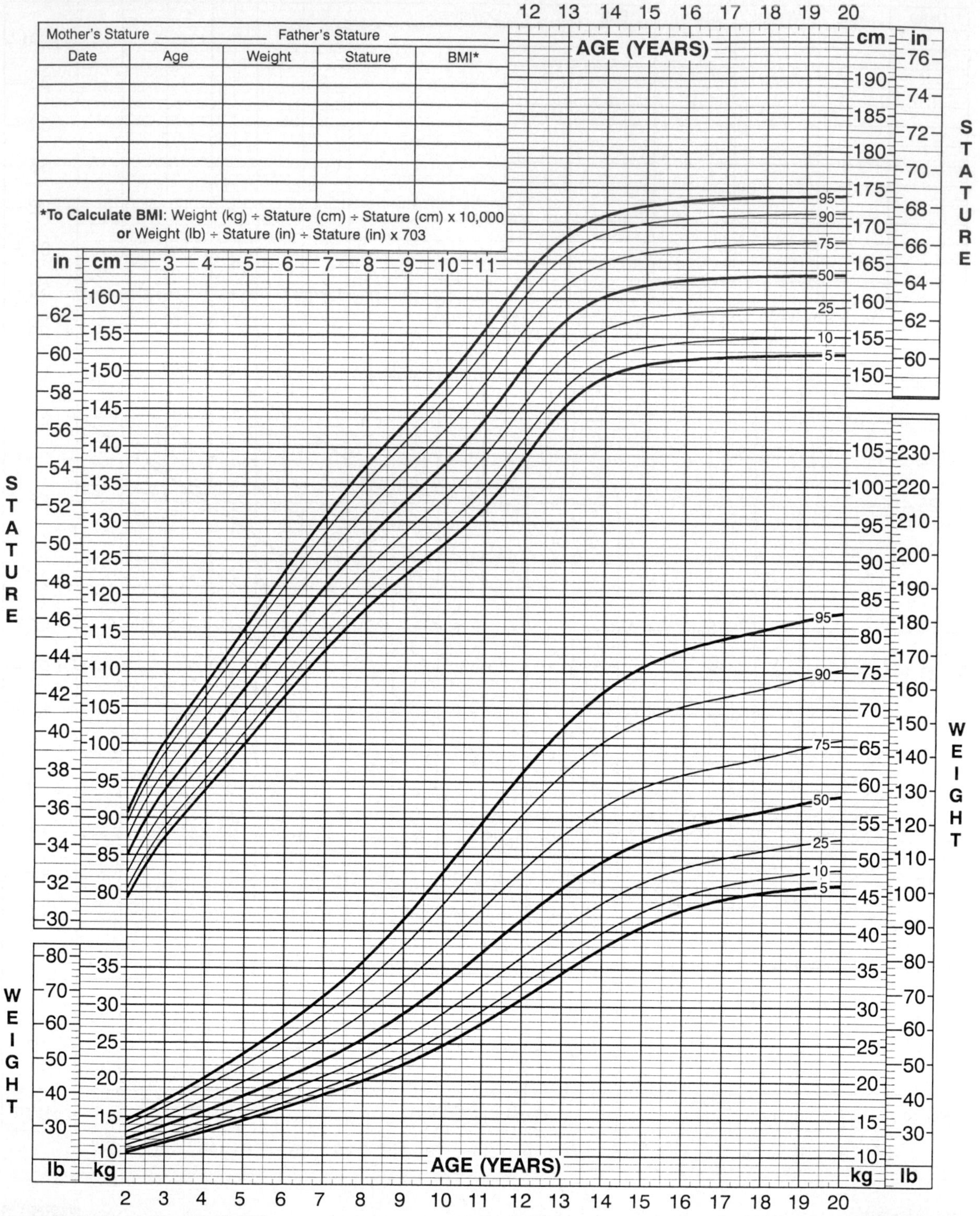

Revised and corrected November 21, 2000.

SOURCE: Developed by the National Center for Health Statistics in collaboration with the National Center for Chronic Disease Prevention and Health Promotion (2000).
http://www.cdc.gov/growthcharts

CDC

2 to 20 years: Girls
Body mass index-for-age percentiles

NAME ____________________

RECORD # ____________

Date	Age	Weight	Stature	BMI*	Comments

***To Calculate BMI**: Weight (kg) ÷ Stature (cm) ÷ Stature (cm) x 10,000
or Weight (lb) ÷ Stature (in) ÷ Stature (in) x 703

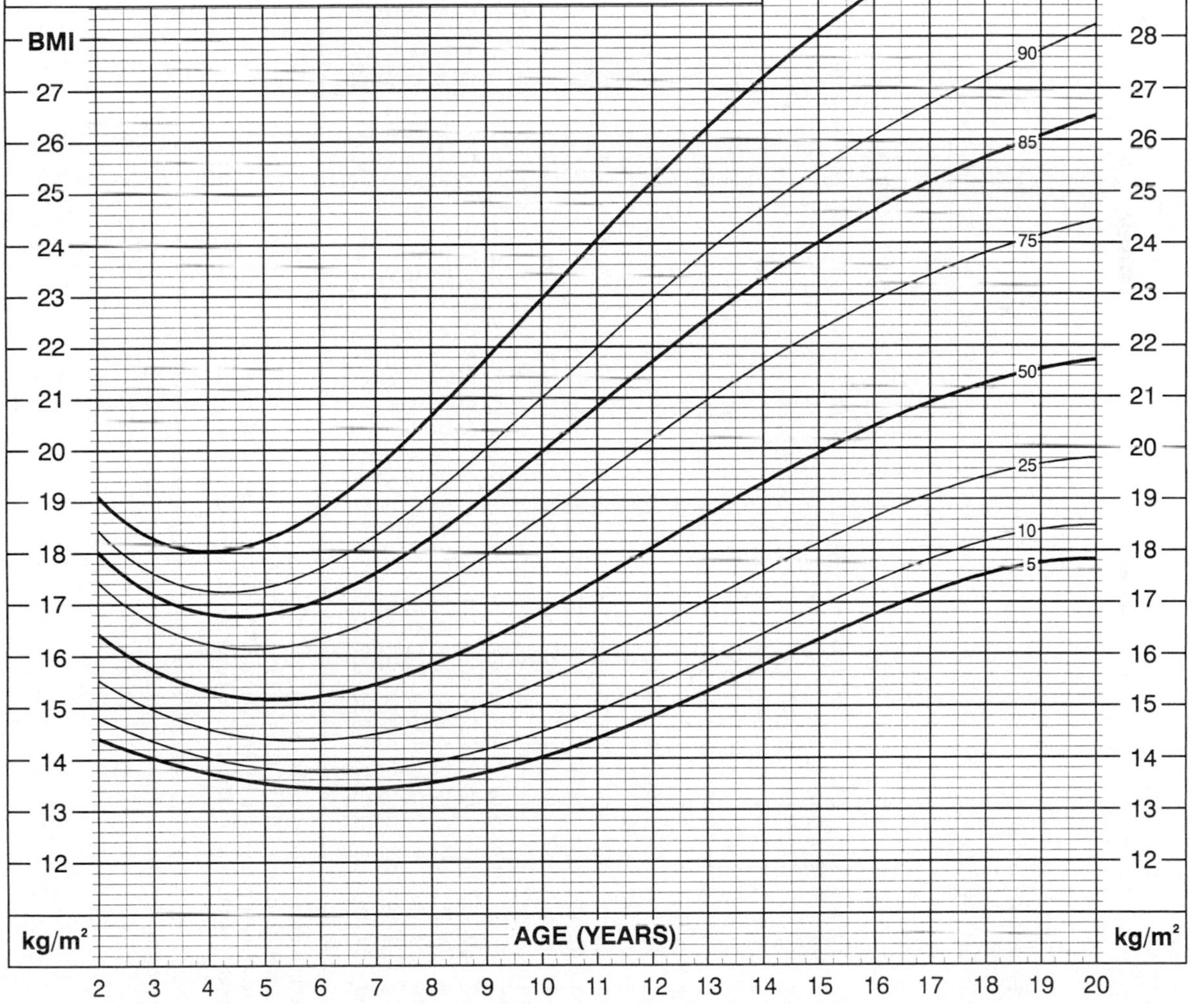

SOURCE: Developed by the National Center for Health Statistics in collaboration with the National Center for Chronic Disease Prevention and Health Promotion (2000).
http://www.cdc.gov/growthcharts

CDC

TABLE 1 Body Mass Index Table

BMI	19	20	21	22	23	24	25	26	27	28	29	30	31	32	33	34	35	36	37	38	39	40	41	42	43	44	45	46	47	48	49	50	51	52	53	54
Height (inches)	***Body weight (pounds)***																																			
58	91	96	100	105	110	115	119	124	129	134	138	143	148	153	158	162	167	172	177	181	186	191	196	201	205	210	215	220	224	229	234	239	244	248	253	258
59	94	99	104	109	114	119	124	128	133	138	143	148	153	158	163	168	173	178	183	188	193	198	203	208	212	217	222	227	232	237	242	247	252	257	262	267
60	97	102	107	112	118	123	128	133	138	143	148	153	158	163	168	174	179	184	189	194	199	204	209	215	220	225	230	235	240	245	250	255	261	266	271	276
61	100	106	111	116	122	127	132	137	143	148	153	158	164	169	174	180	185	190	195	201	206	211	217	222	227	232	238	243	248	254	259	264	269	275	280	285
62	104	109	115	120	126	131	136	142	147	153	158	164	169	175	180	186	191	196	202	207	213	218	224	229	235	240	246	251	256	262	267	273	278	284	289	295
63	107	113	118	124	130	135	141	146	152	158	163	169	175	180	186	191	197	203	208	214	220	225	231	237	242	248	254	259	265	270	278	282	287	293	299	304
64	110	116	122	128	134	140	145	151	157	163	169	174	180	186	192	197	204	209	215	221	227	232	238	244	250	256	262	267	273	279	285	291	296	302	308	314
65	114	120	126	132	138	144	150	156	162	168	174	180	186	192	198	204	210	216	222	228	234	240	246	252	258	264	270	276	282	288	294	300	306	312	318	324
66	118	124	130	136	142	148	155	161	167	173	179	186	192	198	204	210	216	223	229	235	241	247	253	260	266	272	278	284	291	297	303	309	315	322	328	334
67	121	127	134	140	146	153	159	166	172	178	185	191	198	204	211	217	223	230	236	242	249	255	261	268	274	280	287	293	299	306	312	319	325	331	338	344
68	125	131	138	144	151	158	164	171	177	184	190	197	203	210	216	223	230	236	243	249	256	262	269	276	282	289	295	302	308	315	322	328	335	341	348	354
69	128	135	142	149	155	162	169	176	182	189	196	203	209	216	223	230	236	243	250	257	263	270	277	284	291	297	304	311	318	324	331	338	345	351	358	365
70	132	139	146	153	160	167	174	181	188	195	202	209	216	222	229	236	243	250	257	264	271	278	285	292	299	306	313	320	327	334	341	348	355	362	369	376
71	136	143	150	157	165	172	179	186	193	200	208	215	222	229	236	243	250	257	265	272	279	286	293	301	308	315	322	329	338	343	351	358	365	372	379	386
72	140	147	154	162	169	177	184	191	199	206	213	221	228	235	242	250	258	265	272	279	287	294	302	309	316	324	331	338	346	353	361	368	375	383	390	397
73	144	151	159	166	174	182	189	197	204	212	219	227	235	242	250	257	265	272	280	288	295	302	310	318	325	333	340	348	355	363	371	378	386	393	401	408
74	148	155	163	171	179	186	194	202	210	218	225	233	241	249	256	264	272	280	287	295	303	311	319	326	334	342	350	358	365	373	381	389	396	404	412	420
75	152	160	168	176	184	192	200	208	216	224	232	240	248	256	264	272	279	287	295	303	311	319	327	335	343	351	359	367	375	383	391	399	407	415	423	431
76	156	164	172	180	189	197	205	213	221	230	238	246	254	263	271	279	287	295	304	312	320	328	336	344	353	361	369	377	385	394	402	410	418	426	435	443

Calculation of body mass index (BMI) is recommended by the National Heart, Lung, and Blood Institute as a practical means of assessing body fat. Persons with a BMI of 18.5 to 24.9 are considered to be of normal weight. Those with a BMI of 25.0 to 29.9 are overweight. Patients with a BMI of 30.0 to 34.9 or 35.0 to 39.9 are in obesity class I or II, respectively; and those with a BMI of 40 and over are considered extremely obese (obesity class III).

From National Heart, Lung, and Blood Institute (1998). *Clinical guidelines on the identification, evaluation, and treatment of overweight and obesity in adults: The Evidence Report.* Bethesda, MD: National Institutes of Health.

Standard Laboratory Values

APPENDIX F

PREGNANT AND NONPREGNANT WOMEN

VALUES	NONPREGNANT	PREGNANT
Hematologic		
Complete Blood Count (CBC)		
Hemoglobin, g/dL	12–16*	11.5–14*
Hematocrit, PCV, %	37–47	32–42
Red cell volume, mL	1600	1900
Plasma volume, mL	2400	3700
Red blood cell count, million/mm^3	4–5.5	3.75–5.0
White blood cells, total per mm^3	4500–10,000	5000–15,000
Polymorphonuclear cells, %	54–62	60–85
Lymphocytes, %	38–46	15–40
Erythrocyte sedimentation rate, mm/h	≤	30–90
MCHC, g/dL packed RBCs (mean corpuscular hemoglobin concentration)	30–36	No change
MCH (mean corpuscular hemoglobin per picogram)	29–32	No change
MCV/μm^3 (mean corpuscular volume per cubic micrometer)	82–96	No change
Blood Coagulation and Fibrinolytic Activity†		
Factors VII, VIII, IX, X		Increase in pregnancy, return to normal in early puerperium; factor VIII increases during and immediately after delivery
Factors XI, XIII		Decrease in pregnancy
Prothrombin time (protime)	60–70 sec	Slight decrease in pregnancy
Partial thromboplastin time (PTT)	12–14 sec	Slight decrease in pregnancy and again decrease during second and third stage of labor (indicates clotting at placental site)
Bleeding time	1–3 min (Duke) 2–4 min (Ivy)	No appreciable change
Coagulation time	6–10 min (Lee/White)	No appreciable change
Platelets	150,000 to 350,000/mm^3	No significant change until 3–5 days after delivery, then marked increase (may predispose woman to thrombosis) and gradual return to normal
Fibrinolytic activity		Decreases in pregnancy, then abrupt return to normal (protection against thromboembolism)
Fibrinogen	250 mg/dL	400 mg/dL
Mineral and Vitamin Concentrations		
Serum iron, µg	75–150	65–120
Total iron-binding capacity, µg	250–450	300–500
Iron saturation, %	30–40	15–30
Vitamin B_{12}, folic acid, ascorbic acid	Normal	Moderate decrease

(continued)

VALUES	NONPREGNANT	PREGNANT
Serum protein		
Total, g/dL	6.7–8.3	5.5–7.5
Albumin, g/dL	3.5–5.5	3.0–5.0
Globulin, total, g/dL	2.3–3.5	3.0–4.0
Blood sugar		
Fasting, mg/dL	70–80	65
2-hour postprandial, mg/dL	60–110	Under 140 after a 100-g carbohydrate meal is considered normal
Cardiovascular		
Blood pressure, mm Hg	120/80‡	114/65
Peripheral resistance, dyne/s · cm^{-5}	120	100
Venous pressure, cm H_2O		
Femoral	9	24
Antecubital	8	8
Pulse, rate/min	70	80
Stroke volume, mL	65	75
Cardiac output, L/min	4.5	6
Circulation time (arm-tongue), sec	15–16	12–14
Blood volume, mL		
Whole blood	4000	5600
Plasma	2400	3700
Red blood cells	1600	1900
Plasma renin, units/L	3–10	10–80
Chest x-ray studies		
Transverse diameter of heart	—	1–2 cm increase
Left border of heart	—	Straightened
Cardiac volume	—	70-mL increase
Electrocardiogram	—	15° left axis deviation
V_1 and V_2	—	Inverted T-wave
kV_4	—	Low T
III	—	Q + inverted T
aVr	—	Small Q
Hepatic		
Bilirubin total	Not more than 1 mg/dL	Unchanged
Cephalin flocculation	Up to 2+ in 48 h	Positive in 10%
Serum cholesterol	110–300 mg/dL	↑ 60% from 16–32 weeks of pregnancy; remains at this level until after delivery
Thymol turbidity	0–4 units	Positive in 15%
Serum alkaline phosphatase	2–4.5 units (Bodansky)	↑ from week 12 of pregnancy to 6 weeks after delivery
Serum lactate dehydrogenase		Unchanged
Serum glutamic-oxaloacetic transaminase		Unchanged
Serum globulin albumin	1.5–3.0 g/dL 4.5–5.3 g/dL	↑ slight ↓ 3.0 g by late pregnancy
A/G ratio		Decreased
α_2-globulin		Increased
β-globulin		Increased
Serum cholinesterase		Decreased
Leucine aminopeptidase		Increased
Sulfobromophthalein (5 mg/kg)	5% dye or less in 45 min	Somewhat decreased
Renal		
Bladder capacity	1300 mL	1500 mL
Renal plasma flow (RPF), mL/min	490–700	Increase by 25%, to 612–875

(continued)

VALUES	NONPREGNANT	PREGNANT
Glomerular filtration rate (GFR), mL/min	105–132	Increase by 50%, to 160–198
Nonprotein nitrogen (NPN), mg/dL	25–40	Decreases
Blood urea nitrogen (BUN), mg/dL	20–25	Decreases
Serum creatinine, mg/kg/24 hr	20–22	Decreases
Serum uric acid, mg/kg/24 hr	257–750	Decreases
Urine glucose	Negative	Present in 20% of gravidas
Intravenous pyelogram (IVP)	Normal	Slight to moderate hydroureter and hydronephrosis; right kidney larger than left kidney
Miscellaneous		
Total thyroxine concentration	5–12 μg/dL thyroxine	↑ 9–16 μg/dL thyroxine (however, unbound thyroxine not greatly increased)
Ionized calcium		Relatively unchanged
Aldosterone		↑ 1 mg/24 hr by third trimester
Dehydroisoandrosterone	Plasma clearance 6–8 L/24 hr	↑ plasma clearance tenfold to twentyfold

* At sea level. Permanent residents of higher levels (e.g., Denver) require higher levels of hemoglobin.
From Scott, J. R., et al. (2000). *Obstetrics and gynecology*. Philadelphia: Lippincott Williams & Wilkins.
† Pregnancy represents a hypercoagulable state.
‡ For the woman about 20 years of age.
10 years of age: 103/70.
30 years of age: 123/82.
40 years of age: 126/84.

INFANTS AND CHILDREN

The following reference values for laboratory tests represent guidelines only, since the reference range from one institution to the next will vary, depending on the laboratory method used. To simplify the interpretation of laboratory results reported in International System (SI) units, conversion factors (from SI to conventional units) are provided. SI base units are the gram (g), the liter (L), and the mole (mol). Other abbreviations used throughout this table are listed below.

SI Prefixes

FACTOR	PREFIX	SYMBOL
10^{3}	kilo	k
10^{-1}	deci	d
10^{-2}	centi	c
10^{-3}	milli	m
10^{-6}	micro	μ
10^{-9}	nano	n
10^{-12}	pico	p
10^{-15}	femto	f

Abbreviations

CI	confidence interval
d	day
F	female
h	hour
Hb	hemoglobin
M	male
MCHC	mean corpuscular hemoglobin concentration
MCV	mean corpuscular value
mEq	milliequivalent
min	minute
RBC	red blood cell
s	second
SD	standard deviation
U	unit
WBC	white blood cell
yr	year

Blood

TEST	SI REFERENCE RANGE	CONVERSION FACTOR	CONVENTIONAL UNITS REFERENCE RANGE
Adrenocorticotropic hormone (ACTH)	Cord: 130–160 ng/L 1st week: 100–140 Adult 0800 h: 25–100 1800 h: <50		Cord: 130–160 pg/mL 1st week: 100–140 Adult 0800 h: 25–100 1800 h: <50
Alanine aminotransferase (ALT)	<1 yr: 5–28 U/L >1 yr: 820		Same as SI
Albumin	35–50 g/L		3.5–5.0 g/dL
Aldolase	Newborn: <32 U/L Child: <16 Adult: <8		Same as SI
Aldosterone	Newborn: 0.14–1.66 nmol/L 1 wk–1 yr: 0.03–4.43 1–3 yr: 0.14–1.66 3–5 yr: <0.14–2.22 5–7 yr: <0.14–1.39 7–11 yr: 0.14–1.94 11–15 yr: <0.14–1.39	nmol/L × 36.1 = ng/dL	Newborn: 5–60 ng/dL 1 wk–1 yr: 1–160 ng/dL 1–3 yr: 5–60 ng/dL 3–5 yr: <5–80 5–7 yr: <5–50 7–11 yr: 5–70 11–15 yr: <5–50
Alkaline phosphatase	Infant: 150–400 U/L 2–10 yr: 100–300 11–18 yr (M): 50–375 11–18 yr (F): 30–300 Adult: 30–100		Same as SI
α_1–antitrypsin	2–4 g/L		
α–fetoprotein	Fetal: peak of 2–4 g/L Cord: <0.05 g/L >1 yr: <30 μg/L		200–400 mg/dL Fetal: 200–400 mg/dL Cord: <5 >1 yr: <30
Ammonia nitrogen	9–34 μmol/L	μmol/L × 1.4 = μg/dL	13–48 μg/dL
Amylase	Newborn: 5–65 U/L >1 yr: 25–125		Same as SI
Androstenedione	Child: 0.17–1.7 nmol/L Adult (M): 2.4–5.2 Adult (F): 2.7–8.0	nmol/L × 28.7 = ng/dL	Child: 5–50 ng/dL Adult (M): 70–150 Adult (F): 76–228
Angiotensin–converting enzyme	<670 nmol · L^{-1} · S^{-1}	nmol · L^{-1} · S^{-1} × 0.06 = nmol/mL/min	<40 nmol/mL/min
Anion gap [Na – (Cl + HCO_3)]	7–14 mmol/L		7–14 mEq/L
Aspartate amino–transfer (AST)	<1 yr: 15–60 U/L >1 yr: ≤20 U/L		Same as SI
Bicarbonate	<2 yrs: 20–25 mmol/L >2 yrs: 22–26 mmol/L		<2 yrs: 20–25 mEq/L >2 yrs: 22–26
Bilirubin (total)	***Preterm*** / ***Full term*** Cord: <34 / <34 μmol/L 0–1 d: <137 / <103 1–2 d: <205 / <137 3–5 d: <274 / <205 Thereafter: <34 / <17	μmol/L × 0.05848 = mg/dL	***Preterm*** / ***Full term*** Cord: <2 / <2 mg/dL 0–1 d: <8 / <6 1–2 d: <12 / <8 3–5 d: <16 / <12 Thereafter: <2 / <1
Bilirubin (conjugated)	0–3.4 μmol/L	μmol/L × 0.05848 = mg/dL	0–0.2 mg/dL
Calcium (ionized)	1.12–1.23 mmol/L	mmol/L × 4 = mg/dL	4.48–4.92 mg/dL

(continued)

TEST	SI REFERENCE RANGE	CONVERSION FACTOR	CONVENTIONAL UNITS REFERENCE RANGE
Calcium (total)	Preterm <1 wk: 1.5–2.5 mmol/L Term: <1 wk: 1.75–3 Child: 2–2.6 Adult: 2.1–2.6		6–10 mg/dL 7–12 8–10.5 8.5–10.5
Carbon dioxide (CO_2 content)	22–26 mmol/L		22–26 mEq/L
Carbon monoxide (carboxyhemoglobin)	***% total HB*** Nonsmokers: <0.02 Smokers: <0.01 Toxic: >0.20		***Fraction of HB sat*** Nonsmokers: <2 Smokers: <10 Toxic: >20
Carotene	Infant: 0.37–1.30 μmol/L Child: 0.74–2.42 Adult: 1.12–3.72	μmol/L × 53.7 = μg/dL	Infant: 20–70 μg/dL Child: 40–130 Adult: 60–200
Ceruloplasmin	1–12 yr: 300–650 mg/L >12 yr: 150–600 mg/L		1–12 yr: 30–65 mg/dL >12 yr: 15–60
Chloride	94–106 mmol/L		94–106 mEq/L
Cholesterol	Infant: 1.81–4.53 mmol/L Child: 3.11–5.18 Adolescent: 3.11–5.44 Adult: 3.63–6.48	mmol/L × 38.61 = mg/dL	Infant: 53–135 mg/dL Child: 70–175 Adolescent: 140–250 Adult: 140–250
Complement, C_3	1 mo: 0.61–1.30 g/L 6 mo: 0.87–1.36 Adult: 1.11–1.71		1 mo: 61–130 mg/dL 6 mo: 87–136 Adult: 111–171
Complement, C_4	Newborn: 0.16–0.39 g/L Adult: 0.15–0.45 g/L		Newborn: 16–39 mg/dL Adult: 15–45
Complement, total hemolytic (CH 50)	75–160 U/mL		75–160 U/mL
Copper	0–6 mo: 3.1–11 μmol/L 6 yr: 14–30 12 yr: 12.5–25 Adult (M): 11–22 Adult (F): 12.6–24	μmol × 6.353 = μg/dL	0–6 mo: 20–70 μg/dL 6 yr: 90–190 12 yr: 80–160 Adult (M): 70–140 Adult (F): 80–155
Cortisol	0800 h (or pre–ACTH): 225–505 nmol/L Post–ACTH: twice pre–ACTH value	nmol/L × 0.0362 = μg/dL	0800 h (or pre–ACTH): 8–18 μg/dL Post–ACTH: twice pre–ACTH value
Creatine kinase	Newborn: 76–600 U/L Adult (M): 38–174 Adult (F): 96–140		Same as SI
Creatine kinase isoenzymes	***Fraction of total activity*** CK-BB (CK-1): absent or trace CK-MB (CK-2): 0.04–0.06 CK-MM (CK-3): 0.94–0.96		***% Activity*** CK-BB (CK-1): absent or trace CK-MB (CK-2): 4%–6% CK-MM (CK-3): 94%–96%
Creatinine	Newborn: 27–88 μmol/L Infant: 18–35 Child: 27–62 Adolescent: 44–88 Adult (M): 53–106 Adult (F): 44–97	μmol/L × 0.0113 = mg/dL	Newborn: 0.3–1.0 mg/dL Infant: 0.2–0.4 Child: 0.3–0.7 Adolescent: 0.5–1.0 Adult (M): 0.6–1.2 Adult (F): 0.5–1.1
Dehydroepiandrosterone (DHEA)	Child: 3–10 nmol/L Adult (M): 6–15 Adult (F): 7–18	nmol/L × 0.2884 = μg/L	Child: 1–3 μg/L Adult (M): 1.7–4.2 Adult (F): 2–5.2
Dehydroepiandrosterone sulfate (DHEA–S)	1–4 days: <52 μmol/L Child: 1.6–6.6	μmol/L × 0.37 = μg/mL	1–4 days: <20 μg/mL Child: 0.6–2.54

(*continued*)

TEST	SI REFERENCE RANGE	CONVERSION FACTOR	CONVENTIONAL UNITS REFERENCE RANGE
	Males		
Estradiol	Pubertal stage I: 7–29 pmol/L II: 40 III: >73	pmol/L × 0.2723 = pg/mL	2–8 pg/mL 11 >20
	Adult: 29–132		8–36
	Females		
	Pubertal stage I: 0–84 pmol/L II: 0–242 III: 0–385 IV: 73–1101 Follicular: 37–330 Midcycle: 367–1835 Luteal: 184–881		0–23 pg/mL 0–66 0–105 20–300 10–90 100–500 50–240
Free fatty acids	Child: <1.10 mmol/L Adult: 0.3–0.9	mmol/L × 28.25 = mg/dL	Child: <31 mg/dL Adult: 8–25
Ferritin	Child: 7–144 μg/L Adult (M): 30–265 Adult (F): 10–110		Child: 7–144 ng/mL Adult (M): 30–265 Adult (F): 10–110
Fibrinogen	2–4 g/L		200–400 mg/dL
Folate	4–20 nmol/L	nmol/L × 0.4413 = ng/mL	1.8–9.0 ng/mL
Folate (RBCs)	340–1020 nmol/L packed cells	nmol/L × 0.4413 = ng/mL	150–450 ng/mL
Follicle-stimulating hormone (FSH)	Prepubertal: <5 IU/L Adult (M): 1.5–16 Adult (F): 2–17.2		Prepubertal: <5 mIU/mL Adult (M): 1.5–16 Adult (F): 2–17.2
Fructose	55–330 μmol/L	μmol/L × 0.018 = mg/dL	1–6 mg/dL
Galactose	Newborn: 0–1.11 mmol/L Thereafter: <0.28	mmol/L × 18.02 = mg/dL	Newborn: 0–20 mg/dL Thereafter: <5
Gamma glutamyl transferase (GGT)	0–3 wk: 0–130 U/L 3 wk–3 mo: 4–120 3 mo–1 yr (M): 5–65 3 mo–1 yr (F): 5–35 1–15 yr: 0–23 Adult: 0–35		Same as SI
Gastrin	<100 ng/L		<100 pg/mL
Glucagon	50–100 ng/L		50–100 pg/mL
Glucose	Preterm: 1.1–3.6 mmol/L Full term: 1.1–6.1 1 wk–16 yr: 3.3–5.8 >16 yr: 3.9–6.4	mmol/L × 18.02 = mg/dL	Preterm: 20–65 mg/dL Full term: 20–100 1 wk–16 yr: 60–105 >16 yr: 70–115
Haptoglobin	0.4–1.8 g/L		40–180 mg/dL
Hemoglobin A_{1c}	0.039–0.077 fraction of total Hb		3.9%–7.7% of total HB
β-Hydroxybutyrate	<100 μmol/L	μmol/L × 0.01041 = mg/dL	<1 mg/dL
17-Hydroxyprogesterone	Prepubertal (M): 0.3–0.91 nmol/L Prepubertal (F): 0.61–1.52 Adult (M): 0.61–5.45 Adult (F): Follicular: 0.61–2.42 Luteal: 2.42–9.10	nmol/L × 0.33 = ng/mL	Prepubertal (M): 0.1–0.3 ng/mL Prepubertal (F): 0.2–0.5 Adult (M): 0.2–1.8 Adult (F): Follicular: 0.2–0.8 Luteal: 0.8–3.0
Immunoglobulins A, G, M	***IgA***	***IgG***	***IgM***
	Newborn: 0–0.05 g/L 1–3 mo: 0.03–0.66 3–6 mo: 0.04–0.90 6–12 mo: 0.45–2.25	6.4–16 g/L 3.0–10.0 1.4–10.0 4.0–11.5	0.06–0.24 g/L 0.15–1.50 0.15–1.10 0.43–2.25

(continued)

TEST	SI REFERENCE RANGE	CONVERSION FACTOR	CONVENTIONAL UNITS REFERENCE RANGE
	1–2 yr: 0.35–2.40 2–6 yr: 0.40–1.90 6–12 yr: 0.40–2.70 12–16 yr: 0.50–2.32 Adult: 0.70–3.90	3.5–12.0 5.0–13.0 7.0–16.5 7.0–15.5 6.5–15.0	0.36–2.40 0.50–1.99 0.50–2.60 0.45–2.40 0.40–3.4
Immunoglobulin E	Newborn: 0–24 µg/L 6–12 yr: 0–480 Adult: 0–960		Newborn: 0–10 U/mL 6–12 yr: 0–200 Adult: 0–400
Insulin, fasting	3–23 mU/L		3–23 µU/mL
Iron	Newborn: 20–48 µmol/L 4–10 mo: 5.4–12.5 3–19 yr: 9.5–27.0 Adult: 13.0–33.0	µmol/L × 5.587 = µg/dL	Newborn: 110–270 µg/dL 4–10 mo: 30–70 3–10 yr: 53–119 Adult: 72–186
Iron–binding capacity	Newborn: 10.6–31.3 µmol/L Thereafter: 45–72	µmol/L × 5.587 = µg/dL	Newborn: 59–175 µg/dL Thereafter: 250–400
Lactate	Venous: 0.5–2.0 mmol/L Arterial: 0.3–0.8	mmol/L × 9.01 = mg/dL	Venous: 5–18 mg/dL Arterial: 3–7
Lactate dehydrogenase	Newborn: 160–1500 U/L Infant: 150–360 Child: 150–300 Adult: 100–250		Same as SI units
Lactate dehydrogenase isoenzymes		***Fraction of total*** LD 1 (heart): 0.24–0.34 LD 2 (heart, RBCs): 0.35–0.45 LD 3 (muscle): 0.15–0.25 LD 4 (liver, muscle): 0.04–0.10 LD 5 (liver, muscle): 0.01–0.09	
Lead	<1.16 µmol/L	µmol/L × 20.7 = mgm/dL	<24 gmg/dL
Lipids	95th %ile values—mmol/L (mg/dL)		5th %ile values—mmol/L (mg/dL)
	VLDL (Cholesterol)	***LDL (Cholesterol)***	***HDL (Cholesterol)***
	M / *F*	*M* / *F*	*M* / *F*
	5–9 yr: 0.47 (18) / 0.62 (24)	3.34 (129) / 3.62 (140)	0.98 (38) / 0.93 (36)
	10–14 yr: 0.57 (22) / 0.59 (23)	3.41 (132) / 3.52 (136)	0.96 (37) / 0.91 (35)
	15–19 yr: 0.67 (26) / 0.62 (24)	3.36 (130) / 3.49 (135)	0.80 (31) / 0.91 (35)
		mmol/L × 38.61 = mg/dL	
Luteinizing hormone	Prepubertal: <5 IU/L Adult (M): 3.9–18 Adult (F): 2.0–22.6		Prepubertal: <5 mIU/L Adult (M): 3.9–18 Adult (F): 2.0–22.6
Magnesium	0.75–1.0 mmol/L	mmol/L × 2 = mEq/L	1.5–2.0 mEq/L
Methemoglobin	<46 µmol/L	µmol/L × 0.0065 = g/dL	<0.3 gdL
Osmolality	285–295 mmol/kg		285–295 mOsm/kg
Phosphorus	Newborn: 1.36–2.91 mmol/L 1 yr: 1.23–2.00 2–5 yr: 1.13–2.20 Adult: 0.97–1.45	mmol/L × 3.097 = mg/dL	Newborn: 4.2–9.0 mg/dL 1 yr: 3.8–6.2 2–5 yr: 3.5–6.8 Adult: 3.0–4.5
Phytanic acid	<0.003 fraction of total serum fatty acids		<0.3% of total serum fatty acids
Potassium	<10 days: 3.5–6.0 mmol/L >10 days: 3.5–5.0		<10 days: 3.5–6.0 mEq/L >10 days: 3.5–5.0
Progesterone	***Males***		
	Prepubertal: 0.35–0.83 nmol/L Adult: 0.38–0.95	nmol/L × 0.314 = ng/mL	0.11–0.26 ng/mL 0.12–0.30

(continued)

TEST	SI REFERENCE RANGE	CONVERSION FACTOR	CONVENTIONAL UNITS REFERENCE RANGE
	Females		
	Prepubertal: <0.95 Pubertal stage II: <1.46 III: <1.91 IV: 0.16–41.34		≤0.30 ≤0.46 ≤0.60 0.05–13.0
	Follicular: 0.06–2.86 Luteal: 19.08–95.40		0.02–0.9 6.0–30.0
Prolactin	Newborn: <200 μg/L Adult: <20 μg/L		Newborn: <200 ng/mL Adult: <20 ng/mL
Protein, total	Preterm: 40–70 g/L Term newborn: 50–71 1–3 mo: 47–74 3–12 mo: 50–75 1–15 yr: 65–86		Preterm: 4.0–7.0 g/dL Term newborn: 5.0–7.1 1–3 mo: 4.7–7.4 3–12 mo: 5.0–7.5 1–15 yr: 6.5–8.6
Pyruvate	0.03–0.10 mmol/L	mmol/L × 8.81 = mg/dL	0.3–0.9 mg/dL
Renin	Adults: 0.30–1.14 ng · L^{-1} · S^{-1}	ng · L^{-1} · S^{-1} × 3.6 = ng/mL/h	Adults: 1.1–4.1 ng/mL/h
Sodium	135–145 mmol/L		135–145 mEq/L
Somatomedin C	0–2 yr: 220–1000 IU/L 3–5 yr: 270–1600 6–10 yr: 370–2100 11–12 yr: 450–2800 13–14 yr: 1100–4000 15–17 yr: 1000–2900 Thereafter: 460–1500		0–2 yr: 0.22–1.00 U/mL 3–5 yr: 0.27–1.60 6–10 yr: 0.37–2.10 11–12 yr: 0.45–2.80 13–14 yr: 1.10–4.00 15–17 yr: 1.00–2.90 Thereafter: 0.46–1.50
Testosterone, free	Prepubertal: 2.08–13.19 pmol/L Adult (M): 48.6–201 Adult (F): 6.94–25		Prepubertal: 0.06–0.38 ng/dL Adult (M): 1.40–5.79 Adult (F): 0.20–0.73
Testosterone, total	Prepubertal: 0.35–0.70 nmol/L Adult (F): 0.8–2.6 Adult (M): 9.5–30		Prepubertal: 10–20 ng/dL Adult (F): 23–75 Adult (M): 275–875
Thyroid-stimulating hormone (TSH)	Cord 0–17.4 μU/L 1–3 days: 0–13.3 Thereafter: 0–5.5		Cord: 0–17.4 mIU/mL 1–3 days: 0–13.3 Thereafter: 0–5.5
Thyroxine (T_4), total	Cord: 95–168 nmol/L <1 mo: 90–292 1 mo–1 yr: 93–213 1–5 yr: 94–194 5–10 yr: 83–172 10–15 yr: 72–151 Adult: 55–161	nmol/L × 0.0775 = μg/dL	Cord: 7.4–13.0 μg/dL <1 mo: 7.0–22.6 1 mo–1 yr: 7.2–16.5 1–5 yr: 7.3–15.0 5–10 yr: 6.4–13.3 10–15 yr: 5.6–11.7 Adult: 4.3–12.5
Thyroxine (T_4), free	9–22 pmol/L	pmol/L × 0.0777 = ng/dL	0.7–1.7 ng/dL
Transferrin	Newborn: 1.30–2.75 g/L Adult: 2.20–4.00		Newborn: 130–275 mg/dL Adult: 220–440
Triglycerides	***Normal Upper Limits—mmol/L (mg/dL)***		
	Male	***Female***	
	0–4 yr: 1.12 (99) 5–9 yr: 1.14 (101) 10–15 yr: 1.41 (125) 15–19 yr: 1.67 (148)	1.26 (112) 1.19 (105) 1.48 (131) 1.40 (124) mmol/L × 88.55 = mg/dL	

(continued)

TEST	SI REFERENCE RANGE	CONVERSION FACTOR	CONVENTIONAL UNITS REFERENCE RANGE
Triiodothyronine (T_3)	Cord: 0.23–1.16 nmol/L <1 mo: 0.49–3.70 1 mo–1 yr: 1.70–4.31 1–5 yr: 1.62–4.14 5–10 yr: 1.45–3.71 10–15 yr: 1.28–3.31 Adult: 1.08–3.14	nmol/L × 65.1 = ng/dL	Cord: 15–75 ng/dL <1 mo: 32–240 1 mo–1 yr: 110–280 1–5 yr: 105–269 5–10 yr: 94–241 10–15 yr: 83–215 Adult: 70–204
Triiodothyronine resin uptake	0.25–0.35		25%–35%
Urea nitrogen	2–7 mmol/L	mmol/L × 28 = mg/dL	5–20 mg/dL
Uric acid	120–420 µmol/L	µmol/L × 0.0169 = mg/dL	2–7 mg/dL
Vitamin A	Newborn: 1.22–2.62 µmol/L Child: 1.05–2.79 Adult: 1.05–2.27	µmol/L × 28.65 = mg/dL	Newborn: 35–75 µg/dL Child: 30–80 Adult: 30–65
Vitamin B_6	14.6–72.8 nmol/L	nmol/L × 0.247 = ng/mL	3.6–18 ng/mL
Vitamin B_{12}	96–579 pmol/L	pmol/L × 1.355 = pg/mL	130–785 pg/mL
Vitamin C	11.4–113.6 µmol/L	µmol/L × 0.176 = mg/dL	0.2–2.0 mg/dL
Vitamin D_3 (1,25 dihydroxy)	60–108 pmol/L	pmol/L × 0.417 = pg/mL	25–45 pg/mL
Vitamin E	11.6–46.4 µmol/L	µmol/L × 0.043 = mg/dL	0.5–2.0 mg/dL
Zinc	10.7–22.9 µmol/L	µmol/L × 6.54 = µg/dL	70–150 µg/dL

Hematology

	HB (g/DL)		HEMATOCRIT (%)		MCV (fL)		MCHC (g/DL RBC)			WBC (1,000/mm³)		PLATELETS (1,000/mm³)
AGE	*Mean*	*−2 SD*	*Mean*	*−2 SD*	*Mean*	*−2 SD*	*Mean*	*−2 SD*	RETICULOCYTE (%)	*Mean*	*95% CI*	*Mean (Range)*
Term (cord blood)	16.5	13.5	51	42	108	98	33.0	30.0	3.0–7.0	18.1	9.0–30.0	290
1–3 days	18.5	14.5	56	45	108	95	33.0	29.0	1.8–4.6	18.9	9.4–34.0	192
2 weeks	16.6	13.4	53	41	105	88	31.4	28.1		11.4	5.0–20.0	252
1 month	13.9	10.7	44	33	101	91	31.8	28.1	0.1–1.7	10.8	5.0–19.5	
2 months	11.2	9.4	35	28	95	84	31.8	28.3				
6 months	12.6	11.1	36	31	76	68	35.0	32.7	0.7–2.3	11.9	6.0–17.5	
6–24 months	12.0	10.5	36	33	78	70	33.0	30.0		10.6	6.0–17.0	(150–300)
2–6 years	12.5	11.5	37	34	81	75	34.0	31.0	0.5–1.0	8.5	5.0–15.5	(150–300)
6–12 years	13.5	11.5	50	35	86	77	34.0	31.0	0.5–1.0	8.1	4.5–13.5	(150–300)
12–18 years (M)	14.5	13.0	43	36	88	78	34.0	31.0	0.5–1.0	7.8	4.5–13.5	(150–300)
12–18 years (F)	14.0	12.0	41	37	90	78	34.0	31.0	0.5–1.0	7.8	4.5–13.5	(150–300)

Urine

TEST	SI REFERENCE RANGE	CONVERSION FACTOR	CONVENTIONAL UNITS REFERENCE RANGE
Aminolevulinic acid	8–53 µmol/d	µmol/d × 0.131 = mg/d	1–7 mg/d
Calcium	<0.1 mmol/kg/d	mmol/d × 40 = mg/d	<4 mg/kg/d
Copper	<0.6 µmol/d	µmol/d × 63.7 = gmg/d	<40 µg/d
Coproporphyrin	<300 nmol/d	nmol/d × 1.527 = µg/d	<200 µg/d
Cortisol, free	70–340 nmol/d	nmol/d × 0.362 = µg/d	25–125 µg/d
Creatinine	Infant: 71–177 µmol/kg/d Child: 71–194 Adolescent: 71–265	µmol/kg/d × 0.113 = mg/kg/d	Infant: 8–20 mg/kg/d Child: 8–22 Adolescent: 8–30
Cystine	40–260 µmol/d	µmol/d × 0.12 = mg/d	5–31 mg/d
Dehydroepiandrosterone (DHEA)	<5 yr: <0.3 µmol/d 6–9 yr: <0.7 10–15 yr: <1.4 Adult (M): <8.0 Adult (F): <4.2	µmol/d × 0.288 = mg/d	<5 yr: <0.1 mg/d 6–9 yr: <0.2 10–15 yr: <0.4 Adult (M): <2.3 Adult (F): <1.2
Epinephrine	<55 nmol/d	nmol/d × 0.183 = µg/d	<10 µg/d
Fluoride	<50 µmol/d	µmol/d × 0.019 = mg/d	<1 mg/d
Homovanillic acid (HVA)	***mmol/mol/creatinine*** 1–12 mo: 0.75–21.7 1–2 yr: 2.5–14.3 2–5 yr: 0.43–8.4 5–10 yr: 0.31–5.6 10–15 yr: 0.15–7.4 15–18 yr: 0.31–1.24	mmol/mol/creatinine × 1.61 = µg/mg creatinine	***µg/mg creatinine*** 1–12 mo: 1.2–35.0 1–2 yr: 4.0–23.0 2–5 yr: 0.7–13.5 5–10 yr: 0.5–9.0 10–15 yr: 0.25–12.0 15–18 yr: 0.5–2.0
Metanephrines	***mmol/mol/creatinine*** <1 yr: 0.001–2.64 1–2 yr: 0.15–3.09 2–5 yr: 0.20–1.72 5–10 yr: 0.25–1.55 10–15 yr: 0.001–0.38 15–18 yr: 0.03–0.69	mmol/mol creatinine × 1.74 = µg/mg creatinine	***µg/mg creatinine*** <1 yr: 0.001–4.6 1–2 yr: 0.27–5.38 2–5 yr: 0.35–2.99 5–10 yr: 0.43–2.70 10–15 yr: 0.001–1.87 15–18 yr: 0.001–0.67
Norepinephrine	<590 nmol/d	nmol/d × 0.169 = µg/d	<100 µg/d
Osmolality	50–1200 µgmol/kg		50–1200 mOsm/kg
Oxalate	110–440 µmol/d	µmol/d × 0.088 = mg/d	10–40 mg/d
Porphobilinogen	0–8.8 µmol/d	µmol/d × 0.226 = mg/d	0–2 mg/d
Potassium	25–125 mmol/d (varies with diet)		25–125 mEq/d
Pregnanetriol	<7.4 µmol/d	µmol/d × 0.3365 = mg/d	<2.5 mg/d
Protein	10–140 mg/L		1–14 mg/dL
Steroids: 17-hydroxycorticosteroid	Prepubertal: 2.76–15.5 µmol/d Adult (M): 11–33 Adult (F): 11–22	µmol/d × 0.3625 = mg/d	Prepubertal: 1–5.6 mg/d Adult (M): 4–12 Adult (F): 4–8
Steroids: 17-ketosteroids	<1 mo: ≤6.9 µmol/d 1 mo–5 yr: <1.73 6–8 yr: 3.47–6.9 Adult (M): 21–62 Adult (F): 14–45	µmol/d × 0.2884 = mg/d	<1 mo: <2 mg/d 1 mo–5 yr: <0.5 6–8 yr: 1–2 Adult (M): 6–18 Adult (F): 4–13
Uric acid	1.48–4.43 mmol/d	mmol/d × 169 = mg/d	250–750 mg/d
Vanilylmandelic acid (VMA)	***mmol/mol/creatinine*** 1–6 mo: 1.71–9.71 6–12 mo: 1.14–8.57 1–5 yr: 1.14–5.71 5–10 yr: 0.86–4.00 10–15 yr: 0.57–3.43 >15 yr: 0.57–3.43	mmol/mol creatinine × 1.75 = µg/mg	***µg/mg creatinine*** 1–6 mo: 3–7 6–12 mo: 2–15 1–5 yr: 2–10 5–10 yr: 1.5–7 10–15 yr: 1–6 >15 yr: 1–6

Cerebrospinal Fluid

CELL COUNT RANGE

Preterm: 0–25 WBC × 10^6 cells/L (57% polymorphonuclears)
Term: 0–22 WBC × 10^6 cells/L (61% polymorphonuclears)
Child: 0–7 WBC × 10^6 cells/L (0% polymorphonuclears)

CELL COUNT PERCENTILES

	Total WBC			Polymorphonuclears			Monocytes		
	25%	50%	75%	25%	50%	75%	25%	50%	75%
<6 wk	0.50	2.57	5.16	0	0	2.42	0	0.83	2.71
6 wk–3 mo	0.34	1.86	3.75	0	0	0.66	0	0.96	2.78
3–6 mo	0.00	1.11	2.31	0	0	0.40	0	0.43	1.64
6–12 mo	0.41	1.47	3.25	0	0	0.52	0.03	0.93	2.32
>12 mo	0.00	0.68	1.82	0	0	0	0	0.25	1.45

TEST	SI REFERENCE RANGE	CONVENTIONAL UNITS REFERENCE RANGE
Glucose	Preterm: 1.3–3.5 mmol/L Term: 1.9–6.6 Child: 2.2–4.4	Preterm: 24–63 mg/dL Term: 34–119 Child: 40–80
Protein	Preterm: 0.65–1.50 g/L Term: 0.20–1.70 Child: 0.05–0.40	Preterm: 65–150 mg/dL Term: 20–170 Child: 5–40
Pressure	<200 mm H_2O	<200 mm H_2O

(Barone, M. A. [1999]. Laboratory values. In F. A. Oski, et al. [Eds.] *Principles and practice of pediatrics* [3rd ed.]. Philadelphia: Lippincott Williams & Wilkins.)

Pulse, Respiration, and Blood Pressure Values

APPENDIX G

Pulse Rate at Various Ages

AGE	RANGE	AVERAGE
Newborn	70–170	120
1–11 months	80–160	120
2 years	80–130	110
4 years	80–120	100
6 years	75–115	100
8 years	70–110	90
10 years	70–100	90

	GIRLS		BOYS	
	Range	*Average*	*Range*	*Average*
12 years	70–110	90	65–105	85
14 years	65–105	85	60–100	80
16 years	60–100	80	55–95	75
18 years	55–95	75	50–90	70

Normal Blood Pressure for Various Ages

AGE	SYSTOLIC (MEAN ± 2 SD)	DIASTOLIC (MEAN ± 2 SD)
Newborn	80 ± 16	46 ± 16
6 months–1 year	89 ± 29	60 ± 10*
1 year	96 ± 30	66 ± 25*
2 years	99 ± 25	64 ± 25*
3 years	100 ± 25	67 ± 23*
4 years	99 ± 20	65 ± 20*
5–6 years	94 ± 14	55 ± 9
6–7 years	100 ± 15	56 ± 8
8–9 years	105 ± 16	57 ± 9
9–10 years	107 ± 16	57 ± 9
10–11 years	111 ± 17	58 ± 10
11–12 years	113 ± 18	59 ± 10
12–13 years	115 ± 19	59 ± 10
13–14 years	118 ± 19	60 ± 10

* The point of muffling is shown as the diastolic pressure.

Variations in Respirations with Age

AGE	RATE PER MINUTE
Newborn	40–90
1 year	20–40
2 years	20–30
3 years	20–30
5 years	20–25
10 years	17–22
15 years	15–20
20 years	15–20

Average Blood Pressure in Adult American Females

		WHITE WOMEN		BLACK WOMEN	
	Age	*Average (mm Hg)*	*SD*	*Average (mm Hg)*	*SD*
Systolic	Under 20	111.0	13.7	112.7	13.2
	20–29	116.9	13.8	119.1	14.7
	30–39	121.4	16.3	128.1	20.2
	40–49	129.3	19.6	138.3	22.8
Diastolic	Under 20	69.3	9.8	70.0	10.1
	20–29	73.7	7.2	75.4	9.7
	30–39	76.9	10.7	82.0	13.0
	40–49	80.6	11.6	86.9	13.9

SD = standard deviation.
(Adapted from Stamler, J, et al. [1976]. Hypertension screening of one million Americans. *Journal of the American Medical Association, 235*, 2299. Copyright © 1976, American Medical Association.)

Denver Development II*

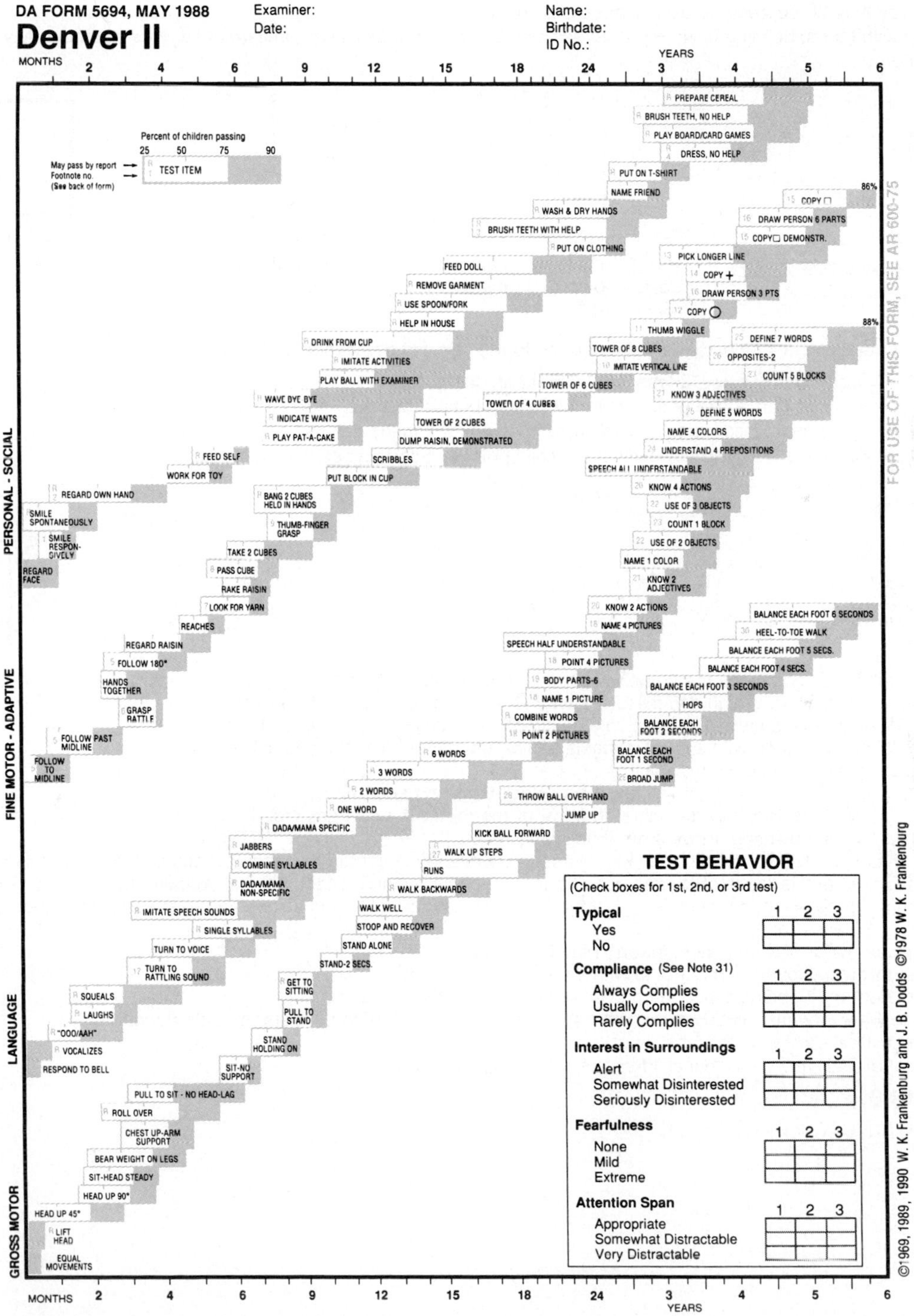

* Denver II test and training materials may be purchased from Denver Developmental Materials, Inc., P.O. Box 6919, Denver CO 80205-0919; phone 303-355-4729.

DIRECTIONS FOR ADMINISTRATION

1. Try to get child to smile by smiling, talking or waving. Do not touch him/her.
2. Child must stare at hand several seconds.
3. Parent may help guide toothbrush and put toothpaste on brush.
4. Child does not have to be able to tie shoes or button/zip in the back.
5. Move yarn slowly in an arc from one side to the other, about 8" above child's face.
6. Pass if child grasps rattle when it is touched to the backs or tips of fingers.
7. Pass if child tries to see where yarn went. Yarn should be dropped quickly from sight from tester's hand without arm movement.
8. Child must transfer cube from hand to hand without help of body, mouth, or table.
9. Pass if child picks up raisin with any part of thumb and finger.
10. Line can vary only 30 degrees or less from tester's line.
11. Make a fist with thumb pointing upward and wiggle only the thumb. Pass if child imitates and does not move any fingers other than the thumb.

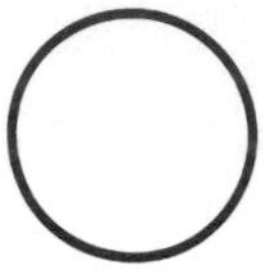

12. Pass any enclosed form. Fail continuous round motions.

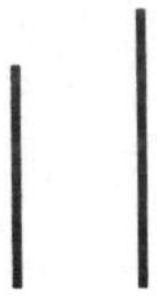

13. Which line is longer? (Not bigger.) Turn paper upside down and repeat. (pass 3 of 3 or 5 of 6)

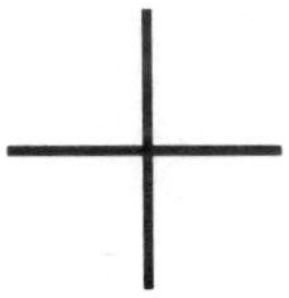

14. Pass any lines crossing near midpoint.

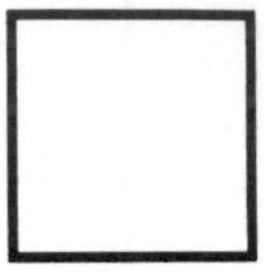

15. Have child copy first. If failed, demonstrate.

When giving items 12, 14, and 15, do not name the forms. Do not demonstrate 12 and 14.

16. When scoring, each pair (2 arms, 2 legs, etc.) counts as one part.
17. Place one cube in cup and shake gently near child's ear, but out of sight. Repeat for other ear.
18. Point to picture and have child name it. (No credit is given for sounds only.)
    If less than 4 pictures are named correctly, have child point to picture as each is named by tester.

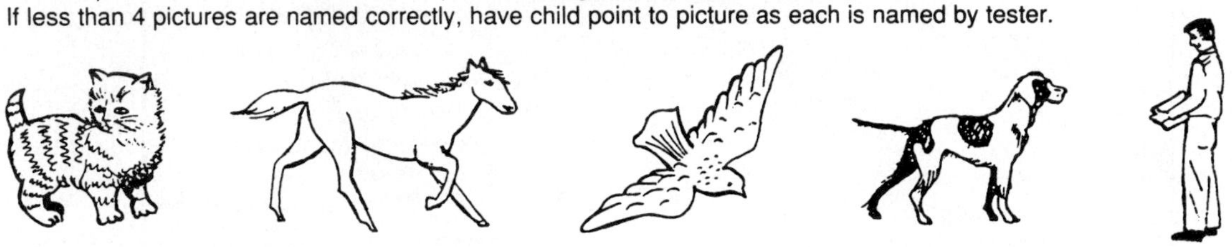

19. Using doll, tell child: Show me the nose, eyes, ears, mouth, hands, feet, tummy, hair. Pass 6 of 8.
20. Using pictures, ask child: Which one flies?... says meow?... talks?... barks?... gallops? Pass 2 of 5, 4 of 5.
21. Ask child: What do you do when you are cold?... tired?... hungry? Pass 2 of 3, 3 of 3.
22. Ask child: What do you do with a cup? What is a chair used for? What is a pencil used for?
    Action words must be included in answers.
23. Pass if child correctly places <u>and</u> says how many blocks are on paper. (1, 5).
24. Tell child: Put block **on** table; **under** table; **in front of** me, **behind** me. Pass 4 of 4.
    (Do not help child by pointing, moving head or eyes.)
25. Ask child: What is a ball?... lake?... desk?... house?... banana?... curtain?... fence?... ceiling? Pass if defined in terms of use, shape, what it is made of, or general category (such as banana is fruit, not just yellow). Pass 5 of 8, 7 of 8.
26. Ask child: If a horse is big, a mouse is __? If fire is hot, ice is __? If the sun shines during the day, the moon shines during the __? Pass 2 of 3.
27. Child may use wall or rail only, not person. May not crawl.
28. Child must throw ball overhand 3 feet to within arm's reach of tester.
29. Child must perform standing broad jump over width of test sheet (8 1/2 inches).
30. Tell child to walk forward,  heel within 1 inch of toe. Tester may demonstrate.
    Child must walk 4 consecutive steps.
31. In the second year, half of normal children are non-compliant.

OBSERVATIONS:

Standard Precautions

APPENDIX I

Use Standard Precautions, or the equivalent, for the care of all patients. *Category IB**

A. Handwashing
   (1) Wash hands after touching blood, body fluids, secretions, excretions, and contaminated items, whether or not gloves are worn. Wash hands immediately after gloves are removed, between patient contacts, and when otherwise indicated to avoid transfer of microorganisms to other patients or environments. It may be necessary to wash hands between tasks and procedures on the same patient to prevent cross-contamination of different body sites. *Category IB*
   (2) Use a plain (nonantimicrobial) soap for routine handwashing. *Category IB*
   (3) Use an antimicrobial agent or a waterless antiseptic agent for specific circumstances (e.g., control of outbreaks or hyperendemic infections), as defined by the infection control program. *Category IB* (See Contact Precautions for additional recommendations on using antimicrobial and antiseptic agents.)

B. Gloves
Wear gloves (clean, nonsterile gloves are adequate) when touching blood, body fluids, secretions, excretions, and contaminated items. Put on clean gloves just before touching mucous membranes and nonintact skin. Change gloves between tasks and procedures on the same patient after contact with material that may contain a high concentration of microorganisms. Remove gloves promptly after use, before touching noncontaminated items and environmental surfaces, and before going to another patient, and wash hands immediately to avoid transfer of microorganisms to other patients or environments. *Category IB*

C. Mask, Eye Protection, Face Shield
Wear a mask and eye protection or a face shield to protect mucous membranes of the eyes, nose, and mouth during procedures and patient-care activities that are likely to generate splashes or sprays of blood, body fluids, secretions, and excretions. *Category IB*

D. Gown
Wear a gown (a clean, nonsterile gown is adequate) to protect skin and to prevent soiling of clothing during procedures and patient-care activities that are likely to generate splashes or sprays of blood, body fluids, secretions, or excretions. Select a gown that is appropriate for the activity and amount of fluid likely to be encountered. Remove a soiled gown as promptly as possible, and wash hands to avoid transfer of microorganisms to other patients or environments. *Category IB*

E. Patient-Care Equipment
Handle used patient-care equipment soiled with blood, body fluids, secretions, and excretions in a manner that prevents skin and mucous membrane exposures, contamination of clothing, and transfer of microorganisms to other patients and environments. Ensure that reusable equipment is not used for the care of another patient until it has been cleaned and reprocessed appropriately. Ensure that single-use items are discarded properly. *Category IB*

F. Environmental Control
Ensure that the hospital has adequate procedures for the routine care, cleaning, and disinfection of environmental surfaces, beds, bedrails, bedside equipment, and other frequently touched surfaces, and ensure that these procedures are being followed. *Category IB*

G. Linen
Handle, transport, and process used linen soiled with blood, body fluids, secretions, and excretions in a manner that prevents skin and mucous membrane exposures and contamination of clothing, and that avoids transfer of microorganisms to other patients and environments. *Category IB*

H. Occupational Health and Bloodborne Pathogens
   (1) Take care to prevent injuries when using needles, scalpels, and other sharp instruments or devices; when handling sharp instruments after procedures; when cleaning used instruments; and when disposing of used needles. Never recap used needles, or otherwise manipulate them using both hands, or use any other technique that involves directing the point of a needle toward any part of the body; rather, use either a one-handed "scoop" technique or a mechanical device designed for holding the needle sheath. Do not remove used needles from disposable syringes by hand, and do not bend, break, or otherwise manipulate used needles by hand. Place used disposable

* *Category IB.* Strongly recommended for all hospitals and reviewed as effective by experts in the field and a consensus of HIC-PAC based on strong rationale and suggestive evidence, even though definitive scientific studies have not been done.

syringes and needles, scalpel blades, and other sharp items in appropriate puncture-resistant containers, which are located as close as practical to the area in which the items were used, and place reusable syringes and needles in a puncture-resistant container for transport to the reprocessing area. *Category IB*

(2) Use mouthpieces, resuscitation bags, or other ventilation devices as an alternative to mouth-to-mouth resuscitation methods in areas where the need for resuscitation is predictable. *Category IB*

I. Patient Placement

Place a patient who contaminates the environment or who does not (or cannot be expected to) assist in maintaining appropriate hygiene or environmental control in a private room. If a private room is not available, consult with infection control professionals regarding patient placement or other alternatives. *Category IB*

(From Guideline for isolation precautions in hospitals developed by the Centers for Disease Control and Prevention and the Hospital Infection Control Practices Advisory Committee [HICPAC], January 1996.)

Recommended Childhood Immunization Schedule, United States, 2002

Recommended Childhood Immunization Schedule United States, 2002

range of recommended ages | catch-up vaccination | preadolescent assessment

<table>
<tr><th>Vaccine ▼ / Age ▶</th><th>Birth</th><th>1 mos</th><th>2 mos</th><th>4 mos</th><th>6 mos</th><th>12 mos</th><th>15 mos</th><th>18 mos</th><th>24 mos</th><th>4-6 yrs</th><th>11-12 yrs</th><th>13-18 yrs</th></tr>
<tr><td rowspan="2">Hepatitis B[1]</td><td>Hep B #1</td><td colspan="2">only if mother HBsAg (-)</td><td></td><td></td><td></td><td></td><td></td><td colspan="4" rowspan="2">Hep B series</td></tr>
<tr><td></td><td colspan="3">Hep B #2</td><td colspan="4">Hep B #3</td></tr>
<tr><td>Diphtheria, Tetanus, Pertussis[2]</td><td></td><td></td><td>DTaP</td><td>DTaP</td><td>DTaP</td><td></td><td colspan="2">DTaP</td><td></td><td>DTaP</td><td>Td</td><td></td></tr>
<tr><td>Haemophilus influenzae Type b[3]</td><td></td><td></td><td>Hib</td><td>Hib</td><td>Hib</td><td colspan="2">Hib</td><td></td><td></td><td></td><td></td><td></td></tr>
<tr><td></td><td></td><td></td><td>IPV</td><td>IPV</td><td colspan="4">IPV</td><td></td><td>IPV</td><td></td><td></td></tr>
<tr><td>Measles, Mumps, Rubella[5]</td><td></td><td></td><td></td><td></td><td></td><td colspan="2">MMR #1</td><td></td><td></td><td>MMR #2</td><td colspan="2">MMR #2</td></tr>
<tr><td>Varicella[6]</td><td></td><td></td><td></td><td></td><td></td><td colspan="3">Varicella</td><td colspan="4">Varicella</td></tr>
<tr><td>Pneumococcal[7]</td><td></td><td></td><td>PCV</td><td>PCV</td><td>PCV</td><td colspan="2">PCV</td><td></td><td colspan="2">PCV</td><td></td><td></td></tr>
<tr><td></td><td></td><td></td><td></td><td></td><td></td><td></td><td></td><td></td><td colspan="4">PPV</td></tr>
<tr><td colspan="13">Vaccines below this line are for selected populations</td></tr>
<tr><td>Hepatitis A[8]</td><td></td><td></td><td></td><td></td><td></td><td></td><td></td><td></td><td colspan="4">Hepatitis A series</td></tr>
<tr><td>Influenza[9]</td><td></td><td></td><td></td><td></td><td colspan="8">Influenza (yearly)</td></tr>
</table>

This schedule indicates the recommended ages for routine administration of currently licensed childhood vaccines, as of December 1, 2001, for children through age 18 years. Any dose not given at the recommended age should be given at any subsequent visit when indicated and feasible. ▭ Indicates age groups that warrant effort to administer those vaccines not previously given. Additional vaccines may be licensed and recommended during the year. Licensed combination vaccines may be used whenever any components of the combination are indicated and the vaccine's other components are not contraindicated. Providers should consult the manufacturers' package inserts for detailed recommendations.

1. Hepatitis B vaccine (Hep B). All infants should receive the first dose of hepatitis B vaccine soon after birth and before hospital discharge; the first dose may also be given by age 2 months if the infant's mother is HBsAg-negative. Only monovalent hepatitis B vaccine can be used for the birth dose. Monovalent or combination vaccine containing Hep B may be used to complete the series; four doses of vaccine may be administered if combination vaccine is used. The second dose should be given at least 4 weeks after the first dose, except for Hib-containing vaccine which cannot be administered before age 6 weeks. The third dose should be given at least 16 weeks after the first dose and at least 8 weeks after the second dose. The last dose in the vaccination series (third or fourth dose) should not be administered before age 6 months.

Infants born to ABsAg-positive mothers should receive hepatitis B vaccine and 0.5 mL hepatitis B immune globulin (HBIG) within 12 hours of birth at separate sites. The second dose is recommended at age 1-2 months and the vaccination series should be completed (third or fourth dose) at age 6 months.

Infants born to mothers whose HBsAg status is unknown should receive hepatitis B vaccine within 12 hours of birth. Maternal blood should be drawn at the time of delivery to determine the mother's HBsAg status; if the HBsAg test is positive, the infant should receive HBIG as soon as possible (no later than age 1 week).

2. Diphtheria and tetanus toxoids and acellular pertussis vaccine (DTaP). The fourth dose of DtaP may be administered as early as age 12 months, provided 6 months have elapsed since the third dose and the child is unlikely to return at age 15-18 months. **Tetanus and diphtheria toxoids (Td)** is recommended at age 11-12 years if at least 5 years have elapsed since the last dose of tetanus and diphtheria toxoid-containing vaccine. Subsequent routine Td boosters are recommended every 10 years.

3. *Haemophilus influenzae* Type b (Hib) conjugate vaccine. Three Hib conjugate vaccines are licensed for infant use. If PRP-OMP (PedvaxHIB® or ComVax® [Merck]) is administered at ages 2 and 4 months, a dose at age 6 months is not required. DTaP/Hib combination products should not be used for primary immunization in infants at age 2, 4,or 6 months, but can be used as boosters following any Hib vaccine.

4. Inactivated poliovirus vaccine (IPV). An all-IPV schedule is recommended for routine childhood poliovirus vaccination in the United States. All children should receive four doses of IPV at age 2 months, 4 months, 6-18 months, and 4-6 years.

5. Measles, mumps, and rubella vaccine (MMR). The second dose of MMR is recommended routinely at age 4-6 years but may be administered during any visit, provided at least 4 weeks have elapsed since the first dose and that both doses are administered beginning at or after age 12 months. Those who have not previously received the second dose should complete the schedule by the visit at 11-12 years.

6. Varicella vaccine. Varicella vaccine is recommended at any visit at or after age 12 months for susceptible children (i.e. those who lack a reliable history of chicken pox). Susceptible persons aged ≥ 13 years should receive two doses, given at least 4 weeks apart.

7. Pneumococcal vaccine. The heptavalent pneumococcal conjugate vaccine (PCV) is recommended for all children aged 2-23 months and for certain children aged 24-59 months. Pneumococcal polysaccharide vaccine (PPV) is recommended in addition to PCV for certain high-risk groups. See *MMWR* 2000;49(RR-9);1-37.

8. Hepatitis A vaccine. Hepatitis A vaccine is recommended for use in selected states and regions, and for certain high-risk groups; consult your local public health authority. See *MMWR* 1999;48(RR-12);1-37.

9.Influenza vaccine. Influenza vaccine is recommended annually for children age≥ 6 months with certain risk factors (including but not limited to asthma, cardiac disease, sickle cell disease, HIV, and diabetes; see *MMRW* 2001;50(RR-4);1-44), and can be administered to all others wishing to obtain immunity. Children aged ≤12 years should receive vaccine in a dosage appropriate for their age (0.25 mL if age 6-35 months or 0.5 mL if aged ≥3 years). Children aged ≤8 years who are receiving influenza vaccine for the first time should receive two doses separated by at least 4 weeks.

For additional information about vaccines, vaccine supply, and contraindications for immunization, please visit the National Immunization Program Website at www.cdc.gov/nip or call the National Immunization Hotline at 800-2332-2522 (English) or 800-232-0233 (Spanish).

Approved by the Advisory Committee on Immunization Practices (www.cdc.gov/nip/acip), the American Academy of Pediatrics (www.aap.org), and the American Academy of Family Physicians (www.aafp.org).

Food Guide Pyramids

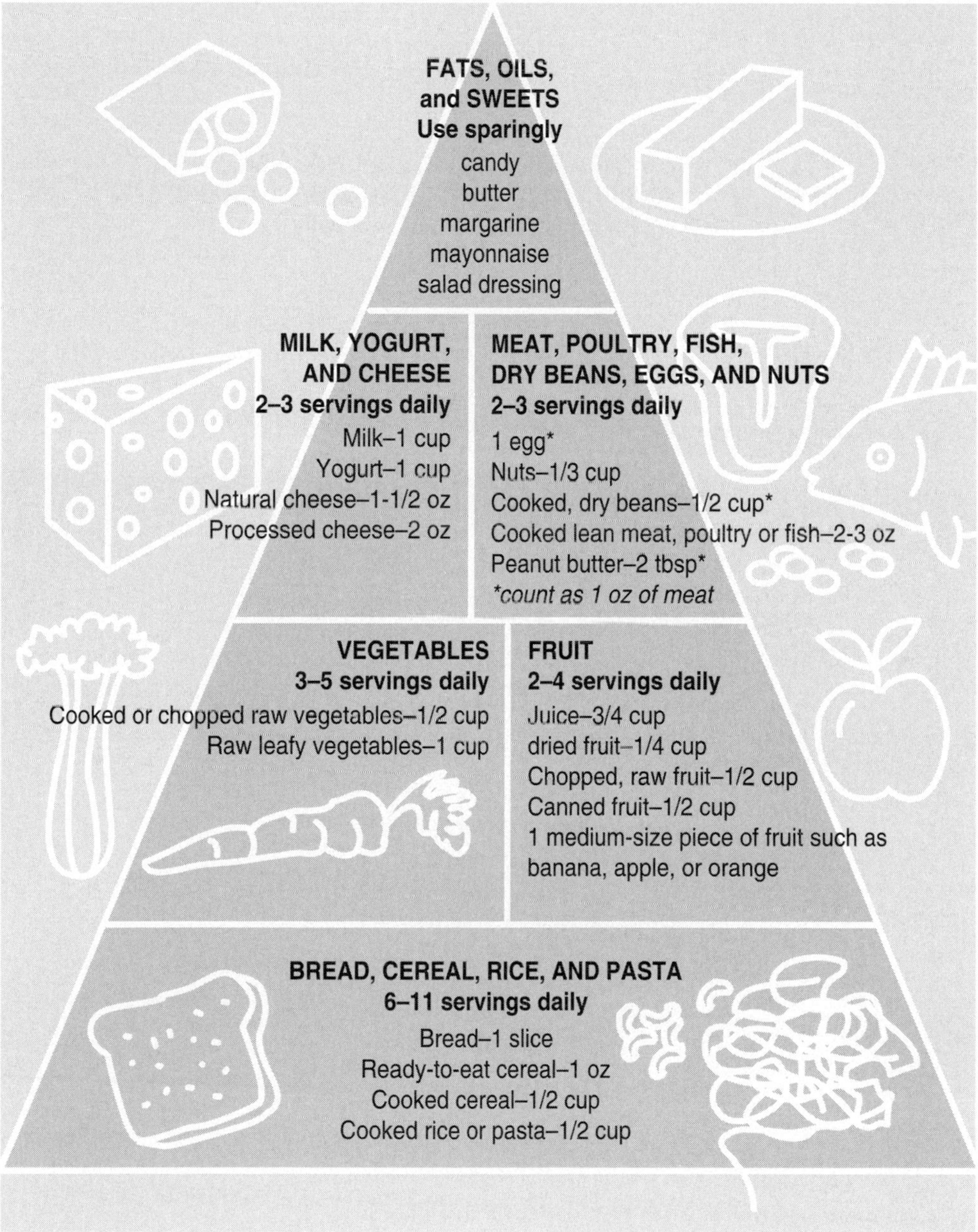

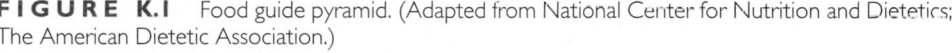

FIGURE K.1 Food guide pyramid. (Adapted from National Center for Nutrition and Dietetics; The American Dietetic Association.)

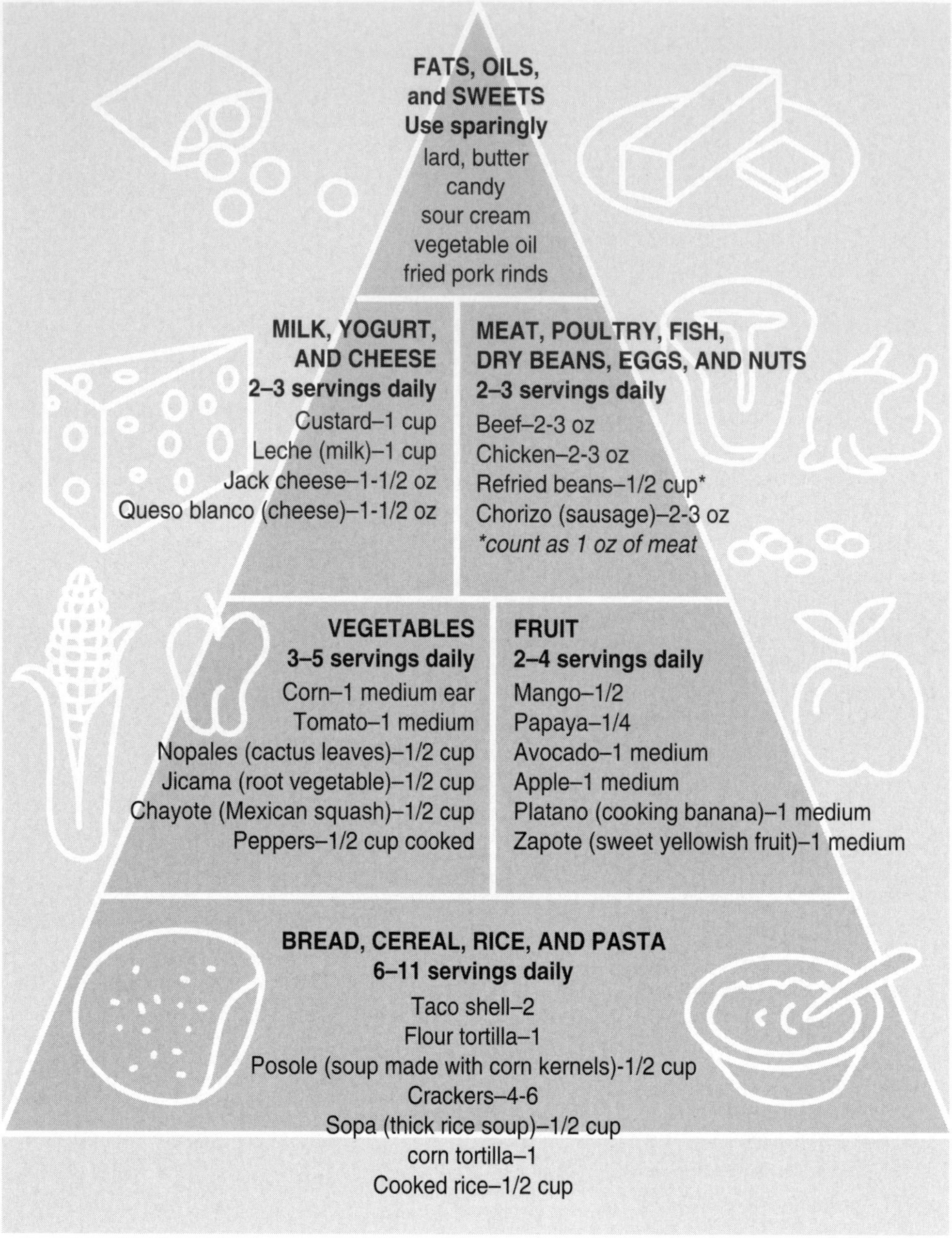
FATS, OILS, and SWEETS
Use sparingly
lard, butter
candy
sour cream
vegetable oil
fried pork rinds
MILK, YOGURT, AND CHEESE
2–3 servings daily
Custard–1 cup
Leche (milk)–1 cup
Jack cheese–1-1/2 oz
Queso blanco (cheese)–1-1/2 oz
MEAT, POULTRY, FISH, DRY BEANS, EGGS, AND NUTS
2–3 servings daily
Beef–2-3 oz
Chicken–2-3 oz
Refried beans–1/2 cup*
Chorizo (sausage)–2-3 oz
*count as 1 oz of meat
VEGETABLES
3–5 servings daily
Corn–1 medium ear
Tomato–1 medium
Nopales (cactus leaves)–1/2 cup
Jicama (root vegetable)–1/2 cup
Chayote (Mexican squash)–1/2 cup
Peppers–1/2 cup cooked
FRUIT
2–4 servings daily
Mango–1/2
Papaya–1/4
Avocado–1 medium
Apple–1 medium
Platano (cooking banana)–1 medium
Zapote (sweet yellowish fruit)–1 medium
BREAD, CEREAL, RICE, AND PASTA
6–11 servings daily
Taco shell–2
Flour tortilla–1
Posole (soup made with corn kernels)-1/2 cup
Crackers–4-6
Sopa (thick rice soup)–1/2 cup
corn tortilla–1
Cooked rice–1/2 cup

FIGURE K.2 Food guide pyramid with popular Mexican fare. (Adapted from National Center for Nutrition and Dietetics; The American Dietetic Association.)

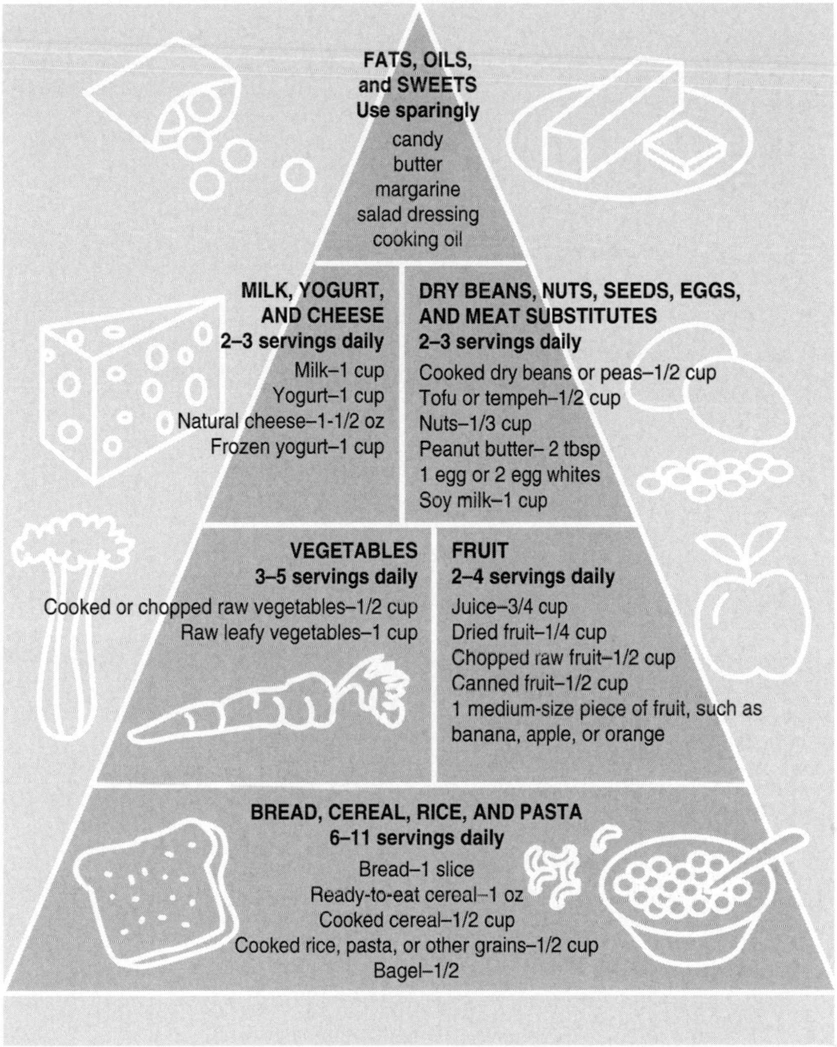

FIGURE K.3 Food guide pyramid for vegetarian meal planning. (Adapted from National Center for Nutrition and Dietetics; The American Dietetic Association.)

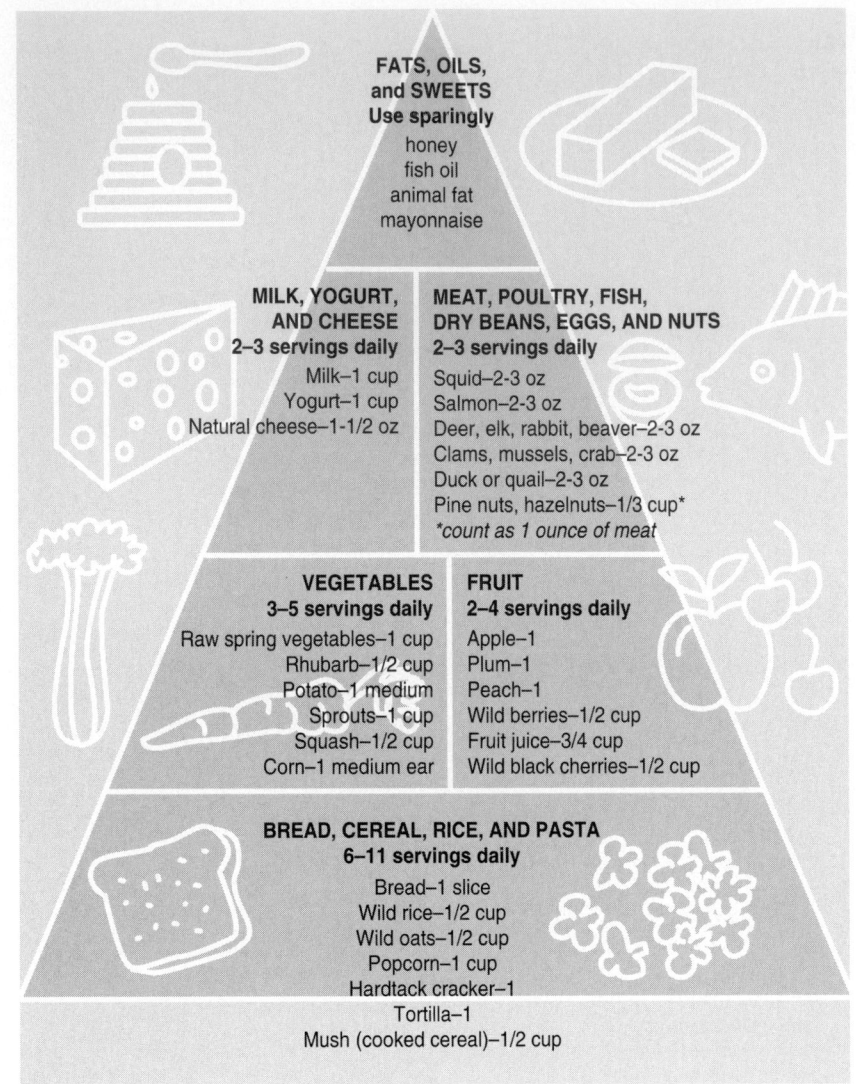

FIGURE K.4 Food guide pyramid with popular Native American Fare. (Adapted from National Center for Nutrition and Dietetics; The American Dietetic Association.)

Care Maps

APPENDIX L

Name: ______________________________

This care path is a guideline and is not intended to create a standard of care. This guideline may be modified based on individual patient's needs.

Prob. #		Day 1/Day of Admission Date:	LOS Day _____ Date:	LOS Day _____ Date:	LOS Day _____ Date:
	ADL	☐ Bedrest ☐ BR/BRP ☐ Wheelchair ☐ Bedside commode ☐ Shower ☐ Up ad lib	☐ Bedrest ☐ BR/BRP ☐ Wheelchair ☐ Bedside commode ☐ Shower ☐ Up ad lib	☐ Bedrest ☐ BR/BRP ☐ Wheelchair ☐ Bedside commode ☐ Shower ☐ Up ad lib	☐ Bedrest ☐ BR/BRP ☐ Wheelchair ☐ Bedside commode ☐ Shower ☐ Up ad lib
	Assessment / Monitor	Maternal assessments: ☐ VS q 4 hours ☐ VS q 4 hours while awake ☐ VS q shift ☐ VS BID Vaginal bleeding Uterine activity Membrane status Vaginal discharge Fetal assessments: ☐ FHR q 4 hours ☐ FHR q shift ☐ Fetal kick counts (DFMR)	Maternal assessments: ☐ VS q 4 hours ☐ VS q 4 hours while awake ☐ VS q shift ☐ VS BID Vaginal bleeding Uterine activity Membrane status Vaginal discharge Fetal assessments: ☐ FHR q 4 hours ☐ FHR q shift ☐ Fetal kick counts (DFMR)	Maternal assessments: ☐ VS q 4 hours ☐ VS q 4 hours while awake ☐ VS q shift ☐ VS BID Vaginal bleeding Uterine activity Membrane status Vaginal discharge Fetal assessments: ☐ FHR q 4 hours ☐ FHR q shift ☐ Fetal kick counts (DFMR)	Maternal assessments: ☐ VS q 4 hours ☐ VS q 4 hours while awake ☐ VS q shift ☐ VS BID Vaginal bleeding Uterine activity Membrane status Vaginal discharge Fetal assessments: ☐ FHR q 4 hours ☐ FHR q shift ☐ Fetal kick counts (DFMR)
	Consults	☐ Perinatal CNS ☐ House officers ☐ NICU staff ☐ Social Services ☐ Pastoral Services	☐ Perinatal CNS ☐ House officers ☐ NICU staff ☐ Social Services ☐ Pastoral Services	☐ Perinatal CNS ☐ House officers ☐ NICU staff ☐ Social Services ☐ Pastoral Services	☐ Perinatal CNS ☐ House officers ☐ NICU staff ☐ Social Services ☐ Pastoral Services
	Procedures/ Tests	Laboratory tests: ☐ CBC ☐ CRP ☐ 24 hour urine ☐ UA for proteinuria Perinatal Center: ☐ NST ☐ Modified BPP	Laboratory tests: ☐ CBC ☐ CRP ☐ 24 hour urine ☐ UA for proteinuria Perinatal Center: ☐ NST ☐ Modified BPP	Laboratory tests: ☐ CBC ☐ CRP ☐ 24 hour urine ☐ UA for proteinuria Perinatal Center: ☐ NST ☐ Modified BPP	Laboratory tests: ☐ CBC ☐ CRP ☐ 24 hour urine ☐ UA for proteinuria Perinatal Center: ☐ NST ☐ Modified BPP
	Treatments				
	Meds/Vs	☐ Prenatal vitamins ☐ Refer to Medication Administration Record	☐ Prenatal vitamins ☐ Refer to Medication Administration Record	☐ Prenatal vitamins ☐ Refer to Medication Administration Record	☐ Prenatal vitamins ☐ Refer to Medication Administration Record
	Nutrition	Regular Diet	Regular Diet	Regular Diet	Regular Diet
	Pt. /Family Education	Purpose and course of tx S&S PTL	Purpose and course of tx S&S PTL	Purpose and course of tx S&S PTL	Purpose and course of tx S&S PTL
	Discharge Planning	Appropriate to clinical and social situation Ongoing reinforcement	Appropriate to clinical and social situation Ongoing reinforcement	Appropriate to clinical and social situation Ongoing reinforcement	Appropriate to clinical and social situation Ongoing reinforcement
	Spiritual/ Psycho/Social/ Emotional Needs	Assess support system Assess family separation anxiety Assist in dealing with high-risk pregnancy Make available information on Pastoral Services Evaluate spiritual needs and respond as appropriate PRN Provide significant sacraments and rituals as requested	Assess support system Assess family separation anxiety Assist in dealing with high-risk pregnancy Assist in developing coping skills Evaluate spiritual needs and respond as appropriate PRN	Assess support system Assess family separation anxiety Assist in dealing with high-risk pregnancy Assist in developing coping skills Evaluate spiritual needs and respond as appropriate PRN	Assess support system Assess family separation anxiety Assist in dealing with high-risk pregnancy Assist in developing coping skills Evaluate spiritual needs and respond as appropriate PRN
Multidisciplinary Team Signatures					

Patient Problems

1. Potential preterm birth
2. Vaginal bleeding
3. Stress related to high-risk pregnancy
4. Stress related to family separation

CARE PATH: Antepartum Complications
Code 089

ST. JOHN'S MERCY MEDICAL CENTER, ST. LOUIS, MO

PATIENT IDENTIFICATION

Name: ______________________________

This care path is a guideline and is not intended to create a standard of care. This guideline may be modified based on individual patient's needs.

Prob. #		Intrapartum	0-4 Hours Date:	4-8 Hours Date:	8-12 Hours Date:	12-24 Hours Date:
3	ADL	Bedrest or ambulation as tolerated	Bedrest or ambulation as tolerated	Up ad lib (assist PRN)	Up ad lib (assist PRN)	Up ad lib (assist PRN)
3	Assessment Monitor	Perinatal Unit admission assessment Ongoing assessments PRN	Immediate postpartum assessments VS Q 15" until stable, then Q 4h VS are WNL	VS Q 4h, VS are WNL Postpartum checks Q 4h - are WNL Assess mother/infant attachment	VS Q 4h, VS are WNL Postpartum checks Q 4h - are WNL Assess mother/infant attachment	VS Q 4h, VS are WNL Postpartum checks Q 4h - are WNL Assess mother/infant attachment
1,2, 4	Consults	Perinatal CNS Anesthesia PRN House officer PRN Resolve PRN NICU staff PRN	→ → → →	Lactation consultant PRN Social Service PRN/ WIC PRN	Lactation consultant PRN Social Service PRN/ WIC	Lactation consultant PRN Social Service PRN/ WIC
3	Procedures/ Tests	Hct PRN	Assess Rubella Titer status Assess need for Rhogam		Rhogam screen PRN	
1	Treatments	External EFM Internal EFM PRN	Ice to perineum Cath PRN	Ice to perineum Cath PRN Supportive bra PRN	Ice to perineum Cath PRN Supportive bra PRN Sitz bath PRN	Ice to perineum Supportive bra PRN Sitz bath PRN
1,2	Meds/IVs	Pain medication IV or IM PRN Alternative D_5 LR/LR when in active labor PRN Epidural/Pudendal/ Pericervical Pitocin augmentation PRN	Pain medication PRN Tucks PRN Anusol PRN Pitocin 20u IV then D/C	Pain medication PRN Tucks PRN Anusol PRN Stool softener PRN	Pain medication PRN Tucks PRN Anusol PRN Stool softener PRN	Pain medication PRN Tucks PRN Anusol PRN Stool softener PRN Rhogam PRN Rubella vaccine PRN
1	Nutrition	Ice chips PRN	Tolerate PO fluids Regular diet	Adequate fluids Regular diet	Adequate fluids Regular diet	Adequate fluids Regular diet
2	Pt./Family Education	EFM Labor support coaching - encourage support person in role	Self peri care/safety issues Perineum care - comfort measures Mother/baby booklet Initiate bottle or breast-feeding Initiate infant care	Bath/cord care and baby care demo Self care reinforcement and demos Discuss normal involution, lochia, fatigue, activity levels, and nutritional needs.	→ → →	Breast pump if indicated
2	Discharge Planning	Mother/baby teaching form	Determine LOS Begin discharge instructions	Continue discharge instructions	→	Assess parent/infant interaction Assess need for home health follow-up Discharge instructions reviewed with mother and S.O.
2,4	Spiritual/ Psycho/ Social/ Emotional Needs	Support patient/S.O. Facilitate a positive childbirth experience	Assess maternal role strengths	Assist mother's transition through tasks of taking on maternal role	→	→
	Multi-disciplinary Team Signatures	______ ______ ______ ______	______ ______ ______ ______	______ ______ ______ ______	______ ______ ______ ______	______ ______ ______ ______

Patient Problems

1. Discomfort/pain
2. Learning needs
3. Potential for instability - postpartum
4. Potential alteration in coping related to childbirth

CARE PATH: VAGINAL BIRTH — DRG# 373

ST. JOHN'S MERCY MEDICAL CENTER, ST. LOUIS, MO

PATIENT IDENTIFICATION

Name: ______________________________

This care path is a guideline and is not intended to create a standard of care. This guideline may be modified based on individual patient's needs.

Prob. No.		Day 1	Day 2	Day 3	Day 4	Day 5
5	ADL	OOB when stable	Up to chair. Up ad lib as tol.	Ambulate in hall TID.		
1,4	Assessment/ Monitor	Head to toe assessment per standards. VS Q 4°.				
3	Consults	Social Service evaluation within 24 hours of admission if appropriate.				
1,4, 5	Procedures/ Tests		Gentamicin peak/ through level around 3rd dose.			
	Treatments	Turn, cough, breathe Q 2 hrs. Accurate I&O. Reinforce drsg., if drsg present. Straight cath/Foley cathether within 8 hrs. post-op if no void.	Daily dressing change as indicated.	→	→	→
	Meds/IVs	• IV antibiotics (as ordered) • PCA as indicated • Antipryetic • Anteimetic • IV fluids	DC PCA basal rate.	DC PCA ↓ IV fluid rate.	Heplock IV	
	Nutrition	NPO except ice chips	Clear liquids as tolerated.	Advance diet to regular for age as tolerated.	→	→
	Pt./ Family Education	Review care expectations with patient & family.				Review S/S infection, dehydration, diet. Activity limitations.
	Discharge Planning	Assess need for intervention necessary for discharge.				Home medications. Wound care.
	Spiritual/ Psycho/ Social/ Emotional/ Develop-mental Needs	Provide information on Pastoral Care Services. Assess spiritual/ emotional needs of patient & family. Notify Child Life & assess individual needs for explanations & coping.	→ →	→ →		
	Multi-disciplinary Team Signatures	____ ____ ____ ____	____ ____ ____ ____	____ ____ ____ ____	____ ____ ____ ____	____ ____ ____ ____

Patient Problems

1. Potential for instability post-op
2. Fluid volume deficit
3. Coping - ineffective/individual
4. Potential for comorbid condition
5. Alteration in mobility
6. Knowledge deficit for caregiver
7. Potential for acute pain

PATIENT IDENTIFICATION

CARE PATH: Pediatric Appendectomy with Complications
Care Path Code: 119

ST. JOHN'S MERCY MEDICAL CENTER, ST. LOUIS, MO

Name: ______________________________

This care path is a guideline and is not intended to create a standard of care. This guideline may be modified based on individual patient's needs.

Prob. No.		Day 1 Admission Day Date: ________	Day 2 Date: ________	Day Date: ________
5, 4	ADL	Activity as tolerated	Activity as tolerated	
1	Assessment/ Monitor	Head to toe assessment per standard VS Q 4 h. BP q shift I&O q shift Daily wts	Head to toe assessment per standard VS Q 4 h. BP q shift I&O q shift Daily wts Reassess need for SaO2 monitoring	Head to toe assessment per standard VS Q 4 h. BP q shift I&O q shift Daily wts VS prior to discharge
4	Consults	Childlife consult	Childlife consult	Physician consult considered if patient not improved (i.e., pulmonary)
4, 1	Procedures/ Tests	CXR (P.P.D. if ordered) Chem 6, CBC, BC	Check C&S results Follow up lab abnormalities	Check C&S results Consider CXR if patient not improved
4	Treatments	See Respiratory Therapy protocol (R.T. to evaluate pulmonary toilet, O2 [sat], bronchodilator) O2 PRN	Respiratory Therapy (see R.T. protocol for patient education) O2 PRN/O2 sat BID/PRN	Discontinue O2/protocol
4, 2	Meds/IVs	I.V. antibiotics (administered within 4 hours after admission) I.V. fluids	I.V. antibiotics - reassess Consider change to I.V. heplock	I.V. antibiotics - reassess and consider switch to oral antibiotics Discontinue I.V. heplock Prescription for home meds
2	Nutrition	Diet as prescribed Encourage fluids	Diet as prescribed Encourage fluids	Diet as prescribed Adequate fluid intake
3, 1	PT./ Family Education	Review care expectations with patient and significant other R.T. to introduce patient education regarding disease process, norms, irritants and therapies	Continue R.T. education per protocol Patient education concerning medication, activities, and nutritional needs	Reinforce patient education and assess understanding Discharge outcomes reviewed with family
3, 5	Discharge Planning	Social Service evaluation within 24 hours of admission if appropriate	⟶ PRN conference with multidisciplinary team	Evaluate need for home equipment (nebulizer), home health care Discharge home if stable and to oral antibiotics Instructions on P.P.D. reading and report to primary physician if done
	Spiritual/Psycho/ Social/Emotional Needs	Provide information on Pastoral Services	Assess spiritual/emotional issues of patient and family as appropriate Contact with faith community PRN Patient care conference PRN Provide sacraments, rituals as requested	Intervention as needed based on spiritual/emotional assessment Patient care conference PRN Provide sacraments/rituals as requested
Multidisciplinary Team Signatures		________	________	________

Patient Problems

1. Gas exchange impaired - ineffective breath pattern
2. Fluid volume deficit
3. Coping - ineffective/individual
4. Potential for comorbid condition
5. Alteration in mobility
6. Knowledge deficit of caregiver

CARE PATH: Pediatric Pneumonia
Care Path Code: 030

ST. JOHN'S MERCY MEDICAL CENTER, ST. LOUIS, MO

PATIENT IDENTIFICATION

Glossary

abortion any interruption of a pregnancy before the fetus is viable (a stage of development that will enable the fetus to survive outside the uterus if born at that time)

absorption transfer of a drug from its point of entry in the body into the bloodstream

abstinence refraining from sexual intercourse

abstract thought final stage in cognitive thought processes; allows problem solving and creating hypotheses

abuse willful injury by one person of another

accommodation adjustment of the eye to focus on a close image (ophthalmology); the ability to adapt thought processes to fit what is perceived (Piaget)

acculturation the process of losing cultural beliefs and values to those of a dominant society

achalasia inability of a muscle to relax, particularly the cardiac sphincter

acrocyanosis cyanosis (blue color) in the feet and hands

acute pain sharp pain, generally occurring abruptly after an injury

acute transplant rejection reaction to a transplanted organ, usually occurring within the first 3 months after transplantation

acyanotic heart disorders heart or circulatory anomalies that involve either a stricture to the flow of blood or a shunt that moves blood from the arterial to the venous system (oxygenated to unoxygenated blood, or **left-to-right shunts**)

adaptability the ability to change one's reaction to stimuli over time

adolescence the time period between 13 years and 18 to 20 years

adrenarche the hormonal changes that occur with puberty

adventitious sounds extra or abnormal breathing sounds

affective learning learning that involves a change in attitude

afterload the resistance against which the cardiac ventricles must pump

afterpains intermittent cramping due to uterine contraction during involution in the postpartal period

aganglionic megacolon (Hirschsprung's disease) absence of ganglionic innervation to the muscle of a section of the bowel

age of viability the earliest age at which fetuses could survive if they were born at that time; generally accepted as 24 weeks, or fetuses weighing more than 400 g

agranulocytes white blood cells without granules in the cell cytoplasm

alleles two like genes

allergen antigen that causes the release of mediating substances causing tissue injury and allergic symptoms

allogeneic transplantation transfer of body tissues from an immune-compatible (histocompatible) donor

allografting transfer of body tissue between two genetically dissimilar individuals

Alport's syndrome a progressive chronic glomerulonephritis inherited as an autosomal dominant disorder

alternative birthing center a setting for birth separate from a hospital

amblyopia reduced vision in one eye; "lazy eye"

amenorrhea absence of a menstrual flow

amniocentesis the withdrawal of amniotic fluid from the uterus by means of introduction of a needle through the abdominal and uterine wall

amnioinfusion enlarging the amount of amniotic fluid by administration of normal saline or lactated Ringer's solution intravaginally into the uterus

amniotic cavity the space in the developing conceptus from which the ectodermal cells develop

amniotic fluid embolism condition in which amniotic fluid is forced into maternal circulation and travels to the lungs as small emboli

amniotic membrane the innermost membrane surrounding the fetus; it secretes amniotic fluid

analgesia a medication that reduces or decreases awareness of pain

anaphylaxis acute hypersensitivity (type I) reaction characterized by extreme vasodilation that leads to circulatory shock and extreme bronchoconstriction that decreases the airway lumens

andrology the branch of medicine that treats the male and diseases specific to the male sex

anesthesia a medication that causes partial or complete loss of sensation

angioedema edema of the skin and subcutaneous tissue.

anhedonia inability to remember the last time when a person felt happy or had a good time

ankle clonus continued motion of the foot

ankyloglossia an abnormal restriction of the tongue caused by an abnormally tight frenulum

anovulation faulty or inadequate production of ova

anteflexion a uterus that is bent forward just above the cervix

anteversion a uterus that is tipped abnormally forward including the cervix

anticipatory grief preparatory phase in which people gradually incorporate the reality of impending death into their thoughts

antigen any foreign substance (molecule) capable of stimulating an immune response

antitoxins antibodies against toxin-producing bacteria

aplastic anemias depression of hematopoietic activity in bone marrow affecting all blood cells

apnea pause in respirations longer than 20 seconds with accompanying bradycardia

apparent life-threatening event (ALTE) infant who is cyanotic and limp in bed but survives after mouth-to-mouth resuscitation by parents

appendicitis inflammation of the appendix

apposition the amount of end-to-end contact of bone fragments

approach a child's response on initial contact with a new stimulus

appropriate for gestational age (AGA) newborn who falls between the 10th and 90th percentile of weight for age regardless of gestational age

areola the pigmented circle surrounding the nipple

arthroscopy direct visualization of a joint with a fiber-optic instrument

aspermia absence of sperm

aspiration inhalation of a foreign object into the airway

aspiration studies studies involving the removal of body fluids by such techniques as lumbar puncture or bone marrow aspiration

assimilation changing a situation or one's perception of it to fit one's thoughts

astereognosis difficulty identifying objects placed in the hand when the eyes are closed

astigmatism congenital or acquired unevenness of the curvature of the cornea

atelectasis collapse of alveoli

atresia complete closure of a body opening

attention span the time interval a person can maintain interest in a topic or object

attitude the degree of head flexion a fetus assumes during labor, or the relation of the fetal parts to each other

audiogram a test to measure hearing

augmentation of labor assisting labor that has started spontaneously to be more effective

auscultation listening with the aid of a stethoscope

autografting transplantation of tissue from one part of the body to another in the same individual

autoimmunity an inability to distinguish self from non-self, causing the immune system to carry out immune responses against normal cells and tissue

autologous transplantation transplantation using the person's own previously removed tissue

automatisms complex purposeless movements, such as lip smacking or fumbling hand movements

autonomic dysreflexia a powerful sympathetic reflex reaction that causes signs of hypertension, tachycardia, flushed face, and severe occipital headache

autonomy independence

azotemia accumulation of nitrogen waste in the bloodstream

B lymphocytes lymphocytes formed in the bone marrow; responsible for antibody formation

baby-bottle syndrome decay of all the upper teeth and the lower posterior teeth, usually due to putting an infant to bed with a bottle

balloon angioplasty procedure usually by way of cardiac catheterization in which a catheter with an uninflated balloon at its tip is inserted and passed through the heart into the stenosed valve. As the balloon is inflated, it breaks valve adhesions and may relieve the stenosis.

ballottement: the sensation of an object rebounding after being pushed by an examining hand; used for pregnancy diagnosis

barium contrast studies x-ray involving the use of barium, a radiopaque substance to outline the gastrointestinal tract

barrier method a method of reproductive life planning in which sperm are prevented from entering the cervix

basal body temperature method a method of natural family planning based on the use of the body temperature on arising

battledore placenta a placenta with the cord inserted marginally rather than centrally

behavior modification a system of rewarding a person for desired behavior and ignoring or punishing the person for undesired behavior

beriberi deficiency of Vitamin B_1 involving tingling and numbness of extremities, heart palpitations, and exhaustion

bicornuate uterus a uterus that has two fundal horns; it may have an accompanying septum

bifidus factor specific growth-promoting factor for the bacteria *Lactobacillus bifidus* whose presence in breast milk interferes with colonization of pathogenic bacteria in the gastrointestinal tract

binge eating episodes of uncontrollable intake of large amounts of food over a specified period of time

binocular vision ability to fuse two images into one

biologic gender a person's chromosomal sexual designation of being male (XY) or female (XX)

biopsy surgical removal of tissue cells for laboratory analysis

birthing bed a bed specifically prepared for birth

birthing chair a chair used in labor and birth

birthing room a specifically prepared room for aiding comfort, safety, and conduct of birth

blastocyst a hollow sphere of cells that forms in early fetal development

blood dyscrasias hematologic disorders

blood plasma liquid portion containing proteins, hormones, enzymes, and electrolytes

body mass index determination of body weight by comparing height to weight (weight divided by height squared)

Bowman's capsule double-walled chamber enclosing the glomerulus of the kidney

Braxton Hicks contractions painless, erratic uterine contractions that occur toward the end of pregnancy. They ready the cervix for labor, but cervical dilation does not occur with them.

breech presentation fetal presentation in which either the buttocks or feet are the first body parts to contact the cervix

broken fluency repetition and prolongation of sounds, syllables, and words

bronchoscopy a procedure in which a bronchoscope, a specially designed tube, is passed through the nose or mouth to observe the larynx, trachea, bronchi, and alveoli

brown fat the special tissue present in newborns to maintain body temperature

bruit a swishing or blowing sound that occurs with turbulent blood flow, such as if there is an outpouching of the aorta

bruxism grinding the teeth during sleep

calendar method a method of natural family planning based on the determination of fertile and nonfertile days each month

calorie counting counting the number of calories that a person ingests in 1 day

caput succedaneum edema of the scalp at the presenting part of the head

cardiac catheterization a procedure in which a small radiopaque catheter is passed through a major vein in the arm, leg, or neck into the heart to secure blood samples or inject dye, to evaluate cardiac function

cardinal movements of labor position changes to keep the smallest diameter of the fetal head (in cephalic presentations) always presenting to the smallest diameter of the birth canal (descent, flexion, internal rotation, extension, external rotation, and expulsion)

caries dental cavities

carpal spasm hand spasm involving abduction of the hand and flexion of the wrist with the thumb positioned across the palm

cartilage connective tissue

case management nursing one nurse being in charge of a patient's care from admission to discharge

catarrhal stage inflammation of the nose and throat during infectious diseases

catatonia immobility

caudal regression syndrome hypoplasia of the lower extremities occurring primarily in infants of diabetic mothers

cavernous hemangioma type of birthmark evidenced as a dilated vascular space

celiac disease sensitivity or immunologic response to protein, particularly the gluten factor of protein found in grains—wheat, rye, oats, and barley

cell-mediated immunity type of immune response due to T-lymphocyte activity

centering focusing on only one aspect of an object or situation

central cyanosis cyanosis of the trunk

central nervous system (CNS) the brain, the spinal cord, and the surrounding membranes or meninges that protect the delicate tissues from normal trauma

cephalhematoma a collection of blood under the periosteum of the skull bone

cephalic presentation fetal presentation in which the head is the body part that first contacts the cervix

cephalocaudal relating to head and tail; progression of development in a fetus and child

cephalopelvic disproportion inability of the fetal head to pass through the maternal pelvis due to a discrepancy in size

cerebrospinal fluid (CSF) the fluid in the subarachnoid space, which serves as a cushion to the spinal cord

cervical cap a latex barrier method of contraception that fits over the uterine cervix

cervical cerclage suturing of the cervix to maintain a pregnancy to prevent premature cervical dilatation

cervical ripening change in cervical consistency from firm to soft

cesarean birth birth accomplished through an abdominal incision into the uterus

Chadwick's sign discolorization of vaginal walls from pink to violet

chain of infection method by which organisms are spread and enter a new individual to cause disease

chemotaxis "calling" leukocytes into the area

chemotherapeutic agent one that is capable of destroying malignant cells

chief concern the reason the parents or patient has come to the health care agency

chloasma extra pigment on the face

choreiform movements aimless movements

choreoathetosis rapid, purposeless movements

choreoid irregular and jerking movements

chorioamnionitis infection of the fetal membranes and amniotic fluid

chorionic membrane the outer fetal membrane

chorionic villi projections of the trophoblast that produce human chorionic gonadotropin and begin osmosis of nutrients to the embryo

chromosome the structure that weaves genes into strands in the nucleus of all body cells

chronic pain pain that lasts for a prolonged period of time (often defined as 6 months' time)

clarifying repeating statements others have made so that you and they can be certain that you understood

class inclusion the ability to understand that objects can belong to more than one classification

classic cesarean incision an incision that is made vertically through both the abdominal skin and the uterus

clean-catch specimen urine specimen obtained after the urinary meatus has been cleaned

cleansing breath a deep breath taken at the beginning and end of breathing exercises during labor that helps prevent hyperventilation

cleft lip failure of the maxillary and median nasal processes to fuse normally

cleft palate an opening of the palate

clinical nurse specialist a nurse prepared at the master's degree level who is capable of acting as a consultant in an area of expertise, as well as serving as a role model, researcher, and teacher of quality nursing care

clubbing a change in the angle between the fingernail and nailbed because of increased capillary growth in the fingertips; a response to hypoxia

coelocentesis the transvaginal aspiration of fluid collected in the extraembryonic cavity early in pregnancy for analysis

cognitive development the acquisition of the ability to think and reason

cognitive learning learning that involves a change in the individual's level of understanding or knowledge

coitus interruptus a method of contraception in which the penis is withdrawn from the vagina before ejaculation.

colonoscopy a procedure in which a colonoscope, a specially designed tube, is passed through the anus to examine the rectum or colon

colostrum a thin, watery, yellow fluid composed of protein, sugar, fat, water, minerals, vitamins, and maternal antibodies that precedes breast milk

comedones the lesions of acne vulgaris; "blackheads"

communication the exchange of ideas between two or more persons

community a limited geographic area in which the residents relate to and interact among themselves

complement a special body protein that is capable of lysing cells; comprised of 20 different proteins that are normally nonfunctional molecules but become active with the immune response

complete miscarriage the entire products of conception (fetus, membranes, and placenta) are expelled spontaneously without any assistance

complete protein a protein that supplies all of the essential amino acids

complex vocal tics repeated use of words or phrases out of context

computed tomography (CT) x-ray procedure in which many views of an organ or body part are made to represent what the organ would look like if it were cut into thin slices

concrete operational thought typical thought pattern of school-age children, preceding abstract thought

conditioned reflex a reflex to respond to a specific stimulus developed by training

condom a latex barrier method of contraception worn on the penis (a male condom) or inserted vaginally (a female condom); provides some protection against STDs as well

conduction transfer of body heat to a cooler solid object in contact with the body

congestive heart failure a condition in which the myocardium of the heart cannot pump and circulate enough blood to supply oxygen and nutrients to body cells.

conjugate vera true conjugate; measurement between the anterior surface of the sacral prominence and the posterior surface of the inferior margin of the symphysis pubis

conjunctivitis commonly called "pink eye" by parents; an infection of the conjunctiva that covers the eye

conscious relaxation deliberate relaxation

conscious sedation a state of depressed consciousness obtained by IV analgesia therapy

consciously controlled breathing deliberately spaced breathing to achieve a desired rate

conservation property of an object that a change in form does not equate to a change in size or amount

constriction ring a simple type of contraction ring that occurs at any point in the myometrium and at any time during labor

contact dermatitis example of a delayed or type IV hypersensitivity response; it is a reaction to skin contact with an allergen (a substance irritating only to the person with prior sensitization)

contraceptive a method or device to prevent the fertilization of the human ovum

contractility the ability of the ventricles to stretch; refers to the force of contraction generated by the myocardial muscle

contraction a rhythmic tightening of the uterus that aids in achieving cervical dilatation and effacement

contrecoup injury an injury resulting from a blow to one side of the skull that causes the brain to rebound and then injure the opposite side

convalescent period interval between when infectious symptoms begin to fade and the child returns to full wellness

convection flow of heat from the body surface to cooler surrounding air

conventional development adult level of moral development (Kohlberg)

coordination of secondary schema stage associated with infant's development of object permanence (Piaget)

coprolalia use of socially unacceptable words, usually obscenities

corona radiata the crown-like grouping of cells that surrounds the ovum immediately after ovulation

cotyledons subdivisions of the maternal surface of the placenta; filled with maternal blood to allow for osmosis of nutrients to the fetal placental villi

couvade syndrome somatic symptoms experienced by the father during pregnancy simulating those of the pregnant mother

couvelaire uterus uteroplacental apoplexy due to blood entering the uterine musculature

crackles the sound of rales

Crohn's disease inflammation of segments of the intestine, affecting any part of the gastrointestinal tract, but most commonly the terminal ileum

crowning the appearance of the fetal head at the perineum just before birth

cryptorchidism failure of one or both testes to descend from the abdominal cavity to the scrotum

culdoscopy the introduction of an endoscope through the posterior vaginal wall to view the pelvic organs

cultural values beliefs generally held by the majority of people in a community or society

culture the learned way of life of a community or society

cutaneous pain pain that arises from superficial structures such as the skin and mucous membrane

cyanosis a blue tinge to the skin indicating hypoxia

cyanotic heart disease cardiac anomaly when blood is shunted from the venous to the arterial system as a result of abnormal communication between the two (deoxygenated blood to oxygenated blood; **right-to-left shunt**)

cystocele a pouching of the bladder into the anterior vaginal wall

cytomegalovirus a member of the herpes virus family; teratogen that can cause extensive damage to a fetus yet causes few symptoms in the woman

cytotoxic (cell-destroying) **response** cells are detected as foreign and immunoglobulins directly attack and destroy the cells without harming surrounding tissue

cytotoxic (killer) **T cells** T lymphocytes that have the specific feature of binding to the surface of antigens and directly destroying the cell membrane and therefore the cell

death end of life; officially determined by unreceptivity and unresponsivity; no spontaneous muscular movement or breath; no reflex response; and a flat electroencephalogram

debridement the removal of foreign material from a burn or wound

decenter to project the self into other peoples' situations and see the world from their viewpoint

decerebrate posturing typical posture occurring when the midbrain is not functional; characterized by rigid extension and adduction of arms and pronation of the wrists with the fingers flexed; legs extended and the feet plantar flexed

decidua basalis the endometrium portion under the implanted blastocyst

decidua capsularis the endometrium portion that covers the blastocyst

decidua vera the endometrium portion that covers the nonimplanted portion of the uterus

deciduous teeth temporary teeth that are replaced by permanent teeth at around age 6 to 7 years

decorticate posturing a child's arms adducted and flexed on the chest with wrists flexed, hands fisted; lower extremities extended and internally rotated; feet plantar flexed; denotes brainstem involvement

deep tendon reflexes neurologic reflexes such as triceps, biceps, patellar, and Achilles reflexes

deep vein thrombosis (DVT) formation of thrombus (blood clot) in the deep veins secondary to stasis, vessel damage, and hypercoagulation

deferred imitation ability to remember an action and imitate it later

dehiscence the separation of a muscle or surgical incision

dehydration an excessive loss of body water

delayed hypersensitivity T-lymphocyte activity occurring solely without an accompanying humoral response

demonstration the showing of a procedure to stimulate learning

dermatoglyphics the study of surface markings of the skin

development an increase in ability (a qualitative change)

developmental care care designed to meet the specific needs of each infant

developmental hip dysplasia (often referred to as *congenital hip dysplasia*) improper formation and function of the hip socket

developmental milestone major marker of normal development

developmental task a skill or a growth responsibility arising at a particular time, the successful achievement of which will provide a foundation for the accomplishment of future tasks

diagonal conjugate distance between the anterior surface of the sacral prominence and the anterior surface of the inferior margin of the symphysis pubis

dialysis separation and removal of solutes from body fluid by diffusion through a semipermeable membrane

diaphragm a mechanical barrier contraceptive device fitted over the cervix in the woman

diaphragmatic excursion distance the diaphragm moves as measured from inspiration to expiration

diaphysis central shaft of a long bone

diastasis recti overstretching and separation of the abdominal musculature

diastole relaxation of the heart chambers

dilatation widening of the opening of the cervix in labor

diplegia (paraplegia); paralysis of the lower extremities

diplopia double vision

direct bilirubin water-soluble end breakdown product of heme that is combined and excreted in bile

direct care a nurse remains in continual attendance or visits frequently and actually administers care

discipline setting rules so people know what is expected

disorganization phase first phase of rape trauma syndrome in which victims feel a combination of humiliation, shame and guilt, embarrassment, anger, and vengefulness

distractibility the ability to shift concentration from one focus to another

distraction (a) a technique that allows the cells of the brain stem that register an impulse as pain to be preoccupied with other stimuli so the pain impulse cannot register; (b) use of an external device to separate opposing bones, thus encouraging new bone growth

distribution movement of a drug through the bloodstream to the specific site of action

dominant gene expressed in preference to the other genes

doula a person without professional experience who guides and assists a woman in labor

drowning asphyxiation because of submersion in a liquid

ductus arteriosus a blood vessel joining the pulmonary artery and aorta in fetal life; closes at birth

ductus venosus a blood vessel joining the umbilical vein and the inferior vena cava in fetal life; closes at birth

dysfunctional labor previously termed *inertia;* occurrence of sluggishness of contractions, or the force of labor

dyskinetic disordered muscle tone

dyslexia reading impairment disorder in which letters or words are reversed

dysmature newborn who is before term or post-term or is under- or overweight for gestational age

dysmenorrhea painful menstruation.

dyspareunia pain on sexual intercourse

dystocia difficult labor

echocardiography ultrasound involving the use of high-frequency sound waves to locate and study the movement and dimensions of the cardiac structures

echolalia repetitive words or phrases spoken by others

eclampsia development of a seizure from hypertension of pregnancy

ecomap a diagram of the family's interactions within the community.

ectoderm: one of the layers of primary germ cell tissue in the embryo

ectomorphic having a slim body build

ectopic pregnancy one in which implantation occurs outside the uterine cavity

effacement thinning of the cervix in labor

effleurage light massage done by the fingertips

egocentrism perceiving that one's thoughts and needs are better or more important than those of others

eighth-month anxiety fear of strangers that peaks during the eighth month

elective termination of pregnancy termination of a pregnancy by medical intervention

Electra complex strong emotional attachment of a preschool girl to her father (Freud)

electrical impulse studies those that include electrical conduction

electrocardiogram (ECG) written record of the electrical voltages generated by the contracting heart

emancipated minor a person before the age of majority who is free from the custody, care, and control of his or her parents and is capable of health care decisions; a pregnant adolescent

embryo the intrauterine growth period from the time following implantation until organogenesis is complete (tenth day to 5 to 8 weeks)

empathy the ability to put yourself in another's place and experience a feeling as that person does

en face position a position in which a caregiver's face and an infant's face look directly at each other

enanthem rash on the mucous membrane

endocervix the inner surface of the cervix

endometriosis abnormal growth of extrauterine endometrial cells, often in the cul-de-sac of the peritoneal cavity, the uterine ligaments, and the ovaries

endometritis an infection of the endometrium, the lining of the uterus

endometrium the inner layer of the uterus that is shed with menstruation

endomorphic having a large body build

endorphins naturally occurring opiate-like substances in the body

endoscopy a procedure in which an endoscope, a specially designed tube, is passed through the mouth to examine the gastrointestinal tract

engagement settling of the fetal head into the pelvis during labor

engorgement breast distention with swelling caused by vascular and lymphatic congestion arising from an increase in the blood and lymph supply to the breasts

engrossment staring at the newborn in the en face position for long intervals

entoderm one of the layers of primary germ cells in the embryo

enucleation eye removal

enuresis involuntary passage of urine past the age when a child should be expected to have attained bladder control

environmental control as many common allergens as possible are removed from the environment

epidural analgesia injection of an analgesic agent into the epidural space just outside the spinal canal, to provide analgesia to the lower body for 12 to 24 hours

epiphyseal plate area where the increase in the length of long bones occurs

epiphysis rounded end portion of a long bone

episiotomy surgical incision of the perineum to prevent tearing and to release pressure on the fetal head with birth

epispadias opening of the urinary meatus on the dorsal or superior surface of the penis

erectile dysfunction impotence; the inability to achieve erection in order to complete a sex act

erosion inflammation of the epithelium of the cervical canal spreading onto the area surrounding the os, giving the cervix a reddened appearance

erythema toxicum newborn rash that usually appears in the 1st to 4th day of life; sometimes called a flea-bite rash

erythroblastosis fetalis see *hemolytic disease of the newborn*

erythroblasts large, nucleated early red blood cells

erythrocytes red blood cells

erythropoietin a hormone produced by the kidneys that stimulates red blood cell development

escharotomy a surgical incision into the hard crust that forms over a burn

esotropia condition in which the eye is always turning in

estimated date of birth the predicted date on which a baby will be born (also estimated date of confinement or EDC)

ethnicity the cultural group into which a person is born

ethnocentrism the belief that one's own values or beliefs are superior to others

evaporation loss of heat through conversion of a liquid to a vapor

evidence-based practice the use of research or controlled investigation of a problem using a scientific method in conjunction with clinical expertise as acquired through experience and practice as a foundation for action

Ewing's sarcoma malignant tumor occurring most often in the bone marrow of the diaphyseal area (mid-shaft) of long bones

exanthem a skin rash

excretion elimination of raw drug or drug metabolites, a process that largely prevents properly administered drugs from becoming toxic

exophthalmos protrusion of the eyeballs

exotoxins poisons produced by some bacteria

exotropia condition in which the eye is always turning outward

expected date of birth: calculated date on which birth can be predicted to occur (EDB)

expiration carbon dioxide–filled air discharged to the outside

exstrophy of the bladder midline closure defect occurring during the embryonic period of gestation (first 8 weeks) and resulting in the bladder lying open and exposed on the abdomen

external cephalic version turning of a fetus from a breech to a cephalic position before birth

extracorporeal membrane oxygenation (ECMO) mechanical means of oxygenating blood

extremely-very-low-birth-weight (EVLBW) infant an infant weighing 500 to 1000 g

extrusion reflex a tongue reflex in infants that expels solid objects from the mouth; fades at 4 months

failure to thrive also called reactive attachment disorder; unique syndrome in which an infant falls below the fifth percentile for weight and height on a standard growth chart or is falling in percentiles on a growth chart

family two or more people who live in the same household (usually), share a common emotional bond, and perform certain interrelated social tasks

family nurse practitioner nurse who provides health care not only to women but all persons throughout the age span; in conjunction with a physician, an FNP can provide prenatal care for the woman with an uncomplicated pregnancy

family nursing the concept that clients do not exist outside a family; the family rather than an individual is considered the client

family of orientation one's birth family: oneself, mother, father, and siblings

family of procreation one's marriage family: oneself, spouse, and children

family theory a way of analyzing problems or concerns from a family's point of view

feedback a reply to communication indicating that the message has been received and interpreted

fertility awareness a method of contraception based on analyzing the consistency of vaginal secretions

fertility rate the proportion of women who could have babies who are having them

fertilization the union of the sperm and ovum

fetal alcohol syndrome condition associated with an infant born to a woman who uses alcohol during pregnancy; infant typically is small for gestational age, cognitively challenged, and has a characteristic craniofacial deformity including short palpebral fissures, thin upper lip, and upturned nose

fetal descent sinking of the fetus in the birth canal just prior to birth (one of six cardinal movements of labor)

fetoscopy the visualization of the fetus by inspection through a fetoscope

fetus the developing structure from the eighth week postfertilization until birth

fibrocystic breast disease benign multiple cysts in the breasts

fine motor development ability to accomplish smaller, more defined body movement; measured by observing or testing prehensile ability

fistula abnormal opening

flat affect not revealing feelings

fluoroscopy a radiologic serial-images technique

focusing helping a person to center on a subject

fomites inanimate objects, such as soil, food, water, bedding, towels, combs, or drinking glasses, that provide a means of infection transmission

foramen ovale an opening between the atria of the heart during intrauterine life

forceps birth birth using forceps (steel double-bladed instruments used to prevent pressure on the fetal head); forceps outlet procedure when the forceps are applied after the fetal head reaches the perineum.

foremilk constantly forming breast milk

formal operational thought final stage of cognitive development, involving the ability to think in abstract terms and use the scientific method to arrive at conclusions

fovea centralis (the center of the macula); an area of closely packed cones on the retinas where color is best perceived

fracture break in the continuity or structure of bone

frenulum the membrane attached to the lower anterior tip of the tongue

gamma globulin serum obtained from the pooled blood of many people; rich in antibodies

gastroesophageal reflux (commonly called achalasia in infants) a neuromuscular disturbance in which the gastroesophageal (cardiac) sphincter and the lower portion of the esophagus are lax, allowing easy regurgitation of gastric contents into the esophagus

gate control theory a theory of how pain impulses can be interrupted before they travel between a site of injury and the brain where the impulse is actually registered as pain

gavage feedings nasogastric tube feedings given to an infant

gender identity: the inner sense of being male or female, which may be the same as or different from biologic gender

gender role the behavior a person conveys about being male or female

genes basic units of heredity that determine both the physical and mental characteristics of people

genetics study of how and why chromosomal disorders occur; the science of heredity

genogram a diagram of family structure depicting essential family relationships; the interactive roles that exist in a family

genome complete set of genes present

genotype actual gene composition

genu valgus knock-knees

geographic tongue term for the rough-appearing tongue surface that often accompanies general symptoms of illness such as fever

gestational age number of weeks fetus remained in utero

gestational trophoblastic disease proliferation and degeneration of the trophoblastic villi

glomerular filtration rate rate at which substances are filtered from the blood to the urine

glomerulonephritis inflammation of the glomeruli of the kidney

glucose tolerance test a test of the body's ability to metabolize carbohydrate by measuring the serum glucose level after ingestion of a fixed amount of glucose

glycogen loading depleting, then replenishing glycogen stores by altering carbohydrate intake, to store extra glycogen for the purpose of sustaining energy through an athletic event

glycosuria excess glucose in the urine

glycosylated hemoglobin measure of the amount of glucose attached to hemoglobin

gonad a sex gland; an ovary in the female; a testis in the male

goniotomy surgical procedure used to treat congenital glaucoma

Goodell's sign softening of the cervix; a probable sign of pregnancy

granulocytes white blood cells with granules in the cell cytoplasm

graphesthesia ability to recognize a shape that has been traced on the skin

gravida number of times a woman has been pregnant, including the present pregnancy; a pregnant woman

grief process regulated steps in grieving

gross motor development ability to accomplish large body movements

growth an increase in size; a quantitative change

gynecology the study of the female reproductive organs and female disorders

gynecomastia enlargement of the breasts; excess development of male breast tissue; a transient occurrence in normal adolescence

hand regard infants holding their hands in front of their face and studying their fingers for long periods of time

hapten formation process whereby a substance, not antigenic in itself, becomes antigenic when combined with a higher-weight molecule, usually a protein

Hawthorne effect an improvement in behavior because of being studied

health fair a display to teach healthful behaviors

Hegar's sign softening of the lower uterine segment; a probable sign of pregnancy

Heinz bodies oddly shaped particles in red blood cells

HELLP syndrome a variation of hypertension of pregnancy named for the common symptoms that occur: *h*emolysis, *e*levated *l*iver enzymes, and *l*ow *p*latelets

helper T cells lymphocytes that stimulate B lymphocytes to divide and mature into plasma cells and begin secretion of immunoglobulins

hemangioma vascular tumor of the skin

hemiplegia paralysis of both extremities on one side

hemochromatosis deposition of iron in body tissues from destruction of red blood cells

hemoglobin a complex protein that is the oxygen-carrying component of red blood cells

hemolysis destruction of red blood cells

hemolytic disease of the newborn condition involving red blood cell destruction in the fetus who is Rh positive and whose mother is Rh negative

hemorrhagic disease of the newborn newborn bleeding disorder resulting from a deficiency of vitamin K

hemosiderosis deposition of iron in body tissues

hepatitis inflammation and infection of the liver

hermaphrodite having both ovaries and testes

heterograft tissue from another species (such as a pig) used as a temporary skin covering

heterosexual an individual whose sexual relations are with persons of the opposite sex

heterozygous trait having two different or unlike genes for a designated characteristic

hiatal hernia intermittent protrusion of the stomach up through the esophageal opening in the diaphragm

high-risk pregnancy one in which a concurrent disorder, pregnancy-related complication, or external factor jeopardizes the health of the mother and/or fetus

hind milk new breast milk formed after the let-down reflex

Homans' sign pain in the calf on dorsiflexion of the foot

home care care of people in their own home, provided by or supervised through a certified home health care or community health care agency

homosexual an individual whose sexual relations are with persons of his or her own sex

homozygous trait having two like genes for a designated characteristic

hordeolum an infection of an eyelash

hormones chemicals produced by ductless glands of the endocrine system

hospice care care of the person with a terminal disease; can be cared for at home

humoral immunity immunity created by antibody production or B-lymphocyte involvement

hydramnios an excessive amount of amniotic fluid (generally over 2,000 mL)

hydrocele collection of fluid in the scrotal sac

hydrocephalus an excess of cerebrospinal fluid (CSF) in the ventricles and subarachnoid spaces of the brain

hydronephrosis enlargement of the pelvis of the kidney with urine as a result of backpressure in the ureter

hydrops fetalis old term for the appearance of a severely involved infant with Rh incompatibility at birth

hyperactivity excess movement

hyperbilirubinemia increased serum bilirubin

hypercholesterolemia greater than usual levels of cholesterol in the blood

hyperfunction overfunction of a gland or organ

hyperglycemia increased blood glucose level

hyperopia farsightedness

hyperplasia an increase in the number of cells of a body part

hyperptyalism excessive secretion of saliva.

hypersensitivity response excessive antigen-antibody response when the invading organism is an allergen rather than a simple immunogen

hypertension elevated blood pressure

hypertonic uterine contractions contractions with an increase in resting tone to more than 15 mm Hg

hypertrophy an increase in the size of an organ because the cells have increased in size rather than number

hypocalcemia decreased serum calcium level

hypodermoclysis subcutaneous infusion

hypofunction underfunction of a gland or organ leading to acute or chronic insufficiency

hypoglycemia decreased blood glucose level

hyposensitization immunotherapy; a process to diminish an allergic response

hypospadias urethral defect in which the urethral opening is not at the end of the penis but on the ventral (lower) aspect of the penis

hypothalamus an organ located in the center of the brain that is the regulator of the autonomic nervous system

hypotonic uterine contractions the number of contractions are low or infrequent (not increasing beyond two or three in a 10-minute period) or ineffective

hypoxemia deficient oxygenation of the blood

hypoxia inadequate oxygenation of body tissue

identity developmental task of adolescence; determining who one is

imminent or **inevitable miscarriage** a threatened miscarriage accompanied by uterine contractions and cervical dilation

immune response body's action plan devised to combat invading organisms or substances by leukocyte and antibody activity

immune serum serum that provides passive immunity

immunity the ability to destroy invading antigens

immunocompetent cells cells capable of resisting foreign invaders

immunogen substance (antigen) that can be readily destroyed by an immune response

immunoglobulins antibodies that bind to and destroy specific antigens

implantation nidation; the attachment of the zygote to the uterine endometrium

imprinting differential expression of genetic material that allows researchers to identify whether the chromosomal material has come from the male or female parent

incest sexual activity between family members

inclusion children with physical or cognitive challenges attending regular schools and classes

incompetent cervix a cervix that dilates and causes birth of a fetus before term

incomplete miscarriage part of the conceptus (usually the fetus) is expelled, but the membranes or placenta is retained in the uterus

incomplete protein a protein that does not contain all of the essential amino acids

incubation period time between the invasion of an organism and the onset of symptoms of infection

indirect care the nurse plans and supervises care given by others, such as home health care aides or parents

induction of labor labor that is artificially started

industry the developmental task of the school-age child, according to Erikson; to learn how to do things well

infant mortality rate percent of infants who die during the first year of life per 1000 births

infantile spasms a form of generalized seizures—"salaam" and "jackknife"—or infantile myoclonic seizures, characterized by very rapid movements

infertility the inability to produce children

inguinal hernia protrusion of a section of the bowel into the inguinal ring

initiative the developmental task of the preschooler, according to Erikson; to learn how to do things

innocent heart murmur heart murmur of no significance; also called insignificant or functional heart murmur

insensible fluid loss fluid loss occurring as a result of evaporation from skin and lungs and from saliva

inspection visual observation to determine health

inspiration delivery of warmed moistened air via the respiratory system to the alveoli

insulin pump an automatic pump about the size of a transistor radio used to deliver insulin continuously

intelligence ability to think abstractly, to adjust to new situations, and to profit from experience

intercostal spaces spaces between the ribs

interferon a protein that protects against viruses

intermittent infusion devices (heparin locks) devices that maintain open venous access for medicine administration, yet allow patients to be free of intravenous tubing so that they can be out of bed and more active

intimate partner abuse abuse by a significant other

intracath a slim, pliable catheter threaded into a vein

intrauterine device (IUD) a contraceptive device inserted into the uterine cavity

intrauterine growth restriction or **retardation (IUGR)** failure to grow at the expected rate in utero

intuitive thought a stage of preschool thinking in which children can only see one characteristic of an object (centering)

intussusception invagination of one portion of the intestine into another

involution the process whereby the reproductive organs return to their nonpregnant state

irritable bowel syndrome presence of either intermittent episodes of loose and normal stools or recurrent abdominal pain

ischial tuberosity diameter distance between the ischial tuberosities, or the transverse diameter of the outlet (the narrowest diameter at that level or the one most apt to cause a misfit)

isoimmunization production of antibodies against Rh-positive blood in a fetus by a woman's immunologic system

jaundice yellowing of the skin

kangaroo care placing a newborn against a parent's skin to transfer heat from the parent to the newborn, thus conserving heat loss

karyotype a visual presentation of chromosomes

keratomalacia necrosis of the cornea with perforation, loss of ocular fluid, and blindness

kernicterus permanent brain cell damage secondary to elevated bilirubin levels

ketoacidosis a lowered serum pH resulting from accumulation of ketones

kinesthesia ability to distinguish movement

Koplik's spots, small, irregular, bright red spots with a blue-white center point, appearing on the buccal membrane with measles

kwashiorkor disease caused by protein deficiency

labile mood sudden mood changes (e.g., crying occurs, followed immediately by giggling or laughing)

labor-delivery-recovery room a hospital room specifically designed to accommodate labor and birth so that a separate delivery room is not needed

labor-delivery-recovery-postpartum room a specifically designed room that serves as the location not only for labor and birth but also for the post-partum recovery period

lactase the enzyme that converts lactose to glucose and galactose

lactiferous sinuses reservoirs for milk located behind the breast nipple

lactoferrin iron-binding protein in breast milk that interferes with growth of pathogenic bacteria

Lamaze method of childbirth a method of childbirth based on conditioned reflexes using paced breathing and relaxation techniques

Landau reflex develops at 3 months; when held in ventral suspension, the infant's head, legs, and spine extend. When the head is depressed, the hips, knees, and elbows flex.

lanugo fine, downy hair that covers a newborn's shoulders, back, and upper arms

laparoscopy examination of the abdominal cavity and organs by insertion of a surgical instrument through the anterior abdominal wall

large-for-gestational-age (LGA) infant an infant who falls above the 90th percentile in weight

latchkey child a child who is without adult supervision for a part of each weekday

latent tetany neuromuscular irritability associated with hypocalcemia

learned helplessness psychological infantilism; phase of intimate partner violence in which the partner is forced to use coping mechanisms such as becoming very obedient and cooperative in a desperate effort to reduce the violence

LeBoyer method a birth method encouraging a quiet, darkened room and maternal-infant bonding

left-to-right shunts heart or circulatory anomalies that involve blood movement from the arterial to the venous system (oxygenated to unoxygenated blood)

Leopold's maneuvers a method of observation and palpation to determine fetal presentation and position

lesbian a female homosexual

let-down reflex collecting sinuses of the mammary glands contract, forcing milk forward through the nipples, thus making it available for the baby

letting-go phase the third phase of the postpartal period in which the woman redefines her new role

leukemia distorted and uncontrolled proliferation of white blood cells (leukocytes)

leukocytes white blood cells

leukopenia a decrease in the number of white blood cells

leukorrhea a whitish, viscous vaginal discharge or an increase in the amount of normal vaginal secretions

libido sexual nature

lie the relationship between the long axis of the fetus and the long axis of the mother

light refraction manner that light is bent as it passes through the lens of the eye

lightening descent of the fetus into the pelvis at about 2 weeks prior to birth; also called engagement

lithotomy position a position with a woman on her back with her thighs flexed and her feet resting in the examining table stirrups

liver transplantation surgical replacement of a malfunctioning liver by a donor liver

lochia uterine flow, consisting of blood, fragments of decidua, white blood cells, mucus, and some bacteria following childbirth

lochia alba colorless or white vaginal discharge occurring about the 10th postpartal day

lochia rubra vaginal discharge consisting almost entirely of blood with only small particles of decidua and mucus, occurring from days 1 to 3 of the postpartal period.

lochia serosa pink or brownish vaginal discharge beginning at about the 4th postpartal day

lordosis forward curve of the spine

low segment incision an incision made horizontally across the abdomen just over the symphysis pubis and also horizontally across the uterus just over the cervix

low-birth-weight infant an infant weighing under 2500 g

lymphokine a substance that contains or prevents migration of antigens

lymphoma malignancy of the lymph or reticuloendothelial system

lysis killing

lysozyme enzyme found in breast milk that apparently actively destroys bacteria by lysing (dissolving) their cell membranes, possibly increasing the effectiveness of antibodies

macronutrient mineral with a daily requirement greater than 100 mg

macrophages mature white blood cells

macrosomia birth weight above the 90th percentile on an intrauterine growth chart for that gestational age

magnetic resonance imaging (MRI) combination of a magnetic field, radio frequency, and computer technology to produce diagnostic images

malleoli rounded prominence on either side of the ankles

malocclusion deviation from normal teeth positioning

mandatory reporters persons who are required to report suspected child abuse when they identify it

manifest tetany muscular twitching and carpopedal spasms from hypocalcemia

mastitis infection of the breast

maternal and child health nursing the full scope of nursing that deals with families during childbearing and childrearing periods

maturation reaching adulthood

McBurney's point one third of the way between the anterior superior iliac crest and the umbilicus; location of the appendix

McDonald's Rule the fundus-to-symphysis distance in cm is equal to the week of gestation between the 20th to 31st week of pregnancy

means of transmission method of spread of pathogens that cause infectious disease

Meckel's diverticulum the remains of a small pouch of the omphalomesenteric (vitelline) duct off the ileum, approximately 18 inches from the ileum–colon junction

meconium a sticky, tarlike, blackish-green, odorless material formed from mucus, vernix, lanugo, hormones, and carbohydrates that accumulates during intra-uterine life in the intestine

meconium plug extremely hard portion of meconium that completely obstructs the intestinal lumen, causing bowel obstruction

megakaryocytes immature thrombocytes

megaloblastic anemia enlarged red blood cells

meiosis type of cell division in which the number of chromosomes in the cell is reduced to the haploid (half) number for reproduction (23 rather than 46 chromosomes)

melasma excessive body pigment on the face that occurs during pregnancy

memory cells B lymphocytes that are responsible for retaining the formula or ability to produce specific immunoglobulins

menarche the first menstrual period

menopause the cessation of ovarian function

menorrhagia an abnormally heavy menstrual flow

mesoderm one of the layers of primary germ cell tissue in the embryo

metabolism conversion of a drug into an active form (biotransformation) or an inactive form (inactivation)

metaphysis thin area between the diaphysis and epiphysis in long bones

metastasis tumors that have extended beyond the original site or have spread systemically

metrorrhagia bleeding between menstrual periods

micronutrient mineral with a daily requirement less than 100 mg

milia pinpoint white papule (a plugged or unopened sebaceous gland) that can be found on the cheek or across the bridge of the nose of newborns

missed miscarriage now more commonly referred to as early pregnancy failure; the fetus dies in utero but is not expelled

mittelschmerz abdominal pain during ovulation from the release of accompanying prostaglandins

molding change in shape of the fetal skull owing to the force of uterine contractions pressing the vertex against the not-yet-dilated cervix

molestation vague term that includes "indecent liberties," such as oral-genital contact, genital fondling and viewing, and masturbation

Mongolian spot collection of pigment cells (melanocytes); slate-gray patches across the sacrum or buttocks and possibly the arms and legs of newborns

monophasic oral contraceptive birth control pills that contain the same amount of estrogen and progestin content in each pill throughout the cycle

Montgomery's tubercles sebaceous glands of the areola of the breast

mood quality a person's usual emotional state

mores customs generally accepted as right to follow by a community or society

mortality rate the number of deaths per 1000 persons

morula the developing blastomere structure as it multiplies rapidly and forms a bumpy surface

motor tics eye blinking, neck jerking, and facial grimacing

multigravida woman who has been pregnant more than once

multipara a woman who has given birth to more than one child past the age of viability

mumps orchitis testicular inflammation and scarring due to the mumps virus

Munchausen syndrome by proxy parent who repeatedly brings a child to a health care facility, reporting symptoms of illness when in fact the child is well

myometrium the muscle layer of the uterus

myopathy disease of the muscular system

myopia nearsightedness

natal teeth teeth present at birth

natural family planning contraception involving no medical devices or chemicals

near drowning a state in which a person has survived drowning

neck righting reflex turning of shoulders, trunk, and pelvis in the same direction when the infant turns the head to the side

necrotizing enterocolitis (NEC) development of necrotic patches in the bowel, interfering with digestion and possibly leading to a paralytic ileus; seen in infants in intensive care nurseries

neonatal nurse practitioner nurse skilled in the care of the newborn, both well and ill

neonatal period the interval from birth to 28 days of age

neonatal teeth teeth erupting in the first 4 weeks of life

neonate a baby in the neonatal period, the first 28 days of life

neoplasm new growth, usually referring to new *abnormal* growth that does not respond to normal growth-control mechanisms

nephrosis altered glomeruli permeability due to fusion of the glomeruli membrane surfaces causing abnormal loss of protein in urine

neural plate the embryonic structure from which the nervous system develops

neuroblastomas tumors that arise from the cells of the sympathetic nervous system

neurons nerve cells

nevus flammeus a macular purple or dark red lesion (sometimes called a *port-wine stain* because of its deep color) that is present at birth.

nociceptors specialized group of sensory receptors for pain

nocturnal emissions ejaculation during sleep

nondisjunction uneven cell division that leads to abnormal chromosome divisions

non–rapid-eye movement (NREM) sleep first stage of sleep; type of sleep that occurs in up to 80% of total sleep time

nonstress test an assessment of fetal well-being determined from examination of the fetal heart rate in relationship to fetal activity

nontherapeutic communication communication that lacks deliberate purpose (e.g., socializing)

normoblast a developmental stage of RBC after erythroblasts

norms customs generally accepted as right to follow by a community or society

nulligravida woman who is not or never has been pregnant

nurse-midwife nurse who assists women with pregnancy and childbearing either independently or in association with an obstetrician; can assume full responsibility for the care and management of women with uncomplicated pregnancies

nursing research controlled investigation of problems that have implications for nursing practice

nutritional marasmus disease caused by deficiency of all food groups, basically a form of starvation

nystagmus rapid, irregular eye movement

obese a body mass index over 29.0 or, in a child, a weight over the 90th percentile on a weight chart

object permanence awareness that an object exists even when it is out of sight

Oedipus complex strong emotional attachment of a preschool boy to his mother (Freud)

oligohydramnios: a decreased amount of amniotic fluid

omphalocele protrusion of abdominal contents through the abdominal wall at the point of the junction of the umbilical cord and abdomen

oncogenic viruses viruses associated with causing cancer due to their ability to change the structure of DNA or RNA

oocyte an immature ovum

operculum the mucous plug formed in the cervical canal during pregnancy

ophthalmia neonatorum eye infection at birth or during the first month, most commonly caused by *Neisseria gonorrhoeae* or *Chlamydia trachomatis*

orchiectomy removal of the testis

orchiopexy surgery to repair undescended testes

orchitis inflammation of the testes

organic heart murmur murmur occurring as the result of heart disease or a congenital defect

organogenesis organ formation

orthopnea position with the head and chest elevated to ease breathing.

orthoptics eye exercises

osteogenic sarcoma malignant tumor of long bone involving rapidly growing bone tissue (mesenchymal-matrix forming cells)

otorrhea discharge from the external ear

overhydration excess body fluid, usually extracellular fluid

overweight a body mass index between 26.1 and 29.0

oxytocin a pituitary hormone that initiates or sustains uterine contractions

pain an unpleasant sensation caused by pressure, injury, or tissue anoxia; whatever the person experiencing it says it is, and existing whenever he or she says it does

pain threshold the point at which the individual reports that a stimulus is painful

pain tolerance the point at which an individual withdraws from a stimulus or seeks relief

palilalia repeating one's own words

palpation an assessment technique that yields information on warmth and edema through touching

pancytopenia reduction of all blood cell components

para number of children above the age of viability a woman has previously birthed

parachute reaction arm extension seen in 6- to 9-month-old infants who are suddenly lowered toward an examining table from ventral suspension, as if to protect themselves from falling

parallel play playing alongside, not with, other children; characteristic of toddlers

paraphrasing restating what a person has said not only to assure the person that you have heard correctly (as in clarifying), but to help explain what the person was trying to say

paraplegia (diplegia) paralysis of the lower extremities

paroxysmal coughing series of expiratory coughs after a deep inspiration

paroxysmal nocturnal dyspnea suddenly waking at night short of breath

passage the birth canal

passenger the fetus

patent urachus failure of the urachus (narrow tube that joins the bladder to the umbilicus in utero) to close properly during embryologic development, leading to the development of a fistula between the bladder and umbilicus

pathologic retraction ring (Bandl's ring) a type of contraction ring that occurs at the juncture of the upper and lower uterine segments; a warning sign that severe dysfunctional labor is occurring

patient-controlled analgesia (PCA) form of administration that allows self-administration of IV boluses of medication, usually opioids, with a medication pump

pedal (foot) spasm foot spasm manifested as the foot is extended, the toes are flexed, and the sole of the foot is cupped

pediatric nurse practitioner an advanced nursing role that specializes in the well care of children

pedophile adult who seeks out children for sexual gratification

pellagra deficiency of niacin involving dermatitis and resembling a sunburn

pelvic inflammatory disease (PID) infection of the pelvic organs: the uterus, fallopian tubes, ovaries, and their supporting structures

peptic ulcer shallow excavation formed in the mucosal wall of the stomach, the pylorus, or the duodenum

perception checking documenting a feeling or emotion

percussion a chest physiotherapy technique that uses a cupped or curved palm against the chest; an assessment technique that helps determine the consistency of tissue beneath the surface area

perimetrium the outer coat of the uterus

perinatal home care health care at home during pregnancy or the neonatal period

periodic respirations irregular breathing pattern typically seen in newborns

periosteum outside sensitive layer covering of central shafts of long bones

peripartal cardiomyopathy myocardial failure apparently due to the effect of the pregnancy on the circulatory system

peripheral nervous system (PNS) the cranial nerves, the spinal nerves, and the somatic and visceral divisions

peritonitis infection of the peritoneal cavity

periventricular leukomalacia (PVL) abnormal formation of the white matter of the brain

permanence the awareness that objects exist when out of sight

permissive reporters people who may, but are not legally required to, report child abuse

petechiae pinpoint, macular, purplish-red spots caused by intradermal or submucous hemorrhage

phagocytosis destruction of invading substances

pharmacokinetics the way a drug is absorbed, distributed throughout the body, metabolized, inactivated, and excreted

phenotype outward appearance or the expression of the genes

phonocardiogram diagram of heart sounds translated into electrical energy by a microphone placed on the chest and then recorded as a diagrammatic representation of heart sounds

photophobia sensitivity to light

physiologic jaundice yellowing of the skin occurring on the 2nd or 3rd day of life as a result of the breakdown of fetal red blood cells

physiologic retraction ring ridge on the inner uterine surface marking the boundary between the upper and lower segments of the uterus during labor

physiologic splitting term to denote closure of the pulmonary valve slightly later than the aortic valve

pica indiscriminate eating of non-food substances

pincer grasp ability to bring the thumb and first finger together to pick up small objects

placenta accreta an unusually deep attachment of the placenta to the uterine myometrium

placenta circumvallata the fetal side of the placenta is covered with chorion membrane

placenta marginata the fold of chorion reaches just to the edge of the placenta

placenta previa low implantation of the placenta.

placenta succenturiata one or more accessory lobes connected to the main placenta by blood vessels

plasma cells B lymphocytes that secrete large quantities of immunoglobulins

play therapy a psychoanalytic technique used by psychiatrists to help children better understand their feelings and thoughts and motivations

plethora marked reddened appearance of the skin

plumbism lead poisoning

pneumothorax the presence of atmospheric air in the pleural space

poikilocytic irregular in shape

point of maximum impulse (PMI) the point on the chest where the apical heartbeat can be heard best

polycystic kidney large, fluid-filled cysts forming in place of normal kidney tissue

polycythemia an increase in the number of red blood cells that results as a compensatory response to insufficient oxygenation of the blood

polydactyly presence of one or more additional fingers

polydipsia excessive thirst

polyuria excessive urination

portal of entry means by which a pathogen can enter a person's body

portal of exit method by which organisms leave an infected person's body to be spread to others

position the relationship of a specific fetal part to the maternal pelvis

positive reinforcement rewarding someone for demonstrating desired behavior

positive signs of pregnancy findings that definitely indicate a pregnancy is present

positron emission tomography (PET) CT scan involving the use of an injectable radioactive contrast medium

postcardiac surgery syndrome febrile illness with pericarditis and pleurisy that appears to be a benign inflammatory response to a surgical procedure, developing at the end of the first postoperative week

postconventional development the mature form of moral reasoning in which standards of conduct are internalized (Kohlberg)

postpartal depression overall feeling of sadness in a woman accompanied by extreme fatigue, an inability to stop crying, increased anxiety about her own or her infant's health, insecurity (unwilling to be left alone or unable to make decisions), psychosomatic symptoms, and either depressive or manic mood fluctuations during the first year following birth

postpartal psychosis psychiatric illness occurring during the postpartum period

postperfusion syndrome a complication after cardiac surgery manifested by fever, splenomegaly, general malaise, maculopapular rash, hepatomegaly, and leukocytosis

post-term infant infant born after the onset of week 43 of pregnancy

post-term pregnancy a pregnancy that exceeds the limit of 42 weeks

post-term syndrome infant who stays in utero past week 42 of pregnancy and demonstrates the characteristics of malnourishment

postural proteinuria also called postural albuminuria; condition in which albumin spills into the urine when children stand upright for an extended period and decreases when resting in the supine position

powers of labor labor contractions

precipitate labor uterine contractions so strong that the woman gives birth with only a few rapidly occurring contractions

preconventional reasoning stage of moral development centering on "niceness" or "fairness"

preeclampsia in pregnancy-induced hypertension, the phase before the pregnant woman experiences a seizure

prehensile ability ability to coordinate hand movements

preload volume of blood in the ventricles at the end of diastole (the point just before contraction)

premature cervical dilatation previously termed an incompetent cervix; refers to a cervix that dilates prematurely and therefore cannot hold a fetus until term

premature ejaculation deposition of sperm before vaginal penetration or the full enjoyment of the sexual partner

premature separation of the placenta also called abruptio placentae; separation of the placenta before birth of the fetus

premenstrual dysphoric disorder (PDD) condition occurring in the luteal phase of the menstrual cycle and relieved by the onset of menses that has both behavioral and physiologic symptoms

preoperational thought period of cognitive development at the end of the toddler stage; the child begins to use assimilation (Piaget)

prereligious stage the infant period of moral reasoning, according to Kohlberg

pressure anesthesia a natural yet simplest form of pain relief for birth that results from the fetal head pressing against the stretched perineum

presumptive signs of pregnancy findings, largely subjective in nature, that suggest but do not confirm that a pregnancy is present

preterm infant infant born before term (less than the full 37th week of pregnancy)

preterm labor labor that occurs before the end of week 37 of gestation

preterm rupture of membranes rupture of fetal membranes with loss of amniotic fluid during pregnancy

priapism persistent, painful erection

primary apnea period of halted respirations during the first few seconds of life

primary circular reaction infant's exploration of objects by grasping them with the hands or by mouthing them

primary engorgement feeling of tension in the breasts on the 3rd or 4th day postpartum

primary infertility no previous conceptions have occurred

primary nursing a nursing pattern in which one nurse assumes complete responsibility for the care of a patient

primigravida a woman during her first pregnancy

primipara a woman who has given birth to one viable infant

probable signs of pregnancy findings, largely objective in nature, that suggest but do not confirm that a pregnancy is present

prodromal period a time between the beginning of nonspecific symptoms and specific infectious symptoms

prolactin an anterior pituitary hormone that acts on the acinar cells of the mammary glands to stimulate the production of milk

proteinuria protein in the urine

prune belly syndrome severe urinary tract dilation that develops as early as intrauterine life from an unknown cause

pseudoanemia the apparent anemia that occurs early in pregnancy due to rapid expansion of blood volume

pseudocyesis false pregnancy

pseudohermaphrodite a child with some external features of both sexes, although only either ovaries or testes (or neither) are present

pseudomenstruation mucous vaginal secretion in female newborns, which is sometimes blood-tinged

psychomotor learning learning that requires a change in an individual's ability to perform a skill

psychoprophylactic method the Lamaze method of childbirth

ptosis drooping of the eyelid

puberty the stage at which a person first becomes capable of sexual reproduction

pudendal nerve block the injection of a local anesthetic near the right and left pudendal nerves at the level of the ischial spine

puerperium the first 6 weeks following childbirth

pulse pressure the gap between systolic and diastolic blood pressure

punishment a consequence that results from a breakdown in discipline (disregarding the rules)

purging self-induced vomiting or the use of laxatives, enemas, or diuretics

purpura hemorrhagic rash or small hemorrhages occurring in the superficial layer of skin

pyloric stenosis hypertrophy or hyperplasia of the muscle surrounding the pyloric sphincter (opening between the lower portion of the stomach and the beginning portion of the intestine, the duodenum), making it difficult for the stomach to empty

pyrosis heartburn

quadriplegia paralysis of all four extremities

quickening the first movement of the fetus perceived by the mother

radiation transfer of body heat to a cooler solid object not in contact with the baby

radiopharmaceuticals radioactive-combined substances that, when given orally or by injection, flow to designated body organs

rales fine crackling lung sound; denotes fluid in alveoli

rape trauma syndrome a form of post-traumatic stress syndrome consisting of two phases: disorganization and reorganization

rapid eye movement (REM) last stage of sleep lasting 10 to 30 minutes in which eyes move in rapid, involuntary motions and respirations are irregular; body turnings, movements, and penile erections may occur

recessive gene gene that is not dominant

rectocele a herniation of the rectum into the posterior vaginal wall

recurrent pregnancy loss having three spontaneous miscarriages that occurred at the same gestation age in three pregnancies

redemonstration returning a demonstration to show competency of the skill

referred pain pain that is perceived at a site distant from its point of origin

reflecting technique for therapeutic communication that involves restating the last word or phrase a person has said

remodeling new bone tissue replacing old bone tissue

reorganization phase second phase of rape trauma syndrome that may last for months or years; rape victims possibly continue to report recurring nightmares, perhaps sexual dysfunction, and continuing inability to relate to men or face new and surprising situations. They may continue to have a great deal of difficulty discussing the rape.

reproductive life planning planning to space children or prevent children from being conceived

reservoir container or place in which organisms grow and reproduce

resorption the breakdown of bone cells

reticulocyte a developmental stage of red blood cells prior to the formation of mature RBCs

retinopathy of prematurity (ROP) an acquired ocular disease that leads to partial or total blindness in children, due to vasoconstriction of immature retinal blood vessels; commonly caused by use of too-high oxygen levels

retractions indentation of intercostal spaces reflecting difficulty breathing

retractors long, metal, curved instruments used to aid birth

retroflexion a uterus that is bent backward just above the cervix

retroversion a uterus that is tipped abnormally backwards

reversibility the ability to retrace steps

review of systems summary of body symptoms as the last step in a health interview

Rh incompatibility an Rh-negative mother (one negative for a D antigen or one with a dd genotype) is carrying a fetus with an Rh-positive blood type (DD or Dd genotype)

rhabdomyosarcoma tumor of striated muscle

rhinorrhea discharge from the nose

rhythmicity a regular rhythm in physiologic functions

rickets deficiency of vitamin D involving poor bone formation

right-to-left shunt cardiac anomaly when blood is shunted from the venous to the arterial system as a result of abnormal communication between the two (deoxygenated blood to oxygenated blood)

ripening softening of the cervix with the approach of labor

role confusion characteristic of people who do not develop a sense of identity; uncertainty about what kind of person one is

role fantasy a method of thinking that changes perceptions to how the child would like things to turn out (magical thinking)

rooming-in a hospital pattern in which infant stays in the room with the mother

sarcomas tumors derived from connective tissue, such as bone and cartilage, muscle, blood vessels, or lymphoid tissue

schemas the means by which thoughts are organized (Piaget)

scope of practice range of activity

scurvy vitamin C deficiency involving muscle tenderness and petecchiae

seborrhea a scaly scalp condition, often called cradle cap

secondary apnea weakening of a newborn's respiratory effort after attempts to initiate respirations with a few strong gasps after 1 to 2 minutes of apnea

secondary circular reaction infant's ability to realize that his or her actions can initiate pleasurable sensations

secondary infertility a couple is unable to conceive at present although they have had a previous viable pregnancy

secondary stuttering stuttering that develops after a child learns to speak without stuttering

sella turcica a depression of the sphenoid bone

sensorimotor stage the period from birth to 2 years of age (Piaget)

sensory deprivation loss of environmental stimuli

sensory overload receiving more stimulation than can be tolerated or processed

septicemia pathogenic organisms in the blood stream

sequestrum dead bone tissue detached from adjoining healthy bone

sexually transmitted diseases (STDs) those spread through sexual contact with an infected partner

shaken baby syndrome repetitive, violent shaking of a small infant by the arms or shoulders causing a whiplash injury to the neck, edema to the brain stem, and distinct retinal hemorrhages

shoulder dystocia an infant's wide shoulders are unable to pass through the outlet of the pelvis

sickle-cell crisis term used to denote a sudden, severe onset of sickling with sickle-cell anemia

sickle-cell trait the existence of hemoglobin AS (normal hemoglobin and abnormal hemoglobin S); a disease carrier

silent rape syndrome long-term effects in victims who do not report rape and receive no counseling

Sim's position turned to the left side with the weight of the uterus resting on the bed

single photon emission computerized tomography (SPECT) CT scan involving the use of an injectable iodine-based contrast medium.

sinus arrhythmia a marked heart rate increase occurring as the child inspires and a marked decrease in heart rate as the child expires

sitz bath small, portable basin that fits on a toilet seat to provide a constant supply of water to the perineal area. It soothes healing tissue and decreases inflammation by vasodilation to the area.

skilled home care care that includes physician-prescribed procedures such as dressing changes, administration of drugs, health teaching, and observation of the client's progress

sleep deprivation lack of adequate amount of sleep leading to difficulty in concentrating and episodes of disorientation and misperception

small-for-gestational-age (SGA) infant an infant who falls below the 10th percentile of weight for age

social smile a definite response (smiling) to an interaction occurring at about 6 weeks of age

somatic pain pain that originates from deep body structures such as muscles or blood vessels

Somogyi phenomenon rebound hyperglycemic response, typically manifested with nighttime hypoglycemia and early morning hyperglycemia

speculum a metal or plastic instrument with movable flat blades used for pelvic examinations

sperm count the number of sperm present in a measured amount of semen

sperm motility whether sperm are seen to be active

spermatogenesis production of sperm cells

spina bifida Latin for "divided spine"; most often used as a collective term for all spinal cord disorders

spontaneous miscarriage pregnancy interruption due to natural causes

stalking repetitive, intrusive, and unwanted actions directed at an individual to gain the individual's attention or evoke fear

station the relationship of the presenting part of the fetus to the level of the ischial spines

status epilepticus a seizure that lasts continuously for more than 30 minutes or a series of seizures from which the child does not return to his or her previous level of consciousness

steatorrhea large, bulky, greasy stools

stenosis narrowing

stereognosis the ability to recognize an object by touch

stereopsis depth perception; the ability to locate an object in space relative to another object

stereotyping applying a fixed conception

strabismus crossed eye

strawberry hemangioma a type of birthmark identified as an elevated area formed by immature capillaries and endothelial cells

striae gravidarum reddish steaks appearing on the abdominal wall during pregnancy

stridor a harsh, strident breath sound on inspiration

stupor lethargy and unresponsiveness

subconjunctival hemorrhage rupture of a conjunctival capillary appearing as a red spot on the sclera, frequently seen in newborns

substance abuse the use of chemicals to improve a mental state or induce euphoria

substance dependent when a person has withdrawal symptoms following discontinuation of the substance, and such activities as abandonment of important activities, spending increased time in activities related to substance use, using substances for a longer time than planned, and continued use despite the existence of worsening problems due to substance use

substitution of meaning also called guided imagery; distraction technique to help a person place another meaning (a non-painful one) on a painful procedure

suppressor T cells T cells that reduce the production of immunoglobulins against a specific antigen and prevent their overproduction

surfactant a lipoprotein secreted by the alveoli cells to reduce surface tension in alveoli

susceptible host individual more prone to infection than others

syndactyly fusing of the fingers

synergeneic transplantation transplantation between a donor and recipient who are genetically identical (i.e., identical twins)

systole contraction of the heart chambers

T lymphocytes lymphocytes that are produced by the bone marrow but mature under the influence of the thymus gland (hence the term *T cells*)

taboos actions that are prohibited in a specific culture

tachypnea an increased respiratory rate

taking-hold phase the second phase of the postpartal period where the woman begins to initiate action

taking-in phase the first phase of the postpartal period experienced when the woman is reflective and plays a largely passive role

teaching plan a design of content to be taught and the teaching-learning techniques to be used

temperament a child's innate behavioral characteristics such as activity level, rhythmicity, tendency to approach or withdraw, and adaptability to situations

teratogen substance that causes fetal harm

teratogenicity capable of causing fetal harm

term infant an infant born after the beginning of week 38 and before week 42 of pregnancy

tertiary circular reaction stage a stage of development in which the child discovers new properties of objects (Piaget)

thelarche breast development changes at puberty

theory a systematic statement of principles that provides a framework for explaining some phenomenon

therapeutic communication an interaction between two people that is planned, has structure, and is helpful and constructive

therapeutic play play technique that can be used by nurses to better understand children's feelings and thoughts and relieve their anxiety

thought stopping technique whereby children are taught to stop anxious thoughts by substituting a positive or relaxing thought

threatened miscarriage pregnancy interruption manifested by vaginal bleeding, initially beginning as scant bleeding, and usually bright red in color

threshold of response the intensity level of stimulation that is necessary to evoke a reaction

threshold sensation the amount of stimulus that results in pain

thrombocytes platelets

thrombocytopenia decreased platelet count

thrombophlebitis inflammation of the lining of a blood vessel with the formation of blood clots

thrush a *Candida* infection that usually appears on the tongue and sides of the cheeks as white or gray patches

thumb opposition ability to bring the thumb and fingers together

tocolytic agent a drug to halt labor

tolerance a state of not responding to an allergen

total parenteral nutrition (TPN) concentrated hypertonic solutions of intravenous fluid containing glucose, vitamins, electrolytes, trace minerals, fat, and protein to meet all of the child's nutritional needs

toxic shock syndrome (TSS) an infection usually caused by toxin-producing strains of *Staphylococcus aureus* organisms

toxoid extract of a toxin with reduced virulence

toxoplasmosis a protozoan infection spread most commonly through contact with uncooked meat; also contracted through handling cat stool in soil or cat litter

tracheostomy an opening into the trachea to create an artificial airway

tracheotomy procedure to create an airway

traction pulling on a body part in one direction against a counterpull exerted in the opposite direction to reduce dislocations and immobilize fractures

transcultural nursing a philosophy of nursing that focuses on the unique cultural beliefs of people

transcutaneous electrical nerve stimulation (TENS) pain relief measure that achieves its effect by counter irritation on nociceptors by use of a light electric current

transillumination holding a bright light such as a flashlight or a specialized light—a Chun gun—against a body part to reveal fluid inside

transition the end of the first stage of labor, just before the woman experiences pushing sensations

transitional stool green and loose stool passed on the 2nd to 3rd day of the newborn's life

transsexual a person of one sex whose perceived identity is of the opposite sex

transvestite a person who engages in the practice of dressing in the clothes of the opposite sex for sexual gratification

triphasic oral contraceptives birth control pills in which the estrogen and progestin content varies throughout the cycle

trophoblast the outer layer of the blastocyst

true conjugate conjugate vera; measurement between the anterior surface of the sacral prominence and the posterior surface of the inferior margin of the symphysis pubis

trust the developmental task of the infant, according to Erikson; learning to love and be loved

tubal ligation a method of contraception in which the fallopian tubes are cauterized, tied, or clamped to prevent sperm from reaching the discharged oocyte

tumor staging procedure by which a malignant tumor's extent and progress are determined

turgor skin characteristic reflecting the amount of fluid in body tissue

tympanocentesis withdrawal of fluid from the middle ear through the tympanic membrane

ulcerative colitis inflammation of continuous intestinal segments, typically the colon and rectum, with the distal colon and rectum most severely affected

ultrasound painless diagnostic procedure in which pictures of internal tissue and organs are produced by high-frequency sound waves

umbilical cord the structure composed of two veins and one artery that connects the placenta to the fetus

umbilical cord prolapse a loop of the umbilical cord slipping down in front of the presenting fetal part

underweight a body mass index under 19.8

urticaria swelling and itching caused by capillary dilatation

uterine atony relaxation of the uterus in the postpartal period

uterine inversion a rare phenomenon in which the uterus turns inside out

vacuum extraction birth of a fetus by means of vacuum pressure

vaginal birth after cesarean birth (VBAC) a birth in a woman who previously had a child by cesarean birth

vaginismus painful, involuntary spasms of the vagina

varicocele abnormal dilation of the veins of the spermatic cord

vascular access port (VAP) small device (infusion port) implanted under the skin, usually on the anterior chest just under the clavicle to allow for circulatory access

vasculitis inflammation of blood vessels

vasectomy a surgical ligation of the vas deferens that results in male sterility

ventral suspension infant's appearance when held in midair on a horizontal plane, supported by a hand under the abdomen

vernix caseosa a white, cream cheese–like substance that serves as a skin lubricant; usually noticeable on a newborn's skin at birth in a term neonate

very-low-birth-weight infant infant weighing less than 1500 g

vesicoureteral reflux retrograde flow of urine from the bladder into the ureters

vibration a chest physiotherapy technique that involves pressing a vibrating hand against a child's chest during exhalation to loosen and raise mucus

visceral pain involves sensations that arise from internal organs such as intestines

vocal tics coughing, throat clearing, snorting, and barking

volvulus a twisting of the bowel causing obstruction

voyeurism the practice of obtaining sexual pleasure by looking at the nude body of another

vulnerable or fragile children children whose parents were told they would die, but who lived and are treated in a cold and unfeeling way—as if they actually did die

vulvovaginitis inflammation of the vulva or vagina

Wharton's jelly the gelatinous substance that gives bulk to the umbilical cord

wheezing whistling expiratory sound

women's health nurse practitioner an advanced practice nurse who specializes in the health care of women

xerophthalmia dry and lusterless conjunctivae caused by vitamin A deficiency

yolk sac the space in the blastocyst from which the hemopoietic system develops

zona pellucida a layer of fluid that surrounds the ovum at ovulation

zygote a fertilized ovum

ANSWERS TO CHECKPOINT QUESTIONS AND WHAT IF? QUESTIONS

Chapter 1: A Framework for Maternal and Child Health Nursing

Checkpoint Question Answers

1. Promotion and maintenance of optimal family health to ensure cycles of optimal childbearing and childrearing is the primary goal of maternal-child health nursing.
2. As children and mothers-to-be exist within families, family-centered care better provides for holistic care.
3. Two other requirements of a profession are that members set their own standards and monitor their practice quality.
4. A philosophy of cost containment and changes in family composition, such as many single-parent families, have had important influences on maternal and child health nursing care.
5. Since the AAP recommended in 1992 that infants be placed on their back or side to sleep, the incidence of SIDS has decreased 44%, greatly lowering the U.S. infant mortality rate.
6. The infant mortality rate is the health statistic most commonly used for international comparison of the health of nations.
7. The Family Medical Leave Act supports family-centered care by mandating that employers with 50 or more employees provide a minimum of 12 weeks' unpaid, job-protected leave to employees who meet set criteria, so the employees may care for a newborn, ill family member, or a personal illness.
8. Empowerment of health care consumers has become increasingly important due to the influence of managed care, a focus on cost containment, and a strengthened focus on health promotion and disease prevention.
9. Family Nurse Practitioners are able to care for the entire family, so are able to form long-term and comprehensive relationships with families.

What If? Question Answers

1. Because the first days of life are the time when bonding between parents first begins, having the infant stay with the mother would be preferred from this standpoint. Unfortunately, this increases cost for the health care agency, so the baby, as a rule, will be discharged home before the mother. Helping the new mother keep in contact with her infant (taking an instant photo of the baby, reserving time for her to talk on the telephone with the baby's temporary caretaker or the baby's father) is an important nursing responsibility.
2. This is not a simple problem because a lot of factors could be playing into it. The first responsibility, therefore, would be to discover the parent's motivation for wanting the child in the hospital. (She doesn't understand that with current antibiotics, the care of children with this disease has been completely modified? She doesn't have anyone to care for the child at home [or is homeless]? She feels too insecure to care for a sick child? Her health insurance only covers in-hospital care?) Once these questions are answered, the task is not simply advocating for hospitalization (or not), but attacking the more basic problem.

Chapter 2: The Childbearing and Childrearing Family

Checkpoint Question Answers

1. A single-parent family offers a child a special parent-child relationship as well as more opportunity for self-reliance and independence
2. A gay couple with a child would most closely resemble a nuclear family (two parents and a child).
3. Most people believe that children who are adopted should be told about the adoption as soon as they are able to understand what this means, or by late preschool age.
4. Small families have fewer child care requirements; however, they also have less experience in childrearing.
5. Children from countries with inadequate health supervision may have a greater risk of illnesses such as hepatitis B and intestinal parasites, as well as growth restriction.
6. If both parents work outside the home, medicine may have to be administered at a time when a parent is home or when getting up, before leaving for work, after school, and at bedtime.
7. A genogram is a diagram that shows family structure, history, and member roles, usually through several generations. An ecomap is a diagram of family and community relationships.
8. The Family APGAR is a screening tool of the family environment.
9. The availability of community transportation impacts a patient's access to health care. If adequate public transportation is not available, a family may have trouble making appointments and may be unable to receive follow-up care or health maintenance.

What If? Question Answers

1. The oldest child in a family marks the family stage. This family, therefore, is a stage 4 (school-age) family. Having children widely spaced can create stress for a family as they try to meet the needs of two widely different interests.
2. As a rule, families with many connections to their community have a ready source of support if a crisis should occur. A family with few connections, therefore, often requires more discharge planning.

Chapter 3: Sociocultural Aspects of Maternal and Child Health Nursing

Checkpoint Question Answers

1. A cultural more is the expected or usual values of a particular group.
2. Stereotyping is the expectation that people will act in a characteristic manner without regard to individual characteristics.
3. Cultural competence is the integration of cultural elements to enhance communication and work effectively with people.
4. Transcultural nursing is a philosophy of nursing that focuses on the unique cultural beliefs of people.
5. Ethnocentrism is the belief that one's values or ways are superior to others.
6. Touch is not universally accepted as a comforting gesture.
7. Time orientation can interfere with health care if the orientation of the family is different from that of the health care provider. For example, if extensive rehabilitation is required, a family that is past oriented may have difficulty coping with the future planning necessary.

What If? Question Answers

1. This situation calls for assessment of why the father is saying he wants no role. If the answer is that he knows nothing about what to do, then teaching him how to be a part of an activity such as tim ing contractions would be helpful. If he does not want to be part of the process because he sees that action as culturally inappropriate, allowing him to sit quietly would be more appropriate. For many women in labor, the very fact that their support person is there is the important consideration, not that the person is actively doing any one thing.
2. The presence or degree of pain can be determined by both verbal and nonverbal communication (facial expression, clenching fists, etc.), so assessing these as well as listening to what a person is saying can help assess whether pain is present or not.

Chapter 4: Reproductive and Sexual Health

Checkpoint Question Answers

1. Testosterone is the hormone that most directly affects growth of male facial hair.
2. The first menstrual period is menarche; beginning breast development is thelarche.
3. Vasectomy involves severing the vas deferens.
4. No. Hymens can be torn by athletic activities such as horseback riding or gymnastics.
5. The junction of the epithelium and mucous membrane is the most frequent site of cervical cancer.
6. Retroversion means the entire uterus is tipped backward. Retroflexion means the body of the uterus is bent sharply back, but the cervix remains in normal position.
7. The pelvic inlet is wider in the transverse diameter. The pelvic outlet is wider in the anteroposterior diameter.
8. The pituitary gland secretes follicle-stimulating hormone (FSH) and luteinizing hormone (LH).
9. Ovulation typically occurs on the 14th day from the end of the cycle.
10. No. Masturbation is a normal characteristic of the preschool age.
11. Up to 50% of adolescents admit to being sexually active.
12. This is good protection for any sexual encounter.

What If? Question Answers

1. Lack of urine output for 6 hours following surgery may occur from dehydration. Assessing whether the woman is receiving adequate intravenous fluid would be important. Observing women for urine output following uterine or fallopian tube surgery is more important than usual because the ureters pass just beneath the fallopian tubes. This means they can be accidentally injured in surgery or, because they are so near the surgery site, be obstructed from local edema.
2. Fetishes such as this are not unusual. Unless there is a reason that the exposure to rubber would interfere with some treatment or procedure being done as a part of the hospitalization, choosing to respect patient privacy in relation to the suitcase's findings would seem to be the best action.

Chapter 5: Reproductive Life Planning

Checkpoint Question Answers

1. No expense or foreign materials are necessary with fertility awareness methods.
2. Using a combination of techniques such as basal body temperature and mucus awareness can be more effective than a single method.
3. Coitus interruptus is usually ineffective because sperm are present even in pre-ejaculation fluid.
4. The estrogen in ovulation suppressants acts to suppress follicle-stimulating and luteinizing hormones, suppressing ovulation. The progesterone action causes a decrease in the permeability of cervical mucus, limiting sperm motility.
5. Nausea, weight gain, headache, breast tenderness, breakthrough bleeding, monilial vaginal infections, mild hypertension, and potential depression are common side effects of ovulation suppressants.
6. Danger signs that a woman taking ovulation suppressants should be instructed to report are pain in the calf of the leg (possibly thrombophlebitis); chest pain (possibly pulmonary embolus), and early signs of pregnancy such as nausea, vomiting, and amenorrhea.
7. Two advantages of subcutaneous implants and IM injections over ovulation suppressants are that no reminders to take them are needed, and they can be used during breastfeeding.
8. Subcutaneous implants are effective for five years, IM injections for 4 to 12 weeks.
9. An IUD interferes with transport of the ova so interferes with fertilization.
10. Advantages of diaphragms are: inexpensive, no hormonal side effects. Disadvantages: preparation time for placement involved; may increase the incidence of urinary tract infection.
11. Nonoxynol-9 is the substance used more often in spermicides to help protect against STDs.
12. Female condoms are not widely used because many women are not aware that they exist. Some women report they are difficult to put in place.
13. A vasectomy is a surgical procedure to cut the vas deferens to prevent passage of spermatozoa.
14. Sharp shoulder pain can occur following a laparoscopy if the carbon dioxide infused during the procedure puts pressure on nerves.
15. Although reversal of these procedures is possible, there is no guarantee that this can be accomplished.
16. Abortion accomplished early in pregnancy has less chance of leading to hemorrhage because the placenta is not well attached.
17. Frequent dilatation of the cervix can lead to an incompetent cervix, or one that dilates so easily that it will not remain contracted during a subsequent pregnancy. Laminaria dilation may be used since this method dilates the cervix gradually.
18. Fever, excessive bleeding or passing of clots, abdominal pain, and severe depression are signals of abortion complications.

What If? Question Answers

1. Diaphragms must be individually fitted to be effective; therefore, they cannot be shared. Sharing one could also lead to spread of infection from one girl to the other.
2. Ovulation suppressants can reduce menstrual pain because they inhibit ovulation. If all the adolescent wants is pain relief, however, use of an over-the-counter NSAID would accomplish this without exposing her to long-term estrogen therapy.

Chapter 6: The Infertile Couple

Checkpoint Question Answers

1. Infertility exists when pregnancy has not occurred after at least 1 year of unprotected coitus.
2. Cryptorchidism can lead to impaired spermatogenesis if not corrected before puberty.
3. Gonorrhea and chlamydia are two organisms commonly associated with PID.
4. Endometriosis can cause dyspareunia; abnormal endothelium may create a pelvic inflammation detrimental to sperm survival.
5. Hysterosalpingography is an x-ray of fallopian tubes to determine patency.
6. Carbon dioxide may accumulate under the diaphragm and cause pressure on nerves. A feeling of abdominal fullness may also be present.
7. AIH is helpful when the male partner has an abnormally low sperm count.
8. Frozen sperm can be matched for physical characteristics; they can allow future childbearing for males undergoing chemotherapy.
9. For GIFT to be successful, the woman must have at least one patent fallopian tube.
10. With GIFT, ova are obtained and, together with sperm, are instilled into the open end of the fallopian tube for fertilization; with ZIFT, the ova and sperm are instilled into the fallopian tube after fertilization in the laboratory.

What If? Question Answers

1. This is a very practical problem as many women today work different shifts and exist without long periods of sustained sleep. In order to detect a pattern for a baseline, this woman probably needs to take her temperature twice a day: on arising in the morning and again on arising after her longest period of sustained sleep in the afternoon. Whichever of these times shows the most constant temperature would be her baseline temperature.
2. This is a legal quandary not yet clearly answered in court. Before couples agree to store sperm in this way, they need to discuss their feelings about this problem so that later there are no misunderstandings about their desires.

Chapter 7: Genetic Assessment and Counseling

Checkpoint Question Answers

1. A phenotype is a person's outward appearance; a genotype is the actual gene composition.
2. There are 23 chromosomes in each sperm.
3. Cystic fibrosis is an example of autosomal recessive inheritance.
4. Only a part of a chromosome needs to be affected, for example, cri-du-chat syndrome involves only one arm.
5. Nondisjunction occurs during meiosis of sperm or ova.
6. Nondisjunction can occur in the X or Y chromosomes, for example, Turner's syndrome.
7. Genetic counseling is best if initiated before the first pregnancy.
8. Persons undergoing genetic counseling need the result of the analysis reported to them accurately and promptly; health care providers should never impose their own values or opinions on the family.
9. Karyotyping is a visual display of a person's chromosomal structure.
10. CVS has been associated with limb reduction syndrome.
11. There is only one functional X chromosome in Turner's syndrome.
12. No, I.Q. ranges from severely to minimally cognitively challenged in Down syndrome.

What If? Question Answers

1. X-linked recessive inherited illnesses are carried by the mother, but the symptoms of these diseases are only apparent in male offspring. Having only boys, therefore, would increase the chance her children would have the disease, not decrease it.
2. This is a true ethical question, so the answer depends on many factors. A major thing to consider would be the length of the pregnancy as this increases the risk to the second child. Other values to weigh would be the value of this pregnancy to the parents, their personal beliefs about abortion, and their philosophy about raising a child who is cognitively challenged.

Chapter 8: The Growing Fetus

Checkpoint Question Answers

1. Currents initiated by the fimbria and muscular contraction of the tube help to propel the ovum through the fallopian tube.
2. Embryo is the term that refers to the conceptus following implantation.
3. Trophoblast cells form the basis for the placenta.
4. Two arteries and one vein are usually found in the umbilical cord.
5. Alcohol can cause fetal alcohol syndrome; nicotine causes vasoconstriction, so can reduce the blood supply to the fetus.
6. Surfactant excretion begins at about 24 weeks' gestation.
7. If a fetal liver is immature, hypoglycemia and hyperbilirubinemia are apt to occur.
8. IgG is the immunoglobulin that crosses the placenta, so can be found in the fetus.
9. Fundal height at 26 weeks would be 26 cm (MacDonald's rule).
10. If no acceleration occurs with fetal movement, the test is rated as nonreactive or abnormal.
11. Before a fetal ultrasound, a woman should drink fluids for 1½ hours prior to the procedure and then not void before the procedure to ensure a full bladder.
12. An elevated alpha-fetoprotein level suggests the fetus has an open lesion such as a spinal lesion.
13. Women need to void prior to amniocentesis to reduce the size of the bladder, which is anterior to the uterus.

What If? Question Answers

1. Nagele's rule is: subtract 3 months and add 7 days from the first day of the last menstrual period. Based on this, the EDB would be December 20th of the next year.
2. The important rule here is that Liz count them three times a day. Doing this after she has eaten has an advantage in that a fetus may be more active at this time because the maternal blood glucose level is higher. Perhaps a bigger question here is, why does a woman report that she snacks constantly rather than eat meals? Is she eating nutritious food or "snack" foods all these times?

Chapter 9: Psychological and Physiologic Changes of Pregnancy

Checkpoint Question Answers

1. Presumptive signs in the first 6 weeks after implantation are breast changes, morning sickness, amenorrhea, frequent urination, and Chadwick's sign. Probable signs in the first 6 weeks are serum lab tests, Goodell's sign, Hegar's sign, and sonographic gestational sac.
2. Laboratory tests for pregnancy are based upon the presence of HCG in the urine or serum in the pregnant woman. Psychotropic drugs, oral contraceptives, proteinuria, postmenopause, and hyperthyroid disease may cause false-positive results.
3. The only three positive signs of pregnancy are demonstration of a fetal heart separate from that of the mother's, fetal movements felt by the examiner, and visualization of the fetus by ultrasound.
4. The view of pregnancy as a time of wellness has influenced the pregnancy and birth experience by encouraging women and families to participate in all aspects of the experience. Also, many family-centered birthing alternatives to the hospital now exist. Overall, childbirth can now be more enjoyable for the woman and family.
5. Individual influences that play a major role in the woman's ability to adapt to pregnancy and parenting include her ability to cope and adapt to new life contingencies, the extent to which she feels secure with people around her, and personal beliefs about pregnancy and mothering.
6. The three psychological tasks of pregnancy include accepting the pregnancy, accepting the baby, and preparing for parenthood.
7. The woman usually begins to think of the fetus as a separate entity after quickening. The partner may have a harder time accepting the pregnancy because he does not undergo physical changes or experience quickening.
8. The tasks involved in preparing for parenthood include reworking developmental tasks, role playing, and fantasy.
9. A woman manifests narcissism by changing her activities to protect her body and the baby. Partners also express narcissism by reducing risk-taking behaviors.
10. Chadwick's sign is discoloration of the vagina. It occurs because of increased blood flow to the pelvis.
11. Braxton Hicks contractions are "practice" contractions that serve as warm-up exercises for labor and increase placental profusion.
12. This changing acid content makes the vagina resistant to bacterial invasion for the length of the pregnancy but, unfortunately, favors the growth of *Candida albicans*, a species of yeast-like fungi.
13. When insulin is less effective during pregnancy, glucose cannot be used as readily so it is freed up for fetal growth.
14. Creatinine clearance is the most effective test of renal function.
15. Melanocyte-stimulating hormone causes increased pigmentation in the woman during pregnancy.

What If? Question Answers

1. You don't really have enough information to draw any conclusion. It's doubtful this is Couvade syndrome, though, because his wife is probably no longer experiencing nausea and vomiting of pregnancy; this typically disappears after the first 3 months of pregnancy.
2. Good advice for women who have morning sickness is to be certain to eat well in the afternoon and evening after their feeling of nausea passes. The answer to fatigue is for women to rest more. Both of these instructions may be meaningless for a homeless woman as she doesn't have access to ready sources of food (only at the time it is served at a nearby shelter) or a place to rest except at night in the shelter. "Walking through" such a woman's day helps to realize what would be opportunities for her.

Chapter 10: Assessing Fetal and Maternal Health: The First Prenatal Visit

Checkpoint Question Answers

1. Listening, counseling, and teaching are three areas of nursing expertise important in prenatal care.
2. Assessments at an initial prenatal visit include an extensive health history and complete physical examination, including pelvic examination and blood and urine specimens.
3. Knowing past illnesses is important as a past condition may become active during or immediately following pregnancy.
4. Abortion is the medical term for a pregnancy terminated before the age of fetal viability.
5. Increased levels of estrogen are thought to account for the nasal congestion of pregnancy.
6. Heart rate can be difficult to hear because of the increase in breast size with pregnancy.
7. Skene's and Bartholin's glands are commonly inspected for enlargement or inflammation at the time of a pelvic exam.
8. The cervical os of a woman who has never been pregnant is typically round and small in contrast to the enlarged and slit-like appearance after birth.
9. Samples for Pap smears are typically taken from the endocervical area, cervical os, and vaginal pool.
10. A gynecoid pelvis is the ideal shape for birth.
11. If the diagonal conjugate measurement is too small (under 12.5 cm), this is most apt to cause a problem with the fit of the fetal head.
12. An ischial tuberosity measurement of at least 11 cm is considered adequate for vaginal birth.

What If? Question Answers

1. If a woman knows nothing about the diseases she had as a child, asking her to question other family members about their memories can be some help. In reality, the only truly important one to know is whether she had German measles (rubella) because of the fetal damage this can cause if contracted during pregnancy. The woman can have a serum titer drawn for this that will confirm whether she has immunity against the illness.
2. Tables in examining room should face away from the door so this problem is avoided. It is also important that women meet the person performing a pelvic examination before they are placed in a lithotomy position on a table so they meet the person at eye level, not from a lesser, vulnerable position.

Chapter 11: Promoting Fetal and Maternal Health

Checkpoint Question Answers

1. Tub bathing is contraindicated if membranes have ruptured or vaginal bleeding is present.
2. Women should use clear tap water (no soap) to clean their breasts as soap can be drying.
3. Women need to maintain safer sex measures during pregnancy to prevent sexually transmitted diseases.
4. Walking is probably the best exercise for women during pregnancy.
5. Supine hypotension syndrome can occur if a pregnant woman rests in a supine position.
6. Women working outside their home may need help planning how to obtain enough rest and adequate nutrition.
7. Mineral oil interferes with absorption of fat-soluble vitamins A, D, E, and K, necessary for fetal growth and maternal health.
8. Decreased serum calcium, increased serum phosphorus, and interference with circulation are all possible causes of leg cramps in pregnancy.
9. Varicosities of the rectal veins result from pressure exerted by the growing uterus on the rectum.
10. Shortness of breath during pregnancy occurs from pressure of the expanding uterus on the diaphragm.
11. A side-lying position and sitting with the feet elevated are both good positions to relieve ankle edema.
12. The most frequent source of exposure to toxoplasmosis is probably uncooked meat, although cat stool in soil or cat litter may also be responsible.
13. Live virus vaccines are contraindicated during pregnancy as the live virus can affect the fetus.
14. Category X is the FDA category for drugs that have proved to be definitely harmful during pregnancy.

What If? Question Answers

1. This is a personal decision, but questions to ask might be whether she is able to obtain a nutritious diet, isn't spending long time periods sitting in one position, and is able to obtain enough rest. If she has resorted to eating fast food, she needs to plan carefully to be certain she obtains enough protein, calcium, and iron. Sitting with her knees sharply bent in an airplane can lead to severe stasis of lower extremities. She needs to consider how fatigued she is at the end of her day and whether she has any opportunity to put up her feet and rest.
2. Your evaluation needs to begin with additional assessment. Urinary tract infections generally have additional symptoms: pain on urination, possibly blood in the urine or a low-grade systemic fever, so asking if any of these is present is important. Asking about the type and amount of vaginal discharge would also be important, as this is a symptom of a normal change in pregnancy but also could be a sexually transmitted disease symptom. Alerting the woman's primary care provider to her concerns would be important to be certain that a clean-catch urine or a vaginal swab for culture is not needed.

Chapter 12: Promoting Nutritional Health During Pregnancy

Checkpoint Question Answers

1. The usual weight gain recommendation during pregnancy is 11.2 to 16 kg (25 to 40 lbs).
2. Women should gain about 1 lb (0.4 kg) per week during the third trimester of pregnancy.
3. A complete protein contains all nine essential amino acids.
4. Linoleic acid is an essential fatty acid that cannot be manufactured by the body.
5. A primary function of folic acid is red blood cell formation.
6. Iron is best absorbed with an acid medium such as orange juice.
7. The best way to obtain a nutrition history is by asking for a 24-hour recall history.
8. Breastfeeding women are eligible for WIC services up to 1 year after birth.
9. Nausea usually disappears by the end of the third month of pregnancy.
10. Pica is the abnormal craving of non-food substances.
11. The risk of cholelithiasis and cardiovascular disease increases with elevated cholesterol levels during pregnancy.
12. Counseling an underweight client can be difficult because you are asking her to change life-long eating habits and she may be nauseated.
13. Vegetarian women are at risk for vitamin B_{12}, calcium, vitamin D, and possibly iron deficiency during pregnancy.
14. Hyperemesis gravidarum can lead to severe dehydration if not treated during pregnancy.
15. Women who continue vomiting during pregnancy may need enteral or parenteral nutrition to avoid dehydration and help ensure fetal growth.

What If? Question Answers

1. Breaking a "coffee habit" is hard, partly because of the caffeine intake and partly because drinking coffee is associated with good conversation and "breaks" from work. Helping a woman see that coffee breaks don't have to include drinking coffee, but could include a fruit or milk drink, helps. Helping her select a restaurant for lunch other than one featuring coffee also helps.
2. The four desserts will probably add pounds. Her action needs to be considered in light of everything else she is eating, however, to be meaningful. It's important for women to understand that a good diet during pregnancy means eating better, not necessarily eating more.

Chapter 13: Preparation for Childbirth and Parenting

Checkpoint Question Answers

1. It is important to strengthen perineal muscles so that they become supple and allow for ready stretching during birth. Tailor sitting and squatting help stretch these muscles.
2. It is important to strengthen abdominal muscles to help restore their normal tone and function quickly after childbirth. Abdominal muscle contractions help strengthen these muscles.
3. A pregnant woman should stop exercising before she is fatigued or if any danger signals of pregnancy appear.
4. The three basic premises of the Lamaze method of childbirth are: (1) pain does not have to occur with contractions if women can relax; (2) sensations such as uterine contractions can be inhibited from reaching the brain cortex and registering as pain; and (3) conditioned reflexes are a positive action used to displace pain sensations in labor.
5. The gating theory of pain refers to gate control mechanisms that can be used to halt the transmission of pain to the spinal cord, stop transmission at the spinal cord, or stop the brain from allowing the sensation to register as pain.
6. Effleurage reduces pain by decreasing sensory stimuli transmission from the abdominal wall. Focusing/imagery helps reduce pain by keeping sensory input from reaching the cortex of the brain.
7. The hospital is the safest setting for a woman with a complication because emergency care is immediately available for both mother and baby.
8. The basic goal of all birth settings is to produce the outcome of a healthy mother and a healthy baby.
9. A doula is a nonmedical person who offers support in labor.

What If? Question Answers

1. Most women appreciate having someone with them whom they know well during labor to both support them and share this very personal experience with them. You might suggest that the woman ask a close family member or friend to fill this role. For women who are alone in labor, a nurse can fill this role.
2. The most important criterion for choosing a place for birth should be a setting that will be safe for mother and baby. Secondary considerations should be enjoyment, ability to actively participate, and cost. Choosing an alternative birth center could be a compromise setting as this could supply safety plus a less structured setting.

Chapter 14: High-Risk Pregnancy: The Woman With a Preexisting or Newly Acquired Illness

Checkpoint Question Answers

1. Women with diabetes and HIV are most apt to develop candidiasis infections during pregnancy.
2. Flagyl (metronidazole) is possibly teratogenic in early pregnancy.

3. Zidovudine (ZVD) administration to the mother can reduce HIV transmission to the fetus.
4. Prescription supplements contain extra folic acid, important for red cell formation and prevention of neural tube defects in the fetus.
5. Fetal effects of folic acid deficiency occur in the first few weeks of fetal development.
6. Women with sickle cell anemia mat not be prescribed iron during pregnancy as they cannot incorporate it into sickled cells and it can accumulate to toxic levels.
7. Women are prone to urinary tract infections during pregnancy because of increased glucose in urine and stasis of urine due to uterine pressure on ureters.
8. Women who have had tuberculosis need increased calcium to prevent healed tuberculosis lesions from becoming reactivated.
9. Women with cystic fibrosis need to take a pancreatic enzyme during pregnancy, as they need this enzyme for digestion.
10. Salicylates are decreased close to birth (1 to 2 weeks) because their use is associated with bleeding defects in the newborn.
11. Hepatitis B is spread through sexual relations or blood products.
12. Phenytoin (Dilantin) is a pregnancy risk category D drug.
13. Digoxin may be taken during pregnancy (pregnancy risk category A).
14. Penicillin is a pregnancy risk category B drug so can be continued during pregnancy.
15. Heparin does not cross the placenta so does not cause a bleeding defect in the fetus.
16. Hyperglycemia can lead to congenital anomalies, especially caudal regression syndrome.
17. Women with diabetes mellitus should exercise consistently during pregnancy to help regulate blood glucose levels.
18. Hypoglycemia can occur at night because insulin administration continues but the woman is not eating.
19. Uterine pressure increases the blood pressure in vessels in lower extremities, increasing the potential loss for blood.
20. Yes. Either ipecac or activated charcoal can be taken safely during pregnancy (pregnancy risk category C).
21. Abused women often cannot support themselves; they are afraid their abuser will follow and kill them.

What If? Question Answers

1. This woman needs to check with her primary care provider for additional guidance. This is a common finding with women who are taking medication for a chronic illness. They abruptly stop taking the medicine when they become pregnant, following the guideline, "Take no medicine during pregnancy." It is one of the reasons that obtaining a thorough health history at a pregnancy's beginning is so important.
2. This woman needs to check with her primary care provider if any salt limitation is required for her particular cardiac problem. During pregnancy, she shouldn't limit her salt intake any further than that. Salt is necessary to regulate and maintain fluid balance, and a large circulatory volume is necessary during pregnancy to supply nutrients to the fetus.

Chapter 15: High-Risk Pregnancy: The Woman Who Develops a Complication of Pregnancy

Checkpoint Question Answers

1. The first symptom of a spontaneous miscarriage is usually painless vaginal spotting.
2. Disseminated intravascular coagulation (DIC) and infection are both potential complications of missed miscarriage.
3. The majority of ectopic pregnancies are located in the ampulla portion of the fallopian tube.
4. Laparotomy with tubal repair is the usual therapy for ruptured ectopic pregnancy. If discovered before rupture, methotrexate or mifepristone can be given to dissolve the implantation and preserve the fallopian tube intact.
5. A placenta that occludes a portion of the cervical os is a partial placenta previa. If it totally occludes the os, it is a complete placenta previa
6. Two complications of placenta previa are postpartal hemorrhage and endometritis.
7. Premature placental separation usually presents first with sharp, stabbing pain high in the fundus.
8. Bedrest and hydration are common first interventions for a woman in preterm labor.
9. Terbutaline is the most common beta-mimetic agent used to halt labor today.
10. The classic symptoms of pregnancy-induced hypertension are hypertension, edema, and proteinurea.
11. Magnesium sulfate is the drug of choice for the prevention of eclampsia.
12. HELLP stands for *h*emolysis, *e*levated *l*iver enzymes, and *l*ow *p*latelets, the symptoms that can complicate a unique form of pregnancy-induced hypertension.
13. Single ovum twins typically have one placenta and two umbilical cords.
14. Hydramnios is present when there is more than 2000 mL of amniotic fluid (sometimes described as polyhydramnios).
15. The chief effect on the fetus from Rh incompatibility is anemia from red blood cell destruction.

What If? Question Answers

1. This is a difficult problem because the woman needs to avoid becoming pregnant again until it is clear that all remnants of the hydatidiform mole have been removed and she is free of the possibility of developing choriocarcinoma. The first step in problem-solving would be not giving her advice but exploring with her what she understands about her condition and risks. When she understands that there are serious health risks involved for her, that birth control is not being advised for her for the sake of birth control but to help prevent a malignancy, her attitude toward using birth control will invariably improve.
2. Heparin cannot be administered orally as it is destroyed by gastrointestinal secretions. Because heparin does not cross the placenta, the newborn should have no more tendency for a blood coagulation disorder at birth than any other infant. The question is a good one to be able to answer because it is often asked by women prescribed the drug.

Chapter 16: Home Care of the Pregnant Client

Checkpoint Question Answers

1. Home care is usually more cost effective unless the family's insurance does not cover the cost of the vis:ts or needed supplies.
2. Home care is most successful when family roles are not disrupted, but strengthened to support whatever new activities or concerns need to be addressed.
3. A first home visit is typically made within 24 hours of discharge from an acute care facility or notice from the ambulatory care facility.
4. To avoid possible fleabites, sit on a non-upholstered chair such as a kitchen chair.
5. Leave immediately or call 911 at any point you feel your safety is threatened.
6. You could refuse food offered at a home visit by saying something like, "I'm trying to cut down on the amount of coffee I drink" or "It's against my agency's policy."
7. Women on bedrest at home may develop constipation from lack of exercise.
8. Encourage pregnant women on home care to drink at least eight full glasses each day to promote kidney function and possibly reduce the possibility of preterm labor.

What If? Question Answers

1. This is a situation that is occurring more and more frequently. The biggest physical problem of caring for women in these situations is that all the accommodations of a home environment (nearby kitchen, bathroom, sense of privacy, etc.) are not necessarily present. The woman may also be only at the setting temporarily, so good follow-up care will need to be planned. The biggest psychosocial problem is often that the woman is not a good problem-solver. This lengthens the time spent in nursing care planning so that outcomes can be optimal.
2. Mice in the house of a newborn baby are a problem that needs to be dealt with because they can carry the potentially deadly hanta virus. Rats in a home can be large enough that they actually attack a

sleeping newborn. The family, therefore, needs to deal with the problem (contacting an exterminator; setting traps, etc.). Working with them to understand the importance of these actions is the nursing responsibility.

Chapter 17: High-Risk Pregnancy: The Woman With Special Needs

Checkpoint Question Answers

1. Factors that contribute to teenage pregnancy are: earlier age of menarche, increased rate of sexual activity, and lack of knowledge about or inability to use contraceptives.
2. Four developmental tasks of adolescence are to establish sense of self-worth and value system, establish long-term relationships, emancipate from parents, and choose a vocation.
3. Pregnancy-induced hypertension, iron deficiency anemia, preterm birth, and cesarean birth are common complications of an adolescent pregnancy.
4. An increased reticulocyte count is a good indication that the girl is actually taking the iron supplement.
5. Blood vessel inelasticity and an already elevated blood pressure may both contribute to PIH in the older woman.
6. Due to inelasticity there may be a decreased ability of the uterus to contract readily, allowing for postpartal hemorrhage.
7. The weight of the fetus can put increased pressure on her buttocks and posterior thighs as she sits in a wheelchair.
8. Autonomic dysreflexia is a severe reaction including headache and high blood pressure that can occur from a stimulus such as a full bladder or labor.
9. Most women with profound hearing losses are concerned that they will not be able to hear their baby cry.
10. Infants need light to develop vision, so visually impaired women may need to be reminded to turn on lights.
11. Cocaine causes severe vasoconstriction that can interfere with placental blood perfusion.
12. A fetus receives about 50% of the drug level circulating in the mother.

What If? Question Answers

1. This diet seems to be almost totally lacking in two important food groups: fruit and vegetables. Unless the liquid drinks are high in protein, it probably also lacks this important nutrition component as well. Many adolescents follow this type of diet because they simply do not know a better nutrition pattern. Help for the adolescent, therefore, would start with assessing what she knows about pregnancy nutrition, then building on her food likes to construct a diet higher in essential pregnancy nutrition.
2. Most women who are drug dependent are able to discuss their dependency with health care providers because they want to know the effect, if any, the drug will have on fetal health. Discovering packets that possibly reveal drug use this way, therefore, presents an opportunity for this type of frank discussion and probably referral for help for the woman so she can break free of the dependency. Ignoring the packets would serve no function and also leave the woman uninformed about possible fetal risk.

Chapter 18: The Labor Process

Checkpoint Question Answers

1. False labor contractions are usually felt initially as abdominal pain that remains confined to the abdomen and groin.
2. Three major signs of true labor are regular contractions, show, and rupture of membranes.
3. Four integrated components of labor are passage, passenger, powers, and psyche.
4. The diameter that is narrowest at the pelvic outlet is the transverse diameter.
5. The anterior fontanelle is at the junction of the coronal and sagittal sutures.
6. The fetal skull diameter that is the widest anteroposterior diameter is the occipitomental diameter.
7. Station refers to the relationship of the fetal presenting part to the level of the ischial spines.
8. A vertex presentation is the ideal presentation.
9. The six cardinal mechanisms of labor are descent, flexion, internal rotation, extension, external rotation, and expulsion.
10. The intensity of the contraction at its strongest point is the acme.
11. Two cervical changes that occur during labor are effacement and dilatation.
12. Three phases of the first stage of labor are the latent phase, active phase, and transition phase.
13. The second stage of labor begins with full cervical dilatation and effacement.
14. Two phases of the third stage of labor are placental separation and placental expulsion.
15. The average increase in systolic blood pressure during a uterine contraction is 15 mm Hg.
16. A pulse over 100 beats per minute is a danger sign of labor.
17. A uterine contraction over 70 seconds has the potential to compromise fetal well-being.
18. Vital signs in labor are usually assessed at least every 4 hours.
19. Leopold's maneuvers are systematic observation and palpation to determine fetal presentation and position.
20. The pH of amniotic fluid is alkaline; pH over 7.5.
21. Before internal electronic fetal monitoring can be used, rupture of membranes and cervical dilatation of at least 3 cm must have occurred.
22. Variable decelerations occur with umbilical cord compression.
23. A late deceleration begins 30 to 40 seconds after the start of a contraction.
24. A full bladder sounds resonant when percussed.
25. Following an amniotomy, prolapse of the umbilical cord may occur.
26. Encourage women not to hold their breath but to breathe out when pushing during the second stage of labor.
27. A midline episiotomy heals more easily with less blood loss than an anterolateral incision.
28. Vital signs are assessed every 15 minutes for the first hour and then according to agency policy.

What If? Question Answers

1. Most people recommend that women lie on their side during labor as this frees up the vena cava, ensuring a good blood supply to the uterus and fetus. Occasionally, a woman will lie on her back after monitors are attached because she believes they will come loose if she turns on her side or not record accurately in that position. As a rule, urge women in labor to assume a side-lying position and assure them that fetal and uterine monitors record accurately in any position.
2. One of the difficulties with having more than one support person in labor is that differences in opinion can arise. In this instance, the person to consult is neither the doula nor the husband, but the woman herself as pain is a subjective sensation, able to be evaluated only by the person experiencing it.

Chapter 19: Providing Comfort During Labor and Birth

Checkpoint Question Answers

1. Pain for the first stage of labor is registered at the levels of T10, T11, T12, and L1.
2. Endorphins and enkephalins are naturally occurring opiates released in response to pain.
3. A non-medical person who acts as a support person in labor is popularly called a doula.
4. Heat applications in labor seem to work most effectively for back pain.
5. Women with ruptured membranes may not be candidates for water immersion because of the risk of infection.
6. Common goals of pharmacologic pain management during labor and birth are relaxation, relief of discomfort, and minimal systemic effects on the woman or her fetus.
7. Systemic meperidine during labor can leave the newborn with severe respiratory depression.
8. Hypotension and a prolonged second phase of labor are two concerns of epidural anesthesia.
9. Spinal anesthesia is placed into the cerebral spinal fluid at the 3rd or 4th lumbar interspace.
10. A pudendal block is a common method to provide relief of perineal pain.
11. Ranitidine (Zantac), metoclopramide (Reglan), or oral antacids are common drugs administered to protect against aspiration with general anesthesia.

12. Epinephrine is the chief hormone released with a stress response.
13. An upright position tends to be most effective in aiding contractions in early labor.

What If? Question Answers

1. Women in labor need to know all of their options to make informed decisions, so this would be the place to start. Gripping a hand tightly can trigger an acupressure point, thereby reducing pain. This also could be a distraction technique.
2. Naloxone hydrochloride is a narcotic antagonist that counteracts the effect of narcotic analgesics. If no narcotic is present when it is given, it acts as a narcotic and will cause depressive symptoms. Because the mother did not receive any narcotic during labor, administration of it to the newborn would be inappropriate. Asking the mother if she has recently used a recreational drug would be appropriate in order to help discover the reason for the newborn's sleepiness.

Chapter 20: Cesarean Birth

Checkpoint Question Answers

1. Intact skin, a primary body defense, is lost with cesarean birth.
2. Vaginal birth results in an average blood loss of 300 to 500 mL; cesarean birth results in an average loss of 500 to 1000 mL
3. Pregnant women can be at surgical risk for poor nutritional status, age variations, altered general health, fluid and electrolyte imbalance, and fear.
4. Lower extremity circulatory stasis can occur readily in women following a cesarean birth because edema from the low pelvic surgery compresses circulation to lower extremities.
5. An indwelling urinary catheter is used to reduce bladder size before surgery.
6. Women receive a gastric emptying, H2 blocker, or acid neutralizer before cesarean surgery to reduce the possibility of aspiration of acid stomach contents. This is necessary because the enlarged uterus puts pressure on the stomach in a supine position and makes her susceptible to esophageal reflux and aspiration.
7. Two types of incision for cesarean birth are a classic (fundal and vertical) and a horizontal low segment incision.
8. Pain, warmth, and redness in the calf suggest a lower extremity thrombosis.
9. Passage of flatus is an excellent indicator that intestinal function has returned following surgery.
10. Postpartum women void approximately 3000 to 5000 mL/24 hrs.

What If? Question Answers

1. Women receiving an epidural anesthesia are not unconscious; therefore, there is little reason that they have to remove contact lenses for anesthesia administration (this would be important if a general anesthesia was anticipated). As seeing her newborn and holding him at birth is important for bonding, not only advocating for this woman but investigating whether this routine policy should be changed would be important.
2. Women are concerned that palpation of their fundal height will cause pain (and if they do not have adequate pain management, that is very true). To reduce discomfort, be certain the woman is receiving optimal pain relief. Explain why the assessment is important and use a gentle touch.

Chapter 21: The Woman Who Develops a Complication During Labor and Birth

Checkpoint Question Answers

1. Hypotonic contractions usually occur during the active phase of labor.
2. A deceleration phase is considered prolonged if it extends beyond 3 hours in a nullipara woman and 1 hour in a multipara woman.
3. The most common cause for arrest of descent in the second stage of labor is cephalopelvic disproportion.
4. A complete uterine rupture produces symptoms of sudden, severe pain during a strong labor contraction, reported as a tearing sensation.
5. The placenta should not be removed with uterine inversion, if still attached, because doing so creates a larger area of bleeding.
6. The best immediate action to take if a prolapsed cord is exposed to room air is to cover any exposed portion with a sterile saline compress to keep it from drying. A second important action is repositioning the mother to take pressure off the cord.
7. The most common birth position for twin fetuses is vertex.
8. A fetal occipitoposterior position causes lower back pain from sacral nerve compression.
9. A post-term male of a multipara is most apt to have shoulder dystocia because such a fetus is most apt to be large.
10. Rickets or an inherited small pelvis are two conditions that can cause pelvic inlet contraction.
11. External cephalic version is a procedure to turn a fetus from a breech to a cephalic position.
12. The first symptoms of water intoxication that can occur with oxytocin induction of labor are headache and vomiting.
13. Fetal blood sampling is a contraindication to vacuum extraction as vacuum extraction may cause scalp bleeding.
14. A typical placenta weights approximately 500 gm.
15. In a battledore placenta, the umbilical cord is inserted marginally rather than centrally.

What If? Question Answers

1. This appears to be a woman who doesn't understand her rights as a patient. The first action, therefore, would be to explore with her those rights (no one will force any therapy on her such as general anesthesia that she doesn't consent to). She also seems to need an explanation of types of anesthesia available for cesarean birth so she can discuss with her doctor why he or she has told her a general anesthetic would be preferable.
2. As this woman had a precipitate birth with her last baby, it is highly probable this may happen again. In light of this, it would seem wise to explore with her other places to stay as she nears her time of expected birth.

Chapter 22: Nursing Care of the Postpartal Woman and Family

Checkpoint Question Answers

1. The three phases of the puerperium identified by Ms. Rubin are the taking in, taking hold, and letting go phases.
2. Women begin to demonstrate a strong interest in child care during the taking hold phase.
3. A mother who relates well to her infant typically uses an "en face" position.
4. Women demonstrate emotional liability during the postpartum period from "baby blues" or a change in hormones.
5. By the 4th day postpartum, a woman's fundus is typically 4 fingerbreadths or 4 cm below the umbilicus.
6. A vaginal birth typically results in a blood loss range from 300 to 500 mL. This causes her hemoglobin to fall 1 to 2 gm.
7. Prolactin is the hormone that stimulates milk production.
8. Lochia immediately after birth should be lochia rubra, or red with small clots.
9. Ice can prevent inflammation and thus decrease pain and edema.
10. Three factors that predispose a woman to infection in the postpartum period are the presence of lochia, proximity of rectum to vagina, and impaired skin integrity related to episiotomy.
11. The best time for self-breast examination is 1 week after menses every month.
12. Talking about their newborn can both help parents clarify their new role and provide a means to assess parent-child bonding.
13. Asking about intimate partner abuse is important at a 6-week checkup because, statistically, this form of abuse increases with stress and care of a new infant can increase stress.
14. By 6 weeks postpartum, a typical cervix is again closed, nearly as it was prepregnancy.

What If? Question Answers

1. These are normal assessment findings for a woman 12 hours postpartum. The first nursing action, therefore, would be to assure Ms. Cooper that these are normal findings. In addition, she needs to be guided to rest to relieve the fatigue and perhaps measures to make her comfortable in the face of diaphoresis.
2. As a rule of thumb, saturating more than one pad an hour is more than the normal amount of lochia flow. The fact that Ms. Cooper is also passing large clots suggests her uterus is not as contracted as it could be. Assessing her fundal height and consistency would be the first assessment needed.

Chapter 23: Nursing Care of the Newborn and Family

Checkpoint Question Answers

1. A newborn loses approximately 5% to 10% (6 to 10 oz) of birth weight during the first few days of life.
2. A typical term newborn head circumference is 34 to 35 cm.
3. Four methods by which a newborn can lose heat are convection, conduction, radiation, and evaporation.
4. A combination of cold receptors, lowered PO_2, and increased PCO_2 help to initiate a newborn's first breath.
5. To elicit a Moro reflex, hold the newborn in a supine position and allow the head to drop back one inch or so.
6. Blueness of hands and feet in a newborn is termed acrocyanosis.
7. Indirect bilirubin is released from the breakdown of red blood cells. It can be detrimental to newborn health if it invades and destroys brain cells.
8. Milia need no therapy; they disappear by 2 to 4 weeks of age as the sebaceous glands mature and drain.
9. The presence of extra digits is termed polydactyly.
10. Apgar scoring assesses heart rate, respiratory effort, muscle tone, reflex irritability, and color.
11. A serum glucose level of less than 40 to 45 mg/100 mL is hypoglycemia in a newborn.
12. Newborns are typically suctioned of oral secretions as soon as the head is born before the first breath.
13. An umbilical cord typically falls off by the 7th to 10th day after birth.
14. Erythromycin ointment is the drug of choice for eye prophylaxis as it is effective against both chlamydia and gonorrhea.
14. Two metabolic screening tests required at birth are tests for phenylketonuria and hypothyroidism. Many states include others as well.
15. A chief danger of male circumcision is bleeding from the incision site.

What If? Question Answers

1. This mother is describing acrocyanosis, a normal finding in newborns because peripheral circulation is not functioning at an optimal level. Assuring her that this is normal in newborns would be helpful.
2. The American Academy of Pediatrics suggests that all newborns receive eye prophylaxis as there is a danger that organisms can enter the amniotic fluid during labor, making infants born by cesarean birth also susceptible to eye infection at birth.
3. Like all decision making, deciding on whether to have an infant circumcised depends on the parent being fully informed. This means supplying her with information on the pros and cons of the procedure. Following this, she doesn't need to be guided; she needs to decide for herself what would be best for her baby—the first of many decisions she will make in this area as a parent.

Chapter 24: Nutritional Needs of the Newborn

Checkpoint Question Answers

1. A 1-month old requires 110 to 120 kcal/kg of body weight (50 to 55 kcal/lb) in 24 hours.
2. Cow's milk is more difficult to digest than human milk or commercial formulas because it contains casein, whose curd is large, tough, and more difficult to digest.
3. Thirty-two percent to 35% of body weight in the newborn is extracellular fluid.
4. Colostrum is the fluid produced in the first 24 hours following birth.
5. Breast milk contains passive antibodies and other ingredients that destroy gram-negative microorganisms in the intestines.
6. A good position to use to burp an infant is sitting the infant on the lap, leaning the baby forward, and supporting the head with the index finger and thumb.
7. An effective method to relieve the discomfort of engorgement is to empty the breasts frequently and apply heat to the breasts.
8. Women who are breastfeeding should increase their calorie intake by about 500 calories.
9. Iron added to newborn formula helps prevent iron deficiency anemia.
10. An 8-lb newborn would require 22 to 24 oz/day (8×2.5 to 3 oz).
11. Two risks of propping bottles for newborns are increased risk for aspiration and the development of otitis media.

What If? Question Answers

1. Breastfeeding an infant is a very personal experience, so is the mother's choice to make. As a rule, it is helpful to urge all mothers to at least try breastfeeding. Some who insist they will not like it are surprised to find how enjoyable and convenient it is. Equally important with this mother would seem to be a discussion of total baby care and other areas she and her husband need to resolve before they can operate as a parent unit.
2. A number of questions come to mind. Where is the baby going to be cared for that is so remote there is not access to a refrigerator? If no refrigeration is available, could she keep the bottle in an ice chest or cool sandwich bag? Milk left unrefrigerated spoils easily and encourages the growth of bacteria.

Chapter 25: Nursing Care of the Woman and Family Experiencing a Postpartal Complication

Checkpoint Question Answers

1. Four major causes of postpartal hemorrhage are uterine atony, lacerations, retained placental fragments, and disseminated intravascular coagulation (DIC).
2. The best emergency measure to increase uterine tone is uterine (fundal) massage.
3. A woman who has retained placental fragments will usually have elevated levels of serum human chorionic gonadotropin hormone.
4. Symptoms of endometritis typically appear on the 3rd or 4th postpartum day.
5. Ambulation encourages drainage of lochia by gravity and prevents pooling of infected secretions from endometritis.
6. A first and important sign of peritonitis is a rigid abdomen (guarding).
7. Signs of femoral thrombophlebitis typically appear around the 10th day postpartum.
8. The antidote for heparin is protamine sulfate.
9. Organisms that cause mastitis can gain entry to the breast through cracked nipples or fissures or from the nasal or oral cavity of the infant.
10. Three typical findings with mastitis are localized breast pain, swelling, and tenderness.
12. Sulfa drugs are not routinely prescribed for breastfeeding women as they are excreted in breast milk and can cause hyperbilirubinemia in the infant.
13. Hallucinations accompany postpartal psychosis; postpartal depression is a sense of overwhelming sadness.

What If? Question Answers

1. This assessment certainly suggests the woman has signs of infection (elevated temperature, foul-smelling lochia, tender abdomen). A referral to her primary care provider would be the next step in care.
2. Some women with a history of thrombophlebitis will need to self-administer heparin during pregnancy to decrease the possibility of thrombophlebitis developing. Women need a referral to the primary care provider to investigate whether this will be necessary. In addition, women need to take precautions against stasis of circulation in their lower extremities: not crossing their legs, not wearing knee high stockings, resting with feet elevated, and ambulating daily.
3. Diuresis begins almost immediately following birth, so by 7 hours post birth most women's bladders are full. A woman may not be aware of the usual sensation of filling, however, because of edema from the birth. Assessing for bladder distention by palpation and percussion would reveal the full bladder. Urging the woman to walk to the bathroom to void would be a second step. If she is unable to void by 8 hours post birth and her bladder is distended, most primary care providers advocate bladder catheterization to relieve bladder pressure.

Chapter 26: Nursing Care of the High-Risk Newborn and Family

Checkpoint Question Answers

1. A first action to take for a newborn who does not spontaneously breathe would be to apply suction to the infant's mouth and nose with a bulb syringe and rub the back.
2. In order to produce sound, a newborn must have good lung expansion.
3. Naloxone (Narcan) is the drug of choice to relieve the effects of a narcotic given to the mother in labor.
4. A newborn's sternum should be depressed about ½ to ¾ inches (1 to 2 cm) for cardiac massage.
5. The optimal range of abdominal skin temperature for a newborn under a radiant heat warmer is 35.5° to 36.5° C (95.9° degrees to 97.7° F).
6. Care in which an infant is held skin to skin is termed kangaroo care.
7. Oral stimulation can be provided for infants during gavage feedings by non-nutritive sucking with a pacifier at feeding time.
8. Cytomegalovirus and toxoplasmosis are common viruses that cross the placenta so can infect an infant in utero.
9. Preterm infants are at high risk for child abuse because they are "special" children or different than anticipated by a parent and are separated from parents at birth.
10. Two findings typical of a small-for-gestational-age infant are increased hematocrit level and increased total red blood cell count (polycythemia).
11. Small-for-gestational-age infants lack subcutaneous fat so may have difficulty maintaining body temperature.
12. A large-for-gestational-age infant may need a cesarean birth because of cephalopelvic disproportion and shoulder dystocia.
13. Even though large sized, sucking may not be effective enough for a large-for-gestational-age infant to obtain an adequate supply of milk.
14. The preterm infant may have difficulty clearing acidosis because of difficulty initiating effective respirations as quickly as the mature infant.
15. A preterm infant produces 40 to 100 mL/kg/day of urine.
16. A preterm infant requires 115 to 140 kcal/kg/day.
17. Preterm infants may show stress by such movements as facial expressions and flailing fingers.
18. Infant immunizations are usually given according to chronologic age or at the point at which the infant would reach 2 months if born term.
19. Respiratory distress syndrome occurs because of lack of surfactant.
20. Pancuronium decreases spontaneous respirations, allowing lower pressure to be used for mechanical ventilation.
21. Meconium is present in the fetal bowel as early as 10 weeks' gestation.
22. Amniotransfusion may be used to help prevent meconium aspiration by diluting amniotic fluid.
23. The peak age for sudden infant death syndrome is between 2 weeks and 1 year of age.
24. Most apnea alarms are set so they sound following apnea of 20 seconds or more or a decrease in heart rate below 80 bpm.
25. Maternal type O and fetal type A blood are blood types most commonly associated with ABO incompatibility.
26. Phototherapy is the method of choice for treating hemolytic disease of the newborn.
27. Bleeding from hemorrhagic disease of the newborn typically occurs between days 2 and 5 of life.
28. The cause of retinopathy of prematurity is exposure of the retinal blood vessels to high concentrations of oxygen.
29. An organism that is a major cause of neonatal infections is beta-hemolytic group B streptococcal infection.
30. Acyclovir is the drug typically used to treat generalized herpesvirus type 2 infection in newborns.
31. Infants of diabetic mothers are fed early to prevent serum glucose from falling too low or hypoglycemia from developing.
32. Withdrawal symptoms for the heroin addicted newborn typically occur within 72 hours of birth.
33. Two characteristic facial features of the newborn with fetal alcohol syndrome are short palpebral fissures and a thin upper lip.

What If? Question Answers

1. Holding a very small newborn can be frightening as the infant seems so delicate. Discussing with the parent how important human contact is for even immature newborns can help them take the first step toward parenting or beginning interaction with their newborn.
2. If power fails while an infant is receiving pancuronium, you would want to initiate respirations immediately by means of a resuscitation bag as the infant cannot do this on his or her own. A second step would be to ready the antidote for pancuronium (an anticholinesterase such as neostigmine) and administer it if prescribed.
3. Infants under bilirubin lights have to wear eye patches to protect their retina against the intense lights. Most sleep soundly during this time. You would want to assure the parents that the majority of newborns sleep between feedings, so this is no different than usual. As long as they talk or sing to the infant during the time they feed their newborn, she should be receiving normal stimulation. It is important not to tap on an Isolette to get the infant's attention, because the sound level this causes inside the Isolette can be extreme.

Chapter 27: Principles of Growth and Development

Checkpoint Question Answers

1. Growth is generally used to denote an increase in physical size or a quantitative change, whereas development is used to denote an increase in skill or the ability to function (a qualitative change).
2. Neurologic and lymphoid tissues grow most rapidly during early childhood.
3. Freud defines libido as instinctual drives within an individual.
4. The toddler who consistently responds to questions with "no" is learning autonomy.
5. The best toys to promote a sense of initiative are those that provide the opportunity and freedom to initiate motor play, such as bikes, paints, and modeling clay.
6. The adolescent must develop a sense of identity.
7. The preschool child is using assimilation when he tells you his broken leg wants to get better.
8. The preschool child is using intuitive thought when he tells you all nurses wear white.
9. The stage of moral reasoning in school-age children is often termed the "nice" or "fair" stage because they engage in actions based on niceness or fairness.
10. Kohlberg's theory of moral development is often criticized for being male-oriented.

What If? Question Answers

1. Children with short attention spans who are not easily distracted are usually described as difficult to care for children. Helping this parent realize that temperament is not a learned quality, but one that is intrinsic, can help him learn to accept and work with his son's actions.
2. This is a common problem as families struggle to match paychecks to the increasing cost of food. Referral to a dietician would probably be helpful to this mother. Helping her understand that protein is important for growth and meat is the best source of this would be helpful as she looks at her week's menus.
3. Preschoolers thrive on free form play, the types that don't necessarily fit well into an orderly household. Suggestions might be for the preschooler to have one spot in the house that is her "messy spot," where she can finger paint, etc. Another might be for her to have a play space outdoors where her activities don't have to be so restricted. Urging the father to solve this problem in conjunction with his daughter is important because it is only one of many they will need to solve together in the years to come.

Chapter 28: The Family With an Infant

Checkpoint Question Answers

1. A usual range for heart rate in infants by the end of the first year is 100 to120 beats per minute.
2. Infants have a greater percentage of extracellular fluid (35% of body weight) compared with the 20% in adults, so they are more prone to dehydration than adults

3. Four positions used to evaluate gross motor development are ventral suspension, prone, sitting, and standing.
4. Infants sit steady without support by approximately 8 months.
5. Infants can pick up small objects using a pincer grasp by 10 months.
6. A typical 12-month-old says two words plus ma-ma and da-da.
7. Children demonstrate they have binocular vision by focusing on and following objects.
8. Most infants demonstrate a social smile by 6 to 8 weeks.
9. Stranger anxiety is typically seen at 8 months of age (often called 8th month anxiety).
10. Infants are ready to play peek-a-boo by around 10 months of age.
11. When infants mouth an object, lack of awareness of what actions he or she can cause is characteristic of the primary circular reaction stage.
12. Object permanence means that an infant realizes an object still exists even when the object is out of sight.
13. Parents instill trust in the infant by making it clear they love the child and establishing some schedule of consistent activity by a consistent caregiver.
14. Aspiration and motor vehicle accidents (also falls) are frequent causes of death in infants.
15. Infants can sleep in bassinets until they can turn over, at approximately 2 months.
16. Solid foods are typically introduced at approximately 6 months of age.
17. Fortified infant cereal is frequently the first solid food introduced.
18. How long to continue breastfeeding is a personal decision; continuing it for 12 months provides a solid foundation for infant nutrition.
19. The cause of colic is unknown, but it may be related to overfeeding or swallowing too much air.
20. Putting the infant to bed with a bottle containing sugar water, formula, milk, or fruit juice, which causes tooth decay, is baby bottle syndrome.
21. Trust is built the same way in physically challenged children as in other infants.

What If? Question Answers

1. If a 10-month-old can pick up a small marble, it probably means he has developed a pincer grasp (opposes the thumb and finger). This is a big developmental step as it means cephalocaudal development has progressed to fine motor control. It also means that the infant can pick up and swallow (and possibly choke on) small objects, so needs to be supervised closely for safety.
2. Always cleaning a plate can lead to overeating in children. A better rule is usually to serve a smaller portion and then allow the child to ask for seconds. Even young children have food preferences and will generally select a balanced diet over a week's time.

Chapter 29: The Family With a Toddler

Checkpoint Question Answers

1. Lordosis of the spine is common during the toddler years.
2. Toddlers have distended abdomens because their abdominal muscles are not yet strong enough to support abdominal contents.
3. The 2-year-old child should master two-word, noun/verb, simple sentences.
4. The typical play pattern of toddlers is parallel play (side-by-side individual play). They enjoy toys they can manipulate and like active, stimulating play.
5. The most common source of lead poisoning is lead paint, which the toddler chews, sucks; or eats from objects such as windowsills, walls, or furniture.
6. It is not generally recommended that fat be restricted from the diet of a child under age 2.
7. In order to toilet train, the child must have control of rectal and urethral sphincters. A good way to know that the child's development has reached this point is to wait until the child is able to walk well independently.
8. Although toddlers can sit well, it is not safe to leave them in a bathtub unsupervised because they can drown or scald themselves with hot water.
9. Parents can best eliminate the toddler's extreme negativism by limiting the number of questions asked and providing him or her with an opportunity to make choices.
10. "Time out" is a technique of teaching children that actions have consequences. Parents select a non-stimulating area, and the child must quietly remain there for a specified amount of time.
11. Toddler temper tantrums are usually best handled by ignoring them.
12. Finger foods are an effective way to encourage autonomy because they can be independently eaten.

What If? Question Answers

1. Saying "no" to a request is a typical toddler response. A better approach to avoid this behavior might be to not give the child a choice or simply announce, "It's time to take medicine now." You could follow this with a secondary choice ("Do you want me to use the red or white spoon?") to allow the child some input into the process.
2. Again, this is a typical toddler response. If the policy of ignoring temper tantrums is to be effective, then ignoring them no matter where they happen is a good policy. Assuming the child will not be hurt by the number of people passing by in the hallway, ignoring the tantrum would still seem to be good advice.

Chapter 30: The Family With a Preschooler

Checkpoint Question Answers

1. Height and weight gain during the preschool years is minimal.
2. Rarely do new teeth develop during this time. Most children have all their deciduous teeth by age 2½.
3. A 3-year-old uses about 900 vocabulary words.
4. If children do not develop a sense of initiative, they may face new situations with a sense of guilt.
5. Preschoolers should wear helmets with bicycles, the same as school-age children.
6. A child who ingests food from all pyramid groups does not need additional supplements.
7. Night grinding is a way to release tension, allowing the child to fall asleep. Children who grind their teeth extensively may have anxiety to a greater degree than the average child.
8. Relating time and space to something the child knows, such as meals, television shows, or a friend's house, is an effective method to minimize separation anxiety.
9. An imaginary friend is normal as long as the imaginary friend does not interfere with other relationships.
10. Bringing a gift for older siblings helps ease sibling rivalry.
11. A parent who is bothered by masturbation might instruct the child that masturbation is a private act, explaining that some things are done in some places and not in others. The parent should not call unnecessary attention to the act as this can increase anxiety and cause increased activity.
12. Respiratory and gastrointestinal infections are frequent in children attending childcare or preschool settings.
13. Broken fluency is a developmental phenomenon that normally fades at the end of the preschool period.

What If? Question Answers

1. Because preschoolers are very concrete in their thinking, they do not generalize well. A child who knows the first rule, therefore, might not know the second statement is actually the same rule.
2. This is a good area to explore with preschoolers because their concept of "stranger" may not be someone they do not know, but someone who looks "strange." When a good-looking man or woman tells them to go with them, therefore, they go willingly with a stranger. Explaining that the word stranger means anyone their parents have not said they can go with solves the problem.

Chapter 31: The Family With a School-Age Child

Checkpoint Question Answers

1. Swelling of rapidly growing lymphatic tissue fills the narrow tube of the appendix, trapping fecal material; this can lead to inflammation.
2. Frontal sinuses develop at about age 6.
3. Supernumerary nipples enlarge with puberty as they are affected by estrogen and androgen.
4. Boys begin to experience nocturnal emissions with puberty as seminal fluid is produced.

5. A 9-year-old gang is typically of the same sex, has a secret code or name, and excludes someone.
6. Boy and Girl Scouts provide constructive activities and strengthen a sense of autonomy. They encourage children to complete small projects, frequently helping to build a sense of industry.
7. Learning class inclusion leads to collecting.
8. Fairness is a step in moral development, according to Kohlberg.
9. A type A school lunch supplies one-third of a child's RDA.
10. Children need additional exercise because school is basically a sit-down activity.
11. If children eat candy, they should eat a type that dissolves fast so it remains in contact with the teeth for only a short time.
12. After it has been established that the child with school phobia is free from illness, he or she should be encouraged to attend school. Counseling for the whole family and addressing a potential conflict are also recommended.
13. A household product frequently abused by school-age children is glue; when sniffed, it produces a temporary giddiness or a "high."
14. Bullies are usually children of above-average size; they can be either boys or girls.

What If? Question Answers

1. The child who does not understand accommodation can make this kind of mistake (because a first action one day led to a second action, he assumes the same action will lead to the same action on a second day).
2. Most parents are confronted with this problem—a child listening more to the advice of friends than parents—in their early school-age child. It is a good topic to discuss with parents of early school-age children so they do not feel threatened, but accepting of the process.
3. School-age children have a great deal of difficulty with this concept, which is why shoplifting is so common with this age child. Frank discussion that the principle is the same helps children understand that stealing is the same no matter who is involved.

Chapter 32: The Family With an Adolescent

Checkpoint Question Answers

1. Growth ceases during adolescence due to closure of the epiphyseal lines of long bones.
2. Apocrine sweat glands are responsible for adolescent body odor.
3. The four main areas in which adolescents must make gains in order to achieve a sense of identity are accepting their changed body image, establishing a value system or what type of person they want to be, making a career decision, and becoming emancipated from their parents.
4. Dressing and acting alike allows adolescents to establish a sense of identity, because they are not excluded from the group. Knowing who they are not is one step in discovering who they are.
5. Parents who suspect their children are sexually active should make sure that they are knowledgeable about safer sex practices.
6. The final stage of cognitive development is formal operations, which involves the ability to think in abstract terms and use the scientific method to arrive at conclusions.
7. Formal reasoning does not protect adolescents from shoplifting because some teens have difficulty envisioning a department store or large corporation as capable of suffering economic loss from stealing.
8. Accidents, most commonly those involving motor vehicles, are the leading cause of death among adolescents.
9. The nutrients most apt to be deficient in the adolescent diet are iron, calcium, and zinc.
10. Adolescents need proportionally more sleep than school-age children to support the growth spurt during this time, which demands the formation of so many new cells.
11. Girls taking tetracycline are apt to develop *Candida vaginitis.*
12. The danger of a very-low-calorie diet for obese adolescents is that such a diet provides insufficient protein and may be deficient in vitamins, potentially leading to inadequate nitrogen balance and in turn impaired growth.
13. The effects of Rohypnol are drowsiness, impaired motor skills, and amnesia.
14. Refer children of alcoholics to Al-Anon or Alateen.
15. Chronic inhalation of cocaine can cause ulceration in the mucous membrane of the nose.
16. An elevated mood can mean an adolescent has worked through and made a decision to commit suicide.
17. Many runaways don't want to return home because a dysfunctional family life is the reason that they left home.

What If? Question Answers

1. As many more people have active exercise programs today than formerly, more and more adolescents are being admitted to the hospital with this concern. Assessing what type of program the adolescent was using and including simple muscle strengthening exercises in an adolescent's plan of care would be important care planning.
2. Many parents are able to find another family member or family friend who can care for an adolescent when the relationship between a teenager and parents becomes unbearable. Other families need referral to a social agency to help them solve this problem. The fact that a family is asking for help is a major forward step toward a workable solution.

Chapter 33: Child Health Assessment

Checkpoint Question Answers

1. Leading questions are questions that supply their own answer.
2. Six areas to explore regarding a chief concern are duration, intensity, frequency, description, associated symptoms, and actions taken.
3. Important areas to consider when eliciting a day history are play, sleep, hygiene, and nutrition.
4. It is important to ask for a family health history because some diseases are inherited.
5. A health history should conclude with "Is there anything more we should know about your child?" or "Is there anything I didn't mention that you want to ask about?"
6. Four techniques used in physical assessment are inspection, palpation, percussion, and auscultation.
7. Blood pressure is included as part of a routine assessment at age 3 years.
8. On a standardized scale, all weights between the 10th and 90th percentile are considered normal.
9. The following factors should be assessed during an examination of the skin: temperature, color, texture, turgor, and presence of any lesions.
10. The red reflex is elicited by shining a bright light into the pupil.
11. Normal ear alignment is determined when a line drawn from the inner canthus of the eye through the outer canthus and then to the ear touches the top of the ear pinna.
12. When a child has epiglottitis, the gag reflex should not be elicited.
13. Edema, erythema, wrinkling, retraction, or dimpling of the skin suggest that a tumor is growing in the deeper layers of breast tissue.
14. The pulmonary heart valve is heard best at the second left intercostal space.
15. Routine scoliosis screening should begin at age 12 years.
16. The preschool E chart is a good type of eye chart for cognitively challenged or non-English-speaking children.
17. Normal conversation is conducted at approximately 50 to 60 dB.
18. Children typically receive DTaP immunizations at 2, 4, and 6 months with a booster dose at 4 to 6 years.
19. Varicella immunization is typically given at 12 to 18 months.

What If? Question Answers

1. Although it is true that the above menu includes foods from the five food groups (hamburger = meat; onion, lettuce, and potatoes = vegetables; tomatoes = fruit; milkshake = dairy products; the bun = grain group), eating hamburger as the main source of protein and iron daily is questionable because of the high fat content in most hamburger. This menu is also very low in fruit. You'd want to make sure the adolescent had additional sources of these at other meals during the day.
2. Ninety-three lbs at 14 years puts this girl's weight in the 10th percentile; a year ago her weight reached the 50th percentile. Growing children, as a rule, never go backward in growth, so the information that this girl has lost 17 lbs in 6 months needs investigation. She may have been dieting vigorously or have developed an eating disorder such as bulimia. Such a drastic weight loss may also signal the onset of illness such as diabetes mellitus, hyperthyroidism, or cancer.

3. Because many families are so mobile today, this is a common situation. As a rule, immunization series are not completely started over; they are picked up at the point most practical (if this mother knew her child had vaccines at 2 months, for example, the child would start with a second DTaP and IVP). An important nursing intervention is to be certain that parents receive a record of their child's immunizations as well as an explanation of what the immunization was and that it is important information for parents to know.

Chapter 34: Communication and Teaching With Children and Families

Checkpoint Question Answers

1. Paraphrasing is documenting words said to you; perception checking documents a feeling or emotion reported to you.
2. Stop talking is the first step in being a good listener.
3. Shortened length of hospital stays and minimized hospital admissions have dramatically changed health teaching by making the window for teaching very narrow.
4. Three types of learning include cognitive, psychomotor, and affective learning.
5. During the school-age years, learning capability is concrete.
6. Motivation to learn or to appreciate how their life will be improved through learning may affect children's emotional readiness to learn. Some factors such as exhaustion, pain, low self-esteem, or distaste for a certain aspect of care must be resolved before children are emotionally ready to learn.
7. Five minutes is the typical attention span of a preschooler.
8. Careful assessment is needed to determine whether formal or informal teaching is the best format for a given situation.
9. Peer learning not only improves knowledge but may also improve attitude and motivation to learn. Children may be more comforted by other children's experiences or may be more willing to accept the advice or solutions of a peer.
10. Trying to modify beliefs or values by behavior modification is unethical.
11. Playing board games is a good technique for school-age children.
12. Children do tend to listen to mass media messages if the messages are attention getting and brief.

What If? Question Answers

1. This is an interesting quandary because you want to support the preschooler's action (Don't speak to strangers), but at the same time you need the child to talk to you to evaluate whether the pain is growing less. A good start would be to talk to the parent and have him or her introduce you to the child and say it's all right to talk to you. That way, you're not a stranger (strangers are not strange; they are people your parents do not know).
2. The answer to this question is ideally "all family members, including the adolescent." It is an example of the way that health teaching affects an entire family, not just the one member receiving the primary instructions.

Chapter 35: Nursing Care of the Ill Child and Family

Checkpoint Question Answers

1. School-age children understand quite a bit about the workings of major body parts. Early grade-school children are able to name the functions of the heart, lungs, and stomach.
2. Newborns are more likely to lose a devastating amount of body water with diarrhea or vomiting because their total body water is composed of approximately 40% of extracellular water and, in turn, much less water is stored in the cells.
3. Useful techniques in preparing preschoolers for hospitalization include allowing the child to bring transitional objects, reading books about hospitalization, and playing or acting out hospitalization and procedures.
4. Height and weight should be measured on hospital admission to determine overall growth and allow for determination of surface area necessary for medicine administration.
5. According to Robertson, the first stage of separation anxiety is protest.
6. As a rule, home care is more cost-effective than hospitalization.
7. A box or additional pillows can be placed under the mattress to elevate the head of a regular bed to a gatch position.
8. To encourage a sense of trust in infants, maintain a schedule as close to their normal routine as possible. To promote a sense of autonomy in ill toddlers and a sense of initiative in preschoolers, allow them to make choices about their care. To promote a sense of industry in school-age children, explain to them about specific procedures and involve them as much as possible in the actual care. To promote a sense of identity in adolescents, help them to participate as much as possible in as many activities as they did before and encourage them to maintain self-care activities and good hygiene.
9. Children accept smaller, fuller glasses of fluid more readily.
10. To ensure that a hospital crib is safe, be sure that side rails are in good repair, fully raised at all times and secured; push bedside stands and tables away from the crib so that the child cannot climb over the rail and use the stand or table as a step down; be sure crib caps are used for small children.
11. Sleepwalking occurs during NREM sleep, probably during the deepest part of stage IV.
12. Children with sensory deprivation lose the ability to make decisions and become easily confused or depressed.
13. Caregivers can make television watching more interactive by playing along with game shows or children's programs such as "Sesame Street" or discussing the characters and plots of a particular show.
14. A cylinder 1 inch in diameter is the most dangerous size for a toy because it totally occludes the trachea if it is aspirated.
15. Therapeutic play allows children to express their feelings about procedures.
16. Therapeutic play can be used either preoperatively (to help prepare the child) or postoperatively (to "debrief" or allow the child to work through anxiety).

What If? Question Answers

1. Children often play with non-typical "toys" such as pots and pans from the cupboard; soft toys such as teddy bears often have missing arms or legs. The purpose of bringing a toy to the hospital is so the child has a familiar, comforting object with him or her. You can assure parents, therefore, that a worn toy is probably the most comforting as it is one well loved.
2. Many 3-year-olds cannot draw a person with more body parts than this. "Centering" often makes them concentrate on one aspect of a drawing (the body parts) but not the color. With only this scant information to guide you, this is a normal drawing for the age group.

Chapter 36: Nursing Care of the Child Undergoing Diagnostic Techniques and Other Therapeutic Modalities

Checkpoint Question Answers

1. School-age children can worry that they will fail a "test," a worry that places unnecessary stress on them.
2. A mummy restraint should be used when a young child needs to be temporarily immobilized.
3. Radioactive iodine will destroy the thyroid if it is not blocked from entering the gland.
4. Endoscopy is direct visualization of the gastrointestinal tract by a fiberoptic tube passed through the mouth or anus. Bronchoscopy is direct visualization of the larynx, trachea, bronchi, and alveoli by a fiberoptic tube passed through the nose or mouth.
5. A blood pressure cuff should be no more than two thirds and no less than half the length of the upper arm.
6. A tympanic thermometer registers in 2 to 3 seconds.
7. The fingertip in an older child and the heel in an infant are appropriate sites for obtaining a capillary puncture.
8. A 24-hour urine should be timed from the time of the discarded urine.
9. Perineal pressure is applied during suprapubic aspiration in girls to block the urethra and prevent loss of urine.
10. A nasogastric tube in an infant is measured from the bridge of the nose to the earlobe to a point halfway between the xiphoid process and the umbilicus.
11. A TPN solution contains approximately twice the amount of glucose normally administered in an intravenous solution, which

may cause dehydration as the body tries to reduce the amount of glucose recognized by the kidneys as excessive and eliminates it.

12. An enema catheter in an infant should be inserted 1 inch.
13. Parents should give acetaminophen rather than acetylsalicylic acid (aspirin) for children's fever because aspirin has been associated with the development of Reye's syndrome (serious liver destruction).

What If? Question Answers

1. Many adolescents try to cover their fear of the unknown by projecting a pseudo-sophisticated attitude. To counteract this, it is often helpful to introduce procedures to this group with a statement such as, "You probably already know this, but let me review it with you." This allows the adolescent to maintain a pretense of knowing everything, but receive an explanation of procedures. It is important that adolescents do understand procedures before they are carried out; otherwise this violates the principle of informed consent.
2. As eating in a restaurant offers more experience than simply the consumption of food, parents should be encouraged to include this type of experience in a child's activities even if the child is not going to eat in the setting. Such an experience builds vocabulary (words like menu, waiter, or waitress), encourages conversational skills, and exposes children to such skills as taking turns.

Chapter 37: Nursing Care of the Child Undergoing Medication Administration and Intravenous Therapy

Checkpoint Question Answers

1. Newborns can have difficulty with distribution of medicine because their peripheral circulation is sluggish; immature liver function may provide a lowered level of plasma proteins to bind to drugs for distribution.
2. To use a nomogram, draw a line from the child's height to the child's weight. The point at which the line crosses the middle column is the child's body surface area.
3. Checking the identification band for a child and comparing it to the name on the medication sheet or medical record is the preferred method for identifying children before medicine administration. In ambulatory settings when children do not have an armband, ask a parent to identify the child for you.
4. Letting children practice swallowing small ice cubes can be an effective way for them to learn to swallow medicine as ice chips melt easily so do not cause distress.
5. Eyedrops should be instilled into the conjunctivae of the lower eyelid.
6. Eardrops should be given at room temperature or slightly warm; cold eardrops cause acute pain.
7. Rectal suppositories should be inserted about a half-inch in infants; an inch in older children.
8. Be certain that transdermal patches are out of sight and away from an area where they would be contaminated by urine.
9. The preferred IM injection site in an infant is the outer aspect of the vastus lateralis muscle of the anterior thigh.
10. Automatic rate infusion pumps, fluid chambers, and mini-droppers are safety devices to ensure the proper rate of fluid administration.
11. Intraosseous infusions are used in emergencies when it is difficult to establish usual IV access or in a child with such extensive burns that the usual sites for IV infusion are unavailable. They may also be used to infuse an antibiotic directly into the bone with bone infection (osteomyelitis).
12. Hypodermoclysis is used when a medicine can infuse over a long time period. It is a technique that parents can institute so can be helpful in home care.

What If? Question Answers

1. This parent may have a misunderstanding of what "no drug" means, so advising her to meet with the school nurse to discuss the problem would be appropriate. In many instances, the "no drug" rule only applies to self-administration of medicine, not to nurse-administered drugs. If the child is not allowed to take medicine to school to self administer, most medicines are not prescribed more than three times a day; the schedule for most medicines can be arranged so the child takes the medicine before school, immediately after returning home, and again at bedtime. These time periods do not fall into exactly even time periods but may be necessary if school rules restrict drug administration during school hours.
2. When instructions with a medicine advise that the medication be taken with a meal, it generally means that the medication is irritating to the stomach lining and taking it with a meal will help reduce the irritation. The point, though, is to be sure that the child eats something with the medicine, not necessarily a full meal. Drinking a glass of milk or eating a snack would both furnish enough food to allow her to give the medicine.

Chapter 38: Pain Management in Children

Checkpoint Question Answers

1. Diffuse body movements; tears; high-pitched, sharp, harsh cry; stiff posture; lack of play; fisting; and guarding are frequent physical findings of infants in pain.
2. To assess pain accurately, use the toddler's terminology.
3. Children are often more adept at imagery because their imaginations are less inhibited than those of adults.
4. With substitution of meaning the child places another, often fantasy meaning on a painful procedure. With thought stopping, the child stops an anxious thought by replacing it with a positive thought.
5. A child's pain management program is optimal if it includes both pharmacologic and non-pharmacologic methods.
6. IM routes are used infrequently with children because they are associated with pain on administration and produce great fear. Children also have limited injection sites.
7. Conscious sedation provides analgesia and blocks anxiety for procedures.
8. Epidural analgesia does not lead to spinal headache as the anesthetic is injected outside the spinal fluid.

What If? Question Answers

1. A child who colors in the entire figure has most likely not understood the directions and is using the figure drawing as a coloring activity, not a pain assessment tool. Some adolescents will do this because they consider the tool "too babyish" for them and respond by using it as a "babyish" coloring activity rather than using it assess their pain.
2. It takes a minimum of an hour for EMLA cream to work. Doing the procedure early, therefore, will cause the child unnecessary pain. Asking the surgeon to respect the hour's time needed for pain relief would be an important nursing role.

Chapter 39: Nursing Care of the Child Born With a Physical Developmental Disorder

Checkpoint Question Answers

1. Cleft lip is more prevalent in males.
2. A child with cleft palate repair should not use a straw because it or any sharp object could tear the suture line.
3. Before surgery, feeding a child with cleft lip is a problem because the infant has difficulty maintaining suction and is at an increased risk for aspiration.
4. The chief danger of tracheoesophageal fistula is aspiration from seepage of fluid from the esophagus into the lungs.
5. The most important consideration in care of the child with omphalocele at birth is protecting the sac covering it from rupturing.
6. Low intermittent nasogastric suction is used for newborns because higher pressure can break down the stomach lining.
7. The most common site for intestinal obstruction in the infant is the duodenum.
8. The best preoperative position for an infant with a diaphragmatic hernia is with the head elevated or turned so the compressed lung is down to allow optimal breathing space.
9. Taping a coin on a newborn's umbilicus to reduce an umbilical hernia can actually cause intestinal obstruction or bowel strangulation.
10. It is important for parents to perform rectal dilatation after surgical repair of an imperforate anus to help keep stenosis from occurring.

11. Changes with increased cranial pressure include increased blood pressure and temperature and decreased pulse and respirations.
12. After a shunting procedure, the infant's bed should be flat or only slightly raised (approximately 30 degrees) to keep excessive CSF from draining.
13. A meningocele sac should be kept moist to keep it from drying and rupturing.
14. Surgery is performed to repair a neural tube defect as soon as possible after birth, usually within 24 hours.
15. Syndactyly describes the condition in which two or more fingers are fused.
16. Passive stretching exercises and encouraging the infant to look in the direction of the affected muscle are important measures to keep the muscle from contracting further.
17. Developmental hip dysplasia is best assessed by examining for hip abduction.
18. The affected hip is abducted and externally rotated.
19. The presence of only streak gonads (small; nonfunctional gonads) results in sterility.
20. The muscles of children with Down syndrome are unusually relaxed; this is often described as a "rag-doll" appearance.

What If? Question Answers

1. One of the problems of detecting bowel obstruction in a newborn who also had meconium staining is that bile-stained emesis and meconium-stained mucus look a great deal alike. Assessing the infant for other signs of bowel obstruction such as a distended abdomen would help reveal the problem.
2. Most authorities believe the child's rights are paramount. The decision varies with each individual child, however, depending on the extent of the defect present and the quality of life that can be anticipated. This family needs referral to the agency's committee on ethical concerns.

Chapter 40: Nursing Care of the Child With a Respiratory Disorder

Checkpoint Question Answers

1. The frontal sinuses and the sphenoid sinuses do not develop until 6 to 8 years of age.
2. After age 2, foreign bodies more often lodge in the right bronchus as the lumen is larger there than on the left.
3. Tachypnea is often the first indicator of airway obstruction.
4. Wheezing is heard most noticeably on expiration, as the lumen of the airway is narrower on expiration.
5. Two noninvasive methods for measuring oxyhemoglobin saturation include pulse oximetry and transcutaneous oxygen monitoring.
6. Tidal volume (TV) denotes the amount of air inhaled or exhaled in a single breath.
7. Nebulizers can feel suffocating because of the water vapor.
8. Instruct children to inhale rather than blow out against the mouthpiece of an incentive spirometer.
9. Gloves should be worn when suctioning a tracheostomy to prevent introducing infection.
10. Covering the opening with a gauze square tied to the child's neck like a bib is a good method to keep crumbs out of a tracheostomy.
11. A capnometer measures the amount of CO_2 in inhaled or exhaled breaths.
12. Pancuronium (Pavulon) may be administered to abolish spontaneous respiratory activity for children on respirators.
13. Children with choanal atresia develop signs of respiratory distress at birth or immediately after they quiet and attempt to breath through their nose.
14. Infants should not be prescribed acetylsalicylic acid (aspirin) because of its association with Reye's syndrome, a fatal liver destruction disease.
15. The palatine tonsils are typically involved with tonsillitis.
16. Subtle signs of post-tonsillectomy bleeding include an increasing pulse rate, frequent swallowing, throat clearing, and a feeling of anxiety.
17. The most effective treatment for laryngitis is for children to rest their voice for at least 24 hours until the inflammation subsides.
18. Never attempt to directly visualize the epiglottis with a tongue blade or obtain a throat culture unless a means of providing an artificial airway is readily available for the child with epiglottitis.
19. A series of five back blows followed by five chest thrusts is considered the most effective method for dislodging an aspirated foreign body in infants.
20. Bronchiolitis is most often seen in children younger than age 2 years, with the highest incidence in winter and spring.
21. Wheezing is the most common presenting symptom in children with asthma.
22. A short-acting beta-2-agonist such as albuterol is the chief medication given for an acute asthma attack.
23. Children with chronic illness, those who have had a splenectomy, or those who are immunocompromised should receive a pneumococcal vaccine.
24. A semi-Fowler's position generally allows for the best lung expansion as it lowers abdominal contents and frees breathing space.
25. Miliary tuberculosis refers to tuberculosis that has spread to other parts of the body than the lungs.
26. A level greater than 60 mEq/dL chloride in sweat is diagnostic of CF.

What If? Question Answers

1. If a child has respiratory secretions in the airway, coughing occurs as a reflex to clear these secretions. You can help initiate this reflex by asking the child to take several deep breaths. This causes the secretions to move and trigger the reflex. Playing "Simon Says" with the child and having Simon say, "Take two deep breaths" also accomplishes this.
2. Unless a child has a blood clotting disorder, most nosebleeds are easy to manage. Parents make the mistake of insisting the child with a nosebleed lie down. This increases the pressure in the broken capillaries in the nose and actually increases the bleeding. Encouraging the child to remain upright decreases pressure in the head. Following this by applying pressure to the nose usually makes the bleeding stop easily.
3. This is a common mistake made by new nurses (assuming the lack of sound shows improvement when it actually means the child's condition is worsening). The second problem here (not enough air is entering the airway to make the sound of stridor) is the major concern. To rule this out, the lungs should be assessed. If good air exchange is present, then the first conclusion (the child's condition is improving) can be made.

Chapter 41: Nursing Care of the Child With a Cardiovascular Disorder

Checkpoint Question Answers

1. Infants with heart disease generally have tachycardia and tachypnea.
2. Organic heart murmur denotes a heart murmur resulting from heart disease.
3. Blood tests help to support the diagnosis of heart disease by ruling out anemia or clotting defects.
4. Routine blood pressure screening begins at age 3 years.
5. Because anemia stresses the heart, an iron supplement is generally given to an infant with congenital heart disease.
6. Children with congenital heart defects need prophylactic antibiotic therapy before oral surgery because streptococcal organisms generally present in the mouth are often involved in infectious endocarditis.
7. Children may experience a temporary tachycardia when a cardiac catheter enters their heart.
8. Cardiac arrhythmias may result from the mechanical action of the catheter having touched the conduction nodes of the heart.
9. After cardiac surgery; children should be encouraged to cough and deep breathe to prevent pooling of secretions in the respiratory system.
10. Children tend to develop hypervolemia after cardiac surgery because of increased production of aldosterone and an increase in antidiuretic hormone secretion from the stress of the procedure.
11. Post-perfusion syndrome is most apt to occur 3 to 12 weeks after surgery.
12. The drug most commonly prescribed for long-term anticoagulation therapy is sodium warfarin.
13. Acute rejection of a transplanted heart occurs in about 7 days.
14. With an atrial septal defect, blood flow is from left to right (oxygenated to unoxygenated).

15. Indomethacin is used to close a patent ductus arteriosus.
16. With total anomalous pulmonary venous return, blood must be shunted across a patent foramen ovale or patent ductus arteriosus to reach the left side.
17. The four defects that present with tetralogy of Fallot include pulmonary stenosis, ventricular septal defect, dextroposition of the aorta, and hypertrophy of the right ventricle.
18. To strengthen heart contractility, digoxin is commonly prescribed.
19. In the child receiving furosemide, be alert for signs of hypokalemia.
20. Rheumatic fever occurs as a result of a group A beta hemolytic streptococcus infection.
21. During the first stage of Kawasaki disease, the primary manifestation is high fever that does not respond to antipyretics.
22. Administration of ampicillin or amoxicillin before ear, nose, throat, tonsil, or mouth surgery or childbirth helps prevent infectious endocarditis.
23. A systolic BP reading above the 95th percentile denotes hypertension.
24. An acceptable level of total cholesterol is 170 mg/dL; for LDL, 110 mg/dL.
25. The most frequent effect of cardiomyopathy is severe dilation of the left or both ventricles, which impairs systolic function and leads to heart failure.
26. Respiratory failure is the most frequent cause of cardiac arrest.
27. A 1:5 ratio of ventilation to compression is used for resuscitation of an infant.

What If? Question Answers

1. This could just be a habitual position the child uses when he is concentrating on a problem, but needs to be investigated as it is just another way for a child to trap blood in his lower extremities, the way younger children use squatting or a knee-chest position to better oxygenate blood with heart disease.
2. First you need to determine that you are certain the child vomited and didn't choke while swallowing, so is spitting up, not vomiting, the medicine. Vomiting is a symptom of digoxin toxicity; if this is what is happening, holding the dose and notifying the child's primary care provider would be the next step. The child needs a serum digoxin level drawn to determine whether the dose needs to be reduced.
3. Ibuprofen has anti-inflammatory action in addition to analgesic and antipyretic actions. In the child with Kawasaki disease, discussed here, the drug is being used for its anti-inflammatory action as well as for pain relief so should be continued.

Chapter 42: Nursing Care of the Child With an Immune Disorder

Checkpoint Question Answers

1. Macrophages and leukocytes are responsible for engulfing, ingesting, and neutralizing pathogens.
2. Two types of lymphocytes produced by bone marrow are type T and B lymphocytes.
3. Maternal transmission of HIV by placental spread is the most common cause of childhood HIV.
4. HIV-positive children are begun on prophylactic TMP/SMZ to prevent *P. carinii* pneumonia.
5. Contact dermatitis results from a type 4 hypersensitivity.
6. Skin testing is done to isolate an antigen to which a child is sensitive.
7. Epinephrine is the first-line drug to treat anaphylaxis.
8. Angioedema occurs where skin is loosely bound by subcutaneous tissue, such as the eyelids, hands, feet, genitalia, and lips.
9. Food allergy is probably the cause of atopic dermatitis in infants.
10. In older children, atopic dermatitis affects flexor surfaces of extremities and dorsal surfaces of wrists and ankles.
11. Food allergies are usually treated with elimination diets.
12. Patch testing is used to identify the allergen of contact dermatitis.

What If? Question Answers

1. Itch-scratch cycles are often associated with times of stress. Final examinations that occur at these times of the year are often the "triggers" for this.
2. This is a typical description of a leather allergy to a new wallet, carried in the back pants pocket. History taking to see if a new wallet was purchased would be important.

Chapter 43: Nursing Care of the Child With an Infectious Disorder

Checkpoint Question Answers

1. Incubation, prodromal, illness, and convalescence are the four stages of an infectious disorder.
2. Reservoir, portal of exit, means of transmission, portal of entry, and susceptible host are five components of the chain of infection.
3. Three categories of transmission-based precautions are airborne, droplet, and contact.
4. Children may interpret the restriction due to infection control precautions as punishment ("time out" or "being grounded" for unwise behavior).
5. The hallmark of roseola is the appearance of a rash immediately after the sharp decline in fever.
6. A discrete, pink-red, maculopapular rash is typically the first sign of rubella noticed by parents.
7. Koplik's spots are found only with rubeola.
8. The four stages of chickenpox lesions are (1) macula, (1) papule, (3) vesicle, and (4) crust.
9. Swelling of mumps is typically located at the parotid gland, just in front of the earlobe.
10. Children with infectious mononucleosis are at risk for splenic rupture upon abdominal palpation.
11. Beta-hemolytic streptococci group A are responsible for scarlet fever.
12. Staphylococci are often the organisms involved in food poisoning episodes in summer months.
13. Massive cell necrosis and inflammation is the result of exotoxin production by diphtheria bacilli.
14. Complications of pertussis include pneumonia, atelectasis, and emphysema.
15. Helminthic infections are transmitted by unclean foods and hands.
16. *Candida albicans* is the organism responsible for thrush.

What If? Question Answers

1. Impetigo is caused by either staphylococcal or streptococcal organisms, pathogens commonly present on children's skin. Impetigo, therefore, is a disease waiting to happen if the child has an open cut. Spread of organisms can occur through sharing objects such as gym towels. Helping parents understand that the disease is easily spread not only helps them understand how their child contracted it but also gives them guidance on how to prevent other family members from contracting it as well.
2. Children with pertussis cough so forcefully and long (paroxysmal coughing) that they can vomit, not from nausea but from the force of the coughing. They can eat again immediately because no nausea is present.

Chapter 44: Nursing Care of the Child With a Hematologic Disorder

Checkpoint Question Answers

1. The hormone responsible for stimulating the production of red blood cells is erythropoietin, produced by the kidneys.
2. The two major forms of white blood cells are granulocytes and agranulocytes.
3. Megakaryocytes is the term used to denote immature platelets.
4. In children the preferred aspiration site for bone marrow is the posterior iliac crest.
5. All potential bone marrow donors are typed for human leukocyte compatibility.
6. The formation and development of white blood cells, platelets, and red blood cells are all affected by aplastic anemia.
7. Iron chelation therapy is needed for hemosiderosis (deposition of iron in body cells), the result of long-term transfusion of packed red cells.
8. Ferrous sulfate is the drug of choice to improve red cell formation and replace iron stores.
9. For absorption of vitamin B_{12} from the intestine, an intrinsic factor must be present in the gastric mucosa.
10. The medical treatment of choice for congenital spherocytosis is generally splenectomy at approximately 5 to 6 years of age.
11. Children with sickle cell anemia need more fluid during the summer months to prevent dehydration, which can lead to sickling.

12. Frontal bossing changes the shape of the skull; the upper teeth protrude and the base of the nose may broaden and flatten.
13. With autoimmune acquired hemolytic anemia, laboratory findings reveal that the red cells are extremely small and round, resembling hereditary spherocytosis.
14. An elevated eosinophil count is frequently associated with allergies.
15. NSAIDs should be avoided in children with ITP because they interfere with blood clotting by preventing the aggregation of platelets at wound sites.
16. The drug of choice for treating DIC is subcutaneous heparin.
17. The coagulation component factor VIII is deficient in hemophilia A.
18. With even minor abrasions, children with hemophilia must have bleeding controlled by administration of factor VIII.

What If? Question Answers

1. This is a problem that can arise because of the magical thinking of children (they believe that what they wish will come true). The reality that all transplantations are not successful should be addressed the first time the topic of transplantation arises, so both the donor and the recipient know this may happen. This prevents the donor feeling that he or she has failed (and possibly has done something wrong to cause this), or that the recipient child has done something wrong to cause this.
2. Children with sickle-cell anemia need to be kept well hydrated, so this solution to bedwetting may not be the best one for this particular child. Reducing, but not eliminating, fluid intake in the evening would be a better program. Urging the parent to talk to the primary care provider about the problem and possibly beginning the child on a specific medication for nocturnal enuresis would be important.

Chapter 45: Nursing Care of the Child With a Gastrointestinal Disorder

Checkpoint Question Answers

1. Interstitial fluid accounts for a greater percentage of body weight in infants than in adults.
2. With isotonic dehydration, the body initially compensates by a shift of interstitial fluid into the blood vessels.
3. A solution is acid or alkaline depending on the proportion of H^+ ions present.
4. Hypokalemia is a frequent secondary problem with vomiting.
5. Although NPO status for a child experiencing vomiting is determined by age, an average of 3 to 6 hours should be sufficient.
6. Because breast milk contains antibodies, breastfeeding best prevents diarrhea in infants.
7. A metabolic acidosis is present with severe diarrhea.
8. Salmonella may be the causative organism if a child develops diarrhea after eating raw eggs.
9. A chest elevated position for 1 hour is the best position after feeding for a child with gastrointestinal reflux.
10. Vomiting almost immediately after feeding that grows increasingly forceful until it is projectile is associated with pyloric stenosis.
11. Fiberoptic endoscopy is the most reliable diagnostic test to confirm peptic ulcer disease.
12. Bowel or stomach perforation, blood loss anemia, and intestinal obstruction are three complications of peptic ulcer disease.
13. Hepatitis A and hepatitis E are transmitted through fecally contaminated water.
14. Hepatitis is considered chronic when it lasts over 6 months.
15. With bile duct obstruction, absorption of fat and fat-soluble vitamins is poor.
16. Children with esophageal varices are at high risk for rupture of varices, which can lead to a large quantity of blood loss.
17. Hypoglycemia is a danger of liver transplant because glucose levels are regulated by the liver, and transplanted organs may not function efficiently at first.
18. Currant jelly–like stools are present with intussusception.
19. Volvulus tends to be a problem of the first 6 months of life.
20. Signs of necrotizing enterocolitis usually appear in the first week of life.
21. The point of sharpest pain with appendicitis is often one-third of the way between the anterior superior iliac crest and the umbilicus (McBurney's point).
22. Steatorrhea; deficiency of fat-soluble vitamins A, D, K, and E; malnutrition; and a distended abdomen are the four most common symptoms of celiac disease.
23. Gluten (the protein of wheat, rye, barley, and oats) must be restricted in a child with celiac disease.
24. A low-residue diet is usually ordered for the child with aganglionic megacolon.
25. The cause of inflammatory bowel disease is probably an alteration in immune system response or an autoimmune process.
26. Kwashiorkor is a disorder of protein deficiency.
27. Calcium cannot be absorbed from the stomach without vitamin D.

What If? Question Answers

1. This question sounds as if a parent has taken a care instruction literally and not as intended. You might want to explain to the parent that "force fluids" doesn't mean he or she should literally force fluids but was intended to mean she should offer fluids frequently. Once the parent is clear on the instruction, then it's time to talk about what offering fluids frequently means and what amount she or he should offer.
2. This is a practical problem because parents do "drop everything" to rush a child to the hospital for appendicitis. Good questions to ask are: Did you leave anything cooking on the stove? Do your other children have safe child care? Did you park your car or leave it by the emergency entrance? Helping the parent look at particular problems this way helps them reduce this situation from "something terrible is happening to me" to one they can handle with support.

Chapter 46: Nursing Care of the Child With a Renal or Urinary Tract Disorder

Checkpoint Question Answers

1. A nephron is the major functioning unit of the kidneys.
2. Creatinine in urine remains constant regardless of the amount of protein in the diet.
3. The presence of UTI is established by urine culture.
4. Cystoscopy is a difficult procedure for many children because it is painful and requires them to lie still for the procedure.
5. To empty urine from a continent urinary reservoir, the parent or child catheterizes the abdominal urethra three or four times daily.
6. The meatus may be near the glans, midway back, or at the base of the penis on the ventral surface in the child with hypospadias.
7. *Escherichia coli* is the organism that most commonly causes UTIs.
8. UTI is a common symptom associated with vesicoureteral reflux.
9. Enuresis is found more commonly in boys.
10. Orthostatic proteinuria is spilling of albumin into the urine when the child stands upright.
11. Acute glomerulonephritis is characterized by a sudden onset of hematuria and proteinuria.
12. Four characteristic symptoms of nephrotic syndrome include (1) proteinuria, (2) edema, (3) low serum albumin, and (4) hyperlipidemia.
13. Oliguria is one of the first symptoms noted with acute renal failure.
14. Children with chronic renal failure are generally placed on low-protein, low-phosphorus diets.
15. It is difficult to transplant adult kidneys into children because of their size.
17. Transplanted kidneys are usually placed in the abdominal cavity rather than the retroperitoneal space.

What If? Question Answers

1. A child who is voiding black urine needs to be seen by a primary care provider as the color is undoubtedly being caused by the addition of old blood. Testing urine by a test strip procedure is the quickest method to determine if blood is present. The urine could also be examined under a microscope for the presence of red blood cells.
2. Dependent edema means that fluid is collecting in lower body parts. Edematous tissue tends to trap and store medicine, so injecting into lower body parts in this child would not be ideal. Giving an injection in the deltoid muscle, therefore, would be better; because it is high on the body, it would be less effected by edema.

Chapter 47: Nursing Care of the Child With a Reproductive Disorder

Checkpoint Question Answers

1. Precocious puberty occurs more often in females than males.
2. Secondary sex characteristics begin in early puberty; girls have until 17 years of age until they are said to have delayed puberty.
3. Males with undescended testes are at a high risk for testicular cancer and infertility if undescended testes are not repaired.
4. The first symptom of testicular torsion is severe scrotal pain.
5. Endometriosis leads to dysmenorrhea because displaced endometrium tissue bleeds and sloughs the same as intrauterine endometrium.
6. Child abuse should be suspected in a young child with vulvovaginitis.
7. Yes. Breast implants are placed in back of breast tissue.
8. Breast cancer could exist concurrently with a fibrocystic breast condition.
9. Candidiasis vaginal infection typically presents with a white, cheese-like discharge, perineal redness, and itching.
10. Gonorrhea is a serious STD because it can lead to infertility in both sexes.

What If? Question Answers

1. All breast tissue, even that under accessory nipples, is susceptible to breast cancer. The girl should include this tissue in self-breast examination. If the tissue is extensive, having it removed would offer her protection against breast cancer and probably an improved cosmetic appearance.
2. Many adolescents are not aware of exactly what immunizations they have had, so they feel confident that they have been immunized against all infectious diseases. They need to be educated that STDs, with the exception of hepatitis B, cannot be immunized against, so they can not only contract these infections but can contract them more than once.

Chapter 48: Nursing Care of the Child With an Endocrine or Metabolic Disorder

Checkpoint Question Answers

1. Following arginine or insulin testing, children may develop severe hypoglycemia.
2. Children with diabetes insipidus may need to use a school lavatory more than others.
3. The most serious effect of congenital hypothyroidism is cognitive impairment.
4. Children with hyperthyroidism are often unable to write or speak clearly; they may have hand tremors, and they also may be unable to sit still during class.
5. Girls who have adrenogenital syndrome at birth are born with masculinized genitalia; the clitoris is enlarged to look like a penis.
6. Aldosterone regulates sodium, so the child becomes dehydrated quickly.
7. Children most frequently develop type I diabetes mellitus.
8. Many children no longer demonstrate symptoms of diabetes for a short time following therapy; this is called a "honeymoon" period.
9. The usual peak time for regular insulin is 2 to 4 hours.
10. Typical symptoms of hypoglycemia are nervousness, weakness, sweating, and tremors.
11. The chief symptom of latent tetany is jitteriness from neuromuscular irritability.
12. Children with glycogen storage disease are unable to break down stored liver glycogen into glucose, so they develop hypoglycemia.

What If? Question Answers

1. Because many people do not understand the great forward strides that have been made in diabetes control, it is not unusual to discover a person who still thinks of people with diabetes as disabled or at least challenged enough not to be able to participate actively in a sports program. Frank discussion with the coach (with the child's permission) would go a long way toward informing him about modern management. Most school systems maintain a board that specifically investigates and advocates for children with illness within the system. Informing the parents how to contact this board and that participation on a sports team is their child's right would make them better informed.
2. Although milk may be nutritious for the average child, it is high in phenylalanine, so is contraindicated for the child with PKU. Investigating why the school wasn't informed of the child's special diet would be in order. Supplying the needed information would be important.

Chapter 49: Nursing Care of the Child With a Neurologic Disorder

Checkpoint Question Answers

1. To test for graphesthesia (ability to recognize a shape that has been traced on the skin), ask a preschooler to close his eyes and then trace first a circle, then a square on the back of his hand; ask him if the shapes are the same or different. For the older child, trace several numbers—for example, 8, 3, 0, and 1—and ask him to identify each one.
2. Cranial nerve XI (accessory) is assessed by asking a child to raise his shoulders against pressure.
3. Deep tendon reflexes diminish in intensity with decreasing level of consciousness or increased intracranial pressure.
4. The intraventricular catheter monitoring method is considered the most accurate.
5. The four types of cerebral palsy are spastic, dyskinetic (athetoid), ataxic, and mixed.
6. Contractures can be prevented with the use of partial leg braces and passive and active exercises. These exercises can be incorporated into play activities.
7. Meningeal irritability is assessed by positive Brudzinski's and Kernig's signs and pain on forward flexion of the neck.
8. Children with bacterial meningitis are placed on respiratory precautions for 24 hours after the start of antibiotic therapy to prevent infection transmission.
9. Enteroviruses are the most frequent cause of encephalitis.
10. Reye's syndrome generally occurs after a viral infection such as varicella (chickenpox) or an upper respiratory infection when the child is given acetylsalicylic acid (aspirin).
11. A common source of botulism spores is honey.
12. A partial seizure with motor signs begins in the fingers and spreads to the wrist, arm, and face.
13. Absence seizures can usually be demonstrated in children by asking them to hyperventilate and count out loud. If they are susceptible to such seizures, they will breathe in and out deeply, possibly 10 times, stop and stare for 3 seconds, then continue to hyperventilate and count, unaware that they paused.
14. Seizures increase at puberty, possibly resulting from glandular changes or sudden growth and the need for an increased medicine dosage, or they may result in part from adolescent rebellion against prescribed medication routines.
15. Breath-holding is a phenomenon that occurs in young children when they are stressed or angry. The child breathes in and, because he is upset, does not breathe out again, or else breathes out and then does not inhale again. As brain cells become anoxic, the child becomes cyanotic and slumps to the floor, momentarily unconscious. With a temper tantrum, a child deliberately attempts to hold his breath and pass out.
16. Loss of autonomic nervous system function would occur during the second recovery phase after spinal cord injury.
17. Spasticity results from the loss of upper level control or transmission of meaningful innervation to the lower muscles.
18. The cervical and thoracolumbar areas of the spine are the ones most likely to sustain injury.

What If? Question Answers

1. If this child is so sleepy, he can't function in school, this parent is probably correct that his dose of phenobarbital is too high. Cutting or ending phenobarbital abruptly or indiscriminately, however, can cause seizures. Bringing the child to have a drug level drawn first the next time she is concerned about the dose would be good advice.
2. These are classic symptoms of autonomic dysreflexia that most often occurs because of a full bladder. Assessing to see whether an indwelling catheter is free flowing would be a crucial first step.

Chapter 50: Nursing Care of the Child With a Disorder of the Eyes or Ears

Checkpoint Question Answers

1. Children with myopia need corrective (concave) lenses to enable them to see at a distance.
2. Nystagmus is rapid, irregular eye movement. It is seen in children with vision-impairing lesions, such as congenital cataracts, and also occurs as a neurologic sign when there is a lesion of the cerebellum or brain stem.
3. Ptosis may be congenital (frequently hereditary and bilateral) or acquired (generally unilateral), such as a result of injury to the third cranial nerve (neurogenic) or to the lid or levator muscle.
4. A cover test or Hirschberg's test will reveal strabismus.
5. Foreign bodies such as sand or dirt can be removed by everting the eyelid and touching the object with a moistened cotton applicator.
6. After a contusion injury, it is important to assess for eye movement to be certain the muscles of eye movement are not damaged.
7. In the infant with congenital glaucoma, the cornea appears enlarged, edematous, and hazy. The infant may have tearing, pain, and photophobia.
8. Vomiting increases intraocular pressure, which could injure the suture line.
9. Children are legally blind if their vision is less than 20/200 on a standard eye chart or their peripheral vision is less than 20 degrees.
10. Sound is a major way in which visually challenged children experience their environment.
11. Acute otitis media is an infection; otitis media with infusion is collection of fluid in the middle ear.
12. It is important to assess for cholesteatoma because, if untreated, it can lead to mastoiditis, meningitis, and possibly facial nerve paralysis.
13. It is important to allow hearing-challenged children to see you before you touch them to avoid frightening them.

What If? Question Answers

1. Fireworks are a major cause of eye injury in children because they are burned by the sparks. You might begin an educational campaign on the importance of adult supervision when lighting fireworks.
2. Many children feel self-conscious about wearing hearing aids. Frank discussion about the benefits the hearing aid provides would go a long way. Pointing out that wearing eyeglasses is really no different might help.

Chapter 51: Nursing Care of the Child With a Musculoskeletal Disorder

Checkpoint Question Answers

1. Increase in the length of long bones occurs at the cartilage segment (the epiphyseal plate).
2. Electromyography studies the electrical activity of skeletal muscle and nerve conduction using needle electrodes inserted into muscle masses.
3. A window may be placed in a cast if an infection, usually identified as a hot spot on the cast surface, is suspected.
4. With crutches, weight bearing is by the arm, not the axilla.
5. Children may have mildly bowed legs as part of normal development (seen most commonly in 2-year-olds).
6. Treatment of Leggs-Calvé-Perthes disease requires a long period of therapy.
7. Osteomyelitis in older children is most often caused by *Staphylococcus aureus.*
8. Synovitis most commonly occurs in the hip joint of children.
9. Scoliosis may be functional (caused by a secondary problem) or structural (a primary deformity).
10. Surgical correction is generally necessary when the degree of curvature is greater than 40 degrees.
11. NSAIDS are the drugs of choice for treating JA.
12. A common non-pharmacologic treatment to reduce pain with juvenile arthritis is application of heat.
13. Myasthenia gravis involves an interference with acetylcholine at the synaptic junctions, leading to symptoms of progressive muscle weakness.
14. Duchenne's disease (pseudohypertrophic) is the most common form of muscular dystrophy.
15. A greenstick fracture is a specific type of fracture that occurs in children whereby the bone is only bent, not broken.
16. Casting an elbow can lead to severe compression of the nerve that crosses there, leading to a permanent contraction of the arm.

What If? Question Answers

1. Children who have exercised in a different way than usual can have pain in muscles the same as adults. An important assessment would be that the pain is truly in the muscle and not in a joint as joint pain is much more apt to be serious.
2. The majority of children with juvenile arthritis will outgrow their symptoms as they reach adulthood. Assessing the child's current image of himself (why he thinks of himself as a cripple) would be important.

Chapter 52: Nursing Care of the Child With a Traumatic Injury

Checkpoint Question Answers

1. In children ages 5 to 9 years, the most frequent types of accidents include motor vehicle accidents, bicycles, drowning, burns, and accidents involving firearms.
2. The Poison Prevention Packaging Act of 1970 that requires safety caps on medicines has decreased the incidence of childhood poisonings.
3. A simple linear skull fracture occurs commonly in the lambdoid suture line.
4. Subdural hematoma is generally bilateral venous bleeding into the space between the dura and arachnoid membrane, occurring when head trauma lacerates minute veins in this area. Epidural hematoma is arterial bleeding into the space between the dura and the skull, occurring when head trauma is severe.
5. A head injury is the most common cause of a coma in children.
6. A Glasgow coma score of 10 indicates moderate trauma.
7. Air under the diaphragm on abdominal x-ray suggests intestinal or gastric rupture.
8. The spleen is the most frequently injured organ in abdominal trauma.
9. Very young children display a mammalian diving reflex when they plunge under cold water.
10. Prophylactic antibiotic therapy may be used after a near-drowning episode to prevent pneumonia and additional airway interference.
11. The specific antidote for acetaminophen poisoning is acetylcysteine (Mucomyst).
12. With caustic and hydrocarbon poisoning, vomiting should not be induced because the substance will cause additional damage when being vomited.
13. A chelating agent is used to remove lead from soft tissue and bone and thus eliminate it in the urine.
14. Children can be poisoned by insecticides (1) by accidental ingestion or (2) through skin or respiratory tract contact when playing in an area that has recently been sprayed with one.
15. A swallowed chicken bone would be removed by esophagoscopy.
16. Sudden warming increases the metabolic rate of cells. Without adequate blood flow to the area because of still-present vasoconstriction from frostbite, additional damage will occur.
17. A second-degree burn involves the entire epidermis.
18. A "rule of nines" is not applicable in children because their body proportions are different from adults.
19. Debridement means removal of foreign bodies from a wound.
20. Autografting implies that tissue has been taken from a donor.

What If? Question Answers

1. The first priority here is to obtain a complete health history, as these symptoms are vague enough that they could be occurring from a number of reasons. If the parents report that the child suffered a head injury, the possibility of a concussion needs to be considered.
2. Prenatal vitamins contain a high dose of iron, so are dangerous to children when swallowed in large amounts. The child can develop gastric bleeding, evidenced either by vomiting blood (within hours) or by blood in the stool (visible by the next day).
3. Small coins do pass readily in children, so usually no intervention needs to be carried out for swallowed pennies. Signs that the obstruction has occurred would be abdominal pain, abdominal distention, and failure to pass stool.

Chapter 53: Nursing Care of the Child With Cancer

Checkpoint Question Answers

1. Metastasis means a neoplastic growth has spread from its primary location to a distant body site.
2. Stage II disease typically implies that cancer cells cannot be totally removed by surgery.
3. Chemotherapeutic agents cause nausea and vomiting because they attack fast-growing cells, such as the cells lining the stomach.
4. Two common side effects of vincristine are constipation and loss of sensation in the fingers.
5. First signs commonly seen in the child with leukemia are fever, bruising, nosebleeds, and fatigue.
6. In children with leukemia and central nervous system involvement, methotrexate is administrated intrathecally (into the spinal cord).
7. The incidence of Hodgkin's disease is highest in adolescents.
8. The first sign of Hodgkin's disease is usually a painless, enlarged lymph node.
9. Parents may dismiss the vomiting that occurs with brain tumors because it is not accompanied by nausea.
10. Straining to have a bowel movement increases intracranial pressure.
11. Usually, the first reported symptom of osteosarcoma is pain near a major joint.
12. Children waiting for surgery for Ewing's sarcoma should not bear weight on the affected leg.
13. An important nursing responsibility for children waiting for surgery for Wilms' tumor is to prevent abdominal palpation in the child.
14. A common finding in children with retinoblastoma is a white pupil.

What If? Question Answers

1. This situation calls for increased education to help the parent understand that although nausea and vomiting imply that the drug is attacking rapidly forming cells, they are extremely uncomfortable sensations and wearing on the child. Helping the parent to see that there are better ways to evaluate chemotherapy effects, such as examining the white blood count, would also be helpful. Being certain that the parent receives information in a timely and helpful manner would be another nursing responsibility.
2. This is a typical way in which Wilms' tumor is first discovered: a parent feels the growth in the infant's abdomen. Discussing that the cause of Wilms' tumor is unknown, but the growth probably arises from an embryonic growth, would help this parent understand that her husband did not cause it. It might even make her appreciate that the fact he found it early may be helpful.

Chapter 54: Nursing Care of the Child With a Cognitive or Mental Health Disorder

Checkpoint Question Answers

1. Four categories of cognitive challenge are mild, moderate, severe, and profound.
2. Children with an IQ of 45 can learn to talk and communicate, but they may have only poor awareness of social conventions. They need supervision and guidance when in stressful settings.
3. To reach optimal level of functioning, areas such as the care setting, health maintenance needs, education, self-care activities, and preparation for adulthood must be addressed.
4. Assessment findings with autism may include social isolation, stereotyped behaviors, resistance to change, abnormal responses to sensory stimuli, insensitivity to pain, inappropriate emotional expressions, poor speech development, and specific, limited intellectual problems.
5. The three major characteristics of ADHD are inattention, impulsivity, and hyperactivity.
6. Problems with sequencing interfere with the child's concept of before and after.
7. Methylphenidate hydrochloride (Ritalin) is most often used to treat ADHD.
8. Therapy for children with conduct disorders focuses on modifying the home environment and training in social and problem-solving skills.
9. Separation anxiety occurs slightly more frequently in girls.
10. Iron deficiency anemia is commonly associated with pica.
11. Anorexia nervosa may occur in boys but is found more frequently in girls.
12. Bulimia refers to recurrent binge eating and purging; anorexia nervosa is an intense preoccupation with food, creating a feeling of revulsion to the point of excessive weight loss.
13. Rumination is a condition most frequently seen in infants.
14. Common symptoms of Tourette's syndrome are complex vocal tics.

What If? Question Answers

1. This is an interesting question because it makes you wonder why the girl is asking. Is she worried she is pregnant? Is she seeking sex education information on where babies come from? Does she need contraceptive information? Did she simply watch a television show last night in which there was a cute baby and is making conversation? Once the unvoiced question (why is she asking) is answered, the answer to the actual question will differ depending on the reason it was raised.
2. Weight loss in children always needs to be investigated, as normally children never lose weight. Exploring whether this girl has been dieting or has any additional symptoms would be important. Her stress level—trying to maintain all those As and be a perfect daughter—also needs to be explored.

Chapter 55: Nursing Care of the Family in Crisis: Abuse and Violence in the Family

Checkpoint Question Answers

1. As few as 10% of child-abusing parents are mentally ill.
2. The triad of child abuse is special parent, special child, and special circumstance.
3. Professional organizations that are helpful for referral are Parents Anonymous and the Child Abuse Prevention Network.
4. Shaken baby syndrome is caused by an adult severely shaking a child, causing a whiplash injury to the neck, edema to the brain stem, and typical retinal hemorrhage.
5. Psychological abuse includes constant belittling or threatening, rejecting, isolating, or exploiting the child.
6. In Munchausen syndrome by proxy, symptoms are those that are not easily detected by physical exam and occur only when the abuser is present.
7. Failure to thrive is defined as a child with weight and height below the 5th percentile.
8. A pedophile is an adult who seeks out children for sexual gratification.
9. Rape is a crime of violence.
10. Abused women may not seek help early in an abusive relationship because they are using denial as a defense mechanism and may have such low self-esteem they do not perceive that anyone would want to help them.
11. The safety of the abused family member should be the priority.

What If? Question Answers

1. This type of "role reversal"—a child comforting a parent—is very typical of child abuse. Listen for it in emergency rooms. It is not diagnostic because some children who are well loved and cared for are so sensitive to their parent's emotions that they also respond this way.
2. This is a legal question depending on how "family" is interpreted. It is usually regarded as incest, however, and definitely rape.

Chapter 56: Nursing Care of the Family Coping With Long-Term or Terminal Illness

Checkpoint Question Answers

1. A grief reaction consists of the stages of denial, anger, bargaining, depression, and acceptance.
2. If at all possible, children with chronic illnesses should attend regular classrooms so they have experiences with their peers.

3. Parents can help siblings by setting aside time for activities with them, as well as explaining the illness and procedures and including them in the care of the ill child.
4. The stage of depression is apt to be the most difficult for parents, as it is the first time they really face what is happening.
5. Anticipatory grief can blunt the hurt of the child's death.
6. The last sense lost with dying is hearing.
7. Organ donations of livers, kidneys, and lungs from children are important because it is difficult to transplant adult organs into children owing to the difference in size.

What If? Question Answers

1. Respite time means time spent doing activities that the parent enjoys. In this example, if cleaning cupboards was what the mother enjoyed and found relaxing, this was an appropriate activity. When helping parents plan for respite time, it is important the activities they choose are those they would enjoy, not necessarily those the health care provider would prefer.
2. These are typical signs of anger that can occur as an expression of grief. Recognizing these in yourself allows you to reassess how involved you are with a patient and seek respite care for yourself.

Index

Note: Page numbers followed by letters *b*, *f*, and *t* indicate boxes, figures, and tables, respectively.

B

C

D

E

F

G

H

J

K

L

M

N

O

P

Q

R

T

U

V

CD-ROM to Accompany PILLITTERI'S MATERNAL & CHILD HEALTH NURSING, 4th EDITION

PROGRAM LICENSE AGREEMENT

Read carefully the following terms and conditions before using the Software. Use of the Software indicates you and, if applicable, your Institution's acceptance of the terms and conditions of this License Agreement. If you do not agree with the terms and conditions, you should promptly return this package to the place you purchased it and your payment will be refunded.

Definitions

As used herein, the following terms shall have the following meanings:

"Software" means the software program contained on the diskette(s) or CD-ROM or preloaded on a workstation and the user documentation, which includes all accompanying printed material.

"Institution" means a nursing or professional school, a single academic organization that does not provide patient care and is located in a single city and has one geographic location/address.

"Geographic location" means a facility at a specific location; geographic locations do not provide for satellite or remote locations that are considered a separate facility.

"Facility" means a health care facility at a specific location that provides patient care and is located in a single city and has one geographic location/address.

"Publisher" means Lippincott Williams & Wilkins, Inc., with its principal office in Philadelphia, Pennsylvania.

"Developer" means the company responsible for developing the software as noted on the product.

License

You are hereby granted a nonexclusive license to use the Software in the United States. This license is not transferable and does not authorize resale or sublicensing without the written approval or an authorized officer of Publisher.

The Publisher retains all rights and title to all copyrights, patents, trademarks, trade secrets, and other proprietary rights in the Software. You may not remove or obscure the copyright notices in or on the Software. You agree to use reasonable efforts to protect the Software from unauthorized use, reproduction, distribution or publication.

Single-User license

If you purchased this Software program at the Single-User License price or a discount of that price, you may use this program on one single-user computer. You may not use the Software in a time-sharing environment or otherwise to provide multiple, simultaneous access. You may not provide or permit access to this program to anyone other than yourself.

Institutional/Facility license

If you purchased the Software at the Institutional or Facility License Price or at a discount of that price, you have purchased the Software for use within your Institution/Facility on a single workstation/computer. You may not provide copies of or remote access to the Software. You may not modify or translate the program or related documentation. You agree to instruct the individuals in your Institution/Facility who will have access to the Software to abide by the terms of this License Agreement. If you or any member of your Institution fail to comply with any of the terms of this License Agreement, this license shall terminate automatically.

Network license

If you purchased the Software at the Network License Price, you may copy the Software for use within your Institution/Facility on an unlimited number of computers within one geographic location/address. You may not provide remote access to the Software over a value-added network or otherwise. You may not provide copies of or remote access to the Software to individuals or entities who are not members of your Institution/Facility. You may not modify or translate the program or related documentation. You agree to instruct the individuals in your Institution/Facility who will have access to the Software to abide by the terms of this License Agreement. If you or any member of your Institution/Facility fail to comply with any of the terms of this License Agreement, this license shall terminate automatically.

Limited warranty

The Publisher warrants that the media on which the Software is furnished shall be free from defects in materials and workmanship under normal use for a period of 90 days from the date of delivery to you, as evidenced by your receipt of purchase.

The Software is sold on a 30-day trial basis. If, for whatever reason, you decide not to keep the software, you may return it for a full refund within 30 days of the invoice date or purchase, as evidenced by your receipt of purchase by returning all parts of the Software and packaging in saleable condition with the original invoice, to the place you purchased it. If the Software is not returned in such condition, you will not be entitled to a refund. When returning the Software, we suggest that you insure all packages for their retail value and mail them by a traceable method.

The Software is a computer assisted instruction (CAI) program that is not intended to provide medical consultation regarding the diagnosis or treatment of any specific patient.

The Software is provided without warranty of any kind, either expressed or implied, including but not limited to any implied warranty of fitness for a particular purpose of merchantability. Neither Publisher nor Developer warrants that the Software will satisfy your requirements or that the Software is free of program or content errors. Neither Publisher nor Developer warrants, guarantees, or makes any representation regarding the use of the Software in terms of accuracy, reliability or completeness, and you rely on the content of the programs solely at your own risk.

The Publisher is not responsible (as a matter of products liability, negligence or otherwise) for any injury resulting from any material contained herein. This Software contains information relating to general principles of patient care that should not be construed as specific instructions for individual patients.

Manufacturers' product information and package inserts should be reviewed for current information, including contraindications, dosages and precautions.

Some states do not allow the exclusion of implied warranties, so the above exclusion may not apply to you. This warranty gives you specific legal rights and you may also have other rights that vary from state to state.

Limitation of remedies

The entire liability of Publisher and Developer and your exclusive remedy shall be: (1) the replacement of any CD which does not meet the limited warranty stated above which is returned to the place you purchased it with your purchase receipt; or (2) if the Publisher or the wholesaler or retailer from whom you purchased the Software is unable to deliver a replacement CD free from defects in material and workmanship, you may terminate this License Agreement by returning the CD, and your money will be refunded.

In no event will Publisher or Developer be liable for any damages, including any damages for personal injury, lost profits, lost savings or other incidental or consequential damages arising out of the use or inability to use the Software or any error or defect in the Software, whether in the database or in the programming, even if the Publisher, Developer, or an authorized wholesaler or retailer has been advised of the possibility of such damage.

Some states do not allow the limitation or exclusion of liability for incidental or consequential damages. The above limitations and exclusions may not apply to you.

General

This License Agreement shall be governed by the laws of the State of Pennsylvania without reference to the conflict of laws provisions thereof, and may only be modified in a written statement signed by an authorized officer of the Publisher. By opening and using the Software, you acknowledge that you have read this License Agreement, understand it, and agree to be bound by its terms and conditions. You further agree that it is a complete and exclusive statement of the agreement between the Institution/Facility and the Publisher, which supersedes any proposal or prior agreement, oral or written, and any other communication between you and Publisher or Developer relative to the subject matter of the License Agreement.

Note

Attach a paid invoice to the License Agreement as proof of purchase.

INSTALLATION INSTRUCTIONS

Student Self-Study CD-ROM to Accompany Pillitteri's Maternal and Child Health Nursing, *4th Edition*

The installation program should automatically start a few seconds after you have inserted the CD-ROM into your CD-ROM drive. Follow the directions on the screen to complete the installation. If the program does *not* automatically start, follow these steps:

1. Open the Start menu and select Run.
2. In Open box, type d:\setup, where d is the letter representing your CD-ROM drive, and press Enter. (If your CD-ROM drive is a letter other than d, substitute that letter.)
3. Follow the directions on the screen to complete the installation.
4. The program will add a shortcut to your desktop.
5. To launch the program, double click on the icon on the Desktop.

SYSTEM REQUIREMENTS

This program will run on any IBM-PC or compatible computer that *minimally* includes:

a Pentium 100 CPU;
32 MB RAM (64 recommended);
Windows 98;
SVGA display supporting 256 colors (16 bit recommended);
12X CD-ROM drive;
800x600 monitor resolution;
mouse;
5 MB of hard-disk space

Note: In order to run this program, you must have Macromedia Flashplayer installed on your PC. If you do not currently have this program installed, it is a free download available at: http://www.macromedia.com/software/flashplayer/.